AMA
AMERICAN MEDICAL ASSOCIATION

AF767293

Dear Valued Customer:

The American Medical Association (AMA) is pleased to bring you the 2008 edition of its high-quality ICD-9-CM coding products. Offering a comprehensive approach to medical diagnosis and procedural coding, the 2008 edition covers significant changes for the upcoming 2008 coding season—including those from the U.S. Department of Health and Human Services that will be in effect from Oct. 1, 2007, through Sept. 30, 2008.

With your 2008 edition, you can feel confident in your coding accuracy and efficiency. In addition, to keep your coding knowledge fully up to date, the AMA provides you with online access to special reports and updates to the ICD-9-CM code set at *www.ama-assn.org/go/cpt* under the heading "ICD-9-CM 2008."

Thank you for your commitment to the AMA's line of coding and reimbursement products. The AMA works hard to build and improve upon the range of services and products we provide today's physicians, their office staff and the health care field at large. With each purchase of an AMA product, you help us continue our mission of helping doctors help patients.

If you have any questions or comments, please do not hesitate to call our customer service department at (800) 621-8335.

Sincerely,

Erica Duke
Marketing manager
American Medical Association

Anthony Frankos
Vice president, Business Products
American Medical Association

Additional AMA resources

Coding and Reimbursement:
CPT® 2008 Professional Edition
CPT® 2008 Standard Edition
CPT® 2008 Electronic Professional Edition
CPT® Changes 2008: An insider's view
CPT® Changes Archives 2000-2008
Principles of CPT® Coding, Fifth Edition
CPT® Assistant Newsletter
CPT® 2008 Express Reference Coding Cards
Coding with Modifiers: A Guide to Correct CPT® and HCPCS Level II Modifier Usage, Third Edition
Medical Record Auditor, Second Edition

Physician ICD-9-CM 2008, Volumes 1 and 2 Full size and Compact
Hospital ICD-9-CM 2008, Volumes 1, 2 and 3 Full size and Compact
Principles of CPT® Coding Workbook, Second Edition
Principles of ICD-9-CM Coding, Third Edition
ICD-9-CM 2008 Express Reference Coding Cards
ICD-9-CM 2008 Data Files

HCPCS 2008 Level II
HCPCS 2008 Level II ASCII Data Files

Medicare RBRVS 2008: The Physicians' Guide
RBRVS Payment Calculator 2008

Practice Management:
AMA Physician's Guide to Financial Planning
Compliance Guide for the Medical Practice: How to Attain and Maintain a Compliant Medical Practice
EHR Implementation: A Step-by-Step Guide for the Medical Practice
Handbook of Medical Office Communication
Maximizing Billing and Collections in the Medical Practice
Technical and Financial Guide to EHR Implementation
The Physician's Guide to Survival and Success in the Medical Practice

To view these and additional resources please visit us at *www.amabookstore.com* or call (800) 621-8335 for a free catalog.

Thank you for purchasing an AMA ICD-9-CM product. We hope you enjoy this exclusive complimentary ICD-10-CM resource.

Introduction to ICD-10-CM

Anticipated changes, differences between ICD-9-CM and ICD-10-CM general organization, conventions comparisons and chapter-by-chapter content review.

AMA
AMERICAN MEDICAL ASSOCIATION

INTRODUCING ICD-10-CM

WHAT IS ICD-10?

Diagnosis coding is the language of reporting why a service was medically necessary for patient care. Payers require accurate reporting of diagnosis coding to explain why a service was provided to the patient. The International Classification of Diseases (ICD) is designed to promote international comparability in the collection, processing, classification, and presentation of mortality statistics. This includes providing a format for reporting causes of death on the death certificate. The reported conditions are then translated into medical codes through use of the classification structure and the selection and modification rules contained in the applicable revision of the ICD, published by the World Health Organization (WHO). These coding rules improve the usefulness of mortality statistics by giving preference to certain categories, by consolidating conditions, and by systematically selecting a single cause of death from a reported sequence of conditions. The single selected cause for tabulation is called the underlying cause of death, and the other reported causes are the nonunderlying causes of death. The combination of underlying and nonunderlying causes is the multiple causes of death.

Beginning the transition to ICD-10-CM and ICD-10-PCS (Procedure Coding System; for hospital inpatient services) is expected to take place around 2008. The new system will provide a significant opportunity to improve the capture of information with our increasingly complex health care delivery system. ICD-10-CM will provide enormous opportunities for documentation improvement processes for health records. This is especially true with physician migration to the electronic medical record. ICD-10-CM will provide greater coding specificity and accuracy for hospitals, physicians, payers, and other health systems to support accurate payment. Detailed, accurate information is vitally important for quality of care and good reporting practices.

All major countries except the United States are currently utilizing

ICD-10, and this difference has created problems in determining national and international comparisons of mortality and morbidity. The United States is currently using ICD-10 for cause of death reporting. This is making statistical analysis and trend comparison difficult because cause of death and disease classification are different.

All health care providers and payers need to begin preparation for the transition from ICD-9-CM to ICD-10-CM now. Key areas that need to be addressed initially are staffing, vendor, and computer technology issues, clinical systems, information management, and the impact on cash flow. ICD-10-CM differs from ICD-9-CM in that it is an alphanumeric coding system with up to 7 digits of specificity.

WHAT IS ICD-10-CM?

The International Classification of Diseases, Tenth Revision, Clinical Modification is called ICD-10-CM. This clinical modification will be the method of reporting diagnoses to payers to support medical necessity for services provided. ICD-10-CM will meet criteria of the Health Insurance Portability and Accountability Act of 1996 (HIPAA) with its alphanumeric structure, which will provide more specific information for ambulatory and managed care, expand injury coding, and describe the clinical picture of the patient more precisely than in ICD-9-CM.

To understand ICD-10-CM, it is important to understand the various agencies involved in the ICD-10-CM implementation process.

The World Health Organization is the agency that maintains an international nomenclature of mortality and morbidity statistics, including cause of death, and public health practices. The original intent of ICD-10, which was adopted in 1994, was to be used as a statistical tool for tracking morbidity and mortality data. The ICD has become the international standard diagnostic classification for many health management purposes. The WHO owns and published the classification in a 3-volume set and is responsible for the development of the adaptation of ICD-10 for use in the United States.

The National Center for Health Statistics (NCHS) is the federal agency responsible for use of the International Statistical Classification of Diseases and Related Health Problems. The NCHS, along with guidance from the Centers for Medicare and Medicaid Services (CMS), revises the ICD-9-CM (current diagnosis coding system). The NCHS is responsible for the development and clinical modification of ICD-10-CM in the United States.

ICD-10 currently is used to code and classify mortality data from death certificates, having replaced ICD-9 for this purpose as of January 1, 1999. ICD-10-CM is planned as the replacement for ICD-9-CM, volumes 1 and 2. The ICD-9-CM system has outgrown its intended level of specificity, which has an impact on the ability to compare data efficiently and precisely for research, clinical support, and appropriate reimbursement.

THE NEED FOR CHANGE

ICD-9-CM has been in use since 1979 and no longer reflects advances in medical treatment. An expandable system is needed. The ICD-9-CM coding standard is in serious crisis. Terminologies and classifications from the 1970s no longer fit with the 21st-century health care system, as numerous conditions and procedures are outdated and inconsistent with current medical knowledge and application. New advances in medicine and medical technology and the growing need for quality data cannot be accommodated. Data incomparability continues to increase globally and within the US due to the use of these antiquated code sets.

The need to replace ICD-9-CM was identified in 1993 and steps were taken by the National Committee on Vital and Health Statistics (NCVHS), the NCHS, and CMS (then the Health Care Financing Administration, or HCFA) to develop a migration plan to ICD-10 for morbidity and mortality coding. Use of ICD-10 for mortality coding in the United States was initiated in 1999; however, while the rest of the industrialized countries are now using their variations of ICD-10 for all reporting, the United States continues with the unsupported ICD-9-CM (the WHO now exclusively supports ICD-10), leading to data incomparability with the rest of the global community.

ICD-9-CM does not meet any of the following criteria:

- Code set standards outlined by HIPAA
- New services and technology that must be acknowledged in CMS payment systems according to the Benefits Improvement and Protection Act of 2000
- Characteristics of a procedural coding system outlined by the NCVHS in 1993

Significant costs are incurred by continued use of severely outdated and limited coding systems. For example, failure of our coding systems to keep pace with medical advances results in the use of vague or incorrect codes often taken from the claims form and thereby requiring excessive reliance on supporting paper documentation (attachments or copies of the health record).

According to the May 4, 2001 *Federal Register*, the ICD-9-CM procedure coding system is limited to a maximum of 10,000 codes, most of which are already assigned. ICD-9-CM has limitations with a 4-digit structure that does not allow for much change. In 1993, the NCVHS indicated to the Department of Health and Human Services (DHHS) that ICD-9-CM was running out of code numbers. Some of the deficiencies in ICD-9-CM include:

- There is insufficient structure for reporting new technology
- It contains duplicate codes and codes that overlap
- It uses outdated terminology
- Sufficient specificity and detail are not available
- Codes for certain types of services are not available

In the DHHS proposed rule for electronic transactions and code sets under HIPAA, ICD-9-CM (*Federal Register*, Vol 63, No. 88), it was noted that ICD-9-CM "lacks the desirable level of flexibility and steps should be taken to improve the flexibility of these code sets or replace them with more flexible options sometime after the year 2000." ICD-9-CM has become outdated and obsolete beyond its original scope.

Providers are consistently required to use multiple coding systems to meet the need for reimbursement, research, profiling, outcomes measurement, and case-mix management.

Some of the pertinent reasons we use coding data today are to:

- Identify fraudulent practices
- Support medical necessity
- Perform research and clinical trials
- Set health policy
- Process claims for reimbursement
- Measure quality and efficacy of care

Progress toward adoption of ICD-10-CM and ICD-10-PCS began well over a decade ago. Extensive work and dedication have gone into developing and evaluating these systems as replacements for ICD-9-CM. While there is significant support for this ICD-9-CM upgrade, there is also a segment of the health care industry, clinging to antiquated legacy systems, that continues to argue for further delay, choosing to forgo the benefits of improved data and information available through 21st-century terminology and impeding progress toward achieving critical US health care goals.

MEETING HIPAA DEMANDS

ICD-10-CM will meet HIPAA criteria with its alphanumeric structure, which will provide more specific information for ambulatory and managed care, expand injury coding, and describe the clinical picture of the patient more precisely than in ICD-9-CM. ICD-10-CM contains an increased number of codes and categories that allow for more specific and accurate representation of current and future medical diagnoses and procedures. ICD-10-CM provides more detailed and clearer clinical descriptions.

OVERVIEW OF THE ICD-10-CM CODING SYSTEM

ICD-10-CM was developed after a thorough evaluation, which included input from a Technical Advisory Panel and consultation with physician groups, clinical coders, and other organizations to ensure accuracy and consistency in coding diagnoses. Some improvements with this clinical modification include the following:

- Addition of information relevant to ambulatory and managed care encounters
- Creation of combination codes for diagnosis/symptoms, which will reduce the number of diagnosis codes required to describe a specific condition
- Expanded injury codes to include code extensions for injuries and external causes of injury
- Additional trimester information
- The addition of up to 7-character incorporation of common fourth- and fifth-digit subclassifications
- Laterality
- Expanded alcohol and substance abuse codes
- Expanded postoperative complication codes
- Greater specificity in code assignment

ICD-10-CM will dramatically affect the way we report diagnoses in the United States. There is not yet an anticipated implementation date for ICD-10-CM. Implementation will be based on the process for adoption of standards under HIPAA. There will be a 2-year implementation window once the final notice to implement has been published in the *Federal Register*.

As part of its responsibilities under HIPAA, the NCVHS monitors the continued effectiveness of the health data standards adopted pursuant to the requirements of HIPAA's administrative simplification provisions.

The ICD has been revised periodically to incorporate changes in the medical field. The Tenth Revision (ICD-10) differs from the Ninth Revision (ICD-9) in a number of respects, although the overall content is similar:

1. ICD-10 is printed in a three-volume set, rather than ICD-9's two-volume set.
2. ICD-10 has alphanumeric categories rather than numeric categories.
3. Some chapters have been rearranged.
4. Some titles have been changed.
5. Conditions have been regrouped.
6. ICD-10 has almost twice as many categories as ICD-9.
7. Minor changes have been made in the coding rules for mortality.

The ICD-10 consists of the following:

1. A tabular list containing cause-of-death titles and codes (Volume 1)
2. Inclusion and exclusion terms for cause-of-death titles (Volume 1)
3. Alphabetical index to diseases and nature of injury
4. External causes of injury
5. Table of drugs and chemicals (Volume 3)
6. Description, guidelines, and coding rules (Volume 2)

The process of converting from ICD-9-CM to ICD-10-CM affects many aspects of the mortality data system, including revision of instruction manuals and medical software. The ICD-10 Clinical Modification (ICD-10-CM) is currently under development. It is intended as a replacement for ICD-9-CM, Volumes 1 and 2 (diagnosis).

LEGISLATIVE ISSUES

While taking into account the diversity of input and lack of industry-wide consensus, NCVHS concludes that it is in the best interests of the country as a whole that ICD-10-CM and ICD-10-PCS be adopted as HIPAA standards for national implementation as replacements for current uses of ICD-9-CM Volumes 1, 2, and 3. As a result, the committee recommended that the Department of Health and Human Services initiate the regulatory process for the concurrent adoption of ICD-10-CM and ICD-10-PCS. The committee further recommends an implementation period of at least 2 years following issuance of a final rule. By issuing a Notice of Proposed Rule Making (NPRM), the department would provide a structured environment in which critical implementation issues may be addressed.

As a result, the Health Information Technology Promotion Act of 2005 passed the House of Representatives on July 27, 2006. HR 4157 was established within the Department of Health and Human Services, Office of the National Coordinator for Health Information Technology. The bill is now in conference committee with the Senate's health information technology bill, S 1418, the Wired for Healthcare Quality Act, with the proposed implementation date for ICD-10 set at October 1, 2010; Section 203 of HR 4157 includes upgrading the ICD codes and coding and documentation of nonmedical information. The bill states:

"The Secretary of Health and Human Services will provide by notice published in the Federal Register for the replacement of the International Classification of Diseases, 9th revision, Clinical Modification (ICD-9-CM) under the regulation promulgated under section 1173(c) of the Social Security Act (42 U.S.C. 1320d-2(c)), including for purposes of part A of title XVIII of such Act, with both of the following:

A. The International Classification of Diseases, 10th revision, Clinical Modification (ICD-10-CM).
B. The International Classification of Diseases, 10th revision, Procedure Coding System (ICD-10-PCS)."

The bill will give the Secretary of Health and Human Services the authority to modify and maintain ICD-10-CM and ICD-10-PCS under the amendments made by section 201. Section 204 of the amendments will develop a strategic plan for coordinating and implementing ICD-10, including replacing ICD-9 with ICD-10. Section 206 of this act also enables the Secretary of Health and Human Service to submit a report to Congress, which evaluates the following:

1. The applicability of health care classification methodologies and codes for purposes beyond the coding of services for diagnostic documentation or billing purposes
2. The usefulness, accuracy, and completeness of such methodologies and codes for such purposes
3. The capacity of such methodologies and codes to produce erroneous or misleading information, with respect to such purposes

A LOOK AT THE ICD-10-CM CONVENTIONS

One of the most common questions asked when looking at ICD-10-CM is, will the conventions be the same or different? Many of the current conventions will be used in ICD-10-CM, which will help make the conversion easier. Many of the same symbols and terminology will carry over to ICD-10-CM as well.

Same Conventions

The following conventions will apply to ICD-10-CM:

Notes: They further define terms, clarify information, or list choices for additional digits.

"With/without" notes are the two options for the final character of a set of codes; the default is always "without." For 5-character codes, a 0 as the fifth-position character represents "without," and 1 represents "with." For 6-character codes, the sixth-position character 1 represents "with" and the 9 represents "without."

Includes: These are notes that further define or provide examples and can apply to the chapter, section, or category. The notes at the beginning of a chapter apply to the entire chapter, the notes at the beginning of the section apply to that entire section, and the notes at the beginning of the category apply to the entire category.

NOS: Not otherwise specified (NOS) is the equivalent of "unspecified." It is used when the information at hand does not permit a more specific code assignment. The coder should ask the physician for more specific information, if available, so that the proper code assignment can be made.

Excludes: These are notes that indicate terms that are to be coded elsewhere. Excludes notes can be located at the beginning of a chapter or section or below a category or subcategory and are always in italics. Excludes notes can be used for three reasons:

1. The condition may have to be coded elsewhere.
2. The code cannot be assigned if the associated condition is present.
3. Additional code(s) may be required to fully explain the condition.

Code First Underlying Disease: This notation is used in those categories not intended as the primary diagnosis. In such cases, the code, title, and instructions appear in italics. The note requires that the underlying cause (etiology) be sequenced first.

NEC: This means not elsewhere classified.

Use an Additional Code: This note appears in categories where further information must be added (by using an additional code) to give a more complete picture of the diagnosis or procedure.

: Colon: A colon is used after an incomplete term that needs one or more of the modifiers that follow to make it assignable to a given category.

( ) Parentheses: Parentheses are used to enclose supplementary words that may be present or absent in the statement of a disease or procedure, without affecting the code number to which it is assigned.

, Comma: Words following a comma are essential modifiers. The term in the inclusion note must be present in the diagnostic statement to qualify the code.

§ Section Mark: A section mark precedes a code to denote a footnote at the bottom of the page. The footnote applies to all codes in the subclassification.

Deleted Conventions

The following conventions found in ICD-9-CM will not be found in ICD-10-CM

} Brace: In ICD-9-CM, a brace was used to enclose a series of terms that modified the statement to the right of the brace. This will not be applicable to ICD-10-CM.

[ ] Brackets: Brackets to enclose synonyms, alternate wording, or explanatory phrases are not required, since level of specificity is 5 to 6 digit subclassifications.

New Conventions

Three new conventions have been added to ICD-10-CM: "And," Excludes1," and "Excludes2."

And: The use of "and" is a new convention. When the term "and" is used in a narrative statement, it represents and/or.

Excludes1: Excludes1 indicates that the code excluded should never be used at the same time as the code above the Excludes1 note. An Excludes1 is used when 2 conditions cannot occur together, such as a congenital form and an acquired form of the same condition.

Example: A 38-year-old woman in her first trimester of pregnancy with a history of benign hypertension presented to the obstetrician-gynecologist for her monthly prenatal visit. She has been on medication for hypertension for 2 years, and her blood pressure is now uncontrolled.

I10 Essential (primary) hypertension

Includes: *high blood pressure hypertension (arterial) (benign) (essential) (malignant) (primary) (systemic)*

Excludes1: *hypertensive disease complicating pregnancy, childbirth and the puerperium (O10-O11, O13-O16)*

Excludes1 instructs the user to go to another code for the excluded condition, so if the patient is pregnant, code I10 is not assigned. The Excludes1 note instructs the user to select the code from O10-O11, or O13-O16.

Here is how the encounter is reported:

O10.01	**Pre-existing essential hypertension complicating pregnancy**
O10.011	**Pre-existing essential hypertension complicating pregnancy, first trimester**

Since the encounter indicates that the patient is in the first trimester, O10.011 is the correct diagnosis for the hypertension complicating the pregnancy.

Excludes2: A type 2 Excludes note represents "Not included here." An Excludes2 note indicates that the condition excluded is not part of the condition represented by the code, but a patient may have both conditions at the same time. When an Excludes2 note appears under a code, it is acceptable to use both the code and the excluded code together.

Example: A patient with hypertension also is diagnosed with bilateral hypertensive retinopathy.

I10 **Essential (primary) hypertension**

Includes: *high blood pressure hypertension (arterial) (benign) (essential) (malignant) (primary) (systemic)*

Excludes2: *essential (primary) hypertension involving vessels of brain (I60-I69)*

essential (primary) hypertension involving vessels of eye (H35.0)

Excludes2 instructs the user that hypertension involving vessels of the eye has a different code than essential hypertension without further specification. If the patient has both systemic hypertension and primary hypertension of the eye, then it would be appropriate to assign a code for both conditions. Diagnosis code I10 is a 3-digit category and would be assigned as the first listed diagnosis followed by the retinopathy.

In the above example, the encounter would be coded as:

I10	**Hypertension**
H35.033	**Hypertensive retinopathy, bilateral**

CHARACTERISTICS OF ICD-10-CM

ICD-10-CM includes expanded disease classifications to include health-related conditions and to provide greater specificity at the sixth-digit and seventh-digit level. Draft guidelines for the use of ICD-10-CM can be found at http://www.cdc.gov/nchs/data/icd9/draft_i10guideln.pdf. ICD-10-CM consists of 3 volumes. Volume 1 contains a listing of alphanumeric codes. Codes can range from 3 to 7 digits of specificity. All 3-digit categories have the same commonalities. Digits beyond the 3 alphanumeric codes define a higher level of specificity.

Example: A patient presented to her internist with a complaint of pain in the right leg. She is taking an over-the-counter pain reliever for the pain, without relief. The physician cannot find the underlying cause of the pain and refers the patient to an orthopedic surgeon for consultation.

M79.6	**Pain in limb, hand, foot, fingers and toes**	
	M79.60	**Pain in limb, unspecified**
	M79.601	**Pain in right arm**
	M79.602	**Pain in left arm**
	M79.603	**Pain in arm, unspecified**
	M79.604	**Pain in right leg**
	M79.605	**Pain in left leg**
	M79.606	**Pain in leg, unspecified**
	M79.609	**Pain in unspecified limb**

Based on the patient encounter, the diagnosis is pain in right leg. The correct ICD-10-CM diagnosis code is M79.604, which is coded to the sixth digit of specificity.

ORGANIZATION OF ICD-10-CM

ICD-10-CM, Volume 1, is composed of 21 chapters, many of which classify diseases by organ or system as ICD-9-CM currently classifies codes. ICD-10-CM, however, has additional special group chapters that are not currently available in ICD-9-CM.

Two new chapters available in ICD-10-CM are:

- Diseases of the Eye and Adnexa
- Disorders of the Ear

The "External Causes of Morbidity and Mortality" and "Factors Influencing Health Status and Contact With Health Services" chapters will no longer be considered supplemental, but will be part of the chapter classifications.

A number of new features in ICD-10-CM will be:

- More complete descriptions
- Postprocedural disorders
- Changes to notes
- Blocks
- Common fourth- and fifth-digit subclassification
- Expanded injury coding
- Information relevant to ambulatory and managed care encounters
- Combination of diagnosis and symptom codes to fully describe a condition

Chapters are further divided into subchapters or "blocks" containing rubrics, which identify conditions that are closely related. A summary of the subchapters is given in each chapter, which indicates an overview of the classification structure.

Three-Character Categories

Notes in ICD-10-CM are similar to those in ICD-9-CM. When a note appears under a 3-digit category code, the note applies to all codes within the category. A note that appears beneath a specific code applies only to that particular code. The following are examples of 3-digit categories:

N17 **Acute renal failure**

Code also associated underlying condition

Excludes1: *posttraumatic renal failure (T79.5)*

N17.0 **Acute renal failure with tubular necrosis**

Acute tubular necrosis Renal tubular necrosis

Tubular necrosis NOS

N18 **Chronic renal failure**

Includes: *chronic uremia diffuse*

sclerosing

glomerulonephritis

Code also associated underlying condition

Excludes1: *Alport syndrome with chronic renal failure (Q87.811)*

chronic renal failure with hypertension (I12.0)

N19 **Unspecified renal failure**

Excludes1: *acute renal failure (N17.-)*

chronic renal failure (N18.-)

extrarenal uremia (R39.2)

prerenal uremia (R39.2)

renal failure with hypertension (I12.0)

renal insufficiency (N28.9)

uremia of newborn (P96.0)

Four-Character Subcategory

Four-digit subcategories define the site, etiology, manifestation, or state of the disease or condition. The 4-digit subcategory includes the 3-digit category plus decimal with an additional digit to further identify the condition to the highest level of specificity.

Example 1:

K44	**Diaphragmatic hernia**	
	Includes:	*hiatus hernia (esophageal) (sliding)*
		paraesophageal hernia
	Excludes1:	*congenital diaphragmatic hernia (Q79.0)*
		congenital hiatus hernia (Q40.1)
K44.0	**Diaphragmatic hernia with obstruction, without gangrene**	
	Diaphragmatic hernia causing obstruction	
	Incarcerated diaphragmatic hernia	
	Irreducible diaphragmatic hernia	
	Strangulated diaphragmatic hernia	
K44.1	**Diaphragmatic hernia with gangrene**	
	Gangrenous diaphragmatic hernia	
K44.9	**Diaphragmatic hernia without obstruction or gangrene**	

Example 2:

L29	**Pruritus**	
	Excludes1:	*neurotic excoriation (L98.1)*
		psychogenic pruritus (F45.8)
L29.0	**Pruritus ani**	
L29.1	**Pruritus scroti**	
L29.2	**Pruritus vulvae**	
L29.3	**Anogenital pruritus, unspecified**	
L29.8	**Other pruritus**	
L29.9	**Pruritus, unspecified**	
	Itch NOS	

Five- or Six-Character Subclassification

In ICD-9-CM, the fifth digit identifies the most precise level of specificity. In ICD-10-CM, a fifth or sixth 6-character subclassification represents the most accurate level of specificity. This addition may identify more specificity regarding the patient's condition or diagnosis. Following are 2 examples of fifth- and sixth-digit specificity:

Example of fifth-digit specificity:

M20.3	**Hallux varus (acquired)**	
	M20.30	**Hallux varus (acquired), unspecified foot**
	M20.31	**Hallux varus (acquired), right foot**
	M20.32	**Hallux varus (acquired), left foot**

Example of sixth-digit specificity:

K50.81	**Crohn's disease of both small and large intestine with complications**	
	K50.811	**Crohn's disease of both small and large intestine with rectal bleeding**
	K50.812	**Crohn's disease of both small and large intestine with intestinal obstruction**
	K50.813	**Crohn's disease of both small and large intestine with fistula**
	K50.814	**Crohn's disease of both small and large intestine with abscess**
	K50.818	**Crohn's disease of both small and large intestine with other complication**
	K50.819	**Crohn's disease of both small and large intestine with unspecified complications**

Alphabetic Index

As with ICD-9-CM, the beginning process when selecting a diagnosis code is to refer to the Alphabetic Index and select the appropriate code from the Tabular List. This also holds true with ICD-10-CM.

The Alphabetic Index is divided into 3 sections and is organized by main terms.

Section 1: Index to Diseases and Nature of Injury

Section 2: Index to External Causes

Section 3: Table of Drugs and Chemicals

The Alphabetic Index is organized in the same manner as ICD-9-CM. Codes are listed by "main term," which describes the disease and/or condition. As with ICD-9-CM, there are exceptions to the rule. Cross-references such as "see" and "see also" are also found in ICD-10-CM. Notes appear in the Alphabetic Index to:

- Define terms
- Provide direction
- Provide coding instructions

Example: A 5-year-old patient was diagnosed by the pediatrician as having lactose intolerance.

The diagnosis is lactose intolerance. To locate the correct category, the main term must be identified. In this example the main term is intolerance.

The following list is from the Alphabetic Index:

Intolerance
carbohydrate K90.4
disaccharide, hereditary E73.0
fat NEC K90.4
  pancreatic K90.3
food K90.4
  dietary counseling and surveillance Z71.3
fructose E74.10
  hereditary E74.12
glucose (-galactose) E74.39
gluten K90.0
lactose E73.9
  specified NEC E73.8
lysine E72.3
milk NEC K90.4
  lactose E73.9
protein K90.4
starch NEC K90.4
sucrose (-isomaltose) E74.31

The following is from the Tabular List:

E73	**Lactose intolerance**	
	E73.0	**Congenital lactase deficiency**
	E73.1	**Secondary lactase deficiency**
	E73.8	**Other lactose intolerance**
	E73.9	**Lactose intolerance, unspecified**

Since the type of lactose intolerance is not specified, the correct code assignment is E73.9.

GENERAL DRAFT ICD-10-CM CODING GUIDELINES

Diagnosis coding in the medical record is the responsibility of the attending physician. A joint effort between the attending physician and the coder is essential in achieving complete and accurate code assignment.

When a code is selected in ICD-10-CM, the first listed diagnosis code should be the reason for the visit documented in the medical record. The code should first be located in the Index and verified in the Tabular List. The instructional notations will appear in both the Index and the Tabular List. As with ICD-9-CM, both the Index and the Tabular List should be used when a diagnosis is assigned in ICD-10-CM. The Index does not always provide the full code, which may include laterality and any applicable extensions only found in the Tabular List. When a dash (-) appears at the end of an index entry, this indicates that additional characters are required.

Signs and Symptoms

As with ICD-9-CM coding, signs and symptoms should not be reported with a confirmed diagnosis if the symptom is integral to the diagnosis. For example, if the patient is experiencing ear pain and the diagnosis is otitis media, the ear pain would be integral to the otitis media and not reported. A symptom code is used with a confirmed diagnosis only when the symptom is not associated with the confirmed diagnosis.

Example: A patient is diagnosed with epigastric pain. The physician referred the patient to a gastroenterologist to rule out ulcer.

The ICD-9-CM and ICD-10-CM codes are compared below.

ICD-9-CM

789.06 **Abdominal pain, epigastric**

ICD-10-CM

R10.13 **Epigastric pain**

Combination Coding

A combination code is a single code to classify 2 diagnoses that includes a diagnosis with an associated sign/symptom or a complication. Combination codes are identified by subterm entries in the Index and by reading the "Includes" and "Exclusion" notes in the Tabular List.

There are many combination codes that include both the etiology and an acute manifestation, in which case the single combination code is assigned as the principal/first listed diagnosis and no sequencing decision is necessary.

The combination code is assigned alone when that code fully identifies the diagnostic conditions involved or when the Index so directs. Multiple codes should not be used when the classification provides a combination code that clearly identifies all of the elements documented in the diagnosis. When the combination code lacks the necessary specificity to fully describe all elements of a diagnosis, an additional code(s) may be used.

Example: A physician diagnosed a patient with rheumatoid arthritis of the right ankle and foot who also had rheumatoid polyneuropathy. The condition is coded in ICD-10-CM using the combination code.

Currently in ICD-9-CM there is no combination code to fully describe the condition, and 2 codes must be used for reporting this diagnosis. With ICD-10-CM a combination code is available.

ICD-9-CM

714.0 **Rheumatoid arthritis**

357.1 **Polyneuropathy in collagen vascular disease**

ICD-10-CM

M05.571 **Rheumatoid polyneuropathy with rheumatoid arthritis of right ankle and foot**

Acute, Subacute, and Chronic Conditions

The draft guidelines for ICD-10-CM are the same as for ICD-9-CM when a patient has an acute/subacute and/or a chronic condition.

The draft ICD-10-CM Guidelines state: "When a condition is documented as both acute, subacute, and chronic and separate codes exist in the Index, both are coded with the acute (subacute) sequenced first followed by the code for the chronic condition."

Example: A patient was diagnosed with acute maxillary sinusitis that is chronic.

In ICD-10-CM, both codes for the acute and chronic condition are reported.

J01 **Acute sinusitis**

Includes: *acute abscess of sinus*
acute empyema of sinus
acute infection of sinus
acute inflammation of sinus
acute suppuration of sinus

Use additional code (B95-B97) to identify infectious agent.

Excludes1: *sinusitis NOS (J32.9)*
Excludes2: *chronic sinusitis (J32.0-J32.8)*

The correct diagnosis coding and reporting is:

J01.00 **Acute maxillary sinusitis, unspecified**

J32.0 **Chronic maxillary sinusitis**

There is an **Excludes2** note that indicates that conditions listed with **Excludes2** are not considered inclusive to a code but may be coexistent and, if present, should be coded as an additional diagnosis.

Acute, Subacute, and Chronic Conditions

The draft guidelines for ICD-10-CM are the same as for ICD-9-CM when a patient has an acute/subacute and/or a chronic condition.

The draft ICD-10-CM Guidelines state: "When a condition is documented as both acute, subacute, and chronic and separate codes exist in the Index, both are coded with the acute (subacute) sequenced first followed by the code for the chronic condition."

Example: A patient was diagnosed with acute maxillary sinusitis that is chronic.

In ICD-10-CM, both codes for the acute and chronic condition are reported.

J01 **Acute sinusitis**

Includes: *acute abscess of sinus*
acute empyema of sinus
acute infection of sinus
acute inflammation of sinus
acute suppuration of sinus

Use additional code (B95-B97) to identify infectious agent.

Excludes1: *sinusitis NOS (J32.9)*
Excludes2: *chronic sinusitis (J32.0-J32.8)*

The correct diagnosis coding and reporting is:

J01.00 **Acute maxillary sinusitis, unspecified**

J32.0 **Chronic maxillary sinusitis**

There is an **Excludes2** note that indicates that conditions listed with **Excludes2** are not considered inclusive to a code but may be coexistent and, if present, should be coded as an additional diagnosis.

Laterality

For bilateral sites, the final character of the codes in ICD-10-CM indicates laterality. The right side is always character 1, the left side character 2. In those cases where a bilateral code is provided, the bilateral character is always 3. An unspecified side code is also provided should the side not be identified in the medical record. The unspecified side is either a character 0 or 9, depending on whether it is a fifth or sixth character.

Example: The patient sees a physician for follow-up for an abscess of a bursa on the left wrist.

M71.03 **Abscess of bursa, wrist**

M71.031 **Abscess of bursa, right wrist**

M71.032 **Abscess of bursa, left wrist**

M71.039 **Abscess of bursa, unspecified wrist**

The correct code selection is M71.032 for this patient encounter.

The code sequenced first on a medical record at the end of an encounter is most important because it defines the main reason for the encounter as determined at the end of the encounter. In the inpatient setting, the first code listed on a medical record is referred to as the principal diagnosis. In all other health care settings it is referred to as the first listed code.

Selection of principal diagnosis/first listed code is based first on the conventions in the classification that provide sequencing instructions. If no sequencing instructions apply, then sequencing is based on the condition(s) that brought the patient into the hospital or physician office and which condition was the primary focus of treatment.

Conditions present on admission that receive treatment, but that do not meet the definition of principal diagnosis, should be coded as additional codes.

Acute Manifestation Versus Underlying Condition

With the Uniform Hospital Discharge Data Set (UHDDS) definition of principal diagnosis in mind, it is generally an underlying condition that precipitates the need for an admission, since treatment of the underlying condition generally resolves any associated acute manifestations and is the primary focus of treatment. If the acute manifestation is immediately life threatening and primary treatment is directed at the acute manifestation, the acute manifestation should be sequenced before the underlying condition. If the acute manifestation is not the primary focus of treatment, the underlying condition should be sequenced first.

Example: A patient is treated by his primary care physician for impetigo manifested by otitis externa.

The underlying condition is the impetigo and the manifestation in this example is the otitis externa. The impetigo is sequenced first, followed by the otitis externa.

L01.00	**Impetigo, unspecified**
H62.41	**Otitis externa in other diseases classified elsewhere, right ear**

This guideline is also based on the fact that the classification has the etiology/manifestation convention that requires that the underlying etiology take sequencing precedence over the acute manifestation.

Two or More Diagnoses That Equally Meet the Definition of Principal Diagnosis/First Listed Diagnosis

When 2 or more confirmed diagnoses equally meet the criteria for principal/first listed diagnosis as determined by the circumstances of admission, diagnostic workup, and/or therapy provided, and the Index, Tabular List, and coding guidelines do not provide sequencing direction, any one of the diagnoses may be sequenced first. This rule also applies to the inpatient and outpatient settings.

Complications of Surgery and Other Medical Care

When the admission is for treatment of a complication resulting from surgery or other medical care, the complication code is sequenced as the first listed code.

Example: A physician performed a spinal puncture on a patient. The patient was doing well after surgery, but later in the evening, he began experiencing weakness and loss of consciousness. The patient was rushed to the emergency department, where the physician met the patient. The physician examined the patient and determined that cerebrospinal fluid was leaking from the puncture site. The physician took the patient into a surgery suite and stopped the leak.

The patient encounter is coded as:

G97.0	**Cerebrospinal fluid leak from spinal puncture**

Selection of Secondary Diagnoses

In most cases, more than 1 code is necessary to fully explain a health care encounter. Though a patient has an encounter for a primary reason (the principal/first listed diagnosis), the additional conditions or reasons for the encounter also need to be coded. These codes are referred to as secondary, additional, or "other" diagnoses. For reporting purposes, the definition of "other diagnoses" is interpreted as additional conditions that affect patient care in terms of requiring clinical evaluation; therapeutic treatment; diagnostic procedures; extended length of hospital stay; or increased nursing care and/or monitoring.

The UHDDS defines "Other Diagnoses" as "all conditions that coexist at the time of admission, that develop subsequently, or that affect the treatment received and/or the length of stay. Diagnoses that relate to an earlier episode which have no bearing on the current hospital stay are to be excluded". UHDDS definitions apply to inpatients in an acute care, short-term, hospital setting. This definition also applies to outpatient encounters."

Previous Conditions

Some physicians include in the diagnostic statement resolved conditions or diagnoses and status-post procedures from previous visits that have no bearing on the current treatment. Such conditions are not to be reported and are coded only if required by the hospital or physician office policy.

For example, if the patient is being treated for hypertension and diabetes during the patient encounter and the patient had pneumonia that resolved 3 months previously and has no bearing on the services rendered at the visit, the pneumonia would not be reported.

Abnormal Test Findings

Abnormal test findings (laboratory, x-ray, pathologic, and other diagnostic results) are not coded and reported unless the physician indicates their clinical significance. If the findings are outside the normal range and the physician has ordered other tests to evaluate the condition or prescribed treatment, it is appropriate to ask the physician whether the abnormal finding should be added.

If the abnormal test finding corresponds to a confirmed diagnosis, it should not be coded in addition to the confirmed diagnosis. A sign or symptom code is to be used as principal/first listed if no definitive diagnosis is established at the time of coding. If the diagnosis is confirmed (eg, an x-ray confirms a fracture, a pathology or laboratory report confirms a diagnosis) before the encounter is coded, the confirmed diagnosis code should be used.

MAPPING ICD-9-CM TO ICD-10-CM

Crosswalking is starting with an already assigned code in one system and then using that information to link to the other system without starting over in the logic stream.

Mappings between ICD-9-CM and ICD-10-CM attempt to find corresponding diagnosis codes between the two code sets, insofar as this is possible. Because the two systems are so different, translating between them the majority of the time can offer only a series of possible compromises rather than the mirror image of one code in the other code set.

Crosswalking and mapping ICD-9-CM to ICD-10-CM will be an important tool in transitioning to ICD-10-CM. The following example correlates ICD-9-CM and ICD-10-CM codes.

Example: A patient with type I diabetes and Kimmelstiel-Wilson disease visited his endocrinologist in follow-up. The codes for this visit are compared below.

ICD-9-CM

250.41	Diabetes with renal manifestations, type I [juvenile type], not stated as uncontrolled
581.81	Nephropathy, not otherwise specified

ICD-10-CM

E10.21	Type 1 diabetes mellitus with diabetic nephropathy
	Type 1 diabetes mellitus with Kimmelstiel-Wilson disease
E8.21	Diabetes mellitus due to underlying condition with diabetic nephropathy

ICD-9-CM combines the eye and ear within the nervous system and sense organs, but ICD-10-CM defines eye and ear in their own chapter.

Example: A patient underwent an initial tympanoplasty (69631) without mastoidectomy in the outpatient hospital surgery department for an attic perforation of the tympanic membrane of the right ear.

The codes for this procedure are compared below.

ICD-9-CM

384.2	Perforation of tympanic membrane	
	384.20	Unspecified perforation of tympanic membrane
	384.21	Central perforation of tympanic membrane
	384.22	Attic perforation of tympanic membrane
	384.23	Other marginal perforation of tympanic membrane
	384.24	Multiple perforations of tympanic membrane
	384.25	Total perforation of tympanic membrane

ICD-10-CM

H72	Perforation of tympanic membrane	
	H72.0	Central perforation of tympanic membrane
	H72.1	Attic perforation of tympanic membrane
	H72.10	Attic perforation of tympanic membrane, unspecified ear
	H72.11	Attic perforation of tympanic membrane, right ear
	H72.12	Attic perforation of tympanic membrane, left ear
	H72.13	Attic perforation of tympanic membrane, bilateral
	H72.2	Other marginal perforations of tympanic membrane

ICD-10-CM is more specific in identifying the ear affected. The example indicates that the procedure was performed on the right ear, which is reported with H72.11 in ICD-10-CM. Among the choices for ICD-9-CM, the most appropriate diagnosis code is 384.22 (attic perforation of the tympanic membrane). ICD-9-CM is not as specific, as it does not identify which ear is affected.

ICD-9-CM

384.22	Attic perforation of tympanic membrane

ICD-10-CM

H72.11	Attic perforation of tympanic membrane, right ear

The draft guidelines specific to this chapter involve complication of care within the body system chapter specific to the organs and structure of that body system. The condition or disease should be sequenced first, followed by a complication code in block H95.

H95	Intraoperative and postprocedural complications and disorders of ear and mastoid process, not elsewhere classified

Example: A patient underwent a revision of the mastoidectomy with apicectomy (69605) for cholesteatoma of the left middle ear and mastoid. During the procedure the patient experienced an intraoperative hemorrhage of the ear and mastoid process. The codes for this procedure are listed below.

ICD-9-CM

385.3	Cholesteatoma of middle ear and mastoid	
	385.30	Unspecified cholesteatoma
	385.31	Cholesteatoma of attic
	385.32	Cholesteatoma of middle ear
	385.33	Cholesteatoma of middle ear and mastoid
	385.35	Diffuse cholesteatosis of middle ear and mastoid

ICD-10-CM

H71.2	Cholesteatoma of mastoid	
	H71.20	Cholesteatoma of mastoid, unspecified ear
	H71.21	Cholesteatoma of mastoid, right ear
	H71.22	Cholesteatoma of mastoid, left ear
	H71.23	Cholesteatoma of mastoid, bilateral

In ICD-10-CM, the diagnosis would be reported with code H71.22 (cholesteatoma of mastoid, left ear) and in ICD-9-CM, with code 385.33 (cholesteatoma of middle ear and mastoid). According to the ICD-10-CM guidelines, the complication is also coded. The options for coding intraoperative and postprocedural complications of the ear (H95.2) are shown below.

H95.2	Intraoperative and postprocedural hemorrhage or hematoma complicating a procedure of the ear and mastoid process
	Excludes1: intraoperative hemorrhage or hematoma due to accidental puncture of laceration during a procedure on the ear (H95.3-) H95.21

Intraoperative hemorrhage of the ear and mastoid process during a procedure of the ear and mastoid process

H95.23	Intraoperative hematoma of the ear and mastoid process during a procedure of the ear and mastoid process

The most appropriate complication code in this block is H95.23, Intraoperative hematoma of the ear and mastoid process during a procedure of the ear and mastoid process.

With ICD-9-CM, the complication would be reported in category 998.1, Hemorrhage or hematoma or seroma complicating a procedure. A fifth digit is required in this category.

998.1	Hemorrhage or hematoma or seroma complicating a procedure
998.11	Hemorrhage complicating a procedure

The following shows the coding comparison between ICD-9-CM and ICD-10-CM:

ICD-9-CM

385.33	Cholesteatoma of middle ear and mastoid
998.11	Hemorrhage complicating a procedure

ICD-10-CM

H71.22	Cholesteatoma of mastoid, left ear
H95.23	Intraoperative hematoma of the ear and mastoid process during a procedure of the ear and mastoid process

Below is a comparison between ICD-9-CM and ICD-10-CM for the diagnosis of low-tension open-angle glaucoma:

ICD-9-CM

365	Glaucoma
365.12	Low-tension open-angle glaucoma

ICD-10-CM

H40-H42	**Glaucoma**	
H40.1	**Open-angle glaucoma**	
H40.12	**Low-tension glaucoma**	
	H40.121	**Low-tension glaucoma, right eye**
	H40.122	**Low-tension glaucoma, left eye**
	H40.123	**Low-tension glaucoma, bilateral**
	H40.129	**Low-tension glaucoma, unspecified eye**

ICD-10-CM more specifically identifies which eye is affected, either right, left, bilateral or unspecified eye, whereas ICD-9-CM identifies only the low-tension open-angle glaucoma without identification of which eye is affected.

The following example shows another comparison of ICD-9-CM and ICD-10-CM.

Example: A patient was involved in an industrial accident and suffered a traumatic cataract of the left eye. After examination, the general ophthalmologist determined that the optic nerve may be damaged in the left eye and sent the patient to a neuro-ophthalmologist for further evaluation. The diagnosis documented in the medical record was total traumatic cataract of the left eye.

In ICD-9-CM the coder must choose the appropriate code from the following options:

366.2x	**Traumatic cataract**
366.20	**Unspecified traumatic cataract**
366.21	**Localized traumatic opacities of cataract**
366.22	**Total traumatic cataract**
366.23	**Partially resolved traumatic cataract**

Within the category H26 in ICD-10-CM, a traumatic cataract is coded to H26.13 with a sixth digit to identify the affected eye if known.

H26.13x	**Total traumatic cataract**
H26.131	**Total traumatic cataract, right eye**
H26.132	**Total traumatic cataract, left eye**
H26.133	**Total traumatic cataract, bilateral**
H26.139	**Total traumatic cataract, unspecified eye**

The following shows the comparison in coding with ICD-9-CM vs ICD-10-CM, demonstrating that ICD-10-CM allows for more specificity.

ICD-9-CM

366.22 **Total traumatic cataract**

ICD-10-CM

H26.132 **Total traumatic cataract, left eye**

Neoplasms

Neoplasm Table

Chapter 2 of ICD-10-CM contains codes for most benign and malignant neoplasms. To properly code neoplasms, the documentation in the medical record must indicate whether the neoplasm is benign, in situ, malignant, or of uncertain histologic behavior. If there is a malignancy, the secondary (metastatic) site should also be reported as it is currently with ICD-9-CM.

As in ICD-9-CM, there is a separate "Neoplasm Table." The codes should be selected from the table. The guidelines in ICD-10-CM state, "If the histology (cell type) of the neoplasm is documented, that term should be referenced first, in the main section of the Index, rather than going immediately to the Neoplasm Table, in order to determine which column in the Neoplasm Table is appropriate."

Example: A physician diagnosed adenocarcinoma of the right breast, lower outer quadrant of the left side, in a 54-year-old woman. The physician's documentation indicated it as the primary site.

The first step is to reference the Alphabetic Index:

Adenocarcinoma (M8140/3) – *see also Neoplasm, malignant*

The Alphabetic Index identifies adenocarcinoma as a malignancy reported by site. The coder then will reference the Neoplasm Table for selection of the correct code.

Excerpt From Neoplasm Table, ICD-10-CM Draft

	Malignant Primary	Malignant Secondary	Malignant Carcinoma in situ	Benign	Uncertain Behavior	Unspecified
Breast central portion (unspecified side)	C50.10	C79.81	D05.90	D24.00	D48.60	D49.3
left side	C50.12	C79.81	D05.92	D24.02	D48.62	D49.3
right side	C50.11	C79.81	D05.91	D24.01	D48.61	D49.3
Ectopic sites (unspecified side)	C50.80	C79.81	D05.90	D24.00	D48.60	D49.3
left side	C50.82	C79.81	D05.92	D24.02	D48.62	D49.3
right side	C50.81	C79.81	D05.91	D24.01	D48.61	D49.3
Inner (unspecified side)	C50.80	C79.81	D05.90	D24.00	D48.60	D49.3
left side	C50.82	C79.81	D05.92	D24.02	D48.62	D49.3
right side	C50.81	C79.81	D05.91	D24.01	D48.61	D49.3
Lower (unspecified side)	C50.80	C79.81	D05.90	D24.00	D48.60	D49.3
left side	C50.82	C79.81	D05.92	D24.02	D48.62	D49.3
right side	C50.81	C79.81	D05.91	D24.01	D48.61	D49.3
Lower inner quadrant (unspecified side)	C50.30	C79.81	D05.90	D24.00	D48.60	D49.3
left side	C50.32	C79.81	D05.92	D24.02	D48.62	D49.3
right side	C50.31	C79.81	D05.91	D24.01	D48.61	D49.3
Lower outer quadrant (unspecified side)	C50.50	C79.81	D05.90	D24.00	D48.60	D49.3
left side	C50.52	C79.81	D05.92	D24.02	D48.62	D49.3
right side	C50.51	C79.81	D05.91	D24.01	D48.61	D49.3

The correct diagnosis code for this example is:

C50.52	**Adenocarcinoma of the left side, lower outer quadrant, malignant, primary site, which is found in the first column.**

The Neoplasm Table provides proper coding based on the histology of the neoplasm by site. The Tabular List should be referenced to verify that the correct code has been selected and a more specific code does not exist.

The following example is from the Tabular List:

C50.50	**Malignant neoplasm of lower-outer quadrant of female breast, unspecified side**
C50.51	**Malignant neoplasm of lower-outer quadrant of right female breast**
C50.52	**Malignant neoplasm of lower-outer quadrant of left female breast**

Use of Pathology Report

The guidelines for ICD-10-CM indicate that a confirmed malignancy diagnosis is not reported without a pathology report on the record to confirm the histologic type of neoplasm. If the pathology report is not in the medical record, the attending physician must confirm the diagnosis in the medical record documentation. The pathology report is not required for encounters such as chemotherapy or radiation therapy.

Morphology Codes

The type of histologic tumor is identified with a morphology code. The Neoplasm Table only distinguishes between malignant, benign, in situ, and uncertain behavior. The morphology code should be included in the medical record when possible. The morphology code can be referenced in the Index under the term for the histology of the neoplasm. This is especially important when coding for the cancer registry.

Neoplasms of Uncertain Behavior vs Unspecified Behavior

A neoplasm of unspecified behavior is coded in category D49, which is only used when documentation does not exist in the medical record to indicate the nature of the neoplasm. If a histologic examination of the specimen was performed, the unspecified behavior code should not be used.

Code categories D37 to D48 include neoplasms of uncertain behavior. These codes are for cases in which, after histologic examination, the pathologist is unable to classify the specimen as benign or malignant or the cell type cannot be determined.

Sequencing of Neoplasm Codes

If the reason for the encounter is for diagnosis of a suspicious lump, skin lesion, or other indication that a malignancy might be present, the code for the sign or symptom is assigned until the diagnosis is confirmed. At the time of coding, if a malignancy has been confirmed for an outpatient visit, the neoplasm code should be assigned.

Example: During a routine examination, the physician found a suspicious mass in the left breast of a female patient who had a history of cancer of the right breast. The physician scheduled a biopsy in the outpatient ambulatory surgery center at the hospital. Since the diagnosis of a malignancy cannot be confirmed at this visit, the breast mass is reported.

The ICD-9-CM to ICD-10-CM comparison is shown below:

ICD-9-CM

611.72 **Lump or mass in breast**

ICD-10-CM

N63 **Unspecified lump in breast**

Includes: nodule(s) NOS in breast

If the reason for the encounter is treatment of the primary neoplasm, the neoplasm is assigned as the principal/first listed diagnosis. The primary site is to be sequenced first, followed by any metastatic sites.

Example: A patient underwent removal of the upper lobe of the lung due to lung cancer after a mass was discovered during a computed tomographic scan.

The comparison between ICD-9-CM and ICD-10-CM is shown below.

ICD-9-CM

162 **Malignant neoplasm of bronchus or lung**

162.3 **Malignant neoplasm of upper lobe, bronchus, or lung**

ICD-10-CM

C34.1 **Malignant neoplasm of upper lobe, bronchus or lung**

C34.10 **Malignant neoplasm of upper lobe, bronchus or lung, unspecified side**

C34.11 **Malignant neoplasm of upper lobe, right bronchus or lung**

C34.12 **Malignant neoplasm of upper lobe, left bronchus or lung**

The correct ICD-10-CM diagnosis code selection would be C34.10 since the side is not specified. Documentation in this example is extremely important, since the specificity in the documentation would indicate either the left or right lobe. It is important to begin encouraging physicians to document details more specifically in order to select the most appropriate diagnosis code. ICD-10-CM also specifies laterality, which ICD-9-CM does not.

When an encounter is for a primary malignancy with metastasis and treatment is directed toward the metastatic (secondary) site(s) only, the metastatic site(s) is designated as the principal/first listed diagnosis. The primary malignancy is coded as an additional code.

Example: A patient was diagnosed with a malignant cancer of the pancreatic duct with metastasis to the liver. The patient was being treated for the liver malignancy.

The comparison between ICD-9-CM and ICD-10-CM is as follows:

ICD-9-CM

First listed diagnosis:

197.7 **Secondary malignant neoplasm of liver**

Primary malignancy:

157.3 **Malignant neoplasm of pancreatic duct**

ICD-10-CM

First listed diagnosis:

C78.7 **Secondary malignant neoplasm of liver**

Primary malignancy:

C25.3 **Malignant neoplasm of pancreatic duct**

When an encounter is for management of a complication associated with the malignancy, such as dehydration, and the treatment is only for the complication, the complication is coded first, followed by the appropriate code(s) for the malignancy.

Example: A patient was admitted to the hospital after chemotherapy for a malignancy of the ethmoidal sinus. The ICD-10-CM codes are as follows:

First listed diagnosis:

E86.0 **Dehydration**

Secondary diagnosis:

C31.1 **Malignant neoplasm of ethmoidal sinus**

An exception to this is anemia due to a neoplasm. Code D63.0, Anemia in neoplastic disease, is a manifestation (secondary) code. Coding conventions require that it be sequenced after the underlying neoplasm code.

Example: A patient was diagnosed with a malignant neoplasm of the frontal lobe. The patient was also anemic because of the tumor.

The following information is from the Tabular List:

D63 **Anemia in chronic diseases classified elsewhere**

D63.0 **Anemia in neoplastic disease**

Code first neoplasm (C00-D49)

First listed diagnosis:

D63.0 **Anemia in neoplastic disease**

Secondary diagnosis:

C71.1 Malignant neoplasm of frontal lobe

When an encounter is for a pathological fracture due to a malignancy, if the focus of treatment is the fracture, a code from subcategory M84.5, Pathological fracture of bone in neoplastic disease, should be sequenced first, followed by the code for the malignancy.

If the focus of treatment is the neoplasm with an associated pathological fracture, the neoplasm code should be sequenced first, followed by a code from M84.5 for the pathological fracture. The "code also" note at M84.5 provides this sequencing instruction.

Example: A patient was treated initially for a pathologic fracture of the right tibia, due to a neoplasm of the right tibia.

The first listed diagnosis would be C76.51, Malignant neoplasm of right lower limb, followed by the code for the pathologic fracture of a bone in neoplastic disease.

The following information is from the Tabular List:

M84.5 Pathologic fracture of bone in neoplastic disease

Code also underlying neoplasm

The following seventh-character extensions are to be added to each code for subcategory M84.5:

a initial encounter for fracture

d subsequent encounter for fracture with routine healing

g subsequent encounter for fracture with delayed healing

j subsequent encounter for fracture with nonunion

m subsequent encounter for fracture with malunion

q sequelae

M84.561a Pathologic fracture of bone in neoplastic disease, right tibia

The codes would be reported in the following sequence:

First listed diagnosis:

C76.51 Malignant neoplasm of right lower limb

Secondary diagnosis:

M84.561a Pathologic fracture of bone in neoplastic disease, right tibia

When an encounter is for pain management due to the malignancy, the pain code R52.02, R52.12, or, R52.22 should be sequenced first, followed by the appropriate neoplasm code(s).

Example: A patient with a malignancy of the frontal lobe of the brain was in acute pain during his follow-up visit. The physician prescribed a drug to relieve the patient's pain.

First listed diagnosis:

R52.02 Acute pain in neoplastic disease

Code also neoplasm

Secondary diagnosis:

C71.1 Malignant neoplasm of frontal lobe

The following is from the Tabular List:

R52.02 Acute pain in neoplastic disease

Code also neoplasm

When the encounter is for treatment of a complication resulting from a surgical procedure performed for the treatment of a malignancy, the complication should be designated as the principal/first listed diagnosis if treatment is directed at resolving the complication.

Example: A patient was treated for sepsis following surgery for the removal of a malignant tumor of the lateral wall of the bladder.

First listed diagnosis:

T81.4a Infection following a procedure, not elsewhere classified

Sepsis following a procedure, not elsewhere classified

Secondary diagnosis:

C67.2 Malignant neoplasm of lateral wall of bladder

According to the Tabular List, the following seventh-character extensions are to be added to each code for category T81:

a initial encounter

d subsequent encounter

q sequelae

When a primary malignancy has been previously excised or eradicated from its site and there is no further treatment directed to that site and no evidence of any existing primary malignancy, a code from category Z85, Personal history of primary and secondary malignant neoplasm, should be used to indicate the former site of the malignancy if no related pathology is discovered.

Any mention of extension, invasion, or metastasis to another site(s) is coded as a secondary malignant neoplasm to the metastatic site(s). The secondary site may be the principal/first listed with the Z85 code used as a secondary code.

Example: A 56-year-old man was seen in follow-up after removal of the prostate 3 years previously for a malignancy.

Z85.46 Personal history of primary malignant neoplasm of prostate

When a primary malignancy has been excised but further treatment, such as additional surgery, radiation therapy, or chemotherapy, is directed to that site, the primary malignancy code, not the Z85 code, should be used until treatment is completed.

Cancer in a Pregnant Patient

When a patient is treated for a malignant neoplasm that complicates pregnancy, childbirth, and the puerperium, a code from subcategory O94.1-, Malignant neoplasm complicating pregnancy, childbirth, and the puerperium, should be used first, followed by the appropriate code to indicate the type of neoplasm.

Example: A 32-year-old woman who was in her second trimester of pregnancy underwent Mohs micrographic surgery for basal cell carcinoma of the lip.

First listed diagnosis:

O94.112 Malignant neoplasm complicating pregnancy, second trimester

Secondary diagnosis:

C44.0 Malignant neoplasm of skin of lip

Malignant neoplasm of basal cell carcinoma of lip

Malignant Neoplasm Without Specification of Site

Code C80, Malignant neoplasm without specification of site, equates to Cancer, unspecified. It is also for disseminated cancer for which no primary site is found. This code should be used only when no determination can be made as to the primary site of a malignancy. It should not be used in place of assigning codes for the primary site and for all known secondary sites.

The following example is from the Tabular List:

C80 Malignant neoplasm without specification of site

Includes: *Cancer unspecified site (primary) (secondary)*
Carcinoma unspecified site (primary) (secondary)
Carcinomatosis unspecified site (primary) (secondary)
Generalized cancer unspecified site (primary) (secondary)
Generalized malignancy unspecified site (primary) (secondary)
Malignancy unspecified site (primary) (secondary)
Malignant cachexia
Multiple cancer unspecified site (primary) (secondary)
Primary site unknown malignant neoplasm's of lymphoid

Encounters for Chemotherapy and Radiation Therapy

As with ICD-9-CM, when an encounter involves the surgical removal of a neoplasm, primary or secondary site, followed by chemotherapy or radiation treatment, chemotherapy, or radiation therapy, the diagnosis should be the first listed diagnosis followed by the malignancy.

If an encounter is solely for the administration of chemotherapy or radiation therapy, code Z51.0, Encounter for radiotherapy session, or Z51.1, Encounter for chemotherapy session for neoplasm, should be the principal/first listed code. If a patient receives both chemotherapy and radiation therapy, both codes should be listed, in either order of sequence.

Example: A patient underwent chemotherapy after an oophorectomy for removal of a malignant tumor of the left ovary.

First listed diagnosis:

Z51.1 Chemotherapy session for neoplasm

Secondary diagnosis:

C56.1 Malignant neoplasm of left ovary

When an encounter is for the purpose of radiotherapy or chemotherapy and the patient develops complications such as uncontrolled nausea and vomiting or dehydration, the principal/first listed code remains the radiation therapy or chemotherapy code. The complications of the treatment should be added as additional codes following code(s) for the malignancy.

Example: A patient was experiencing nausea and vomiting after radiation therapy for treatment of a malignant tumor of the parathyroid gland.

First listed diagnosis:

Z51.0 Encounter for radiotherapy session

Secondary diagnosis:

C75.0 Malignant neoplasm of parathyroid gland

Tertiary diagnosis:

R11.0 Nausea with vomiting

When an encounter is to determine the extent of the malignancy, or for a procedure to treat the malignancy, the primary malignancy or appropriate metastatic site is designated as the principal/first listed diagnosis, even if chemotherapy or radiotherapy is administered.

Example: A physician removed a malignant tumor from the descending colon in the outpatient surgery center. The physician recommended that the patient undergo chemotherapy the same day.

First listed diagnosis:

C18.6 Malignant neoplasm of descending colon

Secondary diagnosis:

Z51.1 Chemotherapy session for neoplasm

When an encounter is for management of the complication of chemotherapy or radiation therapy, and the only treatment is for the complication, the complication is sequenced first, followed by the appropriate code(s) for the malignancy.

Example: The patient was experiencing nausea and vomiting 1 day after chemotherapy to treat the left breast.

First listed diagnosis:

R11.0 Nausea with vomiting

Secondary diagnosis:

C50.32 Malignant neoplasm of lower-inner quadrant of left female breast

Due to the potentially toxic nature of many chemotherapy agents, certain tests may be performed before the administration of chemotherapy as well as during the course of the chemotherapy treatment. The malignancy should be coded as the principal diagnosis for encounters for these tests. The code for long-term (current) use of drug, Z79.82, should be used as a secondary code if the test is being done during the course of chemotherapy treatment.

Injuries and Poisonings

The S codes in ICD-10-CM are used for reporting different types of injuries related to single body regions. In addition, the T codes are used to report injuries to unspecified body regions as well as poisonings and certain other consequences of external causes.

The format of the S section of ICD-10-CM differs from ICD-9-CM in that the blocks cover single body regions with category codes and represent the various types of injuries or specific anatomical parts involved in the injuries.

Example: A 35-year-old man was stabbed in the shoulder during a robbery at a convenience store.

The following codes are from the Tabular List:

S41.03 Puncture wound without foreign body of shoulder

S41.031 Puncture wound without foreign body of right shoulder

S41.032 Puncture wound without foreign body of left shoulder

S41.039 Puncture wound without foreign body of unspecified shoulder

Since in this example the documentation does not specify the right or left shoulder, the unspecified code would be reported as S41.039.

The ICD-10-CM utilizes dummy placeholders, always the letter x. A dummy x is used as a fifth-digit character placeholder at certain 6-character codes to allow for future expansion. The best example of this is at the poisoning codes, categories T36 to T50, and the toxic effect codes, categories T51 to T65.

The sixth character for the codes at categories T36 to T50 always indicates the intent:

- unintentional (accidental)
- intentional self-harm
- assault
- undetermined
- adverse effect
- underdosing

The sixth character for the codes at categories T51 to T65 always indicates the intent. The fifth character x will permit the future expansion of these codes without disturbing the sixth-character structure.

Example: A patient who was experiencing excruciating back pain took 3 tablets of a muscle relaxant at the same time. The directions stated that 1 tablet should be taken every 4 hours. Thirty minutes later, the patient was experiencing nausea with vomiting and severe abdominal pain. The patient presented to the emergency department at the local hospital for treatment. This was the first time the patient had taken an overdose of this medication.

The correct poisoning code is selected from the Tabular List:

T48 **Poisoning by, adverse effect of and underdosing of agents primarily acting on smooth and skeletal muscles and the respiratory system**

The following seventh-character extensions are to be added to each code for category T48:

a initial encounter

d subsequent encounter

q sequelae

T48.1 **Poisoning by, adverse effect of and underdosing of skeletal muscle relaxants [neuromuscular blocking agents]**

T48.1x **Poisoning by, adverse effect of and underdosing of skeletal muscle relaxants [neuromuscular blocking agents]**

T48.1x1 **Poisoning by skeletal muscle relaxants [neuromuscular blocking agents], accidental (unintentional)**

Poisoning by skeletal muscle relaxants [neuromuscular blocking agents] NOS

T48.1x2 **Poisoning by skeletal muscle relaxants [neuromuscular blocking agents], intentional self-harm**

T48.1x3 **Poisoning by skeletal muscle relaxants [neuromuscular blocking agents], assault**

T48.1x4 **Poisoning by skeletal muscle relaxants [neuromuscular blocking agents], undetermined**

T48.1x5 **Adverse effect of skeletal muscle relaxants [neuromuscular blocking agents]**

T48.1x6 **Underdosing of skeletal muscle relaxants [neuromuscular blocking agents]**

The correct poisoning code based on the selection above is T48.1x1. Since this is the first patient encounter related to the poisoning, the seventh digit character extension is a.

External Causes of Morbidity (Y01-Y98)

External causes of morbidity are classified in Chapter 20 of ICD-10-CM. The chapter permits classification of environmental events and circumstances as the cause of injury and other adverse affects. As with ICD-9-CM, these codes are not to be used as the first listed diagnosis, but as a secondary diagnosis when applicable. For many ICD-10-CM Chapter 20 codes, extensions should be added to each of the codes from a category to indicate initial encounter, subsequent encounter, or sequelae of the original injury.

Chapter 20 in ICD-10-CM contains the following blocks:

- V00-V09 Pedestrian injured in transport accident
- V10-V19 Pedal cyclist injured in transport accident
- V20-V29 Motorcycle rider injured in transport accident
- V30-V39 Occupant of three-wheeled motor vehicle injured in transport accident
- V40-V49 Car occupant injured in transport accident
- V50-V59 Occupant of pick-up truck or van injured in transport accident
- V60-V69 Occupant of heavy transport vehicle injured in transport accident
- V70-V79 Bus occupant injured in transport accident
- V80-V89 Other land transport accidents
- V90-V94 Water transport accidents
- V95-V97 Air and space transport accidents
- V98-V99 Other and unspecified transport accidents
- W00-W19 Falls
- W20-W49 Exposure to inanimate mechanical forces
- W50-W64 Exposure to animate mechanical forces
- W65-W74 Accidental drowning and submersion
- W85-W99 Exposure to electric current, radiation and extreme ambient air temperature and pressure
- X00-X09 Exposure to smoke, fire and flames
- X10-X19 Contact with heat and hot substances
- X30-X39 Exposure to forces of nature
- X52, X58 Accidental exposure to other specified factors
- X71-X83 Intentional self-harm
- X92-Y08 Assault
- Y21-Y33 Event of undetermined intent
- Y35-Y38 Legal intervention, operations of war, military operations, and terrorism
- Y62-Y84 Complications of medical and surgical care
- Y62-Y69 Misadventures to patients during surgical and medical care
- Y70-Y82 Medical devices associated with adverse incidents in diagnostic and therapeutic use
- Y83-Y84 Surgical and other medical procedures as the cause of abnormal reaction of the patient, or of later complication, without mention of misadventure at the time of the procedure
- Y90-Y98 Supplementary factors related to causes of morbidity classified elsewhere

Codes from categories V00 to Y35 require an extension to indicate whether the encounter is the initial encounter for treatment, a subsequent encounter for treatment, or the sequelae of an event.

The extensions for these categories are as follows:

a initial encounter

d subsequent encounter

q sequelae

A number of block, category, and subcategory title changes have been made in Chapter 20 of ICD-10-CM compared to ICD-9-CM. ICD-9-CM and ICD-10-CM are compared below.

ICD-9-CM	E880–E888 Accidental falls
ICD-10-CM	W00–X58 Falls

Example: A 3-year-old boy was taken to the emergency department after a fall from a swing on the playground. This was the first time his mother had let him play on the swings in the playground.

In this example only the external cause, not the patient's condition, is identified. Extensions should be added to each code from the category to indicate initial encounter, subsequent encounter, or sequelae of the original injury.

The following codes are from the the Tabular List:

W09 Fall on and from playground equipment

The following seventh-character extensions are to be added to each code from category W09:

- **a** initial encounter
- **d** subsequent encounter
- **q** sequelae

W09.0 Fall on or from playground slide

W09.1 Fall from playground swing

W09.2 Fall on or from jungle gym

W09.8 Fall on or from other playground equipment

The correct code would be W09.1a reported as a secondary code. The a indicates the initial encounter for the fall.

Codes for place of occurrence of the external cause are secondary codes for use with other external cause codes to identify the location of the patient at the time of injury. A place of occurrence code is used only once, at the initial encounter for treatment. Only 1 code from Y92 should be recorded on a medical record. A place of occurrence code should be used in conjunction with an activity code, Y93. A place of occurrence code should be reported as Y92.9 if the place is not stated or is not applicable. Place of occurrence codes are not necessary with poisonings, toxic effects, adverse affects, and underdosing.

Category Y93 identifies the activity. Activity codes are secondary codes for use with other external cause codes to identify the activity of the patient at the time of the injury. An activity code is used only once, at the initial encounter for treatment. Only 1 code from Y93 should be recorded on the medical record. An activity code should be used in conjunction with a place of occurrence code, Y92.

Activity code Y93.9 is used if the activity of the patient is not stated or is not applicable.

Specific seventh-character extensions are required for Y93:

- 1 Non–work-related activity
- 2 Work-related activity
- 3 Student activity
- 4 Military activity

The draft guidelines instruct the user to report extension 2 if a patient is a student but is injured while performing an activity for income.

Example: A 16-year-old boy was injured while playing high school football at the school field during the opening game. A player on the opposing team accidentally stepped on the patient's hand with his cleats. The patient was taken to the local urgent care center for treatment.

When the external cause is coded, the first code will identify the condition or injury, the second code will be the external cause (place of occurrence) (Y92.321), and the third code will be the activity, playing football.

W21.31 Struck by shoe cleats; Stepped on by shoe cleats

Y92.321 Football field as the place of occurrence of the external cause

Y93.0203 Football

External causes are not to be reported as the first listed diagnosis.

Factors Influencing Health Status and Contact With Health Services (Z00–Z99)

In ICD-10-CM, Z codes are similar to V codes in that Z codes represent the reason for encounter, but a corresponding procedure code must be used to identify the specific procedure performed. Categories Z00 through Z99 are provided for occasions when circumstances other than a disease, an injury, or an external cause classifiable to categories A00 through Y89 are recorded as the reason for encounter. These circumstances can arise in 2 main ways:

1. When a person who may or may not be sick encounters the health services for some specific purpose, such as to receive limited care or service for a current condition
   - to donate an organ or tissue
   - to receive a prophylactic vaccination
   - to discuss a problem that is in itself not a disease or injury
2. When some circumstance or problem is present that influences the person's health status but is not in itself a current illness or injury

Example: A 12-month-old infant was seen for her 12-month well-child checkup. The physician examined the patient and found that she was developing normally without problems. Counseling was conducted with the mother and the patient was scheduled to return in 6 months.

The ICD-9-CM and ICD-10-CM codes are compared below.

ICD-9-CM

V20.2 Routine infant or child health check

ICD-10-CM

Z00.10 Encounter for routine child health examination without abnormal findings

Encounter for routine child health examination NOS

Z00.11 Encounter for routine child health examination with abnormal findings

Use additional code to identify abnormal findings

With ICD-10-CM there are 2 diagnosis code choices, 1 for a patient without abnormal findings and 1 for a patient with abnormal findings.

GETTING READY FOR ICD-10-CM

What mechanisms must be in place to prepare for ICD-10-CM in the medical practice? Each medical group, hospital, and practice must begin planning now for ICD-10-CM implementation. It may seem a bit overwhelming, but it can be managed with a step-by-step approach. The following steps are recommended:

1. Form a task force or committee to begin the planning process.
2. Identify potential training needs:
   a. Types of training
   b. Methods of training
   c. Who will conduct training
3. Identify personnel who will need training:
   a. Coding professionals will need a strong background in anatomy and physiology, medial terminology, pharmacology, and medical coding because of the increased level of specificity in ICD-10-CM.
   b. Physician documentation will need more detail in the medical record to adequately code with ICD-10-CM to avoid lost revenue.
   c. Other health care and non–health care professionals will require training.
4. Review information systems/electronic software and billing systems requiring diagnosis or procedure codes (facilities), including, but not limited to:
   a. Billing software
   b. Encoders
   c. Accounting systems
   d. Electronic medical records
   e. Utilization and quality management systems
   f. Performance measurement systems

g. Benefits determination systems

h. Clinical protocols

i. Crosswalks (linking ICD-9 to ICD-10)

5. Address software changes with vendors.
6. Budget for implementation, including:

a. Upgraded or new hardware

b. New software

c. Training cost for clinical and nonclinical staff (everyone will need training)

d. Hiring of consultants or information systems personal to assist with systems change

7. Set up a timetable for implementation.
8. Review charge tickets, superbills, and/or encounter forms for revisions.
9. Attempt to develop crosswalks (linking ICD-9 to ICD-10) for the most common ICD-9-CM codes used in the practice and map the codes to ICD-10-CM.
10. Read articles, newsletters, and professional journals.
11. Monitor the Internet and *Federal Register* for updated information.
12. Anticipate problems prior to implementation.

POTENTIAL IMPACT AFTER IMPLEMENTATION

Some potential problem areas that have been identified by various sources include possible delays in payment from carriers until everyone is fully trained; inaccurate coding, reporting, and processing, increasing delays in payment, denials, and/or rejections; insufficient documentation to assign the diagnosis code; and higher demands on hiring qualified coders and retaining trained coders, which may increase salary costs and benefits.

MORE INFORMATION ON ICD-10-CM

Information can be obtained from the Centers for Disease Control and Prevention web site at:

http://www.cdc.gov/nchs/about/otheract/icd9/abticd10.htm

TEST YOUR KNOWLEDGE

Fill in the blanks:

1. Two new chapters in ICD-10-CM include ____________ and ____________________.
2. The Excludes1 indicates ____________________________.
3. The organization that is responsible for the development and adaptation of ICD-10 for use in the United States is called ____.
4. The pertinent reasons we use coding data today include:

   a. ____

   b. ____

   c. ____

   d. ____

   e. ____

   f. ____

5. The ICD-10 consists of:

   a. ____

   b. ____

   c. ____

   d. ____

   e. ____

   f. ____

6. Chapters are further divided into subchapters referred to as ____.
7. The Alphabetic Index is divided into 3 sections and is organized by main terms. List the 3 sections and the content of each section.

   Section 1: ______________________________

   Section 2: ______________________________

   Section 3: ______________________________

8. Notes appear in the Alphabetic Index to:

   1. ____

   2. ____

   3. ____

9. The draft ICD-10-CM Guidelines state, "When a condition is documented as both acute, subacute, and chronic and separate codes exist in the Index, ____."
10. External causes of mobidity are classified in chapter _____ of ICD-10-CM. The code range for this category is _____-_____.

ANSWER KEY

1. Two new chapters in ICD-10-CM include Diseases of the Eye and Adnexa and Disorders of the Ear.
2. The Excludes1 indicates that the code excluded should never be used at the same time as the code above the Excludes1 note. An Excludes1 is used when 2 conditions cannot occur together, such as a congenital form and an acquired form of the same condition.
3. The organization that is responsible for the development and adaptation of ICD-10 for use in the United States is called The World Health Organization.
4. The pertinent reasons we use coding data today include:

    a. Identifying fraudulent practices

    b. Supporting medical necessity

    c. Conducting research and clinical trials

    d. Setting health policy

    e. Processing claims for reimbursement

    f. Measuring quality and efficacy of care

5. The ICD-10-CM consists of:

    a. A Tabular List containing cause-of-death titles and codes (Volume 1)

    b. Inclusion and exclusion terms for cause-of-death titles (Volume 1)

    c. Alphabetical Index to diseases and nature of injury

    d. External causes of injury

    e. Table of drugs and chemicals (Volume 3)

    f. Description, guidelines, and coding rules (Volume 2)

6. Chapters are further divided into subchapters referred to as blocks.
7. The Alphabetic Index is divided into 3 sections and is organized by main terms. List the 3 sections and the content of each section.

    Section 1: Index to Diseases and Nature of Injury

    Section 2: Index to External Causes

    Section 3: Table of Drugs and Chemicals

8. Notes appear in the Alphabetic Index to:

    1. Define terms

    2. Provide direction

    3. Provide coding instructions

9. The draft ICD-10-CM Guidelines state: "When a condition is documented as both acute, subacute, and chronic and separate codes exist in the Index, both are coded with the acute (subacute) sequenced first followed by the code for the chronic condition."
10. External causes of mobidity are classified in chapter 20 of ICD-10-CM. The code range for this category is Y01-Y98.

International Classification of Diseases

ICD-9-CM 2008

Hospital

Volumes 1, 2 and 3
9th Revision—Clinical Modification

AMA
AMERICAN
MEDICAL
ASSOCIATION

Hospital ICD-9-CM 2008,
Volumes 1, 2 and 3

Printed in the United States of America

Additional copies may be ordered by telephoning the American Medical Association at (800) 621-8335, or visit us at *www.amabookstore.com.*

OP066508 (Spiral)
ISBN: 978-1-57947-902-2
BP29:07-P-058:8/07

Table of Contents

Preface

The *2008 Hospital and Payer Professional ICD-9-CM International Classification of Diseases, Volumes 1, 2 & 3* is the most intuitive and easy-to-use diagnostic coding manual available.

Some of the features you will find in your *2008 Hospital and Payer Professional ICD-9-CM International Classification of Diseases, Volumes 1, 2 & 3* include:

- Full-color anatomical illustrations with facing pages that reference the sections of the ICD-9-CM that are relevant to that body or organ system
- Current accepted national guidelines for diagnostic coding
- A compilation of all ICD-9-CM diagnosis and procedure coding changes for 2008
- Intuitive and nationally-recognized symbols and formats within code descriptions
- Full tabular and alphabetical code lists of all valid ICD-9-CM codes (including V and E codes)
- Intuitive symbols representing codes that require 4th and 5th digits, unspecified and non specific codes, and codes that should not be used as primary diagnoses
- Nationally-accepted symbols within code descriptions that highlight new or revised text
- Symbol legends on every page for coding convenience
- Color-coded page ends to provide easy distinction of disease sections in the Tabular list
- Encyclopedia-style page headers for more efficient referencing
- Government appendices including: morphology of neoplasms; classification of drugs by AHFS list; industrial accidents according to agency; and list of three-digit categories
- Additional symbols denoting age-specific and gender-specific codes, as well as Medicare secondary, and primary/secondary code status.
- Color symbols denote Valid O.R. procedures, Non-O.R. procedures and Nonspecific O.R. procedures
- IPPS compliance symbols to identify important Medicare Code Editor (MCE) edits used to audit claims

Sources

This manual contains ICD-9-CM codes effective for October 1, 2007 through September 30, 2008 as compiled and released by the Department of Health and Human Services (HHS). Many of the symbols, guidelines, and conventions used throughout are derived from the official government release of this information.

Anatomical Illustrations

FAIRMAN STUDIOS
medical & biological illustration & animation

Fairman Studios is an award-winning full-service biocommunications studio serving clients in the Healthcare, Scientific and Biomedical industries. Services include medical and scientific illustration, medical animation, web publishing and interactive design. Fairman Studios: www.fairmanstudios.com

Jessica Jackson received her BFA in Graphic Design from Brigham Young University in 2006. She has been illustrating for over 10 years, adding medical anatomy drawings to her repertoire in 2006.

Introduction to ICD-9-CM

The International Classification of Diseases, 9th Revision, Clinical Modification (ICD-9-CM) is based on the official version of the World Health Organization's 9th Revision, International Classification of Diseases (ICD-9). ICD-9 is designed for the classification of morbidity and mortality information for statistical purposes, and for the indexing of hospital records by disease and operations, for data storage and retrieval. The historical background of the International Classification of Diseases may be found in the Introduction to ICD-9 (*Manual of the International Classification of Diseases, Injuries, and Causes of Death*, World Health Organization, Geneva, Switzerland, 1977).

ICD-9-CM is a clinical modification of the World Health Organization's *International Classification of Diseases, 9th Revision*. The term "clinical" is used to emphasize the modification's intent: to serve as a useful tool in the area of classification of morbidity data for indexing of medical records, medical care review, and ambulatory and other medical care programs, as well as for basic health statistics. To describe the clinical picture of the patient, the codes must be more precise than those needed only for statistical groupings and trend analysis.

THE ICD-9-CM COORDINATION AND MAINTENANCE COMMITTEE

Annual modifications are made to the ICD-9-CM through the ICD-9-CM Coordination and Maintenance Committee (C&M). The Committee is made up of representatives from two Federal Government agencies, the National Center for Health Statistics and the Centers for Medicare and Medicaid Services (CMS). The Committee holds meetings twice a year which are open to the public. Modification proposals submitted to the Committee for consideration are presented at the meetings for public discussion. Those approved modification proposals are incorporated into the official government version of the ICD-9-CM and become effective for use October 1 of the year following their presentation.

CHARACTERISTICS OF ICD-9-CM

ICD-9-CM far exceeds its predecessors in the number of codes provided. The disease classification has been expanded to include health-related conditions and to provide greater specificity at the fifth-digit level of detail. These fifth digits are not optional; they are intended for use in recording the information substantiated in the clinical record.

Volume I of ICD-9-CM contains five appendices:

Appendix A	Morphology of Neoplasms
Appendix B*	Glossary of Mental Disorders (Deleted October 1, 2004)
Appendix C	Classification of Drugs by American Hospital Formulary Service List Number and Their ICD-9-CM Equivalents
Appendix D	Classification of Industrial Accidents According to Agency
Appendix E	List of Three-Digit Categories

These appendices are included as a reference to the user in order to provide further information about the patient's clinical picture, to further define a diagnostic statement, to aid in classifying new drugs, or to reference three-digit categories.

* The American Psychiatric Association (APA) has formally requested that the Glossary of Mental Disorders (previously Appendix B) be removed. It has not been maintained for many years and is no longer accurate. This appendix was deleted October 1, 2004.

Volume 2 of ICD-9-CM contains many diagnostic terms which do not appear in Volume 1 since the index includes most diagnostic terms currently in use.

The Disease Classification

ICD-9-CM is totally compatible with its parent system, ICD-9, thus meeting the need for comparability of morbidity and mortality statistics at the international level. A few fourth-digit codes were created in existing three-digit rubrics only when the necessary detail could not be accommodated by the use of a fifth-digit subclassification. To ensure that each rubric of ICD-9-CM collapses back to its ICD-9 counterpart, the following specifications governed the ICD-9-CM disease classification:

Specifications for the Tabular List

1. Three-digit rubrics and their contents are unchanged from ICD-9.
2. The sequence of three-digit rubrics is unchanged from ICD-9.
3. Unsubdivided three-digit rubrics are subdivided where necessary to:
   a) Add clinical detail
   b) Isolate terms for clinical accuracy
4. The modification in ICD-9-CM is accomplished by the addition of a fifth digit to existing ICD-9 rubrics.
5. The optional dual classification in ICD-9 is modified.
   a) Duplicate rubrics are deleted:
      1) Four-digit manifestation categories duplicating etiology entries.
      2) Manifestation inclusion terms duplicating etiology entries.
   b) Manifestations of diseases are identified, to the extent possible, by creating five-digit codes in the etiology rubrics.
   c) When the manifestation of a disease cannot be included in the etiology rubrics, provision for its identification is made by retaining the ICD-9 rubrics used for classifying manifestations of disease.
6. The format of ICD-9-CM is revised from that used in ICD-9.
   a) American spelling of medical terms is used.
   b) Inclusion terms are indented beneath the titles of codes.
   c) Codes not to be used for principal tabulation of disease are printed with the notation, "Code first underlying disease."

Specifications for the Alphabetic Index

1. Format of the Alphabetic Index follows the format of ICD-9.
2. When two codes are required to indicate etiology and manifestation, the manifestation code appears in brackets (e.g., diabetic cataract 250.5X *[366.41]*). The etiology code is always sequenced first followed by the manifestation code.

How to Use the ICD-9-CM

To code accurately, it is necessary to have a working knowledge of medical terminology and to understand the characteristics, terminology, and conventions of the ICD-9-CM. Transforming verbal descriptions of diseases, injuries, conditions, and procedures into numerical designations (coding) is a complex activity and should not be undertaken without proper training.

Originally, coding was accomplished to provide access to medical records by diagnoses and operations through retrieval for medical research, education, and administration. Medical codes today are utilized to facilitate payment of health services, to evaluate utilization patterns, and to study the appropriateness of healthcare costs. Coding provides the bases for epidemiological studies and research into the quality of healthcare.

Coding must be performed correctly and consistently to produce meaningful statistics to aid in the planning for the health needs of the Nation.

Basic Steps in Coding Diagnoses/Diseases

1. Always consult Volume 2, Alphabetic Index to Diseases first.

   Locate the main entry term. The Alphabetic Index is arranged by condition. Conditions may be expressed as nouns, adjectives, and eponyms. Some conditions have multiple entries under their synonyms. Select the appropriate code.
2. Refer to Volume 1 of the ICD-9-CM locating the selected code.

   Be guided by any exclusion notes or other instructions that would direct the use of a different code from that selected in the Index for a particular diagnosis, condition, or disease.
3. Read and be guided by the conventions used in the Tabular List for Diseases (Volume 1, ICD-9-CM).

   As reference for use by researchers and to maintain comparability with its parent, the ICD-9, a list of three-digit ICD-9-CM categories is given in Appendix E. While these categories form natural statistical groupings, they cannot substitute for the required five-digit ICD-9-CM code.

Monitor ICD-9-CM Usage

It is never good to overuse codes, yet many doctors rely on the "same old, same old" ICD-9-CM diagnoses when coding their services. Coders should double-check the codes to make sure that they are not too generic or overused. Overuse of codes can build profiles that lead to audits or place the practice in an inappropriate peer group. How few is too few? If claims contain only 20 or 25 diagnostic codes, there is probably a need to expand.

The below code list includes some of the most over-reported ICD-9-CM diagnoses:

- 285.9 Anemia, unspecified
- 401.9 Unspecified hypertension
- 429.2 Arteriosclerotic cardiovascular disease
- 724.9 Unspecified disorder of the back
- 784.0 Headache
- 786.09 Shortness of breath
- 786.50 Chest pain
- 789.00 Abdominal pain

The importance of consistent, complete documentation in the medical record cannot be overemphasized. Without such documentation the application of all coding guidelines is a difficult, if not impossible, task. The following are common guidelines for use of ICD-9-CM codes:

- List first, as the principal diagnosis, the ICD-9-CM code for the condition established after study to be chiefly responsible for occasioning the admission of the patient to the hospital for care. Then, additional codes that describe coexisting conditions should be listed.
- Use codes at their highest level of specificity: for example, a three-digit code should be assigned only if there are no four-digit or five-digit codes within the category.
- Code and report chronic diseases treated on an ongoing basis as often as the patient receives treatment and care for the condition(s).
- Abnormal findings (laboratory, x-ray, pathologic, and other diagnostic results) are not coded and reported unless the provider indicates their clinical significance. If the findings are outside the normal range and the attending provider has ordered other tests to evaluate the condition or prescribed treatment, it is appropriate to ask the provider whether the abnormal finding should be added.
- Code all conditions that coexist at the time of admission, that develop subsequently, or that affect the treatment received and/or the length of stay. Diagnoses that relate to an earlier episode which have no bearing on the current hospital stay should not be reported.
- Report as the principal diagnosis the condition, which after study occasioned the admission to the hospital, even though treatment may not have been carried out due to unforeseen circumstances.
- When a symptom(s) is followed by contrasting/comparative diagnoses, the symptom code is sequenced first. All the contrasting/comparative diagnoses should be coded as additional diagnoses.

Frequently Encountered Problem Areas When Choosing the Appropriate Diagnostic Code

The diagnostic code used for billing is not reflective of the problems addressed in the actual progress note.

Medical record reviews should be conducted to determine the accuracy of the diagnostic code choice. Frequently the diagnosis used on a recent admission is simply reported for a subsequent admission when, in fact, the medical record may indicate a different problem was responsible for the admission.

Diagnostic and therapeutic services ordered and performed without adequate documentation of medical necessity in the medical record.

Many payers will only pay for services considered medically necessary. To be considered medically necessary, items and services must have been established as safe and effective. That is, the items and services must be:

- consistent with the symptoms or diagnosis of the illness or injury under treatment; and
- necessary and consistent with generally accepted professional medical standards (i.e., not still experimental or investigational); and
- not furnished primarily for the convenience of the patient, the attending physician, or other physician or supplier; and
- furnished at the most appropriate level which can be provided safely and effectively to the patient.

If services fall into these definitions and there still are problems, prove to insurance carriers through prejustification or the appeals process that the service was medically necessary.

Where a treatment or procedure is neither specifically covered nor excluded in a health plan's policies, carriers must make a coverage determination. This determination is based upon the treatment's/procedures' general acceptance by the professional medical community as an effective and proven treatment for the condition for which it is being used. Most carriers will make payment only when a service is accepted as effective and proven.

Lack of Specificity

A provider simply does not provide a detailed enough diagnosis to pick a good diagnosis code. The most common example of this is the hypertension diagnosis. Code 401.9 is one of the most commonly used codes in the United States. However, this code indicates "unspecified hypertension." It is a poor diagnosis code. Insurance companies usually will not consider it a medically necessary diagnosis and discontinue payment after the first visit. Codes 401.0 and 401.1 are valid and specific codes which indicate malignant and benign hypertension. Providers have to be reminded periodically to document in the medical record enough information regarding the diagnosis to choose an accurate and valid diagnosis.

Basic Steps in Coding Procedures

1. Always consult Volume 3, Alphabetic Index to Procedures first.

   Locate the main entry term. The Alphabetic Index to Procedures is arranged by body system and/or type of procedure being performed.

2. Refer to Volume 3, Tabular List for Procedures of the ICD-9-CM locating the selected code.

   Be guided by any exclusion notes or other instructions that would direct the use of a different code from that selected in the Index for a particular operation, diagnostic or therapeutic procedure.

3. Read and be guided by the conventions used in the Tabular List (Volume 3, ICD-9-CM).

ICD-9-CM Official Conventions

The ICD-9-CM Tabular List for both the Disease and Procedure Classification makes use of certain abbreviations, punctuation, and other conventions which need to be clearly understood for efficient and effective coding.

Abbreviations

NEC Not elsewhere classifiable. The category number for the term including NEC is to be used only when the coder lacks the information necessary to code the term to a more specific category.

NOS Not otherwise specified. This abbreviation is the equivalent of "unspecified."

Punctuation

[ ] Brackets are used to enclose synonyms, alternative wordings, or explanatory phrases.

005.2 Food poisoning due to Clostridium perfringens [C. welchii]

( ) Parentheses are used to enclose supplementary words which may be present or absent in the statement of a disease or procedure without affecting the code number to which it is assigned.

041.6 Proteus (mirabilis) (morganii)

: Colons are used in the Tabular List after an incomplete term which needs one or more of the modifiers which follow in order to make it assignable to a given category.

040.0 Gas gangrene
Gas bacillus infection or gangrene
Infection by Clostridium:
histolyticum
oedematiens
perfringens [welchii]
septicum
sordellii

Other Conventions

The ICD-9-CM uses an indented format for ease in reference

Boldface Boldface type is used for all codes and titles in the tabular list.

Italicized Italicized type is used for all exclusion notes and to identify codes that should not be used for describing the primary diagnosis.

Instructional Notes

These notes appear only in the Tabular List of Diseases

Includes This note appears immediately under a three-digit code title to further define, or give example of, the contents of the category. The includes note in the example below applies only to category 056.

Excludes Terms following the word "*Excludes*" are to be coded elsewhere. The term excludes means "DO NOT CODE HERE". Excludes notes are italicized.

056 Rubella
Includes German measles
Excludes congenital rubella (771.0)

Use additional code

This instruction is placed in the Tabular List in those categories where the user will need to add further information (by using an additional code) to give a more complete picture of the diagnosis or procedure.

094 Neurosyphilis
Use additional code to identify any associated mental disorder

Code first underlying disease

This instructional note is used for those codes not intended to be used as a principal diagnosis, or not to be sequenced before the underlying disease. The note requires that the underlying disease (etiology) be recorded first and the particular manifestation recorded secondarily. This note appears only in the Tabular List.

320.7 *Meningitis in other bacterial diseases classified elsewhere*
Code first underlying disease as:
actinomycosis (039.8)
listeriosis (027.0)
typhoid fever (002.0)
whooping cough (033.0-033.9)

Omit code

"Omit code" is used to instruct the coder that no code is to be assigned. When this instruction is found in the Alphabetic Index to Diseases, the medical term should not be coded as a diagnosis.

Hum, venous - omit code

Comorbidities & Complications Exclusions List

Some codes in the Tabular List for Diseases have a complication and comorbidity diagnosis. Codes that have a complication and comorbidity diagnosis are flagged with the Comorbidity and Complications Exclusions indicator. Any code in the C&C Exclusions list (printed in blue) should be excluded as a secondary diagnosis as it will not be recognized as a comorbidity and complications diagnosis when assigning DRGs. In the following example if 079.88 is the primary diagnosis then 052.2 should not be used as a secondary diagnosis when assigning DRGs as it is excluded.

079.88 Other specified chlamydial infection
C&C Exclusions: 052.2, 053.14, 054.74

Comorbidities & Complications Exclusions Disclaimer

As part of the 2008 Proposed Inpatient Prospective Payment System (IPPS) Rule, the Centers for Medicare and Medicaid Services (CMS) has proposed a new system of DRG classification known as MS-DRGs (Medicare Severity DRGs) to better recognize severity of illness among patients. Part of this effort to create a new classification system of DRGs includes reworking of the list of diagnoses considered complications and a resultant restructuring of the complications and comorbidities (C&C) exclusions list.

Both the proposed MS-DRG classification system and the restructuring of the C&C exclusions list have faced great criticism from influential organizations such as the American Hospital Association (AHA) in the months since their proposal. As time goes by, it appears less and less likely that they will be implemented for 2008. Because this decision is still pending at the time of printing, it has been decided not to update the C&C Exclusion references at this time.

Additional Conventions

New and Revised Text Characters

- ● A bullet denotes a new code, category, or subcategory (Tabular Lists) or line (Alphabetic Indices).
- ▲ A triangle in the Alphabetic Indices denotes a changed code. In the Tabular Lists, the triangle denotes a revised code, category, or subcategory description.
- ►◄ The brace symbols are used in the Alphabetic Indices and Tabular Lists to denote revised text.
- word Underlined words set off text which has been revised or added for 2008. This symbol is relevant only in the 2008 ICD-9-CM code changes table.
- ~~word~~ A word(s) with a strikethrough highlights a word(s) that has been deleted from a particular code description for 2008. This symbol is relevant only in the 2008 ICD-9-CM code changes table.

4th or 5th Digit Required

Specificity and medical necessity are clearly defined by appropriately adding a fourth or fifth digit to the numeric diagnosis code found in a particular ICD-9-CM category. Only the fourth digit symbol is used in the Tabular List of Procedures.

❹ (red) fourth digit required ❺ (red) fifth digit required

Text appearing in red in the Tabular Lists denotes a fourth or fifth digit subclassification that applies to the range of codes specified.

Principle Diagnosis Flags

To facilitate the coding process and add emphasis, we have developed color coded characters regarding the proper use of primary diagnosis codes. These symbols are found only in the Tabular List for Diseases. Keep in mind that some codes may be preceded by multiple characters. ***NOTE:*** *The Medicare Code Editor (MCE) flag for Nonspecific Principal Diagnosis has been deleted for FY2008. Although claims will not be denied for the use of these codes, more precise codes are preferable to give a more complete description of the patient's condition.*

✖ (green) Nonspecific Principal Diagnosis
⦸ (red) Unacceptable Principal Diagnosis
✚ (blue) Manifestation code/Not a principal diagnosis

Operating Room Procedure Flag

These symbols are found only in the Tabular List for Procedures. DRG assignment can be impacted by place of service for certain procedures. The presence of a Valid or Non-OR Procedure symbol is not a clinical determination, but rather an indicator of Medicare Code Editor (MCE) rules for DRG assignment decisions. ***NOTE:*** *The Medicare Code Editor (MCE) flag for Nonspecific O.R. procedures has been deleted for FY2008. Although claims will not be denied for the use of these codes, more precise codes are preferable to give a more complete description of the services provided.*

✖ (red) Non-Operating Room Procedure
✔ (green) Valid Operating Room Procedure
▼ (blue) Nonspecific Valid Operating Room Procedure

Primary/Secondary Diagnosis Only Flag

Primary and Secondary Diagnosis Only flags are those that connect contributing factors to a problem or condition that is being evaluated. A primary diagnosis is the reason a patient presents for evaluation and a secondary diagnosis is a problem or condition that can impact the first diagnosis. V-codes without either symbol can be used as either a primary or secondary diagnosis depending on the circumstances.

1 (blue) Primary Diagnosis Only

V71.1 Observation for suspected malignant neoplasm 1

2 (blue) Secondary Diagnosis Only

V21.31 Low birth weight status, less than 500 grams 2

Medicare Secondary Payer Flag

Medicare as a Secondary Payer flag diagnoses where a patient may have a primary insurance payor that would be billed for services first instead of Medicare.

❷ (blue) Medicare Secondary Payer

958.4 Traumatic shock ❷

Open Biopsy Check

These symbols are found only in the Tabular List for Procedures. DRG assignment for patients who have biopsies performed during their stay is dependent on whether or not the biopsy performed open or closed. Carriers are instructed to audit 10% of all claims with open biopsies reported and to adjust the bills if they determine the biopsy was closed.

⓿ (black) Closed Biopsy ⓪ (black) Open Biopsy

Sex Edits

Sex Edits flag those diagnoses and procedures that are exclusively designated for either a male or female patient. The gender is flagged by the symbol found to the right of the diagnosis or procedure code:

♂ (red) Male **752.61 Hypospadias ♂**
♀ (red) Female **66.69 Other partial salpingectomy ♀**

Age Edits

Age specific edits are utilized as a measure of accuracy on a claim. The specific category of age is determined by the symbol that is found to the right of the diagnosis code:

A (red) Adult (15+ years)

Adult (15+ years) edits flag those diagnoses that are reserved for adults.

790.93 Elevated prostate specific antigen [PSA] A

M (red) Maternity (12-55 years)

Maternity (12-55 years) edits flag those diagnoses used specifically for women that were pregnant.

648.8 Abnormal glucose tolerance M

N (red) Newborn (0 years)

Newborn (0 years) edits flag those diagnoses that are reserved for newborns.

770.6 Transitory tachypnea of newborn N

P (red) Pediatric (0-17 years)

Pediatric (0-17 years) edits flag those diagnoses that are typically designated to a child or adolescent condition.

751.1 Atresia and stenosis of small intestine P

AHA References and Additional Definitions

AHA American Hospital Association's (AHA) *Coding Clinic for ICD-9-CM* references are provided below applicable codes.

DEF Plain English definitions are provided beneath certain codes for clarification.

2008 ICD-9-CM Code Changes

Disease Tabular List (Volume 1)

The new, updated, and deleted ICD-9-CM codes for 2008 have been released. The codes and descriptors have been approved and will be available for use for dates of service on or after October 1, 2007.

	Code	Description
▲	**005.1**	**Botulism food poisoning**
		Synonymous term added
●	**040.4**	**Other specified botulism**
		Synonymous term added
		Excludes note added
●	**040.41**	**Infant botulism**
●	**040.42**	**Wound botulism**
		Synonymous term added
		Use additional code note added
	041	Excludes note term deleted
	049.8	Excludes note added
	054.3	Excludes note added
	057.8	Synonymous terms deleted
		Excludes note added
●	**058**	**Other human herpesvirus**
		Excludes note added
●	**058.1**	**Roseola infantum**
		Synonymous term added
●	**058.10**	**Roseola infantum, unspecified**
		Synonymous term added
●	**058.11**	**Roseola infantum due to human herpesvirus 6**
		Synonymous term added
●	**058.12**	**Roseola infantum due to human herpesvirus 7**
		Synonymous term added
●	**058.2**	**Other human herpesvirus encephalitis**
		Excludes note added
●	**058.21**	**Human herpesvirus 6 encephalitis**
●	**058.29**	**Other human herpesvirus encephalitis**
		Synonymous term added
●	**058.8**	**Other human herpesvirus infections**
●	**058.81**	**Human herpesvirus 6 infection**
●	**058.82**	**Human herpesvirus 7 infection**
●	**058.89**	**Other human herpesvirus infection**
		Synonymous terms added
●	**079.83**	**Parvovirus B19**
		Synonymous terms added
		Excludes note added
	184	Excludes note revised
	193	Synonymous term deleted
▲	**200**	**Lymphosarcoma and reticulosarcoma and other specified malignant tumors of lymphatic tissue**
●	**200.3**	**Marginal zone lymphoma**
		Synonymous terms added
●	**200.30**	**Marginal zone lymphoma, unspecified site, extranodal and solid organ sites**
●	**200.31**	**Marginal zone lymphoma, lymph nodes of head, face, and neck**
●	**200.32**	**Marginal zone lymphoma, intrathoracic lymph nodes**
●	**200.33**	**Marginal zone lymphoma, intra-abdominal lymph nodes**
●	**200.34**	**Marginal zone lymphoma, lymph nodes of axilla and upper limb**
●	**200.35**	**Marginal zone lymphoma, lymph nodes of inguinal region and lower limb**
●	**200.36**	**Marginal zone lymphoma, intrapelvic lymph nodes**
●	**200.37**	**Marginal zone lymphoma, spleen**
●	**200.38**	**Marginal zone lymphoma, lymph nodes of multiple sites**
●	**200.4**	**Mantle cell lymphoma**
●	**200.40**	**Mantle cell lymphoma, unspecified site, extranodal and solid organ sites**
●	**200.41**	**Mantle cell lymphoma, lymph nodes of head, face, and neck**
●	**200.42**	**Mantle cell lymphoma, intrathoracic lymph nodes**
●	**200.43**	**Mantle cell lymphoma, intra-abdominal lymph nodes**
●	**200.44**	**Mantle cell lymphoma, lymph nodes of axilla and upper limb**
●	**200.45**	**Mantle cell lymphoma, lymph nodes of inguinal region and lower limb**
●	**200.46**	**Mantle cell lymphoma, intrapelvic lymph nodes**
●	**200.47**	**Mantle cell lymphoma, spleen**
●	**200.48**	**Mantle cell lymphoma, lymph nodes of multiple sites**
●	**200.5**	**Primary central nervous system lymphoma**
●	**200.50**	**Primary central nervous system lymphoma, unspecified site, extranodal and solid organ sites**
●	**200.51**	**Primary central nervous system lymphoma, lymph nodes of head, face, and neck**
●	**200.52**	**Primary central nervous system lymphoma, intrathoracic lymph nodes**
●	**200.53**	**Primary central nervous system lymphoma, intra-abdominal lymph nodes**
●	**200.54**	**Primary central nervous system lymphoma, lymph nodes of axilla and upper limb**
●	**200.55**	**Primary central nervous system lymphoma, lymph nodes of inguinal region and lower limb**
●	**200.56**	**Primary central nervous system lymphoma, intrapelvic lymph nodes**
●	**200.57**	**Primary central nervous system lymphoma, spleen**
●	**200.58**	**Primary central nervous system lymphoma, lymph nodes of multiple sites**
●	**200.6**	**Anaplastic large cell lymphoma**
●	**200.60**	**Anaplastic large cell lymphoma, unspecified site, extranodal and solid organ sites**
●	**200.61**	**Anaplastic large cell lymphoma, lymph nodes of head, face, and neck**
●	**200.62**	**Anaplastic large cell lymphoma, intrathoracic lymph nodes**
●	**200.63**	**Anaplastic large cell lymphoma, intra-abdominal lymph nodes**
●	**200.64**	**Anaplastic large cell lymphoma, lymph nodes of axilla and upper limb**
●	**200.65**	**Anaplastic large cell lymphoma, lymph nodes of inguinal region and lower limb**
●	**200.66**	**Anaplastic large cell lymphoma, intrapelvic lymph nodes**
●	**200.67**	**Anaplastic large cell lymphoma, spleen**
●	**200.68**	**Anaplastic large cell lymphoma, lymph nodes of multiple sites**
●	**200.7**	**Large cell lymphoma**
●	**200.70**	**Large cell lymphoma, unspecified site, extranodal and solid organ sites**
●	**200.71**	**Large cell lymphoma, lymph nodes of head, face, and neck**
●	**200.72**	**Large cell lymphoma, intrathoracic lymph nodes**
●	**200.73**	**Large cell lymphoma, intra-abdominal lymph nodes**
●	**200.74**	**Large cell lymphoma, lymph nodes of axilla and upper limb**
●	**200.75**	**Large cell lymphoma, lymph nodes of inguinal region and lower limb**
●	**200.76**	**Large cell lymphoma, intrapelvic lymph nodes**
●	**200.77**	**Large cell lymphoma, spleen**
●	**200.78**	**Large cell lymphoma, lymph nodes of multiple sites**
●	**202.7**	**Peripheral T-cell lymphoma**
●	**202.70**	**Peripheral T-cell lymphoma, unspecified site, extranodal and solid organ sites**
●	**202.71**	**Peripheral T-cell lymphoma, lymph nodes of head, face, and neck**
●	**202.72**	**Peripheral T-cell lymphoma, intrathoracic lymph nodes**
●	**202.73**	**Peripheral T-cell lymphoma, intra-abdominal lymph nodes**
●	**202.74**	**Peripheral T-cell lymphoma, lymph nodes of axilla and upper limb**
●	**202.75**	**Peripheral T-cell lymphoma, lymph nodes of inguinal region and lower limb**
●	**202.76**	**Peripheral T-cell lymphoma, intrapelvic lymph nodes**
●	**202.77**	**Peripheral T-cell lymphoma, spleen**
●	**202.78**	**Peripheral T-cell lymphoma, lymph nodes of multiple sites**
	232.5	Excludes note term revised
	233.1	Synonymous term added
●	**233.30**	**Carcinoma in situ of unspecified female genital organ**
●	**233.31**	**Carcinoma in situ of vagina**
		Synonymous terms added
●	**233.32**	**Carcinoma in situ of vulva**
		Synonymous terms added
●	**233.39**	**Carcinoma in situ of other female genital organ**
	250	Excludes note term revised
	250.6	Use additional code note term revised
	255.4	Synonymous terms deleted
●	**255.41**	**Glucocorticoid deficiency**
		Synonymous terms added
●	**255.42**	**Mineralocorticoid deficiency**
		Synonymous term added
		Excludes note added

● = New Code, Category, or Subcategory ▲ = Revised Code, Category, or Subcategory ✖ = Deleted Code, Category, or Subcategory word = New Text ~~word~~ = Deleted Text

	Code	Change
	258.0	Synonymous terms added and deleted
		Use additional code note added
●	258.01	**Multiple endocrine neoplasia [MEN] type I**
		Synonymous term added
●	258.02	**Multiple endocrine neoplasia [MEN] type IIA**
		Synonymous term added
●	258.03	**Multiple endocrine neoplasia [MEN] type IIB**
	268.1	Code first note revised
	276.6	Excludes note term revised
	284.1	Excludes note term revised
	284.8	Synonymous terms deleted
		Use additional code note deleted
●	284.81	**Red cell aplasia (acquired) (adult) (with thymoma)**
		Synonymous term added
●	284.89	**Other specified aplastic anemias**
		Synonymous terms added
		Use additional code note added
	288.0	Use additional code note revised and term added
●	288.66	**Bandemia**
		Synonymous term added
		Excludes note added
	302.5	Synonymous term added
	302.85	Use additional code note added
	315.32	Synonymous term added
		Excludes note added
●	315.34	**Speech and language developmental delay due to hearing loss**
		Use additional code note added
	331	Use additional code note added
	331.1	Use additional code note deleted
	331.3	Synonymous term added
		Excludes note terms added and revised
	331.4	Excludes note terms added and revised
●	331.5	**Idiopathic normal pressure hydrocephalus (INPH)**
		Synonymous term added
		Excludes note added
	331.82	Use additional code note deleted
	353.1	Code first note added
	358.1	Synonymous term deleted
		Code first note term deleted
	359.2	Synonymous terms deleted
		Excludes note added
●	359.21	**Myotonic muscular dystrophy**
		Synonymous terms added
●	359.22	**Myotonia congenita**
		Synonymous terms added
●	359.23	**Myotonic chondrodystrophy**
		Synonymous terms added
●	359.24	**Drug-induced myotonia**
		Use additional code note added
●	359.29	**Other specified myotonic disorder**
		Synonymous terms added
▲	359.3	**~~Familial~~ Periodic paralysis**
		Synonymous terms added
		Excludes note added
	359.5	Code first note term revised
	364.8	Synonymous term deleted
		Excludes note deleted
●	364.81	**Floppy iris syndrome**
		Synonymous term added
		Use additional code note added
●	364.89	**Other disorders of iris and ciliary body**
		Synonymous term added
		Excludes note added
	366.43	Code first note revised
●	388.45	**Acquired auditory processing disorder**
		Synonymous term added
		Excludes note added
	389.0	Excludes note added
●	389.05	**Conductive hearing loss, unilateral**
●	389.06	**Conductive hearing loss, bilateral**
	389.1	Excludes note term added
●	389.13	**Neural hearing loss, unilateral**
▲	389.14	**Central hearing loss~~, bilateral~~**
●	389.17	**Sensory hearing loss, unilateral**
▲	389.18	**Sensorineural hearing loss of combined types~~, bilateral~~**
	389.2	Synonymous term revised
●	389.20	**Mixed hearing loss, unspecified**
●	389.21	**Mixed hearing loss, unilateral**
●	389.22	**Mixed hearing loss, bilateral**
▲	389.7	**Deaf ~~mutism~~<u>nonspeaking</u>, not elsewhere classifiable**
		Synonymous term deleted
	414.0	Use additional code note added
●	414.2	**Chronic total occlusion of coronary artery**
		Synonymous terms added
		Code first note added
		Excludes note added
●	415.12	**Septic pulmonary embolism**
		Synonymous term added
		Code first note added
		Excludes note added
●	423.3	**Cardiac tamponade**
		Code first note added
	425.8	Code first note term revised
	438	Excludes note added
	438.82	Use additional code note added
	440.2	Use additional code note added
●	440.4	**Chronic total occlusion of artery of the extremities**
		Synonymous terms added
		Code first note added
		Excludes note added
	444	Excludes note term added
●	449	**Septic arterial embolism**
		Code first note added
		Use additional code note added
		Excludes note added
	487	Excludes note term added
●	488	**Influenza due to identified avian influenza virus**
		Note added
		Excludes note added
●	525.7	**Endosseous dental implant failure**
●	525.71	**Osseointegration failure of dental implant**
		Synonymous terms added
●	525.72	**Post-osseointegration biological failure of dental implant**
		Synonymous terms added
●	525.73	**Post-osseointegration mechanical failure of dental implant**
		Synonymous terms added
		Excludes note added
●	525.79	**Other endosseous dental implant failure**
		Synonymous term added
	526.4	Excludes note term added
	528.7	Excludes note term revised
	536.3	Code first note added
	565.0	Synonymous term deleted
		Excludes note added
	568.82	Excludes note revised
●	569.43	**Anal sphincter tear (healed) (old)**
		Use additional code note added
		Excludes note added
	572.2	Excludes note added
	585	Code first note revised
	608.22	Synonymous term added
	622.1	Excludes note terms added and deleted
	623.0	Synonymous term added
		Excludes note terms added and revised
	624.0	Synonymous terms deleted
		Excludes note terms added and revised
●	624.01	**Vulvar intraepithelial neoplasia I [VIN I]**
		Synonymous term added
●	624.02	**Vulvar intraepithelial neoplasia II [VIN II]**
		Synonymous term added
●	624.09	**Other dystrophy of vulva**
		Synonymous terms added
	646.3	Excludes note term revised
	654	Excludes note added
	654.8	Synonymous term added
		Excludes note term added
	661.2	Synonymous term added
		Excludes note added
	664.2	Excludes note added
●	664.60	**Anal sphincter tear complicating delivery, not associated with third-degree perineal laceration, unspecified as to episode of care in pregnancy**
		Excludes note added
●	664.61	**Anal sphincter tear complicating delivery, not associated with third-degree perineal laceration, delivered, with or without mention of antepartum condition**
		Excludes note added

● = New Code, Category, or Subcategory ▲ = Revised Code, Category, or Subcategory ✖ = Deleted Code, Category, or Subcategory <u>word</u> = New Text ~~word~~ = Deleted Text

● 664.64 **Anal sphincter tear complicating delivery, not associated with third-degree perineal laceration, postpartum condition or complication**
Excludes note added

666.1 Synonymous term added
Excludes note terms added and revised

731.3 Code first note term revised

● 733.4 **Aseptic necrosis of jaw**
Use additional code note added
Excludes note added

756.4 Excludes note term added

771 Excludes note term added

780.39 Synonymous term added

782.3 Excludes note term revised

784.1 Excludes note term revised

784.99 Synonymous term added
Excludes note added

787.2 Synonymous term deleted
Code first note added

● 787.20 **Dysphagia, unspecified**
Synonymous term added

● 787.21 **Dysphagia, oral phase**

● 787.22 **Dysphagia, oropharyngeal phase**

● 787.23 **Dysphagia, pharyngeal phase**

● 787.24 **Dysphagia, pharyngoesophageal phase**

● 787.29 **Other dysphagia**
Synonymous terms added

789.3 Excludes note term revised

● 789.51 **Malignant ascites**
Code first note added

● 789.59 **Other ascites**

996 Excludes note terms added

996.62 Synonymous term revised
Excludes note added

996.77 Use additional code note added

998.5 Excludes note term revised

999 Use additional code note added

999.3 Use additional code note added

● 999.31 **Infection due to central venous catheter**
Synonymous terms added
Excludes note added

● 999.39 **Infection following other infusion, injection, transfusion, or vaccination**

● V12.53 **Sudden cardiac arrest**
Synonymous term added

● V12.54 **Transient ischemic attack (TIA), and cerebral infarction without residual deficits**
Synonymous terms added
Excludes note added

V13.2 Excludes note term revised

● V13.22 **Personal history of cervical dysplasia**
Synonymous term added
Excludes note added

V16.5 Synonymous term revised

● V16.52 **Family history of neoplasm of bladder**

● V17.41 **Family history of sudden cardiac death (SCD)**
Excludes note added

● V17.49 **Family history of other cardiovascular diseases**
Synonymous term added

● V18.11 **Multiple endocrine neoplasia [MEN] syndrome**

● V18.19 **Other endocrine and metabolic diseases**

V23.2 Excludes note term revised

● V25.04 **Counseling and instruction in natural family planning to avoid pregnancy**

● V26.41 **Procreative counseling and advice using natural family planning**

● V26.49 **Other procreative management counseling and advice**

● V26.81 **Encounter for assisted reproductive fertility procedure cycle**
Synonymous term added
Use additional code note added
Excludes note added

● V26.89 **Other specified procreative management**

● V49.85 **Dual sensory impairment influencing health status**
Synonymous terms added
Code first note added

V58.69 Synonymous term revised

V58.78 Excludes note added

V64.05 Synonymous terms added

V65.4 Excludes note term revised

V68.0 Synonymous terms deleted

● V68.01 **Issue of disability examination certificate**
Use additional code note added

● V68.09 **Other issue of medical certificates**

● V72.12 **Encounter for hearing conservation and treatment**

V72.31 Use additional code note added

● V73.81 **Special screening for human papillomavirus (HPV)**

V74.5 Synonymous terms added
Excludes note added

V76.2 Excludes note term added

V80.3 Excludes note revised

V82.7 Excludes note revised

● V84.81 **Genetic susceptibility to multiple endocrine neoplasia [MEN]**

● V84.89 **Genetic susceptibility to other disease**

● E928.6 **Environmental exposure to harmful algae and toxins**
Synonymous terms added

● E933.6 **Oral bisphosphonates causing adverse effects in therapeutic use**

● E933.7 **Intravenous bisphosphonates causing adverse effects in therapeutic use**

Procedure Tabular List (Volume 3)

▲ 00.18 **Infusion of immunosuppressive antibody therapy ~~during induction phase of solid organ transplantation~~**
Includes note added

● 00.19 **Disruption of blood brain barrier via infusion [BBBD]**
Synonymous term added
Code also note added
Excludes note added

▲ 00.74 **Hip ~~replacement~~ bearing surface, metal-on polyethylene**

▲ 00.75 **Hip ~~replacement~~ bearing surface, metal-on-metal**

▲ 00.76 **Hip ~~replacement~~ bearing surface, ceramic-on ceramic**

▲ 00.77 **Hip ~~replacement~~ bearing surface, ceramic-on polyethylene**

● 00.94 **Intra-operative neurophysiologic monitoring**
Synonymous terms added
Includes note added
Excludes note added

● 01.10 **Intracranial pressure monitoring**
Includes note added

● 01.16 **Intracranial oxygen monitoring**
Includes note added

● 01.17 **Brain temperature monitoring**
Includes note added

01.18 Excludes note terms added

03.09 Code also note added

▲ 07.81 **Other partial excision of thymus**
Synonymous term added
Excludes note term added

▲ 07.82 **Other total excision of thymus**
Synonymous term added
Excludes note added

● 07.83 **Thoracoscopic partial excision of thymus**
Excludes note added

● 07.84 **Thoracoscopic total excision of thymus**
Excludes note added

▲ 07.92 **Other incision of thymus**
Synonymous term added
Excludes note added

● 07.95 **Thoracoscopic incision of thymus**
Excludes note added

● 07.98 **Other and unspecified thoracoscopic operations on thymus**

▲ 07.99 **Other and unspecified operations on thymus**
Synonymous terms added and deleted
Excludes note added

20.99 Synonymous term added

● 32.20 **Thoracoscopic excision of lesion or tissue of lung**
Synonymous term added

32.25 Excludes note added

32.29 Excludes note term added

● 32.3 **Segmental resection of lung**

● 32.30 **Thoracoscopic segmental resection of lung**

● 32.39 **Other and unspecified segmental resection of lung**
Excludes note added

● 32.4 **Lobectomy of lung**
Synonymous term added
Excludes note added

● 32.41 **Thoracoscopic lobectomy of lung**

● 32.49 **Other lobectomy of lung**
Excludes note added

▲	**32.5**	**~~Complete~~ Pneumonectomy**
		Synonymous terms added
●	**32.50**	**Thoracoscopic pneumonectomy**
●	**32.59**	**Other and unspecified pneumonectomy**
		Excludes note added
●	**33.20**	**Thoracoscopic lung biopsy**
		Excludes note added
	33.26	Synonymous terms added
		Excludes note term added
	33.27	Excludes note term added
	34.04	Excludes note added
●	**34.06**	**Thoracoscopic drainage of pleural cavity**
		Synonymous term added
●	**34.20**	**Thoracoscopic pleural biopsy**
▲	**34.24**	**Other pleural biopsy**
		Excludes note added
	34.51	Excludes note added
●	**34.52**	**Thoracoscopic decortication of lung**
▲	**39.8**	**Operations on carotid body, carotid sinus and other vascular bodies**
		Synonymous terms added and deleted
		Excludes note term added
	48.74	Synonymous term added
●	**50.13**	**Transjugular liver biopsy**
		Synonymous term added
		Excludes note added
●	**50.14**	**Laparoscopic liver biopsy**
		Excludes note added
	50.19	Synonymous term deleted
		Excludes note terms added
▲	**53.41**	**Repair of umbilical hernia with graft or prosthesis**
▲	**53.61**	**Incisional hernia repair with graft or prosthesis**
▲	**53.69**	**Repair of other hernia of anterior abdominal wall with graft or prosthesis**
	54	Includes note term revised
		Excludes note term deleted
	70.52	Excludes note added
●	**70.53**	**Repair of cystocele and rectocele with graft or prosthesis**
		Use additional code note added
●	**70.54**	**Repair of cystocele with graft or prosthesis**
		Synonymous term added
		Use additional code note added
●	**70.55**	**Repair of rectocele with graft or prosthesis**
		Synonymous term added
		Use additional code note added
●	**70.63**	**Vaginal construction with graft or prosthesis**
		Use additional code note added
		Excludes note added
●	**70.64**	**Vaginal reconstruction with graft or prosthesis**
		Use additional code note added
		Excludes note added
●	**70.78**	**Vaginal suspension and fixation with graft or prosthesis**
		Use additional code note added
●	**70.93**	**Other operations on cul-de-sac with graft or prosthesis**
		Synonymous term added
		Use additional code note added
●	**70.94**	**Insertion of biological graft**
		Synonymous terms added
		Code first note added
●	**70.95**	**Insertion of synthetic graft or prosthesis**
		Synonymous term added
		Code first note added
	78.6	Synonymous term added
		Excludes note term added
	80.0	Synonymous term added
		Code also note terms revised
		Excludes note added
	81.0	Code also note term added
	81.3	Code also note term added
	81.5	Includes note term deleted
	81.51	Code also note revised
	81.52	Code also note revised
	81.53	Code also note term revised
	84.56	Synonymous term revised
	84.57	Synonymous term revised
✖	~~**84.58**~~	~~**Implantation of interspinous process decompression device**~~
	84.59	Synonymous term deleted
		Excludes note added
●	**84.8**	**Insertion, replacement and revision of posterior spinal motion subcategory preservation device(s)**
		Synonymous term added
		Includes note added
		Code also note added
		Excludes note added
●	**84.80**	**Insertion or replacement of interspinous process device(s)**
		Synonymous terms added
		Excludes note added
●	**84.81**	**Revision of interspinous process device(s)**
		Synonymous term added
		Excludes note added
●	**84.82**	**Insertion or replacement of pedicle-based dynamic stabilization device(s)**
		Excludes note added
●	**84.83**	**Revision of pedicle-based dynamic stabilization device(s)**
		Synonymous term added
		Excludes note added
●	**84.84**	**Insertion or replacement of facet replacement device(s)**
		Synonymous term added
		Excludes note added
●	**84.85**	**Revision of facet replacement device(s)**
		Synonymous term added
		Excludes note added
	86.05	Synonymous term added
	86.6	Excludes note term revised
	86.7	Excludes note term revised
	88.52	Excludes note term added
	88.53	Excludes note term added
	88.54	Excludes note added
	88.55	Excludes note added
	88.56	Excludes note added
	88.57	Excludes note added
●	**88.59**	**Intra-operative fluorescence vascular angiography**
		Synonymous terms added
	92.25	Excludes note added
●	**92.4**	**Intra-operative radiation procedures**
●	**92.41**	**Intra-operative electron radiation therapy**
		Synonymous terms added
	96.7	Excludes note term revised
	97.49	Excludes note added
	98.15	Excludes note added
▲	**99.14**	**Injection or infusion of gamma globulin**
	99.25	Code also note added
	99.29	Excludes note term added

2008 ICD-9-CM Diagnosis Code Crosswalk

The code changes listed on the previous pages will have an effect on coding in 2008. A number of four digit codes have been expanded with fifth-digit subclassifications, requiring a higher level of specificity for proper coding. The addition of 142 new codes increases the need to re-evaluate coding assignments for certain diagnoses.

The crosswalk below provides existing, valid 2007 ICD-9-CM codes with possible 2008 diagnosis code considerations that should be used instead when they are more appropriate.

For example: Code 040.41 *Infant botulism* is a new code for 2008. Codes 005.1 *Botulism* and 771.89 *Other infections specific to the perinatal period* are still valid codes for 2008, and should continue to be used for cases of botulism food poisoning and for perinatal infections that do not have a more specific code assigned to them, respectively. Since infant botulism has been assigned its own specific code (040.41) for 2008, it should no longer be coded to either 005.1 or 771.89.

Only valid codes that require a decision as to whether a new code would be more appropriate to use instead are included. Codes that have been expanded and are no longer valid as a coding option are excluded, as are existing codes that may need a new code assigned in addition.

Previous Code Assignment	New 2008 Code(s) Assignment
005.1	040.41
444.0	449
444.1	449
444.21	449
444.22	449
444.81	449
444.89	449
444.9	449
445.01	449
445.02	449
445.81	449
445.89	449
049.8	058.21, 058.29
054.3	058.21, 058.29
054.9	058.81-058.89
057.8	058.10-058.12
079.89	079.83
193	258.02
197.6	789.51
200.00	200.60, 200.70
200.01	200.61, 200.71
200.02	200.62, 200.72
200.03	200.63, 200.73
200.04	200.64, 200.74
200.05	200.65, 200.75
200.06	200.66, 200.76
200.07	200.67, 200.77
200.08	200.68, 200.78
202.10	202.70
202.11	202.71
202.12	202.72
202.13	202.73
202.14	202.74
202.15	202.75
202.16	202.76
202.17	202.77
202.18	202.78
202.80	200.30, 200.40, 200.50
202.81	200.31, 200.41, 200.51
202.82	200.32, 200.42, 200.52
202.83	200.33, 200.43, 200.53
202.84	200.34, 200.44, 200.54
202.85	200.35, 200.45, 200.55
202.86	200.36, 200.46, 200.56
202.87	200.37, 200.47, 200.57
202.88	200.38, 200.48, 200.58
288.69	288.66
315.31	315.34
315.32	388.45
315.39	315.34
331.3	331.5
415.19	415.12
423.9	423.3
444.21	440.4
444.22	440.4
487.0	488
487.1	488
487.8	488
525.69	525.71-525.79
525.8	525.71-525.79
565.0	569.43
664.20	664.60
664.21	664.61
664.24	664.64
733.49	733.45
771.89	040.41
996.60	999.31
996.62	999.31
996.64	999.31
996.69	999.31
V12.59	V12.53-V12.54
V13.29	V13.22
V16.59	V16.52
V25.09	V25.04
V72.19	V72.12
V73.89	V73.81
E928.8	E928.6
E933.8	E933.6-E933.7

2008 ICD-9-CM Procedure Code Crosswalk

The code changes listed on the previous pages will have an effect on coding in 2008. A number of three digit codes have been expanded with fourth-digit subclassifications, requiring a higher level of specificity for proper procedural coding.

The crosswalk below provides existing, valid 2007 ICD-9-CM procedure codes with possible 2008 code considerations that should be used instead when they are more appropriate.

For example: Code 00.19 *Disruption of blood brain barrier via infusion [BBBD]* is new for 2008. Code 99.29 *Injection or infusion of other therapeutic or prophylactic substance* is still a valid code for 2008, and should continue to be used for injection/infusions that do not have specific codes assigned to them. Since BBBD via infusion has been assigned a specific code (00.19) for 2008, it should no longer be coded as 99.29, although other conditions may continue to be.

Only valid codes that require a decision as to whether a new code would be more appropriate to use instead are included. Codes that have been expanded and are no longer valid as a coding option are excluded, as are existing codes that may need a new code assigned in addition.

Previous Code Assignment	New 2008 Code(s) Assignment
01.18	01.10, 01.16-01.17
07.81	07.83
07.82	07.84
07.92	07.95
07.99	07.98
32.29	32.20
33.28	33.20
34.04	34.06
34.24	34.20
34.51	34.52
39.97	00.19
50.11	50.13
50.19	50.13-50.14
70.50	70.53
70.51	70.54
70.52	70.55
70.61	70.63
70.62	70.64
70.77	70.78
70.92	70.93
78.59	84.80-84.83
84.58	84.80
84.59	84.82, 84.84
88.90	88.59
92.25	92.41
99.29	00.19

Official Coding Guidelines

ICD-9-CM Official Guidelines for Coding and Reporting

Effective November 15, 2006

The guidelines have been updated to include the V Code Table.

The Centers for Medicare and Medicaid Services (CMS) and the National Center for Health Statistics (NCHS), two departments within the U. S. Federal Government's Department of Health and Human Services (DHHS) provide the following guidelines for coding and reporting using the *International Classification of Diseases, 9th Revision, Clinical Modification* (ICD-9-CM). These guidelines should be used as a companion document to the official version of the ICD-9-CM as published on CD-ROM by the U.S. Government Printing Office (GPO).

These guidelines have been approved by the four organizations that make up the Cooperating Parties for the ICD-9-CM: the American Hospital Association (AHA), the American Health Information Management Association (AHIMA), CMS, and NCHS. These guidelines are included on the official government version of the ICD-9-CM, and also appear in "Coding Clinic for ICD-9-CM" published by the AHA.

These guidelines are a set of rules that have been developed to accompany and complement the official conventions and instructions provided within the ICD-9-CM itself. These guidelines are based on the coding and sequencing instructions in Volumes I, II and III of ICD-9-CM, but provide additional instruction. Adherence to these guidelines when assigning ICD-9-CM diagnosis and procedure codes is required under the Health Insurance Portability and Accountability Act (HIPAA). The diagnosis codes (Volumes 1-2) have been adopted under HIPAA for all healthcare settings. Volume 3 procedure codes have been adopted for inpatient procedures reported by hospitals. A joint effort between the healthcare provider and the coder is essential to achieve complete and accurate documentation, code assignment, and reporting of diagnoses and procedures. These guidelines have been developed to assist both the healthcare provider and the coder in identifying those diagnoses and procedures that are to be reported. The importance of consistent, complete documentation in the medical record cannot be overemphasized. Without such documentation accurate coding cannot be achieved. The entire record should be reviewed to determine the specific reason for the encounter and the conditions treated.

The term encounter is used for all settings, including hospital admissions. In the context of these guidelines, the term provider is used throughout the guidelines to mean physician or any qualified health care practitioner who is legally accountable for establishing the patient's diagnosis. Only this set of guidelines, approved by the Cooperating Parties, is official.

The guidelines are organized into sections. Section I includes the structure and conventions of the classification and general guidelines that apply to the entire classification, and chapter-specific guidelines that correspond to the chapters as they are arranged in the classification. Section II includes guidelines for selection of principal diagnosis for non-outpatient settings. Section III includes guidelines for reporting additional diagnoses in non-outpatient settings. Section IV is for outpatient coding and reporting.

Table of Contents

Section I

Conventions, general coding guidelines and chapter specific guidelines

4. **Chapter 4: Diseases of Blood and Blood Forming Organs** (280-289)
   a. Anemia of chronic disease
5. **Chapter 5: Mental Disorders** (290-319)
   Reserved for future guideline expansion
6. **Chapter 6: Diseases of Nervous System and Sense Organs** (320-389)
   a. Pain - Category 338
7. **Chapter 7: Diseases of Circulatory System** (390-459)
   a. Hypertension
   b. Cerebral infarction/stroke/cerebrovascular accident (CVA)
   c. Postoperative cerebrovascular accident
   d. Late Effects of Cerebrovascular Disease
   e. Acute myocardial infarction (AMI)
8. **Chapter 8: Diseases of Respiratory System** (460-519)
   a. Chronic Obstructive Pulmonary Disease [COPD] and Asthma
   b. Chronic Obstructive Pulmonary Disease [COPD] and Bronchitis
9. **Chapter 9: Diseases of Digestive System** (520-579)
   Reserved for future guideline expansion
10. **Chapter 10: Diseases of Genitourinary System** (580-629)
    a. Chronic kidney disease
11. **Chapter 11: Complications of Pregnancy, Childbirth, and the Puerperium** (630-677)
    a. General Rules for Obstetric Cases
    b. Selection of OB Principal or First-listed Diagnosis
    c. Fetal Conditions Affecting the Management of the Mother
    d. HIV Infection in Pregnancy, Childbirth and the Puerperium
    e. Current Conditions Complicating Pregnancy
    f. Diabetes mellitus in pregnancy
    g. Gestational diabetes
    h. Normal Delivery, Code 650
    i. The Postpartum and Peripartum Periods
    j. Code 677, Late effect of complication of pregnancy
    k. Abortions
12. **Chapter 12: Diseases Skin and Subcutaneous Tissue** (680-709)
    Reserved for future guideline expansion
13. **Chapter 13: Diseases of Musculoskeletal and Connective Tissue** (710-739)
    a. Coding of Pathologic Fractures
14. **Chapter 14: Congenital Anomalies** (740-759)
    a. Codes in categories 740-759, Congenital Anomalies
15. **Chapter 15: Newborn (Perinatal) Guidelines** (760-779)
    a. General Perinatal Rules
    b. Use of codes V30-V39
    c. Newborn transfers
    d. Use of category V29
    e. Use of other V codes on perinatal records
    f. Maternal Causes of Perinatal Morbidity
    g. Congenital Anomalies in Newborns
    h. Coding Additional Perinatal Diagnoses
    i. Prematurity and Fetal Growth Retardation
    j. Newborn sepsis
16. **Chapter 16: Signs, Symptoms and Ill-Defined Conditions** (780-799)
17. **Chapter 17: Injury and Poisoning** (800-999)
    a. Coding of Injuries
    b. Coding of Traumatic Fractures
    c. Coding of Burns
    d. Coding of Debridement of Wound, Infection, or Burn
    e. Adverse Effects, Poisoning and Toxic Effects
    f. Complications of care
    g. SIRS due to Non-infectious Process
18. **Classification of Factors Influencing Health Status and Contact with Health Service (Supplemental V01-V86)**
    a. Introduction
    b. V codes use in any healthcare setting
    c. V Codes indicate a reason for an encounter
    d. Categories of V Codes
    e. V Code Table
19. **Supplemental Classification of External Causes of Injury and Poisoning (E-codes, E800-E999)**
    a. General E Code Coding Guidelines
    b. Place of Occurrence Guideline
    c. Adverse Effects of Drugs, Medicinal and Biological Substances Guidelines
    d. Multiple Cause E Code Coding Guidelines
    e. Child and Adult Abuse Guideline
    f. Unknown or Suspected Intent Guideline
    g. Undetermined Cause
    h. Late Effects of External Cause Guidelines
    i. Misadventures and Complications of Care Guidelines
    j. Terrorism Guidelines

Section II

Selection of Principal Diagnosis

A. Codes for symptoms, signs, and ill-defined conditions
B. Two or more interrelated conditions, each potentially meeting the definition for principal diagnosis.
C. Two or more diagnoses that equally meet the definition for principal diagnosis
D. Two or more comparative or contrasting conditions.
E. A symptom(s) followed by contrasting/comparative diagnoses
F. Original treatment plan not carried out
G. Complications of surgery and other medical care
H. Uncertain Diagnosis
I. Admission from Observation Unit
   1. Admission Following Medical Observation
   2. Admission Following Post-Operative Observation
J. Admission from Outpatient Surgery

Section III

Reporting Additional Diagnoses

A. Previous conditions
B. Abnormal findings
C. Uncertain Diagnosis

Section IV

Diagnostic Coding and Reporting Guidelines for Outpatient Services

A. Selection of first-listed condition
B. Codes from 001.0 through V86.1
C. Accurate reporting of ICD-9-CM diagnosis codes
D. Selection of codes 001.0 through 999.9
E. Codes that describe symptoms and signs
F. Encounters for circumstances other than a disease or injury
G. Level of Detail in Coding
   1. ICD-9-CM codes with 3, 4, or 5 digits
   2. Use of full number of digits required for a code
H. ICD-9-CM code for the diagnosis, condition, problem, or other reason for encounter/visit
I. "Probable", "suspected", "questionable", "rule out", or "working diagnosis"
J. Chronic diseases

K. Code all documented conditions that coexist
L. Patients receiving diagnostic services only
M. Patients receiving therapeutic services only
N. Patients receiving preoperative evaluations only
O. Ambulatory surgery
P. Routine outpatient prenatal visits

Appendix I

Present on Admission Reporting Guidelines

Section I

Conventions, general coding guidelines and chapter specific guidelines

The conventions, general guidelines and chapter-specific guidelines are applicable to all health care settings unless otherwise indicated.

A. Conventions for the ICD-9-CM

The conventions for the ICD-9-CM are the general rules for use of the classification independent of the guidelines. These conventions are incorporated within the index and tabular of the ICD-9-CM as instructional notes. The conventions are as follows:

1. Format:

The ICD-9-CM uses an indented format for ease in reference

2. Abbreviations

a. Index abbreviations

NEC "Not elsewhere classifiable" This abbreviation in the index represents "other specified" when a specific code is not available for a condition the index directs the coder to the "other specified" code in the tabular.

b. Tabular abbreviations

NEC "Not elsewhere classifiable" This abbreviation in the tabular represents "other specified". When a specific code is not available for a condition the tabular includes an NEC entry under a code to identify the code as the "other specified" code (See Section I.A.5.a. "Other" codes").

NOS "Not otherwise specified" This abbreviation is the equivalent of unspecified. (See Section I.A.5.b., "Unspecified" codes)

3. Punctuation

[ ] Brackets are used in the tabular list to enclose synonyms, alternative wording or explanatory phrases. Brackets are used in the index to identify manifestation codes. (See Section I.A.6. "Etiology/manifestations")

( ) Parentheses are used in both the index and tabular to enclose supplementary words that may be present or absent in the statement of a disease or procedure without affecting the code number to which it is assigned. The terms within the parentheses are referred to as nonessential modifiers.

: Colons are used in the Tabular list after an incomplete term which needs one or more of the modifiers following the colon to make it assignable to a given category.

4. Includes and Excludes Notes and Inclusion terms

Includes: This note appears immediately under a three-digit code title to further define, or give examples of, the content of the category.

Excludes: An excludes note under a code indicates that the terms excluded from the code are to be coded elsewhere. In some cases the codes for the excluded terms should not be used in conjunction with the code from which it is excluded. An example of this is a congenital condition excluded from an acquired form of the same condition. The congenital and acquired codes should not be used together. In other cases, the excluded terms may be used together with an excluded code. An example of this is when fractures of different bones are coded to different codes. Both codes may be used together if both types of fractures are present.

Inclusion terms: List of terms is included under certain four and five digit codes. These terms are the conditions for which that code number is to be used. The terms may be synonyms of the code title, or, in the case of "other specified" codes, the terms are a list of the various conditions assigned to that code. The inclusion terms are not necessarily exhaustive. Additional terms found only in the index may also be assigned to a code.

5. Other and Unspecified codes

a. "Other" codes
Codes titled "other" or "other specified" (usually a code with a 4th digit 8 or fifth-digit 9 for diagnosis codes) are for use when the information in the medical record provides detail for which a specific code does not exist. Index entries with NEC in the line designate "other" codes in the tabular. These index entries represent specific disease entities for which no specific code exists so the term is included within an "other" code.

b. "Unspecified" codes
Codes (usually a code with a 4th digit 9 or 5th digit 0 for diagnosis codes) titled "unspecified" are for use when the information in the medical record is insufficient to assign a more specific code.

6. Etiology/manifestation convention ("code first", "use additional code" and "in diseases classified elsewhere" notes)

Certain conditions have both an underlying etiology and multiple body system manifestations due to the underlying etiology. For such conditions, the ICD-9-CM has a coding convention that requires the underlying condition be sequenced first followed by the manifestation. Wherever such a combination exists, there is a "use additional code" note at the etiology code, and a "code first" note at the manifestation code. These instructional notes indicate the proper sequencing order of the codes, etiology followed by manifestation.

In most cases the manifestation codes will have in the code title, "in diseases classified elsewhere." Codes with this title are a component of the etiology/ manifestation convention. The code title indicates that it is a manifestation code. "In diseases classified elsewhere" codes are never permitted to be used as first listed or principal diagnosis codes. They must be used in conjunction with an underlying condition code and they must be listed following the underlying condition.

There are manifestation codes that do not have "in diseases classified elsewhere" in the title. For such codes a "use additional code" note will still be present and the rules for sequencing apply.

In addition to the notes in the tabular, these conditions also have a specific index entry structure. In the index both conditions are listed together with the etiology code first followed by the manifestation codes in brackets. The code in brackets is always to be sequenced second.

The most commonly used etiology/manifestation combinations are the codes for Diabetes mellitus, category 250. For each code under category 250 there is a use additional code note for the manifestation that is specific for that particular diabetic manifestation. Should a patient have more than one manifestation of diabetes, more than one code from category 250 may be used with as many manifestation codes as are needed to fully describe the patient's complete diabetic condition. The category 250 diabetes codes should be sequenced first, followed by the manifestation codes.

"Code first" and "Use additional code" notes are also used as sequencing rules in the classification for certain codes that are not part of an etiology/ manifestation combination. See - Section I.B.9. "Multiple coding for a single condition".

7. *"And"*

The word "and" should be interpreted to mean either "and" or "or" when it appears in a title.

8. *"With"*

The word "with" in the alphabetic index is sequenced immediately following the main term, not in alphabetical order.

9. *"See" and "See Also"*

The "see" instruction following a main term in the index indicates that another term should be referenced. It is necessary to go to the main term referenced with the "see" note to locate the correct code.

A "see also" instruction following a main term in the index instructs that there is another main term that may also be referenced that may provide additional index entries that may be useful. It is not necessary to follow the "see also" note when the original main term provides the necessary code.

B. General Coding Guidelines

1. *Use of Both Alphabetic Index and Tabular List*

Use both the Alphabetic Index and the Tabular List when locating and assigning a code. Reliance on only the Alphabetic Index or the Tabular List leads to errors in code assignments and less specificity in code selection.

2. *Locate each term in the Alphabetic Index*

Locate each term in the Alphabetic Index and verify the code selected in the Tabular List. Read and be guided by instructional notations that appear in both the Alphabetic Index and the Tabular List.

3. *Level of Detail in Coding*

Diagnosis and procedure codes are to be used at their highest number of digits available.

ICD-9-CM diagnosis codes are composed of codes with either 3, 4, or 5 digits. Codes with three digits are included in ICD-9-CM as the heading of a category of codes that may be further subdivided by the use of fourth and/or fifth digits, which provide greater detail.

A three-digit code is to be used only if it is not further subdivided. Where fourth-digit subcategories and/or fifth-digit subclassifications are provided, they must be assigned. A code is invalid if it has not been coded to the full number of digits required for that code.

For example, Acute myocardial infarction, code 410, has fourth digits that describe the location of the infarction (e.g., 410.2, Of inferolateral wall), and fifth digits that identify the episode of care. It would be incorrect to report a code in category 410 without a fourth and fifth digit.

ICD-9-CM Volume 3 procedure codes are composed of codes with either 3 or 4 digits. Codes with two digits are included in ICD-9-CM as the heading of a category of codes that may be further subdivided by the use of third and/or fourth digits, which provide greater detail.

4. *Code or codes from 001.0 through V86.1*

The appropriate code or codes from 001.0 through V86.1 must be used to identify diagnoses, symptoms, conditions, problems, complaints or other reason(s) for the encounter/visit.

5. *Selection of codes 001.0 through 999.9*

The selection of codes 001.0 through 999.9 will frequently be used to describe the reason for the admission/encounter. These codes are from the section of ICD-9-CM for the classification of diseases and injuries (e.g., infectious and parasitic diseases; neoplasms; symptoms, signs, and ill-defined conditions, etc.).

6. *Signs and symptoms*

Codes that describe symptoms and signs, as opposed to diagnoses, are acceptable for reporting purposes when a related definitive diagnosis has not been established (confirmed) by the provider. Chapter 16 of ICD-9-CM, Symptoms, Signs, and Ill-defined conditions (codes 780.0 - 799.9) contain many, but not all codes for symptoms.

7. *Conditions that are an integral part of a disease process*

Signs and symptoms that are integral to the disease process should not be assigned as additional codes, unless otherwise instructed by the classification.

8. *Conditions that are not an integral part of a disease process*

Additional signs and symptoms that may not be associated routinely with a disease process should be coded when present.

9. *Multiple coding for a single condition*

In addition to the etiology/manifestation convention that requires two codes to fully describe a single condition that affects multiple body systems, there are other single conditions that also require more than one code. "Use additional code" notes are found in the tabular at codes that are not part of an etiology/manifestation pair where a secondary code is useful to fully describe a condition. The sequencing rule is the same as the etiology/manifestation pair - , "use additional code" indicates that a secondary code should be added.

For example, for infections that are not included in chapter 1, a secondary code from category 041, Bacterial infection in conditions classified elsewhere and of unspecified site, may be required to identify the bacterial organism causing the infection. A "use additional code" note will normally be found at the infectious disease code, indicating a need for the organism code to be added as a secondary code.

"Code first" notes are also under certain codes that are not specifically manifestation codes but may be due to an underlying cause. When a "code first" note is present and an underlying condition is present the underlying condition should be sequenced first.

"Code, if applicable, any causal condition first", notes indicate that this code may be assigned as a principal diagnosis when the causal condition is unknown or not applicable. If a causal condition is known, then the code for that condition should be sequenced as the principal or first-listed diagnosis.

Multiple codes may be needed for late effects, complication codes and obstetric codes to more fully describe a condition. See the specific guidelines for these conditions for further instruction.

10. *Acute and Chronic Conditions*

If the same condition is described as both acute (subacute) and chronic, and separate subentries exist in the Alphabetic Index at the same indentation level, code both and sequence the acute (subacute) code first.

11. *Combination Code*

A combination code is a single code used to classify:

- Two diagnoses, or
- A diagnosis with an associated secondary process (manifestation)
- A diagnosis with an associated complication

Combination codes are identified by referring to subterm entries in the Alphabetic Index and by reading the inclusion and exclusion notes in the Tabular List.

Assign only the combination code when that code fully identifies the diagnostic conditions involved or when the Alphabetic Index so directs. Multiple coding should not be used when the classification provides a combination code that clearly identifies all of the elements documented in the diagnosis. When the combination code lacks necessary specificity in describing the manifestation or complication, an additional code should be used as a secondary code.

12. *Late Effects*

A late effect is the residual effect (condition produced) after the acute phase of an illness or injury has terminated. There is no time limit on when a late effect code can be used. The residual may be apparent early, such as in cerebrovascular accident cases, or it may occur months or years later, such as that due to a previous injury. Coding of late effects generally requires two codes sequenced in the following order: The condition or nature of the late effect is sequenced first. The late effect code is sequenced second.

An exception to the above guidelines are those instances where the code for late effect is followed by a manifestation code identified in the Tabular List and title, or the late effect code has been expanded (at the fourth and fifth-digit levels) to include the manifestation(s). The code for the acute phase of an illness or injury that led to the late effect is never used with a code for the late effect.

13. *Impending or Threatened Condition*

Code any condition described at the time of discharge as "impending" or "threatened" as follows:

- If it did occur, code as confirmed diagnosis.
- If it did not occur, reference the Alphabetic Index to determine if the condition has a subentry term for "impending" or "threatened" and also reference main term entries for "Impending" and for "Threatened."
- If the subterms are listed, assign the given code.
- If the subterms are not listed, code the existing underlying condition(s) and not the condition described as impending or threatened.

C. Chapter-Specific Coding Guidelines

In addition to general coding guidelines, there are guidelines for specific diagnoses and/or conditions in the classification. Unless otherwise indicated, these guidelines apply to all health care settings. Please refer to Section II for guidelines on the selection of principal diagnosis.

1. *Chapter 1: Infectious and Parasitic Diseases (001-139)*

a. Human Immunodeficiency Virus (HIV) Infections

1. Code only confirmed cases

Code only confirmed cases of HIV infection/illness. This is an exception to the hospital inpatient guideline Section II, H.

In this context, "confirmation" does not require documentation of positive serology or culture for HIV; the provider's diagnostic statement that the patient is HIV positive, or has an HIV-related illness is sufficient.

2. Selection and sequencing of HIV codes

a. Patient admitted for HIV-related condition

If a patient is admitted for an HIV-related condition, the principal diagnosis should be 042, followed by additional diagnosis codes for all reported HIV-related conditions.

b. Patient with HIV disease admitted for unrelated condition

If a patient with HIV disease is admitted for an unrelated condition (such as a traumatic injury), the code for the unrelated condition (e.g., the nature of injury code) should be the principal diagnosis. Other diagnoses would be 042 followed by additional diagnosis codes for all reported HIV-related conditions.

c. Whether the patient is newly diagnosed

Whether the patient is newly diagnosed or has had previous admissions/encounters for HIV conditions is irrelevant to the sequencing decision.

d. Asymptomatic human immunodeficiency virus

V08 Asymptomatic human immunodeficiency virus [HIV] infection, is to be applied when the patient without any documentation of symptoms is listed as being "HIV positive," "known HIV," "HIV test positive," or similar terminology. Do not use this code if the term "AIDS" is used or if the patient is treated for any HIV-related illness or is described as having any condition(s) resulting from his/her HIV positive status; use 042 in these cases.

e. Patients with inconclusive HIV serology

Patients with inconclusive HIV serology, but no definitive diagnosis or manifestations of the illness, may be assigned code 795.71, Inconclusive serologic test for Human Immunodeficiency Virus [HIV].

f. Previously diagnosed HIV-related illness

Patients with any known prior diagnosis of an HIV-related illness should be coded to 042. Once a patient has developed an HIV-related illness, the patient should always be assigned code 042 on every subsequent admission/encounter. Patients previously diagnosed with any HIV illness (042) should never be assigned to 795.71 or V08.

g. HIV Infection in Pregnancy, Childbirth and the Puerperium

During pregnancy, childbirth or the puerperium, a patient admitted (or presenting for a health care encounter) because of an HIV-related illness should receive a principal diagnosis code of 647.6X, Other specified infectious and parasitic diseases in the mother classifiable elsewhere, but complicating the pregnancy, childbirth or the puerperium, followed by 042 and the code(s) for the HIV-related illness(es). Codes from Chapter 15 always take sequencing priority.

Patients with asymptomatic HIV infection status admitted (or presenting for a health care encounter) during pregnancy, childbirth, or the puerperium should receive codes of 647.6X and V08.

h. Encounters for testing for HIV

If a patient is being seen to determine his/her HIV status, use code V73.89, Screening for other specified viral disease. Use code V69.8, Other problems related to lifestyle, as a secondary code if an asymptomatic patient is in a known high risk group for HIV. Should a patient with signs or symptoms or illness, or a confirmed HIV related diagnosis be tested for HIV, code the signs and symptoms or the diagnosis. An additional counseling code V65.44 may be used if counseling is provided during the encounter for the test.

When a patient returns to be informed of his/her HIV test results use code V65.44, HIV counseling, if the results of the test are negative.

If the results are positive but the patient is asymptomatic use code V08, Asymptomatic HIV infection. If the results are positive and the patient is symptomatic use code 042, HIV infection, with codes for the HIV related symptoms or diagnosis. The HIV counseling code may also be used if counseling is provided for patients with positive test results.

b. Septicemia, Systemic Inflammatory Response Syndrome (SIRS), Sepsis, Severe Sepsis, and Septic Shock

1. SIRS, Septicemia, and Sepsis

a. The terms septicemia and sepsis are often used interchangeably by providers, however they are not considered synonymous terms. The following descriptions are provided for reference but do not preclude querying the provider for clarification about terms used in the documentation:

i. Septicemia generally refers to a systemic disease associated with the presence of pathological microorganisms or toxins in the blood, which can include bacteria, viruses, fungi or other organisms.

ii. Systemic inflammatory response syndrome (SIRS) generally refers to the systemic response to infection, trauma/burns, or other insult (such as cancer) with symptoms including fever, tachycardia, tachypnea, and leukocytosis.
iii. Sepsis generally refers to SIRS due to infection.
iv. Severe sepsis generally refers to sepsis with associated acute organ dysfunction.

b. The coding of SIRS, sepsis and severe sepsis requires a minimum of 2 codes: a code for the underlying cause (such as infection or trauma) and a code from subcategory 995.9 Systemic inflammatory response syndrome (SIRS).
i. The code for the underlying cause (such as infection or trauma) must be sequenced before the code from subcategory 995.9 Systemic inflammatory response syndrome (SIRS).
ii. Sepsis and severe sepsis require a code for the systemic infection (038.xx, 112.5, etc.) and either code 995.91, Sepsis, or 995.92, Severe sepsis. If the causal organism is not documented, assign code 038.9, Unspecified septicemia.
iii. Severe sepsis requires additional code(s) for the associated acute organ dysfunction(s).
iv. If a patient has sepsis with multiple organ dysfunctions, follow the instructions for coding severe sepsis.
v. Either the term sepsis or SIRS must be documented to assign a code from subcategory 995.9.
vi. See Section I.C.17.g, Injury and poisoning, for information regarding systemic inflammatory response syndrome (SIRS) due to trauma/burns and other non-infectious processes.

c. Due to the complex nature of sepsis and severe sepsis, some cases may require querying the provider prior to assignment of the codes.

2. *Sequencing sepsis and severe sepsis*

a. Sepsis and severe sepsis as principal diagnosis
If sepsis or severe sepsis is present on admission, and meets the definition of principal diagnosis, the systemic infection code (e.g., 038.xx, 112.5, etc) should be assigned as the principal diagnosis, followed by code 995.91, Sepsis or 995.92, Severe sepsis as required by the sequencing rules in the Tabular List. Codes from subcategory 995.9 can never be assigned as a principal diagnosis. A code should also be assigned for any localized infection, if present.

b. Sepsis and severe sepsis as secondary diagnoses
When sepsis or severe sepsis develops during the encounter (it was not present on admission), the systemic infection code and codes 995.91 and 995.92 should be assigned as secondary diagnoses.

c. Documentation unclear as to whether sepsis or severe sepsis is present on admission
Sepsis or severe sepsis may be present on admission but the diagnosis may not be confirmed until sometime after admission. If the documentation is not clear whether the sepsis or severe sepsis was present on admission, the provider should be queried.

3. *Sepsis/SIRS with Localized Infection*
If the reason for admission is both sepsis, severe sepsis, or SIRS and a localized infection, such as pneumonia or cellulitis, a code for the systemic infection (038.xx, 112.5, etc) should be assigned first, then code 995.91 or 995.92, followed by the code for the localized infection. If the patient is admitted with a localized infection, such as pneumonia, and sepsis/SIRS doesn't develop until after admission, see guideline 2b).
Note: The term urosepsis is a nonspecific term. If that is the only term documented then only code 599.0 should be assigned based on the default for the term in the ICD-9-CM index, in addition to the code for the causal organism if known.

4. *Bacterial Sepsis and Septicemia*
In most cases, it will be a code from category 038, Septicemia, that will be used in conjunction with a code from subcategory 995.9 such as the following:

a. Streptococcal sepsis
If the documentation in the record states streptococcal sepsis, codes 038.0, Streptococcal sepsis, and code 995.91 should be used, in that sequence.

b. Streptococcal septicemia
If the documentation states streptococcal septicemia, only code 038.0 should be assigned, however, the provider should be queried whether the patient has sepsis, an infection with SIRS.

5. *Acute organ dysfunction that is not clearly associated with the sepsis*
If a patient has sepsis and an acute organ dysfunction, but the medical record documentation indicates that the acute organ dysfunction is related to a medical condition other than the sepsis, do not assign code 995.92, Severe sepsis. An acute organ dysfunction must be associated with the sepsis in order to assign the severe sepsis code. If the documentation is not clear as to whether an acute organ dysfunction is related to the sepsis or another medical condition, query the provider.

6. *Septic shock*

a. Sequencing of septic shock
Septic shock generally refers to circulatory failure associated with severe sepsis, and, therefore, it represents a type of acute organ dysfunction. For all cases of septic shock, the code for the systemic infection should be sequenced first, followed by codes 995.92 and 785.52. Any additional codes for other acute organ dysfunctions should also be assigned. As noted in the sequencing instructions in the Tabular List, the code for septic shock cannot be assigned as a principal diagnosis.

b. Septic Shock without documentation of severe sepsis
Septic shock indicates the presence of severe sepsis. Code 995.92, Severe sepsis, must be assigned with code 785.52, Septic shock, even if the term severe sepsis is not documented in the record. The "use additional code" note and the "code first" note in the tabular support this guideline.

7. *Sepsis and septic shock complicating abortion and pregnancy*
Sepsis and septic shock complicating abortion, ectopic pregnancy, and molar pregnancy are classified to category codes in Chapter 11 (630-639). See section I.C.11.

8. *Negative or inconclusive blood cultures*
Negative or inconclusive blood cultures do not preclude a diagnosis of septicemia or sepsis in patients with clinical evidence of the condition, however, the provider should be queried.

9. *Newborn sepsis*
See Section I.C.15.j for information on the coding of newborn sepsis.

10. *Sepsis due to a Postprocedural Infection*
Sepsis resulting from a postprocedural infection is a complication of care. For such cases the postprocedural infection, such as code 998.59, Other postoperative infection, or 674.3x, Other complications of obstetrical

surgical wounds, should be coded first followed by the appropriate sepsis codes (systemic infection code and either code 995.91or 995.92). An additional code(s) for any acute organ dysfunction should also be assigned for cases of severe sepsis.

11. *External cause of injury codes with SIRS*
Refer to Section I.C.19.a.7 for instruction on the use of external cause of injury codes with codes for SIRS resulting from trauma.

12. *Sepsis and Severe Sepsis Associated with Noninfectious Process*
In some cases, a non-infectious process, such as trauma, may lead to an infection which can result in sepsis or severe sepsis. If sepsis or severe sepsis is documented as associated with a non-infectious condition, such as a burn or serious injury, and this condition meets the definition for principal diagnosis, the code for the non-infectious condition should be sequenced first, followed by the code for the systemic infection and either code 995.91, Sepsis, or 995.92, Severe sepsis. Additional codes for any associated acute organ dysfunction(s) should also be assigned for cases of severe sepsis. If the sepsis or severe sepsis meets the definition of principal diagnosis, the systemic infection and sepsis codes should be sequenced before the non-infectious condition. See Section I.C.1.b.2)(a) for guidelines pertaining to sepsis or severe sepsis as the principal diagnosis. When both the associated non-infectious condition and the sepsis or severe sepsis meet the definition of principal diagnosis, either may be assigned as principal diagnosis.
Only one SIRS code, representing the sepsis or severe sepsis, should be assigned for patients with sepsis or severe sepsis associated with trauma or other non-infectious condition. Do not assign codes 995.93, Systemic inflammatory response syndrome due to non-infectious process without acute organ dysfunction, or 995.94, Systemic inflammatory response syndrome due to noninfectious process with acute organ dysfunction, in addition to 995.91, Sepsis, or 995.92, Severe sepsis, if the patient has sepsis or severe sepsis associated with a non-infectious condition.
See Section I.C.17.g for information on the coding of SIRS due to trauma/burns or other non-infectious disease processes.

2. ***Chapter 2: Neoplasms (140-239)***

General guidelines

Chapter 2 of the ICD-9-CM contains the codes for most benign and all malignant neoplasms. Certain benign neoplasms, such as prostatic adenomas, may be found in the specific body system chapters. To properly code a neoplasm it is necessary to determine from the record if the neoplasm is benign, in-situ, malignant, or of uncertain histologic behavior. If malignant, any secondary (metastatic) sites should also be determined.

The neoplasm table in the Alphabetic Index should be referenced first. However, if the histological term is documented, that term should be referenced first, rather than going immediately to the Neoplasm Table, in order to determine which column in the Neoplasm Table is appropriate. For example, if the documentation indicates "adenoma," refer to the term in the Alphabetic Index to review the entries under this term and the instructional note to "see also neoplasm, by site, benign." The table provides the proper code based on the type of neoplasm and the site. It is important to select the proper column in the table that corresponds to the type of neoplasm. The tabular should then be referenced to verify that the correct code has been selected from the table and that a more specific site code does not exist.

See Section I. C. 18.d.4. for information regarding V codes for genetic susceptibility to cancer.

a. **Treatment directed at the malignancy**
If the treatment is directed at the malignancy, designate the malignancy as the principal diagnosis.

b. **Treatment of secondary site**
When a patient is admitted because of a primary neoplasm with metastasis and treatment is directed toward the secondary site only, the secondary neoplasm is designated as the principal diagnosis even though the primary malignancy is still present.

c. **Coding and sequencing of complications**
Coding and sequencing of complications associated with the malignancies or with the therapy thereof are subject to the following guidelines:

1. *Anemia associated with malignancy*
When admission/encounter is for management of an anemia associated with the malignancy, and the treatment is only for anemia, the appropriate anemia code (such as code 285.22, Anemia in neoplastic disease) is designated at the principal diagnosis and is followed by the appropriate code(s) for the malignancy.
Code 285.22 may also be used as a secondary code if the patient suffers from anemia and is being treated for the malignancy.

2. *Anemia associated with chemotherapy, immunotherapy, and radiation therapy*
When the admission/encounter is for management of an anemia associated with chemotherapy, immunotherapy, or radiotherapy and the only treatment is for the anemia, the anemia is sequenced first followed by code E933.1. The appropriate neoplasm code should be assigned as an additional code.

3. *Management of dehydration due to the malignancy*
When the admission/encounter is for management of dehydration due to the malignancy or the therapy, or a combination of both, and only the dehydration is being treated (intravenous rehydration), the dehydration is sequenced first, followed by the code(s) for the malignancy.

4. *Treatment of a complication resulting from a surgical procedure*
When the admission/encounter is for treatment of a complication resulting from a surgical procedure, designate the complication as the principal or first-listed diagnosis if treatment is directed at resolving the complication.

d. **Primary malignancy previously excised**
When a primary malignancy has been previously excised or eradicated from its site and there is no further treatment directed to that site and there is no evidence of any existing primary malignancy, a code from category V10, Personal history of malignant neoplasm, should be used to indicate the former site of the malignancy. Any mention of extension, invasion, or metastasis to another site is coded as a secondary malignant neoplasm to that site. The secondary site may be the principal or first-listed with the V10 code used as a secondary code.

e. **Admissions/Encounters involving chemotherapy, immunotherapy, and radiation therapy**

1. *Episode of care involves surgical removal of neoplasm*
When an episode of care involves the surgical removal of a neoplasm, primary or secondary site, followed by adjunct chemotherapy or radiation treatment, the neoplasm code should be assigned as principal or first-listed diagnosis, using codes in the 140-198 series or where appropriate in the 200-203 series.

2. *Patient admission/encounter solely for administration of chemotherapy, immunotherapy and radiation therapy*
If a patient admission/encounter is solely for the administration of chemotherapy, immunotherapy or radiation therapy assign code V58.0, Encounter for radiation therapy, or V58.11, Encounter for antineoplastic chemotherapy, or V58.12, Encounter for antineoplastic immunotherapy as the first-listed or principal diagnosis. If a patient receives more than one of these therapies during

the same admission more than one of these codes may be assigned, in any sequence.

3. *Patient admitted for radiotherapy/chemotherapy and develops complications*
   When a patient is admitted for the purpose of radiotherapy, immunotherapy or chemotherapy and develops complications such as uncontrolled nausea and vomiting or dehydration, the principal or first-listed diagnosis is V58.0, Encounter for radiotherapy, or V58.11, Encounter for antineoplastic chemotherapy, or V58.12, Encounter for antineoplastic immunotherapy followed by any codes for the complications.
   See Section I.C.18.d.8. for additional information regarding aftercare V codes.

f. Admission/encounter to determine extent of malignancy
When the reason for admission/encounter is to determine the extent of the malignancy, or for a procedure such as paracentesis or thoracentesis, the primary malignancy or appropriate metastatic site is designated as the principal or first-listed diagnosis, even though chemotherapy or radiotherapy is administered.

g. Symptoms, signs, and ill-defined conditions listed in Chapter 16
Symptoms, signs, and ill-defined conditions listed in Chapter 16 characteristic of, or associated with, an existing primary or secondary site malignancy cannot be used to replace the malignancy as principal or first-listed diagnosis, regardless of the number of admissions or encounters for treatment and care of the neoplasm.
See section I.C.18.d.14, Encounter for prophylactic organ removal

h. Admission/encounter for pain control/management
See Section I.C.6.a.5 for information on coding admission/ encounter for pain control/management.

3. Chapter 3: Endocrine, Nutritional, and Metabolic Diseases and Immunity Disorders (240-279)

a. Diabetes mellitus
Codes under category 250, Diabetes mellitus, identify complications/manifestations associated with diabetes mellitus. A fifth-digit is required for all category 250 codes to identify the type of diabetes mellitus and whether the diabetes is controlled or uncontrolled.

1. *Fifth-digits for category 250:*
   The following are the fifth-digits for the codes under category 250:
   - 0 type II or unspecified type, not stated as uncontrolled
   - 1 type I, [juvenile type], not stated as uncontrolled
   - 2 type II or unspecified type, uncontrolled
   - 3 type I, [juvenile type], uncontrolled

   The age of a patient is not the sole determining factor, though most type I diabetics develop the condition before reaching puberty. For this reason type I diabetes mellitus is also referred to as juvenile diabetes.
2. *Type of diabetes mellitus not documented*
   If the type of diabetes mellitus is not documented in the medical record the default is type II.
3. *Diabetes mellitus and the use of insulin*
   All type I diabetics must use insulin to replace what their bodies do not produce. However, the use of insulin does not mean that a patient is a type I diabetic. Some patients with type II diabetes mellitus are unable to control their blood sugar through diet and oral medication alone and do require insulin. If the documentation in a medical record does not indicate the type of diabetes but does indicate that the patient uses insulin, the appropriate fifth-digit for type II must be used. For type II patients who routinely use insulin, code V58.67, Long-term (current) use of insulin, should also be assigned to indicate that the patient uses insulin. Code V58.67 should not be assigned if insulin is given temporarily to bring a type II patient's blood sugar under control during an encounter.
4. *Assigning and sequencing diabetes codes and associated conditions*
   When assigning codes for diabetes and its associated conditions, the code(s) from category 250 must be sequenced before the codes for the associated conditions. The diabetes codes and the secondary codes that correspond to them are paired codes that follow the etiology/manifestation convention of the classification (See Section I.A.6., Etiology/manifestation convention). Assign as many codes from category 250 as needed to identify all of the associated conditions that the patient has. The corresponding secondary codes are listed under each of the diabetes codes.
   a. Diabetic retinopathy/diabetic macular edema
      Diabetic macular edema, code 362.07, is only present with diabetic retinopathy. Another code from subcategory 362.0, Diabetic retinopathy, must be used with code 362.07. Codes under subcategory 362.0 are diabetes manifestation codes, so they must be used following the appropriate diabetes code.
5. *Diabetes mellitus in pregnancy and gestational diabetes*
   a. For diabetes mellitus complicating pregnancy, see Section I.C.11.f., Diabetes mellitus in pregnancy.
   b. For gestational diabetes, see Section I.C.11, g., Gestational diabetes.
6. *Insulin pump malfunction*
   a. Underdose of insulin due insulin pump failure
      An underdose of insulin due to an insulin pump failure should be assigned 996.57, Mechanical complication due to insulin pump, as the principal or first listed code, followed by the appropriate diabetes mellitus code based on documentation.
   b. Overdose of insulin due to insulin pump failure
      The principal or first listed code for an encounter due to an insulin pump malfunction resulting in an overdose of insulin, should also be 996.57, Mechanical complication due to insulin pump, followed by code 962.3, Poisoning by insulins and antidiabetic agents, and the appropriate diabetes mellitus code based on documentation.

4. Chapter 4: Diseases of Blood and Blood Forming Organs (280-289)

a. Anemia of chronic disease
Subcategory 285.2, Anemia in chronic illness, has codes for anemia in chronic kidney disease, code 285.21; anemia in neoplastic disease, code 285.22; and anemia in other chronic illness, code 285.29. These codes can be used as the principal/ first listed code if the reason for the encounter is to treat the anemia. They may also be used as secondary codes if treatment of the anemia is a component of an encounter, but not the primary reason for the encounter. When using a code from subcategory 285 it is also necessary to use the code for the chronic condition causing the anemia.

1. *Anemia in chronic kidney disease*
   When assigning code 285.21, Anemia in chronic kidney disease. It is also necessary to assign a code from category 585, Chronic kidney disease, to indicate the stage of chronic kidney disease. See I.C.10.a. Chronic kidney disease (CKD)
2. *Anemia in neoplastic disease*
   When assigning code 285.22, Anemia in neoplastic disease, it is also necessary to assign the neoplasm code that is responsible for the anemia. Code 285.22 is for use for

anemia that is due to the malignancy, not for anemia due to antineoplastic chemotherapy drugs, which is an adverse effect.

See I.C.2.c.1 Anemia associated with malignancy

See I.C.2.c.2 Anemia associated with chemotherapy, immunotherapy and radiation therapy

See I.C.17.e.1. Adverse effects

5. *Chapter 5: Mental Disorders (290-319)*

Reserved for future guideline expansion

6. *Chapter 6: Diseases of Nervous System and Sense Organs (320-389)*

a. Pain - Category 338

1. *General coding information*

Codes in category 338 may be used in conjunction with codes from other categories and chapters to provide more detail about acute or chronic pain and neoplasm-related pain. If the pain is not specified as acute or chronic, do not assign codes from category 338, except for post-thoracotomy pain, postoperative pain or neoplasm related pain.

A code from subcategories 338.1 and 338.2 should not be assigned if the underlying (definitive) diagnosis is known, unless the reason for the encounter is pain control/ management and not management of the underlying condition.

a. Category 338 Codes as Principal or First-Listed Diagnosis Category 338 codes are acceptable as principal diagnosis or the first-listed code for reporting purposes:
   - When the related definitive diagnosis has not been established (confirmed) by the provider, or
   - When pain control or pain management is the reason for the admission/encounter (e.g., a patient with displaced intervertebral disc, nerve impingement and severe back pain presents for injection of steroid into the spinal canal). The underlying cause of the pain should be reported as an additional diagnosis, if known.

b. Use of Category 338 Codes in Conjunction with Site Specific Pain Codes

   i Assigning Category 338 Codes and Site-Specific Pain Codes Codes from category 338 may be used in conjunction with codes that identify the site of pain (including codes from chapter 16) if the category 338 code provides additional information. For example, if the code describes the site of the pain, but does not fully describe whether the pain is acute or chronic, then both codes should be assigned.

   ii. Sequencing of Category 338 Codes with Site-Specific Pain Codes The sequencing of category 338 codes with site-specific pain codes (including chapter 16 codes), is dependent on the circumstances of the encounter/admission as follows:
   - If the encounter is for pain control or pain management, assign the code from category 338 followed by the code identifying the specific site of pain (e.g., encounter for painmanagement for acute neck pain from trauma is assigned code 338.11, Acute pain due to trauma, followed by code 723.1, Cervicalgia, to identify the site of pain).
   - If the encounter is for any other reason except pain control or pain management, and a related definitive diagnosis has not been established (confirmed) by the provider, assign the code for the specific site of pain first, followed by the appropriate code from category 338.

2. *Pain due to devices*

Pain associated with devices or foreign bodies left in a surgical site is assigned to the appropriate code(s) found in Chapter 17, Injury and Poisoning (for example painful retained suture).

3. *Postoperative Pain*

Post-thoracotomy pain and other postoperative pain are classified to subcategories 338.1 and 338.2, depending on whether the pain is acute or chronic. The default for post-thoracotomy and other postoperative pain not specified as acute or chronic is the code for the acute form.

Postoperative pain not associated with a specific postoperative complication is assigned to the appropriate postoperative pain code in category 338.

Postoperative pain associated with a specific postoperative complication (such as a device left in the body) is assigned to the appropriate code(s) found in Chapter 17, Injury and Poisoning. Since the complication represents the underlying (definitive) diagnosis associated with the pain, no additional code should be assigned from category 338. If pain control/ management is the reason for the encounter, a code from category 338 should be assigned as the principal or first-listed diagnosis in accordance with Section I.C.6.a.1.a above.

Postoperative pain may be reported as the principal or first-listed diagnosis when the stated reason for the admission/ encounter is documented as postoperative pain control/ management.

Postoperative pain may be reported as a secondary diagnosis code when a patient presents for outpatient surgery and develops an unusual or inordinate amount of postoperative pain.

Routine or expected postoperative pain immediately after surgery should not be coded.

The provider's documentation should be used to guide the coding of postoperative pain, as well as Section III. Reporting Additional Diagnoses and Section IV. Diagnostic Coding and Reporting in the Outpatient Setting.

See Section II.I.2 for information on sequencing of diagnoses for patients admitted to hospital inpatient care following post-operative observation.

See Section II.J for information on sequencing of diagnoses for patients admitted to hospital inpatient care from outpatient surgery.

See Section IV.A.2 for information on sequencing of diagnoses for patients admitted for observation.

4. *Chronic pain*

Chronic pain is classified to subcategory 338.2. There is no time frame defining when pain becomes chronic pain. The provider's documentation should be used to guide use of these codes.

5. *Neoplasm Related Pain*

Code 338.3 is assigned to pain documented as being related, associated or due to cancer, primary or secondary malignancy, or tumor. This code is assigned regardless of whether the pain is acute or chronic.

This code may be assigned as the principal or first-listed code when the stated reason for the admission/encounter is documented as pain control/pain management. The underlying neoplasm should be reported as an additional diagnosis.

When the reason for the admission/encounter is management of the neoplasm and the pain associated with the neoplasm is also documented, code 338.3 may be assigned as an additional diagnosis.

See Section I.C.2 for instructions on the sequencing of neoplasms for all other stated reasons for the admission/encounter (except for pain control/pain management).

6. *Chronic pain syndrome*
This condition is different than the term "chronic pain," and therefore this code should only be used when the provider has specifically documented this condition.

7. ***Chapter 7: Diseases of Circulatory System (390-459)***

a. **Hypertension**
Hypertension Table
The Hypertension Table, found under the main term, "Hypertension", in the Alphabetic Index, contains a complete listing of all conditions due to or associated with hypertension and classifies them according to malignant, benign, and unspecified.

1. *Hypertension, Essential, or NOS*
Assign hypertension (arterial) (essential) (primary) (systemic) (NOS) to category code 401 with the appropriate fourth digit to indicate malignant (.0), benign (.1), or unspecified (.9). Do not use either .0 malignant or .1 benign unless medical record documentation supports such a designation.

2. *Hypertension with Heart Disease*
Heart conditions (425.8, 429.0-429.3, 429.8, 429.9) are assigned to a code from category 402 when a causal relationship is stated (due to hypertension) or implied (hypertensive). Use an additional code from category 428 to identify the type of heart failure in those patients with heart failure. More than one code from category 428 may be assigned if the patient has systolic or diastolic failure and congestive heart failure.
The same heart conditions (425.8, 429.0-429.3, 429.8, 429.9) with hypertension, but without a stated casual relationship, are coded separately. Sequence according to the circumstances of the admission/encounter.

3. *Hypertensive Chronic Kidney Disease with Chronic Renal Failure*
Assign codes from category 403, Hypertensive kidney disease, when conditions classified to categories 585-587 are present. Unlike hypertension with heart disease, ICD-9-CM presumes a cause-and-effect relationship and classifies chronic kidney disease (CKD) with hypertension as hypertensive chronic kidney disease.
Fifth digits for category 403 should be assigned as follows:
   - 0 with CKD stage I through stage IV, or unspecified.
   - 1 with CKD stage V or end stage renal disease.

The appropriate code from category 585, Chronic kidney disease, should be used as a secondary code with a code from category 403 to identify the stage of chronic kidney disease.
See Section I.C.10.a for information on the coding of chronic kidney disease.

4. *Hypertensive Heart and Chronic Kidney Disease*
Assign codes from combination category 404, Hypertensive heart and chronic kidney disease, when both hypertensive kidney disease and hypertensive heart disease are stated in the diagnosis. Assume a relationship between the hypertension and the chronic kidney disease, whether or not the condition is so designated. Assign an additional code from category 428, to identify the type of heart failure. More than one code from category 428 may be assigned if the patient has systolic or diastolic failure and congestive heart failure.
Fifth digits for category 404 should be assigned as follows:
   - 0 without heart failure and with chronic kidney disease (CKD) stage I through stage IV, or unspecified
   - 1 with heart failure and with CKD stage I through stage IV, or unspecified
   - 2 without heart failure and with CKD stage V or end stage renal disease
   - 3 with heart failure and with CKD stage V or end stage renal disease

The appropriate code from category 585, Chronic kidney disease, should be used as a secondary code with a code from category 404 to identify the stage of kidney disease. See Section I.C.10.a for information on the coding of chronic kidney disease.

5. *Hypertensive Cerebrovascular Disease*
First assign codes from 430-438, Cerebrovascular disease, then the appropriate hypertension code from categories 401-405.

6. *Hypertensive Retinopathy*
Two codes are necessary to identify the condition. First assign the code from subcategory 362.11, Hypertensive retinopathy, then the appropriate code from categories 401-405 to indicate the type of hypertension.

7. *Hypertension, Secondary*
Two codes are required: one to identify the underlying etiology and one from category 405 to identify the hypertension. Sequencing of codes is determined by the reason for admission/encounter.

8. *Hypertension, Transient*
Assign code 796.2, Elevated blood pressure reading without diagnosis of hypertension, unless patient has an established diagnosis of hypertension. Assign code 642.3x for transient hypertension of pregnancy.

9. *Hypertension, Controlled*
Assign appropriate code from categories 401-405. This diagnostic statement usually refers to an existing state of hypertension under control by therapy.

10. *Hypertension, Uncontrolled*
Uncontrolled hypertension may refer to untreated hypertension or hypertension not responding to current therapeutic regimen. In either case, assign the appropriate code from categories 401-405 to designate the stage and type of hypertension. Code to the type of hypertension.

11. *Elevated Blood Pressure*
For a statement of elevated blood pressure without further specificity, assign code 796.2, Elevated blood pressure reading without diagnosis of hypertension, rather than a code from category 401.

b. **Cerebral infarction/stroke/cerebrovascular accident (CVA)**
The terms stroke and CVA are often used interchangeably to refer to a cerebral infarction. The terms stroke, CVA, and cerebral infarction NOS are all indexed to the default code 434.91, Cerebral artery occlusion, unspecified, with infarction. Code 436, Acute, but ill-defined, cerebrovascular disease, should not be used when the documentation states stroke or CVA.

c. **Postoperative cerebrovascular accident**
A cerebrovascular hemorrhage or infarction that occurs as a result of medical intervention is coded to 997.02, Iatrogenic cerebrovascular infarction or hemorrhage. Medical record documentation should clearly specify the cause- and-effect relationship between the medical intervention and the cerebrovascular accident in order to assign this code. A secondary code from the code range 430-432 or from a code from subcategories 433 or 434 with a fifth digit of "1" should also be used to identify the type of hemorrhage or infarct. This guideline conforms to the use additional code note instruction at category 997. Code 436, Acute, but ill-defined, cerebrovascular disease, should not be used as a secondary code with code 997.02.

d. **Late Effects of Cerebrovascular Disease**

1. *Category 438, Late Effects of Cerebrovascular disease*
Category 438 is used to indicate conditions classifiable to categories 430-437 as the causes of late effects (neurologic deficits), themselves classified elsewhere. These "late effects" include neurologic deficits that persist after initial onset of conditions classifiable to 430-437. The neurologic deficits caused by cerebrovascular disease may be present from the onset or may arise at any time after the onset of the condition classifiable to 430-437.
2. *Codes from category 438 with codes from 430-437*
Codes from category 438 may be assigned on a health care record with codes from 430-437, if the patient has a current cerebrovascular accident (CVA) and deficits from an old CVA.
3. *Code V12.59*
Assign code V12.59 (and not a code from category 438) as an additional code for history of cerebrovascular disease when no neurologic deficits are present.

e. **Acute myocardial infarction (AMI)**

1. *ST elevation myocardial infarction (STEMI) and non ST elevation myocardial infarction (NSTEMI)*
The ICD-9-CM codes for acute myocardial infarction (AMI) identify the site, such as anterolateral wall or true posterior wall. Subcategories 410.0-410.6 and 410.8 are used for ST elevation myocardial infarction (STEMI). Subcategory 410.7, Subendocardial infarction, is used for non ST elevation myocardial infarction (NSTEMI) and nontransmural MIs.
2. *Acute myocardial infarction, unspecified*
Subcategory 410.9 is the default for the unspecified term acute myocardial infarction. If only STEMI or transmural MI without the site is documented, query the provider as to the site, or assign a code from subcategory 410.9.
3. *AMI documented as nontransmural or subendocardial but site provided*
If an AMI is documented as nontransmural or subendocardial, but the site is provided, it is still coded as a subendocardial AMI. If NSTEMI evolves to STEMI, assign the STEMI code. If STEMI converts to NSTEMI due to thrombolytic therapy, it is still coded as STEMI.

8. ***Chapter 8: Diseases of Respiratory System (460-519)***

a. **Chronic Obstructive Pulmonary Disease [COPD] and Asthma**

1. *Conditions that comprise COPD and Asthma*
The conditions that comprise COPD are obstructive chronic bronchitis, subcategory 491.2, and emphysema, category 492. All asthma codes are under category 493, Asthma. Code 496, Chronic airway obstruction, not elsewhere classified, is a nonspecific code that should only be used when the documentation in a medical record does not specify the type of COPD being treated.
2. *Acute exacerbation of chronic obstructive bronchitis and asthma*
The codes for chronic obstructive bronchitis and asthma distinguish between uncomplicated cases and those in acute exacerbation. An acute exacerbation is a worsening or a decompensation of a chronic condition. An acute exacerbation is not equivalent to an infection superimposed on a chronic condition, though an exacerbation may be triggered by an infection.
3. *Overlapping nature of the conditions that comprise COPD and asthma*
Due to the overlapping nature of the conditions that make up COPD and asthma, there are many variations in the way these conditions are documented. Code selection must be based on the terms as documented. When selecting the correct code for the documented type of COPD and asthma, it is essential to first review the index, and then verify the code in the tabular list. There are many instructional notes under the different COPD subcategories and codes. It is important that all such notes be reviewed to assure correct code assignment.
4. *Acute exacerbation of asthma and status asthmaticus*
An acute exacerbation of asthma is an increased severity of the asthma symptoms, such as wheezing and shortness of breath. Status asthmaticus refers to a patient's failure to respond to therapy administered during an asthmatic episode and is a life threatening complication that requires emergency care. If status asthmaticus is documented by the provider with any type of COPD or with acute bronchitis, the status asthmaticus should be sequenced first. It supersedes any type of COPD including that with acute exacerbation or acute bronchitis. It is inappropriate to assign an asthma code with 5th digit 2, with acute exacerbation, together with an asthma code with 5th digit 1, with status asthmatics. Only the 5th digit 1 should be assigned.

b. **Chronic Obstructive Pulmonary Disease [COPD] and Bronchitis**

1. *Acute bronchitis with COPD*
Acute bronchitis, code 466.0, is due to an infectious organism. When acute bronchitis is documented with COPD, code 491.22, Obstructive chronic bronchitis with acute bronchitis, should be assigned. It is not necessary to also assign code 466.0. If a medical record documents acute bronchitis with COPD with acute exacerbation, only code 491.22 should be assigned. The acute bronchitis included in code 491.22 supersedes the acute exacerbation. If a medical record documents COPD with acute exacerbation without mention of acute bronchitis, only code 491.21 should be assigned.

c. **Acute Respiratory Failure**

1. *Acute respiratory failure as principal diagnosis*
Code 518.81, Acute respiratory failure, may be assigned as a principal diagnosis when it is the condition established after study to be chiefly responsible for occasioning the admission to the hospital, and the selection is supported by the Alphabetic Index and Tabular List. However, chapter-specific coding guidelines (such as obstetrics, poisoning, HIV, newborn) that provide sequencing direction take precedence.
2. *Acute respiratory failure as secondary diagnosis* Respiratory failure may be listed as a secondary diagnosis if it occurs after admission, or if it is present on admission, but does not meet the definition of principal diagnosis.
3. *Sequencing of acute respiratory failure and another acute condition*
When a patient is admitted with respiratory failure and another acute condition, (e.g., myocardial infarction, cerebrovascular accident), the principal diagnosis will not be the same in every situation. Selection of the principal diagnosis will be dependent on the circumstances of admission. If both the respiratory failure and the other acute condition are equally responsible for occasioning the admission to the hospital, and there are no chapter-specific sequencing rules, the guideline regarding two or more diagnoses that equally meet the definition for principal diagnosis (Section II, C.) may be applied in these situations. If the documentation is not clear as to whether acute respiratory failure and another condition are equally responsible for occasioning the admission, query the provider for clarification.

9. *Chapter 9: Diseases of Digestive System (520-579)*

Reserved for future guideline expansion

10. *Chapter 10: Diseases of Genitourinary System (580-629)*

a. Chronic kidney disease

1. *Stages of chronic kidney disease (CKD)*
   The ICD-9-CM classifies CKD based on severity. The severity of CKD is designated by stages I-V. Stage II, code 585.2, equates to mild CKD; stage III, code 585.3, equates to moderate CKD; and stage IV, code 585.4, equates to severe CKD. Code 585.6, End stage renal disease (ESRD), is assigned when the provider has documented end-stage-renal disease (ESRD).
   If both a stage of CKD and ESRD are documented, assign code 585.6 only.
2. *Chronic kidney disease and kidney transplant status*
   Patients who have undergone kidney transplant may still have some form of CKD, because the kidney transplant may not fully restore kidney function. Therefore, the presence of CKD alone does not constitute a transplant complication. Assign the appropriate 585 code for the patient's stage of CKD and code V42.0. If a transplant complication such as failure or rejection is documented, see section I.C.17.f.1.b for information on coding complications of a kidney transplant. If the documentation is unclear as to whether the patient has a complication of the transplant, query the provider.
3. *Chronic kidney disease with other conditions*
   Patients with CKD may also suffer from other serious conditions, most commonly diabetes mellitus and hypertension. The sequencing of the CKD code in relationship to codes for other contributing conditions is based on the conventions in the tabular list. See I.C.3.a.4 for sequencing instructions for diabetes.
   See I.C.4.a.1. for anemia in CKD.
   See I.C.7.a.3 for hypertensive chronic kidney disease.
   See I.C.17.f.1.b. Transplant complications, for instructions on coding of documented rejection or failure.

11. *Chapter 11: Complications of Pregnancy, Childbirth, and the Puerperium (630-677)*

a. General Rules for Obstetric Cases

1. *Codes from chapter 11 and sequencing priority*
   Obstetric cases require codes from chapter 11, codes in the range 630-677, Complications of Pregnancy, Childbirth, and the Puerperium. Chapter 11 codes have sequencing priority over codes from other chapters. Additional codes from other chapters may be used in conjunction with chapter 11 codes to further specify conditions. Should the provider document that the pregnancy is incidental to the encounter, then code V22.2 should be used in place of any chapter 11 codes. It is the provider's responsibility to state that the condition being treated is not affecting the pregnancy.
2. *Chapter 11 codes used only on the maternal record*
   Chapter 11 codes are to be used only on the maternal record, never on the record of the newborn.
3. *Chapter 11 fifth-digits*
   Categories 640-648, 651-676 have required fifth-digits, which indicate whether the encounter is antepartum, postpartum and whether a delivery has also occurred.
4. *Fifth-digits, appropriate for each code*
   The fifth-digits, which are appropriate for each code number, are listed in brackets under each code. The fifth-digits on each code should all be consistent with each other. That is, should a delivery occur all of the fifth-digits should indicate the delivery.

b. Selection of OB Principal or First-listed Diagnosis

1. *Routine outpatient prenatal visits*
   For routine outpatient prenatal visits when no complications are present codes V22.0, Supervision of normal first pregnancy, and V22.1, Supervision of other normal pregnancy, should be used as the first-listed diagnoses. These codes should not be used in conjunction with chapter 11 codes.
2. *Prenatal outpatient visits for high-risk patients*
   For prenatal outpatient visits for patients with high-risk pregnancies, a code from category V23, Supervision of high-risk pregnancy, should be used as the principal or first-listed diagnosis. Secondary chapter 11 codes may be used in conjunction with these codes if appropriate.
3. *Episodes when no delivery occurs*
   In episodes when no delivery occurs, the principal diagnosis should correspond to the principal complication of the pregnancy, which necessitated the encounter. Should more than one complication exist, all of which are treated or monitored, any of the complications codes may be sequenced first.
4. *When a delivery occurs*
   When a delivery occurs, the principal diagnosis should correspond to the main circumstances or complication of the delivery. In cases of cesarean delivery, the selection of the principal diagnosis should correspond to the reason the cesarean delivery was performed unless the reason for admission/encounter was unrelated to the condition resulting in the cesarean delivery.
5. *Outcome of delivery*
   An outcome of delivery code, V27.0-V27.9, should be included on every maternal record when a delivery has occurred. These codes are not to be used on subsequent records or on the newborn record.

c. Fetal Conditions Affecting the Management of the Mother

1. *Codes from category 655*
   Known or suspected fetal abnormality affecting management of the mother, and category 656, Other fetal and placental problems affecting the management of the mother, are assigned only when the fetal condition is actually responsible for modifying the management of the mother, i.e., by requiring diagnostic studies, additional observation, special care, or termination of pregnancy. The fact that the fetal condition exists does not justify assigning a code from this series to the mother's record.
2. *In utero surgery*
   In cases when surgery is performed on the fetus, a diagnosis code from category 655, Known or suspected fetal abnormalities affecting management of the mother, should be assigned identifying the fetal condition. Procedure code 75.36, Correction of fetal defect, should be assigned on the hospital inpatient record.
   No code from Chapter 15, the perinatal codes, should be used on the mother's record to identify fetal conditions. Surgery performed in utero on a fetus is still to be coded as an obstetric encounter.

d. HIV Infection in Pregnancy, Childbirth and the Puerperium

During pregnancy, childbirth or the puerperium, a patient admitted because of an HIV-related illness should receive a principal diagnosis of 647.6X, Other specified infectious and parasitic diseases in the mother classifiable elsewhere, but complicating the pregnancy, childbirth or the puerperium, followed by 042 and the code(s) for the HIV-related illness(es). Patients with asymptomatic HIV infection status admitted during pregnancy, childbirth, or the puerperium should receive codes of 647.6X and V08.

e. Current Conditions Complicating Pregnancy
Assign a code from subcategory 648.x for patients that have current conditions when the condition affects the management of the pregnancy, childbirth, or the puerperium. Use additional secondary codes from other chapters to identify the conditions, as appropriate.

f. Diabetes mellitus in pregnancy
Diabetes mellitus is a significant complicating factor in pregnancy. Pregnant women who are diabetic should be assigned code 648.0x, Diabetes mellitus complicating pregnancy, and a secondary code from category 250, Diabetes mellitus, to identify the type of diabetes.
Code V58.67, Long-term (current) use of insulin, should also be assigned if the diabetes mellitus is being treated with insulin.

g. Gestational diabetes
Gestational diabetes can occur during the second and third trimester of pregnancy in women who were not diabetic prior to pregnancy. Gestational diabetes can cause complications in the pregnancy similar to those of pre-existing diabetes mellitus. It also puts the woman at greater risk of developing diabetes after the pregnancy. Gestational diabetes is coded to 648.8x, Abnormal glucose tolerance. Codes 648.0x and 648.8x should never be used together on the same record.
Code V58.67, Long-term (current) use of insulin, should also be assigned if the gestational diabetes is being treated with insulin.

h. Normal Delivery, Code 650

1. *Normal delivery*
Code 650 is for use in cases when a woman is admitted for a full-term normal delivery and delivers a single, healthy infant without any complications antepartum, during the delivery, or postpartum during the delivery episode. Code 650 is always a principal diagnosis. It is not to be used if any other code from chapter 11 is needed to describe a current complication of the antenatal, delivery, or perinatal period. Additional codes from other chapters may be used with code 650 if they are not related to or are in any way complicating the pregnancy.
2. *Normal delivery with resolved antepartum complication*
Code 650 may be used if the patient had a complication at some point during her pregnancy, but the complication is not present at the time of the admission for delivery.
3. *V27.0, Single liveborn, outcome of delivery*
V27.0, Single liveborn, is the only outcome of delivery code appropriate for use with 650.

i. The Postpartum and Peripartum Periods

1. *Postpartum and peripartum periods*
The postpartum period begins immediately after delivery and continues for six weeks following delivery. The peripartum period is defined as the last month of pregnancy to five months postpartum.
2. *Postpartum complication*
A postpartum complication is any complication occurring within the six-week period.
3. *Pregnancy-related complications after 6 week period*
Chapter 11 codes may also be used to describe pregnancy-related complications after the six-week period should the provider document that a condition is pregnancy related.
4. *Postpartum complications occurring during the same admission as delivery*
Postpartum complications that occur during the same admission as the delivery are identified with a fifth digit of "2." Subsequent admissions/encounters for postpartum complications should be identified with a fifth digit of "4."
5. *Admission for routine postpartum care following delivery outside hospital*
When the mother delivers outside the hospital prior to admission and is admitted for routine postpartum care and no complications are noted, code V24.0, Postpartum care and examination immediately after delivery, should be assigned as the principal diagnosis.
6. *Admission following delivery outside hospital with postpartum conditions*
A delivery diagnosis code should not be used for a woman who has delivered prior to admission to the hospital. Any postpartum conditions and/or postpartum procedures should be coded.

j. Code 677, Late effect of complication of pregnancy

1. *Code 677*
Code 677, Late effect of complication of pregnancy, childbirth, and the puerperium is for use in those cases when an initial complication of a pregnancy develops a sequelae requiring care or treatment at a future date.
2. *After the initial postpartum period*
This code may be used at any time after the initial postpartum period.
3. *Sequencing of Code 677*
This code, like all late effect codes, is to be sequenced following the code describing the sequelae of the complication.

k. Abortions

1. *Fifth-digits required for abortion categories*
Fifth-digits are required for abortion categories 634-637. Fifth-digit 1, incomplete, indicates that all of the products of conception have not been expelled from the uterus. Fifth-digit 2, complete, indicates that all products of conception have been expelled from the uterus prior to the episode of care.
2. *Code from categories 640-648 and 651-659*
A code from categories 640-648 and 651-659 may be used as additional codes with an abortion code to indicate the complication leading to the abortion.
Fifth digit 3 is assigned with codes from these categories when used with an abortion code because the other fifth digits will not apply. Codes from the 660-669 series are not to be used for complications of abortion.
3. *Code 639 for complications*
Code 639 is to be used for all complications following abortion. Code 639 cannot be assigned with codes from categories 634-638.
4. *Abortion with Liveborn Fetus*
When an attempted termination of pregnancy results in a liveborn fetus assign code 644.21, Early onset of delivery, with an appropriate code from category V27, Outcome of Delivery. The procedure code for the attempted termination of pregnancy should also be assigned.
5. *Retained Products of Conception following an abortion*
Subsequent admissions for retained products of conception following a spontaneous or legally induced abortion are assigned the appropriate code from category 634, Spontaneous abortion, or 635 Legally induced abortion, with a fifth digit of "1" (incomplete). This advice is appropriate even when the patient was discharged previously with a discharge diagnosis of complete abortion.

12. Chapter 12: Diseases Skin and Subcutaneous Tissue (680709)
Reserved for future guideline expansion

13. Chapter 13: Diseases of Musculoskeletal and Connective Tissue (710-739)

a. Coding of Pathologic Fractures

1. Acute Fractures vs. Aftercare

Pathologic fractures are reported using subcategory 733.1, when the fracture is newly diagnosed. Subcategory 733.1 may be used while the patient is receiving active treatment for the fracture. Examples of active treatment are: surgical treatment, emergency department encounter, evaluation and treatment by a new physician.

Fractures are coded using the aftercare codes (subcategories V54.0, V54.2, V54.8 or V54.9) for encounters after the patient has completed active treatment of the fracture and is receiving routine care for the fracture during the healing or recovery phase. Examples of fracture aftercare are: cast change or removal, removal of external or internal fixation device, medication adjustment, and follow up visits following fracture treatment.

Care for complications of surgical treatment for fracture repairs during the healing or recovery phase should be coded with the appropriate complication codes. Care of complications of fractures, such as malunion and nonunion, should be reported with the appropriate codes.

See Section I. C. 17.b for information on the coding of traumatic fractures.

14. Chapter 14: Congenital Anomalies (740-759)

a. Codes in categories 740-759, Congenital Anomalies

Assign an appropriate code(s) from categories 740-759, Congenital Anomalies, when an anomaly is documented. A congenital anomaly may be the principal/first listed diagnosis on a record or a secondary diagnosis.

When a congenital anomaly does not have a unique code assignment, assign additional code(s) for any manifestations that may be present.

When the code assignment specifically identifies the congenital anomaly, manifestations that are an inherent component of the anomaly should not be coded separately. Additional codes should be assigned for manifestations that are not an inherent component.

Codes from Chapter 14 may be used throughout the life of the patient. If a congenital anomaly has been corrected, a personal history code should be used to identify the history of the anomaly. Although present at birth, a congenital anomaly may not be identified until later in life. Whenever the condition is diagnosed by the physician, it is appropriate to assign a code from codes 740-759.

For the birth admission, the appropriate code from category V30, Liveborn infants, according to type of birth should be sequenced as the principal diagnosis, followed by any congenital anomaly codes, 740-759.

15. Chapter 15: Newborn (Perinatal) Guidelines (760-779)

For coding and reporting purposes the perinatal period is defined as before birth through the 28th day following birth. The following guidelines are provided for reporting purposes. Hospitals may record other diagnoses as needed for internal data use.

a. General Perinatal Rules

1. Chapter 15 Codes

They are never for use on the maternal record. Codes from Chapter 11, the obstetric chapter, are never permitted on the newborn record. Chapter 15 code may be used throughout the life of the patient if the condition is still present.

2. Sequencing of perinatal codes

Generally, codes from Chapter 15 should be sequenced as the principal/first-listed diagnosis on the newborn record, with the exception of the appropriate V30 code for the birth episode, followed by codes from any other chapter that provide additional detail. The "use additional code" note at the beginning of the chapter supports this guideline. If the index does not provide a specific code for a perinatal condition, assign code 779.89, Other specified conditions originating in the perinatal period, followed by the code from another chapter that specifies the condition. Codes for signs and symptoms may be assigned when a definitive diagnosis has not been established.

3. Birth process or community acquired conditions

If a newborn has a condition that may be either due to the birth process or community acquired and the documentation does not indicate which it is, the default is due to the birth process and the code from Chapter 15 should be used. If the condition is community-acquired, a code from Chapter 15 should not be assigned.

4. Code all clinically significant conditions

All clinically significant conditions noted on routine newborn examination should be coded. A condition is clinically significant if it requires:

- clinical evaluation; or
- herapeutic treatment; or
- diagnostic procedures; or
- extended length of hospital stay; or
- increased nursing care and/or monitoring; or
- has implications for future health care needs

Note: The perinatal guidelines listed above are the same as the general coding guidelines for "additional diagnoses", except for the final point regarding implications for future health care needs. Codes should be assigned for conditions that have been specified by the provider as having implications for future health care needs. Codes from the perinatal chapter should not be assigned unless the provider has established a definitive diagnosis.

b. Use of codes V30-V39

When coding the birth of an infant, assign a code from categories V30-V39, according to the type of birth. A code from this series is assigned as a principal diagnosis, and assigned only once to a newborn at the time of birth.

c. Newborn transfers

If the newborn is transferred to another institution, the V30 series is not used at the receiving hospital.

d. Use of category V29

1. Assigning a code from category V29

Assign a code from category V29, Observation and evaluation of newborns and infants for suspected conditions not found, to identify those instances when a healthy newborn is evaluated for a suspected condition that is determined after study not to be present. Do not use a code from category V29 when the patient has identified signs or symptoms of a suspected problem; in such cases, code the sign or symptom.

A code from category V29 may also be assigned as a principal code for readmissions or encounters when the V30 code no longer applies. Codes from category V29 are for use only for healthy newborns and infants for which no condition after study is found to be present.

2. V29 code on a birth record

A V29 code is to be used as a secondary code after the V30, Outcome of delivery, code.

e. Use of other V codes on perinatal records

V codes other than V30 and V29 may be assigned on a perinatal or newborn record code. The codes may be used as a principal or first-listed diagnosis for specific types of encounters or for readmissions or encounters when the V30 code no longer applies. See Section I.C.18 for information regarding the assignment of V codes.

f. **Maternal Causes of Perinatal Morbidity**
Codes from categories 760-763, Maternal causes of perinatal morbidity and mortality, are assigned only when the maternal condition has actually affected the fetus or newborn. The fact that the mother has an associated medical condition or experiences some complication of pregnancy, labor or delivery does not justify the routine assignment of codes from these categories to the newborn record.

g. **Congenital Anomalies in Newborns**
For the birth admission, the appropriate code from category V30, Liveborn infants according to type of birth, should be used, followed by any congenital anomaly codes, categories 740-759. Use additional secondary codes from other chapters to specify conditions associated with the anomaly, if applicable. Also, see Section I.C.14 for information on the coding of congenital anomalies.

h. **Coding Additional Perinatal Diagnoses**

1. *Assigning codes for conditions that require treatment*
Assign codes for conditions that require treatment or further investigation, prolong the length of stay, or require resource utilization.
2. *Codes for conditions specified as having implications for future health care needs*
Assign codes for conditions that have been specified by the provider as having implications for future health care needs. Note: This guideline should not be used for adult patients.
3. *Codes for newborn conditions originating in the perinatal period*
Assign a code for newborn conditions originating in the perinatal period (categories 760-779), as well as complications arising during the current episode of care classified in other chapters, only if the diagnoses have been documented by the responsible provider at the time of transfer or discharge as having affected the fetus or newborn.

i. **Prematurity and Fetal Growth Retardation**
Providers utilize different criteria in determining prematurity. A code for prematurity should not be assigned unless it is documented. The 5th digit assignment for codes from category 764 and subcategories 765.0 and 765.1 should be based on the recorded birth weight and estimated gestational age.
A code from subcategory 765.2, Weeks of gestation, should be assigned as an additional code with category 764 and codes from 765.0 and 765.1 to specify weeks of gestation as documented by the provider in the record.

j. **Newborn sepsis**
Code 771.81, Septicemia [sepsis] of newborn, should be assigned with a secondary code from category 041, Bacterial infections in conditions classified elsewhere and of unspecified site, to identify the organism. It is not necessary to use a code from subcategory 995.9, Systemic inflammatory response syndrome (SIRS), on a newborn record. A code from category 038, Septicemia, should not be used on a newborn record. Code 771.81 describes the sepsis.

16. *Chapter 16: Signs, Symptoms and Ill-Defined Conditions (780-799)*
Reserved for future guideline expansion

17. *Chapter 17: Injury and Poisoning (800-999)*

a. **Coding of Injuries**
When coding injuries, assign separate codes for each injury unless a combination code is provided, in which case the combination code is assigned. Multiple injury codes are provided in ICD-9-CM, but should not be assigned unless information for a more specific code is not available. These codes are not to be used for normal, healing surgical wounds or to identify complications of surgical wounds.
The code for the most serious injury, as determined by the provider and the focus of treatment, is sequenced first.

1. *Superficial injuries*
Superficial injuries such as abrasions or contusions are not coded when associated with more severe injuries of the same site.
2. *Primary injury with damage to nerves/blood vessels*
When a primary injury results in minor damage to peripheral nerves or blood vessels, the primary injury is sequenced first with additional code(s) from categories 950-957, Injury to nerves and spinal cord, and/or 900-904, Injury to blood vessels. When the primary injury is to the blood vessels or nerves, that injury should be sequenced first.

b. **Coding of Fractures**
The principles of multiple coding of injuries should be followed in coding fractures. Fractures of specified sites are coded individually by site in accordance with both the provisions within categories 800-829 and the level of detail furnished by medical record content. Combination categories for multiple fractures are provided for use when there is insufficient detail in the medical record (such as trauma cases transferred to another hospital), when the reporting form limits the number of codes that can be used in reporting pertinent clinical data, or when there is insufficient specificity at the fourth-digit or fifth-digit level. More specific guidelines are as follows:

1. *Acute Fractures vs. Aftercare*
Traumatic fractures are coded using the acute fracture codes (800-829) while the patient is receiving active treatment for the fracture. Examples of active treatment are: surgical treatment, emergency department encounter, and evaluation and treatment by a new physician.
Fractures are coded using the aftercare codes (subcategories V54.0, V54.1, V54.8, or V54.9) for encounters after the patient has completed active treatment of the fracture and is receiving routine care for the fracture during the healing or recovery phase. Examples of fracture aftercare are: cast change or removal, removal of external or internal fixation device, medication adjustment, and follow up visits following fracture treatment.
Care for complications of surgical treatment for fracture repairs during the healing or recovery phase should be coded with the appropriate complication codes.
Care of complications of fractures, such as malunion and nonunion, should be reported with the appropriate codes.
Pathologic fractures are not coded in the 800-829 range, but instead are assigned to subcategory 733.1. See Section I.C.13.a for additional information.
2. *Multiple fractures of same limb*
Multiple fractures of same limb classifiable to the same three-digit or four-digit category are coded to that category.
3. *Multiple unilateral or bilateral fractures of same bone*
Multiple unilateral or bilateral fractures of same bone(s) but classified to different fourth-digit subdivisions (bone part) within the same three-digit category are coded individually by site.
4. *Multiple fracture categories 819 and 828*
Multiple fracture categories 819 and 828 classify bilateral fractures of both upper limbs (819) and both lower limbs (828), but without any detail at the fourth-digit level other than open and closed type of fractures.
5. *Multiple fractures sequencing*
Multiple fractures are sequenced in accordance with the severity of the fracture. The provider should be asked to list the fracture diagnoses in the order of severity.

c. **Coding of Burns**

Current burns (940-948) are classified by depth, extent and by agent (E code). Burns are classified by depth as first degree (erythema), second degree (blistering), and third degree (full-thickness involvement).

1. ***Sequencing of burn and related condition codes***

   Sequence first the code that reflects the highest degree of burn when more than one burn is present.

   a. When the reason for the admission or encounter is for treatment of external multiple burns, sequence first the code that reflects the burn of the highest degree.

   b. When a patient has both internal and external burns, the circumstances of admission govern the selection of the principal diagnosis or first-listed diagnosis.

   c. When a patient is admitted for burn injuries and other related conditions such as smoke inhalation and/or respiratory failure, the circumstances of admission govern the selection of the principal or first-listed diagnosis.

2. ***Burns of the same local site***

   Classify burns of the same local site (three-digit category level, 940-947) but of different degrees to the subcategory identifying the highest degree recorded in the diagnosis.

3. ***Non-healing burns***

   Non-healing burns are coded as acute burns.

   Necrosis of burned skin should be coded as a non-healed burn.

4. ***Code 958.3, Posttraumatic wound infection***

   Assign code 958.3, Posttraumatic wound infection, not elsewhere classified, as an additional code for any documented infected burn site.

5. ***Assign separate codes for each burn site***

   When coding burns, assign separate codes for each burn site. Category 946 Burns of Multiple specified sites, should only be used if the location of the burns are not documented. Category 949, Burn, unspecified, is extremely vague and should rarely be used.

6. ***Assign codes from category 948, Burns***

   Burns classified according to extent of body surface involved, when the site of the burn is not specified or when there is a need for additional data. It is advisable to use category 948 as additional coding when needed to provide data for evaluating burn mortality, such as that needed by burn units. It is also advisable to use category 948 as an additional code for reporting purposes when there is mention of a third-degree burn involving 20 percent or more of the body surface.

   In assigning a code from category 948:

   - Fourth-digit codes are used to identify the percentage of total body surface involved in a burn (all degree).
   - Fifth-digits are assigned to identify the percentage of body surface involved in third-degree burn.
   - Fifth-digit zero (0) is assigned when less than 10 percent or when no body surface is involved in a third-degree burn.

   Category 948 is based on the classic "rule of nines" in estimating body surface involved: head and neck are assigned nine percent, each arm nine percent, each leg 18 percent, the anterior trunk 18 percent, posterior trunk 18 percent, and genitalia one percent. Providers may change these percentage assignments where necessary to accommodate infants and children who have proportionately larger heads than adults and patients who have large buttocks, thighs, or abdomen that involve burns.

7. ***Encounters for treatment of late effects of burns***

   Encounters for the treatment of the late effects of burns (i.e., scars or joint contractures) should be coded to the residual condition (sequelae) followed by the appropriate late effect code (906.5-906.9). A late effect E code may also be used, if desired.

8. ***Sequelae with a late effect code and current burn***

   When appropriate, both a sequelae with a late effect code, and a current burn code may be assigned on the same record (when both a current burn and sequelae of an old burn exist).

d. **Coding of Debridement of Wound, Infection, or Burn**

Excisional debridement involves an excisional debridement (surgical removal or cutting away), as opposed to a mechanical (brushing, scrubbing, washing) debridement.

For coding purposes, excisional debridement is assigned to code 86.22.

Nonexcisional debridement is assigned to code 86.28.

e. **Adverse Effects, Poisoning and Toxic Effects**

The properties of certain drugs, medicinal and biological substances or combinations of such substances, may cause toxic reactions. The occurrence of drug toxicity is classified in ICD-9-CM as follows:

1. ***Adverse Effect***

When the drug was correctly prescribed and properly administered, code the reaction plus the appropriate code from the E930-E949 series. Codes from the E930-E949 series must be used to identify the causative substance for an adverse effect of drug, medicinal and biological substances, correctly prescribed and properly administered. The effect, such as tachycardia, delirium, gastrointestinal hemorrhaging, vomiting, hypokalemia, hepatitis, renal failure, or respiratory failure, is coded and followed by the appropriate code from the E930-E949 series.

Adverse effects of therapeutic substances correctly prescribed and properly administered (toxicity, synergistic reaction, side effect, and idiosyncratic reaction) may be due to (1) differences among patients, such as age, sex, disease, and genetic factors, and (2) drug-related factors, such as type of drug, route of administration, duration of therapy, dosage, and bioavailability.

2. ***Poisoning***

   a. Error was made in drug prescription

      Errors made in drug prescription or in the administration of the drug by provider, nurse, patient, or other person, use the appropriate poisoning code from the 960-979 series.

   b. Overdose of a drug intentionally taken

      If an overdose of a drug was intentionally taken or administered and resulted in drug toxicity, it would be coded as a poisoning (960-979 series).

   c. Nonprescribed drug taken with correctly prescribed and properly administered drug

      If a nonprescribed drug or medicinal agent was taken in combination with a correctly prescribed and properly administered drug, any drug toxicity or other reaction resulting from the interaction of the two drugs would be classified as a poisoning.

   d. Sequencing of poisoning

      When coding a poisoning or reaction to the improper use of a medication (e.g., wrong dose, wrong substance, wrong route of administration) the poisoning code is sequenced first, followed by a code for the manifestation. If there is also a diagnosis of drug abuse or dependence to the substance, the abuse or dependence is coded as an additional code.

      See Section I.C.3.a.6.b. if poisoning is the result of insulin pump malfunctions and Section I.C.19 for general use of E-codes.

3. *Toxic Effects*
   a. Toxic effect codes
   When a harmful substance is ingested or comes in contact with a person, this is classified as a toxic effect. The toxic effect codes are in categories 980-989.
   b. Sequencing toxic effect codes
   A toxic effect code should be sequenced first, followed by the code(s) that identify the result of the toxic effect.
   c. External cause codes for toxic effects
   An external cause code from categories E860-E869 for accidental exposure, codes E950.6 or E950.7 for intentional self-harm, category E962 for assault, or categories E980-E982, for undetermined, should also be assigned to indicate intent.

f. Complications of care

1. *Transplant complications*
   a. Transplant complications other than kidney
   Codes under subcategory 996.8, Complications of transplanted organ, are for use for both complications and rejection of transplanted organs. A transplant complication code is only assigned if the complication affects the function of the transplanted organ. Two codes are required to fully describe a transplant complication, the appropriate code from subcategory 996.8 and a secondary code that identifies the complication.
   Pre-existing conditions or conditions that develop after the transplant are not coded as complications unless they affect the function of the transplanted organs.
   Post-transplants surgical complications that do not relate to the function of the transplanted organ are classified to the specific complication. For example, a surgical wound dehiscence would be coded to the wound dehiscence, not as a transplant complication.
   Post-transplant patients who are seen for treatment unrelated to the transplanted organ should be assigned a code from category V42, Organ or tissue replaced by transplant, to identify the transplant status of the patient. A code from category V42 should never be used with a code from subcategory 996.8.
   b. Kidney transplant complications
   Code 996.81 should be assigned for documented complications of a kidney transplant, such as transplant failure or rejection. Code 996.81 should not be assigned for post kidney transplant patients who have chronic kidney (CKD) unless a transplant complication such as transplant failure or rejection is documented. If the documentation is unclear as to whether the patient has a complication of the transplant, query the provider.
   For patients with CKD following a kidney transplant, but who do not have a complication such as failure or rejection, see section I.C.10.a.2, Chronic kidney disease and kidney transplant status.

g. SIRS due to Non-infectious Process

The systemic inflammatory response syndrome (SIRS) can develop as a result of certain non-infectious disease processes, such as trauma, malignant neoplasm, or pancreatitis. When SIRS is documented with a noninfectious condition, and no subsequent infection is documented, the code for the underlying condition, such as an injury, should be assigned, followed by code 995.93, Systemic inflammatory response syndrome due to noninfectious process without acute organ dysfunction, or 995.94, Systemic inflammatory response syndrome due to non-infectious process with acute organ dysfunction. If an acute organ dysfunction is documented, the appropriate code(s) for the associated acute organ dysfunction(s) should be assigned in addition to code 995.94. If acute organ dysfunction is documented, but it cannot be determined if the acute organ dysfunction is associated with SIRS or due to another condition (e.g., directly due to the trauma), the provider should be queried.

When the non-infectious condition has led to an infection that results in SIRS, see Section I.C.1.b.11 for the guideline for sepsis and severe sepsis associated with a non-infectious process.

18. *Classification of Factors Influencing Health Status and Contact with Health Service (Supplemental V01-V86)*

Note: The chapter specific guidelines provide additional information about the use of V codes for specified encounters.

a. Introduction

ICD-9-CM provides codes to deal with encounters for circumstances other than a disease or injury. The Supplementary Classification of Factors Influencing Health Status and Contact with Health Services (V01.0-V86.1) is provided to deal with occasions when circumstances other than a disease or injury (codes 001-999) are recorded as a diagnosis or problem.

There are four primary circumstances for the use of V codes:

1. *A person who is not currently sick encounters the health services for some specific reason, such as to act as an organ donor, to receive prophylactic care, such as inoculations or health screenings, or to receive counseling on health related issues.*
2. *A person with a resolving disease or injury, or a chronic, long-term condition requiring continuous care, encounters the health care system for specific aftercare of that disease or injury (e.g., dialysis for renal disease; chemotherapy for malignancy; cast change). A diagnosis/symptom code should be used whenever a current, acute, diagnosis is being treated or a sign or symptom is being studied.*
3. *Circumstances or problems influence a person's health status but are not in themselves a current illness or injury.*
4. *Newborns, to indicate birth status*

b. V codes use in any healthcare setting

V codes are for use in any healthcare setting. V codes may be used as either a first listed (principal diagnosis code in the inpatient setting) or secondary code, depending on the circumstances of the encounter. Certain V codes may only be used as first listed, others only as secondary codes. See Section I.C.18.e, V Code Table.

c. V Codes indicate a reason for an encounter

They are not procedure codes. A corresponding procedure code must accompany a V code to describe the procedure performed.

d. Categories of V Codes

1. *Contact/Exposure*
   Category V01 indicates contact with or exposure to communicable diseases. These codes are for patients who do not show any sign or symptom of a disease but have been exposed to it by close personal contact with an infected individual or are in an area where a disease is epidemic. These codes may be used as a first listed code to explain an encounter for testing, or, more commonly, as a secondary code to identify a potential risk.
2. *Inoculations and vaccinations*
   Categories V03-V06 are for encounters for inoculations and vaccinations. They indicate that a patient is being seen to receive a prophylactic inoculation against a disease. The injection itself must be represented by the appropriate procedure code. A code from V03-V06 may be used as a secondary code if the inoculation is given as a routine part of preventive health care, such as a well-baby visit.

3. *Status*

Status codes indicate that a patient is either a carrier of a disease or has the sequelae or residual of a past disease or condition. This includes such things as the presence of prosthetic or mechanical devices resulting from past treatment.

A status code is informative, because the status may affect the course of treatment and its outcome. A status code is distinct from a history code. The history code indicates that the patient no longer has the condition.

A status code should not be used with a diagnosis code from one of the body system chapters, if the diagnosis code includes the information provided by the status code. For example, code V42.1, Heart transplant status, should not be used with code 996.83, Complications of transplanted heart. The status code does not provide additional information. The complication code indicates that the patient is a heart transplant patient.

The status V codes/categories are:

V02	Carrier or suspected carrier of infectious diseases Carrier status indicates that a person harbors the specific organisms of a disease without manifest symptoms and is capable of transmitting the infection.
V08	Asymptomatic HIV infection status This code indicates that a patient has tested positive for HIV but has manifested no signs or symptoms of the disease.
V09	Infection with drug-resistant microorganisms This category indicates that a patient has an infection that is resistant to drug treatment. Sequence the infection code first.
V21	Constitutional states in development
V22.2	Pregnant state, incidental This code is a secondary code only for use when the pregnancy is in no way complicating the reason for visit. Otherwise, a code from the obstetric chapter is required.
V26.5x	Sterilization status
V42	Organ or tissue replaced by transplant
V43	Organ or tissue replaced by other means
V44	Artificial opening status
V45	Other postsurgical states
V46	Other dependence on machines
V49.6	Upper limb amputation status
V49.7	Lower limb amputation status
V49.81	Postmenopausal status
V49.82	Dental sealant status
V49.83	Awaiting organ transplant status
V58.6	Long-term (current) drug use This subcategory indicates a patient's continuous use of a prescribed drug (including such things as aspirin therapy) for the long-term treatment of a condition or for prophylactic use. It is not for use for patients who have addictions to drugs. Assign a code from subcategory V58.6, Long-term (current) drug use, if the patient is receiving a medication for an extended period as a prophylactic measure (such as for the prevention of deep vein thrombosis) or as treatment of a chronic condition (such as arthritis) or a disease requiring a lengthy course of treatment (such as cancer). Do not assign a code from subcategory V58.6 for medication being administered for a brief period of time to treat an acute illness or injury (such as a course of antibiotics to treat acute bronchitis).
V83	Genetic carrier status Genetic carrier status indicates that a person carries a gene, associated with a particular disease, which may be passed to offspring who may develop that disease. The person does not have the disease and is not at risk of developing the disease.
V84	Genetic susceptibility status Genetic susceptibility indicates that a person has a gene that increases the risk of that person developing the disease. Codes from category V84, Genetic susceptibility to disease, should not be used as principal or first-listed codes. If the patient has the condition to which he/she is susceptible, and that condition is the reason for the encounter, the code for the current condition should be sequenced first. If the patient is being seen for follow-up after completed treatment for this condition, and the condition no longer exists, a follow-up code should be sequenced first, followed by the appropriate personal history and genetic susceptibility codes. If the purpose of the encounter is genetic counseling associated with procreative management, a code from subcategory V26.3, Genetic counseling and testing, should be assigned as the first-listed code, followed by a code from category V84. Additional codes should be assigned for any applicable family or personal history. See Section I.C. 18.d.14 for information on prophylactic organ removal due to a genetic susceptibility.
V86	Estrogen receptor status

Note: Categories V42-V46, and subcategories V49.6, V49.7 are for use only if there are no complications or malfunctions of the organ or tissue replaced, the amputation site or the equipment on which the patient is dependent. These are always secondary codes.

4. *History (of)*

There are two types of history V codes, personal and family. Personal history codes explain a patient's past medical condition that no longer exists and is not receiving any treatment, but that has the potential for recurrence, and therefore may require continued monitoring. The exceptions to this general rule are category V14, Personal history of allergy to medicinal agents, and subcategory V15.0, Allergy, other than to medicinal agents. A person who has had an allergic episode to a substance or food in the past should always be considered allergic to the substance.

Family history codes are for use when a patient has a family member(s) who has had a particular disease that causes the patient to be at higher risk of also contracting the disease. Personal history codes may be used in conjunction with follow-up codes and family history codes may be used in conjunction with screening codes to explain the need for a test or procedure. History codes are also acceptable on any medical record regardless of the reason for visit. A history of an illness, even if no longer present, is important information that may alter the type of treatment ordered.

The history V code categories are:

V10	Personal history of malignant neoplasm
V12	Personal history of certain other diseases
V13	Personal history of other diseases Except: V13.4, Personal history of arthritis, and V13.6, Personal history of congenital

	malformations. These conditions are life-long so are not true history codes.
V14	Personal history of allergy to medicinal agents
V15	Other personal history presenting hazards to health Except: V15.7, Personal history of contraception.
V16	Family history of malignant neoplasm
V17	Family history of certain chronic disabling diseases
V18	Family history of certain other specific diseases
V19	Family history of other conditions

5. *Screening*

Screening is the testing for disease or disease precursors in seemingly well individuals so that early detection and treatment can be provided for those who test positive for the disease. Screenings that are recommended for many subgroups in a population include: routine mammograms for women over 40, a fecal occult blood test for everyone over 50, an amniocentesis to rule out a fetal anomaly for pregnant women over 35, because the incidence of breast cancer and colon cancer in these subgroups is higher than in the general population, as is the incidence of Down's syndrome in older mothers.

The testing of a person to rule out or confirm a suspected diagnosis because the patient has some sign or symptom is a diagnostic examination, not a screening. In these cases, the sign or symptom is used to explain the reason for the test.

A screening code may be a first listed code if the reason for the visit is specifically the screening exam. It may also be used as an additional code if the screening is done during an office visit for other health problems. A screening code is not necessary if the screening is inherent to a routine examination, such as a pap smear done during a routine pelvic examination.

Should a condition be discovered during the screening then the code for the condition may be assigned as an additional diagnosis.

The V code indicates that a screening exam is planned. A procedure code is required to confirm that the screening was performed.

The screening V code categories:

V28	Antenatal screening
V73-V82	Special screening examinations

6. *Observation*

There are two observation V code categories. They are for use in very limited circumstances when a person is being observed for a suspected condition that is ruled out. The observation codes are not for use if an injury or illness or any signs or symptoms related to the suspected condition are present. In such cases the diagnosis/symptom code is used with the corresponding E code to identify any external cause.

The observation codes are to be used as principal diagnosis only. The only exception to this is when the principal diagnosis is required to be a code from the V30, Live born infant, category. Then the V29 observation code is sequenced after the V30 code. Additional codes may be used in addition to the observation code but only if they are unrelated to the suspected condition being observed.

The observation V code categories:

V29	Observation and evaluation of newborns for suspected condition not found For the birth encounter, a code from category V30 should be sequenced before the V29 code.
V71	Observation and evaluation for suspected condition not found

7. *Aftercare*

Aftercare visit codes cover situations when the initial treatment of a disease or injury has been performed and the patient requires continued care during the healing or recovery phase, or for the long-term consequences of the disease. The aftercare V code should not be used if treatment is directed at a current, acute disease or injury. The diagnosis code is to be used in these cases. Exceptions to this rule are codes V58.0, Radiotherapy, and codes from subcategory V58.1, Encounter for chemotherapy and immunotherapy for neoplastic conditions. These codes are to be first listed, followed by the diagnosis code when a patient's encounter is solely to receive radiation therapy or chemotherapy for the treatment of a neoplasm. Should a patient receive both chemotherapy and radiation therapy during the same encounter code V58.0 and V58.1 may be used together on a record with either one being sequenced first.

The aftercare codes are generally first listed to explain the specific reason for the encounter. An aftercare code may be used as an additional code when some type of aftercare is provided in addition to the reason for admission and no diagnosis code is applicable. An example of this would be the closure of a colostomy during an encounter for treatment of another condition.

Certain aftercare V code categories need a secondary diagnosis code to describe the resolving condition or sequelae, for others, the condition is inherent in the code title.

Additional V code aftercare category terms include, fitting and adjustment, and attention to artificial openings.

Status V codes may be used with aftercare V codes to indicate the nature of the aftercare. For example code V45.81, Aortocoronary bypass status, may be used with code V58.73, Aftercare following surgery of the circulatory system, NEC, to indicate the surgery for which the aftercare is being performed. Also, a transplant status code may be used following code V58.44, Aftercare following organ transplant, to identify the organ transplanted. A status code should not be used when the aftercare code indicates the type of status, such as using V55.0, Attention to tracheostomy with V44.0, Tracheostomy status.

The aftercare V category/codes:

V52	Fitting and adjustment of prosthetic device and implant
V53	Fitting and adjustment of other device
V54	Other orthopedic aftercare
V55	Attention to artificial openings
V56	Encounter for dialysis and dialysis catheter care
V57	Care involving the use of rehabilitation procedures
V58.0	Radiotherapy
V58.11	Encounter for antineoplastic chemotherapy
V58.12	Encounter for antineoplastic immunotherapy
V58.3	Attention to surgical dressings and sutures
V58.41	Encounter for planned post-operative wound closure
V58.42	Aftercare, surgery, neoplasm
V58.43	Aftercare, surgery, trauma
V58.44	Aftercare involving organ transplant
V58.49	Other specified aftercare following surgery
V58.7x	Aftercare following surgery
V58.81	Fitting and adjustment of vascular catheter
V58.82	Fitting and adjustment of non-vascular catheter
V58.83	Monitoring therapeutic drug
V58.89	Other specified aftercare

8. *Follow-up*

The follow-up codes are used to explain continuing surveillance following completed treatment of a disease, condition, or injury. They imply that the condition has been fully treated and no longer exists. They should not be confused with aftercare codes that explain current treatment for a healing condition or its sequelae. Follow-up codes may be used in conjunction with history codes to provide the full picture of the healed condition and its treatment. The follow-up code is sequenced first, followed by the history code.

A follow-up code may be used to explain repeated visits. Should a condition be found to have recurred on the follow-up visit, then the diagnosis code should be used in place of the follow-up code.

The follow-up V code categories:

V24	Postpartum care and evaluation
V67	Follow-up examination

9. *Donor*

Category V59 is the donor codes. They are used for living individuals who are donating blood or other body tissue. These codes are only for individuals donating for others, not for self donations. They are not for use to identify cadaveric donations.

10. *Counseling*

Counseling V codes are used when a patient or family member receives assistance in the aftermath of an illness or injury, or when support is required in coping with family or social problems. They are not necessary for use in conjunction with a diagnosis code when the counseling component of care is considered integral to standard treatment.

The counseling V categories/codes:

V25.0	General counseling and advice for contraceptive management
V26.3	Genetic counseling
V26.4	General counseling and advice for procreative management
V61	Other family circumstances
V65.1	Person consulted on behalf of another person
V65.3	Dietary surveillance and counseling
V65.4	Other counseling, not elsewhere classified

11. *Obstetrics and related conditions*

See Section I.C.11., the Obstetrics guidelines for further instruction on the use of these codes.

V codes for pregnancy are for use in those circumstances when none of the problems or complications included in the codes from the Obstetrics chapter exist (a routine prenatal visit or postpartum care). Codes V22.0, Supervision of normal first pregnancy, and V22.1, Supervision of other normal pregnancy, are always first listed and are not to be used with any other code from the OB chapter.

The outcome of delivery, category V27, should be included on all maternal delivery records. It is always a secondary code.

V codes for family planning (contraceptive) or procreative management and counseling should be included on an obstetric record either during the pregnancy or the postpartum stage, if applicable.

Obstetrics and related conditions V code categories:

V22	Normal pregnancy
V23	Supervision of high-risk pregnancy Except: V23.2, Pregnancy with history of abortion. Code 646.3, Habitual aborter, from the OB chapter is required to indicate a history of abortion during a pregnancy.
V24	Postpartum care and evaluation
V25	Encounter for contraceptive management Except V25.0x (See Section I.C.18.d.11, Counseling)
V26	Procreative management Except V26.5x, Sterilization status, V26.3 and V26.4 (See Section I.C.18.d.11., Counseling)
V27	Outcome of delivery
V28	Antenatal screening (See Section I.C.18.d.6., Screening)

12. *Newborn, infant and child*

See Section I.C.15, the Newborn guidelines for further instruction on the use of these codes.

Newborn V code categories:

V20	Health supervision of infant or child
V29	Observation and evaluation of newborns for suspected condition not found (See Section I.C.18.d.7, Observation).
V30-V39	Liveborn infant according to type of birth

13. *Routine and administrative examinations*

The V codes allow for the description of encounters for routine examinations, such as, a general check-up, or, examinations for administrative purposes, such as, a pre-employment physical. The codes are for use as first listed codes only, and are not to be used if the examination is for diagnosis of a suspected condition or for treatment purposes. In such cases the diagnosis code is used. During a routine exam, should a diagnosis or condition be discovered, it should be coded as an additional code. Pre-existing and chronic conditions and history codes may also be included as additional codes as long as the examination is for administrative purposes and not focused on any particular condition.

Pre-operative examination V codes are for use only in those situations when a patient is being cleared for surgery and no treatment is given.

The V codes categories/code for routine and administrative examinations:

V20.2	Routine infant or child health check Any injections given should have a corresponding procedure code.
V70	General medical examination
V72	Special investigations and examinations Codes V72.5 and V72.6 may be used if the reason for the patient encounter is for routine laboratory/radiology testing in the absence of any signs, symptoms, or associated diagnosis. If routine testing is performed during the same encounter as a test to evaluate a sign, symptom, or diagnosis, it is appropriate to assign both the V code and the code describing the reason for the non-routine test.

14. *Miscellaneous V codes*

The miscellaneous V codes capture a number of other health care encounters that do not fall into one of the other categories.

Certain of these codes identify the reason for the encounter, others are for use as additional codes that provide useful information on circumstances that may affect a patient's care and treatment.

Miscellaneous V code categories/codes:

V07	Need for isolation and other prophylactic measures
V50	Elective surgery for purposes other than remedying health states
V58.5	Orthodontics
V60	Housing, household, and economic circumstances

V62 Other psychosocial circumstances
V63 Unavailability of other medical facilities for care
V64 Persons encountering health services for specific procedures, not carried out
V66 Convalescence and Palliative Care
V68 Encounters for administrative purposes
V69 Problems related to lifestyle
V85 Body Mass Index

15. Nonspecific V codes

Certain V codes are so non-specific, or potentially redundant with other codes in the classification, that there can be little justification for their use in the inpatient setting. Their use in the outpatient setting should be limited to those instances when there is no further documentation to permit more precise coding. Otherwise, any sign or symptom or any other reason for visit that is captured in another code should be used.

Nonspecific V code categories/codes:

V11 Personal history of mental disorder
A code from the mental disorders chapter, with an in remission fifth-digit, should be used.
V13.4 Personal history of arthritis
V13.6 Personal history of congenital malformations
V15.7 Personal history of contraception
V23.2 Pregnancy with history of abortion
V40 Mental and behavioral problems
V41 Problems with special senses and other special functions
V47 Other problems with internal organs
V48 Problems with head, neck, and trunk
V49 Problems with limbs and other problems

Exceptions:

V49.6 Upper limb amputation status
V49.7 Lower limb amputation status
V49.81 Postmenopausal status
V49.82 Dental sealant status
V49.83 Awaiting organ transplant status
V51 Aftercare involving the use of plastic surgery
V58.2 Blood transfusion, without reported diagnosis
V58.9 Unspecified aftercare
V72.5 Radiological examination, NEC
V72.6 Laboratory examination
Codes V72.5 and V72.6 are not to be used if any sign or symptoms, or reason for a test is documented. See Section IV.K. and Section IV.L. of the Outpatient guidelines.

V Code Table

1st Dx only - Generally for use as first listed only but may be used as additional if patient has more than one encounter on one day

1st or add'l Dx only - These codes may be used as first listed or additional codes

Add'l Dx only - These codes are only for use as additional codes

Non-spec Dx only - These codes are primarily for use in the nonacute setting and should be limited to encounters for which no sign or symptom or reason for visit is documented in the record. Their use may be as either a first listed or additional code.

Code(s)	Description	1st Dx only	1st or add'l Dx only	Add'l Dx only	Non-spec Dx only
V01.X	Contact with or exposure to communicable diseases		X		
V02.X	Carrier or suspected carrier of infectious diseases		X		
V03.X	Need for prophylactic vaccination and inoculation against bacterial diseases		X		
V04.X	Need for prophylactic vaccination and inoculation against certain diseases		X		
V05.X	Need for prophylactic vaccination and inoculation against single diseases		X		
V06.X	Need for prophylactic vaccination and inoculation against combinations of diseases		X		
V07.X	Need for isolation and other prophylactic measures		X		
V08	Asymptomatic HIV infection status		X		
V09.X	Infection with drug resistant organisms			X	
V10.X	Personal history of malignant neoplasm		X		
V11.X	Personal history of mental disorder				X
V12.X	Personal history of certain other diseases		X		
V13.0X	Personal history of other disorders of urinary system		X		
V13.1	Personal history of trophoblastic disease		X		
V13.2X	Personal history of other genital system and obstetric disorders		X		
V13.3	Personal history of diseases of skin and subcutaneous tissue		X		
V13.4	Personal history of arthritis				X
V13.5	Personal history of other musculoskeletal disorders		X		
V13.61	Personal history of hypospadias			X	
V13.69	Personal history of congenital malformations				X
V13.7	Personal history of perinatal problems		X		
V13.8	Personal history of other specified diseases		X		

Code(s)	Description	1st Dx only	1st or add'l Dx only	Add'l Dx only	Non-spec Dx only
V13.9	Personal history of unspecified disease				X
V14.X	Personal history of allergy to medicinal agents			X	
V15.0X	Personal history of allergy, other than to medicinal agents			X	
V15.1	Personal history of surgery to heart and great vessels			X	
V15.2	Personal history of surgery to other major organs			X	
V15.3	Personal history of irradiation			X	
V15.4X	Personal history of psychological trauma			X	
V15.5	Personal history of injury			X	
V15.6	Personal history of poisoning			X	
V15.7	Personal history of contraception				X
V15.81	Personal history of noncompliance with medical treatment			X	
V15.82	Personal history of tobacco use			X	
V15.84	Personal history of exposure to asbestos			X	
V15.85	Personal history of exposure to potentially hazardous body fluids			X	
V15.86	Personal history of exposure to lead			X	
V15.87	Personal history of extracorporeal membrane oxygenation [ECMO]			X	
V15.88	History of fall		X		
V15.89	Other specified personal history presenting hazards to health			X	
V16.X	Family history of malignant neoplasm		X		
V17.X	Family history of certain chronic disabling diseases		X		
V18.X	Family history of certain other specific conditions		X		
V19.X	Family history of other conditions		X		
V20.X	Health supervision of infant or child	X			
V21.X	Constitutional states in development			X	
V22.0	Supervision of normal first pregnancy	X			
V22.1	Supervision of other normal pregnancy	X			
V22.2	Pregnancy state, incidental			X	
V23.X	Supervision of high-risk pregnancy		X		
V24.X	Postpartum care and examination	X			
V25.X	Encounter for contraceptive management		X		

Code(s)	Description	1st Dx only	1st or add'l Dx only	Add'l Dx only	Non-spec Dx only
V26.0	Tuboplasty or vasoplasty after previous sterilization		X		
V26.1	Artificial insemination		X		
V26.2X	Procreative management investigation and testing		X		
V26.3X	Procreative management, genetic counseling and testing		X		
V26.4	Procreative management, genetic counseling and advice		X		
V26.5X	Procreative management, sterilization status			X	
V26.8	Other specified procreative management		X		
V26.9	Unspecified procreative management		X		
V27.X	Outcome of delivery			X	
V28.X	Encounter for antenatal screening of mother		X		
V29.X	Observation and evaluation of newborns for suspected condition not found	X			
V30.X	Single liveborn	X			
V31.X	Twin, mate liveborn	X			
V32.X	Twin, mate stillborn	X			
V33.X	Twin, unspecified	X			
V34.X	Other multiple, mates all liveborn	X			
V35.X	Other multiple, mates all stillborn	X			
V36.X	Other multiple, mates live- and stillborn	X			
V37.X	Other multiple, unspecified	X			
V39.X	Unspecified	X			
V40.0	Mental and behavioral problems				X
V41.X	Problems with special senses and other special functions				X
V42.X	Organ or tissue replaced by transplant			X	
V43.0	Organ or tissue replaced by other means, eye globe			X	
V43.1	Organ or tissue replaced by other means, lens			X	
V43.21	Organ or tissue replaced by other means, heart assist device			X	
V43.22	Fully implantable artificial heart status		X		
V43.3	Organ or tissue replaced by other means, heart valve			X	
V43.4	Organ or tissue replaced by other means, blood vessel			X	
V43.5	Organ or tissue replaced by other means, bladder			X	
V43.6X	Organ or tissue replaced by other means, joint			X	
V43.7	Organ or tissue replaced by other means, limb			X	
V43.8X	Other organ or tissue replaced by other means			X	

Code(s)	Description	1st Dx only	1st or add'l Dx only	Add'l Dx only	Non-spec Dx only
V44.X	Artificial opening status			X	
V45.0X	Cardiac device in situ			X	
V45.1	Renal dialysis status			X	
V45.2	Presence of cerebrospinal fluid drainage device			X	
V45.3	Intestinal bypass or anastomosis status			X	
V45.4	Arthrodesis status			X	
V45.5X	Presence of contraceptive device			X	
V45.6X	States following surgery of eye and adnexa			X	
V45.7X	Acquired absence of organ		X		
V45.8X	Other postprocedural status			X	
V46.0	Other dependence on machines, aspirator			X	
V46.11	Dependence on respiratory, status			X	
V46.12	Encounter for respirator dependence during power failure	X			
V46.13	Encounter for weaning from respirator [ventilator]	X			
V46.14	Mechanical complication of respirator [ventilator]		X		
V46.2	Other dependence on machines, supplemental oxygen			X	
V46.8	Other dependence on other enabling machines			X	
V46.9	Unspecified machine dependence				X
V47.X	Other problems with internal organs				X
V48.X	Problems with head, neck and trunk				X
V49.0	Deficiencies of limbs				X
V49.1	Mechanical problems with limbs				X
V49.2	Motor problems with limbs				X
V49.3	Sensory problems with limbs				X
V49.4	Disfigurements of limbs				X
V49.5	Other problems with limbs				X
V49.6X	Upper limb amputation status		X		
V49.7X	Lower limb amputation status		X		
V49.81	Asymptomatic postmenopausal status (age-related) (natural)		X		
V49.82	Dental sealant status			X	
V49.83	Awaiting organ transplant status			X	
V49.84	Bed confinement status		X		
V49.89	Other specified conditions influencing health status		X		
V49.9	Unspecified condition influencing health status				X
V50.X	Elective surgery for purposes other than remedying health states		X		
V51	Aftercare involving the use of plastic surgery				X
V52.X	Fitting and adjustment of prosthetic device and implant		X		
V53.X	Fitting and adjustment of other device		X		
V54.X	Other orthopedic aftercare		X		
V55.X	Attention to artificial openings		X		
V56.0	Extracorporeal dialysis	X			
V56.1	Encounter for fitting and adjustment of extracorporeal dialysis catheter		X		
V56.2	Encounter for fitting and adjustment of peritoneal dialysis catheter		X		
V56.3X	Encounter for adequacy testing for dialysis		X		
V56.8	Encounter for other dialysis and dialysis catheter care		X		
V57.X	Care involving use of rehabilitation procedures	X			
V58.0	Radiotherapy	X			
V58.11	Encounter for antineoplastic chemotherapy	X			
V58.12	Encounter for antineoplastic immunotherapy	X			
V58.2	Blood transfusion without reported diagnosis				X
V58.3X	Attention to dressings and sutures		X		
V58.4X	Other aftercare following surgery		X		
V58.5	Encounter for orthodontics				X
V58.6X	Long term (current) drug use			X	
V58.7X	Aftercare following surgery to specified body systems, not elsewhere classified		X		
V58.8X	Other specified procedures and aftercare		X		
V58.9	Unspecified aftercare				X
V59.X	Donors	X			
V60.X	Housing, household, and economic circumstances			X	
V61.X	Other family circumstances		X		
V62.X	Other psychosocial circumstances			X	
V63.X	Unavailability of other medical facilities for care		X		
V64.X	Persons encountering health services for specified procedure, not carried out			X	
V65.X	Other persons seeking consultation without complaint or sickness		X		
V66.0	Convalescence and palliative care following surgery	X			
V66.1	Convalescence and palliative care following radiotherapy	X			

Code(s)	Description	1st Dx only	1st or add'l Dx only	Add'l Dx only	Non-spec Dx only
V66.2	Convalescence and palliative care following chemotherapy	X			
V66.3	Convalescence and palliative care following psychotherapy and other treatment for mental disorder	X			
V66.4	Convalescence and palliative care following treatment of fracture	X			
V66.5	Convalescence and palliative care following other treatment	X			
V66.6	Convalescence and palliative care following combined treatment	X			
V66.7	Encounter for palliative care			X	
V66.9	Unspecified convalescence	X			
V67.X	Follow-up examination		X		
V68.X	Encounters for administrative purposes	X			
V69.X	Problems related to lifestyle		X		
V70.0	Routine general medical examination at a health care facility	X			
V70.1	General psychiatric examination, requested by the authority	X			
V70.2	General psychiatric examination, other and unspecified	X			
V70.3	Other medical examination for administrative purposes	X			
V70.4	Examination for medicolegal reasons	X			
V70.5	Health examination of defined subpopulations	X			
V70.6	Health examination in population surveys	X			
V70.7	Examination of participant in clinical trial		X		
V70.8	Other specified general medical examinations	X			
V70.9	Unspecified general medical examination	X			
V71.X	Observation and evaluation for suspected conditions not found	X			
V72.0	Examination of eyes and vision		X		
V72.1X	Examination of ears and hearing		X		
V72.2	Dental examination		X		
V72.3X	Gynecological examination		X		
V72.4X	Pregnancy examination or test		X		
V72.5	Radiological examination, NEC		X		
V72.6	Laboratory examination		X		
V72.7	Diagnostic skin and sensitization tests		X		
V72.81	Preoperative cardiovascular examination		X		
V72.82	Preoperative respiratory examination		X		
V72.83	Other specified preoperative examination		X		
V72.84	Preoperative examination, unspecified		X		
V72.85	Other specified examination		X		
V72.86	Encounter for blood typing		X		
V72.9	Unspecified examination				X
V73.X	Special screening examination for viral and chlamydial diseases		X		
V74.X	Special screening examination for bacterial and spirochetal diseases		X		
V75.X	Special screening examination for other infectious diseases		X		
V76.X	Special screening examination for malignant neoplasms		X		
V77.X	Special screening examination for endocrine, nutritional, metabolic and immunity disorders		X		
V78.X	Special screening examination for disorders of blood and blood-forming organs		X		
V79.X	Special screening examination for mental disorders and developmental handicaps		X		
V80.X	Special screening examination for neurological, eye, and ear diseases		X		
V81.X	Special screening examination for cardiovascular, respiratory, and genitourinary diseases		X		
V82.X	Special screening examination for other conditions		X		
V83.X	Genetic carrier status		X		
V84.X	Genetic susceptibility to disease			X	
V85.X	Body mass index			X	
V86.X	Estrogen receptor status			X	

19. ***Supplemental Classification of External Causes of Injury and Poisoning (E-codes, E800-E999)***

Introduction: These guidelines are provided for those who are currently collecting E codes in order that there will be standardization in the process. If your institution plans to begin collecting E codes, these guidelines are to be applied. The use of E codes is supplemental to the application of ICD-9-CM diagnosis codes. E codes are never to be recorded as principal diagnoses (first-listed in non-inpatient setting) and are not required for reporting to CMS.

External causes of injury and poisoning codes (E codes) are intended to provide data for injury research and evaluation of injury prevention strategies. E codes capture how the injury or poisoning happened (cause), the intent (unintentional or accidental; or intentional, such as suicide or assault), and the place where the event occurred.

Some major categories of E codes include:

- transport accidents
- poisoning and adverse effects of drugs, medicinal substances and
- biologicals
- accidental falls
- accidents caused by fire and flames
- accidents due to natural and environmental factors
- late effects of accidents, assaults or self injury
- assaults or purposely inflicted injury
- suicide or self inflicted injury

These guidelines apply for the coding and collection of E codes from records in hospitals, outpatient clinics, emergency departments, other ambulatory care settings and provider offices, and nonacute care settings, except when other specific guidelines apply.

a. General E Code Coding Guidelines

1. *Used with any code in the range of 001-V84.8*
   An E code may be used with any code in the range of 001-V84.8, which indicates an injury, poisoning, or adverse effect due to an external cause.
2. *Assign the appropriate E code for all initial treatments*
   Assign the appropriate E code for the initial encounter of an injury, poisoning, or adverse effect of drugs, not for subsequent treatment.
   External cause of injury codes (E-codes) may be assigned while the acute fracture codes are still applicable.
   See Section I.C.17.b.1 for coding of acute fractures.
3. *Use the full range of E codes*
   Use the full range of E codes to completely describe the cause, the intent and the place of occurrence, if applicable, for all injuries, poisonings, and adverse effects of drugs.
4. *Assign as many E codes as necessary*
   Assign as many E codes as necessary to fully explain each cause. If only one E code can be recorded, assign the E code most related to the principal diagnosis.
5. *The selection of the appropriate E code*
   The selection of the appropriate E code is guided by the Index to External Causes, which is located after the alphabetical index to diseases and by Inclusion and Exclusion notes in the Tabular List.
6. *E code can never be a principal diagnosis*
   An E code can never be a principal (first listed) diagnosis.
7. *External cause code(s) with systemic inflammatory* response syndrome (SIRS)
   An external cause code is not appropriate with a code from subcategory 995.9, unless the patient also has an injury, poisoning, or adverse effect of drugs.

b. Place of Occurrence Guideline

Use an additional code from category E849 to indicate the Place of Occurrence for injuries and poisonings. The Place of Occurrence describes the place where the event occurred and not the patient's activity at the time of the event.
Do not use E849.9 if the place of occurrence is not stated.

c. Adverse Effects of Drugs, Medicinal and Biological Substances Guidelines

1. *Do not code directly from the Table of Drugs*
   Do not code directly from the Table of Drugs and Chemicals. Always refer back to the Tabular List.
2. *Use as many codes as necessary to describe*
   Use as many codes as necessary to describe completely all drugs, medicinal or biological substances.
3. *If the same E code would describe the causative agent*
   If the same E code would describe the causative agent for more than one adverse reaction, assign the code only once.
4. *If two or more drugs, medicinal or biological substances*
   If two or more drugs, medicinal or biological substances are reported, code each individually unless the combination code is listed in the Table of Drugs and Chemicals. In that case, assign the E code for the combination.
5. *When a reaction results from the interaction of a drug(s)*
   When a reaction results from the interaction of a drug(s) and alcohol, use poisoning codes and E codes for both.
6. *If the reporting format limits the number of E codes*
   If the reporting format limits the number of E codes that can be used in reporting clinical data, code the one most related to the principal diagnosis. Include at least one from each category (cause, intent, place) if possible.
   If there are different fourth digit codes in the same three digit category, use the code for "Other specified" of that category. If there is no "Other specified" code in that category, use the appropriate "Unspecified" code in that category.
   If the codes are in different three digit categories, assign the appropriate E code for other multiple drugs and medicinal substances.
7. *Codes from the E930-E949 series*
   Codes from the E930-E949 series must be used to identify the causative substance for an adverse effect of drug, medicinal and biological substances, correctly prescribed and properly administered. The effect, such as tachycardia, delirium, gastrointestinal hemorrhaging, vomiting, hypokalemia, hepatitis, renal failure, or respiratory failure, is coded and followed by the appropriate code from the E930-E949 series.

d. Multiple Cause E Code Coding Guidelines

If two or more events cause separate injuries, an E code should be assigned for each cause. The first listed E code will be selected in the following order:

- E codes for child and adult abuse take priority over all other E codes. See Section I.C.19.e., Child and Adult abuse guidelines
- E codes for terrorism events take priority over all other E codes except child and adult abuse
- E codes for cataclysmic events take priority over all other E codes except child and adult abuse and terrorism.
- E codes for transport accidents take priority over all other E codes except cataclysmic events and child and adult abuse and terrorism.

The first-listed E code should correspond to the cause of the most serious diagnosis due to an assault, accident, or self-harm, following the order of hierarchy listed above.

e. Child and Adult Abuse Guideline

1. *Intentional injury*
   When the cause of an injury or neglect is intentional child or adult abuse, the first listed E code should be assigned from categories E960-E968, Homicide and injury purposely inflicted by other persons, (except category E967). An E code from category E967, Child and adult battering and other maltreatment, should be added as an additional code to identify the perpetrator, if known.
2. *Accidental intent*
   In cases of neglect when the intent is determined to be accidental E code E904.0, Abandonment or neglect of infant and helpless person, should be the first listed E code.

f. Unknown or Suspected Intent Guideline

1. *If the intent (accident, self-harm, assault) of the cause of an injury or poisoning is unknown*
   If the intent (accident, self-harm, assault) of the cause of an injury or poisoning is unknown or unspecified, code the intent as undetermined E980-E989.

2. *If the intent (accident, self-harm, assault) of the cause of an injury or poisoning is questionable*
   If the intent (accident, self-harm, assault) of the cause of an injury or poisoning is questionable, probable or suspected, code the intent as undetermined E980-E989.

g. **Undetermined Cause**
When the intent of an injury or poisoning is known, but the cause is unknown, use codes: E928.9, Unspecified accident, E958.9, Suicide and self-inflicted injury by unspecified means, and E968.9, Assault by unspecified means.
These E codes should rarely be used, as the documentation in the medical record, in both the inpatient outpatient and other settings, should normally provide sufficient detail to determine the cause of the injury.

h. **Late Effects of External Cause Guidelines**
1. *Late effect E codes*
   Late effect E codes exist for injuries and poisonings but not for adverse effects of drugs, misadventures and surgical complications.
2. *Late effect E codes (E929, E959, E969, E977, E989, or E999.1)*
   A late effect E code (E929, E959, E969, E977, E989, or E999.1) should be used with any report of a late effect or sequela resulting from a previous injury or poisoning (905-909).
3. *Late effect E code with a related current injury*
   A late effect E code should never be used with a related current nature of injury code.
4. *Use of late effect E codes for subsequent visits*
   Use a late effect E code for subsequent visits when a late effect of the initial injury or poisoning is being treated. There is no late effect E code for adverse effects of drugs. Do not use a late effect E code for subsequent visits for follow-up care (e.g., to assess healing, to receive rehabilitative therapy) of the injury or poisoning when no late effect of the injury has been documented.

i. **Misadventures and Complications of Care Guidelines**
1. *Code range E870-E876*
   Assign a code in the range of E870-E876 if misadventures are stated by the provider.
2. *Code range E878-E879*
   Assign a code in the range of E878-E879 if the provider attributes an abnormal reaction or later complication to a surgical or medical procedure, but does not mention misadventure at the time of the procedure as the cause of the reaction.

j. **Terrorism Guidelines**
1. *Cause of injury identified by the Federal Government (FBI) as terrorism*
   When the cause of an injury is identified by the Federal Government (FBI) as terrorism, the first-listed E-code should be a code from category E979, Terrorism. The definition of terrorism employed by the FBI is found at the inclusion note at E979. The terrorism E-code is the only E-code that should be assigned. Additional E codes from the assault categories should not be assigned.
2. *Cause of an injury is suspected to be the result of terrorism*
   When the cause of an injury is suspected to be the result of terrorism a code from category E979 should not be assigned. Assign a code in the range of E codes based circumstances on the documentation of intent and mechanism.
3. *Code E979.9, Terrorism, secondary effects*
   Assign code E979.9, Terrorism, secondary effects, for conditions occurring subsequent to the terrorist event. This code should not be assigned for conditions that are due to the initial terrorist act.
4. *Statistical tabulation of terrorism codes*
   For statistical purposes these codes will be tabulated within the category for assault, expanding the current category from E960-E969 to include E979 and E999.1.

Section II

Selection of Principal Diagnosis

The circumstances of inpatient admission always govern the selection of principal diagnosis. The principal diagnosis is defined in the Uniform Hospital Discharge Data Set (UHDDS) as "that condition established after study to be chiefly responsible for occasioning the admission of the patient to the hospital for care."

The UHDDS definitions are used by hospitals to report inpatient data elements in a standardized manner. These data elements and their definitions can be found in the July 31, 1985, Federal Register (Vol. 50, No, 147), pp. 31038-40.

Since that time the application of the UHDDS definitions has been expanded to include all non-outpatient settings (acute care, short term, long term care and psychiatric hospitals; home health agencies; rehab facilities; nursing homes, etc).

In determining principal diagnosis the coding conventions in the ICD-9-CM, Volumes I and II take precedence over these official coding guidelines. (See Section I.A., Conventions for the ICD-9-CM).

The importance of consistent, complete documentation in the medical record cannot be overemphasized. Without such documentation the application of all coding guidelines is a difficult, if not impossible, task.

A. ***Codes for symptoms, signs, and ill-defined conditions***
Codes for symptoms, signs, and ill-defined conditions from Chapter 16 are not to be used as principal diagnosis when a related definitive diagnosis has been established.

B. ***Two or more interrelated conditions, each potentially meeting the definition for principal diagnosis***
When there are two or more interrelated conditions (such as diseases in the same ICD-9-CM chapter or manifestations characteristically associated with a certain disease) potentially meeting the definition of principal diagnosis, either condition may be sequenced first, unless the circumstances of the admission, the therapy provided, the Tabular List, or the Alphabetic Index indicate otherwise.

C. ***Two or more diagnoses that equally meet the definition for principal diagnosis***
In the unusual instance when two or more diagnoses equally meet the criteria for principal diagnosis as determined by the circumstances of admission, diagnostic workup and/or therapy provided, and the Alphabetic Index, Tabular List, or another coding guidelines does not provide sequencing direction, any one of the diagnoses may be sequenced first.

D. ***Two or more comparative or contrasting conditions***
In those rare instances when two or more contrasting or comparative diagnoses are documented as "either/or" (or similar terminology), they are coded as if the diagnoses were confirmed and the diagnoses are sequenced according to the circumstances of the admission. If no further determination can be made as to which diagnosis should be principal, either diagnosis may be sequenced first.

E. ***A symptom(s) followed by contrasting/comparative diagnoses***
When a symptom(s) is followed by contrasting/comparative diagnoses, the symptom code is sequenced first. All the contrasting/comparative diagnoses should be coded as additional diagnoses.

F. ***Original treatment plan not carried out***
Sequence as the principal diagnosis the condition, which after study occasioned the admission to the hospital, even though treatment may not have been carried out due to unforeseen circumstances.

G. Complications of surgery and other medical care

When the admission is for treatment of a complication resulting from surgery or other medical care, the complication code is sequenced as the principal diagnosis. If the complication is classified to the 996-999 series and the code lacks the necessary specificity in describing the complication, an additional code for the specific complication should be assigned.

H. Uncertain Diagnosis

If the diagnosis documented at the time of discharge is qualified as "probable", "suspected", "likely", "questionable", "possible", or "still to be ruled out", or other similar terms indicating uncertainty, code the condition as if it existed or was established. The bases for these guidelines are the diagnostic workup, arrangements for further workup or observation, and initial therapeutic approach that correspond most closely with the established diagnosis.

Note: This guideline is applicable only to short-term, acute, long-term care and psychiatric hospitals.

I. Admission from Observation Unit

1. Admission Following Medical Observation

When a patient is admitted to an observation unit for a medical condition, which either worsens or does not improve, and is subsequently admitted as an inpatient of the same hospital for this same medical condition, the principal diagnosis would be the medical condition which led to the hospital admission.

2. Admission Following Post-Operative Observation

When a patient is admitted to an observation unit to monitor a condition (or complication) that develops following outpatient surgery, and then is subsequently admitted as an inpatient of the same hospital, hospitals should apply the Uniform Hospital Discharge Data Set (UHDDS) definition of principal diagnosis as "that condition established after study to be chiefly responsible for occasioning the admission of the patient to the hospital for care."

J. Admission from Outpatient Surgery

When a patient receives surgery in the hospital's outpatient surgery department and is subsequently admitted for continuing inpatient care at the same hospital, the following guidelines should be followed in selecting the principal diagnosis for the inpatient admission:

- If the reason for the inpatient admission is a complication, assign the complication as the principal diagnosis.
- If no complication, or other condition, is documented as the reason for the inpatient admission, assign the reason for the outpatient surgery as the principal diagnosis.
- If the reason for the inpatient admission is another condition unrelated to the surgery, assign the unrelated condition as the principal diagnosis.

Section III

Reporting Additional Diagnoses

GENERAL RULES FOR OTHER (ADDITIONAL) DIAGNOSES

For reporting purposes the definition for "other diagnoses" is interpreted as additional conditions that affect patient care in terms of requiring:

- clinical evaluation; or
- therapeutic treatment; or
- diagnostic procedures; or
- extended length of hospital stay; or
- increased nursing care and/or monitoring.

The UHDDS item #11-b defines Other Diagnoses as "all conditions that coexist at the time of admission, that develop subsequently, or that affect the treatment received and/or the length of stay. Diagnoses that relate to an earlier episode which have no bearing on the current hospital stay are to be excluded." UHDDS definitions apply to inpatients in acute care, short-term, long term care and psychiatric hospital setting. The UHDDS definitions are used by acute care short-term hospitals to report inpatient data elements in a standardized manner. These data elements and their definitions can be found in the July 31, 1985, Federal Register (Vol. 50, No, 147), pp. 31038-40.

Since that time the application of the UHDDS definitions has been expanded to include all non—outpatient settings (acute care, short term, long term care and psychiatric hospitals; home health agencies; rehab facilities; nursing homes, etc).

The following guidelines are to be applied in designating "other diagnoses" when neither the Alphabetic Index nor the Tabular List in ICD-9-CM provide direction. The listing of the diagnoses in the patient record is the responsibility of the attending provider.

A. Previous conditions

If the provider has included a diagnosis in the final diagnostic statement, such as the discharge summary or the face sheet, it should ordinarily be coded. Some providers include in the diagnostic statement resolved conditions or diagnoses and status-post procedures from previous admission that have no bearing on the current stay. Such conditions are not to be reported and are coded only if required by hospital policy.

However, history codes (V10-V19) may be used as secondary codes if the historical condition or family history has an impact on current care or influences treatment.

B. Abnormal findings

Abnormal findings (laboratory, x-ray, pathologic, and other diagnostic results) are not coded and reported unless the provider indicates their clinical significance. If the findings are outside the normal range and the attending provider has ordered other tests to evaluate the condition or prescribed treatment, it is appropriate to ask the provider whether the abnormal finding should be added.

Please note: This differs from the coding practices in the outpatient setting for coding encounters for diagnostic tests that have been interpreted by a provider.

C. Uncertain Diagnosis

If the diagnosis documented at the time of discharge is qualified as "probable", "suspected", "likely", "questionable", "possible", or "still to be ruled out", or other similar terms indicating uncertainty, code the condition as if it existed or was established. The bases for these guidelines are the diagnostic workup, arrangements for further workup or observation, and initial therapeutic approach that correspond most closely with the established diagnosis.

Note: This guideline is applicable only to short-term, acute, long-term care and psychiatric hospitals.

Section IV

Diagnostic Coding and Reporting Guidelines for Outpatient Services

These coding guidelines for outpatient diagnoses have been approved for use by hospitals/ providers in coding and reporting hospital-based outpatient services and provider-based office visits.

Information about the use of certain abbreviations, punctuation, symbols, and other conventions used in the ICD-9-CM Tabular List (code numbers and titles), can be found in Section IA of these guidelines, under "Conventions Used in the Tabular List." Information about the correct sequence to use in finding a code is also described in Section I.

The terms encounter and visit are often used interchangeably in describing outpatient service contacts and, therefore, appear together in these guidelines without distinguishing one from the other.

Though the conventions and general guidelines apply to all settings, coding guidelines for outpatient and provider reporting of diagnoses will vary in a number of instances from those for inpatient diagnoses, recognizing that:

The Uniform Hospital Discharge Data Set (UHDDS) definition of principal diagnosis applies only to inpatients in acute, short-term, long-term care and psychiatric hospitals.

Coding guidelines for inconclusive diagnoses (probable, suspected, rule out, etc.) were developed for inpatient reporting and do not apply to outpatients.

A. *Selection of first-listed condition*

In the outpatient setting, the term first-listed diagnosis is used in lieu of principal diagnosis.

In determining the first-listed diagnosis the coding conventions of ICD-9-CM, as well as the general and disease specific guidelines take precedence over the outpatient guidelines.

Diagnoses often are not established at the time of the initial encounter/visit. It may take two or more visits before the diagnosis is confirmed.

The most critical rule involves beginning the search for the correct code assignment through the Alphabetic Index. Never begin searching initially in the Tabular List as this will lead to coding errors.

1. **Outpatient Surgery**
   When a patient presents for outpatient surgery, code the reason for the surgery as the first-listed diagnosis (reason for the encounter), even if the surgery is not performed due to a contraindication.
2. **Observation Stay**
   When a patient is admitted for observation for a medical condition, assign a code for the medical condition as the first-listed diagnosis. When a patient presents for outpatient surgery and develops complications requiring admission to observation, code the reason for the surgery as the first reported diagnosis (reason for the encounter), followed by codes for the complications as secondary diagnoses.

B. *Codes from 001.0 through V86.1*

The appropriate code or codes from 001.0 through V86.1 must be used to identify diagnoses, symptoms, conditions, problems, complaints, or other reason(s) for the encounter/visit.

C. *Accurate reporting of ICD-9-CM diagnosis codes*

For accurate reporting of ICD-9-CM diagnosis codes, the documentation should describe the patient's condition, using terminology which includes specific diagnoses as well as symptoms, problems, or reasons for the encounter. There are ICD-9-CM codes to describe all of these.

D. *Selection of codes 001.0 through 999.9*

The selection of codes 001.0 through 999.9 will frequently be used to describe the reason for the encounter. These codes are from the section of ICD-9-CM for the classification of diseases and injuries (e.g. infectious and parasitic diseases; neoplasms; symptoms, signs, and ill-defined conditions, etc.).

E. *Codes that describe symptoms and signs*

Codes that describe symptoms and signs, as opposed to diagnoses, are acceptable for reporting purposes when a diagnosis has not been established (confirmed) by the provider. Chapter 16 of ICD-9-CM, Symptoms, Signs, and Ill-defined conditions (codes 780.0 - 799.9) contain many, but not all codes for symptoms.

F. *Encounters for circumstances other than a disease or injury*

ICD-9-CM provides codes to deal with encounters for circumstances other than a disease or injury. The Supplementary Classification of factors Influencing Health Status and Contact with Health Services (V01.0- V86.1) is provided to deal with occasions when circumstances other than a disease or injury are recorded as diagnosis or problems.

G. Level of Detail in Coding

1. **ICD-9-CM codes with 3, 4, or 5 digits**
   ICD-9-CM is composed of codes with either 3, 4, or 5 digits. Codes with three digits are included in ICD-9-CM as the heading of a category of codes that may be further subdivided by the use of fourth and/or fifth digits, which provide greater specificity.
2. **Use of full number of digits required for a code**
   A three-digit code is to be used only if it is not further subdivided. Where fourth-digit subcategories and/or fifth-digit subclassifications are provided, they must be assigned. A code is invalid if it has not been coded to the full number of digits required for that code. See also discussion under Section I.b.3., General Coding Guidelines, Level of Detail in Coding.

H. *ICD-9-CM code for the diagnosis, condition, problem, or other reason for encounter/visit*

List first the ICD-9-CM code for the diagnosis, condition, problem, or other reason for encounter/visit shown in the medical record to be chiefly responsible for the services provided. List additional codes that describe any coexisting conditions. In some cases the first-listed diagnosis may be a symptom when a diagnosis has not been established (confirmed) by the physician.

I. *Uncertain diagnosis*

Do not code diagnoses documented as "probable", "suspected," "questionable," "rule out," or "working diagnosis" or other similar terms indicating uncertainty. Rather, code the condition(s) to the highest degree of certainty for that encounter/visit, such as symptoms, signs, abnormal test results, or other reason for the visit. Please note: This differs from the coding practices used by short-term, acute care, long-term care and psychiatric hospitals.

J. *Chronic diseases*

Chronic diseases treated on an ongoing basis may be coded and reported as many times as the patient receives treatment and care for the condition(s)

K. *Code all documented conditions that coexist*

Code all documented conditions that coexist at the time of the encounter/visit, and require or affect patient care treatment or management. Do not code conditions that were previously treated and no longer exist. However, history codes (V10-V19) may be used as secondary codes if the historical condition or family history has an impact on current care or influences treatment.

L. *Patients receiving diagnostic services only*

For patients receiving diagnostic services only during an encounter/visit, sequence first the diagnosis, condition, problem, or other reason for encounter/visit shown in the medical record to be chiefly responsible for the outpatient services provided during the encounter/visit. Codes for other diagnoses (e.g., chronic conditions) may be sequenced as additional diagnoses.

For encounters for routine laboratory/radiology testing in the absence of any signs, symptoms, or associated diagnosis, assign V72.5 and V72.6. If routine testing is performed during the same encounter as a test to evaluate a sign, symptom, or diagnosis, it is appropriate to assign both the V code and the code describing the reason for the non-routine test.

For outpatient encounters for diagnostic tests that have been interpreted by a physician, and the final report is available at the time of coding, code any confirmed or definitive diagnosis(es) documented in the interpretation. Do not code related signs and symptoms as additional diagnoses.

Please note: This differs from the coding practice in the hospital inpatient setting regarding abnormal findings on test results.

M. *Patients receiving therapeutic services only*

For patients receiving therapeutic services only during an encounter/visit, sequence first the diagnosis, condition, problem, or other reason for encounter/visit shown in the medical record to be chiefly responsible for the outpatient services provided during the encounter/visit. Codes for other diagnoses (e.g., chronic conditions) may be sequenced as additional diagnoses.

The only exception to this rule is that when the primary reason for the admission/encounter is chemotherapy, radiation therapy, or rehabilitation, the appropriate V code for the service is listed first, and the diagnosis or problem for which the service is being performed listed second.

N. Patients receiving preoperative evaluations only

For patients receiving preoperative evaluations only, sequence first a code from category V72.8, Other specified examinations, to describe the pre-op consultations. Assign a code for the condition to describe the reason for the surgery as an additional diagnosis. Code also any findings related to the pre-op evaluation.

O. Ambulatory surgery

For ambulatory surgery, code the diagnosis for which the surgery was performed. If the postoperative diagnosis is known to be different from the preoperative diagnosis at the time the diagnosis is confirmed, select the postoperative diagnosis for coding, since it is the most definitive.

P. Routine outpatient prenatal visits

For routine outpatient prenatal visits when no complications are present, codes V22.0, Supervision of normal first pregnancy, or V22.1, Supervision of other normal pregnancy, should be used as the principal diagnosis. These codes should not be used in conjunction with chapter 11 codes.

Appendix I

Present on Admission Reporting Guidelines

[Added to the Official Coding Guidelines October 1, 2006]

Introduction

These guidelines are to be used as a supplement to the ICD-9-CM Official Guidelines for Coding and Reporting to facilitate the assignment of the Present on Admission (POA) indicator for each diagnosis and external cause of injury code reported on claim forms (UB-04 and 837 Institutional).

These guidelines are not intended to replace any guidelines in the main body of the ICD-9-CM Official Guidelines for Coding and Reporting. The POA guidelines are not intended to provide guidance on when a condition should be coded, but rather, how to apply the POA indicator to the final set of diagnosis codes that have been assigned in accordance with Sections I, II, and III of the official coding guidelines. Subsequent to the assignment of the ICD-9-CM codes, the POA indicator should then be assigned to those conditions that have been coded.

As stated in the Introduction to the ICD-9-CM Official Guidelines for Coding and Reporting, a joint effort between the healthcare provider and the coder is essential to achieve complete and accurate documentation, code assignment, and reporting of diagnoses and procedures. The importance of consistent, complete documentation in the medical record cannot be overemphasized. Medical record documentation from any provider involved in the care and treatment of the patient may be used to support the determination of whether a condition was present on admission or not. In the context of the official coding guidelines, the term "provider" means a physician or any qualified healthcare practitioner who is legally accountable for establishing the patient's diagnosis.

General Reporting Requirements

All claims involving inpatient admissions to general acute care hospitals or other facilities that are subject to a law or regulation mandating collection of present on admission information.

Present on admission is defined as present at the time the order for inpatient admission occurs — conditions that develop during an outpatient encounter, including emergency department, observation, or outpatient surgery, are considered as present on admission.

POA indicator is assigned to principal and secondary diagnoses (as defined in Section II of the Official Guidelines for Coding and Reporting) and the external cause of injury codes.

Issues related to inconsistent, missing, conflicting or unclear documentation must still be resolved by the provider.

If a condition would not be coded and reported based on UHDDS definitions and current official coding guidelines, then the POA indicator would not be reported.

Reporting Options

Y - Yes

N - No

U - Unknown

W – Clinically undetermined

Unreported/Not used – (Exempt from POA reporting)

Reporting Definitions

Y = present at the time of inpatient admission

N = not present at the time of inpatient admission

U = documentation is insufficient to determine if condition is present on admission

W = provider is unable to clinically determine whether condition was present on admission or not

Assigning the POA Indicator

Condition is on the "Exempt from Reporting" list

Leave the "present on admission" field blank if the condition is on the list of ICD-9-CM codes for which this field is not applicable. This is the only circumstance in which the field may be left blank.

POA Explicitly Documented

Assign Y for any condition the provider explicitly documents as being present on admission.

Assign N for any condition the provider explicitly documents as not present at the time of admission.

Conditions diagnosed prior to inpatient admission

Assign "Y" for conditions that were diagnosed prior to admission (example: hypertension, diabetes mellitus, asthma)

Conditions diagnosed during the admission but clearly present before admission

Assign "Y" for conditions diagnosed during the admission that were clearly present but not diagnosed until after admission occurred.

Diagnoses subsequently confirmed after admission are considered present on admission if at the time of admission they are documented as suspected, possible, rule out, differential diagnosis, or constitute an underlying cause of a symptom that is present at the time of admission.

Condition develops during outpatient encounter prior to inpatient admission

Assign Y for any condition that develops during an outpatient encounter prior to a written order for inpatient admission.

Documentation does not indicate whether condition was present on admission

Assign "U" when the medical record documentation is unclear as to whether the condition was present on admission. "U" should not be routinely assigned and used only in very limited circumstances. Coders are encouraged to query the providers when the documentation is unclear.

Documentation states that it cannot be determined whether the condition was or was not present on admission

Assign "W" when the medical record documentation indicates that it cannot be clinically determined whether or not the condition was present on admission.

Chronic condition with acute exacerbation during the admission

If the code is a combination code that identifies both the chronic condition and the acute exacerbation, see POA guidelines pertaining to combination codes.

If the combination code only identifies the chronic condition and not the acute exacerbation (e.g., acute exacerbation of CHF), assign "Y."

Conditions documented as possible, probable, suspected, or rule out at the time of discharge

If the final diagnosis contains a possible, probable, suspected, or rule out diagnosis, and this diagnosis was suspected at the time of inpatient admission, assign "Y."

If the final diagnosis contains a possible, probable, suspected, or rule out diagnosis, and this diagnosis was based on symptoms or clinical findings that were not present on admission, assign "N".

Conditions documented as impending or threatened at the time of discharge

If the final diagnosis contains an impending or threatened diagnosis, and this diagnosis is based on symptoms or clinical findings that were present on admission, assign "Y".

If the final diagnosis contains an impending or threatened diagnosis, and this diagnosis is based on symptoms or clinical findings that were not present on admission, assign "N".

Acute and Chronic Conditions

Assign "Y" for acute conditions that are present at time of admission and N for acute conditions that are not present at time of admission.

Assign "Y" for chronic conditions, even though the condition may not be
diagnosed until after admission.

If a single code identifies both an acute and chronic condition, see the POA guidelines for combination codes.

Combination Codes

Assign "N" if any part of the combination code was not present on admission (e.g., obstructive chronic bronchitis with acute exacerbation and the exacerbation was not present on admission; gastric ulcer that does not start bleeding until after admission; asthma patient develops status asthmaticus after admission)

Assign "Y" if all parts of the combination code were present on admission (e.g., patient with diabetic nephropathy is admitted with uncontrolled diabetes)

If the final diagnosis includes comparative or contrasting diagnoses, and both were present, or suspected, at the time of admission, assign "Y".

For infection codes that include the causal organism, assign "Y" if the infection (or signs of the infection) was present on admission, even though the culture results may not be known until after admission (e.g., patient is admitted with pneumonia and the provider documents pseudomonas as the causal organism a few days later).

Obstetrical conditions

Whether or not the patient delivers during the current hospitalization does not affect assignment of the POA indicator. The determining factor for POA assignment is whether the pregnancy complication or obstetrical condition described by the code was present at the time of admission or not.

If the pregnancy complication or obstetrical condition was present on admission (e.g., patient admitted in preterm labor), assign "Y".

If the pregnancy complication or obstetrical condition was not present on admission (e.g., 2nd degree laceration during delivery, postpartum hemorrhage that occurred during current hospitalization, fetal distress develops after admission), assign "N".

If the obstetrical code includes more than one diagnosis and any of the diagnoses identified by the code were not present on admission assign "N".

(e.g., Code 642.7, Pre-eclampsia or eclampsia superimposed on preexisting hypertension).

If the obstetrical code includes information that is not a diagnosis, do not consider that information in the POA determination.

(e.g. Code 652.1x, Breech or other malpresentation successfully converted to cephalic presentation should be reported as present on admission if the fetus was breech on admission but was converted to cephalic presentation after admission (since the conversion to cephalic presentation does not represent a diagnosis, the fact that the conversion occurred after admission has no bearing on the POA determination).

Perinatal conditions

Newborns are not considered to be admitted until after birth. Therefore, any condition present at birth or that developed in utero is considered present at admission and should be assigned "Y". This includes conditions that occur during delivery (e.g., injury during delivery, meconium aspiration, exposure to streptococcus B in the vaginal canal).

Congenital conditions and anomalies

Assign "Y" for congenital conditions and anomalies. Congenital conditions are always considered present on admission.

External cause of injury codes

Assign "Y" for any E code representing an external cause of injury or poisoning that occurred prior to inpatient admission (e.g., patient fell out of bed at home, patient fell out of bed in emergency room prior to admission)

Assign "N" for any E code representing an external cause of injury or poisoning that occurred during inpatient hospitalization (e.g., patient fell out of hospital bed during hospital stay, patient experienced an adverse reaction to a medication administered after inpatient admission)

Categories and Codes Exempt from Diagnosis Present on Admission Requirement

Note: "Diagnosis present on admission" for these code categories are exempt because they represent circumstances regarding the healthcare encounter or factors influencing health status that do not represent a current disease or injury or are always present on admission

137-139	Late effects of infectious and parasitic diseases
268.1	Rickets, late effect
326	Late effects of intracranial abscess or pyogenic infection
438	Late effects of cerebrovascular disease
650	Normal delivery
660.7	Failed forceps or vacuum extractor, unspecified
677	Late effect of complication of pregnancy, childbirth, and the puerperium
905-909	Late effects of injuries, poisonings, toxic effects, and other external causes
V02	Carrier or suspected carrier of infectious diseases
V03	Need for prophylactic vaccination and inoculation against bacterial diseases
V04	Need for prophylactic vaccination and inoculation against certain viral diseases
V05	Need for other prophylactic vaccination and inoculation against single diseases
V06	Need for prophylactic vaccination and inoculation against combinations of diseases
V07	Need for isolation and other prophylactic measures
V10	Personal history of malignant neoplasm
V11	Personal history of mental disorder
V12	Personal history of certain other diseases
V13	Personal history of other diseases
V14	Personal history of allergy to medicinal agents

V15	Other personal history presenting hazards to health
V16	Family history of malignant neoplasm
V17	Family history of certain chronic disabling diseases
V18	Family history of certain other specific conditions
V19	Family history of other conditions
V20	Health supervision of infant or child
V21	Constitutional states in development
V22	Normal pregnancy
V23	Supervision of high-risk pregnancy
V24	Postpartum care and examination
V25	Encounter for contraceptive management
V26	Procreative management
V27	Outcome of delivery
V28	Antenatal screening
V29	Observation and evaluation of newborns for suspected condition not found
V30-V39	Liveborn infants according to type of birth
V42	Organ or tissue replaced by transplant
V43	Organ or tissue replaced by other means
V44	Artificial opening status
V45	Other postprocedural states
V46	Other dependence on machines
V49.60-V49.77	Upper and lower limb amputation status
V49.81-V49.84	Other specified conditions influencing health status
V50	Elective surgery for purposes other than remedying health states
V51	Aftercare involving the use of plastic surgery
V52	Fitting and adjustment of prosthetic device and implant
V53	Fitting and adjustment of other device
V54	Other orthopedic aftercare
V55	Attention to artificial openings
V56	Encounter for dialysis and dialysis catheter care
V57	Care involving use of rehabilitation procedures
V58	Encounter for other and unspecified procedures and aftercare
V59	Donors
V60	Housing, household, and economic circumstances
V61	Other family circumstances
V62	Other psychosocial circumstances
V64	Persons encountering health services for specific procedures, not carried out
V65	Other persons seeking consultation
V66	Convalescence and palliative care
V67	Follow-up examination
V68	Encounters for administrative purposes
V69	Problems related to lifestyle
V70	General medical examination
V71	Observation and evaluation for suspected condition not found
V72	Special investigations and examinations
V73	Special screening examination for viral and chlamydial diseases
V74	Special screening examination for bacterial and spirochetal diseases
V75	Special screening examination for other infectious diseases
V76	Special screening for malignant neoplasms
V77	Special screening for endocrine, nutritional, metabolic, and immunity disorders
V78	Special screening for disorders of blood and blood-forming organs
V79	Special screening for mental disorders and developmental handicaps
V80	Special screening for neurological, eye, and ear diseases
V81	Special screening for cardiovascular, respiratory, and genitourinary diseases
V82	Special screening for other conditions
V83	Genetic carrier status
V84	Genetic susceptibility to disease
V85	Body Mass Index
V86	Estrogen receptor status
E800-E807	Railway accidents
E810-E819	Motor vehicle traffic accidents
E820-E825	Motor vehicle nontraffic accidents
E826-E829	Other road vehicle accidents
E830-E838	Water transport accidents
E840-E845	Air and space transport accidents
E846-E848	Vehicle accidents not elsewhere classifiable
E849.0-E849.6	Place of occurrence
E849.8-E849.9	Place of occurrence
E883.1	Accidental fall into well
E883.2	Accidental fall into storm drain or manhole
E884.0	Fall from playground equipment
E884.1	Fall from cliff
E885.0	Fall from (nonmotorized) scooter
E885.1	Fall from roller skates
E885.2	Fall from skateboard
E885.3	Fall from skis
E885.4	Fall from snowboard
E886.0	Fall on same level from collision, pushing, or shoving, by or with other person, in sports
E890.0-E89.9	Conflagration in private dwelling
E893.0	Accident caused by ignition of clothing, from controlled fire in private dwelling
E893.2	Accident caused by ignition of clothing, from controlled fire not in building or structure
E894	Ignition of highly inflammable material
E895	Accident caused by controlled fire in private dwelling
E897	Accident caused by controlled fire not in building or structure
E898.0-E898.1	Accident caused by other specified fire and flames
E917.0	Striking against or struck accidentally by objects or persons, in sports without subsequent fall
E917.1	Striking against or struck accidentally by objects or persons, caused by a crowd, by collective fear or panic without subsequent fall
E917.2	Striking against or struck accidentally by objects or persons, in running water without subsequent fall
E917.5	Striking against or struck accidentally by objects or persons, object in sports with subsequent fall
E917.6	Striking against or struck accidentally by objects or persons, caused by a crowd, by collective fear or panic with subsequent fall
E919	Accidents caused by machinery
E921.0-E921.9	Accident caused by explosion of pressure vessel
E922.0-E922.9	Accident caused by firearm and air gun missile
E924.1	Caustic and corrosive substances
E926.2	Visible and ultraviolet light sources
E927	Overexertion and strenuous movements
E928.0-E928.8	Other and unspecified environmental and accidental causes
E929.0-E929.9	Late effects of accidental injury
E959	Late effects of self-inflicted injury
E970-E978	Legal intervention

E979	Terrorism
E981.0-E980.9	Poisoning by gases in domestic use, undetermined whether accidentally or purposely inflicted
E982.0-E982.9	Poisoning by other gases, undetermined whether accidentally or purposely inflicted
E985.0-E985.7	Injury by firearms, air guns and explosives, undetermined whether accidentally or purposely inflicted
E987.0	Falling from high place, undetermined whether accidentally or purposely inflicted, residential premises
E987.2	Falling from high place, undetermined whether accidentally or purposely inflicted, natural sites
E989	Late effects of injury, undetermined whether accidentally or purposely inflicted
E990-E999	Injury resulting from operations of war

POA Examples

General Medical Surgical

1. Patient is admitted for diagnostic work-up for cachexia. The final diagnosis is malignant neoplasm of lung with metastasis.
   Assign "Y" on the POA field for the malignant neoplasm. The malignant neoplasm was clearly present on admission, although it was not diagnosed until after the admission occurred.
2. A patient undergoes outpatient surgery. During the recovery period, the patient develops atrial fibrillation and the patient is subsequently admitted to the hospital as an inpatient.
   Assign "Y" on the POA field for the atrial fibrillation since it developed prior to a written order for inpatient admission.
3. A patient is treated in observation and while in Observation, the patient falls out of bed and breaks a hip. The patient is subsequently admitted as an inpatient to treat the hip fracture.
   Assign "Y" on the POA field for the hip fracture since it developed prior to a written order for inpatient admission.
4. A patient with known congestive heart failure is admitted to the hospital after he develops decompensated congestive heart failure.
   Assign "Y" on the POA field for the congestive heart failure. The ICD-9-CM code identifies the chronic condition and does not specify the acute exacerbation.
5. A patient undergoes inpatient surgery. After surgery, the patient develops fever and is treated aggressively. The physician's final diagnosis documents "possible postoperative infection following surgery."
   Assign "N" on the POA field for the postoperative infection since final diagnoses that contain the terms "possible", "probable", "suspected" or "rule out" and that are based on symptoms or clinical findings that were not present on admission should be reported as "N".
6. A patient with severe cough and difficulty breathing was diagnosed during his hospitalization to have lung cancer.
   Assign "Y" on the POA field for the lung cancer. Even though the cancer was not diagnosed until after admission, it is a chronic condition that was clearly present before the patient's admission.
7. A patient is admitted to the hospital for a coronary artery bypass surgery. Postoperatively he developed a pulmonary embolism.
   Assign "N" on the POA field for the pulmonary embolism. This is an acute condition that was not present on admission.
8. A patient is admitted with a known history of coronary atherosclerosis, status post myocardial infarction five years ago is now admitted for treatment of impending myocardial infarction. The final diagnosis is documented as "impending myocardial infarction."
   Assign "Y" to the impending myocardial infarction because the condition is present on admission.
9. A patient with diabetes mellitus developed uncontrolled diabetes on day 3 of the hospitalization.
   Assign "N" to the diabetes code because the "uncontrolled" component of the code was not present on admission.
10. A patient is admitted with high fever and pneumonia. The patient rapidly deteriorates and becomes septic. The discharge diagnosis lists sepsis and pneumonia. The documentation is unclear as to whether the sepsis was present on admission or developed shortly after admission.
    Query the physician as to whether the sepsis was present on admission, developed shortly after admission, or it cannot be clinically determined as to whether it was present on admission or not.
11. A patient is admitted for repair of an abdominal aneurysm. However, the aneurysm ruptures after hospital admission.
    Assign "N" for the ruptured abdominal aneurysm. Although the aneurysm was present on admission, the "ruptured" component of the code description did not occur until after admission.
12. A patient with viral hepatitis B progresses to hepatic coma after admission.
    Assign "N" for the viral hepatitis B with hepatic coma because part of the code description did not develop until after admission.
13. A patient with a history of varicose veins and ulceration of the left lower extremity strikes the area against the side of his hospital bed during an inpatient hospitalization. It bleeds profusely. The final diagnosis lists varicose veins with ulcer and hemorrhage.
    Assign "Y" for the varicose veins with ulcer. Although the hemorrhage occurred after admission, the code description for varicose veins with ulcer does not mention hemorrhage.

Obstetrics

1. A female patient was admitted to the hospital and underwent a normal delivery.
   Leave the "present on admission" (POA) field blank. Code 650, Normal delivery, is on the "exempt from reporting" list.
2. Patient admitted in late pregnancy due to excessive vomiting and dehydration. During admission patient goes into premature labor
   Assign "Y" for the excessive vomiting and the dehydration.
   Assign "N" for the premature labor
3. Patient admitted in active labor. During the stay, a breast abscess is noted when mother attempted to breast feed. Provider is unable to determine whether the abscess was present on admission
   Assign "W" for the breast abscess.
4. Patient admitted in active labor. After 12 hours of labor it is noted that the infant is in fetal distress and a Cesarean section is performed
   Assign "N" for the fetal distress.

Newborn

1. A single liveborn infant was delivered in the hospital via Cesarean section. The physician documented fetal bradycardia during labor in the final diagnosis in the newborn record.
   Assign " Y" because the bradycardia developed prior to the newborn admission (birth).
2. A newborn developed diarrhea which was believed to be due to the hospital baby formula.
   Assign " N" because the diarrhea developed after admission.

Anatomy Color Plates

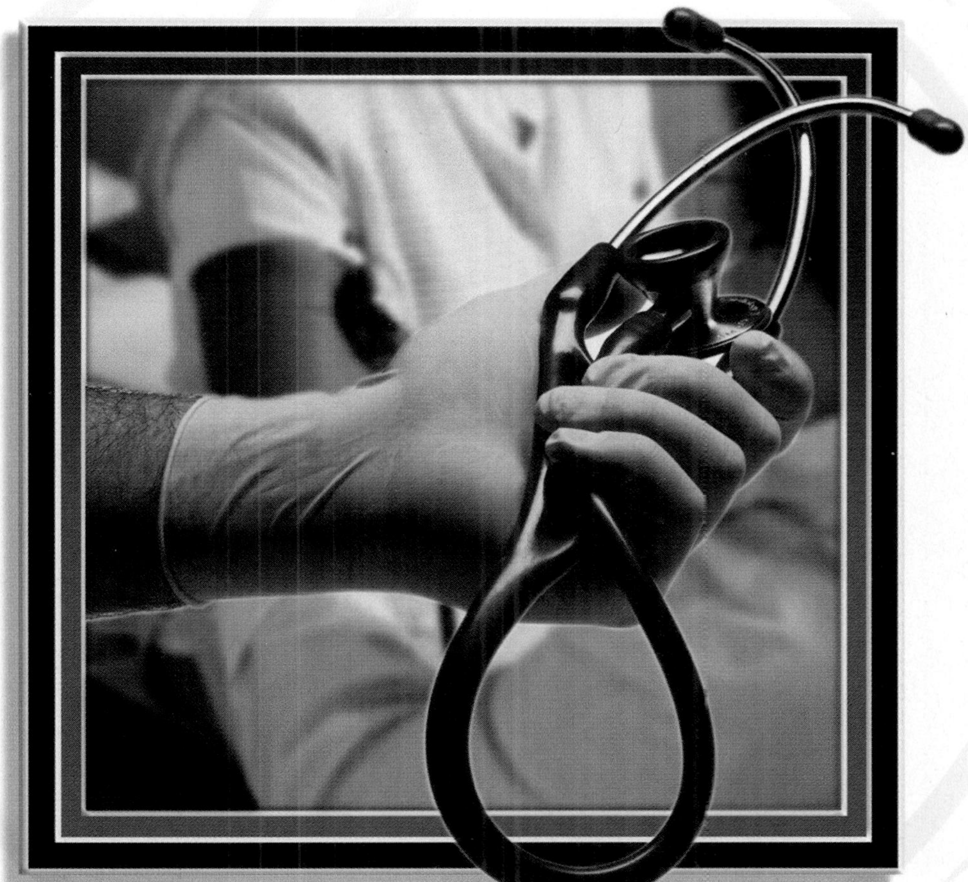

Anatomical Illustrations

Introduction

Without a strong background in or reference materials regarding human anatomy and physiology, it would be impossible to adequately code medical diagnoses. The following pages have been created as a reference for beginning and seasoned coders alike.

These precise, full-color anatomical illustrations, in conjunction with the facing pages that provide page and section references, have been designed to facilitate diagnostic coding.

Each left-hand facing page contains a list of the most common diagnostic categories used when treating the body or organ system on the corresponding right-hand facing page.

These diagnoses are presented with their three-digit category shown in parentheses () and the page in Volume 1 of the ICD-9-CM (the Tabular List) on which the hierarchy of codes for that diagnosis family begins.

Body/Organ System — Page

Skin and Subcutaneous Tissue – Male, Anterior View

Male Figure
(Anterior View)

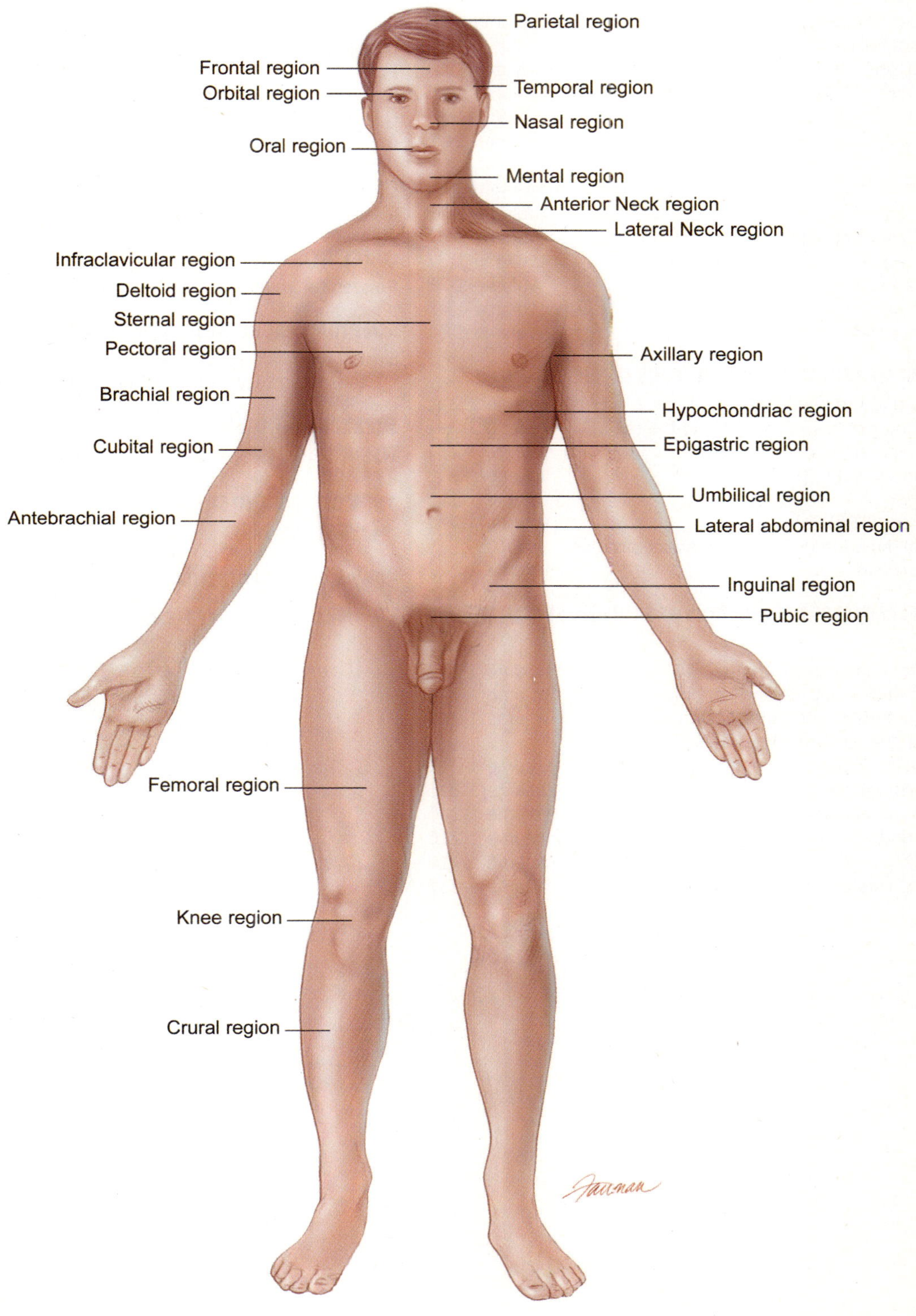

Skin and Subcutaneous Tissue – Female, Anterior View

Female Figure
(Anterior View)

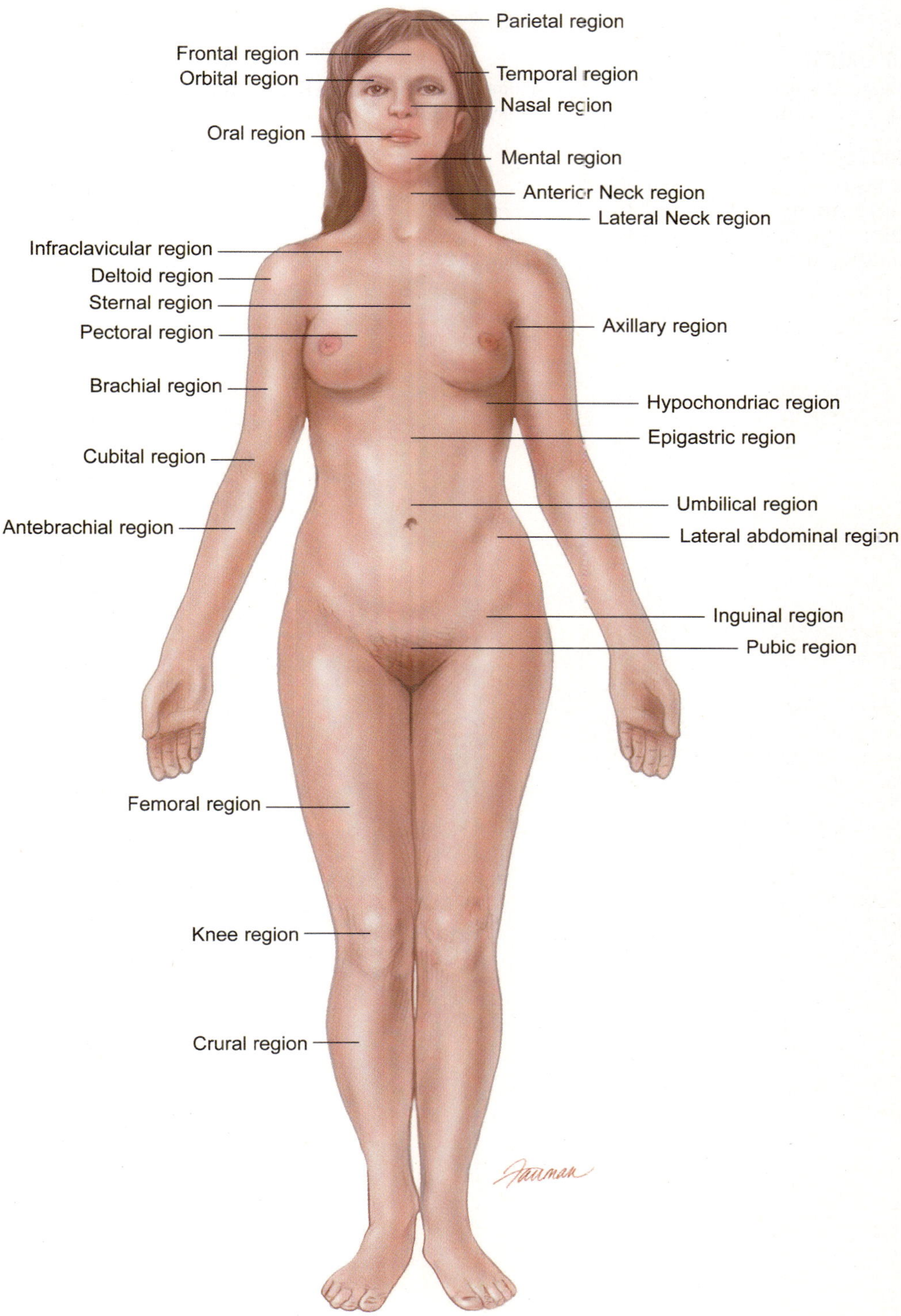

Female Breast

Female Breast

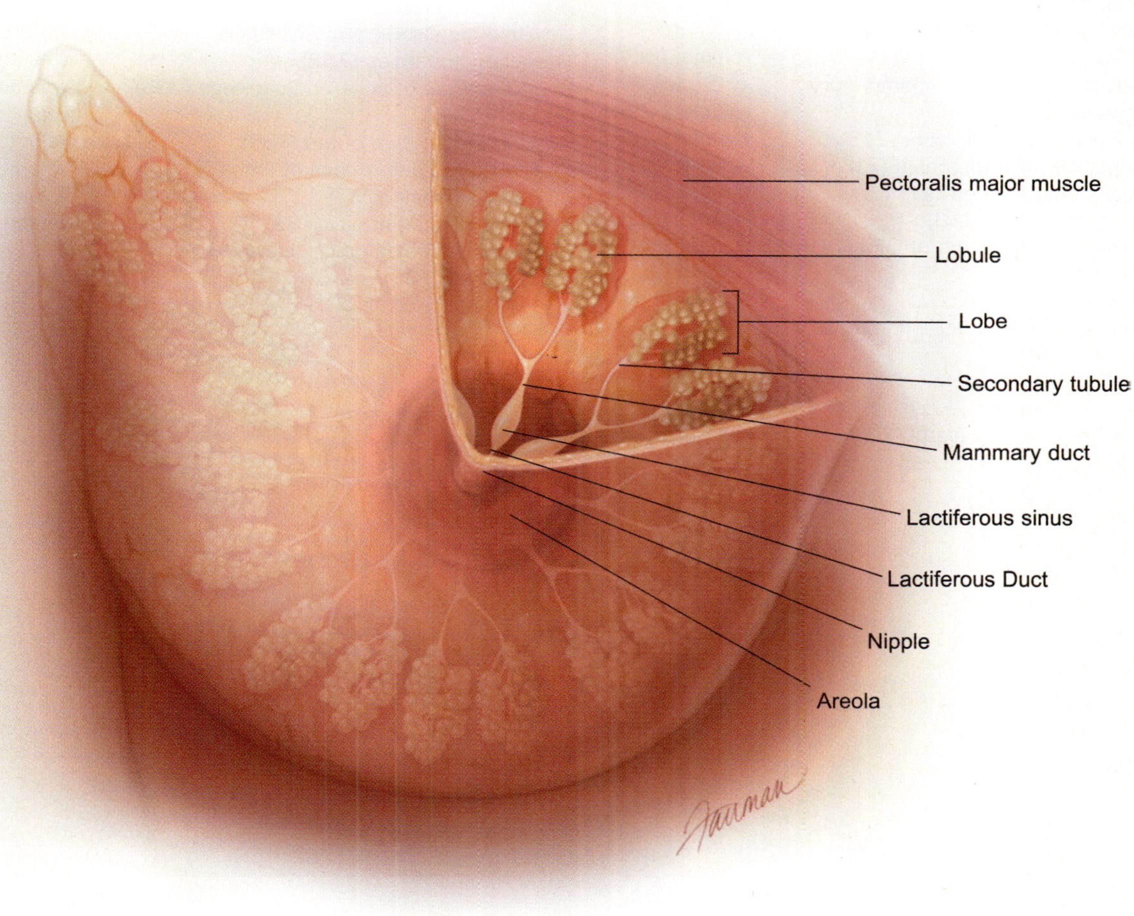

Muscular System and Connective Tissue – Anterior View

Muscular System
(Anterior View)

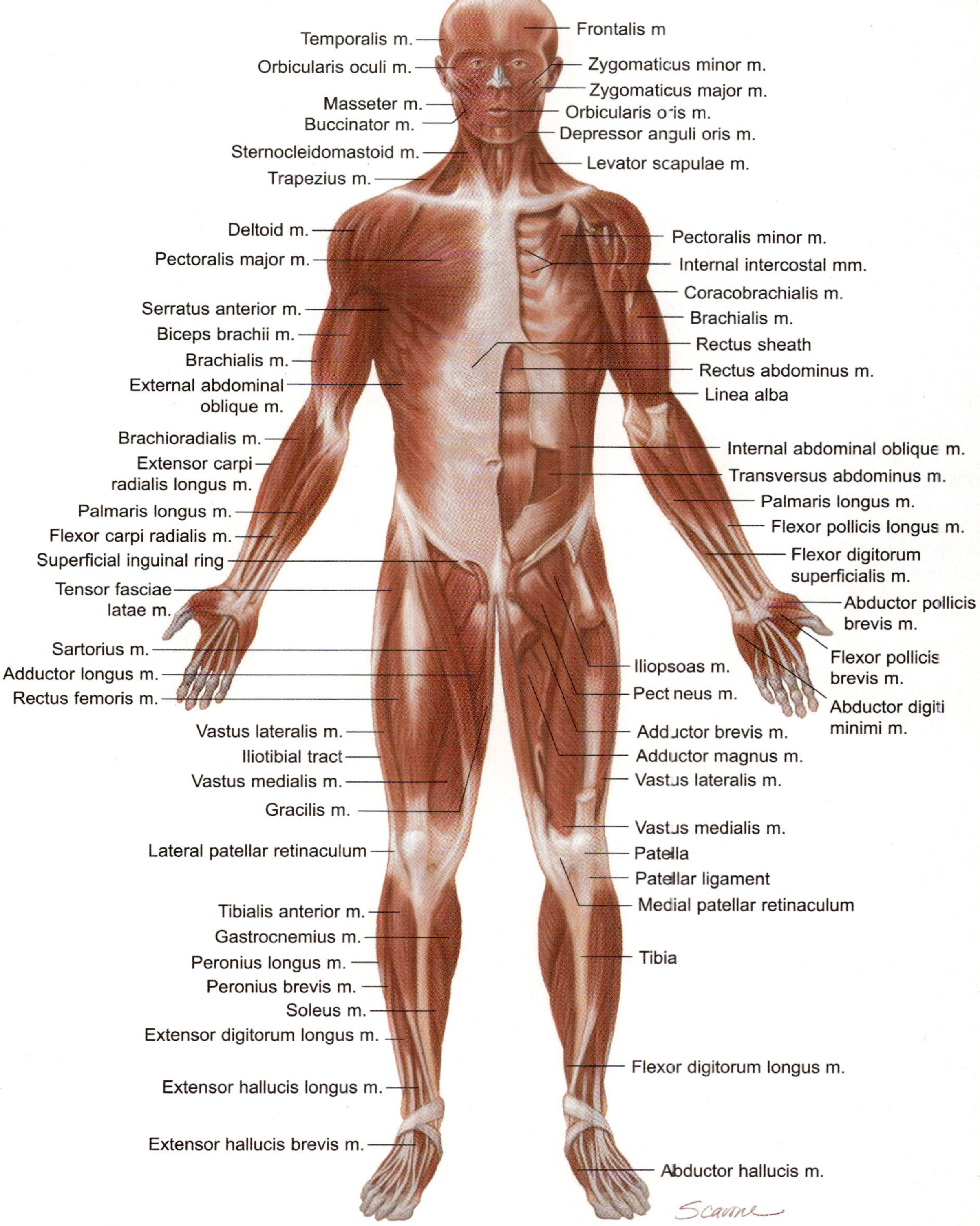

Muscular System and Connective Tissue – Posterior View

Muscular System
(Posterior View)

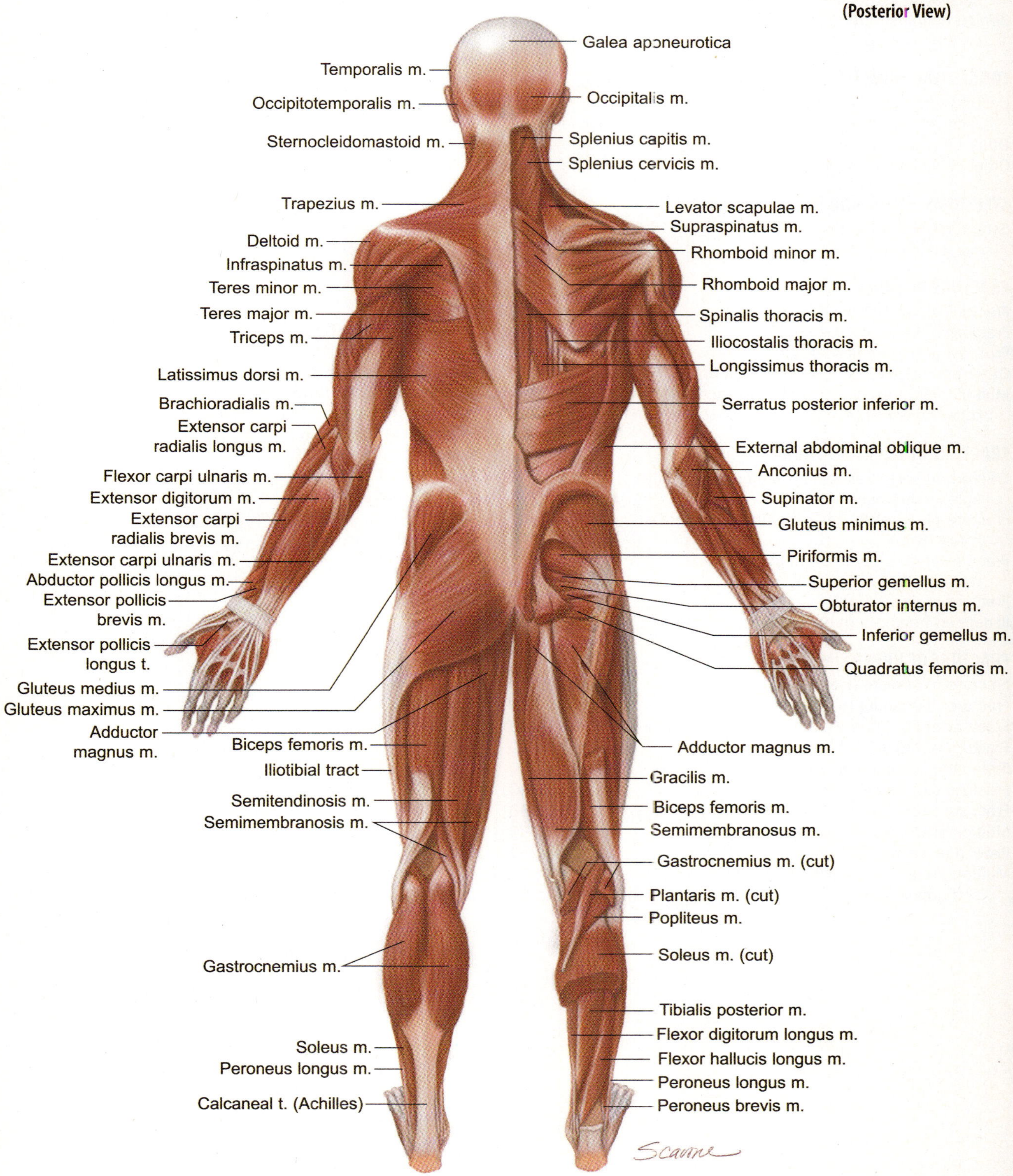

Skeletal System – Anterior View

Skeletal System

(Anterior View)

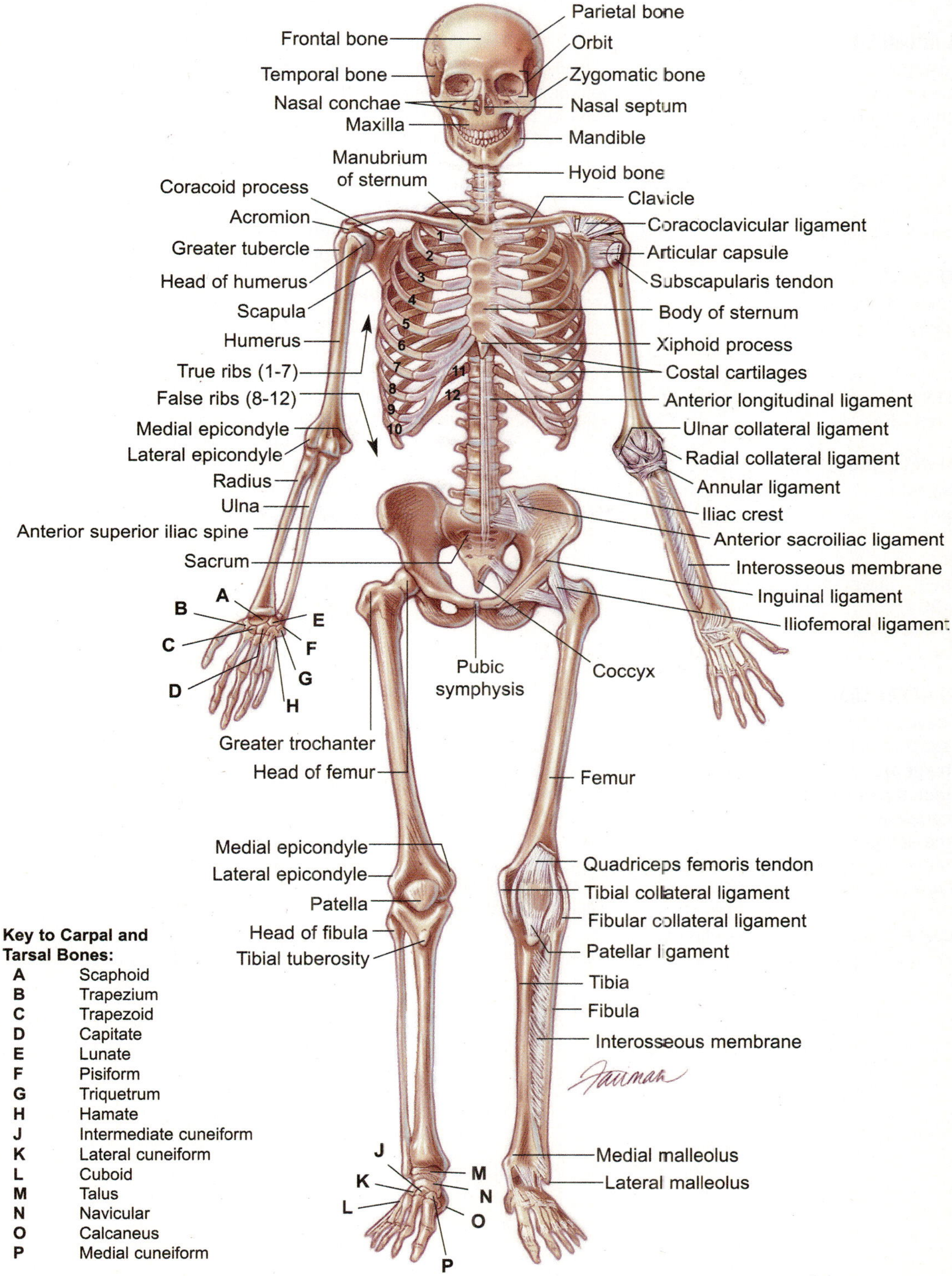

Key to Carpal and Tarsal Bones:

A	Scaphoid
B	Trapezium
C	Trapezoid
D	Capitate
E	Lunate
F	Pisiform
G	Triquetrum
H	Hamate
J	Intermediate cuneiform
K	Lateral cuneiform
L	Cuboid
M	Talus
N	Navicular
O	Calcaneus
P	Medial cuneiform

Skeletal System – Posterior View

Skeletal System
(Posterior View)

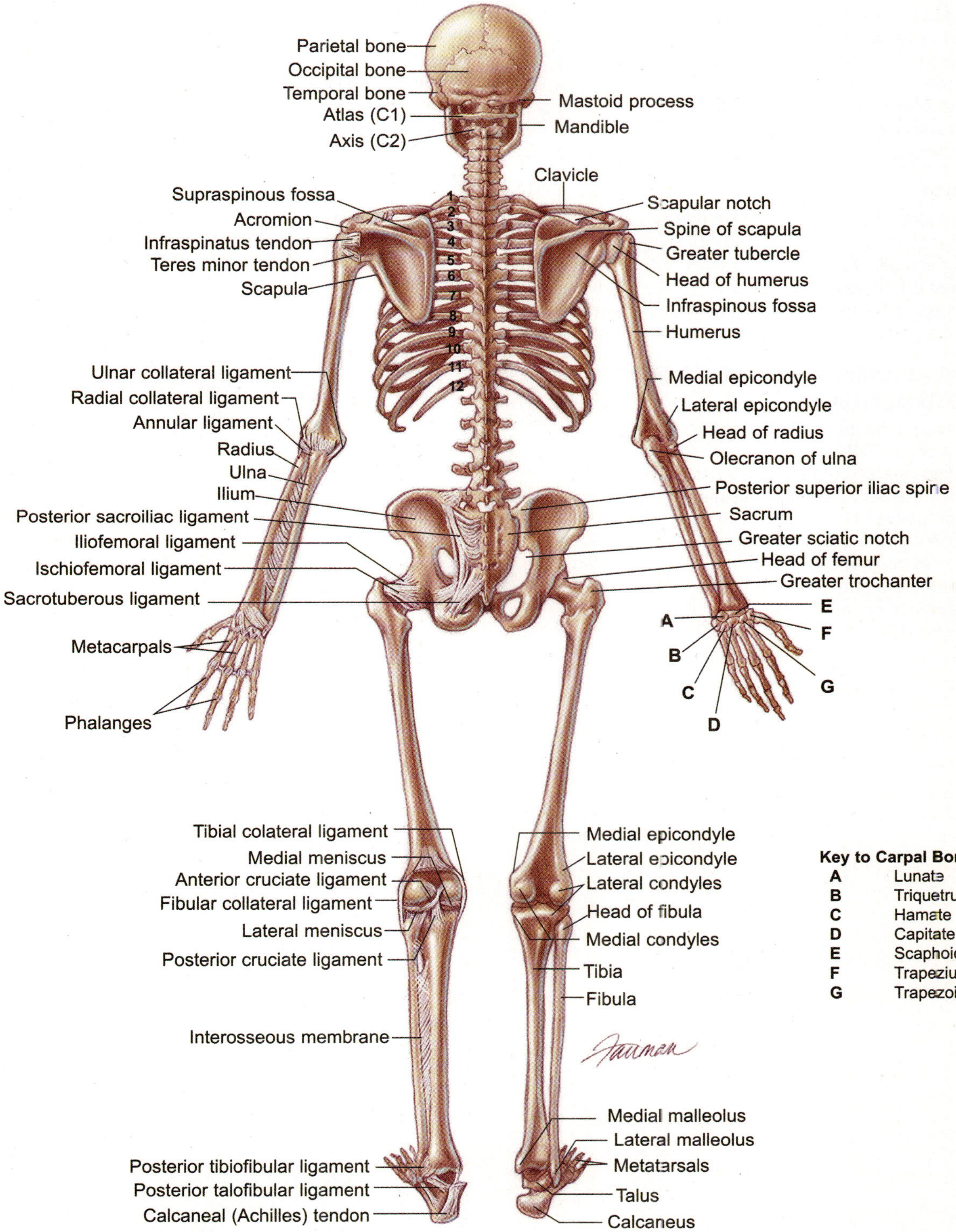

Key to Carpal Bones:

A	Lunate
B	Triquetrum
C	Hamate
D	Capitate
E	Scaphoid
F	Trapezium
G	Trapezoid

Skeletal System – Spinal Column

Skeletal System
(Vertebral Column – Left Lateral View)

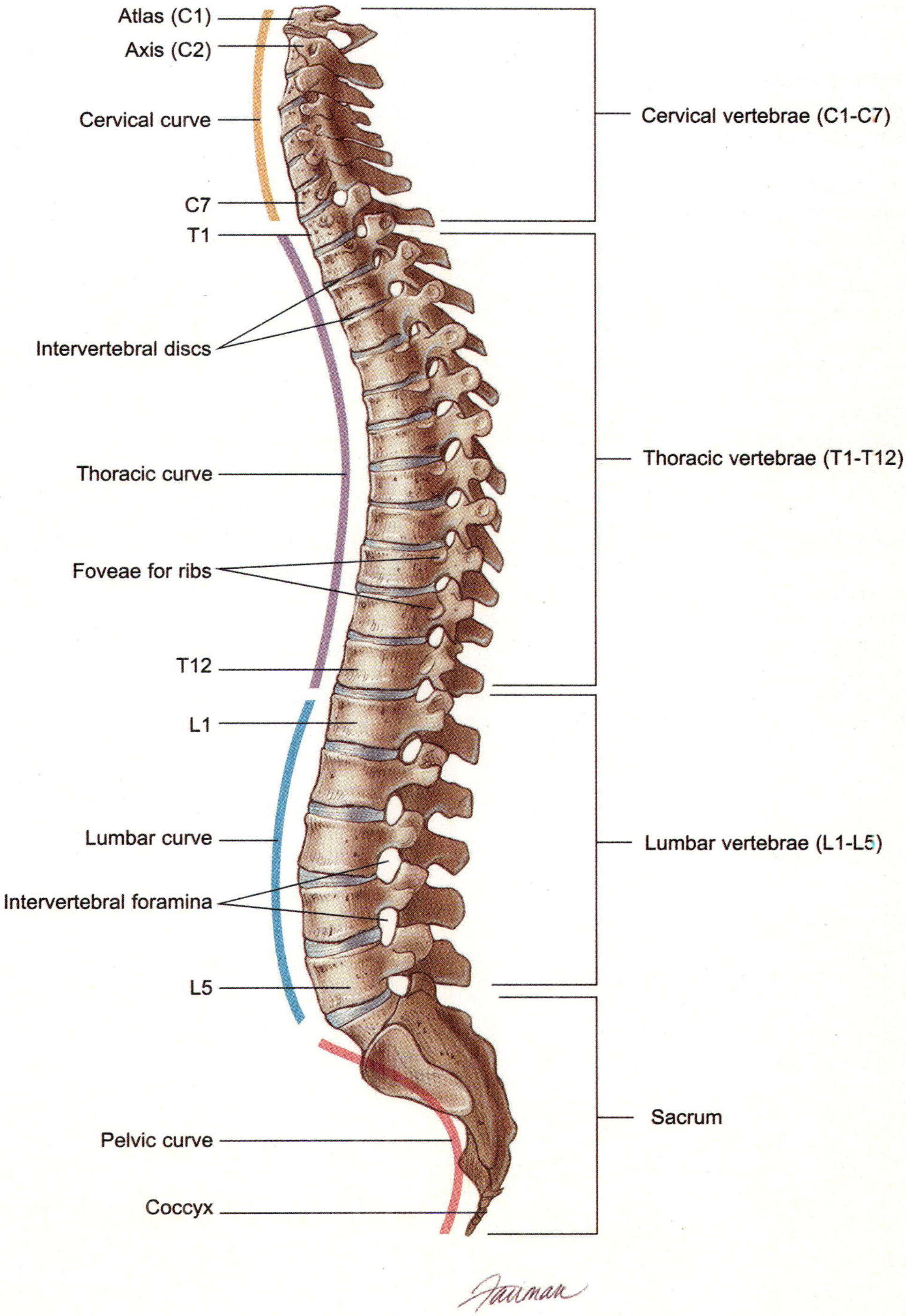

Musculoskeletal System – Shoulder and Elbow

Shoulder and Elbow

(Anterior View)

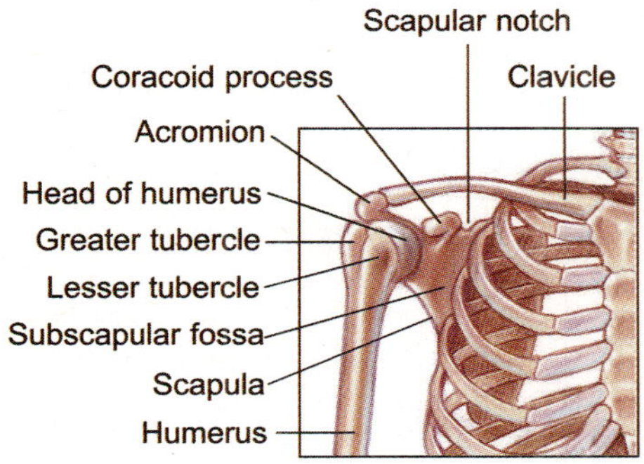

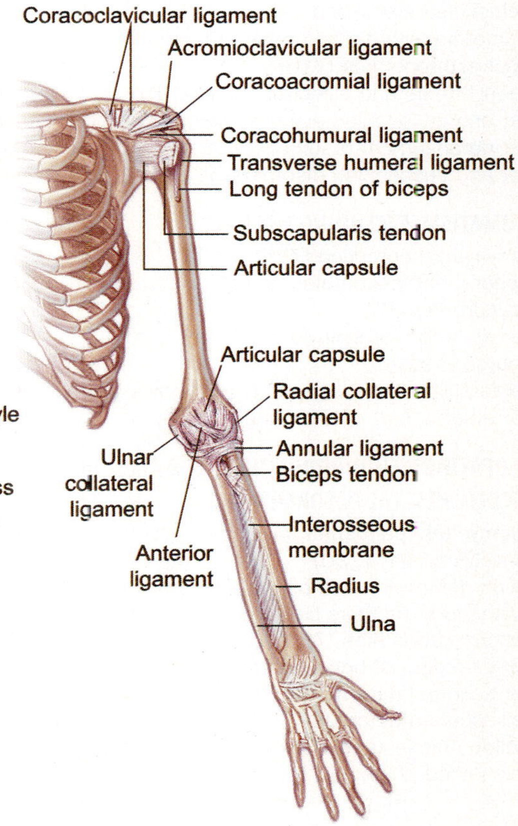

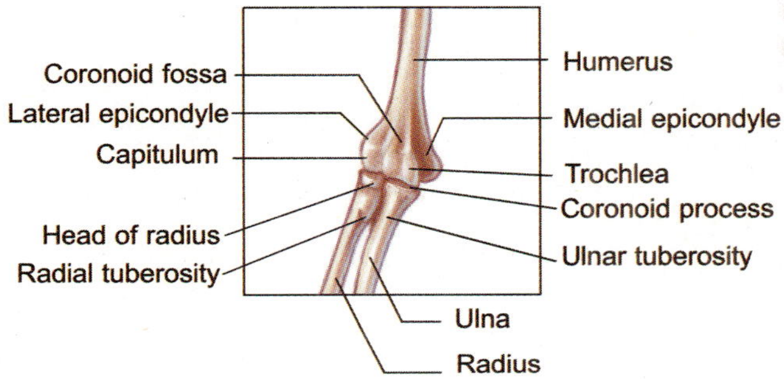

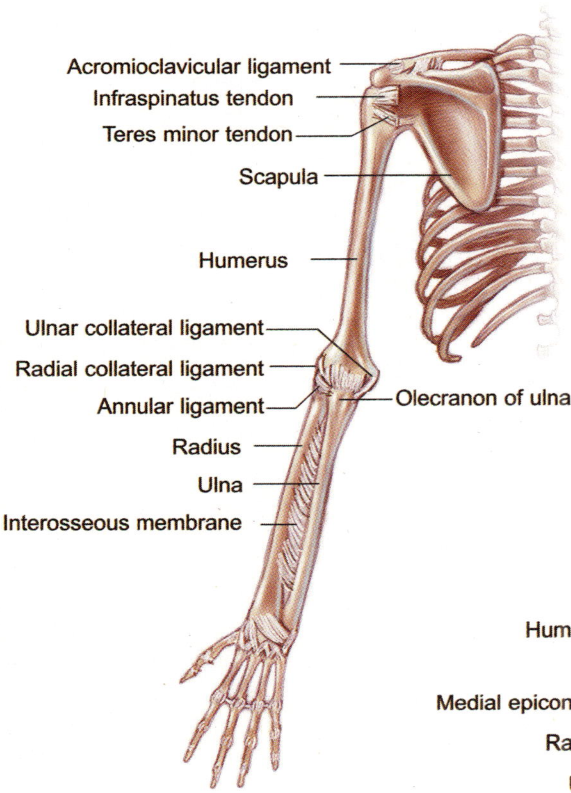

(Posterior View)

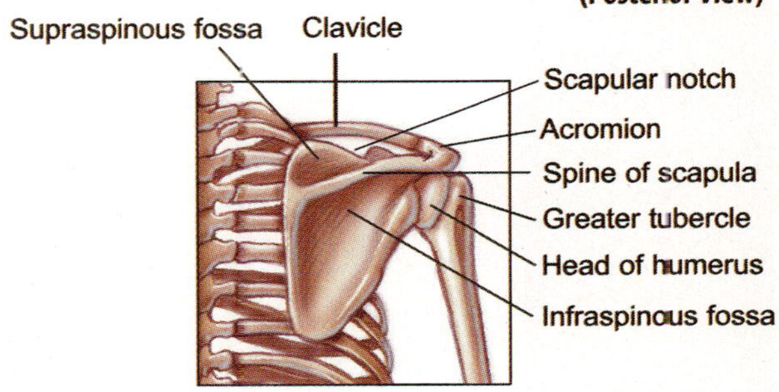

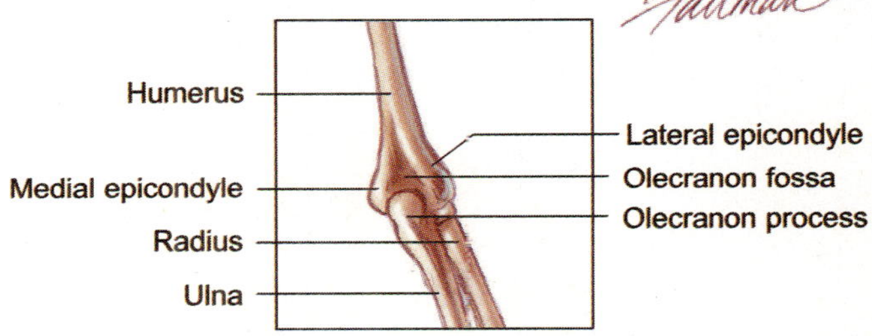

Musculoskeletal System – Hand and Wrist

Musculoskeletal System – Hand and Wrist

(Dorsal and Palmar Views)

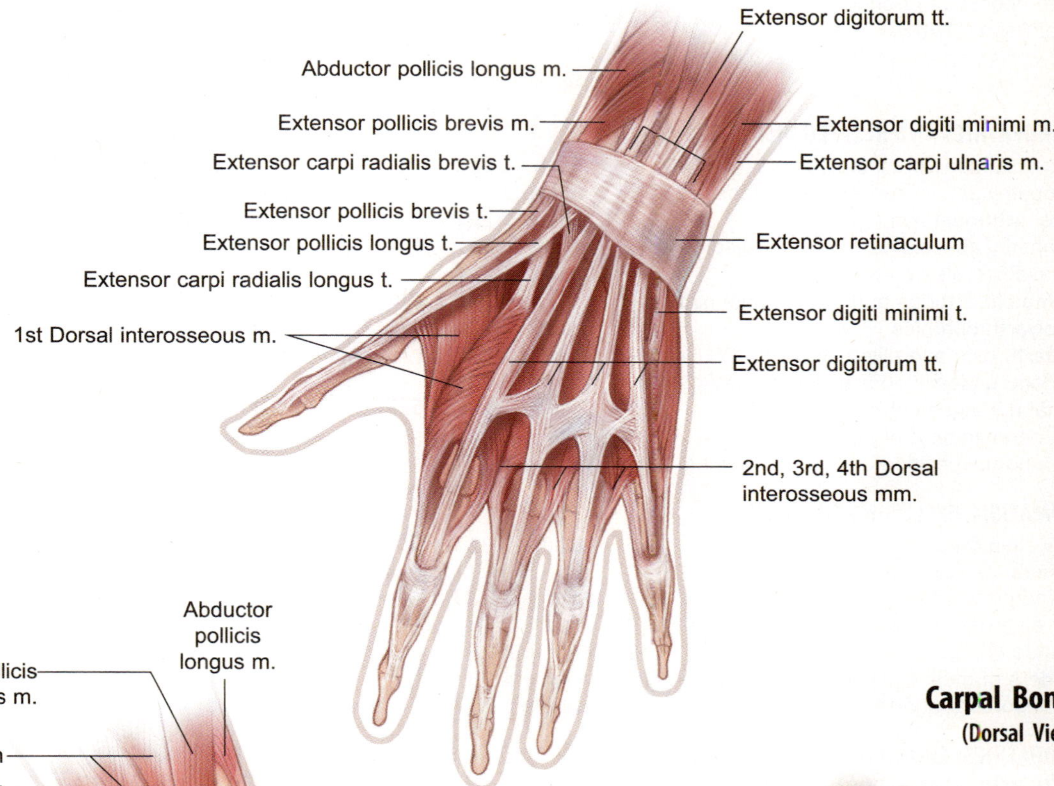

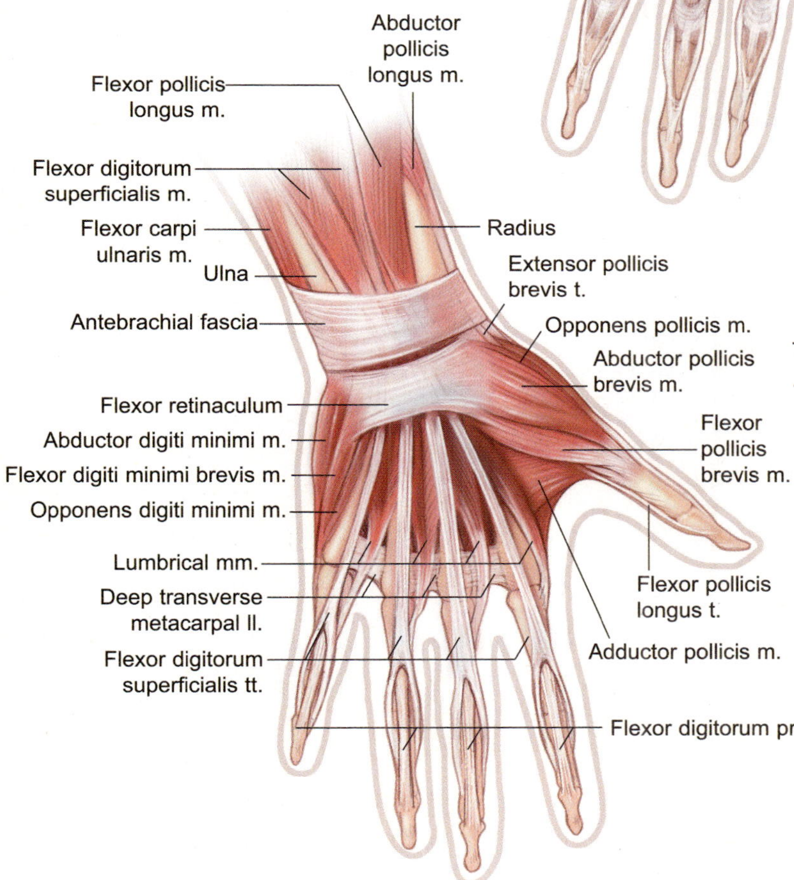

Carpal Bones

(Dorsal View)

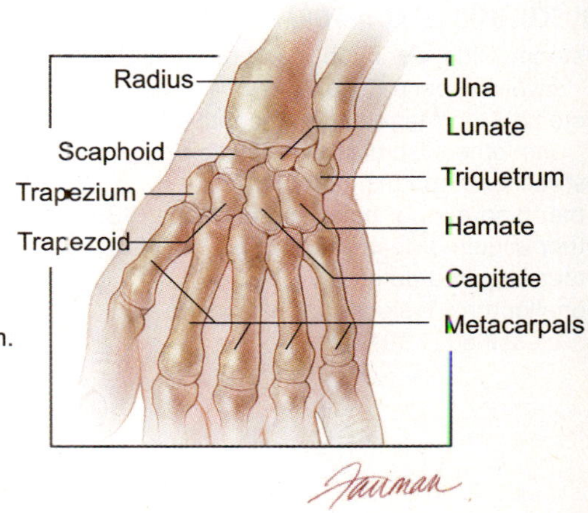

Musculoskeletal System – Hip and Knee

Anatomy Color Plates

Musculoskeletal System – Hip and Knee

(Anterior and Posterior Views)

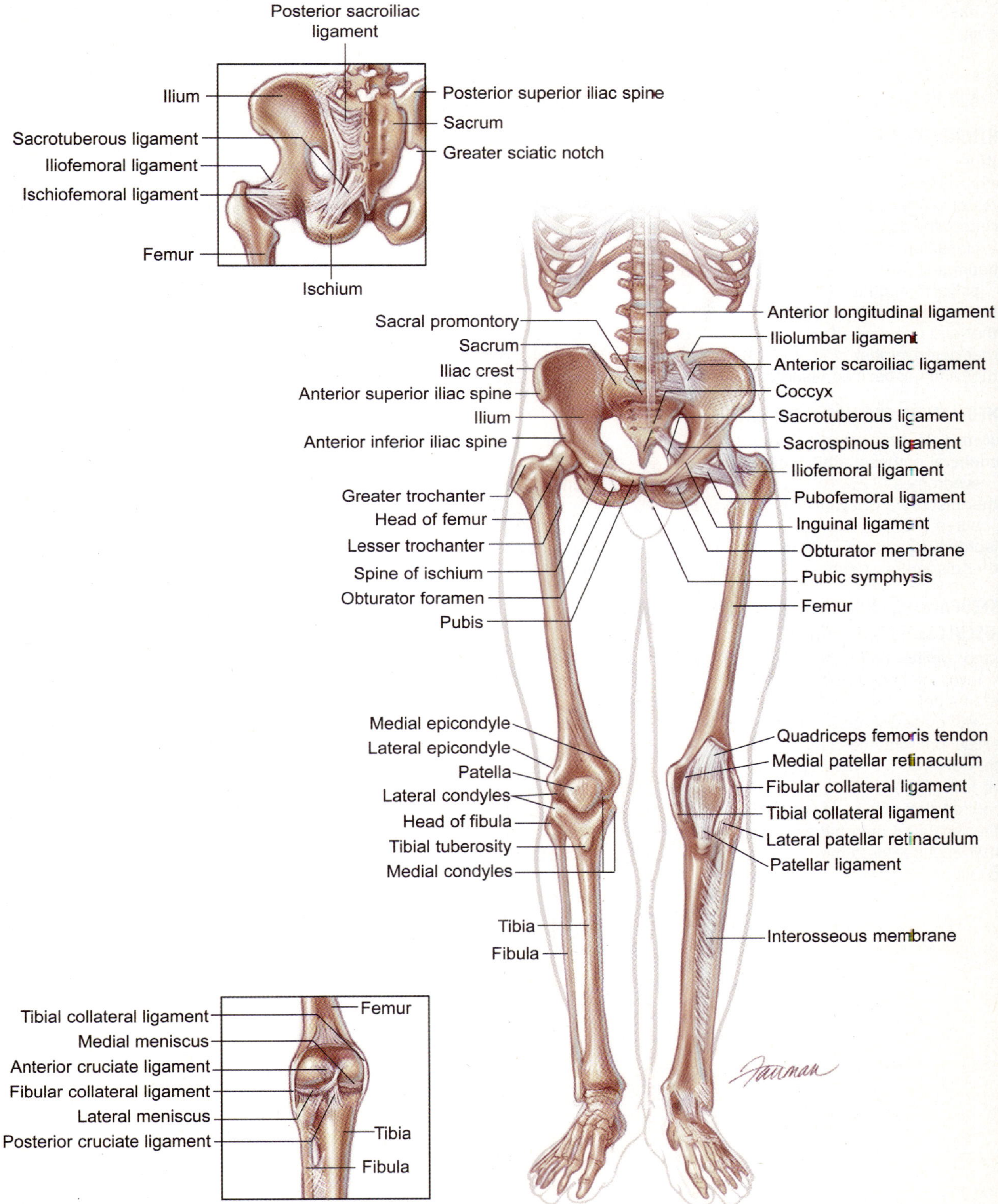

Musculoskeletal System – Foot and Ankle

Musculoskeletal System – Foot and Ankle

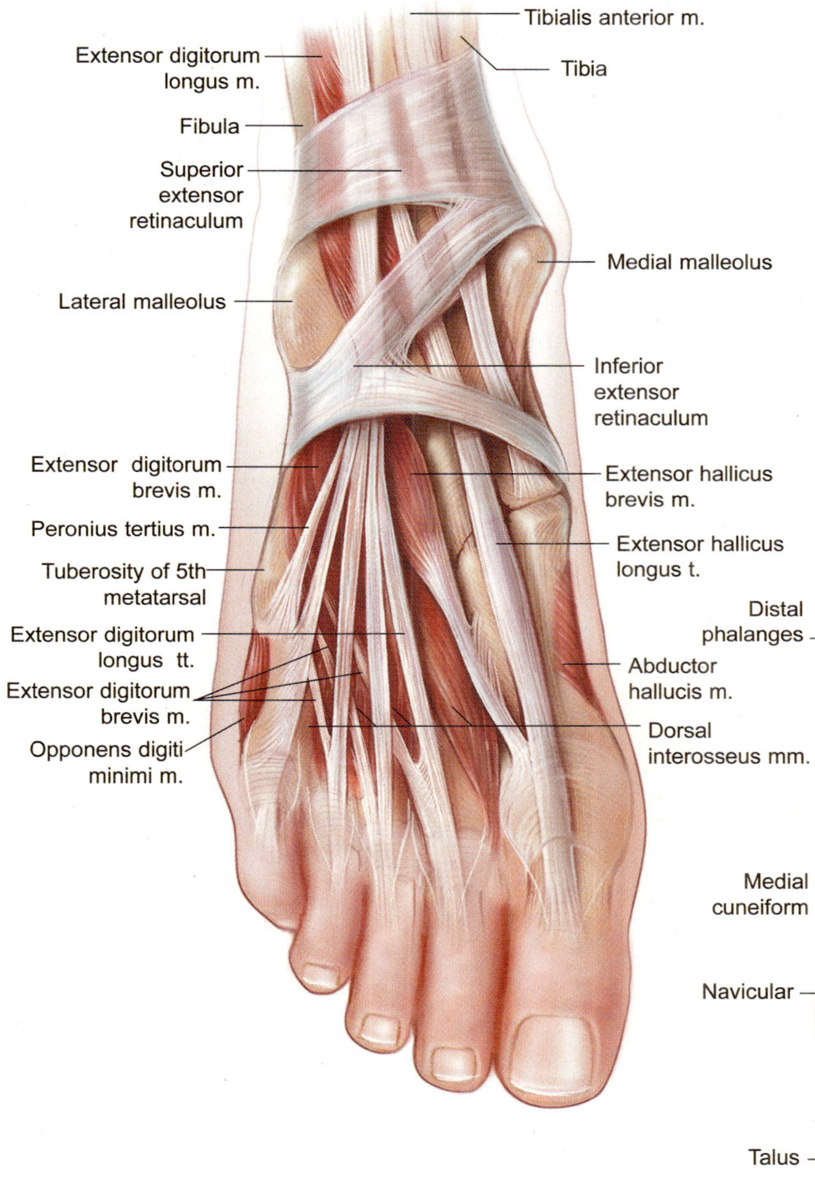

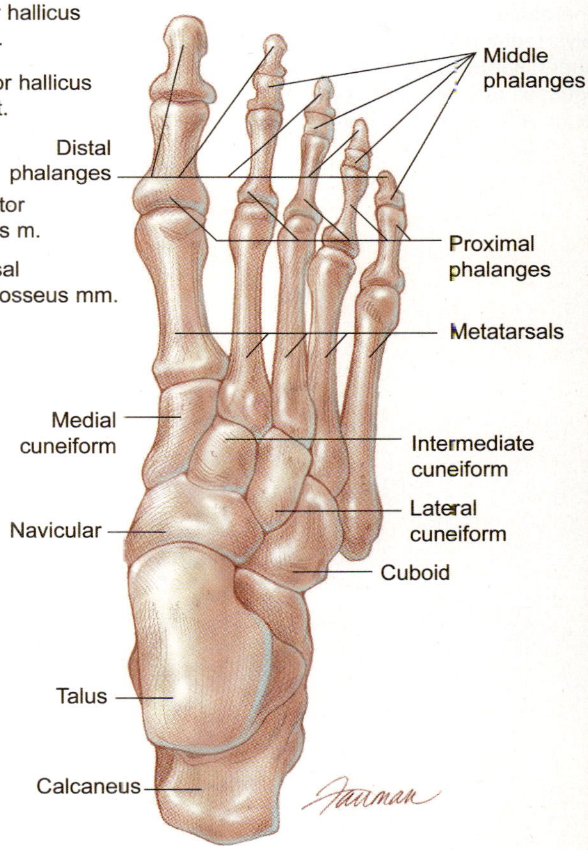

Vascular System

Vascular System

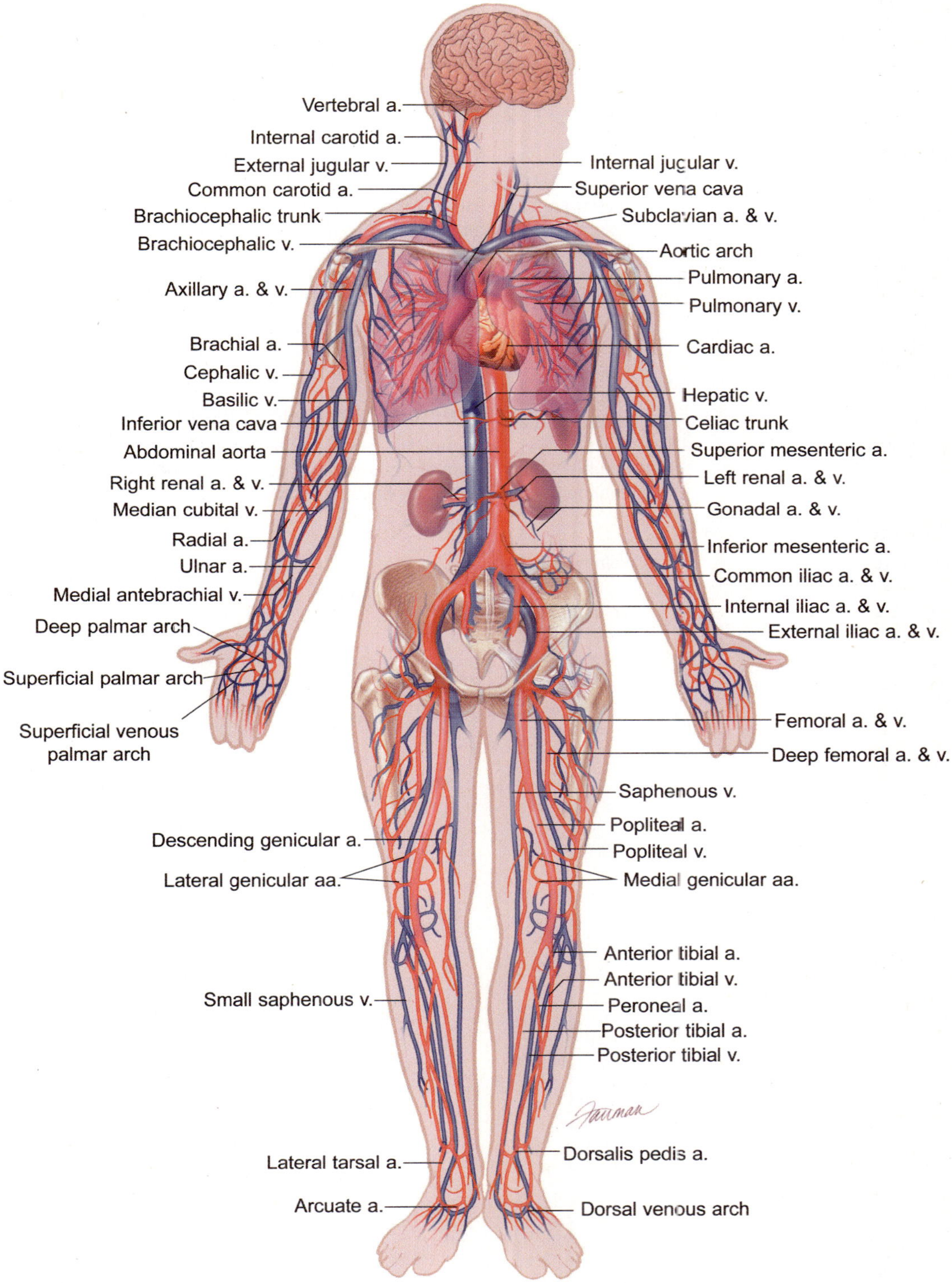

Heart and Pericardium

Heart
(External View)

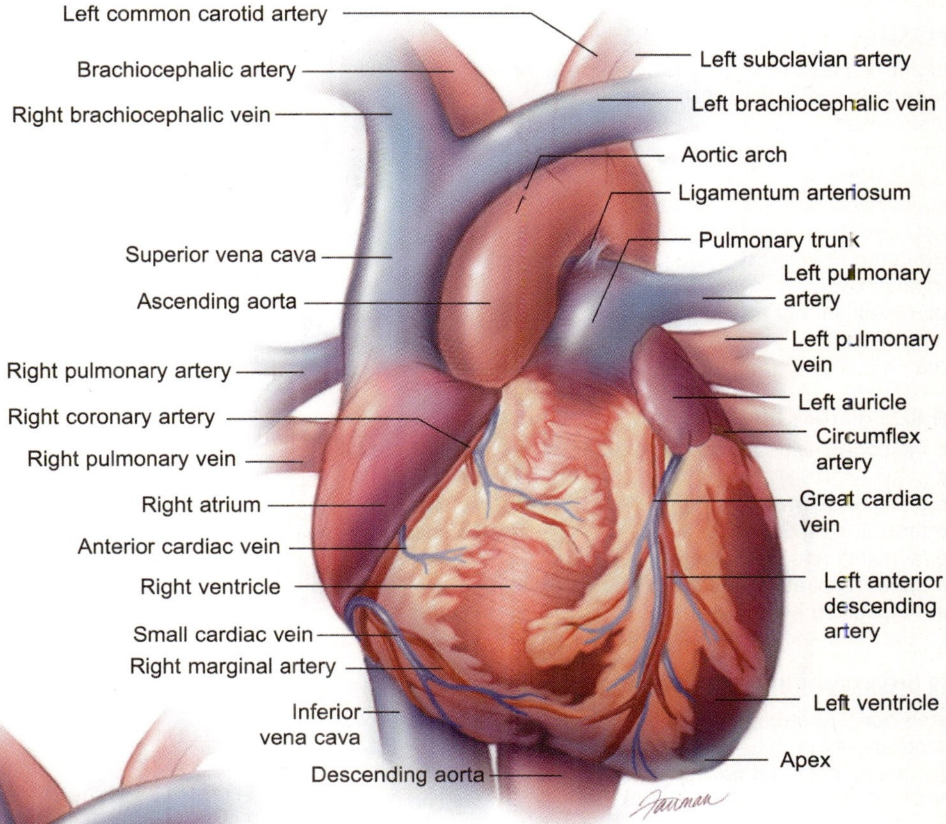

Heart
(Internal View)

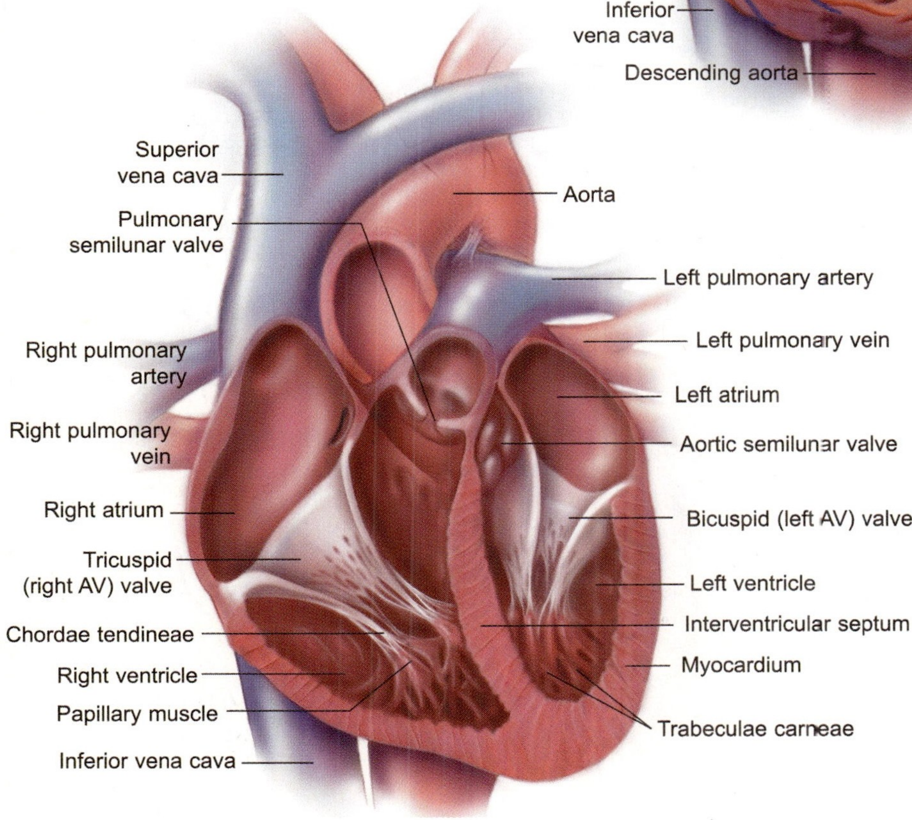

Respiratory System

Respiratory System

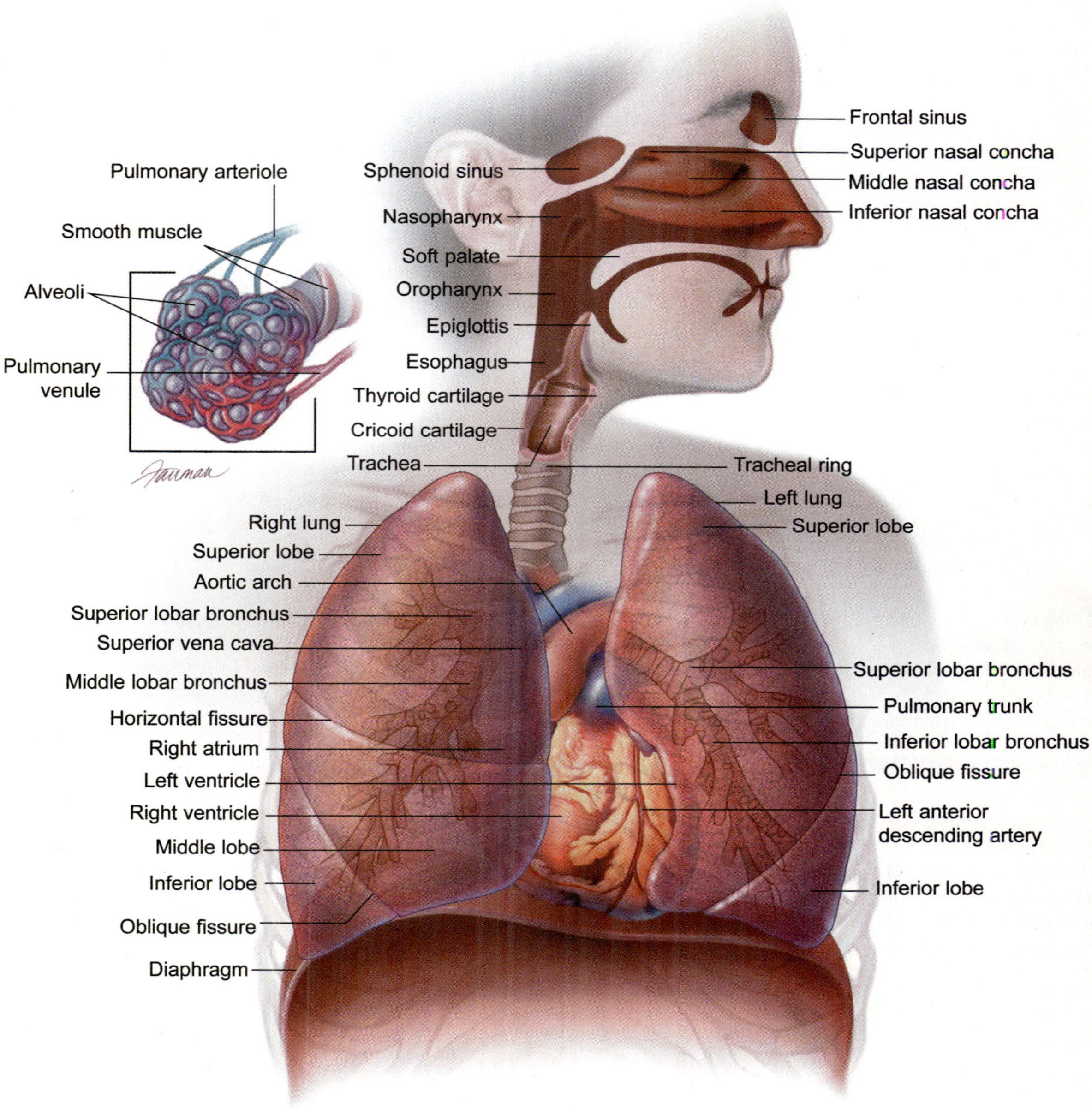

Digestive System

NEOPLASM OF DIGESTIVE ORGANS AND PERITONEUM

DISEASES OF ESOPHAGUS, STOMACH, AND DUODENUM

APPENDICITIS

HERNIA OF ABDOMINAL CAVITY

NONINFECTIOUS ENTERITIS AND COLITIS

OTHER DISEASES OF INTESTINES AND PERITONEUM

OTHER DISEASES OF DIGESTIVE SYSTEM

CONGENITAL ANOMALIES

SYMPTOMS, SIGNS, AND ILL DEFINED CONDITIONS

Digestive System

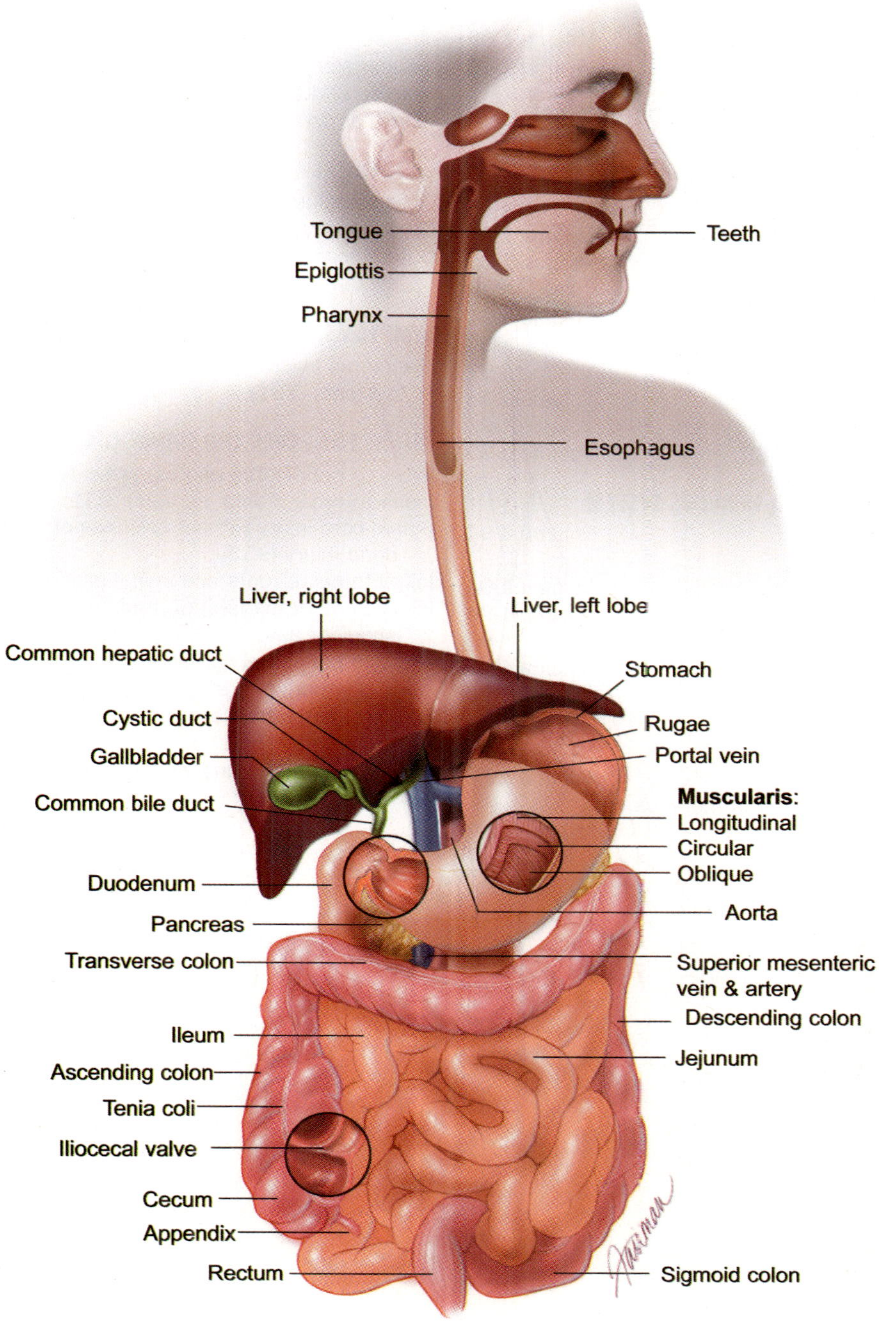

Nervous System

Nervous System

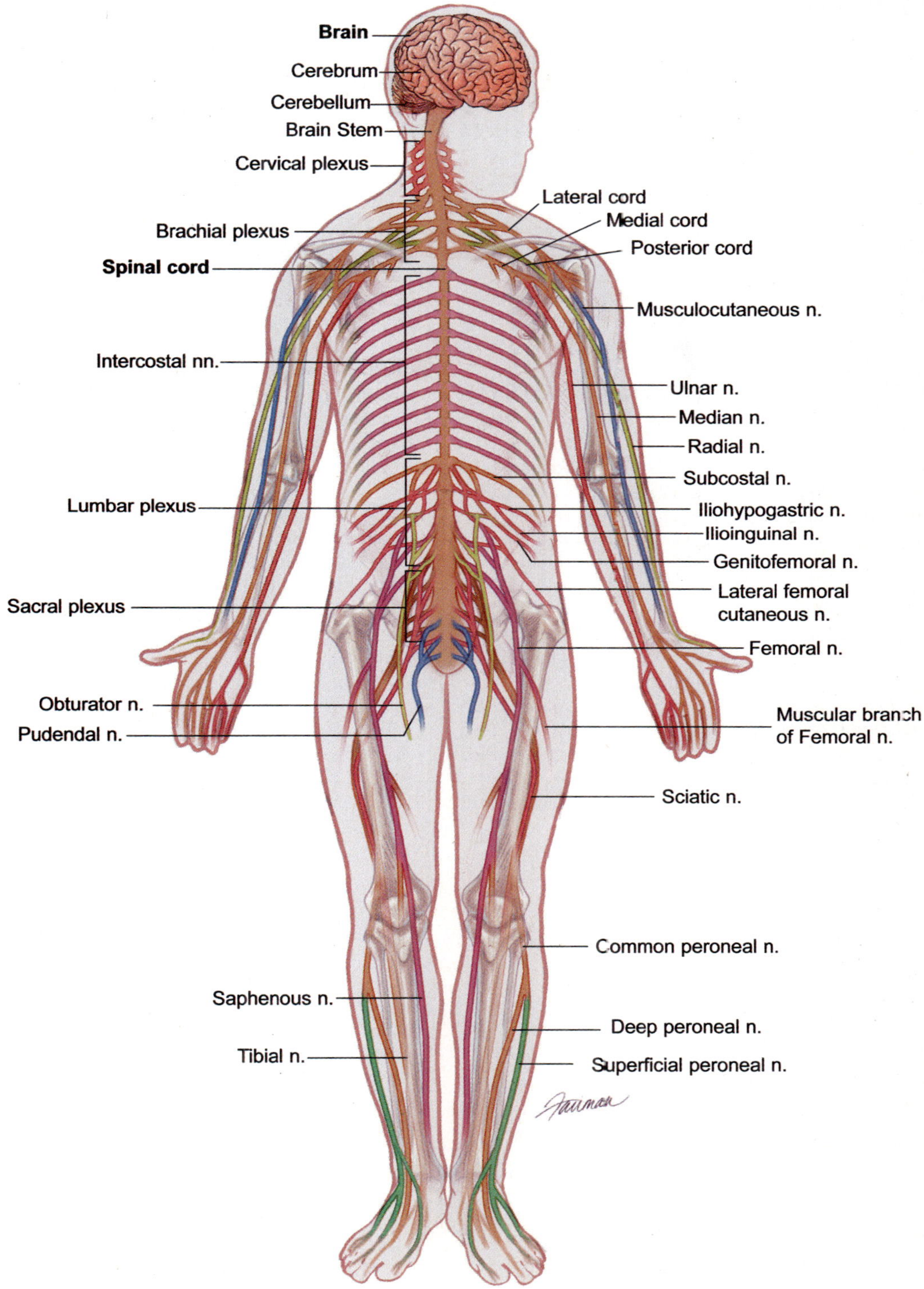

Brain

Brain
(Inferior View)

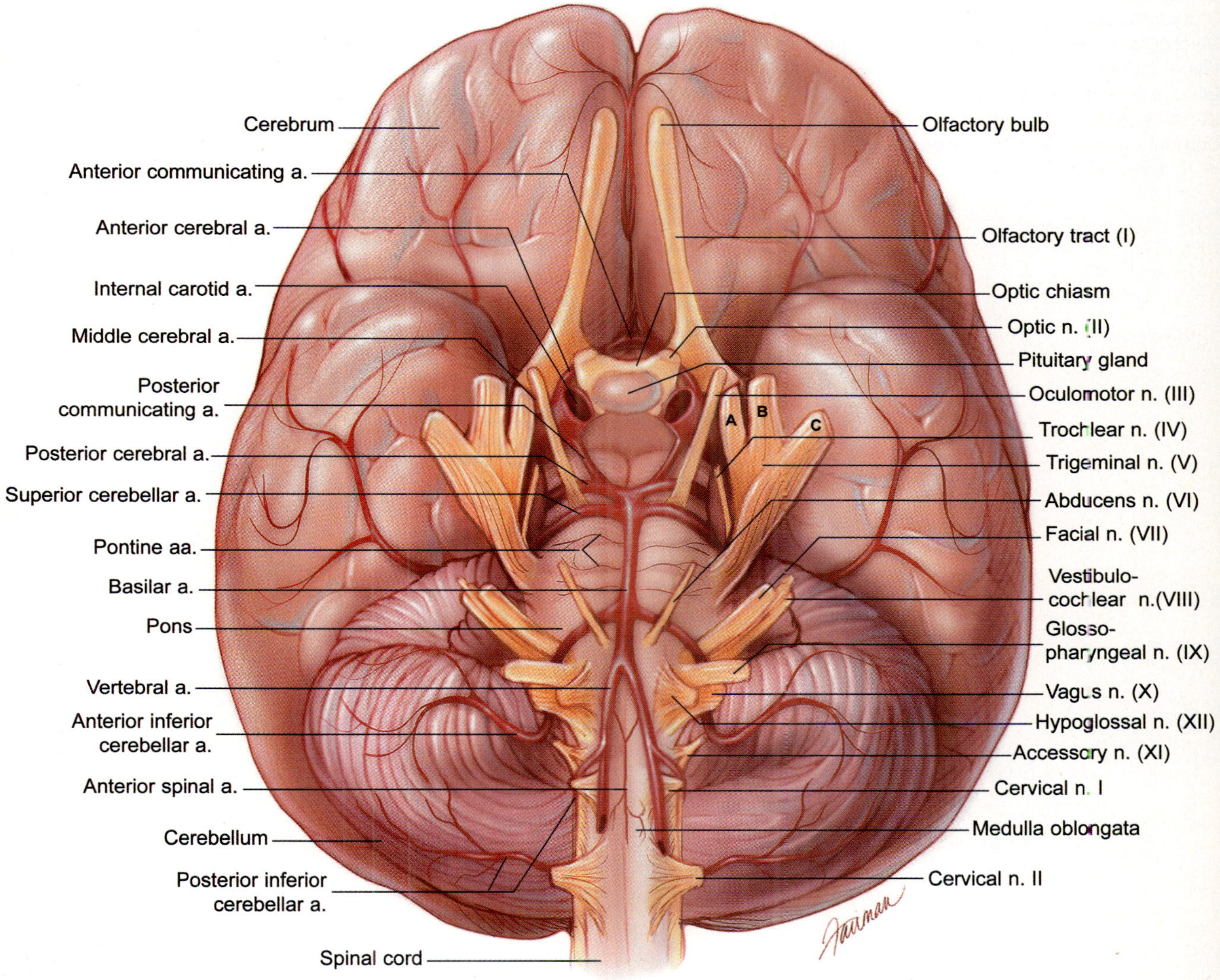

Trigeminal Nerve (V) branches:
- **A** Ophthalmic branch
- **B** Maxillary branch
- **C** Mandibular branch

Eye and Ocular Adnexa

DISORDERS OF THE EYE AND ADNEXA

DISORDERS OF THE EYE AND ADNEXA - CONTINUED

CONGENITAL ANOMALIES

The Right Eye
(Transverse Section)

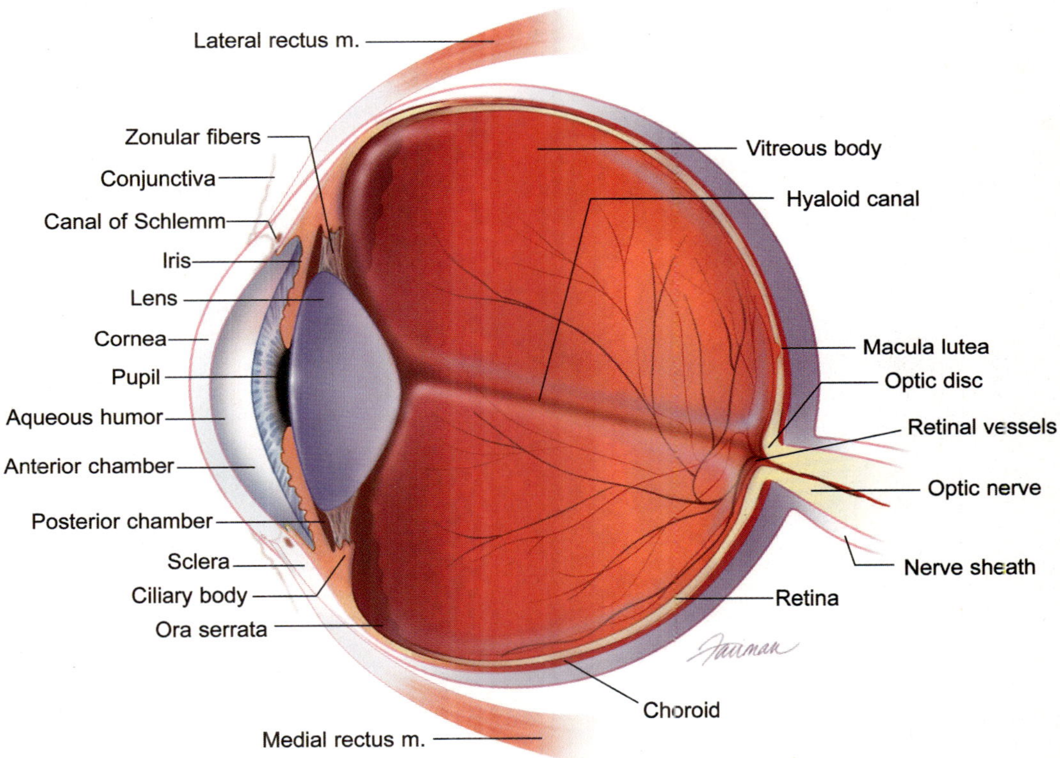

Ear

The Right Ear

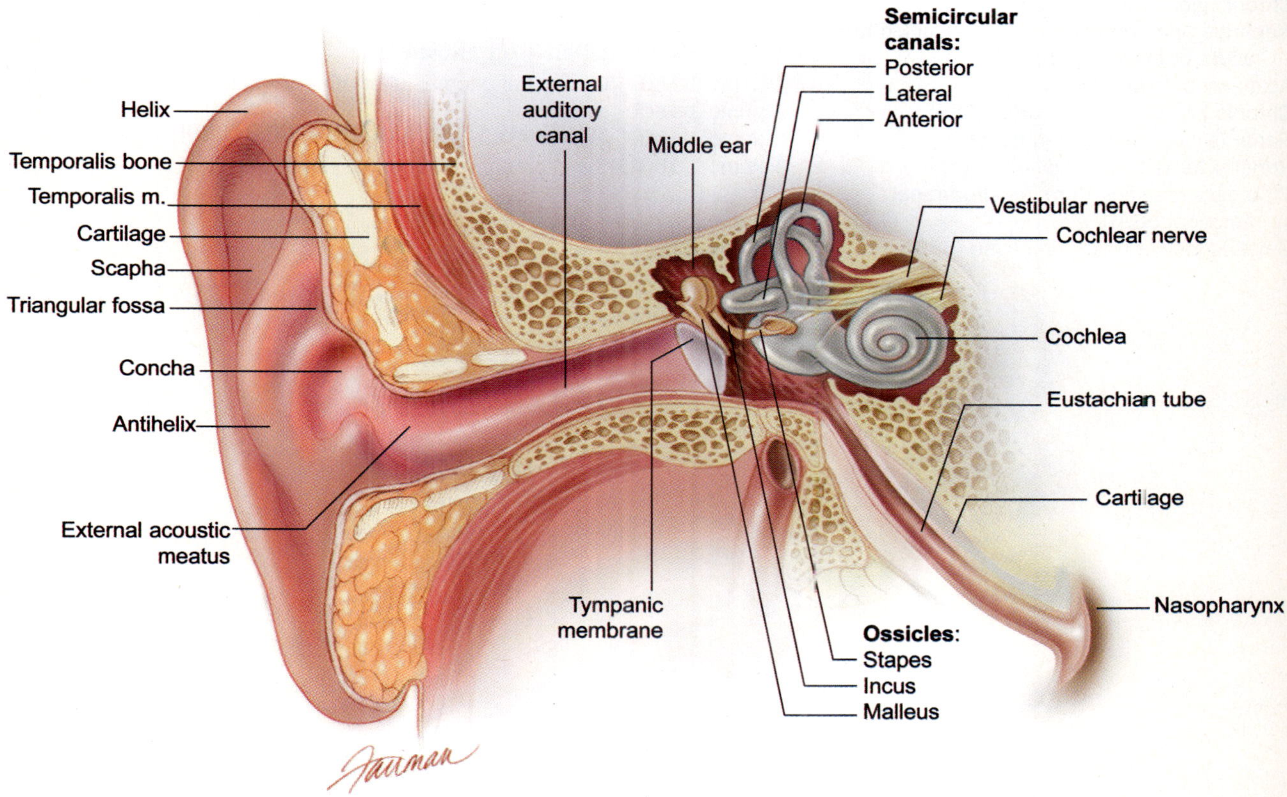

Urinary System

Urinary System

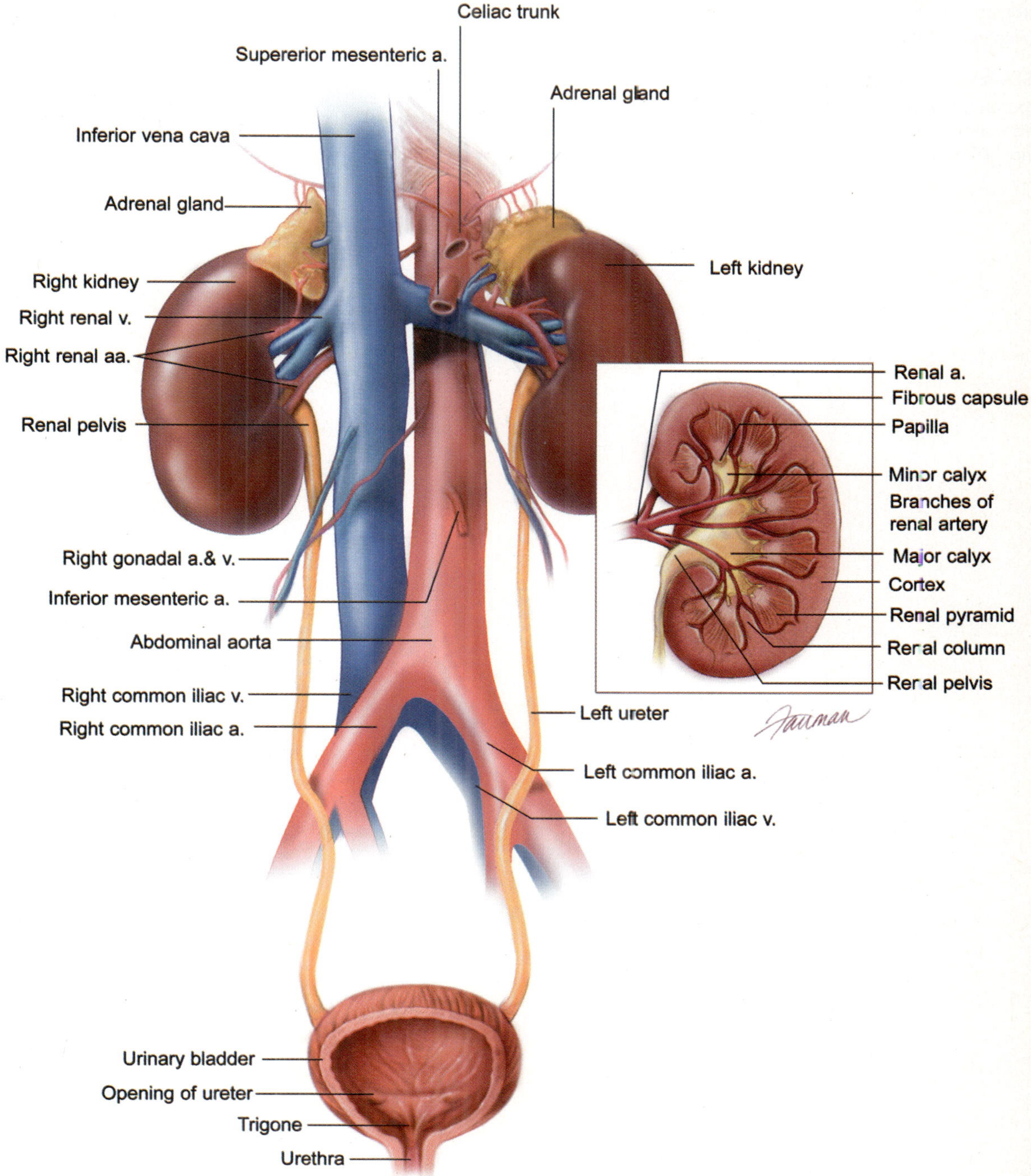

Male Genital System

Male Genital System

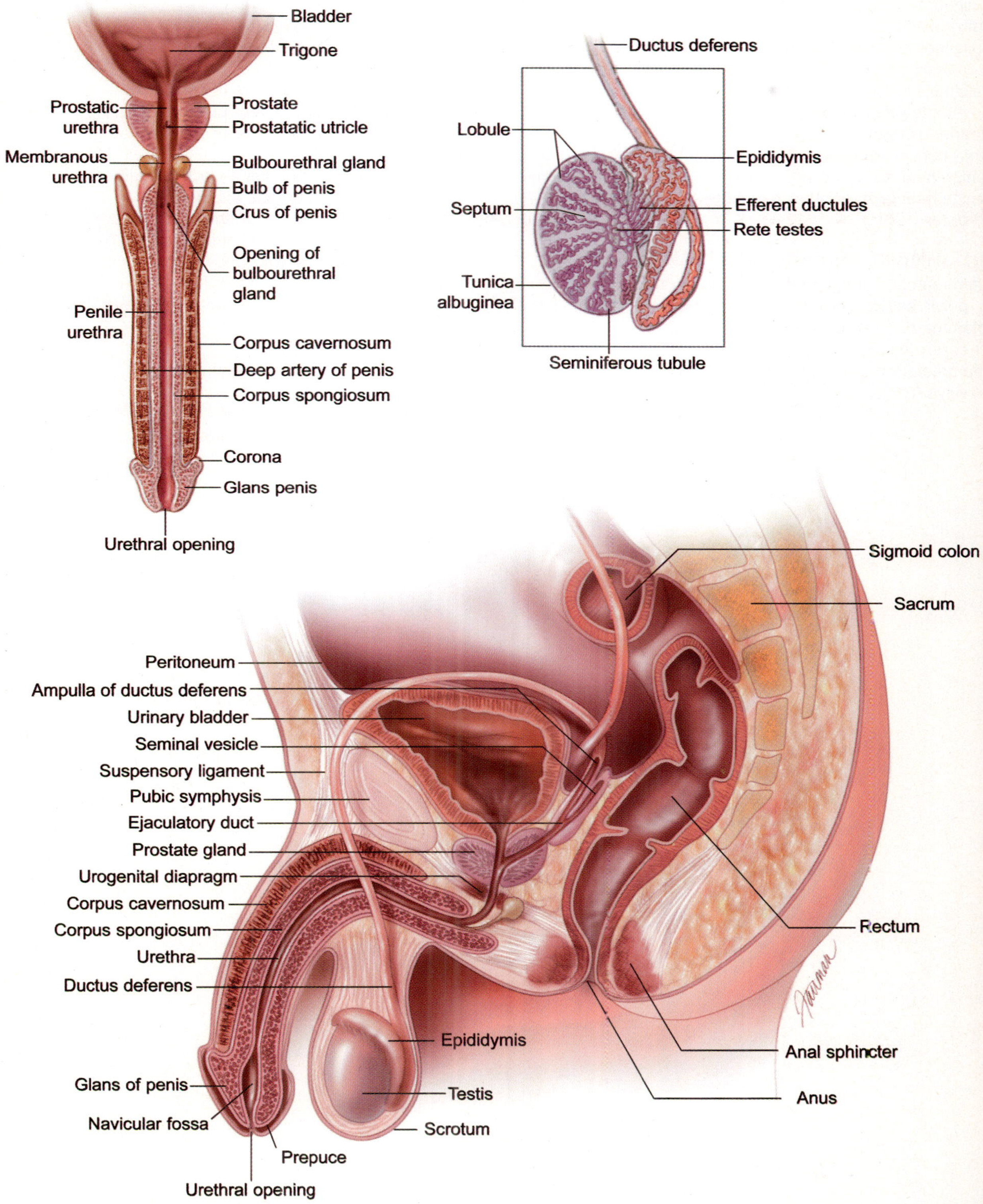

Female Genital System

Female Genital System

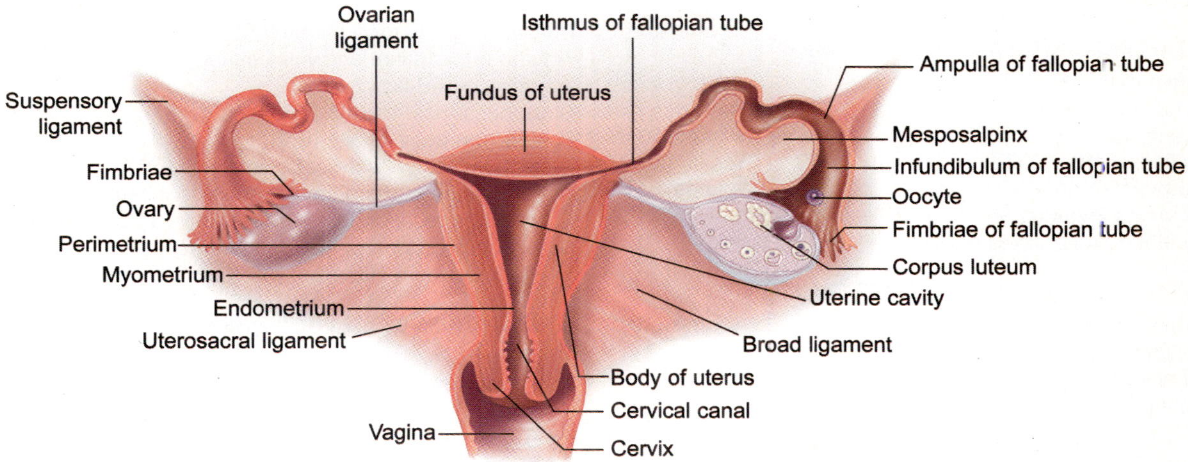

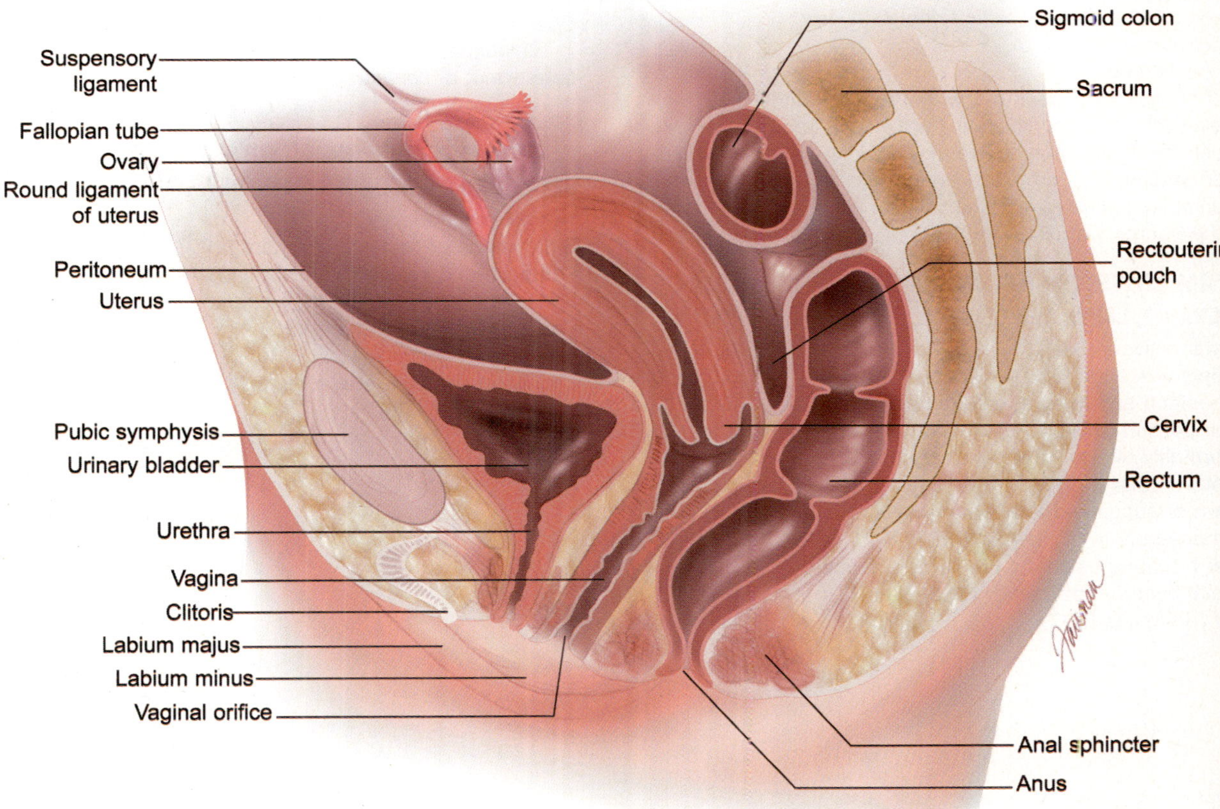

Female Reproductive System – Pregnancy

ECTOPIC AND MOLAR PREGNANCY

OTHER PREGNANCY WITH ABORTIVE OUTCOME

COMPLICATIONS MAINLY RELATED TO PREGNANCY

NORMAL DELIVERY, AND OTHER INDICATIONS FOR CARE IN PREGNANCY, LABOR AND DELIVERY

COMPLICATIONS OCCURRING MAINLY IN THE COURSE OF LABOR AND DELIVERY

COMPLICATIONS OF THE PUERPERIUM

PERSONS ENCOUNTERING HEALTH SERVICES IN CIRCUMSTANCES RELATED TO REPRODUCTION AND DEVELOPMENT

Female Reproductive System – Pregnancy
(Lateral View)

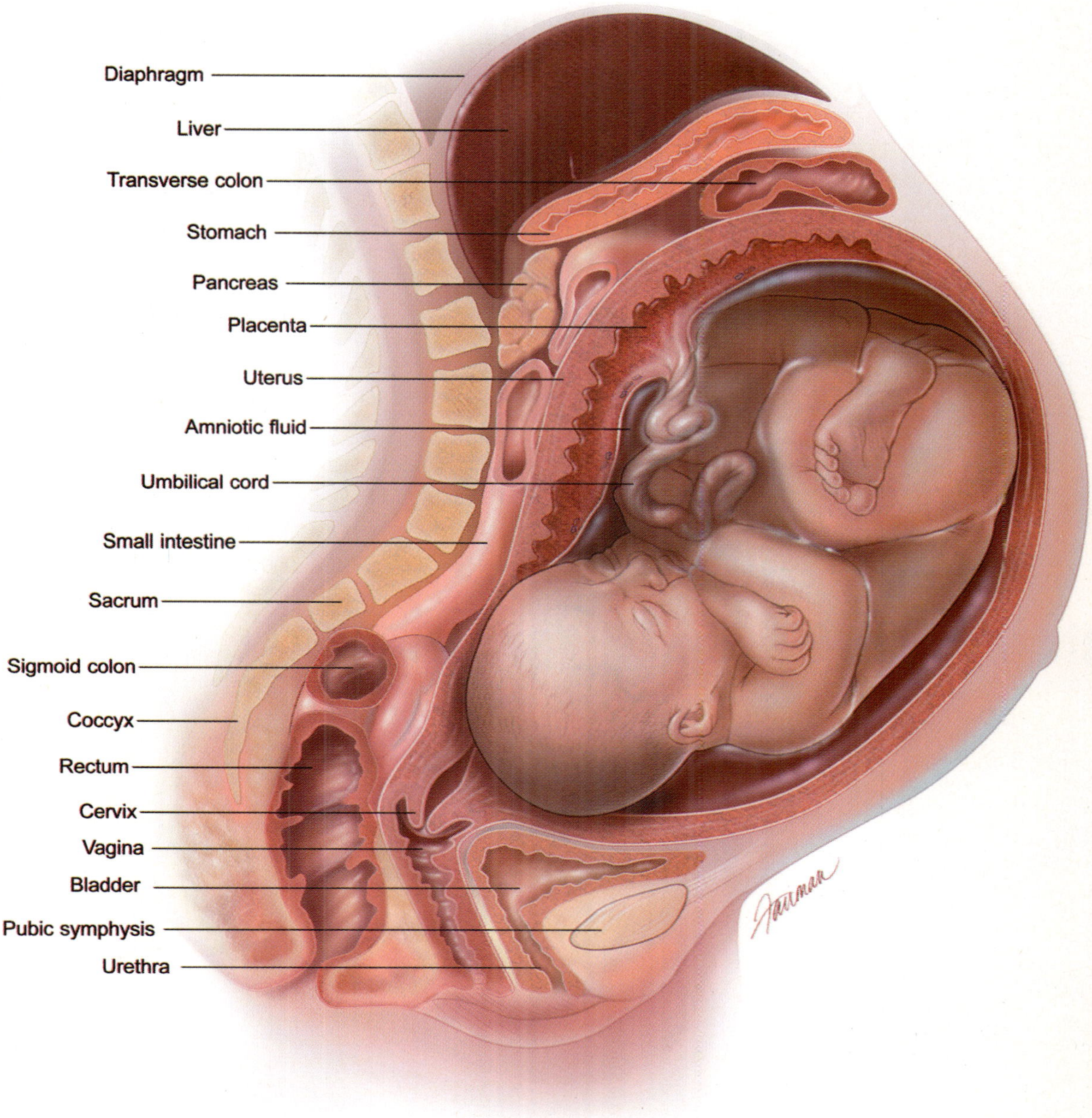

Alphabetic Index to Diseases

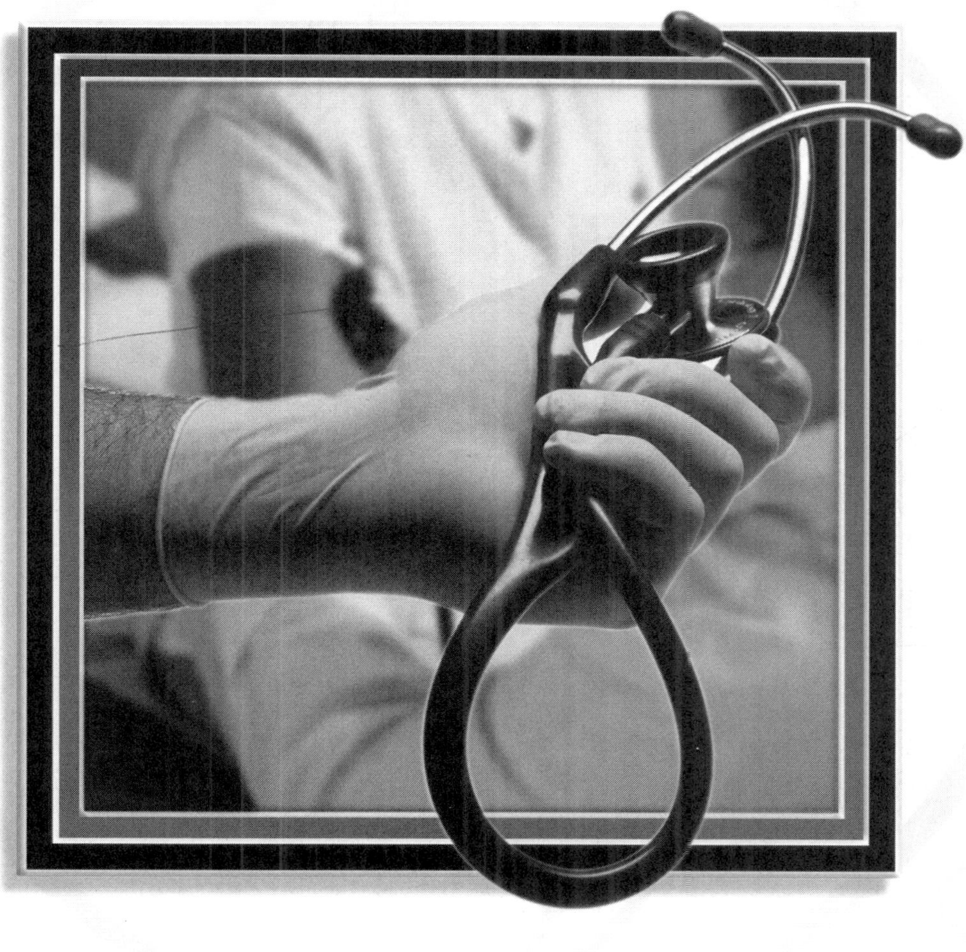

Volume 2 • Section 1

A

- **AAT** (alpha-1 antitrypsin) **deficiency** 273.4
- **AAV** (disease) (illness) (infection) – *see* Human immunodeficiency virus (disease) (illness) (infection)
- **Abactio** – *see* Abortion, induced
- **Abactus venter** – *see* Abortion, induced
- **Abarognosis** 781.99
- **Abasia** (-astasia) 307.9
  - atactica 781.3
  - choreic 781.3
  - hysterical 300.11
  - paroxysmal trepidant 781.3
  - spastic 781.3
  - trembling 781.3
  - trepidans 781.3
- **Abderhalden-Kaufmann-Lignac syndrome** (cystinosis) 270.0
- **Abdomen, abdominal** – *see also* condition
  - accordion 306.4
  - acute 789.0❺
  - angina 557.1
  - burst 868.00
  - convulsive equivalent (*see also* Epilepsy) 345.5❺
  - heart 746.87
  - muscle deficiency syndrome 756.79
  - obstipum 756.79
- **Abdominalgia** 789.0❺
  - periodic 277.31
- **Abduction contracture, hip or other joint** – *see* Contraction, joint
- **Abercrombie's syndrome** (amyloid degeneration) 277.39
- **Aberrant** (congenital) – *see also* Malposition, congenital
  - adrenal gland 759.1
  - blood vessel NEC 747.60
    - arteriovenous NEC 747.60
    - cerebrovascular 747.81
    - gastrointestinal 747.61
    - lower limb 747.64
    - renal 747.62
    - spinal 747.82
    - upper limb 747.63
  - breast 757.6
  - endocrine gland NEC 759.2
  - gastrointestinal vessel (peripheral) 747.61
  - hepatic duct 751.69
  - lower limb vessel (peripheral) 747.64
  - pancreas 751.7
  - parathyroid gland 759.2
  - peripheral vascular vessel NEC 747.60
  - pituitary gland (pharyngeal) 759.2
  - renal blood vessel 747.62
  - sebaceous glands, mucous membrane, mouth 750.26
  - spinal vessel 747.82
  - spleen 759.0
  - testis (descent) 752.51
  - thymus gland 759.2
  - thyroid gland 759.2
  - upper limb vessel (peripheral) 747.63
- **Aberratio**
  - lactis 757.6
  - testis 752.51
- **Aberration** – *see also* Anomaly
  - chromosome – *see* Anomaly, chromosome(s)
  - distantial 368.9
  - mental (*see also* Disorder, mental, nonpsychotic) 300.9
- **Abetalipoproteinemia** 272.5
- **Abionarce** 780.79
- **Abiotrophy** 799.89
- **Ablatio**
  - placentae – *see* Placenta, ablatio
  - retinae (*see also* Detachment, retina) 361.9
- **Ablation**
  - pituitary (gland) (with hypofunction) 253.7
  - placenta – *see* Placenta, ablatio
  - uterus 621.8
- **Ablepharia, ablepharon, ablephary** 743.62
- **Ablepsia** – *see* Blindness
- **Ablepsy** – *see* Blindness
- **Ablutomania** 300.3
- **Abnormal, abnormality, abnormalities** – *see also* Anomaly
  - acid-base balance 276.4
    - fetus or newborn – *see* Distress, fetal
  - adaptation curve, dark 368.63
  - alveolar ridge 525.9
  - amnion 658.9❺
    - affecting fetus or newborn 762.9
  - anatomical relationship NEC 759.9
  - apertures, congenital, diaphragm 756.6
  - auditory perception NEC 388.40
  - autosomes NEC 758.5
    - 13 758.1
    - 18 758.2
    - 21 or 22 758.0
    - D_1 758.1
    - E_3 758.2
    - G 758.0
  - ballistocardiogram 794.39
  - basal metabolic rate (BMR) 794.7
  - biosynthesis, testicular androgen 257.2
  - blood level (of)
    - cobalt 790.6
    - copper 790.6
    - iron 790.6
    - lead 790.6
    - lithium 790.6
    - magnesium 790.6
    - mineral 790.6
    - zinc 790.6
  - blood pressure
    - elevated (without diagnosis of hypertension) 796.2
    - low (*see also* Hypotension) 458.9
      - reading (incidental) (isolated) (nonspecific) 796.3
  - blood sugar 790.29 ●
  - bowel sounds 787.5
  - breathing behavior – *see* Respiration
  - caloric test 794.19
  - cervix (acquired) NEC 622.9
    - congenital 752.40
    - in pregnancy or childbirth 654.6❺
      - causing obstructed labor 660.2❺
        - affecting fetus or newborn 763.1
  - chemistry, blood NEC 790.6
  - chest sounds 786.7
  - chorion 658.9❺
    - affecting fetus or newborn 762.9
  - chromosomal NEC 758.89
    - analysis, nonspecific result 795.2
    - autosomes (*see also* Abnormal, autosomes NEC) 758.5
    - fetal, (suspected) affecting management of pregnancy 655.1❺
    - sex 758.81
  - clinical findings NEC 796.4
  - communication – *see* Fistula
  - configuration of pupils 379.49
  - coronary
    - artery 746.85
    - vein 746.9
  - cortisol-binding globulin 255.8
  - course, Eustachian tube 744.24
  - dentofacial NEC 524.9
    - functional 524.50
    - specified type NEC 524.89
  - development, developmental NEC 759.9
    - bone 756.9
    - central nervous system 742.9
  - direction, teeth 524.30
  - Dynia (*see also* Defect, coagulation) 286.9
  - Ebstein 746.2
  - echocardiogram 793.2
  - echoencephalogram 794.01
  - echogram NEC – *see* Findings, abnormal, structure
  - electrocardiogram (ECG) (EKG) 794.31
  - electroencephalogram (EEG) 794.02
  - electromyogram (EMG) 794.17
    - ocular 794.14
  - electro-oculogram (EOG) 794.12
  - electroretinogram (ERG) 794.11
  - erythrocytes 289.9
    - congenital, with perinatal jaundice 282.9 *[774.0]*
  - Eustachian valve 746.9
  - excitability under minor stress 301.9
  - fat distribution 782.9
  - feces 787.7
  - fetal heart rate – *see* Distress, fetal

Abnormal, abnormality, abnormalities – *continued*

  - fetus NEC
    - affecting management of pregnancy – *see* Pregnancy, management affected by, fetal
    - causing disproportion 653.7❺
      - affecting fetus or newborn 763.1
      - causing obstructed labor 660.1❺
        - affecting fetus or newborn 763.1
  - findings without manifest disease – *see* Findings, abnormal
  - fluid
    - amniotic 792.3
    - cerebrospinal 792.0
    - peritoneal 792.9
    - pleural 792.9
    - synovial 792.9
    - vaginal 792.9
  - forces of labor NEC 661.9❺
    - affecting fetus or newborn 763.7
  - form, teeth 520.2
  - function studies
    - auditory 794.15
    - bladder 794.9
    - brain 794.00
    - cardiovascular 794.30
    - endocrine NEC 794.6
    - kidney 794.4
    - liver 794.8
    - nervous system
      - central 794.00
      - peripheral 794.19
    - oculomotor 794.14
    - pancreas 794.9
    - placenta 794.9
    - pulmonary 794.2
    - retina 794.11
    - special senses 794.19
    - spleen 794.9
    - thyroid 794.5
    - vestibular 794.16
  - gait 781.2
    - hysterical 300.11
  - gastrin secretion 251.5
  - globulin
    - cortisol-binding 255.8
    - thyroid-binding 246.8
  - glucagon secretion 251.4
  - glucose 790.29
    - fetus or newborn 775.0
    - in pregnancy, childbirth, or puerperium 648.8❺
    - non-fasting 790.29
  - gravitational (G) forces or states 994.9
  - hair NEC 704.2
  - hard tissue formation in pulp 522.3
  - head movement 781.0
  - heart
    - rate
      - fetus, affecting liveborn infant
        - before the onset of labor 763.81
        - during labor 763.82
        - unspecified as to time of onset 763.83
      - intrauterine
        - before the onset of labor 763.81
        - during labor 763.82
        - unspecified as to time of onset 763.83
      - newborn
        - before the onset of labor 763.81
        - during labor 763.82
        - unspecified as to time of onset 763.83
    - shadow 793.2
    - sounds NEC 785.3
  - hemoglobin (*see also* Disease, hemoglobin) 282.7
    - trait – *see* Trait, hemoglobin, abnormal
  - hemorrhage, uterus – *see* Hemorrhage, uterus
  - histology NEC 795.4
  - increase in
    - appetite 783.6
    - development 783.9
  - involuntary movement 781.0
  - jaw closure 524.51
  - karyotype 795.2
  - knee jerk 796.1
  - labor NEC 661.9❺
    - affecting fetus or newborn 763.7
  - laboratory findings – *see* Findings, abnormal
  - length, organ or site, congenital – *see* Distortion
  - loss of height 781.91
  - loss of weight 783.21
  - lung shadow 793.1

AAT – Abnormal, abnormality, abnormalities

- **Abnormal, abnormality, abnormalities** – *continued*
  - mammogram 793.80
    - calcification 793.89
    - calculus 793.89
    - microcalcification 793.81
  - Mantoux test 795.5
  - membranes (fetal)
    - affecting fetus or newborn 762.9
    - complicating pregnancy 658.8❺
  - menstruation – *see* Menstruation
  - metabolism (*see also* condition) 783.9
  - movement 781.0
    - disorder NEC 333.90
      - sleep related, unspecified 780.58
      - specified NEC 333.99
    - head 781.0
    - involuntary 781.0
    - specified type NEC 333.99
  - muscle contraction, localized 728.85
  - myoglobin (Aberdeen) (Annapolis) 289.9
  - narrowness, eyelid 743.62
  - optokinetic response 379.57
  - organs or tissues of pelvis NEC
    - in pregnancy or childbirth 654.9❺
      - affecting fetus or newborn 763.89
      - causing obstructed labor 660.2❺
        - affecting fetus or newborn 763.1
  - origin – *see* Malposition, congenital
  - palmar creases 757.2
  - Papanicolaou (smear)
    - cervix 795.00
      - with
        - atypical squamous cells
          - cannot exclude high grade squamous intraepithelial lesion (ASC-H) 795.02
          - favor benign (ASCUS favor benign) 795.01
          - favor dysplasia (ASCUS favor dysplasia) 795.02
          - of undetermined significance (ASC-US)795.01
        - cytologic evidence of malignancy 795.06
        - high grade squamous intraepithelial lesion (HGSIL) 795.04
        - low grade squamous intraepithelial lesion (LGSIL) 795.03
      - nonspecific finding NEC 795.09
    - other site 795.1
  - parturition
    - affecting fetus or newborn 763.9
    - mother – *see* Delivery, complicated
  - pelvis (bony) – *see* Deformity, pelvis
  - percussion, chest 786.7
  - periods (grossly) (*see also* Menstruation) 626.9
  - phonocardiogram 794.39
  - placenta – *see* Placenta, abnormal
  - plantar reflex 796.1
  - plasma protein – *see* Deficiency, plasma, protein
  - pleural folds 748.8
  - position – *see also* Malposition
    - gravid uterus 654.4❺
      - causing obstructed labor 660.2❺
        - affecting fetus or newborn 763.1
  - posture NEC 781.92
  - presentation (fetus) – *see* Presentation, fetus, abnormal
  - product of conception NEC 631
  - puberty – *see* Puberty
  - pulmonary
    - artery 747.3
    - function, newborn 770.89
    - test results 794.2
    - ventilation, newborn 770.89
      - hyperventilation 786.01
  - pulsations in neck 785.1
  - pupil reflexes 379.40
  - quality of milk 676.8❺
  - radiological examination 793.99
    - abdomen NEC 793.6
    - biliary tract 793.3
    - breast 793.89
      - mammogram NOS 793.80
      - mammographic
        - calcification 793.89
        - calculus 793.89
        - microcalcification 793.81
    - gastrointestinal tract 793.4
    - genitourinary organs 793.5
    - head 793.0
- **Abnormal, abnormality, abnormalities** – *continued*
  - radiological examination – *continued*
    - image test inconclusive due to excess body fat 793.91
    - intrathoracic organ NEC 793.2
    - lung (field) 793.1
    - musculoskeletal system 793.7
    - retroperitoneum 793.6
    - skin and subcutaneous tissue 793.99
    - skull 793.0
  - red blood cells 790.09
    - morphology 790.09
    - volume 790.09
  - reflex NEC 796.1
  - renal function test 794.4
  - respiration signs – *see* Respiration
  - response to nerve stimulation 794.10
  - retinal correspondence 368.34
  - rhythm, heart – *see also* Arrhythmia
    - fetus – *see* Distress, fetal
  - saliva 792.4
  - scan
    - brain 794.09
    - kidney 794.4
    - liver 794.8
    - lung 794.2
    - thyroid 794.5
  - secretion
    - gastrin 251.5
    - glucagon 251.4
  - semen 792.2
  - serum level (of)
    - acid phosphatase 790.5
    - alkaline phosphatase 790.5
    - amylase 790.5
    - enzymes NEC 790.5
    - lipase 790.5
  - shape
    - cornea 743.41
    - gallbladder 751.69
    - gravid uterus 654.4❺
      - affecting fetus or newborn 763.89
      - causing obstructed labor 660.2❺
        - affecting fetus or newborn 763.1
    - head (*see also* Anomaly, skull) 756.0
    - organ or site, congenital NEC – *see* Distortion
  - sinus venosus 747.40
  - size
    - fetus, complicating delivery 653.5❺
      - causing obstructed labor 660.1❺
    - gallbladder 751.69
    - head (*see also* Anomaly, skull) 756.0
    - organ or site, congenital NEC – *see* Distortion
    - teeth 520.2
  - skin and appendages, congenital NEC 757.9
  - soft parts of pelvis – *see* Abnormal, organs or tissues of pelvis
  - spermatozoa 792.2
  - sputum (amount) (color) (excessive) (odor) (purulent) 786.4
  - stool NEC 787.7
    - bloody 578.1
      - occult 792.1
    - bulky 787.7
    - color (dark) (light) 792.1
    - content (fat) (mucus) (pus) 792.1
    - occult blood 792.1
  - synchondrosis 756.9
  - test results without manifest disease – *see* Findings, abnormal
  - thebesian valve 746.9
  - thermography – *see* Findings, abnormal, structure
  - threshold, cones or rods (eye) 368.63
  - thyroid-binding globulin 246.8
  - thyroid product 246.8
  - toxicology (findings) NEC 796.0
  - tracheal cartilage (congenital) 748.3
  - transport protein 273.8
  - ultrasound results – *see* Findings, abnormal, structure
  - umbilical cord
    - affecting fetus or newborn 762.6
    - complicating delivery 663.9❺
    - specified NEC 663.8❺
  - union
    - cricoid cartilage and thyroid cartilage 748.3
    - larynx and trachea 748.3
    - thyroid cartilage and hyoid bone 748.3
  - urination NEC 788.69
    - psychogenic 306.53
- **Abnormal, abnormality, abnormalities** – *continued*
  - urination – *continued*
    - stream
      - intermittent 788.61
      - slowing 788.62
      - splitting 788.61
      - weak 788.62
    - urgency 788.63
  - urine (constituents) NEC 791.9
  - uterine hemorrhage (*see also* Hemorrhage, uterus) 626.9
    - climacteric 627.0
    - postmenopausal 627.1
  - vagina (acquired) (congenital)
    - in pregnancy or childbirth 654.7❺
      - affecting fetus or newborn 763.89
      - causing obstructed labor 660.2❺
        - affecting fetus or newborn 763.1
  - vascular sounds 785.9
  - vectorcardiogram 794.39
  - visually evoked potential (VEP) 794.13
  - vulva (acquired) (congenital)
    - in pregnancy or childbirth 654.8❺
      - affecting fetus or newborn 763.89
      - causing obstructed labor 660.2❺
        - affecting fetus or newborn 763.1
  - weight
    - gain 783.1
      - of pregnancy 646.1❺
        - with hypertension – *see* Toxemia, of pregnancy
    - loss 783.21
  - x-ray examination – *see* Abnormal, radiological examination
- **Abnormally formed uterus** – *see* Anomaly, uterus
- **Abnormity (any organ or part)** – *see* Anomaly
- **ABO**
  - hemolytic disease 773.1
  - incompatibility reaction 999.6
- **Abocclusion** 524.20
- **Abolition, language** 784.69
- **Aborter, habitual or recurrent** NEC
  - without current pregnancy 629.81
  - current abortion (*see also* Abortion, spontaneous) 634.9❺
    - affecting fetus or newborn 761.8
  - observation in current pregnancy 646.3❺
- **Abortion** (complete) (incomplete) (inevitable) (with retained products of conception) 637.9❺

  Note – Use the following fifth-digit subclassification with categories 634-637:

  0 unspecified
  1 incomplete
  2 complete

  - with
    - complication(s) (any) following previous abortion – *see* category 639❹
    - damage to pelvic organ (laceration) (rupture) (tear) 637.2❺
    - embolism (air) (amniotic fluid) (blood clot) (pulmonary) (pyemic) (septic) (soap) 637.6❺
    - genital tract and pelvic infection 637.0❺
    - hemorrhage, delayed or excessive 637.1❺
    - metabolic disorder 637.4❺
    - renal failure (acute) 637.3❺
    - sepsis (genital tract) (pelvic organ) 637.0❺
      - urinary tract 637.7❺
    - shock (postoperative) (septic) 637.5❺
    - specified complication NEC 637.7❺
    - toxemia 637.3❺
    - unspecified complication(s) 637.8❺
    - urinary tract infection 637.7❺
  - accidental – *see* Abortion, spontaneous
  - artificial – *see* Abortion, induced
  - attempted (failed) – *see* Abortion, failed
  - criminal – *see* Abortion, illegal
  - early – *see* Abortion, spontaneous
  - elective – *see* Abortion, legal
  - failed (legal) 638.9
    - with
      - damage to pelvic organ (laceration) (rupture) (tear) 638.2
      - embolism (air) (amniotic fluid) (blood clot) (pulmonary) (pyemic) (septic) (soap) 638.6
      - genital tract and pelvic infection 638.0
      - hemorrhage, delayed or excessive 638.1
      - metabolic disorder 638.4
      - renal failure (acute) 638.3

Abortion – *continued*
failed – *continued*
with – *continued*
sepsis (genital tract) (pelvic organ) 638.0
urinary tract 638.7
shock (postoperative) (septic) 638.5
specified complication NEC 638.7
toxemia 638.3
unspecified complication(s) 638.8
urinary tract infection 638.7
fetal indication – *see* Abortion, legal
fetus 779.6
following threatened abortion – *see* Abortion, by type
habitual or recurrent (care during pregnancy) 646.3❺
with current abortion (*see also* Abortion, spontaneous) 634.9❺
affecting fetus or newborn 761.8
without current pregnancy 629.81
homicidal – *see* Abortion, illegal
illegal 636.9❺
with
damage to pelvic organ (laceration) (rupture) (tear) 636.2❺
embolism (air) (amniotic fluid) (blood clot) (pulmonary) (pyemic) (septic) (soap) 636.6❺
genital tract and pelvic infection 636.0❺
hemorrhage, delayed or excessive 636.1❺
metabolic disorder 636.4❺
renal failure 636.3❺
sepsis (genital tract) (pelvic organ) 636.0❺
urinary tract 636.7❺
shock (postoperative) (septic) 636.5❺
specified complication NEC 636.7❺
toxemia 636.3❺
unspecified complication(s) 636.8❺
urinary tract infection 636.7❺
fetus 779.6
induced 637.9❺
illegal – *see* Abortion, illegal
legal indications – *see* Abortion, legal
medical indications – *see* Abortion, legal
therapeutic – *see* Abortion, legal
late – *see* Abortion, spontaneous
legal (legal indication) (medical indication) (under medical supervision) 635.9❺
with
damage to pelvic organ (laceration) (rupture) (tear) 635.2❺
embolism (air) (amniotic fluid) (blood clot) (pulmonary) (pyemic) (septic) (soap) 635.6❺
genital tract and pelvic infection 635.0❺
hemorrhage, delayed or excessive 635.1❺
metabolic disorder 635.4❺
renal failure (acute) 635.3❺
sepsis (genital tract) (pelvic organ) 635.0❺
urinary tract 635.7❺
shock (postoperative) (septic) 635.5❺
specified complication NEC 635.7❺
toxemia 635.3❺
unspecified complication(s) 635.8❺
urinary tract infection 635.7❺
fetus 779.6
medical indication – *see* Abortion, legal
mental hygiene problem – *see* Abortion, legal
missed 632
operative – *see* Abortion, legal
psychiatric indication – *see* Abortion, legal
recurrent – *see* Abortion, spontaneous
self-induced – *see* Abortion, illegal
septic – *see* Abortion, by type, with sepsis
spontaneous 634.9❺
with
damage to pelvic organ (laceration) (rupture) (tear) 634.2❺
embolism (air) (amniotic fluid) (blood clot) (pulmonary) (pyemic) (septic) (soap) 634.6❺
genital tract and pelvic infection 634.0❺
hemorrhage, delayed or excessive 634.1❺
metabolic disorder 634.4❺
renal failure 634.3❺
sepsis (genital tract) (pelvic organ) 634.0❺
urinary tract 634.7❺
shock (postoperative) (septic) 634.5❺
specified complication NEC 634.7❺
toxemia 634.3❺
unspecified complication(s) 634.8❺
urinary tract infection 634.7❺

Abortion – *continued*
spontaneous – *continued*
fetus 761.8
threatened 640.0❺
affecting fetus or newborn 762.1
surgical – *see* Abortion, legal
therapeutic – *see* Abortion, legal
threatened 640.0❺
affecting fetus or newborn 762.1
tubal – *see* Pregnancy, tubal
voluntary – *see* Abortion, legal
Abortus fever 023.9
Aboulomania 301.6
Abrachia 755.20
Abrachiatism 755.20
Abrachiocephalia 759.89
Abrachiocephalus 759.89
Abrami's disease (acquired hemolytic jaundice) 283.9
Abramov-Fiedler myocarditis (acute isolated myocarditis) 422.91
Abrasion – *see also* Injury, superficial, by site
cornea 918.1
dental 521.20
extending into
dentine 521.22
pulp 521.23
generalized 521.25
limited to enamel 521.21
localized 521.24
teeth, tooth (dentifrice) (habitual) (hard tissues) (occupational) (ritual) (traditional) (wedge defect) (*see also* Abrasion, dental) 521.20
Abrikossov's tumor (M9580/0) – *see also* Neoplasm, connective tissue, benign
malignant (M9580/3) – *see* Neoplasm, connective tissue, malignant
Abrism 988.8
Abruption, placenta – *see* Placenta, abruptio
Abruptio placentae – *see* Placenta, abruptio
Abscess (acute) (chronic) (infectional) (lymphangitic) (metastatic) (multiple) (pyogenic) (septic) (with lymphangitis) (*see also* Cellulitis) 682.9
abdomen, abdominal
cavity 567.22
wall 682.2
abdominopelvic 567.22
accessory sinus (chronic) (*see also* Sinusitis) 473.9
adrenal (capsule) (gland) 255.8
alveolar 522.5
with sinus 522.7
amebic 006.3
bladder 006.8
brain (with liver or lung abscess) 006.5
liver (without mention of brain or lung abscess) 006.3
with
brain abscess (and lung abscess) 006.5
lung abscess 006.4
lung (with liver abscess) 006.4
with brain abscess 006.5
seminal vesicle 006.8
specified site NEC 006.8
spleen 006.8
anaerobic 040.0
ankle 682.6
anorectal 566
antecubital space 682.3
antrum (chronic) (Highmore) (*see also* Sinusitis, maxillary) 473.0
anus 566
apical (tooth) 522.5
with sinus (alveolar) 522.7
appendix 540.1
areola (acute) (chronic) (nonpuerperal) 611.0
puerperal, postpartum 675.1❺
arm (any part, above wrist) 682.3
artery (wall) 447.2
atheromatous 447.2
auditory canal (external) 380.10
auricle (ear) (staphylococcal) (streptococcal) 380.10
axilla, axillary (region) 682.3
lymph gland or node 683
back (any part) 682.2
Bartholin's gland 616.3
with
abortion – *see* Abortion, by type, with sepsis

Abscess – *continued*
Bartholin's gland – *continued*
with – *continued*
ectopic pregnancy (*see also* categories 633.0-633.9) 639.0
molar pregnancy (*see also* categories 630-632) 639.0
complicating pregnancy or puerperium 646.6❺
following
abortion 639.0
ectopic or molar pregnancy 639.0
bartholinian 616.3
Bezold's 383.01
bile, biliary, duct or tract (*see also* Cholecystitis) 576.8
bilharziasis 120.1
bladder (wall) 595.89
amebic 006.8
bone (subperiosteal) (*see also* Osteomyelitis) 730.0❺
accessory sinus (chronic) (*see also* Sinusitis) 473.9
acute 730.0❺
chronic or old 730.1❺
jaw (lower) (upper) 526.4
mastoid – *see* Mastoiditis, acute
petrous (*see also* Petrositis) 383.20
spinal (tuberculous) (*see also* Tuberculosis) 015.0❺ *[730.88]*
nontuberculous 730.08
bowel 569.5
brain (any part) 324.0
amebic (with liver or lung abscess) 006.5
cystic 324.0
late effect – *see* category 326
otogenic 324.0
tuberculous (*see also* Tuberculosis) 013.3❺
breast (acute) (chronic) (nonpuerperal) 611.0
newborn 771.5
puerperal, postpartum 675.1❺
tuberculous (*see also* Tuberculosis) 017.9❺
broad ligament (chronic) (*see also* Disease, pelvis, inflammatory) 614.4
acute 614.3
Brodie's (chronic) (localized) (*see also* Osteomyelitis) 730.1❺
bronchus 519.19
buccal cavity 528.3
bulbourethral gland 597.0
bursa 727.89
pharyngeal 478.29
buttock 682.5
canaliculus, breast 611.0
canthus 372.20
cartilage 733.99
cecum 569.5
with appendicitis 540.1
cerebellum, cerebellar 324.0
late effect – *see* category 326
cerebral (embolic) 324.0
late effect – *see* category 326
cervical (neck region) 682.1
lymph gland or node 683
stump (*see also* Cervicitis) 616.0
cervix (stump) (uteri) (*see also* Cervicitis) 616.0
cheek, external 682.0
inner 528.3
chest 510.9
with fistula 510.0
wall 682.2
chin 682.0
choroid 363.00
ciliary body 364.3
circumtonsillar 475
cold (tuberculous) – *see also* Tuberculosis, abscess
articular – *see* Tuberculosis, joint
colon (wall) 569.5
colostomy or enterostomy 569.61
conjunctiva 372.00
connective tissue NEC 682.9
cornea 370.55
with ulcer 370.00
corpus
cavernosum 607.2
luteum (*see also* Salpingo-oophoritis) 614.2
Cowper's gland 597.0
cranium 324.0
cul-de-sac (Douglas') (posterior) (*see also* Disease, pelvis, inflammatory) 614.4
acute 614.3

Abscess – *continued*
- dental 522.5
  - with sinus (alveolar) 522.7
- dentoalveolar 522.5
  - with sinus (alveolar) 522.7
- diaphragm, diaphragmatic 567.22
- digit NEC 681.9
- Douglas' cul-de-sac or pouch (*see also* Disease, pelvis, inflammatory) 614.4
  - acute 614.3
- Dubois' 090.5
- ductless gland 259.8
- ear
  - acute 382.00
  - external 380.10
  - inner 386.30
  - middle – *see* Otitis media
- elbow 682.3
- endamebic – *see* Abscess, amebic
- entamebic – *see* Abscess, amebic
- enterostomy 569.61
- epididymis 604.0
- epidural 324.9
  - brain 324.0
  - late effect – *see* category 326
  - spinal cord 324.1
- epiglottis 478.79
- epiploon, epiploic 567.22
- erysipelatous (*see also* Erysipelas) 035
- esophagostomy 530.86
- esophagus 530.19
- ethmoid (bone) (chronic) (sinus) (*see also* Sinusitis, ethmoidal) 473.2
- external auditory canal 380.10
- extradural 324.9
  - brain 324.0
  - late effect – *see* category 326
  - spinal cord 324.1
- extraperitoneal – *see* Abscess, peritoneum
- eye 360.00
- eyelid 373.13
- face (any part, except eye) 682.0
- fallopian tube (*see also* Salpingo-oophoritis) 614.2
- fascia 728.89
- fauces 478.29
- fecal 569.5
- femoral (region) 682.6
- filaria, filarial (*see also* Infestation, filarial) 125.9
- finger (any) (intrathecal) (periosteal) (subcutaneous) (subcuticular) 681.00
- fistulous NEC 682.9
- flank 682.2
- foot (except toe) 682.7
- forearm 682.3
- forehead 682.0
- frontal (sinus) (chronic) (*see also* Sinusitis, frontal) 473.1
- gallbladder (*see also* Cholecystitis, acute) 575.0
- gastric 535.0❺
- genital organ or tract NEC
  - female 616.9
    - with
      - abortion – *see* Abortion, by type, with sepsis
      - ectopic pregnancy (*see also* categories 633.0-633.9) 639.0
      - molar pregnancy (*see also* categories 630-632) 639.0
    - following
      - abortion 639.0
      - ectopic or molar pregnancy 639.0
    - puerperal, postpartum, childbirth 670❹
  - male 608.4
- genitourinary system, tuberculous (*see also* Tuberculosis) 016.9❺
- gingival 523.30
- gland, glandular (lymph) (acute) NEC 683
- glottis 478.79
- gluteal (region) 682.5
- gonorrheal NEC (*see also* Gonococcus) 098.0
- groin 682.2
- gum 523.30
- hand (except finger or thumb) 682.4
- head (except face) 682.8
- heart 429.89
- heel 682.7
- helminthic (*see also* Infestation, by specific parasite) 128.9
- hepatic 572.0
  - amebic (*see also* Abscess, liver, amebic) 006.3
  - duct 576.8
- hip 682.6
  - tuberculous (active) (*see also* Tuberculosis) 015.1❺
- ileocecal 540.1
- ileostomy (bud) 569.61
- iliac (region) 682.2
  - fossa 540.1
- iliopsoas 567.31
  - tuberculous (*see also* Tuberculosis) 015.0 *[730.88]*
- infraclavicular (fossa) 682.3
- inguinal (region) 682.2
  - lymph gland or node 683
- intersphincteric (anus) 566
- intestine, intestinal 569.5
  - rectal 566
- intra-abdominal (*see also* Abscess, peritoneum) 567.22
  - postoperative 998.59
- intracranial 324.0
  - late effect – *see* category 326
- intramammary – *see* Abscess, breast
- intramastoid (*see also* Mastoiditis, acute) 383.00
- intraorbital 376.01
- intraperitoneal 567.22
- intraspinal 324.1
  - late effect – *see* category 326
- intratonsillar 475
- iris 364.3
- ischiorectal 566
- jaw (bone) (lower) (upper) 526.4
  - skin 682.0
- joint (*see also* Arthritis, pyogenic) 711.0❺
  - vertebral (tuberculous) (*see also* Tuberculosis) 015.0❺ *[730.88]*
    - nontuberculous 724.8
- kidney 590.2
  - with
    - abortion – *see* Abortion, by type, with urinary tract infection
    - calculus 592.0
    - ectopic pregnancy (*see also* categories 633.0-633.9) 639.8
    - molar pregnancy (*see also* categories 630-632) 639.8
  - complicating pregnancy or puerperium 646.6❺
    - affecting fetus or newborn 760.1
  - following
    - abortion 639.8
    - ectopic or molar pregnancy 639.8
- knee 682.6
  - joint 711.06
  - tuberculous (active) (*see also* Tuberculosis) 015.2❺
- labium (majus) (minus) 616.4
  - complicating pregnancy, childbirth, or puerperium 646.6❺
- lacrimal (passages) (sac) (*see also* Dacryocystitis) 375.30
  - caruncle 375.30
  - gland (*see also* Dacryoadenitis) 375.00
- lacunar 597.0
- larynx 478.79
- lateral (alveolar) 522.5
  - with sinus 522.7
- leg, except foot 682.6
- lens 360.00
- lid 373.13
- lingual 529.0
  - tonsil 475
- lip 528.5
- Littre's gland 597.0
- liver 572.0
  - amebic 006.3
    - with
      - brain abscess (and lung abscess) 006.5
      - lung abscess 006.4
  - due to Entamoeba histolytica 006.3
  - dysenteric (*see also* Abscess, liver, amebic) 006.3
  - pyogenic 572.0
  - tropical (*see also* Abscess, liver, amebic) 006.3
- loin (region) 682.2
- lumbar (tuberculous) (*see also* Tuberculosis) 015.0❺ *[730.88]*
  - nontuberculous 682.2
- lung (miliary) (putrid) 513.0
  - amebic (with liver abscess) 006.4
    - with brain abscess 006.5
- lymph, lymphatic, gland or node (acute) 683
  - any site, except mesenteric 683
  - mesentery 289.2
- lymphangitic, acute – *see* Cellulitis
- malar 526.4
- mammary gland – *see* Abscess, breast
- marginal (anus) 566
- mastoid (process) (*see also* Mastoiditis, acute) 383.00
  - subperiosteal 383.01
- maxilla, maxillary 526.4
  - molar (tooth) 522.5
    - with sinus 522.7
  - premolar 522.5
  - sinus (chronic) (*see also* Sinusitis, maxillary) 473.0
- mediastinum 513.1
- meibomian gland 373.12
- meninges (*see also* Meningitis) 320.9
- mesentery, mesenteric 567.22
- mesosalpinx (*see also* Salpingo-oophoritis) 614.2
- milk 675.1❺
- Monro's (psoriasis) 696.1
- mons pubis 682.2
- mouth (floor) 528.3
- multiple sites NEC 682.9
- mural 682.2
- muscle 728.89
  - psoas 567.31
- myocardium 422.92
- nabothian (follicle) (*see also* Cervicitis) 616.0
- nail (chronic) (with lymphangitis) 681.9
  - finger 681.02
  - toe 681.11
- nasal (fossa) (septum) 478.19
  - sinus (chronic) (*see also* Sinusitis) 473.9
- nasopharyngeal 478.29
- nates 682.5
- navel 682.2
  - newborn NEC 771.4
- neck (region) 682.1
  - lymph gland or node 683
- nephritic (*see also* Abscess, kidney) 590.2
- nipple 611.0
  - puerperal, postpartum 675.0❺
- nose (septum) 478.19
  - external 682.0
- omentum 567.22
- operative wound 998.59
- orbit, orbital 376.01
- ossifluent – *see* Abscess, bone
- ovary, ovarian (corpus luteum) (*see also* Salpingo-oophoritis) 614.2
- oviduct (*see also* Salpingo-oophoritis) 614.2
- palate (soft) 528.3
  - hard 526.4
- palmar (space) 682.4
- pancreas (duct) 577.0
- paradontal 523.30
- parafrenal 607.2
- parametric, parametrium (chronic) (*see also* Disease, pelvis, inflammatory) 614.4
  - acute 614.3
- paranephric 590.2
- parapancreatic 577.0
- parapharyngeal 478.22
- pararectal 566
- parasinus (*see also* Sinusitis) 473.9
- parauterine (*see also* Disease, pelvis, inflammatory) 614.4
  - acute 614.3
- paravaginal (*see also* Vaginitis) 616.10
- parietal region 682.8
- parodontal 523.30
- parotid (duct) (gland) 527.3
  - region 528.3
- parumbilical 682.2
  - newborn 771.4
- pectoral (region) 682.2
- pelvirectal 567.22
- pelvis, pelvic
  - female (chronic) (*see also* Disease, pelvis, inflammatory) 614.4
    - acute 614.3
  - male, peritoneal (cellular tissue) – *see* Abscess, peritoneum
  - tuberculous (*see also* Tuberculosis) 016.9❺

Abscess – *continued*
- penis 607.2
  - gonococcal (acute) 098.0
    - chronic or duration of 2 months or over 098.2
- perianal 566
- periapical 522.5
  - with sinus (alveolar) 522.7
- periappendiceal 540.1
- pericardial 420.99
- pericecal 540.1
- pericemental 523.30
- pericholecystic (*see also* Cholecystitis, acute) 575.0
- pericoronal 523.30
- peridental 523.30
- perigastric 535.0❺
- perimetric (*see also* Disease, pelvis, inflammatory) 614.4
  - acute 614.3
- perinephric, perinephritic (*see also* Abscess, kidney) 590.2
- perineum, perineal (superficial) 682.2
  - deep (with urethral involvement) 597.0
  - urethra 597.0
- periodontal (parietal) 523.31
  - apical 522.5
- periosteum, periosteal (*see also* Periostitis) 730.3❺
  - with osteomyelitis (*see also* Osteomyelitis) 730.2❺
    - acute or subacute 730.0❺
    - chronic or old 730.1❺
- peripleuritic 510.9
  - with fistula 510.0
- periproctic 566
- periprostatic 601.2
- perirectal (staphylococcal) 566
- perirenal (tissue) (*see also* Abscess, kidney) 590.2
- perisinuous (nose) (*see also* Sinusitis) 473.9
- peritoneum, peritoneal (perforated) (ruptured) 567.22
  - with
    - abortion – *see* Abortion, by type, with sepsis
    - appendicitis 540.1
    - ectopic pregnancy (*see also* categories 633.0-633.9) 639.0
    - molar pregnancy (*see also* categories 630-632) 639.0
  - following
    - abortion 639.0
    - ectopic or molar pregnancy 639.0
  - pelvic, female (*see also* Disease, pelvis, inflammatory) 614.4
    - acute 614.3
  - postoperative 998.59
  - puerperal, postpartum, childbirth 670❹
  - tuberculous (*see also* Tuberculosis) 014.0❺
- peritonsillar 475
- perityphlic 540.1
- periureteral 593.89
- periurethral 597.0
  - gonococcal (acute) 098.0
    - chronic or duration of 2 months or over 098.2
- periuterine (*see also* Disease, pelvis, inflammatory) 614.4
  - acute 614.3
- perivesical 595.89
- pernicious NEC 682.9
- petrous bone – *see* Petrositis
- phagedenic NEC 682.9
  - chancroid 099.0
- pharynx, pharyngeal (lateral) 478.29
- phlegmonous NEC 682.9
- pilonidal 685.0
- pituitary (gland) 253.8
- pleura 510.9
  - with fistula 510.0
- popliteal 682.6
- postanal 566
- postcecal 540.1
- postlaryngeal 478.79
- postnasal 478.19
- postpharyngeal 478.24
- posttonsillar 475
- posttyphoid 002.0
- Pott's (*see also* Tuberculosis) 015.0❺ *[730.88]*
- pouch of Douglas (chronic) (*see also* Disease, pelvis, inflammatory) 614.4
- premammary – *see* Abscess, breast

Abscess – *continued*
- prepatellar 682.6
- prostate (*see also* Prostatitis) 601.2
  - gonococcal (acute) 098.12
    - chronic or duration of 2 months or over 098.32
- psoas 567.31
  - tuberculous (*see also* Tuberculosis) 015.0❺ *[730.88]*
- pterygopalatine fossa 682.8
- pubis 682.2
- puerperal – *see* Puerperal, abscess, by site
- pulmonary – *see* Abscess, lung
- pulp, pulpal (dental) 522.0
  - finger 681.01
  - toe 681.10
- pyemic – *see* septicemia
- pyloric valve 535.0❺
- rectovaginal septum 569.5
- rectovesical 595.89
- rectum 566
- regional NEC 682.9
- renal (*see also* Abscess, kidney) 590.2
- retina 363.00
- retrobulbar 376.01
- retrocecal 567.22
- retrolaryngeal 478.79
- retromammary – *see* Abscess, breast
- retroperineal 682.2
- retroperitoneal 567.38
  - postprocedural 998.59
- retropharyngeal 478.24
  - tuberculous (*see also* Tuberculosis) 012.8❺
- retrorectal 566
- retrouterine (*see also* Disease, pelvis, inflammatory) 614.4
  - acute 614.3
- retrovesical 595.89
- root, tooth 522.5
  - with sinus (alveolar) 522.7
- round ligament (*see also* Disease, pelvis, inflammatory) 614.4
  - acute 614.3
- rupture (spontaneous) NEC 682.9
- sacrum (tuberculous) (*see also* Tuberculosis) 015.0❺ *[730.88]*
  - nontuberculous 730.08
- salivary duct or gland 527.3
- scalp (any part) 682.8
- scapular 730.01
- sclera 379.09
- scrofulous (*see also* Tuberculosis) 017.2❺
- scrotum 608.4
- seminal vesicle 608.0
  - amebic 006.8
- septal, dental 522.5
  - with sinus (alveolar) 522.7
- septum (nasal) 478.19
- serous (*see also* Periostitis) 730.3❺
- shoulder 682.3
- side 682.2
- sigmoid 569.5
- sinus (accessory) (chronic) (nasal) (*see also* Sinusitis) 473.9
  - intracranial venous (any) 324.0
    - late effect – *see* category 326
- Skene's duct or gland 597.0
- skin NEC 682.9
  - tuberculous (primary) (*see also* Tuberculosis) 017.0❺
- sloughing NEC 682.9
- specified site NEC 682.8
  - amebic 006.8
- spermatic cord 608.4
- sphenoidal (sinus) (*see also* Sinusitis, sphenoidal) 473.3
- spinal
  - cord (any part) (staphylococcal) 324.1
    - tuberculous (*see also* Tuberculosis) 013.5❺
  - epidural 324.1
- spine (column) (tuberculous) (*see also* Tuberculosis) 015.0❺ *[730.88]*
  - nontuberculous 730.08
- spleen 289.59
  - amebic 006.8
- staphylococcal NEC 682.9
- stitch 998.59
- stomach (wall) 535.0❺
- strumous (tuberculous) (*see also* Tuberculosis) 017.2❺

Abscess – *continued*
- subarachnoid 324.9
  - brain 324.0
  - cerebral 324.0
  - late effect – *see* category 326
  - spinal cord 324.1
- subareolar – *see also* Abscess, breast
  - puerperal, postpartum 675.1❺
- subcecal 540.1
- subcutaneous NEC 682.9
- subdiaphragmatic 567.22
- subdorsal 682.2
- subdural 324.9
  - brain 324.0
  - late effect – *see* category 326
  - spinal cord 324.1
- subgaleal 682.8
- subhepatic 567.22
- sublingual 528.3
  - gland 527.3
- submammary – *see* Abscess, breast
- submandibular (region) (space) (triangle) 682.0
  - gland 527.3
- submaxillary (region) 682.0
  - gland 527.3
- submental (pyogenic) 682.0
  - gland 527.3
- subpectoral 682.2
- subperiosteal – *see* Abscess, bone
- subperitoneal 567.22
- subphrenic – *see also* Abscess, peritoneum 567.22
  - postoperative 998.59
- subscapular 682.2
- subungual 681.9
- suburethral 597.0
- sudoriparous 705.89
- suppurative NEC 682.9
- supraclavicular (fossa) 682.3
- suprahepatic 567.22
- suprapelvic (*see also* Disease, pelvis, inflammatory) 614.4
  - acute 614.3
- suprapubic 682.2
- suprarenal (capsule) (gland) 255.8
- sweat gland 705.89
- syphilitic 095.8
- teeth, tooth (root) 522.5
  - with sinus (alveolar) 522.7
  - supporting structures NEC 523.30
- temple 682.0
- temporal region 682.0
- temporosphenoidal 324.0
  - late effect – *see* category 326
- tendon (sheath) 727.89
- testicle – *see* Orchitis
- thecal 728.89
- thigh (acquired) 682.6
- thorax 510.9
  - with fistula 510.0
- throat 478.29
- thumb (intrathecal) (periosteal) (subcutaneous) (subcuticular) 681.00
- thymus (gland) 254.1
- thyroid (gland) 245.0
- toe (any) (intrathecal) (periosteal) (subcutaneous) (subcuticular) 681.10
- tongue (staphylococcal) 529.0
- tonsil(s) (lingual) 475
- tonsillopharyngeal 475
- tooth, teeth (root) 522.5
  - with sinus (alveolar) 522.7
  - supporting structures NEC 523.30
- trachea 478.9
- trunk 682.2
- tubal (*see also* Salpingo-oophoritis) 614.2
- tuberculous – *see* Tuberculosis, abscess
- tubo-ovarian (*see also* Salpingo-oophoritis) 614.2
- tunica vaginalis 608.4
- umbilicus NEC 682.2
  - newborn 771.4
- upper arm 682.3
- upper respiratory 478.9
- urachus 682.2
- urethra (gland) 597.0
- urinary 597.0
- uterus, uterine (wall) (*see also* Endometritis) 615.9
  - ligament (*see also* Disease, pelvis, inflammatory) 614.4
    - acute 614.3
  - neck (*see also* Cervicitis) 616.0

❹ Fourth-Digit Required   ❺ Fifth-Digit Required   *[code]* Manifestation Code   ►◄ Revised Text   ● New Line   ▲ Revised Code

- **Abscess** – *continued*
  - uvula 528.3
  - vagina (wall) (*see also* Vaginitis) 616.10
  - vaginorectal (*see also* Vaginitis) 616.10
  - vas deferens 608.4
  - vermiform appendix 540.1
  - vertebra (column) (tuberculous) (*see also* Tuberculosis) 015.0❺ *[730.88]*
    - nontuberculous 730.0❺
  - vesical 595.89
  - vesicouterine pouch (*see also* Disease, pelvis, inflammatory) 614.4
  - vitreous (humor) (pneumococcal) 360.04
  - vocal cord 478.5
  - von Bezold's 383.01
  - vulva 616.4
    - complicating pregnancy, childbirth, or puerperium 646.6❺
  - vulvovaginal gland (*see also* Vaginitis) 616.3
  - web-space 682.4
  - wrist 682.4
- **Absence** (organ or part) (complete or partial)
  - acoustic nerve 742.8
  - adrenal (gland) (congenital) 759.1
    - acquired V45.79
  - albumin (blood) 273.8
  - alimentary tract (complete) (congenital) (partial) 751.8
    - lower 751.5
    - upper 750.8
  - alpha-fucosidase 271.8
  - alveolar process (acquired) 525.8
    - congenital 750.26
  - anus, anal (canal) (congenital) 751.2
  - aorta (congenital) 747.22
  - aortic valve (congenital) 746.89
  - appendix, congenital 751.2
  - arm (acquired) V49.60
    - above elbow V49.66
    - below elbow V49.65
    - congenital (*see also* Deformity, reduction, upper limb) 755.20
      - lower – *see* Absence, forearm, congenital
      - upper (complete) (partial) (with absence of distal elements, incomplete) 755.24
        - with
          - complete absence of distal elements 755.21
          - forearm (incomplete) 755.23
  - artery (congenital) (peripheral) NEC (*see also* Anomaly, peripheral vascular system) 747.60
    - brain 747.81
    - cerebral 747.81
    - coronary 746.85
    - pulmonary 747.3
    - umbilical 747.5
  - atrial septum 745.69
  - auditory canal (congenital) (external) 744.01
  - auricle (ear) (with stenosis or atresia of auditory canal), congenital 744.01
  - bile, biliary duct (common) or passage (congenital) 751.61
  - bladder (acquired) V45.74
    - congenital 753.8
  - bone (congenital) NEC 756.9
    - marrow 284.9
      - acquired (secondary) 284.89 ▲
      - congenital 284.09
      - hereditary 284.09
      - idiopathic 284.9
    - skull 756.0
  - bowel sounds 787.5
  - brain 740.0
    - specified part 742.2
  - breast(s) (acquired) V45.71
    - congenital 757.6
  - broad ligament (congenital) 752.19
  - bronchus (congenital) 748.3
  - calvarium, calvaria (skull) 756.0
  - canaliculus lacrimalis, congenital 743.65
  - carpal(s) (congenital) (complete) (partial) (with absence of distal elements, incomplete) (*see also* Deformity, reduction, upper limb) 755.28
    - with complete absence of distal elements 755.21
  - cartilage 756.9
  - caudal spine 756.13
  - cecum (acquired) (postoperative) (posttraumatic) V45.72
    - congenital 751.2
  - cementum 520.4
- **Absence** – *continued*
  - cerebellum (congenital) (vermis) 742.2
  - cervix (acquired) (uteri) V45.77
    - congenital 752.49
  - chin, congenital 744.89
  - cilia (congenital) 743.63
    - acquired 374.89
  - circulatory system, part NEC 747.89
  - clavicle 755.51
  - clitoris (congenital) 752.49
  - coccyx, congenital 756.13
  - cold sense (*see also* Disturbance, sensation) 782.0
  - colon (acquired) (postoperative) V45.72
    - congenital 751.2
  - congenital
    - lumen – *see* Atresia
    - organ or site NEC – *see* Agenesis
    - septum – *see* Imperfect, closure
  - corpus callosum (congenital) 742.2
  - cricoid cartilage 748.3
  - diaphragm (congenital) (with hernia) 756.6
    - with obstruction 756.6
  - digestive organ(s) or tract, congenital (complete) (partial) 751.8
    - acquired V45.79
    - lower 751.5
    - upper 750.8
  - ductus arteriosus 747.89
  - duodenum (acquired) (postoperative) V45.72
    - congenital 751.1
  - ear, congenital 744.09
    - acquired V45.79
    - auricle 744.01
    - external 744.01
    - inner 744.05
    - lobe, lobule 744.21
    - middle, except ossicles 744.03
      - ossicles 744.04
    - ossicles 744.04
  - ejaculatory duct (congenital) 752.89
  - endocrine gland NEC (congenital) 759.2
  - epididymis (congenital) 752.89
    - acquired V45.77
  - epiglottis, congenital 748.3
  - epileptic (atonic) (typical) (*see also* Epilepsy) 345.0❺
  - erythrocyte 284.9
  - erythropoiesis 284.9
    - congenital 284.01
  - esophagus (congenital) 750.3
  - Eustachian tube (congenital) 744.24
  - extremity (acquired)
    - congenital (*see also* Deformity, reduction) 755.4
    - lower V49.70
    - upper V49.60
  - extrinsic muscle, eye 743.69
  - eye (acquired) V45.78
    - adnexa (congenital) 743.69
    - congenital 743.00
    - muscle (congenital) 743.69
  - eyelid (fold), congenital 743.62
    - acquired 374.89
  - face
    - bones NEC 756.0
    - specified part NEC 744.89
  - fallopian tube(s) (acquired) V45.77
    - congenital 752.19
  - femur, congenital (complete) (partial) (with absence of distal elements, incomplete) (*see also* Deformity, reduction, lower limb) 755.34
    - with
      - complete absence of distal elements 755.31
      - tibia and fibula (incomplete) 755.33
  - fibrin 790.92
  - fibrinogen (congenital) 286.3
    - acquired 286.6
  - fibula, congenital (complete) (partial) (with absence of distal elements, incomplete) (*see also* Deformity, reduction, lower limb) 755.37
    - with
      - complete absence of distal elements 755.31
      - tibia 755.35
        - with
          - complete absence of distal elements 755.31
          - femur (incomplete) 755.33
            - with complete absence of distal elements 755.31
- **Absence** – *continued*
  - finger (acquired) V49.62
    - congenital (complete) (partial) (*see also* Deformity, reduction, upper limb) 755.29
      - meaning all fingers (complete) (partial) 755.21
      - transverse 755.21
  - fissures of lungs (congenital) 748.5
  - foot (acquired) V49.73
    - congenital (complete) 755.31
  - forearm (acquired) V49.65
    - congenital (complete) (partial) (with absence of distal elements, incomplete) (*see also* Deformity, reduction, upper limb) 755.25
      - with
        - complete absence of distal elements (hand and fingers) 755.21
        - humerus (incomplete) 755.23
  - fovea centralis 743.55
  - fucosidase 271.8
  - gallbladder (acquired) V45.79
    - congenital 751.69
  - gamma globulin (blood) 279.00
  - genital organs
    - acquired V45.77
    - congenital
      - female 752.89
        - external 752.49
        - internal NEC 752.89
      - male 752.89
        - penis 752.69
  - genitourinary organs, congenital NEC 752.89
  - glottis 748.3
  - gonadal, congenital NEC 758.6
  - hair (congenital) 757.4
    - acquired – *see* Alopecia
  - hand (acquired) V49.63
    - congenital (complete) (*see also* Deformity, reduction, upper limb) 755.21
  - heart (congenital) 759.89
    - acquired – *see* Status, organ replacement
  - heat sense (*see also* Disturbance, sensation) 782.0
  - humerus, congenital (complete) (partial) (with absence of distal elements, incomplete) (*see also* Deformity, reduction, upper limb) 755.24
    - with
      - complete absence of distal elements 755.21
      - radius and ulna (incomplete) 755.23
  - hymen (congenital) 752.49
  - ileum (acquired) (postoperative) (posttraumatic) V45.72
    - congenital 751.1
  - immunoglobulin, isolated NEC 279.03
    - IgA 279.01
    - IgG 279.03
    - IgM 279.02
  - incus (acquired) 385.24
    - congenital 744.04
  - internal ear (congenital) 744.05
  - intestine (acquired) (small) V45.72
    - congenital 751.1
      - large 751.2
    - large V45.72
      - congenital 751.2
  - iris (congenital) 743.45
  - jaw – *see* Absence, mandible
  - jejunum (acquired) V45.72
    - congenital 751.1
  - joint, congenital NEC 755.8
  - kidney(s) (acquired) V45.73
    - congenital 753.0
  - labium (congenital) (majus) (minus) 752.49
  - labyrinth, membranous 744.05
  - lacrimal apparatus (congenital) 743.65
  - larynx (congenital) 748.3
  - leg (acquired) V49.70
    - above knee V49.76
    - below knee V49.75
    - congenital (partial) (unilateral) (*see also* Deformity, reduction, lower limb) 755.31
      - lower (complete) (partial) (with absence of distal elements, incomplete) 755.35
        - with
          - complete absence of distal elements (foot and toes) 755.31
          - thigh (incomplete) 755.33
            - with complete absence of distal elements 755.31
      - upper – *see* Absence, femur

- **Absence** – *continued*
  - lens (congenital) 743.35
    - acquired 379.31
  - ligament, broad (congenital) 752.19
  - limb (acquired)
    - congenital (complete) (partial) (*see also* Deformity, reduction) 755.4
      - lower 755.30
        - complete 755.31
        - incomplete 755.32
        - longitudinal – *see* Deficiency, lower limb, longitudinal
        - transverse 755.31
      - upper 755.20
        - complete 755.21
        - incomplete 755.22
        - longitudinal – *see* Deficiency, upper limb, longitudinal
        - transverse 755.21
    - lower NEC V49.70
    - upper NEC V49.60
  - lip 750.26
  - liver (congenital) (lobe) 751.69
  - lumbar (congenital) (vertebra) 756.13
    - isthmus 756.11
    - pars articularis 756.11
  - lumen – *see* Atresia
  - lung (bilateral) (congenital) (fissure) (lobe) (unilateral) 748.5
    - acquired (any part) V45.76
  - mandible (congenital) 524.09
  - maxilla (congenital) 524.09
  - menstruation 626.0
  - metacarpal(s), congenital (complete) (partial) (with absence of distal elements, incomplete) (*see also* Deformity, reduction, upper limb) 755.28
    - with all fingers, complete 755.21
  - metatarsal(s), congenital (complete) (partial) (with absence of distal elements, incomplete) (*see also* Deformity, reduction, lower limb) 755.38
    - with complete absence of distal elements 755.31
  - muscle (congenital) (pectoral) 756.81
    - ocular 743.69
  - musculoskeletal system (congenital) NEC 756.9
  - nail(s) (congenital) 757.5
  - neck, part 744.89
  - nerve 742.8
  - nervous system, part NEC 742.8
  - neutrophil 288.00
  - nipple (congenital) 757.6
  - nose (congenital) 748.1
    - acquired 738.0
  - nuclear 742.8
  - ocular muscle (congenital) 743.69
  - organ
    - of Corti (congenital) 744.05
    - or site
      - acquired V45.79
      - congenital NEC 759.89
  - osseous meatus (ear) 744.03
  - ovary (acquired) V45.77
    - congenital 752.0
  - oviduct (acquired) V45.77
    - congenital 752.19
  - pancreas (congenital) 751.7
    - acquired (postoperative) (posttraumatic) V45.79
  - parathyroid gland (congenital) 759.2
  - parotid gland(s) (congenital) 750.21
  - patella, congenital 755.64
  - pelvic girdle (congenital) 755.69
  - penis (congenital) 752.69
    - acquired V45.77
  - pericardium (congenital) 746.89
  - perineal body (congenital) 756.81
  - phalange(s), congenital 755.4
    - lower limb (complete) (intercalary) (partial) (terminal) (*see also* Deformity, reduction, lower limb) 755.39
      - meaning all toes (complete) (partial) 755.31
      - transverse 755.31
    - upper limb (complete) (intercalary) (partial) (terminal) (*see also* Deformity, reduction, upper limb) 755.29
      - meaning all digits (complete) (partial) 755.21
      - transverse 755.21
  - pituitary gland (congenital) 759.2
  - postoperative – *see* Absence, by site, acquired

- **Absence** – *continued*
  - prostate (congenital) 752.89
    - acquired V45.77
  - pulmonary
    - artery 747.3
    - trunk 747.3
    - valve (congenital) 746.01
    - vein 747.49
  - punctum lacrimale (congenital) 743.65
  - radius, congenital (complete) (partial) (with absence of distal elements, incomplete) 755.26
    - with
      - complete absence of distal elements 755.21
      - ulna 755.25
        - with
          - complete absence of distal elements 755.21
          - humerus (incomplete) 755.23
  - ray, congenital 755.4
    - lower limb (complete) (partial) (*see also* Deformity, reduction, lower limb) 755.38
      - meaning all rays 755.31
      - transverse 755.31
    - upper limb (complete) (partial) (*see also* Deformity, reduction, upper limb) 755.28
      - meaning all rays 755.21
      - transverse 755.21
  - rectum (congenital) 751.2
    - acquired V45.79
  - red cell 284.9
    - acquired (secondary) 284.81 ▲
    - congenital 284.01
    - hereditary 284.01
    - idiopathic 284.9
  - respiratory organ (congenital) NEC 748.9
  - rib (acquired) 738.3
    - congenital 756.3
  - roof of orbit (congenital) 742.0
  - round ligament (congenital) 752.89
  - sacrum, congenital 756.13
  - salivary gland(s) (congenital) 750.21
  - scapula 755.59
  - scrotum, congenital 752.89
  - seminal tract or duct (congenital) 752.89
    - acquired V45.77
  - septum (congenital) – *see also* Imperfect, closure, septum
    - atrial 745.69
      - and ventricular 745.7
    - between aorta and pulmonary artery 745.0
    - ventricular 745.3
      - and atrial 745.7
  - sex chromosomes 758.81
  - shoulder girdle, congenital (complete) (partial) 755.59
  - skin (congenital) 757.39
  - skull bone 756.0
    - with
      - anencephalus 740.0
      - encephalocele 742.0
      - hydrocephalus 742.3
        - with spina bifida (*see also* Spina bifida) 741.0❺
      - microcephalus 742.1
  - spermatic cord (congenital) 752.89
  - spinal cord 742.59
  - spine, congenital 756.13
  - spleen (congenital) 759.0
    - acquired V45.79
  - sternum, congenital 756.3
  - stomach (acquired) (partial) (postoperative) V45.75
    - with postgastric surgery syndrome 564.2
    - congenital 750.7
  - submaxillary gland(s) (congenital) 750.21
  - superior vena cava (congenital) 747.49
  - tarsal(s), congenital (complete) (partial) (with absence of distal elements, incomplete) (*see also* Deformity, reduction, lower limb) 755.38
  - teeth, tooth (congenital) 520.0
    - with abnormal spacing 524.30
    - acquired 525.10
      - with malocclusion 524.30
      - due to
        - caries 525.13
        - extraction 525.10
        - periodontal disease 525.12
        - trauma 525.11
  - tendon (congenital) 756.81
  - testis (congenital) 752.89
    - acquired V45.77

- **Absence** – *continued*
  - thigh (acquired) 736.89
  - thumb (acquired) V49.61
    - congenital 755.29
  - thymus gland (congenital) 759.2
  - thyroid (gland) (surgical) 246.8
    - with hypothyroidism 244.0
    - cartilage, congenital 748.3
    - congenital 243
  - tibia, congenital (complete) (partial) (with absence of distal elements, incomplete) (*see also* Deformity, reduction, lower limb) 755.36
    - with
      - complete absence of distal elements 755.31
      - fibula 755.35
        - with
          - complete absence of distal elements 755.31
          - femur (incomplete) 755.33
            - with complete absence of distal elements 755.31
  - toe (acquired) V49.72
    - congenital (complete) (partial) 755.39
      - meaning all toes 755.31
      - transverse 755.31
    - great V49.71
  - tongue (congenital) 750.11
  - tooth, teeth (congenital) 520.0
    - with abnormal spacing 524.30
    - acquired 525.10
      - with malocclusion 524.30
      - due to
        - caries 525.13
        - extraction 525.10
        - periodontal disease 525.12
        - trauma 525.11
  - trachea (cartilage) (congenital) (rings) 748.3
  - transverse aortic arch (congenital) 747.21
  - tricuspid valve 746.1
  - ulna, congenital (complete) (partial) (with absence of distal elements, incomplete) (*see also* Deformity, reduction, upper limb) 755.27
    - with
      - complete absence of distal elements 755.21
      - radius 755.25
        - with
          - complete absence of distal elements 755.21
          - humerus (incomplete) 755.23
  - umbilical artery (congenital) 747.5
  - ureter (congenital) 753.4
    - acquired V45.74
  - urethra, congenital 753.8
    - acquired V45.74
  - urinary system, part NEC, congenital 753.8
    - acquired V45.74
  - uterus (acquired) V45.77
    - congenital 752.3
  - uvula (congenital) 750.26
  - vagina, congenital 752.49
    - acquired V45.77
  - vas deferens (congenital) 752.89
    - acquired V45.77
  - vein (congenital) (peripheral) NEC (*see also* Anomaly, peripheral vascular system) 747.60
    - brain 747.81
    - great 747.49
    - portal 747.49
    - pulmonary 747.49
  - vena cava (congenital) (inferior) (superior) 747.49
  - ventral horn cell 742.59
  - ventricular septum 745.3
  - vermis of cerebellum 742.2
  - vertebra, congenital 756.13
  - vulva, congenital 752.49
- **Absentia epileptica** (*see also* Epilepsy) 345.0❺
- **Absinthemia** (*see also* Dependence) 304.6❺
- **Absinthism** (*see also* Dependence) 304.6❺
- **Absorbent system disease** 459.89
- **Absorption**
  - alcohol, through placenta or breast milk 760.71
  - antibiotics, through placenta or breast milk 760.74
  - anticonvulsants, through placenta or breast milk 760.77
  - antifungals, through placenta or breast milk 760.74
  - anti-infective, through placenta or breast milk 760.74
  - antimetabolics, through placenta or breast milk 760.78

Absorption – *continued*
  chemical NEC 989.9
    specified chemical or substance – *see* Table of Drugs and Chemicals
    through placenta or breast milk (fetus or newborn) 760.70
      alcohol 760.71
      anticonvulsants 760.77
      antifungals 760.74
      anti-infective agents 760.74
      antimetabolics 760.78
      cocaine 760.75
      "crack" 760.75
      diethylstilbestrol [DES] 760.76
      hallucinogenic agents 760.73
      medicinal agents NEC 760.79
      narcotics 760.72
      obstetric anesthetic or analgesic drug 763.5
      specified agent NEC 760.79
      suspected, affecting management of pregnancy 655.5❺
  cocaine, through placenta or breast milk 760.75
  drug NEC (*see also* Reaction, drug)
    through placenta or breast milk (fetus or newborn) 760.70
      alcohol 760.71
      anticonvulsants 760.77
      antifungals 760.74
      anti-infective agents 760.74
      antimetabolics 760.78
      cocaine 760.75
      "crack" 760.75
      diethylstilbestrol (DES) 760.76
      hallucinogenic agents 760.73
      medicinal agents NEC 760.79
      narcotics 760.72
      obstetric anesthetic or analgesic drug 763.5
      specified agent NEC 760.79
      suspected, affecting management of pregnancy 655.5❺
  fat, disturbance 579.8
  hallucinogenic agents, through placenta or breast milk 760.73
  immune sera, through placenta or breast milk 760.79
  lactose defect 271.3
  medicinal agents NEC, through placenta or breast milk 760.79
  narcotics, through placenta or breast milk 760.72
  noxious substance – *see* Absorption, chemical
  protein, disturbance 579.8
  pus or septic, general – *see* Septicemia
  quinine, through placenta or breast milk 760.74
  toxic substance – *see* Absorption, chemical
  uremic – *see* Uremia
Abstinence symptoms or syndrome
  alcohol 291.81
  drug 292.0
Abt-Letterer-Siwe syndrome (acute histiocytosis X) (M9722/3) 202.5❺
Abulia 799.89
Abulomania 301.6
Abuse
  adult 995.80
    emotional 995.82
    multiple forms 995.85
    neglect (nutritional) 995.84
    physical 995.81
    psychological 995.82
    sexual 995.83
  alcohol (*see also* Alcoholism) 305.0❺
    dependent 303.9❺
    nondependent 305.0❺
  child 995.50
    counseling
      perpetrator
        non-parent V62.83
        parent V61.22
      victim V61.21
    emotional 995.51
    multiple forms 995.59
    neglect (nutritional) 995.52
    physical 995.54
      shaken infant syndrome 995.55
    psychological 995.51
    sexual 995.53

Abuse – *continued*
  drugs, nondependent 305.9❺

Note – Use the following fifth-digit subclassification with the following codes: 305.0, 305.2-305.9:
0 unspecified
1 continuous
2 episodic
3 in remission

    amphetamine type 305.7❺
    antidepressants 305.8❺
    anxiolytic 305.4❺
    barbiturates 305.4❺
    caffeine 305.9❺
    cannabis 305.2❺
    cocaine type 305.6❺
    hallucinogens 305.3❺
    hashish 305.2❺
    hypnotic 305.4❺
    inhalant 305.9❺
    LSD 305.3❺
    marijuana 305.2❺
    mixed 305.9❺
    morphine type 305.5❺
    opioid type 305.5❺
    phencyclidine (PCP) 305.9❺
    sedative 305.4❺
    specified NEC 305.9❺
    tranquilizers 305.4❺
  spouse 995.80
  tobacco 305.1
Acalcerosis 275.40
Acalcicosis 275.40
Acalculia 784.69
  developmental 315.1
Acanthocheilonemiasis 125.4
Acanthocytosis 272.5
Acanthokeratodermia 701.1
Acantholysis 701.8
  bullosa 757.39
Acanthoma (benign) (M8070/0) – *see also* Neoplasm, by site, benign
  malignant (M8070/3) – *see* Neoplasm, by site, malignant
Acanthosis (acquired) (nigricans) 701.2
  adult 701.2
  benign (congenital) 757.39
  congenital 757.39
  glycogenic
    esophagus 530.89
  juvenile 701.2
  tongue 529.8
Acanthrocytosis 272.5
Acapnia 276.3
Acarbia 276.2
Acardia 759.89
Arcadiacus amorphus 759.89
Acardiotrophia 429.1
Acardius 759.89
Acariasis 133.9
  sarcoptic 133.0
Acaridiasis 133.9
Acarinosis 133.9
Acariosis 133.9
Acarodermatitis 133.9
  urticarioides 133.9
Acarophobia 300.29
Acatalasemia 277.89
Acatalasia 277.89
Acatamathesia 784.69
Acataphasia 784.5
Acathisia 781.0
  due to drugs 333.99
Acceleration, accelerated
  atrioventricular conduction 426.7
  idioventricular rhythm 427.89
Accessory (congenital)
  adrenal gland 759.1
  anus 751.5
  appendix 751.5
  atrioventricular conduction 426.7
  auditory ossicles 744.04
  auricle (ear) 744.1
  autosome(s) NEC 758.5
    21 or 22 758.0
  biliary duct or passage 751.69

Accessory – *continued*
  bladder 753.8
  blood vessels (peripheral) (congenital) NEC (*see also* Anomaly, peripheral vascular system) 747.60
    cerebral 747.81
    coronary 746.85
  bone NEC 756.9
    foot 755.67
  breast tissue, axilla 757.6
  carpal bones 755.56
  cecum 751.5
  cervix 752.49
  chromosome(s) NEC 758.5
    13-15 758.1
    16-18 758.2
    21 or 22 758.0
    autosome(s) NEC 758.5
    D_1 758.1
    E_3 758.2
    G 758.0
    sex 758.81
  coronary artery 746.85
  cusp(s), heart valve NEC 746.89
    pulmonary 746.09
  cystic duct 751.69
  digits 755.00
  ear (auricle) (lobe) 744.1
  endocrine gland NEC 759.2
  external os 752.49
  eyelid 743.62
  eye muscle 743.69
  face bone(s) 756.0
  fallopian tube (fimbria) (ostium) 752.19
  fingers 755.01
  foreskin 605
  frontonasal process 756.0
  gallbladder 751.69
  genital organ(s)
    female 752.89
      external 752.49
      internal NEC 752.89
    male NEC 752.89
      penis 752.69
  genitourinary organs NEC 752.89
  heart 746.89
    valve NEC 746.89
      pulmonary 746.09
  hepatic ducts 751.69
  hymen 752.49
  intestine (large) (small) 751.5
  kidney 753.3
  lacrimal canal 743.65
  leaflet, heart valve NEC 746.89
    pulmonary 746.09
  ligament, broad 752.19
  liver (duct) 751.69
  lobule (ear) 744.1
  lung (lobe) 748.69
  muscle 756.82
  navicular of carpus 755.56
  nervous system, part NEC 742.8
  nipple 757.6
  nose 748.1
  organ or site NEC – *see* Anomaly, specified type NEC
  ovary 752.0
  oviduct 752.19
  pancreas 751.7
  parathyroid gland 759.2
  parotid gland (and duct) 750.22
  pituitary gland 759.2
  placental lobe – *see* Placenta, abnormal
  preauricular appendage 744.1
  prepuce 605
  renal arteries (multiple) 747.62
  rib 756.3
    cervical 756.2
  roots (teeth) 520.2
  salivary gland 750.22
  sesamoids 755.8
  sinus – *see* condition
  skin tags 757.39
  spleen 759.0
  sternum 756.3
  submaxillary gland 750.22
  tarsal bones 755.67
  teeth, tooth 520.1
    causing crowding 524.31
  tendon 756.89
  thumb 755.01
  thymus gland 759.2

Accessory – *continued*
- thyroid gland 759.2
- toes 755.02
- tongue 750.13
- tragus 744.1
- ureter 753.4
- urethra 753.8
- urinary organ or tract NEC 753.8
- uterus 752.2
- vagina 752.49
- valve, heart NEC 746.89
  - pulmonary 746.09
- vertebra 756.19
- vocal cords 748.3
- vulva 752.49

Accident, accidental – *see also* condition
- birth NEC 767.9
- cardiovascular (*see also* Disease, cardiovascular) 429.2
- cerebral (*see also* Disease, cerebrovascular, acute) 434.91
- cerebrovascular (current) (CVA) (*see also* Disease, cerebrovascular, acute) 434.91
  - aborted 434.91 ●
  - embolic 434.11
  - healed or old V12.54 ▲
  - hemorrhagic – *see* Hemorrhage, brain
  - impending 435.9
  - ischemic 434.91
  - late effect – *see* Late effect(s) (of) cerebrovascular disease
  - postoperative 997.02
  - thrombotic 434.01
- coronary (*see also* Infarct, myocardium) 410.9❺
- craniovascular (*see also* Disease, cerebrovascular, acute) 436
- during pregnancy, to mother, affecting fetus or newborn 760.5
- heart, cardiac (*see also* Infarct, myocardium) 410.9❺
- intrauterine 779.89
- vascular – *see* Disease, cerebrovascular, acute

Accommodation
- disorder of 367.51
  - drug-induced 367.89
  - toxic 367.89
- insufficiency of 367.4
- paralysis of 367.51
  - hysterical 300.11
- spasm of 367.53

Accouchement – *see* Delivery

Accreta placenta (without hemorrhage) 667.0❺
- with hemorrhage 666.0❺

Accretio cordis (nonrheumatic) 423.1

Accretions on teeth 523.6

Accumulation secretion, prostate 602.8

Acephalia, acephalism, acephaly 740.0

Acephalic 740.0

Acephalobrachia 759.89

Acephalocardia 759.89

Acephalocardius 759.89

Acephalochiria 759.89

Acephalochirus 759.89

Acephalogaster 759.89

Acephalostomus 759.89

Acephalothorax 759.89

Acephalus 740.0

Acetonemia 790.6
- diabetic 250.1❺

Acetonglycosuria 982.8

Acetonuria 791.6

Achalasia 530.0
- cardia 530.0
- digestive organs congenital NEC 751.8
- esophagus 530.0
- pelvirectal 751.3
- psychogenic 306.4
- pylorus 750.5
- sphincteral NEC 564.89

Achard-Thiers syndrome (adrenogenital) 255.2

Ache(s) – *see* Pain

Acheilia 750.26

Acheiria 755.21

Achillobursitis 726.71

Achillodynia 726.71

Achlorhydria, achlorhydric 536.0
- anemia 280.9

Achlorhydria, achlorhydric – *continued*
- diarrhea 536.0
- neurogenic 536.0
- postvagotomy 564.2
- psychogenic 306.4
- secondary to vagotomy 564.2

Achloroblepsia 368.52

Achloropsia 368.52

Acholia 575.8

Acholuric jaundice (familial) (splenomegalic) (*see also* Spherocytosis) 282.0
- acquired 283.9

Achondroplasia 756.4

Achrestic anemia 281.8

Achroacytosis, lacrimal gland 375.00
- tuberculous (*see also* Tuberculosis) 017.3❺

Achroma, cutis 709.00

Achromate (congenital) 368.54

Achromatopia 368.54

Achromatopsia (congenital) 368.54

Achromia
- congenital 270.2
- parasitica 111.0
- unguium 703.8

Achylia
- gastrica 536.8
  - neurogenic 536.3
  - psychogenic 306.4
- pancreatica 577.1

Achylosis 536.8

Acid
- burn – *see also* Burn, by site
  - from swallowing acid – *see* Burn, internal organs
- deficiency
  - amide nicotinic 265.2
  - amino 270.9
  - ascorbic 267
  - folic 266.2
  - nicotinic (amide) 265.2
  - pantothenic 266.2
- intoxication 276.2
- peptic disease 536.8
- stomach 536.8
  - psychogenic 306.4

Acidemia 276.2
- arginosuccinic 270.6
- fetal
  - affecting management of pregnancy 656.3❺
  - before onset of labor, in liveborn infant 768.2
  - during labor and delivery, in liveborn infant 768.3
  - intrauterine 656.3❺
  - unspecified as to time of onset, in liveborn infant 768.4
- newborn 775.81
- pipecolic 270.7

Acidity, gastric (high) (low) 536.8
- psychogenic 306.4

Acidocytopenia 288.59

Acidocytosis 288.3

Acidopenia 288.59

Acidosis 276.2
- diabetic 250.1❺
- fetal, affecting newborn 775.81
- fetal, affecting management of pregnancy 656.8❺
- kidney tubular 588.89
- lactic 276.2
- metabolic NEC 276.2
  - with respiratory acidosis 276.4
    - of newborn 775.81
  - late, of newborn 775.7
- newborn 775.81
- renal
  - hyperchloremic 588.89
  - tubular (distal) (proximal) 588.89
- respiratory 276.2
  - complicated by
    - metabolic acidosis 276.4
      - of newborn 775.81
    - metabolic alkalosis 276.4

Aciduria 791.9
- arginosuccinic 270.6
- beta-aminoisobutyric (BAIB) 277.2
- glutaric
  - type I 270.7
  - type II (type IIA, IIB, IIC) 277.85

Aciduria – *continued*
- glutaric – *continued*
  - type III 277.86
- glycolic 271.8
- methylmalonic 270.3
  - with glycinemia 270.7
- organic 270.9
- orotic (congenital) (hereditary) (pyrimidine deficiency) 281.4

Acladiosis 111.8
- skin 111.8

Aclasis
- diaphyseal 756.4
- tarsoepiphyseal 756.59

Acleistocardia 745.5

Aclusion 524.4

Acmesthesia 782.0

Acne (pustular) (vulgaris) 706.1
- agminata (*see also* Tuberculosis) 017.0❺
- artificialis 706.1
- atrophica 706.0
- cachecticorum (Hebra) 706.1
- conglobata 706.1
- conjunctiva 706.1
- cystic 706.1
- decalvans 704.09
- erythematosa 695.3
- eyelid 706.1
- frontalis 706.0
- indurata 706.1
- keloid 706.1
- lupoid 706.0
- necrotic, necrotica 706.0
  - miliaris 704.8
- neonatal 706.1
- nodular 706.1
- occupational 706.1
- papulosa 706.1
- rodens 706.0
- rosacea 695.3
- scorbutica 267
- scrofulosorum (Bazin) (*see also* Tuberculosis) 017.0❺
- summer 692.72
- tropical 706.1
- varioliformis 706.0

Acneiform drug eruptions 692.3

Acnitis (primary) (*see also* Tuberculosis) 017.0❺

Acomia 704.00

Acontractile bladder 344.61

Aconuresis (*see also* Incontinence) 788.30

Acosta's disease 993.2

Acousma 780.1

Acoustic – *see* condition

Acousticophobia 300.29

Acquired – *see* condition

Acquired immune deficiency syndrome – *see* Human immunodeficiency virus (disease) (illness) (infection)

Acquired immunodeficiency syndrome – *see* Human immunodeficiency virus (disease) (illness) (infection)

Acragnosis 781.99

Acrania 740.0

Acroagnosis 781.99

Acroasphyxia, chronic 443.89

Acrobrachycephaly 756.0

Acrobystiolith 608.89

Acrobystitis 607.2

Acrocephalopolysyndactyly 755.55

Acrocephalosyndactyly 755.55

Acrocephaly 756.0

Acrochondrohyperplasia 759.82

Acrocyanosis 443.89
- newborn 770.83
  - meaning transient blue hands and feet - *omit code*

Acrodermatitis 686.8
- atrophicans (chronica) 701.8
- continua (Hallopeau) 696.1
- enteropathica 686.8
- Hallopeau's 696.1
- perstans 696.1
- pustulosa continua 696.1
- recalcitrant pustular 696.1

Acrodynia 985.0

Accessory – Acrodynia

Acrodysplasia 755.55
Acrohyperhidrosis (*see also* Hyperhidrosis) 780.8
Acrokeratosis verruciformis 757.39
Acromastitis 611.0
Acromegaly, acromegalia (skin) 253.0
Acromelalgia 443.82
Acromicria, acromikria 756.59
Acronyx 703.0
Acropachy, thyroid (*see also* Thyrotoxicosis) 242.9❺
Acropachyderma 757.39
Acroparesthesia 443.89
simple (Schultz's type) 443.89
vasomotor (Nothnagel's type) 443.89
Acropathy thyroid (*see also* Thyrotoxicosis) 242.9❺
Acrophobia 300.29
Acroposthitis 607.2
Acroscleriasis (*see also* Scleroderma) 710.1
Acroscleroderma (*see also* Scleroderma) 710.1
Acrosclerosis (*see also* Scleroderma) 710.1
Acrosphacelus 785.4
Acrosphenosyndactylia 755.55
Acrospiroma, eccrine (M8402/0) – *see* Neoplasm, skin, benign
Acrostealgia 732.9
Acrosyndactyly (*see also* Syndactylism) 755.10
Acrotrophodynia 991.4
Actinic – *see also* condition
cheilitis (due to sun) 692.72
chronic NEC 692.74
due to radiation, except from sun 692.82
conjunctivitis 370.24
dermatitis (due to sun) (*see also* Dermatitis, actinic) 692.70
due to
roentgen rays or radioactive substance 692.82
ultraviolet radiation, except from sun 692.82
sun NEC 692.70
elastosis solare 692.74
granuloma 692.73
keratitis 370.24
ophthalmia 370.24
reticuloid 692.73
Actinobacillosis, general 027.8
Actinobacillus
lignieresii 027.8
mallei 024
muris 026.1
Actinocutitis NEC (*see also* Dermatitis, actinic) 692.70
Actinodermatitis NEC (*see also* Dermatitis, actinic) 692.70
Actinomyces
israelii (infection) – *see* Actinomycosis
muris-ratti (infection) 026.1
Actinomycosis, actinomycotic 039.9
with
pneumonia 039.1
abdominal 039.2
cervicofacial 039.3
cutaneous 039.0
pulmonary 039.1
specified site NEC 039.8
thoracic 039.1
Actinoneuritis 357.89
Action, heart
disorder 427.9
postoperative 997.1
irregular 427.9
postoperative 997.1
psychogenic 306.2
Active – *see* condition
Activity decrease, functional 780.99
Acute – *see also* condition
abdomen NEC 789.0❺
gallbladder (*see also* Cholecystitis, acute) 575.0
Acyanoblepsia 368.53
Acyanopsia 368.53
Acystia 753.8
Acystinervia – *see* Neurogenic, bladder
Acystineuria – *see* Neurogenic, bladder
Adactylia, adactyly (congenital) 755.4
lower limb (complete) (intercalary) (partial) (terminal) (*see also* Deformity, reduction, lower limb) 755.39
meaning all digits (complete) (partial) 755.31
transverse (complete) (partial) 755.31
upper limb (complete) (intercalary) (partial) (terminal) (*see also* Deformity, reduction, upper limb) 755.29
meaning all digits (complete) (partial) 755.21
transverse (complete) (partial) 755.21
Adair-Dighton syndrome (brittle bones and blue sclera, deafness) 756.51
Adamantinoblastoma (M9310/0) – *see* Ameloblastoma
Adamantinoma (M9310/0) – *see* Ameloblastoma
Adamantoblastoma (M9310/0) – *see* Ameloblastoma
Adams-Stokes (-Morgagni) disease or syndrome (syncope with heart block) 426.9
Adaptation reaction (*see also* Reaction, adjustment) 309.9
Addiction – *see also* Dependence
absinthe 304.6❺
alcoholic (ethyl) (methyl) (wood) 303.9❺
complicating pregnancy, childbirth, or puerperium 648.4❺
affecting fetus or newborn 760.71
suspected damage to fetus affecting management of pregnancy 655.4❺
drug (*see also* Dependence) 304.9❺
ethyl alcohol 303.9❺
heroin 304.0❺
hospital 301.51
methyl alcohol 303.9❺
methylated spirit 303.9❺
morphine (-like substances) 304.0❺
nicotine 305.1
opium 304.0❺
tobacco 305.1
wine 303.9❺
Addison's
anemia (pernicious) 281.0
disease (bronze) (primary adrenal insufficiency) 255.41 ▲
tuberculous (*see also* Tuberculosis) 017.6❺
keloid (morphea) 701.0
melanoderma (adrenal cortical hypofunction) 255.41 ▲
Addison-Biermer anemia (pernicious) 281.0
Addison-Gull disease – *see* Xanthoma
Addisonian crisis or melanosis (acute adrenocortical insufficiency) 255.41 ▲
Additional – *see also* Accessory
chromosome(s) 758.5
13-15 758.1
16-18 758.2
21 758.0
autosome(s) NEC 758.5
sex 758.81
Adduction contracture, hip or other joint – *see* Contraction, joint
ADEM (acute disseminated encephalomyelitis) (postinfectious) 136.9 *[323.61]*
infectious 136.9 *[323.61]*
noninfectious 323.81
Adenasthenia gastrica 536.0
Aden fever 061
Adenitis (*see also* Lymphadenitis) 289.3
acute, unspecified site 683
epidemic infectious 075
axillary 289.3
acute 683
chronic or subacute 289.1
Bartholin's gland 616.89
bulbourethral gland (*see also* Urethritis) 597.89
cervical 289.3
acute 683
chronic or subacute 289.1
chancroid (Ducrey's bacillus) 099.0
chronic (any lymph node, except mesenteric) 289.1
mesenteric 289.2
Cowper's gland (*see also* Urethritis) 597.89
epidemic, acute 075
gangrenous 683
gonorrheal NEC 098.89
groin 289.3
acute 683
chronic or subacute 289.1
Adenitis – *continued*
infectious 075
inguinal (region) 289.3
acute 683
chronic or subacute 289.1
lymph gland or node, except mesenteric 289.3
acute 683
chronic or subacute 289.1
mesenteric (acute) (chronic) (nonspecific) (subacute) 289.2
mesenteric (acute) (chronic) (nonspecific) (subacute) 289.2
due to Pasteurella multocida (P. septica) 027.2
parotid gland (suppurative) 527.2
phlegmonous 683
salivary duct or gland (any) (recurring) (suppurative) 527.2
scrofulous (*see also* Tuberculosis) 017.2❺
septic 289.3
Skene's duct or gland (*see also* Urethritis) 597.89
strumous, tuberculous (*see also* Tuberculosis) 017.2❺
subacute, unspecified site 289.1
sublingual gland (suppurative) 527.2
submandibular gland (suppurative) 527.2
submaxillary gland (suppurative) 527.2
suppurative 683
tuberculous – *see* Tuberculosis, lymph gland
urethral gland (*see also* Urethritis) 597.89
venereal NEC 099.8
Wharton's duct (suppurative) 527.2
Adenoacanthoma (M8570/3) – *see* Neoplasm, by site malignant
Adenoameloblastoma (M9300/0) 213.1
upper jaw (bone) 213.0
Adenocarcinoma (M8140/3) – *see also* Neoplasm, by site, malignant

Note – The list of adjectival modifiers below is not exhaustive. A description of adenocarcinoma that does not appear in this list should be coded in the same manner as carcinoma with that description. Thus, "mixed acidophil-basophil adenocarcinoma," should be coded in the same manner as "mixed acidophil-basophil carcinoma," which appears in the list under "Carcinoma."

Except where otherwise indicated, the morphological varieties of adenocarcinoma in the list below should be coded by site as for "Neoplasm, malignant."

with
apocrine metaplasia (M8573/3)
cartilaginous (and osseous) metaplasia (M8571/3)
osseous (and cartilaginous) metaplasia (M8571/3)
spindle cell metaplasia (M8572/3)
squamous metaplasia (M8570/3)
acidophil (M8280/3)
specified site – *see* Neoplasm, by site, malignant
unspecified site 194.3
acinar (M8550/3)
acinic cell (M8550/3)
adrenal cortical (M8370/3) 194.0
alveolar (M8251/3)
and
epidermoid carcinoma, mixed (M8560/3)
squamous cell carcinoma, mixed (M8560/3)
apocrine (M8401/3)
breast – *see* Neoplasm, breast, malignant
specified site NEC – *see* Neoplasm, skin, malignant
unspecified site 173.9
basophil (M8300/3)
specified site – *see* Neoplasm, by site, malignant
unspecified site 194.3
bile duct type (M8160/3)
liver 155.1
specified site NEC – *see* Neoplasm, by site, malignant
unspecified site 155.1
bronchiolar (M8250/3) – *see* Neoplasm, lung, malignant
ceruminous (M8420/3) 173.2

Adenocarcinoma – *continued*
- chromophobe (M8270/3)
  - specified site – *see* Neoplasm, by site, malignant
  - unspecified site 194.3
- clear cell (mesonephroid type) (M8310/3)
- colloid (M8480/3)
- cylindroid type (M8200/3)
- diffuse type (M8145/3)
  - specified site – *see* Neoplasm, by site, malignant
  - unspecified site 151.9
- duct (infiltrating) (M8500/3)
  - with Paget's disease (M8541/3) – *see* Neoplasm, breast, malignant
  - specified site – *see* Neoplasm, by site, malignant
  - unspecified site 174.9
- embryonal (M9070/3)
- endometrioid (M8380/3) – *see* Neoplasm, by site, malignant
- eosinophil (M8280/3)
  - specified site – *see* Neoplasm, by site, malignant
  - unspecified site 194.3
- follicular (M8330/3)
  - and papillary (M8340/3) 193
  - moderately differentiated type (M8332/3) 193
  - pure follicle type (M8331/3) 193
  - specified site – *see* Neoplasm, by site, malignant
  - trabecular type (M8332/3) 193
  - unspecified type 193
  - well differentiated type (M8331/3) 193
- gelatinous (M8480/3)
- granular cell (M8320/3)
- Hürthle cell (M8290/3) 193
- in
  - adenomatous
    - polyp (M8210/3)
    - polyposis coli (M8220/3) 153.9
  - polypoid adenoma (M8210/3)
  - tubular adenoma (M8210/3)
  - villous adenoma (M8261/3)
- infiltrating duct (M8500/3)
  - with Paget's disease (M8541/3) – *see* Neoplasm, breast, malignant
  - specified site – *see* Neoplasm, by site, malignant
  - unspecified site 174.9
- inflammatory (M8530/3)
  - specified site – *see* Neoplasm, by site, malignant
  - unspecified site 174.9
- in situ (M8140/2) – *see* Neoplasm, by site, in situ
- intestinal type (M8144/3)
  - specified site – *see* Neoplasm, by site, malignant
  - unspecified site 151.9
- intraductal (noninfiltrating) (M8500/2)
  - papillary (M8503/2)
    - specified site – *see* Neoplasm, by site, in situ
    - unspecified site 233.0
  - specified site – *see* Neoplasm, by site, in situ
  - unspecified site 233.0
- islet cell (M8150/3)
  - and exocrine, mixed (M8154/3)
    - specified site – *see* Neoplasm, by site, malignant
    - unspecified site 157.9
  - pancreas 157.4
  - specified site NEC – *see* Neoplasm, by site, malignant
  - unspecified site 157.4
- lobular (M8520/3)
  - specified site – *see* Neoplasm, by site, malignant
  - unspecified site 174.9
- medullary (M8510/3)
- mesonephric (M9110/3)
- mixed cell (M8323/3)
- mucinous (M8480/3)
- mucin-producing (M8481/3)
- mucoid (M8480/3) – *see also* Neoplasm, by site, malignant
  - cell (M8300/3)
    - specified site – *see* Neoplasm, by site, malignant
    - unspecified site 194.3
- nonencapsulated sclerosing (M8350/3) 193
- oncocytic (M8290/3)
- oxyphilic (M8290/3)

Adenocarcinoma – *continued*
- papillary (M8260/3)
  - and follicular (M8340/3) 193
  - intraductal (noninfiltrating) (M8503/2)
    - specified site – *see* Neoplasm, by site, in situ
    - unspecified site 233.0
  - serous (M8460/3)
    - specified site – *see* Neoplasm, by site, malignant
    - unspecified site 183.0
- papillocystic (M8450/3)
  - specified site – *see* Neoplasm, by site, malignant
  - unspecified site 183.0
- pseudomucinous (M8470/3)
  - specified site – *see* Neoplasm, by site, malignant
  - unspecified site 183.0
- renal cell (M8312/3) 189.0
- sebaceous (M8410/3)
- serous (M8441/3) – *see also* Neoplasm, by site, malignant
  - papillary
    - specified site – *see* Neoplasm, by site, malignant
    - unspecified site 183.0
- signet ring cell (M8490/3)
- superficial spreading (M8143/3)
- sweat gland (M8400/3) – *see* Neoplasm, skin, malignant
- trabecular (M8190/3)
- tubular (M8211/3)
- villous (M8262/3)
- water-clear cell (M8322/3) 194.1

Adenofibroma (M9013/0)
- clear cell (M8313/0) – *see* Neoplasm, by site, benign
- endometrioid (M8381/0) 220
  - borderline malignancy (M8381/1) 236.2
  - malignant (M8381/3) 183.0
- mucinous (M9015/0)
  - specified site – *see* Neoplasm, by site, benign
  - unspecified site 220
- prostate 600.20
  - with
    - other lower urinary tract symptoms (LUTS) 600.21
    - urinary
      - obstruction 600.21
      - retention 600.21
- serous (M9014/0)
  - specified site – *see* Neoplasm, by site, benign
  - unspecified site 220
- specified site – *see* Neoplasm, by site, benign
- unspecified site 220

Adenofibrosis
- breast 610.2
- endometroid 617.0

Adenoiditis 474.01
- acute 463
- chronic 474.01
  - with chronic tonsillitis 474.02

Adenoids (congenital) (of nasal fossa) 474.9
- hypertrophy 474.12
- vegetations 474.2

Adenolipomatosis (symmetrical) 272.8

Adenolymphoma (M8561/0)
- specified site – *see* Neoplasm, by site, benign
- unspecified 210.2

Adenoma (sessile) (M8140/0) – *see also* Neoplasm, by site, benign

Note – Except where otherwise indicated, the morphological varieties of adenoma in the list below should be coded by site as for "Neoplasm, benign."

- acidophil (M8280/0)
  - specified site – *see* Neoplasm, by site, benign
  - unspecified site 227.3
- acinar (cell) (M8550/0)
- acinic cell (M8550/0)
- adrenal (cortex) (cortical) (functioning) (M8370/0) 227.0
  - clear cell type (M8373/0) 227.0
  - compact cell type (M8371/0) 227.0
  - glomerulosa cell type (M8374/0) 227.0
  - heavily pigmented variant (M8372/0) 227.0
  - mixed cell type (M8375/0) 227.0
- alpha cell (M8152/0)
  - pancreas 211.7

Adenoma – *continued*
- alpha cell – *continued*
  - specified site NEC – *see* Neoplasm, by site, benign
  - unspecified site 211.7
- alveolar (M8251/0)
- apocrine (M8401/0)
  - breast 217
  - specified site NEC – *see* Neoplasm, skin, benign
  - unspecified site 216.9
- basal cell (M8147/0)
- basophil (M8300/0)
  - specified site – *see* Neoplasm, by site, benign
  - unspecified site 227.3
- beta cell (M8151/0)
  - pancreas 211.7
  - specified site NEC – *see* Neoplasm, by site, benign
  - unspecified site 211.7
- bile duct (M8160/0) 211.5
- black (M8372/0) 227.0
- bronchial (M8140/1) 235.7
  - carcinoid type (M8240/3) – *see* Neoplasm, lung, malignant
  - cylindroid type (M8200/3) – *see* Neoplasm, lung, malignant
- ceruminous (M8420/0) 216.2
- chief cell (M8321/0) 227.1
- chromophobe (M8270/0)
  - specified site – *see* Neoplasm, by site, benign
  - unspecified site 227.3
- clear cell (M8310/0)
- colloid (M8334/0)
  - specified site – *see* Neoplasm, by site, benign
  - unspecified site 226
- cylindroid type, bronchus (M8200/3) – *see* Neoplasm, lung, malignant
- duct (M8503/0)
- embryonal (M8191/0)
- endocrine, multiple (M8360/1)
  - single specified site – *see* Neoplasm, by site, uncertain behavior
  - two or more specified sites 237.4
  - unspecified site 237.4
- endometrioid (M8380/0) – *see also* Neoplasm, by site, benign
  - borderline malignancy (M8380/1) – *see* Neoplasm, by site, uncertain behavior
- eosinophil (M8280/0)
  - specified site – *see* Neoplasm, by site, benign
  - unspecified site 227.3
- fetal (M8333/0)
  - specified site – *see* Neoplasm, by site, benign
  - unspecified site 226
- follicular (M8330/0)
  - specified site – *see* Neoplasm, by site, benign
  - unspecified site 226
- hepatocellular (M8170/0) 211.5
- Hürthle cell (M8290/0) 226
- intracystic papillary (M8504/0)
- islet cell (functioning) (M8150/0)
  - pancreas 211.7
  - specified site NEC – *see* Neoplasm, by site, benign
  - unspecified site 211.7
- liver cell (M8170/0) 211.5
- macrofollicular (M8334/0)
  - specified site NEC – *see* Neoplasm, by site, benign
  - unspecified site 226
- malignant, malignum (M8140/3) – *see* Neoplasm, by site, malignant
- mesonephric (M9110/0)
- microfollicular (M8333/0)
  - specified site – *see* Neoplasm, by site, benign
  - unspecified site 226
- mixed cell (M8323/0)
- monomorphic (M8146/0)
- mucinous (M8480/0)
- mucoid cell (M8300/0)
  - specified site – *see* Neoplasm, by site, benign
  - unspecified site 227.3
- multiple endocrine (M8360/1)
  - single specified site – *see* Neoplasm, by site, uncertain behavior
  - two or more specified sites 237.4
  - unspecified site 237.4
- nipple (M8506/0) 217
- oncocytic (M8290/0)
- oxyphilic (M8290/0)

Adenocarcinoma – Adenoma

- **Adenoma** – *continued*
  - papillary (M8260/0) – *see also* Neoplasm, by site, benign
    - intracystic (M8504/0)
  - papillotubular (M8263/0)
  - Pick's tubular (M8640/0)
    - specified site – *see* Neoplasm, by site, benign
    - unspecified site
      - female 220
      - male 222.0
  - pleomorphic (M8940/0)
  - polypoid (M8210/0)
  - prostate (benign) 600.20
    - with
      - other lower urinary tract symptoms (LUTS) 600.21
      - urinary
        - obstruction 600.21
        - retention 600.21
  - rete cell 222.0
  - sebaceous, sebaceum (gland) (senile) (M8410/0) – *see also* Neoplasm, skin, benign
    - disseminata 759.5
  - Sertoli cell (M8640/0)
    - specified site – *see* Neoplasm, by site, benign
    - unspecified site
      - female 220
      - male 222.0
  - skin appendage (M8390/0) – *see* Neoplasm, skin, benign
  - sudoriferous gland (M8400/0) – *see* Neoplasm, skin, benign
  - sweat gland or duct (M8400/0) – *see* Neoplasm, skin, benign
  - testicular (M8640/0)
    - specified site – *see* Neoplasm, by site, benign
    - unspecified site
      - female 220
      - male 222.0
  - thyroid 226
  - trabecular (M8190/0)
  - tubular (M8211/0) – *see also* Neoplasm, by site, benign
    - papillary (M8460/3)
    - Pick's (M8640/0)
      - specified site – *see* Neoplasm, by site, benign
      - unspecified site
        - female 220
        - male 222.0
  - tubulovillous (M8263/0)
  - villoglandular (M8263/0)
  - villous (M8261/1) – *see* Neoplasm, by site, uncertain behavior
  - water-clear cell (M8322/0) 227.1
  - wolffian duct (M9110/0)
- **Adenomatosis** (M8220/0)
  - endocrine (multiple) (M8360/1)
    - single specified site – *see* Neoplasm, by site, uncertain behavior
    - two or more specified sites 237.4
    - unspecified site 237.4
  - erosive of nipple (M8506/0) 217
  - pluriendocrine – *see* Adenomatosis, endocrine
  - pulmonary (M8250/1) 235.7
    - malignant (M8250/3) – *see* Neoplasm, lung, malignant
  - specified site – *see* Neoplasm, by site, benign
  - unspecified site 211.3
- **Adenomatous**
  - cyst, thyroid (gland) – *see* Goiter, nodular
  - goiter (nontoxic) (*see also* Goiter, nodular) 241.9
    - toxic or with hyperthyroidism 242.3❺
- **Adenomyoma** (M8932/0) – *see also* Neoplasm, by site, benign
  - prostate 600.20
    - with
      - other lower urinary tract symptoms (LUTS) 600.21
      - urinary
        - obstruction 600.21
        - retention 600.21
- **Adenomyometritis** 617.0
- **Adenomyosis** (uterus) (internal) 617.0
- **Adenopathy** (lymph gland) 785.6
  - inguinal 785.6
  - mediastinal 785.6
  - mesentery 785.6
  - syphilitic (secondary) 091.4
- **Adenopathy** – *continued*
  - tracheobronchial 785.6
    - tuberculous (*see also* Tuberculosis) 012.1❺
      - primary, progressive 010.8❺
  - tuberculous (*see also* Tuberculosis, lymph gland) 017.2❺
    - tracheobronchial 012.1❺
      - primary, progressive 010.8❺
- **Adenopharyngitis** 462
- **Adenophlegmon** 683
- **Adenosalpingitis** 614.1
- **Adenosarcoma** (M8960/3) 189.0
- **Adenosclerosis** 289.3
- **Adenosis**
  - breast (sclerosing) 610.2
  - vagina, congenital 752.49
- **Adentia** (complete) (partial) (*see also* Absence, teeth) 520.0
- **Adherent**
  - labium (minus) 624.4
  - pericardium (nonrheumatic) 423.1
    - rheumatic 393
  - placenta 667.0❺
    - with hemorrhage 666.0❺
  - prepuce 605
  - scar (skin) NEC 709.2
  - tendon in scar 709.2
- **Adhesion(s), adhesive** (postinfectional) (postoperative)
  - abdominal (wall) (*see also* Adhesions, peritoneum) 568.0
  - amnion to fetus 658.8❺
    - affecting fetus or newborn 762.8
  - appendix 543.9
  - arachnoiditis – *see* Meningitis
  - auditory tube (Eustachian) 381.89
  - bands – *see also* Adhesions, peritoneum
    - cervix 622.3
    - uterus 621.5
  - bile duct (any) 576.8
  - bladder (sphincter) 596.8
  - bowel (*see also* Adhesions, peritoneum) 568.0
  - cardiac 423.1
    - rheumatic 398.99
  - cecum (*see also* Adhesions, peritoneum) 568.0
  - cervicovaginal 622.3
    - congenital 752.49
    - postpartal 674.8❺
      - old 622.3
  - cervix 622.3
  - clitoris 624.4
  - colon (*see also* Adhesions, peritoneum) 568.0
  - common duct 576.8
  - congenital – *see also* Anomaly, specified type NEC
    - fingers (*see also* Syndactylism, fingers) 755.11
    - labium (majus) (minus) 752.49
    - omental, anomalous 751.4
    - ovary 752.0
    - peritoneal 751.4
    - toes (*see also* Syndactylism, toes) 755.13
    - tongue (to gum or roof of mouth) 750.12
  - conjunctiva (acquired) (localized) 372.62
    - congenital 743.63
    - extensive 372.63
  - cornea – *see* Opacity, cornea
  - cystic duct 575.8
  - diaphragm (*see also* Adhesions, peritoneum) 568.0
  - due to foreign body – *see* Foreign body
  - duodenum (*see also* Adhesions, peritoneum) 568.0
    - with obstruction 537.3
  - ear, middle – *see* Adhesions, middle ear
  - epididymis 608.89
  - epidural – *see* Adhesions, meninges
  - epiglottis 478.79
  - Eustachian tube 381.89
  - eyelid 374.46
    - postoperative 997.99
      - surgically created V45.69
  - gallbladder (*see also* Disease, gallbladder) 575.8
  - globe 360.89
  - heart 423.1
    - rheumatic 398.99
  - ileocecal (coil) (*see also* Adhesions, peritoneum) 568.0
  - ileum (*see also* Adhesions, peritoneum) 568.0
- **Adhesion(s), adhesive** – *continued*
  - intestine (postoperative) (*see also* Adhesions, peritoneum) 568.0
    - with obstruction 560.81
      - with hernia – *see also* Hernia, by site, with obstruction
        - gangrenous – *see* Hernia, by site, with gangrene
  - intra-abdominal (*see also* Adhesions, peritoneum) 568.0
  - iris 364.70
    - to corneal graft 996.79
  - joint (*see also* Ankylosis) 718.5❺
  - kidney 593.89
  - labium (majus) (minus), congenital 752.49
  - liver 572.8
  - lung 511.0
  - mediastinum 519.3
  - meninges 349.2
    - cerebral (any) 349.2
      - congenital 742.4
    - congenital 742.8
    - spinal (any) 349.2
      - congenital 742.59
    - tuberculous (cerebral) (spinal) (*see also* Tuberculosis, meninges) 013.0❺
  - mesenteric (*see also* Adhesions, peritoneum) 568.0
  - middle ear (fibrous) 385.10
    - drum head 385.19
      - to
        - incus 385.11
        - promontorium 385.13
        - stapes 385.12
    - specified NEC 385.19
  - nasal (septum) (to turbinates) 478.19
  - nerve NEC 355.9
    - spinal 355.9
      - root 724.9
        - cervical NEC 723.4
        - lumbar NEC 724.4
        - lumbosacral 724.4
        - thoracic 724.4
  - ocular muscle 378.60
  - omentum (*see also* Adhesions, peritoneum) 568.0
  - organ or site, congenital NEC – *see* Anomaly, specified type NEC
  - ovary 614.6
    - congenital (to cecum, kidney, or omentum) 752.0
  - parauterine 614.6
  - parovarian 614.6
  - pelvic (peritoneal)
    - female (postoperative) (postinfection) 614.6
    - male (postoperative) (postinfection) (*see also* Adhesions, peritoneum) 568.0
    - postpartal (old) 614.6
    - tuberculous (*see also* Tuberculosis) 016.9❺
  - penis to scrotum (congenital) 752.69
  - periappendiceal (*see also* Adhesions, peritoneum) 568.0
  - pericardium (nonrheumatic) 423.1
    - rheumatic 393
    - tuberculous (*see also* Tuberculosis) 017.9❺ *[420.0]*
  - pericholecystic 575.8
  - perigastric (*see also* Adhesions, peritoneum) 568.0
  - periovarian 614.6
  - periprostatic 602.8
  - perirectal (*see also* Adhesions, peritoneum) 568.0
  - perirenal 593.89
  - peritoneum, peritoneal (fibrous) (postoperative) 568.0
    - with obstruction (intestinal) 560.81
      - with hernia – *see also* Hernia, by site, with obstruction
        - gangrenous – *see* Hernia, by site, with gangrene
      - duodenum 537.3
    - congenital 751.4
    - female (postoperative) (postinfective) 614.6
    - pelvic, female 614.6
    - pelvic, male 568.0
    - postpartal, pelvic 614.6
    - to uterus 614.6
  - peritubal 614.6
  - periureteral 593.89
  - periuterine 621.5
  - perivesical 596.8

Adenoma – Adhesion(s), adhesive

Adhesion(s), adhesive – *continued*
- perivesicular (seminal vesicle) 608.89
- pleura, pleuritic 511.0
  - tuberculous (*see also* Tuberculosis, pleura) 012.0❺
- pleuropericardial 511.0
- postoperative (gastrointestinal tract) (*see also* Adhesions, peritoneum)
  - pelvic female 614.9
  - pelvic, male 568.0
  - eyelid 997.99
    - surgically created V45.69
  - urethra 598.2
- postpartal, old 624.4
- preputial, prepuce 605
- pulmonary 511.0
- pylorus (*see also* Adhesions, peritoneum) 568.0
- Rosenmüller's fossa 478.29
- sciatic nerve 355.0
- seminal vesicle 608.89
- shoulder (joint) 726.0
- sigmoid flexure (*see also* Adhesions, peritoneum) 568.0
- spermatic cord (acquired) 608.89
  - congenital 752.89
- spinal canal 349.2
  - nerve 355.9
    - root 724.9
      - cervical NEC 723.4
      - lumbar NEC 724.4
      - lumbosacral 724.4
      - thoracic 724.4
- stomach (*see also* Adhesions, peritoneum) 568.0
- subscapular 726.2
- tendonitis 726.90
  - shoulder 726.0
- testicle 608.89
- tongue (congenital) (to gum or roof of mouth) 750.12
  - acquired 529.8
- trachea 519.19
- tubo-ovarian 614.6
- tunica vaginalis 608.89
- ureter 593.89
- uterus 621.5
  - to abdominal wall 614.6
    - in pregnancy or childbirth 654.4❺
      - affecting fetus or newborn 763.89
- vagina (chronic) (postoperative) (postradiation) 623.2
- vaginitis (congenital) 752.49
- vesical 596.8
- vitreous 379.29

Adie (-Holmes) **syndrome** (tonic pupillary reaction) 379.46

Adiponecrosis neonatorum 778.1

Adiposa dolorosa 272.8

Adiposalgia 272.8

Adiposis 278.0❺
- cerebralis 253.8
- dolorosa 272.8
- tuberosa simplex 272.8

Adiposity 278.02
- heart (*see also* Degeneration, myocardial) 429.1
- localized 278.1

Adiposogenital dystrophy 253.8

Adjustment
- prosthesis or other device – *see* Fitting of
- reaction – *see* Reaction, adjustment

Administration, prophylactic
- antibiotics V07.39
- antitoxin, any V07.2
- antivenin V07.2
- chemotherapeutic agent NEC V07.39
- chemotherapy NEC V07.39
- diphtheria antitoxin V07.2
- fluoride V07.31
- gamma globulin V07.2
- immune sera (gamma globulin) V07.2
- passive immunization agent V07.2
- RhoGAM V07.2

Admission (encounter)
- as organ donor – *see* Donor
- by mistake V68.9
- for
  - adequacy testing (for)
    - hemodialysis V56.31
    - peritoneal dialysis V56.32

Admission – *continued*
- for – *continued*
  - adjustment (of)
    - artificial
      - arm (complete) (partial) V52.0
      - eye V52.2
      - leg (complete) (partial) V52.1
    - brain neuropacemaker V53.02
    - breast
      - implant V52.4
      - prosthesis V52.4
    - cardiac device V53.39
      - defibrillator, automatic implantable V53.32
      - pacemaker V53.31
        - carotid sinus V53.39
    - catheter
      - non-vascular V58.82
      - vascular V58.81
    - cerebral ventricle (communicating) shunt V53.01
    - colostomy belt V55.3
    - contact lenses V53.1
    - cystostomy device V53.6
    - dental prosthesis V52.3
    - device, unspecified type V53.90
      - abdominal V53.5
      - cardiac V53.39
        - defibrillator, automatic implantable V53.32
        - pacemaker V53.31
      - carotid sinus V53.39
      - cerebral ventricle (communicating) shunt V53.01
      - insulin pump V53.91
      - intrauterine contraceptive V25.1
      - nervous system V53.09
      - orthodontic V53.4
      - other device V53.99
      - prosthetic V52.9
        - breast V52.4
        - dental V52.3
        - eye V52.2
        - specified type NEC V52.8
      - special senses V53.09
      - substitution
        - auditory V53.09
        - nervous system V53.09
        - visual V53.09
      - urinary V53.6
    - dialysis catheter
      - extracorporeal V56.1
      - peritoneal V56.2
    - diaphragm (contraceptive) V25.02
    - growth rod V54.02
    - hearing aid V53.2
    - ileostomy device V55.2
    - intestinal appliance or device NEC V53.5
    - intrauterine contraceptive device V25.1
    - neuropacemaker (brain) (peripheral nerve) (spinal cord) V53.02
    - orthodontic device V53.4
    - orthopedic (device) V53.7
      - brace V53.7
      - cast V53.7
      - shoes V53.7
    - pacemaker
      - brain V53.02
      - cardiac V53.31
      - carotid sinus V53.39
      - peripheral nerve V53.02
      - spinal cord V53.02
    - prosthesis V52.9
      - arm (complete) (partial) V52.0
      - breast V52.4
      - dental V52.3
      - eye V52.2
      - leg (complete) (partial) V52.1
      - specified type NEC V52.8
    - spectacles V53.1
    - wheelchair V53.8
  - adoption referral or proceedings V68.89
  - aftercare (*see also* Aftercare) V58.9
    - cardiac pacemaker V53.31
    - chemotherapy V58.11
    - dialysis
      - extracorporeal (renal) V56.0
      - peritoneal V56.8
      - renal V56.0
    - fracture (*see also* Aftercare, fracture) V54.9
    - medical NEC V58.89
    - organ transplant V58.44

Admission – *continued*
- for – *continued*
  - aftercare – *continued*
    - orthopedic V54.9
      - specified care NEC V54.89
    - pacemaker device
      - brain V53.02
      - cardiac V53.31
      - carotid sinus V53.39
      - nervous system V53.02
      - spinal cord V53.02
    - postoperative NEC V58.49
      - wound closure, planned V58.41
    - postpartum
      - immediately after delivery V24.0
      - routine follow-up V24.2
    - postradiation V58.0
    - radiation therapy V58.0
    - removal of
      - non-vascular catheter V58.82
      - vascular catheter V58.81
    - specified NEC V58.89
    - surgical NEC V58.49
      - wound closure, planned V58.41
  - antineoplastic
    - chemotherapy V58.11
    - immunotherapy V58.12
  - artificial insemination V26.1
  - assisted reproductive fertility procedure cycle V26.81 ●
  - attention to artificial opening (of) V55.9
    - artificial vagina V55.7
    - colostomy V55.3
    - cystostomy V55.5
    - enterostomy V55.4
    - gastrostomy V55.1
    - ileostomy V55.2
    - jejunostomy V55.4
    - nephrostomy V55.6
    - specified site NEC V55.8
      - intestinal tract V55.4
      - urinary tract V55.6
    - tracheostomy V55.0
    - ureterostomy V55.6
    - urethrostomy V55.6
  - battery replacement
    - cardiac pacemaker V53.31
  - blood typing V72.86
    - Rh typing V72.86
  - boarding V65.0
  - breast
    - augmentation or reduction V50.1
    - removal, prophylactic V50.41
  - change of
    - cardiac pacemaker (battery) V53.31
    - carotid sinus pacemaker V53.39
    - catheter in artificial opening – *see* Attention to, artificial, opening
    - drains V58.49
    - dressing
      - wound V58.30
        - nonsurgical V58.30
        - surgical V58.31
    - fixation device
      - external V54.89
      - internal V54.01
    - Kirschner wire V54.89
    - neuropacemaker device (brain) (peripheral nerve) (spinal cord) V53.02
    - nonsurgical wound dressing V58.30
    - pacemaker device
      - brain V53.02
      - cardiac V53.31
      - carotid sinus V53.39
      - nervous system V53.02
    - plaster cast V54.89
    - splint, external V54.89
    - Steinmann pin V54.89
    - surgical wound dressing V58.31
    - traction device V54.89
    - wound packing V58.30
      - nonsurgical V58.30
      - surgical V58.31
  - checkup only V70.0
  - chemotherapy, antineoplastic V58.11
  - circumcision, ritual or routine (in absence of medical indication) V50.2
  - clinical research investigation (control) (normal comparison) (participant) V70.7
  - closure of artificial opening – *see* Attention to, artificial, opening

Adhesion(s), adhesive – Admission

- **Admission** – *continued*
  - for – *continued*
    - contraceptive
      - counseling V25.09
        - emergency V25.03
        - postcoital V25.03
      - management V25.9
        - specified type NEC V25.8
    - convalescence following V66.9
      - chemotherapy V66.2
      - psychotherapy V66.3
      - radiotherapy V66.1
      - surgery V66.0
      - treatment (for) V66.5
        - combined V66.6
        - fracture V66.4
        - mental disorder NEC V66.3
        - specified condition NEC V66.5
    - cosmetic surgery NEC V50.1
      - following healed injury or operation V51
    - counseling (*see also* Counseling) V65.40
      - without complaint or sickness V65.49
      - contraceptive management V25.09
        - emergency V25.03
        - postcoital V25.03
      - dietary V65.3
      - exercise V65.41
      - for
        - nonattending third party V65.19
        - pediatric pre-birth visit for expectant mother V65.11
        - victim of abuse
          - child V61.21
          - partner or spouse V61.11
      - genetic V26.33
      - gonorrhea V65.45
      - HIV V65.44
      - human immunodeficiency virus V65.44
      - injury prevention V65.43
      - insulin pump training V65.46
      - natural family planning ●
        - procreative V26.41 ●
        - to avoid pregnancy V25.04 ●
      - procreative management V26.49 ▲
        - using natural family planning V26.41 ●
      - sexually transmitted disease NEC V65.45
        - HIV V65.44
      - specified reason NEC V65.49
      - substance use and abuse V65.42
      - syphilis V65.45
      - victim of abuse
        - child V61.21
        - partner or spouse V61.11
    - desensitization to allergens V07.1
    - dialysis V56.0
      - catheter
        - fitting and adjustment
          - extracorporeal V56.1
          - peritoneal V56.2
        - removal or replacement
          - extracorporeal V56.1
          - peritoneal V56.2
      - extracorporeal (renal) V56.0
      - peritoneal V56.8
      - renal V56.0
    - dietary surveillance and counseling V65.3
    - drug monitoring, therapeutic V58.83
    - ear piercing V50.3
    - elective surgery
      - breast
        - augmentation or reduction V50.1
        - removal, prophylactic V50.41
      - circumcision, ritual or routine (in absence of medical indication) V50.2
      - cosmetic NEC V50.1
        - following healed injury or operation V51
      - ear piercing V50.3
      - face-lift V50.1
      - hair transplant V50.0
      - plastic
        - cosmetic NEC V50.1
        - following healed injury or operation V51
      - prophylactic organ removal V50.49
        - breast V50.41
        - ovary V50.42
      - repair of scarred tissue (following healed injury or operation) V51
      - specified type NEC V50.8
    - end-of-life care V66.7
    - examination (*see also* Examination) V70.9
      - administrative purpose NEC V70.3
      - adoption V70.3

- **Admission** – *continued*
  - for – *continued*
    - examination – *continued*
      - allergy V72.7
      - at health care facility V70.0
      - athletic team V70.3
      - camp V70.3
      - cardiovascular, preoperative V72.81
      - clinical research investigation (control) (participant) V70.7
      - dental V72.2
      - developmental testing (child) (infant) V20.2
      - donor (potential) V70.8
      - driver's license V70.3
      - ear V72.19
      - employment V70.5
      - eye V72.0
      - follow-up (routine) – *see* Examination, follow-up
      - for admission to
        - old age home V70.3
        - school V70.3
      - general V70.9
        - specified reason NEC V70.8
      - gynecological V72.31
      - health supervision (child) (infant) V20.2
      - hearing V72.19
        - following failed hearing screening V72.11
      - immigration V70.3
      - infant, routine V20.2
      - insurance certification V70.3
      - laboratory V72.6
      - marriage license V70.3
      - medical (general) (*see also* Examination, medical) V70.9
      - medicolegal reasons V70.4
      - naturalization V70.3
      - pelvic (annual) (periodic) V72.31
      - postpartum checkup V24.2
      - pregnancy (possible) (unconfirmed) V72.40
        - negative result V72.41
        - positive result V72.42
      - preoperative V72.84
        - cardiovascular V72.81
        - respiratory V72.82
        - specified NEC V72.83
      - preprocedural V72.84
        - cardiovascular V72.81
        - general physical V72.83
        - respiratory V72.82
        - specified NEC V72.83
      - prison V70.3
      - psychiatric (general) V70.2
        - requested by authority V70.1
      - radiological NEC V72.5
      - respiratory, preoperative V72.82
      - school V70.3
      - screening – *see* Screening
      - skin hypersensitivity V72.7
      - specified type NEC V72.85
      - sport competition V70.3
      - vision V72.0
      - well baby and child care V20.2
    - exercise therapy V57.1
    - face-lift, cosmetic reason V50.1
    - fitting (of)
      - artificial
        - arm (complete) (partial) V52.0
        - eye V52.2
        - leg (complete) (partial) V52.1
      - biliary drainage tube V58.82
      - brain neuropacemaker V53.02
      - breast V52.4
        - implant V52.4
        - prosthesis V52.4
      - cardiac pacemaker V53.31
      - catheter
        - non-vascular V58.82
        - vascular V58.81
      - cerebral ventricle (communicating) shunt V53.01
      - chest tube V58.82
      - colostomy belt V55.2
      - contact lenses V53.1
      - cystostomy device V53.6
      - dental prosthesis V52.3
      - device, unspecified type V53.90
        - abdominal V53.5
        - cerebral ventricle (communicating) shunt V53.01
        - insulin pump V53.91
        - intrauterine contraceptive V25.1

- **Admission** – *continued*
  - for – *continued*
    - fitting – *continued*
      - device, unspecified type – *continued*
        - nervous system V53.09
        - orthodontic V53.4
        - other device V53.99
        - prosthetic V52.9
          - breast V52.4
          - dental V52.3
          - eye V52.2
        - special senses V53.09
        - substitution
          - auditory V53.09
          - nervous system V53.09
          - visual V53.09
      - diaphragm (contraceptive) V25.02
      - fistula (sinus tract) drainage tube V58.82
      - growth rod V54.02
      - hearing aid V53.2
      - ileostomy device V55.2
      - intestinal appliance or device NEC V53.5
      - intrauterine contraceptive device V25.1
      - neuropacemaker (brain) (peripheral nerve) (spinal cord) V53.02
      - orthodontic device V53.4
      - orthopedic (device) V53.7
        - brace V53.7
        - cast V53.7
        - shoes V53.7
      - pacemaker
        - brain V53.02
        - cardiac V53.31
        - carotid sinus V53.39
        - spinal cord V53.02
      - pleural drainage tube V58.82
      - prosthesis V52.9
        - arm (complete) (partial) V52.0
        - breast V52.4
        - dental V52.3
        - eye V52.2
        - leg (complete) (partial) V52.1
        - specified type NEC V52.8
      - spectacles V53.1
      - wheelchair V53.8
    - follow-up examination (routine) (following) V67.9
      - cancer chemotherapy V67.2
      - chemotherapy V67.2
      - high-risk medication NEC V67.51
      - injury NEC V67.59
      - psychiatric V67.3
      - psychotherapy V67.3
      - radiotherapy V67.1
      - specified surgery NEC V67.09
      - surgery V67.00
        - vaginal pap smear V67.01
      - treatment (for) V67.9
        - combined V67.6
        - fracture V67.4
        - involving high-risk medication NEC V67.51
        - mental disorder V67.3
        - specified NEC V67.59
    - hair transplant, for cosmetic reason V50.0
    - health advice, education, or instruction V65.4
    - hearing conservation and treatment V72.12 ●
    - hormone replacement therapy (postmenopausal) V07.4
    - hospice care V66.7
    - immunotherapy, antineoplastic V58.12
    - insertion (of)
      - subdermal implantable contraceptive V25.5
    - insulin pump titration V53.91
    - insulin pump training V65.46
    - intrauterine device
      - insertion V25.1
      - management V25.42
    - investigation to determine further disposition V63.8
    - in vitro fertilization cycle V26.81 ●
    - isolation V07.0
    - issue of
      - disability examination certificate V68.01 ●
      - medical certificate NEC V68.09 ▲
      - repeat prescription NEC V68.1
        - contraceptive device NEC V25.49
    - kidney dialysis V56.0
    - lengthening of growth rod V54.02
    - mental health evaluation V70.2
      - requested by authority V70.1

- **Admission** – *continued*
  - for – *continued*
    - vaccination, prophylactic – *continued*
      - influenza V04.81
        - with
          - Streptococcus pneumoniae [pneumococcus] V06.6
      - Leishmaniasis V05.2
      - measles alone V04.2
      - measles-mumps-rubella (MMR) V06.4
      - mumps alone V04.6
        - with measles and rubella (MMR) V06.4
      - not done because of contraindication V64.09
      - pertussis alone V03.6
      - plague V03.3
      - pneumonia V03.82
      - poliomyelitis V04.0
        - with diphtheria-tetanus-pertussis (DTP polio) V06.3
      - rabies V04.5
      - respiratory syncytial virus (RSV) V04.82
      - rubella alone V04.3
        - with measles and mumps (MMR) V06.4
      - smallpox V04.1
      - specified type NEC V05.8
      - Streptococcus pneumoniae [pneumococcus] V03.82
        - with
          - influenza V06.6
      - tetanus toxoid alone V03.7
        - with diphtheria [Td] [DT] V06.5
          - and pertussis (DTP) (DTaP)V06.1
      - tuberculosis (BCG) V03.2
      - tularemia V03.4
      - typhoid alone V03.1
        - with diphtheria-tetanus-pertussis (TAB + DTP) V06.2
      - typhoid-paratyphoid alone (TAB) V03.1
      - typhus V05.8
      - varicella (chicken pox) V05.4
      - viral encephalitis, arthropod-borne V05.0
      - viral hepatitis V05.3
      - yellow fever V04.4
    - vasectomy V25.2
    - vasoplasty for previous sterilization V26.0
    - vision examination V72.0
    - vocational therapy V57.22
    - waiting period for admission to other facility V63.2
      - undergoing social agency investigation V63.8
    - well baby and child care V20.2
    - x-ray of chest
      - for suspected tuberculosis V71.2
      - routine V72.5
- **Adnexitis** (suppurative) (*see also* Salpingo-oophoritis) 614.2
- **Adolescence** NEC V21.2
- **Adoption**
  - agency referral V68.89
  - examination V70.3
  - held for V68.89
- **Adrenal gland** – *see* condition
- **Adrenalism** 255.9
  - tuberculous (*see also* Tuberculosis) 017.6❺
- **Adrenalitis, adrenitis** 255.8
  - meningococcal hemorrhagic 036.3
- **Adrenarche, precocious** 259.1
- **Adrenocortical syndrome** 255.2
- **Adrenogenital syndrome** (acquired) (congenital) 255.2
  - iatrogenic, fetus or newborn 760.79
- **Adrenoleukodystrophy** 277.86
  - neonatal 277.86
  - x-linked 277.86
- **Adrenomyeloneuropathy** 277.86
- **Adventitious bursa** – *see* Bursitis
- **Adynamia** (episodica) (hereditary) (periodic) 359.3
- **Adynamic**
  - ileus or intestine (*see also* Ileus) 560.1
  - ureter 753.22
- **Aeration lung, imperfect, newborn** 770.5
- **Aerobullosis** 993.3
- **Aerocele** – *see* Embolism, air
- **Aerodermectasia**
  - subcutaneous (traumatic) 958.7
    - surgical 998.81
  - surgical 998.81
- **Aerodontalgia** 993.2
- **Aeroembolism** 993.3
- **Aerogenes capsulatus infection** (*see also* Gangrene, gas) 040.0
- **Aero-otitis media** 993.0
- **Aerophagy, aerophagia** 306.4
  - psychogenic 306.4
- **Aerosinusitis** 993.1
- **Aerotitis** 993.0
- **Affection, affections** – *see also* Disease
  - sacroiliac (joint), old 724.6
  - shoulder region NEC 726.2
- **Afibrinogenemia** 286.3
  - acquired 286.6
  - congenital 286.3
  - postpartum 666.3❺
- **African**
  - sleeping sickness 086.5
  - tick fever 087.1
  - trypanosomiasis 086.5
    - Gambian 086.3
    - Rhodesian 086.4
- **Aftercare** V58.9
  - amputation stump V54.89
  - artificial openings – *see* Attention to, artificial, opening
  - blood transfusion without reported diagnosis V58.2
  - breathing exercise V57.0
  - cardiac device V53.39
    - defibrillator, automatic implantable V53.32
    - pacemaker V53.31
      - carotid sinus V53.39
  - carotid sinus pacemaker V53.39
  - cerebral ventricle (communicating) shunt V53.01
  - chemotherapy session (adjunctive) (maintenance) V58.11
  - defibrillator, automatic implantable cardiac V53.32
  - exercise (remedial) (therapeutic) V57.1
    - breathing V57.0
  - extracorporeal dialysis (intermittent) (treatment) V56.0
  - following surgery NEC V58.49
    - for
      - injury V58.43
      - neoplasm V58.42
      - organ transplant V58.44
      - trauma V58.43
    - joint replacement V54.81
    - of
      - circulatory system V58.73
      - digestive system V58.75
      - genital organs V58.76
      - genitourinary system V58.76
      - musculoskeletal system V58.78
      - nervous system V58.72
      - oral cavity V58.75
      - respiratory system V58.74
      - sense organs V58.71
      - skin V58.77
      - subcutaneous tissue V58.77
      - teeth V58.75
      - urinary system V58.76
    - spinal – *see* Aftercare, following surgery, of, specified body system ●
    - wound closure, planned V58.41
  - fracture V54.9
    - healing V54.89
      - pathologic
        - ankle V54.29
        - arm V54.20
          - lower V54.22
          - upper V54.21
        - finger V54.29
        - foot V54.29
        - hand V54.29
        - hip V54.23
        - leg V54.24
          - lower V54.26
          - upper V54.25
        - pelvis V54.29
        - specified site NEC V54.29
        - toe(s) V54.29
        - vertebrae V54.27
        - wrist V54.29
      - traumatic
        - ankle V54.19
        - arm V54.10
          - lower V54.12
          - upper V54.11
- **Aftercare** – *continued*
  - fracture – *continued*
    - healing – *continued*
      - traumatic – *continued*
        - finger V54.19
        - foot V54.19
        - hand V54.19
        - hip V54.13
        - leg V54.14
          - lower V54.16
          - upper V54.15
        - pelvis V54.19
        - specified site NEC V54.19
        - toe(s) V54.19
        - vertebrae V54.17
        - wrist V54.19
    - removal of
      - external fixation device V54.89
      - internal fixation device V54.01
    - specified care NEC V54.89
  - gait training V57.1
    - for use of artificial limb(s) V57.81
  - internal fixation device V54.09
  - involving
    - dialysis (intermittent) (treatment)
      - extracorporeal V56.0
      - peritoneal V56.8
      - renal V56.0
    - gait training V57.1
      - for use of artificial limb(s) V57.81
    - growth rod
      - adjustment V54.02
      - lengthening V54.02
    - internal fixation device V54.09
    - orthoptic training V57.4
    - orthotic training V57.81
    - radiotherapy session V58.0
    - removal of
      - drains V58.49
      - dressings
        - wound V58.30
          - nonsurgical V58.30
          - surgical V58.31
      - fixation device
        - external V54.89
        - internal V54.01
      - fracture plate V54.01
      - nonsurgical wound dressing V58.30
      - pins V54.01
      - plaster cast V54.89
      - rods V54.01
      - screws V54.01
      - staples V58.32
      - surgical wound dressings V58.31
      - sutures V58.32
      - traction device, external V54.89
      - wound packing V58.30
        - nonsurgical V58.30
        - surgical V58.31
  - neuropacemaker (brain) (peripheral nerve) (spinal cord) V53.02
  - occupational therapy V57.21
  - orthodontic V58.5
  - orthopedic V54.9
    - change of external fixation or traction device V54.89
    - following joint replacement V54.81
    - internal fixation device V54.09
    - removal of fixation device
      - external V54.89
      - internal V54.01
    - specified care NEC V54.89
  - orthoptic training V57.4
  - orthotic training V57.81
  - pacemaker
    - brain V53.02
    - cardiac V53.31
    - carotid sinus V53.39
    - peripheral nerve V53.02
    - spinal cord V53.02
  - peritoneal dialysis (intermittent) (treatment) V56.8
  - physical therapy NEC V57.1
    - breathing exercises V57.0
  - radiotherapy session V58.0
  - rehabilitation procedure V57.9
    - breathing exercises V57.0
    - multiple types V57.89
    - occupational V57.21
    - orthoptic V57.4
    - orthotic V57.81
    - physical therapy NEC V57.1

Aftercare – *continued*
- rehabilitation procedure – *continued*
  - remedial exercises V57.1
  - specified type NEC V57.89
  - speech V57.3
  - therapeutic exercises V57.1
  - vocational V57.22
- renal dialysis (intermittent) (treatment) V56.0
- specified type NEC V58.89
  - removal of non-vascular cathether V58.82
  - removal of vascular catheter V58.81
- speech therapy V57.3
- stump, amputation V54.89
- vocational rehabilitation V57.22

After-cataract 366.50
- obscuring vision 366.53
- specified type, not obscuring vision 366.52

Agalactia 676.4❺

Agammaglobulinemia 279.00
- with lymphopenia 279.2
- acquired (primary) (secondary) 279.06
- Bruton's X-linked 279.04
- infantile sex-linked (Bruton's) (congenital) 279.04
- Swiss-type 279.2

Aganglionosis (bowel) (colon) 751.3

Age (old) (*see also* Senile) 797

Agenesis – *see also* Absence, by site, congenital
- acoustic nerve 742.8
- adrenal (gland) 759.1
- alimentary tract (complete) (partial) NEC 751.8
  - lower 751.2
  - upper 750.8
- anus, anal (canal) 751.2
- aorta 747.22
- appendix 751.2
- arm (complete) (partial) (*see also* Deformity, reduction, upper limb) 755.20
- artery (peripheral) NEC (*see also* Anomaly, peripheral vascular system) 747.60
  - brain 747.81
  - coronary 746.85
  - pulmonary 747.3
  - umbilical 747.5
- auditory (canal) (external) 744.01
- auricle (ear) 744.01
- bile, biliary duct or passage 751.61
- bone NEC 756.9
- brain 740.0
  - specified part 742.2
- breast 757.6
- bronchus 748.3
- canaliculus lacrimalis 743.65
- carpus NEC (*see also* Deformity, reduction, upper limb) 755.28
- cartilage 756.9
- cecum 751.2
- cerebellum 742.2
- cervix 752.49
- chin 744.89
- cilia 743.63
- circulatory system, part NEC 747.89
- clavicle 755.51
- clitoris 752.49
- coccyx 756.13
- colon 751.2
- corpus callosum 742.2
- cricoid cartilage 748.3
- diaphragm (with hernia) 756.6
- digestive organ(s) or tract (complete) (partial) NEC 751.8
  - lower 751.2
  - upper 750.8
- ductus arteriosus 747.89
- duodenum 751.1
- ear NEC 744.09
  - auricle 744.01
  - lobe 744.21
- ejaculatory duct 752.89
- endocrine (gland) NEC 759.2
- epiglottis 748.3
- esophagus 750.3
- Eustachian tube 744.24
- extrinsic muscle, eye 743.69
- eye 743.00
  - adnexa 743.69
- eyelid (fold) 743.62
- face
  - bones NEC 756.0
  - specified part NEC 744.89
- fallopian tube 752.19

Agenesis – *continued*
- femur NEC (*see also* Absence, femur, congenital) 755.34
- fibula NEC (*see also* Absence, fibula, congenital) 755.37
- finger NEC (*see also* Absence, finger, congenital) 755.29
- foot (complete) (*see also* Deformity, reduction, lower limb) 755.31
- gallbladder 751.69
- gastric 750.8
- genitalia, genital (organ)
  - female 752.89
    - external 752.49
    - internal NEC 752.89
  - male 752.89
    - penis 752.69
- glottis 748.3
- gonadal 758.6
- hair 757.4
- hand (complete) (*see also* Deformity, reduction, upper limb) 755.21
- heart 746.89
  - valve NEC 746.89
    - aortic 746.89
    - mitral 746.89
    - pulmonary 746.01
- hepatic 751.69
- humerus NEC (*see also* Absence, humerus, congenital) 755.24
- hymen 752.49
- ileum 751.1
- incus 744.04
- intestine (small) 751.1
  - large 751.2
- iris (dilator fibers) 743.45
- jaw 524.09
- jejunum 751.1
- kidney(s) (partial) (unilateral) 753.0
- labium (majus) (minus) 752.49
- labyrinth, membranous 744.05
- lacrimal apparatus (congenital) 743.65
- larynx 748.3
- leg NEC (*see also* Deformity, reduction, lower limb) 755.30
- lens 743.35
- limb (complete) (partial) (*see also* Deformity, reduction) 755.4
  - lower NEC 755.30
  - upper 755.20
- lip 750.26
- liver 751.69
- lung (bilateral) (fissures) (lobe) (unilateral) 748.5
- mandible 524.09
- maxilla 524.09
- metacarpus NEC 755.28
- metatarsus NEC 755.38
- muscle (any) 756.81
- musculoskeletal system NEC 756.9
- nail(s) 757.5
- neck, part 744.89
- nerve 742.8
- nervous system, part NEC 742.8
- nipple 757.6
- nose 748.1
- nuclear 742.8
- organ
  - of Corti 744.05
  - or site not listed – *see* Anomaly, specified type NEC
- osseous meatus (ear) 744.03
- ovary 752.0
- oviduct 752.19
- pancreas 751.7
- parathyroid (gland) 759.2
- patella 755.64
- pelvic girdle (complete) (partial) 755.69
- penis 752.69
- pericardium 746.89
- perineal body 756.81
- pituitary (gland) 759.2
- prostate 752.89
- pulmonary
  - artery 747.3
  - trunk 747.3
  - vein 747.49
- punctum lacrimale 743.65
- radioulnar NEC (*see also* Absence, forearm, congenital) 755.25
- radius NEC (*see also* Absence, radius, congenital) 755.26
- rectum 751.2

Agenesis – *continued*
- renal 753.0
- respiratory organ NEC 748.9
- rib 756.3
- roof of orbit 742.0
- round ligament 752.89
- sacrum 756.13
- salivary gland 750.21
- scapula 755.59
- scrotum 752.89
- seminal duct or tract 752.89
- septum
  - atrial 745.69
  - between aorta and pulmonary artery 745.0
  - ventricular 745.3
- shoulder girdle (complete) (partial) 755.59
- skull (bone) 756.0
  - with
    - anencephalus 740.0
    - encephalocele 742.0
    - hydrocephalus 742.3
      - with spina bifida (*see also* Spina bifida) 741.0❺
    - microcephalus 742.1
- spermatic cord 752.89
- spinal cord 742.59
- spine 756.13
  - lumbar 756.13
    - isthmus 756.11
    - pars articularis 756.11
- spleen 759.0
- sternum 756.3
- stomach 750.7
- tarsus NEC 755.38
- tendon 756.81
- testicular 752.89
- testis 752.89
- thymus (gland) 759.2
- thyroid (gland) 243
  - cartilage 748.3
- tibia NEC (*see also* Absence, tibia, congenital) 755.36
- tibiofibular NEC 755.35
- toe (complete) (partial) (*see also* Absence, toe, congenital) 755.39
- tongue 750.11
- trachea (cartilage) 748.3
- ulna NEC (*see also* Absence, ulna, congenital) 755.27
- ureter 753.4
- urethra 753.8
- urinary tract NEC 753.8
- uterus 752.3
- uvula 750.26
- vagina 752.49
- vas deferens 752.89
- vein(s) (peripheral) NEC (*see also* Anomaly, peripheral vascular system) 747.60
  - brain 747.81
  - great 747.49
  - portal 747.49
  - pulmonary 747.49
- vena cava (inferior) (superior) 747 49
- vermis of cerebellum 742.2
- vertebra 756.13
  - lumbar 756.13
    - isthmus 756.11
    - pars articularis 756.11
- vulva 752.49

Ageusia (*see also* Disturbance, sensation) 781.1

Aggressiveness 301.3

Aggressive outburst (*see also* Disturbance, conduct) 312.0❺
- in children or adolescents 313.9

Aging skin 701.8

Agitated – *see* condition

Agitation 307.9
- catatonic (*see also* Schizophrenia) 295.2❺

Aglossia (congenital) 750.11

Aglycogenosis 271.0

Agnail (finger) (with lymphangitis) 681.02

Agnosia (body image) (tactile) 784.69
- verbal 784.69
  - auditory 784.69
    - secondary to organic lesion 784.69
  - developmental 315.8
  - secondary to organic lesion 784.69
  - visual 784.69
    - developmental 315.8
    - secondary to organic lesion 784.69

- **Agnosia** – *continued*
  - visual 368.16
    - developmental 315.31
- **Agoraphobia** 300.22
  - with panic disorder 300.21
- **Agrammatism** 784.69
- **Agranulocytopenia** (*see also* Agranulocytosis) 288.09
- **Agranulocytosis** (angina) 288.09
  - chronic 288.09
  - cyclical 288.02
  - genetic 288.01
  - infantile 288.01
  - periodic 288.02
  - pernicious 288.09
- **Agraphia** (absolute) 784.69
  - with alexia 784.61
  - developmental 315.39
- **Agrypnia** (*see also* Insomnia) 780.52
- **Ague** (*see also* Malaria) 084.6
  - brass-founders' 985.8
  - dumb 084.6
  - tertian 084.1
- **Agyria** 742.2
- **Ahumada-del Castillo syndrome** (nonpuerperal galactorrhea and amenorrhea) 253.1
- **AIDS** 042
- **AIDS-associated retrovirus** (disease) (illness) 042
  - infection – *see* Human immunodeficiency virus, infection
- **AIDS-associated virus** (disease) (illness) 042
  - infection – *see* Human immunodeficiency virus, infection
- **AIDS-like disease** (illness) (syndrome) 042
- **AIDS-related complex** 042
- **AIDS-related conditions** 042
- **AIDS-related virus** (disease) (illness) 042
  - infection – *see* Human immunodeficiency virus, infection
- **AIDS virus** (disease) (illness) 042
  - infection – *see* Human immunodeficiency virus, infection
- **Ailment, heart** – *see* Disease, heart
- **Ailurophobia** 300.29
- **Ainhum** (disease) 136.0
- **Air**
  - anterior mediastinum 518.1
  - compressed, disease 993.3
  - embolism (any site) (artery) (cerebral) 958.0
    - with
      - abortion – *see* Abortion, by type, with embolism
      - ectopic pregnancy (*see also* categories 633.0-633.9) 639.6
      - molar pregnancy (*see also* categories 630-632) 639.6
    - due to implanted device – *see* Complications, due to (presence of) any device, implant, or graft classified to 996.0-996.5 NEC
    - following
      - abortion 639.6
      - ectopic or molar pregnancy 639.6
      - infusion, perfusion, or transfusion 999.1
    - in pregnancy, childbirth, or puerperium 673.0❺
    - traumatic 958.0
  - hunger 786.09
    - psychogenic 306.1
  - leak (lung) (pulmonary) (thorax) 512.8
    - iatrogenic 512.1
    - postoperative 512.1
  - rarefied, effects of – *see* Effect, adverse, high altitude
  - sickness 994.6
- **Airplane sickness** 994.6
- **Akathisia, acathisia** 781.0
  - due to drugs 333.99
  - neuroleptic-induced acute 333.99
- **Akinesia algeria** 352.6
- **Akiyami** 100.89
- **Akureyri disease** (epidemic neuromyasthenia) 049.8
- **Alacrima** (congenital) 743.65
- **Alactasia** (hereditary) 271.3
- **Alagille syndrome** 759.89
- **Alalia** 784.3
  - developmental 315.31
    - receptive-expressive 315.32
  - secondary to organic lesion 784.3
- **Alaninemia** 270.8
- **Alastrim** 050.1
- **Albarrán's disease** (colibacilluria) 791.9
- **Albers-Schönberg's disease** (marble bones) 756.52
- **Albert's disease** 726.71
- **Albinism, albino** (choroid) (cutaneous) (eye) (generalized) (isolated) (ocular) (oculocutaneous) (partial) 270.2
- **Albinismus** 270.2
- **Albright** (-Martin) (-Bantam) **disease** (pseudohypoparathyroidism) 275.49
- **Albright** (-McCune) (-Sternberg) **syndrome** (osteitis fibrosa disseminata) 756.59
- **Albuminous** – *see* condition
- **Albuminuria, albuminuric** (acute) (chronic) (subacute) 791.0
  - Bence-Jones 791.0
  - cardiac 785.9
  - complicating pregnancy, childbirth, or puerperium 646.2❺
    - with hypertension – *see* Toxemia, of pregnancy
    - affecting fetus or newborn 760.1
  - cyclic 593.6
  - gestational 646.2❺
  - gravidarum 646.2❺
    - with hypertension – *see* Toxemia, of pregnancy
    - affecting fetus or newborn 760.1
  - heart 785.9
  - idiopathic 593.6
  - orthostatic 593.6
  - postural 593.6
  - pre-eclamptic (mild) 642.4❺
    - affecting fetus or newborn 760.0
    - severe 642.5❺
      - affecting fetus or newborn 760.0
  - recurrent physiologic 593.6
  - scarlatinal 034.1
- **Albumosuria** 791.0
  - Bence-Jones 791.0
  - myelopathic (M9730/3) 203.0❺
- **Alcaptonuria** 270.2
- **Alcohol, alcoholic**
  - abstinence 291.81
  - acute intoxication 305.0❺
    - with dependence 303.0❺
  - addiction (*see also* Alcoholism) 303.9❺
    - maternal
      - with suspected fetal damage affecting management of pregnancy 655.4❺
      - affecting fetus or newborn 760.71
  - amnestic disorder, persisting 291.1
  - anxiety 291.89
  - brain syndrome, chronic 291.2
  - cardiopathy 425.5
  - chronic (*see also* Alcoholism) 303.9❺
  - cirrhosis (liver) 571.2
  - delirium 291.0
    - acute 291.0
    - chronic 291.1
    - tremens 291.0
    - withdrawal 291.0
  - dementia NEC 291.2
  - deterioration 291.2
  - drunkenness (simple) 305.0❺
  - hallucinosis (acute) 291.3
  - induced
    - circadian rhythm sleep disorder 291.82
    - hypersomnia 291.82
    - insomnia 291.82
    - mental disorder 291.9
      - anxiety 291.89
      - mood 291.89
      - sexual 291.89
      - sleep 291.92
      - specified type 291.89
    - parasomnia 291.82
    - persisting
      - amnestic disorder 291.1
      - dementia 291.2
    - psychotic disorder
      - with
        - delusions 291.5
        - hallucinations 291.3
    - sleep disorder 291.82
  - insanity 291.9
- **Alcohol, alcoholic** – *continued*
  - intoxication (acute) 305.0❺
    - with dependence 303.0❺
    - pathological 291.4
  - jealousy 291.5
  - Korsakoff's, Korsakov's, Korsakow's 291.1
  - liver NEC 571.3
    - acute 571.1
    - chronic 571.2
  - mania (acute) (chronic) 291.9
  - mood 291.89
  - paranoia 291.5
  - paranoid (type) psychosis 291.5
  - pellagra 265.2
  - poisoning, accidental (acute) NEC 980.9
    - specified type of alcohol – *see* Table of Drugs and Chemicals
  - psychosis (*see also* Psychosis, alcoholic) 291.9
    - Korsakoff's, Korsakov's, Korsakow's 291.1
    - polyneuritic 291.1
      - with
        - delusions 291.5
        - hallucinations 291.3
  - related disorder 291.9
  - withdrawal symptoms, syndrome NEC 291.81
    - delirium 291.0
    - hallucinosis 291.3
- **Alcoholism** 303.9❺

  Note – Use the following fifth-digit subclassification with category 303:

0	*unspecified*
1	*continuous*
2	*episodic*
3	*in remission*

  - with psychosis (*see also* Psychosis, alcoholic) 291.9
  - acute 303.0❺
  - chronic 303.9❺
    - with psychosis 291.9
  - complicating pregnancy, childbirth, or puerperium 648.4❺
    - affecting fetus or newborn 760.71
  - history V11.3
  - Korsakoff's, Korsakov's, Korsakow's 291.1
  - suspected damage to fetus affecting management of pregnancy 655.4❺
- **Alder's anomaly or syndrome** (leukocyte granulation anomaly) 288.2
- **Alder-Reilly anomaly** (leukocyte granulation) 288.2
- **Aldosteronism** (primary) 255.10
  - congenital 255.10
  - familial type I 255.11
  - glucocorticoid-remediable 255.11
  - secondary 255.14
- **Aldosteronoma** (M8370/1) 237.2
- **Aldrich** (-Wiskott) **syndrome** (eczema-thrombocytopenia) 279.12
- **Aleppo boil** 085.1
- **Aleukemic** – *see* condition
- **Aleukia**
  - congenital 288.09
  - hemorrhagica 284.9
    - acquired (secondary) 284.89 ▲
    - congenital 284.09
    - idiopathic 284.9
  - splenica 289.4
- **Alexia** (congenital) (developmental) 315.01
  - secondary to organic lesion 784.61
- **Algoneurodystrophy** 733.7
- **Algophobia** 300.29
- **Alibert's disease** (mycosis fungoides) (M9700/3) 202.1❺
- **Alibert-Bazin disease** (M9700/3) 202.1❺
- **Alice in Wonderland syndrome** 293.89
- **Alienation, mental** (*see also* Psychosis) 298.9
- **Alkalemia** 276.3
- **Alkalosis** 276.3
  - metabolic 276.3
    - with respiratory acidosis 276.4
  - respiratory 276.3
- **Alkaptonuria** 270.2
- **Allen-Masters syndrome** 620.6
- **Allergic bronchopulmonary aspergillosis** 518.6
- **Allergy, allergic** (reaction) 995.3
  - air-borne substance (*see also* Fever, hay) 477.9
    - specified allergen NEC 477.8

Agnosia – Allergy, allergic

Allergy, allergic – *continued*
  alveolitis (extrinsic) 495.9
    due to
      Aspergillus clavatus 495.4
      cryptostroma corticale 495.6
      organisms (fungal, thermophilic actinomycete, other) growing in ventilation (air conditioning systems) 495.7
    specified type NEC 495.8
  anaphylactic shock 999.4
    due to food – *see* Anaphylactic shock, due to, food
  angioneurotic edema 995.1
  animal (cat) (dog) (epidermal) 477.8
    dander, animal (cat) (dog) 477.2
    hair, animal (cat) (dog) 477.2
  arthritis (*see also* Arthritis, allergic) 716.2❺
  asthma – *see* Asthma
  bee sting (anaphylactic shock) 989.5
  biological – *see* Allergy, drug
  bronchial asthma – *see* Asthma
  conjunctivitis (eczematous) 372.14
  dander, animal (cat) (dog) 477.2
  dandruff 477.8
  dermatitis (venenata) – *see* Dermatitis
  diathesis V15.09
  drug, medicinal substance, and biological (any) (correct medicinal substance properly administered) (external) (internal) 995.27
    wrong substance given or taken NEC 977.9
      specified drug or substance – *see* Table of Drugs and Chemicals
  dust (house) (stock) 477.8
  eczema – *see* Eczema
  endophthalmitis 360.19
  epidermal (animal) 477.8
  existing dental restorative material 525.66●
  feathers 477.8
  food (any) (ingested) 693.1
    atopic 691.8
    in contact with skin 692.5
  gastritis 535.4❺
  gastroenteritis 558.3
  gastrointestinal 558.3
  grain 477.0
  grass (pollen) 477.0
    asthma (*see also* Asthma) 493.0❺
    hay fever 477.0
  hair, animal (cat) (dog) 477.8
  hay fever (grass) (pollen) (ragweed) (tree) (*see also* Fever, hay) 477.9
  history (of) V15.09
    to
      eggs V15.03
      food additives V15.05
      insect bite V15.06
      latex V15.07
      milk products V15.02
      nuts V15.05
        peanuts V15.01
      radiographic dye V15.08
      seafood V15.04
      specified food NEC V15.05
      spider bite V15.06
  horse serum – *see* Allergy, serum
  inhalant 477.9
    dust 477.8
    pollen 477.0
    specified allergen other than pollen 477.8
  kapok 477.8
  medicine – *see* Allergy, drug
  migraine 346.2❺
  milk protein 558.3
  pannus 370.62
  pneumonia 518.3
  pollen (any) (hay fever) 477.0
    asthma (*see also* Asthma) 493.0❺
  primrose 477.0
  primula 477.0
  purpura 287.0
  ragweed (pollen) (Senecio jacobae) 477.0
    asthma (*see also* Asthma) 493.0❺
    hay fever 477.0
  respiratory (*see also* Allergy, inhalant) 477.9
    due to
      drug – *see* Allergy, drug
      food – *see* Allergy, food
  rhinitis (*see also* Fever, hay) 477.9
    due to food 477.1
  rose 477.0
  Senecio jacobae 477.0

Allergy, allergic – *continued*
  serum (prophylactic) (therapeutic) 999.5
    anaphylactic shock 999.4
  shock (anaphylactic) (due to adverse effect of correct medicinal substance properly administered) 995.0
    food – *see* Anaphylactic shock, due to, food
    from serum or immunization 999.5
      anaphylactic 999.4
  sinusitis (*see also* Fever, hay) 477.9
  skin reaction 692.9
    specified substance – *see* Dermatitis, due to
  tree (any) (hay fever) (pollen) 477.0
    asthma (*see also* Asthma) 493.0❺
  upper respiratory (*see also* Fever, hay) 477.9
  urethritis 597.89
  urticaria 708.0
  vaccine – *see* Allergy, serum
Allescheriosis 117.6
Alligator skin disease (ichthyosis congenita) 757.1
  acquired 701.1
Allocheiria, allochiria (*see also* Disturbance, sensation) 782.0
Almeida's disease (Brazilian blastomycosis) 116.1
Alopecia (atrophicans) (pregnancy) (premature) (senile) 704.00
  adnata 757.4
  areata 704.01
  celsi 704.01
  cicatrisata 704.09
  circumscripta 704.01
  congenital, congenitalis 757.4
  disseminata 704.01
  effluvium (telogen) 704.02
  febrile 704.09
  generalisata 704.09
  hereditaria 704.09
  marginalis 704.01
  mucinosa 704.09
  postinfectional 704.09
  seborrheica 704.09
  specific 091.82
  syphilitic (secondary) 091.82
  telogen effluvium 704.02
  totalis 704.09
  toxica 704.09
  universalis 704.09
  x-ray 704.09
Alpers' disease 330.8
Alpha-lipoproteinemia 272.4
Alpha thalassemia 282.49
Alphos 696.1
Alpine sickness 993.2
Alport's syndrome (hereditary hematurianephropathy-deafness) 759.89
Alteration (of), altered
  awareness 780.09
    transient 780.02
  consciousness 780.09
    persistent vegetative state 780.03
    transient 780.02
  mental status 780.97
    amnesia (retrograde) 780.93
    memory loss 780.93
Alternaria (infection) 118
Alternating – *see* condition
Altitude, high (effects) – *see* Effect, adverse, high altitude
Aluminosis (of lung) 503
Alvarez syndrome (transient cerebral ischemia) 435.9
Alveolar capillary block syndrome 516.3
Alveolitis
  allergic (extrinsic) 495.9
    due to organisms (fungal, thermophilic actinomycete, other) growing in ventilation (air conditioning systems) 495.7
    specified type NEC 495.8
  due to
    Aspergillus clavatus 495.4
    Cryptostroma corticale 495.6
  fibrosing (chronic) (cryptogenic) (lung) 516.3
    idiopathic 516.3
    rheumatoid 714.81
  jaw 526.5
  sicca dolorosa 526.5
Alveolus, alveolar – *see* condition
Alymphocytosis (pure) 279.2

Alymphoplasia, thymic 279.2
Alzheimer's
  dementia (senile)
    with behavioral disturbance 331.0 *[294.11]*
    without behavioral disturbance 331.0 *[294.10]*
  disease or sclerosis 331.0
    with dementia – *see* Alzheimer's, dementia
Amastia (*see also* Absence, breast) 611.8
Amaurosis (acquired) (congenital) (*see also* Blindness) 369.00
  fugax 362.34
  hysterical 300.11
  Leber's (congenital) 362.76
  tobacco 377.34
  uremic – *see* Uremia
Amaurotic familial idiocy (infantile) (juvenile) (late) 330.1
Ambisexual 752.7
Amblyopia (acquired) (congenital) (partial) 368.00
  color 368.59
    acquired 368.55
  deprivation 368.02
  ex anopsia 368.00
  hysterical 300.11
  nocturnal 368.60
    vitamin A deficiency 264.5
  refractive 368.03
  strabismic 368.01
  suppression 368.01
  tobacco 377.34
  toxic NEC 377.34
  uremic – *see* Uremia
Ameba, amebic (histolytica) – *see also* Amebiasis
  abscess 006.3
    bladder 006.8
    brain (with liver and lung abscess) 006.5
    liver 006.3
      with
        brain abscess (and lung abscess) 006.5
        lung abscess 006.4
    lung (with liver abscess) 006.4
      with brain abscess 006.5
    seminal vesicle 006.8
    spleen 006.8
  carrier (suspected of) V02.2
  meningoencephalitis
    due to Naegleria (gruberi) 136.2
    primary 136.2
Amebiasis NEC 006.9
  with
    brain abscess (with liver or lung abscess) 006.5
    liver abscess (without mention of brain or lung abscess) 006.3
    lung abscess (with liver abscess) 006.4
      with brain abscess 006.5
  acute 006.0
  bladder 006.8
  chronic 006.1
  cutaneous 006.6
  cutis 006.6
  due to organism other than Entamoeba histolytica 007.8
  hepatic (*see also* Abscess, liver, amebic) 006.3
  nondysenteric 006.2
  seminal vesicle 006.8
  specified
    organism NEC 007.8
    site NEC 006.8
Ameboma 006.8
Amelia 755.4
  lower limb 755.31
  upper limb 755.21
Ameloblastoma (M9310/0) 213.1
  jaw (bone) (lower) 213.1
    upper 213.0
  long bones (M9261/3) – *see* Neoplasm, bone, malignant
  malignant (M9310/3) 170.1
    jaw (bone) (lower) 170.1
      upper 170.0
  mandible 213.1
  tibial (M9261/3) 170.7
Amelogenesis imperfecta 520.5
  nonhereditaria (segmentalis) 520.4
Amenorrhea (primary) (secondary) 626.0
  due to ovarian dysfunction 256.8
  hyperhormonal 256.8

Allergy, allergic – Amenorrhea

Amentia (*see also* Retardation, mental) 319
- Meynert's (nonalcoholic) 294.0
  - alcoholic 291.1
- nevoid 759.6

American
- leishmaniasis 085.5
- mountain tick fever 066.1
- trypanosomiasis – *see* Trypanosomiasis, American

Ametropia (*see also* Disorder, accommodation) 367.9
Amianthosis 501
Amimia 784.69
Amino acid
- deficiency 270.9
  - anemia 281.4
- metabolic disorder (*see also* Disorder, amino acid) 270.9

Aminoaciduria 270.9
- imidazole 270.5

Amnesia (retrograde) 780.93
- auditory 784.69
  - developmental 315.31
  - secondary to organic lesion 784.69
- dissociative 300.12
- hysterical or dissociative type 300.12
- psychogenic 300.12
- transient global 437.7

Amnestic (confabulatory) **syndrome** 294.0
- alcohol-induced persisting 291.1
- drug-induced persisting 292.83
- posttraumatic 294.0

Amniocentesis screening (for) V28.2
- alphafetoprotein level, raised V28.1
- chromosomal anomalies V28.0

Amnion, amniotic – *see also* condition
- nodosum 658.8❺

Amnionitis (complicating pregnancy) 658.4❺
- affecting fetus or newborn 762.7

Amoral trends 301.7
Amotio retinae (*see also* Detachment, retina) 361.9
Ampulla
- lower esophagus 530.89
- phrenic 530.89

Amputation
- any part of fetus, to facilitate delivery 763.89
- cervix (supravaginal) (uteri) 622.8
  - in pregnancy or childbirth 654.6❺
    - affecting fetus or newborn 763.89
- clitoris – *see* Wound, open, clitoris
- congenital
  - lower limb 755.31
  - upper limb 755.21
- neuroma (traumatic) – *see also* Injury, nerve, by site
  - surgical complication (late) 997.61
- penis – *see* Amputation, traumatic, penis
- status (without complication) – *see* Absence, by site, acquired
- stump (surgical) (posttraumatic)
  - abnormal, painful, or with complication (late) 997.60
  - healed or old NEC – *see also* Absence, by site, acquired
    - lower V49.70
    - upper V49.60
- traumatic (complete) (partial)

> *Note – "Complicated" includes traumatic amputation with delayed healing, delayed treatment, foreign body, or infection.*

  - arm 887.4
    - at or above elbow 887.2
      - complicated 887.3
    - below elbow 887.0
      - complicated 887.1
    - both (bilateral) (any level(s)) 887.6
      - complicated 887.7
    - complicated 887.5
  - finger(s) (one or both hands) 886.0
    - with thumb(s) 885.0
      - complicated 885.1
    - complicated 886.1
  - foot (except toe(s) only) 896.0
    - and other leg 897.6
      - complicated 897.7
    - both (bilateral) 896.2
      - complicated 896.3
    - complicated 896.1
    - toe(s) only (one or both feet) 895.0
      - complicated 895.1

Amputation – *continued*
- traumatic – *continued*
  - genital organ(s) (external) NEC 878.8
    - complicated 878.9
  - hand (except finger(s) only) 887.0
    - and other arm 887.6
      - complicated 887.7
    - both (bilateral) 887.6
      - complicated 887.7
    - complicated 887.1
    - finger(s) (one or both hands) 886.0
      - with thumb(s) 885.0
        - complicated 885.1
      - complicated 886.1
    - thumb(s) (with fingers of either hand) 885.0
      - complicated 885.1
  - head 874.9
  - late effect – *see* Late, effects (of), amputation
  - leg 897.4
    - and other foot 897.6
      - complicated 897.7
    - at or above knee 897.2
      - complicated 897.3
    - below knee 897.0
      - complicated 897.1
    - both (bilateral) 897.6
      - complicated 897.7
    - complicated 897.5
  - lower limb(s) except toe(s) – *see* Amputation, traumatic, leg
  - nose – *see* Wound, open, nose
  - penis 878.0
    - complicated 878.1
  - sites other than limbs – *see* Wound, open, by site
  - thumb(s) (with finger(s) of either hand) 885.0
    - complicated 885.1
  - toe(s) (one or both feet) 895.0
    - complicated 895.1
  - upper limb(s) – *see* Amputation traumatic, arm

Amputee (bilateral) (old) – *see also* Absence, by site, acquired V49.70
Amusia 784.69
- developmental 315.39
- secondary to organic lesion 784.69

Amyelencephalus 740.0
Amyelia 742.59
Amygdalitis – *see* Tonsillitis
Amygdalolith 474.8
Amyloid disease or degeneration 277.30
- heart 277.39 *[425.7]*

Amyloidosis (familial) (general) (generalized) (genetic) (primary) 277.39
- with lung involvement 277.39 *[517.8]*
- cardiac, hereditary 277.39
- heart 277.39 *[425.7]*
- nephropathic 277.39 *[583.81]*
- neuropathic (Portuguese) (Swiss) 277.39 *[357.4]*
- pulmonary 277.39 *[517.8]*
- secondary 277.39
- systemic, inherited 277.39

Amylopectinosis (brancher enzyme deficiency) 271.0
Amylophagia 307.52
Amyoplasia, congenita 756.89
Amyotonia 728.2
- congenita 358.8

Amyotrophia, amyotrophy, amyotrophic 728.2
- congenita 756.89
- diabetic 250.6❺ *[353.1]* ▲
- lateral sclerosis (syndrome) 335.20
- neuralgic 353.5
- sclerosis (lateral) 335.20
- spinal progressive 335.21

Anacidity, gastric 536.0
- psychogenic 306.4

Anaerosis of newborn 770.88
Analbuminemia 273.8
Analgesia (*see also* Anesthesia) 782.0
Analphalipoproteinemia 272.5
Anaphylactic shock or reaction (correct substance properly administered) 995.0
- due to
  - food 995.60
    - additives 995.66
    - crustaceans 995.62
    - eggs 995.68
    - fish 995.65
    - fruits 995.63

Anaphylactic shock or reaction – *continued*
- due to – *continued*
  - food – *continued*
    - milk products 995.67
    - nuts (tree) 995.64
    - peanuts 995.61
    - seeds 995.64
    - specified NEC 995.69
    - tree nuts 995.64
    - vegetables 995.63
  - immunization 999.4
  - overdose or wrong substance given or taken 977.9
    - specified drug – *see* Table of Drugs and Chemicals
  - serum 999.4
- following sting(s) 989.5
- purpura 287.0
- serum 999.4

Anaphylactoid shock or reaction – *see* Anaphylactic shock
Anaphylaxis – *see* Anaphylactic shock
Anaplasia, cervix 622.10
Anarthria 784.5
Anarthritic rheumatoid disease 446.5
Anasarca 782.3
- cardiac (*see also* Failure, heart) 428.0
- fetus or newborn 778.0
- lung 514
- nutritional 262
- pulmonary 514
- renal (*see also* Nephrosis) 581.9

Anaspadias 752.62
Anastomosis
- aneurysmal – *see* Aneurysm
- arteriovenous, congenital NEC (*see also* Anomaly, arteriovenous) 747.60
  - ruptured, of brain (*see also* Hemorrhage, subarachnoid) 430
- intestinal 569.89
  - complicated NEC 997.4
    - involving urinary tract 997.5
- retinal and choroidal vessels 743.58
  - acquired 362.17

Anatomical narrow angle (glaucoma) 365.02
Ancylostoma (infection) (infestation) 126.9
- americanus 126.1
- braziliense 126.2
- caninum 126.8
- ceylanicum 126.3
- duodenale 126.0
- Necator americanus 126.1

Ancylostomiasis (intestinal) 126.9
- ancylostoma
  - americanus 126.1
  - caninum 126.8
  - ceylanicum 126.3
  - duodenale 126.0
- braziliense 126.2
- Necator americanus 126.1

Anders' disease or syndrome (adiposis tuberosa simplex) 272.8
Andersen's glycogen storage disease 271.0
Anderson's disease 272.7
Andes disease 993.2
Andrews' disease (bactérid) 686.8
Androblastoma (M8630/1)
- benign (M8630/0)
  - specified site – *see* Neoplasm, by site, benign
  - unspecified site
    - female 220
    - male 222.0
- malignant (M8630/3)
  - specified site – *see* Neoplasm, by site, malignant
  - unspecified site
    - female 183.0
    - male 186.9
- specified site – *see* Neoplasm, by site, uncertain behavior
- tubular (M8640/0)
  - with lipid storage (M8641/0)
    - specified site – *see* Neoplasm, by site, benign
    - unspecified site
      - female 220
      - male 222.0
  - specified site – *see* Neoplasm, by site, benign

Amentia – Androblastoma

Androblastoma – *continued*
- tubular – *continued*
  - unspecified site
    - female 220
    - male 222.0
- unspecified site
  - female 236.2
  - male 236.4

Android pelvis 755.69
- with disproportion (fetopelvic) 653.3❺
  - affecting fetus or newborn 763.1
  - causing obstructed labor 660.1❺
    - affecting fetus or newborn 763.1

Anectasis, pulmonary (newborn or fetus) 770.5

Anemia 285.9
- with
  - disorder of
    - anaerobic glycolysis 282.3
    - pentose phosphate pathway 282.2
  - koilonychia 280.9
- 6-phosphogluconic dehydrogenase deficiency 282.2
- achlorhydric 280.9
- achrestic 281.8
- Addison's (pernicious) 281.0
- Addison-Biermer (pernicious) 281.0
- agranulocytic 288.09
- amino acid deficiency 281.4
- aplastic 284.9
  - acquired (secondary) 284.81 ▲
  - congenital 284.01
  - constitutional 284.01
  - due to
    - chronic systemic disease 284.89 ▲
    - drugs 284.89 ▲
    - infection 284.89 ▲
    - radiation 284.89 ▲
  - idiopathic 284.9
  - myxedema 244.9
  - of or complicating pregnancy 648.2❺
  - red cell (acquired) ▶(adult)◀ (with thymoma) 284.81 ▲
    - congenital 284.01
    - pure 284.01
  - specified type NEC 284.89 ▲
  - toxic (paralytic) 284.89 ▲
- aregenerative 284.9
  - congenital 284.01
- asiderotic 280.9
- atypical (primary) 285.9
- autohemolysis of Selwyn and Dacie (type I) 282.2
- autoimmune hemolytic 283.0
- Baghdad Spring 282.2
- Balantidium coli 007.0
- Biermer's (pernicious) 281.0
- blood loss (chronic) 280.0
  - acute 285.1
- bothriocephalus 123.4
- brickmakers' (*see also* Ancylostomiasis) 126.9
- cerebral 437.8
- childhood 282.9
- chlorotic 280.9
- chronica congenita aregenerativa 284.01
- chronic simple 281.9
- combined system disease NEC 281.0 *[336.2]*
  - due to dietary deficiency 281.1 *[336.2]*
- complicating pregnancy or childbirth 648.2❺
- congenital (following fetal blood loss) 776.5
  - aplastic 284.01
  - due to isoimmunization NEC 773.2
  - Heinz-body 282.7
  - hereditary hemolytic NEC 282.9
  - nonspherocytic
    - type I 282.2
    - type II 282.3
  - pernicious 281.0
  - spherocytic (*see also* Spherocytosis) 282.0
- Cooley's (erythroblastic) 282.49
- crescent – *see* Disease, sickle-cell
- cytogenic 281.0
- Dacie's (nonspherocytic)
  - type I 282.2
  - type II 282.3
- Davidson's (refractory) 284.9
- deficiency 281.9
  - 2, 3 diphosphoglycurate mutase 282.3
  - 2, 3 PG 282.3
  - 6-PGD 282.2
  - 6-phosphogluronic dehydrogenase 282.2
  - amino acid 281.4
  - combined B_{12} and folate 281.3

Anemia – *continued*
- deficiency – *continued*
  - enzyme, drug-induced (hemolytic) 282.2
  - erythrocytic glutathione 282.2
  - folate 281.2
    - dietary 281.2
    - drug-induced 281.2
  - folic acid 281.2
    - dietary 281.2
    - drug-induced 281.2
  - G-6-PD 282.2
  - GGS-R 282.2
  - glucose-6-phosphate dehydrogenase (G-6-PD) 282.2
  - glucose-phosphate isomerase 282.3
  - glutathione peroxidase 282.2
  - glutathione reductase 282.2
  - glyceraldehyde phosphate dehydrogenase 282.3
  - GPI 282.3
  - G SH 282.2
  - hexokinase 282.3
  - iron (Fe) 280.9
    - specified NEC 280.8
  - nutritional 281.9
    - with
      - poor iron absorption 280.9
      - specified deficiency NEC 281.8
    - due to inadequate dietary iron intake 280.1
    - specified type NEC 281.8
  - of or complicating pregnancy 648.2❺
  - pentose phosphate pathway 282.2
  - PFK 282.3
  - phosphofructo-aldolase 282.3
  - phosphofructokinase 282.3
  - phosphoglycerate kinase 282.3
  - PK 282.3
  - protein 281.4
  - pyruvate kinase (PK) 282.3
  - TPI 282.3
  - triosephosphate isomerase 282.3
  - vitamin B_{12} NEC 281.1
    - dietary 281.1
    - pernicious 281.0
- Diamond-Blackfan (congenital hypoplastic) 284.01
- dibothriocephalus 123.4
- dimorphic 281.9
- diphasic 281.8
- diphtheritic 032.89
- Diphyllobothrium 123.4
- drepanocytic (*see also* Disease, sickle-cell) 282.60
- due to
  - blood loss (chronic) 280.0
    - acute 285.1
  - defect of Embden-Meyerhof pathway glycolysis 282.3
  - disorder of glutathione metabolism 282.2
  - fetal blood loss 776.5
  - fish tapeworm (D. latum) infestation 123.4
  - glutathione metabolism disorder 282.2
  - hemorrhage (chronic) 280.0
    - acute 285.1
  - hexose monophosphate (HMP) shunt deficiency 282.2
  - impaired absorption 280.9
  - loss of blood (chronic) 280.0
    - acute 285.1
  - myxedema 244.9
  - Necator americanus 126.1
  - prematurity 776.6
  - selective vitamin B12 malabsorption with proteinuria 281.1
- Dyke-Young type (secondary) (symptomatic) 283.9
- dyserythropoietic (congenital) (types I, II, III) 285.8
- dyshemopoietic (congenital) 285.8
- Egypt (*see also* Ancylostomiasis) 126.9
- elliptocytosis (*see also* Elliptocytosis) 282.1
- enzyme deficiency, drug-induced 282.2
- epidemic (*see also* Ancylostomiasis) 126.9
- EPO resistant 285.21
- erythroblastic
  - familial 282.49
  - fetus or newborn (*see also* Disease, hemolytic) 773.2
    - late 773.5
- erythrocytic glutathione deficiency 282.2
- erythropoietin-resistant (EPO resistant anemia) 285.21

Anemia – *continued*
- essential 285.9
- Faber's (achlorhydric anemia) 280.9
- factitious (self-induced bloodletting) 280.0
- familial erythroblastic (microcytic) 282.49
- Fanconi's (congenital pancytopenia) 284.09
- favism 282.2
- fetal, following blood loss 776.5
- fetus or newborn
  - due to
    - ABO
      - antibodies 773.1
      - incompatibility, maternal/fetal 773.1
      - isoimmunization 773.1
    - Rh
      - antibodies 773.0
      - incompatibility, maternal/fetal 773.0
      - isoimmunization 773.0
  - following fetal blood loss 776.5
- fish tapeworm (D. latum) infestation 123.4
- folate (folic acid) deficiency 281.2
  - dietary 281.2
  - drug-induced 281.2
- folate malabsorption, congenital 281.2
- folic acid deficiency 281.2
  - dietary 281.2
  - drug-induced 281.2
- G-6-PD 282.2
- general 285.9
- glucose-6-phosphate dehydrogenase deficiency 282.2
- glutathione-reductase deficiency 282.2
- goat's milk 281.2
- granulocytic 288.09
- Heinz-body, congenital 282.7
- hemoglobin deficiency 285.9
- hemolytic 283.9
  - acquired 283.9
    - with hemoglobinuria NEC 283.2
    - autoimmune (cold type) (idiopathic) (primary) (secondary) (symptomatic) (warm type) 283.0
    - due to
      - cold reactive antibodies 283.0
      - drug exposure 283.0
      - warm reactive antibodies 283.0
    - fragmentation 283.19
    - idiopathic (chronic) 283.9
    - infectious 283.19
      - autoimmune 283.0
    - non-autoimmune 283.10
    - toxic 283.19
    - traumatic cardiac 283.19
  - acute 283.9
    - due to enzyme deficiency NEC 282.3
    - fetus or newborn (*see also* Disease, hemolytic) 773.2
      - late 773.5
    - Lederer's (acquired infectious hemolytic anemia) 283.19
  - autoimmune (acquired) 283.0
  - chronic 282.9
    - idiopathic 283.9
  - cold type (secondary) (symptomatic) 283.0
  - congenital (spherocytic) (*see also* Spherocytosis) 282.0
    - nonspherocytic – *see* Anemia, hemolytic, nonspherocytic, congenital
  - drug-induced 283.0
    - enzyme deficiency 282.2
  - due to
    - cardiac conditions 283.19
    - drugs 283.0
    - enzyme deficiency NEC 282.3
      - drug-induced 282.2
    - presence of shunt or other internal prosthetic device 283.19
    - thrombotic thrombocytopenic purpura 446.6
  - elliptocytotic (*see also* Elliptocytosis) 282.1
  - familial 282.9
  - hereditary 282.9
    - due to enzyme deficiency NEC 282.3
    - specified NEC 282.8
  - idiopathic (chronic) 283.9
  - infectious (acquired) 283.19
  - mechanical 283.19
  - microangiopathic 283.19
  - nonautoimmune 283.10
  - nonspherocytic
    - congenital or hereditary NEC 282.3
      - glucose-6-phosphate dehydrogenase deficiency 282.2

Anemia – *continued*
nonspherocytic – *continued*
congenital or hereditary – *continued*
pyruvate kinase (PK) deficiency 282.3
type I 282.2
type II 282.3
type I 282.2
type II 282.3
of or complicating pregnancy 648.2❺
resulting from presence of shunt or other internal prosthetic device 283.19
secondary 283.19
autoimmune 283.0
sickle-cell – *see* Disease, sickle-cell
Stransky-Regala type (Hb-E) (*see also* Disease, hemoglobin) 282.7
symptomatic 283.19
autoimmune 283.0
toxic (acquired) 283.19
uremic (adult) (child) 283.11
warm type (secondary) (symptomatic) 283.0
hemorrhagic (chronic) 280.0
acute 285.1
HEMPAS 285.8
hereditary erythroblast multinuclearity-positive acidified serum test 285.8
Herrick's (hemoglobin S disease) 282.61
hexokinase deficiency 282.3
high A_2 282.49
hookworm (*see also* Ancylostomiasis) 126.9
hypochromic (idiopathic) (microcytic) (normoblastic) 280.9
with iron loading 285.0
due to blood loss (chronic) 280.0
acute 285.1
familial sex linked 285.0
pyridoxine-responsive 285.0
hypoplasia, red blood cells 284.81 ▲
congenital or familial 284.01
hypoplastic (idiopathic) 284.9
congenital 284.01
familial 284.01
of childhood 284.09
idiopathic 285.9
hemolytic, chronic 283.9
in
chronic illness NEC 285.29
chronic kidney disease 285.21
end-stage renal disease 285.21
neoplastic disease 285.22
infantile 285.9
infective, infectional 285.9
intertropical (*see also* Ancylostomiasis) 126.9
iron (Fe) deficiency 280.9
due to blood loss (chronic) 280.0
acute 285.1
of or complicating pregnancy 648.2❺
specified NEC 280.8
Jaksch's (pseudoleukemia infantum) 285.8
Joseph-Diamond-Blackfan (congenital hypoplastic) 284.01
labyrinth 386.50
Lederer's (acquired infectious hemolytic anemia) 283.19
leptocytosis (hereditary) 282.49
leukoerythroblastic 284.2
macrocytic 281.9
nutritional 281.2
of or complicating pregnancy 648.2❺
tropical 281.2
malabsorption (familial), selective B12 with proteinuria 281.1
malarial (*see also* Malaria) 084.6
malignant (progressive) 281.0
malnutrition 281.9
marsh (*see also* Malaria) 084.6
Mediterranean (with hemoglobinopathy) 282.49
megaloblastic 281.9
combined B12 and folate deficiency 281.3
nutritional (of infancy) 281.2
of infancy 281.2
of or complicating pregnancy 648.2❺
refractory 281.3
specified NEC 281.3
megalocytic 281.9
microangiopathic hemolytic 283.19
microcytic (hypochromic) 280.9
due to blood loss (chronic) 280.0
acute 285.1
familial 282.49
hypochromic 280.9
microdrepanocytosis 282.49

Anemia – *continued*
miners' (*see also* Ancylostomiasis) 126.9
myelopathic 285.8
myelophthisic (normocytic) 284.2
newborn (*see also* Disease, hemolytic) 773.2
due to isoimmunization (*see also* Disease, hemolytic) 773.2
late, due to isoimmunization 773.5
posthemorrhagic 776.5
nonregenerative 284.9
nonspherocytic hemolytic – *see* Anemia, hemolytic, nonspherocytic
normocytic (infectional) (not due to blood loss) 285.9
due to blood loss (chronic) 280.0
acute 285.1
myelophthisic 284.2
nutritional (deficiency) 281.9
with
poor iron absorption 280.9
specified deficiency NEC 281.8
due to inadequate dietary iron intake 280.1
megaloblastic (of infancy) 281.2
of childhood 282.9
of chronic
disease NEC 285.29
illness NEC 285.29
of or complicating pregnancy 648.2❺
affecting fetus or newborn 760.8
of prematurity 776.6
orotic aciduric (congenital) (hereditary) 281.4
osteosclerotic 289.89
ovalocytosis (hereditary) (*see also* Elliptocytosis) 282.1
pentose phosphate pathway deficiency 282.2
pernicious (combined system disease) (congenital) (dorsolateral spinal degeneration) (juvenile) (myelopathy) (neuropathy) (posterior sclerosis) (primary) (progressive) (spleen) 281.0
of or complicating pregnancy 648.2❺
pleochromic 285.9
of sprue 281.8
portal 285.8
posthemorrhagic (chronic) 280.0
acute 285.1
newborn 776.5
postoperative
due to ▶(acute)◀ blood loss 285.1
chronic blood loss 280.0 ●
other 285.9
postpartum 648.2❺
pressure 285.9
primary 285.9
profound 285.9
progressive 285.9
malignant 281.0
pernicious 281.0
protein-deficiency 281.4
pseudoleukemica infantum 285.8
puerperal 648.2❺
pure red cell 284.81 ▲
congenital 284.01
pyridoxine-responsive (hypochromic) 285.0
pyruvate kinase (PK) deficiency 282.3
refractoria sideroblastica 238.72
refractory (primary) 238.72
with
excess
blasts-1 (RAEB-1) 238.73
blasts-2 (RAEB-2) 238.73
hemochromatosis 238.72
ringed sideroblasts (RARS) 238.72
megaloblastic 281.3
sideroblastic 238.72
sideropenic 280.9
Rietti-Greppi-Micheli (thalassemia minor) 282.49
scorbutic 281.8
secondary (to) 285.9
blood loss (chronic) 280.0
acute 285.1
hemorrhage 280.0
acute 285.1
inadequate dietary iron intake 280.1
semiplastic 284.9
septic 285.9
sickle-cell (*see also* Disease, sickle-cell) 282.60
sideroachrestic 285.0

Anemia – *continued*
sideroblastic (acquired) (any type) (congenital) (drug-induced) (due to disease) (hereditary) (primary) (secondary) (sex-linked hypochromic) (vitamin B_6 responsive) 285.0
refractory 238.72
sideropenic (refractory) 280.9
due to blood loss (chronic) 280.0
acute 285.1
simple chronic 281.9
specified type NEC 285.8
spherocytic (hereditary) (*see also* Spherocytosis) 282.0
splenic 285.8
familial (Gaucher's) 272.7
splenomegalic 285.8
stomatocytosis 282.8
syphilitic 095.8
target cell (oval) 282.49
thalassemia 282.49
thrombocytopenic (*see also* Thrombocytopenia) 287.5
toxic 284.89 ▲
triosephosphate isomerase deficiency 282.3
tropical, macrocytic 281.2
tuberculous (*see also* Tuberculosis) 017.9❺
Vegan's 281.1
vitamin
B_6-responsive 285.0
B_{12} deficiency (dietary) 281.1
pernicious 281.0
von Jaksch's (pseudoleukemia infantum) 285.8
Witts' (achlorhydric anemia) 280.9
Zuelzer (-Ogden) (nutritional megaloblastic anemia) 281.2

Anencephalus, anencephaly 740.0
fetal, affecting management of pregnancy 655.0❺

Anergasia (*see also* Psychosis, organic) 294.9
senile 290.0

Anesthesia, anesthetic 782.0
complication or reaction NEC 995.22
due to
correct substance properly administered 995.22
overdose or wrong substance given 968.4
specified anesthetic – *see* Table of Drugs and Chemicals
cornea 371.81
death from
correct substance properly administered 995.4
during delivery 668.9❺
overdose or wrong substance given 968.4
specified anesthetic – *see* Table of Drugs and Chemicals
eye 371.81
functional 300.11
hyperesthetic, thalamic 338.0
hysterical 300.11
local skin lesion 782.0
olfactory 781.1
sexual (psychogenic) 302.72
shock
due to
correct substance properly administered 995.4
overdose or wrong substance given 968.4
specified anesthetic – *see* Table of Drugs and Chemicals
skin 782.0
tactile 782.0
testicular 608.9
thermal 782.0

Anetoderma (maculosum) 701.3

Aneuploidy NEC 758.5

Aneurin deficiency 265.1

Aneurysm (anastomotic) (artery) (cirsoid) (diffuse) (false) (fusiform) (multiple) (ruptured) (saccular) (varicose) 442.9
abdominal (aorta) 441.4
ruptured 441.3
syphilitic 093.0
aorta, aortic (nonsyphilitic) 441.9
abdominal 441.4
dissecting 441.02
ruptured 441.3
syphilitic 093.0
arch 441.2
ruptured 441.1
arteriosclerotic NEC 441.9
ruptured 441.5

Aneurysm – *continued*
- aorta, aortic – *continued*
  - ascending 441.2
    - ruptured 441.1
  - congenital 747.29
  - descending 441.9
    - abdominal 441.4
      - ruptured 441.3
    - ruptured 441.5
    - thoracic 441.2
      - ruptured 441.1
  - dissecting 441.00
    - abdominal 441.02
    - thoracic 441.01
    - thoracoabdominal 441.03
  - due to coarctation (aorta) 747.10
  - ruptured 441.5
  - sinus, right 747.29
  - syphilitic 093.0
  - thoracoabdominal 441.7
    - ruptured 441.6
  - thorax, thoracic (arch) (nonsyphilitic) 441.2
    - dissecting 441.01
    - ruptured 441.1
    - syphilitic 093.0
  - transverse 441.2
    - ruptured 441.1
  - valve (heart) (*see also* Endocarditis, aortic) 424.1
- arteriosclerotic NEC 442.9
  - cerebral 437.3
    - ruptured (*see also* Hemorrhage, subarachnoid) 430
- arteriovenous (congenital) (peripheral) NEC (*see also* Anomaly, arteriovenous) 747.60
  - acquired NEC 447.0
    - brain 437.3
      - ruptured (*see also* Hemorrhage, subarachnoid) 430
    - coronary 414.11
    - pulmonary 417.0
  - brain (cerebral) 747.81
    - ruptured (*see also* Hemorrhage, subarachnoid) 430
  - coronary 746.85
  - pulmonary 747.3
  - retina 743.58
  - specified site NEC 747.89
    - acquired 447.0
  - traumatic (*see also* Injury, blood vessel, by site) 904.9
- basal – *see* Aneurysm, brain
- berry (congenital) (ruptured) (*see also* Hemorrhage, subarachnoid) 430
- brain 437.3
  - arteriosclerotic 437.3
    - ruptured (*see also* Hemorrhage, subarachnoid) 430
  - arteriovenous 747.81
    - acquired 437.3
      - ruptured (*see also* Hemorrhage, subarachnoid) 430
    - ruptured (*see also* Hemorrhage, subarachnoid) 430
  - berry (congenital) (ruptured) (*see also* Hemorrhage, subarachnoid) 430
  - congenital 747.81
    - ruptured (*see also* Hemorrhage, subarachnoid) 430
  - meninges 437.3
    - ruptured (*see also* Hemorrhage, subarachnoid) 430
  - miliary (congenital) (ruptured) (*see also* Hemorrhage, subarachnoid) 430
  - mycotic 421.0
    - ruptured (*see also* Hemorrhage, subarachnoid) 430
  - nonruptured 437.3
  - ruptured (*see also* Hemorrhage, subarachnoid) 430
    - syphilitic 094.87
  - syphilitic (hemorrhage) 094.87
  - traumatic – *see* Injury, intracranial
- cardiac (false) (*see also* Aneurysm, heart) 414.10
- carotid artery (common) (external) 442.81
  - internal (intracranial portion) 437.3
    - extracranial portion 442.81
    - ruptured into brain (*see also* Hemorrhage, subarachnoid) 430
  - syphilitic 093.89
    - intracranial 094.87

Aneurysm – *continued*
- cavernous sinus (*see also* Aneurysm, brain) 437.3
  - arteriovenous 747.81
    - ruptured (*see also* Hemorrhage, subarachnoid) 430
  - congenital 747.81
    - ruptured (*see also* Hemorrhage, subarachnoid) 430
- celiac 442.84
- central nervous system, syphilitic 094.89
- cerebral – *see* Aneurysm, brain
- chest – *see* Aneurysm, thorax
- circle of Willis (*see also* Aneurysm, brain) 437.3
  - congenital 747.81
    - ruptured (*see also* Hemorrhage, subarachnoid) 430
  - ruptured (*see also* Hemorrhage, subarachnoid) 430
- common iliac artery 442.2
- congenital (peripheral) NEC 747.60
  - brain 747.81
    - ruptured (*see also* Hemorrhage, subarachnoid) 430
  - cerebral – *see* Aneurysm, brain, congenital
  - coronary 746.85
  - gastrointestinal 747.61
  - lower limb 747.64
  - pulmonary 747.3
  - renal 747.62
  - retina 743.58
  - specified site NEC 747.89
  - spinal 747.82
  - upper limb 747.63
- conjunctiva 372.74
- conus arteriosus (*see also* Aneurysm, heart) 414.10
- coronary (arteriosclerotic) (artery) (vein) (*see also* Aneurysm, heart) 414.11
  - arteriovenous 746.85
  - congenital 746.85
  - syphilitic 093.89
- cylindrical 441.9
  - ruptured 441.5
  - syphilitic 093.9
- dissecting 442.9
  - aorta 441.00
    - abdominal 441.02
    - thoracic 441.01
    - thoracoabdominal 441.03
  - syphilitic 093.9
- ductus arteriosus 747.0
- embolic – *see* Embolism, artery
- endocardial, infective (any valve) 421.0
- femoral 442.3
- gastroduodenal 442.84
- gastroepiploic 442.84
- heart (chronic or with a stated duration of over 8 weeks) (infectional) (wall) 414.10
  - acute or with a stated duration of 8 weeks or less (*see also* Infarct, myocardium) 410.9❺
  - congenital 746.89
  - valve – *see* Endocarditis
- hepatic 442.84
- iliac (common) 442.2
- infective (any valve) 421.0
- innominate (nonsyphilitic) 442.89
  - syphilitic 093.89
- interauricular septum (*see also* Aneurysm, heart) 414.10
- interventricular septum (*see also* Aneurysm, heart) 414.10
- intracranial – *see* Aneurysm, brain
- intrathoracic (nonsyphilitic) 441.2
  - ruptured 441.1
  - syphilitic 093.0
- jugular vein 453.8
- lower extremity 442.3
- lung (pulmonary artery) 417.1
- malignant 093.9
- mediastinal (nonsyphilitic) 442.89
  - syphilitic 093.89
- miliary (congenital) (ruptured) (*see also* Hemorrhage, subarachnoid) 430
- mitral (heart) (valve) 424.0
- mural (arteriovenous) (heart) (*see also* Aneurysm, heart) 414.10
- mycotic, any site 421.0
  - ruptured, brain (*see also* Hemorrhage, subarachnoid) 430
  - without endocarditis – *see* Aneurysm, by site

Aneurysm – *continued*
- myocardium (*see also* Aneurysm heart) 414.10
- neck 442.81
- pancreaticoduodenal 442.84
- patent ductus arteriosus 747.0
- peripheral NEC 442.89
  - congenital NEC (*see also* Aneurysm, congenital) 747.60
- popliteal 442.3
- pulmonary 417.1
  - arteriovenous 747.3
    - acquired 417.0
  - syphilitic 093.89
  - valve (heart) (*see also* Endocarditis, pulmonary) 424.3
- racemose 442.9
  - congenital (peripheral) NEC 747.60
- radial 442.0
- Rasmussen's (*see also* Tuberculosis) 011.2❺
- renal 442.1
- retinal (acquired) 362.17
  - congenital 743.58
  - diabetic 250.5❺ *[362.01]*
- sinus, aortic (of Valsalva) 747.29
- specified site NEC 442.89
- spinal (cord) 442.89
  - congenital 747.82
  - syphilitic (hemorrhage) 094.89
- spleen, splenic 442.83
- subclavian 442.82
  - syphilitic 093.89
- superior mesenteric 442.84
- syphilitic 093.9
  - aorta 093.0
  - central nervous system 094.89
  - congenital 090.5
  - spine, spinal 094.89
- thoracoabdominal 441.7
  - ruptured 441.6
- thorax, thoracic (arch) (nonsyphilitic) 441.2
  - dissecting 441.0❺
  - ruptured 441.1
  - syphilitic 093.0
- traumatic (complication) (early) – *see* Injury, blood vessel, by site
- tricuspid (heart) (valve) – *see* Endocarditis, tricuspid
- ulnar 442.0
- upper extremity 442.0
- valve, valvular – *see* Endocarditis
- venous 456.8
  - congenital NEC (*see also* Aneurysm, congenital) 747.60
- ventricle (arteriovenous) (*see also* Aneurysm, heart) 414.10
- visceral artery NEC 442.84

Angiectasis 459.89

Angiectopia 459.9

Angiitis 447.6
- allergic granulomatous 446.4
- hypersensitivity 446.20
  - Goodpasture's syndrome 446.21
  - specified NEC 446.29
- necrotizing 446.0
- Wegener's (necrotizing respiratory granulomatosis) 446.4

Angina (attack) (cardiac) (chest) (effort) (heart) (pectoris) (syndrome) (vasomotor) 413.9
- abdominal 557.1
- accelerated 411.1
- agranulocytic 288.03
- aphthous 074.0
- catarrhal 462
- crescendo 411.1
- croupous 464.4
- cruris 443.9
  - due to atherosclerosis NEC (*see also* Arteriosclerosis, extremities) 440.20
- decubitus 413.0
- diphtheritic (membranous) 032.0
- erysipelatous 034.0
- erythematous 462
- exudative, chronic 476.0
- faucium 478.29
- gangrenous 462
  - diphtheritic 032.0
- infectious 462
- initial 411.1
- intestinal 557.1
- ludovici 528.3
- Ludwig's 528.3

Aneurysm – Angina

- **Angina** – *continued*
  - malignant 462
    - diphtheritic 032.0
  - membranous 464.4
    - diphtheritic 032.0
  - mesenteric 557.1
  - monocytic 075
  - nocturnal 413.0
  - phlegmonous 475
    - diphtheritic 032.0
  - preinfarctional 411.1
  - Prinzmetal's 413.1
  - progressive 411.1
  - pseudomembranous 101
  - psychogenic 306.2
  - pultaceous, diphtheritic 032.0
  - scarlatinal 034.1
  - septic 034.0
  - simple 462
  - stable NEC 413.9
  - staphylococcal 462
  - streptococcal 034.0
  - stridulous, diphtheritic 032.3
  - syphilitic 093.9
    - congenital 090.5
  - tonsil 475
  - trachealis 464.4
  - unstable 411.1
  - variant 413.1
  - Vincent's 101
- **Angioblastoma** (M9161/1) – *see* Neoplasm, connective tissue, uncertain behavior
- **Angiocholecystitis** (*see also* Cholecystitis, acute) 575.0
- **Angiocholitis** (*see also* Cholecystitis, acute) 576.1
- **Angiodysgensis spinalis** 336.1
- **Angiodysplasia** (intestinalis) (intestine) 569 84
  - with hemorrhage 569.85
  - duodenum 537.82
    - with hemorrhage 537.83
  - stomach 537.82
    - with hemorrhage 537.83
- **Angioedema** (allergic) (any site) (with urticaria) 995.1
  - hereditary 277.6
- **Angioendothelioma** (M9130/1) – *see also* Neoplasm, by site, uncertain behavior
  - benign (M9130/0) (*see also* Hemangioma, by site) 228.00
  - bone (M9260/3) – *see* Neoplasm, bone, malignant
  - Ewing's (M9260/3) – *see* Neoplasm, bone, malignant
  - nervous system (M9130/0) 228.09
- **Angiofibroma** (M9160/0) – *see also* Neoplasm, by site, benign
  - juvenile (M9160/0) 210.7
    - specified site – *see* Neoplasm, by site, benign
    - unspecified site 210.7
- **Angiohemophilia** (A) (B) 286.4
- **Angioid streaks** (choroid) (retina) 363.43
- **Angiokeratoma** (M9141/0) – *see also* Neoplasm, skin, benign
  - corporis diffusum 272.7
- **Angiokeratosis**
  - diffuse 272.7
- **Angioleiomyoma** (M8894/0) – *see* Neoplasm, connective tissue, benign
- **Angioleucitis** 683
- **Angiolipoma** (M8861/0) (*see also* Lipoma, by site) 214.9
  - infiltrating (M8861/1) – *see* Neoplasm, connective tissue, uncertain behavior
- **Angioma** (M9120/0) (*see also* Hemangioma, by site) 228.00
  - capillary 448.1
  - hemorrhagicum hereditaria 448.0
  - malignant (M9120/3) – *see* Neoplasm, connective tissue, malignant
  - pigmentosum et atrophicum 757.33
  - placenta – *see* Placenta, abnormal
  - plexiform (M9131/0) – *see* Hemangioma, by site
  - senile 448.1
  - serpiginosum 709.1
  - spider 448.1
  - stellate 448.1
- **Angiomatosis** 757.32
  - bacillary 083.8
  - corporis diffusum universale 272.7
  - cutaneocerebral 759.6
- **Angiomatosis** – *continued*
  - encephalocutaneous 759.6
  - encephalofacial 759.6
  - encephalotrigeminal 759.6
  - hemorrhagic familial 448.0
  - hereditary familial 448.0
  - heredofamilial 448.0
  - meningo-oculofacial 759.6
  - multiple sites 228.09
  - neuro-oculocutaneous 759.6
  - retina (Hippel's disease) 759.6
  - retinocerebellosa 759.6
  - retinocerebral 759.6
  - systemic 228.09
- **Angiomyolipoma** (M8860/0)
  - specified site – *see* Neoplasm, connective tissue, benign
  - unspecified site 223.0
- **Angiomyoliposarcoma** (M8860/3) – *see* Neoplasm, connective tissue, malignant
- **Angiomyoma** (M8894/0) – *see* Neoplasm, connective tissue, benign
- **Angiomyosarcoma** (M8894/3) – *see* Neoplasm, connective tissue, malignant
- **Angioneurosis** 306.2
- **Angioneurotic edema** (allergic) (any site) (with urticaria) 995.1
  - hereditary 277.6
- **Angiopathia, angiopathy** 459.9
  - diabetic (peripheral) 250.7❺ *[443.81]*
  - peripheral 443.9
    - diabetic 250.7❺ *[443.81]*
    - specified type NEC 443.89
  - retinae syphilitica 093.89
  - retinalis (juvenilis) 362.18
    - background 362.10
    - diabetic 250.5❺ *[362.01]*
    - proliferative 362.29
    - tuberculous (*see also* Tuberculosis) 017.3❺ *[362.18]*
- **Angiosarcoma** (M9120/3) – *see* Neoplasm, connective tissue, malignant
- **Angiosclerosis** – *see* Arteriosclerosis
- **Angioscotoma, enlarged** 368.42
- **Angiospasm** 443.9
  - brachial plexus 353.0
  - cerebral 435.9
  - cervical plexus 353.2
  - nerve
    - arm 354.9
      - axillary 353.0
      - median 354.1
      - ulnar 354.2
    - autonomic (*see also* Neuropathy, peripheral, autonomic) 337.9
    - axillary 353.0
    - leg 355.8
      - plantar 355.6
    - lower extremity – *see* Angiospasm, nerve, leg
    - median 354.1
    - peripheral NEC 355.9
    - spinal NEC 355.9
    - sympathetic (*see also* Neuropathy, peripheral, autonomic) 337.9
    - ulnar 354.2
    - upper extremity – *see* Angiospasm, nerve, arm
  - peripheral NEC 443.9
  - traumatic 443.9
    - foot 443.9
    - leg 443.9
  - vessel 443.9
- **Angiospastic disease or edema** 443.9
- **Angle's**
  - class I 524.21
  - class II 524.22
  - class III 524.23
- **Anguillulosis** 127.2
- **Angulation**
  - cecum (*see also* Obstruction, intestine) 560.9
  - coccyx (acquired) 738.6
    - congenital 756.19
  - femur (acquired) 736.39
    - congenital 755.69
  - intestine (large) (small) (*see also* Obstruction, intestine) 560.9
  - sacrum (acquired) 738.5
    - congenital 756.19
  - sigmoid (flexure) (*see also* Obstruction, intestine) 560.9
- **Angulation** – *continued*
  - spine (*see also* Curvature, spine) 737.9
  - tibia (acquired) 736.89
    - congenital 755.69
  - ureter 593.3
  - wrist (acquired) 736.09
    - congenital 755.59
- **Angulus infectiosus** 686.8
- **Anhedonia** 780.99 ▲
- **Anhidrosis** (lid) (neurogenic) (thermogenic) 705.0
- **Anhydration** 276.51
  - with
    - hypernatremia 276.0
    - hyponatremia 276.1
- **Anhydremia** 276.52
  - with
    - hypernatremia 276.0
    - hyponatremia 276.1
- **Anidrosis** 705.0
- **Aniridia** (congenital) 743.45
- **Anisakiasis** (infection) (infestation) 127.1
- **Anisakis larva infestation** 127.1
- **Aniseikonia** 367.32
- **Anisocoria** (pupil) 379.41
  - congenital 743.46
- **Anisocytosis** 790.09
- **Anisometropia** (congenital) 367.31
- **Ankle** – *see* condition
- **Ankyloblepharon** (acquired) (eyelid) 374.46
  - filiforme (adnatum) (congenital) 743.62
  - total 743.62
- **Ankylodactly** (*see also* Syndactylism) 755.10
- **Ankyloglossia** 750.0
- **Ankylosis** (fibrous) (osseous) 718.50
  - ankle 718.57
  - any joint, produced by surgical fusion V45.4
  - cricoarytenoid (cartilage) (joint) (larynx) 478.79
  - dental 521.6
  - ear ossicle NEC 385.22
    - malleus 385.21
  - elbow 718.52
  - finger 718.54
  - hip 718.55
  - incostapedial joint (infectional) 385.22
  - joint, produced by surgical fusion NEC V45.4
  - knee 718.56
  - lumbosacral (joint) 724.6
  - malleus 385.21
  - multiple sites 718.59
  - postoperative (status) V45.4
  - sacroiliac (joint) 724.6
  - shoulder 718.51
  - specified site NEC 718.58
  - spine NEC 724.9
  - surgical V45.4
  - teeth, tooth (hard tissues) 521.6
  - temporomandibular joint 524.61
  - wrist 718.53
- **Ankylostoma** – *see* Ancylostoma
- **Ankylostomiasis** (intestinal) – *see* Ancylostomiasis
- **Ankylurethria** (*see also* Stricture, urethra) 598.9
- **Annular** – *see also* condition
  - detachment, cervix 622.8
  - organ or site, congenital NEC – *see* Distortion
  - pancreas (congenital) 751.7
- **Anodontia** (complete) (partial) (vera) 520.0
  - with abnormal spacing 524.30
  - acquired 525.10
    - causing malocclusion 524.30
    - due to
      - caries 525.13
      - extraction 525.10
      - periodontal disease 525.12
      - trauma 525.11
- **Anomaly, anomalous** (congenital) (unspecified type) 759.9
  - abdomen 759.9
  - abdominal wall 756.70
  - acoustic nerve 742.9
  - adrenal (gland) 759.1
  - Alder (-Reilly) (leukocyte granulation) 288.2
  - alimentary tract 751.9
    - lower 751.5
    - specified type NEC 751.8
    - upper (any part, except tongue) 750.9
      - tongue 750.10
        - specified type NEC 750.19

Anomaly, anomalous – *continued*
- alveolar 524.70
  - ridge (process) 525.8
  - specified NEC 524.79
- ankle (joint) 755.69
- anus, anal (canal) 751.5
- aorta, aortic 747.20
  - arch 747.21
  - coarctation (postductal) (preductal) 747.10
  - cusp or valve NEC 746.9
  - septum 745.0
  - specified type NEC 747.29
- aorticopulmonary septum 745.0
- apertures, diaphragm 756.6
- appendix 751.5
- aqueduct of Sylvius 742.3
  - with spina bifida (*see also* Spina bifida) 741.0❺
- arm 755.50
  - reduction (*see also* Deformity, reduction, upper limb) 755.20
- arteriovenous (congenital) (peripheral) NEC 747.60
  - brain 747.81
  - cerebral 747.81
  - coronary 746.85
  - gastrointestinal 747.61
    - acquired – *see* Angiodysplasia
  - lower limb 747.64
  - renal 747.62
  - specified site NEC 747.69
  - spinal 747.82
  - upper limb 747.63
- artery (*see also* Anomaly, peripheral vascular system) NEC 747.60
  - brain 747.81
  - cerebral 747.81
  - coronary 746.85
  - eye 743.9
  - pulmonary 747.3
  - renal 747.62
  - retina 743.9
  - umbilical 747.5
- arytenoepiglottic folds 748.3
- atrial
  - bands 746.9
  - folds 746.9
  - septa 745.5
- atrioventricular
  - canal 745.69
  - common 745.69
  - conduction 426.7
  - excitation 426.7
  - septum 745.4
- atrium – *see* Anomaly, atrial
- auditory canal 744.3
  - specified type NEC 744.29
    - with hearing impairment 744.02
- auricle
  - ear 744.3
    - causing impairment of hearing 744.02
  - heart 746.9
    - septum 745.5
- autosomes, autosomal NEC 758.5
- Axenfeld's 743.44
- back 759.9
- band
  - atrial 746.9
  - heart 746.9
  - ventricular 746.9
- Bartholin's duct 750.9
- biliary duct or passage 751.60
  - atresia 751.61
- bladder (neck) (sphincter) (trigone) 753.9
  - specified type NEC 753.8
- blood vessel 747.9
  - artery – *see* Anomaly, artery
  - peripheral vascular – *see* Anomaly, peripheral vascular system
  - vein – *see* Anomaly, vein
- bone NEC 756.9
  - ankle 755.69
  - arm 755.50
  - chest 756.3
  - cranium 756.0
  - face 756.0
  - finger 755.50
  - foot 755.67
  - forearm 755.50
  - frontal 756.0
  - head 756.0
  - hip 755.63

Anomaly, anomalous – *continued*
- bone – *continued*
  - leg 755.60
  - lumbosacral 756.10
  - nose 748.1
  - pelvic girdle 755.60
  - rachitic 756.4
  - rib 756.3
  - shoulder girdle 755.50
  - skull 756.0
    - with
      - anencephalus 740.0
      - encephalocele 742.0
      - hydrocephalus 742.3
        - with spina bifida (*see also* Spina bifida) 741.0❺
      - microcephalus 742.1
  - toe 755.66
- brain 742.9
  - multiple 742.4
  - reduction 742.2
  - specified type NEC 742.4
  - vessel 747.81
- branchial cleft NEC 744.49
  - cyst 744.42
  - fistula 744.41
  - persistent 744.41
  - sinus (external) (internal) 744.41
- breast 757.9
- broad ligament 752.10
  - specified type NEC 752.19
- bronchus 748.3
- bulbar septum 745.0
- bulbus cordis 745.9
  - persistent (in left ventricle) 745.8
- bursa 756.9
- canal of Nuck 752.9
- canthus 743.9
- capillary NEC (*see also* Anomaly, peripheral vascular system) 747.60
- cardiac 746.9
  - septal closure 745.9
    - acquired 429.71
  - valve NEC 746.9
    - pulmonary 746.00
    - specified type NEC 746.89
- cardiovascular system 746.9
  - complicating pregnancy, childbirth, or puerperium 648.5❺
- carpus 755.50
- cartilage, trachea 748.3
- cartilaginous 756.9
- caruncle, lacrimal, lachrymal 743.9
- cascade stomach 750.7
- cauda equina 742.59
- cecum 751.5
- cerebral – *see also* Anomaly, brain vessels 747.81
- cerebrovascular system 747.81
- cervix (uterus) 752.40
  - with doubling of vagina and uterus 752.2
  - in pregnancy or childbirth 654.6❺
    - affecting fetus or newborn 763.89
    - causing obstructed labor 660.2❺
      - affecting fetus or newborn 763.1
- Chédiak-Higashi (-Steinbrinck) (congenital gigantism of peroxidase granules) 288.2
- cheek 744.9
- chest (wall) 756.3
- chin 744.9
  - specified type NEC 744.89
- chordae tendineae 746.9
- choroid 743.9
  - plexus 742.9
- chromosomes, chromosomal 758.9
  - 13 (13-15) 758.1
  - 18 (16-18) 758.2
  - 21 or 22 758.0
  - autosomes NEC (*see also* Abnormal, autosomes) 758.5
    - deletion 758.39
  - Christchurch 758.39
  - D_1 758.1
  - E_3 758.2
  - G 758.0
  - mitochondrial 758.9
  - mosaics 758.89
  - sex 758.81
    - complement, XO 758.6
    - complement, XXX 758.81
    - complement, XXY 758.7
    - complement, XYY 758.81

Anomaly, anomalous – *continued*
- chromosomes, chromosomal – *continued*
  - sex – *continued*
    - gonadal dysgenesis 758.6
    - Klinefelter's 758.7
    - Turner's 758.6
  - trisomy 21 758.0
- cilia 743.9
- circulatory system 747.9
  - specified type NEC 747.89
- clavicle 755.51
- clitoris 752.40
- coccyx 756.10
- colon 751.5
- common duct 751.60
- communication
  - coronary artery 746.85
  - left ventricle with right atrium 745.4
- concha (ear) 744.3
- connection
  - renal vessels with kidney 747.62
  - total pulmonary venous 747.41
- connective tissue 756.9
  - specified type NEC 756.89
- cornea 743.9
  - shape 743.41
  - size 743.41
  - specified type NEC 743.49
- coronary
  - artery 746.85
  - vein 746.89
- cranium – *see* Anomaly, skull
- cricoid cartilage 748.3
- cushion, endocardial 745.60
  - specified type NEC 745.69
- cystic duct 751.60
- dental arch 524.20
  - specified NEC 524.29
- dental arch relationship 524.20
  - Angle's class I 524.21
  - Angle's class II 524.22
  - Angle's class III 524.23
  - articulation
    - anterior 524.27
    - posterior 524.27
    - reverse 524.27
  - disto-occlusion 524.22
    - division I 524.22
    - division II 524.22
  - excessive horizontal overlap 524.26
  - interarch distance (excessive) (inadequate) 524.28
  - mesio-occlusion 524.23
  - neutro-occlusion 524.21
  - open
    - anterior occlusal relationship 524.25
    - posterior occlusal relationship 524.25
  - specified NEC 524.29
- dentition 520.6
- dentofacial NEC 524.9
  - functional 524.50
  - specified type NEC 524.89
- dermatoglyphic 757.2
- Descemet's membrane 743.9
  - specified type NEC 743.49
- development
  - cervix 752.40
  - vagina 752.40
  - vulva 752.40
- diaphragm, diaphragmatic (apertures) NEC 756.6
- digestive organ(s) or system 751.9
  - lower 751.5
  - specified type NEC 751.8
  - upper 750.9
- distribution, coronary artery 746.85
- ductus
  - arteriosus 747.0
  - Botalli 747.0
- duodenum 751.5
- dura 742.9
  - brain 742.4
  - spinal cord 742.59
- ear 744.3
  - causing impairment of hearing 744.00
    - specified type NEC 744.09
  - external 744.3
    - causing impairment of hearing 744.02
    - specified type NEC 744.29
  - inner (causing impairment of hearing) 744.05
  - middle, except ossicles (causing impairment of hearing) 744.03
    - ossicles 744.04

Anomaly, anomalous – *continued*
  ear – *continued*
    ossicles 744.04
    prominent auricle 744.29
    specified type NEC 744.29
      with hearing impairment 744.09
  Ebstein's (heart) 746.2
    tricuspid valve 746.2
  ectodermal 757.9
  Eisenmenger's (ventricular septal defect) 745.4
  ejaculatory duct 752.9
    specified type NEC 752.89
  elbow (joint) 755.50
  endocardial cushion 745.60
    specified type NEC 745.69
  endocrine gland NEC 759.2
  epididymis 752.9
  epiglottis 748.3
  esophagus 750.9
    specified type NEC 750.4
  Eustachian tube 744.3
    specified type NEC 744.24
  eye (any part) 743.9
    adnexa 743.9
      specified type NEC 743.69
    anophthalmos 743.00
    anterior
      chamber and related structures 743.9
        angle 743.9
          specified type NEC 743.44
        specified type NEC 743.44
      segment 743.9
        combined 743.48
        multiple 743.48
        specified type NEC 743.49
    cataract (*see also* Cataract) 743.30
    glaucoma (*see also* Buphthalmia) 743 20
    lid 743.9
      specified type NEC 743.63
    microphthalmos (*see also* Microphthalmos) 743.10
    posterior segment 743.9
      specified type NEC 743.59
      vascular 743.58
      vitreous 743.9
        specified type NEC 743.51
    ptosis (eyelid) 743.61
    retina 743.9
      specified type NEC 743.59
    sclera 743.9
      specified type NEC 743.47
    specified type NEC 743.8
  eyebrow 744.89
  eyelid 743.9
    specified type NEC 743.63
  face (any part) 744.9
    bone(s) 756.0
    specified type NEC 744.89
  fallopian tube 752.10
    specified type NEC 752.19
  fascia 756.9
    specified type NEC 756.89
  femur 755.60
  fibula 755.60
  finger 755.50
    supernumerary 755.01
    webbed (*see also* Syndactylism, fingers) 755.11
  fixation, intestine 751.4
  flexion (joint) 755.9
    hip or thigh (*see also* Dislocation, hip, congenital) 754.30
  folds, heart 746.9
  foot 755.67
  foramen
    Botalli 745.5
    ovale 745.5
  forearm 755.50
  forehead (*see also* Anomaly, skull) 756.0
  form, teeth 520.2
  fovea centralis 743.9
  frontal bone (*see also* Anomaly, skull) 756.0
  gallbladder 751.60
  Gartner's duct 752.41
  gastrointestinal tract 751.9
    specified type NEC 751.8
    vessel 747.61
  genitalia, genital organ(s) or system
    female 752.9
      external 752.40
        specified type NEC 752.49
      internal NEC 752.9

Anomaly, anomalous – *continued*
  genitalia, genital organ(s) or system – *continued*
    male (external and internal) 752.9
      epispadias 752.62
      hidden penis 752.65
      hydrocele, congenital 778.6
      hypospadias 752.61
      micropenis 752.64
      testis, undescended 752.51
        retractile 752.52
    specified type NEC 752.89
  genitourinary NEC 752.9
  Gerbode 745.4
  globe (eye) 743.9
  glottis 748.3
  granulation or granulocyte, genetic 288.2
    constitutional 288.2
    leukocyte 288.2
  gum 750.9
  gyri 742.9
  hair 757.9
    specified type NEC 757.4
  hand 755.50
  hard tissue formation in pulp 522.3
  head (*see also* Anomaly, skull) 756.0
  heart 746.9
    auricle 746.9
    bands 746.9
    fibroelastosis cordis 425.3
    folds 746.9
    malposition 746.87
    maternal, affecting fetus or newborn 760.3
    obstructive NEC 746.84
    patent ductus arteriosus (Botalli) 747.0
    septum 745.9
      acquired 429.71
      aortic 745.0
      aorticopulmonary 745.0
      atrial 745.5
      auricular 745.5
      between aorta and pulmonary artery 745.0
      endocardial cushion type 745.60
        specified type NEC 745.69
      interatrial 745.5
      interventricular 745.4
        with pulmonary stenosis or atresia, dextraposition of aorta, and hypertrophy of right ventricle 745.2
        acquired 429.71
      specified type NEC 745.8
      ventricular 745.4
        with pulmonary stenosis or atresia, dextraposition of aorta, and hypertrophy of right ventricle 745.2
        acquired 429.71
    specified type NEC 746.89
    tetralogy of Fallot 745.2
    valve NEC 746.9
      aortic 746.9
        atresia 746.89
        bicuspid valve 746.4
        insufficiency 746.4
        specified type NEC 746.89
        stenosis 746.3
          subaortic 746.81
          supravalvular 747.22
      mitral 746.9
        atresia 746.89
        insufficiency 746.6
        specified type NEC 746.89
        stenosis 746.5
      pulmonary 746.00
        atresia 746.01
        insufficiency 746.09
        stenosis 746.02
          infundibular 746.83
          subvalvular 746.83
      tricuspid 746.9
        atresia 746.1
        stenosis 746.1
    ventricle 746.9
  heel 755.67
  Hegglin's 288.2
  hemianencephaly 740.0
  hemicephaly 740.0
  hemicrania 740.0
  hepatic duct 751.60
  hip (joint) 755.63
  hourglass
    bladder 753.8
    gallbladder 751.69
    stomach 750.7

Anomaly, anomalous – *continued*
  humerus 755.50
  hymen 752.40
  hypersegmentation of neutrophils, hereditary 288.2
  hypophyseal 759.2
  ileocecal (coil) (valve) 751.5
  ileum (intestine) 751.5
  ilium 755.60
  integument 757.9
    specified type NEC 757.8
  interarch distance (excessive) (inadequate) 524.28
  intervertebral cartilage or disc 756.10
  intestine (large) (small) 751.5
    fixational type 751.4
  iris 743.9
    specified type NEC 743.46
  ischium 755.60
  jaw NEC 524.9
    closure 524.51
    size (major) NEC 524.00
    specified type NEC 524.89
  jaw-cranial base relationship 524.10
    specified NEC 524.19
  jejunum 751.5
  joint 755.9
    hip
      dislocation (*see also* Dislocation, hip, congenital) 754.30
      predislocation (*see also* Subluxation, congenital, hip) 754.32
      preluxation (*see also* Subluxation, congenital, hip) 754.32
      subluxation (*see also* Subluxation, congenital, hip) 754.32
    lumbosacral 756.10
      spondylolisthesis 756.12
      spondylosis 756.11
    multiple arthrogryposis 754.89
    sacroiliac 755.69
  Jordan's 288.2
  kidney(s) (calyx) (pelvis) 753.9
    vessel 747.62
  Klippel-Feil (brevicollis) 756.16
  knee (joint) 755.64
  labium (majus) (minus) 752.40
  labyrinth, membranous (causing impairment of hearing) 744.05
  lacrimal
    apparatus, duct or passage 743.9
      specified type NEC 743.65
    gland 743.9
      specified type NEC 743.64
  Langdon Down (mongolism) 758.0
  larynx, laryngeal (muscle) 748.3
    web, webbed 748.2
  leg (lower) (upper) 755.60
    reduction NEC (*see also* Deformity, reduction, lower limb) 755.30
  lens 743.9
    shape 743.36
    specified type NEC 743.39
  leukocytes, genetic 288.2
    granulation (constitutional) 288.2
  lid (fold) 743.9
  ligament 756.9
    broad 752.10
    round 752.9
  limb, except reduction deformity 755.8
    lower 755.60
      reduction deformity (*see also* Deformity, reduction, lower limb) 755.30
      specified type NEC 755.69
    upper 755.50
      reduction deformity (*see also* Deformity, reduction, upper limb) 755.20
      specified type NEC 755.59
  lip 750.9
    harelip (*see also* Cleft, lip) 749.10
    specified type NEC 750.26
  liver (duct) 751.60
    atresia 751.69
  lower extremity 755.60
    vessel 747.64
  lumbosacral (joint) (region) 756.10
  lung (fissure) (lobe) NEC 748.60
    agenesis 748.5
    specified type NEC 748.69
  lymphatic system 759.9
  Madelung's (radius) 755.54

Anomaly, anomalous – *continued*
- mandible 524.9
  - size NEC 524.00
- maxilla 524.90
  - size NEC 524.00
- May (-Hegglin) 288.2
- meatus urinarius 753.9
  - specified type NEC 753.8
- meningeal bands or folds, constriction of 742.8
- meninges 742.9
  - brain 742.4
  - spinal 742.59
- meningocele (*see also* Spina bifida) 741.9❺
  - acquired 349.2
- mesentery 751.9
- metacarpus 755.50
- metatarsus 755.67
- middle ear, except ossicles (causing impairment of hearing) 744.03
  - ossicles 744.04
- mitral (leaflets) (valve) 746.9
  - atresia 746.89
  - insufficiency 746.6
  - specified type NEC 746.89
  - stenosis 746.5
- mouth 750.9
  - specified type NEC 750.26
- multiple NEC 759.7
  - specified type NEC 759.89
- muscle 756.9
  - eye 743.9
    - specified type NEC 743.69
  - specified type NEC 756.89
- musculoskeletal system, except limbs 756.9
  - specified type NEC 756.9
- nail 757.9
  - specified type NEC 757.5
- narrowness, eyelid 743.62
- nasal sinus or septum 748.1
- neck (any part) 744.9
  - specified type NEC 744.89
- nerve 742.9
  - acoustic 742.9
    - specified type NEC 742.8
  - optic 742.9
    - specified type NEC 742.8
  - specified type NEC 742.8
- nervous system NEC 742.9
  - brain 742.9
    - specified type NEC 742.4
  - specified type NEC 742.8
- neurological 742.9
- nipple 757.6
- nonteratogenic NEC 754.89
- nose, nasal (bone) (cartilage) (septum) (sinus) 748.1
- ocular muscle 743.9
- omphalomesenteric duct 751.0
- opening, pulmonary veins 747.49
- optic
  - disc 743.9
    - specified type NEC 743.57
  - nerve 742.9
- opticociliary vessels 743.9
- orbit (eye) 743.9
  - specified type NEC 743.66
- organ
  - of Corti (causing impairment of hearing) 744.05
  - or site 759.9
    - specified type NEC 759.89
- origin
  - both great arteries from same ventricle 745.11
  - coronary artery 746.85
  - innominate artery 747.69
  - left coronary artery from pulmonary artery 746.85
  - pulmonary artery 747.3
  - renal vessels 747.62
  - subclavian artery (left) (right) 747.21
- osseous meatus (ear) 744.03
- ovary 752.0
- oviduct 752.10
- palate (hard) (soft) 750.9
  - cleft (*see also* Cleft, palate) 749.00
- pancreas (duct) 751.7
- papillary muscles 746.9
- parathyroid gland 759.2
- paraurethral ducts 753.9
- parotid (gland) 750.9
- patella 755.64
- Pelger-Huët (hereditary hyposegmentation) 288.2

Anomaly, anomalous – *continued*
- pelvic girdle 755.60
  - specified type NEC 755.69
- pelvis (bony) 755.60
  - complicating delivery 653.0❺
  - rachitic 268.1
    - fetal 756.4
- penis (glans) 752.69
- pericardium 746.89
- peripheral vascular system NEC 747.60
  - gastrointestinal 747.61
  - lower limb 747.64
  - renal 747.62
  - specified site NEC 747.69
  - spinal 747.82
  - upper limb 747.63
- Peter's 743.44
- pharynx 750.9
  - branchial cleft 744.41
  - specified type NEC 750.29
- Pierre Robin 756.0
- pigmentation 709.00
  - congenital 757.33
  - specified NEC 709.09
- pituitary (gland) 759.2
- pleural folds 748.8
- portal vein 747.40
- position tooth, teeth 524.30
  - crowding 524.31
  - displacement 524.30
    - horizontal 524.33
    - vertical 524.34
  - distance
    - interocclusal
      - excessive 524.37
      - insufficient 524.36
  - excessive spacing 524.32
  - rotation 524.35
  - specified NEC 524.39
- preauricular sinus 744.46
- prepuce 752.9
- prostate 752.9
- pulmonary 748.60
  - artery 747.3
  - circulation 747.3
  - specified type NEC 748.69
  - valve 746.00
    - atresia 746.01
    - insufficiency 746.09
    - specified type NEC 746.09
    - stenosis 746.02
      - infundibular 746.83
      - subvalvular 746.83
  - vein 747.40
  - venous
    - connection 747.49
      - partial 747.42
      - total 747.41
    - return 747.49
      - partial 747.42
      - total (TAPVR) (complete) (subdiaphragmatic) (supradiaphragmatic) 747.41
- pupil 743.9
- pylorus 750.9
  - hypertrophy 750.5
  - stenosis 750.5
- rachitic, fetal 756.4
- radius 755.50
- rectovaginal (septum) 752.40
- rectum 751.5
- refraction 367.9
- renal 753.9
  - vessel 747.62
- respiratory system 748.9
  - specified type NEC 748.8
- rib 756.3
  - cervical 756.2
- Rieger's 743.44
- rings, trachea 748.3
- rotation – *see also* Malrotation
  - hip or thigh (*see also* Subluxation, congenital, hip) 754.32
- round ligament 752.9
- sacroiliac (joint) 755.69
- sacrum 756.10
- saddle
  - back 754.2
  - nose 754.0
    - syphilitic 090.5
- salivary gland or duct 750.9
  - specified type NEC 750.26

Anomaly, anomalous – *continued*
- scapula 755.50
- sclera 743.9
  - specified type NEC 743.47
- scrotum 752.9
- sebaceous gland 757.9
- seminal duct or tract 752.9
- sense organs 742.9
  - specified type NEC 742.8
- septum
  - heart – *see* Anomaly, heart, septum
  - nasal 748.1
- sex chromosomes NEC (*see also* Anomaly, chromosomes) 758.81
- shoulder (girdle) (joint) 755.50
  - specified type NEC 755.59
- sigmoid (flexure) 751.5
- sinus of Valsalva 747.29
- site NEC 759.9
- skeleton generalized NEC 756.50
- skin (appendage) 757.9
  - specified type NEC 757.39
- skull (bone) 756.0
  - with
    - anencephalus 740.0
    - encephalocele 742.0
    - hydrocephalus 742.3
      - with spina bifida (*see also* Spina bifida) 741.0❺
    - microcephalus 742.1
- specified type NEC
  - adrenal (gland) 759.1
  - alimentary tract (complete) (partial) 751.8
    - lower 751.5
    - upper 750.8
  - ankle 755.69
  - anus, anal (canal) 751.5
  - aorta, aortic 747.29
    - arch 747.21
  - appendix 751.5
  - arm 755.59
  - artery (peripheral) NEC (*see also* Anomaly, peripheral vascular system) 747.60
    - brain 747.81
    - coronary 746.85
    - eye 743.58
    - pulmonary 747.3
    - retinal 743.58
    - umbilical 747.5
  - auditory canal 744.29
    - causing impairment of hearing 744.02
  - bile duct or passage 751.69
  - bladder 753.8
    - neck 753.8
  - bone(s) 756.9
    - arm 755.59
    - face 756.0
    - leg 755.69
    - pelvic girdle 755.69
    - shoulder girdle 755.59
    - skull 756.0
      - with
        - anencephalus 740.0
        - encephalocele 742.0
        - hydrocephalus 742.3
          - with spina bifida (*see also* Spina bifida) 741.0❺
        - microcephalus 742.1
  - brain 742.4
  - breast 757.6
  - broad ligament 752.19
  - bronchus 748.3
  - canal of Nuck 752.89
  - cardiac septal closure 745.8
  - carpus 755.59
  - cartilaginous 756.9
  - cecum 751.5
  - cervix 752.49
  - chest (wall) 756.3
  - chin 744.89
  - ciliary body 743.46
  - circulatory system 747.89
  - clavicle 755.51
  - clitoris 752.49
  - coccyx 756.19
  - colon 751.5
  - common duct 751.69
  - connective tissue 756.89
  - cricoid cartilage 748.3
  - cystic duct 751.69
  - diaphragm 756.6

Anomaly, anomalous – Anomaly, anomalous

- **Anomaly, anomalous** – *continued*
  - specified type – *continued*
    - digestive organ(s) or tract 751.8
      - lower 751.5
      - upper 750.8
    - duodenum 751.5
    - ear 744.29
      - auricle 744.29
        - causing impairment of hearing 744.02
      - causing impairment of hearing 744.09
      - inner (causing impairment of hearing) 744.05
      - middle, except ossicles 744.03
        - ossicles 744.04
    - ejaculatory duct 752.89
    - endocrine 759.2
    - epiglottis 748.3
    - esophagus 750.4
    - Eustachian tube 744.24
    - eye 743.8
      - lid 743.63
      - muscle 743.69
    - face 744.89
      - bone(s) 756.0
    - fallopian tube 752.19
    - fascia 756.89
    - femur 755.69
    - fibula 755.69
    - finger 755.59
    - foot 755.67
    - fovea centralis 743.55
    - gallbladder 751.69
    - Gartner's duct 752.89
    - gastrointestinal tract 751.8
    - genitalia, genital organ(s)
      - female 752.89
        - external 752.49
        - internal NEC 752.89
      - male 752.89
        - penis 752.69
        - scrotal transposition 752.81
    - genitourinary tract NEC 752.89
    - glottis 748.3
    - hair 757.4
    - hand 755.59
    - heart 746.89
      - valve NEC 746.89
        - pulmonary 746.09
    - hepatic duct 751.69
    - hydatid of Morgagni 752.89
    - hymen 752.49
    - integument 757.8
    - intestine (large) (small) 751.5
      - fixational type 751.4
    - iris 743.46
    - jejunum 751.5
    - joint 755.8
    - kidney 753.3
    - knee 755.64
    - labium (majus) (minus) 752.49
    - labyrinth, membranous 744.05
    - larynx 748.3
    - leg 755.69
    - lens 743.39
    - limb, except reduction deformity 755.8
      - lower 755.69
        - reduction deformity (*see also* Deformity, reduction, lower limb) 755.30
      - upper 755.59
        - reduction deformity (*see also* Deformity, reduction, upper limb) 755.20
    - lip 750.26
    - liver 751.69
    - lung (fissure) (lobe) 748.69
    - meatus urinarius 753.8
    - metacarpus 755.59
    - mouth 750.26
    - muscle 756.89
      - eye 743.69
    - musculoskeletal system, except limbs 756.9
    - nail 757.5
    - neck 744.89
    - nerve 742.8
      - acoustic 742.8
      - optic 742.8
    - nervous system 742.8
    - nipple 757.6
    - nose 748.1
    - organ NEC 759.89
      - of Corti 744.05
    - osseous meatus (ear) 744.03
    - ovary 752.0

- **Anomaly, anomalous** – *continued*
  - specified type – *continued*
    - oviduct 752.19
    - pancreas 751.7
    - parathyroid 759.2
    - patella 755.64
    - pelvic girdle 755.69
    - penis 752.69
    - pericardium 746.89
    - peripheral vascular system NEC (*see also* Anomaly, peripheral vascular system) 747.60
    - pharynx 750.29
    - pituitary 759.2
    - prostate 752.89
    - radius 755.59
    - rectum 751.5
    - respiratory system 748.8
    - rib 756.3
    - round ligament 752.89
    - sacrum 756.19
    - salivary duct or gland 750.26
    - scapula 755.59
    - sclera 743.47
    - scrotum 752.89
      - transposition 752.81
    - seminal duct or tract 752.89
    - shoulder girdle 755.59
    - site NEC 759.89
    - skin 757.39
    - skull (bone(s)) 756.0
      - with
        - anencephalus 740.0
        - encephalocele 742.0
        - hydrocephalus 742.3
          - with spina bifida (*see also* Spina bifida) 741.0❺
        - microcephalus 742.1
    - specified organ or site NEC 759.89
    - spermatic cord 752.89
    - spinal cord 742.59
    - spine 756.19
    - spleen 759.0
    - sternum 756.3
    - stomach 750.7
    - tarsus 755.67
    - tendon 756.89
    - testis 752.89
    - thorax (wall) 756.3
    - thymus 759.2
    - thyroid (gland) 759.2
      - cartilage 748.3
    - tibia 755.69
    - toe 755.66
    - tongue 750.19
    - trachea (cartilage) 748.3
    - ulna 755.59
    - urachus 753.7
    - ureter 753.4
      - obstructive 753.29
    - urethra 753.8
      - obstructive 753.6
    - urinary tract 753.8
    - uterus 752.3
    - uvula 750.26
    - vagina 752.49
    - vascular NEC (*see also* Anomaly, peripheral vascular system) 747.60
      - brain 747.81
    - vas deferens 752.89
    - vein(s) (peripheral) NEC (*see also* Anomaly, peripheral vascular system) 747.60
      - brain 747.81
      - great 747.49
      - portal 747.49
      - pulmonary 747.49
    - vena cava (inferior) (superior) 747.49
    - vertebra 756.19
    - vulva 752.49
  - spermatic cord 752.9
  - spine, spinal 756.10
    - column 756.10
    - cord 742.9
      - meningocele (*see also* Spina bifida) 741.9❺
      - specified type NEC 742.59
      - spina bifida (*see also* Spina bifida) 741.9❺
      - vessel 747.82
    - meninges 742.59
    - nerve root 742.9
  - spleen 759.0
  - Sprengel's 755.52

- **Anomaly, anomalous** – *continued*
  - sternum 756.3
  - stomach 750.9
    - specified type NEC 750.7
  - submaxillary gland 750.9
  - superior vena cava 747.40
  - talipes – *see* Talipes
  - tarsus 755.67
    - with complete absence of distal elements 755.31
  - teeth, tooth NEC 520.9
    - position 524.30
      - crowding 524.31
      - displacement 524.30
        - horizontal 524.33
        - vertical 524.34
      - distance
        - interocclusal
          - excessive 524.37
          - insufficient 524.36
      - excessive spacing 524.32
      - rotation 524.35
      - specified NEC 524.39
    - spacing 524.30
  - tendon 756.9
    - specified type NEC 756.89
  - termination
    - coronary artery 746.85
  - testis 752.9
  - thebesian valve 746.9
  - thigh 755.60
    - flexion (*see also* Subluxation, congenital, hip) 754.32
  - thorax (wall) 756.3
  - throat 750.9
  - thumb 755.50
    - supernumerary 755.01
  - thymus gland 759.2
  - thyroid (gland) 759.2
    - cartilage 748.3
  - tibia 755.60
    - saber 090.5
  - toe 755.66
    - supernumerary 755.02
    - webbed (*see also* Syndactylism, toes) 755.13
  - tongue 750.10
    - specified type NEC 750.19
  - trachea, tracheal 748.3
    - cartilage 748.3
    - rings 748.3
  - tragus 744.3
  - transverse aortic arch 747.21
  - trichromata 368.59
  - trichromatopsia 368.59
  - tricuspid (leaflet) (valve) 746.9
    - atresia 746.1
    - Ebstein's 746.2
    - specified type NEC 746.89
    - stenosis 746.1
  - trunk 759.9
  - Uhl's (hypoplasia of myocardium, right ventricle) 746.84
  - ulna 755.50
  - umbilicus 759.9
    - artery 747.5
  - union, trachea with larynx 748.3
  - unspecified site 759.9
  - upper extremity 755.50
    - vessel 747.63
  - urachus 753.7
    - specified type NEC 753.7
  - ureter 753.9
    - obstructive 753.20
    - specified type NEC 753.4
      - obstructive 753.29
  - urethra (valve) 753.9
    - obstructive 753.6
    - specified type NEC 753.8
  - urinary tract or system (any part, except urachus) 753.9
    - specified type NEC 753.8
    - urachus 753.7
  - uterus 752.3
    - with only one functioning horn 752.3
    - in pregnancy or childbirth 654.0❺
      - affecting fetus or newborn 763.89
      - causing obstructed labor 660.2❺
        - affecting fetus or newborn 763.1
  - uvula 750.9
  - vagina 752.40
  - valleculae 748.3

Anomaly, anomalous – *continued*
valve (heart) NEC 746.9
formation, ureter 753.29
pulmonary 746.00
specified type NEC 746.89
vascular NEC (*see also* Anomaly, peripheral vascular system) 747.60
ring 747.21
vas deferens 752.9
vein(s) (peripheral) NEC (*see also* Anomaly, peripheral vascular system) 747.60
brain 747.81
cerebral 747.81
coronary 746.89
great 747.40
specified type NEC 747.49
portal 747.40
pulmonary 747.40
retina 743.9
vena cava (inferior) (superior) 747.40
venous return (pulmonary) 747.49
partial 747.42
total 747.41
ventricle, ventricular (heart) 746.9
bands 746.9
folds 746.9
septa 745.4
vertebra 756.10
vesicourethral orifice 753.9
vessels NEC (*see also* Anomaly, peripheral vascular system) 747.60
optic papilla 743.9
vitelline duct 751.0
vitreous humor 743.9
specified type NEC 743.51
vulva 752.40
wrist (joint) 755.50
Anomia 784.69
Anonychia 757.5
acquired 703.8
Anophthalmos, anophthalmus (clinical) (congenital) (globe) 743.00
acquired V45.78
Anopsia (altitudinal) (quadrant) 368.46
Anorchia 752.89
Anorchism, anorchidism 752.89
Anorexia 783.0
hysterical 300.11
nervosa 307.1
Anosmia (*see also* Disturbance, sensation) 781.1
hysterical 300.11
postinfectional 478.9
psychogenic 306.7
traumatic 951.8
Anosognosia 780.99
Anosphrasia 781.1
Anosteoplasia 756.50
Anotia 744.09
Anovulatory cycle 628.0
Anoxemia 799.02
newborn 770.88
Anoxia 799.02
altitude 993.2
cerebral 348.1
with
abortion – *see* Abortion, by type, with specified complication NEC
ectopic pregnancy (*see also* categories 633.0-633.9) 639.8
molar pregnancy (*see also* categories 630-632) 639.8
complicating
delivery (cesarean) (instrumental) 669.4❺
ectopic or molar pregnancy 639.8
obstetric anesthesia or sedation 668.2❺
during or resulting from a procedure 997.01
following
abortion 639.8
ectopic or molar pregnancy 639.8
newborn (*see also* Distress, fetal, liveborn infant) 770.88
due to drowning 994.1
fetal, affecting newborn 770.88
heart – *see* Insufficiency, coronary
high altitude 993.2
intrauterine
fetal death (before onset of labor) 768.0
during labor 768.1

Anoxia – *continued*
intrauterine – *continued*
liveborn infant – *see* Distress, fetal, liveborn infant
myocardial – *see* Insufficiency, coronary
newborn 768.9
mild or moderate 768.6
severe 768.5
pathological 799.02
Anteflexion – *see* Anteversion
Antenatal
care, normal pregnancy V22.1
first V22.0
screening of mother (for) V28.9
based on amniocentesis NEC V28.2
chromosomal anomalies V28.0
raised alphafetoprotein levels V28.1
chromosomal anomalies V28.0
fetal growth retardation using ultrasonics V28.4
isoimmunization V28.5
malformations using ultrasonics V28.3
raised alphafetoprotein levels in amniotic fluid V28.1
specified condition NEC V28.8
Streptococcus B V28.6
Antepartum – *see* condition
Anterior – *see also* condition
spinal artery compression syndrome 721.1
Antero-occlusion 524.24
Anteversion
cervix – *see* Anteversion, uterus
femur (neck), congenital 755.63
uterus, uterine (cervix) (postinfectional) (postpartal, old) 621.6
congenital 752.3
in pregnancy or childbirth 654.4❺
affecting fetus or newborn 763.89
causing obstructed labor 660.2❺
affecting fetus or newborn 763.1
Anthracosilicosis (occupational) 500
Anthracosis (lung) (occupational) 500
lingua 529.3
Anthrax 022.9
with pneumonia 022.1 *[484.5]*
colitis 022.2
cutaneous 022.0
gastrointestinal 022.2
intestinal 022.2
pulmonary 022.1
respiratory 022.1
septicemia 022.3
specified manifestation NEC 022.8
Anthropoid pelvis 755.69
with disproportion (fetopelvic) 653.2❺
affecting fetus or newborn 763.1
causing obstructed labor 660.1❺
affecting fetus or newborn 763.1
Anthropophobia 300.29
Antibioma, breast 611.0
Antibodies
maternal (blood group) (*see also* Incompatibility) 656.2❺
anti-D, cord blood 656.1❺
fetus or newborn 773.0
Antibody deficiency syndrome
agammaglobulinemic 279.00
congenital 279.04
hypogammaglobulinemic 279.00
Anticoagulant, circulating (*see also* Circulating anticoagulants) 286.5
Antimongolism syndrome 758.39
Antimonial cholera 985.4
Antisocial personality 301.7
Antithrombinemia (*see also* Circulating anticoagulants) 286.5
Antithromboplastinemia (*see also* Circulating anticoagulants) 286.5
Antithromboplastinogenemia (*see also* Circulating anticoagulants) 286.5
Antitoxin complication or reaction – *see* Complications, vaccination
Anton (-Babinski) **syndrome** (hemiasomatognosia) 307.9
Antritis (chronic) 473.0
maxilla 473.0
acute 461.0
stomach 535.4❺

Antrum, antral – *see* condition
Anuria 788.5
with
abortion – *see* Abortion, by type, with renal failure
ectopic pregnancy (*see also* categories 633.0-633.9) 639.3
molar pregnancy (*see also* categories 630-632) 639.3
calculus (impacted) (recurrent) 592.9
kidney 592.0
ureter 592.1
congenital 753.3
due to a procedure 997.5
following
abortion 639.3
ectopic or molar pregnancy 639.3
newborn 753.3
postrenal 593.4
puerperal, postpartum, childbirth 669.3❺
specified as due to a procedure 997.5
sulfonamide
correct substance properly administered 788.5
overdose or wrong substance given or taken 961.0
traumatic (following crushing) 958.5
Anus, anal – *see* condition
Anusitis 569.49
Anxiety (neurosis) (reaction) (state) 300.00
alcohol-induced 291.89
depression 300.4
drug-induced 292.89
due to or associated with physical condition 293.84
generalized 300.02
hysteria 300.20
in
acute stress reaction 308.0
transient adjustment reaction 309.24
panic type 300.01
separation, abnormal 309.21
syndrome (organic) (transient) 293 84
Aorta, aortic – *see* condition
Aortectasia 441.9
Aortitis (nonsyphilitic) 447.6
arteriosclerotic 440.0
calcific 447.6
Döhle-Heller 093.1
luetic 093.1
rheumatic (*see also* Endocarditis, acute, rheumatic) 391.1
rheumatoid – *see* Arthritis, rheumatoid
specific 093.1
syphilitic 093.1
congenital 090.5
Apathetic thyroid storm (*see also* Thyrotoxicosis) 242.9❺
Apepsia 536.8
achlorhydric 536.0
psychogenic 306.4
Aperistalsis, esophagus 530.0
Apert's syndrome (acrocephalosyndactyly) 755.55
Apert-Gallais syndrome (adrenogenital) 255.2
Apertognathia 524.20
Aphagia 787.20 ▲
psychogenic 307.1
Aphakia (acquired) (bilateral) (postoperative) (unilateral) 379.31
congenital 743.35
Aphalangia (congenital) 755.4
lower limb (complete) (intercalary) (partial) (terminal) 755.39
meaning all digits (complete) (partial) 755.31
transverse 755.31
upper limb (complete) (intercalary) (partial) (terminal) 755.29
meaning all digits (complete) (partial) 755.21
transverse 755.21
Aphasia (amnestic) (ataxic) (auditory) (Broca's) (choreatic) (classic) (expressive) (global) (ideational) (ideokinetic) (ideomotor) (jargon) (motor) (nominal) (receptive) (semantic) (sensory) (syntactic) (verbal) (visual) (Wernicke's) 784.3
developmental 315.31
syphilis, tertiary 094.89
uremic – *see* Uremia
Aphemia 784.3
uremic – *see* Uremia

Anomaly, anomalous – Aphemia

- **Aphonia** 784.41
  - clericorum 784.49
  - hysterical 300.11
  - organic 784.41
  - psychogenic 306.1
- **Aphthae, aphthous** – *see also* condition
  - Bednar's 528.2
  - cachectic 529.0
  - epizootic 078.4
  - fever 078.4
  - oral 528.2
  - stomatitis 528.2
  - thrush 112.0
  - ulcer (oral) (recurrent) 528.2
    - genital organ(s) NEC
      - female 616.50 ▲
      - male 608.89
    - larynx 478.79
- **Apical** – *see* condition
- **Apical ballooning syndrome** 429.83
- **Aplasia** – *see also* Agenesis
  - alveolar process (acquired) 525.8
    - congenital 750.26
  - aorta (congenital) 747.22
  - aortic valve (congenital) 746.89
  - axialis extracorticalis (congenital) 330.0
  - bone marrow (myeloid) 284.9
    - acquired (secondary) 284.89 ▲
    - congenital 284.01
    - idiopathic 284.9
  - brain 740.0
    - specified part 742.2
  - breast 757.6
  - bronchus 748.3
  - cementum 520.4
  - cerebellar 742.2
  - congenital (pure) red cell 284.01
  - corpus callosum 742.2
  - erythrocyte 284.81 ▲
    - congenital 284.01
  - extracortical axial 330.0
  - eye (congenital) 743.00
  - fovea centralis (congenital) 743.55
  - germinal (cell) 606.0
  - iris 743.45
  - labyrinth, membranous 744.05
  - limb (congenital) 755.4
    - lower NEC 755.30
    - upper NEC 755.20
  - lung (bilateral) (congenital) (unilateral) 748.5
  - nervous system NEC 742.8
  - nuclear 742.8
  - ovary 752.0
  - Pelizaeus-Merzbacher 330.0
  - prostate (congenital) 752.89
  - red cell (with thymoma) ▶(adult)◀ 284.81 ▲
    - acquired (secondary) 284.81 ▲
    - congenital 284.01
    - hereditary 284.01
    - of infants 284.01
    - primary 284.01
    - pure 284.01
  - round ligament (congenital) 752.89
  - salivary gland 750.21
  - skin (congenital) 757.39
  - spinal cord 742.59
  - spleen 759.0
  - testis (congenital) 752.89
  - thymic, with immunodeficiency 279.2
  - thyroid 243
  - uterus 752.3
  - ventral horn cell 742.59
- **Apleuria** 756.3
- **Apnea, apneic** (spells) 786.03
  - newborn, neonatorum 770.81
    - essential 770.81
    - obstructive 770.82
    - primary 770.81
    - sleep 770.81
    - specified NEC 770.82
  - psychogenic 306.1
  - sleep, unspecified 780.57
    - with
      - hypersomnia, unspecified 780.53
      - hyposomnia, unspecified 780.51
      - insomnia, unspecified 780.51
      - sleep disturbance 780.57
    - central, in conditions classified elsewhere 327.27
    - obstructive (adult) (pediatric) 327.23

- **Apnea, apneic** – *continued*
  - sleep – *continued*
    - organic 327.20
      - other 327.29
    - primary central 327.21
- **Apneumatosis newborn** 770.4
- **Apodia** 755.31
- **Apophysitis** (bone) (*see also* Osteochondrosis) 732.9
  - calcaneus 732.5
  - juvenile 732.6
- **Apoplectiform convulsions** (*see also* Disease, cerebrovascular, acute) 436
- **Apoplexia, apoplexy, apoplectic** (*see also* Disease, cerebrovascular, acute) 436
  - abdominal 569.89
  - adrenal 036.3
  - attack 436
  - basilar (*see also* Disease, cerebrovascular, acute) 436
  - brain (*see also* Disease, cerebrovascular, acute) 436
  - bulbar (*see also* Disease, cerebrovascular, acute) 436
  - capillary (*see also* Disease, cerebrovascular, acute) 436
  - cardiac (*see also* Infarct, myocardium) 410.9❺
  - cerebral (*see also* Disease, cerebrovascular, acute) 436
  - chorea (*see also* Disease, cerebrovascular, acute) 436
  - congestive (*see also* Disease, cerebrovascular, acute) 436
    - newborn 767.4
  - embolic (*see also* Embolism, brain) 434.1❺
  - fetus 767.0
  - fit (*see also* Disease, cerebrovascular, acute) 436
  - healed or old V12.54 ▲
  - heart (auricle) (ventricle) (*see also* Infarct, myocardium) 410.9❺
  - heat 992.0
  - hemiplegia (*see also* Disease, cerebrovascular, acute) 436
  - hemorrhagic (stroke) (*see also* Hemorrhage, brain) 432.9
  - ingravescent (*see also* Disease, cerebrovascular, acute) 436
  - late effect – *see* Late effect(s) (of) cerebrovascular disease
  - lung – *see* Embolism, pulmonary
  - meninges, hemorrhagic (*see also* Hemorrhage, subarachnoid) 430
  - neonatorum 767.0
  - newborn 767.0
  - pancreatitis 577.0
  - placenta 641.2❺
  - progressive (*see also* Disease, cerebrovascular, acute) 436
  - pulmonary (artery) (vein) – *see* Embolism, pulmonary
  - sanguineous (*see also* Disease, cerebrovascular, acute) 436
  - seizure (*see also* Disease, cerebrovascular, acute) 436
  - serous (*see also* Disease, cerebrovascular, acute) 436
  - spleen 289.59
  - stroke (*see also* Disease, cerebrovascular, acute) 436
  - thrombotic (*see also* Thrombosis, brain) 434.0❺
  - uremic – *see* Uremia
  - uteroplacental 641.2❺
- **Appendage**
  - fallopian tube (cyst of Morgagni) 752.11
  - intestine (epiploic) 751.5
  - preauricular 744.1
  - testicular (organ of Morgagni) 752.89
- **Appendicitis** 541
  - with
    - perforation, peritonitis (generalized), or rupture 540.0
      - with peritoneal abscess 540.1
    - peritoneal abscess 540.1
  - acute (catarrhal) (fulminating) (gangrenous) (inflammatory) (obstructive) (retrocecal) (suppurative) 540.9
    - with
      - perforation, peritonitis, or rupture 540.0
        - with peritoneal abscess 540.1
      - peritoneal abscess 540.1

- **Appendicitis** – *continued*
  - amebic 006.8
  - chronic (recurrent) 542
  - exacerbation – *see* Appendicitis, acute
  - fulminating – *see* Appendicitis, acute
  - gangrenous – *see* Appendicitis, acute
  - healed (obliterative) 542
  - interval 542
  - neurogenic 542
  - obstructive 542
  - pneumococcal 541
  - recurrent 542
  - relapsing 542
  - retrocecal 541
  - subacute (adhesive) 542
  - subsiding 542
  - suppurative – *see* Appendicitis, acute
  - tuberculous (*see also* Tuberculosis) 014.8❺
- **Appendiclausis** 543.9
- **Appendicolithiasis** 543.9
- **Appendicopathia oxyurica** 127.4
- **Appendix, appendicular** – *see also* condition
  - Morgagni (male) 752.89
    - fallopian tube 752.11
- **Appetite**
  - depraved 307.52
  - excessive 783.6
    - psychogenic 307.51
  - lack or loss (*see also* Anorexia) 783.0
    - nonorganic origin 307.59
  - perverted 307.52
    - hysterical 300.11
- **Apprehension, apprehensiveness** (abnormal) (state) 300.00
  - specified type NEC 300.09
- **Approximal wear** 521.10
- **Apraxia** (classic) (ideational) (ideokinetic) (ideomotor) (motor) 784.69
  - oculomotor, congenital 379.51
  - verbal 784.69
- **Aptyalism** 527.7
- **Aqueous misdirection** 365.83
- **Arabicum elephantiasis** (*see also* Infestation, filarial) 125.9
- **Arachnidism** 989.5
- **Arachnitis** – *see* Meningitis
- **Arachnodactyly** 759.82
- **Arachnoidism** 989.5
- **Arachnoiditis** (acute) (adhesive) (basic) (brain) (cerebrospinal) (chiasmal) (chronic) (spinal) (*see also* Meningitis) 322.9
  - meningococcal (chronic) 036.0
  - syphilitic 094.2
  - tuberculous (*see also* Tuberculosis, meninges) 013.0❺
- **Araneism** 989.5
- **Arboencephalitis, Australian** 062.4
- **Arborization block** (heart) 426.6
- **Arbor virus, arbovirus** (infection) NEC 066.9
- **ARC** 042
- **Arches** – *see* condition
- **Arcuatus uterus** 752.3
- **Arcus** (cornea)
  - juvenilis 743.43
    - interfering with vision 743.42
  - senilis 371.41
- **Arc-welders' lung** 503
- **Arc-welders' syndrome** (photokeratitis) 370.24
- **Areflexia** 796.1
- **Areola** – *see* condition
- **Argentaffinoma** (M8241/1) – *see also* Neoplasm, by site, uncertain behavior
  - benign (M8241/0) – *see* Neoplasm, by site, benign
  - malignant (M8241/3) – *see* Neoplasm, by site, malignant
  - syndrome 259.2
- **Argentinian hemorrhagic fever** 078.7
- **Arginosuccinicaciduria** 270.6
- **Argonz-Del Castillo syndrome** (nonpuerperal galactorrhea and amenorrhea) 253.1
- **Argyll-Robertson phenomenon, pupil, or syndrome** (syphilitic) 094.89
  - atypical 379.45
  - nonluetic 379.45
  - nonsyphilitic 379.45

Aphonia – Argyll-Robertson phenomenon, pupil, or syndrome

Argyll-Robertson phenomenon, pupil, or syndrome – *continued*
- reversed 379.45

Argyria, argyriasis NEC 985.8
- conjunctiva 372.55
- cornea 371.16
- from drug or medicinal agent
  - correct substance properly administered 709.09
  - overdose or wrong substance given or taken 961.2

Arhinencephaly 742.2

Arias-Stella phenomenon 621.30

Ariboflavinosis 266.0

Arizona enteritis 008.1

Arm – *see* condition

Armenian disease 277.31

Arnold-Chiari obstruction or syndrome (*see also* Spina bifida) 741.0❺
- type I 348.4
- type II (*see also* Spina bifida) 741.0❺
- type III 742.0
- type IV 742.2

Arousals
- confusional 327.41

Arrest, arrested
- active phase of labor 661.1❺
  - affecting fetus or newborn 763.7
- any plane in pelvis
  - complicating delivery 660.1❺
    - affecting fetus or newborn 763.1
- bone marrow (*see also* Anemia, aplastic) 284.9
- cardiac 427.5
  - with
    - abortion – *see* Abortion, by type, with specified complication NEC
    - ectopic pregnancy (*see also* categories 633.0-633.9) 639.8
    - molar pregnancy (*see also* categories 630-632) 639.8
  - complicating
    - anesthesia
      - correct substance properly administered 427.5
      - obstetric 668.1❺
      - overdose or wrong substance given 968.4
        - specified anesthetic – *see* Table of Drugs and Chemicals
    - delivery (cesarean) (instrumental) 669.4❺
    - ectopic or molar pregnancy 639.8
    - surgery (nontherapeutic) (therapeutic) 997.1
  - fetus or newborn 779.85
  - following
    - abortion 639.8
    - ectopic or molar pregnancy 639.8
  - personal history, successfully rescucitated V12.53 ●
  - postoperative (immediate) 997.1
    - long-term effect of cardiac surgery 429.4
- cardiorespiratory (*see also* Arrest, cardiac) 427.5
- deep transverse 660.3❺
  - affecting fetus or newborn 763.1
- development or growth
  - bone 733.91
  - child 783.40
  - fetus 764.9❺
    - affecting management of pregnancy 656.5❺
  - tracheal rings 748.3
- epiphyseal 733.91
- granulopoiesis 288.09
- heart – *see* Arrest, cardiac
- respiratory 799.1
  - newborn 770.87
- sinus 426.6
- transverse (deep) 660.3❺
  - affecting fetus or newborn 763.1

Arrhenoblastoma (M8630/1)
- benign (M8630/0)
  - specified site – *see* Neoplasm, by site, benign
  - unspecified site
    - female 220
    - male 222.0
- malignant (M8630/3)
  - specified site – *see* Neoplasm, by site, malignant
  - unspecified site
    - female 183.0
    - male 186.9

Arrhenoblastoma – *continued*
- specified site – *see* Neoplasm, by site, uncertain behavior
- unspecified site
  - female 236.2
  - male 236.4

Arrhinencephaly 742.2
- due to
  - trisomy 13 (13-15) 758.1
  - trisomy 18 (16-18) 758.2

Arrhythmia (auricle) (cardiac) (cordis) (gallop rhythm) (juvenile) (nodal) (reflex) (sinus) (supraventricular) (transitory) (ventricle) 427.9
- bigeminal rhythm 427.89
- block 426.9
- bradycardia 427.89
- contractions, premature 427.60
- coronary sinus 427.89
- ectopic 427.89
- extrasystolic 427.60
- postoperative 997.1
- psychogenic 306.2
- vagal 780.2

Arrillaga-Ayerza syndrome (pulmonary artery sclerosis with pulmonary hypertension) 416.0

Arsenical
- dermatitis 692.4
- keratosis 692.4
- pigmentation 985.1
  - from drug or medicinal agent
    - correct substance properly administered 709.09
    - overdose or wrong substance given or taken 961.1

Arsenism 985.1
- from drug or medicinal agent
  - correct substance properly administered 692.4
  - overdose or wrong substance given or taken 961.1

Arterial – *see* condition

Arteriectasis 447.8

Arteriofibrosis – *see* Arteriosclerosis

Arteriolar sclerosis – *see* Arteriosclerosis

Arteriolith – *see* Arteriosclerosis

Arteriolitis 447.6
- necrotizing, kidney 447.5
- renal – *see* Hypertension, kidney

Arteriolosclerosis – *see* Arteriosclerosis

Arterionephrosclerosis (*see also* Hypertension, kidney) 403.90

Arteriopathy 447.9

Arteriosclerosis, arteriosclerotic (artery) (deformans) (diffuse) (disease) (endarteritis) (general) (obliterans) (obliterative) (occlusive) (senile) (with calcification) 440.9
- with
  - gangrene 440.24
  - psychosis (*see also* Psychosis, arteriosclerotic) 290.40
  - ulceration 440.23
- aorta 440.0
- arteries of extremities – *see* Arteriosclerosis, extremities
- basilar (artery) (*see also* Occlusion, artery, basilar) 433.0❺
- brain 437.0
- bypass graft
  - coronary artery 414.05
    - autologous artery (gastroepiploic) (internal mammary) 414.04
    - autologous vein 414.02
    - nonautologous biological 414.03
    - of transplanted heart 414.07
  - extremity 440.30
    - autologous vein 440.31
    - nonautologous biological 440.32
- cardiac – *see* Arteriosclerosis, coronary
- cardiopathy – *see* Arteriosclerosis, coronary
- cardiorenal (*see also* Hypertension, cardiorenal) 404.90
- cardiovascular (*see also* Disease, cardiovascular) 429.2
- carotid (artery) (common) (internal) (*see also* Occlusion, artery, carotid) 433.1❺
- central nervous system 437.0
- cerebral 437.0
  - late effect – *see* Late effect(s) (of) cerebrovascular disease
- cerebrospinal 437.0

Arteriosclerosis, arteriosclerotic – *continued*
- cerebrovascular 437.0
- coronary (artery) 414.00
  - graft – *see* Arteriosclerosis, bypass graft
  - native artery 414.01
    - of transplanted heart 414.06
  - of transplanted heart 414.06
- extremities (native artery) NEC 440.20
  - bypass graft 440.30
    - autologous vein 440.31
    - nonautologous biological 440.32
  - claudication (intermittent) 440.21
    - and
      - gangrene 440.24
      - rest pain 440.22
        - and
          - gangrene 440.24
          - ulceration 440.23
            - and gangrene 440.24
      - ulceration 440.23
        - and gangrene 440.24
  - gangrene 440.24
  - rest pain 440.22
    - and
      - gangrene 440.24
      - ulceration 440.23
        - and gangrene 440.24
  - specified site NEC 440.29
  - ulceration 440.23
    - and gangrene 440.24
- heart (disease) – *see also* Arteriosclerosis, coronary
  - valve 424.99
    - aortic 424.1
    - mitral 424.0
    - pulmonary 424.3
    - tricuspid 424.2
- kidney (*see also* Hypertension, kidney) 403.90
- labyrinth, labyrinthine 388.00
- medial NEC (*see also* Arteriosclerosis, extremities) 440.20
- mesentery (artery) 557.1
- Mönckeberg's (*see also* Arteriosclerosis, extremities) 440.20
- myocarditis 429.0
- nephrosclerosis (*see also* Hypertension, kidney) 403.90
- peripheral (of extremities) – *see* Arteriosclerosis, extremities
- precerebral 433.9❺
  - specified artery NEC 433.8❺
- pulmonary (idiopathic) 416.0
- renal (*see also* Hypertension, kidney) 403.90
  - arterioles (*see also* Hypertension, kidney) 403.90
  - artery 440.1
- retinal (vascular) 440.8 *[362.13]*
- specified artery NEC 440.8
  - with gangrene 440.8 *[785.4]*
- spinal (cord) 437.0
- vertebral (artery) (*see also* Occlusion, artery, vertebral) 433.2❺

Arteriospasm 443.9

Arteriovenous – *see* condition

Arteritis 447.6
- allergic (*see also* Angiitis, hypersensitivity) 446.20
- aorta (nonsyphilitic) 447.6
  - syphilitic 093.1
- aortic arch 446.7
- brachiocephalica 446.7
- brain 437.4
  - syphilitic 094.89
- branchial 446.7
- cerebral 437.4
  - late effect – *see* Late effect(s) (of) cerebrovascular disease
  - sphylitic 094.89
- coronary (artery) – *see also* Arteriosclerosis, coronary
  - rheumatic 391.9
    - chronic 398.99
  - syphilitic 093.89
- cranial (left) (right) 446.5
- deformans – *see* Arteriosclerosis
- giant cell 446.5
- necrosing or necrotizing 446.0
- nodosa 446.0
- obliterans – *see also* Arteriosclerosis
  - subclaviocarotica 446.7
- pulmonary 417.8

Arteritis – *continued*
- retina 362.18
- rheumatic – *see* Fever, rheumatic
- senile – *see* Arteriosclerosis
- suppurative 447.2
- syphilitic (general) 093.89
  - brain 094.89
  - coronary 093.89
  - spinal 094.89
- temporal 446.5
- young female, syndrome 446.7

Artery, arterial – *see* condition

Arthralgia (*see also* Pain, joint) 719.4❺
- allergic (*see also* Pain, joint) 719.4❺
- in caisson disease 993.3
- psychogenic 307.89
- rubella 056.71
- Salmonella 003.23
- temporomandibular joint 524.62

Arthritis, arthritic (acute) (chronic) (subacute) 716.9
- meaning Osteoarthritis – *see* Osteoarthrosis

Note – Use the following fifth-digit subclassification with categories 711-712, 715-716:

0	*site unspecified*
1	*shoulder region*
2	*upper arm*
3	*forearm*
4	*hand*
5	*pelvic region and thigh*
6	*lower leg*
7	*ankle and foot*
8	*other specified sites*
9	*multiple sites*

- allergic 716.2❺
- ankylosing (crippling) (spine) 720.0 *[713.2]*
  - sites other than spine 716.9❺
- atrophic 714.0
  - spine 720.9
- back (*see also* Arthritis, spine) 721.90
- Bechterew's (ankylosing spondylitis) 720.0
- blennorrhagic 098.50 *[711.6]*
- cervical, cervicodorsal (*see also* Spondylosis, cervical) 721.0
- Charcôt's 094.0 *[713.5]*
  - diabetic 250.6❺ *[713.5]*
  - syringomyelic 336.0 *[713.5]*
  - tabetic 094.0 *[713.5]*
- chylous (*see also* Filariasis) 125.9 *[711.7]*❺
- climacteric NEC 716.3❺
- coccyx 721.8
- cricoarytenoid 478.79
- crystal (-induced) – *see* Arthritis, due to crystals
- deformans (*see also* Osteoarthrosis) 715.9❺
  - spine 721.90
    - with myelopathy 721.91
- degenerative (*see also* Osteoarthrosis) 715.9❺
  - idiopathic 715.09
  - polyarticular 715.09
  - spine 721.90
    - with myelopathy 721.91
- dermatoarthritis, lipoid 272.8 *[713.0]*
- due to or associated with
  - acromegaly 253.0 *[713.0]*
  - actinomycosis 039.8 *[711.4]*❺
  - amyloidosis 277.39 *[713.7]*
  - bacterial disease NEC 040.89 *[711.4]*❺
  - Behçet's syndrome 136.1 *[711.2]*❺
  - blastomycosis 116.0 *[711.6]*❺
  - brucellosis (*see also* Brucellosis) 023.9 *[711.4]*❺
  - caisson disease 993.3
  - coccidioidomycosis 114.3 *[711.6]*❺
  - coliform (Escherichia coli) 711.0❺
  - colitis, ulcerative - (*see also* Colitis, ulcerative) 556.9 *[713.1]*
  - cowpox 051.0 *[711.5]*❺
  - crystals -(*see also* Gout)
    - dicalcium phosphate 275.49 *[712.1]*
    - pyrophosphate 275.49 *[712.2]*
    - specified NEC 275.49 *[712.8]*
  - dermatoarthritis, lipoid 272.8 *[713.0]*
  - dermatological disorder NEC 709.9 *[713.3]*
  - diabetes 250.6❺ *[713.5]*
  - diphtheria 032.89 *[711.4]*❺
  - dracontiasis 125.7 *[711.7]*❺
  - dysentery 009.0 *[711.3]*❺
  - endocrine disorder NEC 259.9 *[713.0]*

Arthritis, arthritic – *continued*
- due to or associated with – *continued*
  - enteritis NEC 009.1 *[711.3]*❺
    - infectious (*see also* Enteritis, infectious) 009.0 *[711.3]*❺
      - specified organism NEC 008.8 *[711.3]*❺
    - regional (*see also* Enteritis, regional) 555.9 *[713.1]*
    - specified organism NEC 008.8 *[711.3]*❺
  - epiphyseal slip, nontraumatic (old) 716.8❺
  - erysipelas 035 *[711.4]*❺
  - erythema
    - epidemic 026.1
    - multiforme 695.1 *[713.3]*
    - nodosum 695.2 *[713.3]*
  - Escherichia coli 711.0❺
  - filariasis NEC 125.9 *[711.7]*
  - gastrointestinal condition NEC 569.9 *[713.1]*
  - glanders 024 *[711.4]*❺
  - Gonococcus 098.50
  - gout 274.0
  - H. influenzae 711.0❺
  - helminthiasis NEC 128.9 *[711.7]*❺
  - hematological disorder NEC 289.9 *[713.2]*
  - hemochromatosis 275.0 *[713.0]*
  - hemoglobinopathy NEC (*see also* Disease, hemoglobin) 282.7 *[713.2]*
  - hemophilia (*see also* Hemophilia) 286.0 *[713.2]*
  - hemophilus influenzae (H. influenzae) 711.0❺
  - Henoch (-Schönlein) purpura 287.0 *[713.6]*
  - histoplasmosis NEC (*see also* Histoplasmosis) 115.99 *[711.6]*❺
  - human parvovirus 079.83 *[711.5]*❺ ●
  - hyperparathyroidism 252.00 *[713.0]*
  - hypersensitivity reaction NEC 995.3 *[713.6]*
  - hypogammaglobulinemia (*see also* Hypogammaglobulinemia) 279.00 *[713.0]*
  - hypothyroidism NEC 244.9 *[713.0]*
  - infection (*see also* Arthritis, infectious) 711.9❺
  - infectious disease NEC 136.9 *[711.8]*❺
  - leprosy (*see also* Leprosy) 030.9 *[711.4]*❺
  - leukemia NEC (M9800/3) 208.9❺ *[713.2]*
  - lipoid dermatoarthritis 272.8 *[713.0]*
  - Lyme disease 088.81 *[711.8]*❺
  - Mediterranean fever, familial 277.31 *[713.7]*
  - meningococcal infection 036.82
  - metabolic disorder NEC 277.9 *[713.0]*
  - multiple myelomatosis (M9730/3) 203.0❺ *[713.2]*
  - mumps 072.79 *[711.5]*❺
  - mycobacteria 031.8 *[711.4]*❺
  - mycosis NEC 117.9 *[711.6]*❺
  - neurological disorder NEC 349.9 *[713.5]*
  - ochronosis 270.2 *[713.0]*
  - O'nyong nyong 066.3 *[711.5]*❺
  - parasitic disease NEC 136.9 *[711.8]*❺
  - paratyphoid fever (*see also* Fever, paratyphoid) 002.9 *[711.3]*❺
  - parvovirus B19 079.83 *[711.5]*❺ ●
  - Pneumococcus 711.0❺
  - poliomyelitis (*see also* Poliomyelitis) 045.9❺ *[711.5]*❺
  - Pseudomonas 711.0❺
  - psoriasis 696.0
  - pyogenic organism (E. coli) (H. influenzae) (Pseudomonas) (Streptococcus) 711.0❺
  - rat-bite fever 026.1 *[711.4]*❺
  - regional enteritis (*see also* Enteritis, regional) 555.9 *[713.1]*
  - Reiter's disease 099.3 *[711.1]*❺
  - respiratory disorder NEC 519.9 *[713.4]*
  - reticulosis, malignant (M9720/3) 202.3❺ *[713.2]*
  - rubella 056.71
  - salmonellosis 003.23
  - sarcoidosis 135 *[713.7]*
  - serum sickness 999.5 *[713.6]*
  - Staphylococcus 711.0❺
  - Streptococcus 711.0❺
  - syphilis (*see also* Syphilis) 094.0 *[711.4]*❺
  - syringomyelia 336.0 *[713.5]*
  - thalassemia 282.49 *[713.2]*
  - tuberculosis (*see also* Tuberculosis, arthritis) 015.9❺ *[711.4]*❺
  - typhoid fever 002.0 *[711.3]*❺
  - ulcerative colitis - (*see also* Colitis, ulcerative) 556.9 *[713.1]*

Arthritis, arthritic – *continued*
- due to or associated with – *continued*
  - urethritis
    - nongonococcal (*see also* Urethritis, nongonococcal) 099.40 *[711.1]*❺
    - nonspecific (*see also* Urethritis, nongonococcal) 099.40 *[711.1]*❺
    - Reiter's 099.3 *[711.1]*❺
  - viral disease NEC 079.99 *[711.5]*❺
- erythema epidemic 026.1
- gonococcal 098.50
- gouty (acute) 274.0
- hypertrophic (*see also* Osteoarthrosis) 715.9❺
  - spine 721.90
    - with myelopathy 721.91
- idiopathic, blennorrheal 099.3
- in caisson disease 993.3 *[713.8]*
- infectious or infective (acute) (chronic) (subacute) NEC 711.9❺
  - nonpyogenic 711.9❺
  - spine 720.9
- inflammatory NEC 714.9
- juvenile rheumatoid (chronic) (polyarticular) 714.30
  - acute 714.31
  - monoarticular 714.33
  - pauciarticular 714.32
- lumbar (*see also* Spondylosis, lumbar) 721.3
- meningococcal 036.82
- menopausal NEC 716.3❺
- migratory – *see* Fever, rheumatic
- neuropathic (Charcôt's) 094.0 *[713.5]*
  - diabetic 250.6❺ *[713.5]*
  - nonsyphilitic NEC 349.9 *[713.5]*
  - syringomyelic 336.0 *[713.5]*
  - tabetic 094.0 *[713.5]*
- nodosa (*see also* Osteoarthrosis) 715.9❺
  - spine 721.90
    - with myelopathy 721.91
- nonpyogenic NEC 716.9❺
  - spine 721.90
    - with myelopathy 721.91
- ochronotic 270.2 *[713.0]*
- palindromic (*see also* Rheumatism, palindromic) 719.3❺
- pneumococcal 711.0❺
- postdysenteric 009.0 *[711.3]*❺
- postrheumatic, chronic (Jaccoud's) 714.4
- primary progressive 714.0
  - spine 720.9
- proliferative 714.0
  - spine 720.0
- psoriatic 696.0
- purulent 711.0❺
- pyogenic or pyemic 711.0❺
- rheumatic 714.0
  - acute or subacute – *see* Fever, rheumatic
  - chronic 714.0
  - spine 720.9
- rheumatoid (nodular) 714.0
  - with
    - splenoadenomegaly and leukopenia 714.1
    - visceral or systemic involvement 714.2
  - aortitis 714.89
  - carditis 714.2
  - heart disease 714.2
  - juvenile (chronic) (polyarticular) 714.30
    - acute 714.31
    - monoarticular 714.33
    - pauciarticular 714.32
  - spine 720.0
- rubella 056.71
- sacral, sacroiliac, sacrococcygeal (*see also* Spondylosis, sacral) 721.3
- scorbutic 267
- senile or senescent (*see also* Osteoarthrosis) 715.9❺
  - spine 721.90
    - with myelopathy 721.91
- septic 711.0❺
- serum (nontherapeutic) (therapeutic) 999.5 *[713.6]*
- specified form NEC 716.8❺
- spine 721.90
  - with myelopathy 721.91
  - atrophic 720.9
  - degenerative 721.90
    - with myelopathy 721.91
  - hypertrophic (with deformity) 721.90
    - with myelopathy 721.91
  - infectious or infective NEC 720.9
  - Marie-Strümpell 720.0

Arthritis, arthritic – *continued*
- spine – *continued*
  - nonpyogenic 721.90
    - with myelopathy 721.91
  - pyogenic 720.9
  - rheumatoid 720.0
  - traumatic (old) 721.7
  - tuberculous (*see also* Tuberculosis) 015.0❺ *[720.81]*
- staphylococcal 711.0❺
- streptococcal 711.0❺
- suppurative 711.0❺
- syphilitic 094.0 *[713.5]*
  - congenital 090.49 *[713.5]*
- syphilitica deformans (Charcôt) 094.0 *[713.5]*
- temporomandibular joint 524.69
- thoracic (*see also* Spondylosis, thoracic) 721.2
- toxic of menopause 716.3❺
- transient 716.4❺
- traumatic (chronic) (old) (post) 716.1❺
  - current injury – *see* nature of injury
- tuberculous (*see also* Tuberculosis, arthritis) 015.9❺ *[711.4]*❺
- urethritica 099.3 *[711.1]*❺
- urica, uratic 274.0
- venereal 099.3 *[711.1]*❺
- vertebral (*see also* Arthritis, spine) 721.90
- villous 716.8❺
- von Bechterew's 720.0

Arthrocele (*see also* Effusion, joint) 719.0❺

Arthrochondritis – *see* Arthritis

Arthrodesis status V45.4

Arthrodynia (*see also* Pain, joint) 719.4❺
- psychogenic 307.89

Arthrodysplasia 755.9

Arthrofibrosis, joint (*see also* Ankylosis) 718.5❺

Arthrogryposis 728.3
- multiplex, congenita 754.89

Arthrokatadysis 715.35

Arthrolithiasis 274.0

Arthro-onychodysplasia 756.89

Arthro-osteo-onychodysplasia 756.89

Arthropathy (*see also* Arthritis) 716.9❺

Note – Use the following fifth-digit subclassification with categories 711-712, 716:

0	*site unspecified*
1	*shoulder region*
2	*upper arm*
3	*forearm*
4	*hand*
5	*pelvic region and thigh*
6	*lower leg*
7	*ankle and foot*
8	*other specified sites*
9	*multiple sites*

- Behçet's 136.1 *[711.2]*❺
- Charcôt's 094.0 *[713.5]*
  - diabetic 250.6❺ *[713.5]*
  - syringomyelic 336.0 *[713.5]*
  - tabetic 094.0 *[713.5]*
- crystal (-induced) – *see* Arthritis, due to crystals
- gouty 274.0
- neurogenic, neuropathic (Charcôt's) (tabetic) 094.0 *[713.5]*
  - diabetic 250.6❺ *[713.5]*
  - nonsyphilitic NEC 349.9 *[713.5]*
  - syringomyelic 336.0 *[713.5]*
- postdysenteric NEC 009.0 *[711.3]*❺
- postrheumatic, chronic (Jaccoud's) 714.4
- psoriatic 696.0
- pulmonary 731.2
- specified NEC 716.8❺
- syringomyelia 336.0 *[713.5]*
- tabes dorsalis 094.0 *[713.5]*
- tabetic 094.0 *[713.5]*
- transient 716.4❺
- traumatic 716.1❺
- uric acid 274.0

Arthrophyte (*see also* Loose, body, joint) 718.1❺

Arthrophytis 719.80
- ankle 719.87
- elbow 719.82
- foot 719.87
- hand 719.84
- hip 719.85
- knee 719.86
- multiple sites 719.89
- pelvic region 719.85

Arthrophytis – *continued*
- shoulder (region) 719.81
- specified site NEC 719.88
- wrist 719.83

Arthropyosis (*see also* Arthritis, pyogenic) 711.0❺

Arthroscopic surgical procedure converted to open procedure V64.43

Arthrosis (deformans) (degenerative) (*see also* Osteoarthrosis) 715.9❺
- Charcôt's 094.0 *[713.5]*
- polyarticular 715.09
- spine (*see also* Spondylosis) 721.90

Arthus phenomenon 995.21
- due to
  - correct substance properly administered 995.21
  - overdose or wrong substance given or taken 977.9
    - specified drug – *see* Table of Drugs and Chemicals
- serum 999.5

Articular – *see also* condition
- disc disorder (reducing or non-reducing) 524.63
- spondylolisthesis 756.12

Articulation
- anterior 524.27
- posterior 524.27
- reverse 524.27

Artificial
- device (prosthetic) – *see* Fitting, device
- insemination V26.1
- menopause (states) (symptoms) (syndrome) 627.4
- opening status (functioning) (without complication) V44.9
  - anus (colostomy) V44.3
  - colostomy V44.3
  - cystostomy V44.50
    - appendico-vesicostomy V44.52
    - cutaneous-vesicostomy V44.51
    - specifed type NEC V44.59
  - enterostomy V44.4
  - gastrostomy V44.1
  - ileostomy V44.2
  - intestinal tract NEC V44.4
  - jejunostomy V44.4
  - nephrostomy V44.6
  - specified site NEC V44.8
  - tracheostomy V44.0
  - ureterostomy V44.6
  - urethrostomy V44.6
  - urinary tract NEC V44.6
  - vagina V44.7
  - vagina status V44.7

ARV (disease) (illness) (infection) – *see* Human immunodeficiency virus (disease) (illness) (infection)

Arytenoid – *see* condition

Asbestosis (occupational) 501

Asboe-Hansen's disease (incontinentia pigmenti) 757.33

Ascariasis (intestinal) (lung) 127.0

Ascaridiasis 127.0

Ascaridosis 127.0

Ascaris 127.0
- lumbricoides (infestation) 127.0
- pneumonia 127.0

Ascending – *see* condition

ASC-H (atypical squamous cells cannot exclude high grade squamous intraepithelial lesion) 795.02

Aschoff's bodies (*see also* Myocarditis, rheumatic) 398.0

Ascites 789.59 ▲
- abdominal NEC 789.59 ▲
- cancerous (M8000/6) 789.51 ▲
- cardiac 428.0
- chylous (nonfilarial) 457.8
  - filarial (*see also* Infestation, filarial) 125.9
- congenital 778.0
- due to S. japonicum 120.2
- fetal, causing fetopelvic disproportion 653.7❺
- heart 428.0
- joint (*see also* Effusion, joint) 719.0❺
- malignant (M8000/6) 789.51 ▲
- pseudochylous 789.59 ▲
- syphilitic 095.2
- tuberculous (*see also* Tuberculosis) 014.0❺

Ascorbic acid (vitamin C) deficiency (scurvy) 267

ASC-US (atypical squamous cells of undetermined significance) 795.01

ASCVD (arteriosclerotic cardiovascular disease) 429.2

Aseptic – *see* condition

Asherman's syndrome 621.5

Asialia 527.7

Asiatic cholera (*see also* Cholera) 001.9

Asocial personality or trends 301.7

Asomatognosia 781.8

Aspergillosis 117.3
- with pneumonia 117.3 *[484.6]*
- allergic bronchopulmonary 518.6
- nonsyphilitic NEC 117.3

Aspergillus (flavus) (fumigatus) (infection) (terreus) 117.3

Aspermatogenesis 606.0

Aspermia (testis) 606.0

Asphyxia, asphyxiation (by) 799.01
- antenatal – *see* Distress, fetal
- bedclothes 994.7
- birth (*see also* Asphyxia, newborn) 768.9
- bunny bag 994.7
- carbon monoxide 986
- caul (*see also* Asphyxia, newborn) 768.9
- cave-in 994.7
  - crushing – *see* Injury, internal, intrathoracic organs
- constriction 994.7
- crushing – *see* Injury, internal, intrathoracic organs
- drowning 994.1
- fetal, affecting newborn 768.9
- food or foreign body (in larynx) 933.1
  - bronchioles 934.8
  - bronchus (main) 934.1
  - lung 934.8
  - nasopharynx 933.0
  - nose, nasal passages 932
  - pharynx 933.0
  - respiratory tract 934.9
    - specified part NEC 934.8
  - throat 933.0
  - trachea 934.0
- gas, fumes, or vapor NEC 987.9
  - specified – *see* Table of Drugs and Chemicals
- gravitational changes 994.7
- hanging 994.7
- inhalation – *see* Inhalation
- intrauterine
  - fetal death (before onset of labor) 768.0
    - during labor 768.1
  - liveborn infant – *see* Distress, fetal, liveborn infant
- local 443.0
- mechanical 994.7
  - during birth (*see also* Distress, fetal) 768.9
- mucus 933.1
  - bronchus (main) 934.1
  - larynx 933.1
  - lung 934.8
  - nasal passages 932
  - newborn 770.18
  - pharynx 933.0
  - respiratory tract 934.9
    - specified part NEC 934.8
  - throat 933.0
  - trachea 934.0
  - vaginal (fetus or newborn) 770.18
- newborn 768.9
  - with neurologic involvement 768.5
  - blue 768.6
  - livida 768.6
  - mild or moderate 768.6
  - pallida 768.5
  - severe 768.5
  - white 768.5
- pathological 799.01
- plastic bag 994.7
- postnatal (*see also* Asphyxia, newborn) 768.9
  - mechanical 994.7
- pressure 994.7
- reticularis 782.61
- strangulation 994.7
- submersion 994.1
- traumatic NEC – *see* Injury, internal, intrathoracic organs
- vomiting, vomitus – *see* Asphyxia, food or foreign body

Arthritis, arthritic – Asphyxia, asphyxiation

Aspiration
  acid pulmonary (syndrome) 997.3
    obstetric 668.0❺
  amniotic fluid 770.13
    with respiratory symptoms 770.14
  bronchitis 507.0
  clear amniotic fluid 770.13
    with
      pneumonia 770.14
      pneumonitis 770.14
      respiratory symptoms 770.14
  contents of birth canal 770.17
    with respiratory symptoms 770.18
  fetal 770.10
    blood 770.15
      with
        pneumonia 770.16
        pneumonitis 770.16
    pneumonitis 770.18
  food, foreign body, or gasoline (with asphyxiation) – *see* Asphyxia, food or foreign body
  meconium 770.11
    with
      pneumonia 770.12
      pneumonitis 770.12
      respiratory symptoms 770.12
    below vocal cords 770.11
      with respiratory symptoms 770.12
  mucus 933.1
    into
      bronchus (main) 934.1
      lung 934.8
      respiratory tract 934.9
        specified part NEC 934.8
      trachea 934.0
    newborn 770.17
    vaginal (fetus or newborn) 770.17
  newborn 770.10
    with respiratory symptoms 770.18
    blood 770.15
      with
        pneumonia 770.16
        pneumonitis 770.16
        respiratory symptoms 770.16
  pneumonia 507.0
    fetus or newborn 770.18
      meconium 770.12
  pneumonitis 507.0
    fetus or newborn 770.18
      meconium 770.12
    obstetric 668.0❺
  postnatal stomach contents 770.85
    with
      pneumonia 770.86
      pneumonitis 770.86
      respiratory symptoms 770.86
  syndrome of newborn (massive) 770.18
    meconium 770.12
  vernix caseosa 770.17
Asplenia 759.0
  with mesocardia 746.87
Assam fever 085.0
Assimilation, pelvis
  with disproportion 653.2❺
    affecting fetus or newborn 763.1
    causing obstructed labor 660.1❺
      affecting fetus or newborn 763.1
Assmann's focus (*see also* Tuberculosis) 011.0❺
Astasia (-abasia) 307.9
  hysterical 300.11
Asteatosis 706.8
  cutis 706.8
Astereognosis 780.99
Asterixis 781.3
  in liver disease 572.8
Asteroid hyalitis 379.22
Asthenia, asthenic 780.79
  cardiac (*see also* Failure, heart) 428.9
    psychogenic 306.2
  cardiovascular (*see also* Failure, heart) 428.9
    psychogenic 306.2
  heart (*see also* Failure, heart) 428.9
    psychogenic 306.2
  hysterical 300.11
  myocardial (*see also* Failure, heart) 428.9
    psychogenic 306.2
  nervous 300.5
  neurocirculatory 306.2
  neurotic 300.5
  psychogenic 300.5

Asthenia, asthenic – *continued*
  psychoneurotic 300.5
  psychophysiologic 300.5
  reaction, psychoneurotic 300.5
  senile 797
  Stiller's 780.79
  tropical anhidrotic 705.1
Asthenopia 368.13
  accommodative 367.4
  hysterical (muscular) 300.11
  psychogenic 306.7
Asthenospermia 792.2
Asthma, asthmatic (bronchial) (catarrh) (spasmodic) 493.9❺

Note – Use the following fifth digit subclassification with category 493:
0 unspecified
1 with status asthmaticus
2 with (acute) exacerbation

  with
    chronic obstructive pulmonary disease (COPD) 493.2❺
    hay fever 493.0❺
    rhinitis, allergic 493.0❺
  allergic 493.9❺
    stated cause (external allergen) 493.0❺
  atopic 493.0❺
  cardiac (*see also* Failure, ventricular, left) 428.1
  cardiobronchial (*see also* Failure, ventricular, left) 428.1
  cardiorenal (*see also* Hypertension, cardiorenal) 404.90
  childhood 493.0❺
  Colliers' 500
  cough variant 493.82
  croup 493.9❺
  detergent 507.8
  due to
    detergent 507.8
    inhalation of fumes 506.3
    internal immunological process 493.0❺
  endogenous (intrinsic) 493.1❺
  eosinophilic 518.3
  exercise induced bronchospasm 493.81
  exogenous (cosmetics) (dander or dust) (drugs) (dust) (feathers) (food) (hay) (platinum) (pollen) 493.0❺
  extrinsic 493.0❺
  grinders' 502
  hay 493.0❺
  heart (*see also* Failure, ventricular, left) 428.1
  IgE 493.0
  infective 493.1❺
  intrinsic 493.1❺
  Kopp's 254.8
  late-onset 493.1❺
  meat-wrappers' 506.9
  Millar's (laryngismus stridulus) 478.75
  millstone makers' 502
  miners' 500
  Monday morning 504
  New Orleans (epidemic) 493.0❺
  platinum 493.0❺
  pneumoconiotic (occupational) NEC 505
  potters' 502
  psychogenic 316 *[493.9]*❺
  pulmonary eosinophilic 518.3
  red cedar 495.8
  Rostan's (*see also* Failure, ventricular, left) 428.1
  sandblasters' 502
  sequoiosis 495.8
  stonemasons' 502
  thymic 254.8
  tuberculous (*see also* Tuberculosis, pulmonary) 011.9❺
  Wichmann's (laryngismus stridulus) 478.75
  wood 495.8
Astigmatism (compound) (congenital) 367.20
  irregular 367.22
  regular 367.21
Astroblastoma (M9430/3)
  nose 748.1
  specified site – *see* Neoplasm, by site, malignant
  unspecified site 191.9
Astrocytoma (cystic) (M9400/3)
  anaplastic type (M9401/3)
    specified site – *see* Neoplasm, by site, malignant
    unspecified site 191.9

Astrocytoma – *continued*
  fibrillary (M9420/3)
    specified site – *see* Neoplasm, by site, malignant
    unspecified site 191.9
  fibrous (M9420/3)
    specified site – *see* Neoplasm, by site, malignant
    unspecified site 191.9
  gemistocytic (M9411/3)
    specified site – *see* Neoplasm, by site, malignant
    unspecified site 191.9
  juvenile (M9421/3)
    specified site – *see* Neoplasm, by site, malignant
    unspecified site 191.9
  nose 748.1
  pilocytic (M9421/3)
    specified site – *see* Neoplasm, by site, malignant
    unspecified site 191.9
  piloid (M9421/3)
    specified site – *see* Neoplasm, by site, malignant
    unspecified site 191.9
  protoplasmic (M9410/3)
    specified site – *see* Neoplasm, by site, malignant
    unspecified site 191.9
  specified site – *see* Neoplasm, by site, malignant
  subependymal (M9383/1) 237.5
    giant cell (M9384/1) 237.5
  unspecified site 191.9
Astroglioma (M9400/3)
  nose 748.1
  specified site – *see* Neoplasm, by site, malignant
  unspecified site 191.9
Asymbolia 784.60
Asymmetrical breathing 786.09
Asymmetry – *see also* Distortion
  chest 786.9
  face 754.0
  jaw NEC 524.12
    maxillary 524.11
  pelvis with disproportion 653.0❺
    affecting fetus or newborn 763.1
    causing obstructed labor 660.1❺
      affecting fetus or newborn 763.1
Asynergia 781.3
Asynergy 781.3
  ventricular 429.89
Asystole (heart) (*see also* Arrest, cardiac) 427.5
At risk for falling V15.88
Ataxia, ataxy, ataxic 781.3
  acute 781.3
  brain 331.89
  cerebellar 334.3
    hereditary (Marie's) 334.2
    in
      alcoholism 303.9❺ *[334.4]*
      myxedema (*see also* Myxedema) 244.9 *[334.4]*
      neoplastic disease NEC 239.9 *[334.4]*
  cerebral 331.89
  family, familial 334.2
    cerebral (Marie's) 334.2
    spinal (Friedreich's) 334.0
  Friedreich's (heredofamilial) (spinal) 334.0
  frontal lobe 781.3
  gait 781.2
    hysterical 300.11
  general 781.3
  hereditary NEC 334.2
    cerebellar 334.2
    spastic 334.1
    spinal 334.0
  heredofamilial (Marie's) 334.2
  hysterical 300.11
  locomotor (progressive) 094.0
    diabetic 250.6❺ *[337.1]*
  Marie's (cerebellar) (heredofamilial) 334.2
  nonorganic origin 307.9
  partial 094.0
  postchickenpox 052.7
  progressive locomotor 094.0
  psychogenic 307.9
  Sanger-Brown's 334.2
  spastic 094.0
    hereditary 334.1

- **Ataxia, ataxy, ataxic** – *continued*
  - spastic – *continued*
    - syphilitic 094.0
  - spinal
    - hereditary 334.0
    - progressive locomotor 094.0
  - telangiectasia 334.8
- **Ataxia-telangiectasia** 334.8
- **Atelectasis** (absorption collapse) (complete) (compression) (massive) (partial) (postinfective) (pressure collapse) (pulmonary) (relaxation) 518.0
  - newborn (congenital) (partial) 770.5
    - primary 770.4
  - primary 770.4
  - tuberculous (*see also* Tuberculosis, pulmonary) 011.9❺
- **Ateleiosis, ateliosis** 253.3
- **Atelia** – *see* Distortion
- **Ateliosis** 253.3
- **Atelocardia** 746.9
- **Atelomyelia** 742.59
- **Athelia** 757.6
- **Atheroembolism**
  - extremity
    - lower 445.02
    - upper 445.01
  - kidney 445.81
  - specified site NEC 445.89
- **Atheroma, atheromatous** (*see also* Arteriosclerosis) 440.9
  - aorta, aortic 440.0
    - valve (*see also* Endocarditis, aortic) 424.1
  - artery – *see* Arteriosclerosis
  - basilar (artery) (*see also* Occlusion, artery, basilar) 433.0❺
  - carotid (artery) (common) (internal) (*see also* Occlusion, artery, carotid) 433.1❺
  - cerebral (arteries) 437.0
  - coronary (artery) – *see* Arteriosclerosis, coronary
  - degeneration – *see* Arteriosclerosis
  - heart, cardiac – *see* Arteriosclerosis, coronary
  - mitral (valve) 424.0
  - myocardium, myocardial – *see* Arteriosclerosis, coronary
  - pulmonary valve (heart) (*see also* Endocarditis, pulmonary) 424.3
  - skin 706.2
  - tricuspid (heart) (valve) 424.2
  - valve, valvular – *see* Endocarditis
  - vertebral (artery) (*see also* Occlusion, artery, vertebral) 433.2❺
- **Atheromatosis** – *see also* Arteriosclerosis
  - arterial, congenital 272.8
- **Atherosclerosis** – *see* Arteriosclerosis
- **Athetosis** (acquired) 781.0
  - bilateral 333.79
  - congenital (bilateral) 333.6
  - double 333.71
  - unilateral 781.0
- **Athlete's**
  - foot 110.4
  - heart 429.3
- **Athletic team examination** V70.3
- **Athrepsia** 261
- **Athyrea** (acquired) (*see also* Hypothyroidism) 244.9
  - congenital 243
- **Athyreosis** (congenital) 243
  - acquired – *see* Hypothyroidism
- **Athyroidism** (acquired) (*see also* Hypothyroidism) 244.9
  - congenital 243
- **Atmospheric pyrexia** 992.0
- **Atonia, atony, atonic**
  - abdominal wall 728.2
  - bladder (sphincter) 596.4
    - neurogenic NEC 596.54
      - with cauda equina syndrome 344.61
  - capillary 448.9
  - cecum 564.89
    - psychogenic 306.4
  - colon 564.89
    - psychogenic 306.4
  - congenital 779.89
  - dyspepsia 536.3
    - psychogenic 306.4
  - intestine 564.89
    - psychogenic 306.4
- **Atonia, atony, atonic** – *continued*
  - stomach 536.3
    - neurotic or psychogenic 306.4
    - psychogenic 306.4
  - uterus 661.2 ❺▲
    - with hemorrhage ▶(postpartum)◀ 666.1❺
    - without hemorrhage
      - intrapartum 661.2 ❺●
      - postpartum 669.8 ❺●
    - affecting fetus or newborn 763.7
  - vesical 596.4
- **Atopy** NEC V15.09
- **Atransferrinemia, congenital** 273.8
- **Atresia, atretic** (congenital) 759.89
  - alimentary organ or tract NEC 751.8
    - lower 751.2
    - upper 750.8
  - ani, anus, anal (canal) 751.2
  - aorta 747.22
    - with hypoplasia of ascending aorta and defective development of left ventricle (with mitral valve atresia) 746.7
    - arch 747.11
    - ring 747.21
  - aortic (orifice) (valve) 746.89
    - arch 747.11
  - aqueduct of Sylvius 742.3
    - with spina bifida (*see also* Spina bifida) 741.0❺
  - artery NEC (*see also* Atresia, blood vessel) 747.60
    - cerebral 747.81
    - coronary 746.85
    - eye 743.58
    - pulmonary 747.3
    - umbilical 747.5
  - auditory canal (external) 744.02
  - bile, biliary duct (common) or passage 751.61
    - acquired (*see also* Obstruction, biliary) 576.2
  - bladder (neck) 753.6
  - blood vessel (peripheral) NEC 747.60
    - cerebral 747.81
    - gastrointestinal 747.61
    - lower limb 747.64
    - pulmonary artery 747.3
    - renal 747.62
    - spinal 747.82
    - upper limb 747.63
  - bronchus 748.3
  - canal, ear 744.02
  - cardiac
    - valve 746.89
      - aortic 746.89
      - mitral 746.89
      - pulmonary 746.01
      - tricuspid 746.1
  - cecum 751.2
  - cervix (acquired) 622.4
    - congenital 752.49
    - in pregnancy or childbirth 654.6❺
      - affecting fetus or newborn 763.89
      - causing obstructed labor 660.2❺
        - affecting fetus or newborn 763.1
  - choana 748.0
  - colon 751.2
  - cystic duct 751.61
    - acquired 575.8
      - with obstruction (*see also* Obstruction, gallbladder) 575.2
  - digestive organs NEC 751.8
  - duodenum 751.1
  - ear canal 744.02
  - ejaculatory duct 752.89
  - epiglottis 748.3
  - esophagus 750.3
  - Eustachian tube 744.24
  - fallopian tube (acquired) 628.2
    - congenital 752.19
  - follicular cyst 620.0
  - foramen of
    - Luschka 742.3
      - with spina bifida (*see also* Spina bifida) 741.0❺
    - Magendie 742.3
      - with spina bifida (*see also* Spina bifida) 741.0❺
  - gallbladder 751.69
  - genital organ
    - external
      - female 752.49
- **Atresia, atretic** – *continued*
  - genital organ – *continued*
    - external – *continued*
      - male NEC 752.89
        - penis 752.69
    - internal
      - female 752.89
      - male 752.89
  - glottis 748.3
  - gullet 750.3
  - heart
    - valve NEC 746.89
      - aortic 746.89
      - mitral 746.89
      - pulmonary 746.01
      - tricuspid 746.1
  - hymen 752.42
    - acquired 623.3
    - postinfective 623.3
  - ileum 751.1
  - intestine (small) 751.1
    - large 751.2
  - iris, filtration angle (*see also* Buphthalmia) 743.20
  - jejunum 751.1
  - kidney 753.3
  - lacrimal, apparatus 743.65
    - acquired – *see* Stenosis, lacrimal
  - larynx 748.3
  - ligament, broad 752.19
  - lung 748.5
  - meatus urinarius 753.6
  - mitral valve 746.89
    - with atresia or hypoplasia of aortic orifice or valve, with hypoplasia of ascending aorta and defective development of left ventricle 746.7
  - nares (anterior) (posterior) 748.0
  - nasolacrimal duct 743.65
  - nasopharynx 748.8
  - nose, nostril 748.0
    - acquired 738.0
  - organ or site NEC – *see* Anomaly, specified type NEC
  - osseous meatus (ear) 744.03
  - oviduct (acquired) 628.2
    - congenital 752.19
  - parotid duct 750.23
    - acquired 527.8
  - pulmonary (artery) 747.3
    - valve 746.01
    - vein 747.49
  - pulmonic 746.01
  - pupil 743.46
  - rectum 751.2
  - salivary duct or gland 750.23
    - acquired 527.8
  - sublingual duct 750.23
    - acquired 527.8
  - submaxillary duct or gland 750.23
    - acquired 527.8
  - trachea 748.3
  - tricuspid valve 746.1
  - ureter 753.29
  - ureteropelvic junction 753.21
  - ureterovesical orifice 753.22
  - urethra (valvular) 753.6
  - urinary tract NEC 753.29
  - uterus 752.3
    - acquired 621.8
  - vagina (acquired) 623.2
    - congenital 752.49
    - postgonococcal (old) 098.2
    - postinfectional 623.2
    - senile 623.2
  - vascular NEC (*see also* Atresia, blood vessel) 747.60
    - cerebral 747.81
  - vas deferens 752.89
  - vein NEC (*see also* Atresia, blood vessel) 747.60
    - cardiac 746.89
    - great 747.49
    - portal 747.49
    - pulmonary 747.49
  - vena cava (inferior) (superior) 747.49
  - vesicourethral orifice 753.6
  - vulva 752.49
    - acquired 624.8
- **Atrichia, atrichosis** 704.00
  - congenital (universal) 757.4
- **Atrioventricularis commune** 745.69

Atrophy, atrophic – *continued*
- optic nerve (ascending) (descending) (infectional) (nonfamilial) (papillomacular bundle) (postretinal) (secondary NEC) (simple) 377.10
  - associated with retinal dystrophy 377.13
  - dominant hereditary 377.16
  - glaucomatous 377.14
  - hereditary (dominant) (Leber's) 377.16
  - Leber's (hereditary) 377.16
  - partial 377.15
  - postinflammatory 377.12
  - primary 377.11
  - syphilitic 094.84
    - congenital 090.49
    - tabes dorsalis 094.0
- orbit 376.45
- ovary (senile), acquired 620.3
- oviduct (senile), acquired 620.3
- palsy, diffuse 335.20
- pancreas (duct) (senile) 577.8
- papillary muscle 429.81
- paralysis 355.9
- parotid gland 527.0
- patches skin 701.3
  - senile 701.8
- penis 607.89
- pharyngitis 472.1
- pharynx 478.29
- pluriglandular 258.8
- polyarthritis 714.0
- prostate 602.2
- pseudohypertrophic 359.1
- renal (*see also* Sclerosis, renal) 587
- reticulata 701.8
- retina (*see also* Degeneration, retina) 362.60
  - hereditary (*see also* Dystrophy, retina) 362.70
- rhinitis 472.0
- salivary duct or gland 527.0
- scar NEC 709.2
- sclerosis, lobar (of brain) 331.0
  - with dementia
    - with behavioral disturbance 331.0 *[294.11]*
    - without behavioral disturbance 331.0 *[294.10]*
- scrotum 608.89
- seminal vesicle 608.89
- senile 797
  - degenerative, of skin 701.3
- skin (patches) (senile) 701.8
- spermatic cord 608.89
- spinal (cord) 336.8
  - acute 336.8
  - muscular (chronic) 335.10
    - adult 335.19
    - familial 335.11
    - juvenile 335.10
  - paralysis 335.10
    - acute (*see also* Poliomyelitis, with paralysis) 045.1❺
- spine (column) 733.99
- spleen (senile) 289.59
- spots (skin) 701.3
  - senile 701.8
- stomach 537.89
- striate and macular 701.3
  - syphilitic 095.8
- subcutaneous 701.9
  - due to injection 999.9
- sublingual gland 527.0
- submaxillary gland 527.0
- Sudeck's 733.7
- suprarenal (autoimmune) (capsule) (gland) 255.41 ▲
  - with hypofunction 255.41 ▲
- tarso-orbital fascia, congenital 743.66
- testis 608.3
- thenar, partial 354.0
- throat 478.29
- thymus (fat) 254.8
- thyroid (gland) 246.8
  - with
    - cretinism 243
    - myxedema 244.9
  - congenital 243
- tongue (senile) 529.8
  - papillae 529.4
  - smooth 529.4
- trachea 519.19
- tunica vaginalis 608.89
- turbinate 733.99

Atrophy, atrophic – *continued*
- tympanic membrane (nonflaccid) 384.82
  - flaccid 384.81
- ulcer (*see also* Ulcer, skin) 707.9
- upper respiratory tract 478.9
- uterus, uterine (acquired) (senile) 621.8
  - cervix 622.8
  - due to radiation (intended effect) 621.8
- vagina (senile) 627.3
- vascular 459.89
- vas deferens 608.89
- vertebra (senile) 733.99
- vulva (primary) (senile) 624.1
- Werdnig-Hoffmann 335.0
- yellow (acute) (congenital) (liver) (subacute) (*see also* Necrosis, liver) 570
  - chronic 571.8
  - resulting from administration of blood, plasma, serum, or other biological substance (within 8 months of administration) – *see* Hepatitis, viral

Attack
- akinetic (*see also* Epilepsy) 345.0❺
- angina – *see* Angina
- apoplectic (*see also* Disease, cerebrovascular, acute) 436
- benign shuddering 333.93
- bilious – *see* Vomiting
- cataleptic 300.11
- cerebral (*see also* Disease, cerebrovascular, acute) 436
- coronary (*see also* Infarct, myocardium) 410.9❺
- cyanotic, newborn 770.83
- epileptic (*see also* Epilepsy) 345.9❺
- epileptiform 780.39
- heart (*see also* Infarct, myocardium) 410.9❺
- hemiplegia (*see also* Disease, cerebrovascular, acute) 436
- hysterical 300.11
- Jacksonian (*see also* Epilepsy) 345.5❺
- myocardium, myocardial (*see also* Infarct, myocardium) 410.9❺
- myoclonic (*see also* Epilepsy) 345.1❺
- panic 300.01
- paralysis (*see also* Disease, cerebrovascular, acute) 436
- paroxysmal 780.39
- psychomotor (*see also* Epilepsy) 345.4❺
- salaam (*see also* Epilepsy) 345.6❺
- schizophreniform (*see also* Schizophrenia) 295.4❺
- sensory and motor 780.39
- syncope 780.2
- toxic, cerebral 780.39
- transient ischemic (TIA) 435.9
- unconsciousness 780.2
  - hysterical 300.11
- vasomotor 780.2
- vasovagal (idiopathic) (paroxysmal) 780.2

Attention to
- artificial
  - opening (of) V55.9
    - digestive tract NEC V55.4
    - specified site NEC V55.8
    - urinary tract NEC V55.6
  - vagina V55.7
- colostomy V55.3
- cystostomy V55.5
- dressing
  - wound V58.30
    - nonsurgical V58.30
    - surgical V58.31
- gastrostomy V55.1
- ileostomy V55.2
- jejunostomy V55.4
- nephrostomy V55.6
- surgical dressings V58.31
- sutures V58.32
- tracheostomy V55.0
- ureterostomy V55.6
- urethrostomy V55.6

Attrition
- gum (*see also* Recession, gingival) 523.20
- teeth (hard tissues) 521.10
  - excessive 521.10
    - extending into
      - dentine 521.12
      - pulp 521.13
    - generalized 521.15
    - limited to enamel 521.11
    - localized 521.14

Atypical – *see also* condition
- cells
  - endocervical 795.00
  - endometrial 795.00
  - glandular 795.00
- distribution, vessel (congenital) (peripheral) NEC 747.60
- endometrium 621.9
- kidney 593.89

Atypism, cervix 622.10

Audible tinnitus (*see also* Tinnitus) 388.30

Auditory – *see* condition

Audry's syndrome (acropachyderma) 757.39

Aujeszky's disease 078.89

Aura, jacksonian (*see also* Epilepsy) 345.5❺

Aurantiasis, cutis 278.3

Auricle, auricular – *see* condition

Auriculotemporal syndrome 350.8

Australian
- Q fever 083.0
- X disease 062.4

Autism, autistic (child) (infantile) 299.0❺

Autodigestion 799.89

Autoerythrocyte sensitization 287.2

Autographism 708.3

Autoimmune
- cold sensitivity 283.0
- disease NEC 279.4
- hemolytic anemia 283.0
- thyroiditis 245.2

Autoinfection, septic – *see* Septicemia

Autointoxication 799.89

Automatism 348.8
- epileptic (*see also* Epilepsy) 345.4❺
- paroxysmal, idiopathic (*see also* Epilepsy) 345.4❺

Autonomic, autonomous
- bladder 596.54
  - neurogenic 596.54
    - with cauda equina 344.61
- dysreflexia 337.3
- faciocephalalgia (*see also* Neuropathy, peripheral, autonomic) 337.9
- hysterical seizure 300.11
- imbalance (*see also* Neuropathy, peripheral, autonomic 337.9

Autophony 388.40

Autosensitivity, erythrocyte 287.2

Autotopagnosia 780.99

Autotoxemia 799.89

Autumn – *see* condition

Avellis' syndrome 344.89

Aviators
- disease or sickness (*see also* Effect, adverse, high altitude) 993.2
- ear 993.0
- effort syndrome 306.2

Avitaminosis (multiple NEC) (*see also* Deficiency, vitamin) 269.2
- A 264.9
- B 266.9
  - with
    - beriberi 265.0
    - pellagra 265.2
- B_1 265.1
- B_2 266.0
- B_6 266.1
- B_{12} 266.2
- C (with scurvy) 267
- D 268.9
  - with
    - osteomalacia 268.2
    - rickets 268.0
- E 269.1
- G 266.0
- H 269.1
- K 269.0
- multiple 269.2
- nicotinic acid 265.2
- P 269.1

Avulsion (traumatic) 879.8
- blood vessel – *see* Injury, blood vessel, by site
- cartilage – *see also* Dislocation, by site
  - knee, current (*see also* Tear, meniscus) 836.2
  - symphyseal (inner), complicating delivery 665.6❺
- complicated 879.9

❹ Fourth-Digit Required ❺ Fifth-Digit Required *[code]* Manifestation Code ▶◀ Revised Text ● New Line ▲ Revised Code

Avulsion – *continued*
  diaphragm – *see* Injury, internal, diaphragm
  ear – *see* Wound, open, ear
  epiphysis of bone – *see* Fracture, by site
  external site other than limb – *see* Wound, open, by site
  eye 871.3
  fingernail – *see* Wound, open, finger
  fracture – *see* Fracture, by site
  genital organs, external – *see* Wound, open, genital organs
  head (intracranial) NEC – *see also* Injury, intracranial, with open intracranial wound
    complete 874.9
    external site NEC 873.8
      complicated 873.9
  internal organ or site – *see* Injury, internal, by site
  joint – *see also* Dislocation, by site
    capsule – *see* Sprain, by site
  ligament – *see* Sprain, by site
  limb – *see also* Amputation, traumatic, by site
    skin and subcutaneous tissue – *see* Wound, open, by site
  muscle – *see* Sprain, by site
  nerve (root) – *see* Injury, nerve, by site
  scalp – *see* Wound, open, scalp
  skin and subcutaneous tissue – *see* Wound, open, by site
  symphyseal cartilage (inner), complicating delivery 665.6❺
  tendon – *see also* Sprain, by site
    with open wound – *see* Wound, open, by site
  toenail – *see* Wound, open, toe(s)
  tooth 873.63
    complicated 873.73
Awaiting organ transplant status V49.83
Awareness of heart beat 785.1
Axe grinders' disease 502
Axenfeld's anomaly or syndrome 743.44
Axilla, axillary – *see also* condition
  breast 757.6
Axonotmesis – *see* Injury, nerve, by site
Ayala's disease 756.89
Ayerza's disease or syndrome (pulmonary artery sclerosis with pulmonary hypertension) 416.0
Azoospermia 606.0
Azorean disease (of the nervous system) 334.8
Azotemia 790.6
  meaning uremia (*see also* Uremia) 586
Aztec ear 744.29
Azygos lobe, lung (fissure) 748.69

B

Baader's syndrome (erythema multiforme exudativum) 695.1
Baastrup's syndrome 721.5
Babesiasis 088.82
Babesiosis 088.82
Babington's disease (familial hemorrhagic telangiectasia) 448.0
Babinski's syndrome (cardiovascular syphilis) 093.89
Babinski-Fröhlich syndrome (adiposogenital dystrophy) 253.8
Babinski-Nageotte syndrome 344.89
Bacillary – *see* condition
Bacilluria 791.9
  asymptomatic, in pregnancy or puerperium 646.5❺
  tuberculous (*see also* Tuberculosis) 016.9❺
Bacillus – *see also* Infection, bacillus
  abortus infection 023.1
  anthracis infection 022.9
  coli
    infection 041.4
      generalized 038.42
      intestinal 008.00
    pyemia 038.42
    septicemia 038.42
  Flexner's 004.1
  fusiformis infestation 101
  mallei infection 024
  Shiga's 004.0
Bacillus – *continued*
  suipestifer infection (*see also* Infection, Salmonella) 003.9
Back – *see* condition
Backache (postural) 724.5
  psychogenic 307.89
  sacroiliac 724.6
Backflow (pyelovenous) (*see also* Disease, renal) 593.9
Backknee (*see also* Genu, recurvatum) 736.5
Bacteremia 790.7
  newborn 771.83
Bacteria
  in blood (*see also* Bacteremia) 790.7
  in urine (*see also* Bacteriuria) 791.9
Bacterial – *see* condition
Bactericholia (*see also* Cholecystitis, acute) 575.0
Bacterid, bacteride (Andrews' pustular) 686.8
Bacteriuria, bacteruria 791.9
  with
    urinary tract infection 599.0
  asymptomatic 791.9
    in pregnancy or puerperium 646.5❺
      affecting fetus or newborn 760.1
Bad
  breath 784.99
  heart – *see* Disease, heart
  trip (*see also* Abuse, drugs, nondependent) 305.3❺
Baehr-Schiffrin disease (thrombotic thrombocytopenic purpura) 446.6
Baelz's disease (cheilitis glandularis apostematosa) 528.5
Baerensprung's disease (eczema marginatum) 110.3
Bagassosis (occupational) 495.1
Baghdad boil 085.1
Bagratuni's syndrome (temporal arteritis) 446.5
Baker's
  cyst (knee) 727.51
    tuberculous (*see also* Tuberculosis) 015.2❺
  itch 692.89
Bakwin-Krida syndrome (craniometaphyseal dysplasia) 756.89
Balanitis (circinata) (gangraenosa) (infectious) (vulgaris) 607.1
  amebic 006.8
  candidal 112.2
  chlamydial 099.53
  due to Ducrey's bacillus 099.0
  erosiva circinata et gangraenosa 607.1
  gangrenous 607.1
  gonococcal (acute) 098.0
    chronic or duration of 2 months or over 098.2
  nongonococcal 607.1
  phagedenic 607.1
  venereal NEC 099.8
  xerotica obliterans 607.81
Balanoposthitis 607.1
  chlamydial 099.53
  gonococcal (acute) 098.0
    chronic or duration of 2 months or over 098.2
  ulcerative NEC 099.8
Balanorrhagia – *see* Balanitis
Balantidiasis 007.0
Balantidiosis 007.0
Balbuties, balbutio 307.0
Bald
  patches on scalp 704.00
  tongue 529.4
Baldness (*see also* Alopecia) 704.00
Balfour's disease (chloroma) 205.3❺
Balint's syndrome (psychic paralysis of visual fixation) 368.16
Balkan grippe 083.0
Ball
  food 938
  hair 938
Ballantyne (-Runge) **syndrome** (postmaturity) 766.22
Balloon disease (*see also* Effect, adverse, high altitude) 993.2
Ballooning posterior leaflet syndrome 424.0
Baló's disease or concentric sclerosis 341.1
Bamberger's disease (hypertrophic pulmonary osteoarthropathy) 731.2
Bamberger-Marie disease (hypertrophic pulmonary osteoarthropathy) 731.2
Bamboo spine 720.0
Bancroft's filariasis 125.0
Band(s)
  adhesive (*see also* Adhesions, peritoneum) 568.0
  amniotic 658.8❺
    affecting fetus or newborn 762.8
  anomalous or congenital – *see also* Anomaly, specified type NEC
    atrial 746.9
    heart 746.9
    intestine 751.4
    omentum 751.4
    ventricular 746.9
  cervix 622.3
  gallbladder (congenital) 751.69
  intestinal (adhesive) (*see also* Adhesions, peritoneum) 568.0
    congenital 751.4
  obstructive (*see also* Obstruction, intestine) 560.81
  periappendiceal (congenital) 751.4
  peritoneal (adhesive) (*see also* Adhesions, peritoneum) 568.0
    with intestinal obstruction 560.81
    congenital 751.4
  uterus 621.5
  vagina 623.2
Bandemia (without diagnosis of specific infection) 288.66 ●
Bandl's ring (contraction)
  complicating delivery 661.4❺
    affecting fetus or newborn 763.7
Bang's disease (Brucella abortus) 023.1
Bangkok hemorrhagic fever 065.4
Bannister's disease 995.1
Bantam-Albright-Martin disease (pseudohypoparathyroidism) 275.49
Banti's disease or syndrome (with cirrhosis) (with portal hypertension) – *see* Cirrhosis, liver
Bar
  calcaneocuboid 755.67
  calcaneonavicular 755.67
  cubonavicular 755.67
  prostate 600.90
    with
      other lower urinary tract symptoms (LUTS) 600.91
      urinary
        obstruction 600.91
        retention 600.91
  talocalcaneal 755.67
Baragnosis 780.99
Barasheh, barashek 266.2
Barcoo disease or rot (*see also* Ulcer, skin) 707.9
Bard-Pic syndrome (carcinoma, head of pancreas) 157.0
Bärensprung's disease (eczema marginatum) 110.3
Baritosis 503
Barium lung disease 503
Barlow's syndrome (meaning mitral valve prolapse) 424.0
Barlow (-Möller) **disease or syndrome** (meaning infantile scurvy) 267
Barodontalgia 993.2
Baron Münchausen syndrome 301.51
Barosinusitis 993.1
Barotitis 993.0
Barotrauma 993.2
  odontalgia 993.2
  otitic 993.0
  sinus 993.1
Barraquer's disease or syndrome (progressive lipodystrophy) 272.6
Barré-Guillain syndrome 357.0
Barré-Liéou syndrome (posterior cervical sympathetic) 723.2
Barrel chest 738.3
Barrett's esophagus 530.85
Barrett's syndrome or ulcer (chronic peptic ulcer of esophagus) 530.85
Bársony-Polgár syndrome (corkscrew esophagus) 530.5
Bársony-Teschendorf syndrome (corkscrew esophagus) 530.5

Barth syndrome 759.89
Bartholin's
adenitis (*see also* Bartholinitis) 616.89
gland – *see* condition
Bartholinitis (suppurating) 616.89
gonococcal (acute) 098.0
chronic or duration of 2 months or over 098.2
Bartonellosis 088.0
Bartter's syndrome (secondary hyperaldosteronism with juxtaglomerular hyperplasia) 255.13
Basal – *see* condition
Basan's (hidrotic) **ectodermal dysplasia** 757.31
Baseball finger 842.13
Basedow's disease or syndrome (exophthalmic goiter) 242.0❺
Basic – *see* condition
Basilar – *see* condition
Bason's (hidrotic) **ectodermal dysplasia** 757.31
Basopenia 288.59
Basophilia 288.65
Basophilism (corticoadrenal) (Cushing's) (pituitary) (thymic) 255.0
Bassen-Kornzweig syndrome (abetalipoproteinemia) 272.5
Bat ear 744.29
Bateman's
disease 078.0
purpura (senile) 287.2
Bathing cramp 994.1
Bathophobia 300.23
Batten's disease, retina 330.1 *[362.71]*
Batten-Mayou disease 330.1 *[362.71]*
Batten-Steinert syndrome 359.21 ▲
Battered
adult (syndrome) 995.81
baby or child (syndrome) 995.54
spouse (syndrome) 995.81
Battey mycobacterium infection 031.0
Battledore placenta – *see* Placenta, abnormal
Battle exhaustion (*see also* Reaction, stress, acute) 308.9
Baumgarten-Cruveilhier (cirrhosis) **disease, or syndrome** 571.5
Bauxite
fibrosis (of lung) 503
workers' disease 503
Bayle's disease (dementia paralytica) 094.1
Bazin's disease (primary) (*see also* Tuberculosis) 017.1❺
Beach ear 380.12
Beaded hair (congenital) 757.4
Beals syndrome 759.82
Beard's disease (neurasthenia) 300.5
Bearn-Kunkel (-Slater) **syndrome** (lupoid hepatitis) 571.49
Beat
elbow 727.2
hand 727.2
knee 727.2
Beats
ectopic 427.60
escaped, heart 427.60
postoperative 997.1
premature (nodal) 427.60
atrial 427.61
auricular 427.61
postoperative 997.1
specified type NEC 427.69
supraventricular 427.61
ventricular 427.69
Beau's
disease or syndrome (*see also* Degeneration, myocardial) 429.1
lines (transverse furrows on fingernails) 703.8
Bechterew's disease (ankylosing spondylitis) 720.0
Bechterew-Strümpell-Marie syndrome (ankylosing spondylitis) 720.0
Beck's syndrome (anterior spinal artery occlusion) 433.8❺
Becker's
disease
idiopathic mural endomyocardial disease 425.2 ●
myotonia congenita, recessive form 359.22 ●
Becker's – *continued*
dystrophy 359.22 ▲
Beckwith (-Wiedemann) **syndrome** 759.89
Bed confinement status V49.84
Bedclothes, asphyxiation or suffocation by 994.7
Bednar's aphthae 528.2
Bedsore 707.00
with gangrene 707.00 *[785.4]*
Bedwetting (*see also* Enuresis) 788.36
Beer-drinkers' heart (disease) 425.5
Bee sting (with allergic or anaphylactic shock) 989.5
Begbie's disease (exophthalmic goiter) 242.0❺
Behavior disorder, disturbance – *see also* Disturbance, conduct
antisocial, without manifest psychiatric disorder
adolescent V71.02
adult V71.01
child V71.02
dyssocial, without manifest psychiatric disorder
adolescent V71.02
adult V71.01
child V71.02
high-risk- *see* problem
Behçet's syndrome 136.1
Behr's disease 362.50
Beigel's disease or morbus (white piedra) 111.2
Bejel 104.0
Bekhterev's disease (ankylosing spondylitis) 720.0
Bekhterev-Strümpell-Marie syndrome (ankylosing spondylitis) 720.0
Belching (*see also* Eructation) 787.3
Bell's
disease (*see also* Psychosis, affective) 296.0❺
mania (*see also* Psychosis, affective) 296.0❺
palsy, paralysis 351.0
infant 767.5
newborn 767.5
syphilitic 094.89
spasm 351.0
Bence-Jones albuminuria, albuminosuria, or proteinuria 791.0
Bends 993.3
Benedikt's syndrome (paralysis) 344.89
Benign – *see also* condition
cellular changes, cervix 795.09
prostate
hyperplasia 600.20
with
other lower urinary tract symptoms (LUTS) 600.21
urinary
obstruction 600.21
retention 600.21
neoplasm 222.2
Bennett's
disease (leukemia) 208.9❺
fracture (closed) 815.01
open 815.11
Benson's disease 379.22
Bent
back (hysterical) 300.11
nose 738.0
congenital 754.0
Bereavement V62.82
as adjustment reaction 309.0
Berger's paresthesia (lower limb) 782.0
Bergeron's disease (hysteroepilepsy) 300.11
Beriberi (acute) (atrophic) (chronic) (dry) (subacute) (wet) 265.0
with polyneuropathy 265.0 *[357.4]*
heart (disease) 265.0 *[425.7]*
leprosy 030.1
neuritis 265.0 *[357.4]*
Berlin's disease or edema (traumatic) 921.3
Berloque dermatitis 692.72
Bernard-Horner syndrome (*see also* Neuropathy, peripheral, autonomic) 337.9
Bernard-Sergent syndrome (acute adrenocortical insufficiency) 255.41 ▲
Bernard-Soulier disease or thrombopathy 287.1
Bernhardt's disease or paresthesia 355.1
Bernhardt-Roth disease or syndrome (parasthesia) 355.1
Bernheim's syndrome (*see also* Failure, heart) 428.0
Bertielliasis 123.8
Bertolotti's syndrome (sacralization of fifth lumbar vertebra) 756.15
Berylliosis (acute) (chronic) (lung) (occupational) 503
Besnier's
lupus pernio 135
prurigo (atopic dermatitis) (infantile eczema) 691.8
Besnier-Boeck disease or sarcoid 135
Besnier-Boeck-Schaumann disease (sarcoidosis) 135
Best's disease 362.76
Bestiality 302.1
Beta-adrenergic hyperdynamic circulatory state 429.82
Beta-aminoisobutyric aciduria 277.2
Beta-mercaptolactate-cysteine disulfiduria 270.0
Beta thalassemia (major) (minor) (mixed) 282.49
Beurmann's disease (sporotrichosis) 117.1
Bezoar 938
intestine 936
stomach 935.2
Bezold's abscess (*see also* Mastoiditis) 383.01
Bianchi's syndrome (aphasia-apraxia-alexia) 784.69
Bicornuate or bicornis uterus 752.3
in pregnancy or childbirth 654.0❺
with obstructed labor 660.2❺
affecting fetus or newborn 763.1
affecting fetus or newborn 763.89
Bicuspid aortic valve 746.4
Biedl-Bardet syndrome 759.89
Bielschowsky's disease 330.1
Bielschowsky-Jansky
amaurotic familial idiocy 330.1
disease 330.1
Biemond's syndrome (obesity, polydactyly, and mental retardation) 759.89
Biermer's anemia or disease (pernicious anemia) 281.0
Biett's disease 695.4
Bifid (congenital) – *see also* Imperfect, closure
apex, heart 746.89
clitoris 752.49
epiglottis 748.3
kidney 753.3
nose 748.1
patella 755.64
scrotum 752.89
toe 755.66
tongue 750.13
ureter 753.4
uterus 752.3
uvula 749.02
with cleft lip (*see also* Cleft, palate, with cleft lip) 749.20
Biforis uterus (suprasimplex) 752.3
Bifurcation (congenital) – *see also* Imperfect, closure
gallbladder 751.69
kidney pelvis 753.3
renal pelvis 753.3
rib 756.3
tongue 750.13
trachea 748.3
ureter 753.4
urethra 753.8
uvula 749.02
with cleft lip (*see also* Cleft, palate, with cleft lip) 749.20
vertebra 756.19
Bigeminal pulse 427.89
Bigeminy 427.89
Big spleen syndrome 289.4
Bilateral – *see* condition
Bile duct – *see* condition
Bile pigments in urine 791.4
Bilharziasis (*see also* Schistosomiasis) 120.9
chyluria 120.0
cutaneous 120.3
galacturia 120.0
hematochyluria 120.0
intestinal 120.1
lipemia 120.9
lipuria 120.0
Oriental 120.2
piarhemia 120.9
pulmonary 120.2
tropical hematuria 120.0

Barth syndrome – Bilharziasis

- **Bilharziasis** – *continued*
  - vesical 120.0
- **Biliary** – *see* condition
- **Bilious** (attack) – *see also* Vomiting
  - fever, hemoglobinuric 084.8
- **Bilirubinuria** 791.4
- **Biliuria** 791.4
- **Billroth's disease**
  - meningocele (*see also* Spina bifida) 741.9❺
- **Bilobate placenta** – *see* Placenta, abnormal
- **Bilocular**
  - heart 745.7
  - stomach 536.8
- **Bing-Horton syndrome** (histamine cephalgia) 346.2❺
- **Binswanger's disease or dementia** 290.12
- **Biörck** (-Thorson) **syndrome** (malignant carcinoid) 259.2
- **Biparta, bipartite** – *see also* Imperfect, closure
  - carpal scaphoid 755.59
  - patella 755.64
  - placenta – *see* Placenta, abnormal
  - vagina 752.49
- **Bird**
  - face 756.0
  - fanciers' lung or disease 495.2
- **Bird's disease** (oxaluria) 271.8
- **Birth**
  - abnormal fetus or newborn 763.9
  - accident, fetus or newborn – *see* Birth, injury
  - complications in mother – *see* Delivery, complicated
  - compression during NEC 767.9
  - defect – *see* Anomaly
  - delayed, fetus 763.9
  - difficult NEC, affecting fetus or newborn 763.9
  - dry, affecting fetus or newborn 761.1
  - forced, NEC, affecting fetus or newborn 763.89
  - forceps, affecting fetus or newborn 763.2
  - hematoma of sternomastoid 767.8
  - immature 765.1❺
    - extremely 765.0❺
  - inattention, after or at 995.52
  - induced, affecting fetus or newborn 763.89
  - infant – *see* Newborn
  - injury NEC 767.9
    - adrenal gland 767.8
    - basal ganglia 767.0
    - brachial plexus (paralysis) 767.6
    - brain (compression) (pressure) 767.0
    - cerebellum 767.0
    - cerebral hemorrhage 767.0
    - conjunctiva 767.8
    - eye 767.8
    - fracture
      - bone, any except clavicle or spine 767.3
      - clavicle 767.2
      - femur 767.3
      - humerus 767.3
      - long bone 767.3
      - radius and ulna 767.3
      - skeleton NEC 767.3
      - skull 767.3
      - spine 767.4
      - tibia and fibula 767.3
    - hematoma 767.8
      - liver (subcapsular) 767.8
      - mastoid 767.8
      - skull 767.19
      - sternomastoid 767.8
      - testes 767.8
      - vulva 767.8
    - intracranial (edema) 767.0
    - laceration
      - brain 767.0
      - by scalpel 767.8
      - peripheral nerve 767.7
    - liver 767.8
    - meninges
      - brain 767.0
      - spinal cord 767.4
    - nerves (cranial, peripheral) 767.7
      - brachial plexus 767.6
      - facial 767.5
    - paralysis 767.7
      - brachial plexus 767.6
      - Erb (-Duchenne) 767.6
      - facial nerve 767.5
      - Klumpke (-Déjérine) 767.6

- **Birth** – *continued*
  - injury – *continued*
    - paralysis – *continued*
      - radial nerve 767.6
      - spinal (cord) (hemorrhage) (laceration) (rupture) 767.4
    - rupture
      - intracranial 767.0
      - liver 767.8
      - spinal cord 767.4
      - spleen 767.8
      - viscera 767.8
    - scalp 767.19
    - scalpel wound 767.8
    - skeleton NEC 767.3
    - specified NEC 767.8
    - spinal cord 767.4
    - spleen 767.8
    - subdural hemorrhage 767.0
    - tentorial, tear 767.0
    - testes 767.8
    - vulva 767.8
  - instrumental, NEC, affecting fetus or newborn 763.2
  - lack of care, after or at 995.52
  - multiple
    - affected by maternal complications of pregnancy 761.5
    - healthy liveborn – *see* Newborn, multiple
  - neglect, after or at 995.52
  - newborn – *see* Newborn
  - palsy or paralysis NEC 767.7
  - precipitate, fetus or newborn 763.6
  - premature (infant) 765.1❺
  - prolonged, affecting fetus or newborn 763.9
  - retarded, fetus or newborn 763.9
  - shock, newborn 779.89
  - strangulation or suffocation
    - due to aspiration of clear amniotic fluid 770.13
      - with respiratory symptoms 770.14
    - mechanical 767.8
  - trauma NEC 767.9
  - triplet
    - affected by maternal complications of pregnancy 761.5
    - healthy liveborn – *see* Newborn, multiple
  - twin
    - affected by maternal complications of pregnancy 761.5
    - healthy liveborn – *see* Newborn, twin
  - ventouse, affecting fetus or newborn 763.3
- **Birthmark** 757.32
- **Bisalbuminemia** 273.8
- **Biskra button** 085.1
- **Bite(s)**
  - with intact skin surface – *see* Contusion
  - animal – *see* Wound, open, by site
    - intact skin surface – *see* Contusion
  - centipede 989.5
  - chigger 133.8
  - fire ant 989.5
  - flea – *see* Injury, superficial, by site
  - human (open wound) – *see also* Wound, open, by site
    - intact skin surface – *see* Contusion
  - insect
    - nonvenomous – *see* Injury, superficial, by site
    - venomous 989.5
  - mad dog (death from) 071
  - open
    - anterior 524.24
    - posterior 524.25
  - poisonous 989.5
  - red bug 133.8
  - reptile 989.5
    - nonvenomous – *see* Wound, open, by site
  - snake 989.5
    - nonvenomous – *see* Wound, open, by site
  - spider (venomous) 989.5
    - nonvenomous – *see* Injury, superficial, by site
  - venomous 989.5
- **Biting**
  - cheek or lip 528.9
  - nail 307.9
- **Black**
  - death 020.9
  - eye NEC 921.0
  - hairy tongue 529.3
  - heel 924.20
  - lung disease 500
  - palm 923.20

- **Blackfan-Diamond anemia or syndrome** (congenital hypoplastic anemia) 284.01
- **Blackhead** 706.1
- **Blackout** 780.2
- **Blackwater fever** 084.8
- **Bladder** – *see* condition
- **Blast**
  - blindness 921.3
  - concussion – *see* Blast, injury
  - injury 869.0
    - with open wound into cavity 869.1
    - abdomen or thorax – *see* Injury, internal, by site
    - brain (*see also* Concussion, brain) 850.9
      - with skull fracture – *see* Fracture, skull
    - ear (acoustic nerve trauma) 951.5
      - with perforation, tympanic membrane – *see* Wound, open, ear, drum
    - lung (*see also* Injury, internal, lung) 861.20
    - otitic (explosive) 388.11
- **Blastomycosis, blastomycotic** (chronic) (cutaneous) (disseminated) (lung) (pulmonary) (systemic) 116.0
  - Brazilian 116.1
  - European 117.5
  - keloidal 116.2
  - North American 116.0
  - primary pulmonary 116.0
  - South American 116.1
- **Bleb(s)** 709.8
  - emphysematous (bullous) (diffuse) (lung) (ruptured) (solitary) 492.0
  - filtering, eye (postglaucoma) (status) V45.69
    - with complication 997.99
    - postcataract extraction (complication) 997.99
  - lung (ruptured) 492.0
    - congenital 770.5
  - subpleural (emphysematous) 492.0
- **Bleeder** (familial) (hereditary) (*see also* Defect, coagulation) 286.9
  - nonfamilial 286.9
- **Bleeding** (*see also* Hemorrhage) 459.0
  - anal 569.3
  - anovulatory 628.0
  - atonic, following delivery 666.1❺
  - capillary 448.9
  - due to subinvolution 621.1
    - puerperal 666.2❺
  - ear 388.69
  - excessive, associated with menopausal onset 627.0
  - familial (*see also* Defect, coagulation) 286.9
  - following intercourse 626.7
  - gastrointestinal 578.9
  - gums 523.8
  - hemorrhoids – *see* Hemorrhoids, bleeding
  - intermenstrual
    - irregular 626.6
    - regular 626.5
  - intraoperative 998.11
  - irregular NEC 626.4
  - menopausal 627.0
  - mouth 528.9
  - nipple 611.79
  - nose 784.7
  - ovulation 626.5
  - postclimacteric 627.1
  - postcoital 626.7
  - postmenopausal 627.1
    - following induced menopause 627.4
  - postoperative 998.11
  - preclimacteric 627.0
  - puberty 626.3
    - excessive, with onset of menstrual periods 626.3
  - rectum, rectal 569.3
  - tendencies (*see also* Defect, coagulation) 286.9
  - throat 784.8
  - umbilical stump 772.3
  - umbilicus 789.9
  - unrelated to menstrual cycle 626.6
  - uterus, uterine 626.9
    - climacteric 627.0
    - dysfunctional 626.8
    - functional 626.8
    - unrelated to menstrual cycle 626.6
  - vagina, vaginal 623.8
    - functional 626.8
  - vicarious 625.8
- **Blennorrhagia, blennorrhagic** – *see* Blennorrhea

Blennorrhea (acute) 098.0
  adultorum 098.40
  alveolaris 523.40
  chronic or duration of 2 months or over 098.2
  gonococcal (neonatorum) 098.40
  inclusion (neonatal) (newborn) 771.6
  neonatorum 098.40
Blepharelosis (*see also* Entropion) 374.00
Blepharitis (eyelid) 373.00
  angularis 373.01
  ciliaris 373.00
    with ulcer 373.01
  marginal 373.00
    with ulcer 373.01
  scrofulous (*see also* Tuberculosis) 017.3❺ *[373.00]*
  squamous 373.02
  ulcerative 373.01
Blepharochalasis 374.34
  congenital 743.62
Blepharoclonus 333.81
Blepharoconjunctivitis (*see also* Conjunctivitis) 372.20
  angular 372.21
  contact 372.22
Blepharophimosis (eyelid) 374.46
  congenital 743.62
Blepharoplegia 374.89
Blepharoptosis 374.30
  congenital 743.61
Blepharopyorrhea 098.49
Blepharospasm 333.81
  due to drugs 333.85
Blessig's cyst 362.62
Blighted ovum 631
Blind
  bronchus (congenital) 748.3
  eye – *see also* Blindness
    hypertensive 360.42
    hypotensive 360.41
  loop syndrome (postoperative) 579.2
  sac, fallopian tube (congenital) 752.19
  spot, enlarged 368.42
  tract or tube (congenital) NEC – *see* Atresia
Blindness (acquired) (congenital) (both eyes) 369.00
  with deafness V49.85 ●
  blast 921.3
    with nerve injury – *see* Injury, nerve, optic
  Bright's – *see* Uremia
  color (congenital) 368.59
    acquired 368.55
    blue 368.53
    green 368.52
    red 368.51
    total 368.54
  concussion 950.9
  cortical 377.75
  day 368.10
    acquired 368.10
    congenital 368.10
    hereditary 368.10
    specified type NEC 368.10
  due to
    injury NEC 950.9
    refractive error – *see* Error, refractive
  eclipse (total) 363.31
  emotional 300.11
  hysterical 300.11
  legal (both eyes) (USA definition) 369.4
    with impairment of better (less impaired) eye
      near-total 369.02
        with
          lesser eye impairment 369.02
            near-total 369.04
            total 369.03
      profound 369.05
        with
          lesser eye impairment 369.05
            near-total 369.07
            profound 369.08
            total 369.06
      severe 369.21
        with
          lesser eye impairment 369.21
            blind 369.11
            near-total 369.13
            profound 369.14
            severe 369.22
            total 369.12

Blindness – *continued*
  legal – *continued*
    with impairment of better (less impaired) eye - *continued*
      total
        with lesser eye impairment
          total 369.01
  mind 784.69
  moderate
    both eyes 369.25
      with impairment of lesser eye (specified as)
        blind, not further specified 369.15
        low vision, not further specified 369.23
        near-total 369.17
        profound 369.18
        severe 369.24
        total 369.16
    one eye 369.74
      with vision of other eye (specified as)
        near-normal 369.75
        normal 369.76
  near-total
    both eyes 369.04
      with impairment of lesser eye (specified as)
        blind, not further specified 369.02
        total 369.03
    one eye 369.64
      with vision of other eye (specified as)
        near-normal 369.65
        normal 369.66
  night 368.60
    acquired 368.62
    congenital (Japanese) 368.61
    hereditary 368.61
    specified type NEC 368.69
    vitamin A deficiency 264.5
  nocturnal – *see* Blindness, night
  one eye 369.60
    with low vision of other eye 369.10
  profound
    both eyes 369.08
      with impairment of lesser eye (specified as)
        blind, not further specified 369.05
        near-total 369.07
        total 369.06
    one eye 369.67
      with vision of other eye (specified as)
        near-normal 369.68
        normal 369.69
  psychic 784.69
  severe
    both eyes 369.22
      with impairment of lesser eye (specified as)
        blind, not further specified 369.11
        low vision, not further specified 369.21
        near-total 369.13
        profound 369.14
        total 369.12
    one eye 369.71
      with vision of other eye (specified as)
        near-normal 369.72
        normal 369.73
  snow 370.24
  sun 363.31
  temporary 368.12
  total
    both eyes 369.01
    one eye 369.61
      with vision of other eye (specified as)
        near-normal 369.62
        normal 369.63
  transient 368.12
  traumatic NEC 950.9
  word (developmental) 315.01
    acquired 784.61
    secondary to organic lesion 784.61
Blister – *see also* Injury, superficial, by site
  beetle dermatitis 692.89
  due to burn – *see* Burn, by site, second degree
  fever 054.9
  multiple, skin, nontraumatic 709.8
Bloating 787.3
Bloch-Siemens syndrome (incontinentia pigmenti) 757.33
Bloch-Stauffer dyshormonal dermatosis 757.33
Bloch-Sulzberger disease or syndrome (incontinentia pigmenti) (melanoblastosis) 757.33
Block
  alveolar capillary 516.3
  arborization (heart) 426.6
  arrhythmic 426.9

Block – *continued*
  atrioventricular (AV) (incomplete) (partial) 426.10
    with
      2:1 atrioventricular response block 426.13
      atrioventricular dissociation 426.0
    first degree (incomplete) 426.11
    second degree (Mobitz type I) 426.13
      Mobitz (type II) 426.12
    third degree 426.0
    complete 426.0
      congenital 746.86
    congenital 746.86
    Mobitz (incomplete)
      type I (Wenckebach's) 426.13
      type II 426.12
    partial 426.13
  auriculoventricular (*see also* Block, atrioventricular) 426.10
    complete 426.0
      congenital 746.86
    congenital 746.86
  bifascicular (cardiac) 426.53
  bundle branch (complete) (false) (incomplete) 426.50
    bilateral 426.53
    left (complete) (main stem) 426.3
      with right bundle branch block 426.53
      anterior fascicular 426.2
        with
          posterior fascicular block 426.3
          right bundle branch block 426.52
      hemiblock 426.2
      incomplete 426.2
        with right bundle branch block 426.53
      posterior fascicular 426.2
        with
          anterior fascicular block 426.3
          right bundle branch block 426.51
    right 426.4
      with
        left bundle branch block (incomplete) (main stem) 426.53
        left fascicular block 426.53
          anterior 426.52
          posterior 426.51
    Wilson's type 426.4
  cardiac 426.9
  conduction 426.9
    complete 426.0
  Eustachian tube (*see also* Obstruction, Eustachian tube) 381.60
  fascicular (left anterior) (left posterior) 426.2
  foramen Magendie (acquired) 331.3
    congenital 742.3
      with spina bifida (*see also* Spina bifida) 741.0❺
  heart 426.9
    first degree (atrioventricular) 426.11
    second degree (atrioventricular) 426.13
    third degree (atrioventricular) 426.0
    bundle branch (complete) (false) (incomplete) 426.50
      bilateral 426.53
      left (*see also* Block, bundle branch, left) 426.3
      right (*see also* Block, bundle branch, right) 426.4
    complete (atrioventricular) 426.0
    congenital 746.86
    incomplete 426.13
    intra-atrial 426.6
    intraventricular NEC 426.6
    sinoatrial 426.6
    specified type NEC 426.6
  hepatic vein 453.0
  intraventricular (diffuse) (myofibrillar) 426.6
    bundle branch (complete) (false) (incomplete) 426.50
      bilateral 426.53
      left (*see also* Block, bundle branch, left) 426.3
      right (*see also* Block, bundle branch, right) 426.4
  kidney (*see also* Disease, renal) 593.9
    postcystoscopic 997.5
  myocardial (*see also* Block, heart) 426.9
  nodal 426.10
  optic nerve 377.49
  organ or site (congenital) NEC – *see* Atresia
  parietal 426.6
  peri-infarction 426.6
  portal (vein) 452

Blennorrhea – Block

- **Block** – *continued*
  - sinoatrial 426.6
  - sinoauricular 426.6
  - spinal cord 336.9
  - trifascicular 426.54
  - tubal 628.2
  - vein NEC 453.9
- **Blocq's disease or syndrome** (astasia-abasia) 307.9
- **Blood**
  - constituents, abnormal NEC 790.6
  - disease 289.9
    - specified NEC 289.89
  - donor V59.01
    - other blood components V59.09
    - stem cells V59.02
    - whole blood V59.01
  - dyscrasia 289.9
    - with
      - abortion – *see* Abortion, by type, with hemorrhage, delayed or excessive
      - ectopic pregnancy (*see also* categories 633.0-633.9) 639.1
      - molar pregnancy (*see also* categories 630-632) 639.1
    - fetus or newborn NEC 776.9
    - following
      - abortion 639.1
      - ectopic or molar pregnancy 639.1
    - puerperal, postpartum 666.3❺
  - flukes NEC (*see also* Infestation, Schistosoma) 120.9
  - in
    - feces (*see also* Melena) 578.1
      - occult 792.1
    - urine (*see also* Hematuria) 599.7
  - mole 631
  - occult 792.1
  - poisoning (*see also* Septicemia) 038.9
  - pressure
    - decreased, due to shock following injury 958.4
    - fluctuating 796.4
    - high (*see also* Hypertension) 401.9
      - incidental reading (isolated) (nonspecific), without diagnosis of hypertension 796.2
    - low (*see also* Hypotension) 458.9
      - incidental reading (isolated) (nonspecific), without diagnosis of hypotension 796.3
  - spitting (*see also* Hemoptysis) 786.3
  - staining cornea 371.12
  - transfusion
    - without reported diagnosis V58.2
    - donor V59.01
      - stem cells V59.02
    - reaction or complication – *see* Complications, transfusion
  - tumor – *see* Hematoma
  - vessel rupture – *see* Hemorrhage
  - vomiting (*see also* Hematemesis) 578.0
- **Blood-forming organ disease** 289.9
- **Bloodgood's disease** 610.1
- **Bloodshot eye** 379.93
- **Bloom** (-Machacek) (-Torre) **syndrome** 757.39
- **Blotch, palpebral** 372.55
- **Blount's disease** (tibia vara) 732.4
- **Blount-Barber syndrome** (tibia vara) 732.4
- **Blue**
  - baby 746.9
  - bloater 491.20
    - with
      - acute bronchitis 491.22
      - exacerbation (acute) 491.21
  - diaper syndrome 270.0
  - disease 746.9
  - dome cyst 610.0
  - drum syndrome 381.02
  - sclera 743.47
    - with fragility of bone and deafness 756.51
  - toe syndrome 445.02
- **Blueness** (*see also* Cyanosis) 782.5
- **Blurring, visual** 368.8
- **Blushing** (abnormal) (excessive) 782.62
- **BMI** (body mass index)
  - adult
    - 25.0-25.9 V85.21
    - 26.0-26.9 V85.22
    - 27.0-27.9 V85.23
    - 28.0-28.9 V85.24
    - 29.0-29.9 V85.25
    - 30.0-30.9 V85.30
    - 31.0-31.9 V85.31
- **BMI** – *continued*
  - adult – *continued*
    - 32.0-32.9 V85.32
    - 33.0-33.9 V85.33
    - 34.0-34.9 V85.34
    - 35.0-35.9 V85.35
    - 36.0-36.9 V85.36
    - 37.0-37.9 V85.37
    - 38.0-38.9 V85.38
    - 39.0-39.9 V85.39
    - 40 and over V85.4
    - between 19-24 V85.1
    - less than 19 V85.0
  - pediatric
    - 5th percentile to less than 85th percentile for age V85.52
    - 85th percentile to less than 95th percentile for age V85.53
    - greater than or equal to 95th percentile for age V85.54
    - less than 5th percentile for age V85.51
- **Boarder, hospital** V65.0
  - infant V65.0
- **Bockhart's impetigo** (superficial folliculitis) 704.8
- **Bodechtel-Guttmann disease** (subacute sclerosing panencephalitis) 046.2
- **Boder-Sedgwick syndrome** (ataxia-telangiectasia) 334.8
- **Body, bodies**
  - Aschoff (*see also* Myocarditis, rheumatic) 398.0
  - asteroid, vitreous 379.22
  - choroid, colloid (degenerative) 362.57
    - hereditary 362.77
  - cytoid (retina) 362.82
  - drusen (retina) (*see also* Drusen) 362.57
    - optic disc 377.21
  - fibrin, pleura 511.0
  - foreign – *see* Foreign body
  - Hassall-Henle 371.41
  - loose
    - joint (*see also* Loose, body, joint) 718.1❺
      - knee 717.6
    - knee 717.6
    - sheath, tendon 727.82
  - Mallory's 034.1
  - mass index (BMI)
    - adult
      - 25.0-25.9 V85.21
      - 26.0-26.9 V85.22
      - 27.0-27.9 V85.23
      - 28.0-28.9 V85.24
      - 29.0-29.9 V85.25
      - 30.0-30.9 V85.30
      - 31.0-31.9 V85.31
      - 32.0-32.9 V85.32
      - 33.0-33.9 V85.33
      - 34.0-34.9 V85.34
      - 35.0-35.9 V85.35
      - 36.0-36.9 V85.36
      - 37.0-37.9 V85.37
      - 38.0-38.9 V85.38
      - 39.0-39.9 V85.39
      - 40 and over V85.4
      - between 19-24 V85.1
      - less than 19 V85.0
    - pediatric
      - 5th percentile to less than 85th percentile for age V85.52
      - 85th percentile to less than 95th percentile for age V85.53
      - greater than or equal to 95th percentile for age V85.54
      - less than 5th percentile for age V85.51
  - Mooser 081.0
  - Negri 071
  - rice (joint) (*see also* Loose, body, joint) 718.1❺
    - knee 717.6
  - rocking 307.3
- **Boeck's**
  - disease (sarcoidosis) 135
  - lupoid (miliary) 135
  - sarcoid 135
- **Boerhaave's syndrome** (spontaneous esophageal rupture) 530.4
- **Boggy**
  - cervix 622.8
  - uterus 621.8
- **Boil** (*see also* Carbuncle) 680.9
  - abdominal wall 680.2
  - Aleppo 085.1
- **Boil** – *continued*
  - ankle 680.6
  - anus 680.5
  - arm (any part, above wrist) 680.3
  - auditory canal, external 680.0
  - axilla 680.3
  - back (any part) 680.2
  - Baghdad 085.1
  - breast 680.2
  - buttock 680.5
  - chest wall 680.2
  - corpus cavernosum 607.2
  - Delhi 085.1
  - ear (any part) 680.0
  - eyelid 373.13
  - face (any part, except eye) 680.0
  - finger (any) 680.4
  - flank 680.2
  - foot (any part) 680.7
  - forearm 680.3
  - Gafsa 085.1
  - genital organ, male 608.4
  - gluteal (region) 680.5
  - groin 680.2
  - hand (any part) 680.4
  - head (any part, except face) 680.8
  - heel 680.7
  - hip 680.6
  - knee 680.6
  - labia 616.4
  - lacrimal (*see also* Dacryocystitis) 375.30
    - gland (*see also* Dacryoadenitis) 375.00
    - passages (duct) (sac) (*see also* Dacryocystitis) 375.30
  - leg, any part, except foot 680.6
  - multiple sites 680.9
  - natal 085.1
  - neck 680.1
  - nose (external) (septum) 680.0
  - orbit, orbital 376.01
  - partes posteriores 680.5
  - pectoral region 680.2
  - penis 607.2
  - perineum 680.2
  - pinna 680.0
  - scalp (any part) 680.8
  - scrotum 608.4
  - seminal vesicle 608.0
  - shoulder 680.3
  - skin NEC 680.9
  - specified site NEC 680.8
  - spermatic cord 608.4
  - temple (region) 680.0
  - testis 608.4
  - thigh 680.6
  - thumb 680.4
  - toe (any) 680.7
  - tropical 085.1
  - trunk 680.2
  - tunica vaginalis 608.4
  - umbilicus 680.2
  - upper arm 680.3
  - vas deferens 608.4
  - vulva 616.4
  - wrist 680.4
- **Bold hives** (*see also* Urticaria) 708.9
- **Bolivian hemorrhagic fever** 078.7
- **Bombé, iris** 364.74
- **Bomford-Rhoads anemia** (refractory) 238.72
- **Bone** – *see* condition
- **Bonnevie-Ullrich syndrome** 758.6
- **Bonnier's syndrome** 386.19
- **Bonvale Dam fever** 780.79
- **Bony block of joint** 718.80
  - ankle 718.87
  - elbow 718.82
  - foot 718.87
  - hand 718.84
  - hip 718.85
  - knee 718.86
  - multiple sites 718.89
  - pelvic region 718.85
  - shoulder (region) 718.81
  - specified site NEC 718.88
  - wrist 718.83
- **Borderline**
  - intellectual functioning V62.89
  - pelvis 653.1❺
    - with obstruction during labor 660.1❺
      - affecting fetus or newborn 763.1

Block – Borderline

Borderline – *continued*
  psychosis (*see also* Schizophrenia) 295.5⑤
    of childhood (*see also* Psychosis, childhood) 299.8⑤
  schizophrenia (*see also* Schizophrenia) 295.5⑤
Borna disease 062.9
Bornholm disease (epidemic pleurodynia) 074.1
Borrelia vincentii (mouth) (pharynx) (tonsils) 101
Bostock's catarrh (*see also* Fever, hay) 477.9
Boston exanthem 048
Botalli, ductus (patent) (persistent) 747.0
Bothriocephalus latus infestation 123.4
Botulism 005.1
  food poisoning 005.1 ●
  infant 040.41 ●
  non-foodborne 040.42 ●
  wound 040.42 ▲
Bouba (*see also* Yaws) 102.9
Bouffée délirante 298.3
Bouillaud's disease or syndrome (rheumatic heart disease) 391.9
Bourneville's disease (tuberous sclerosis) 759.5
Boutonneuse fever 082.1
Boutonniere
  deformity (finger) 736.21
  hand (intrinsic) 736.21
Bouveret (-Hoffmann) **disease or syndrome** (paroxysmal tachycardia) 427.2
Bovine heart – *see* Hypertrophy, cardiac
Bowel – *see* condition
Bowen's
  dermatosis (precancerous) (M8081/2) – *see* Neoplasm, skin, in situ
  disease (M8081/2) – *see* Neoplasm, skin, in situ
  epithelioma (M8081/2) – *see* Neoplasm, skin, in situ
  type
    epidermoid carcinoma in situ (M8081/2) – *see* Neoplasm, skin, in situ
    intraepidermal squamous cell carcinoma (M8081/2) – *see* Neoplasm, skin, in situ
Bowing
  femur 736.89
    congenital 754.42
  fibula 736.89
    congenital 754.43
  forearm 736.09
    away from midline (cubitus valgus) 736.01
    toward midline (cubitus varus) 736.02
  leg(s), long bones, congenital 754.44
  radius 736.09
    away from midline (cubitus valgus) 736.01
    toward midline (cubitus varus) 736.02
  tibia 736.89
    congenital 754.43
Bowleg(s) 736.42
  congenital 754.44
  rachitic 268.1
Boyd's dysentery 004.2
Brachial – *see* condition
Brachman-de Lange syndrome (Amsterdam dwarf, mental retardation, and brachycephaly) 759.89
Brachycardia 427.89
Brachycephaly 756.0
Brachymorphism and ectopia lentis 759.89
Bradley's disease (epidemic vomiting) 078.82
Bradycardia 427.89
  chronic (sinus) 427.81
  newborn 779.81
  nodal 427.89
  postoperative 997.1
  reflex 337.0
  sinoatrial 427.89
    with paroxysmal tachyarrhythmia or tachycardia 427.81
    chronic 427.81
  sinus 427.89
    with paroxysmal tachyarrhythmia or tachycardia 427.81
    chronic 427.81
    persistent 427.81
    severe 427.81
  tachycardia syndrome 427.81
  vagal 427.89
Bradypnea 786.09
Brailsford's disease 732.3
  radial head 732.3

Brailsford's disease – *continued*
  tarsal scaphoid 732.5
Brailsford-Morquio disease or syndrome (mucopolysaccharidosis IV) 277.5
Brain – *see also* condition
  death 348.8
  syndrome (acute) (chronic) (nonpsychotic) (organic) (with neurotic reaction) (with behavioral reaction) (*see also* Syndrome, brain) 310.9
    with
      presenile brain disease 290.10
      psychosis, psychotic reaction (*see also* Psychosis, organic) 294.9
    congenital (*see also* Retardation, mental) 319
Branched-chain amino-acid disease 270.3
Branchial – *see* condition
Brandt's syndrome (acrodermatitis enteropathica) 686.8
Brash (water) 787.1
Brass-founders' ague 985.8
Bravais-Jacksonian epilepsy (*see also* Epilepsy) 345.5⑤
Braxton Hicks contractions 644.1⑤
Braziers' disease 985.8
Brazilian
  blastomycosis 116.1
  leishmaniasis 085.5
BRBPR (bright red blood per rectum) 569.3
Break
  cardiorenal – *see* Hypertension, cardiorenal
  retina (*see also* Defect, retina) 361.30
Breakbone fever 061
Breakdown
  device, implant, or graft – *see* Complications, mechanical
  nervous (*see also* Disorder, mental, nonpsychotic) 300.9
  perineum 674.2⑤
Breast – *see* condition
Breast feeding difficulties 676.8⑤
Breath
  foul 784.99
  holder, child 312.81
  holding spells 786.9
  shortness 786.05
Breathing
  asymmetrical 786.09
  bronchial 786.09
  exercises V57.0
  labored 786.09
  mouth 784.99
    causing malocclusion 524.59
  periodic 786.09
    high altitude 327.22
  tic 307.20
Breathlessness 786.09
Breda's disease (*see also* Yaws) 102.9
Breech
  delivery, affecting fetus or newborn 763.0
  extraction, affecting fetus or newborn 763.0
  presentation (buttocks) (complete) (frank) 652.2⑤
    with successful version 652.1⑤
    before labor, affecting fetus or newborn 761.7
    during labor, affecting fetus or newborn 763.0
Breisky's disease (kraurosis vulvae) 624.09 ●
Brennemann's syndrome (acute mesenteric lymphadenitis) 289.2
Brenner's
  tumor (benign) (M9000/0) 220
    borderline malignancy (M9000/1) 236.2
    malignant (M9000/3) 183.0
    proliferating (M9000/1) 236.2
Bretonneau's disease (diphtheritic malignant angina) 032.0
Breus' mole 631
Brevicollis 756.16
Bricklayers' itch 692.89
Brickmakers' anemia 126.9
Bridge
  myocardial 746.85
Bright red blood per rectum (BRBPR) 569.3
Bright's
  blindness – *see* Uremia

Bright's – *continued*
  disease (*see also* Nephritis) 583 9
    arteriosclerotic (*see also* Hypertension, kidney) 403.90
Brill's disease (recrudescent typhus) 081.1
  flea-borne 081.0
  louse-borne 081.1
Brill-Symmers disease (follicular lymphoma) (M9690/3) 202.0⑤
Brill-Zinsser disease (recrudescent typhus) 081.1
Brinton's disease (linitis plastica) (M8142/3) 151.9
Brion-Kayser disease (*see also* Fever paratyphoid) 002.9
Briquet's disorder or syndrome 300.81
Brissaud's
  infantilism (infantile myxedema) 244.9
  motor-verbal tic 307.23
Brissaud-Meige syndrome (infantile myxedema) 244.9
Brittle
  bones (congenital) 756.51
  nails 703.8
    congenital 757.5
Broad – *see also* condition
  beta disease 272.2
  ligament laceration syndrome 620 6
Brock's syndrome (atelectasis due to enlarged lymph nodes) 518.0
Brocq's disease 691.8
  atopic (diffuse) neurodermatitis 691.8
  lichen simplex chronicus 698.3
  parakeratosis psoriasiformis 696.2
  parapsoriasis 696.2
Brocq-Duhring disease (dermatitis herpetiformis) 694.0
Brodie's
  abscess (localized) (chronic) (*see also* Osteomyelitis) 730.1⑤
  disease (joint) (*see also* Osteomyelitis) 730.1⑤
Broken
  arches 734
    congenital 755.67
  back – *see* Fracture, vertebra, by site
  bone – *see* Fracture, by site
  compensation – *see* Disease, heart
  heart syndrome 429.83
  implant or internal device – *see* listing under Complications, mechanical
  neck – *see* Fracture, vertebra, cervical
  nose 802.0
    open 802.1
  tooth, teeth 873.63
    complicated 873.73
Bromhidrosis 705.89
Bromidism, bromism
  acute 967.3
    correct substance properly administered 349.82
    overdose or wrong substance given or taken 967.3
  chronic (*see also* Dependence) 304.1⑤
Bromidrosiphobia 300.23
Bromidrosis 705.89
Bronchi, bronchial – *see* condition
Bronchiectasis (cylindrical) (diffuse) (fusiform) (localized) (moniliform) (postinfectious) (recurrent) (saccular) 494.0
  with acute exacerbation 494.1
  congenital 748.61
  tuberculosis (*see also* Tuberculosis) 011.5⑤
Bronchiolectasis – *see* Bronchiectasis
Bronchiolitis (acute) (infectious) (subacute) 466.19
  with
    bronchospasm or obstruction 466.19
    influenza, flu, or grippe 487.1
  catarrhal (acute) (subacute) 466.19
  chemical 506.0
    chronic 506.4
  chronic (obliterative) 491.8
  due to external agent – *see* Bronchitis, acute, due to
  fibrosa obliterans 491.8
  influenzal 487.1
  obliterans 491.8
    with organizing pneumonia (B.O.O.P.) 516.8
    status post lung transplant 996.84
  obliterative (chronic) (diffuse) (subacute) 491.8
    due to fumes or vapors 506.4

- **Bronchiolitis** – *continued*
  - respiratory syncytial virus 466.11
  - vesicular – *see* Pneumonia, broncho-
- **Bronchitis** (diffuse) (hypostatic) (infectious) (inflammatory) (simple) 490
  - with
    - emphysema – *see* Emphysema
    - influenza, flue, or grippe 487.1
    - obstruction airway, chronic 491.20
      - with
        - acute bronchitis 491.22
        - exacerbation (acute) 491.21
    - tracheitis 490
      - acute or subacute 466.0
        - with bronchospasm or obstruction 466.0
      - chronic 491.8
  - acute or subacute 466.0
    - with
      - bronchospasm 466.0
      - obstruction 466.0
      - tracheitis 466.0
    - chemical (due to fumes or vapors) 506.0
    - due to
      - fumes or vapors 506.0
      - radiation 508.8
  - allergic (acute) (*see also* Asthma) 493.9⑤
  - arachidic 934.1
  - aspiration 507.0
    - due to fumes or vapors 506.0
  - asthmatic (acute) 493.90
    - with
      - acute exacerbation 493.92
      - status asthmaticus 493.91
    - chronic 493.2
  - capillary 466.19
    - with bronchospasm or obstruction 466.19
    - chronic 491.8
  - caseous (*see also* Tuberculosis) 011.3⑤
  - Castellani's 104.8
  - catarrhal 490
    - acute – *see* Bronchitis, acute
    - chronic 491.0
  - chemical (acute) (subacute) 506.0
    - chronic 506.4
    - due to fumes or vapors (acute) (subactue) 506.0
      - chronic 506.4
  - chronic 491.9
    - with
      - tracheitis (chronic) 491.8
    - asthmatic 493.2
    - catarrhal 491.0
    - chemical (due to fumes and vapors) 506.4
    - due to
      - fumes or vapors (chemical) (inhalation) 506.4
      - radiation 508.8
      - tobacco smoking 491.0
    - mucopurulent 491.1
    - obstructive 491.20
      - with
        - acute bronchitis 491.22
        - exacerbation (acute) 491.21
    - purulent 491.1
    - simple 491.0
    - specified type NEC 491.8
  - croupous 466.0
    - with bronchospasm or obstruction 466.0
    - due to fumes or vapors 506.0
  - emphysematous 491.20
    - with
      - acute bronchitis 491.22
      - exacerbation (acute) 491.21
  - exudative 466.0
  - fetid (chronic) (recurrent) 491.1
  - fibrinous, acute or subacute 466.0
    - with bronchospasm or obstruction 466.0
  - grippal 487.1
  - influenzal 487.1
  - membranous, acute or subactue 466.0
    - with bronchospasm or obstruction 466.0
  - moulders' 502
  - mucopurulent (chronic) (recurrent) 491.1
    - acute or subacute 466.0
  - obliterans 491.8
  - obstructive (chronic) 491.20
    - with
      - acute bronchitis 491.22
      - exacerbation (acute) 491.21
  - pituitous 491.1
  - plastic (inflammatory) 466.0
- **Bronchitis** – *continued*
  - pneumococcal, acute or subacute 466.0
    - with bronchospasm or obstruction 466.0
  - pseudomembranous 466.0
  - purulent (chronic) (recurrent) 491.1
    - acute or subacute 466.0
      - with bronchospasm or obstruction 466.0
  - putrid 491.1
  - scrofulous (*see also* Tuberculosis) 011.3⑤
  - senile 491.9
  - septic, acute or subacute 466.0
    - with bronchospasm or obstruction 466.0
  - smokers' 491.0
  - spirochetal 104.8
  - suffocative, acute or subacute 466.0
  - summer (*see also* Asthma) 493.9⑤
  - suppurative (chronic) 491.1
    - acute or subacute 466.0
  - tuberculous (*see also* Tuberculosis) 011.3
  - ulcerative 491.8
    - Vincent's 101
  - Vincent's 101
  - viral, acute or subacute 466.0
- **Bronchoalveolitis** 485
- **Bronchoaspergillosis** 117.3
- **Bronchocele**
  - meaning
    - dilatation of bronchus 519.19
    - goiter 240.9
- **Bronchogenic carcinoma** 162.9
- **Bronchohemisporosis** 117.9
- **Broncholithiasis** 518.89
  - tuberculous (*see also* Tuberculosis) 011.3⑤
- **Bronchomalacia** 748.3
- **Bronchomoniliasis** 112.89
- **Bronchomycosis** 112.89
- **Bronchonocardiosis** 039.1
- **Bronchopleuropneumonia** – *see* Pneumonia, broncho-
- **Bronchopneumonia** – *see* Pneumonia, broncho-
- **Bronchopneumonitis** – *see* Pneumonia, broncho-
- **Bronchopulmonary** – *see* condition
- **Bronchopulmonitis** – *see* Pneumonia, broncho-
- **Bronchorrhagia** 786.3
  - newborn 770.3
  - tuberculous (*see also* Tuberculosis) 011.3⑤
- **Bronchorrhea** (chronic) (purulent) 491.0
  - acute 466.0
- **Bronchospasm** 519.11
  - with
    - asthma – *see* Asthma
    - bronchiolitis, acute 466.19
      - due to respiratory syncytial virus 466.11
    - bronchitis – *see* Bronchitis
    - chronic obstructive pulmonary disease (COPD) 496
    - emphysema – *see* Emphysema
      - due to external agent – *see* Condition, respiratory, acute, due to
  - acute 519.11
  - exercise induced 493.81
- **Bronchospirochetosis** 104.8
- **Bronchostenosis** 519.19
- **Bronchus** – *see* condition
- **Bronze, bronzed**
  - diabetes 275.0
  - disease (Addison's) (skin) 255.41 ▲
    - tuberculous (*see also* Tuberculosis) 017.6⑤
- **Brooke's disease or tumor** (M8100/0) – *see* Neoplasm, skin, benign
- **Brown's tendon sheath syndrome** 378.61
- **Brown enamel of teeth** (hereditary) 520.5
- **Brown-Séquard's paralysis** (syndrome) 344.89
- **Brow presentation complicating delivery** 652.4⑤
- **Brucella, brucellosis** (infection) 023.9
  - abortus 023.1
  - canis 023.3
  - dermatitis, skin 023.9
  - melitensis 023.0
  - mixed 023.8
  - suis 023.2
- **Bruck's disease** 733.99
- **Bruck-de Lange disease or syndrome** (Amsterdam dwarf, mental retardation, and brachycephaly) 759.89
- **Brugada syndrome** 746.89
- **Brug's filariasis** 125.1
- **Brugsch's syndrome** (acropachyderma) 757.39
- **Bruhl's disease** (splenic anemia with fever) 285.8
- **Bruise** (skin surface intact) – *see also* Contusion
  - with
    - fracture - Fracture, by site
    - open wound – *see* Wound, open, by site
  - internal organ (abdomen, chest, or pelvis) – *see* Injury, internal, by site
  - umbilical cord 663.6⑤
    - affecting fetus or newborn 762.6
- **Bruit** 785.9
  - arterial (abdominal) (carotid) 785.9
  - supraclavicular 785.9
- **Brushburn** – *see* Injury, superficial, by site
- **Bruton's X-linked agammaglobulinemia** 279.04
- **Bruxism** 306.8
  - sleep related 327.53
- **Bubbly lung syndrome** 770.7
- **Bubo** 289.3
  - blennorrhagic 098.89
  - chancroidal 099.0
  - climatic 099.1
  - due to Hemophilus ducreyi 099.0
  - gonococcal 098.89
  - indolent NEC 099.8
  - inguinal NEC 099.8
    - chancroidal 099.0
    - climatic 099.1
    - due to H. ducreyi 099.0
  - scrofulous (*see also* Tuberculosis) 017.2⑤
  - soft chancre 099.0
  - suppurating 683
  - syphilitic 091.0
    - congenital 090.0
  - tropical 099.1
  - venereal NEC 099.8
  - virulent 099.0
- **Bubonic plague** 020.0
- **Bubonocele** – *see* Hernia, inguinal
- **Buccal** – *see* condition
- **Buchanan's disease** (juvenile osteochondrosis of iliac crest) 732.1
- **Buchem's syndrome** (hyperostosis corticalis) 733.3
- **Buchman's disease** (osteochondrosis, juvenile) 732.1
- **Bucket handle fracture** (semilunar cartilage) (*see also* Tear, meniscus) 836.2
- **Budd-Chiari syndrome** (hepatic vein thrombosis) 453.0
- **Budgerigar-fanciers' disease or lung** 495.2
- **Büdinger-Ludloff-Läwen disease** 717.89
- **Buerger's disease** (thromboangiitis obliterans) 443.1
- **Bulbar** – *see* condition
- **Bulbus cordis** 745.9
  - persistent (in left ventricle) 745.8
- **Bulging fontanels** (congenital) 756.0
- **Bulimia** 783.6
  - nervosa 307.51
  - nonorganic origin 307.51
- **Bulky uterus** 621.2
- **Bulla(e)** 709.8
  - lung (emphysematous) (solitary) 492.0
- **Bullet wound** – *see also* Wound, open, by site
  - fracture – *see* Fracture, by site, open
  - internal organ (abdomen, chest, or pelvis) – *see* Injury, internal, by site, with open wound
  - intracranial – *see* Laceration, brain, with open wound
- **Bullis fever** 082.8
- **Bullying** (*see also* Disturbance, conduct) 312.0⑤
- **Bundle**
  - branch block (complete) (false) (incomplete) 426.50
    - bilateral 426.53
    - left (*see also* Block, bundle branch, left) 426.3
      - hemiblock 426.2
    - right (*see also* Block, bundle branch, right) 426.4
  - of His – *see* condition
  - of Kent syndrome (anomalous atrioventricular excitation) 426.7
- **Bungpagga** 040.81
- **Bunion** 727.1
- **Bunionette** 727.1
- **Bunyamwera fever** 066.3

- **Buphthalmia, buphthalmos** (congenital) 743.20
  - associated with
    - keratoglobus, congenital 743.22
    - megalocornea 743.22
    - ocular anomalies NEC 743.22
  - isolated 743.21
  - simple 743.21
- **Bürger-Grütz disease or syndrome** (essential familial hyperlipemia) 272.3
- **Buried roots** 525.3
- **Burke's syndrome** 577.8
- **Burkitt's**
  - tumor (M9750/3) 200.2❺
  - type malignant, lymphoma, lymphoblastic, or undifferentiated (M9750/3) 200.2❺
- **Burn** (acid) (cathode ray) (caustic) (chemical) (electric heating appliance) (electricity) (fire) (flame) (hot liquid or object) (irradiation) (lime) (radiation) (steam) (thermal) (x-ray) 949.0

Note – Use the following fifth-digit subclassification with category 948 to indicate the percent of body surface with third degree burn:

0 less than 10 percent or unspecified
1 10-19 percent
2 20-29 percent
3 30-39 percent
4 40-49 percent
5 50-59 percent
6 60-69 percent
7 70-79 percent
8 80-89 percent
9 90 percent or more of body surface

  - with
    - blisters – *see* Burn, by site, second degree
    - erythema – *see* Burn, by site, first degree
    - skin loss (epidermal) – *see also* Burn, by site, second degree
      - full thickness – *see also* Burn, by site, third degree
        - with necrosis of underlying tissues – *see* Burn, by site, third degree, deep
  - first degree – *see* Burn, by site, first degree
  - second degree – *see* Burn, by site, second degree
  - third degree – *see also* Burn, by site, third degree
    - deep – *see* Burn, by site, third degree, deep
  - abdomen, abdominal (muscle) (wall) 942.03
    - with
      - trunk – *see* Burn, trunk, multiple sites
    - first degree 942.13
    - second degree 942.23
    - third degree 942.33
      - deep 942.43
        - with loss of body part 942.53
  - ankle 945.03
    - with
      - lower limb(s) – *see* Burn, leg, multiple sites
    - first degree 945.13
    - second degree 945.23
    - third degree 945.33
      - deep 945.43
        - with loss of body part 945.53
  - anus – *see* Burn, trunk, specified site NEC
  - arm(s) 943.00
    - first degree 943.10
    - second degree 943.20
    - third degree 943.30
      - deep 943.40
        - with loss of body part 943.50
    - lower – *see* Burn, forearm(s)
    - multiple sites, except hand(s) or wrist(s) 943.09
      - first degree 943.19
      - second degree 943.29
      - third degree 943.39
        - deep 943.49
          - with loss of body part 943.59
    - upper 943.03
      - first degree 943.13
      - second degree 943.23
      - third degree 943.33
        - deep 943.43
          - with loss of body part 943.53
  - auditory canal (external) – *see* Burn, ear
  - auricle (ear) – *see* Burn, ear
  - axilla 943.04
    - with
      - upper limb(s), except hand(s) or wrist(s) – *see* Burn, arm(s), multiple sites
    - first degree 943.14

Burn – *continued*
  - axilla – *continued*
    - second degree 943.24
    - third degree 943.34
      - deep 943.44
        - with loss of body part 943.54
  - back 942.04
    - with
      - trunk – *see* Burn, trunk, multiple sites
    - first degree 942.14
    - second degree 942.24
    - third degree 942.34
      - deep 942.44
        - with loss of body part 942.54
  - biceps
    - brachii – *see* Burn, arm(s), upper
    - femoris – *see* Burn, thigh
  - breast(s) 942.01
    - with
      - trunk – *see* Burn, trunk, multiple sites
    - first degree 942.11
    - second degree 942.21
    - third degree 942.31
      - deep 942.41
        - with loss of body part 942.51
  - brow – *see* Burn, forehead
  - buttock(s) – *see* Burn, back
  - canthus (eye) 940.1
    - chemical 940.0
  - cervix (uteri) 947.4
  - cheek (cutaneous) 941.07
    - with
      - face or head – *see* Burn, head, multiple sites
    - first degree 941.17
    - second degree 941.27
    - third degree 941.37
      - deep 941.47
        - with loss of body part 941.57
  - chest wall (anterior) 942.02
    - with
      - trunk – *see* Burn, trunk, multiple sites
    - first degree 942.12
    - second degree 942.22
    - third degree 942.32
      - deep 942.42
        - with loss of body part 942.52
  - chin 941.04
    - with
      - face or head – *see* Burn, head, multiple sites
    - first degree 941.14
    - second degree 941.24
    - third degree 941.34
      - deep 941.44
        - with loss of body part 941.54
  - clitoris – *see* Burn, genitourinary organs, external
  - colon 947.3
  - conjunctiva (and cornea) 940.4
    - chemical
      - acid 940.3
      - alkaline 940.2
  - cornea (and conjunctiva) 940.4
    - chemical
      - acid 940.3
      - alkaline 940.2
  - costal region – *see* Burn, chest wall
  - due to ingested chemical agent – *see* Burn, internal organs
  - ear (auricle) (canal) (drum) (external) 941.01
    - with
      - face or head – *see* Burn, head, multiple sites
    - first degree 941.11
    - second degree 941.21
    - third degree 941.31
      - deep 941.41
        - with loss of a body part 941.51
  - elbow 943.02
    - with
      - hand(s) and wrist(s) – *see* Burn, multiple specified sites
      - upper limb(s), except hand(s) or wrist(s) – *see also* Burn, arm(s), multiple sites
    - first degree 943.12
    - second degree 943.22
    - third degree 943.32
      - deep 943.42
        - with loss of body part 943.52
  - electricity, electric current – *see* Burn, by site
  - entire body – *see* Burn, multiple, specified sites
  - epididymis – *see* Burn, genitourinary organs, external
  - epigastric region – *see* Burn, abdomen

Burn – *continued*
  - epiglottis 947.1
  - esophagus 947.2
  - extent (percent of body surface)
    - less than 10 percent 948.0❺
    - 10-19 percent 948.1❺
    - 20-29 percent 948.2❺
    - 30-39 percent 948.3❺
    - 40-49 percent 948.4❺
    - 50-59 percent 948.5❺
    - 60-69 percent 948.6❺
    - 70-79 percent 948.7❺
    - 80-89 percent 948.8❺
    - 90 percent or more 948.9❺
  - extremity
    - lower – *see* Burn, leg
    - upper – *see* Burn, arm(s)
  - eye(s) (and adnexa) (only) 940.9
    - with
      - face, head, or neck 941.02
        - first degree 941.12
        - second degree 941.22
        - third degree 941.32
          - deep 941.42
            - with loss of body part 941.52
      - other sites (classifiable to more than one category in 940-945) – *see* Burn, multiple, specified sites
      - resulting rupture and destruction of eyeball 940.5
    - specified part – *see* Burn, by site
  - eyeball – *see also* Burn, eye
    - with resulting rupture and destruction of eyeball 940.5
  - eyelid(s) 940.1
    - chemical 940.0
  - face – *see* Burn, head
  - finger (nail) (subungual) 944.01
    - with
      - hand(s) – *see* Burn, hand(s), multiple sites
      - other sites – *see* Burn, multiple, specified sites
      - thumb 944.04
        - first degree 944.14
        - second degree 944.24
        - third degree 944.34
          - deep 944.44
            - with loss of body part 944.54
    - first degree 944.11
    - second degree 944.21
    - third degree 944.31
      - deep 944.41
        - with loss of body part 944.51
    - multiple (digits) 944.03
      - with thumb – *see* Burn, finger, with thumb
      - first degree 944.13
      - second degree 944.23
      - third degree 944.33
        - deep 944.43
          - with loss of body part 944.53
  - flank – *see* Burn, abdomen
  - foot 945.02
    - with
      - lower limb(s) – *see* Burn, leg, multiple sites
    - first degree 945.12
    - second degree 945.22
    - third degree 945.32
      - deep 945.42
        - with loss of body part 945.52
  - forearm(s) 943.01
    - with
      - upper limb(s), except hand(s) or wrist(s) – *see* Burn, arm(s), multiple sites
    - first degree 943.11
    - second degree 943.21
    - third degree 943.31
      - deep 943.41
        - with loss of body part 943.51
  - forehead 941.07
    - with
      - face or head – *see* Burn, head, multiple sites
    - first degree 941.17
    - second degree 941.27
    - third degree 941.37
      - deep 941.47
        - with loss of body part 941.57
  - fourth degree – *see* Burn, by site, third degree, deep
  - friction – *see* Injury, superficial, by site
  - from swallowing caustic or corrosive substance NEC – *see* Burn, internal organs
  - full thickness – *see* Burn, by site, third degree

Buphthalmia, buphthalmos – Burn

- **Burn** – *continued*
  - gastrointestinal tract 947.3
  - genitourinary organs
    - external 942.05
      - with
        - trunk – *see* Burn, trunk, multiple sites
      - first degree 942.15
      - second degree 942.25
      - third degree 942.35
        - deep 942.45
          - with loss of body part 942.55
    - internal 947.8
  - globe (eye) – *see* Burn, eyeball
  - groin – *see* Burn, abdomen
  - gum 947.0
  - hand(s) (phalanges) (and wrist) 944.00
    - first degree 944.10
    - second degree 944.20
    - third degree 944.30
      - deep 944.40
        - with loss of body part 944.50
    - back (dorsal surface) 944.06
      - first degree 944.16
      - second degree 944.26
      - third degree 944.36
        - deep 944.46
          - with loss of body part 944.56
    - multiple sites 944.08
      - first degree 944.18
      - second degree 944.28
      - third degree 944.38
        - deep 944.48
          - with loss of body part 944.58
  - head (and face) 941.00
    - eye(s) only 940.9
      - specified part – *see* Burn, by site
    - first degree 941.10
    - second degree 941.20
    - third degree 941.30
      - deep 941.40
        - with loss of body part 941.50
    - multiple sites 941.09
      - with eyes – *see* Burn, eyes, with face, head, or neck
      - first degree 941.19
      - second degree 941.29
      - third degree 941.39
        - deep 941.49
          - with loss of body part 941.59
  - heel – *see* Burn, foot
  - hip – *see* Burn, trunk, specified site NEC
  - iliac region – *see* Burn, trunk, specified site NEC
  - infected 958.3
  - inhalation (*see also* Burn, internal organs) 947.9
  - internal organs 947.9
    - from caustic or corrosive substance (swallowing) NEC 947.9
    - specified NEC (*see also* Burn, by site) 947.8
  - interscapular region – *see* Burn, back
  - intestine (large) (small) 947.3
  - iris – *see* Burn, eyeball
  - knee 945.05
    - with
      - lower limb(s) – *see* Burn, leg, multiple sites
    - first degree 945.15
    - second degree 945.25
    - third degree 945.35
      - deep 945.45
        - with loss of body part 945.55
  - labium (majus) (minus) – *see* Burn, genitourinary organs, external
  - lacrimal apparatus, duct, gland, or sac 940.1
    - chemical 940.0
  - larynx 947.1
  - late effect – *see* Late, effects (of), burn
  - leg 945.00
    - first degree 945.10
    - second degree 945.20
    - third degree 945.30
      - deep 945.40
        - with loss of body part 945.50
    - lower 945.04
      - with other part(s) of lower limb(s) – *see* Burn, leg, multiple sites
      - first degree 945.14
      - second degree 945.24
      - third degree 945.34
        - deep 945.44
          - with loss of body part 945.54
    - multiple sites 945.09
      - first degree 945.19
      - second degree 945.29

- **Burn** – *continued*
  - leg – *continued*
    - multiple sites – *continued*
      - third degree 945.39
        - deep 945.49
          - with loss of body part 945.59
    - upper – *see* Burn, thigh
  - lightning – *see* Burn, by site
  - limb(s)
    - lower (including foot or toe(s)) – *see* Burn, leg
    - upper (except wrist and hand) – *see* Burn, arm(s)
  - lip(s) 941.03
    - with
      - face or head – *see* Burn, head, multiple sites
    - first degree 941.13
    - second degree 941.23
    - third degree 941.33
      - deep 941.43
        - with loss of body part 941.53
  - lumbar region – *see* Burn, back
  - lung 947.1
  - malar region – *see* Burn, cheek
  - mastoid region – *see* Burn, scalp
  - membrane, tympanic – *see* Burn, ear
  - midthoracic region – *see* Burn, chest wall
  - mouth 947.0
  - multiple (*see also* Burn, unspecified) 949.0
    - specified sites classifiable to more than one category in 940-945 946.0
      - first degree 946.1
      - second degree 946.2
      - third degree 946.3
        - deep 946.4
          - with loss of body part 946.5
  - muscle, abdominal – *see* Burn, abdomen
  - nasal (septum) – *see* Burn, nose
  - neck 941.08
    - with
      - face or head – *see* Burn, head, multiple sites
    - first degree 941.18
    - second degree 941.28
    - third degree 941.38
      - deep 941.48
        - with loss of body part 941.58
  - nose (septum) 941.05
    - with
      - face or head – *see* Burn, head, multiple sites
    - first degree 941.15
    - second degree 941.25
    - third degree 941.35
      - deep 941.45
        - with loss of body part 941.55
  - occipital region – *see* Burn, scalp
  - orbit region 940.1
    - chemical 940.0
  - oronasopharynx 947.0
  - palate 947.0
  - palm(s) 944.05
    - with
      - hand(s) and wrist(s) – *see* Burn, hand(s), multiple sites
    - first degree 944.15
    - second degree 944.25
    - third degree 944.35
      - deep 944.45
        - with loss of a body part 944.55
  - parietal region – *see* Burn, scalp
  - penis – *see* Burn, genitourinary organs, external
  - perineum – *see* Burn, genitourinary organs, external
  - periocular area 940.1
    - chemical 940.0
  - pharynx 947.0
  - pleura 947.1
  - popliteal space – *see* Burn, knee
  - prepuce – *see* Burn, genitourinary organs, external
  - pubic region – *see* Burn, genitourinary organs, external
  - pudenda – *see* Burn, genitourinary organs, external
  - rectum 947.3
  - sac, lacrimal 940.1
    - chemical 940.0
  - sacral region – *see* Burn, back
  - salivary (ducts) (glands) 947.0
  - scalp 941.06
    - with
      - face or neck – *see* Burn, head, multiple sites
    - first degree 941.16
    - second degree 941.26

- **Burn** – *continued*
  - scalp – *continued*
    - third degree 941.36
      - deep 941.46
        - with loss of body part 941.56
  - scapular region 943.06
    - with
      - upper limb(s), except hand(s) or wrist(s) – *see* Burn, arm(s), multiple sites
    - first degree 943.16
    - second degree 943.26
    - third degree 943.36
      - deep 943.46
        - with loss of body part 943.56
  - sclera – *see* Burn, eyeball
  - scrotum – *see* Burn, genitourinary organs, external
  - septum, nasal – *see* Burn, nose
  - shoulder(s) 943.05
    - with
      - hand(s) and wrist(s) – *see* Burn, multiple, specified sites
      - upper limb(s), except hand(s) or wrist(s) – *see* Burn, arm(s), multiple sites
    - first degree 943.15
    - second degree 943.25
    - third degree 943.35
      - deep 943.45
        - with loss of body part 943.55
  - skin NEC (*see also* Burn, unspecified) 949.0
  - skull – *see* Burn, head
  - small intestine 947.3
  - sternal region – *see* Burn, chest wall
  - stomach 947.3
  - subconjunctival – *see* Burn, conjunctiva
  - subcutaneous – *see* Burn, by site, third degree
  - submaxillary region – *see* Burn, head
  - submental region – *see* Burn, chin
  - sun – *see* Sunburn
  - supraclavicular fossa – *see* Burn, neck
  - supraorbital – *see* Burn, forehead
  - temple – *see* Burn, scalp
  - temporal region – *see* Burn, scalp
  - testicle – *see* Burn, genitourinary organs, external
  - testis – *see* Burn, genitourinary organs, external
  - thigh 945.06
    - with
      - lower limb(s) – *see* Burn, leg, multiple sites
    - first degree 945.16
    - second degree 945.26
    - third degree 945.36
      - deep 945.46
        - with loss of body part 945.56
  - thorax (external) – *see* Burn, chest wall
  - throat 947.0
  - thumb(s) (nail) (subungual) 944.02
    - with
      - finger(s) – *see* Burn, finger, with other sites, thumb
      - hand(s) and wrist(s) – *see* Burn, hand(s), multiple sites
    - first degree 944.12
    - second degree 944.22
    - third degree 944.32
      - deep 944.42
        - with loss of body part 944.52
  - toe (nail) (subungual) 945.01
    - with
      - lower limb(s) – *see* Burn, leg, multiple sites
    - first degree 945.11
    - second degree 945.21
    - third degree 945.31
      - deep 945.41
        - with loss of body part 945.51
  - tongue 947.0
  - tonsil 947.0
  - trachea 947.1
  - trunk 942.00
    - first degree 942.10
    - second degree 942.20
    - third degree 942.30
      - deep 942.40
        - with loss of body part 942.50
    - multiple sites 942.09
      - first degree 942.19
      - second degree 942.29
      - third degree 942.39
        - deep 942.49
          - with loss of body part 942.59
    - specified site NEC 942.09
      - first degree 942.19
      - second degree 942.29

- **Burn** – *continued*
  - trunk – *continued*
    - specified site – *continued*
      - third degree 942.39
        - deep 942.49
          - with loss of body part 942.59
  - tunica vaginalis – *see* Burn, genitourinary organs, external
  - tympanic membrane – *see* Burn, ear
  - tympanum – *see* Burn, ear
  - ultraviolet 692.82
  - unspecified site (multiple) 949.0
    - with extent of body surface involved specified
      - less than 10 percent 948.0❺
      - 10-19 percent 948.1❺
      - 20-29 percent 948.2❺
      - 30-39 percent 948.3❺
      - 40-49 percent 948.4❺
      - 50-59 percent 948.5❺
      - 60-69 percent 948.6❺
      - 70-79 percent 948.7❺
      - 80-89 percent 948.8❺
      - 90 percent or more 948.9❺
    - first degree 949.1
    - second degree 949.2
    - third degree 949.3
      - deep 949.4
        - with loss of body part 949.5
  - uterus 947.4
  - uvula 947.0
  - vagina 947.4
  - vulva – *see* Burn, genitourinary organs, external
  - wrist(s) 944.07
    - with
      - hand(s) – *see* Burn, hand(s), multiple sites
    - first degree 944.17
    - second degree 944.27
    - third degree 944.37
      - deep 944.47
        - with loss of body part 944.57
- **Burnett's syndrome** (milk-alkali) 275.42
- **Burnier's syndrome** (hypophyseal dwarfism) 253.3
- **Burning**
  - feet syndrome 266.2
  - sensation (*see also* Disturbance, sensation) 782.0
  - tongue 529.6
- **Burns' disease** (osteochondrosis, lower ulna) 732.3
- **Bursa** – *see also* condition
  - pharynx 478.29
- **Bursitis** NEC 727.3
  - Achilles tendon 726.71
  - adhesive 726.90
    - shoulder 726.0
  - ankle 726.79
  - buttock 726.5
  - calcaneal 726.79
  - collateral ligament
    - fibular 726.63
    - tibial 726.62
  - Duplay's 726.2
  - elbow 726.33
  - finger 726.8
  - foot 726.79
  - gonococcal 098.52
  - hand 726.4
  - hip 726.5
  - infrapatellar 726.69
  - ischiogluteal 726.5
  - knee 726.60
  - occupational NEC 727.2
  - olecranon 726.33
  - pes anserinus 726.61
  - pharyngeal 478.29
  - popliteal 727.51
  - prepatellar 726.65
  - radiohumeral 727.3
  - scapulohumeral 726.19
    - adhesive 726.0
  - shoulder 726.10
    - adhesive 726.0
  - subacromial 726.19
    - adhesive 726.0
  - subcoracoid 726.19
  - subdeltoid 726.19
    - adhesive 726.0
  - subpatellar 726.69
  - syphilitic 095.7
  - Thornwaldt's, Tornwaldt's (pharyngeal) 478.29
  - toe 726.79
  - trochanteric area 726.5
- **Bursitis** – *continued*
  - wrist 726.4
- **Burst stitches or sutures** (complication of surgery) (external) 998.32
  - internal 998.31
- **Buruli ulcer** 031.1
- **Bury's disease** (erythema elevatum diutinum) 695.89
- **Buschke's disease or scleredema** (adultorum) 710.1
- **Busquet's disease** (osteoperiostitis) (*see also* Osteomyelitis) 730.1❺
- **Busse-Buschke disease** (cryptococcosis) 117.5
- **Buttock** – *see* condition
- **Button**
  - Biskra 085.1
  - Delhi 085.1
  - oriental 085.1
- **Buttonhole hand** (intrinsic) 736.21
- **Bwamba fever** (encephalitis) 066.3
- **Byssinosis** (occupational) 504
- **Bywaters' syndrome** 958.5

C

- **Cacergasia** 300.9
- **Cachexia** 799.4
  - cancerous – *see also* Neoplasm, by site, malignant 799.4
  - cardiac – *see* Disease, heart
  - dehydration 276.51
    - with
      - hypernatremia 276.0
      - hyponatremia 276.1
  - due to malnutrition 799.4
  - exophthalmic 242.0❺
  - heart – *see* Disease, heart
  - hypophyseal 253.2
  - hypopituitary 253.2
  - lead 984.9
    - specified type of lead – *see* Table of Drugs and Chemicals
  - malaria 084.9
  - malignant – *see also* Neoplasm, by site, malignant 799.4
  - marsh 084.9
  - nervous 300.5
  - old age 797
  - pachydermic – *see* Hypothyroidism
  - paludal 084.9
  - pituitary (postpartum) 253.2
  - renal (*see also* Disease, renal) 593.9
  - saturnine 984.9
    - specified type of lead – *see* Table of Drugs and Chemicals
  - senile 797
  - Simmonds' (pituitary cachexia) 253.2
  - splenica 289.59
  - strumipriva (*see also* Hypothyroidism) 244.9
  - tuberculous NEC (*see also* Tuberculosis) 011.9❺
- **Café au lait spots** 709.09
- **Caffey's disease or syndrome** (infantile cortical hyperostosis) 756.59
- **Caisson disease** 993.3
- **Caked breast** (puerperal, postpartum) 676.2❺
- **Cake kidney** 753.3
- **Calabar swelling** 125.2
- **Calcaneal spur** 726.73
- **Calcaneoapophysitis** 732.5
- **Calcaneonavicular bar** 755.67
- **Calcareous** – *see* condition
- **Calcicosis** (occupational) 502
- **Calciferol** (vitamin D) **deficiency** 268.9
  - with
    - osteomalacia 268.2
    - rickets (*see also* Rickets) 268.0
- **Calcification**
  - adrenal (capsule) (gland) 255.41 ▲
    - tuberculous (*see also* Tuberculosis) 017.6❺
  - aorta 440.0
  - artery (annular) – *see* Arteriosclerosis
  - auricle (ear) 380.89
  - bladder 596.8
    - due to S. hematobium 120.0
- **Calcification** – *continued*
  - brain (cortex) – *see* Calcification, cerebral
  - bronchus 519.19
  - bursa 727.82
  - cardiac (*see also* Degeneration, myocardial) 429.1
  - cartilage (postinfectional) 733.99
  - cerebral (cortex) 348.8
    - artery 437.0
  - cervix (uteri) 622.8
  - choroid plexus 349.2
  - conjunctiva 372.54
  - corpora cavernosa (penis) 607.89
  - cortex (brain) – *see* Calcification, cerebral
  - dental pulp (nodular) 522.2
  - dentinal papilla 520.4
  - disc, intervertebral 722.90
    - cervical, cervicothoracic 722.91
    - lumbar, lumbosacral 722.93
    - thoracic, thoracolumbar 722.92
  - fallopian tube 620.8
  - falx cerebri – *see* Calcification, cerebral
  - fascia 728.89
  - gallbladder 575.8
  - general 275.40
  - heart (*see also* Degeneration, myocardial) 429.1
    - valve – *see* Endocarditis
  - intervertebral cartilage or disc (postinfectional) 722.90
    - cervical, cervicothoracic 722.91
    - lumbar, lumbosacral 722.93
    - thoracic, thoracolumbar 722.92
  - intracranial – *see* Calcification, cerebral
  - intraspinal ligament 728.89
  - joint 719.80
    - ankle 719.87
    - elbow 719.82
    - foot 719.87
    - hand 719.84
    - hip 719.85
    - knee 719.86
    - multiple sites 719.89
    - pelvic region 719.85
    - shoulder (region) 719.81
    - specified site NEC 719.88
    - wrist 719.83
  - kidney 593.89
    - tuberculous (*see also* Tuberculosis) 016.0❺
  - larynx (senile) 478.79
  - lens 366.8
  - ligament 728.89
    - intraspinal 728.89
    - knee (medial collateral) 717.89
  - lung 518.89
    - active 518.89
    - postinfectional 518.89
    - tuberculous (*see also* Tuberculosis, pulmonary) 011.9❺
  - lymph gland or node (postinfectional) 289.3
    - tuberculous (*see also* Tuberculosis, lymph gland) 017.2❺
  - mammographic 793.89
  - massive (paraplegic) 728.10
  - medial (*see also* Arteriosclerosis, extremities) 440.20
  - meninges (cerebral) 349.2
  - metastatic 275.40
  - Mönckeberg's – *see* Arteriosclerosis
  - muscle 728.10
    - heterotopic, postoperative 728.13
  - myocardium, myocardial (*see also* Degeneration, myocardial) 429.1
  - ovary 620.8
  - pancreas 577.8
  - penis 607.89
  - periarticular 728.89
  - pericardium (*see also* Pericarditis) 423.8
  - pineal gland 259.8
  - pleura 511.0
    - postinfectional 518.89
    - tuberculous (*see also* Tuberculosis, pleura) 012.0❺
  - pulp (dental) (nodular) 522.2
  - renal 593.89
  - Rider's bone 733.99
  - sclera 379.16
  - semilunar cartilage 717.89
  - spleen 289.59
  - subcutaneous 709.3
  - suprarenal (capsule) (gland) 255.41 ▲
  - tendon (sheath) 727.82
    - with bursitis, synovitis or tenosynovitis 727.82

Calcification – *continued*
  trachea 519.19
  ureter 593.89
  uterus 621.8
  vitreous 379.29
Calcified – *see also* Calcification
  hematoma NEC 959.9
Calcinosis (generalized) (interstitial) (tumoral) (universalis) 275.49
  circumscripta 709.3
  cutis 709.3
  intervertebralis 275.49 *[722.90]*
  Raynaud's
    phenomenonsclerodactylytelangiectasis (CRST) 710.1
Calciphylaxis (*see also* Calcification, by site) 275.49
Calcium
  blood
    high (*see also* Hypercalcemia) 275.42
    low (*see also* Hypocalcemia) 275.41
  deposits – *see also* Calcification, by site
    in bursa 727.82
    in tendon (sheath) 727.82
      with bursitis, synovitis or tenosynovitis 727.82
  salts or soaps in vitreous 379.22
Calciuria 791.9
Calculi – *see* Calculus
Calculosis, intrahepatic – *see* Choledocholithiasis
Calculus, calculi, calculous 592.9
  ampulla of Vater – *see* Choledocholithiasis
  anuria (impacted) (recurrent) 592.0
  appendix 543.9
  bile duct (any) – *see* Choledocholithiasis
  biliary – *see* Cholelithiasis
  bilirubin, multiple – *see* Cholelithiasis
  bladder (encysted) (impacted) (urinary) 594.1
    diverticulum 594.0
  bronchus 518.89
  calyx (kidney) (renal) 592.0
    congenital 753.3
  cholesterol (pure) (solitary) – *see* Cholelithiasis
  common duct (bile) – *see* Choledocholithiasis
  conjunctiva 372.54
  cystic 594.1
    duct – *see* Cholelithiasis
  dental 523.6
    subgingival 523.6
    supragingival 523.6
  epididymis 608.89
  gallbladder – *see also* Cholelithiasis
    congenital 751.69
  hepatic (duct) – *see* Choledocholithiasis
  intestine (impaction) (obstruction) 560.39
  kidney (impacted) (multiple) (pelvis) (recurrent) (staghorn) 592.0
    congenital 753.3
  lacrimal (passages) 375.57
  liver (impacted) – *see* Choledocholithiasis
  lung 518.89
  mammographic 793.89
  nephritic (impacted) (recurrent) 592.0
  nose 478.19
  pancreas (duct) 577.8
  parotid gland 527.5
  pelvis, encysted 592.0
  prostate 602.0
  pulmonary 518.89
  renal (impacted) (recurrent) 592.0
    congenital 753.3
  salivary (duct) (gland) 527.5
  seminal vesicle 608.89
  staghorn 592.0
  Stensen's duct 527.5
  sublingual duct or gland 527.5
    congenital 750.26
  submaxillary duct, gland, or region 527.5
  suburethral 594.8
  tonsil 474.8
  tooth, teeth 523.6
  tunica vaginalis 608.89
  ureter (impacted) (recurrent) 592.1
  urethra (impacted) 594.2
  urinary (duct) (impacted) (passage) (tract) 592.9
    lower tract NEC 594.9
      specified site 594.8
  vagina 623.8
  vesical (impacted) 594.1
  Wharton's duct 527.5
Caliectasis 593.89
California
  disease 114.0
  encephalitis 062.5
Caligo cornea 371.03
Callositas, callosity (infected) 700
Callus (infected) 700
  bone 726.91
  excessive, following fracture – *see also* Late, effect (of), fracture
Calvé (-Perthes) **disease** (osteochondrosis, femoral capital) 732.1
Calvities (*see also* Alopecia) 704.00
Cameroon fever (*see also* Malaria) 084.6
Camptocormia 300.11
Camptodactyly (congenital) 755.59
Camurati-Engelmann disease (diaphyseal sclerosis) 756.59
Canal – *see* condition
Canaliculitis (lacrimal) (acute) 375.31
  Actinomyces 039.8
  chronic 375.41
Canavan's disease 330.0
Cancer (M8000/3) – *see also* Neoplasm, by site, malignant

Note – The term "cancer" when modified by an adjective or adjectival phrase indicating a morphological type should be coded in the same manner as "carcinoma" with that adjective or phrase. Thus, "squamous-cell cancer" should be coded in the same manner as "squamous-cell carcinoma," which appears in the list under "Carcinoma."

  bile duct type (M8160/3), liver 155.1
  hepatocellular (M8170/3) 155.0
Cancerous (M8000/3 – *see* Neoplasm, by site, malignant
Cancerphobia 300.29
Cancrum oris 528.1
Candidiasis, candidal 112.9
  with pneumonia 112.4
  balanitis 112.2
  congenital 771.7
  disseminated 112.5
  endocarditis 112.81
  esophagus 112.84
  intertrigo 112.3
  intestine 112.85
  lung 112.4
  meningitis 112.83
  mouth 112.0
  nails 112.3
  neonatal 771.7
  onychia 112.3
  otitis externa 112.82
  otomycosis 112.82
  paronychia 112.3
  perionyxis 112.3
  pneumonia 112.4
  pneumonitis 112.4
  skin 112.3
  specified site NEC 112.89
  systemic 112.5
  urogenital site NEC 112.2
  vagina 112.1
  vulva 112.1
  vulvovaginitis 112.1
Candidiosis – *see* Candidiasis
Candiru infection or infestation 136.8
Canities (premature) 704.3
  congenital 757.4
Canker (mouth) (sore) 528.2
  rash 034.1
Cannabinosis 504
Canton fever 081.9
Cap
  cradle 690.11
Capillariasis 127.5
Capillary – *see* condition
Caplan's syndrome 714.81
Caplan-Colinet syndrome 714.81
Capsule – *see* condition
Capsulitis (joint) 726.90
  adhesive (shoulder)726.0
  hip 726.5
  knee 726.60
Capsulitis – *continued*
  labyrinthine 387.8
  thyroid 245.9
  wrist 726.4
Caput
  crepitus 756.0
  medusae 456.8
  succedaneum 767.19
Carapata disease 087.1
Carate – *see* Pinta
Carbohydrate-deficient glycoprotein syndrome (CDGS) 271.8
Carboxyhemoglobinemia 986
Carbuncle 680.9
  abdominal wall 680.2
  ankle 680.6
  anus 680.5
  arm (any part, above wrist) 680.3
  auditory canal, external 680.0
  axilla 680.3
  back (any part) 680.2
  breast 680.2
  buttock 680.5
  chest wall 680.2
  corpus cavernosum 607.2
  ear (any part) (external) 680.0
  eyelid 373.13
  face (any part, except eye) 680.0
  finger (any) 680.4
  flank 680.2
  foot (any part) 680.7
  forearm 680.3
  genital organ (male) 608.4
  gluteal (region) 680.5
  groin 680.2
  hand (any part) 680.4
  head (any part, except face) 680.8
  heel 680.7
  hip 680.6
  kidney (*see also* Abscess, kidney) 590.2
  knee 680.6
  labia 616.4
  lacrimal
    gland (*see also* Dacryoadenitis) 375.00
    passages (duct) (sac) (*see also* Dacryocystitis) 375.30
  leg, any part except foot 680.6
  lower extremity, any part except foot 680.6
  malignant 022.0
  multiple sites 680.9
  neck 680.1
  nose (external) (septum) 680.0
  orbit, orbital 376.01
  partes posteriores 680.5
  pectoral region 680.2
  penis 607.2
  perineum 680.2
  pinna 680.0
  scalp (any part) 680.8
  scrotum 608.4
  seminal vesicle 608.0
  shoulder 680.3
  skin NEC 680.9
  specified site NEC 680.8
  spermatic cord 608.4
  temple (region) 680.0
  testis 608.4
  thigh 680.6
  thumb 680.4
  toe (any) 680.7
  trunk 680.2
  tunica vaginalis 608.4
  umbilicus 680.2
  upper arm 680.3
  urethra 597.0
  vas deferens 608.4
  vulva 616.4
  wrist 680.4
Carbunculus (*see also* Carbuncle) 680.9
Carcinoid (tumor) (M8240/1) – *see also* Neoplasm, by site, uncertain behavior
  and struma ovarii (M9091/1) 236.2
  argentaffin (M8241/1) – *see* Neoplasm, by site uncertain behavior
    malignant (M8241/3) – *see* Neoplasm, by site, malignant
  benign (M9091/0) 220
  composite (M8244/3) – *see* Neoplasm, by site, malignant

Carcinoid – *continued*
- goblet cell (M8243/3) – *see* Neoplasm, by site, malignant
- malignant (M8240/3) – *see* Neoplasm, by site, malignant
- nonargentaffin (M8242/1) – *see also* Neoplasm, by site, uncertain behavior
  - malignant (M8242/3) – *see* Neoplasm, by site, malignant
- strumal (M9091/1) 236.2
- syndrome (intestinal) (metastatic) 259.2
- type bronchial adenoma (M8240/3) – *see* Neoplasm, lung, malignant

Carcinoidosis 259.2

Carcinoma (M8010/3) – *see also* Neoplasm, by site, malignant

Note – Except where otherwise indicated, the morphological varieties of carcinoma in the list below should be coded by site as for "Neoplasm, malignant."

- with
  - apocrine metaplasia (M8573/3)
  - cartilaginous (and osseous) metaplasia (M8571/3)
  - osseous (and cartilaginous) metaplasia (M8571/3)
  - productive fibrosis (M8141/3)
  - spindle cell metaplasia (M8572/3)
  - squamous metaplasia (M8570/3)
- acidophil (M8280/3)
  - specified site – *see* Neoplasm, by site, malignant
  - unspecified site 194.3
- acidophil-basophil, mixed (M8281/3)
  - specified site – *see* Neoplasm, by site, malignant
  - unspecified site 194.3
- acinar (cell) (M8550/3)
- acinic cell (M8550/3)
- adenocystic (M8200/3)
- adenoid
  - cystic (M8200/3)
  - squamous cell (M8075/3)
- adenosquamous (M8560/3)
- adnexal (skin) (M8390/3) – *see* Neoplasm, skin, malignant
- adrenal cortical (M8370/3) 194.0
- alveolar (M8251/3)
  - cell (M8250/3) – *see* Neoplasm, lung, malignant
- anaplastic type (M8021/3)
- apocrine (M8401/3)
  - breast – *see* Neoplasm, breast, malignant
  - specified site NEC – *see* Neoplasm, skin, malignant
  - unspecified site 173.9
- basal cell (pigmented) (M8090/3) – *see also* Neoplasm, skin, malignant
  - fibro-epithelial type (M8093/3) – *see* Neoplasm, skin, malignant
  - morphea type (M8092/3) – *see* Neoplasm, skin, malignant
  - multicentric (M8091/3) – *see* Neoplasm, skin, malignant
- basaloid (M8123/3)
- basal-squamous cell, mixed (M8094/3) – *see* Neoplasm, skin, malignant
- basophil (M8300/3)
  - specified site – *see* Neoplasm, by site, malignant
  - unspecified site 194.3
- basophil-acidophil, mixed (M8281/3)
  - specified site – *see* Neoplasm, by site, malignant
  - unspecified site 194.3
- basosquamous (M8094/3) – *see* Neoplasm, skin, malignant
- bile duct type (M8160/3)
  - and hepatocellular, mixed (M8180/3) 155.0
  - liver 155.1
  - specified site NEC – *see* Neoplasm, by site, malignant
  - unspecified site 155.1
- branchial or branchiogenic 146.8
- bronchial or bronchogenic – *see* Neoplasm, lung, malignant
- bronchiolar (terminal) (M8250/3) – *see* Neoplasm, lung, malignant
- bronchiolo-alveolar (M8250/3) – *see* Neoplasm, lung, malignant
- bronchogenic (epidermoid) 162.9

Carcinoma – *continued*
- C cell (M8510/3)
  - specified site – *see* Neoplasm, by site, malignant
  - unspecified site 193
- ceruminous (M8420/3) 173.2
- chorionic (M9100/3)
  - specified site – *see* Neoplasm, by site, malignant
  - unspecified site
    - female 181
    - male 186.9
- chromophobe (M8270/3)
  - specified site – *see* Neoplasm, by site, malignant
  - unspecified site 194.3
- clear cell (mesonephroid type) (M8310/3)
- cloacogenic (M8124/3)
  - specified site – *see* Neoplasm, by site, malignant
  - unspecified site 154.8
- colloid (M8480/3)
- cribriform (M8201/3)
- cylindroid type (M8200/3)
- diffuse type (M8145/3)
  - specified site – *see* Neoplasm, by site, malignant
  - unspecified site 151.9
- duct (cell) (M8500/3)
  - with Paget's disease (M8541/3) – *see* Neoplasm, breast, malignant
  - infiltrating (M8500/3)
    - specified site – *see* Neoplasm, by site, malignant
    - unspecified site 174.9
- ductal (M8500/3)
- ductular, infiltrating (M8521/3)
- embryonal (M9070/3)
  - and teratoma, mixed (M9081/3)
  - combined with choriocarcinoma (M9101/3) – *see* Neoplasm, by site, malignant
  - infantile type (M9071/3)
  - liver 155.0
  - polyembryonal type (M9072/3)
- endometrioid (M8380/3)
- eosinophil (M8280/3)
  - specified site – *see* Neoplasm, by site, malignant
  - unspecified site 194.3
- epidermoid (M8070/3) – *see also* Carcinoma, squamous cell
  - and adenocarcinoma, mixed (M8560/3)
  - in situ, Bowen's type (M8081/2) – *see* Neoplasm, skin, in situ
    - intradermal – *see* Neoplasm, skin, in situ
- fibroepithelial type basal cell (M8093/3) – *see* Neoplasm, skin, malignant
- follicular (M8330/3)
  - and papillary (mixed) (M8340/3) 193
  - moderately differentiated type (M8332/3) 193
  - pure follicle type (M8331/3) 193
  - specified site – *see* Neoplasm, by site, malignant
  - trabecular type (M8332/3) 193
  - unspecified site 193
  - well differentiated type (M8331/3) 193
- gelatinous (M8480/3)
- giant cell (M8031/3)
  - and spindle cell (M8030/3)
- granular cell (M8320/3)
- granulosa cell (M8620/3) 183.0
- hepatic cell (M8170/3) 155.0
- hepatocellular (M8170/3) 155.0
  - and bile duct, mixed (M8180/3) 155.0
- hepatocholangiolitic (M8180/3) 155.0
- Hürthle cell (thyroid) 193
- hypernephroid (M8311/3)
- in
  - adenomatous
    - polyp (M8210/3)
    - polyposis coli (M8220/3) 153.9
  - pleomorphic adenoma (M8940/3)
  - polypoid adenoma (M8210/3)
  - situ (M8010/3) – *see* Carcinoma, in situ
  - tubular adenoma (M8210/3)
  - villous adenoma (M8261/3)
- infiltrating duct (M8500/3)
  - with Paget's disease (M8541/3) – *see* Neoplasm, breast, malignant
  - specified site – *see* Neoplasm, by site, malignant
  - unspecified site 174.9

Carcinoma – *continued*
- inflammatory (M8530/3)
  - specified site – *see* Neoplasm, by site, malignant
  - unspecified site 174.9
- in situ (M8010/2) – *see also* Neoplasm, by site, in situ
  - epidermoid (M8070/2) – *see also* Neoplasm, by site, in situ
    - with questionable stromal invasion (M8076/2)
      - specified site – *see* Neoplasm, by site, in situ
      - unspecified site 233.1
    - Bowen's type (M8081/2) – *see* Neoplasm, skin, in situ
  - intraductal (M8500/2)
    - specified site – *see* Neoplasm, by site, in situ
    - unspecified site 233.0
  - lobular (M8520/2)
    - specified site – *see* Neoplasm, by site, in situ
    - unspecified site 233.0
  - papillary (M8050/2) – *see* Neoplasm, by site, in situ
  - squamous cell (M8070/2) – *see also* Neoplasm, by site, in situ
    - with questionable stromal invasion (M8076/2)
      - specified site – *see* Neoplasm, by site, in situ
      - unspecified site 233.1
  - transitional cell (M8120/2) – *see* Neoplasm, by site, in situ
- intestinal type (M8144/3)
  - specified site – *see* Neoplasm, by site, malignant
  - unspecified site 151.9
- intraductal (noninfiltrating) (M8500/2)
  - papillary (M8503/2)
    - specified site – *see* Neoplasm, by site, in situ
    - unspecified site 233.0
  - specified site – *see* Neoplasm, by site, in situ
  - unspecified site 233.0
- intraepidermal (M8070/2) – *see also* Neoplasm, skin, in situ
  - squamous cell, Bowen's type (M8081/2) – *see* Neoplasm, skin, in situ
- intraepithelial (M8010/2) – *see also* Neoplasm, by site, in situ
  - squamous cell (M8072/2) – *see* Neoplasm, by site, in situ
- intraosseous (M9270/3) 170.1
  - upper jaw (bone) 170.0
- islet cell (M8150/3)
  - and exocrine, mixed (M8154/3)
    - specified site – *see* Neoplasm, by site, malignant
    - unspecified site 157.9
  - pancreas 157.4
  - specified site NEC – *see* Neoplasm, by site, malignant
  - unspecified site 157.4
- juvenile, breast (M8502/3) – *see* Neoplasm, breast, malignant
- Kulchitsky's cell (carcinoid tumor of intestine) 259.2
- large cell (M8012/3)
  - squamous cell, non-keratinizing type (M8072/3)
- Leydig cell (testis) (M8650/3)
  - specified site – *see* Neoplasm, by site, malignant
  - unspecified site 186.9
    - female 183.0
    - male 186.9
- liver cell (M8170/3) 155.0
- lobular (infiltrating) (M8520/3)
  - noninfiltrating (M8520/3)
    - specified site – *see* Neoplasm, by site, in situ
    - unspecified site 233.0
  - specified site – *see* Neoplasm, by site, malignant
  - unspecified site 174.9
- lymphoepithelial (M8082/3)
- medullary (M8510/3)
  - with
    - amyloid stroma (M8511/3)
      - specified site – *see* Neoplasm, by site, malignant
      - unspecified site 193

Carcinoid – Carcinoma

Carcinoma – *continued*
medullary – *continued*
with – *continued*
lymphoid stroma (M8512/3)
specified site – *see* Neoplasm, by site, malignant
unspecified site 174.9
mesometanephric (M9110/3)
mesonephric (M9110/3)
metastatic (M8010/6) – *see* Metastasis, cancer
metatypical (M8095/3) – *see* Neoplasm, skin, malignant
morphea type basal cell (M8092/3) – *see* Neoplasm, skin, malignant
mucinous (M8480/3)
mucin-producing (M8481/3)
mucin-secreting (M8481/3)
mucoepidermoid (M8430/3)
mucoid (M8480/3)
cell (M8300/3)
specified site – *see* Neoplasm, by site, malignant
unspecified site 194.3
mucous (M8480/3)
nonencapsulated sclerosing (M8350/3) 193
noninfiltrating
intracystic (M8504/2) – *see* Neoplasm, by site, in situ
intraductal (M8500/2)
papillary (M8503/2)
specified site – *see* Neoplasm, by site, in situ
unspecified site 233.0
specified site – *see* Neoplasm, by site, in situ
unspecified site 233.0
lobular (M8520/2)
specified site – *see* Neoplasm, by site, in situ
unspecified site 233.0
oat cell (M8042/3)
specified site – *see* Neoplasm, by site, malignant
unspecified site 162.9
odontogenic (M9270/3) 170.1
upper jaw (bone) 170.0
onocytic (M8290/3)
oxyphilic (M8290/3)
papillary (M8050/3)
and follicular (mixed) (M8340/3) 193
epidermoid (M8052/3)
intraductal (noninfiltrating) (M8503/2)
specified site – *see* Neoplasm, by site, in situ
unspecified site 233.0
serous (M8460/3)
specified site – *see* Neoplasm, by site, malignant
surface (M8461/3)
specified site – *see* Neoplasm, by site, malignant
unspecified site 183.0
unspecified site 183.0
squamous cell (M8052/3)
transitional cell (M8130/3)
papillocystic (M8450/3)
specified site – *see* Neoplasm, by site, malignant
unspecified site 183.0
parafollicular cell (M8510/3)
specified site – *see* Neoplasm, by site, malignant
unspecified site 193
pleomorphic (M8022/3)
polygonal cell (M8034/3)
prickle cell (M8070/3)
pseudoglandular, squamous cell (M8075/3)
pseudomucinous (M8470/3)
specified site – *see* Neoplasm, by site, malignant
unspecified site 183.0
pseudosarcomatous (M8033/3)
regaud type (M8082/3) – *see* Neoplasm, nasopharynx, malignant
renal cell (M8312/3) 189.0
reserve cell (M8041/3)
round cell (M8041/3)
Schmincke (M8082/3) – *see* Neoplasm, nasopharynx, malignant
Schneiderian (M8121/3)
specified site – *see* Neoplasm, by site, malignant
unspecified site 160.0
scirrhous (M8141/3)

Carcinoma – *continued*
sebaceous (M8410/3) – *see* Neoplasm, skin, malignant
secondary (M8010/6) – *see* Neoplasm, by site, malignant, secondary
secretory, breast (M8502/3) – *see* Neoplasm, breast, malignant
serous (M8441/3)
papillary (M8460/3)
specified site – *see* Neoplasm, by site, malignant
unspecified site 183.0
surface, papillary (M8461/3)
specified site – *see* Neoplasm, by site, malignant
unspecified site 183.0
Sertoli cell (M8640/3)
specified site – *see* Neoplasm, by site, malignant
unspecified site 186.9
signet ring cell (M8490/3)
metastatic (M8490/6) – *see* Neoplasm, by site, secondary
simplex (M8231/3)
skin appendage (M8390/3) – *see* Neoplasm, skin, malignant
small cell (M8041/3)
fusiform cell type (M8043/3)
squamous cell, nonkeratinizing type (M8073/3)
solid (M8230/3)
with amyloid stroma (M8511/3)
specified site – *see* Neoplasm, by site, malignant
unspecified site 193
spheroidal cell (M8035/3)
spindle cell (M8032/3)
and giant cell (M8030/3)
spinous cell (M8070/3)
squamous (cell) (M8070/3)
adenoid type (M8075/3)
and adenocarcinoma, mixed (M8560/3)
intraepidermal, Bowen's type – *see* Neoplasm, skin, in situ
keratinizing type (large cell) (M8071/3)
large cell, nonkeratinizing type (M8072/3)
microinvasive (M8076/3)
specified site – *see* Neoplasm, by site, malignant
unspecified site 180.9
nonkeratinizing type (M8072/3)
papillary (M8052/3)
pseudoglandular (M8075/3)
small cell, nonkeratinizing type (M8073/3)
spindle cell type (M8074/3)
verrucous (M8051/3)
superficial spreading (M8143/3)
sweat gland (M8400/3) – *see* Neoplasm, skin, malignant
theca cell (M8600/3) 183.0
thymic (M8580/3) 164.0
trabecular (M8190/3)
transitional (cell) (M8120/3)
papillary (M8130/3)
spindle cell type (M8122/3)
tubular (M8211/3)
undifferentiated type (M8020/3)
urothelial (M8120/3)
ventriculi 151.9
verrucous (epidermoid) (squamous cell) (M8051/3)
villous (M8262/3)
water-clear cell (M8322/3) 194.1
wolffian duct (M9110/3)

Carcinomaphobia 300.29

Carcinomatosis
peritonei (M8010/6) 197.6
specified site NEC (M8010/3) – *see* Neoplasm, by site, malignant
unspecified site (M8010/6) 199.0

Carcinosarcoma (M8980/3) – *see also* Neoplasm, by site, malignant
embryonal type (M8981/3) – *see* Neoplasm, by site, malignant

Cardia, cardial – *see* condition

Cardiac – *see also* condition
death – *see* Disease, heart
device
defibrillator, automatic implantable V45.02
in situ NEC V45.00

Cardiac – *continued*
device – *continued*
pacemaker
cardiac
fitting or adjustment V53.31
in situ V45.01
carotid sinus
fitting or adjustment V53.39
in situ V45.09
pacemaker – *see* Cardiac, device, pacemaker
tamponade 423.3 ▲

Cardialgia (*see also* Pain, precordial) 786.51

Cardiectasis – *see* Hypertrophy, cardiac

Cardiochalasia 530.81

Cardiomalacia (*see also* Degeneration, myocardial) 429.1

Cardiomegalia glycogenica diffusa 271.0

Cardiomegaly (*see also* Hypertrophy, cardiac) 429.3
congenital 746.89
glycogen 271.0
hypertensive (*see also* Hypertension, heart) 402.90
idiopathic 425.4

Cardiomyoliposis (*see also* Degeneration, myocardial) 429.1

Cardiomyopathy (congestive) (constrictive) (familial) (infiltrative) (obstructive) (restrictive) (sporadic) 425.4
alcoholic 425.5
amyloid 277.39 *[425.7]*
beriberi 265.0 *[425.7]*
cobalt-beer 425.5
congenital 425.3
due to
amyloidosis 277.39 *[425.7]*
beriberi 265.0 *[425.7]*
cardiac glycogenosis 271.0 *[425.7]*
Chagas' disease 086.0
Friedreich's ataxia 334.0 *[425.8]*
hypertension – *see* Hypertension, with, heart involvement
mucopolysaccharidosis 277.5 *[425.7]*
myotonia atrophica 359.21 ▲ *[425.8]*
progressive muscular dystrophy 359.1 *[425.8]*
sarcoidosis 135 *[425.8]*
glycogen storage 271.0 *[425.7]*
hypertensive – *see* Hypertension, with, heart involvement
hypertrophic
nonobstructive 425.4
obstructive 425.1
congenital 746.84
idiopathic (concentric) 425.4
in
Chagas' disease 086.0
sarcoidosis 135 *[425.8]*
ischemic 414.8
metabolic NEC 277.9 *[425.7]*
amyloid 277.39 *[425.7]*
thyrotoxic (*see also* Thyrotoxicosis) 242.9❺ *[425.7]*
thyrotoxicosis (*see also* Thyrotoxicosis) 242.9❺ *[425.7]*
newborn 425.4
congenital 425.3
nutritional 269.9 *[425.7]*
beriberi 265.0 *[425.7]*
obscure of Africa 425.2
peripartum 674.5❺
postpartum 674.5❺
primary 425.4
secondary 425.9
stress induced 429.83
takotsubo 429.83
thyrotoxic (*see also* Thyrotoxicosis) 242.9❺ *[425.7]*
toxic NEC 425.9
tuberculous (*see also* Tuberculosis) 017.9❺ *[425.8]*

Cardionephritis – *see* Hypertension, cardiorenal

Cardionephropathy – *see* Hypertension, cardiorenal

Cardionephrosis – *see* Hypertension, cardiorenal

Cardioneurosis 306.2

Cardiopathia nigra 416.0

Cardiopathy (*see also* Disease, heart) 429.9
hypertensive (*see also* Hypertension, heart) 402.90
idiopathic 425.4
mucopolysaccharidosis 277.5 *[425.7]*

Cardiopericarditis (*see also* Pericarditis) 423.9
Cardiophobia 300.29
Cardioptosis 746.87
Cardiorenal – *see* condition
Cardiorrhexis (*see also* Infarct, myocardium) 410.9❺
Cardiosclerosis – *see* Arteriosclerosis, coronary
Cardiosis – *see* Disease, heart
Cardiospasm (esophagus) (reflex) (stomach) 530.0
congenital 750.7
Cardiostenosis – *see* Disease, heart
Cardiosymphysis 423.1
Cardiothyrotoxicosis – *see* Hyperthyroidism
Cardiovascular – *see* condition
Carditis (acute) (bacterial) (chronic) (subacute) 429.89
Coxsackie 074.20
hypertensive (*see also* Hypertension, heart) 402.90
meningococcal 036.40
rheumatic – *see* Disease, heart, rheumatic
rheumatoid 714.2
Care (of)
child (routine) V20.1
convalescent following V66.9
chemotherapy V66.2
medical NEC V66.5
psychotherapy V66.3
radiotherapy V66.1
surgery V66.0
surgical NEC V66.0
treatment (for) V66.5
combined V66.6
fracture V66.4
mental disorder NEC V66.3
specified type NEC V66.5
end-of-life V66.7
family member (handicapped) (sick)
creating problem for family V61.49
provided away from home for holiday relief V60.5
unavailable, due to
absence (person rendering care) (sufferer) V60.4
inability (any reason) of person rendering care V60.4
holiday relief V60.5
hospice V66.7
lack of (at or after birth) (infant) (child) 995.52
adult 995.84
lactation of mother V24.1
palliative V66.7
postpartum
immediately after delivery V24.0
routine follow-up V24.2
prenatal V22.1
first pregnancy V22.0
high-risk pregnancy V23.9
specified problem NEC V23.8❺
terminal V66.7
unavailable, due to
absence of person rendering care V60.4
inability (any reason) of person rendering care V60.4
well baby V20.1
Caries (bone) (*see also* Tuberculosis, bone) 015.9❺ *[730.8]*❺
arrested 521.04
cementum 521.03
cerebrospinal (tuberculous) 015.0❺ *[730.88]*
dental (acute) (chronic) (incipient) (infected) 521.00
with pulp exposure 521.03
extending to
dentine 521.02
pulp 521.03
other specified NEC 521.09
pit and fissure 521.06
primary
pit and fissure origin 521.06
root ▶surface◀ 521.08
smooth surface origin 521.07
root surface 521.08
smooth surface 521.07
dentin (acute) (chronic) 521.02
enamel (acute) (chronic) (incipient) 521.01
external meatus 380.89
hip (*see also* Tuberculosis) 015.1❺ *[730.85]*
initial 521.01

Caries – *continued*
knee 015.2❺ *[730.86]*
labyrinth 386.8
limb NEC 015.7❺ *[730.88]*
mastoid (chronic) (process) 383.1
middle ear 385.89
nose 015.7❺ *[730.88]*
orbit 015.7❺ *[730.88]*
ossicle 385.24
petrous bone 383.20
sacrum (tuberculous) 015.0❺ *[730.88]*
spine, spinal (column) (tuberculous) 015.0❺ *[730.88]*
syphilitic 095.5
congenital 090.0 *[730.8]*❺
teeth (internal) 521.00
initial 521.01
vertebra (column) (tuberculous) 015.0❺ *[730.88]*
Carini's syndrome (ichthyosis congenita) 757.1
Carious teeth 521.00
Carneous mole 631
Carnosinemia 270.5
Carotid body or sinus syndrome 337.0
Carotidynia 337.0
Carotinemia (dietary) 278.3
Carotinosis (cutis) (skin) 278.3
Carpal tunnel syndrome 354.0
Carpenter's syndrome 759.89
Carpopedal spasm (*see also* Tetany) 781.7
Carpoptosis 736.05
Carrier (suspected) of
amebiasis V02.2
bacterial disease (meningococcal, staphylococcal) NEC V02.59
cholera V02.0
cystic fibrosis gene V83.81
defective gene V83.89
diphtheria V02.4
dysentery (bacillary) V02.3
amebic V02.2
Endamoeba histolytica V02.2
gastrointestinal pathogens NEC V02.3
genetic defect V83.89
gonorrhea V02.7
group B streptococcus V02.51
HAA (hepatitis Australian-antigen) V02.61
hemophilia A (asymptomatic) V83.01
symptomatic V83.02
hepatitis V02.60
Australian-antigen (HAA) V02.61
B V02.61
C V02.62
specified type NEC V02.69
serum V02.61
viral V02.60
infective organism NEC V02.9
malaria V02.9
paratyphoid V02.3
Salmonella V02.3
typhosa V02.1
serum hepatitis V02.61
Shigella V02.3
Staphylococcus NEC V02.59
Streptococcus NEC V02.52
group B V02.51
typhoid V02.1
venereal disease NEC V02.8
Carrión's disease (Bartonellosis) 088.0
Car sickness 994.6
Carter's
relapsing fever (Asiatic) 087.0
Cartilage – *see* condition
Caruncle (inflamed)
abscess, lacrimal (*see also* Dacryocystitis) 375.30
conjunctiva 372.00
acute 372.00
eyelid 373.00
labium (majus) (minus) 616.89
lacrimal 375.30
urethra (benign) 599.3
vagina (wall) 616.89
Cascade stomach 537.6
Caseation lymphatic gland (*see also* Tuberculosis) 017.2❺
Caseous
bronchitis – *see* Tuberculosis, pulmonary

Caseous – *continued*
meningitis 013.0❺
pneumonia – *see* Tuberculosis, pulmonary
Cassidy (-Scholte) **syndrome** (malignant carcinoid) 259.2
Castellani's bronchitis 104.8
Castleman's tumor or lymphoma (mediastinal lymph node hyperplasia) 785.6
Castration, traumatic 878.2
complicated 878.3
Casts in urine 791.7
Cat scratch – *see also* Injury, superficial
Cat's ear 744.29
Catalepsy 300.11
catatonic (acute) (*see also* Schizophrenia) 295.2❺
hysterical 300.11
schizophrenic (*see also* Schizophrenia) 295.2❺
Cataphasia 307.0
Cataplexy (idiopathic) *see also* Narcolepsy
Cataract (anterior cortical) (anterior polar) (black) (capsular) (central) (cortical) (hypermature) (immature) (incipient) (mature) 366.9
anterior
and posterior axial embryonal 743.33
pyramidal 743.31
subcapsular polar
infantile, juvenile, or presenile 366.01
senile 366.13
associated with
calcinosis 275.40 *[366.42]*
craniofacial dysostosis 756.0 *[366.44]*
galactosemia 271.1 *[366.44]*
hypoparathyroidism 252.1 *[366.42]*
myotonic disorders 359.21 ▲ *[366.43]*
neovascularization 366.33
blue dot 743.39
cerulean 743.39
complicated NEC 366.30
congenital 743.30
capsular or subcapsular 743.31
cortical 743.32
nuclear 743.33
specified type NEC 743.39
total or subtotal 743.34
zonular 743.32
coronary (congenital) 743.39
acquired 366.12
cupuliform 366.14
diabetic 250.5❺ *[366.41]*
drug-induced 366.45
due to
chalcosis 360.24 *[366.34]*
chronic choroiditis (*see also* Choroiditis) 363.20 *[366.32]*
degenerative myopia 360.21 *[366.34]* ▲
glaucoma (*see also* Glaucoma) 365.9 *[366.31]*
infection, intraocular NEC 366.32
inflammatory ocular disorder NEC 366.32
iridocyclitis, chronic 364.10 *[366.33]*
pigmentary retinal dystrophy 362.74 *[366.34]* ▲
radiation 366.46
electric 366.46
glassblowers' 366.46
heat ray 366.46
heterochromic 366.33
in eye disease NEC 366.30
infantile (*see also* Cataract, juvenile) 366.00
intumescent 366.12
irradiational 366.46
juvenile 366.00
anterior subcapsular polar 366.01
combined forms 366.09
cortical 366.03
lamellar 366.03
nuclear 366.04
posterior subcapsular polar 366.02
specified NEC 366.09
zonular 366.03
lamellar 743.32
infantile juvenile, or presenile 366.03
morgagnian 366.18
myotonic 359.21 ▲ *[366.43]*
myxedema 244.9 *[366.44]*
nuclear 366.16
posterior, polar (capsular) 743.31
infantile, juvenile, or presenile 366.02
senile 366.14
presenile (*see also* Cataract, juvenile) 366.00

❹ Fourth-Digit Required ❺ Fifth-Digit Required *[code]* Manifestation Code ▶◀ Revised Text ● New Line ▲ Revised Code

- **Cataract** – *continued*
  - punctate
    - acquired 366.12
    - congenital 743.39
  - secondary (membrane) 366.50
    - obscuring vision 366.53
    - specified type, not obscuring vision 366.52
  - senile 366.10
    - anterior subcapsular polar 366.13
    - combined forms 366.19
    - cortical 366.15
    - hypermature 366.18
    - immature 366.12
    - incipient 366.12
    - mature 366.17
    - nuclear 366.16
    - posterior subcapsular polar 366.14
    - specified NEC 366.19
    - total or subtotal 366.17
  - snowflake 250.5❺ *[366.41]*
  - specified NEC 366.8
  - subtotal (senile) 366.17
    - congenital 743.34
  - sunflower 360.24 *[366.34]*
  - tetanic NEC 252.1 *[366.42]*
  - total (mature) (senile) 366.17
    - congenital 743.34
    - localized 366.21
    - traumatic 366.22
  - toxic 366.45
  - traumatic 366.20
    - partially resolved 366.23
    - total 366.22
  - zonular (perinuclear) 743.32
    - infantile, juvenile, or presenile 366.03
- **Cataracta** 366.10
  - brunescens 366.16
  - cerulea 743.39
  - complicata 366.30
  - congenita 743.30
  - coralliformis 743.39
  - coronaria (congenital) 743.39
    - acquired 366.12
  - diabetic 250.5❺ *[366.41]*
  - floriformis 360.24 *[366.34]*
  - membranacea
    - accreta 366.50
    - congenita 743.39
  - nigra 366.16
- **Catarrh, catarrhal** (inflammation) (*see also* condition) 460
  - acute 460
  - asthma, asthmatic (*see also* Asthma) 493.9❺
  - Bostock's (*see also* Fever, hay) 477.9
  - bowel – *see* Enteritis
  - bronchial 490
    - acute 466.0
    - chronic 491.0
    - subacute 466.0
  - cervix, cervical (canal) (uteri) – *see* Cervicitis
  - chest (*see also* Bronchitis) 490
  - chronic 472.0
  - congestion 472.0
  - conjunctivitis 372.03
  - due to syphilis 095.9
    - congenital 090.0
  - enteric – *see* Enteritis
  - epidemic 487.1
  - Eustachian 381.50
  - eye (acute) (vernal) 372.03
  - fauces (*see also* Pharyngitis) 462
  - febrile 460
  - fibrinous acute 466.0
  - gastroenteric – *see* Enteritis
  - gastrointestinal – *see* Enteritis
  - gingivitis 523.00
  - hay (*see also* Fever, hay) 477.9
  - infectious 460
  - intestinal – *see* Enteritis
  - larynx (*see also* Laryngitis, chronic) 476.0
  - liver 070.1
    - with hepatic coma 070.0
  - lung (*see also* Bronchitis) 490
    - acute 466.0
    - chronic 491.0
  - middle ear (chronic) – *see* Otitis media, chronic
  - mouth 528.00
  - nasal (chronic) (*see also* Rhinitis) 472.0
    - acute 460
  - nasobronchial 472.2
  - nasopharyngeal (chronic) 472.2
    - acute 460
- **Catarrh, catarrhal** – *continued*
  - nose – *see* Catarrh, nasal
  - ophthalmia 372.03
  - pneumococcal, acute 466.0
  - pulmonary (*see also* Bronchitis) 490
    - acute 466.0
    - chronic 491.0
  - spring (eye) 372.13
  - suffocating (*see also* Asthma) 493.9❺
  - summer (hay) (*see also* Fever, hay) 477.9
  - throat 472.1
  - tracheitis 464.10
    - with obstruction 464.11
  - tubotympanal 381.4
    - acute (*see also* Otitis media, acute, nonsuppurative) 381.00
    - chronic 381.10
  - vasomotor (*see also* Fever, hay) 477.9
  - vesical (bladder) – *see* Cystitis
- **Catarrhus aestivus** (*see also* Fever, hay) 477.9
- **Catastrophe, cerebral** (*see also* Disease, cerebrovascular, acute) 436
- **Catatonia, catatonic** (acute) 781.99
  - with
    - affective psychosis – *see* Psychosis, affective
  - agitation 295.2❺
  - dementia (praecox) 295.2❺
  - due to or associated with physical condition 293.89
  - excitation 295.2❺
  - excited type 295.2❺
  - in conditions classified elsewhere 293.89
  - schizophrenia 295.2❺
  - stupor 295.2❺
- **Cat-scratch**
  - disease or fever 078.3
- **Cauda equina** – *see also* condition
  - syndrome 344.60
- **Cauliflower ear** 738.7
- **Caul over face** 768.9
- **Causalgia** 355.9
  - lower limb 355.71
  - upper limb 354.4
- **Cause**
  - external, general effects NEC 994.9
  - not stated 799.9
  - unknown 799.9
- **Caustic burn** – *see also* Burn, by site
  - from swallowing caustic or corrosive substance – *see* Burn, internal organs
- **Cavare's disease** (familial periodic paralysis) 359.3
- **Cave-in, injury**
  - crushing (severe) (*see also* Crush, by site) 869.1
  - suffocation 994.7
- **Cavernitis** (penis) 607.2
  - lymph vessel – *see* Lymphangioma
- **Cavernositis** 607.2
- **Cavernous** – *see* condition
- **Cavitation of lung** (*see also* Tuberculosis) 011.2❺
  - nontuberculous 518.89
  - primary, progressive 010.8❺
- **Cavity**
  - lung – *see* Cavitation of lung
  - optic papilla 743.57
  - pulmonary – *see* Cavitation of lung
  - teeth 521.00
  - vitreous (humor) 379.21
- **Cavovarus foot, congenital** 754.59
- **Cavus foot** (congenital) 754.71
  - acquired 736.73
- **Cazenave's**
  - disease (pemphigus) NEC 694.4
  - lupus (erythematosus) 695.4
- **CDGS** (carbohydrate-deficient glycoprotein syndrome) 271.8
- **Cecitis** – *see* Appendicitis
- **Cecocele** – *see* Hernia
- **Cecum** – *see* condition
- **Celiac**
  - artery compression syndrome 447.4
  - disease 579.0
  - infantilism 579.0
- **Cell, cellular** – *see also* condition
  - anterior chamber (eye) (positive aqueous ray) 364.04
- **Cellulitis** (diffuse) (with lymphangitis) (*see also* Abscess) 682.9
  - abdominal wall 682.2
  - anaerobic (*see also* Gas gangrene) 040.0
  - ankle 682.6
  - anus 566
  - areola 611.0
  - arm (any part, above wrist) 682.3
  - auditory canal (external) 380.10
  - axilla 682.3
  - back (any part) 682.2
  - breast 611.0
    - postpartum 675.1❺
  - broad ligament (*see also* Disease, pelvis, inflammatory) 614.4
    - acute 614.3
  - buttock 682.5
  - cervical (neck region) 682.1
  - cervix (uteri) (*see also* Cervicitis) 616.0
  - cheek, external 682.0
    - internal 528.3
  - chest wall 682.2
  - chronic NEC 682.9
  - colostomy 569.61
  - corpus cavernosum 607.2
  - digit 681.9
  - Douglas' cul-de-sac or pouch (chronic) (*see also* Disease, pelvis, inflammatory) 614.4
    - acute 614.3
  - drainage site (following operation) 998.59
  - ear, external 380.10
  - enterostomy 569.61
  - erysipelar (*see also* Erysipelas) 035
  - esophagostomy 530.86
  - eyelid 373.13
  - face (any part, except eye) 682.0
  - finger (intrathecal) (periosteal) (subcutaneous) (subcuticular) 681.00
  - flank 682.2
  - foot (except toe) 682.7
  - forearm 682.3
  - gangrenous (*see also* Gangrene) 785.4
  - genital organ NEC
    - female – *see* Abscess, genital organ, female
    - male 608.4
  - glottis 478.71
  - gluteal (region) 682.5
  - gonococcal NEC 098.0
  - groin 682.2
  - hand (except finger or thumb) 682.4
  - head (except face) NEC 682.8
  - heel 682.7
  - hip 682.6
  - jaw (region) 682.0
  - knee 682.6
  - labium (majus) (minus) (*see also* Vulvitis) 616.10
  - larynx 478.71
  - leg, except foot 682.6
  - lip 528.5
  - mammary gland 611.0
  - mouth (floor) 528.3
  - multiple sites NEC 682.9
  - nasopharynx 478.21
  - navel 682.2
    - newborn NEC 771.4
  - neck (region) 682.1
  - nipple 611.0
  - nose 478.19
    - external 682.0
  - orbit, orbital 376.01
  - palate (soft) 528.3
  - pectoral (region) 682.2
  - pelvis, pelvic
    - with
      - abortion – *see* Abortion, by type, with sepsis
      - ectopic pregnancy (*see also* categories 633.0-633.9) 639.0
      - molar pregnancy (*see also* categories 630-632) 639.0
    - female (*see also* Disease, pelvis, inflammatory) 614.4
      - acute 614.3
    - following
      - abortion 639.0
      - ectopic or molar pregnancy 639.0
    - male 567.21
    - puerperal, postpartum, childbirth 670❹
  - penis 607.2
  - perineal, perineum 682.2
  - perirectal 566
  - peritonsillar 475
  - periurethral 597.0

Note – For malignant change occurring in a neoplasm, use the appropriate M code with behavior digit/3 e.g., malignant change in uterine fibroid M8890/3. For malignant change occurring in a nonneoplastic condition (e.g., gastric ulcer) use the M code M8000/3.

- **Change(s)** (of) – *continued*
  - scleral 379.19
    - degenerative 379.16
  - senile (*see also* Senility) 797
  - sensory (*see also* Disturbance, sensation) 782.0
  - skin texture 782.8
  - spinal cord 336.9
  - splint, external V54.89
  - subdermal implantable contraceptive V25.5
  - suture V58.32
  - traction device V54.89
  - trophic 355.9
    - arm NEC 354.9
    - leg NEC 355.8
    - lower extremity NEC 355.8
    - upper extremity NEC 354.9
  - vascular 459.9
  - vasomotor 443.9
  - voice 784.49
    - psychogenic 306.1
  - wound packing V58.30
    - nonsurgical V58.30
    - surgical V58.31
- **Changing sleep-work schedule, affecting sleep** 327.36
- **Changuinola fever** 066.0
- **Chapping skin** 709.8
- **Character**
  - depressive 301.12
- **Charcôt's**
  - arthropathy 094.0 *[713.5]*
  - cirrhosis – *see* Cirrhosis, biliary
  - disease 094.0
    - spinal cord 094.0
  - fever (biliary) (hepatic) (intermittent) – *see* Choledocholithiasis
  - joint (disease) 094.0 *[713.5]*
    - diabetic 250.6❺ *[713.5]*
    - syringomyelic 336.0 *[713.5]*
  - syndrome (intermittent claudication) 443.9
    - due to atherosclerosis 440.21
- **Charcôt-Marie-Tooth disease, paralysis, or syndrome** 356.1
- **CHARGE association** (syndrome) 759.89
- **Charleyhorse** (quadriceps) 843.8
  - muscle, except quadriceps – *see* Sprain, by site
- **Charlouis' disease** (*see also* Yaws) 102.9
- **Chauffeur's fracture** – *see* Fracture, ulna, lower end
- **Cheadle** (-Möller) (-Barlow) **disease or syndrome** (infantile scurvy) 267
- **Checking (of)**
  - contraceptive device (intrauterine) V25.42
  - device
    - fixation V54.89
      - external V54.89
      - internal V54.09
    - traction V54.89
  - Kirschner wire V54.89
  - plaster cast V54.89
  - splint, external V54.89
- **Checkup**
  - following treatment – *see* Examination
  - health V70.0
  - infant (not sick) V20.2
  - newborn, routine
    - initial V20.2
    - subsequent V20.2
  - pregnancy (normal) V22.1
    - first V22.0
    - high-risk pregnancy V23.9
      - specified problem NEC V23.8❺
- **Chédiak-Higashi** (-Steinbrinck) anomaly, disease, or syndrome (congenital gigantism of peroxidase granules) 288.2
- **Cheek** – *see also* condition
  - biting 528.9
- **Cheese itch** 133.8
- **Cheese washers' lung** 495.8
- **Cheilitis** 528.5
  - actinic (due to sun) 692.72
    - chronic NEC 692.74
      - due to radiation, except from sun 692.82
    - due to radiation, except from sun 692.82
  - acute 528.5
  - angular 528.5
  - catarrhal 528.5
  - chronic 528.5
  - exfoliative 528.5
  - gangrenous 528.5
- **Cheilitis** – *continued*
  - glandularis apostematosa 528.5
  - granulomatosa 351.8
  - infectional 528.5
  - membranous 528.5
  - Miescher's 351.8
  - suppurative 528.5
  - ulcerative 528.5
  - vesicular 528.5
- **Cheilodynia** 528.5
- **Cheilopalatoschisis** (*see also* Cleft, palate, with cleft lip) 749.20
- **Cheilophagia** 528.9
- **Cheiloschisis** (*see also* Cleft, lip) 749.10
- **Cheilosis** 528.5
  - with pellagra 265.2
  - angular 528.5
  - due to
    - dietary deficiency 266.0
    - vitamin deficiency 266.0
- **Cheiromegaly** 729.89
- **Cheiropompholyx** 705.81
- **Cheloid** (*see also* Keloid) 701.4
- **Chemical burn** – *see also* Burn, by site
  - from swallowing chemical – *see* Burn, internal organs
- **Chemodectoma** (M8693/1) – *see* Paraganglioma, nonchromaffin
- **Chemoprophylaxis** NEC V07.39
- **Chemosis, conjunctiva** 372.73
- **Chemotherapy**
  - convalescence V66.2
  - encounter (for) V58.11
  - maintenance V58.11
  - prophylactic NEC V07.39
    - fluoride V07.31
- **Cherubism** 526.89
- **Chest** – *see* condition
- **Cheyne-Stokes respiration** (periodic) 786.04
- **Chiari's**
  - disease or syndrome (hepatic vein thrombosis) 453.0
  - malformation
    - type I 348.4
    - type II (*see also* Spina bifida) 741.0❺
    - type III 742.0
    - type IV 742.2
  - network 746.89
- **Chiari-Frommel syndrome** 676.6❺
- **Chicago disease** (North American blastomycosis) 116.0
- **Chickenpox** (*see also* Varicella) 052.9
  - exposure to V01.71
  - vaccination and inoculation (prophylactic) V05.4
- **Chiclero ulcer** 085.4
- **Chiggers** 133.8
- **Chignon** 111.2
  - fetus or newborn (from vacuum extraction) 767.19
- **Chigoe disease** 134.1
- **Chikungunya fever** 066.3
- **Chilaiditi's syndrome** (subphrenic displacement, colon) 751.4
- **Chilblains** 991.5
  - lupus 991.5
- **Child**
  - behavior causing concern V61.20
- **Childbed fever** 670❹
- **Childbirth** – *see also* Delivery
  - puerperal complications – *see* Puerperal
- **Childhood, period of rapid growth** V21.0
- **Chill(s)** 780.99
  - with fever 780.6
  - congestive 780.99
    - in malarial regions 084.6
  - septic – *see* Septicemia
  - urethral 599.84
- **Chilomastigiasis** 007.8
- **Chin** – *see* condition
- **Chinese dysentery** 004.9
- **Chiropractic dislocation** (*see also* Lesion, nonallopathic, by site) 739.9
- **Chitral fever** 066.0
- **Chlamydia, chlamydial** – *see* condition
- **Chloasma** 709.09
  - cachecticorum 709.09
  - eyelid 374.52
    - congenital 757.33
    - hyperthyroid 242.0❺
  - gravidarum 646.8❺
  - idiopathic 709.09
  - skin 709.09
  - symptomatic 709.09
- **Chloroma** (M9930/3) 205.3❺
- **Chlorosis** 280.9
  - Egyptian (*see also* Ancylostomiasis) 126.9
  - miners' (*see also* Ancylostomiasis) 126.9
- **Chlorotic anemia** 280.9
- **Chocolate cyst** (ovary) 617.1
- **Choked**
  - disk or disc – *see* Papilledema
  - on food, phlegm, or vomitus NEC (*see also* Asphyxia, food) 933.1
  - phlegm 933.1
  - while vomiting NEC (*see also* Asphyxia, food) 933.1
- **Chokes** (resulting from bends) 993.3
- **Choking sensation** 784.99
- **Cholangiectasis** (*see also* Disease, gallbladder) 575.8
- **Cholangiocarcinoma** (M8160/3)
  - and hepatocellular carcinoma, combined (M8180/3) 155.0
  - liver 155.1
  - specified site NEC – *see* Neoplasm, by site, malignant
  - unspecified site 155.1
- **Cholangiohepatitis** 575.8
  - due to fluke infestation 121.1
- **Cholangiohepatoma** (M8180/3) 155.0
- **Cholangiolitis** (acute) (chronic) (extrahepatic) (gangrenous) 576.1
  - intrahepatic 575.8
  - paratyphoidal (*see also* Fever, paratyphoid) 002.9
  - typhoidal 002.0
- **Cholangioma** (M8160/0) 211.5
  - malignant – *see* Cholangiocarcinoma
- **Cholangitis** (acute) (ascending) (catarrhal) (chronic) (infective) (malignant) (primary) (recurrent) (sclerosing) (secondary) (stenosing) (suppurative) 576.1
  - chronic nonsuppurative destructive 571.6
  - nonsuppurative destructive (chronic) 571.6
- **Cholecystdocholithiasis** – *see* Choledocholithiasis
- **Cholecystitis** 575.10
  - with
    - calculus, stones in
      - bile duct (common) (hepatic) – *see* Choledocholithiasis
      - gallbladder – *see* Cholelithiasis
  - acute 575.0
  - acute and chronic 575.12
  - chronic 575.11
  - emphysematous (acute) (*see also* Cholecystitis, acute) 575.0
  - gangrenous (*see also* Cholecystitis, acute) 575.0
  - paratyphoidal, current (*see also* Fever, paratyphoid) 002.9
  - suppurative (*see also* Cholecystitis, acute) 575.0
  - typhoidal 002.0
- **Choledochitis** (suppurative) 576.1
- **Choledocholith** – *see* Choledocholithiasis
- **Choledocholithiasis** 574.5❺

  Note – Use the following fifth-digit subclassification with category 574:
  0 without mention of obstruction
  1 with obstruction

  - with
    - cholecystitis 574.4❺
      - acute 574.3❺
      - chronic 574.4❺
    - cholelithiasis 574.9❺
      - with
        - cholecystitis 574.7❺
          - acute 574.6❺
            - and chronic 574.8❺
          - chronic 574.7❺

Cholelithiasis (impacted) (multiple) 574.2⑤

Note – Use the following fifth-digit subclassification with category 574:
0 without mention of obstruction
1 with obstruction

with
  cholecystitis 574.1⑤
    acute 574.0⑤
    chronic 574.1⑤
  choledocholithiasis 574.9⑤
    with
      cholecystitis 574.7⑤
        acute 574.6⑤
          and chronic 574.8⑤
        chronic cholecystitis 574.7⑤

Cholemia (*see also* Jaundice) 782.4
  familial 277.4
  Gilbert's (familial nonhemolytic) 277.4
Cholemic gallstone – *see* Cholelithiasis
Choleperitoneum, choleperitonitis (*see also* Disease, gallbladder) 567.81
Cholera (algid) (Asiatic) (asphyctic) (epidemic) (gravis) (Indian) (malignant) (morbus) (pestilential) (spasmodic) 001.9
  antimonial 985.4
  carrier (suspected) of V02.0
  classical 001.0
  contact V01.0
  due to
    Vibrio
      cholerae (Inaba, Ogawa, Hikojima serotypes) 001.0
        el tor 001.1
  el tor 001.1
  exposure to V01.0
  vaccination, prophylactic (against) V03.0
Cholerine (*see also* Cholera) 001.9
Cholestasis 576.8
  due to total parenteral nutrition (TPN) 573.8
Cholesteatoma (ear) 385.30
  attic (primary) 385.31
  diffuse 385.35
  external ear (canal) 380.21
  marginal (middle ear) 385.32
    with involvement of mastoid cavity 385.33
    secondary (with middle ear involvement) 385.33
  mastoid cavity 385.30
  middle ear (secondary) 385.32
    with involvement of mastoid cavity 385.33
  postmastoidectomy cavity (recurrent) 383.32
  primary 385.31
  recurrent, postmastoidectomy cavity 383.32
  secondary (middle ear) 385.32
    with involvement of mastoid cavity 385.33
Cholesteatosis (middle ear) (*see also* Cholesteatoma) 385.30
  diffuse 385.35
Cholesteremia 272.0
Cholesterin
  granuloma, middle ear 385.82
  in vitreous 379.22
Cholesterol
  deposit
    retina 362.82
    vitreous 379.22
  elevated (high) 272.0 ●
    with elevated (high) triglycerides 272.2 ●
  imbibition of gallbladder (*see also* Disease, gallbladder) 575.6
Cholesterolemia 272.0
  essential 272.0
  familial 272.0
  hereditary 272.0
Cholesterosis, cholesterolosis (gallbladder) 575.6
  with
    cholecystitis – *see* Cholecystitis
    cholelithiasis – *see* Cholelithiasis
  middle ear (*see also* Cholesteatoma) 385.30
Cholocolic fistula (*see also* Fistula, gallbladder) 575.5
Choluria 791.4
Chondritis (purulent) 733.99
  auricle 380.03
  costal 733.6
    Tietze's 733.6
  patella, posttraumatic 717.7
  pinna 380.03

Chondritis – *continued*
  posttraumatica patellae 717.7
  tuberculous (active) (*see also* Tuberculosis) 015.9⑤
    intervertebral 015.0⑤ *[730.88]*
Chondroangiopathia calcarea seu punctate 756.59
Chondroblastoma (M9230/0) – *see also* Neoplasm, bone, benign
  malignant (M9230/3) – *see* Neoplasm, bone, malignant
Chondrocalcinosis (articular) (crystal deposition) (dihydrate) (*see also* Arthritis, due to, crystals) 275.49 *[712.3]*⑤
  due to
    calcium pyrophosphate 275.49 *[712.2]*⑤
    dicalcium phosphate crystals 275.49 *[712.1]*⑤
    pyrophosphate crystals 275.49 *[712.2]*⑤
Chondrodermatitis nodularis helicis 380.00
Chondrodysplasia 756.4
  angiomatose 756.4
  calcificans congenita 756.59
  epiphysialis punctata 756.59
  hereditary deforming 756.4
  rhizomelic punctata 277.86
Chondrodystrophia (fetalis) 756.4
  calcarea 756.4
  calcificans congenita 756.59
  fetalis hypoplastica 756.59
  hypoplastica calcinosa 756.59
  punctata 756.59
  tarda 277.5
Chondrodystrophy (familial) (hypoplastic) 756.4
  myotonic (congenital) 359.23 ●
Chondroectodermal dysplasia 756.55
Chondrolysis 733.99
Chondroma (M9220/0) – *see also* Neoplasm cartilage, benign
  juxtacortical (M9221/0) – *see* Neoplasm, bone, benign
  periosteal (M9221/0) – *see* Neoplasm, bone, benign
Chondromalacia 733.92
  epiglottis (congenital) 748.3
  generalized 733.92
  knee 717.7
  larynx (congenital) 748.3
  localized, except patella 733.92
  patella, patellae 717.7
  systemic 733.92
  tibial plateau 733.92
  trachea (congenital) 748.3
Chondromatosis (M9220/1) – *see* Neoplasm, cartilage, uncertain behavior
Chondromyxosarcoma (M9220/3) – *see* Neoplasm, cartilage, malignant
Chondro-osteodysplasia (Morquio-Brailsford type) 277.5
Chondro-osteodystrophy 277.5
Chondro-osteoma (M9210/0) – *see* Neoplasm, bone, benign
Chondropathia tuberosa 733.6
Chondrosarcoma (M9220/3) – *see also* Neoplasm, cartilage, malignant
  juxtacortical (M9221/3) – *see* Neoplasm, bone, malignant
  mesenchymal (M9240/3) – *see* Neoplasm, connective tissue, malignant
Chordae tendineae rupture (chronic) 429.5
Chordee (nonvenereal) 607.89
  congenital 752.63
  gonococcal 098.2
Chorditis (fibrinous) (nodosa) (tuberosa) 478.5
Chordoma (M9370/3) – *see* Neoplasm, by site, malignant
Chorea (gravis) (minor) (spasmodic) 333.5
  with
    heart involvement – *see* Chorea with rheumatic heart disease
    rheumatic heart disease (chronic, inactive, or quiescent) (conditions classifiable to 393-398) – *see* rheumatic heart condition involved,
      active or acute (conditions classifiable to 391) 392.0
  acute – *see* Chorea, Sydenham's

Chorea – *continued*
  apoplectic (*see also* Disease, cerebrovascular, acute) 436
  chronic 333.4
  electric 049.8
  gravidarum – *see* Eclampsia, pregnancy
  habit 307.22
  hereditary 333.4
  Huntington's 333.4
  posthemiplegic 344.89
  pregnancy – *see* Eclampsia, pregnancy
  progressive 333.4
    chronic 333.4
    hereditary 333.4
  rheumatic (chronic) 392.9
    with heart disease or involvement – *see* Chorea, with rheumatic heart disease
  senile 333.5
  Sydenham's 392.9
    with heart involvement – *see* Chorea, with rheumatic heart disease
    nonrheumatic 333.5
  variabilis 307.23
Choreoathetosis (paroxysmal) 333.5
Chorioadenoma (destruens) (M9100/1) 236.1
Chorioamnionitis 658.4⑤
  affecting fetus or newborn 762.7
Chorioangioma (M9120/0) 219.8
Choriocarcinoma (M9100/3)
  combined with
    embryonal carcinoma (M9101/3) – *see* Neoplasm, by site, malignant
    teratoma (M9101/3) – *see* Neoplasm, by site, malignant
  specified site – *see* Neoplasm, by site, malignant
  unspecified site
    female 181
    male 186.9
Chorioencephalitis, lymphocytic (acute) (serous) 049.0
Chorioepithelioma (M9100/3) – *see* Choriocarcinoma
Choriomeningitis (acute) (benign) (lymphocytic) (serous) 049.0
Chorionepithelioma (M9100/3) – *see* Choriocarcinoma
Chorionitis (*see also* Scleroderma) 710.1
Chorioretinitis 363.20
  disseminated 363.10
    generalized 363.13
    in
      neurosyphilis 094.83
      secondary syphilis 091.51
    peripheral 363.12
    posterior pole 363.11
    tuberculous (*see also* Tuberculosis) 017.3⑤ *[363.13]*
  due to
    histoplasmosis (*see also* Histoplasmosis) 115.92
    toxoplasmosis (acquired) 130.2
      congenital (active) 771.2
  focal 363.00
    juxtapapillary 363.01
    peripheral 363.04
    posterior pole NEC 363.03
  juxtapapillaris, juxtapapillary 363.01
  progressive myopia (degeneration) 360.21
  syphilitic (secondary) 091.51
    congenital (early) 090.0 *[363.13]*
      late 090.5 *[363.13]*
    late 095.8 *[363.13]*
  tuberculous (*see also* Tuberculosis) 017.3⑤ *[363.13]*
Choristoma – *see* Neoplasm, by site, benign
Choroid – *see* condition
Choroideremia, choroidermia (initial stage) (late stage) (partial or total atrophy) 363.55
Choroiditis (*see also* Chorioretinitis) 363.20
  leprous 030.9 *[363.13]*
  senile guttate 363.41
  sympathetic 360.11
  syphilitic (secondary) 091.51
    congenital (early) 090.0 *[363.13]*
      late 090.5 *[363.13]*
    late 095.8 *[363.13]*
  Tay's 363.41
  tuberculous (*see also* Tuberculosis) 017.3⑤ *[363.13]*

Choroidopathy – Cirrhosis, cirrhotic

- **Choroidopathy** NEC 363.9
  - degenerative (*see also* Degeneration, choroid) 363.40
  - hereditary (*see also* Dystrophy, choroid) 363.50
  - specified type NEC 363.8
- **Choroidoretinitis** – *see* Chorioretinitis
- **Choroidosis, central serous** 362.41
- **Choroidretinopathy, serous** 362.41
- **Christian's syndrome** (chronic histiocytosis X) 277.89
- **Christian-Weber disease** (nodular nonsuppurative panniculitis) 729.30
- **Christmas disease** 286.1
- **Chromaffinoma** (M8700/0) – *see also* Neoplasm, by site, benign
  - malignant (M8700/3) – *see* Neoplasm, by site, malignant
- **Chromatopsia** 368.59
- **Chromhidrosis, chromidrosis** 705.89
- **Chromoblastomycosis** 117.2
- **Chromomycosis** 117.2
- **Chromophytosis** 111.0
- **Chromotrichomycosis** 111.8
- **Chronic** – *see* condition
- **Churg-Strauss syndrome** 446.4
- **Chyle cyst, mesentery** 457.8
- **Chylocele** (nonfilarial) 457.8
  - filarial (*see also* Infestation, filarial) 125.9
  - tunica vaginalis (nonfilarial) 608.84
    - filarial (*see also* Infestation, filarial) 125.9
- **Chylomicronemia** (fasting) (with hyperprebetalipoproteinemia) 272.3
- **Chylopericardium** (acute) 420.90
- **Chylothorax** (nonfilarial) 457.8
  - filarial (*see also* Infestation, filarial) 125.9
- **Chylous**
  - ascites 457.8
  - cyst of peritoneum 457.8
  - hydrocele 603.9
  - hydrothorax (nonfilarial) 457.8
    - filarial (*see also* Infestation, filarial) 125.9
- **Chyluria** 791.1
  - bilharziasis 120.0
  - due to
    - Brugia (malayi) 125.1
    - Wuchereria (bancrofti) 125.0
      - malayi 125.1
  - filarial (*see also* Infestation, filarial) 125.9
  - filariasis (*see also* Infestation, filarial) 125.9
  - nonfilarial 791.1
- **Cicatricial** (deformity) – *see* Cicatrix
- **Cicatrix** (adherent) (contracted) (painful) (vicious) 709.2
  - adenoid 474.8
  - alveolar process 525.8
  - anus 569.49
  - auricle 380.89
  - bile duct (*see also* Disease, biliary) 576.8
  - bladder 596.8
  - bone 733.99
  - brain 348.8
  - cervix (postoperative) (postpartal) 622.3
    - in pregnancy or childbirth 654.6❺
      - causing obstructed labor 660.2❺
  - chorioretinal 363.30
    - disseminated 363.35
    - macular 363.32
    - peripheral 363.34
    - posterior pole NEC 363.33
  - choroid – *see* Cicatrix, chorioretinal
  - common duct (*see also* Disease, biliary) 576.8
  - congenital 757.39
  - conjunctiva 372.64
  - cornea 371.00
    - tuberculous (*see also* Tuberculosis) 017.3❺ *[372.15]*
  - duodenum (bulb) 537.3
  - esophagus 530.3
  - eyelid 374.46
    - with
      - ectropion – *see* Ectropion
      - entropion – *see* Entropion
  - hypopharynx 478.29
  - knee, semilunar cartilage 717.5
  - lacrimal
    - canaliculi 375.53
    - duct
      - acquired 375.56

- **Cicatrix** – *continued*
  - lacrimal – *continued*
    - duct – *continued*
      - neonatal 375.55
    - punctum 375.52
    - sac 375.54
  - larynx 478.79
  - limbus (cystoid) 372.64
  - lung 518.89
  - macular 363.32
    - disseminated 363.35
    - peripheral 363.34
  - middle ear 385.89
  - mouth 528.9
  - muscle 728.89
  - nasolacrimal duct
    - acquired 375.56
    - neonatal 375.55
  - nasopharynx 478.29
  - palate (soft) 528.9
  - penis 607.89
  - prostate 602.8
  - rectum 569.49
  - retina 363.30
    - disseminated 363.35
    - macular 363.32
    - peripheral 363.34
    - posterior pole NEC 363.33
  - semilunar cartilage – *see* Derangement, meniscus
  - seminal vesicle 608.89
  - skin 709.2
    - infected 686.8
    - postinfectional 709.2
    - tuberculous (*see also* Tuberculosis) 017.0❺
  - specified site NEC 709.2
  - throat 478.29
  - tongue 529.8
  - tonsil (and adenoid) 474.8
  - trachea 478.9
  - tuberculous NEC (*see also* Tuberculosis) 011.9❺
  - ureter 593.89
  - urethra 599.84
  - uterus 621.8
  - vagina 623.4
    - in pregnancy or childbirth 654.7❺
      - causing obstructed labor 660.2❺
  - vocal cord 478.5
  - wrist, constricting (annular) 709.2
- **CIDP** (chronic inflammatory demyelinating polyneuropathy) 357.81 ●
- **CIN I** [cervical intraepithelial neoplasia I] 622.11
- **CIN II** [cervical intraepithelial neoplasia II] 622.12
- **CIN III** [cervical intraepithelial neoplasia III] 233.1
- **Cinchonism**
  - correct substance properly administered 386.9
  - overdose or wrong substance given or taken 961.4
- **Circine herpes** 110.5
- **Circle of Willis** – *see* condition
- **Circular** – *see also* condition
  - hymen 752.49
- **Circulating anticoagulants** 286.5
  - following childbirth 666.3❺
  - postpartum 666.3❺
- **Circulation**
  - collateral (venous), any site 459.89
  - defective 459.9
    - congenital 747.9
    - lower extremity 459.89
  - embryonic 747.9
  - failure 799.89
    - fetus or newborn 779.89
    - peripheral 785.59
  - fetal, persistent 747.83
  - heart, incomplete 747.9
- **Circulatory system** – *see* condition
- **Circulus senilis** 371.41
- **Circumcision**
  - in absence of medical indication V50.2
  - ritual V50.2
  - routine V50.2
- **Circumscribed** – *see* condition
- **Circumvallata placenta** – *see* Placenta, abnormal
- **Cirrhosis, cirrhotic** 571.5
  - with alcoholism 571.2
  - alcoholic (liver) 571.2
  - atrophic (of liver) – *see* Cirrhosis, portal
  - Baumgarten-Cruveilhier 571.5

- **Cirrhosis, cirrhotic** – *continued*
  - biliary (cholangiolitic) (cholangitic) (cholestatic) (extrahepatic) (hypertrophic) (intrahepatic) (nonobstructive) (obstructive) (pericholangiolitic) (posthepatic) (primary) (secondary) (xanthomatous) 571.6
    - due to
      - clonorchiasis 121.1
      - flukes 121.3
  - brain 331.9
  - capsular – *see* Cirrhosis, portal
  - cardiac 571.5
    - alcoholic 571.2
  - central (liver) – *see* Cirrhosis, liver
  - Charcôt's 571.6
  - cholangiolitic – *see* Cirrhosis, biliary
  - cholangitic – *see* Cirrhosis, biliary
  - cholestatic – *see* Cirrhosis, biliary
  - clitoris (hypertrophic) 624.2
  - coarsely nodular 571.5
  - congestive (liver) – *see* Cirrhosis, cardiac
  - Cruveilhier-Baumgarten 571.5
  - cryptogenic (of liver) 571.5
    - alcoholic 571.2
  - dietary (*see also* Cirrhosis, portal) 571.5
  - due to
    - bronzed diabetes 275.0
    - congestive hepatomegaly – *see* Cirrhosis, cardiac
    - cystic fibrosis 277.00
    - hemochromatosis 275.0
    - hepatolenticular degeneration 275.1
    - passive congestion (chronic) – *see* Cirrhosis, cardiac
    - Wilson's disease 275.1
    - xanthomatosis 272.2
  - extrahepatic (obstructive) – *see* Cirrhosis, biliary
  - fatty 571.8
    - alcoholic 571.0
  - florid 571.2
  - Glisson's – *see* Cirrhosis, portal
  - Hanot's (hypertrophic) – *see* Cirrhosis, biliary
  - hepatic – *see* Cirrhosis, liver
  - hepatolienal – *see* Cirrhosis, liver
  - hobnail – *see* Cirrhosis, portal
  - hypertrophic – *see also* Cirrhosis, liver
    - biliary – *see* Cirrhosis, biliary
    - Hanot's – *see* Cirrhosis, biliary
  - infectious NEC – *see* Cirrhosis, portal
  - insular – *see* Cirrhosis, portal
  - intrahepatic (obstructive) (primary) (secondary) – *see* Cirrhosis, biliary
  - juvenile (*see also* Cirrhosis, portal) 571.5
  - kidney (*see also* Sclerosis, renal) 587
  - Laennec's (of liver) 571.2
    - nonalcoholic 571.5
  - liver (chronic) (hepatolienal) (hypertrophic) (nodular) (splenomegalic) (unilobar) 571.5
    - with alcoholism 571.2
    - alcoholic 571.2
    - congenital (due to failure of obliteration of umbilical vein) 777.8
    - cryptogenic 571.5
      - alcoholic 571.2
    - fatty 571.8
      - alcoholic 571.0
    - macronodular 571.5
      - alcoholic 571.2
    - micronodular 571.5
      - alcoholic 571.2
    - nodular, diffuse 571.5
      - alcoholic 571.2
    - pigmentary 275.0
    - portal 571.5
      - alcoholic 571.2
    - postnecrotic 571.5
      - alcoholic 571.2
    - syphilitic 095.3
  - lung (chronic) (*see also* Fibrosis, lung) 515
  - macronodular (of liver) 571.5
    - alcoholic 571.2
  - malarial 084.9
  - metabolic NEC 571.5
  - micronodular (of liver) 571.5
    - alcoholic 571.2
  - monolobular – *see* Cirrhosis, portal
  - multilobular – *see* Cirrhosis, portal
  - nephritis (*see also* Sclerosis, renal) 587
  - nodular – *see* Cirrhosis, liver
  - nutritional (fatty) 571.5
  - obstructive (biliary) (extrahepatic) (intrahepatic) – *see* Cirrhosis, biliary

❹ Fourth-Digit Required ❺ Fifth-Digit Required *[code]* Manifestation Code ▶◀ Revised Text ● New Line ▲ Revised Code

- **Cirrhosis, cirrhotic** – *continued*
  - ovarian 620.8
  - paludal 084.9
  - pancreas (duct) 577.8
  - pericholangiolitic – *see* Cirrhosis, biliary
  - periportal – *see* Cirrhosis, portal
  - pigment, pigmentary (of liver) 275.0
  - portal (of liver) 571.5
    - alcoholic 571.2
  - posthepatitic (*see also* Cirrhosis, postnecrotic) 571.5
  - postnecrotic (of liver) 571.5
    - alcoholic 571.2
  - primary (intrahepatic) – *see* Cirrhosis, biliary
  - pulmonary (*see also* Fibrosis, lung) 515
  - renal (*see also* Sclerosis, renal) 587
  - septal (*see also* Cirrhosis, postnecrotic) 571.5
  - spleen 289.51
  - splenomegalic (of liver) – *see* Cirrhosis, liver
  - stasis (liver) – *see* Cirrhosis, liver
  - stomach 535.4❺
  - Todd's (*see also* Cirrhosis, biliary) 571.6
  - toxic (nodular) – *see* Cirrhosis, postnecrotic
  - trabecular – *see* Cirrhosis, postnecrotic
  - unilobar – *see* Cirrhosis, liver
  - vascular (of liver) – *see* Cirrhosis, liver
  - xanthomatous (biliary) (*see also* Cirrhosis, biliary) 571.6
    - due to xanthomatosis (familial) (metabolic) (primary) 272.2
- **Cistern, subarachnoid** 793.0
- **Citrullinemia** 270.6
- **Citrullinuria** 270.6
- **Ciuffini-Pancoast tumor** (M8010/3) (carcinoma, pulmonary apex) 162.3
- **Civatte's disease or poikiloderma** 709.09
- **Clam diggers' itch** 120.3
- **Clap** – *see* Gonorrhea
- **Clark's paralysis** 343.9
- **Clarke-Hadfield syndrome** (pancreatic infantilism) 577.8
- **Clastothrix** 704.2
- **Claude's syndrome** 352.6
- **Claude Bernard-Horner syndrome** (*see also* Neuropathy, peripheral, autonomic) 337.9
- **Claudication, intermittent** 443.9
  - cerebral (artery) (*see also* Ischemia, cerebral, transient) 435.9
  - due to atherosclerosis 440.21
  - spinal cord (arteriosclerotic) 435.1
    - syphilitic 094.89
  - spinalis 435.1
  - venous (axillary) 453.8
- **Claudicatio venosa intermittens** 453.8
- **Claustrophobia** 300.29
- **Clavus** (infected) 700
- **Clawfoot** (congenital) 754.71
  - acquired 736.74
- **Clawhand** (acquired) 736.06
  - congenital 755.59
- **Clawtoe** (congenital) 754.71
  - acquired 735.5
- **Clay eating** 307.52
- **Clay shovelers' fracture** – *see* Fracture, vertebra, cervical
- **Cleansing of artificial opening** (*see also* Attention to artificial opening) V55.9
- **Cleft** (congenital) – *see also* Imperfect, closure
  - alveolar process 525.8
  - branchial (persistent) 744.41
    - cyst 744.42
  - clitoris 752.49
  - cricoid cartilage, posterior 748.3
  - facial (*see also* Cleft, lip) 749.10
  - lip 749.10
    - with cleft palate 749.20
      - bilateral (lip and palate) 749.24
        - with unilateral lip or palate 749.25
        - complete 749.23
        - incomplete 749.24
      - unilateral (lip and palate) 749.22
        - with bilateral lip or palate 749.25
        - complete 749.21
        - incomplete 749.22
    - bilateral 749.14
      - with cleft palate, unilateral 749.25
      - complete 749.13
      - incomplete 749.14
- **Cleft** – *continued*
  - lip – *continued*
    - unilateral 749.12
      - with cleft palate, bilateral 749.25
      - complete 749.11
      - incomplete 749.12
  - nose 748.1
  - palate 749.00
    - with cleft lip 749.20
      - bilateral (lip and palate) 749.24
        - with unilateral lip or palate 749.25
        - complete 749.23
        - incomplete 749.24
      - unilateral (lip and palate) 749.22
        - with bilateral lip or palate 749.25
        - complete 749.21
        - incomplete 749.22
    - bilateral 749.04
      - with cleft lip, unilateral 749.25
      - complete 749.03
      - incomplete 749.04
    - unilateral 749.02
      - with cleft lip, bilateral 749.25
      - complete 749.01
      - incomplete 749.02
  - penis 752.69
  - posterior, cricoid cartilage 748.3
  - scrotum 752.89
  - sternum (congenital) 756.3
  - thyroid cartilage (congenital) 748.3
  - tongue 750.13
  - uvula 749.02
    - with cleft lip (*see also* Cleft, lip, with cleft palate) 749.20
  - water 366.12
- **Cleft hand** (congenital) 755.58
- **Cleidocranial dysostosis** 755.59
- **Cleidotomy, fetal** 763.89
- **Cleptomania** 312.32
- **Clérambault's syndrome** 297.8
  - erotomania 302.89
- **Clergyman's sore throat** 784.49
- **Click, clicking**
  - systolic syndrome 785.2
- **Clifford's syndrome** (postmaturity) 766.22
- **Climacteric** (*see also* Menopause) 627.2
  - arthritis NEC (*see also* Arthritis, climacteric) 716.3❺
  - depression (*see also* Psychosis, affective) 296.2❺
  - disease 627.2
    - recurrent episode 296.3❺
    - single episode 296.2❺
  - female (symptoms) 627.2
  - male (symptoms) (syndrome) 608.89
  - melancholia (*see also* Psychosis, affective) 296.2❺
    - recurrent episode 296.3❺
    - single episode 296.2❺
  - paranoid state 297.2
  - paraphrenia 297.2
  - polyarthritis NEC 716.39
    - male 608.89
  - symptoms (female) 627.2
- **Clinical research investigation** (control) (participant) V70.7
- **Clinodactyly** 755.59
- **Clitoris** – *see* condition
- **Cloaca, persistent** 751.5
- **Clonorchiasis** 121.1
- **Clonorchiosis** 121.1
- **Clonorchis infection, liver** 121.1
- **Clonus** 781.0
- **Closed bite** 524.20
- **Closed surgical procedure converted to open procedure**
  - arthroscopic V64.43
  - laparoscopic V64.41
  - thoracoscopic V64.42
- **Closure**
  - artificial opening (*see also* Attention to artificial opening) V55.9
  - congenital, nose 748.0
  - cranial sutures, premature 756.0
  - defective or imperfect NEC – *see* Imperfect, closure
  - fistula, delayed – *see* Fistula
  - fontanelle, delayed 756.0
  - foramen ovale, imperfect 745.5
- **Closure** – *continued*
  - hymen 623.3
  - interauricular septum, defective 745.5
  - interventricular septum, defective 745.4
  - lacrimal duct 375.56
    - congenital 743.65
    - neonatal 375.55
  - nose (congenital) 748.0
    - acquired 738.0
  - vagina 623.2
  - valve – *see* Endocarditis
  - vulva 624.8
- **Clot** (blood)
  - artery (obstruction) (occlusion) (*see also* Embolism) 444.9
  - atrial appendage 429.89
  - bladder 596.7
  - brain (extradural or intradural) (*see also* Thrombosis, brain) 434.0❺
    - late effect – *see* Late effect(s) (of) cerebrovascular disease
  - circulation 444.9
  - heart (*see also* Infarct, myocardium) 410.9❺
    - without myocardial infarction 429.89
  - vein (*see also* Thrombosis) 453.9
- **Clotting defect** NEC (*see also* Defect, coagulation) 286.9
- **Clouded state** 780.09
  - epileptic (*see also* Epilepsy) 345.9❺
  - paroxysmal (idiopathic) (*see also* Epilepsy) 345.9❺
- **Clouding**
  - corneal graft 996.51
- **Cloudy**
  - antrum, antra 473.0
  - dialysis effluent 792.5
- **Clouston's** (hidrotic) ectodermal dysplasia 757.31
- **Clubbing of fingers** 781.5
- **Clubfinger** 736.29
  - acquired 736.29
  - congenital 754.89
- **Clubfoot** (congenital) 754.70
  - acquired 736.71
  - equinovarus 754.51
  - paralytic 736.71
- **Club hand** (congenital) 754.89
  - acquired 736.07
- **Clubnail** (acquired) 703.8
  - congenital 757.5
- **Clump kidney** 753.3
- **Clumsiness** 781.3
  - syndrome 315.4
- **Cluttering** 307.0
- **Clutton's joints** 090.5
- **Coagulation, intravascular** (diffuse) (disseminated) (*see also* Fibrinolysis) 286.6
  - newborn 776.2
- **Coagulopathy** (*see also* Defect, coagulation) 286.9
  - consumption 286.6
  - intravascular (disseminated) NEC 286.6
    - newborn 776.2
- **Coalition**
  - calcaneoscaphoid 755.67
  - calcaneus 755.67
  - tarsal 755.67
- **Coal miners'**
  - elbow 727.2
  - lung 500
- **Coal workers' lung or pneumoconiosis** 500
- **Coarctation**
  - aorta (postductal) (preductal) 747.10
  - pulmonary artery 747.3
- **Coated tongue** 529.3
- **Coats' disease** 362.12
- **Cocainism** (*see also* Dependence) 304.2❺
- **Coccidioidal granuloma** 114.3
- **Coccidioidomycosis** 114.9
  - with pneumonia 114.0
  - cutaneous (primary) 114.1
  - disseminated 114.3
  - extrapulmonary (primary) 114.1
  - lung 114.5
    - acute 114.0
    - chronic 114.4
    - primary 114.0
  - meninges 114.2

Cirrhosis, cirrhotic – Coccidioidomycosis

Coccidioidomycosis – *continued*
  primary (pulmonary) 114.0
    acute 114.0
  prostate 114.3
  pulmonary 114.5
    acute 114.0
    chronic 114.4
    primary 114.0
  specified site NEC 114.3
Coccidioidosis 114.9
  lung 114.5
    acute 114.0
    chronic 114.4
    primary 114.0
  meninges 114.2
Coccidiosis (colitis) (diarrhea) (dysentery) 007.2
Cocciuria 791.9
Coccus in urine 791.9
Coccydynia 724.79
Coccygodynia 724.79
Coccyx – *see* condition
Cochin-China
  diarrhea 579.1
    anguilluliasis 127.2
  ulcer 085.1
Cock's peculiar tumor 706.2
Cockayne's disease or syndrome (microcephaly and dwarfism) 759.89
Cockayne-Weber syndrome (epidermolysis bullosa) 757.39
Cocked-up toe 735.2
Codman's tumor (benign chondroblastoma) (M9230/0) – *see* Neoplasm, bone, benign
Coenurosis 123.8
Coffee workers' lung 495.8
Cogan's syndrome 370.52
  congenital oculomotor apraxia 379.51
  nonsyphilitic interstitial keratitis 370.52
Coiling, umbilical cord – *see* Complications, umbilical cord
Coitus, painful (female) 625.0
  male 608.89
  psychogenic 302.76
Cold 460
  with influenza, flu, or grippe 487.1
  abscess – *see also* Tuberculosis, abscess
    articular – *see* Tuberculosis, joint
  agglutinin
    disease (chronic) or syndrome 283.0
    hemoglobinuria 283.0
      paroxysmal (cold) (nocturnal) 283.2
  allergic (*see also* Fever, hay) 477.9
  bronchus or chest – *see* Bronchitis
    with grippe or influenza 487.1
  common (head) 460
    vaccination, prophylactic (against) V04.7
  deep 464.10
  effects of 991.9
    specified effect NEC 991.8
  excessive 991.9
    specified effect NEC 991.8
  exhaustion from 991.8
  exposure to 991.9
    specified effect NEC 991.8
  grippy 487.1
  head 460
  injury syndrome (newborn) 778.2
  intolerance 780.99
  on lung – *see* Bronchitis
  rose 477.0
  sensitivity, autoimmune 283.0
  virus 460
Coldsore (*see also* Herpes, simplex) 054.9
Colibacillosis 041.4
  generalized 038.42
Colibacilluria 791.9
Colic (recurrent) 789.0❺
  abdomen 789.0❺
    psychogenic 307.89
  appendicular 543.9
  appendix 543.9
  bile duct – *see* Choledocholithiasis
  biliary – *see* Cholelithiasis
  bilious – *see* Cholelithiasis
  common duct – *see* Choledocholithiasis
  Devonshire NEC 984.9
    specified type of lead – *see* Table of Drugs and Chemicals
Colic – *continued*
  flatulent 787.3
  gallbladder or gallstone – *see* Cholelithiasis
  gastric 536.8
  hepatic (duct) – *see* Choledocholithiasis
  hysterical 300.11
  infantile 789.0❺
  intestinal 789.0❺
  kidney 788.0
  lead NEC 984.9
    specified type of lead – *see* Table of Drugs and Chemicals
  liver (duct) – *see* Choledocholithiasis
  mucous 564.9
    psychogenic 316 *[564.9]*
  nephritic 788.0
  painter's NEC 984.9
  pancreas 577.8
  psychogenic 306.4
  renal 788.0
  saturnine NEC 984.9
    specified type of lead – *see* Table of Drugs and Chemicals
  spasmodic 789.0❺
  ureter 788.0
  urethral 599.84
    due to calculus 594.2
  uterus 625.8
    menstrual 625.3
  vermicular 543.9
  virus 460
  worm NEC 128.9
Colicystitis (*see also* Cystitis) 595.9
Colitis (acute) (catarrhal) (croupous) (cystica superficialis) (exudative) (hemorrhagic) (noninfectious) (phlegmonous) (presumed noninfectious) 558.9
  adaptive 564.9
  allergic 558.3
  amebic (*see also* Amebiasis) 006.9
    nondysenteric 006.2
  anthrax 022.2
  bacillary (*see also* Infection, Shigella) 004.9
  balantidial 007.0
  chronic 558.9
    ulcerative (*see also* Colitis, ulcerative) 556.9
  coccidial 007.2
  dietetic 558.9
  due to radiation 558.1
  functional 558.9
  gangrenous 009.0
  giardial 007.1
  granulomatous 555.1
  gravis (*see also* Colitis, ulcerative) 556.9
  infectious (*see also* Enteritis, due to, specific organism) 009.0
    presumed 009.1
  ischemic 557.9
    acute 557.0
    chronic 557.1
    due to mesenteric artery insufficiency 557.1
  membranous 564.9
    psychogenic 316 *[564.9]*
  mucous 564.9
    psychogenic 316 *[564.9]*
  necrotic 009.0
  polyposa (*see also* Colitis, ulcerative) 556.9
  protozoal NEC 007.9
  pseudomembranous 008.45
  pseudomucinous 564.9
  regional 555.1
  segmental 555.1
  septic (*see also* Enteritis, due to, specific organism) 009.0
  spastic 564.9
    psychogenic 316 *[564.9]*
  Staphylococcus 008.41
    food 005.0
  thromboulcerative 557.0
  toxic 558.2
  transmural 555.1
  trichomonal 007.3
  tuberculous (ulcerative) 014.8❺
  ulcerative (chronic) (idiopathic) (nonspecific) 556.9
    entero- 556.0
    fulminant 557.0
    ileo- 556.1
    left-sided 556.5
    procto- 556.2
    proctosigmoid 556.3
Colitis – *continued*
  ulcerative – *continued*
    psychogenic 316 *[556]*❹
    specified NEC 556.8
    universal 556.6
Collagen disease NEC 710.9
  nonvascular 710.9
  vascular (allergic) (*see also* Angiitis, hypersensitivity) 446.20
Collagenosis (*see also* Collagen disease) 710.9
  cardiovascular 425.4
  mediastinal 519.3
Collapse 780.2
  adrenal 255.8
  cardiorenal (*see also* Hypertension, cardiorenal) 404.90
  cardiorespiratory 785.51
    fetus or newborn 779.85
  cardiovascular (*see also* Disease, heart) 785.51
    fetus or newborn 779.85
  circulatory (peripheral) 785.59
    with
      abortion – *see* Abortion, by type, with shock
      ectopic pregnancy (*see also* categories 633.0-633.9) 639.5
      molar pregnancy (*see also* categories 630-632) 639.5
    during or after labor and delivery 669.1❺
    fetus or newborn 779.85
    following
      abortion 639.5
      ectopic or molar pregnancy 639.5
  during or after labor and delivery 669.1❺
    fetus or newborn 779.89
  external ear canal 380.50
    secondary to
      inflammation 380.53
      surgery 380.52
      trauma 380.51
  general 780.2
  heart – *see* Disease, heart
  heat 992.1
  hysterical 300.11
  labyrinth, membranous (congenital) 744.05
  lung (massive) (*see also* Atelectasis) 518.0
    pressure, during labor 668.0❺
  myocardial – *see* Disease, heart
  nervous (*see also* Disorder, mental, nonpsychotic) 300.9
  neurocirculatory 306.2
  nose 738.0
  postoperative (cardiovascular) 998.0
  pulmonary (*see also* Atelectasis) 518.0
    fetus or newborn 770.5
      partial 770.5
      primary 770.4
  thorax 512.8
    iatrogenic 512.1
    postoperative 512.1
  trachea 519.19
  valvular – *see* Endocarditis
  vascular (peripheral) 785.59
    with
      abortion – *see* Abortion, by type, with shock
      ectopic pregnancy (*see also* categories 633.0-633.9) 639.5
      molar pregnancy (*see also* categories 630-632) 639.5
    cerebral (*see also* Disease, cerebrovascular, acute) 436
    during or after labor and delivery 669.1❺
    fetus or newborn 779.89
    following
      abortion 639.5
      ectopic or molar pregnancy 639.5
  vasomotor 785.59
  vertebra 733.13
Collateral – *see also* condition
  circulation (venous) 459.89
  dilation, veins 459.89
Colles' fracture (closed) (reversed) (separation) 813.41
  open 813.51
Collet's syndrome 352.6
Collet-Sicard syndrome 352.6
Colliculitis urethralis (*see also* Urethritis) 597.89
Colliers'
  asthma 500
  lung 500
  phthisis (*see also* Tuberculosis) 011.4❺

Collodion baby (ichthyosis congenita) 757.1
Colloid milium 709.3
Coloboma NEC 743.49
  choroid 743.59
  fundus 743.52
  iris 743.46
  lens 743.36
  lids 743.62
  optic disc (congenital) 743.57
    acquired 377.23
  retina 743.56
  sclera 743.47
Coloenteritis – *see* Enteritis
Colon – *see* condition
Coloptosis 569.89
Color
  amblyopia NEC 368.59
    acquired 368.55
  blindness NEC (congenital) 368.59
    acquired 368.55
Colostomy
  attention to V55.3
  fitting or adjustment V55.3
  malfunctioning 569.62
  status V44.3
Colpitis (*see also* Vaginitis) 616.10
Colpocele 618.6
Colpocystitis (*see also* Vaginitis) 616.10
Colporrhexis 665.4❺
Colpospasm 625.1
Column, spinal, vertebral – *see* condition
Coma 780.01
  apoplectic (*see also* Disease, cerebrovascular, acute) 436
  diabetic (with ketoacidosis) 250.3❺
    hyperosmolar 250.2❺
  eclamptic (*see also* Eclampsia) 780.39
  epileptic 345.3
  hepatic 572.2
  hyperglycemic 250.2
  hyperosmolar (diabetic) (nonketotic) 250.2❺
  hypoglycemic 251.0
    diabetic 250.3❺
  insulin 250.3
    hyperosmolar 250.2
    nondiabetic 251.0
    organic hyperinsulinism 251.0
  Kussmaul's (diabetic) 250.3❺
  liver 572.2
  newborn 779.2
  prediabetic 250.2❺
  uremic – *see* Uremia
Combat fatigue (*see also* Reaction, stress, acute) 308.9
Combined – *see* condition
Comedo 706.1
Comedocarcinoma (M8501/3) – *see also* Neoplasm, breast, malignant
  noninfiltrating (M8501/2)
    specified site – *see* Neoplasm, by site, in situ
    unspecified site 233.0
Comedomastitis 610.4
Comedones 706.1
  lanugo 757.4
Comma bacillus, carrier (suspected) of V02.3
Comminuted fracture – *see* Fracture, by site
Common
  aortopulmonary trunk 745.0
  atrioventricular canal (defect) 745.69
  atrium 745.69
  cold (head) 460
    vaccination, prophylactic (against) V04.7
  truncus (arteriosus) 745.0
  ventricle 745.3
Commotio (current)
  cerebri (*see also* Concussion, brain) 850.9
    with skull fracture – *see* Fracture, skull, by site
  retinae 921.3
  spinalis – *see* Injury, spinal, by site
Commotion (current)
  brain (without skull fracture) (*see also* Concussion, brain) 850.9
    with skull fracture – *see* Fracture, skull, by site
  spinal cord – *see* Injury, spinal, by site
Communication
  abnormal – *see also* Fistula
    between
      base of aorta and pulmonary artery 745.0

Communication – *continued*
  abnormal – *continued*
    between – *continued*
      left ventricle and right atrium 745.4
      pericardial sac and pleural sac 748.8
      pulmonary artery and pulmonary vein 747.3
    congenital, between uterus and anterior abdominal wall 752.3
      bladder 752.3
      intestine 752.3
      rectum 752.3
  left ventricular-right atrial 745.4
  pulmonary artery-pulmonary vein 747.3
Compartment syndrome – *see* Syndrome, compartment
Compensation
  broken – *see* Failure, heart
  failure – *see* Failure, heart
  neurosis, psychoneurosis 300.11
Complaint – *see also* Disease
  bowel, functional 564.9
    psychogenic 306.4
  intestine, functional 564.9
    psychogenic 306.4
  kidney (*see also* Disease, renal) 593.9
  liver 573.9
  miners' 500
Complete – *see* condition
Complex
  cardiorenal (*see also* Hypertension, cardiorenal) 404.90
  castration 300.9
  Costen's 524.60
  ego-dystonic homosexuality 302.0
  Eisenmenger's (ventricular septal defect) 745.4
  homosexual, ego-dystonic 302.0
  hypersexual 302.89
  inferiority 301.9
  jumped process
    spine – *see* Dislocation, vertebra
  primary, tuberculosis (*see also* Tuberculosis) 010.0❺
  Taussig-Bing (transposition, aorta and overriding pulmonary artery) 745.11
Complications
  abortion NEC – *see* categories 634-639
  accidental puncture or laceration during a procedure 998.2
  amputation stump (late) (surgical) 997.60
    traumatic – *see* Amputation, traumatic
  anastomosis (and bypass) – *see also* Complications, due to (presence of) any device, implant, or graft classified to 996.0-996.5 NEC
    hemorrhage NEC 998.11
    intestinal (internal) NEC 997.4
      involving urinary tract 997.5
    mechanical – *see* Complications, mechanical, graft
    urinary tract (involving intestinal tract) 997.5
  anesthesia, anesthetic NEC (*see also* Anesthesia, complication) 995.22
    in labor and delivery 668.9❺
      affecting fetus or newborn 763.5
      cardiac 668.1❺
      central nervous system 668.2❺
      pulmonary 668.0❺
      specified type NEC 668.8❺
  aortocoronary (bypass) graft 996.03
    atherosclerosis – *see* Arteriosclerosis, coronary
    embolism 996.72
    occlusion NEC 996.72
    thrombus 996.72
  arthroplasty (*see also* Complications, prosthetic joint) 996.49
  artificial opening
    cecostomy 569.60
    colostomy 569.6❺
    cystostomy 997.5
    enterostomy 569.60
    esophagostomy 530.87
      infection 530.86
      mechanical 530.87
    gastrostomy 536.40
    ileostomy 569.60
    jejunostomy 569.60
    nephrostomy 997.5
    tracheostomy 519.00
    ureterostomy 997.5
    urethrostomy 997.5

Complications – *continued*
  bariatric surgery 997.4
  bile duct implant (prosthetic) NEC 996.79
    infection or inflammation 996.69
    mechanical 996.59
  bleeding (intraoperative) (postoperative) 998.11
  blood vessel graft 996.1
    aortocoronary 996.03
      atherosclerosis – *see* Arteriosclerosis, coronary
      embolism 996.72
      occlusion NEC 996.72
      thrombus 996.72
    atherosclerosis – *see* Arteriosclerosis, extremities
    embolism 996.74
    occlusion NEC 996.74
    thrombus 996.74
  bone growth stimulator NEC 996.78
    infection or inflammation 996.67
  bone marrow transplant 996.85
  breast implant (prosthetic) NEC 996.79
    infection or inflammation 996.69
    mechanical 996.54
  bypass – *see also* Complications, anastomosis
    aortocoronary 996.03
      atherosclerosis – *see* Arteriosclerosis, coronary
      embolism 996.72
      occlusion NEC 996.72
      thrombus 996.72
    carotid artery 996.1
      atherosclerosis – *see* Arteriosclerosis, coronary
      embolism 996.74
      occlusion NEC 996.74
      thrombus 996.74
  cardiac (*see also* Disease, heart) 429.9
    device, implant, or graft NEC 996.72
      infection or inflammation 996.61
      long-term effect 429.4
      mechanical (*see also* Complications, mechanical, by type) 996.00
      valve prosthesis 996.71
        infection or inflammation 996.61
    postoperative NEC 997.1
      long-term effect 429.4
  cardiorenal (*see also* Hypertension, cardiorenal) 404.90
  carotid artery bypass graft 996.1
    atherosclerosis – *see* Arteriosclerosis, coronary
    embolism 996.74
    occlusion NEC 996.74
    thrombus 996.74
  cataract fragments in eye 998.82
  catheter device NEC – *see also* Complications, due to (presence of) any device, implant, or graft classified to 996.0-996.5 NEC
    mechanical – *see* Complications, mechanical, catheter
  cecostomy 569.60
  cesarean section wound 674.3❺
  chemotherapy (antineoplastic) 995.29 ●
  chin implant (prosthetic) NEC 996.79
    infection or inflammation 996.69
    mechanical 996.59
  colostomy (enterostomy) 569.60
    specified type NEC 569.69
  contraceptive device, intrauterine NEC 996.76
    infection 996.65
    inflammation 996.65
    mechanical 996.32
  cord (umbilical) – *see* Complications, umbilical cord
  cornea
    due to
      contact lens 371.82
  coronary (artery) bypass (graft) NEC 996.03
    atherosclerosis – *see* Arteriosclerosis, coronary
    embolism 996.72
    infection or inflammation 996.61
    mechanical 996.03
    occlusion NEC 996.72
    specified type NEC 996.72
    thrombus 996.72
  cystostomy 997.5
  delivery 669.9❺
    procedure (instrumental) (manual) (surgical) 669.4❺
    specified type NEC 669.8❺

Complications – *continued*
- dialysis (hemodialysis) (peritoneal) (renal) NEC 999.9
  - catheter NEC – *see also* Complications, due to (presence of) any device, implant, or graft classified to 996.0-996.5 NEC
    - infection or inflammation 996.62
      - peritoneal 996.68
    - mechanical 996.1
      - peritoneal 996.56
- drug NEC 995.29 ●
- due to (presence of) any device, implant, or graft classified to 996.0-996.5 NEC 996.70
  - with infection or inflammation – *see* Complications, infection or inflammation, due to (presence of) any device, implant, or graft classified to 996.0-996.5 NEC
  - arterial NEC 996.74
    - coronary NEC 996.03
      - atherosclerosis – *see* Arteriosclerosis, coronary
      - embolism 996.72
      - occlusion NEC 996.72
      - specified type NEC 996.72
      - thrombus 996.72
    - renal dialysis 996.73
  - arteriovenous fistula or shunt NEC 996.74
  - bone growth stimulator 996.78
  - breast NEC 996.79
  - cardiac NEC 996.72
    - defibrillator 996.72
    - pacemaker 996.72
    - valve prosthesis 996.71
  - catheter NEC 996.79
    - spinal 996.75
    - urinary, indwelling 996.76
    - vascular NEC 996.74
      - renal dialysis 996.73
    - ventricular shunt 996.75
  - coronary (artery) bypass (graft) NEC 996.03
    - atherosclerosis – *see* Arteriosclerosis, coronary
    - embolism 996.72
    - occlusion NEC 996.72
    - thrombus 996.72
  - electrodes
    - brain 996.75
    - heart 996.72
  - esophagostomy 530.87
  - gastrointestinal NEC 996.79
  - genitourinary NEC 996.76
  - heart valve prosthesis NEC 996.71
  - infusion pump 996.74
  - insulin pump 996.57
  - internal
    - joint prosthesis 996.77
    - orthopedic NEC 996.78
    - specified type NEC 996.79
  - intrauterine contraceptive device NEC 996.76
  - joint prosthesis, internal NEC 996.77
  - mechanical – *see* Complications, mechanical
  - nervous system NEC 996.75
  - ocular lens NEC 996.79
  - orbital NEC 996.79
  - orthopedic NEC 996.78
    - joint, internal 996.77
    - renal dialysis 996.73
  - specified type NEC 996.79
  - urinary catheter, indwelling 996.76
  - vascular NEC 996.74
  - ventricular shunt 996.75
- during dialysis NEC 999.9
- ectopic or molar pregnancy NEC 639.9
- electroshock therapy NEC 999.9
- enterostomy 569.60
  - specified type NEC 569.69
- esophagostomy 530.87
  - infection 530.86
  - mechanical 530.87
- external (fixation) device with internal component(s) NEC 996.78
  - infection or inflammation 996.67
  - mechanical 996.49
- extracorporeal circulation NEC 999.9
- eye implant (prosthetic) NEC 996.79
  - infection or inflammation 996.69
  - mechanical
    - ocular lens 996.53
    - orbital globe 996.59
- gastrointestinal, postoperative NEC (*see also* Complications, surgical procedures) 997.4

Complications – *continued*
- gastrostomy 536.40
  - specified type NEC 536.49
- genitourinary device, implant or graft NEC 996.76
  - infection or inflammation 996.65
    - urinary catheter, indwelling 996.64
  - mechanical (*see also* Complications, mechanical, by type) 996.30
  - specified NEC 996.39
- graft (bypass) (patch) – *see also* Complications, due to (presence of) any device, implant, or graft classified to 996.0-996.5 NEC
  - bone marrow 996.85
  - corneal NEC 996.79
    - infection or inflammation 996.69
    - rejection or reaction 996.51
  - mechanical – *see* Complications, mechanical, graft
  - organ (immune or nonimmune cause) (partial) (total) 996.80
    - bone marrow 996.85
    - heart 996.83
    - intestines 996.87
    - kidney 996.81
    - liver 996.82
    - lung 996.84
    - pancreas 996.86
    - specified NEC 996.89
  - skin NEC 996.79
    - infection or inflammation 996.69
    - rejection 996.52
      - artificial 996.55
      - decellularized allodermis 996.55
- heart – *see also* Disease, heart transplant (immune or nonimmune cause) 996.83
- hematoma (intraoperative) (postoperative) 998.12
- hemorrhage (intraoperative) (postoperative) 998.11
- hyperalimentation therapy NEC 999.9
- immunization (procedure) – *see* Complications, vaccination
- implant – *see also* Complications, due to (presence of) any device, implant, or graft classified to 996.0-996.5 NEC
  - dental placement, hemorrhagic 525.71 ●
  - mechanical, – *see* Complications, mechanical, implant
- infection and inflammation
  - due to (presence of) any device, implant or graft classified to 996.0-996.5 NEC 996.60
    - arterial NEC 996.62
      - coronary 996.61
      - renal dialysis 996.62
    - arteriovenous fistula or shunt 996.62
    - artificial heart 996.61
    - bone growth stimulator 996.67
    - breast 996.69
    - cardiac 996.61
    - catheter NEC 996.69
      - central venous 999.31 ●
      - Hickman 999.31 ●
      - peripherally inserted central (PICC) 999.31 ●
      - peritoneal 996.68
      - spinal 996.63
      - triple lumen 999.31 ●
      - urinary, indwelling 996.64
      - vascular ▶(arterial) (dialysis) (peripheral venous)◀ NEC 996.62
      - ventricular shunt 996.63
    - central venous catheter 999.31 ●
    - coronary artery bypass 996.61
    - electrodes
      - brain 996.63
      - heart 996.61
    - gastrointestinal NEC 996.69
    - genitourinary NEC 996.65
      - indwelling urinary catheter 996.64
    - heart assist device 996.61
    - heart valve 996.61
    - Hickman catheter 999.31 ●
    - infusion pump 996.62
    - insulin pump 996.69
    - intrauterine contraceptive device 996.65
    - joint prosthesis, internal 996.66
    - ocular lens 996.69
    - orbital (implant) 996.69
    - orthopedic NEC 996.67
      - joint, internal 996.66
    - peripherally inserted central catheter (PICC) 999.31 ●

Complications – *continued*
- infection and inflammation – *continued*
  - due to (presence of) any device, implant or graft classified to 996.0-996.5 - *continued*
    - specified type NEC 996.69
    - triple lumen catheter 999.31 ●
    - urinary catheter, indwelling 996.64
    - ventricular shunt 996.63
- infusion (procedure) 999.9
  - blood – *see* Complications, transfusion
  - infection NEC 999.39 ▲
  - sepsis NEC 999.39 ▲
- inhalation therapy NEC 999.9
- injection (procedure) 999.9
  - drug reaction (*see also* Reaction, drug) 995.27
  - infection NEC 999.39 ▲
  - sepsis NEC 999.39 ▲
  - serum (prophylactic) (therapeutic) – *see* Complications, vaccination
  - vaccine (any) – *see* Complications, vaccination
- inoculation (any) – *see* Complications, vaccination
- insulin pump 996.57
- internal device (catheter) (electronic) (fixation) (prosthetic) – *see also* Complications, due to (presence of) any device, implant, or graft classified to 996.0-996.5 NEC
  - mechanical – *see* Complications, mechanical
- intestinal transplant (immune or nonimmune cause) 996.87
- intraoperative bleeding or hemorrhage 998.11
- intrauterine contraceptive device (*see also* Complications, contraceptive device) 996.76
  - with fetal damage affecting management of pregnancy 655.8❺
  - infection or inflammation 996.65
- jejunostomy 569.60
- kidney transplant (immune or nonimmune cause) 996.81
- labor 669.9❺
  - specified condition NEC 669.8❺
- liver transplant (immune or nonimmune cause) 996.82
- lumbar puncture 349.0
- mechanical
  - anastomosis – *see* Complications, mechanical, graft
  - artificial heart 996.09
  - bypass – *see* Complications, mechanical, graft
  - catheter NEC 996.59
    - cardiac 996.09
    - cystostomy 996.39
    - dialysis (hemodialysis) 996.1
      - peritoneal 996.56
    - during a procedure 998.2
    - urethral, indwelling 996.31
  - colostomy 569.62
  - device NEC 996.59
    - balloon (counterpulsation), intra-aortic 996.1
    - cardiac 996.00
      - automatic implantable defibrillator 996.04
      - long-term effect 429.4
      - specified NEC 996.09
    - contraceptive, intrauterine 996.32
    - counterpulsation, intra-aortic 996.1
    - fixation, external, with internal components 996.49
    - fixation, internal (nail, rod, plate) 996.40
    - genitourinary 996.30
      - specified NEC 996.39
    - insulin pump 996.57
    - nervous system 996.2
    - orthopedic, internal 996.40
      - prosthetic joint (*see also* Complications, mechanical, device, orthopedic, prosthetic, joint) 996.47
    - prosthetic NEC 996.59
      - joint (*see also* Complications, prosthetic joint) 996.47
        - articular bearing surface wear 996.46
        - aseptic loosening 996.41
        - breakage 996.43
        - dislocation 996.42
        - failure 996.43
        - fracture 996.43
          - around prosthetic 996.44
          - peri-prosthetic 996.44
        - instability 996.42
        - loosening 996.41
        - peri-prosthetic osteolysis 996.45
        - subluxation 996.42
        - wear 996.46

Complications – *continued*
mechanical – *continued*
device – *continued*
umbrella, vena cava 996.1
vascular 996.1
dorsal column stimulator 996.2
electrode NEC 996.59
brain 996.2
cardiac 996.01
spinal column 996.2
enterostomy 569.62
esophagostomy 530.87
fistula, arteriovenous, surgically created 996.1
gastrostomy 536.42
graft NEC 996.52
aortic (bifurcation) 996.1
aortocoronary bypass 996.03
blood vessel NEC 996.1
bone 996.49
cardiac 996.00
carotid artery bypass 996.1
cartilage 996.49
corneal 996.51
coronary bypass 996.03
decellularized allodermis 996.55
genitourinary 996.30
specified NEC 996.39
muscle 996.49
nervous system 996.2
organ (immune or nonimmune cause) 996.80
heart 996.83
intestines 996.87
kidney 996.81
liver 996.82
lung 996.84
pancreas 996.86
specified NEC 996.89
orthopedic, internal 996.49
peripheral nerve 996.2
prosthetic NEC 996.59
skin 996.52
artificial 996.55
specified NEC 996.59
tendon 996.49
tissue NEC 996.52
tooth 996.59
ureter, without mention of resection 996.39
vascular 996.1
heart valve prosthesis 996.02
long-term effect 429.4
implant NEC 996.59
cardiac 996.00
automatic implantable defibrillator 996.04
long-term effect 429.4
specified NEC 996.09
electrode NEC 996.59
brain 996.2
cardiac 996.01
spinal column 996.2
genitourinary 996.30
nervous system 996.2
orthopedic, internal 996.49
prosthetic NEC 996.59
in
bile duct 996.59
breast 996.54
chin 996.59
eye
ocular lens 996.53
orbital globe 996.59
vascular 996.1
insulin pump 996.57
nonabsorbable surgical material 996.59
pacemaker NEC 996.59
brain 996.2
cardiac 996.01
nerve (phrenic) 996.2
patch – *see* Complications, mechanical, graft
prosthesis NEC 996.59
bile duct 996.59
breast 996.54
chin 996.59
ocular lens 996.53
reconstruction, vas deferens 996.39
reimplant NEC 996.59
extremity (*see also* Complications, reattached, extremity) 996.90
organ (*see also* Complications, transplant, organ, by site) 996.80
repair – *see* Complications, mechanical, graft

Complications – *continued*
mechanical – *continued*
respirator [ventilator] V46.14
shunt NEC 996.59
arteriovenous, surgically created 996.1
ventricular (communicating) 996.2
stent NEC 996.59
tracheostomy 519.02
vas deferens reconstruction 996.39
ventilator [respirator] V46.14
medical care NEC 999.9
cardiac NEC 997.1
gastrointestinal NEC 997.4
nervous system NEC 997.00
peripheral vascular NEC 997.2
respiratory NEC 997.3
urinary NEC 997.5
vascular
mesenteric artery 997.71
other vessels 997.79
peripheral vessels 997.2
renal artery 997.72
nephrostomy 997.5
nervous system
device, implant, or graft NEC 349.1
mechanical 996.2
postoperative NEC 997.00
obstetric 669.9❺
procedure (instrumental) (manual) (surgical) 669.4❺
specified NEC 669.8❺
surgical wound 674.3❺
ocular lens implant NEC 996.79
infection or inflammation 996.69
mechanical 996.53
organ transplant – *see* Complications, transplant, organ, by site
orthopedic device, implant, or graft
internal (fixation) (nail) (plate) (rod) NEC 996.78
infection or inflammation 996.67
joint prosthesis 996.77
infection or inflammation 996.66
mechanical 996.40
pacemaker (cardiac) 996.72
infection or inflammation 996.61
mechanical 996.01
pancreas transplant (immune or nonimmune cause) 996.86
perfusion NEC 999.9
perineal repair (obstetrical) 674.3❺
disruption 674.2❺
pessary (uterus) (vagina) – *see* Complications, contraceptive device
phototherapy 990
postcystoscopic 997.5
postmastoidectomy NEC 383.30
postoperative – *see* Complications, surgical procedures
pregnancy NEC 646.9❺
affecting fetus or newborn 761.9
prosthetic device, internal – *see also* Complications, due to (presence of) any device, implant or graft classified to 996.0-996.5 NEC
mechanical NEC (*see also* Complications, mechanical) 996.59
puerperium NEC (*see also* Puerperal) 674.9❺
puncture, spinal 349.0
pyelogram 997.5
radiation 990
radiotherapy 990
reattached
body part, except extremity 996.99
extremity (infection) (rejection) 996.90
arm(s) 996.94
digit(s) (hand) 996.93
foot 996.95
finger(s) 996.93
foot 996.95
forearm 996.91
hand 996.92
leg 996.96
lower NEC 996.96
toe(s) 996.95
upper NEC 996.94
reimplant NEC – *see also* Complications, due to (presence of) any device, implant, or graft classified to 996.0-996.5 NEC
bone marrow 996.85

Complications – *continued*
reimplant – *continued*
extremity (*see also* Complications, reattached, extremity) 996.90
due to infection 996.90
mechanical – *see* Complications, mechanical, reimplant
organ (immune or nonimmune cause) (partial) (total) (*see also* Complications, transplant, organ, by site) 996.80
renal allograft 996.81
renal dialysis – *see* Complications, dialysis
respirator [ventilator], mechanical V46.14
respiratory 519.9
device, implant or graft NEC 996.79
infection or inflammation 996.69
mechanical 996.59
distress syndrome, adult, following trauma or surgery 518.5
insufficiency, acute, postoperative 518.5
postoperative NEC 997.3
therapy NEC 999.9
sedation during labor and delivery 668.9❺
affecting fetus or newborn 763.5
cardiac 668.1❺
central nervous system 668.2❺
pulmonary 668.0❺
specified type NEC 668.8❺
seroma (intraoperative) (postoperative) (noninfected) 998.13
infected 998.51
shunt – *see also* Complications, due to (presence of) any device, implant, or graft classified to 996.0-996.5 NEC
mechanical – *see* Complications, mechanical, shunt
specified body system NEC
device, implant, or graft – *see* Complications, due to (presence of) any device, implant, or graft classified to 996.0-996.5 NEC
postoperative NEC 997.99
spinal puncture or tap 349.0
stoma, external
gastrointestinal tract
colostomy 569.60
enterostomy 569.60
esophagostomy 530.87
infection 530.86
mechanical 530.87
gastrostomy 536.40
urinary tract 997.5
stomach banding 997.4
stomach stapling 997.4
surgical procedures 998.9
accidental puncture or laceration 998.2
amputation stump (late) 997.60
anastomosis – *see* Complications, anastomosis
burst stitches or sutures (external) 998.32
internal 998.31
cardiac 997.1
long-term effect following cardiac surgery 429.4
catheter device – *see* Complications, catheter device
cataract fragments in eye 998.82
cecostomy malfunction 569.62
colostomy malfunction 569.62
cystostomy malfunction 997.5
dehiscence (of incision) (external) 998.32
internal 998.31
dialysis NEC (*see also* Complications, dialysis) 999.9
disruption
anastomosis (internal) – *see* Complications, mechanical, graft
internal suture (line) 998.31
wound (external) 998.32
internal 998.31
dumping syndrome (postgastrectomy) 564.2
elephantiasis or lymphedema 997.99
postmastectomy 457.0
emphysema (surgical) 998.81
enterostomy malfunction 569.62
esophagostomy malfunction 530.87
evisceration 998.32
fistula (persistent postoperative) 998.6
foreign body inadvertently left in wound (sponge) (suture) (swab) 998.4

Complications – Complications

- **Complications** – *continued*
  - surgical procedures – *continued*
    - from nonabsorbable surgical material (Dacron) (mesh) (permanent suture) (reinforcing) (Teflon) – *see* Complications due to (presence of) any device, implant or graft classified to 996.0-996.5 NEC
    - gastrointestinal NEC 997.4
    - gastrostomy malfunction 536.42
    - hematoma 998.12
    - hemorrhage 998.11
    - ileostomy malfunction 569.62
    - internal prosthetic device NEC (*see also* Complications, internal device) 996.70
      - hemolytic anemia 283.19
      - infection or inflammation 996.60
      - malfunction – *see* Complications, mechanical
      - mechanical complication – *see* Complications, mechanical
      - thrombus 996.70
    - jejunostomy malfunction 569.62
    - nervous system NEC 997.00
    - obstruction, internal anastomosis – *see* Complications, mechanical, graft
    - other body system NEC 997.99
    - peripheral vascular NEC 997.2
    - postcardiotomy syndrome 429.4
    - postcholecystectomy syndrome 576.0
    - postcommissurotomy syndrome 429.4
    - postgastrectomy dumping syndrome 564.2
    - postmastectomy lymphedema syndrome 457.0
    - postmastoidectomy 383.30
      - cholesteatoma, recurrent 383.32
      - cyst, mucosal 383.31
      - granulation 383.33
      - inflammation, chronic 383.33
    - postvagotomy syndrome 564.2
    - postvalvulotomy syndrome 429.4
    - reattached extremity (infection) (rejection) (*see also* Complications, reattached extremity) 996.90
    - respiratory NEC 997.3
    - seroma 998.13
    - shock (endotoxic) (hypovolemic) (septic) 998.0
    - shunt, prosthetic (thrombus) – *see also* Complications, due to (presence of) any device, implant, or graft classified to 996.0-996.5 NEC
      - hemolytic anemia 283.19
    - specified complication NEC 998.89
    - stitch abscess 998.59
    - transplant – *see* Complications, graft
    - ureterostomy malfunction 997.5
    - urethrostomy malfunction 997.5
    - urinary NEC 997.5
    - vascular
      - mesenteric artery 997.71
      - other vessels 997.79
      - peripheral vessels 997.2
      - renal artery 997.72
    - wound infection 998.59
  - therapeutic misadventure NEC 999.9
    - surgical treatment 998.9
  - tracheostomy 519.00
  - transfusion (blood) (lymphocytes) (plasma) NEC 999.8
    - acute lung injury (TRALI) 518.7
    - atrophy, liver, yellow, subacute (within 8 months of administration) – *see* Hepatitis, viral
    - bone marrow 996.85
    - embolism
      - air 999.1
      - thrombus 999.2
    - hemolysis NEC 999.8
      - bone marrow 996.85
    - hepatitis (serum) (type B) (within 8 months after administration) – *see* Hepatitis, viral
    - incompatibility reaction (ABO) (blood group) 999.6
      - Rh (factor) 999.7
    - infection 999.39 ▲
    - jaundice (serum) (within 8 months after administration) – *see* Hepatitis, viral
    - sepsis 999.39 ▲
    - shock or reaction NEC 999.8
      - bone marrow 996.85
    - subacute yellow atrophy of liver (within 8 months after administration) – *see* Hepatitis, viral
    - thromboembolism 999.2

- **Complications** – *continued*
  - transplant NEC – *see also* Complications, due to (presence of) any device, implant, or graft classified to 996.0-996.5 NEC
    - bone marrow 996.85
    - organ (immune or nonimmune cause) (partial) (total) 996.80
      - bone marrow 996.85
      - heart 996.83
      - intestines 996.87
      - kidney 996.81
      - liver 996.82
      - lung 996.84
      - pancreas 996.86
      - specified NEC 996.89
  - trauma NEC (early) 958.8
  - ultrasound therapy NEC 999.9
  - umbilical cord
    - affecting fetus or newborn 762.6
    - complicating delivery 663.9⑤
      - affecting fetus or newborn 762.6
      - specified type NEC 663.8⑤
  - urethral catheter NEC 996.76
    - infection or inflammation 996.64
    - mechanical 996.31
  - urinary, postoperative NEC 997.5
  - vaccination 999.9
    - anaphylaxis NEC 999.4
    - cellulitis 999.39 ▲
    - encephalitis or encephalomyelitis 323.51
    - hepatitis (serum) (type B) (within 8 months after administration) – *see* Hepatitis, viral
    - infection (general) (local) NEC 999.39 ▲
    - jaundice (serum) (within 8 months after administration) – *see* Hepatitis, viral
    - meningitis 997.09 *[321.8]*
    - myelitis 323.52
    - protein sickness 999.5
    - reaction (allergic) 999.5
      - Herxheimer's 995.0
      - serum 999.5
    - sepsis 999.39 ▲
    - serum intoxication, sickness, rash, or other serum reaction NEC 999.5
    - shock (allergic) (anaphylactic) 999.4
    - subacute yellow atrophy of liver (within 8 months after administration) – *see* Hepatitis, viral
    - vaccinia (generalized) 999.0
      - localized 999.39 ▲
  - vascular
    - device, implant, or graft NEC 996.74
      - infection or inflammation 996.62
      - mechanical NEC 996.1
        - cardiac (*see also* Complications, mechanical, by type) 996.00
    - following infusion, perfusion, or transfusion 999.2
    - postoperative NEC 997.2
      - mesenteric artery 997.71
      - other vessels 997.79
      - peripheral vessels 997.2
      - renal artery 997.72
  - ventilation therapy NEC 999.9
  - ventilator [respirator], mechanical V46.14
- **Compound presentation, complicating delivery** 652.8⑤
  - causing obstructed labor 660.0⑤
- **Compressed air disease** 993.3
- **Compression**
  - with injury – *see* specific injury
  - arm NEC 354.9
  - artery 447.1
    - celiac, syndrome 447.4
  - brachial plexus 353.0
  - brain (stem) 348.4
    - due to
      - contusion, brain – *see* Contusion, brain
      - injury NEC – *see also* Hemorrhage, brain, traumatic
        - birth – *see* Birth, injury, brain
      - laceration, brain – *see* Laceration, brain
    - osteopathic 739.0
  - bronchus 519.19
  - by cicatrix – *see* Cicatrix
  - cardiac 423.9
  - cauda equina 344.60
    - with neurogenic bladder 344.61
  - celiac (artery) (axis) 447.4
  - cerebral – *see* Compression, brain
  - cervical plexus 353.2

- **Compression** – *continued*
  - cord (umbilical) – *see* Compression, umbilical cord
  - cranial nerve 352.9
    - second 377.49
    - third (partial) 378.51
      - total 378.52
    - fourth 378.53
    - fifth 350.8
    - sixth 378.54
    - seventh 351.8
  - divers' squeeze 993.3
  - duodenum (external) (*see also* Obstruction, duodenum) 537.3
  - during birth 767.9
  - esophagus 530.3
    - congenital, external 750.3
  - Eustachian tube 381.63
  - facies (congenital) 754.0
  - fracture – *see* Fracture, by site
  - heart – *see* Disease, heart
  - intestine (*see also* Obstruction, intestine) 560.9
    - with hernia – *see* Hernia, by site, with obstruction
  - laryngeal nerve, recurrent 478.79
  - leg NEC 355.8
  - lower extremity NEC 355.8
  - lumbosacral plexus 353.1
  - lung 518.89
  - lymphatic vessel 457.1
  - medulla – *see* Compression, brain
  - nerve NEC – *see also* Disorder, nerve
    - arm NEC 354.9
    - autonomic nervous system (*see also* Neuropathy, peripheral, autonomic) 337.9
    - axillary 353.0
    - cranial NEC 352.9
    - due to displacement of intervertebral disc 722.2
      - with myelopathy 722.70
      - cervical 722.0
        - with myelopathy 722.71
      - lumbar, lumbosacral 722.10
        - with myelopathy 722.73
      - thoracic, thoracolumbar 722.11
        - with myelopathy 722.72
    - iliohypogastric 355.79
    - ilioinguinal 355.79
    - leg NEC 355.8
    - lower extremity NEC 355.8
    - median (in carpal tunnel) 354.0
    - obturator 355.79
    - optic 377.49
    - plantar 355.6
    - posterior tibial (in tarsal tunnel) 355.5
    - root (by scar tissue) NEC 724.9
      - cervical NEC 723.4
      - lumbar NEC 724.4
      - lumbosacral 724.4
      - thoracic 724.4
    - saphenous 355.79
    - sciatic (acute) 355.0
    - sympathetic 337.9
    - traumatic – *see* Injury, nerve
    - ulnar 354.2
    - upper extremity NEC 354.9
  - peripheral – *see* Compression, nerve
  - spinal (cord) (old or nontraumatic) 336.9
    - by displacement of intervertebral disc – *see* Displacement, intervertebral disc
    - nerve
      - root NEC 724.9
        - postoperative 722.80
          - cervical region 722.81
          - lumbar region 722.83
          - thoracic region 722.82
        - traumatic – *see* Injury, nerve, spinal
      - traumatic – *see* Injury, nerve, spinal
    - spondylogenic 721.91
      - cervical 721.1
      - lumbar, lumbosacral 721.42
      - thoracic 721.41
    - traumatic – *see also* Injury, spinal, by site
      - with fracture, vertebra – *see* Fracture, vertebra, by site, with spinal cord injury
  - spondylogenic – *see* Compression, spinal cord, spondylogenic
  - subcostal nerve (syndrome) 354.8
  - sympathetic nerve NEC 337.9
  - syndrome 958.5
  - thorax 512.8
    - iatrogenic 512.1

Compression – *continued*
thorax – *continued*
postoperative 512.1
trachea 519.19
congenital 748.3
ulnar nerve (by scar tissue) 354.2
umbilical cord
affecting fetus or newborn 762.5
cord prolapsed 762.4
complicating delivery 663.2❺
cord around neck 663.1❺
cord prolapsed 663.0❺
upper extremity NEC 354.9
ureter 593.3
urethra – *see* Stricture, urethra
vein 459.2
vena cava (inferior) (superior) 459.2
vertebral NEC – *see* Compression, spinal (cord)
Compulsion, compulsive
eating 307.51
neurosis (obsessive) 300.3
personality 301.4
states (mixed) 300.3
swearing 300.3
in Gilles de la Tourette's syndrome 307.23
tics and spasms 307.22
water drinking NEC (syndrome) 307.9
Concato's disease (pericardial polyserositis) 423.2
peritoneal 568.82
pleural – *see* Pleurisy
Concavity, chest wall 738.3
Concealed
hemorrhage NEC 459.0
penis 752.65
Concentric fading 368.12
Concern (normal) **about sick person in family** V61.49
Concrescence (teeth) 520.2
Concretio cordis 423.1
rheumatic 393
Concretion – *see also* Calculus
appendicular 543.9
canaliculus 375.57
clitoris 624.8
conjunctiva 372.54
eyelid 374.56
intestine (impaction) (obstruction) 560.39
lacrimal (passages) 375.57
prepuce (male) 605
female (clitoris) 624.8
salivary gland (any) 527.5
seminal vesicle 608.89
stomach 537.89
tonsil 474.8
Concussion (current) 850.9
with
loss of consciousness 850.5
brief (less than one hour)
30 minutes or less 850.11
31-59 minutes 850.12
moderate (1-24 hours) 850.2
prolonged (more than 24 hours) (with complete recovery) (with return to pre-existing conscious level) 850.3
without return to pre-existing conscious level 850.4
mental confusion or disorientation (without loss of consciousness) 850.0
with loss of consciousness – *see* Concussion, with, loss of consciousness
without loss of consciousness 850.0
blast (air) (hydraulic) (immersion) (underwater) 869.0
with open wound into cavity 869.1
abdomen or thorax – *see* Injury, internal, by site
brain – *see* Concussion, brain
ear (acoustic nerve trauma) 951.5
with perforation, tympanic membrane – *see* Wound, open, ear drum
thorax – *see* Injury, internal, intrathoracic organs NEC
brain or cerebral (without skull fracture) 850.9
with
loss of consciousness 850.5
brief (less than one hour)
30 minutes or less 850.11
31-59 minutes 850.12
moderate (1-24 hours) 850.2

Concussion – *continued*
brain or cerebral – *continued*
with – *continued*
loss of consciousness – *continued*
prolonged (more than 24 hours) (with complete recovery) (with return to pre-existing conscious level) 850.3
without return to pre-existing conscious level 850.4
mental confusion or disorientation (without loss of consciousness) 850.0
with loss of consciousness – *see* Concussion, brain, with, loss of consciousness
skull fracture – *see* Fracture, skull, by site
without loss of consciousness 850.0
cauda equina 952.4
cerebral – *see* Concussion, brain
conus medullaris (spine) 952.4
hydraulic – *see* Concussion, blast
internal organs – *see* Injury, internal, by site
labyrinth – *see* Injury, intracranial
ocular 921.3
osseous labyrinth – *see* Injury, intracranial
spinal (cord) – *see also* Injury, spinal, by site
due to
broken
back – *see* Fracture, vertebra, by site, with spinal cord injury
neck – *see* Fracture, vertebra, cervical, with spinal cord injury
fracture, fracture dislocation, or compression fracture of spine or vertebra – *see* Fracture, vertebra, by site, with spinal cord injury
syndrome 310.2
underwater blast – *see* Concussion, blast
Condition – *see also* Disease
psychiatric 298.9
respiratory NEC 519.9
acute or subacute NEC 519.9
due to
external agent 508.9
specified type NEC 508.8
fumes or vapors (chemical) (inhalation) 506.3
radiation 508.0
chronic NEC 519.9
due to
external agent 508.9
specified type NEC 508.8
fumes or vapors (chemical) (inhalation) 506.4
radiation 508.1
due to
external agent 508.9
specified type NEC 508.8
fumes or vapors (chemical) inhalation 506.9
Conduct disturbance (*see also* Disturbance, conduct) 312.9
adjustment reaction 309.3
hyperkinetic 314.2
Condyloma NEC 078.10
acuminatum 078.11
gonorrheal 098.0
latum 091.3
syphilitic 091.3
congenital 090.0
venereal, syphilitic 091.3
Confinement – *see* Delivery
Conflagration – *see also* Burn, by site
asphyxia (by inhalation of smoke, gases, fumes, or vapors) 987.9
specified agent – *see* Table of Drugs and Chemicals
Conflict
family V61.9
specified circumstance NEC V61.8
interpersonal NEC V62.81
marital V61.10
involving divorce or estrangement V61.0
parent-child V61.20
partner V61.10
Confluent – *see* condition
Confusion, confused (mental) (state) (*see also* State, confusional) 298.9
acute 293.0
epileptic 293.0
postoperative 293.9
psychogenic 298.2

Confusion, confused – *continued*
reactive (from emotional stress, psychological trauma) 298.2
subacute 293.1
Confusional arousals 327.41
Congelation 991.9
Congenital – *see also* condition
aortic septum 747.29
generalized fibromatosis (CGF) 759.89
intrinsic factor deficiency 281.0
malformation – *see* Anomaly
Congestion, congestive
asphyxia, newborn 768.9
bladder 596.8
bowel 569.89
brain (*see also* Disease, cerebrovascular NEC) 437.8
malarial 084.9
breast 611.79
bronchi 519.19
bronchial tube 519.19
catarrhal 472.0
cerebral – *see* Congestion, brain
cerebrospinal – *see* Congestion, brain
chest 786.9 ▲
chill 780.99
malarial (*see also* Malaria) 084.6
circulatory NEC 459.9
conjunctiva 372.71
due to disturbance of circulation 459.9
duodenum 537.3
enteritis – *see* Enteritis
eye 372.71
fibrosis syndrome (pelvic) 625.5
gastroenteritis – *see* Enteritis
general 799.89
glottis 476.0
heart (*see also* Failure, heart) 428.0
hepatic 573.0
hypostatic (lung) 514
intestine 569.89
intracranial – *see* Congestion, brain
kidney 593.89
labyrinth 386.50
larynx 476.0
liver 573.0
lung 786.9 ▲
active or acute (*see also* Pneumonia) 486
congenital 770.0
chronic 514
hypostatic 514
idiopathic, acute 518.5
passive 514
malaria, malarial (brain) (fever) (*see also* Malaria) 084.6
medulla – *see* Congestion, brain
nasal 478.19
nose 478.19 ●
orbit, orbital 376.33
inflammatory (chronic) 376.10
acute 376.00
ovary 620.8
pancreas 577.8
pelvic, female 625.5
pleural 511.0
prostate (active) 602.1
pulmonary – *see* Congestion, lung
renal 593.89
retina 362.89
seminal vesicle 608.89
spinal cord 336.1
spleen 289.51
chronic 289.51
stomach 537.89
trachea 464.11
urethra 599.84
uterus 625.5
with subinvolution 621.1
viscera 799.89
Congestive – *see* Congestion
Conical
cervix 622.6
cornea 371.60
teeth 520.2
Conjoined twins 759.4
causing disproportion (fetopelvic) 653.7❺
Conjugal maladjustment V61.10
involving divorce or estrangement V61.0
Conjunctiva – *see* condition

Compression – Conjunctiva

- **Conjunctivitis** (exposure) (infectious) (nondiphtheritic) (pneumococcal) (pustular) (staphylococcal) (streptococcal) NEC 372.30
  - actinic 370.24
  - acute 372.00
    - atopic 372.05
    - contagious 372.03
    - follicular 372.02
    - hemorrhagic (viral) 077.4
  - adenoviral (acute) 077.3
  - allergic (chronic) 372.14
    - with hay fever 372.05
  - anaphylactic 372.05
  - angular 372.03
  - Apollo (viral) 077.4
  - atopic 372.05
  - blennorrhagic (neonatorum) 098.40
  - catarrhal 372.03
  - chemical 372.01
    - allergic 372.05
    - meaning corrosion – *see* Burn, conjunctiva
  - chlamydial 077.98
    - due to
      - Chlamydia trachomatis – *see* Trachoma
      - paratrachoma 077.0
  - chronic 372.10
    - allergic 372.14
    - follicular 372.12
    - simple 372.11
    - specified type NEC 372.14
    - vernal 372.13
  - diphtheritic 032.81
  - due to
    - dust 372.05
    - enterovirus type 70 077.4
    - erythema multiforme 695.1 *[372.33]*
    - filariasis (*see also* Filariasis) 125.9 *[372.15]*
    - mucocutaneous
      - disease NEC 372.33
      - leishmaniasis 085.5 *[372.15]*
    - Reiter's disease 099.3 *[372.33]*
    - syphilis 095.8 *[372.10]*
    - toxoplasmosis (acquired) 130.1
      - congenital (active) 771.2
    - trachoma – *see* Trachoma
  - dust 372.05
  - eczematous 370.31
  - epidemic 077.1
    - hemorrhagic 077.4
  - follicular (acute) 372.02
    - adenoviral (acute) 077.3
    - chronic 372.12
  - glare 370.24
  - gonococcal (neonatorum) 098.40
  - granular (trachomatous) 076.1
    - late effect 139.1
  - hemorrhagic (acute) (epidemic) 077.4
  - herpetic (simplex) 054.43
    - zoster 053.21
  - inclusion 077.0
  - infantile 771.6
  - influenzal 372.03
  - Koch-Weeks 372.03
  - light 372.05
  - medicamentosa 372.05
  - membranous 372.04
  - meningococcic 036.89
  - Morax-Axenfeld 372.02
  - mucopurulent NEC 372.03
  - neonatal 771.6
    - gonococcal 098.40
  - Newcastle's 077.8
  - nodosa 360.14
  - of Beal 077.3
  - parasitic 372.15
    - filariasis (*see also* Filariasis) 125.9 *[372.15]*
    - mucocutaneous leishmaniasis 085.5 *[372.15]*
  - Parinaud's 372.02
  - petrificans 372.39
  - phlyctenular 370.31
  - pseudomembranous 372.04
    - diphtheritic 032.81
  - purulent 372.03
  - Reiter's 099.3 *[372.33]*
  - rosacea 695.3 *[372.31]*
  - serous 372.01
    - viral 077.99
  - simple chronic 372.11
  - specified NEC 372.39
  - sunlamp 372.04
  - swimming pool 077.0

- **Conjunctivitis** – *continued*
  - trachomatous (follicular) 076.1
    - acute 076.0
    - late effect 139.1
  - traumatic NEC 372.39
  - tuberculous (*see also* Tuberculosis) 017.3❺ *[370.31]*
  - tularemic 021.3
  - tularensis 021.3
  - vernal 372.13
    - limbar 372.13 *[370.32]*
  - viral 077.99
    - acute hemorrhagic 077.4
    - specified NEC 077.8
- **Conjunctoblepharitis** – *see* Conjunctivitis
- **Conjunctivochalasis** 372.81
- **Conn** (-Louis) **syndrome** (primary aldosteronism) 255.12
- **Connective tissue** – *see* condition
- **Conradi** (-Hünermann) **syndrome or disease** (chondrodysplasia calcificans congenita) 756.59
- **Consanguinity** V19.7
- **Consecutive** – *see* condition
- **Consolidated lung** (base) – *see* Pneumonia, lobar
- **Constipation** 564.00
  - atonic 564.09
  - drug induced
    - correct substance properly administered 564.09
    - overdose or wrong substance given or taken 977.9
      - specified drug – *see* Table of Drugs and Chemicals
  - neurogenic 564.09
  - other specified NEC 564.09
  - outlet dysfunction 564.02
  - psychogenic 306.4
  - simple 564.00
  - slow transit 564.01
  - spastic 564.09
- **Constitutional** – *see also* condition
  - arterial hypotension (*see also* Hypotension) 458.9
  - obesity 278.00
    - morbid 278.01
  - psychopathic state 301.9
  - short stature in childhood 783.43
  - state, developmental V21.9
    - specified development NEC V21.8
  - substandard 301.6
- **Constitutionally substandard** 301.6
- **Constriction**
  - anomalous, meningeal bands or folds 742.8
  - aortic arch (congenital) 747.10
  - asphyxiation or suffocation by 994.7
  - bronchus 519.19
  - canal, ear (*see also* Stricture, ear canal, acquired) 380.50
  - duodenum 537.3
  - gallbladder (*see also* Obstruction, gallbladder) 575.2
    - congenital 751.69
  - intestine (*see also* Obstruction, intestine) 560.9
  - larynx 478.74
    - congenital 748.3
  - meningeal bands or folds, anomalous 742.8
  - organ or site, congenital NEC – *see* Atresia
  - prepuce (congenital) 605
  - pylorus 537.0
    - adult hypertrophic 537.0
    - congenital or infantile 750.5
    - newborn 750.5
  - ring (uterus) 661.4❺
    - affecting fetus or newborn 763.7
  - spastic – *see also* Spasm
    - ureter 593.3
    - urethra – *see* Stricture, urethra
  - stomach 537.89
  - ureter 593.3
  - urethra – *see* Stricture, urethra
  - visual field (functional) (peripheral) 368.45
- **Constrictive** – *see* condition
- **Consultation** V65.9
  - medical – *see also* Counseling, medical
  - specified reason NEC V65.8
  - without complaint or sickness V65.9
    - feared complaint unfounded V65.5
    - specified reason NEC V65.8

- **Consumption** – *see* Tuberculosis
- **Contact**
  - with
    - AIDS virus V01.79
    - anthrax V01.81
    - cholera V01.0
    - communicable disease V01.9
      - specified type NEC V01.89
      - viral NEC V01.79
    - Escherichia coli (E. coli) V01.83
    - German measles V01.4
    - gonorrhea V01.6
    - HIV V01.79
    - human immunodeficiency virus V01.79
    - meningococcus V01.84
    - parasitic disease NEC V01.89
    - poliomyelitis V01.2
    - rabies V01.5
    - rubella V01.4
    - SARS-associated coronavirus V01.82
    - smallpox V01.3
    - syphilis V01.6
    - tuberculosis V01.1
    - varicella V01.71
    - venereal disease V01.6
    - viral disease NEC V01.79
  - dermatitis – *see* Dermatitis
- **Contamination, food** (*see also* Poisoning, food) 005.9
- **Contraception, contraceptive**
  - advice NEC V25.09
    - family planning V25.09
    - fitting of diaphragm V25.02
    - prescribing or use of
      - oral contraceptive agent V25.01
      - specified agent NEC V25.02
  - counseling NEC V25.09
    - emergency V25.03
    - family planning V25.09
    - fitting of diaphragm V25.02
    - prescribing or use of
      - oral contraceptive agent V25.01
        - emergency V25.03
        - postcoital V25.03
      - specified agent NEC V25.02
  - device (in situ) V45.59
    - causing menorrhagia 996.76
    - checking V25.42
    - complications 996.32
    - insertion V25.1
    - intrauterine V45.51
    - reinsertion V25.42
    - removal V25.42
    - subdermal V45.52
  - fitting of diaphragm V25.02
  - insertion
    - intrauterine contraceptive device V25.1
    - subdermal implantable V25.5
  - maintenance V25.40
    - examination V25.40
      - intrauterine device V25.42
      - oral contraceptive V25.41
      - specified method NEC V25.49
      - subdermal implantable V25.43
    - intrauterine device V25.42
    - oral contraceptive V25.41
    - specified method NEC V25.49
    - subdermal implantable V25.43
  - management NEC V25.49
  - prescription
    - oral contraceptive agent V25.01
      - emergency V25.03
      - postcoital V25.03
      - repeat V25.41
    - specified agent NEC V25.02
      - repeat V25.49
  - sterilization V25.2
  - surveillance V25.40
    - intrauterine device V25.42
    - oral contraceptive agent V25.41
    - specified method NEC V25.49
    - subdermal implantable V25.43
- **Contraction, contracture, contracted**
  - Achilles tendon (*see also* Short, tendon, Achilles) 727.81
  - anus 564.89
  - axilla 729.9
  - bile duct (*see also* Disease, biliary) 576.8
  - bladder 596.8
    - neck or sphincter 596.0
  - bowel (*see also* Obstruction, intestine) 560.9

Contraction, contracture, contracted – *continued*
  Braxton Hicks 644.1❺
  bronchus 519.19
  burn (old) – *see* Cicatrix
  cecum (*see also* Obstruction, intestine) 560.9
  cervix (*see also* Stricture, cervix) 622.4
    congenital 752.49
  cicatricial – *see* Cicatrix
  colon (*see also* Obstruction, intestine) 560.9
  conjunctiva trachomatous, active 076.1
    late effect 139.1
  Dupuytren's 728.6
  eyelid 374.41
  eye socket (after enucleation) 372.64
  face 729.9
  fascia (lata) (postural) 728.89
    Dupuytren's 728.6
    palmar 728.6
    plantar 728.71
  finger NEC 736.29
    congenital 755.59
    joint (*see also* Contraction, joint) 718.44
  flaccid, paralytic
    joint (*see also* Contraction, joint) 718.4❺
    muscle 728.85
      ocular 378.50
  gallbladder (*see also* Obstruction, gallbladder) 575.2
  hamstring 728.89
    tendon 727.81
  heart valve – *see* Endocarditis
  Hicks' 644.1❺
  hip (*see also* Contraction, joint) 718.4❺
  hourglass
    bladder 596.8
      congenital 753.8
    gallbladder (*see also* Obstruction, gallbladder) 575.2
      congenital 751.69
    stomach 536.8
      congenital 750.7
      psychogenic 306.4
    uterus 661.4❺
      affecting fetus or newborn 763.7
  hysterical 300.11
  infantile (*see also* Epilepsy) 345.6❺
  internal os (*see also* Stricture, cervix) 622.4
  intestine (*see also* Obstruction, intestine) 560.9
  joint (abduction) (acquired) (adduction) (flexion) (rotation) 718.40
    ankle 718.47
    congenital NEC 755.8
      generalized or multiple 754.89
        lower limb joints 754.89
      hip (*see also* Subluxation, congenital, hip) 754.32
      lower limb (including pelvic girdle) not involving hip 754.89
      upper limb (including shoulder girdle) 755.59
    elbow 718.42
    foot 718.47
    hand 718.44
    hip 718.45
    hysterical 300.11
    knee 718.46
    multiple sites 718.49
    pelvic region 718.45
    shoulder (region) 718.41
    specified site NEC 718.48
    wrist 718.43
  kidney (granular) (secondary) (*see also* Sclerosis, renal) 587
    congenital 753.3
    hydronephritic 591
    pyelonephritic (*see also* Pyelitis, chronic) 590.00
    tuberculous (*see also* Tuberculosis) 016.0❺
  ligament 728.89
    congenital 756.89
  liver – *see* Cirrhosis, liver
  muscle (postinfectional) (postural) NEC 728.85
    congenital 756.89
      sternocleidomastoid 754.1
    extraocular 378.60
    eye (extrinsic) (*see also* Strabismus) 378.9
      paralytic (*see also* Strabismus, paralytic) 378.50
    flaccid 728.85
    hysterical 300.11
    ischemic (Volkmann's) 958.6
    paralytic 728.85
    posttraumatic 958.6

Contraction, contracture, contracted – *continued*
  muscle – *continued*
    psychogenic 306.0
      specified as conversion reaction 300.11
  myotonic 728.85
  neck (*see also* Torticollis) 723.5
    congenital 754.1
    psychogenic 306.0
  ocular muscle (*see also* Strabismus) 378.9
    paralytic (*see also* Strabismus, paralytic) 378.50
  organ or site, congenital NEC – *see* Atresia
  outlet (pelvis) – *see* Contraction, pelvis
  palmar fascia 728.6
  paralytic
    joint (*see also* Contraction, joint) 718.4❺
    muscle 728.85
      ocular (*see also* Strabismus, paralytic) 378.50
  pelvis (acquired) (general) 738.6
    affecting fetus or newborn 763.1
    complicating delivery 653.1❺
      causing obstructed labor 660.1❺
      generally contracted 653.1❺
        causing obstructed labor 660.1❺
      inlet 653.2❺
        causing obstructed labor 660.1❺
      midpelvic 653.8❺
        causing obstructed labor 660.1❺
      midplane 653.8❺
        causing obstructed labor 660.1❺
      outlet 653.3❺
        causing obstructed labor 660.1❺
  plantar fascia 728.71
  premature
    atrial 427.61
    auricular 427.61
    auriculoventricular 427.61
    heart (junctional) (nodal) 427.60
    supraventricular 427.61
    ventricular 427.69
  prostate 602.8
  pylorus (*see also* Pylorospasm) 537.81
  rectosigmoid (*see also* Obstruction, intestine) 560.9
  rectum, rectal (sphincter) 564.89
    psychogenic 306.4
  ring (Bandl's) 661.4❺
    affecting fetus or newborn 763.7
  scar – *see* Cicatrix
  sigmoid (*see also* Obstruction, intestine) 560.9
  socket, eye 372.64
  spine (*see also* Curvature, spine) 737.9
  stomach 536.8
    hourglass 536.8
      congenital 750.7
      psychogenic 306.4
    psychogenic 306.4
  tendon (sheath) (*see also* Short, tendon) 727.81
  toe 735.8
  ureterovesical orifice (postinfectional) 593.3
  urethra 599.84
  uterus 621.8
    abnormal 661.9❺
      affecting fetus or newborn 763.7
    clonic, hourglass or tetanic 661.4❺
      affecting fetus or newborn 763.7
    dyscoordinate 661.4❺
      affecting fetus or newborn 763.7
    hourglass 661.4❺
      affecting fetus or newborn 763.7
    hypotonic NEC 661.2❺
      affecting fetus or newborn 763.7
    incoordinate 661.4❺
      affecting fetus or newborn 763.7
    inefficient or poor 661.2❺
      affecting fetus or newborn 763.7
    irregular 661.2❺
      affecting fetus or newborn 763.7
    tetanic 661.4❺
      affecting fetus or newborn 763.7
  vagina (outlet) 623.2
  vesical 596.8
    neck or urethral orifice 596.0
  visual field, generalized 368.45
  Volkmann's (ischemic) 958.6

Contusion (skin surface intact) 924.9
  with
    crush injury – *see* Crush
    dislocation – *see* Dislocation, by site
    fracture – *see* Fracture, by site

Contusion – *continued*
  with – *continued*
    internal injury – *see also* Injury internal, by site
      heart – *see* Contusion, cardiac
      kidney – *see* Contusion, kidney
      liver – *see* Contusion, liver
      lung – *see* Contusion, lung
      spleen – *see* Contusion, spleen
    intracranial injury – *see* Injury, intracranial
    nerve injury – *see* Injury, nerve
    open wound – *see* Wound, open, by site
  abdomen, abdominal (muscle) (wall) 922.2
    organ(s) NEC 868.00
  adnexa, eye NEC 921.9
  ankle 924.21
    with other parts of foot 924.20
  arm 923.9
    lower (with elbow) 923.10
    upper 923.03
      with shoulder or axillary region 923.09
  auditory canal (external) (meatus) (and other part(s) of neck, scalp, or face, except eye) 920
  auricle, ear (and other part(s) of neck, scalp, or face except eye) 920
  axilla 923.02
    with shoulder or upper arm 923.09
  back 922.31
  bone NEC 924.9
  brain (cerebral) (membrane) (with hemorrhage) 851.8❺

Note – Use the following fifth-digit subclassification with categories 851-854:
0 unspecified state of consciousness
1 with no loss of consciousness
2 with brief [less than one hour] loss of consciousness
3 with moderate [1-24 hours] loss of consciousness
4 with prolonged [more than 24 hours] loss of consciousness and return to pre-existing conscious level
5 with prolonged [more than 24 hours] loss of consciousness, without return to pre-existing conscious level
Use fifth-digit 5 to designate when a patient is unconscious and dies before regaining consciousness, regardless of the duration of the loss of consciousness
6 with loss of consciousness of unspecified duration
9 with concussion, unspecified

    with
      open intracranial wound 851.9❺
      skull fracture – *see* Fracture, skull, by site
    cerebellum 851.4❺
      with open intracranial wound 851.5❺
    cortex 851.0❺
      with open intracranial wound 851.1❺
    occipital lobe 851.4❺
      with open intracranial wound 851.5❺
    stem 851.4❺
      with open intracranial wound 851.5❺
  breast 922.0
  brow (and other part(s) of neck, scalp, or face, except eye) 920
  buttock 922.32
  canthus 921.1
  cardiac 861.01
    with open wound into thorax 861.11
  cauda equina (spine) 952.4
  cerebellum – *see* Contusion, brain, cerebellum
  cerebral – *see* Contusion, brain
  cheek(s) (and other part(s) of neck, scalp, or face, except eye) 920
  chest (wall) 922.1
  chin (and other part(s) of neck, scalp, or face, except eye) 920
  clitoris 922.4
  conjunctiva 921.1
  conus medullaris (spine) 952.4
  cornea 921.3
  corpus cavernosum 922.4
  cortex (brain) (cerebral) – *see* Contusion, brain, cortex
  costal region 922.1
  ear (and other part(s) of neck, scalp, or face except eye) 920
  elbow 923.11
    with forearm 923.10
  epididymis 922.4

Contusion – *continued*
  epigastric region 922.2
  eye NEC 921.9
  eyeball 921.3
  eyelid(s) (and periocular area) 921.1
  face (and neck, or scalp, any part, except eye) 920
  femoral triangle 922.2
  fetus or newborn 772.6
  finger(s) (nail) (subungual) 923.3
  flank 922.2
  foot (with ankle) (excluding toe(s)) 924.20
  forearm (and elbow) 923.10
  forehead (and other part(s) of neck, scalp, or face, except eye) 920
  genital organs, external 922.4
  globe (eye) 921.3
  groin 922.2
  gum(s) (and other part(s) of neck, scalp, or face, except eye) 920
  hand(s) (except fingers alone) 923.20
  head (any part, except eye) (and face) (and neck) 920
  heart – *see* Contusion, cardiac
  heel 924.20
  hip 924.01
    with thigh 924.00
  iliac region 922.2
  inguinal region 922.2
  internal organs (abdomen, chest, or pelvis) NEC – *see* Injury, internal, by site
  interscapular region 922.33
  iris (eye) 921.3
  kidney 866.01
    with open wound into cavity 866.11
  knee 924.11
    with lower leg 924.10
  labium (majus) (minus) 922.4
  lacrimal apparatus, gland, or sac 921.1
  larynx (and other part(s) of neck, scalp, or face, except eye) 920
  late effect – *see* Late, effects (of), contusion
  leg 924.5
    lower (with knee) 924.10
  lens 921.3
  lingual (and other part(s) of neck, scalp, or face, except eye) 920
  lip(s) (and other part(s) of neck, scalp, or face, except eye) 920
  liver 864.01
    with
      laceration – *see* Laceration, liver
      open wound into cavity 864.11
  lower extremity 924.5
    multiple sites 924.4
  lumbar region 922.31
  lung 861.21
    with open wound into thorax 861.31
  malar region (and other part(s) of neck, scalp, or face, except eye) 920
  mandibular joint (and other part(s) of neck, scalp, or face, except eye) 920
  mastoid region (and other part(s) of neck, scalp, or face, except eye) 920
  membrane, brain – *see* Contusion, brain
  midthoracic region 922.1
  mouth (and other part(s) of neck, scalp, or face, except eye) 920
  multiple sites (not classifiable to same three-digit category) 924.8
    lower limb 924.4
    trunk 922.8
    upper limb 923.8
  muscle NEC 924.9
  myocardium – *see* Contusion, cardiac
  nasal (septum) (and other part(s) of neck, scalp, or face, except eye) 920
  neck (and scalp, or face, any part, except eye) 920
  nerve – *see* Injury, nerve, by site
  nose (and other part(s) of neck, scalp or face, except eye) 920
  occipital region (scalp) (and neck or face, except eye) 920
    lobe – *see* Contusion, brain, occipital lobe
  orbit (region) (tissues) 921.2
  palate (soft) (and other part(s) of neck, scalp, or face, except eye) 920
  parietal region (scalp) (and neck, or face, except eye) 920
    lobe – *see* Contusion, brain
  penis 922.4

Contusion – *continued*
  pericardium – *see* Contusion, cardiac
  perineum 922.4
  periocular area 921.1
  pharynx (and other part(s) of neck, scalp, or face, except eye) 920
  popliteal space (*see also* Contusion, knee) 924.11
  prepuce 922.4
  pubic region 922.4
  pudenda 922.4
  pulmonary – *see* Contusion, lung
  quadriceps femoralis 924.00
  rib cage 922.1
  sacral region 922.32
  salivary ducts or glands (and other part(s) of neck, scalp, or face, except eye) 920
  scalp (and neck, or face any part, except eye) 920
  scapular region 923.01
    with shoulder or upper arm 923.09
  sclera (eye) 921.3
  scrotum 922.4
  shoulder 923.00
    with upper arm or axillar regions 923.09
  skin NEC 924.9
  skull 920
  spermatic cord 922.4
  spinal cord – *see also* Injury, spinal, by site
    cauda equina 952.4
    conus medullaris 952.4
  spleen 865.01
    with open wound into cavity 865.11
  sternal region 922.1
  stomach – *see* Injury, internal, stomach
  subconjunctival 921.1
  subcutaneous NEC 924.9
  submaxillary region (and other part(s) of neck, scalp, or face, except eye) 920
  submental region (and other part(s) of neck, scalp, or face, except eye) 920
  subperiosteal NEC 924.9
  supraclavicular fossa (and other part(s) of neck, scalp, or face, except eye) 920
  supraorbital (and other part(s) of neck, scalp, or face, except eye) 920
  temple (region) (and other part(s) of neck, scalp, or face, except eye) 920
  testis 922.4
  thigh (and hip) 924.00
  thorax 922.1
    organ – *see* Injury, internal, intrathoracic
  throat (and other part(s) of neck, scalp, or face, except eye) 920
  thumb(s) (nail) (subungual) 923.3
  toe(s) (nail) (subungual) 924.3
  tongue (and other part(s) of neck, scalp, or face, except eye) 920
  trunk 922.9
    multiple sites 922.8
    specified site – *see* Contusion, by site
  tunica vaginalis 922.4
  tympanum (membrane) (and other part(s) of neck, scalp, or face, except eye) 920
  upper extremity 923.9
    multiple sites 923.8
  uvula (and other part(s) of neck, scalp, or face, except eye) 920
  vagina 922.4
  vocal cord(s) (and other part(s) of neck, scalp, or face, except eye) 920
  vulva 922.4
  wrist 923.21
    with hand(s), except finger(s) alone 923.20
Conus (any type) (congenital) 743.57
  acquired 371.60
  medullaris syndrome 336.8
Convalescence (following) V66.9
  chemotherapy V66.2
  medical NEC V66.5
  psychotherapy V66.3
  radiotherapy V66.1
  surgery NEC V66.0
  treatment (for) NEC V66.5
    combined V66.6
    fracture V66.4
    mental disorder NEC V66.3
    specified disorder NEC V66.5
Conversion
  closed surgical procedure to open procedure
    arthroscopic V64.43

Conversion – *continued*
  closed surgical procedure to open procedure- *continued*
    laparoscopic V64.41
    thoracoscopic V64.42
  hysteria, hysterical, any type 300.11
  neurosis, any 300.11
  reaction, any 300.11
Converter, tuberculosis (test reaction) 795.5
Convulsions (idiopathic) 780.39
  apoplectiform (*see also* Disease, cerebrovascular, acute) 436
  brain 780.39
  cerebral 780.39
  cerebrospinal 780.39
  due to trauma NEC – *see* Injury, intracranial
  eclamptic (*see also* Eclampsia) 780.39
  epileptic (*see also* Epilepsy) 345.9❺
  epileptiform (*see also* Seizure, epileptiform) 780.39
  epileptoid (*see also* Seizure, epileptiform) 780.39
  ether
    anesthetic
      correct substance properly administered 780.39
      overdose or wrong substance given 968.2
    other specified type – *see* Table of Drugs and Chemicals
  febrile (simple) 780.31
    complex 780.32
  generalized 780.39
  hysterical 300.11
  infantile 780.39
    epilepsy – *see* Epilepsy
  internal 780.39
  Jacksonian (*see also* Epilepsy) 345.5❺
  myoclonic 333.2
  newborn 779.0
  paretic 094.1
  pregnancy (nephritic) (uremic) – *see* Eclampsia, pregnancy
  psychomotor (*see also* Epilepsy) 345.4❺
  puerperal, postpartum – *see* Eclampsia, pregnancy
  recurrent 780.39
    epileptic – *see* Epilepsy
  reflex 781.0
  repetitive 780.39
    epileptic – *see* Epilepsy
  Salaam (*see also* Epilepsy) 345.6❺
  scarlatinal 034.1
  spasmodic 780.39
  tetanus, tetanic (*see also* Tetanus) 037
  thymic 254.8
  uncinate 780.39
  uremic 586
Convulsive – *see also* Convulsions
  disorder or state 780.39
    epileptic – *see* Epilepsy
  equivalent, abdominal (*see also* Epilepsy) 345.5❺
Cooke-Apert-Gallais syndrome (adrenogenital) 255.2
Cooley's anemia (erythroblastic) 282.49
Coolie itch 126.9
Cooper's
  disease 610.1
  hernia – *see* Hernia, Cooper's
Coordination disturbance 781.3
Copper wire arteries, retina 362.13
Copra itch 133.8
Coprolith 560.39
Coprophilia 302.89
Coproporphyria, hereditary 277.1
Coprostasis 560.39
  with hernia – *see also* Hernia, by site, with obstruction
    gangrenous – *see* Hernia, by site, with gangrene
Cor
  biloculare 745.7
  bovinum – *see* Hypertrophy, cardiac
  bovis – *see also* Hypertrophy, cardiac
  pulmonale (chronic) 416.9
    acute 415.0
  triatriatum, triatrium 746.82
  triloculare 745.8
    biatriatum 745.3
    biventriculare 745.69
Corbus' disease 607.1

Cord – *see also* condition
- around neck (tightly) (with compression)
  - affecting fetus or newborn 762.5
  - complicating delivery 663.1❺
    - without compression 663.3❺
      - affecting fetus or newborn 762.6
- bladder NEC 344.61
  - tabetic 094.0
- prolapse
  - affecting fetus or newborn 762.4
  - complicating delivery 663.0❺

Cord's angiopathy (*see also* Tuberculosis) 017.3❺ *[362.18]*
Cordis ectopia 746.87
Corditis (spermatic) 608.4
Corectopia 743.46
Cori type glycogen storage disease – *see* Disease, glycogen storage
Cork-handlers' disease or lung 495.3
Corkscrew esophagus 530.5
Corlett's pyosis (impetigo) 684
Corn (infected) 700
Cornea – *see also* condition
- donor V59.5
- guttata (dystrophy) 371.57
- plana 743.41

Cornelia de Lange's syndrome (Amsterdam dwarf, mental retardation, and brachycephaly) 759.89
Cornual gestation or pregnancy – *see* Pregnancy, cornual
Cornu cutaneum 702.8
Coronary (artery) – *see also* condition
- arising from aorta or pulmonary trunk 746.85

Corpora – *see also* condition
- amylacea (prostate) 602.8
- cavernosa – *see* condition

Corpulence (*see also* Obesity) 278.0❺
Corpus – *see* condition
Corrigan's disease – *see* Insufficiency, aortic
Corrosive burn – *see* Burn, by site
Corsican fever (*see also* Malaria) 084.6
Cortical – *see also* condition
- blindness 377.75
- necrosis, kidney (bilateral) 583.6

Corticoadrenal – *see* condition
Corticosexual syndrome 255.2
Coryza (acute) 460
- with grippe or influenza 487.1
- syphilitic 095.8
  - congenital (chronic) 090.0

Costen's syndrome or complex 524.60
Costiveness (*see also* Constipation) 564.00
Costochondritis 733.6
Cotard's syndrome (paranoia) 297.1
Cot death 798.0
Cotungo's disease 724.3
Cough 786.2
- with hemorrhage (*see also* Hemoptysis) 786.3
- affected 786.2
- bronchial 786.2
  - with grippe or influenza 487.1
- chronic 786.2
- epidemic 786.2
- functional 306.1
- hemorrhagic 786.3
- hysterical 300.11
- laryngeal, spasmodic 786.2
- nervous 786.2
- psychogenic 306.1
- smokers' 491.0
- tea tasters' 112.89

Counseling NEC V65.40
- without complaint or sickness V65.49
- abuse victim NEC V62.89
  - child V61.21
  - partner V61.11
  - spouse V61.11
- child abuse, maltreatment, or neglect V61.21
- contraceptive NEC V25.09
  - device (intrauterine) V25.02
  - maintenance V25.40
    - intrauterine contraceptive device V25.42
    - oral contraceptive (pill) V25.41
    - specified type NEC V25.49
    - subdermal implantable V25.43
  - management NEC V25.9

Counseling – *continued*
- contraceptive – *continued*
  - oral contraceptive (pill) V25.01
    - emergency V25.03
    - postcoital V25.03
  - prescription NEC V25.02
    - oral contraceptive (pill) V25.01
      - emergency V25.03
      - postcoital V25.03
      - repeat prescription V25.41
    - repeat prescription V25.40
  - subdermal implantable V25.43
  - surveillance NEC V25.40
- dietary V65.3
- exercise V65.41
- expectant mother, pediatric pre-birth visit V65.11
- explanation of
  - investigation finding NEC V65.49
  - medication NEC V65.49
- family planning V25.09
  - natural ●
    - procreative V26.41 ●
    - to avoid pregnancy V25.04 ●
- for nonattending third party V65.19
- genetic V26.33
- gonorrhea V65.45
- health (advice) (education) (instruction) NEC V65.49
- HIV V65.44
- human immunodeficiency virus V65.44
- injury prevention V65.43
- insulin pump training V65.46
- marital V61.10
- medical (for) V65.9
  - boarding school resident V60.6
  - condition not demonstrated V65.5
  - feared complaint and no disease found V65.5
  - institutional resident V60.6
  - on behalf of another V65.19
  - person living alone V60.3
- natural family planning ●
  - procreative V26.41 ●
  - to avoid pregnancy V25.04 ●
- parent-child conflict V61.20
  - specified problem NEC V61.29
- partner abuse
  - perpetrator V61.12
  - victim V61.11
- pediatric pre-birth visit for expectant mother V65.11
- perpetrator of
  - child abuse V62.83
    - parental V61.22
  - partner abuse V61.12
  - spouse abuse V61.12
- procreative V65.49
- sex NEC V65.49
  - transmitted disease NEC V65.45
    - HIV V65.44
- specified reason NEC V65.49
- spousal abuse
  - perpetrator V61.12
  - victim V61.11
- substance use and abuse V65.42
- syphilis V65.45
- victim (of)
  - abuse NEC V62.89
  - child abuse V61.21
  - partner abuse V61.11
  - spousal abuse V61.11

Coupled rhythm 427.89
Couvelaire uterus (complicating delivery) – *see* Placenta, separation
Cowper's gland – *see* condition
Cowperitis (*see also* Urethritis) 597.89
- gonorrheal (acute) 098.0
  - chronic or duration of 2 months or over 098.2

Cowpox (abortive) 051.0
- due to vaccination 999.0
- eyelid 051.0 *[373.5]*
  - postvaccination 999.0 *[373.5]*

Coxa
- plana 732.1
- valga (acquired) 736.31
  - congenital 755.61
  - late effect of rickets 268.1
- vara (acquired) 736.32
  - congenital 755.62
  - late effect of rickets 268.1

Coxae malum senilis 715.25
Coxalgia (nontuberculous) 719.45
- tuberculous (*see also* Tuberculosis) 015.1❺ *[730.85]*

Coxalgic pelvis 736.30
Coxitis 716.65
Coxsackie (infection) (virus) 079.2
- central nervous system NEC 048
- endocarditis 074.22
- enteritis 008.67
- meningitis (aseptic) 047.0
- myocarditis 074.23
- pericarditis 074.21
- pharyngitis 074.0
- pleurodynia 074.1
- specific disease NEC 074.8

Crabs, meaning pubic lice 132.2
Crack baby 760.75
Cracked
- nipple 611.2
  - puerperal, postpartum 676.1❺
- tooth 521.81

Cradle cap 690.11
Craft neurosis 300.89
Craigiasis 007.8
Cramp(s) 729.82
- abdominal 789.0❺
- bathing 994.1
- colic 789.0❺
  - psychogenic 306.4
- due to immersion 994.1
- extremity (lower) (upper) NEC 729.82
- fireman 992.2
- heat 992.2
- hysterical 300.11
- immersion 994.1
- intestinal 789.0❺
  - psychogenic 306.4
- linotypist's 300.89
  - organic 333.84
- muscle (extremity) (general) 729.82
  - due to immersion 994.1
  - hysterical 300.11
- occupational (hand) 300.89
  - organic 333.84
- psychogenic 307.89
- salt depletion 276.1
- sleep related leg 327.52
- stoker 992.2
- stomach 789.0❺
- telegraphers' 300.89
  - organic 333.84
- typists' 300.89
  - organic 333.84
- uterus 625.8
  - menstrual 625.3
- writers' 333.84
  - organic 333.84
  - psychogenic 300.89

Cranial – *see* condition
Cranioclasis, fetal 763.89
Craniocleidodysostosis 755.59
Craniofenestria (skull) 756.0
Craniolacunia (skull) 756.0
Craniopagus 759.4
Craniopathy, metabolic 733.3
Craniopharyngeal – *see* condition
Craniopharyngioma (M9350/1) 237.0
Craniorachischisis (totalis) 740.1
Cranioschisis 756.0
Craniostenosis 756.0
Craniosynostosis 756.0
Craniotabes (cause unknown) 733.3
- rachitic 268.1
- syphilitic 090.5

Craniotomy, fetal 763.89
Cranium – *see* condition
Craw-craw 125.3
CRBSI (catheter-related bloodstream infection) 999.31 ●
Creaking joint 719.60
- ankle 719.67
- elbow 719.62
- foot 719.67
- hand 719.64
- hip 719.65
- knee 719.66
- multiple sites 719.69

Creaking joint – *continued*
- pelvic region 719.65
- shoulder (region) 719.61
- specified site NEC 719.68
- wrist 719.63

Creeping
- eruption 126.9
- palsy 335.21
- paralysis 335.21

Crenated tongue 529.8
Creotoxism 005.9
Crepitus
- caput 756.0
- joint 719.60
  - ankle 719.67
  - elbow 719.62
  - foot 719.67
  - hand 719.64
  - hip 719.65
  - knee 719.66
  - multiple sites 719.69
  - pelvic region 719.65
  - shoulder (region) 719.61
  - specified site NEC 719.68
  - wrist 719.63

Crescent or conus choroid, congenital 743.57
Cretin, cretinism (athyrotic) (congenital) (endemic) (metabolic) (nongoitrous) (sporadic) 243
- goitrous (sporadic) 246.1
- pelvis (dwarf type) (male type) 243
  - with disproportion (fetopelvic) 653.1❺
    - affecting fetus or newborn 763.1
    - causing obstructed labor 660.1❺
      - affecting fetus or newborn 763.1
- pituitary 253.3

Cretinoid degeneration 243
Creutzfeldt-Jakob disease (syndrome) (new variant) 046.1
- with dementia
  - with behavioral disturbance 046.1 *[294.11]*
  - without behavioral disturbance 046.1 *[294.10]*

Crib death 798.0
Cribriform hymen 752.49
Cri-du-chat syndrome 758.31
Crigler-Najjar disease or syndrome (congenital hyperbilirubinemia) 277.4
Crimean hemorrhagic fever 065.0
Criminalism 301.7
Crisis
- abdomen 789.0❺
- Addisonian (acute adrenocortical insufficiency) 255.41 ▲
- adrenal (cortical) 255.41 ▲
- asthmatic – *see* Asthma
- brain, cerebral (*see also* Disease, cerebrovascular, acute) 436
- celiac 579.0
- Dietl's 593.4
- emotional NEC 309.29
  - acute reaction to stress 308.0
  - adjustment reaction 309.9
  - specific to childhood or adolescence 313.9
- gastric (tabetic) 094.0
- glaucomatocyclitic 364.22
- heart (*see also* Failure, heart) 428.9
- hypertensive – *see* Hypertension
- nitritoid
  - correct substance properly administered 458.29
  - overdose or wrong substance given or taken 961.1
- oculogyric 378.87
  - psychogenic 306.7
- Pel's 094.0
- psychosexual identity 302.6
- rectum 094.0
- renal 593.81
- sickle cell 282.62
- stomach (tabetic) 094.0
- tabetic 094.0
- thyroid (*see also* Thyrotoxicosis) 242.9❺
- thyrotoxic (*see also* Thyrotoxicosis) 242.9❺
- vascular – *see* Disease, cerebrovascular, acute

Crocq's disease (acrocyanosis) 443.89
Crohn's disease (*see also* Enteritis, regional) 555.9
Cronkhite-Canada syndrome 211.3
Crooked septum, nasal 470
Cross
- birth (of fetus) complicating delivery 652.3❺
  - with successful version 652.1❺
  - causing obstructed labor 660.0❺
- bite, anterior or posterior 524.27
- eye (*see also* Esotropia) 378.00

Crossed ectopia of kidney 753.3
Crossfoot 754.50
Croup, croupous (acute) (angina) (catarrhal) (infective) (inflammatory) (laryngeal) (membranous) (nondiphtheritic) (pseudomembranous) 464.4
- asthmatic (*see also* Asthma) 493.9❺
- bronchial 466.0
- diphtheritic (membranous) 032.3
- false 478.75
- spasmodic 478.75
  - diphtheritic 032.3
- stridulous 478.75
  - diphtheritic 032.3

Crouzon's disease (craniofacial dysostosis) 756.0
Crowding, teeth 524.31
CRST syndrome (cutaneous systemic sclerosis) 710.1
Cruchet's disease (encephalitis lethargica) 049.8
Cruelty in children (*see also* Disturbance, conduct) 312.9
Crural ulcer (*see also* Ulcer, lower extremity) 707.10
Crush, crushed, crushing (injury) 929.9
- abdomen 926.19
  - internal – *see* Injury, internal, abdomen
- ankle 928.21
  - with other parts of foot 928.20
- arm 927.9
  - lower (and elbow) 927.10
  - upper 927.03
    - with shoulder or axillary region 927.09
- axilla 927.02
  - with shoulder or upper arm 927.09
- back 926.11
- breast 926.19
- buttock 926.12
- cheek 925.1
- chest – *see* Injury, internal, chest
- ear 925.1
- elbow 927.11
  - with forearm 927.10
- face 925.1
- finger(s) 927.3
  - with hand(s) 927.20
    - and wrist(s) 927.21
- flank 926.19
- foot, excluding toe(s) alone (with ankle) 928.20
- forearm (and elbow) 927.10
- genitalia, external (female) (male) 926.0
  - internal – *see* Injury, internal, genital organ NEC
- hand, except finger(s) alone (and wrist) 927.20
- head – *see* Fracture, skull, by site
- heel 928.20
- hip 928.01
  - with thigh 928.00
- internal organ (abdomen, chest, or pelvis) – *see* Injury, internal, by site
- knee 928.11
  - with leg, lower 928.10
- labium (majus) (minus) 926.0
- larynx 925.2
- late effect – *see* Late, effects (of), crushing
- leg 928.9
  - lower 928.10
    - and knee 928.11
  - upper 928.00
- limb
  - lower 928.9
    - multiple sites 928.8
  - upper 927.9
    - multiple sites 927.8
- multiple sites NEC 929.0
- neck 925.2
- nerve – *see* Injury, nerve, by site
- nose 802.0
  - open 802.1
- penis 926.0
- pharynx 925.2
- scalp 925.1
- scapular region 927.01
  - with shoulder or upper arm 927.09
- scrotum 926.0
- shoulder 927.00
  - with upper arm or axillary region 927.09

Crush, crushed, crushing – *continued*
- skull or cranium – *see* Fracture, skull, by site
- spinal cord – *see* Injury, spinal, by site
- syndrome (complication of trauma) 958.5
- testis 926.0
- thigh (with hip) 928.00
- throat 925.2
- thumb(s) (and fingers) 927.3
- toe(s) 928.3
  - with foot 928.20
    - and ankle 928.21
- tonsil 925.2
- trunk 926.9
  - chest – *see* Injury, internal, intrathoracic organs NEC
  - internal organ – *see* Injury, internal, by site
  - multiple sites 926.8
  - specified site NEC 926.19
- vulva 926.0
- wrist 927.21
  - with hand(s), except fingers alone 927.20

Crusta lactea 690.11
Crusts 782.8
Crutch paralysis 953.4
Cruveilhier's disease 335.21
Cruveilhier-Baumgarten cirrhosis, disease, or syndrome 571.5
Cruz-Chagas disease (*see also* Trypanosomiasis) 086.2
Crying
- constant, continuous
  - adolescent 780.95
  - adult 780.95
  - baby 780.92
  - child 780.95
  - infant 780.92
  - newborn 780.92
- excessive
  - adolescent 780.95
  - adult 780.95
  - baby 780.92
  - child 780.95
  - infant 780.92
  - newborn 780.92

Cryoglobulinemia (mixed) 273.2
Crypt (anal) (rectal) 569.49
Cryptitis (anal) (rectal) 569.49
Cryptococcosis (European) (pulmonary) (systemic) 117.5
Cryptococcus 117.5
- epidermicus 117.5
- neoformans, infection by 117.5

Cryptopapillitis (anus) 569.49
Cryptophthalmos (eyelid) 743.06
Cryptorchid, cryptorchism, cryptorchidism 752.51
Cryptosporidiosis 007.4
Cryptotia 744.29
Crystallopathy
- calcium pyrophosphate (*see also* Arthritis) 275.49 *[712.2]*
- dicalcium phosphate (*see also* Arthritis) 275.49 *[712.1]*
- gouty 274.0
- pyrophosphate NEC (*see also* Arthritis) 275.49 *[712.2]*
- uric acid 274.0

Crystalluria 791.9
Csillag's disease (lichen sclerosus et atrophicus) 701.0
Cuban itch 050.1
Cubitus
- valgus (acquired) 736.01
  - congenital 755.59
  - late effect of rickets 268.1
- varus (acquired) 736.02
  - congenital 755.59
  - late effect of rickets 268.1

Cultural deprivation V62.4
Cupping of optic disc 377.14
Curling's ulcer – *see* Ulcer, duodenum
Curling esophagus 530.5
Curschmann (-Batten) (-Steinert) **disease or syndrome** 359.21 ▲
Curvature
- organ or site, congenital NEC – *see* Distortion
- penis (lateral) 752.69

Curvature – *continued*
- Pott's (spinal) (*see also* Tuberculosis) 015.0❺ *[737.43]*
- radius, idiopathic, progressive (congenital) 755.54
- spine (acquired) (angular) (idiopathic) (incorrect) (postural) 737.9
  - congenital 754.2
  - due to or associated with
    - Charcôt-Marie-Tooth disease 356.1 *[737.40]*
    - mucopolysaccharidosis 277.5 *[737.40]*
    - neurofibromatosis 237.71 *[737.40]*
    - osteitis
      - deformans 731.0 *[737.40]*
      - fibrosa cystica 252.01 *[737.40]*
    - osteoporosis (*see also* Osteoporosis) 733.00 *[737.40]*
    - poliomyelitis (*see also* Poliomyelitis) 138 *[737.40]*
    - tuberculosis (Pott's curvature) (*see also* Tuberculosis) 015.0❺ *[737.43]*
  - kyphoscoliotic (*see also* Kyphoscoliosis) 737.30
  - kyphotic (*see also* Kyphosis) 737.10
  - late effect of rickets 268.1 *[737.40]*
  - Pott's 015.0❺ *[737.40]*
  - scoliotic (*see also* Scoliosis) 737.30
  - specified NEC 737.8
  - tuberculous 015.0❺ *[737.40]*

Cushing's
- basophilism, disease, or syndrome (iatrogenic) (idiopathic) (pituitary basophilism) (pituitary dependent) 255.0
- ulcer – *see* Ulcer, peptic

Cushingoid due to steroid therapy
- correct substance properly administered 255.0
- overdose or wrong substance given or taken 962.0

Cut (external) – *see* Wound, open, by site

Cutaneous – *see also* condition
- hemorrhage 782.7
- horn (cheek) (eyelid) (mouth) 702.8
- larva migrans 126.9

Cutis – *see also* condition
- hyperelastic 756.83
  - acquired 701.8
- laxa 756.83
  - senilis 701.8
- marmorata 782.61
- osteosis 709.3
- pendula 756.83
  - acquired 701.8
- rhomboidalis nuchae 701.8
- verticis gyrata 757.39
  - acquired 701.8

Cyanopathy, newborn 770.83

Cyanosis 782.5
- autotoxic 289.7
- common atrioventricular canal 745.69
- congenital 770.83
- conjunctiva 372.71
- due to
  - endocardial cushion defect 745.60
  - nonclosure, foramen botalli 745.5
  - patent foramen botalli 745.5
  - persistent foramen ovale 745.5
- enterogenous 289.7
- fetus or newborn 770.83
- ostium primum defect 745.61
- paroxysmal digital 443.0
- retina, retinal 362.10

Cycle
- anovulatory 628.0
- menstrual, irregular 626.4

Cyclencephaly 759.89

Cyclical vomiting 536.2
- psychogenic 306.4

Cyclitic membrane 364.74

Cyclitis (*see also* Iridocyclitis) 364.3
- acute 364.00
  - primary 364.01
  - recurrent 364.02
- chronic 364.10
  - in
    - sarcoidosis 135 *[364.11]*
    - tuberculosis (*see also* Tuberculosis) 017.3❺ *[364.11]*
- Fuchs' heterochromic 364.21
- granulomatous 364.10
- lens induced 364.23

Cyclitis – *continued*
- nongranulomatous 364.00
- posterior 363.21
- primary 364.01
- recurrent 364.02
- secondary (noninfectious) 364.04
  - infectious 364.03
- subacute 364.00
  - primary 364.01
  - recurrent 364.02

Cyclokeratitis – *see* Keratitis

Cyclophoria 378.44

Cyclopia, cyclops 759.89

Cycloplegia 367.51

Cyclospasm 367.53

Cyclosporiasis 007.5

Cyclothymia 301.13

Cyclothymic personality 301.13

Cyclotropia 378.33

Cyesis – *see* Pregnancy

Cylindroma (M8200/3) – *see also* Neoplasm, by site, malignant
- eccrine dermal (M8200/0) – *see* Neoplasm, skin, benign
- skin (M8200/0) – *see* Neoplasm, skin, benign

Cylindruria 791.7

Cyllosoma 759.89

Cynanche
- diphtheritic 032.3
- tonsillaris 475

Cynorexia 783.6

Cyphosis – *see* Kyphosis

Cyprus fever (*see also* Brucellosis) 023.9

Cyriax's syndrome (slipping rib) 733.99

Cyst (mucus) (retention) (serous) (simple)

> *Note – In general, cysts are not neoplastic and are classified to the appropriate category for disease of the specified anatomical site. This generalization does not apply to certain types of cysts which are neoplastic in nature, for example, dermoid, nor does it apply to cysts of certain structures, for example, branchial cleft, which are classified as developmental anomalies.*
>
> *The following listing includes some of the most frequently reported sites of cysts as well as qualifiers which indicate the type of cyst. The latter qualifiers usually are not repeated under the anatomical sites. Since the code assignment for a given site may vary depending upon the type of cyst, the coder should refer to the listings under the specified type of cyst before consideration is given to the site.*

- accessory, fallopian tube 752.11
- adenoid (infected) 474.8
- adrenal gland 255.8
  - congenital 759.1
- air, lung 518.89
- allantoic 753.7
- alveolar process (jaw bone) 526.2
- amnion, amniotic 658.8❺
- anterior chamber (eye) 364.60
  - exudative 364.62
  - implantation (surgical) (traumatic) 364.61
  - parasitic 360.13
- anterior nasopalatine 526.1
- antrum 478.19
- anus 569.49
- apical (periodontal) (tooth) 522.8
- appendix 543.9
- arachnoid, brain 348.0
- arytenoid 478.79
- auricle 706.2
- Baker's (knee) 727.51
  - tuberculous (*see also* Tuberculosis) 015.2❺
- Bartholin's gland or duct 616.2
- bile duct (*see also* Disease, biliary) 576.8
- bladder (multiple) (trigone) 596.8
- Blessig's 362.62
- blood, endocardial (*see also* Endocarditis) 424.90
- blue dome 610.0
- bone (local) 733.20
  - aneurysmal 733.22
  - jaw 526.2
    - developmental (odontogenic) 526.0

Cyst – *continued*
- bone – *continued*
  - jaw – *continued*
    - fissural 526.1
    - latent 526.89
  - solitary 733.21
  - unicameral 733.21
- brain 348.0
  - congenital 742.4
  - hydatid (*see also* Echinococcus) 122.9
  - third ventricle (colloid) 742.4
- branchial (cleft) 744.42
- branchiogenic 744.42
- breast (benign) (blue dome) (pedunculated) (solitary) (traumatic) 610.0
  - involution 610.4
  - sebaceous 610.8
- broad ligament (benign) 620.8
  - embryonic 752.11
- bronchogenic (mediastinal) (sequestration) 518.89
  - congenital 748.4
- buccal 528.4
- bulbourethral gland (Cowper's) 599.89
- bursa, bursal 727.49
  - pharyngeal 478.26
- calcifying odontogenic (M9301/0) 213.1
  - upper jaw (bone) 213.0
- canal of Nuck (acquired) (serous) 629.1
  - congenital 752.41
- canthus 372.75
- carcinomatous (M8010/3) – *see* Neoplasm, by site, malignant
- cartilage (joint) – *see* Derangement, joint
- cauda equina 336.8
- cavum septi pellucidi NEC 348.0
- celomic (pericardium) 746.89
- cerebellopontine (angle) – *see* Cyst, brain
- cerebellum – *see* Cyst, brain
- cerebral – *see* Cyst, brain
- cervical lateral 744.42
- cervix 622.8
  - embryonal 752.41
  - nabothian (gland) 616.0
- chamber, anterior (eye) 364.60
  - exudative 364.62
  - implantation (surgical) (traumatic) 364.61
  - parasitic 360.13
- chiasmal, optic NEC (*see also* Lesion, chiasmal) 377.54
- chocolate (ovary) 617.1
- choledochal (congenital) 751.69
  - acquired 576.8
- choledochus 751.69
- chorion 658.8❺
- choroid plexus 348.0
- chyle, mesentery 457.8
- ciliary body 364.60
  - exudative 364.64
  - implantation 364.61
  - primary 364.63
- clitoris 624.8
- coccyx (*see also* Cyst, bone) 733.20
- colloid
  - third ventricle (brain) 742.4
  - thyroid gland – *see* Goiter
- colon 569.89
- common (bile) duct (*see also* Disease, biliary) 576.8
- congenital NEC 759.89
  - adrenal glands 759.1
  - epiglottis 748.3
  - esophagus 750.4
  - fallopian tube 752.11
  - kidney 753.10
    - multiple 753.19
    - single 753.11
  - larynx 748.3
  - liver 751.62
  - lung 748.4
  - mediastinum 748.8
  - ovary 752.0
  - oviduct 752.11
  - pancreas 751.7
  - periurethral (tissue) 753.8
  - prepuce NEC 752.69
    - penis 752.69
  - sublingual 750.26
  - submaxillary gland 750.26
  - thymus (gland) 759.2
  - tongue 750.19
  - ureterovesical orifice 753.4

Curvature – Cyst

- **Cyst** – *continued*
  - congenital – *continued*
    - vulva 752.41
  - conjunctiva 372.75
  - cornea 371.23
  - corpora quadrigemina 348.0
  - corpus
    - albicans (ovary) 620.2
    - luteum (ruptured) 620.1
  - Cowper's gland (benign) (infected) 599.89
  - cranial meninges 348.0
  - craniobuccal pouch 253.8
  - craniopharyngeal pouch 253.8
  - cystic duct (*see also* Disease, gallbladder) 575.8
  - Cysticercus (any site) 123.1
  - Dandy-Walker 742.3
    - with spina bifida (*see also* Spina bifida) 741.0❺
  - dental 522.8
    - developmental 526.0
    - eruption 526.0
    - lateral periodontal 526.0
    - primordial (keratocyst) 526.0
    - root 522.8
  - dentigerous 526.0
    - mandible 526.0
    - maxilla 526.0
  - dermoid (M9084/0) – *see also* Neoplasm, by site, benign
    - with malignant transformation (M9084/3) 183.0
    - implantation
      - external area or site (skin) NEC 709.8
      - iris 364.61
      - skin 709.8
      - vagina 623.8
      - vulva 624.8
    - mouth 528.4
    - oral soft tissue 528.4
    - sacrococcygeal 685.1
      - with abscess 685.0
  - developmental of ovary, ovarian 752.0
  - dura (cerebral) 348.0
    - spinal 349.2
  - ear (external) 706.2
  - echinococcal (*see also* Echinococcus) 122.9
  - embryonal
    - cervix uteri 752.41
    - genitalia, female external 752.41
    - uterus 752.3
    - vagina 752.41
  - endometrial 621.8
    - ectopic 617.9
  - endometrium (uterus) 621.8
    - ectopic – *see* Endometriosis
  - enteric 751.5
  - enterogenous 751.5
  - epidermal (inclusion) (*see also* Cyst, skin) 706.2
  - epidermoid (inclusion) (*see also* Cyst, skin) 706.2
    - mouth 528.4
    - not of skin – *see* Cyst, by site
    - oral soft tissue 528.4
  - epididymis 608.89
  - epiglottis 478.79
  - epiphysis cerebri 259.8
  - epithelial (inclusion) (*see also* Cyst, skin) 706.2
  - epoophoron 752.11
  - eruption 526.0
  - esophagus 530.89
  - ethmoid sinus 478.19
  - eye (retention) 379.8
    - congenital 743.03
    - posterior segment, congenital 743.54
  - eyebrow 706.2
  - eyelid (sebaceous) 374.84
    - infected 373.13
    - sweat glands or ducts 374.84
  - falciform ligament (inflammatory) 573.8
  - fallopian tube 620.8
  - female genital organs NEC 629.89
  - fimbrial (congenital) 752.11
  - fissural (oral region) 526.1
  - follicle (atretic) (graafian) (ovarian) 620.0
    - nabothian (gland) 616.0
  - follicular (atretic) (ovarian) 620.0
    - dentigerous 526.0
  - frontal sinus 478.19
  - gallbladder or duct 575.8
  - ganglion 727.43
  - Gartner's duct 752.41
  - gas, of mesentery 568.89
  - gingiva 523.8

- **Cyst** – *continued*
  - gland of moll 374.84
  - globulomaxillary 526.1
  - graafian follicle 620.0
  - granulosal lutein 620.2
  - hemangiomatous (M9121/0) (*see also* Hemangioma) 228.00
  - hydatid (*see also* Echinococcus) 122.9
    - fallopian tube (Morgagni) 752.11
    - liver NEC 122.8
    - lung NEC 122.9
    - Morgagni 752.89
      - fallopian tube 752.11
    - specified site NEC 122.9
  - hymen 623.8
    - embryonal 752.41
  - hypopharynx 478.26
  - hypophysis, hypophyseal (duct) (recurrent) 253.8
    - cerebri 253.8
  - implantation (dermoid)
    - anterior chamber (eye) 364.61
    - external area or site (skin) NEC 709.8
    - iris 364.61
    - vagina 623.8
    - vulva 624.8
  - incisor, incisive canal 526.1
  - inclusion (epidermal) (epithelial) (epidermoid) (mucous) (squamous) (*see also* Cyst, skin) 706.2
    - not of skin – *see* Neoplasm, by site, benign
  - intestine (large) (small) 569.89
  - intracranial – *see* Cyst, brain
  - intraligamentous 728.89
    - knee 717.89
  - intrasellar 253.8
  - iris (idiopathic) 364.60
    - exudative 364.62
    - implantation (surgical) (traumatic) 364.61
    - miotic pupillary 364.55
    - parasitic 360.13
  - Iwanoff's 362.62
  - jaw (bone) (aneurysmal) (extravasation) (hemorrhagic) (traumatic) 526.2
    - developmental (odontogenic) 526.0
    - fissural 526.1
  - keratin 706.2
  - kidney (congenital) 753.10
    - acquired 593.2
    - calyceal (*see also* Hydronephrosis) 591
    - multiple 753.19
    - pyelogenic (*see also* Hydronephrosis) 591
    - simple 593.2
    - single 753.11
    - solitary (not congenital) 593.2
  - labium (majus) (minus) 624.8
    - sebaceous 624.8
  - lacrimal
    - apparatus 375.43
    - gland or sac 375.12
  - larynx 478.79
  - lens 379.39
    - congenital 743.39
  - lip (gland) 528.5
  - liver 573.8
    - congenital 751.62
    - hydatid (*see also* Echinococcus) 122.8
      - granulosis 122.0
      - multilocularis 122.5
  - lung 518.89
    - congenital 748.4
    - giant bullous 492.0
  - lutein 620.1
  - lymphangiomatous (M9173/0) 228.1
  - lymphoepithelial
    - mouth 528.4
    - oral soft tissue 528.4
  - macula 362.54
  - malignant (M8000/3) – *see* Neoplasm, by site, malignant
  - mammary gland (sweat gland) (*see also* Cyst, breast) 610.0
  - mandible 526.2
    - dentigerous 526.0
    - radicular 522.8
  - maxilla 526.2
    - dentigerous 526.0
    - radicular 522.8
  - median
    - anterior maxillary 526.1
    - palatal 526.1
  - mediastinum (congenital) 748.8

- **Cyst** – *continued*
  - meibomian (gland) (retention) 373.2
    - infected 373.12
  - membrane, brain 348.0
  - meninges (cerebral) 348.0
    - spinal 349.2
  - meniscus knee 717.5
  - mesentery, mesenteric (gas) 568.89
    - chyle 457.8
    - gas 568.89
  - mesonephric duct 752.89
  - mesothelial
    - peritoneum 568.89
    - pleura (peritoneal) 568.89
  - milk 611.5
  - miotic pupillary (iris) 364.55
  - Morgagni (hydatid) 752.89
    - fallopian tube 752.11
  - mouth 528.4
  - mullerian duct 752.89
  - multilocular (ovary) (M8000/1) 239.5
  - myometrium 621.8
  - nabothian (follicle) (ruptured) 616.0
  - nasal sinus 478.19
  - nasoalveolar 528.4
  - nasolabial 528.4
  - nasopalatine (duct) 526.1
    - anterior 526.1
  - nasopharynx 478.26
  - neoplastic (M8000/1) – *see also* Neoplasm, by site, unspecified nature
    - benign (M8000/0) – *see* Neoplasm, by site, benign
    - uterus 621.8
  - nervous system – *see* Cyst, brain
  - neuroenteric 742.59
  - neuroepithelial ventricle 348.0
  - nipple 610.0
  - nose 478.19
    - skin of 706.2
  - odontogenic, developmental 526.0
  - omentum (lesser) 568.89
    - congenital 751.8
  - oral soft tissue (dermoid) (epidermoid) (lymphoepithelial) 528.4
  - ora serrata 361.19
  - orbit 376.81
  - ovary, ovarian (twisted) 620.2
    - adherent 620.2
    - chocolate 617.1
    - corpus
      - albicans 620.2
      - luteum 620.1
    - dermoid (M9084/0) 220
    - developmental 752.0
    - due to failure of involution NEC 620.2
    - endometrial 617.1
    - follicular (atretic) (graafian) (hemorrhagic) 620.0
    - hemorrhagic 620.2
    - in pregnancy or childbirth 654.4❺
      - affecting fetus or newborn 763.89
      - causing obstructed labor 660.2❺
        - affecting fetus or newborn 763.1
    - multilocular (M8000/1) 239.5
    - pseudomucinous (M8470/0) 220
    - retention 620.2
    - serous 620.2
    - theca lutein 620.2
    - tuberculous (*see also* Tuberculosis) 016.6❺
    - unspecified 620.2
  - oviduct 620.8
  - palatal papilla (jaw) 526.1
  - palate 526.1
    - fissural 526.1
    - median (fissural) 526.1
  - palatine, of papilla 526.1
  - pancreas, pancreatic 577.2
    - congenital 751.7
    - false 577.2
    - hemorrhagic 577.2
    - true 577.2
  - paranephric 593.2
  - para ovarian 752.11
  - paraphysis, cerebri 742.4
  - parasitic NEC 136.9
  - parathyroid (gland) 252.8
  - paratubal (fallopian) 620.8
  - paraurethral duct 599.89
  - paroophoron 752.11
  - parotid gland 527.6
    - mucous extravasation or retention 527.6

- **Cyst** – *continued*
  - parovarian 752.11
  - pars planus 364.60
    - exudative 364.64
    - primary 364.63
  - pelvis, female
    - in pregnancy or childbirth 654.4❺
      - affecting fetus or newborn 763.89
      - causing obstructed labor 660.2❺
        - affecting fetus or newborn 763.1
  - penis (sebaceous) 607.89
  - periapical 522.8
  - pericardial (congenital) 746.89
    - acquired (secondary) 423.8
  - pericoronal 526.0
  - perineural (Tarlov's) 355.9
  - periodontal 522.8
    - lateral 526.0
  - peripancreatic 577.2
  - peripelvic (lymphatic) 593.2
  - peritoneum 568.89
    - chylous 457.8
  - pharynx (wall) 478.26
  - pilonidal (infected) (rectum) 685.1
    - with abscess 685.0
    - malignant (M9084/3) 173.5
  - pituitary (duct) (gland) 253.8
  - placenta (amniotic) – *see* Placenta, abnormal
  - pleura 519.8
  - popliteal 727.51
  - porencephalic 742.4
    - acquired 348.0
  - postanal (infected) 685.1
    - with abscess 685.0
  - posterior segment of eye, congenital 743.54
  - postmastoidectomy cavity 383.31
  - preauricular 744.47
  - prepuce 607.89
    - congenital 752.69
  - primordial (jaw) 526.0
  - prostate 600.3
  - pseudomucinous (ovary) (M8470/0) 220
  - pudenda (sweat glands) 624.8
  - pupillary, miotic 364.55
    - sebaceous 624.8
  - radicular (residual) 522.8
  - radiculodental 522.8
  - ranular 527.6
  - Rathke's pouch 253.8
  - rectum (epithelium) (mucous) 569.49
  - renal – *see* Cyst, kidney
  - residual (radicular) 522.8
  - retention (ovary) 620.2
  - retina 361.19
    - macular 362.54
    - parasitic 360.13
    - primary 361.13
    - secondary 361.14
  - retroperitoneal 568.89
  - sacrococcygeal (dermoid) 685.1
    - with abscess 685.0
  - salivary gland or duct 527.6
    - mucous extravasation or retention 527.6
  - Sampson's 617.1
  - sclera 379.19
  - scrotum (sebaceous) 706.2
    - sweat glands 706.2
  - sebaceous (duct) (gland) 706.2
    - breast 610.8
    - eyelid 374.84
    - genital organ NEC
      - female 629.89
      - male 608.89
    - scrotum 706.2
  - semilunar cartilage (knee) (multiple) 717.5
  - seminal vesicle 608.89
  - serous (ovary) 620.2
  - sinus (antral) (ethmoidal) (frontal) (maxillary) (nasal) (sphenoidal) 478.19
  - Skene's gland 599.89
  - skin (epidermal) (epidermoid, inclusion) (epithelial) (inclusion) (retention) (sebaceous) 706.2
    - breast 610.8
    - eyelid 374.84
    - genital organ NEC
      - female 629.89
      - male 608.89
    - neoplastic 216.3
    - scrotum 706.2
    - sweat gland or duct 705.89

- **Cyst** – *continued*
  - solitary
    - bone 733.21
    - kidney 593.2
  - spermatic cord 608.89
  - sphenoid sinus 478.19
  - spinal meninges 349.2
  - spine (*see also* Cyst, bone) 733.20
  - spleen NEC 289.59
    - congenital 759.0
    - hydatid (*see also* Echinococcus) 122.9
  - spring water (pericardium) 746.89
  - subarachnoid 348.0
    - intrasellar 793.0
  - subdural (cerebral) 348.0
    - spinal cord 349.2
  - sublingual gland 527.6
    - mucous extravasation or retention 527.6
  - submaxillary gland 527.6
    - mucous extravasation or retention 527.6
  - suburethral 599.89
  - suprarenal gland 255.8
  - suprasellar – *see* Cyst, brain
  - sweat gland or duct 705.89
  - sympathetic nervous system 337.9
  - synovial 727.40
    - popliteal space 727.51
  - Tarlov's 355.9
  - tarsal 373.2
  - tendon (sheath) 727.42
  - testis 608.89
  - theca-lutein (ovary) 620.2
  - Thornwaldt's, Tornwaldt's 478.26
  - thymus (gland) 254.8
  - thyroglossal (duct) (infected) (persistent) 759.2
  - thyroid (gland) 246.2
    - adenomatous – *see* Goiter, nodular
    - colloid (*see also* Goiter) 240.9
  - thyrolingual duct (infected) (persistent) 759.2
  - tongue (mucous) 529.8
  - tonsil 474.8
  - tooth (dental root) 522.8
  - tubo-ovarian 620.8
    - inflammatory 614.1
  - tunica vaginalis 608.89
  - turbinate (nose) (*see also* Cyst, bone) 733.20
  - Tyson's gland (benign) (infected) 607.89
  - umbilicus 759.89
  - urachus 753.7
  - ureter 593.89
  - ureterovesical orifice 593.89
    - congenital 753.4
  - urethra 599.84
  - urethral gland (Cowper's) 599.89
  - uterine
    - ligament 620.8
      - embryonic 752.11
    - tube 620.8
  - uterus (body) (corpus) (recurrent) 621.8
    - embryonal 752.3
  - utricle (ear) 386.8
    - prostatic 599.89
  - utriculus masculinus 599.89
  - vagina, vaginal (squamous cell) (wall) 623.8
    - embryonal 752.41
    - implantation 623.8
    - inclusion 623.8
  - vallecula, vallecular 478.79
  - ventricle, neuroepithelial 348.0
  - verumontanum 599.89
  - vesical (orifice) 596.8
  - vitreous humor 379.29
  - vulva (sweat glands) 624.8
    - congenital 752.41
    - implantation 624.8
    - inclusion 624.8
    - sebaceous gland 624.8
  - vulvovaginal gland 624.8
  - Wolffian 752.89

- **Cystadenocarcinoma** (M8440/3) – *see also* Neoplasm, by site, malignant
  - bile duct type (M8161/3) 155.1
  - endometrioid (M8380/3) – *see* Neoplasm, by site, malignant
  - mucinous (M8470/3)
    - papillary (M8471/3)
      - specified site – *see* Neoplasm, by site, malignant
      - unspecified site 183.0
    - specified site – *see* Neoplasm, by site, malignant
    - unspecified site 183.0

- **Cystadenocarcinoma** – *continued*
  - papillary (M8450/3)
    - mucinous (M8471/3)
      - specified site – *see* Neoplasm, by site, malignant
      - unspecified site 183.0
    - pseudomucinous (M8471/3)
      - specified site – *see* Neoplasm, by site, malignant
      - unspecified site 183.0
    - serous (M8460/3)
      - specified site – *see* Neoplasm, by site, malignant
      - unspecified site 183.0
    - specified site – *see* Neoplasm, by site, malignant
    - unspecified 183.0
  - pseudomucinous (M8470/3)
    - papillary (M8471/3)
      - specified site – *see* Neoplasm, by site, malignant
      - unspecified site 183.0
    - specified site – *see* Neoplasm, by site, malignant
    - unspecified site 183.0
  - serous (M8441/3)
    - papillary (M8460/3)
      - specified site – *see* Neoplasm, by site, malignant
      - unspecified site 183.0
    - specified site – *see* Neoplasm, by site, malignant
    - unspecified site 183.0
- **Cystadenofibroma** (M9013/0)
  - clear cell (M8313/0) – *see* Neoplasm, by site, benign
  - endometrioid (M8381/0) 220
    - borderline malignancy (M8381/1) 236.2
    - malignant (M8381/3) 183.0
  - mucinous (M9015/0)
    - specified site – *see* Neoplasm, by site, benign
    - unspecified site 220
  - serous (M9014/0)
    - specified site – *see* Neoplasm, by site, benign
    - unspecified site 220
  - specified site – *see* Neoplasm, by site, benign
  - unspecified site 220
- **Cystadenoma** (M8440/0) – *see also* Neoplasm, by site, benign
  - bile duct (M8161/0) 211.5
  - endometrioid (M8380/0) – *see also* Neoplasm, by site, benign
    - borderline malignancy (M8380/1) – *see* Neoplasm, by site, uncertain behavior
  - malignant (M8440/3) – *see* Neoplasm, by site, malignant
  - mucinous (M8470/0)
    - borderline malignancy (M8470/1)
      - specified site – *see* Neoplasm, uncertain behavior
      - unspecified site 236.2
    - papillary (M8471/0)
      - borderline malignancy (M8471/1)
        - specified site – *see* Neoplasm, by site, uncertain behavior
        - unspecified site 236.2
      - specified site – *see* Neoplasm, by site, benign
      - unspecified site 220
    - specified site – *see* Neoplasm, by site, benign
    - unspecified site 220
  - papillary (M8450/0)
    - borderline malignancy (M8450/1)
      - specified site – *see* Neoplasm, by site, uncertain behavior
      - unspecified site 236.2
    - lymphomatosum (M8561/0) 210.2
    - mucinous (M8471/0)
      - borderline malignancy (M8471/1)
        - specified site – *see* Neoplasm, by site, uncertain behavior
        - unspecified site 236.2
      - specified site – *see* Neoplasm, by site, benign
      - unspecified site 220
    - pseudomucinous (M8471/0)
      - borderline malignancy (M8471/1)
        - specified site – *see* Neoplasm, by site uncertain behavior
        - unspecified site 236.2
      - specified site – *see* Neoplasm, by site, benign

Cyst – Cystadenoma

Cystadenoma – *continued*
papillary – *continued*
pseudomucinous – *continued*
unspecified site 220
serous (M8460/0)
borderline malignancy (M8460/1)
specified site – *see* Neoplasm, by site, uncertain behavior
unspecified site 236.2
specified site – *see* Neoplasm, by site, benign
unspecified site 220
specified site – *see* Neoplasm, by site, benign
unspecified site 220
pseudomucinous (M8470/0)
borderline malignancy (M8470/1)
specified site – *see* Neoplasm, by site uncertain behavior
unspecified site 236.2
papillary (M8471/0)
borderline malignancy (M8471/1)
specified site – *see* Neoplasm, by site uncertain behavior
unspecified site 236.2
specified site – *see* Neoplasm, by site, benign
unspecified site 220
specified site – *see* Neoplasm, by site, benign
unspecified site 220
serous (M8441/0)
borderline malignancy (M8441/1)
specified site – *see* Neoplasm, by site, uncertain behavior
unspecified site 236.2
papillary (M8460/0)
borderline malignancy (M8460/1)
specified site – *see* Neoplasm, by site, uncertain behavior
unspecified site 236.2
specified site – *see* Neoplasm, by site, benign
unspecified site 220
specified site – *see* Neoplasm, by site, benign
unspecified site 220
thyroid 226
Cystathioninemia 270.4
Cystathioninuria 270.4
Cystic – *see also* condition
breast, chronic 610.1
corpora lutea 620.1
degeneration, congenital
brain 742.4
kidney (*see also* Cystic, disease, kidney) 753.10
disease
breast, chronic 610.1
kidney, congenital 753.10
medullary 753.16
multiple 753.19
polycystic – *see* Polycystic, kidney
single 753.11
specified NEC 753.19
liver, congenital 751.62
lung 518.89
congenital 748.4
pancreas, congenital 751.7
semilunar cartilage 717.5
duct – *see* condition
eyeball, congenital 743.03
fibrosis (pancreas) 277.00
with
manifestations
gastrointestinal 277.03
pulmonary 277.02
specified NEC 277.09
meconium ileus 277.01
pulmonary exacerbation 277.02
hygroma (M9173/0) 228.1
kidney, congenital 753.10
medullary 753.16
multiple 753.19
polycystic – *see* Polycystic, kidney
single 753.11
specified NEC 753.19
liver, congenital 751.62
lung 518.89
congenital 748.4
mass – *see* Cyst
mastitis, chronic 610.1
ovary 620.2
pancreas, congenital 751.7

Cysticerciasis 123.1
Cysticercosis (mammary) (subretinal) 123.1
Cysticercus 123.1
cellulosae infestation 123.1
Cystinosis (malignant) 270.0
Cystinuria 270.0
Cystitis (bacillary) (colli) (diffuse) (exudative) (hemorrhagic) (purulent) (recurrent) (septic) (suppurative) (ulcerative) 595.9
with
abortion – *see* Abortion, by type, with urinary tract infection
ectopic pregnancy (*see also* categories 633.0-633.9) 639.8
fibrosis 595.1
leukoplakia 595.1
malakoplakia 595.1
metaplasia 595.1
molar pregnancy (*see also* categories 630-632) 639.8
actinomycotic 039.8 *[595.4]*
acute 595.0
of trigone 595.3
allergic 595.89
amebic 006.8 *[595.4]*
bilharzial 120.9 *[595.4]*
blennorrhagic (acute) 098.11
chronic or duration of 2 months or more 098.31
bullous 595.89
calculous 594.1
chlamydial 099.53
chronic 595.2
interstitial 595.1
of trigone 595.3
complicating pregnancy, childbirth, or puerperium 646.6❺
affecting fetus or newborn 760.1
cystic(a) 595.81
diphtheritic 032.84
echinococcal
granulosus 122.3 *[595.4]*
multilocularis 122.6 *[595.4]*
emphysematous 595.89
encysted 595.81
follicular 595.3
following
abortion 639.8
ectopic or molar pregnancy 639.8
gangrenous 595.89
glandularis 595.89
gonococcal (acute) 098.11
chronic or duration of 2 months or more 098.31
incrusted 595.89
interstitial 595.1
irradiation 595.82
irritation 595.89
malignant 595.89
monilial 112.2
of trigone 595.3
panmural 595.1
polyposa 595.89
prostatic 601.3
radiation 595.82
Reiter's (abacterial) 099.3
specified NEC 595.89
subacute 595.2
submucous 595.1
syphilitic 095.8
trichomoniasis 131.09
tuberculous (*see also* Tuberculosis) 016.1❺
ulcerative 595.1
Cystocele
female (without uterine prolapse) 618.01
with uterine prolapse 618.4
complete 618.3
incomplete 618.2
lateral 618.02
midline 618.01
paravaginal 618.02
in pregnancy or childbirth 654.4❺
affecting fetus or newborn 763.89
causing obstructed labor 660.2❺
affecting fetus or newborn 763.1
male 596.8
Cystoid
cicatrix limbus 372.64
degeneration macula 362.53
Cystolithiasis 594.1

Cystoma (M8440/0) – *see also* Neoplasm, by site, benign
endometrial, ovary 617.1
mucinous (M8470/0)
specified site – *see* Neoplasm, by site, benign
unspecified site 220
serous (M8441/0)
specified site – *see* Neoplasm, by site, benign
unspecified site 220
simple (ovary) 620.2
Cystoplegia 596.53
Cystoptosis 596.8
Cystopyelitis (*see also* Pyelitis) 590.80
Cystorrhagia 596.8
Cystosarcoma phyllodes (M9020/1) 238.3
benign (M9020/0) 217
malignant (M9020/3) – *see* Neoplasm, breast, malignant
Cystostomy status V44.50
with complication 997.5
appendico-vesicostomy V44.52
cutaneous-vesicostomy V44.51
specifed type NEC V44.59
Cystourethritis (*see also* Urethritis) 597.89
Cystourethrocele (*see also* Cystocele)
female (without uterine prolapse) 618.09
with uterine prolapse 618.4
complete 618.3
incomplete 618.2
male 596.8
Cytomegalic inclusion disease 078.5
congenital 771.1
Cytomycosis, reticuloendothelial (*see also* Histoplasmosis, American) 115.00
Cytopenia 289.9
refractory
with
multilineage dysplasia (RCMD) 238.72
and ringed sideroblasts (RCMD-RS) 238.72

D

Daae (-Finsen) **disease** (epidemic pleurodynia) 074.1
Dabney's grip 074.1
Da Costa's syndrome (neurocirculatory asthenia) 306.2
Dacryoadenitis, dacryadenitis 375.00
acute 375.01
chronic 375.02
Dacryocystitis 375.30
acute 375.32
chronic 375.42
neonatal 771.6
phlegmonous 375.33
syphilitic 095.8
congenital 090.0
trachomatous, active 076.1
late effect 139.1
tuberculous (*see also* Tuberculosis) 017.3❺
Dacryocystoblenorrhea 375.42
Dacryocystocele 375.43
Dacryolith, dacryolithiasis 375.57
Dacryoma 375.43
Dacryopericystitis (acute) (subacute) 375.32
chronic 375.42
Dacryops 375.11
Dacryosialadenopathy, atrophic 710.2
Dacryostenosis 375.56
congenital 743.65
Dactylitis
bone (*see also* Osteomyelitis) 730.2❺
sickle-cell 282.62
Hb-C 282.64
Hb-SS 282.62
specified NEC 282.69
syphilitic 095.5
tuberculous (*see also* Tuberculosis) 015.5❺
Dactylolysis spontanea 136.0
Dactylosymphysis (*see also* Syndactylism) 755.10
Damage
arteriosclerotic – *see* Arteriosclerosis
brain 348.9
anoxic, hypoxic 348.1
during or resulting from a procedure 997.01

Decompensation – Deferentitis

Defibrination syndrome (*see also* Fibrinolysis) 286.6

Deficiency, deficient
- 3-beta-hydroxysteroid dehydrogenase 255.2
- 6-phosphogluconic dehydrogenase (anemia) 282.2
- 11-beta-hydroxylase 255.2
- 17-alpha-hydroxylase 255.2
- 18-hydroxysteroid dehydrogenase 255.2
- 20-alpha-hydroxylase 255.2
- 21-hydroxylase 255.2
- AAT (alpha-1 antitrypsin) 273.4
- abdominal muscle syndrome 756.79
- accelerator globulin (Ac G) (blood) (*see also* Defect, coagulation) 286.3
- AC globulin (congenital) (*see also* Defect, coagulation) 286.3
  - acquired 286.7
- activating factor (blood) (*see also* Defect, coagulation) 286.3
- adenohypophyseal 253.2
- adenosine deaminase 277.2
- aldolase (hereditary) 271.2
- alpha-1-antitrypsin 273.4
- alpha-1-trypsin inhibitor 273.4
- alpha-fucosidase 271.8
- alpha-lipoprotein 272.5
- alpha-mannosidase 271.8
- amino acid 270.9
- anemia – *see* Anemia, deficiency
- aneurin 265.1
  - with beriberi 265.0
- antibody NEC 279.00
- antidiuretic hormone 253.5
- antihemophilic
  - factor (A) 286.0
    - B 286.1
    - C 286.2
  - globulin (AHG) NEC 286.0
- antithrombin III 289.81
- antitrypsin 273.4
- argininosuccinate synthetase or lyase 270.6
- ascorbic acid (with scurvy) 267
- autoprothrombin
  - I (*see also* Defect, coagulation) 286.3
  - II 286.1
  - C (*see also* Defect, coagulation) 286.3
- bile salt 579.8
- biotin 266.2
- biotinidase 277.6
- bradykinase-1 277.6
- brancher enzyme (amylopectinosis) 271.0
- calciferol 268.9
  - with
    - osteomalacia 268.2
    - rickets (*see also* Rickets) 268.0
- calcium 275.40
  - dietary 269.3
- calorie, severe 261
- carbamyl phosphate synthetase 270.6
- cardiac (*see also* Insufficiency, myocardial) 428.0
- carnitine 277.81
  - due to
    - hemodialysis 277.83
    - inborn errors of metabolism 277.82
    - valproic acid therapy 277.83
  - iatrogenic 277.83
  - palmitoyltransferase (CPT1, CPT2) 277.85
  - palmityl transferase (CPT1, CPT2) 277.85
  - primary 277.81
  - secondary 277.84
- carotene 264.9
- Carr factor (*see also* Defect, coagulation) 286.9
- central nervous system 349.9
- ceruloplasmin 275.1
- cevitamic acid (with scurvy) 267
- choline 266.2
- Christmas factor 286.1
- chromium 269.3
- citrin 269.1
- clotting (blood) (*see also* Defect, coagulation) 286.9
- coagulation factor NEC 286.9
  - with
    - abortion – *see* Abortion, by type, with hemorrhage
    - ectopic pregnancy (*see also* categories 634-638) 639.1
    - molar pregnancy (*see also* categories 630-632) 639.1
  - acquired (any) 286.7
  - antepartum or intrapartum 641.3⑤
    - affecting fetus or newborn 762.1

Deficiency, deficient – *continued*
- coagulation factor – *continued*
  - complicating pregnancy, childbirth, or puerperium 649.3⑤
  - due to
    - liver disease 286.7
    - vitamin K deficiency 286.7
  - newborn, transient 776.3
  - postpartum 666.3⑤
  - specified type NEC 286.3
- color vision (congenital) 368.59
  - acquired 368.55
- combined glucocorticoid and mineralocorticoid 255.41 ●
- combined, two or more coagulation factors (*see also* Defect, coagulation) 286.9
- complement factor NEC 279.8
- contact factor (*see also* Defect, coagulation) 286.3
- copper NEC 275.1
- corticoadrenal 255.41 ▲
- craniofacial axis 756.0
- cyanocobalamin (vitamin B_{12}) 266.2
- debrancher enzyme (limit dextrinosis) 271.0
- desmolase 255.2
- diet 269.9
- dihydrofolate reductase 281.2
- dihydropteridine reductase 270.1
- disaccharidase (intestinal) 271.3
- disease NEC 269.9
- ear(s) V48.8
- edema 262
- endocrine 259.9
- enzymes, circulating NEC (*see also* Deficiency, by specific enzyme) 277.6
- ergosterol 268.9
  - with
    - osteomalacia 268.2
    - rickets (*see also* Rickets) 268.0
- erythrocytic glutathione (anemia) 282.2
- eyelid(s) V48.8
- factor (*see also* Defect, coagulation) 286.9
  - I (congenital) (fibrinogen) 286.3
    - antepartum or intrapartum 641.3⑤
      - affecting fetus or newborn 762.1
    - newborn, transient 776.3
    - postpartum 666.3⑤
  - II (congenital) (prothrombin) 286.3
  - V (congenital) (labile) 286.3
  - VII (congenital) (stable) 286.3
  - VIII (congenital) (functional) 286.0
    - with
      - functional defect 286.0
      - vascular defect 286.4
  - IX (Christmas) (congenital) (functional) 286.1
  - X (congenital) (Stuart-Prower) 286.3
  - XI (congenital) (plasma thromboplastin antecedent) 286.2
  - XII (congenital) (Hageman) 286.3
  - XIII (congenital) (fibrin stabilizing) 286.3
  - hageman 286.3
  - multiple (congenital) 286.9
    - acquired 286.7
- fibrinase (*see also* Defect, coagulation) 286.3
- fibrinogen (congenital) (*see also* Defect, coagulation) 286.3
  - acquired 286.6
- fibrin-stabilizing factor (congenital) (*see also* Defect, coagulation) 286.3
  - acquired 286.7
- finger – *see* Absence, finger
- fletcher factor (*see also* Defect, coagulation) 286.9
- fluorine 269.3
- folate, anemia 281.2
- folic acid (vitamin BC) 266.2
  - anemia 281.2
- follicle-stimulating hormone (FSH) 253.4
- fructokinase 271.2
- fructose-1, 6-diphosphate 271.2
- fructose-1-phosphate aldolase 271.2
- FSH (follicle-stimulating hormone) 253.4
- fucosidase 271.8
- galactokinase 271.1
- galactose-1-phosphate uridyl transferase 271.1
- gamma globulin in blood 279.00
- glass factor (*see also* Defect, coagulation) 286.3
- glucocorticoid 255.41 ▲
- glucose-6-phosphatase 271.0
- glucose-6-phosphate dehydrogenase anemia 282.2
- glucuronyl transferase 277.4

Deficiency, deficient – *continued*
- glutathione-reductase (anemia) 282.2
- glycogen synthetase 271.0
- growth hormone 253.3
- Hageman factor (congenital) (*see also* Defect, coagulation) 286.3
- head V48.0
- hemoglobin (*see also* Anemia) 285.9
- hepatophosphorylase 271.0
- hexose monophosphate (HMP) shunt 282.2
- HGH (human growth hormone) 253.3
- HG-PRT 277.2
- homogentisic acid oxidase 270.2
- hormone – *see also* Deficiency, by specific hormone
  - anterior pituitary (isolated) (partial) NEC 253.4
    - growth (human) 253.3
  - follicle-stimulating 253.4
  - growth (human) (isolated) 253.3
  - human growth 253.3
  - interstitial cell-stimulating 253.4
  - luteinizing 253.4
  - melanocyte-stimulating 253.4
  - testicular 257.2
- human growth hormone 253.3
- humoral 279.00
  - with
    - hyper-IgM 279.05
      - autosomal recessive 279.05
      - X-linked 279.05
    - increased IgM 279.05
  - congenital hypogammaglobulinemia 279.04
    - non-sex-linked 279.06
  - selective immunoglobulin NEC 279.03
    - IgA 279.01
    - IgG 279.03
    - IgM 279.02
      - increased 279.05
  - specified NEC 279.09
- hydroxylase 255.2
- hypoxanthine-guanine phosphoribosyltransferase (HG-PRT) 277.2
- ICSH (interstitial cell-stimulating hormone) 253.4
- immunity NEC 279.3
  - cell-mediated 279.10
    - with
      - hyperimmunoglobulinemia 279.2
      - thrombocytopenia and eczema 279.12
    - specified NEC 279.19
  - combined (severe) 279.2
    - syndrome 279.2
  - common variable 279.06
  - humoral NEC 279.00
  - IgA (secretory) 279.01
  - IgG 279.03
  - IgM 279.02
- immunoglobulin, selective NEC 279.03
  - IgA 279.01
  - IgG 279.03
  - IgM 279.02
- inositol (B complex) 266.2
- interferon 279.4
- internal organ V47.0
- interstitial cell-stimulating hormone (ICSH) 253.4
- intrinsic factor (Castle's) (congenital) 281.0
- intrinsic (urethral) sphincter (ISD) 599.82
- invertase 271.3
- iodine 269.3
- iron, anemia 280.9
- labile factor (congenital) (*see also* Defect, coagulation) 286.3
  - acquired 286.7
- lacrimal fluid (acquired) 375.15
  - congenital 743.64
- lactase 271.3
- Laki-Lorand factor (*see also* Defect, coagulation) 286.3
- lecithin-cholesterol acyltranferase 272.5
- LH (luteinizing hormone) 253.4
- limb V49.0
  - lower V49.0
    - congenital (*see also* Deficiency, lower limb, congenital) 755.30
  - upper V49.0
    - congenital (*see also* Deficiency, upper limb, congenital) 755.20
- lipocaic 577.8
- lipoid (high-density) 272.5
- lipoprotein (familial) (high-density) 272.5
- liver phosphorylase 271.0
- long chain 3-hydroxyacyl CoA dehydrogenase (LCHAD) 277.85

Deficiency, deficient – *continued*
- long chain/very long chain acyl CoA dehydrogenase (LCAD, VLCAD) 277.85
- lower limb V49.0
  - congenital 755.30
    - with complete absence of distal elements 755.31
    - longitudinal (complete) (partial) (with distal deficiencies, incomplete) 755.32
      - with complete absence of distal elements 755.31
      - combined femoral, tibial, fibular (incomplete) 755.33
      - femoral 755.34
      - fibular 755.37
      - metatarsal(s) 755.38
      - phalange(s) 755.39
        - meaning all digits 755.31
      - tarsal(s) 755.38
      - tibia 755.36
      - tibiofibular 755.35
    - transverse 755.31
- luteinizing hormone (LH) 253.4
- lysosomal alpha-1, 4 glucosidase 271.0
- magnesium 275.2
- mannosidase 271.8
- medium chain acyl CoA dehydrogenase (MCAD) 277.85
- melanocyte-stimulating hormone (MSH) 253.4
- menadione (vitamin K) 269.0
  - newborn 776.0
- mental (familial) (hereditary) (*see also* Retardation, mental) 319
- methylenetetrahydrofolate reductase (MTHFR) 270.4 ●
- mineral NEC 269.3
- mineralocorticoid 255.42 ●
- molybdenum 269.3
- moral 301.7
- multiple, syndrome 260
- myocardial (*see also* Insufficiency, myocardial) 428.0
- myophosphorylase 271.0
- NADH (DPNH) -methemoglobin-reductase (congenital) 289.7
- NADH diaphorase or reductase (congenital) 289.7
- neck V48.1
- niacin (amide) (-tryptophan) 265.2
- nicotinamide 265.2
- nicotinic acid (amide) 265.2
- nose V48.8
- number of teeth (*see also* Anodontia) 520.0
- nutrition, nutritional 269.9
  - specified NEC 269.8
- ornithine transcarbamylase 270.6
- ovarian 256.39
- oxygen (*see also* Anoxia) 799.02
- pantothenic acid 266.2
- parathyroid (gland) 252.1
- phenylalanine hydroxylase 270.1
- phosphoenolpyruvate carboxykinase 271.8
- phosphofructokinase 271.2
- phosphoglucomutase 271.0
- phosphohexosisomerase 271.0
- phosphomannomutase 271.8
- phosphomannose isomerase 271.8
- phosphomannosyl mutase 271.8
- phosphorylase kinase, liver 271.0
- pituitary (anterior) 253.2
  - posterior 253.5
- placenta – *see* Placenta, insufficiency
- plasma
  - cell 279.00
  - protein (paraproteinemia) (pyroglobulinemia) 273.8
    - gamma globulin 279.00
  - thromboplastin
    - antecedent (PTA) 286.2
    - component (PTC) 286.1
- platelet NEC 287.1
  - constitutional 286.4
- polyglandular 258.9
- potassium (K) 276.8
- proaccelerin (congenital) (*see also* Defect, congenital) 286.3
  - acquired 286.7
- proconvertin factor (congenital) (*see also* Defect, coagulation) 286.3
  - acquired 286.7
- prolactin 253.4
- protein 260
  - anemia 281.4

Deficiency, deficient – *continued*
- protein – *continued*
  - C 289.81
  - plasma – *see* Deficiency, plasma, protein
  - S 289.81
- prothrombin (congenital) (*see also* Defect, coagulation) 286.3
  - acquired 286.7
- Prower factor (*see also* Defect, coagulation) 286.3
- PRT 277.2
- pseudocholinesterase 289.89
- psychobiological 301.6
- PTA 286.2
- PTC 286.1
- purine nucleoside phosphorylase 277.2
- pyracin (alpha) (beta) 266.1
- pyridoxal 266.1
- pyridoxamine 266.1
- pyridoxine (derivatives) 266.1
- pyruvate carboxylase 271.8
- pyruvate dehydrogenase 271.8
- pyruvate kinase (PK) 282.3
- riboflavin (vitamin B_2) 266.0
- saccadic eye movements 379.57
- salivation 527.7
- salt 276.1
- secretion
  - ovary 256.39
  - salivary gland (any) 527.7
  - urine 788.5
- selenium 269.3
- serum
  - antitrypsin, familial 273.4
  - protein (congenital) 273.8
- short chain acyl CoA dehydrogenase (SCAD) 277.85
- short stature homeobox gene (SHOX) ●
  - with ●
    - dyschondrosteosis 756.89 ●
    - short stature (idiopathic) 783.43 ●
    - Turner's syndrome 758.6 ●
- smooth pursuit movements (eye) 379.58
- sodium (Na) 276.1
- SPCA (*see also* Defect, coagulation) 286.3
- specified NEC 269.8
- stable factor (congenital) (*see also* Defect, coagulation) 286.3
  - acquired 286.7
- Stuart (-Prower) factor (*see also* Defect, coagulation) 286.3
- sucrase 271.3
- sucrase-isomaltase 271.3
- sulfite oxidase 270.0
- syndrome, multiple 260
- thiamine, thiaminic (chloride) 265.1
- thrombokinase (*see also* Defect, coagulation) 286.3
  - newborn 776.0
- thrombopoieten 287.39
- thymolymphatic 279.2
- thyroid (gland) 244.9
- tocopherol 269.1
- toe – *see* Absence, toe
- tooth bud (*see also* Anodontia) 520.0
- trunk V48.1
- UDPG-glycogen transferase 271.0
- upper limb V49.0
  - congenital 755.20
    - with complete absence of distal elements 755.21
    - longitudinal (complete) (partial) (with distal deficiencies, incomplete) 755.22
      - carpal(s) 755.28
      - combined humeral, radial, ulnar (incomplete) 755.23
      - humeral 755.24
      - metacarpal(s) 755.28
      - phalange(s) 755.29
        - meaning all digits 755.21
      - radial 755.26
      - radioulnar 755.25
      - ulnar 755.27
    - transverse (complete) (partial) 755.21
- vascular 459.9
- vasopressin 253.5
- viosterol (*see also* Deficiency, calciferol) 268.9

Deficiency, deficient – *continued*
- vitamin (multiple) NEC 269.2
  - A 264.9
    - with
      - Bitôt's spot 264.1
        - corneal 264.2
          - with corneal ulceration 264.3
      - keratomalacia 264.4
      - keratosis, follicular 264.8
      - night blindness 264.5
      - scar of cornea, xerophthalmic 264.6
      - specified manifestation NEC 264.8
        - ocular 264.7
    - xeroderma 264.8
    - xerophthalmia 264.7
    - xerosis
      - conjunctival 264.0
        - with Bitôt's spot 264.1
      - corneal 264.2
        - with corneal ulceration 264.3
  - B (complex) NEC 266.9
    - with
      - beriberi 265.0
      - pellagra 265.2
    - specified type NEC 266.2
  - B_1 NEC 265.1
    - beriberi 265.0
  - B_2 266.0
  - B_6 266.1
  - B_{12} 266.2
  - B_9 (folic acid) 266.2
  - C (ascorbic acid) (with scurvy) 267
  - D (calciferol) (ergosterol) 268.9
    - with
      - osteomalacia 268.2
      - rickets (*see also* Rickets) 268.0
  - E 269.1
  - folic acid 266.2
  - G 266.0
  - H 266.2
  - K 269.0
    - of newborn 776.0
  - nicotinic acid 265.2
  - P 269.1
  - PP 265.2
  - specified NEC 269.1
- zinc 269.3

Deficient – *see also* Deficiency
- blink reflex 374.45
- craniofacial axis 756.0
- number of teeth (*see also* Anodontia) 520.0
- secretion of urine 788.5

Deficit
- neurologic NEC 781.99
  - due to
    - cerebrovascular lesion (*see also* Disease, cerebrovascular, acute) 436
      - late effect – *see* Late effect(s) (of) cerebrovascular disease
    - transient ischemic attack 435.9
  - ischemic ●
    - reversible (RIND) 434.91 ●
      - history of (personal) V12.54 ●
      - prolonged (PRIND) 434.91 ●
        - history of (personal) V12.54 ●
- oxygen 799.02

Deflection
- radius 736.09
- septum (acquired) (nasal) (nose) 470
- spine – *see* Curvature, spine
- turbinate (nose) 470

Defluvium
- capillorum (*see also* Alopecia) 704.00
- ciliorum 374.55
- unguium 703.8

Deformity 738.9
- abdomen, congenital 759.9
- abdominal wall
  - acquired 738.8
  - congenital 756.70
  - muscle deficiency syndrome 756.79
- acquired (unspecified site) 738.9
  - specified site NEC 738.8
- adrenal gland (congenital) 759.1
- alimentary tract, congenital 751.9
  - lower 751.5
  - specified type NEC 751.8
  - upper (any part, except tongue) 750.9
    - specified type NEC 750.8
    - tongue 750.10
      - specified type NEC 750.19

Deformity – *continued*
  ankle (joint) (acquired) 736.70
    abduction 718.47
    congenital 755.69
    contraction 718.47
    specified NEC 736.79
  anus (congenital) 751.5
    acquired 569.49
  aorta (congenital) 747.20
    acquired 447.8
    arch 747.21
      acquired 447.8
    coarctation 747.10
  aortic
    arch 747.21
      acquired 447.8
    cusp or valve (congenital) 746.9
      acquired (*see also* Endocarditis, aortic) 424.1
    ring 747.21
  appendix 751.5
  arm (acquired) 736.89
    congenital 755.50
  arteriovenous (congenital) (peripheral) NEC 747.60
    gastrointestinal 747.61
    lower limb 747.64
    renal 747.62
    specified NEC 747.69
    spinal 747.82
    upper limb 747.63
  artery (congenital) (peripheral) NEC (*see also* Deformity, vascular) 747.60
    acquired 447.8
    cerebral 747.81
    coronary (congenital) 746.85
      acquired (*see also* Ischemia, heart) 414.9
    retinal 743.9
    umbilical 747.5
  atrial septal (congenital) (heart) 745.5
  auditory canal (congenital) (external) (*see also* Deformity, ear) 744.3
    acquired 380.50
  auricle
    ear (congenital) (*see also* Deformity, ear) 744.3
      acquired 380.32
    heart (congenital) 746.9
  back (acquired) – *see* Deformity, spine
  Bartholin's duct (congenital) 750.9
  bile duct (congenital) 751.60
    acquired 576.8
      with calculus, choledocholithiasis, or stones – *see* Choledocholithiasis
  biliary duct or passage (congenital) 751.60
    acquired 576.8
      with calculus, choledocholithiasis, or stones – *see* Choledocholithiasis
  bladder (neck) (sphincter) (trigone) (acquired) 596.8
    congenital 753.9
  bone (acquired) NEC 738.9
    congenital 756.9
    turbinate 738.0
  boutonniere (finger) 736.21
  brain (congenital) 742.9
    acquired 348.8
    multiple 742.4
    reduction 742.2
    vessel (congenital) 747.81
  breast (acquired) 611.8
    congenital 757.9
  bronchus (congenital) 748.3
    acquired 519.19
  bursa, congenital 756.9
  canal of Nuck 752.9
  canthus (congenital) 743.9
    acquired 374.89
  capillary (acquired) 448.9
    congenital NEC (*see also* Deformity, vascular) 747.60
  cardiac – *see* Deformity, heart
  cardiovascular system (congenital) 746.9
  caruncle, lacrimal (congenital) 743.9
    acquired 375.69
  cascade, stomach 537.6
  cecum (congenital) 751.5
    acquired 569.89
  cerebral (congenital) 742.9
    acquired 348.8
  cervix (acquired) (uterus) 622.8
    congenital 752.40

Deformity – *continued*
  cheek (acquired) 738.19
    congenital 744.9
  chest (wall) (acquired) 738.3
    congenital 754.89
    late effect of rickets 268.1
  chin (acquired) 738.19
    congenital 744.9
  choroid (congenital) 743.9
    acquired 363.8
    plexus (congenital) 742.9
      acquired 349.2
  cicatricial – *see* Cicatrix
  cilia (congenital) 743.9
    acquired 374.89
  circulatory system (congenital) 747.9
  clavicle (acquired) 738.8
    congenital 755.51
  clitoris (congenital) 752.40
    acquired 624.8
  clubfoot – *see* Clubfoot
  coccyx (acquired) 738.6
    congenital 756.10
  colon (congenital) 751.5
    acquired 569.89
  concha (ear) (congenital) (*see also* Deformity, ear) 744.3
    acquired 380.32
  congenital, organ or site not listed (*see also* Anomaly) 759.9
  cornea (congenital) 743.9
    acquired 371.70
  coronary artery (congenital) 746.85
    acquired (*see also* Ischemia, heart) 414.9
  cranium (acquired) 738.19
    congenital (*see also* Deformity, skull, congenital) 756.0
  cricoid cartilage (congenital) 748.3
    acquired 478.79
  cystic duct (congenital) 751.60
    acquired 575.8
  Dandy-Walker 742.3
    with spina bifida (*see also* Spina bifida) 741.0❺
  diaphragm (congenital) 756.6
    acquired 738.8
  digestive organ(s) or system (congenital) NEC 751.9
    specified type NEC 751.8
  ductus arteriosus 747.0
  duodenal bulb 537.89
  duodenum (congenital) 751.5
    acquired 537.89
  dura (congenital) 742.9
    brain 742.4
      acquired 349.2
    spinal 742.59
      acquired 349.2
  ear (congenital) 744.3
    acquired 380.32
    auricle 744.3
      causing impairment of hearing 744.02
    causing impairment of hearing 744.00
    external 744.3
      causing impairment of hearing 744.02
    internal 744.05
    lobule 744.3
    middle 744.03
      ossicles 744.04
    ossicles 744.04
  ectodermal (congenital) NEC 757.9
    specified type NEC 757.8
  ejaculatory duct (congenital) 752.9
    acquired 608.89
  elbow (joint) (acquired) 736.00
    congenital 755.50
    contraction 718.42
  endocrine gland NEC 759.2
  epididymis (congenital) 752.9
    acquired 608.89
    torsion 608.24
  epiglottis (congenital) 748.3
    acquired 478.79
  esophagus (congenital) 750.9
    acquired 530.89
  Eustachian tube (congenital) NEC 744.3
    specified type NEC 744.24
  extremity (acquired) 736.9
    congenital, except reduction deformity 755.9
      lower 755.60
      upper 755.50
    reduction – *see* Deformity, reduction

Deformity – *continued*
  eye (congenital) 743.9
    acquired 379.8
    muscle 743.9
  eyebrow (congenital) 744.89
  eyelid (congenital) 743.9
    acquired 374.89
    specified type NEC 743.62
  face (acquired) 738.19
    congenital (any part) 744.9
      due to intrauterine malposition and pressure 754.0
  fallopian tube (congenital) 752.10
    acquired 620.8
  femur (acquired) 736.89
    congenital 755.60
  fetal
    with fetopelvic disproportion 653.7❺
      affecting fetus or newborn 763.1
    causing obstructed labor 660.1❺
      affecting fetus or newborn 763.1
    known or suspected, affecting management of pregnancy 655.9❺
  finger (acquired) 736.20
    boutonniere type 736.21
    congenital 755.50
    flexion contracture 718.44
    swan neck 736.22
  flexion (joint) (acquired) 736.9
    congenital NEC 755.9
    hip or thigh (acquired) 736.39
      congenital (*see also* Subluxation, congenital, hip) 754.32
  foot (acquired) 736.70
    cavovarus 736.75
      congenital 754.59
    congenital NEC 754.70
      specified type NEC 754.79
    valgus (acquired) 736.79
      congenital 754.60
        specified type NEC 754.69
    varus (acquired) 736.79
      congenital 754.50
        specified type NEC 754.59
  forearm (acquired) 736.00
    congenital 755.50
  forehead (acquired) 738.19
    congenital (*see also* Deformity, skull, congenital) 756.0
  frontal bone (acquired) 738.19
    congenital (*see also* Deformity, skull, congenital) 756.0
  gallbladder (congenital) 751.60
    acquired 575.8
  gastrointestinal tract (congenital) NEC 751.9
    acquired 569.89
    specified type NEC 751.8
  genitalia, genital organ(s) or system NEC
    congenital 752.9
    female (congenital) 752.9
      acquired 629.89
      external 752.40
      internal 752.9
    male (congenital) 752.9
      acquired 608.89
  globe (eye) (congenital) 743.9
    acquired 360.89
  gum (congenital) 750.9
    acquired 523.9
  gunstock 736.02
  hand (acquired) 736.00
    claw 736.06
    congenital 755.50
    minus (and plus) (intrinsic) 736.09
    pill roller (intrinsic) 736.09
    plus (and minus) (intrinsic) 736.09
    swan neck (intrinsic) 736.09
  head (acquired) 738.10
    congenital (*see also* Deformity, skull, congenital) 756.0
    specified NEC 738.19
  heart (congenital) 746.9
    auricle (congenital) 746.9
    septum 745.9
      auricular 745.5
      specified type NEC 745.8
      ventricular 745.4
    valve (congenital) NEC 746.9
      acquired – *see* Endocarditis
      pulmonary (congenital) 746.00
      specified type NEC 746.89
    ventricle (congenital) 746.9

Deformity – *continued*
heel (acquired) 736.76
congenital 755.67
hepatic duct (congenital) 751.60
acquired 576.8
with calculus, choledocholithiasis, or stones – *see* Choledocholithiasis
hip (joint) (acquired) 736.30
congenital NEC 755.63
flexion 718.45
congenital (*see also* Subluxation, congenital, hip) 754.32
hourglass – *see* Contraction, hourglass
humerus (acquired) 736.89
congenital 755.50
hymen (congenital) 752.40
hypophyseal (congenital) 759.2
ileocecal (coil) (valve) (congenital) 751.5
acquired 569.89
ileum (intestine) (congenital) 751.5
acquired 569.89
ilium (acquired) 738.6
congenital 755.60
integument (congenital) 757.9
intervertebral cartilage or disc (acquired) – *see also* Displacement, intervertebral disc
congenital 756.10
intestine (large) (small) (congenital) 751.5
acquired 569.89
iris (acquired) 364.75
congenital 743.9
prolapse 364.89 ▲
ischium (acquired) 738.6
congenital 755.60
jaw (acquired) (congenital) NEC 524.9
due to intrauterine malposition and pressure 754.0
joint (acquired) NEC 738.8
congenital 755.9
contraction (abduction) (adduction) (extension) (flexion) – *see* Contraction, joint
kidney(s) (calyx) (pelvis) (congenital) 753.9
acquired 593.89
vessel 747.62
acquired 459.9
Klippel-Feil (brevicollis) 756.16
knee (acquired) NEC 736.6
congenital 755.64
labium (majus) (minus) (congenital) 752.40
acquired 624.8
lacrimal apparatus or duct (congenital) 743.9
acquired 375.69
larynx (muscle) (congenital) 748.3
acquired 478.79
web (glottic) (subglottic) 748.2
leg (lower) (upper) (acquired) NEC 736.89
congenital 755.60
reduction – *see* Deformity, reduction, lower limb
lens (congenital) 743.9
acquired 379.39
lid (fold) (congenital) 743.9
acquired 374.89
ligament (acquired) 728.9
congenital 756.9
limb (acquired) 736.9
congenital, except reduction deformity 755.9
lower 755.60
reduction (*see also* Deformity, reduction, lower limb) 755.30
upper 755.50
reduction (*see also* Deformity, reduction, lower limb) 755.20
specified NEC 736.89
lip (congenital) NEC 750.9
acquired 528.5
specified type NEC 750.26
liver (congenital) 751.60
acquired 573.8
duct (congenital) 751.60
acquired 576.8
with calculus, choledocholithiasis, or stones – *see* Choledocholithiasis
lower extremity – *see* Deformity, leg
lumbosacral (joint) (region) (congenital) 756.10
acquired 738.5
lung (congenital) 748.60
acquired 518.89
specified type NEC 748.69
lymphatic system, congenital 759.9
Madelung's (radius) 755.54
maxilla (acquired) (congenital) 524.9

Deformity – *continued*
meninges or membrane (congenital) 742.9
brain 742.4
acquired 349.2
spinal (cord) 742.59
acquired 349.2
mesentery (congenital) 751.9
acquired 568.89
metacarpus (acquired) 736.00
congenital 755.50
metatarsus (acquired) 736.70
congenital 754.70
middle ear, except ossicles (congenital) 744.03
ossicles 744.04
mitral (leaflets) (valve) (congenital) 746.9
acquired – *see* Endocarditis, mitral
Ebstein's 746.89
parachute 746.5
specified type NEC 746.89
stenosis, congenital 746.5
mouth (acquired) 528.9
congenital NEC 750.9
specified type NEC 750.26
multiple, congenital NEC 759.7
specified type NEC 759.89
muscle (acquired) 728.9
congenital 756.9
specified type NEC 756.89
sternocleidomastoid (due to intrauterine malposition and pressure) 754.1
musculoskeletal system, congenital NEC 756.9
specified type NEC 756.9
nail (acquired) 703.9
congenital 757.9
nasal – *see* Deformity, nose
neck (acquired) NEC 738.2
congenital (any part) 744.9
sternocleidomastoid 754.1
nervous system (congenital) 742.9
nipple (congenital) 757.9
acquired 611.8
nose, nasal (cartilage) (acquired) 738.0
bone (turbinate) 738.0
congenital 748.1
bent 754.0
squashed 754.0
saddle 738.0
syphilitic 090.5
septum 470
congenital 748.1
sinus (wall) (congenital) 748.1
acquired 738.0
syphilitic (congenital) 090.5
late 095.8
ocular muscle (congenital) 743.9
acquired 378.60
opticociliary vessels (congenital) 743.9
orbit (congenital) (eye) 743.9
acquired NEC 376.40
associated with craniofacial deformities 376.44
due to
bone disease 376.43
surgery 376.47
trauma 376.47
organ of Corti (congenital) 744.05
ovary (congenital) 752.0
acquired 620.8
oviduct (congenital) 752.10
acquired 620.8
palate (congenital) 750.9
acquired 526.89
cleft (congenital) (*see also* Cleft, palate) 749.00
hard, acquired 526.89
soft, acquired 528.9
pancreas (congenital) 751.7
acquired 577.8
parachute, mitral valve 746.5
parathyroid (gland) 759.2
parotid (gland) (congenital) 750.9
acquired 527.8
patella (acquired) 736.6
congenital 755.64
pelvis, pelvic (acquired) (bony) 738.6
with disproportion (fetopelvic) 653.0❺
affecting fetus or newborn 763.1
causing obstructed labor 660.1❺
affecting fetus or newborn 763.1
congenital 755.60
rachitic (late effect) 268.1

Deformity – *continued*
penis (glans) (congenital) 752.9
acquired 607.89
pericardium (congenital) 746.9
acquired – *see* Pericarditis
pharynx (congenital) 750.9
acquired 478.29
Pierre Robin (congenital) 756.0
pinna (acquired) 380.32
congenital 744.3
pituitary (congenital) 759.2
pleural folds (congenital) 748.8
portal vein (congenital) 747.40
posture – *see* Curvature, spine
prepuce (congenital) 752.9
acquired 607.89
prostate (congenital) 752.9
acquired 602.8
pulmonary valve – *see* Endocarditis, pulmonary
pupil (congenital) 743.9
acquired 364.75
pylorus (congenital) 750.9
acquired 537.89
rachitic (acquired), healed or old 268.1
radius (acquired) 736.00
congenital 755.50
reduction – *see* Deformity, reduction, upper limb
rectovaginal septum (congenital) 752.40
acquired 623.8
rectum (congenital) 751.5
acquired 569.49
reduction (extremity) (limb) 755.4
brain 742.2
lower limb 755.30
with complete absence of distal elements 755.31
longitudinal (complete) (partial) (with distal deficiencies, incomplete) 755.32
with complete absence of distal elements 755.31
combined femoral, tibial, fibular (incomplete) 755.33
femoral 755.34
fibular 755.37
metatarsal(s) 755.38
phalange(s) 755.39
meaning all digits 755.31
tarsal(s) 755.38
tibia 755.36
tibiofibular 755.35
transverse 755.31
upper limb 755.20
with complete absence of distal elements 755.21
longitudinal (complete) (partial) (with distal deficiencies, incomplete) 755.22
with complete absence of distal elements 755.21
carpal(s) 755.28
combined humeral, radial, ulnar (incomplete) 755.23
humeral 755.24
metacarpal(s) 755.28
phalange(s) 755.29
meaning all digits 755.21
radial 755.26
radioulnar 755.25
ulnar 755.27
transverse (complete) (partial) 755.21
renal – *see* Deformity, kidney
respiratory system (congenital) 748.9
specified type NEC 748.8
rib (acquired) 738.3
congenital 756.3
cervical 756.2
rotation (joint) (acquired) 736.9
congenital 755.9
hip or thigh 736.39
congenital (*see also* Subluxation, congenital, hip) 754.32
sacroiliac joint (congenital) 755.69
acquired 738.5
sacrum (acquired) 738.5
congenital 756.10
saddle
back 737.8
nose 738.0
syphilitic 090.5
salivary gland or duct (congenital) 750.9
acquired 527.8

Deformity – *continued*
- scapula (acquired) 736.89
  - congenital 755.50
- scrotum (congenital) 752.9
  - acquired 608.89
- sebaceous gland, acquired 706.8
- seminal tract or duct (congenital) 752.9
  - acquired 608.89
- septum (nasal) (acquired) 470
  - congenital 748.1
- shoulder (joint) (acquired) 736.89
  - congenital 755.50
    - specified type NEC 755.59
  - contraction 718.41
- sigmoid (flexure) (congenital) 751.5
  - acquired 569.89
- sinus of Valsalva 747.29
- skin (congenital) 757.9
  - acquired NEC 709.8
- skull (acquired) 738.19
  - congenital 756.0
    - with
      - anencephalus 740.0
      - encephalocele 742.0
      - hydrocephalus 742.3
        - with spina bifida (*see also* Spina bifida) 741.0❺
      - microcephalus 742.1
    - due to intrauterine malposition and pressure 754.0
- soft parts, organs or tissues (of pelvis)
  - in pregnancy or childbirth NEC 654.9❺
    - affecting fetus or newborn 763.89
    - causing obstructed labor 660.2❺
      - affecting fetus or newborn 763.1
- spermatic cord (congenital) 752.9
  - acquired 608.89
    - torsion 608.22
      - extravaginal 608.21
      - intravaginal 608.22
- spinal
  - column – *see* Deformity, spine
  - cord (congenital) 742.9
    - acquired 336.8
    - vessel (congenital) 747.82
  - nerve root (congenital) 742.9
    - acquired 724.9
- spine (acquired) NEC 738.5
  - congenital 756.10
    - due to intrauterine malposition and pressure 754.2
  - kyphoscoliotic (*see also* Kyphoscoliosis) 737.30
  - kyphotic (*see also* Kyphosis) 737.10
  - lordotic (*see also* Lordosis) 737.20
  - rachitic 268.1
  - scoliotic (*see also* Scoliosis) 737.30
- spleen
  - acquired 289.59
  - congenital 759.0
- Sprengel's (congenital) 755.52
- sternum (acquired) 738.3
  - congenital 756.3
- stomach (congenital) 750.9
  - acquired 537.89
- submaxillary gland (congenital) 750.9
  - acquired 527.8
- swan neck (acquired)
  - finger 736.22
  - hand 736.09
- talipes – *see* Talipes
- teeth, tooth NEC 520.9
- testis (congenital) 752.9
  - acquired 608.89
    - torsion 608.20
- thigh (acquired) 736.89
  - congenital 755.60
- thorax (acquired) (wall) 738.3
  - congenital 754.89
  - late effect of rickets 268.1
- thumb (acquired) 736.20
  - congenital 755.50
- thymus (tissue) (congenital) 759.2
- thyroid (gland) (congenital) 759.2
  - cartilage 748.3
    - acquired 478.79
- tibia (acquired) 736.89
  - congenital 755.60
  - saber 090.5
- toe (acquired) 735.9
  - congenital 755.66
  - specified NEC 735.8

Deformity – *continued*
- tongue (congenital) 750.10
  - acquired 529.8
- tooth, teeth NEC 520.9
- trachea (rings) (congenital) 748.3
  - acquired 519.19
- transverse aortic arch (congenital) 747.21
- tricuspid (leaflets) (valve) (congenital) 746.9
  - acquired – *see* Endocarditis, tricuspid
  - atresia or stenosis 746.1
  - specified type NEC 746.89
- trunk (acquired) 738.3
  - congenital 759.9
- ulna (acquired) 736.00
  - congenital 755.50
- upper extremity – *see* Deformity, arm
- urachus (congenital) 753.7
- ureter (opening) (congenital) 753.9
  - acquired 593.89
- urethra (valve) (congenital) 753.9
  - acquired 599.84
- urinary tract or system (congenital) 753.9
  - urachus 753.7
- uterus (congenital) 752.3
  - acquired 621.8
- uvula (congenital) 750.9
  - acquired 528.9
- vagina (congenital) 752.40
  - acquired 623.8
- valve, valvular (heart) (congenital) 746.9
  - acquired – *see* Endocarditis
  - pulmonary 746.00
  - specified type NEC 746.89
- vascular (congenital) (peripheral) NEC 747.60
  - acquired 459.9
  - gastrointestinal 747.61
  - lower limb 747.64
  - renal 747.62
  - specified site NEC 747.69
  - spinal 747.82
  - upper limb 747.63
- vas deferens (congenital) 752.9
  - acquired 608.89
- vein (congenital) NEC (*see also* Deformity, vascular) 747.60
  - brain 747.81
  - coronary 746.9
  - great 747.40
- vena cava (inferior) (superior) (congenital) 747.40
- vertebra – *see* Deformity, spine
- vesicourethral orifice (acquired) 596.8
  - congenital NEC 753.9
    - specified type NEC 753.8
- vessels of optic papilla (congenital) 743.9
- visual field (contraction) 368.45
- vitreous humor (congenital) 743.9
  - acquired 379.29
- vulva (congenital) 752.40
  - acquired 624.8
- wrist (joint) (acquired) 736.00
  - congenital 755.50
  - contraction 718.43
  - valgus 736.03
    - congenital 755.59
  - varus 736.04
    - congenital 755.59

Degeneration, degenerative
- adrenal (capsule) (gland) 255.8
  - with hypofunction 255.41 ▲
  - fatty 255.8
  - hyaline 255.8
  - infectional 255.8
  - lardaceous 277.39
- amyloid (any site) (general) 277.39
- anterior cornua, spinal cord 336.8
- aorta, aortic 440.0
  - fatty 447.8
  - valve (heart) (*see also* Endocarditis, aortic) 424.1
- arteriovascular – *see* Arteriosclerosis
- artery, arterial (atheromatous) (calcareous) – *see also* Arteriosclerosis
  - amyloid 277.39
  - lardaceous 277.39
  - medial NEC (*see also* Arteriosclerosis, extremities) 440.20
- articular cartilage NEC (*see also* Disorder, cartilage, articular) 718.0❺
  - elbow 718.02
  - knee 717.5
  - patella 717.7
  - shoulder 718.01

Degeneration, degenerative – *continued*
- articular cartilage – *continued*
  - spine (*see also* Spondylosis) 721.90
- atheromatous – *see* Arteriosclerosis
- bacony (any site) 277.39
- basal nuclei or ganglia NEC 333.0
- bone 733.90
- brachial plexus 353.0
- brain (cortical) (progressive) 331.9
  - arteriosclerotic 437.0
  - childhood 330.9
    - specified type NEC 330.8
  - congenital 742.4
  - cystic 348.0
    - congenital 742.4
  - familial NEC 331.89
  - grey matter 330.8
  - heredofamilial NEC 331.89
  - in
    - alcoholism 303.9❺ *[331.7]*
    - beriberi 265.0 *[331.7]*
    - cerebrovascular disease 437.9 *[331.7]*
    - congenital hydrocephalus 742.3 *[331.7]*
      - with spina bifida (*see also* Spina bifida) 741.0❺ *[331.7]*
    - Fabry's disease 272.7 *[330.2]*
    - Gaucher's disease 272.7 *[330.2]*
    - Hunter's disease or syndrome 277.5 *[330.3]*
    - lipidosis
      - cerebral 330.1
      - generalized 272.7 *[330.2]*
    - mucopolysaccharidosis 277.5 *[330.3]*
    - myxedema (*see also* Myxedema) 244.9 *[331.7]*
    - neoplastic disease NEC (M8000/1) 239.9 *[331.7]*
    - Niemann-Pick disease 272.7 *[330.2]*
    - sphingolipidosis 272.7 *[330.2]*
    - vitamin B_{12} deficiency 266.2 *[331.7]*
  - motor centers 331.89
  - senile 331.2
  - specified type NEC 331.89
- breast – *see* Disease, breast
- Bruch's membrane 363.40
- bundle of His 426.50
  - left 426.3
  - right 426.4
- calcareous NEC 275.49
- capillaries 448.9
  - amyloid 277.39
  - fatty 448.9
  - lardaceous 277.39
- cardiac (brown) (calcareous) (fatty) (fibrous) (hyaline) (mural) (muscular) (pigmentary) (senile) (with arteriosclerosis) (*see also* Degeneration, myocardial) 429.1
  - valve, valvular – *see* Endocarditis
- cardiorenal (*see also* Hypertension, cardiorenal) 404.90
- cardiovascular (*see also* Disease, cardiovascular) 429.2
  - renal (*see also* Hypertension, cardiorenal) 404.90
- cartilage (joint) – *see* Derangement, joint
- cerebellar NEC 334.9
  - primary (hereditary) (sporadic) 334.2
- cerebral – *see* Degeneration, brain
- cerebromacular 330.1
- cerebrovascular 437.1
  - due to hypertension 437.2
  - late effect – *see* Late effect(s) (of) cerebrovascular disease
- cervical plexus 353.2
- cervix 622.8
  - due to radiation (intended effect) 622.8
    - adverse effect or misadventure 622.8
- changes, spine or vertebra (*see also* Spondylosis) 721.90
- chitinous 277.39
- chorioretinal 363.40
  - congenital 743.53
  - hereditary 363.50
- choroid (colloid) (drusen) 363.40
  - hereditary 363.50
  - senile 363.41
    - diffuse secondary 363.42
- cochlear 386.8
- collateral ligament (knee) (medial) 717.82
  - lateral 717.81
- combined (spinal cord) (subacute) 266.2 *[336.2]*
  - with anemia (pernicious) 281.0 *[336.2]*
    - due to dietary deficiency 281.1 *[336.2]*

Degeneration, degenerative – *continued*
- combined – *continued*
  - due to vitamin B_{12} deficiency anemia (dietary) 281.1 *[336.2]*
- conjunctiva 372.50
  - amyloid 277.39 *[372.50]*
- cornea 371.40
  - calcerous 371.44
  - familial (hereditary) (*see also* Dystrophy, cornea) 371.50
    - macular 371.55
    - reticular 371.54
  - hyaline (of old scars) 371.41
  - marginal (Terrien's) 371.48
  - mosaic (shagreen) 371.41
  - nodular 371.46
  - peripheral 371.48
  - senile 371.41
- cortical (cerebellar) (parenchymatous) 334.2
  - alcoholic 303.9❺ *[334.4]*
  - diffuse, due to arteriopathy 437.0
- corticostriatal-spinal 334.8
- cretinoid 243
- cruciate ligament (knee) (posterior) 717.84
  - anterior 717.83
- cutis 709.3
  - amyloid 277.39
- dental pulp 522.2
- disc disease – *see* Degeneration, intervertebral disc
- dorsolateral (spinal cord) – *see* Degeneration, combined
- endocardial 424.90
- extrapyramidal NEC 333.90
- eye NEC 360.40
  - macular (*see also* Degeneration, macula) 362.50
    - congenital 362.75
    - hereditary 362.76
- fatty (diffuse) (general) 272.8
  - liver 571.8
    - alcoholic 571.0
  - localized site – *see* Degeneration, by site, fatty
  - placenta – *see* Placenta, abnormal
- globe (eye) NEC 360.40
  - macular – *see* Degeneration, macula
- grey matter 330.8
- heart (brown) (calcareous) (fatty) (fibrous) (hyaline) (mural) (muscular) (pigmentary) (senile) (with arteriosclerosis) (*see also* Degeneration, myocardial) 429.1
  - amyloid 277.39 *[425.7]*
  - atheromatous – *see* Arteriosclerosis, coronary
  - gouty 274.82
  - hypertensive (*see also* Hypertension, heart) 402.90
  - ischemic 414.9
  - valve, valvular – *see* Endocarditis
- hepatolenticular (Wilson's) 275.1
- hepatorenal 572.4
- heredofamilial
  - brain NEC 331.89
  - spinal cord NEC 336.8
- hyaline (diffuse) (generalized) 728.9
  - localized – *see also* Degeneration, by site
    - cornea 371.41
    - keratitis 371.41
- hypertensive vascular – *see* Hypertension
- infrapatellar fat pad 729.31
- internal semilunar cartilage 717.3
- intervertebral disc 722.6
  - with myelopathy 722.70
  - cervical, cervicothoracic 722.4
    - with myelopathy 722.71
  - lumbar, lumbosacral 722.52
    - with myelopathy 722.73
  - thoracic, thoracolumbar 722.51
    - with myelopathy 722.72
- intestine 569.89
  - amyloid 277.39
  - lardaceous 277.39
- iris (generalized) (*see also* Atrophy, iris) 364.59
  - pigmentary 364.53
  - pupillary margin 364.54
- ischemic – *see* Ischemia
- joint disease (*see also* Osteoarthrosis) 715.9❺
  - multiple sites 715.09
  - spine (*see also* Spondylosis) 721.90
- kidney (*see also* Sclerosis, renal) 587
  - amyloid 277.39 *[583.81]*

Degeneration, degenerative – *continued*
- kidney – *continued*
  - cyst, cystic (multiple) (solitary) 593.2
    - congenital (*see also* Cystic, disease, kidney) 753.10
  - fatty 593.89
  - fibrocystic (congenital) 753.19
  - lardaceous 277.39 *[583.81]*
  - polycystic (congenital) 753.12
    - adult type (APKD) 753.13
    - autosomal dominant 753.13
    - autosomal recessive 753.14
    - childhood type (CPKD) 753.14
    - infantile type 753.14
  - waxy 277.39 *[583.81]*
- Kuhnt-Junius (retina) 362.52
- labyrinth, osseous 386.8
- lacrimal passages, cystic 375.12
- lardaceous (any site) 277.39
- lateral column (posterior), spinal cord (*see also* Degeneration, combined) 266.2 *[336.2]*
- lattice 362.63
- lens 366.9
  - infantile, juvenile, or presenile 366.00
  - senile 366.10
- lenticular (familial) (progressive) (Wilson's) (with cirrhosis of liver) 275.1
  - striate artery 437.0
- lethal ball, prosthetic heart valve 996.02
- ligament
  - collateral (knee) (medial) 717.82
    - lateral 717.81
  - cruciate (knee) (posterior) 717.84
    - anterior 717.83
- liver (diffuse) 572.8
  - amyloid 277.39
  - congenital (cystic) 751.62
  - cystic 572.8
    - congenital 751.62
  - fatty 571.8
    - alcoholic 571.0
  - hypertrophic 572.8
  - lardaceous 277.39
  - parenchymatous, acute or subacute (*see also* Necrosis, liver) 570
  - pigmentary 572.8
  - toxic (acute) 573.8
  - waxy 277.39
- lung 518.89
- lymph gland 289.3
  - hyaline 289.3
  - lardaceous 277.39
- macula (acquired) (senile) 362.50
  - atrophic 362.51
  - Best's 362.76
  - congenital 362.75
  - cystic 362.54
  - cystoid 362.53
  - disciform 362.52
  - dry 362.51
  - exudative 362.52
  - familial pseudoinflammatory 362.77
  - hereditary 362.76
  - hole 362.54
  - juvenile (Stargardt's) 362.75
  - nonexudative 362.51
  - pseudohole 362.54
  - wet 362.52
- medullary – *see* Degeneration, brain
- membranous labyrinth, congenital (causing impairment of hearing) 744.05
- meniscus – *see* Derangement, joint
- microcystoid 362.62
- mitral – *see* Insufficiency, mitral
- Mönckeberg's (*see also* Arteriosclerosis, extremities) 440.20
- moral 301.7
- motor centers, senile 331.2
- mural (*see also* Degeneration, myocardial) 429.1
  - heart, cardiac (*see also* Degeneration, myocardial) 429.1
  - myocardium, myocardial (*see also* Degeneration, myocardial) 429.1
- muscle 728.9
  - fatty 728.9
  - fibrous 728.9
  - heart (*see also* Degeneration, myocardial) 429.1
  - hyaline 728.9
- muscular progressive 728.2
- myelin, central nervous system NEC 341.9

Degeneration, degenerative – *continued*
- myocardium, myocardial (brown) (calcareous) (fatty) (fibrous) (hyaline) (mural) (muscular) (pigmentary) (senile) (with arteriosclerosis) 429.1
  - with rheumatic fever (conditions classifiable to 390) 398.0
    - active, acute, or subacute 391.2
      - with chorea 392.0
    - inactive or quiescent (with chorea) 398.0
  - amyloid 277.39 *[425.7]*
  - congenital 746.89
  - fetus or newborn 779.89
  - gouty 274.82
  - hypertensive (*see also* Hypertension, heart) 402.90
  - ischemic 414.8
  - rheumatic (*see also* Degeneration, myocardium, with rheumatic fever) 398.0
  - syphilitic 093.82
- nasal sinus (mucosa) (*see also* Sinusitis) 473.9
  - frontal 473.1
  - maxillary 473.0
- nerve – *see* Disorder, nerve
- nervous system 349.89
  - amyloid 277.39 *[357.4]*
  - autonomic (*see also* Neuropathy, peripheral, autonomic) 337.9
  - fatty 349.89
  - peripheral autonomic NEC (*see also* Neuropathy, peripheral, autonomic) 337.9
- nipple 611.9
- nose 478.19
- oculoacousticocerebral, congenital (progressive) 743.8
- olivopontocerebellar (familial) (hereditary) 333.0
- osseous labyrinth 386.8
- ovary 620.8
  - cystic 620.2
  - microcystic 620.2
- pallidal, pigmentary (progressive) 333.0
- pancreas 577.8
  - tuberculous (*see also* Tuberculosis) 017.9❺
- papillary muscle 429.81
- paving stone 362.61
- penis 607.89
- peritoneum 568.89
- pigmentary (diffuse) (general)
  - localized – *see* Degeneration, by site
  - pallidal (progressive) 333.0
  - secondary 362.65
- pineal gland 259.8
- pituitary (gland) 253.8
- placenta (fatty) (fibrinoid) (fibroid) – *see* Placenta, abnormal
- popliteal fat pad 729.31
- posterolateral (spinal cord) (*see also* Degeneration, combined) 266.2 *[336.2]*
- pulmonary valve (heart) (*see also* Endocarditis, pulmonary) 424.3
- pulp (tooth) 522.2
- pupillary margin 364.54
- renal (*see also* Sclerosis, renal) 587
  - fibrocystic 753.19
  - polycystic 753.12
    - adult type (APKD) 753.13
    - autosomal dominant 753.13
    - autosomal recessive 753.14
    - childhood type (CPKD) 753.14
    - infantile type 753.14
- reticuloendothelial system 289.89
- retina (peripheral) 362.60
  - with retinal defect (*see also* Detachment, retina, with retinal defect) 361.00
  - cystic (senile) 362.50
  - cystoid 362.53
  - hereditary (*see also* Dystrophy, retina) 362.70
    - cerebroretinal 362.71
    - congenital 362.75
    - juvenile (Stargardt's) 362.75
    - macula 362.76
  - Kuhnt-Junius 362.52
  - lattice 362.63
  - macular (*see also* Degeneration, macula) 362.50
  - microcystoid 362.62
  - palisade 362.63
  - paving stone 362.61
  - pigmentary (primary) 362.74
    - secondary 362.65
  - posterior pole (*see also* Degeneration, macula) 362.50

Degeneration, degenerative – *continued*
- retina – *continued*
  - secondary 362.66
  - senile 362.60
    - cystic 362.53
    - reticular 362.64
- saccule, congenital (causing impairment of hearing) 744.05
- sacculocochlear 386.8
- senile 797
  - brain 331.2
  - cardiac, heart, or myocardium (*see also* Degeneration, myocardial) 429.1
  - motor centers 331.2
  - reticule 362.64
  - retina, cystic 362.50
  - vascular – *see* Arteriosclerosis
- silicone rubber poppet (prosthetic valve) 996.02
- sinus (cystic) (*see also* Sinusitis) 473.9
  - polypoid 471.1
- skin 709.3
  - amyloid 277.39
  - colloid 709.3
- spinal (cord) 336.8
  - amyloid 277.39
  - column 733.90
  - combined (subacute) (*see also* Degeneration, combined) 266.2 *[336.2]*
    - with anemia (pernicious) 281.0 *[336.2]*
  - dorsolateral (*see also* Degeneration, combined) 266.2 *[336.2]*
  - familial NEC 336.8
  - fatty 336.8
  - funicular (*see also* Degeneration, combined) 266.2 *[336.2]*
  - heredofamilial NEC 336.8
  - posterolateral (*see also* Degeneration, combined) 266.2 *[336.2]*
  - subacute combined – *see* Degeneration, combined
  - tuberculous (*see also* Tuberculosis) 013.8❺
- spine 733.90
- spleen 289.59
  - amyloid 277.39
  - lardaceous 277.39
- stomach 537.89
  - lardaceous 277.39
- strionigral 333.0
- sudoriparous (cystic) 705.89
- suprarenal (capsule) (gland) 255.8
  - with hypofunction 255.41 ▲
- sweat gland 705.89
- synovial membrane (pulpy) 727.9
- tapetoretinal 362.74
  - adult or presenile form 362.50
- testis (postinfectional) 608.89
- thymus (gland) 254.8
  - fatty 254.8
  - lardaceous 277.39
- thyroid (gland) 246.8
- tricuspid (heart) (valve) – *see* Endocarditis, tricuspid
- tuberculous NEC (*see also* Tuberculosis) 011.9❺
- turbinate 733.90
- uterus 621.8
  - cystic 621.8
- vascular (senile) – *see also* Arteriosclerosis
  - hypertensive – *see* Hypertension
- vitreoretinal (primary) 362.73
  - secondary 362.66
- vitreous humor (with infiltration) 379.21
- Wallerian NEC – *see* Disorder, nerve
- waxy (any site) 277.39
- Wilson's hepatolenticular 275.1

Deglutition
- paralysis 784.99
  - hysterical 300.11
- pneumonia 507.0

Degos' disease or syndrome 447.8

Degradation disorder, branched-chain amino-acid 270.3

Dehiscence
- anastomosis – *see* Complications, anastomosis
- cesarean wound 674.1❺
- episiotomy 674.2❺
- operation wound 998.32
  - internal 998.31
- perineal wound (postpartum) 674.2❺

Dehiscence – *continued*
- postoperative 998.32
  - abdomen 998.32
    - internal 998.31
  - internal 998.31
- uterine wound 674.1❺

Dehydration (cachexia) 276.51
- with
  - hypernatremia 276.0
  - hyponatremia 276.1
- newborn 775.5

Deiters' nucleus syndrome 386.19

Déjérine's disease 356.0

Déjérine-Klumpke paralysis 767.6

Déjérine-Roussy syndrome 338.0

Déjérine-Sottas disease or neuropathy (hypertrophic) 356.0

Déjérine-Thomas atrophy or syndrome 333.0

de Lange's syndrome (Amsterdam dwarf, mental retardation, and brachycephaly) 759.89

Delay, delayed
- adaptation, cones or rods 368.63
- any plane in pelvis
  - affecting fetus or newborn 763.1
  - complicating delivery 660.1❺
- birth or delivery NEC 662.1❺
  - affecting fetus or newborn 763.9
  - second twin, triplet, or multiple mate 662.3❺
- closure – *see also* Fistula
  - cranial suture 756.0
  - fontanel 756.0
- coagulation NEC 790.92
- conduction (cardiac) (ventricular) 426.9
- delivery NEC 662.1❺
  - second twin, triplet, etc. 662.3❺
    - affecting fetus or newborn 763.89
- development
  - in childhood 783.40
    - physiological 783.40
  - intellectual NEC 315.9
  - learning NEC 315.2
  - reading 315.00
  - sexual 259.0
  - speech 315.39
    - and language due to hearing loss 315.34 ●
    - associated with hyperkinesis 314.1
  - spelling 315.09
- gastric emptying 536.8
- menarche 256.39
  - due to pituitary hypofunction 253.4
- menstruation (cause unknown) 626.8
- milestone in childhood 783.42
- motility – *see* Hypomotility
- passage of meconium (newborn) 777.1
- primary respiration 768.9
- puberty 259.0
- separation of umbilical cord 779.83
- sexual maturation, female 259.0

Del Castillo's syndrome (germinal aplasia) 606.0

Deleage's disease 359.89

Deletion syndrome
- 5p 758.31
- 22q11.2 758.32
- autosomal NEC 758.39
- constitutional 5q deletion 758.39

Delhi (boil) (button) (sore) 085.1

Delinquency (juvenile) 312.9
- group (*see also* Disturbance, conduct) 312.2❺
- neurotic 312.4

Delirium, delirious 780.09
- acute (psychotic) 293.0
- alcoholic 291.0
  - acute 291.0
  - chronic 291.1
- alcoholicum 291.0
- chronic (*see also* Psychosis) 293.89
  - due to or associated with physical condition – *see* Psychosis, organic
- drug-induced 292.81
- due to conditions classified elsewhere 293.0
- eclamptic (*see also* Eclampsia) 780.39
- exhaustion (*see also* Reaction, stress, acute) 308.9
- hysterical 300.11
- in
  - presenile dementia 290.11
  - senile dementia 290.3
- induced by drug 292.81

Delirium, delirious – *continued*
- manic, maniacal (acute) (*see also* Psychosis, affective) 296.0❺
  - recurrent episode 296.1❺
  - single episode 296.0❺
- puerperal 293.9
- senile 290.3
- subacute (psychotic) 293.1
- thyroid (*see also* Thyrotoxicosis) 242.9❺
- traumatic – *see also* Injury, intracranial
  - with
    - lesion, spinal cord – *see* Injury, spinal, by site
    - shock, spinal – *see* Injury, spinal, by site
- tremens (impending) 291.0
- uremic – *see* Uremia
- withdrawal
  - alcoholic (acute) 291.0
    - chronic 291.1
  - drug 292.0

Delivery

Note – Use the following fifth-digit subclassification with categories 640-648, 651-676:

0 unspecified as to episode of care
1 delivered, with or without mention of antepartum condition
2 delivered, with mention of postpartum complication
3 antepartum condition or complication
4 postpartum condition or complication

- breech (assisted) (buttocks) (complete) (frank) (spontaneous) 652.2❺
  - affecting fetus or newborn 763.0
  - extraction NEC 669.6❺
- cesarean (for) 669.7❺
  - abnormal
    - cervix 654.6❺
    - pelvic organs of tissues 654.9❺
    - pelvis (bony) (major) NEC 653.0❺
    - presentation or position 652.9❺
      - in multiple gestation 652.6❺
    - size, fetus 653.5❺
    - soft parts (of pelvis) 654.9❺
    - uterus, congenital 654.0❺
    - vagina 654.7❺
    - vulva 654.8❺
  - abruptio placentae 641.2❺
  - acromion presentation 652.8❺
  - affecting fetus or newborn 763.4❺
  - anteversion, cervix or uterus 654.4❺
  - atony, uterus 661.2❺ ▲
    - with hemorrhage 666.1 ❺ ●
  - bicornis or bicornuate uterus 654.0❺
  - breech presentation (buttocks) (complete) (frank)652.2❺
  - brow presentation 652.4❺
  - cephalopelvic disproportion (normally formed fetus) 653.4❺
  - chin presentation 652.4❺
  - cicatrix of cervix 654.6❺
  - contracted pelvis (general) 653.1❺
    - inlet 653.2❺
    - outlet 653.3❺
  - cord presentation or prolapse 663.0❺
  - cystocele 654.4❺
  - deformity (acquired) (congenital)
    - pelvic organs or tissues NEC 654.9❺
    - pelvis (bony) NEC 653.0❺
  - displacement, uterus NEC 654.4❺
  - disproportion NEC 653.9❺
  - distress
    - fetal 656.8❺
    - maternal 669.0❺
  - eclampsia 642.6❺
  - face presentation 652.4❺
  - failed
    - forceps 660.7❺
    - trial of labor NEC 660.6❺
    - vacuum extraction 660.7❺
    - ventouse 660.7❺
  - fetal deformity 653.7❺
  - fetal-maternal hemorrhage 656.0❺
  - fetus, fetal
    - distress 656.8❺
    - prematurity 656.8❺
  - fibroid (tumor) (uterus) 654.1❺
  - footling 652.8❺
    - with successful version 652.1❺
  - hemorrhage (antepartum) (intrapartum) NEC 641.9❺
  - hydrocephalic fetus 653.6❺

Degeneration, degenerative – Delivery

Delivery – *continued*
- cesarean – *continued*
  - incarceration of uterus 654.3❺
  - incoordinate uterine action 661.4❺
  - inertia, uterus 661.2❺
    - primary 661.0❺
    - secondary 661.1❺
  - lateroversion, uterus or cervix 654.4❺
  - mal lie 652.9❺
  - malposition
    - fetus 652.9❺
      - in multiple gestation 652.6❺
    - pelvic organs or tissues NEC 654.9❺
    - uterus NEC or cervix 654.4❺
  - malpresentation NEC 652.9❺
    - in multiple gestation 652.6❺
  - maternal
    - diabetes mellitus 648.0❺
    - heart disease NEC 648.6❺
  - meconium in liquor 656.8❺
    - staining only 792.3
  - oblique presentation 652.3❺
  - oversize fetus 653.5❺
  - pelvic tumor NEC 654.9❺
  - placental insufficiency 656.5❺
  - placenta previa 641.0❺
    - with hemorrhage 641.1❺
  - poor dilation, cervix 661.0❺
  - pre-eclampsia 642.4❺
    - severe 642.5❺
  - previous
    - cesarean delivery, section 654.2❺
    - surgery (to)
      - cervix 654.6❺
      - gynecological NEC 654.9❺
      - rectum 654.8
      - uterus NEC 654.9❺
        - previous cesarean delivery, section 654.2❺
      - vagina 654.7❺
  - prolapse
    - arm or hand 652.7❺
    - uterus 654.4❺
  - prolonged labor 662.1❺
  - rectocele 654.4❺
  - retroversion, uterus or cervix 654.3❺
  - rigid
    - cervix 654.6❺
    - pelvic floor 654.4❺
    - perineum 654.8❺
    - vagina 654.7❺
    - vulva 654.8❺
  - sacculation, pregnant uterus 654.4❺
  - scar(s)
    - cervix 654.6❺
    - cesarean delivery, section 654.2❺
    - uterus NEC 654.9❺
      - due to previous cesarean delivery, section 654.2❺
  - Shirodkar suture in situ 654.5❺
  - shoulder presentation 652.8❺
  - stenosis or stricture, cervix 654.6❺
  - transverse presentation or lie 652.3❺
  - tumor, pelvic organs or tissues NEC 654.4❺
  - umbilical cord presentation or prolapse 663.0❺
- completely normal case – *see* category 650
- complicated (by) NEC 669.9❺
  - abdominal tumor, fetal 653.7❺
    - causing obstructed labor 660.1❺
  - abnormal, abnormality of
    - cervix 654.6❺
      - causing obstructed labor 660.2❺
    - forces of labor 661.9❺
    - formation of uterus 654.0❺
    - pelvic organs or tissues 654.9❺
      - causing obstructed labor 660.2❺
    - pelvis (bony) (major) NEC 653.0❺
      - causing obstructed labor 660.1❺
    - presentation or position NEC 652.9❺
      - causing obstructed labor 660.0❺
    - size, fetus 653.5❺
      - causing obstructed labor 660.1❺
    - soft parts (of pelvis) 654.9❺
      - causing obstructed labor 660.2❺
    - uterine contractions NEC 661.9❺
    - uterus (formation) 654.0❺
      - causing obstructed labor 660.2❺
    - vagina 654.7❺
      - causing obstructed labor 660.2❺
  - abnormally formed uterus (any type) (congenital) 654.0❺

Delivery – *continued*
- complicated (by) – *continued*
  - abnormally formed uterus – *continued*
    - causing obstructed labor 660.2❺
  - acromion presentation 652.8❺
    - causing obstructed labor 660.0❺
  - adherent placenta 667.0❺
    - with hemorrhage 666.0❺
  - adhesions, uterus (to abdominal wall) 654.4❺
  - advanced maternal age NEC 659.6❺
    - multigravida 659.6❺
    - primigravida 659.5❺
  - air embolism 673.0❺
  - amnionitis 658.4❺
  - amniotic fluid embolism 673.1❺
  - anesthetic death 668.9❺
  - annular detachment, cervix 665.3❺
  - antepartum hemorrhage – *see* Delivery, complicated, hemorrhage
  - anteversion, cervix or uterus 654.4❺
    - causing obstructed labor 660.2❺
  - apoplexy 674.0❺
    - placenta 641.2❺
  - arrested active phase 661.1❺
  - asymmetrical pelvis bone 653.0❺
    - causing obstructed labor 660.1❺
  - atony, uterus with hemorrhage (hypotonic) (inertia) 666.1❺
    - hypertonic 661.4❺
  - Bandl's ring 661.4❺
  - Battledore placenta – *see* Placenta, abnormal
  - bicornis or bicornuate uterus 654.0❺
    - causing obstructed labor 660.2❺
  - birth injury to mother NEC 665.9❺
  - bleeding (*see also* Delivery, complicated, hemorrhage) 641.9❺
  - breech presentation (assisted) (buttocks) (complete) (frank) (spontaneous) 652.2❺
    - with successful version 652.1❺
  - brow presentation 652.4❺
  - cephalopelvic disproportion (normally formed fetus) 653.4❺
    - causing obstructed labor 660.1❺
  - cerebral hemorrhage 674.0❺
  - cervical dystocia 661.2❺▲
  - chin presentation 652.4❺
    - causing obstructed labor 660.0❺
  - cicatrix
    - cervix 654.6❺
      - causing obstructed labor 660.2❺
    - vagina 654.7❺
      - causing obstructed labor 660.2❺
  - coagulation defect 649.3❺
  - colporrhexis 665.4❺
    - with perineal laceration 664.0❺
  - compound presentation 652.8❺
    - causing obstructed labor 660.0❺
  - compression of cord (umbilical) 663.2❺
    - around neck 663.1❺
    - cord prolapsed 663.0❺
  - contraction, contracted pelvis 653.1❺
    - causing obstructed labor 660.1❺
    - general 653.1❺
      - causing obstructed labor 660.1❺
    - inlet 653.2❺
      - causing obstructed labor 660.1❺
    - midpelvic 653.8❺
      - causing obstructed labor 660.1❺
    - midplane 653.8❺
      - causing obstructed labor 660.1❺
    - outlet 653.3❺
      - causing obstructed labor 660.1❺
  - contraction ring 661.4❺
  - cord (umbilical) 663.9❺
    - around neck, tightly or with compression 663.1❺
      - without compression 663.3❺
    - bruising 663.6❺
    - complication NEC 663.9❺
      - specified type NEC 663.8❺
    - compression NEC 663.2❺
    - entanglement NEC 663.3❺
      - with compression 663.2❺ forelying 663.0❺
    - hematoma 663.6❺
    - marginal attachment 663.8❺
    - presentation 663.0❺
    - prolapse (complete) (occult) (partial) 663.0❺
    - short 663.4❺
    - specified complication NEC 663.8❺
    - thrombosis (vessels) 663.6❺

Delivery – *continued*
- complicated (by) – *continued*
  - cord – *continued*
    - vascular lesion 663.6❺
    - velamentous insertion 663.8❺
  - Couvelaire uterus 641.2❺
  - cretin pelvis (dwarf type) (male type) 653.1❺
    - causing obstructed labor 660.1❺
  - crossbirth 652.3❺
    - with successful version 652.1❺
    - causing obstructed labor 660.0❺
  - cyst (Gartner's duct) 654.7❺
  - cystocele 654.4❺
    - causing obstructed labor 660.2❺
  - death of fetus (near term) 656.4❺
    - early (before 22 completed weeks gestation) 632
  - deformity (acquired) (congenital)
    - fetus 653.7❺
      - causing obstructed labor 660.1❺
    - pelvic organs or tissues NEC 654.9❺
      - causing obstructed labor 660.2❺
    - pelvis (bony) NEC 653.0❺
      - causing obstructed labor 660.1❺
  - delay, delayed
    - delivery in multiple pregnancy 662.3❺
      - due to locked mates 660.5❺
    - following rupture of membranes (spontaneous) 658.2❺
      - artificial 658.3❺
  - depressed fetal heart tones 659.7❺
  - diastasis recti 665.8❺
  - dilatation
    - bladder 654.4❺
      - causing obstructed labor 660.2❺
    - cervix, incomplete, poor or slow 661.0❺
  - diseased placenta 656.7❺
  - displacement uterus NEC 654.4❺
    - causing obstructed labor 660.2❺
  - disproportion NEC 653.9❺
    - causing obstructed labor 660.1❺
  - disruptio uteri – *see* Delivery, complicated, rupture, uterus
  - distress
    - fetal 656.8❺
    - maternal 669.0❺
  - double uterus (congenital) 654.0❺
    - causing obstructed labor 660.2❺
  - dropsy amnion 657❹
  - dysfunction, uterus 661.9❺
    - hypertonic 661.4❺
    - hypotonic 661.2❺
      - primary 661.0❺
      - secondary 661.1❺
    - incoordinate 661.4❺
  - dystocia
    - cervical 661.2❺▲
    - fetal – *see* Delivery, complicated, abnormal, presentation
    - maternal – *see* Delivery, complicated, prolonged labor
    - pelvic – *see* Delivery, complicated, contraction pelvis
    - positional 652.8❺
    - shoulder girdle 660.4❺
  - eclampsia 642.6❺
  - ectopic kidney 654.4❺
    - causing obstructed labor 660.2❺
  - edema, cervix 654.6❺
    - causing obstructed labor 660.2❺
  - effusion, amniotic fluid 658.1❺
  - elderly multigravida 659.6❺
  - elderly primigravida 659.5❺
  - embolism (pulmonary) 673.2❺
    - air 673.0❺
    - amniotic fluid 673.1❺
    - blood-clot 673.2❺
    - cerebral 674.0❺
    - fat 673.8❺
    - pyemic 673.3❺
    - septic 673.3❺
  - entanglement, umbilical cord 663.3❺
    - with compression 663.2❺
    - around neck (with compression) 663.1❺
  - eversion, cervix or uterus 665.2❺
  - excessive
    - fetal growth 653.5❺
      - causing obstructed labor 660.1❺
    - size of fetus 653.5❺
      - causing obstructed labor 660.1❺
  - face presentation 652.4❺
    - causing obstructed labor 660.0❺

- **Delivery** – *continued*
  - complicated (by) – *continued*
    - face presentation – *continued*
      - to pubes 660.3❺
    - failure, fetal head to enter pelvic brim 652.5❺
      - causing obstructed labor 660.0❺
    - female genital mutilation 660.8❺
    - fetal
      - acid-base balance 656.8❺
      - death (near term) NEC 656.4❺
        - early (before 22 completed weeks gestation) 632
      - deformity 653.7❺
        - causing obstructed labor 660.1❺
      - distress 656.8❺
      - heart rate or rhythm 659.7❺
      - reduction of multiple fetuses reduced to single fetus 651.7❺
    - fetopelvic disproportion 653.4❺
      - causing obstructed labor 660.1❺
    - fever during labor 659.2❺
    - fibroid (tumor) (uterus) 654.1❺
      - causing obstructed labor 660.2❺
    - fibromyomata 654.1❺
      - causing obstructed labor 660.2❺
    - forelying umbilical cord 663.0❺
    - fracture of coccyx 665.6❺
    - hematoma 664.5❺
      - broad ligament 665.7❺
      - ischial spine 665.7❺
      - pelvic 665.7❺
      - perineum 664.5❺
      - soft tissues 665.7❺
      - subdural 674.0❺
      - umbilical cord 663.6❺
      - vagina 665.7❺
      - vulva or perineum 664.5❺
    - hemorrhage (uterine) (antepartum) (intrapartum) (pregnancy) 641.9❺
      - accidental 641.2❺
      - associated with
        - afibrinogenemia 641.3❺
        - coagulation defect 641.3❺
          - hyperfibrinolysis 641.3❺
          - hypofibrinogenemia 641.3❺
      - cerebral 674.0❺
      - due to
        - low-lying placenta 641.1❺
        - placenta previa 641.1❺
        - premature separation of placenta (normally implanted) 641.2❺
        - retained placenta 666.0❺
        - trauma 641.8❺
        - uterine leiomyoma 641.8❺
      - marginal sinus rupture 641.2❺
      - placenta NEC 641.9❺
      - postpartum (atonic) (immediate) (within 24 hours) 666.1❺
        - with retained or trapped placenta 666.0❺
        - delayed 666.2❺
        - secondary 666.2❺
        - third stage 666.0❺
    - hourglass contraction, uterus 661.4❺
    - hydramnios 657❹
    - hydrocephalic fetus 653.6❺
      - causing obstructed labor 660.1❺
    - hydrops fetalis 653.7❺
      - causing obstructed labor 660.1❺
    - hypertension – *see* Hypertension, complicating pregnancy
    - hypertonic uterine dysfunction 661.4❺
    - hypotonic uterine dysfunction 661.2❺
    - impacted shoulders 660.4❺
    - incarceration, uterus 654.3❺
      - causing obstructed labor 660.2❺
    - incomplete dilation (cervix) 661.0❺
    - incoordinate uterus 661.4❺
    - indication NEC 659.9❺
      - specified type NEC 659.8❺
    - inertia, uterus 661.2❺
      - hypertonic 661.4❺
      - hypotonic 661.2❺
      - primary 661.0❺
      - secondary 661.1❺
    - infantile
      - genitalia 654.4❺
        - causing obstructed labor 660.2❺
      - uterus (os) 654.4❺
        - causing obstructed labor 660.2❺
    - injury (to mother) NEC 665.9❺

- **Delivery** – *continued*
  - complicated (by) – *continued*
    - intrauterine fetal death (near term) NEC 656.4❺
      - early (before 22 completed weeks gestation) 632
    - inversion, uterus 665.2❺
    - kidney, ectopic 654.4❺
      - causing obstructed labor 660.2❺
    - knot (true), umbilical cord 663.2❺
    - labor, premature (before 37 completed weeks gestation) 644.2❺
    - laceration 664.9❺
      - anus (sphincter) ▶(healed) (old)◀ 654.8 ❺▲
        - with mucosa 664.3❺
        - not associated with third-degree perineal laceration 664.6 ❺●
      - bladder (urinary) 665.5❺
      - bowel 665.5❺
      - central 664.4❺
      - cervix (uteri) 665.3❺
      - fourchette 664.0❺
      - hymen 664.0❺
      - labia (majora) (minora) 664.0❺
      - pelvic
        - floor 664.1❺
        - organ NEC 665.5❺
      - perineum, perineal 664.4❺
        - first degree 664.0❺
        - second degree 664.1❺
        - third degree 664.2❺
        - fourth degree 664.3❺
        - central 664.4❺
        - extensive NEC 664.4❺
        - muscles 664.1❺
        - skin 664.0❺
        - slight 664.0❺
      - peritoneum 665.5❺
      - periurethral tissue 664.8❺▲
      - rectovaginal (septum) (without perineal laceration) 665.4❺
        - with perineum 664.2❺
          - with anal or rectal mucosa 664.3❺
      - skin (perineum) 664.0❺
      - specified site or type NEC 664.8❺
      - sphincter ani ▶(healed) (old)◀ 654.8 ❺▲
        - with mucosa 664.3❺
        - not associated with third-degree perineal laceration 664.6 ❺●
      - urethra 665.5❺
      - uterus 665.1❺
        - before labor 665.0❺
      - vagina, vaginal (deep) (high) (sulcus) (wall) (without perineal laceration) 665.4❺
        - with perineum 664.0❺
        - muscles, with perineum 664.1❺
      - vulva 664.0❺
    - lateroversion, uterus or cervix 654.4❺
      - causing obstructed labor 660.2❺
    - locked mates 660.5❺
    - low implantation of placenta – *see* Delivery, complicated, placenta, previa
    - mal lie 652.9❺
    - malposition
      - fetus NEC 652.9❺
        - causing obstructed labor 660.0❺
      - pelvic organs or tissues NEC 654.9❺
        - causing obstructed labor 660.2❺
      - placenta 641.1❺
        - without hemorrhage 641.0❺
      - uterus NEC or cervix 654.4❺
        - causing obstructed labor 660.2❺
    - malpresentation 652.9❺
      - causing obstructed labor 660.0❺
    - marginal sinus (bleeding) (rupture) 641.2❺
    - maternal hypotension syndrome 669.2❺
    - meconium in liquor 656.8❺
    - membranes, retained – *see* Delivery, complicated, placenta, retained
    - mentum presentation 652.4❺
      - causing obstructed labor 660.0❺
    - metrorrhagia (myopathia) – *see* Delivery, complicated, hemorrhage
    - metrorrhexis – *see* Delivery, complicated, rupture, uterus
    - multiparity (grand) 659.4❺
    - myelomeningocele, fetus 653.7❺
      - causing obstructed labor 660.1❺
    - Nägele's pelvis 653.0❺
      - causing obstructed labor 660.1❺

- **Delivery** – *continued*
  - complicated (by) – *continued*
    - nonengagement, fetal head 652.5❺
      - causing obstructed labor 660.0❺
    - oblique presentation 652.3❺
      - causing obstructed labor 660.0❺
    - obstetric
      - shock 669.1❺
      - trauma NEC 665.9❺
    - obstructed labor 660.9❺
      - due to
        - abnormality of pelvic organs or tissues (conditions classifiable to 654.0-654.9) 660.2❺
        - deep transverse arrest 660.3❺
        - impacted shoulders 660.4❺
        - locked twins 660.5❺
        - malposition and malpresentation of fetus (conditions classifiable to 652.0-652.9) 660.0❺
        - persistent occipitoposterior 660.3❺
        - shoulder dystocia 660.4❺
    - occult prolapse of umbilical cord 663.0❺
    - oversize fetus 653.5❺
      - causing obstructed labor 660.1❺
    - pathological retraction ring, uterus 661.4❺
    - pelvic
      - arrest (deep) (high) (of fetal head) (transverse) 660.3❺
      - deformity (bone) – *see also* Deformity, pelvis, with disproportion
        - soft tissue 654.9❺
          - causing obstructed labor 660.2❺
      - tumor NEC 654.9❺
        - causing obstructed labor 660.2❺
    - penetration, pregnant uterus by instrument 665.1❺
    - perforation – *see* Delivery, complicated, laceration
    - persistent
      - hymen 654.8❺
        - causing obstructed labor 660.2❺
      - occipitoposterior 660.3❺
    - placenta, placental
      - ablatio 641.2❺
      - abnormality 656.7❺
        - with hemorrhage 641.2❺
      - abruptio 641.2❺
      - accreta 667.0❺
        - with hemorrhage 666.0❺
      - adherent (without hemorrhage) 667.0❺
        - with hemorrhage 666.0❺
      - apoplexy 641.2❺
      - battledore – *see* Placenta, abnormal
      - detachment (premature) 641.2❺
      - disease 656.7❺
      - hemorrhage NEC 641.9❺
      - increta (without hemorrhage) 667.0❺
        - with hemorrhage 666.0❺
      - low (implantation) 641.1❺
        - without hemorrhage 641.0❺
      - malformation 656.7❺
        - with hemorrhage 641.2❺
      - malposition 641.1❺
        - without hemorrhage 641.0❺
      - marginal sinus rupture 641.2❺
      - percreta 667.0❺
        - with hemorrhage 666.0❺
      - premature separation 641.2❺
      - previa (central) (lateral) (marginal) (partial) 641.1❺
        - without hemorrhage 641.0❺
      - retained (with hemorrhage) 666.0❺
        - without hemorrhage 667.0❺
      - rupture of marginal sinus 641.2❺
      - separation (premature) 641.2❺
      - trapped 666.0❺
        - without hemorrhage 667.0❺
      - vicious insertion 641.1❺
    - polyhydramnios 657❹
    - polyp, cervix 654.6❺
      - causing obstructed labor 660.2❺
    - precipitate labor 661.3❺
    - premature
      - labor (before 37 completed weeks gestation) 644.2❺
      - rupture, membranes 658.1❺
        - delayed delivery following 658.2❺
    - presenting umbilical cord 663.0❺
    - previous
      - cesarean delivery, section 654.2❺

❹ Fourth-Digit Required ❺ Fifth-Digit Required *[code]* Manifestation Code ▶◀ Revised Text ● New Line ▲ Revised Code

Delivery – Delivery

- **Delivery** – *continued*
  - complicated (by) – *continued*
    - previous – *continued*
      - surgery
        - cervix 654.6❺
          - causing obstructed labor 660.2❺
        - gynecological NEC 654.9❺
          - causing obstructed labor 660.2❺
        - perineum 654.8❺
        - rectum 654.8
        - uterus NEC 654.9❺
          - due to previous cesarean delivery, section 654.2❺
        - vagina 654.7❺
          - causing obstructed labor 660.2❺
        - vulva 654.8❺
    - primary uterine inertia 661.0❺
    - primipara, elderly or old 659.5❺
    - prolapse
      - arm or hand 652.7❺
        - causing obstructed labor 660.0❺
      - cord (umbilical) 663.0❺
      - fetal extremity 652.8❺
      - foot or leg 652.8❺
        - causing obstructed labor 660.0❺
      - umbilical cord (complete) (occult) (partial) 663.0❺
      - uterus 654.4❺
        - causing obstructed labor 660.2❺
    - prolonged labor 662.1❺
      - first stage 662.0❺
      - second stage 662.2❺
      - active phase 661.2❺
      - due to
        - cervical dystocia 661.2❺ ▲
        - contraction ring 661.4❺
        - tetanic uterus 661.4❺
        - uterine inertia 661.2❺
          - primary 661.0❺
          - secondary 661.1❺
      - latent phase 661.0❺
    - pyrexia during labor 659.2❺
    - rachitic pelvis 653.2❺
      - causing obstructed labor 660.1❺
    - rectocele 654.4❺
      - causing obstructed labor 660.2❺
    - retained membranes or portions of placenta 666.2❺
      - without hemorrhage 667.1❺
    - retarded (prolonged) birth 662.1❺
    - retention secundines (with hemorrhage) 666.2❺
      - without hemorrhage 667.1❺
    - retroversion, uterus or cervix 654.3❺
      - causing obstructed labor 660.2❺
    - rigid
      - cervix 654.6❺
        - causing obstructed labor 660.2❺
      - pelvic floor 654.4❺
        - causing obstructed labor 660.2❺
      - perineum or vulva 654.8❺
        - causing obstructed labor 660.2❺
      - vagina 654.7❺
        - causing obstructed labor 660.2❺
    - Robert's pelvis 653.0❺
      - causing obstructed labor 660.1❺
    - rupture – *see also* Delivery, complicated, laceration
      - bladder (urinary) 665.5❺
      - cervix 665.3❺
      - marginal sinus 641.2❺
      - membranes, premature 658.1❺
      - pelvic organ NEC 665.5❺
      - perineum (without mention of other laceration) – *see* Delivery, complicated, laceration, perineum
      - peritoneum 665.5❺
      - urethra 665.5❺
      - uterus (during labor) 665.1❺
        - before labor 665.0❺
    - sacculation, pregnant uterus 654.4❺
    - sacral teratomas, fetal 653.7❺
      - causing obstructed labor 660.1❺
    - scar(s)
      - cervix 654.6❺
        - causing obstructed labor 660.2❺
      - cesarean delivery, section 654.2❺
        - causing obstructed labor 660.2❺
      - perineum 654.8❺
        - causing obstructed labor 660.2❺
      - uterus NEC 654.9❺
        - causing obstructed labor 660.2

- **Delivery** – *continued*
  - complicated (by) – *continued*
    - scar(s) – *continued*
      - uterus – *continued*
        - due to previous cesarean delivery, section 654.2❺
      - vagina 654.7❺
        - causing obstructed labor 660.2❺
      - vulva 654.8❺
        - causing obstructed labor 660.2❺
    - scoliotic pelvis 653.0❺
      - causing obstructed labor 660.1❺
    - secondary uterine inertia 661.1❺
    - secundines, retained – *see* Delivery, complicated, placenta, retained
    - separation
      - placenta (premature) 641.2❺
      - pubic bone 665.6❺
      - symphysis pubis 665.6❺
    - septate vagina 654.7❺
      - causing obstructed labor 660.2❺
    - shock (birth) (obstetric) (puerperal) 669.1❺
    - short cord syndrome 663.4❺
    - shoulder
      - girdle dystocia 660.4❺
      - presentation 652.8❺
        - causing obstructed labor 660.0❺
    - Siamese twins 653.7❺
      - causing obstructed labor 660.1❺
    - slow slope active phase 661.2❺
    - spasm
      - cervix 661.4❺
      - uterus 661.4❺
    - spondylolisthesis, pelvis 653.3❺
      - causing obstructed labor 660.1❺
    - spondylolysis (lumbosacral) 653.3❺
      - causing obstructed labor 660.1❺
    - spondylosis 653.0❺
      - causing obstructed labor 660.1❺
    - stenosis or stricture
      - cervix 654.6❺
        - causing obstructed labor 660.2❺
      - vagina 654.7❺
        - causing obstructed labor 660.2❺
    - sudden death, unknown cause 669.9❺
    - tear (pelvic organ) (*see also* Delivery, complicated, laceration) 664.9❺
      - anal sphincter (healed) (old) 654.8❺ ●
        - not associated with third-degree perineal laceration 664.6❺ ●
    - teratomas, sacral, fetal 653.7❺
      - causing obstructed labor 660.1❺
    - tetanic uterus 661.4❺
    - tipping pelvis 653.0❺
      - causing obstructed labor 660.1❺
    - transverse
      - arrest (deep) 660.3❺
      - presentation or lie 652.3❺
        - with successful version 652.1❺
        - causing obstructed labor 660.0❺
    - trauma (obstetrical) NEC 665.9❺
    - tumor
      - abdominal, fetal 653.7❺
        - causing obstructed labor 660.1❺
      - pelvic organs or tissues NEC 654.9❺
        - causing obstructed labor 660.2❺
    - umbilical cord (*see also* Delivery, complicated, cord) 663.9❺
      - around neck tightly, or with compression 663.1❺
      - entanglement NEC 663.3❺
        - with compression 663.2❺
      - prolapse (complete) (occult) (partial) 663.0❺
    - unstable lie 652.0❺
      - causing obstructed labor 660.0❺
    - uterine
      - inertia (*see also* Delivery, complicated, inertia, uterus) 661.2❺
      - spasm 661.4❺
    - vasa previa 663.5❺
    - velamentous insertion of cord 663.8❺
    - young maternal age 659.8❺
  - delayed NEC 662.1❺
    - following rupture of membranes (spontaneous) 658.2❺
      - artificial 658.3❺
    - second twin, triplet, etc. 662.3❺
  - difficult NEC 669.9❺
    - previous, affecting management of pregnancy or childbirth V23.49
    - specified type NEC 669.8❺

- **Delivery** – *continued*
  - early onset (spontaneous) 644.2❺
  - footling 652.8❺
    - with successful version 652.1❺
  - forceps NEC 669.5❺
    - affecting fetus or newborn 763.2❺
  - missed (at or near term) 656.4❺
  - multiple gestation NEC 651.9❺
    - with fetal loss and retention of one or more fetus(es) 651.6❺
    - following (elective) fetal reduction 651.7❺
    - specified type NEC 651.8❺
      - with fetal loss and retention of one or more fetus(es) 651.6❺
      - following (elective) fetal reduction 651.7❺
  - nonviable infant 656.4❺
  - normal – *see* category 650
  - precipitate 661.3❺
    - affecting fetus or newborn 763.6
  - premature NEC (before 37 completed weeks gestation) 644.2❺
    - previous, affecting management of pregnancy V23.41
  - quadruplet NEC 651.2❺
    - with fetal loss and retention of one or more fetus(es) 651.5❺
    - following (elective) fetal reduction 651.7❺
  - quintuplet NEC 651.8❺
    - with fetal loss and retention of one or more fetus(es) 651.6❺
    - following (elective) fetal reduction 651.7❺
  - sextuplet NEC 651.8❺
    - with fetal loss and retention of one or more fetus(es) 651.6❺
    - following (elective) fetal reduction 651.7❺
  - specified complication NEC 669.8❺
  - stillbirth (near term) NEC 656.4❺
    - early (before 22 completed weeks gestation) 632
  - term pregnancy (live birth) NEC – *see* category 650
    - stillbirth NEC 656.4❺
  - threatened premature 644.2❺
  - triplets NEC 651.1❺
    - with fetal loss and retention of one or more fetus(es) 651.4❺
    - delayed delivery (one or more mates) 662.3❺
    - following (elective) fetal reduction 651.7❺
    - locked mates 660.5❺
  - twins NEC 651.0❺
    - with fetal loss and retention of one fetus 651.3❺
    - delayed delivery (one or more mates) 662.3❺
    - following (elective) fetal reduction 651.7❺
    - locked mates 660.5❺
  - uncomplicated – *see* category 650
  - vacuum extractor NEC 669.5❺
    - affecting fetus or newborn 763.3
  - ventouse NEC 669.5❺
    - affecting fetus or newborn 763.3
- **Dellen, cornea** 371.41
- **Delusions** (paranoid) 297.9
  - grandiose 297.1
  - parasitosis 300.29
  - systematized 297.1
- **Dementia** 294.8
  - alcohol-induced persisting (*see also* Psychosis, alcoholic) 291.2
  - Alzheimer's – *see* Alzheimer's, dementia
  - arteriosclerotic (simple type) (uncomplicated) 290.40
    - with
      - acute confusional state 290.41
      - delirium 290.41
      - delusional features 290.42
      - delusions 290.42
      - depressed mood 290.43
      - depressive features 290.43
    - depressed type 290.43
    - paranoid type 290.42
  - Binswanger's 290.12
  - catatonic (acute) (*see also* Schizophrenia) 295.2❺
  - congenital (*see also* Retardation, mental) 319
  - degenerative 290.9
    - presenile-onset – *see* Dementia, presenile
    - senile-onset – *see* Dementia, senile
  - developmental (*see also* Schizophrenia) 295.9❺
  - dialysis 294.8
    - transient 293.9

Dementia – *continued*
- drug-induced persisting (*see also* Psychosis, drug) 292.82
- due to or associated with condition(s) classified elsewhere
  - Alzheimer's
    - with behavioral disturbance 331.0 *[294.11]*
    - without behavioral disturbance 331.0 *[294.10]*
  - cerebral lipidoses
    - with behavioral disturbance 330.1 *[294.11]*
    - without behavioral disturbance 330.1 *[294.10]*
  - epilepsy
    - with behavioral disturbance 345.9❺ *[294.11]*
    - without behavioral disturbance 345.9❺ *[294.10]*
  - hepatolenticular degeneration
    - with behavioral disturbance 275.1 *[294.11]*
    - without behavioral disturbance 275.1 *[294.10]*
  - HIV
    - with behavioral disturbance 042 *[294.11]*
    - without behavioral disturbance 042 *[294.10]*
  - Huntington's chorea
    - with behavioral disturbance 333.4 *[294.11]*
    - without behavioral disturbance 333.4 *[294.10]*
  - Jakob-Creutzfeldt disease (new variant)
    - with behavioral disturbance 046.1 *[294.11]*
    - without behavioral disturbance 046.1 *[294.10]*
  - Lewy bodies
    - with behavioral disturbance 331.82 *[294.11]*
    - without behavioral disturbance 331.82 *[294.10]*
  - multiple sclerosis
    - with behavioral disturbance 340 *[294.11]*
    - without behavioral disturbance 340 *[294.10]*
  - neurosyphilis
    - with behavioral disturbance 094.9 *[294.11]*
    - without behavioral disturbance 094.9 *[294.10]*
  - Parkinsonism
    - with behavioral disturbance 331.82 *[294.11]*
    - without behavioral disturbance 331.82 *[294.10]*
  - Pelizaeus-Merzbacher disease
    - with behavioral disturbance 333.0 *[294.11]*
    - without behavioral disturbance 333.0 *[294.10]*
  - Pick's disease
    - with behavioral disturbance 331.11 *[294.11]*
    - without behavioral disturbance 331.11 *[294.10]*
  - polyarteritis nodosa
    - with behavioral disturbance 446.0 *[294.11]*
    - without behavioral disturbance 446.0 *[294.10]*
  - syphilis
    - with behavioral disturbance 094.1 *[294.11]*
    - without behavioral disturbance 094.1 *[294.10]*
  - Wilson's disease
    - with behavioral disturbance 275.1 *[294.11]*
    - without behavioral disturbance 275.1 *[294.10]*
- frontal 331.19
  - with behavioral disturbance 331.19 *[294.11]*
  - without behavioral disturbance 331.19 *[294.10]*
- frontotemporal 331.19
  - with behavioral disturbance 331.19 *[294.11]*
  - without behavioral disturbance 331.19 *[294.10]*
- hebephrenic (acute) 295.1❺
- Heller's (infantile psychosis) (*see also* Psychosis, childhood) 299.1❺
- idiopathic 290.9
  - presenile-onset – *see* Dementia, presenile
  - senile-onset – *see* Dementia, senile
- in
  - arteriosclerotic brain disease 290.40
  - senility 290.0
- induced by drug 292.82
- infantile, infantilia (*see also* Psychosis, childhood) 299.0❺
- Lewy body 331.82
  - with behavioral disturbance 331.82 *[294.11]*
  - without behavioral disturbance 331.82 *[294.10]*

Dementia – *continued*
- multi-infarct (cerebrovascular) (*see also* Dementia, arteriosclerotic) 290.40
- old age 290.0
- paralytica, paralytic 094.1
  - juvenilis 090.40
  - syphilitic 094.1
    - congenital 090.40
  - tabetic form 094.1
- paranoid (*see also* Schizophrenia) 295.3❺
- paraphrenic (*see also* Schizophrenia) 295.3❺
- paretic 094.1
- praecox (*see also* Schizophrenia) 295.9❺
- presenile 290.10
  - with
    - acute confusional state 290.11
    - delirium 290.11
    - delusional features 290.12
    - depressive features 290.13
  - depressed type 290.13
  - paranoid type 290.12
  - simple type 290.10
  - uncomplicated 290.10
- primary (acute) (*see also* Schizophrenia) 295.0❺
- progressive, syphilitic 094.1
- puerperal – *see* Psychosis, puerperal
- schizophrenic (*see also* Schizophrenia) 295.9❺
- senile 290.0
  - with
    - acute confusional state 290.3
    - delirium 290.3
    - delusional features 290.20
    - depressive features 290.21
  - depressed type 290.21
  - exhaustion 290.0
  - paranoid type 290.20
- simple type (acute) (*see also* Schizophrenia) 295.0
- simplex (acute) (*see also* Schizophrenia) 295.0
- syphilitic 094.1
- uremic – *see* Uremia
- vascular 290.40
  - with
    - delirium 290.41
    - delusions 290.42
    - depressed mood 290.43

Demerol dependence (*see also* Dependence) 304.0❺

Demineralization, ankle (*see also* Osteoporosis) 733.00

Demodex folliculorum (infestation) 133.8

de Morgan's spots (senile angiomas) 448.1

Demyelinating
- polyneuritis, chronic inflammatory 357.81

Demyelination, demyelinization
- central nervous system 341.9
  - specified NEC 341.8
- corpus callosum (central) 341.8
- global 340

Dengue (fever) 061
- sandfly 061
- vaccination, prophylactic (against) V05.1
- virus hemorrhagic fever 065.4

Dens
- evaginatus 520.2
- in dente 520.2
- invaginatus 520.2

Density
- increased, bone (disseminated) (generalized) (spotted) 733.99
- lung (nodular) 518.89

Dental – *see also* condition
- examination only V72.2

Dentia praecox 520.6

Denticles (in pulp) 522.2

Dentigerous cyst 526.0

Dentin
- irregular (in pulp) 522.3
- opalescent 520.5
- secondary (in pulp) 522.3
- sensitive 521.89

Dentinogenesis imperfecta 520.5

Dentinoma (M9271/0) 213.1
- upper jaw (bone) 213.0

Dentition 520.7
- abnormal 520.6
- anomaly 520.6
- delayed 520.6

Dentition – *continued*
- difficult 520.7
- disorder of 520.6
- precocious 520.6
- retarded 520.6

Denture sore (mouth) 528.9

Dependence

> *Note – Use the following fifth-digit subclassification with category 304:*
> *0 unspecified*
> *1 continuous*
> *2 episodic*
> *3 in remission*

- with
  - withdrawal symptoms
    - alcohol 291.81
    - drug 292.0
- 14-hydroxy-dihydromorphinone 304.0❺
- absinthe 304.6❺
- acemorphan 304.0❺
- acetanilid(e) 304.6❺
- acetophenetidin 304.6❺
- acetorphine 304.0❺
- acetyldihydrocodeine 304.0❺
- acetyldihydrocodeinone 304.0❺
- Adalin 304.1❺
- Afghanistan black 304.3❺
- agrypnal 304.1❺
- alcohol, alcoholic (ethyl) (methyl) (wood) 303.9❺
  - maternal, with suspected fetal damage affecting management of pregnancy 655.4❺
- allobarbitone 304.1❺
- allonal 304.1❺
- allylisopropylacetylurea 304.1❺
- alphaprodine (hydrochloride) 304.0❺
- Alurate 304.1❺
- Alvodine 304.0❺
- amethocaine 304.6❺
- amidone 304.0❺
- amidopyrine 304.6❺
- aminopyrine 304.6❺
- amobarbital 304.1❺
- amphetamine(s) (type) (drugs classifiable to 969.7) 304.4❺
- amylene hydrate 304.6❺
- amylobarbitone 304.1❺
- amylocaine 304.6❺
- Amytal (sodium) 304.1❺
- analgesic (drug) NEC 304.6❺
  - synthetic with morphine-like effect 304.0❺
- anesthetic (agent) (drug) (gas) (general) (local) NEC 304.6❺
- Angel dust 304.6❺
- anileridine 304.0❺
- antipyrine 304.6❺
- anxiolytic 304.1❺
- aprobarbital 304.1❺
- aprobarbitone 304.1❺
- atropine 304.6❺
- Avertin (bromide) 304.6❺
- barbenyl 304.1❺
- barbital(s) 304.1❺
- barbitone 304.1❺
- barbiturate(s) (compounds) (drugs classifiable to 967.0) 304.1❺
- barbituric acid (and compounds) 304.1❺
- benzedrine 304.4❺
- benzylmorphine 304.0❺
- Beta-chlor 304.1❺
- bhang 304.3❺
- blue velvet 304.0❺
- Brevital 304.1❺
- bromal (hydrate) 304.1❺
- bromide(s) NEC 304.1❺
- bromine compounds NEC 304.1❺
- bromisovalum 304.1❺
- bromoform 304.1❺
- Bromo-seltzer 304.1❺
- bromural 304.1❺
- butabarbital (sodium) 304.1❺
- butabarpal 304.1❺
- butallylonal 304.1❺
- butethal 304.1❺
- buthalitone (sodium) 304.1❺
- Butisol 304.1❺
- butobarbitone 304.1❺
- butyl chloral (hydrate) 304.1❺
- caffeine 304.4
- cannabis (indica) (sativa) (resin) (derivatives) (type) 304.3❺

Dementia – Dependence

- **Dependence** – *continued*
  - carbamazepine 304.6⑤
  - Carbrital 304.1⑤
  - carbromal 304.1⑤
  - carisoprodol 304.6⑤
  - Catha (edulis) 304.4⑤
  - chloral (betaine) (hydrate) 304.1⑤
  - chloralamide 304.1⑤
  - chloralformamide 304.1⑤
  - chloralose 304.1⑤
  - chlordiazepoxide 304.1⑤
  - Chloretone 304.1⑤
  - chlorobutanol 304.1⑤
  - chlorodyne 304.1⑤
  - chloroform 304.6⑤
  - Cliradon 304.0⑤
  - coca (leaf) and derivatives 304.2⑤
  - cocaine 304.2⑤
    - hydrochloride 304.2⑤
    - salt (any) 304.2⑤
  - codeine 304.0⑤
  - combination of drugs (excluding morphine or opioid type drug) NEC 304.8⑤
    - morphine or opioid type drug with any other drug 304.7⑤
  - croton-chloral 304.1⑤
  - cyclobarbital 304.1⑤
  - cyclobarbitone 304.1⑤
  - dagga 304.3⑤
  - Delvinal 304.1⑤
  - Demerol 304.0⑤
  - desocodeine 304.0⑤
  - desomorphine 304.0⑤
  - desoxyephedrine 304.4⑤
  - DET 304.5⑤
  - dexamphetamine 304.4⑤
  - dexedrine 304.4⑤
  - dextromethorphan 304.0⑤
  - dextromoramide 304.0⑤
  - dextronorpseudoephedrine 304.4⑤
  - dextrorphan 304.0⑤
  - diacetylmorphine 304.0⑤
  - Dial 304.1⑤
  - diallylbarbituric acid 304.1⑤
  - diamorphine 304.0⑤
  - diazepam 304.1⑤
  - dibucaine 304.6⑤
  - dichloroethane 304.6⑤
  - diethyl barbituric acid 304.1⑤
  - diethylsulfone-diethylmethane 304.1⑤
  - difencloxazine 304.0⑤
  - dihydrocodeine 304.0⑤
  - dihydrocodeinone 304.0⑤
  - dihydrohydroxycodeinone 304.0⑤
  - dihydroisocodeine 304.0⑤
  - dihydromorphine 304.0⑤
  - dihydromorphinone 304.0⑤
  - dihydroxcodeinone 304.0⑤
  - Dilaudid 304.0⑤
  - dimenhydrinate 304.6⑤
  - dimethylmeperidine 304.0⑤
  - dimethyltriptamine 304.5⑤
  - Dionin 304.0⑤
  - diphenoxylate 304.6⑤
  - dipipanone 304.0⑤
  - d-lysergic acid diethylamide 304.5⑤
  - DMT 304.5⑤
  - Dolophine 304.0⑤
  - DOM 304.2⑤
  - doriden 304.1⑤
  - dormiral 304.1⑤
  - Dormison 304.1⑤
  - Dromoran 304.0⑤
  - drug NEC 304.9
    - analgesic NEC 304.6⑤
    - combination (excluding morphine or opioid type drug) NEC 304.8⑤
      - morphine or opioid type drug with any other drug 304.7⑤
    - complicating pregnancy, childbirth or puerperium 648.3⑤
      - affecting fetus or newborn 779.5
    - hallucinogenic 304.5⑤
    - hypnotic NEC 304.1⑤
    - narcotic NEC 304.9⑤
    - psychostimulant NEC 304.4⑤
    - sedative 304.1⑤
    - soporific NEC 304.1⑤
    - specified type NEC 304.6⑤
    - suspected damage to fetus affecting management of pregnancy 655.5⑤
    - synthetic, with morphine-like effect 304.0⑤

- **Dependence** – *continued*
  - drug – *continued*
    - tranquilizing 304.1⑤
  - duboisine 304.6⑤
  - ectylurea 304.1⑤
  - Endocaine 304.6⑤
  - Equanil 304.1⑤
  - Eskabarb 304.1⑤
  - ethchlorvynol 304.1⑤
  - ether (ethyl) (liquid) (vapor) (vinyl) 304.6⑤
  - ethidene 304.6⑤
  - ethinamate 304.1⑤
  - ethoheptazine 304.6⑤
  - ethyl
    - alcohol 303.9⑤
    - bromide 304.6⑤
    - carbamate 304.6⑤
    - chloride 304.6⑤
    - morphine 304.0⑤
  - ethylene (gas) 304.6⑤
    - dichloride 304.6⑤
  - ethylidene chloride 304.6⑤
  - etilfen 304.1⑤
  - etorphine 304.0⑤
  - etoval 304.1⑤
  - eucodal 304.0⑤
  - euneryl 304.1⑤
  - Evipal 304.1⑤
  - Evipan 304.1⑤
  - fentanyl 304.0⑤
  - ganja 304.3⑤
  - gardenal 304.1⑤
  - gardenpanyl 304.1⑤
  - gelsemine 304.6⑤
  - Gelsemium 304.6⑤
  - Gemonil 304.1⑤
  - glucochloral 304.1⑤
  - glue (airplane) (sniffing) 304.6⑤
  - glutethimide 304.1⑤
  - hallucinogenics 304.5⑤
  - hashish 304.3⑤
  - headache powder NEC 304.6⑤
  - Heavenly Blue 304.5⑤
  - hedonal 304.1⑤
  - hemp 304.3⑤
  - heptabarbital 304.1⑤
  - Heptalgin 304.0⑤
  - heptobarbitone 304.1⑤
  - heroin 304.0⑤
    - salt (any) 304.0⑤
  - hexethal (sodium) 304.1⑤
  - hexobarbital 304.1⑤
  - Hycodan 304.0⑤
  - hydrocodone 304.0⑤
  - hydromorphinol 304.0⑤
  - hydromorphinone 304.0⑤
  - hydromorphone 304.0⑤
  - hydroxycodeine 304.0⑤
  - hypnotic NEC 304.1⑤
  - Indian hemp 304.3⑤
  - inhalant 304.6⑤
  - intranarcon 304.1⑤
  - Kemithal 304.1⑤
  - ketobemidone 304.0⑤
  - khat 304.4⑤
  - kif 304.3⑤
  - Lactuca (virosa) extract 304.1⑤
  - lactucarium 304.1⑤
  - laudanum 304.0⑤
  - Lebanese red 304.3⑤
  - Leritine 304.0⑤
  - lettuce opium 304.1⑤
  - Levanil 304.1⑤
  - Levo-Dromoran 304.0⑤
  - levo-iso-methadone 304.0⑤
  - levorphanol 304.0⑤
  - Librium 304.1⑤
  - Lomotil 304.6⑤
  - Lotusate 304.1⑤
  - LSD (-25) (and derivatives) 304.5⑤
  - Luminal 304.1⑤
  - lysergic acid 304.5⑤
    - amide 304.5⑤
  - maconha 304.3
  - magic mushroom 304.5⑤
  - marihuana 304.3⑤
  - MDA (methylene dioxyamphetamine) 304.4⑤
  - Mebaral 304.1⑤
  - Medinal 304.1⑤
  - Medomin 304.1⑤
  - megahallucinogenics 304.5⑤
  - meperidine 304.0⑤

- **Dependence** – *continued*
  - mephobarbital 304.1⑤
  - meprobamate 304.1⑤
  - mescaline 304.5⑤
  - methadone 304.0⑤
  - methamphetamine(s) 304.4⑤
  - methaqualone 304.1⑤
  - metharbital 304.1⑤
  - methitural 304.1⑤
  - methobarbitone 304.1⑤
  - methohexital 304.1⑤
  - methopholine 304.6⑤
  - methyl
    - alcohol 303.9⑤
    - bromide 304.6⑤
    - morphine 304.0⑤
    - sulfonal 304.1⑤
  - methylated spirit 303.9⑤
  - methylbutinol 304.6⑤
  - methyldihydromorphinone 304.0⑤
  - methylene
    - chloride 304.6⑤
    - dichloride 304.6⑤
    - dioxyamphetamine (MDA) 304.4⑤
  - methylparafynol 304.1⑤
  - methylphenidate 304.4⑤
  - methyprylone 304.1⑤
  - metopon 304.0⑤
  - Miltown 304.1⑤
  - morning glory seeds 304.5⑤
  - morphinan(s) 304.0⑤
  - morphine (sulfate) (sulfite) (type) (drugs classifiable to 965.00-965.09) 304.0⑤
  - morphine or opioid type drug (drugs classifiable to 965.00-965.09) with any other drug 304.7⑤
  - morphinol(s) 304.0⑤
  - morphinon 304.0⑤
  - morpholinylethylmorphine 304.0⑤
  - mylomide 304.1⑤
  - myristicin 304.5⑤
  - narcotic (drug) NEC 304.9⑤
  - nealbarbital 304.1⑤
  - nealbarbitone 304.1⑤
  - Nembutal 304.1⑤
  - Neonal 304.1⑤
  - Neraval 304.1⑤
  - Neravan 304.1⑤
  - neurobarb 304.1⑤
  - nicotine 305.1⑤
  - Nisentil 304.0⑤
  - nitrous oxide 304.6⑤
  - Noctec 304.1⑤
  - Noludar 304.1⑤
  - nonbarbiturate sedatives and tranquilizers with similar effect 304.1⑤
  - noptil 304.1⑤
  - normorphine 304.0⑤
  - noscapine 304.0⑤
  - Novocaine 304.6⑤
  - Numorphan 304.0⑤
  - nunol 304.1⑤
  - Nupercaine 304.6⑤
  - Oblivon 304.1⑤
  - on
    - aspirator V46.0
    - hemodialysis V45.1
    - hyperbaric chamber V46.8
    - iron lung V46.11
    - machine (enabling) V46.9
      - specified type NEC V46.8
    - peritoneal dialysis V45.1
    - Possum (patient-operated-selector-mechanism) V46.8
    - renal dialysis machine V45.1
    - respirator [ventilator] V46.11
      - encounter
        - during
          - mechanical failure V46.14
          - power failure V46.12
        - for weaning V46.13
    - supplemental oxygen V46.2
  - opiate 304.0⑤
  - opioids 304.0⑤
  - opioid type drug 304.0⑤
    - with any other drug 304.7⑤
  - opium (alkaloids) (derivatives) (tincture) 304.0⑤
  - ortal 304.1⑤
  - polysubstance 304.8⑤
  - oxazepam 304.1⑤
  - oxycodone 304.0⑤
  - oxymorphone 304.0⑤

Dependence – Dependence

Dependence – *continued*
- Palfium 304.0❺
- Panadol 304.6❺
- pantopium 304.0❺
- pantopon 304.0❺
- papaverine 304.0❺
- paracetamol 304.6❺
- paracodin 304.0❺
- paraldehyde 304.1❺
- paregoric 304.0❺
- Parzone 304.0❺
- PCP (phencyclidine) 304.6❺
- Pearly Gates 304.5❺
- pentazocine 304.0❺
- pentobarbital 304.1❺
- pentobarbitone (sodium) 304.1❺
- Pentothal 304.1❺
- Percaine 304.6❺
- Percodan 304.0❺
- Perichlor 304.1❺
- Pernocton 304.1❺
- Pernoston 304.1❺
- peronine 304.0❺
- pethidine (hydrochloride) 304.0❺
- petrichloral 304.1❺
- peyote 304.5❺
- Phanodorn 304.1❺
- phenacetin 304.6❺
- phenadoxone 304.0❺
- phenaglycodol 304.1❺
- phenazocine 304.0❺
- phencyclidine 304.6❺
- phenmetrazine 304.4❺
- phenobal 304.1❺
- phenobarbital 304.1❺
- phenobarbitone 304.1❺
- phenomorphan 304.0❺
- phenonyl 304.1❺
- phenoperidine 304.0❺
- pholcodine 304.0❺
- piminodine 304.0❺
- Pipadone 304.0❺
- Pitkin's solution 304.6❺
- Placidyl 304.1❺
- polysubstance 304.8❺
- Pontocaine 304.6❺
- pot 304.3❺
- potassium bromide 304.1❺
- Preludin 304.4❺
- Prinadol 304.0❺
- probarbital 304.1❺
- procaine 304.6❺
- propanal 304.1❺
- propoxyphene 304.6❺
- psilocibin 304.5❺
- psilocin 304.5❺
- psilocybin 304.5❺
- psilocyline 304.5❺
- psilocyn 304.5❺
- psychedelic agents 304.5❺
- psychostimulant NEC 304.4❺
- psychotomimetic agents 304.5❺
- pyrahexyl 304.3❺
- Pyramidon 304.6❺
- quinalbarbitone 304.1❺
- racemoramide 304.0❺
- racemorphan 304.0❺
- Rela 304.6❺
- scopolamine 304.6❺
- secobarbital 304.1❺
- Seconal 304.1❺
- sedative NEC 304.1
  - nonbarbiturate with barbiturate effect 304.1❺
- Sedormid 304.1❺
- sernyl 304.1❺
- sodium bromide 304.1❺
- Soma 304.6❺
- Somnal 304.1❺
- Somnos 304.1❺
- Soneryl 304.1❺
- soporific (drug) NEC 304.1❺
- specified drug NEC 304.6❺
- speed 304.4❺
- spinocaine 304.6❺
- stovaine 304.6❺
- STP 304.5❺
- stramonium 304.6❺
- Sulfonal 304.1❺
- sulfonethylmethane 304.1❺
- sulfonmethane 304.1❺
- Surital 304.1❺
- synthetic drug with morphine-like effect 304.0❺

Dependence – *continued*
- talbutal 304.1❺
- tetracaine 304.6
- tetrahydrocannabinol 304.3❺
- tetronal 304.1❺
- THC 304.3❺
- thebacon 304.0❺
- thebaine 304.0❺
- thiamil 304.1❺
- thiamylal 304.1❺
- thiopental 304.1❺
- tobacco 305.1❺
- toluene, toluol 304.6❺
- tranquilizer NEC 304.1❺
  - nonbarbiturate with barbiturate effect 304.1❺
- tribromacetaldehyde 304.6❺
- tribromethanol 304.6❺
- tribromomethane 304.6❺
- trichloroethanol 304.6❺
- trichoroethyl phosphate 304.1❺
- triclofos 304.1❺
- Trional 304.1❺
- Tuinal 304.1❺
- Turkish green 304.3❺
- urethan(e) 304.6❺
- Valium 304.1❺
- Valmid 304.1❺
- veganin 304.0❺
- veramon 304.1❺
- Veronal 304.1❺
- versidyne 304.6❺
- vinbarbital 304.1❺
- vinbarbitone 304.1❺
- vinyl bitone 304.1❺
- vitamin B_6 266.1
- wine 303.9
- Zactane 304.6

Dependency
- passive 301.6
- reactions 301.6

Depersonalization (episode, in neurotic state) (neurotic) (syndrome) 300.6

Depletion
- carbohydrates 271.9
- complement factor 279.8
- extracellular fluid 276.52
- plasma 276.52
- potassium 276.8
  - nephropathy 588.89
- salt or sodium 276.1
  - causing heat exhaustion or prostration 992.4
  - nephropathy 593.9
- volume 276.50
  - extracellular fluid 276.52
  - plasma 276.52

Deposit
- argentous, cornea 371.16
- bone, in Boeck's sarcoid 135
- calcareous, calcium – *see* Calcification
- cholesterol
  - retina 362.82
  - skin 709.3
  - vitreous (humor) 379.22
- conjunctival 372.56
- cornea, corneal NEC 371.10
  - argentous 371.16
  - in
    - cystinosis 270.0 *[371.15]*
    - mucopolysaccharidosis 277.5 *[371.15]*
- crystalline, vitreous (humor) 379.22
- hemosiderin, in old scars of cornea 371.11
- metallic, in lens 366.45
- skin 709.3
- teeth, tooth (betel) (black) (green) (materia alba) (orange) (soft) (tobacco) 523.6
- urate, in kidney (*see also* Disease, renal) 593.9

Depraved appetite 307.52

Depression 311
- acute (*see also* Psychosis, affective) 296.2❺
  - recurrent episode 296.3❺
  - single episode 296.2❺
- agitated (*see also* Psychosis, affective) 296.2❺
  - recurrent episode 296.3❺
  - single episode 296.2❺
- anaclitic 309.21
- anxiety 300.4
- arches 734
  - congenital 754.61
- autogenous (*see also* Psychosis, affective) 296.2❺
  - recurrent episode 296.3❺

Depression – *continued*
- autogenous – *continued*
  - single episode 296.2❺
- basal metabolic rate (BMR) 794.7
- bone marrow 289.9
- central nervous system 799.1
  - newborn 779.2
- cerebral 331.9
  - newborn 779.2
- cerebrovascular 437.8
  - newborn 779.2
- chest wall 738.3
- endogenous (*see also* Psychosis, affective) 296.2❺
  - recurrent episode 296.3❺
  - single episode 296.2❺
- functional activity 780.99
- hysterical 300.11
- involutional, climacteric, or menopausal (*see also* Psychosis, affective) 296.2❺
  - recurrent episode 296.3❺
  - single episode 296.2❺
- manic (*see also* Psychosis, affective) 296.80
- medullary 348.8
  - newborn 779.2
- mental 300.4
- metatarsal heads – *see* Depression, arches
- metatarsus – *see* Depression, arches
- monopolar (*see also* Psychosis, affective) 296.2❺
  - recurrent episode 296.3❺
  - single episode 296.2❺
- nervous 300.4
- neurotic 300.4
- nose 738.0
- postpartum 648.4❺
- psychogenic 300.4
  - reactive 298.0
- psychoneurotic 300.4
- psychotic (*see also* Psychosis, affective) 296.2❺
  - reactive 298.0
  - recurrent episode 296.3❺
  - single episode 296.2❺
- reactive 300.4
  - neurotic 300.4
  - psychogenic 298.0
  - psychoneurotic 300.4
  - psychotic 298.0
- recurrent 296.3❺
- respiratory center 348.8
  - newborn 770.89
- scapula 736.89
- senile 290.21
- situational (acute) (brief) 309.0
  - prolonged 309.1
- skull 754.0
- sternum 738.3
- visual field 368.40

Depressive reaction – *see also* Reaction, depressive
- acute (transient) 309.0
  - with anxiety 309.28
- prolonged 309.1
- situational (acute) 309.0
  - prolonged 309.1

Deprivation
- cultural V62.4
- emotional V62.89
  - affecting
    - adult 995.82
    - infant or child 995.51
- food 994.2
  - specific substance NEC 269.8
- protein (familial) (kwashiorkor) 260
- sleep V69.4
- social V62.4
  - affecting
    - adult 995.82
    - infant or child 995.51
- symptoms, syndrome
  - alcohol 291.81
  - drug 292.0
- vitamins (*see also* Deficiency, vitamin) 269.2
- water 994.3

de Quervain's
- disease (tendon sheath) 727.04
- thyroiditis (subacute granulomatous thyroiditis) 245.1

- **Derangement**
  - ankle (internal) 718.97
    - current injury (*see also* Dislocation, ankle) 837.0
    - recurrent 718.37
  - cartilage (articular) NEC (*see also* Disorder, cartilage, articular) 718.0❺
    - knee 717.9
      - recurrent 718.36
    - recurrent 718.3❺
  - collateral ligament (knee) (medial) (tibial) 717.82
    - current injury 844.1
      - lateral (fibular) 844.0
    - lateral (fibular) 717.81
      - current injury 844.0
  - cruciate ligament (knee) (posterior) 717.84
    - anterior 717.83
      - current injury 844.2
    - current injury 844.2
  - elbow (internal) 718.92
    - current injury (*see also* Dislocation, elbow) 832.00
    - recurrent 718.32
  - gastrointestinal 536.9
  - heart – *see* Disease, heart
  - hip (joint) (internal) (old) 718.95
    - current injury (*see also* Dislocation, hip) 835.00
    - recurrent 718.35
  - intervertebral disc – *see* Displacement, intervertebral disc
  - joint (internal) 718.90
    - ankle 718.97
    - current injury – *see also* Dislocation, by site
      - knee, meniscus or cartilage (*see also* Tear, meniscus) 836.2
    - elbow 718.92
    - foot 718.97
    - hand 718.94
    - hip 718.95
    - knee 717.9
    - multiple sites 718.99
    - pelvic region 718.95
    - recurrent 718.30
      - ankle 718.37
      - elbow 718.32
      - foot 718.37
      - hand 718.34
      - hip 718.35
      - knee 718.36
      - multiple sites 718.39
      - pelvic region 718.35
      - shoulder (region) 718.31
      - specified site NEC 718.38
      - temporomandibular (old) 524.69
      - wrist 718.33
    - shoulder (region) 718.91
    - specified site NEC 718.98
    - spine NEC 724.9
    - temporomandibular 524.69
    - wrist 718.93
  - knee (cartilage) (internal) 717.9
    - current injury (*see also* Tear, meniscus) 836.2
    - ligament 717.89
      - capsular 717.85
      - collateral – *see* Derangement, collateral ligament
      - cruciate – *see* Derangement, cruciate ligament
      - specified NEC 717.85
    - recurrent 718.36
  - low back NEC 724.9
  - meniscus NEC (knee) 717.5
    - current injury (*see also* Tear, meniscus) 836.2
    - lateral 717.40
      - anterior horn 717.42
      - posterior horn 717.43
      - specified NEC 717.49
    - medial 717.3
      - anterior horn 717.1
      - posterior horn 717.2
    - recurrent 718.3❺
    - site other than knee – *see* Disorder, cartilage, articular
  - mental (*see also* Psychosis) 298.9
  - rotator cuff (recurrent) (tear) 726.10
    - current 840.4
  - sacroiliac (old) 724.6
    - current – *see* Dislocation, sacroiliac
  - semilunar cartilage (knee) 717.5
    - current injury 836.2
      - lateral 836.1

- **Derangement** – *continued*
  - semilunar cartilage – *continued*
    - current injury – *continued*
      - medial 836.0
    - recurrent 718.3❺
  - shoulder (internal) 718.91
    - current injury (*see also* Dislocation, shoulder) 831.00
    - recurrent 718.31
  - spine (recurrent) NEC 724.9
    - current – *see* Dislocation, spine
  - temporomandibular (internal) (joint) (old) 524.69
    - current – *see* Dislocation, jaw
- **Dercum's disease or syndrome** (adiposis dolorosa) 272.8
- **Derealization** (neurotic) 300.6
- **Dermal** – *see* condition
- **Dermaphytid** – *see* Dermatophytosis
- **Dermatergosis** – *see* Dermatitis
- **Dermatitis** (allergic) (contact) (occupational) (venenata) 692.9
  - ab igne 692.82
  - acneiform 692.9
  - actinic (due to sun) 692.70
    - acute 692.72
    - chronic NEC 692.74
    - other than from sun NEC 692.82
  - ambustionis
    - due to
      - burn or scald – *see* Burn, by site
      - sunburn (*see also* Sunburn) 692.71
  - amebic 006.6
  - ammonia 691.0
  - anaphylactoid NEC 692.9
  - arsenical 692.4
  - artefacta 698.4
    - psychogenic 316 *[698.4]*
  - asthmatic 691.8
  - atopic (allergic) (intrinsic) 691.8
    - psychogenic 316 *[691.8]*
  - atrophicans 701.8
    - diffusa 701.8
    - maculosa 701.3
  - berlock, berloque 692.72
  - blastomycetic 116.0
  - blister beetle 692.89
  - Brucella NEC 023.9
  - bullosa 694.9
    - striata pratensis 692.6
  - bullous 694.9
    - mucosynechial, atrophic 694.60
      - with ocular involvement 694.61
    - seasonal 694.8
  - calorica
    - due to
      - burn or scald – *see* Burn, by site
      - cold 692.89
      - sunburn (*see also* Sunburn) 692.71
  - caterpillar 692.89
  - cercarial 120.3
  - combustionis
    - due to
      - burn or scald – *see* Burn, by site
      - sunburn (*see also* Sunburn) 692.71
  - congelationis 991.5
  - contusiformis 695.2
  - diabetic 250.8❺
  - diaper 691.0
  - diphtheritica 032.85
  - due to
    - acetone 692.2
    - acids 692.4
    - adhesive plaster 692.4
    - alcohol (skin contact) (substances classifiable to 980.0-980.9) 692.4
      - taken internally 693.8
    - alkalis 692.4
    - allergy NEC 692.9
    - ammonia (household) (liquid) 692.4
    - animal
      - dander (cat) (dog) 692.84
      - hair (cat) (dog) 692.84
    - arnica 692.3
    - arsenic 692.4
      - taken internally 693.8
    - blister beetle 692.89
    - cantharides 692.3
    - carbon disulphide 692.2
    - caterpillar 692.89
    - caustics 692.4

- **Dermatitis** – *continued*
  - due to – *continued*
    - cereal (ingested) 693.1
      - contact with skin 692.5
    - chemical(s) NEC 692.4
      - internal 693.8
      - irritant NEC 692.4
        - taken internally 693.8
    - chlorocompounds 692.2
    - coffee (ingested) 693.1
      - contact with skin 692.5
    - cold weather 692.89
    - cosmetics 692.81
    - cyclohexanes 692.2
    - dander, animal (cat) (dog) 692.84
    - deodorant 692.81
    - detergents 692.0
    - dichromate 692.4
    - drugs and medicinals (correct substance properly administered) (internal use) 693.0
      - external (in contact with skin) 692.3
        - wrong substance given or taken 976.9
          - specified substance – *see* Table of Drugs and Chemicals
      - wrong substance given or taken 977.9
        - specified substance – *see* Table of Drugs and Chemicals
    - dyes 692.89
      - hair 692.89
    - epidermophytosis – *see* Dermatophytosis
    - esters 692.2
    - external irritant NEC 692.9
      - specified agent NEC 692.89
    - eye shadow 692.81
    - fish (ingested) 693.1
      - contact with skin 692.5
    - flour (ingested) 693.1
      - contact with skin 692.5
    - food (ingested) 693.1
      - in contact with skin 692.5
    - fruit (ingested) 693.1
      - contact with skin 692.5
    - fungicides 692.3
    - furs 692.84
    - glycols 692.2
    - greases NEC 692.1
    - hair, animal (cat) (dog) 692.84
    - hair dyes 692.89
    - hot
      - objects and materials – *see* Burn, by site
      - weather or places 692.89
    - hydrocarbons 692.2
    - infrared rays, except from sun 692.82
      - solar NEC (*see also* Dermatitis, due to, sun) 692.70
    - ingested substance 693.9
      - drugs and medicinals (*see also* Dermatitis, due to, drugs and medicinals) 693.0
      - food 693.1
      - specified substance NEC 693.8
    - ingestion or injection of chemical 693.8
      - drug (correct substance properly administered) 693.0
      - wrong substance given or taken 977.9
        - specified substance – *see* Table of Drugs and Chemicals
    - insecticides 692.4
    - internal agent 693.9
      - drugs and medicinals (*see also* Dermatitis, due to, drugs and medicinals) 693.0
      - food (ingested) 693.1
        - in contact with skin 692.5
      - specified agent NEC 693.8
    - iodine 692.3
    - iodoform 692.3
    - irradiation 692.82
    - jewelry 692.83
    - keratolytics 692.3
    - ketones 692.2
    - lacquer tree (Rhus verniciflua) 692.6
    - light (sun) NEC (*see also* Dermatitis, due to, sun) 692.70
      - other 692.82
    - low temperature 692.89
    - mascara 692.81
    - meat (ingested) 693.1
      - contact with skin 692.5
    - mercury, mercurials 692.3
    - metals 692.83
    - milk (ingested) 693.1
      - contact with skin 692.5
    - Neomycin 692.3

Dermatitis – *continued*
- due to – *continued*
  - nylon 692.4
  - oils NEC 692.1
  - paint solvent 692.2
  - pediculocides 692.3
  - petroleum products (substances classifiable to 981) 692.4
  - phenol 692.3
  - photosensitiveness, photosensitivity (sun) 692.72
    - other light 692.82
  - plants NEC 692.6
  - plasters, medicated (any) 692.3
  - plastic 692.4
  - poison
    - ivy (Rhus toxicodendron) 692.6
    - oak (Rhus diversiloba) 692.6
    - plant or vine 692.6
    - sumac (Rhus venenata) 692.6
    - vine (Rhus radicans) 692.6
  - preservatives 692.89
  - primrose (primula) 692.6
  - primula 692.6
  - radiation 692.82
    - sun NEC (*see also* Dermatitis, due to, sun) 692.70
    - tanning bed 692.82
  - radioactive substance 692.82
  - radium 692.82
  - ragweed (Senecio jacobae) 692.6
  - Rhus (diversiloba) (radicans) (toxicodendron) (venenata) (verniciflua) 692.6
  - rubber 692.4
  - scabicides 692.3
  - Senecio jacobae 692.6
  - solar radiation – *see* Dermatitis, due to, sun
  - solvents (any) (substances classifiable to (982.0-982.8) 692.2
    - chlorocompound group 692.2
    - cyclohexane group 692.2
    - ester group 692.2
    - glycol group 692.2
    - hydrocarbon group 692.2
    - ketone group 692.2
    - paint 692.2
  - specified agent NEC 692.89
  - sun 692.70
    - acute 692.72
    - chronic NEC 692.74
    - specified NEC 692.79
  - sunburn (*see also* Sunburn) 692.71
  - sunshine NEC (*see also* Dermatitis, due to, sun) 692.70
  - tanning bed 692.82
  - tetrachlorethylene 692.2
  - toluene 692.2
  - topical medications 692.3
  - turpentine 692.2
  - ultraviolet rays, except from sun 692.82
    - sun NEC (*see also* Dermatitis, due to, sun) 692.70
  - vaccine or vaccination (correct substance properly administered) 693.0
    - wrong substance given or taken
      - bacterial vaccine 978.8
        - specified – *see* Table of Drugs and Chemicals
      - other vaccines NEC 979.9
        - specified – *see* Table of Drugs and Chemicals
  - varicose veins (*see also* Varicose, vein, inflamed or infected) 454.1
  - x-rays 692.82
- dyshydrotic 705.81
- dysmenorrheica 625.8
- eczematoid NEC 692.9
  - infectious 690.8
- eczematous NEC 692.9
- epidemica 695.89
- erysipelatosa 695.81
- escharotica – *see* Burn, by site
- exfoliativa, exfoliative 695.89
  - generalized 695.89
  - infantum 695.81
  - neonatorum 695.81
- eyelid 373.31
  - allergic 373.32
  - contact 373.32
  - eczematous 373.31
  - herpes (zoster) 053.20
    - simplex 054.41

Dermatitis – *continued*
- eyelid – *continued*
  - infective 373.5
    - due to
      - actinomycosis 039.3 *[373.5]*
      - herpes
        - simplex 054.41
        - zoster 053.20
      - impetigo 684 *[373.5]*
      - leprosy (*see also* Leprosy) 030.0 *[373.4]*
      - lupus vulgaris (tuberculous) (*see also* Tuberculosis) 017.0❺ *[373.4]*
      - mycotic dermatitis (*see also* Dermatomycosis) 111.9 *[373.5]*
      - vaccinia 051.0 *[373.5]*
        - postvaccination 999.0 *[373.5]*
    - yaws (*see also* Yaws) 102.9 *[373.4]*
- facta, factitia 698.4
  - psychogenic 316 *[698.4]*
- ficta 698.4
  - psychogenic 316 *[698.4]*
- flexural 691.8
- follicularis 704.8
- friction 709.8
- fungus 111.9
  - specified type NEC 111.8
- gangrenosa, gangrenous (infantum) (*see also* Gangrene) 785.4
- gestationis 646.8❺
- gonococcal 098.89
- gouty 274.89
- harvest mite 133.8
- heat 692.89
- herpetiformis (bullous) (erythematous) (pustular) (vesicular) 694.0
  - juvenile 694.2
  - senile 694.5
- hiemalis 692.89
- hypostatic, hypostatica 454.1
  - with ulcer 454.2
- impetiginous 684
- infantile (acute) (chronic) (intertriginous) (intrinsic) (seborrheic) 690.12
- infectiosa eczematoides 690.8
- infectious (staphylococcal) (streptococcal) 686.9
  - eczematoid 690.8
- infective eczematoid 690.8
- Jacquet's (diaper dermatitis) 691.0
- leptus 133.8
- lichenified NEC 692.9
- lichenoid, chronic 701.0
- lichenoides purpurica pigmentosa 709.1
- meadow 692.6
- medicamentosa (correct substance properly administered) (internal use) (*see also* Dermatitis, due to, drugs or medicinals) 693.0
  - due to contact with skin 692.3
- mite 133.8
- multiformis 694.0
  - juvenile 694.2
  - senile 694.5
- napkin 691.0
- neuro 698.3
- neurotica 694.0
- nummular NEC 692.9
- osteatosis, osteatotic 706.8
- papillaris capillitii 706.1
- pellagrous 265.2
- perioral 695.3
- perstans 696.1
- photosensitivity (sun) 692.72
  - other light 692.82
- pigmented purpuric lichenoid 709.1
- polymorpha dolorosa 694.0
- primary irritant 692.9
- pruriginosa 694.0
- pruritic NEC 692.9
- psoriasiform nodularis 696.2
- psychogenic 316
- purulent 686.00
- pustular contagious 051.2
- pyococcal 686.00
- pyocyaneus 686.09
- pyogenica 686.00
- radiation 692.82
- repens 696.1
- Ritter's (exfoliativa) 695.81
- Schamberg's (progressive pigmentary dermatosis) 709.09
- schistosome 120.3
- seasonal bullous 694.8

Dermatitis – *continued*
- seborrheic 690.10
  - infantile 690.12
- sensitization NEC 692.9
- septic (*see also* Septicemia) 686.00
  - gonococcal 098.89
- solar, solare NEC (*see also* Dermatitis, due to, sun) 692.70
- stasis 459.81
  - due to
    - postphlebitic syndrome 459.12
      - with ulcer 459.13
    - varicose veins – *see* Varicose
  - ulcerated or with ulcer (varicose) 454.2
- sunburn (*see also* Sunburn) 692.71
- suppurative 686.00
- traumatic NEC 709.8
- trophoneurotica 694.0
- ultraviolet, except from sun 692.82
  - due to sun NEC (*see also* Dermatitis, due to, sun) 692.70
- varicose 454.1
  - with ulcer 454.2
- vegetans 686.8
- verrucosa 117.2
- xerotic 706.8

Dermatoarthritis, lipoid 272.8 *[713.0]*

Dermatochalasia, dermatochalasis 374.87

Dermatofibroma (lenticulare) (M8832/0) – *see also* Neoplasm, skin, benign
- protuberans (M8832/1) – *see* Neoplasm, skin, uncertain behavior

Dermatofibrosarcoma (protuberans) (M8832/3) – *see* Neoplasm, skin, malignant

Dermatographia 708.3

Dermatolysis (congenital) (exfoliativa) 757.39
- acquired 701.8
- eyelids 374.34
- palpebrarum 374.34
- senile 701.8

Dermatomegaly NEC 701.8

Dermatomucomyositis 710.3

Dermatomycosis 111.9
- furfuracea 111.0
- specified type NEC 111.8

Dermatomyositis (acute) (chronic) 710.3

Dermatoneuritis of children 985.0

Dermatophiliasis 134.1

Dermatophytide – *see* Dermatophytosis

Dermatophytosis (Epidermophyton) (infection) (microsporum) (tinea) (Trichophyton) 110.9
- beard 110.0
- body 110.5
- deep seated 110.6
- fingernails 110.1
- foot 110.4
- groin 110.3
- hand 110.2
- nail 110.1
- perianal (area) 110.3
- scalp 110.0
- scrotal 110.8
- specified site NEC 110.8
- toenails 110.1
- vulva 110.8

Dermatopolyneuritis 985.0

Dermatorrhexis 756.83
- acquired 701.8

Dermatosclerosis (*see also* Scleroderma) 710.1
- localized 701.0

Dermatosis 709.9
- Andrews' 686.8
- atopic 691.8
- Bowen's (M8081/2) – *see* Neoplasm, skin, in situ
- bullous 694.9
  - specified type NEC 694.8
- erythematosquamous 690.8
- exfoliativa 695.89
- factitial 698.4
- gonococcal 098.89
- herpetiformis 694.0
  - juvenile 694.2
  - senile 694.5
- hysterical 300.11
- linear IgA 694.8
- menstrual NEC 709.8
- neutrophilic, acute febrile 695.89
- occupational (*see also* Dermatitis) 692.9
- papulosa nigra 709.8

Dermatosis – *continued*
pigmentary NEC 709.00
progressive 709.09
Schamberg's 709.09
Siemens-Bloch 757.33
progressive pigmentary 709.09
psychogenic 316
pustular subcorneal 694.1
Schamberg's (progressive pigmentary) 709.09
senile NEC 709.3
specified NEC 702.8
Unna's (seborrheic dermatitis) 690.10
Dermographia 708.3
Dermographism 708.3
Dermoid (cyst) (M9084/0) – *see also* Neoplasm, by site, benign
with malignant transformation (M9084/3) 183.0
Dermopathy
infiltrative, with thyrotoxicosis 242.0❺
senile NEC 709.3
Dermophytosis – *see* Dermatophytosis
Descemet's membrane – *see* condition
Descemetocele 371.72
Descending – *see* condition
Descensus uteri (complete) (incomplete) (partial) (without vaginal wall prolapse) 618.1
with mention of vaginal wall prolapse – *see* Prolapse, uterovaginal
Desensitization to allergens V07.1
Desert
rheumatism 114.0
sore (*see also* Ulcer, skin) 707.9
Desertion (child) (newborn) 995.52
adult 995.84
Desmoid (extra-abdominal) (tumor) (M8821/1) – *see also* Neoplasm, connective tissue, uncertain behavior
abdominal (M8822/1) – *see* Neoplasm, connective tissue, uncertain behavior
Despondency 300.4
Desquamative dermatitis NEC 695.89
Destruction
articular facet (*see also* Derangement, joint) 718.9❺
vertebra 724.9
bone 733.90
syphilitic 095.5
joint (*see also* Derangement, joint) 718.9❺
sacroiliac 724.6
kidney 593.89
live fetus to facilitate birth NEC 763.89
ossicles (ear) 385.24
rectal sphincter 569.49
septum (nasal) 478.19
tuberculous NEC (*see also* Tuberculosis) 011.9❺
tympanic membrane 384.82
tympanum 385.89
vertebral disc – *see* Degeneration, intervertebral disc
Destructiveness (*see also* Disturbance, conduct) 312.9
adjustment reaction 309.3
Detachment
cartilage – *see also* Sprain, by site
knee – *see* Tear, meniscus
cervix, annular 622.8
complicating delivery 665.3❺
choroid (old) (postinfectional) (simple) (spontaneous) 363.70
hemorrhagic 363.72
serous 363.71
knee, medial meniscus (old) 717.3
current injury 836.0
ligament – *see* Sprain, by site
placenta (premature) – *see* Placenta, separation
retina (recent) 361.9
with retinal defect (rhegmatogenous) 361.00
giant tear 361.03
multiple 361.02
partial
with
giant tear 361.03
multiple defects 361.02
retinal dialysis (juvenile) 361.04
single defect 361.01
retinal dialysis (juvenile) 361.04
single 361.01
subtotal 361.05

Detachment – *continued*
retina – *continued*
with retinal defect – *continued*
total 361.05
delimited (old) (partial) 361.06
old
delimited 361.06
partial 361.06
total or subtotal 361.07
pigment epithelium (RPE) (serous) 362.42
exudative 362.42
hemorrhagic 362.43
rhegmatogenous (*see also* Detachment, retina, with retinal defect) 361.00
serous (without retinal defect) 361.2
specified type NEC 361.89
traction (with vitreoretinal organization) 361.81
vitreous humor 379.21
Detergent asthma 507.8
Deterioration
epileptic
with behavioral disturbance 345.9 *[294.11]*
without behavioral disturbance 345.9 *[294.10]*
heart, cardiac (*see also* Degeneration, myocardial) 429.1
mental (*see also* Psychosis) 298.9
myocardium, myocardial (*see also* Degeneration, myocardial) 429.1
senile (simple) 797
transplanted organ – *see* Complications, transplant, organ, by site
de Toni-Fanconi syndrome (cystinosis) 270.0
Deuteranomaly 368.52
Deuteranopia (anomalous trichromat) (complete) (incomplete) 368.52
Deutschländer's disease – *see* Fracture, foot
Development
abnormal, bone 756.9
arrested 783.40
bone 733.91
child 783.40
due to malnutrition (protein-calorie) 263.2
fetus or newborn 764.9❺
tracheal rings (congenital) 748.3
defective, congenital – *see also* Anomaly
cauda equina 742.59
left ventricle 746.9
with atresia or hypoplasia of aortic orifice or valve with hypoplasia of ascending aorta 746.7
in hypoplastic left heart syndrome 746.7
delayed (*see also* Delay, development) 783.40
arithmetical skills 315.1
language (skills) 315.31
and speech due to hearing loss 315.34 ●
expressive 315.31
mixed receptive-expressive 315.32
learning skill, specified NEC 315.2
mixed skills 315.5
motor coordination 315.4
reading 315.00
specified
learning skill NEC 315.2
type NEC, except learning 315.8
speech 315.39
and language due to hearing loss 315.34 ●
associated with hyperkinesia 314.1
phonological 315.39
spelling 315.09
written expression 315.2
imperfect, congenital – *see also* Anomaly
heart 746.9
lungs 748.60
improper (fetus or newborn) 764.9❺
incomplete (fetus or newborn) 764.9❺
affecting management of pregnancy 656.5❺
bronchial tree 748.3
organ or site not listed – *see* Hypoplasia
respiratory system 748.9
sexual, precocious NEC 259.1
tardy, mental (*see also* Retardation, mental) 319
Developmental – *see* condition
Devergie's disease (pityriasis rubra pilaris) 696.4
Deviation
conjugate (eye) 378.87
palsy 378.81
spasm, spastic 378.82
esophagus 530.89
eye, skew 378.87
mandible, opening and closing 524.53

Deviation – *continued*
midline (jaw) (teeth) 524.29
specified site NEC – *see* Malposition
occlusal plane 524.76
organ or site, congenital NEC – *see* Malposition, congenital
septum (acquired) (nasal) 470
congenital 754.0
sexual 302.9
bestiality 302.1
coprophilia 302.89
ego-dystonic
homosexuality 302.0
lesbianism 302.0
erotomania 302.89
Clérambault's 297.8
exhibitionism (sexual) 302.4
fetishism 302.81
transvestic 302.3
frotteurism 302.89
homosexuality, ego-dystonic 302.0
pedophilic 302.2
lesbianism, ego-dystonic 302.0
masochism 302.83
narcissism 302.89
necrophilia 302.89
nymphomania 302.89
pederosis 302.2
pedophilia 302.2
sadism 302.84
sadomasochism 302.84
satyriasis 302.89
specified type NEC 302.89
transvestic fetishism 302.3
transvestism 302.3
voyeurism 302.82
zoophilia (erotica) 302.1
teeth, midline 524.29
trachea 519.19
ureter (congenital) 753.4
Devic's disease 341.0
Device
cerebral ventricle (communicating) in situ V45.2
contraceptive – *see* Contraceptive, device
drainage, cerebrospinal fluid V45.2
Devil's
grip 074.1
pinches (purpura simplex) 287.2
Devitalized tooth 522.9
Devonshire colic 984.9
specified type of lead – *see* Table of Drugs and Chemicals
Dextraposition, aorta 747.21
with ventricular septal defect, pulmonary stenosis or atresia, and hypertrophy of right ventricle 745.2
in tetralogy of Fallot 745.2
Dextratransposition, aorta 745.11
Dextrinosis, limit (debrancher enzyme deficiency) 271.0
Dextrocardia (corrected) (false) (isolated) (secondary) (true) 746.87
with
complete transposition of viscera 759.3
situs inversus 759.3
Dextroversion, kidney (left) 753.3
Dhobie itch 110.3
Diabetes, diabetic (brittle) (congenital) (familial) (mellitus) (poorly controlled) (severe) (slight) (without complication) 250.0❺

Note – Use the following fifth-digit subclassification with category 250:
0 type II or unspecified type, not stated as uncontrolled
Fifth-digit 0 is for use for type II, patients, even if the patient requires insulin
1 type I [juvenile type], not stated as uncontrolled
2 type II or unspecified type, uncontrolled
Fifth-digit 2 is for use for type II, patients, even if the patient requires insulin
3 type I [juvenile type], uncontrolled

with
coma (with ketoacidosis) 250.3❺
hyperosmolar (nonketotic) 250.2❺

Dermatosis – Diabetes, diabetic

- **Diabetes, diabetic** – *continued*
  - with – *continued*
    - complication NEC 250.9❺
      - specified NEC 250.8❺
    - gangrene 250.7❺ *[785.4]*
    - hyperosmolarity 250.2❺
    - ketosis, ketoacidosis 250.1❺
    - osteomyelitis 250.8❺ *[731.8]*
    - specified manifestations NEC 250.8❺
  - acetonemia 250.1❺
  - acidosis 250.1❺
  - amyotrophy 250.6❺ *[353.1]*▲
  - angiopathy, peripheral 250.7❺ *[443.81]*
  - asymptomatic 790.29
  - autonomic neuropathy (peripheral) 250.6❺ *[337.1]*
  - bone change 250.8❺ *[731.8]*
  - bronze, bronzed 275.0
  - cataract 250.5❺ *[366.41]*
  - chemical 790.29
    - complicating pregnancy, childbirth, or puerperium 648.8❺
  - coma (with ketoacidosis) 250.3❺
    - hyperglycemic 250.3❺
    - hyperosmolar (nonketotic) 250.2❺
    - hypoglycemic 250.3❺
    - insulin 250.3❺
  - complicating pregnancy, childbirth, or puerperium (maternal) 648.0❺
    - affecting fetus or newborn 775.0
  - complication NEC 250.9❺
    - specified NEC 250.8❺
  - dorsal sclerosis 250.6❺ *[340]*
  - dwarfism-obesity syndrome 258.1
  - gangrene 250.7❺ *[785.4]*
  - gastroparesis 250.6❺ *[536.3]*
  - gestational 648.8❺
    - complicating pregnancy, childbirth, or puerperium 648.8❺
  - glaucoma 250.5❺ *[365.44]*
  - glomerulosclerosis (intercapillary) 250.4❺ *[581.81]*
  - glycogenosis, secondary 250.8❺ *[259.8]*
  - hemochromatosis 275.0
  - hyperosmolar coma 250.2❺
  - hyperosmolarity 250.2❺
  - hypertension-nephrosis syndrome 250.4❺ *[581.81]*
  - hypoglycemia 250.8❺
  - hypoglycemic shock 250.8❺
  - insipidus 253.5
    - nephrogenic 588.1
    - pituitary 253.5
    - vasopressin-resistant 588.1
  - intercapillary glomerulosclerosis 250.4❺ *[581.81]*
  - iritis 250.5❺ *[364.42]*
  - ketosis, ketoacidosis 250.1❺
  - Kimmelstiel (-Wilson) disease or syndrome (intercapillary glomerulosclerosis) 250.4❺ *[581.81]*
  - Lancereaux's (diabetes mellitus with marked emaciation) 250.8❺ *[261]*
  - latent (chemical) 790.29
    - complicating pregnancy, childbirth, or puerperium 648.8❺
  - lipoidosis 250.8❺ *[272.7]*
  - macular edema 250.5❺ *[362.07]*
  - maternal
    - with manifest disease in the infant 775.1
      - affecting fetus or newborn 775.0
  - microaneurysms, retinal 250.5❺ *[362.01]*
  - mononeuropathy 250.6❺ *[355.9]*
  - neonatal, transient 775.1
  - nephropathy 250.4❺ *[583.81]*
  - nephrosis (syndrome) 250.4❺ *[581.81]*
  - neuralgia 250.6❺ *[357.2]*
  - neuritis 250.6❺ *[357.2]*
  - neurogenic arthropathy 250.6❺ *[713.5]*
  - neuropathy 250.6❺ *[357.2]*
  - nonclinical 790.29
  - osteomyelitis 250.8❺ *[731.8]*
  - peripheral autonomic neuropathy 250.6❺ *[337.1]*
  - phosphate 275.3
  - polyneuropathy 250.6❺ *[357.2]*
  - renal (true) 271.4
  - retinal
    - edema 250.5❺ *[362.07]*
    - hemorrhage 250.5❺ *[362.01]*
    - microaneurysms 250.5❺ *[362.01]*
  - retinitis 250.5❺ *[362.01]*

- **Diabetes, diabetic** – *continued*
  - retinopathy 250.5❺ *[362.01]*
    - background 250.5❺ *[362.01]*
    - nonproliferative 250.5❺ *[362.03]*
      - mild 250.5❺ *[362.04]*
      - moderate 250.5❺ *[362.05]*
      - severe 250.5❺ *[362.06]*
    - proliferative 250.5❺ *[362.02]*
  - steroid induced
    - correct substance properly administered 251.8
    - overdose or wrong substance given or taken 962.0
  - stress 790.29
  - subclinical 790.29
  - subliminal 790.29
  - sugar 250.0❺
  - ulcer (skin) 250.8❺ *[707.9]*
    - lower extremity 250.8❺ *[707.10]*
      - ankle 250.8 *[707.13]*
      - calf 250.8 *[707.12]*
      - foot 250.8 *[707.15]*
      - heel 250.8 *[707.14]*
      - knee 250.8 *[707.19]*
      - specified site NEC 250.8 *[707.19]*
      - thigh 250.8 *[707.11]*
      - toes 250.8 *[707.15]*
    - specified site NEC 250.8❺ *[707.8]*
  - xanthoma 250.8❺ *[272.2]*
- **Diacyclothrombopathia** 287.1
- **Diagnosis deferred** 799.9
- **Dialysis** (intermittent) (treatment)
  - anterior retinal (juvenile) (with detachment) 361.04
  - extracorporeal V56.0
  - hemodialysis V56.0
    - status only V45.1
  - peritoneal V56.8
    - status only V45.1
  - renal V56.0
    - status only V45.1
  - specified type NEC V56.8
- **Diamond-Blackfan anemia or syndrome** (congenital hypoplastic anemia) 284.01
- **Diamond-Gardener syndrome** (autoerythrocyte sensitization) 287.2
- **Diaper rash** 691.0
- **Diaphoresis** (excessive) NEC (*see also* Hyperhidrosis) 780.8
- **Diaphragm** – *see* condition
- **Diaphragmalgia** 786.52
- **Diaphragmitis** 519.4
- **Diaphyseal aclasis** 756.4
- **Diaphysitis** 733.99
- **Diarrhea, diarrheal** (acute) (autumn) (bilious) (bloody) (catarrhal) (choleraic) (chronic) (gravis) (green) (infantile) (lienteric) (noninfectious) (presumed noninfectious) (putrefactive) (secondary) (sporadic) (summer) (symptomatic) (thermic) 787.91
  - achlorhydric 536.0
  - allergic 558.3
  - amebic (*see also* Amebiasis) 006.9
    - with abscess – *see* Abscess, amebic
    - acute 006.0
    - chronic 006.1
    - nondysenteric 006.2
  - bacillary – *see* Dysentery, bacillary
  - bacterial NEC 008.5
  - balantidial 007.0
  - bile salt-induced 579.8
  - cachectic NEC 787.91
  - chilomastix 007.8
  - choleriformis 001.1
  - coccidial 007.2
  - Cochin-China 579.1
    - anguilluliasis 127.2
    - psilosis 579.1
  - Dientamoeba 007.8
  - dietetic 787.91
  - due to
    - achylia gastrica 536.8
    - Aerobacter aerogenes 008.2❺
    - Bacillus coli – *see* Enteritis, E. coli
    - bacteria NEC 008.5
    - bile salts 579.8
    - Capillaria
      - hepatica 128.8
      - philippinensis 127.5
    - Clostridium perfringens (C) (F) 008.46

- **Diarrhea, diarrheal** – *continued*
  - due to – *continued*
    - Enterobacter aerogenes 008.2❺
    - enterococci 008.49
    - Escherichia coli – *see* Enteritis, E. coli
    - Giardia lamblia 007.1
    - Heterophyes heterophyes 121.6
    - irritating foods 787.91
    - Metagonimus yokogawai 121.5
    - Necator americanus 126.1
    - Paracolobactrum arizonae 008.1
    - Paracolon bacillus NEC 008.47
      - Arizona 008.1
    - Proteus (bacillus) (mirabilis) (Morganii) 008.3
    - Pseudomonas aeruginosa 008.42
    - S. japonicum 120.2
    - specified organism NEC 008.8
      - bacterial 008.49
      - viral NEC 008.69
    - Staphylococcus 008.41
    - Streptococcus 008.49
      - anaerobic 008.46
    - Strongyloides stercoralis 127.2
    - Trichuris trichiuria 127.3
    - virus NEC (*see also* Enteritis, viral) 008.69
  - dysenteric 009.2
    - due to specified organism NEC 008.8
  - dyspeptic 787.91
  - endemic 009.3
    - due to specified organism NEC 008.8
  - epidemic 009.2
    - due to specified organism NEC 008.8
  - fermentative 787.91
  - flagellate 007.9
  - Flexner's (ulcerative) 004.1
  - functional 564.5
    - following gastrointestinal surgery 564.4
    - psychogenic 306.4
  - giardial 007.1
  - Giardia lamblia 007.1
  - hill 579.1
  - hyperperistalsis (nervous) 306.4
  - infectious 009.2
    - due to specified organism NEC 008.8
    - presumed 009.3
  - inflammatory 787.91
    - due to specified organism NEC 008.8
  - malarial (*see also* Malaria) 084.6
  - mite 133.8
  - mycotic 117.9
  - nervous 306.4
  - neurogenic 564.5
  - parenteral NEC 009.2
  - postgastrectomy 564.4
  - postvagotomy 564.4
  - prostaglandin induced 579.8
  - protozoal NEC 007.9
  - psychogenic 306.4
  - septic 009.2
    - due to specified organism NEC 008.8
  - specified organism NEC 008.8
    - bacterial 008.49
    - viral NEC 008.69
  - Staphylococcus 008.41
  - Streptococcus 008.49
    - anaerobic 008.46
  - toxic 558.2
  - travelers' 009.2
    - due to specified organism NEC 008.8
  - trichomonal 007.3
  - tropical 579.1
  - tuberculous 014.8❺
  - ulcerative (chronic) (*see also* Colitis, ulcerative) 556.9
  - viral (*see also* Enteritis, viral) 008.8
  - zymotic NEC 009.2
- **Diastasis**
  - cranial bones 733.99
    - congenital 756.0
  - joint (traumatic) – *see* Dislocation, by site
  - muscle 728.84
    - congenital 756.89
  - recti (abdomen) 728.84
    - complicating delivery 665.8❺
    - congenital 756.79
- **Diastema, teeth, tooth** 524.30
- **Diastematomyelia** 742.51
- **Diataxia, cerebral, infantile** 343.0
- **Diathesis**
  - allergic V15.09
  - bleeding (familial) 287.9

Diathesis – *continued*
  cystine (familial) 270.0
  gouty 274.9
  hemorrhagic (familial) 287.9
    newborn NEC 776.0
  oxalic 271.8
  scrofulous (*see also* Tuberculosis) 017.2❺
  spasmophilic (*see also* Tetany) 781.7
  ulcer 536.9
  uric acid 274.9
Diaz's disease or osteochondrosis 732.5
Dibothriocephaliasis 123.4
  larval 123.5
Dibothriocephalus (infection) (infestation) (latus) 123.4
  larval 123.5
Dicephalus 759.4
Dichotomy, teeth 520.2
Dichromat, dichromata (congenital) 368.59
Dichromatopsia (congenital) 368.59
Dichuchwa 104.0
Dicroceliasis 121.8
Didelphys, didelphic (*see also* Double uterus) 752.2
Didymitis (*see also* Epididymitis) 604.90
Died – *see also* Death
  without
    medical attention (cause unknown) 798.9
    sign of disease 798.2
Dientamoeba diarrhea 007.8
Dietary
  inadequacy or deficiency 269.9
  surveillance and counseling V65.3
Dietl's crisis 593.4
Dieulafoy's lesion (hemorrhagic)
  of
    duodenum 537.84
    esophagus 530.82
    intestine 569.86
    stomach 537.84
Difficult
  birth, affecting fetus or newborn 763.9
  delivery NEC 669.9❺
Difficulty
  feeding 783.3
    adult 783.3
    breast 676.8❺
    child 783.3
    elderly 783.3
    infant 783.3
    newborn 779.3
    nonorganic (infant) NEC 307.59
  mechanical, gastroduodenal stoma 537.89
  reading 315.00
  specific, spelling 315.09
  swallowing (*see also* Dysphagia) 787.20 ▲
  walking 719.7❺
Diffuse – *see* condition
Diffused ganglion 727.42
Di George's syndrome (thymic hypoplasia) 279.11
Digestive – *see* condition
Di Guglielmo's disease or syndrome (M9841/3) 207.0❺
Diktyoma (M9051/3) – *see* Neoplasm, by site, malignant
Dilaceration, tooth 520.4
Dilatation
  anus 564.89
    venule – *see* Hemorrhoids
  aorta (focal) (general) (*see also* Aneurysm, aorta) 441.9
    congenital 747.29
    infectional 093.0
    ruptured 441.5
    syphilitic 093.0
  appendix (cystic) 543.9
  artery 447.8
  bile duct (common) (cystic) (congenital) 751.69
    acquired 576.8
  bladder (sphincter) 596.8
    congenital 753.8
    in pregnancy or childbirth 654.4❺
      causing obstructed labor 660.2❺
        affecting fetus or newborn 763.1
  blood vessel 459.89
  bronchus, bronchi 494.0
    with acute exacerbation 494.1
  calyx (due to obstruction) 593.89

Dilatation – *continued*
  capillaries 448.9
  cardiac (acute) (chronic) (*see also* Hypertrophy, cardiac) 429.3
    congenital 746.89
      valve NEC 746.89
        pulmonary 746.09
    hypertensive (*see also* Hypertension, heart) 402.90
  cavum septi pellucidi 742.4
  cecum 564.89
    psychogenic 306.4
  cervix (uteri) – *see also* Incompetency, cervix
    incomplete, poor, slow
      affecting fetus or newborn 763.7
      complicating delivery 661.0❺
        affecting fetus or newborn 763.7
  colon 564.7
    congenital 751.3
    due to mechanical obstruction 560.89
    psychogenic 306.4
  common bile duct (congenital) 751.69
    acquired 576.8
      with calculus, choledocholithiasis, or stones – *see* Choledocholithiasis
  cystic duct 751.69
    acquired (any bile duct) 575.8
  duct, mammary 610.4
  duodenum 564.89
  esophagus 530.89
    congenital 750.4
    due to
      achalasia 530.0
      cardiospasm 530.0
  Eustachian tube, congenital 744.24
  fontanel 756.0
  gallbladder 575.8
    congenital 751.69
  gastric 536.8
    acute 536.1
    psychogenic 306.4
  heart (acute) (chronic) (*see also* Hypertrophy, cardiac) 429.3
    congenital 746.89
    hypertensive (*see also* Hypertension, heart) 402.90
    valve – *see also* Endocarditis
      congenital 746.89
  ileum 564.89
    psychogenic 306.4
  inguinal rings – *see* Hernia, inguinal
  jejunum 564.89
    psychogenic 306.4
  kidney (calyx) (collecting structures) (cystic) (parenchyma) (pelvis) 593.89
  lacrimal passages 375.69
  lymphatic vessel 457.1
  mammary duct 610.4
  Meckel's diverticulum (congenital) 751.0
  meningeal vessels, congenital 742.8
  myocardium (acute) (chronic) (*see also* Hypertrophy, cardiac) 429.3
  organ or site, congenital NEC – *see* Distortion
  pancreatic duct 577.8
  pelvis, kidney 593.89
  pericardium – *see* Pericarditis
  pharynx 478.29
  prostate 602.8
  pulmonary
    artery (idiopathic) 417.8
      congenital 747.3
    valve, congenital 746.09
  pupil 379.43
  rectum 564.89
  renal 593.89
  saccule vestibularis, congenital 744.05
  salivary gland (duct) 527.8
  sphincter ani 564.89
  stomach 536.8
    acute 536.1
    psychogenic 306.4
  submaxillary duct 527.8
  trachea, congenital 748.3
  ureter (idiopathic) 593.89
    congenital 753.20
    due to obstruction 593.5
  urethra (acquired) 599.84
  vasomotor 443.9
  vein 459.89
  ventricular, ventricle (acute) (chronic) (*see also* Hypertrophy, cardiac) 429.3
    cerebral, congenital 742.4

Dilatation – *continued*
  ventricular, ventricle – *continued*
    hypertensive (*see also* Hypertension, heart) 402.90
  venule 459.89
    anus – *see* Hemorrhoids
  vesical orifice 596.8
Dilated, dilation – *see* Dilatation
Diminished
  hearing (acuity) (*see also* Deafness) 389.9
  pulse pressure 785.9
  vision NEC 369.9
  vital capacity 794.2
Diminuta taenia 123.6
Diminution, sense or sensation (cold) (heat) (tactile) (vibratory) (*see also* Disturbance, sensation) 782.0
Dimitri-Sturge-Weber disease (encephalocutaneous angiomatosis) 759.6
Dimple
  parasacral 685.1
    with abscess 685.0
  pilonidal 685.1
    with abscess 685.0
  postanal 685.1
    with abscess 685.0
Dioctophyma renale (infection) (infestation) 128.8
Dipetalonemiasis 125.4
Diphallus 752.69
Diphtheria, diphtheritic (gangrenous) (hemorrhagic) 032.9
  carrier (suspected) of V02.4
  cutaneous 032.85
  cystitis 032.84
  faucial 032.0
  infection of wound 032.85
  inoculation (anti) (not sick) V03.5
  laryngeal 032.3
  myocarditis 032.82
  nasal anterior 032.2
  nasopharyngeal 032.1
  neurological complication 032.89
  peritonitis 032.83
  specified site NEC 032.89
Diphyllobothriasis (intestine) 123.4
  larval 123.5
Diplacusis 388.41
Diplegia (upper limbs) 344.2
  brain or cerebral 437.8
  congenital 343.0
  facial 351.0
    congenital 352.6
  infantile or congenital (cerebral) (spastic) (spinal) 343.0
  lower limbs 344.1
  syphilitic, congenital 090.49
Diplococcus, diplococcal – *see* condition
Diplomyelia 742.59
Diplopia 368.2
  refractive 368.15
Dipsomania (*see also* Alcoholism) 303.9❺
  with psychosis (*see also* Psychosis, alcoholic) 291.9
Dipylidiasis 123.8
  intestine 123.8
Direction, teeth, abnormal 524.30
Dirt-eating child 307.52
Disability
  heart – *see* Disease, heart
  learning NEC 315.2
  special spelling 315.09
Disarticulation (*see also* Derangement, joint) 718.9❺
  meaning
    amputation
      status – *see* Absence, by site
      traumatic – *see* Amputation, traumatic
    dislocation, traumatic or congenital – *see* Dislocation
Disaster, cerebrovascular (*see also* Disease, cerebrovascular, acute) 436
Discharge
  anal NEC 787.99
  breast (female) (male) 611.79
  conjunctiva 372.89
  continued locomotor idiopathic (*see also* Epilepsy) 345.5❺

❹ Fourth-Digit Required ❺ Fifth-Digit Required *[code]* Manifestation Code ▶◀ Revised Text ● New Line ▲ Revised Code

Diathesis – Discharge

Discharge – *continued*
- diencephalic autonomic idiopathic (*see also* Epilepsy) 345.5❺
- ear 388.60
  - blood 388.69
  - cerebrospinal fluid 388.61
- excessive urine 788.42
- eye 379.93
- nasal 478.19
- nipple 611.79
- patterned motor idiopathic (*see also* Epilepsy) 345.5❺
- penile 788.7
- postnasal – *see* Sinusitis
- sinus, from mediastinum 510.0
- umbilicus 789.9
- urethral 788.7
  - bloody 599.84
- vaginal 623.5

Discitis 722.90
- cervical, cervicothoracic 722.91
- lumbar, lumbosacral 722.93
- thoracic, thoracolumbar 722.92

Discogenic syndrome – *see* Displacement, intervertebral disc

Discoid
- kidney 753.3
- meniscus, congenital 717.5
- semilunar cartilage 717.5

Discoloration
- mouth 528.9
- nails 703.8
- teeth 521.7
  - due to
    - drugs 521.7
    - metals (copper) (silver) 521.7
    - pulpal bleeding 521.7
  - during formation 520.8
  - extrinsic 523.6
  - intrinsic posteruptive 521.7

Discomfort
- chest 786.59
- visual 368.13

Discomycosis – *see* Actinomycosis

Discontinuity, ossicles, ossicular chain 385.23

Discrepancy
- centric occlusion
  - maximum intercuspation 524.55
  - of teeth 524.55
- leg length (acquired) 736.81
  - congenital 755.30
- uterine size-date 649.6❺

Discrimination
- political V62.4
- racial V62.4
- religious V62.4
- sex V62.4

Disease, diseased – *see also* Syndrome
- Abrami's (acquired hemolytic jaundice) 283.9
- absorbent system 459.89
- accumulation – *see* Thesaurismosis
- acid-peptic 536.8
- Acosta's 993.2
- Adams-Stokes (-Morgagni) (syncope with heart block) 426.9
- Addison's (bronze) (primary adrenal insufficiency) 255.41 ▲
  - anemia (pernicious) 281.0
  - tuberculous (*see also* Tuberculosis) 017.6❺
- Addison-Gull – *see* Xanthoma
- adenoids (and tonsils) (chronic) 474.9
- adrenal (gland) (capsule) (cortex) 255.9
  - hyperfunction 255.3
  - hypofunction 255.41 ▲
  - specified type NEC 255.8
- ainhum (dactylolysis spontanea) 136.0
- akamushi (scrub typhus) 081.2
- Akureyri (epidemic neuromyasthenia) 049.8
- Albarrán's (colibacilluria) 791.9
- Albers-Schönberg's (marble bones) 756.52
- Albert's 726.71
- Albright (-Martin) (-Bantam) 275.49
- Alibert's (mycosis fungoides) (M9700/3) 202.1❺
- Alibert-Bazin (M9700/3) 202.1❺
- alimentary canal 569.9
- alligator skin (ichthyosis congenita) 757.1
  - acquired 701.1
- Almeida's (Brazilian blastomycosis) 116.1
- Alpers' 330.8

Disease, diseased – *continued*
- alpine 993.2
- altitude 993.2
- alveoli, teeth 525.9
- Alzheimer's – *see* Alzheimer's
- amyloid (any site) 277.30
- anarthritic rheumatoid 446.5
- Anders' (adiposis tuberosa simplex) 272.8
- Andersen's (glycogenosis IV) 271.0
- Anderson's (angiokeratoma corporis diffusum) 272.7
- Andes 993.2
- Andrews' (bacterid) 686.8
- angiopastic, angiospasmodic 443.9
  - cerebral 435.9
    - with transient neurologic deficit 435.9
  - vein 459.89
- anterior
  - chamber 364.9
  - horn cell 335.9
    - specified type NEC 335.8
- antral (chronic) 473.0
  - acute 461.0
- anus NEC 569.49
- aorta (nonsyphilitic) 447.9
  - syphilitic NEC 093.89
- aortic (heart) (valve) (*see also* Endocarditis, aortic) 424.1
- Apollo 077.4
- aponeurosis 726.90
- appendix 543.9
- aqueous (chamber) 364.9
- arc-welders' lung 503
- Armenian 277.31
- Arnold-Chiari (*see also* Spina bifida) 741.0❺
- arterial 447.9
  - occlusive (*see also* Occlusion, by site) 444.22
    - with embolus or thrombus – *see* Occlusion, by site
    - due to stricture or stenosis 447.1
  - specified type NEC 447.8
- arteriocardiorenal (*see also* Hypertension, cardiorenal) 404.90
- arteriolar (generalized) (obliterative) 447.90
  - specified type NEC 447.8
- arteriorenal – *see* Hypertension, kidney
- arteriosclerotic – *see also* Arteriosclerosis
  - cardiovascular 429.2
  - coronary – *see* Arteriosclerosis, coronary
  - heart – *see* Arteriosclerosis, coronary
  - vascular – *see* Arteriosclerosis
- artery 447.9
  - cerebral 437.9
  - coronary – *see* Arteriosclerosis, coronary
  - specified type NEC 447.8
- arthropod-borne NEC 088.9
  - specified type NEC 088.89
- Asboe-Hansen's (incontinentia pigmenti) 757.33
- atticoantral, chronic (with posterior or superior marginal perforation of ear drum) 382.2
- auditory canal, ear 380.9
- Aujeszky's 078.89
- auricle, ear NEC 380.30
- Australian X 062.4
- autoimmune NEC 279.4
  - hemolytic (cold type) (warm type) 283.0
  - parathyroid 252.1
  - thyroid 245.2
- aviators' (*see also* Effect, adverse, high altitude) 993.2
- ax(e)-grinders' 502
- Ayala's 756.89
- Ayerza's (pulmonary artery sclerosis with pulmonary hypertension) 416.0
- Azorean (of the nervous system) 334.8
- Babington's (familial hemorrhagic telangiectasia) 448.0
- back bone NEC 733.90
- bacterial NEC 040.89
  - zoonotic NEC 027.9
    - specified type NEC 027.8
- Baehr-Schiffrin (thrombotic thrombocytopenic purpura) 446.6
- Baelz's (cheilitis glandularis apostematosa) 528.5
- Baerensprung's (eczema marginatum) 110.3
- Balfour's (chloroma) 205.3❺
- balloon (*see also* Effect, adverse, high altitude) 993.2
- Baló's 341.1
- Bamberger (-Marie) (hypertrophic pulmonary osteoarthropathy) 731.2

Disease, diseased – *continued*
- Bang's (Brucella abortus) 023.1
- Bannister's 995.1
- Banti's (with cirrhosis) (with portal hypertension) – *see* Cirrhosis, liver
- Barcoo (*see also* Ulcer, skin) 707.9
- barium lung 503
- Barlow (-Möller) (infantile scurvy) 267
- barometer makers' 985.0
- Barraquer (-Simons) (progressive lipodystrophy) 272.6
- basal ganglia 333.90
  - degenerative NEC 333.0
  - specified NEC 333.89
- Basedow's (exophthalmic goiter) 242.0❺
- basement membrane NEC 583.89
  - with
    - pulmonary hemorrhage (Goodpasture's syndrome) 446.21 *[583.81]*
- Bateman's 078.0
  - purpura (senile) 287.2
- Batten's 330.1 *[362.71]*
- Batten-Mayou (retina) 330.1 *[362.71]*
- Batten-Steinert 359.21 ▲
- Battey 031.0
- Baumgarten-Cruveilhier (cirrhosis of liver) 571.5
- bauxite-workers' 503
- Bayle's (dementia paralytica) 094.1
- Bazin's (primary) (*see also* Tuberculosis) 017.1❺
- Beard's (neurasthenia) 300.5
- Beau's (*see also* Degeneration, myocardial) 429.1
- Bechterew's (ankylosing spondylitis) 720.0
- Becker's
  - idiopathic mural endomyocardial disease 425.2 ●
  - myotonia congenita, recessive form 359.22 ●
- Begbie's (exophthalmic goiter) 242.0❺
- Behr's 362.50
- Beigel's (white piedra) 111.2
- Bekhterev's (ankylosing spondylitis) 720.0
- Bell's (*see also* Psychosis, affective) 296.0❺
- Bennett's (leukemia) 208.9❺
- Benson's 379.22
- Bergeron's (hysteroepilepsy) 300.11
- Berlin's 921.3
- Bernard-Soulier (thrombopathy) 287.1
- Bernhardt (-Roth) 355.1
- beryllium 503
- Besnier-Boeck (-Schaumann) (sarcoidosis) 135
- Best's 362.76
- Beurmann's (sporotrichosis) 117.1
- Bielschowsky (-Jansky) 330.1
- Biermer's (pernicious anemia) 281.0
- Biett's (discoid lupus erythematosus) 695.4
- bile duct (*see also* Disease, biliary) 576.9
- biliary (duct) (tract) 576.9
  - with calculus, choledocholithiasis, or stones – *see* Choledocholithiasis
- Billroth's (meningocele) (*see also* Spina bifida) 741.9❺
- Binswanger's 290.12
- Bird's (oxaluria) 271.8
- bird fanciers' 495.2
- black lung 500
- bladder 596.9
  - specified NEC 596.8
- bleeder's 286.0
- Bloch-Sulzberger (incontinentia pigmenti) 757.33
- Blocq's (astasia-abasia) 307.9
- blood (-forming organs) 289.9
  - specified NEC 289.89
  - vessel 459.9
- Bloodgood's 610.1
- Blount's (tibia vara) 732.4
- blue 746.9
- Bodechtel-Guttmann (subacute sclerosing panencephalitis) 046.2
- Boeck's (sarcoidosis) 135
- bone 733.90
  - fibrocystic NEC 733.29
    - jaw 526.2
  - marrow 289.9
  - Paget's (osteitis deformans) 731.0
  - specified type NEC 733.99
  - von Recklinghausen's (osteitis fibrosa cystica) 252.01
- Bonfils' – *see* Disease, Hodgkin's
- Borna 062.9
- Bornholm (epidemic pleurodynia) 074.1
- Bostock's (*see also* Fever, hay) 477.9

Discharge – Disease, diseased

Disease, diseased – *continued*
- Bouchard's (myopathic dilatation of the stomach) 536.1
- Bouillaud's (rheumatic heart disease) 391.9
- Bourneville (-Brissaud) (tuberous sclerosis) 759.5
- Bouveret (-Hoffmann) (paroxysmal tachycardia) 427.2
- bowel 569.9
  - functional 564.9
    - psychogenic 306.4
- Bowen's (M8081/2) – *see* Neoplasm, skin, in situ
- Bozzolo's (multiple myeloma) (M9730/3) 203.0❺
- Bradley's (epidemic vomiting) 078.82
- Brailsford's 732.3
  - radius, head 732.3
  - tarsal, scaphoid 732.5
- Brailsford-Morquio (mucopolysaccharidosis IV) 277.5
- brain 348.9
  - Alzheimer's 331.0
    - with dementia – *see* Alzheimer's, dementia
  - arterial, artery 437.9
  - arteriosclerotic 437.0
  - congenital 742.9
  - degenerative – *see* Degeneration, brain
  - inflammatory – *see also* Encephalitis
    - late effect – *see* category 326
  - organic 348.9
    - arteriosclerotic 437.0
  - parasitic NEC 123.9
  - Pick's 331.11
    - with dementia
      - with behavioral disturbance 331.11 *[294.11]*
      - without behavioral disturbance 331.11 *[294.10]*
  - senile 331.2
- braziers' 985.8
- breast 611.9
  - cystic (chronic) 610.1
  - fibrocystic 610.1
  - inflammatory 611.0
  - Paget's (M8540/3) 174.0
  - puerperal, postpartum NEC 676.3❺
  - specified NEC 611.8
- Breda's (*see also* Yaws) 102.9
- Breisky's (kraurosis vulvae) 624.09 ▲
- Bretonneau's (diphtheritic malignant angina) 032.0
- Bright's (*see also* Nephritis) 583.9
  - arteriosclerotic (*see also* Hypertension, kidney) 403.90
- Brill's (recrudescent typhus) 081.1
  - flea-borne 081.0
  - louse-borne 081.1
- Brill-Symmers (follicular lymphoma) (M9690/3) 202.0❺
- Brill-Zinsser (recrudescent typhus) 081.1
- Brinton's (leather bottle stomach) (M8142/3) 151.9
- Brion-Kayser (*see also* Fever, paratyphoid) 002.9
- broad
  - beta 272.2
  - ligament, noninflammatory 620.9
    - specified NEC 620.8
- Brocq's 691.8
  - meaning
    - atopic (diffuse) neurodermatitis 691.8
    - dermatitis herpetiformis 694.0
    - lichen simplex chronicus 698.3
    - parapsoriasis 696.2
    - prurigo 698.2
- Brocq-Duhring (dermatitis herpetiformis) 694.0
- Brodie's (joint) (*see also* Osteomyelitis) 730.1❺
- bronchi 519.19
- bronchopulmonary 519.19
- bronze (Addison's) 255.41 ▲
  - tuberculous (*see also* Tuberculosis) 017.6❺
- Brown-Séquard 344.89
- Bruck's 733.99
- Bruck-de Lange (Amsterdam dwarf, mental retardation, and brachycephaly) 759.89
- Bruhl's (splenic anemia with fever) 285.8
- Bruton's (X-linked agammaglobulinemia) 279.04
- buccal cavity 528.9
- Buchanan's (juvenile osteochondrosis, iliac crest) 732.1
- Buchman's (osteochondrosis juvenile) 732.1
- Budgerigar-Fanciers' 495.2
- Budinger-Ludloff-Läwen 717.89
- Büerger's (thromboangiitis obliterans) 443.1

Disease, diseased – *continued*
- Bürger-Grütz (essential familial hyperlipemia) 272.3
- Burns' (lower ulna) 732.3
- bursa 727.9
- Bury's (erythema elevatum diutinum) 695.89
- Buschke's 710.1
- Busquet's (*see also* Osteomyelitis) 730.1❺
- Busse-Buschke (cryptococcosis) 117.5
- C_2 (*see also* Alcoholism) 303.9❺
- Caffey's (infantile cortical hyperostosis) 756.59
- caisson 993.3
- calculous 592.9
- California 114.0
- Calvé (-Perthes) (osteochondrosis, femoral capital) 732.1
- Camurati-Engelmann (diaphyseal sclerosis) 756.59
- Canavan's 330.0
- capillaries 448.9
- Carapata 087.1
- cardiac – *see* Disease, heart
- cardiopulmonary, chronic 416.9
- cardiorenal (arteriosclerotic) (hepatic) (hypertensive) (vascular) (*see also* Hypertension, cardiorenal) 404.90
- cardiovascular (arteriosclerotic) 429.2
  - congenital 746.9
  - hypertensive (*see also* Hypertension, heart) 402.90
    - benign 402.10
    - malignant 402.00
  - renal (*see also* Hypertension, cardiorenal) 404.90
  - syphilitic (asymptomatic) 093.9
- carotid gland 259.8
- Carrión's (Bartonellosis) 088.0
- cartilage NEC 733.90
  - specified NEC 733.99
- Castellani's 104.8
- cat-scratch 078.3
- Cavare's (familial periodic paralysis) 359.3
- Cazenave's (pemphigus) 694.4
- cecum 569.9
- celiac (adult) 579.0
  - infantile 579.0
- cellular tissue NEC 709.9
- central core 359.0
- cerebellar, cerebellum – *see* Disease, brain
- cerebral (*see also* Disease, brain) 348.9
  - arterial, artery 437.9
  - degenerative – *see* Degeneration, brain
- cerebrospinal 349.9
- cerebrovascular NEC 437.9
  - acute 436
    - embolic – *see* Embolism, brain
    - late effect – *see* Late effect(s) (of) cerebrovascular disease
    - puerperal, postpartum, childbirth 674.0❺
    - thrombotic – *see* Thrombosis, brain
  - arteriosclerotic 437.0
  - embolic – *see* Embolism, brain
  - ischemic, generalized NEC 437.1
  - late effect – *see* Late effect(s) (of) cerebrovascular disease
  - occlusive 437.1
  - puerperal, postpartum, childbirth 674.0❺
  - specified type NEC 437.8
  - thrombotic – *see* Thrombosis, brain
- ceroid storage 272.7
- cervix (uteri)
  - inflammatory 616.0 ▲
  - noninflammatory 622.9
    - specified NEC 622.8
- Chabert's 022.9
- Chagas' (*see also* Trypanosomiasis, American) 086.2
- Chandler's (osteochondritis dissecans, hip) 732.7
- Charcôt's (joint) 094.0 *[713.5]*
  - spinal cord 094.0
- Charcôt-Marie-Tooth 356.1
- Charlouis' (*see also* Yaws) 102.9
- Cheadle (-Möller) (-Barlow) (infantile scurvy) 267
- Chédiak-Steinbrinck (-Higashi) (congenital gigantism of peroxidase granules) 288.2
- cheek, inner 528.9
- chest 519.9
- Chiari's (hepatic vein thrombosis) 453.0
- Chicago (North American blastomycosis) 116.0
- chignon (white piedra) 111.2
- chigoe, chigo (jigger) 134.1
- childhood granulomatous 288.1

Disease, diseased – *continued*
- Chinese liver fluke 121.1
- chlamydial NEC 078.88
- cholecystic (*see also* Disease, gallbladder) 575.9
- choroid 363.9
  - degenerative (*see also* Degeneration, choroid) 363.40
  - hereditary (*see also* Dystrophy, choroid) 363.50
  - specified type NEC 363.8
- Christian's (chronic histiocytosis X) 277.89
- Christian-Weber (nodular nonsuppurative panniculitis) 729.30
- Christmas 286.1
- ciliary body 364.9
  - specified NEC 364.89 ●
- circulatory (system) NEC 459.9
  - chronic, maternal, affecting fetus or newborn 760.3
  - specified NEC 459.89
  - syphilitic 093.9
    - congenital 090.5
- Civatte's (poikiloderma) 709.09
- climacteric 627.2
  - male 608.89
- coagulation factor deficiency (congenital) (*see also* Defect, coagulation) 286.9
- Coats' 362.12
- coccidioidal pulmonary 114.5
  - acute 114.0
  - chronic 114.4
  - primary 114.0
  - residual 114.4
- Cockayne's (microcephaly and dwarfism) 759.89
- Cogan's 370.52
- cold
  - agglutinin 283.0
    - or hemoglobinuria 283.0
      - paroxysmal (cold) (nocturnal) 283.2
  - hemagglutinin (chronic) 283.0
- collagen NEC 710.9
  - nonvascular 710.9
  - specified NEC 710.8
  - vascular (allergic) (*see also* Angiitis, hypersensitivity) 446.20
- colon 569.9
  - functional 564.9
    - congenital 751.3
  - ischemic 557.0
- combined system (of spinal cord) 266.2 *[336.2]*
  - with anemia (pernicious) 281.0 *[336.2]*
- compressed air 993.3
- Concato's (pericardial polyserositis) 423.2
  - peritoneal 568.82
  - pleural – *see* Pleurisy
- congenital NEC 799.89
- conjunctiva 372.9
  - chlamydial 077.98
    - specified NEC 077.8
  - specified type NEC 372.89
  - viral 077.99
    - specified NEC 077.8
- connective tissue, diffuse (*see also* Disease, collagen) 710.9
- Conor and Bruch's (boutonneuse fever) 082.1
- Conradi (-Hünermann) 756.59
- Cooley's (erythroblastic anemia) 282.49
- Cooper's 610.1
- Corbus' 607.1
- cork-handlers' 495.3
- cornea (*see also* Keratopathy) 371.9
- coronary (*see also* Ischemia, heart) 414.9
  - congenital 746.85
  - ostial, syphilitic 093.20
    - aortic 093.22
    - mitral 093.21
    - pulmonary 093.24
    - tricuspid 093.23
- Corrigan's – *see* Insufficiency, aortic
- Cotugno's 724.3
- Coxsackie (virus) NEC 074.8
- cranial nerve NEC 352.9
- Creutzfeldt-Jakob (new variant) 046.1
  - with dementia
    - with behavioral disturbance 046.1 *[294.11]*
    - without behavioral disturbance 046.1 *[294.10]*
- Crigler-Najjar (congenital hyperbilirubinemia) 277.4
- Crocq's (acrocyanosis) 443.89
- Crohn's (intestine) (*see also* Enteritis, regional) 555.9

Disease, diseased – *continued*
- Crouzon's (craniofacial dysostosis) 756.0
- Cruchet's (encephalitis lethargica) 049.8
- Cruveilhier's 335.21
- Cruz-Chagas (*see also* Trypanosomiasis, American) 086.2
- crystal deposition (*see also* Arthritis, due to, crystals) 712.9❺
- Csillag's (lichen sclerosus et atrophicus) 701.0
- Curschmann's 359.21 ▲
- Cushing's (pituitary basophilism) 255.0
- cystic
  - breast (chronic) 610.1
  - kidney, congenital (*see also* Cystic, disease, kidney) 753.10
  - liver, congenital 751.62
  - lung 518.89
    - congenital 748.4
  - pancreas 577.2
    - congenital 751.7
  - renal, congenital (*see also* Cystic, disease, kidney) 753.10
  - semilunar cartilage 717.5
- cysticercus 123.1
- cystine storage (with renal sclerosis) 270.0
- cytomegalic inclusion (generalized) 078.5
  - with
    - pneumonia 078.5 *[484.1]*
  - congenital 771.1
- Daae (-Finsen) (epidemic pleurodynia) 074.1
- dancing 297.8
- Danielssen's (anesthetic leprosy) 030.1
- Darier's (congenital) (keratosis follicularis) 757.39
  - erythema annulare centrifugum 695.0
  - vitamin A deficiency 264.8
- Darling's (histoplasmosis) (*see also* Histoplasmosis, American) 115.00
- Davies' 425.0
- de Beurmann-Gougerot (sporotrichosis) 117.1
- Débove's (splenomegaly) 789.2
- deer fly (*see also* Tularemia) 021.9
- deficiency 269.9
- degenerative – *see also* Degeneration
  - disc – *see* Degeneration, intervertebral disc
- degos' 447.8
- Déjérine (-Sottas) 356.0
- Déleage's 359.89
- demyelinating, demyelinizating (brain stem) (central nervous system) 341.9
  - multiple sclerosis 340
  - specified NEC 341.8
- de Quervain's (tendon sheath) 727.04
  - thyroid (subacute granulomatous thyroiditis) 245.1
- Dercum's (adiposis dolorosa) 272.8
- Deutschländer's – *see* Fracture, foot
- Devergie's (pityriasis rubra pilaris) 696.4
- Devic's 341.0
- diaphorase deficiency 289.7
- diaphragm 519.4
- diarrheal, infectious 009.2
- diatomaceous earth 502
- Diaz's (osteochondrosis astragalus) 732.5
- digestive system 569.9
- Di Guglielmo's (erythemic myelosis) (M9841/3) 207.0❺
- Dimitri-Sturge-Weber (encephalocutaneous angiomatosis) 759.6
- disc, degenerative – *see* Degeneration, intervertebral disc
- discogenic (*see also* Disease, intervertebral disc) 722.90
- diverticular – *see* Diverticula
- Down's (mongolism) 758.0
- Dubini's (electric chorea) 049.8
- Dubois' (thymus gland) 090.5
- Duchenne's 094.0
  - locomotor ataxia 094.0
  - muscular dystrophy 359.1
  - paralysis 335.22
  - pseudohypertrophy, muscles 359.1
- Duchenne-Griesinger 359.1
- ductless glands 259.9
- Duhring's (dermatitis herpetiformis) 694.0
- Dukes (-Filatov) 057.8
- duodenum NEC 537.9
  - specified NEC 537.89
- Duplay's 726.2
- Dupré's (meningism) 781.6
- Dupuytren's (muscle contracture) 728.6
- Durand-Nicolas-Favre (climatic bubo) 099.1

Disease, diseased – *continued*
- Duroziez's (congenital mitral stenosis) 746.5
- Dutton's (trypanosomiasis) 086.9
- Eales' 362.18
- ear (chronic) (inner) NEC 388.9
  - middle 385.9
    - adhesive (*see also* Adhesions, middle ear) 385.10
    - specified NEC 385.89
- Eberth's (typhoid fever) 002.0
- Ebstein's
  - heart 746.2
  - meaning diabetes 250.4❺ *[581.81]*
- Echinococcus (*see also* Echinococcus) 122.9
- ECHO virus NEC 078.89
- Economo's (encephalitis lethargica) 049.8
- Eddowes' (brittle bones and blue sclera) 756.51
- Edsall's 992.2
- Eichstedt's (pityriasis versicolor) 111.0
- Ellis-van Creveld (chondroectodermal dysplasia) 756.55
- endocardium – *see* Endocarditis
- endocrine glands or system NEC 259.9
  - specified NEC 259.8
- endomyocardial, idiopathic mural 425.2
- Engel-von Recklinghausen (osteitis fibrosa cystica) 252.01
- Engelmann's (diaphyseal sclerosis) 756.59
- English (rickets) 268.0
- Engman's (infectious eczematoid dermatitis) 690.8
- enteroviral, enterovirus NEC 078.89
  - central nervous system NEC 048
- epidemic NEC 136.9
- epididymis 608.9
- epigastric, functional 536.9
  - psychogenic 306.4
- Erb (-Landouzy) 359.1
- Erb-Goldflam 358.00
- Erichsen's (railway spine) 300.16
- esophagus 530.9
  - functional 530.5
  - psychogenic 306.4
- Eulenburg's (congenital paramyotonia) 359.29 ▲
- Eustachian tube 381.9
- Evans' (thrombocytopenic purpura) 287.32
- external auditory canal 380.9
- extrapyramidal NEC 333.90
- eye 379.90
  - anterior chamber 364.9
  - inflammatory NEC 364.3
  - muscle 378.9
- eyeball 360.9
- eyelid 374.9
- eyeworm of Africa 125.2
- Fabry's (angiokeratoma corporis diffusum) 272.7
- facial nerve (seventh) 351.9
  - newborn 767.5
- Fahr-Volhard (malignant nephrosclerosis) 403.00
- fallopian tube, noninflammatory 620.9
  - specified NEC 620.8
- familial periodic 277.31
  - paralysis 359.3
- Fanconi's (congenital pancytopenia) 284.09
- Farber's (disseminated lipogranulomatosis) 272.8
- fascia 728.9
  - inflammatory 728.9
- Fauchard's (periodontitis) 523.40
- Favre-Durand-Nicolas (climatic bubo) 099.1
- Favre-Racouchot (elastoidosis cutanea nodularis) 701.8
- Fede's 529.0
- Feer's 985.0
- Felix's (juvenile osteochondrosis, hip) 732.1
- Fenwick's (gastric atrophy) 537.89
- Fernels' (aortic aneurysm) 441.9
- fibrocaseous, of lung (*see also* Tuberculosis, pulmonary) 011.9❺
- fibrocystic – *see also* Fibrocystic, disease
  - newborn 277.01
- Fiedler's (leptospiral jaundice) 100.0
- fifth 057.0
- Filatoff's (infectious mononucleosis) 075
- Filatov's (infectious mononucleosis) 075
- file-cutters' 984.9
  - specified type of lead – *see* Table of Drugs and Chemicals
- filterable virus NEC 078.89
- fish skin 757.1
  - acquired 701.1
- Flajani (-Basedow) (exophthalmic goiter) 242.0❺
- Flatau-Schilder 341.1

Disease, diseased – *continued*
- flax-dressers' 504
- Fleischner's 732.3
- flint 502
- fluke – *see* Infestation, fluke
- Følling's (phenylketonuria) 270.1
- foot and mouth 078.4
- foot process 581.3
- Forbes' (glycogenosis III) 271.0
- Fordyce's (ectopic sebaceous glands) (mouth) 750.26
- Fordyce-Fox (apocrine miliaria) 705.82
- Fothergill's
  - meaning scarlatina anginosa 034.1
  - neuralgia (*see also* Neuralgia, trigeminal) 350.1
- Fournier's 608.83
- fourth 057.8
- Fox (-Fordyce) (apocrine miliaria) 705.82
- Francis' (*see also* Tularemia) 021.9
- Franklin's (heavy chain) 273.2
- Frei's (climatic bubo) 099.1
- Freiberg's (flattening metatarsal) 732.5
- Friedländer's (endarteritis obliterans) – *see* Arteriosclerosis
- Friedreich's
  - combined systemic or ataxia 334.0
  - facial hemihypertrophy 756.0
  - myoclonia 333.2
- Fröhlich's (adiposogenital dystrophy) 253.8
- Frommel's 676.6❺
- frontal sinus (chronic) 473.1
  - acute 461.1
- Fuller's earth 502
- fungus, fungous NEC 117.9
- Gaisböck's (polycythemia hypertonica) 289.0
- gallbladder 575.9
  - congenital 751.60
- Gamna's (siderotic splenomegaly) 289.51
- Gamstorp's (adynamia episodica hereditaria) 359.3
- Gandy-Nanta (siderotic splenomegaly) 289.51
- Gannister (occupational) 502
- Garré's (*see also* Osteomyelitis) 730.1❺
- gastric (*see also* Disease, stomach) 537.9
- gastrointestinal (tract) 569.9
  - amyloid 277.39
  - functional 536.9
    - psychogenic 306.4
- Gaucher's (adult) (cerebroside lipidosis) (infantile) 272.7
- Gayet's (superior hemorrhagic polioencephalitis) 265.1
- Gee (-Herter) (-Heubner) (-Thaysen) (nontropical sprue) 579.0
- generalized neoplastic (M8000/6) 199.0
- genital organs NEC
  - female 629.9
    - specified NEC 629.89
  - male 608.9
- Gerhardt's (erythromelalgia) 443.82
- Gerlier's (epidemic vertigo) 078.81
- Gibert's (pityriasis rosea) 696.3
- Gibney's (perispondylitis) 720.9
- Gierke's (glycogenosis I) 271.0
- Gilbert's (familial nonhemolytic jaundice) 277.4
- Gilchrist's (North American blastomycosis) 116.0
- Gilford (-Hutchinson) (progeria) 259.8
- Gilles de la Tourette's (motor-verbal tic) 307.23
- Giovannini's 117.9
- gland (lymph) 289.9
- Glanzmann's (hereditary hemorrhagic thrombasthenia) 287.1
- glassblowers' 527.1
- Glénard's (enteroptosis) 569.89
- Glisson's (*see also* Rickets) 268.0
- glomerular
  - membranous, idiopathic 581.1
  - minimal change 581.3
- glycogen storage (Andersen's) (Cori types 1-7) (Forbes') (McArdle-Schmid-Pearson) (Pompe's) (types I-VII) 271.0
  - cardiac 271.0 *[425.7]*
  - generalized 271.0
  - glucose-6-phosphatase deficiency 271.0
  - heart 271.0 *[425.7]*
  - hepatorenal 271.0
  - liver and kidneys 271.0
  - myocardium 271.0 *[425.7]*
  - von Gierke's (glycogenosis I) 271.0
- Goldflam-Erb 358.00
- Goldscheider's (epidermolysis bullosa) 757.39

Disease, diseased – *continued*
- Goldstein's (familial hemorrhagic telangiectasia) 448.0
- gonococcal NEC 098.0
- Goodall's (epidemic vomiting) 078.82
- Gordon's (exudative enteropathy) 579.8
- Gougerot's (trisymptomatic) 709.1
- Gougerot-Carteaud (confluent reticulate papillomatosis) 701.8
- Gougerot-Hailey-Hailey (benign familial chronic pemphigus) 757.39
- graft-versus-host (bone marrow) 996.85
  - due to organ transplant NEC – *see* Complications, transplant, organ
- grain-handlers' 495.8
- Grancher's (splenopneumonia) – *see* Pneumonia
- granulomatous (childhood) (chronic) 288.1
- graphite lung 503
- Graves' (exophthalmic goiter) 242.0❺
- Greenfield's 330.0
- green monkey 078.89
- Griesinger's (*see also* Ancylostomiasis) 126.9
- grinders' 502
- Grisel's 723.5
- Gruby's (tinea tonsurans) 110.0
- Guertin's (electric chorea) 049.8
- Guillain-Barré 357.0
- Guinon's (motor-verbal tic) 307.23
- Gull's (thyroid atrophy with myxedema) 244.8
- Gull and Sutton's – *see* Hypertension, kidney
- gum NEC 523.9
- Günther's (congenital erythropoietic porphyria) 277.1
- gynecological 629.9
  - specified NEC 629.89
- H 270.0
- Haas' 732.3
- Habermann's (acute parapsoriasis varioliformis) 696.2
- Haff 985.1
- Hageman (congenital factor XII deficiency) (*see also* Defect, congenital) 286.3
- Haglund's (osteochondrosis os tibiale externum) 732.5
- Hagner's (hypertrophic pulmonary osteoarthropathy) 731.2
- Hailey-Hailey (benign familial chronic pemphigus) 757.39
- hair (follicles) NEC 704.9
  - specified type NEC 704.8
- Hallervorden-Spatz 333.0
- Hallopeau's (lichen sclerosus et atrophicus) 701.0
- Hamman's (spontaneous mediastinal emphysema) 518.1
- hand, foot, and mouth 074.3
- Hand-Schüller-Christian (chronic histiocytosis X) 277.89
- Hanot's – *see* Cirrhosis, biliary
- Hansen's (leprosy) 030.9
  - benign form 030.1
  - malignant form 030.0
- Harada's 363.22
- Harley's (intermittent hemoglobinuria) 283.2
- Hart's (pellagra-cerebellar ataxia-renal aminoaciduria) 270.0
- Hartnup (pellagra-cerebellar ataxia-renal aminoaciduria) 270.0
- Hashimoto's (struma lymphomatosa) 245.2
- Hb – *see* Disease, hemoglobin
- heart (organic) 429.9
  - with
    - acute pulmonary edema (*see also* Failure, ventricular, left) 428.1
      - hypertensive 402.91
        - with renal failure 404.92
        - benign 402.11
          - with renal failure 404.12
        - malignant 402.01
          - with renal failure 404.02
    - kidney disease – see Hypertension, cardiorenal
    - rheumatic fever (conditions classifiable to 390)
      - active 391.9
        - with chorea 392.0
      - inactive or quiescent (with chorea) 398.90
  - amyloid 277.39 *[425.7]*
  - aortic (valve) (*see also* Endocarditis, aortic) 424.1
  - arteriosclerotic or sclerotic (minimal) (senile) – *see* Arteriosclerosis, coronary

Disease, diseased – *continued*
- heart – *continued*
  - artery, arterial – *see* Arteriosclerosis, coronary
  - atherosclerotic – *see* Arteriosclerosis, coronary
  - beer drinkers' 425.5
  - beriberi 265.0 *[425.7]*
  - black 416.0
  - congenital NEC 746.9
    - cyanotic 746.9
    - maternal, affecting fetus or newborn 760.3
    - specified type NEC 746.89
  - congestive (*see also* Failure, heart) 428.0
  - coronary 414.9
  - cryptogenic 429.9
  - due to
    - amyloidosis 277.39 *[425.7]*
    - beriberi 265.0 *[425.7]*
    - cardiac glycogenosis 271.0 *[425.7]*
    - Friedreich's ataxia 334.0 *[425.8]*
    - gout 274.82
    - mucopolysaccharidosis 277.5 *[425.7]*
    - myotonia atrophica 359.21 ▲ *[425.8]*
    - progressive muscular dystrophy 359.1 *[425.8]*
    - sarcoidosis 135 *[425.8]*
  - fetal 746.9
    - inflammatory 746.89
  - fibroid (*see also* Myocarditis) 429.0
  - functional 427.9
    - postoperative 997.1
    - psychogenic 306.2
  - glycogen storage 271.0 *[425.7]*
  - gonococcal NEC 098.85
  - gouty 274.82
  - hypertensive (*see also* Hypertension, heart) 402.90
    - benign 402.10
    - malignant 402.00
  - hyperthyroid (*see also* Hyperthyroidism) 242.9❺ *[425.7]*
  - incompletely diagnosed – *see* Disease, heart
  - ischemic (chronic) (*see also* Ischemia, heart) 414.9
    - acute (*see also* Infarct, myocardium) 410.9
      - without myocardial infarction 411.89
        - with coronary (artery) occlusion 411.81
    - asymptomatic 412
    - diagnosed on ECG or other special investigation but currently presenting no symptoms 412
  - kyphoscoliotic 416.1
  - mitral (*see also* Endocarditis, mitral) 394.9
  - muscular (*see also* Degeneration, myocardial) 429.1
  - postpartum 674.8❺
  - psychogenic (functional) 306.2
  - pulmonary (chronic) 416.9
    - acute 415.0
    - specified NEC 416.8
  - rheumatic (chronic) (inactive) (old) (quiescent) (with chorea) 398.90
    - active or acute 391.9
      - with chorea (active) (rheumatic) (Sydenham's) 392.0
      - specified type NEC 391.8
    - maternal, affecting fetus or newborn 760.3
  - rheumatoid – *see* Arthritis, rheumatoid
  - sclerotic – *see* Arteriosclerosis, coronary
  - senile (*see also* Myocarditis) 429.0
  - specified type NEC 429.89
  - syphilitic 093.89
    - aortic 093.1
      - aneurysm 093.0
    - asymptomatic 093.89
    - congenital 090.5
  - thyroid (gland) (*see also* Hyperthyroidism) 242.9❺ *[425.7]*
  - thyrotoxic (*see also* Thyrotoxicosis) 242.9❺ *[425.7]*
  - tuberculous (*see also* Tuberculosis) 017.9❺ *[425.8]*
  - valve, valvular (obstructive) (regurgitant) – *see also* Endocarditis
    - congenital NEC (*see also* Anomaly, heart, valve) 746.9
      - pulmonary 746.00
      - specified type NEC 746.89
  - vascular – *see* Disease, cardiovascular
- heavy-chain (gamma G) 273.2
- Heberden's 715.04
- Hebra's
  - dermatitis exfoliativa 695.89

Disease, diseased – *continued*
- Hebra's – *continued*
  - erythema multiforme exudativum 695.1
  - pityriasis
    - maculata et circinata 696.3
    - rubra 695.89
      - pilaris 696.4
  - prurigo 698.2
- Heerfordt's (uveoparotitis) 135
- Heidenhain's 290.10
  - with dementia 290.10
- Heilmeyer-Schöner (M9842/3) 207.1❺
- Heine-Medin (*see also* Poliomyelitis) 045.9❺
- Heller's (*see also* Psychosis, childhood) 299.1❺
- Heller-Döhle (syphilitic aortitis) 093.1
- hematopoietic organs 289.9
- hemoglobin (Hb) 282.7
  - with thalassemia 282.49
  - abnormal (mixed) NEC 282.7
    - with thalassemia 282.49
  - AS genotype 282.5
  - Bart's 282.49
  - C (Hb-C) 282.7
    - with other abnormal hemoglobin NEC 282.7
    - elliptocytosis 282.7
    - Hb-S (without crisis) 282.63
      - with
        - crisis 282.64
          - vaso-occlusive pain 282.64
    - sickle-cell (without crisis)282.63
      - with
        - crisis 282.64
          - vaso-occlusive pain 282.64
    - thalassemia 282.49
  - constant spring 282.7
  - D (Hb-D) 282.7
    - with other abnormal hemoglobin NEC 282.7
    - Hb-S (without crisis) 282.68
      - with crisis 282.69
    - sickle-cell (without crisis) 282.68
      - with crisis 282.69
    - thalassemia 282.49
  - E (Hb-E) 282.7
    - with other abnormal hemoglobin NEC 282.7
    - Hb-S (without crisis) 282.68
      - with crisis 282.69
    - sickle-cell (without crisis) 282.68
      - with crisis 282.69
    - thalassemia 282.49
  - elliptocytosis 282.7
  - F (Hb-F) 282.7
  - G (Hb-G) 282.7
  - H (Hb-H) 282.49
  - hereditary persistence, fetal (HPFH) ("Swiss variety") 282.7
  - high fetal gene 282.7
  - I thalassemia 282.49
  - M 289.7
  - S – *see also* Disease, sickle-cell, Hb-S
    - thalassemia (without crisis) 282.41
      - with
        - crisis 282.42
          - vaso-occlusive pain 282.42
  - spherocytosis 282.7
  - unstable, hemolytic 282.7
  - Zurich (Hb-Zurich) 282.7
- hemolytic (fetus) (newborn) 773.2
  - autoimmune (cold type) (warm type) 283.0
  - due to or with
    - incompatibility
      - ABO (blood group) 773.1
      - blood (group) (Duffy) (Kell) (Kidd) (Lewis) (M) (S) NEC 773.2
      - Rh (blood group) (factor) 773.0
    - Rh negative mother 773.0
  - unstable hemoglobin 282.7
- hemorrhagic 287.9
  - newborn 776.0
- Henoch (-Schönlein) (purpura nervosa) 287.0
- hepatic – *see* Disease, liver
- hepatolenticular 275.1
- heredodegenerative NEC
  - brain 331.89
  - spinal cord 336.8
- Hers' (glycogenosis VI) 271.0
- Herter (-Gee) (-Heubner) (nontropical sprue) 579.0
- Herxheimer's (diffuse idiopathic cutaneous atrophy) 701.8
- Heubner's 094.89
- Heubner-Herter (nontropical sprue) 579.0

Disease, diseased – Disease, diseased

Disease, diseased – *continued*
- high fetal gene or hemoglobin thalassemia 282.49
- Hildenbrand's (typhus) 081.9
- hip (joint) NEC 719.95
  - congenital 755.63
  - suppurative 711.05
  - tuberculous (*see also* Tuberculosis) 015.1❺ *[730.85]*
- Hippel's (retinocerebral angiomatosis) 759.6
- Hirschfeld's (acute diabetes mellitus) (*see also* Diabetes) 250.0❺
- Hirschsprung's (congenital megacolon) 751.3
- His (-Werner) (trench fever) 083.1
- HIV 042
- Hodgkin's (M9650/3) 201.9❺

Note – Use the following fifth-digit subclassification with category 201:
- *0 unspecified site*
- *1 lymph nodes of head, face, and neck*
- *2 intrathoracic lymph nodes*
- *3 intra-abdominal lymph nodes*
- *4 lymph nodes of axilla and upper limb*
- *5 lymph nodes of inguinal region and lower limb*
- *6 intrapelvic lymph nodes*
- *7 spleen*
- *8 lymph nodes of multiple sites*

-
  - lymphocytic
    - depletion (M9653/3) 201.7❺
      - diffuse fibrosis (M9654/3) 201.7❺
      - reticular type (M9655/3) 201.7❺
    - predominance (M9651/3) 201.4❺
  - lymphocytic-histiocytic predominance (M9651/3) 201.4❺
  - mixed cellularity (M9652/3) 201.6❺
  - nodular sclerosis (M9656/3) 201.5❺
    - cellular phase (M9657/3) 201.5❺
- Hodgson's 441.9
  - ruptured 441.5
- Hoffa (-Kastert) (liposynovitis prepatellaris) 272.8
- Holla (*see also* Spherocytosis) 282.0
- homozygous-Hb-S 282.61
- hoof and mouth 078.4
- hookworm (*see also* Ancylostomiasis) 126.9
- Horton's (temporal arteritis) 446.5
- host-versus-graft (immune or nonimmune cause) 996.80
  - bone marrow 996.85
  - heart 996.83
  - intestines 996.87
  - kidney 996.81
  - liver 996.82
  - lung 996.84
  - pancreas 996.86
  - specified NEC 996.89
- HPFH (hereditary persistence of fetal hemoglobin) ("Swiss variety") 282.7
- Huchard's (continued arterial hypertension) 401.9
- Huguier's (uterine fibroma) 218.9
- human immunodeficiency (virus) 042
- hunger 251.1
- Hunt's
  - dyssynergia cerebellaris myoclonica 334.2
  - herpetic geniculate ganglionitis 053.11
- Huntington's 333.4
- Huppert's (multiple myeloma) (M9730/3) 203.0❺
- Hurler's (mucopolysaccharidosis I) 277.5
- Hutchinson's, meaning
  - angioma serpiginosum 709.1
  - cheiropompholyx 705.81
  - prurigo estivalis 692.72
- Hutchinson-Boeck (sarcoidosis) 135
- Hutchinson-Gilford (progeria) 259.8
- hyaline (diffuse) (generalized) 728.9
  - membrane (lung) (newborn) 769
- hydatid (*see also* Echinococcus) 122.9
- Hyde's (prurigo nodularis) 698.3
- hyperkinetic (*see also* Hyperkinesia) 314.9
  - heart 429.82
- hypertensive (*see also* Hypertension) 401.9
- hypophysis 253.9
  - hyperfunction 253.1
  - hypofunction 253.2
- Iceland (epidemic neuromyasthenia) 049.8
- I cell 272.7
- ill-defined 799.89
- immunologic NEC 279.9
- immunoproliferative 203.8❺

Disease, diseased – *continued*
- inclusion 078.5
  - salivary gland 078.5
- infancy, early NEC 779.9
- infective NEC 136.9
- inguinal gland 289.9
- internal semilunar cartilage, cystic 717.5
- intervertebral disc 722.90
  - with myelopathy 722.70
  - cervical, cervicothoracic 722.91
    - with myelopathy 722.71
  - lumbar, lumbosacral 722.93
    - with myelopathy 722.73
  - thoracic, thoracolumbar 722.92
    - with myelopathy 722.72
- intestine 569.9
  - functional 564.9
    - congenital 751.3
    - psychogenic 306.4
  - lardaceous 277.39
  - organic 569.9
  - protozoal NEC 007.9
- iris 364.9
  - specified NEC 364.89 ●
- iron
  - metabolism 275.0
  - storage 275.0
- Isambert's (*see also* Tuberculosis, larynx) 012.3❺
- Iselin's (osteochondrosis, fifth metatarsal) 732.5
- island (scrub typhus) 081.2
- itai-itai 985.5
- Jadassohn's (maculopapular erythroderma) 696.2
- Jadassohn-Pellizari's (anetoderma) 701.3
- Jakob-Creutzfeldt (new variant) 046.1
  - with dementia
    - with behavioral disturbance 046.1 *[294.11]*
    - without behavioral disturbance 046.1 *[294.10]*
- Jaksch (-Luzet) (pseudoleukemia infantum) 285.8
- Janet's 300.89
- Jansky-Bielschowsky 330.1
- jaw NEC 526.9
  - fibrocystic 526.2
- Jensen's 363.05
- Jeune's (asphyxiating thoracic dystrophy) 756.4
- Jigger 134.1
- Johnson-Stevens (erythema multiforme exudativum) 695.1
- joint NEC 719.9❺
  - ankle 719.97
  - Charcôt 094.0 *[713.5]*
  - degenerative (*see also* Osteoarthrosis) 715.9❺
    - multiple 715.09
    - spine (*see also* Spondylosis) 721.90
  - elbow 719.92
  - foot 719.97
  - hand 719.94
  - hip 719.95
  - hypertrophic (chronic) (degenerative) (*see also* Osteoarthrosis) 715.9❺
    - spine (*see also* Spondylosis) 721.90
  - knee 719.96
  - Luschka 721.90
  - multiple sites 719.99
  - pelvic region 719.95
  - sacroiliac 724.6
  - shoulder (region) 719.91
  - specified site NEC 719.98
  - spine NEC 724.9
    - pseudarthrosis following fusion 733.82
    - sacroiliac 724.6
  - wrist 719.93
- Jourdain's (acute gingivitis) 523.00
- Jüngling's (sarcoidosis) 135
- Kahler (-Bozzolo) (multiple myeloma) (M9730/3) 203.0❺
- Kalischer's 759.6
- Kaposi's 757.33
  - lichen ruber 697.8
    - acuminatus 696.4
    - moniliformis 697.8
  - xeroderma pigmentosum 757.33
- Kaschin-Beck (endemic polyarthritis) 716.00
  - ankle 716.07
  - arm 716.02
    - lower (and wrist) 716.03
    - upper (and elbow) 716.02
  - foot (and ankle) 716.07
  - forearm (and wrist) 716.03
  - hand 716.04

Disease, diseased – *continued*
- Kaschin-Beck – *continued*
  - leg 716.06
    - lower 716.06
    - upper 716.05
  - multiple sites 716.09
  - pelvic region (hip) (thigh) 716.05
  - shoulder region 716.01
  - specified site NEC 716.08
- Katayama 120.2
- Kawasaki 446.1
- Kedani (scrub typhus) 081.2
- kidney (functional) (pelvis) (*see also* Disease, renal) 593.9
  - chronic 585.9
    - requiring chronic dialysis 585.6
    - stage
      - I 585.1
      - II (mild) 585.2
      - III (moderate) 585.3
      - IV (severe) 585.4
      - V 585.5
  - cystic (congenital) 753.10
    - multiple 753.19
    - single 753.11
    - specified NEC 753.19
  - fibrocystic (congenital) 753.19
  - in gout 274.10
  - polycystic (congenital) 753.12
    - adult type (APKD) 753.13
    - autosomal dominant 753.13
    - autosomal recessive 753.14
    - childhood type (CPKD) 753.14
    - infantile type 753.14
- Kienböck's (carpal lunate) (wrist) 732.3
- Kimmelstiel (-Wilson) (intercapillary glomerulosclerosis) 250.4❺ *[581.81]*
- Kinnier Wilson's (hepatolenticular degeneration) 275.1
- kissing 075
- Kleb's (*see also* Nephritis) 583.9
- Klinger's 446.4
- Klippel's 723.8
- Klippel-Feil (brevicollis) 756.16
- Knight's 911.1
- Köbner's (epidermolysis bullosa) 757.39
- Koenig-Wichmann (pemphigus) 694.4
- Köhler's
  - first (osteoarthrosis juvenilis) 732.5
  - second (Freiberg's infraction, metatarsal head) 732.5
  - patellar 732.4
  - tarsal navicular (bone) (osteoarthrosis juvenilis) 732.5
- Köhler-Freiberg (infraction, metatarsal head) 732.5
- Köhler-Mouchet (osteoarthrosis juvenilis) 732.5
- Köhler-Pellegrini-Stieda (calcification, knee joint) 726.62
- Kok 759.89
- König's (osteochondritis dissecans) 732.7
- Korsakoff's (nonalcoholic) 294.0
  - alcoholic 291.1
- Kostmann's (infantile genetic agranulocytosis) 288.01
- Krabbe's 330.0
- Kraepelin-Morel (*see also* Schizophrenia) 295.9❺
- Kraft-Weber-Dimitri 759.6
- Kufs' 330.1
- Kugelberg-Welander 335.11
- Kuhnt-Junius 362.52
- Kümmell's (-Verneuil) (spondylitis) 721.7
- Kundrat's (lymphosarcoma) 200.1❺
- kuru 046.0
- Kussmaul (-Meier) (polyarteritis nodosa) 446.0
- Kyasanur Forest 065.2
- Kyrle's (hyperkeratosis follicularis in cutem penetrans) 701.1
- labia
  - inflammatory 616.10 ▲
  - noninflammatory 624.9
    - specified NEC 624.8
- labyrinth, ear 386.8
- lacrimal system (apparatus) (passages) 375.9
  - gland 375.00
  - specified NEC 375.89
- Lafora's 333.2
- Lagleyze-von Hippel (retinocerebral angiomatosis) 759.6
- Lancereaux-Mathieu (leptospiral jaundice) 100.0
- Landry's 357.0

- **Disease, diseased** – *continued*
  - Lane's 569.89
  - lardaceous (any site) 277.39
  - Larrey-Weil (leptospiral jaundice) 100.0
  - Larsen (-Johansson) (juvenile osteopathia patellae) 732.4
  - larynx 478.70
  - Lasègue's (persecution mania) 297.9
  - Leber's 377.16
  - Lederer's (acquired infectious hemolytic anemia) 283.19
  - Legg's (capital femoral osteochondrosis) 732.1
  - Legg-Calvé-Perthes (capital femoral osteochondrosis) 732.1
  - Legg-Calvé-Waldenström (femoral capital osteochondrosis) 732.1
  - Legg-Perthes (femoral capital osteochrondosis) 732.1
  - Legionnaires' 482.84
  - Leigh's 330.8
  - Leiner's (exfoliative dermatitis) 695.89
  - Leloir's (lupus erythematosus) 695.4
  - Lenegre's 426.0
  - lens (eye) 379.39
  - Leriche's (osteoporosis, posttraumatic) 733.7
  - Letterer-Siwe (acute histiocytosis X) (M9722/3) 202.5❺
  - Lev's (acquired complete heart block) 426.0
  - Lewandowski's (*see also* Tuberculosis) 017.0❺
  - Lewandowski-Lutz (epidermodysplasia verruciformis) 078.19
  - Lewy body 331.82
    - with dementia
      - with behavioral disturbance 331.82 *[294.11]*
      - without behavioral disturbance 331.82 *[294.10]*
  - Leyden's (periodic vomiting) 536.2
  - Libman-Sacks (verrucous endocarditis) 710.0 *[424.91]*
  - Lichtheim's (subacute combined sclerosis with pernicious anemia) 281.0 *[336.2]*
  - ligament 728.9
  - light chain 203.0❺
  - Lightwood's (renal tubular acidosis) 588.89
  - Lignac's (cystinosis) 270.0
  - Lindau's (retinocerebral angiomatosis) 759.6
  - Lindau-von Hippel (angiomatosis retinocerebellosa) 759.6
  - lip NEC 528.5
  - lipidosis 272.7
  - lipoid storage NEC 272.7
  - Lipschütz's 616.50
  - Little's – *see* Palsy, cerebral
  - liver 573.9
    - alcoholic 571.3
      - acute 571.1
      - chronic 571.3
    - chronic 571.9
      - alcoholic 571.3
    - cystic, congenital 751.62
    - drug-induced 573.3
    - due to
      - chemicals 573.3
      - fluorinated agents 573.3
      - hypersensitivity drugs 573.3
      - isoniazids 573.3
    - end stage NEC 572.8 ●
      - due to hepatitis – *see* Hepatitis ●
    - fibrocystic (congenital) 751.62
    - glycogen storage 271.0
    - organic 573.9
    - polycystic (congenital) 751.62
  - Lobo's (keloid blastomycosis) 116.2
  - Lobstein's (brittle bones and blue sclera) 756.51
  - locomotor system 334.9
  - Lorain's (pituitary dwarfism) 253.3
  - Lou Gehrig's 335.20
  - Lucas-Championnière (fibrinous bronchitis) 466.0
  - Ludwig's (submaxillary cellulitis) 528.3
  - luetic – *see* Syphilis
  - lumbosacral region 724.6
  - lung NEC 518.89
    - black 500
    - congenital 748.60
    - cystic 518.89
      - congenital 748.4
    - fibroid (chronic) (*see also* Fibrosis, lung) 515
    - fluke 121.2
      - oriental 121.2
    - in
      - amyloidosis 277.39 *[517.8]*
      - polymyositis 710.4 *[517.8]*

- **Disease, diseased** – *continued*
  - lung – *continued*
    - in – *continued*
      - sarcoidosis 135 *[517.8]*
      - Sjögren's syndrome 710.2 *[517.8]*
      - syphilis 095.1
      - systemic lupus erythematosus 710.0 *[517.8]*
      - systemic sclerosis 710.1 *[517.2]*
    - interstitial (chronic) 515
      - acute 136.3
    - nonspecific, chronic 496
    - obstructive (chronic) (COPD) 496
      - with
        - acute
          - bronchitis 491.22
          - exacerbation (acute) 491.21
        - alveolitis, allergic (*see also* Alveolitis, allergic) 495.9
        - asthma (chronic) (obstructive) 493.2❺
        - bronchiectasis 494.0
          - with acute exacerbation 494.1
        - bronchitis (chronic) 491.20
          - with
            - acute bronchitis 491.22
            - exacerbation (acute) 491.21
        - decompensated 491.21
          - with exacerbation 491.21
        - emphysema NEC 492.8
      - diffuse (with fibrosis) 496
    - polycystic 518.89
      - asthma (chronic) (obstructive) 493.2❺
      - congenital 748.4
    - purulent (cavitary) 513.0
    - restrictive 518.89
    - rheumatoid 714.81
      - diffuse interstitial 714.81
    - specified NEC 518.89
  - Lutembacher's (atrial septal defect with mitral stenosis) 745.5
  - Lutz-Miescher (elastosis perforans serpiginosa) 701.1
  - Lutz-Splendore-de Almeida (Brazilian blastomycosis) 116.1
  - Lyell's (toxic epidermal necrolysis) 695.1
    - due to drug
      - correct substance properly administered 695.1
      - overdose or wrong substance given or taken 977.9
        - specific drug – *see* Table of Drugs and Chemicals
  - Lyme 088.81
  - lymphatic (gland) (system) 289.9
    - channel (noninfective) 457.9
    - vessel (noninfective) 457.9
      - specified NEC 457.8
  - lymphoproliferative (chronic) (M9970/1) 238.79
  - Machado-Joseph 334.8
  - Madelung's (lipomatosis) 272.8
  - Madura (actinomycotic) 039.9
    - mycotic 117.4
  - Magitot's 526.4
  - Majocchi's (purpura annularis telangiectodes) 709.1
  - malarial (*see also* Malaria) 084.6
  - Malassez's (cystic) 608.89
  - Malibu 919.8
    - infected 919.9
  - malignant (M8000/3) – *see also* Neoplasm, by site, malignant
    - previous, affecting management of pregnancy V23.8❺
  - Manson's 120.1
  - maple bark 495.6
  - maple syrup (urine) 270.3
  - Marburg (virus) 078.89
  - Marchiafava (-Bignami) 341.8
  - Marfan's 090.49
    - congenital syphilis 090.49
    - meaning Marfan's syndrome 759.82
  - Marie-Bamberger (hypertrophic pulmonary osteoarthropathy) (secondary) 731.2
    - primary or idiopathic (acropachyderma) 757.39
    - pulmonary (hypertrophic osteoarthropathy) 731.2
  - Marie-Strümpell (ankylosing spondylitis) 720.0
  - Marion's (bladder neck obstruction) 596.0
  - Marsh's (exophthalmic goiter) 242.0❺
  - Martin's 715.27
  - mast cell 757.33
    - systemic (M9741/3) 202.6❺

- **Disease, diseased** – *continued*
  - mastoid (*see also* Mastoiditis) 383.9
    - process 385.9
  - maternal, unrelated to pregnancy NEC, affecting fetus or newborn 760.9
  - Mathieu's (leptospiral jaundice) 100.0
  - Mauclaire's 732.3
  - Mauriac's (erythema nodosum syphiliticum) 091.3❺
  - Maxcy's 081.0
  - McArdle (-Schmid-Pearson) (glycogenosis V) 271.0
  - mediastinum NEC 519.3
  - Medin's (*see also* Poliomyelitis) 045.9❺
  - Mediterranean (with hemoglobinopathy) 282.49
  - medullary center (idiopathic) (respiratory) 348.8
  - Meige's (chronic hereditary edema) 757.0
  - Meleda 757.39
  - Ménétrier's (hypertrophic gastritis) 535.2❺
  - Ménière's (active) 386.00
    - cochlear 386.02
    - cochleovestibular 386.01
    - inactive 386.04
    - in remission 386.04
    - vestibular 386.03
  - meningeal – *see* Meningitis
  - mental (*see also* Psychosis) 298.9
  - Merzbacher-Pelizaeus 330.0
  - mesenchymal 710.9
  - mesenteric embolic 557.0
  - metabolic NEC 277.9
  - metal polishers' 502
  - metastatic – *see* Metastasis
  - Mibelli's 757.39
  - microdrepanocytic 282.49
  - microvascular - *code to condition*
  - Miescher's 709.3
  - Mikulicz's (dryness of mouth, absent or decreased lacrimation) 527.1
  - Milkman (-Looser) (osteomalacia with pseudofractures) 268.2
  - Miller's (osteomalacia) 268.2
  - Mills' 335.29
  - Milroy's (chronic hereditary edema) 757.0
  - Minamata 985.0
  - Minor's 336.1
  - Minot's (hemorrhagic disease, newborn) 776.0
  - Minot-von Willebrand-Jürgens (angiohemophilia) 286.4
  - Mitchell's (erythromelalgia) 443.82
  - mitral – *see* Endocarditis, mitral
  - Mljet (mal de Meleda) 757.39
  - Möbius', Moebius' 346.8❺
  - Möeller's 267
  - Möller (-Barlow) (infantile scurvy) 267
  - Mönckeberg's (*see also* Arteriosclerosis, extremities) 440.20
  - Mondor's (thrombophlebitis of breast) 451.89
  - Monge's 993.2
  - Morel-Kraepelin (*see also* Schizophrenia) 295.9❺
  - Morgagni's (syndrome) (hyperostosis frontalis interna) 733.3
  - Morgagni-Adams-Stokes (syncope with heart block) 426.9
  - Morquio (-Brailsford) (-Ullrich) (mucopolysaccharidosis IV) 277.5
  - Morton's (with metatarsalgia) 355.6
  - Morvan's 336.0
  - motor neuron (bulbar) (mixed type) 335.20
  - Mouchet's (juvenile osteochondrosis, foot) 732.5
  - mouth 528.9
  - Moyamoya 437.5
  - Mucha's (acute parapsoriasis varioliformis) 696.2
  - mu-chain 273.2
  - mucolipidosis (I) (II) (III) 272.7
  - Münchmeyer's (exostosis luxurians) 728.11
  - Murri's (intermittent hemoglobinuria) 283.2
  - muscle 359.9
    - inflammatory 728.9
    - ocular 378.9
  - musculoskeletal system 729.9
  - mushroom workers' 495.5
  - Myà's (congenital dilation, colon) 751.3
  - mycotic 117.9
  - myeloproliferative (chronic) (M9960/1) 238.79
  - myocardium, myocardial (*see also* Degeneration, myocardial) 429.1
    - hypertensive (*see also* Hypertension, heart) 402.90
    - primary (idiopathic) 425.4
  - myoneural 358.9
  - Naegeli's 287.1

❹ Fourth-Digit Required   ❺ Fifth-Digit Required   *[code]* Manifestation Code   ►◄ Revised Text   ● New Line   ▲ Revised Code

Disease, diseased – *continued*
  nail 703.9
    specified type NEC 703.8
  Nairobi sheep 066.1
  nasal 478.19
    cavity NEC 478.19
    sinus (chronic) – *see* Sinusitis
  navel (newborn) NEC 779.89
    delayed separation of umbilical cord 779.83
  nemaline body 359.0
  neoplastic, generalized (M8000/6) 199.0
  nerve – *see* Disorder, nerve
  nervous system (central) 349.9
    autonomic, peripheral (*see also* Neuropathy, peripheral, autonomic) 337.9
    congenital 742.9
    inflammatory – *see* Encephalitis
    parasympathetic (*see also* Neuropathy, peripheral, autonomic) 337.9
    peripheral NEC 355.9
    specified NEC 349.89
    sympathetic (*see also* Neuropathy, peripheral, autonomic) 337.9
    vegetative (*see also* Neuropathy, peripheral, autonomic) 337.9
  Nettleship's (urticaria pigmentosa) 757.33
  Neumann's (pemphigus vegetans) 694.4
  neurologic (central) NEC (*see also* Disease, nervous system) 349.9
    peripheral NEC 355.9
  neuromuscular system NEC 358.9
  Newcastle 077.8
  Nicolas (-Durand) -Favre (climatic bubo) 099.1
  Niemann-Pick (lipid histiocytosis) 272.7
  nipple 611.9
    Paget's (M8540/3) 174.0
  Nishimoto (-Takeuchi) 437.5
  nonarthropod-borne NEC 078.89
    central nervous system NEC 049.9
    enterovirus NEC 078.89
  nonautoimmune hemolytic NEC 283.10
  Nonne-Milroy-Meige (chronic hereditary edema) 757.0
  Norrie's (congenital progressive oculoacousticocerebral degeneration) 743.8
  nose 478.19
  nucleus pulposus – *see* Disease, intervertebral disc
  nutritional 269.9
    maternal, affecting fetus or newborn 760.4
  oasthouse, urine 270.2
  obliterative vascular 447.1
  Odelberg's (juvenile osteochondrosis) 732.1
  Oguchi's (retina) 368.61
  Ohara's (*see also* Tularemia) 021.9
  Ollier's (chondrodysplasia) 756.4
  Opitz's (congestive splenomegaly) 289.51
  Oppenheim's 358.8
  Oppenheim-Urbach (necrobiosis lipoidica diabeticorum) 250.8❺ *[709.3]*
  optic nerve NEC 377.49
  orbit 376.9
    specified NEC 376.89
  Oriental liver fluke 121.1
  Oriental lung fluke 121.2
  Ormond's 593.4
  Osgood's tibia (tubercle) 732.4
  Osgood-Schlatter 732.4
  Osler (-Vaquez) (polycythemia vera) (M9950/1) 238.4
  Osler-Rendu (familial hemorrhagic telangiectasia) 448.0
  osteofibrocystic 252.01
  Otto's 715.35
  outer ear 380.9
  ovary (noninflammatory) NEC 620.9
    cystic 620.2
    polycystic 256.4
    specified NEC 620.8
  Owren's (congenital) (*see also* Defect, coagulation) 286.3
  Paas' 756.59
  Paget's (osteitis deformans) 731.0
    with infiltrating duct carcinoma of the breast (M8541/3) – *see* Neoplasm, breast, malignant
    bone 731.0
      osteosarcoma in (M9184/3) – *see* Neoplasm, bone, malignant
    breast (M8540/3) 174.0

Disease, diseased – *continued*
  Paget's – *continued*
    extramammary (M8542/3) – *see also* Neoplasm, skin, malignant
      anus 154.3
        skin 173.5
    malignant (M8540/3)
      breast 174.0
      specified site NEC (M8542/3) – *see* Neoplasm, skin, malignant
      unspecified site 174.0
    mammary (M8540/3) 174.0
    nipple (M8540/3) 174.0
  palate (soft) 528.9
  Paltauf-Sternberg 201.9❺
  pancreas 577.9
    cystic 577.2
      congenital 751.7
    fibrocystic 277.00
  Panner's 732.3
    capitellum humeri 732.3
    head of humerus 732.3
    tarsal navicular (bone) (osteochondrosis) 732.5
  panvalvular – *see* Endocarditis, mitral
  parametrium 629.9
  parasitic NEC 136.9
    cerebral NEC 123.9
    intestinal NEC 129
    mouth 112.0
    skin NEC 134.9
    specified type – *see* Infestation
    tongue 112.0
  parathyroid (gland) 252.9
    specified NEC 252.8
  Parkinson's 332.0
  parodontal 523.9
  Parrot's (syphilitic osteochondritis) 090.0
  Parry's (exophthalmic goiter) 242.0❺
  Parson's (exophthalmic goiter) 242.0❺
  Pavy's 593.6
  Paxton's (white piedra) 111.2
  Payr's (splenic flexure syndrome) 569.89
  pearl-workers' (chronic osteomyelitis) (*see also* Osteomyelitis) 730.1❺
  Pel-Ebstein – *see* Disease, Hodgkin's
  Pelizaeus-Merzbacher 330.0
    with dementia
      with behavioral disturbance 330.0 *[294.11]*
      without behavioral disturbance 330.0 *[294.10]*
  Pellegrini-Stieda (calcification, knee joint) 726.62
  pelvis, pelvic
    female NEC 629.9
      specified NEC 629.89
    gonococcal (acute) 098.19
      chronic or duration of 2 months or over 098.39
    infection (*see also* Disease, pelvis, inflammatory) 614.9
    inflammatory (female) (PID) 614.9
      with
        abortion – *see* Abortion, by type, with sepsis
        ectopic pregnancy (*see also* categories 633.0-633.9) 639.0
        molar pregnancy (*see also* categories 630-632) 639.0
      acute 614.3
      chronic 614.4
      complicating pregnancy 646.6❺
        affecting fetus or newborn 760.8
      following
        abortion 639.0
        ectopic or molar pregnancy 639.0
      peritonitis (acute) 614.5
        chronic NEC 614.7
      puerperal, postpartum, childbirth 670❹
      specified NEC 614.8
    organ, female NEC 629.9
      specified NEC 629.89
    peritoneum, female NEC 629.9
      specified NEC 629.89
  penis 607.9
    inflammatory 607.2
  peptic NEC 536.9
    acid 536.8
  periapical tissues NEC 522.9
  pericardium 423.9
    specified type NEC 423.8

Disease, diseased – *continued*
  perineum
    female
      inflammatory 616.9
        specified NEC 616.89
      noninflammatory 624.9
        specified NEC 624.8
    male (inflammatory) 682.2
  periodic (familial) (Reimann's) NEC 277.31
    paralysis 359.3
  periodontal NEC 523.9
    specified NEC 523.8
  periosteum 733.90
  peripheral
    arterial 443.9
    autonomic nervous system (*see also* Neuropathy, autonomic) 337.9
    nerve NEC (*see also* Neuropathy) 356.9
      multiple – *see* Polyneuropathy
    vascular 443.9
      specified type NEC 443.89
  peritoneum 568.9
    pelvic, female 629.9
      specified NEC 629.89
  Perrin-Ferraton (snapping hip) 719.65
  persistent mucosal (middle ear) (with posterior or superior marginal perforation of ear drum) 382.2
  Perthes' (capital femoral osteochondrosis) 732.1
  Petit's (*see also* Hernia, lumbar) 553.8
  Peutz-Jeghers 759.6
  Peyronie's 607.85
  Pfeiffer's (infectious mononucleosis) 075
  pharynx 478.20
  Phocas' 610.1
  photochromogenic (acid-fast bacilli) (pulmonary) 031.0
    nonpulmonary 031.9
  Pick's
    brain 331.11
      with dementia
        with behavioral disturbance 331.11 *[294.11]*
        without behavioral disturbance 331.11 *[294.10]*
    cerebral atrophy 331.11
      with dementia
        with behavioral disturbance 331.11 *[294.11]*
        without behavioral disturbance 331.11 *[294.10]*
    lipid histiocytosis 272.7
    liver (pericardial pseudocirrhosis of liver) 423.2
    pericardium (pericardial pseudocirrhosis of liver) 423.2
    polyserositis (pericardial pseudocirrhosis of liver) 423.2
  Pierson's (osteochondrosis) 732.1
  pigeon fanciers' or breeders' 495.2
  pineal gland 259.8
  pink 985.0
  Pinkus' (lichen nitidus) 697.1
  pinworm 127.4
  pituitary (gland) 253.9
    hyperfunction 253.1
    hypofunction 253.2
  pituitary snuff-takers' 495.8
  placenta
    affecting fetus or newborn 762.2
    complicating pregnancy or childbirth 656.7❺
  pleura (cavity) (*see also* Pleurisy) 511.0
  Plummer's (toxic nodular goiter) 242.3❺
  pneumatic
    drill 994.9
    hammer 994.9
  policeman's 729.2
  Pollitzer's (hidradenitis suppurativa) 705.83
  polycystic (congenital) 759.89
    kidney or renal 753.12
      adult type (APKD) 753.13
      autosomal dominant 753.13
      autosomal recessive 753.14
      childhood type (CPKD) 753.14
      infantile type 753.14
    liver or hepatic 751.62
    lung or pulmonary 518.89
      congenital 748.4
    ovary, ovaries 256.4
    spleen 759.0
  Pompe's (glycogenosis II) 271.0
  Poncet's (tuberculous rheumatism) (*see also* Tuberculosis) 015.9❺

Disease, diseased – *continued*
- Posada-Wernicke 114.9
- Potain's (pulmonary edema) 514
- Pott's (*see also* Tuberculosis) 015.0❺ *[730.88]*
  - osteomyelitis 015.0❺ *[730.88]*
  - paraplegia 015.0❺ *[730.88]*
  - spinal curvature 015.0❺ *[737.43]*
  - spondylitis 015.0❺ *[720.81]*
- Potter's 753.0
- Poulet's 714.2
- pregnancy NEC (*see also* Pregnancy) 646.9❺
- Preiser's (osteoporosis) 733.09
- Pringle's (tuberous sclerosis) 759.5
- Profichet's 729.9
- prostate 602.9
  - specified type NEC 602.8
- protozoal NEC 136.8
  - intestine, intestinal NEC 007.9
- pseudo-Hurler's (mucolipidosis III) 272.7
- psychiatric (*see also* Psychosis) 298.9
- psychotic (*see also* Psychosis) 298.9
- Puente's (simple glandular cheilitis) 528.5
- puerperal NEC (*see also* Puerperal) 674.9❺
- pulmonary – *see also* Disease, lung
  - amyloid 277.39 *[517.8]*
  - artery 417.9
  - circulation, circulatory 417.9
    - specified NEC 417.8
  - diffuse obstructive (chronic) 496
    - with
      - acute bronchitis 491.22
      - asthma (chronic) (obstructive) 493.2❺
      - exacerbation NEC (acute) 491.21
  - heart (chronic) 416.9
    - specified NEC 416.8
  - hypertensive (vascular) 416.0
    - cardiovascular 416.0
  - obstructive diffuse (chronic) 496
    - with
      - acute bronchitis 491.22
      - asthma (chronic) (obstructive) 493.2❺
      - bronchitis (chronic) 491.20
        - with
          - exacerbation (acute) 491.21
        - acute 491.22
      - decompensated 491.21
        - with exacerbation 491.21
      - exacerbation NEC (acute) 491.21
  - valve (*see also* Endocarditis, pulmonary) 424.3
- pulp (dental) NEC 522.9
- pulseless 446.7
- Putnam's (subacute combined sclerosis with pernicious anemia) 281.0 *[336.2]*
- Pyle (-Cohn) (craniometaphyseal dysplasia) 756.89
- pyramidal tract 333.90
- Quervain's
  - tendon sheath 727.04
  - thyroid (subacute granulomatous thyroiditis) 245.1
- Quincke's – *see* Edema, angioneurotic
- Quinquaud (acne decalvans) 704.09
- rag sorters' 022.1
- Raynaud's (paroxysmal digital cyanosis) 443.0
- reactive airway – *see* Asthma
- Recklinghausen's (M9540/1) 237.71
  - bone (osteitis fibrosa cystica) 252.01
- Recklinghausen-Applebaum (hemochromatosis) 275.0
- Reclus' (cystic) 610.1
- rectum NEC 569.49
- Refsum's (heredopathia atactica polyneuritiformis) 356.3
- Reichmann's (gastrosuccorrhea) 536.8
- Reimann's (periodic) 277.31
- Reiter's 099.3
- renal (functional) (pelvis)(*see also* Disease, kidney) 593.9
  - with
    - edema (*see also* Nephrosis) 581.9
    - exudative nephritis 583.89
    - lesion of interstitial nephritis 583.89
    - stated generalized cause – *see* Nephritis
  - acute 593.9
  - basement membrane NEC 583.89
    - with pulmonary hemorrhage (Goodpasture's syndrome) 446.21 *[583.81]*
  - chronic (*see also* Disease, kidney, chronic) 585.9

Disease, diseased – *continued*
- renal – *continued*
  - complicating pregnancy or puerperium NEC 646.2❺
    - with hypertension – *see* Toxemia, of pregnancy
    - affecting fetus or newborn 760.1
  - cystic, congenital (*see also* Cystic, disease, kidney) 753.10
  - diabetic 250.4❺ *[583.81]*
  - due to
    - amyloidosis 277.39 *[583.81]*
    - diabetes mellitus 250.4❺ *[583.81]*
    - systemic lupus erythematosis 710.0 *[583.81]*
  - end-stage 585.6
  - exudative 583.89
  - fibrocystic (congenital) 753.19
  - gonococcal 098.19 *[583.81]*
  - gouty 274.10
  - hypertensive (*see also* Hypertension, kidney) 403.90
  - immune complex NEC 583.89
  - interstitial (diffuse) (focal) 583.89
  - lupus 710.0 *[583.81]*
  - maternal, affecting fetus or newborn 760.1
    - hypertensive 760.0
  - phosphate-losing (tubular) 588.0
  - polycystic (congenital) 753.12
    - adult type (APKD) 753.13
    - autosomal dominant 753.13
    - autosomal recessive 753.14
    - childhood type (CPKD) 753.14
    - infantile type 753.14
  - specified lesion or cause NEC (*see also* Glomerulonephritis) 583.89
  - subacute 581.9
  - syphilitic 095.4
  - tuberculous (*see also* Tuberculosis) 016.0❺ *[583.81]*
  - tubular (*see also* Nephrosis, tubular) 584.5
- Rendu-Osler-Weber (familial hemorrhagic telangiectasia) 448.0
- renovascular (arteriosclerotic) (*see also* Hypertension, kidney) 403.90
- respiratory (tract) 519.9
  - acute or subacute (upper) NEC 465.9
    - due to fumes or vapors 506.3
    - multiple sites NEC 465.8
    - noninfectious 478.9
    - streptococcal 034.0
  - chronic 519.9
    - arising in the perinatal period 770.7
    - due to fumes or vapors 506.4
  - due to
    - aspiration of liquids or solids 508.9
    - external agents NEC 508.9
      - specified NEC 508.8
    - fumes or vapors 506.9
      - acute or subacute NEC 506.3
      - chronic 506.4
  - fetus or newborn NEC 770.9
  - obstructive 496
  - specified type NEC 519.8
  - upper (acute) (infectious) NEC 465.9
    - multiple sites NEC 465.8
    - noninfectious NEC 478.9
    - streptococcal 034.0
- retina, retinal NEC 362.9
  - Batten's or Batten-Mayou 330.1 *[362.71]*
  - degeneration 362.89
  - vascular lesion 362.17
- rheumatic (*see also* Arthritis) 716.8❺
  - heart – *see* Disease, heart, rheumatic
- rheumatoid (heart) – *see* Arthritis, rheumatoid
- rickettsial NEC 083.9
  - specified type NEC 083.8
- Riedel's (ligneous thyroiditis) 245.3
- Riga (-Fede) (cachectic aphthae) 529.0
- Riggs' (compound periodontitis) 523.40
- Ritter's 695.81
- Rivalta's (cervicofacial actinomycosis) 039.3
- Robles' (onchocerciasis) 125.3 *[360.13]*
- Roger's (congenital interventricular septal defect) 745.4
- Rokitansky's (*see also* Necrosis, liver) 570
- Romberg's 349.89
- Rosenthal's (factor XI deficiency) 286.2
- Rossbach's (hyperchlorhydria) 536.8
  - psychogenic 306.4
- Roth (-Bernhardt) 355.1

Disease, diseased – *continued*
- Runeberg's (progressive pernicious anemia) 281.0
- Rust's (tuberculous spondylitis) (*see also* Tuberculosis) 015.0❺ *[720.81]*
- Rustitskii's (multiple myeloma) (M9730/3) 203.0❺
- Ruysch's (Hirschsprung's disease) 751.3
- Sachs (-Tay) 330.1
- sacroiliac NEC 724.6
- salivary gland or duct NEC 527.9
  - inclusion 078.5
    - streptococcal 034.0
  - virus 078.5
- Sander's (paranoia) 297.1
- Sandhoff's 330.1
- sandworm 126.9
- Savill's (epidemic exfoliative dermatitis) 695.89
- Schamberg's (progressive pigmentary dermatosis) 709.09
- Schaumann's (sarcoidosis) 135
- Schenck's (sporotrichosis) 117.1
- Scheuermann's (osteochondrosis) 732.0
- Schilder (-Flatau) 341.1
- Schimmelbusch's 610.1
- Schlatter's tibia (tubercle) 732.4
- Schlatter-Osgood 732.4
- Schmorl's 722.30
  - cervical 722.39
  - lumbar, lumbosacral 722.32
  - specified region NEC 722.39
  - thoracic, thoracolumbar 722.31
- Scholz's 330.0
- Schönlein (-Henoch) (purpura rheumatica) 287.0
- Schottmüller's (*see also* Fever, paratyphoid) 002.9
- Schüller-Christian (chronic histiocytosis X) 277.89
- Schultz's (agranulocytosis) 288.09
- Schwalbe-Ziehen-Oppenheimer 333.6
- Schwartz-Jampel 359.23 ●
- Schweninger-Buzzi (macular atrophy) 701.3
- sclera 379.19
- scrofulous (*see also* Tuberculosis) 017.2❺
- scrotum 608.9
- sebaceous glands NEC 706.9
- Secretan's (posttraumatic edema) 782.3
- semilunar cartilage, cystic 717.5
- seminal vesicle 608.9
- Senear-Usher (pemphigus erythematosus) 694.4
- serum NEC 999.5
- Sever's (osteochondrosis calcaneum) 732.5
- sexually transmitted – *see* Disease, venereal ●
- Sézary's (reticulosis) (M9701/3) 202.2❺
- Shaver's (bauxite pneumoconiosis) 503
- Sheehan's (postpartum pituitary necrosis) 253.2
- shimamushi (scrub typhus) 081.2
- shipyard 077.1
- sickle-cell 282.60
  - with
    - crisis 282.62
    - Hb-S disease 282.61
    - other abnormal hemoglobin (Hb-D) (Hb-E) (Hb-G) (Hb-J) (Hb-K) (Hb-O) (Hb-P) (high fetal gene) (without crisis) 282.68
      - with crisis 282.69
  - elliptocytosis 282.60
  - Hb-C (without crisis) 282.63
    - with
      - crisis 282.64
      - vaso-occlusive pain 282.64
  - Hb-S 282.61
    - with
      - crisis 282.62
      - Hb-C (without crisis)282.63
        - with
          - crisis 282.64
          - vaso-occlusive pain 282.64
      - other abnormal hemoglobin (Hb-D) (Hb-E) (Hb-G) (Hb-J) (Hb-K) (Hb-O) (Hb-P) (high fetal gene) (without crisis) 282.68
        - with crisis 282.69
  - spherocytosis 282.60
  - thalassemia (without crisis)282.41
    - with
      - crisis 282.42
      - vaso-occlusive pain 282.42
- Siegal-Cattan-Mamou (periodic) 277.31
- silo fillers' 506.9
- Simian B 054.3
- Simmonds' (pituitary cachexia) 253.2
- Simons' (progressive lipodystrophy) 272.6

Disease, diseased – Disease, diseased

Disease, diseased – *continued*
- Sinding-Larsen (juvenile osteopathia patellae) 732.4
- sinus – *see also* Sinusitis
  - brain 437.9
  - specified NEC 478.19
- Sirkari's 085.0
- sixth ▶(*see also* Exanthem subitum)◀ 058.10 ▲
- Sjögren (-Gougerot) 710.2
  - with lung involvement 710.2 *[517.8]*
- Skevas-Zerfus 989.5
- skin NEC 709.9
  - due to metabolic disorder 277.9
  - specified type NEC 709.8
- sleeping (*see also* Narcolepsy) 347.00
  - meaning sleeping sickness (*see also* Trypanosomiasis) 086.5
- small vessel 443.9
- Smith-Strang (oasthouse urine) 270.2
- Sneddon-Wilkinson (subcorneal pustular dermatosis) 694.1
- South African creeping 133.8
- Spencer's (epidemic vomiting) 078.82
- Spielmeyer-Stock 330.1
- Spielmeyer-Vogt 330.1
- spine, spinal 733.90
  - combined system (*see also* Degeneration, combined) 266.2 *[336.2]*
    - with pernicious anemia 281.0 *[336.2]*
  - cord NEC 336.9
    - congenital 742.9
  - demyelinating NEC 341.8
  - joint (*see also* Disease, joint, spine) 724.9
  - tuberculous 015.0❺ *[730.8]*❺
- spinocerebellar 334.9
  - specified NEC 334.8
- spleen (organic) (postinfectional) 289.50
  - amyloid 277.39
  - lardaceous 277.39
  - polycystic 759.0
  - specified NEC 289.59
- sponge divers' 989.5
- Stanton's (melioidosis) 025
- Stargardt's 362.75
- Startle 759.89
- Steinert's 359.21 ▲
- Sternberg's – *see* Disease, Hodgkin's
- Stevens-Johnson (erythema multiforme exudativum) 695.1
- Sticker's (erythema infectiosum) 057.0
- Stieda's (calcification, knee joint) 726.62
- Still's (juvenile rheumatoid arthritis) 714.30
- Stiller's (asthenia) 780.79
- Stokes' (exophthalmic goiter) 242.0❺
- Stokes-Adams (syncope with heart block) 426.9
- Stokvis (-Talma) (enterogenous cyanosis) 289.7
- stomach NEC (organic) 537.9
  - functional 536.9
    - psychogenic 306.4
  - lardaceous 277.39
- stonemasons' 502
- storage
  - glycogen (*see also* Disease, glycogen storage) 271.0
  - lipid 272.7
  - mucopolysaccharide 277.5
- striatopallidal system 333.90
  - specified NEC 333.89
- Strümpell-Marie (ankylosing spondylitis) 720.0
- Stuart's (congenital factor X deficiency) (*see also* Defect, coagulation) 286.3
- Stuart-Prower (congenital factor X deficiency) (*see also* Defect, coagulation) 286.3
- Sturge (-Weber) (-Dimitri) (encephalocutaneous angiomatosis) 759.6
- Stuttgart 100.89
- Sudeck's 733.7
- supporting structures of teeth NEC 525.9
- suprarenal (gland) (capsule) 255.9
  - hyperfunction 255.3
  - hypofunction 255.41 ▲
- Sutton's 709.09
- Sutton and Gull's – *see* Hypertension, kidney
- sweat glands NEC 705.9
  - specified type NEC 705.89
- sweating 078.2
- Sweeley-Klionsky 272.4
- Swift (-Feer) 985.0
- swimming pool (bacillus) 031.1
- swineherd's 100.89
- Sylvest's (epidemic pleurodynia) 074.1

Disease, diseased – *continued*
- Symmers (follicular lymphoma) (M9690/3) 202.0❺
- sympathetic nervous system (*see also* Neuropathy, peripheral, autonomic) 337.9
- synovium 727.9
- syphilitic – *see* Syphilis
- systemic tissue mast cell (M9741/3) 202.6❺
- Taenzer's 757.4
- Takayasu's (pulseless) 446.7
- Talma's 728.85
- Tangier (familial high-density lipoprotein deficiency) 272.5
- Tarral-Besnier (pityriasis rubra pilaris) 696.4
- Tay-Sachs 330.1
- Taylor's 701.8
- tear duct 375.69
- teeth, tooth 525.9
  - hard tissues 521.9
    - specified NEC 521.89
  - pulp NEC 522.9
- tendon 727.9
  - inflammatory NEC 727.9
- terminal vessel 443.9
- testis 608.9
- Thaysen-Gee (nontropical sprue) 579.0
- Thomsen's 359.22 ▲
- Thomson's (congenital poikiloderma) 757.33
- Thornwaldt's, Tornwaldt's (pharyngeal bursitis) 478.29
- throat 478.20
  - septic 034.0
- thromboembolic (*see also* Embolism) 444.9
- thymus (gland) 254.9
  - specified NEC 254.8
- thyroid (gland) NEC 246.9
  - heart (*see also* Hyperthyroidism) 242.9❺ *[425.7]*
  - lardaceous 277.39
  - specified NEC 246.8
- Tietze's 733.6
- Tommaselli's
  - correct substance properly administered 599.7
  - overdose or wrong substance given or taken 961.4
- tongue 529.9
- tonsils, tonsillar (and adenoids) (chronic) 474.9
  - specified NEC 474.8
- tooth, teeth 525.9
  - hard tissues 521.9
    - specified NEC 521.89
  - pulp NEC 522.9
- Tornwaldt's (pharyngeal bursitis) 478.29
- Tourette's 307.23
- trachea 519.19
- tricuspid – *see* Endocarditis, tricuspid
- triglyceride-storage, type I, II, III 272.7
- triple vessel – *see* Arteriosclerosis, coronary
- trisymptomatic, Gougerot's 709.1
- trophoblastic (*see also* Hydatidiform mole) 630
  - previous, affecting management of pregnancy V23.1
- tsutsugamushi (scrub typhus) 081.2
- tube (fallopian), noninflammatory 620.9
  - specified NEC 620.8
- tuberculous NEC (*see also* Tuberculosis) 011.9❺
- tubo-ovarian
  - inflammatory (*see also* Salpingo-oophoritis) 614.2
  - noninflammatory 620.9
    - specified NEC 620.8
- tubotympanic, chronic (with anterior perforation of ear drum) 382.1
- tympanum 385.9
- Uhl's 746.84
- umbilicus (newborn) NEC 779.89
  - delayed separation 779.83
- Underwood's (sclerema neonatorum) 778.1
- undiagnosed 799.9
- Unna's (seborrheic dermatitis) 690.18
- unstable hemoglobin hemolytic 282.7
- Unverricht (-Lundborg) 333.2
- Urbach-Oppenheim (necrobiosis lipoidica diabeticorum) 250.8❺ *[709.3]*
- Urbach-Wiethe (lipoid proteinosis) 272.8
- ureter 593.9
- urethra 599.9
  - specified type NEC 599.84
- urinary (tract) 599.9
  - bladder 596.9
    - specified NEC 596.8

Disease, diseased – *continued*
- urinary – *continued*
  - maternal, affecting fetus or newborn 760.1
- Usher-Senear (pemphigus erythematosus) 694.4
- uterus (organic) 621.9
  - infective (*see also* Endometritis) 615.9
  - inflammatory (*see also* Endometritis) 615.9
  - noninflammatory 621.9
    - specified type NEC 621.8
- uveal tract
  - anterior 364.9
  - posterior 363.9
- vagabonds' 132.1
- vagina, vaginal
  - inflammatory 616.10 ▲
  - noninflammatory 623.9
    - specified NEC 623.8
- Valsuani's (progressive pernicious anemia, puerperal) 648.2❺
  - complicating pregnancy or puerperium 648.2❺
- valve, valvular – *see* Endocarditis
- van Bogaert-Nijssen (-Peiffer) 330.0
- van Creveld-von Gierke (glycogenosis I) 271.0
- van den Bergh's (enterogenous cyanosis) 289.7
- van Neck's (juvenile osteochondrosis) 732.1
- Vaquez (-Osler) (polycythemia vera) (M9950/1) 238.4
- vascular 459.9
  - arteriosclerotic – *see* Arteriosclerosis
  - hypertensive – *see* Hypertension
  - obliterative 447.1
    - peripheral 443.9
  - occlusive 459.9
  - peripheral (occlusive) 443.9
    - in diabetes mellitus 250.7❺ *[443.81]*
    - specified type NEC 443.89
- vas deferens 608.9
- vasomotor 443.9
- vasospastic 443.9
- vein 459.9
- venereal 099.9
  - chlamydial NEC 099.50
    - anus 099.52
    - bladder 099.53
    - cervix 099.53
    - epididymis 099.54
    - genitourinary NEC 099.55
      - lower 099.53
      - specified NEC 099.54
    - pelvic inflammatory disease 099.54
    - perihepatic 099.56
    - peritoneum 099.56
    - pharynx 099.51
    - rectum 099.52
    - specified site NEC 099.59
    - testis 099.54
    - vagina 099.53
    - vulva 099.53
  - fifth 099.1
  - sixth 099.1
  - complicating pregnancy, childbirth, or puerperium 647.2❺
  - specified nature or type NEC 099.8
    - chlamydial – *see* Disease, venereal, chlamydial
- Verneuil's (syphilitic bursitis) 095.7
- Verse's (calcinosis intervertebralis) 275.49 *[722.90]*
- vertebra, vertebral NEC 733.90
  - disc – *see* Disease, Intervertebral disc
- vibration NEC 994.9
- Vidal's (lichen simplex chronicus) 698.3
- Vincent's (trench mouth) 101
- Virchow's 733.99
- virus (filterable) NEC 078.89
  - arbovirus NEC 066.9
  - arthropod-borne NEC 066.9
  - central nervous system NEC 049.9
    - specified type NEC 049.8
  - complicating pregnancy, childbirth, or puerperium 647.6❺
  - contact (with) V01.79
    - varicella V01.71
  - exposure to V01.79
    - varicella V01.71
  - Marburg 078.89
  - maternal
    - with fetal damage affecting management of pregnancy 655.3❺

Disease, diseased – Disease, diseased

- **Disease, diseased** – *continued*
  - virus – *continued*
    - nonarthropod-borne NEC 078.89
      - central nervous system NEC 049.9
        - specified NEC 049.8
    - vaccination, prophylactic (against) V04.89
  - vitreous 379.29
  - vocal cords NEC 478.5
  - Vogt's (Cecile) 333.71
  - Vogt-Spielmeyer 330.1
  - Volhard-Fahr (malignant nephrosclerosis) 403.00
  - Volkmann's
    - acquired 958.6
  - von Bechterew's (ankylosing spondylitis) 720.0
  - von Economo's (encephalitis lethargica) 049.8
  - von Eulenburg's (congenital paramyotonia) 359.29 ▲
  - von Gierke's (glycogenosis I) 271.0
  - von Graefe's 378.72
  - von Hippel's (retinocerebral angiomatosis) 759.6
  - von Hippel-Lindau (angiomatosis retinocerebellosa) 759.6
  - von Jaksch's (pseudoleukemia infantum) 285.8
  - von Recklinghausen's (M9540/1) 237.71
    - bone (osteitis fibrosa cystica) 252.01
  - von Recklinghausen-Applebaum (hemochromatosis) 275.0
  - von Willebrand (-Jürgens) (angiohemophilia) 286.4
  - von Zambusch's (lichen sclerosus et atrophicus) 701.0
  - Voorhoeve's (dyschondroplasia) 756.4
  - Vrolik's (osteogenesis imperfecta) 756.51
  - vulva
    - inflammatory 616.10 ▲
    - noninflammatory 624.9
      - specified NEC 624.8
  - Wagner's (colloid milium) 709.3
  - Waldenström's (osteochondrosis capital femoral) 732.1
  - Wallgren's (obstruction of splenic vein with collateral circulation) 459.89
  - Wardrop's (with lymphangitis) 681.9
    - finger 681.02
    - toe 681.11
  - Wassilieff's (leptospiral jaundice) 100.0
  - wasting NEC 799.4
    - due to malnutrition 261
    - paralysis 335.21
  - Waterhouse-Friderichsen 036.3
  - waxy (any site) 277.39
  - Weber-Christian (nodular nonsuppurative panniculitis) 729.30
  - Wegner's (syphilitic osteochondritis) 090.0
  - Weil's (leptospiral jaundice) 100.0
    - of lung 100.0
  - Weir Mitchell's (erythromelalgia) 443.82
  - Werdnig-Hoffmann 335.0
  - Werlhof's (*see also* Purpura, thrombocytopenic) 287.39
  - Wermer's 258.01 ▲
  - Werner's (progeria adultorum) 259.8
  - Werner-His (trench fever) 083.1
  - Werner-Schultz (agranulocytosis) 288.09
  - Wernicke's (superior hemorrhagic polioencephalitis) 265.1
  - Wernicke-Posadas 114.9
  - Whipple's (intestinal lipodystrophy) 040 2
  - whipworm 127.3
  - white
    - blood cell 288.9
      - specified NEC 288.8
    - spot 701.0
  - White's (congenital) (keratosis follicularis) 757.39
  - Whitmore's (melioidosis) 025
  - Widal-Abrami (acquired hemolytic jaundice) 283.9
  - Wilkie's 557.1
  - Wilkinson-Sneddon (subcorneal pustular dermatosis) 694.1
  - Willis' (diabetes mellitus) (*see also* Diabetes) 250.0❺
  - Wilson's (hepatolenticular degeneration) 275.1
  - Wilson-Brocq (dermatitis exfoliativa) 695.89
  - winter vomiting 078.82
  - Wise's 696.2
  - Wohlfart-Kugelberg-Welander 335.11
  - Woillez's (acute idiopathic pulmonary congestion) 518.5
  - Wolman's (primary familial xanthomatosis) 272.7
  - wool-sorters' 022.1
  - Zagari's (xerostomia) 527.7
  - Zahorsky's (exanthem subitum) 058.10 ▲
  - Ziehen-Oppenheim 333.6

- **Disease, diseased** – *continued*
  - zoonotic, bacterial NEC 027.9
    - specified type NEC 027.8
- **Disfigurement** (due to scar) 709.2
  - head V48.6
  - limb V49.4
  - neck V48.7
  - trunk V48.7
- **Disgerminoma** – *see* Dysgerminoma
- **Disinsertion, retina** 361.04
- **Disintegration, complete, of the body** 799.89
  - traumatic 869.1
- **Disk kidney** 753.3
- **Dislocatable hip, congenital** (*see also* Dislocation, hip, congenital) 754.30
- **Dislocation** (articulation) (closed) (displacement) (simple) (subluxation) 839.8

Note – "Closed" includes simple, complete, partial, uncomplicated, and unspecified dislocation.

"Open" includes dislocation specified as infected or compound and dislocation with foreign body.

"Chronic," "habitual," "old," or "recurrent" dislocations should be coded as indicated under the entry "Dislocation, recurrent"; and "pathological" as indicated under the entry "Dislocation, pathological."

For late effect of dislocation see Late, effect, dislocation.

  - with fracture – *see* Fracture, by site
  - acromioclavicular (joint) (closed) 831.04
    - open 831.14
  - anatomical site (closed)
    - specified NEC 839.69
      - open 839.79
    - unspecified or ill-defined 839.8
      - open 839.9
  - ankle (scaphoid bone) (closed) 837.0
    - open 837.1
  - arm (closed) 839.8
    - open 839.9
  - astragalus (closed) 837.0
    - open 837.1
  - atlanto-axial (closed) 839.01
    - open 839.11
  - atlas (closed) 839.01
    - open 839.11
  - axis (closed) 839.02
    - open 839.12
  - back (closed) 839.8
    - open 839.9
  - Bell-Daly 723.8
  - breast bone (closed) 839.61
    - open 839.71
  - capsule, joint – *see* Dislocation, by site
  - carpal (bone) – *see* Dislocation, wrist
  - carpometacarpal (joint) (closed) 833.04
    - open 833.14
  - cartilage (joint) – *see also* Dislocation, by site
    - knee – *see* Tear, meniscus
  - cervical, cervicodorsal, or cervicothoracic (spine) (vertebra) – *see* Dislocation, vertebra, cervical
  - chiropractic (*see also* Lesion, nonallopathic) 739.9
  - chondrocostal – *see* Dislocation, costochondral
  - chronic – *see* Dislocation, recurrent
  - clavicle (closed) 831.04
    - open 831.14
  - coccyx (closed) 839.41
    - open 839.51
  - collar bone (closed) 831.04
    - open 831.14
  - compound (open) NEC 839.9
  - congenital NEC 755.8
    - hip (*see also* Dislocation, hip, congenital) 754.30
    - lens 743.37
    - rib 756.3
    - sacroiliac 755.69
    - spine NEC 756.19
    - vertebra 756.19
  - coracoid (closed) 831.09
    - open 831.19
  - costal cartilage (closed) 839.69
    - open 839.79
  - costochondral (closed) 839.69
    - open 839.79

- **Dislocation** – *continued*
  - cricoarytenoid articulation (closed) 839.69
    - open 839.79
  - cricothyroid (cartilage) articulation (closed) 839.69
    - open 839.79
  - dorsal vertebrae (closed) 839.21
    - open 839.31
  - ear ossicle 385.23
  - elbow (closed) 832.00
    - anterior (closed) 832.01
      - open 832.11
    - congenital 754.89
    - divergent (closed) 832.09
      - open 832.19
    - lateral (closed) 832.04
      - open 832.14
    - medial (closed) 832.03
      - open 832.13
    - open 832.10
    - posterior (closed) 832.02
      - open 832.12
    - recurrent 718.32
    - specified type NEC 832.09
      - open 832.19
  - eye 360.81
    - lateral 376.36
  - eyeball 360.81
    - lateral 376.36
  - femur
    - distal end (closed) 836.50
      - anterior 836.52
        - open 836.62
      - lateral 836.53
        - open 836.63
      - medial 836.54
        - open 836.64
      - open 836.60
      - posterior 836.51
        - open 836.61
    - proximal end (closed) 835.00
      - anterior (pubic) 835.03
        - open 835.13
      - obturator 835.02
        - open 835.12
      - open 835.10
      - posterior 835.01
        - open 835.11
  - fibula
    - distal end (closed) 837.0
      - open 837.1
    - proximal end (closed) 836.59
      - open 836.69
  - finger(s) (phalanx) (thumb) (closed) 834.00
    - interphalangeal (joint) 834.02
      - open 834.12
    - metacarpal (bone), distal end 834.01
      - open 834.11
    - metacarpophalangeal (joint) 834.01
      - open 834.11
    - open 834.10
    - recurrent 718.34
  - foot (closed) 838.00
    - open 838.10
    - recurrent 718.37
  - forearm (closed) 839.8
    - open 839.9
  - fracture – *see* Fracture, by site
  - glenoid (closed) 831.09
    - open 831.19
  - habitual – *see* Dislocation, recurrent
  - hand (closed) 839.8
    - open 839.9
  - hip (closed) 835.00
    - anterior 835.03
      - obturator 835.02
        - open 835.12
      - open 835.13
    - congenital (unilateral) 754.30
      - with subluxation of other hip 754.35
      - bilateral 754.31
    - developmental 718.75
    - open 835.10
    - posterior 835.01
      - open 835.11
    - recurrent 718.35
  - humerus (closed) 831.00
    - distal end (*see also* Dislocation, elbow) 832.00
    - open 831.10

- **Dislocation** – *continued*
  - humerus – *continued*
    - proximal end (closed) 831.00
      - anterior (subclavicular) (subcoracoid) (subglenoid) (closed) 831.01
        - open 831.11
      - inferior (closed) 831.03
        - open 831.13
      - open 831.10
      - posterior (closed) 831.02
        - open 831.12
  - implant – *see* Complications, mechanical
  - incus 385.23
  - infracoracoid (closed) 831.01
    - open 831.11
  - innominate (pubic junction) (sacral junction) (closed) 839.69
    - acetabulum (*see also* Dislocation, hip) 835.00
    - open 839.79
  - interphalangeal (joint)
    - finger or hand (closed) 834.02
      - open 834.12
    - foot or toe (closed) 838.06
      - open 838.16
  - jaw (cartilage) (meniscus) (closed) 830.0
    - open 830.1
    - recurrent 524.69
  - joint NEC (closed) 839.8
    - developmental 718.7❺
    - open 839.9
    - pathological – *see* Dislocation, pathological
    - recurrent – *see* Dislocation, recurrent
  - knee (closed) 836.50
    - anterior 836.51
      - open 836.61
    - congenital (with genu recurvatum) 754.41
    - habitual 718.36
    - lateral 836.54
      - open 836.64
    - medial 836.53
      - open 836.63
    - old 718.36
    - open 836.60
    - posterior 836.52
      - open 836.62
    - recurrent 718.36
    - rotatory 836.59
      - open 836.69
  - lacrimal gland 375.16
  - leg (closed) 839.8
    - open 839.9
  - lens (crystalline) (complete) (partial) 379.32
    - anterior 379.33
    - congenital 743.37
    - ocular implant 996.53
    - posterior 379.34
    - traumatic 921.3
  - ligament – *see* Dislocation, by site
  - lumbar (vertebrae) (closed) 839.20
    - open 839.30
  - lumbosacral (vertebrae) (closed) 839.20
    - congenital 756.19
    - open 839.30
  - mandible (closed) 830.0
    - open 830.1
  - maxilla (inferior) (closed) 830.0
    - open 830.1
  - meniscus (knee) – *see also* Tear, meniscus
    - other sites – *see* Dislocation, by site
  - metacarpal (bone)
    - distal end (closed) 834.01
      - open 834.11
    - proximal end (closed) 833.05
      - open 833.15
  - metacarpophalangeal (joint) (closed) 834.01
    - open 834.11
  - metatarsal (bone) (closed) 838.04
    - open 838.14
  - metatarsophalangeal (joint) (closed) 838.05
    - open 838.15
  - midcarpal (joint) (closed) 833.03
    - open 833.13
  - midtarsal (joint) (closed) 838.02
    - open 838.12
  - Monteggia's – *see* Dislocation, hip
  - multiple locations (except fingers only or toes only) (closed) 839.8
    - open 839.9
  - navicular (bone) foot (closed) 837.0
    - open 837.1
  - neck (*see also* Dislocation, vertebra, cervical) 839.00

- **Dislocation** – *continued*
  - Nélaton's – *see* Dislocation, ankle
  - nontraumatic (joint) – *see* Dislocation, pathological
  - nose (closed) 839.69
    - open 839.79
  - not recurrent, not current injury – *see* Dislocation, pathological
  - occiput from atlas (closed) 839.01
    - open 839.11
  - old – *see* Dislocation, recurrent
  - open (compound) NEC 839.9
  - ossicle, ear 385.23
  - paralytic (flaccid) (spastic) – *see* Dislocation, pathological
  - patella (closed) 836.3
    - congenital 755.64
    - open 836.4
  - pathological NEC 718.20
    - ankle 718.27
    - elbow 718.22
    - foot 718.27
    - hand 718.24
    - hip 718.25
    - knee 718.26
    - lumbosacral joint 724.6
    - multiple sites 718.29
    - pelvic region 718.25
    - sacroiliac 724.6
    - shoulder (region) 718.21
    - specified site NEC 718.28
    - spine 724.8
      - sacroiliac 724.6
    - wrist 718.23
  - pelvis (closed) 839.69
    - acetabulum (*see also* Dislocation, hip) 835.00
    - open 839.79
  - phalanx
    - foot or toe (closed) 838.09
      - open 838.19
    - hand or finger (*see also* Dislocation, finger) 834.00
  - postpoliomyelitic – *see* Dislocation, pathological
  - prosthesis, internal – *see* Complications, mechanical
  - radiocarpal (joint) (closed) 833.02
    - open 833.12
  - radioulnar (joint)
    - distal end (closed) 833.01
      - open 833.11
    - proximal end (*see also* Dislocation, elbow) 832.00
  - radius
    - distal end (closed) 833.00
      - open 833.10
    - proximal end (closed) 832.01
      - open 832.11
  - recurrent (*see also* Derangement, joint, recurrent) 718.3❺
    - elbow 718.32
    - hip 718.35
    - joint NEC 718.38
    - knee 718.36
    - lumbosacral (joint) 724.6
    - patella 718.36
    - sacroiliac 724.6
    - shoulder 718.31
    - temporomandibular 524.69
  - rib (cartilage) (closed) 839.69
    - congenital 756.3
    - open 839.79
  - sacrococcygeal (closed) 839.42
    - open 839.52
  - sacroiliac (joint) (ligament) (closed) 839.42
    - congenital 755.69
    - open 839.52
    - recurrent 724.6
  - sacrum (closed) 839.42
    - open 839.52
  - scaphoid (bone)
    - ankle or foot (closed) 837.0
      - open 837.1
    - wrist (closed) (*see also* Dislocation, wrist) 833.00
      - open 833.10
  - scapula (closed) 831.09
    - open 831.19
  - semilunar cartilage, knee – *see* Tear, meniscus
  - septal cartilage (nose) (closed) 839.69
    - open 839.79
  - septum (nasal) (old) 470
  - sesamoid bone – *see* Dislocation, by site

- **Dislocation** – *continued*
  - shoulder (blade) (ligament) (closed) 831.00
    - anterior (subclavicular) (subcoracoid) (subglenoid) (closed) 831.01
      - open 831.11
    - chronic 718.31
    - inferior 831.03
      - open 831.13
    - open 831.10
    - posterior (closed) 831.02
      - open 831.12
    - recurrent 718.31
  - skull – *see* Injury, intracranial
  - Smith's – *see* Dislocation, foot
  - spine (articular process) (*see also* Dislocation, vertebra) (closed) 839.40
    - atlanto-axial (closed) 839.01
      - open 839.11
      - recurrent 723.8
    - cervical, cervicodorsal, cervicothoracic (closed) (*see also* Dislocation, vertebrae, cervical) 839.00
      - open 839.10
      - recurrent 723.8
    - coccyx 839.41
      - open 839.51
    - congenital 756.19
    - due to birth trauma 767.4
    - open 839.50
    - recurrent 724.9
    - sacroiliac 839.42
      - recurrent 724.6
    - sacrum (sacrococcygeal) (sacroiliac) 839.42
      - open 839.52
  - spontaneous – *see* Dislocation, pathological
  - sternoclavicular (joint) (closed) 839.61
    - open 839.71
  - sternum (closed) 839.61
    - open 839.71
  - subastragalar – *see* Dislocation, foot
  - subglenoid (closed) 831.01
    - open 831.11
  - symphysis
    - jaw (closed) 830.0
      - open 830.1
    - mandibular (closed) 830.0
      - open 830.1
    - pubis (closed) 839.69
      - open 839.79
  - tarsal (bone) (joint) 838.01
    - open 838.11
  - tarsometatarsal (joint) 838.03
    - open 838.13
  - temporomandibular (joint) (closed) 830.0
    - open 830.1
    - recurrent 524.69
  - thigh
    - distal end (*see also* Dislocation, femur, distal end) 836.50
    - proximal end (*see also* Dislocation, hip) 835.00
  - thoracic (vertebrae) (closed) 839.21
    - open 839.31
  - thumb(s) (*see also* Dislocation, finger) 834.00
  - thyroid cartilage (closed) 839.69
    - open 839.79
  - tibia
    - distal end (closed) 837.0
      - open 837.1
    - proximal end (closed) 836.50
      - anterior 836.51
        - open 836.61
      - lateral 836.54
        - open 836.64
      - medial 836.53
        - open 836.63
      - open 836.60
      - posterior 836.52
        - open 836.62
      - rotatory 836.59
        - open 836.69
  - tibiofibular
    - distal (closed) 837.0
      - open 837.1
    - superior (closed) 836.59
      - open 836.69
  - toe(s) (closed) 838.09
    - open 838.19
  - trachea (closed) 839.69
    - open 839.79
  - ulna
    - distal end (closed) 833.09
      - open 833.19

- **Dislocation** – *continued*
  - ulna – *continued*
    - proximal end – *see* Dislocation, elbow
  - vertebra (articular process) (body) (closed) (traumatic) 839.40
    - cervical, cervicodorsal or cervicothoracic (closed) 839.00
      - first (atlas) 839.01
        - open 839.11
      - second (axis) 839.02
        - open 839.12
      - third 839.03
        - open 839.13
      - fourth 839.04
        - open 839.14
      - fifth 839.05
        - open 839.15
      - sixth 839.06
        - open 839.16
      - seventh 839.07
        - open 839.17
      - congenital 756.19
      - multiple sites 839.08
        - open 839.18
      - open 839.10
    - congenital 756.19
    - dorsal 839.21
      - open 839.31
      - recurrent 724.9
    - lumbar, lumbosacral 839.20
      - open 839.30
    - non-traumatic – *see* Displacement, intervertebral disc
    - open NEC 839.50
    - recurrent 724.9
    - specified region NEC 839.49
      - open 839.59
    - thoracic 839.21
      - open 839.31
  - wrist (carpal bone) (scaphoid) (semilunar) (closed) 833.00
    - carpometacarpal (joint) 833.04
      - open 833.14
    - metacarpal bone, proximal end 833.05
      - open 833.15
    - midcarpal (joint) 833.03
      - open 833.13
    - open 833.10
    - radiocarpal (joint) 833.02
      - open 833.12
    - radioulnar (joint) 833.01
      - open 833.11
    - recurrent 718.33
    - specified site NEC 833.09
      - open 833.19
  - xiphoid cartilage (closed) 839.61
    - open 839.71
- **Dislodgement**
  - artificial skin graft 996.55
  - decellularized allodermis graft 996.55
- **Disobedience, hostile** (covert) (overt) (*see also* Disturbance, conduct) 312.0❺
- **Disorder** – *see also* Disease
  - academic underachievement, childhood and adolescence 313.83
  - accommodation 367.51
    - drug-induced 367.89
    - toxic 367.89
  - adjustment (*see also* Reaction, adjustment) 309.9
    - with
      - anxiety 309.24
      - anxiety and depressed mood 309.28
      - depressed mood 309.0
      - disturbance of conduct 309.3
      - disturbance of emotions and conduct 309.4
  - adrenal (capsule) (cortex) (gland) 255.9
    - specified type NEC 255.8
  - adrenogenital 255.2
  - affective (*see also* Psychosis, affective) 296.90
    - atypical 296.81
  - aggressive, unsocialized (*see also* Disturbance, conduct) 312.0❺
  - alcohol, alcoholic (*see also* Alcohol) 291.9
  - allergic – *see* Allergy
  - amino acid (metabolic) (*see also* Disturbance, metabolism, amino acid) 270.9
    - albinism 270.2
    - alkaptonuria 270.2
    - argininosuccinicaciduria 270.6
    - beta-amino-isobutyricaciduria 277.2
- **Disorder** – *continued*
  - amino acid – *continued*
    - cystathioninuria 270.4
    - cystinosis 270.0
    - cystinuria 270.0
    - glycinuria 270.0
    - homocystinuria 270.4
    - imidazole 270.5
    - maple syrup (urine) disease 270.3
    - neonatal, transitory 775.89
    - oasthouse urine disease 270.2
    - ochronosis 270.2
    - phenylketonuria 270.1
    - phenylpyruvic oligophrenia 270.1
    - purine NEC 277.2
    - pyrimidine NEC 277.2
    - renal transport NEC 270.0
    - specified type NEC 270.8
    - transport NEC 270.0
      - renal 270.0
    - xanthinuria 277.2
  - amnestic (*see also* Amnestic syndrome) 294.8
    - alcohol-induced persisting 291.1
    - drug-induced persisting 292.83
    - in conditions classified elsewhere 294.0
  - anaerobic glycolysis with anemia 282.3
  - anxiety (*see also* Anxiety) 300.00
    - due to or associated with physical condition 293.84
  - arteriole 447.9
    - specified type NEC 447.8
  - artery 447.9
    - specified type NEC 447.8
  - articulation – *see* Disorder, joint
  - Asperger's 299.8❺
  - attachment of infancy or early childhood 313.89
  - attention deficit 314.00
    - with hyperactivity 314.01
    - predominantly
      - combined hyperactive/inattentive 314.01
      - hyperactive/impulsive 314.01
      - inattentive 314.00
    - residual type 314.8
  - auditory processing disorder 388.45 ●
    - acquired 388.45 ●
    - developmental 315.32 ●
  - autistic 299.0❺
  - autoimmune NEC 279.4
    - hemolytic (cold type) (warm type) 283.0
    - parathyroid 252.1
    - thyroid 245.2
  - avoidant, childhood or adolescence 313.21
  - balance
    - acid-base 276.9
      - mixed (with hypercapnia) 276.4
    - electrolyte 276.9
    - fluid 276.9
  - behavior NEC (*see also* Disturbance, conduct) 312.9
    - disruptive 312.9
  - bilirubin excretion 277.4
  - bipolar (affective) (alternating) 296.80

    Note – Use the following fifth-digit subclassification with categories 296.0-296.6:

    0 unspecified
    1 mild
    2 moderate
    3 severe, without mention of psychotic behavior
    4 severe, specified as with psychotic behavior
    5 in partial or unspecified remission
    6 in full remission

    - atypical 296.7
    - mixed 296.6❺
    - specified type NEC 296.89
    - type I 296.7
      - most recent episode (or current)❺
        - depressed 296.5❺
        - hypomaniac 296.4❺
        - manic 296.4❺
        - mixed 296.6❺
        - unspecified 296.7
      - single manic episode 296.0❺
    - type II (recurrent major depressive episodes with hypomania) 296.89
  - bladder 596.9
    - functional NEC 596.59
    - specified NEC 596.8
  - bleeding 286.9 ●
- **Disorder** – *continued*
  - bone NEC 733.90
    - specified NEC 733.99
  - brachial plexus 353.0
  - branched-chain amino-acid degradation 270.3
  - breast 611.9
    - puerperal, postpartum 676.3❺
    - specified NEC 611.8
  - Briquet's 300.81
  - bursa 727.9
    - shoulder region 726.10
  - carbohydrate metabolism, congenital 271.9
  - cardiac, functional 427.9
    - postoperative 997.1
    - psychogenic 306.2
  - cardiovascular, psychogenic 306.2
  - cartilage NEC 733.90
    - articular 718.00
      - ankle 718.07
      - elbow 718.02
      - foot 718.07
      - hand 718.04
      - hip 718.05
      - knee 717.9
      - multiple sites 718.09
      - pelvic region 718.05
      - shoulder region 718.01
      - specified
        - site NEC 718.08
        - type NEC 733.99
      - wrist 718.03
  - catatonic – *see* Catatonia
  - central auditory processing 315.32
    - acquired 388.45 ●
    - developmental 315.32 ●
  - cervical region NEC 723.9
  - cervical root (nerve) NEC 353.2
  - character NEC (*see also* Disorder, personality) 301.9
  - ciliary body 364.9 ●
    - specified NEC 364.89 ●
  - coagulation (factor) (*see also* Defect, coagulation) 286.9
    - factor VIII (congenital) (functional) 286.0
    - factor IX (congenital) (functional) 286.1
    - neonatal, transitory 776.3
  - coccyx 724.70
    - specified NEC 724.79
  - cognitive 294.9
  - colon 569.9
    - functional 564.9
      - congenital 751.3
  - communication 307.9
  - conduct (*see also* Disturbance, conduct) 312.9
    - adjustment reaction 309.3
    - adolescent onset type 312.82
    - childhood onset type 312.81
    - compulsive 312.30
      - specified type NEC 312.39
    - hyperkinetic 314.2
    - onset unspecified 312.89
    - socialized (type) 312.20
      - aggressive 312.23
      - unaggressive 312.21
    - specified NEC 312.89
  - conduction, heart 426.9
    - specified NEC 426.89
  - conflict
    - sexual orientation 302.0
  - congenital
    - glycosylation (CDG) 271.8
  - convulsive (secondary) (*see also* Convulsions) 780.39
    - due to injury at birth 767.0
    - idiopathic 780.39
  - coordination 781.3
  - cornea NEC 371.89
    - due to contact lens 371.82
  - corticosteroid metabolism NEC 255.2
  - cranial nerve – *see* Disorder, nerve, cranial
  - cyclothymic 301.13
  - degradation, branched-chain amino acid 270.3
  - delusional 297.1
  - dentition 520.6
  - depersonalization 300.6
  - depressive NEC 311
    - atypical 296.82
    - major (*see also* Psychosis, affective) 296.2❺
      - recurrent episode 296.3❺
      - single episode 296.2❺
  - development, specific 315.9
    - associated with hyperkinesia 314.1

Dislocation – Disorder

Disorder – *continued*
- development, specific – *continued*
  - coordination 315.4
  - language 315.31
    - and speech due to hearing loss 315.34 ●
  - learning 315.2
    - arithmetical 315.1
    - reading 315.00
  - mixed 315.5
  - motor coordination 315.4
  - specified type NEC 315.8
  - speech 315.39
    - and language due to hearing loss 315.34 ●
- diaphragm 519.4
- digestive 536.9
  - fetus or newborn 777.9
    - specified NEC 777.8
  - psychogenic 306.4
- disintegrative, childhood 299.1❺
- dissociative 300.15
  - identity 300.14
  - nocturnal 307.47
- drug-related 292.9
- dysmorphic body 300.7
- dysthymic 300.4
- ear 388.9
  - degenerative NEC 388.00
  - external 380.9
    - specified 380.89
  - pinna 380.30
  - specified type NEC 388.8
  - vascular NEC 388.00
- eating NEC 307.50
- electrolyte NEC 276.9
  - with
    - abortion – *see* Abortion, by type, with metabolic disorder
    - ectopic pregnancy (*see also* categories 633.0-633.9) 639.4
    - molar pregnancy (*see also* categories 630-632) 639.4
  - acidosis 276.2
    - metabolic 276.2
    - respiratory 276.2
  - alkalosis 276.3
    - metabolic 276.3
    - respiratory 276.3
  - following
    - abortion 639.4
    - ectopic or molar pregnancy 639.4
  - neonatal, transitory NEC 775.5
- emancipation as adjustment reaction 309.22
- emotional (*see also* Disorder, mental, nonpsychotic) V40.9
- endocrine 259.9
  - specified type NEC 259.8
- esophagus 530.9
  - functional 530.5
  - psychogenic 306.4
- explosive
  - intermittent 312.34
  - isolated 312.35
- expressive language 315.31
- eye 379.90
  - globe – *see* Disorder, globe
  - ill-defined NEC 379.99
  - limited duction NEC 378.63
  - specified NEC 379.8
- eyelid 374.9
  - degenerative 374.50
  - sensory 374.44
  - specified type NEC 374.89
  - vascular 374.85
- factitious (with combined psychological and physical signs and symptoms) (with predominately physical signs and symptoms) 300.19
  - with predominately psychological signs and symptoms 300.16
- factor, coagulation (*see also* Defect, coagulation) 286.9
  - VIII (congenital) (functional) 286.0
  - IX (congenital) (functional) 286.1
- fascia 728.9
- fatty acid oxidation 277.85
- feeding – *see* Feeding
- female sexual arousal 302.72
- fluid NEC 276.9
- gastric (functional) 536.9
  - motility 536.8
  - psychogenic 306.4
  - secretion 536.8

Disorder – *continued*
- gastrointestinal (functional) NEC 536.9
  - newborn (neonatal) 777.9
    - specified NEC 777.8
  - psychogenic 306.4
- gender (child) 302.6
  - adult 302.85
- gender identity (childhood) 302.6
  - adolescents 302.85
  - adults (-life) 302.85
- genitourinary system, psychogenic 306.50
- globe 360.9
  - degenerative 360.20
    - specified NEC 360.29
  - specified type NEC 360.89
- hearing – *see also* Deafness
  - conductive type (air) (*see also* Deafness, conductive) 389.00
  - mixed conductive and sensorineural 389.20 ▲
    - bilateral 389.22 ●
    - unilateral 389.21 ●
  - nerve
    - bilateral 389.12 ●
    - unilateral 389.13 ●
  - perceptive (*see also* Deafness, perceptive) 389.10
  - sensorineural type NEC (*see also* Deafness, sensorineural) 389.10
- heart action 427.9
  - postoperative 997.1
- hematological, transient neonatal 776.9
  - specified type NEC 776.8
- hematopoietic organs 289.9
- hemorrhagic NEC 287.9
  - due to intrinsic circulating anticoagulants 286.5
  - specified type NEC 287.8
- hemostasis (*see also* Defect, coagulation) 286.9
- homosexual conflict 302.0
- hypomanic (chronic) 301.11
- identity
  - childhood and adolescence 313.82
    - gender 302.6
- immune mechanism (immunity) 279.9
  - single complement (C1-C9) 279.8
  - specified type NEC 279.8
- impulse control (*see also* Disturbance, conduct, compulsive) 312.30
- infant sialic acid storage 271.8
- integument, fetus or newborn 778.9
  - specified type NEC 778.8
- interactional psychotic (childhood) (*see also* Psychosis, childhood) 299.1❺
- intermittent explosive 312.34
- intervertebral disc 722.90
  - cervical, cervicothoracic 722.91
  - lumbar, lumbosacral 722.93
  - thoracic, thoracolumbar 722.92
- intestinal 569.9
  - functional NEC 564.9
    - congenital 751.3
    - postoperative 564.4
  - psychogenic 306.4
- introverted, of childhood and adolescence 313.22
- involuntary emotional expression (IEED) 310.8 ●
- iris 364.9 ●
  - specified NEC 364.89 ●
- iron, metabolism 275.0
- isolated explosive 312.35
- joint NEC 719.90
  - ankle 719.97
  - elbow 719.92
  - foot 719.97
  - hand 719.94
  - hip 719.95
  - knee 719.96
  - multiple sites 719.99
  - pelvic region 719.95
  - psychogenic 306.0
  - shoulder (region) 719.91
  - specified site NEC 719.98
  - temporomandibular 524.60
    - sounds on opening or closing 524.64
    - specified NEC 524.69
  - wrist 719.93
- kidney 593.9
  - functional 588.9
    - specified NEC 588.89
- labyrinth, labyrinthine 386.9
  - specified type NEC 386.8
- lactation 676.9❺

Disorder – *continued*
- language (developmental) (expressive) 315.31
  - mixed receptive-expressive 315.32
- learning 315.9
- ligament 728.9
- ligamentous attachments, peripheral – *see also* Enthesopathy
  - spine 720.1
- limb NEC 729.9
  - psychogenic 306.0
- lipid
  - metabolism, congenital 272.9
  - storage 272.7
- lipoprotein deficiency (familial) 272.5
- low back NEC 724.9
  - psychogenic 306.0
- lumbosacral
  - plexus 353.1
  - root (nerve) NEC 353.4
- lymphoproliferative (chronic) NEC (M9970/1) 238.79
- major depressive (*see also* Psychosis, affective) 296.2❺
  - recurrent episode 296.3❺
  - single episode 296.2❺
- male erectile 607.84
  - nonorganic origin 302.72
- manic (*see also* Psychosis, affective) 296.0❺
  - atypical 296.81
- mathematics 315.1
- meniscus NEC (*see also* Disorder, cartilage, articular) 718.0❺
- menopausal 627.9
  - specified NEC 627.8
- menstrual 626.9
  - psychogenic 306.52
  - specified NEC 626.8
- mental (nonpsychotic) 300.9
  - affecting management of pregnancy, childbirth, or puerperium 648.4❺
  - drug-induced 292.9
    - hallucinogen persisting perception 292.89
    - specified type NEC 292.89
  - due to or associated with
    - alcoholism 291.9
    - drug consumption NEC 292.9
      - specified type NEC 292.89
    - physical condition NEC 293.9
  - induced by drug 292.9
    - specified type NEC 292.89
  - neurotic (*see also* Neurosis) 300.9
  - of infancy, childhood or adolesence 313.9
  - persistent
    - other
      - due to conditions classified elsewhere 294.8
    - unspecified
      - due to conditions classified elsewhere 293.9
  - presenile 310.1
    - psychotic NEC 290.10
  - previous, affecting management of pregnancy V23.8❺
  - psychoneurotic (*see also* Neurosis) 300.9
  - psychotic (*see also* Psychosis) 298.9
    - brief 298.8
    - senile 290.20
  - specific, following organic brain damage 310.9
    - cognitive or personality change of other type 310.1
    - frontal lobe syndrome 310.0
    - postconcussional syndrome 310.2
    - specified type NEC 310.8
  - transient
    - in conditions classified elsewhere 293.9
- metabolism NEC 277.9
  - with
    - abortion – *see* Abortion, by type, with metabolic disorder
    - ectopic pregnancy (*see also* categories 633.0-633.9) 639.4
    - molar pregnancy (*see also* categories 630-632) 639.4
  - alkaptonuria 270.2
  - amino acid (*see also* Disorder, amino acid) 270.9
    - specified type NEC 270.8
  - ammonia 270.6
  - arginine 270.6
  - argininosuccinic acid 270.6
  - basal 794.7
  - bilirubin 277.4

Disorder – Disorder

Disorder – *continued*
metabolism – *continued*
calcium 275.40
carbohydrate 271.9
specified type NEC 271.8
cholesterol 272.9
citrulline 270.6
copper 275.1
corticosteroid 255.2
cystine storage 270.0
cystinuria 270.0
fat 272.9
fatty acid oxidation 277.85
following
abortion 639.4
ectopic or molar pregnancy 639.4
fructosemia 271.2
fructosuria 271.2
fucosidosis 271.8
galactose-1-phosphate uridyl transferase 271.1
glutamine 270.7
glycine 270.7
glycogen storage NEC 271.0
hepatorenal 271.0
hemochromatosis 275.0
in labor and delivery 669.0⑤
iron 275.0
lactose 271.3
lipid 272.9
specified type NEC 272.8
storage 272.7
lipoprotein – *see also* Hyperlipemia
deficiency (familial) 272.5
lysine 270.7
magnesium 275.2
mannosidosis 271.8
mineral 275.9
specified type NEC 275.8
mitochondrial 277.87
mucopolysaccharide 277.5
nitrogen 270.9
ornithine 270.6
oxalosis 271.8
pentosuria 271.8
phenylketonuria 270.1
phosphate 275.3
phosphorus 275.3
plasma protein 273.9
specified type NEC 273.8
porphyrin 277.1
purine 277.2
pyrimidine 277.2
serine 270.7
sodium 276.9
specified type NEC 277.89
steroid 255.2
threonine 270.7
urea cycle 270.6
xylose 271.8
micturition NEC 788.69
psychogenic 306.53
misery and unhappiness, of childhood and adolescence 313.1
mitochondrial metabolism 277.87
mitral valve 424.0
mood (*see also* Disorder, bipolar) 296.90
episodic 296.30
specified NEC 296.99
in conditions classified elsewhere 293.83
motor tic 307.20
chronic 307.22
transient (childhood) 307.21
movement NEC 333.90
hysterical 300.11
medication-induced 333.90
periodic limb 327.51
sleep related, unspecified 780.58
other organic 327.59
specified type NEC 333.99
stereotypic 307.3
mucopolysaccharide 277.5
muscle 728.9
psychogenic 306.0
specified type NEC 728.3
muscular attachments, peripheral – *see also* Enthesopathy
spine 720.1
musculoskeletal system NEC 729.9
psychogenic 306.0
myeloproliferative (chronic) NEC (M9960/1) 238.79

Disorder – *continued*
myoneural 358.9
due to lead 358.2
specified type NEC 358.8
toxic 358.2
myotonic 359.29 ▲
neck region NEC 723.9
nerve 349.9
abducens NEC 378.54
accessory 352.4
acoustic 388.5
auditory 388.5
auriculotemporal 350.8
axillary 353.0
cerebral – *see* Disorder, nerve, cranial
cranial 352.9
first 352.0
second 377.49
third
partial 378.51
total 378.52
fourth 378.53
fifth 350.9
sixth 378.54
seventh NEC 351.9
eighth 388.5
ninth 352.2
tenth 352.3
eleventh 352.4
twelfth 352.5
multiple 352.6
entrapment – *see* Neuropathy, entrapment
facial 351.9
specified NEC 351.8
femoral 355.2
glossopharyngeal NEC 352.2
hypoglossal 352.5
iliohypogastric 355.79
ilioinguinal 355.79
intercostal 353.8
lateral
cutaneous of thigh 355.1
popliteal 355.3
lower limb NEC 355.8
medial, popliteal 355.4
median NEC 354.1
obturator 355.79
oculomotor
partial 378.51
total 378.52
olfactory 352.0
optic 377.49
hypoplasia 377.43
ischemic 377.41
nutritional 377.33
toxic 377.34
peroneal 355.3
phrenic 354.8
plantar 355.6
pneumogastric 352.3
posterior tibial 355.5
radial 354.3
recurrent laryngeal 352.3
root 353.9
specified NEC 353.8
saphenous 355.79
sciatic NEC 355.0
specified NEC 355.9
lower limb 355.79
upper limb 354.8
spinal 355.9
sympathetic NEC 337.9
trigeminal 350.9
specified NEC 350.8
trochlear 378.53
ulnar 354.2
upper limb NEC 354.9
vagus 352.3
nervous system NEC 349.9
autonomic (peripheral) (*see also* Neuropathy, peripheral, autonomic) 337.9
cranial 352.9
parasympathetic (*see also* Neuropathy, peripheral, autonomic) 337.9
specified type NEC 349.89
sympathetic (*see also* Neuropathy, peripheral, autonomic) 337.9
vegetative (*see also* Neuropathy, peripheral, autonomic) 337.9
neurohypophysis NEC 253.6
neurological NEC 781.99
peripheral NEC 355.9

Disorder – *continued*
neuromuscular NEC 358.9
hereditary NEC 359.1
specified NEC 358.8
toxic 358.2
neurotic 300.9
specified type NEC 300.89
neutrophil, polymorphonuclear (functional) 288.1
nightmare 307.47
night terror 307.46
obsessive-compulsive 300.3
oppositional defiant, childhood and adolescence 313.81
optic
chiasm 377.54
associated with
inflammatory disorders 377.54
neoplasm NEC 377.52
pituitary 377.51
pituitary disorders 377.51
vascular disorders 377.53
nerve 377.49
radiations 377.63
tracts 377.63
orbit 376.9
specified NEC 376.89
orgasmic
female 302.73
male 302.74
overanxious, of childhood and adolescence 313.0
oxidation, fatty acid 277.85
pancreas, internal secretion (other than diabetes mellitus) 251.9
specified type NEC 251.8
panic 300.01
with agoraphobia 300.21
papillary muscle NEC 429.81
paranoid 297.9
induced 297.3
shared 297.3
parathyroid 252.9
specified type NEC 252.8
paroxysmal, mixed 780.39
pentose phosphate pathway with anemia 282.2
periodic limb movement 327.51
peroxisomal 277.86
personality 301.9
affective 301.10
aggressive 301.3
amoral 301.7
anancastic, anankastic 301.4
antisocial 301.7
asocial 301.7
asthenic 301.6
avoidant 301.82
borderline 301.83
compulsive 301.4
cyclothymic 301.13
dependent-passive 301.6
dyssocial 301.7
emotional instability 301.59
epileptoid 301.3
explosive 301.3
following organic brain damage 310.1
histrionic 301.50
hyperthymic 301.11
hypomanic (chronic) 301.11
hypothymic 301.12
hysterical 301.50
immature 301.89
inadequate 301.6
introverted 301.21
labile 301.59
moral deficiency 301.7
narcissistic 301.81
obsessional 301.4
obsessive-compulsive 301.4
overconscientious 301.4
paranoid 301.0
passive (-dependent) 301.6
passive-aggressive 301.84
pathological NEC 301.9
pseudosocial 301.7
psychopathic 301.9
schizoid 301.20
introverted 301.21
schizotypal 301.22
schizotypal 301.22
seductive 301.59
type A 301.4
unstable 301.59

Disorder – *continued*
- pervasive developmental 299.9❺
  - childhood-onset 299.8❺
  - specified NEC 299.8❺
- phonological 315.39
- pigmentation, choroid (congenital) 743.53
- pinna 380.30
  - specified type NEC 380.39
- pituitary, thalamic 253.9
  - anterior NEC 253.4
  - iatrogenic 253.7
  - postablative 253.7
  - specified NEC 253.8
- pityriasis-like NEC 696.8
- platelets (blood) 287.1
- polymorphonuclear neutrophils (functional) 288.1
- porphyrin metabolism 277.1
- postmenopausal 627.9
  - specified type NEC 627.8
- posttraumatic stress 309.81
  - acute 309.81
  - brief 309.81
  - chronic 309.81
- post-traumatic stress (PTSD) 309.81
- premenstrual dysphoric (PMDD) 625.4
- psoriatic-like NEC 696.8
- psychic, with diseases classified elsewhere 316
- psychogenic NEC (*see also* condition) 300.9
  - allergic NEC
    - respiratory 306.1
  - anxiety 300.00
    - atypical 300.00
    - generalized 300.02
  - appetite 307.59
  - articulation, joint 306.0
  - asthenic 300.5
  - blood 306.8
  - cardiovascular (system) 306.2
  - compulsive 300.3
  - cutaneous 306.3
  - depressive 300.4
  - digestive (system) 306.4
  - dysmenorrheic 306.52
  - dyspneic 306.1
  - eczematous 306.3
  - endocrine (system) 306.6
  - eye 306.7
  - feeding 307.59
  - functional NEC 306.9
  - gastric 306.4
  - gastrointestinal (system) 306.4
  - genitourinary (system) 306.50
  - heart (function) (rhythm) 306.2
  - hemic 306.8
  - hyperventilatory 306.1
  - hypochondriacal 300.7
  - hysterical 300.10
  - intestinal 306.4
  - joint 306.0
  - learning 315.2
  - limb 306.0
  - lymphatic (system) 306.8
  - menstrual 306.52
  - micturition 306.53
  - monoplegic NEC 306.0
  - motor 307.9
  - muscle 306.0
  - musculoskeletal 306.0
  - neurocirculatory 306.2
  - obsessive 300.3
  - occupational 300.89
  - organ or part of body NEC 306.9
  - organs of special sense 306.7
  - paralytic NEC 306.0
  - phobic 300.20
  - physical NEC 306.9
  - pruritic 306.3
  - rectal 306.4
  - respiratory (system) 306.1
  - rheumatic 306.0
  - sexual (function) 302.70
    - specified type NEC 302.79
  - sexual orientation conflict 302.0
  - skin (allergic) (eczematous) (pruritic) 306.3
  - sleep 307.40
    - initiation or maintenance 307.41
      - persistent 307.42
      - transient 307.41
    - movement 780.58
    - sleep terror 307.46
    - specified type NEC 307.49
  - specified part of body NEC 306.8

Disorder – *continued*
- psychogenic – *continued*
  - stomach 306.4
- psychomotor NEC 307.9
  - hysterical 300.11
- psychoneurotic (*see also* Neurosis) 300.9
  - mixed NEC 300.89
- psychophysiologic (*see also* Disorder, psychosomatic) 306.9
- psychosexual identity (childhood) 302.6
  - adult-life 302.85
- psychosomatic NEC 306.9
  - allergic NEC
    - respiratory 306.1
  - articulation, joint 306.0
  - cardiovascular (system) 306.2
  - cutaneous 306.3
  - digestive (system) 306.4
  - dysmenorrheic 306.52
  - dyspneic 306.1
  - endocrine (system) 306.6
  - eye 306.7
  - gastric 306.4
  - gastrointestinal (system) 306.4
  - genitourinary (system) 306.50
  - heart (functional) (rhythm) 306.2
  - hyperventilatory 306.1
  - intestinal 306.4
  - joint 306.0
  - limb 306.0
  - lymphatic (system) 306.8
  - menstrual 306.52
  - micturition 306.53
  - monoplegic NEC 306.0
  - muscle 306.0
  - musculoskeletal 306.0
  - neurocirculatory 306.2
  - organs of special sense 306.7
  - paralytic NEC 306.0
  - pruritic 306.3
  - rectal 306.4
  - respiratory (system) 306.1
  - rheumatic 306.0
  - sexual (function) 302.70
    - specified type NEC 302.79
  - skin 306.3
  - specified part of body NEC 306.8
  - stomach 306.4
- psychotic (*see also* Psychosis) 298.9
  - brief 298.8
- purine metabolism NEC 277.2
- pyrimidine metabolism NEC 277.2
- reactive attachment of infancy or early childhood 313.89
- reading, developmental 315.00
- reflex 796.1
- REM sleep behavior 327.42
- renal function, impaired 588.9
  - specified type NEC 588.89
- renal transport NEC 588.89
- respiration, respiratory NEC 519.9
  - due to
    - aspiration of liquids or solids 508.9
    - inhalation of fumes or vapors 506.9
  - psychogenic 306.1
- retina 362.9
  - specified type NEC 362.89
- rumination 307.53
- sacroiliac joint NEC 724.6
- sacrum 724.6
- schizo-affective (*see also* Schizophrenia) 295.7❺
- schizoid, childhood or adolescence 313.22
- schizophreniform 295.4❺
- schizotypal personality 301.22
- secretion, thyrocalcitonin 246.0
- seizure 345.9
  - recurrent 345.9
    - epileptic – *see* Epilepsy
- sense of smell 781.1
  - psychogenic 306.7
- separation anxiety 309.21
- sexual (*see also* Deviation, sexual) 302.9
  - aversion 302.79
  - desire, hypoactive 302.71
  - function, psychogenic 302.70
- shyness, of childhood and adolescence 313.21
- single complement (C1-C9) 279.8
- skin NEC 709.9
  - fetus or newborn 778.9
    - specified type 778.8

Disorder – *continued*
- skin – *continued*
  - psychogenic (allergic) (eczematous) (pruritic) 306.3
  - specified type NEC 709.8
  - vascular 709.1
- sleep 780.50
  - with apnea – *see* Apnea, sleep
  - alcohol-induced 291.82
  - arousal 307.46
    - confusional 327.41
  - circadian rhythm 327.30
    - advanced sleep phase type 327.32
    - alcohol-induced 291.82
    - delayed sleep phase type 327.31
    - drug-induced 292.85
    - free running type 327.34
    - in conditions classified elsewhere 327.37
    - irregular sleep wake type 327.33
    - jet lag type 327.35
    - other 327.39
    - shift work type 327.36
  - drug-induced 292.85
  - initiation or maintenance (*see also* Insomnia) 780.52
    - nonorganic origin (transient) 307.41
      - persistent 307.42
  - nonorganic origin 307.40
    - specified type NEC 307.49
  - organic specified type NEC 327.8
  - periodic limb movement 327.51
  - specified NEC 780.59
  - wake
    - cycle – *see* Disorder, sleep, circadian rhythm
    - schedule – *see* Disorder, sleep, circadian rhythm
- social, of childhood and adolescence 313.22
- soft tissue 729.9
- somatization 300.81
- somatoform (atypical) (undifferentiated) 300.82
  - severe 300.81
  - specified type NEC 300.89
- speech NEC 784.5
  - nonorganic origin 307.9
- spine NEC 724.9
  - ligamentous or muscular attachments, peripheral 720.1
- steroid metabolism NEC 255.2
- stomach (functional) (*see also* Disorder, gastric) 536.9
  - psychogenic 306.4
- storage, iron 275.0
- stress (*see also* Reaction, stress, acute) 308.3
  - posttraumatic
    - acute 309.81
    - brief 309.81
    - chronic (motor or vocal) 309.81
- substitution 300.11
- suspected – *see* Observation
- synovium 727.9
- temperature regulation, fetus or newborn 778.4
- temporomandibular joint NEC 524.60
  - sounds on opening or closing 524.64
  - specified NEC 524.69
- tendon 727.9
  - shoulder region 726.10
- thoracic root (nerve) NEC 353.3
- thyrocalcitonin secretion 246.0
- thyroid (gland) NEC 246.9
  - specified type NEC 246.8
- tic 307.20
  - chronic (motor or vocal) 307.22
  - motor-verbal 307.23
  - organic origin 333.1
  - transient (of childhood) 307.21
- tooth NEC 525.9
  - development NEC 520.9
    - specified type NEC 520.8
  - eruption 520.6
  - specified type NEC 525.8
- Tourette's 307.23
- transport, carbohydrate 271.9
  - specified type NEC 271.8
- tubular, phosphate-losing 588.0
- tympanic membrane 384.9
- unaggressive, unsocialized (*see also* Disturbance, conduct) 312.1❺
- undersocialized, unsocialized (*see also* Disturbance, conduct)
  - aggressive (type) 312.0❺
  - unaggressive (type) 312.1❺

Disorder – *continued*
vision, visual NEC 368.9
binocular NEC 368.30
cortex 377.73
associated with
inflammatory disorders 377.73
neoplasms 377.71
vascular disorders 377.72
pathway NEC 377.63
associated with
inflammatory disorders 377.63
neoplasms 377.61
vascular disorders 377.62
vocal tic
chronic 307.22
wakefulness (*see also* Hypersomnia) 780.54
nonorganic origin (transient) 307.43
persistent 307.44
written expression 315.2
Disorganized globe 360.29
Displacement, displaced

Note – For acquired displacement of bones, cartilage, joints, tendons, due to injury, see also Dislocation.

Displacements at ages under one year should be considered congenital, provided there is no indication the condition was acquired after birth.

acquired traumatic of bone, cartilage, joint, tendon NEC (without fracture) (*see also* Dislocation) 839.8
with fracture – *see* Fracture, by site
adrenal gland (congenital) 759.1
alveolus and teeth, vertical 524.75
appendix, retrocecal (congenital) 751.5
auricle (congenital) 744.29
bladder (acquired) 596.8
congenital 753.8
brachial plexus (congenital) 742.8
brain stem, caudal 742.4
canaliculus lacrimalis 743.65
cardia, through esophageal hiatus 750.6
cerebellum, caudal 742.4
cervix – *see* Displacement, uterus
colon (congenital) 751.4
device, implant, or graft – *see* Complications, mechanical
epithelium
columnar of cervix 622.10
cuboidal, beyond limits of external os (uterus) 752.49
esophageal mucosa into cardia of stomach, congenital 750.4
esophagus (acquired) 530.89
congenital 750.4
eyeball (acquired) (old) 376.36
congenital 743.8
current injury 871.3
lateral 376.36
fallopian tube (acquired) 620.4
congenital 752.19
opening (congenital) 752.19
gallbladder (congenital) 751.69
gastric mucosa 750.7
into
duodenum 750.7
esophagus 750.7
Meckel's diverticulum, congenital 750.7
globe (acquired) (lateral) (old) 376.36
current injury 871.3
graft
artificial skin graft 996.55
decellularized allodermis graft 996.55
heart (congenital) 746.87
acquired 429.89
hymen (congenital) (upward) 752.49
internal prosthesis NEC – *see* Complications, mechanical
intervertebral disc (with neuritis, radiculitis, sciatica, or other pain) 722.2
with myelopathy 722.70
cervical, cervicodorsal, cervicothoracic 722.0
with myelopathy 722.71
due to major trauma – *see* Dislocation, vertebra, cervical
due to trauma – *see* Dislocation, vertebra
lumbar, lumbosacral 722.10
with myelopathy 722.73
due to major trauma – *see* Dislocation, vertebra, lumbar

Displacement, displaced – *continued*
intervertebral disc – *continued*
thoracic, thoracolumbar 722.11
with myelopathy 722.72
due to major trauma – *see* Dislocation, vertebra, thoracic
intrauterine device 996.32
kidney (acquired) 593.0
congenital 753.3
lacrimal apparatus or duct (congenital) 743.65
macula (congenital) 743.55
Meckel's diverticulum (congenital) 751.0
nail (congenital) 757.5
acquired 703.8
opening of Wharton's duct in mouth 750.26
organ or site, congenital NEC – *see* Malposition, congenital
ovary (acquired) 620.4
congenital 752.0
free in peritoneal cavity (congenital) 752.0
into hernial sac 620.4
oviduct (acquired) 620.4
congenital 752.19
parathyroid (gland) 252.8
parotid gland (congenital) 750.26
punctum lacrimale (congenital) 743.65
sacroiliac (congenital) (joint) 755.69
current injury – *see* Dislocation, sacroiliac
old 724.6
spine (congenital) 756.19
spleen, congenital 759.0
stomach (congenital) 750.7
acquired 537.89
subglenoid (closed) 831.01
sublingual duct (congenital) 750.26
teeth, tooth 524.30
horizontal 524.33
vertical 524.34
tongue (congenital) (downward) 750.19
trachea (congenital) 748.3
ureter or ureteric opening or orifice (congenital) 753.4
uterine opening of oviducts or fallopian tubes 752.19
uterus, uterine (*see also* Malposition, uterus) 621.6
congenital 752.3
ventricular septum 746.89
with rudimentary ventricle 746.89
xyphoid bone (process) 738.3
Disproportion 653.9❺
affecting fetus or newborn 763.1
caused by
conjoined twins 653.7❺
contraction, pelvis (general) 653.1❺
inlet 653.2❺
midpelvic 653.8❺
midplane 653.8❺
outlet 653.3❺
fetal
ascites 653.7❺
hydrocephalus 653.6❺
hydrops 653.7❺
meningomyelocele 653.7❺
sacral teratoma 653.7❺
tumor 653.7❺
hydrocephalic fetus 653.6❺
pelvis, pelvic, abnormality (bony) NEC 653.0❺
unusually large fetus 653.5❺
causing obstructed labor 660.1❺
cephalopelvic, normally formed fetus 653.4❺
causing obstructed labor 660.1❺
fetal NEC 653.5❺
causing obstructed labor 660.1❺
fetopelvic, normally formed fetus 653.4❺
causing obstructed labor 660.1❺
mixed maternal and fetal origin, normally, formed fetus 653.4❺
pelvis, pelvic (bony) NEC 653.1❺
causing obstructed labor 660.1❺
specified type NEC 653.8❺
Disruption
cesarean wound 674.1❺
family V61.0
gastrointestinal anastomosis 997.4
ligament(s) – *see also* Sprain
knee
current injury – *see* Dislocation, knee
old 717.89
capsular 717.85
collateral (medial) 717.82
lateral 717.81

Disruption – *continued*
ligament(s) – *continued*
knee – *continued*
old – *continued*
cruciate (posterior) 717.84
anterior 717.83
specified site NEC 717.85
marital V61.10
involving divorce or estrangement V61.0
operation wound (external) 998.32
internal 998.31
organ transplant, anastomosis site – *see* Complications, transplant, organ, by site
ossicles, ossicular chain 385.23
traumatic – *see* Fracture, skull, base
parenchyma
liver (hepatic) – *see* Laceration, liver, major
spleen – *see* Laceration, spleen, parenchyma, massive
phase-shift, of 24 hour sleep wake cycle, unspecified 780.55
nonorganic origin 307.45
sleep wake cycle (24 hour)(unspecified) 780.55
circadian rhythm 327.33
nonorganic origin 307.45
suture line (external) 998.32
internal 998.31
wound
cesarean operation 674.1❺
episiotomy 674.2❺
operation 998.32
cesarean 674.1❺
internal 998.31
perineal (obstetric) 674.2❺
uterine 674.1❺
Disruptio uteri – *see also* Rupture, uterus
complicating delivery – *see* Delivery, complicated, rupture, uterus
Dissatisfaction with
employment V62.2
school environment V62.3
Dissecting – *see* condition
Dissection
aorta 441.00
abdominal 441.02
thoracic 441.01
thoracoabdominal 441.03
artery, arterial
carotid 443.21
coronary 414.12
iliac 443.22
renal 443.23
specified NEC 443.29
vertebral 443.24
vascular 459.9
wound – *see* Wound, open, by site
Disseminated – *see* condition
Dissociated personality NEC 300.15
Dissociation
auriculoventricular or atrioventricular (any degree) (AV) 426.89
with heart block 426.0
interference 426.89
isorhythmic 426.89
rhythm
atrioventricular (AV) 426.89
interference 426.89
Dissociative
identity disorder 300.14
reaction NEC 300.15
Dissolution, vertebra (*see also* Osteoporosis) 733.00
Distention
abdomen (gaseous) 787.3
bladder 596.8
cecum 569.89
colon 569.89
gallbladder 575.8
gaseous (abdomen) 787.3
intestine 569.89
kidney 593.89
liver 573.9
seminal vesicle 608.89
stomach 536.8
acute 536.1
psychogenic 306.4
ureter 593.5
uterus 621.8
Distichia, distichiasis (eyelid) 743.63
Distoma hepaticum infestation 121.3

Distomiasis 121.9
  bile passages 121.3
    due to Clonorchis sinensis 121.1
  hemic 120.9
  hepatic (liver) 121.3
    due to Clonorchis sinensis (clonorchiasis) 121.1
  intestinal 121.4
  liver 121.3
    due to Clonorchis sinensis 121.1
  lung 121.2
  pulmonary 121.2
Distomolar (fourth molar) 520.1
  causing crowding 524.31
Disto-occlusion (division I) (division II) 524.22
Distortion (congenital)
  adrenal (gland) 759.1
  ankle (joint) 755.69
  anus 751.5
  aorta 747.29
  appendix 751.5
  arm 755.59
  artery (peripheral) NEC (*see also* Distortion, peripheral vascular system) 747.60
    cerebral 747.81
    coronary 746.85
    pulmonary 747.3
    retinal 743.58
    umbilical 747.5
  auditory canal 744.29
    causing impairment of hearing 744.02
  bile duct or passage 751.69
  bladder 753.8
  brain 742.4
  bronchus 748.3
  cecum 751.5
  cervix (uteri) 752.49
  chest (wall) 756.3
  clavicle 755.51
  clitoris 752.49
  coccyx 756.19
  colon 751.5
  common duct 751.69
  cornea 743.41
  cricoid cartilage 748.3
  cystic duct 751.69
  duodenum 751.5
  ear 744.29
    auricle 744.29
      causing impairment of hearing 744.02
    causing impairment of hearing 744.09
    external 744.29
      causing impairment of hearing 744.02
    inner 744.05
    middle, except ossicles 744.03
      ossicles 744.04
    ossicles 744.04
  endocrine (gland) NEC 759.2
  epiglottis 748.3
  Eustachian tube 744.24
  eye 743.8
    adnexa 743.69
  face bone(s) 756.0
  fallopian tube 752.19
  femur 755.69
  fibula 755.69
  finger(s) 755.59
  foot 755.67
  gallbladder 751.69
  genitalia, genital organ(s)
    female 752.89
      external 752.49
      internal NEC 752.89
    male 752.89
      penis 752.69
  glottis 748.3
  gyri 742.4
  hand bone(s) 755.59
  heart (auricle) (ventricle) 746.89
    valve (cusp) 746.89
  hepatic duct 751.69
  humerus 755.59
  hymen 752.49
  ileum 751.5
  intestine (large) (small) 751.5
    with anomalous adhesions, fixation or malrotation 751.4
  jaw NEC 524.89
  jejunum 751.5
  kidney 753.3
  knee (joint) 755.64
Distortion – *continued*
  labium (majus) (minus) 752.49
  larynx 748.3
  leg 755.69
  lens 743.36
  liver 751.69
  lumbar spine 756.19
    with disproportion (fetopelvic) 653.0❺
      affecting fetus or newborn 763.1
      causing obstructed labor 660.1❺
  lumbosacral (joint) (region) 756.19
  lung (fissures) (lobe) 748.69
  nerve 742.8
  nose 748.1
  organ
    of Corti 744.05
    of site not listed – *see* Anomaly, specified type NEC
  ossicles, ear 744.04
  ovary 752.0
  oviduct 752.19
  pancreas 751.7
  parathyroid (gland) 759.2
  patella 755.64
  peripheral vascular system NEC 747.60
    gastrointestinal 747.61
    lower limb 747.64
    renal 747.62
    spinal 747.82
    upper limb 747.63
  pituitary (gland) 759.2
  radius 755.59
  rectum 751.5
  rib 756.3
  sacroiliac joint 755.69
  sacrum 756.19
  scapula 755.59
  shoulder girdle 755.59
  site not listed – *see* Anomaly, specified type NEC
  skull bone(s) 756.0
    with
      anencephalus 740.0
      encephalocele 742.0
      hydrocephalus 742.3
        with spina bifida (*see also* Spina bifida) 741.0❺
      microcephalus 742.1
  spinal cord 742.59
  spine 756.19
  spleen 759.0
  sternum 756.3
  thorax (wall) 756.3
  thymus (gland) 759.2
  thyroid (gland) 759.2
    cartilage 748.3
  tibia 755.69
  toe(s) 755.66
  tongue 750.19
  trachea (cartilage) 748.3
  ulna 755.59
  ureter 753.4
    causing obstruction 753.20
  urethra 753.8
    causing obstruction 753.6
  uterus 752.3
  vagina 752.49
  vein (peripheral) NEC (*see also* Distortion, peripheral vascular system) 747.60
    great 747.49
    portal 747.49
    pulmonary 747.49
  vena cava (inferior) (superior) 747.49
  vertebra 756.19
  visual NEC 368.15
    shape or size 368.14
  vulva 752.49
  wrist (bones) (joint) 755.59
Distress
  abdomen 789.0❺
  colon 564.9❺
  emotional V40.9
  epigastric 789.0❺
  fetal (syndrome) 768.4
    affecting management of pregnancy or childbirth 656.8❺
    liveborn infant 768.4
      first noted
        before onset of labor 768.2
        during labor and delivery 768.3
    stillborn infant (death before onset of labor) 768.0
      death during labor 768.1
Distress – *continued*
  gastrointestinal (functional) 536.9
    psychogenic 306.4
  intestinal (functional) NEC 564.9
    psychogenic 306.4
  intrauterine – *see* Distress, fetal
  leg 729.5
  maternal 669.0❺
  mental V40.9
  respiratory 786.09
    acute (adult) 518.82
    adult syndrome (following shock, surgery, or trauma) 518.5
      specified NEC 518.82
    fetus or newborn 770.89
    syndrome (idiopathic) (newborn) 769
  stomach 536.9
    psychogenic 306.4
Distribution vessel, atypical NEC 747.60
  coronary artery 746.85
  spinal 747.82
Districhiasis 704.2
Disturbance – *see also* Disease
  absorption NEC 579.9
    calcium 269.3
    carbohydrate 579.8
    fat 579.8
    protein 579.8
    specified type NEC 579.8
    vitamin (*see also* Deficiency, vitamin) 269.2
  acid-base equilibrium 276.9
  activity and attention, simple, with hyperkinesis 314.01
  amino acid (metabolic) (*see also* Disorder, amino acid) 270.9
    imidazole 270.5
    maple syrup (urine) disease 270.3
    transport 270.0
  assimilation, food 579.9
  attention, simple 314.00
    with hyperactivity 314.01
  auditory, nerve, except deafness 388.5
  behavior (*see also* Disturbance, conduct) 312.9
  blood clotting (hypoproteinemia) (mechanism) (*see also* Defect, coagulation) 286.9
  central nervous system NEC 349.9
  cerebral nerve NEC 352.9
  circulatory 459.9
  conduct 312.9
    adjustment reaction 309.3
    adolescent onset type 312.82
    childhood onset type 312.81

Note – Use the following fifth-digit subclassification with categories 312.0-312.2:
0 unspecified
1 mild
2 moderate
3 severe

    compulsive 312.30
      intermittent explosive disorder 312.34
      isolated explosive disorder 312.35
      kleptomania 312.32
      pathological gambling 312.31
      pyromania 312.33
    hyperkinetic 314.2
    intermittent explosive 312.34
    isolated explosive 312.35
    mixed with emotions 312.4
    socialized (type) 312.20
      aggressive 312.23
      unaggressive 312.21
    specified type NEC 312.89
    undersocialized, unsocialized
      aggressive (type) 312.0❺
      unaggressive (type) 312.1❺
  coordination 781.3
  cranial nerve NEC 352.9
  deep sensibility – *see* Disturbance, sensation
  digestive 536.9
    psychogenic 306.4
  electrolyte – *see* Imbalance, electrolyte
  emotions specific to childhood or adolescence 313.9
    with
      academic underachievement 313.83
      anxiety and fearfulness 313.0
      elective mutism 313.23
      identity disorder 313.82
      jealousy 313.3
      misery and unhappiness 313.1

Distomiasis – Disturbance

Diverticula, diverticulosis, diverticulum – Drug

- **Drug** – *continued*
  - hypersensitivity 995.27
  - induced
    - circadian rhythm sleep disorder 292.85
    - hypersomnia 292.85
    - insomnia 292.85
    - mental disorder 292.9
      - anxiety 292.89
      - mood 292.84
      - sexual 292.89
      - sleep 292.85
      - specified type 292.89
    - parasomnia 292.85
    - persisting
      - amnestic disorder 292.83
      - dementia 292.82
    - psychotic disorder
      - with
        - delusions 292.11
        - hallucinations 292.12
    - sleep disorder 292.85
  - intoxication 292.89
  - overdose – *see* Table of Drugs and Chemicals
  - poisoning – *see* Table of Drugs and Chemicals
  - therapy (maintenance) status NEC
    - chemotherapy, antineoplastic V58.11
    - immunotherapy, antineoplastic V58.12
    - long-term (current) use V58.69
      - antibiotics V58.62
      - anticoagulants V58.61
      - anti-inflammatories, non-steroidal (NSAID) V58.64
      - antiplatelets V58.63
      - antithrombotics V58.63
      - aspirin V58.66
      - high-risk medications NEC V58.69 ●
      - insulin V58.67
      - steroids V58.65
  - wrong substance given or taken in error – *see* Table of Drugs and Chemicals
- **Drunkenness** (*see also* Abuse, drugs, nondependent) 305.0❺
  - acute in alcoholism (*see also* Alcoholism) 303.0❺
  - chronic (*see also* Alcoholism) 303.9❺
  - pathologic 291.4
  - simple (acute) 305.0❺
    - in alcoholism 303.0❺
  - sleep 307.47
- **Drusen**
  - optic disc or papilla 377.21
  - retina (colloid) (hyaloid degeneration) 362.57
    - hereditary 362.77
- **Drusenfieber** 075
- **Dry, dryness** – *see also* condition
  - eye 375.15
    - syndrome 375.15
  - larynx 478.79
  - mouth 527.7
  - nose 478.19
  - skin syndrome 701.1
  - socket (teeth) 526.5
  - throat 478.29
- **DSAP** (disseminated superficial actinic porokeratosis) 692.75
- **Duane's retraction syndrome** 378.71
- **Duane-Stilling-Türk syndrome** (ocular retraction syndrome) 378.71
- **Dubin-Johnson disease or syndrome** 277.4
- **Dubini's disease** (electric chorea) 049.8
- **Dubois' abscess or disease** 090.5
- **Duchenne's**
  - disease 094.0
    - locomotor ataxia 094.0
    - muscular dystrophy 359.1
    - pseudohypertrophy, muscles 359.1
  - paralysis 335.22
  - syndrome 335.22
- **Duchenne-Aran myelopathic, muscular atrophy** (nonprogressive) (progressive) 335.21
- **Duchenne-Griesinger disease** 359.1
- **Ducrey's**
  - bacillus 099.0
  - chancre 099.0
  - disease (chancroid) 099.0
- **Duct, ductus** – *see* condition
- **Duengero** 061
- **Duhring's disease** (dermatitis herpetiformis) 694.0
- **Dukes** (-Filatov) disease 057.8
- **Dullness**
  - cardiac (decreased) (increased) 785.3
- **Dumb ague** (*see also* Malaria) 084.6
- **Dumbness** (*see also* Aphasia) 784.3
- **Dumdum fever** 085.0
- **Dumping syndrome** (postgastrectomy) 564.2
  - nonsurgical 536.8
- **Duodenitis** (nonspecific) (peptic) 535.60
  - with hemorrhage 535.61
  - due to
    - strongyloides stercoralis 127.2
- **Duodenocholangitis** 575.8
- **Duodenum, duodenal** – *see* condition
- **Duplay's disease, periarthritis, or syndrome** 726.2
- **Duplex** – *see also* Accessory
  - kidney 753.3
  - placenta – *see* Placenta, abnormal
  - uterus 752.2
- **Duplication** – *see also* Accessory
  - anus 751.5
  - aortic arch 747.21
  - appendix 751.5
  - biliary duct (any) 751.69
  - bladder 753.8
  - cecum 751.5
    - and appendix 751.5
  - clitoris 752.49
  - cystic duct 751.69
  - digestive organs 751.8
  - duodenum 751.5
  - esophagus 750.4
  - fallopian tube 752.19
  - frontonasal process 756.0
  - gallbladder 751.69
  - ileum 751.5
  - intestine (large) (small) 751.5
  - jejunum 751.5
  - kidney 753.3
  - liver 751.69
  - nose 748.1
  - pancreas 751.7
  - penis 752.69
  - respiratory organs NEC 748.9
  - salivary duct 750.22
  - spinal cord (incomplete) 742.51
  - stomach 750.7
  - ureter 753.4
  - vagina 752.49
  - vas deferens 752.89
  - vocal cords 748.3
- **Dupré's disease or syndrome** (meningism) 781.6
- **Dupuytren's**
  - contraction 728.6
  - disease (muscle contracture) 728.6
  - fracture (closed) 824.4
    - ankle (closed) 824.4
      - open 824.5
    - fibula (closed) 824.4
      - open 824.5
    - open 824.5
    - radius (closed) 813.42
      - open 813.52
  - muscle contracture 728.6
- **Durand-Nicolas-Favre disease** (climatic bubo) 099.1
- **Duroziez's disease** (congenital mitral stenosis) 746.5
- **Dust**
  - conjunctivitis 372.05
  - reticulation (occupational) 504
  - disease (trypanosomiasis) 086.9
- **Dutton's**
  - relapsing fever (West African) 087.1
- **Dwarf, dwarfism** 259.4
  - with infantilism (hypophyseal) 253.3
  - achondroplastic 756.4
  - Amsterdam 759.89
  - bird-headed 759.89
  - congenital 259.4
  - constitutional 259.4
  - hypophyseal 253.3
  - infantile 259.4
  - Levi type 253.3
  - Lorain-Levi (pituitary) 253.3
  - Lorain type (pituitary) 253.3
  - metatropic 756.4
  - nephrotic-glycosuric, with hypophosphatemic rickets 270.0
  - nutritional 263.2
  - ovarian 758.6
  - pancreatic 577.8
- **Dwarf, dwarfism** – *continued*
  - pituitary 253.3
  - polydystrophic 277.5
  - primordial 253.3
  - psychosocial 259.4
  - renal 588.0
    - with hypertension – *see* Hypertension, kidney
  - Russell's (uterine dwarfism and craniofacial dysostosis) 759.89
- **Dyke-Young anemia or syndrome** (acquired macrocytic hemolytic anemia) (secondary) (symptomatic) 283.9
- **Dynia abnormality** (*see also* Defect, coagulation) 286.9
- **Dysacousis** 388.40
- **Dysadrenocortism** 255.9
  - hyperfunction 255.3
  - hypofunction 255.41 ▲
- **Dysarthria** 784.5
- **Dysautonomia** (*see also* Neuropathy, peripheral, autonomic) 337.9
  - familial 742.8
- **Dysbarism** 993.3
- **Dysbasia** 719.7❺
  - angiosclerotica intermittens 443.9
    - due to atherosclerosis 440.21
  - hysterical 300.11
  - lordotica (progressiva) 333.6
  - nonorganic origin 307.9
  - psychogenic 307.9
- **Dysbetalipoproteinemia** (familial) 272.2
- **Dyscalculia** 315.1
- **Dyschezia** (*see also* Constipation) 564.00
- **Dyschondroplasia** (with hemangiomata) 756.4
  - Voorhoeve's 756.4
- **Dyschondrosteosis** 756.59
- **Dyschromia** 709.00
- **Dyscollagenosis** 710.9
- **Dyscoria** 743.41
- **Dyscraniopyophalangy** 759.89
- **Dyscrasia**
  - blood 289.9
    - with antepartum hemorrhage 641.3❺
    - fetus or newborn NEC 776.9
    - hemorrhage, subungual 287.8
    - puerperal, postpartum 666.3❺
  - ovary 256.8
  - plasma cell 273.9
  - pluriglandular 258.9
  - polyglandular 258.9
- **Dysdiadochokinesia** 781.3
- **Dysectasia, vesical neck** 596.8
- **Dysendocrinism** 259.9
- **Dysentery, dysenteric** (bilious) (catarrhal) (diarrhea) (epidemic) (gangrenous) (hemorrhagic) (infectious) (sporadic) (tropical) (ulcerative) 009.0
  - abscess, liver (*see also* Abscess, amebic) 006.3
  - amebic (*see also* Amebiasis) 006.9
    - with abscess – *see* Abscess, amebic
    - acute 006.0
    - carrier (suspected) of V02.2
    - chronic 006.1
  - arthritis (*see also* Arthritis, due to, dysentery) 009.0 *[711.3]*❺
    - bacillary 004.9 *[711.3]*❺
  - asylum 004.9
  - bacillary 004.9
    - arthritis 004.9 *[711.3]*❺
    - boyd 004.2
    - flexner 004.1
    - schmitz (-Stutzer) 004.0
    - shiga 004.0
    - shigella 004.9
      - group A 004.0
      - group B 004.1
      - group C 004.2
      - group D 004.3
      - specified type NEC 004.8
    - sonne 004.3
    - specified type NEC 004.8
  - bacterium 004.9
  - balantidial 007.0
  - balantidium coli 007.0
  - Boyd's 004.2
  - Chilomastix 007.8
  - Chinese 004.9
  - choleriform 001.1

Dysentery, dysenteric – *continued*
  coccidial 007.2
  Dientamoeba fragilis 007.8
  due to specified organism NEC – *see* Enteritis, due to, by organism
  Embadomonas 007.8
  Endolimax nana – *see* Dysentery, amebic
  Entamoba, entamebic – *see* Dysentery, amebic
  Flexner's 004.1
  Flexner-Boyd 004.2
  giardial 007.1
  Giardia lamblia 007.1
  Hiss-Russell 004.1
  lamblia 007.1
  leishmanial 085.0
  malarial (*see also* Malaria) 084.6
  metazoal 127.9
  Monilia 112.89
  protozoal NEC 007.9
  Russell's 004.8
  salmonella 003.0
  schistosomal 120.1
  Schmitz (-Stutzer) 004.0
  Shiga 004.0
  Shigella NEC (*see also* Dysentery, bacillary) 004.9
    boydii 004.2
    dysenteriae 004.0
      schmitz 004.0
      shiga 004.0
    flexneri 004.1
    group A 004.0
    group B 004.1
    group C 004.2
    group D 004.3
    Schmitz 004.0
    Shiga 004.0
    Sonnei 004.3
  Sonne 004.3
  strongyloidiasis 127.2
  trichomonal 007.3
  tuberculous (*see also* Tuberculosis) 014.8❺
  viral (*see also* Enteritis, viral) 008.8
Dysequilibrium 780.4
Dysesthesia 782.0
  hysterical 300.11
Dysfibrinogenemia (congenital) (*see also* Defect, coagulation) 286.3
Dysfunction
  adrenal (cortical) 255.9
    hyperfunction 255.3
    hypofunction 255.41 ▲
  associated with sleep stages or arousal from sleep 780.56
    nonorganic origin 307.47
  bladder NEC 596.59
  bleeding, uterus 626.8
  brain, minimal (*see also* Hyperkinesia) 314.9
  cerebral 348.30
  colon 564.9
    psychogenic 306.4
  colostomy or enterostomy 569.62
  cystic duct 575.8
  diastolic 429.9
    with heart failure – *see* Failure, heart
    due to
      cardiomyopathy – *see* Cardiomyopathy
      hypertension – *see* Hypertension, heart
  endocrine NEC 259.9
  endometrium 621.8
  enteric stoma 569.62
  enterostomy 569.62
  erectile 607.84
    nonorganic origin 302.72
  esophagostomy 530.87
  Eustachian tube 381.81
  gallbladder 575.8
  gastrointestinal 536.9
  gland, glandular NEC 259.9
  heart 427.9
    postoperative (immediate) 997.1
      long-term effect of cardiac surgery 429.4
  hemoglobin 289.89
  hepatic 573.9
  hepatocellular NEC 573.9
  hypophysis 253.9
    hyperfunction 253.1
    hypofunction 253.2
    posterior lobe 253.6
      hypofunction 253.5
  kidney (*see also* Disease, renal) 593.9

Dysfunction – *continued*
  labyrinthine 386.50
    specified NEC 386.58
  liver 573.9
    constitutional 277.4
  minimal brain (child) (*see also* Hyperkinesia) 314.9
  ovary, ovarian 256.9
    hyperfunction 256.1
      estrogen 256.0
    hypofunction 256.39
      postablative 256.2
    postablative 256.2
    specified NEC 256.8
  papillary muscle 429.81
    with myocardial infarction 410.8❺
  parathyroid 252.8
    hyperfunction 252.00
    hypofunction 252.1
  pineal gland 259.8
  pituitary (gland) 253.9
    hyperfunction 253.1
    hypofunction 253.2
    posterior 253.6
      hypofunction 253.5
  placental – *see* Placenta, insufficiency
  platelets (blood) 287.1
  polyglandular 258.9
    specified NEC 258.8
  psychosexual 302.70
    with
      dyspareunia (functional) (psychogenic) 302.76
      frigidity 302.72
      impotence 302.72
      inhibition
        orgasm
          female 302.73
          male 302.74
        sexual
          desire 302.71
          excitement 302.72
      premature ejaculation 302.75
      sexual aversion 302.79
      specified disorder NEC 302.79
      vaginismus 306.51
  pylorus 537.9
  rectum 564.9
    psychogenic 306.4
  segmental (*see also* Dysfunction, somatic) 739.9
  senile 797
  sexual 302.70
  sinoatrial node 427.81
  somatic 739.9
    abdomen 739.9
    acromioclavicular 739.7
    cervical 739.1
    cervicothoracic 739.1
    costochondral 739.8
    costovertebral 739.8
    extremities
      lower 739.6
      upper 739.7
    head 739.0
    hip 739.5
    lumbar, lumbosacral 739.3
    occipitocervical 739.0
    pelvic 739.5
    pubic 739.5
    rib cage 739.8
    sacral 739.4
    sacrococcygeal 739.4
    sacroiliac 739.4
    specified site NEC 739.9
    sternochondral 739.8
    sternoclavicular 739.7
    temporomandibular 739.0
    thoracic, thoracolumbar 739.2
  stomach 536.9
    psychogenic 306.4
  suprarenal 255.9
    hyperfunction 255.3
    hypofunction 255.41 ▲
  symbolic NEC 784.60
    specified type NEC 784.69
  systolic 429.9
    with heart failure – *see* Failure, heart
  temporomandibular (joint) (joint-pain-syndrome) NEC 524.60
    sounds on opening or closing 524.64
    specified NEC 524.69

Dysfunction – *continued*
  testicular 257.9
    hyperfunction 257.0
    hypofunction 257.2
    specified type NEC 257.8
  thymus 254.9
  thyroid 246.9
    complicating pregnancy, childbirth, or puerperium 648.1❺
    hyperfunction – *see* Hyperthyroidism
    hypofunction – *see* Hypothyroidism
  uterus, complicating delivery 661.9❺
    affecting fetus or newborn 763.7
    hypertonic 661.4❺
    hypotonic 661.2❺
      primary 661.0❺
      secondary 661.1❺
  velopharyngeal (acquired) 528.9
    congenital 750.29
  ventricular 429.9
    with congestive heart failure (*see also* Failure, heart) 428.0
    due to
      cardiomyopathy – *see* Cardiomyopathy
      hypertension – *see* Hypertension, heart
    left, reversible following sudden emotional stress 429.83
  vesicourethral NEC 596.59
  vestibular 386.50
    specified type NEC 386.58
Dysgammaglobulinemia 279.06
Dysgenesis
  gonadal (due to chromosomal anomaly) 758.6
    pure 752.7
  kidney(s) 753.0
  ovarian 758.6
  renal 753.0
  reticular 279.2
  seminiferous tubules 758.6
  tidal platelet 287.31
Dysgerminoma (M9060/3)
  specified site – *see* Neoplasm, by site, malignant
  unspecified site
    female 183.0
    male 186.9
Dysgeusia 781.1
Dysgraphia 781.3
Dyshidrosis 705.81
Dysidrosis 705.81
Dysinsulinism 251.8
Dyskaryotic cervical smear 795.09
Dyskeratosis (*see also* Keratosis) 701.1
  bullosa hereditaria 757.39
  cervix 622.10
  congenital 757.39
  follicularis 757.39
    vitamin A deficiency 264.8
  gingiva 523.8
  oral soft tissue NEC 528.79
  tongue 528.79
  uterus NEC 621.8
Dyskinesia 781.3
  biliary 575.8
  esophagus 530.5
  hysterical 300.11
  intestinal 564.89
  neuroleptic-induced tardive 333.85
  nonorganic origin 307.9
  orofacial 333.82
    due to drugs 333.85
  psychogenic 307.9
  subacute, due to drugs 333.85
  tardive (oral) 333.85
Dyslalia 784.5
  developmental 315.39
Dyslexia 784.61
  developmental 315.02
  secondary to organic lesion 784.61
Dyslipidemia 272.4
Dysmaturity (*see also* Immaturity) 765.1❺
  lung 770.4
  pulmonary 770.4
Dysmenorrhea (essential) (exfoliative) (functional) (intrinsic) (membranous) (primary) (secondary) 625.3
  psychogenic 306.52
Dysmetabolic syndrome X 277.7
Dysmetria 781.3
Dysmorodystrophia mesodermalis congenita 759.82

- **Dysnomia** 784.3
- **Dysorexia** 783.0
  - hysterical 300.11
- **Dysostosis**
  - cleidocranial, cleidocranialis 755.59
  - craniofacial 756.0
  - Fairbank's (idiopathic familial generalized osteophytosis) 756.50
  - mandibularis 756.0
  - mandibulofacial, incomplete 756.0
  - multiplex 277.5
  - orodigitofacial 759.89
- **Dyspareunia** (female) 625.0
  - male 608.89
  - psychogenic 302.76
- **Dyspepsia** (allergic) (congenital) (fermentative) (flatulent) (functional) (gastric) (gastrointestinal) (neurogenic) (occupational) (reflex) 536.8
  - acid 536.8
  - atonic 536.3
    - psychogenic 306.4
  - diarrhea 787.91
    - psychogenic 306.4
  - intestinal 564.89
    - psychogenic 306.4
  - nervous 306.4
  - neurotic 306.4
  - psychogenic 306.4
- **Dysphagia** 787.20 ▲
  - cervical 787.29 ●
  - functional 300.11
  - hysterical 300.11
  - nervous 300.11
  - neurogenic 787.29 ●
  - oral phase 787.21 ●
  - oropharyngeal phase 787.22 ●
  - pharyngeal phase 787.23 ●
  - pharyngoesophageal phase 787.24 ●
  - psychogenic 306.4
  - sideropenic 280.8
  - spastica 530.5
  - specified NEC 787.29 ●
- **Dysphagocytosis, congenital** 288.1
- **Dysphasia** 784.5
- **Dysphonia** 784.49
  - clericorum 784.49
  - functional 300.11
  - hysterical 300.11
  - psychogenic 306.1
  - spastica 478.79
- **Dyspigmentation** – *see also* Pigmentation
  - eyelid (acquired) 374.52
- **Dyspituitarism** 253.9
  - hyperfunction 253.1
  - hypofunction 253.2
  - posterior lobe 253.6
- **Dysplasia** – *see also* Anomaly
  - artery
    - fibromuscular NEC 447.8
      - carotid 447.8
      - renal 447.3
  - bladder 596.8
  - bone (fibrous) NEC 733.29
    - diaphyseal, progressive 756.59
    - jaw 526.89
    - monostotic 733.29
    - polyostotic 756.54
    - solitary 733.29
  - brain 742.9
  - bronchopulmonary, fetus or newborn 770.7
  - cervix (uteri) 622.10
    - cervical intraepithelial neoplasia I [CIN I] 622.11
    - cervical intraepithelial neoplasia II [CIN II] 622.12
    - cervical intraepithelial neoplasia III [CIN III] 233.1
    - CIN I 622.11
    - CIN II 622.12
    - CIN III 233.1
    - mild 622.11
    - moderate 622.12
    - severe 233.1
  - chondroectodermal 756.55
  - chondromatose 756.4
  - colon 211.3
  - craniocarpotarsal 759.89
  - craniometaphyseal 756.89
  - dentinal 520.5
  - diaphyseal, progressive 756.59

- **Dysplasia** – *continued*
  - ectodermal (anhidrotic) (Bason) (Clouston's) (congenital) (Feinmesser) (hereditary) (hidrotic) (Marshall) (Robinson's) 757.31
  - epiphysealis 756.9
    - multiplex 756.56
    - punctata 756.59
  - epiphysis 756.9
    - multiple 756.56
  - epithelial
    - epiglottis 478.79
    - uterine cervix 622.10
  - erythroid NEC 289.89
  - eye (*see also* Microphthalmos) 743.10
  - familial metaphyseal 756.89
  - fibromuscular, artery NEC 447.8
    - carotid 447.8
    - renal 447.3
  - fibrous
    - bone NEC 733.29
    - diaphyseal, progressive 756.59
    - jaw 526.89
    - monostotic 733.29
    - polyostotic 756.54
    - solitary 733.29
  - high grade, focal – *see* Neoplasm, by site, benign
  - hip (congenital) 755.63
    - with dislocation (*see also* Dislocation, hip, congenital) 754.30
  - hypohidrotic ectodermal 757.31
  - joint 755.8
  - kidney 753.15
  - leg 755.69
  - linguofacialis 759.89
  - lung 748.5
  - macular 743.55
  - mammary (benign) (gland) 610.9
    - cystic 610.1
    - specified type NEC 610.8
  - metaphyseal 756.9
    - familial 756.89
  - monostotic fibrous 733.29
  - muscle 756.89
  - myeloid NEC 289.89
  - nervous system (general) 742.9
  - neuroectodermal 759.6
  - oculoauriculovertebral 756.0
  - oculodentodigital 759.89
  - olfactogenital 253.4
  - osteo-onycho-arthro (hereditary) 756.89
  - periosteum 733.99
  - polyostotic fibrous 756.54
  - progressive diaphyseal 756.59
  - prostate 602.3
    - intraepithelial neoplasia I [PIN I] 602.3
    - intraepithelial neoplasia II [PIN II] 602.3
    - intraepithelial neoplasia III [PIN III] 233.4
  - renal 753.15
  - renofacialis 753.0
  - retinal NEC 743.56
  - retrolental 362.21
  - spinal cord 742.9
  - thymic, with immunodeficiency 279.2
  - vagina 623.0
    - severe 233.31 ●
  - vocal cord 478.5
  - vulva 624.8
    - intraepithelial neoplasia I [VIN I] 624.01 ▲
    - intraepithelial neoplasia II [VIN II] 624.02 ▲
    - intraepithelial neoplasia III [VIN III] 233.32 ▲
    - mild 624.01 ●
    - moderate 624.02 ●
    - severe 233.32 ●
    - VIN I 624.01 ▲
    - VIN II 624.02 ▲
    - VIN III 233.32 ▲
- **Dyspnea** (nocturnal) (paroxysmal) 786.09
  - asthmatic (bronchial) (*see also* Asthma) 493.9❺
    - with bronchitis (*see also* Asthma) 493.9❺
      - chronic 493.2
    - cardiac (*see also* Failure, ventricular, left) 428.1
  - cardiac (*see also* Failure, ventricular, left) 428.1
  - functional 300.11
  - hyperventilation 786.01
  - hysterical 300.11
  - Monday morning 504
  - newborn 770.89
  - psychogenic 306.1
  - uremic – *see* Uremia
- **Dyspraxia** 781.3
  - syndrome 315.4

- **Dysproteinemia** 273.8
  - transient with copper deficiency 281.4
- **Dysprothrombinemia** (constitutional) (*see also* Defect, coagulation) 286.3
- **Dysreflexia, autonomic** 337.3
- **Dysrhythmia**
  - cardiac 427.9
    - postoperative (immediate) 997.1
      - long-term effect of cardiac surgery 429.4
    - specified type NEC 427.89
  - cerebral or cortical 348.30
- **Dyssecretosis, mucoserous** 710.2
- **Dyssocial reaction, without manifest psychiatric** disorder
  - adolescent V71.02
  - adult V71.01
  - child V71.02
- **Dyssomnia** NEC 780.56
  - nonorganic origin 307.47
- **Dyssplenism** 289.4
- **Dyssynergia**
  - biliary (*see also* Disease, biliary) 576.8
  - cerebellaris myoclonica 334.2
  - detrusor sphincter (bladder) 596.55
  - ventricular 429.89
- **Dystasia, hereditary areflexic** 334.3
- **Dysthymia** 300.4
- **Dysthymic disorder** 300.4
- **Dysthyroidism** 246.9
- **Dystocia** 660.9❺
  - affecting fetus or newborn 763.1
  - cervical 661.2❺ ▲
    - affecting fetus or newborn 763.7
  - contraction ring 661.4❺
    - affecting fetus or newborn 763.7
  - fetal 660.9❺
    - abnormal size 653.5❺
    - affecting fetus or newborn 763.1
    - deformity 653.7❺
  - maternal 660.9❺
    - affecting fetus or newborn 763.1
  - positional 660.0❺
    - affecting fetus or newborn 763.1
  - shoulder (girdle) 660.4❺
    - affecting fetus or newborn 763.1
  - uterine NEC 661.4❺
    - affecting fetus or newborn 763.7
- **Dystonia**
  - acute
    - due to drugs 333.72
    - neuroleptic-induced acute 333.72
  - deformans progressiva 333.6
  - lenticularis 333.6
  - musculorum deformans 333.6
  - torsion (idiopathic) 333.6
    - acquired 333.79
    - fragments (of) 333.89
    - genetic 333.6
    - symptomatic 333.79
- **Dystonic**
  - movements 781.0
- **Dystopia kidney** 753.3
- **Dystrophy, dystrophia** 783.9
  - adiposogenital 253.8
  - asphyxiating thoracic 756.4
  - Becker's type 359.22 ▲
  - brevicollis 756.16
  - Bruch's membrane 362.77
  - cervical (sympathetic) NEC 337.0
  - chondro-osseus with punctate epiphyseal dysplasia 756.59
  - choroid (hereditary) 363.50
    - central (areolar) (partial) 363.53
      - total (gyrate) 363.54
    - circinate 363.53
    - circumpapillary (partial) 363.51
      - total 363.52
    - diffuse
      - partial 363.56
      - total 363.57
    - generalized
      - partial 363.56
      - total 363.57
    - gyrate
      - central 363.54
      - generalized 363.57
    - helicoid 363.52
    - peripapillary – *see* Dystrophy, choroid, circumpapillary

Dysnomia – Dystrophy, dystrophia

Ectopic, ectopia – Effect, adverse

Ectopic, ectopia – *continued*
- testis 752.51
- thyroid 759.2
- ureter 753.4
- ventricular beats 427.69
- vesicae 753.5

Ectrodactyly 755.4
- finger (*see also* Absence, finger, congenital) 755.29
- toe (*see also* Absence, toe, congenital) 755.39

Ectromelia 755.4
- lower limb 755.30
- upper limb 755.20

Ectropion 374.10
- anus 569.49
- cervix 622.0
  - with mention of cervicitis 616.0
- cicatricial 374.14
- congenital 743.62
- eyelid 374.10
  - cicatricial 374.14
  - congenital 743.62
  - mechanical 374.12
  - paralytic 374.12
  - senile 374.11
  - spastic 374.13
- iris (pigment epithelium) 364.54
- lip (congenital) 750.26
  - acquired 528.5
- mechanical 374.12
- paralytic 374.12
- rectum 569.49
- senile 374.11
- spastic 374.13
- urethra 599.84
- uvea 364.54

Eczema (acute) (allergic) (chronic) (erythematous) (fissum) (occupational) (rubrum) (squamous) 692.9
- asteatotic 706.8
- atopic 691.8
- contact NEC 692.9
- dermatitis NEC 692.9
- due to specified cause – *see* Dermatitis, due to
- dyshidrotic 705.81
- external ear 380.22
- flexural 691.8
- gouty 274.89
- herpeticum 054.0
- hypertrophicum 701.8
- hypostatic – *see* Varicose, vein
- impetiginous 684
- infantile (acute) (chronic) (due to any substance) (intertriginous) (seborrheic) 690.12
- intertriginous NEC 692.9
  - infantile 690.12
- intrinsic 691.8
- lichenified NEC 692.9
- marginatum 110.3
- nummular 692.9
- pustular 686.8
- seborrheic 690.18
  - infantile 690.12
- solare 692.72
- stasis (lower extremity) 454.1
  - ulcerated 454.2
- vaccination, vaccinatum 999.0
- varicose (lower extremity) – *see* Varicose, vein
- verrucosum callosum 698.3

Eczematoid, exudative 691.8

Eddowes' syndrome (brittle bones and blue sclera) 756.51

Edema, edematous 782.3
- with nephritis (*see also* Nephrosis) 581.9
- allergic 995.1
- angioneurotic (allergic) (any site) (with urticaria) 995.1
  - hereditary 277.6
- angiospastic 443.9
- Berlin's (traumatic) 921.3
- brain 348.5
  - due to birth injury 767.8
  - fetus or newborn 767.8
- cardiac (*see also* Failure, heart) 428.0
- cardiovascular (*see also* Failure, heart) 428.0
- cerebral – *see* Edema, brain
- cerebrospinal vessel – *see* Edema, brain
- cervix (acute) (uteri) 622.8
  - puerperal, postpartum 674.8❺
- chronic hereditary 757.0

Edema, edematous – *continued*
- circumscribed, acute 995.1
  - hereditary 277.6
- complicating pregnancy (gestational) 646.1❺
  - with hypertension – *see* Toxemia, of pregnancy
- conjunctiva 372.73
- connective tissue 782.3
- cornea 371.20
  - due to contact lenses 371.24
  - idiopathic 371.21
  - secondary 371.22
- cystoid macular 362.53
- due to
  - lymphatic obstruction – *see* Edema, lymphatic
  - salt retention 276.0
- epiglottis – *see* Edema, glottis
- essential, acute 995.1
  - hereditary 277.6
- extremities, lower – *see* Edema, legs
- eyelid NEC 374.82
- familial, hereditary (legs) 757.0
- famine 262
- fetus or newborn 778.5
- genital organs
  - female 629.89
  - male 608.86
- gestational 646.1❺
  - with hypertension – *see* Toxemia, of pregnancy
- glottis, glottic, glottides (obstructive) (passive) 478.6
  - allergic 995.1
    - hereditary 277.6
  - due to external agent – *see* Condition, respiratory, acute, due to specified agent
- heart (*see also* Failure, heart) 428.0
  - newborn 779.89
- heat 992.7
- hereditary (legs) 757.0
- inanition 262
- infectious 782.3
- intracranial 348.5
  - due to injury at birth 767.8
- iris 364.89 ▲
- joint (*see also* Effusion, joint) 719.0❺
- larynx (*see also* Edema, glottis) 478.6
- legs 782.3
  - due to venous obstruction 459.2
  - hereditary 757.0
- localized 782.3
  - due to venous obstruction 459.2
    - lower extremity 459.2
- lower extremities – *see* Edema, legs
- lung 514
  - acute 518.4
    - with heart disease or failure (*see also* Failure, ventricular, left) 428.1
      - congestive 428.0
    - chemical (due to fumes or vapors) 506.1
    - due to
      - external agent(s) NEC 508.9
        - specified NEC 508.8
      - fumes and vapors (chemical) (inhalation) 506.1
      - radiation 508.0
  - chemical (acute) 506.1
    - chronic 506.4
  - chronic 514
    - chemical (due to fumes or vapors) 506.4
    - due to
      - external agent(s) NEC 508.9
        - specified NEC 508.8
      - fumes or vapors (chemical) (inhalation) 506.4
      - radiation 508.1
  - due to
    - external agent 508.9
      - specified NEC 508.8
    - high altitude 993.2
    - near drowning 994.1
  - postoperative 518.4
  - terminal 514
- lymphatic 457.1
  - due to mastectomy operation 457.0
- macula 362.83
  - cystoid 362.53
  - diabetic 250.5❺ *[362.07]*
- malignant (*see also* Gangrene, gas) 040.0
- Milroy's 757.0
- nasopharynx 478.25
- neonatorum 778.5
- nutritional (newborn) 262
  - with dyspigmentation, skin and hair 260

Edema, edematous – *continued*
- optic disc or nerve – *see* Papilledema
- orbit 376.33
  - circulatory 459.89
- palate (soft) (hard) 528.9
- pancreas 577.8
- penis 607.83
- periodic 995.1
  - hereditary 277.6
- pharynx 478.25
- pitting 782.3
- pulmonary – *see* Edema, lung
- Quincke's 995.1
  - hereditary 277.6
- renal (*see also* Nephrosis) 581.9
- retina (localized) (macular) (peripheral) 362.83
  - cystoid 362.53
  - diabetic 250.5❺ *[362.07]*
- salt 276.0
- scrotum 608.86
- seminal vesicle 608.86
- spermatic cord 608.86
- spinal cord 336.1
- starvation 262
- stasis (*see also* Hypertension, venous) 459.30
- subconjunctival 372.73
- subglottic (*see also* Edema, glottis) 478.6
- supraglottic (*see also* Edema, glottis) 478.6
- testis 608.86
- toxic NEC 782.3
- traumatic NEC 782.3
- tunica vaginalis 608.86
- vas deferens 608.86
- vocal cord – *see* Edema, glottis
- vulva (acute) 624.8

Edentia (complete) (partial) (*see also* Absence, tooth) 520.0
- acquired (*see also* Edentulism) 525.40
  - due to
    - caries 525.13
    - extraction 525.10
    - periodontal disease 525.12
    - specified NEC 525.19
    - trauma 525.11
- causing malocclusion 524.30
- congenital (deficiency of tooth buds) 520.0

Edentulism 525.40
- complete 525.40
  - class I 525.41
  - class II 525.42
  - class III 525.43
  - class IV 525.44
- partial 525.50
  - class I 525.51
  - class II 525.52
  - class III 525.53
  - class IV 525.54

Edsall's disease 992.2

Educational handicap V62.3

Edwards' syndrome 758.2

Effect, adverse NEC
- abnormal gravitational (G) forces or states 994.9
- air pressure – *see* Effect, adverse, atmospheric pressure
- altitude (high) – *see* Effect, adverse, high altitude
- anesthetic
  - in labor and delivery NEC 668.9❺
    - affecting fetus or newborn 763.5
- antitoxin – *see* Complications, vaccination
- atmospheric pressure 993.9
  - due to explosion 993.4
  - high 993.3
  - low – *see* Effect, adverse, high altitude
  - specified effect NEC 993.8
- biological, correct substance properly administered (*see also* Effect, adverse, drug) 995.20
- blood (derivatives) (serum) (transfusion) – *see* Complications, transfusion
- chemical substance NEC 989.9
  - specified – *see* Table of Drugs and Chemicals
- cobalt, radioactive (*see also* Effect, adverse, radioactive substance) 990
- cold (temperature) (weather) 991.9
  - chilblains 991.5
  - frostbite – *see* Frostbite
  - specified effect NEC 991.8
- drugs and medicinals 995.20
  - correct substance properly administered 995.20

Effect, adverse – *continued*
- drugs and medicinals – *continued*
  - overdose or wrong substance given or taken 977.9
    - specified drug – *see* Table of Drugs and Chemicals
- electric current (shock) 994.8
  - burn – *see* Burn, by site
- electricity (electrocution) (shock) 994.8
  - burn – *see* Burn, by site
- exertion (excessive) 994.5
- exposure 994.9
  - exhaustion 994.4
- external cause NEC 994.9
- fallout (radioactive) NEC 990
- fluoroscopy NEC 990
- foodstuffs
  - allergic reaction (*see also* Allergy, food) 693.1
  - anaphylactic shock due to food NEC 995.60
  - noxious 988.9
    - specified type NEC (*see also* Poisoning, by name of noxious foodstuff) 988.8
- gases, fumes, or vapors – *see* Table of Drugs and Chemicals
- glue (airplane) sniffing 304.6❺
- heat – *see* Heat
- high altitude NEC 993.2
  - anoxia 993.2
  - on
    - ears 993.0
    - sinuses 993.1
  - polycythemia 289.0
- hot weather – *see* Heat
- hunger 994.2
- immersion, foot 991.4
- immunization – *see* Complications, vaccination
- immunological agents – *see* Complications, vaccination
- implantation (removable) of isotope or radium NEC 990
- infrared (radiation) (rays) NEC 990
  - burn – *see* Burn, by site
  - dermatitis or eczema 692.82
- infusion – *see* Complications, infusion
- ingestion or injection of isotope (therapeutic) NEC 990
- irradiation NEC (*see also* Effect, adverse, radiation) 990
- isotope (radioactive) NEC 990
- lack of care (child) (infant) (newborn) 995.52
  - adult 995.84
- lightning 994.0
  - burn – *see* Burn, by site
- Lirugin – *see* Complications, vaccination
- medicinal substance, correct, properly administered (*see also* Effect, adverse, drugs) 995.20
- mesothorium NEC 990
- motion 994.6
- noise, inner ear 388.10
- other drug, medicinal and biological substance 995.29
- overheated places – *see* Heat
- polonium NEC 990
- psychosocial, of work environment V62.1
- radiation (diagnostic) (fallout) (infrared) (natural source) (therapeutic) (tracer) (ultraviolet) (x-ray) NEC 990
  - with pulmonary manifestations
    - acute 508.0
    - chronic 508.1
  - dermatitis or eczema 692.82
    - due to sun NEC (*see also* Dermatitis, due to, sun) 692.70
  - fibrosis of lungs 508.1
  - maternal with suspected damage to fetus affecting management of pregnancy 655.6❺
  - pneumonitis 508.0
- radioactive substance NEC 990
  - dermatitis or eczema 692.82
- radioactivity NEC 990
- radiotherapy NEC 990
  - dermatitis or eczema 692.82
- radium NEC 990
- reduced temperature 991.9
  - frostbite – *see* Frostbite
  - immersion, foot (hand) 991.4
  - specified effect NEC 991.8
- roentgenography NEC 990
- roentgenoscopy NEC 990
- roentgen rays NEC 990

Effect, adverse – *continued*
- serum (prophylactic) (therapeutic) NEC 999.5
- specified NEC 995.89
  - external cause NEC 994.9
- strangulation 994.7
- submersion 994.1
- teletherapy NEC 990
- thirst 994.3
- transfusion – *see* Complications, transfusion
- ultraviolet (radiation) (rays) NEC 990
  - burn – *see also* Burn, by site
    - from sun (*see also* Sunburn) 692.71
  - dermatitis or eczema 692.82
    - due to sun NEC (*see also* Dermatitis, due to, sun) 692.70
- uranium NEC 990
- vaccine (any) – *see* Complications, vaccination
- weightlessness 994.9
- whole blood – *see also* Complications, transfusion
  - overdose or wrong substance given (*see also* Table of Drugs and Chemicals) 964.7
- working environment V62.1
  - x-rays NEC 990
  - dermatitis or eczema 692.82

Effect, remote
- of cancer – *see* condition

Effects, late – *see* Late, effect (of)

Effluvium, telogen 704.02

Effort
- intolerance 306.2
- syndrome (aviators) (psychogenic) 306.2

Effusion
- amniotic fluid (*see also* Rupture, membranes, premature) 658.1❺
- brain (serous) 348.5
- bronchial (*see also* Bronchitis) 490
- cerebral 348.5
- cerebrospinal (*see also* Meningitis) 322.9
  - vessel 348.5
- chest – *see* Effusion, pleura
- intracranial 348.5
- joint 719.00
  - ankle 719.07
  - elbow 719.02
  - foot 719.07
  - hand 719.04
  - hip 719.05
  - knee 719.06
  - multiple sites 719.09
  - pelvic region 719.05
  - shoulder (region) 719.01
  - specified site NEC 719.08
  - wrist 719.03
- meninges (*see also* Meningitis) 322.9
- pericardium, pericardial (*see also* Pericarditis) 423.9
  - acute 420.90
- peritoneal (chronic) 568.82
- pleura, pleurisy, pleuritic, pleuropericardial 511.9
  - bacterial, nontuberculous 511.1
  - fetus or newborn 511.9
  - malignant 197.2
  - nontuberculous 511.9
    - bacterial 511.1
  - pneumococcal 511.1
  - staphylococcal 511.1
  - streptococcal 511.1
  - traumatic 862.29
    - with open wound 862.39
  - tuberculous (*see also* Tuberculosis, pleura) 012.0❺
    - primary progressive 010.1❺
- pulmonary – *see* Effusion, pleura
- spinal (*see also* Meningitis) 322.9
- thorax, thoracic – *see* Effusion, pleura

Egg (oocyte) (ovum)
- donor V59.70
  - over age 35 V59.73
    - anonymous recipient V59.73
    - designated recipient V59.74
  - under age 35 V59.71
    - anonymous recipient V59.71
    - designated recipient V59.72

Eggshell nails 703.8
- congenital 757.5

Ego-dystonic
- homosexuality 302.0
- lesbianism 302.0
- sexual orientation 302.0

Egyptian splenomegaly 120.1

Ehlers-Danlos syndrome 756.83

Ehrlichiosis 082.40
- chaffeensis 082.41
- specified type NEC 082.49

Eichstedt's disease (pityriasis versicolor) 111.0

Eisenmenger's complex or syndrome (ventricular septal defect) 745.4

Ejaculation, semen
- painful 608.89
  - psychogenic 306.59
- premature 302.75
- retrograde 608.87

Ekbom syndrome (restless legs) 333.94

Ekman's syndrome (brittle bones and blue sclera) 756.51

Elastic skin 756.83
- acquired 701.8

Elastofibroma (M8820/0) – *see* Neoplasm, connective tissue, benign

Elastoidosis
- cutanea nodularis 701.8
- cutis cystica et comedonica 701.8

Elastoma 757.39
- juvenile 757.39
- Miescher's (elastosis perforans serpiginosa) 701.1

Elastomyofibrosis 425.3

Elastosis 701.8
- atrophicans 701.8
- perforans serpiginosa 701.1
- reactive perforating 701.1
- senilis 701.8
- solar (actinic) 692.74

Elbow – *see* condition

Electric
- current, electricity, effects (concussion) (fatal) (nonfatal) (shock) 994.8
  - burn – *see* Burn, by site
- feet (foot) syndrome 266.2

Electrocution 994.8

Electrolyte imbalance 276.9
- with
  - abortion – *see* Abortion, by type, with metabolic disorder
  - ectopic pregnancy (*see also* categories 633.0-633.9) 639.4
  - hyperemesis gravidarum (before 22 completed weeks gestation) 643.1❺
  - molar pregnancy (*see also* categories 630-632) 639.4
- following
  - abortion 639.4
  - ectopic or molar pregnancy 639.4

Elephant man syndrome 237.71

Elephantiasis (nonfilarial) 457.1
- arabicum (*see also* Infestation, filarial) 125.9
- congenita hereditaria 757.0
- congenital (any site) 757.0
- due to
  - Brugia (malayi) 125.1
  - mastectomy operation 457.0
  - Wuchereria (bancrofti) 125.0
    - malayi 125.1
- eyelid 374.83
- filarial (*see also* Infestation, filarial) 125.9
- filariensis (*see also* Infestation, filarial) 125.9
- gingival 523.8
- glandular 457.1
- graecorum 030.9
- lymphangiectatic 457.1
- lymphatic vessel 457.1
  - due to mastectomy operation 457.0
- neuromatosa 237.71
- postmastectomy 457.0
- scrotum 457.1
- streptococcal 457.1
- surgical 997.99
  - postmastectomy 457.0
- telangiectodes 457.1
- vulva (nonfilarial) 624.8

Elevated – *see* Elevation

Elevation
- 17-ketosteroids 791.9
- acid phosphatase 790.5
- alkaline phosphatase 790.5
- amylase 790.5
- antibody titers 795.79

Effect, adverse – Elevation

- **Elevation** – *continued*
  - basal metabolic rate (BMR) 794.7
  - blood pressure (*see also* Hypertension) 401.9
    - reading (incidental) (isolated) (nonspecific), no diagnosis of hypertension 796.2
  - blood sugar 790.29 ●
  - body temperature (of unknown origin) (*see also* Pyrexia) 780.6
  - C-reactive protein (CRP) 790.95
  - cancer antigen 125 [CA 125] 795.82
  - carcinoembryonic antigen [CEA] 795.81
  - cholesterol 272.0 ●
    - with triglycerides 272.2 ●
  - conjugate, eye 378.81
  - CRP (C-reactive protein) 790.95
  - diaphragm, congenital 756.6
  - glucose
    - fasting 790.21
    - tolerance test 790.22
  - immunoglobulin level 795.79
  - indolacetic acid 791.9
  - lactic acid dehydrogenase (LDH) level 790.4
  - leukocytes 288.60
  - lipase 790.5
  - lipoprotein a level 272.8
  - liver function text (LFT) 790.6
    - alkaline phosphatase 790.5
    - aminotransferase 790.4
    - bilirubin 782.4
    - hepatic enzyme NEC 790.5
    - lactate dehydrogenase 790.4
  - lymphocytes 288.61
  - prostate specific antigen (PSA) 790.93
  - renin 790.99
    - in hypertension (*see also* Hypertension, renovascular) 405.91
  - Rh titer 999.7
  - scapula, congenital 755.52
  - sedimentation rate 790.1
  - SGOT 790.4
  - SGPT 790.4
  - transaminase 790.4
  - triglycerides 272.1 ●
    - with cholesterol 272.2 ●
  - vanillylmandelic acid 791.9
  - venous pressure 459.89
  - VMA 791.9
  - white blood cell count 288.60
    - specified NEC 288.69
- **Elliptocytosis** (congenital) (hereditary) 282.1
  - Hb-C (disease) 282.7
  - hemoglobin disease 282.7
  - sickle-cell (disease) 282.60
    - trait 282.5
- **Ellis-van Creveld disease or syndrome** (chondroectodermal dysplasia) 756.55
- **Ellison-Zollinger syndrome** (gastric hypersecretion with pancreatic islet cell tumor) 251.5
- **Elongation, elongated** (congenital) – *see also* Distortion
  - bone 756.9
  - cervix (uteri) 752.49
    - acquired 622.6
    - hypertrophic 622.6
  - colon 751.5
  - common bile duct 751.69
  - cystic duct 751.69
  - frenulum, penis 752.69
  - labia minora, acquired 624.8
  - ligamentum patellae 756.89
  - petiolus (epiglottidis) 748.3
  - styloid bone (process) 733.99
  - tooth, teeth 520.2
  - uvula 750.26
    - acquired 528.9
- **Elschnig bodies or pearls** 366.51
- **el tor cholera** 001.1
- **Emaciation** (due to malnutrition) 261
- **Emancipation disorder** 309.22
- **Embadomoniasis** 007.8
- **Embarrassment heart, cardiac** – *see* Disease, heart
- **Embedded tooth, teeth** 520.6
  - root only 525.3
- **Embolic** – *see* condition
- **Embolism** 444.9
  - with
    - abortion – *see* Abortion, by type, with embolism
    - ectopic pregnancy (*see also* categories 633.0-633.9) 639.6

- **Embolism** – *continued*
  - with – *continued*
    - molar pregnancy (*see also* categories 630-632) 639.6
  - air (any site) 958.0
    - with
      - abortion – *see* Abortion, by type, with embolism
      - ectopic pregnancy (*see also* categories 633.0-633.9) 639.6
      - molar pregnancy (*see also* categories 630-632) 639.6
    - due to implanted device – *see* Complications, due to (presence of) any device, implant, or graft classified to 996.0-996.5 NEC
    - following
      - abortion 639.6
      - ectopic or molar pregnancy 639.6
      - infusion, perfusion, or transfusion 999.1
    - in pregnancy, childbirth, or puerperium 673.0❺
    - traumatic 958.0
  - amniotic fluid (pulmonary) 673.1❺
    - with
      - abortion – *see* Abortion, by type, with embolism
      - ectopic pregnancy (*see also* categories 633.0-633.9) 639.6
      - molar pregnancy (*see also* categories 630-632) 639.6
    - following
      - abortion 639.6
      - ectopic or molar pregnancy 639.6
  - aorta, aortic 444.1
    - abdominal 444.0
    - bifurcation 444.0
    - saddle 444.0
    - thoracic 444.1
  - artery 444.9
    - auditory, internal 433.8❺
    - basilar (*see also* Occlusion, artery, basilar) 433.0❺
    - bladder 444.89
    - carotid (common) (internal) (*see also* Occlusion, artery, carotid) 433.1❺
    - cerebellar (anterior inferior) (posterior inferior) (superior) 433.8❺
    - cerebral (*see also* Embolism, brain) 434.1❺
    - choroidal (anterior) 433.8❺
    - communicating posterior 433.8❺
    - coronary (*see also* Infarct, myocardium) 410.9❺
      - without myocardial infarction 411.81
    - extremity 444.22
      - lower 444.22
      - upper 444.21
    - hypophyseal 433.8❺
    - mesenteric (with gangrene) 557.0
    - ophthalmic (*see also* Occlusion, retina) 362.30
    - peripheral 444.22
    - pontine 433.8❺
    - precerebral NEC – *see* Occlusion, artery, precerebral
    - pulmonary – *see* Embolism, pulmonary
    - pyemic 449 ●
      - pulmonary 415.12 ●
    - renal 593.81
    - retinal (*see also* Occlusion, retina) 362.30
    - septic 449 ●
      - pulmonary 415.12 ●
    - specified site NEC 444.89
    - vertebral (*see also* Occlusion, artery, vertebral) 433.2❺
  - auditory, internal 433.8❺
  - basilar (artery) (*see also* Occlusion, artery, basilar) 433.0❺
  - birth, mother – *see* Embolism, obstetrical
  - blood-clot
    - with
      - abortion – *see* Abortion, by type, with embolism
      - ectopic pregnancy (*see also* categories 633.0-633.9) 639.6
      - molar pregnancy (*see also* categories 630-632) 639.6
    - following
      - abortion 639.6
      - ectopic or molar pregnancy 639.6
    - in pregnancy, childbirth, or puerperium 673.2❺

- **Embolism** – *continued*
  - brain 434.1❺
    - with
      - abortion – *see* Abortion, by type, with embolism
      - ectopic pregnancy (*see also* categories 633.0-633.9) 639.6
      - molar pregnancy (*see also* categories 630-632) 639.6
    - following
      - abortion 639.6
      - ectopic or molar pregnancy 639.6
    - late effect – *see* Late effect(s) (of) cerebrovascular disease
    - puerperal, postpartum, childbirth 674.0❺
  - capillary 448.9
  - cardiac (*see also* Infarct, myocardium) 410.9❺
  - carotid (artery) (common) (internal) (*see also* Occlusion, artery, carotid) 433.1❺
  - cavernous sinus (venous) – *see* Embolism, intracranial venous sinus
  - cerebral (*see also* Embolism, brain) 434.1❺
  - cholesterol – *see* Atheroembolism
  - choroidal (anterior) (artery) 433.8❺
  - coronary (artery or vein) (systemic) (*see also* Infarct, myocardium) 410.9❺
    - without myocardial infarction 411.81
  - due to (presence of) any device, implant, or graft classifiable to 996.0-996.5 – *see* Complications, due to (presence of) any device, implant, or graft classified to 996.0-996.5 NEC
  - encephalomalacia (*see also* Embolism, brain) 434.1❺
  - extremities 444.22
    - lower 444.22
    - upper 444.21
  - eye 362.30
  - fat (cerebral) (pulmonary) (systemic) 958.1
    - with
      - abortion – *see* Abortion, by type, with embolism
      - ectopic pregnancy (*see also* categories 633.0-633.9) 639.6
      - molar pregnancy (*see also* categories 630-632) 639.6
    - complicating delivery or puerperium 673.8❺
    - following
      - abortion 639.6
      - ectopic or molar pregnancy 639.6
    - in pregnancy, childbirth, or the puerperium 673.8❺
  - femoral (artery) 444.22
    - vein 453.8
      - deep 453.41
  - following
    - abortion 639.6
    - ectopic or molar pregnancy 639.6
    - infusion, perfusion, or transfusion
      - air 999.1
      - thrombus 999.2
  - heart (fatty) (*see also* Infarct, myocardium) 410.9❺
  - hepatic (vein) 453.0
  - iliac (artery) 444.81
  - iliofemoral 444.81
  - in pregnancy, childbirth, or puerperium (pulmonary) – *see* Embolism, obstetrical
  - intestine (artery) (vein) (with gangrene) 557.0
  - intracranial (*see also* Embolism, brain) 434.1❺
    - venous sinus (any) 325
      - late effect – *see* category 326
      - nonpyogenic 437.6
        - in pregnancy or puerperium 671.5❺
  - kidney (artery) 593.81
  - lateral sinus (venous) – *see* Embolism, intracranial venous sinus
  - longitudinal sinus (venous) – *see* Embolism, intracranial venous sinus
  - lower extremity 444.22
  - lung (massive) – *see* Embolism, pulmonary
  - meninges (*see also* Embolism, brain) 434.1❺
  - mesenteric (artery) (with gangrene) 557.0
  - multiple NEC 444.9
  - obstetrical (pulmonary) 673.2❺
    - air 673.0❺
    - amniotic fluid (pulmonary) 673.1❺
    - blood-clot 673.2❺
    - cardiac 674.8❺
    - fat 673.8❺
    - heart 674.8❺
    - pyemic 673.3❺

Embolism – *continued*
- obstetrical – *continued*
  - septic 673.3❺
  - specified NEC 674.8❺
- ophthalmic (*see also* Occlusion, retina) 362.30
- paradoxical NEC 444.9
- penis 607.82
- peripheral arteries NEC 444.22
  - lower 444.22
  - upper 444.21
- pituitary 253.8
- popliteal (artery) 444.22
- portal (vein) 452
- postoperative NEC 997.2
  - cerebral 997.02
  - mesenteric artery 997.71
  - other vessels 997.79
  - peripheral vascular 997.2
  - pulmonary 415.11
    - septic 415.12 ●
  - renal artery 997.72
- precerebral artery (*see also* Occlusion, artery, precerebral) 433.9❺
- puerperal – *see* Embolism, obstetrical
- pulmonary (artery) (vein) 415.1❺
  - with
    - abortion – *see* Abortion, by type, with embolism
    - ectopic pregnancy (*see also* categories 633.0-633.9) 639.6
    - molar pregnancy (*see also* categories 630-632) 639.6
  - following
    - abortion 639.6
    - ectopic or molar pregnancy 639.6
  - iatrogenic 415.11
  - in pregnancy, childbirth, or puerperium – *see* Embolism, obstetrical
  - postoperative 415.11
  - septic 415.12 ●
- pyemic (multiple) ▶(*see also* Septicemia)◀ 415.12 ▲
  - with
    - abortion – *see* Abortion, by type, with embolism
    - ectopic pregnancy (*see also* categories 633.0-633.9) 639.6
    - molar pregnancy (*see also* categories 630-632) 639.6
  - Aerobacter aerogenes 415.12 ▲
  - enteric gram-negative bacilli 415.12 ▲
  - Enterobacter aerogenes 415.12 ▲
  - Escherichia coli 415.12 ▲
  - following
    - abortion 639.6
    - ectopic or molar pregnancy 639.6
  - Hemophilus influenzae 415.12 ▲
  - pneumococcal 415.12 ▲
  - Proteus vulgaris 415.12 ▲
  - Pseudomonas (aeruginosa) 415.12 ▲
  - puerperal, postpartum, childbirth (any organism) 673.3❺
  - Serratia 415.12 ▲
  - specified organism NEC 415.12 ▲
  - staphylococcal 415.12 ▲
    - aureus 415.12 ▲
    - specified organism NEC 415.12 ▲
  - streptococcal 415.12 ▲
- renal (artery) 593.81
  - vein 453.3
- retina, retinal (*see also* Occlusion, retina) 362.30
- saddle (aorta) 444.0
- septic 415.12 ●
  - arterial 449 ●
- septicemic – *see* Embolism, pyemic
- sinus – *see* Embolism, intracranial venous sinus
- soap
  - with
    - abortion – *see* Abortion, by type, with embolism
    - ectopic pregnancy (*see also* categories 633.0-633.9) 639.6
    - molar pregnancy (*see also* categories 630-632) 639.6
  - following
    - abortion 639.6
    - ectopic or molar pregnancy 639.6
- spinal cord (nonpyogenic) 336.1
  - in pregnancy or puerperium 671.5❺
  - pyogenic origin 324.1
    - late effect – *see* category 326
- spleen, splenic (artery) 444.89

Embolism – *continued*
- thrombus (thromboembolism) following infusion, perfusion, or transfusion 999.2
- upper extremity 444.21
- vein 453.9
  - with inflammation or phlebitis – *see* Thrombophlebitis
  - cerebral (*see also* Embolism, brain) 434.1❺
  - coronary (*see also* Infarct, myocardium) 410.9❺
    - without myocardial infarction 411.81
  - hepatic 453.0
  - lower extremity 453.8
    - deep 453.40
      - calf 453.42
      - distal (lower leg) 453.42
      - femoral 453.41
      - iliac 453.41
      - lower leg 453.42
      - peroneal 453.42
      - popliteal 453.41
      - proximal (upper leg) 453.41
      - thigh 453.41
      - tibial 453.42
  - mesenteric (with gangrene) 557.0
  - portal 452
  - pulmonary – *see* Embolism, pulmonary
  - renal 453.3
  - specified NEC 453.8
    - with inflammation or phlebitis – *see* Thrombophlebitis
- vena cava (inferior) (superior) 453.2
- vessels of brain (*see also* Embolism, brain) 434.1❺

Embolization – *see* Embolism

Embolus – *see* Embolism

Embryoma (M9080/1) – *see also* Neoplasm, by site, uncertain behavior
- benign (M9080/0) – *see* Neoplasm, by site, benign
- kidney (M8960/3) 189.0
- liver (M8970/3) 155.0
- malignant (M9080/3) – *see also* Neoplasm, by site, malignant
  - kidney (M8960/3) 189.0
  - liver (M8970/3) 155.0
  - testis (M9070/3) 186.9
    - undescended 186.0
- testis (M9070/3) 186.9
  - undescended 186.0

Embryonic
- circulation 747.9
- heart 747.9
- vas deferens 752.89

Embryopathia NEC 759.9

Embryotomy, fetal 763.89

Embryotoxon 743.43
- interfering with vision 743.42

Emesis – *see also* Vomiting
- gravidarum – *see* Hyperemesis, gravidarum

Emissions, nocturnal (semen) 608.89

Emotional
- crisis – *see* Crisis, emotional
- disorder (*see also* Disorder, mental) 300.9
- instability (excessive) 301.3
- overlay – *see* Reaction, adjustment
- upset 300.9

Emotionality, pathological 301.3

Emotogenic disease (*see also* Disorder, psychogenic) 306.9

Emphysema (atrophic) (centriacinar) (centrilobular) (chronic) (diffuse) (essential) (hypertrophic) (interlobular) (lung) (obstructive) (panlobular) (paracicatricial) (paracinar) (postural) (pulmonary) (senile) (subpleural) (traction) (unilateral) (unilobular) (vesicular) 492.8
- with bronchitis
  - chronic 491.20
    - with
      - acute bronchitis 491.22
      - exacerbation (acute) 491.21
- bullous (giant) 492.0
- cellular tissue 958.7
  - surgical 998.81
- compensatory 518.2
- congenital 770.2
- conjunctiva 372.89
- connective tissue 958.7
  - surgical 998.81

Emphysema – *continued*
- due to fumes or vapors 506.4
- eye 376.89
- eyelid 374.85
  - surgical 998.81
  - traumatic 958.7
- fetus or newborn (interstitial) (mediastinal) (unilobular) 770.2
- heart 416.9
- interstitial 518.1
  - congenital 770.2
  - fetus or newborn 770.2
- laminated tissue 958.7
  - surgical 998.81
- mediastinal 518.1
  - fetus or newborn 770.2
- newborn (interstitial) (mediastinal) (unilobular) 770.2
- obstructive diffuse with fibrosis 492.8
- orbit 376.89
- subcutaneous 958.7
  - due to trauma 958.7
  - nontraumatic 518.1
  - surgical 998.81
- surgical 998.81
- thymus (gland) (congenital) 254.8
- traumatic 958.7
- tuberculous (*see also* Tuberculosis, pulmonary) 011.9❺

Employment examination (certification) V70.5

Empty sella (turcica) **syndrome** 253.8

Empyema (chest) (diaphragmatic) (double) (encapsulated) (general) (interlobar) (lung) (medial) (necessitatis) (perforating chest wall) (pleura) (pneumococcal) (residual) (sacculated) (streptococcal) (supradiaphragmatic) 510.9
- with fistula 510.0
- accessory sinus (chronic) (*see also* Sinusitis) 473.9
- acute 510.9
  - with fistula 510.0
- antrum (chronic) (*see also* Sinusitis, maxillary) 473.0
- brain (any part) (*see also* Abscess, brain) 324.0
- ethmoidal (sinus) (chronic) (*see also* Sinusitis, ethmoidal) 473.2
- extradural (*see also* Abscess, extradural) 324.9
- frontal (sinus) (chronic) (*see also* Sinusitis, frontal) 473.1
- gallbladder (*see also* Cholecystitis, acute) 575.0
- mastoid (process) (acute) (*see also* Mastoiditis, acute) 383.00
- maxilla, maxillary 526.4
  - sinus (chronic) (*see also* Sinusitis, maxillary) 473.0
- nasal sinus (chronic) (*see also* Sinusitis) 473.9
- sinus (accessory) (nasal) (*see also* Sinusitis) 473.9
- sphenoidal (chronic) (sinus) (*see also* Sinusitis, sphenoidal) 473.3
- subarachnoid (*see also* Abscess, extradural) 324.9
- subdural (*see also* Abscess, extradural) 324.9
- tuberculous (*see also* Tuberculosis, pleura) 012.0❺
- ureter (*see also* Ureteritis) 593.89
- ventricular (*see also* Abscess, brain) 324.0

Enameloma 520.2

Encephalitis (bacterial) (chronic) (hemorrhagic) (idiopathic) (nonepidemic) (spurious) (subacute) 323.9
- acute – *see also* Encephalitis, viral
  - disseminated (postinfectious) NEC 136.9 *[323.61]*
    - postimmunization or postvaccination 323.51
  - inclusional 049.8
  - inclusion body 049.8
  - necrotizing 049.8
- arboviral, arbovirus NEC 064
- arthropod-borne (*see also* Encephalitis, viral, arthropod-borne) 064
- Australian X 062.4
- Bwamba fever 066.3
- California (virus) 062.5
- Central European 063.2
- Czechoslovakian 063.2
- Dawson's (inclusion body) 046.2
- diffuse sclerosing 046.2
- due to
  - actinomycosis 039.8 *[323.41]*
  - cat-scratch disease 078.3 *[323.01]*

Encephalitis – *continued*
due to – *continued*
human herpesvirus 6 058.21 ●
human herpesvirus 7 058.29 ●
human herpesvirus NEC 058.29 ●
infection classified elsewhere 136.9 *[323.41]*
infectious mononucleosis 075 *[323.01]*
malaria (*see also* Malaria) 084.6 *[323.2]*
Negishi virus 064
ornithosis 073.7 *[323.01]*
prophylactic inoculation against smallpox 323.51
rickettsiosis (*see also* Rickettsiosis) 083.9 *[323.1]*
rubella 056.01
toxoplasmosis (acquired) 130.0
congenital (active) 771.2 *[323.41]*
typhus (fever) (*see also* Typhus) 081.9 *[323.1]*
vaccination (smallpox) 323.51
Eastern equine 062.2
endemic 049.8
epidemic 049.8
equine (acute) (infectious) (viral) 062.9
Eastern 062.2
Venezuelan 066.2
Western 062.1
Far Eastern 063.0
following vaccination or other immunization procedure 323.51
herpes 054.3
human herpesvirus 6 058.21 ●
human herpesvirus 7 058.29 ●
human herpesvirus NEC 058.29 ●
ilheus (virus) 062.8
inclusion body 046.2
infectious (acute) (virus) NEC 049.8
influenzal 487.8 *[323.41]*
lethargic 049.8
Japanese (B type) 062.0
La Crosse 062.5
Langat 063.8
late effect – *see* Late, effect, encephalitis
lead 984.9 *[323.71]*
lethargic (acute) (infectious) (influenzal) 049.8
lethargica 049.8
louping ill 063.1
lupus 710.0 *[323.81]*
lymphatica 049.0
Mengo 049.8
meningococcal 036.1
mumps 072.2
Murray Valley 062.4
myoclonic 049.8
Negishi virus 064
otitic NEC 382.4 *[323.41]*
parasitic NEC 123.9 *[323.41]*
periaxialis (concentrica) (diffusa) 341.1
postchickenpox 052.0
postexanthematous NEC 057.9 *[323.62]*
postimmunization 323.51
postinfectious NEC 136.9 *[323.62]*
postmeasles 055.0
posttraumatic 323.81
postvaccinal (smallpox) 323.51
postvaricella 052.0
postviral NEC 079.99 *[323.62]*
postexanthematous 057.9 *[323.62]*
specified NEC 057.8 *[323.62]*
Powassan 063.8
progressive subcortical (Binswanger's) 290.12
Rasmussen 323.81
Rio Bravo 049.8
rubella 056.01
Russian
autumnal 062.0
spring-summer type (taiga) 063.0
saturnine 984.9 *[323.71]*
Semliki Forest 062.8
serous 048
slow-acting virus NEC 046.8
specified cause NEC 323.81
St. Louis type 062.3
subacute sclerosing 046.2
subcorticalis chronica 290.12
summer 062.0
suppurative 324.0
syphilitic 094.81
congenital 090.41
tick-borne 063.9
torula, torular 117.5 *[323.41]*
toxic NEC 989.9 *[323.71]*

Encephalitis – *continued*
toxoplasmic (acquired) 130.0
congenital (active) 771.2 *[323.41]*
trichinosis 124 *[323.41]*
Trypanosomiasis (*see also* Trypanosomiasis) 086.9 *[323.2]*
tuberculous (*see also* Tuberculosis) 013.6❺
type B (Japanese) 062.0
type C 062.3
van Bogaert's 046.2
Venezuelan 066.2
Vienna type 049.8
viral, virus 049.9
arthropod-borne NEC 064
mosquito-borne 062.9
Australian X disease 062.4
California virus 062.5
Eastern equine 062.2
Ilheus virus 062.8
Japanese (B type) 062.0
Murray Valley 062.4
specified type NEC 062.8
St. Louis 062.3
type B 062.0
type C 062.3
Western equine 062.1
tick-borne 063.9
biundulant 063.2
Central European 063.2
Czechoslovakian 063.2
diphasic meningoencephalitis 063.2
Far Eastern 063.0
Langat 063.8
louping ill 063.1
Powassan 063.8
Russian spring-summer (taiga) 063.0
specified type NEC 063.8
vector unknown 064
slow acting NEC 046.8
specified type NEC 049.8
vaccination, prophylactic (against) V05.0
von Economo's 049.8
Western equine 062.1
West Nile type 066.41

Encephalocele 742.0
orbit 376.81

Encephalocystocele 742.0

Encephalomalacia (brain) (cerebellar) (cerebral) (cerebrospinal) (*see also* Softening, brain) 434.9❺
due to
hemorrhage (*see also* Hemorrhage, brain) 431
recurrent spasm of artery 435.9
embolic (cerebral) (*see also* Embolism, brain) 434.1❺
subcorticalis chronicus arteriosclerotica 290.12
thrombotic (*see also* Thrombosis, brain) 434.0❺

Encephalomeningitis – *see* Meningoencephalitis

Encephalomeningocele 742.0

Encephalomeningomyelitis – *see* Meningoencephalitis

Encephalomeningopathy (*see also* Meningoencephalitis) 349.9

Encephalomyelitis (chronic) (granulomatous) (hemorrhagic necrotizing, acute) (myalgic, benign) (*see also* Encephalitis) 323.9
abortive disseminated 049.8
acute disseminated (ADEM)(postinfectious) 136.9 *[323.61]*
infectious 136.9 *[323.61]*
noninfectious 323.81
postimmunization 323.51
due to
cat-scratch disease 078.3 *[323.01]*
infectious mononucleosis 075 *[323.01]*
ornithosis 073.7 *[323.01]*
vaccination (any) 323.51
equine (acute) (infectious) 062.9
Eastern 062.2
Venezuelan 066.2
Western 062.1
funicularis infectiosa 049.8
late effect – *see* Late, effect, encephalitis
Munch-Peterson's 049.8
postchickenpox 052.0
postimmunization 323.51
postmeasles 055.0
postvaccinal (smallpox) 323.51
rubella 056.01
specified cause NEC 323.81

Encephalomyelitis – *continued*
syphilitic 094.81
West Nile 066.41

Encephalomyelocele 742.0

Encephalomyelomeningitis – *see* Meningoencephalitis

Encephalomyeloneuropathy 349.9

Encephalomyelopathy 349.9
subacute necrotizing (infantile) 330.8

Encephalomyeloradiculitis (acute) 357.0

Encephalomyeloradiculoneuritis (acute) 357.0

Encephalomyeloradiculopathy 349.9

Encephalomyocarditis 074.23

Encephalopathia hyperbilirubinemica, newborn 774.7
due to isoimmunization (conditions classifiable to 773.0-773.2) 773.4

Encephalopathy (acute) 348.30
alcoholic 291.2
anoxic – *see* Damage, brain, anoxic
arteriosclerotic 437.0
late effect – *see* Late effect(s) (of) cerebrovascular disease
bilirubin, newborn 774.7
due to isoimmunization 773.4
congenital 742.9
demyelinating (callosal) 341.8
due to
birth injury (intracranial) 767.8
dialysis 294.8
transient 293.9
hyperinsulinism – *see* Hyperinsulinism
influenza (virus) 487.8
lack of vitamin (*see also* Deficiency, vitamin) 269.2
nicotinic acid deficiency 291.2
serum (nontherapeutic) (therapeutic) 999.5
syphilis 094.81
trauma (postconcussional) 310.2
current (*see also* Concussion, brain) 850.9
with skull fracture – *see* Fracture, skull, by site, with intracranial injury
vaccination 323.51
hepatic 572.2
hyperbilirubinemic, newborn 774.7
due to isoimmunization (conditions classifiable to 773.0-773.2) 773.4
hypertensive 437.2
hypoglycemic 251.2
hypoxic – *see* also Damage, brain, anoxic
ischemic (HIE) 768.7
infantile cystic necrotizing (congenital) 341.8
lead 984.9 *[323.71]*
leukopolio 330.0
metabolic (*see also* Delirium) 348.31
toxic 349.82
necrotizing
hemorrhagic 323.61
subacute 330.8
other specified type NEC 348.39
pellagrous 265.2
portal-systemic 572.2
postcontusional 310.2
posttraumatic 310.2
saturnine 984.9 *[323.71]*
septic 348.31
spongioform, subacute (viral) 046.1
subacute
necrotizing 330.8
spongioform 046.1
viral, spongioform 046.1
subcortical progressive (Schilder) 341.1
chronic (Binswanger's) 290.12
toxic 349.82
metabolic 349.82
traumatic (postconcussional) 310.2
current (*see also* Concussion, brain) 850.9
with skull fracture – *see* Fracture, skull, by site, with intracranial injury
vitamin B deficiency NEC 266.9
Wernicke's (superior hemorrhagic polioencephalitis) 265.1

Encephalorrhagia (*see also* Hemorrhage, brain) 432.9
healed or old V12.54 ▲
late effect – *see* Late effect(s) (of) cerebrovascular disease

Encephalosis, posttraumatic 310.2

Encephalitis – Encephalosis, posttraumatic

Enchondroma (M9220/0) – *see also* Neoplasm, bone, benign
multiple, congenital 756.4
Enchondromatosis (cartilaginous) (congenital) (multiple) 756.4
Enchondroses, multiple (cartilaginous) (congenital) 756.4
Encopresis (*see also* Incontinence, feces) 787.6
nonorganic origin 307.7
Encounter for – *see also* Admission for
administrative purpose only V68.9
referral of patient without examination or treatment V68.81
specified purpose NEC V68.89
chemotherapy, antineoplastic V58.11
dialysis
extracorporeal (renal) V56.0
peritoneal V56.8
disability examination V68.01 ●
end-of-life care V66.7
hospice care V66.7
immunotherapy, antineoplastic V58.12
palliative care V66.7
paternity testing V70.4
radiotherapy V58.0
respirator [ventilator] dependence
during
mechanical failure V46.14
power failure V46.12
for weaning V46.13
screening mammogram NEC V76.12
for high-risk patient V76.11
terminal care V66.7
weaning from respirator [ventilator] V46.13
Encystment – *see* Cyst
End-of-life care V66.7
Endamebiasis – *see* Amebiasis
Endamoeba – *see* Amebiasis
Endarteritis (bacterial, subacute) (infective) (septic) 447.6
brain, cerebral or cerebrospinal 437.4
late effect – *see* Late effect(s) (of) cerebrovascular disease
coronary (artery) – *see* Arteriosclerosis, coronary
deformans – *see* Arteriosclerosis
embolic (*see also* Embolism) 444.9
obliterans – *see also* Arteriosclerosis
pulmonary 417.8
pulmonary 417.8
retina 362.18
senile – *see* Arteriosclerosis
syphilitic 093.89
brain or cerebral 094.89
congenital 090.5
spinal 094.89
tuberculous (*see also* Tuberculosis) 017.9⑤
Endemic – *see* condition
Endocarditis (chronic) (indeterminate) (interstitial) (marantis) (nonbacterial thrombotic) (residual) (sclerotic) (sclerous) (senile) (valvular) 424.90
with
rheumatic fever (conditions classifiable to 390)
active – *see* Endocarditis, acute, rheumatic
inactive or quiescent (with chorea) 397.9
acute or subacute 421.9
rheumatic (aortic) (mitral) (pulmonary) (tricuspid) 391.1
with chorea (acute) (rheumatic) (Sydenham's) 392.0
aortic (heart) (nonrheumatic) (valve) 424.1
with
mitral (valve) disease 396.9
active or acute 391.1
with chorea (acute) (rheumatic) (Sydenham's) 392.0
bacterial 421.0
rheumatic fever (conditions classifiable to 390)
active – *see* Endocarditis, acute, rheumatic
inactive or quiescent (with chorea) 395.9
with mitral disease 396.9
acute or subacute 421.9
arteriosclerotic 424.1
congenital 746.89
hypertensive 424.1
rheumatic (chronic) (inactive) 395.9
with mitral (valve) disease 396.9
active or acute 391.1
with chorea (acute) (rheumatic) (Sydenham's) 392.0

Endocarditis – *continued*
aortic – *continued*
rheumatic – *continued*
active or acute 391.1
with chorea (acute) (rheumatic) (Sydenham's) 392.0
specified cause, except rheumatic 424.1
syphilitic 093.22
arteriosclerotic or due to arteriosclerosis 424.99
atypical verrucous (Libman-Sacks) 710.0 *[424.91]*
bacterial (acute) (any valve) (chronic) (subacute) 421.0
blastomycotic 116.0 *[421.1]*
candidal 112.81
congenital 425.3
constrictive 421.0
Coxsackie 074.22
due to
blastomycosis 116.0 *[421.1]*
candidiasis 112.81
coxsackie (virus) 074.22
disseminated lupus erythematosus 710.0 *[424.91]*
histoplasmosis (*see also* Histoplasmosis) 115.94
hypertension (benign) 424.99
moniliasis 112.81
prosthetic cardiac valve 996.61
Q fever 083.0 *[421.1]*
serratia marcescens 421.0
typhoid (fever) 002.0 *[421.1]*
fetal 425.3
gonococcal 098.84
hypertensive 424.99
infectious or infective (acute) (any valve) (chronic) (subacute) 421.0
lenta (acute) (any valve) (chronic) (subacute) 421.0
Libman-Sacks 710.0 *[424.91]*
Loeffler's (parietal fibroplastic) 421.0
malignant (acute) (any valve) (chronic) (subacute) 421.0
meningococcal 036.42
mitral (chronic) (double) (fibroid) (heart) (inactive) (valve) (with chorea) 394.9
with
aortic (valve) disease 396.9
active or acute 391.1
with chorea (acute) (rheumatic) (Sydenham's) 392.0
rheumatic fever (conditions classifiable to 390)
active – *see* Endocarditis, acute, rheumatic
inactive or quiescent (with chorea) 394.9
with aortic valve disease 396.9
active or acute 391.1
with chorea (acute) (rheumatic) (Sydenham's) 392.0
bacterial 421.0
arteriosclerotic 424.0
congenital 746.89
hypertensive 424.0
nonrheumatic 424.0
acute or subacute 421.9
syphilitic 093.21
monilial 112.81
mycotic (acute) (any valve) (chronic) (subacute) 421.0
pneumococcic (acute) (any valve) (chronic) (subacute) 421.0
pulmonary (chronic) (heart) (valve) 424.3
with
rheumatic fever (conditions classifiable to 390)
active – *see* Endocarditis, acute, rheumatic
inactive or quiescent (with chorea) 397.1
acute or subacute 421.9
rheumatic 391.1
with chorea (acute) (rheumatic) (Sydenham's) 392.0
arteriosclerotic or due to arteriosclerosis 424.3
congenital 746.09
hypertensive or due to hypertension (benign) 424.3
rheumatic (chronic) (inactive) (with chorea) 397.1
active or acute 391.1
with chorea (acute) (rheumatic) (Sydenham's) 392.0
syphilitic 093.24

Endocarditis – *continued*
purulent (acute) (any valve) (chronic) (subacute) 421.0
rheumatic (chronic) (inactive) (with chorea) 397.9
active or acute (aortic) (mitral) (pulmonary) (tricuspid) 391.1
with chorea (acute) (rheumatic) (Sydenham's) 392.0
septic (acute) (any valve) (chronic) (subacute) 421.0
specified cause, except rheumatic 424.99
streptococcal (acute) (any valve) (chronic) (subacute) 421.0
subacute – *see* Endocarditis, acute
suppurative (any valve) (acute) (chronic) (subacute) 421.0
syphilitic NEC 093.20
toxic (*see also* Endocarditis, acute) 421.9
tricuspid (chronic) (heart) (inactive) (rheumatic) (valve) (with chorea) 397.0
with
rheumatic fever (conditions classifiable to 390)
active – *see* Endocarditis, acute, rheumatic
inactive or quiescent (with chorea) 397.0
active or acute 391.1
with chorea (acute) (rheumatic) (Sydenham's) 392.0
arteriosclerotic 424.2
congenital 746.89
hypertensive 424.2
nonrheumatic 424.2
acute or subacute 421.9
specified cause, except rheumatic 424.2
syphilitic 093.23
tuberculous (*see also* Tuberculosis) 017.9⑤ *[424.91]*
typhoid 002.0 *[421.1]*
ulcerative (acute) (any valve) (chronic) (subacute) 421.0
vegetative (acute) (any valve) (chronic) (subacute) 421.0
verrucous (acute) (any valve) (chronic) (subacute) NEC 710.0 *[424.91]*
nonbacterial 710.0 *[424.91]*
nonrheumatic 710.0 *[424.91]*
Endocardium, endocardial – *see also* condition
cushion defect 745.60
specified type NEC 745.69
Endocervicitis (*see also* Cervicitis) 616.0
due to
intrauterine (contraceptive) device 996.65
gonorrheal (acute) 098.15
chronic or duration of 2 months or over 098.35
hyperplastic 616.0
syphilitic 095.8
trichomonal 131.09
tuberculous (*see also* Tuberculosis) 016.7⑤
Endocrine – *see* condition
Endocrinopathy, pluriglandular 258.9
Endodontitis 522.0
Endomastoiditis (*see also* Mastoiditis) 383.9
Endometrioma 617.9
Endometriosis 617.9
appendix 617.5
bladder 617.8
bowel 617.5
broad ligament 617.3
cervix 617.0
colon 617.5
cul-de-sac (Douglas') 617.3
exocervix 617.0
fallopian tube 617.2
female genital organ NEC 617.8
gallbladder 617.8
in scar of skin 617.6
internal 617.0
intestine 617.5
lung 617.8
myometrium 617.0
ovary 617.1
parametrium 617.3
pelvic peritoneum 617.3
peritoneal (pelvic) 617.3
rectovaginal septum 617.4
rectum 617.5
round ligament 617.3
skin 617.6
specified site NEC 617.8
stromal (M8931/1) 236.0
umbilicus 617.8

Enchondroma – Endometriosis

- **Endometriosis** – *continued*
  - uterus 617.0
    - internal 617.0
  - vagina 617.4
  - vulva 617.8
- **Endometritis** (nonspecific) (purulent) (septic) (suppurative) 615.9
  - with
    - abortion – *see* Abortion, by type, with sepsis
    - ectopic pregnancy (*see also* categories 633.0-633.9) 639.0
    - molar pregnancy (*see also* categories 630-632) 639.0
  - acute 615.0
  - blennorrhagic 098.16
    - acute 098.16
    - chronic or duration of 2 months or over 098.36
  - cervix, cervical (*see also* Cervicitis) 616.0
    - hyperplastic 616.0
  - chronic 615.1
  - complicating pregnancy 646.6❺
    - affecting fetus or newborn 760.8
  - decidual 615.9
  - following
    - abortion 639.0
    - ectopic or molar pregnancy 639.0
  - gonorrheal (acute) 098.16
    - chronic or duration of 2 months or over 098.36
  - hyperplastic (*see also* Hyperplasia, endometrium) 621.30
    - cervix 616.0
  - polypoid – *see* Endometritis, hyperplastic
  - puerperal, postpartum, childbirth 670❹
  - senile (atrophic) 615.9
  - subacute 615.0
  - tuberculous (*see also* Tuberculosis) 016.7❺
- **Endometrium** – *see* condition
- **Endomyocardiopathy, South African** 425.2
- **Endomyocarditis** – *see* Endocarditis
- **Endomyofibrosis** 425.0
- **Endomyometritis** (*see also* Endometritis) 615.9
- **Endopericarditis** – *see* Endocarditis
- **Endoperineuritis** – *see* Disorder, nerve
- **Endophlebitis** (*see also* Phlebitis) 451.9
  - leg 451.2
    - deep (vessels) 451.19
    - superficial (vessels) 451.0
  - portal (vein) 572.1
  - retina 362.18
  - specified site NEC 451.89
  - syphilitic 093.89
- **Endophthalmia** (*see also* Endophthalmitis) 360.00
  - gonorrheal 098.42
- **Endophthalmitis** (globe) (infective) (metastatic) (purulent) (subacute) 360.00
  - acute 360.01
  - bleb associated 379.63
  - chronic 360.03
  - parasitic 360.13
  - phacoanaphylactic 360.19
  - specified type NEC 360.19
  - sympathetic 360.11
- **Endosalpingioma** (M9111/1) 236.2
- **Endosalpingiosis** 629.89 ●
- **Endosteitis** – *see* Osteomyelitis
- **Endothelioma, bone** (M9260/3) – *see* Neoplasm, bone, malignant
- **Endotheliosis** 287.8
  - hemorrhagic infectional 287.8
- **Endotoxemia** - *code to condition*
- **Endotoxic shock** 785.52
- **Endotrachelitis** (*see also* Cervicitis) 616.0
- **Enema rash** 692.89
- **Engel-von Recklinghausen disease or syndrome** (osteitis fibrosa cystica) 252.01
- **Engelmann's disease** (diaphyseal sclerosis) 756.59
- **English disease** (*see also* Rickets) 268.0
- **Engman's disease** (infectious eczematoid dermatitis) 690.8
- **Engorgement**
  - breast 611.79
    - newborn 778.7
    - puerperal, postpartum 676.2❺
  - liver 573.9
  - lung 514
  - pulmonary 514
  - retina, venous 362.37
  - stomach 536.8
- **Engorgement** – *continued*
  - venous, retina 362.37
- **Enlargement, enlarged** – *see also* Hypertrophy
  - abdomen 789.3❺
  - adenoids 474.12
    - and tonsils 474.10
  - alveolar process or ridge 525.8
  - apertures of diaphragm (congenital) 756.6
  - blind spot, visual field 368.42
  - gingival 523.8
  - heart, cardiac (*see also* Hypertrophy, cardiac) 429.3
  - lacrimal gland, chronic 375.03
  - liver (*see also* Hypertrophy, liver) 789.1
  - lymph gland or node 785.6
  - orbit 376.46
  - organ or site, congenital NEC – *see* Anomaly, specified type NEC
  - parathyroid (gland) 252.01
  - pituitary fossa 793.0
  - prostate (simple) (soft) 600.00
    - with
      - other lower urinary tract symptoms (LUTS) 600.01
      - urinary
        - obstruction 600.01
        - retention 600.01
  - sella turcica 793.0
  - spleen (*see also* Splenomegaly) 789.2
    - congenital 759.0
  - thymus (congenital) (gland) 254.0
  - thyroid (gland) (*see also* Goiter) 240.9
  - tongue 529.8
  - tonsils 474.11
    - and adenoids 474.10
  - uterus 621.2
- **Enophthalmos** 376.50
  - due to
    - atrophy of orbital tissue 376.51
    - surgery 376.52
    - trauma 376.52
- **Enostosis** 526.89
- **Entamebiasis** – *see* Amebiasis
- **Entamebic** – *see* Amebiasis
- **Entanglement, umbilical cord(s)** 663.3❺
  - with compression 663.2❺
  - affecting fetus or newborn 762.5
  - around neck with compression 663.1❺
  - twins in monoamniotic sac 663.2❺
- **Enteralgia** 789.0❺
- **Enteric** – *see* condition
- **Enteritis** (acute) (catarrhal) (choleraic) (chronic) (congestive) (diarrheal) (exudative) (follicular) (hemorrhagic) (infantile) (lienteric) (noninfectious) (perforative) (phlegmonous) (presumed noninfectious) (pseudomembranous) 558.9
  - adaptive 564.9
  - aertrycke infection 003.0
  - allergic 558.3
  - amebic (*see also* Amebiasis) 006.9
    - with abscess – *see* Abscess, amebic
    - acute 006.0
      - with abscess – *see* Abscess, amebic
      - nondysenteric 006.2
    - chronic 006.1
      - with abscess – *see* Abscess, amebic
      - nondysenteric 006.2
    - nondysenteric 006.2
  - anaerobic (cocci) (gram-negative) (gram-positive) (mixed) NEC 008.46
  - bacillary NEC 004.9
  - bacterial NEC 008.5
    - specified NEC 008.49
  - Bacteroides (fragilis) (melaninogeniscus) (oralis) 008.46
  - Butyrivibrio (fibriosolvens) 008.46
  - Campylobacter 008.43
  - Candida 112.85
  - Chilomastix 007.8
  - choleriformis 001.1
  - chronic 558.9
    - ulcerative (*see also* Colitis, ulcerative) 556.9
  - cicatrizing (chronic) 555.0
  - Clostridium
    - botulinum 005.1
    - difficile 008.45
    - haemolyticum 008.46
    - novyi 008.46
    - perfringens (C) (F) 008.46
- **Enteritis** – *continued*
  - Clostridium – *continued*
    - specified type NEC 008.46
  - coccidial 007.2
  - dietetic 558.9
  - due to
    - achylia gastrica 536.8
    - adenovirus 008.62
    - Aerobacter aerogenes 008.2❺
    - anaerobes (*see also* Enteritis, anaerobic) 008.46
    - Arizona (bacillus) 008.1
    - astrovirus 008.66
    - Bacillus coli – *see* Enteritis, E. coli
    - bacteria NEC 008.5❺
      - specified NEC 008.49
    - Bacteroides (*see also* Enteritis, Bacteroides) 008.46
    - Butyrivibrio (fibriosolvens) 008.46
    - Calcivirus 008.65
    - Camplyobacter 008.43
    - Clostridium – *see* Enteritis, Clostridium
    - Cockle agent 008.64
    - Coxsackie (virus) 008.67
    - Ditchling agent 008.64
    - ECHO virus 008.67
    - Enterobacter aerogenes 008.2❺
    - enterococci 008.49
    - enterovirus NEC 008.67
    - Escherichia coli – *see* Enteritis, E. coli 008.0❺
    - Eubacterium 008.46
    - Fusobacterium (nucleatum) 008.46
    - gram-negative bacteria NEC 008.47
      - anaerobic NEC 008.46
    - Hawaii agent 008.63
    - irritating foods 558.9
    - Klebsiella aerogenes 008.47
    - Marin County agent 008.66
    - Montgomery County agent 008.63
    - Norwalk-like agent 008.63
    - Norwalk virus 008.63
    - Otofuke agent 008.63
    - Paracolobactrum arizonae 008.1
    - paracolon bacillus NEC 008.47
      - arizona 008.1
    - Paramatta agent 008.64
    - Peptococcus 008.46
    - Peptostreptococcus 008.46
    - Proprionibacterium 008.46
    - Proteus (bacillus) (mirabilis) (morganii) 008.3
    - Pseudomonas aeruginosa 008.42
    - Rotavirus 008.61
    - Sapporo agent 008.63
    - small round virus (SRV) NEC 008.64
      - featureless NEC 008.63
      - structured NEC 008.63
    - Snow Mountain (SM) agent 008.63
    - specified
      - bacteria NEC 008.49
      - organism, nonbacterial NEC 008.8
      - virus NEC 008.69
    - Staphylococcus 008.41
    - Streptococcus 008.49
      - anaerobic 008.46
    - Taunton agent 008.63
    - Torovirus 008.69
    - Treponema 008.46
    - Veillonella 008.46
    - virus 008.8
      - specified type NEC 008.69
    - Wollan (W) agent 008.64
    - Yersinia enterocolitica 008.44
  - dysentery – *see* Dysentery
  - E. coli 008.00
    - enterohemorrhagic 008.04
    - enteroinvasive 008.03
    - enteropathogenic 008.01
    - enterotoxigenic 008.02
    - specified type NEC 008.09
  - el tor 001.1
  - embadomonial 007.8
  - epidemic 009.0
  - Eubacterium 008.46
  - fermentative 558.9
  - fulminant 557.0
  - Fusobacterium (nucleatum) 008.46
  - gangrenous (*see also* Enteritis, due to, by organism) 009.0
  - giardial 007.1
  - gram-negative bacteria NEC 008.47
    - anaerobic NEC 008.46

Endometriosis – Enteritis

Enteritis – *continued*
- infectious NEC (*see also* Enteritis, due to, by organism) 009.0
  - presumed 009.1
- influenzal 487.8
- ischemic 557.9
  - acute 557.0
  - chronic 557.1
  - due to mesenteric artery insufficiency 557.1
- membranous 564.9
- mucous 564.9
- myxomembranous 564.9
- necrotic (*see also* Enteritis, due to, by organism) 009.0
- necroticans 005.2
- necrotizing of fetus or newborn 777.5
- neurogenic 564.9
- newborn 777.8
  - necrotizing 777.5
- parasitic NEC 129
- paratyphoid (fever) (*see also* Fever, paratyphoid) 002.9
- Peptococcus 008.46
- Peptostreptococcus 008.46
- Proprionibacterium 008.46
- protozoal NEC 007.9
- radiation 558.1 ●
- regional (of) 555.9
  - intestine
    - large (bowel, colon, or rectum) 555.1
      - with small intestine 555.2
    - small (duodenum, ileum, or jejunum) 555.0
      - with large intestine 555.2
- Salmonella infection 003.0
- salmonellosis 003.0
- segmental (*see also* Enteritis, regional) 555.9
- septic (*see also* Enteritis, due to, by organism) 009.0
- Shigella 004.9
- simple 558.9
- spasmodic 564.9
- spastic 564.9
- staphylococcal 008.41
  - due to food 005.0
- streptococcal 008.49
  - anaerobic 008.46
- toxic 558.2
- Treponema (denticola) (macrodentium) 008.46
- trichomonal 007.3
- tuberculous (*see also* Tuberculosis) 014.8❺
- typhosa 002.0
- ulcerative (chronic) (*see also* Colitis, ulcerative) 556.9
- Veillonella 008.46
- viral 008.8
  - adenovirus 008.62
  - enterovirus 008.67
  - specified virus NEC 008.69
- Yersinia enterocolitica 008.44
- zymotic 009.0

Enteroarticular syndrome 099.3

Enterobiasis 127.4

Enterobius vermicularis 127.4

Enterocele (*see also* Hernia) 553.9
- pelvis, pelvic (acquired) (congenital) 618.6
- vagina, vaginal (acquired) (congenital) 618.6

Enterocolitis – *see also* Enteritis
- fetus or newborn 777.8
  - necrotizing 777.5
- fulminant 557.0
- granulomatous 555.2
- hemorrhagic (acute) 557.0
  - chronic 557.1
- necrotizing (acute) (membranous) 557.0
- primary necrotizing 777.5
- pseudomembranous 008.45
- radiation 558.1
  - newborn 777.5
- ulcerative 556.0

Enterocystoma 751.5

Enterogastritis – *see* Enteritis

Enterogenous cyanosis 289.7

Enterolith, enterolithiasis (impaction) 560.39
- with hernia – *see also* Hernia, by site, with obstruction
  - gangrenous – *see* Hernia, by site, with gangrene

Enteropathy 569.9
- exudative (of Gordon) 579.8
- gluten 579.0
- hemorrhagic, terminal 557.0

Enteropathy – *continued*
- protein-losing 579.8

Enteroperitonitis (*see also* Peritonitis) 567.9

Enteroptosis 569.89

Enterorrhagia 578.9

Enterospasm 564.9
- psychogenic 306.4

Enterostenosis (*see also* Obstruction, intestine) 560.9

Enterostomy status V44.4
- with complication 569.60

Enthesopathy 726.90
- ankle and tarsus 726.70
- elbow region 726.30
  - specified NEC 726.39
- hip 726.5
- knee 726.60
- peripheral NEC 726.8
- shoulder region 726.10
  - adhesive 726.0
- spinal 720.1
- wrist and carpus 726.4

Entrance, air into vein – *see* Embolism, air

Entrapment, nerve – *see* Neuropathy, entrapment

Entropion (eyelid) 374.00
- cicatricial 374.04
- congenital 743.62
- late effect of trachoma (healed) 139.1
- mechanical 374.02
- paralytic 374.02
- senile 374.01
- spastic 374.03

Enucleation of eye (current) (traumatic) 871.3

Enuresis 788.30
- habit disturbance 307.6
- nocturnal 788.36
  - psychogenic 307.6
- nonorganic origin 307.6
- psychogenic 307.6

Enzymopathy 277.9

Eosinopenia 288.59

Eosinophilia 288.3
- allergic 288.3
- hereditary 288.3
- idiopathic 288.3
- infiltrative 518.3
- Loeffler's 518.3
- myalgia syndrome 710.5
- pulmonary (tropical) 518.3
- secondary 288.3
- tropical 518.3

Eosinophilic – *see also* condition
- fasciitis 728.89
- granuloma (bone) 277.89
- infiltration lung 518.3

Ependymitis (acute) (cerebral) (chronic) (granular) (*see also* Meningitis) 322.9

Ependymoblastoma (M9392/3)
- specified site – *see* Neoplasm, by site, malignant
- unspecified site 191.9

Ependymoma (epithelial) (malignant) (M9391/3)
- anaplastic type (M9392/3)
  - specified site – *see* Neoplasm, by site, malignant
  - unspecified site 191.9
- benign (M9391/0)
  - specified site – *see* Neoplasm, by site, benign
  - unspecified site 225.0
- myxopapillary (M9394/1) 237.5
- papillary (M9393/1) 237.5
- specified site – *see* Neoplasm, by site, malignant
- unspecified site 191.9

Ependymopathy 349.2
- spinal cord 349.2

Ephelides, ephelis 709.09

Ephemeral fever (*see also* Pyrexia) 780.6

Epiblepharon (congenital) 743.62

Epicanthus, epicanthic fold (congenital) (eyelid) 743.63

Epicondylitis (elbow) (lateral) 726.32
- medial 726.31

Epicystitis (*see also* Cystitis) 595.9

Epidemic – *see* condition

Epidermidalization, cervix – *see* condition

Epidermidization, cervix – *see* condition

Epidermis, epidermal – *see* condition

Epidermization, cervix – *see* condition

Epidermodysplasia verruciformis 078.19

Epidermoid
- cholesteatoma – *see* Cholesteatoma
- inclusion (*see also* Cyst, skin) 706.2

Epidermolysis
- acuta (combustiformis) (toxica) 695.1
- bullosa 757.39
- necroticans combustiformis 695.1
  - due to drug
    - correct substance properly administered 695.1
    - overdose or wrong substance given or taken 977.9
      - specified drug – *see* Table of Drugs and Chemicals

Epidermophytid – *see* Dermatophytosis

Epidermophytosis (infected) – *see* Dermatophytosis

Epidermosis, ear (middle) (*see also* Cholesteatoma) 385.30

Epididymis – *see* condition

Epididymitis (nonvenereal) 604.90
- with abscess 604.0
- acute 604.99
- blennorrhagic (acute) 098.0
  - chronic or duration of 2 months or over 098.2
- caseous (*see also* Tuberculosis) 016.4❺
- chlamydial 099.54
- diphtheritic 032.89 *[604.91]*
- filarial 125.9 *[604.91]*
- gonococcal (acute) 098.0
  - chronic or duration of 2 months or over 098.2
- recurrent 604.99
- residual 604.99
- syphilitic 095.8 *[604.91]*
- tuberculous (*see also* Tuberculosis) 016.4❺

Epididymo-orchitis (*see also* Epididymitis) 604.90
- with abscess 604.0
- chlamydial 099.54
- gonococcal (acute) 098.13
  - chronic or duration of 2 months or over 098.33

Epidural – *see* condition

Epigastritis (*see also* Gastritis) 535.5❺

Epigastrium, epigastric – *see* condition

Epigastrocele (*see also* Hernia, epigastric) 553.29

Epiglottiditis (acute) 464.30
- with obstruction 464.31
- chronic 476.1
- viral 464.30
  - with obstruction 464.31

Epiglottis – *see* condition

Epiglottitis (acute) 464.30
- with obstruction 464.31
- chronic 476.1
- viral 464.30
  - with obstruction 464.31

Epignathus 759.4

Epilepsia
- partialis continua (*see also* Epilepsy) 345.7❺
- procursiva (*see also* Epilepsy) 345.8❺

Epilepsy, epileptic (idiopathic) 345.9❺

Note – use the following fifth-digit subclassifications with categories 345.0, 345.1, 345.4-345.9

0 without mention of intractable epilepsy

1 with intractable epilepsy

- abdominal 345.5❺
- absence (attack) 345.0❺
- akinetic 345.0❺
  - psychomotor 345.4❺
- automatism 345.4❺
- autonomic diencephalic 345.5❺
- brain 345.9❺
- Bravais-Jacksonian 345.5❺
- cerebral 345.9❺
- climacteric 345.9❺
- clonic 345.1❺
- clouded state 345.9❺
- coma 345.3
- communicating 345.4❺
- complicating pregnancy, childbirth, or the puerperium 649.4❺
- congenital 345.9❺
- convulsions 345.9❺
- cortical (focal) (motor) 345.5❺
- cursive (running) 345.8❺
- cysticercosis 123.1
- deterioration
  - with behavioral disturbance 345.9❺ *[294.11]*

Epilepsy, epileptic – *continued*
  deterioration – *continued*
    without behavioral disturbance 345.9❺ *[294.10]*
  due to syphilis 094.89
  equivalent 345.5❺
  fit 345.9❺
  focal (motor) 345.5❺
  gelastic 345.8❺
  generalized 345.9❺
    convulsive 345.1❺
    flexion 345.1❺
    nonconvulsive 345.0❺
  grand mal (idiopathic) 345.1❺
  Jacksonian (motor) (sensory) 345.5❺
  Kojevnikoff's, Kojevnikov's, Kojewnikoff's 345.7❺
  laryngeal 786.2
  limbic system 345.4❺
  localization related (focal) (partial) and epileptic syndromes
    with
      complex partial seizures 345.4
      simple partial seizures 345.5
  major (motor) 345.1❺
  minor 345.0❺
  mixed (type) 345.9❺
  motor partial 345.5❺
  musicogenic 345.1❺
  myoclonus, myoclonic 345.1❺
    progressive (familial) 333.2
  nonconvulsive, generalized 345.0❺
  parasitic NEC 123.9
  partial (focalized) 345.5❺
    with
      impairment of consciousness 345.4❺
      memory and ideational disturbances 345.4❺
    abdominal type 345.5❺
    motor type 345.5❺
    psychomotor type 345.4❺
    psychosensory type 345.4❺
    secondarily generalized 345.4❺
    sensory type 345.5❺
    somatomotor type 345.5❺
    somatosensory type 345.5❺
    temporal lobe type 345.4❺
    visceral type 345.5❺
    visual type 345.5❺
    without impairment of consciousness 345.5
  peripheral 345.9❺
  petit mal 345.0❺
  photokinetic 345.8❺
  progressive myoclonic (familial) 333.2
  psychic equivalent 345.5❺
  psychomotor 345.4❺
  psychosensory 345.4❺
  reflex 345.1❺
  seizure 345.9❺
  senile 345.9❺
  sensory-induced 345.5❺
  sleep (*see also* Narcolepsy) 347.00
  somatomotor type 345.5❺
  somatosensory 345.5❺
  specified type NEC 345.8❺
  status (grand mal) 345.3
    focal motor 345.7❺
    petit mal 345.2
    psychomotor 345.7❺
    temporal lobe 345.7❺
  symptomatic 345.9❺
  temporal lobe 345.4❺
  tonic (-clonic) 345.1❺
  traumatic (injury unspecified) 907.0
    injury specified – *see* Late, effect (of) specified injury
  twilight 293.0
  uncinate (gyrus) 345.4❺
  unverricht (-Lundborg) (familial myoclonic) 333.2
  visceral 345.5❺
  visual 345.5❺
Epileptiform
  convulsions 780.39
  seizure 780.39
Epiloia 759.5
Epimenorrhea 626.2
Epipharyngitis (*see also* Nasopharyngitis) 460
Epiphora 375.20
  due to
    excess lacrimation 375.21
    insufficient drainage 375.22
Epiphyseal arrest 733.91
  femoral head 732.2
Epiphyseolysis, epiphysiolysis (*see also* Osteochondrosis) 732.9
Epiphysitis (*see also* Osteochondrosis) 732.9
  juvenile 732.6
  marginal (Scheuermann's) 732.0
  os calcis 732.5
  syphilitic (congenital) 090.0
  vertebral (Scheuermann's) 732.0
Epiplocele (*see also* Hernia) 553.9
Epiploitis (*see also* Peritonitis) 567.9
Epiplosarcomphalocele (*see also* Hernia, umbilicus) 553.1
Episcleritis 379.00
  gouty 274.89 *[379.09]*
  nodular 379.02
  periodica fugax 379.01
    angioneurotic – *see* Edema, angioneurotic
  specified NEC 379.09
  staphylococcal 379.00
  suppurative 379.00
  syphilitic 095.0
  tuberculous (*see also* Tuberculosis) 017.3❺ *[379.09]*
Episode
  brain (*see also* Disease, cerebrovascular, acute) 436
  cerebral (*see also* Disease, cerebrovascular, acute) 436
  depersonalization (in neurotic state) 300.6
  hyporesponsive 780.09
  psychotic (*see also* Psychosis) 298.9
    organic, transient 293.9
  schizophrenic (acute) NEC (*see also* Schizophrenia) 295.4❺
Epispadias
  female 753.8
  male 752.62
Episplenitis 289.59
Epistaxis (multiple) 784.7
  hereditary 448.0
  vicarious menstruation 625.8
Epithelioma (malignant) (M8011/3) – *see also* Neoplasm, by site, malignant
  adenoides cysticum (M8100/0) – *see* Neoplasm, skin, benign
  basal cell (M8090/3) – *see* Neoplasm, skin, malignant
  benign (M8011/0) – *see* Neoplasm, by site, benign
  Bowen's (M8081/2) – *see* Neoplasm, skin, in situ
  calcifying (benign) (Malherbe's) (M8110/0) – *see* Neoplasm, skin, benign
  external site – *see* Neoplasm, skin, malignant
  intraepidermal, Jadassohn (M8096/0) – *see* Neoplasm, skin, benign
  squamous cell (M8070/3) – *see* Neoplasm, by site, malignant
Epitheliopathy
  pigment, retina 363.15
  posterior multifocal placoid (acute) 363.15
Epithelium, epithelial – *see* condition
Epituberculosis (allergic) (with atelectasis) (*see also* Tuberculosis) 010.8❺
Eponychia 757.5
Epstein's
  nephrosis or syndrome (*see also* Nephrosis) 581.9
  pearl (mouth) 528.4
Epstein-Barr infection (viral) 075
  chronic 780.79 *[139.8]*
Epulis (giant cell) (gingiva) 523.8
Equinia 024
Equinovarus (congenital) 754.51
  acquired 736.71
Equivalent
  convulsive (abdominal) (*see also* Epilepsy) 345.5❺
  epileptic (psychic) (*see also* Epilepsy) 345.5❺
Erb's
  disease 359.1
  palsy, paralysis (birth) (brachial) (newborn) 767.6
    spinal (spastic) syphilitic 094.89
  pseudohypertrophic muscular dystrophy 359.1
Erb (-Duchenne) **paralysis** (birth injury) (newborn) 767.6
Erb-Goldflam disease or syndrome 358.00
Erdheim's syndrome (acromegalic macrospondylitis) 253.0
Erection, painful (persistent) 607.3
Ergosterol deficiency (vitamin D) 268.9
  with
    osteomalacia 268.2
    rickets (*see also* Rickets) 268.0
Ergotism (ergotized grain) 988.2
  from ergot used as drug (migraine therapy)
    correct substance properly administered 349.82
    overdose or wrong substance given or taken 975.0
Erichsen's disease (railway spine) 300.16
Erlacher-Blount syndrome (tibia vara) 732.4
Erosio interdigitalis blastomycetica 112.3
Erosion
  arteriosclerotic plaque – *see* Arteriosclerosis, by site
  artery NEC 447.2
    without rupture 447.8
  bone 733.99
  bronchus 519.19
  cartilage (joint) 733.99
  cervix (uteri) (acquired) (chronic) (congenital) 622.0
    with mention of cervicitis 616.0
  cornea (recurrent) (*see also* Keratitis) 371.42
    traumatic 918.1
  dental (idiopathic) (occupational) 521.30
    extending into
      dentine 521.32
      pulp 521.33
    generalized 521.35
    limited to enamel 521.31
    localized 521.34
  duodenum, postpyloric – *see* Ulcer, duodenum
  esophagus 530.89
  gastric 535.4❺
  intestine 569.89
  lymphatic vessel 457.8
  pylorus, pyloric (ulcer) 535.4❺
  sclera 379.16
  spine, aneurysmal 094.89
  spleen 289.59
  stomach 535.4❺
  teeth (idiopathic) (occupational) (*see also* Erosion, dental) 521.30
    due to
      medicine 521.30
      persistent vomiting 521.30
  urethra 599.84
  uterus 621.8
  vertebra 733.99
Erotomania 302.89
  Clerambault's 297.8
Error
  in diet 269.9
  refractive 367.9
    astigmatism (*see also* Astigmatism) 367.20
    drug-induced 367.89
    hypermetropia 367.0
    hyperopia 367.0
    myopia 367.1
    presbyopia 367.4
    toxic 367.89
Eructation 787.3
  nervous 306.4
  psychogenic 306.4
Eruption
  creeping 126.9
  drug – *see* Dermatitis, due to, drug
  Hutchinson, summer 692.72
  Kaposi's varicelliform 054.0
  napkin (psoriasiform) 691.0
  polymorphous
    light (sun) 692.72
      other source 692.82
  psoriasiform, napkin 691.0
  recalcitrant pustular 694.8
  ringed 695.89
  skin (*see also* Dermatitis) 782.1
    creeping (meaning hookworm) 126.9
    due to
      chemical(s) NEC 692.4
        internal use 693.8
      drug – *see* Dermatitis, due to, drug
      prophylactic inoculation or vaccination against disease – *see* Dermatitis, due to, vaccine

- **Eruption** – *continued*
  - skin – *continued*
    - due to – *continued*
      - smallpox vaccination NEC – *see* Dermatitis, due to, vaccine
    - erysipeloid 027.1
    - feigned 698.4
    - hutchinson, summer 692.72
    - Kaposi's, varicelliform 054.0
      - vaccinia 999.0
    - lichenoid, axilla 698.3
    - polymorphous, due to light 692.72
    - toxic NEC 695.0
    - vesicular 709.8
  - teeth, tooth
    - accelerated 520.6
    - delayed 520.6
    - difficult 520.6
    - disturbance of 520.6
    - in abnormal sequence 520.6
    - incomplete 520.6
    - late 520.6
    - natal 520.6
    - neonatal 520.6
    - obstructed 520.6
    - partial 520.6
    - persistent primary 520.6
    - premature 520.6
    - prenatal 520.6
  - vesicular 709.8
- **Erysipelas** (gangrenous) (infantile) (newborn) (phlegmonous) (suppurative) 035
  - external ear 035 *[380.13]*
  - puerperal, postpartum, childbirth 670⑤
- **Erysipelatoid** (Rosenbach's) 027.1
- **Erysipeloid** (Rosenbach's) 027.1
- **Erythema, erythematous** (generalized) 695.9
  - ab igne – *see* Burn, by site, first degree
  - annulare (centrifugum) (rheumaticum) 695.0
  - arthriticum epidemicum 026.1
  - brucellum (*see also* Brucellosis) 023.9
  - bullosum 695.1
  - caloricum – *see* Burn, by site, first degree
  - chronicum migrans 088.81
  - circinatum 695.1
  - diaper 691.0
  - due to
    - chemical (contact) NEC 692.4
      - internal 693.8
    - drug (internal use) 693.0
      - contact 692.3
  - elevatum diutinum 695.89
  - endemic 265.2
  - epidemic, arthritic 026.1
  - figuratum perstans 695.0
  - gluteal 691.0
  - gyratum (perstans) (repens) 695.1
  - heat – *see* Burn, by site, first degree
  - ichthyosiforme congenitum 757.1
  - induratum (primary) (scrofulosorum) (*see also* Tuberculosis) 017.1⑤
    - nontuberculous 695.2
  - infantum febrile 057.8
  - infectional NEC 695.9
  - infectiosum 057.0
  - inflammation NEC 695.9
  - intertrigo 695.89
  - iris 695.1
  - lupus (discoid) (localized) (*see also* Lupus, erythematosus) 695.4
  - marginatum 695.0
    - rheumaticum – *see* Fever, rheumatic
  - medicamentosum – *see* Dermatitis, due to, drug
  - migrans 529.1
    - chronicum 088.81
  - multiforme 695.1
    - bullosum 695.1
    - conjunctiva 695.1
    - exudativum (Hebra) 695.1
    - pemphigoides 694.5
  - napkin 691.0
  - neonatorum 778.8
  - nodosum 695.2
    - tuberculous (*see also* Tuberculosis) 017.1⑤
  - nummular, nummulare 695.1
  - palmar 695.0
  - palmaris hereditarium 695.0
  - pernio 991.5
  - perstans solare 692.72
  - rash, newborn 778.8
  - scarlatiniform (exfoliative) (recurrent) 695.0
- **Erythema, erythematous** – *continued*
  - simplex marginatum 057.8
  - solare (*see also* Sunburn) 692.71
  - streptogenes 696.5
  - toxic, toxicum NEC 695.0
    - newborn 778.8
  - tuberculous (primary) (*see also* Tuberculosis) 017.0⑤
  - venenatum 695.0
- **Erythematosus** – *see* condition
- **Erythematous** – *see* condition
- **Erythermalgia** (primary) 443.82
- **Erythralgia** 443.82
- **Erythrasma** 039.0
- **Erythredema** 985.0
  - polyneuritica 985.0
  - polyneuropathy 985.0
- **Erythremia** (acute) (M9841/3) 207.0⑤
  - chronic (M9842/3) 207.1⑤
  - secondary 289.0
- **Erythroblastopenia** (acquired) 284.89 ▲
  - congenital 284.01
- **Erythroblastophthisis** 284.01
- **Erythroblastosis** (fetalis) (newborn) 773.2
  - due to
    - ABO
      - antibodies 773.1
      - incompatibility, maternal/fetal 773.1
      - isoimmunization 773.1
    - Rh
      - antibodies 773.0
      - incompatibility, maternal/fetal 773.0
      - isoimmunization 773.0
- **Erythrocyanosis** (crurum) 443.89
- **Erythrocythemia** – *see* Erythremia
- **Erythrocytopenia** 285.9
- **Erythrocytosis** (megalosplenic)
  - familial 289.6
  - oval, hereditary (*see also* Elliptocytosis) 282.1
  - secondary 289.0
  - stress 289.0
- **Erythroderma** (*see also* Erythema) 695.9
  - desquamativa (in infants) 695.89
  - exfoliative 695.89
  - ichthyosiform, congenital 757.1
  - infantum 695.89
  - maculopapular 696.2
  - neonatorum 778.8
  - psoriaticum 696.1
  - secondary 695.9
- **Erythrodysesthesia, palmar plantar** (PPE) 693.0 ●
- **Erythrogenesis imperfecta** 284.09
- **Erythroleukemia** (M9840/3) 207.0⑤
- **Erythromelalgia** 443.82
- **Erythromelia** 701.8
- **Erythropenia** 285.9
- **Erythrophagocytosis** 289.9
- **Erythrophobia** 300.23
- **Erythroplakia**
  - oral mucosa 528.79
  - tongue 528.79
- **Erythroplasia** (Queyrat) (M8080/2)
  - specified site – *see* Neoplasm, skin, in situ
  - unspecified site 233.5
- **Erythropoiesis, idiopathic ineffective** 285.0
- **Escaped beats, heart** 427.60
  - postoperative 997.1
- **Esoenteritis** – *see* Enteritis
- **Esophagalgia** 530.89
- **Esophagectasis** 530.89
  - due to cardiospasm 530.0
- **Esophagismus** 530.5
- **Esophagitis** (alkaline) (chemical) (chronic) (infectional) (necrotic) (peptic) (postoperative) (regurgitant) 530.10
  - acute 530.12
  - candidal 112.84
  - reflux 530.11
  - specified NEC 530.19
  - tuberculous (*see also* Tuberculosis) 017.8⑤
  - ulcerative 530.19
- **Esophagocele** 530.6
- **Esophagodynia** 530.89
- **Esophagomalacia** 530.89
- **Esophagoptosis** 530.89
- **Esophagospasm** 530.5
- **Esophagostenosis** 530.3
- **Esophagostomiasis** 127.7
- **Esophagostomy**
  - complication 530.87
    - infection 530.86
    - malfunctioning 530.87
    - mechanical 530.87
- **Esophagotracheal** – *see* condition
- **Esophagus** – *see* condition
- **Esophoria** 378.41
  - convergence, excess 378.84
  - divergence, insufficiency 378.85
- **Esotropia** (nonaccommodative) 378.00
  - accommodative 378.35
  - alternating 378.05
    - with
      - A pattern 378.06
      - specified noncomitancy NEC 378.08
      - V pattern 378.07
      - X pattern 378.08
      - Y pattern 378.08
    - intermittent 378.22
  - intermittent 378.20
    - alternating 378.22
    - monocular 378.21
  - monocular 378.01
    - with
      - A pattern 378.02
      - specified noncomitancy NEC 378.04
      - V pattern 378.03
      - X pattern 378.04
      - Y pattern 378.04
    - intermittent 378.21
- **Espundia** 085.5
- **Essential** – *see* condition
- **Esterapenia** 289.89
- **Esthesioneuroblastoma** (M9522/3) 160.0
- **Esthesioneurocytoma** (M9521/3) 160.0
- **Esthesioneuroepithelioma** (M9523/3) 160.0
- **Esthiomene** 099.1
- **Estivo-autumnal**
  - fever 084.0
  - malaria 084.0
- **Estrangement** V61.0
- **Estriasis** 134.0
- **Ethanolaminuria** 270.8
- **Ethanolism** (*see also* Alcoholism) 303.9⑤
- **Ether dependence, dependency** (*see also* Dependence) 304.6⑤
- **Etherism** (*see also* Dependence) 304.6⑤
- **Ethmoid, ethmoidal** – *see* condition
- **Ethmoiditis** (chronic) (nonpurulent) (purulent) (*see also* Sinusitis, ethmoidal) 473.2
  - influenzal 487.1
  - Woakes' 471.1
- **Ethylism** (*see also* Alcoholism) 303.9⑤
- **Eulenburg's disease** (congenital paramyotonia) 359.29 ▲
- **Eunuchism** 257.2
- **Eunuchoidism** 257.2
  - hypogonadotropic 257.2
- **European blastomycosis** 117.5
- **Eustachian** – *see* condition
- **Euthyroid sick syndrome** 790.94
- **Euthyroidism** 244.9
- **Evaluation**
  - fetal lung maturity 659.8
  - for suspected condition (*see also* Observation) V71.9
    - abuse V71.81
    - exposure
      - anthrax V71.82
      - biologic agent NEC V71.83
      - SARS V71.83
    - neglect V71.81
    - newborn – *see* Observation, suspected, condition, newborn
    - specified condition NEC V71.89
  - mental health V70.2
    - requested by authority V70.1
  - nursing care V63.8
  - social service V63.8
- **Evans' syndrome** (thrombocytopenic purpura) 287.32
- **Eventration**
  - colon into chest – *see* Hernia, diaphragm
  - diaphragm (congenital) 756.6

Eruption – Eventration

④ Fourth-Digit Required ⑤ Fifth-Digit Required *[code]* Manifestation Code ▶◀ Revised Text ● New Line ▲ Revised Code

Eversion
- bladder 596.8
- cervix (uteri) 622.0
  - with mention of cervicitis 616.0
- foot NEC 736.79
  - congenital 755.67
- lacrimal punctum 375.51
- punctum lacrimale (postinfectional) (senile) 375.51
- ureter (meatus) 593.89
- urethra (meatus) 599.84
- uterus 618.1
  - complicating delivery 665.2❺
    - affecting fetus or newborn 763.89
  - puerperal, postpartum 674.8❺

Evidence
- of malignancy
  - cytologic
    - without histologic confirmation 795.06

Evisceration
- birth injury 767.8
- bowel (congenital) – *see* Hernia, ventral
- congenital (*see also* Hernia, ventral) 553.29
- operative wound 998.32
- traumatic NEC 869.1
  - eye 871.3

Evulsion – *see* Avulsion

Ewing's
- angioendothelioma (M9260/3) – *see* Neoplasm, bone, malignant
- sarcoma (M9260/3) – *see* Neoplasm, bone, malignant
- tumor (M9260/3) – *see* Neoplasm, bone, malignant

Exaggerated lumbosacral angle (with impinging spine) 756.12

Examination (general) (routine) (of) (for) V70.9
- allergy V72.7
- annual V70.0
- cardiovascular preoperative V72.81
- cervical Papanicolaou smear V76.2
  - as a part of routine gynecological examination V72.31
  - to confirm findings of recent normal smear following initial abnormal smear V72.32
- child care (routine) V20.2
- clinical research investigation (normal control patient) (participant) V70.7
- dental V72.2
- developmental testing (child) (infant) V20.2
- donor (potential) V70.8
- ear V72.19
- eye V72.0
- following
  - accident (motor vehicle) V71.4
  - alleged rape or seduction (victim or culprit) V71.5
  - inflicted injury (victim or culprit) NEC V71.6
  - rape or seduction, alleged (victim or culprit) V71.5
  - treatment (for) V67.9
    - combined V67.6
    - fracture V67.4
    - involving high-risk medication NEC V67.51
    - mental disorder V67.3
    - specified condition NEC V67.59
- follow-up (routine) (following) V67.9
  - cancer chemotherapy V67.2
  - chemotherapy V67.2
  - disease NEC V67.59
  - high-risk medication NEC V67.51
  - injury NEC V67.59
  - population survey V70.6
  - postpartum V24.2
  - psychiatric V67.3
  - psychotherapy V67.3
  - radiotherapy V67.1
  - specified surgery NEC V67.09
  - surgery V67.00
    - vaginal pap smear V67.01
- gynecological V72.31
  - for contraceptive maintenance V25.40
    - intrauterine device V25.42
    - pill V25.41
    - specified method NEC V25.49
- health (of)
  - armed forces personnel V70.5
  - checkup V70.0
  - child, routine V20.2
  - defined subpopulation NEC V70.5
  - inhabitants of institutions V70.5

Examination – *continued*
- health (of) – *continued*
  - occupational V70.5
  - pre-employment screening V70.5
  - preschool children V70.5
    - for admission to school V70.3
  - prisoners V70.5
    - for entrance into prison V70.3
  - prostitutes V70.5
  - refugees V70.5
  - school children V70.5
  - students V70.5
- hearing V72.19
  - following failed hearing screening V72.11
- infant V20.2
- laboratory V72.6
- lactating mother V24.1
- medical (for) (of) V70.9
  - administrative purpose NEC V70.3
  - admission to
    - old age home V70.3
    - prison V70.3
    - school V70.3
  - adoption V70.3
  - armed forces personnel V70.5
  - at health care facility V70.0
  - camp V70.3
  - child, routine V20.2
  - clinical research investigation(control) (normal comparison) (participant) V70.7
  - defined subpopulation NEC V70.5
  - donor (potential) V70.8
  - driving license V70.3
  - general V70.9
    - routine V70.0
    - specified reason NEC V70.8
  - immigration V70.3
  - inhabitants of institutions V70.5
  - insurance certification V70.3
  - marriage V70.3
  - medicolegal reasons V70.4
  - naturalization V70.3
  - occupational V70.5
  - population survey V70.6
  - pre-employment V70.5
  - preschool children V70.5
    - for admission to school V70.3
  - prison V70.3
  - prisoners V70.5
    - for entrance into prison V70.3
  - prostitutes V70.5
  - refugees V70.5
  - school children V70.5
  - specified reason NEC V70.8
  - sport competition V70.3
  - students V70.5
- medicolegal reason V70.4
- pelvic (annual) (periodic) V72.31
- periodic (annual) (routine) V70.0
- postpartum
  - immediately after delivery V24.0
  - routine follow-up V24.2
- pregnancy (unconfirmed) (possible) V72.40
  - negative result V72.41
  - positive result V72.42
- prenatal V22.1
  - first pregnancy V22.0
  - high-risk pregnancy V23.9
    - specified problem NEC V23.8❺
- preoperative V72.84
  - cardiovascular V72.81
  - respiratory V72.82
  - specified NEC V72.83
- preprocedural V72.84
  - cardiovascular V72.81
  - general physical V72.83
  - respiratory V72.82
  - specified NEC V72.83
- psychiatric V70.2
  - follow-up not needing further care V67.3
  - requested by authority V70.1
- radiological NEC V72.5
- respiratory preoperative V72.82
- screening – *see* Screening
- sensitization V72.7
- skin V72.7
  - hypersensitivity V72.7
- special V72.9
- specified type or reason NEC V72.85
  - preoperative V72.83
    - specified NEC V72.83
- teeth V72.2

Examination – *continued*
- vaginal Papanicolaou smear V76.47
  - following hysterectomy for malignant condition V67.01
- victim or culprit following
  - alleged rape or seduction V71.5
  - inflicted injury NEC V71.6
- vision V72.0
- well baby V20.2

Exanthem, exanthema (*see also* Rash) 782.1
- Boston 048
- epidemic, with meningitis 048
- lichenoid psoriasiform 696.2
- subitum 058.10 ▲
  - due to ●
    - human herpesvirus 6 058.11 ●
    - human herpesvirus 7 058.12 ●
- viral, virus NEC 057.9
  - specified type NEC 057.8

Excess, excessive, excessively
- alcohol level in blood 790.3
- carbohydrate tissue, localized 278.1
- carotene (dietary) 278.3
- cold 991.9
  - specified effect NEC 991.8
- convergence 378.84
- crying 780.95
  - of
    - adolescent 780.95
    - adult 780.95
    - baby 780.92
    - child 780.95
    - infant (baby) 780.92
    - newborn 780.92
- development, breast 611.1
- diaphoresis (*see also* Hyperhidrosis) 780.8
- distance, interarch 524.28
- divergence 378.85
- drinking (alcohol) NEC (*see also* Abuse, drugs, nondependent) 305.0❺
  - continual (*see also* Alcoholism) 303.9❺
  - habitual (*see also* Alcoholism) 303.9❺
- eating 783.6
- eyelid fold (congenital) 743.62
- fat 278.02
  - in heart (*see also* Degeneration, myocardial) 429.1
  - tissue, localized 278.1
- foreskin 605
- gas 787.3
- gastrin 251.5
- glucagon 251.4
- heat (*see also* Heat) 992.9
- horizontal
  - overjet 524.26
  - overlap 524.26
- interarch distance 524.28
- intermaxillary vertical dimension 524.37
- interocclusal distance of teeth 524.37
- large
  - colon 564.7
    - congenital 751.3
  - fetus or infant 766.0
    - with obstructed labor 660.1❺
      - affecting management of pregnancy 656.6❺
    - causing disproportion 653.5❺
  - newborn (weight of 4500 grams or more) 766.0
  - organ or site, congenital NEC – *see* Anomaly, specified type NEC
- lid fold (congenital) 743.62
- long
  - colon 751.5
  - organ or site, congenital NEC – *see* Anomaly, specified type NEC
  - umbilical cord (entangled)
    - affecting fetus or newborn 762.5
    - in pregnancy or childbirth 663.3❺
      - with compression 663.2❺
- menstruation 626.2
- number of teeth 520.1
  - causing crowding 524.31
- nutrients (dietary) NEC 783.6
- potassium (K) 276.7
- salivation (*see also* Ptyalism) 527.7
- secretion – *see also* Hypersecretion
  - milk 676.6❺
  - sputum 786.4
  - sweat (*see also* Hyperhidrosis) 780.8

- **Excess, excessive, excessively** – *continued*
  - short
    - organ or site, congenital NEC – *see* Anomaly, specified type NEC
    - umbilical cord
      - affecting fetus or newborn 762.6
      - in pregnancy or childbirth 663.4❺
  - skin NEC 701.9
    - eyelid 743.62
      - acquired 374.30
  - sodium (Na) 276.0
  - spacing of teeth 524.32
  - sputum 786.4
  - sweating (*see also* Hyperhidrosis) 780.8
  - tearing (ducts) (eye) (*see also* Epiphora) 375.20
  - thirst 783.5
    - due to deprivation of water 994.3
  - tuberosity 524.07
  - vitamin
    - A (dietary) 278.2
      - administered as drug (chronic) (prolonged excessive intake) 278.2
        - reaction to sudden overdose 963.5
    - D (dietary) 278.4
      - administered as drug (chronic) (prolonged excessive intake) 278.4
        - reaction to sudden overdose 963.5
  - weight 278.02
    - gain 783.1
      - of pregnancy 646.1❺
    - loss 783.21
- **Excitability, abnormal, under minor stress** 309.29
- **Excitation**
  - catatonic (*see also* Schizophrenia) 295.2❺
  - psychogenic 298.1
  - reactive (from emotional stress, psychological trauma) 298.1
- **Excitement**
  - manic (*see also* Psychosis, affective) 296.0❺
    - recurrent episode 296.1❺
    - single episode 296.0❺
  - mental, reactive (from emotional stress, psychological trauma) 298.1
  - state, reactive (from emotional stress, psychological trauma) 298.1
- **Excluded pupils** 364.76
- **Excoriation** (traumatic) (*see also* Injury, superficial, by site) 919.8
  - neurotic 698.4
- **Excyclophoria** 378.44
- **Excyclotropia** 378.33
- **Exencephalus, exencephaly** 742.0
- **Exercise**
  - breathing V57.0
  - remedial NEC V57.1
  - therapeutic NEC V57.1
- **Exfoliation, teeth due to systemic causes** 525.0
- **Exfoliative** – *see also* condition
  - dermatitis 695.89
- **Exhaustion, exhaustive** (physical NEC) 780.79
  - battle (*see also* Reaction, stress, acute) 308.9
  - cardiac (*see also* Failure, heart) 428.9
  - delirium (*see also* Reaction, stress, acute) 308.9
  - due to
    - cold 991.8
    - excessive exertion 994.5
    - exposure 994.4
  - fetus or newborn 779.89
  - heart (*see also* Failure, heart) 428.9
  - heat 992.5
    - due to
      - salt depletion 992.4
      - water depletion 992.3
  - manic (*see also* Psychosis, affective) 296.0❺
    - recurrent episode 296.1❺
    - single episode 296.0❺
  - maternal, complicating delivery 669.8❺
    - affecting fetus or newborn 763.89
  - mental 300.5
  - myocardium, myocardial (*see also* Failure, heart) 428.9
  - nervous 300.5
  - old age 797
  - postinfectional NEC 780.79
  - psychogenic 300.5
  - psychosis (*see also* Reaction, stress, acute) 308.9
  - senile 797
    - dementia 290.0
- **Exhibitionism** (sexual) 302.4
- **Exomphalos** 756.79
- **Exophoria** 378.42
  - convergence, insufficiency 378.83
  - divergence, excess 378.85
- **Exophthalmic**
  - cachexia 242.0❺
  - goiter 242.0❺
  - ophthalmoplegia 242.0❺ *[376.22]*
- **Exophthalmos** 376.30
  - congenital 743.66
  - constant 376.31
  - endocrine NEC 259.9 *[376.22]*
  - hyperthyroidism 242.0❺ *[376.21]*
  - intermittent NEC 376.34
  - malignant 242.0❺ *[376.21]*
  - pulsating 376.35
    - endocrine NEC 259.9 *[376.22]*
  - thyrotoxic 242.0❺ *[376.21]*
- **Exostosis** 726.91
  - cartilaginous (M9210/0) – *see* Neoplasm, bone, benign
  - congenital 756.4
  - ear canal, external 380.81
  - gonococcal 098.89
  - hip 726.5
  - intracranial 733.3
  - jaw (bone) 526.81
  - luxurians 728.11
  - multiple (cancellous) (congenital) (hereditary) 756.4
  - nasal bones 726.91
  - orbit, orbital 376.42
  - osteocartilaginous (M9210/0) – *see* Neoplasm, bone, benign
  - spine 721.8
    - with spondylosis – *see* Spondylosis
  - syphilitic 095.5
  - wrist 726.4
- **Exotropia** 378.10
  - alternating 378.15
    - with
      - A pattern 378.16
      - specified noncomitancy NEC 378.18
      - V pattern 378.17
      - X pattern 378.18
      - Y pattern 378.18
    - intermittent 378.24
  - intermittent 378.20
    - alternating 378.24
    - monocular 378.23
  - monocular 378.11
    - with
      - A pattern 378.12
      - specified noncomitancy NEC 378.14
      - V pattern 378.13
      - X pattern 378.14
      - Y pattern 378.14
    - intermittent 378.23
- **Explanation of**
  - investigation finding V65.4
  - medication V65.4
- **Exposure** 994.9
  - cold 991.9
    - specified effect NEC 991.8
  - effects of 994.9
  - exhaustion due to 994.4
  - to
    - AIDS virus V01.79
    - anthrax V01.81
    - asbestos V15.84
    - body fluids (hazardous) V15.85
    - cholera V01.0
    - communicable disease V01.9
      - specified type NEC V01.89
    - Escherichia coli (E. coli) V01.83
    - German measles V01.4
    - gonorrhea V01.6
    - hazardous body fluids V15.85
    - HIV V01.79
    - human immunodeficiency virus V01.79
    - lead V15.86
    - meningococcus V01.84
    - parasitic disease V01.89
    - poliomyelitis V01.2
    - potentially hazardous body fluids V15.85
    - rabies V01.5
    - rubella V01.4
    - SARS-associated coronavirus V01.82
    - smallpox V01.3
    - syphilis V01.6
    - tuberculosis V01.1
- **Exposure** – *continued*
  - to – *continued*
    - varicella V01.71
    - venereal disease V01.6
    - viral disease NEC V01.79
      - varicella V01.71
- **Exsanguination, fetal** 772.0
- **Exstrophy**
  - abdominal content 751.8
  - bladder (urinary) 753.5
- **Extensive** – *see* condition
- **Extra** – *see also* Accessory
  - rib 756.3
    - cervical 756.2
- **Extraction**
  - with hook 763.89
  - breech NEC 669.6❺
    - affecting fetus or newborn 763.0
  - cataract postsurgical V45.61
  - manual NEC 669.8❺
    - affecting fetus or newborn 763.89
- **Extrasystole** 427.60
  - atrial 427.61
  - postoperative 997.1
  - ventricular 427.69
- **Extrauterine gestation or pregnancy** – *see* Pregnancy, ectopic
- **Extravasation**
  - blood 459.0
    - lower extremity 459.0
  - chyle into mesentery 457.8
  - pelvicalyceal 593.4
  - pyelosinus 593.4
  - urine 788.8
    - from ureter 788.8
- **Extremity** – *see* condition
- **Extrophy** – *see* Exstrophy
- **Extroversion**
  - bladder 753.5
  - uterus 618.1
    - complicating delivery 665.2❺
      - affecting fetus or newborn 763.89
    - postpartal (old) 618.1
- **Extruded tooth** 524.34
- **Extrusion**
  - alveolus and teeth 524.75
  - breast implant (prosthetic) 996.54
  - device, implant, or graft – *see* Complications, mechanical
  - eye implant (ball) (globe) 996.59
  - intervertebral disc – *see* Displacement, intervertebral disc
  - lacrimal gland 375.43
  - mesh (reinforcing) 996.59
  - ocular lens implant 996.53
  - prosthetic device NEC – *see* Complications, mechanical
  - vitreous 379.26
- **Exudate, pleura** – *see* Effusion, pleura
- **Exudates, retina** 362.82
- **Exudative** – *see* condition
- **Eye, eyeball, eyelid** – *see* condition
- **Eyestrain** 368.13
- **Eyeworm disease of Africa** 125.2

F

- **Faber's anemia or syndrome** (achlorhydric anemia) 280.9
- **Fabry's disease** (angiokeratoma corporis diffusum) 272.7
- **Face, facial** – *see* condition
- **Facet of cornea** 371.44
- **Faciocephalalgia, autonomic** (*see also* Neuropathy, peripheral, autonomic) 337.9
- **Facioscapulohumeral myopathy** 359.1
- **Factitious disorder, illness** – *see* Illness, factitious
- **Factor**
  - deficiency – *see* Deficiency, factor
  - psychic, associated with diseases classified elsewhere 316
  - risk – *see* problem
- **Fahr-Volhard disease** (malignant nephrosclerosis) 403.00

Failure, failed
  adenohypophyseal 253.2
  attempted abortion (legal) (*see also* Abortion, failed) 638.9
  bone marrow (anemia) 284.9
    acquired (secondary) 284.89 ▲
    congenital 284.09
    idiopathic 284.9
  cardiac (*see also* Failure, heart) 428.9
    newborn 779.89
  cardiorenal (chronic) 428.9
    hypertensive (*see also* Hypertension, cardiorenal) 404.93
  cardiorespiratory 799.1
    specified during or due to a procedure 997.1
      long-term effect of cardiac surgery 429.4
  cardiovascular (chronic) 428.9
  cerebrovascular 437.8
  cervical dilation in labor 661.0❺
    affecting fetus or newborn 763.7
  circulation, circulatory 799.89
    fetus or newborn 779.89
    peripheral 785.50
  compensation – *see* Disease, heart
  congestive (*see also* Failure, heart) 428.0
  coronary (*see also* Insufficiency, coronary) 411.89
  dental implant 525.79 ●
    due to ●
      lack of attached gingiva 525.72 ●
      occlusal trauma (caused by poor prosthetic design) 525.72 ●
      parafunctional habits 525.72 ●
      periodontal infection (peri-implantitis) 525.72 ●
      poor oral hygiene 525.72 ●
    endosseous NEC 525.79 ●
    osseointegration 525.71 ●
      due to ●
        complications of systemic disease 525.71 ●
        poor bone quality 525.71 ●
      iatrogenic 525.71 ●
    post-osseointegration ●
      biological 525.72 ●
        iatrogenic 525.72 ●
      due to complications of systemic disease 525.72 ●
      mechanical 525.73 ●
    pre-integration 525.71 ●
    pre-osseointegration 525.71 ●
  dental prosthesis causing loss of dental implant 525.73 ●
  dental restoration
    marginal integrity 525.61
    periodontal anatomical integrity 525.65
  descent of head (at term) 652.5❺
    affecting fetus or newborn 763.1
    in labor 660.0❺
      affecting fetus or newborn 763.1
  device, implant, or graft – *see* Complications, mechanical
  engagement of head NEC 652.5❺
    in labor 660.0❺
  extrarenal 788.9
  fetal head to enter pelvic brim 652.5❺
    affecting fetus or newborn 763.1
    in labor 660.0❺
      affecting fetus or newborn 763.1
  forceps NEC 660.7❺
    affecting fetus or newborn 763.1
  fusion (joint) (spinal) 996.49
  growth in childhood 783.43
  heart (acute) (sudden) 428.9
    with
      abortion – *see* Abortion, by type, with specified complication NEC
      acute pulmonary edema (*see also* Failure, ventricular, left) 428.1
        with congestion (*see also* Failure, heart) 428.0
      decompensated (*see also* Failure, heart) 428.0
      dilation – *see* Disease, heart
      ectopic pregnancy (*see also* categories 633.0-633.9) 639.8
      molar pregnancy (*see also* categories 630-632) 639.8
    arteriosclerotic 440.9
    combined left-right sided 428.0
    combined systolic and diastolic 428.40
      acute 428.41

Failure, failed – *continued*
  heart – *continued*
    combined systolic and diastolic – *continued*
      acute on chronic 428.43
      chronic 428.42
    compensated (*see also* Failure, heart) 428.0
    complicating
      abortion – *see* Abortion, by type, with specified complication NEC
      delivery (cesarean) (instrumental) 669.4❺
      ectopic pregnancy (*see also* categories 633.0-633.9) 639.8
      molar pregnancy (*see also* categories 630-632) 639.8
      obstetric anesthesia or sedation 668.1❺
      surgery 997.1
    congestive (compensated) (decompensated) (*see also* Failure, heart) 428.0
      with rheumatic fever (conditions classifiable to 390)
        active 391.8
        inactive or quiescent (with chorea) 398.91
      fetus or newborn 779.89
      hypertensive (*see also* Hypertension, heart) 402.91
        with renal disease (*see also* Hypertension, cardiorenal) 404.91
          with renal failure 404.93
        benign 402.11
        malignant 402.01
      rheumatic (chronic) (inactive) (with chorea) 398.91
        active or acute 391.8
          with chorea (Sydenham's) 392.0
    decompensated (*see also* Failure, heart) 428.0
    degenerative (*see also* Degeneration, myocardial) 429.1
    diastolic 428.30
      acute 428.31
      acute on chronic 428.33
      chronic 428.32
    due to presence of (cardiac) prosthesis 429.4
    fetus or newborn 779.89
    following
      abortion 639.8
      cardiac surgery 429.4
      ectopic or molar pregnancy 639.8
    high output NEC 428.9
    hypertensive (*see also* Hypertension, heart) 402.91
      with renal disease (*see also* Hypertension, cardiorenal) 404.91
        with renal failure 404.93
      benign 402.11
      malignant 402.01
    left (ventricular) (*see also* Failure, ventricular, left) 428.1
      with right-sided failure (*see also* Failure, heart) 428.0
    low output (syndrome) NEC 428.9
    organic – *see* Disease, heart
    postoperative (immediate) 997.1
      long term effect of cardiac surgery 429.4
    rheumatic (chronic) (congestive) (inactive) 398.91
    right (secondary to left heart failure, conditions classifiable to 428.1) (ventricular) (*see also* Failure, heart) 428.0
    senile 797
    specified during or due to a procedure 997.1
      long-term effect of cardiac surgery 429.4
    systolic 428.20
      acute 428.21
      acute on chronic 428.23
      chronic 428.22
    thyrotoxic (*see also* Thyrotoxicosis) 242.9❺ *[425.7]*
    valvular – *see* Endocarditis
  hepatic 572.8
    acute 570
    due to a procedure 997.4
  hepatorenal 572.4
  hypertensive heart (*see also* Hypertension, heart) 402.91
    benign 402.11
    malignant 402.01
  induction (of labor) 659.1❺
    abortion (legal) (*see also* Abortion, failed) 638.9
    affecting fetus or newborn 763.89
    by oxytocic drugs 659.1❺
    instrumental 659.0❺

Failure, failed – *continued*
  induction (of labor) – *continued*
    mechanical 659.0❺
    medical 659.1❺
    surgical 659.0❺
  initial alveolar expansion, newborn 770.4
  involution, thymus (gland) 254.8
  kidney – *see* Failure, renal
  lactation 676.4❺
  Leydig's cell, adult 257.2
  liver 572.8
    acute 570
  medullary 799.89
  mitral – *see* Endocarditis, mitral
  myocardium, myocardial (*see also* Failure, heart) 428.9
    chronic (*see also* Failure, heart) 428.0
    congestive (*see also* Failure, heart) 428.0
  ovarian (primary) 256.39
    iatrogenic 256.2
    postablative 256.2
    postirradiation 256.2
    postsurgical 256.2
  ovulation 628.0
  prerenal 788.9
  renal 586
    with
      abortion – *see* Abortion, by type, with renal failure
      ectopic pregnancy (*see also* categories 633.0-633.9) 639.3
      edema (*see also* Nephrosis) 581.9
      hypertension (*see also* Hypertension, kidney) 403.91
      hypertensive heart disease (conditions classifiable to 402) 404.92
        with heart failure 404.93
        benign 404.12
          with heart failure 404.13
        malignant 404.02
          with heart failure 404.03
      molar pregnancy (*see also* categories 630-632) 639.3
      tubular necrosis (acute) 584.5
    acute 584.9
      with lesion of
        necrosis
          cortical (renal) 584.6
          medullary (renal) (papillary) 584.7
          tubular 584.5
        specified pathology NEC 584.8
    chronic 585.9
      hypertensive or with hypertension (*see also* Hypertension, kidney) 403.91
    due to a procedure 997.5
    following
      abortion 639.3
      crushing 958.5
      ectopic or molar pregnancy 639.3
      labor and delivery (acute) 669.3❺
    hypertensive (*see also* Hypertension, kidney) 403.91
    puerperal, postpartum 669.3❺
  respiration, respiratory 518.81
    acute 518.81
    acute and chronic 518.84
    center 348.8
      newborn 770.84
    chronic 518.83
    due to trauma, surgery or shock 518.5
    newborn 770.84
  rotation
    cecum 751.4
    colon 751.4
    intestine 751.4
    kidney 753.3
  segmentation – *see also* Fusion
    fingers (*see also* Syndactylism, fingers) 755.11
    toes (*see also* Syndactylism, toes) 755.13
  seminiferous tubule, adult 257.2
  senile (general) 797
    with psychosis 290.20
  testis, primary (seminal) 257.2
  to progress 661.2❺
  to thrive
    adult 783.7
    child 783.41
  transplant 996.80
    bone marrow 996.85
    organ (immune or nonimmune cause) 996.80
      bone marrow 996.85
      heart 996.83

Failure, failed – *continued*
- transplant – *continued*
  - organ – *continued*
    - intestines 996.87
    - kidney 996.81
    - liver 996.82
    - lung 996.84
    - pancreas 996.86
    - specified NEC 996.89
  - skin 996.52
    - artificial 996.55
    - decellularized allodermis 996.55
    - temporary allograft or pigskin graft - omit code
- trial of labor NEC 660.6❺
  - affecting fetus or newborn 763.1
- tubal ligation 998.89
- urinary 586
- vacuum extraction
  - abortion – *see* Abortion, failed
  - delivery NEC 660.7❺
    - affecting fetus or newborn 763.1
- vasectomy 998.89
- ventouse NEC 660.7❺
  - affecting fetus or newborn 763.1
- ventricular (*see also* Failure, heart) 428.9
  - left 428.1
    - with rheumatic fever (conditions classifiable to 390)
      - active 391.8
        - with chorea 392.0
      - inactive or quiescent (with chorea) 398.91
    - hypertensive (*see also* Hypertension, heart) 402.91
      - benign 402.11
      - malignant 402.01
    - rheumatic (chronic) (inactive) (with chorea) 398.91
      - active or acute 391.8
        - with chorea 392.0
  - right (*see also* Failure, heart) 428.0
- vital centers, fetus or newborn 779.8❺
- weight gain in childhood 783.41

Fainting (fit) (spell) 780.2

Falciform hymen 752.49

Fall, maternal, affecting fetus or newborn 760.5

Fallen arches 734

Falling, any organ or part – *see* Prolapse

Fallopian
- insufflation
  - fertility testing V26.21
  - following sterilization reversal V26.22
- tube – *see* condition

Fallot's
- pentalogy 745.2
- tetrad or tetralogy 745.2
- triad or trilogy 746.09

Fallout, radioactive (adverse effect) NEC 990

False – *see also* condition
- bundle branch block 426.50
- bursa 727.89
- croup 478.75
- joint 733.82
- labor (pains) 644.1❺
- opening, urinary, male 752.69
- passage, urethra (prostatic) 599.4
- positive
  - serological test for syphilis 795.6
  - Wassermann reaction 795.6
- pregnancy 300.11

Family, familial – *see also* condition
- disruption V61.0
- hemophagocytic
  - lymphohistiocytosis 288.4
  - reticulosis 288.4
- Li-Fraumeni (syndrome) V84.01
- planning advice V25.09
  - natural ●
    - procreative V26.41 ●
    - to avoid pregnancy V25.04 ●
- problem V61.9
  - specified circumstance NEC V61.8
- retinoblastoma (syndrome) 190.5

Famine 994.2
- edema 262

Fanconi's anemia (congenital pancytopenia) 284.09

Fanconi (-de Toni) (-Debré) **syndrome** (cystinosis) 270.0

Farber (-Uzman) **syndrome or disease** (disseminated lipogranulomatosis) 272.8

Farcin 024

Farcy 024

Farmers'
- lung 495.0
- skin 692.74

Farsightedness 367.0

Fascia – *see* condition

Fasciculation 781.0

Fasciculitis optica 377.32

Fasciitis 729.4
- eosinophilic 728.89
- necrotizing 728.86
- nodular 728.79
- perirenal 593.4
- plantar 728.71
- pseudosarcomatous 728.79
- traumatic (old) NEC 728.79
  - current – *see* Sprain, by site

Fasciola hepatica infestation 121.3

Fascioliasis 121.3

Fasciolopsiasis (small intestine) 121.4

Fasciolopsis (small intestine) 121.4

Fast pulse 785.0

Fat
- embolism (cerebral) (pulmonary) (systemic) 958.1
  - with
    - abortion – *see* Abortion, by type, with embolism
    - ectopic pregnancy (*see also* categories 633.0-633.9) 639.6
    - molar pregnancy (*see also* categories 630-632) 639.6
  - complicating delivery or puerperium 673.8❺
  - following
    - abortion 639.6
    - ectopic or molar pregnancy 639.6
  - in pregnancy, childbirth, or the puerperium 673.8❺
- excessive 278.02
  - in heart (*see also* Degeneration, myocardial) 429.1
- general 278.02
- hernia, herniation 729.30
  - eyelid 374.34
  - knee 729.31
  - orbit 374.34
  - retro-orbital 374.34
  - retropatellar 729.31
  - specified site NEC 729.39
- indigestion 579.8
- in stool 792.1
- localized (pad) 278.1
  - heart (*see also* Degeneration, myocardial) 429.1
  - knee 729.31
  - retropatellar 729.31
- necrosis – *see also* Fatty, degeneration
  - breast (aseptic) (segmental) 611.3
  - mesentery 567.82
  - omentum 567.82
  - peritoneum 567.82
- pad 278.1

Fatal syncope 798.1

Fatigue 780.79
- auditory deafness (*see also* Deafness) 389.9
- chronic 780.7❺
- chronic, syndrome 780.71
- combat (*see also* Reaction, stress, acute) 308.9
- during pregnancy 646.8❺
- general 780.79
  - psychogenic 300.5
- heat (transient) 992.6
- muscle 729.89
- myocardium (*see also* Failure, heart) 428.9
- nervous 300.5
- neurosis 300.5
- operational 300.89
- postural 729.89
- posture 729.89
- psychogenic (general) 300.5
- senile 797
- syndrome NEC 300.5
  - chronic 780.71
- undue 780.79
- voice 784.49

Fatness 278.02

Fatty – *see also* condition
- apron 278.1
- degeneration (diffuse) (general) NEC 272.8
  - localized – *see* Degeneration, by site, fatty
  - placenta – *see* Placenta, abnormal
- heart (enlarged) (*see also* Degeneration, myocardial) 429.1
- infiltration (diffuse) (general) (*see also* Degeneration, by site, fatty) 272.8
  - heart (enlarged) (*see also* Degeneration, myocardial) 429.1
- liver 571.8
  - alcoholic 571.0
- necrosis – *see* Degeneration, fatty
- phanerosis 272.8

Fauces – *see* condition

Fauchard's disease (periodontitis) 523.40

Faucitis 478.29

Faulty – *see also* condition
- position of teeth 524.30

Favism (anemia) 282.2

Favre-Racouchot disease (elastoidosis cutanea nodularis) 701.8

Favus 110.9
- beard 110.0
- capitis 110.0
- corporis 110.5
- eyelid 110.8
- foot 110.4
- hand 110.2
- scalp 110.0
- specified site NEC 110.8

Fear, fearfulness (complex) (reaction) 300.20
- child 313.0
- of
  - animals 300.29
  - closed spaces 300.29
  - crowds 300.29
  - eating in public 300.23
  - heights 300.29
  - open spaces 300.22
    - with panic attacks 300.21
  - public speaking 300.23
  - streets 300.22
    - with panic attacks 300.21
  - travel 300.22
    - with panic attacks 300.21
  - washing in public 300.23
- transient 308.0

Feared complaint unfounded V65.5

Febricula (continued) (simple) (*see also* Pyrexia) 780.6

Febrile (*see also* Pyrexia) 780.6
- convulsion (simple) 780.31
  - complex 780.32
- seizure (simple) 780.31
  - atypical 780.32
  - complex 780.32
  - complicated 780.32

Febris (*see also* Fever) 780.6
- aestiva (*see also* Fever, hay) 477.9
- flava (*see also* Fever, yellow) 060.9
- melitensis 023.0
- pestis (*see also* Plague) 020.9
- puerperalis 672❺
- recurrens (*see also* Fever, relapsing) 087.9
  - pediculo vestimenti 087.0
- rubra 034.1
- typhoidea 002.0
- typhosa 002.0

Fecal – *see* condition

Fecalith (impaction) 560.39
- with hernia – *see also* Hernia, by site, with obstruction
  - gangrenous – *see* Hernia, by site, with gangrene
- appendix 543.9
- congenital 777.1

Fede's disease 529.0

Feeble-minded 317

Feeble rapid pulse due to shock following injury 958.4

Feeding
- faulty (elderly) (infant) 783.3
  - newborn 779.3
- formula check V20.2
- improper (elderly) (infant) 783.3
  - newborn 779.3
- problem (elderly)(infant) 783.3
  - newborn 779.3

- **Feeding** – *continued*
  - nonorganic origin 307.59
- **Feeling of foreign body in throat** 784.99 ●
- **Feer's disease** 985.0
- **Feet** – *see* condition
- **Feigned illness** V65.2
- **Feil-Klippel syndrome** (brevicollis) 756.16
- **Feinmesser's** (hidrotic) **ectodermal dysplasia** 757.31
- **Felix's disease** (juvenile osteochondrosis, hip) 732.1
- **Felon** (any digit) (with lymphangitis) 681.01
  - herpetic 054.6
- **Felty's syndrome** (rheumatoid arthritis with splenomegaly and leukopenia) 714.1
- **Feminism in boys** 302.6
- **Feminization, testicular** 259.5
  - with pseudohermaphroditism, male 259.5
- **Femoral hernia** – *see* Hernia, femoral
- **Femora vara** 736.32
- **Femur, femoral** – *see* condition
- **Fenestrata placenta** – *see* Placenta, abnormal
- **Fenestration, fenestrated** – *see also* Imperfect, closure
  - aorta-pulmonary 745.0
  - aorticopulmonary 745.0
  - aortopulmonary 745.0
  - cusps, heart valve NEC 746.89
    - pulmonary 746.09
  - hymen 752.49
  - pulmonic cusps 746.09
- **Fenwick's disease** 537.89
- **Fermentation** (gastric) (gastrointestinal) (stomach) 536.8
  - intestine 564.89
    - psychogenic 306.4
  - psychogenic 306.4
- **Fernell's disease** (aortic aneurysm) 441.9
- **Fertile eunuch syndrome** 257.2
- **Fertility, meaning multiparity** – *see* Multiparity
- **Fetal alcohol syndrome** 760.71
- **Fetalis uterus** 752.3
- **Fetid**
  - breath 784.99
  - sweat 705.89
- **Fetishism** 302.81
  - transvestic 302.3
- **Fetomaternal hemorrhage**
  - affecting management of pregnancy 656.0❺
  - fetus or newborn 772.0
- **Fetus, fetal** – *see also* condition
  - papyraceous 779.89
  - type lung tissue 770.4
- **Fever** 780.6
  - with chills 780.6
    - in malarial regions (*see also* Malaria) 084.6
  - abortus NEC 023.9
  - aden 061
  - African tick-borne 087.1
  - American
    - mountain tick 066.1
    - spotted 082.0
  - and ague (*see also* Malaria) 084.6
  - aphthous 078.4
  - arbovirus hemorrhagic 065.9
  - Assam 085.0
  - Australian A or Q 083.0
  - Bangkok hemorrhagic 065.4
  - biliary, Charcôt's intermittent – *see* Choledocholithiasis
  - bilious, hemoglobinuric 084.8
  - blackwater 084.8
  - blister 054.9
  - Bonvale Dam 780.79
  - boutonneuse 082.1
  - brain 323.9
    - late effect – *see* category 326
  - breakbone 061
  - Bullis 082.8
  - Bunyamwera 066.3
  - Burdwan 085.0
  - Bwamba (encephalitis) 066.3
  - Cameroon (*see also* Malaria) 084.6
  - Canton 081.9
  - catarrhal (acute) 460
    - chronic 472.0
  - cat-scratch 078.3
  - cerebral 323.9
    - late effect – *see* category 326

- **Fever** – *continued*
  - cerebrospinal (meningococcal) (*see also* Meningitis, cerebrospinal) 036.0
  - Chagres 084.0
  - Chandipura 066.8
  - changuinola 066.0
  - Charcôt's (biliary) (hepatic) (intermittent) *see* Choledocholithiasis
  - Chikungunya (viral) 066.3
    - hemorrhagic 065.4
  - childbed 670❹
  - Chitral 066.0
  - Colombo (*see also* Fever, paratyphoid) 002.9
  - Colorado tick (virus) 066.1
  - congestive
    - malarial (*see also* Malaria) 084.6
    - remittent (*see also* Malaria) 084.6
  - Congo virus 065.0
  - continued 780.6
    - malarial 084.0
  - Corsican (*see also* Malaria) 084.6
  - Crimean hemorrhagic 065.0
  - Cyprus (*see also* Brucellosis) 023.9
  - dandy 061
  - deer fly (*see also* Tularemia) 021.9
  - dehydration, newborn 778.4
  - dengue (virus) 061
    - hemorrhagic 065.4
  - desert 114.0
  - due to heat 992.0
  - Dumdum 085.0
  - enteric 002.0
  - ephemeral (of unknown origin) (*see also* Pyrexia) 780.6
  - epidemic, hemorrhagic of the Far East 065.0
  - erysipelatous (*see also* Erysipelas) 035
  - estivo-autumnal (malarial) 084.0
  - etiocholanolone 277.31
  - famine – *see also* Fever, relapsing
    - meaning typhus – *see* Typhus
  - Far Eastern hemorrhagic 065.0
  - five day 083.1
  - Fort Bragg 100.89
  - gastroenteric 002.0
  - gastromalarial (*see also* Malaria) 084.6
  - Gibraltar (*see also* Brucellosis) 023.9
  - glandular 075
  - Guama (viral) 066.3
  - Haverhill 026.1
  - hay (allergic) (with rhinitis) 477.9
    - with
      - asthma (bronchial) (*see also* Asthma) 493.0❺
    - due to
      - dander, animal (cat) (dog) 477.2
      - dust 477.8
      - fowl 477.8
      - hair, animal (cat) (dog) 477.2
      - pollen, any plant or tree 477.0
      - specified allergen other than pollen 477.8
  - heat (effects) 992.0
  - hematuric, bilious 084.8
  - hemoglobinuric (malarial) 084.8
    - bilious 084.8
  - hemorrhagic (arthropod-borne) NEC 065.9
    - with renal syndrome 078.6
    - arenaviral 078.7
    - Argentine 078.7
    - Bangkok 065.4
    - Bolivian 078.7
    - Central Asian 065.0
    - chikungunya 065.4
    - Crimean 065.0
    - dengue (virus) 065.4
    - Ebola 065.8
    - epidemic 078.6
      - of Far East 065.0
    - Far Eastern 065.0
    - Junin virus 078.7
    - Korean 078.6
    - Kyasanur forest 065.2
    - Machupo virus 078.7
    - mite-borne NEC 065.8
    - mosquito-borne 065.4
    - Omsk 065.1
    - Philippine 065.4
    - Russian (Yaroslav) 078.6
    - Singapore 065.4
    - Southeast Asia 065.4
    - Thailand 065.4
    - tick-borne NEC 065.3

- **Fever** – *continued*
  - hepatic (*see also* Cholecystitis) 575.8
    - intermittent (Charcôt's) – *see* Choledocholithiasis
  - herpetic (*see also* Herpes) 054.9
  - hyalomma tick 065.0
  - icterohemorrhagic 100.0
  - inanition 780.6
    - newborn 778.4
  - infective NEC 136.9
  - intermittent (bilious) (*see also* Malaria) 084.6
    - hepatic (Charcôt) – *see* Choledocholithiasis
    - of unknown origin (*see also* Pyrexia) 780.6
    - pernicious 084.0
  - iodide
    - correct substance properly administered 780.6
    - overdose or wrong substance given or taken 975.5
  - Japanese river 081.2
  - jungle yellow 060.0
  - Junin virus, hemorrhagic 078.7
  - Katayama 120.2
  - Kedani 081.2
  - Kenya 082.1
  - Korean hemorrhagic 078.6
  - Lassa 078.89
  - Lone Star 082.8
  - lung – *see* Pneumonia
  - Machupo virus, hemorrhagic 078.7
  - malaria, malarial (*see also* Malaria) 084.6
  - Malta (*see also* Brucellosis) 023.9
  - Marseilles 082.1
  - marsh (*see also* Malaria) 084.6
  - Mayaro (viral) 066.3
  - Mediterranean (*see also* Brucellosis) 023.9
    - familial 277.31
    - tick 082.1
  - meningeal – *see* Meningitis
  - metal fumes NEC 985.8
  - Meuse 083.1
  - Mexican – *see* Typhus, Mexican
  - Mianeh 087.1
  - miasmatic (*see also* Malaria) 084.6
  - miliary 078.2
  - milk, female 672❹
  - mill 504
  - mite-borne hemorrhagic 065.8
  - Monday 504
  - mosquito-borne NEC 066.3
    - hemorrhagic NEC 065.4
  - mountain 066.1
    - meaning
      - Rocky Mountain spotted 082.0
      - undulant fever (*see also* Brucellosis) 023.9
    - tick (American) 066.1
  - Mucambo (viral) 066.3
  - mud 100.89
  - Neapolitan (*see also* Brucellosis) 023.9
  - neutropenic 288.00
  - nine-mile 083.0
  - nonexanthematous tick 066.1
  - North Asian tick-borne typhus 082.2
  - Omsk hemorrhagic 065.1
  - O'nyong nyong (viral) 066.3
  - Oropouche (viral) 066.3
  - Oroya 088.0
  - paludal (*see also* Malaria) 084.6
  - Panama 084.0
  - pappataci 066.0
  - paratyphoid 002.9
    - A 002.1
    - B (Schottmüller's) 002.2
    - C (Hirschfeld) 002.3
  - parrot 073.9
  - periodic 277.31
  - pernicious, acute 084.0
  - persistent (of unknown origin) (*see also* Pyrexia) 780.6
  - petechial 036.0
  - pharyngoconjunctival 077.2
    - adenoviral type 3 077.2
  - Philippine hemorrhagic 065.4
  - phlebotomus 066.0
  - Piry 066.8
  - Pixuna (viral) 066.3
  - Plasmodium ovale 084.3
  - pleural (*see also* Pleurisy) 511.0
  - pneumonic – *see* Pneumonia
  - polymer fume 987.8
  - postoperative 998.89
    - due to infection 998.59
  - pretibial 100.89

- **Fever** – *continued*
  - puerperal, postpartum 672❹
  - putrid – *see* Septicemia
  - pyemic – *see* Septicemia
  - Q 083.0
    - with pneumonia 083.0 *[484.8]*
  - quadrilateral 083.0
  - quartan (malaria) 084.2
  - Queensland (coastal) 083.0
    - seven-day 100.89
  - Quintan (A) 083.1
  - quotidian 084.0
  - rabbit (*see also* Tularemia) 021.9
  - rat-bite 026.9
    - due to
      - Spirillum minor or minus 026.0
      - Spirochaeta morsus muris 026.0
      - Streptobacillus moniliformis 026.1
  - recurrent – *see* Fever, relapsing
  - relapsing 087.9
    - Carter's (Asiatic) 087.0
    - Dutton's (West African) 087.1
    - Koch's 087.9
    - louse-borne (epidemic) 087.0
    - Novy's (American) 087.1
    - Obermeyer's (European) 087.0
    - spirillum NEC 087.9
    - tick-borne (endemic) 087.1
  - remittent (bilious) (congestive) (gastric) (*see also* Malaria) 084.6
  - rheumatic (active) (acute) (chronic) (subacute) 390
    - with heart involvement 391.9
      - carditis 391.9
      - endocarditis (aortic) (mitral) (pulmonary) (tricuspid) 391.1
      - multiple sites 391.8
      - myocarditis 391.2
      - pancarditis, acute 391.8
      - pericarditis 391.0
      - specified type NEC 391.8
      - valvulitis 391.1
    - inactive or quiescent with cardiac hypertrophy 398.99
      - carditis 398.90
      - endocarditis 397.9
        - aortic (valve) 395.9
          - with mitral (valve) disease 396.9
        - mitral (valve) 394.9
          - with aortic (valve) disease 396.9
        - pulmonary (valve) 397.1
        - tricuspid (valve) 397.0
      - heart conditions (classifiable to 429.3, 429.6, 429.9) 398.99
        - failure (congestive) (conditions classifiable to 428.0, 428.9) 398.91
      - left ventricular failure (conditions classifiable to 428.1) 398.91
      - myocardial degeneration (conditions classifiable to 429.1) 398.0
      - myocarditis (conditions classifiable to 429.0) 398.0
      - pancarditis 398.99
      - pericarditis 393
  - Rift Valley (viral) 066.3
  - Rocky Mountain spotted 082.0
  - rose 477.0
  - Ross river (viral) 066.3
  - Russian hemorrhagic 078.6
  - sandfly 066.0
  - San Joaquin (valley) 114.0
  - Sao Paulo 082.0
  - scarlet 034.1
  - septic – *see* Septicemia
  - seven-day 061
    - Japan 100.89
    - Queensland 100.89
  - shin bone 083.1
  - Singapore hemorrhagic 065.4
  - solar 061
  - sore 054.9
  - South African tick-bite 087.1
  - Southeast Asia hemorrhagic 065.4
  - spinal – *see* Meningitis
  - spirillary 026.0
  - splenic (*see also* Anthrax) 022.9
  - spotted (Rocky Mountain) 082.0
    - American 082.0
    - Brazilian 082.0
    - Colombian 082.0
    - meaning
      - cerebrospinal meningitis 036.0

- **Fever** – *continued*
  - spotted – *continued*
    - meaning – *continued*
      - typhus 082.9
  - spring 309.23
  - steroid
    - correct substance properly administered 780.6
    - overdose or wrong substance given or taken 962.0
  - streptobacillary 026.1
  - subtertian 084.0
  - Sumatran mite 081.2
  - sun 061
  - swamp 100.89
  - sweating 078.2
  - swine 003.8
  - sylvatic yellow 060.0
  - Tahyna 062.5
  - tertian – *see* Malaria, tertian
  - Thailand hemorrhagic 065.4
  - thermic 992.0
  - three day 066.0
    - with Coxsackie exanthem 074.8
  - tick
    - American mountain 066.1
    - Colorado 066.1
    - Kemerovo 066.1
    - Mediterranean 082.1
    - mountain 066.1
    - nonexanthematous 066.1
    - Quaranfil 066.1
  - tick-bite NEC 066.1
  - tick-borne NEC 066.1
    - hemorrhagic NEC 065.3
  - transitory of newborn 778.4
  - trench 083.1
  - tsutsugamushi 081.2
  - typhogastric 002.0
  - typhoid (abortive) (ambulant) (any site) (hemorrhagic) (infection) (intermittent) (malignant) (rheumatic) 002.0
  - typhomalarial (*see also* Malaria) 084.6
  - typhus – *see* Typhus
  - undulant (*see also* Brucellosis) 023.9
  - unknown origin (*see also* Pyrexia) 780.6
  - uremic – *see* Uremia
  - uveoparotid 135
  - valley (Coccidioidomycosis) 114.0
  - Venezuelan equine 066.2
  - Volhynian 083.1
  - Wesselsbron (viral) 066.3
  - West
    - African 084.8
    - Nile (viral) 066.40
      - with
        - cranial nerve disorders 066.42
        - encephalitis 066.41
        - optic neuritis 066.42
        - other complications 066.49
        - other neurologic manifestations 066.42
        - polyradiculitis 066.42
  - Whitmore's 025
  - Wolhynian 083.1
  - worm 128.9
  - Yaroslav hemorrhagic 078.6
  - yellow 060.9
    - jungle 060.0
    - sylvatic 060.0
    - urban 060.1
    - vaccination, prophylactic (against) V04.4
  - Zika (viral) 066.3
- **Fibrillation**
  - atrial (established) (paroxysmal) 427.31
  - auricular (atrial) (established) 427.31
  - cardiac (ventricular) 427.41
  - coronary (*see also* Infarct, myocardium) 410.9❺
  - heart (ventricular) 427.41
  - muscular 728.9
  - postoperative 997.1
  - ventricular 427.41
- **Fibrin**
  - ball or bodies, pleural (sac) 511.0
  - chamber, anterior (eye) (gelatinous exudate) 364.04
- **Fibrinogenolysis** (hemorrhagic) – *see* Fibrinolysis
- **Fibrinogenopenia** (congenital) (hereditary) (*see also* Defect, coagulation) 286.3
  - acquired 286.6

- **Fibrinolysis** (acquired) (hemorrhagic) (pathologic) 286.6
  - with
    - abortion – *see* Abortion, by type, with hemorrhage, delayed or excessive
    - ectopic pregnancy (*see also* categories 633.0-633.9) 639.1
    - molar pregnancy (*see also* categories 630-632) 639.1
  - antepartum or intrapartum 641.3❺
    - affecting fetus or newborn 762.1
  - following
    - abortion 639.1
    - ectopic or molar pregnancy 639.1
  - newborn, transient 776.2
  - postpartum 666.3❺
- **Fibrinopenia** (hereditary) (*see also* Defect, coagulation) 286.3
  - acquired 286.6
- **Fibrinopurulent** – *see* condition
- **Fibrinous** – *see* condition
- **Fibroadenoma** (M9010/0)
  - cellular intracanalicular (M9020/0) 217
  - giant (intracanalicular) (M9020/0) 217
  - intracanalicular (M9011/0)
    - cellular (M9020/0) 217
    - giant (M9020/0) 217
    - specified site – *see* Neoplasm, by site, benign
    - unspecified site 217
  - juvenile (M9030/0) 217
  - pericanicular (M9012/0)
    - specified site – *see* Neoplasm, by site, benign
    - unspecified site 217
  - phyllodes (M9020/0) 217
  - prostate 600.20
    - with
      - other lower urinary tract symptoms (LUTS) 600.21
      - urinary
        - obstruction 600.21
        - retention 600.21
  - specified site – *see* Neoplasm, by site, benign
  - unspecified site 217
- **Fibroadenosis, breast** (chronic) (cystic) (diffuse) (periodic) (segmental) 610.2
- **Fibroangioma** (M9160/0) – *see also* Neoplasm, by site, benign
  - juvenile (M9160/0)
    - specified site – *see* Neoplasm, by site, benign
    - unspecified site 210.7
- **Fibrocellulitis progressiva ossificans** 728.11
- **Fibrochondrosarcoma** (M9220/3) – *see* Neoplasm, cartilage, malignant
- **Fibrocystic**
  - disease 277.00
    - bone NEC 733.29
    - breast 610.1
    - jaw 526.2
    - kidney (congenital) 753.19
    - liver 751.62
    - lung 518.89
      - congenital 748.4
    - pancreas 277.00
  - kidney (congenital) 753.19
- **Fibrodysplasia ossificans multiplex** (progressiva) 728.11
- **Fibroelastosis** (cordis) (endocardial) (endomyocardial) 425.3
- **Fibroid** (tumor) (M8890/0) – *see also* Neoplasm, connective tissue, benign
  - disease, lung (chronic) (*see also* Fibrosis, lung) 515
  - heart (disease) (*see also* Myocarditis) 429.0
  - induration, lung (chronic) (*see also* Fibrosis, lung) 515
  - in pregnancy or childbirth 654.1❺
    - affecting fetus or newborn 763.89
    - causing obstructed labor 660.2❺
      - affecting fetus or newborn 763.1
  - liver – *see* Cirrhosis, liver
  - lung (*see also* Fibrosis, lung) 515
  - pneumonia (chronic) (*see also* Fibrosis, lung) 515
  - uterus (M8890/0) (*see also* Leiomyoma, uterus) 218.9
- **Fibrolipoma** (M8851/0) (*see also* Lipoma, by site) 214.9
- **Fibroliposarcoma** (M8850/3) – *see* Neoplasm, connective tissue, malignant

❹ Fourth-Digit Required ❺ Fifth-Digit Required *[code]* Manifestation Code ▶◀ Revised Text ● New Line ▲ Revised Code

- **Fibroma** (M8810/0) – *see also* Neoplasm, connective tissue, benign
  - ameloblastic (M9330/0) 213.1
    - upper jaw (bone) 213.0
  - bone (nonossifying) 733.99
    - ossifying (M9262/0) – *see* Neoplasm, bone, benign
  - cementifying (M9274/0) – *see* Neoplasm, bone, benign
  - chondromyxoid (M9241/0) – *see* Neoplasm, bone, benign
  - desmoplastic (M8823/1) – *see* Neoplasm, connective tissue, uncertain behavior
  - facial (M8813/0) – *see* Neoplasm, connective tissue, benign
  - invasive (M8821/1) – *see* Neoplasm, connective tissue, uncertain behavior
  - molle (M8851/0) (*see also* Lipoma, by site) 214.9
  - myxoid (M8811/0) – *see* Neoplasm, connective tissue, benign
  - nasopharynx, nasopharyngeal (juvenile) (M9160/0) 210.7
  - nonosteogenic (nonossifying) – *see* Dysplasia, fibrous
  - odontogenic (M9321/0) 213.1
    - upper jaw (bone) 213.0
  - ossifying (M9262/0) – *see* Neoplasm, bone, benign
  - periosteal (M8812/0) – *see* Neoplasm, bone, benign
  - prostate 600.20
    - with
      - other lower urinary tract symptoms (LUTS) 600.21
      - urinary
        - obstruction 600.21
        - retention 600.21
  - soft (M8851/0) (*see also* Lipoma, by site) 214.9
- **Fibromatosis** 728.79
  - abdominal (M8822/1) – *see* Neoplasm, connective tissue, uncertain behavior
  - aggressive (M8821/1) – *see* Neoplasm, connective tissue, uncertain behavior
  - congenital generalized (CGF) 759.89
  - Dupuytren's 728.6
  - gingival 523.8
  - plantar fascia 728.71
  - proliferative 728.79
  - pseudosarcomatous (proliferative) (subcutaneous) 728.79
  - subcutaneous pseudosarcomatous (proliferative) 728.79
- **Fibromyalgia** 729.1
- **Fibromyoma** (M8890/0) – *see also* Neoplasm, connective tissue, benign
  - uterus (corpus) (*see also* Leiomyoma, uterus) 218.9
    - in pregnancy or childbirth 654.1❺
      - affecting fetus or newborn 763.89
      - causing obstructed labor 660.2❺
        - affecting fetus or newborn 763.1
- **Fibromyositis** (*see also* Myositis) 729.1
  - scapulohumeral 726.2
- **Fibromyxolipoma** (M8852/0) (*see also* Lipoma, by site) 214.9
- **Fibromyxoma** (M8811/0) – *see* Neoplasm, connective tissue, benign
- **Fibromyxosarcoma** (M8811/3) – *see* Neoplasm, connective tissue, malignant
- **Fibro-odontoma, ameloblastic** (M9290/0) 213.1
  - upper jaw (bone) 213.0
- **Fibro-osteoma** (M9262/0) – *see* Neoplasm, bone, benign
- **Fibroplasia, retrolental** 362.21
- **Fibropurulent** – *see* condition
- **Fibrosarcoma** (M8810/3) – *see also* Neoplasm, connective tissue, malignant
  - ameloblastic (M9330/3) 170.1
    - upper jaw (bone) 170.0
  - congenital (M8814/3) – *see* Neoplasm, connective tissue, malignant
  - fascial (M8813/3) – *see* Neoplasm, connective tissue, malignant
  - infantile (M8814/3) – *see* Neoplasm, connective tissue, malignant
  - odontogenic (M9330/3) 170.1
    - upper jaw (bone) 170.0

Fibrosarcoma – *continued*

  - periosteal (M8812/3) – *see* Neoplasm, bone, malignant
- **Fibrosclerosis**
  - breast 610.3
  - corpora cavernosa (penis) 607.89
  - familial multifocal NEC 710.8
  - multifocal (idiopathic) NEC 710.8
  - penis (corpora cavernosa) 607.89
- **Fibrosis, fibrotic**
  - adrenal (gland) 255.8
  - alveolar (diffuse) 516.3
  - amnion 658.8❺
  - anal papillae 569.49
  - anus 569.49
  - appendix, appendiceal, noninflammatory 543.9
  - arteriocapillary – *see* Arteriosclerosis
  - bauxite (of lung) 503
  - biliary 576.8
    - due to Clonorchis sinensis 121.1
  - bladder 596.8
    - interstitial 595.1
    - localized submucosal 595.1
    - panmural 595.1
  - bone, diffuse 756.59
  - breast 610.3
  - capillary – *see also* Arteriosclerosis
    - lung (chronic) (*see also* Fibrosis, lung) 515
  - cardiac (*see also* Myocarditis) 429.0
  - cervix 622.8
  - chorion 658.8❺
  - corpus cavernosum 607.89
  - cystic (of pancreas) 277.00
    - with
      - manifestations
        - gastrointestinal 277.03
        - pulmonary 277.02
        - specified NEC 277.09
      - meconium ileus 277.01
      - pulmonary exacerbation 277.02
  - due to (presence of) any device, implant, or graft – *see* Complications, due to (presence of) any device, implant, or graft classified to 996.0-996.5 NEC
  - ejaculatory duct 608.89
  - endocardium (*see also* Endocarditis) 424.90
  - endomyocardial (African) 425.0
  - epididymis 608.89
  - eye muscle 378.62
  - graphite (of lung) 503
  - heart (*see also* Myocarditis) 429.0
  - hepatic – *see also* Cirrhosis, liver
    - due to Clonorchis sinensis 121.1
  - hepatolienal – *see* Cirrhosis, liver
  - hepatosplenic – *see* Cirrhosis, liver
  - infrapatellar fat pad 729.31
  - interstitial pulmonary, newborn 770.7
  - intrascrotal 608.89
  - kidney (*see also* Sclerosis, renal) 587
  - liver – *see* Cirrhosis, liver
  - lung (atrophic) (capillary) (chronic) (confluent) (massive) (perialveolar) (peribronchial) 515
    - with
      - anthracosilicosis (occupational) 500
      - anthracosis (occupational) 500
      - asbestosis (occupational) 501
      - bagassosis (occupational) 495.1
      - bauxite 503
      - berylliosis (occupational) 503
      - byssinosis (occupational) 504
      - calcicosis (occupational) 502
      - chalicosis (occupational) 502
      - dust reticulation (occupational) 504
      - farmers' lung 495.0
      - gannister disease (occupational) 502
      - graphite 503
      - pneumonoconiosis (occupational) 505
      - pneumosiderosis (occupational) 503
      - siderosis (occupational) 503
      - silicosis (occupational) 502
      - tuberculosis (*see also* Tuberculosis) 011.4❺
    - diffuse (idiopathic) (interstitial) 516.3
    - due to
      - bauxite 503
      - fumes or vapors (chemical) (inhalation) 506.4
      - graphite 503
    - following radiation 508.1
    - postinflammatory 515
    - silicotic (massive) (occupational) 502
    - tuberculous (*see also* Tuberculosis) 011.4❺

Fibrosis, fibrotic – *continued*

  - lymphatic gland 289.3
  - median bar 600.90
    - with
      - other lower urinary tract symptoms (LUTS) 600.91
      - urinary
        - obstruction 600.91
        - retention 600.91
  - mediastinum (idiopathic) 519.3
  - meninges 349.2
  - muscle NEC 728.2
    - iatrogenic (from injection) 999.9
  - myocardium, myocardial (*see also* Myocarditis) 429.0
  - oral submucous 528.8
  - ovary 620.8
  - oviduct 620.8
  - pancreas 577.8
    - cystic 277.00
      - with
        - manifestations
          - gastrointestinal 277.03
          - pulmonary 277.02
          - specified NEC 277.09
        - meconium ileus 277.01
        - pulmonary exacerbation 277.02
  - penis 607.89
  - periappendiceal 543.9
  - periarticular (*see also* Ankylosis) 718.5❺
  - pericardium 423.1
  - perineum, in pregnancy or childbirth 654.8❺
    - affecting fetus or newborn 763.89
    - causing obstructed labor 660.2❺
      - affecting fetus or newborn 763.1
  - perineural NEC 355.9
    - foot 355.6
  - periureteral 593.89
  - placenta – *see* Placenta, abnormal
  - pleura 511.0
  - popliteal fat pad 729.31
  - preretinal 362.56
  - prostate (chronic) 600.90
    - with
      - other lower urinary tract symptoms (LUTS) 600.91
      - urinary
        - obstruction 600.91
        - retention 600.91
  - pulmonary (chronic) (*see also* Fibrosis, lung) 515
    - alveolar capillary block 516.3
    - interstitial
      - diffuse (idiopathic) 516.3
      - newborn 770.7
  - radiation – *see* Effect, adverse, radiation
  - rectal sphincter 569.49
  - retroperitoneal, idiopathic 593.4
  - sclerosing mesenteric (idiopathic) 567.82
  - scrotum 608.89
  - seminal vesicle 608.89
  - senile 797
  - skin NEC 709.2
  - spermatic cord 608.89
  - spleen 289.59
    - bilharzial (*see also* Schistosomiasis) 120.9
  - subepidermal nodular (M8832/0) – *see* Neoplasm, skin, benign
  - submucous NEC 709.2
    - oral 528.8
    - tongue 528.8
  - syncytium – *see* Placenta, abnormal
  - testis 608.89
    - chronic, due to syphilis 095.8
  - thymus (gland) 254.8
  - tunica vaginalis 608.89
  - ureter 593.89
  - urethra 599.84
  - uterus (nonneoplastic) 621.8
    - bilharzial (*see also* Schistosomiasis) 120.9
    - neoplastic (*see also* Leiomyoma, uterus) 218.9
  - vagina 623.8
  - valve, heart (*see also* Endocarditis) 424.90
  - vas deferens 608.89
  - vein 459.89
    - lower extremities 459.89
  - vesical 595.1
- **Fibrositis** (periarticular) (rheumatoid) 729.0
  - humeroscapular region 726.2
  - nodular, chronic
    - Jaccoud's 714.4
    - rheumatoid 714.4
  - ossificans 728.11

- **Fibrositis** – *continued*
  - scapulohumeral 726.2
- **Fibrothorax** 511.0
- **Fibrotic** – *see* Fibrosis
- **Fibrous** – *see* condition
- **Fibroxanthoma** (M8831/0) – *see also* Neoplasm, connective tissue, benign
  - atypical (M8831/1) – *see* Neoplasm, connective tissue, uncertain behavior
  - malignant (M8831/3) – *see* Neoplasm, connective tissue, malignant
- **Fibroxanthosarcoma** (M8831/3) – *see* Neoplasm, connective tissue, malignant
- **Fiedler's**
  - disease (leptospiral jaundice) 100.0
  - myocarditis or syndrome (acute isolated myocarditis) 422.91
- **Fiessinger-Leroy** (-Reiter) **syndrome** 099.3
- **Fiessinger-Rendu syndrome** (erythema muliforme exudativum) 695.1
- **Fifth disease** (eruptive) 057.0
  - venereal 099.1
- **Filaria, filarial** – *see* Infestation, filarial
- **Filariasis** (*see also* Infestation, filarial) 125.9
  - bancroftian 125.0
  - brug's 125.1
  - due to
    - bancrofti 125.0
    - Brugia (Wuchereria) (malayi) 125.1
    - loa loa 125.2
    - malayi 125.1
    - organism NEC 125.6
    - Wuchereria (bancrofti) 125.0
      - malayi 125.1
  - Malayan 125.1
  - ozzardi 125.5
  - specified type NEC 125.6
- **Filatoff's, Filatov's, Filatow's disease** (infectious mononucleosis) 075
- **File-cutters' disease** 984.9
  - specified type of lead – *see* Table of Drugs and Chemicals
- **Filling defect**
  - biliary tract 793.3
  - bladder 793.5
  - duodenum 793.4
  - gallbladder 793.3
  - gastrointestinal tract 793.4
  - intestine 793.4
  - kidney 793.5
  - stomach 793.4
  - ureter 793.5
- **Filtering bleb, eye** (postglaucoma) (status) V45.69
  - with complication or rupture 997.99
  - postcataract extraction (complication) 997.99
- **Fimbrial cyst** (congenital) 752.11
- **Fimbriated hymen** 752.49
- **Financial problem affecting care** V60.2
- **Findings, abnormal, without diagnosis** (examination) (laboratory test) 796.4
  - 17-ketosteroids, elevated 791.9
  - acetonuria 791.6
  - acid phosphatase 790.5
  - albumin-globulin ratio 790.99
  - albuminuria 791.0
  - alcohol in blood 790.3
  - alkaline phosphatase 790.5
  - amniotic fluid 792.3
  - amylase 790.5
  - antenatal screening 796.5
  - anisocytosis 790.09
  - anthrax, positive 795.31
  - antibody titers, elevated 795.79
  - anticardiolipin antibody 795.79
  - antigen-antibody reaction 795.79
  - antiphospholipid antibody 795.79
  - bacteriuria 791.9
  - ballistocardiogram 794.39
  - bicarbonate 276.9
  - bile in urine 791.4
  - bilirubin 277.4
  - bleeding time (prolonged) 790.92
  - blood culture, positive 790.7
  - blood gas level (arterial) 790.91
  - blood sugar level 790.29
    - high 790.29
      - fasting glucose 790.21
      - glucose tolerance test 790.22
- **Findings, abnormal, without diagnosis** – *continued*
  - blood sugar level – *continued*
    - low 251.2
  - C-reactive protein (CRP) 790.95
  - calcium 275.40
  - cancer antigen 125 [CA 125] 795.82
  - carbonate 276.9
  - carcinoembryonic antigen [CEA] 795.81
  - casts, urine 791.7
  - catecholamines 791.9
  - cells, urine 791.7
  - cerebrospinal fluid (color) (content) (pressure) 792.0
  - cervical
    - high risk human papillomavirus (HPV) DNA test positive 795.05
    - low risk human papillomavirus (HPV) DNA test positive 795.09
  - chloride 276.9
  - cholesterol 272.9
    - high 272.0 ●
      - with high triglycerides 272.2 ●
  - chromosome analysis 795.2
  - chyluria 791.1
  - circulation time 794.39
  - cloudy dialysis effluent 792.5
  - cloudy urine 791.9
  - coagulation study 790.92
  - cobalt, blood 790.6
  - color of urine (unusual) NEC 791.9
  - copper, blood 790.6
  - crystals, urine 791.9
  - culture, positive NEC 795.39
    - blood 790.7
    - HIV V08
    - human immunodeficiency virus V08
    - nose 795.39
    - skin lesion NEC 795.39
    - spinal fluid 792.0
    - sputum 795.39
    - stool 792.1
    - throat 795.39
    - urine 791.9
    - viral
      - human immunodeficiency V08
    - wound 795.39
  - echocardiogram 793.2
  - echoencephalogram 794.01
  - echogram NEC – *see* Findings, abnormal, structure
  - electrocardiogram (ECG) (EKG) 794.31
  - electroencephalogram (EEG) 794.02
  - electrolyte level, urinary 791.9
  - electromyogram (EMG) 794.17
    - ocular 794.14
  - electro-oculogram (EOG) 794.12
  - electroretinogram (ERG) 794.11
  - enzymes, serum NEC 790.5
  - fibrinogen titer coagulation study 790.92
  - filling defect – *see* Filling defect
  - function study NEC 794.9
    - auditory 794.15
    - bladder 794.9
    - brain 794.00
    - cardiac 794.30
    - endocrine NEC 794.6
      - thyroid 794.5
    - kidney 794.4
    - liver 794.8
    - nervous system
      - central 794.00
      - peripheral 794.19
    - oculomotor 794.14
    - pancreas 794.9
    - placenta 794.9
    - pulmonary 794.2
    - retina 794.11
    - special senses 794.19
    - spleen 794.9
    - vestibular 794.16
  - gallbladder, nonvisualization 793.3
  - glucose 790.29
    - elevated
      - fasting 790.21
      - tolerance test 790.22
  - glycosuria 791.5
  - heart
    - shadow 793.2
    - sounds 785.3
  - hematinuria 791.2
  - hematocrit
    - drop (precipitous) 790.01
- **Findings, abnormal, without diagnosis** – *continued*
  - hematocrit – *continued*
    - elevated 282.7
    - low 285.9
  - hematologic NEC 790.99
  - hematuria 599.7
  - hemoglobin
    - elevated 282.7
    - low 285.9
  - hemoglobinuria 791.2
  - histological NEC 795.4
  - hormones 259.9
  - immunoglobulins, elevated 795.79
  - indolacetic acid, elevated 791.9
  - iron 790.6
  - karyotype 795.2
  - ketonuria 791.6
  - lactic acid dehydrogenase (LDH) 790.4
  - lead 790.6
  - lipase 790.5
  - lipids NEC 272.9
  - lithium, blood 790.6
  - liver function test 790.6
  - lung field (coin lesion) (shadow) 793.1
  - magnesium, blood 790.6
  - mammogram 793.80
    - calcification 793.89
    - calculus 793.89
    - microcalcification 793.81
  - mediastinal shift 793.2
  - melanin, urine 791.9
  - microbiologic NEC 795.39
  - mineral, blood NEC 790.6
  - myoglobinuria 791.3
  - nasal swab, anthrax 795.31
  - neonatal screening 796.6
  - nitrogen derivatives, blood 790.6
  - nonvisualization of gallbladder 793.3
  - nose culture, positive 795.39
  - odor of urine (unusual) NEC 791.9
  - oxygen saturation 790.91
  - Papanicolaou (smear) 795.1
    - cervix 795.00
      - with
        - atypical squamous cells
          - cannot exclude high grade squamous intraepithelial lesion (ASC-H) 795.02
          - of undetermined significance (ASC-US) 795.01
        - cytologic evidence of malignancy 795.06
        - high grade squamous intraepithelial lesion (HGSIL) 795.04
        - low grade squamous intraepithelial lesion (LGSIL) 795.03
      - dyskaryotic 795.09
      - nonspecific finding NEC 795.09
    - other site 795.1
  - peritoneal fluid 792.9
  - phonocardiogram 794.39
  - phosphorus 275.3
  - pleural fluid 792.9
  - pneumoencephalogram 793.0
  - PO_2-oxygen ratio 790.91
  - poikilocytosis 790.09
  - potassium
    - deficiency 276.8
    - excess 276.7
  - PPD 795.5
  - prostate specific antigen (PSA) 790.93
  - protein, serum NEC 790.99
  - proteinuria 791.0
  - prothrombin time (prolonged) (partial) (PT) (PTT) 790.92
  - pyuria 791.9
  - radiologic (x-ray) 793.99
    - abdomen 793.6
    - biliary tract 793.3
    - breast 793.89
      - abnormal mammogram NOS 793.80
      - mammographic
        - calcification 793.89
        - calculus 793.89
        - microcalcification 793.81
    - gastrointestinal tract 793.4
    - genitourinary organs 793.5
    - head 793.0
    - image test inconclusive due to excess body fat 793.91
    - intrathoracic organs NEC 793.2
    - lung 793.1
    - musculoskeletal 793.7

Findings, abnormal, without diagnosis – *continued*
- radiologic – *continued*
  - placenta 793.99
  - retroperitoneum 793.6
  - skin 793.99
  - skull 793.0
  - subcutaneous tissue 793.99
- red blood cell 790.09
  - count 790.09
  - morphology 790.09
  - sickling 790.09
  - volume 790.09
- saliva 792.4
- scan NEC 794.9
  - bladder 794.9
  - bone 794.9
  - brain 794.09
  - kidney 794.4
  - liver 794.8
  - lung 794.2
  - pancreas 794.9
  - placental 794.9
  - spleen 794.9
  - thyroid 794.5
- sedimentation rate, elevated 790.1
- semen 792.2
- serological (for)
  - human immunodeficiency virus (HIV)
    - inconclusive 795.71
    - positive V08
  - syphilis – *see* Findings, serology for syphilis
- serology for syphilis
  - false positive 795.6
  - positive 097.1
    - false 795.6
    - follow-up of latent syphilis – *see* Syphilis, latent
    - only finding – *see* Syphilis, latent
- serum 790.99
  - blood NEC 790.99
  - enzymes NEC 790.5
  - proteins 790.99
- SGOT 790.4
- SGPT 790.4
- sickling of red blood cells 790.09
- skin test, positive 795.79
  - tuberculin (without active tuberculosis) 795.5
- sodium 790.6
  - deficiency 276.1
  - excess 276.0
- spermatozoa 792.2
- spinal fluid 792.0
  - culture, positive 792.0
- sputum culture, positive 795.39
  - for acid-fast bacilli 795.39
- stool NEC 792.1
  - bloody 578.1
    - occult 792.1
  - color 792.1
  - culture, positive 792.1
  - occult blood 792.1
- stress test 794.39
- structure, body (echogram) (thermogram) (ultrasound) (x-ray) NEC 793.99
  - abdomen 793.6
  - breast 793.89
    - abnormal mammogram 793.80
    - mammographic
      - calcification 793.89
      - calculus 793.89
      - microcalcification 793.81
  - gastrointestinal tract 793.4
  - genitourinary organs 793.5
  - head 793.0
    - echogram (ultrasound) 794.01
  - intrathoracic organs NEC 793.2
  - lung 793.1
  - musculoskeletal 793.7
  - placenta 793.99
  - retroperitoneum 793.6
  - skin 793.99
  - subcutaneous tissue NEC 793.99
- synovial fluid 792.9
- thermogram – *see* Findings, abnormal, structure
- throat culture, positive 795.39
- thyroid (function) 794.5
  - metabolism (rate) 794.5
  - scan 794.5
  - uptake 794.5
- total proteins 790.99
- toxicology (drugs) (heavy metals) 796.0
- transaminase (level) 790.4
- triglycerides 272.9
  - high 272.1 ●
    - with high cholesterol 272.2 ●
- tuberculin skin test (without active tuberculosis) 795.5
- tumor markers NEC 795.89
- ultrasound – *see also* Findings, abnormal, structure
  - cardiogram 793.2
- uric acid, blood 790.6
- urine, urinary constituents 791.9
  - acetone 791.6
  - albumin 791.0
  - bacteria 791.9
  - bile 791.4
  - blood 599.7
  - casts or cells 791.7
  - chyle 791.1
  - culture, positive 791.9
  - glucose 791.5
  - hemoglobin 791.2
  - ketone 791.6
  - protein 791.0
  - pus 791.9
  - sugar 791.5
- vaginal fluid 792.9
- vanillylmandelic acid, elevated 791.9
- vectorcardiogram (VCG) 794.39
- ventriculogram (cerebral) 793.0
- VMA, elevated 791.9
- Wassermann reaction
  - false positive 795.6
  - positive 097.1
    - follow-up of latent syphilis – *see* Syphilis, latent
    - only finding – *see* Syphilis, latent
- white blood cell 288.9
  - count 288.9
    - elevated 288.60
    - low 288.50
  - differential 288.9
  - morphology 288.9
- wound culture 795.39
- xerography 793.89
- zinc, blood 790.6

Finger – *see* condition

Finnish type nephrosis (congenital) 759.89 ●

Fire, St. Anthony's (*see also* Erysipelas) 035

Fish
- hook stomach 537.89
- meal workers' lung 495.8

Fisher's syndrome 357.0

Fissure, fissured
- abdominal wall (congenital) 756.79
- anus, anal 565.0
  - congenital 751.5
- buccal cavity 528.9
- clitoris (congenital) 752.49
- ear, lobule (congenital) 744.29
- epiglottis (congenital) 748.3
- larynx 478.79
  - congenital 748.3
- lip 528.5
  - congenital (*see also* Cleft, lip) 749.10
- nipple 611.2
  - puerperal, postpartum 676.1❺
- palate (congenital) (*see also* Cleft, palate) 749.00
- postanal 565.0
- rectum 565.0
- skin 709.8
  - streptococcal 686.9
- spine (congenital) (*see also* Spina bifida) 741.9❺
- sternum (congenital) 756.3
- tongue (acquired) 529.5
  - congenital 750.13

Fistula (sinus) 686.9
- abdomen (wall) 569.81
  - bladder 596.2
  - intestine 569.81
  - ureter 593.82
  - uterus 619.2
- abdominorectal 569.81
- abdominosigmoidal 569.81
- abdominothoracic 510.0
- abdominouterine 619.2
  - congenital 752.3
- abdominovesical 596.2
- accessory sinuses (*see also* Sinusitis) 473.9
- actinomycotic – *see* Actinomycosis
- alveolar
  - antrum (*see also* Sinusitis, maxillary) 473.0
  - process 522.7
- anorectal 565.1
- antrobuccal (*see also* Sinusitis, maxillary) 473.0
- antrum (*see also* Sinusitis, maxillary) 473.0
- anus, anal (infectional) (recurrent) 565.1
  - congenital 751.5
  - tuberculous (*see also* Tuberculosis) 014.8❺
- aortic sinus 747.29
- aortoduodenal 447.2
- appendix, appendicular 543.9
- arteriovenous (acquired) 447.0
  - brain 437.3
    - congenital 747.81
      - ruptured (*see also* Hemorrhage, subarachnoid) 430
    - ruptured (*see also* Hemorrhage, subarachnoid) 430
  - cerebral 437.3
    - congenital 747.81
  - congenital (peripheral) 747.60
    - brain – *see* Fistula, arteriovenous, brain, congenital
    - coronary 746.85
    - gastrointestinal 747.61
    - lower limb 747.64
    - pulmonary 747.3
    - renal 747.62
    - specified site NEC 747.69
    - upper limb 747.63
  - coronary 414.19
    - congenital 746.85
  - heart 414.19
  - pulmonary (vessels) 417.0
    - congenital 747.3
  - surgically created (for dialysis) V45.1
    - complication NEC 996.73
      - atherosclerosis – *see* Arteriosclerosis, extremities
      - embolism 996.74
      - infection or inflammation 996.62
      - mechanical 996.1
      - occlusion NEC 996.74
      - thrombus 996.74
  - traumatic – *see* Injury, blood vessel, by site
- artery 447.2
- aural 383.81
  - congenital 744.49
- auricle 383.81
  - congenital 744.49
- Bartholin's gland 619.8
- bile duct (*see also* Fistula, biliary) 576.4
- biliary (duct) (tract) 576.4
  - congenital 751.69
- bladder (neck) (sphincter) 596.2
  - into seminal vesicle 596.2
- bone 733.99
- brain 348.8
  - arteriovenous – *see* Fistula, arteriovenous, brain
- branchial (cleft) 744.41
- branchiogenous 744.41
- breast 611.0
  - puerperal, postpartum 675.1❺
- bronchial 510.0
- bronchocutaneous, bronchomediastinal, bronchopleural, bronchopleuromediastinal (infective) 510.0
  - tuberculous (*see also* Tuberculosis) 011.3❺
- bronchoesophageal 530.84
  - congenital 750.3
- buccal cavity (infective) 528.3
- canal, ear 380.89
- carotid-cavernous
  - congenital 747.81
    - with hemorrhage 430
  - traumatic 900.82
    - with hemorrhage (*see also* Hemorrhage, brain, traumatic) 853.0❺
    - late effect 908.3
- cecosigmoidal 569.81
- cecum 569.81
- cerebrospinal (fluid) 349.81
- cervical, lateral (congenital) 744.41
- cervicoaural (congenital) 744.49
- cervicosigmoidal 619.1
- cervicovesical 619.0
- cervix 619.8
- chest (wall) 510.0

Fistula – *continued*
- cholecystocolic (*see also* Fistula, gallbladder) 575.5
- cholecystocolonic (*see also* Fistula, gallbladder) 575.5
- cholecystoduodenal (*see also* Fistula, gallbladder) 575.5
- cholecystoenteric (*see also* Fistula, gallbladder) 575.5
- cholecystogastric (*see also* Fistula, gallbladder) 575.5
- cholecystointestinal (*see also* Fistula, gallbladder) 575.5
- choledochoduodenal 576.4
- cholocolic (*see also* Fistula, gallbladder) 575.5
- coccyx 685.1
  - with abscess 685.0
- colon 569.81
- colostomy 569.69
- colovaginal (acquired) 619.1
- common duct (bile duct) 576.4
- congenital, NEC – *see* Anomaly, specified type NEC
- cornea, causing hypotony 360.32
- coronary, arteriovenous 414.19
  - congenital 746.85
- costal region 510.0
- cul-de-sac, Douglas' 619.8
- cutaneous 686.9
- cystic duct (*see also* Fistula, gallbladder) 575.5
  - congenital 751.69
- dental 522.7
- diaphragm 510.0
  - bronchovisceral 510.0
  - pleuroperitoneal 510.0
  - pulmonoperitoneal 510.0
- duodenum 537.4
- ear (canal) (external) 380.89
- enterocolic 569.81
- enterocutaneous 569.81
- enteroenteric 569.81
- entero-uterine 619.1
  - congenital 752.3
- enterovaginal 619.1
  - congenital 752.49
- enterovesical 596.1
- epididymis 608.89
  - tuberculous (*see also* Tuberculosis) 016.4❺
- esophagobronchial 530.89
  - congenital 750.3
- esophagocutaneous 530.89
- esophagopleurocutaneous 530.89
- esophagotracheal 530.84
  - congenital 750.3
- esophagus 530.89
  - congenital 750.4
- ethmoid (*see also* Sinusitis, ethmoidal) 473.2
- eyeball (cornea) (sclera) 360.32
- eyelid 373.11
- fallopian tube (external) 619.2
- fecal 569.81
  - congenital 751.5
- from periapical lesion 522.7
- frontal sinus (*see also* Sinusitis, frontal) 473.1
- gallbladder 575.5
  - with calculus, cholelithiasis, stones (*see also* Cholelithiasis) 574.2❺
  - congenital 751.69
- gastric 537.4
- gastrocolic 537.4
  - congenital 750.7
  - tuberculous (*see also* Tuberculosis) 014.8❺
- gastroenterocolic 537.4
- gastroesophageal 537.4
- gastrojejunal 537.4
- gastrojejunocolic 537.4
- genital
  - organs
    - female 619.9
      - specified site NEC 619.8
    - male 608.89
  - tract-skin (female) 619.2
- hepatopleural 510.0
- hepatopulmonary 510.0
- horseshoe 565.1
- ileorectal 569.81
- ileosigmoidal 569.81
- ileostomy 569.69
- ileovesical 596.1
- ileum 569.81
- in ano 565.1
  - tuberculous (*see also* Tuberculosis) 014.8❺
- inner ear (*see also* Fistula, labyrinth) 386.40
- intestine 569.81
- intestinocolonic (abdominal) 569.81
- intestinoureteral 593.82
- intestinouterine 619.1
- intestinovaginal 619.1
  - congenital 752.49
- intestinovesical 596.1
- involving female genital tract 619.9
  - digestive-genital 619.1
  - genital tract-skin 619.2
  - specified site NEC 619.8
  - urinary-genital 619.0
- ischiorectal (fossa) 566
- jejunostomy 569.69
- jejunum 569.81
- joint 719.80
  - ankle 719.87
  - elbow 719.82
  - foot 719.87
  - hand 719.84
  - hip 719.85
  - knee 719.86
  - multiple sites 719.89
  - pelvic region 719.85
  - shoulder (region) 719.81
  - specified site NEC 719.88
  - tuberculous – *see* Tuberculosis, joint
  - wrist 719.83
- kidney 593.89
- labium (majus) (minus) 619.8
- labyrinth, labyrinthine NEC 386.40
  - combined sites 386.48
  - multiple sites 386.48
  - oval window 386.42
  - round window 386.41
  - semicircular canal 386.43
- lacrimal, lachrymal (duct) (gland) (sac) 375.61
- lacrimonasal duct 375.61
- laryngotracheal 748.3
- larynx 478.79
- lip 528.5
  - congenital 750.25
- lumbar, tuberculous (*see also* Tuberculosis) 015.0❺ *[730.8]*❺
- lung 510.0
- lymphatic (node) (vessel) 457.8
- mamillary 611.0
- mammary (gland) 611.0
  - puerperal, postpartum 675.1❺
- mastoid (process) (region) 383.1
- maxillary (*see also* Sinusitis, maxillary) 473.0
- mediastinal 510.0
- mediastinobronchial 510.0
- mediastinocutaneous 510.0
- middle ear 385.89
- mouth 528.3
- nasal 478.19
  - sinus (*see also* Sinusitis) 473.9
- nasopharynx 478.29
- nipple – *see* Fistula, breast
- nose 478.19
- oral (cutaneous) 528.3
  - maxillary (*see also* Sinusitis, maxillary) 473.0
  - nasal (with cleft palate) (*see also* Cleft, palate) 749.00
- orbit, orbital 376.10
- oro-antral (*see also* Sinusitis, maxillary) 473.0
- oval window (internal ear) 386.42
- oviduct (external) 619.2
- palate (hard) 526.89
  - soft 528.9
- pancreatic 577.8
- pancreaticoduodenal 577.8
- parotid (gland) 527.4
  - region 528.3
- pelvoabdominointestinal 569.81
- penis 607.89
- perianal 565.1
- pericardium (pleura) (sac) (*see also* Pericarditis) 423.8
- pericecal 569.81
- perineal – *see* Fistula, perineum
- perineorectal 569.81
- perineosigmoidal 569.81
- perineo-urethroscrotal 608.89
- perineum, perineal (with urethral involvement) NEC 599.1
  - tuberculous (*see also* Tuberculosis) 017.9❺
  - ureter 593.82
- perirectal 565.1
  - tuberculous (*see also* Tuberculosis) 014.8❺
- peritoneum (*see also* Peritonitis) 567.22
- periurethral 599.1
- pharyngo-esophageal 478.29
- pharynx 478.29
  - branchial cleft (congenital) 744.41
- pilonidal (infected) (rectum) 685.1
  - with abscess 685.0
- pleura, pleural, pleurocutaneous, pleuroperitoneal 510.0
  - stomach 510.0
  - tuberculous (*see also* Tuberculosis) 012.0❺
- pleuropericardial 423.8
- postauricular 383.81
- postoperative, persistent 998.6
- preauricular (congenital) 744.46
- prostate 602.8
- pulmonary 510.0
  - arteriovenous 417.0
    - congenital 747.3
  - tuberculous (*see also* Tuberculosis, pulmonary) 011.9❺
- pulmonoperitoneal 510.0
- rectolabial 619.1
- rectosigmoid (intercommunicating) 569.81
- rectoureteral 593.82
- rectourethral 599.1
  - congenital 753.8
- rectouterine 619.1
  - congenital 752.3
- rectovaginal 619.1
  - congenital 752.49
  - old, postpartal 619.1
  - tuberculous (*see also* Tuberculosis) 014.8❺
- rectovesical 596.1
  - congenital 753.8
- rectovesicovaginal 619.1
- rectovulvar 619.1
  - congenital 752.49
- rectum (to skin) 565.1
  - tuberculous (*see also* Tuberculosis) 014.8❺
- renal 593.89
- retroauricular 383.81
- round window (internal ear) 386.41
- salivary duct or gland 527.4
  - congenital 750.24
- sclera 360.32
- scrotum (urinary) 608.89
  - tuberculous (*see also* Tuberculosis) 016.5❺
- semicircular canals (internal ear) 386.43
- sigmoid 569.81
  - vesicoabdominal 596.1
- sigmoidovaginal 619.1
  - congenital 752.49
- skin 686.9
  - ureter 593.82
  - vagina 619.2
- sphenoidal sinus (*see also* Sinusitis, sphenoidal) 473.3
- splenocolic 289.59
- stercoral 569.81
- stomach 537.4
- sublingual gland 527.4
  - congenital 750.24
- submaxillary
  - gland 527.4
    - congenital 750.24
  - region 528.3
- thoracic 510.0
  - duct 457.8
- thoracicoabdominal 510.0
- thoracicogastric 510.0
- thoracicointestinal 510.0
- thoracoabdominal 510.0
- thoracogastric 510.0
- thorax 510.0
- thyroglossal duct 759.2
- thyroid 246.8
- trachea (congenital) (external) (internal) 748.3
- tracheoesophageal 530.84
  - congenital 750.3
  - following tracheostomy 519.09
- traumatic
  - arteriovenous (*see also* Injury, blood vessel, by site) 904.9
    - brain – *see* Injury, intracranial
- tuberculous – *see* Tuberculosis, by site
- typhoid 002.0
- umbilical 759.89
- umbilico-urinary 753.8

Fistula – *continued*
  urachal, urachus 753.7
  ureter (persistent) 593.82
  ureteroabdominal 593.82
  ureterocervical 593.82
  ureterorectal 593.82
  ureterosigmoido-abdominal 593.82
  ureterovaginal 619.0
  ureterovesical 596.2
  urethra 599.1
    congenital 753.8
    tuberculous (*see also* Tuberculosis) 016.3❺
  urethroperineal 599.1
  urethroperineovesical 596.2
  urethrorectal 599.1
    congenital 753.8
  urethroscrotal 608.89
  urethrovaginal 619.0
  urethrovesical 596.2
  urethrovesicovaginal 619.0
  urinary (persistent) (recurrent) 599.1
  uteroabdominal (anterior wall) 619.2
    congenital 752.3
  uteroenteric 619.1
  uterofecal 619.1
  uterointestinal 619.1
    congenital 752.3
  uterorectal 619.1
    congenital 752.3
  uteroureteric 619.0
  uterovaginal 619.8
  uterovesical 619.0
    congenital 752.3
  uterus 619.8
  vagina (wall) 619.8
    postpartal, old 619.8
  vaginocutaneous (postpartal) 619.2
  vaginoileal (acquired) 619.1
  vaginoperineal 619.2
  vesical NEC 596.2
  vesicoabdominal 596.2
  vesicocervicovaginal 619.0
  vesicocolic 596.1
  vesicocutaneous 596.2
  vesicoenteric 596.1
  vesicointestinal 596.1
  vesicometrorectal 619.1
  vesicoperineal 596.2
  vesicorectal 596.1
    congenital 753.8
  vesicosigmoidal 596.1
  vesicosigmoidovaginal 619.1
  vesicoureteral 596.2
  vesicoureterovaginal 619.0
  vesicourethral 596.2
  vesicourethrorectal 596.1
  vesicouterine 619.0
    congenital 752.3
  vesicovaginal 619.0
  vulvorectal 619.1
    congenital 752.49
Fit 780.39
  apoplectic (*see also* Disease, cerebrovascular, acute) 436
    late effect – *see* Late effect(s) (of) cerebrovascular disease
  epileptic (*see also* Epilepsy) 345.9❺
  fainting 780.2
  hysterical 300.11
  newborn 779.0
Fitting (of)
  artificial
    arm (complete) (partial) V52.0
    breast V52.4
    eye(s) V52.2
    leg(s) (complete) (partial) V52.1
  brain neuropacemaker V53.02
  cardiac pacemaker V53.31
  carotid sinus pacemaker V53.39
  cerebral ventricle (communicating) shunt V53.01
  colostomy belt V55.3
  contact lenses V53.1
  cystostomy device V53.6
  defibrillator, automatic implantable cardiac V53.32
  dentures V52.3
  device, unspecified type V53.90
    abdominal V53.5
    cardiac
      defibrillator, automatic implantable V53.32
      pacemaker V53.31
      specified NEC V53.39

Fitting – *continued*
  device, unspecified type – *continued*
    cerebral ventricle (communicating) shunt V53.01
    insulin pump V53.91
    intrauterine contraceptive V25.1
    nervous system V53.09
    orthodontic V53.4
    orthoptic V53.1
    other device V53.99
    prosthetic V52.9
      breast V52.4
      dental V52.3
      eye V52.2
      specified type NEC V52.8
    special senses V53.09
    substitution
      auditory V53.09
      nervous system V53.09
      visual V53.09
    urinary V53.6
  diaphragm (contraceptive) V25.02
  glasses (reading) V53.1
  growth rod V54.02
  hearing aid V53.2
  ileostomy device V55.2
  intestinal appliance or device NEC V53.5
  intrauterine contraceptive device V25.1
  neuropacemaker (brain) (peripheral nerve) (spinal cord) V53.02
  orthodontic device V53.4
  orthopedic (device) V53.7
    brace V53.7
    cast V53.7
    corset V53.7
    shoes V53.7
  pacemaker (cardiac) V53.31
    brain V53.02
    carotid sinus V53.39
    peripheral nerve V53.02
    spinal cord V53.02
  prosthesis V52.9
    arm (complete) (partial) V52.0
    breast V52.4
    dental V52.3
    eye V52.2
    leg (complete) (partial) V52.1
    specified type NEC V52.8
  spectacles V53.1
  wheelchair V53.8
Fitz's syndrome (acute hemorrhagic pancreatitis) 577.0
Fitz-Hugh and Curtis syndrome 098.86
  due to
    Chlamydia trachomatis 099.56
    Neisseria gonorrhoeae (gonococcal peritonitis) 098.86
Fixation
  joint – *see* Ankylosis
  larynx 478.79
  pupil 364.76
  stapes 385.22
    deafness (*see also* Deafness, conductive) 389.04
  uterus (acquired) – *see* Malposition, uterus
  vocal cord 478.5
Flaccid – *see also* condition
  foot 736.79
  forearm 736.09
  palate, congenital 750.26
Flail
  chest 807.4
    newborn 767.3
  joint (paralytic) 718.80
    ankle 718.87
    elbow 718.82
    foot 718.87
    hand 718.84
    hip 718.85
    knee 718.86
    multiple sites 718.89
    pelvic region 718.85
    shoulder (region) 718.81
    specified site NEC 718.88
    wrist 718.83
Flajani (-Basedow) syndrome or disease (exophthalmic goiter) 242.0❺
Flap, liver 572.8
Flare, anterior chamber (aqueous) (eye) 364.04
Flashback phenomena (drug) (hallucinogenic) 292.89

Flat
  chamber (anterior) (eye) 360.34
  chest, congenital 754.89
  electroencephalogram (EEG) 348.8
  foot (acquired) (fixed type) (painful) (postural) (spastic) 734
    congenital 754.61
      rocker bottom 754.61
      vertical talus 754.61
    rachitic 268.1
    rocker bottom (congenital) 754.61
    vertical talus, congenital 754.61
  organ or site, congenital NEC – *see* Anomaly, specified type NEC
  pelvis 738.6
    with disproportion (fetopelvic) 653.2❺
      affecting fetus or newborn 763.1
      causing obstructed labor 660.1❺
        affecting fetus or newborn 763.1
    congenital 755.69
Flatau-Schilder disease 341.1
Flattening
  head, femur 736.39
  hip 736.39
  lip (congenital) 744.89
  nose (congenital) 754.0
    acquired 738.0
Flatulence 787.3
Flatus 787.3
  vaginalis 629.89
Flax dressers' disease 504
Flea bite – *see* Injury, superficial, by site
Fleischer (-Kayser) **ring** (corneal pigmentation) 275.1 *[371.14]*
Fleischner's disease 732.3
Fleshy mole 631
Flexibilitas cerea (*see also* Catalepsy) 300.11
Flexion
  cervix – *see* Flexion, uterus
  contracture, joint (*see also* Contraction, joint) 718.4❺
  deformity, joint (*see also* Contraction, joint) 736.9
    hip, congenital (*see also* Subluxation, congenital, hip) 754.32
  uterus (*see also* Malposition, uterus) 621.6
Flexner's
  bacillus 004.1
  diarrhea (ulcerative) 004.1
  dysentery 004.1
Flexner-Boyd dysentery 004.2
Flexure – *see* condition
Floater, vitreous 379.24
Floating
  cartilage (joint) (*see also* Disorder, cartilage, articular) 718.0❺
    knee 717.6
  gallbladder (congenital) 751.69
  kidney 593.0
    congenital 753.3
  liver (congenital) 751.69
  rib 756.3
  spleen 289.59
Flooding 626.2
Floor – *see* condition
Floppy
  infant NEC 781.99
  iris syndrome 364.81 ●
  valve syndrome (mitral) 424.0
Flu – *see also* Influenza
  gastric NEC 008.8
Fluctuating blood pressure 796.4
Fluid
  abdomen 789.59 ▲
  chest (*see also* Pleurisy, with effusion) 511.9
  heart (*see also* Failure, heart) 428.0
  joint (*see also* Effusion, joint) 719.0❺
  loss (acute) 276.50
    with
      hypernatremia 276.0
      hyponatremia 276.1
  lung – *see also* Edema, lung
    encysted 511.8
  peritoneal cavity 789.59 ▲
    malignant 789.51 ●
  pleural cavity (*see also* Pleurisy, with effusion) 511.9
  retention 276.6

Flukes NEC (*see also* Infestation, fluke) 121.9
  blood NEC (*see also* Infestation, Schistosoma) 120.9
  liver 121.3
Fluor (albus) (vaginalis) 623.5
  trichomonal (Trichomonas vaginalis) 131.00
Fluorosis (dental) (chronic) 520.3
Flushing 782.62
  menopausal 627.2
Flush syndrome 259.2
Flutter
  atrial or auricular 427.32
  heart (ventricular) 427.42
    atrial 427.32
  impure 427.32
  postoperative 997.1
  ventricular 427.42
Flux (bloody) (serosanguineous) 009.0
Focal – *see* condition
Fochier's abscess – *see* Abscess, by site
Focus, Assmann's (*see also* Tuberculosis) 011.0❺
Fogo selvagem 694.4
Foix-Alajouanine syndrome 336.1
Folds, anomalous – *see also* Anomaly, specified type NEC
  Bowman's membrane 371.31
  Descemet's membrane 371.32
  epicanthic 743.63
  heart 746.89
  posterior segment of eye, congenital 743.54
Folie a deux 297.3
Follicle
  cervix (nabothian) (ruptured) 616.0
  graafian, ruptured, with hemorrhage 620.0
  nabothian 616.0
Folliclis (primary) (*see also* Tuberculosis) 017.0❺
Follicular – *see also* condition
  cyst (atretic) 620.0
Folliculitis 704.8
  abscedens et suffodiens 704.8
  decalvans 704.09
  gonorrheal (acute) 098.0
    chronic or duration of 2 months or more 098.2
  keloid, keloidalis 706.1
  pustular 704.8
  ulerythematosa reticulata 701.8
Folliculosis, conjunctival 372.02
Følling's disease (phenylketonuria) 270.1
Follow-up (examination) (routine) (following) V67.9
  cancer chemotherapy V67.2
  chemotherapy V67.2
  fracture V67.4
  high-risk medication V67.51
  injury NEC V67.59
  postpartum
    immediately after delivery V24.0
    routine V24.2
  psychiatric V67.3
  psychotherapy V67.3
  radiotherapy V67.1
  specified condition NEC V67.59
  specified surgery NEC V67.09
  surgery V67.00
    vaginal pap smear V67.01
  treatment V67.9
    combined NEC V67.6
    fracture V67.4
    involving high-risk medication NEC V67.51
    mental disorder V67.3
    specified NEC V67.59
Fong's syndrome (hereditary osteoonychodysplasia) 756.89
Food
  allergy 693.1
  anaphylactic shock – *see* Anaphylactic shock, due to food
  asphyxia (from aspiration or inhalation) (*see also* Asphyxia, food) 933.1
  choked on (*see also* Asphyxia, food) 933.1
  deprivation 994.2
    specified kind of food NEC 269.8
  intoxication (*see also* Poisoning, food) 005.9
  lack of 994.2
  poisoning (*see also* Poisoning, food) 005.9
  refusal or rejection NEC 307.59
  strangulation or suffocation (*see also* Asphyxia, food) 933.1
  toxemia (*see also* Poisoning, food) 005.9
Foot – *see also* condition
  and mouth disease 078.4
  process disease 581.3
Foramen ovale (nonclosure) (patent) (persistent) 745.5
Forbes' (glycogen storage) **disease** 271.0
Forbes-Albright syndrome (nonpuerperal amenorrhea and lactation associated with pituitary tumor) 253.1
Forced birth or delivery NEC 669.8❺
  affecting fetus or newborn NEC 763.89
Forceps
  delivery NEC 669.5❺
    affecting fetus or newborn 763.2
Fordyce's disease (ectopic sebaceous glands) (mouth) 750.26
Fordyce-Fox disease (apocrine miliaria) 705.82
Forearm – *see* condition
Foreign body

Note – For foreign body with open wound or other injury, see Wound, open, or the type of injury specified.

  accidentally left during a procedure 998.4
  anterior chamber (eye) 871.6
    magnetic 871.5
      retained or old 360.51
    retained or old 360.61
  ciliary body (eye) 871.6
    magnetic 871.5
      retained or old 360.52
    retained or old 360.62
  entering through orifice (current) (old)
    accessory sinus 932
    air passage (upper) 933.0
      lower 934.8
    alimentary canal 938
    alveolar process 935.0
    antrum (Highmore) 932
    anus 937
    appendix 936
    asphyxia due to (*see also* Asphyxia, food) 933.1
    auditory canal 931
    auricle 931
    bladder 939.0
    bronchioles 934.8
    bronchus (main) 934.1
    buccal cavity 935.0
    canthus (inner) 930.1
    cecum 936
    cervix (canal) uterine 939.1
    coil, ileocecal 936
    colon 936
    conjunctiva 930.1
    conjunctival sac 930.1
    cornea 930.0
    digestive organ or tract NEC 938
    duodenum 936
    ear (external) 931
    esophagus 935.1
    eye (external) 930.9
      combined sites 930.8
      intraocular – *see* Foreign body, by site
      specified site NEC 930.8
    eyeball 930.8
      intraocular – *see* Foreign body, intraocular
    eyelid 930.1
      retained or old 374.86
    frontal sinus 932
    gastrointestinal tract 938
    genitourinary tract 939.9
    globe 930.8
      penetrating 871.6
        magnetic 871.5
          retained or old 360.50
        retained or old 360.60
    gum 935.0
    Highmore's antrum 932
    hypopharynx 933.0
    ileocecal coil 936
    ileum 936
    inspiration (of) 933.1
    intestine (large) (small) 936
    lacrimal apparatus, duct, gland, or sac 930.2
    larynx 933.1
    lung 934.8
    maxillary sinus 932
    mouth 935.0
    nasal sinus 932

Foreign body – *continued*
  entering through orifice – *continued*
    nasopharynx 933.0
    nose (passage) 932
    nostril 932
    oral cavity 935.0
    palate 935.0
    penis 939.3
    pharynx 933.0
    pyriform sinus 933.0
    rectosigmoid 937
      junction 937
    rectum 937
    respiratory tract 934.9
      specified part NEC 934.8
    sclera 930.1
    sinus 932
      accessory 932
      frontal 932
      maxillary 932
      nasal 932
      pyriform 933.0
    small intestine 936
    stomach (hairball) 935.2
    suffocation by (*see also* Asphyxia, food) 933.1
    swallowed 938
      tongue 933.0
    tear ducts or glands 930.2
    throat 933.0
    tongue 935.0
      swallowed 933.0
    tonsil, tonsillar 933.0
      fossa 933.0
    trachea 934.0
    ureter 939.0
    urethra 939.0
    uterus (any part) 939.1
    vagina 939.2
    vulva 939.2
    wind pipe 934.0
  feeling of, in throat 784.99 ●
  granuloma (old) 728.82
    bone 733.99
    in operative wound (inadvertently left) 998.4
      due to surgical material intentionally left – *see* Complications, due to (presence of) any device, implant, or graft classified to 996.0-996.5 NEC
    muscle 728.82
    skin 709.4
    soft tissue NEC 709.4
    subcutaneous tissue 709.4
  in
    bone (residual) 733.99
    open wound – *see* Wound, open, by site complicated
    soft tissue (residual) 729.6
  inadvertently left in operation wound (causing adhesions, obstruction, or perforation) 998.4
  ingestion, ingested NEC 938
  inhalation or inspiration (*see also* Asphyxia, food) 933.1
  internal organ, not entering through an orifice – *see* Injury, internal, by site, with open wound
  intraocular (nonmagnetic) 871.6
    combined sites 871.6
      magnetic 871.5
        retained or old 360.59
      retained or old 360.69
    magnetic 871.5
      retained or old 360.50
    retained or old 360.60
    specified site NEC 871.6
      magnetic 871.5
        retained or old 360.59
      retained or old 360.69
  iris (nonmagnetic) 871.6
    magnetic 871.5
      retained or old 360.52
    retained or old 360.62
  lens (nonmagnetic) 871.6
    magnetic 871.5
      retained or old 360.53
    retained or old 360.63
  lid, eye 930.1
  ocular muscle 870.4
    retained or old 376.6
  old or residual
    bone 733.99
    eyelid 374.86
    middle ear 385.83

Flukes – Foreign body

- **Foreign body** – *continued*
  - old or residual – *continued*
    - muscle 729.6
      - ocular 376.6
    - retrobulbar 376.6
    - skin 729.6
      - with granuloma 709.4
    - soft tissue 729.6
      - with granuloma 709.4
    - subcutaneous tissue 729.6
      - with granuloma 709.4
  - operation wound, left accidentally 998.4
  - orbit 870.4
    - retained or old 376.6
  - posterior wall, eye 871.6
    - magnetic 871.5
      - retained or old 360.55
    - retained or old 360.65
  - respiratory tree 934.9
    - specified site NEC 934.8
  - retained (old) (nonmagnetic) (in)
    - anterior chamber (eye) 360.61
      - magnetic 360.51
    - ciliary body 360.62
      - magnetic 360.52
    - eyelid 374.86
    - globe 360.60
      - magnetic 360.50
    - intraocular 360.60
      - magnetic 360.50
      - specified site NEC 360.69
        - magnetic 360.59
    - iris 360.62
      - magnetic 360.52
    - lens 360.63
      - magnetic 360.53
    - muscle 729.6
    - orbit 376.6
    - posterior wall of globe 360.65
      - magnetic 360.55
    - retina 360.65
      - magnetic 360.55
    - retrobulbar 376.6
    - skin 729.6
      - with granuloma 709.4
    - soft tissue 729.6
      - with granuloma 709.4
    - subcutaneous tissue 729.6
      - with granuloma 709.4
    - vitreous 360.64
      - magnetic 360.54
  - retina 871.6
    - magnetic 871.5
      - retained or old 360.55
    - retained or old 360.65
  - superficial, without major open wound (*see also* Injury, superficial, by site) 919.6
  - swallowed NEC 938
  - throat, feeling of 784.99 ●
  - vitreous (humor) 871.6
    - magnetic 871.5
      - retained or old 360.54
    - retained or old 360.64
- **Forking, aqueduct of Sylvius** 742.3
  - with spina bifida (*see also* Spina bifida) 741.0❺
- **Formation**
  - bone in scar tissue (skin) 709.3
  - connective tissue in vitreous 379.25
  - Elschnig pearls (postcataract extraction) 366.51
  - hyaline in cornea 371.49
  - sequestrum in bone (due to infection) (*see also* Osteomyelitis) 730.1❺
  - valve
    - colon, congenital 751.5
    - ureter (congenital) 753.29
- **Formication** 782.0
- **Fort Bragg fever** 100.89
- **Fossa** – *see also* condition
  - pyriform – *see* condition
- **Foster-Kennedy syndrome** 377.04
- **Fothergill's**
  - disease, meaning scarlatina anginosa 034.1
  - neuralgia (*see also* Neuralgia, trigeminal) 350.1
- **Foul breath** 784.99
- **Found dead** (cause unknown) 798.9
- **Foundling** V20.0
- **Fournier's disease** (idiopathic gangrene) 608.83
- **Fourth**
  - cranial nerve – *see* condition
  - disease 057.8
- **Fourth** – *continued*
  - molar 520.1
- **Foville's syndrome** 344.89
- **Fox's**
  - disease (apocrine miliaria) 705.82
  - impetigo (contagiosa) 684
- **Fox-Fordyce disease** (apocrine miliaria) 705.82
- **Fracture** (abduction) (adduction) (avulsion) (compression) (crush) (dislocation) (oblique) (separation) (closed) 829.0

  Note – For fracture of any of the following sites with fracture of other bonessee Fracture, multiple.

  "Closed" includes the following descriptions of fractures, with or without delayed healing, unless they are specified as open or compound:

  comminuted
  depressed
  elevated
  fissured
  greenstick
  impacted
  linear
  simple
  slipped epiphysis
  spiral
  unspecified

  "Open" includes the following descriptions of fractures, with or without delayed healing:

  compound
  infected
  missile
  puncture
  with foreign body

  For late effect of fracture, see Late, effect, fracture, by site.

  - with
    - internal injuries in same region (conditions classifiable to 860-869) – *see also* Injury, internal, by site
      - pelvic region – *see* Fracture, pelvis
  - acetabulum (with visceral injury) (closed) 808.0
    - open 808.1
  - acromion (process) (closed) 811.01
    - open 811.11
  - alveolus (closed) 802.8
    - open 802.9
  - ankle (malleolus) (closed) 824.8
    - bimalleolar (Dupuytren's) (Pott's) 824.4
      - open 824.5
    - bone 825.21
      - open 825.31
    - lateral malleolus only (fibular) 824.2
      - open 824.3
    - medial malleolus only (tibial) 824.0
      - open 824.1
    - open 824.9
    - pathologic 733.16
    - talus 825.21
      - open 825.31
    - trimalleolar 824.6
      - open 824.7
  - antrum – *see* Fracture, skull, base
  - arm (closed) 818.0
    - and leg(s) (any bones) 828.0
      - open 828.1
    - both (any bones) (with rib(s)) (with sternum) 819.0
      - open 819.1
    - lower 813.80
      - open 813.90
    - open 818.1
    - upper – *see* Fracture, humerus
  - astragalus (closed) 825.21
    - open 825.31
  - atlas – *see* Fracture, vertebra, cervical, first
  - axis – *see* Fracture, vertebra, cervical, second
  - back – *see* Fracture, vertebra, by site
  - Barton's – *see* Fracture, radius, lower end
  - basal (skull) – *see* Fracture, skull, base
  - Bennett's (closed) 815.01
    - open 815.11
  - bimalleolar (closed) 824.4
    - open 824.5
  - bone (closed) NEC 829.0
    - birth injury NEC 767.3
    - open 829.1
- **Fracture** – *continued*
  - bone – *continued*
    - pathological NEC (*see also* Fracture, pathologic) 733.10
    - stress NEC (*see also* Fracture, stress) 733.95
  - boot top – *see* Fracture, fibula
  - boxers' – *see* Fracture, metacarpal bone(s)
  - breast bone – *see* Fracture, sternum
  - bucket handle (semilunar cartilage) – *see* Tear, meniscus
  - burst – *see* Fracture, traumatic, by site ●
  - bursting – *see* Fracture, phalanx, hand, distal
  - calcaneus (closed) 825.0
    - open 825.1
  - capitate (bone) (closed) 814.07
    - open 814.17
  - capitellum (humerus) (closed) 812.49
    - open 812.59
  - carpal bone(s) (wrist NEC) (closed) 814.00
    - open 814.10
    - specified site NEC 814.09
      - open 814.19
  - cartilage, knee (semilunar) – *see* Tear, meniscus
  - cervical – *see* Fracture, vertebra, cervical
  - chauffeur's – *see* Fracture, ulna, lower end
  - chisel – *see* Fracture, radius, upper end
  - clavicle (interligamentous part) (closed) 810.00
    - acromial end 810.03
      - open 810.13
    - due to birth trauma 767.2
    - open 810.10
    - shaft (middle third) 810.02
      - open 810.12
    - sternal end 810.01
      - open 810.11
  - clayshovelers' – *see* Fracture, vertebra, cervical
  - coccyx – *see also* Fracture, vertebra, coccyx
    - complicating delivery 665.6❺
  - collar bone – *see* Fracture, clavicle
  - Colles' (reversed) (closed) 813.41
    - open 813.51
  - comminuted – *see* Fracture, by site
  - compression – *see also* Fracture, by site
    - nontraumatic – *see* Fracture, pathologic
  - congenital 756.9
  - coracoid process (closed) 811.02
    - open 811.12
  - coronoid process (ulna) (closed) 813.02
    - mandible (closed) 802.23
      - open 802.33
    - open 813.12
  - corpus cavernosum penis 959.13
  - costochondral junction – *see* Fracture, rib
  - costosternal junction – *see* Fracture, rib
  - cranium – *see* Fracture, skull, by site
  - cricoid cartilage (closed) 807.5
    - open 807.6
  - cuboid (ankle) (closed) 825.23
    - open 825.33
  - cuneiform
    - foot (closed) 825.24
      - open 825.34
    - wrist (closed) 814.03
      - open 814.13
  - dental implant 525.73 ●
  - dental restorative material
    - with loss of material 525.64
    - without loss of material 525.63
  - due to
    - birth injury – *see* Birth injury, fracture
    - gunshot – *see* Fracture, by site, open
    - neoplasm – *see* Fracture, pathologic
    - osteoporosis – *see* Fracture, pathologic
  - Dupuytren's (ankle) (fibula) (closed) 824.4
    - open 824.5
    - radius 813.42
      - open 813.52
  - Duverney's – *see* Fracture, ilium
  - elbow – *see also* Fracture, humerus, lower end
    - olecranon (process) (closed) 813.01
      - open 813.11
    - supracondylar (closed) 812.41
      - open 812.51
  - ethmoid (bone) (sinus) – *see* Fracture, skull, base
  - face bone(s) (closed) NEC 802.8
    - with
      - other bone(s) – *see* Fracture, multiple, skull
      - skull – *see also* Fracture, skull
        - involving other bones – *see* Fracture, multiple, skull
    - open 802.9
  - fatigue – *see* Fracture, march

Vertical side tab: Foreign body – Fracture

- **Fracture** – *continued*
  - femur, femoral (closed) 821.00
    - cervicotrochanteric 820.03
      - open 820.13
    - condyles, epicondyles 821.21
      - open 821.31
    - distal end – *see* Fracture, femur, lower end
    - epiphysis (separation)
      - capital 820.01
        - open 820.11
      - head 820.01
        - open 820.11
      - lower 821.22
        - open 821.32
      - trochanteric 820.01
        - open 820.11
      - upper 820.01
        - open 820.11
    - head 820.09
      - open 820.19
    - lower end or extremity (distal end) (closed) 821.20
      - condyles, epicondyles 821.21
        - open 821.31
      - epiphysis (separation) 821.22
        - open 821.32
      - multiple sites 821.29
        - open 821.39
      - open 821.30
      - specified site NEC 821.29
        - open 821.39
      - supracondylar 821.23
        - open 821.33
      - T-shaped 821.21
        - open 821.31
    - neck (closed) 820.8
      - base (cervicotrochanteric) 820.03
        - open 820.13
      - extracapsular 820.20
        - open 820.30
      - intertrochanteric (section) 820.21
        - open 820.31
      - intracapsular 820.00
        - open 820.10
      - intratrochanteric 820.21
        - open 820.31
      - midcervical 820.02
        - open 820.12
      - open 820.9
      - pathologic 733.14
        - specified part NEC 733.15
      - specified site NEC 820.09
        - open 820.19
      - transcervical 820.02
        - open 820.12
      - transtrochanteric 820.20
        - open 820.30
    - open 821.10
    - pathologic 733.14
      - specified part NEC 733.15
    - peritrochanteric (section) 820.20
      - open 820.30
    - shaft (lower third) (middle third) (upper third) 821.01
      - open 821.11
    - subcapital 820.09
      - open 820.19
    - subtrochanteric (region) (section) 820.22
      - open 820.32
    - supracondylar 821.23
      - open 821.33
    - transepiphyseal 820.01
      - open 820.11
    - trochanter (greater) (lesser) (*see also* Fracture, femur, neck, by site) 820.20
      - open 820.30
    - T-shaped, into knee joint 821.21
      - open 821.31
    - upper end 820.8
      - open 820.9
  - fibula (closed) 823.81
    - with tibia 823.82
      - open 823.92
    - distal end 824.8
      - open 824.9
    - epiphysis
      - lower 824.8
        - open 824.9
      - upper – *see* Fracture, fibula, upper end
    - head – *see* Fracture, fibula, upper end
    - involving ankle 824.2
      - open 824.3

- **Fracture** – *continued*
  - fibula – *continued*
    - lower end or extremity 824.8
      - open 824.9
    - malleolus (external) (lateral) 824.2
      - open 824.3
    - open NEC 823.91
    - pathologic 733.16
    - proximal end – *see* Fracture, fibula, upper end
    - shaft 823.21
      - with tibia 823.22
        - open 823.32
      - open 823.31
    - stress 733.93
    - torus 823.41
      - with tibia 823.42
    - upper end or extremity (epiphysis) (head) (proximal end) (styloid) 823.01
      - with tibia 823.02
        - open 823.12
      - open 823.11
  - finger(s), of one hand (closed) (*see also* Fracture, phalanx, hand) 816.00
    - with
      - metacarpal bone(s), of same hand 817.0
        - open 817.1
      - thumb of same hand 816.03
        - open 816.13
    - open 816.10
  - foot, except toe(s) alone (closed) 825.20
    - open 825.30
  - forearm (closed) NEC 813.80
    - lower end (distal end) (lower epiphysis) 813.40
      - open 813.50
    - open 813.90
    - shaft 813.20
      - open 813.30
    - upper end (proximal end) (upper epiphysis) 813.00
      - open 813.10
  - fossa, anterior, middle, or posterior – *see* Fracture, skull, base
  - frontal (bone) – *see also* Fracture, skull, vault
    - sinus – *see* Fracture, skull, base
  - Galeazzi's – *see* Fracture, radius, lower end
  - glenoid (cavity) (fossa) (scapula) (closed) 811.03
    - open 811.13
  - Gosselin's – *see* Fracture, ankle
  - greenstick – *see* Fracture, by site
  - grenade-throwers' – *see* Fracture, humerus, shaft
  - gutter – *see* Fracture, skull, vault
  - hamate (closed) 814.08
    - open 814.18
  - hand, one (closed) 815.00
    - carpals 814.00
      - open 814.10
      - specified site NEC 814.09
        - open 814.19
    - metacarpals 815.00
      - open 815.10
    - multiple, bones of one hand 817.0
      - open 817.1
    - open 815.10
    - phalanges (*see also* Fracture, phalanx, hand) 816.00
      - open 816.10
  - healing
    - aftercare (*see also* Aftercare, fracture) V54.89
    - change of cast V54.89
    - complications – *see* condition
    - convalescence V66.4
    - removal of
      - cast V54.89
      - fixation device
        - external V54.89
        - internal V54.01
  - heel bone (closed) 825.0
    - open 825.1
  - hip (closed) (*see also* Fracture, femur, neck) 820.8
    - open 820.9
    - pathologic 733.14
  - humerus (closed) 812.20
    - anatomical neck 812.02
      - open 812.12
    - articular process (*see also* Fracture humerus, condyle(s)) 812.44
      - open 812.54
    - capitellum 812.49
      - open 812.59

- **Fracture** – *continued*
  - humerus – *continued*
    - condyle(s) 812.44
      - lateral (external) 812.42
        - open 812.52
      - medial (internal epicondyle) 812.43
        - open 812.53
      - open 812.54
    - distal end – *see* Fracture, humerus, lower end
    - epiphysis
      - lower (*see also* Fracture, humerus, condyle(s)) 812.44
        - open 812.54
      - upper 812.09
        - open 812.19
    - external condyle 812.42
      - open 812.52
    - great tuberosity 812.03
      - open 812.13
    - head 812.09
      - open 812.19
    - internal epicondyle 812.43
      - open 812.53
    - lesser tuberosity 812.09
      - open 812.19
    - lower end or extremity (distal end) (*see also* Fracture, humerus, by site) 812.40
      - multiple sites NEC 812.49
        - open 812.59
      - open 812.50
      - specified site NEC 812.49
        - open 812.59
    - neck 812.01
      - open 812.11
    - open 812.30
    - pathologic 733.11
    - proximal end – *see* Fracture, humerus, upper end
    - shaft 812.21
      - open 812.31
    - supracondylar 812.41
      - open 812.51
    - surgical neck 812.01
      - open 812.11
    - trochlea 812.49
      - open 812.59
    - T-shaped 812.44
      - open 812.54
    - tuberosity – *see* Fracture, humerus, upper end
    - upper end or extremity (proximal end) (*see also* Fracture, humerus, by site) 812.00
      - open 812.10
      - specified site NEC 812.09
        - open 812.19
  - hyoid bone (closed) 807.5
    - open 807.6
  - hyperextension – *see* Fracture, radius, lower end
  - ilium (with visceral injury) (closed) 808.41
    - open 808.51
  - impaction, impacted – *see* Fracture, by site
  - incus – *see* Fracture, skull, base
  - innominate bone (with visceral injury) (closed) 808.49
    - open 808.59
  - instep, of one foot (closed) 825.20
    - with toe(s) of same foot 827.0
      - open 827.1
    - open 825.30
  - insufficiency – *see* Fracture, pathologic, by site ●
  - internal
    - ear – *see* Fracture, skull, base
    - semilunar cartilage, knee – *see* Tear, meniscus, medial
  - intertrochanteric – *see* Fracture, femur, neck, intertrochanteric
  - ischium (with visceral injury) (closed) 808.42
    - open 808.52
  - jaw (bone) (lower) (closed) (*see also* Fracture, mandible) 802.20
    - angle 802.25
      - open 802.35
    - open 802.30
    - upper – *see* Fracture, maxilla
  - knee
    - cap (closed) 822.0
      - open 822.1
    - cartilage (semilunar) – *see* Tear, meniscus
  - labyrinth (osseous) – *see* Fracture, skull, base
  - larynx (closed) 807.5
    - open 807.6
  - late effect – *see* Late, effects (of), fracture
  - Le Fort's – *see* Fracture, maxilla

Fracture – *continued*
- leg (closed) 827.0
  - with rib(s) or sternum 828.0
    - open 828.1
  - both (any bones) 828.0
    - open 828.1
  - lower – *see* Fracture, tibia
  - open 827.1
  - upper – *see* Fracture, femur
- limb
  - lower (multiple) (closed) NEC 827.0
    - open 827.1
  - upper (multiple) (closed) NEC 818.0
    - open 818.1
- long bones, due to birth trauma – *see* Birth injury, fracture
- lumbar – *see* Fracture, vertebra, lumbar
- lunate bone (closed) 814.02
  - open 814.12
- malar bone (closed) 802.4
  - open 802.5
- Malgaigne's (closed) 808.43
  - open 808.53
- malleolus (closed) 824.8
  - bimalleolar 824.4
    - open 824.5
  - lateral 824.2
    - and medial – *see also* Fracture, malleolus, bimalleolar
      - with lip of tibia – *see* Fracture, malleolus, trimalleolar
    - open 824.3
  - medial (closed) 824.0
    - and lateral – *see also* Fracture, malleolus, bimalleolar
      - with lip of tibia – *see* Fracture, malleolus, trimalleolar
    - open 824.1
  - open 824.9
  - trimalleolar (closed) 824.6
    - open 824.7
- malleus – *see* Fracture, skull, base
- malunion 733.81
- mandible (closed) 802.20
  - angle 802.25
    - open 802.35
  - body 802.28
    - alveolar border 802.27
      - open 802.37
    - open 802.38
    - symphysis 802.26
      - open 802.36
  - condylar process 802.21
    - open 802.31
  - coronoid process 802.23
    - open 802.33
  - multiple sites 802.29
    - open 802.39
  - open 802.30
  - ramus NEC 802.24
    - open 802.34
  - subcondylar 802.22
    - open 802.32
- manubrium – *see* Fracture, sternum
- march 733.95
  - fibula 733.93
  - metatarsals 733.94
  - tibia 733.93
- maxilla, maxillary (superior) (upper jaw) (closed) 802.4
  - inferior – *see* Fracture, mandible
  - open 802.5
- meniscus, knee – *see* Tear, meniscus
- metacarpus, metacarpal (bone(s)), of one hand (closed) 815.00
  - with phalanx, phalanges, hand (finger(s)) (thumb) of same hand 817.0
    - open 817.1
  - base 815.02
    - first metacarpal 815.01
      - open 815.11
    - open 815.12
    - thumb 815.01
      - open 815.11
  - multiple sites 815.09
    - open 815.19
  - neck 815.04
    - open 815.14
  - open 815.10
  - shaft 815.03
    - open 815.13

Fracture – *continued*
- metatarsus, metatarsal (bone(s)), of one foot (closed) 825.25
  - with tarsal bone(s) 825.29
    - open 825.39
  - open 825.35
- Monteggia's (closed) 813.03
  - open 813.13
- Moore's – *see* Fracture, radius, lower end
- multangular bone (closed)
  - larger 814.05
    - open 814.15
  - smaller 814.06
    - open 814.16
- multiple (closed) 829.0

Note – Multiple fractures of sites classifiable to the same three-or four-digit category are coded to that category, except for sites classifiable to 810-818 or 820-827 in different limbs.

Multiple fractures of sites classifiable to different fourth-digit subdivisions within the same three-digit category should be dealt with according to coding rules.

Multiple fractures of sites classifiable to different three-digit categories (identifiable from the listing under "Fracture"), and of sites classifiable to 810-818 or 820-827 in different limbs should be coded according to the following list, which should be referred to in the following priority order: skull or face bones, pelvis or vertebral column, legs, arms.

  - arm (multiple bones in same arm except in hand alone) (sites classifiable to 810-817 with sites classifiable to a different three-digit category in 810-817 in same arm) (closed) 818.0
    - open 818.1
  - arms, both or arm(s) with rib(s) or sternum (sites classifiable to 810-818 with sites classifiable to same range of categories in other limb or to 807) (closed) 819.0
    - open 819.1
  - bones of trunk NEC (closed) 809.0
    - open 809.1
  - hand, metacarpal bone(s) with phalanx or phalanges of same hand (sites classifiable to 815 with sites classifiable to 816 in same hand) (closed) 817.0
    - open 817.1
  - leg (multiple bones in same leg) (sites classifiable to 820-826 with sites classifiable to a different three-digit category in that range in same leg) (closed) 827.0
    - open 827.1
  - legs, both or leg(s) with arm(s), rib(s), or sternum (sites classifiable to 820-827 with sites classifiable to same range of categories in other leg or to 807 or 810-819) (closed) 828.0
    - open 828.1
  - open 829.1
  - pelvis with other bones except skull or face bones (sites classifiable to 808 with sites classifiable to 805-807 or 810-829) (closed) 809.0
    - open 809.1

Fracture – *continued*
- multiple – *continued*
  - skull, specified or unspecified bones, or face bone(s) with any other bone(s) (sites classifiable to 800-803 with sites classifiable to 805-829) (closed) 804.0❺

Note – Use the following fifth-digit subclassification with categories 800, 801, 803, and 804:

0 unspecified state of consciousness
1 with no loss of consciousness
2 with brief [less than one hour] loss of consciousness
3 with moderate [1-24 hours] loss of consciousness
4 with prolonged [more than 24 hours] loss of consciousness and return to pre-existing conscious level
5 with prolonged [more than 24 hours] loss of consciousness, without return to pre-existing conscious level

Use fifth-digit 5 to designate when a patient is unconscious and dies before regaining consciousness, regardless of the duration of the loss of consciousness

6 with loss of consciousness of unspecified duration
9 with concussion, unspecified

    - with
      - contusion, cerebral 804.1❺
      - epidural hemorrhage 804.2❺
      - extradural hemorrhage 804.2❺
      - hemorrhage (intracranial) NEC 804.3❺
      - intracranial injury NEC 804.4❺
      - laceration, cerebral 804.1❺
      - subarachnoid hemorrhage 804.2❺
      - subdural hemorrhage 804.2❺
    - open 804.5❺
      - with
        - contusion, cerebral 804.6❺
        - epidural hemorrhage 804.7❺
        - extradural hemorrhage 804.7❺
        - hemorrhage (intracranial) NEC 804.8❺
        - intracranial injury NEC 804.9❺
        - laceration, cerebral 804.6❺
        - subarachnoid hemorrhage 804.7❺
        - subdural hemorrhage 804.7❺
  - vertebral column with other bones, except skull or face bones (sites classifiable to 805 or 806 with sites classifiable to 807-808 or 810-829) (closed) 809.0
    - open 809.1
- nasal (bone(s)) (closed) 802.0
  - open 802.1
  - sinus – *see* Fracture, skull, base
- navicular
  - carpal (wrist) (closed) 814.01
    - open 814.11
  - tarsal (ankle) (closed) 825.22
    - open 825.32
- neck – *see* Fracture, vertebra, cervical
- neural arch – *see* Fracture, vertebra, by site
- nonunion 733.82
- nose, nasal, (bone) (septum) (closed) 802.0
  - open 802.1
- occiput – *see* Fracture, skull, base
- odontoid process – *see* Fracture, vertebra, cervical
- olecranon (process) (ulna) (closed) 813.01
  - open 813.11
- open 829.1
- orbit, orbital (bone) (region) (closed) 802.8
  - floor (blow-out) 802.6
    - open 802.7
  - open 802.9
  - roof – *see* Fracture, skull, base
  - specified part NEC 802.8
    - open 802.9
- os
  - calcis (closed) 825.0
    - open 825.1
  - magnum (closed) 814.07
    - open 814.17
  - pubis (with visceral injury) (closed) 808.2
    - open 808.3
  - triquetrum (closed) 814.03
    - open 814.13
- osseous
  - auditory meatus – *see* Fracture, skull, base

Fracture – *continued*
osseous – *continued*
labyrinth – *see* Fracture, skull, base ossicles, auditory (incus) (malleus) (stapes) – *see* Fracture, skull, base
osteoporotic – *see* Fracture, pathologic
palate (closed) 802.8
open 802.9
paratrooper – *see* Fracture, tibia, lower end
parietal bone – *see* Fracture, skull, vault
parry – *see* Fracture, Monteggia's
patella (closed) 822.0
open 822.1
pathologic (cause unknown) 733.10
ankle 733.16
femur (neck) 733.14
specified NEC 733.15
fibula 733.16
hip 733.14
humerus 733.11
radius (distal) 733.12
specified site NEC 733.19
tibia 733.16
ulna 733.12
vertebrae (collapse) 733.13
wrist 733.12
pedicle (of vertebral arch) – *see* Fracture, vertebra, by site
pelvis, pelvic (bone(s)) (with visceral injury) (closed) 808.8
multiple (with disruption of pelvic circle) 808.43
open 808.53
open 808.9
rim (closed) 808.49
open 808.59
peritrochanteric (closed) 820.20
open 820.30
phalanx, phalanges, of one
foot (closed) 826.0
with bone(s) of same lower limb 827.0
open 827.1
open 826.1
hand (closed) 816.00
with metacarpal bone(s) of same hand 817.0
open 817.1
distal 816.02
open 816.12
middle 816.01
open 816.11
multiple sites NEC 816.03
open 816.13
open 816.10
proximal 816.01
open 816.11
pisiform (closed) 814.04
open 814.14
pond – *see* Fracture, skull, vault
Pott's (closed) 824.4
open 824.5
prosthetic device, internal – *see* Complications, mechanical
pubis (with visceral injury) (closed) 808.2
open 808.3
Quervain's (closed) 814.01
open 814.11
radius (alone) (closed) 813.81
with ulna NEC 813.83
open 813.93
distal end – *see* Fracture, radius, lower end
epiphysis
lower – *see* Fracture, radius, lower end
upper – *see* Fracture, radius, upper end
head – *see* Fracture, radius, upper end
lower end or extremity (distal end) (lower epiphysis) 813.42
with ulna (lower end) 813.44
open 813.54
open 813.52
torus 813.45
neck – *see* Fracture, radius, upper end
open NEC 813.91
pathologic 733.12
proximal end – *see* Fracture, radius, upper end
shaft (closed) 813.21
with ulna (shaft) 813.23
open 813.33
open 813.31
upper end 813.07
with ulna (upper end) 813.08
open 813.18

Fracture – *continued*
radius – *continued*
upper end – *continued*
epiphysis 813.05
open 813.15
head 813.05
open 813.15
multiple sites 813.07
open 813.17
neck 813.06
open 813.16
open 813.17
specified site NEC 813.07
open 813.17
ramus
inferior or superior (with visceral injury) (closed) 808.2
open 808.3
ischium – *see* Fracture, ischium
mandible 802.24
open 802.34
rib(s) (closed) 807.0

Note – Use the following fifth-digit subclassification with categories 807.0-807.1:

0	*rib(s), unspecified*
1	*one rib*
2	*two ribs*
3	*three ribs*
4	*four ribs*
5	*five ribs*
6	*six ribs*
7	*seven ribs*
8	*eight or more ribs*
9	*multiple ribs, unspecified*

with flail chest (open) 807.4
open 807.1❺
root, tooth 873.63
complicated 873.73
sacrum – *see* Fracture, vertebra, sacrum
scaphoid
ankle (closed) 825.22
open 825.32
wrist (closed) 814.01
open 814.11
scapula (closed) 811.00
acromial, acromion (process) 811.01
open 811.11
body 811.09
open 811.19
coracoid process 811.02
open 811.12
glenoid (cavity) (fossa) 811.03
open 811.13
neck 811.03
open 811.13
open 811.10
semilunar
bone, wrist (closed) 814.02
open 814.12
cartilage (interior) (knee) – *see* Tear, meniscus
sesamoid bone – *see* Fracture, by site
shepherd's (closed) 825.21
open 825.31
shoulder – *see also* Fracture, humerus, upper end
blade – *see* Fracture, scapula
silverfork – *see* Fracture, radius, lower end
sinus (ethmoid) (frontal) (maxillary) (nasal) (sphenoidal) – *see* Fracture, skull, base
Skillern's – *see* Fracture, radius, shaft

Fracture – *continued*
skull (multiple NEC) (with face bones) (closed) 803.0❺

Note – Use the following fifth-digit subclassification with categories 800, 801, 803, and 804:

0	*unspecified state of consciousness*
1	*with no loss of consciousness*
2	*with brief [less than one hour] loss of consciousness*
3	*with moderate [1-24 hours] loss of consciousness*
4	*with prolonged [more than 24 hours] loss of consciousness and return to pre-existing conscious level*
5	*with prolonged [more than 24 hours] loss of consciousness, without return to pre-existing conscious level*

Use fifth-digit 5 to designate when a patient is unconscious and dies before regaining consciousness, regardless of the duration of the loss of consciousness

6	*with loss of consciousness of unspecified duration*
9	*with concussion, unspecified*

with
contusion, cerebral 803.1❺
epidural hemorrhage 803.2❺
extradural hemorrhage 803.2❺
hemorrhage (intracranial) NEC 803.3❺
intracranial injury NEC 803.4❺
laceration, cerebral 803.1❺
other bones – *see* Fracture, multiple, skull
subarachnoid hemorrhage 803.2❺
subdural hemorrhage 803.2❺
base (antrum) (ethmoid bone) (fossa) (internal ear) (nasal sinus) (occiput) (sphenoid) (temporal bone) (closed) 801.0❺
with
contusion, cerebral 801.1❺
epidural hemorrhage 801.2❺
extradural hemorrhage 801.2❺
hemorrhage (intracranial) NEC 801.3❺
intracranial injury NEC 801.4❺
laceration, cerebral 801.1❺
subarachnoid hemorrhage 801.2❺
subdural hemorrhage 801.2❺
open 801.5❺
with
contusion, cerebral 801.6❺
epidural hemorrhage 801.7❺
extradural hemorrhage 801.7❺
hemorrhage (intracranial) NEC 801.8❺
intracranial injury NEC 801.9❺
laceration, cerebral 801.6❺
subarachnoid hemorrhage 801.7❺
subdural hemorrhage 801.7❺
birth injury 767.3
face bones – *see* Fracture, face bones
open 803.5❺
with
contusion, cerebral 803.6❺
epidural hemorrhage 803.7❺
extradural hemorrhage 803.7❺
hemorrhage (intracranial) NEC 803.8❺
intracranial injury NEC 803.9❺
laceration, cerebral 803.6❺
subarachnoid hemorrhage 803.7❺
subdural hemorrhage 803.7❺
vault (frontal bone) (parietal bone) (vertex) (closed) 800.0❺
with
contusion, cerebral 800.1❺
epidural hemorrhage 800.2❺
extradural hemorrhage 800.2❺
hemorrhage (intracranial) NEC 800.3❺
intracranial injury NEC 800.4❺
laceration, cerebral 800.1❺
subarachnoid hemorrhage 800.2❺
subdural hemorrhage 800.2❺
open 800.5❺
with
contusion, cerebral 800.6❺
epidural hemorrhage 800.7❺
extradural hemorrhage 800.7❺
hemorrhage (intracranial) NEC 800.8❺
intracranial injury NEC 800.9❺
laceration, cerebral 800.6❺
subarachnoid hemorrhage 800.7❺
subdural hemorrhage 800.7❺

- **Fracture** – *continued*
  - Smith's 813.41
    - open 813.51
  - sphenoid (bone) (sinus) – *see* Fracture, skull, base
  - spine – *see also* Fracture, vertebra, by site due to birth trauma 767.4
  - spinous process – *see* Fracture, vertebra, by site
  - spontaneous – *see* Fracture, pathologic
  - sprinters' – *see* Fracture, ilium
  - stapes – *see* Fracture, skull, base
  - stave – *see also* Fracture, metacarpus, metacarpal bone(s)
    - spine – *see* Fracture, tibia, upper end
  - sternum (closed) 807.2
    - with flail chest (open) 807.4
    - open 807.3
  - Stieda's – *see* Fracture, femur, lower end
  - stress 733.95
    - fibula 733.93
    - metatarsals 733.94
    - specified site NEC 733.95
    - tibia 733.93
  - styloid process
    - metacarpal (closed) 815.02
      - open 815.12
    - radius – *see* Fracture, radius, lower end
    - temporal bone – *see* Fracture, skull, base
    - ulna – *see* Fracture, ulna, lower end
  - supracondylar, elbow 812.41
    - open 812.51
  - symphysis pubis (with visceral injury) (closed) 808.2
    - open 808.3
  - talus (ankle bone) (closed) 825.21
    - open 825.31
  - tarsus, tarsal bone(s) (with metatarsus) of one foot (closed) NEC 825.29
    - open 825.39
  - temporal bone (styloid) – *see* Fracture, skull, base
  - tendon – *see* Sprain, by site
  - thigh – *see* Fracture, femur, shaft
  - thumb (and finger(s)) of one hand (closed) (*see also* Fracture, phalanx, hand) 816.00
    - with metacarpal bone(s) of same hand 817.0
      - open 817.1
    - metacarpal(s) – *see* Fracture, metacarpus
    - open 816.10
  - thyroid cartilage (closed) 807.5
    - open 807.6
  - tibia (closed) 823.80
    - with fibula 823.82
      - open 823.92
    - condyles – *see* Fracture, tibia, upper end
    - distal end 824.8
      - open 824.9
    - epiphysis
      - lower 824.8
        - open 824.9
      - upper – *see* Fracture, tibia, upper end
    - head (involving knee joint) – *see* Fracture, tibia, upper end
    - intercondyloid eminence – *see* Fracture, tibia, upper end
    - involving ankle 824.0
      - open 824.1
    - lower end or extremity (anterior lip) (posterior lip) 824.8
      - open 824.9
    - malleolus (internal) (medial) 824.0
      - open 824.1
    - open NEC 823.90
    - pathologic 733.16
    - proximal end – *see* Fracture, tibia, upper end
    - shaft 823.20
      - with fibula 823.22
        - open 823.32
      - open 823.30
    - spine – *see* Fracture, tibia, upper end
    - stress 733.93
    - torus 823.40
      - with tibia 823.42
    - tuberosity – *see* Fracture, tibia, upper end
    - upper end or extremity (condyle) (epiphysis) (head) (spine) (proximal end) (tuberosity) 823.00
      - with fibula 823.02
        - open 823.12
      - open 823.10
  - toe(s), of one foot (closed) 826.0
    - with bone(s) of same lower limb 827.0
      - open 827.1

- **Fracture** – *continued*
  - toe – *continued*
    - open 826.1
  - tooth (root) 873.63
    - complicated 873.73
  - torus
    - fibula 823.41
      - with tibia 823.42
    - radius 813.45
    - tibia 823.40
      - with fibula 823.42
  - trachea (closed) 807.5
    - open 807.6
  - transverse process – *see* Fracture, vertebra, by site
  - trapezium (closed) 814.05
    - open 814.15
  - trapezoid bone (closed) 814.06
    - open 814.16
  - trimalleolar (closed) 824.6
    - open 824.7
  - triquetral (bone) (closed) 814.03
    - open 814.13
  - trochanter (greater) (lesser) (closed) (*see also* Fracture, femur, neck, by site) 820.20
    - open 820.30
  - trunk (bones) (closed) 809.0
    - open 809.1
  - tuberosity (external) – *see* Fracture, by site
  - ulna (alone) (closed) 813.82
    - with radius NEC 813.83
      - open 813.93
    - coronoid process (closed) 813.02
      - open 813.12
    - distal end – *see* Fracture, ulna, lower end
    - epiphysis
      - lower – *see* Fracture, ulna, lower end
      - upper – *see* Fracture, ulna, upper, end
    - head – *see* Fracture, ulna, lower end
    - lower end (distal end) (head) (lower epiphysis) (styloid process) 813.43
      - with radius (lower end) 813.44
        - open 813.54
      - open 813.53
    - olecranon process (closed) 813.01
      - open 813.11
    - open NEC 813.92
    - pathologic 733.12
    - proximal end – *see* Fracture, ulna, upper end
    - shaft 813.22
      - with radius (shaft) 813.23
        - open 813.33
      - open 813.32
    - styloid process – *see* Fracture, ulna, lower end
    - transverse – *see* Fracture, ulna, by site
    - upper end (epiphysis) 813.04
      - with radius (upper end) 813.08
        - open 813.18
      - multiple sites 813.04
        - open 813.14
      - open 813.14
      - specified site NEC 813.04
        - open 813.14
  - unciform (closed) 814.08
    - open 814.18
  - vertebra, vertebral (back) (body) (column) (neural arch) (pedicle) (spine) (spinous process) (transverse process) (closed) 805.8
    - with
      - hematomyelia – *see* Fracture, vertebra, by site, with spinal cord injury
      - injury to
        - cauda equina – *see* Fracture, vertebra, sacrum, with spinal cord injury
        - nerve – *see* Fracture, vertebra, by site, with spinal cord injury
      - paralysis – *see* Fracture, vertebra, by site, with spinal cord injury
      - paraplegia – *see* Fracture, vertebra, by site, with spinal cord injury
      - quadriplegia – *see* Fracture, vertebra, by site, with spinal cord injury
      - spinal concussion – *see* Fracture, vertebra, by site, with spinal cord injury

- **Fracture** – *continued*
  - vertebra, vertebral – *continued*
    - with – *continued*
      - spinal cord injury (closed) NEC 806.8

Note – Use the following fifth-digit subclassification with categories 806.0-806.3:

C1-C4 or unspecified level and D1-D6 (T1-T6) or unspecified level with:

0 unspecified spinal cord injury
1 complete lesion of cord
2 anterior cord syndrome
3 central cord syndrome
4 specified injury NEC

C5-C7 level and D7-D12 level with:

5 unspecified spinal cord injury
6 complete lesion of cord
7 anterior cord syndrome
8 central cord syndrome
9 specified injury NEC

-
        - cervical 806.0❺
          - open 806.1❺
        - dorsal, dorsolumbar 806.2❺
          - open 806.3❺
        - open 806.9
        - thoracic, thoracolumbar 806.2❺
          - open 806.3❺
    - atlanto-axial – *see* Fracture, vertebra, cervical
    - cervical (hangman) (teardrop) (closed) 805.00
      - with spinal cord injury – *see* Fracture, vertebra, with spinal cord injury, cervical
      - first (atlas) 805.01
        - open 805.11
      - second (axis) 805.02
        - open 805.12
      - third 805.03
        - open 805.13
      - fourth 805.04
        - open 805.14
      - fifth 805.05
        - open 805.15
      - sixth 805.06
        - open 805.16
      - seventh 805.07
        - open 805.17
      - multiple sites 805.08
        - open 805.18
      - open 805.10
    - chronic 733.13 ●
    - coccyx (closed) 805.6
      - with spinal cord injury (closed) 806.60
        - cauda equina injury 806.62
          - complete lesion 806.61
            - open 806.71
          - open 806.72
        - open 806.70
        - specified type NEC 806.69
          - open 806.79
      - open 805.7
    - collapsed 733.13
    - compression, not due to trauma 733.13
    - dorsal (closed) 805.2
      - with spinal cord injury – *see* Fracture, vertebra, with spinal cord injury, dorsal
      - open 805.3
    - dorsolumbar (closed) 805.2
      - with spinal cord injury – *see* Fracture, vertebra, with spinal cord injury, dorsal
      - open 805.3
    - due to osteoporosis 733.13
    - fetus or newborn 767.4
    - lumbar (closed) 805.4
      - with spinal cord injury (closed) 806.4
        - open 806.5
      - open 805.5
    - nontraumatic 733.13
    - open NEC 805.9
    - pathologic (any site) 733.13
    - sacrum (closed) 805.6
      - with spinal cord injury 806.60
        - cauda equina injury 806.62
          - complete lesion 806.61
            - open 806.71
          - open 806.72
        - open 806.70
        - specified type NEC 806.69
          - open 806.79
      - open 805.7

Fracture – *continued*
- vertebra, vertebral – *continued*
  - site unspecified (closed) 805.8
    - with spinal cord injury (closed) 806.8
      - open 806.9
    - open 805.9
  - stress (any site) 733.95
  - thoracic (closed) 805.2
    - with spinal cord injury – *see* Fracture, vertebra, with spinal cord injury, thoracic
    - open 805.3
- vertex – *see* Fracture, skull, vault
- vomer (bone) 802.0
  - open 802.1
- Wagstaffe's – *see* Fracture, ankle
- wrist (closed) 814.00
  - open 814.10
  - pathologic 733.12
- xiphoid (process) – *see* Fracture, sternum
- zygoma (zygomatic arch) (closed) 802.4
  - open 802.5

Fragile X syndrome 759.83

Fragilitas
- crinium 704.2
- hair 704.2
- ossium 756.51
  - with blue sclera 756.51
- unguium 703.8
  - congenital 757.5

Fragility
- bone 756.51
  - with deafness and blue sclera 756.51
- capillary (hereditary) 287.8
- hair 704.2
- nails 703.8

Fragmentation – *see* Fracture, by site

Frambesia, frambesial (tropica) (*see also* Yaws) 102.9
- initial lesion or ulcer 102.0
- primary 102.0

Frambeside
- gummatous 102.4
- of early yaws 102.2

Frambesioma 102.1

Franceschetti's syndrome (mandibulofacial dysostosis) 756.0

Francis' disease (*see also* Tularemia) 021.9

Frank's essential thrombocytopenia (*see also* Purpura, thrombocytopenic) 287.39

Franklin's disease (heavy chain) 273.2

Fraser's syndrome 759.89

Freckle 709.09
- malignant melanoma in (M8742/3) – *see* Melanoma
- melanotic (of Hutchinson) (M8742/2) – *see* Neoplasm, skin, in situ

Freeman-Sheldon syndrome 759.89

Freezing 991.9
- specified effect NEC 991.8

Frei's disease (climatic bubo) 099.1

Freiberg's
- disease (osteochondrosis, second metatarsal) 732.5
- infraction of metatarsal head 732.5
- osteochondrosis 732.5

Fremitus, friction, cardiac 785.3

Frenulum linguae 750.0

Frenum
- external os 752.49
- tongue 750.0

Frequency (urinary) NEC 788.41
- micturition 788.41
- nocturnal 788.43
- polyuria 788.42
- psychogenic 306.53

Frey's syndrome (auriculotemporal syndrome) 705.22

Friction
- burn (*see also* Injury, superficial, by site) 919.0
- fremitus, cardiac 785.3
- precordial 785.3
- sounds, chest 786.7

Friderichsen-Waterhouse syndrome or disease 036.3

Friedländer's
- B (bacillus) NEC (*see also* condition) 041.3
  - sepsis or septicemia 038.49
- disease (endarteritis obliterans) – *see* Arteriosclerosis

Friedreich's
- ataxia 334.0
- combined systemic disease 334.0
- disease 333.2
  - combined systemic 334.0
- myoclonia 333.2
- sclerosis (spinal cord) 334.0

Friedrich-Erb-Arnold syndrome (acropachyderma) 757.39

Frigidity 302.72
- psychic or psychogenic 302.72

Fröhlich's disease or syndrome (adiposogenital dystrophy) 253.8

Froin's syndrome 336.8

Frommel's disease 676.6❺

Frommel-Chiari syndrome 676.6❺

Frontal – *see also* condition
- lobe syndrome 310.0

Frostbite 991.3
- face 991.0
- foot 991.2
- hand 991.1
- specified site NEC 991.3

Frotteurism 302.89

Frozen 991.9
- pelvis 620.8
- shoulder 726.0

Fructosemia 271.2

Fructosuria (benign) (essential) 271.2

Fuchs'
- black spot (myopic) 360.21
- corneal dystrophy (endothelial) 371.57
- heterochromic cyclitis 364.21

Fucosidosis 271.8

Fugue 780.99
- dissociative 300.13
- hysterical (dissociative) 300.13
- reaction to exceptional stress (transient) 308.1

Fukuhara syndrome 277.87

Fuller Albright's syndrome (osteitis fibrosa disseminata) 756.59

Fuller's earth disease 502

Fulminant, fulminating – *see* condition

Functional – *see* condition

Functioning
- borderline intellectual V62.89

Fundus – *see also* condition
- flavimaculatus 362.76

Fungemia 117.9

Fungus, fungous
- cerebral 348.8
- disease NEC 117.9
- infection – *see* Infection, fungus
- testis (*see also* Tuberculosis) 016.5❺ *[608.81]*

Funiculitis (acute) 608.4
- chronic 608.4
- endemic 608.4
- gonococcal (acute) 098.14
  - chronic or duration of 2 months or over 098.34
- tuberculous (*see also* Tuberculosis) 016.5❺

F.U.O. (*see also* Pyrexia) 780.6

Funnel
- breast (acquired) 738.3
  - congenital 754.81
  - late effect of rickets 268.1
- chest (acquired) 738.3
  - congenital 754.81
  - late effect of rickets 268.1
- pelvis (acquired) 738.6
  - with disproportion (fetopelvic) 653.3❺
    - affecting fetus or newborn 763.1
    - causing obstructed labor 660.1❺
      - affecting fetus or newborn 763.1
  - congenital 755.69
  - tuberculous (*see also* Tuberculosis) 016.9❺

Furfur 690.18
- microsporon 111.0

Furor, paroxysmal (idiopathic) (*see also* Epilepsy) 345.8❺

Furriers' lung 495.8

Furrowed tongue 529.5
- congenital 750.13

Furrowing nail(s) (transverse) 703.8
- congenital 757.5

Furuncle 680.9
- abdominal wall 680.2

Furuncle – *continued*
- ankle 680.6
- anus 680.5
- arm (any part, above wrist) 680.3
- auditory canal, external 680.0
- axilla 680.3
- back (any part) 680.2
- breast 680.2
- buttock 680.5
- chest wall 680.2
- corpus cavernosum 607.2
- ear (any part) 680.0
- eyelid 373.13
- face (any part, except eye) 680.0
- finger (any) 680.4
- flank 680.2
- foot (any part) 680.7
- forearm 680.3
- gluteal (region) 680.5
- groin 680.2
- hand (any part) 680.4
- head (any part, except face) 680.8
- heel 680.7
- hip 680.6
- kidney (*see also* Abscess, kidney) 590.2
- knee 680.6
- labium (majus) (minus) 616.4
- lacrimal
  - gland (*see also* Dacryoadenitis) 375.00
  - passages (duct) (sac) (*see also* Dacryocystitis) 375.30
- leg, any part except foot 680.6
- malignant 022.0
- multiple sites 680.9
- neck 680.1
- nose (external) (septum) 680.0
- orbit 376.01
- partes posteriores 680.5
- pectoral region 680.2
- penis 607.2
- perineum 680.2
- pinna 680.0
- scalp (any part) 680.8
- scrotum 608.4
- seminal vesicle 608.0
- shoulder 680.3
- skin NEC 680.9
- specified site NEC 680.8
- spermatic cord 608.4
- temple (region) 680.0
- testis 604.90
- thigh 680.6
- thumb 680.4
- toe (any) 680.7
- trunk 680.2
- tunica vaginalis 608.4
- umbilicus 680.2
- upper arm 680.3
- vas deferens 608.4
- vulva 616.4
- wrist 680.4

Furunculosis (*see also* Furuncle) 680.9
- external auditory meatus 680.0 *[380.13]*

Fusarium (infection) 118

Fusion, fused (congenital)
- anal (with urogenital canal) 751.5
- aorta and pulmonary artery 745.0
- astragaloscaphoid 755.67
- atria 745.5
- atrium and ventricle 745.69
- auditory canal 744.02
- auricles, heart 745.5
- binocular, with defective stereopsis 368.33
- bone 756.9
- cervical spine – *see* Fusion, spine
- choanal 748.0
- commissure, mitral valve 746.5
- cranial sutures, premature 756.0
- cusps, heart valve NEC 746.89
  - mitral 746.5
  - tricuspid 746.89
- ear ossicles 744.04
- fingers (*see also* Syndactylism, fingers) 755.11
- hymen 752.42
- hymeno-urethral 599.89
  - causing obstructed labor 660.1❺
    - affecting fetus or newborn 763.1
- joint (acquired) – *see also* Ankylosis
  - congenital 755.8
- kidneys (incomplete) 753.3
- labium (majus) (minus) 752.49

- **Fusion, fused** – *continued*
  - larynx and trachea 748.3
  - limb 755.8
    - lower 755.69
    - upper 755.59
  - lobe, lung 748.5
  - lumbosacral (acquired) 724.6
    - congenital 756.15
    - surgical V45.4
  - nares (anterior) (posterior) 748.0
  - nose, nasal 748.0
  - nostril(s) 748.0
  - organ or site NEC – *see* Anomaly, specified type NEC
  - ossicles 756.9
    - auditory 744.04
  - pulmonary valve segment 746.02
  - pulmonic cusps 746.02
  - ribs 756.3
  - sacroiliac (acquired) (joint) 724.6
    - congenital 755.69
    - surgical V45.4
  - skull, imperfect 756.0
  - spine (acquired) 724.9
    - arthrodesis status V45.4
    - congenital (vertebra) 756.15
    - postoperative status V45.4
  - sublingual duct with submaxillary duct at opening in mouth 750.26
  - talonavicular (bar) 755.67
  - teeth, tooth 520.2
  - testes 752.89
  - toes (*see also* Syndactylism, toes) 755.13
  - trachea and esophagus 750.3
  - twins 759.4
  - urethral-hymenal 599.89
  - vagina 752.49
  - valve cusps – *see* Fusion, cusps, heart valve
  - ventricles, heart 745.4
  - vertebra (arch) – *see* Fusion, spine
  - vulva 752.49
- **Fusospirillosis** (mouth) (tongue) (tonsil) 101
- **Fussy infant** (baby) 780.91

G

- **Gafsa boil** 085.1
- **Gain, weight** (abnormal) (excessive) (*see also* Weight, gain) 783.1
- **Gaisböck's disease or syndrome** (polycythemia hypertonica) 289.0
- **Gait**
  - abnormality 781.2
    - hysterical 300.11
  - ataxic 781.2
    - hysterical 300.11
  - disturbance 781.2
    - hysterical 300.11
  - paralytic 781.2
  - scissor 781.2
  - spastic 781.2
  - staggering 781.2
    - hysterical 300.11
- **Galactocele** (breast) (infected) 611.5
  - puerperal, postpartum 676.8❺
- **Galactophoritis** 611.0
  - puerperal, postpartum 675.2❺
- **Galactorrhea** 676.6❺
  - not associated with childbirth 611.6
- **Galactosemia** (classic) (congenital) 271.1
- **Galactosuria** 271.1
- **Galacturia** 791.1
  - bilharziasis 120.0
- **Galen's vein** – *see* condition
- **Gallbladder** – *see also* condition
  - acute (*see also* Disease, gallbladder) 575.0
- **Gall duct** – *see* condition
- **Gallop rhythm** 427.89
- **Gallstone** (cholemic) (colic) (impacted) – *see also* Cholelithiasis
  - causing intestinal obstruction 560.31
- **Gambling, pathological** 312.31
- **Gammaloidosis** 277.39
- **Gammopathy** 273.9
  - macroglobulinemia 273.3
  - monoclonal (benign) (essential) (idiopathic) (with lymphoplasmacytic dyscrasia) 273.1
- **Gamna's disease** (siderotic splenomegaly) 289.51
- **Gampsodactylia** (congenital) 754.71
- **Gamstorp's disease** (adynamia episodica hereditaria) 359.3
- **Gandy-Nanta disease** (siderotic splenomegaly) 289.51
- **Gang activity, without manifest psychiatric disorder** V71.09
  - adolescent V71.02
  - adult V71.01
  - child V71.02
- **Gangliocytoma** (M9490/0) – *see* Neoplasm, connective tissue, benign
- **Ganglioglioma** (M9505/1) – *see* Neoplasm, by site, uncertain behavior
- **Ganglion** 727.43
  - joint 727.41
  - of yaws (early) (late) 102.6
  - periosteal (*see also* Periostitis) 730.3❺
  - tendon sheath (compound) (diffuse) 727.42
  - tuberculous (*see also* Tuberculosis) 015.9❺
- **Ganglioneuroblastoma** (M9490/3) – *see* Neoplasm, connective tissue, malignant
- **Ganglioneuroma** (M9490/0) – *see also* Neoplasm, connective tissue, benign
  - malignant (M9490/3) – *see* Neoplasm, connective tissue, malignant
- **Ganglioneuromatosis** (M9491/0) – *see* Neoplasm, connective tissue, benign
- **Ganglionitis**
  - fifth nerve (*see also* Neuralgia, trigeminal) 350.1
  - gasserian 350.1
  - geniculate 351.1
    - herpetic 053.11
    - newborn 767.5
  - herpes zoster 053.11
  - herpetic geniculate (Hunt's syndrome) 053.11
- **Gangliosidosis** 330.1
- **Gangosa** 102.5
- **Gangrene, gangrenous** (anemia) (artery) (cellulitis) (dermatitis) (dry) (infective) (moist) (pemphigus) (septic) (skin) (stasis) (ulcer) 785.4
  - with
    - arteriosclerosis (native artery) 440.24
      - bypass graft 440.30
        - autologous vein 440.31
        - nonautologous biological 440.32
    - diabetes (mellitus) 250.7❺ *[785.4]*
  - abdomen (wall) 785.4
  - adenitis 683
  - alveolar 526.5
  - angina 462
    - diphtheritic 032.0
  - anus 569.49
  - appendices epiploicae – *see* Gangrene, mesentery
  - appendix – *see* Appendicitis, acute
  - arteriosclerotic – *see* Arteriosclerosis, with, gangrene
  - auricle 785.4
  - Bacillus welchii (*see also* Gangrene, gas) 040.0
  - bile duct (*see also* Cholangitis) 576.8
  - bladder 595.89
  - bowel – *see* Gangrene, intestine
  - cecum – *see* Gangrene, intestine
  - Clostridium perfringens or welchii (*see also* Gangrene, gas) 040.0
  - colon – *see* Gangrene, intestine
  - connective tissue 785.4
  - cornea 371.40
  - corpora cavernosa (infective) 607.2
    - noninfective 607.89
  - cutaneous, spreading 785.4
  - decubital (*see also* Decubitus) 707.00 *[785.4]*
  - diabetic (any site) 250.7❺ *[785.4]*
  - dropsical 785.4
  - emphysematous (*see also* Gangrene, gas) 040.0
  - epidemic (ergotized grain) 988.2
  - epididymis (infectional) (*see also* Epididymitis) 604.99
  - erysipelas (*see also* Erysipelas) 035
  - extremity (lower) (upper) 785.4
  - gallbladder or duct (*see also* Cholecystitis, acute) 575.0
  - gas (bacillus) 040.0
    - with
      - abortion – *see* Abortion, by type, with sepsis
      - ectopic pregnancy (*see also* categories 633.0-633.9) 639.0
      - molar pregnancy (*see also* categories 630-632) 639.0
    - following
      - abortion 639.0
      - ectopic or molar pregnancy 639.0
    - puerperal, postpartum, childbirth 670❹
  - glossitis 529.0
  - gum 523.8
  - hernia – *see* Hernia, by site, with gangrene
  - hospital noma 528.1
  - intestine, intestinal (acute) (hemorrhagic) (massive) 557.0
    - with
      - hernia – *see* Hernia, by site, with gangrene
      - mesenteric embolism or infarction 557.0
      - obstruction (*see also* Obstruction, intestine) 560.9
  - laryngitis 464.00
    - with obstruction 464.01
  - liver 573.8
  - lung 513.0
    - spirochetal 104.8
  - lymphangitis 457.2
  - Meleney's (cutaneous) 686.09
  - mesentery 557.0
    - with
      - embolism or infarction 557.0
      - intestinal obstruction (*see also* Obstruction, intestine) 560.9
  - mouth 528.1
  - noma 528.1
  - orchitis 604.90
  - ovary (*see also* Salpingo-oophoritis) 614.2
  - pancreas 577.0
  - penis (infectional) 607.2
    - noninfective 607.89
  - perineum 785.4
  - pharynx 462
    - septic 034.0
  - pneumonia 513.0
  - Pott's 440.24
  - presenile 443.1
  - pulmonary 513.0
  - pulp, tooth 522.1
  - quinsy 475
  - Raynaud's (symmetric gangrene) 443.0 *[785.4]*
  - rectum 569.49
  - retropharyngeal 478.24
  - rupture – *see* Hernia, by site, with gangrene
  - scrotum 608.4
    - noninfective 608.83
  - senile 440.24
  - sore throat 462
  - spermatic cord 608.4
    - noninfective 608.89
  - spine 785.4
  - spirochetal NEC 104.8
  - spreading cutaneous 785.4
  - stomach 537.89
  - stomatitis 528.1
  - symmetrical 443.0 *[785.4]*
  - testis (infectional) (*see also* Orchitis) 604.99
    - noninfective 608.89
  - throat 462
    - diphtheritic 032.0
  - thyroid (gland) 246.8
  - tonsillitis (acute) 463
  - tooth (pulp) 522.1
  - tuberculous NEC (*see also* Tuberculosis) 011.9❺
  - tunica vaginalis 608.4
    - noninfective 608.89
  - umbilicus 785.4
  - uterus (*see also* Endometritis) 615.9
  - uvulitis 528.3
  - vas deferens 608.4
    - noninfective 608.89
  - vulva (*see also* Vulvitis) 616.10
- **Gannister disease** (occupational) 502
  - with tuberculosis – *see* Tuberculosis, pulmonary
- **Ganser's syndrome, hysterical** 300.16
- **Gardner-Diamond syndrome** (autoerythrocyte sensitization) 287.2
- **Gargoylism** 277.5

Garré's
  disease (*see also* Osteomyelitis) 730.1❺
  osteitis (sclerosing) (*see also* Osteomyelitis) 730.1❺
  osteomyelitis (*see also* Osteomyelitis) 730.1❺
Garrod's pads, knuckle 728.79
Gartner's duct
  cyst 752.41
  persistent 752.41
Gas 787.3 ▲
  asphyxia, asphyxiation, inhalation, poisoning, suffocation NEC 987.9
    specified gas – *see* Table of Drugs and Chemicals
  bacillus gangrene or infection – *see* Gas, gangrene
  cyst, mesentery 568.89
  excessive 787.3
  gangrene 040.0
    with
      abortion – *see* Abortion, by type, with sepsis
      ectopic pregnancy (*see also* categories 633.0-633.9) 639.0
      molar pregnancy (*see also* categories 630-632) 639.0
    following
      abortion 639.0
      ectopic or molar pregnancy 639.0
    puerperal, postpartum, childbirth 670❹
  on stomach 787.3
  pains 787.3
Gastradenitis 535.0
Gastralgia 536.8
  psychogenic 307.89
Gastrectasis, gastrectasia 536.1
  psychogenic 306.4
Gastric – *see* condition
Gastrinoma (M8153/1)
  malignant (M8153/3)
    pancreas 157.4
    specified site NEC – *see* Neoplasm, by site, malignant
    unspecified site 157.4
  specified site – *see* Neoplasm, by site, uncertain behavior
  unspecified site 235.5
Gastritis 535.5❺

Note – Use the following fifth-digit subclassification for category 535:
0 without mention of hemorrhage
1 with hemorrhage

  acute 535.0❺
  alcoholic 535.3❺
  allergic 535.4❺
  antral 535.4❺
  atrophic 535.1❺
  atrophic-hyperplastic 535.1❺
  bile-induced 535.4❺
  catarrhal 535.0❺
  chronic (atrophic) 535.1❺
  cirrhotic 535.4❺
  corrosive (acute) 535.4❺
  dietetic 535.4❺
  due to diet deficiency 269.9 *[535.4]*
  eosinophilic 535.4❺
  erosive 535.4❺
  follicular 535.4❺
    chronic 535.1❺
  giant hypertrophic 535.2❺
  glandular 535.4❺
    chronic 535.1❺
  hypertrophic (mucosa) 535.2❺
    chronic giant 211.1
  irritant 535.4❺
  nervous 306.4
  phlegmonous 535.0❺
  psychogenic 306.4
  sclerotic 535.4❺
  spastic 536.8
  subacute 535.0❺
  superficial 535.4❺
  suppurative 535.0❺
  toxic 535.4❺
  tuberculous (*see also* Tuberculosis) 017.9❺
Gastrocarcinoma (M8010/3) 151.9
Gastrocolic – *see* condition
Gastrocolitis – *see* Enteritis
Gastrodisciasis 121.8
Gastroduodenitis (*see also* Gastritis) 535.5❺
  catarrhal 535.0❺
  infectional 535.0❺
  virus, viral 008.8
    specified type NEC 008.69
Gastrodynia 536.8
Gastroenteritis (acute) (catarrhal) (congestive) (hemorrhagic) (noninfectious) (*see also* Enteritis) 558.9
  aertrycke infection 003.0
  allergic 558.3
  chronic 558.9
    ulcerative (*see also* Colitis, ulcerative) 556.9
  dietetic 558.9
  due to
    food poisoning (*see also* Poisoning, food) 005.9
    radiation 558.1
  epidemic 009.0
  functional 558.9
  infectious (*see also* Enteritis, due to, by organism) 009.0
    presumed 009.1
  salmonella 003.0
  septic (*see also* Enteritis, due to, by organism) 009.0
  toxic 558.2
  tuberculous (*see also* Tuberculosis) 014.8❺
  ulcerative (*see also* Colitis, ulcerative) 556.9
  viral NEC 008.8
    specified type NEC 008.69
  zymotic 009.0
Gastroenterocolitis – *see* Enteritis
Gastroenteropathy, protein-losing 579.8
Gastroenteroptosis 569.89
Gastroesophageal laceration-hemorrhage syndrome 530.7
Gastroesophagitis 530.19
Gastrohepatitis (*see also* Gastritis) 535.5❺
Gastrointestinal – *see* condition
Gastrojejunal – *see* condition
Gastrojejunitis (*see also* Gastritis) 535.5❺
Gastrojejunocolic – *see* condition
Gastroliths 537.89
Gastromalacia 537.89
Gastroparalysis 536.3
  diabetic 250.6❺ *[536.3]*
Gastroparesis 536.3
  diabetic 250.6❺ *[536.3]*
Gastropathy 537.9
  congestive portal 537.89 ●
  erythematous 535.5
  exudative 579.8
  portal hypertensive 537.89 ●
Gastroptosis 537.5
Gastrorrhagia 578.0
Gastrorrhea 536.8
  psychogenic 306.4
Gastroschisis (congenital) 756.79
  acquired 569.89
Gastrospasm (neurogenic) (reflex) 536.8
  neurotic 306.4
  psychogenic 306.4
Gastrostaxis 578.0
Gastrostenosis 537.89
Gastrostomy
  attention to V55.1
  complication 536.40
    specified type 536.49
  infection 536.41
  malfunctioning 536.42
  status V44.1
Gastrosuccorrhea (continuous) (intermittent) 536.8
  neurotic 306.4
  psychogenic 306.4
Gaucher's
  disease (adult) (cerebroside lipidosis) (infantile) 272.7
  hepatomegaly 272.7
  splenomegaly (cerebroside lipidosis) 272.7
GAVE (gastric antral vascular ectasia) 537.82 ●
  with hemorrhage 537.83 ●
  without hemorrhage 537.82 ●
Gayet's disease (superior hemorrhagic polioencephalitis) 265.1
Gayet-Wernicke's syndrome (superior hemorrhagic polioencephalitis) 265.1
Gee (-Herter) (-Heubner) (-Thaysen) **disease or syndrome** (nontropical sprue) 579.0
Gélineau's syndrome (*see also* Narcolepsy) 347.00
Gemination, teeth 520.2
Gemistocytoma (M9411/3)
  specified site – *see* Neoplasm, by site, malignant
  unspecified site 191.9
General, generalized – *see* condition
Genetic
  susceptibility to
    MEN (multiple endocrine neoplasia) V84.81 ●
    neoplasia ●
      multiple endocrine [MEN] V84.81 ●
    neoplasm
      malignant, of
        breast V84.01
        endometrium V84.04
        other V84.09
        ovary V84.02
        prostate V84.03
    ▶specified◀ disease ▶NEC◀ V84.89 ▲
Genital – *see* condition
  warts 078.19
Genito-anorectal syndrome 099.1
Genitourinary system – *see* condition
Genu
  congenital 755.64
  extrorsum (acquired) 736.42
    congenital 755.64
    late effects of rickets 268.1
  introrsum (acquired) 736.41
    congenital 755.64
    late effects of rickets 268.1
  rachitic (old) 268.1
  recurvatum (acquired) 736.5
    congenital 754.40
      with dislocation of knee 754.41
    late effects of rickets 268.1
  valgum (acquired) (knock-knee) 736.41
    congenital 755.64
    late effects of rickets 268.1
  varum (acquired) (bowleg) 736.42
    congenital 755.64
    late effect of rickets 268.1
Geographic tongue 529.1
Geophagia 307.52
Geotrichosis 117.9
  intestine 117.9
  lung 117.9
  mouth 117.9
Gephyrophobia 300.29
Gerbode defect 745.4
Gerhardt's
  disease (erythromelalgia) 443.82
  syndrome (vocal cord paralysis) 478.30
Gerlier's disease (epidemic vertigo) 078.81
German measles 056.9
  exposure to V01.4
Germinoblastoma (diffuse) (M9614/3) 202.8❺
  follicular (M9692/3) 202.0❺
Germinoma (M9064/3) – *see* Neoplasm, by site, malignant
Gerontoxon 371.41
Gerstmann's syndrome (finger agnosia) 784.69
Gestation (period) – *see also* Pregnancy
  ectopic NEC (*see also* Pregnancy, ectopic) 633.90
    with intrauterine pregnancy 633.91
Gestational proteinuria 646.2❺
  with hypertension – *see* Toxemia, of pregnancy
Ghon tubercle primary infection (*see also* Tuberculosis) 010.0❺
Ghost
  teeth 520.4
  vessels, cornea 370.64
Ghoul hand 102.3
Gianotti Crosti syndrome 057.8
  due to known virus – *see* Infection, virus
  due to unknown virus 057.8
Giant
  cell
    epulis 523.8
    peripheral (gingiva) 523.8
    tumor, tendon sheath 727.02
  colon (congenital) 751.3
  esophagus (congenital) 750.4

- **Giant** – *continued*
  - kidney 753.3
  - urticaria 995.1
    - hereditary 277.6
- **Giardia lamblia infestation** 007.1
- **Giardiasis** 007.1
- **Gibert's disease** (pityriasis rosea) 696.3
- **Gibraltar fever** – *see* Brucellosis
- **Giddiness** 780.4
  - hysterical 300.11
  - psychogenic 306.9
- **Gierke's disease** (glycogenosis I) 271.0
- **Gigantism** (cerebral) (hypophyseal) (pituitary) 253.0
- **Gilbert's disease or cholemia** (familial nonhemolytic jaundice) 277.4
- **Gilchrist's disease** (North American blastomycosis) 116.0
- **Gilford** (-Hutchinson) **disease or syndrome** (progeria) 259.8
- **Gilles de la Tourette's disease** (motor-verbal tic) 307.23
- **Gillespie's syndrome** (dysplasia oculodentodigitalis) 759.89
- **Gingivitis** 523.10
  - acute 523.00
    - necrotizing 101
    - non-plaque induced 523.01
    - plaque induced 523.00
  - catarrhal 523.00
  - chronic 523.10
    - non-plaque induced 523.11
  - desquamative 523.10
  - expulsiva 523.40
  - hyperplastic 523.10
  - marginal, simple 523.10
  - necrotizing, acute 101
  - non-plaque induced 523.11
  - pellagrous 265.2
  - plaque induced 523.10
  - ulcerative 523.10
    - acute necrotizing 101
  - Vincent's 101
- **Gingivoglossitis** 529.0
- **Gingivopericementitis** 523.40
- **Gingivosis** 523.10
- **Gingivostomatitis** 523.10
  - herpetic 054.2
- **Giovannini's disease** 117.9
- **GISA** (glycopeptide intermediate staphylococcus aureus) V09.8
- **Gland, glandular** – *see* condition
- **Glanders** 024
- **Glanzmann** (-Naegeli) **disease or thrombasthenia** 287.1
- **Glassblowers' disease** 527.1
- **Glaucoma** (capsular) (inflammatory) (noninflammatory) (primary) 365.9
  - with increased episcleral venous pressure 365.82
  - absolute 360.42
  - acute 365.22
    - narrow angle 365.22
    - secondary 365.60
  - angle closure 365.20
    - acute 365.22
    - chronic 365.23
    - intermittent 365.21
    - interval 365.21
    - residual stage 365.24
    - subacute 365.21
  - borderline 365.00
  - chronic 365.11
    - noncongestive 365.11
    - open angle 365.11
    - simple 365.11
  - closed angle – *see* Glaucoma, angle closure
  - congenital 743.20
    - associated with other eye anomalies 743.22
    - simple 743.21
  - congestive – *see* Glaucoma, narrow angle
  - corticosteroid-induced (glaucomatous stage) 365.31
    - residual stage 365.32
  - hemorrhagic 365.60
  - hypersecretion 365.81
  - in or with
    - aniridia 743.45 *[365.42]*
- **Glaucoma** – *continued*
  - in or with – *continued*
    - Axenfeld's anomaly 743.44 *[365.41]*
    - concussion of globe 921.3 *[365.65]*
    - congenital syndromes NEC 759.89 *[365.44]*
    - dislocation of lens
      - anterior 379.33 *[365.59]*
      - posterior 379.34 *[365.59]*
    - disorder of lens NEC 365.59
    - epithelial down-growth 364.61 *[365.64]*
    - glaucomatocyclitic crisis 364.22 *[365.62]*
    - hypermature cataract 366.18 *[365.51]*
    - hyphema 364.41 *[365.63]*
    - inflammation, ocular 365.62
    - iridocyclitis 364.3 *[365.62]*
    - iris
      - anomalies NEC 743.46 *[365.42]*
      - atrophy, essential 364.51 *[365.42]*
      - bombé 364.74 *[365.61]*
      - rubeosis 364.42 *[365.63]*
    - microcornea 743.41 *[365.43]*
    - neurofibromatosis 237.71 *[365.44]*
    - ocular
      - cysts NEC 365.64
      - disorders NEC 365.60
      - trauma 365.65
      - tumors NEC 365.64
    - postdislocation of lens
      - anterior 379.33 *[365.59]*
      - posterior 379.34 *[365.59]*
    - pseudoexfoliation of capsule 366.11 *[365.52]*
    - pupillary block or seclusion 364.74 *[365.61]*
    - recession of chamber angle 364.77 *[365.65]*
    - retinal vein occlusion 362.35 *[365.63]*
    - Rieger's anomaly or syndrome 743.44 *[365.41]*
    - rubeosis of iris 364.42 *[365.63]*
    - seclusion of pupil 364.74 *[365.61]*
    - spherophakia 743.36 *[365.59]*
    - Sturge-Weber (-Dimitri) syndrome 759.6 *[365.44]*
    - systemic syndrome NEC 365.44
    - tumor of globe 365.64
    - vascular disorders NEC 365.63
  - infantile 365.14
    - congenital 743.20
      - associated with other eye anomalies 743.22
      - simple 743.21
  - juvenile 365.14
  - low tension 365.12
  - malignant 365.83
  - narrow angle (primary) 365.20
    - acute 365.22
    - chronic 365.23
    - intermittent 365.21
    - interval 365.21
    - residual stage 365.24
    - subacute 365.21
  - newborn 743.20
    - associated with other eye anomalies 743.22
    - simple 743.21
  - noncongestive (chronic) 365.11
  - nonobstructive (chronic) 365.11
  - obstructive 365.60
    - due to lens changes 365.59
  - open angle 365.10
    - with
      - borderline intraocular pressure 365.01
      - cupping of optic discs 365.01
    - primary 365.11
    - residual stage 365.15
  - phacolytic 365.51
    - with hypermature cataract 366.18 *[365.51]*
  - pigmentary 365.13
  - postinfectious 365.60
  - pseudoexfoliation 365.52
    - with pseudoexfoliation of capsule 366.11 *[365.52]*
  - secondary NEC 365.60
  - simple (chronic) 365.11
  - simplex 365.11
  - steroid responders 365.03
  - suspect 365.00
  - syphilitic 095.8
  - traumatic NEC 365.65
    - newborn 767.8
  - tuberculous (*see also* Tuberculosis) 017.3❺ *[365.62]*
  - wide angle (*see also* Glaucoma, open angle) 365.10
- **Glaucomatous flecks** (subcapsular) 366.31
- **Glazed tongue** 529.4
- **Gleet** 098.2
- **Glénard's disease or syndrome** (enteroptosis) 569.89
- **Glinski-Simmonds syndrome** (pituitary cachexia) 253.2
- **Glioblastoma** (multiforme) (M9440/3)
  - with sarcomatous component (M9442/3)
    - specified site – *see* Neoplasm, by site, malignant
    - unspecified site 191.9
  - giant cell (M9441/3)
    - specified site – *see* Neoplasm, by site, malignant
    - unspecified site 191.9
  - specified site – *see* Neoplasm, by site, malignant
  - unspecified site 191.9
- **Glioma** (malignant) (M9380/3)
  - astrocytic (M9400/3)
    - specified site – *see* Neoplasm, by site, malignant
    - unspecified site 191.9
  - mixed (M9382/3)
    - specified site – *see* Neoplasm, by site, malignant
    - unspecified site 191.9
  - nose 748.1
  - specified site NEC – *see* Neoplasm, by site, malignant
  - subependymal (M9383/1) 237.5
  - unspecified site 191.9
- **Gliomatosis cerebri** (M9381/3) 191.0
- **Glioneuroma** (M9505/1) – *see* Neoplasm, by site, uncertain behavior
- **Gliosarcoma** (M9380/3)
  - specified site – *see* Neoplasm, by site, malignant
  - unspecified site 191.9
- **Gliosis** (cerebral) 349.89
  - spinal 336.0
- **Glisson's**
  - cirrhosis – *see* Cirrhosis, portal
  - disease (*see also* Rickets) 268.0
- **Glissonitis** 573.3
- **Globinuria** 791.2
- **Globus** 306.4
  - hystericus 300.11
- **Glomangioma** (M8712/0) (*see also* Hemangioma) 228.00
- **Glomangiosarcoma** (M8710/3) – *see* Neoplasm, connective tissue, malignant
- **Glomerular nephritis** (*see also* Nephritis) 583.9
- **Glomerulitis** (*see also* Nephritis) 583.9
- **Glomerulonephritis** (*see also* Nephritis) 583.9
  - with
    - edema (*see also* Nephrosis) 581.9
    - lesion of
      - exudative nephritis 583.89
      - interstitial nephritis (diffuse) (focal) 583.89
      - necrotizing glomerulitis 583.4
        - acute 580.4
        - chronic 582.4
      - renal necrosis 583.9
        - cortical 583.6
        - medullary 583.7
      - specified pathology NEC 583.89
        - acute 580.89
        - chronic 582.89
    - necrosis, renal 583.9
      - cortical 583.6
      - medullary (papillary) 583.7
    - specified pathology or lesion NEC 583.89
  - acute 580.9
    - with
      - exudative nephritis 580.89
      - interstitial nephritis (diffuse) (focal) 580.89
      - necrotizing glomerulitis 580.4
    - extracapillary with epithelial crescents 580.4
    - poststreptococcal 580.0
    - proliferative (diffuse) 580.0
    - rapidly progressive 580.4
    - specified pathology NEC 580.89
  - arteriolar (*see also* Hypertension, kidney) 403.90
  - arteriosclerotic (*see also* Hypertension, kidney) 403.90
  - ascending (*see also* Pyelitis) 590.80
  - basement membrane NEC 583.89
    - with
      - pulmonary hemorrhage (Goodpasture's syndrome) 446.21 *[583.81]*

Glomerulonephritis – *continued*
- chronic 582.9
  - with
    - exudative nephritis 582.89
    - interstitial nephritis (diffuse) (focal) 582.89
    - necrotizing glomerulitis 582.4
    - specified pathology or lesion NEC 582.89
- chronic
  - endothelial 582.2
  - extracapillary with epithelial crescents 582.4
  - hypocomplementemic persistent 582.2
  - lobular 582.2
  - membranoproliferative 582.2
  - membranous 582.1
    - and proliferative (mixed) 582.2
    - sclerosing 582.1
  - mesangiocapillary 582.2
  - mixed membranous and proliferative 582.2
  - proliferative (diffuse) 582.0
  - rapidly progressive 582.4
  - sclerosing 582.1
- cirrhotic – *see* Sclerosis, renal
- desquamative – *see* Nephrosis
- due to or associated with
  - amyloidosis 277.39 *[583.81]*
    - with nephrotic syndrome 277.39 *[581.81]*
    - chronic 277.39 *[582.81]*
  - diabetes mellitus 250.4❺ *[583.81]*
    - with nephrotic syndrome 250.4❺ *[581.81]*
  - diphtheria 032.89 *[580.81]*
  - gonococcal infection (acute) 098.19 *[583.81]*
    - chronic or duration of 2 months or over 098.39 *[583.81]*
  - infectious hepatitis 070.9 *[580.81]*
  - malaria (with nephrotic syndrome) 084.9 *[581.81]*
  - mumps 072.79 *[580.81]*
  - polyarteritis (nodosa) (with nephrotic syndrome) 446.0 *[581.81]*
  - specified pathology NEC 583.89
    - acute 580.89
    - chronic 582.89
  - streptotrichosis 039.8 *[583.81]*
  - subacute bacterial endocarditis 421.0 *[580.81]*
  - syphilis (late) 095.4
    - congenital 090.5 *[583.81]*
    - early 091.69 *[583.81]*
  - systemic lupus erythematosus 710.0 *[583.81]*
    - with nephrotic syndrome 710.0 *[581.81]*
    - chronic 710.0 *[582.81]*
  - tuberculosis (*see also* Tuberculosis) 016.0❺ *[583.81]*
  - typhoid fever 002.0 *[580.81]*
- extracapillary with epithelial crescents 583.4
  - acute 580.4
  - chronic 582.4
- exudative 583.89
  - acute 580.89
  - chronic 582.89
- focal (*see also* Nephritis) 583.9
  - embolic 580.4
- granular 582.89
- granulomatous 582.89
- hydremic (*see also* Nephrosis) 581.9
- hypocomplementemic persistent 583.2
  - with nephrotic syndrome 581.2
  - chronic 582.2
- immune complex NEC 583.89
- infective (*see also* Pyelitis) 590.80
- interstitial (diffuse) (focal) 583.89
  - with nephrotic syndrome 581.89
  - acute 580.89
  - chronic 582.89
- latent or quiescent 582.9
- lobular 583.2
  - with nephrotic syndrome 581.2
  - chronic 582.2
- membranoproliferative 583.2
  - with nephrotic syndrome 581.2
  - chronic 582.2
- membranous 583.1
  - with nephrotic syndrome 581.1
  - and proliferative (mixed) 583.2
    - with nephrotic syndrome 581.2
    - chronic 582.2
  - chronic 582.1
  - sclerosing 582.1
    - with nephrotic syndrome 581.1
- mesangiocapillary 583.2
  - with nephrotic syndrome 581.2
  - chronic 582.2
- minimal change 581.3

Glomerulonephritis – *continued*
- mixed membranous and proliferative 583.2
  - with nephrotic syndrome 581.2
  - chronic 582.2
- necrotizing 583.4
  - acute 580.4
  - chronic 582.4
- nephrotic (*see also* Nephrosis) 581.9
- old – *see* Glomerulonephritis, chronic
- parenchymatous 581.89
- poststreptococcal 580.0
- proliferative (diffuse) 583.0
  - with nephrotic syndrome 581.0
  - acute 580.0
  - chronic 582.0
- purulent (*see also* Pyelitis) 590.80
- quiescent – *see* Nephritis, chronic
- rapidly progressive 583.4
  - acute 580.4
  - chronic 582.4
- sclerosing membranous (chronic) 582.1
  - with nephrotic syndrome 581.1
- septic (*see also* Pyelitis) 590.80
- specified pathology or lesion NEC 583.89
  - with nephrotic syndrome 581.89
  - acute 580.89
  - chronic 582.89
- suppurative (acute) (disseminated) (*see also* Pyelitis) 590.80
- toxic – *see* Nephritis, acute
- tubal, tubular – *see* Nephrosis, tubular
- type II (Ellis) – *see* Nephrosis
- vascular – *see* Hypertension, kidney

Glomerulosclerosis (*see also* Sclerosis, renal) 587
- focal 582.1
  - with nephrotic syndrome 581.1
- intercapillary (nodular) (with diabetes) 250.4❺ *[581.81]*

Glossagra 529.6

Glossalgia 529.6

Glossitis 529.0
- areata exfoliativa 529.1
- atrophic 529.4
- benign migratory 529.1
- gangrenous 529.0
- Hunter's 529.4
- median rhomboid 529.2
- Moeller's 529.4
- pellagrous 265.2

Glossocele 529.8

Glossodynia 529.6
- exfoliativa 529.4

Glossoncus 529.8

Glossophytia 529.3

Glossoplegia 529.8

Glossoptosis 529.8

Glossopyrosis 529.6

Glossotrichia 529.3

Glossy skin 701.9

Glottis – *see* condition

Glottitis – *see* Glossitis

Glucagonoma (M8152/0)
- malignant (M8152/3)
  - pancreas 157.4
  - specified site NEC – *see* Neoplasm, by site, malignant
  - unspecified site 157.4
- pancreas 211.7
- specified site NEC – *see* Neoplasm, by site, benign
- unspecified site 211.7

Glucoglycinuria 270.7

Glue ear syndrome 381.20

Glue sniffing (airplane glue) (*see also* Dependence) 304.6❺

Glycinemia (with methylmalonic acidemia) 270.7

Glycinuria (renal) (with ketosis) 270.0

Glycogen
- infiltration (*see also* Disease, glycogen storage) 271.0
- storage disease (*see also* Disease, glycogen storage) 271.0

Glycogenosis (*see also* Disease, glycogen storage) 271.0
- cardiac 271.0 *[425.7]*
- Cori, types I-VII 271.0
- diabetic, secondary 250.8❺ *[259.8]*
- diffuse (with hepatic cirrhosis) 271.0

Glycogenosis – *continued*
- generalized 271.0
- glucose-6-phosphatase deficiency 271.0
- hepatophosphorylase deficiency 271.0
- hepatorenal 271.0
- myophosphorylase deficiency 271.0

Glycopenia 251.2

Glycopeptide
- intermediate staphylococcus aureus (GISA) V09.8
- resistant
  - enterococcus V09.8
  - staphylococcus aureus (GRSA) V09.8

Glycoprolinuria 270.8

Glycosuria 791.5
- renal 271.4

Gnathostoma (spinigerum) (infection) (infestation) 128.1
- wandering swellings from 128.1

Gnathostomiasis 128.1

Goiter (adolescent) (colloid) (diffuse) (dipping) (due to iodine deficiency) (endemic) (euthyroid) (heart) (hyperplastic) (internal) (intrathoracic) (juvenile) (mixed type) (nonendemic) (parenchymatous) (plunging) (sporadic) (subclavicular) (substernal) 240.9
- with
  - hyperthyroidism (recurrent) (*see also* Goiter, toxic) 242.0❺
  - thyrotoxicosis (*see also* Goiter, toxic) 242.0❺
- adenomatous (*see also* Goiter, nodular) 241.9
- cancerous (M8000/3) 193
- complicating pregnancy, childbirth, or puerperium 648.1❺
- congenital 246.1
- cystic (*see also* Goiter, nodular) 241.9
- due to enzyme defect in synthesis of thyroid hormone (butane-insoluble iodine) (coupling) (deiodinase) (iodide trapping or organification) (iodotyrosine dehalogenase) (peroxidase) 246.1
- dyshormonogenic 246.1
- exophthalmic (*see also* Goiter, toxic) 242.0❺
- familial (with deaf-mutism) 243
- fibrous 245.3
- lingual 759.2
- lymphadenoid 245.2
- malignant (M8000/3) 193
- multinodular (nontoxic) 241.1
  - toxic or with hyperthyroidism (*see also* Goiter, toxic) 242.2❺
- nodular (nontoxic) 241.9
  - with
    - hyperthyroidism (*see also* Goiter, toxic) 242.3❺
    - thyrotoxicosis (*see also* Goiter, toxic) 242.3❺
  - endemic 241.9
  - exophthalmic (diffuse) (*see also* Goiter, toxic) 242.0❺
  - multinodular (nontoxic) 241.1
  - sporadic 241.9
  - toxic (*see also* Goiter, toxic) 242.3❺
  - uninodular (nontoxic) 241.0
- nontoxic (nodular) 241.9
  - multinodular 241.1
  - uninodular 241.0
- pulsating (*see also* Goiter, toxic) 242.0❺
- simple 240.0
- toxic 242.0❺

  Note – Use the following fifth-digit subclassification with category 242:
  0 without mention of thyrotoxic crisis or storm
  1 with mention of thyrotoxic crisis or storm

  - adenomatous 242.3❺
    - multinodular 242.2❺
    - uninodular 242.1❺
  - multinodular 242.2❺
  - nodular 242.3❺
    - multinodular 242.2❺
    - uninodular 242.1❺
  - uninodular 242.1❺
- uninodular (nontoxic) 241.0
  - toxic or with hyperthyroidism (*see also* Goiter, toxic) 242.1❺

Goldberg (-Maxwell) (-Morris) **syndrome** (testicular feminization) 259.5

Glomerulonephritis – Goldberg syndrome

- **Goldblatt's**
  - hypertension 440.1
  - kidney 440.1
- **Goldenhar's syndrome** (oculoauriculovertebral dysplasia) 756.0
- **Goldflam-Erb disease or syndrome** 358.00
- **Goldscheider's disease** (epidermolysis bullosa) 757.39
- **Goldstein's disease** (familial hemorrhagic telangiectasia) 448.0
- **Golfer's elbow** 726.32
- **Goltz-Gorlin syndrome** (dermal hypoplasia) 757.39
- **Gonadoblastoma** (M9073/1)
  - specified site – *see* Neoplasm, by site uncertain behavior
  - unspecified site
    - female 236.2
    - male 236.4
- **Gonecystitis** (*see also* Vesiculitis) 608.0
- **Gongylonemiasis** 125.6
  - mouth 125.6
- **Goniosynechiae** 364.73
- **Gonococcemia** 098.89
- **Gonococcus, gonococcal** (disease) (infection) (*see also* condition) 098.0
  - anus 098.7
  - bursa 098.52
  - chronic NEC 098.2
  - complicating pregnancy, childbirth, or puerperium 647.1❺
    - affecting fetus or newborn 760.2
  - conjunctiva, conjunctivitis (neonatorum) 098.40
  - dermatosis 098.89
  - endocardium 098.84
  - epididymo-orchitis 098.13
    - chronic or duration of 2 months or over 098.33
  - eye (newborn) 098.40
  - fallopian tube (chronic) 098.37
    - acute 098.17
  - genitourinary (acute) (organ) (system) (tract) (*see also* Gonorrhea) 098.0
    - lower 098.0
      - chronic 098.2
    - upper 098.10
      - chronic 098.30
  - heart NEC 098.85
  - joint 098.50
  - keratoderma 098.81
  - keratosis (blennorrhagica) 098.81
  - lymphatic (gland) (node) 098.89
  - meninges 098.82
  - orchitis (acute) 098.13
    - chronic or duration of 2 months or over 098.33
  - pelvis (acute) 098.19
    - chronic or duration of 2 months or over 098.39
  - pericarditis 098.83
  - peritonitis 098.86
  - pharyngitis 098.6
  - pharynx 098.6
  - proctitis 098.7
  - pyosalpinx (chronic) 098.37
    - acute 098.17
  - rectum 098.7
  - septicemia 098.89
  - skin 098.89
  - specified site NEC 098.89
  - synovitis 098.51
  - tendon sheath 098.51
  - throat 098.6
  - urethra (acute) 098.0
    - chronic or duration of 2 months or over 098.2
  - vulva (acute) 098.0
    - chronic or duration of 2 months or over 098.2
- **Gonocytoma** (M9073/1)
  - specified site – *see* Neoplasm, by site, uncertain behavior
  - unspecified site
    - female 236.2
    - male 236.4
- **Gonorrhea** 098.0
  - acute 098.0
  - Bartholin's gland (acute) 098.0
    - chronic or duration of 2 months or over 098.2
  - bladder (acute) 098.11
    - chronic or duration of 2 months or over 098.31
  - carrier (suspected of) V02.7
  - cervix (acute) 098.15
    - chronic or duration of 2 months or over 098.35
  - chronic 098.2

Gonorrhea – *continued*

  - complicating pregnancy, childbirth, or puerperium 647.1❺
    - affecting fetus or newborn 760.2
  - conjunctiva, conjunctivitis (neonatorum) 098.40
  - contact V01.6
  - Cowper's gland (acute) 098.0
    - chronic or duration of 2 months or over 098.2
  - duration of 2 months or over 098.2
  - exposure to V01.6
  - fallopian tube (chronic) 098.37
    - acute 098.17
  - genitourinary (acute) (organ) (system) (tract) 098.0
    - chronic 098.2
    - duration of 2 months or over 098.2
  - kidney (acute) 098.19
    - chronic or duration of 2 months or over 098.39
  - ovary (acute) 098.19
    - chronic or duration of 2 months or over 098.39
  - pelvis (acute) 098.19
    - chronic or duration of 2 months or over 098.39
  - penis (acute) 098.0
    - chronic or duration of 2 months or over 098.2
  - prostate (acute) 098.12
    - chronic or duration of 2 months or over 098.32
  - seminal vesicle (acute) 098.14
    - chronic or duration of 2 months or over 098.34
  - specified site NEC – *see* Gonococcus
  - spermatic cord (acute) 098.14
    - chronic or duration of 2 months or over 098.34
  - urethra (acute) 098.0
    - chronic or duration of 2 months or over 098.2
  - vagina (acute) 098.0
    - chronic or duration of 2 months or over 098.2
  - vas deferens (acute) 098.14
    - chronic or duration of 2 months or over 098.34
  - vulva (acute) 098.0
    - chronic or duration of 2 months or over 098.2
- **Good's syndrome** 279.06
- **Goodpasture's syndrome** (pneumorenal) 446.21
- **Gopalan's syndrome** (burning feet) 266.2
- **Gordon's disease** (exudative enteropathy) 579.8
- **Gorlin-Chaudhry-Moss syndrome** 759.89
- **Gougerot's syndrome** (trisymptomatic) 709.1
- **Gougerot-Blum syndrome** (pigmented purpuric lichenoid dermatitis) 709.1
- **Gougerot-Carteaud disease or syndrome** (confluent reticulate papillomatosis) 701.8
- **Gougerot-Hailey-Hailey disease** (benign familial chronic pemphigus) 757.39
- **Gougerot** (-Houwer)-**Sjögren syndrome** (keratoconjunctivitis sicca) 710.2
- **Gouley's syndrome** (constrictive pericarditis) 423.2
- **Goundou** 102.6
- **Gout, gouty** 274.9
  - with specified manifestations NEC 274.89
  - arthritis (acute) 274.0
  - arthropathy 274.0
  - degeneration, heart 274.82
  - diathesis 274.9
  - eczema 274.89
  - episcleritis 274.89 *[379.09]*
  - external ear (tophus) 274.81
  - glomerulonephritis 274.10
  - iritis 274.89 *[364.11]*
  - joint 274.0
  - kidney 274.10
  - lead 984.9
    - specified type of lead – *see* Table of Drugs and Chemicals
  - nephritis 274.10
  - neuritis 274.89 *[357.4]*
  - phlebitis 274.89 *[451.9]*
  - rheumatic 714.0
  - saturnine 984.9
    - specified type of lead – *see* Table of Drugs and Chemicals
  - spondylitis 274.0
  - synovitis 274.0
  - syphilitic 095.8
  - tophi 274.0
    - ear 274.81
    - heart 274.82
    - specified site NEC 274.82
- **Gowers'**
  - muscular dystrophy 359.1
  - syndrome (vasovagal attack) 780.2
- **Gowers-Paton-Kennedy syndrome** 377.04
- **Gradenigo's syndrome** 383.02
- **Graft-versus-host disease** (bone marrow) 996.85
  - due to organ transplant NEC – *see* Complications, transplant, organ
- **Graham Steell's murmur** (pulmonic regurgitation) (*see also* Endocarditis, pulmonary) 424.3
- **Grain-handlers' disease or lung** 495.8
- **Grain mite** (itch) 133.8
- **Grand**
  - mal (idiopathic) (*see also* Epilepsy) 345.1❺
    - hysteria of Charcôt 300.11
    - nonrecurrent or isolated 780.39
  - multipara
    - affecting management of labor and delivery 659.4❺
    - status only (not pregnant) V61.5
- **Granite workers' lung** 502
- **Granular** – *see also* condition
  - inflammation, pharynx 472.1
  - kidney (contracting) (*see also* Sclerosis, renal) 587
  - liver – *see* Cirrhosis, liver
  - nephritis – *see* Nephritis
- **Granulation tissue, abnormal** – *see also* Granuloma
  - abnormal or excessive 701.5
  - postmastoidectomy cavity 383.33
  - postoperative 701.5
  - skin 701.5
- **Granulocytopenia, granulocytopenic** (primary) 288.00
  - malignant 288.09
- **Granuloma** NEC 686.1
  - abdomen (wall) 568.89
    - skin (pyogenicum) 686.1
      - from residual foreign body 709.4
  - annulare 695.89
  - anus 569.49
  - apical 522.6
  - appendix 543.9
  - aural 380.23
  - beryllium (skin) 709.4
    - lung 503
  - bone (*see also* Osteomyelitis) 730.1❺
    - eosinophilic 277.89
    - from residual foreign body 733.99
  - canaliculus lacrimalis 375.81
  - cerebral 348.8
  - cholesterin, middle ear 385.82
  - coccidioidal (progressive) 114.3
    - lung 114.4
    - meninges 114.2
    - primary (lung) 114.0
  - colon 569.89
  - conjunctiva 372.61
  - dental 522.6
  - ear, middle (cholesterin) 385.82
    - with otitis media – *see* Otitis media
  - eosinophilic 277.89
    - bone 277.89
    - lung 277.89
    - oral mucosa 528.9
  - exuberant 701.5
  - eyelid 374.89
  - facial
    - lethal midline 446.3
    - malignant 446.3
  - faciale 701.8
  - fissuratum (gum) 523.8
  - foot NEC 686.1
  - foreign body (in soft tissue) NEC 728.82
    - bone 733.99
    - in operative wound 998.4
    - muscle 728.82
    - skin 709.4
    - subcutaneous tissue 709.4
  - fungoides 202.1❺
  - gangraenescens 446.3
  - giant cell (central) (jaw) (reparative) 526.3
    - gingiva 523.8
    - peripheral (gingiva) 523.8
  - gland (lymph) 289.3
  - Hodgkin's (M9661/3) 201.1❺
  - ileum 569.89
  - infectious NEC 136.9
  - inguinale (Donovan) 099.2
    - venereal 099.2
  - intestine 569.89
  - iridocyclitis 364.10
  - jaw (bone) 526.3
    - reparative giant cell 526.3

Goldblatt's – Granuloma

Granuloma – *continued*
  kidney (*see also* Infection, kidney) 590.9
  lacrimal sac 375.81
  larynx 478.79
  lethal midline 446.3
  lipid 277.89
  lipoid 277.89
  liver 572.8
  lung (infectious) (*see also* Fibrosis, lung) 515
    coccidioidal 114.4
    eosinophilic 277.89
  lymph gland 289.3
  Majocchi's 110.6
  malignant, face 446.3
  mandible 526.3
  mediastinum 519.3
  midline 446.3
  monilial 112.3
  muscle 728.82
    from residual foreign body 728.82
  nasal sinus (*see also* Sinusitis) 473.9
  operation wound 998.59
    foreign body 998.4
    stitch (external) 998.89
      internal wound 998.89
    talc 998.7
  oral mucosa, eosinophilic or pyogenic 528.9
  orbit, orbital 376.11
  paracoccidioidal 116.1
  penis, venereal 099.2
  periapical 522.6
  peritoneum 568.89
    due to ova of helminths NEC (*see also* Helminthiasis) 128.9
  postmastoidectomy cavity 383.33
  postoperative – *see* Granuloma, operation wound
  prostate 601.8
  pudendi (ulcerating) 099.2
  pudendorum (ulcerative) 099.2
  pulp, internal (tooth) 521.49
  pyogenic, pyogenicum (skin) 686.1
    maxillary alveolar ridge 522.6
    oral mucosa 528.9
  rectum 569.49
  reticulohistiocytic 277.89
  rubrum nasi 705.89
  sarcoid 135
  Schistosoma 120.9
  septic (skin) 686.1
  silica (skin) 709.4
  sinus (accessory) (infectional) (nasal) (*see also* Sinusitis) 473.9
  skin (pyogenicum) 686.1
    from foreign body or material 709.4
  sperm 608.89
  spine
    syphilitic (epidural) 094.89
    tuberculous (*see also* Tuberculosis) 015.0❺ *[730.88]*
  stitch (postoperative) 998.89
    internal wound 998.89
  suppurative (skin) 686.1
  suture (postoperative) 998.89
    internal wound 998.89
  swimming pool 031.1
  tracheostomy 519.09
  talc 728.82
    in operation wound 998.7
  telangiectaticum (skin) 686.1
  trichophyticum 110.6
  tropicum 102.4
  umbilicus 686.1
    newborn 771.4
  urethra 599.84
  uveitis 364.10
  vagina 099.2
  venereum 099.2
  vocal cords 478.5
  Wegener's (necrotizing respiratory granulomatosis) 446.4
Granulomatosis NEC 686.1
  disciformis chronica et progressiva 709.3
  infantiseptica 771.2
  lipoid 277.89
  lipophagic, intestinal 040.2
  miliary 027.0
  necrotizing, respiratory 446.4
  progressive, septic 288.1
  Wegener's (necrotizing respiratory) 446.4
Granulomatous tissue – *see* Granuloma
Granulosis rubra nasi 705.89
Graphite fibrosis (of lung) 503
Graphospasm 300.89
  organic 333.84
Grating scapula 733.99
Gravel (urinary) (*see also* Calculus) 592.9
Graves' disease (exophthalmic goiter) (*see also* Goiter, toxic) 242.0❺
Gravis – *see* condition
Grawitz's tumor (hypernephroma) (M8312/3) 189.0
Grayness, hair (premature) 704.3
  congenital 757.4
Gray or grey syndrome (chloramphenicol) (newborn) 779.4
Greenfield's disease 330.0
Green sickness 280.9
Greenstick fracture – *see* Fracture, by site
Grief 309.0 ●
Greig's syndrome (hypertelorism) 756.0
Griesinger's disease (*see also* Ancylostomiasis) 126.9
Grinders'
  asthma 502
  lung 502
  phthisis (*see also* Tuberculosis) 011.4❺
Grinding, teeth 306.8
Grip
  Dabney's 074.1
  devil's 074.1
Grippe, grippal – *see also* Influenza
  Balkan 083.0
  intestinal 487.8
  summer 074.8
Grippy cold 487.1
Grisel's disease 723.5
Groin – *see* condition
Grooved
  nails (transverse) 703.8
  tongue 529.5
    congenital 750.13
Ground itch 126.9
Growing pains, children 781.99
Growth (fungoid) (neoplastic) (new) (M8000/1) – *see also* Neoplasm, by site, unspecified nature
  adenoid (vegetative) 474.12
    benign (M8000/0) – *see* Neoplasm, by site, benign
  fetal, poor 764.9❺
    affecting management of pregnancy 656.5❺
  malignant (M8000/3) – *see* Neoplasm, by site, malignant
  rapid, childhood V21.0
  secondary (M8000/6) – *see* Neoplasm, by site, malignant, secondary
GRSA (glycopeptide resistant staphylococcus aureus) V09.8
Gruber's hernia – *see* Hernia, Gruber's
Gruby's disease (tinea tonsurans) 110.0
G-trisomy 758.0
Guama fever 066.3
Gubler (-Millard) **paralysis or syndrome** 344.89
Guérin-Stern syndrome (arthrogryposis multiplex congenita) 754.89
Guertin's disease (electric chorea) 049.8
Guillain-Barré disease or syndrome 357.0
Guinea worms (infection) (infestation) 125.7
Guinon's disease (motor-verbal tic) 307.23
Gull's disease (thyroid atrophy with myxedema) 244.8
Gull and Sutton's disease – *see* Hypertension, kidney
Gum – *see* condition
Gumboil 522.7
Gumma (syphilitic) 095.9
  artery 093.89
    cerebral or spinal 094.89
  bone 095.5
    of yaws (late) 102.6
  brain 094.89
  cauda equina 094.89
  central nervous system NEC 094.9
  ciliary body 095.8 *[364.11]*
  congenital 090.5
    testis 090.5
  eyelid 095.8 *[373.5]*
  heart 093.89
  intracranial 094.89
Gumma – *continued*
  iris 095.8 *[364.11]*
  kidney 095.4
  larynx 095.8
  leptomeninges 094.2
  liver 095.3
  meninges 094.2
  myocardium 093.82
  nasopharynx 095.8
  neurosyphilitic 094.9
  nose 095.8
  orbit 095.8
  palate (soft) 095.8
  penis 095.8
  pericardium 093.81
  pharynx 095.8
  pituitary 095.8
  scrofulous (*see also* Tuberculosis) 017.0❺
  skin 095.8
  specified site NEC 095.8
  spinal cord 094.89
  tongue 095.8
  tonsil 095.8
  trachea 095.8
  tuberculous (*see also* Tuberculosis) 017.0❺
  ulcerative due to yaws 102.4
  ureter 095.8
  yaws 102.4
    bone 102.6
Gunn's syndrome (jaw-winking syndrome) 742.8
Gunshot wound – *see also* Wound, open, by site
  fracture – *see* Fracture, by site, open
  internal organs (abdomen, chest, or pelvis) – *see* Injury, internal, by site, with open wound
  intracranial – *see* Laceration, brain, with open intracranial wound
Günther's disease or syndrome (congenital erythropoietic porphyria) 277.1
Gustatory hallucination 780.1
Gynandrism 752.7
Gynandroblastoma (M8632/1)
  specified site – *see* Neoplasm, by site, uncertain behavior
  unspecified site
    female 236.2
    male 236.4
Gynandromorphism 752.7
Gynatresia (congenital) 752.49
Gynecoid pelvis, male 738.6
Gynecological examination V72.31
  for contraceptive maintenance V25.40
Gynecomastia 611.1
Gynephobia 300.29
Gyrate scalp 757.39

H

Haas' disease (osteochondrosis head of humerus) 732.3
Habermann's disease (acute parapsoriasis varioliformis) 696.2
Habit, habituation
  chorea 307.22
    disturbance, child 307.9
  drug (*see also* Dependence) 304.9❺
  laxative (*see also* Abuse, drugs, nondependent) 305.9❺
  spasm 307.20
    chronic 307.22
    transient (of childhood) 307.21
  tic 307.20
    chronic 307.22
    transient (of childhood) 307.21
  use of
    nonprescribed drugs (*see also* Abuse, drugs, nondependent) 305.9❺
    patent medicines (*see also* Abuse, drugs, nondependent) 305.9❺
  vomiting 536.2
Hadfield-Clarke syndrome (pancreatic infantilism) 577.8
Haff disease 985.1
Hageman factor defect, deficiency, or disease (*see also* Defect, coagulation) 286.3

Granuloma – Hageman factor defect, deficiency, or disease

Haglund's disease (osteochondrosis os tibiale externum) 732.5
Haglund-Läwen-Fründ syndrome 717.89
Hagner's disease (hypertrophic pulmonary osteoarthropathy) 731.2
Hag teeth, tooth 524.39
Hailey-Hailey disease (benign familial chronic pemphigus) 757.39
Hair – *see also* condition
  plucking 307.9
Hairball in stomach 935.2
Hairy black tongue 529.3
Half vertebra 756.14
Halitosis 784.99
Hallermann-Streiff syndrome 756.0
Hallervorden-Spatz disease or syndrome 333.0
Hallopeau's
  acrodermatitis (continua) 696.1
  disease (lichen sclerosis et atrophicus) 701.0
Hallucination (auditory) (gustatory) (olfactory) (tactile) 780.1
  alcohol-induced 291.3
  drug-induced 292.12
  visual 368.16
Hallucinosis 298.9
  alcohol induced (acute) 291.3
  drug-induced 292.12
Hallus – *see* Hallux
Hallux 735.9
  limitus 735.8 ●
  malleus (acquired) 735.3
  rigidus (acquired) 735.2
    congenital 755.66
    late effects of rickets 268.1
  valgus (acquired) 735.0
    congenital 755.66
  varus (acquired) 735.1
    congenital 755.66
Halo, visual 368.15
Hamartoblastoma 759.6
Hamartoma 759.6
  epithelial (gingival), odontogenic, central, or peripheral (M9321/0) 213.1
    upper jaw (bone) 213.0
  vascular 757.32
Hamartosis, hamartoses NEC 759.6
Hamman's disease or syndrome (spontaneous mediastinal emphysema) 518.1
Hamman-Rich syndrome (diffuse interstitial pulmonary fibrosis) 516.3
Hammer toe (acquired) 735.4
  congenital 755.66
  late effects of rickets 268.1
Hand – *see* condition
Hand-Schüller-Christian disease or syndrome (chronic histiocytosis x) 277.89
Hand-foot syndrome 693.0 ▲
Hanging (asphyxia) (strangulation) (suffocation) 994.7
Hangnail (finger) (with lymphangitis) 681.02
Hangover (alcohol) (*see also* Abuse, drugs, nondependent) 305.0❺
Hanot's cirrhosis or disease – *see* Cirrhosis, biliary
Hanot-Chauffard (-Troisier) **syndrome** (bronze diabetes) 275.0
Hansen's disease (leprosy) 030.9
  benign form 030.1
  malignant form 030.0
Harada's disease or syndrome 363.22
Hard chancre 091.0
Hard firm prostate 600.10
  with
    urinary
      obstruction 600.11
      retention 600.11
Hardening
  artery – *see* Arteriosclerosis
  brain 348.8
  liver 571.8
Hare's syndrome (M8010/3) (carcinoma, pulmonary apex) 162.3
Harelip (*see also* Cleft, lip) 749.10
Harkavy's syndrome 446.0
Harlequin (fetus) 757.1
  color change syndrome 779.89
Harley's disease (intermittent hemoglobinuria) 283.2
Harris'
  lines 733.91
  syndrome (organic hyperinsulinism) 251.1
Hart's disease or syndrome (pellagra-cerebellar ataxia-renal aminoaciduria) 270.0
Hartmann's pouch (abnormal sacculation of gallbladder neck) 575.8
  of intestine V44.3
    attention to V55.3
Hartnup disease (pellagra-cerebellar ataxia-renal aminoaciduria) 270.0
Harvester lung 495.0
Hashimoto's disease or struma (struma lymphomatosa) 245.2
Hassall-Henle bodies (corneal warts) 371.41
Haut mal (*see also* Epilepsy) 345.1❺
Haverhill fever 026.1
Hawaiian wood rose dependence 304.5❺
Hawkins' keloid 701.4
Hay
  asthma (*see also* Asthma) 493.0❺
  fever (allergic) (with rhinitis) 477.9
    with asthma (bronchial) (*see also* Asthma) 493.0❺
    allergic, due to grass, pollen, ragweed, or tree 477.0
    conjunctivitis 372.05
    due to
      dander, animal (cat) (dog) 477.8
      dust 477.8
      fowl 477.8
      hair, animal (cat) (dog) 477.2
      pollen 477.0
      specified allergen other than pollen 477.8
Hayem-Faber syndrome (achlorhydric anemia) 280.9
Hayem-Widal syndrome (acquired hemolytic jaundice) 283.9
Haygarth's nodosities 715.04
Hazard-Crile tumor (M8350/3) 193
Hb (abnormal)
  disease – *see* Disease, hemoglobin
  trait – *see* Trait
H disease 270.0
Head – *see also* condition
  banging 307.3
Headache 784.0
  allergic 346.2❺
  cluster 346.2❺
  due to
    loss, spinal fluid 349.0
    lumbar puncture 349.0
    saddle block 349.0
  emotional 307.81
  histamine 346.2❺
  lumbar puncture 349.0
  menopausal 627.2
  migraine 346.9❺
  nonorganic origin 307.81
  postspinal 349.0
  psychogenic 307.81
  psychophysiologic 307.81
  sick 346.1❺
  spinal 349.0
    complicating labor and delivery 668.8
    postpartum 668.8
  spinal fluid loss 349.0
  tension 307.81
  vascular 784.0
    migraine type 346.9❺
  vasomotor 346.9❺
Health
  advice V65.4
  audit V70.0
  checkup V70.0
  education V65.4
  hazard (*see also* History of) V15.9
    falling V15.88
    specified cause NEC V15.89
  instruction V65.4
  services provided because (of)
    boarding school residence V60.6
    holiday relief for person providing home care V60.5
    inadequate
      housing V60.1
      resources V60.2
    lack of housing V60.0
Health – *continued*
  services provided because (of) – *continued*
    no care available in home V60.4
    person living alone V60.3
    poverty V60.3
    residence in institution V60.6
    specified cause NEC V60.8
    vacation relief for person providing home care V60.5
Healthy
  donor (*see also* Donor) V59.9
  infant or child
    accompanying sick mother V65.0
    receiving care V20.1
  person
    accompanying sick relative V65.0
    admitted for sterilization V25.2
    receiving prophylactic inoculation or vaccination (*see also* Vaccination, prophylactic) V05.9
Hearing
  conservation and treatment V72.12 ●
  examination V72.19 ●
    following failed hearing screening V72.11 ●
Heart – *see* condition
Heartburn 787.1
  psychogenic 306.4
Heat (effects) 992.9
  apoplexy 992.0
  burn – *see also* Burn, by site
    from sun (*see also* Sunburn) 692.71
  collapse 992.1
  cramps 992.2
  dermatitis or eczema 692.89
  edema 992.7
  erythema – *see* Burn, by site
  excessive 992.9
    specified effect NEC 992.8
  exhaustion 992.5
    anhydrotic 992.3
    due to
      salt (and water) depletion 992.4
      water depletion 992.3
  fatigue (transient) 992.6
  fever 992.0
  hyperpyrexia 992.0
  prickly 705.1
  prostration – *see* Heat, exhaustion
  pyrexia 992.0
  rash 705.1
  specified effect NEC 992.8
  stroke 992.0
  sunburn (*see also* Sunburn) 692.71
  syncope 992.1
Heavy-chain disease 273.2
Heavy-for-dates (fetus or infant) 766.1
  4500 grams or more 766.0
  exceptionally 766.0
Hebephrenia, hebephrenic (acute) (*see also* Schizophrenia) 295.1❺
  dementia (praecox) (*see also* Schizophrenia) 295.1❺
  schizophrenia (*see also* Schizophrenia) 295.1❺
Heberden's
  disease or nodes 715.04
  syndrome (angina pectoris) 413.9
Hebra's disease
  dermatitis exfoliativa 695.89
  erythema multiforme exudativum 695.1
  pityriasis 695.89
    maculata et circinata 696.3
    rubra 695.89
      pilaris 696.4
  prurigo 698.2
Hebra, nose 040.1
Hedinger's syndrome (malignant carcinoid) 259.2
Heel – *see* condition
Heerfordt's disease or syndrome (uveoparotitis) 135
Hegglin's anomaly or syndrome 288.2
Heidenhain's disease 290.10
  with dementia 290.10
Heilmeyer-Schoner disease (M9842/3) 207.1❺
Heine-Medin disease (*see also* Poliomyelitis) 045.9❺
Heinz-body anemia, congenital 282.7
Heller's disease or syndrome (infantile psychosis) (*see also* Psychosis, childhood) 299.1❺
H.E.L.L.P. 642.5❺

Haglund's disease – H.E.L.L.P.

- **Helminthiasis** (*see also* Infestation, by specific parasite) 128.9
  - Ancylostoma (*see also* Ancylostoma) 126.9
  - intestinal 127.9
    - mixed types (types classifiable to more than one of the categories 120.0-127.7) 127.8
    - specified type 127.7
  - mixed types (intestinal) (types classifiable to more than one of the categories 120.0-127.7) 127.8
  - Necator americanus 126.1
  - specified type NEC 128.8
  - Trichinella 124
- **Heloma** 700
- **Hemangioblastoma** (M9161/1) – *see also* Neoplasm, connective tissue, uncertain behavior
  - malignant (M9161/3) – *see* Neoplasm, connective tissue, malignant
- **Hemangioblastomatosis, cerebelloretinal** 759.6
- **Hemangioendothelioma** (M9130/1) – *see also* Neoplasm, by site, uncertain behavior
  - benign (M9130/0) 228.00
  - bone (diffuse) (M9130/3) – *see* Neoplasm, bone, malignant
  - malignant (M9130/3) – *see* Neoplasm, connective tissue, malignant
  - nervous system (M9130/0) 228.09
- **Hemangioendotheliosarcoma** (M9130/3) – *see* Neoplasm, connective tissue, malignant
- **Hemangiofibroma** (M9160/0) – *see* Neoplasm, by site, benign
- **Hemangiolipoma** (M8861/0) – *see* Lipoma
- **Hemangioma** (M9120/0) 228.00
  - arteriovenous (M9123/0) – *see* Hemangioma, by site
  - brain 228.02
  - capillary (M9131/0) – *see* Hemangioma, by site
  - cavernous (M9121/0) – *see* Hemangioma, by site
  - central nervous system NEC 228.09
  - choroid 228.09
  - heart 228.09
  - infantile (M9131/0) – *see* Hemangioma, by site
  - intra-abdominal structures 228.04
  - intracranial structures 228.02
  - intramuscular (M9132/0) – *see* Hemangioma, by site
  - iris 228.09
  - juvenile (M9131/0) – *see* Hemangioma, by site
  - malignant (M9120/3) – *see* Neoplasm, connective tissue, malignant
  - meninges 228.09
    - brain 228.02
    - spinal cord 228.09
  - peritoneum 228.04
  - placenta – *see* Placenta, abnormal
  - plexiform (M9131/0) – *see* Hemangioma, by site
  - racemose (M9123/0) – *see* Hemangioma, by site
  - retina 228.03
  - retroperitoneal tissue 228.04
  - sclerosing (M8832/0) – *see* Neoplasm, skin, benign
  - simplex (M9131/0) – *see* Hemangioma, by site
  - skin and subcutaneous tissue 228.01
  - specified site NEC 228.09
  - spinal cord 228.09
  - venous (M9122/0) – *see* Hemangioma, by site
  - verrucous keratotic (M9142/0) – *see* Hemangioma, by site
- **Hemangiomatosis** (systemic) 757.32
  - involving single site – *see* Hemangioma
- **Hemangiopericytoma** (M9150/1) – *see also* Neoplasm, connective tissue, uncertain behavior
  - benign (M9150/0) – *see* Neoplasm, connective tissue, benign
  - malignant (M9150/3) – *see* Neoplasm, connective tissue, malignant
- **Hemangiosarcoma** (M9120/3) – *see* Neoplasm, connective tissue, malignant
- **Hemarthrosis** (nontraumatic) 719.10
  - ankle 719.17
  - elbow 719.12
  - foot 719.17
  - hand 719.14
  - hip 719.15
  - knee 719.16
  - multiple sites 719.19
  - pelvic region 719.15
  - shoulder (region) 719.11
- **Hemarthrosis** – *continued*
  - specified site NEC 719.18
  - traumatic – *see* Sprain, by site
  - wrist 719.13
- **Hematemesis** 578.0
  - with ulcer – *see* Ulcer, by site, with hemorrhage
  - due to S. japonicum 120.2
  - Goldstein's (familial hemorrhagic telangiectasia) 448.0
  - newborn 772.4
    - due to swallowed maternal blood 777.3
- **Hematidrosis** 705.89
- **Hematinuria** (*see also* Hemoglobinuria) 791.2
  - malarial 084.8
  - paroxysmal 283.2
- **Hematite miners' lung** 503
- **Hematobilia** 576.8
- **Hematocele** (congenital) (diffuse) (idiopathic) 608.83
  - broad ligament 620.7
  - canal of Nuck 629.0
  - cord, male 608.83
  - fallopian tube 620.8
  - female NEC 629.0
  - ischiorectal 569.89
  - male NEC 608.83
  - ovary 629.0
  - pelvis, pelvic
    - female 629.0
      - with ectopic pregnancy (*see also* Pregnancy, ectopic) 633.90
        - with intrauterine pregnancy 633.91
    - male 608.83
  - periuterine 629.0
  - retrouterine 629.0
  - scrotum 608.83
  - spermatic cord (diffuse) 608.83
  - testis 608.84
  - traumatic – *see* Injury, internal, pelvis
  - tunica vaginalis 608.83
  - uterine ligament 629.0
  - uterus 621.4
  - vagina 623.6
  - vulva 624.5
- **Hematocephalus** 742.4
- **Hematochezia** (*see also* Melena) 578.1
- **Hematochyluria** (*see also* Infestation, filarial) 125.9
- **Hematocolpos** 626.8
- **Hematocornea** 371.12
- **Hematogenous** – *see* condition
- **Hematoma** (skin surface intact) (traumatic) – *see also* Contusion

Note – Hematomas are coded according to origin and the nature and site of the hematoma or the accompanying injury. Hematomas of unspecified origin are coded as injuries of the sites involved, except:

(a) hematomas of genital organs which are coded as diseases of the organ involved unless they complicate pregnancy or delivery

(b) hematomas of the eye which are coded as diseases of the eye.

For late effect of hematoma classifiable to 920-924 see Late, effect, contusion.

  - with
    - crush injury – *see* Crush
    - fracture – *see* Fracture, by site
    - injury of internal organs – *see also* Injury, internal, by site
      - kidney – *see* Hematoma, kidney, traumatic
      - liver – *see* Hematoma, liver, traumatic
      - spleen – *see* Hematoma, spleen
    - nerve injury – *see* Injury, nerve
    - open wound – *see* Wound, open, by site
    - skin surface intact – *see* Contusion
  - abdomen (wall) – *see* Contusion, abdomen
  - amnion 658.8❺
  - aorta, dissecting 441.00
    - abdominal 441.02
  - aorta, dissecting
    - thoracic 441.01
    - thoracoabdominal 441.03
  - arterial (complicating trauma) 904.9
    - specified site – *see* Injury, blood vessel, by site
  - auricle (ear) 380.31
  - birth injury 767.8
    - skull 767.19
- **Hematoma** – *continued*
  - brain (traumatic) 853.0❺

Note – Use the following fifth-digit subclassification with categories 851-854:

0 unspecified state of consciousness
1 with no loss of consciousness
2 with brief [less than one hour] loss of consciousness
3 with moderate [1-24 hours] loss of consciousness
4 with prolonged [more than 24 hours] loss of consciousness and return to pre-existing conscious level
5 with prolonged [more than 24 hours] loss of consciousness, without return to pre-existing conscious level

Use fifth-digit 5 to designate when a patient is unconscious and dies before regaining consciousness, regardless of the duration of the loss of consciousness

6 with loss of consciousness of unspecified duration
9 with concussion, unspecified

    - with
      - cerebral
        - contusion – *see* Contusion, brain
        - laceration – *see* Laceration, brain
      - open intracranial wound 853.1❺
      - skull fracture – *see* Fracture, skull, by site
    - extradural or epidural 852.4❺
      - with open intracranial wound 852.5❺
      - fetus or newborn 767.0
      - nontraumatic 432.0
    - fetus or newborn NEC 767.0
    - nontraumatic (*see also* Hemorrhage, brain) 431
      - epidural or extradural 432.0
      - newborn NEC 772.8
      - subarachnoid, arachnoid, or meningeal (*see also* Hemorrhage, subarachnoid) 430
      - subdural (*see also* Hemorrhage, subdural) 432.1
    - subarachnoid, arachnoid, or meningeal 852.0❺
      - with open intracranial wound 852.1❺
      - fetus or newborn 772.2
      - nontraumatic (*see also* Hemorrhage, subarachnoid) 430
    - subdural 852.2❺
      - with open intracranial wound 852.3❺
      - fetus or newborn (localized) 767.0
      - nontraumatic (*see also* Hemorrhage, subdural) 432.1
  - breast (nontraumatic) 611.8
  - broad ligament (nontraumatic) 620.7
    - complicating delivery 665.7❺
    - traumatic – *see* Injury, internal, broad ligament
  - calcified NEC 959.9
  - capitis 920
    - due to birth injury 767.19
    - newborn 767.19
  - cerebral – *see* Hematoma, brain
  - cesarean section wound 674.3❺
  - chorion – *see* Placenta, abnormal
  - complicating delivery (perineum) (vulva) 664.5❺
    - pelvic 665.7❺
    - vagina 665.7❺
  - corpus
    - cavernosum (nontraumatic) 607.82
    - luteum (nontraumatic) (ruptured) 620.1
  - dura (mater) – *see* Hematoma, brain, subdural
  - epididymis (nontraumatic) 608.83
  - epidural (traumatic) – *see also* Hematoma, brain, extradural
    - spinal – *see* Injury, spinal, by site
  - episiotomy 674.3❺
  - external ear 380.31
  - extradural – *see also* Hematoma, brain, extradural
    - fetus or newborn 767.0
    - nontraumatic 432.0
      - fetus or newborn 767.0
  - fallopian tube 620.8
  - genital organ (nontraumatic)
    - female NEC 629.89
    - male NEC 608.83
    - traumatic (external site) 922.4
      - internal – *see* Injury, internal, genital organ
  - graafian follicle (ruptured) 620.0
  - internal organs (abdomen, chest, or pelvis) – *see also* Injury, internal, by site
    - kidney – *see* Hematoma, kidney, traumatic

- **Hematoma** – *continued*
  - internal organs – *continued*
    - liver – *see* Hematoma, liver, traumatic
    - spleen – *see* Hematoma, spleen
  - intracranial – *see* Hematoma, brain
  - kidney, cystic 593.81
    - traumatic 866.01
      - with open wound into cavity 866.11
  - labia (nontraumatic) 624.5
  - lingual (and other parts of neck, scalp, or face, except eye) 920
  - liver (subcapsular) 573.8
    - birth injury 767.8
    - fetus or newborn 767.8
    - traumatic NEC 864.01
      - with
        - laceration – *see* Laceration, liver
        - open wound into cavity 864.11
  - mediastinum – *see* Injury, internal, mediastinum
  - meninges, meningeal (brain) – *see also* Hematoma, brain, subarachnoid
    - spinal – *see* Injury, spinal, by site
  - mesosalpinx (nontraumatic) 620.8
    - traumatic – *see* Injury, internal, pelvis
  - muscle (traumatic) – *see* Contusion, by site
  - nasal (septum) (and other part(s) of neck, scalp, or face, except eye) 920
  - obstetrical surgical wound 674.3❺
  - orbit, orbital (nontraumatic) 376.32
    - traumatic 921.2
  - ovary (corpus luteum) (nontraumatic) 620.1
    - traumatic – *see* Injury, internal, ovary
  - pelvis (female) (nontraumatic) 629.89
    - complicating delivery 665.7❺
    - male 608.83
    - traumatic – *see also* Injury, internal, pelvis
      - specified organ NEC (*see also* Injury, internal, pelvis) 867.6
  - penis (nontraumatic) 607.82
  - pericranial (and neck, or face any part, except eye) 920
    - due to injury at birth 767.19
  - perineal wound (obstetrical) 674.3❺
    - complicating delivery 664.5❺
  - perirenal, cystic 593.81
  - pinna 380.31
  - placenta – *see* Placenta, abnormal
  - postoperative 998.12
  - retroperitoneal (nontraumatic) 568.81
    - traumatic – *see* Injury, internal, retroperitoneum
  - retropubic, male 568.81
  - scalp (and neck, or face any part, except eye) 920
    - fetus or newborn 767.19
  - scrotum (nontraumatic) 608.83
    - traumatic 922.4
  - seminal vesicle (nontraumatic) 608.83
    - traumatic – *see* Injury, internal, seminal, vesicle
  - spermatic cord – *see also* Injury, internal, spermatic cord
    - nontraumatic 608.83
  - spinal (cord) (meninges) – *see also* Injury, spinal, by site
    - fetus or newborn 767.4
    - nontraumatic 336.1
  - spleen 865.01
    - with
      - laceration – *see* Laceration, spleen
      - open wound into cavity 865.11
  - sternocleidomastoid, birth injury 767.8
  - sternomastoid, birth injury 767.8
  - subarachnoid – *see also* Hematoma, brain, subarachnoid
    - fetus or newborn 772.2
    - nontraumatic (*see also* Hemorrhage, subarachnoid) 430
      - newborn 772.2
  - subdural – *see also* Hematoma, brain, subdural
    - fetus or newborn (localized) 767.0
    - nontraumatic (*see also* Hemorrhage, subdural) 432.1
  - subperiosteal (syndrome) 267
    - traumatic – *see* Hematoma, by site
  - superficial, fetus or newborn 772.6
  - syncytium – *see* Placenta, abnormal
  - testis (nontraumatic) 608.83
    - birth injury 767.8
    - traumatic 922.4
  - tunica vaginalis (nontraumatic) 608.83
  - umbilical cord 663.6❺
    - affecting fetus or newborn 762.6

- **Hematoma** – *continued*
  - uterine ligament (nontraumatic) 620.7
    - traumatic – *see* Injury, internal, pelvis
  - uterus 621.4
    - traumatic – *see* Injury, internal, pelvis
  - vagina (nontraumatic) (ruptured) 623.6
    - complicating delivery 665.7❺
    - traumatic 922.4
  - vas deferens (nontraumatic) 608.83
    - traumatic – *see* Injury, internal, vas deferens
  - vitreous 379.23
  - vocal cord 920
  - vulva (nontraumatic) 624.5
    - complicating delivery 664.5❺
    - fetus or newborn 767.8
    - traumatic 922.4
- **Hematometra** 621.4
- **Hematomyelia** 336.1
  - with fracture of vertebra (*see also* Fracture, vertebra, by site, with spinal cord injury) 806.8
  - fetus or newborn 767.4
- **Hematomyelitis** 323.9
  - late effect – *see* category 326
- **Hematoperitoneum** (*see also* Hemoperitoneum) 568.81
- **Hematopneumothorax** (*see also* Hemothorax) 511.8
- **Hematopoiesis, cyclic** 288.02
- **Hematoporphyria** (acquired) (congenital) 277.1
- **Hematoporphyrinuria** (acquired) (congenital) 277.1
- **Hematorachis, hematorrhachis** 336.1
  - fetus or newborn 767.4
- **Hematosalpinx** 620.8
  - with
    - ectopic pregnancy (*see also* categories 633.0-633.9) 639.2
    - molar pregnancy (*see also* categories 630-632) 639.2
  - infectional (*see also* Salpingo-oophoritis) 614.2
- **Hematospermia** 608.82
- **Hematothorax** (*see also* Hemothorax) 511.8
- **Hematotympanum** 381.03
- **Hematuria** (benign) (essential) (idiopathic) 599.7
  - due to S. hematobium 120.0
  - endemic 120.0
  - intermittent 599.7
  - malarial 084.8
  - paroxysmal 599.7
  - sulfonamide
    - correct substance properly administered 599.7
    - overdose or wrong substance given or taken 961.0
  - tropical (bilharziasis) 120.0
  - tuberculous (*see also* Tuberculosis) 016.9❺
- **Hematuric bilious fever** 084.8
- **Hemeralopia** 368.10
- **Hemiabiotrophy** 799.89
- **Hemi-akinesia** 781.8
- **Hemianalgesia** (*see also* Disturbance, sensation) 782.0
- **Hemianencephaly** 740.0
- **Hemianesthesia** (*see also* Disturbance, sensation) 782.0
- **Hemianopia, hemianopsia** (altitudinal) (homonymous) 368.46
  - binasal 368.47
  - bitemporal 368.47
  - heteronymous 368.47
  - syphilitic 095.8
- **Hemiasomatognosia** 307.9
- **Hemiathetosis** 781.0
- **Hemiatrophy** 799.89
  - cerebellar 334.8
  - face 349.89
    - progressive 349.89
  - fascia 728.9
  - leg 728.2
  - tongue 529.8
- **Hemiballism**(us) 333.5
- **Hemiblock** (cardiac) (heart) (left) 426.2
- **Hemicardia** 746.89
- **Hemicephalus, hemicephaly** 740.0
- **Hemichorea** 333.5
- **Hemicrania** 346.9❺
  - congenital malformation 740.0
- **Hemidystrophy** – *see* Hemiatrophy
- **Hemiectromelia** 755.4
- **Hemihypalgesia** (*see also* Disturbance, sensation) 782.0
- **Hemihypertrophy** (congenital) 759.89
  - cranial 756.0
- **Hemihypesthesia** (*see also* Disturbance, sensation) 782.0
- **Hemi-inattention** 781.8
- **Hemimelia** 755.4
  - lower limb 755.30
    - paraxial (complete) (incomplete) (intercalary) (terminal) 755.32
      - fibula 755.37
      - tibia 755.36
    - transverse (complete) (partial) 755.31
  - upper limb 755.20
    - paraxial (complete) (incomplete) (intercalary) (terminal) 755.22
      - radial 755.26
      - ulnar 755.27
    - transverse (complete) (partial) 755.21
- **Hemiparalysis** (*see also* Hemiplegia) 342.9❺
- **Hemiparesis** (*see also* Hemiplegia) 342.9❺
- **Hemiparesthesia** (*see also* Disturbance, sensation) 782.0
- **Hemiplegia** 342.9❺
  - acute (*see also* Disease, cerebrovascular, acute) 436
  - alternans facialis 344.89
  - apoplectic (*see also* Disease, cerebrovascular, acute) 436
    - late effect or residual
      - affecting
        - dominant side 438.21
        - nondominant side 438.22
        - unspecified side 438.20
  - arteriosclerotic 437.0
    - late effect or residual
      - affecting
        - dominant side 438.21
        - nondominant side 438.22
        - unspecified side 438.20
  - ascending (spinal) NEC 344.89
  - attack (*see also* Disease, cerebrovascular, acute) 436
  - brain, cerebral (current episode) 437.8
    - congenital 343.1
  - cerebral – *see* Hemiplegia, brain
  - congenital (cerebral) (spastic) (spinal) 343.1
  - conversion neurosis (hysterical) 300.11
  - cortical – *see* Hemiplegia, brain
  - due to
    - arteriosclerosis 437.0
      - late effect or residual
        - affecting
          - dominant side 438.21
          - nondominant side 438.22
          - unspecified side 438.20
    - cerebrovascular lesion (*see also* Disease, cerebrovascular, acute) 436
      - late effect
        - affecting
          - dominant side 438.21
          - nondominant side 438.22
          - unspecified side 438.20
  - embolic (current) (*see also* Embolism, brain) 434.1❺
    - late effect
      - affecting
        - dominant side 438.21
        - nondominant side 438.22
        - unspecified side 438.20
  - flaccid 342.0
  - hypertensive (current episode) 437.8
  - infantile (postnatal) 343.4
  - late effect
    - birth injury, intracranial or spinal 343.4
    - cerebrovascular lesion – *see* Late effect(s) (of) cerebrovascular disease
    - viral encephalitis 139.0
  - middle alternating NEC 344.89
  - newborn NEC 767.0
  - seizure (current episode) (*see also* Disease, cerebrovascular, acute) 436
  - spastic 342.1❺
    - congenital or infantile 343.1
  - specified NEC 342.8

Hemiplegia – *continued*
thrombotic (current) (*see also* Thrombosis, brain) 434.0❺
late effect – *see* Late effect(s) (of) cerebrovascular disease
Hemisection, spinal cord – *see* Fracture, vertebra, by site, with spinal cord injury
Hemispasm 781.0
facial 781.0
Hemispatial neglect 781.8
Hemisporosis 117.9
Hemitremor 781.0
Hemivertebra 756.14
Hemobilia 576.8
Hemocholecyst 575.8
Hemochromatosis (acquired) (diabetic) (hereditary) (liver) (myocardium) (primary idiopathic) (secondary) 275.0
with refractory anemia 238.72
Hemodialysis V56.0
Hemoglobin – *see also* condition
abnormal (disease) – *see* Disease, hemoglobin
AS genotype 282.5
fetal, hereditary persistence 282.7
high-oxygen-affinity 289.0
low NEC 285.9
S (Hb-S), heterozygous 282.5
Hemoglobinemia 283.2
due to blood transfusion NEC 999.8
bone marrow 996.85
paroxysmal 283.2
Hemoglobinopathy (mixed) (*see also* Disease, hemoglobin) 282.7
with thalassemia 282.49
sickle-cell 282.60
with thalassemia (without crisis) 282.41
with
crisis 282.42
vaso-occlusive pain 282.42
Hemoglobinuria, hemoglobinuric 791.2
with anemia, hemolytic, acquired (chronic) NEC 283.2
cold (agglutinin) (paroxysmal) (with Raynaud's syndrome) 283.2
due to
exertion 283.2
hemolysis (from external causes) NEC 283.2
exercise 283.2
fever (malaria) 084.8
infantile 791.2
intermittent 283.2
malarial 084.8
march 283.2
nocturnal (paroxysmal) 283.2
paroxysmal (cold) (nocturnal) 283.2
Hemolymphangioma (M9175/0) 228.1
Hemolysis
fetal – *see* Jaundice, fetus or newborn
intravascular (disseminated) NEC 286.6
with
abortion – *see* Abortion, by type, with hemorrhage, delayed or excessive
ectopic pregnancy (*see also* categories 633.0-633.9) 639.1
hemorrhage of pregnancy 641.3❺
affecting fetus or newborn 762.1
molar pregnancy (*see also* categories 630-632) 639.1
acute 283.2
following
abortion 639.1
ectopic or molar pregnancy 639.1
neonatal – *see* Jaundice, fetus or newborn
transfusion NEC 999.8
bone marrow 996.85
Hemolytic – *see also* condition
anemia – *see* Anemia, hemolytic
uremic syndrome 283.11
Hemometra 621.4
Hemopericardium (with effusion) 423.0
newborn 772.8
traumatic (*see also* Hemothorax, traumatic) 860.2
with open wound into thorax 860.3
Hemoperitoneum 568.81
infectional (*see also* Peritonitis) 567.29
traumatic – *see* Injury, internal, peritoneum
Hemophagocytic syndrome 288.4
infection-associated 288.4
Hemophilia (familial) (hereditary) 286.0
A 286.0
carrier (asymptomatic) V83.01
symptomatic V83.02
acquired 286.5
B (Leyden) 286.1
C 286.2
calcipriva (*see also* Fibrinolysis) 286.7
classical 286.0
nonfamilial 286.7
secondary 286.5
vascular 286.4
Hemophilus influenzae NEC 041.5
arachnoiditis (basic) (brain) (spinal) 320.0
late effect – *see* category 326
bronchopneumonia 482.2
cerebral ventriculitis 320.0
late effect – *see* category 326
cerebrospinal inflammation 320.0
late effect – *see* category 326
infection NEC 041.5
leptomeningitis 320.0
late effect – *see* category 326
meningitis (cerebral) (cerebrospinal) (spinal) 320.0
late effect – *see* category 326
meningomyelitis 320.0
late effect – *see* category 326
pachymeningitis (adhesive) (fibrous) (hemorrhagic) (hypertrophic) (spinal) 320.0
late effect – *see* category 326
pneumonia (broncho-) 482.2
Hemophthalmos 360.43
Hemopneumothorax (*see also* Hemothorax) 511.8
traumatic 860.4
with open wound into thorax 860.5
Hemoptysis 786.3
due to Paragonimus (westermani) 121.2
newborn 770.3
tuberculous (*see also* Tuberculosis, pulmonary) 011.9❺
Hemorrhage, hemorrhagic (nontraumatic) 459.0
abdomen 459.0
accidental (antepartum) 641.2❺
affecting fetus or newborn 762.1
adenoid 474.8
adrenal (capsule) (gland) (medulla) 255.41 ▲
newborn 772.5
after labor – *see* Hemorrhage, postpartum
alveolar
lung, newborn 770.3
process 525.8
alveolus 525.8
amputation stump (surgical) 998.11
secondary, delayed 997.69
anemia (chronic) 280.0
acute 285.1
antepartum – *see* Hemorrhage, pregnancy
anus (sphincter) 569.3
apoplexy (stroke) 432.9
arachnoid – *see* Hemorrhage, subarachnoid
artery NEC 459.0
brain (*see also* Hemorrhage, brain) 431
middle meningeal – *see* Hemorrhage, subarachnoid
basilar (ganglion) (*see also* Hemorrhage, brain) 431
bladder 596.8
blood dyscrasia 289.9
bowel 578.9
newborn 772.4
brain (miliary) (nontraumatic)431
with
birth injury 767.0
arachnoid – *see* Hemorrhage, subarachnoid
due to
birth injury 767.0
rupture of aneurysm (congenital) (*see also* Hemorrhage, subarachnoid) 430
mycotic 431
syphilis 094.89
epidural or extradural – *see* Hemorrhage, extradural
fetus or newborn (anoxic) (hypoxic) (due to birth trauma) (nontraumatic) 767.0
intraventricular 772.10
grade I 772.11
grade II 772.12
grade III 772.13
Hemorrhage, hemorrhagic – *continued*
brain – *continued*
fetus or newborn – *continued*
intraventricular – *continued*
grade IV 772.14
iatrogenic 997.02
postoperative 997.02
puerperal, postpartum, childbirth 674.0❺
stem 431
subarachnoid, arachnoid, or meningeal – *see* Hemorrhage, subarachnoid
subdural – *see* Hemorrhage, subdural
traumatic NEC 853.0❺

Note – Use the following fifth-digit subclassification with categories 851-854:
0 unspecified state of consciousness
1 with no loss of consciousness
2 with brief [less than one hour] loss of consciousness
3 with moderate [1-24 hours] loss of consciousness
4 with prolonged [more than 24 hours] loss of consciousness and return to pre-existing conscious level
5 with prolonged [more than 24 hours] loss of consciousness, without return to pre-existing conscious level
Use fifth-digit 5 to designate when a patient is unconscious and dies before regaining consciousness, regardless of the duration of the loss of consciousness
6 with loss of consciousness of unspecified duration
9 with concussion, unspecified

with
cerebral
contusion – *see* Contusion, brain
laceration – *see* Laceration, brain
open intracranial wound 853.1❺
skull fracture – *see* Fracture, skull, by site
extradural or epidural 852.4❺
with open intracranial wound 852.5❺
subarachnoid 852.0❺
with open intracranial wound 852.1❺
subdural 852.2❺
with open intracranial wound 852.3❺
breast 611.79
bronchial tube – *see* Hemorrhage, lung
bronchopulmonary – *see* Hemorrhage, lung
bronchus (cause unknown) (*see also* Hemorrhage, lung) 786.3
bulbar (*see also* Hemorrhage, brain) 431
bursa 727.89
capillary 448.9
primary 287.8
capsular – *see* Hemorrhage, brain
cardiovascular 429.89
cecum 578.9
cephalic (*see also* Hemorrhage, brain) 431
cerebellar (*see also* Hemorrhage, brain) 431
cerebellum (*see also* Hemorrhage, brain) 431
cerebral (*see also* Hemorrhage, brain) 431
fetus or newborn (anoxic) (traumatic) 767.0
cerebromeningeal (*see also* Hemorrhage, brain) 431
cerebrospinal (*see also* Hemorrhage, brain) 431
cerebrovascular accident – *see* Hemorrhage, brain
cerebrum (*see also* Hemorrhage, brain) 431
cervix (stump) (uteri) 622.8
cesarean section wound 674.3❺
chamber, anterior (eye) 364.41
childbirth – *see* Hemorrhage, complicating, delivery
choroid 363.61
expulsive 363.62
ciliary body 364.41
cochlea 386.8
colon – *see* Hemorrhage, intestine
complicating
delivery 641.9❺
affecting fetus or newborn 762.1
associated with
afibrinogenemia 641.3❺
affecting fetus or newborn 763.89
coagulation defect 641.3❺
affecting fetus or newborn 763.89
hyperfibrinolysis 641.3❺
affecting fetus or newborn 763.89

Hemiplegia – Hemorrhage, hemorrhagic

- **Hemorrhage, hemorrhagic** – *continued*
  - complicating – *continued*
    - delivery – *continued*
      - associated with – *continued*
        - hypofibrinogenemia 641.3❺
          - affecting fetus or newborn 763.89
      - due to
        - low-lying placenta 641.1❺
          - affecting fetus or newborn 762.0
        - placenta previa 641.1❺
          - affecting fetus or newborn 762.0
        - premature separation of placenta 641.2❺
          - affecting fetus or newborn 762.1
        - retained
          - placenta 666.0❺
          - secundines 666.2❺
        - trauma 641.8❺
          - affecting fetus or newborn 763.89
        - uterine leiomyoma 641.8❺
          - affecting fetus or newborn 763.89
    - surgical procedure 998.11
  - complication(s) ●
    - of dental implant placement 525.71 ●
  - concealed NEC 459.0
  - congenital 772.9
  - conjunctiva 372.72
    - newborn 772.8
  - cord, newborn 772.0
    - slipped ligature 772.3
    - stump 772.3
  - corpus luteum (ruptured) 620.1
  - cortical (*see also* Hemorrhage, brain) 431
  - cranial 432.9
  - cutaneous 782.7
    - newborn 772.6
  - cyst, pancreas 577.2
  - cystitis – *see* Cystitis
  - delayed
    - with
      - abortion – *see* Abortion, by type, with hemorrhage, delayed or excessive
      - ectopic pregnancy (*see also* categories 633.0-633.9) 639.1
      - molar pregnancy (*see also* categories 630-632) 639.1
    - following
      - abortion 639.1
      - ectopic or molar pregnancy 639.1
    - postpartum 666.2❺
  - diathesis (familial) 287.9
    - newborn 776.0
  - disease 287.9
    - newborn 776.0
    - specified type NEC 287.8
  - disorder 287.9
    - due to intrinsic circulating anticoagulants 286.5
    - specified type NEC 287.8
  - due to
    - any device, implant, or graft (presence of) classifiable to 996.0-996.5 – *see* Complications, due to (presence of) any device, implant, or graft classified to 996.0-996.5 NEC
    - intrinsic circulating anticoagulant 286.5
  - duodenum, duodenal 537.89
    - ulcer – *see* Ulcer, duodenum, with hemorrhage
  - dura mater – *see* Hemorrhage, subdural
  - endotracheal – *see* Hemorrhage, lung
  - epicranial subaponeurotic (massive) 767.11
  - epidural – *see* Hemorrhage, extradural
  - episiotomy 674.3❺
  - esophagus 530.82
    - varix (*see also* Varix, esophagus, bleeding) 456.0
  - excessive
    - with
      - abortion – *see* Abortion, by type, with hemorrhage, delayed or excessive
      - ectopic pregnancy (*see also* categories 633.0-633.9) 639.1
      - molar pregnancy (*see also* categories 630-632) 639.1
    - following
      - abortion 639.1
      - ectopic or molar pregnancy 639.1
  - external 459.0
  - extradural (traumatic) – *see also* Hemorrhage, brain, traumatic, extradural
    - birth injury 767.0
    - fetus or newborn (anoxic) (traumatic) 767.0

- **Hemorrhage, hemorrhagic** – *continued*
  - extradural – *continued*
    - nontraumatic 432.0
  - eye 360.43
    - chamber (anterior) (aqueous) 364.41
    - fundus 362.81
  - eyelid 374.81
  - fallopian tube 620.8
  - fetomaternal 772.0
    - affecting management of pregnancy or puerperium 656.0❺
  - fetus, fetal 772.0
    - from
      - cut end of co-twin's cord 772.0
      - placenta 772.0
      - ruptured cord 772.0
      - vasa previa 772.0
    - into
      - co-twin 772.0
      - mother's circulation 772.0
        - affecting management of pregnancy or puerperium 656.0❺
  - fever (*see also* Fever, hemorrhagic) 065.9
    - with renal syndrome 078.6
    - arthropod-borne NEC 065.9
    - Bangkok 065.4
    - Crimean 065.0
    - dengue virus 065.4
    - epidemic 078.6
    - Junin virus 078.7
    - Korean 078.6
    - Machupo virus 078.7
    - mite-borne 065.8
    - mosquito-borne 065.4
    - Philippine 065.4
    - Russian (Yaroslav) 078.6
    - Singapore 065.4
    - Southeast Asia 065.4
    - Thailand 065.4
    - tick-borne NEC 065.3
  - fibrinogenolysis (*see also* Fibrinolysis) 286.6
  - fibrinolytic (acquired) (*see also* Fibrinolysis) 286.6
  - fontanel 767.19
  - from tracheostomy stoma 519.09
  - fundus, eye 362.81
  - funis
    - affecting fetus or newborn 772.0
    - complicating delivery 663.8❺
  - gastric (*see also* Hemorrhage, stomach) 578.9
  - gastroenteric 578.9
    - newborn 772.4
  - gastrointestinal (tract) 578.9
    - newborn 772.4
  - genitourinary (tract) NEC 599.89
  - gingiva 523.8
  - globe 360.43
  - gravidarum – *see* Hemorrhage, pregnancy
  - gum 523.8
  - heart 429.89
  - hypopharyngeal (throat) 784.8
  - intermenstrual 626.6
    - irregular 626.6
    - regular 626.5
  - internal (organs) 459.0
    - capsule (*see also* Hemorrhage brain) 431
    - ear 386.8
    - newborn 772.8
  - intestine 578.9
    - congenital 772.4
    - newborn 772.4
  - into
    - bladder wall 596.7
    - bursa 727.89
    - corpus luysii (*see also* Hemorrhage, brain) 431
  - intra-abdominal 459.0
    - during or following surgery 998.11
  - intra-alveolar, newborn (lung) 770.3
  - intracerebral (*see also* Hemorrhage, brain) 431
  - intracranial NEC 432.9
    - puerperal, postpartum, childbirth 674.0❺
    - traumatic – *see* Hemorrhage, brain, traumatic
  - intramedullary NEC 336.1
  - intraocular 360.43
  - intraoperative 998.11
  - intrapartum – *see* Hemorrhage, complicating, delivery
  - intrapelvic
    - female 629.89
    - male 459.0
  - intraperitoneal 459.0
  - intrapontine (*see also* Hemorrhage, brain) 431

- **Hemorrhage, hemorrhagic** – *continued*
  - intrauterine 621.4
    - complicating delivery – *see* Hemorrhage, complicating, delivery
    - in pregnancy or childbirth – *see* Hemorrhage, pregnancy
    - postpartum (*see also* Hemorrhage, postpartum) 666.1❺
  - intraventricular (*see also* Hemorrhage, brain) 431
    - fetus or newborn (anoxic) (traumatic) 772.10
      - grade I 772.11
      - grade II 772.12
      - grade III 772.13
      - grade IV 772.14
  - intravesical 596.7
  - iris (postinfectional) (postinflammatory) (toxic) 364.41
  - joint (nontraumatic) 719.10
    - ankle 719.17
    - elbow 719.12
    - foot 719.17
    - forearm 719.13
    - hand 719.14
    - hip 719.15
    - knee 719.16
    - lower leg 719.16
    - multiple sites 719.19
    - pelvic region 719.15
    - shoulder (region) 719.11
    - specified site NEC 719.18
    - thigh 719.15
    - upper arm 719.12
    - wrist 719.13
  - kidney 593.81
  - knee (joint) 719.16
  - labyrinth 386.8
  - leg NEC 459.0
  - lenticular striate artery (*see also* Hemorrhage, brain) 431
  - ligature, vessel 998.11
  - liver 573.8
  - lower extremity NEC 459.0
  - lung 786.3
    - newborn 770.3
    - tuberculous (*see also* Tuberculosis, pulmonary) 011.9❺
  - malaria 084.8
  - marginal sinus 641.2❺
  - massive subaponeurotic, birth injury 767.11
  - maternal, affecting fetus or newborn 762.1
  - mediastinum 786.3
  - medulla (*see also* Hemorrhage, brain) 431
  - membrane (brain) (*see also* Hemorrhage, subarachnoid) 430
    - spinal cord – *see* Hemorrhage, spinal cord
  - meninges, meningeal (brain) (middle) (*see also* Hemorrhage, subarachnoid) 430
    - spinal cord – *see* Hemorrhage, spinal cord
  - mesentery 568.81
  - metritis 626.8
  - midbrain (*see also* Hemorrhage, brain) 431
  - mole 631
  - mouth 528.9
  - mucous membrane NEC 459.0
    - newborn 772.8❺
  - muscle 728.89
  - nail (subungual) 703.8
  - nasal turbinate 784.7
    - newborn 772.8
  - nasopharynx 478.29
  - navel, newborn 772.3
  - newborn 772.9
    - adrenal 772.5
    - alveolar (lung) 770.3
    - brain (anoxic) (hypoxic) (due to birth trauma) 767.0
    - cerebral (anoxic) (hypoxic) (due to birth trauma) 767.0
    - conjunctiva 772.8
    - cutaneous 772.6
    - diathesis 776.0
    - due to vitamin K deficiency 776.0
    - epicranial subaponeurotic (massive) 767.11
    - gastrointestinal 772.4
    - internal (organs) 772.8
    - intestines 772.4
    - intra-alveolar (lung) 770.3
    - intracranial (from any perinatal cause) 767.0
    - intraventricular (from any perinatal cause) 772.10
      - grade I 772.11
      - grade II 772.12

Hemorrhage, hemorrhagic – *continued*
newborn – *continued*
intraventricular – *continued*
grade III 772.13
grade IV 772.14
lung 770.3
pulmonary (massive) 770.3
spinal cord, traumatic 767.4
stomach 772.4
subaponeurotic (massive) 767.11
subarachnoid (from any perinatal cause) 772.2
subconjunctival 772.8
subgaleal 767.11
umbilicus 772.0
slipped ligature 772.3
vasa previa 772.0
nipple 611.79
nose 784.7
newborn 772.8
obstetrical surgical wound 674.3❺
omentum 568.89
newborn 772.4
optic nerve (sheath) 377.42
orbit 376.32
ovary 620.1
oviduct 620.8
pancreas 577.8
parathyroid (gland) (spontaneous) 252.8
parturition – *see* Hemorrhage, complicating, delivery
penis 607.82
pericardium, pericarditis 423.0
perineal wound (obstetrical) 674.3❺
peritoneum, peritoneal 459.0
peritonsillar tissue 474.8
after operation on tonsils 998.11
due to infection 475
petechial 782.7
pituitary (gland) 253.8
placenta NEC 641.9❺
affecting fetus or newborn 762.1
from surgical or instrumental damage 641.8❺
affecting fetus or newborn 762.1
previa 641.1❺
affecting fetus or newborn 762.0
pleura – *see* Hemorrhage, lung
polioencephalitis, superior 265.1
polymyositis – *see* Polymyositis
pons (*see also* Hemorrhage, brain) 431
pontine (*see also* Hemorrhage, brain) 431
popliteal 459.0
postcoital 626.7
postextraction (dental) 998.11
postmenopausal 627.1
postnasal 784.7
postoperative 998.11
postpartum (atonic) (following delivery of placenta) 666.1❺
delayed or secondary (after 24 hours) 666.2❺
retained placenta 666.0❺
third stage 666.0❺
pregnancy (concealed) 641.9❺
accidental 641.2❺
affecting fetus or newborn 762.1
affecting fetus or newborn 762.1
before 22 completed weeks gestation 640.9❺
affecting fetus or newborn 762.1
due to
abruptio placenta 641.2❺
affecting fetus or newborn 762.1
afibrinogenemia or other coagulation defect (conditions classifiable to 286.0-286.9) 641.3❺
affecting fetus or newborn 762.1
coagulation defect 641.3❺
affecting fetus or newborn 762.1
hyperfibrinolysis 641.3❺
affecting fetus or newborn 762.1
hypofibrinogenemia 641.3❺
affecting fetus or newborn 762.1
leiomyoma, uterus 641.8❺
affecting fetus or newborn 762.1
low-lying placenta 641.1❺
affecting fetus or newborn 762.1
marginal sinus (rupture) 641.2❺
affecting fetus or newborn 762.1
placenta previa 641.1❺
affecting fetus or newborn 762.0
premature separation of placenta (normally implanted) 641.2❺
affecting fetus or newborn 762.1

Hemorrhage, hemorrhagic – *continued*
pregnancy – *continued*
due to – *continued*
threatened abortion 640.0❺
affecting fetus or newborn 762.1
trauma 641.8❺
affecting fetus or newborn 762.1
early (before 22 completed weeks gestation) 640.9❺
affecting fetus or newborn 762.1
previous, affecting management of pregnancy or childbirth V23.49
unavoidable – *see* Hemorrhage, pregnancy, due to placenta previa
prepartum (mother) – *see* Hemorrhage, pregnancy
preretinal, cause unspecified 362.81
prostate 602.1
puerperal (*see also* Hemorrhage, postpartum) 666.1❺
pulmonary – *see also* Hemorrhage, lung
newborn (massive) 770.3
renal syndrome 446.21
purpura (primary) (*see also* Purpura, thrombocytopenic) 287.39
rectum (sphincter) 569.3
recurring, following initial hemorrhage at time of injury 958.2
renal 593.81
pulmonary syndrome 446.21
respiratory tract (*see also* Hemorrhage, lung) 786.3
retina, retinal (deep) (superficial) (vessels) 362.81
diabetic 250.5❺ *[362.01]*
due to birth injury 772.8
retrobulbar 376.89
retroperitoneal 459.0
retroplacental (*see also* Placenta, separation) 641.2❺
scalp 459.0
due to injury at birth 767.19
scrotum 608.83
secondary (nontraumatic) 459.0
following initial hemorrhage at time of injury 958.2
seminal vesicle 608.83
skin 782.7
newborn 772.6
spermatic cord 608.83
spinal (cord) 336.1
aneurysm (ruptured) 336.1
syphilitic 094.89
due to birth injury 767.4
fetus or newborn 767.4
spleen 289.59
spontaneous NEC 459.0
petechial 782.7
stomach 578.9
newborn 772.4
ulcer – *see* Ulcer, stomach, with hemorrhage
subaponeurotic, newborn 767.11
massive (birth injury) 767.11
subarachnoid (nontraumatic) 430
fetus or newborn (anoxic) (traumatic) 772.2
puerperal, postpartum, childbirth 674.0❺
traumatic – *see* Hemorrhage, brain, traumatic, subarachnoid
subconjunctival 372.72
due to birth injury 772.8
newborn 772.8
subcortical (*see also* Hemorrhage, brain) 431
subcutaneous 782.7
subdiaphragmatic 459.0
subdural (nontraumatic) 432.1
due to birth injury 767.0
fetus or newborn (anoxic) (hypoxic) (due to birth trauma) 767.0
puerperal, postpartum, childbirth 674.0❺
spinal 336.1
traumatic – *see* Hemorrhage, brain, traumatic, subdural
subgaleal 767.11
subhyaloid 362.81
subperiosteal 733.99
subretinal 362.81
subtentorial (*see also* Hemorrhage, subdural) 432.1
subungual 703.8
due to blood dyscrasia 287.8
suprarenal (capsule) (gland) 255.41 ▲
fetus or newborn 772.5

Hemorrhage, hemorrhagic – *continued*
tentorium (traumatic) – *see also* Hemorrhage, brain, traumatic
fetus or newborn 767.0
nontraumatic – *see* Hemorrhage, subdural
testis 608.83
thigh 459.0
third stage 666.0❺
thorax – *see* Hemorrhage, lung
throat 784.8
thrombocythemia 238.71
thymus (gland) 254.8
thyroid (gland) 246.3
cyst 246.3
tongue 529.8
tonsil 474.8
postoperative 998.11
tooth socket (postextraction) 998.11
trachea – *see* Hemorrhage, lung
traumatic – *see also* nature of injury
brain – *see* Hemorrhage, brain traumatic
recurring or secondary (following initial hemorrhage at time of injury) 958.2
tuberculous NEC (*see also* Tuberculosis, pulmonary) 011.9❺
tunica vaginalis 608.83
ulcer – *see* Ulcer, by site, with hemorrhage
umbilicus, umbilical cord 772.0
after birth, newborn 772.3
complicating delivery 663.8❺
affecting fetus or newborn 772.0
slipped ligature 772.3
stump 772.3
unavoidable (due to placenta previa) 641.1❺
affecting fetus or newborn 762.0
upper extremity 459.0
urethra (idiopathic) 599.84
uterus, uterine (abnormal) 626.9
climacteric 627.0
complicating delivery – *see* Hemorrhage, complicating, delivery
due to
intrauterine contraceptive device 996.76
perforating uterus 996.32
functional or dysfunctional 626.8
in pregnancy – *see* Hemorrhage, pregnancy
intermenstrual 626.6
irregular 626.6
regular 626.5
postmenopausal 627.1
postpartum (*see also* Hemorrhage, postpartum) 666.1❺
prepubertal 626.8
pubertal 626.3
puerperal (immediate) 666.1❺
vagina 623.8
vasa previa 663.5❺
affecting fetus or newborn 772.0
vas deferens 608.83
ventricular (*see also* Hemorrhage, brain) 431
vesical 596.8
viscera 459.0
newborn 772.8
vitreous (humor) (intraocular) 379.23
vocal cord 478.5
vulva 624.8

Hemorrhoids (anus) (rectum) (without complication) 455.6
bleeding, prolapsed, strangulated, or ulcerated NEC 455.8
external 455.5
internal 455.2
complicated NEC 455.8
complicating pregnancy and puerperium 671.8❺
external 455.3
with complication NEC 455.5
bleeding, prolapsed, strangulated, or ulcerated 455.5
thrombosed 455.4
internal 455.0
with complication NEC 455.2
bleeding, prolapsed, strangulated, or ulcerated 455.2
thrombosed 455.1
residual skin tag 455.9
sentinel pile 455.9
thrombosed NEC 455.7
external 455.4
internal 455.1

Hemosalpinx 620.8

Hemosiderosis – Hernia, hernial

Hernia, hernial – *continued*
- diaphragm, diaphragmatic 553.3
  - with
    - gangrene (obstructed) 551.3
    - obstruction 552.3
      - and gangrene 551.3
  - congenital 756.6
  - due to gross defect of diaphragm 756.6
  - traumatic 862.0
    - with open wound into cavity 862.1
- direct (inguinal) – *see* Hernia, inguinal
- disc, intervertebral – *see* Displacement, intervertebral disc
- diverticulum, intestine 553.9
  - with
    - gangrene (obstructed) 551.9
    - obstruction 552.9
      - and gangrene 551.9
- double (inguinal) – *see* Hernia, inguinal
- due to adhesion with obstruction 560.81
- duodenojejunal 553.8
  - with
    - gangrene (obstructed) 551.8
    - obstruction 552.8
      - and gangrene 551.8
- en glissade – *see* Hernia, inguinal
- enterostomy (stoma) 569.69
- epigastric 553.29
  - with
    - gangrene (obstruction) 551.29
    - obstruction 552.29
      - and gangrene 551.29
  - recurrent 553.21
    - with
      - gangrene (obstructed) 551.21
      - obstruction 552.21
        - and gangrene 551.21
- esophageal hiatus (sliding) 553.3
  - with
    - gangrene (obstructed) 551.3
    - obstruction 552.3
      - and gangrene 551.3
  - congenital 750.6
- external (inguinal) – *see* Hernia, inguinal
- fallopian tube 620.4
- fascia 728.89
- fat 729.30
  - eyelid 374.34
  - orbital 374.34
  - pad 729.30
    - eye, eyelid 374.34
    - knee 729.31
    - orbit 374.34
    - popliteal (space) 729.31
    - specified site NEC 729.39
- femoral (unilateral) 553.00
  - with
    - gangrene (obstructed) 551.00
    - obstruction 552.00
      - with gangrene 551.0❺
  - bilateral 553.02
    - gangrenous (obstructed) 551.02
    - obstructed 552.02
      - with gangrene 551.02
    - recurrent 553.03
      - gangrenous (obstructed) 551.03
      - obstructed 552.03
        - with gangrene 551.03
  - recurrent (unilateral) 553.01
    - bilateral 553.03
      - gangrenous (obstructed) 551.03
      - obstructed 552.03
        - with gangrene 551.03
    - gangrenous (obstructed) 551.01
    - obstructed 552.01
      - with gangrene 551.01
- foramen
  - Bochdalek 553.3
    - with
      - gangrene (obstructed) 551.3
      - obstruction 552.3
        - and gangrene 551.3
    - congenital 756.6
  - magnum 348.4
  - Morgagni, Morgagnian 553.3
    - with
      - gangrene 551.3
      - obstruction 552.3
        - and gangrene 551.3
      - congenital 756.6

Hernia, hernial – *continued*
- funicular (umbilical) 553.1
  - with
    - gangrene (obstructed) 551.1
    - obstruction 552.1
      - and gangrene 551.1
  - spermatic cord – *see* Hernia, inguinal
- gangrenous – *see* Hernia, by site, with gangrene
- gastrointestinal tract 553.9
  - with
    - gangrene (obstructed) 551.9
    - obstruction 552.9
      - and gangrene 551.9
- gluteal – *see* Hernia, femoral
- Gruber's (internal mesogastric) 553.8
  - with
    - gangrene (obstructed) 551.8
    - obstruction 552.8
      - and gangrene 551.8
- Hesselbach's 553.8
  - with
    - gangrene (obstructed) 551.8
    - obstruction 552.8
      - and gangrene 551.8
- hiatal (esophageal) (sliding) 553.3
  - with
    - gangrene (obstructed) 551.3
    - obstruction 552.3
      - and gangrene 551.3
  - congenital 750.6
- incarcerated (*see also* Hernia, by site, with obstruction) 552.9
  - gangrenous (*see also* Hernia, by site, with gangrene) 551.9
- incisional 553.21
  - with
    - gangrene (obstructed) 551.21
    - obstruction 552.21
      - and gangrene 551.21
  - lumbar – *see* Hernia, lumbar
  - recurrent 553.21
    - with
      - gangrene (obstructed) 551.21
      - obstruction 552.21
        - and gangrene 551.21
- indirect (inguinal) – *see* Hernia, inguinal
- infantile – *see* Hernia, inguinal
- infrapatellar fat pad 729.31
- inguinal (direct) (double) (encysted) (external) (funicular) (indirect) (infantile) (internal) (interstitial) (oblique) (scrotal) (sliding) 550.9❺

  Note – Use the following fifth-digit subclassification with category 550:

0	*unilateral or unspecified (not specified as recurrent)*
1	*unilateral or unspecified, recurrent*
2	*bilateral (not specified as recurrent)*
3	*bilateral, recurrent*

  - with
    - gangrene (obstructed) 550.0❺
    - obstruction 550.1❺
      - and gangrene 550.0❺
- internal 553.8
  - with
    - gangrene (obstructed) 551.8
    - obstruction 552.8
      - and gangrene 551.8
  - inguinal – *see* Hernia, inguinal
- interstitial 553.9
  - with
    - gangrene (obstructed) 551.9
    - obstruction 552.9
      - and gangrene 551.9
  - inguinal – *see* Hernia, inguinal
- intervertebral cartilage or disc – *see* Displacement, intervertebral disc
- intestine, intestinal 553.9
  - with
    - gangrene (obstructed) 551.9
    - obstruction 552.9
      - and gangrene 551.9
- intra-abdominal 553.9
  - with
    - gangrene (obstructed) 551.9
    - obstruction 552.9
      - and gangrene 551.9
- intraparietal 553.9
  - with
    - gangrene (obstructed) 551.9

Hernia, hernial – *continued*
- intraparietal – *continued*
  - with – *continued*
    - obstruction 552.9
      - and gangrene 551.9
- iris 364.89 ▲
  - traumatic 871.1
- irreducible (*see also* Hernia, by site, with obstruction) 552.9
  - gangrenous (with obstruction) (*see also* Hernia, by site, with gangrene) 551.9
- ischiatic 553.8
  - with
    - gangrene (obstructed) 551.8
    - obstruction 552.8
      - and gangrene 551.8
- ischiorectal 553.8
  - with
    - gangrene (obstructed) 551.8
    - obstruction 552.8
      - and gangrene 551.8
- lens 379.32
  - traumatic 871.1
- linea
  - alba – *see* Hernia, epigastric
  - semilunaris – *see* Hernia, spigelian
- Littre's (diverticular) 553.9
  - with
    - gangrene (obstructed) 551.9
    - obstruction 552.9
      - and gangrene 551.9
- lumbar 553.8
  - with
    - gangrene (obstructed) 551.8
    - obstruction 552.8
      - and gangrene 551.8
  - intervertebral disc 722.10
- lung (subcutaneous) 518.89
  - congenital 748.69
- mediastinum 519.3
- mesenteric (internal) 553.8
  - with
    - gangrene (obstructed) 551.8
    - obstruction 552.8
      - and gangrene 551.8
- mesocolon 553.8
  - with
    - gangrene (obstructed) 551.8
    - obstruction 552.8
      - and gangrene 551.8
- muscle (sheath) 728.89
- nucleus pulposus – *see* Displacement, intervertebral disc
- oblique (inguinal) – *see* Hernia, inguinal
- obstructive (*see also* Hernia, by site, with obstruction) 552.9
  - gangrenous (with obstruction) (*see also* Hernia, by site, with gangrene) 551.9
- obturator 553.8
  - with
    - gangrene (obstructed) 551.8
    - obstruction 552.8
      - and gangrene 551.8
- omental 553.8
  - with
    - gangrene (obstructed) 551.8
    - obstruction 552.8
      - and gangrene 551.8
- orbital fat (pad) 374.34
- ovary 620.4
- oviduct 620.4
- paracolostomy (stoma) 569.69
- paraduodenal 553.8
  - with
    - gangrene (obstructed) 551.8
    - obstruction 552.8
      - and gangrene 551.8
- paraesophageal 553.3
  - with
    - gangrene (obstructed) 551.3
    - obstruction 552.3
      - and gangrene 551.3
  - congenital 750.6
- parahiatal 553.3
  - with
    - gangrene (obstructed) 551.3
    - obstruction 552.3
      - and gangrene 551.3
- paraumbilical 553.1
  - with
    - gangrene (obstructed) 551.1

- **Hernia, hernial** – *continued*
  - paraumbilical – *continued*
    - with – *continued*
      - obstruction 552.1
        - and gangrene 551.1
  - parietal 553.9
    - with
      - gangrene (obstructed) 551.9
      - obstruction 552.9
        - and gangrene 551.9
  - perineal 553.8
    - with
      - gangrene (obstructed) 551.8
      - obstruction 552.8
        - and gangrene 551.8
  - peritoneal sac, lesser 553.8
    - with
      - gangrene (obstructed) 551.8
      - obstruction 552.8
        - and gangrene 551.8
  - popliteal fat pad 729.31
  - postoperative 553.21
    - with
      - gangrene (obstructed) 551.21
      - obstruction 552.21
        - and gangrene 551.21
  - pregnant uterus 654.4❺
  - prevesical 596.8
  - properitoneal 553.8
    - with
      - gangrene (obstructed) 551.8
      - obstruction 552.8
        - and gangrene 551.8
  - pudendal 553.8
    - with
      - gangrene (obstructed) 551.8
      - obstruction 552.8
        - and gangrene 551.8
  - rectovaginal 618.6
  - retroperitoneal 553.8
    - with
      - gangrene (obstructed) 551.8
      - obstruction 552.8
        - and gangrene 551.8
  - Richter's (parietal) 553.9
    - with
      - gangrene (obstructed) 551.9
      - obstruction 552.9
        - and gangrene 551.9
  - Rieux's, Riex's (retrocecal) 553.8
    - with
      - gangrene (obstructed) 551.8
      - obstruction 552.8
        - and gangrene 551.8
  - sciatic 553.8
    - with
      - gangrene (obstructed) 551.8
      - obstruction 552.8
        - and gangrene 551.8
  - scrotum, scrotal – *see* Hernia, inguinal
  - sliding (inguinal) – *see also* Hernia, inguinal
    - hiatus – *see* Hernia, hiatal
  - spigelian 553.29
    - with
      - gangrene (obstructed) 551.29
      - obstruction 552.29
        - and gangrene 551.29
  - spinal (*see also* Spina bifida) 741.9❺
    - with hydrocephalus 741.0❺
  - strangulated (*see also* Hernia, by site, with obstruction) 552.9
    - gangrenous (with obstruction) (*see also* Hernia, by site, with gangrene) 551.9
  - supraumbilicus (linea alba) – *see* Hernia, epigastric
  - tendon 727.9
  - testis (nontraumatic) 550.9
    - meaning
      - scrotal hernia 550.9
      - symptomatic late syphilis 095.8
  - Treitz's (fossa) 553.8
    - with
      - gangrene (obstructed) 551.8
      - obstruction 552.8
        - and gangrene 551.8
  - tunica
    - albuginea 608.89
    - vaginalis 752.89
  - umbilicus, umbilical 553.1
    - with
      - gangrene (obstructed) 551.1
      - obstruction 552.1
        - and gangrene 551.1
  - ureter 593.89
    - with obstruction 593.4
  - uterus 621.8
    - pregnant 654.4❺
  - vaginal (posterior) 618.6
  - Velpeau's (femoral) (*see also* Hernia, femoral) 553.00
  - ventral 553.20
    - with
      - gangrene (obstructed) 551.20
      - obstruction 552.20
        - and gangrene 551.20
    - incisional 553.21
    - recurrent 553.21
      - with
        - gangrene (obstructed) 551.21
        - obstruction 552.21
          - and gangrene 551.21
  - vesical
    - congenital (female) (male) 756.71
    - female (*see also* Cystocele, female) 618.01
    - male 596.8
  - vitreous (into anterior chamber) 379.21
    - traumatic 871.1
- **Herniation** – *see also* Hernia
  - brain (stem) 348.4
  - cerebral 348.4
  - gastric mucosa (into duodenal bulb) 537.89
  - mediastinum 519.3
  - nucleus pulposus – *see* Displacement, intervertebral disc
- **Herpangina** 074.0
- **Herpes, herpetic** 054.9
  - auricularis (zoster) 053.71
    - simplex 054.73
  - blepharitis (zoster) 053.20
    - simplex 054.41
  - circinate 110.5
  - circinatus 110.5
    - bullous 694.5
  - conjunctiva (simplex) 054.43
    - zoster 053.21
  - cornea (simplex) 054.43
    - disciform (simplex) 054.43
    - zoster 053.21
  - encephalitis 054.3
  - eye (zoster) 053.29
    - simplex 054.40
  - eyelid (zoster) 053.20
    - simplex 054.41
  - febrilis 054.9
  - fever 054.9
  - geniculate ganglionitis 053.11
  - genital, genitalis 054.10
    - specified site NEC 054.19
  - gestationis 646.8❺
  - gingivostomatitis 054.2
  - iridocyclitis (simplex) 054.44
    - zoster 053.22
  - iris (any site) 695.1
  - iritis (simplex) 054.44
  - keratitis (simplex) 054.43
    - dendritic 054.42
    - disciform 054.43
    - interstitial 054.43
    - zoster 053.21
  - keratoconjunctivitis (simplex) 054.43
    - zoster 053.21
  - labialis 054.9
    - meningococcal 036.89
  - lip 054.9
  - meningitis (simplex) 054.72
    - zoster 053.0
  - ophthalmicus (zoster) 053.20
    - simplex 054.40
  - otitis externa (zoster) 053.71
    - simplex 054.73
  - penis 054.13
  - perianal 054.10
  - pharyngitis 054.79
  - progenitalis 054.10
  - scrotum 054.19
  - septicemia 054.5❺
  - simplex 054.9
    - complicated 054.8
      - ophthalmic 054.40
        - specified NEC 054.49
      - specified NEC 054.79
    - congenital 771.2
    - external ear 054.73
    - keratitis 054.43
      - dendritic 054.42
    - meningitis 054.72
    - myelitis 054.74
    - neuritis 054.79
    - specified complication NEC 054.79
      - ophthalmic 054.49
    - visceral 054.71
  - stomatitis 054.2
  - tonsurans 110.0
    - maculosus (of Hebra) 696.3
  - visceral 054.71
  - vulva 054.12
  - vulvovaginitis 054.11
  - whitlow 054.6
  - zoster 053.9
    - auricularis 053.71
    - complicated 053.8
      - specified NEC 053.79
    - conjunctiva 053.21
    - cornea 053.21
    - ear 053.71
    - eye 053.29
    - geniculate 053.11
    - keratitis 053.21
      - interstitial 053.21
    - myelitis 053.14
    - neuritis 053.10
    - ophthalmicus(a) 053.20
    - oticus 053.71
    - otitis externa 053.71
    - specified complication NEC 053.79
    - specified site NEC 053.9
  - zosteriform, intermediate type 053.9
- **Herrick's**
  - anemia (hemoglobin S disease) 282.61
  - syndrome (hemoglobin S disease) 282.61
- **Hers' disease** (glycogenosis VI) 271.0
- **Herter's infantilism** (nontropical sprue) 579.0
- **Herter** (-Gee) **disease or syndrome** (nontropical sprue) 579.0
- **Herxheimer's disease** (diffuse idiopathic cutaneous atrophy) 701.8
- **Herxheimer's reaction** 995.0
- **Hesitancy, urinary** 788.64
- **Hesselbach's hernia** – *see* Hernia, Hesselbach's
- **Heterochromia** (congenital) 743.46
  - acquired 364.53
  - cataract 366.33
  - cyclitis 364.21
  - hair 704.3
  - iritis 364.21
  - retained metallic foreign body 360.62
    - magnetic 360.52
  - uveitis 364.21
- **Heterophoria** 378.40
  - alternating 378.45
  - vertical 378.43
- **Heterophyes, small intestine** 121.6
- **Heterophyiasis** 121.6
- **Heteropsia** 368.8
- **Heterotopia, heterotopic** – *see also* Malposition, congenital
  - cerebralis 742.4
  - pancreas, pancreatic 751.7
  - spinalis 742.59
- **Heterotropia** 378.30
  - intermittent 378.20
    - vertical 378.31
  - vertical (constant) (intermittent) 378.31
- **Heubner's disease** 094.89
- **Heubner-Herter disease or syndrome** (nontropical sprue) 579.0
- **Hexadactylism** 755.0❺
- **Heyd's syndrome** (hepatorenal) 572.4
- **HGSIL** (high grade squamous intraepithelial lesion) ▶(cytologic finding) (Pap smear finding)◀ 795.04
  - biopsy finding - *code to* CIN II or CIN III ●
- **Hibernoma** (M8880/0) – *see* Lipoma

- **Hiccough** 786.8
  - epidemic 078.89
  - psychogenic 306.1
- **Hiccup** (*see also* Hiccough) 786.8
- **Hicks** (-Braxton) **contractures** 644.1⑤
- **Hidden penis** 752.65
- **Hidradenitis** (axillaris) (suppurative) 705.83
- **Hidradenoma** (nodular) (M8400/0) – *see also* Neoplasm, skin, benign
  - clear cell (M8402/0) – *see* Neoplasm, skin, benign
  - papillary (M8405/0) – *see* Neoplasm, skin, benign
- **Hidrocystoma** (M8404/0) – *see* Neoplasm, skin, benign
- **HIE** (hypoxic-ischemic encephalopathy) 768.7
- **High**
  - A_2 anemia 282.49
  - altitude effects 993.2
    - anoxia 993.2
    - on
      - ears 993.0
      - sinuses 993.1
    - polycythemia 289.0
  - arch
    - foot 755.67
    - palate 750.26
  - artery (arterial) tension (*see also* Hypertension) 401.9
    - without diagnosis of hypertension 796.2
  - basal metabolic rate (BMR) 794.7
  - blood pressure (*see also* Hypertension) 401.9
    - incidental reading (isolated) (nonspecific), no diagnosis of hypertension 796.2
  - cholesterol 272.0 ●
    - with high triglycerides 272.2 ●
  - compliance bladder 596.4
  - diaphragm (congenital) 756.6
  - frequency deafness (congenital) (regional) 389.8
  - head at term 652.5⑤
    - affecting fetus or newborn 763.1
  - output failure (cardiac) (*see also* Failure, heart) 428.9
  - oxygen-affinity hemoglobin 289.0
  - palate 750.26
  - risk
    - behavior – *see* problem
    - cervical, human papillomavirus (HPV) DNA test positive 795.05
    - family situation V61.9
      - specified circumstance NEC V61.8
    - individual NEC V62.89
    - infant NEC V20.1
    - patient taking drugs (prescribed) V67.51
      - nonprescribed (*see also* Abuse, drugs, nondependent) 305.9⑤
    - pregnancy V23.9
      - inadequate prenatal care V23.7
      - specified problem NEC V23.8⑤
  - temperature (of unknown origin) (*see also* Pyrexia) 780.6
  - thoracic rib 756.3
  - triglycerides 272.1 ●
    - with high cholesterol 272.2 ●
- **Hildenbrand's disease** (typhus) 081.9
- **Hilger's syndrome** 337.0
- **Hill diarrhea** 579.1
- **Hilliard's lupus** (*see also* Tuberculosis) 017.0⑤
- **Hilum** – *see* condition
- **Hip** – *see* condition
- **Hippel's disease** (retinocerebral angiomatosis) 759.6
- **Hippus** 379.49
- **Hirschfeld's disease** (acute diabetes mellitus) (*see also* Diabetes) 250.0⑤
- **Hirschsprung's disease or megacolon** (congenital) 751.3
- **Hirsuties** (*see also* Hypertrichosis) 704.1
- **Hirsutism** (*see also* Hypertrichosis) 704.1
- **Hirudiniasis** (external) (internal) 134.2
- **His-Werner disease** (trench fever) 083.1
- **Hiss-Russell dysentery** 004.1
- **Histamine cephalgia** 346.2⑤
- **Histidinemia** 270.5
- **Histidinuria** 270.5
- **Histiocytic syndromes** 288.4
- **Histiocytoma** (M8832/0) – *see also* Neoplasm, skin, benign
  - fibrous (M8830/0) – *see also* Neoplasm, skin, benign
    - atypical (M8830/1) – *see* Neoplasm, connective tissue, uncertain behavior
    - malignant (M8830/3) – *see* Neoplasm, connective tissue, malignant
- **Histiocytosis** (acute) (chronic) (subacute) 277.89
  - acute differentiated progressive (M9722/3) 202.5⑤
  - cholesterol 277.89
  - essential 277.89
  - lipid, lipoid (essential) 272.7
  - lipochrome (familial) 288.1
  - malignant (M9720/3) 202.3⑤
  - X (chronic) 277.89
    - acute (progressive) (M9722/3) 202.5⑤
- **Histoplasmosis** 115.90
  - with
    - endocarditis 115.94
    - meningitis 115.91
    - pericarditis 115.93
    - pneumonia 115.95
    - retinitis 115.92
    - specified manifestation NEC 115.99
  - African (due to Histoplasma duboisii) 115.10
    - with
      - endocarditis 115.14
      - meningitis 115.11
      - pericarditis 115.13
      - pneumonia 115.15
      - retinitis 115.12
      - specified manifestation NEC 115.19
  - American (due to Histoplasma capsulatum) 115.00
    - with
      - endocarditis 115.04
      - meningitis 115.01
      - pericarditis 115.03
      - pneumonia 115.05
      - retinitis 115.02
      - specified manifestation NEC 115.09
  - Darling's – *see* Histoplasmosis, American
  - large form (*see also* Histoplasmosis, African) 115.10
  - lung 115.05
  - small form (*see also* Histoplasmosis, American) 115.00
- **History** (personal) **of**
  - abuse
    - emotional V15.42
    - neglect V15.42
    - physical V15.41
    - sexual V15.41
  - affective psychosis V11.1
  - alcoholism V11.3
    - specified as drinking problem (*see also* Abuse, drugs, nondependent) 305.0⑤
  - allergy to
    - analgesic agent NEC V14.6
    - anesthetic NEC V14.4
    - antibiotic agent NEC V14.1
      - penicillin V14.0
    - anti-infective agent NEC V14.3
    - diathesis V15.09
    - drug V14.9
      - specified type NEC V14.8
    - eggs V15.03
    - food additives V15.05
    - insect bite V15.06
    - latex V15.07
    - medicinal agents V14.9
      - specified type NEC V14.8
    - milk products V15.02
    - narcotic agent NEC V14.5
    - nuts V15.05
      - peanuts V15.01
    - penicillin V14.0
    - radiographic dye V15.08
    - seafood V15.04
    - serum V14.7
    - specified food NEC V15.05
    - specified nonmedicinal agents NEC V15.09
    - spider bite V15.06
    - sulfa V14.2
    - sulfonamides V14.2
    - therapeutic agent NEC V15.09
    - vaccine V14.7
  - anemia V12.3
  - arrest, sudden cardiac V12.53 ●

History – *continued*

  - arthritis V13.4
  - attack, transient ischemic (TIA) V12.54 ●
  - benign neoplasm of brain V12.41
  - blood disease V12.3
  - calculi, urinary V13.01
  - cardiovascular disease V12.50
    - myocardial infarction 412
  - child abuse V15.41
  - cigarette smoking V15.82
  - circulatory system disease V12.50
    - myocardial infarction 412
  - congenital malformation V13.69
  - contraception V15.7
  - death, sudden, successfully resuscitated V12.53 ●
  - deficit ●
    - prolonged reversible ischemic neurologic (PRIND) V12.54 ●
    - reversible ischemic neurologic (RIND) V12.54 ●
  - diathesis, allergic V15.09
  - digestive system disease V12.70
    - peptic ulcer V12.71
    - polyps, colonic V12.72
    - specified NEC V12.79
  - disease (of) V13.9
    - blood V12.3
    - blood-forming organs V12.3
    - cardiovascular system V12.50
    - circulatory system V12.50
      - specified NEC V12.59 ●
    - digestive system V12.70
      - peptic ulcer V12.71
      - polyps, colonic V12.72
      - specified NEC V12.79
    - infectious V12.00
      - malaria V12.03
      - poliomyelitis V12.02
      - specified NEC V12.09
      - tuberculosis V12.01
    - parasitic V12.00
      - specified NEC V12.09
    - respiratory system V12.60
      - pneumonia V12.61
      - specified NEC V12.69
    - skin V13.3
    - specified site NEC V13.8
    - subcutaneous tissue V13.3
    - trophoblastic V13.1
      - affecting management of pregnancy V23.1
  - disorder (of) V13.9
    - endocrine V12.2
    - genital system V13.29
    - hematological V12.3
    - immunity V12.2
    - mental V11.9
      - affective type V11.1
      - manic-depressive V11.1
      - neurosis V11.2
      - schizophrenia V11.0
      - specified type NEC V11.8
    - metabolic V12.2
    - musculoskeletal NEC V13.5
    - nervous system V12.40
      - specified type NEC V12.49
    - obstetric V13.29
      - affecting management of current pregnancy V23.49
        - pre-term labor V23.41
      - pre-term labor V13.21
    - sense organs V12.40
      - specified type NEC V12.49
    - specified site NEC V13.8
    - urinary system V13.00
      - calculi V13.01
      - infection V13.02
      - nephrotic syndrome V13.03
      - specified NEC V13.09
  - drug use
    - nonprescribed (*see also* Abuse, drugs, nondependent) 305.9⑤
    - patent (*see also* Abuse, drugs, nondependent) 305.9⑤
  - dysplasia ●
    - cervical (conditions classifiable to 622.10-622.12) V13.22 ●
  - effect NEC of external cause V15.89
  - embolism (pulmonary) V12.51
  - emotional abuse V15.42
  - encephalitis V12.42
  - endocrine disorder V12.2

- **History** – *continued*
  - extracorporeal membrane oxygenation (ECMO) V15.87
  - falling V15.88
  - family
    - allergy V19.6
    - anemia V18.2
    - arteriosclerosis V17.49 ▲
    - arthritis V17.7
    - asthma V17.5
    - blindness V19.0
    - blood disorder NEC V18.3
    - cardiovascular disease V17.49 ▲
    - carrier, genetic disease V18.9
    - cerebrovascular disease V17.1
    - chronic respiratory condition NEC V17.6
    - colonic polyps V18.51
    - congenital anomalies V19.5
    - consanguinity V19.7
    - coronary artery disease V17.3
    - cystic fibrosis V18.19 ▲
    - deafness V19.2
    - diabetes mellitus V18.0
    - digestive disorders V18.59
    - disease or disorder (of)
      - allergic V19.6
      - blood NEC V18.3
      - cardiovascular NEC V17.49 ▲
      - cerebrovascular V17.1
      - colonic polyps V18.51
      - coronary artery V17.3
      - death, sudden cardiac (SCD) V17.41 ●
      - digestive V18.59
      - ear NEC V19.3
      - endocrine V18.19 ▲
        - multiple neoplasia [MEN] syndrome V18.11 ●
      - eye NEC V19.1
      - genitourinary NEC V18.7
      - hypertensive V17.49 ▲
      - infectious V18.8
      - ischemic heart V17.3
      - kidney V18.69
        - polycystic V18.61
      - mental V17.0
      - metabolic V18.19 ▲
      - musculoskeletal NEC V17.89
        - osteoporosis V17.81
      - neurological NEC V17.2
      - parasitic V18.8
      - psychiatric condition V17.0
      - skin condition V19.4
    - ear disorder NEC V19.3
    - endocrine disease V18.19 ▲
      - multiple neoplasia [MEN] syndrome V18.11 ●
    - epilepsy V17.2
    - eye disorder NEC V19.1
    - genetic disease carrier V18.9
    - genitourinary disease NEC V18.7
    - glomerulonephritis V18.69
    - gout V18.19 ▲
    - hay fever V17.6
    - hearing loss V19.2
    - hematopoietic neoplasia V16.7
    - Hodgkin's disease V16.7
    - Huntington's chorea V17.2
    - hydrocephalus V19.5
    - hypertension V17.49 ▲
    - infarction, myocardial V17.3 ●
    - infectious disease V18.8
    - ischemic heart disease V17.3
    - kidney disease V18.69
      - polycystic V18.61
    - leukemia V16.6
    - lymphatic malignant neoplasia NEC V16.7
    - malignant neoplasm (of) NEC V16.9
      - anorectal V16.0
      - anus V16.0
      - appendix V16.0
      - bladder V16.52 ▲
      - bone V16.8
      - brain V16.8
      - breast V16.3
        - male V16.8
      - bronchus V16.1
      - cecum V16.0
      - cervix V16.49
      - colon V16.0
      - duodenum V16.0
      - esophagus V16.0
      - eye V16.8

- **History** – *continued*
  - family – *continued*
    - malignant neoplasm – *continued*
      - gallbladder V16.0
      - gastrointestinal tract V16.0
      - genital organs V16.40
      - hemopoietic NEC V16.7
      - ileum V16.0
      - ilium V16.8
      - intestine V16.0
      - intrathoracic organs NEC V16.2
      - kidney V16.51
      - larynx V16.2
      - liver V16.0
      - lung V16.1
      - lymphatic NEC V16.7
      - ovary V16.41
      - oviduct V16.41
      - pancreas V16.0
      - penis V16.49
      - prostate V16.42
      - rectum V16.0
      - respiratory organs NEC V16.2
      - skin V16.8
      - specified site NEC V16.8
      - stomach V16.0
      - testis V16.43
      - trachea V16.1
      - ureter V16.59
      - urethra V16.59
      - urinary organs V16.59
      - uterus V16.49
      - vagina V16.49
      - vulva V16.49
    - MEN (multiple endocrine neoplasia syndrome) V18.11 ●
    - mental retardation V18.4
    - metabolic disease NEC V18.19 ▲
    - mongolism V19.5
    - multiple
      - endocrine neoplasia [MEN] syndrome V18.11 ●
      - myeloma V16.7 ●
    - musculoskeletal disease NEC V17.89
      - osteoporosis V17.81
    - myocardial infarction V17.3 ●
    - nephritis V18.69
    - nephrosis V18.69
    - osteoporosis V17.81
    - parasitic disease V18.8
    - polycystic kidney disease V18.61
    - psychiatric disorder V17.0
    - psychosis V17.0
    - retardation, mental V18.4
    - retinitis pigmentosa V19.1
    - schizophrenia V17.0
    - skin conditions V19.4
    - specified condition NEC V19.8
    - stroke (cerebrovascular) V17.1
    - sudden cardiac death (SCD) V17.41 ●
    - visual loss V19.0
  - genital system disorder V13.29
    - pre-term labor V13.21
  - health hazard V15.9
    - falling V15.88
    - specified cause NEC V15.89
  - hepatitis
    - B V12.09
    - C V12.09
  - Hodgkin's disease V10.72
  - hypospadias V13.61 ●
  - immunity disorder V12.2
  - infarction, cerebral, without residual deficits V12.54 ●
  - infection
    - central nervous system V12.42
    - urinary (tract) V13.02
  - infectious disease V12.00
    - malaria V12.03
    - poliomyelitis V12.02
    - specified NEC V12.09
    - tuberculosis V12.01
  - injury NEC V15.5
  - insufficient prenatal care V23.7
  - irradiation V15.3
  - leukemia V10.60
    - lymphoid V10.61
    - monocytic V10.63
    - myeloid V10.62
    - specified type NEC V10.69
  - little or no prenatal care V23.7

- **History** – *continued*
  - low birth weight (*see also* Status, low birth weight) V21.30
  - lymphosarcoma V10.71
  - malaria V12.03
  - malignant neoplasm (of) V10.9
    - accessory sinus V10.22
    - adrenal V10.88
    - anus V10.06
    - bile duct V10.09
    - bladder V10.51
    - bone V10.81
    - brain V10.85
    - breast V10.3
    - bronchus V10.11
    - cervix uteri V10.41
    - colon V10.05
    - connective tissue NEC V10.89
    - corpus uteri V10.42
    - digestive system V10.00
      - specified part NEC V10.09
    - duodenum V10.09
    - endocrine gland NEC V10.88
    - epididymis V10.48
    - esophagus V10.03
    - eye V10.84
    - fallopian tube V10.44
    - female genital organ V10.40
      - specified site NEC V10.44
    - gallbladder V10.09
    - gastrointestinal tract V10.00
    - gum V10.02
    - hematopoietic NEC V10.79
    - hypopharynx V10.02
    - ileum V10.09
    - intrathoracic organs NEC V10.20
    - jejunum V10.09
    - kidney V10.52
    - large intestine V10.05
    - larynx V10.21
    - lip V10.02
    - liver V10.07
    - lung V10.11
    - lymphatic NEC V10.79
    - lymph glands or nodes NEC V10.79
    - male genital organ V10.45
      - specified site NEC V10.49
    - mediastinum V10.29
    - melanoma (of skin) V10.82
    - middle ear V10.22
    - mouth V10.02
      - specified part NEC V10.02
    - nasal cavities V10.22
    - nasopharynx V10.02
    - nervous system NEC V10.86
    - nose V10.22
    - oropharynx V10.02
    - ovary V10.43
    - pancreas V10.09
    - parathyroid V10.88
    - penis V10.49
    - pharynx V10.02
    - pineal V10.88
    - pituitary V10.88
    - placenta V10.44
    - pleura V10.29
    - prostate V10.46
    - rectosigmoid junction V10.06
    - rectum V10.06
    - renal pelvis V10.53
    - respiratory organs NEC V10.20
    - salivary gland V10.02
    - skin V10.83
      - melanoma V10.82
    - small intestine NEC V10.09
    - soft tissue NEC V10.89
    - specified site NEC V10.89
    - stomach V10.04
    - testis V10.47
    - thymus V10.29
    - thyroid V10.87
    - tongue V10.01
    - trachea V10.12
    - ureter V10.59
    - urethra V10.59
    - urinary organ V10.50
    - uterine adnexa V10.44
    - uterus V10.42
    - vagina V10.44
    - vulva V10.44
  - manic-depressive psychosis V11.1
  - meningitis V12.42

History – *continued*
- mental disorder V11.9
  - affective type V11.1
  - manic-depressive V11.1
  - neurosis V11.2
  - schizophrenia V11.0
  - specified type NEC V11.8
- metabolic disorder V12.2
- musculoskeletal disorder NEC V13.5
- myocardial infarction 412
- neglect (emotional) V15.42
- nephrotic syndrome V13.03
- nervous system disorder V12.40
  - specified type NEC V12.49
- neurosis V11.2
- noncompliance with medical treatment V15.81
- nutritional deficiency V12.1
- obstetric disorder V13.29
  - affecting management of current pregnancy V23.49
    - pre-term labor V23.41
  - pre-term labor V13.21
- parasitic disease V12.00
  - specified NEC V12.09
- perinatal problems V13.7
  - low birth weight (*see also* Status, low birth weight) V21.30
- physical abuse V15.41
- poisoning V15.6
- poliomyelitis V12.02
- polyps, colonic V12.72
- poor obstetric V13.29
  - affecting management of current pregnancy V23.49
    - pre-term labor V23.41
  - pre-term labor V13.21
- prolonged reversible ischemic neurologic deficit (PRIND) V12.54 ●
- psychiatric disorder V11.9
  - affective type V11.1
  - manic-depressive V11.1
  - neurosis V11.2
  - schizophrenia V11.0
  - specified type NEC V11.8
- psychological trauma V15.49
  - emotional abuse V15.42
  - neglect V15.42
  - physical abuse V15.41
  - rape V15.41
- psychoneurosis V11.2
- radiation therapy V15.3
- rape V15.41
- respiratory system disease V12.60
  - pneumonia V12.61
  - specified NEC V12.69
- reticulosarcoma V10.71
- reversible ischemic neurologic deficit (RIND) V12.54 ●
- schizophrenia V11.0
- skin disease V13.3
- smoking (tobacco) V15.82
- stroke without residual deficits V12.54 ●
- subcutaneous tissue disease V13.3
- sudden ●
  - cardiac ●
    - arrest V12.53 ●
    - death (successfully resuscitated) V12.53 ●
- surgery (major) to
  - great vessels V15.1
  - heart V15.1
  - major organs NEC V15.2
- syndrome, nephrotic V13.03
- thrombophlebitis V12.52
- thrombosis V12.51
- tobacco use V15.82
- trophoblastic disease V13.1
  - affecting management of pregnancy V23.1
- tuberculosis V12.01
- ulcer, peptic V12.71
- urinary system disorder V13.00
  - calculi V13.01
  - infection V13.02
  - nephrotic syndrome V13.03
  - specified NEC V13.09

HIV infection (disease) (illness) – *see* Human immunodeficiency virus (disease) (illness) (infection)

Hives (bold) (*see also* Urticaria) 708.9

Hoarseness 784.49

Hobnail liver – *see* Cirrhosis, portal

Hobo, hoboism V60.0

Hodgkin's
- disease (M9650/3) 201.9⑤
  - lymphocytic
    - depletion (M9653/3) 201.7⑤
      - diffuse fibrosis (M9654/3) 201.7⑤
      - reticular type (M9655/3) 201.7⑤
    - predominance (M9651/3) 201.4⑤
  - lymphocytic-histiocytic predominance (M9651/3) 201.4⑤
  - mixed cellularity (M9652/3) 201.6⑤
  - nodular sclerosis (M9656/3) 201.5⑤
    - cellular phase (M9657/3) 201.5⑤
- granuloma (M9661/3) 201.1⑤
- lymphogranulomatosis (M9650/3) 201.9⑤
- lymphoma (M9650/3) 201.9⑤
- lymphosarcoma (M9650/3) 201.9⑤
- paragranuloma (M9660/3) 201.0⑤
- sarcoma (M9662/3) 201.2⑤

Hodgson's disease (aneurysmal dilatation of aorta) 441.9
- ruptured 441.5

Hodi-potsy 111.0

Hoffa (-Kastert) **disease or syndrome** (liposynovitis prepatellaris) 272.8

Hoffmann's syndrome 244.9 *[359.5]*

Hoffmann-Bouveret syndrome (paroxysmal tachycardia) 427.2

Hole
- macula 362.54
- optic disc, crater-like 377.22
- retina (macula) 362.54
  - round 361.31
    - with detachment 361.01

Holla disease (*see also* Spherocytosis) 282.0

Holländer-Simons syndrome (progressive lipodystrophy) 272.6

Hollow foot (congenital) 754.71
- acquired 736.73

Holmes' syndrome (visual disorientation) 368.16

Holoprosencephaly 742.2
- due to
  - trisomy 13 758.1
  - trisomy 18 758.2

Holthouse's hernia – *see* Hernia, inguinal

Homesickness 309.89

Homocystinemia 270.4

Homocystinuria 270.4

Homologous serum jaundice (prophylactic) (therapeutic) – *see* Hepatitis, viral

Homosexuality - omit code
- ego-dystonic 302.0
- pedophilic 302.2
- problems with 302.0

Homozygous Hb-S disease 282.61

Honeycomb lung 518.89
- congenital 748.4

Hong Kong ear 117.3

HOOD (hereditary osteo-onychodysplasia) 756.89

Hooded
- clitoris 752.49
- penis 752.69

Hookworm (anemia) (disease) (infestation) – *see* Ancylostomiasis

Hoppe-Goldflam syndrome 358.00

Hordeolum (external) (eyelid) 373.11
- internal 373.12

Horn
- cutaneous 702.8
  - cheek 702.8
  - eyelid 702.8
  - penis 702.8
- iliac 756.89
- nail 703.8
  - congenital 757.5
- papillary 700

Horner's
- syndrome (*see also* Neuropathy, peripheral, autonomic) 337.9
  - traumatic 954.0
- teeth 520.4

Horseshoe kidney (congenital) 753.3

Horton's
- disease (temporal arteritis) 446.5
- headache or neuralgia 346.2⑤

Hospice care V66.7

Hospitalism (in children) NEC 309.83

Hourglass contraction, contracture
- bladder 596.8
- gallbladder 575.2
  - congenital 751.69
- stomach 536.8
  - congenital 750.7
  - psychogenic 306.4
- uterus 661.4⑤
  - affecting fetus or newborn 763.7

Household circumstance affecting care V60.9
- specified type NEC V60.8

Housemaid's knee 727.2

Housing circumstance affecting care V60.9
- specified type NEC V60.8

Huchard's disease (continued arterial hypertension) 401.9

Hudson-Stähli lines 371.11

Huguier's disease (uterine fibroma) 218.9

Hum, venous - omit code

Human bite (open wound) - (*see also* Wound, open, by site)
- intact skin surface – *see* Contusion

Human immunodeficiency virus (disease) (illness) 042
- infection V08
  - with symptoms, symptomatic 042

Human immunodeficiency virus-2 infection 079.53

Human immunovirus (disease) (illness) (infection) – *see* Human immunodeficiency virus (disease) (illness) (infection)

Human papillomavirus 079.4
- cervical
  - high risk, DNA test positive 795.05
  - low risk, DNA test positive 795.09

Human parvovirus 079.83 ●

Human T-cell lymphotrophic virus I infection 079.51

Human T-cell lymphotrophic virus II infection 079.52

Human T-cell lymphotropic virus-III (disease) (illness) (infection) – *see* Human immunodeficiency virus (disease) (illness) (infection)

HTLV-I infection 079.51

HTLV-II infection 079.52

HTLV-III (disease) (illness) (infection) – *see* Human immunodeficiency virus (disease) (illness) (infection)

HTLV-III/LAV (disease) (illness) (infection) – *see* Human immunodeficiency virus (disease) (illness) (infection)

Humpback (acquired) 737.9
- congenital 756.19

Hunchback (acquired) 737.9
- congenital 756.19

Hunger 994.2
- air, psychogenic 306.1
- disease 251.1

Hunner's ulcer (*see also* Cystitis) 595.1

Hunt's
- neuralgia 053.11
- syndrome (herpetic geniculate ganglionitis) 053.11
  - dyssynergia cerebellaris myoclonica 334.2

Hunter's glossitis 529.4

Hunter (-Hurler) syndrome (mucopolysaccharidosis II) 277.5

Hunterian chancre 091.0

Huntington's
- chorea 333.4
- disease 333.4

Huppert's disease (multiple myeloma) (M9730/3) 203.0⑤

Hurler (-Hunter) **disease or syndrome** (mucopolysaccharidosis II) 277.5

Hürthle cell
- adenocarcinoma (M8290/3) 193
- adenoma (M8290/0) 226
- carcinoma (M8290/3) 193
- tumor (M8290/0) 226

Hutchinson's
- disease meaning
  - angioma serpiginosum 709.1
  - cheiropompholyx 705.81
  - prurigo estivalis 692.72
  - summer eruption, or summer prurigo 692.72
- incisors 090.5

Hutchinson's – *continued*
melanotic freckle (M8742/2) – *see also* Neoplasm, skin, in situ
malignant melanoma in (M8742/3) – *see* Melanoma
teeth or incisors (congenital syphilis) 090.5
Hutchinson-Boeck disease or syndrome (sarcoidosis) 135
Hutchinson-Gilford disease or syndrome (progeria) 259.8
Hyaline
degeneration (diffuse) (generalized) 728.9
localized – *see* Degeneration, by site
membrane (disease) (lung) (newborn) 769
Hyalinosis cutis et mucosae 272.8
Hyalin plaque, sclera, senile 379.16
Hyalitis (asteroid) 379.22
syphilitic 095.8
Hydatid
cyst or tumor – *see also* Echinococcus
fallopian tube 752.11
mole – *see* Hydatidiform mole
Morgagni (congenital) 752.89
fallopian tube 752.11
Hydatidiform mole (benign) (complicating pregnancy) (delivered) (undelivered) 630
invasive (M9100/1) 236.1
malignant (M9100/1) 236.1
previous, affecting management of pregnancy V23.1
Hydatidosis – *see* Echinococcus
Hyde's disease (prurigo nodularis) 698.3
Hydradenitis 705.83
Hydradenoma (M8400/0) – *see* Hidradenoma
Hydralazine lupus or syndrome
correct substance properly administered 695.4
overdose or wrong substance given or taken 972.6
Hydramnios 657❹
affecting fetus or newborn 761.3
Hydrancephaly 742.3
with spina bifida (*see also* Spina bifida) 741.0❺
Hydranencephaly 742.3
with spina bifida (*see also* Spina bifida) 741.0❺
Hydrargyrism NEC 985.0
Hydrarthrosis (*see also* Effusion, joint) 719.0❺
gonococcal 098.50
intermittent (*see also* Rheumatism, palindromic) 719.3❺
of yaws (early) (late) 102.6
syphilitic 095.8
congenital 090.5
Hydremia 285.9
Hydrencephalocele (congenital) 742.0
Hydrencephalomeningocele (congenital) 742.0
Hydroa 694.0
aestivale 692.72
gestationis 646.8❺
herpetiformis 694.0
pruriginosa 694.0
vacciniforme 692.72
Hydroadenitis 705.83
Hydrocalycosis (*see also* Hydronephrosis) 591
congenital 753.29
Hydrocalyx (*see also* Hydronephrosis) 591
Hydrocele (calcified) (chylous) (idiopathic) (infantile) (inguinal canal) (recurrent) (senile) (spermatic cord) (testis) (tunica vaginalis) 603.9
canal of Nuck (female) 629.1
male 603.9
congenital 778.6
encysted 603.0
congenital 778.6
female NEC 629.89
infected 603.1
round ligament 629.89
specified type NEC 603.8
congenital 778.6
spinalis (*see also* Spina bifida) 741.9❺
vulva 624.8
Hydrocephalic fetus
affecting management or pregnancy 655.0❺
causing disproportion 653.6❺
with obstructed labor 660.1❺
affecting fetus or newborn 763.1

Hydrocephalus (acquired) (external) (internal) (malignant) (noncommunicating) (obstructive) (recurrent) 331.4
aqueduct of Sylvius stricture 742.3
with spina bifida (*see also* Spina bifida) 741.0❺
chronic 742.3
with spina bifida (*see also* Spina bifida) 741.0❺
communicating 331.3
congenital (external) (internal) 742.3
with spina bifida (*see also* Spina bifida) 741.0❺
due to
stricture of aqueduct of Sylvius 742.3
with spina bifida (*see also* Spina bifida) 741.0❺
toxoplasmosis (congenital) 771.2
fetal affecting management of pregnancy 655.0❺
foramen Magendie block (acquired) 331.3
congenital 742.3
with spina bifida (*see also* Spina bifida) 741.0❺
newborn 742.3
with spina bifida (*see also* Spina bifida) 741.0❺
normal pressure 331.5 ●
idiopathic (INPH) 331.5 ●
secondary 331.3 ●
otitic 348.2
syphilitic, congenital 090.49
tuberculous (*see also* Tuberculosis) 013.8❺
Hydrocolpos (congenital) 623.8
Hydrocystoma (M8404/0) – *see* Neoplasm, skin, benign
Hydroencephalocele (congenital) 742.0
Hydroencephalomeningocele (congenital) 742.0
Hydrohematopneumothorax (*see also* Hemothorax) 511.8
Hydromeningitis – *see* Meningitis
Hydromeningocele (spinal) (*see also* Spina bifida) 741.9❺
cranial 742.0
Hydrometra 621.8
Hydrometrocolpos 623.8
Hydromicrocephaly 742.1
Hydromphalus (congenital) (since birth) 757.39
Hydromyelia 742.53
Hydromyelocele (*see also* Spina bifida) 741.9❺
Hydronephrosis 591
atrophic 591
congenital 753.29
due to S. hematobium 120.0
early 591
functionless (infected) 591
infected 591
intermittent 591
primary 591
secondary 591
tuberculous (*see also* Tuberculosis) 016.0❺
Hydropericarditis (*see also* Pericarditis) 423.9
Hydropericardium (*see also* Pericarditis) 423.9
Hydroperitoneum 789.59 ▲
Hydrophobia 071
Hydrophthalmos (*see also* Buphthalmia) 743.20
Hydropneumohemothorax (*see also* Hemothorax) 511.8
Hydropneumopericarditis (*see also* Pericarditis) 423.9
Hydropneumopericardium (*see also* Pericarditis) 423.9
Hydropneumothorax 511.8
nontuberculous 511.8
bacterial 511.1
pneumococcal 511.1
staphylococcal 511.1
streptococcal 511.1
traumatic 860.0
with open wound into thorax 860.1
tuberculous (*see also* Tuberculosis, pleura) 012.0❺
Hydrops 782.3
abdominis 789.59 ▲
amnii (complicating pregnancy) (*see also* Hydramnios) 657❹

Hydrops – *continued*
articulorum intermittens (*see also* Rheumatism, palindromic) 719.3❺
cardiac (*see also* Failure, heart) 428.0
congenital – *see* Hydrops, fetalis
endolymphatic (*see also* Disease, Ménière's) 386.00
fetal(is) or newborn 778.0
due to isoimmunization 773.3
not due to isoimmunization 778.0
gallbladder 575.3
idiopathic (fetus or newborn) 778.0
joint (*see also* Effusion, joint) 719.0❺
labyrinth (*see also* Disease, Ménière's) 386.00
meningeal NEC 331.4
nutritional 262
pericardium – *see* Pericarditis
pleura (*see also* Hydrothorax) 511.8
renal (*see also* Nephrosis) 581.9
spermatic cord (*see also* Hydrocele) 603.9
Hydropyonephrosis (*see also* Pyelitis) 590.80
chronic 590.00
Hydrorachis 742.53
Hydrorrhea (nasal) 478.19
gravidarum 658.1❺
pregnancy 658.1❺
Hydrosadenitis 705.83
Hydrosalpinx (fallopian tube) (follicularis) 614.1
Hydrothorax (double) (pleural) 511.8
chylous (nonfilarial) 457.8
filaria (*see also* Infestation, filarial) 125.9
nontuberculous 511.8
bacterial 511.1
pneumococcal 511.1
staphylococcal 511.1
streptococcal 511.1
traumatic 862.29
with open wound into thorax 862.39
tuberculous (*see also* Tuberculosis, pleura) 012.0❺
Hydroureter 593.5
congenital 753.22
Hydroureteronephrosis (*see also* Hydronephrosis) 591
Hydrourethra 599.84
Hydroxykynureninuria 270.2
Hydroxyprolinemia 270.8
Hydroxyprolinuria 270.8
Hygroma (congenital) (cystic) (M9173/0) 228.1
prepatellar 727.3
subdural – *see* Hematoma, subdural
Hymen – *see* condition
Hymenolepiasis (diminuta) (infection) (infestation) (nana) 123.6
Hymenolepsis (diminuta) (infection) (infestation) (nana) 123.6
Hypalgesia (*see also* Disturbance, sensation) 782.0
Hyperabduction syndrome 447.8
Hyperacidity, gastric 536.8
psychogenic 306.4
Hyperactive, hyperactivity 314.01 ▲
basal cell, uterine cervix 622.10
bladder 596.51
bowel (syndrome) 564.9
sounds 787.5
cervix epithelial (basal) 622.10
child 314.01
colon 564.9
gastrointestinal 536.8
psychogenic 306.4
intestine 564.9
labyrinth (unilateral) 386.51
with loss of labyrinthine reactivity 386.58
bilateral 386.52
nasal mucous membrane 478.19
stomach 536.8
thyroid (gland) (*see also* Thyrotoxicosis) 242.9❺
Hyperacusis 388.42
Hyperadrenalism (cortical) 255.3
medullary 255.6
Hyperadrenocorticism 255.3
congenital 255.2
iatrogenic
correct substance properly administered 255.3
overdose or wrong substance given or taken 962.0
Hyperaffectivity 301.11

- **Hyperaldosteronism** (atypical) (hyperplastic) (normoaldosteronal) (normotensive) (primary) 255.10
  - secondary 255.14
- **Hyperalgesia** (*see also* Disturbance, sensation) 782.0
- **Hyperalimentation** 783.6
  - carotene 278.3
  - specified NEC 278.8
  - vitamin A 278.2
  - vitamin D 278.4
- **Hyperaminoaciduria** 270.9
  - arginine 270.6
  - citrulline 270.6
  - cystine 270.0
  - glycine 270.0
  - lysine 270.7
  - ornithine 270.6
  - renal (types I, II, III) 270.0
- **Hyperammonemia** (congenital) 270.6
- **Hyperamnesia** 780.99
- **Hyperamylasemia** 790.5
- **Hyperaphia** 782.0
- **Hyperazotemia** 791.9
- **Hyperbetalipoproteinemia** (acquired) (essential) (familial) (hereditary) (primary) (secondary) 272.0
  - with prebetalipoproteinemia 272.2
- **Hyperbilirubinemia** 782.4
  - congenital 277.4
  - constitutional 277.4
  - neonatal (transient) (*see also* Jaundice, fetus or newborn) 774.6
    - of prematurity 774.2
- **Hyperbilirubinemica encephalopathia, newborn** 774.7
  - due to isoimmunization 773.4
- **Hypercalcemia, hypercalcemic** (idiopathic) 275.42
  - nephropathy 588.89
- **Hypercalcinuria** 275.40
- **Hypercapnia** 786.09
  - with mixed acid-based disorder 276.4
  - fetal, affecting newborn 770.89
- **Hypercarotinemia** 278.3
- **Hypercementosis** 521.5
- **Hyperchloremia** 276.9
- **Hyperchlorhydria** 536.8
  - neurotic 306.4
  - psychogenic 306.4
- **Hypercholesterinemia** – *see* Hypercholesterolemia
- **Hypercholesterolemia** 272.0
  - with hyperglyceridemia, endogenous 272.2
  - essential 272.0
  - familial 272.0
  - hereditary 272.0
  - primary 272.0
  - pure 272.0
- **Hypercholesterolosis** 272.0
- **Hyperchylia gastrica** 536.8
  - psychogenic 306.4
- **Hyperchylomicronemia** (familial) (with hyperbetalipoproteinemia) 272.3
- **Hypercoagulation syndrome** (primary) 289.81
  - secondary 289.82
- **Hypercorticosteronism**
  - correct substance properly administered 255.3
  - overdose or wrong substance given or taken 962.0
- **Hypercortisonism**
  - correct substance properly administered 255.3
  - overdose or wrong substance given or taken 962.0
- **Hyperdynamic beta-adrenergic state or syndrome** (circulatory) 429.82
- **Hyperekplexia** 759.89
- **Hyperelectrolytemia** 276.9
- **Hyperemesis** 536.2
  - arising during pregnancy – *see* Hyperemesis, gravidarum
  - gravidarum (mild) (before 22 completed weeks gestation) 643.0❺
    - with
      - carbohydrate depletion 643.1❺
      - dehydration 643.1❺
      - electrolyte imbalance 643.1❺
      - metabolic disturbance 643.1❺
- **Hyperemesis** – *continued*
  - gravidarum – *continued*
    - affecting fetus or newborn 761.8
    - severe (with metabolic disturbance) 643.1❺
  - psychogenic 306.4
- **Hyperemia** (acute) 780.99
  - anal mucosa 569.49
  - bladder 596.7
  - cerebral 437.8
  - conjunctiva 372.71
  - ear, internal, acute 386.30
  - enteric 564.89
  - eye 372.71
  - eyelid (active) (passive) 374.82
  - intestine 564.89
  - iris 364.41
  - kidney 593.81
  - labyrinth 386.30
  - liver (active) (passive) 573.8
  - lung 514
  - ovary 620.8
  - passive 780.99
  - pulmonary 514
  - renal 593.81
  - retina 362.89
  - spleen 289.59
  - stomach 537.89
- **Hyperesthesia** (body surface) (*see also* Disturbance sensation) 782.0
  - larynx (reflex) 478.79
    - hysterical 300.11
  - pharynx (reflex) 478.29
- **Hyperestrinism** 256.0
- **Hyperestrogenism** 256.0
- **Hyperestrogenosis** 256.0
- **Hyperexplexia** 759.89
- **Hyperextension, joint** 718.80
  - ankle 718.87
  - elbow 718.82
  - foot 718.87
  - hand 718.84
  - hip 718.85
  - knee 718.86
  - multiple sites 718.89
  - pelvic region 718.85
  - shoulder (region) 718.81
  - specified site NEC 718.88
  - wrist 718.83
- **Hyperfibrinolysis** – *see* Fibrinolysis
- **Hyperfolliculinism** 256.0
- **Hyperfructosemia** 271.2
- **Hyperfunction**
  - adrenal (cortex) 255.3
    - androgenic, acquired benign 255.3
    - medulla 255.6
    - virilism 255.2
  - corticoadrenal NEC 255.3
  - labyrinth – *see* Hyperactive, labyrinth
  - medulloadrenal 255.6
  - ovary 256.1
    - estrogen 256.0
  - pancreas 577.8
  - parathyroid (gland) 252.00
  - pituitary (anterior) (gland) (lobe) 253.1
  - testicular 257.0
- **Hypergammaglobulinemia** 289.89
  - monoclonal, benign (BMH) 273.1
  - polyclonal 273.0
  - Waldenström's 273.0
- **Hyperglobulinemia** 273.8
- **Hyperglycemia** 790.29
  - maternal
    - affecting fetus or newborn 775.0
    - manifest diabetes in infant 775.1
  - postpancreatectomy (complete) (partial) 251.3
- **Hyperglyceridemia** 272.1
  - endogenous 272.1
  - essential 272.1
  - familial 272.1
  - hereditary 272.1
  - mixed 272.3
  - pure 272.1
- **Hyperglycinemia** 270.7
- **Hypergonadism**
  - ovarian 256.1
  - testicular (infantile) (primary) 257.0
- **Hyperheparinemia** (*see also* Circulating anticoagulants) 286.5
- **Hyperhidrosis, hyperidrosis** 705.21
  - axilla 705.21
  - face 705.21
  - focal (localized) 705.21
    - primary 705.21
      - axilla 705.21
      - face 705.21
      - palms 705.21
      - soles 705.21
    - secondary 705.22
      - axilla 705.22
      - face 705.22
      - palms 705.22
      - soles 705.22
  - generalized 780.8
  - palms 705.21
  - psychogenic 306.3
  - secondary 780.8
  - soles 705.21
- **Hyperhistidinemia** 270.5
- **Hyperinsulinism** (ectopic) (functional) (organic) NEC 251.1
  - iatrogenic 251.0
  - reactive 251.2
  - spontaneous 251.2
  - therapeutic misadventure (from administration of insulin) 962.3
- **Hyperiodemia** 276.9
- **Hyperirritability** (cerebral), in newborn 779.1
- **Hyperkalemia** 276.7
- **Hyperkeratosis** (*see also* Keratosis) 701.1
  - cervix 622.2
  - congenital 757.39
  - cornea 371.89
  - due to yaws (early) (late) (palmar or plantar) 102.3
  - eccentrica 757.39
  - figurata centrifuga atrophica 757.39
  - follicularis 757.39
    - in cutem penetrans 701.1
  - limbic (cornea) 371.89
  - palmoplantaris climacterica 701.1
  - pinta (carate) 103.1
  - senile (with pruritus) 702.0
  - tongue 528.79
  - universalis congenita 757.1
  - vagina 623.1
  - vocal cord 478.5
  - vulva 624.09 ▲
- **Hyperkinesia, hyperkinetic** (disease) (reaction) (syndrome) 314.9
  - with
    - attention deficit – *see* Disorder, attention deficit
    - conduct disorder 314.2
    - developmental delay 314.1
    - simple disturbance of activity and attention 314.01
    - specified manifestation NEC 314.8
  - heart (disease) 429.82
  - of childhood or adolescence NEC 314.9
- **Hyperlacrimation** (*see also* Epiphora) 375.20
- **Hyperlipemia** (*see also* Hyperlipidemia) 272.4
- **Hyperlipidemia** 272.4
  - carbohydrate-induced 272.1
  - combined 272.4
  - endogenous 272.1
  - exogenous 272.3
  - fat-induced 272.3
  - group
    - A 272.0
    - B 272.1
    - C 272.2
    - D 272.3
  - mixed 272.2
  - specified type NEC 272.4
- **Hyperlipidosis** 272.7
  - hereditary 272.7
- **Hyperlipoproteinemia** (acquired) (essential) (familial) (hereditary) (primary) (secondary) 272.4
  - Fredrickson type
    - I 272.3
    - IIa 272.0
    - IIb 272.2
    - III 272.2
    - IV 272.1
    - V 272.3
  - low-density-lipoid-type (LDL) 272.0
  - very-low-density-lipoid-type [VLDL] 272.1
- **Hyperlucent lung, unilateral** 492.8

- **Hyperluteinization** 256.1
- **Hyperlysinemia** 270.7
- **Hypermagnesemia** 275.2
  - neonatal 775.5
- **Hypermaturity** (fetus or newborn)
  - post term infant 766.21
  - prolonged gestation infant 766.22
- **Hypermenorrhea** 626.2
- **Hypermetabolism** 794.7
- **Hypermethioninemia** 270.4
- **Hypermetropia** (congenital) 367.0
- **Hypermobility**
  - cecum 564.9
  - coccyx 724.71
  - colon 564.9
    - psychogenic 306.4
  - ileum 564.89
  - joint (acquired) 718.80
    - ankle 718.87
    - elbow 718.82
    - foot 718.87
    - hand 718.84
    - hip 718.85
    - knee 718.86
    - multiple sites 718.89
    - pelvic region 718.85
    - shoulder (region) 718.81
    - specified site NEC 718.88
    - wrist 718.83
  - kidney, congenital 753.3
  - meniscus (knee) 717.5
  - scapula 718.81
  - stomach 536.8
    - psychogenic 306.4
  - syndrome 728.5
  - testis, congenital 752.52
  - urethral 599.81
- **Hypermotility**
  - gastrointestinal 536.8
  - intestine 564.9
    - psychogenic 306.4
  - stomach 536.8
- **Hypernasality** 784.49
- **Hypernatremia** 276.0
  - with water depletion 276.0
- **Hypernephroma** (M8312/3) 189.0
- **Hyperopia** 367.0
- **Hyperorexia** 783.6
- **Hyperornithinemia** 270.6
- **Hyperosmia** (*see also* Disturbance, sensation) 781.1
- **Hyperosmolality** 276.0
- **Hyperosteogenesis** 733.99
- **Hyperostosis** 733.99
  - calvarial 733.3
  - cortical 733.3
    - infantile 756.59
  - frontal, internal of skull 733.3
  - interna frontalis 733.3
  - monomelic 733.99
  - skull 733.3
    - congenital 756.0
  - vertebral 721.8
    - with spondylosis – *see* Spondylosis
    - ankylosing 721.6
- **Hyperovarianism** 256.1
- **Hyperovarism, hyperovaria** 256.1
- **Hyperoxaluria** (primary) 271.8
- **Hyperoxia** 987.8
- **Hyperparathyroidism** 252.00
  - ectopic 259.3
  - other 252.08
  - primary 252.01
  - secondary (of renal origin) 588.81
    - non-renal 252.02
  - tertiary 252.08
- **Hyperpathia** (*see also* Disturbance, sensation) 782.0
  - psychogenic 307.80
- **Hyperperistalsis** 787.4
  - psychogenic 306.4
- **Hyperpermeability, capillary** 448.9
- **Hyperphagia** 783.6
- **Hyperphenylalaninemia** 270.1
- **Hyperphoria** 378.40
  - alternating 378.45
- **Hyperphosphatemia** 275.3
- **Hyperpiesia** (*see also* Hypertension) 401.9
- **Hyperpiesis** (*see also* Hypertension) 401.9
- **Hyperpigmentation** – *see* Pigmentation
- **Hyperpinealism** 259.8
- **Hyperpipecolatemia** 270.7
- **Hyperpituitarism** 253.1
- **Hyperplasia, hyperplastic**
  - adenoids (lymphoid tissue) 474.12
    - and tonsils 474.10
  - adrenal (capsule) (cortex) (gland) 255.8
    - with
      - sexual precocity (male) 255.2
      - virilism, adrenal 255.2
      - virilization (female) 255.2
    - congenital 255.2
    - due to excess ACTH (ectopic) (pituitary) 255.0
    - medulla 255.8
  - alpha cells (pancreatic)
    - with
      - gastrin excess 251.5
      - glucagon excess 251.4
  - appendix (lymphoid) 543.0
  - artery, fibromuscular NEC 447.8
    - carotid 447.8
    - renal 447.3
  - bone 733.99
    - marrow 289.9
  - breast (*see also* Hypertrophy, breast) 611.1
  - carotid artery 447.8
  - cementation, cementum (teeth) (tooth) 521.5
  - cervical gland 785.6
  - cervix (uteri) 622.10
    - basal cell 622.10
    - congenital 752.49
    - endometrium 622.10
    - polypoid 622.10
  - chin 524.05
  - clitoris, congenital 752.49
  - dentin 521.5
  - endocervicitis 616.0
  - endometrium, endometrial (adenomatous) (atypical) (cystic) (glandular) (polypoid) (uterus) 621.30
    - with atypia 621.33
    - without atypia
      - complex 621.32
      - simple 621.31
    - cervix 622.10
  - epithelial 709.8
    - focal, oral, including tongue 528.79
    - mouth (focal) 528.79
    - nipple 611.8
    - skin 709.8
    - tongue (focal) 528.79
    - vaginal wall 623.0
  - erythroid 289.9
  - fascialis ossificans (progressiva) 728.11
  - fibromuscular, artery NEC 447.8
    - carotid 447.8
    - renal 447.3
  - genital
    - female 629.89
    - male 608.89
  - gingiva 523.8
  - glandularis
    - cystica uteri 621.30
    - endometrium (uterus) 621.30
    - interstitialis uteri 621.30
  - granulocytic 288.69
  - gum 523.8
  - hymen, congenital 752.49
  - islands of Langerhans 251.1
  - islet cell (pancreatic) 251.9
    - alpha cells
      - with excess
        - gastrin 251.5
        - glucagon 251.4
    - beta cells 251.1
  - juxtaglomerular (complex) (kidney) 593.89
  - kidney (congenital) 753.3
  - liver (congenital) 751.69
  - lymph node (gland) 785.6
  - lymphoid (diffuse) (nodular) 785.6
    - appendix 543.0
    - intestine 569.89
  - mandibular 524.02
    - alveolar 524.72
    - unilateral condylar 526.89
  - Marchand multiple nodular (liver) – *see* Cirrhosis, postnecrotic
  - maxillary 524.01
    - alveolar 524.71
  - medulla, adrenal 255.8

Hyperplasia, hyperplastic – *continued*

  - myometrium, myometrial 621.2
  - nose (lymphoid) (polypoid) 478.19
  - oral soft tissue (inflammatory) (irritative) (mucosa) NEC 528.9
    - gingiva 523.8
    - tongue 529.8
  - organ or site, congenital NEC – *see* Anomaly, specified type NEC
  - ovary 620.8
  - palate, papillary 528.9
  - pancreatic islet cells 251.9
    - alpha
      - with excess
        - gastrin 251.5
        - glucagon 251.4
    - beta 251.1
  - parathyroid (gland) 252.01
  - persistent, vitreous (primary) 743.51
  - pharynx (lymphoid) 478.29
  - prostate 600.90
    - with
      - other lower urinary tract symptoms (LUTS) 600.91
      - urinary
        - obstruction 600.91
        - retention 600.91
    - adenofibromatous 600.20
      - with
        - other lower urinary tract symptoms (LUTS) 600.21
        - urinary
          - obstruction 600.21
          - retention 600.21
    - nodular 600.10
      - with
        - urinary
          - obstruction 600.11
          - retention 600.11
  - renal artery (fibromuscular) 447.3
  - reticuloendothelial (cell) 289.9
  - salivary gland (any) 527.1
  - Schimmelbusch's 610.1
  - suprarenal (capsule) (gland) 255.8
  - thymus (gland) (persistent) 254.0
  - thyroid (*see also* Goiter) 240.9
    - primary 242.0❺
    - secondary 242.2❺
  - tonsil (lymphoid tissue) 474.11
    - and adenoids 474.10
  - urethrovaginal 599.89
  - uterus, uterine (myometrium) 621.2
    - endometrium (*see also* Hyperplasia, endometrium) 621.30
  - vitreous (humor), primary persistent 743.51
  - vulva 624.3
  - zygoma 738.11
- **Hyperpnea** (*see also* Hyperventilation) 786.01
- **Hyperpotassemia** 276.7
- **Hyperprebetalipoproteinemia** 272.1
  - with chylomicronemia 272.3
  - familial 272.1
- **Hyperprolactinemia** 253.1
- **Hyperprolinemia** 270.8
- **Hyperproteinemia** 273.8
- **Hyperprothrombinemia** 289.89
- **Hyperpselaphesia** 782.0
- **Hyperpyrexia** 780.6
  - heat (effects of) 992.0
  - malarial (*see also* Malaria) 084.6
  - malignant, due to anesthetic 995.86
  - rheumatic – *see* Fever, rheumatic
  - unknown origin (*see also* Pyrexia) 780.6
- **Hyperreactor, vascular** 780.2
- **Hyperreflexia** 796.1
  - bladder, autonomic 596.54
    - with cauda equina 344.61
  - detrusor 344.61
- **Hypersalivation** (*see also* Ptyalism) 527.7
- **Hypersarcosinemia** 270.8
- **Hypersecretion**
  - ACTH 255.3
  - androgens (ovarian) 256.1
  - calcitonin 246.0
  - corticoadrenal 255.3
  - cortisol 255.0
  - estrogen 256.0
  - gastric 536.8
    - psychogenic 306.4
  - gastrin 251.5

Hypersecretion – *continued*
- glucagon 251.4
- hormone
  - ACTH 255.3
  - anterior pituitary 253.1
  - growth NEC 253.0
  - ovarian androgen 256.1
  - testicular 257.0
  - thyroid stimulating 242.8❺
- insulin – *see* Hyperinsulinism
- lacrimal glands (*see also* Epiphora) 375.20
- medulloadrenal 255.6
- milk 676.6❺
- ovarian androgens 256.1
- pituitary (anterior) 253.1
- salivary gland (any) 527.7
- testicular hormones 257.0
- thyrocalcitonin 246.0
- upper respiratory 478.9

Hypersegmentation, hereditary 288.2
- eosinophils 288.2
- neutrophil nuclei 288.2

Hypersensitive, hypersensitiveness, hypersensitivity – *see also* Allergy
- angiitis 446.20
  - specified NEC 446.29
- carotid sinus 337.0
- colon 564.9
  - psychogenic 306.4
- DNA (deoxyribonucleic acid) NEC 287.2
- drug (*see also* Allergy, drug) 995.27
- esophagus 530.89
- insect bites – *see* Injury, superficial, by site
- labyrinth 386.58
- pain (*see also* Disturbance, sensation) 782.0
- pneumonitis NEC 495.9
- reaction (*see also* Allergy) 995.3
  - upper respiratory tract NEC 478.8
- stomach (allergic) (nonallergic) 536.8
  - psychogenic 306.4

Hypersomatotropism (classic) 253.0

Hypersomnia, unspecified 780.54
- with sleep apnea, unspecified 780.53
- alcohol-induced 291.82
- drug-induced 292.85

Hypersomnia, unspecified – *continued*
- due to
  - medical condition classified elsewhere 327.14
  - mental disorder 327.15
- idiopathic
  - with long sleep time 327.11
  - without long sleep time 327.12
- menstrual related 327.13
- nonorganic origin 307.43
  - persistent (primary) 307.44
  - transient 307.43
- organic 327.10
  - other 327.19
- primary 307.44
- recurrent 327.13

Hypersplenia 289.4

Hypersplenism 289.4

Hypersteatosis 706.3

Hyperstimulation, ovarian 256.1

Hypersuprarenalism 255.3

Hypersusceptibility – *see* Allergy

Hyper-TBG-nemia 246.8

Hypertelorism 756.0
- orbit, orbital 376.41

Hypersecretion – Hypertelorism

	Malignant	Benign	Unspecified
Hypertension, hypertensive (arterial) (arteriolar) (crisis) (degeneration) (disease) (essential) (fluctuating) (idiopathic) (intermittent) (labile) (low renin) (orthostatic) (paroxysmal) (primary) (systemic) (uncontrolled) (vascular)	401.0	401.1	401.9
with			
chronic kidney disease			
stage I through stage IV, or unspecified	403.00	403.10	403.90
stage V or end stage renal disease	403.01	403.11	403.91
heart involvement (conditions classifiable to 429.0-429.3, 429.8, 429.9 due to hypertension) (*see also* Hypertension, heart)	402.00	402.10	402.90
with kidney involvement – *see* Hypertension, cardiorenal			
renal involvement (only conditions classifiable to 585, 586, 587) (excludes conditions classifiable to 584) (*see also* Hypertension, kidney)	403.00	403.10	403.90
renal sclerosis or failure	403.00	403.10	403.90
with heart involvement – *see* Hypertension, cardiorenal			
failure (and sclerosis) (*see also* Hypertension, kidney)	403.01	403.11	403.91
sclerosis without failure (*see also* Hypertension, kidney)	403.00	403.10	403.90
accelerated – (*see also* Hypertension, by type, malignant)	401.0	–	–
antepartum – *see* Hypertension, complicating pregnancy, childbirth, or the puerperium			
cardiorenal (disease)	404.00	404.10	404.90
with			
chronic kidney disease			
stage I through stage IV, or unspecified	404.00	404.10	404.90
and heart failure	404.01	404.11	404.91
stage V or end stage renal disease	404.02	404.12	404.92
and heart failure	404.03	404.13	404.93
heart failure	404.01	404.11	404.91
and chronic kidney disease	404.01▲	404.11▲	404.91▲
stage I through stage IV, or unspecified	404.01▲	404.11▲	404.91▲
stage V or end stage renal disease	404.03	404.13	404.93
cardiovascular disease (arteriosclerotic) (sclerotic)	402.00	402.10	402.90
with			
heart failure	402.01	402.11	402.91
renal involvement (conditions classifiable to 403) (*see also* Hypertension, cardiorenal)	404.00	404.10	404.90
cardiovascular renal (disease) (sclerosis) (*see also* Hypertension, cardiorenal)	404.00	404.10	404.90
cerebrovascular disease NEC	437.2	437.2	437.2
complicating pregnancy, childbirth, or the puerperium	642.2❺	642.0	642.9❺
with			
albuminuria (and edema) (mild)	–	–	642.4❺
severe	–	–	642.5❺
chronic kidney disease	642.2❺	642.2❺	642.2❺
and heart disease	642.2❺	642.2❺	642.2❺
edema (mild)	–	–	642.4❺
severe	–	–	642.5❺
heart disease	642.2❺	642.2❺	642.2❺
and chronic kidney disease	642.2❺	642.2❺	642.2❺
renal disease	642.2❺	642.2❺	642.2❺
and heart disease	642.2❺	642.2❺	642.2❺

	Malignant	Benign	Unspecified
Hypertension, hypertensive – *continued*			
complicating pregnancy, childbirth, or the puerperium – *continued*			
chronic	642.2❺	642.0❺	642.0❺
with pre-eclampsia or eclampsia	642.7❺	642.7❺	642.7❺
fetus or newborn	760.0	760.0	760.0
essential	–	642.0	642.0❺
with pre-eclampsia or eclampsia	–	642.7❺	642.7❺
fetus or newborn	760.0	760.0	760.0
gestational	–	–	642.3❺
pre-existing	642.2❺	642.0	642.0❺
with pre-eclampsia or eclampsia	642.7❺	642.7❺	642.7❺
fetus or newborn	760.0	760.0	760.0
secondary to renal disease	642.1❺	642.1❺	642.1❺
with pre-eclampsia or eclampsia	642.7❺	642.7❺	642.7❺
fetus or newborn	760.0	760.0	760.0
transient	–	–	642.3❺
due to			
aldosteronism, primary	405.09	405.19	405.99
brain tumor	405.09	405.19	405.99
bulbar poliomyelitis	405.09	405.19	405.99
calculus			
kidney	405.09	405.19	405.99
ureter	405.09	405.19	405.99
coarctation, aorta	405.09	405.19	405.99
Cushing's disease	405.09	405.19	405.99
glomerulosclerosis (*see also* Hypertension, kidney)	403.00	403.10	403.90
periarteritis nodosa	405.09	405.19	405.99
pheochromocytoma	405.09	405.19	405.99
polycystic kidney(s)	405.09	405.19	405.99
polycythemia	405.09	405.19	405.99
porphyria	405.09	405.19	405.99
pyelonephritis	405.09	405.19	405.99
renal (artery)			
aneurysm	405.01	405.11	405.91
anomaly	405.01	405.11	405.91
embolism	405.01	405.11	405.91
fibromuscular hyperplasia	405.01	405.11	405.91
occlusion	405.01	405.11	405.91
stenosis	405.01	405.11	405.91
thrombosis	405.01	405.11	405.91
encephalopathy	437.2	437.2	437.2
gestational (transient) NEC	–	–	642.3❺
Goldblatt's	440.1	440.1	440.1
heart (disease) (conditions classifiable to 429.0-429.3, 429.8, 429.9 due to hypertension)	402.00	402.10	402.90
with heart failure	402.01	402.11	402.91
hypertensive kidney disease (conditions classifiable to 403) (*see also* Hypertension, cardiorenal)	404.00	404.10	404.90
renal sclerosis (*see also* Hypertension, cardiorenal)	404.00	404.10	404.90
intracranial, benign	–	348.2	–
intraocular	–	–	365.04
kidney	403.00	403.10	403.90
with			
chronic kidney disease			
stage I through stage IV, or unspecified	403.00	403.10	403.90
stage V or end stage renal disease	403.01	403.11	403.91
heart involvement (conditions classifiable to 429.0-429.3, 429.8, 429.9 due to hypertension) (*see also* Hypertension, cardiorenal)	404.00	404.10	404.90

	Malignant	Benign	Unspecified
Hypertension, hypertensive – *continued*			
kidney – *continued*			
with – *continued*			
hypertensive heart (disease) (conditions classifiable to 402) (*see also* Hypertension, cardiorenal)	404.00	404.10	404.90
lesser circulation	–	–	416.0
necrotizing	401.0	–	–
ocular	–	–	365.04
of newborn	–	–	747.83
portal (due to chronic liver disease)	–	–	572.3
postoperative			997.91
psychogenic	–	–	306.2
puerperal, postpartum – *see* Hypertension, complicating pregnancy, childbirth, or the puerperium			
pulmonary (artery)	–	–	416.8
with cor pulmonale (chronic)	–	–	416.8
acute	–	–	415.0
idiopathic	–	–	416.0
primary	–	–	416.0
secondary	–	–	416.8
renal (disease) (*see also* Hypertension, kidney)	403.00	403.10	403.90
renovascular NEC	405.01	405.11	405.91
secondary NEC	405.09	405.19	405.99
due to			
aldosteronism, primary	405.09	405.19	405.99
brain tumor	405.09	405.19	405.99
bulbar poliomyelitis	405.09	405.19	405.99
calculus			
kidney	405.09	405.19	405.99
ureter	405.09	405.19	405.99

	Malignant	Benign	Unspecified
Hypertension, hypertensive – *continued*			
secondary NEC – *continued*			
due to – *continued*			
coarctation, aorta	405.09	405.19	405.99
Cushing's disease	405.09	405.19	405.99
glomerulosclerosis (*see also* Hypertension, kidney)	403.00	403.10	403.90
periarteritis nodosa	405.09	405.19	405.99
pheochromocytoma	405.09	405.19	405.99
polycystic kidney(s)	405.09	405.19	405.99
polycythemia	405.09	405.19	405.99
porphyria	405.09	405.19	405.99
pyelonephritis	405.09	405.19	405.99
renal (artery)			
aneurysm	405.01	405.11	405.91
anomaly	405.01	405.11	405.91
embolism	405.01	405.11	405.91
fibromuscular hyperplasia	405.01	405.11	405.91
occlusion	405.01	405.11	405.91
stenosis	405.01	405.11	405.91
thrombosis	405.01	405.11	405.91
transient	–	–	796.2
of pregnancy	–	–	642.3❺
venous, chronic (asymptomatic) (idiopathic)	–	–	459.3
with			
complication, NEC	–	–	459.39
inflammation	–	–	459.32
with ulcer	–	–	459.33
ulcer	–	–	459.31
with inflammation	–	–	459.33
due to ●			
deep vein thrombosis (*see also* Syndrome, postphlebitic) ●	–	–	459.10

Hyperthecosis, ovary 256.8
Hyperthermia (of unknown origin) (*see also* Pyrexia) 780.6
  malignant (due to anesthesia) 995.86
  newborn 778.4
Hyperthymergasia (*see also* Psychosis, affective) 296.0❺
  reactive (from emotional stress, psychological trauma) 298.1
  recurrent episode 296.1❺
  single episode 296.0❺
Hyperthymism 254.8
Hyperthyroid (recurrent) – *see* Hyperthyroidism
Hyperthyroidism (latent) (preadult) (recurrent) (without goiter) 242.9❺

Note – Use the following fifth-digit subclassification with category 242:
0 without mention of thyrotoxic crisis or storm
1 with mention of thyrotoxic crisis or storm

  with
    goiter (diffuse) 242.0❺
      adenomatous 242.3❺
        multinodular 242.2❺
        uninodular 242.1❺
      nodular 242.3❺
        multinodular 242.2❺
        uninodular 242.1❺
    thyroid nodule 242.1❺
  complicating pregnancy, childbirth, or puerperium 648.1❺
  neonatal (transient) 775.3
Hypertonia – *see* Hypertonicity
Hypertonicity
  bladder 596.51
  fetus or newborn 779.89
  gastrointestinal (tract) 536.8
  infancy 779.89
    due to electrolyte imbalance 779.89
  muscle 728.85
  stomach 536.8
    psychogenic 306.4
  uterus, uterine (contractions) 661.4❺
    affecting fetus or newborn 763.7
Hypertony – *see* Hypertonicity
Hypertransaminemia 790.4
Hypertrichosis 704.1
  congenital 757.4
  eyelid 374.54
  lanuginosa 757.4
    acquired 704.1
Hypertriglyceridemia, essential 272.1
Hypertrophy, hypertrophic
  adenoids (infectional) 474.12
    and tonsils (faucial) (infective) (lingual) (lymphoid) 474.10
  adrenal 255.8
  alveolar process or ridge 525.8
  anal papillae 569.49
  apocrine gland 705.82
  artery NEC 447.8
    carotid 447.8
    congenital (peripheral) NEC 747.60
      gastrointestinal 747.61
      lower limb 747.64
      renal 747.62
      specified NEC 747.69
      spinal 747.82
      upper limb 747.63
    renal 447.3
  arthritis (chronic) (*see also* Osteoarthrosis) 715.9❺
    spine (*see also* Spondylosis) 721.90
  arytenoid 478.79
  asymmetrical (heart) 429.9
  auricular – *see* Hypertrophy, cardiac
  Bartholin's gland 624.8
  bile duct 576.8
  bladder (sphincter) (trigone) 596.8
  blind spot, visual field 368.42
  bone 733.99
  brain 348.8
  breast 611.1
    cystic 610.1
    fetus or newborn 778.7
    fibrocystic 610.1
    massive pubertal 611.1
    puerperal, postpartum 676.3❺

Hypertrophy, hypertrophic – *continued*
  breast – *continued*
    senile (parenchymatous) 611.1
  cardiac (chronic) (idiopathic) 429.3
    with
      rheumatic fever (conditions classifiable to 390)
        active 391.8
          with chorea 392.0
        inactive or quiescent (with chorea) 398.99
    congenital NEC 746.89
    fatty (*see also* Degeneration, myocardial) 429.1
    hypertensive (*see also* Hypertension, heart) 402.90
    rheumatic (with chorea) 398.99
      active or acute 391.8
        with chorea 392.0
    valve (*see also* Endocarditis) 424.90
      congenital NEC 746.89
  cartilage 733.99
  cecum 569.89
  cervix (uteri) 622.6
    congenital 752.49
    elongation 622.6
  clitoris (cirrhotic) 624.2
    congenital 752.49
  colon 569.89
    congenital 751.3
  conjunctiva, lymphoid 372.73
  cornea 371.89
  corpora cavernosa 607.89
  duodenum 537.89
  endometrium (uterus) (*see also* Hyperplasia, endometrium) 621.30
    cervix 622.6
  epididymis 608.89
  esophageal hiatus (congenital) 756.6
    with hernia – *see* Hernia, diaphragm
  eyelid 374.30
  falx, skull 733.99
  fat pad 729.30
    infrapatellar 729.31
    knee 729.31
    orbital 374.34
    popliteal 729.31
    prepatellar 729.31
    retropatellar 729.31
    specified site NEC 729.39
  foot (congenital) 755.67
  frenum, frenulum (tongue) 529.8
    linguae 529.8
    lip 528.5
  gallbladder or cystic duct 575.8
  gastric mucosa 535.2❺
  gingiva 523.8
  gland, glandular (general) NEC 785.6
  gum (mucous membrane) 523.8
  heart (idiopathic) – *see also* Hypertrophy, cardiac
    valve – *see also* Endocarditis
      congenital NEC 746.89
  hemifacial 754.0
  hepatic – *see* Hypertrophy, liver
  hiatus (esophageal) 756.6
  hilus gland 785.6
  hymen, congenital 752.49
  ileum 569.89
  infrapatellar fat pad 729.31
  intestine 569.89
  jejunum 569.89
  kidney (compensatory) 593.1
    congenital 753.3
  labial frenulum 528.5
  labium (majus) (minus) 624.3
  lacrimal gland, chronic 375.03
  ligament 728.9
    spinal 724.8
  linguae frenulum 529.8
  lingual tonsil (infectional) 474.11
  lip (frenum) 528.5
    congenital 744.81
  liver 789.1
    acute 573.8
    cirrhotic – *see* Cirrhosis, liver
    congenital 751.69
    fatty – *see* Fatty, liver
  lymph gland 785.6
    tuberculous – *see* Tuberculosis, lymph gland
  mammary gland – *see* Hypertrophy, breast
  maxillary frenulum 528.5
  Meckel's diverticulum (congenital) 751.0
  medial meniscus, acquired 717.3

Hypertrophy, hypertrophic – *continued*
  median bar 600.90
    with
      other lower urinary tract symptoms (LUTS) 600.91
      urinary
        obstruction 600.91
        retention 600.91
  mediastinum 519.3
  meibomian gland 373.2
  meniscus, knee, congenital 755.64
  metatarsal head 733.99
  metatarsus 733.99
  mouth 528.9
  mucous membrane
    alveolar process 523.8
    nose 478.19
    turbinate (nasal) 478.0
  muscle 728.9
  muscular coat, artery NEC 447.8
    carotid 447.8
    renal 447.3
  myocardium (*see also* Hypertrophy, cardiac) 429.3
    idiopathic 425.4
  myometrium 621.2
  nail 703.8
    congenital 757.5
  nasal 478.19
    alae 478.19
    bone 738.0
    cartilage 478.19
    mucous membrane (septum) 478.19
    sinus (*see also* Sinusitis) 473.9
    turbinate 478.0
  nasopharynx, lymphoid (infectional) (tissue) (wall) 478.29
  neck, uterus 622.6
  nipple 611.1
  normal aperture diaphragm (congenital) 756.6
  nose (*see also* Hypertrophy, nasal) 478.19
  orbit 376.46
  organ or site, congenital NEC – *see* Anomaly, specified type NEC
  osteoarthropathy (pulmonary) 731.2
  ovary 620.8
  palate (hard) 526.89
    soft 528.9
  pancreas (congenital) 751.7
  papillae
    anal 569.49
    tongue 529.3
  parathyroid (gland) 252.01
  parotid gland 527.1
  penis 607.89
  phallus 607.89
    female (clitoris) 624.2
  pharyngeal tonsil 474.12
  pharyngitis 472.1
  pharynx 478.29
    lymphoid (infectional) (tissue) (wall) 478.29
  pituitary (fossa) (gland) 253.8
  popliteal fat pad 729.31
  preauricular (lymph) gland (Hampstead) 785.6
  prepuce (congenital) 605
    female 624.2
  prostate (asymptomatic) (early) (recurrent) 600.90
    with
      other lower urinary tract symptoms (LUTS) 600.91
      urinary
        obstruction 600.91
        retention 600.91
    adenofibromatous 600.20
      with
        other lower urinary tract symptoms (LUTS) 600.21
        urinary
          obstruction 600.21
          retention 600.21
    benign 600.00
      with
        other lower urinary tract symptoms (LUTS) 600.01
        urinary
          obstruction 600.01
          retention 600.01
    congenital 752.89
  pseudoedematous hypodermal 757.0
  pseudomuscular 359.1
  pylorus (muscle) (sphincter) 537.0
    congenital 750.5

Hypertrophy, hypertrophic – *continued*
  pylorus – *continued*
    infantile 750.5
  rectal sphincter 569.49
  rectum 569.49
  renal 593.1
  rhinitis (turbinate) 472.0
  salivary duct or gland 527.1
    congenital 750.26
  scaphoid (tarsal) 733.99
  scar 701.4
  scrotum 608.89
  sella turcica 253.8
  seminal vesicle 608.89
  sigmoid 569.89
  skin condition NEC 701.9
  spermatic cord 608.89
  spinal ligament 724.8
  spleen – *see* Splenomegaly
  spondylitis (spine) (*see also* Spondylosis) 721.90
  stomach 537.89
  subaortic stenosis (idiopathic) 425.1
  sublingual gland 527.1
    congenital 750.26
  submaxillary gland 527.1
  suprarenal (gland) 255.8
  tendon 727.9
  testis 608.89
    congenital 752.89
  thymic, thymus (congenital) (gland) 254.0
  thyroid (gland) (*see also* Goiter) 240.9
    primary 242.0❺
    secondary 242.2❺
  toe (congenital) 755.65
    acquired 735.8
  tongue 529.8
    congenital 750.15
    frenum 529.8
    papillae (foliate) 529.3
  tonsil (faucial) (infective) (lingual) (lymphoid) 474.11
    with
      adenoiditis 474.01
      tonsillitis 474.00
        and adenoiditis 474.02
    and adenoids 474.10
  tunica vaginalis 608.89
  turbinate (mucous membrane) 478.0
  ureter 593.89
  urethra 599.84
  uterus 621.2
    puerperal, postpartum 674.8❺
  uvula 528.9
  vagina 623.8
  vas deferens 608.89
  vein 459.89
  ventricle, ventricular (heart) (left) (right) – *see also* Hypertrophy, cardiac
    congenital 746.89
    due to hypertension (left) (right) (*see also* Hypertension, heart) 402.90
      benign 402.10
      malignant 402.00
    right with ventricular septal defect, pulmonary stenosis or atresia, and dextraposition of aorta 745.2
  verumontanum 599.89
  vesical 596.8
  vocal cord 478.5
  vulva 624.3
    stasis (nonfilarial) 624.3
Hypertropia (intermittent) (periodic) 378.31
Hypertyrosinemia 270.2
Hyperuricemia 790.6
Hypervalinemia 270.3
Hyperventilation (tetany) 786.01
  hysterical 300.11
  psychogenic 306.1
  syndrome 306.1
Hyperviscidosis 277.00
Hyperviscosity (of serum) (syndrome) NEC 273.3
  polycythemic 289.0
  sclerocythemic 282.8
Hypervitaminosis (dietary) NEC 278.8
  A (dietary) 278.2
  D (dietary) 278.4
  from excessive administration or use of vitamin preparations (chronic) 278.8
    reaction to sudden overdose 963.5
    vitamin A 278.2
      reaction to sudden overdose 963.5

Hypervitaminosis – *continued*
  from excessive administration or use of vitamin preparations – *continued*
    vitamin D 278.4
      reaction to sudden overdose 963.5
    vitamin K
      correct substance properly administered 278.8
      overdose or wrong substance given or taken 964.3
Hypervolemia 276.6
Hypesthesia (*see also* Disturbance, sensation) 782.0
  cornea 371.81
Hyphema (anterior chamber) (ciliary body) (iris) 364.41
  traumatic 921.3
Hyphemia – *see* Hyphema
Hypoacidity, gastric 536.8
  psychogenic 306.4
Hypoactive labyrinth (function) – *see* Hypofunction, labyrinth
Hypoadrenalism 255.41 ▲
  tuberculous (*see also* Tuberculosis) 017.6❺
Hypoadrenocorticism 255.41 ▲
  pituitary 253.4
Hypoalbuminemia 273.8
Hypoaldosteronism 255.42 ▲
Hypoalphalipoproteinemia 272.5
Hypobarism 993.2
Hypobaropathy 993.2
Hypobetalipoproteinemia (familial) 272.5
Hypocalcemia 275.41
  cow's milk 775.4
  dietary 269.3
  neonatal 775.4
  phosphate-loading 775.4
Hypocalcification, teeth 520.4
Hypochloremia 276.9
Hypochlorhydria 536.8
  neurotic 306.4
  psychogenic 306.4
Hypocholesteremia 272.5
Hypochondria (reaction) 300.7
Hypochondriac 300.7
Hypochondriasis 300.7
Hypochromasia blood cells 280.9
Hypochromic anemia 280.9
  due to blood loss (chronic) 280.0
    acute 285.1
  microcytic 280.9
Hypocoagulability (*see also* Defect, coagulation) 286.9
Hypocomplementemia 279.8
Hypocythemia (progressive) 284.9
Hypodontia (*see also* Anodontia) 520.0
Hypoeosinophilia 288.59
Hypoesthesia (*see also* Disturbance, sensation) 782.0
  cornea 371.81
  tactile 782.0
Hypoestrinism 256.39
Hypoestrogenism 256.39
Hypoferremia 280.9
  due to blood loss (chronic) 280.0
Hypofertility
  female 628.9
  male 606.1
Hypofibrinogenemia 286.3
  acquired 286.6
  congenital 286.3
Hypofunction
  adrenal (gland) 255.41 ▲
    cortex 255.41 ▲
    medulla 255.5
    specified NEC 255.5
  cerebral 331.9
  corticoadrenal NEC 255.41 ▲
  intestinal 564.89
  labyrinth (unilateral) 386.53
    with loss of labyrinthine reactivity 386.55
    bilateral 386.54
      with loss of labyrinthine reactivity 386.56
  Leydig cell 257.2
  ovary 256.39
    postablative 256.2

Hypofunction – *continued*
  pituitary (anterior) (gland) (lobe) 253.2
    posterior 253.5
  testicular 257.2
    iatrogenic 257.1
    postablative 257.1
    postirradiation 257.1
    postsurgical 257.1
Hypogammaglobulinemia 279.00
  acquired primary 279.06
  non-sex-linked, congenital 279.06
  sporadic 279.06
  transient of infancy 279.09
Hypogenitalism (congenital) (female) (male) 752.89
  penis 752.69
Hypoglycemia (spontaneous) 251.2
  coma 251.0
    diabetic 250.3❺
  diabetic 250.8❺
  due to insulin 251.0
    therapeutic misadventure 962.3
  familial (idiopathic) 251.2
  following gastrointestinal surgery 579.3
  infantile (idiopathic) 251.2
  in infant of diabetic mother 775.0
  leucine-induced 270.3
  neonatal 775.6
  reactive 251.2
  specified NEC 251.1
Hypoglycemic shock 251.0
  diabetic 250.8❺
  due to insulin 251.0
  functional (syndrome) 251.1
Hypogonadism
  female 256.39
  gonadotrophic (isolated) 253.4
  hypogonadotropic (isolated) (with anosmia) 253.4
  isolated 253.4
  male 257.2
    hereditary familial (Reifenstein s syndrome) 259.5
  ovarian (primary) 256.39
  pituitary (secondary) 253.4
  testicular (primary) (secondary) 257.2
Hypohidrosis 705.0
Hypohidrotic ectodermal dysplasia 757.31
Hypoidrosis 705.0
Hypoinsulinemia, postsurgical 251.3
  postpancreatectomy (complete) (partial) 251.3
Hypokalemia 276.8
Hypokinesia 780.99
Hypoleukia splenica 289.4
Hypoleukocytosis 288.50
Hypolipidemia 272.5
Hypolipoproteinemia 272.5
Hypomagnesemia 275.2
  neonatal 775.4
Hypomania, hypomanic reaction (*see also* Psychosis, affective) 296.0❺
  recurrent episode 296.1❺
  single episode 296.0❺
Hypomastia (congenital) 757.6
Hypomenorrhea 626.1
Hypometabolism 783.9
Hypomotility
  gastrointestinal tract 536.8
    psychogenic 306.4
  intestine 564.89
    psychogenic 306.4
  stomach 536.8
    psychogenic 306.4
Hyponasality 784.49
Hyponatremia 276.1
Hypo-ovarianism 256.39
Hypo-ovarism 256.39
Hypoparathyroidism (idiopathic) (surgically induced) 252.1
  neonatal 775.4
Hypopharyngitis 462
Hypophoria 378.40
Hypophosphatasia 275.3
Hypophosphatemia (acquired) (congenital) (familial) 275.3
  renal 275.3
Hypophyseal, hypophysis – *see also* condition
  dwarfism 253.3
  gigantism 253.0

Hypertrophy, hypertrophic – Hypophyseal, hypophysis

- **Hypopyrexia** 780.99
- **Hyporeflex** 796.1
- **Hyporeninemia, extreme** 790.99
  - in primary aldosteronism 255.10
- **Hyporesponsive episode** 780.09
- **Hyposecretion**
  - ACTH 253.4
  - ovary 256.39
    - postablative 256.2
  - salivary gland (any) 527.7
- **Hyposegmentation of neutrophils, hereditary** 288.2
- **Hyposiderinemia** 280.9
- **Hyposmolality** 276.1
  - syndrome 276.1
- **Hyposomatotropism** 253.3
- **Hyposomnia, unspecified** (*see also* Insomnia) 780.52
  - with sleep apnea, unspecified 780.51
- **Hypospadias** (male) 752.61
  - female 753.8
- **Hypospermatogenesis** 606.1
- **Hyposphagma** 372.72
- **Hyposplenism** 289.59
- **Hypostasis, pulmonary** 514
- **Hypostatic** – *see* condition
- **Hyposthenuria** 593.89
- **Hyposuprarenalism** 255.41 ▲
- **Hypo-TBG-nemia** 246.8
- **Hypotension** (arterial) (constitutional) 458.9
  - chronic 458.1
  - iatrogenic 458.29
  - maternal, syndrome (following labor and delivery) 669.2❺
  - of hemodialysis 458.21
  - orthostatic (chronic) 458.0
    - dysautonomic-dyskinetic syndrome 333.0
  - permanent idiopathic 458.1
  - postoperative 458.29
  - postural 458.0
  - specified type NEC 458.8
  - transient 796.3
- **Hypothermia** (accidental) 991.6
  - anesthetic 995.89
  - newborn NEC 778.3
  - not associated with low environmental temperature 780.99
- **Hypothymergasia** (*see also* Psychosis, affective) 296.2❺
  - recurrent episode 296.3❺
  - single episode 296.2❺
- **Hypothyroidism** (acquired) 244.9
  - complicating pregnancy, childbirth, or puerperium 648.1❺
  - congenital 243
  - due to
    - ablation 244.1
      - radioactive iodine 244.1
      - surgical 244.0
    - iodine (administration) (ingestion) 244.2
      - radioactive 244.1
    - irradiation therapy 244.1
    - p-aminosalicylic acid (PAS) 244.3
    - phenylbutazone 244.3
    - resorcinol 244.3
    - specified cause NEC 244.8
    - surgery 244.0
  - goitrous (sporadic) 246.1
  - iatrogenic NEC 244.3
  - iodine 244.2
  - pituitary 244.8
  - postablative NEC 244.1
  - postsurgical 244.0
  - primary 244.9
  - secondary NEC 244.8
  - specified cause NEC 244.8
  - sporadic goitrous 246.1
- **Hypotonia, hypotonicity, hypotony** 781.3
  - benign congenital 358.8
  - bladder 596.4
  - congenital 779.89
    - benign 358.8
  - eye 360.30
    - due to
      - fistula 360.32
      - ocular disorder NEC 360.33
    - following loss of aqueous or vitreous 360.33
    - primary 360.31
  - infantile muscular (benign) 359.0
  - muscle 728.9
- **Hypotonia, hypotonicity, hypotony** – *continued*
  - uterus, uterine (contractions) – *see* Inertia, uterus
- **Hypotrichosis** 704.09
  - congenital 757.4
  - lid (congenital) 757.4
    - acquired 374.55
  - postinfectional NEC 704.09
- **Hypotropia** 378.32
- **Hypoventilation** 786.09
  - congenital central alveolar syndrome 327.25
  - idiopathic sleep related nonobstructive alveolar 327.24
  - sleep relate, in conditions classifiable elsewhere 327.26
- **Hypovitaminosis** (*see also* Deficiency, vitamin) 269.2
- **Hypovolemia** 276.52
  - surgical shock 998.0
  - traumatic (shock) 958.4
- **Hypoxemia** (*see also* Anoxia) 799.02
  - sleep related, in conditions classifiable elsewhere 327.26
- **Hypoxia** (*see also* Anoxia) 799.02
  - cerebral 348.1
    - during or resulting from a procedure 997.01
    - newborn 770.88
      - mild or moderate 768.6
      - severe 768.5
  - fetal, affecting newborn 770.88
  - intrauterine – *see* Distress, fetal
  - myocardial (*see also* Insufficiency, coronary) 411.89
    - arteriosclerotic – *see* Arteriosclerosis, coronary
  - newborn 770.88
  - sleep related 327.24
- **Hypoxic-ischemic encephalopathy** (HIE) 768.7
- **Hypsarrhythmia** (*see also* Epilepsy) 345.6❺
- **Hysteralgia, pregnant uterus** 646.8❺
- **Hysteria, hysterical** 300.10
  - anxiety 300.20
  - Charcôt's gland 300.11
  - conversion (any manifestation) 300.11
  - dissociative type NEC 300.15
  - psychosis, acute 298.1
- **Hysteroepilepsy** 300.11
- **Hysterotomy, affecting fetus or newborn** 763.89

I

- **Iatrogenic syndrome of excess cortisol** 255.0
- **Iceland disease** (epidemic neuromyasthenia) 049.8
- **Ichthyosis** (congenita) 757.1
  - acquired 701.1
  - fetalis gravior 757.1
  - follicularis 757.1
  - hystrix 757.39
  - lamellar 757.1
  - lingual 528.6
  - palmaris and plantaris 757.39
  - simplex 757.1
  - vera 757.1
  - vulgaris 757.1
- **Ichthyotoxism** 988.0
  - bacterial (*see also* Poisoning, food) 005.9
- **Icteroanemia, hemolytic** (acquired) 283.9
  - congenital (*see also* Spherocytosis) 282.0
- **Icterus** (*see also* Jaundice) 782.4
  - catarrhal – *see* Icterus, infectious
  - conjunctiva 782.4
    - newborn 774.6
  - epidemic – *see* Icterus, infectious
  - febrilis – *see* Icterus, infectious
  - fetus or newborn – *see* Jaundice, fetus or newborn
  - gravis (*see also* Necrosis, liver) 570
    - complicating pregnancy 646.7❺
      - affecting fetus or newborn 760.8
    - fetus or newborn NEC 773.0
    - obstetrical 646.7❺
      - affecting fetus or newborn 760.8
  - hematogenous (acquired) 283.9
  - hemolytic (acquired) 283.9
    - congenital (*see also* Spherocytosis) 282.0
  - hemorrhagic (acute) 100.0
    - leptospiral 100.0
    - newborn 776.0
    - spirochetal 100.0
- **Icterus** – *continued*
  - infectious 070.1
    - with hepatic coma 070.0
    - leptospiral 100.0
    - spirochetal 100.0
  - intermittens juvenilis 277.4
  - malignant (*see also* Necrosis, liver) 570
  - neonatorum (*see also* Jaundice, fetus or newborn) 774.6
  - pernicious (*see also* Necrosis, liver) 570
  - spirochetal 100.0
- **Ictus solaris, solis** 992.0
- **Ideation**
  - suicidal V62.84
- **Identity disorder** 313.82
  - dissociative 300.14
  - gender role (child) 302.6
    - adult 302.85
  - psychosexual (child) 302.6
    - adult 302.85
- **Idioglossia** 307.9
- **Idiopathic** – *see* condition
- **Idiosyncrasy** (*see also* Allergy) 995.3
  - drug, medicinal substance, and biological – *see* Allergy, drug
- **Idiot, idiocy** (congenital) 318.2
  - amaurotic (Bielschowsky) (-Jansky) (family) (infantile (late)) (juvenile (late)) (Vogt-Spielmeyer) 330.1
  - microcephalic 742.1
  - Mongolian 758.0
  - oxycephalic 756.0
- **Id reaction** (due to bacteria) 692.89
- **IEED** (involuntary emotional expression disorder) 310.8 ●
- **IFIS** (intraoperative floppy iris syndrome) 364.81 ●
- **IgE asthma** 493.0❺
- **Ileitis** (chronic) (*see also* Enteritis) 558.9
  - infectious 009.0
  - noninfectious 558.9
  - regional (ulcerative) 555.0
    - with large intestine 555.2
  - segmental 555.0
    - with large intestine 555.2
  - terminal (ulcerative) 555.0
    - with large intestine 555.2
- **Ileocolitis** (*see also* Enteritis) 558.9
  - infectious 009.0
  - regional 555.2
  - ulcerative 556.1
- **Ileostomy status** V44.2
  - with complication 569.60
- **Ileotyphus** 002.0
- **Ileum** – *see* condition
- **Ileus** (adynamic) (bowel) (colon) (inhibitory) (intestine) (neurogenic) (paralytic) 560.1
  - arteriomesenteric duodenal 537.2
  - due to gallstone (in intestine) 560.31
  - duodenal, chronic 537.2
  - following gastrointestinal surgery 997.4
  - gallstone 560.31
  - mechanical (*see also* Obstruction intestine) 560.9
  - meconium 777.1
    - due to cystic fibrosis 277.01
  - myxedema 564.89
  - postoperative 997.4
  - transitory, newborn 777.4
- **Iliac** – *see* condition
- **Iliotibial band friction syndrome** 728 89
- **Ill, louping** 063.1
- **Illegitimacy** V61.6
- **Illness** – *see also* Disease
  - factitious 300.19
    - with
      - combined psychological and physical signs and symptoms 300.19
      - physical symptoms 300.19
      - predominantly
        - physical signs and symptoms 300.19
        - psychological symptoms 300.16
    - chronic (with physical symptoms) 301.51
  - heart – *see* Disease, heart
  - manic-depressive (*see also* Psychosis, affective) 296.80
  - mental (*see also* Disorder, mental) 300.9

- **Imbalance** 781.2
  - autonomic (*see also* Neuropathy, peripheral, autonomic) 337.9
  - electrolyte 276.9
    - with
      - abortion – *see* Abortion, by type, with metabolic disorder
      - ectopic pregnancy (*see also* categories 633.0-633.9) 639.4
      - hyperemesis gravidarum (before 22 completed weeks gestation) 643.1❺
      - molar pregnancy (*see also* categories 630-632) 639.4
    - following
      - abortion 639.4
      - ectopic or molar pregnancy 639.4
    - neonatal, transitory NEC 775.5
  - endocrine 259.9
  - eye muscle NEC 378.9
    - heterophoria – *see* Heterophoria
  - glomerulotubular NEC 593.89
  - hormone 259.9
  - hysterical (*see also* Hysteria) 300.10
  - labyrinth NEC 386.50
  - posture 729.9
  - sympathetic (*see also* Neuropathy, peripheral, autonomic) 337.9
- **Imbecile, imbecility** 318.0
  - moral 301.7
  - old age 290.9
  - senile 290.9
  - specified IQ – *see* IQ
  - unspecified IQ 318.0
- **Imbedding, intrauterine device** 996.32
- **Imbibition, cholesterol** (gallbladder) 575.6
- **Imerslund** (-Gräsbeck) **syndrome** (anemia due to familial selective vitamin B_{12} malabsorption) 281.1
- **Iminoacidopathy** 270.8
- **Iminoglycinuria, familial** 270.8
- **Immature** – *see also* Immaturity
  - personality 301.89
- **Immaturity** 765.1❺
  - extreme 765.0❺
  - fetus or infant light-for-dates – *see* Light-for-dates
  - lung, fetus or newborn 770.4
  - organ or site NEC – *see* Hypoplasia
  - pulmonary, fetus or newborn 770.4
  - reaction 301.89
  - sexual (female) (male) 259.0
- **Immersion** 994.1
  - foot 991.4
  - hand 991.4
- **Immobile, immobility**
  - intestine 564.89
  - joint – *see* Ankylosis
  - syndrome (paraplegic) 728.3
- **Immunization**
  - ABO
    - affecting management of pregnancy 656.2❺
      - fetus or newborn 773.1
  - complication – *see* Complications, vaccination
  - Rh factor
    - affecting management of pregnancy 656.1❺
      - fetus or newborn 773.0
    - from transfusion 999.7
- **Immunodeficiency** 279.3
  - with
    - adenosine-deaminase deficiency 279.2
    - defect, predominant
      - B-cell 279.00
      - T-cell 279.10
    - hyperimmunoglobulinemia 279.2
    - lymphopenia, hereditary 279.2
    - thrombocytopenia and eczema 279.12
    - thymic
      - aplasia 279.2
      - dysplasia 279.2
  - autosomal recessive, Swiss-type 279.2
  - common variable 279.06
  - severe combined (SCID) 279.2
  - to Rh factor
    - affecting management of pregnancy 656.1❺
      - fetus or newborn 773.0
  - X-linked, with increased IgM 279.05
- **Immunotherapy, prophylactic** V07.2
  - antineoplastic V58.12
- **Impaction, impacted**
  - bowel, colon, rectum 560.30
    - with hernia – *see also* Hernia, by site, with obstruction
      - gangrenous – *see* Hernia, by site, with gangrene
    - by
      - calculus 560.39
      - gallstone 560.31
    - fecal 560.39
    - specified type NEC 560.39
  - calculus – *see* Calculus
  - cerumen (ear) (external) 380.4
  - cuspid 520.6
  - dental 520.6
  - fecal, feces 560.39
    - with hernia – *see also* Hernia, by site, with obstruction
      - gangrenous – *see* Hernia, by site, with gangrene
  - fracture – *see* Fracture, by site
  - gallbladder – *see* Cholelithiasis
  - gallstone(s) – *see* Cholelithiasis
    - in intestine (any part) 560.31
  - intestine(s) 560.30
    - with hernia – *see also* Hernia, by site, with obstruction
      - gangrenous – *see* Hernia, by site, with gangrene
    - by
      - calculus 560.39
      - gallstone 560.31
    - fecal 560.39
    - specified type NEC 560.39
  - intrauterine device (IUD) 996.32
  - molar 520.6
  - shoulder 660.4❺
    - affecting fetus or newborn 763.1
  - tooth, teeth 520.6
  - turbinate 733.99
- **Impaired, impairment** (function)
  - arm V49.1
    - movement, involving
      - musculoskeletal system V49.1
      - nervous system V49.2
  - auditory discrimination 388.43
  - back V48.3
  - body (entire) V49.89
  - cognitive, mild, so stated 331.83
  - combined visual hearing V49.85 ●
  - dual sensory V49.85 ●
  - glucose
    - fasting 790.21
    - tolerance test (oral) 790.22
  - hearing (*see also* Deafness) 389.9
    - combined with visual impairment V49.85 ●
  - heart – *see* Disease, heart
  - kidney (*see also* Disease, renal) 593.9
    - disorder resulting from 588.9
      - specified NEC 588.89
  - leg V49.1
    - movement, involving
      - musculoskeletal system V49.1
      - nervous system V49.2
  - limb V49.1
    - movement, involving
      - musculoskeletal system V49.1
      - nervous system V49.2
  - liver 573.8
  - mastication 524.9
  - mild cognitive, so stated 331.83
  - mobility
    - ear ossicles NEC 385.22
    - incostapedial joint 385.22
    - malleus 385.21
  - myocardium, myocardial (*see also* Insufficiency, myocardial) 428.0
  - neuromusculoskeletal NEC V49.89
    - back V48.3
    - head V48.2
    - limb V49.2
    - neck V48.3
    - spine V48.3
    - trunk V48.3
  - rectal sphincter 787.99
  - renal (*see also* Disease, renal) 593.9
    - disorder resulting from 588.9
      - specified NEC 588.89
  - spine V48.3
  - vision NEC 369.9
    - both eyes NEC 369.3

Impaired, impairment – *continued*

- vision – *continued*
  - combined with hearing impairment V49.85 ●
  - moderate 369.74
    - both eyes 369.25
      - with impairment of lesser eye (specified as)
        - blind, not further specified 369.15
        - low vision, not further specified 369.23
        - near-total 369.17
        - profound 369.18
        - severe 369.24
        - total 369.16
    - one eye 369.74
      - with vision of other eye (specified as)
        - near-normal 369.75
        - normal 369.76
  - near-total 369.64
    - both eyes 369.04
      - with impairment of lesser eye (specified as)
        - blind, not further specified 369.02
        - total 369.03
    - one eye 369.64
      - with vision of other eye (specified as)
        - near-normal 369.65
        - normal 369.66
  - one eye 369.60
    - with low vision of other eye 369.10
  - profound 369.67
    - both eyes 369.08
      - with impairment of lesser eye (specified as)
        - blind, not further specified 369.05
        - near-total 369.07
        - total 369.06
    - one eye 369.67
      - with vision of other eye (specified as)
        - near-normal 369.68
        - normal 369.69
  - severe 369.71
    - both eyes 369.22
      - with impairment of lesser eye (specified as)
        - blind, not further specified 369.11
        - low vision, not further specified 369.21
        - near-total 369.13
        - profound 369.14
        - total 369.12
    - one eye 369.71
      - with vision of other eye (specified as)
        - near-normal 369.72
        - normal 369.73
  - total
    - both eyes 369.01
    - one eye 369.61
      - with vision of other eye (specified as)
        - near-normal 369.62
        - normal 369.63
- **Impaludism** – *see* Malaria
- **Impediment, speech** NEC 784.5
  - psychogenic 307.9
  - secondary to organic lesion 784.5
- **Impending**
  - cerebrovascular accident or attack 435.9
  - coronary syndrome 411.1
  - delirium tremens 291.0
  - myocardial infarction 411.1
- **Imperception, auditory** (acquired) (congenital) 389.9
- **Imperfect**
  - aeration, lung (newborn) 770.5
  - closure (congenital)
    - alimentary tract NEC 751.8
      - lower 751.5
      - upper 750.8
    - atrioventricular ostium 745.69
    - atrium (secundum) 745.5
      - primum 745.61
    - branchial cleft or sinus 744.41
    - choroid 743.59
    - cricoid cartilage 748.3
    - cusps, heart valve NEC 746.89
      - pulmonary 746.09
    - ductus
      - arteriosus 747.0
      - Botalli 747.0
    - ear drum 744.29
      - causing impairment of hearing 744.03
    - endocardial cushion 745.60
    - epiglottis 748.3

Imperfect – *continued*
closure – *continued*
esophagus with communication to bronchus or trachea 750.3
Eustachian valve 746.89
eyelid 743.62
face, facial (*see also* Cleft, lip) 749.10
foramen
Botalli 745.5
ovale 745.5
genitalia, genital organ(s) or system
female 752.89
external 752.49
internal NEC 752.89
uterus 752.3
male 752.89
penis 752.69
glottis 748.3
heart valve (cusps) NEC 746.89
interatrial ostium or septum 745.5
interauricular ostium or septum 745.5
interventricular ostium or septum 745.4
iris 743.46
kidney 753.3
larynx 748.3
lens 743.36
lip (*see also* Cleft, lip) 749.10
nasal septum or sinus 748.1
nose 748.1
omphalomesenteric duct 751.0
optic nerve entry 743.57
organ or site NEC – *see* Anomaly, specified type, by site
ostium
interatrial 745.5
interauricular 745.5
interventricular 745.4
palate (*see also* Cleft, palate) 749.00
preauricular sinus 744.46
retina 743.56
roof of orbit 742.0
sclera 743.47
septum
aortic 745.0
aorticopulmonary 745.0
atrial (secundum) 745.5
primum 745.61
between aorta and pulmonary artery 745.0
heart 745.9
interatrial (secundum) 745.5
primum 745.61
interauricular (secundum) 745.5
primum 745.61
interventricular 745.4
with pulmonary stenosis or atresia, dextraposition of aorta, and hypertrophy of right ventricle 745.2
in tetralogy of Fallot 745.2
nasal 748.1
ventricular 745.4
with pulmonary stenosis or atresia, dextraposition of aorta, and hypertrophy of right ventricle 745.2
in tetralogy of Fallot 745.2
skull 756.0
with
anencephalus 740.0
encephalocele 742.0
hydrocephalus 742.3
with spina bifida (*see also* Spina bifida) 741.0❺
microcephalus 742.1
spine (with meningocele) (*see also* Spina bifida) 741.90
thyroid cartilage 748.3
trachea 748.3
tympanic membrane 744.29
causing impairment of hearing 744.03
uterus (with communication to bladder, intestine, or rectum) 752.3
uvula 749.02
with cleft lip (*see also* Cleft, palate, with cleft lip) 749.20
vitelline duct 751.0
development – *see* Anomaly, by site
erection 607.84
fusion – *see* Imperfect, closure
inflation lung (newborn) 770.5
intestinal canal 751.5
poise 729.9
rotation – *see* Malrotation
septum, ventricular 745.4

Imperfectly descended testis 752.51
Imperforate (congenital) – *see also* Atresia
anus 751.2
bile duct 751.61
cervix (uteri) 752.49
esophagus 750.3
hymen 752.42
intestine (small) 751.1
large 751.2
jejunum 751.1
pharynx 750.29
rectum 751.2
salivary duct 750.23
urethra 753.6
urinary meatus 753.6
vagina 752.49
Impervious (congenital) – *see also* Atresia
anus 751.2
bile duct 751.61
esophagus 750.3
intestine (small) 751.1
large 751.5
rectum 751.2
urethra 753.6
Impetiginization of other dermatoses 684
Impetigo (any organism) (any site) (bullous) (circinate) (contagiosa) (neonatorum) (simplex) 684
Bockhart's (superficial folliculitis) 704.8
external ear 684 *[380.13]*
eyelid 684 *[373.5]*
Fox's (contagiosa) 684
furfuracea 696.5
herpetiformis 694.3
nonobstetrical 694.3
staphylococcal infection 684
ulcerative 686.8
vulgaris 684
Impingement, soft tissue between teeth 524.89
anterior 524.81
posterior 524.82
Implant, endometrial 617.9
Implantation
anomalous – *see also* Anomaly, specified type, by site
ureter 753.4
cyst
external area or site (skin) NEC 709.8
iris 364.61
vagina 623.8
vulva 624.8
dermoid (cyst)
external area or site (skin) NEC 709.8
iris 364.61
vagina 623.8
vulva 624.8
placenta, low or marginal – *see* Placenta previa
Impotence (sexual) 607.84
organic origin NEC 607.84
psychogenic 302.72
Impoverished blood 285.9
Impression, basilar 756.0
Imprisonment V62.5
Improper
development, infant 764.9❺
Improperly tied umbilical cord (causing hemorrhage) 772.3
Impulses, obsessional 300.3
Impulsive neurosis 300.3
Inaction, kidney (*see also* Disease, renal) 593.9
Inactive – *see* condition
Inadequate, inadequacy
aesthetics of dental restoration 525.67
biologic 301.6
cardiac and renal – *see* Hypertension, cardiorenal
constitutional 301.6
development
child 783.40
fetus 764.9❺
affecting management of pregnancy 656.5❺
genitalia
after puberty NEC 259.0
congenital – *see* Hypoplasia, genitalia
lungs 748.5
organ or site NEC – *see* Hypoplasia, by site
dietary 269.9
distance, interarch 524.28
education V62.3

Inadequate, inadequacy – *continued*
environment
economic problem V60.2
household condition NEC V60.1
poverty V60.2
unemployment V62.0
functional 301.6
household care, due to
family member
handicapped or ill V60.4
temporarily away from home V60.4
on vacation V60.5
technical defects in home V60.1
temporary absence from home of person rendering care V60.4
housing (heating) (space) V60.1
interarch distance 524.28
material resources V60.2
mental (*see also* Retardation, mental) 319
nervous system 799.2
personality 301.6
prenatal care in current pregnancy V23.7
pulmonary
function 786.09
newborn 770.89
ventilation, newborn 770.89
respiration 786.09
newborn 770.89
sample, Papanicolaou smear 795.08
social 301.6
Inanition 263.9
with edema 262
due to
deprivation of food 994.2
malnutrition 263.9
fever 780.6
Inappropriate secretion
ACTH 255.0
antidiuretic hormone (ADH) (excessive) 253.6
deficiency 253.5
ectopic hormone NEC 259.3
pituitary (posterior) 253.6
Inattention after or at birth 995.52
Inborn errors of metabolism – *see* Disorder, metabolism
Incarceration, incarcerated
bubonocele – *see also* Hernia, inguinal, with obstruction
gangrenous – *see* Hernia, inguinal, with gangrene
colon (by hernia) – *see also* Hernia, by site with obstruction
gangrenous – *see* Hernia, by site, with gangrene
enterocele 552.9
gangrenous 551.9
epigastrocele 552.29
gangrenous 551.29
epiplocele 552.9
gangrenous 551.9
exomphalos 552.1
gangrenous 551.1
fallopian tube 620.8
hernia – *see also* Hernia, by site, with obstruction
gangrenous – *see* Hernia, by site, with gangrene
iris, in wound 871.1
lens, in wound 871.1
merocele (*see also* Hernia, femoral, with obstruction) 552.00
omentum (by hernia) – *see also* Hernia, by site, with obstruction
gangrenous – *see* Hernia, by site, with gangrene
omphalocele 756.79
rupture (meaning hernia) (*see also* Hernia, by site, with obstruction) 552.9
gangrenous (*see also* Hernia, by site, with gangrene) 551.9
sarcoepiplocele 552.9
gangrenous 551.9
sarcoepiplomphalocele 552.1
with gangrene 551.1
uterus 621.8
gravid 654.3❺
causing obstructed labor 660.2❺
affecting fetus or newborn 763.1
Incident, cerebrovascular (*see also* Disease, cerebrovascular, acute) 436
Incineration (entire body) (from fire, conflagration, electricity, or lightning) – *see* Burn, multiple, specified sites

Imperfect – Incineration

- **Incised wound**
  - external – *see* Wound, open, by site
  - internal organs (abdomen, chest, or pelvis) – *see* Injury, internal, by site, with open wound
- **Incision, incisional**
  - hernia – *see* Hernia, incisional
  - surgical, complication – *see* Complications, surgical procedures
  - traumatic
    - external – *see* Wound, open, by site
    - internal organs (abdomen, chest, or pelvis) – *see* Injury, internal, by site, with open wound
- **Inclusion**
  - azurophilic leukocytic 288.2
  - blennorrhea (neonatal) (newborn) 771.6
  - cyst – *see* Cyst, skin
  - gallbladder in liver (congenital) 751.69
- **Incompatibility**
  - ABO
    - affecting management of pregnancy 656.2⑤
    - fetus or newborn 773.1
    - infusion or transfusion reaction 999.6
  - blood (group) (Duffy) (E) (K(ell)) (Kidd) (Lewis) (M) (N) (P) (S) NEC
    - affecting management of pregnancy 656.2⑤
    - fetus or newborn 773.2
    - infusion or transfusion reaction 999.6
  - contour of existing restoration of tooth
    - with oral health 525.65
  - marital V61.10
    - involving divorce or estrangement V61.0
  - Rh (blood group) (factor)
    - affecting management of pregnancy 656.1⑤
    - fetus or newborn 773.0
    - infusion or transfusion reaction 999.7
  - Rhesus – *see* Incompatibility, Rh
- **Incompetency, incompetence, incompetent**
  - annular
    - aortic (valve) (*see also* Insufficiency, aortic) 424.1
    - mitral (valve) - (*see also* Insufficiency, mitral) 424.0
    - pulmonary valve (heart) (*see also* Endocarditis, pulmonary) 424.3
  - aortic (valve) (*see also* Insufficiency, aortic) 424.1
    - syphilitic 093.22
  - cardiac (orifice) 530.0
    - valve – *see* Endocarditis
  - cervix, cervical (os) 622.5
    - in pregnancy 654.5⑤
      - affecting fetus or newborn 761.0
  - esophagogastric (junction) (sphincter) 530.0
  - heart valve, congenital 746.89
  - mitral (valve) – *see* Insufficiency, mitral
  - papillary muscle (heart) 429.81
  - pelvic fundus
    - pubocervical tissue 618.81
    - rectovaginal tissue 618.82
  - pulmonary valve (heart) (*see also* Endocarditis, pulmonary) 424.3
    - congenital 746.09
  - tricuspid (annular) (rheumatic) (valve) (*see also* Endocarditis, tricuspid) 397.0
  - valvular – *see* Endocarditis
  - vein, venous (saphenous) (varicose) (*see also* Varicose, vein) 454.9
  - velopharyngeal (closure)
    - acquired 528.9
    - congenital 750.29
- **Incomplete** – *see also* condition
  - bladder emptying 788.21
  - expansion lungs (newborn) 770.5
  - gestation (liveborn) – *see* Immaturity
  - rotation – *see* Malrotation
- **Incontinence** 788.30
  - without sensory awareness 788.34
  - anal sphincter 787.6
  - continuous leakage 788.37
  - feces 787.6
    - due to hysteria 300.11
    - nonorganic origin 307.7
  - hysterical 300.11
  - mixed (male) (female) (urge and stress) 788.33
  - overflow 788.38
  - paradoxical 788.39
  - rectal 787.6
  - specified NEC 788.39
  - stress (female) 625.6
    - male NEC 788.32
- **Incontinence** – *continued*
  - urethral sphincter 599.84
  - urge 788.31
    - and stress (male) (female) 788.33
  - urine 788.30
    - active 788.30
    - male 788.30
      - stress 788.32
        - and urge 788.33
    - neurogenic 788.39
    - nonorganic origin 307.6
    - stress (female) 625.6
      - male NEC 788.32
    - urge 788.31
      - and stress 788.33
- **Incontinentia pigmenti** 757.33
- **Incoordinate**
  - uterus (action) (contractions) 661.4⑤
    - affecting fetus or newborn 763.7
- **Incoordination**
  - esophageal-pharyngeal (newborn) 787.24 ▲
  - muscular 781.3
  - papillary muscle 429.81
- **Increase, increased**
  - abnormal, in development 783.9
  - androgens (ovarian) 256.1
  - anticoagulants (antithrombin) (anti-VIIIa) (anti-IXa) (anti-Xa) (anti-XIa) 286.5
    - postpartum 666.3⑤
  - cold sense (*see also* Disturbance, sensation) 782.0
  - estrogen 256.0
  - function
    - adrenal (cortex) 255.3
      - medulla 255.6
    - pituitary (anterior) (gland) (lobe) 253.1
      - posterior 253.6
  - heat sense (*see also* Disturbance, sensation) 782.0
  - intracranial pressure 781.99
    - injury at birth 767.8
  - light reflex of retina 362.13
  - permeability, capillary 448.9
  - pressure
    - intracranial 781.99
      - injury at birth 767.8
    - intraocular 365.00
  - pulsations 785.9
  - pulse pressure 785.9
  - sphericity, lens 743.36
  - splenic activity 289.4
  - venous pressure 459.89
    - portal 572.3
- **Incrustation, cornea, lead, or zinc** 930.0
- **Incyclophoria** 378.44
- **Incyclotropia** 378.33
- **Indeterminate sex** 752.7
- **India rubber skin** 756.83
- **Indicanuria** 270.2
- **Indigestion** (bilious) (functional) 536.8
  - acid 536.8
  - catarrhal 536.8
  - due to decomposed food NEC 005.9
  - fat 579.8
  - nervous 306.4
  - psychogenic 306.4
- **Indirect** – *see* condition
- **Indolent bubo** NEC 099.8
- **Induced**
  - abortion – *see* Abortion, induced
  - birth, affecting fetus or newborn 763.89
  - delivery – *see* Delivery
  - labor – *see* Delivery
- **Induration, indurated**
  - brain 348.8
  - breast (fibrous) 611.79
    - puerperal, postpartum 676.3⑤
  - broad ligament 620.8
  - chancre 091.0
    - anus 091.1
    - congenital 090.0
    - extragenital NEC 091.2
  - corpora cavernosa (penis) (plastic) 607.89
  - liver (chronic) 573.8
    - acute 573.8
  - lung (black) (brown) (chronic) (fibroid) (*see also* Fibrosis, lung) 515
    - essential brown 275.0 *[516.1]*
  - penile 607.89
- **Induration, indurated** – *continued*
  - phlebitic – *see* Phlebitis
  - skin 782.8
  - stomach 537.89
- **Induratio penis plastica** 607.89
- **Industrial** – *see* condition
- **Inebriety** (*see also* Abuse, drugs, nondependent) 305.0⑤
- **Inefficiency**
  - kidney (*see also* Disease, renal) 593.9
  - thyroid (acquired) (gland) 244.9
- **Inelasticity, skin** 782.8
- **Inequality, leg** (acquired) (length) 736.81
  - congenital 755.30
- **Inertia**
  - bladder 596.4
    - neurogenic 596.54
      - with cauda equina syndrome 344.61
  - stomach 536.8
    - psychogenic 306.4
  - uterus, uterine 661.2⑤
    - affecting fetus or newborn 763.7
    - primary 661.0⑤
    - secondary 661.1⑤
  - vesical 596.4
    - neurogenic 596.54
      - with cauda equina 344.61
- **Infant** – *see also* condition
  - excessive crying of 780.92
  - fussy (baby) 780.91
  - held for adoption V68.89
  - newborn – *see* Newborn
  - post-term (gestation period over 40 completed weeks to 42 completed weeks) 766.21
  - prolonged gestation of (period over 42 completed weeks) 766.22
  - syndrome of diabetic mother 775.0
- **"Infant Hercules" syndrome** 255.2
- **Infantile** – *see also* condition
  - genitalia, genitals 259.0
    - in pregnancy or childbirth NEC 654.4⑤
      - affecting fetus or newborn 763.89
      - causing obstructed labor 660.2⑤
        - affecting fetus or newborn 763.1
  - heart 746.9
  - kidney 753.3
  - lack of care 995.52
  - macula degeneration 362.75
  - melanodontia 521.05
  - os, uterus (*see also* Infantile, genitalia) 259.0
  - pelvis 738.6
    - with disproportion (fetopelvic) 653.1⑤
      - affecting fetus or newborn 763.1
      - causing obstructed labor 660.1⑤
        - affecting fetus or newborn 763.1
  - penis 259.0
  - testis 257.2
  - uterus (*see also* Infantile, genitalia) 259.0
  - vulva 752.49
- **Infantilism** 259.9
  - with dwarfism (hypophyseal) 253.3
  - Brissaud's (infantile myxedema) 244.9
  - celiac 579.0
  - Herter's (nontropical sprue) 579.0
  - hypophyseal 253.3
  - hypothalamic (with obesity) 253.8
  - idiopathic 259.9
  - intestinal 579.0
  - pancreatic 577.8
  - pituitary 253.3
  - renal 588.0
  - sexual (with obesity) 259.0
- **Infants, healthy liveborn** – *see* Newborn
- **Infarct, infarction**
  - adrenal (capsule) (gland) 255.41 ▲
  - amnion 658.8⑤
  - anterior (with contiguous portion of intraventricular septum) NEC (*see also* Infarct, myocardium) 410.1⑤
  - appendices epiploicae 557.0
  - bowel 557.0
  - brain (stem) 434.91
    - embolic (*see also* Embolism, brain) 434.11
    - healed or old without residuals V12.54 ▲
    - iatrogenic 997.02
    - lacunar 434.91
    - late effect – *see* Late effect(s) (of) cerebrovascular disease
    - postoperative 997.02
    - puerperal, postpartum, childbirth 674.0⑤

Infarct, infarction – *continued*
  brain – *continued*
    thrombotic (*see also* Thrombosis, brain) 434.01
  breast 611.8
  Brewer's (kidney) 593.81
  cardiac (*see also* Infarct, myocardium) 410.9❺
  cerebellar (*see also* Infarct, brain) 434.91
    embolic (*see also* Embolism, brain) 434.11
  cerebral (*see also* Infarct, brain) 434.91
    aborted 434.91 ●
    embolic (*see also* Embolism, brain) 434.11
    thrombotic (*see also* Infarct, brain) 434.01
  chorion 658.8❺
  colon (acute) (agnogenic) (embolic) (hemorrhagic) (nonocclusive) (nonthrombotic) (occlusive) (segmental) (thrombotic) (with gangrene) 557.0
  coronary artery (*see also* Infarct, myocardium) 410.9❺
  cortical 434.91
  embolic (*see also* Embolism) 444.9
  fallopian tube 620.8
  gallbladder 575.8
  heart (*see also* Infarct, myocardium) 410.9❺
  hepatic 573.4
  hypophysis (anterior lobe) 253.8
  impending (myocardium) 411.1
  intestine (acute) (agnogenic) (embolic) (hemorrhagic) (nonocclusive) (nonthrombotic) (occlusive) (thrombotic) (with gangrene) 557.0
  kidney 593.81
  lacunar 434.91
  liver 573.4
  lung (embolic) (thrombotic) 415.1❺
    with
      abortion – *see* Abortion, by type, with, embolism
      ectopic pregnancy (*see also* categories 633.0-633.9) 639.6
      molar pregnancy (*see also* categories 630-632) 639.6
    following
      abortion 639.6
      ectopic or molar pregnancy 639.6
    iatrogenic 415.11
    in pregnancy, childbirth, or puerperium – *see* Embolism, obstetrical
    postoperative 415.11
    septic 415.12 ●
  lymph node or vessel 457.8
  medullary (brain) – *see* Infarct, brain
  meibomian gland (eyelid) 374.85
  mesentery, mesenteric (embolic) (thrombotic) (with gangrene) 557.0
    with symptoms after 8 weeks from date of infarction 414.8
    non-ST elevation (NSTEMI) 410.7❺
    ST elevation (STEMI) 410.9❺
      anterior (wall) 410.1❺
      anterolateral (wall) 410.0❺
      inferior (wall) 410.4❺
      inferolateral (wall) 410.2❺
      inferoposterior wall 410.3❺
      lateral wall 410.5❺
      posterior (strictly) (true) (wall) 410.6❺
      specified site NEC 410.8❺
  midbrain – *see* Infarct, brain
  myocardium, myocardial (acute or with a stated duration of 8 weeks or less) (with hypertension) 410.9❺

Note – Use the following fifth-digit subclassification with category 410:
0 episode unspecified
1 initial episode
2 subsequent episode without recurrence

    with symptoms after 8 weeks from date of infarction 414.8
    anterior (wall) (with contiguous portion of intraventricular septum) NEC 410.1❺
    anteroapical (with contiguous portion of intraventricular septum) 410.1❺
    anterolateral (wall) 410.0❺
    anteroseptal (with contiguous portion of intraventricular septum) 410.1❺
    apical-lateral 410.5❺
    atrial 410.8❺
    basal-lateral 410.5❺

Infarct, infarction – *continued*
  myocardium, myocardial – *continued*
    chronic (with symptoms after 8 weeks from date of infarction) 414.8
    diagnosed on ECG, but presenting no symptoms 412
    diaphragmatic wall (with contiguous portion of intraventricular septum) 410.4❺
    healed or old, currently presenting no symptoms 412
    high lateral 410.5❺
    impending 411.1
    inferior (wall) (with contiguous portion of intraventricular septum) 410.4❺
    inferolateral (wall) 410.2❺
    inferoposterior wall 410.3❺
    intraoperative 997.1 ●
    lateral wall 410.5❺
    non-Q wave 410.7❺ ●
    nontransmural 410.7❺
    papillary muscle 410.8❺
    past (diagnosed on ECG or other special investigation, but currently presenting no symptoms) 412
      with symptoms NEC 414.8
    posterior (strictly) (true) (wall) 410.6❺
    posterobasal 410.6❺
    posteroinferior 410.3❺
    posterolateral 410.5❺
    postprocedural 997.1 ●
    previous, currently presenting no symptoms 412
    Q wave (*see also* Infarct, myocardium, by site) 410.9❺ ●
    septal 410.8❺
    specified site NEC 410.8❺
    subendocardial 410.7❺
    syphilitic 093.82
  non-ST elevation myocardial infarction (NSTEMI) 410.7❺
  nontransmural 410.7❺
  omentum 557.0
  ovary 620.8
  pancreas 577.8
  papillary muscle (*see also* Infarct, myocardium) 410.8❺
  parathyroid gland 252.8
  pituitary (gland) 253.8
  placenta (complicating pregnancy) 656.7❺
    affecting fetus or newborn 762.2
  pontine – *see* Infarct, brain
  posterior NEC (*see also* Infarct, myocardium) 410.6❺
  prostate 602.8
  pulmonary (artery) (hemorrhagic) (vein) 415.1❺
    with
      abortion – *see* Abortion, by type, with embolism
      ectopic pregnancy (*see also* categories 633.0-633.9) 639.6
      molar pregnancy (*see also* categories 630-632) 639.6
    following
      abortion 639.6
      ectopic or molar pregnancy 639.6
    iatrogenic 415.11
    in pregnancy, childbirth, or puerperium – *see* Embolism, obstetrical
    postoperative 415.11
    septic 415.12 ●
  renal 593.81
    embolic or thrombotic 593.81
  retina, retinal 362.84
    with occlusion – *see* Occlusion, retina
  spinal (acute) (cord) (embolic) (nonembolic) 336.1
  spleen 289.59
    embolic or thrombotic 444.89
  subchorionic – *see* Infarct, placenta
  subendocardial (*see also* Infarct, myocardium) 410.7❺
  suprarenal (capsule) (gland) 255.41 ▲
  syncytium – *see* Infarct, placenta
  testis 608.83
  thrombotic (*see also* Thrombosis) 453.9
    artery, arterial – *see* Embolism
  thyroid (gland) 246.3
  ventricle (heart) (*see also* Infarct, myocardium) 410.9❺
Infecting – *see* condition
Infection, infected, infective (opportunistic) 136.9
  with lymphangitis – *see* Lymphangitis
  abortion – *see* Abortion, by type, with, sepsis

Infection, infected, infective – *continued*
  abscess (skin) – *see* Abscess, by site
  Absidia 117.7
  Acanthocheilonema (perstans) 125.4
    streptocerca 125.6
  accessory sinus (chronic) (*see also* Sinusitis) 473.9
  Achorion – *see* Dermatophytosis
  Acremonium falciforme 117.4
  acromioclavicular (joint) 711.91
  actinobacillus
    lignieresii 027.8
    mallei 024
    muris 026.1
  actinomadura – *see* Actinomycosis
  Actinomyces (israelii) – *see also* Actinomycosis
    muris-ratti 026.1
  Actinomycetales (actinomadura) (Actinomyces) (Nocardia) (Streptomyces) – *see* Actinomycosis
  actinomycotic NEC (*see also* Actinomycosis) 039.9
  adenoid (chronic) 474.01
    acute 463
    and tonsil (chronic) 474.02
      acute or subacute 463
  adenovirus NEC 079.0
    in diseases classified elsewhere – *see* category 079❹
    unspecified nature or site 079.0
  Aerobacter aerogenes NEC 041.85
    enteritis 008.2
  aerogenes capsulatus (*see also* Gangrene, gas) 040.0
  aertrycke (*see also* Infection, Salmonella) 003.9
  ajellomyces dermatitidis 116.0
  alimentary canal NEC (*see also* Enteritis, due to, by organism) 009.0
  Allescheria boydii 117.6
  Alternaria 118
  alveolus, alveolar (process) (pulpal origin) 522.4
  ameba, amebic (histolytica) (*see also* Amebiasis) 006.9
    acute 006.0
    chronic 006.1
    free-living 136.2
    hartmanni 007.8
    specified
      site NEC 006.8
      type NEC 007.8
  amniotic fluid or cavity 658.4❺
    affecting fetus or newborn 762.7
  anaerobes (cocci) (gram-negative) (gram-positive) (mixed) NEC 041.84
  anal canal 569.49
  Ancylostoma braziliense 126.2
  angiostrongylus cantonensis 128.8
  anisakiasis 127.1
  Anisakis larva 127.1
  anthrax (*see also* Anthrax) 022.9
  antrum (chronic) (*see also* Sinusitis, maxillary) 473.0
  anus (papillae) (sphincter) 569.49
  arbor virus NEC 066.9
  arbovirus NEC 066.9
  argentophil-rod 027.0
  Ascaris lumbricoides 127.0
  ascomycetes 117.4
  Aspergillus (flavus) (fumigatus) (terreus) 117.3
  atypical
    acid-fast (bacilli) (*see also* Mycobacterium, atypical) 031.9
    mycobacteria (*see also* Mycobacterium, atypical) 031.9
  auditory meatus (circumscribed) (diffuse) (external) (*see also* Otitis, externa) 380.10
  auricle (ear) (*see also* Otitis, externa) 380.10
  axillary gland 683
  Babesiasis 088.82
  Babesiosis 088.82
  Bacillus NEC 041.89
    abortus 023.1
    anthracis (*see also* Anthrax) 022.9
    cereus (food poisoning) 005.89
    coli – *see* Infection, Escherichia coli
    coliform NEC 041.85
    Ducrey's (any location) 099.0
    Flexner's 004.1
    Friedländer's NEC 041.3
    fusiformis 101
    gas (gangrene) (*see also* Gangrene, gas) 040.0
    mallei 024

Infarct, infarction – Infection, infected, infective

- **Infection, infected, infective** – *continued*
  - Bacillus – *continued*
    - melitensis 023.0
    - paratyphoid, paratyphosus 002.9
      - A 002.1
      - B 002.2
      - C 002.3
    - Schmorl's 040.3
    - Shiga 004.0
    - suipestifer (*see also* Infection, Salmonella) 003.9
    - swimming pool 031.1
    - typhosa 002.0
    - welchii (*see also* Gangrene, gas) 040.0
    - Whitmore's 025
  - bacterial NEC 041.9
    - specified NEC 041.89
      - anaerobic NEC 041.84
      - gram-negative NEC 041.85
        - anaerobic NEC 041.84
  - Bacterium
    - paratyphosum 002.9
      - A 002.1
      - B 002.2
      - C 002.3
    - typhosum 002.9
  - Bacteroides (fragilis) (melaninogenicus) (oralis) NEC 041.82
  - balantidium coli 007.0
  - Bartholin's gland 616.89
  - Basidiobolus 117.7
  - Bedsonia 079.98
    - specified NEC 079.88
  - bile duct 576.1
  - bladder (*see also* Cystitis) 595.9
  - Blastomyces, blastomycotic 116.0
    - brasiliensis 116.1
    - dermatitidis 116.0
    - European 117.5
    - Loboi 116.2
    - North American 116.0
    - South American 116.1
  - bleb
    - postprocedural 379.60
      - stage 1 379.61
      - stage 2 379.62
      - stage 3 379.63
  - blood stream – *see* ▶*also*◀ Septicemia
    - catheter-related (CRBSI) 999.31 ●
  - bone 730.9❺
    - specified – *see* Osteomyelitis
  - Bordetella 033.9
    - bronchiseptica 033.8
    - parapertussis 033.1
    - pertussis 033.0
  - Borrelia
    - bergdorfi 088.81
    - vincentii (mouth) (pharynx) (tonsil) 101
  - brain (*see also* Encephalitis) 323.9
    - late effect – *see* category 326
    - membranes - (*see also* Meningitis) 322.9
    - septic 324.0
      - late effect – *see* category 326
      - meninges (*see also* Meningitis) 320.9
  - branchial cyst 744.42
  - breast 611.0
    - puerperal, postpartum 675.2❺
      - with nipple 675.9❺
        - specified type NEC 675.8❺
      - nonpurulent 675.2❺
      - purulent 675.1❺
  - bronchus (*see also* Bronchitis) 490
    - fungus NEC 117.9
  - Brucella 023.9
    - abortus 023.1
    - canis 023.3
    - melitensis 023.0
    - mixed 023.8
    - suis 023.2
  - Brugia (Wuchereria) malayi 125.1
  - bursa – *see* Bursitis
  - buttocks (skin) 686.9
  - Candida (albicans) (tropicalis) (*see also* Candidiasis) 112.9
    - congenital 771.7
  - Candiru 136.8
  - Capillaria
    - hepatica 128.8
    - philippinensis 127.5
  - cartilage 733.99
  - catheter-related bloodstream (CRBSI) 999.31 ●
  - cat liver fluke 121.0

- **Infection, infected, infective** – *continued*
  - cellulitis – *see* Cellulitis, by site
  - Cephalosporum falciforme 117.4
  - Cercomonas hominis (intestinal) 007.3
  - cerebrospinal (*see also* Meningitis) 322.9
    - late effect – *see* category 326
  - cervical gland 683
  - cervix (*see also* Cervicitis) 616.0
  - cesarean section wound 674.3❺
  - Chilomastix (intestinal) 007.8
  - Chlamydia 079.98
    - specified NEC 079.88
  - Cholera (*see also* Cholera) 001.9
  - chorionic plate 658.8❺
  - Cladosporium
    - bantianum 117.8
    - carrionii 117.2
    - mansoni 111.1
    - trichoides 117.8
    - wernecki 111.1
  - Clonorchis (sinensis) (liver) 121.1
  - Clostridium (haemolyticum) (novyi) NEC 041.84
    - botulinum 005.1
    - histolyticum (*see also* Gangrene, gas) 040.0
    - oedematiens (*see also* Gangrene, gas) 040.0
    - perfringens 041.83
      - due to food 005.2
    - septicum (*see also* Gangrene, gas) 040.0
    - sordellii (*see also* Gangrene, gas) 040.0
    - welchii (*see also* Gangrene, gas) 040.0
      - due to food 005.2
  - Coccidioides (immitis) (*see also* Coccidioidomycosis) 114.9
  - coccus NEC 041.89
  - colon (*see also* Enteritis, due to, by organism) 009.0
    - bacillus – *see* Infection, Escherichia coli
  - colostomy or enterostomy 569.61
  - common duct 576.1
  - complicating pregnancy, childbirth, or puerperium NEC 647.9❺
    - affecting fetus or newborn 760.2
  - Condiobolus 117.7
  - congenital NEC 771.89
    - Candida albicans 771.7
    - chronic 771.2
    - cytomegalovirus 771.1
    - hepatitis, viral 771.2
    - herpes simplex 771.2
    - listeriosis 771.2
    - malaria 771.2
    - poliomyelitis 771.2
    - rubella 771.0
    - toxoplasmosis 771.2
    - tuberculosis 771.2
    - urinary (tract) 771.82
    - vaccinia 771.2
  - coronavirus 079.89
    - SARS-associated 079.82
  - corpus luteum (*see also* Salpingo-oophoritis) 614.2
  - Corynebacterium diphtheriae – *see* Diphtheria
  - Coxsackie (*see also* Coxsackie) 079.2
    - endocardium 074.22
    - heart NEC 074.20
    - in diseases classified elsewhere – *see* category 079❹
    - meninges 047.0
    - myocardium 074.23
    - pericardium 074.21
    - pharynx 074.0
    - specified disease NEC 074.8
    - unspecified nature or site 079.2
  - Cryptococcus neoformans 117.5
  - Cryptosporidia 007.4
  - Cunninghamella 117.7
  - cyst – *see* Cyst
  - Cysticercus cellulosae 123.1
  - cytomegalovirus 078.5
    - congenital 771.1
  - dental (pulpal origin) 522.4
  - deuteromycetes 117.4
  - Dicrocoelium dendriticum 121.8
  - Dipetalonema (perstans) 125.4
    - streptocerca 125.6
  - diphtherial – *see* Diphtheria
  - Diphyllobothrium (adult) (latum) (pacificum) 123.4
    - larval 123.5
  - Diplogonoporus (grandis) 123.8
  - Dipylidium (caninum) 123.8
  - Dirofilaria 125.6
  - dog tapeworm 123.8

- **Infection, infected, infective** – *continued*
  - Dracunculus medinensis 125.7
  - Dreschlera 118
    - hawaiiensis 117.8
  - Ducrey's bacillus (any site) 099.0
  - due to or resulting from
    - central venous catheter 999.31 ●
    - device, implant, or graft (any) (presence of) – *see* Complications, infection and inflammation, due to (presence of) any device, implant, or graft classified to 996.0-996.5 NEC
    - injection, inoculation, infusion, transfusion, or vaccination (prophylactic) (therapeutic) 999.39 ▲
    - injury NEC – *see* Wound, open, by site, complicated
    - surgery 998.59
  - duodenum 535.6❺
  - ear – *see also* Otitis
    - external (*see also* Otitis, externa) 380.10
    - inner (*see also* Labyrinthitis) 386.30
    - middle – *see* Otitis, media
  - Eaton's agent NEC 041.81
  - Eberthella typhosa 002.0
  - Ebola 078.89
  - echinococcosis 122.9
  - Echinococcus (*see also* Echinococcus) 122.9
  - Echinostoma 121.8
  - ECHO virus 079.1
    - in diseases classified elsewhere – *see* category 079❹
    - unspecified nature or site 079.1
  - Ehrlichiosis 082.40
    - chaffeensis 082.41
    - specified type NEC 082.49
  - Endamoeba – *see* Infection, ameba
  - endocardium (*see also* Endocarditis) 421.0
  - endocervix (*see also* Cervicitis) 616.0
  - Entamoeba – *see* Infection, ameba
  - enteric (*see also* Enteritis, due to, by organism) 009.0
  - Enterobacter aerogenes NEC 041.85
  - Enterobacter sakazakii 041.85
  - Enterobius vermicularis 127.4
  - enterococcus NEC 041.04
  - enterovirus NEC 079.89
    - central nervous system NEC 048
    - enteritis 008.67
    - meningitis 047.9
  - Entomophthora 117.7
  - Epidermophyton – *see* Dermatophytosis
  - epidermophytosis – *see* Dermatophytosis
  - episiotomy 674.3❺
  - Epstein-Barr virus 075
    - chronic 780.79 *[139.8]*
  - erysipeloid 027.1
  - Erysipelothrix (insidiosa) (rhusiopathiae) 027.1
  - erythema infectiosum 057.0
  - Escherichia coli NEC 041.4
    - enteritis – *see* Enteritis, E. coli
    - generalized 038.42
    - intestinal – *see* Enteritis, E. coli
  - esophagostomy 530.86
  - ethmoidal (chronic) (sinus) (*see also* Sinusitis, ethmoidal) 473.2
  - Eubacterium 041.84
  - Eustachian tube (ear) 381.50
    - acute 381.51
    - chronic 381.52
  - exanthema subitum ▶(*see also* Exanthem subitum)◀ 058.10 ▲
  - external auditory canal (meatus) (*see also* Otitis, externa) 380.10
  - eye NEC 360.00
  - eyelid 373.9
    - specified NEC 373.8
  - fallopian tube (*see also* Salpingo-oophoritis) 614.2
  - fascia 728.89
  - Fasciola
    - gigantica 121.3
    - hepatica 121.3
  - Fasciolopsis (buski) 121.4
  - fetus (intra-amniotic) – *see* Infection, congenital
  - filarial – *see* Infestation, filarial
  - finger (skin) 686.9
    - abscess (with lymphangitis) 681.00
      - pulp 681.01
    - cellulitis (with lymphangitis) 681.00
    - distal closed space (with lymphangitis) 681.00

❹ Fourth-Digit Required   ❺ Fifth-Digit Required   *[code]* Manifestation Code   ▶◀ Revised Text   ● New Line   ▲ Revised Code

- **Infection, infected, infective** – *continued*
  - finger – *continued*
    - nail 681.02
      - fungus 110.1
  - fish tapeworm 123.4
    - larval 123.5
  - flagellate, intestinal 007.9
  - fluke – *see* Infestation, fluke
  - focal
    - teeth (pulpal origin) 522.4
    - tonsils 474.00
      - and adenoids 474.02
  - Fonsecaea
    - compactum 117.2
    - pedrosoi 117.2
  - food (*see also* Poisoning, food) 005.9
  - foot (skin) 686.9
    - fungus 110.4
  - Francisella tularensis (*see also* Tularemia) 021.9
  - frontal sinus (chronic) (*see also* Sinusitis, frontal) 473.1
  - fungus NEC 117.9
    - beard 110.0
    - body 110.5
    - dermatiacious NEC 117.8
    - foot 110.4
    - groin 110.3
    - hand 110.2
    - nail 110.1
    - pathogenic to compromised host only 118
    - perianal (area) 110.3
    - scalp 110.0
    - scrotum 110.8
    - skin 111.9
      - foot 110.4
      - hand 110.2
    - toenails 110.1
    - trachea 117.9
  - Fusarium 118
  - Fusobacterium 041.84
  - gallbladder (*see also* Cholecystitis, acute) 575.0
  - Gardnerella vaginalis 041.89
  - gas bacillus (*see also* Gas, gangrene) 040.0
  - gastric (*see also* Gastritis) 535.5❺
  - Gastrodiscoides hominis 121.8
  - gastroenteric (*see also* Enteritis, due to, by organism) 009.0
  - gastrointestinal (*see also* Enteritis, due to, by organism) 009.0
  - gastrostomy 536.41
  - generalized NEC (*see also* Septicemia) 038.9
  - genital organ or tract NEC
    - female 614.9
      - with
        - abortion – *see* Abortion, by type, with sepsis
        - ectopic pregnancy (*see also* categories 633.0-633.9) 639.0
        - molar pregnancy (*see also* categories 630-632) 639.0
      - complicating pregnancy 646.6❺
        - affecting fetus or newborn 760.8
      - following
        - abortion 639.0
        - ectopic or molar pregnancy 639.0
      - puerperal, postpartum, childbirth 670❹
        - minor or localized 646.6❺
          - affecting fetus or newborn 760.8
    - male 608.4
  - genitourinary tract NEC 599.0
  - Ghon tubercle, primary (*see also* Tuberculosis) 010.0❺
  - Giardia lamblia 007.1
  - gingival (chronic) 523.10
    - acute 523.00
    - Vincent's 101
  - glanders 024
  - Glenosporopsis amazonica 116.2
  - Gnathostoma spinigerum 128.1
  - Gongylonema 125.6
  - gonococcal NEC (*see also* Gonococcus) 098.0
  - gram-negative bacilli NEC 041.85
    - anaerobic 041.84
  - guinea worm 125.7
  - gum (*see also* Infection, gingival) 523.10
  - Hantavirus 079.81
  - heart 429.89
  - Helicobacter pylori (H. pylori) 041.86
  - helminths NEC 128.9
    - intestinal 127.9
      - mixed (types classifiable to more than one category in 120.0-127.7) 127.8

- **Infection, infected, infective** – *continued*
  - helminths – *continued*
    - intestinal – *continued*
      - specified type NEC 127.7
    - specified type NEC 128.8
  - Hemophilus influenzae NEC 041.5
    - generalized 038.41
  - Herpes (simplex) (*see also* Herpes, simplex) 054.9
    - congenital 771.2
    - zoster (*see also* Herpes, zoster) 053.9
      - eye NEC 053.29
  - Heterophyes heterophyes 121.6
  - Histoplasma (*see also* Histoplasmosis) 115.90
    - capsulatum (*see also* Histoplasmosis, American) 115.00
    - duboisii (*see also* Histoplasmosis, African) 115.10
  - HIV V08
    - with symptoms, symptomatic 042
  - hookworm (*see also* Ancylostomiasis) 126.9
  - human herpesvirus 6 058.81 ●
  - human herpesvirus 7 058.82 ●
  - human herpesvirus 8 058.89 ●
  - human herpesvirus NEC 058.89 ●
  - human immunodeficiency virus V08
    - with symptoms, symptomatic 042
  - human papillomavirus 079.4
  - hydrocele 603.1
  - hydronephrosis 591
  - Hymenolepis 123.6
  - hypopharynx 478.29
  - inguinal glands 683
    - due to soft chancre 099.0
  - intestine, intestinal (*see also* Enteritis, due to, by organism) 009.0
  - intrauterine (*see also* Endometritis) 615.9
    - complicating delivery 646.6❺
  - isospora belli or hominis 007.2
  - Japanese B encephalitis 062.0
  - jaw (bone) (acute) (chronic) (lower) (subacute) (upper) 526.4
  - joint – *see* Arthritis, infectious or infective
  - Kaposi's sarcoma-associated herpesvirus 058.89 ●
  - kidney (cortex) (hematogenous) 590.9
    - with
      - abortion – *see* Abortion, by type, with urinary tract infection
      - calculus 592.0
      - ectopic pregnancy (*see also* categories 633.0-633.9) 639.8
      - molar pregnancy (*see also* categories 630-632) 639.8
    - complicating pregnancy or puerperium 646.6❺
      - affecting fetus or newborn 760.1
    - following
      - abortion 639.8
      - ectopic or molar pregnancy 639.8
    - pelvis and ureter 590.3
  - Klebsiella pneumoniae NEC 041.3
  - knee (skin) NEC 686.9
    - joint – *see* Arthritis, infectious
  - Koch's (*see also* Tuberculosis, pulmonary) 011.9❺
  - labia (majora) (minora) (*see also* Vulvitis) 616.10
  - lacrimal
    - gland (*see also* Dacryoadenitis) 375.00
    - passages (duct) (sac) (*see also* Dacryocystitis) 375.30
  - larynx NEC 478.79
  - leg (skin) NEC 686.9
  - Leishmania (*see also* Leishmaniasis) 085.9
    - braziliensis 085.5
    - donovani 085.0
    - Ethiopica 085.3
    - furunculosa 085.1
    - infantum 085.0
    - Mexicana 085.4
    - tropica (minor) 085.1
      - major 085.2
  - Leptosphaeria senegalensis 117.4
  - leptospira (*see also* Leptospirosis) 100.9
    - Australis 100.89
    - Bataviae 100.89
    - pyrogenes 100.89
    - specified type NEC 100.89
  - leptospirochetal NEC (*see also* Leptospirosis) 100.9
  - Leptothrix – *see* Actinomycosis
  - Listeria monocytogenes (listeriosis) 027.0
    - congenital 771.2

- **Infection, infected, infective** – *continued*
  - liver fluke – *see* Infestation, fluke, liver
  - Loa loa 125.2
    - eyelid 125.2 *[373.6]*
  - Loboa loboi 116.2
  - local, skin (staphylococcal) (streptococcal) NEC 686.9
    - abscess – *see* Abscess, by site
    - cellulitis – *see* Cellulitis, by site
    - ulcer (*see also* Ulcer, skin) 707.9
  - Loefflerella
    - mallei 024
    - whitmori 025
  - lung 518.89
    - atypical Mycobacterium 031.0
      - tuberculous (*see also* Tuberculosis, pulmonary) 011.9❺
    - basilar 518.89
    - chronic 518.89
    - fungus NEC 117.9
    - spirochetal 104.8
    - virus – *see* Pneumonia, virus
  - lymph gland (axillary) (cervical) (inguinal) 683
    - mesenteric 289.2
  - lymphoid tissue, base of tongue or posterior pharynx, NEC 474.00
  - madurella
    - grisea 117.4
    - mycetomii 117.4
  - major
    - with
      - abortion – *see* Abortion, by type, with sepsis
      - ectopic pregnancy (*see also* categories 633.0-633.9) 639.0
      - molar pregnancy (*see also* categories 630-632) 639.0
    - following
      - abortion 639.0
      - ectopic or molar pregnancy 639.0
    - puerperal, postpartum, childbirth 670❹
  - malarial – *see* Malaria
  - Malassezia furfur 111.0
  - Malleomyces
    - mallei 024
    - pseudomallei 025
  - mammary gland 611.0
    - puerperal, postpartum 675.2❺
  - Mansonella (ozzardi) 125.5
  - mastoid (suppurative) – *see* Mastoiditis
  - maxilla, maxillary 526.4
    - sinus (chronic) (*see also* Sinusitis, maxillary) 473.0
  - mediastinum 519.2
  - medina 125.7
  - meibomian
    - cyst 373.12
    - gland 373.12
  - melioidosis 025
  - meninges (*see also* Meningitis) 320.9
  - meningococcal (*see also* condition) 036.9
    - brain 036.1
    - cerebrospinal 036.0
    - endocardium 036.42
    - generalized 036.2
    - meninges 036.0
    - meningococcemia 036.2
    - specified site NEC 036.89
  - mesenteric lymph nodes or glands NEC 289.2
  - Metagonimus 121.5
  - metatarsophalangeal 711.97
  - microorganism resistant to drugs – *see* Resistance (to), drugs by microorganisms
  - Microsporidia 136.8
  - microsporum, microsporic – *see* Dermatophytosis
  - Mima polymorpha NEC 041.85
  - mixed flora NEC 041.89
  - Monilia (*see also* Candidiasis) 112.9
    - neonatal 771.7
  - monkeypox 057.8
  - Monosporium apiospermum 117.6
  - mouth (focus) NEC 528.9
    - parasitic 136.9
  - Mucor 117.7
  - muscle NEC 728.89
  - mycelium NEC 117.9
  - mycetoma
    - actinomycotic NEC (*see also* Actinomycosis) 039.9
    - mycotic NEC 117.4
  - Mycobacterium, mycobacterial (*see also* Mycobacterium) 031.9
  - Mycoplasma NEC 041.81

Infection, infected, infective

❹ Fourth-Digit Required ❺ Fifth-Digit Required *[code]* Manifestation Code ▶◀ Revised Text ● New Line ▲ Revised Code

Infection, infected, infective – *continued*
- mycotic NEC 117.9
  - pathogenic to compromised host only 118
  - skin NEC 111.9
  - systemic 117.9
- myocardium NEC 422.90
- nail (chronic) (with lymphangitis) 681.9
  - finger 681.02
    - fungus 110.1
  - ingrowing 703.0
  - toe 681.11
    - fungus 110.1
- nasal sinus (chronic) (*see also* Sinusitis) 473.9
- nasopharynx (chronic) 478.29
  - acute 460
- navel 686.9
  - newborn 771.4
- Neisserian – *see* Gonococcus
- Neotestudina rosatii 117.4
- newborn, generalized 771.89
- nipple 611.0
  - puerperal, postpartum 675.0❺
    - with breast 675.9❺
      - specified type NEC 675.8❺
- Nocardia – *see* Actinomycosis
- nose 478.19
- nostril 478.19
- obstetrical surgical wound 674.3❺
- Oesophagostomum (apiostomum) 127.7
- Oestrus ovis 134.0
- Oidium albicans (*see also* Candidiasis) 112.9
- Onchocerca (volvulus) 125.3
  - eye 125.3 *[360.13]*
  - eyelid 125.3 *[373.6]*
- operation wound 998.59
- Opisthorchis (felineus) (tenuicollis) (viverrini) 121.0
- orbit 376.00
  - chronic 376.10
- ovary (*see also* Salpingo-oophoritis) 614.2
- Oxyuris vermicularis 127.4
- pancreas 577.0
- Paracoccidioides brasiliensis 116.1
- Paragonimus (westermani) 121.2
- parainfluenza virus 079.89
- parameningococcus NEC 036.9
  - with meningitis 036.0
- parasitic NEC 136.9
- paratyphoid 002.9
  - type A 002.1
  - type B 002.2
  - type C 002.3
- paraurethral ducts 597.89
- parotid gland 527.2
- Pasteurella NEC 027.2
  - multocida (cat-bite) (dog-bite) 027.2
  - pestis (*see also* Plague) 020.9
  - pseudotuberculosis 027.2
  - septica (cat-bite) (dog-bite) 027.2
  - tularensis (*see also* Tularemia) 021.9
- pelvic, female (*see also* Disease, pelvis, inflammatory) 614.9
- penis (glans) (retention) NEC 607.2
  - herpetic 054.13
- Peptococcus 041.84
- Peptostreptococcus 041.84
- periapical (pulpal origin) 522.4
- peridental 523.30
- perineal wound (obstetrical) 674.3❺
- periodontal 523.31
- periorbital 376.00
  - chronic 376.10
- perirectal 569.49
- perirenal (*see also* Infection, kidney) 590.9
- peritoneal (*see also* Peritonitis) 567.9
- periureteral 593.89
- periurethral 597.89
- Petriellidium boydii 117.6
- pharynx 478.29
  - Coxsackie virus 074.0
  - phlegmonous 462
  - posterior, lymphoid 474.00
- Phialophora
  - gougerotii 117.8
  - jeanselmei 117.8
  - verrucosa 117.2
- Piedraia hortai 111.3
- pinna, acute 380.11
- pinta 103.9
  - intermediate 103.1
  - late 103.2
  - mixed 103.3

Infection, infected, infective – *continued*
- pinta – *continued*
  - primary 103.0
- pinworm 127.4
- pityrosporum furfur 111.0
- pleuropneumonia-like organisms NEC (PPLO) 041.81
- pneumococcal NEC 041.2
  - generalized (purulent) 038.2
- Pneumococcus NEC 041.2
- postoperative wound 998.59
- posttraumatic NEC 958.3
- postvaccinal 999.39 ▲
- prepuce NEC 607.1
- Proprionibacterium 041.84
- prostate (capsule) (*see also* Prostatitis) 601.9
- Proteus (mirabilis) (morganii) (vulgaris) NEC 041.6
  - enteritis 008.3
- protozoal NEC 136.8
  - intestinal NEC 007.9
- Pseudomonas NEC 041.7
  - mallei 024
  - pneumonia 482.1
  - pseudomallei 025
- psittacosis 073.9
- puerperal, postpartum (major) 670❹
  - minor 646.6❺
- pulmonary – *see* Infection, lung
- purulent – *see* Abscess
- putrid, generalized – *see* Septicemia
- pyemic – *see* Septicemia
- Pyrenochaeta romeroi 117.4
- Q fever 083.0
- rabies 071
- rectum (sphincter) 569.49
- renal (*see also* Infection, kidney) 590.9
  - pelvis and ureter 590.3
- resistant to drugs – *see* Resistance (to), drugs by microorganisms
- respiratory 519.8
  - chronic 519.8
  - influenzal (acute) (upper) 487.1
  - lung 518.89
  - rhinovirus 460
  - syncytial virus 079.6
  - upper (acute) (infectious) NEC 465.9
    - with flu, grippe, or influenza 487.1
    - influenzal 487.1
    - multiple sites NEC 465.8
    - streptococcal 034.0
    - viral NEC 465.9
- respiratory syncytial virus (RSV) 079.6
- resulting from presence of shunt or other internal prosthetic device – *see* Complications, infection and inflammation, due to (presence of) any device, implant, or graft classified to 996.0-996.5 NEC
- retroperitoneal 567.39
- retrovirus 079.50
  - human immunodeficiency virus type 2 [HIV 2] 079.53
  - human T-cell lymphotrophic virus type I [HTLV-I] 079.51
  - human T-cell lymphotrophic virus type II [HTLV-II] 079.52
  - specified NEC 079.59
- Rhinocladium 117.1
- Rhinosporidium (seeberi) 117.0
- rhinovirus
  - in diseases classified elsewhere – *see* category 079❹
  - unspecified nature or site 079.3
- Rhizopus 117.7
- rickettsial 083.9
- rickettsialpox 083.2
- rubella (*see also* Rubella) 056.9
  - congenital 771.0
- Saccharomyces (*see also* Candidiasis) 112.9
- Saksenaea 117.7
- salivary duct or gland (any) 527.2
- Salmonella (aertrycke) (callinarum) (choleraesuis) (enteritidis) (suipestifer) (typhimurium) 003.9
  - with
    - arthritis 003.23
    - gastroenteritis 003.0
    - localized infection 003.20
      - specified type NEC 003.29
    - meningitis 003.21
    - osteomyelitis 003.24
    - pneumonia 003.22
    - septicemia 003.1
    - specified manifestation NEC 003.8

Infection, infected, infective – *continued*
- Salmonella – *continued*
  - due to food (poisoning) (any serotype) (*see also* Poisoning, food, due to, Salmonella)
  - hirschfeldii 002.3
  - localized 003.20
    - specified type NEC 003.29
  - paratyphi 002.9
    - A 002.1
    - B 002.2
    - C 002.3
  - schottmuelleri 002.2
  - specified type NEC 003.8
  - typhi 002.0
  - typhosa 002.0
- saprophytic 136.8
- Sarcocystis, lindemanni 136.5
- SARS-associated coronavirus 079.82
- scabies 133.0
- Schistosoma – *see* Infestation, Schistosoma
- Schmorl's bacillus 040.3
- scratch or other superficial injury – *see* Injury, superficial, by site
- scrotum (acute) NEC 608.4
- secondary, burn or open wound (dislocation) (fracture) 958.3
- seminal vesicle (*see also* Vesiculitis) 608.0
- septic
  - generalized – *see* Septicemia
  - localized, skin (*see also* Abscess) 682.9
- septicemic – *see* Septicemia
- seroma 998.51
- Serratia (marcescens) 041.85
  - generalized 038.44
- sheep liver fluke 121.3
- Shigella 004.9
  - boydii 004.2
  - dysenteriae 004.0
  - Flexneri 004.1
  - Group
    - A 004.0
    - B 004.1
    - C 004.2
    - D 004.3
  - Schmitz (-Stutzer) 004.0
  - Schmitzii 004.0
  - Shiga 004.0
  - Sonnei 004.3
  - specified type NEC 004.8
- Sin Nombre virus 079.81
- sinus (*see also* Sinusitis) 473.9
  - pilonidal 685.1
    - with abscess 685.0
  - skin NEC 686.9
- Skene's duct or gland (*see also* Urethritis) 597.89
- skin (local) (staphylococcal) (streptococcal) NEC 686.9
  - abscess – *see* Abscess, by site
  - cellulitis – *see* Cellulitis, by site
  - due to fungus 111.9
    - specified type NEC 111.8
  - mycotic 111.9
    - specified type NEC 111.8
  - ulcer (*see also* Ulcer, skin) 707.9
- slow virus 046.9
  - specified condition NEC 046.8
- Sparganum (mansoni) (proliferum) 123.5
- spermatic cord NEC 608.4
- sphenoidal (chronic) (sinus) (*see also* Sinusitis, sphenoidal) 473.3
- Spherophorus necrophorus 040.3
- spinal cord NEC (*see also* Encephalitis) 323.9
  - abscess 324.1
    - late effect – *see* category 326
  - late effect – *see* category 326
  - meninges – *see* Meningitis
  - streptococcal 320.2
- Spirillum
  - minus or minor 026.0
  - morsus muris 026.0
  - obermeieri 087.0
- spirochetal NEC 104.9
  - lung 104.8
  - specified nature or site NEC 104.8
- spleen 289.59
- Sporothrix schenckii 117.1
- Sporotrichum (schenckii) 117.1
- Sporozoa 136.8
- staphylococcal NEC 041.10
  - aureus 041.11
  - food poisoning 005.0

Infection, infected, infective – *continued*
- staphylococcal – *continued*
  - generalized (purulent) 038.10
    - aureus 038.11
    - specified organism NEC 038.19
  - pneumonia 482.40
    - aureus 482.41
    - specified type NEC 482.49
  - septicemia 038.10
    - aureus 038.11
    - specified organism NEC 038.19
  - specified NEC 041.19
- steatoma 706.2
- Stellantchasmus falcatus 121.6
- Streptobacillus moniliformis 026.1
- streptococcal NEC 041.00
  - generalized (purulent) 038.0
  - group
    - A 041.01
    - B 041.02
    - C 041.03
    - D [enterococcus] 041.04
    - G 041.05
  - pneumonia – *see* Pneumonia, streptococcal 482.3❺
  - septicemia 038.0
  - sore throat 034.0
  - specified NEC 041.09
- Streptomyces – *see* Actinomycosis
- streptotrichosis – *see* Actinomycosis
- Strongyloides (stercoralis) 127.2
- stump (amputation) (posttraumatic) (surgical) 997.62
  - traumatic – *see* Amputation, traumatic, by site, complicated
- subcutaneous tissue, local NEC 686.9
- submaxillary region 528.9
- suipestifer (*see also* Infection, Salmonella) 003.9
- swimming pool bacillus 031.1
- syphilitic – *see* Syphilis
- systemic – *see* Septicemia
- Taenia – *see* Infestation, Taenia
- Taeniarhynchus saginatus 123.2
- tapeworm – *see* Infestation, tapeworm
- tendon (sheath) 727.89
- Ternidens diminutus 127.7
- testis (*see also* Orchitis) 604.90
- thigh (skin) 686.9
- threadworm 127.4
- throat 478.29
  - pneumococcal 462
  - staphylococcal 462
  - streptococcal 034.0
  - viral NEC (*see also* Pharyngitis) 462
- thumb (skin) 686.9
  - abscess (with lymphangitis) 681.00
    - pulp 681.01
  - cellulitis (with lymphangitis) 681.00
  - nail 681.02
- thyroglossal duct 529.8
- toe (skin) 686.9
  - abscess (with lymphangitis) 681.10
  - cellulitis (with lymphangitis) 681.10
  - nail 681.11
    - fungus 110.1
- tongue NEC 529.0
  - parasitic 112.0
- tonsil (faucial) (lingual) (pharyngeal) 474.00
  - acute or subacute 463
  - and adenoid 474.02
  - tag 474.00
- tooth, teeth 522.4
  - periapical (pulpal origin) 522.4
  - peridental 523.30
  - periodontal 523.31
  - pulp 522.0
  - socket 526.5
- Torula histolytica 117.5
- Toxocara (cani) (cati) (felis) 128.0
- Toxoplasma gondii (*see also* Toxoplasmosis) 130.9
- trachea, chronic 491.8
  - fungus 117.9
- traumatic NEC 958.3
- trematode NEC 121.9
- trench fever 083.1
- Treponema
  - denticola 041.84
  - macrodenticum 041.84
  - pallidum (*see also* Syphilis) 097.9
- Trichinella (spiralis) 124

Infection, infected, infective – *continued*
- Trichomonas 131.9
  - bladder 131.09
  - cervix 131.09
  - hominis 007.3
  - intestine 007.3
  - prostate 131.03
  - specified site NEC 131.8
  - urethra 131.02
  - urogenitalis 131.00
  - vagina 131.01
  - vulva 131.01
- Trichophyton, trichophytid – *see* Dermatophytosis
- Trichosporon (beigelii) cutaneum 111.2
- Trichostrongylus 127.6
- Trichuris (trichiuria) 127.3
- Trombicula (irritans) 133.8
- Trypanosoma (*see also* Trypanosomiasis) 086.9
  - cruzi 086.2
- tubal (*see also* Salpingo-oophoritis) 614.2
- tuberculous NEC (*see also* Tuberculosis) 011.9❺
- tubo-ovarian (*see also* Salpingo-oophoritis) 614.2
- tunica vaginalis 608.4
- tympanic membrane – *see* Myringitis
- typhoid (abortive) (ambulant) (bacillus) 002.0
- typhus 081.9
  - flea-borne (endemic) 081.0
  - louse-borne (epidemic) 080
  - mite-borne 081.2
  - recrudescent 081.1
  - tick-borne 082.9
    - African 082.1
    - North Asian 082.2
- umbilicus (septic) 686.9
  - newborn NEC 771.4
- ureter 593.89
- urethra (*see also* Urethritis) 597.80
- urinary (tract) NEC 599.0
  - with
    - abortion – *see* Abortion, by type, with urinary tract infection
    - ectopic pregnancy (*see also* categories 633.0-633.9) 639.8
    - molar pregnancy (*see also* categories 630-632) 639.8
  - candidal 112.2
  - complicating pregnancy, childbirth, or puerperium 646.6❺
    - affecting fetus or newborn 760.1
    - asymptomatic 646.5❺
      - affecting fetus or newborn 760.1
  - diplococcal (acute) 098.0
    - chronic 098.2
  - due to Trichomonas (vaginalis) 131.00
  - following
    - abortion 639.8
    - ectopic or molar pregnancy 639.8
  - gonococcal (acute) 098.0
    - chronic or duration of 2 months or over 098.2
  - newborn 771.82
  - trichomonal 131.00
  - tuberculous (*see also* Tuberculosis) 016.3❺
- uterus, uterine (*see also* Endometritis) 615.9
- utriculus masculinus NEC 597.89
- vaccination 999.39 ▲
- vagina (granulation tissue) (wall) (*see also* Vaginitis) 616.10
- varicella 052.9
- varicose veins – *see* Varicose, veins
- variola 050.9
  - major 050.0
  - minor 050.1
- vas deferens NEC 608.4
- Veillonella 041.84
- verumontanum 597.89
- vesical (*see also* Cystitis) 595.9
- Vibrio
  - cholerae 001.0
    - El Tor 001.1
  - parahaemolyticus (food poisoning) 005.4
  - vulnificus 041.85
- Vincent's (gums) (mouth) (tonsil) 101
- virus, viral 079.99
  - adenovirus
    - in diseases classified elsewhere – *see* category 079❹
    - unspecified nature or site 079.0
  - central nervous system NEC 049.9
    - enterovirus 048
      - meningitis 047.9
        - specified type NEC 047.8

Infection, infected, infective – *continued*
- virus, viral – *continued*
  - central nervous system – *continued*
    - slow virus 046.9
      - specified condition NEC 046.8
  - chest 519.8
  - conjunctivitis 077.99
    - specified type NEC 077.89
  - coronavirus 079.89
    - SARS-associated 079.82
  - Coxsackie (*see also* Infection, Coxsackie) 079.2
  - Ebola 065.8
  - ECHO
    - in diseases classified elsewhere – *see* category 079❹
    - unspecified nature or site 079.1
  - encephalitis 049.9
    - arthropod-borne NEC 064
    - tick-borne 063.9
      - specified type NEC 063.8
  - enteritis NEC (*see also* Enteritis, viral) 008.8
  - exanthem NEC 057.9
  - Hantavirus 079.81
  - human papilloma 079.4
  - in diseases classified elsewhere – *see* category 079❹
  - intestine (*see also* Enteritis, viral) 008.8
  - lung – *see* Pneumonia, viral
  - respiratory syncytial (RSV) 079.6
  - retrovirus 079.50
  - rhinovirus
    - in diseases classified elsewhere – *see* category 079❹
    - unspecified nature or site 079.3
  - salivary gland disease 078.5
  - slow 046.9
    - specified condition NEC 046.8
  - specified type NEC 079.89
    - in diseases classified elsewhere – *see* category 079❹
  - unspecified nature or site 079.99
  - warts NEC 078.10
- vulva (*see also* Vulvitis) 616.10
- whipworm 127.3
- Whitmore's bacillus 025
- wound (local) (posttraumatic) NEC 958.3
  - with
    - dislocation – *see* Dislocation, by site, open
    - fracture – *see* Fracture, by site, open
    - open wound – *see* Wound, open, by site, complicated
  - postoperative 998.59
  - surgical 998.59
- Wuchereria 125.0
  - bancrofti 125.0
  - malayi 125.1
- yaws – *see* Yaws
- yeast (*see also* Candidiasis) 112.9
- yellow fever (*see also* Fever, yellow) 060.9
- Yersinia pestis (*see also* Plague) 020.9
- Zeis' gland 373.12
- zoonotic bacterial NEC 027.9
- Zopfia senegalensis 117.4

Infective, infectious – *see* condition

Inferiority complex 301.9
- constitutional psychopathic 301.9

Infertility
- female 628.9
  - age related 628.8
  - associated with
    - adhesions, peritubal 614.6 *[628.2]*
    - anomaly
      - cervical mucus 628.4
      - congenital
        - cervix 628.4
        - fallopian tube 628.2
        - uterus 628.3
        - vagina 628.4
    - anovulation 628.0
    - dysmucorrhea 628.4
    - endometritis, tuberculous (*see also* Tuberculosis) 016.7❺ *[628.3]*
    - Stein-Leventhal syndrome 256.4 *[628.0]*
  - due to
    - adiposogenital dystrophy 253.8 *[628.1]*
    - anterior pituitary disorder NEC 253.4 *[628.1]*
      - hyperfunction 253.1 *[628.1]*
    - cervical anomaly 628.4
    - fallopian tube anomaly 628.2
    - ovarian failure 256.39 *[628.0]*

Infection, infected, infective – Infertility

Infertility – Infestation

Infestation – *continued*
- tapeworm – *continued*
  - fish 123.4
    - larval 123.5
  - pork 123.0
  - rat 123.6
- Ternidens diminutus 127.7
- Tetranychus molestissimus 133.8
- threadworm 127.4
- tongue 112.0
- Toxocara (cani) (cati) (felis) 128.0
- trematode(s) NEC 121.9
- Trichina spiralis 124
- Trichinella spiralis 124
- Trichocephalus 127.3
- Trichomonas 131.9
  - bladder 131.09
  - cervix 131.09
  - intestine 007.3
  - prostate 131.03
  - specified site NEC 131.8
  - urethra (female) (male) 131.02
  - urogenital 131.00
  - vagina 131.01
  - vulva 131.01
- Trichophyton – *see* Dermatophytosis
- Trichostrongylus instabilis 127.6
- Trichuris (trichiuria) 127.3
- Trombicula (irritans) 133.8
- Trypanosoma – *see* Trypanosomiasis
- Tunga penetrans 134.1
- Uncinaria americana 126.1
- whipworm 127.3
- worms NEC 128.9
  - intestinal 127.9
- Wuchereria 125.0
  - bancrofti 125.0
  - malayi 125.1

Infiltrate, infiltration
- with an iron compound 275.0
- amyloid (any site) (generalized) 277.39
- calcareous (muscle) NEC 275.49
  - localized – *see* Degeneration, by site
- calcium salt (muscle) 275.49
- corneal (*see also* Edema, cornea) 371.20
- eyelid 373.9
- fatty (diffuse) (generalized) 272.8
  - localized – *see* Degeneration, by site, fatty
- glycogen, glycogenic (*see also* Disease, glycogen storage) 271.0
- heart, cardiac
  - fatty (*see also* Degeneration, myocardial) 429.1
  - glycogenic 271.0 *[425.7]*
- inflammatory in vitreous 379.29
- kidney (*see also* Disease, renal) 593.9
- leukemic (M9800/3) – *see* Leukemia
- liver 573.8
  - fatty – *see* Fatty, liver
  - glycogen (*see also* Disease, glycogen storage) 271.0
- lung (*see also* Infiltrate, pulmonary) 518.3
  - eosinophilic 518.3
  - x-ray finding only 793.1
- lymphatic (*see also* Leukemia, lymphatic) 204.9⑤
  - gland, pigmentary 289.3
- muscle, fatty 728.9
- myelogenous (*see also* Leukemia, myeloid) 205.9⑤
- myocardium, myocardial
  - fatty (*see also* Degeneration, myocardial) 429.1
  - glycogenic 271.0 *[425.7]*
- pulmonary 518.3
  - with
    - eosinophilia 518.3
    - pneumonia – *see* Pneumonia, by type
    - x-ray finding only 793.1
- Ranke's primary (*see also* Tuberculosis) 010.0⑤
- skin, lymphocytic (benign) 709.8
- thymus (gland) (fatty) 254.8
- urine 788.8
- vitreous humor 379.29

Infirmity 799.89
- senile 797

Inflammation, inflamed, inflammatory (with exudation)
- abducens (nerve) 378.54
- accessory sinus (chronic) (*see also* Sinusitis) 473.9
- adrenal (gland) 255.8
- alimentary canal – *see* Enteritis

Inflammation, inflamed, inflammatory – *continued*
- alveoli (teeth) 526.5
  - scorbutic 267
- amnion – *see* Amnionitis
- anal canal 569.49
- antrum (chronic) (*see also* Sinusitis, maxillary) 473.0
- anus 569.49
- appendix (*see also* Appendicitis) 541
- arachnoid – *see* Meningitis
- areola 611.0
  - puerperal, postpartum 675.0⑤
- areolar tissue NEC 686.9
- artery – *see* Arteritis
- auditory meatus (external) (*see also* Otitis, externa) 380.10
- Bartholin's gland 616.89
- bile duct or passage 576.1
- bladder (*see also* Cystitis) 595.9
- bleb
  - postprocedural 379.60
    - stage 1 379.61
    - stage 2 379.62
    - stage 3 379.63
- bone – *see* Osteomyelitis
- bowel (*see also* Enteritis) 558.9
- brain (*see also* Encephalitis) 323.9
  - late effect – *see* category 326
  - membrane – *see* Meningitis
- breast 611.0
  - puerperal, postpartum 675.2⑤
- broad ligament (*see also* Disease, pelvis, inflammatory) 614.4
  - acute 614.3
- bronchus – *see* Bronchitis
- bursa – *see* Bursitis
- capsule
  - liver 573.3
  - spleen 289.59
- catarrhal (*see also* Catarrh) 460
  - vagina 616.10
- cecum (*see also* Appendicitis) 541
- cerebral (*see also* Encephalitis) 323.9
  - late effect – *see* category 326
  - membrane – *see* Meningitis
- cerebrospinal (*see also* Meningitis) 322.9
  - late effect – *see* category 326
  - meningococcal 036.0
  - tuberculous (*see also* Tuberculosis) 013.6⑤
- cervix (uteri) (*see also* Cervicitis) 616.0
- chest 519.9
- choroid NEC (*see also* Choroiditis) 363.20
- cicatrix (tissue) – *see* Cicatrix
- colon (*see also* Enteritis) 558.9
  - granulomatous 555.1
  - newborn 558.9
- connective tissue (diffuse) NEC 728.9
- cornea (*see also* Keratitis) 370.9
  - with ulcer (*see also* Ulcer, cornea) 370.00
- corpora cavernosa (penis) 607.2
- cranial nerve – *see* Disorder, nerve, cranial
- diarrhea – *see* Diarrhea
- disc (intervertebral) (space) 722.90
  - cervical, cervicothoracic 722.91
  - lumbar, lumbosacral 722.93
  - thoracic, thoracolumbar 722.92
- Douglas' cul-de-sac or pouch (chronic) (*see also* Disease, pelvis, inflammatory) 614.4
  - acute 614.3
- due to (presence of) any device, implant, or graft classifiable to 996.0-996.5 – *see* Complications, infection and inflammation, due to (presence of) any device, implant, or graft classified to 996.0-996.5 NEC
- duodenum 535.6⑤
- dura mater – *see* Meningitis
- ear – *see also* Otitis
  - external (*see also* Otitis, externa) 380.10
  - inner (*see also* Labyrinthitis) 386.30
  - middle – *see* Otitis media
- esophagus 530.10
- ethmoidal (chronic) (sinus) (*see also* Sinusitis, ethmoidal) 473.2
- Eustachian tube (catarrhal) 381.50
  - acute 381.51
  - chronic 381.52
- extrarectal 569.49
- eye 379.99
- eyelid 373.9
  - specified NEC 373.8
- fallopian tube (*see also* Salpingo-oophoritis) 614.2

Inflammation, inflamed, inflammatory – *continued*
- fascia 728.9
- fetal membranes (acute) 658.4⑤
  - affecting fetus or newborn 762.7
- follicular, pharynx 472.1
- frontal (chronic) (sinus) (*see also* Sinusitis, frontal) 473.1
- gallbladder (*see also* Cholecystitis, acute) 575.0
- gall duct (*see also* Cholecystitis) 575.10
- gastrointestinal (*see also* Enteritis) 558.9
- genital organ (diffuse) (internal)
  - female 614.9
    - with
      - abortion – *see* Abortion, by type, with sepsis
      - ectopic pregnancy (*see also* categories 633.0-633.9) 639.0
      - molar pregnancy (*see also* categories 630-632) 639.0
    - complicating pregnancy, childbirth, or puerperium 646.6⑤
      - affecting fetus or newborn 760.8
    - following
      - abortion 639.0
      - ectopic or molar pregnancy 639.0
  - male 608.4
- gland (lymph) (*see also* Lymphadenitis) 289.3
- glottis (*see also* Laryngitis) 464.00
  - with obstruction 464.01
- granular, pharynx 472.1
- gum 523.10
- heart (*see also* Carditis) 429.89
- hepatic duct 576.8
- hernial sac – *see* Hernia, by site
- ileum (*see also* Enteritis) 558.9
  - terminal or regional 555.0
    - with large intestine 555.2
- intervertebral disc 722.90
  - cervical, cervicothoracic 722.91
  - lumbar, lumbosacral 722.93
  - thoracic, thoracolumbar 722.92
- intestine (*see also* Enteritis) 558.9
- jaw (acute) (bone) (chronic) (lower) (suppurative) (upper) 526.4
- jejunum – *see* Enteritis
- joint NEC (*see also* Arthritis) 716.9⑤
  - sacroiliac 720.2
- kidney (*see also* Nephritis) 583.9
- knee (joint) 716.66
  - tuberculous (active) (*see also* Tuberculosis) 015.2⑤
- labium (majus) (minus) (*see also* Vulvitis) 616.10
- lacrimal
  - gland (*see also* Dacryoadenitis) 375.00
  - passages (duct) (sac) (*see also* Dacryocystitis) 375.30
- larynx (*see also* Laryngitis) 464.00
  - with obstruction 464.01
  - diphtheritic 032.3
- leg NEC 686.9
- lip 528.5
- liver (capsule) (*see also* Hepatitis) 573.3
  - acute 570
  - chronic 571.40
  - suppurative 572.0
- lung (acute) (*see also* Pneumonia) 486
  - chronic (interstitial) 518.89
- lymphatic vessel (*see also* Lymphangitis) 457.2
- lymph node or gland (*see also* Lymphadenitis) 289.3
- mammary gland 611.0
  - puerperal, postpartum 675.2⑤
- maxilla, maxillary 526.4
  - sinus (chronic) (*see also* Sinusitis, maxillary) 473.0
- membranes of brain or spinal cord – *see* Meningitis
- meninges – *see* Meningitis
- mouth 528.00
- muscle 728.9
- myocardium (*see also* Myocarditis) 429.0
- nasal sinus (chronic) (*see also* Sinusitis) 473.9
- nasopharynx – *see* Nasopharyngitis
- navel 686.9
  - newborn NEC 771.4
- nerve NEC 729.2
- nipple 611.0
  - puerperal, postpartum 675.0⑤
- nose 478.19
  - suppurative 472.0
- oculomotor nerve 378.51
- optic nerve 377.30

Infestation – Inflammation, inflamed, inflammatory

Inflammation, inflamed, inflammatory – *continued*
- orbit (chronic) 376.10
  - acute 376.00
  - chronic 376.10
- ovary (*see also* Salpingo-oophoritis) 614.2
- oviduct (*see also* Salpingo-oophoritis) 614.2
- pancreas – *see* Pancreatitis
- parametrium (chronic) (*see also* Disease, pelvis, inflammatory) 614.4
  - acute 614.3
- parotid region 686.9
  - gland 527.2
- pelvis, female (*see also* Disease, pelvis, inflammatory) 614.9
- penis (corpora cavernosa) 607.2
- perianal 569.49
- pericardium (*see also* Pericarditis) 423.9
- perineum (female) (male) 686.9
- perirectal 569.49
- peritoneum (*see also* Peritonitis) 567.9
- periuterine (*see also* Disease, pelvis, inflammatory) 614.9
- perivesical (*see also* Cystitis) 595.9
- petrous bone (*see also* Petrositis) 383.20
- pharynx (*see also* Pharyngitis) 462
  - follicular 472.1
  - granular 472.1
- pia mater – *see* Meningitis
- pleura – *see* Pleurisy
- postmastoidectomy cavity 383.30
  - chronic 383.33
- prostate (*see also* Prostatitis) 601.9
- rectosigmoid – *see* Rectosigmoiditis
- rectum (*see also* Proctitis) 569.49
- respiratory, upper (*see also* Infection, respiratory, upper) 465.9
  - chronic, due to external agent – *see* Condition, respiratory, chronic, due to, external agent
  - due to
    - fumes or vapors (chemical) (inhalation) 506.2
    - radiation 508.1
- retina (*see also* Retinitis) 363.20
- retrocecal (*see also* Appendicitis) 541
- retroperitoneal (*see also* Peritonitis) 567.9
- salivary duct or gland (any) (suppurative) 527.2
- scorbutic, alveoli, teeth 267
- scrotum 608.4
- sigmoid – *see* Enteritis
- sinus (*see also* Sinusitis) 473.9
- Skene's duct or gland (*see also* Urethritis) 597.89
- skin 686.9
- spermatic cord 608.4
- sphenoidal (sinus) (*see also* Sinusitis, sphenoidal) 473.3
- spinal
  - cord (*see also* Encephalitis) 323.9
    - late effect – *see* category 326
  - membrane – *see* Meningitis
  - nerve – *see* Disorder, nerve
- spine (*see also* Spondylitis) 720.9
- spleen (capsule) 289.59
- stomach – *see* Gastritis
- stricture, rectum 569.49
- subcutaneous tissue NEC 686.9
- suprarenal (gland) 255.8
- synovial (fringe) (membrane) – *see* Bursitis
- tendon (sheath) NEC 726.90
- testis (*see also* Orchitis) 604.90
- thigh 686.9
- throat (*see also* Sore throat) 462
- thymus (gland) 254.8
- thyroid (gland) (*see also* Thyroiditis) 245.9
- tongue 529.0
- tonsil – *see* Tonsillitis
- trachea – *see* Tracheitis
- trochlear nerve 378.53
- tubal (*see also* Salpingo-oophoritis) 614.2
- tuberculous NEC (*see also* Tuberculosis) 011.9❺
- tubo-ovarian (*see also* Salpingo-oophoritis) 614.2
- tunica vaginalis 608.4
- tympanic membrane – *see* Myringitis
- umbilicus, umbilical 686.9
  - newborn NEC 771.4
- uterine ligament (*see also* Disease, pelvis, inflammatory) 614.4
  - acute 614.3
- uterus (catarrhal) (*see also* Endometritis) 615.9
- uveal tract (anterior) (*see also* Iridocyclitis) 364.3
  - posterior – *see* Chorioretinitis
  - sympathetic 360.11
- vagina (*see also* Vaginitis) 616.10
- vas deferens 608.4
- vein (*see also* Phlebitis) 451.9
  - thrombotic 451.9
    - cerebral (*see also* Thrombosis, brain) 434.0❺
    - leg 451.2
      - deep (vessels) NEC 451.19
      - superficial (vessels) 451.0
    - lower extremity 451.2
      - deep (vessels) NEC 451.19
      - superficial (vessels) 451.0
- vocal cord 478.5
- vulva (*see also* Vulvitis) 616.10

Inflation, lung imperfect (newborn) 770.5

Influenza, influenzal 487.1
- with
  - bronchitis 487.1
  - bronchopneumonia 487.0
  - cold (any type) 487.1
  - digestive manifestations 487.8
  - hemoptysis 487.1
  - involvement of
    - gastrointestinal tract 487.8
    - nervous system 487.8
  - laryngitis 487.1
  - manifestations NEC 487.8
    - respiratory 487.1
      - pneumonia 487.0
  - pharyngitis 487.1
  - pneumonia (any form classifiable to 480-483, 485-486) 487.0
  - respiratory manifestations NEC 487.1
  - sinusitis 487.1
  - sore throat 487.1
  - tonsillitis 487.1
  - tracheitis 487.1
  - upper respiratory infection (acute) 487.1
- abdominal 487.8
- Asian 487.1
- bronchial 487.1
- bronchopneumonia 487.0
- catarrhal 487.1
- due to identified avian influenza virus 488 ●
- epidemic 487.1
- gastric 487.8
- intestinal 487.8
- laryngitis 487.1
- maternal affecting fetus or newborn 760.2
  - manifest influenza in infant 771.2
- pharyngitis 487.1
- pneumonia (any form) 487.0
- respiratory (upper) 487.1
- stomach 487.8
- vaccination, prophylactic (against) V04.81

Influenza-like disease 487.1

Infraction, Freiberg's (metatarsal head) 732.5

Infraeruption, teeth 524.34

Infusion complication, misadventure, or reaction – *see* Complication, infusion

Ingestion
- chemical – *see* Table of Drugs and Chemicals
- drug or medicinal substance
  - overdose or wrong substance given or taken 977.9
    - specified drug – *see* Table of Drugs and Chemicals
- foreign body NEC (*see also* Foreign body) 938

Ingrowing
- hair 704.8
- nail (finger) (toe) (infected) 703.0

Inguinal – *see also* condition
- testis 752.51

Inhalation
- carbon monoxide 986
- flame
  - mouth 947.0
  - lung 947.1
- food or foreign body (*see also* Asphyxia, food or foreign body) 933.1
- gas, fumes, or vapor (noxious) 987.9
  - specified agent – *see* Table of Drugs and Chemicals
- liquid or vomitus (*see also* Asphyxia, food or foreign body) 933.1
  - lower respiratory tract NEC 934.9
- meconium (fetus or newborn) 770.11
  - with respiratory symptoms 770.12
- mucus (*see also* Asphyxia, mucus) 933.1

Inhalation – *continued*
- oil (causing suffocation) (*see also* Asphyxia, food or foreign body) 933.1
- pneumonia – *see* Pneumonia, aspiration
- smoke 987.9
- steam 987.9
- stomach contents or secretions (*see also* Asphyxia, food or foreign body) 933.1
  - in labor and delivery 668.0❺

Inhibition, inhibited
- academic as adjustment reaction 309.23
- orgasm
  - female 302.73
  - male 302.74
- sexual
  - desire 302.71
  - excitement 302.72
- work as adjustment reaction 309.23

Inhibitor, systemic lupus erythematosus (presence of) 286.5

Iniencephalus, iniencephaly 740.2

Injected eye 372.74

Injury 959.9

Note – For abrasion, insect bite (nonvenomous), blister, or scratch, see Injury, superficial.

For laceration, traumatic rupture, tear, or penetrating wound of internal organs, such as heart, lung, liver, kidney, pelvic organs, whether or not accompanied by open wound in the same region, see Injury, internal.

For nerve injury, see Injury, nerve.

For late effect of injuries classifiable to 850-854, 860-869, 900-919, 950-959, see Late, effect, injury, by type.

- abdomen, abdominal (viscera) – *see also* Injury, internal, abdomen
  - muscle or wall 959.12
- acoustic, resulting in deafness 951.5
- adenoid 959.09
- adrenal (gland) – *see* Injury, internal, adrenal
- alveolar (process) 959.09
- ankle (and foot) (and knee) (and leg, except thigh) 959.7
- anterior chamber, eye 921.3
- anus 959.19
- aorta (thoracic) 901.0
  - abdominal 902.0
- appendix – *see* Injury, internal, appendix
- arm, upper (and shoulder) 959.2
- artery (complicating trauma) (*see also* Injury, blood vessel, by site) 904.9
  - cerebral or meningeal (*see also* Hemorrhage, brain, traumatic, subarachnoid) 852.0❺
- auditory canal (external) (meatus) 959.09
- auricle, auris, ear 959.09
- axilla 959.2
- back 959.19
- bile duct – *see* Injury, internal, bile duct
- birth – *see also* Birth, injury
  - canal NEC, complicating delivery 665.9❺
- bladder (sphincter) – *see* Injury, internal, bladder
- blast (air) (hydraulic) (immersion) (underwater) NEC 869.0
  - with open wound into cavity NEC 869.1
  - abdomen or thorax – *see* Injury, internal, by site
  - brain – *see* Concussion, brain
  - ear (acoustic nerve trauma) 951.5
    - with perforation of tympanic membrane – *see* Wound, open, ear, drum
- blood vessel NEC 904.9
  - abdomen 902.9
    - multiple 902.87
    - specified NEC 902.89
  - aorta (thoracic) 901.0
    - abdominal 902.0
  - arm NEC 903.9
  - axillary 903.00
    - artery 903.1
    - vein 903.02
  - azygos vein 901.89
  - basilic vein 903.1
  - brachial (artery) (vein) 903.1
  - bronchial 901.89
  - carotid artery 900.00
    - common 900.01
    - external 900.02
    - internal 900.03

Injury – *continued*
  blood vessel – *continued*
    celiac artery 902.20
      specified branch NEC 902.24
    cephalic vein (arm) 903.1
    colica dextra 902.26
    cystic
      artery 902.24
      vein 902.39
    deep plantar 904.6
    digital (artery) (vein) 903.5
    due to accidental puncture or laceration during procedure 998.2
    extremity
      lower 904.8
        multiple 904.7
        specified NEC 904.7
      upper 903.9
        multiple 903.8
        specified NEC 903.8
    femoral
      artery (superficial) 904.1
        above profunda origin 904.0
        common 904.0
      vein 904.2
    gastric
      artery 902.21
      vein 902.39
    head 900.9
      intracranial – *see* Injury, intracranial
      multiple 900.82
      specified NEC 900.89
    hemiazygos vein 901.89
    hepatic
      artery 902.22
      vein 902.11
    hypogastric 902.59
      artery 902.51
      vein 902.52
    ileocolic
      artery 902.26
      vein 902.31
    iliac 902.50
      artery 902.53
      specified branch NEC 902.59
      vein 902.54
    innominate
      artery 901.1
      vein 901.3
    intercostal (artery) (vein) 901.81
    jugular vein (external) 900.81
      internal 900.1
    leg NEC 904.8
    mammary (artery) (vein) 901.82
    mesenteric
      artery 902.20
        inferior 902.27
        specified branch NEC 902.29
        superior (trunk) 902.25
          branches, primary 902.26
      vein 902.39
        inferior 902.32
        superior (and primary subdivisions) 902.31
    neck 900.9
      multiple 900.82
      specified NEC 900.89
    ovarian 902.89
      artery 902.81
      vein 902.82
    palmar artery 903.4
    pelvis 902.9
      multiple 902.87
      specified NEC 902.89
    plantar (deep) (artery) (vein) 904.6
    popliteal 904.40
      artery 904.41
      vein 904.42
    portal 902.33
    pulmonary 901.40
      artery 901.41
      vein 901.42
    radial (artery) (vein) 903.2
    renal 902.40
      artery 902.41
      specified NEC 902.49
      vein 902.42
    saphenous
      artery 904.7
      vein (greater) (lesser) 904.3
    splenic
      artery 902.23
      vein 902.34

Injury – *continued*
  blood vessel – *continued*
    subclavian
      artery 901.1
      vein 901.3
    suprarenal 902.49
    thoracic 901.9
      multiple 901.83
      specified NEC 901.89
    tibial 904.50
      artery 904.50
        anterior 904.51
        posterior 904.53
      vein 904.50
        anterior 904.52
        posterior 904.54
    ulnar (artery) (vein) 903.3
    uterine 902.59
      artery 902.55
      vein 902.56
    vena cava
      inferior 902.10
        specified branches NEC 902.19
      superior 901.2
  brachial plexus 953.4
    newborn 767.6
  brain NEC (*see also* Injury, intracranial) 854.0❺
  breast 959.19
  broad ligament – *see* Injury, internal, broad ligament
  bronchus, bronchi – *see* Injury, internal, bronchus
  brow 959.09
  buttock 959.19
  canthus, eye 921.1
  cathode ray 990
  cauda equina 952.4
    with fracture, vertebra – *see* Fracture, vertebra, sacrum
  cavernous sinus (*see also* Injury, intracranial) 854.0❺
  cecum – *see* Injury, internal, cecum
  celiac ganglion or plexus 954.1
  cerebellum (*see also* Injury, intracranial) 854.0❺
  cervix (uteri) – *see* Injury, internal, cervix
  cheek 959.09
  chest – *see* Injury, internal, chest
    wall 959.11
  childbirth – *see also* Birth, injury
    maternal NEC 665.9❺
  chin 959.09
  choroid (eye) 921.3
  clitoris 959.14
  coccyx 959.19
    complicating delivery 665.6❺
  colon – *see* Injury, internal, colon
  common duct – *see* Injury, internal, common duct
  conjunctiva 921.1
    superficial 918.2
  cord
    spermatic – *see* Injury, internal, spermatic cord
    spinal – *see* Injury, spinal, by site
  cornea 921.3
    abrasion 918.1
    due to contact lens 371.82
    penetrating – *see* Injury, eyeball, penetrating
    superficial 918.1
      due to contact lens 371.82
  cortex (cerebral) (*see also* Injury, intracranial) 854.0❺
    visual 950.3
  costal region 959.11
  costochondral 959.11
  cranial
    bones – *see* Fracture, skull, by site
    cavity (*see also* Injury, intracranial) 854.0❺
    nerve – *see* Injury, nerve, cranial
  crushing – *see* Crush
  cutaneous sensory nerve
    lower limb 956.4
    upper limb 955.5❺
  delivery – *see also* Birth, injury
    maternal NEC 665.9❺
  Descemet's membrane – *see* Injury, eyeball, penetrating
  diaphragm – *see* Injury, internal, diaphragm
  diffuse axonal – *see* Injury, intracranial
  duodenum – *see* Injury, internal, duodenum
  ear (auricle) (canal) (drum) (external) 959.09
  elbow (and forearm) (and wrist) 959.3
  epididymis 959.14
  epigastric region 959.12
  epiglottis 959.09

Injury – *continued*
  epiphyseal, current – *see* Fracture, by site
  esophagus – *see* Injury, internal, esophagus
  Eustachian tube 959.09
  extremity (lower) (upper) NEC 959.8
  eye 921.9
    penetrating eyeball – *see* Injury, eyeball, penetrating
    superficial 918.9
  eyeball 921.3
    penetrating 871.7
      with
        partial loss (of intraocular tissue) 871.2
        prolapse or exposure (of intraocular tissue) 871.1
      without prolapse 871.0
      foreign body (nonmagnetic) 871.6
        magnetic 871.5
    superficial 918.9
  eyebrow 959.09
  eyelid(s) 921.1
    laceration – *see* Laceration, eyelid
    superficial 918.0
  face (and neck) 959.09
  fallopian tube – *see* Injury, internal, fallopian tube
  fingers(s) (nail) 959.5
  flank 959.19
  foot (and ankle) (and knee) (and leg, except thigh) 959.7
  forceps NEC 767.9
    scalp 767.19
  forearm (and elbow) (and wrist) 959.3
  forehead 959.09
  gallbladder – *see* Injury, internal, gallbladder
  gasserian ganglion 951.2
  gastrointestinal tract – *see* Injury, internal, gastrointestinal tract
  genital organ(s)
    with
      abortion – *see* Abortion, by type, with, damage to pelvic organs
      ectopic pregnancy (*see also* categories 633.0-633.9) 639.2
      molar pregnancy (*see also* categories 630-632) 639.2
    external 959.14
      fracture of corpus cavernosum penis 959.13
    following
      abortion 639.2
      ectopic or molar pregnancy 639.2
    internal – *see* Injury, internal, genital organs
    obstetrical trauma NEC 665.9❺
      affecting fetus or newborn 763.89
  gland
    lacrimal 921.1
      laceration 870.8
    parathyroid 959.09
    salivary 959.09
    thyroid 959.09
  globe (eye) (*see also* Injury, eyeball) 921.3
  grease gun – *see* Wound, open, by site, complicated
  groin 959.19
  gum 959.09
  hand(s) (except fingers) 959.4
  head NEC 959.01
    with
      loss of consciousness 850.5
      skull fracture – *see* Fracture, skull, by site
  heart – *see* Injury, internal, heart
  heel 959.7
  hip (and thigh) 959.6
  hymen 959.14
  hyperextension (cervical) (vertebra) 847.0
  ileum – *see* Injury, internal, ileum
  iliac region 959.19
  infrared rays NEC 990
  instrumental (during surgery) 998.2
    birth injury – *see* Birth, injury
    nonsurgical (*see also* Injury, by site) 959.9
    obstetrical 665.9❺
      affecting fetus or newborn 763.89
      bladder 665.5❺
      cervix 665.3❺
      high vaginal 665.4❺
      perineal NEC 664.9❺
      urethra 665.5❺
      uterus 665.5❺

Injury – Injury

- **Injury** – *continued*
  - internal 869.0

Note – For injury of internal organ(s) by foreign body entering through a natural orifice (e.g., inhaled, ingested, or swallowed) – see Foreign body, entering through orifice.

For internal injury of any of the following sites with internal injury of any other of the sites – see Injury, internal, multiple.

    - with
      - fracture
        - pelvis – *see* Fracture, pelvis
        - specified site, except pelvis – *see* Injury, internal, by site
      - open wound into cavity 869.1
    - abdomen, abdominal (viscera) NEC 868.00
      - with
        - fracture, pelvis – *see* Fracture, pelvis
        - open wound into cavity 868.10
      - specified site NEC 868.09
        - with open wound into cavity 868.19
    - adrenal (gland) 868.01
      - with open wound into cavity 868.11
    - aorta (thoracic) 901.0
      - abdominal 902.0
    - appendix 863.85
      - with open wound into cavity 863.95
    - bile duct 868.02
      - with open wound into cavity 868.12
    - bladder (sphincter) 867.0
      - with
        - abortion – *see* Abortion, by type, with, damage to pelvic organs
        - ectopic pregnancy (*see also* categories 633.0-633.9) 639.2
        - molar pregnancy (*see also* categories 630-632) 639.2
        - open wound into cavity 867.1
      - following
        - abortion 639.2
        - ectopic or molar pregnancy 639.2
      - obstetrical trauma 665.5❺
        - affecting fetus or newborn 763.89
    - blood vessel – *see* Injury, blood vessel, by site
    - broad ligament 867.6
      - with open wound into cavity 867.7
    - bronchus, bronchi 862.21
      - with open wound into cavity 862.31
    - cecum 863.89
      - with open wound into cavity 863.99
    - cervix (uteri) 867.4
      - with
        - abortion – *see* Abortion, by type, with damage to pelvic organs
        - ectopic pregnancy (*see also* categories 633.0-633.9) 639.2
        - molar pregnancy (*see also* categories 630-632) 639.2
        - open wound into cavity 867.5
      - following
        - abortion 639.2
        - ectopic or molar pregnancy 639.2
      - obstetrical trauma 665.3❺
        - affecting fetus or newborn 763.89
    - chest (*see also* Injury, internal, intrathoracic organs) 862.8
      - with open wound into cavity 862.9
    - colon 863.40
      - with
        - open wound into cavity 863.50
        - rectum 863.46
          - with open wound into cavity 863.56
      - ascending (right) 863.41
        - with open wound into cavity 863.51
      - descending (left) 863.43
        - with open wound into cavity 863.53
      - multiple sites 863.46
        - with open wound into cavity 863.56
      - sigmoid 863.44
        - with open wound into cavity 863.54
      - specified site NEC 863.49
        - with open wound into cavity 863.59
      - transverse 863.42
        - with open wound into cavity 863.52
    - common duct 868.02
      - with open wound into cavity 868.12
    - complicating delivery 665.9❺
      - affecting fetus or newborn 763.89
    - diaphragm 862.0
      - with open wound into cavity 862.1

- **Injury** – *continued*
  - internal – *continued*
    - duodenum 863.21
      - with open wound into cavity 863.31
    - esophagus (intrathoracic) 862.22
      - with open wound into cavity 862.32
      - cervical region 874.4
        - complicated 874.5
    - fallopian tube 867.6
      - with open wound into cavity 867.7
    - gallbladder 868.02
      - with open wound into cavity 868.12
    - gastrointestinal tract NEC 863.80
      - with open wound into cavity 863.90
    - genital organ NEC 867.6
      - with open wound into cavity 867.7
    - heart 861.00
      - with open wound into thorax 861.10
    - ileum 863.29
      - with open wound into cavity 863.39
    - intestine NEC 863.89
      - with open wound into cavity 863.99
      - large NEC 863.40
        - with open wound into cavity 863.50
      - small NEC 863.20
        - with open wound into cavity 863.30
    - intra-abdominal (organ) 868.00
      - with open wound into cavity 868.10
      - multiple sites 868.09
        - with open wound into cavity 868.19
      - specified site NEC 868.09
        - with open wound into cavity 868.19
    - intrathoracic organs (multiple) 862.8
      - with open wound into cavity 862.9
      - diaphragm (only) – *see* Injury, internal, diaphragm
      - heart (only) – *see* Injury, internal, heart
      - lung (only) – *see* Injury, internal, lung
      - specified site NEC 862.29
        - with open wound into cavity 862.39
    - intrauterine (*see also* Injury, internal, uterus) 867.4
      - with open wound into cavity 867.5
    - jejunum 863.29
      - with open wound into cavity 863.39
    - kidney (subcapsular) 866.00
      - with
        - disruption of parenchyma (complete) 866.03
          - with open wound into cavity 866.13
        - hematoma (without rupture of capsule) 866.01
          - with open wound into cavity 866.11
        - laceration 866.02
          - with open wound into cavity 866.12
        - open wound into cavity 866.10
    - liver 864.00
      - with
        - contusion 864.01
          - with open wound into cavity 864.11
        - hematoma 864.01
          - with open wound into cavity 864.11
        - laceration 864.05
          - with open wound into cavity 864.15
          - major (disruption of hepatic parenchyma) 864.04
            - with open wound into cavity 864.14
          - minor (capsule only) 864.02
            - with open wound into cavity 864.12
          - moderate (involving parenchyma) 864.03
            - with open wound into cavity 864.13
            - multiple 864.04
          - stellate 864.04
            - with open wound into cavity 864.14
        - open wound into cavity 864.10
    - lung 861.20
      - with open wound into thorax 861.30
      - hemopneumothorax – *see* Hemopneumothorax, traumatic
      - hemothorax – *see* Hemothorax, traumatic
      - pneumohemothorax – *see* Pneumohemothorax, traumatic
      - pneumothorax – *see* Pneumothorax, traumatic
      - transfusion related, acute (TRALI) 518.7
    - mediastinum 862.29
      - with open wound into cavity 862.39
    - mesentery 863.89
      - with open wound into cavity 863.99
    - mesosalpinx 867.6
      - with open wound into cavity 867.7

- **Injury** – *continued*
  - internal – *continued*
    - multiple 869.0

Note – Multiple internal injuries of sites classifiable to the same three- or four-digit category should be classified to that category.

Multiple injuries classifiable to different fourth-digit subdivisions of 861._ (heart and lung injuries) should be dealt with according to coding rules.

      - internal 869.0
        - with open wound into cavity 869.1
      - intra-abdominal organ (sites classifiable to 863-868)
        - with
          - intrathoracic organ(s) (sites classifiable to 861-862) 869.0
            - with open wound into cavity 869.1
          - other intra-abdominal organ(s) (sites classifiable to 863-868, except where classifiable to the same three-digit category) 868.09
            - with open wound into cavity 868.19
      - intrathoracic organ (sites classifiable to 861-862)
        - with
          - intra-abdominal organ(s) (sites classifiable to 863-868) 869.0
            - with open wound into cavity 869.1
          - open wound into cavity 862.9
        - other intrathoracic organs(s) (sites classifiable to 861-862, except where classifiable to the same three-digit category) 862.8
    - myocardium – *see* Injury, internal, heart
    - ovary 867.6
      - with open wound into cavity 867.7
    - pancreas (multiple sites) 863.84
      - with open wound into cavity 863.94
      - body 863.82
        - with open wound into cavity 863.92
      - head 863.81
        - with open wound into cavity 863.91
      - tail 863.83
        - with open wound into cavity 863.93
    - pelvis, pelvic (organs) (viscera) 867.8
      - with
        - fracture, pelvis – *see* Fracture, pelvis
        - open wound into cavity 867.9
      - specified site NEC 867.6
        - with open wound into cavity 867.7
    - peritoneum 868.03
      - with open wound into cavity 868.13
    - pleura 862.29
      - with open wound into cavity 862.39
    - prostate 867.6
      - with open wound into cavity 867.7
    - rectum 863.45
      - with
        - colon 863.46
          - with open wound into cavity 863.56
        - open wound into cavity 863.55
    - retroperitoneum 868.04
      - with open wound into cavity 868.14
    - round ligament 867.6
      - with open wound into cavity 867.7
    - seminal vesicle 867.6
      - with open wound into cavity 867.7
    - spermatic cord 867.6
      - with open wound into cavity 867.7
      - scrotal – *see* Wound, open, spermatic cord
    - spleen 865.00
      - with
        - disruption of parenchyma (massive) 865.04
          - with open wound into cavity 865.14
        - hematoma (without rupture of capsule) 865.01
          - with open wound into cavity 865.11
        - open wound into cavity 865.10
        - tear, capsular 865.02
          - with open wound into cavity 865.12
          - extending into parenchyma 865.03
            - with open wound into cavity 865.13
    - stomach 863.0
      - with open wound into cavity 863.1
    - suprarenal gland (multiple) 868.01
      - with open wound into cavity 868.11

- **Injury** – *continued*
  - internal – *continued*
    - thorax, thoracic (cavity) (organs) (multiple) (*see also* Injury, internal, intrathoracic organs) 862.8
      - with open wound into cavity 862.9
    - thymus (gland) 862.29
      - with open wound into cavity 862.39
    - trachea (intrathoracic) 862.29
      - with open wound into cavity 862.39
      - cervical region (*see also* Wound, open, trachea) 874.02
    - ureter 867.2
      - with open wound into cavity 867.3
    - urethra (sphincter) 867.0
      - with
        - abortion – *see* Abortion, by type, with, damage to pelvic organs
        - ectopic pregnancy (*see also* categories 633.0-633.9) 639.2
        - molar pregnancy (*see also* categories 630-632) 639.2
        - open wound into cavity 867.1
      - following
        - abortion 639.2
        - ectopic or molar pregnancy 639.2
      - obstetrical trauma 665.5⑤
        - affecting fetus or newborn 763.89
    - uterus 867.4
      - with
        - abortion – *see* Abortion, by type, with, damage to pelvic organs
        - ectopic pregnancy (*see also* categories 633.0-633.9) 639.2
        - molar pregnancy (*see also* categories 630-632) 639.2
        - open wound into cavity 867.5
      - following
        - abortion 639.2
        - ectopic or molar pregnancy 639.2
      - obstetrical trauma NEC 665.5⑤
        - affecting fetus or newborn 763.89
    - vas deferens 867.6
      - with open wound into cavity 867.7
    - vesical (sphincter) 867.0
      - with open wound into cavity 867.1
    - viscera (abdominal) (*see also* Injury, internal, multiple) 868.00
      - with
        - fracture, pelvis – *see* Fracture, pelvis
        - open wound into cavity 868.10
      - thoracic NEC (*see also* Injury, internal, intrathoracic organs) 862.8
        - with open wound into cavity 862.9
  - interscapular region 959.19
  - intervertebral disc 959.19
  - intestine – *see* Injury, internal, intestine
  - intra-abdominal (organs) NEC – *see* Injury, internal, intra-abdominal
  - intracranial 854.0⑤

    Note – Use the following fifth-digit subclassification with categories 851-854:

    0 unspecified state of consciousness
    1 with no loss of consciousness
    2 with brief [less than one hour] loss of consciousness
    3 with moderate [1-24 hours] loss of consciousness
    4 with prolonged [more than 24 hours] loss of consciousness and return to pre-existing conscious level
    5 with prolonged [more than 24 hours] loss of consciousness, without return to pre-existing conscious level

    Use fifth-digit 5 to designate when a patient is unconscious and dies before regaining consciousness, regardless of the duration of the loss of consciousness

    6 with loss of consciousness of unspecified duration
    9 with concussion, unspecified

    - with
      - open intracranial wound 854.1⑤
      - skull fracture – *see* Fracture, skull, by site
    - contusion 851.8⑤
      - with open intracranial wound 851.9⑤
      - brain stem 851.4⑤
        - with open intracranial wound 851.5⑤
      - cerebellum 851.4⑤
        - with open intracranial wound 851.5⑤

- **Injury** – *continued*
  - intracranial – *continued*
    - contusion – *continued*
      - cortex (cerebral) 851.0⑤
        - with open intracranial wound 851.2⑤
    - hematoma – *see* Injury, intracranial, hemorrhage
    - hemorrhage 853.0⑤
      - with
        - laceration – *see* Injury, intracranial, laceration
        - open intracranial wound 853.1⑤
      - extradural 852.4⑤
        - with open intracranial wound 852.5⑤
      - subarachnoid 852.0⑤
        - with open intracranial wound 852.1⑤
      - subdural 852.2⑤
        - with open intracranial wound 852.3⑤
    - laceration 851.8⑤
      - with open intracranial wound 851.9⑤
      - brain stem 851.6⑤
        - with open intracranial wound 851.7⑤
      - cerebellum 851.6⑤
        - with open intracranial wound 851.7⑤
      - cortex (cerebral) 851.2⑤
        - with open intracranial wound 851.3⑤
  - intraocular – *see* Injury, eyeball, penetrating
  - intrathoracic organs (multiple) – *see* Injury, internal, intrathoracic organs
  - intrauterine – *see* Injury, internal, intrauterine
  - iris 921.3
    - penetrating – *see* Injury, eyeball, penetrating
  - jaw 959.09
  - jejunum – *see* Injury, internal, jejunum
  - joint NEC 959.9
    - old or residual 718.80
      - ankle 718.87
      - elbow 718.82
      - foot 718.87
      - hand 718.84
      - hip 718.85
      - knee 718.86
      - multiple sites 718.89
      - pelvic region 718.85
      - shoulder (region) 718.81
      - specified site NEC 718.88
      - wrist 718.83
  - kidney – *see* Injury, internal, kidney
  - knee (and ankle) (and foot) (and leg, except thigh) 959.7
  - labium (majus) (minus) 959.14
  - labyrinth, ear 959.09
  - lacrimal apparatus, gland, or sac 921.1
    - laceration 870.8
  - larynx 959.09
  - late effect – *see* Late, effects (of), injury
  - leg, except thigh (and ankle) (and foot) (and knee) 959.7
    - upper or thigh 959.6
  - lens, eye 921.3
    - penetrating – *see* Injury, eyeball, penetrating
  - lid, eye – *see* Injury, eyelid
  - lip 959.09
  - liver – *see* Injury, internal, liver
  - lobe, parietal – *see* Injury, intracranial
  - lumbar (region) 959.19
    - plexus 953.5
  - lumbosacral (region) 959.19
    - plexus 953.5
  - lung – *see* Injury, internal, lung
  - malar region 959.09
  - mastoid region 959.09
  - maternal, during pregnancy, affecting fetus or newborn 760.5
  - maxilla 959.09
  - mediastinum – *see* Injury, internal, mediastinum
  - membrane
    - brain (*see also* Injury, intracranial) 854.0⑤
    - tympanic 959.09
  - meningeal artery – *see* Hemorrhage, brain, traumatic, subarachnoid
  - meninges (cerebral) – *see* Injury, intracranial
  - mesenteric
    - artery – *see* Injury, blood vessel, mesenteric, artery
    - plexus, inferior 954.1
    - vein – *see* Injury, blood vessel, mesenteric, vein
  - mesentery – *see* Injury, internal, mesentery
  - mesosalpinx – *see* Injury, internal, mesosalpinx
  - middle ear 959.09
  - midthoracic region 959.11
  - mouth 959.09

- **Injury** – *continued*
  - multiple (sites not classifiable to the same four-digit category in 959.0-959.7) 959.8
    - internal 869.0
      - with open wound into cavity 869.1
  - musculocutaneous nerve 955.4
  - nail
    - finger 959.5
    - toe 959.7
  - nasal (septum) (sinus) 959.09
  - nasopharynx 959.09
  - neck (and face) 959.09
  - nerve 957.9
    - abducens 951.3
    - abducent 951.3
    - accessory 951.6
    - acoustic 951.5
    - ankle and foot 956.9
    - anterior crural, femoral 956.1
    - arm (*see also* Injury, nerve, upper limb) 955.9
    - auditory 951.5
    - axillary 955.0
    - brachial plexus 953.4
    - cervical sympathetic 954.0
    - cranial 951.9
      - first or olfactory 951.8
      - second or optic 950.0
      - third or oculomotor 951.0
      - fourth or trochlear 951.1
      - fifth or trigeminal 951.2
      - sixth or abducens 951.3
      - seventh or facial 951.4
      - eighth, acoustic, or auditory 951.5
      - ninth or glossopharyngeal 951.8
      - tenth, pneumogastric, or vagus 951.8
      - eleventh or accessory 951.6
      - twelfth or hypoglossal 951.7
      - newborn 767.7
    - cutaneous sensory
      - lower limb 956.4
      - upper limb 955.5⑤
    - digital (finger) 955.6
      - toe 956.5
    - facial 951.4
      - newborn 767.5
    - femoral 956.1
    - finger 955.9
    - foot and ankle 956.9
    - forearm 955.9
    - glossopharyngeal 951.8
    - hand and wrist 955.9
    - head and neck, superficial 957.0
    - hypoglossal 951.7
    - involving several parts of body 957.8
    - leg (*see also* Injury, nerve, lower limb) 956.9
    - lower limb 956.9
      - multiple 956.8
      - specified site NEC 956.5
    - lumbar plexus 953.5
    - lumbosacral plexus 953.5
    - median 955.1
      - forearm 955.1
      - wrist and hand 955.1
    - multiple (in several parts of body) (sites not classifiable to the same three-digit category) 957.8
    - musculocutaneous 955.4
    - musculospiral 955.3
      - upper arm 955.3
    - oculomotor 951.0
    - olfactory 951.8
    - optic 950.0
    - pelvic girdle 956.9
      - multiple sites 956.8
      - specified site NEC 956.5
    - peripheral 957.9
      - multiple (in several regions) (sites not classifiable to the same three-digit category) 957.8
      - specified site NEC 957.1
    - peroneal 956.3
      - ankle and foot 956.3
      - lower leg 956.3
    - plantar 956.5
    - plexus 957.9
      - celiac 954.1
      - mesenteric, inferior 954.1
      - spinal 953.9
        - brachial 953.4
        - lumbosacral 953.5
        - multiple sites 953.8
      - sympathetic NEC 954.1

Injury – *continued*
nerve – *continued*
pneumogastric 951.8
radial 955.3
wrist and hand 955.3
sacral plexus 953.5
sciatic 956.0
thigh 956.0
shoulder girdle 955.9
multiple 955.8
specified site NEC 955.7
specified site NEC 957.1
spinal 953.9
plexus – *see* Injury, nerve, plexus, spinal
root 953.9
cervical 953.0
dorsal 953.1
lumbar 953.2
multiple sites 953.8
sacral 953.3
splanchnic 954.1
sympathetic NEC 954.1
cervical 954.0
thigh 956.9
tibial 956.5
ankle and foot 956.2
lower leg 956.5
posterior 956.2
toe 956.9
trigeminal 951.2
trochlear 951.1
trunk, excluding shoulder and pelvic girdles 954.9
specified site NEC 954.8
sympathetic NEC 954.1
ulnar 955.2
forearm 955.2
wrist (and hand) 955.2
upper limb 955.9
multiple 955.8
specified site NEC 955.7
vagus 951.8
wrist and hand 955.9
nervous system, diffuse 957.8
nose (septum) 959.09
obstetrical NEC 665.9❺
affecting fetus or newborn 763.89
occipital (region) (scalp) 959.09
lobe (*see also* Injury, intracranial) 854.0❺
optic 950.9
chiasm 950.1
cortex 950.3
nerve 950.0
pathways 950.2
orbit, orbital (region) 921.2
penetrating 870.3
with foreign body 870.4
ovary – *see* Injury, internal, ovary
paint gun – *see* Wound, open, by site, complicated
palate (soft) 959.09
pancreas – *see* Injury, internal, pancreas
parathyroid (gland) 959.09
parietal (region) (scalp) 959.09
lobe – *see* Injury, intracranial
pelvic
floor 959.19
complicating delivery 664.1❺
affecting fetus or newborn 763.89
joint or ligament, complicating delivery 665.6❺
affecting fetus or newborn 763.89
organs – *see also* Injury, internal, pelvis
with
abortion – *see* Abortion, by type, with damage to pelvic organs
ectopic pregnancy (*see also* categories 633.0-633.9) 639.2
molar pregnancy (*see also* categories 633.0-633.9) 639.2
following
abortion 639.2
ectopic or molar pregnancy 639.2
obstetrical trauma 665.5❺
affecting fetus or newborn 763.89
pelvis 959.19
penis 959.14
fracture of corpus cavernosum 959.13
perineum 959.14
peritoneum – *see* Injury, internal, peritoneum

Injury – *continued*
periurethral tissue
with
abortion – *see* Abortion, by type, with damage to pelvic organs
ectopic pregnancy (*see also* categories 633.0-633.9) 639.2
molar pregnancy (*see also* categories 630-632) 639.2
complicating delivery 665.5❺
affecting fetus or newborn 763.89
following
abortion 639.2
ectopic or molar pregnancy 639.2
phalanges
foot 959.7
hand 959.5
pharynx 959.09
pleura – *see* Injury, internal, pleura
popliteal space 959.7
post-cardiac surgery (syndrome) 429.4
prepuce 959.14
prostate – *see* Injury, internal, prostate
pubic region 959.19
pudenda 959.14
radiation NEC 990
radioactive substance or radium NEC 990
rectovaginal septum 959.14
rectum – *see* Injury, internal, rectum
retina 921.3
penetrating – *see* Injury, eyeball, penetrating
retroperitoneal – *see* Injury, internal, retroperitoneum
roentgen rays NEC 990
round ligament – *see* Injury, internal, round ligament
sacral (region) 959.19
plexus 953.5
sacroiliac ligament NEC 959.19
sacrum 959.19
salivary ducts or glands 959.09
scalp 959.09
due to birth trauma 767.19
fetus or newborn 767.19
scapular region 959.2
sclera 921.3
penetrating – *see* Injury, eyeball, penetrating
superficial 918.2
scrotum 959.14
seminal vesicle – *see* Injury, internal, seminal vesicle
shoulder (and upper arm) 959.2
sinus
cavernous (*see also* Injury, intracranial) 854.0❺
nasal 959.09
skeleton NEC, birth injury 767.3
skin NEC 959.9
skull – *see* Fracture, skull, by site
soft tissue (of external sites) (severe) – *see* Wound, open, by site
specified site NEC 959.8
spermatic cord – *see* Injury, internal, spermatic cord
spinal (cord) 952.9
with fracture, vertebra – *see* Fracture, vertebra, by site, with spinal cord injury
cervical (C_1-C_4) 952.00
with
anterior cord syndrome 952.02
central cord syndrome 952.03
complete lesion of cord 952.01
incomplete lesion NEC 952.04
posterior cord syndrome 952.04
C_5-C_7 level 952.05
with
anterior cord syndrome 952.07
central cord syndrome 952.08
complete lesion of cord 952.06
incomplete lesion NEC 952.09
posterior cord syndrome 952.09
specified type NEC 952.09
specified type NEC 952.04
dorsal (D_1-D_6) (T_1-T_6) (thoracic) 952.10
with
anterior cord syndrome 952.12
central cord syndrome 952.13
complete lesion of cord 952.11
incomplete lesion NEC 952.14
posterior cord syndrome 952.14

Injury – *continued*
spinal – *continued*
dorsal – *continued*
D_7-D_{12} level (T_7-T_{12}) 952.15
with
anterior cord syndrome 952.17
central cord syndrome 952.18
complete lesion of cord 952.16
incomplete lesion NEC 952.19
posterior cord syndrome 952.19
specified type NEC 952.19
specified type NEC 952.14
lumbar 952.2
multiple sites 952.8
nerve (root) NEC – *see* Injury, nerve, spinal, root
plexus 953.9
brachial 953.4
lumbosacral 953.5
multiple sites 953.8
sacral 952.3
thoracic (*see also* Injury, spinal, dorsal) 952.10
spleen – *see* Injury, internal, spleen
stellate ganglion 954.1
sternal region 959.11
stomach – *see* Injury, internal, stomach
subconjunctival 921.1
subcutaneous 959.9
subdural – *see* Injury, intracranial
submaxillary region 959.09
submental region 959.09
subungual
fingers 959.5
toes 959.7
superficial 919❹

Note – Use the following fourth-digit subdivisions with categories 910-919:
.0 abrasion or friction burn without mention of infection
.1 abrasion or friction burn, infected
.2 blister without mention of infection
.3 blister, infected
.4 insect bite, nonvenomous, without mention of infection
.5 insect bite, nonvenomous, infected
.6 superficial foreign body (splinter) without major open wound and without mention of infection
.7 superficial foreign body (splinter) without major open wound, infected
.8 other and unspecified superficial injury without mention of infection
.9 other and unspecified superficial injury, infected

For late effects of superficial injury, see category 906.2.

abdomen, abdominal (muscle) (wall) (and other part(s) of trunk) 911❹
ankle (and hip, knee, leg, or thigh) 916❹
anus (and other part(s) of trunk) 911❹
arm 913❹
upper (and shoulder) 912❹
auditory canal (external) (meatus) (and other part(s) of face, neck, or scalp, except eye) 910❹
axilla (and upper arm) 912❹
back (and other part(s) of trunk) 911❹
breast (and other part(s) of trunk) 911❹
brow (and other part(s) of face, neck, or scalp, except eye) 910❹
buttock (and other part(s) of trunk) 911❹
canthus, eye 918.0
cheek(s) (and other part(s) of face, neck, or scalp, except eye) 910❹
chest wall (and other part(s) of trunk) 911❹
chin (and other part(s) of face, neck, or scalp, except eye) 910❹
clitoris (and other part(s) of trunk) 911❹
conjunctiva 918.2
cornea 918.1
due to contact lens 371.82
costal region (and other part(s) of trunk) 911❹
ear(s) (auricle) (canal) (drum) (external) (and other part(s) of face, neck, or scalp, except eye) 910❹
elbow (and forearm) (and wrist) 913❹
epididymis (and other part(s) of trunk) 911❹
epigastric region (and other part(s) of trunk) 911❹
epiglottis (and other part(s) of face, neck, or scalp, except eye) 910❹

- **Injury** – *continued*
  - superficial – *continued*
    - eye(s) (and adnexa) NEC 918.9
    - eyelid(s) (and periocular area) 918.0
    - face (any part(s), except eye) (and neck or scalp) 910❹
    - finger(s) (nail) (any) 915❹
    - flank (and other part(s) of trunk) 911❹
    - foot (phalanges) (and toe(s)) 917❹
    - forearm (and elbow) (and wrist) 913❹
    - forehead (and other part(s) of face, neck, or scalp, except eye) 910❹
    - globe (eye) 918.9
    - groin (and other part(s) of trunk) 911❹
    - gums(s) (and other part(s) of face, neck, or scalp, except eye) 910❹
    - hand(s) (except fingers alone) 914❹
    - head (and other part(s) of face, neck, or scalp, except eye) 910❹
    - heel (and foot or toe) 917❹
    - hip (and ankle, knee, leg, or thigh) 916❹
    - iliac region (and other part(s) of trunk) 911❹
    - interscapular region (and other part(s) of trunk) 911❹
    - iris 918.9
    - knee (and ankle, hip, leg, or thigh) 916❹
    - labium (majus) (minus) (and other part(s) of trunk) 911❹
    - lacrimal (apparatus) (gland) (sac) 918.0
    - leg (lower) (upper) (and ankle, hip, knee, or thigh) 916❹
    - lip(s) (and other part(s) of face, neck, or scalp, except eye) 910❹
    - lower extremity (except foot) 916❹
    - lumbar region (and other part(s) of trunk) 911❹
    - malar region (and other part(s) of face, neck, or scalp, except eye) 910❹
    - mastoid region (and other part(s) of face, neck, or scalp, except eye) 910❹
    - midthoracic region (and other part(s) of trunk) 911❹
    - mouth (and other part(s) of face, neck, or scalp, except eye) 910❹
    - multiple sites (not classifiable to the same three-digit category) 919❹
    - nasal (septum) (and other part(s) of face, neck, or scalp, except eye) 910❹
    - neck (and face or scalp, any part(s), except eye) 910❹
    - nose (septum) (and other part(s) of face, neck, or scalp, except eye) 910❹
    - occipital region (and other part(s) of face, neck, or scalp, except eye) 910❹
    - orbital region 918.0
    - palate (soft) (and other part(s) of face, neck, or scalp, except eye) 910❹
    - parietal region (and other part(s) of face, neck, or scalp, except eye) 910❹
    - penis (and other part(s) of trunk) 911❹
    - perineum (and other part(s) of trunk) 911❹
    - periocular area 918.0
    - pharynx (and other part(s) of face, neck, or scalp, except eye) 910❹
    - popliteal space (and ankle, hip, leg, or thigh) 916❹
    - prepuce (and other part(s) of trunk) 911❹
    - pubic region (and other part(s) of trunk) 911❹
    - pudenda (and other part(s) of trunk) 911❹
    - sacral region (and other part(s) of trunk) 911❹
    - salivary (ducts) (glands) (and other part(s) of face, neck, or scalp, except eye) 910❹
    - scalp (and other part(s) of face or neck, except eye) 910❹
    - scapular region (and upper arm) 912❹
    - sclera 918.2
    - scrotum (and other part(s) of trunk) 911❹
    - shoulder (and upper arm) 912❹
    - skin NEC 919❹
    - specified site(s) NEC 919❹
    - sternal region (and other part(s) of trunk) 911❹
    - subconjunctival 918.2
    - subcutaneous NEC 919❹
    - submaxillary region (and other part(s) of face, neck, or scalp, except eye) 910❹
    - submental region (and other part(s) of face, neck, or scalp, except eye) 910❹
    - supraclavicular fossa (and other part(s) of face, neck, or scalp, except eye) 910❹
    - supraorbital 918.0
    - temple (and other part(s) of face, neck, or scalp, except eye) 910❹
    - temporal region (and other part(s) of face, neck, or scalp, except eye) 910❹
    - testis (and other part(s) of trunk) 911❹
    - thigh (and ankle, hip, knee, or leg) 916❹
    - thorax, thoracic (external) (and other part(s) of trunk) 911❹
    - throat (and other part(s) of face, neck, or scalp, except eye) 910❹
    - thumb(s) (nail) 915❹
    - toe(s) (nail) (subungual) (and foot) 917❹
    - tongue (and other part(s) of face, neck, or scalp, except eye) 910❹
    - tooth, teeth (*see also* Abrasion, dental) 521.20
    - trunk (any part(s)) 911❹
    - tunica vaginalis (and other part(s) of trunk) 911❹
    - tympanum, tympanic membrane (and other part(s) of face, neck, or scalp, except eye) 910❹
    - upper extremity NEC 913❹
    - uvula (and other part(s) of face, neck, or scalp, except eye) 910❹
    - vagina (and other part(s) of trunk) 911❹
    - vulva (and other part(s) of trunk) 911❹
    - wrist (and elbow) (and forearm) 913❹
  - supraclavicular fossa 959.19
  - supraorbital 959.09
  - surgical complication (external or internal site) 998.2
  - symphysis pubis 959.19
    - complicating delivery 665.6❺
      - affecting fetus or newborn 763.89
  - temple 959.09
  - temporal region 959.09
  - testis 959.14
  - thigh (and hip) 959.6
  - thorax, thoracic (external) 959.11
    - cavity – *see* Injury, internal, thorax
    - internal – *see* Injury, internal, intrathoracic organs
  - throat 959.09
  - thumb(s) (nail) 959.5
  - thymus – *see* Injury, internal, thymus
  - thyroid (gland) 959.09
  - toe (nail) (any) 959.7
  - tongue 959.09
  - tonsil 959.09
  - tooth NEC 873.63
    - complicated 873.73
  - trachea – *see* Injury, internal, trachea
  - trunk 959.19
  - tunica vaginalis 959.14
  - tympanum, tympanic membrane 959.09
  - ultraviolet rays NEC 990
  - ureter – *see* Injury, internal, ureter
  - urethra (sphincter) – *see* Injury, internal, urethra
  - uterus – *see* Injury, internal, uterus
  - uvula 959.09
  - vagina 959.14
  - vascular – *see* Injury, blood vessel
  - vas deferens – *see* Injury, internal, vas deferens
  - vein (*see also* Injury, blood vessel, by site) 904.9
  - vena cava
    - inferior 902.10
    - superior 901.2
  - vesical (sphincter) – *see* Injury, internal, vesical
  - viscera (abdominal) – *see* Injury, internal, viscera
    - with fracture, pelvis – *see* Fracture, pelvis
  - visual 950.9
    - cortex 950.3
  - vitreous (humor) 871.2
  - vulva 959.14
  - whiplash (cervical spine) 847.0
  - wringer – *see* Crush, by site
  - wrist (and elbow) (and forearm) 959.3
  - x-ray NEC 990
- **Inoculation** – *see also* Vaccination
  - complication or reaction – *see* Complication, vaccination
- **INPH** (idiopathic normal pressure hydrocephalus) 331.5 ●
- **Insanity, insane** (*see also* Psychosis) 298.9
  - adolescent (*see also* Schizophrenia) 295.9❺
  - alternating (*see also* Psychosis, affective, circular) 296.7
  - confusional 298.9
    - acute 293.0
    - subacute 293.1
  - delusional 298.9
  - paralysis, general 094.1
    - progressive 094.1
  - paresis, general 094.1
  - senile 290.20
- **Insect**
  - bite – *see* Injury, superficial, by site
  - venomous, poisoning by 989.5
- **Insemination, artificial** V26.1
- **Insensitivity**
  - adrenocorticotropin hormone (ACTH) 255.41 ●
  - androgen 259.5
    - partial 259.5
- **Insertion**
  - cord (umbilical) lateral or velamentous 663.8❺
    - affecting fetus or newborn 762.6
  - intrauterine contraceptive device V25.1
  - placenta, vicious – *see* Placenta, previa
  - subdermal implantable contraceptive V25.5
  - velamentous, umbilical cord 663.8❺
    - affecting fetus or newborn 762.6
- **Insolation** 992.0
  - meaning sunstroke 992.0
- **Insomnia**, unspecified 780.52
  - with sleep apnea, unspecified 780.51
  - adjustment 307.41
  - alcohol-induced 291.82
  - behavioral, of childhood V69.5
  - drug-induced 292.85
  - due to
    - medical condition classified elsewhere 327.01
    - mental disorder 327.02
  - idiopathic 307.42
  - nonorganic origin 307.41
    - persistent (primary) 307.42
    - transient 307.41
  - organic 327.00
    - other 327.09
  - paradoxical 307.42
  - primary 307.42
  - psychophysiological 307.42
  - subjective complaint 307.49
- **Inspiration**
  - food or foreign body (*see also* Asphyxia, food or foreign body) 933.1
  - mucus (*see also* Asphyxia, mucus) 933.1
- **Inspissated bile syndrome, newborn** 774.4
- **Instability**
  - detrusor 596.59
  - emotional (excessive) 301.3
  - joint (posttraumatic) 718.80
    - ankle 718.87
    - elbow 718.82
    - foot 718.87
    - hand 718.84
    - hip 718.85
    - knee 718.86
    - lumbosacral 724.6
    - multiple sites 718.89
    - pelvic region 718.85
    - sacroiliac 724.6
    - shoulder (region) 718.81
    - specified site NEC 718.88
    - wrist 718.83
  - lumbosacral 724.6
  - nervous 301.89
  - personality (emotional) 301.59
  - thyroid, paroxysmal 242.9❺
  - urethral 599.83
  - vasomotor 780.2
- **Insufficiency, insufficient**
  - accommodation 367.4
  - adrenal (gland) (acute) (chronic) 255.41 ▲
    - medulla 255.5
    - primary 255.41 ▲
    - specified site NEC 255.5
  - adrenocortical 255.41 ▲
  - anterior (occlusal) guidance 524.54
  - anus 569.49
  - aortic (valve) 424.1
    - with
      - mitral (valve) disease 396.1
        - insufficiency, incompetence, or regurgitation 396.3
        - stenosis or obstruction 396.1

Insufficiency, insufficient – *continued*
- aortic – *continued*
  - with – *continued*
    - stenosis or obstruction 424.1
      - with mitral (valve) disease 396.8
  - congenital 746.4
  - rheumatic 395.1
    - with
      - mitral (valve) disease 396.1
        - insufficiency, incompetence, or regurgitation 396.3
        - stenosis or obstruction 396.1
      - stenosis or obstruction 395.2
        - with mitral (valve) disease 396.8
  - specified cause NEC 424.1
  - syphilitic 093.22
- arterial 447.1
  - basilar artery 435.0
  - carotid artery 435.8
  - cerebral 437.1
  - coronary (acute or subacute) 411.89
  - mesenteric 557.1
  - peripheral 443.9
  - precerebral 435.9
  - vertebral artery 435.1
  - vertebrobasilar 435.3
- arteriovenous 459.9
- basilar artery 435.0
- biliary 575.8
- cardiac (*see also* Insufficiency, myocardial) 428.0
  - complicating surgery 997.1
  - due to presence of (cardiac) prosthesis 429.4
  - postoperative 997.1
    - long-term effect of cardiac surgery 429.4
  - specified during or due to a procedure 997.1
    - long-term effect of cardiac surgery 429.4
- cardiorenal (*see also* Hypertension, cardiorenal) 404.90
- cardiovascular (*see also* Disease, cardiovascular) 429.2
  - renal (*see also* Hypertension, cardiorenal) 404.90
- carotid artery 435.8
- cerebral (vascular) 437.9
- cerebrovascular 437.9
  - with transient focal neurological signs and symptoms 435.9
  - acute 437.1
    - with transient focal neurological signs and symptoms 435.9
- circulatory NEC 459.9
  - fetus or newborn 779.89
- convergence 378.83
- coronary (acute or subacute) 411.89
  - chronic or with a stated duration of over 8 weeks 414.8
- corticoadrenal 255.41 ▲
- dietary 269.9
- divergence 378.85
- food 994.2
- gastroesophageal 530.89
- gonadal
  - ovary 256.39
  - testis 257.2
- gonadotropic hormone secretion 253.4
- heart – *see also* Insufficiency, myocardial
  - fetus or newborn 779.89
  - valve (*see also* Endocarditis) 424.90
    - congenital NEC 746.89
- hepatic 573.8
- idiopathic autonomic 333.0
- interocclusal distance of teeth (ridge) 524.36
- kidney
  - acute 593.9
  - chronic 585.9
- labyrinth, labyrinthine (function) 386.53
  - bilateral 386.54
  - unilateral 386.53
- lacrimal 375.15
- liver 573.8
- lung (acute) (*see also* Insufficiency, pulmonary) 518.82
  - following trauma, surgery, or shock 518.5
  - newborn 770.89
- mental (congenital) (*see also* Retardation, mental) 319
- mesenteric 557.1
- mitral (valve) 424.0
  - with
    - aortic (valve) disease 396.3
      - insufficiency, incompetence, or regurgitation 396.3

Insufficiency, insufficient – *continued*
- mitral – *continued*
  - with – *continued*
    - aortic (valve) disease – *continued*
      - stenosis or obstruction 396.2
    - obstruction or stenosis 394.2
      - with aortic valve disease 396.8
  - congenital 746.6
  - rheumatic 394.1
    - with
      - aortic (valve) disease 396.3
        - insufficiency, incompetence, or regurgitation 396.3
        - stenosis or obstruction 396.2
      - obstruction or stenosis 394.2
        - with aortic valve disease 396.8
    - active or acute 391.1
      - with chorea, rheumatic (Sydenham's) 392.0
  - specified cause, except rheumatic 424.0
- muscle
  - heart – *see* Insufficiency, myocardial
  - ocular (*see also* Strabismus) 378.9
- myocardial, myocardium (with arteriosclerosis) 428.0
  - with rheumatic fever (conditions classifiable to 390)
    - active, acute, or subacute 391.2
      - with chorea 392.0
    - inactive or quiescent (with chorea) 398.0
  - congenital 746.89
  - due to presence of (cardiac) prosthesis 429.4
  - fetus or newborn 779.89
  - following cardiac surgery 429.4
  - hypertensive (*see also* Hypertension, heart) 402.91
    - benign 402.11
    - malignant 402.01
  - postoperative 997.1
    - long-term effect of cardiac surgery 429.4
  - rheumatic 398.0
    - active, acute, or subacute 391.2
      - with chorea (Sydenham's) 392.0
  - syphilitic 093.82
- nourishment 994.2
- organic 799.89
- ovary 256.39
  - postablative 256.2
- pancreatic 577.8
- parathyroid (gland) 252.1
- peripheral vascular (arterial) 443.9
- pituitary (anterior) 253.2
  - posterior 253.5
- placental – *see* Placenta, insufficiency
- platelets 287.5
- prenatal care in current pregnancy V23.7
- progressive pluriglandular 258.9
- pseudocholinesterase 289.89
- pulmonary (acute) 518.82
  - following
    - shock 518.5
    - surgery 518.5
    - trauma 518.5
  - newborn 770.89
  - valve (*see also* Endocarditis, pulmonary) 424.3
    - congenital 746.09
- pyloric 537.0
- renal 593.9
  - acute 593.9
  - chronic 585.9
  - due to a procedure 997.5
- respiratory 786.09
  - acute 518.82
    - following shock, surgery, or trauma 518.5
  - newborn 770.89
- rotation – *see* Malrotation
- suprarenal 255.41 ▲
  - medulla 255.5
- tarso-orbital fascia, congenital 743.66
- tear film 375.15
- testis 257.2
- thyroid (gland) (acquired) – *see also* Hypothyroidism
  - congenital 243
- tricuspid (*see also* Endocarditis, tricuspid) 397.0
  - congenital 746.89
  - syphilitic 093.23
- urethral sphincter 599.84
- valve, valvular (heart) (*see also* Endocarditis) 424.90
- vascular 459.9
  - intestine NEC 557.9

Insufficiency, insufficient – *continued*
- vascular – *continued*
  - mesenteric 557.1
  - peripheral 443.9
  - renal (*see also* Hypertension, kidney) 403.90
- velopharyngeal
  - acquired 528.9
  - congenital 750.29
- venous (peripheral) 459.81
- ventricular – *see* Insufficiency, myocardial
- vertebral artery 435.1
- vertebrobasilar artery 435.3
- weight gain during pregnancy 646.8❺
- zinc 269.3

Insufflation
- fallopian
  - fertility testing V26.21
  - following sterilization reversal V26.22
- meconium 770.11
  - with respiratory symptoms 770.12

Insular – *see* condition

Insulinoma (M8151/0)
- malignant (M8151/3)
  - pancreas 157.4
  - specified site – *see* Neoplasm, by site, malignant
  - unspecified site 157.4
- pancreas 211.7
- specified site – *see* Neoplasm, by site, benign
- unspecified site 211.7

Insuloma – *see* Insulinoma

Insult
- brain 437.9
  - acute 436
- cerebral 437.9
  - acute 436
- cerebrovascular 437.9
  - acute 436
- vascular NEC 437.9
  - acute 436

Insurance examination (certification) V70.3

Intemperance (*see also* Alcoholism) 303.9❺

Interception of pregnancy (menstrual extraction) V25.3

Interference
- balancing side 524.56
- non-working side 524.56

Intermenstrual
- bleeding 626.6
  - irregular 626.6
  - regular 626.5
- hemorrhage 626.6
  - irregular 626.6
  - regular 626.5
- pain(s) 625.2

Intermittent – *see* condition

Internal – *see* condition

Interproximal wear 521.10

Interruption
- aortic arch 747.11
- bundle of His 426.50
- fallopian tube (for sterilization) V25.2
- phase-shift, sleep cycle 307.45
- repeated REM-sleep 307.48
- sleep
  - due to perceived environmental disturbances 307.48
  - phase-shift, of 24-hour sleep-wake cycle 307.45
  - repeated REM-sleep type 307.48
- vas deferens (for sterilization) V25.2

Intersexuality 752.7

Interstitial – *see* condition

Intertrigo 695.89
- labialis 528.5

Intervertebral disc – *see* condition

Intestine, intestinal – *see also* condition
- flu 487.8

Intolerance
- carbohydrate NEC 579.8
- cardiovascular exercise, with pain (at rest) (with less than ordinary activity) (with ordinary activity) V47.2
- cold 780.99
- dissacharide (hereditary) 271.3
- drug
  - correct substance properly administered 995.27

- **Intolerance** – *continued*
  - drug – *continued*
    - wrong substance given or taken in error 977.9
      - specified drug – *see* Table of Drugs and Chemicals
  - effort 306.2
  - fat NEC 579.8
  - foods NEC 579.8
  - fructose (hereditary) 271.2
  - glucose (-galactose) (congenital) 271.3
  - gluten 579.0
  - lactose (hereditary) (infantile) 271.3
  - lysine (congenital) 270.7
  - milk NEC 579.8
  - protein (familial) 270.7
  - starch NEC 579.8
  - sucrose (-isomaltose) (congenital) 271.3
- **Intoxicated** NEC (*see also* Alcoholism) 305.0❺
- **Intoxication**
  - acid 276.2
  - acute
    - alcoholic 305.0❺
      - with alcoholism 303.0❺
      - hangover effects 305.0❺
    - caffeine 305.9❺
    - hallucinogenic (*see also* Abuse, drugs, nondependent) 305.3❺
  - alcohol (acute) 305.0❺
    - with alcoholism 303.0❺
    - hangover effects 305.0❺
    - idiosyncratic 291.4
    - pathological 291.4
  - alimentary canal 558.2
  - ammonia (hepatic) 572.2
  - caffeine 305.9
  - chemical – *see also* Table of Drugs and Chemicals
    - via placenta or breast milk 760.70
      - alcohol 760.71
      - anticonvulsants 760.77
      - antifungals 760.74
      - anti-infective agents 760.74
      - antimetabolics 760.78
      - cocaine 760.75
      - "crack" 760.75
      - hallucinogenic agents NEC 760.73
      - medicinal agents NEC 760.79
      - narcotics 760.72
      - obstetric anesthetic or analgesic drug 763.5
      - specified agent NEC 760.79
      - suspected, affecting management of pregnancy 655.5❺
  - cocaine, through placenta or breast milk 760.75
  - delirium
    - alcohol 291.0
    - drug 292.81
  - drug 292.89
    - with delirium 292.81
    - correct substance properly administered (*see also* Allergy, drug) 995.27
    - newborn 779.4
    - obstetric anesthetic or sedation 668.9❺
      - affecting fetus or newborn 763.5
    - overdose or wrong substance given or taken – *see* Table of Drugs and Chemicals
    - pathologic 292.2
    - specific to newborn 779.4
    - via placenta or breast milk 760.70
      - alcohol 760.71
      - anticonvulsants 760.77
      - antifungals 760.74
      - anti-infective agents 760.74
      - antimetabolics 760.78
      - cocaine 760.75
      - "crack" 760.75
      - hallucinogenic agents 760.73
      - medicinal agents NEC 760.79
      - narcotics 760.72
      - obstetric anesthetic or analgesic drug 763.5
      - specified agent NEC 760.79
      - suspected, affecting management of pregnancy 655.5❺
  - enteric – *see* Intoxication, intestinal
  - fetus or newborn, via placenta or breast milk 760.70
    - alcohol 760.71
    - anticonvulsants 760.77
    - antifungals 760.74
    - anti-infective agents 760.74
    - antimetabolics 760.78
    - cocaine 760.75
    - "crack" 760.75
    - hallucinogenic agents 760.73

- **Intoxication** – *continued*
  - fetus or newborn, via placenta or breast milk - *continued*
    - medicinal agents NEC 760.79
    - narcotics 760.72
    - obstetric anesthetic or analgesic drug 763.5
    - specified agent NEC 760.79
    - suspected, affecting management of pregnancy 655.5❺
  - food – *see* Poisoning, food
  - gastrointestinal 558.2
  - hallucinogenic (acute) 305.3❺
  - hepatocerebral 572.2
  - idiosyncratic alcohol 291.4
  - intestinal 569.89
    - due to putrefaction of food 005.9
  - methyl alcohol (*see also* Alcoholism) 305.0❺
    - with alcoholism 303.0❺
  - non-foodborne due to toxins of Clostridium botulinum [C. botulinum] – *see* Botulism ●
  - pathologic 291.4
    - drug 292.2
  - potassium (K) 276.7
  - septic
    - with
      - abortion – *see* Abortion, by type, with sepsis
      - ectopic pregnancy (*see also* categories 633.0-633.9) 639.0
      - molar pregnancy (*see also* categories 630-632) 639.0
    - during labor 659.3❺
    - following
      - abortion 639.0
      - ectopic or molar pregnancy 639.0
    - generalized – *see* Septicemia
    - puerperal, postpartum, childbirth 670❹
  - serum (prophylactic) (therapeutic) 999.5
  - uremic – *see* Uremia
  - water 276.6
- **Intracranial** – *see* condition
- **Intrahepatic gallbladder** 751.69
- **Intraligamentous** – *see also* condition
  - pregnancy – *see* Pregnancy, cornual
- **Intraocular** – *see also* condition
  - sepsis 360.00
- **Intrathoracic** – *see also* condition
  - kidney 753.3
  - stomach – *see* Hernia, diaphragm
- **Intrauterine contraceptive device**
  - checking V25.42
  - insertion V25.1
  - in situ V45.51
  - management V25.42
  - prescription V25.02
    - repeat V25.42
  - reinsertion V25.42
  - removal V25.42
- **Intraventricular** – *see* condition
- **Intrinsic deformity** – *see* Deformity
- **Intruded tooth** 524.34
- **Intrusion, repetitive, of sleep** (due to environmental disturbances) (with atypical polysomnographic features) 307.48
- **Intumescent, lens** (eye) NEC 366.9
  - senile 366.12
- **Intussusception** (colon) (enteric) (intestine) (rectum) 560.0
  - appendix 543.9
  - congenital 751.5
  - fallopian tube 620.8
  - ileocecal 560.0
  - ileocolic 560.0
  - ureter (obstruction) 593.4
- **Invagination**
  - basilar 756.0
  - colon or intestine 560.0
- **Invalid** (since birth) 799.89
- **Invalidism** (chronic) 799.89
- **Inversion**
  - albumin-globulin (A-G) ratio 273.8
  - bladder 596.8
  - cecum (*see also* Intussusception) 560.0
  - cervix 622.8
  - nipple 611.79
    - congenital 757.6
    - puerperal, postpartum 676.3❺
  - optic papilla 743.57
  - organ or site, congenital NEC – *see* Anomaly, specified type NEC

- **Inversion** – *continued*
  - sleep rhythm 327.39
    - nonorganic origin 307.45
  - testis (congenital) 752.51
  - uterus (postinfectional) (postpartal, old) 621.7
    - chronic 621.7
    - complicating delivery 665.2❺
      - affecting fetus or newborn 763.89
  - vagina – *see* Prolapse, vagina
- **Investigation**
  - allergens V72.7
  - clinical research (control) (normal comparison) (participant) V70.7
- **Inviability** – *see* Immaturity
- **Involuntary movement, abnormal** 781 0
- **Involution, involutional** – *see also* condition
  - breast, cystic or fibrocystic 610.1
  - depression (*see also* Psychosis, affective) 296.2❺
    - recurrent episode 296.3❺
    - single episode 296.2❺
  - melancholia (*see also* Psychosis, affective) 296.2
    - recurrent episode 296.3
    - single episode 296.2
  - ovary, senile 620.3
  - paranoid state (reaction) 297.2
  - paraphrenia (climacteric) (menopause) 297.2
  - psychosis 298.8
  - thymus failure 254.8
- **IQ**
  - under 20 318.2
  - 20-34 318.1
  - 35-49 318.0
  - 50-70 317
- **IRDS** 769
- **Irideremia** 743.45
- **Iridis rubeosis** 364.42
  - diabetic 250.5❺ *[364.42]*
- **Iridochoroiditis** (panuveitis) 360.12
- **Iridocyclitis** NEC 364.3
  - acute 364.00
    - primary 364.01
    - recurrent 364.02
  - chronic 364.10
    - in
      - lepromatous leprosy 030.0 *[364.11]*
      - sarcoidosis 135 *[364.11]*
      - tuberculosis (*see also* Tuberculosis) 017.3❺ *[364.11]*
  - due to allergy 364.04
  - endogenous 364.01
  - gonococcal 098.41
  - granulomatous 364.10
  - herpetic (simplex) 054.44
    - zoster 053.22
  - hypopyon 364.05
  - lens induced 364.23
  - nongranulomatous 364.00
  - primary 364.01
  - recurrent 364.02
  - rheumatic 364.10
  - secondary 364.04
    - infectious 364.03
    - noninfectious 364.04
  - subacute 364.00
    - primary 364.01
    - recurrent 364.02
  - sympathetic 360.11
  - syphilitic (secondary) 091.52
  - tuberculous (chronic) (*see also* Tuberculosis) 017.3❺ *[364.11]*
- **Iridocyclochoroiditis** (panuveitis) 360.12
- **Iridodialysis** 364.76
- **Iridodonesis** 364.89 ▲
- **Iridoplegia** (complete) (partial) (reflex) 379.49
- **Iridoschisis** 364.52
- **Iris** – *see* condition
- **Iritis** 364.3
  - acute 364.00
    - primary 364.01
    - recurrent 364.02
  - chronic 364.10
    - in
      - sarcoidosis 135 *[364.11]*
      - tuberculosis (*see also* Tuberculosis) 017.3❺ *[364.11]*
  - diabetic 250.5❺ *[364.42]*
  - due to
    - allergy 364.04

Intolerance – Iritis

❹ Fourth-Digit Required ❺ Fifth-Digit Required *[code]* Manifestation Code ▶◀ Revised Text ● New Line ▲ Revised Code

- **Iritis** – *continued*
  - due to – *continued*
    - herpes simplex 054.44
    - leprosy 030.0 *[364.11]*
  - endogenous 364.01
  - gonococcal 098.41
  - gouty 274.89 *[364.11]*
  - granulomatous 364.10
  - hypopyon 364.05
  - lens induced 364.23
  - nongranulomatous 364.00
  - papulosa 095.8 *[364.11]*
  - primary 364.01
  - recurrent 364.02
  - rheumatic 364.10
  - secondary 364.04
    - infectious 364.03
    - noninfectious 364.04
  - subacute 364.00
    - primary 364.01
    - recurrent 364.02
  - sympathetic 360.11
  - syphilitic (secondary) 091.52
    - congenital 090.0 *[364.11]*
    - late 095.8 *[364.11]*
  - tuberculous (*see also* Tuberculosis) 017.3❺ *[364.11]*
  - uratic 274.89 *[364.11]*
- **Iron**
  - deficiency anemia 280.9
  - metabolism disease 275.0
  - storage disease 275.0
- **Iron-miners' lung** 503
- **Irradiated enamel** (tooth, teeth) 521.89
- **Irradiation**
  - burn – *see* Burn, by site
  - effects, adverse 990
- **Irreducible, irreducibility** – *see* condition
- **Irregular, irregularity**
  - action, heart 427.9
  - alveolar process 525.8
  - bleeding NEC 626.4
  - breathing 786.09
  - colon 569.89
  - contour of cornea 743.41
    - acquired 371.70
  - dentin in pulp 522.3
  - eye movements NEC 379.59
  - menstruation (cause unknown) 626.4
  - periods 626.4
  - prostate 602.9
  - pupil 364.75
  - respiratory 786.09
  - septum (nasal) 470
  - shape, organ or site, congenital NEC – *see* Distortion
  - sleep-wake rhythm (non-24-hour) 327.39
    - nonorganic origin 307.45
  - vertebra 733.99
- **Irritability** (nervous) 799.2
  - bladder 596.8
    - neurogenic 596.54
      - with cauda equina syndrome 344.61
  - bowel (syndrome) 564.1
  - bronchial (*see also* Bronchitis) 490
  - cerebral, newborn 779.1
  - colon 564.1
    - psychogenic 306.4
  - duodenum 564.89
  - heart (psychogenic) 306.2
  - ileum 564.89
  - jejunum 564.89
  - myocardium 306.2
  - rectum 564.89
  - stomach 536.9
    - psychogenic 306.4
  - sympathetic (nervous system) (*see also* Neuropathy, peripheral, autonomic) 337.9
  - urethra 599.84
  - ventricular (heart) (psychogenic) 306.2
- **Irritable** – *see* Irritability
- **Irritation**
  - anus 569.49
  - axillary nerve 353.0
  - bladder 596.8
  - brachial plexus 353.0
  - brain (traumatic) (*see also* Injury, intracranial) 854.0❺
    - nontraumatic – *see* Encephalitis
  - bronchial (*see also* Bronchitis) 490
- **Irritation** – *continued*
  - cerebral (traumatic) (*see also* Injury, intracranial) 854.0❺
    - nontraumatic – *see* Encephalitis
  - cervical plexus 353.2
  - cervix (*see also* Cervicitis) 616.0
  - choroid, sympathetic 360.11
  - cranial nerve – *see* Disorder, nerve, cranial
  - digestive tract 536.9
    - psychogenic 306.4
  - gastric 536.9
    - psychogenic 306.4
  - gastrointestinal (tract) 536.9
    - functional 536.9
    - psychogenic 306.4
  - globe, sympathetic 360.11
  - intestinal (bowel) 564.9
  - labyrinth 386.50
  - lumbosacral plexus 353.1
  - meninges (traumatic) (*see also* Injury, intracranial) 854.0❺
    - nontraumatic – *see* Meningitis
  - myocardium 306.2
  - nerve – *see* Disorder, nerve
  - nervous 799.2
  - nose 478.19
  - penis 607.89
  - perineum 709.9
  - peripheral
    - autonomic nervous system (*see also* Neuropathy, peripheral, autonomic) 337.9
    - nerve – *see* Disorder, nerve
  - peritoneum (*see also* Peritonitis) 567.9
  - pharynx 478.29
  - plantar nerve 355.6
  - spinal (cord) (traumatic) – *see also* Injury, spinal, by site
    - nerve – *see also* Disorder, nerve
      - root NEC 724.9
      - traumatic – *see* Injury, nerve, spinal
    - nontraumatic – *see* Myelitis
  - stomach 536.9
    - psychogenic 306.4
  - sympathetic nerve NEC (*see also* Neuropathy, peripheral, autonomic) 337.9
  - ulnar nerve 354.2
  - vagina 623.9
- **Isambert's disease** 012.3❺
- **Ischemia, ischemic** 459.9
  - basilar artery (with transient neurologic deficit) 435.0
  - bone NEC 733.40
  - bowel (transient) 557.9
    - acute 557.0
    - chronic 557.1
    - due to mesenteric artery insufficiency 557.1
  - brain – *see also* Ischemia, cerebral
    - recurrent focal 435.9
  - cardiac (*see also* Ischemia, heart) 414.9
  - cardiomyopathy 414.8
  - carotid artery (with transient neurologic deficit) 435.8
  - cerebral (chronic) (generalized) 437.1
    - arteriosclerotic 437.0
    - intermittent (with transient neurologic deficit) 435.9
    - newborn 779.2
    - puerperal, postpartum, childbirth 674.0❺
    - recurrent focal (with transient neurologic deficit) 435.9
    - transient (with transient neurologic deficit) 435.9
  - colon 557.9
    - acute 557.0
    - chronic 557.1
    - due to mesenteric artery insufficiency 557.1
  - coronary (chronic) (*see also* Ischemia, heart) 414.9
  - heart (chronic or with a stated duration of over 8 weeks) 414.9
    - acute or with a stated duration of 8 weeks or less (*see also* Infarct, myocardium) 410.9❺
      - without myocardial infarction 411.89
        - with coronary (artery) occlusion 411.81
    - subacute 411.89
  - intestine (transient) 557.9
    - acute 557.0
    - chronic 557.1
    - due to mesenteric artery insufficiency 557.1
  - kidney 593.81
  - labyrinth 386.50
- **Ischemia, ischemic** – *continued*
  - muscles, leg 728.89
  - myocardium, myocardial (chronic or with a stated duration of over 8 weeks) 414.8
    - acute (*see also* Infarct, myocardium) 410.9❺
      - without myocardial infarction 411.89
        - with coronary (artery) occlusion 411.81
  - renal 593.81
  - retina, retinal 362.84
  - small bowel 557.9
    - acute 557.0
    - chronic 557.1
    - due to mesenteric artery insufficiency 557.1
  - spinal cord 336.1
  - subendocardial (*see also* Insufficiency, coronary) 411.89
  - vertebral artery (with transient neurologic deficit) 435.1
- **Ischialgia** (*see also* Sciatica) 724.3
- **Ischiopagus** 759.4
- **Ischium, ischial** – *see* condition
- **Ischomenia** 626.8
- **Ischuria** 788.5
- **Iselin's disease or osteochondrosis** 732.5
- **Islands of**
  - parotid tissue in
    - lymph nodes 750.26
    - neck structures 750.26
  - submaxillary glands in
    - fascia 750.26
    - lymph nodes 750.26
    - neck muscles 750.26
- **Islet cell tumor, pancreas** (M8150/0) 211.7
- **Isoimmunization** NEC (*see also* Incompatibility) 656.2❺
  - anti-E 656.2 ●❺
  - fetus or newborn 773.2
    - ABO blood groups 773.1
    - Rhesus (Rh) factor 773.0
- **Isolation** V07.0
  - social V62.4
- **Isosporosis** 007.2
- **Issue**
  - medical certificate NEC V68.09 ▲
    - cause of death V68.09 ▲
    - disability examination V68.01 ●
    - fitness V68.09 ▲
    - incapacity V68.09 ▲
  - repeat prescription NEC V68.1
    - appliance V68.1
    - contraceptive V25.40
      - device NEC V25.49
        - intrauterine V25.42
        - specified type NEC V25.49
      - pill V25.41
    - glasses V68.1
    - medicinal substance V68.1
- **Itch** (*see also* Pruritus) 698.9
  - bakers' 692.89
  - barbers' 110.0
  - bricklayers' 692.89
  - cheese 133.8
  - clam diggers' 120.3
  - coolie 126.9
  - copra 133.8
  - Cuban 050.1
  - dew 126.9
  - dhobie 110.3
  - eye 379.99
  - filarial (*see also* Infestation, filarial) 125.9
  - grain 133.8
  - grocers' 133.8
  - ground 126.9
  - harvest 133.8
  - jock 110.3
  - Malabar 110.9
    - beard 110.0
    - foot 110.4
    - scalp 110.0
  - meaning scabies 133.0
  - Norwegian 133.0
  - perianal 698.0
  - poultrymen's 133.8
  - sarcoptic 133.0
  - scrub 134.1
  - seven year V61.10
    - meaning scabies 133.0
  - straw 133.8
  - swimmers' 120.3
  - washerwoman's 692.4

Iritis – Itch

Itch – *continued*
  water 120.3
  winter 698.8
Itsenko-Cushing syndrome (pituitary basophilism) 255.0
Ivemark's syndrome (asplenia with congenital heart disease) 759.0
Ivory bones 756.52
Ixodes 134.8
Ixodiasis 134.8

J

Jaccoud's nodular fibrositis, chronic (Jaccoud's syndrome) 714.4
Jackson's
  membrane 751.4
  paralysis or syndrome 344.89
  veil 751.4
Jacksonian
  epilepsy (*see also* Epilepsy) 345.5⑤
  seizures (focal) (*see also* Epilepsy) 345.5⑤
Jacob's ulcer (M8090/3) – *see* Neoplasm, skin, malignant, by site
Jacquet's dermatitis (diaper dermatitis) 691.0
Jadassohn's
  blue nevus (M8780/0) – *see* Neoplasm, skin, benign
  disease (maculopapular erythroderma) 696.2
  intraepidermal epithelioma (M8096/0) – *see* Neoplasm, skin, benign
Jadassohn-Lewandowski syndrome (pachyonychia congenita) 757.5
Jadassohn-Pellizari's disease (anetoderma) 701.3
Jadassohn-Tièche nevus (M8780/0) – *see* Neoplasm, skin, benign
Jaffe-Lichtenstein (-Uehlinger) **syndrome** 252.01
Jahnke's syndrome (encephalocutaneous angiomatosis) 759.6
Jakob-Creutzfeldt disease (syndrome) (new variant) 046.1
  with dementia
    with behavioral disturbance 046.1 *[294.11]*
    without behavioral disturbance 046.1 *[294.10]*
Jaksch (-Luzet) **disease or syndrome** (pseudoleukemia infantum) 285.8
Jamaican
  neuropathy 349.82
  paraplegic tropical ataxic-spastic syndrome 349.82
Janet's disease (psychasthenia) 300.89
Janiceps 759.4
Jansky-Bielschowsky amaurotic familial idiocy 330.1
Japanese
  B-type encephalitis 062.0
  river fever 081.2
  seven-day fever 100.89
Jaundice (yellow) 782.4
  acholuric (familial) (splenomegalic) (*see also* Spherocytosis) 282.0
    acquired 283.9
  breast milk 774.39
  catarrhal (acute) 070.1
    with hepatic coma 070.0
    chronic 571.9
    epidemic – *see* Jaundice, epidemic
  cholestatic (benign) 782.4
  chronic idiopathic 277.4
  epidemic (catarrhal) 070.1
    with hepatic coma 070.0
    leptospiral 100.0
    spirochetal 100.0
  febrile (acute) 070.1
    with hepatic coma 070.0
    leptospiral 100.0
    spirochetal 100.0
  fetus or newborn 774.6
    due to or associated with
      ABO
        antibodies 773.1
        incompatibility, maternal/fetal 773.1
        isoimmunization 773.1
      absence or deficiency of enzyme system for bilirubin conjugation (congenital) 774.39
      blood group incompatibility NEC 773.2

Jaundice – *continued*
  fetus or newborn – *continued*
    due to or associated with – *continued*
      breast milk inhibitors to conjugation 774.39
        associated with preterm delivery 774.2
      bruising 774.1
      Crigler-Najjar syndrome 277.4 *[774.31]*
      delayed conjugation 774.30
        associated with preterm delivery 774.2
        development 774.39
      drugs or toxins transmitted from mother 774.1
      G-6-PD deficiency 282.2 *[774.0]*
      galactosemia 271.1 *[774.5]*
      Gilbert's syndrome 277.4 *[774.31]*
      hepatocellular damage 774.4
      hereditary hemolytic anemia (*see also* Anemia, hemolytic) 282.9 *[774.0]*
      hypothyroidism, congenital 243 *[774.31]*
      incompatibility, maternal/fetal NEC 773.2
      infection 774.1
      inspissated bile syndrome 774.4
      isoimmunization NEC 773.2
      mucoviscidosis 277.01 *[774.5]*
      obliteration of bile duct, congenital 751.61 *[774.5]*
      polycythemia 774.1
      preterm delivery 774.2
      red cell defect 282.9 *[774.0]*
      Rh
        antibodies 773.0
        incompatibility, maternal/fetal 773.0
        isoimmunization 773.0
      spherocytosis (congenital) 282.0 *[774.0]*
      swallowed maternal blood 774.1
    physiological NEC 774.6
  from injection, inoculation, infusion, or transfusion (blood) (plasma) (serum) (other substance) (onset within 8 months after administration) – *see* Hepatitis, viral
  Gilbert's (familial nonhemolytic) 277.4
  hematogenous 283.9
  hemolytic (acquired) 283.9
    congenital (*see also* Spherocytosis) 282.0
  hemorrhagic (acute) 100.0
    leptospiral 100.0
    newborn 776.0
    spirochetal 100.0
  hepatocellular 573.8
  homologous (serum) – *see* Hepatitis, viral
  idiopathic, chronic 277.4
  infectious (acute) (subacute) 070.1
    with hepatic coma 070.0
    leptospiral 100.0
    spirochetal 100.0
  leptospiral 100.0
  malignant (*see also* Necrosis, liver) 570
  newborn (physiological) (*see also* Jaundice, fetus or newborn) 774.6
  nonhemolytic, congenital familial (Gilbert's) 277.4
  nuclear, newborn (*see also* Kernicterus of newborn) 774.7
  obstructive NEC (*see also* Obstruction, biliary) 576.8
  postimmunization – *see* Hepatitis, viral
  posttransfusion – *see* Hepatitis, viral
  regurgitation (*see also* Obstruction, biliary) 576.8
  serum (homologous) (prophylactic) (therapeutic) – *see* Hepatitis, viral
  spirochetal (hemorrhagic) 100.0
  symptomatic 782.4
    newborn 774.6
Jaw – *see* condition
Jaw-blinking 374.43
  congenital 742.8
Jaw-winking phenomenon or syndrome 742.8
Jealousy
  alcoholic 291.5
  childhood 313.3
  sibling 313.3
Jejunitis (*see also* Enteritis) 558.9
Jejunostomy status V44.4
Jejunum, jejunal – *see* condition
Jensen's disease 363.05
Jericho boil 085.1
Jerks, myoclonic 333.2
Jervell-Lange-Nielsen syndrome 426.82
Jeune's disease or syndrome (asphyxiating thoracic dystrophy) 756.4
Jigger disease 134.1

Job's syndrome (chronic granulomatous disease) 288.1
Jod-Basedow phenomenon 242.8⑤
Johnson-Stevens disease (erythema multiforme exudativum) 695.1
Joint – *see also* condition
  Charcôt's 094.0 *[713.5]*
  false 733.82
  flail – *see* Flail, joint
  mice- *see* Loose, body, joint, by site
  sinus to bone 730.9⑤
  von Gies' 095.8
Jordan's anomaly or syndrome 288.2
Josephs-Diamond-Blackfan anemia (congenital hypoplastic) 284.01
Joubert syndrome 759.89
Jumpers' knee 727.2
Jungle yellow fever 060.0
Jungling's disease (sarcoidosis) 135
Junin virus hemorrhagic fever 078.7
Juvenile – *see also* condition
  delinquent 312.9
    group (*see also* Disturbance, conduct) 312.2⑤
    neurotic 312.4

K

Kabuki syndrome 759.89
Kahler (-Bozzolo) **disease** (multiple myeloma) (M9730/3) 203.0⑤
Kakergasia 300.9
Kakke 265.0
Kala-azar (Indian) (infantile) (Mediterranean) (Sudanese) 085.0
Kalischer's syndrome (encephalocutaneous angiomatosis) 759.6
Kallmann's syndrome (hypogonadotropic hypogonadism with anosmia) 253.4
Kanner's syndrome (autism) (*see also* Psychosis, childhood) 299.0⑤
Kaolinosis 502
Kaposi's
  disease 757.33
    lichen ruber 696.4
      acuminatus 696.4
      moniliformis 697.8
    xeroderma pigmentosum 757.33
  sarcoma (M9140/3) 176.9
    adipose tissue 176.1
    aponeurosis 176.1
    artery 176.1
    associated herpesvirus infection 058.89 ●
    blood vessel 176.1
    bursa 176.1
    connective tissue 176.1
    external genitalia 176.8
    fascia 176.1
    fatty tissue 176.1
    fibrous tissue 176.1
    gastrointestinal tract NEC 176.3
    ligament 176.1
    lung 176.4
    lymph
      gland(s) 176.5
      node(s) 176.5
    lymphatic(s) NEC 176.1
    muscle (skeletal) 176.1
    oral cavity NEC 176.8
    palate 176.2
    scrotum 176.8
    skin 176.0
    soft tissue 176.1
    specified site NEC 176.8
    subcutaneous tissue 176.1
    synovia 176.1
    tendon (sheath) 176.1
    vein 176.1
    vessel 176.1
    viscera NEC 176.9
    vulva 176.8
  varicelliform eruption 054.0
    vaccinia 999.0
Kartagener's syndrome or triad (sinusitis, bronchiectasis, situs inversus) 759.3

Kasabach-Merritt syndrome (capillary hemangioma associated with thrombocytopenic purpura) 287.39

Kaschin-Beck disease (endemic polyarthritis) – *see* Disease, Kaschin-Beck

Kast's syndrome (dyschondroplasia with hemangiomas) 756.4

Katatonia – *see* Catatonia ❺

Katayama disease or fever 120.2

Kathisophobia 781.0

Kawasaki disease 446.1

Kayser-Fleischer ring (cornea) (pseudosclerosis) 275.1 *[371.14]*

Kaznelson's syndrome (congenital hypoplastic anemia) 284.01

Kearns-Sayre syndrome 277.87

Kedani fever 081.2

Kelis 701.4

Kelly (-Patterson) **syndrome** (sideropenic dysphagia) 280.8

Keloid, cheloid 701.4
- Addison's (morphea) 701.0
- cornea 371.00
- Hawkins' 701.4
- scar 701.4

Keloma 701.4

Kenya fever 082.1

Keratectasia 371.71
- congenital 743.41

Keratinization NEC
- alveolar ridge mucosa
  - excessive 528.72
  - minimal 528.71

Keratitis (nodular) (nonulcerative) (simple) (zonular) NEC 370.9
- with ulceration (*see also* Ulcer, cornea) 370.00
- actinic 370.24
- arborescens 054.42
- areolar 370.22
- bullosa 370.8
- deep – *see* Keratitis, interstitial
- dendritic(a) 054.42
- desiccation 370.34
- diffuse interstitial 370.52
- disciform(is) 054.43
  - varicella 052.7 *[370.44]*
- epithelialis vernalis 372.13 *[370.32]*
- exposure 370.34
- filamentary 370.23
- gonococcal (congenital) (prenatal) 098.43
- herpes, herpetic (simplex) NEC 054.43
  - zoster 053.21
- hypopyon 370.04
- in
  - chickenpox 052.7 *[370.44]*
  - exanthema (*see also* Exanthem) 057.9 *[370.44]*
  - paravaccinia (*see also* Paravaccinia) 051.9 *[370.44]*
  - smallpox (*see also* Smallpox) 050.9 *[370.44]*
  - vernal conjunctivitis 372.13 *[370.32]*
- interstitial (nonsyphilitic) 370.50
  - with ulcer (*see also* Ulcer, cornea) 370.00
  - diffuse 370.52
  - herpes, herpetic (simplex) 054.43
    - zoster 053.21
  - syphilitic (congenital) (hereditary) 090.3
  - tuberculous (*see also* Tuberculosis) 017.3❺ *[370.59]*
- lagophthalmic 370.34
- macular 370.22
- neuroparalytic 370.35
- neurotrophic 370.35
- nummular 370.22
- oyster-shuckers' 370.8
- parenchymatous – *see* Keratitis, interstitial
- petrificans 370.8
- phlyctenular 370.31
- postmeasles 055.71
- punctata, punctate 370.21
  - leprosa 030.0 *[370.21]*
  - profunda 090.3
  - superficial (Thygeson's) 370.21
- purulent 370.8
- pustuliformis profunda 090.3
- rosacea 695.3 *[370.49]*
- sclerosing 370.54
- specified type NEC 370.8

Keratitis – *continued*
- stellate 370.22
- striate 370.22
- superficial 370.20
  - with conjunctivitis (*see also* Keratoconjunctivitis) 370.40
  - punctate (Thygeson's) 370.21
- suppurative 370.8
- syphilitic (congenital) (prenatal) 090.3
- trachomatous 076.1
  - late effect 139.1
- tuberculous (phlyctenular) (*see also* Tuberculosis) 017.3❺ *[370.31]*
- ulcerated (*see also* Ulcer, cornea) 370.00
- vesicular 370.8
- welders' 370.24
- xerotic (*see also* Keratomalacia) 371.45
  - vitamin A deficiency 264.4

Keratoacanthoma 238.2

Keratocele 371.72

Keratoconjunctivitis (*see also* Keratitis) 370.40
- adenovirus type 8 077.1
- epidemic 077.1
- exposure 370.34
- gonococcal 098.43
- herpetic (simplex) 054.43
  - zoster 053.21
- in
  - chickenpox 052.7 *[370.44]*
  - exanthema (*see also* Exanthem) 057.9 *[370.44]*
  - paravaccinia (*see also* Paravaccinia) 051.9 *[370.44]*
  - smallpox (*see also* Smallpox) 050.9 *[370.44]*
- infectious 077.1
- neurotrophic 370.35
- phlyctenular 370.31
- postmeasles 055.71
- shipyard 077.1
- sicca (Sjögren's syndrome) 710.2
  - not in Sjögren's syndrome 370.33
- specified type NEC 370.49
- tuberculous (phlyctenular) (*see also* Tuberculosis) 017.3❺ *[370.31]*

Keratoconus 371.60
- acute hydrops 371.62
- congenital 743.41
- stable 371.61

Keratocyst (dental) 526.0

Keratoderma, keratodermia (congenital) (palmaris et plantaris) (symmetrical) 757.39
- acquired 701.1
- blennorrhagica 701.1
  - gonococcal 098.81
- climacterium 701.1
- eccentrica 757.39
- gonorrheal 098.81
- punctata 701.1
- tylodes, progressive 701.1

Keratodermatocele 371.72

Keratoglobus 371.70
- congenital 743.41
  - associated with buphthalmos 743.22

Keratohemia 371.12

Keratoiritis (*see also* Iridocyclitis) 364.3
- syphilitic 090.3
- tuberculous (*see also* Tuberculosis) 017.3❺ *[364.11]*

Keratolysis exfoliativa (congenital) 757.39
- acquired 695.89
- neonatorum 757.39

Keratoma 701.1
- congenital 757.39
- malignum congenitale 757.1
- palmaris et plantaris hereditarium 757.39
- senile 702.0

Keratomalacia 371.45
- vitamin A deficiency 264.4

Keratomegaly 743.41

Keratomycosis 111.1
- nigricans (palmaris) 111.1

Keratopathy 371.40
- band (*see also* Keratitis) 371.43
- bullous (*see also* Keratitis) 371.23
- degenerative (*see also* Degeneration, cornea) 371.40
  - hereditary (*see also* Dystrophy, cornea) 371.50
- discrete colliquative 371.49

Keratoscleritis, tuberculous (*see also* Tuberculosis) 017.3❺ *[370.31]*

Keratosis 701.1
- actinic 702.0
- arsenical 692.4
- blennorrhagica 701.1
  - gonococcal 098.81
- congenital (any type) 757.39
- ear (middle) (*see also* Cholesteatoma) 385.30
- female genital (external) 629.89
- follicular, vitamin A deficiency 264.8
- follicularis 757.39
  - acquired 701.1
  - congenital (acneiformis) (Siemens') 757.39
  - spinulosa (decalvans) 757.39
  - vitamin A deficiency 264.8
- gonococcal 098.81
- larynx, laryngeal 478.79
- male genital (external) 608.89
- middle ear (*see also* Cholesteatoma) 385.30
- nigricans 701.2
  - congenital 757.39
- obturans 380.21
- oral epithelium
  - residual ridge mucosa
    - excessive 528.72
    - minimal 528.71
- palmaris et plantaris (symmetrical) 757.39
- penile 607.89
- pharyngeus 478.29
- pilaris 757.39
  - acquired 701.1
- punctata (palmaris et plantaris) 701.1
- scrotal 608.89
- seborrheic 702.19
  - inflamed 702.11
- senilis 702.0
- solar 702.0
- suprafollicularis 757.39
- tonsillaris 478.29
- vagina 623.1
- vegetans 757.39
- vitamin A deficiency 264.8

Kerato-uveitis (*see also* Iridocyclitis) 364.3

Keraunoparalysis 994.0

Kerion (celsi) 110.0

Kernicterus of newborn (not due to isoimmunization) 774.7
- due to isoimmunization (conditions classifiable to 773.0-773.2) 773.4

Ketoacidosis 276.2
- diabetic 250.1❺

Ketonuria 791.6
- branched-chain, intermittent 270.3

Ketosis 276.2
- diabetic 250.1❺

Kidney – *see* condition

Kienböck's
- disease 732.3
  - adult 732.8
- osteochondrosis 732.3

Kimmelstiel (-Wilson) **disease or syndrome** (intercapillary glomerulosclerosis) 250.4❺ *[581.81]*

Kink, kinking
- appendix 543.9
- artery 447.1
- cystic duct, congenital 751.61
- hair (acquired) 704.2
- ileum or intestine (*see also* Obstruction, intestine) 560.9
- Lane's (*see also* Obstruction, intestine) 560.9
- organ or site, congenital NEC – *see* Anomaly, specified type NEC, by site
- ureter (pelvic junction) 593.3
  - congenital 753.20
- vein(s) 459.2
  - caval 459.2
  - peripheral 459.2

Kinnier Wilson's disease (hepatolenticular degeneration) 275.1

Kissing
- osteophytes 721.5
- spine 721.5
- vertebra 721.5

Klauder's syndrome (erythema multiforme exudativum) 695.1

Klebs' disease (*see also* Nephritis) 583.9

Kasabach-Merritt syndrome – Klebs' disease

Klein-Waardenburg syndrome (ptosis - epicanthus) 270.2
Kleine-Levin syndrome 327.13
Kleptomania 312.32
Klinefelter's syndrome 758.7
Klinger's disease 446.4
Klippel's disease 723.8
Klippel-Feil disease or syndrome (brevicollis) 756.16
Klippel-Trenaunay syndrome 759.89
Klumpke (-Déjérine) **palsy, paralysis** (birth) (newborn) 767.6
Klüver-Bucy (-Terzian) **syndrome** 310.0
Knee – *see* condition
Knifegrinders' rot (*see also* Tuberculosis) 011.4❺
Knock-knee (acquired) 736.41
  congenital 755.64
Knot
  intestinal, syndrome (volvulus) 560.2
  umbilical cord (true) 663.2❺
    affecting fetus or newborn 762.5
Knots, surfer 919.8
  infected 919.9
Knotting (of)
  hair 704.2
  intestine 560.2
Knuckle pads (Garrod's) 728.79
Köbner's disease (epidermolysis bullosa) 757.39
Koch's
  infection (*see also* Tuberculosis, pulmonary) 011.9❺
  relapsing fever 087.9
Koch-Weeks conjunctivitis 372.03
Koenig-Wichman disease (pemphigus) 694.4
Köhler's disease (osteochondrosis) 732.5
  first (osteochondrosis juvenilis) 732.5
  second (Freiburg's infarction, metatarsal head) 732.5
  patellar 732.4
  tarsal navicular (bone) (osteoarthosis juvenilis) 732.5
Köhler-Mouchet disease (osteoarthrosis juvenilis) 732.5
Köhler-Pellegrini-Stieda disease or syndrome (calcification, knee joint) 726.62
Koilonychia 703.8
  congenital 757.5
Kojevnikov's, Kojewnikoff's epilepsy (*see also* Epilepsy) 345.7❺
König's
  disease (osteochondritis dissecans) 732.7
  syndrome 564.89
Koniophthisis (*see also* Tuberculosis) 011.4❺
Koplik's spots 055.9
Kopp's asthma 254.8
Korean hemorrhagic fever 078.6
Korsakoff (-Wernicke) **disease, psychosis, or syndrome** (nonalcoholic) 294.0
  alcoholic 291.1
Korsakov's disease – *see* Korsakoff's disease
Korsakow's disease – *see* Korsakoff's disease
Kostmann's disease or syndrome (infantile genetic agranulocytosis) 288.01
Krabbe's
  disease (leukodystrophy) 330.0
  syndrome
    congenital muscle hypoplasia 756.89
    cutaneocerebral angioma 759.6
Kraepelin-Morel disease (*see also* Schizophrenia) 295.9❺
Kraft-Weber-Dimitri disease 759.6
Kraurosis
  ani 569.49
  penis 607.0
  vagina 623.8
  vulva 624.09 ▲
Kreotoxism 005.9
Krukenberg's
  spindle 371.13
  tumor (M8490/6) 198.6
Kufs' disease 330.1
Kugelberg-Welander disease 335.11
Kuhnt-Junius degeneration or disease 362.52
Kulchitsky's cell carcinoma (carcinoid tumor of intestine) 259.2
Kümmell's disease or spondylitis 721.7
Kundrat's disease (lymphosarcoma) 200.1❺
Kunekune – *see* Dermatophytosis
Kunkel syndrome (lupoid hepatitis) 571.49
Kupffer cell sarcoma (M9124/3) 155.0
Kuru 046.0
Kussmaul's
  coma (diabetic) 250.3❺
  disease (polyarteritis nodosa) 446.0
  respiration (air hunger) 786.09
Kwashiorkor (marasmus type) 260
Kyasanur Forest disease 065.2
Kyphoscoliosis, kyphoscoliotic (acquired) (*see also* Scoliosis) 737.30
  congenital 756.19
  due to radiation 737.33
  heart (disease) 416.1
  idiopathic 737.30
    infantile
      progressive 737.32
      resolving 737.31
  late effect of rickets 268.1 *[737.43]*
  specified NEC 737.39
  thoracogenic 737.34
  tuberculous (*see also* Tuberculosis) 015.0❺ *[737.43]*
Kyphosis, kyphotic (acquired) (postural) 737.10
  adolescent postural 737.0
  congenital 756.19
  dorsalis juvenilis 732.0
  due to or associated with
    Charcôt-Marie-Tooth disease 356.1 *[737.41]*
    mucopolysaccharidosis 277.5 *[737.41]*
    neurofibromatosis 237.71 *[737.41]*
    osteitis
      deformans 731.0 *[737.41]*
      fibrosa cystica 252.01 *[737.41]*
    osteoporosis (*see also* Osteoporosis) 733.0❺ *[737.41]*
    poliomyelitis (*see also* Poliomyelitis) 138 *[737.41]*
    radiation 737.11
    tuberculosis (*see also* Tuberculosis) 015.0❺ *[737.41]*
  Kümmell's 721.7
  late effect of rickets 268.1 *[737.41]*
  Morquio-Brailsford type (spinal) 277.5 *[737.41]*
  pelvis 738.6
  postlaminectomy 737.12
  specified cause NEC 737.19
  syphilitic, congenital 090.5 *[737.41]*
  tuberculous (*see also* Tuberculosis) 015.0❺ *[737.41]*
Kyrle's disease (hyperkeratosis follicularis in cutem penetrans) 701.1

L

Labia, labium – *see* condition
Labiated hymen 752.49
Labile
  blood pressure 796.2
  emotions, emotionality 301.3
  vasomotor system 443.9
Labioglossal paralysis 335.22
Labium leporinum (*see also* Cleft, lip) 749.10
Labor (*see also* Delivery)
  with complications – *see* Delivery, complicated
  abnormal NEC 661.9❺
    affecting fetus or newborn 763.7
  arrested active phase 661.1❺
    affecting fetus or newborn 763.7
  desultory 661.2❺
    affecting fetus or newborn 763.7
  dyscoordinate 661.4❺
    affecting fetus or newborn 763.7
  early onset (22-36 weeks gestation) 644.2❺
  failed
    induction 659.1❺
      mechanical 659.0❺
      medical 659.1❺
      surgical 659.0❺
    trial (vaginal delivery) 660.6❺
  false 644.1❺
  forced or induced, affecting fetus or newborn 763.89
Labor – *continued*
  hypertonic 661.4❺
    affecting fetus or newborn 763.7
  hypotonic 661.2❺
    affecting fetus or newborn 763.7
    primary 661.0❺
      affecting fetus or newborn 763.7
    secondary 661.1❺
      affecting fetus or newborn 763.7
  incoordinate 661.4❺
    affecting fetus or newborn 763.7
  irregular 661.2❺
    affecting fetus or newborn 763.7
  long – *see* Labor, prolonged
  missed (at or near term) 656.4❺
  obstructed NEC 660.9❺
    affecting fetus or newborn 763.1
    due to female genital mutilation 660.8❺
    specified cause NEC 660.8❺
      affecting fetus or newborn 763.1
  pains, spurious 644.1❺
  precipitate 661.3❺
    affecting fetus or newborn 763.6
  premature 644.2❺
    threatened 644.0❺
  prolonged or protracted 662.1❺
    affecting fetus or newborn 763.89
    first stage 662.0❺
      affecting fetus or newborn 763.89
    second stage 662.2❺
      affecting fetus or newborn 763.89
  threatened NEC 644.1❺
  undelivered 644.1❺
Labored breathing (*see also* Hyperventilation) 786.09
Labyrinthitis (inner ear) (destructive) (latent) 386.30
  circumscribed 386.32
  diffuse 386.31
  focal 386.32
  purulent 386.33
  serous 386.31
  suppurative 386.33
  syphilitic 095.8
  toxic 386.34
  viral 386.35
Laceration – *see also* Wound, open, by site
  accidental, complicating surgery 998.2
  Achilles tendon 845.09
    with open wound 892.2
  anus (sphincter) 879.6
    with
      abortion – *see* Abortion, by type, with damage to pelvic organs
      ectopic pregnancy (*see also* categories 633.0-633.9) 639.2
      molar pregnancy (*see also* categories 630-632) 639.2
    complicated 879.7
    complicating delivery ▶(healed) (old)◀ 654.8❺ ▲
      with laceration of anal or rectal mucosa 664.3❺
      not associated with third-degree perineal laceration 664.6❺ ●
    following
      abortion 639.2
      ectopic or molar pregnancy 639.2
    nontraumatic, nonpuerperal ▶(healed) (old)◀ 569.43 ▲
  bladder (urinary)
    with
      abortion – *see* Abortion, by type, with damage to pelvic organs
      ectopic pregnancy (*see also* categories 633.0-633.9) 639.2
      molar pregnancy (*see also* categories 630-632) 639.2
    following
      abortion 639.2
      ectopic or molar pregnancy 639.2
    obstetrical trauma 665.5❺
  blood vessel – *see* Injury, blood vessel, by site
  bowel
    with
      abortion – *see* Abortion, by type, with damage to pelvic organs
      ectopic pregnancy (*see also* categories 633.0-633.9) 639.2
      molar pregnancy (*see also* categories 630-632) 639.2

Klein-Waardenburg syndrome – Laceration

Laceration – *continued*
  bowel – *continued*
    following
      abortion 639.2
      ectopic or molar pregnancy 639.2
    obstetrical trauma 665.5❺
  brain (cerebral) (membrane) (with hemorrhage)
      851.8❺

Note – Use the following fifth-digit subclassification with categories 851-854:

0	*unspecified state of consciousness*
1	*with no loss of consciousness*
2	*with brief [less than one hour] loss of consciousness*
3	*with moderate [1-24 hours] loss of consciousness*
4	*with prolonged [more than 24 hours] loss of consciousness and return to pre-existing conscious level*
5	*with prolonged [more than 24 hours] loss of consciousness, without return to pre-existing conscious level*

Use fifth-digit 5 to designate when a patient is unconscious and dies before regaining consciousness, regardless of the duration of the loss of consciousness

6	*with loss of consciousness of unspecified duration*
9	*with concussion, unspecified*

    with
      open intracranial wound 851.9❺
      skull fracture – *see* Fracture, skull, by site
    cerebellum 851.6❺
      with open intracranial wound 851.7❺
    cortex 851.2❺
      with open intracranial wound 851.3❺
    during birth 767.0
    stem 851.6❺
      with open intracranial wound 851.7❺
  broad ligament
    with
      abortion – *see* Abortion, by type, with damage to pelvic organs
      ectopic pregnancy (*see also* categories 633.0-633.9) 639.2
      molar pregnancy (*see also* categories 630-632) 639.2
    following
      abortion 639.2
      ectopic or molar pregnancy 639.2
    nontraumatic 620.6
    obstetrical trauma 665.6❺
    syndrome (nontraumatic) 620.6
  capsule, joint – *see* Sprain, by site
  cardiac – *see* Laceration, heart
  causing eversion of cervix uteri (old) 622.0
  central, complicating delivery 664.4❺
  cerebellum – *see* Laceration, brain, cerebellum
  cerebral – *see also* Laceration, brain
    during birth 767.0
  cervix (uteri)
    with
      abortion – *see* Abortion, by type, with damage to pelvic organs
      ectopic pregnancy (*see also* categories 633.0-633.9) 639.2
      molar pregnancy (*see also* categories 630-632) 639.2
    following
      abortion 639.2
      ectopic or molar pregnancy 639.2
    nonpuerperal, nontraumatic 622.3
    obstetrical trauma (current) 665.3❺
    old (postpartal) 622.3
    traumatic – *see* Injury, internal, cervix
  chordae heart 429.5
  complicated 879.9
  cornea – *see* Laceration, eyeball
    superficial 918.1
  cortex (cerebral) – *see* Laceration, brain, cortex
  esophagus 530.89
  eye(s) – *see* Laceration, ocular
  eyeball NEC 871.4
    with prolapse or exposure of intraocular tissue 871.1
    penetrating – *see* Penetrating wound, eyeball
    specified as without prolapse of intraocular tissue 871.0
  eyelid NEC 870.8
    full thickness 870.1
      involving lacrimal passages 870.2

Laceration – *continued*
  eyelid – *continued*
    skin (and periocular area) 870.0
      penetrating – *see* Penetrating wound, orbit
  fourchette
    with
      abortion – *see* Abortion, by type, with damage to pelvic organs
      ectopic pregnancy (*see also* categories 633.0-633.9) 639.2
      molar pregnancy (*see also* categories 630-632) 639.2
    complicating delivery 664.0❺
    following
      abortion 639.2
      ectopic or molar pregnancy 639.2
  heart (without penetration of heart chambers) 861.02
    with
      open wound into thorax 861.12
      penetration of heart chambers 861.03
        with open wound into thorax 861.13
  hernial sac – *see* Hernia, by site
  internal organ (abdomen) (chest) (pelvis) NEC – *see* Injury, internal, by site
  kidney (parenchyma) 866.02
    with
      complete disruption of parenchyma (rupture) 866.03
        with open wound into cavity 866.13
      open wound into cavity 866.12
  labia
    complicating delivery 664.0❺
  ligament – *see also* Sprain, by site
    with open wound – *see* Wound, open, by site
  liver 864.05
    with open wound into cavity 864.15
    major (disruption of hepatic parenchyma) 864.04
      with open wound into cavity 864.14
    minor (capsule only) 864.02
      with open wound into cavity 864.12
    moderate (involving parenchyma without major disruption) 864.03
      with open wound into cavity 864.13
      multiple 864.04
        with open wound into cavity 864.14
    stellate 864.04
      with open wound into cavity 864.14
  lung 861.22
    with open wound into thorax 861.32
  meninges – *see* Laceration, brain
  meniscus (knee) (*see also* Tear, meniscus) 836.2
    old 717.5
    site other than knee – *see also* Sprain, by site
      old NEC (*see also* Disorder, cartilage, articular) 718.0❺
  muscle – *see also* Sprain, by site
    with open wound – *see* Wound, open, by site
  myocardium – *see* Laceration, heart
  nerve – *see* Injury, nerve, by site
  ocular NEC (*see also* Laceration, eyeball) 871.4
    adnexa NEC 870.8
      penetrating 870.3
        with foreign body 870.4
  orbit (eye) 870.8
    penetrating 870.3
      with foreign body 870.4
  pelvic
    floor (muscles)
      with
        abortion – *see* Abortion, by type, with damage to pelvic organs
        ectopic pregnancy (*see also* categories 633.0-633.9) 639.2
        molar pregnancy (*see also* categories 630-632) 639.2
      complicating delivery 664.1❺
      following
        abortion 639.2
        ectopic or molar pregnancy 639.2
      nonpuerperal 618.7
      old (postpartal) 618.7
    organ NEC
      with
        abortion – *see* Abortion, by type, with damage to pelvic organs
        ectopic pregnancy (*see also* categories 633.0-633.9) 639.2
        molar pregnancy (*see also* categories 630-632) 639.2

Laceration – *continued*
  pelvic – *continued*
    organ – *continued*
      complicating delivery 665.5❺
        affecting fetus or newborn 763.89
      following
        abortion 639.2
        ectopic or molar pregnancy 639.2
      obstetrical trauma 665.5❺
  perineum, perineal (old) (postpartal) 618.7
    with
      abortion – *see* Abortion, by type, with damage to pelvic floor
      ectopic pregnancy (*see also* categories 633.0-633.9) 639.2
      molar pregnancy (*see also* categories 630-632) 639.2
    complicating delivery 664.4❺
      first degree 664.0❺
      second degree 664.1❺
      third degree 664.2❺
      fourth degree 664.3❺
      central 664.4❺
      involving
        anal sphincter ▶(healed) (old)◀ 654.8❺▲
          not associated with third-degree perineal laceration 664.6❺●
        fourchette 664.0❺
        hymen 664.0❺
        labia 664.0❺
        pelvic floor 664.1❺
        perineal muscles 664.1❺
        rectovaginal with septum 664.2❺
          with anal mucosa 664.3❺
        skin 664.0❺
        sphincter (anal) ▶(healed) (old)◀ 654.8❺▲
          with anal mucosa 664.3❺
          not associated with third-degree perineal laceration 664.6❺●
        vagina 664.0❺
        vaginal muscles 664.1❺
        vulva 664.0❺
      secondary 674.2❺
    following
      abortion 639.2
      ectopic or molar pregnancy 639.2
    male 879.6
      complicated 879.7
    muscles, complicating delivery 664.1❺
    nonpuerperal, current injury 879.6
      complicated 879.7
    secondary (postpartal) 674.2❺
  peritoneum
    with
      abortion – *see* Abortion, by type, with damage to pelvic organs
      ectopic pregnancy (*see also* categories 633.0-633.9) 639.2
      molar pregnancy (*see also* categories 630-632) 639.2
    following
      abortion 639.2
      ectopic or molar pregnancy 639.2
    obstetrical trauma 665.5❺
  periurethral tissue
    with
      abortion – *see* Abortion, by type, with damage to pelvic organs
      ectopic pregnancy (*see also* categories 633.0-633.9) 639.2
      molar pregnancy (*see also* categories 630-632) 639.2
    following
      abortion 639.2
      ectopic or molar pregnancy 639.2
    obstetrical trauma 665.5❺
  rectovaginal (septum)
    with
      abortion – *see* Abortion, by type, with damage to pelvic organs
      ectopic pregnancy (*see also* categories 633.0-633.9) 639.2
      molar pregnancy (*see also* categories 630-632) 639.2
    complicating delivery 665.4❺
      with perineum 664.2❺
        involving anal or rectal mucosa 664.3❺
    following
      abortion 639.2
      ectopic or molar pregnancy 639.2

Laceration – *continued*
  rectovaginal (septum) – *continued*
    nonpuerperal 623.4
    old (postpartal) 623.4
  spinal cord (meninges) – *see also* Injury, spinal, by site
    due to injury at birth 767.4
    fetus or newborn 767.4
  spleen 865.09
    with
      disruption of parenchyma (massive) 865.04
        with open wound into cavity 865.14
      open wound into cavity 865.19
    capsule (without disruption of parenchyma) 865.02
      with open wound into cavity 865.12
    parenchyma 865.03
      with open wound into cavity 865.13
      massive disruption (rupture) 865.04
        with open wound into cavity 865.14
  tendon 848.9
    with open wound – *see* Wound, open, by site
    Achilles 845.09
      with open wound 892.2
    lower limb NEC 844.9
      with open wound NEC 894.2
    upper limb NEC 840.9
      with open wound NEC 884.2
  tentorium cerebelli – *see* Laceration, brain, cerebellum
  tongue 873.64
    complicated 873.74
  urethra
    with
      abortion – *see* Abortion, by type, with damage to pelvic organs
      ectopic pregnancy (*see also* categories 633.0-633.9) 639.2
      molar pregnancy (*see also* categories 630-632) 639.2
    following
      abortion 639.2
      ectopic or molar pregnancy 639.2
    nonpuerperal, nontraumatic 599.84
    obstetrical trauma 665.5❺
  uterus
    with
      abortion – *see* Abortion, by type, with damage to pelvic organs
      ectopic pregnancy (*see also* categories 633.0-633.9) 639.2
      molar pregnancy (*see also* categories 630-632) 639.2
    following
      abortion 639.2
      ectopic or molar pregnancy 639.2
    nonpuerperal, nontraumatic 621.8
    obstetrical trauma NEC 665.5❺
    old (postpartal) 621.8
  vagina
    with
      abortion – *see* Abortion, by type, with damage to pelvic organs
      ectopic pregnancy (*see also* categories 633.0-633.9) 639.2
      molar pregnancy (*see also* categories 630-632) 639.2
      perineal involvement, complicating delivery 664.0❺
    complicating delivery 665.4❺
      first degree 664.0❺
      second degree 664.1❺
      third degree 664.2❺
      fourth degree 664.3❺
      high 665.4❺
      muscles 664.1❺
      sulcus 665.4❺
      wall 665.4❺
    following
      abortion 639.2
      ectopic or molar pregnancy 639.2
    nonpuerperal, nontraumatic 623.4
    old (postpartal) 623.4
  valve, heart – *see* Endocarditis
  vulva
    with
      abortion – *see* Abortion, by type, with damage to pelvic organs
      ectopic pregnancy (*see also* categories 633.0-633.9) 639.2
      molar pregnancy (*see also* categories 630-632) 639.2

Laceration – *continued*
  vulva – *continued*
    complicating delivery 664.0❺
    following
      abortion 639.2
      ectopic or molar pregnancy 639.2
    nonpuerperal, nontraumatic 624.4
    old (postpartal) 624.4
Lachrymal – *see* condition
Lachrymonasal duct – *see* condition
Lack of
  adequate intermaxillary vertical dimension 524.36
  appetite (*see also* Anorexia) 783.0
  care
    in home V60.4
    of adult 995.84
    of infant (at or after birth) 995.52
  coordination 781.3
  development – *see also* Hypoplasia
    physiological in childhood 783.40
  education V62.3
  energy 780.79
  financial resources V60.2
  food 994.2
    in environment V60.8
  growth in childhood 783.43
  heating V60.1
  housing (permanent) (temporary) V60.0
    adequate V60.1
  material resources V60.2
  medical attention 799.89
  memory (*see also* Amnesia) 780.93
    mild, following organic brain damage 310.1
  ovulation 628.0
  person able to render necessary care V60.4
  physical exercise V69.0
  physiologic development in childhood 783.40
  posterior occlusal support 524.57
  prenatal care in current pregnancy V23.7
  shelter V60.0
  sleep V69.4
  water 994.3
Lacrimal – *see* condition
Lacrimation, abnormal (*see also* Epiphora) 375.20
Lacrimonasal duct – *see* condition
Lactation, lactating (breast) (puerperal) (postpartum)
  defective 676.4❺
  disorder 676.9❺
    specified type NEC 676.8❺
  excessive 676.6❺
  failed 676.4❺
  mastitis NEC 675.2❺
  mother (care and/or examination) V24.1
  nonpuerperal 611.6
  suppressed 676.5❺
Lacticemia 271.3
  excessive 276.2
Lactosuria 271.3
Lacunar skull 756.0
Laennec's cirrhosis (alcoholic) 571.2
  nonalcoholic 571.5
Lafora's disease 333.2
Lag, lid (nervous) 374.41
Lagleyze-von Hippel disease (retinocerebral angiomatosis) 759.6
Lagophthalmos (eyelid) (nervous) 374.20
  cicatricial 374.23
  keratitis (*see also* Keratitis) 370.34
  mechanical 374.22
  paralytic 374.21
La grippe – *see* Influenza
Lahore sore 085.1
Lakes, venous (cerebral) 437.8
Laki-Lorand factor deficiency (*see also* Defect, coagulation) 286.3
Lalling 307.9
Lambliasis 007.1
Lame back 724.5
Lancereaux's diabetes (diabetes mellitus with marked emaciation) 250.8❺ *[261]*
Landouzy-Déjérine dystrophy (fascioscapulohumeral atrophy) 359.1
Landry's disease or paralysis 357.0
Landry-Guillain-Barré syndrome 357.0
Lane's
  band 751.4

Lane's – *continued*
  disease 569.89
  kink (*see also* Obstruction, intestine) 560.9
Langdon Down's syndrome (mongolism) 758.0
Language abolition 784.69
Lanugo (persistent) 757.4
Laparoscopic surgical procedure converted to open procedure V64.41
Lardaceous
  degeneration (any site) 277.39
  disease 277.39
  kidney 277.39 *[583.81]*
  liver 277.39
Large
  baby (regardless of gestational age) 766.1
    exceptionally (weight of 4500 grams or more) 766.0
    of diabetic mother 775.0
  ear 744.22
  fetus – *see also* Oversize, fetus
    causing disproportion 653.5❺
      with obstructed labor 660.1❺
  for dates
    fetus or newborn (regardless of gestational age) 766.1
      affecting management of pregnancy 656.6❺
      exceptionally (weight of 4500 grams or more) 766.0
  physiological cup 743.57
  stature 783.9
  waxy liver 277.39
  white kidney – *see* Nephrosis
Larsen's syndrome (flattened facies and multiple congenital dislocations) 755.8
Larsen-Johansson disease (juvenile osteopathia patellae) 732.4
Larva migrans
  cutaneous NEC 126.9
    ancylostoma 126.9
  of Diptera in vitreous 128.0
  visceral NEC 128.0
Laryngeal – *see also* condition
  syncope 786.2
Laryngismus (acute) (infectious) (stridulous) 478.75
  congenital 748.3
  diphtheritic 032.3
Laryngitis (acute) (edematous) (fibrinous) (gangrenous) (infective) (infiltrative) (malignant) (membranous) (phlegmonous) (pneumococcal) (pseudomembranous) (septic) (subglottic) (suppurative) (ulcerative) (viral) 464.00
  with
    influenza, flu, or grippe 487.1
    obstruction 464.01
    tracheitis (*see also* Laryngotracheitis) 464.20
      with obstruction 464.21
      acute 464.20
        with obstruction 464.21
      chronic 476.1
  atrophic 476.0
  Borrelia vincentii 101
  catarrhal 476.0
  chronic 476.0
    with tracheitis (chronic) 476.1
    due to external agent – *see* Condition, respiratory, chronic, due to
  diphtheritic (membranous) 032.3
  due to external agent – *see* Inflammation, respiratory, upper, due to
  H. influenzae 464.00
    with obstruction 464.01
  Hemophilus influenzae 464.00
    with obstruction 464.01
  hypertrophic 476.0
  influenzal 487.1
  pachydermic 478.79
  sicca 476.0
  spasmodic 478.75
    acute 464.00
      with obstruction 464.01
  streptococcal 034.0
  stridulous 478.75
  syphilitic 095.8
    congenital 090.5
  tuberculous (*see also* Tuberculosis, larynx) 012.3❺
  Vincent's 101
Laryngocele (congenital) (ventricular) 748.3
Laryngofissure 478.79
  congenital 748.3

Laryngomalacia (congenital) 748.3
Laryngopharyngitis (acute) 465.0
chronic 478.9
due to external agent – *see* Condition, respiratory, chronic, due to
due to external agent – *see* Inflammation, respiratory, upper, due to
septic 034.0
Laryngoplegia (*see also* Paralysis, vocal cord) 478.30
Laryngoptosis 478.79
Laryngospasm 478.75
due to external agent – *see* Condition, respiratory, acute, due to
Laryngostenosis 478.74
congenital 748.3
Laryngotracheitis (acute) (infectional) (viral) (*see also* Laryngitis) 464.20
with obstruction 464.21
atrophic 476.1
Borrelia vincenti 101
catarrhal 476.1
chronic 476.1
due to external agent – *see* Condition, respiratory, chronic, due to
diphtheritic (membranous) 032.3
due to external agent – *see* Inflammation, respiratory, upper, due to
H. influenzae 464.20
with obstruction 464.21
hypertrophic 476.1
influenzal 487.1
pachydermic 478.75
sicca 476.1
spasmodic 478.75
acute 464.20
with obstruction 464.21
streptococcal 034.0
stridulous 478.75
syphilitic 095.8
congenital 090.5
tuberculous (*see also* Tuberculosis, larynx) 012.3❺
Vincent's 101
Laryngotracheobronchitis (*see also* Bronchitis) 490
acute 466.0
chronic 491.8
viral 466.0
Laryngotracheobronchopneumonitis – *see* Pneumonia, broncho-
Larynx, laryngeal – *see* condition
Lasègue's disease (persecution mania) 297.9
Lassa fever 078.89
Lassitude (*see also* Weakness) 780.79
Late – *see also* condition
effect(s) (of) – *see also* condition
abscess
intracranial or intraspinal (conditions classifiable to 324) – *see* category 326
adverse effect of drug, medicinal or biological substance 909.5
allergic reaction 909.9
amputation
postoperative (late) 997.60
traumatic (injury classifiable to 885-887 and 895-897) 905.9
burn (injury classifiable to 948-949) 906.9
extremities NEC (injury classifiable to 943 or 945) 906.7
hand or wrist (injury classifiable to 944) 906.6
eye (injury classifiable to 940) 906.5
face, head, and neck (injury classifiable to 941) 906.5
specified site NEC (injury classifiable to 942 and 946-947) 906.8
cerebrovascular disease (conditions classifiable to 430-437) 438.9
with
alterations of sensations 438.6
aphasia 438.11
apraxia 438.81
ataxia 438.84
cognitive deficits 438.0
disturbances of vision 438.7
dysphagia 438.82
dysphasia 438.12

Late – *continued*
effect – *continued*
cerebrovascular disease – *continued*
with – *continued*
facial droop 438.83
facial weakness 438.83
hemiplegia/hemiparesis
affecting
dominant side 438.21
nondomiant side 438.22
unspecified side 438.20
monoplegia of lower limb
affecting
dominant side 438.41
nondominant side 438.42
unspecified side 438.40
monoplegia of upper limb
affecting
dominant side 438.31
nondominant side 438.32
unspecified side 438.30
paralytic syndrome NEC
affecting
bilateral 438.53
dominant side 438.51
nondominant side 438.52
unspecified side 438.50
speech and language deficit 438.10
specified type NEC 438.19
vertigo 438.85
specified type NEC 438.89
childbirth complication(s) 677
complication(s) of
childbirth 677
delivery 677
pregnancy 677
puerperium 677
surgical and medical care (conditions classifiable to 996-999) 909.3
trauma (conditions classifiable to 958) 908.6
contusion (injury classifiable to 920-924) 906.3
crushing (injury classifiable to 925-929) 906.4
delivery complication(s) 677
dislocation (injury classifiable to 830-839) 905.6
encephalitis or encephalomyelitis (conditions classifiable to 323) – *see* category 326
in infectious diseases 139.8
viral (conditions classifiable to 049.8, 049.9, 062-064) 139.0
external cause NEC (conditions classifiable to 995) 909.9
certain conditions classifiable to categories 991-994 909.4
foreign body in orifice (injury classifiable to 930-939) 908.5
fracture (multiple) (injury classifiable to 828-829) 905.5
extremity
lower (injury classifiable to 821-827) 905.4
neck of femur (injury classifiable to 820) 905.3
upper (injury classifiable to 810-819) 905.2
face and skull (injury classifiable to 800-804) 905.0
skull and face (injury classifiable to 800-804) 905.0
spine and trunk (injury classifiable to 805 and 807-809) 905.1
with spinal cord lesion (injury classifiable to 806) 907.2
infection
pyogenic, intracranial – *see* category 326
infectious diseases (conditions classifiable to 001-136) NEC 139.8
injury (injury classifiable to 959) 908.9
blood vessel 908.3
abdomen and pelvis (injury classifiable to 902) 908.4
extremity (injury classifiable to 903-904) 908.3
head and neck (injury classifiable to 900) 908.3
intracranial (injury classifiable to 850-854) 907.0
with skull fracture 905.0
thorax (injury classifiable to 901) 908.4

Late – *continued*
effect – *continued*
injury – *continued*
internal organ NEC (injury classifiable to 867 and 869) 908.2
abdomen (injury classifiable to 863-866 and 868) 908.1
thorax (injury classifiable to 860-862) 908.0
intracranial (injury classifiable to 850-854) 907.0
with skull fracture (injury classifiable to 800-801 and 803-804) 905.0
nerve NEC (injury classifiable to 957) 907.9
cranial (injury classifiable to 950-951) 907.1
peripheral NEC (injury classifiable to 957) 907.9
lower limb and pelvic girdle (injury classifiable to 956) 907.5
upper limb and shoulder girdle (injury classifiable to 955) 907.4
roots and plexus(es), spinal (injury classifiable to 953) 907.3
trunk (injury classifiable to 954) 907.3
spinal
cord (injury classifiable to 806 and 952) 907.2
nerve root(s) and plexus(es) (injury classifiable to 953) 907.3
superficial (injury classifiable to 910-919) 906.2
tendon (tendon injury classifiable to 840-848, 880-884 with .2, and 890-894 with .2) 905.8
meningitis
bacterial (conditions classifiable to 320) – *see* category 326
unspecified cause (conditions classifiable to 322) – *see* category 326
myelitis (*see also* Late, effect(s) (of), encephalitis) – *see* category 326
parasitic diseases (conditions classifiable to 001-136 NEC) 139.8
phlebitis or thrombophlebitis of intracranial venous sinuses (conditions classifiable to 325) – *see* category 326
poisoning due to drug, medicinal or biological substance (conditions classifiable to 960-979) 909.0
poliomyelitis, acute (conditions classifiable to 045) 138
pregnancy complication(s) 677
puerperal complication(s) 677
radiation (conditions classifiable to 990) 909.2
rickets 268.1
sprain and strain without mention of tendon injury (injury classifiable to 840-848, except tendon injury) 905.7
tendon involvement 905.8
toxic effect of
drug, medicinal or biological substance (conditions classifiable to 960-979) 909.0
nonmedical substance (conditions classifiable to 980-989) 909.1
trachoma (conditions classifiable to 076) 139.1
tuberculosis 137.0
bones and joints (conditions classifiable to 015) 137.3
central nervous system (conditions classifiable to 013) 137.1
genitourinary (conditions classifiable to 016) 137.2
pulmonary (conditions classifiable to 010-012) 137.0
specified organs NEC (conditions classifiable to 014, 017-018) 137.4
viral encephalitis (conditions classifiable to 049.8, 049.9, 062-064) 139.0
wound, open
extremity (injury classifiable to 880-884 and 890-894, except .2) 906.1
tendon (injury classifiable to 880-884 with .2 and 890-894 with .2) 905.8
head, neck, and trunk (injury classifiable to 870-879) 906.0
infant
post-term (gestation period over 40 completed weeks to 42 completed weeks) 766.21
prolonged gestation (period over 42 completed weeks) 766.22

Latent – *see* condition
Lateral – *see* condition
Laterocession – *see* Lateroversion
Lateroflexion – *see* Lateroversion
Lateroversion
cervix – *see* Lateroversion, uterus
uterus, uterine (cervix) (postinfectional) (postpartal, old) 621.6
congenital 752.3
in pregnancy or childbirth 654.4❺
affecting fetus or newborn 763.89
Lathyrism 988.2
Launois' syndrome (pituitary gigantism) 253.0
Launois-Bensaude's lipomatosis 272.8
Launois-Cleret syndrome (adiposogenital dystrophy) 253.8
Laurence-Moon-Biedl syndrome (obesity, polydactyly, and mental retardation) 759.89
LAV (disease) (illness) (infection) – *see* Human immunodeficiency virus (disease) (illness) (infection)
LAV/HTLV-III (disease) (illness) (infection) – *see* Human immunodeficiency virus (disease) (illness) (infection)
Lawford's syndrome (encephalocutaneous angiomatosis) 759.6
Lax, laxity – *see also* Relaxation
ligament 728.4
skin (acquired) 701.8
congenital 756.83
Laxative habit (*see also* Abuse, drugs, nondependent) 305.9❺
Lazy leukocyte syndrome 288.09
LCAD (long chain/very long chain acyl CoA dehydrogenase deficiency, VLCAD) 277.85
LCHAD (long chain 3-hydroxyacyl CoA dehydrogenase deficiency) 277.85
Lead – *see also* condition
exposure to V15.86
incrustation of cornea 371.15
poisoning 984.9
specified type of lead – *see* Table of Drugs and Chemicals
Lead miners' lung 503
Leakage
amniotic fluid 658.1❺
with delayed delivery 658.2❺
affecting fetus or newborn 761.1
bile from drainage tube (T tube) 997.4
blood (microscopic), fetal, into maternal circulation 656.0❺
affecting management of pregnancy or puerperium 656.0❺
device, implant, or graft – *see* Complications, mechanical
spinal fluid at lumbar puncture site 997.09
urine, continuous 788.37
Leaky heart – *see* Endocarditis
Learning defect, specific NEC (strephosymbolia) 315.2
Leather bottle stomach (M8142/3) 151.9
Leber's
congenital amaurosis 362.76
optic atrophy (hereditary) 377.16
Lederer's anemia or disease (acquired infectious hemolytic anemia) 283.19
Lederer-Brill syndrome (acquired infectious hemolytic anemia) 283.19
Leeches (aquatic) (land) 134.2
Left-sided neglect 781.8
Leg – *see* condition
Legal investigation V62.5
Legg (-Calvé)-**Perthes disease or syndrome** (osteochondrosis, femoral capital) 732.1
Legionnaires' disease 482.84
Leigh's disease 330.8
Leiner's disease (exfoliative dermatitis) 695.89
Leiofibromyoma (M8890/0) – *see also* Leiomyoma
uterus (cervix) (corpus) (*see also* Leiomyoma, uterus) 218.9
Leiomyoblastoma (M8891/1) – *see* Neoplasm, connective tissue, uncertain behavior
Leiomyofibroma (M8890/0) – *see also* Neoplasm, connective tissue, benign
uterus (cervix) (corpus) (*see also* Leiomyoma, uterus) 218.9
Leiomyoma (M8890/0) – *see also* Neoplasm, connective tissue, benign
bizarre (M8893/0) – *see* Neoplasm, connective tissue, benign
cellular (M8892/1) – *see* Neoplasm, connective tissue, uncertain behavior
epithelioid (M8891/1) – *see* Neoplasm, connective tissue, uncertain behavior
prostate (polypoid) 600.20
with
other lower urinary tract symptoms (LUTS) 600.21
urinary
obstruction 600.21
retention 600.21
uterus (cervix) (corpus) 218.9
interstitial 218.1
intramural 218.1
submucous 218.0
subperitoneal 218.2
subserous 218.2
vascular (M8894/0) – *see* Neoplasm, connective tissue, benign
Leiomyomatosis (intravascular) (M8890/1) – *see* Neoplasm, connective tissue, uncertain behavior
Leiomyosarcoma (M8890/3) – *see also* Neoplasm, connective tissue, malignant
epithelioid (M8891/3) – *see* Neoplasm, connective tissue, malignant
Leishmaniasis 085.9
American 085.5
cutaneous 085.4
mucocutaneous 085.5
Asian desert 085.2
Brazilian 085.5
cutaneous 085.9
acute necrotizing 085.2
American 085.4
Asian desert 085.2
diffuse 085.3
dry form 085.1
Ethiopian 085.3
eyelid 085.5 *[373.6]*
late 085.1
lepromatous 085.3
recurrent 085.1
rural 085.2
ulcerating 085.1
urban 085.1
wet form 085.2
zoonotic form 085.2
dermal – *see also* Leishmaniasis, cutaneous
post kala-azar 085.0
eyelid 085.5 *[373.6]*
infantile 085.0
Mediterranean 085.0
mucocutaneous (American) 085.5
naso-oral 085.5
nasopharyngeal 085.5
Old World 085.1
tegumentaria diffusa 085.4
vaccination, prophylactic (against) V05.2
visceral (Indian) 085.0
Leishmanoid, dermal – *see also* Leishmaniasis, cutaneous
post kala-azar 085.0
Leloir's disease 695.4
Lemiere syndrome 451.89
Lenegre's disease 426.0
Lengthening, leg 736.81
Lennox-Gastaut syndrome 345.0❺
with tonic seizures 345.1
Lennox's syndrome (*see also* Epilepsy) 345.0❺
Lens – *see* condition
Lenticonus (anterior) (posterior) (congenital) 743.36
Lenticular degeneration, progressive 275.1
Lentiglobus (posterior) (congenital) 743.36
Lentigo (congenital) 709.09
juvenile 709.09
Maligna (M8742/2) – *see also* Neoplasm, skin, in situ
melanoma (M8742/3) – *see* Melanoma
senile 709.09
Leonine leprosy 030.0
Leontiasis
ossium 733.3
syphilitic 095.8
congenital 090.5
Léopold-Lévi's syndrome (paroxysmal thyroid instability) 242.9❺
Lepore hemoglobin syndrome 282.49
Lepothrix 039.0
Lepra 030.9
Willan's 696.1
Leprechaunism 259.8
Lepromatous leprosy 030.0
Leprosy 030.9
anesthetic 030.1
beriberi 030.1
borderline (group B) (infiltrated) (neuritic) 030.3
cornea (*see also* Leprosy, by type) 030.9 *[371.89]*
dimorphous (group B) (infiltrated) (lepromatous) (neuritic) (tuberculoid) 030.3
eyelid 030.0 *[373.4]*
indeterminate (group I) (macular) (neuritic) (uncharacteristic) 030.2
leonine 030.0
lepromatous (diffuse) (infiltrated) (macular) (neuritic) (nodular) (type L) 030.0
macular (early) (neuritic) (simple) 030.2
maculoanesthetic 030.1
mixed 030.0
neuro 030.1
nodular 030.0
primary neuritic 030.3
specified type or group NEC 030.8
tubercular 030.1
tuberculoid (macular) (maculoanesthetic) (major) (minor) (neuritic) (type T) 030.1
Leptocytosis, hereditary 282.49
Leptomeningitis (chronic) (circumscribed) (hemorrhagic) (nonsuppurative) – *see also* Meningitis) 322.9
aseptic 047.9
adenovirus 049.1
Coxsackie virus 047.0
ECHO virus 047.1
enterovirus 047.9
lymphocytic choriomeningitis 049.0
epidemic 036.0
late effect – *see* category 326
meningococcal 036.0
pneumococcal 320.1
syphilitic 094.2
tuberculous (*see also* Tuberculosis, meninges) 013.0❺
Leptomeningopathy (*see also* Meningitis) 322.9
Leptospiral – *see* condition
Leptospirochetal – *see* condition
Leptospirosis 100.9
autumnalis 100.89
canicula 100.89
grippotyphosa 100.89
hebdomidis 100.89
icterohemorrhagica 100.0
nanukayami 100.89
pomona 100.89
Weil's disease 100.0
Leptothricosis – *see* Actinomycosis
Leptothrix infestation – *see* Actinomycosis
Leptotricosis – *see* Actinomycosis
Leptus dermatitis 133.8
Léris pleonosteosis 756.89
Léri-Weill syndrome 756.59
Leriche's syndrome (aortic bifurcation occlusion) 444.0
Lermoyez's syndrome (*see also* Disease, Ménière's) 386.00
Lesbianism - omit code
ego-dystonic 302.0
problems with 302.0
Lesch-Nyhan syndrome (hypoxanthine-guanine-phosphoribosyltransferase deficiency) 277.2
Lesion(s)
abducens nerve 378.54
alveolar process 525.8
anorectal 569.49
aortic (valve) – *see* Endocarditis, aortic
auditory nerve 388.5
basal ganglion 333.90
bile duct (*see also* Disease, biliary) 576.8

Latent – Lesion(s)

Lesion(s) – *continued*
- bladder 596.9
- bone 733.90
- brachial plexus 353.0
- brain 348.8
  - congenital 742.9
  - vascular (*see also* Lesion, cerebrovascular) 437.9
    - degenerative 437.1
    - healed or old without residuals V12.54 ▲
    - hypertensive 437.2
    - late effect – *see* Late effect(s) (of) cerebrovascular disease
- buccal 528.9
- calcified – *see* Calcification
- canthus 373.9
- carate – *see* Pinta, lesions
- cardia 537.89
- cardiac – *see also* Disease, heart
  - congenital 746.9
  - valvular – *see* Endocarditis
- cauda equina 344.60
  - with neurogenic bladder 344.61
- cecum 569.89
- cerebral – *see* Lesion, brain
- cerebrovascular (*see also* Disease, cerebrovascular NEC) 437.9
  - degenerative 437.1
  - healed or old without residuals V12.54 ▲
  - hypertensive 437.2
  - specified type NEC 437.8
- cervical root (nerve) NEC 353.2
- chiasmal 377.54
  - associated with
    - inflammatory disorders 377.54
    - neoplasm NEC 377.52
      - pituitary 377.51
    - pituitary disorders 377.51
    - vascular disorders 377.53
- chorda tympani 351.8
- coin, lung 793.1
- colon 569.89
- congenital – *see* Anomaly
- conjunctiva 372.9
- coronary artery (*see also* Ischemia, heart) 414.9
- cranial nerve 352.9
  - first 352.0
  - second 377.49
  - third
    - partial 378.51
    - total 378.52
  - fourth 378.53
  - fifth 350.9
  - sixth 378.54
  - seventh 351.9
  - eighth 388.5
  - ninth 352.2
  - tenth 352.3
  - eleventh 352.4
  - twelfth 352.5
- cystic – *see* Cyst
- degenerative – *see* Degeneration
- dermal (skin) 709.9
- Dieulafoy (hemorrhagic)
  - of
    - duodenum 537.84
    - intestine 569.86
    - stomach 537.84
- duodenum 537.89
  - with obstruction 537.3
- eyelid 373.9
- gasserian ganglion 350.8
- gastric 537.89
- gastroduodenal 537.89
- gastrointestinal 569.89
- glossopharyngeal nerve 352.2
- heart (organic) – *see also* Disease, heart
  - vascular – *see* Disease, cardiovascular
- helix (ear) 709.9
- high grade myelodysplastic syndrome 238.73
- hyperchromic, due to pinta (carate) 103.1
- hyperkeratotic (*see also* Hyperkeratosis) 701.1
- hypoglossal nerve 352.5
- hypopharynx 478.29
- hypothalamic 253.9
- ileocecal coil 569.89
- ileum 569.89
- iliohypogastric nerve 355.79
- ilioinguinal nerve 355.79
- in continuity – *see* Injury, nerve, by site
- inflammatory – *see* Inflammation
- intestine 569.89
- intracerebral – *see* Lesion, brain
- intrachiasmal (optic) (*see also* Lesion, chiasmal) 377.54
- intracranial, space-occupying NEC 784.2
- joint 719.90
  - ankle 719.97
  - elbow 719.92
  - foot 719.97
  - hand 719.94
  - hip 719.95
  - knee 719.96
  - multiple sites 719.99
  - pelvic region 719.95
  - sacroiliac (old) 724.6
  - shoulder (region) 719.91
  - specified site NEC 719.98
  - wrist 719.93
- keratotic (*see also* Keratosis) 701.1
- kidney (*see also* Disease, renal) 593.9
- laryngeal nerve (recurrent) 352.3
- leonine 030.0
- lip 528.5
- liver 573.8
- low grade myelodysplastic syndrome 238.72
- lumbosacral
  - plexus 353.1
  - root (nerve) NEC 353.4
- lung 518.89
  - coin 793.1
- maxillary sinus 473.0
- mitral – *see* Endocarditis, mitral
- motor cortex 348.8
- nerve (*see also* Disorder, nerve) 355.9
- nervous system 349.9
  - congenital 742.9
- nonallopathic NEC 739.9
  - in region (of)
    - abdomen 739.9
    - acromioclavicular 739.7
    - cervical, cervicothoracic 739.1
    - costochondral 739.8
    - costovertebral 739.8
    - extremity
      - lower 739.6
      - upper 739.7
    - head 739.0
    - hip 739.5
    - lower extremity 739.6
    - lumbar, lumbosacral 739.3
    - occipitocervical 739.0
    - pelvic 739.5
    - pubic 739.5
    - rib cage 739.8
    - sacral, sacrococcygeal, sacroiliac 739.4
    - sternochondral 739.8
    - sternoclavicular 739.7
    - thoracic, thoracolumbar 739.2
    - upper extremity 739.7
- nose (internal) 478.19
- obstructive – *see* Obstruction
- obturator nerve 355.79
- occlusive
  - artery – *see* Embolism, artery
- organ or site NEC – *see* Disease, by site
- osteolytic 733.90
- paramacular, of retina 363.32
- peptic 537.89
- periodontal, due to traumatic occlusion 523.8
- perirectal 569.49
- peritoneum (granulomatous) 568.89
- pigmented (skin) 709.00
- pinta – *see* Pinta, lesions
- polypoid – *see* Polyp
- prechiasmal (optic) (*see also* Lesion, chiasmal) 377.54
- primary – *see also* Syphilis, primary
  - carate 103.0
  - pinta 103.0
  - yaws 102.0
- pulmonary 518.89
  - valve (*see also* Endocarditis, pulmonary) 424.3
- pylorus 537.89
- radiation NEC 990
- radium NEC 990
- rectosigmoid 569.89
- retina, retinal – *see also* Retinopathy
  - vascular 362.17
- retroperitoneal 568.89
- romanus 720.1
- sacroiliac (joint) 724.6
- salivary gland 527.8
  - benign lymphoepithelial 527.8
- saphenous nerve 355.79
- secondary – *see* Syphilis, secondary
- sigmoid 569.89
- sinus (accessory) (nasal) (*see also* Sinusitis) 473.9
- skin 709.9
  - suppurative 686.00
- SLAP (superior glenoid labrum) 840.7
- space-occupying, intracranial NEC 784.2
- spinal cord 336.9
  - congenital 742.9
  - traumatic (complete) (incomplete) (transverse) – *see also* Injury, spinal, by site
    - with
      - broken
        - back – *see* Fracture, vertebra, by site, with spinal cord injury
        - neck – *see* Fracture, vertebra, cervical, with spinal cord injury
      - fracture, vertebra – *see* Fracture, vertebra, by site, with spinal cord injury
- spleen 289.50
- stomach 537.89
- superior glenoid labrum (SLAP) 840.7
- syphilitic – *see* Syphilis
- tertiary – *see* Syphilis, tertiary
- thoracic root (nerve) 353.3
- tonsillar fossa 474.9
- tooth, teeth 525.8
  - white spot 521.01
- traumatic NEC (*see also* nature and site of injury) 959.9
- tricuspid (valve) – *see* Endocarditis, tricuspid
- trigeminal nerve 350.9
- ulcerated or ulcerative – *see* Ulcer
- uterus NEC 621.9
- vagina 623.8
- vagus nerve 352.3
- valvular – *see* Endocarditis
- vascular 459.9
  - affecting central nervous system (*see also* Lesion, cerebrovascular) 437.9
  - following trauma (*see also* Injury, blood vessel, by site) 904.9
  - retina 362.17
  - traumatic – *see* Injury, blood vessel, by site
  - umbilical cord 663.6❺
    - affecting fetus or newborn 762.6
- visual
  - cortex NEC (*see also* Disorder, visual, cortex) 377.73
  - pathway NEC (*see also* Disorder, visual, pathway) 377.63
- warty – *see* Verruca
- white spot, on teeth 521.01
- x-ray NEC 990

Lethargic – *see* condition

Lethargy 780.79

Letterer-Siwe disease (acute histiocytosis X) (M9722/3) 202.5❺

Leucinosis 270.3

Leucocoria 360.44

Leucosarcoma (M9850/3) 207.8❺

Leukasmus 270.2

Leukemia, leukemic (congenital) (M9800/3) 208.9❺

Note – Use the following fifth-digit subclassification for categories 203-208:
0 without mention of remission
1 with remission

- acute NEC (M9801/3) 208.0❺
- aleukemic NEC (M9804/3) 208.8❺
  - granulocytic (M9864/3) 205.8❺
- basophilic (M9870/3) 205.1❺
- blast (cell) (M9801/3) 208.0❺
- blastic (M9801/3) 208.0❺
  - granulocytic (M9861/3) 205.0❺
- chronic NEC (M9803/3) 208.1❺
- compound (M9810/3) 207.8❺
- eosinophilic (M9880/3) 205.1❺
- giant cell (M9910/3) 207.2❺
- granulocytic (M9860/3) 205.9❺
  - acute (M9861/3) 205.0❺
  - aleukemic (M9864/3) 205.8❺
  - blastic (M9861/3) 205.0❺
  - chronic (M9863/3) 205.1❺
  - subacute (M9862/3) 205.2❺

Leukemia, leukemic – *continued*
  granulocytic – *continued*
    subleukemic (M9864/3) 205.8❺
  hairy cell (M9940/3) 202.4❺
  hemoblastic (M9801/3) 208.0❺
  histiocytic (M9890/3) 206.9❺
  lymphatic (M9820/3) 204.9❺
    acute (M9821/3) 204.0❺
    aleukemic (M9824/3) 204.8❺
    chronic (M9823/3) 204.1❺
    subacute (M9822/3) 204.2❺
    subleukemic (M9824/3) 204.8❺
  lymphoblastic (M9821/3) 204.0❺
  lymphocytic (M9820/3) 204.9❺
    acute (M9821/3) 204.0❺
    aleukemic (M9824/3) 204.8❺
    chronic (M9823/3) 204.1❺
    subacute (M9822/3) 204.2❺
    subleukemic (M9824/3) 204.8❺
  lymphogenous (M9820/3) – *see* Leukemia, lymphoid
  lymphoid (M9820/3) 204.9❺
    acute (M9821/3) 204.0❺
    aleukemic (M9824/3) 204.8❺
    blastic (M9821/3) 204.0❺
    chronic (M9823/3) 204.1❺
    subacute (M9822/3) 204.2❺
    subleukemic (M9824/3) 204.8❺
  lymphosarcoma cell (M9850/3) 207.8❺
  mast cell (M9900/3) 207.8❺
  megakaryocytic (M9910/3) 207.2❺
  megakaryocytoid (M9910/3) 207.2❺
  mixed (cell) (M9810/3) 207.8❺
  monoblastic (M9891/3) 206.0❺
  monocytic (Schilling-type) (M9890/3) 206.9❺
    acute (M9891/3) 206.0❺
    aleukemic (M9894/3) 206.8❺
    chronic (M9893/3) 206.1❺
    Naegeli-type (M9863/3) 205.1❺
    subacute (M9892/3) 206.2❺
    subleukemic (M9894/3) 206.8❺
  monocytoid (M9890/3) 206.9❺
    acute (M9891/3) 206.0❺
    aleukemic (M9894/3) 206.8❺
    chronic (M9893/3) 206.1❺
    myelogenous (M9863/3) 205.1❺
    subacute (M9892/3) 206.2❺
    subleukemic (M9894/3) 206.8❺
  monomyelocytic (M9860/3) – *see* Leukemia, myelomonocytic
  myeloblastic (M9861/3) 205.0❺
  myelocytic (M9863/3) 205.1❺
    acute (M9861/3) 205.0❺
  myelogenous (M9860/3) 205.9❺
    acute (M9861/3) 205.0❺
    aleukemic (M9864/3) 205.8❺
    chronic (M9863/3) 205.1❺
    monocytoid (M9863/3) 205.1❺
    subacute (M9862/3) 205.2❺
    subleukemic (M9864) 205.8❺
  myeloid (M9860/3) 205.9❺
    acute (M9861/3) 205.0❺
    aleukemic (M9864/3) 205.8❺
    chronic (M9863/3) 205.1❺
    subacute (M9862/3) 205.2❺
    subleukemic (M9864/3) 205.8❺
  myelomonocytic (M9860/3) 205.9❺
    acute (M9861/3) 205.0❺
    chronic (M9863/3) 205.1❺
  Naegeli-type monocytic (M9863/3) 205.1❺
  neutrophilic (M9865/3) 205.1❺
  plasma cell (M9830/3) 203.1❺
  plasmacytic (M9830/3) 203.1❺
  prolymphocytic (M9825/3) – *see* Leukemia, lymphoid
  promyelocytic, acute (M9866/3) 205.0❺
  Schilling-type monocytic (M9890/3) – *see* Leukemia, monocytic
  stem cell (M9801/3) 208.0❺
  subacute NEC (M9802/3) 208.2❺
  subleukemic NEC (M9804/3) 208.8❺
  thrombocytic (M9910/3) 207.2❺
  undifferentiated (M9801/3) 208.0❺
Leukemoid reaction (basophilic) (lymphocytic) (monocytic) (myelocytic) (neutrophilic) 288.62
Leukoclastic vasculitis 446.29
Leukocoria 360.44
Leukocythemia – *see* Leukemia
Leukocytopenia 288.50
Leukocytosis 288.60
  basophilic 288.8
Leukocytosis – *continued*
  eosinophilic 288.3
  lymphocytic 288.8
  monocytic 288.8
  neutrophilic 288.8
Leukoderma 709.09
  syphilitic 091.3
    late 095.8
Leukodermia (*see also* Leukoderma) 709.09
Leukodystrophy (cerebral) (globoid cell) (metachromatic) (progressive) (sudanophilic) 330.0
Leukoedema, mouth or tongue 528.79
Leukoencephalitis
  acute hemorrhagic (postinfectious) NEC 136.9 *[323.61]*
    postimmunization or postvaccinal 323.51
  subacute sclerosing 046.2
    van Bogaert's 046.2
  van Bogaert's (sclerosing) 046.2
Leukoencephalopathy (*see also* Encephalitis) 323.9
  acute necrotizing hemorrhagic (postinfectious) 136.9 *[323.61]*
    postimmunization or postvaccinal 323.51
  metachromatic 330.0
  multifocal (progressive) 046.3
  progressive multifocal 046.3
Leukoerythroblastosis 289.9
Leukoerythrosis 289.0
Leukokeratosis (*see also* Leukoplakia) 702.8
  mouth 528.6
  nicotina palati 528.79
  tongue 528.6
Leukokoria 360.44
Leukokraurosis vulva, vulvae 624.09 ▲
Leukolymphosarcoma (M9850/3) 207.8❺
Leukoma (cornea) (interfering with central vision) 371.03
  adherent 371.04
Leukomalacia, periventricular 779.7
Leukomelanopathy, hereditary 288.2
Leukonychia (punctata) (striata) 703.8
  congenital 757.5
Leukopathia
  unguium 703.8
    congenital 757.5
Leukopenia 288.50
  basophilic 288.59
  cyclic 288.02
  eosinophilic 288.59
  familial 288.59
  malignant (*see also* Agranulocytosis) 288.09
  periodic 288.02
  transitory neonatal 776.7
Leukopenic – *see* condition
Leukoplakia 702.8
  anus 569.49
  bladder (postinfectional) 596.8
  buccal 528.6
  cervix (uteri) 622.2
  esophagus 530.83
  gingiva 528.6
  kidney (pelvis) 593.89
  larynx 478.79
  lip 528.6
  mouth 528.6
  oral soft tissue (including tongue) (mucosa) 528.6
  palate 528.6
  pelvis (kidney) 593.89
  penis (infectional) 607.0
  rectum 569.49
  syphilitic 095.8
  tongue 528.6
  tonsil 478.29
  ureter (postinfectional) 593.89
  urethra (postinfectional) 599.84
  uterus 621.8
  vagina 623.1
  vesical 596.8
  vocal cords 478.5
  vulva 624.09 ▲
Leukopolioencephalopathy 330.0
Leukorrhea (vagina) 623.5
  due to Trichomonas (vaginalis) 131.00
  trichomonal (Trichomonas vaginalis) 131.00
Leukosarcoma (M9850/3) 207.8❺
Leukosis (M9800/3) – *see* Leukemia
Lev's disease or syndrome (acquired complete heart block) 426.0
Levi's syndrome (pituitary dwarfism) 253.3
Levocardia (isolated) 746.87
  with situs inversus 759.3
Levulosuria 271.2
Lewandowski's disease (primary) (*see also* Tuberculosis) 017.0❺
Lewandowski-Lutz disease (epidermodysplasia verruciformis) 078.19
Lewy body dementia 331.82
Lewy body disease 331.82
Leyden's disease (periodic vomiting) 536.2
Leyden-Möbius dystrophy 359.1
Leydig cell
  carcinoma (M8650/3)
    specified site – *see* Neoplasm, by site, malignant
    unspecified site
      female 183.0
      male 186.9
  tumor (M8650/1)
    benign (M8650/0)
      specified site – *see* Neoplasm, by site, benign
      unspecified site
        female 220
        male 222.0
    malignant (M8650/3)
      specified site – *see* Neoplasm, by site, malignant
      unspecified site
        female 183.0
        male 186.9
    specified site – *see* Neoplasm, by site, uncertain behavior
    unspecified site
      female 236.2
      male 236.4
Leydig-Sertoli cell tumor (M8631/0)
  specified site – *see* Neoplasm, by site, benign
  unspecified site
    female 220
    male 222.0
LGSIL (low grade squamous intraepithelial lesion) 795.03
Liar, pathologic 301.7
Libman-Sacks disease or syndrome 710.0 *[424.91]*
Lice (infestation) 132.9
  body (pediculus corporis) 132.1
  crab 132.2
  head (pediculus capitis) 132.0
  mixed (classifiable to more than one of the categories 132.0-132.2) 132.3
  pubic (pediculus pubis) 132.2
Lichen 697.9
  albus 701.0
  annularis 695.89
  atrophicus 701.0
  corneus obtusus 698.3
  myxedematous 701.8
  nitidus 697.1
  pilaris 757.39
    acquired 701.1
  planopilaris 697.0
  planus (acute) (chronicus) (hypertrophic) (verrucous) 697.0
    morphoeicus 701.0
    sclerosus (et atrophicus) 701.0
  ruber 696.4
    acuminatus 696.4
    moniliformis 697.8
    obtusus corneus 698.3
    of Wilson 697.0
    planus 697.0
  sclerosus (et atrophicus) 701.0
  scrofulosus (primary) (*see also* Tuberculosis) 017.0❺
  simplex (Vidal's) 698.3
    chronicus 698.3
    circumscriptus 698.3
  spinulosus 757.39
    mycotic 117.9
  striata 697.8
  urticatus 698.2
Lichenification 698.3
  nodular 698.3
Lichenoides tuberculosis (primary) (*see also* Tuberculosis) 017.0❺

Leukemia, leukemic – Lichenoides tuberculosis

Lichtheim's disease or syndrome (subacute combined sclerosis with pernicious anemia) 281.0 *[336.2]*
Lien migrans 289.59
Lientery (*see also* Diarrhea) 787.91
  infectious 009.2
Life circumstance problem NEC V62.89
Li-Fraumeni cancer syndrome V84.01
Ligament – *see* condition
Light-for-dates (infant) 764.0❺
  with signs of fetal malnutrition 764.1❺
  affecting management of pregnancy 656.5❺
Light-headedness 780.4
Lightning (effects) (shock) (stroke) (struck by) 994.0
  burn – *see* Burn, by site
  foot 266.2
Lightwood's disease or syndrome (renal tubular acidosis) 588.89
Lignac's disease (cystinosis) 270.0
Lignac (-de Toni) (-Fanconi) (-Debré) **syndrome** (cystinosis) 270.0
Lignac (-Fanconi) **syndrome** (cystinosis) 270.0
Ligneous thyroiditis 245.3
Likoff's syndrome (angina in menopausal women) 413.9
Limb – *see* condition
Limitation of joint motion (*see also* Stiffness, joint) 719.5❺
  sacroiliac 724.6
Limit dextrinosis 271.0
Limited
  cardiac reserve – *see* Disease, heart
  duction, eye NEC 378.63
  mandibular range of motion 524.52
Lindau's disease (retinocerebral angiomatosis) 759.6
Lindau (-von Hippel) **disease** (angiomatosis retinocerebellosa) 759.6
Linea corneae senilis 371.41
Lines
  Beau's (transverse furrows on fingernails) 703.8
  Harris' 733.91
  Hudson-Stähli 371.11
  Stähli's 371.11
Lingua
  geographical 529.1
  nigra (villosa) 529.3
  plicata 529.5
    congenital 750.13
  tylosis 528.6
Lingual (tongue) – *see also* condition
  thyroid 759.2
Linitis (gastric) 535.4❺
  plastica (M8142/3) 151.9
Lioderma essentialis (cum melanosis et telangiectasia) 757.33
Lip – *see also* condition
  biting 528.9
Lipalgia 272.8
Lipedema – *see* Edema
Lipemia (*see also* Hyperlipidemia) 272.4
  retina, retinalis 272.3
Lipidosis 272.7
  cephalin 272.7
  cerebral (infantile) (juvenile) (late) 330.1
  cerebroretinal 330.1 *[362.71]*
  cerebroside 272.7
  cerebrospinal 272.7
  chemically-induced 272.7
  cholesterol 272.7
  diabetic 250.8❺ *[272.7]*
  dystopic (hereditary) 272.7
  glycolipid 272.7
  hepatosplenomegalic 272.3
  hereditary, dystopic 272.7
  sulfatide 330.0
Lipoadenoma (M8324/0 – *see* Neoplasm, by site, benign
Lipoblastoma (M8881/0) – *see* Lipoma, by site
Lipoblastomatosis (M8881/0) – *see* Lipoma, by site
Lipochondrodystrophy 277.5
Lipochrome histiocytosis (familial) 288.1
Lipodystrophia progressiva 272.6
Lipodystrophy (progressive) 272.6
  insulin 272.6
  intestinal 040.2
Lipodystrophy – *continued*
  mesenteric 567.82
Lipofibroma (M8851/0) – *see* Lipoma, by site
Lipoglycoproteinosis 272.8
Lipogranuloma, sclerosing 709.8
Lipogranulomatosis (disseminated) 272.8
  kidney 272.8
Lipoid – *see also* condition
  histiocytosis 272.7
    essential 272.7
  nephrosis (*see also* Nephrosis) 581.3
  proteinosis of Urbach 272.8
Lipoidemia (*see also* Hyperlipidemia) 272.4
Lipoidosis (*see also* Lipidosis) 272.7
Lipoma (M8850/0) 214.9
  breast (skin) 214.1
  face 214.0
  fetal (M8881/0) – *see also* Lipoma, by site
    fat cell (M8880/0) – *see* Lipoma, by site
  infiltrating (M8856/0) – *see* Lipoma, by site
  intra-abdominal 214.3
  intramuscular (M8856/0) – *see* Lipoma, by site
  intrathoracic 214.2
  kidney 214.3
  mediastinum 214.2
  muscle 214.8
  peritoneum 214.3
  retroperitoneum 214.3
  skin 214.1
    face 214.0
  spermatic cord 214.4
  spindle cell (M8857/0) – *see* Lipoma, by site
  stomach 214.3
  subcutaneous tissue 214.1
    face 214.0
  thymus 214.2
  thyroid gland 214.2
Lipomatosis (dolorosa) 272.8
  epidural 214.8
  fetal (M8881/0) – *see* Lipoma, by site
  Launois-Bensaude's 272.8
Lipomyohemangioma (M8860/0)
  specified site – *see* Neoplasm, connective tissue, benign
  unspecified site 223.0
Lipomyoma (M8860/0)
  specified site – *see* Neoplasm, connective tissue, benign
  unspecified site 223.0
Lipomyxoma (M8852/0) – *see* Lipoma, by site
Lipomyxosarcoma (M8852/3) – *see* Neoplasm, connective tissue, malignant
Lipophagocytosis 289.89
Lipoproteinemia (alpha) 272.4
  broad-beta 272.2
  floating-beta 272.2
  hyper-pre-beta 272.1
Lipoproteinosis (Rossle-Urbach-Wiethe) 272.8
Liposarcoma (M8850/3) – *see also* Neoplasm, connective tissue, malignant
  differentiated type (M8851/3) – *see* Neoplasm, connective tissue, malignant
  embryonal (M8852/3) – *see* Neoplasm, connective tissue, malignant
  mixed type (M8855/3) – *see* Neoplasm, connective tissue, malignant
  myxoid (M8852/3) – *see* Neoplasm, connective tissue, malignant
  pleomorphic (M8854/3) – *see* Neoplasm, connective tissue, malignant
  round cell (M8853/3) – *see* Neoplasm, connective tissue, malignant
  well differentiated type (M8851/3) – *see* Neoplasm, connective tissue, malignant
Liposynovitis prepatellaris 272.8
Lipping
  cervix 622.0
  spine (*see also* Spondylosis) 721.90
  vertebra (*see also* Spondylosis) 721.90
Lip pits (mucus), congenital 750.25
Lipschütz disease or ulcer 616.50
Lipuria 791.1
  bilharziasis 120.0
Liquefaction, vitreous humor 379.21
Lisping 307.9
Lissauer's paralysis 094.1
Lissencephalia, lissencephaly 742.2
Listerellose 027.0
Listeriose 027.0
Listeriosis 027.0
  congenital 771.2
  fetal 771.2
  suspected fetal damage affecting management of pregnancy 655.4❺
Listlessness 780.79
Lithemia 790.6
Lithiasis – *see also* Calculus
  hepatic (duct) – *see* Choledocholithiasis
  urinary 592.9
Lithopedion 779.9
  affecting management of pregnancy 656.8❺
Lithosis (occupational) 502
  with tuberculosis – *see* Tuberculosis, pulmonary
Lithuria 791.9
Litigation V62.5
Little
  league elbow 718.82
  stroke syndrome 435.9
Little's disease – *see* Palsy, cerebral
Littre's
  gland – *see* condition
  hernia – *see* Hernia, Littre's
Littritis (*see also* Urethritis) 597.89
Livedo 782.61
  annularis 782.61
  racemose 782.61
  reticularis 782.61
Live flesh 781.0
Liver – *see also* condition
  donor V59.6
Livida, asphyxia
  newborn 768.6
Living
  alone V60.3
    with handicapped person V60.4
Lloyd's syndrome 258.1
Loa loa 125.2
Loasis 125.2
Lobe, lobar – *see* condition
Lobo's disease or blastomycosis 116.2
Lobomycosis 116.2
Lobotomy syndrome 310.0
Lobstein's disease (brittle bones and blue sclera) 756.51
Lobster-claw hand 755.58
Lobulation (congenital) – *see also* Anomaly, specified type NEC, by site
  kidney, fetal 753.3
  liver, abnormal 751.69
  spleen 759.0
Lobule, lobular – *see* condition
Local, localized – *see* condition
Locked bowel or intestine (*see also* Obstruction, intestine) 560.9
Locked-in state 344.81
Locked twins 660.5❺
  affecting fetus or newborn 763.1
Locking
  joint (*see also* Derangement, joint) 718.90
  knee 717.9
Lockjaw (*see also* Tetanus) 037
Locomotor ataxia (progressive) 094.0
Löffler's
  endocarditis 421.0
  eosinophilia or syndrome 518.3
  pneumonia 518.3
  syndrome (eosinophilic pneumonitis) 518.3
Löfgren's syndrome (sarcoidosis) 135
Loiasis 125.2
  eyelid 125.2 *[373.6]*
Loneliness V62.89
Lone star fever 082.8
Long labor 662.1❺
  affecting fetus or newborn 763.89
  first stage 662.0❺
  second stage 662.2❺
Longitudinal stripes or grooves, nails 703.8
  congenital 757.5
Long-term (current) **drug use** V58.69
  antibiotics V58.62
  anticoagulants V58.61
  anti-inflammatories, non-steroidal (NSAID) V58.64

Lichtheim's disease or syndrome – Long-term drug use

- **Long-term** (current) **drug use** – *continued*
  - antiplatelets/antithrombotics V58.63
  - aspirin V58.66
  - high-risk medications NEC V58.69 ●
  - insulin V58.67
  - pain killers V58.69 ●
    - anti-inflammatories, non-steroidal (NSAID) V58.64 ●
    - aspirin V58.66 ●
  - steroids V58.65
  - tamoxifen V58.69 ●
- **Loop**
  - intestine (*see also* Volvulus) 560.2
  - intrascleral nerve 379.29
  - vascular on papilla (optic) 743.57
- **Loose** – *see also* condition
  - body
    - in tendon sheath 727.82
    - joint 718.10
      - ankle 718.17
      - elbow 718.12
      - foot 718.17
      - hand 718.14
      - hip 718.15
      - knee 717.6
      - multiple sites 718.19
      - pelvic region 718.15
      - prosthetic implant – *see* Complications, mechanical
      - shoulder (region) 718.11
      - specified site NEC 718.18
      - wrist 718.13
  - cartilage (joint) (*see also* Loose, body, joint) 718.1❺
    - knee 717.6
  - facet (vertebral) 724.9
  - prosthetic implant – *see* Complications, mechanical
  - sesamoid, joint (*see also* Loose, body, joint) 718.1❺
  - tooth, teeth 525.8
- **Loosening epiphysis** 732.9
- **Looser** (-Debray)-**Milkman syndrome** (osteomalacia with pseudofractures) 268.2
- **Lop ear** (deformity) 744.29
- **Lorain's disease or syndrome** (pituitary dwarfism) 253.3
- **Lorain-Levi syndrome** (pituitary dwarfism) 253.3
- **Lordosis** (acquired) (postural) 737.20
  - congenital 754.2
  - due to or associated with
    - Charcôt-Marie-Tooth disease 356.1 *[737.42]*
    - mucopolysaccharidosis 277.5 *[737.42]*
    - neurofibromatosis 237.71 *[737.42]*
    - osteitis
      - deformans 731.0 *[737.42]*
      - fibrosa cystica 252.01 *[737.42]*
    - osteoporosis (*see also* Osteoporosis) 733.00 *[737.42]*
    - poliomyelitis (*see also* Poliomyelitis) 138 *[737.42]*
    - tuberculosis (*see also* Tuberculosis) 015.0❺ *[737.42]*
  - late effect of rickets 268.1 *[737.42]*
  - postlaminectomy 737.21
  - postsurgical NEC 737.22
  - rachitic 268.1 *[737.42]*
  - specified NEC 737.29
  - tuberculous (*see also* Tuberculosis) 015.0❺ *[737.42]*
- **Loss**
  - appetite 783.0
    - hysterical 300.11
    - nonorganic origin 307.59
    - psychogenic 307.59
  - blood – *see* Hemorrhage
  - central vision 368.41
  - consciousness 780.09
    - transient 780.2
  - control, sphincter, rectum 787.6
    - nonorganic origin 307.7
  - ear ossicle, partial 385.24
  - elasticity, skin 782.8
  - extremity or member, traumatic, current – *see* Amputation, traumatic
  - fluid (acute) 276.50
    - with
      - hypernatremia 276.0
      - hyponatremia 276.1
    - fetus or newborn 775.5
- **Loss** – *continued*
  - hair 704.00
  - hearing – *see also* Deafness
    - central 389.14
    - conductive (air) 389.00
      - with sensorineural hearing loss 389.20 ▲
        - bilateral 389.22 ●
        - unilateral 389.21 ●
      - bilateral 389.06 ●
      - combined types 389.08
      - external ear 389.01
      - inner ear 389.04
      - middle ear 389.03
      - multiple types 389.08
      - tympanic membrane 389.02
      - unilateral 389.05 ●
    - mixed conductive and sensorineural 389.20 ●
      - bilateral 389.22 ●
      - unilateral 389.21 ●
    - mixed type 389.20 ▲
      - bilateral 389.22 ●
      - unilateral 389.21 ●
    - nerve
      - bilateral 389.12 ●
      - unilateral 389.13 ●
    - neural
      - bilateral 389.12 ●
      - unilateral 389.13 ●
    - noise-induced 388.12
    - perceptive NEC (*see also* Loss, hearing, sensorineural) 389.10
    - sensorineural 389.10
      - with conductive hearing loss 389.20 ▲
        - bilateral 389.22 ●
        - unilateral 389.21 ●
      - asymmetrical 389.16
      - bilateral 389.18 ●
      - central 389.14
      - neural
        - bilateral 389.12 ●
        - unilateral 389.13 ●
      - sensory
        - bilateral 389.11 ●
        - unilateral 389.17 ●
      - unilateral 389.15
    - sensory
      - bilateral 389.11 ●
      - unilateral 389.17 ●
    - specified type NEC 389.8
    - sudden NEC 388.2
  - height 781.91
  - labyrinthine reactivity (unilateral) 386.55
    - bilateral 386.56
  - memory (*see also* Amnesia) 780.93
    - mild, following organic brain damage 310.1
  - mind (*see also* Psychosis) 298.9
  - occlusal vertical dimension 524.37
  - organ or part – *see* Absence, by site, acquired
  - sensation 782.0
  - sense of
    - smell (*see also* Disturbance, sensation) 781.1
    - taste (*see also* Disturbance, sensation) 781.1
    - touch (*see also* Disturbance, sensation) 781.1
  - sight (acquired) (complete) (congenital) – *see* Blindness
  - spinal fluid
    - headache 349.0
  - substance of
    - bone (*see also* Osteoporosis) 733.00
    - cartilage 733.99
      - ear 380.32
    - vitreous (humor) 379.26
  - tooth, teeth
    - acquired 525.10
      - due to
        - caries 525.13
        - extraction 525.10
        - periodontal disease 525.12
        - specified NEC 525.19
        - trauma 525.11
  - vision, visual (*see also* Blindness) 369.9
    - both eyes (*see also* Blindness, both eyes) 369.3
    - complete (*see also* Blindness, both eyes) 369.00
    - one eye 369.8
    - sudden 368.11
    - transient 368.12
  - vitreous 379.26
  - voice (*see also* Aphonia) 784.41
  - weight (cause unknown) 783.21
- **Lou Gehrig's disease** 335.20
- **Louis-Bar syndrome** (ataxia-telangiectasia) 334.8
- **Louping ill** 063.1
- **Lousiness** – *see* Lice
- **Low**
  - back syndrome 724.2
  - basal metabolic rate (BMR) 794.7
  - birthweight 765.1❺
    - extreme (less than 1000 grams) 765.0❺
    - for gestational age 764.0❺
    - status (*see also* Status, low birth weight) V21.30
  - bladder compliance 596.52
  - blood pressure (*see also* Hypotension) 458.9
    - reading (incidental) (isolated) (nonspecific) 796.3
  - cardiac reserve – *see* Disease, heart
  - compliance bladder 596.52
  - frequency deafness – *see* Disorder, hearing
  - function – *see also* Hypofunction
    - kidney (*see also* Disease, renal) 593.9
    - liver 573.9
  - hemoglobin 285.9
  - implantation, placenta – *see* Placenta, previa
  - insertion, placenta – *see* Placenta, previa
  - lying
    - kidney 593.0
    - organ or site, congenital – *see* Malposition, congenital
    - placenta – *see* Placenta, previa
  - output syndrome (cardiac) (*see also* Failure, heart) 428.9
  - platelets (blood) (*see also* Thrombocytopenia) 287.5
  - reserve, kidney (*see also* Disease, renal) 593.9
  - risk
    - cervical, human papillomavirus (HPV) DNA test positive 795.09
  - salt syndrome 593.9
  - tension glaucoma 365.12
  - vision 369.9
    - both eyes 369.20
    - one eye 369.70
- **Lowe** (-Terrey-MacLachlan) **syndrome** (oculocerebrorenal dystrophy) 270.8
- **Lower extremity** – *see* condition
- **Lown** (-Ganong)-**Levine syndrome** (short P-R interval, normal QRS complex, and paroxysmal supraventricular tachycardia) 426.81
- **LSD reaction** (*see also* Abuse, drugs, nondependent) 305.3❺
- **L-shaped kidney** 753.3
- **Lucas-Championnière disease** (fibrinous bronchitis) 466.0
- **Lucey-Driscoll syndrome** (jaundice due to delayed conjugation) 774.30
- **Ludwig's**
  - angina 528.3
  - disease (submaxillary cellulitis) 528.3
- **Lues** (venerea), luetic – *see* Syphilis
- **Luetscher's syndrome** (dehydration) 276.51
- **Lumbago** 724.2
  - due to displacement, intervertebral disc 722.10
- **Lumbalgia** 724.2
  - due to displacement, intervertebral disc 722.10
- **Lumbar** – *see* condition
- **Lumbarization, vertebra** 756.15
- **Lumbermen's itch** 133.8
- **Lump** – *see also* Mass
  - abdominal 789.3❺
  - breast 611.72
  - chest 786.6
  - epigastric 789.3❺
  - head 784.2
  - kidney 753.3
  - liver 789.1
  - lung 786.6
  - mediastinal 786.6
  - neck 784.2
  - nose or sinus 784.2
  - pelvic 789.3❺
  - skin 782.2
  - substernal 786.6
  - throat 784.2
  - umbilicus 789.3❺
- **Lunacy** (*see also* Psychosis) 298.9
- **Lunatomalacia** 732.3
- **Lung** – *see also* condition
  - donor V59.8

Lymphoma – *continued*
  compound (M9613/3) 200.8❺
  convoluted cell type (lymphoblastic) (M9602/3) 202.8❺
  diffuse NEC (M9590/3) 202.8❺
    large B cell 202.8❺ ●
  follicular (giant) (M9690/3) 202.0❺
    center cell (diffuse) (M9615/3) 202.8❺
      cleaved (diffuse) (M9623/3) 202.8❺
        follicular (M9695/3) 202.0❺
      non-cleaved (diffuse) (M9633/3) 202.8❺
        follicular (M9698/3) 202.0❺
    centroblastic-centrocytic (M9692/3) 202.0❺
    centroblastic type (M9697/3) 202.0❺
    lymphocytic
      intermediate differentiation (M9694/3) 202.0❺
      poorly differentiated (M9696/3) 202.0❺
    mixed (cell type) (lymphocytic-histiocytic) (small cell and large cell) (M9691/3) 202.0❺
  germinocytic (M9622/3) 202.8❺
  giant, follicular or follicle (M9690/3) 202.0❺
  histiocytic (diffuse) (M9640/3) 200.0❺
    nodular (M9642/3) 200.0❺
    pleomorphic cell type (M9641/3) 200.0❺
  Hodgkin's (M9650/3) (*see also* Disease, Hodgkin's) 201.9❺
  immunoblastic (type) (M9612/3) 200.8❺
  large cell (M9640/3) 200.7❺ ▲
    anaplastic 200.6❺ ●
    nodular (M9642/3) 200.0❺
    pleomorphic cell type (M9641/3) 200.0❺
  lymphoblastic (diffuse) (M9630/3) 200.1❺
    Burkitt's type (M9750/3) 200.2❺
    convoluted cell type (M9602/3) 202.8❺
  lymphocytic (cell type) (diffuse) (M9620/3) 200.1❺
    with plasmacytoid differentiation, diffuse (M9611/3) 200.8❺
    intermediate differentiation (diffuse) (M9621/3) 200.1❺
      follicular (M9694/3) 202.0❺
      nodular (M9694/3) 202.0❺
    nodular (M9690/3) 202.0❺
    poorly differentiated (diffuse) (M9630/3) 200.1❺
      follicular (M9696/3) 202.0❺
      nodular (M9696/3) 202.0❺
    well differentiated (diffuse) (M9620/3) 200.1❺
      follicular (M9693/3) 202.0❺
      nodular (M9693/3) 202.0❺
  lymphocytic-histiocytic, mixed (diffuse) (M9613/3) 200.8❺
    follicular (M9691/3) 202.0❺
    nodular (M9691/3) 202.0❺
  lymphoplasmacytoid type (M9611/3) 200.8❺
  lymphosarcoma type (M9610/3) 200.1❺
  macrofollicular (M9690/3) 202.0❺
  mantle cell 200.4❺ ●
  marginal zone 200.3❺ ●
    extranodal B-cell 200.3❺ ●
    nodal B-cell 200.3❺ ●
    splenic B-cell 200.3❺ ●
  mixed cell type (diffuse) (M9613/3) 200.8❺
    follicular (M9691/3) 202.0❺
    nodular (M9691/3) 202.0❺
  nodular (M9690/3) 202.0❺
    histiocytic (M9642/3) 200.0❺
    lymphocytic (M9690/3) 202.0❺
      intermediate differentiation (M9694/3) 202.0❺
      poorly differentiated (M9696/3) 202.0❺
    mixed (cell type) (lymphocytic-histiocytic) (small cell and large cell) (M9691/3) 202.0❺
  non-Hodgkin's type NEC (M9591/3) 202.8❺
  peripheral T-cell 202.7❺ ●
  primary central nervous system 200.5❺ ●
  reticulum cell (type) (M9640/3) 200.0❺
  small cell and large cell, mixed (diffuse) (M9613/3) 200.8❺
    follicular (M9691/3) 202.0❺
    nodular (9691/3) 202.0❺
  stem cell (type) (M9601/3) 202.8❺
  T-cell 202.1❺
    peripheral 202.7❺ ●
  undifferentiated (cell type) (non-Burkitt's) (M9600/3) 202.8❺
    Burkitt's type (M9750/3) 200.2❺
Lymphomatosis (M9590/3) – *see also* Lymphoma
  granulomatous 099.1
Lymphopathia
  venereum 099.1
  veneris 099.1
Lymphopenia 288.51
  familial 279.2
Lymphoreticulosis, benign (of inoculation) 078.3
Lymphorrhea 457.8
Lymphosarcoma (M9610/3) 200.1❺
  diffuse (M9610/3) 200.1❺
    with plasmacytoid differentiation (M9611/3) 200.8❺
    lymphoplasmacytic (M9611/3) 200.8❺
  follicular (giant) (M9690/3) 202.0❺
    lymphoblastic (M9696/3) 202.0❺
    lymphocytic, intermediate differentiation (M9694/3) 202.0❺
    mixed cell type (M9691/3) 202.0❺
  giant follicular (M9690/3) 202.0❺
  Hodgkin's (M9650/3) 201.9❺
  immunoblastic (M9612/3) 200.8❺
  lymphoblastic (diffuse) (M9630/3) 200.1❺
    follicular (M9696/3) 202.0❺
    nodular (M9696/3) 202.0❺
  lymphocytic (diffuse) (M9620/3) 200.1❺
    intermediate differentiation (diffuse) (M9621/3) 200.1❺
      follicular (M9694/3) 202.0❺
      nodular (M9694/3) 202.0❺
  mixed cell type (diffuse) (M9613/3) 200.8❺
    follicular (M9691/3) 202.0❺
    nodular (M9691/3) 202.0❺
  nodular (M9690/3) 202.0❺
    lymphoblastic (M9696/3) 202.0❺
    lymphocytic, intermediate differentiation (M9694/3) 202.0❺
    mixed cell type (M9691/3) 202.0❺
  prolymphocytic (M9631/3) 200.1❺
  reticulum cell (M9640/3) 200.0❺
Lymphostasis 457.8
Lypemania (*see also* Melancholia) 296.2❺
Lyssa 071

M

Macacus ear 744.29
Maceration
  fetus (cause not stated) 779.9
  wet feet, tropical (syndrome) 991.4
Machado-Joseph disease 334.8
Machupo virus hemorrhagic fever 078.7
Macleod's syndrome (abnormal transradiancy, one lung) 492.8
Macrocephalia, macrocephaly 756.0
Macrocheilia (congenital) 744.81
Macrochilia (congenital) 744.81
Macrocolon (congenital) 751.3
Macrocornea 743.41
  associated with buphthalmos 743.22
Macrocytic – *see* condition
Macrocytosis 289.89
Macrodactylia, macrodactylism (fingers) (thumbs) 755.57
  toes 755.65
Macrodontia 520.2
Macroencephaly 742.4
Macrogenia 524.05
Macrogenitosomia (female) (male) (praecox) 255.2
Macrogingivae 523.8
Macroglobulinemia (essential) (idiopathic) (monoclonal) (primary) (syndrome) (Waldenström's) 273.3
Macroglossia (congenital) 750.15
  acquired 529.8
Macrognathia, macrognathism (congenital) 524.00
  mandibular 524.02
    alveolar 524.72
  maxillary 524.01
    alveolar 524.71
Macrogyria (congenital) 742.4
Macrohydrocephalus (*see also* Hydrocephalus) 331.4
Macromastia (*see also* Hypertrophy, breast) 611.1
Macrophage activation syndrome 288.4
Macropsia 368.14
Macrosigmoid 564.7
  congenital 751.3
Macrospondylitis, acromegalic 253.0
Macrostomia (congenital) 744.83
Macrotia (external ear) (congenital) 744.22
Macula
  cornea, corneal
    congenital 743.43
      interfering with vision 743.42
    interfering with central vision 371.03
    not interfering with central vision 371.02
  degeneration (*see also* Degeneration, macula) 362.50
    hereditary (*see also* Dystrophy, retina) 362.70
  edema, cystoid 362.53
Maculae ceruleae 132.1
Macules and papules 709.8
Maculopathy, toxic 362.55
Madarosis 374.55
Madelung's
  deformity (radius) 755.54
  disease (lipomatosis) 272.8
  lipomatosis 272.8
Madness (*see also* Psychosis) 298.9
  myxedema (acute) 293.0
    subacute 293.1
Madura
  disease (actinomycotic) 039.9
    mycotic 117.4
  foot (actinomycotic) 039.4
    mycotic 117.4
Maduromycosis (actinomycotic) 039.9
  mycotic 117.4
Maffucci's syndrome (dyschondroplasia with hemangiomas) 756.4
Magenblase syndrome 306.4
Main en griffe (acquired) 736.06
  congenital 755.59
Maintenance
  chemotherapy regimen or treatment V58.11
  dialysis regimen or treatment
    extracorporeal (renal) V56.0
    peritoneal V56.8
    renal V56.0
  drug therapy or regimen
    chemotherapy, antineoplastic V58.11
    immunotherapy, antineoplastic V58.12
  external fixation NEC V54.89
  radiotherapy V58.0
  traction NEC V54.89
Majocchi's
  disease (purpura annularis telangiectodes) 709.1
  granuloma 110.6
Major – *see* condition
Mal
  cerebral (idiopathic) (*see also* Epilepsy) 345.9❺
  comital (*see also* Epilepsy) 345.9❺
  de los pintos (*see also* Pinta) 103.9
  de Meleda 757.39
  de mer 994.6
  lie – *see* Presentation, fetal
  perforant (*see also* Ulcer, lower extremity) 707.15
Malabar itch 110.9
  beard 110.0
  foot 110.4
  scalp 110.0
Malabsorption 579.9
  calcium 579.8
  carbohydrate 579.8
  disaccharide 271.3
  drug-induced 579.8
  due to bacterial overgrowth 579.8
  fat 579.8
  folate, congenital 281.2
  galactose 271.1
  glucose-galactose (congenital) 271.3
  intestinal 579.9
  isomaltose 271.3
  lactose (hereditary) 271.3
  methionine 270.4
  monosaccharide 271.8
  postgastrectomy 579.3
  postsurgical 579.3
  protein 579.8
  sucrose (-isomaltose) (congenital) 271.3
  syndrome 579.9
    postgastrectomy 579.3
    postsurgical 579.3

- **Malacia, bone** 268.2
  - juvenile (*see also* Rickets) 268.0
  - Kienböck's (juvenile) (lunate) (wrist) 732.3
    - adult 732.8
- **Malacoplakia**
  - bladder 596.8
  - colon 569.89
  - pelvis (kidney) 593.89
  - ureter 593.89
  - urethra 599.84
- **Malacosteon** 268.2
  - juvenile (*see also* Rickets) 268.0
- **Maladaptation** – *see* Maladjustment
- **Maladie de Roger** 745.4
- **Maladjustment**
  - conjugal V61.10
    - involving divorce or estrangement V61.0
  - educational V62.3
  - family V61.9
    - specified circumstance NEC V61.8
  - marital V61.10
    - involving divorce or estrangement V61.0
  - occupational V62.2
  - simple, adult (*see also* Reaction, adjustment) 309.9
  - situational acute (*see also* Reaction, adjustment) 309.9
  - social V62.4
- **Malaise** 780.79
- **Malakoplakia** – *see* Malacoplakia
- **Malaria, malarial** (fever) 084.6
  - algid 084.9
  - any type, with
    - algid malaria 084.9
    - blackwater fever 084.8
    - fever
      - blackwater 084.8
      - hemoglobinuric (bilious) 084.8
    - hemoglobinuria, malarial 084.8
    - hepatitis 084.9 *[573.2]*
    - nephrosis 084.9 *[581.81]*
    - pernicious complication NEC 084.9
      - cardiac 084.9
      - cerebral 084.9
  - cardiac 084.9
  - carrier (suspected) of V02.9
  - cerebral 084.9
  - complicating pregnancy, childbirth, or puerperium 647.4❺
  - congenital 771.2
  - congestion, congestive 084.6
    - brain 084.9
  - continued 084.0
  - estivo-autumnal 084.0
  - falciparum (malignant tertian) 084.0
  - hematinuria 084.8
  - hematuria 084.8
  - hemoglobinuria 084.8
  - hemorrhagic 084.6
  - induced (therapeutically) 084.7
    - accidental – *see* Malaria, by type
  - liver 084.9 *[573.2]*
  - malariae (quartan) 084.2
  - malignant (tertian) 084.0
  - mixed infections 084.5
  - monkey 084.4
  - ovale 084.3
  - pernicious, acute 084.0
  - Plasmodium, P.
    - falciparum 084.0
    - malariae 084.2
    - ovale 084.3
    - vivax 084.1
  - quartan 084.2
  - quotidian 084.0
  - recurrent 084.6
    - induced (therapeutically) 084.7
      - accidental – *see* Malaria, by type
  - remittent 084.6
  - specified types NEC 084.4
  - spleen 084.6
  - subtertian 084.0
  - tertian (benign) 084.1
    - malignant 084.0
  - tropical 084.0
  - typhoid 084.6
  - vivax (benign tertian) 084.1
- **Malassez's disease** (testicular cyst) 608.89
- **Malassimilation** 579.9
- **Maldescent, testis** 752.51
- **Maldevelopment** – *see also* Anomaly, by site
  - brain 742.9
  - colon 751.5
  - hip (joint) 755.63
    - congenital dislocation (*see also* Dislocation, hip, congenital) 754.30
  - mastoid process 756.0
  - middle ear, except ossicles 744.03
    - ossicles 744.04
  - newborn (not malformation) 764.9❺
  - ossicles, ear 744.04
  - spine 756.10
  - toe 755.66
- **Male type pelvis** 755.69
  - with disproportion (fetopelvic) 653.2❺
    - affecting fetus or newborn 763.1
    - causing obstructed labor 660.1❺
      - affecting fetus or newborn 763.1
- **Malformation** (congenital) – *see also* Anomaly
  - bone 756.9
  - bursa 756.9
  - Chiari
    - type I 348.4
    - type II (*see also* Spina bifida) 741.0❺
    - type III 742.0
    - type IV 742.2
  - circulatory system NEC 747.9
    - specified type NEC 747.89
  - cochlea 744.05
  - digestive system NEC 751.9
    - lower 751.5
    - specified type NEC 751.8
    - upper 750.9
  - eye 743.9
  - gum 750.9
  - heart NEC 746.9
    - specified type NEC 746.89
    - valve 746.9
  - internal ear 744.05
  - joint NEC 755.9
    - specified type NEC 755.8
  - Mondini's (congenital) (malformation, cochlea) 744.05
  - muscle 756.9
  - nervous system (central) 742.9
  - pelvic organs or tissues
    - in pregnancy or childbirth 654.9❺
      - affecting fetus or newborn 763.89
      - causing obstructed labor 660.2❺
        - affecting fetus or newborn 763.1
  - placenta (*see also* Placenta, abnormal) 656.7❺
  - respiratory organs 748.9
    - specified type NEC 748.8
  - Rieger's 743.44
  - sense organs NEC 742.9
    - specified type NEC 742.8
  - skin 757.9
    - specified type NEC 757.8
  - spinal cord 742.9
  - teeth, tooth NEC 520.9
  - tendon 756.9
  - throat 750.9
  - umbilical cord (complicating delivery) 663.9❺
    - affecting fetus or newborn 762.6
  - umbilicus 759.9
  - urinary system NEC 753.9
    - specified type NEC 753.8
- **Malfunction** – *see also* Dysfunction
  - arterial graft 996.1
  - cardiac pacemaker 996.01
  - catheter device – *see* Complications, mechanical, catheter
  - colostomy 569.62
    - valve 569.62
  - cystostomy 997.5
  - device, implant, or graft NEC – *see* Complications, mechanical
  - enteric stoma 569.62
  - enterostomy 569.62
  - esophagostomy 530.87
  - gastroenteric 536.8
  - gastrostomy 536.42
  - ileostomy
    - valve 569.62
  - nephrostomy 997.5
  - pacemaker – *see* Complications, mechanical, pacemaker
  - prosthetic device, internal – *see* Complications, mechanical
  - tracheostomy 519.02
- **Malfunction** – *continued*
  - valve
    - colostomy 569.62
    - ileostomy 569.62
  - vascular graft or shunt 996.1
- **Malgaigne's fracture** (closed) 808.43
  - open 808.53
- **Malherbe's**
  - calcifying epithelioma (M8110/0) – *see* Neoplasm, skin, benign
  - tumor (M8110/0) – *see* Neoplasm, skin, benign
- **Malibu disease** 919.8
  - infected 919.9
- **Malignancy** (M8000/3) – *see* Neoplasm, by site, malignant
- **Malignant** – *see* condition
- **Malingerer, malingering** V65.2
- **Mallet, finger** (acquired) 736.1
  - congenital 755.59
  - late effect of rickets 268.1
- **Malleus** 024
- **Mallory's bodies** 034.1
- **Mallory-Weiss syndrome** 530.7
- **Malnutrition** (calorie) 263.9
  - complicating pregnancy 648.9❺
  - degree
    - first 263.1
    - second 263.0
    - third 262
    - mild 263.1
    - moderate 263.0
    - severe 261
      - protein-calorie 262
  - fetus 764.2❺
    - "light-for-dates" 764.1❺
  - following gastrointestinal surgery 579.3
  - intrauterine or fetal 764.2❺
    - fetus or infant "light-for-dates" 764.1❺
  - lack of care, or neglect (child) (infant) 995.52
    - adult 995.84
  - malignant 260
  - mild 263.1
  - moderate 263.0
  - protein 260
  - protein-calorie 263.9
    - severe 262
    - specified type NEC 263.8
  - severe 261
    - protein-calorie NEC 262
- **Malocclusion** (teeth) 524.4
  - Angle's class I 524.21
  - Angle's class II 524.22
  - Angle's class III 524.23
  - due to
    - abnormal swallowing 524.59
    - accessory teeth (causing crowding) 524.31
    - dentofacial abnormality NEC 524.89
    - impacted teeth (causing crowding) 520.6
    - missing teeth 524.30
    - mouth breathing 524.59
    - sleep postures 524.59
    - supernumerary teeth (causing crowding) 524.31
    - thumb sucking 524.59
    - tongue, lip, or finger habits 524.59
  - temporomandibular (joint) 524.69
- **Malposition**
  - cardiac apex (congenital) 746.87
  - cervix – *see* Malposition, uterus
  - congenital
    - adrenal (gland) 759.1
    - alimentary tract 751.8
      - lower 751.5
      - upper 750.8
    - aorta 747.21
    - appendix 751.5
    - arterial trunk 747.29
    - artery (peripheral) NEC (*see also* Malposition, congenital, peripheral vascular system) 747.60
      - coronary 746.85
      - pulmonary 747.3
    - auditory canal 744.29
      - causing impairment of hearing 744.02
    - auricle (ear) 744.29
      - causing impairment of hearing 744.02
      - cervical 744.43
    - biliary duct or passage 751.69
    - bladder (mucosa) 753.8
      - exteriorized or extroverted 753.5

- **Malposition** – *continued*
  - congenital – *continued*
    - brachial plexus 742.8
    - brain tissue 742.4
    - breast 757.6
    - bronchus 748.3
    - cardiac apex 746.87
    - cecum 751.5
    - clavicle 755.51
    - colon 751.5
    - digestive organ or tract NEC 751.8
      - lower 751.5
      - upper 750.8
    - ear (auricle) (external) 744.29
      - ossicles 744.04
    - endocrine (gland) NEC 759.2
    - epiglottis 748.3
    - Eustachian tube 744.24
    - eye 743.8
    - facial features 744.89
    - fallopian tube 752.19
    - finger(s) 755.59
      - supernumerary 755.01
    - foot 755.67
    - gallbladder 751.69
    - gastrointestinal tract 751.8
    - genitalia, genital organ(s) or tract
      - female 752.89
        - external 752.49
        - internal NEC 752.89
      - male 752.89
        - penis 752.69
        - scrotal transposition 752.81
    - glottis 748.3
    - hand 755.59
    - heart 746.87
      - dextrocardia 746.87
        - with complete transposition of viscera 759.3
    - hepatic duct 751.69
    - hip (joint) (*see also* Dislocation, hip, congenital) 754.30
    - intestine (large) (small) 751.5
      - with anomalous adhesions, fixation, or malrotation 751.4
    - joint NEC 755.8
    - kidney 753.3
    - larynx 748.3
    - limb 755.8
      - lower 755.69
      - upper 755.59
    - liver 751.69
    - lung (lobe) 748.69
    - nail(s) 757.5
    - nerve 742.8
    - nervous system NEC 742.8
    - nose, nasal (septum) 748.1
    - organ or site NEC – *see* Anomaly, specified type NEC, by site
    - ovary 752.0
    - pancreas 751.7
    - parathyroid (gland) 759.2
    - patella 755.64
    - peripheral vascular system 747.60
      - gastrointestinal 747.61
      - lower limb 747.64
      - renal 747.62
      - specified NEC 747.69
      - spinal 747.82
      - upper limb 747.63
    - pituitary (gland) 759.2
    - respiratory organ or system NEC 748.9
    - rib (cage) 756.3
      - supernumerary in cervical region 756.2
    - scapula 755.59
    - shoulder 755.59
    - spinal cord 742.59
    - spine 756.19
    - spleen 759.0
    - sternum 756.3
    - stomach 750.7
    - symphysis pubis 755.69
    - testis (undescended)752.51
    - thymus (gland) 759.2
    - thyroid (gland) (tissue) 759.2
      - cartilage 748.3
    - toe(s) 755.66
      - supernumerary 755.02
    - tongue 750.19
    - trachea 748.3
    - uterus 752.3
- **Malposition** – *continued*
  - congenital – *continued*
    - vein(s) (peripheral) NEC (*see also* Malposition, congenital, peripheral vascular system) 747.60
      - great 747.49
      - portal 747.49
      - pulmonary 747.49
    - vena cava (inferior) (superior) 747.49
  - device, implant, or graft – *see* Complications, mechanical
  - fetus NEC (*see also* Presentation, fetal) 652.9❺
    - with successful version 652.1❺
    - affecting fetus or newborn 763.1
    - before labor, affecting fetus or newborn 761.7
    - causing obstructed labor 660.0❺
    - in multiple gestation (one fetus or more) 652.6❺
      - with locking 660.5❺
      - causing obstructed labor 660.0❺
  - gallbladder (*see also* Disease, gallbladder) 575.8
  - gastrointestinal tract 569.89
    - congenital 751.8
  - heart (*see also* Malposition, congenital, heart) 746.87
  - intestine 569.89
    - congenital 751.5
  - pelvic organs or tissues
    - in pregnancy or childbirth 654.4❺
      - affecting fetus or newborn 763.89
      - causing obstructed labor 660.2❺
        - affecting fetus or newborn 763.1
  - placenta – *see* Placenta, previa
  - stomach 537.89
    - congenital 750.7
  - tooth, teeth 524.30
    - with impaction 520.6
  - uterus (acquired) (acute) (adherent) (any degree) (asymptomatic) (postinfectional) (postpartal, old) 621.6
    - anteflexion or anteversion (*see also* Anteversion, uterus) 621.6
    - congenital 752.3
    - flexion 621.6
      - lateral (*see also* Lateroversion, uterus) 621.6
    - in pregnancy or childbirth 654.4❺
      - affecting fetus or newborn 763.89
      - causing obstructed labor 660.2❺
        - affecting fetus or newborn 763.1
    - inversion 621.6
    - lateral (flexion) (version) (*see also* Lateroversion, uterus) 621.6
    - lateroflexion (*see also* Lateroversion, uterus) 621.6
    - lateroversion (*see also* Lateroversion, uterus) 621.6
    - retroflexion or retroversion (*see also* Retroversion, uterus) 621.6
- **Malposture** 729.9
- **Malpresentation, fetus** (*see also* Presentation, fetal) 652.9❺
- **Malrotation**
  - cecum 751.4
  - colon 751.4
  - intestine 751.4
  - kidney 753.3
- **MALT** (mucosa associated lymphoid tissue) 200.3❺ ●
- **Malta fever** (*see also* Brucellosis) 023.9
- **Maltosuria** 271.3
- **Maltreatment** (of)
  - adult 995.80
    - emotional 995.82
    - multiple forms 995.85
    - neglect (nutritional) 995.84
    - physical 995.81
    - psychological 995.82
    - sexual 995.83
  - child 995.50
    - emotional 995.51
    - multiple forms 995.59
    - neglect (nutritional) 995.52
    - physical 995.54
      - shaken infant syndrome 995.55
    - psychological 995.51
    - sexual 995.53
  - spouse (*see also* Maltreatment, adult) 995.80
- **Malt workers' lung** 495.4
- **Malum coxae senilis** 715.25
- **Malunion, fracture** 733.81
- **Mammillitis** (*see also* Mastitis) 611.0
  - puerperal, postpartum 675.2❺
- **Mammitis** (*see also* Mastitis) 611.0
  - puerperal, postpartum 675.2❺
- **Mammographic**
  - calcification 793.89
  - calculus 793.89
  - microcalcification 793.81
- **Mammoplasia** 611.1
- **Management**
  - contraceptive V25.9
    - specified type NEC V25.8
  - procreative V26.9
    - specified type NEC V26.89 ▲
- **Mangled** NEC (*see also* nature and site of injury) 959.9
- **Mania** (monopolar) (*see also* Psychosis, affective) 296.0❺
  - alcoholic (acute) (chronic) 291.9
  - Bell's – *see* Mania, chronic
  - chronic 296.0❺
    - recurrent episode 296.1❺
    - single episode 296.0❺
  - compulsive 300.3
  - delirious (acute) 296.0❺
    - recurrent episode 296.1❺
    - single episode 296.0❺
  - epileptic (*see also* Epilepsy) 345.4❺
  - hysterical 300.10
  - inhibited 296.89
  - puerperal (after delivery) 296.0❺
    - recurrent episode 296.1❺
    - single episode 296.0❺
  - recurrent episode 296.1❺
  - senile 290.8
  - single episode 296.0❺
  - stupor 296.89
  - stuporous 296.89
  - unproductive 296.89
- **Manic-depressive insanity, psychosis, reaction, or syndrome** (*see also* Psychosis, affective) 296.80
  - circular (alternating) 296.7
    - currently
      - depressed 296.5❺
      - episode unspecified 296.7
      - hypomanic, previously depressed 296.4❺
      - manic 296.4❺
    - mixed 296.6❺
  - depressed (type), depressive 296.2❺
    - atypical 296.82
    - recurrent episode 296.3❺
    - single episode 296.2❺
  - hypomanic 296.0❺
    - recurrent episode 296.1❺
    - single episode 296.0❺
  - manic 296.0❺
    - atypical 296.81
    - recurrent episode 296.1❺
    - single episode 296.0❺
  - mixed NEC 296.89
  - perplexed 296.89
  - stuporous 296.89
- **Manifestations, rheumatoid**
  - lungs 714.81
  - pannus – *see* Arthritis, rheumatoid
  - subcutaneous nodules – *see* Arthritis, rheumatoid
- **Mankowsky's syndrome** (familial dysplastic osteopathy) 731.2
- **Mannoheptulosuria** 271.8
- **Mannosidosis** 271.8
- **Manson's**
  - disease (schistosomiasis) 120.1
  - pyosis (pemphigus contagiosus) 684
  - schistosomiasis 120.1
- **Mansonellosis** 125.5
- **Manual** – *see* condition
- **Maple bark disease** 495.6
- **Maple bark-strippers' lung** 495.6
- **Maple syrup** (urine) **disease or syndrome** 270.3
- **Marable's syndrome** (celiac artery compression) 447.4
- **Marasmus** 261
  - brain 331.9
  - due to malnutrition 261
  - intestinal 569.89
  - nutritional 261
  - senile 797

Marasmus – *continued*
- tuberculous NEC (*see also* Tuberculosis) 011.9❺

Marble
- bones 756.52
- skin 782.61

Marburg disease (virus) 078.89

March
- foot 733.94
- hemoglobinuria 283.2

Marchand multiple nodular hyperplasia (liver) 571.5

Marchesani (-Weill) **syndrome** (brachymorphism and ectopia lentis) 759.89

Marchiafava (-Bignami) **disease or syndrome** 341.8

Marchiafava-Micheli syndrome (paroxysmal nocturnal hemoglobinuria) 283.2

Marcus Gunn's syndrome (jaw-winking syndrome) 742.8

Marfan's
- congenital syphilis 090.49
- disease 090.49
- syndrome (arachnodactyly) 759.82
  - meaning congenital syphilis 090.49
    - with luxation of lens 090.49 *[379.32]*

Marginal
- implantation, placenta – *see* Placenta, previa
- placenta – *see* Placenta, previa
- sinus (hemorrhage) (rupture) 641.2❺
  - affecting fetus or newborn 762.1

Marie's
- cerebellar ataxia 334.2
- syndrome (acromegaly) 253.0

Marie-Bamberger disease or syndrome (hypertrophic) (pulmonary) (secondary) 731.2
- idiopathic (acropachyderma) 757.39
- primary (acropachyderma) 757.39

Marie-Charcôt-Tooth neuropathic atrophy, muscle 356.1

Marie-Strümpell arthritis or disease (ankylosing spondylitis) 720.0

Marihuana, marijuana
- abuse (*see also* Abuse, drugs, nondependent) 305.2❺
- dependence (*see also* Dependence) 304.3❺

Marion's disease (bladder neck obstruction) 596.0

Marital conflict V61.10

Mark
- port wine 757.32
- raspberry 757.32
- strawberry 757.32
- stretch 701.3
- tattoo 709.09

Maroteaux-Lamy syndrome (mucopolysaccharidosis VI) 277.5

Marriage license examination V70.3

Marrow (bone)
- arrest 284.9
- megakaryocytic 287.30
- poor function 289.9

Marseilles fever 082.1

Marsh's disease (exophthalmic goiter) 242.0❺

Marshall's (hidrotic) ectodermal dysplasia 757.31

Marsh fever (*see also* Malaria) 084.6

Martin's disease 715.27

Martin-Albright syndrome (pseudohypoparathyroidism) 275.49

Martorell-Fabre syndrome (pulseless disease) 446.7

Masculinization, female, with adrenal hyperplasia 255.2

Masculinovoblastoma (M8670/0) 220

Masochism 302.83

Masons' lung 502

Mass
- abdominal 789.3❺
- anus 787.99
- bone 733.90
- breast 611.72
- cheek 784.2
- chest 786.6
- cystic – *see* Cyst
- ear 388.8
- epigastric 789.3❺
- eye 379.92
- female genital organ 625.8
- gum 784.2
- head 784.2
- intracranial 784.2

Mass – *continued*
- joint 719.60
  - ankle 719.67
  - elbow 719.62
  - foot 719.67
  - hand 719.64
  - hip 719.65
  - knee 719.66
  - multiple sites 719.69
  - pelvic region 719.65
  - shoulder (region) 719.61
  - specified site NEC 719.68
  - wrist 719.63
- kidney (*see also* Disease, kidney) 593.9
- lung 786.6
- lymph node 785.6
- malignant (M8000/3) – *see* Neoplasm, by site, malignant
- mediastinal 786.6
- mouth 784.2
- muscle (limb) 729.89
- neck 784.2
- nose or sinus 784.2
- palate 784.2
- pelvis, pelvic 789.3❺
- penis 607.89
- perineum 625.8
- rectum 787.99
- scrotum 608.89
- skin 782.2
- specified organ NEC – *see* Disease of specified organ or site
- splenic 789.2
- substernal 786.6
  - thyroid (*see also* Goiter) 240.9
- superficial (localized) 782.2
- testes 608.89
- throat 784.2
- tongue 784.2
- umbilicus 789.3❺
- uterus 625.8
- vagina 625.8
- vulva 625.8

Massive – *see* condition

Mastalgia 611.71
- psychogenic 307.89

Mast cell
- disease 757.33
  - systemic (M9741/3) 202.6❺
- leukemia (M9900/3) 207.8❺
- sarcoma (M9742/3) 202.6❺
- tumor (M9740/1) 238.5
  - malignant (M9740/3) 202.6❺

Masters-Allen syndrome 620.6

Mastitis (acute) (adolescent) (diffuse) (interstitial) (lobular) (nonpuerperal) (nonsuppurative) (parenchymatous) (phlegmonous) (simple) (subacute) (suppurative) 611.0
- chronic (cystic) (fibrocystic) 610.1
- cystic 610.1
  - Schimmelbusch's type 610.1
- fibrocystic 610.1
- infective 611.0
- lactational 675.2❺
- lymphangitis 611.0
- neonatal (noninfective) 778.7
  - infective 771.5
- periductal 610.4
- plasma cell 610.4
- puerperal, postpartum, (interstitial) (nonpurulent) (parenchymatous) 675.2❺
  - purulent 675.1❺
  - stagnation 676.2❺
- puerperalis 675.2❺
- retromammary 611.0
  - puerperal, postpartum 675.1❺
- submammary 611.0
  - puerperal, postpartum 675.1❺

Mastocytoma (M9740/1) 238.5
- malignant (M9740/3) 202.6❺

Mastocytosis 757.33
- malignant (M9741/3) 202.6❺
- systemic (M9741/3) 202.6❺

Mastodynia 611.71
- psychogenic 307.89

Mastoid – *see* condition

Mastoidalgia (*see also* Otalgia) 388.70

Mastoiditis (coalescent) (hemorrhagic) (pneumococcal) (streptococcal) (suppurative) 383.9
- acute or subacute 383.00
  - with
    - Gradenigo's syndrome 383.02
    - petrositis 383.02
    - specified complication NEC 383.02
    - subperiosteal abscess 383.01
- chronic (necrotic) (recurrent) 383.1
- tuberculous (*see also* Tuberculosis) 015.6❺

Mastopathy, mastopathia 611.9
- chronica cystica 610.1
- diffuse cystic 610.1
- estrogenic 611.8
- ovarian origin 611.8

Mastoplasia 611.1

Masturbation 307.9

Maternal condition, affecting fetus or newborn
- acute yellow atrophy of liver 760.8
- albuminuria 760.1
- anesthesia or analgesia 763.5
- blood loss 762.1
- chorioamnionitis 762.7
- circulatory disease, chronic (conditions classifiable to 390-459, 745-747) 760.3
- congenital heart disease (conditions classifiable to 745-746) 760.3
- cortical necrosis of kidney 760.1
- death 761.6
- diabetes mellitus 775.0
  - manifest diabetes in the infant 775.1
- disease NEC 760.9
  - circulatory system, chronic (conditions classifiable to 390-459, 745-747) 760.3
  - genitourinary system (conditions classifiable to 580-599) 760.1
  - respiratory (conditions classifiable to 490-519, 748) 760.3
- eclampsia 760.0
- hemorrhage NEC 762.1
- hepatitis acute, malignant, or subacute 760.8
- hyperemesis (gravidarum) 761.8
- hypertension (arising during pregnancy) (conditions classifiable to 642) 760.0
- infection
  - disease classifiable to 001-136 760.2
  - genital tract NEC 760.8
  - urinary tract 760.1
- influenza 760.2
  - manifest influenza in the infant 771.2
- injury (conditions classifiable to 800-996) 760.5
- malaria 760.2
  - manifest malaria in infant or fetus 771.2
- malnutrition 760.4
- necrosis of liver 760.8
- nephritis (conditions classifiable to 580-583) 760.1
- nephrosis (conditions classifiable to 581) 760.1
- noxious substance transmitted via breast milk or placenta 760.70
  - alcohol 760.71
  - anticonvulsants 760.77
  - antifungals 760.74
  - anti-infective agents 760.74
  - antimetabolics 760.78
  - cocaine 760.75
  - "crack" 760.75
  - diethylstilbestrol [DES] 760.76
  - hallucinogenic agents 760.73
  - medicinal agents NEC 760.79
  - narcotics 760.72
  - obstetric anesthetic or analgesic drug 760.72
  - specified agent NEC 760.79
- nutritional disorder (conditions classifiable to 260-269) 760.4
- operation unrelated to current delivery 760.6
- pre-eclampsia 760.0
- pyelitis or pyelonephritis, arising during pregnancy (conditions classifiable to 590) 760.1
- renal disease or failure 760.1
- respiratory disease, chronic (conditions classifiable to 490-519, 748) 760.3
- rheumatic heart disease (chronic) (conditions classifiable to 393-398) 760.3
- rubella (conditions classifiable to 056) 760.2
  - manifest rubella in the infant or fetus 771.0
- surgery unrelated to current delivery 760.6
  - to uterus or pelvic organs 763.89

Marasmus – Maternal condition, affecting fetus or newborn

Maternal condition, affecting fetus or newborn – Melanoma

Melanoma – *continued*
- auditory canal (external) 172.2
- auricle (ear) 172.2
- auricular canal (external) 172.2
- axilla 172.5
- axillary fold 172.5
- back 172.5
- balloon cell (M8722/3) – *see* Melanoma, by site
- benign (M8720/0) – *see* Neoplasm, skin, benign
- breast (female) (male) 172.5
- brow 172.3
- buttock 172.5
- canthus (eye) 172.1
- cheek (external) 172.3
- chest wall 172.5
- chin 172.3
- choroid 190.6
- conjunctiva 190.3
- ear (external) 172.2
- epithelioid cell (M8771/3) – *see also* Melanoma, by site
  - and spindle cell, mixed (M8775/3) – *see* Melanoma, by site
- external meatus (ear) 172.2
- eye 190.9
- eyebrow 172.3
- eyelid (lower) (upper) 172.1
- face NEC 172.3
- female genital organ (external) NEC 184.4
- finger 172.6
- flank 172.5
- foot 172.7
- forearm 172.6
- forehead 172.3
- foreskin 187.1
- gluteal region 172.5
- groin 172.5
- hand 172.6
- heel 172.7
- helix 172.2
- hip 172.7
- in
  - giant pigmented nevus (M8761/3) – *see* Melanoma, by site
  - Hutchinson's melanotic freckle (M8742/3) – *see* Melanoma, by site
  - junctional nevus (M8740/3) – *see* Melanoma, by site
  - precancerous melanosis (M8741/3) – *see* Melanoma, by site
- interscapular region 172.5
- iris 190.0
- jaw 172.3
- juvenile (M8770/0) – *see* Neoplasm, skin, benign
- knee 172.7
- labium
  - majus 184.1
  - minus 184.2
- lacrimal gland 190.2
- leg 172.7
- lip (lower) (upper) 172.0
- liver 197.7
- lower limb NEC 172.7
- male genital organ (external) NEC 187.9
- meatus, acoustic (external) 172.2
- meibomian gland 172.1
- metastatic
  - of or from specified site – *see* Melanoma, by site
  - site not of skin – *see* Neoplasm, by site, malignant, secondary
  - to specified site – *see* Neoplasm, by site, malignant, secondary
  - unspecified site 172.9
- nail 172.9
  - finger 172.6
  - toe 172.7
- neck 172.4
- nodular (M8721/3) – *see* Melanoma, by site
- nose, external 172.3
- orbit 190.1
- penis 187.4
- perianal skin 172.5
- perineum 172.5
- pinna 172.2
- popliteal (fossa) (space) 172.7
- prepuce 187.1
- pubes 172.5
- pudendum 184.4
- retina 190.5
- scalp 172.4
- scrotum 187.7

Melanoma – *continued*
- septum nasal (skin) 172.3
- shoulder 172.6
- skin NEC 172.8
- spindle cell (M8772/3) – *see also* Melanoma, by site
  - type A (M8773/3) 190.0
  - type B (M8774/3) 190.0
- submammary fold 172.5
- superficial spreading (M8743/3) – *see* Melanoma, by site
- temple 172.3
- thigh 172.7
- toe 172.7
- trunk NEC 172.5
- umbilicus 172.5
- upper limb NEC 172.6
- vagina vault 184.0
- vulva 184.4

Melanoplakia 528.9

Melanosarcoma (M8720/3) – *see also* Melanoma
- epithelioid cell (M8771/3) – *see* Melanoma

Melanosis 709.09
- Addisonian (primary adrenal insufficiency) 255.41 ▲
  - tuberculous (*see also* Tuberculosis) 017.6❺
- adrenal 255.41 ▲
- colon 569.89
- conjunctiva 372.55
  - congenital 743.49
- corii degenerativa 757.33
- cornea (presenile) (senile) 371.12
  - congenital 743.43
    - interfering with vision 743.42
  - prenatal 743.43
    - interfering with vision 743.42
- eye 372.55
  - congenital 743.49
- jute spinners' 709.09
- lenticularis progressiva 757.33
- liver 573.8
- precancerous (M8741/2) – *see also* Neoplasm, skin, in situ
  - malignant melanoma in (M8741/3) – *see* Melanoma
- Riehl's 709.09
- sclera 379.19
  - congenital 743.47
- suprarenal 255.41 ▲
- tar 709.09
- toxic 709.09

Melanuria 791.9

MELAS syndrome (mitochondrial encephalopathy, lactic acidosis and stroke-like episodes) 277.87

Melasma 709.09
- adrenal (gland) 255.41 ▲
- suprarenal (gland) 255.41 ▲

Melena 578.1
- due to
  - swallowed maternal blood 777.3
  - ulcer – *see* Ulcer, by site, with hemorrhage
- newborn 772.4
  - due to swallowed maternal blood 777.3

Meleney's
- gangrene (cutaneous) 686.09
- ulcer (chronic undermining) 686.09

Melioidosis 025

Melitensis, febris 023.0

Melitococcosis 023.0

Melkersson (-Rosenthal) **syndrome** 351.8

Mellitus, diabetes – *see* Diabetes

Melorheostosis (bone) (leri) 733.99

Meloschisis 744.83

Melotia 744.29

Membrana
- capsularis lentis posterior 743.39
- epipapillaris 743.57

Membranacea placenta – *see* Placenta, abnormal

Membranaceous uterus 621.8

Membrane, membranous – *see also* condition
- folds, congenital – *see* Web
- Jackson's 751.4
- over face (causing asphyxia), fetus or newborn 768.9
- premature rupture – *see* Rupture, membranes, premature
- pupillary 364.74
  - persistent 743.46

Membrane, membranous – *continued*
- retained (complicating delivery) (with hemorrhage) 666.2❺
  - without hemorrhage 667.1❺
- secondary (eye) 366.50
- unruptured (causing asphyxia) 768.9
- vitreous humor 379.25

Membranitis, fetal 658.4❺
- affecting fetus or newborn 762.7

Memory disturbance, loss or lack (*see also* Amnesia) 780.93
- mild, following organic brain damage 310.1

MEN (multiple endocrine neoplasia) **syndromes** ●
- type I 258.01 ●
- type IIA 258.02 ●
- type IIB 258.03 ●

Menadione (vitamin K) **deficiency** 269.0

Menarche, precocious 259.1

Mendacity, pathologic 301.7

Mende's syndrome (ptosis-epicanthus) 270.2

Mendelson's syndrome (resulting from a procedure) 997.3
- obstetric 668.0❺

Ménétrier's disease or syndrome (hypertrophic gastritis) 535.2❺

Ménière's disease, syndrome, or vertigo 386.00
- cochlear 386.02
- cochleovestibular 386.01
- inactive 386.04
- in remission 386.04
- vestibular 386.03

Meninges, meningeal – *see* condition

Meningioma (M9530/0) – *see also* Neoplasm, meninges, benign
- angioblastic (M9535/0) – *see* Neoplasm, meninges, benign
- angiomatous (M9534/0) – *see* Neoplasm, meninges, benign
- endotheliomatous (M9531/0) – *see* Neoplasm, meninges, benign
- fibroblastic (M9532/0) – *see* Neoplasm, meninges, benign
- fibrous (M9532/0) – *see* Neoplasm, meninges, benign
- hemangioblastic (M9535/0) – *see* Neoplasm, meninges, benign
- hemangiopericytic (M9536/0) – *see* Neoplasm, meninges, benign
- malignant (M9530/3) – *see* Neoplasm, meninges, malignant
- meningiothelial (M9531/0) – *see* Neoplasm, meninges, benign
- meningotheliomatous (M9531/0) – *see* Neoplasm, meninges, benign
- mixed (M9537/0) – *see* Neoplasm, meninges, benign
- multiple (M9530/1) 237.6
- papillary (M9538/1) 237.6
- psammomatous (M9533/0) – *see* Neoplasm, meninges, benign
- syncytial (M9531/0) – *see* Neoplasm, meninges, benign
- transitional (M9537/0) – *see* Neoplasm, meninges, benign

Meningiomatosis (diffuse) (M9530/1) 237.6

Meningism (*see also* Meningismus) 781.6

Meningismus (infectional) (pneumococcal) 781.6
- due to serum or vaccine 997.09 *[321.8]*
- influenzal NEC 487.8

Meningitis (basal) (basic) (basilar) (brain) (cerebral) (cervical) (congestive) (diffuse) (hemorrhagic) (infantile) (membranous) (metastatic) (nonspecific) (pontine) (progressive) (simple) (spinal) (subacute) (sympathetica) (toxic) 322.9
- abacterial NEC (*see also* Meningitis, aseptic) 047.9
- actinomycotic 039.8 *[320.7]*
- adenoviral 049.1
- Aerobacter aerogenes 320.82
- anaerobes (cocci) (gram-negative) (gram-positive) (mixed) (NEC) 320.81
- arbovirus NEC 066.9 *[321.2]*
  - specified type NEC 066.8 *[321.2]*
- aseptic (acute) NEC 047.9
  - adenovirus 049.1
  - Coxsackie virus 047.0
  - due to
    - adenovirus 049.1
    - Coxsackie virus 047.0

Meningitis – *continued*
aseptic – *continued*
due to – *continued*
ECHO virus 047.1
enterovirus 047.9
mumps 072.1
poliovirus (*see also* Poliomyelitis) 045.2❺ *[321.2]*
ECHO virus 047.1
herpes (simplex) virus 054.72
zoster 053.0
leptospiral 100.81
lymphocytic choriomeningitis 049.0
noninfective 322.0
Bacillus pyocyaneus 320.89
bacterial NEC 320.9
anaerobic 320.81
gram-negative 320.82
anaerobic 320.81
Bacteroides (fragilis) (oralis) (melaninogenicus) 320.81
cancerous (M8000/6) 198.4
candidal 112.83
carcinomatous (M8010/6) 198.4
caseous (*see also* Tuberculosis, meninges) 013.0❺
cerebrospinal (acute) (chronic) (diplococcal) (endemic) (epidemic) (fulminant) (infectious) (malignant) (meningococcal) (sporadic) 036.0
carrier (suspected) of V02.59
chronic NEC 322.2
clear cerebrospinal fluid NEC 322.0
Clostridium (haemolyticum) (novyi) NEC 320.81
coccidioidomycosis 114.2
Coxsackie virus 047.0
cryptococcal 117.5 *[321.0]*
diplococcal 036.0
gram-negative 036.0
gram-positive 320.1
Diplococcus pneumoniae 320.1
due to
actinomycosis 039.8 *[320.7]*
adenovirus 049.1
coccidiomycosis 114.2
enterovirus 047.9
specified NEC 047.8
histoplasmosis (*see also* Histoplasmosis) 115.91
Listerosis 027.0 *[320.7]*
Lyme disease 088.81 *[320.7]*
moniliasis 112.83
mumps 072.1
neurosyphilis 094.2
nonbacterial organisms NEC 321.8
oidiomycosis 112.83
poliovirus (*see also* Poliomyelitis) 045.2❺ *[321.2]*
preventive immunization, inoculation, or vaccination 997.09 *[321.8]*
sarcoidosis 135 *[321.4]*
sporotrichosis 117.1 *[321.1]*
syphilis 094.2
acute 091.81
congenital 090.42
secondary 091.81
trypanosomiasis (*see also* Trypanosomiasis) 086.9 *[321.3]*
whooping cough 033.9 *[320.7]*
E. coli 320.82
ECHO virus 047.1
endothelial-leukocytic, benign, recurrent 047.9
Enterobacter aerogenes 320.82
enteroviral 047.9
specified type NEC 047.8
enterovirus 047.9
specified NEC 047.8
eosinophilic 322.1
epidemic NEC 036.0
Escherichia coli (E. coli) 320.82
Eubacterium 320.81
fibrinopurulent NEC 320.9
specified type NEC 320.89
Friedländer (bacillus) 320.82
fungal NEC 117.9 *[321.1]*
Fusobacterium 320.81
gonococcal 098.82
gram-negative bacteria NEC 320.82
anaerobic 320.81
cocci 036.0
specified NEC 320.82
gram-negative cocci NEC 036.0
specified NEC 320.82

Meningitis – *continued*
gram-positive cocci NEC 320.9
H. influenzae 320.0
herpes (simplex) virus 054.72
zoster 053.0
infectious NEC 320.9
influenzal 320.0
Klebsiella pneumoniae 320.82
late effect – *see* Late, effect, meningitis
leptospiral (aseptic) 100.81
Listerella (monocytogenes) 027.0 *[320.7]*
Listeria monocytogenes 027.0 *[320.7]*
lymphocytic (acute) (benign) (serous) 049.0
choriomeningitis virus 049.0
meningococcal (chronic) 036.0
Mima polymorpha 320.82
Mollaret's 047.9
monilial 112.83
mumps (virus) 072.1
mycotic NEC 117.9 *[321.1]*
Neisseria 036.0
neurosyphilis 094.2
nonbacterial NEC (*see also* Meningitis, aseptic) 047.9
nonpyogenic NEC 322.0
oidiomycosis 112.83
ossificans 349.2
Peptococcus 320.81
PeptoStreptococcus 320.81
pneumococcal 320.1
poliovirus (*see also* Poliomyelitis) 045.2❺ *[321.2]*
Proprionibacterium 320.81
Proteus morganii 320.82
Pseudomonas (aeruginosa) (pyocyaneus) 320.82
purulent NEC 320.9
specified organism NEC 320.89
pyogenic NEC 320.9
specified organism NEC 320.89
Salmonella 003.21
septic NEC 320.9
specified organism NEC 320.89
serosa circumscripta NEC 322.0
serous NEC (*see also* Meningitis, aseptic) 047.9
lymphocytic 049.0
syndrome 348.2
Serratia (marcescens) 320.82
specified organism NEC 320.89
sporadic cerebrospinal 036.0
sporotrichosis 117.1 *[321.1]*
staphylococcal 320.3
sterile 997.09
streptococcal (acute) 320.2
suppurative 320.9
specified organism NEC 320.89
syphilitic 094.2
acute 091.81
congenital 090.42
secondary 091.81
torula 117.5 *[321.0]*
traumatic (complication of injury) 958.8
Treponema (denticola) (macrodenticum) 320.81
trypanosomiasis 086.1 *[321.3]*
tuberculous (*see also* Tuberculosis, meninges) 013.0❺
typhoid 002.0 *[320.7]*
Veillonella 320.81
Vibrio vulnificus 320.82
viral, virus NEC (*see also* Meningitis, aseptic) 047.9
Wallgren's (*see also* Meningitis, aseptic) 047.9

Meningocele (congenital) (spinal) (*see also* Spina bifida) 741.9❺
acquired (traumatic) 349.2
cerebral 742.0
cranial 742.0

Meningocerebritis – *see* Meningoencephalitis

Meningococcemia (acute) (chronic) 036.2

Meningococcus, meningococcal (*see also* condition) 036.9
adrenalitis, hemorrhagic 036.3
carditis 036.40
carrier (suspected) of V02.59
cerebrospinal fever 036.0
encephalitis 036.1
endocarditis 036.42
exposure to V01.84
infection NEC 036.9
meningitis (cerebrospinal) 036.0
myocarditis 036.43
optic neuritis 036.81

Meningococcus, meningococcal – *continued*
pericarditis 036.41
septicemia (chronic) 036.2

Meningoencephalitis (*see also* Encephalitis) 323.9
acute NEC 048
bacterial, purulent, pyogenic, or septic – *see* Meningitis
chronic NEC 094.1
diffuse NEC 094.1
diphasic 063.2
due to
actinomycosis 039.8 *[320.7]*
blastomycosis NEC (*see also* Blastomycosis) 116.0 *[323.41]*
free-living amebae 136.2
Listeria monocytogenes 027.0 *[320.7]*
Lyme disease 088.81 *[320.7]*
mumps 072.2
Naegleria (amebae) (gruberi) (organisms) 136.2
rubella 056.01
sporotrichosis 117.1 *[321.1]*
toxoplasmosis (acquired) 130.0
congenital (active) 771.2 *[323.41]*
Trypanosoma 086.1 *[323.2]*
epidemic 036.0
herpes 054.3
herpetic 054.3
H. influenzae 320.0
infectious (acute) 048
influenzal 320.0
late effect – *see* category 326
Listeria monocytogenes 027.0 *[320.7]*
lymphocytic (serous) 049.0
mumps 072.2
parasitic NEC 123.9 *[323.41]*
pneumococcal 320.1
primary amebic 136.2
rubella 056.01
serous 048
lymphocytic 049.0
specific 094.2
staphylococcal 320.3
streptococcal 320.2
syphilitic 094.2
toxic NEC 989.9 *[323.71]*
due to
carbon tetrachloride 987.8 *[323.71]*
hydroxyquinoline derivatives poisoning 961.3 *[323.71]*
lead 984.9 *[323.71]*
mercury 985.0 *[323.71]*
thallium 985.8 *[323.71]*
toxoplasmosis (acquired) 130.0
trypanosomic 086.1 *[323.2]*
tuberculous (*see also* Tuberculosis, meninges) 013.0❺
virus NEC 048

Meningoencephalocele 742.0
syphilitic 094.89
congenital 090.49

Meningoencephalomyelitis (*see also* Meningoencephalitis) 323.9
acute NEC 048
disseminated (postinfectious) 136.9 *[323.61]*
postimmunization or postvaccination 323.51
due to
actinomycosis 039.8 *[320.7]*
torula 117.5 *[323.41]*
toxoplasma or toxoplasmosis (acquired) 130.0
congenital (active) 771.2 *[323.41]*
late effect – *see* category 326

Meningoencephalomyelopathy (*see also* Meningoencephalomyelitis) 349.9

Meningoencephalopathy (*see also* Meningoencephalitis) 348.39

Meningoencephalopoliomyelitis (*see also* Poliomyelitis, bulbar) 045.0❺
late effect 138

Meningomyelitis (*see also* Meningoencephalitis) 323.9
blastomycotic NEC (*see also* Blastomycosis) 116.0 *[323.41]*
due to
actinomycosis 039.8 *[320.7]*
blastomycosis (*see also* Blastomycosis) 116.0 *[323.41]*
Meningococcus 036.0
sporotrichosis 117.1 *[323.41]*
torula 117.5 *[323.41]*
late effect – *see* category 326

Meningitis – Meningomyelitis

Meningomyelitis – *continued*
- lethargic 049.8
- meningococcal 036.0
- syphilitic 094.2
- tuberculous (*see also* Tuberculosis, meninges) 013.0❺

Meningomyelocele (*see also* Spina bifida) 741.9❺
- syphilitic 094.89

Meningomyeloneuritis – *see* Meningoencephalitis
Meningoradiculitis – *see* Meningitis
Meningovascular – *see* condition
Meniscocytosis 282.60
Menkes' syndrome – *see* Syndrome, Menkes'
Menolipsis 626.0
Menometrorrhagia 626.2
Menopause, menopausal (symptoms) (syndrome) 627.2
- arthritis (any site) NEC 716.3❺
- artificial 627.4
- bleeding 627.0
- crisis 627.2
- depression (*see also* Psychosis, affective) 296.2❺
  - agitated 296.2❺
    - recurrent episode 296.3❺
    - single episode 296.2❺
  - psychotic 296.2❺
    - recurrent episode 296.3❺
    - single episode 296.2❺
  - recurrent episode 296.3
  - single episode 296.2
- melancholia (*see also* Psychosis, affective) 296.2
  - recurrent episode 296.3
  - single episode 296.2
- paranoid state 297.2
- paraphrenia 297.2
- postsurgical 627.4
- premature 256.31
  - postirradiation 256.2
  - postsurgical 256.2
- psychoneurosis 627.2
- psychosis NEC 298.8
- surgical 627.4
- toxic polyarthritis NEC 716.39

Menorrhagia (primary) 626.2
- climacteric 627.0
- menopausal 627.0
- postclimacteric 627.1
- postmenopausal 627.1
- preclimacteric 627.0
- premenopausal 627.0
- puberty (menses retained) 626.3

Menorrhalgia 625.3
Menoschesis 626.8
Menostaxis 626.2
Menses, retention 626.8
Menstrual – *see also* Menstruation
- cycle, irregular 626.4
- disorders NEC 626.9
- extraction V25.3
- fluid, retained 626.8
- molimen 625.4
- period, normal V65.5
- regulation V25.3

Menstruation
- absent 626.0
- anovulatory 628.0
- delayed 626.8
- difficult 625.3
- disorder 626.9
  - psychogenic 306.52
  - specified NEC 626.8
- during pregnancy 640.8❺
- excessive 626.2
- frequent 626.2
- infrequent 626.1
- irregular 626.4
- latent 626.8
- membranous 626.8
- painful (primary) (secondary) 625.3
  - psychogenic 306.52
- passage of clots 626.2
- precocious 626.8
- protracted 626.8
- retained 626.8
- retrograde 626.8
- scanty 626.1
- suppression 626.8
- vicarious (nasal) 625.8

Mentagra (*see also* Sycosis) 704.8
Mental – *see also* condition
- deficiency (*see also* Retardation, mental) 319
- deterioration (*see also* Psychosis) 298.9
- disorder (*see also* Disorder, mental) 300.9
- exhaustion 300.5
- insufficiency (congenital) (*see also* Retardation, mental) 319
- observation without need for further medical care NEC V71.09
- retardation (*see also* Retardation, mental) 319
- subnormality (*see also* Retardation, mental) 319
  - mild 317
  - moderate 318.0
  - profound 318.2
  - severe 318.1
- upset (*see also* Disorder, mental) 300.9

Meralgia paresthetica 355.1
Mercurial – *see* condition
Mercurialism NEC 985.0
Merergasia 300.9
MERFF 758.89
Merkel cell tumor – *see* Neoplasm, by site, malignant
Merocele (*see also* Hernia, femoral) 553.00
Meromelia 755.4
- lower limb 755.30
  - intercalary 755.32
    - femur 755.34
      - tibiofibular (complete) (incomplete) 755.33
    - fibula 755.37
    - metartarsal(s) 755.38
    - tarsal(s) 755.38
    - tibia 755.36
    - tibiofibular 755.35
  - terminal (complete) (partial) (transverse) 755.31
    - longitudinal 755.32
      - metatarsal(s) 755.38
      - phalange(s) 755.39
      - tarsal(s) 755.38
  - transverse 755.31
- upper limb 755.20
  - intercalary 755.22
    - carpal(s) 755.28
    - humeral 755.24
      - radioulnar (complete) (incomplete) 755.23
    - metacarpal(s) 755.28
    - phalange(s) 755.29
    - radial 755.26
    - radioulnar 755.25
    - ulnar 755.27
  - terminal (complete) (partial) (transverse) 755.21
    - longitudinal 755.22
      - carpal(s) 755.28
      - metacarpal(s) 755.28
      - phalange(s) 755.29
  - transverse 755.21

Merosmia 781.1
MERRF syndrome (myoclonus with epilepsy and with ragged red fibers) 277.87
Merycism – *see also* Vomiting
- psychogenic 307.53

Merzbacher-Pelizaeus disease 330.0
Mesaortitis – *see* Aortitis
Mesarteritis – *see* Arteritis
Mesencephalitis (*see also* Encephalitis) 323.9
- late effect – *see* category 326

Mesenchymoma (M8990/1) – *see also* Neoplasm, connective tissue, uncertain behavior
- benign (M8990/0) – *see* Neoplasm, connective tissue, benign
- malignant (M8990/3) – *see* Neoplasm, connective tissue, malignant

Mesenteritis
- retractile 567.82
- sclerosing 567.82

Mesentery, mesenteric – *see* condition
Mesiodens, mesiodentes 520.1
- causing crowding 524.31

Mesio-occlusion 524.23
Mesocardia (with asplenia) 746.87
Mesocolon – *see* condition
Mesonephroma (malignant) (M9110/3) – *see also* Neoplasm, by site, malignant
- benign (M9110/0) – *see* Neoplasm, by site, benign

Mesophlebitis – *see* Phlebitis
Mesostromal dysgenesis 743.51
Mesothelioma (malignant) (M9050/3) – *see also* Neoplasm, by site, malignant
- benign (M9050/0) – *see* Neoplasm, by site, benign
- biphasic type (M9053/3) – *see also* Neoplasm, by site, malignant
  - benign (M9053/0) – *see* Neoplasm, by site, benign
- epithelioid (M9052/3) – *see also* Neoplasm, by site, malignant
  - benign (M9052/0) – *see* Neoplasm, by site, benign
- fibrous (M9051/3) – *see also* Neoplasm, by site, malignant
  - benign (M9051/0) – *see* Neoplasm, by site, benign

Metabolic syndrome 277.7
Metabolism disorder 277.9
- specified type NEC 277.89

Metagonimiasis 121.5
Metagonimus infestation (small intestine) 121.5
Metal
- pigmentation (skin) 709.00
- polishers' disease 502

Metalliferous miners' lung 503
Metamorphopsia 368.14
Metaplasia
- bone, in skin 709.3
- breast 611.8
- cervix - omit code
- endometrium (squamous) 621.8
- esophagus 530.85
- intestinal, of gastric mucosa 537.89
- kidney (pelvis) (squamous) (*see also* Disease, renal) 593.89
- myelogenous 289.89
- myeloid 289.89
  - agnogenic 238.76
  - megakaryocytic 238.76
- spleen 289.59
- squamous cell
  - amnion 658.8❺
  - bladder 596.8
  - trachea 519.19
  - tracheobronchial tree 519.19
  - uterus 621.8
    - cervix – *see* condition

Metastasis, metastatic
- abscess – *see* Abscess
- calcification 275.40
- cancer, neoplasm, or disease
  - from specified site (M8000/3) – *see* Neoplasm, by site, malignant
  - to specified site (M8000/6) – *see* Neoplasm, by site, secondary
- deposits (in) (M8000/6) – *see* Neoplasm, by site, secondary
- pneumonia 038.8 *[484.8]*
- spread (to) (M8000/6) – *see* Neoplasm, by site, secondary

Metatarsalgia 726.70
- anterior 355.6
- due to Freiberg's disease 732.5
- Morton's 355.6

Metatarsus, metatarsal – *see also* condition
- abductus valgus (congenital) 754.60
- adductus varus (congenital) 754.53
- primus varus 754.52
- valgus (adductus) (congenital) 754.60
- varus (abductus) (congenital) 754.53
  - primus 754.52

Methemoglobinemia 289.7
- acquired (with sulfhemoglobinemia) 289.7
- congenital 289.7
- enzymatic 289.7
- Hb-M disease 289.7
- hereditary 289.7
- toxic 289.7

Methemoglobinuria (*see also* Hemoglobinuria) 791.2
Methicillin-resistant staphylococcus aureus (MRSA) V09.0
Methioninemia 270.4

Metritis (catarrhal) (septic) (suppurative) (*see also* Endometritis) 615.9
  blennorrhagic 098.16
    chronic or duration of 2 months or over 098.36
  cervical (*see also* Cervicitis) 616.0
  gonococcal 098.16
    chronic or duration of 2 months or over 098.36
  hemorrhagic 626.8
  puerperal, postpartum, childbirth 670❹
  tuberculous (*see also* Tuberculosis) 016.7❺
Metropathia hemorrhagica 626.8
Metroperitonitis (*see also* Peritonitis, pelvic, female) 614.5
Metrorrhagia 626.6
  arising during pregnancy – *see* Hemorrhage, pregnancy
  postpartum NEC 666.2❺
  primary 626.6
  psychogenic 306.59
  puerperal 666.2❺
Metrorrhexis – *see* Rupture, uterus
Metrosalpingitis (*see also* Salpingo-oophoritis) 614.2
Metrostaxis 626.6
Metrovaginitis (*see also* Endometritis) 615.9
  gonococcal (acute) 098.16
    chronic or duration of 2 months or over 098.36
Mexican fever – *see* Typhus, Mexican
Meyenburg-Altherr-Uehlinger syndrome 733.99
Meyer-Schwickerath and Weyers syndrome (dysplasia oculodentodigitalis) 759.89
Meynert's amentia (nonalcoholic) 294.0
  alcoholic 291.1
Mibelli's disease 757.39
Mice, joint (*see also* Loose, body, joint) 718.1❺
  knee 717.6
Micheli-Rietti syndrome (thalassemia minor) 282.49
Michotte's syndrome 721.5
Micrencephalon, micrencephaly 742.1
Microalbuminuria 791.0
Microaneurysm, retina 362.14
  diabetic 250.5❺ *[362.01]*
Microangiopathy 443.9
  diabetic (peripheral) 250.7❺ *[443.81]*
    retinal 250.5❺ *[362.01]*
  peripheral 443.9
    diabetic 250.7❺ *[443.81]*
  retinal 362.18
    diabetic 250.5❺ *[362.01]*
  thrombotic 446.6
    Moschcowitz's (thrombotic thrombocytopenic purpura) 446.6
Microcalcification, mammographic 793.81
Microcephalus, microcephalic, microcephaly 742.1
  due to toxoplasmosis (congenital) 771.2
Microcheilia 744.82
Microcolon (congenital) 751.5
Microcornea (congenital) 743.41
Microcytic – *see* condition
Microdeletions NEC 758.33
Microdontia 520.2
Microdrepanocytosis (thalassemia-Hb-S disease) 282.49
Microembolism
  atherothrombotic – *see* Atheroembolism
  retina 362.33
Microencephalon 742.1
Microfilaria streptocerca infestation 125.3
Microgastria (congenital) 750.7
Microgenia 524.0❺
Microgenitalia (congenital) 752.89
  penis 752.64
Microglioma (M9710/3)
  specified site – *see* Neoplasm, by site, malignant
  unspecified site 191.9
Microglossia (congenital) 750.16
Micrognathia, micrognathism (congenital) 524.00
  mandibular 524.04
    alveolar 524.74
  maxillary 524.03
    alveolar 524.73
Microgyria (congenital) 742.2
Microinfarct, heart (*see also* Insufficiency, coronary) 411.89
Microlithiasis, alveolar, pulmonary 516.2
Micromyelia (congenital) 742.59
Micropenis 752.64
Microphakia (congenital) 743.36
Microphthalmia (congenital) (*see also* Microphthalmos) 743.10
Microphthalmos (congenital) 743.10
  associated with eye and adnexal anomalies NEC 743.12
  due to toxoplasmosis (congenital) 771.2
  isolated 743.11
  simple 743.11
  syndrome 759.89
Micropsia 368.14
Microsporidiosis 136.8
Microsporon furfur infestation 111.0
Microsporosis (*see also* Dermatophytosis) 110.9
  nigra 111.1
Microstomia (congenital) 744.84
Microthelia 757.6
Microthromboembolism – *see* Embolism
Microtia (congenital) (external ear) 744.23
Microtropia 378.34
Micturition
  disorder NEC 788.69
    psychogenic 306.53
  frequency 788.41
    psychogenic 306.53
  nocturnal 788.43
  painful 788.1
    psychogenic 306.53
Middle
  ear – *see* condition
  lobe (right) syndrome 518.0
Midplane – *see* condition
Miescher's disease 709.3
  cheilitis 351.8
  granulomatosis disciformis 709.3
Miescher-Leder syndrome or granulomatosis 709.3
Mieten's syndrome 759.89
Migraine (idiopathic) 346.9❺
  with aura 346.0❺
  abdominal (syndrome) 346.2❺
  allergic (histamine) 346.2❺
  atypical 346.1❺
  basilar 346.2❺
  classical 346.0❺
  common 346.1❺
  hemiplegic 346.8❺
  lower-half 346.2❺
  menstrual 625.4
  ophthalmic 346.8❺
  ophthalmoplegic 346.8❺
  retinal 346.2❺
  variant 346.2❺
Migrant, social V60.0
Migratory, migrating – *see also* condition
  person V60.0
  testis, congenital 752.52
Mikulicz's disease or syndrome (dryness of mouth, absent or decreased lacrimation) 527.1
Milian atrophia blanche 701.3
Miliaria (crystallina) (rubra) (tropicalis) 705.1
  apocrine 705.82
Miliary – *see* condition
Milium (*see also* Cyst, sebaceous) 706.2
  colloid 709.3
  eyelid 374.84
Milk
  crust 690.11
  excess secretion 676.6❺
  fever, female 672❺
  poisoning 988.8
  retention 676.2❺
  sickness 988.8
  spots 423.1
Milkers' nodes 051.1
Milk-leg (deep vessels) 671.4❺
  complicating pregnancy 671.3❺
  nonpuerperal 451.19
  puerperal, postpartum, childbirth 671.4❺
Milkman (-Looser) **disease or syndrome** (osteomalacia with pseudofractures) 268.2
Milky urine (*see also* Chyluria) 791.1
Millar's asthma (laryngismus stridulus) 478.75
Millard-Gubler paralysis or syndrome 344.89
Millard-Gubler-Foville paralysis 344.89
Miller's disease (osteomalacia) 268.2
Miller-Dieker syndrome 758.33
Miller Fisher's syndrome 357.0
Milles' syndrome (encephalocutaneous angiomatosis) 759.6
Mills' disease 335.29
Millstone makers' asthma or lung 502
Milroy's disease (chronic hereditary edema) 757.0
Miners' – *see also* condition
  asthma 500
  elbow 727.2
  knee 727.2
  lung 500
  nystagmus 300.89
  phthisis (*see also* Tuberculosis) 011.4❺
  tuberculosis (*see also* Tuberculosis) 011.4❺
Minkowski-Chauffard syndrome (*see also* Spherocytosis) 282.0
Minor – *see* condition
Minor's disease 336.1
Minot's disease (hemorrhagic disease, newborn) 776.0
Minot-von Willebrand (-Jürgens) **disease or syndrome** (angiohemophilia) 286.4
Minus (and plus) **hand** (intrinsic) 736.09
Miosis (persistent) (pupil) 379.42
Mirizzi's syndrome (hepatic duct stenosis) (*see also* Obstruction, biliary) 576.2
  with calculus, cholelithiasis, or stones – *see* Choledocholithiasis
Mirror writing 315.09
  secondary to organic lesion 784.69
Misadventure (prophylactic) (therapeutic) (*see also* Complications) 999.9
  administration of insulin 962.3
  infusion – *see* Complications, infusion
  local applications (of fomentations, plasters, etc.) 999.9
    burn or scald – *see* Burn, by site
  medical care (early) (late) NEC 999.9
    adverse effect of drugs or chemicals – *see* Table of Drugs and Chemicals
    burn or scald – *see* Burn, by site
  radiation NEC 990
  radiotherapy NEC 990
  surgical procedure (early) (late) – *see* Complications, surgical procedure
  transfusion – *see* Complications, transfusion
  vaccination or other immunological procedure – *see* Complications, vaccination
Misanthropy 301.7
Miscarriage – *see* Abortion, spontaneous
Mischief, malicious, child (*see also* Disturbance, conduct) 312.0❺
Misdirection
  aqueous 365.83
Mismanagement, feeding 783.3
Misplaced, misplacement
  kidney (*see also* Disease, renal) 593.0
    congenital 753.3
  organ or site, congenital NEC – *see* Malposition, congenital
Missed
  abortion 632
  delivery (at or near term) 656.4❺
  labor (at or near term) 656.4❺
Missing – *see also* Absence
  teeth (acquired) 525.10
    congenital (*see also* Anodontia) 520.0
    due to
      caries 525.13
      extraction 525.10
      periodontal disease 525.12
      specified NEC 525.19
      trauma 525.11
  vertebrae (congenital) 756.13
Misuse of drugs NEC (*see also* Abuse, drug, nondependent) 305.9❺
Mitchell's disease (erythromelalgia) 443.82
Mite(s)
  diarrhea 133.8
  grain (itch) 133.8
  hair follicle (itch) 133.8
  in sputum 133.8
Mitochondrial encephalopathy, lactic acidosis and stroke-like episodes (MELAS syndrome) 277.87

Mitochondrial neurogastrointestinal encephalopathy syndrome (MNGIE) 277.87
Mitral – *see* condition
Mittelschmerz 625.2
Mixed – *see* condition
Mljet disease (mal de Meleda) 757.39
Mobile, mobility
  cecum 751.4
  coccyx 733.99
  excessive – *see* Hypermobility
  gallbladder 751.69
  kidney 593.0
    congenital 753.3
  organ or site, congenital NEC – *see* Malposition, congenital
  spleen 289.59
Mobitz heart block (atrioventricular) 426.10
  type I (Wenckebach's) 426.13
  type II 426.12
Möbius'
  disease 346.8❺
  syndrome
    congenital oculofacial paralysis 352.6
    ophthalmoplegic migraine 346.8❺
Moeller (-Barlow) **disease** (infantile scurvy) 267
  glossitis 529.4
Mohr's syndrome (types I and II) 759.89
Mola destruens (M9100/1) 236.1
Molarization, premolars 520.2
Molar pregnancy 631
  hydatidiform (delivered) (undelivered) 630
Mold(s) in vitreous 117.9
Molding, head (during birth) - omit code
Mole (pigmented) (M8720/0) – *see also* Neoplasm, skin, benign
  blood 631
  Breus' 631
  cancerous (M8720/3) – *see* Melanoma
  carneous 631
  destructive (M9100/1) 236.1
  ectopic – *see* Pregnancy, ectopic
  fleshy 631
  hemorrhagic 631
  hydatid, hydatidiform (benign) (complicating pregnancy) (delivered) (undelivered) (*see also* Hydatidiform mole) 630
    invasive (M9100/1) 236.1
    malignant (M9100/1) 236.1
    previous, affecting management of pregnancy V23.1
  invasive (hydatidiform) (M9100/1) 236.1
  malignant
    meaning
      malignant hydatidiform mole (9100/1) 236.1
      melanoma (M8720/3) – *see* Melanoma
  nonpigmented (M8730/0) – *see* Neoplasm, skin, benign
  pregnancy NEC 631
  skin (M8720/0) – *see* Neoplasm, skin, benign
  tubal – *see* Pregnancy, tubal
  vesicular (*see also* Hydatidiform mole) 630
Molimen, molimina (menstrual) 625.4
Mollaret's meningitis 047.9
Mollities (cerebellar) (cerebral) 437.8
  ossium 268.2
Molluscum
  contagiosum 078.0
  epitheliale 078.0
  fibrosum (M8851/0) – *see* Lipoma, by site
  pendulum (M8851/0) – *see* Lipoma, by site
Mönckeberg's arteriosclerosis, degeneration, disease, or sclerosis (*see also* Arteriosclerosis, extremities) 440.20
Monday fever 504
Monday morning dyspnea or asthma 504
Mondini's malformation (cochlea) 744.05
Mondor's disease (thrombophlebitis of breast) 451.89
Mongolian, mongolianism, mongolism, mongoloid 758.0
  spot 757.33
Monilethrix (congenital) 757.4
Monilia infestation – *see* Candidiasis
Moniliasis – *see also* Candidiasis
  neonatal 771.7
  vulvovaginitis 112.1
Monkeypox 057.8
Monoarthritis 716.60
  ankle 716.67
  arm 716.62
    lower (and wrist) 716.63
    upper (and elbow) 716.62
  foot (and ankle) 716.67
  forearm (and wrist) 716.63
  hand 716.64
  leg 716.66
    lower 716.66
    upper 716.65
  pelvic region (hip) (thigh) 716.65
  shoulder (region) 716.61
  specified site NEC 716.68
Monoblastic – *see* condition
Monochromatism (cone) (rod) 368.54
Monocytic – *see* condition
Monocytopenia 288.59
Monocytosis (symptomatic) 288.63
Monofixation syndrome 378.34
Monomania (*see also* Psychosis) 298.9
Mononeuritis 355.9
  cranial nerve – *see* Disorder, nerve, cranial
  femoral nerve 355.2
  lateral
    cutaneous nerve of thigh 355.1
    popliteal nerve 355.3
  lower limb 355.8
    specified nerve NEC 355.79
  medial popliteal nerve 355.4
  median nerve 354.1
  multiplex 354.5
  plantar nerve 355.6
  posterior tibial nerve 355.5
  radial nerve 354.3
  sciatic nerve 355.0
  ulnar nerve 354.2
  upper limb 354.9
    specified nerve NEC 354.8
  vestibular 388.5
Mononeuropathy (*see also* Mononeuritis) 355.9
  diabetic NEC 250.6❺ *[355.9]*
    lower limb 250.6❺ *[355.8]*
    upper limb 250.6❺ *[354.9]*
  iliohypogastric nerve 355.79
  ilioinguinal nerve 355.79
  obturator nerve 355.79
  saphenous nerve 355.79
Mononucleosis, infectious 075
  with hepatitis 075 *[573.1]*
Monoplegia 344.5
  brain (current episode) (*see also* Paralysis, brain) 437.8
    fetus or newborn 767.8
  cerebral (current episode) (*see also* Paralysis, brain) 437.8
  congenital or infantile (cerebral) (spastic) (spinal) 343.3
  embolic (current) (*see also* Embolism, brain) 434.1❺
    late effect – *see* Late effect(s) (of) cerebrovascular disease
  infantile (cerebral) (spastic) (spinal) 343.3
  lower limb 344.30
    affecting
      dominant side 344.31
      nondominant side 344.32
    due to late effect of cerebrovascular accident-*see* Late effect(s) (of) cerebrovascular accident
  newborn 767.8
  psychogenic 306.0
    specified as conversion reaction 300.11
  thrombotic (current) (*see also* Thrombosis, brain) 434.0❺
    late effect – *see* Late effect(s) (of) cerebrovascular disease
  transient 781.4
  upper limb 344.40
    affecting
      dominant side 344.41
      nondominant side 344.42
    due to late effect of cerebrovascular accident-*see* Late effect(s) (of) cerebrovascular accident
Monorchism, monorchidism 752.89
Monteggia's fracture (closed) 813.03
  open 813.13
Mood swings
  brief compensatory 296.99
Mood swings – *continued*
  rebound 296.99
Moore's syndrome (*see also* Epilepsy) 345.5❺
Mooren's ulcer (cornea) 370.07
Mooser-Neill reaction 081.0
Mooser bodies 081.0
Moral
  deficiency 301.7
  imbecility 301.7
Morax-Axenfeld conjunctivitis 372.03
Morbilli (*see also* Measles) 055.9
Morbus
  anglicus, anglorum 268.0
  Beigel 111.2
  caducus (*see also* Epilepsy) 345.9❺
  caeruleus 746.89
  celiacus 579.0
  comitialis (*see also* Epilepsy) 345.9❺
  cordis – *see also* Disease, heart
    valvulorum – *see* Endocarditis
  coxae 719.95
    tuberculous (*see also* Tuberculosis) 015.1❺
  hemorrhagicus neonatorum 776.0
  maculosus neonatorum 772.6
  renum 593.0
  senilis (*see also* Osteoarthrosis) 715.9❺
Morel-Kraepelin disease (*see also* Schizophrenia) 295.9❺
Morel-Moore syndrome (hyperostosis frontalis interna) 733.3
Morel-Morgagni syndrome (hyperostosis frontalis interna) 733.3
Morgagni
  cyst, organ, hydatid, or appendage 752.89
    fallopian tube 752.11
  disease or syndrome (hyperostosis frontalis interna) 733.3
Morgagni-Adams-Stokes syndrome (syncope with heart block) 426.9
Morgagni-Stewart-Morel syndrome (hyperostosis frontalis interna) 733.3
Moria (*see also* Psychosis) 298.9
Morning sickness 643.0❺
Moron 317
Morphea (guttate) (linear) 701.0
Morphine dependence (*see also* Dependence) 304.0❺
Morphinism (*see also* Dependence) 304.0❺
Morphinomania (*see also* Dependence) 304.0❺
Morphoea 701.0
Morquio (-Brailsford) (-Ullrich) **disease or syndrome** (mucopolysaccharidosis IV) 277.5
  kyphosis 277.5
Morris syndrome (testicular feminization) 259.5
Morsus humanus (open wound) – *see also* Wound, open, by site
  skin surface intact – *see* Contusion
Mortification (dry) (moist) (*see also* Gangrene) 785.4
Morton's
  disease 355.6
  foot 355.6
  metatarsalgia (syndrome) 355.6
  neuralgia 355.6
  neuroma 355.6
  syndrome (metatarsalgia) (neuralgia) 355.6
  toe 355.6
Morvan's disease 336.0
Mosaicism, mosaic (chromosomal) 758.9
  autosomal 758.5
  sex 758.81
Moschcowitz's syndrome (thrombotic thrombocytopenic purpura) 446.6
Mother yaw 102.0
Motion sickness (from travel, any vehicle) (from roundabouts or swings) 994.6
Mottled teeth (enamel) (endemic) (nonendemic) 520.3
Mottling enamel (endemic) (nonendemic) (teeth) 520.3
Mouchet's disease 732.5
Mould(s) (in vitreous) 117.9
Moulders'
  bronchitis 502
  tuberculosis (*see also* Tuberculosis) 011.4❺

- **Mounier-Kuhn syndrome** 748.3
  - with
    - acute exacerbation 494.1
    - bronchiectasis 494.0
      - with (acute) exacerbation 494.1
  - acquired 519.19
    - with bronchiectasis 494.0
      - with (acute) exacerbation 494.1
- **Mountain**
  - fever – *see* Fever, mountain
  - sickness 993.2
    - with polycythemia, acquired 289.0
    - acute 289.0
  - tick fever 066.1
- **Mouse, joint** (*see also* Loose, body, joint) 718.1❺
  - knee 717.6
- **Mouth** – *see* condition
- **Movable**
  - coccyx 724.71
  - kidney (*see also* Disease, renal) 593.0
    - congenital 753.3
  - organ or site, congenital NEC – *see* Malposition, congenital
  - spleen 289.59
- **Movement**
  - abnormal (dystonic) (involuntary) 781.0
  - decreased fetal 655.7❺
  - paradoxical facial 374.43
- **Moya Moya disease** 437.5
- **Mozart's ear** 744.29
- **MRSA** (methicillin-resistant staphylococcus aureus) V09.0
- **Mucha's disease** (acute parapsoriasis varioliformis) 696.2
- **Mucha-Haberman syndrome** (acute parapsoriasis varioliformis) 696.2
- **Mu-chain disease** 273.2
- **Mucinosis** (cutaneous) (papular) 701.8
- **Mucocele**
  - appendix 543.9
  - buccal cavity 528.9
  - gallbladder (*see also* Disease, gallbladder) 575.3
  - lacrimal sac 375.43
  - orbit (eye) 376.81
  - salivary gland (any) 527.6
  - sinus (accessory) (nasal) 478.19
  - turbinate (bone) (middle) (nasal) 478.19
  - uterus 621.8
- **Mucocutaneous lymph node syndrome** (acute) (febrile) (infantile) 446.1
- **Mucoenteritis** 564.9
- **Mucolipidosis I, II, III** 272.7
- **Mucopolysaccharidosis** (types 1-6) 277.5
  - cardiopathy 277.5 *[425.7]*
- **Mucormycosis** (lung) 117.7
- **Mucosa associated lymphoid tissue** (MALT) 200.3❺●
- **Mucositis** – *see also* Inflammation, by site 528.00
  - cervix (ulcerative) 616.81
  - due to
    - antineoplastic therapy (ulcerative) 528.01
    - other drugs (ulcerative) 528.02
    - specified NEC 528.09
  - gastrointestinal (ulcerative) 538
  - nasal (ulcerative) 478.11
  - necroticans agranulocytica (*see also* Agranulocytosis) 288.09
  - ulcerative 528.00
  - vagina (ulcerative) 616.81
  - vulva (ulcerative) 616.81
- **Mucous** – *see also* condition
  - patches (syphilitic) 091.3
    - congenital 090.0
- **Mucoviscidosis** 277.00
  - with meconium obstruction 277.01
- **Mucus**
  - asphyxia or suffocation (*see also* Asphyxia, mucus) 933.1
    - newborn 770.18
  - in stool 792.1
  - plug (*see also* Asphyxia, mucus) 933.1
    - aspiration, of newborn 770.17
    - tracheobronchial 519.19
      - newborn 770.18
- **Muguet** 112.0
- **Mulberry molars** 090.5
- **Mullerian mixed tumor** (M8950/3) – *see* Neoplasm, by site, malignant
- **Multicystic kidney** 753.19
- **Multilobed placenta** – *see* Placenta, abnormal
- **Multinodular prostate** 600.10
  - with
    - urinary
      - obstruction 600.11
      - retention 600.11
- **Multiparity** V61.5
  - affecting
    - fetus or newborn 763.89
    - management of
      - labor and delivery 659.4❺
      - pregnancy V23.3
  - requiring contraceptive management (*see also* Contraception) V25.9
- **Multipartita placenta** – *see* Placenta, abnormal
- **Multiple, multiplex** – *see also* condition
  - birth
    - affecting fetus or newborn 761.5
    - healthy liveborn – *see* Newborn, multiple
  - digits (congenital) 755.00
    - fingers 755.01
    - toes 755.02
  - organ or site NEC – *see* Accessory
  - personality 300.14
  - renal arteries 747.62
- **Mumps** 072.9
  - with complication 072.8
    - specified type NEC 072.79
  - encephalitis 072.2
  - hepatitis 072.71
  - meningitis (aseptic) 072.1
  - meningoencephalitis 072.2
  - oophoritis 072.79
  - orchitis 072.0
  - pancreatitis 072.3
  - polyneuropathy 072.72
  - vaccination, prophylactic (against) V04.6
- **Mumu** (*see also* Infestation, filarial) 125.9
- **Münchausen syndrome** 301.51
- **Münchmeyer's disease or syndrome** (exostosis luxurians) 728.11
- **Mural** – *see* condition
- **Murmur** (cardiac) (heart) (nonorganic) (organic) 785.2
  - abdominal 787.5
  - aortic (valve) (*see also* Endocarditis, aortic) 424.1
  - benign - omit code
  - cardiorespiratory 785.2
  - diastolic – *see* condition
  - Flint (*see also* Endocarditis, aortic) 424.1
  - functional - omit code
  - Graham Steell (pulmonic regurgitation) (*see also* Endocarditis, pulmonary) 424.3
  - innocent - omit code
  - insignificant - omit code
  - midsystolic 785.2
  - mitral (valve) – *see* Stenosis
  - physiologic – *see* condition
  - presystolic, mitral – *see* Insufficiency, mitral
  - pulmonic (valve) (*see also* Endocarditis, pulmonary) 424.3
  - Still's (vibratory) - omit code
  - systolic (valvular) – *see* condition
  - tricuspid (valve) – *see* Endocarditis, tricuspid
  - undiagnosed 785.2
  - valvular – *see* condition
  - vibratory - omit code
- **Murri's disease** (intermittent hemoglobinuria) 283.2
- **Muscae volitantes** 379.24
- **Muscle, muscular** – *see* condition
- **Musculoneuralgia** 729.1
- **Mushrooming hip** 718.95
- **Mushroom workers'** (pickers') **lung** 495.5
- **Mutation**
  - factor V leiden 289.81
  - prothrombin gene 289.81
- **Mutism** (*see also* Aphasia) 784.3
  - akinetic 784.3
  - deaf (acquired) (congenital) 389.7
  - hysterical 300.11
  - selective (elective) 313.23
    - adjustment reaction 309.83
- **Myà's disease** (congenital dilation, colon) 751.3
- **Myalgia** (intercostal) 729.1
  - eosinophilia syndrome 710.5
- **Myalgia** (intercostal) – *continued*
  - epidemic 074.1
    - cervical 078.89
  - psychogenic 307.89
  - traumatic NEC 959.9
- **Myasthenia** 358.00
  - cordis – *see* Failure, heart
  - gravis 358.00
    - with exacerbation (acute) 358.01
    - in crisis 358.01
    - neonatal 775.2
    - pseudoparalytica 358.00
  - stomach 536.8
    - psychogenic 306.4
  - syndrome
    - in
      - botulism 005.1 *[358.1]*
      - diabetes mellitus 250.6❺ *[358.1]*
      - hypothyroidism (*see also* Hypothyroidism) 244.9 *[358.1]*
      - malignant neoplasm NEC 199.1 *[358.1]*
      - pernicious anemia 281.0 *[358.1]*
      - thyrotoxicosis (*see also* Thyrotoxicosis) 242.9❺ *[358.1]*
- **Myasthenic** 728.87
- **Mycelium infection** NEC 117.9
- **Mycetismus** 988.1
- **Mycetoma** (actinomycotic) 039.9
  - bone 039.8
    - mycotic 117.4
  - foot 039.4
    - mycotic 117.4
  - madurae 039.9
    - mycotic 117.4
  - maduromycotic 039.9
    - mycotic 117.4
  - mycotic 117.4
  - nocardial 039.9
- **Mycobacteriosis** – *see* Mycobacterium
- **Mycobacterium, mycobacterial** (infection) 031.9
  - acid-fast (bacilli) 031.9
  - anonymous (*see also* Mycobacterium, atypical) 031.9
  - atypical (acid-fast bacilli) 031.9
    - cutaneous 031.1
    - pulmonary 031.0
      - tuberculous (*see also* Tuberculosis, pulmonary) 011.9❺
    - specified site NEC 031.8
  - avium 031.0
    - intracellulare complex bacteremia (MAC) 031.2
  - balnei 031.1
  - Battey 031.0
  - cutaneous 031.1
  - disseminated 031.2
    - avium-intracellulare complex (DMAC) 031.2
  - fortuitum 031.0
  - intracellulare (battey bacillus) 031.0
  - kakerifu 031.8
  - kansasii 031.0
  - kasongo 031.8
  - leprae – *see* Leprosy
  - luciflavum 031.0
  - marinum 031.1
  - pulmonary 031.0
    - tuberculous (*see also* Tuberculosis, pulmonary) 011.9❺
  - scrofulaceum 031.1
  - tuberculosis (human, bovine) – *see also* Tuberculosis
    - avian type 031.0
  - ulcerans 031.1
  - xenopi 031.0
- **Mycosis, mycotic** 117.9
  - cutaneous NEC 111.9
  - ear 111.8 *[380.15]*
  - fungoides (M9700/3) 202.1❺
  - mouth 112.0
  - pharynx 117.9
  - skin NEC 111.9
  - stomatitis 112.0
  - systemic NEC 117.9
  - tonsil 117.9
  - vagina, vaginitis 112.1
- **Mydriasis** (persistent) (pupil) 379.43
- **Myelatelia** 742.59
- **Myelinoclasis, perivascular, acute** (postinfectious) NEC 136.9 *[323.61]*
  - postimmunization or postvaccinal 323.51
- **Myelinosis, central pontine** 341.8

Mounier-Kuhn syndrome – Myelinosis, central pontine

- **Myelitis** (ascending) (cerebellar) (childhood) (chronic) (descending) (diffuse) (disseminated) (pressure) (progressive) (spinal cord) (subacute) (*see also* Encephalitis) 323.9
  - acute (transverse) 341.20
    - idiopathic 341.22
    - in conditions classified elsewhere 341.21
  - due to
    - infection classified elsewhere 136.9 *[323.42]*▲
    - specified cause NEC 323.82
    - vaccination (any) 323.52
    - viral diseases classified elsewhere 323.02
  - herpes simplex 054.74
  - herpes zoster 053.14
  - late effect – *see* category 326
  - optic neuritis in 341.0
  - postchickenpox 052.2
  - postimmunization 323.52
  - postinfectious 136.9 *[323.63]*▲
  - postvaccinal 323.52
  - postvaricella 052.2
  - syphilitic (transverse) 094.89
  - toxic 989.9 *[323.72]*▲
  - transverse 323.82
    - acute 341.20
      - idiopathic 341.22
      - in conditions classified elsewhere 341.21
    - idiopathic 341.22
  - tuberculous (*see also* Tuberculosis) 013.6❺
  - virus 049.9
- **Myeloblastic** – *see* condition
- **Myelocele** (*see also* Spina bifida) 741.9❺
  - with hydrocephalus 741.0❺
- **Myelocystocele** (*see also* Spina bifida) 741.9❺
- **Myelocytic** – *see* condition
- **Myelocytoma** 205.1❺
- **Myelodysplasia** (spinal cord) 742.59
  - meaning myelodysplastic syndrome – *see* Syndrome, myelodysplastic
- **Myeloencephalitis** – *see* Encephalitis
- **Myelofibrosis** 289.83
  - with myeloid metaplasia 238.76
  - idiopathic (chronic) 238.76
  - megakaryocytic 238.79
  - primary 238.76
  - secondary 289.83
- **Myelogenous** – *see* condition
- **Myeloid** – *see* condition
- **Myelokathexis** 288.09
- **Myeloleukodystrophy** 330.0
- **Myelolipoma** (M8870/0) – *see* Neoplasm, by site, benign
- **Myeloma** (multiple) (plasma cell) (plasmacytic) (M9730/3) 203.0❺
  - monostotic (M9731/1) 238.6
  - solitary (M9731/1) 238.6
- **Myelomalacia** 336.8
- **Myelomata, multiple** (M9730/3) 203.0❺
- **Myelomatosis** (M9730/3) 203.0❺
- **Myelomeningitis** – *see* Meningoencephalitis
- **Myelomeningocele** (spinal cord) (*see also* Spina bifida) 741.9❺
  - fetal, causing fetopelvic disproportion 653.7❺
- **Myelo-osteo-musculodysplasia hereditaria** 756.89
- **Myelopathic** – *see* condition
- **Myelopathy** (spinal cord) 336.9
  - cervical 721.1
  - diabetic 250.6❺ *[336.3]*
  - drug-induced 336.8
  - due to or with
    - carbon tetrachloride 987.8 *[323.72]*
    - degeneration or displacement, intervertebral disc 722.70
      - cervical, cervicothoracic 722.71
      - lumbar, lumbosacral 722.73
      - thoracic, thoracolumbar 722.72
    - hydroxyquinoline derivatives 961.3 *[323.72]*
    - infection – *see* Encephalitis
    - intervertebral disc disorder 722.70
      - cervical, cervicothoracic 722.71
      - lumbar, lumbosacral 722.73
      - thoracic, thoracolumbar 722.72
    - lead 984.9 *[323.72]*
    - mercury 985.0 *[323.72]*
    - neoplastic disease (*see also* Neoplasm, by site) 239.9 *[336.3]*
    - pernicious anemia 281.0 *[336.3]*

- **Myelopathy** – *continued*
  - due to or with – *continued*
    - spondylosis 721.91
      - cervical 721.1
      - lumbar, lumbosacral 721.42
      - thoracic 721.41
    - thallium 985.8 *[323.72]*
  - lumbar, lumbosacral 721.42
  - necrotic (subacute) 336.1
  - radiation-induced 336.8
  - spondylogenic NEC 721.91
    - cervical 721.1
    - lumbar, lumbosacral 721.42
    - thoracic 721.41
  - thoracic 721.41
  - toxic NEC 989.9 *[323.72]*
  - transverse (*see also* Myelitis) 323.82
  - vascular 336.1
- **Myelophthisis** 284.2
- **Myeloproliferative disease** (M9960/1) 238.79
- **Myeloradiculitis** (*see also* Polyneuropathy) 357.0
- **Myeloradiculodysplasia** (spinal) 742.59
- **Myelosarcoma** (M9930/3) 205.3❺
- **Myelosclerosis** 289.89
  - with myeloid metaplasia (M9961/1) 238.76
  - disseminated, of nervous system 340
  - megakaryocytic (M9961/1) 238.79
- **Myelosis** (M9860/3) (*see also* Leukemia, myeloid) 205.9❺
  - acute (M9861/3) 205.0❺
  - aleukemic (M9864/3) 205.8❺
  - chronic (M9863/3) 205.1❺
  - erythremic (M9840/3) 207.0❺
    - acute (M9841/3) 207.0❺
  - megakaryocytic (M9920/3) 207.2❺
  - nonleukemic (chronic) 288.8
  - subacute (M9862/3) 205.2❺
- **Myesthenia** – *see* Myasthenia
- **Myiasis** (cavernous) 134.0
  - orbit 134.0 *[376.13]*
- **Myoadenoma, prostate** 600.20
  - with
    - other lower urinary tract symptoms (LUTS) 600.21
    - urinary
      - obstruction 600.21
      - retention 600.21
- **Myoblastoma**
  - granular cell (M9580/0) – *see also* Neoplasm, connective tissue, benign
    - malignant (M9580/3) – *see* Neoplasm, connective tissue, malignant
  - tongue (M9580/0) 210.1
- **Myocardial** – *see* condition
- **Myocardiopathy** (congestive) (constrictive) (familial) (hypertrophic nonobstructive) (idiopathic) (infiltrative) (obstructive) (primary) (restrictive) (sporadic) 425.4
  - alcoholic 425.5
  - amyloid 277.39 *[425.7]*
  - beriberi 265.0 *[425.7]*
  - cobalt-beer 425.5
  - due to
    - amyloidosis 277.39 *[425.7]*
    - beriberi 265.0 *[425.7]*
    - cardiac glycogenosis 271.0 *[425.7]*
    - Chagas' disease 086.0
    - Friedreich's ataxia 334.0 *[425.8]*
    - influenza 487.8 *[425.8]*
    - mucopolysaccharidosis 277.5 *[425.7]*
    - myotonia atrophica 359.21 ▲ *[425.8]*
    - progressive muscular dystrophy 359.1 *[425.8]*
    - sarcoidosis 135 *[425.8]*
  - glycogen storage 271.0 *[425.7]*
  - hypertrophic obstructive 425.1
  - metabolic NEC 277.9 *[425.7]*
  - nutritional 269.9 *[425.7]*
  - obscure (African) 425.2
  - peripartum 674.5❺
  - postpartum 674.5❺
  - secondary 425.9
  - thyrotoxic (*see also* Thyrotoxicosis) 242.9❺ *[425.7]*
  - toxic NEC 425.9

- **Myocarditis** (fibroid) (interstitial) (old) (progressive) (senile) (with arteriosclerosis) 429.0
  - with
    - rheumatic fever (conditions classifiable to 390) 398.0
      - active (*see also* Myocarditis, acute, rheumatic) 391.2
      - inactive or quiescent (with chorea) 398.0
  - active (nonrheumatic) 422.90
    - rheumatic 391.2
      - with chorea (acute) (rheumatic) (Sydenham's) 392.0
  - acute or subacute (interstitial) 422.90
    - due to Streptococcus (beta-hemolytic) 391.2
    - idiopathic 422.91
    - rheumatic 391.2
      - with chorea (acute) (rheumatic) (Sydenham's) 392.0
    - specified type NEC 422.99
  - aseptic of newborn 074.23
  - bacterial (acute) 422.92
  - chagasic 086.0
  - chronic (interstitial) 429.0
  - congenital 746.89
  - constrictive 425.4
  - Coxsackie (virus) 074.23
  - diphtheritic 032.82
  - due to or in
    - Coxsackie (virus) 074.23
    - diphtheria 032.82
    - epidemic louse-borne typhus 080 *[422.0]*
    - influenza 487.8 *[422.0]*
    - Lyme disease 088.81 *[422.0]*
    - scarlet fever 034.1 *[422.0]*
    - toxoplasmosis (acquired) 130.3
    - tuberculosis (*see also* Tuberculosis) 017.9❺ *[422.0]*
    - typhoid 002.0 *[422.0]*
    - typhus NEC 081.9 *[422.0]*
  - eosinophilic 422.91
  - epidemic of newborn 074.23
  - Fiedler's (acute) (isolated) (subacute) 422.91
  - giant cell (acute) (subacute) 422.91
  - gonococcal 098.85
  - granulomatous (idiopathic) (isolated) (nonspecific) 422.91
  - hypertensive (*see also* Hypertension, heart) 402.90
  - idiopathic 422.91
    - granulomatous 422.91
  - infective 422.92
  - influenzal 487.8 *[422.0]*
  - isolated (diffuse) (granulomatous) 422.91
  - malignant 422.99
  - meningococcal 036.43
  - nonrheumatic, active 422.90
  - parenchymatous 422.90
  - pneumococcal (acute) (subacute) 422.92
  - rheumatic (chronic) (inactive) (with chorea) 398.0
    - active or acute 391.2
      - with chorea (acute) (rheumatic) (Sydenham's) 392.0
  - septic 422.92
  - specific (giant cell) (productive) 422.91
  - staphylococcal (acute) (subacute) 422.92
  - suppurative 422.92
  - syphilitic (chronic) 093.82
  - toxic 422.93
    - rheumatic (*see also* Myocarditis, acute rheumatic) 391.2
  - tuberculous (*see also* Tuberculosis) 017.9❺ *[422.0]*
  - typhoid 002.0 *[422.0]*
  - valvular – *see* Endocarditis
  - viral, except Coxsackie 422.91
    - Coxsackie 074.23
    - of newborn (Coxsackie) 074.23
- **Myocardium, myocardial** – *see* condition
- **Myocardosis** (*see also* Cardiomyopathy) 425.4
- **Myoclonia** (essential) 333.2
  - epileptica 333.2
  - Friedrich's 333.2
  - massive 333.2
- **Myoclonic**
  - epilepsy, familial (progressive) 333.2
  - jerks 333.2
- **Myoclonus** (familial essential) (multifocal) (simplex) 333.2
  - with epilepsy and with ragged red fibers (MERRF syndrome) 277.87
  - facial 351.8

Myelitis – Myoclonus

N

④ Fourth-Digit Required ⑤ Fifth-Digit Required *[code]* Manifestation Code ►◄ Revised Text ● New Line ▲ Revised Code

Narrowing – *continued*
artery – *continued*
cerebellar 433.8❺
choroidal 433.8❺
communicating posterior 433.8❺
coronary – *see also* Arteriosclerosis, coronary
congenital 746.85
due to syphilis 090.5
hypophyseal 433.8❺
pontine 433.8❺
precerebral NEC 433.9❺
multiple or bilateral 433.3❺
specified NEC 433.8❺
vertebral 433.2❺
with other precerebral artery 433.3❺
bilateral 433.3❺
auditory canal (external) (*see also* Stricture, ear canal, acquired) 380.50
cerebral arteries 437.0
cicatricial – *see* Cicatrix
congenital – *see* Anomaly, congenital
coronary artery – *see* Narrowing, artery, coronary
ear, middle 385.22
Eustachian tube (*see also* Obstruction, Eustachian tube) 381.60
eyelid 374.46
congenital 743.62
intervertebral disc or space NEC – *see* Degeneration, intervertebral disc
joint space, hip 719.85
larynx 478.74
lids 374.46
congenital 743.62
mesenteric artery (with gangrene) 557.0
palate 524.89
palpebral fissure 374.46
retinal artery 362.13
ureter 593.3
urethra (*see also* Stricture, urethra) 598.9
Narrowness, abnormal, eyelid 743.62
Nasal – *see* condition
Nasolacrimal – *see* condition
Nasopharyngeal – *see also* condition
bursa 478.29
pituitary gland 759.2
torticollis 723.5
Nasopharyngitis (acute) (infective) (subacute) 460
chronic 472.2
due to external agent – *see* Condition, respiratory, chronic, due to
due to external agent – *see* Condition, respiratory, due to
septic 034.0
streptococcal 034.0
suppurative (chronic) 472.2
ulcerative (chronic) 472.2
Nasopharynx, nasopharyngeal – *see* condition
Natal tooth, teeth 520.6
Nausea (*see also* Vomiting) 787.02
with vomiting 787.01
epidemic 078.82
gravidarum – *see* Hyperemesis, gravidarum
marina 994.6
Naval – *see* condition
Neapolitan fever (*see also* Brucellosis) 023.9
Near-syncope 780.2
Nearsightedness 367.1
Nebécourt's syndrome 253.3
Nebula, cornea (eye) 371.01
congenital 743.43
interfering with vision 743.42
Necator americanus infestation 126.1
Necatoriasis 126.1
Neck – *see* condition
Necrencephalus (*see also* Softening, brain) 437.8
Necrobacillosis 040.3
Necrobiosis 799.89
brain or cerebral (*see also* Softening, brain) 437.8
lipoidica 709.3
diabeticorum 250.8❺ *[709.3]*
Necrodermolysis 695.1
Necrolysis, toxic epidermal 695.1
due to drug
correct substance properly administered 695.1
overdose or wrong substance given or taken 977.9
specified drug – *see* Table of Drugs and Chemicals
Necrophilia 302.89

Necrosis, necrotic
adrenal (capsule) (gland) 255.8
antrum, nasal sinus 478.19
aorta (hyaline) (*see also* Aneurysm, aorta) 441.9
cystic medial 441.00
abdominal 441.02
thoracic 441.01
thoracoabdominal 441.03
ruptured 441.5
arteritis 446.0
artery 447.5
aseptic, bone 733.40
femur (head) (neck) 733.42
medial condyle 733.43
humoral head 733.41
jaw 733.45 ●
medial femoral condyle 733.43
specific site NEC 733.49
talus 733.44
avascular, bone NEC (*see also* Necrosis, aseptic, bone) 733.40
bladder (aseptic) (sphincter) 596.8
bone (*see also* Osteomyelitis) 730.1❺
acute 730.0❺
aseptic or avascular 733.40
femur (head) (neck) 733.42
medial condyle 733.43
humoral head 733.41
jaw 733.45 ●
medial femoral condyle 733.43
specified site NEC 733.49
talus 733.44
ethmoid 478.19
ischemic 733.40
jaw 526.4
aseptic 733.45 ●
marrow 289.89
Paget's (osteitis deformans) 731.0
tuberculous – *see* Tuberculosis, bone
brain (softening) (*see also* Softening, brain) 437.8
breast (aseptic) (fat) (segmental) 611.3
bronchus, bronchi 519.19
central nervous system NEC (*see also* Softening, brain) 437.8
cerebellar (*see also* Softening, brain) 437.8
cerebral (softening) (*see also* Softening, brain) 437.8
cerebrospinal (softening) (*see also* Softening, brain) 437.8
colon 557.0 ●
cornea (*see also* Keratitis) 371.40
cortical, kidney 583.6
cystic medial (aorta) 441.00
abdominal 441.02
thoracic 441.01
thoracoabdominal 441.03
dental 521.09
pulp 522.1
due to swallowing corrosive substance – *see* Burn, by site
ear (ossicle) 385.24
esophagus 530.89
ethmoid (bone) 478.19
eyelid 374.50
fat, fatty (generalized) (*see also* Degeneration, fatty) 272.8
abdominal wall 567.82
breast (aseptic) (segmental) 611.3
intestine 569.89
localized – *see* Degeneration, by site, fatty
mesentery 567.82
omentum 567.82
pancreas 577.8
peritoneum 567.82
skin (subcutaneous) 709.3
newborn 778.1
femur (aseptic) (avascular) 733.42
head 733.42
medial condyle 733.43
neck 733.42
gallbladder (*see also* Cholecystitis, acute) 575.0
gangrenous 785.4
gastric 537.89
glottis 478.79
heart (myocardium) – *see* Infarct, myocardium
hepatic (*see also* Necrosis, liver) 570
hip (aseptic) (avascular) 733.42
intestine (acute) (hemorrhagic) (massive) 557.0
ischemic 785.4
jaw 526.4
aseptic 733.45 ●
kidney (bilateral) 583.9
acute 584.9

Necrosis, necrotic – *continued*
kidney (bilateral) – *continued*
cortical 583.6
acute 584.6
with
abortion – *see* Abortion, by type, with renal failure
ectopic pregnancy (*see also* categories 633.0-633.9) 639.3
molar pregnancy (*see also* categories 630-632) 639.3
complicating pregnancy 646.2❺
affecting fetus or newborn 760.1
following labor and delivery 669.3❺
medullary (papillary) (*see also* Pyelitis) 590.80
in
acute renal failure 584.7
nephritis, nephropathy 583.7
papillary (*see also* Pyelitis) 590.80
in
acute renal failure 584.7
nephritis, nephropathy 583.7
tubular 584.5
with
abortion – *see* Abortion, by type, with renal failure
ectopic pregnancy (*see also* categories 633.0-633.9) 639.3
molar pregnancy (*see also* categories 630-632) 639.3
complicating
abortion 639.3
ectopic or molar pregnancy 639.3
pregnancy 646.2❺
affecting fetus or newborn 760.1
following labor and delivery 669.3❺
traumatic 958.5
larynx 478.79
liver (acute) (congenital) (diffuse) (massive) (subacute) 570
with
abortion – *see* Abortion, by type, with specified complication NEC
ectopic pregnancy (*see also* categories 633.0-633.9) 639.8
molar pregnancy (*see also* categories 630-632) 639.8
complicating pregnancy 646.7❺
affecting fetus or newborn 760.8
following
abortion 639.8
ectopic or molar pregnancy 639.8
obstetrical 646.7❺
postabortal 639.8
puerperal, postpartum 674.8❺
toxic 573.3
lung 513.0
lymphatic gland 683
mammary gland 611.3
mastoid (chronic) 383.1
mesentery 557.0
fat 567.82
mitral valve – *see* Insufficiency, mitral
myocardium, myocardial – *see* Infarct, myocardium
nose (septum) 478.19
omentum 557.0
with mesenteric infarction 557.0
fat 567.82
orbit, orbital 376.10
ossicles, ear (aseptic) 385.24
ovary (*see also* Salpingo-oophoritis) 614.2
pancreas (aseptic) (duct) (fat) 577.8
acute 577.0
infective 577.0
papillary, kidney (*see also* Pyelitis) 590.80
perineum 624.8
peritoneum 557.0
with mesenteric infarction 557.0
fat 567.82
pharynx 462
in granulocytopenia 288.09
phosphorus 983.9
pituitary (gland) (postpartum) (Sheehan) 253.2
placenta (*see also* Placenta, abnormal) 656.7❺
pneumonia 513.0
pulmonary 513.0
pulp (dental) 522.1
pylorus 537.89
radiation – *see* Necrosis, by site
radium – *see* Necrosis, by site
renal – *see* Necrosis, kidney
sclera 379.19
scrotum 608.89

Neoplasm, abdomen, abdominal – Neoplasm, bile or biliary

	Malignant					
	Primary	Secondary	Ca in situ	Benign	Uncertain Behavior	Unspecified
Neoplasm, neoplastic	199.1	199.1	234.9	229.9	238.9	239.9

Notes:

1. *The list below gives the code numbers for neoplasms by anatomical site. For each site there are six possible code numbers according to whether the neoplasm in question is malignant, benign, in situ, of uncertain behavior, or of unspecified nature. The description of the neoplasm will often indicate which of the six columns is appropriate; e.g., malignant melanoma of skin, benign fibroadenoma of breast, carcinoma in situ of cervix uteri.*

   Where such descriptors are not present, the remainder of the Index should be consulted where guidance is given to the appropriate column for each morphological (histological) variety listed; e.g., Mesonephroma – see Neoplasm, malignant; Embryoma – see also Neoplasm, uncertain behavior; Disease, Bowen's – see Neoplasm, skin, in situ. However, the guidance in the Index can be overridden if one of the descriptors mentioned above is present; e.g., malignant adenoma of colon is coded to 153.9 and not to 211.3 as the adjective "malignant" overrides the Index entry "Adenoma - see also Neoplasm, benign."

2. *Sites marked with the sign * (e.g., face NEC*) should be classified to malignant neoplasm of skin of these sites if the variety of neoplasm is a squamous cell carcinoma or an epidermoid carcinoma and to benign neoplasm of skin of these sites if the variety of neoplasm is a papilloma (any type).*

	Primary	Secondary	Ca in situ	Benign	Uncertain Behavior	Unspecified
abdomen, abdominal	195.2	198.89	234.8	229.8	238.8	239.8
cavity	195.2	198.89	234.8	229.8	238.8	239.8
organ	195.2	198.89	234.8	229.8	238.8	239.8
viscera	195.2	198.89	234.8	229.8	238.8	239.8
wall	173.5	198.2	232.5	216.5	238.2	239.2
connective tissue	171.5	198.89	–	215.5	238.1	239.2
abdominopelvic	195.8	198.89	234.8	229.8	238.8	239.8
accessory sinus - *see* Neoplasm, sinus						
acoustic nerve	192.0	198.4	–	225.1	237.9	239.7
acromion (process)	170.4	198.5	–	213.4	238.0	239.2
adenoid (pharynx) (tissue)	147.1	198.89	230.0	210.7	235.1	239.0
adipose tissue (*see also* Neoplasm, connective tissue)	171.9	198.89	–	215.9	238.1	239.2
adnexa (uterine)	183.9	198.82	233.39▲	221.8	236.3	239.5
adrenal (cortex) (gland) (medulla)	194.0	198.7	234.8	227.0	237.2	239.7
ala nasi (external)	173.3	198.2	232.3	216.3	238.2	239.2
alimentary canal or tract NEC	159.9	197.8	230.9	211.9	235.5	239.0
alveolar	143.9	198.89	230.0	210.4	235.1	239.0
mucosa	143.9	198.89	230.0	210.4	235.1	239.0
lower	143.1	198.89	230.0	210.4	235.1	239.0
upper	143.0	198.89	230.0	210.4	235.1	239.0
ridge or process	170.1	198.5	–	213.1	238.0	239.2
carcinoma	143.9	–	–	–	–	–
lower	143.1	–	–	–	–	–
upper	143.0	–	–	–	–	–
lower	170.1	198.5	–	213.1	238.0	239.2
mucosa	143.9	198.89	230.0	210.4	235.1	239.0
lower	143.1	198.89	230.0	210.4	235.1	239.0
upper	143.0	198.89	230.0	210.4	235.1	239.0
upper	170.0	198.5	–	213.0	238.0	239.2
sulcus	145.1	198.89	230.0	210.4	235.1	239.0
alveolus	143.9	198.89	230.0	210.4	235.1	239.0
lower	143.1	198.89	230.0	210.4	235.1	239.0
upper	143.0	198.89	230.0	210.4	235.1	239.0
ampulla of Vater	156.2	197.8	230.8	211.5	235.3	239.0
ankle NEC*	195.5	198.89	232.7	229.8	238.8	239.8
anorectum, anorectal (junction)	154.8	197.5	230.7	211.4	235.2	239.0
antecubital fossa or space*	195.4	198.89	232.6	229.8	238.8	239.8
antrum (Highmore) (maxillary)	160.2	197.3	231.8	212.0	235.9	239.1
pyloric	151.2	197.8	230.2	211.1	235.2	239.0

	Malignant					
	Primary	Secondary	Ca in situ	Benign	Uncertain Behavior	Unspecified
Neoplasm, neoplastic *– continued*						
antrum *– continued*						
tympanicum	160.1	197.3	231.8	212.0	235.9	239.1
anus, anal	154.3	197.5	230.6	211.4	235.5	239.0
canal	154.2	197.5	230.5	211.4	235.5	239.0
contiguous sites with rectosigmoid junction or rectum	154.8	–	–	–	–	–
margin	173.5	198.2	232.5	216.5	238.2	239.2
skin	173.5	198.2	232.5	216.5	238.2	239.2
sphincter	154.2	197.5	230.5	211.4	235.5	239.0
aorta (thoracic)	171.4	198.89	–	215.4	238.1	239.2
abdominal	171.5	198.89	–	215.5	238.1	239.2
aortic body	194.6	198.89	–	227.6	237.3	239.7
aponeurosis	171.9	198.89	–	215.9	238.1	239.2
palmar	171.2	198.89	–	215.2	238.1	239.2
plantar	171.3	198.89	–	215.3	238.1	239.2
appendix	153.5	197.5	230.3	211.3	235.2	239.0
arachnoid (cerebral)	192.1	198.4	–	225.2	237.6	239.7
spinal	192.3	198.4	–	225.4	237.6	239.7
areola (female)	174.0	198.81	233.0	217	238.3	239.3
male	175.0	198.81	233.0	217	238.3	239.3
arm NEC*	195.4	198.89	232.6	229.8	238.8	239.8
artery - *see* Neoplasm, connective tissue						
aryepiglottic fold	148.2	198.89	230.0	210.8	235.1	239.0
hypopharyngeal aspect	148.2	198.89	230.0	210.8	235.1	239.0
laryngeal aspect	161.1	197.3	231.0	212.1	235.6	239.1
marginal zone	148.2	198.89	230.0	210.8	235.1	239.0
arytenoid (cartilage)	161.3	197.3	231.0	212.1	235.6	239.1
fold - *see* Neoplasm, aryepiglottic						
atlas	170.2	198.5	–	213.2	238.0	239.2
atrium, cardiac	164.1	198.89	–	212.7	238.8	239.8
auditory						
canal (external) (skin)	173.2	198.2	232.2	216.2	238.2	239.2
internal	160.1	197.3	231.8	212.0	235.9	239.1
nerve	192.0	198.4	–	225.1	237.9	239.7
tube	160.1	197.3	231.8	212.0	235.9	239.1
opening	147.2	198.89	230.0	210.7	235.1	239.0
auricle, ear	173.2	198.2	232.2	216.2	238.2	239.2
cartilage	171.0	198.89	–	215.0	238.1	239.2
auricular canal (external)	173.2	198.2	232.2	216.2	238.2	239.2
internal	160.1	197.3	231.8	212.0	235.9	239.1
autonomic nerve or nervous system NEC	171.9	198.89	–	215.9	238.1	239.2
axilla, axillary	195.1	198.89	234.8	229.8	238.8	239.8
fold	173.5	198.2	232.5	216.5	238.2	239.2
back NEC*	195.8	198.89	232.5	229.8	238.8	239.8
Bartholin's gland	184.1	198.82	233.32▲	221.2	236.3	239.5
basal ganglia	191.0	198.3	–	225.0	237.5	239.6
basis pedunculi	191.7	198.3	–	225.0	237.5	239.6
bile or biliary (tract)	156.9	197.8	230.8	211.5	235.3	239.0
canaliculi (biliferi) (intrahepatic)	155.1	197.8	230.8	211.5	235.3	239.0
canals, interlobular	155.1	197.8	230.8	211.5	235.3	239.0
contiguous sites	156.8	–	–	–	–	–
duct or passage (common) (cystic) (extrahepatic)	156.1	197.8	230.8	211.5	235.3	239.0
contiguous sites with gallbladder	156.8	–	–	–	–	–
interlobular	155.1	197.8	230.8	211.5	235.3	239.0
intrahepatic	155.1	197.8	230.8	211.5	235.3	239.0
and extrahepatic	156.9	197.8	230.8	211.5	235.3	239.0

	Malignant					
	Primary	Secondary	Ca in situ	Benign	Uncertain Behavior	Unspecified
Neoplasm, neoplastic – *continued*						
bladder (urinary)	188.9	198.1	233.7	223.3	236.7	239.4
contiguous sites	188.8	–	–	–	–	–
dome	188.1	198.1	233.7	223.3	236.7	239.4
neck	188.5	198.1	233.7	223.3	236.7	239.4
orifice	188.9	198.1	233.7	223.3	236.7	239.4
ureteric	188.6	198.1	233.7	223.3	236.7	239.4
urethral	188.5	198.1	233.7	223.3	236.7	239.4
sphincter	188.8	198.1	233.7	223.3	236.7	239.4
trigone	188.0	198.1	233.7	223.3	236.7	239.4
urachus	188.7	–	233.7	223.3	236.7	239.4
wall	188.9	198.1	233.7	223.3	236.7	239.4
anterior	188.3	198.1	233.7	223.3	236.7	239.4
lateral	188.2	198.1	233.7	223.3	236.7	239.4
posterior	188.4	198.1	233.7	223.3	236.7	239.4
blood vessel - *see* Neoplasm, connective tissue						
bone (periosteum)	170.9	198.5	–	213.9	238.0	239.2

Note: Carcinomas and adenocarcinomas, of any type other than intraosseous or odontogenic, of the sites listed under "Neoplasm, bone" should be considered as constituting metastatic spread from an unspecified primary site and coded to 198.5 for morbidity coding and to 199.1 for underlying cause of death coding.

	Primary	Secondary	Ca in situ	Benign	Uncertain Behavior	Unspecified
acetabulum	170.6	198.5	–	213.6	238.0	239.2
acromion (process)	170.4	198.5	–	213.4	238.0	239.2
ankle	170.8	198.5	–	213.8	238.0	239.2
arm NEC	170.4	198.5	–	213.4	238.0	239.2
astragalus	170.8	198.5	–	213.8	238.0	239.2
atlas	170.2	198.5	–	213.2	238.0	239.2
axis	170.2	198.5	–	213.2	238.0	239.2
back NEC	170.2	198.5	–	213.2	238.0	239.2
calcaneus	170.8	198.5	–	213.8	238.0	239.2
calvarium	170.0	198.5	–	213.0	238.0	239.2
carpus (any)	170.5	198.5	–	213.5	238.0	239.2
cartilage NEC	170.9	198.5	–	213.9	238.0	239.2
clavicle	170.3	198.5	–	213.3	238.0	239.2
clivus	170.0	198.5	–	213.0	238.0	239.2
coccygeal vertebra	170.6	198.5	–	213.6	238.0	239.2
coccyx	170.6	198.5	–	213.6	238.0	239.2
costal cartilage	170.3	198.5	–	213.3	238.0	239.2
costovertebral joint	170.3	198.5	–	213.3	238.0	239.2
cranial	170.0	198.5	–	213.0	238.0	239.2
cuboid	170.8	198.5	–	213.8	238.0	239.2
cuneiform	170.9	198.5	–	213.9	238.0	239.2
ankle	170.8	198.5	–	213.8	238.0	239.2
wrist	170.5	198.5	–	213.5	238.0	239.2
digital	170.9	198.5	–	213.9	238.0	239.2
finger	170.5	198.5	–	213.5	238.0	239.2
toe	170.8	198.5	–	213.8	238.0	239.2
elbow	170.4	198.5	–	213.4	238.0	239.2
ethmoid (labyrinth)	170.0	198.5	–	213.0	238.0	239.2
face	170.0	198.5	–	213.0	238.0	239.2
lower jaw	170.1	198.5	–	213.1	238.0	239.2
femur (any part)	170.7	198.5	–	213.7	238.0	239.2
fibula (any part)	170.7	198.5	–	213.7	238.0	239.2
finger (any)	170.5	198.5	–	213.5	238.0	239.2
foot	170.8	198.5	–	213.8	238.0	239.2
forearm	170.4	198.5	–	213.4	238.0	239.2
frontal	170.0	198.5	–	213.0	238.0	239.2
hand	170.5	198.5	–	213.5	238.0	239.2
heel	170.8	198.5	–	213.8	238.0	239.2
hip	170.6	198.5	–	213.6	238.0	239.2
humerus (any part)	170.4	198.5	–	213.4	238.0	239.2
hyoid	170.0	198.5	–	213.0	238.0	239.2
ilium	170.6	198.5	–	213.6	238.0	239.2
innominate	170.6	198.5	–	213.6	238.0	239.2

	Malignant					
	Primary	Secondary	Ca in situ	Benign	Uncertain Behavior	Unspecified
Neoplasm, neoplastic – *continued*						
bone – *continued*						
intervertebral cartilage or disc	170.2	198.5	–	213.2	238.0	239.2
ischium	170.6	198.5	–	213.6	238.0	239.2
jaw (lower)	170.1	198.5	–	213.1	238.0	239.2
upper	170.0	198.5	–	213.0	238.0	239.2
knee	170.7	198.5	–	213.7	238.0	239.2
leg NEC	170.7	198.5	–	213.7	238.0	239.2
limb NEC	170.9	198.5	–	213.9	238.0	239.2
lower (long bones)	170.7	198.5	–	213.7	238.0	239.2
short bones	170.8	198.5	–	213.8	238.0	239.2
upper (long bones)	170.4	198.5	–	213.4	238.0	239.2
short bones	170.5	198.5	–	213.5	238.0	239.2
long	170.9	198.5	–	213.9	238.0	239.2
lower limbs NEC	170.7	198.5	–	213.7	238.0	239.2
upper limbs NEC	170.4	198.5	–	213.4	238.0	239.2
malar	170.0	198.5	–	213.0	238.0	239.2
mandible	170.1	198.5	–	213.1	238.0	239.2
marrow NEC	202.9❺	198.5	–	–	–	238.79
mastoid	170.0	198.5	–	213.0	238.0	239.2
maxilla, maxillary (superior)	170.0	198.5	–	213.0	238.0	239.2
inferior	170.1	198.5	–	213.1	238.0	239.2
metacarpus (any)	170.5	198.5	–	213.5	238.0	239.2
metatarsus (any)	170.8	198.5	–	213.8	238.0	239.2
navicular (ankle)	170.8	198.5	–	213.8	238.0	239.2
hand	170.5	198.5	–	213.5	238.0	239.2
nose, nasal	170.0	198.5	–	213.0	238.0	239.2
occipital	170.0	198.5	–	213.0	238.0	239.2
orbit	170.0	198.5	–	213.0	238.0	239.2
parietal	170.0	198.5	–	213.0	238.0	239.2
patella	170.8	198.5	–	213.8	238.0	239.2
pelvic	170.6	198.5	–	213.6	238.0	239.2
phalanges	170.9	198.5	–	213.9	238.0	239.2
foot	170.8	198.5	–	213.8	238.0	239.2
hand	170.5	198.5	–	213.5	238.0	239.2
pubic	170.6	198.5	–	213.6	238.0	239.2
radius (any part)	170.4	198.5	–	213.4	238.0	239.2
rib	170.3	198.5	–	213.3	238.0	239.2
sacral vertebra	170.6	198.5	–	213.6	238.0	239.2
sacrum	170.6	198.5	–	213.6	238.0	239.2
scaphoid (of hand)	170.5	198.5	–	213.5	238.0	239.2
of ankle	170.8	198.5	–	213.8	238.0	239.2
scapula (any part)	170.4	198.5	–	213.4	238.0	239.2
sella turcica	170.0	198.5	–	213.0	238.0	239.2
short	170.9	198.5	–	213.9	238.0	239.2
lower limb	170.8	198.5	–	213.8	238.0	239.2
upper limb	170.5	198.5	–	213.5	238.0	239.2
shoulder	170.4	198.5	–	213.4	238.0	239.2
skeleton, skeletal NEC	170.9	198.5	–	213.9	238.0	239.2
skull	170.0	198.5	–	213.0	238.0	239.2
sphenoid	170.0	198.5	–	213.0	238.0	239.2
spine, spinal (column)	170.2	198.5	–	213.2	238.0	239.2
coccyx	170.6	198.5	–	213.6	238.0	239.2
sacrum	170.6	198.5	–	213.6	238.0	239.2
sternum	170.3	198.5	–	213.3	238.0	239.2
tarsus (any)	170.8	198.5	–	213.8	238.0	239.2
temporal	170.0	198.5	–	213.0	238.0	239.2
thumb	170.5	198.5	–	213.5	238.0	239.2
tibia (any part)	170.7	198.5	–	213.7	238.0	239.2
toe (any)	170.8	198.5	–	213.8	238.0	239.2
trapezium	170.5	198.5	–	213.5	238.0	239.2
trapezoid	170.5	198.5	–	213.5	238.0	239.2
turbinate	170.0	198.5	–	213.0	238.0	239.2
ulna (any part)	170.4	198.5	–	213.4	238.0	239.2
unciform	170.5	198.5	–	213.5	238.0	239.2

Neoplasm, bladder – Neoplasm, bone

Neoplasm, bone – Neoplasm, cartilage

	Malignant					
	Primary	Secondary	Ca in situ	Benign	Uncertain Behavior	Unspecified
Neoplasm, neoplastic – *continued*						
bone – *continued*						
vertebra (column)	170.2	198.5	–	213.2	238.0	239.2
coccyx	170.6	198.5	–	213.6	238.0	239.2
sacrum	170.6	198.5	–	213.6	238.0	239.2
vomer	170.0	198.5	–	213.0	238.0	239.2
wrist	170.5	198.5	–	213.5	238.0	239.2
xiphoid process	170.3	198.5	–	213.3	238.0	239.2
zygomatic	170.0	198.5	–	213.0	238.0	239.2
book-leaf (mouth)	145.8	198.89	230.0	210.4	235.1	239.0
bowel - *see* Neoplasm, intestine						
brachial plexus	171.2	198.89	–	215.2	238.1	239.2
brain NEC	191.9	198.3	–	225.0	237.5	239.6
basal ganglia	191.0	198.3	–	225.0	237.5	239.6
cerebellopontine angle	191.6	198.3	–	225.0	237.5	239.6
cerebellum NOS	191.6	198.3	–	225.0	237.5	239.6
cerebrum	191.0	198.3	–	225.0	237.5	239.6
choroid plexus	191.5	198.3	–	225.0	237.5	239.6
contiguous sites	191.8	–	–	–	–	–
corpus callosum	191.8	198.3	–	225.0	237.5	239.6
corpus striatum	191.0	198.3	–	225.0	237.5	239.6
cortex (cerebral)	191.0	198.3	–	225.0	237.5	239.6
frontal lobe	191.1	198.3	–	225.0	237.5	239.6
globus pallidus	191.0	198.3	–	225.0	237.5	239.6
hippocampus	191.2	198.3	–	225.0	237.5	239.6
hypothalamus	191.0	198.3	–	225.0	237.5	239.6
internal capsule	191.0	198.3	–	225.0	237.5	239.6
medulla oblongata	191.7	198.3	–	225.0	237.5	239.6
meninges	192.1	198.4	–	225.2	237.6	239.7
midbrain	191.7	198.3	–	225.0	237.5	239.6
occipital lobe	191.4	198.3	–	225.0	237.5	239.6
parietal lobe	191.3	198.3	–	225.0	237.5	239.6
peduncle	191.7	198.3	–	225.0	237.5	239.6
pons	191.7	198.3	–	225.0	237.5	239.6
stem	191.7	198.3	–	225.0	237.5	239.6
tapetum	191.8	198.3	–	225.0	237.5	239.6
temporal lobe	191.2	198.3	–	225.0	237.5	239.6
thalamus	191.0	198.3	–	225.0	237.5	239.6
uncus	191.2	198.3	–	225.0	237.5	239.6
ventricle (floor)	191.5	198.3	–	225.0	237.5	239.6
branchial (cleft) (vestiges)	146.8	198.89	230.0	210.6	235.1	239.0
breast (connective tissue) (female) (glandular tissue) (soft parts)	174.9	198.81	233.0	217	238.3	239.3
areola	174.0	198.81	233.0	217	238.3	239.3
male	175.0	198.81	233.0	217	238.3	239.3
axillary tail	174.6	198.81	233.0	217	238.3	239.3
central portion	174.1	198.81	233.0	217	238.3	239.3
contiguous sites	174.8	–	–	–	–	–
ectopic sites	174.8	198.81	233.0	217	238.3	239.3
inner	174.8	198.81	233.0	217	238.3	239.3
lower	174.8	198.81	233.0	217	238.3	239.3
lower-inner quadrant	174.3	198.81	233.0	217	238.3	239.3
lower-outer quadrant	174.5	198.81	233.0	217	238.3	239.3
male	175.9	198.81	233.0	217	238.3	239.3
areola	175.0	198.81	233.0	217	238.3	239.3
ectopic tissue	175.9	198.81	233.0	217	238.3	239.3
nipple	175.0	198.81	233.0	217	238.3	239.3
mastectomy site (skin)	173.5	198.2	–	–	–	–
specified as breast tissue	174.8	198.81	–	–	–	–
midline	174.8	198.81	233.0	217	238.3	239.3
nipple	174.0	198.81	233.0	217	238.3	239.3
male	175.0	198.81	233.0	217	238.3	239.3

	Malignant					
	Primary	Secondary	Ca in situ	Benign	Uncertain Behavior	Unspecified
Neoplasm, neoplastic – *continued*						
breast – *continued*						
outer	174.8	198.81	233.0	217	238.3	239.3
skin	173.5	198.2	232.5	216.5	238.2	239.2
tail (axillary)	174.6	198.81	233.0	217	238.3	239.3
upper	174.8	198.81	233.0	217	238.3	239.3
upper-inner quadrant	174.2	198.81	233.0	217	238.3	239.3
upper–outer quadrant	174.4	198.81	233.0	217	238.3	239.3
broad ligament	183.3	198.82	233.39▲	221.0	236.3	239.5
bronchiogenic, bronchogenic (lung)	162.9	197.0	231.2	212.3	235.7	239.1
bronchiole	162.9	197.0	231.2	212.3	235.7	239.1
bronchus	162.9	197.0	231.2	212.3	235.7	239.1
carina	162.2	197.0	231.2	212.3	235.7	239.1
contiguous sites with lung or trachea	162.8	–	–	–	–	–
lower lobe of lung	162.5	197.0	231.2	212.3	235.7	239.1
main	162.2	197.0	231.2	212.3	235.7	239.1
middle lobe of lung	162.4	197.0	231.2	212.3	235.7	239.1
upper lobe of lung	162.3	197.0	231.2	212.3	235.7	239.1
brow	173.3	198.2	232.3	216.3	238.2	239.2
buccal (cavity)	145.9	198.89	230.0	210.4	235.1	239.0
commissure	145.0	198.89	230.0	210.4	235.1	239.0
groove (lower) (upper)	145.1	198.89	230.0	210.4	235.1	239.0
mucosa	145.0	198.89	230.0	210.4	235.1	239.0
sulcus (lower) (upper)	145.1	198.89	230.0	210.4	235.1	239.0
bulbourethral gland	189.3	198.1	233.9	223.81	236.99	239.5
bursa - *see* Neoplasm, connective tissue						
buttock NEC*	195.3	198.89	232.5	229.8	238.8	239.8
calf*	195.5	198.89	232.7	229.8	238.8	239.8
calvarium	170.0	198.5	–	213.0	238.0	239.2
calyx, renal	189.1	198.0	233.9	223.1	236.91	239.5
canal						
anal	154.2	197.5	230.5	211.4	235.5	239.0
auditory (external)	173.2	198.2	232.2	216.2	238.2	239.2
auricular (external)	173.2	198.2	232.2	216.2	238.2	239.2
canaliculi, biliary (biliferi) (intrahepatic)	155.1	197.8	230.8	211.5	235.3	239.0
canthus (eye) (inner) (outer)	173.1	198.2	232.1	216.1	238.2	239.2
capillary - *see* Neoplasm, connective tissue						
caput coli	153.4	197.5	230.3	211.3	235.2	239.0
cardia (gastric)	151.0	197.8	230.2	211.1	235.2	239.0
cardiac orifice (stomach)	151.0	197.8	230.2	211.1	235.2	239.0
cardio–esophageal junction	151.0	197.8	230.2	211.1	235.2	239.0
cardio–esophagus	151.0	197.8	230.2	211.1	235.2	239.0
carina (bronchus)	162.2	197.0	231.2	212.3	235.7	239.1
carotid (artery)	171.0	198.89	–	215.0	238.1	239.2
body	194.5	198.89	–	227.5	237.3	239.7
carpus (any bone)	170.5	198.5	–	213.5	238.0	239.2
cartilage (articular) (joint) NEC - *see also* Neoplasm, bone	170.9	198.5	–	213.9	238.0	239.2
arytenoid	161.3	197.3	231.0	212.1	235.6	239.1
auricular	171.0	198.89	–	215.0	238.1	239.2
bronchi	162.2	197.3	–	212.3	235.7	239.1
connective tissue - *see* Neoplasm, connective tissue						
costal	170.3	198.5	–	213.3	238.0	239.2
cricoid	161.3	197.3	231.0	212.1	235.6	239.1
cuneiform	161.3	197.3	231.0	212.1	235.6	239.1
ear (external)	171.0	198.89	–	215.0	238.1	239.2
ensiform	170.3	198.5	–	213.3	238.0	239.2

	Malignant					
	Primary	Secondary	Ca in situ	Benign	Uncertain Behavior	Unspecified
Neoplasm, neoplastic – *continued*						
cartilage – *continued*						
epiglottis	161.1	197.3	231.0	212.1	235.6	239.1
anterior surface	146.4	198.89	230.0	210.6	235.1	239.0
eyelid	171.0	198.89	–	215.0	238.1	239.2
intervertebral	170.2	198.5	–	213.2	238.0	239.2
larynx, laryngeal	161.3	197.3	231.0	212.1	235.6	239.1
nose, nasal	160.0	197.3	231.8	212.0	235.9	239.1
pinna	171.0	198.89	–	215.0	238.1	239.2
rib	170.3	198.5	–	213.3	238.0	239.2
semilunar (knee)	170.7	198.5	–	213.7	238.0	239.2
thyroid	161.3	197.3	231.0	212.1	235.6	239.1
trachea	162.0	197.3	231.1	212.2	235.7	239.1
cauda equina	192.2	198.3	–	225.3	237.5	239.7
cavity						
buccal	145.9	198.89	230.0	210.4	235.1	239.0
nasal	160.0	197.3	231.8	212.0	235.9	239.1
oral	145.9	198.89	230.0	210.4	235.1	239.0
peritoneal	158.9	197.6	–	211.8	235.4	239.0
tympanic	160.1	197.3	231.8	212.0	235.9	239.1
cecum	153.4	197.5	230.3	211.3	235.2	239.0
central						
nervous system - *see* Neoplasm, nervous system						
white matter	191.0	198.3	–	225.0	237.5	239.6
cerebellopontine (angle)	191.6	198.3	–	225.0	237.5	239.6
cerebellum, cerebellar	191.6	198.3	–	225.0	237.5	239.6
cerebrum, cerebral (cortex) (hemisphere) (white matter)	191.0	198.3	–	225.0	237.5	239.6
meninges	192.1	198.4	–	225.2	237.6	239.7
peduncle	191.7	198.3	–	225.0	237.5	239.6
ventricle (any)	191.5	198.3	–	225.0	237.5	239.6
cervical region	195.0	198.89	234.8	229.8	238.8	239.8
cervix (cervical) (uteri) (uterus)	180.9	198.82	233.1	219.0	236.0	239.5
canal	180.0	198.82	233.1	219.0	236.0	239.5
contiguous sites	180.8	–	–	–	–	–
endocervix (canal) (gland)	180.0	198.82	233.1	219.0	236.0	239.5
exocervix	180.1	198.82	233.1	219.0	236.0	239.5
external os	180.1	198.82	233.1	219.0	236.0	239.5
internal os	180.0	198.82	233.1	219.0	236.0	239.5
nabothian gland	180.0	198.82	233.1	219.0	236.0	239.5
squamocolumnar junction	180.8	198.82	233.1	219.0	236.0	239.5
stump	180.8	198.82	233.1	219.0	236.0	239.5
cheek	195.0	198.89	234.8	229.8	238.8	239.8
external	173.3	198.2	232.3	216.3	238.2	239.2
inner aspect	145.0	198.89	230.0	210.4	235.1	239.0
internal	145.0	198.89	230.0	210.4	235.1	239.0
mucosa	145.0	198.89	230.0	210.4	235.1	239.0
chest (wall) NEC	195.1	198.89	234.8	229.8	238.8	239.8
chiasma opticum	192.0	198.4	–	225.1	237.9	239.7
chin	173.3	198.2	232.3	216.3	238.2	239.2
choana	147.3	198.89	230.0	210.7	235.1	239.0
cholangiole	155.1	197.8	230.8	211.5	235.3	239.0
choledochal duct	156.1	197.8	230.8	211.5	235.3	239.0
choroid	190.6	198.4	234.0	224.6	238.8	239.8
plexus	191.5	198.3	–	225.0	237.5	239.6
ciliary body	190.0	198.4	234.0	224.0	238.8	239.8
clavicle	170.3	198.5	–	213.3	238.0	239.2
clitoris	184.3	198.82	233.32▲	221.2	236.3	239.5
clivus	170.0	198.5	–	213.0	238.0	239.2
cloacogenic zone	154.8	197.5	230.7	211.4	235.5	239.0
coccygeal						
body or glomus	194.6	198.89	–	227.6	237.3	239.7

	Malignant					
	Primary	Secondary	Ca in situ	Benign	Uncertain Behavior	Unspecified
Neoplasm, neoplastic – *continued*						
coccygeal – *continued*						
vertebra	170.6	198.5	–	213.6	233.0	239.2
coccyx	170.6	198.5	–	213.6	233.0	239.2
colon - *see also* Neoplasm, intestine, large and rectum	154.0	197.5	230.4	211.4	235.2	239.0
column, spinal - *see* Neoplasm, spine						
columnella	173.3	198.2	232.3	216.3	238.2	239.2
commissure						
labial, lip	140.6	198.89	230.0	210.4	235.1	239.0
laryngeal	161.0	197.3	231.0	212.1	235.6	239.1
common (bile) duct	156.1	197.8	230.8	211.5	235.3	239.0
concha	173.2	198.2	232.2	216.2	238.2	239.2
nose	160.0	197.3	231.8	212.0	235.9	239.1
conjunctiva	190.3	198.4	234.0	224.3	238.8	239.8
connective tissue NEC	171.9	198.89	–	215.9	238.1	239.2

Note: For neoplasms of connective tissue (blood vessel, bursa, fascia, ligament, muscle, peripheral nerves, sympathetic and parasympathetic nerves and ganglia, synovia, tendon, etc.) or of morphological types that indicate connective tissue, code according to the list under "Neoplasm, connective tissue;" for sites that do not appear in this list, code to neoplasm of that site; e.g.,

- *liposarcoma, shoulder 171.2*
- *leiomyosarcoma, stomach 151.9*
- *neurofibroma, chest wall 215.4*

Morphological types that indicate connective tissue appear in their proper place in the alphabetic index with the instruction "see Neoplasm, connective tissue"

	Primary	Secondary	Ca in situ	Benign	Uncertain Behavior	Unspecified
abdomen	171.5	198.89	–	215.5	238.1	239.2
abdominal wall	171.5	198.89	–	215.5	238.1	239.2
ankle	171.3	198.89	–	215.3	238.1	239.2
antecubital fossa or space	171.2	198.89	–	215.2	238.1	239.2
arm	171.2	198.89	–	215.2	238.1	239.2
auricle (ear)	171.0	198.89	–	215.0	238.1	239.2
axilla	171.4	198.89	–	215.4	238.1	239.2
back	171.7	198.89	–	215.7	238.1	239.2
breast (female) (*see also* Neoplasm, breast)	174.9	198.81	233.0	217	238.3	239.3
male	175.9	198.81	233.0	217	238.3	239.3
buttock	171.6	198.89	–	215.6	238.1	239.2
calf	171.3	198.89	–	215.3	238.1	239.2
cervical region	171.0	198.89	–	215.0	238.1	239.2
cheek	171.0	198.89	–	215.0	238.1	239.2
chest (wall)	171.4	198.89	–	215.4	238.1	239.2
chin	171.0	198.89	–	215.0	238.1	239.2
contiguous sites	171.8	–	–	–	–	–
diaphragm	171.4	198.89	–	215.4	238.1	239.2
ear (external)	171.0	198.89	–	215.0	238.1	239.2
elbow	171.2	198.89	–	215.2	238.1	239.2
extrarectal	171.6	198.89	–	215.6	238.1	239.2
extremity	171.8	198.89	–	215.8	238.1	239.2
lower	171.3	198.89	–	215.3	238.1	239.2
upper	171.2	198.89	–	215.2	238.1	239.2
eyelid	171.0	198.89	–	215.0	238.1	239.2
face.	171.0	198.89	–	215.0	238.1	239.2
finger	171.2	198.89	–	215.2	238.1	239.2
flank	171.7	198.89	–	215.7	238.1	239.2
foot.	171.3	198.89	–	215.3	238.1	239.2
forearm	171.2	198.89	–	215.2	238.1	239.2
forehead	171.0	198.89	–	215.0	238.1	239.2
gastric	171.5	198.89	–	215.5	238.1	–
gastrointestinal	171.5	198.89	–	215.5	238.1	–
gluteal region	171.6	198.89	–	215.6	238.1	239.2
great vessels NEC	171.4	198.89	–	215.4	238.1	239.2
groin	171.6	198.89	–	215.6	238.1	239.2

Neoplasm, cartilage – Neoplasm, connective tissue

	Malignant					
	Primary	Secondary	Ca in situ	Benign	Uncertain Behavior	Unspecified
Neoplasm, neoplastic – *continued*						
connective tissue – *continued*						
hand	171.2	198.89	–	215.2	238.1	239.2
head	171.0	198.89	–	215.0	238.1	239.2
heel	171.3	198.89	–	215.3	238.1	239.2
hip	171.3	198.89	–	215.3	238.1	239.2
hypochondrium	171.5	198.89	–	215.5	238.1	239.2
iliopsoas muscle	171.6	198.89	–	215.5	238.1	239.2
infraclavicular region	171.4	198.89	–	215.4	238.1	239.2
inguinal (canal) (region)	171.6	198.89	–	215.6	238.1	239.2
intestinal	171.5	198.89	–	215.5	238.1	–
intrathoracic	171.4	198.89	–	215.4	238.1	239.2
ischorectal fossa	171.6	198.89	–	215.6	238.1	239.2
jaw	143.9	198.89	230.0	210.4	235.1	239.0
knee	171.3	198.89	–	215.3	238.1	239.2
leg	171.3	198.89	–	215.3	238.1	239.2
limb NEC	171.9	198.89	–	215.8	238.1	239.2
lower	171.3	198.89	–	215.3	238.1	239.2
upper	171.2	198.89	–	215.2	238.1	239.2
nates	171.6	198.89	–	215.6	238.1	239.2
neck	171.0	198.89	–	215.0	238.1	239.2
orbit	190.1	198.4	234.0	224.1	238.8	239.8
pararectal	171.6	198.89	–	215.6	238.1	239.2
para-urethral	171.6	198.89	–	215.6	238.1	239.2
paravaginal	171.6	198.89	–	215.6	238.1	239.2
pelvis (floor)	171.6	198.89	–	215.6	238.1	239.2
pelvo-abdominal	171.8	198.89	–	215.8	238.1	239.2
perirectal (tissue)	171.6	198.89	–	215.6	238.1	239.2
periurethral (tissue)	171.6	198.89	–	215.6	238.1	239.2
popliteal fossa or space	171.3	198.89	–	215.3	238.1	239.2
presacral	171.6	198.89	–	215.6	238.1	239.2
psoas muscle	171.5	198.89	–	215.5	238.1	239.2
pterygoid fossa	171.0	198.89	–	215.0	238.1	239.2
rectovaginal septum or wall	171.6	198.89	–	215.6	238.1	239.2
rectovesical	171.6	198.89	–	215.6	238.1	239.2
retroperitoneum	158.0	197.6	–	211.8	235.4	239.0
sacrococcygeal region	171.6	198.89	–	215.6	238.1	239.2
scalp	171.0	198.89	–	215.0	238.1	239.2
scapular region	171.4	198.89	–	215.4	238.1	239.2
shoulder	171.2	198.89	–	215.2	238.1	239.2
skin (dermis) NEC	173.9	198.2	232.9	216.9	238.2	239.2
stomach	171.5	198.89	–	215.5	238.1	–
submental	171.0	198.89	–	215.0	238.1	239.2
supraclavicular region	171.0	198.89	–	215.0	238.1	239.2
temple	171.0	198.89	–	215.0	238.1	239.2
temporal region	171.0	198.89	–	215.0	238.1	239.2
thigh	171.3	198.89	–	215.3	238.1	239.2
thoracic (duct) (wall)	171.4	198.89	–	215.4	238.1	239.2
thorax	171.4	198.89	–	215.4	238.1	239.2
thumb	171.2	198.89	–	215.2	238.1	239.2
toe	171.3	198.89	–	215.3	238.1	239.2
trunk	171.7	198.89	–	215.7	238.1	239.2
umbilicus	171.5	198.89	–	215.5	238.1	239.2
vesicorectal	171.6	198.89	–	215.6	238.1	239.2
wrist	171.2	198.89	–	215.2	238.1	239.2
conus medullaris	192.2	198.3	–	225.3	237.5	239.7
cord (true) (vocal)	161.0	197.3	231.0	212.1	235.6	239.1
false	161.1	197.3	231.0	212.1	235.6	239.1
spermatic	187.6	198.82	233.6	222.8	236.6	239.5
spinal (cervical) (lumbar) (thoracic)	192.2	198.3	–	225.3	237.5	239.7
cornea (limbus)	190.4	198.4	234.0	224.4	238.8	239.8
Neoplasm, neoplastic – *continued*						
corpus						
albicans	183.0	198.6	233.39▲	220	236.2	239.5
callosum, brain	191.8	198.3	–	225.0	237.5	239.6
cavernosum	187.3	198.82	233.5	222.1	236.6	239.5
gastric	151.4	197.8	230.2	211.1	235.2	239.0
penis	187.3	198.82	233.5	222.1	236.6	239.5
striatum, cerebrum	191.0	198.3	–	225.0	237.5	239.6
uteri	182.0	198.82	233.2	219.1	236.0	239.5
isthmus	182.1	198.82	233.2	219.1	236.0	239.5
cortex						
adrenal	194.0	198.7	234.8	227.0	237.2	239.7
cerebral	191.0	198.3	–	225.0	237.5	239.6
costal cartilage	170.3	198.5	–	213.3	238.0	239.2
costovertebral joint	170.3	198.5	–	213.3	238.0	239.2
Cowper's gland	189.3	198.1	233.9	223.81	236.99	239.5
cranial (fossa, any)	191.9	198.3	–	225.0	237.5	239.6
meninges	192.1	198.4	–	225.2	237.6	239.7
nerve (any)	192.0	198.4	–	225.1	237.9	239.7
craniobuccal pouch	194.3	198.89	234.8	227.3	237.0	239.7
craniopharyngeal (duct) (pouch)	194.3	198.89	234.8	227.3	237.0	239.7
cricoid	148.0	198.89	230.0	210.8	235.1	239.0
cartilage	161.3	197.3	231.0	212.1	235.6	239.1
cricopharynx	148.0	198.89	230.0	210.8	235.1	239.0
crypt of Morgagni	154.8	197.5	230.7	211.4	235.2	239.0
crystalline lens	190.0	198.4	234.0	224.0	238.8	239.8
cul-de-sac (Douglas')	158.8	197.6	–	211.8	235.4	239.0
cuneiform cartilage	161.3	197.3	231.0	212.1	235.6	239.1
cutaneous - *see* Neoplasm, skin						
cutis - *see* Neoplasm, skin						
cystic (bile) duct (common)	156.1	197.8	230.8	211.5	235.3	239.0
dermis - *see* Neoplasm, skin						
diaphragm	171.4	198.89	–	215.4	238.1	239.2
digestive organs, system, tube, or tract NEC	159.9	197.8	230.9	211.9	235.5	239.0
contiguous sites with peritoneum	159.8	–	–	–	–	–
disc, intervertebral	170.2	198.5	–	213.2	238.0	239.2
disease, generalized	199.0	199.0	234.9	229.9	238.9	199.0
disseminated	199.0	199.0	234.9	229.9	238.9	199.0
Douglas' cul-de-sac or pouch	158.8	197.6	–	211.8	235.4	239.0
duodenojejunal junction	152.8	197.4	230.7	211.2	235.2	239.0
duodenum	152.0	197.4	230.7	211.2	235.2	239.0
dura (cranial) (mater)	192.1	198.4	–	225.2	237.6	239.7
cerebral	192.1	198.4	–	225.2	237.6	239.7
spinal	192.3	198.4	–	225.4	237.6	239.7
ear (external)	173.2	198.2	232.2	216.2	238.2	239.2
auricle or auris	173.2	198.2	232.2	216.2	238.2	239.2
canal, external	173.2	198.2	232.2	216.2	238.2	239.2
cartilage	171.0	198.89	–	215.0	238.1	239.2
external meatus	173.2	198.2	232.2	216.2	238.2	239.2
inner	160.1	197.3	231.8	212.0	235.9	239.8
lobule	173.2	198.2	232.2	216.2	238.2	239.2
middle	160.1	197.3	231.8	212.0	235.9	239.8
contiguous sites with accessory sinuses or nasal cavities	160.8	–	–	–	–	–
skin	173.2	198.2	232.2	216.2	238.2	239.2
earlobe	173.2	198.2	232.2	216.2	238.2	239.2
ejaculatory duct	187.8	198.82	233.6	222.8	236.6	239.5
elbow NEC*	195.4	198.89	232.6	229.8	238.8	239.8

❹ Fourth-Digit Required ❺ Fifth-Digit Required ►◄ Revised Text ● New Line ▲ Revised Code

	Malignant Primary	Malignant Secondary	Malignant Ca in situ	Benign	Uncertain Behavior	Unspecified
Neoplasm, neoplastic – *continued*						
endocardium	164.1	198.89	–	212.7	238.8	239.8
endocervix (canal) (gland)	180.0	198.82	233.1	219.0	236.0	239.5
endocrine gland NEC	194.9	198.89	–	227.9	237.4	239.7
pluriglandular NEC	194.8	198.89	234.8	227.8	237.4	239.7
endometrium (gland) (stroma)	182.0	198.82	233.2	219.1	236.0	239.5
ensiform cartilage	170.3	198.5	–	213.3	238.0	239.2
enteric - *see* Neoplasm, intestine						
ependyma (brain)	191.5	198.3	–	225.0	237.5	239.6
epicardium	164.1	198.89	–	212.7	238.8	239.8
epididymis	187.5	198.82	233.6	222.3	236.6	239.5
epidural	192.9	198.4	–	225.9	237.9	239.7
epiglottis	161.1	197.3	231.0	212.1	235.6	239.1
anterior aspect or surface	146.4	198.89	230.0	210.6	235.1	239.0
cartilage	161.3	197.3	231.0	212.1	235.6	239.1
free border (margin)	146.4	198.89	230.0	210.6	235.1	239.0
junctional region	146.5	198.89	230.0	210.6	235.1	239.0
posterior (laryngeal) surface	161.1	197.3	231.0	212.1	235.6	239.1
suprahyoid portion	161.1	197.3	231.0	212.1	235.6	239.1
esophagogastric junction	151.0	197.8	230.2	211.1	235.2	239.0
esophagus	150.9	197.8	230.1	211.0	235.5	239.0
abdominal	150.2	197.8	230.1	211.0	235.5	239.0
cervical	150.0	197.8	230.1	211.0	235.5	239.0
contiguous sites	150.8	–	–	–	–	–
distal (third)	150.5	197.8	230.1	211.0	235.5	239.0
lower (third)	150.5	197.8	230.1	211.0	235.5	239.0
middle (third).	150.4	197.8	230.1	211.0	235.5	239.0
proximal (third)	150.3	197.8	230.1	211.0	235.5	239.0
specified part NEC	150.8	197.8	230.1	211.0	235.5	239.0
thoracic	150.1	197.8	230.1	211.0	235.5	239.0
upper (third)	150.3	197.8	230.1	211.0	235.5	239.0
ethmoid (sinus)	160.3	197.3	231.8	212.0	235.9	239.1
bone or labyrinth	170.0	198.5	–	213.0	238.0	239.2
Eustachian tube	160.1	197.3	231.8	212.0	235.9	239.1
exocervix	180.1	198.82	233.1	219.0	236.0	239.5
external						
meatus (ear)	173.2	198.2	232.2	216.2	238.2	239.2
os, cervix uteri	180.1	198.82	233.1	219.0	236.0	239.5
extradural	192.9	198.4	–	225.9	237.9	239.7
extrahepatic (bile) duct	156.1	197.8	230.8	211.5	235.3	239.0
contiguous sites with gallbladder	156.8	–	–	–	–	–
extraocular muscle	190.1	198.4	234.0	224.1	238.8	239.8
extrarectal	195.3	198.89	234.8	229.8	238.8	239.8
extremity*	195.8	198.89	232.8	229.8	238.8	239.8
lower*	195.5	198.89	232.7	229.8	238.8	239.8
upper*	195.4	198.89	232.6	229.8	238.8	239.8
eye NEC	190.9	198.4	234.0	224.9	238.8	239.8
contiguous sites	190.8	–	–	–	–	–
specified sites NEC	190.8	198.4	234.0	224.8	238.8	239.8
eyeball	190.0	198.4	234.0	224.0	238.8	239.8
eyebrow	173.3	198.2	232.3	216.3	238.2	239.2
eyelid (lower) (skin) (upper)	173.1	198.2	232.1	216.1	238.2	239.2
cartilage	171.0	198.89	–	215.0	238.1	239.2
face NEC*	195.0	198.89	232.3	229.8	238.8	239.8
Fallopian tube (accessory)	183.2	198.82	233.39▲	221.0	236.3	239.5
falx (cerebella) (cerebri)	192.1	198.4	–	225.2	237.6	239.7
fascia - *see also* Neoplasm, connective tissue						
palmar	171.2	198.89	–	215.2	238.1	239.2
plantar	171.3	198.89	–	215.3	238.1	239.2

	Malignant Primary	Malignant Secondary	Malignant Ca in situ	Benign	Uncertain Behavior	Unspecified
Neoplasm, neoplastic – *continued*						
fatty tissue - *see* Neoplasm, connective tissue						
fauces, faucial NEC	146.9	198.89	230.0	210.6	235.1	239.0
pillars	146.2	198.89	230.0	210.6	235.1	239.0
tonsil	146.0	198.89	230.0	210.5	235.1	239.0
femur (any part)	170.7	198.5	–	213.7	238.0	239.2
fetal membrane	181	198.82	233.2	219.8	236.1	239.5
fibrous tissue - *see* Neoplasm, connective tissue						
fibula (any part)	170.7	198.5	–	213.7	238.0	239.2
filum terminale	192.2	198.3	–	225.3	237.5	239.7
finger NEC*	195.4	198.89	232.6	229.8	238.8	239.8
flank NEC*	195.8	198.89	232.5	229.8	238.8	239.8
follicle, nabothian	180.0	198.82	233.1	219.0	236.0	239.5
foot NEC*	195.5	198.89	232.7	229.8	238.8	239.8
forearm NEC*	195.4	198.89	232.6	229.8	238.8	239.8
forehead (skin)	173.3	198.2	232.3	216.3	238.2	239.2
foreskin	187.1	198.82	233.5	222.1	236.6	239.5
fornix						
pharyngeal	147.3	198.89	230.0	210.7	235.1	239.0
vagina	184.0	198.82	233.31▲	221.1	236.3	239.5
fossa (of)						
anterior (cranial)	191.9	198.3	–	225.0	237.5	239.6
cranial	191.9	198.3	–	225.0	237.5	239.6
ischiorectal	195.3	198.89	234.8	229.8	238.8	239.8
middle (cranial)	191.9	198.3	–	225.0	237.5	239.6
pituitary	194.3	198.89	234.8	227.3	237.0	239.7
posterior (cranial)	191.9	198.3	–	225.0	237.5	239.6
pterygoid	171.0	198.89	–	215.0	238.1	239.2
pyriform	148.1	198.89	230.0	210.8	235.1	239.0
Rosenmüller	147.2	198.89	230.0	210.7	235.1	239.0
tonsillar	146.1	198.89	230.0	210.6	235.1	239.0
fourchette	184.4	198.82	233.32▲	221.2	236.3	239.5
frenulum						
labii - *see* Neoplasm, lip, internal						
linguae	141.3	198.89	230.0	210.1	235.1	239.0
frontal						
bone	170.0	198.5	–	213.0	238.0	239.2
lobe, brain	191.1	198.3	–	225.0	237.5	239.6
meninges	192.1	198.4	–	225.2	237.6	239.7
pole	191.1	198.3	–	225.0	237.5	239.6
sinus	160.4	197.3	231.8	212.0	235.9	239.1
fundus						
stomach	151.3	197.8	230.2	211.1	235.2	239.0
uterus	182.0	198.82	233.2	219.1	236.0	239.5
gall duct (extrahepatic)	156.1	197.8	230.8	211.5	235.3	239.0
intrahepatic	155.1	197.8	230.8	211.5	235.3	239.0
gallbladder	156.0	197.8	230.8	211.5	235.3	239.0
contiguous sites with extrahepatic bile ducts	156.8	–	–	–	–	–
ganglia (*see also* Neoplasm, connective tissue)	171.9	198.89	–	215.9	238.1	239.2
basal	191.0	198.3	–	225.0	237.5	239.6
ganglion (*see also* Neoplasm, connective tissue)	171.9	198.89	–	215.9	238.1	239.2
cranial nerve	192.0	198.4	–	225.1	237.9	239.7
Gartner's duct	184.0	198.82	233.31▲	221.1	236.3	239.5
gastric - *see* Neoplasm, stomach						
gastrocolic	159.8	197.8	230.9	211.9	235.5	239.0
gastroesophageal junction	151.0	197.8	230.2	211.1	235.2	239.0

Neoplasm, endocardium – Neoplasm, gastroesophageal junction

	Malignant					
	Primary	Secondary	Ca in situ	Benign	Uncertain Behavior	Unspecified
Neoplasm, neoplastic – *continued*						
gastrointestinal (tract) NEC	159.9	197.8	230.9	211.9	235.5	239.0
generalized	199.0	199.0	234.9	229.9	238.9	199.0
genital organ or tract						
female NEC	184.9	198.82	233.39▲	221.9	236.3	239.5
contiguous sites	184.8	–	–	–	–	–
specified site NEC	184.8	198.82	233.39▲	221.8	236.3	239.5
male NEC	187.9	198.82	233.6	222.9	236.6	239.5
contiguous sites	187.8	–	–	–	–	–
specified site NEC	187.8	198.82	233.6	222.8	236.6	239.5
genitourinary tract						
female	184.9	198.82	233.39▲	221.9	236.3	239.5
male	187.9	198.82	233.6	222.9	236.6	239.5
gingiva (alveolar) (marginal)	143.9	198.89	230.0	210.4	235.1	239.0
lower	143.1	198.89	230.0	210.4	235.1	239.0
mandibular	143.1	198.89	230.0	210.4	235.1	239.0
maxillary	143.0	198.89	230.0	210.4	235.1	239.0
upper	143.0	198.89	230.0	210.4	235.1	239.0
gland, glandular (lymphatic) (system) - *see also* Neoplasm, lymph gland						
endocrine NEC	194.9	198.89	–	227.9	237.4	239.7
salivary - *see* Neoplasm, salivary, gland						
glans penis	187.2	198.82	233.5	222.1	236.6	239.5
globus pallidus	191.0	198.3	–	225.0	237.5	239.6
glomus						
coccygeal	194.6	198.89	–	227.6	237.3	239.7
jugularis	194.6	198.89	–	227.6	237.3	239.7
glosso–epiglottic fold(s)	146.4	198.89	230.0	210.6	235.1	239.0
glossopalatine fold	146.2	198.89	230.0	210.6	235.1	239.0
glossopharyngeal sulcus	146.1	198.89	230.0	210.6	235.1	239.0
glottis	161.0	197.3	231.0	212.1	235.6	239.1
gluteal region*	195.3	198.89	232.5	229.8	238.8	239.8
great vessels NEC	171.4	198.89	–	215.4	238.1	239.2
groin NEC	195.3	198.89	232.5	229.8	238.8	239.8
gum	143.9	198.89	230.0	210.4	235.1	239.0
contiguous sites	143.8	–	–	–	–	–
lower	143.1	198.89	230.0	210.4	235.1	239.0
upper	143.0	198.89	230.0	210.4	235.1	239.0
hand NEC*	195.4	198.89	232.6	229.8	238.8	239.8
head NEC*	195.0	198.89	232.4	229.8	238.8	239.8
heart	164.1	198.89	–	212.7	238.8	239.8
contiguous sites with mediastinum or thymus	164.8	–	–	–	–	–
heel NEC*	195.5	198.89	232.7	229.8	238.8	239.8
helix	173.2❺	198.2	232.2	216.2	238.2	239.2
hematopoietic, hemopoietic tissue NEC	202.8	198.89	–	–	–	238.79
hemisphere, cerebral	191.0	198.3	–	225.0	237.5	239.6
hemorrhoidal zone	154.2	197.5	230.5	211.4	235.5	239.0
hepatic	155.2	197.7	230.8	211.5	235.3	239.0
duct (bile)	156.1	197.8	230.8	211.5	235.3	239.0
flexure (colon)	153.0	197.5	230.3	211.3	235.2	239.0
primary	155.0	–	–	–	–	–
hilus of lung	162.2	197.0	231.2	212.3	235.7	239.1
hip NEC*	195.5	198.89	232.7	229.8	238.8	239.8
hippocampus, brain	191.2	198.3	–	225.0	237.5	239.6
humerus (any part)	170.4	198.5	–	213.4	238.0	239.2
hymen	184.0	198.82	233.31▲	221.1	236.3	239.5

	Malignant					
	Primary	Secondary	Ca in situ	Benign	Uncertain Behavior	Unspecified
Neoplasm, neoplastic – *continued*						
hypopharynx, hypopharyngeal NEC	148.9	198.89	230.0	210.8	235.1	239.0
contiguous sites	148.8	–	–	–	–	–
postcricoid region	148.0	198.89	230.0	210.8	235.1	239.0
posterior wall	148.3	198.89	230.0	210.8	235.1	239.0
pyriform fossa (sinus)	148.1	198.89	230.0	210.8	235.1	239.0
specified site NEC	148.8	198.89	230.0	210.8	235.1	239.0
wall	148.9	198.89	230.0	210.8	235.1	239.0
posterior	148.3	198.89	230.0	210.8	235.1	239.0
hypophysis	194.3	198.89	234.8	227.3	237.0	239.7
hypothalamus	191.0	198.3	–	225.0	237.5	239.6
ileocecum, ileocecal (coil) (junction) (valve)	153.4	197.5	230.3	211.3	235.2	239.0
ileum	152.2	197.4	230.7	211.2	235.2	239.0
ilium	170.6	198.5	–	213.6	238.0	239.2
immunoproliferative NEC	203.8❺	–	–	–	–	–
infraclavicular (region)*	195.1	198.89	232.5	229.8	238.8	239.8
inguinal (region)*	195.3	198.89	232.5	229.8	238.8	239.8
insula	191.0	198.3	–	225.0	237.5	239.6
insular tissue (pancreas)	157.4	197.8	230.9	211.7	235.5	239.0
brain	191.0	198.3	–	225.0	237.5	239.6
interarytenoid fold	148.2	198.89	230.0	210.8	235.1	239.0
hypopharyngeal aspect	148.2	198.89	230.0	210.8	235.1	239.0
laryngeal aspect	161.1	197.3	231.0	212.1	235.6	239.1
marginal zone	148.2	198.89	230.0	210.8	235.1	239.0
interdental papillae	143.9	198.89	230.0	210.4	235.1	239.0
lower	143.1	198.89	230.0	210.4	235.1	239.0
upper	143.0	198.89	230.0	210.4	235.1	239.0
internal						
capsule	191.0	198.3	–	225.0	237.5	239.6
os (cervix)	180.0	198.82	233.1	219.0	236.0	239.5
intervertebral cartilage or disc	170.2	198.5	–	213.2	238.0	239.2
intestine, intestinal	159.0	197.8	230.7	211.9	235.2	239.0
large	153.9	197.5	230.3	211.3	235.2	239.0
appendix	153.5	197.5	230.3	211.3	235.2	239.0
caput coli	153.4	197.5	230.3	211.3	235.2	239.0
cecum	153.4	197.5	230.3	211.3	235.2	239.0
colon	153.9	197.5	230.3	211.3	235.2	239.0
and rectum	154.0	197.5	230.4	211.4	235.2	239.0
ascending	153.6	197.5	230.3	211.3	235.2	239.0
caput	153.4	197.5	230.3	211.3	235.2	239.0
contiguous sites	153.8	–	–	–	–	–
descending	153.2	197.5	230.3	211.3	235.2	239.0
distal	153.2	197.5	230.3	211.3	235.2	239.0
left	153.2	197.5	230.3	211.3	235.2	239.0
pelvic	153.3	197.5	230.3	211.3	235.2	239.0
right	153.6	197.5	230.3	211.3	235.2	239.0
sigmoid (flexure)	153.3	197.5	230.3	211.3	235.2	239.0
transverse	153.1	197.5	230.3	211.3	235.2	239.0
contiguous sites	153.8	–	–	–	–	–
hepatic flexure	153.0	197.5	230.3	211.3	235.2	239.0
ileocecum, ileocecal (coil) (valve)	153.4	197.5	230.3	211.3	235.2	239.0
sigmoid flexure (lower) (upper)	153.3	197.5	230.3	211.3	235.2	239.0
splenic flexure	153.7	197.5	230.3	211.3	235.2	239.0
small	152.9	197.4	230.7	211.2	235.2	239.0
contiguous sites	152.8	–	–	–	–	–
duodenum	152.0	197.4	230.7	211.2	235.2	239.0
ileum	152.2	197.4	230.7	211.2	235.2	239.0
jejunum	152.1	197.4	230.7	211.2	235.2	239.0
tract NEC	159.0	197.8	230.7	211.9	235.2	239.0

	Malignant					
	Primary	Secondary	Ca in situ	Benign	Uncertain Behavior	Unspecified
Neoplasm, neoplastic *– continued*						
intra-abdominal	195.2	198.89	234.8	229.8	238.8	239.8
intracranial NEC	191.9	198.3	–	225.0	237.5	239.6
intrahepatic (bile) duct	155.1	197.8	230.8	211.5	235.3	239.0
intraocular	190.0	198.4	234.0	224.0	238.8	239.8
intraorbital	190.1	198.4	234.0	224.1	238.8	239.8
intrasellar	194.3	198.89	234.8	227.3	237.0	239.7
intrathoracic (cavity) (organs NEC)	195.1	198.89	234.8	229.8	238.8	239.8
contiguous sites with respiratory organs	165.8	–	–	–	–	–
iris	190.0	198.4	234.0	224.0	238.8	239.8
ischiorectal (fossa)	195.3	198.89	234.8	229.8	238.8	239.8
ischium	170.6	198.5	–	213.6	238.0	239.2
island of Reil	191.0	198.3	–	225.0	237.5	239.6
islands or islets of Langerhans	157.4	197.8	230.9	211.7	235.5	239.0
isthmus uteri	182.1	198.82	233.2	219.1	236.0	239.5
jaw	195.0	198.89	234.8	229.8	238.8	239.8
bone	170.1	198.5	–	213.1	238.0	239.2
carcinoma	143.9	–	–	–	–	–
lower	143.1	–	–	–	–	–
upper	143.0	–	–	–	–	–
lower	170.1	198.5	–	213.1	238.0	239.2
upper	170.0	198.5	–	213.0	238.0	239.2
carcinoma (any type) (lower) (upper)	195.0	–	–	–	–	–
skin	173.3	198.2	232.3	216.3	238.2	239.2
soft tissues	143.9	198.89	230.0	210.4	235.1	239.0
lower	143.1	198.89	230.0	210.4	235.1	239.0
upper	143.0	198.89	230.0	210.4	235.1	239.0
jejunum	152.1	197.4	230.7	211.2	235.2	239.0
joint NEC (*see also* Neoplasm, bone)	170.9	198.5	–	213.9	238.0	239.2
acromioclavicular	170.4	198.5	–	213.4	238.0	239.2
bursa or synovial membrane - *see* Neoplasm, connective tissue						
costovertebral	170.3	198.5	–	213.3	238.0	239.2
sternocostal	170.3	198.5	–	213.3	238.0	239.2
temporomandibular	170.1	198.5	–	213.1	238.0	239.2
junction						
anorectal	154.8	197.5	230.7	211.4	235.5	239.0
cardioesophageal	151.0	197.8	230.2	211.1	235.2	239.0
esophagogastric	151.0	197.8	230.2	211.1	235.2	239.0
gastroesophageal	151.0	197.8	230.2	211.1	235.2	239.0
hard and soft palate	145.5	198.89	230.0	210.4	235.1	239.0
ileocecal	153.4	197.5	230.3	211.3	235.2	239.0
pelvirectal	154.0	197.5	230.4	211.4	235.2	239.0
pelviureteric	189.1	198.0	233.9	223.1	236.91	239.5
rectosigmoid	154.0	197.5	230.4	211.4	235.2	239.0
squamocolumnar, of cervix	180.8	198.82	233.1	219.0	236.0	239.5
kidney (parenchymal)	189.0	198.0	233.9	223.0	236.91	239.5
calyx	189.1	198.0	233.9	223.1	236.91	239.5
hilus	189.1	198.0	233.9	223.1	236.91	239.5
pelvis	189.1	198.0	233.9	223.1	236.91	239.5
knee NEC*	195.5	198.89	232.7	229.8	238.8	239.8
labia (skin)	184.4	198.82	233.32▲	221.2	236.3	239.5
majora	184.1	198.82	233.32▲	221.2	236.3	239.5
minora	184.2	198.82	233.32▲	221.2	236.3	239.5
labial - *see also* Neoplasm, lip						
sulcus (lower) (upper)	145.1	198.89	230.0	210.4	235.1	239.0
labium (skin)	184.4	198.82	233.32▲	221.2	236.3	239.5
majus	184.1	198.82	233.32▲	221.2	236.3	239.5
Neoplasm, neoplastic *– continued*						
labium *– continued*						
minus	184.2	198.82	233.32▲	221.2	236.3	239.5
lacrimal						
canaliculi	190.7	198.4	234.0	224.7	238.8	239.8
duct (nasal)	190.7	198.4	234.0	224.7	238.8	239.8
gland	190.2	198.4	234.0	224.2	238.8	239.8
punctum	190.7	198.4	234.0	224.7	238.8	239.8
sac	190.7	198.4	234.0	224.7	238.8	239.8
Langerhans, islands or islets	157.4	197.8	230.9	211.7	235.5	239.0
laryngopharynx	148.9	198.89	230.0	210.8	235.1	239.0
larynx, laryngeal NEC	161.9	197.3	231.0	212.1	235.6	239.1
aryepiglottic fold	161.1	197.3	231.0	212.1	235.6	239.1
cartilage (arytenoid) (cricoid) (cuneiform) (thyroid)	161.3	197.3	231.0	212.1	235.6	239.1
commissure (anterior) (posterior)	161.0	197.3	231.0	212.1	235.6	239.1
contiguous sites	161.8	–	–	–	–	–
extrinsic NEC	161.1	197.3	231.0	212.1	235.6	239.1
meaning hypopharynx	148.9	198.89	230.0	210.8	235.1	239.0
interarytenoid fold	161.1	197.3	231.0	212.1	235.6	239.1
intrinsic	161.0	197.3	231.0	212.1	235.6	239.1
ventricular band	161.1	197.3	231.0	212.1	235.6	239.1
leg NEC*	195.5	198.89	232.7	229.8	238.8	239.8
lens, crystalline	190.0	198.4	234.0	224.0	238.8	239.8
lid (lower) (upper)	173.1	198.2	232.1	216.1	238.2	239.2
ligament - *see also* Neoplasm, connective tissue						
broad	183.3	198.82	233.39▲	221.0	236.3	239.5
Mackenrodt's	183.8	198.82	233.39▲	221.8	236.3	239.5
non-uterine - *see* Neoplasm, connective tissue						
round	183.5	198.82	–	221.0	236.3	239.5
sacro-uterine	183.4	198.82	–	221.0	236.3	239.5
uterine	183.4	198.82	–	221.0	236.3	239.5
utero-ovarian	183.8	198.82	233.39▲	221.8	236.3	239.5
uterosacral	183.4	198.82	–	221.0	236.3	239.5
limb*	195.8	198.89	232.8	229.8	238.8	239.8
lower*	195.5	198.89	232.7	229.8	238.8	239.8
upper*	195.4	198.89	232.6	229.8	238.8	239.8
limbus of cornea	190.4	198.4	234.0	224.4	238.8	239.8
lingual NEC (*see also* Neoplasm, tongue)	141.9	198.89	230.0	210.1	235.1	239.0
lingula, lung	162.3	197.0	231.2	212.3	235.7	239.1
lip (external) (lipstick area) (vermillion border)	140.9	198.89	230.0	210.0	235.1	239.0
buccal aspect - *see* Neoplasm, lip, internal						
commissure	140.6	198.89	230.0	210.4	235.1	239.0
contiguous sites	140.8	–	–	–	–	–
with oral cavity or pharynx	149.8	–	–	–	–	–
frenulum - *see* Neoplasm, lip, internal						
inner aspect - *see* Neoplasm, lip, internal						
internal (buccal) (frenulum) (mucosa) (oral)	140.5	198.89	230.0	210.0	235.1	239.0
lower	140.4	198.89	230.0	210.0	235.1	239.0
upper	140.3	198.89	230.0	210.0	235.1	239.0

Neoplasm, intra-abdominal – Neoplasm, lip

	Malignant					
	Primary	Secondary	Ca in situ	Benign	Uncertain Behavior	Unspecified
Neoplasm, neoplastic *– continued*						
lip – *continued*						
lower	140.1	198.89	230.0	210.0	235.1	239.0
internal (buccal) (frenulum) (mucosa) (oral)	140.4	198.89	230.0	210.0	235.1	239.0
mucosa - *see* Neoplasm, lip, internal						
oral aspect - *see* Neoplasm, lip, internal						
skin (commissure) (lower) (upper)	173.0	198.2	232.0	216.0	238.2	239.2
upper	140.0	198.89	230.0	210.0	235.1	239.0
internal (buccal) (frenulum) (mucosa) (oral)	140.3	198.89	230.0	210.0	235.1	239.0
liver	155.2	197.7	230.8	211.5	235.3	239.0
primary	155.0	–	–	–	–	–
lobe						
azygos	162.3	197.0	231.2	212.3	235.7	239.1
frontal	191.1	198.3	–	225.0	237.5	239.6
lower	162.5	197.0	231.2	212.3	235.7	239.1
middle	162.4	197.0	231.2	212.3	235.7	239.1
occipital	191.4	198.3	–	225.0	237.5	239.6
parietal	191.3	198.3	–	225.0	237.5	239.6
temporal	191.2	198.3	–	225.0	237.5	239.6
upper	162.3	197.0	231.2	212.3	235.7	239.1
lumbosacral plexus	171.6	198.4	–	215.6	238.1	239.2
lung	162.9	197.0	231.2	212.3	235.7	239.1
azygos lobe	162.3	197.0	231.2	212.3	235.7	239.1
carina	162.2	197.0	231.2	212.3	235.7	239.1
contiguous sites with bronchus or trachea	162.8	–	–	–	–	–
hilus	162.2	197.0	231.2	212.3	235.7	239.1
linqula	162.3	197.0	231.2	212.3	235.7	239.1
lobe NEC	162.9	197.0	231.2	212.3	235.7	239.1
lower lobe	162.5	197.0	231.2	212.3	235.7	239.1
main bronchus	162.2	197.0	231.2	212.3	235.7	239.1
middle lobe	162.4	197.0	231.2	212.3	235.7	239.1
upper lobe	162.3	197.0	231.2	212.3	235.7	239.1
lymph, lymphatic						
channel NEC (*see also* Neoplasm, connective tissue)	171.9	198.89	–	215.9	238.1	239.2
gland (secondary)	–	196.9	–	229.0	238.8	239.8
abdominal	–	196.2	–	229.0	238.8	239.8
aortic	–	196.2	–	229.0	238.8	239.8
arm	–	196.3	–	229.0	238.8	239.8
auricular (anterior) (posterior)	–	196.0	–	229.0	238.8	239.8
axilla, axillary	–	196.3	–	229.0	238.8	239.8
brachial	–	196.3	–	229.0	238.8	239.8
bronchial	–	196.1	–	229.0	238.8	239.8
bronchopulmonary	–	196.1	–	229.0	238.8	239.8
celiac	–	196.2	–	229.0	238.8	239.8
cervical	–	196.0	–	229.0	238.8	239.8
cervicofacial	–	196.0	–	229.0	238.8	239.8
Cloquet	–	196.5	–	229.0	238.8	239.8
colic	–	196.2	–	229.0	238.8	239.8
common duct	–	196.2	–	229.0	238.8	239.8
cubital	–	196.3	–	229.0	238.8	239.8
diaphragmatic	–	196.1	–	229.0	238.8	239.8
epigastric, inferior	–	196.6	–	229.0	238.8	239.8
epitrochlear	–	196.3	–	229.0	238.8	239.8
esophageal	–	196.1	–	229.0	238.8	239.8

	Malignant					
	Primary	Secondary	Ca in situ	Benign	Uncertain Behavior	Unspecified
Neoplasm, neoplastic *– continued*						
lymph, lymphatic *– continued*						
gland – *continued*						
face	–	196.0	–	229.0	238.8	239.8
femoral	–	196.5	–	229.0	238.8	239.8
gastric	–	196.2	–	229.0	238.8	239.8
groin	–	196.5	–	229.0	238.8	239.8
head	–	196.0	–	229.0	238.8	239.8
hepatic	–	196.2	–	229.0	238.8	239.8
hypogastric	–	196.6	–	229.0	238.8	239.8
ileocolic	–	196.2	–	229.0	238.8	239.8
iliac	–	196.6	–	229.0	238.8	239.8
infraclavicular	–	196.3	–	229.0	238.8	239.8
inguina, inguinal	–	196.5	–	229.0	238.8	239.8
innominate	–	196.1	–	229.0	238.8	239.8
intercostal	–	196.1	–	229.0	238.8	239.8
intestinal	–	196.2	–	229.0	238.8	239.8
intrabdominal	–	196.2	–	229.0	238.8	239.8
intrapelvic	–	196.6	–	229.0	238.8	239.8
intrathoracic	–	196.1	–	229.0	238.8	239.9
jugular	–	196.0	–	229.0	238.8	239.8
leg	–	196.5	–	229.0	238.8	239.8
limb						
lower	–	196.5	–	229.0	238.8	239.8
upper	–	196.3	–	229.0	238.8	239.8
lower limb	–	196.5	–	229.0	238.8	238.9
lumbar	–	196.2	–	229.0	238.8	239.8
mandibular	–	196.0	–	229.0	238.8	239.8
mediastinal	–	196.1	–	229.0	238.8	239.8
mesenteric (inferior) (superior)	–	196.2	–	229.0	238.8	239.8
midcolic	–	196.2	–	229.0	238.8	239.8
multiple sites in categories 196.0-196.6	–	196.8	–	229.0	238.8	239.8
neck	–	196.0	–	229.0	238.8	239.8
obturator	–	196.6	–	229.0	238.8	239.8
occipital	–	196.0	–	229.0	238.8	239.8
pancreatic	–	196.2	–	229.0	238.8	239.8
para–aortic	–	196.2	–	229.0	238.8	239.8
paracervical	–	196.6	–	229.0	238.8	239.8
parametrial	–	196.6	–	229.0	238.8	239.8
parasternal	–	196.1	–	229.0	238.8	239.8
parotid	–	196.0	–	229.0	238.8	239.8
pectoral	–	196.3	–	229.0	238.8	239.8
pelvic	–	196.6	–	229.0	238.8	239.8
peri–aortic	–	196.2	–	229.0	238.8	239.8
peripancreatic	–	196.2	–	229.0	238.8	239.8
popliteal	–	196.5	–	229.0	238.8	239.8
porta hepatis	–	196.2	–	229.0	238.8	239.8
portal	–	196.2	–	229.0	238.8	239.8
preauricular	–	196.0	–	229.0	238.8	239.8
prelaryngeal	–	196.0	–	229.0	238.8	239.8
presymphysial	–	196.6	–	229.0	238.8	239.8
pretracheal	–	196.0	–	229.0	238.8	239.8
primary (any site) NEC	202.9❺	–	–	–	–	–
pulmonary (hiler)	–	196.1	–	229.0	238.8	239.8
pyloric	–	196.2	–	229.0	238.8	239.8
retroperitoneal	–	196.2	–	229.0	238.8	239.8
retropharyngeal	–	196.0	–	229.0	238.8	239.8
Rosenmüller's	–	196.5	–	229.0	238.8	239.8
sacral	–	196.6	–	229.0	238.8	239.8
scalene	–	196.0	–	229.0	238.8	239.8
site NEC	–	196.9	–	229.0	238.8	239.8
splenic (hilar)	–	196.2	–	229.0	238.8	239.8
subclavicular	–	196.3	–	229.0	238.8	239.8

❹ Fourth-Digit Required ❺ Fifth-Digit Required ►◄ Revised Text ● New Line ▲ Revised Code

	Malignant					
	Primary	Secondary	Ca in situ	Benign	Uncertain Behavior	Unspecified
Neoplasm, neoplastic – *continued*						
lymph, lymphatic – *continued*						
gland – *continued*						
subinguinal	–	196.5	–	229.0	238.8	239.8
sublingual	–	196.0	–	229.0	238.8	239.8
submandibular	–	196.0	–	229.0	238.8	239.8
submaxillary	–	196.0	–	229.0	238.8	239.8
submental	–	196.0	–	229.0	238.8	239.8
subscapular	–	196.3	–	229.0	238.8	239.8
supraclavicular	–	196.0	–	229.0	238.8	239.8
thoracic	–	196.1	–	229.0	238.8	239.8
tibial	–	196.5	–	229.0	238.8	239.8
tracheal	–	196.1	–	229.0	238.8	239.8
tracheobronchial	–	196.1	–	229.0	238.8	239.8
upper limb	–	196.3	–	229.0	238.8	239.8
Virchow's	–	196.0	–	229.0	238.8	239.8
vessel (*see also* Neoplasm, connective tissue)	171.9	198.89	–	215.9	238.1	239.2
Mackenrodt's ligament	183.8	198.82	233.39▲	221.8	236.3	239.5
malar	170.0	198.5	–	213.0	238.0	239.2
region - *see* Neoplasm, cheek						
mammary gland - *see* Neoplasm, breast						
mandible	170.1	198.5	–	213.1	238.0	239.2
alveolar						
mucosa	143.1	198.89	230.0	210.4	235.1	239.0
ridge or process	170.1	198.5	–	213.1	238.0	239.2
carcinoma	143.1	–	–	–	–	–
carcinoma	143.1	–	–	–	–	–
marrow (bone) NEC	202.9❺	198.5	–	–	–	238.79
mastectomy site (skin)	173.5	198.2	–	–	–	–
specified as breast tissue	174.8	198.81	–	–	–	–
mastoid (air cells) (antrum) (cavity)	160.1	197.3	231.8	212.0	235.9	239.1
bone or process	170.0	198.5	–	213.0	238.0	239.2
maxilla, maxillary (superior)	170.0	198.5	–	213.0	238.0	239.2
alveolar						
mucosa	143.0	198.89	230.0	210.4	235.1	239.0
ridge or process	170.0	198.5	–	213.0	238.0	239.2
carcinoma	143.0	–	–	–	–	–
antrum	160.2	197.3	231.8	212.0	235.9	239.1
carcinoma	143.0	–	–	–	–	–
inferior - *see* Neoplasm, mandible						
sinus	160.2	197.3	231.8	212.0	235.9	239.1
meatus						
external (ear)	173.2	198.2	232.2	216.2	238.2	239.2
Meckel's diverticulum	152.3	197.4	230.7	211.2	235.2	239.0
mediastinum, mediastinal	164.9	197.1	–	212.5	235.8	239.8
anterior	164.2	197.1	–	212.5	235.8	239.8
contiguous sites with heart and thymus	164.8	–	–	–	–	–
posterior	164.3	197.1	–	212.5	235.8	239.8
medulla						
adrenal	194.0	198.7	234.8	227.0	237.2	239.7
oblongata	191.7	198.3	–	225.0	237.5	239.6
meibomian gland	173.1	198.2	232.1	216.1	238.2	239.2
melanoma - *see* Melanoma						

	Malignant					
	Primary	Secondary	Ca in situ	Benign	Uncertain Behavior	Unspecified
Neoplasm, neoplastic – *continued*						
meninges (brain) (cerebral) (cranial) (intracranial)	192.1	198.4	–	225.2	237.6	239.7
spinal (cord)	192.3	198.4	–	225.4	237.6	239.7
meniscus, knee joint (lateral) (medial)	170.7	198.5	–	213.7	238.0	239.2
mesentery, mesenteric	158.8	197.6	–	211.8	235.4	239.0
mesoappendix	158.8	197.6	–	211.8	235.4	239.0
mesocolon	158.8	197.6	–	211.8	235.4	239.0
mesopharynx - *see* Neoplasm, oropharynx						
mesosalpinx	183.3	198.82	233.39▲	221.0	236.3	239.5
mesovarium	183.3	198.82	233.39▲	221.0	236.3	239.5
metacarpus (any bone)	170.5	198.5	–	213.5	238.0	239.2
metastatic NEC - *see also* Neoplasm, by site, secondary	–	199.1	–	–	–	–
metatarsus (any bone)	170.8	198.5	–	213.8	238.0	239.2
midbrain	191.7	198.3	–	225.0	237.5	239.6
milk duct - *see* Neoplasm, breast						
mons						
pubis	184.4	198.82	233.32▲	221.2	236.3	239.5
veneris	184.4	198.82	233.32▲	221.2	236.3	239.5
motor tract	192.9	198.4	–	225.9	237.9	239.7
brain	191.9	198.3	–	225.0	237.5	239.6
spinal	192.2	198.3	–	225.3	237.5	239.7
mouth	145.9	198.89	230.0	210.4	235.1	239.0
contiguous sites	145.8	–	–	–	–	–
floor	144.9	198.89	230.0	210.3	235.1	239.0
anterior portion	144.0	198.89	230.0	210.3	235.1	239.0
contiguous sites	144.8	–	–	–	–	–
lateral portion	144.1	198.89	230.0	210.3	235.1	239.0
roof	145.5	198.89	230.0	210.4	235.1	239.0
specified part NEC	145.8	198.89	230.0	210.4	235.1	239.0
vestibule	145.1	198.89	230.0	210.4	235.1	239.0
mucosa						
alveolar (ridge or process)	143.9	198.89	230.0	210.4	235.1	239.0
lower	143.1	198.89	230.0	210.4	235.1	239.0
upper	143.0	198.89	230.0	210.4	235.1	239.0
buccal	145.0	198.89	230.0	210.4	235.1	239.0
cheek	145.0	198.89	230.0	210.4	235.1	239.0
lip - *see* Neoplasm, lip, internal						
nasal	160.0	197.3	231.8	212.0	235.9	239.1
oral	145.0	198.89	230.0	210.4	235.1	239.0
Müllerian duct						
female	184.8	198.82	233.39▲	221.8	236.3	239.5
male	187.8	198.82	233.6	222.8	236.6	239.5
multiple sites NEC	199.0	199.0	234.9	229.9	238.9	199.0
muscle - *see also* Neoplasm, connective tissue						
extraocular	190.1	198.4	234.0	224.1	238.8	239.8
myocardium	164.1	198.89	–	212.7	238.8	239.8
myometrium	182.0	198.82	233.2	219.1	236.0	239.5
myopericardium	164.1	198.89	–	212.7	238.8	239.8
nabothian gland (follicle)	180.0	198.82	233.1	219.0	236.0	239.5
nail	173.9	198.2	232.9	216.9	238.2	239.2
finger	173.6	198.2	232.6	216.6	238.2	239.2
toe	173.7	198.2	232.7	216.7	238.2	239.2
nares, naris (anterior) (posterior)	160.0	197.3	231.8	212.0	235.9	239.1
nasal - *see* Neoplasm, nose						
nasolabial groove	173.3	198.2	232.3	216.3	238.2	239.2
nasolacrimal duct	190.7	198.4	234.0	224.7	238.8	239.8

Neoplasm, lymph, lymphatic – Neoplasm, nasolacrimal duct

❹ Fourth-Digit Required ❺ Fifth-Digit Required ▶◀ Revised Text ● New Line ▲ Revised Code

Neoplasm, nasopharynx, nasopharyngeal – Neoplasm, palpebra

	Malignant					
	Primary	Secondary	Ca in situ	Benign	Uncertain Behavior	Unspecified
Neoplasm, neoplastic – *continued*						
nasopharynx, nasopharyngeal	147.9	198.89	230.0	210.7	235.1	239.0
contiguous sites	147.8	–	–	–	–	–
floor	147.3	198.89	230.0	210.7	235.1	239.0
roof	147.0	198.89	230.0	210.7	235.1	239.0
specified site NEC	147.8	198.89	230.0	210.7	235.1	239.0
wall	147.9	198.89	230.0	210.7	235.1	239.0
anterior	147.3	198.89	230.0	210.7	235.1	239.0
lateral	147.2	198.89	230.0	210.7	235.1	239.0
posterior	147.1	198.89	230.0	210.7	235.1	239.0
superior	147.0	198.89	230.0	210.7	235.1	239.0
nates	173.5	198.2	232.5	216.5	238.2	239.2
neck NEC*	195.0	198.89	234.8	229.8	238.8	239.8
nerve (autonomic) (ganglion) (parasympathetic) (peripheral) (sympathetic) *see also* Neoplasm, connective tissue						
abducens	192.0	198.4	–	225.1	237.9	239.7
accessory (spinal)	192.0	198.4	–	225.1	237.9	239.7
acoustic	192.0	198.4	–	225.1	237.9	239.7
auditory	192.0	198.4	–	225.1	237.9	239.7
brachial	171.2	198.89	–	215.2	238.1	239.2
cranial (any)	192.0	198.4	–	225.1	237.9	239.7
facial	192.0	198.4	–	225.1	237.9	239.7
femoral	171.3	198.89	–	215.3	238.1	239.2
glossopharyngeal	192.0	198.4	–	225.1	237.9	239.7
hypoglossal	192.0	198.4	–	225.1	237.9	239.7
intercostal	171.4	198.89	–	215.4	238.1	239.2
lumbar	171.7	198.89	–	215.7	238.1	239.2
median	171.2	198.89	–	215.2	238.1	239.2
obturator	171.3	198.89	–	215.3	238.1	239.2
oculomotor	192.0	198.4	–	225.1	237.9	239.7
olfactory	192.0	198.4	–	225.1	237.9	239.7
optic	192.0	198.4	–	225.1	237.9	239.7
peripheral NEC	171.9	198.89	–	215.9	238.1	239.2
radial	171.2	198.89	–	215.2	238.1	239.2
sacral	171.6	198.89	–	215.6	238.1	239.2
sciatic	171.3	198.89	–	215.3	238.1	239.2
spinal NEC	171.9	198.89	–	215.9	238.1	239.2
trigeminal	192.0	198.4	–	225.1	237.9	239.7
trochlear	192.0	198.4	–	225.1	237.9	239.7
ulnar	171.2	198.89	–	215.2	238.1	239.2
vagus	192.0	198.4	–	225.1	237.9	239.7
nervous system (central) NEC	192.9	198.4	–	225.9	237.9	239.7
autonomic NEC	171.9	198.89	–	215.9	238.1	239.2
brain - *see also* Neoplasm, brain						
membrane or meninges	192.1	198.4	–	225.2	237.6	239.7
contiguous sites	192.8	–	–	–	–	–
parasympathetic NEC	171.9	198.89	–	215.9	238.1	239.2
sympathetic NEC	171.9	198.89	–	215.9	238.1	239.2
nipple (female)	174.0	198.81	233.0	217	238.3	239.3
male	175.0	198.81	233.0	217	238.3	239.3
nose, nasal	195.0	198.89	234.8	229.8	238.8	239.8
ala (external)	173.3	198.2	232.3	216.3	238.2	239.2
bone	170.0	198.5	–	213.0	238.0	239.2
cartilage	160.0	197.3	231.8	212.0	235.9	239.1
cavity	160.0	197.3	231.8	212.0	235.9	239.1
contiguous sites with accessory sinuses or middle ear	160.8	–	–	–	–	–
choana	147.3	198.89	230.0	210.7	235.1	239.0

	Malignant					
	Primary	Secondary	Ca in situ	Benign	Uncertain Behavior	Unspecified
Neoplasm, neoplastic – *continued*						
nose, nasal – *continued*						
external (skin)	173.3	198.2	232.3	216.3	238.2	239.2
fossil	160.0	197.3	231.8	212.0	235.9	239.1
internal	160.0	197.3	231.8	212.0	235.9	239.1
mucosa	160.0	197.3	231.8	212.0	235.9	239.1
septum	160.0	197.3	231.8	212.0	235.9	239.1
posterior margin	147.3	198.89	230.0	210.7	235.1	239.0
sinus - *see* Neoplasm, sinus						
skin	173.3	198.2	232.3	216.3	238.2	239.2
turbinate (mucosa)	160.0	197.3	231.8	212.0	235.9	239.1
bone	170.0	198.5	–	2130.0	238.0	239.2
vestibule	160.0	197.3	231.8	212.0	235.9	239.1
nostril	160.0	197.3	231.8	212.0	235.9	239.1
nucleus pulposus	170.2	198.5	–	213.2	238.0	230.2
occipital						
bone	170.0	198.5	–	213.0	238.0	239.2
lobe or pole, brain	191.4	198.3	–	225.0	237.5	239.6
odontogenic - *see* Neoplasm, jaw bone						
oesophagus - *see* Neoplasm, esophagus						
olfactory nerve or bulb	192.0	198.4	–	225.1	237.9	239.7
olive (brain)	191.7	198.3	–	225.0	237.5	239.6
omentum	158.8	197.6	–	211.8	235.4	239.0
operculum (brain)	191.0	198.3	–	225.0	237.5	239.6
optic nerve, chiasm, or tract	192.0	198.4	–	225.1	237.9	239.7
oral (cavity)	145.9	198.89	230.0	210.4	235.1	239.0
contiguous sites with lip or pharynx	149.8	–	–	–	–	–
ill-defined	149.9	198.89	230.0	210.4	235.1	239.0
mucosa	145.9	198.89	230.0	210.4	235.1	239.0
orbit	190.1	198.4	234.0	224.1	238.8	239.8
bone	170.0	198.5	–	213.0	238.0	239.2
eye	190.1	198.4	234.0	224.1	238.8	239.8
soft parts	190.1	198.4	234.0	224.1	238.8	239.8
organ of Zuckerkandl	194.6	198.89	–	227.6	237.3	239.7
oropharynx	146.9	198.89	230.0	210.6	235.1	239.0
branchial cleft (vestige)	146.8	198.89	230.0	210.6	235.1	239.0
contiguous sites	146.8	–	–	–	–	–
junctional region	146.5	198.89	230.0	210.6	235.1	239.0
lateral wall	146.6	198.89	230.0	210.6	235.1	239.0
pillars of fauces	146.2	198.89	230.0	210.6	235.1	239.0
posterior wall	146.7	198.89	230.0	210.6	235.1	239.0
specified part NEC	146.8	198.89	230.0	210.6	235.1	239.0
vallecula	146.3	198.89	230.0	210.6	235.1	239.0
os						
external	180.1	198.82	233.1	219.0	236.0	239.5
internal	180.0	198.82	233.1	219.0	236.0	239.5
ovary	183.0	198.6	233.39▲	220	236.2	239.5
oviduct	183.2	198.82	233.39▲	221.0	236.3	239.5
palate	145.5	198.89	230.0	210.4	235.1	239.0
hard	145.2	198.89	230.0	210.4	235.1	239.0
junction of hard and soft palate	145.5	198.89	230.0	210.4	235.1	239.0
soft	145.3	198.89	230.0	210.4	235.1	239.0
nasopharyngeal surface	147.3	198.89	230.0	210.7	235.1	239.0
posterior surface	147.3	198.89	230.0	210.7	235.1	239.0
superior surface	147.3	198.89	230.0	210.7	235.1	239.0
palatoglossal arch	146.2	198.89	230.0	210.6	235.1	239.0
palatopharyngeal arch	146.2	198.89	230.0	210.6	235.1	239.0
pallium	191.0	198.3	–	225.0	237.5	239.6
palpebra	173.1	198.2	232.1	216.1	238.2	239.2

❹ Fourth-Digit Required ❺ Fifth-Digit Required ▶◀ Revised Text ● New Line ▲ Revised Code

	Malignant					
	Primary	Secondary	Ca in situ	Benign	Uncertain Behavior	Unspecified
Neoplasm, neoplastic – *continued*						
pancreas	157.9	197.8	230.9	211.6	235.5	239.0
body	157.1	197.8	230.9	211.6	235.5	239.0
contiguous sites	157.8	–	–	–	–	–
duct (of Santorini) (of Wirsung)	157.3	197.8	230.9	211.6	235.5	239.0
ectopic tissue	157.8	197.8				
head	157.0	197.8	230.9	211.6	235.5	239.0
islet cells	157.4	197.8	230.9	211.7	235.5	239.0
neck	157.8	197.8	230.9	211.6	235.5	239.0
tail	157.2	197.8	230.9	211.6	235.5	239.0
para-aortic body	194.6	198.89	–	227.6	237.3	239.7
paraganglion NEC	194.6	198.89	–	227.6	237.3	239.7
parametrium	183.4	198.82	–	221.0	236.3	239.5
paranephric	158.0	197.6	–	211.8	235.4	239.0
pararectal	195.3	198.89	–	229.8	238.8	239.8
parasagittal (region)	195.0	198.89	234.8	229.8	238.8	239.8
parasellar	192.9	198.4	–	225.9	237.9	239.7
parathyroid (gland)	194.1	198.89	234.8	227.1	237.4	239.7
paraurethral	195.3	198.89	–	229.8	238.8	239.8
gland	189.4	198.1	233.9	223.89	236.99	239.5
paravaginal	195.3	198.89	–	229.8	238.8	239.8
parenchyma, kidney	189.0	198.0	233.9	223.0	236.91	239.5
parietal						
bone	170.0	198.5	–	213.0	238.0	239.2
lobe, brain	191.3	198.3	–	225.0	237.5	239.6
paroophoron	183.3	198.82	233.39▲	221.0	236.3	239.5
parotid (duct) (gland)	142.0	198.89	230.0	210.2	235.0	239.0
parovarium	183.3	198.82	233.39▲	221.0	236.3	239.5
patella	170.8	198.5	–	213.8	238.0	239.2
peduncle, cerebral	191.7	198.3	–	225.0	237.5	239.6
pelvirectal junction	154.0	197.5	230.4	211.4	235.2	239.0
pelvis, pelvic	195.3	198.89	234.8	229.8	238.8	239.8
bone	170.6	198.5	–	213.6	238.0	239.2
floor	195.3	198.89	234.8	229.8	238.8	239.8
renal	189.1	198.0	233.9	223.1	236.91	239.5
viscera	195.3	198.89	234.8	229.8	238.8	239.8
wall	195.3	198.89	234.8	229.8	238.8	239.8
pelvo-abdominal	195.8	198.89	234.8	229.8	238.8	239.8
penis	187.4	198.82	233.5	222.1	236.6	239.5
body	187.3	198.82	233.5	222.1	236.6	239.5
corpus (cavernosum)	187.3	198.82	233.5	222.1	236.6	239.5
glans	187.2	198.82	233.5	222.1	236.6	239.5
skin NEC	187.4	198.82	233.5	222.1	236.6	239.5
periadrenal (tissue)	158.0	197.6	–	211.8	235.4	239.0
perianal (skin)	173.5	198.2	232.5	216.5	238.2	239.2
pericardium	164.1	198.89	–	212.7	238.9	239.8
perinephric	158.0	197.6	–	211.8	235.4	239.0
perineum	195.3	198.89	234.8	229.8	238.8	239.8
periodontal tissue NEC	143.9	198.89	230.0	210.4	235.1	239.0
periosteum - *see* Neoplasm, bone						
peripancreatic	158.0	197.6	–	211.8	235.4	239.0
peripheral nerve NEC	171.9	198.89	–	215.9	238.1	239.2
perirectal (tissue)	195.3	198.89	–	229.8	238.8	239.8
perirenal (tissue)	158.0	197.6	–	211.8	235.4	239.0
peritoneum, peritoneal (cavity)	158.9	197.6	–	211.8	235.4	239.0
contiguous sites	158.8	–	–	–	–	–
with digestive organs	159.8	–	–	–	–	–
parietal	158.8	197.6	–	211.8	235.4	239.0
pelvic	158.8	197.6	–	211.8	235.4	239.0
specified part NEC	158.8	197.6	–	211.8	235.4	239.0
peritonsillar (tissue)	195.0	198.89	234.8	229.8	238.8	239.8
periurethral tissue	195.3	198.89	–	229.8	238.8	239.8
phalanges	170.9	198.5	–	213.9	238.0	239.2
foot	170.8	198.5	–	213.8	238.0	239.2

	Malignant					
	Primary	Secondary	Ca in situ	Benign	Uncertain Behavior	Unspecified
Neoplasm, neoplastic – *continued*						
phalanges – *continued*						
hand	170.5	198.5	–	213.5	238.0	239.2
pharynx, pharyngeal	149.0	198.89	230.0	210.9	235.1	239.0
bursa	147.1	198.89	230.0	210.7	235.1	239.0
fornix	147.3	198.89	230.0	210.7	235.1	239.0
recess	147.2	198.89	230.0	210.7	235.1	239.0
region	149.0	198.89	230.0	210.9	235.1	239.0
tonsil	147.1	198.89	230.0	210.7	235.1	239.0
wall (lateral) (posterior)	149.0	198.89	230.0	210.9	235.1	239.0
pia mater (cerebral) (cranial)	192.1	198.4	–	225.2	237.6	239.7
spinal	192.3	198.4	–	225.4	237.6	239.7
pillars of fauces	146.2	198.89	230.0	210.6	235.1	239.0
pineal (body) (gland)	194.4	198.89	234.8	227.4	237.1	239.7
pinna (ear) NEC	173.2	198.2	232.2	216.2	238.2	239.2
cartilage	171.0	198.89	–	215.0	238.1	239.2
piriform fossa or sinus	148.1	198.89	230.0	210.8	235.1	239.0
pituitary (body) (fossa) (gland) (lobe)	194.3	198.89	234.8	227.3	237.0	239.7
placenta	181	198.82	233.2	219.8	236.1	239.5
pleura, pleural (cavity)	163.9	197.2	–	212.4	235.8	239.1
contiguous sites	163.8	–	–	–	–	–
parietal	163.0	197.2	–	212.4	235.8	239.1
visceral	163.1	197.2	–	212.4	235.8	239.1
plexus						
brachial	171.2	198.89	–	215.2	238.1	239.2
cervical	171.0	198.89	–	215.0	238.1	239.2
choroid	191.5	198.3	–	225.0	237.5	239.6
lumbosacral	171.6	198.89	–	215.6	238.1	239.2
sacral	171.6	198.89	–	215.6	238.1	239.2
pluri-endocrine	194.8	198.89	234.8	227.8	237.4	239.7
pole						
frontal	191.1	198.3	–	225.0	237.5	239.6
occipital	191.4	198.3	–	225.0	237.5	239.6
pons (varolii)	191.7	198.3	–	225.0	237.5	239.6
popliteal fossa or space*	195.5	198.89	234.8	229.8	238.8	239.8
postcricoid (region)	148.0	198.89	230.0	210.8	235.1	239.0
posterior fossa (cranial)	191.9	198.3	–	225.0	237.5	239.6
postnasal space	147.9	198.89	230.0	210.7	235.1	239.0
prepuce	187.1	198.82	233.5	222.1	236.6	239.5
prepylorus	151.1	197.8	230.2	211.1	235.2	239.0
presacral (region)	195.3	198.89	–	229.8	238.8	239.8
prostate (gland)	185	198.82	233.4	222.2	236.5	239.5
utricle	189.3	198.1	233.9	223.81	236.99	239.5
pterygoid fossa	171.0	198.89	–	215.0	238.1	239.2
pubic bone	170.6	198.5	–	213.6	238.0	239.2
pudenda, pudendum (female)	184.4	198.82	233.32▲	221.2	236.3	239.5
pulmonary	162.9	197.0	231.2	212.3	235.7	239.1
putamen	191.0	198.3	–	225.0	237.5	239.6
pyloric						
antrum	151.2	197.8	230.2	211.1	235.2	239.0
canal	151.1	197.8	230.2	211.1	235.2	239.0
pylorus	151.1	197.8	230.2	211.1	235.2	239.0
pyramid (brain)	191.7	198.3	–	225.0	237.5	239.6
pyriform fossa or sinus	148.1	198.89	230.0	210.8	235.1	239.0
radius (any part)	170.4	198.5	–	213.4	238.0	239.2
Rathke's pouch	194.3	198.89	234.8	227.3	237.0	239.7
rectosigmoid (colon) (junction)	154.0	197.5	230.4	211.4	235.2	239.0
contiguous sites with anus or rectum	154.8	–	–	–	–	–
rectouterine pouch	158.8	197.6	–	211.8	235.4	239.0
rectovaginal septum or wall	195.3	198.89	234.8	229.8	238.8	239.8
rectovesical septum	195.3	198.89	234.8	229.8	238.8	239.8

Neoplasm, pancreas – Neoplasm, rectovesical septum

	Malignant					
	Primary	Secondary	Ca in situ	Benign	Uncertain Behavior	Unspecified
Neoplasm, neoplastic – *continued*						
rectum (ampulla)	154.1	197.5	230.4	211.4	235.2	239.0
and colon	154.0	197.5	230.4	211.4	235.2	239.0
contiguous sites with anus or rectosigmoid junction	154.8	–	–	–	–	–
renal	189.0	198.0	233.9	223.0	236.91	239.5
calyx	189.1	198.0	233.9	223.1	236.91	239.5
hilus	189.1	198.0	233.9	223.1	236.91	239.5
parenchyma	189.0	198.0	233.9	223.0	236.91	239.5
pelvis	189.1	198.0	233.9	223.1	236.91	239.5
respiratory						
organs or system NEC	165.9	197.3	231.9	212.9	235.9	239.1
contiguous sites with intrathoracic organs	165.8	–	–	–	–	–
specified sites NEC	165.8	197.3	231.8	212.8	235.9	239.1
tract NEC	165.9	197.3	231.9	212.9	235.9	239.1
upper	165.0	197.3	231.9	212.9	235.9	239.1
retina	190.5	198.4	234.0	224.5	238.8	239.8
retrobulbar	190.1	198.4	–	224.1	238.8	239.8
retrocecal	158.0	197.6	–	211.8	235.4	239.0
retromolar (area) (traingle) (trigone)	145.6	198.89	230.0	210.4	235.1	239.0
retro-orbital	195.0	198.89	234.8	229.8	238.8	239.8
retroperitoneal (space) (tissue)	158.0	197.6	–	211.8	235.4	239.0
contiguous sites	158.8	–	–	–	–	–
retroperitoneum	158.0	197.6	–	211.8	235.4	239.0
contiguous sites	158.8	–	–	–	–	–
retropharyngeal	149.0	198.89	230.0	210.9	235.1	239.0
retrovesical (septum)	195.3	198.89	234.8	229.8	238.8	239.8
rhinencephalon	191.0	198.3	–	225.0	237.5	239.6
rib	170.3	198.5	–	213.3	238.0	239.2
Rosenmüller's fossa	147.2	198.89	230.0	210.7	235.1	239.0
round ligament	183.5	198.82	–	221.0	236.3	239.5
sacrococcyx, sacrococcygeal	170.6	198.5	–	213.6	238.0	239.2
region	195.3	198.89	234.8	229.8	238.8	239.8
sacrouterine ligament	183.4	198.82	–	221.0	236.3	239.5
sacrum, sacral (vertebra)	170.6	198.5	–	213.6	238.0	239.2
salivary gland or duct (major)	142.9	198.89	230.0	210.2	235.0	239.0
contiguous sites	142.8	–	–	–	–	–
minor NEC	145.9	198.89	230.0	210.4	235.1	239.0
parotid	142.0	198.89	230.0	210.2	235.0	239.0
pluriglandular	142.8	198.89	230.0	210.2	235.0	239.0
sublingual	142.2	198.89	230.0	210.2	235.0	239.0
submandibular	142.1	198.89	230.0	210.2	235.0	239.0
submaxillary	142.1	198.89	230.0	210.2	235.0	239.0
salpinx (uterine)	183.2	198.82	233.39▲	221.0	236.3	239.5
Santorini's duct	157.3	197.8	230.9	211.6	235.5	239.0
scalp	173.4	198.2	232.4	216.4	238.2	239.2
scapula (any part)	170.4	198.5	–	213.4	238.0	239.2
scapular region	195.1	198.89	234.8	229.8	238.8	239.8
scar NEC (*see also* Neoplasm, skin)	173.9	198.2	232.9	216.9	238.2	239.2
sciatic nerve	171.3	198.89	–	215.3	238.1	239.2
sclera	190.0	198.4	234.0	224.0	238.8	239.8
scrotum (skin)	187.7	198.82	233.6	222.4	236.6	239.5
sebaceous gland - *see* Neoplasm, skin						
sella turcica	194.3	198.89	234.8	227.3	237.0	239.7
bone	170.0	198.5	–	213.0	238.0	239.2

	Malignant					
	Primary	Secondary	Ca in situ	Benign	Uncertain Behavior	Unspecified
Neoplasm, neoplastic – *continued*						
semilunar cartilage (knee)	170.7	198.5	–	213.7	238.0	239.2
seminal vesicle	187.8	198.82	233.6	222.8	236.6	239.5
septum						
nasal	160.0	197.3	231.8	212.0	235.9	239.1
posterior margin	147.3	198.89	230.0	210.7	235.1	239.0
rectovaginal	195.3	198.89	234.8	229.8	238.8	239.8
rectovesical	195.3	198.89	234.8	229.8	238.8	239.8
urethrovaginal	184.9	198.82	233.39▲	221.9	236.3	239.5
vesicovaginal	184.9	198.82	233.39▲	221.9	236.3	239.5
shoulder NEC*	195.4	198.89	232.6	229.8	238.8	239.8
sigmoid flexure (lower) (upper)	153.3	197.5	230.3	211.3	235.2	239.0
sinus (accessory)	160.9	197.3	231.8	212.0	235.9	239.1
bone (any)	170.0	198.5	–	213.0	238.0	239.2
contiguous sites with middle ear or nasal cavities	160.8	–	–	–	–	–
ethmoidal	160.3	197.3	231.8	212.0	235.9	239.1
frontal	160.4	197.3	231.8	212.0	235.9	239.1
maxillary	160.2	197.3	231.8	212.0	235.9	239.1
nasal, paranasal NEC	160.9	197.3	231.8	212.0	235.9	239.1
pyriform	148.1	198.89	230.0	210.8	235.1	239.0
sphenoidal	160.5	197.3	231.8	212.0	235.9	239.1
skeleton, skeletal NEC	170.9	198.5	–	213.9	238.0	239.2
Skene's gland	189.4	198.1	233.9	223.89	236.99	239.5
skin NEC	173.9	198.2	232.9	216.9	238.2	239.2
abdominal wall	173.5	198.2	232.5	216.5	238.2	239.2
ala nasi	173.3	198.2	232.3	216.3	238.2	239.2
ankle	173.7	198.2	232.7	216.7	238.2	239.2
antecubital space	173.6	198.2	232.6	216.6	238.2	239.2
anus	173.5	198.2	232.5	216.5	238.2	239.2
arm	173.6	198.2	232.6	216.6	238.2	239.2
auditory canal (external)	173.2	198.2	232.2	216.2	238.2	239.2
auricle (ear)	173.2	198.2	232.2	216.2	238.2	239.2
auricular canal (external)	173.2	198.2	232.2	216.2	238.2	239.2
axilla, axillary fold	173.5	198.2	232.5	216.5	238.2	239.2
back	173.5	198.2	232.5	216.5	238.2	239.2
breast	173.5	198.2	232.5	216.5	238.2	239.2
brow	173.3	198.2	232.3	216.3	238.2	239.2
buttock	173.5	198.2	232.5	216.5	238.2	239.2
calf	173.7	198.2	232.7	216.7	238.2	239.2
canthus (eye) (inner) (outer)	173.1	198.2	232.1	216.1	238.2	239.2
cervical region	173.4	198.2	232.4	216.4	238.2	239.2
cheek (external)	173.3	198.2	232.3	216.3	238.2	239.2
chest (wall)	173.5	198.2	232.5	216.5	238.2	239.2
chin	173.3	198.2	232.3	216.3	238.2	239.2
clavicular area	173.5	198.2	232.5	216.5	238.2	239.2
clitoris	184.3	198.82	233.32▲	221.2	236.3	239.5
columnella	173.3	198.2	232.3	216.3	238.2	239.2
concha	173.2	198.2	232.2	216.2	238.2	239.2
contiguous sites	173.8	–	–	–	–	–
ear (external)	173.2	198.2	232.2	216.2	238.2	239.2
elbow	173.6	198.2	232.6	216.6	238.2	239.2
eyebrow	173.3	198.2	232.3	216.3	238.2	239.2
eyelid	173.1	198.2	232.1	216.1	238.2	239.2
face NEC	173.3	198.2	232.3	216.3	238.2	239.2
female genital organs (external)	184.4	198.82	233.30▲	221.2	236.3	239.5
clitoris	184.3	198.82	233.32▲	221.2	236.3	239.5
labium NEC	184.4	198.82	233.32▲	221.2	236.3	239.5
majus	184.1	198.82	233.32▲	221.2	236.3	239.5
minus	184.2	198.82	233.32▲	221.2	236.3	239.5
pudendum	184.4	198.82	233.32▲	221.2	236.3	239.5
vulva	184.4	198.82	233.32▲	221.2	236.3	239.5

	Malignant					
	Primary	Secondary	Ca in situ	Benign	Uncertain Behavior	Unspecified
Neoplasm, neoplastic – *continued*						
skin – *continued*						
finger	173.6	198.2	232.6	216.6	238.2	239.2
flank	173.5	198.2	232.5	216.5	238.2	239.2
foot	173.7	198.2	232.7	216.7	238.2	239.2
forearm	173.6	198.2	232.6	216.6	238.2	239.2
forehead	173.3	198.2	232.3	216.3	238.2	239.2
glabella	173.3	198.2	232.3	216.3	238.2	239.2
gluteal region	173.5	198.2	232.5	216.5	238.2	239.2
groin	173.5	198.2	232.5	216.5	238.2	239.2
hand	173.6	198.2	232.6	216.6	238.2	239.2
head NEC	173.4	198.2	232.4	216.4	238.2	239.2
heel	173.7	198.2	232.7	216.7	238.2	239.2
helix	173.2	198.2	232.2	216.2	238.2	239.2
hip	173.7	198.2	232.7	216.7	238.2	239.2
infraclavicular region	173.5	198.2	232.5	216.5	238.2	239.2
inguinal region	173.5	198.2	232.5	216.5	238.2	239.2
jaw	173.3	198.2	232.3	216.3	238.2	239.2
knee	173.7	198.2	232.7	216.7	238.2	239.2
labia						
majora	184.1	198.82	233.32▲	221.2	236.3	239.5
minora	184.2	198.82	233.32▲	221.2	236.3	239.5
leg	173.7	198.2	232.7	216.7	238.2	239.2
lid (lower) (upper)	173.1	198.2	232.1	216.1	238.2	239.2
limb NEC	173.9	198.2	232.9	216.9	238.2	239.5
lower	173.7	198.2	232.7	216.7	238.2	239.2
upper	173.6	198.2	232.6	216.6	238.2	239.2
lip (lower) (upper)	173.0	198.2	232.0	216.0	238.2	239.2
male genital organs	187.9	198.82	233.6	222.9	236.6	239.5
penis	187.4	198.82	233.5	222.1	236.6	239.5
prepuce	187.1	198.82	233.5	222.1	236.6	239.5
scrotum	187.7	198.82	233.6	222.4	236.6	239.5
mastectomy site	173.5	198.2	–	–	–	–
specified as breast tissue	174.8	198.81	–	–	–	–
meatus, acoustic (external)	173.2	198.2	232.2	216.2	238.2	239.2
nates	173.5	198.2	232.5	216.5	238.2	239.2
neck	173.4	198.2	232.4	216.4	238.2	239.2
nose (external)	173.3	198.2	232.3	216.3	238.2	239.2
palm	173.6	198.2	232.6	216.6	238.2	239.2
palpebra	173.1	198.2	232.1	216.1	238.2	239.2
penis NEC	187.4	198.82	233.5	222.1	236.6	239.5
perianal	173.5	198.2	232.5	216.5	238.2	239.2
perineum	173.5	198.2	232.5	216.5	238.2	239.2
pinna	173.2	198.2	232.2	216.2	238.2	239.2
plantar	173.7	198.2	232.7	216.7	238.2	239.2
popliteal fossa or space	173.7	198.2	232.7	216.7	238.2	239.2
prepuce	187.1	198.82	233.5	222.1	236.6	239.5
pubes	173.5	198.2	232.5	216.5	238.2	239.2
sacrococcygeal region	173.5	198.2	232.5	216.5	238.2	239.2
scalp	173.4	198.2	232.4	216.4	238.2	239.2
scapular region	173.5	198.2	232.5	216.5	238.2	239.2
scrotum	187.7	198.82	233.6	222.4	236.6	239.5
shoulder	173.6	198.2	232.6	216.6	238.2	239.2
sole (foot)	173.7	198.2	232.7	216.7	238.2	239.2
specified sites NEC	173.8	198.2	232.8	216.8	232.8	239.2
submammary fold	173.5	198.2	232.5	216.5	238.2	239.2
supraclavicular region	173.4	198.2	232.4	216.4	238.2	239.2
temple	173.3	198.2	232.3	216.3	238.2	239.2
thigh	173.7	198.2	232.7	216.7	238.2	239.2
thoracic wall	173.5	198.2	232.5	216.5	238.2	239.2
thumb	173.6	198.2	232.6	216.6	238.2	239.2
toe	173.7	198.2	232.7	216.7	238.2	239.2
tragus	173.2	198.2	232.2	216.2	238.2	239.2
trunk	173.5	198.2	232.5	216.5	238.2	239.2
umbilicus	173.5	198.2	232.5	216.5	238.2	239.2
Neoplasm, neoplastic – *continued*						
skin – *continued*						
vulva	184.4	198.82	233.32▲	221.2	236.3	239.5
wrist	173.6	198.2	232.6	216.6	238.2	239.2
skull	170.0	198.5	–	213.0	238.0	239.2
soft parts or tissues - *see* Neoplasm, connective tissue						
specified site NEC	195.8	198.89	234.8	229.8	238.8	239.8
spermatic cord	187.6	198.82	233.6	222.8	236.6	239.5
sphenoid	160.5	197.3	231.8	212.0	235.9	239.1
bone	170.0	198.5	–	213.0	238.0	239.2
sinus	160.5	197.3	231.8	212.0	235.9	239.1
sphincter						
anal	154.2	197.5	230.5	211.4	235.5	239.0
of Oddi	156.1	197.8	230.8	211.5	235.3	239.0
spine, spinal (column)	170.2	198.5	–	213.2	238.0	239.2
bulb	191.7	198.3	–	225.0	237.5	239.6
coccyx	170.6	198.5	–	213.6	238.0	239.2
cord (cervical) (lumbar) (sacral) (thoracic)	192.2	198.3	–	225.3	237.5	239.7
dura mater	192.3	198.4	–	225.4	237.6	239.7
lumbosacral	170.2	198.5	–	213.2	238.0	239.2
membrane	192.3	198.4	–	225.4	237.6	239.7
meninges	192.3	198.4	–	225.4	237.6	239.7
nerve (root)	171.9	198.89	–	215.9	238.1	239.2
pia mater	192.3	198.4	–	225.4	237.6	239.7
root	171.9	198.89	–	215.9	238.1	239.2
sacrum	170.6	198.5	–	213.6	238.0	239.2
spleen, splenic NEC	159.1	197.8	230.9	211.9	235.5	239.0
flexure (colon)	153.7	197.5	230.3	211.3	235.2	239.0
stem, brain	191.7	198.3	–	225.0	237.5	239.6
Stensen's duct	142.0	198.89	230.0	210.2	235.0	239.0
sternum	170.3	198.5	–	213.3	238.0	239.2
stomach	151.9	197.8	230.2	211.1	235.2	239.0
antrum (pyloric)	151.2	197.8	230.2	211.1	235.2	239.0
body	151.4	197.8	230.2	211.1	235.2	239.0
cardia	151.0	197.8	230.2	211.1	235.2	239.0
cardiac orifice	151.0	197.8	230.2	211.1	235.2	239.0
contiguous sites	151.8	–	–	–	–	–
corpus	151.4	197.8	230.2	211.1	235.2	239.0
fundus	151.3	197.8	230.2	211.1	235.2	239.0
greater curvature NEC	151.6	197.8	230.2	211.1	235.2	239.0
lesser curvature NEC	151.5	197.8	230.2	211.1	235.2	239.0
prepylorus	151.1	197.8	230.2	211.1	235.2	239.0
pylorus	151.1	197.8	230.2	211.1	235.2	239.0
wall NEC	151.9	197.8	230.2	211.1	235.2	239.0
anterior NEC	151.8	197.8	230.2	211.1	235.2	239.0
posterior NEC	151.8	197.8	230.2	211.1	235.2	239.0
stroma, endometrial	182.0	198.82	233.2	219.1	236.0	239.5
stump, cervical	180.8	198.82	233.1	219.0	236.0	239.5
subcutaneous (nodule) (tissue) NEC - *see* Neoplasm, connective tissue						
subdural	192.1	198.4	–	225.2	237.6	239.7
subglottis, subglottic	161.2	197.3	231.0	212.1	235.6	239.1
sublingual	144.9	198.89	230.0	210.3	235.1	239.0
gland or duct	142.2	198.89	230.0	210.2	235.0	239.0
submandibular gland	142.1	198.89	230.0	210.2	235.0	239.0
submaxillary gland or duct	142.1	198.89	230.0	210.2	235.0	239.0
submental	195.0	198.89	234.8	229.8	238.8	239.8
subpleural	162.9	197.0	–	212.3	235.7	239.1
substernal	164.2	197.1	–	212.5	235.8	239.8

Neoplasm, skin – Neoplasm, substernal

	Malignant					
	Primary	Secondary	Ca in situ	Benign	Uncertain Behavior	Unspecified
Neoplasm, neoplastic – *continued*						
sudoriferous, sudoriparous gland, site unspecified	173.9	198.2	232.9	216.9	238.2	239.2
specified site - *see* Neoplasm, skin						
supraclavicular region	195.0	198.89	234.8	229.8	238.8	239.8
supraglottis	161.1	197.3	231.0	212.1	235.6	239.1
suprarenal (capsule) (cortex) (gland) (medulla)	194.0	198.7	234.8	227.0	237.2	239.7
suprasellar (region)	191.9	198.3	–	225.0	237.5	239.6
sweat gland (apocrine) (eccrine), site unspecified	173.9	198.2	232.9	216.9	238.2	239.2
specified site - *see* Neoplasm, skin						
sympathetic nerve or nervous system NEC	171.9	198.89	–	215.9	238.1	239.2
symphysis pubis	170.6	198.5	–	213.6	238.0	239.2
synovial membrane - *see* Neoplasm, connective tissue						
tapetum, brain	191.8	198.3	–	225.0	237.5	239.6
tarsus (any bone)	170.8	198.5	–	213.8	238.0	239.2
temple (skin)	173.3	198.2	232.3	216.3	238.2	239.2
temporal						
bone	170.0	198.5	–	213.0	238.0	239.2
lobe or pole	191.2	198.3	–	225.0	237.5	239.6
region	195.0	198.89	234.8	229.8	238.8	239.8
skin	173.3	198.2	232.3	216.3	238.2	239.2
tendon (sheath) - *see* Neoplasm, connective tissue						
tentorium (cerebelli)	192.1	198.4	–	225.2	237.6	239.7
testis, testes (descended) (scrotal)	186.9	198.82	233.6	222.0	236.4	239.5
ectopic	186.0	198.82	233.6	222.0	236.4	239.5
retained	186.0	198.82	233.6	222.0	236.4	239.5
undescended	186.0	198.82	233.6	222.0	236.4	239.5
thalamus	191.0	198.3	–	225.0	237.5	239.6
thigh NEC*	195.5	198.89	234.8	229.8	238.8	239.8
thorax, thoracic (cavity) (organs NEC)	195.1	198.89	234.8	229.8	238.8	239.8
duct	171.4	198.89	–	215.4	238.1	239.2
wall NEC	195.1	198.89	234.8	229.8	238.8	239.8
throat	149.0	198.89	230.0	210.9	235.1	239.0
thumb NEC*	195.4	198.89	232.6	229.8	238.8	239.8
thymus (gland)	164.0	198.89	–	212.6	235.8	239.8
contiguous sites with heart and mediastinum	164.8	–	–	–	–	–
thyroglossal duct	193	198.89	234.8	226	237.4	239.7
thyroid (gland)	193	198.89	234.8	226	237.4	239.7
cartilage	161.3	197.3	231.0	212.1	235.6	239.1
tibia (any part)	170.7	198.5	–	213.7	238.0	239.2
toe NEC*	195.5	198.89	232.7	229.8	238.8	239.8
tongue	141.9	198.89	230.0	210.1	235.1	239.0
anterior (two-thirds) NEC	141.4	198.89	230.0	210.1	235.1	239.0
dorsal surface	141.1	198.89	230.0	210.1	235.1	239.0
ventral surface	141.3	198.89	230.0	210.1	235.1	239.0
base (dorsal surface)	141.0	198.89	230.0	210.1	235.1	239.0
border (lateral)	141.2	198.89	230.0	210.1	235.1	239.0
contiguous sites	141.8	–	–	–	–	–
dorsal surface NEC	141.1	198.89	230.0	210.1	235.1	239.0
fixed part NEC	141.0	198.89	230.0	210.1	235.1	239.0
foreamen cecum	141.1	198.89	230.0	210.1	235.1	239.0

	Malignant					
	Primary	Secondary	Ca in situ	Benign	Uncertain Behavior	Unspecified
Neoplasm, neoplastic – *continued*						
tongue – *continued*						
frenulum linguae	141.3	198.89	230.0	210.1	235.1	239.0
junctional zone	141.5	198.89	230.0	210.1	235.1	239.0
margin (lateral)	141.2	198.89	230.0	210.1	235.1	239.0
midline NEC	141.1	198.89	230.0	210.1	235.1	239.0
mobile part NEC	141.4	198.89	230.0	210.1	235.1	239.0
posterior (third)	141.0	198.89	230.0	210.1	235.1	239.0
root	141.0	198.89	230.0	210.1	235.1	239.0
surface (dorsal)	141.1	198.89	230.0	210.1	235.1	239.0
base	141.0	198.89	230.0	210.1	235.1	239.0
ventral	141.3	198.89	230.0	210.1	235.1	239.0
tip	141.2	198.89	230.0	210.1	235.1	239.0
tonsil	141.6	198.89	230.0	210.1	235.1	239.0
tonsil	146.0	198.89	230.0	210.5	235.1	239.0
fauces, faucial	146.0	198.89	230.0	210.5	235.1	239.0
lingual	141.6	198.89	230.0	210.1	235.1	239.0
palatine	146.0	198.89	230.0	210.5	235.1	239.0
pharyngeal	147.1	198.89	230.0	210.7	235.1	239.0
pillar (anterior) (posterior)	146.2	198.89	230.0	210.6	235.1	239.0
tonsillar fossa	146.1	198.89	230.0	210.6	235.1	239.0
tooth socket NEC	143.9	198.89	230.0	210.4	235.1	239.0
trachea (cartilage) (mucosa)	162.0	197.3	231.1	212.2	235.7	239.1
contiguous sites with bronchus or lung	162.8	–	–	–	–	–
tracheobronchial	162.8	197.3	231.1	212.2	235.7	239.1
contiguous sites with lung	162.8	–	–	–	–	–
tragus	173.2	198.2	232.2	216.2	238.2	239.2
trunk NEC*	195.8	198.89	232.5	229.8	238.8	239.8
tubo-ovarian	183.8	198.82	233.39▲	221.8	236.3	239.5
tunica vaginalis	187.8	198.82	233.6	222.8	236.6	239.5
turbinate (bone)	170.0	198.5	–	213.0	238.0	239.2
nasal	160.0	197.3	231.8	212.0	235.9	239.1
tympanic cavity	160.1	197.3	231.8	212.0	235.9	239.1
ulna (any part)	170.4	198.5	–	213.4	238.0	239.2
umbilicus, umbilical	173.5	198.2	232.5	216.5	238.2	239.2
uncus, brain	191.2	198.3	–	225.0	237.5	239.6
unknown site or unspecified	199.1	199.1	234.9	229.9	238.9	239.9
urachus	188.7	198.1	233.7	223.3	236.7	239.4
ureter, ureteral	189.2	198.1	233.9	223.2	236.9	239.5
orifice (bladder)	188.6	198.1	233.7	223.3	236.7	239.4
ureter-bladder (junction)	188.6	198.1	233.7	223.3	236.7	239.4
urethra, urethral (gland)	189.3	198.1	233.9	223.81	236.99	239.5
orifice, internal	188.5	198.1	233.7	223.3	236.7	239.4
urethrovaginal (septum)	184.9	198.82	233.39▲	221.9	236.3	239.5
urinary organ or system NEC	189.9	198.1	233.9	223.9	236.99	239.5
bladder - *see* Neoplasm, bladder						
contiguous sites	189.8	–	–	–	–	–
specified sites NEC	189.8	198.1	233.9	223.89	236.99	239.5
utero-ovarian	183.8	198.82	233.39▲	221.8	236.3	239.5
ligament	183.3	198.82	–	221.0	236.3	239.5
uterosacral ligament	183.4	198.82	–	221.0	236.3	239.5
uterus, uteri, uterine	179	198.82	233.2	219.9	236.0	239.5
adnexa NEC	183.9	198.82	233.39▲	221.8	236.3	239.5
contiguous sites	183.8	–	–	–	–	–
body	182.0	198.82	233.2	219.1	236.0	239.5
contiguous sites	182.8	–	–	–	–	–
cervix	180.9	198.82	233.1	219.0	236.0	239.5
cornu	182.0	198.82	233.2	219.1	236.0	239.5
corpus	182.0	198.82	233.2	219.1	236.0	239.5

❹ Fourth-Digit Required ❺ Fifth-Digit Required ►◄ Revised Text ● New Line ▲ Revised Code

	Malignant					
	Primary	Secondary	Ca in situ	Benign	Uncertain Behavior	Unspecified
Neoplasm, neoplastic – *continued*						
uterus, uteri, uterine – *continued*						
endocervix (canal) (gland)	180.0	198.82	233.1	219.0	236.0	239.5
endometrium	182.0	198.82	233.2	219.1	236.0	239.5
exocervix	180.1	198.82	233.1	219.0	236.0	239.5
external os	180.1	198.82	233.1	219.0	236.0	239.5
fundus	182.0	198.82	233.2	219.1	236.0	239.5
internal os	180.0	198.82	233.1	219.0	236.0	239.5
isthmus	182.1	198.82	233.2	219.1	236.0	239.5
ligament	183.4	198.82	–	221.0	236.3	239.5
broad	183.3	198.82	233.39▲	221.0	236.3	239.5
round	183.5	198.82	–	221.0	236.3	239.5
lower segment	182.1	198.82	233.2	219.1	236.0	239.5
myometrium	182.0	198.82	233.2	219.1	236.0	239.5
squamocolumnar junction	180.8	198.82	233.1	219.0	236.0	239.5
tube	183.2	198.82	233.39▲	221.0	236.3	239.5
utricle, prostatic	189.3	198.1	233.9	223.81	236.99	239.5
uveal tract	190.0	198.4	234.0		238.8	239.8
uvula	145.4	198.89	230.0	210.4	235.1	239.0
vagina, vaginal (fornix) (vault) (wall)	184.0	198.82	233.31▲	221.1	236.3	239.5
vaginovesical	184.9	198.82	233.39▲	221.9	236.3	239.5
septum	194.9	198.82	233.39▲	221.9	236.3	239.5
vallecula (epigiottis)	146.3	198.89	230.0	210.6	235.1	239.0
vascular - *see* Neoplasm, connective tissue						
vas deferens	187.6	198.82	233.6	222.8	236.6	239.5
Vater's ampulla	156.2	197.8	230.8	211.5	235.3	239.0
vein, venous - *see* Neoplasm, connective tissue						
vena cava (abdominal) (inferior)	171.5	198.89	–	215.5	238.1	239.2
superior	171.4	198.89	–	215.4	238.1	239.2
ventricle (cerebral) (floor) (fourth) (lateral) (third)	191.5	198.3	–	225.0	237.5	239.6
cardiac (left) (right)	164.1	198.89	–	212.7	238.8	239.8
ventricular band of larynx	161.1	197.3	231.0	212.1	235.6	239.1
ventriculus - *see* Neoplasm, stomach						

	Malignant					
	Primary	Secondary	Ca in situ	Benign	Uncertain Behavior	Unspecified
Neoplasm, neoplastic – *continued*						
vermillion border - *see* Neoplasm, lip						
vermis, cerebellum	191.6	198.3	–	225.0	237.5	239.6
vertebra (column)	170.2	198.5	–	213.2	238.0	239.2
coccyx	170.6	198.5	–	213.6	238.0	239.2
sacrum	170.6	198.5	–	213.6	238.0	239.2
vesical - *see* Neoplasm, bladder						
vesicle, seminal	187.8	198.82	233.6	222.8	236.6	239.5
vesicocervical tissue	184.9	198.82	233.39▲	221.9	236.3	239.5
vesicorectal	195.3	198.89	234.8	229.8	238.8	239.8
vesicovaginal	184.9	198.82	233.39▲	221.9	236.3	239.5
septum	184.9	198.82	233.39▲	221.9	236.3	239.5
vessel (blood) - *see* Neoplasm, connective tissue						
vestibular gland, greater	184.1	198.82	233.32▲	221.2	236.3	239.5
vestibule						
mouth	145.1	198.89	230.0	210.4	235.1	239.0
nose	160.0	197.3	231.8	212.0	235.9	239.1
Virchow's gland	–	196.0	–	229.0	238.8	239.8
viscera NEC	195.8	198.89	234.8	229.8	238.8	239.8
vocal cords (true)	161.0	197.3	231.0	212.1	235.6	239.1
false	161.1	197.3	231.0	212.1	235.6	239.1
vomer	170.0	198.5	–	213.0	238.0	239.2
vulva	184.4	198.82	233.32▲	221.2	236.3	239.5
vulvovaginal gland	184.4	198.82	233.32▲	221.2	236.3	239.5
Waldeyer's ring	149.1	198.89	230.0	210.9	235.1	239.0
Wharton's duct	142.1	198.89	230.0	210.2	235.0	239.0
white matter (central) (cerebral)	191.0	198.3	–	225.0	237.5	239.6
windpipe	162.0	197.3	231.1	212.2	235.7	239.1
Wirsung's duct	157.3	197.8	230.9	211.6	235.5	239.0
wolffian (body) (duct)						
female	184.8	198.82	233.39▲	221.8	236.3	239.5
male	187.8	198.82	233.6	222.8	236.6	239.5
womb - *see* Neoplasm, uterus						
wrist NEC*	195.4	198.89	232.6	229.8	238.8	239.8
xiphoid process	170.3	198.5	–	213.3	238.0	239.2
Zuckerkandl's organ	194.6	198.89	–	227.6	237.3	239.7

Neoplasm, uterus, uteri, uterine – Neoplasm, Zuckerkandl's organ

- **Neovascularization**
  - choroid 362.16
  - ciliary body 364.42
  - cornea 370.60
    - deep 370.63
    - localized 370.61
  - iris 364.42
  - retina 362.16
  - subretinal 362.16
- **Nephralgia** 788.0
- **Nephritis, nephritic** (albuminuric) (azotemic) (congenital) (degenerative) (diffuse) (disseminated) (epithelial) (familial) (focal) (granulomatous) (hemorrhagic) (infantile) (nonsuppurative, excretory) (uremic) 583.9
  - with
    - edema – *see* Nephrosis
    - lesion of
      - glomerulonephritis
        - hypocomplementemic persistent 583.2
          - with nephrotic syndrome 581.2
          - chronic 582.2
        - lobular 583.2
          - with nephrotic syndrome 581.2
          - chronic 582.2
        - membranoproliferative 583.2
          - with nephrotic syndrome 581.2
          - chronic 582.2
        - membranous 583.1
          - with nephrotic syndrome 581.1
          - chronic 582.1
        - mesangiocapillary 583.2
          - with nephrotic syndrome 581.2
          - chronic 582.2
        - mixed membranous and proliferative 583.2
          - with nephrotic syndrome 581.2
          - chronic 582.2
        - proliferative (diffuse) 583.0
          - with nephrotic syndrome 581.0
          - acute 580.0
          - chronic 582.0
        - rapidly progressive 583.4
          - acute 580.4
          - chronic 582.4
      - interstitial nephritis (diffuse) (focal) 583.89
        - with nephrotic syndrome 581.89
        - acute 580.89
        - chronic 582.89
      - necrotizing glomerulitis 583.4
        - acute 580.4
        - chronic 582.4
      - renal necrosis 583.9
        - cortical 583.6
        - medullary 583.7
      - specified pathology NEC 583.89
        - with nephrotic syndrome 581.89
        - acute 580.89
        - chronic 582.89
    - necrosis, renal 583.9
      - cortical 583.6
      - medullary (papillary) 583.7
    - nephrotic syndrome (*see also* Nephrosis) 581.9
    - papillary necrosis 583.7
    - specified pathology NEC 583.89
  - acute 580.9
    - extracapillary with epithelial crescents 580.4
    - hypertensive (*see also* Hypertension, kidney) 403.90
    - necrotizing 580.4
    - poststreptococcal 580.0
    - proliferative (diffuse) 580.0
    - rapidly progressive 580.4
    - specified pathology NEC 580.89
  - amyloid 277.39 *[583.81]*
    - chronic 277.39 *[582.81]*
  - arteriolar (*see also* Hypertension, kidney) 403.90
  - arteriosclerotic (*see also* Hypertension, kidney) 403.90
  - ascending (*see also* Pyelitis) 590.80
  - atrophic 582.9
  - basement membrane NEC 583.89
    - with pulmonary hemorrhage (Goodpasture's syndrome) 446.21 *[583.81]*
  - calculous, calculus 592.0
  - cardiac (*see also* Hypertension, kidney) 403.90
  - cardiovascular (*see also* Hypertension, kidney) 403.90
  - chronic 582.9
    - arteriosclerotic (*see also* Hypertension, kidney) 403.90

- **Nephritis, nephritic** – *continued*
  - chronic – *continued*
    - hypertensive (*see also* Hypertension, kidney) 403.90
  - cirrhotic (*see also* Sclerosis, renal) 587
  - complicating pregnancy, childbirth, or puerperium 646.2❺
    - with hypertension 642.1❺
      - affecting fetus or newborn 760.0
    - affecting fetus or newborn 760.1
  - croupous 580.9
  - desquamative – *see* Nephrosis
  - due to
    - amyloidosis 277.39 *[583.81]*
      - chronic 277.39 *[582.81]*
    - arteriosclerosis (*see also* Hypertension, kidney) 403.90
    - diabetes mellitus 250.4❺ *[583.81]*
      - with nephrotic syndrome 250.4❺ *[581.81]*
    - diphtheria 032.89 *[580.81]*
    - gonococcal infection (acute) 098.19 *[583.81]*
      - chronic or duration of 2 months or over 098.39 *[583.81]*
    - gout 274.10
    - infectious hepatitis 070.9 *[580.81]*
    - mumps 072.79 *[580.81]*
    - specified kidney pathology NEC 583.89
      - acute 580.89
      - chronic 582.89
    - streptotrichosis 039.8 *[583.81]*
    - subacute bacterial endocarditis 421.0 *[580.81]*
    - systemic lupus erythematosus 710.0 *[583.81]*
      - chronic 710.0 *[582.81]*
    - typhoid fever 002.0 *[580.81]*
  - endothelial 582.2
  - end state (chronic) (terminal) NEC 585.6
  - epimembranous 581.1
  - exudative 583.89
    - with nephrotic syndrome 581.89
    - acute 580.89
    - chronic 582.89
  - gonococcal (acute) 098.19 *[583.81]*
    - chronic or duration of 2 months or over 098.39 *[583.81]*
  - gouty 274.10
  - hereditary (Alport's syndrome) 759.89
  - hydremic – *see* Nephrosis
  - hypertensive (*see also* Hypertension, kidney) 403.90
  - hypocomplementemic persistent 583.2
    - with nephrotic syndrome 581.2
    - chronic 582.2
  - immune complex NEC 583.89
  - infective (*see also* Pyelitis) 590.80
  - interstitial (diffuse) (focal) 583.89
    - with nephrotic syndrome 581.89
    - acute 580.89
    - chronic 582.89
  - latent or quiescent – *see* Nephritis, chronic
  - lead 984.9
    - specified type of lead – *see* Table of Drugs and Chemicals
  - lobular 583.2
    - with nephrotic syndrome 581.2
    - chronic 582.2
  - lupus 710.0 *[583.81]*
    - acute 710.0 *[581.81]*
    - chronic 710.0 *[582.81]*
  - membranoproliferative 583.2
    - with nephrotic syndrome 581.2
    - chronic 582.2
  - membranous 583.1
    - with nephrotic syndrome 581.1
    - chronic 582.1
  - mesangiocapillary 583.2
    - with nephrotic syndrome 581.2
    - chronic 582.2
  - minimal change 581.3
  - mixed membranous and proliferative 583.2
    - with nephrotic syndrome 581.2
    - chronic 582.2
  - necrotic, necrotizing 583.4
    - acute 580.4
    - chronic 582.4
  - nephrotic – *see* Nephrosis
  - old – *see* Nephritis, chronic
  - parenchymatous 581.89
  - polycystic 753.12
    - adult type (APKD) 753.13
    - autosomal dominant 753.13
    - autosomal recessive 753.14
    - childhood type (CPKD) 753.14

- **Nephritis, nephritic** – *continued*
  - polycystic – *continued*
    - infantile type 753.14
  - poststreptococcal 580.0
  - pregnancy – *see* Nephritis, complicating pregnancy
  - proliferative 583.0
    - with nephrotic syndrome 581.0
    - acute 580.0
    - chronic 582.0
  - purulent (*see also* Pyelitis) 590.80
  - rapidly progressive 583.4
    - acute 580.4
    - chronic 582.4
  - salt-losing or salt-wasting (*see also* Disease, renal) 593.9
  - saturnine 584.9
    - specified type of lead – *see* Table of Drugs and Chemicals
  - septic (*see also* Pyelitis) 590.80
  - specified pathology NEC 583.89
    - acute 580.89
    - chronic 582.89
  - staphylococcal (*see also* Pyelitis) 590.80
  - streptotrichosis 039.8 *[583.81]*
  - subacute (*see also* Nephrosis) 581.9
  - suppurative (*see also* Pyelitis) 590.80
  - syphilitic (late) 095.4
    - congenital 090.5 *[583.81]*
    - early 091.69 *[583.81]*
  - terminal (chronic) (end-stage) NEC 585.6
  - toxic – *see* Nephritis, acute
  - tubal, tubular – *see* Nephrosis, tubular
  - tuberculous (*see also* Tuberculosis) 016.0❺ *[583.81]*
  - type II (Ellis) – *see* Nephrosis
  - vascular – *see also* Hypertension, kidney
  - war 580.9
- **Nephroblastoma** (M8960/3) 189.0
  - epithelial (M8961/3) 189.0
  - mesenchymal (M8962/3) 189.0
- **Nephrocalcinosis** 275.49
- **Nephrocystitis, pustular** (*see also* Pyelitis) 590.80
- **Nephrolithiasis** (congenital) (pelvis) (recurrent) 592.0
  - uric acid 274.11
- **Nephroma** (M8960/3) 189.0
  - mesoblastic (M8960/1) 236.9❺
- **Nephronephritis** (*see also* Nephrosis) 581.9
- **Nephronopthisis** 753.16
- **Nephropathy** (*see also* Nephritis) 583.9
  - with
    - exudative nephritis 583.89
    - interstitial nephritis (diffuse) (focal) 583.89
    - medullary necrosis 583.7
    - necrosis 583.9
      - cortical 583.6
      - medullary or papillary 583.7
    - papillary necrosis 583.7
    - specified lesion or cause NEC 583.89
  - analgesic 583.89
    - with medullary necrosis, acute 584.7
  - arteriolar (*see also* Hypertension, kidney) 403.90
  - arteriosclerotic (*see also* Hypertension, kidney) 403.90
  - complicating pregnancy 646.2❺
  - diabetic 250.4❺ *[583.81]*
  - gouty 274.10
    - specified type NEC 274.19
  - hereditary amyloid 277.31
  - hypercalcemic 588.89
  - hypertensive (*see also* Hypertension, kidney) 403.90
  - hypokalemic (vacuolar) 588.89
  - IgA 583.9
  - obstructive 593.89
    - congenital 753.20
  - phenacetin 584.7
  - phosphate-losing 588.0
  - potassium depletion 588.89
  - proliferative (*see also* Nephritis, proliferative) 583.0
  - protein-losing 588.89
  - salt-losing or salt-wasting (*see also* Disease, renal) 593.9
  - sickle-cell (*see also* Disease, sickle-cell) 282.60 *[583.81]*
  - toxic 584.5
  - vasomotor 584.5
  - water-losing 588.89
- **Nephroptosis** (*see also* Disease, renal) 593.0
  - congenital (displaced) 753.3

Neovascularization – Nephroptosis

- **Neurosis, neurotic** – *continued*
  - gastric 306.4
  - gastrointestinal 306.4
  - genitourinary 306.50
  - heart 306.2
  - hypochondriacal 300.7
  - hysterical 300.10
    - conversion type 300.11
    - dissociative type 300.15
  - impulsive 300.3
  - incoordination 306.0
    - larynx 306.1
    - vocal cord 306.1
  - intestine 306.4
  - larynx 306.1
    - hysterical 300.11
    - sensory 306.1
  - menopause, unspecified type 627.2
  - mixed NEC 300.89
  - musculoskeletal 306.0
  - obsessional 300.3
    - phobia 300.3
  - obsessive-compulsive 300.3
  - occupational 300.89
  - ocular 306.7
  - oral 307.0
  - organ (*see also* Disorder, psychosomatic) 306.9
  - pharynx 306.1
  - phobic 300.20
  - posttraumatic (acute) (situational) 309.81
    - chronic 309.81
  - psychasthenic (type) 300.89
  - railroad 300.16
  - rectum 306.4
  - respiratory 306.1
  - rumination 306.4
  - senile 300.89
  - sexual 302.70
  - situational 300.89
  - specified type NEC 300.89
  - state 300.9
    - with depersonalization episode 300.6
  - stomach 306.4
  - vasomotor 306.2
  - visceral 306.4
  - war 300.16
- **Neurospongioblastosis diffusa** 759.5
- **Neurosyphilis** (arrested) (early) (inactive) (late) (latent) (recurrent) 094.9
  - with ataxia (cerebellar) (locomotor) (spastic) (spinal) 094.0
  - acute meningitis 094.2
  - aneurysm 094.89
  - arachnoid (adhesive) 094.2
  - arteritis (any artery) 094.89
  - asymptomatic 094.3
  - congenital 090.40
  - dura (mater) 094.89
  - general paresis 094.1
  - gumma 094.9
  - hemorrhagic 094.9
  - juvenile (asymptomatic) (meningeal) 090.40
  - leptomeninges (aseptic) 094.2
  - meningeal 094.2
  - meninges (adhesive) 094.2
  - meningovascular (diffuse) 094.2
  - optic atrophy 094.84
  - parenchymatous (degenerative) 094.1
  - paresis (*see also* Paresis, general) 094.1
  - paretic (*see also* Paresis, general) 094.1
  - relapse 094.9
  - remission in (sustained) 094.9
  - serological 094.3
  - specified nature or site NEC 094.89
  - tabes (dorsalis) 094.0
    - juvenile 090.40
  - tabetic 094.0
    - juvenile 090.40
  - taboparesis 094.1
    - juvenile 090.40
  - thrombosis 094.89
  - vascular 094.89
- **Neurotic** (*see also* Neurosis) 300.9
  - excoriation 698.4
    - psychogenic 306.3
- **Neurotmesis** – *see* Injury, nerve, by site
- **Neurotoxemia** – *see* Toxemia
- **Neutro-occlusion** 524.21
- **Neutropenia, neutropenic** (idiopathic) (pernicious) (primary) 288.00
  - chronic 288.09
    - hypoplastic 288.09
  - congenital (nontransient) 288.01
  - cyclic 288.02
  - drug induced 288.03
  - due to infection 288.04
  - fever 288.00
  - genetic 288.01
  - immune 288.09
  - infantile 288.01
  - malignant 288.09
  - neonatal, transitory (isoimmune) (maternal transfer) 776.7
  - periodic 288.02
  - splenic 289.53
  - splenomegaly 289.53
  - toxic 288.09
- **Neutrophilia, hereditary giant** 288.2
- **Nevocarcinoma** (M8720/3) – *see* Melanoma
- **Nevus** (M8720/0) – *see also* Neoplasm, skin, benign

  Note – Except where otherwise indicated, varieties of nevus in the list below that are followed by a morphology code number (M____/0) should be coded by site as for "Neoplasm, skin, benign."

  - acanthotic 702.8
  - achromic (M8730/0)
  - amelanotic (M8730/0)
  - anemic, anemicus 709.09
  - angiomatous (M9120/0) (*see also* Hemangioma) 228.00
  - araneus 448.1
  - avasculosus 709.09
  - balloon cell (M8722/0)
  - bathing trunk (M8761/1) 238.2
  - blue (M8780/0)
    - cellular (M8790/0)
    - giant (M8790/0)
    - Jadassohn's (M8780/0)
    - malignant (M8780/3) – *see* Melanoma
  - capillary (M9131/0) (*see also* Hemangioma) 228.00
  - cavernous (M9121/0) (*see also* Hemangioma) 228.00
  - cellular (M8720/0)
    - blue (M8790/0)
  - comedonicus 757.33
  - compound (M8760/0)
  - conjunctiva (M8720/0) 224.3
  - dermal (8750/0)
    - and epidermal (M8760/0)
  - epithelioid cell (and spindle cell) (M8770/0)
  - flammeus 757.32
    - osteohypertrophic 759.89
  - hairy (M8720/0)
  - halo (M8723/0)
  - hemangiomatous (M9120/0) (*see also* Hemangioma) 228.00
  - intradermal (M8750/0)
  - intraepidermal (M8740/0)
  - involuting (M8724/0)
  - Jadassohn's (blue) (M8780/0)
  - junction, junctional (M8740/0)
    - malignant melanoma in (M8740/3) – *see* Melanoma
  - juvenile (M8770/0)
  - lymphatic (M9170/0) 228.1
  - magnocellular (M8726/0)
    - specified site – *see* Neoplasm, by site, benign
    - unspecified site 224.0
  - malignant (M8720/3) – *see* Melanoma
  - meaning hemangioma (M9120/0) (*see also* Hemangioma) 228.00
  - melanotic (pigmented) (M8720/0)
  - multiplex 759.5
  - nonneoplastic 448.1
  - nonpigmented (M8730/0)
  - nonvascular (M8720/0)
  - oral mucosa, white sponge 750.26
  - osteohypertrophic, flammeus 759.89
  - papillaris (M8720/0)
  - papillomatosus (M8720/0)
  - pigmented (M8720/0)
    - giant (M8761/1) – *see also* Neoplasm, skin, uncertain behavior
      - malignant melanoma in (M8761/3) – *see* Melanoma
    - systematicus 757.33
  - pilosus (M8720/0)
  - port wine 757.32
  - sanguineous 757.32
  - sebaceous (senile) 702.8
  - senile 448.1
  - spider 448.1
  - spindle cell (and epithelioid cell) (M8770/0)
  - stellar 448.1
  - strawberry 757.32
  - syringocystadenomatous papilliferous (M8406/0)
  - unius lateris 757.33
  - Unna's 757.32
  - vascular 757.32
  - verrucous 757.33
  - white sponge (oral mucosa) 750.26
- **Newborn** (infant) (liveborn)
  - affected by maternal abuse of drugs (gestational) (via placenta) (via breast milk) (*see also* Noxious, substances transmitted through placenta or breast milk (affecting fetus or newborn)) 760.70
  - apnea 770.81
    - obstructive 770.82
    - specified NEC 770.82
  - cardiomyopathy 425.4
    - congenital 425.3
  - convulsion 779.0
  - electrolyte imbalance NEC (transitory) 775.5
  - gestation
    - 24 completed weeks 765.22
    - 25-26 completed weeks 765.23
    - 27-28 completed weeks 765.24
    - 29-30 completed weeks 765.25
    - 31-32 completed weeks 765.26
    - 33-34 completed weeks 765.27
    - 35-36 completed weeks 765.28
    - 37 or more completed weeks 765.29
    - less than 24 completed weeks 765.21
    - unspecified completed weeks 765.20
  - infection 771.89
    - candida 771.7
    - mastitis 771.5
    - specified NEC 771.89
    - urinary tract 771.82
  - mastitis 771.5
  - multiple NEC
    - born in hospital (without mention of cesarean delivery or section) V37.00
      - with cesarean delivery or section V37.01
    - born outside hospital
      - hospitalized V37.1
      - not hospitalized V37.2
    - mates all liveborn
      - born in hospital (without mention of cesarean delivery or section) V34.00
        - with cesarean delivery or section V34.01
      - born outside hospital
        - hospitalized V34.1
        - not hospitalized V34.2
    - mates all stillborn
      - born in hospital (without mention of cesarean delivery or section) V35.00
        - with cesarean delivery or section V35.01
      - born outside hospital
        - hospitalized V35.1
        - not hospitalized V35.2
    - mates liveborn and stillborn
      - born in hospital (without mention of cesarean delivery or section) V36.00
        - with cesarean delivery or section V36.01
      - born outside hospital
        - hospitalized V36.1
        - not hospitalized V36.2
  - omphalitis 771.4
  - seizure 779.0
  - sepsis 771.81
  - single
    - born in hospital (without mention of cesarean delivery or section) V30.00
      - with cesarean delivery or section V30.01
    - born outside hospital
      - hospitalized V30.1
      - not hospitalized V30.2
  - specified condition NEC 779.89
  - twin NEC
    - born in hospital (without mention of cesarean delivery or section) V33.00
      - with cesarean delivery or section V33.01
    - born outside hospital
      - hospitalized V33.1
      - not hospitalized V33.2

Neurosis, neurotic – Newborn

- **Newborn** – *continued*
  - twin – *continued*
    - mate liveborn
      - born in hospital V31.0❺
      - born outside hospital
        - hospitalized V31.1
        - not hospitalized V31.2
    - mate stillborn
      - born in hospital V32.0❺
      - born outside hospital
        - hospitalized V32.1
        - not hospitalized V32.2
  - unspecified as to single or multiple birth
    - born in hospital (without mention of cesarean delivery or section) V39.00
      - with cesarean delivery or section V39.01
    - born outside hospital
      - hospitalized V39.1
      - not hospitalized V39.2
- **Newcastle's conjunctivitis or disease** 077.8
- **Nezelof's syndrome** (pure alymphocytosis) 279.13
- **Niacin** (amide) **deficiency** 265.2
- **Nicolas-Durand-Favre disease** (climatic bubo) 099.1
- **Nicolas-Favre disease** (climatic bubo) 099.1
- **Nicotinic acid** (amide) **deficiency** 265.2
- **Niemann-Pick disease** (lipid histiocytosis) (splenomegaly) 272.7
- **Night**
  - blindness (*see also* Blindness, night) 368.60
    - congenital 368.61
    - vitamin A deficiency 264.5
  - cramps 729.82
  - sweats 780.8
  - terrors, child 307.46
- **Nightmare** 307.47
  - REM-sleep type 307.47
- **Nipple** – *see* condition
- **Nisbet's chancre** 099.0
- **Nishimoto** (-Takeuchi) **disease** 437.5
- **Nitritoid crisis or reaction** – *see* Crisis, nitritoid
- **Nitrogen retention, extrarenal** 788.9
- **Nitrosohemoglobinemia** 289.89
- **Njovera** 104.0
- **No**
  - diagnosis 799.9
  - disease (found) V71.9
  - room at the inn V65.0
- **Nocardiasis** – *see* Nocardiosis
- **Nocardiosis** 039.9
  - with pneumonia 039.1
  - lung 039.1
  - specified type NEC 039.8
- **Nocturia** 788.43
  - psychogenic 306.53
- **Nocturnal** – *see also* condition
  - dyspnea (paroxysmal) 786.09
  - emissions 608.89
  - enuresis 788.36
    - psychogenic 307.6
  - frequency (micturition) 788.43
    - psychogenic 306.53
- **Nodal rhythm disorder** 427.89
- **Nodding of head** 781.0
- **Node(s)** – *see also* Nodules
  - Heberden's 715.04
  - larynx 478.79
  - lymph – *see* condition
  - milkers' 051.1
  - Osler's 421.0
  - rheumatic 729.89
  - Schmorl's 722.30
    - lumbar, lumbosacral 722.32
    - specified region NEC 722.39
    - thoracic, thoracolumbar 722.31
  - singers' 478.5
  - skin NEC 782.2
  - tuberculous – *see* Tuberculosis, lymph gland
  - vocal cords 478.5
- **Nodosities, Haygarth's** 715.04
- **Nodule(s), nodular**
  - actinomycotic (*see also* Actinomycosis) 039.9
  - arthritic – *see* Arthritis, nodosa
  - cutaneous 782.2
  - Haygarth's 715.04
  - inflammatory – *see* Inflammation
  - juxta-articular 102.7
    - syphilitic 095.7
    - yaws 102.7
- **Nodule(s), nodular** – *continued*
  - larynx 478.79
  - lung, solitary 518.89
    - emphysematous 492.8
  - milkers' 051.1
  - prostate 600.10
    - with
      - urinary
        - obstruction 600.11
        - retention 600.11
  - rheumatic 729.89
  - rheumatoid – *see* Arthritis rheumatoid
  - scrotum (inflammatory) 608.4
  - singers' 478.5
  - skin NEC 782.2
  - solitary, lung 518.89
    - emphysematous 492.8
  - subcutaneous 782.2
  - thyroid (gland) (nontoxic) (uninodular) 241.0
    - with
      - hyperthyroidism 242.1❺
      - thyrotoxicosis 242.1❺
    - toxic or with hyperthyroidism 242.1❺
  - vocal cords 478.5
- **Noma** (gangrenous) (hospital) (infective) 528.1
  - auricle (*see also* Gangrene) 785.4
  - mouth 528.1
  - pudendi (*see also* Vulvitis) 616.10
  - vulvae (*see also* Vulvitis) 616.10
- **Nomadism** V60.0
- **Non-adherence**
  - artificial skin graft 996.55
  - decellularized allodermis graft 996.55
- **Non-autoimmune hemolytic anemia** NEC 283.10
- **Nonclosure** – *see also* Imperfect, closure
  - ductus
    - arteriosus 747.0
    - Botalli 747.0
  - Eustachian valve 746.89
  - foramen
    - Botalli 745.5
    - ovale 745.5
- **Noncompliance with medical treatment** V15.81
- **Nondescent** (congenital) – *see also* Malposition, congenital
  - cecum 751.4
  - colon 751.4
  - testis 752.51
- **Nondevelopment**
  - brain 742.1
    - specified part 742.2
  - heart 746.89
  - organ or site, congenital NEC – *see* Hypoplasia
- **Nonengagement**
  - head NEC 652.5❺
    - in labor 660.1❺
      - affecting fetus or newborn 763.1
- **Nonexanthematous tick fever** 066.1
- **Nonexpansion, lung** (newborn) NEC 770.4
- **Nonfunctioning**
  - cystic duct (*see also* Disease, gallbladder) 575.8
  - gallbladder (*see also* Disease, gallbladder) 575.8
  - kidney (*see also* Disease, renal) 593.9
  - labyrinth 386.58
- **Nonhealing**
  - stump (surgical) 997.69
  - wound, surgical 998.83
- **Nonimplantation of ovum, causing infertility** 628.3
- **Noninsufflation, fallopian tube** 628.2
- **Nonne-Milroy-Meige syndrome** (chronic hereditary edema) 757.0
- **Nonovulation** 628.0
- **Nonpatent fallopian tube** 628.2
- **Nonpneumatization, lung** NEC 770.4
- **Nonreflex bladder** 596.54
  - with cauda equina 344.61
- **Nonretention of food** – *see* Vomiting
- **Nonrotation** – *see* Malrotation
- **Nonsecretion, urine** (*see also* Anuria) 788.5
  - newborn 753.3
- **Nonunion**
  - fracture 733.82
  - organ or site, congenital NEC – *see* Imperfect, closure
  - symphysis pubis, congenital 755.69
  - top sacrum, congenital 756.19
- **Nonviability** 765.0❺
- **Nonvisualization, gallbladder** 793.3
- **Nonvitalized tooth** 522.9
- **Non-working side interference** 524.56
- **Normal**
  - delivery – *see* category 650
  - menses V65.5
  - state (feared complaint unfounded) V65.5
- **Normoblastosis** 289.89
- **Normocytic anemia** (infectional) 285.9
  - due to blood loss (chronic) 280.0
    - acute 285.1
- **Norrie's disease** (congenital) (progressive oculoacousticocerebral degeneration) 743.8
- **North American blastomycosis** 116.0
- **Norwegian itch** 133.0
- **Nose, nasal** – *see* condition
- **Nosebleed** 784.7
- **Nosomania** 298.9
- **Nosophobia** 300.29
- **Nostalgia** 309.89
- **Notch of iris** 743.46
- **Notched lip, congenital** (*see also* Cleft, lip) 749.10
- **Notching nose, congenital** (tip) 748.1
- **Nothnagel's**
  - syndrome 378.52
  - vasomotor acroparesthesia 443.89
- **Novy's relapsing fever** (American) 087.1
- **Noxious**
  - foodstuffs, poisoning by
    - fish 988.0
    - fungi 988.1
    - mushrooms 988.1
    - plants (food) 988.2
    - shellfish 988.0
    - specified type NEC 988.8
    - toadstool 988.1
  - substances transmitted through placenta or breast milk (affecting fetus or newborn) 760.70
    - acetretin 760.78
    - alcohol 760.71
    - aminopterin 760.78
    - antiandrogens 760.79
    - anticonvulsant 760.77
    - antifungal 760.74
    - anti-infective agents 760.74
    - antimetabolic 760.78
    - atorvastatin 760.78
    - carbamazepine 760.77
    - cocaine 760.75
    - "crack" 760.75
    - diethylstilbestrol (DES) 760.76
    - divalproex sodium 760.77
    - endocrine disrupting chemicals 760.79
    - estrogens 760.79
    - etretinate 760.78
    - fluconazole 760.74
    - fluvastatin 760.78
    - hallucinogenic agents NEC 760.73
    - hormones 760.79
    - lithium 760.79
    - lovastatin 760.78
    - medicinal agents NEC 760.79
    - methotrexate 760.78
    - misoprostil 760.79
    - narcotics 760.72
    - obstetric anesthetic or analgesic 763.5
    - phenobarbital 760.77
    - phenytoin 760.77
    - pravastatin 760.78
    - progestins 760.79
    - retinoic acid 760.78
    - simvastatin 760.78
    - solvents 760.79
    - specified agent NEC 760.79
    - statins 760.78
    - suspected, affecting management of pregnancy 655.5❺
    - tetracycline 760.74
    - thalidomide 760.79
    - trimethadione 760.77
    - valproate 760.77
    - valproic acid 760.77
    - vitamin A 760.78
- **Nuchal hitch** (arm) 652.8
- **Nucleus pulposus** – *see* condition
- **Numbness** 782.0
- **Nuns' knee** 727.2

- **Nursemaid's**
  - elbow 832.0❺
  - shoulder 831.0❺
- **Nutmeg liver** 573.8
- **Nutrition, deficient or insufficient** (particular kind of food) 269.9
  - due to
    - insufficient food 994.2
    - lack of
      - care (child) (infant) 995.52
        - adult 995.84
      - food 994.2
- **Nyctalopia** (*see also* Blindness, night) 368.60
  - vitamin A deficiency 264.5
- **Nycturia** 788.43
  - psychogenic 306.53
- **Nymphomania** 302.89
- **Nystagmus** 379.50
  - associated with vestibular system disorders 379.54
  - benign paroxysmal positional 386.11
  - central positional 386.2
  - congenital 379.51
  - deprivation 379.53
  - dissociated 379.55
  - latent 379.52
  - miners' 300.89
  - positional
    - benign paroxysmal 386.11
    - central 386.2
  - specified NEC 379.56
  - vestibular 379.54
  - visual deprivation 379.53

O

- **Oasthouse urine disease** 270.2
- **Obermeyer's relapsing fever** (European) 087.0
- **Obesity** (constitutional) (exogenous) (familial) (nutritional) (simple) 278.00
  - adrenal 255.8
  - complicating pregnancy, childbirth, or puerperium 649.1❺
  - due to hyperalimentation 278.00
  - endocrine NEC 259.9
  - endogenous 259.9
  - Fröhlich's (adiposogenital dystrophy) 253.8
  - glandular NEC 259.9
  - hypothyroid (*see also* Hypothyroidism) 244.9
  - morbid 278.01
  - of pregnancy 649.1❺
  - pituitary 253.8
  - severe 278.01
  - thyroid (*see also* Hypothyroidism) 244.9
- **Oblique** – *see also* condition
  - lie before labor, affecting fetus or newborn 761.7
- **Obliquity, pelvis** 738.6
- **Obliteration**
  - abdominal aorta 446.7
  - appendix (lumen) 543.9
  - artery 447.1
  - ascending aorta 446.7
  - bile ducts 576.8
    - with calculus, choledocholithiasis, or stones – *see* Choledocholithiasis
    - congenital 751.61
      - jaundice from 751.61 *[774.5]*
  - common duct 576.8
    - with calculus, choledocholithiasis, or stones – *see* Choledocholithiasis
    - congenital 751.61
  - cystic duct 575.8
    - with calculus, choledocholithiasis, or stones – *see* Choledocholithiasis
  - disease, arteriolar 447.1
  - endometrium 621.8
  - eye, anterior chamber 360.34
  - fallopian tube 628.2
  - lymphatic vessel 457.1
    - postmastectomy 457.0
  - organ or site, congenital NEC – *see* Atresia
  - placental blood vessels – *see* Placenta, abnormal
  - supra-aortic branches 446.7
  - ureter 593.89
  - urethra 599.84
  - vein 459.9
  - vestibule (oral) 525.8
- **Observation** (for) V71.9
  - without need for further medical care V71.9
  - accident NEC V71.4
    - at work V71.3
  - criminal assault V71.6
  - deleterious agent ingestion V71.89
  - disease V71.9
    - cardiovascular V71.7
    - heart V71.7
    - mental V71.09
    - specified condition NEC V71.89
  - foreign body ingestion V71.89
  - growth and development variations V21.8
  - injuries (accidental) V71.4
    - inflicted NEC V71.6
      - during alleged rape or seduction V71.5
  - malignant neoplasm, suspected V71.1
  - postpartum
    - immediately after delivery V24.0
    - routine follow-up V24.2
  - pregnancy
    - high-risk V23.9
      - specified problem NEC V23.8❺
    - normal (without complication) V22.1
      - with nonobstetric complication V22.2
      - first V22.0
  - rape or seduction, alleged V71.5
    - injury during V71.5
  - suicide attempt, alleged V71.89
  - suspected (undiagnosed) (unproven)
    - abuse V71.81
    - cardiovascular disease V71.7
    - child or wife battering victim V71.6
    - concussion (cerebral) V71.6
    - condition NEC V71.89
      - infant – *see* Observation, suspected, condition, newborn
      - newborn V29.9
        - cardiovascular disease V29.8
        - congenital anomaly V29.8
        - genetic V29.3
        - infectious V29.0
        - ingestion foreign object V29.8
        - injury V29.8
        - metabolic V29.3
        - neoplasm V29.8
        - neurological V29.1
        - poison, poisoning V29.8
        - respiratory V29.2
        - specified NEC V29.8
    - exposure
      - anthrax V71.82
      - biologic agent NEC V71.83
      - SARS V71.83
    - infectious disease not requiring isolation V71.89
    - malignant neoplasm V71.1
    - mental disorder V71.09
    - neglect V71.81
    - neoplasm
      - benign V71.89
      - malignant V71.1
    - specified condition NEC V71.89
    - tuberculosis V71.2
  - tuberculosis, suspected V71.2
- **Obsession, obsessional** 300.3
  - ideas and mental images 300.3
  - impulses 300.3
  - neurosis 300.3
  - phobia 300.3
  - psychasthenia 300.3
  - ruminations 300.3
  - state 300.3
  - syndrome 300.3
- **Obsessive-compulsive** 300.3
  - neurosis 300.3
  - personality 301.4
  - reaction 300.3
- **Obstetrical trauma NEC** (complicating delivery) 665.9❺
  - with
    - abortion – *see* Abortion, by type, with damage to pelvic organs
    - ectopic pregnancy (*see also* categories 633.0-633.9) 639.2
    - molar pregnancy (*see also* categories 630-632) 639.2
  - affecting fetus or newborn 763.89
  - following
    - abortion 639.2
    - ectopic or molar pregnancy 639.2
- **Obstipation** (*see also* Constipation) 564.00
  - psychogenic 306.4
- **Obstruction, obstructed, obstructive**
  - airway NEC 519.8
    - with
      - allergic alveolitis NEC 495.9
      - asthma NEC (*see also* Asthma) 493.9❺
      - bronchiectasis 494.0
        - with acute exacerbation 494.1
      - bronchitis (*see also* Bronchitis, with, obstruction) 491.20
      - emphysema NEC 492.8
    - chronic 496
      - with
        - allergic alveolitis NEC 495.5
        - asthma NEC (*see also* Asthma) 493.2❺
        - bronchiectasis 494.0
          - with acute exacerbation 494.1
        - bronchitis (chronic) (*see also* Bronchitis, chronic, obstructive) 491.20
        - emphysema NEC 492.8
    - due to
      - bronchospasm 519.11
      - foreign body 934.9
      - inhalation of fumes or vapors 506.9
      - laryngospasm 478.75
  - alimentary canal (*see also* Obstruction, intestine) 560.9
  - ampulla of Vater 576.2
    - with calculus, cholelithiasis, or stones – *see* Choledocholithiasis
  - aortic (heart) (valve) (*see also* Stenosis, aortic) 424.1
    - rheumatic (*see also* Stenosis, aortic, rheumatic) 395.0
  - aortoiliac 444.0
  - aqueduct of Sylvius 331.4
    - congenital 742.3
      - with spina bifida (*see also* Spina bifida) 741.0❺
  - Arnold-Chiari (*see also* Spina bifida) 741.0❺
  - artery (*see also* Embolism, artery) 444.9
    - basilar (complete) (partial) (*see also* Occlusion, artery, basilar) 433.0❺
    - carotid (complete) (partial) (*see also* Occlusion, artery, carotid) 433.1❺
    - precerebral – *see* Occlusion, artery, precerebral NEC
    - retinal (central) (*see also* Occlusion, retina) 362.30
    - vertebral (complete) (partial) (*see also* Occlusion, artery, vertebral) 433.2❺
  - asthma (chronic) (with obstructive pulmonary disease) 493.2❺
  - band (intestinal) 560.81
  - bile duct or passage (*see also* Obstruction, biliary) 576.2
    - congenital 751.61
      - jaundice from 751.61 *[774.5]*
  - biliary (duct) (tract) 576.2
    - with calculus 574.51
      - with cholecystitis (chronic) 574.41
        - acute 574.31
    - congenital 751.61
      - jaundice from 751.61 *[774.5]*
    - gallbladder 575.2
      - with calculus 574.21
        - with cholecystitis (chronic) 574.11
          - acute 574.01
  - bladder neck (acquired) 596.0
    - congenital 753.6
  - bowel (*see also* Obstruction, intestine) 560.9
  - bronchus 519.19
  - canal, ear (*see also* Stricture, ear canal, acquired) 380.50
  - cardia 537.89
  - caval veins (inferior) (superior) 459.2
  - cecum (*see also* Obstruction, intestine) 560.9
  - circulatory 459.9
  - colon (*see also* Obstruction, intestine) 560.9
    - sympathicotonic 560.89
  - common duct (*see also* Obstruction, biliary) 576.2
    - congenital 751.61
  - coronary (artery) (heart) - (*see* also Arteriosclerosis, coronary)
    - acute (*see also* Infarct, myocardium) 410.9❺
      - without myocardial infarction 411.81
  - cystic duct (*see also* Obstruction, gallbladder) 575.2
    - congenital 751.61

Nursemaid's – Obstruction, obstructed, obstructive

Obstruction, obstructed, obstructive – *continued*
- device, implant, or graft – *see* Complications, due to (presence of) any device, implant, or graft classified to 996.0-996.5 NEC
- due to foreign body accidentally left in operation wound 998.4
- duodenum 537.3
  - congenital 751.1
  - due to
    - compression NEC 537.3
    - cyst 537.3
    - intrinsic lesion or disease NEC 537.3
    - scarring 537.3
    - torsion 537.3
    - ulcer 532.91
    - volvulus 537.3
- ejaculatory duct 608.89
- endocardium 424.90
  - arteriosclerotic 424.99
  - specified cause, except rheumatic 424.99
- esophagus 530.3
- eustachian tube (complete) (partial) 381.60
  - cartilaginous
    - extrinsic 381.63
    - intrinsic 381.62
  - due to
    - cholesteatoma 381.61
    - osseous lesion NEC 381.61
    - polyp 381.61
  - osseous 381.61
- fallopian tube (bilateral) 628.2
- fecal 560.39
  - with hernia – *see also* Hernia, by site, with obstruction
    - gangrenous – *see* Hernia, by site, with gangrene
- foramen of Monro (congenital) 742.3
  - with spina bifida (*see also* Spina bifida) 741.0❺
- foreign body – *see* Foreign body
- gallbladder 575.2
  - with calculus, cholelithiasis, or stones 574.21
    - with cholecystitis (chronic) 574.11
      - acute 574.01
  - congenital 751.69
    - jaundice from 751.69 *[774.5]*
- gastric outlet 537.0
- gastrointestinal (*see also* Obstruction, intestine) 560.9
- glottis 478.79
- hepatic 573.8
  - duct (*see also* Obstruction, biliary) 576.2
    - congenital 751.61
- icterus (*see also* Obstruction, biliary) 576.8
  - congenital 751.61
- ileocecal coil (*see also* Obstruction, intestine) 560.9
- ileum (*see also* Obstruction, intestine) 560.9
- iliofemoral (artery) 444.81
- internal anastomosis – *see* Complications, mechanical, graft
- intestine (mechanical) (neurogenic) (paroxysmal) (postinfectional) (reflex) 560.9
  - with
    - adhesions (intestinal) (peritoneal) 560.81
    - hernia – *see also* Hernia, by site, with obstruction
      - gangrenous – *see* Hernia, by site, with gangrene
  - adynamic (*see also* Ileus) 560.1
  - by gallstone 560.31
  - congenital or infantile (small) 751.1
    - large 751.2
  - due to
    - Ascaris lumbricoides 127.0
    - mural thickening 560.89
    - procedure 997.4
      - involving urinary tract 997.5
  - impaction 560.39
  - infantile – *see* Obstruction, intestine, congenital
  - newborn
    - due to
      - fecaliths 777.1
      - inspissated milk 777.2
      - meconium (plug) 777.1
        - in mucoviscidosis 277.01
    - transitory 777.4
  - specified cause NEC 560.89
  - transitory, newborn 777.4
  - volvulus 560.2
- intracardiac ball valve prosthesis 996.02

Obstruction, obstructed, obstructive – *continued*
- jaundice (*see also* Obstruction, biliary) 576.8
  - congenital 751.61
- jejunum (*see also* Obstruction, intestine) 560.9
- kidney 593.89
- labor 660.9❺
  - affecting fetus or newborn 763.1
  - by
    - bony pelvis (conditions classifiable to 653.0-653.9) 660.1❺
    - deep transverse arrest 660.3❺
    - impacted shoulder 660.4❺
    - locked twins 660.5❺
    - malposition (fetus) (conditions classifiable to 652.0-652.9) 660.0❺
      - head during labor 660.3❺
    - persistent occipitoposterior position 660.3❺
    - soft tissue, pelvic (conditions classifiable to 654.0-654.9) 660.2❺
- lacrimal
  - canaliculi 375.53
  - congenital 743.65
  - punctum 375.52
  - sac 375.54
- lacrimonasal duct 375.56
  - congenital 743.65
  - neonatal 375.55
- lacteal, with steatorrhea 579.2
- laryngitis (*see also* Laryngitis) 464.01
- larynx 478.79
  - congenital 748.3
- liver 573.8
  - cirrhotic (*see also* Cirrhosis, liver) 571.5
- lung 518.89
  - with
    - asthma – *see* Asthma
    - bronchitis (chronic) 491.20❺
    - emphysema NEC 492.8
  - airway, chronic 496
  - chronic NEC 496
    - with
      - asthma (chronic) (obstructive) 493.2❺
  - disease, chronic 496
    - with
      - asthma (chronic) (obstructive) 493.2❺
  - emphysematous 492.8
- lymphatic 457.1
- meconium
  - fetus or newborn 777.1
    - in mucoviscidosis 277.01
  - newborn due to fecaliths 777.1
- mediastinum 519.3
- mitral (rheumatic) – *see* Stenosis, mitral
- nasal 478.19
  - duct 375.56
    - neonatal 375.55
  - sinus – *see* Sinusitis
- nasolacrimal duct 375.56
  - congenital 743.65
  - neonatal 375.55
- nasopharynx 478.29
- nose 478.19
- organ or site, congenital NEC – *see* Atresia
- pancreatic duct 577.8
- parotid gland 527.8
- pelviureteral junction (*see also* Obstruction, ureter) 593.4
- pharynx 478.29
- portal (circulation) (vein) 452
- prostate 600.90
  - with
    - other lower urinary tract symptoms (LUTS) 600.91
    - urinary
      - obstruction 600.91
      - retention 600.91
  - valve (urinary) 596.0
- pulmonary
  - valve (heart) (*see also* Endocarditis, pulmonary) 424.3
  - vein, isolated 747.49
- pyemic – *see* Septicemia
- pylorus (acquired) 537.0
  - congenital 750.5
  - infantile 750.5
- rectosigmoid (*see also* Obstruction, intestine) 560.9
- rectum 569.49
- renal 593.89
- respiratory 519.8
  - chronic 496

Obstruction, obstructed, obstructive – *continued*
- retinal (artery) (vein) (central) (*see also* Occlusion, retina) 362.30
- salivary duct (any) 527.8
  - with calculus 527.5
- sigmoid (*see also* Obstruction, intestine) 560.9
- sinus (accessory) (nasal) (*see also* Sinusitis) 473.9
- Stensen's duct 527.8
- stomach 537.89
  - acute 536.1
  - congenital 750.7
- submaxillary gland 527.8
  - with calculus 527.5
- thoracic duct 457.1
- thrombotic – *see* Thrombosis
- tooth eruption 520.6
- trachea 519.19
- tracheostomy airway 519.09
- tricuspid – *see* Endocarditis, tricuspid
- upper respiratory, congenital 748.8
- ureter (functional) 593.4
  - congenital 753.20
  - due to calculus 592.1
- ureteropelvic junction, congenital 753.21
- ureterovesical junction, congenital 753.22
- urethra 599.60
  - congenital 753.6
- urinary (moderate) 599.60
  - organ or tract (lower) 599.60
    - due to
      - benign prostatic hypertrophy (BPH) – *see* category 600
    - specified NEC 599.69
      - due to
        - benign prostatic hypertrophy (BPH) – *see* category 600
  - prostatic valve 596.0
  - specified NEC 599.69
    - due to
      - benign prostatic hypertrophy (BPH) – *see* category 600
- uropathy 599.60
- uterus 621.8
- vagina 623.2
- valvular – *see* Endocarditis
- vascular graft or shunt 996.1
  - atherosclerosis – *see* Arteriosclerosis, coronary
  - embolism 996.74
  - occlusion NEC 996.74
  - thrombus 996.74
- vein, venous 459.2
  - caval (inferior) (superior) 459.2
  - thrombotic – *see* Thrombosis
- vena cava (inferior) (superior) 459.2
- ventricular shunt 996.2
- vesical 596.0
- vesicourethral orifice 596.0
- vessel NEC 459.9

Obturator – *see* condition

Occlusal
- plane deviation 524.76
- wear, teeth 521.10

Occlusion
- anus 569.49
  - congenital 751.2
  - infantile 751.2
- aortoiliac (chronic) 444.0
- aqueduct of Sylvius 331.4
  - congenital 742.3
    - with spina bifida (*see also* Spina bifida) 741.0❺
- arteries of extremities, lower 444.22
  - without thrombus or embolus (*see also* Arteriosclerosis, extremities) 440.20
  - due to stricture or stenosis 447.1
  - upper 444.21
    - without thrombus or embolus (*see also* Arteriosclerosis, extremities) 440.20
    - due to stricture or stenosis 447.1
- artery NEC (*see also* Embolism, artery) 444.9
  - auditory, internal 433.8❺
  - basilar 433.0❺
    - with other precerebral artery 433.3❺
    - bilateral 433.3❺
  - brain or cerebral (*see also* Infarct, brain) 434.9❺
  - carotid 433.1❺
    - with other precerebral artery 433.3❺
    - bilateral 433.3❺

Obstruction, obstructed, obstructive – Occlusion

Occlusion – *continued*
  artery – *continued*
    cerebellar (anterior inferior) (posterior inferior) (superior) 433.8❺
    cerebral (*see also* Infarct, brain) 434.9❺
    choroidal (anterior) 433.8❺
    chronic total ●
      coronary 414.2 ●
      extremity(ies) 440.4 ●
    communicating posterior 433.8❺
    complete ●
      coronary 414.2 ●
      extremity(ies) 440.4 ●
    coronary (thrombotic) (*see also* Infarct, myocardium) 410.9❺
      acute 410.9❺
        without myocardial infarction 411.81
      chronic total 414.2 ●
      complete 414.2 ●
      healed or old 412
      total 414.2 ●
    extremity(ies) ●
      chronic total 440.4 ●
      complete 440.4 ●
      total 440.4 ●
    hypophyseal 433.8❺
    iliac 444.81
    mesenteric (embolic) (thrombotic) (with gangrene) 557.0
    pontine 433.8❺
    precerebral NEC 433.9❺
      late effect – *see* Late effect(s) (of) cerebrovascular disease
      multiple or bilateral 433.3❺
      puerperal, postpartum, childbirth 674.0❺
      specified NEC 433.8❺
    renal 593.81
    retinal – *see* Occlusion, retina, artery
    spinal 433.8❺
    vertebral 433.2❺
      with other precerebral artery 433.3❺
      bilateral 433.3❺
  basilar (artery) – *see* Occlusion, artery, basilar
  bile duct (any) (*see also* Obstruction, biliary) 576.2
  bowel (*see also* Obstruction, intestine) 560.9
  brain (artery) (vascular) (*see also* Infarct, brain) 434.9❺
  breast (duct) 611.8
  carotid (artery) (common) (internal) – *see* Occlusion, artery, carotid
  cerebellar (anterior inferior) (artery) (posterior inferior) (superior) 433.8❺
  cerebral (artery) (*see also* Infarct, brain) 434.9❺
  cerebrovascular (*see also* Infarct, brain) 434.9❺
    diffuse 437.0
  cervical canal (*see also* Stricture, cervix) 622.4
    by falciparum malaria 084.0
  cervix (uteri) (*see also* Stricture, cervix) 622.4
  choanal 748.0
  choroidal (artery) 433.8❺
  colon (*see also* Obstruction, intestine) 560.9
  communicating posterior artery 433.8❺
  coronary (artery) (thrombotic) (*see also* Infarct, myocardium) 410.9❺
    acute 410.9❺
      without myocardial infarction 411.81
    healed or old 412
  cystic duct (*see also* Obstruction, gallbladder) 575.2
    congenital 751.69
  disto
    division I 524.22
    division II 524.22
  embolic – *see* Embolism
  fallopian tube 628.2
    congenital 752.19
  gallbladder (*see also* Obstruction, gallbladder) 575.2
    congenital 751.69
      jaundice from 751.69 *[744.5]*
  gingiva, traumatic 523.8
  hymen 623.3
    congenital 752.42
  hypophyseal (artery) 433.8❺
  iliac (artery) 444.81
  intestine (*see also* Obstruction, intestine) 560.9
  kidney 593.89
  lacrimal apparatus – *see* Stenosis, lacrimal
  lung 518.89
  lymph or lymphatic channel 457.1
  mammary duct 611.8

Occlusion – *continued*
  mesenteric artery (embolic) (thrombotic) (with gangrene) 557.0
  nose 478.1
    congenital 748.0
  organ or site, congenital NEC – *see* Atresia
  oviduct 628.2
    congenital 752.19
  periodontal, traumatic 523.8
  peripheral arteries (lower extremity) 444.22
    without thrombus or embolus (*see also* Arteriosclerosis, extremities) 440.20
    due to stricture or stenosis 447.1
    upper extremity 444.21
      without thrombus or embolus (*see also* Arteriosclerosis, extremities) 440.20
      due to stricture or stenosis 447.1
  pontine (artery) 433.8❺
  posterior lingual, of mandibular teeth 524.29
  precerebral artery – *see* Occlusion, artery, precerebral NEC
  puncta lacrimalia 375.52
  pupil 364.74
  pylorus (*see also* Stricture, pylorus) 537.0
  renal artery 593.81
  retina, retinal (vascular) 362.30
    artery, arterial 362.30
      branch 362.32
      central (total) 362.31
      partial 362.33
      transient 362.34
      tributary 362.32
    vein 362.30
      branch 362.36
      central (total) 362.35
      incipient 362.37
      partial 362.37
      tributary 362.36
  spinal artery 433.8❺
  stent
    coronary 996.72
  teeth (mandibular) (posterior lingual) 524.29
  thoracic duct 457.1
  tubal 628.2
  ureter (complete) (partial) 593.4
    congenital 753.29
  urethra (*see also* Stricture, urethra) 598.9
    congenital 753.6
  uterus 621.8
  vagina 623.2
  vascular NEC 459.9
  vein – *see* Thrombosis
  vena cava (inferior) (superior) 453.2
  ventricle (brain) NEC 331.4
  vertebral (artery) – *see* Occlusion, artery, vertebral
  vessel (blood) NEC 459.9
  vulva 624.8
Occlusio pupillae 364.74
Occupational
  problems NEC V62.2
  therapy V57.21
Ochlophobia 300.29
Ochronosis (alkaptonuric) (congenital) (endogenous) 270.2
  with chloasma of eyelid 270.2
Ocular muscle – *see also* condition
  myopathy 359.1
  torticollis 781.93
Oculoauriculovertebral dysplasia 756.0
Oculogyric
  crisis or disturbance 378.87
    psychogenic 306.7
Oculomotor syndrome 378.81
Oddi's sphincter spasm 576.5
Odelberg's disease (juvenile osteochondrosis) 732.1
Odontalgia 525.9
Odontoameloblastoma (M9311/0) 213.1
  upper jaw (bone) 213.0
Odontoclasia 521.05
Odontoclasis 873.63
  complicated 873.73
Odontodysplasia, regional 520.4
Odontogenesis imperfecta 520.5
Odontoma (M9280/0) 213.1
  ameloblastic (M9311/0) 213.1
    upper jaw (bone) 213.0
  calcified (M9280/0) 213.1
    upper jaw (bone) 213.0

Odontoma – *continued*
  complex (M9282/0) 213.1
    upper jaw (bone) 213.0
  compound (M9281/0) 213.1
    upper jaw (bone) 213.0
  fibroameloblastic (M9290/0) 213.1
    upper jaw (bone) 213.0
  follicular 526.0
    upper jaw (bone) 213.0
Odontomyelitis (closed) (open) 522.0
Odontonecrosis 521.09
Odontorrhagia 525.8
Odontosarcoma, ameloblastic (M9290/3) 170.1
  upper jaw (bone) 170.0
Odynophagia 787.20 ▲
Oesophagostomiasis 127.7
Oesophagostomum infestation 127.7
Oestriasis 134.0
Ogilvie's syndrome (sympathicotonic colon obstruction) 560.89
Oguchi's disease (retina) 368.61
Ohara's disease (*see also* Tularemia) 021.9
Oidiomycosis (*see also* Candidiasis) 112.9
Oidiomycotic meningitis 112.83
Oidium albicans infection (*see also* Candidiasis) 112.9
Old age 797
  dementia (of) 290.0
Olfactory – *see* condition
Oligemia 285.9
Oligergasia (*see also* Retardation, mental) 319
Oligoamnios 658.0❺
  affecting fetus or newborn 761.2
Oligoastrocytoma, mixed (M9382/3)
  specified site – *see* Neoplasm, by site, malignant
  unspecified site 191.9
Oligocythemia 285.9
Oligodendroblastoma (M9460/3)
  specified site – *see* Neoplasm, by site, malignant
  unspecified site 191.9
Oligodendroglioma (M9450/3)
  anaplastic type (M9451/3)
    specified site – *see* Neoplasm, by site, malignant
    unspecified site 191.9
  specified site – *see* Neoplasm, by site, malignant
  unspecified site 191.9
Oligodendroma – *see* Oligodendroglioma
Oligodontia (*see also* Anodontia) 520.0
Oligoencephalon 742.1
Oligohydramnios 658.0❺
  affecting fetus or newborn 761.2
  due to premature rupture of membranes 658.1❺
    affecting fetus or newborn 761.2
Oligohydrosis 705.0
Oligomenorrhea 626.1
Oligophrenia (*see also* Retardation, mental) 319
  phenylpyruvic 270.1
Oligospermia 606.1
Oligotrichia 704.09
  congenita 757.4
Oliguria 788.5
  with
    abortion – *see* Abortion, by type, with renal failure
    ectopic pregnancy (*see also* categories 633.0-633.9) 639.3
    molar pregnancy (*see also* categories 630-632) 639.3
  complicating
    abortion 639.3
    ectopic or molar pregnancy 639.3
    pregnancy 646.2❺
      with hypertension – *see* Toxemia, of pregnancy
  due to a procedure 997.5
  following labor and delivery 669.3❺
  heart or cardiac – *see* Failure, heart
  puerperal, postpartum 669.3❺
  specified due to a procedure 997.5
Ollier's disease (chondrodysplasia) 756.4
Omentitis (*see also* Peritonitis) 567.9
Omentocele (*see also* Hernia, omental) 553.8
Omentum, omental – *see* condition
Omphalitis (congenital) (newborn) 771.4
  not of newborn 686.9

Occlusion – Omphalitis

Omphalitis – *continued*
  tetanus 771.3
Omphalocele 756.79
Omphalomesenteric duct, persistent 751.0
Omphalorrhagia, newborn 772.3
Omsk hemorrhagic fever 065.1
Onanism 307.9
Onchocerciasis 125.3
  eye 125.3 *[360.13]*
Onchocercosis 125.3
Oncocytoma (M8290/0) – *see* Neoplasm, by site, benign
Ondine's curse 348.8
Oneirophrenia (*see also* Schizophrenia) 295.4❺
Onychauxis 703.8
  congenital 757.5
Onychia (with lymphangitis) 681.9
  dermatophytic 110.1
  finger 681.02
  toe 681.11
Onychitis (with lymphangitis) 681.9
  finger 681.02
  toe 681.11
Onychocryptosis 703.0
Onychodystrophy 703.8
  congenital 757.5
Onychogryphosis 703.8
Onychogryposis 703.8
Onycholysis 703.8
Onychomadesis 703.8
Onychomalacia 703.8
Onychomycosis 110.1
  finger 110.1
  toe 110.1
Onycho-osteodysplasia 756.89
Onychophagy 307.9
Onychoptosis 703.8
Onychorrhexis 703.8
  congenital 757.5
Onychoschizia 703.8
Onychotrophia (*see also* Atrophy, nail) 703.8
O'Nyong Nyong fever 066.3
Onyxis (finger) (toe) 703.0
Onyxitis (with lymphangitis) 681.9
  finger 681.02
  toe 681.11
Oocyte (egg) (ovum)
  donor V59.70
    over age 35 V59.73
      anonymous recipient V59.73
      designated recipient V59.74
    under age 35 V59.71
      anonymous recipient V59.71
      designated recipient V59.72
Oophoritis (cystic) (infectional) (interstitial) (*see also* Salpingo-oophoritis) 614.2
  complicating pregnancy 646.6❺
  fetal (acute) 752.0
  gonococcal (acute) 098.19
    chronic or duration of 2 months or over 098.39
  tuberculous (*see also* Tuberculosis) 016.6❺
Opacity, opacities
  cornea 371.00
    central 371.03
    congenital 743.43
      interfering with vision 743.42
    degenerative (*see also* Degeneration, cornea) 371.40
    hereditary (*see also* Dystrophy, cornea) 371.50
    inflammatory (*see also* Keratitis) 370.9
    late effect of trachoma (healed) 139.1
    minor 371.01
    peripheral 371.02
  enamel (fluoride) (nonfluoride) (teeth) 520.3
  lens (*see also* Cataract) 366.9
  snowball 379.22
  vitreous (humor) 379.24
    congenital 743.51
Opalescent dentin (hereditary) 520.5
Open, opening
  abnormal, organ or site, congenital – *see* Imperfect, closure
  angle with
    borderline intraocular pressure 365.01
    cupping of discs 365.01
Open, opening – *continued*
  bite
    anterior 524.24 ●
    posterior 524.25 ●
  false – *see* Imperfect, closure
  margin on tooth restoration 525.61
  restoration margins 525.61
  wound – *see* Wound, open, by site
Operation
  causing mutilation of fetus 763.89
  destructive, on live fetus, to facilitate birth 763.89
  for delivery, fetus or newborn 763.89
  maternal, unrelated to current delivery, affecting fetus or newborn 760.6
Operational fatigue 300.89
Operative – *see* condition
Operculitis (chronic) 523.40
  acute 523.30
Operculum, retina 361.32
  with detachment 361.01
Ophiasis 704.01
Ophthalmia (*see also* Conjunctivitis) 372.30
  actinic rays 370.24
  allergic (acute) 372.05
    chronic 372.14
  blennorrhagic (neonatorum) 098.40
  catarrhal 372.03
  diphtheritic 032.81
  Egyptian 076.1
  electric, electrica 370.24
  gonococcal (neonatorum) 098.40
  metastatic 360.11
  migraine 346.8❺
  neonatorum, newborn 771.6
    gonococcal 098.40
  nodosa 360.14
  phlyctenular 370.31
    with ulcer (*see also* Ulcer, cornea) 370.00
  sympathetic 360.11
Ophthalmitis – *see* Ophthalmia
Ophthalmocele (congenital) 743.66
Ophthalmoneuromyelitis 341.0
Ophthalmopathy, infiltrative with thyrotoxicosis 242.0❺
Ophthalmoplegia (*see also* Strabismus) 378.9
  anterior internuclear 378.86
  ataxia-areflexia syndrome 357.0
  bilateral 378.9
  diabetic 250.5❺ *[378.86]*
  exophthalmic 242.0❺ *[376.22]*
  external 378.55
    progressive 378.72
    total 378.56
  internal (complete) (total) 367.52
  internuclear 378.86
  migraine 346.8❺
  painful 378.55
  Parinaud's 378.81
  progressive external 378.72
  supranuclear, progressive 333.0
  total (external) 378.56
    internal 367.52
  unilateral 378.9
Opisthognathism 524.00
Opisthorchiasis (felineus) (tenuicollis) (viverrini) 121.0
Opisthotonos, opisthotonus 781.0
Opitz's disease (congestive splenomegaly) 289.51
Opiumism (*see also* Dependence) 304.0❺
Oppenheim's disease 358.8
Oppenheim-Urbach disease or syndrome (necrobiosis lipoidica diabeticorum) 250.8❺ *[709.3]*
Opsoclonia 379.59
Optic nerve – *see* condition
Orbit – *see* condition
Orchioblastoma (M9071/3) 186.9
Orchitis (nonspecific) (septic) 604.90
  with abscess 604.0
  blennorrhagic (acute) 098.13
    chronic or duration of 2 months or over 098.33
  diphtheritic 032.89 *[604.91]*
  filarial 125.9 *[604.91]*
  gangrenous 604.99
  gonococcal (acute) 098.13
    chronic or duration of 2 months or over 098.33
  mumps 072.0
  parotidea 072.0
Orchitis – *continued*
  suppurative 604.99
  syphilitic 095.8 *[604.91]*
  tuberculous (*see also* Tuberculosis) 016.5❺ *[608.81]*
Orf 051.2
Organic – *see also* condition
  heart – *see* Disease, heart
  insufficiency 799.89
Oriental
  bilharziasis 120.2
  schistosomiasis 120.2
  sore 085.1
Orientation
  ego-dystonic sexual 302.0
Orifice – *see* condition
Origin, both great vessels from right ventricle 745.11
Ormond's disease or syndrome 593.4
Ornithosis 073.9
  with
    complication 073.8
      specified NEC 073.7
    pneumonia 073.0
    pneumonitis (lobular) 073.0
Orodigitofacial dysostosis 759.89
Oropouche fever 066.3
Orotaciduria, oroticaciduria (congenital) (hereditary) (pyrimidine deficiency) 281.4
Oroya fever 088.0
Orthodontics V58.5
  adjustment V53.4
  aftercare V58.5
  fitting V53.4
Orthopnea 786.02
Os, uterus – *see* condition
Osgood-Schlatter
  disease 732.4
  osteochondrosis 732.4
Osler's
  disease (M9950/1) (polycythemia vera) 238.4
  nodes 421.0
Osler-Rendu disease (familial hemorrhagic telangiectasia) 448.0
Osler-Vaquez disease (M9950/1) (polycythemia vera) 238.4
Osler-Weber-Rendu syndrome (familial hemorrhagic telangiectasia) 448.0
Osmidrosis 705.89
Osseous – *see* condition
Ossification
  artery – *see* Arteriosclerosis
  auricle (ear) 380.39
  bronchus 519.19
  cardiac (*see also* Degeneration, myocardial) 429.1
  cartilage (senile) 733.99
  coronary – *see* Arteriosclerosis, coronary
  diaphragm 728.10
  ear 380.39
    middle (*see also* Otosclerosis) 387.9
  falx cerebri 349.2
  fascia 728.10
  fontanel
    defective or delayed 756.0
    premature 756.0
  heart (*see also* Degeneration, myocardial) 429.1
    valve – *see* Endocarditis
  larynx 478.79
  ligament
    posterior longitudinal 724.8
      cervical 723.7
  meninges (cerebral) 349.2
    spinal 336.8
  multiple, eccentric centers 733.99
  muscle 728.10
    heterotopic, postoperative 728.13
  myocardium, myocardial (*see also* Degeneration, myocardial) 429.1
  penis 607.81
  periarticular 728.89
  sclera 379.16
  tendon 727.82
  trachea 519.19
  tympanic membrane (*see also* Tympanosclerosis) 385.00
  vitreous (humor) 360.44

- **Osteitis** (*see also* Osteomyelitis) 730.2❺
  - acute 730.0❺
  - alveolar 526.5
  - chronic 730.1❺
  - condensans (ilii) 733.5
  - deformans (Paget's) 731.0
    - due to or associated with malignant neoplasm (*see also* Neoplasm, bone, malignant) 170.9 *[731.1]*
  - due to yaws 102.6
  - fibrosa NEC 733.29
    - cystica (generalisata) 252.01
    - disseminata 756.59
    - osteoplastica 252.01
  - fragilitans 756.51
  - Garré's (sclerosing) 730.1❺
  - infectious (acute) (subacute) 730.0❺
    - chronic or old 730.1❺
  - jaw (acute) (chronic) (lower) (neonatal) (suppurative) (upper) 526.4
  - parathyroid 252.01
  - petrous bone (*see also* Petrositis) 383.20
  - pubis 733.5
  - sclerotic, nonsuppurative 730.1❺
  - syphilitic 095.5
  - tuberculosa
    - cystica (of Jüngling) 135
    - multiplex cystoides 135
- **Osteoarthritica spondylitis** (spine) (*see also* Spondylosis) 721.90
- **Osteoarthritis** (*see also* Osteoarthrosis) 715.9❺
  - distal interphalangeal 715.9❺
  - hyperplastic 731.2
  - interspinalis (*see also* Spondylosis) 721.90
  - spine, spinal NEC (*see also* Spondylosis) 721.90
- **Osteoarthropathy** (*see also* Osteoarthrosis) 715.9❺
  - chronic idiopathic hypertrophic 757.39
  - familial idiopathic 757.39
  - hypertrophic pulmonary 731.2
    - secondary 731.2
  - idiopathic hypertrophic 757.39
  - primary hypertrophic 731.2
  - pulmonary hypertrophic 731.2
  - secondary hypertrophic 731.2
- **Osteoarthrosis** (degenerative) (hypertrophic) (rheumatoid) 715.9❺

Note – Use the following fifth-digit subclassification with category 715:

0	*site unspecified*
1	*shoulder region*
2	*upper arm*
3	*forearm*
4	*hand*
5	*pelvic region and thigh*
6	*lower leg*
7	*ankle and foot*
8	*other specified sites except spine*
9	*multiple sites*

  - Deformans alkaptonurica 270.2
  - generalized 715.09
  - juvenilis (Köhler's) 732.5
  - localized 715.3❺
    - idiopathic 715.1❺
    - primary 715.1❺
    - secondary 715.2❺
  - multiple sites, not specified as generalized 715.89
  - polyarticular 715.09
  - spine (*see also* Spondylosis) 721.90
  - temporomandibular joint 524.69
- **Osteoblastoma** (M9200/0) – *see* Neoplasm, bone, benign
- **Osteochondritis** (*see also* Osteochondrosis) 732.9
  - dissecans 732.7
    - hip 732.7
  - ischiopubica 732.1
  - multiple 756.59
  - syphilitic (congenital) 090.0
- **Osteochondrodermodysplasia** 756.59
- **Osteochondrodystrophy** 277.5
  - deformans 277.5
  - familial 277.5
  - fetalis 756.4
- **Osteochondrolysis** 732.7
- **Osteochondroma** (M9210/0) – *see also* Neoplasm, bone, benign
  - multiple, congenital 756.4
- **Osteochondromatosis** (M9210/1) 238.0
  - synovial 727.82
- **Osteochondromyxosarcoma** (M9180/3) – *see* Neoplasm, bone, malignant
- **Osteochondropathy** NEC 732.9
- **Osteochondrosarcoma** (M9180/3) – *see* Neoplasm, bone, malignant
- **Osteochondrosis** 732.9
  - acetabulum 732.1
  - adult spine 732.8
  - astragalus 732.5
  - Blount's 732.4
  - Buchanan's (juvenile osteochondrosis of iliac crest) 732.1
  - Buchman's (juvenile osteochondrosis) 732.1
  - Burns' 732.3
  - calcaneus 732.5
  - capitular epiphysis (femur) 732.1
  - carpal
    - lunate (wrist) 732.3
    - scaphoid 732.3
  - coxae juvenilis 732.1
  - deformans juvenilis (coxae) (hip) 732.1
    - Scheuermann's 732.0
    - spine 732.0
    - tibia 732.4
    - vertebra 732.0
  - Diaz's (astragalus) 732.5
  - dissecans (knee) (shoulder) 732.7
  - femoral capital epiphysis 732.1
  - femur (head) (juvenile) 732.1
  - foot (juvenile) 732.5
  - Freiberg's (disease) (second metatarsal) 732.5
  - Haas' 732.3
  - Haglund's (os tibiale externum) 732.5
  - hand (juvenile) 732.3
  - head of
    - femur 732.1
    - humerus (juvenile) 732.3
  - hip (juvenile) 732.1
  - humerus (juvenile) 732.3
  - iliac crest (juvenile) 732.1
  - ilium (juvenile) 732.1
  - ischiopubic synchondrosis 732.1
  - Iselin's (osteochondrosis fifth metatarsal) 732.5
  - juvenile, juvenilis 732.6
    - arm 732.3
    - capital femoral epiphysis 732.1
    - capitellum humeri 732.3
    - capitular epiphysis 732.1
    - carpal scaphoid 732.3
    - clavicle, sternal epiphysis 732.6
    - coxae 732.1
    - deformans 732.1
    - foot 732.5
    - hand 732.3
    - hip and pelvis 732.1
    - lower extremity, except foot 732.4
    - lunate, wrist 732.3
    - medial cuneiform bone 732.5
    - metatarsal (head) 732.5
    - metatarsophalangeal 732.5
    - navicular, ankle 732.5
    - patella 732.4
    - primary patellar center (of Köhler) 732.4
    - specified site NEC 732.6
    - spine 732.0
    - tarsal scaphoid 732.5
    - tibia (epiphysis) (tuberosity) 732.4
    - upper extremity 732.3
    - vertebra (body) (Calvé) 732.0
      - epiphyseal plates (of Scheuermann) 732.0
  - Kienböck's (disease) 732.3
  - Köhler's (disease) (navicular, ankle) 732.5
    - patellar 732.4
    - tarsal navicular 732.5
  - Legg-Calvé-Perthes (disease) 732.1
  - lower extremity (juvenile) 732.4
  - lunate bone 732.3
  - Mauclaire's 732.3
  - metacarpal heads (of Mauclaire) 732.3
  - metatarsal (fifth) (head) (second) 732.5
  - navicular, ankle 732.5
  - os calcis 732.5
  - Osgood-Schlatter 732.4
  - os tibiale externum 732.5
  - Panner's 732.3
  - patella (juvenile) 732.4
  - patellar center
    - primary (of Köhler) 732.4
    - secondary (of Sinding-Larsen) 732.4
  - pelvis (juvenile) 732.1
  - Pierson's 732.1
  - radial head (juvenile) 732.3
  - Scheuermann's 732.0
  - Sever's (calcaneum) 732.5
  - Sinding-Larsen (secondary patellar center) 732.4
  - spine (juvenile) 732.0
    - adult 732.8
  - symphysis pubis (of Pierson) (juvenile) 732.1
  - syphilitic (congenital) 090.0
  - tarsal (navicular) (scaphoid) 732.5
  - tibia (proximal) (tubercle) 732.4
  - tuberculous – *see* Tuberculosis, bone
  - ulna 732.3
  - upper extremity (juvenile) 732.3
  - van Neck's (juvenile osteochondrosis) 732.1
  - vertebral (juvenile) 732.0
    - adult 732.8
- **Osteoclastoma** (M9250/1) 238.0
  - malignant (M9250/3) – *see* Neoplasm, bone, malignant
- **Osteocopic pain** 733.90
- **Osteodynia** 733.90
- **Osteodystrophy**
  - azotemic 588.0
  - chronica deformans hypertrophica 731.0
  - congenital 756.50
    - specified type NEC 756.59
  - deformans 731.0
  - fibrosa localisata 731.0
  - parathyroid 252.01
  - renal 588.0
- **Osteofibroma** (M9262/0) – *see* Neoplasm, bone, benign
- **Osteofibrosarcoma** (M9182/3) – *see* Neoplasm, bone, malignant
- **Osteogenesis imperfecta** 756.51
- **Osteogenic** – *see* condition
- **Osteoma** (M9180/0) – *see also* Neoplasm, bone, benign
  - osteoid (M9191/0) – *see also* Neoplasm, bone, benign
    - giant (M9200/0) – *see* Neoplasm, bone, benign
- **Osteomalacia** 268.2
  - chronica deformans hypertrophica 731.0
  - due to vitamin D deficiency 268.2
  - infantile (*see also* Rickets) 268.0
  - juvenile (*see also* Rickets) 268.0
  - pelvis 268.2
  - vitamin D-resistant 275.3
- **Osteomalacic bone** 268.2
- **Osteomalacosis** 268.2
- **Osteomyelitis** (general) (infective) (localized) (neonatal) (purulent) (pyogenic) (septic) (staphylococcal) (streptococcal) (suppurative) (with periostitis) 730.2❺

Note – Use the following fifth-digit subclassification with category 730:

0	*site unspecified*
1	*shoulder region*
2	*upper arm*
3	*forearm*
4	*hand*
5	*pelvic region and thigh*
6	*lower leg*
7	*ankle and foot*
8	*other specified sites*
9	*multiple sites*

  - acute or subacute 730.0❺
  - chronic or old 730.1❺
  - due to or associated with
    - diabetes mellitus 250.8❺ *[731.8]*
    - tuberculosis (*see also* Tuberculosis, bone) 015.9❺ *[730.8]*❺
      - limb bones 015.5❺ *[730.8]*❺
      - specified bones NEC 015.7❺ *[730.8]*❺
      - spine 015.0❺ *[730.8]*❺
    - typhoid 002.0 *[730.8]*❺
  - Garré's 730.1❺
  - jaw (acute) (chronic) (lower) (neonatal) (suppurative) (upper) 526.4
  - nonsuppurating 730.1❺
  - orbital 376.03
  - petrous bone (*see also* Petrositis) 383.20
  - Salmonella 003.24
  - sclerosing, nonsuppurative 730.1❺
  - sicca 730.1❺

- **Osteomyelitis** – *continued*
  - syphilitic 095.5
    - congenital 090.0 *[730.8]*❺
  - tuberculous – *see* Tuberculosis, bone
  - typhoid 002.0 *[730.8]*❺
- **Osteomyelofibrosis** 289.89
- **Osteomyelosclerosis** 289.89
- **Osteonecrosis** 733.40
  - meaning osteomyelitis 730.1
- **Osteo-onycho-arthro dysplasia** 756.89
- **Osteo-onychodysplasia, hereditary** 756.89
- **Osteopathia**
  - condensans disseminata 756.53
  - hyperostotica multiplex infantilis 756.59
  - hypertrophica toxica 731.2
  - striata 756.4
- **Osteopathy resulting from poliomyelitis** (*see also* Poliomyelitis) 045.9❺ *[730.7]*
  - familial dysplastic 731.2
- **Osteopecilia** 756.53
- **Osteopenia** 733.90
- **Osteoperiostitis** (*see also* Osteomyelitis) 730.2❺
  - ossificans toxica 731.2
  - toxica ossificans 731.2
- **Osteopetrosis** (familial) 756.52
- **Osteophyte** – *see* Exostosis
- **Osteophytosis** – *see* Exostosis
- **Osteopoikilosis** 756.53
- **Osteoporosis** (generalized) 733.00
  - circumscripta 731.0
  - disuse 733.03
  - drug-induced 733.09
  - idiopathic 733.02
  - postmenopausal 733.01
  - posttraumatic 733.7
  - screening V82.81
  - senile 733.01
  - specified type NEC 733.09
- **Osteoporosis-osteomalacia syndrome** 268.2
- **Osteopsathyrosis** 756.51
- **Osteoradionecrosis, jaw** 526.89
- **Osteosarcoma** (M9180/3) – *see also* Neoplasm, bone, malignant
  - chondroblastic (M9181/3) – *see* Neoplasm, bone, malignant
  - fibroblastic (M9182/3) – *see* Neoplasm, bone, malignant
  - in Paget's disease of bone (M9184/3) – *see* Neoplasm, bone, malignant
  - juxtacortical (M9190/3) – *see* Neoplasm, bone malignant
  - parosteal (M9190/3) – *see* Neoplasm, bone, malignant
  - telangiectatic (M9183/3) – *see* Neoplasm, bone, malignant
- **Osteosclerosis** 756.52
  - fragilis (generalisata) 756.52
- **Osteosclerotic anemia** 289.89
- **Osteosis**
  - acromegaloid 757.39
  - cutis 709.3
  - parathyroid 252.01
  - renal fibrocystic 588.0
- **Österreicher-Turner syndrome** 756.89
- **Ostium**
  - atrioventriculare commune 745.69
  - primum (arteriosum) (defect) (persistent) 745.61
  - secundum (arteriosum) (defect) (patent) (persistent) 745.5
- **Ostrum-Furst syndrome** 756.59
- **Otalgia** 388.70
  - otogenic 388.71
  - referred 388.72
- **Othematoma** 380.31
- **Otitic hydrocephalus** 348.2
- **Otitis** 382.9
  - with effusion 381.4
    - purulent 382.4
    - secretory 381.4
    - serous 381.4
    - suppurative 382.4
  - acute 382.9
  - adhesive (*see also* Adhesions, middle ear) 385.10
  - chronic 382.9
    - with effusion 381.3
    - mucoid, mucous (simple) 381.20
- **Otitis** – *continued*
  - chronic – *continued*
    - purulent 382.3
    - secretory 381.3
    - serous 381.10
    - suppurative 382.3
  - diffuse parasitic 136.8
  - externa (acute) (diffuse) (hemorrhagica) 380.10
    - actinic 380.22
    - candidal 112.82
      - chemical 380.22
      - chronic 380.23
      - mycotic – *see* Otitis, externa, mycotic
      - specified type NEC 380.23
    - circumscribed 380.10
    - contact 380.22
    - due to
      - erysipelas 035 *[380.13]*
      - impetigo 684 *[380.13]*
      - seborrheic dermatitis 690.10 *[380.13]*
    - eczematoid 380.22
    - furuncular 680.0 *[380.13]*
    - infective 380.10
      - chronic 380.16
    - malignant 380.14
    - mycotic (chronic) 380.15
      - due to
        - aspergillosis 117.3 *[380.15]*
        - moniliasis 112.82
        - otomycosis 111.8 *[380.15]*
    - reactive 380.22
    - specified type NEC 380.22
    - tropical 111.8 *[380.15]*
  - insidiosa (*see also* Otosclerosis) 387.9
  - interna (*see also* Labyrinthitis) 386.30
  - media (hemorrhagic) (staphylococcal) (streptococcal) 382.9
    - acute 382.9
      - with effusion 381.00
      - allergic 381.04
        - mucoid 381.05
        - sanguineous 381.06
        - serous 381.04
      - catarrhal 381.00
      - exudative 381.00
      - mucoid 381.02
        - allergic 381.05
      - necrotizing 382.00
        - with spontaneous rupture of ear drum 382.01
        - in
          - influenza 487.8 *[382.02]*
          - measles 055.2
          - scarlet fever 034.1 *[382.02]*
      - nonsuppurative 381.00
      - purulent 382.00
        - with spontaneous rupture of ear drum 382.01
      - sanguineous 381.03
        - allergic 381.06
      - secretory 381.01
      - seromucinous 381.02
      - serous 381.01
        - allergic 381.04
      - suppurative 382.00
        - with spontaneous rupture of ear drum 382.01
        - due to
          - influenza 487.8 *[382.02]*
          - scarlet fever 034.1 *[382.02]*
      - transudative 381.00
    - adhesive (*see also* Adhesions, middle ear) 385.10
    - allergic 381.4
      - acute 381.04
        - mucoid 381.05
        - sanguineous 381.06
        - serous 381.04
      - chronic 381.3
    - catarrhal 381.4
      - acute 381.00
      - chronic (simple) 381.10
    - chronic 382.9
      - with effusion 381.3
      - adhesive (*see also* Adhesions, middle ear) 385.10
      - allergic 381.3
      - atticoantral, suppurative (with posterior or superior marginal perforation of ear drum) 382.2
      - benign suppurative (with anterior perforation of ear drum) 382.1
- **Otitis** – *continued*
  - media – *continued*
    - chronic – *continued*
      - catarrhal 381.10
      - exudative 381.3
      - mucinous 381.20
      - mucoid, mucous (simple) 381.20
      - mucosanguineous 381.29
      - nonsuppurative 381.3
      - purulent 382.3
      - secretory 381.3
      - seromucinous 381.3
      - serosanguineous 381.19
      - serous (simple) 381.10
      - suppurative 382.3
        - atticoantral (with posterior or superior marginal perforation of ear drum) 382.2
        - benign (with anterior perforation of ear drum) 382.1
        - tuberculous (*see also* Tuberculosis) 017.4❺
        - tubotympanic 382.1
      - transudative 381.3
    - exudative 381.4
      - acute 381.00
      - chronic 381.3
    - fibrotic (*see also* Adhesions, middle ear) 385.10
    - mucoid, mucous 381.4
      - acute 381.02
      - chronic (simple) 381.20
    - mucosanguineous, chronic 381.29
    - nonsuppurative 381.4
      - acute 381.00
      - chronic 381.3
    - postmeasles 055.2
    - purulent 382.4
      - acute 382.00
        - with spontaneous rupture of ear drum 382.01
      - chronic 382.3
    - sanguineous, acute 381.03
      - allergic 381.06
    - secretory 381.4
      - acute or subacute 381.01
      - chronic 381.3
    - seromucinous 381.4
      - acute or subacute 381.02
      - chronic 381.3
    - serosanguineous, chronic 381.19
    - serous 381.4
      - acute or subacute 381.01
      - chronic (simple) 381.10
    - subacute – *see* Otitis, media, acute
    - suppurative 382.4
      - acute 382.00
        - with spontaneous rupture of ear drum 382.01
      - chronic 382.3
        - atticoantral 382.2
        - benign 382.1
        - tuberculous (*see also* Tuberculosis) 017.4❺
        - tubotympanic 382.1
    - transudative 381.4
      - acute 381.00
      - chronic 381.3
    - tuberculous (*see also* Tuberculosis 017.4❺
  - postmeasles 055.2
- **Otoconia** 386.8
- **Otolith syndrome** 386.19
- **Otomycosis** 111.8 *[380.15]*
  - in
    - aspergillosis 117.3 *[380.15]*
    - moniliasis 112.82
- **Otopathy** 388.9
- **Otoporosis** (*see also* Otosclerosis) 387.9
- **Otorrhagia** 388.69
  - traumatic – *see* nature of injury
- **Otorrhea** 388.60
  - blood 388.69
  - cerebrospinal (fluid) 388.61
- **Otosclerosis** (general) 387.9
  - cochlear (endosteal) 387.2
  - involving
    - otic capsule 387.2
    - oval window
      - nonobliterative 387.0
      - obliterative 387.1

Otosclerosis – *continued*
    - round window 387.2
  - nonobliterative 387.0
  - obliterative 387.1
  - specified type NEC 387.8

Otospongiosis (*see also* Otosclerosis) 387.9
Otto's disease or pelvis 715.35
Outburst, aggressive (*see also* Disturbance, conduct) 312.0❺
  - in children or adolescents 313.9

Outcome of delivery
  - multiple birth NEC V27.9
    - all liveborn V27.5
    - all stillborn V27.7
    - some liveborn V27.6
    - unspecified V27.9
  - single V27.9
    - liveborn V27.0
    - stillborn V27.1
  - twins V27.9
    - both liveborn V27.2
    - both stillborn V27.4
    - one liveborn, one stillborn V27.3

Outlet – *see also* condition
  - syndrome (thoracic) 353.0

Outstanding ears (bilateral) 744.29
Ovalocytosis (congenital) (hereditary) (*see also* Elliptocytosis) 282.1
Ovarian – *see also* condition
  - pregnancy – *see* Pregnancy, ovarian
  - remnant syndrome 620.8
  - vein syndrome 593.4

Ovaritis (cystic) (*see also* Salpingo-oophoritis) 614.2
Ovary, ovarian – *see* condition
Overactive – *see also* Hyperfunction
  - bladder 596.51
  - eye muscle (*see also* Strabismus) 378.9
  - hypothalamus 253.8
  - thyroid (*see also* Thyrotoxicosis) 242.9❺

Overactivity, child 314.01
Overbite (deep) (excessive) (horizontal) (vertical) 524.29
Overbreathing (*see also* Hyperventilation) 786.01
Overconscientious personality 301.4
Overdevelopment – *see also* Hypertrophy
  - breast (female) (male) 611.1
  - nasal bones 738.0
  - prostate, congenital 752.89

Overdistention – *see* Distention
Overdose overdosage (drug) 977.9
  - specified drug or substance – *see* Table of Drugs and Chemicals

Overeating 783.6
  - with obesity 278.0❺
  - nonorganic origin 307.51

Overexertion (effects) (exhaustion) 994.5
Overexposure (effects) 994.9
  - exhaustion 994.4

Overfeeding (*see also* Overeating) 783.6
Overfill, endodontic 526.62
Overgrowth, bone NEC 733.99
Overhanging
  - tooth restoration 525.62
  - unrepairable, dental restorative materials 525.62

Overheated (effects) (places) – *see* Heat
Overinhibited child 313.0
Overjet 524.29
  - excessive horizontal 524.26

Overlaid, overlying (suffocation) 994.7
Overlap
  - excessive horizontal 524.26

Overlapping toe (acquired) 735.8
  - congenital (fifth toe) 755.66

Overload
  - fluid 276.6
  - potassium (K) 276.7
  - sodium (Na) 276.0

Overnutrition (*see also* Hyperalimentation) 783.6
Overproduction – *see also* Hypersecretion
  - ACTH 255.3
  - cortisol 255.0
  - growth hormone 253.0
  - thyroid-stimulating hormone (TSH) 242.8❺

Overriding
  - aorta 747.21

Overriding – *continued*
  - finger (acquired) 736.29
    - congenital 755.59
  - toe (acquired) 735.8
    - congenital 755.66

Oversize
  - fetus (weight of 4500 grams or more) 766.0
    - affecting management of pregnancy 656.6❺
    - causing disproportion 653.5❺
      - with obstructed labor 660.1❺
        - affecting fetus or newborn 763.1

Overstimulation, ovarian 256.1
Overstrained 780.79
  - heart – *see* Hypertrophy, cardiac

Overweight (*see also* Obesity) 278.02
Overwork 780.79
Oviduct – *see* condition
Ovotestis 752.7
Ovulation (cycle)
  - failure or lack of 628.0
  - pain 625.2

Ovum
  - blighted 631
  - donor V59.70
    - over age 35 V59.73
      - anonymous recipient V59.73
      - designated recipient V59.74
    - under age 35 V59.71
      - anonymous recipient V59.71
      - designated recipient V59.72
  - dropsical 631
  - pathologic 631

Owren's disease or syndrome (parahemophilia) (*see also* Defect, coagulation) 286.3
Oxalosis 271.8
Oxaluria 271.8
Ox heart – *see* Hypertrophy, cardiac
OX syndrome 758.6
Oxycephaly, oxycephalic 756.0
  - syphilitic, congenital 090.0

Oxyuriasis 127.4
Oxyuris vermicularis (infestation) 127.4
Ozena 472.0

P

Pacemaker syndrome 429.4
Pachyderma, pachydermia 701.8
  - laryngis 478.5
  - laryngitis 478.79
  - larynx (verrucosa) 478.79

Pachydermatitis 701.8
Pachydermatocele (congenital) 757.39
  - acquired 701.8

Pachydermatosis 701.8
Pachydermoperiostitis
  - secondary 731.2

Pachydermoperiostosis
  - primary idiopathic 757.39
  - secondary 731.2

Pachymeningitis (adhesive) (basal) (brain) (cerebral) (cervical) (chronic) (circumscribed) (external) (fibrous) (hemorrhagic) (hypertrophic) (internal) (purulent) (spinal) (suppurative) (*see also* Meningitis) 322.9
  - gonococcal 098.82

Pachyonychia (congenital) 757.5
  - acquired 703.8

Pachyperiosteodermia
  - primary or idiopathic 757.39
  - secondary 731.2

Pachyperiostosis
  - primary or idiopathic 757.39
  - secondary 731.2

Pacinian tumor (M9507/0) – *see* Neoplasm, skin, benign
Pads, knuckle or Garrod's 728.79
Paget's disease (osteitis deformans) 731.0
  - with infiltrating duct carcinoma of the breast (M8541/3) – *see* Neoplasm, breast, malignant

Paget's disease – *continued*
  - bone 731.0
    - osteosarcoma in (M9184/3) – *see* Neoplasm, bone, malignant
  - breast (M8540/3) 174.0
  - extramammary (M8542/3) – *see also* Neoplasm, skin, malignant
    - anus 154.3
      - skin 173.5
  - malignant (M8540/3)
    - breast 174.0
    - specified site NEC (M8542/3) – *see* Neoplasm, skin, malignant
    - unspecified site 174.0
  - mammary (M8540/3) 174.0
  - necrosis of bone 731.0
  - nipple (M8540/3) 174.0
  - osteitis deformans 731.0

Paget-Schroetter syndrome (intermittent venous claudication) 453.8
Pain(s) ▶(*see also* Painful)◀ 780.96
  - abdominal 789.0❺
  - acute 338.19
    - due to trauma 338.11
    - postoperative 338.18
      - post-thoracotomy 338.12
  - adnexa (uteri) 625.9
  - alimentary, due to vascular insufficiency 557.9
  - anginoid (*see also* Pain, precordial) 786.51
  - anus 569.42
  - arch 729.5
  - arm 729.5
  - axillary 729.5
  - back (postural) 724.5
    - low 724.2
    - psychogenic 307.89
  - bile duct 576.9
  - bladder 788.9
  - bone 733.90
  - breast 611.71
    - psychogenic 307.89
  - broad ligament 625.9
  - cancer associated 338.3
  - cartilage NEC 733.90
  - cecum 789.0❺
  - cervicobrachial 723.3
  - chest (central) 786.50
    - atypical 786.59
    - midsternal 786.51
    - musculoskeletal 786.59
    - noncardiac 786.59
    - substernal 786.51
    - wall (anterior) 786.52
  - chronic 338.29
    - associated with significant psychosocial dysfunction 338.4
    - due to trauma 338.21
    - postoperative 338.28
      - post-thoracotomy 338.22
    - syndrome 338.4
  - coccyx 724.79
  - colon 789.0❺
  - common duct 576.9
  - coronary – *see* Angina
  - costochondral 786.52
  - diaphragm 786.52
  - due to (presence of) any device, implant, or graft classifiable to 996.0-996.5 – *see* Complications, due to (presence of) any device, implant, or graft classified to 996.0-996.5 NEC
  - malignancy (primary) (secondary) 338.3
  - ear (*see also* Otalgia) 388.70
  - epigastric, epigastrium 789.0❺
  - extremity (lower) (upper) 729.5
  - eye 379.91
  - face, facial 784.0
    - atypical 350.2
    - nerve 351.8
  - false (labor) 644.1❺
  - female genital organ NEC 625.9
    - psychogenic 307.89
  - finger 729.5
  - flank 789.0❺
  - foot 729.5
  - gallbladder 575.9
  - gas (intestinal) 787.3
  - gastric 536.8
  - generalized 780.96
  - genital organ
    - female 625.9
    - male 608.9

Otosclerosis – Pain(s)

Pain(s) – *continued*
- genital organ – *continued*
  - psychogenic 307.89
- groin 789.0❺
- growing 781.99
- hand 729.5
- head (*see also* Headache) 784.0
- heart (*see also* Pain, precordial) 786.51
- infraorbital (*see also* Neuralgia, trigeminal) 350.1
- intermenstrual 625.2
- jaw 526.9
- joint 719.40
  - ankle 719.47
  - elbow 719.42
  - foot 719.47
  - hand 719.44
  - hip 719.45
  - knee 719.46
  - multiple sites 719.49
  - pelvic region 719.45
  - psychogenic 307.89
  - shoulder (region) 719.41
  - specified site NEC 719.48
  - wrist 719.43
- kidney 788.0
- labor, false or spurious 644.1❺
- laryngeal 784.1
- leg 729.5
- limb 729.5
- low back 724.2
- lumbar region 724.2
- mastoid (*see also* Otalgia) 388.70
- maxilla 526.9
- menstrual 625.3 ●
- metacarpophalangeal (joint) 719.44
- metatarsophalangeal (joint) 719.47
- mouth 528.9
- muscle 729.1
  - intercostal 786.59
- musculoskeletal (*see also* Pain, by site) 729.1
- nasal 478.19
- nasopharynx 478.29
- neck NEC 723.1
  - psychogenic 307.89
- neoplasm related (acute) (chronic) 338.3
- nerve NEC 729.2
- neuromuscular 729.1
- nose 478.19
- ocular 379.91
- ophthalmic 379.91
- orbital region 379.91
- osteocopic 733.90
- ovary 625.9
  - psychogenic 307.89
- over heart (*see also* Pain, precordial) 786.51
- ovulation 625.2
- pelvic (female) 625.9
  - male NEC 789.0❺
    - psychogenic 307.89
  - psychogenic 307.89
- penis 607.9
  - psychogenic 307.89
- pericardial (*see also* Pain, precordial) 786.51
- perineum
  - female 625.9
  - male 608.9
- pharynx 478.29
- pleura, pleural, pleuritic 786.52
- postoperative 338.18
  - acute 338.18
  - chronic 338.28
- post-thoracotomy 338.12
  - acute 338.12
  - chronic 338.22
- preauricular 388.70
- precordial (region) 786.51
  - psychogenic 307.89
- premenstrual 625.4 ●
- psychogenic 307.80
  - cardiovascular system 307.89
  - gastrointestinal system 307.89
  - genitourinary system 307.89
  - heart 307.89
  - musculoskeletal system 307.89
  - respiratory system 307.89
  - skin 306.3
- radicular (spinal) (*see also* Radiculitis) 729.2
- rectum 569.42
- respiration 786.52
- retrosternal 786.51
- rheumatic NEC 729.0
  - muscular 729.1

Pain(s) – *continued*
- rib 786.50
- root (spinal) (*see also* Radiculitis) 729.2
- round ligament (stretch) 625.9
- sacroiliac 724.6
- sciatic 724.3
- scrotum 608.9
  - psychogenic 307.89
- seminal vesicle 608.9
- sinus 478.19
- skin 782.0
- spermatic cord 608.9
- spinal root (*see also* Radiculitis) 729.2
- stomach 536.8
  - psychogenic 307.89
- substernal 786.51
- temporomandibular (joint) 524.62
- temporomaxillary joint 524.62
- testis 608.9
  - psychogenic 307.89
- thoracic spine 724.1
  - with radicular and visceral pain 724.4
- throat 784.1
- tibia 733.90
- toe 729.5
- tongue 529.6
- tooth 525.9
- total hip replacement 996.77 ●
- total knee replacement 996.77 ●
- trigeminal (*see also* Neuralgia, trigeminal) 350.1
- tumor associated 338.3
- umbilicus 789.0❺
- ureter 788.0
- urinary (organ) (system) 788.0
- uterus 625.9
  - psychogenic 307.89
- vagina 625.9
- vertebrogenic (syndrome) 724.5
- vesical 788.9
- vulva 625.9
- xiphoid 733.90

Painful – *see also* Pain
- arc syndrome 726.19
- coitus
  - female 625.0
  - male 608.89
  - psychogenic 302.76
- ejaculation (semen) 608.89
  - psychogenic 302.79
- erection 607.3
- feet syndrome 266.2
- menstruation 625.3
  - psychogenic 306.52
- micturition 788.1
- ophthalmoplegia 378.55
- respiration 786.52
- scar NEC 709.2
- urination 788.1
- wire sutures 998.89

Painters' colic 984.9
- specified type of lead – *see* Table of Drugs and Chemicals

Palate – *see* condition

Palatoplegia 528.9

Palatoschisis (*see also* Cleft, palate) 749.00

Palilalia 784.69

Palindromic arthritis (*see also* Rheumatism, palindromic) 719.3❺

Palliative care V66.7

Pallor 782.61
- temporal, optic disc 377.15

Palmar – *see also* condition
- fascia – *see* condition

Palpable
- cecum 569.89
- kidney 593.89
- liver 573.9
- lymph nodes 785.6
- ovary 620.8
- prostate 602.9
- spleen (*see also* Splenomegaly) 789.2
- uterus 625.8

Palpitation (heart) 785.1
- psychogenic 306.2

Palsy (*see also* Paralysis) 344.9
- atrophic diffuse 335.20
- Bell's 351.0
  - newborn 767.5
- birth 767.7

Palsy – *continued*
- brachial plexus 353.0
  - fetus or newborn 767.6
- brain – *see also* Palsy, cerebral
  - noncongenital or noninfantile 344.89
    - due to vascular lesion – *see* category 438❹
    - late effect – *see* Late effect(s) (of) cerebrovascular disease
  - syphilitic 094.89
    - congenital 090.49
- bulbar (chronic) (progressive) 335.22
  - pseudo NEC 335.23
  - supranuclear NEC 344.8❺
- cerebral (congenital) (infantile) (spastic) 343.9
  - athetoid 333.71
  - diplegic 343.0
    - due to previous vascular lesion – *see* category 438❹
    - late effect – *see* Late effect(s) (of) cerebrovascular disease
  - hemiplegic 343.1
  - monoplegic 343.3
  - noncongenital or noninfantile 437.8
    - due to previous vascular lesion – *see* category 438❹
    - late effect – *see* Late effect(s) (of) cerebrovascular disease
  - paraplegic 343.0
  - quadriplegic 343.2
  - spastic, not congenital or infantile 344.8❺
  - syphilitic 094.89
    - congenital 090.49
  - tetraplegic 343.2
- cranial nerve – *see also* Disorder, nerve, cranial
  - multiple 352.6
- creeping 335.21
- divers' 993.3
- Erb's (birth injury) 767.6
- facial 351.0
  - newborn 767.5
- glossopharyngeal 352.2
- Klumpke (-Déjérine) 767.6
- lead 984.9
  - specified type of lead – *see* Table of Drugs and Chemicals
- median nerve (tardy) 354.0
- peroneal nerve (acute) (tardy) 355.3
- progressive supranuclear 333.0
- pseudobulbar NEC 335.23
- radial nerve (acute) 354.3
- seventh nerve 351.0
  - newborn 767.5
- shaking (*see also* Parkinsonism) 332.0
- spastic (cerebral) (spinal) 343.9
  - hemiplegic 343.1
- specified nerve NEC – *see* Disorder, nerve
- supranuclear NEC 356.8
  - progressive 333.0
- ulnar nerve (tardy) 354.2
- wasting 335.21

Paltauf-Sternberg disease 201.9❺

Paludism – *see* Malaria

Panama fever 084.0

Panaris (with lymphangitis) 681.9
- finger 681.02
- toe 681.11

Panaritium (with lymphangitis) 681.9
- finger 681.02
- toe 681.11

Panarteritis (nodosa) 446.0
- brain or cerebral 437.4

Pancake heart 793.2
- with cor pulmonale (chronic) 416.9

Pancarditis (acute) (chronic) 429.89
- with
  - rheumatic
    - fever (active) (acute) (chronic) (subacute) 391.8
      - inactive or quiescent 398.99
- rheumatic, acute 391.8
  - chronic or inactive 398.99

Pancoast's syndrome or tumor (carcinoma, pulmonary apex) (M8010/3) 162.3

Pancoast-Tobias syndrome (M8010/3) (carcinoma, pulmonary apex) 162.3

Pancolitis 556.6

Pancreas, pancreatic – *see* condition

Pancreatitis 577.0
- acute (edematous) (hemorrhagic) (recurrent) 577.0

❹ Fourth-Digit Required ❺ Fifth-Digit Required *[code]* Manifestation Code ▶◀ Revised Text ● New Line ▲ Revised Code

Pancreatitis – *continued*
- annular 577.0
- apoplectic 577.0
- calcereous 577.0
- chronic (infectious) 577.1
  - recurrent 577.1
- cystic 577.2
- fibrous 577.8
- gangrenous 577.0
- hemorrhagic (acute) 577.0
- interstitial (chronic) 577.1
  - acute 577.0
- malignant 577.0
- mumps 072.3
- painless 577.1
- recurrent 577.1
- relapsing 577.1
- subacute 577.0
- suppurative 577.0
- syphilitic 095.8

Pancreatolithiasis 577.8

Pancytolysis 289.9

Pancytopenia (acquired) 284.1
- with malformations 284.09
- congenital 284.09

Panencephalitis – *see also* Encephalitis
- subacute, sclerosing 046.2

Panhematopenia 284.81 ▲
- congenital 284.09
- constitutional 284.09
- splenic, primary 289.4

Panhemocytopenia 284.81 ▲
- congenital 284.09
- constitutional 284.09

Panhypogonadism 257.2

Panhypopituitarism 253.2
- prepubertal 253.3

Panic (attack) (state) 300.01
- reaction to exceptional stress (transient) 308.0

Panmyelopathy, familial constitutional 284.09

Panmyelophthisis 284.2
- acquired (secondary) 284.81 ▲
- congenital 284.2
- idiopathic 284.9

Panmyelosis (acute) (M9951/1) 238.79

Panner's disease 732.3
- capitellum humeri 732.3
- head of humerus 732.3
- tarsal navicular (bone) (osteochondrosis) 732.5

Panneuritis endemica 265.0 *[357.4]*

Panniculitis 729.30
- back 724.8
- knee 729.31
- neck 723.6
- mesenteric 567.82
- nodular, nonsuppurative 729.30
- sacral 724.8
- specified site NEC 729.39

Panniculus adiposus (abdominal) 278.1

Pannus (corneal) 370.62
- abdominal (symptomatic) 278.1
- allergic eczematous 370.62
- degenerativus 370.62
- keratic 370.62
- rheumatoid – *see* Arthritis, rheumatoid
- trachomatosus, trachomatous (active) 076.1 *[370.62]*
  - late effect 139.1

Panophthalmitis 360.02

Panotitis – *see* Otitis media

Pansinusitis (chronic) (hyperplastic) (nonpurulent) (purulent) 473.8
- acute 461.8
- due to fungus NEC 117.9
- tuberculous (*see also* Tuberculosis) 012.8❺

Panuveitis 360.12
- sympathetic 360.11

Panvalvular disease – *see* Endocarditis, mitral

Papageienkrankheit 073.9

Papanicolaou smear
- cervix (screening test) V76.2
  - as part of gynecological examination V72.31
  - for suspected malignant neoplasm V76.2
    - no disease found V71.1
  - inadequate sample 795.08
  - nonspecific abnormal finding 795.00
    - with
      - atypical squamous cells - changes of undetermined significance
        - cannot exclude high grade squamous intraepithelial lesion (ASC-H) 795.02
        - of undetermined significance (ASC-US) 795.01
      - cytologic evidence of malignancy 795.06
      - high grade squamous intraepithelial lesion (HGSIL) 795.04
      - low grade squamous intraepithelial lesion (LGSIL) 795.03
    - nonspecific finding NEC 795.09
    - to confirm findings of recent normal smear following initial abnormal smear V72.32
  - unsatisfactory 795.08
- other specified site – *see also* Screening, malignant neoplasm
  - for suspected malignant neoplasm – *see also* Screening, malignant neoplasm
    - no disease found V71.1
  - nonspecific abnormal finding 795.1
- vagina V76.47
  - following hysterectomy for malignant condition V67.01

Papilledema 377.00
- associated with
  - decreased ocular pressure 377.02
  - increased intracranial pressure 377.01
  - retinal disorder 377.03
- choked disc 377.00
- infectional 377.00

Papillitis 377.31
- anus 569.49
- chronic lingual 529.4
- necrotizing, kidney 584.7
- optic 377.31
- rectum 569.49
- renal, necrotizing 584.7
- tongue 529.0

Papilloma (M8050/0) – *see also* Neoplasm, by site, benign

Note – Except where otherwise indicated, the morphological varieties of papilloma in the list below should be coded by site as for "Neoplasm, benign".

- acuminatum (female) (male) 078.1❺
- bladder (urinary) (transitional cell) (M8120/1) 236.7
  - benign (M8120/0) 223.3
- choroid plexus (M9390/0) 225.0
  - anaplastic type (M9390/3) 191.5
  - malignant (M9390/3) 191.5
- ductal (M8503/0)
- dyskeratotic (M8052/0)
- epidermoid (M8052/0)
- hyperkeratotic (M8052/0)
- intracystic (M8504/0)
- intraductal (M8503/0)
- inverted (M8053/0)
- keratotic (M8052/0)
- parakeratotic (M8052/0)
- pinta (primary) 103.0
- renal pelvis (transitional cell) (M8120/1) 236.99
  - benign (M8120/0) 223.1
- Schneiderian (M8121/0)
  - specified site – *see* Neoplasm, by site, benign
  - unspecified site 212.0
- serous surface (M8461/0)
  - borderline malignancy (M8461/1)
    - specified site – *see* Neoplasm, by site, uncertain behavior
    - unspecified site 236.2
  - specified site – *see* Neoplasm, by site, benign
  - unspecified site 220
- squamous (cell) (M8052/0)
- transitional (cell) (M8120/0)
  - bladder (urinary) (M8120/1) 236.7
  - inverted type (M8121/1) – *see* Neoplasm, by site, uncertain behavior
  - renal pelvis (M8120/1) 236.91
  - ureter (M8120/1) 236.91
- ureter (transitional cell) (M8120/1) 236.91
  - benign (M8120/0) 223.2
- urothelial (M8120/1) – *see* Neoplasm, by site, uncertain behavior
- verrucous (M8051/0)
- villous (M8261/1) – *see* Neoplasm, by site, uncertain behavior
- yaws, plantar or palmar 102.1

Papillomata, multiple, of yaws 102.1

Papillomatosis (M8060/0) – *see also* Neoplasm, by site, benign
- confluent and reticulate 701.8
- cutaneous 701.8
- ductal, breast 610.1
- Gougerot-Carteaud (confluent reticulate) 701.8
- intraductal (diffuse) (M8505/0) – *see* Neoplasm, by site, benign
- subareolar duct (M8506/0) 217

Papillon-Léage and Psaume syndrome (orodigitofacial dysostosis) 759.89

Papule 709.8
- carate (primary) 103.0
- fibrous, of nose (M8724/0) 216.3
- pinta (primary) 103.0

Papulosis, malignant 447.8

Papyraceous fetus 779.89
- complicating pregnancy 646.0❺

Paracephalus 759.7

Parachute mitral valve 746.5

Paracoccidioidomycosis 116.1
- mucocutaneous-lymphangitic 116.1
- pulmonary 116.1
- visceral 116.1

Paracoccidiomycosis – *see* Paracoccidioidomycosis

Paracusis 388.40

Paradentosis 523.5

Paradoxical facial movements 374.43

Paraffinoma 999.9

Paraganglioma (M8680/1)
- adrenal (M8700/0) 227.0
  - malignant (M8700/3) 194.0
- aortic body (M8691/1) 237.3
  - malignant (M8691/3) 194.6
- carotid body (M8692/1) 237.3
  - malignant (M8692/3) 194.5
- chromaffin (M8700/0) – *see also* Neoplasm, by site, benign
  - malignant (M8700/3) – *see* Neoplasm, by site, malignant
- extra-adrenal (M8693/1)
  - malignant (M8693/3)
    - specified site – *see* Neoplasm, by site, malignant
    - unspecified site 194.6
  - specified site – *see* Neoplasm, by site, uncertain behavior
  - unspecified site 237.3
- glomus jugulare (M8690/1) 237.3
  - malignant (M8690/3) 194.6
- jugular (M8690/1) 237.3
- malignant (M8680/3)
  - specified site – *see* Neoplasm, by site, malignant
  - unspecified site 194.6
- nonchromaffin (M8693/1)
  - malignant (M8693/3)
    - specified site – *see* Neoplasm, by site, malignant
    - unspecified site 194.6
  - specified site – *see* Neoplasm, by site, uncertain behavior
  - unspecified site 237.3
- parasympathetic (M8682/1)
  - specified site – *see* Neoplasm, by site, uncertain behavior
  - unspecified site 237.3
- specified site – *see* Neoplasm, by site, uncertain behavior
- sympathetic (M8681/1)
  - specified site – *see* Neoplasm, by site, uncertain behavior
  - unspecified site 237.3
- unspecified site 237.3

Parageusia 781.1
- psychogenic 306.7

Paragonimiasis 121.2

Paragranuloma, Hodgkin's (M9660/3) 201.0❺

Parahemophilia (*see also* Defect, coagulation) 286.3

Parakeratosis 690.8
- psoriasiformis 696.2
- variegata 696.2

Paralysis, paralytic (complete) (incomplete) 344.9
with
broken
back – *see* Fracture, vertebra, by site, with spinal cord injury
neck – *see* Fracture, vertebra, cervical, with spinal cord injury
fracture, vertebra – *see* Fracture, vertebra, by site, with spinal cord injury
syphilis 094.89
abdomen and back muscles 355.9
abdominal muscles 355.9
abducens (nerve) 378.54
abductor 355.9
lower extremity 355.8
upper extremity 354.9
accessory nerve 352.4
accommodation 367.51
hysterical 300.11
acoustic nerve 388.5
agitans 332.0
arteriosclerotic 332.0
alternating 344.89
oculomotor 344.89
amyotrophic 335.20
ankle 355.8
anterior serratus 355.9
anus (sphincter) 569.49
apoplectic (current episode) (*see also* Disease, cerebrovascular, acute) 436
late effect – *see* Late effect(s) (of) cerebrovascular disease
arm 344.40
affecting
dominant side 344.41
nondominant side 344.42
both 344.2
due to old CVA – *see* category 438❹
hysterical 300.11
late effect – *see* Late effect(s) (of) cerebrovascular disease
psychogenic 306.0
transient 781.4
traumatic NEC (*see also* Injury, nerve, upper limb) 955.9
arteriosclerotic (current episode) 437.0
late effect – *see* Late effect(s) (of) cerebrovascular disease
ascending (spinal), acute 357.0
associated, nuclear 344.89
asthenic bulbar 358.00
ataxic NEC 334.9
general 094.1
athetoid 333.71
atrophic 356.9
infantile, acute (*see also* Poliomyelitis, with paralysis) 045.1❺
muscle NEC 355.9
progressive 335.21
spinal (acute) (*see also* Poliomyelitis, with paralysis) 045.1❺
attack (*see also* Disease, cerebrovascular, acute) 436
axillary 353.0
Babinski-Nageotte's 344.89
Bell's 351.0
newborn 767.5
Benedikt's 344.89
birth (injury) 767.7
brain 767.0
intracranial 767.0
spinal cord 767.4
bladder (sphincter) 596.53
neurogenic 596.54
with cauda equina syndrome 344.61
puerperal, postpartum, childbirth 665.5❺
sensory 596.54
with cauda equina 344.61
spastic 596.54
with cauda equina 344.61
bowel, colon, or intestine (*see also* Ileus) 560.1
brachial plexus 353.0
due to birth injury 767.6
newborn 767.6
brain
congenital – *see* Palsy, cerebral
current episode 437.8
due to previous vascular lesion – *see* 438❹
diplegia 344.2
late effect – *see* Late effect(s) (of) cerebrovascular disease

Paralysis, paralytic – *continued*
brain – *continued*
hemiplegia 342.9
due to previous vascular lesion – *see* category 438❹
late effect – *see* Late effect(s) (of) cerebrovascular disease
infantile – *see* Palsy, cerebral
monoplegia – *see also* Monoplegia
due to previous vascular lesion – *see* category 438❹
late effect – *see* Late effect(s) (of) cerebrovascular disease
paraplegia 344.1
quadriplegia – *see* Quadriplegia
syphilitic, congenital 090.49
triplegia 344.89
bronchi 519.19
Brown-Séquard's 344.89
bulbar (chronic) (progressive) 335.22
infantile (*see also* Poliomyelitis, bulbar) 045.0❺
poliomyelitic (*see also* Poliomyelitis, bulbar) 045.0❺
pseudo 335.23
supranuclear 344.89
bulbospinal 358.00
cardiac (*see also* Failure, heart) 428.9
cerebral
current episode 437.8
spastic, infantile – *see* Palsy, cerebral
cerebrocerebellar 437.8
diplegic infantile 343.0
cervical
plexus 353.2
sympathetic NEC 337.0
Céstan-Chenais 344.89
Charcôt-Marie-Tooth type 356.1
childhood – *see* Palsy, cerebral
Clark's 343.9
colon (*see also* Ileus) 560.1
compressed air 993.3
compression
arm NEC 354.9
cerebral – *see* Paralysis, brain
leg NEC 355.8
lower extremity NEC 355.8
upper extremity NEC 354.9
congenital (cerebral) (spastic) (spinal) – *see* Palsy, cerebral
conjugate movement (of eye) 378.81
cortical (nuclear) (supranuclear) 378.81
convergence 378.83
cordis (*see also* Failure, heart) 428.9
cortical (*see also* Paralysis, brain) 437.8
cranial or cerebral nerve (*see also* Disorder, nerve, cranial) 352.9
creeping 335.21
crossed leg 344.89
crutch 953.4
deglutition 784.99
hysterical 300.11
dementia 094.1
descending (spinal) NEC 335.9
diaphragm (flaccid) 519.4
due to accidental section of phrenic nerve during procedure 998.2
digestive organs NEC 564.89
diplegic – *see* Diplegia
divergence (nuclear) 378.85
divers' 993.3
Duchenne's 335.22
due to intracranial or spinal birth injury – *see* Palsy, cerebral
embolic (current episode) (*see also* Embolism, brain) 434.1❺
late effect – *see* Late effect(s) (of) cerebrovascular disease
enteric (*see also* Ileus) 560.1
with hernia – *see* Hernia, by site, with obstruction
Erb's syphilitic spastic spinal 094.89
Erb (-Duchenne) (birth) (newborn) 767.6
esophagus 530.8❺
essential, infancy (*see also* Poliomyelitis) 045.9❺
extremity
lower – *see* Paralysis, leg
spastic (hereditary) 343.3
noncongenital or noninfantile 344.1
transient (cause unknown) 781.4
upper – *see* Paralysis, arm

Paralysis, paralytic – *continued*
eye muscle (extrinsic) 378.55
intrinsic 367.51
facial (nerve) 351.0
birth injury 767.5
congenital 767.5
following operation NEC 998.2
newborn 767.5
familial 359.3
periodic 359.3
spastic 334.1
fauces 478.29
finger NEC 354.9
foot NEC 355.8
gait 781.2
gastric nerve 352.3
gaze 378.81
general 094.1
ataxic 094.1
insane 094.1
juvenile 090.40
progressive 094.1
tabetic 094.1
glossopharyngeal (nerve) 352.2
glottis (*see also* Paralysis, vocal cord) 478.30
gluteal 353.4
Gubler (-Millard) 344.89
hand 354.9
hysterical 300.11
psychogenic 306.0
heart (*see also* Failure, heart) 428.9
hemifacial, progressive 349.89
hemiplegic – *see* Hemiplegia
hyperkalemic periodic (familial) 359.3
hypertensive (current episode) 437.8
hypoglossal (nerve) 352.5
hypokalemic periodic 359.3
Hyrtl's sphincter (rectum) 569.49
hysterical 300.11
ileus (*see also* Ileus) 560.1
infantile (*see also* Poliomyelitis) 045.9❺
atrophic acute 045.1❺
bulbar 045.0❺
cerebral – *see* Palsy, cerebral
paralytic 045.1❺
progressive acute 045.9❺
spastic – *see* Palsy, cerebral
spinal 045.9❺
infective (*see also* Poliomyelitis) 045.9❺
inferior nuclear 344.9
insane, general or progressive 094.1
internuclear 378.86
interosseous 355.9
intestine (*see also* Ileus) 560.1
intracranial (current episode) (*see also* Paralysis, brain) 437.8
due to birth injury 767.0
iris 379.49
due to diphtheria (toxin) 032.81 *[379.49]*
ischemic, Volkmann's (complicating trauma) 958.6
isolated sleep, recurrent 327.43
Jackson's 344.8❺
jake 357.7
Jamaica ginger (jake) 357.7
juvenile general 090.40
Klumpke (-Déjérine) (birth) (newborn) 767.6
labioglossal (laryngeal) (pharyngeal) 335.22
Landry's 357.0
laryngeal nerve (recurrent) (superior) (*see also* Paralysis, vocal cord) 478.30
larynx (*see also* Paralysis, vocal cord) 478.30
due to diphtheria (toxin) 032.3
late effect
due to
birth injury, brain or spinal (cord) – *see* Palsy, cerebral
edema, brain or cerebral – *see* Paralysis, brain
lesion
cerebrovascular – *see* category 438❹
late effect – *see* Late effect(s) (of) cerebrovascular disease
spinal (cord) – *see* Paralysis, spinal
lateral 335.24
lead 984.9
specified type of lead – *see* Table of Drugs and Chemicals
left side – *see* Hemiplegia
leg 344.30
affecting
dominant side 344.31

Paralysis, paralytic – Paralysis, paralytic

- **Paralysis, paralytic** – *continued*
  - leg – *continued*
    - affecting – *continued*
      - nondominant side 344.32
    - both (*see also* Paraplegia) 344.1
    - crossed 344.89
    - hysterical 300.11
    - psychogenic 306.0
    - transient or transitory 781.4
      - traumatic NEC (*see also* Injury, nerve, lower limb) 956.9
  - levator palpebrae superioris 374.31
  - limb NEC 344.5
    - all four – *see* Quadriplegia
    - quadriplegia – *see* Quadriplegia
  - lip 528.5
  - Lissauer's 094.1
  - local 355.9
  - lower limb – *see also* Paralysis, leg
    - both (*see also* Paraplegia) 344.1
  - lung 518.89
    - newborn 770.89
  - median nerve 354.1
  - medullary (tegmental) 344.89
  - mesencephalic NEC 344.89
    - tegmental 344.89
  - middle alternating 344.89
  - Millard-Gubler-Foville 344.89
  - monoplegic – *see* Monoplegia
  - motor NEC 344.9
    - cerebral – *see* Paralysis, brain
    - spinal – *see* Paralysis, spinal
  - multiple
    - cerebral – *see* Paralysis, brain
    - spinal – *see* Paralysis, spinal
  - muscle (flaccid) 359.9
    - due to nerve lesion NEC 355.9
    - eye (extrinsic) 378.55
      - intrinsic 367.51
      - oblique 378.51
    - iris sphincter 364.89 ▲
    - ischemic (complicating trauma) (Volkmann's) 958.6
    - pseudohypertrophic 359.1
  - muscular (atrophic) 359.9
    - progressive 335.21
  - musculocutaneous nerve 354.9
  - musculospiral 354.9
  - nerve – *see also* Disorder, nerve
    - third or oculomotor (partial) 378.51
      - total 378.52
    - fourth or trochlear 378.53
    - sixth or abducens 378.54
    - seventh or facial 351.0
      - birth injury 767.5
      - due to
        - injection NEC 999.9
        - operation NEC 997.09
      - newborn 767.5
    - accessory 352.4
    - auditory 388.5
    - birth injury 767.7
    - cranial or cerebral (*see also* Disorder, nerve, cranial) 352.9
    - facial 351.0
      - birth injury 767.5
      - newborn 767.5
    - laryngeal (*see also* Paralysis, vocal cord) 478.30
    - newborn 767.7
    - phrenic 354.8
      - newborn 767.7
    - radial 354.3
      - birth injury 767.6
      - newborn 767.6
    - syphilitic 094.89
    - traumatic NEC (*see also* Injury, nerve, by site) 957.9
    - trigeminal 350.9
    - ulnar 354.2
  - newborn NEC 767.0
  - normokalemic periodic 359.3
  - obstetrical, newborn 767.7
  - ocular 378.9
  - oculofacial, congenital 352.6
  - oculomotor (nerve) (partial) 378.51
    - alternating 344.89
    - external bilateral 378.55
    - total 378.52
  - olfactory nerve 352.0
  - palate 528.9
  - palatopharyngolaryngeal 352.6

- **Paralysis, paralytic** – *continued*
  - paratrigeminal 350.9
  - periodic (familial) (hyperkalemic) (hypokalemic) (normokalemic) ▶(potassium sensitive)◀ (secondary) 359.3
  - peripheral
    - autonomic nervous system – *see* Neuropathy, peripheral, autonomic
    - nerve NEC 355.9
  - peroneal (nerve) 355.3
  - pharynx 478.29
  - phrenic nerve 354.8
  - plantar nerves 355.6
  - pneumogastric nerve 352.3
  - poliomyelitis (current) (*see also* Poliomyelitis, with paralysis) 045.1❺
    - bulbar 045.0❺
  - popliteal nerve 355.3
  - pressure (*see also* Neuropathy, entrapment) 355.9
  - progressive 335.21
    - atrophic 335.21
    - bulbar 335.22
    - general 094.1
    - hemifacial 349.89
    - infantile, acute (*see also* Poliomyelitis) 045.9❺
    - multiple 335.20
  - pseudobulbar 335.23
  - pseudohypertrophic 359.1
    - muscle 359.1
  - psychogenic 306.0
  - pupil, pupillary 379.49
  - quadriceps 355.8
  - quadriplegic (*see also* Quadriplegia) 344.0
  - radial nerve 354.3
    - birth injury 767.6
  - rectum (sphincter) 569.49
  - rectus muscle (eye) 378.55
  - recurrent
    - isolated sleep 327.43
    - laryngeal nerve (*see also* Paralysis, vocal cord) 478.30
  - respiratory (muscle) (system) (tract) 786.09
    - center NEC 344.89
      - fetus or newborn 770.87
    - congenital 768.9
    - newborn 768.9
  - right side – *see* Hemiplegia
  - Saturday night 354.3
  - saturnine 984.9
    - specified type of lead – *see* Table of Drugs and Chemicals
  - sciatic nerve 355.0
  - secondary – *see* Paralysis, late effect
  - seizure (cerebral) (current episode) (*see also* Disease, cerebrovascular, acute) 436
    - late effect – *see* Late effect(s) (of) cerebrovascular disease
  - senile NEC 344.9
  - serratus magnus 355.9
  - shaking (*see also* Parkinsonism) 332.0
  - shock (*see also* Disease, cerebrovascular, acute) 436
    - late effect – *see* Late effect(s) (of) cerebrovascular disease
  - shoulder 354.9
  - soft palate 528.9
  - spasmodic – *see* Paralysis, spastic
  - spastic 344.9
    - cerebral infantile – *see* Palsy, cerebral
    - congenital (cerebral) – *see* Palsy, cerebral
    - familial 334.1
    - hereditary 334.1
    - infantile 343.9
    - noncongenital or noninfantile, cerebral 344.9
    - syphilitic 094.0
      - spinal 094.89
  - sphincter, bladder (*see also* Paralysis, bladder) 596.53
  - spinal (cord) NEC 344.1
    - accessory nerve 352.4
    - acute (*see also* Poliomyelitis) 045.9❺
    - ascending acute 357.0
    - atrophic (acute) (*see also* Poliomyelitis, with paralysis) 045.1❺
      - spastic, syphilitic 094.89
    - congenital NEC 343.9
    - hemiplegic – *see* Hemiplegia
    - hereditary 336.8
    - infantile (*see also* Poliomyelitis) 045.9❺
    - late effect NEC 344.89

- **Paralysis, paralytic** – *continued*
  - spinal (cord) – *continued*
    - monoplegic – *see* Monoplegia
    - nerve 355.9
    - progressive 335.10
    - quadriplegic – *see* Quadriplegia
    - spastic NEC 343.9
    - traumatic – *see* Injury, spinal, by site
  - sternomastoid 352.4
  - stomach 536.3
    - diabetic 250.6 *[536.3]*
    - nerve (nondiabetic) 352.3
  - stroke (current episode) – *see* Infarct, brain
    - late effect – *see* Late effect(s) (of) cerebrovascular disease
  - subscapularis 354.8
  - superior nuclear NEC 334.9
  - supranuclear 356.8
  - sympathetic
    - cervical NEC 337.0
    - nerve NEC (*see also* Neuropathy, peripheral, autonomic) 337.9
    - nervous system – *see* Neuropathy, peripheral, autonomic
  - syndrome 344.9
    - specified NEC 344.89
  - syphilitic spastic spinal (Erb's) 094.89
  - tabetic general 094.1
  - thigh 355.8
  - throat 478.29
    - diphtheritic 032.0
    - muscle 478.29
  - thrombotic (current episode) (*see also* Thrombosis, brain) 434.0❺
    - late effect – *see* Late effect(s) (of) cerebrovascular disease
    - old – *see* category 438❹
  - thumb NEC 354.9
  - tick (-bite) 989.5
  - Todd's (postepileptic transitory paralysis) 344.89
  - toe 355.6
  - tongue 529.8
  - transient
    - arm or leg NEC 781.4
    - traumatic NEC (*see also* Injury, nerve, by site) 957.9
  - trapezius 352.4
  - traumatic, transient NEC (*see also* Injury, nerve, by site) 957.9
  - trembling (*see also* Parkinsonism) 332.0
  - triceps brachii 354.9
  - trigeminal nerve 350.9
  - trochlear nerve 378.53
  - ulnar nerve 354.2
  - upper limb – *see also* Paralysis, arm
    - both (*see also* Diplegia) 344.2
  - uremic – *see* Uremia
  - uveoparotitic 135
  - uvula 528.9
    - hysterical 300.11
    - postdiphtheritic 032.0
  - vagus nerve 352.3
  - vasomotor NEC 337.9
  - velum palati 528.9
  - vesical (*see also* Paralysis, bladder) 596.53
  - vestibular nerve 388.5
  - visual field, psychic 368.16
  - vocal cord 478.30
    - bilateral (partial) 478.33
      - complete 478.34
    - complete (bilateral) 478.34
    - unilateral (partial) 478.31
      - complete 478.32
  - Volkmann's (complicating trauma) 958.6
  - wasting 335.21
  - Weber's 344.89
  - wrist NEC 354.9
- **Paramedial orifice, urethrovesical** 753.8
- **Paramenia** 626.9
- **Parametritis** (chronic) (*see also* Disease, pelvis, inflammatory) 614.4
  - acute 614.3
  - puerperal, postpartum, childbirth 670❹
- **Parametrium, parametric** – *see* condition
- **Paramnesia** (*see also* Amnesia) 780.93
- **Paramolar** 520.1
  - causing crowding 524.31
- **Paramyloidosis** 277.30
- **Paramyoclonus multiplex** 333.2

Paralysis, paralytic – Paramyoclonus multiplex

- **Paramyotonia** 359.29 ▲
  - congenita ▶(of von Eulenburg)◀ 359.29 ▲
- **Paraneoplastic syndrome**- *see* condition
- **Parangi** (*see also* Yaws) 102.9
- **Paranoia** 297.1
  - alcoholic 291.5
  - querulans 297.8
  - senile 290.20
- **Paranoid**
  - dementia (*see also* Schizophrenia) 295.3❺
    - praecox (acute) 295.3❺
    - senile 290.20
  - personality 301.0
  - psychosis 297.9
    - alcoholic 291.5
    - climacteric 297.2
    - drug-induced 292.11
    - involutional 297.2
    - menopausal 297.2
    - protracted reactive 298.4
    - psychogenic 298.4
      - acute 298.3
    - senile 290.20
  - reaction (chronic) 297.9
    - acute 298.3
  - schizophrenia (acute) (*see also* Schizophrenia) 295.3❺
  - state 297.9
    - alcohol-induced 291.5
    - climacteric 297.2
    - drug-induced 292.11
    - due to or associated with
      - arteriosclerosis (cerebrovascular) 290.42
      - presenile brain disease 290.12
      - senile brain disease 290.20
    - involutional 297.2
    - menopausal 297.2
    - senile 290.20
    - simple 297.0
    - specified type NEC 297.8
  - tendencies 301.0
  - traits 301.0
  - trends 301.0
  - type, psychopathic personality 301.0
- **Paraparesis** (*see also* ▶Paraplegia◀) 344.1 ▲
- **Paraphasia** 784.3
- **Paraphilia** (*see also* Deviation, sexual) 302.9
- **Paraphimosis** (congenital) 605
  - chancroidal 099.0
- **Paraphrenia, paraphrenic** (late) 297.2
  - climacteric 297.2
  - dementia (*see also* Schizophrenia) 295.3❺
  - involutional 297.2
  - menopausal 297.2
  - schizophrenia (acute) (*see also* Schizophrenia) 295.3❺
- **Paraplegia** 344.1
  - with
    - broken back – *see* Fracture, vertebra, by site, with spinal cord injury
    - fracture, vertebra – *see* Fracture, vertebra, by site, with spinal cord injury
  - ataxic – *see* Degeneration, combined, spinal cord
  - brain (current episode) (*see also* Paralysis, brain) 437.8
  - cerebral (current episode) (*see also* Paralysis, brain) 437.8
  - congenital or infantile (cerebral) (spastic) (spinal) 343.0
  - cortical – *see* Paralysis, brain
  - familial spastic 334.1
  - functional (hysterical) 300.11
  - hysterical 300.11
  - infantile 343.0
  - late effect 344.1
  - Pott's (*see also* Tuberculosis) 015.0❺ *[730.88]*
  - psychogenic 306.0
  - spastic
    - Erb's spinal 094.89
    - hereditary 334.1
    - not infantile or congenital 344.1
  - spinal (cord)
    - traumatic NEC – *see* Injury, spinal, by site
  - syphilitic (spastic) 094.89
  - traumatic NEC – *see* Injury, spinal, by site
- **Paraproteinemia** 273.2
  - benign (familial) 273.1
  - monoclonal 273.1
  - secondary to malignant or inflammatory disease 273.1
- **Parapsoriasis** 696.2
  - en plaques 696.2
  - guttata 696.2
  - lichenoides chronica 696.2
  - retiformis 696.2
  - varioliformis (acuta) 696.2
- **Parascarlatina** 057.8
- **Parasitic** – *see also* condition
  - disease NEC (*see also* Infestation, parasitic) 136.9
    - contact V01.89
    - exposure to V01.89
    - intestinal NEC 129
    - skin NEC 134.9
  - stomatitis 112.0
  - sycosis 110.0
    - beard 110.0
    - scalp 110.0
  - twin 759.4
- **Parasitism** NEC 136.9
  - intestinal NEC 129
  - skin NEC 134.9
  - specified – *see* Infestation
- **Parasitophobia** 300.29
- **Parasomnia** 307.47
  - alcohol-induced 291.82
  - drug-induced 292.85
  - nonorganic origin 307.47
  - organic 327.40
    - in conditions classified elsewhere 327.44
    - other 327.49
- **Paraspadias** 752.69
- **Paraspasm facialis** 351.8
- **Parathyroid gland** – *see* condition
- **Parathyroiditis** (autoimmune) 252.1
- **Parathyroprival tetany** 252.1
- **Paratrachoma** 077.0
- **Paratyphilitis** (*see also* Appendicitis) 541
- **Paratyphoid** (fever) – *see* Fever, paratyphoid
- **Paratyphus** – *see* Fever, paratyphoid
- **Paraurethral duct** 753.8
- **Para-urethritis** 597.89
  - gonococcal (acute) 098.0
    - chronic or duration of 2 months or over 098.2
- **Paravaccinia** NEC 051.9
  - milkers' node 051.1
- **Paravaginitis** (*see also* Vaginitis) 616.10
- **Parencephalitis** (*see also* Encephalitis) 323.9
  - late effect – *see* category 326
- **Parergasia** 298.9
- **Paresis** (*see also* Paralysis) 344.9
  - accommodation 367.51
  - bladder (spastic) (sphincter) (*see also* Paralysis, bladder) 596.53
    - tabetic 094.0
  - bowel, colon, or intestine (*see also* Ileus) 560.1
  - brain or cerebral – *see* Paralysis, brain
  - extrinsic muscle, eye 378.55
  - general 094.1
    - arrested 094.1
    - brain 094.1
    - cerebral 094.1
    - insane 094.1
    - juvenile 090.40
      - remission 090.49
    - progressive 094.1
    - remission (sustained) 094.1
    - tabetic 094.1
  - heart (*see also* Failure, heart) 428.9
  - infantile (*see also* Poliomyelitis) 045.9❺
  - insane 094.1
  - juvenile 090.40
  - late effect – *see* Paralysis, late effect
  - luetic (general) 094.1
  - peripheral progressive 356.9
  - pseudohypertrophic 359.1
  - senile NEC 344.9
  - stomach 536.3
    - diabetic 250.6 *[536.3]*
  - syphilitic (general) 094.1
    - congenital 090.40
  - transient, limb 781.4
  - vesical (sphincter) NEC 596.53
- **Paresthesia** (*see also* Disturbance, sensation) 782.0
  - Berger's (paresthesia of lower limb) 782.0
  - Bernhardt 355.1
  - Magnan's 782.0
- **Paretic** – *see* condition
- **Parinaud's**
  - conjunctivitis 372.02
  - oculoglandular syndrome 372.02
  - ophthalmoplegia 378.81
  - syndrome (paralysis of conjugate upward gaze) 378.81
- **Parkes Weber and Dimitri syndrome** (encephalocutaneous angiomatosis) 759.6
- **Parkinson's disease, syndrome, or tremor** – *see* Parkinsonism
- **Parkinsonism** (arteriosclerotic) (idiopathic) (primary) 332.0
  - associated with orthostatic hypotension (idiopathic) (symptomatic) 333.0
  - due to drugs 332.1
  - neuroleptic-induced 332.1
  - secondary 332.1
  - syphilitic 094.82
- **Parodontitis** 523.40
- **Parodontosis** 523.5
- **Paronychia** (with lymphangitis) 681.9
  - candidal (chronic) 112.3
  - chronic 681.9
    - candidal 112.3
    - finger 681.02
    - toe 681.11
  - finger 681.02
  - toe 681.11
  - tuberculous (primary) (*see also* Tuberculosis) 017.0❺
- **Parorexia** NEC 307.52
  - hysterical 300.11
- **Parosmia** 781.1
  - psychogenic 306.7
- **Parotid gland** – *see* condition
- **Parotiditis** (*see also* Parotitis) 527.2
  - epidemic 072.9
  - infectious 072.9
- **Parotitis** 527.2
  - allergic 527.2
  - chronic 527.2
  - epidemic (*see also* Mumps) 072.9
  - infectious (*see also* Mumps) 072.9
  - noninfectious 527.2
  - nonspecific toxic 527.2
  - not mumps 527.2
  - postoperative 527.2
  - purulent 527.2
  - septic 527.2
  - suppurative (acute) 527.2
  - surgical 527.2
  - toxic 527.2
- **Paroxysmal** – *see also* condition
  - dyspnea (nocturnal) 786.09
- **Parrot's disease** (syphilitic osteochondritis) 090.0
- **Parrot fever** 073.9
- **Parry's disease or syndrome** (exophthalmic goiter) 242.0❺
- **Parry-Romberg syndrome** 349.89
- **Parson's disease** (exophthalmic goiter) 242.0❺
- **Parsonage-Aldren-Turner syndrome** 353.5
- **Parsonage-Turner syndrome** 353.5
- **Pars planitis** 363.21
- **Particolored infant** 757.39
- **Parturition** – *see* Delivery
- **Parvovirus** 079.83 ●
  - B19 079.83 ●
  - human 079.83 ●
- **Passage**
  - false, urethra 599.4
  - meconium noted during delivery 763.84
  - of sounds or bougies (*see also* Attention to artificial opening) V55.9
- **Passive** – *see* condition
- **Pasteurella septica** 027.2
- **Pasteurellosis** (*see also* Infection, Pasteurella) 027.2
- **PAT** (paroxysmal atrial tachycardia) 427.0
- **Patau's syndrome** (trisomy D1) 758.1
- **Patch**
  - herald 696.3
- **Patches**
  - mucous (syphilitic) 091.3
    - congenital 090.0
  - smokers' (mouth) 528.6
- **Patellar** – *see* condition
- **Patellofemoral syndrome** 719.46

Perforation, perforative – *continued*
- ethmoidal sinus (*see also* Sinusitis, ethmoidal) 473.2
- foreign body (external site) – *see also* Wound, open, by site, complicated
  - internal site, by ingested object – *see* Foreign body
- frontal sinus (*see also* Sinusitis, frontal) 473.1
- gallbladder or duct (*see also* Disease, gallbladder) 575.4
- gastric (ulcer) – *see* Ulcer, stomach, with perforation
- heart valve – *see* Endocarditis
- ileum (*see also* Perforation, intestine) 569.83
- instrumental
  - external – *see* Wound, open, by site
  - pregnant uterus, complicating delivery 665.9❺
  - surgical (accidental) (blood vessel) (nerve) (organ) 998.2
- intestine 569.83
  - with
    - abortion – *see* Abortion, by type, with damage to pelvic organs
    - ectopic pregnancy (*see also* categories 633.0-633.9) 639.2
    - molar pregnancy (*see also* categories 630-632) 639.2
  - fetus or newborn 777.6
  - obstetrical trauma 665.5❺
  - ulcerative NEC 569.83
- jejunum, jejunal 569.83
  - ulcer – *see* Ulcer, gastrojejunal, with perforation
- mastoid (antrum) (cell) 383.89
- maxillary sinus (*see also* Sinusitis, maxillary) 473.0
- membrana tympani – *see* Perforation, tympanum
- nasal
  - septum 478.19
    - congenital 748.1
    - syphilitic 095.8
  - sinus (*see also* Sinusitis) 473.9
    - congenital 748.1
- palate (hard) 526.89
  - soft 528.9
    - syphilitic 095.8
  - syphilitic 095.8
- palatine vault 526.89
  - syphilitic 095.8
    - congenital 090.5
- pelvic
  - floor
    - with
      - abortion – *see* Abortion, by type, with damage to pelvic organs
      - ectopic pregnancy (*see also* categories 633.0-633.9) 639.2
      - molar pregnancy (*see also* categories 630-632) 639.2
    - obstetrical trauma 664.1❺
  - organ
    - with
      - abortion – *see* Abortion, by type, with damage to pelvic organs
      - ectopic pregnancy (*see also* categories 633.0-633.9) 639.2
      - molar pregnancy (*see also* categories 630-632) 639.2
    - following
      - abortion 639.2
      - ectopic or molar pregnancy 639.2
    - obstetrical trauma 665.5❺
- perineum – *see* Laceration, perineum
- periurethral tissue
  - with
    - abortion – *see* Abortion, by type, with damage to pelvic organs
    - ectopic pregnancy (*see also* categories 630-632) 639.2
    - molar pregnancy (*see also* categories 630-632) 639.2
- pharynx 478.29
- pylorus, pyloric (ulcer) – *see* Ulcer, stomach, with perforation
- rectum 569.49
- root canal space 526.61
- sigmoid 569.83
- sinus (accessory) (chronic) (nasal) (*see also* Sinusitis) 473.9
- sphenoidal sinus (*see also* Sinusitis, sphenoidal) 473.3
- stomach (due to ulcer) – *see* Ulcer, stomach, with perforation

Perforation, perforative – *continued*
- surgical (accidental) (by instrument) (blood vessel) (nerve) (organ) 998.2
- traumatic
  - external – *see* Wound, open, by site
  - eye (*see also* Penetrating wound, ocular) 871.7
  - internal organ – *see* Injury, internal, by site
- tympanum (membrane) (persistent posttraumatic) (postinflammatory) 384.20
  - with
    - otitis media- *see* Otitis media
  - attic 384.22
  - central 384.21
  - healed 384.81
  - marginal NEC 384.23
  - multiple 384.24
  - pars flaccida 384.22
  - total 384.25
  - traumatic – *see* Wound, open, ear, drum
- typhoid, gastrointestinal 002.0
- ulcer – *see* Ulcer, by site, with perforation
- ureter 593.89
- urethra
  - with
    - abortion – *see* Abortion, by type, with damage to pelvic organs
    - ectopic pregnancy (*see also* categories 633.0-633.9) 639.2
    - molar pregnancy (*see also* categories 630-632) 639.2
  - following
    - abortion 639.2
    - ectopic or molar pregnancy 639.2
  - obstetrical trauma 665.5❺
- uterus – *see also* Injury, internal, uterus
  - with
    - abortion – *see* Abortion, by type, with damage to pelvic organs
    - ectopic pregnancy (*see also* categories 633.0-633.9) 639.2
    - molar pregnancy (*see also* categories 630-632) 639.2
  - by intrauterine contraceptive device 996.32
  - following
    - abortion 639.2
    - ectopic or molar pregnancy 639.2
  - obstetrical trauma – *see* Injury, internal, uterus, obstetrical trauma
- uvula 528.9
  - syphilitic 095.8
- vagina – *see* Laceration, vagina
- viscus NEC 799.89
  - traumatic 868.00
    - with open wound into cavity 868.10

Periadenitis mucosa necrotica recurrens 528.2

Periangiitis 446.0

Periantritis 535.4❺

Periappendicitis (acute) (*see also* Appendicitis) 541

Periarteritis (disseminated) (infectious) (necrotizing) (nodosa) 446.0

Periarthritis (joint) 726.90
- Duplay's 726.2
- gonococcal 098.50
- humeroscapularis 726.2
- scapulohumeral 726.2
- shoulder 726.2
- wrist 726.4

Periarthrosis (angioneural) – *see* Periarthritis

Peribronchitis 491.9
- tuberculous (*see also* Tuberculosis) 011.3❺

Pericapsulitis, adhesive (shoulder) 726.0

Pericarditis (granular) (with decompensation) (with effusion) 423.9
- with
  - rheumatic fever (conditions classifiable to 390)
    - active (*see also* Pericarditis, rheumatic) 391.0
    - inactive or quiescent 393
- actinomycotic 039.8 *[420.0]*
- acute (nonrheumatic) 420.90
  - with chorea (acute) (rheumatic) (Sydenham's) 392.0
  - bacterial 420.99
  - benign 420.91
  - hemorrhagic 420.90
  - idiopathic 420.91
  - infective 420.90
  - nonspecific 420.91

Pericarditis – *continued*
- acute – *continued*
  - rheumatic 391.0
    - with chorea (acute) (rheumatic) (Sydenham's) 392.0
  - sicca 420.90
  - viral 420.91
- adhesive or adherent (external) (internal) 423.1
  - acute – *see* Pericarditis, acute
  - rheumatic (external) (internal) 393
- amebic 006.8 *[420.0]*
- bacterial (acute) (subacute) (with serous or seropurulent effusion) 420.99
- calcareous 423.2
- cholesterol (chronic) 423.8
  - acute 420.90
- chronic (nonrheumatic) 423.8
  - rheumatic 393
- constrictive 423.2
- Coxsackie 074.21
- due to
  - actinomycosis 039.8 *[420.0]*
  - amebiasis 006.8 *[420.0]*
  - Coxsackie (virus) 074.21
  - histoplasmosis (*see also* Histoplasmosis) 115.93
  - nocardiosis 039.8 *[420.0]*
  - tuberculosis (*see also* Tuberculosis) 017.9❺ *[420.0]*
- fibrinocaseous (*see also* Tuberculosis) 017.9❺ *[420.0]*
- fibrinopurulent 420.99
- fibrinous – *see* Pericarditis, rheumatic
- fibropurulent 420.99
- fibrous 423.1
- gonococcal 098.83
- hemorrhagic 423.0
- idiopathic (acute) 420.91
- infective (acute) 420.90
- meningococcal 036.41
- neoplastic (chronic) 423.8
  - acute 420.90
- nonspecific 420.91
- obliterans, obliterating 423.1
- plastic 423.1
- pneumococcal (acute) 420.99
- postinfarction 411.0
- purulent (acute) 420.99
- rheumatic (active) (acute) (with effusion) (with pneumonia) 391.0
  - with chorea (acute) (rheumatic) (Sydenham's) 392.0
  - chronic or inactive (with chorea) 393
- septic (acute) 420.99
- serofibrinous – *see* Pericarditis, rheumatic
- staphylococcal (acute) 420.99
- streptococcal (acute) 420.99
- suppurative (acute) 420.99
- syphilitic 093.81
- tuberculous (acute) (chronic) (*see also* Tuberculosis) 017.9❺ *[420.0]*
- uremic 585.9 *[420.0]*
- viral (acute) 420.91

Pericardium, pericardial – *see* condition

Pericellulitis (*see also* Cellulitis) 682.9

Pericementitis 523.40
- acute 523.30
- chronic (suppurative) 523.40

Pericholecystitis (*see also* Cholecystitis) 575.10

Perichondritis
- auricle 380.00
  - acute 380.01
  - chronic 380.02
- bronchus 491.9
- ear (external) 380.00
  - acute 380.01
  - chronic 380.02
- larynx 478.71
  - syphilitic 095.8
  - typhoid 002.0 *[478.71]*
- nose 478.19
- pinna 380.00
  - acute 380.01
  - chronic 380.02
- trachea 478.9

Periclasia 523.5

Pericolitis 569.89

Pericoronitis (chronic) 523.40
- acute 523.30

Pericystitis (*see also* Cystitis) 595.9

❹ Fourth-Digit Required ❺ Fifth-Digit Required *[code]* Manifestation Code ▶◀ Revised Text ● New Line ▲ Revised Code

Pericytoma (M9150/1) – *see also* Neoplasm, connective tissue, uncertain behavior
benign (M9150/0) – *see* Neoplasm, connective tissue, benign
malignant (M9150/3) – *see* Neoplasm, connective tissue, malignant
Peridacryocystitis, acute 375.32
Peridiverticulitis (*see also* Diverticulitis) 562.11
Periduodenitis 535.6❺
Periendocarditis (*see also* Endocarditis) 424.90
acute or subacute 421.9
Periepididymitis (*see also* Epididymitis) 604.90
Perifolliculitis (abscedens) 704.8
capitis, abscedens et suffodiens 704.8
dissecting, scalp 704.8
scalp 704.8
superficial pustular 704.8
Perigastritis (acute) 535.0❺
Perigastrojejunitis (acute) 535.0❺
Perihepatitis (acute) 573.3
chlamydial 099.56
gonococcal 098.86
Peri-ileitis (subacute) 569.89
Perilabyrinthitis (acute) – *see* Labyrinthitis
Perimeningitis – *see* Meningitis
Perimetritis (*see also* Endometritis) 615.9
Perimetrosalpingitis (*see also* Salpingo-oophoritis) 614.2
Perineocele 618.05
Perinephric – *see* condition
Perinephritic – *see* condition
Perinephritis (*see also* Infection, kidney) 590.9
purulent (*see also* Abscess, kidney) 590.2
Perineum, perineal – *see* condition
Perineuritis NEC 729.2
Periodic – *see also* condition
disease (familial) 277.31
edema 995.1
hereditary 277.6
fever 277.31
limb movement disorder 327.51
paralysis (familial) 359.3
peritonitis 277.31
polyserositis 277.31
somnolence (*see also* Narcolepsy) 347.00
Periodontal
cyst 522.8
pocket 523.8
Periodontitis (chronic) (complex) (compound) (simplex) 523.40
acute 523.33
aggressive 523.30
generalized 523.32
localized 523.31
apical 522.6
acute (pulpal origin) 522.4
generalized 523.42
localized 523.41
Periodontoclasia 523.5
Periodontosis 523.5
Periods – *see also* Menstruation
heavy 626.2
irregular 626.4
Perionychia (with lymphangitis) 681.9
finger 681.02
toe 681.11
Perioophoritis (*see also* Salpingo-oophoritis) 614.2
Periorchitis (*see also* Orchitis) 604.90
Periosteum, periosteal – *see* condition
Periostitis (circumscribed) (diffuse) (infective) 730.3❺

Note – Use the following fifth-digit subclassification with category 730:

0	*site unspecified*
1	*shoulder region*
2	*upper arm*
3	*forearm*
4	*hand*
5	*pelvic region and thigh*
6	*lower leg*
7	*ankle and foot*
8	*other specified sites*
9	*multiple sites*

with osteomyelitis (*see also* Osteomyelitis) 730.2❺
acute or subacute 730.0❺

Periostitis – *continued*
with osteomyelitis – *continued*
chronic or old 730.1❺
albuminosa, albuminosus 730.3❺
alveolar 526.5
alveolodental 526.5
dental 526.5
gonorrheal 098.89
hyperplastica, generalized 731.2
jaw (lower) (upper) 526.4
monomelic 733.99
orbital 376.02
syphilitic 095.5
congenital 090.0 *[730.8]*❺
secondary 091.61
tuberculous (*see also* Tuberculosis, bone) 015.9❺ *[730.8]*❺
yaws (early) (hypertrophic) (late) 102.6
Periostosis (*see also* Periostitis) 730.3❺
with osteomyelitis (*see also* Osteomyelitis) 730.2❺
acute or subacute 730.0❺
chronic or old 730.1❺
hyperplastic 756.59
Peripartum cardiomyopathy 674.5❺
Periphlebitis (*see also* Phlebitis) 451.9
lower extremity 451.2
deep (vessels) 451.19
superficial (vessels) 451.0
portal 572.1
retina 362.18
superficial (vessels) 451.0
tuberculous (*see also* Tuberculosis) 017.9❺
retina 017.3❺ *[362.18]*
Peripneumonia – *see* Pneumonia
Periproctitis 569.49
Periprostatitis (*see also* Prostatitis) 601.9
Perirectal – *see* condition
Perirenal – *see* condition
Perisalpingitis (*see also* Salpingo-oophoritis) 614.2
Perisigmoiditis 569.89
Perisplenitis (infectional) 289.59
Perispondylitis – *see* Spondylitis
Peristalsis reversed or visible 787.4
Peritendinitis (*see also* Tenosynovitis) 726.90
adhesive (shoulder) 726.0
Perithelioma (M9150/1) – *see* Pericytoma
Peritoneum, peritoneal – *see also* condition
equilibration test V56.32
Peritonitis (acute) (adhesive) (fibrinous) (hemorrhagic) (idiopathic) (localized) (perforative) (primary) (with adhesions) (with effusion) 567.9
with or following
abortion – *see* Abortion, by type, with sepsis
abscess 567.21
appendicitis 540.0
with peritoneal abscess 540.1
ectopic pregnancy (*see also* categories 633.0-633.9) 639.0
molar pregnancy (*see also* categories 630-632) 639.0
aseptic 998.7
bacterial 567.29
spontaneous 567.23
bile, biliary 567.81
chemical 998.7
chlamydial 099.56
chronic proliferative 567.89
congenital NEC 777.6
diaphragmatic 567.22
diffuse NEC 567.29
diphtheritic 032.83
disseminated NEC 567.29
due to
bile 567.81
foreign
body or object accidentally left during a procedure (instrument) (sponge) (swab) 998.4
substance accidentally left during a procedure (chemical) (powder) (talc) 998.7
talc 998.7
urine 567.89
fibrinopurulent 567.29
fibrinous 567.29
fibrocaseous (*see also* Tuberculosis) 014.0❺
fibropurulent 567.29

Peritonitis – *continued*
general, generalized (acute) 567.21
gonococcal 098.86
in infective disease NEC 136.9 *[567.0]*
meconium (newborn) 777.6
pancreatic 577.8
paroxysmal, benign 277.31
pelvic
female (acute) 614.5
chronic NEC 614.7
with adhesions 614.6
puerperal, postpartum, childbirth 670❹
male (acute) 567.21
periodic (familial) 277.31
phlegmonous 567.29
pneumococcal 567.1
postabortal 639.0
proliferative, chronic 567.89
puerperal, postpartum, childbirth 670❹
purulent 567.29
septic 567.29
spontaneous bacterial 567.23
staphylococcal 567.29
streptococcal 567.29
subdiaphragmatic 567.29
subphrenic 567.29
suppurative 567.29
syphilitic 095.2
congenital 090.0 *[567.0]*
talc 998.7
tuberculous (*see also* Tuberculosis) 014.0❺
urine 567.89
Peritonsillar – *see* condition
Peritonsillitis 475
Perityphlitis (*see also* Appendicitis) 541
Periureteritis 593.89
Periurethral – *see* condition
Periurethritis (gangrenous) 597.89
Periuterine – *see* condition
Perivaginitis (*see also* Vaginitis) 616.10
Perivasculitis, retinal 362.18
Perivasitis (chronic) 608.4
Periventricular leukomalacia 779.7
Perivesiculitis (seminal) (*see also* Vesiculitis) 608.0
Perlèche 686.8
due to
moniliasis 112.0
riboflavin deficiency 266.0
Pernicious – *see* condition
Pernio, perniosis 991.5
Persecution
delusion 297.9
social V62.4
Perseveration (tonic) 784.69
Persistence, persistent (congenital) 759.89
anal membrane 751.2
arteria stapedia 744.04
atrioventricular canal 745.69
bloody ejaculate 792.2
branchial cleft 744.41
bulbus cordis in left ventricle 745.8
canal of Cloquet 743.51
capsule (opaque) 743.51
cilioretinal artery or vein 743.51
cloaca 751.5
communication – *see* Fistula, congenital
convolutions
aortic arch 747.21
fallopian tube 752.19
oviduct 752.19
uterine tube 752.19
double aortic arch 747.21
ductus
arteriosus 747.0
Botalli 747.0
fetal
circulation 747.83
form of cervix (uteri) 752.49
hemoglobin (hereditary) ("Swiss variety") 282.7
pulmonary hypertension 747.83
foramen
Botalli 745.5
ovale 745.5
Gartner's duct 752.41
hemoglobin, fetal (hereditary) (HPFH) 282.7
hyaloid
artery (generally incomplete) 743.51
system 743.51

Persistence, persistent – Pharyngoconjunctivitis, viral

Persistence, persistent – *continued*
- hymen (tag)
  - in pregnancy or childbirth 654.8❺
    - causing obstructed labor 660.2❺
- lanugo 757.4
- left
  - posterior cardinal vein 747.49
  - root with right arch of aorta 747.21
  - superior vena cava 747.49
- Meckel's diverticulum 751.0
- mesonephric duct 752.89
  - fallopian tube 752.11
- mucosal disease (middle ear) (with posterior or superior marginal perforation of ear drum) 382.2
- nail(s), anomalous 757.5
- occiput, anterior or posterior 660.3❺
  - fetus or newborn 763.1
- omphalomesenteric duct 751.0
- organ or site NEC – *see* Anomaly, specified type NEC
- ostium
  - atrioventriculare commune 745.69
  - primum 745.61
  - secundum 745.5
- ovarian rests in fallopian tube 752.19
- pancreatic tissue in intestinal tract 751.5
- primary (deciduous)
  - teeth 520.6
  - vitreous hyperplasia 743.51
- pulmonary hypertension 747.83
- pupillary membrane 743.46
  - iris 743.46
  - Rhesus (Rh) titer 999.7
- right aortic arch 747.21
- sinus
  - urogenitalis 752.89
  - venosus with imperfect incorporation in right auricle 747.49
- thymus (gland) 254.8
  - hyperplasia 254.0
- thyroglossal duct 759.2
- thyrolingual duct 759.2
- truncus arteriosus or communis 745.0
- tunica vasculosa lentis 743.39
- umbilical sinus 753.7
- urachus 753.7
- vegetative state 780.03
- vitelline duct 751.0
- Wolffian duct 752.89

Person (with)
- admitted for clinical research, as participant or control subject V70.7
- awaiting admission to adequate facility elsewhere V63.2
  - undergoing social agency investigation V63.8
- concern (normal) about sick person in family V61.49
- consulting on behalf of another V65.19
  - pediatric pre-birth visit for expectant mother V65.11
- feared
  - complaint in whom no diagnosis was made V65.5
  - condition not demonstrated V65.5
- feigning illness V65.2
- healthy, accompanying sick person V65.0
- living (in)
  - alone V60.3
  - boarding school V60.6
  - residence remote from hospital or medical care facility V63.0
  - residential institution V60.6
  - without
    - adequate
      - financial resources V60.2
      - housing (heating) (space) V60.1
    - housing (permanent) (temporary) V60.0
    - material resources V60.2
    - person able to render necessary care V60.4
    - shelter V60.0
- medical services in home not available V63.1
- on waiting list V63.2
  - undergoing social agency investigation V63.8
- sick or handicapped in family V61.49
- "worried well" V65.5

Personality
- affective 301.10
- aggressive 301.3
- amoral 301.7
- anancastic, anankastic 301.4
- antisocial 301.7

Personality – *continued*
- asocial 301.7
- asthenic 301.6
- avoidant 301.82
- borderline 301.83
- change 310.1
- compulsive 301.4
- cycloid 301.13
- cyclothymic 301.13
- dependent 301.6
- depressive (chronic) 301.12
- disorder, disturbance NEC 301.9
  - with
    - antisocial disturbance 301.7
    - pattern disturbance NEC 301.9
    - sociopathic disturbance 301.7
    - trait disturbance 301.9
- dual 300.14
- dyssocial 301.7
- eccentric 301.89
  - "haltlose" type 301.89
- emotionally unstable 301.59
- epileptoid 301.3
- explosive 301.3
- fanatic 301.0
- histrionic 301.50
- hyperthymic 301.11
- hypomanic 301.11
- hypothymic 301.12
- hysterical 301.50
- immature 301.89
- inadequate 301.6
- labile 301.59
- masochistic 301.89
- morally defective 301.7
- multiple 300.14
- narcissistic 301.81
- obsessional 301.4
- obsessive-compulsive 301.4
- overconscientious 301.4
- paranoid 301.0
- passive (-dependent) 301.6
- passive-aggressive 301.84
- pathologic NEC 301.9
- pattern defect or disturbance 301.9
- pseudosocial 301.7
- psychoinfantile 301.59
- psychoneurotic NEC 301.89
- psychopathic 301.9
  - with
    - amoral trend 301.7
    - antisocial trend 301.7
    - asocial trend 301.7
    - pathologic sexuality (*see also* Deviation, sexual) 302.9
  - mixed types 301.9
- schizoid 301.20
  - introverted 301.21
  - schizotypal 301.22
- type A 301.4
- unstable (emotional) 301.59

Perthes' disease (capital femoral osteochondrosis) 732.1

Pertussis (*see also* Whooping cough) 033.9
- vaccination, prophylactic (against) V03.6

Peruvian wart 088.0

Perversion, perverted
- appetite 307.52
  - hysterical 300.11
- function
  - pineal gland 259.8
  - pituitary gland 253.9
    - anterior lobe
      - deficient 253.2
      - excessive 253.1
    - posterior lobe 253.6
  - placenta – *see* Placenta, abnormal
- sense of smell or taste 781.1
  - psychogenic 306.7
- sexual (*see also* Deviation, sexual) 302.9

Pervious, congenital – *see also* Imperfect, closure
- ductus arteriosus 747.0

Pes (congenital) (*see also* Talipes) 754.70
- abductus (congenital) 754.60
  - acquired 736.79
- acquired NEC 736.79
  - planus 734
- adductus (congenital) 754.79
  - acquired 736.79
- cavus 754.71
  - acquired 736.73

Pes – *continued*
- planovalgus (congenital) 754.69
  - acquired 736.79
- planus (acquired) (any degree) 734
  - congenital 754.61
  - rachitic 268.1
- valgus (congenital) 754.61
  - acquired 736.79
- varus (congenital) 754.50
  - acquired 736.79

Pest (*see also* Plague) 020.9

Pestis (*see also* Plague) 020.9
- bubonica 020.0
- fulminans 020.0
- minor 020.8
- pneumonica – *see* Plague, pneumonic

Petechia, petechiae 782.7
- fetus or newborn 772.6

Petechial
- fever 036.0
- typhus 081.9

Petges-Cléjat or Petges-Clégat syndrome (poikilodermatomyositis) 710.3

Petit's
- disease (*see also* Hernia, lumbar) 553.8

Petit mal (idiopathic) (*see also* Epilepsy) 345.0❺
- status 345.2

Petrellidosis 117.6

Petrositis 383.20
- acute 383.21
- chronic 383.22

Peutz-Jeghers disease or syndrome 759.6

Peyronie's disease 607.85

Pfeiffer's disease 075

Phacentocele 379.32
- traumatic 921.3

Phacoanaphylaxis 360.19

Phacocele (old) 379.32
- traumatic 921.3

Phaehyphomycosis 117.8

Phagedena (dry) (moist) (*see also* Gangrene) 785.4
- arteriosclerotic 440.24
- geometric 686.09
- penis 607.89
- senile 440.24
- sloughing 785.4
- tropical (*see also* Ulcer, skin) 707.9
- vulva 616.50

Phagedenic – *see also* condition
- abscess – *see also* Abscess
  - chancroid 099.0
- bubo NEC 099.8
- chancre 099.0
- ulcer (tropical) (*see also* Ulcer, skin) 707.9

Phagomania 307.52

Phakoma 362.89

Phantom limb (syndrome) 353.6

Pharyngeal – *see also* condition
- arch remnant 744.41
- pouch syndrome 279.11

Pharyngitis (acute) (catarrhal) (gangrenous) (infective) (malignant) (membranous) (phlegmonous) (pneumococcal) (pseudomembranous) (simple) (staphylococcal) (subacute) (suppurative) (ulcerative) (viral) 462
- with influenza, flu, or grippe 487.1
- aphthous 074.0
- atrophic 472.1
- chlamydial 099.51
- chronic 472.1
- Coxsackie virus 074.0
- diphtheritic (membranous) 032.0
- follicular 472.1
- fusospirochetal 101
- gonococcal 098.6
- granular (chronic) 472.1
- herpetic 054.79
- hypertrophic 472.1
- infectional, chronic 472.1
- influenzal 487.1
- lymphonodular, acute 074.8
- septic 034.0
- streptococcal 034.0
- tuberculous (*see also* Tuberculosis) 012.8❺
- vesicular 074.0

Pharyngoconjunctival fever 077.2

Pharyngoconjunctivitis, viral 077.2

Pharyngolaryngitis (acute) 465.0
  chronic 478.9
  septic 034.0
Pharyngoplegia 478.29
Pharyngotonsillitis 465.8
  tuberculous 012.8❺
Pharyngotracheitis (acute) 465.8
  chronic 478.9
Pharynx, pharyngeal – *see* condition
Phase of life problem NEC V62.89
Phenomenon
  Arthus 995.21
  flashback (drug) 292.89
  jaw-winking 742.8
  Jod-Basedow 242.8❺
  L. E. cell 710.0
  lupus erythematosus cell 710.0
  Pelger-Huët (hereditary hyposegmentation) 288.2
  Raynaud's (paroxysmal digital cyanosis) (secondary) 443.0
  Reilly's (*see also* Neuropathy, peripheral, autonomic) 337.9
  vasomotor 780.2
  vasospastic 443.9
  vasovagal 780.2
  Wenckebach's, heart block (second degree) 426.13
Phenylketonuria (PKU) 270.1
Phenylpyruvicaciduria 270.1
Pheochromoblastoma (M8700/3)
  specified site – *see* Neoplasm, by site, malignant
  unspecified site 194.0
Pheochromocytoma (M8700/0)
  malignant (M8700/3)
    specified site – *see* Neoplasm, by site, malignant
    unspecified site 194.0
  specified site – *see* Neoplasm, by site, benign
  unspecified site 227.0
Phimosis (congenital) 605
  chancroidal 099.0
  due to infection 605
Phlebectasia (*see also* Varicose, vein) 454.9
  congenital NEC 747.6❺
  esophagus (*see also* Varix, esophagus) 456.1
    with hemorrhage (*see also* Varix, esophagus, bleeding) 456.0
Phlebitis (infective) (pyemic) (septic) (suppurative) 451.9
  antecubital vein 451.82
  arm NEC 451.84
    axillary vein 451.89
    basilic vein 451.82
    deep 451.83
    superficial 451.82
  axillary vein 451.89
  basilic vein 451.82
  blue 451.9
  brachial vein 451.83
  breast, superficial 451.89
  cavernous (venous) sinus – *see* Phlebitis, intracranial sinus
  cephalic vein 451.82
  cerebral (venous) sinus – *see* Phlebitis, intracranial sinus
  chest wall, superficial 451.89
  complicating pregnancy or puerperium 671.9❺
    affecting fetus or newborn 760.3
  cranial (venous) sinus – *see* Phlebitis, intracranial sinus
  deep (vessels) 451.19
    femoral vein 451.11
    specified vessel NEC 451.19
  due to implanted device – *see* Complications, due to (presence of) any device, implant, or graft classified to 996.0-996.5 NEC
  during or resulting from a procedure 997.2
  femoral vein (deep) (superficial) 451.11
  femoropopliteal 451.19
  following infusion, perfusion, or transfusion 999.2
  gouty 274.89 *[451.9]*
  hepatic veins 451.89
  iliac vein 451.81
  iliofemoral 451.11
  intracranial sinus (any) (venous) 325
    late effect – *see* category 326
    nonpyogenic 437.6
      in pregnancy or puerperium 671.5❺
  jugular vein 451.89

Phlebitis – *continued*
  lateral (venous) sinus – *see* Phlebitis, intracranial sinus
  leg 451.2
    deep (vessels) 451.19
      specified vessel NEC 451.19
    superficial (vessels) 451.0
      femoral vein 451.11
  longitudinal sinus – *see* Phlebitis, intracranial sinus
  lower extremity 451.2
    deep (vessels) 451.19
      specified vessel NEC 451.19
    superficial (vessels) 451.0
      femoral vein 451.11
  migrans, migrating (superficial) 453.1
  pelvic
    with
      abortion – *see* Abortion, by type, with sepsis
      ectopic pregnancy (*see also* categories 633.0-633.9) 639.0
      molar pregnancy (*see also* categories 630-632) 639.0
    following
      abortion 639.0
      ectopic or molar pregnancy 639.0
    puerperal, postpartum 671.4❺
  popliteal vein 451.19
  portal (vein) 572.1
  postoperative 997.2
  pregnancy 671.9❺
    deep 671.3❺
    specified type NEC 671.5❺
    superficial 671.2❺
  puerperal, postpartum, childbirth 671.9❺
    deep 671.4❺
    lower extremities 671.2❺
    pelvis 671.4❺
    specified site NEC 671.5❺
    superficial 671.2❺
  radial vein 451.83
  retina 362.18
  saphenous (great) (long) 451.0
    accessory or small 451.0
  sinus (meninges) – *see* Phlebitis, intracranial sinus
  specified site NEC 451.89
  subclavian vein 451.89
  syphilitic 093.89
  tibial vein 451.19
  ulcer, ulcerative 451.9
    leg 451.2
      deep (vessels) 451.19
        specified vessel NEC 451.19
      superficial (vessels) 451.0
        femoral vein 451.11
    lower extremity 451.2
      deep (vessels) 451.19
        femoral vein 451.11
        specified vessel NEC 451.19
      superficial (vessels) 451.0
  ulnar vein 451.83
  umbilicus 451.89
  upper extremity – *see* Phlebitis, arm
    deep (veins) 451.83
      brachial vein 451.83
      radial vein 451.83
      ulnar vein 451.83
    superficial (veins) 451.82
      antecubital vein 451.82
      basilic vein 451.82
      cephalic vein 451.82
  uterus (septic) (*see also* Endometritis) 615.9
  varicose (leg) (lower extremity) (*see also* Varicose, vein) 454.1
Phlebofibrosis 459.89
Phleboliths 459.89
Phlebosclerosis 459.89
Phlebothrombosis – *see* Thrombosis
Phlebotomus fever 066.0
Phlegm, choked on 933.1
Phlegmasia
  alba dolens (deep vessels) 451.19
    complicating pregnancy 671.3❺
    nonpuerperal 451.19
    puerperal, postpartum, childbirth 671.4❺
  cerulea dolens 451.19
Phlegmon (*see also* Abscess) 682.9
  erysipelatous (*see also* Erysipelas) 035
  iliac 682.2
    fossa 540.1
  throat 478.29

Phlegmonous – *see* condition
Phlyctenulosis (allergic) (keratoconjunctivitis) (nontuberculous) 370.31
  cornea 370.31
    with ulcer (*see also* Ulcer, cornea) 370.00
  tuberculous (*see also* Tuberculosis) 017.3❺ *[370.31]*
Phobia, phobic (reaction) 300.20
  animal 300.29
  isolated NEC 300.29
  obsessional 300.3
  simple NEC 300.29
  social 300.23
  specified NEC 300.29
  state 300.20
Phocas' disease 610.1
Phocomelia 755.4
  lower limb 755.32
    complete 755.33
    distal 755.35
    proximal 755.34
  upper limb 755.22
    complete 755.23
    distal 755.25
    proximal 755.24
Phoria (*see also* Heterophoria) 378.40
Phosphate-losing tubular disorder 588.0
Phosphatemia 275.3
Phosphaturia 275.3
Photoallergic response 692.72
Photocoproporphyria 277.1
Photodermatitis (sun) 692.72
  light other than sun 692.82
Photokeratitis 370.24
Photo-ophthalmia 370.24
Photophobia 368.13
Photopsia 368.15
Photoretinitis 363.31
Photoretinopathy 363.31
Photosensitiveness (sun) 692.72
  light other than sun 692.82
Photosensitization skin (sun) 692.72
  light other than sun 692.82
Phototoxic response 692.72
Phrenitis 323.9
Phrynoderma 264.8
Phthiriasis (pubis) (any site) 132.2
  with any infestation classifiable to 132.0 and 132.1 132.3
Phthirus infestation – *see* Phthiriasis
Phthisis (*see also* Tuberculosis) 011.9❺
  bulbi (infectional) 360.41
  colliers' 011.4❺
  cornea 371.05
  eyeball (due to infection) 360.41
  millstone makers' 011.4❺
  miners' 011.4❺
  potters' 011.4❺
  sandblasters' 011.4❺
  stonemasons' 011.4❺
Phycomycosis 117.7
Physalopteriasis 127.7
Physical therapy NEC V57.1
  breathing exercises V57.0
Physiological cup, optic papilla
  borderline, glaucoma suspect 365.00
  enlarged 377.14
  glaucomatous 377.14
Phytobezoar 938
  intestine 936
  stomach 935.2
Pian (*see also* Yaws) 102.9
Pianoma 102.1
Piarhemia, piarrhemia (*see also* Hyperlipemia) 272.4
  bilharziasis 120.9
Pica 307.52
  hysterical 300.11
Pick's
  cerebral atrophy 331.11
    with dementia
      with behavioral disturbance 331.11 *[294.11]*
      without behavioral disturbance 331.11 *[294.10]*

- **Pick's** – *continued*
  - disease
    - brain 331.11
      - dementia in
        - with behavioral disturbance 331.11 *[294.11]*
        - without behavioral disturbance 331.11 *[294.10]*
    - lipid histiocytosis 272.7
    - liver (pericardial pseudocirrhosis of liver) 423.2
    - pericardium (pericardial pseudocirrhosis of liver) 423.2
  - polyserositis (pericardial pseudocirrhosis of liver) 423.2
  - syndrome
    - heart (pericardial pseudocirrhosis of liver) 423.2
    - liver (pericardial pseudocirrhosis of liver) 423.2
  - tubular adenoma (M8640/0)
    - specified site – *see* Neoplasm, by site, benign
    - unspecified site
      - female 220
      - male 222.0
- **Pick-Herxheimer syndrome** (diffuse idiopathic cutaneous atrophy) 701.8
- **Pick-Niemann disease** (lipid histiocytosis) 272.7
- **Pickwickian syndrome** (cardiopulmonary obesity) 278.8
- **Piebaldism, classic** 709.09
- **Piedra** 111.2
  - beard 111.2
    - black 111.3
    - white 111.2
  - black 111.3
  - scalp 111.3
    - black 111.3
    - white 111.2
  - white 111.2
- **Pierre Marie's syndrome** (pulmonary hypertrophic osteoarthropathy) 731.2
- **Pierre Marie-Bamberger syndrome** (hypertrophic pulmonary osteoarthropathy) 731.2
- **Pierre Mauriac's syndrome** (diabetes-dwarfism-obesity) 258.1
- **Pierre Robin deformity or syndrome** (congenital) 756.0
- **Pierson's disease or osteochondrosis** 732.1
- **Pigeon**
  - breast or chest (acquired) 738.3
    - congenital 754.82
    - rachitic (*see also* Rickets) 268.0
  - breeders' disease or lung 495.2
  - fanciers' disease or lung 495.2
  - toe 735.8
- **Pigmentation** (abnormal) 709.00
  - anomalies NEC 709.00
    - congenital 757.33
    - specified NEC 709.09
  - conjunctiva 372.55
  - cornea 371.10
    - anterior 371.11
    - posterior 371.13
    - stromal 371.12
  - lids (congenital) 757.33
    - acquired 374.52
  - limbus corneae 371.10
  - metals 709.00
  - optic papilla, congenital 743.57
  - retina (congenital) (grouped) (nevoid) 743.53
    - acquired 362.74
  - scrotum, congenital 757.33
- **Piles** – *see* Hemorrhoids
- **Pili**
  - annulati or torti (congenital) 757.4
  - incarnati 704.8
- **Pill roller hand** (intrinsic) 736.09
- **Pilomatrixoma** (M8110/0) – *see* Neoplasm, skin, benign
- **Pilonidal** – *see* condition
- **Pimple** 709.8
- **PIN I** (prostatic intraepithelial neoplasia I) 602.3
- **PIN II** (prostatic intraepithelial neoplasia II) 602.3
- **PIN III** (prostatic intraepithelial neoplasia III) 233.4
- **Pinched nerve** – *see* Neuropathy, entrapment
- **Pineal body or gland** – *see* condition
- **Pinealoblastoma** (M9362/3) 194.4
- **Pinealoma** (M9360/1) 237.1
  - malignant (M9360/3) 194.4
- **Pineoblastoma** (M9362/3) 194.4
- **Pineocytoma** (M9361/1) 237.1
- **Pinguecula** 372.51
- **Pinhole meatus** (*see also* Stricture, urethra) 598.9
- **Pink**
  - disease 985.0
  - eye 372.03
  - puffer 492.8
- **Pinkus' disease** (lichen nitidus) 697.1
- **Pinpoint**
  - meatus (*see also* Stricture, urethra) 598.9
  - os (uteri) (*see also* Stricture, cervix) 622.4
- **Pinselhaare** (congenital) 757.4
- **Pinta** 103.9
  - cardiovascular lesions 103.2
  - chancre (primary) 103.0
  - erythematous plaques 103.1
  - hyperchromic lesions 103.1
  - hyperkeratosis 103.1
  - lesions 103.9
    - cardiovascular 103.2
    - hyperchromic 103.1
    - intermediate 103.1
    - late 103.2
    - mixed 103.3
    - primary 103.0
    - skin (achromic) (cicatricial) (dyschromic) 103.2
      - hyperchromic 103.1
      - mixed (achromic and hyperchromic) 103.3
  - papule (primary) 103.0
  - skin lesions (achromic) (cicatricial) (dyschromic) 103.2
    - hyperchromic 103.1
    - mixed (achromic and hyperchromic) 103.3
  - vitiligo 103.2
- **Pintid** 103.0
- **Pinworms** (disease) (infection) (infestation) 127.4
- **Piry fever** 066.8
- **Pistol wound** – *see* Gunshot wound
- **Pit, lip** (mucus), congenital 750.25
- **Pitchers' elbow** 718.82
- **Pithecoid pelvis** 755.69
  - with disproportion (fetopelvic) 653.2❺
    - affecting fetus or newborn 763.1
    - causing obstructed labor 660.1❺
- **Pithiatism** 300.11
- **Pitted** – *see also* Pitting
  - teeth 520.4
- **Pitting** (edema) (*see also* Edema) 782.3
  - lip 782.3
  - nail 703.8
    - congenital 757.5
- **Pituitary gland** – *see* condition
- **Pituitary snuff-takers' disease** 495.8
- **Pityriasis** 696.5
  - alba 696.5
  - capitis 690.11
  - circinata (et maculata) 696.3
  - Hebra's (exfoliative dermatitis) 695.89
  - lichenoides et varioliformis 696.2
  - maculata (et circinata) 696.3
  - nigra 111.1
  - pilaris 757.39
    - acquired 701.1
    - Hebra's 696.4
  - rosea 696.3
  - rotunda 696.3
  - rubra (Hebra) 695.89
    - pilaris 696.4
  - sicca 690.18
  - simplex 690.18
  - specified type NEC 696.5
  - streptogenes 696.5
  - versicolor 111.0
    - scrotal 111.0
- **Placenta, placental**
  - ablatio 641.2❺
    - affecting fetus or newborn 762.1
  - abnormal, abnormality 656.7❺
    - with hemorrhage 641.8❺
      - affecting fetus or newborn 762.1
    - affecting fetus or newborn 762.2
  - abruptio 641.2❺
    - affecting fetus or newborn 762.1
  - accessory lobe – *see* Placenta, abnormal
  - accreta (without hemorrhage) 667.0❺
    - with hemorrhage 666.0❺
  - adherent (without hemorrhage) 667.0❺
    - with hemorrhage 666.0❺
  - apoplexy – *see* Placenta, separation
  - battledore – *see* Placenta, abnormal
  - bilobate – *see* Placenta, abnormal
  - bipartita – *see* Placenta, abnormal
  - carneous mole 631
  - centralis – *see* Placenta, previa
  - circumvallata – *see* Placenta, abnormal
  - cyst (amniotic) – *see* Placenta, abnormal
  - deficiency – *see* Placenta, insufficiency
  - degeneration – *see* Placenta, insufficiency
  - detachment (partial) (premature) (with hemorrhage) 641.2❺
    - affecting fetus or newborn 762.1
  - dimidiata – *see* Placenta, abnormal
  - disease 656.7❺
    - affecting fetus or newborn 762.2
  - duplex – *see* Placenta, abnormal
  - dysfunction – *see* Placenta, insufficiency
  - fenestrata – *see* Placenta, abnormal
  - fibrosis – *see* Placenta, abnormal
  - fleshy mole 631
  - hematoma – *see* Placenta, abnormal
  - hemorrhage NEC – *see* Placenta, separation
  - hormone disturbance or malfunction – *see* Placenta, abnormal
  - hyperplasia – *see* Placenta, abnormal
  - increta (without hemorrhage) 667.0❺
    - with hemorrhage 666.0❺
  - infarction 656.7❺
    - affecting fetus or newborn 762.2
  - insertion, vicious – *see* Placenta, previa
  - insufficiency
    - affecting
      - fetus or newborn 762.2
      - management of pregnancy 656.5❺
  - lateral – *see* Placenta, previa
  - low implantation or insertion – *see* Placenta, previa
  - low-lying – *see* Placenta, previa
  - malformation – *see* Placenta, abnormal
  - malposition – *see* Placenta, previa
  - marginalis, marginata – *see* Placenta, previa
  - marginal sinus (hemorrhage) (rupture) 641.2❺
    - affecting fetus or newborn 762.1
  - membranacea – *see* Placenta, abnormal
  - multilobed – *see* Placenta, abnormal
  - multipartita – *see* Placenta, abnormal
  - necrosis – *see* Placenta, abnormal
  - percreta (without hemorrhage) 667.0❺
    - with hemorrhage 666.0❺
  - polyp 674.4❺
  - previa (central) (centralis) (complete) (lateral) (marginal) (marginalis) (partial) (partialis) (total) (with hemorrhage) 641.1❺
    - affecting fetus or newborn 762.0
    - noted
      - before labor, without hemorrhage (with cesarean delivery) 641.0❺
      - during pregnancy (without hemorrhage) 641.0❺
    - without hemorrhage (before labor and delivery) (during pregnancy) 641.0❺
  - retention (with hemorrhage) 666.0❺
    - fragments, complicating puerperium (delayed hemorrhage) 666.2❺
      - without hemorrhage 667.1❺
    - postpartum, puerperal 666.2❺
    - without hemorrhage 667.0❺
  - separation (normally implanted) (partial) (premature) (with hemorrhage) 641.2❺
    - affecting fetus or newborn 762.1
  - septuplex – *see* Placenta, abnormal
  - small – *see* Placenta, insufficiency
  - softening (premature) – *see* Placenta, abnormal
  - spuria – *see* Placenta, abnormal
  - succenturiata – *see* Placenta, abnormal
  - syphilitic 095.8
  - transfusion syndromes 762.3
  - transmission of chemical substance – *see* Absorption, chemical, through placenta
  - trapped (with hemorrhage) 666.0❺
    - without hemorrhage 667.0❺
  - trilobate – *see* Placenta, abnormal
  - tripartita – *see* Placenta, abnormal
  - triplex – *see* Placenta, abnormal
  - varicose vessel – *see* Placenta, abnormal
  - vicious insertion – *see* Placenta, previa

Placentitis
  affecting fetus or newborn 762.7
  complicating pregnancy 658.4❺
Plagiocephaly (skull) 754.0
Plague 020.9
  abortive 020.8
  ambulatory 020.8
  bubonic 020.0
  cellulocutaneous 020.1
  lymphatic gland 020.0
  pneumonic 020.5
    primary 020.3
    secondary 020.4
  pulmonary – *see* Plague, pneumonic
  pulmonic – *see* Plague, pneumonic
  septicemic 020.2
  tonsillar 020.9
    septicemic 020.2
  vaccination, prophylactic (against) V03.3
Planning, family V25.09
  contraception V25.9
  natural ●
    procreative V26.41 ●
    to avoid pregnancy V25.04 ●
  procreation V26.49 ▲
    natural V26.41●
Plaque
  artery, arterial – *see* Arteriosclerosis
  calcareous – *see* Calcification
  Hollenhorst's (retinal) 362.33
  tongue 528.6
Plasma cell myeloma 203.0❺
Plasmacytoma, plasmocytoma (solitary) (M9731/1) 238.6
  benign (M9731/0) – *see* Neoplasm, by site, benign
  malignant (M9731/3) 203.8❺
Plasmacytopenia 288.59
Plasmacytosis 288.64
Plaster ulcer (*see also* Decubitus) 707.00
Platybasia 756.0
Platyonchia (congenital) 757.5
  acquired 703.8
Platypelloid pelvis 738.6
  with disproportion (fetopelvic) 653.2❺
    affecting fetus or newborn 763.1
    causing obstructed labor 660.1❺
      affecting fetus or newborn 763.1
  congenital 755.69
Platyspondylia 756.19
Plethora 782.62
  newborn 776.4
Pleura, pleural – *see* condition
Pleuralgia 786.52
Pleurisy (acute) (adhesive) (chronic) (costal) (diaphragmatic) (double) (dry) (fetid) (fibrinous) (fibrous) (interlobar) (latent) (lung) (old) (plastic) (primary) (residual) (sicca) (sterile) (subacute) (unresolved) (with adherent pleura) 511.0
  with
    effusion (without mention of cause) 511.9
      bacterial, nontuberculous 511.1
      nontuberculous NEC 511.9
        bacterial 511.1
      pneumococcal 511.1
      specified type NEC 511.8
      staphylococcal 511.1
      streptococcal 511.1
      tuberculous (*see also* Tuberculosis, pleura) 012.0❺
        primary, progressive 010.1❺
    influenza, flu, or grippe 487.1
    tuberculosis – *see* Pleurisy, tuberculous
  encysted 511.8
  exudative (*see also* Pleurisy, with effusion) 511.9
    bacterial, nontuberculous 511.1
  fibrinopurulent 510.9
    with fistula 510.0
  fibropurulent 510.9
    with fistula 510.0
  hemorrhagic 511.8
  influenzal 487.1
  pneumococcal 511.0
    with effusion 511.1
  purulent 510.9
    with fistula 510.0
  septic 510.9
    with fistula 510.0
Pleurisy – *continued*
  serofibrinous (*see also* Pleurisy, with effusion) 511.9
    bacterial, nontuberculous 511.1
  seropurulent 510.9
    with fistula 510.0
  serous (*see also* Pleurisy, with effusion) 511.9
    bacterial, nontuberculous 511.1
  staphylococcal 511.0
    with effusion 511.1
  streptococcal 511.0
    with effusion 511.1
  suppurative 510.9
    with fistula 510.0
  traumatic (post) (current) 862.29
    with open wound into cavity 862.39
  tuberculous (with effusion) (*see also* Tuberculosis, pleura) 012.0❺
    primary, progressive 010.1❺
Pleuritis sicca – *see* Pleurisy
Pleurobronchopneumonia (*see also* Pneumonia, broncho-) 485
Pleurodynia 786.52
  epidemic 074.1
  viral 074.1
Pleurohepatitis 573.8
Pleuropericarditis (*see also* Pericarditis) 423.9
  acute 420.90
Pleuropneumonia (acute) (bilateral) (double) (septic) (*see also* Pneumonia) 486
  chronic (*see also* Fibrosis, lung) 515
Pleurorrhea (*see also* Hydrothorax) 511.8
Plexitis, brachial 353.0
Plica
  knee 727.83
  polonica 132.0
  tonsil 474.8
Plicae dysphonia ventricularis 784.49
Plicated tongue 529.5
  congenital 750.13
Plug
  bronchus NEC 519.19
  meconium (newborn) NEC 777.1
  mucus – *see* Mucus, plug
Plumbism 984.9
  specified type of lead – *see* Table of Drugs and Chemicals
Plummer's disease (toxic nodular goiter) 242.3❺
Plummer-Vinson syndrome (sideropenic dysphagia) 280.8
Pluricarential syndrome of infancy 260
Plurideficiency syndrome of infancy 260
Plus (and minus) **hand** (intrinsic) 736.09
PMDD (premenstrual dysphoric disorder) 625.4
PMS 625.4
Pneumathemia – *see* Air, embolism, by type
Pneumatic drill or hammer disease 994.9
Pneumatocele (lung) 518.89
  intracranial 348.8
  tension 492.0
Pneumatosis
  cystoides intestinalis 569.89
  peritonei 568.89
  pulmonum 492.8
Pneumaturia 599.84
Pneumoblastoma (M8981/3) – *see* Neoplasm, lung, malignant
Pneumocephalus 348.8
Pneumococcemia 038.2
Pneumococcus, pneumococcal – *see* condition
Pneumoconiosis (due to) (inhalation of) 505
  aluminum 503
  asbestos 501
  bagasse 495.1
  bauxite 503
  beryllium 503
  carbon electrode makers' 503
  coal
    miners' (simple) 500
    workers' (simple) 500
  cotton dust 504
  diatomite fibrosis 502
  dust NEC 504
    inorganic 503
    lime 502
    marble 502
    organic NEC 504
Pneumoconiosis – *continued*
  fumes or vapors (from silo) 506.9
  graphite 503
  hard metal 503
  mica 502
  moldy hay 495.0
  rheumatoid 714.81
  silica NEC 502
    and carbon 500
  silicate NEC 502
  talc 502
Pneumocystis carinii pneumonia 136.3
Pneumocystis jiroveci pneumonia 136.3
Pneumocystosis 136.3
  with pneumonia 136.3
Pneumoenteritis 025
Pneumohemopericardium (*see also* Pericarditis) 423.9
Pneumohemothorax (*see also* Hemothorax) 511.8
  traumatic 860.4
    with open wound into thorax 860.5
Pneumohydropericardium (*see also* Pericarditis) 423.9
Pneumohydrothorax (*see also* Hydrothorax) 511.8
Pneumomediastinum 518.1
  congenital 770.2
  fetus or newborn 770.2
Pneumomycosis 117.9
Pneumonia (acute) (Alpenstich) (benign) (bilateral) (brain) (cerebral) (circumscribed) (congestive) (creeping) (delayed resolution) (double) (epidemic) (fever) (flash) (fulminant) (fungoid) (granulomatous) (hemorrhagic) (incipient) (infantile) (infectious) (infiltration) (insular) (intermittent) (latent) (lobe) (migratory) (newborn) (organized) (overwhelming) (primary) (progressive) (pseudolobar) (purulent) (resolved) (secondary) (senile) (septic) (suppurative) (terminal) (true) (unresolved) (vesicular) 486
  with influenza, flu, or grippe 487.0
  adenoviral 480.0
  adynamic 514
  alba 090.0
  allergic 518.3
  alveolar – *see* Pneumonia, lobar
  anaerobes 482.81
  anthrax 022.1 *[484.5]*
  apex, apical – *see* Pneumonia, lobar
  ascaris 127.0 *[484.8]*
  aspiration 507.0
    due to
      aspiration of microorganisms
        bacterial 482.9
          specified type NEC 482.89
        specified organism NEC 483.8
          bacterial NEC 482.89
        viral 480.9
          specified type NEC 480.8
      food (regurgitated) 507.0
      gastric secretions 507.0
      milk 507.0
      oils, essences 507.1
      solids, liquids NEC 507.8
      vomitus 507.0
    fetal 770.18
      due to
        blood 770.16
        clear amniotic fluid 770.14
        meconium 770.12
        postnatal stomach contents 770.86
    newborn 770.18
      due to
        blood 770.16
        clear amniotic fluid 770.14
        meconium 770.12
        postnatal stomach contents 770.86
  asthenic 514
  atypical (disseminated) (focal) (primary) 486
    with influenza 487.0
  bacillus 482.9
    specified type NEC 482.89
  bacterial 482.9
    specified type NEC 482.89
  Bacteroides (fragilis) (oralis) (melaninogenicus) 482.81
  basal, basic, basilar – *see* Pneumonia, lobar

- **Pneumonia** – *continued*
  - broncho-, bronchial (confluent) (croupous) (diffuse) (disseminated) (hemorrhagic) (involving lobes) (lobar) (terminal) 485
    - with influenza 487.0
    - allergic 518.3
    - aspiration (*see also* Pneumonia, aspiration) 507.0
    - bacterial 482.9
      - specified type NEC 482.89
    - capillary 466.19
      - with bronchospasm or obstruction 466.19
    - chronic (*see also* Fibrosis, lung) 515
    - congenital (infective) 770.0
    - diplococcal 481
    - Eaton's agent 483.0
    - Escherichia coli (E. coli) 482.82
    - Friedländer's bacillus 482.0
    - Hemophilus influenzae 482.2
    - hiberno-vernal 083.0 *[484.8]*
    - hypostatic 514
    - influenzal 487.0
    - inhalation (*see also* Pneumonia, aspiration) 507.0
      - due to fumes or vapors (chemical) 506.0
    - Klebsiella 482.0
    - lipid 507.1
      - endogenous 516.8
    - Mycoplasma (pneumoniae) 483.0
    - ornithosis 073.0
    - pleuropneumonia-like organisms (PPLO) 483.0
    - pneumococcal 481
    - Proteus 482.83
    - Pseudomonas 482.1
    - specified organism NEC 483.8
      - bacterial NEC 482.89
    - staphylococcal 482.40
      - aureus 482.41
      - specified type NEC 482.49
    - streptococcal – *see* Pneumonia, streptococcal
    - typhoid 002.0 *[484.8]*
    - viral, virus (*see also* Pneumonia, viral) 480.9
  - Butyrivibrio (fibriosolvens) 482.81
  - Candida 112.4
  - capillary 466.19
    - with bronchospasm or obstruction 466.19
  - caseous (*see also* Tuberculosis) 011.6❺
  - catarrhal – *see* Pneumonia, broncho-
  - central – *see* Pneumonia, lobar
  - Chlamydia, chlamydial 483.1
    - pneumoniae 483.1
    - psittaci 073.0
    - specified type NEC 483.1
    - trachomatis 483.1
  - cholesterol 516.8
  - chronic (*see also* Fibrosis, lung) 515
  - cirrhotic (chronic) (*see also* Fibrosis, lung) 515
  - Clostridium (haemolyticum) (novyi) NEC 482.81
  - confluent – *see* Pneumonia, broncho-
  - congenital (infective) 770.0
    - aspiration 770.18
  - croupous – *see* Pneumonia, lobar
  - cytomegalic inclusion 078.5 *[484.1]*
  - deglutition (*see also* Pneumonia, aspiration) 507.0
  - desquamative interstitial 516.8
  - diffuse – *see* Pneumonia, broncho-
  - diplococcal, diplococcus (broncho-) (lobar) 481
  - disseminated (focal) – *see* Pneumonia, broncho-
  - due to
    - adenovirus 480.0
    - anaerobes 482.81
    - Bacterium anitratum 482.83
    - Chlamydia, chlamydial 483.1
      - pneumoniae 483.1
      - psittaci 073.0
      - specified type NEC 483.1
      - trachomatis 483.1
    - coccidioidomycosis 114.0
    - Diplococcus (pneumoniae) 481
    - Eaton's agent 483.0
    - Escherichia coli (E. coli) 482.82
    - Friedländer's bacillus 482.0
    - fumes or vapors (chemical) (inhalation) 506.0
    - fungus NEC 117.9 *[484.7]*
      - coccidioidomycosis 114.0
    - Hemophilus influenzae (H. influenzae) 482.2
    - Herellea 482.83
    - influenza 487.0
    - Klebsiella pneumoniae 482.0
    - Mycoplasma (pneumoniae) 483.0
    - parainfluenza virus 480.2

- **Pneumonia** – *continued*
  - due to – *continued*
    - pleuropneumonia-like organism (PPLO) 483.0
    - Pneumococcus 481
    - Pneumocystis carinii 136.3
    - Pneumocystis jiroveci 136.3
    - Proteus 482.83
    - Pseudomonas 482.1
    - respiratory syncytial virus 480.1
    - rickettsia 083.9 *[484.8]*
    - SARS-associated coronavirus 480.3
    - specified
      - bacteria NEC 482.89
      - organism NEC 483.8
      - virus NEC 480.8
    - Staphylococcus 482.40
      - aureus 482.41
      - specified type NEC 482.49
    - Streptococcus – *see also* Pneumonia, streptococcal
      - pneumoniae 481
    - virus (*see also* Pneumonia, viral) 480.9
  - Eaton's agent 483.0
  - embolic, embolism (*see* Embolism, pulmonary) 415.1❺
  - eosinophilic 518.3
  - Escherichia coli (E. coli) 482.82
  - Eubacterium 482.81
  - fibrinous – *see* Pneumonia, lobar
  - fibroid (chronic) (*see also* Fibrosis, lung) 515
  - fibrous (*see also* Fibrosis, lung) 515
  - Friedländer's bacillus 482.0
  - fusobacterium (nucleatum) 482.81
  - gangrenous 513.0
  - giant cell (*see also* Pneumonia, viral) 480.9
  - gram-negative bacteria NEC 482.83
    - anaerobic 482.81
  - grippal 487.0
  - Hemophilus influenzae (bronchial) (lobar) 482.2
  - hypostatic (broncho-) (lobar) 514
  - in
    - actinomycosis 039.1
    - anthrax 022.1 *[484.5]*
    - aspergillosis 117.3 *[484.6]*
    - candidiasis 112.4
    - coccidioidomycosis 114.0
    - cytomegalic inclusion disease 078.5 *[484.1]*
    - histoplasmosis (*see also* Histoplasmosis) 115.95
    - infectious disease NEC 136.9 *[484.8]*
    - measles 055.1
    - mycosis, systemic NEC 117.9 *[484.7]*
    - nocardiasis, nocardiosis 039.1
    - ornithosis 073.0
    - pneumocystosis 136.3
    - psittacosis 073.0
    - Q fever 083.0 *[484.8]*
    - salmonellosis 003.22
    - toxoplasmosis 130.4
    - tularemia 021.2
    - typhoid (fever) 002.0 *[484.8]*
    - varicella 052.1
    - whooping cough (*see also* Whooping cough) 033.9 *[484.3]*
  - infective, acquired prenatally 770.0
  - influenzal (broncho) (lobar) (virus) 487.0
  - inhalation (*see also* Pneumonia, aspiration) 507.0
    - fumes or vapors (chemical) 506.0
  - interstitial 516.8
    - with influenzal 487.0
    - acute 136.3
    - chronic (*see also* Fibrosis, lung) 515
    - desquamative 516.8
    - hypostatic 514
    - lipoid 507.1
    - lymphoid 516.8
    - plasma cell 136.3
    - Pseudomonas 482.1
  - intrauterine (infective) 770.0
    - aspiration 770.18
      - blood 770.16
      - clear amniotic fluid 770.14
      - meconium 770.12
      - postnatal stomach contents 770.86
  - Klebsiella pneumoniae 482.0
  - Legionnaires' 482.84
  - lipid, lipoid (exogenous) (interstitial) 507.1
    - endogenous 516.8
  - lobar (diplococcal) (disseminated) (double) (interstitial) (pneumococcal, any type) 481
    - with influenza 487.0

- **Pneumonia** – *continued*
  - lobar – *continued*
    - bacterial 482.9
      - specified type NEC 482.89
    - chronic (*see also* Fibrosis, lung) 515
    - Escherichia coli (E. coli) 482.82
    - Friedländer's bacillus 482.0
    - Hemophilus influenzae (H. influenzae) 482.2
    - hypostatic 514
    - influenzal 487.0
    - Klebsiella 482.0
    - ornithosis 073.0
    - Proteus 482.83
    - Pseudomonas 482.1
    - psittacosis 073.0
    - specified organism NEC 483.8
      - bacterial NEC 482.89
    - staphylococcal 482.40
      - aureus 482.41
      - specified type NEC 482.49
    - streptococcal – *see* Pneumonia, streptococcal
    - viral, virus (*see also* Pneumonia, viral) 480.9
  - lobular (confluent) – *see* Pneumonia, broncho-
  - Löffler's 518.3
  - massive – *see* Pneumonia, lobar
  - meconium aspiration 770.12
  - metastatic NEC 038.8 *[484.8]*
  - Mycoplasma (pneumoniae) 483.0
  - necrotic 513.0
  - nitrogen dioxide 506.9
  - orthostatic 514
  - parainfluenza virus 480.2
  - parenchymatous (*see also* Fibrosis, lung) 515
  - passive 514
  - patchy – *see* Pneumonia, broncho
  - Peptococcus 482.81
  - Peptostreptococcus 482.81
  - plasma cell 136.3
  - pleurolobar – *see* Pneumonia, lobar
  - pleuropneumonia-like organism (PPLO) 483.0
  - pneumococcal (broncho) (lobar) 481
  - Pneumocystis (carinii) (jiroveci) 136.3
  - postinfectional NEC 136.9 *[484.8]*
  - postmeasles 055.1
  - postoperative 997.3
  - primary atypical 486
  - Proprionibacterium 482.81
  - Proteus 482.83
  - Pseudomonas 482.1
  - psittacosis 073.0
  - radiation 508.0
  - respiratory syncytial virus 480.1
  - resulting from a procedure 997.3
  - rheumatic 390 *[517.1]*
  - Salmonella 003.22
  - SARS-associated coronavirus 480.3
  - segmented, segmental – *see* Pneumonia, broncho-
  - Serratia (marcascens) 482.83
  - specified
    - bacteria NEC 482.89
    - organism NEC 483.8
    - virus NEC 480.8
  - spirochetal 104.8 *[484.8]*
  - staphylococcal (broncho) (lobar) 482.40
    - aureus 482.41
    - specified type NEC 482.49
  - static, stasis 514
  - streptococcal (broncho) (lobar) NEC 482.30
    - Group
      - A 482.31
      - B 482.32
      - specified NEC 482.39
    - pneumoniae 481
    - specified type NEC 482.39
  - Streptococcus pneumoniae 481
  - traumatic (complication) (early) (secondary) 958.8
  - tuberculous (any) (*see also* Tuberculosis) 011.6❺
  - tularemic 021.2
  - TWAR agent 483.1
  - varicella 052.1
  - Veillonella 482.81
  - ventilator associated 999.9 ●
  - viral, virus (broncho) (interstitial) (lobar) 480.9
    - with influenza, flu, or grippe 487.0
    - adenoviral 480.0
    - parainfluenza 480.2
    - respiratory syncytial 480.1
    - SARS-associated coronavirus 480.3
    - specified type NEC 480.8
  - white (congenital) 090.0

Pneumonic – *see* condition

Pneumonitis (acute) (primary) (*see also* Pneumonia) 486
- allergic 495.9
  - specified type NEC 495.8
- aspiration 507.0
  - due to fumes or gases 506.0
  - fetal 770.18
    - due to
      - blood 770.16
      - clear amniotic fluid 770.14
      - meconium 770.12
      - postnatal stomach contents 770.86
  - newborn 770.18
    - due to
      - blood 770.16
      - clear amniotic fluid 770.14
      - meconium 770.12
      - postnatal stomach contents 770.86
  - obstetric 668.0❺
- chemical 506.0
  - due to fumes or gases 506.0
- cholesterol 516.8
- chronic (*see also* Fibrosis, lung) 515
- congenital rubella 771.0
- crack 506.0
- due to
  - crack (cocaine) 506.0
  - fumes or vapors 506.0
  - inhalation
    - food (regurgitated), milk, vomitus 507.0
    - oils, essences 507.1
    - saliva 507.0
    - solids, liquids NEC 507.8
  - toxoplasmosis (acquired) 130.4
    - congenital (active) 771.2 *[484.8]*
- eosinophilic 518.3
- fetal aspiration 770.18
  - due to
    - blood 770.16
    - clear amniotic fluid 770.14
    - meconium 770.12
    - postnatal stomach contents 770.86
- hypersensitivity 495.9
- interstitial (chronic) (*see also* Fibrosis, lung) 515
  - lymphoid 516.8
- lymphoid, interstitial 516.8
- meconium aspiration 770.12
- postanesthetic
  - correct substance properly administered 507.0
  - obstetric 668.0❺
  - overdose or wrong substance given 968.4
    - specified anesthetic – *see* Table of Drugs and Chemicals
- postoperative 997.3
  - obstetric 668.0❺
- radiation 508.0
- rubella, congenital 771.0
- "ventilation" 495.7
- wood-dust 495.8

Pneumonoconiosis – *see* Pneumoconiosis

Pneumoparotid 527.8

Pneumopathy NEC 518.89
- alveolar 516.9
  - specified NEC 516.8
- due to dust NEC 504
- parietoalveolar 516.9
  - specified condition NEC 516.8

Pneumopericarditis (*see also* Pericarditis) 423.9
- acute 420.90

Pneumopericardium – *see also* Pericarditis
- congenital 770.2
- fetus or newborn 770.2
- traumatic (post) (*see also* Pneumothorax, traumatic) 860.0
  - with open wound into thorax 860.1

Pneumoperitoneum 568.89
- fetus or newborn 770.2

Pneumophagia (psychogenic) 306.4

Pneumopleurisy, pneumopleuritis (*see also* Pneumonia) 486

Pneumopyopericardium 420.99

Pneumopyothorax (*see also* Pyopneumothorax) 510.9
- with fistula 510.0

Pneumorrhagia 786.3
- newborn 770.3
- tuberculous (*see also* Tuberculosis, pulmonary) 011.9❺

Pneumosiderosis (occupational) 503

Pneumothorax (acute) (chronic) 512.8
- congenital 770.2
- due to operative injury of chest wall or lung 512.1
  - accidental puncture or laceration 512.1
- fetus or newborn 770.2
- iatrogenic 512.1
- postoperative 512.1
- spontaneous 512.8
  - fetus or newborn 770.2
  - tension 512.0
- sucking 512.8
  - iatrogenic 512.1
  - postoperative 512.1
- tense valvular, infectional 512.0
- tension 512.0
  - iatrogenic 512.1
  - postoperative 512.1
  - spontaneous 512.0
- traumatic 860.0
  - with
    - hemothorax 860.4
      - with open wound into thorax 860.5
    - open wound into thorax 860.1
- tuberculous (*see also* Tuberculosis) 011.7❺

Pocket(s)
- endocardial (*see also* Endocarditis) 424.90
- periodontal 523.8

Podagra 274.9

Podencephalus 759.89

Poikilocytosis 790.09

Poikiloderma 709.09
- Civatte's 709.09
- congenital 757.33
- vasculare atrophicans 696.2

Poikilodermatomyositis 710.3

Pointed ear 744.29

Poise imperfect 729.9

Poisoned – *see* Poisoning

Poisoning (acute) – *see also* Table of Drugs and Chemicals
- Bacillus, B.
  - aertrycke (*see also* Infection, Salmonella) 003.9
  - botulinus 005.1
  - cholerae (suis) (*see also* Infection, Salmonella) 003.9
  - paratyphosus (*see also* Infection, Salmonella) 003.9
  - suipestifer (*see also* Infection, Salmonella) 003.9
- bacterial toxins NEC 005.9
- berries, noxious 988.2
- blood (general) – *see* Septicemia
- botulism 005.1
- bread, moldy, mouldy – *see* Poisoning, food
- Ciguatera 988.0 ●
- damaged meat – *see* Poisoning, food
- death-cap (Amanita phalloides) (Amanita verna) 988.1
- decomposed food – *see* Poisoning, food
- diseased food – *see* Poisoning, food
- drug – *see* Table of Drugs and Chemicals
- epidemic, fish, meat, or other food – *see* Poisoning, food
- fava bean 282.2
- fish (bacterial) – *see also* Poisoning, food
  - noxious 988.0
- food (acute) (bacterial) (diseased) (infected) NEC 005.9
  - due to
    - bacillus
      - aertrycke (*see also* Poisoning, food, due to Salmonella) 003.9
      - botulinus 005.1
      - cereus 005.89
      - choleraesuis (*see also* Poisoning, food, due to Salmonella) 003.9
      - paratyphosus (*see also* Poisoning, food, due to Salmonella) 003.9
      - suipestifer (*see also* Poisoning, food, due to Salmonella) 003.9
    - Clostridium 005.3
      - botulinum 005.1
      - perfringens 005.2
      - welchii 005.2
    - Salmonella (aertrycke) (callinarum) (choleraesuis) (enteritidis) (paratyphi) (suipestifer) 003.9
      - with
        - gastroenteritis 003.0

Poisoning – *continued*
- food – *continued*
  - due to – *continued*
    - Salmonella – *continued*
      - with – *continued*
        - localized infection(s) (*see also* Infection, Salmonella) 003.20
        - septicemia 003.1
        - specified manifestation NEC 003.8
    - specified bacterium NEC 005.89
    - Staphylococcus 005.0
    - Streptococcus 005.8❺
    - Vibrio parahaemolyticus 005.4
    - Vibrio vulnificus 005.81
  - noxious or naturally toxic 988.0
    - berries 988.2
    - fish 988.0
    - mushroom 988.1
    - plants NEC 988.2
- ice cream – *see* Poisoning, food
- ichthyotoxism (bacterial) 005.9
- kreotoxism, food 005.9
- malarial – *see* Malaria
- meat – *see* Poisoning, food
- mushroom (noxious) 988.1
- mussel – *see also* Poisoning, food
  - noxious 988.0
- noxious foodstuffs (*see also* Poisoning, food, noxious) 988.9
  - specified type NEC 988.8
- plants, noxious 988.2
- pork – *see also* Poisoning, food
  - specified NEC 988.8
  - Trichinosis 124
- ptomaine – *see* Poisoning, food
- putrefaction, food – *see* Poisoning, food
- radiation 508.0
- Salmonella (*see also* Infection, Salmonella) 003.9
- sausage – *see also* Poisoning, food
  - Trichinosis 124
- saxitoxin 988.0
- shellfish – *see also* Poisoning, food
  - noxious ▶(amnesic) (azaspiracic) (diarrheic) (neurotoxic) (paralytic)◀ 988.0
- Staphylococcus, food 005.0
- toxic, from disease NEC 799.89
- truffles – *see* Poisoning, food
- uremic – *see* Uremia
- uric acid 274.9
- water 276.6 ●

Poison ivy, oak, sumac or other plant dermatitis 692.6

Poker spine 720.0

Policeman's disease 729.2

Polioencephalitis (acute) (bulbar) (*see also* Poliomyelitis, bulbar) 045.0❺
- inferior 335.22
- influenzal 487.8
- superior hemorrhagic (acute) (Wernicke's) 265.1
- Wernicke's (superior hemorrhagic) 265.1

Polioencephalomyelitis (acute) (anterior) (bulbar) (*see also* Polioencephalitis) 045.0❺

Polioencephalopathy, superior hemorrhagic 265.1
- with
  - beriberi 265.0
  - pellagra 265.2

Poliomeningoencephalitis – *see* Meningoencephalitis

Poliomyelitis (acute) (anterior) (epidemic) 045.9

Note – Use the following fifth-digit subclassification with category 045:
0 poliovirus, unspecified type
1 poliovirus, type I
2 poliovirus, type II
3 poliovirus, type III

- with
  - paralysis 045.1❺
    - bulbar 045.0❺
- abortive 045.2❺
- ascending 045.9❺
  - progressive 045.9❺
- bulbar 045.0❺
- cerebral 045.0❺
- chronic 335.21
- congenital 771.2
- contact V01.2
- deformities 138
- exposure to V01.2
- late effect 138
- nonepidemic 045.9❺

- **Poliomyelitis** – *continued*
  - nonparalytic 045.2❺
  - old with deformity 138
  - posterior, acute 053.19
  - residual 138
  - sequelae 138
  - spinal, acute 045.9❺
  - syphilitic (chronic) 094.89
  - vaccination, prophylactic (against) V04.0
- **Poliosis** (eyebrow) (eyelashes) 704.3
  - circumscripta (congenital) 757.4
    - acquired 704.3
  - congenital 757.4
- **Pollakiuria** 788.4❺
  - psychogenic 306.53
- **Pollinosis** 477.0
- **Pollitzer's disease** (hidradenitis suppurativa) 705.83
- **Polyadenitis** (*see also* Adenitis) 289.3
  - malignant 020.0
- **Polyalgia** 729.9
- **Polyangiitis** (essential) 446.0
- **Polyarteritis** (nodosa) (renal) 446.0
- **Polyarthralgia** 719.49
  - psychogenic 306.0
- **Polyarthritis, polyarthropathy** NEC 716.59
  - due to or associated with other specified conditions – *see* Arthritis, due to or associated with
  - endemic (*see also* Disease, Kaschin-Beck) 716.0❺
  - inflammatory 714.9
    - specified type NEC 714.89
  - juvenile (chronic) 714.30
    - acute 714.31
  - migratory – *see* Fever, rheumatic
  - rheumatic 714.0
    - fever (acute) – *see* Fever, rheumatic
- **Polycarential syndrome of infancy** 260
- **Polychondritis** (atrophic) (chronic) (relapsing) 733.99
- **Polycoria** 743.46
- **Polycystic** (congenital) (disease) 759.89
  - degeneration, kidney – *see* Polycystic, kidney
  - kidney (congenital) 753.12
    - adult type (APKD) 753.13
    - autosomal dominant 753.13
    - autosomal recessive 753.14
    - childhood type (CPKD) 753.14
    - infantile type 753.14
  - liver 751.62
  - lung 518.89
    - congenital 748.4
  - ovary, ovaries 256.4
  - spleen 759.0
- **Polycythemia** (primary) (rubra) (vera) (M9950/1) 238.4
  - acquired 289.0
  - benign 289.0
    - familial 289.6
  - due to
    - donor twin 776.4
    - fall in plasma volume 289.0
    - high altitude 289.0
    - maternal-fetal transfusion 776.4
    - stress 289.0
  - emotional 289.0
  - erythropoietin 289.0
  - familial (benign) 289.6
  - Gaisböck's (hypertonica) 289.0
  - high altitude 289.0
  - hypertonica 289.0
  - hypoxemic 289.0
  - neonatorum 776.4
  - nephrogenous 289.0
  - relative 289.0
  - secondary 289.0
  - spurious 289.0
  - stress 289.0
- **Polycytosis cryptogenica** 289.0
- **Polydactylism, polydactyly** 755.00
  - fingers 755.01
  - toes 755.02
- **Polydipsia** 783.5
- **Polydystrophic oligophrenia** 277.5
- **Polyembryoma** (M9072/3) – *see* Neoplasm, by site, malignant
- **Polygalactia** 676.6❺
- **Polyglandular**
  - deficiency 258.9
- **Polyglandular** – *continued*
  - dyscrasia 258.9
  - dysfunction 258.9
  - syndrome 258.8
- **Polyhydramnios** (*see also* Hydramnios) 657❺
- **Polymastia** 757.6
- **Polymenorrhea** 626.2
- **Polymicrogyria** 742.2
- **Polymyalgia** 725
  - arteritica 446.5
  - rheumatica 725
- **Polymyositis** (acute) (chronic) (hemorrhagic) 710.4
  - with involvement of
    - lung 710.4 *[517.8]*
    - skin 710.3
  - ossificans (generalisata) (progressiva) 728.19
  - Wagner's (dermatomyositis) 710.3
- **Polyneuritis, polyneuritic** (*see also* Polyneuropathy) 356.9
  - alcoholic 357.5
    - with psychosis 291.1
  - cranialis 352.6
  - demyelinating, chronic inflammatory ▶(CIDP)◀ 357.81
  - diabetic 250.6❺ *[357.2]*
  - due to lack of vitamin NEC 269.2 *[357.4]*
  - endemic 265.0 *[357.4]*
  - erythredema 985.0
  - febrile 357.0
  - hereditary ataxic 356.3
  - idiopathic, acute 357.0
  - infective (acute) 357.0
  - nutritional 269.9 *[357.4]*
  - postinfectious 357.0
- **Polyneuropathy** (peripheral) 356.9
  - alcoholic 357.5
  - amyloid 277.39 *[357.4]*
  - arsenical 357.7
  - critical illness 357.82
  - demyelinating, chronic inflammatory (CIDP) 357.81 ●
  - diabetic 250.6❺ *[357.2]*
  - due to
    - antitetanus serum 357.6
    - arsenic 357.7
    - drug or medicinal substance 357.6
      - correct substance properly administered 357.6
      - overdose or wrong substance given or taken 977.9
        - specified drug – *see* Table of Drugs and Chemicals
    - lack of vitamin NEC 269.2 *[357.4]*
    - lead 357.7
    - organophosphate compounds 357.7
    - pellagra 265.2 *[357.4]*
    - porphyria 277.1 *[357.4]*
    - serum 357.6
    - toxic agent NEC 357.7
  - hereditary 356.0
  - idiopathic 356.9
    - progressive 356.4
  - in
    - amyloidosis 277.39 *[357.4]*
    - avitaminosis 269.2 *[357.4]*
      - specified NEC 269.1 *[357.4]*
    - beriberi 265.0 *[357.4]*
    - collagen vascular disease NEC 710.9 *[357.1]*
    - deficiency
      - B-complex NEC 266.2 *[357.4]*
      - vitamin B 266.9 *[357.4]*
      - vitamin B6 266.1 *[357.4]*
    - diabetes 250.6❺ *[357.2]*
    - diphtheria (*see also* Diphtheria) 032.89 *[357.4]*
    - disseminated lupus erythematosus 710.0 *[357.1]*
    - herpes zoster 053.13
    - hypoglycemia 251.2 *[357.4]*
    - malignant neoplasm (M8000/3) NEC 199.1 *[357.3]*
    - mumps 072.72
    - pellagra 265.2 *[357.4]*
    - polyarteritis nodosa 446.0 *[357.1]*
    - porphyria 277.1 *[357.4]*
    - rheumatoid arthritis 714.0 *[357.1]*
    - sarcoidosis 135 *[357.4]*
    - uremia 585.9 *[357.4]*
  - lead 357.7
  - nutritional 269.9 *[357.4]*
    - specified NEC 269.8 *[357.4]*
  - postherpetic 053.13
- **Polyneuropathy** – *continued*
  - progressive 356.4
  - sensory (hereditary) 356.2
  - specified NEC 356.8 ●
- **Polyonychia** 757.5
- **Polyopia** 368.2
  - refractive 368.15
- **Polyorchism, polyorchidism** (three testes) 752.89
- **Polyorrhymenitis** (peritoneal) (*see also* Polyserositis) 568.82
  - pericardial 423.2
- **Polyostotic fibrous dysplasia** 756.54
- **Polyotia** 744.1
- **Polyp, polypus**

Note – Polyps of organs or sites that do not appear in the list below should be coded to the residual category for diseases of the organ or site concerned.

  - accessory sinus 471.8
  - adenoid tissue 471.0
  - adenomatous (M8210/0) – *see also* Neoplasm, by site, benign
    - adenocarcinoma in (M8210/3) – *see* Neoplasm, by site, malignant
    - carcinoma in (M8210/3) – *see* Neoplasm, by site, malignant
    - multiple (M8221/0) – *see* Neoplasm, by site, benign
  - antrum 471.8
  - anus, anal (canal) (nonadenomatous) 569.0
    - adenomatous 211.4
  - Bartholin's gland 624.6
  - bladder (M8120/1) 236.7
  - broad ligament 620.8
  - cervix (uteri) 622.7
    - adenomatous 219.0
    - in pregnancy or childbirth 654.6❺
      - affecting fetus or newborn 763.89
      - causing obstructed labor 660.2❺
    - mucous 622.7
    - nonneoplastic 622.7
  - choanal 471.0
  - cholesterol 575.6
  - clitoris 624.6
  - colon (M8210/0) (*see also* Polyp, adenomatous) 211.3
  - corpus uteri 621.0
  - dental 522.0
  - ear (middle) 385.30
  - endometrium 621.0
  - ethmoidal (sinus) 471.8
  - fallopian tube 620.8
  - female genital organs NEC 624.8
  - frontal (sinus) 471.8
  - gallbladder 575.6
  - gingiva 523.8
  - gum 523.8
  - labia 624.6
  - larynx (mucous) 478.4
  - malignant (M8000/3) – *see* Neoplasm, by site, malignant
  - maxillary (sinus) 471.8
  - middle ear 385.30
  - myometrium 621.0
  - nares
    - anterior 471.9
    - posterior 471.0
  - nasal (mucous) 471.9
    - cavity 471.0
    - septum 471.9
  - nasopharyngeal 471.0
  - neoplastic (M8210/0) – *see* Neoplasm, by site, benign
  - nose (mucous) 471.9
  - oviduct 620.8
  - paratubal 620.8
  - pharynx 478.29
    - congenital 750.29
  - placenta, placental 674.4❺
  - prostate 600.20
    - with
      - other lower urinary tract symptoms (LUTS) 600.21
      - urinary
        - obstruction 600.21
        - retention 600.21
  - pudenda 624.6
  - pulp (dental) 522.0
  - rectosigmoid 211.4

Poliomyelitis – Polyp, polypus

Potter's – *continued*
syndrome (with renal agenesis) 753.0
Pouch
bronchus 748.3
Douglas' – *see* condition
esophagus, esophageal (congenital) 750.4
acquired 530.6
gastric 537.1
Hartmann's (abnormal sacculation of gallbladder neck) 575.8
of intestine V44.3
attention to V55.3
pharynx, pharyngeal (congenital) 750.27
Poulet's disease 714.2
Poultrymen's itch 133.8
Poverty V60.2
PPE (palmar plantar erythrodysesthesia) 693.0 ●
Prader-Labhart-Willi-Fanconi syndrome (hypogenital dystrophy with diabetic tendency) 759.81
Prader-Willi syndrome (hypogenital dystrophy with diabetic tendency) 759.81
Preachers' voice 784.49
Pre-AIDS – *see* Human immunodeficiency virus (disease) (illness) (infection)
Preauricular appendage 744.1
Prebetalipoproteinemia (acquired) (essential) (familial) (hereditary) (primary) (secondary) 272.1
with chylomicronemia 272.3
Precipitate labor 661.3❺
affecting fetus or newborn 763.6
Preclimacteric bleeding 627.0
menorrhagia 627.0
Precocious
adrenarche 259.1
menarche 259.1
menstruation 626.8
pubarche 259.1
puberty NEC 259.1
sexual development NEC 259.1
thelarche 259.1
Precocity, sexual (constitutional) (cryptogenic) (female) (idiopathic) (male) NEC 259.1
with adrenal hyperplasia 255.2
Precordial pain 786.51
psychogenic 307.89
Predeciduous teeth 520.2
Prediabetes, prediabetic 790.29
complicating pregnancy, childbirth, or puerperium 648.8❺
fetus or newborn 775.89
Predislocation status of hip, at birth (*see also* Subluxation, congenital, hip) 754.32
Pre-eclampsia (mild) 642.4❺
with pre-existing hypertension 642.7❺
affecting fetus or newborn 760.0
severe 642.5❺
superimposed on pre-existing hypertensive disease 642.7❺
Preeruptive color change, teeth, tooth 520.8
Preexcitation 426.7
atrioventricular conduction 426.7
ventricular 426.7
Preglaucoma 365.00
Pregnancy (single) (uterine) (without sickness) V22.2

Note – Use the following fifth-digit subclassification with categories 640-648, 651-676:

0 unspecified as to episode of care
1 delivered, with or without mention of antepartum condition
2 delivered, with mention of postpartum complication
3 antepartum condition or complication
4 postpartum condition or complication

abdominal (ectopic) 633.00
with intrauterine pregnancy 633.01
affecting fetus or newborn 761.4
abnormal NEC 646.9❺
ampullar – *see* Pregnancy, tubal
broad ligament – *see* Pregnancy, cornual
cervical – *see* Pregnancy, cornual
combined (extrauterine and intrauterine) – *see* Pregnancy, cornual
complicated (by) 646.9
abnormal, abnormality NEC 646.9❺
cervix 654.6❺

Pregnancy – *continued*
complicated (by) – *continued*
abnormal, abnormality – *continued*
cord (umbilical) 663.9❺
glucose tolerance (conditions classifiable to 790.21-790.29) 648.8❺
injury 648.9❺
obstetrical NEC 665.9❺
obstetrical trauma NEC 665.9❺
pelvic organs or tissues NEC 654.9❺
pelvis (bony) 653.0❺
perineum or vulva 654.8❺
placenta, placental (vessel) 656.7❺
position
cervix 654.4❺
placenta 641.1❺
without hemorrhage 641.0❺
uterus 654.4❺
size, fetus 653.5❺
uterus (congenital) 654.0❺
abscess or cellulitis
bladder 646.6❺
genitourinary tract (conditions classifiable to 590, 595, 597, 599.0, 614.0-614.5, 614.7-614.9, 615) 646.6❺
kidney 646.6❺
urinary tract NEC 646.6❺
adhesion, pelvic peritoneal 648.9❺
air embolism 673.0❺
albuminuria 646.2❺
with hypertension – *see* Toxemia, of pregnancy
amnionitis 658.4❺
amniotic fluid embolism 673.1❺
anemia (conditions classifiable to 280-285) 648.2❺
appendicitis 648.9❺
atrophy, yellow (acute) (liver) (subacute) 646.7❺
bacilluria, asymptomatic 646.5❺
bacteriuria, asymptomatic 646.5❺
bariatric surgery status 649.2❺
bicornis or bicornuate uterus 654.0❺
biliary problems 646.8
bone and joint disorders (conditions classifiable to 720-724 or conditions affecting lower limbs classifiable to 711-719, 725-738) 648.7❺
breech presentation (buttocks) (complete) (frank) 652.2❺
with successful version 652.1❺
cardiovascular disease (conditions classifiable to 390-398, 410-429) 648.6❺
congenital (conditions classifiable to 745-747) 648.5❺
cerebrovascular disorders (conditions classifiable to 430-434, 436-437) 674.0❺
cervicitis (conditions classifiable to 616.0) 646.6❺
chloasma (gravidarum) 646.8❺
cholelithiasis 646.8
chorea (gravidarum) – *see* Eclampsia, pregnancy
coagulation defect 649.3❺
contraction, pelvis (general) 653.1
inlet 653.2❺
outlet 653.3❺
convulsions (eclamptic) (uremic) 642.6❺
with pre-existing hypertension 642.7❺
current disease or condition (nonobstetric)
abnormal glucose tolerance 648.8❺
anemia 648.2❺
bone and joint (lower limb) 648.7❺
cardiovascular 648.6❺
congenital 648.5❺
cerebrovascular 674.0❺
diabetic 648.0❺
drug dependence 648.3❺
genital organ or tract 646.6❺
female genital mutilation 648.9❺
gonorrheal 647.1❺
hypertensive 642.2❺
chronic kidney 642.2❺
renal 642.1❺
infectious 647.9❺
specified type NEC 647.8❺
liver 646.7❺
malarial 647.4❺
nutritional deficiency 648.9❺
parasitic NEC 647.8❺
periodontal disease 648.9❺

Pregnancy – *continued*
complicated (by) – *continued*
current disease or condition (nonobstetric) - *continued*
renal 646.2❺
hypertensive 642.1❺
rubella 647.5❺
specified condition NEC 648.9❺
syphilitic 647.0❺
thyroid 648.1❺
tuberculous 647.3❺
urinary 646.6❺
venereal 647.2❺
viral NEC 647.6❺
cystitis 646.6❺
cystocele 654.4❺
death of fetus (near term) 656.4❺
early pregnancy (before 22 completed weeks gestation) 632
deciduitis 646.6❺
decreased fetal movements 655.7
diabetes (mellitus) (conditions classifiable to 250) 648.0❺
disorders of liver 646.7❺
displacement, uterus NEC 654.4❺
disproportion – *see* Disproportion
double uterus 654.0❺
drug dependence (conditions classifiable to 304) 648.3❺
dysplasia, cervix 654.6❺
early onset of delivery (spontaneous) 644.2❺
eclampsia, eclamptic (coma) (convulsions) (delirium) (nephritis) (uremia) 642.6❺
with pre-existing hypertension 642.7❺
edema 646.1❺
with hypertension – *see* Toxemia, of pregnancy
effusion, amniotic fluid 658.1❺
delayed delivery following 658.2❺
embolism
air 673.0❺
amniotic fluid 673.1❺
blood-clot 673.2❺
cerebral 674.0❺
pulmonary NEC 673.2❺
pyemic 673.3❺
septic 673.3❺
emesis (gravidarum) – *see* Pregnancy, complicated, vomiting
endometritis (conditions classifiable to 615.0-615.9) 670❺ ▲
decidual 646.6❺
epilepsy 649.4❺
excessive weight gain NEC 646.1❺
face presentation 652.4❺
failure, fetal head to enter pelvic brim 652.5❺
false labor (pains) 644.1❺
fatigue 646.8❺
fatty metamorphosis of liver 646.7❺
female genital mutilation 648.9❺
fetal
death (near term) 656.4❺
early (before 22 completed weeks gestation) 632
deformity 653.7❺
distress 656.8❺
reduction of multiple fetuses reduced to single fetus 651.7
fibroid (tumor) (uterus) 654.1❺
footling presentation 652.8❺
with successful version 652.1❺
gallbladder disease 646.8
gastric banding status 649.2❺
gastric bypass status for obesity 649.2❺
goiter 648.1❺
gonococcal infection (conditions classifiable to 098) 647.1❺
gonorrhea (conditions classifiable to 098) 647.1❺
hemorrhage 641.9❺
accidental 641.2❺
before 22 completed weeks gestation NEC 640.9❺
cerebrovascular 674.0❺
due to
afibrinogenemia or other coagulation defect (conditions classifiable to 286.0-286.9) 641.3❺
leiomyoma, uterine 641.8❺
marginal sinus (rupture) 641.2❺
premature separation, placenta 641.2❺
trauma 641.8❺

Pregnancy – *continued*
- complicated (by) – *continued*
  - hemorrhage – *continued*
    - early (before 22 completed weeks gestation) 640.9❺
    - threatened abortion 640.0❺
    - unavoidable 641.1❺
  - hepatitis (acute) (malignant) (subacute) 646.7❺
    - viral 647.6❺
  - herniation of uterus 654.4❺
  - high head at term 652.5❺
  - hydatidiform mole (delivered) (undelivered) 630
  - hydramnios 657❺
  - hydrocephalic fetus 653.6❺
  - hydrops amnii 657❺
  - hydrorrhea 658.1❺
  - hyperemesis (gravidarum) – *see* Hyperemesis, gravidarum
  - hypertension – *see* Hypertension, complicating pregnancy
  - hypertensive
    - chronic kidney disease 642.2❺
    - heart and chronic kidney disease 642.2❺
    - heart and renal disease 642.2❺
    - heart disease 642.2❺
    - renal disease 642.2❺
  - hypertensive heart and chronic kidney disease 642.2❺
  - hyperthyroidism 648.1❺
  - hypothyroidism 648.1❺
  - hysteralgia 646.8❺
  - icterus gravis 646.7❺
  - incarceration, uterus 654.3❺
  - incompetent cervix (os) 654.5❺
  - infection 647.9❺
    - amniotic fluid 658.4❺
    - bladder 646.6❺
    - genital organ (conditions classifiable to 614.0-614.5, 614.7-614.9, 615) 646.6❺
    - kidney (conditions classifiable to 590.0-590.9) 646.6❺
    - urinary (tract) 646.6❺
      - asymptomatic 646.5❺
  - infective and parasitic diseases NEC 647.8❺
  - inflammation
    - bladder 646.6❺
    - genital organ (conditions classifiable to 614.0-614.5, 614.7-614.9, 615) 646.6❺
    - urinary tract NEC 646.6❺
  - injury 648.9❺
    - obstetrical NEC 665.9❺
  - insufficient weight gain 646.8❺
  - intrauterine fetal death (near term) NEC 656.4❺
    - early (before 22 completed weeks gestation) 632
  - malaria (conditions classifiable to 084) 647.4❺
  - malformation, uterus (congenital) 654.0❺
  - malnutrition (conditions classifiable to 260-269) 648.9❺
  - malposition
    - fetus – *see* Pregnancy, complicated, malpresentation
    - uterus or cervix 654.4❺
  - malpresentation 652.9❺
    - with successful version 652.1❺
    - in multiple gestation 652.6❺
    - specified type NEC 652.8❺
  - marginal sinus hemorrhage or rupture 641.2❺
  - maternal obesity syndrome 646.1❺
  - menstruation 640.8❺
  - mental disorders (conditions classifiable to 290-303, 305.0, 305.2-305.9, 306-316, 317-319) 648.4❺
  - mentum presentation 652.4❺
  - missed
    - abortion 632
    - delivery (at or near term) 656.4❺
    - labor (at or near term) 656.4❺
  - necrosis
    - genital organ or tract (conditions classifiable to 614.0-614.5, 614.7-614.9, 615) 646.6❺
    - liver (conditions classifiable to 570) 646.7❺
    - renal, cortical 646.2❺
  - nephritis or nephrosis (conditions classifiable to 580-589) 646.2❺
    - with hypertension 642.1❺

Pregnancy – *continued*
- complicated (by) – *continued*
  - nephropathy NEC 646.2❺
  - neuritis (peripheral) 646.4❺
  - nutritional deficiency (conditions classifiable to 260-269) 648.9❺
  - obesity 649.1❺
    - surgery status 649.2❺
  - oblique lie or presentation 652.3❺
    - with successful version 652.1❺
  - obstetrical trauma NEC 665.9❺
  - oligohydramnios NEC 658.0❺
  - onset of contractions before 37 weeks 644.0❺
  - oversize fetus 653.5❺
  - papyraceous fetus 646.0❺
  - patent cervix 654.5❺
  - pelvic inflammatory disease (conditions classifiable to 614.0-614.5, 614.7-614.9, 615) 646.6❺
  - pelvic peritoneal adhesion 648.9❺
  - placenta, placental
    - abnormality 656.7❺
    - abruptio or ablatio 641.2❺
    - detachment 641.2❺
    - disease 656.7❺
    - infarct 656.7❺
    - low implantation 641.1❺
      - without hemorrhage 641.0❺
    - malformation 656.7❺
    - malposition 641.1❺
      - without hemorrhage 641.0❺
    - marginal sinus hemorrhage 641.2❺
    - previa 641.1❺
      - without hemorrhage 641.0❺
    - separation (premature) (undelivered) 641.2❺
  - placentitis 658.4❺
  - polyhydramnios 657❺
  - postmaturity
    - post-term 645.1❺
    - prolonged 645.2❺
  - prediabetes 648.8❺
  - pre-eclampsia (mild) 642.4❺
    - severe 642.5❺
    - superimposed on pre-existing hypertensive disease 642.7❺
  - premature rupture of membranes 658.1❺
    - with delayed delivery 658.2❺
  - previous
    - infertility V23.0
    - nonobstetric condition V23.8❺
    - poor obstetrical history V23.49
    - premature delivery V23.41
    - trophoblastic disease (conditions classifiable to 630) V23.1
  - prolapse, uterus 654.4❺
  - proteinuria (gestational) 646.2❺
    - with hypertension – *see* Toxemia, of pregnancy
  - pruritus (neurogenic) 646.8❺
  - psychosis or psychoneurosis 648.4❺
  - ptyalism 646.8❺
  - pyelitis (conditions classifiable to 590.0-590.9) 646.6❺
  - renal disease or failure NEC 646.2❺
    - with secondary hypertension 642.1❺
    - hypertensive 642.2❺
  - retention, retained dead ovum 631
  - retroversion, uterus 654.3❺
  - Rh immunization, incompatibility, or sensitization 656.1❺
  - rubella (conditions classifiable to 056) 647.5❺
  - rupture
    - amnion (premature) 658.1❺
      - with delayed delivery 658.2❺
    - marginal sinus (hemorrhage) 641.2❺
    - membranes (premature) 658.1❺
      - with delayed delivery 658.2❺
    - uterus (before onset of labor) 665.0❺
  - salivation (excessive) 646.8❺
  - salpingo-oophoritis (conditions classifiable to 614.0-614.2) 646.6❺
  - septicemia (conditions classifiable to 038.0-038.9) 647.8❺
    - postpartum 670❹
    - puerperal 670❹
  - smoking 649.0❺
  - spasms, uterus (abnormal) 646.8❺
  - specified condition NEC 646.8❺
  - spotting 649.5❺

Pregnancy – *continued*
- complicated (by) – *continued*
  - spurious labor pains 644.1❺
  - status post
    - bariatric surgery 649.2❺
    - gastric banding 649.2❺
    - gastric bypass for obesity 649.2❺
    - obesity surgery 649.2❺
  - superfecundation 651.9❺
  - superfetation 651.9❺
  - syphilis (conditions classifiable to 090-097) 647.0❺
  - threatened
    - abortion 640.0❺
    - premature delivery 644.2❺
    - premature labor 644.0❺
  - thrombophlebitis (superficial) 671.2❺
    - deep 671.3❺
  - thrombosis 671.9❺
    - venous (superficial) 671.2❺
      - deep 671.3❺
  - thyroid dysfunction (conditions classifiable to 240-246) 648.1❺
  - thyroiditis 648.1❺
  - thyrotoxicosis 648.1❺
  - tobacco use disorder 649.0❺
  - torsion of uterus 654.4❺
  - toxemia – *see* Toxemia, of pregnancy
  - transverse lie or presentation 652.3❺
    - with successful version 652.1❺
  - trauma 648.9❺
    - obstetrical 665.9❺
  - tuberculosis (conditions classifiable to 010-018) 647.3❺
  - tumor
    - cervix 654.6❺
    - ovary 654.4❺
    - pelvic organs or tissue NEC 654.4❺
    - uterus (body) 654.1❺
      - cervix 654.6❺
    - vagina 654.7❺
    - vulva 654.8❺
  - unstable lie 652.0❺
  - uremia – *see* Pregnancy, complicated, renal disease
  - urethritis 646.6❺
  - vaginitis or vulvitis (conditions classifiable to 616.1) 646.6❺
  - varicose
    - placental vessels 656.7❺
    - veins (legs) 671.0❺
      - perineum 671.1❺
      - vulva 671.1❺
  - varicosity, labia or vulva 671.1❺
  - venereal disease NEC (conditions classifiable to 099) 647.2❺
  - viral disease NEC (conditions classifiable to 042, 050-055, 057-079) 647.6❺
  - vomiting (incoercible) (pernicious) (persistent) (uncontrollable) (vicious) 643.9❺
    - due to organic disease or other cause 643.8❺
    - early – *see* Hyperemesis, gravidarum
    - late (after 22 completed weeks gestation) 643.2❺
  - young maternal age 659.8❺
- complications NEC 646.9❺
- cornual 633.80
  - with intrauterine pregnancy 633.81
  - affecting fetus or newborn 761.4
- death, maternal NEC 646.9❺
- delivered – *see* Delivery
- ectopic (ruptured) NEC 633.90
  - with intrauterine pregnancy 633.91
  - abdominal – *see* Pregnancy, abdominal
  - affecting fetus or newborn 761.4
  - combined (extrauterine and intrauterine) – *see* Pregnancy, cornual
  - ovarian – *see* Pregnancy, ovarian
  - specified type NEC 633.80
    - with intrauterine pregnancy 633.81
    - affecting fetus or newborn 761.4
  - tubal – *see* Pregnancy, tubal
- examination, pregnancy
  - negative result V72.41
  - not confirmed V72.40
  - positive result V72.42
- extrauterine – *see* Pregnancy, ectopic
- fallopian – *see* Pregnancy, tubal
- false 300.11
  - labor (pains) 644.1❺
- fatigue 646.8❺

Pregnancy – Pregnancy

- **Pregnancy** – *continued*
  - illegitimate V61.6
  - incidental finding V22.2
  - in double uterus 654.0❺
  - interstitial – *see* Pregnancy, cornual
  - intraligamentous – *see* Pregnancy, cornual
  - intramural – *see* Pregnancy, cornual
  - intraperitoneal – *see* Pregnancy, abdominal
  - isthmian – *see* Pregnancy, tubal
  - management affected by
    - abnormal, abnormality
      - fetus (suspected) 655.9❺
        - specified NEC 655.8❺
      - placenta 656.7❺
    - advanced maternal age NEC 659.6❺
      - multigravida 659.6❺
      - primigravida 659.5❺
    - antibodies (maternal)
      - anti-c 656.1❺
      - anti-d 656.1❺
      - anti-e 656.1❺
      - blood group (ABO) 656.2❺
        - Rh(esus) 656.1❺
    - appendicitis 648.9❺
    - bariatric surgery status 649.2❺
    - coagulation defect 649.3❺
    - elderly multigravida 659.6❺
    - elderly primigravida 659.5❺
    - epilepsy 649.4❺
    - fetal (suspected)
      - abnormality 655.9❺
        - acid-base balance 656.8❺
        - heart rate or rhythm 659.7❺
        - specified NEC 655.8❺
      - acidemia 656.3❺
      - anencephaly 655.0❺
      - bradycardia 659.7❺
      - central nervous system malformation 655.0❺
      - chromosomal abnormalities (conditions classifiable to 758.0-758.9) 655.1❺
      - damage from
        - drugs 655.5❺
          - obstetric, anesthetic, or sedative 655.5❺
        - environmental toxins 655.8❺
        - intrauterine contraceptive device 655.8❺
        - maternal
          - alcohol addiction 655.4❺
          - disease NEC 655.4❺
          - drug use 655.5❺
          - listeriosis 655.4❺
          - rubella 655.3❺
          - toxoplasmosis 655.4❺
          - viral infection 655.3❺
        - radiation 655.6❺
      - death (near term) 656.4❺
        - early (before 22 completed weeks gestation) 632
      - distress 656.8❺
      - excessive growth 656.6❺
      - growth retardation 656.5❺
      - hereditary disease 655.2❺
      - hydrocephalus 655.0❺
      - intrauterine death 656.4❺
      - poor growth 656.5❺
      - spina bifida (with myelomeningocele) 655.0❺
    - fetal-maternal hemorrhage 656.0❺
    - gastric banding status 649.2❺
    - gastric bypass status for obesity 649.2❺
    - hereditary disease in family (possibly) affecting fetus 655.2❺
    - incompatibility, blood groups (ABO) 656.2❺
      - Rh(esus) 656.1❺
    - insufficient prenatal care V23.7
    - intrauterine death 656.4❺
    - isoimmunization (ABO) 656.2❺
      - Rh(esus) 656.1❺
    - large-for-dates fetus 656.6❺
    - light-for-dates fetus 656.5❺
    - meconium in liquor 656.8❺
    - mental disorder (conditions classifiable to 290-303, 305.0, 305.2-305.9, 306-316, 317-319) 648.4❺
    - multiparity (grand) 659.4❺
    - obesity 649.1❺
      - surgery status 649.2❺
    - poor obstetric history V23.49
      - pre-term labor V23.41
    - postmaturity
      - post-term 645.1❺

- **Pregnancy** – *continued*
  - management affected by – *continued*
    - postmaturity – *continued*
      - prolonged 645.2❺
    - post-term pregnancy 645.1❺
    - previous
      - abortion V23.2
        - habitual 646.3❺
      - cesarean delivery 654.2❺
      - difficult delivery V23.49
      - forceps delivery V23.49
      - habitual abortions 646.3❺
      - hemorrhage, antepartum or postpartum V23.49
      - hydatidiform mole V23.1
      - infertility V23.0
      - malignancy NEC V23.8❺
      - nonobstetrical conditions V23.8❺
      - premature delivery V23.41
      - trophoblastic disease (conditions in 630) V23.1
      - vesicular mole V23.1
    - prolonged pregnancy 645.2❺
    - small-for-dates fetus 656.5❺
    - smoking 649.0❺
    - spotting 649.5❺
    - tobacco use disorder 649.0❺
    - young maternal age 659.8❺
  - maternal death NEC 646.9❺
  - mesometric (mural) – *see* Pregnancy, cornual
  - molar 631
    - hydatidiform (*see also* Hydatidiform mole) 630
      - previous, affecting management of pregnancy V23.1
    - previous, affecting management of pregnancy V23.49
  - multiple NEC 651.9❺
    - with fetal loss and retention of one or more fetus(es) 651.6❺
    - affecting fetus or newborn 761.5
    - following (elective) fetal reduction 651.7
    - specified type NEC 651.8❺
      - with fetal loss and retention of one or more fetus(es) 651.6❺
      - following (elective) fetal reduction 651.7
  - mural – *see* Pregnancy, cornual
  - observation NEC V22.1
    - first pregnancy V22.0
    - high-risk V23.9
      - specified problem NEC V23.8❺
  - ovarian 633.20
    - with intrauterine pregnancy 633.21
    - affecting fetus or newborn 761.4
  - possible, not (yet) confirmed V72.40
  - postmature
    - post-term 645.1❺
    - prolonged 645.2❺
  - post-term 645.1❺
  - prenatal care only V22.1
    - first pregnancy V22.0
    - high-risk V23.9
      - specified problem NEC V23.8❺
  - prolonged 645.2❺
  - quadruplet NEC 651.2❺
    - with fetal loss and retention of one or more fetus(es) 651.5❺
    - affecting fetus or newborn 761.5
    - following (elective) fetal reduction 651.7
  - quintuplet NEC 651.8❺
    - with fetal loss and retention of one or more fetus(es) 651.6❺
    - affecting fetus or newborn 761.5
    - following (elective) fetal reduction 651.7
  - sextuplet NEC 651.8❺
    - with fetal loss and retention of one or more fetus(es) 651.6❺
    - affecting fetus or newborn 761.5
    - following (elective) fetal reduction 651.7
  - spurious 300.11
  - superfecundation NEC 651.9❺
    - with fetal loss and retention of one or more fetus(es) 651.6❺
    - following (elective) fetal reduction 651.7
  - superfetation NEC 651.9❺
    - with fetal loss and retention of one or more fetus(es) 651.6❺
    - following (elective) fetal reduction 651.7
  - supervision (of) (for) – *see also* Pregnancy, management affected by
    - elderly
      - multigravida V23.82
      - primigravida V23.81

- **Pregnancy** – *continued*
  - supervision (of) (for) – *continued*
    - high-risk V23.9
      - insufficient prenatal care V23.7
      - specified problem NEC V23.8❺
    - multiparity V23.3
    - normal NEC V22.1
      - first V22.0
    - poor
      - obstetric history V23.49
        - pre-term labor V23.41
      - reproductive history V23.5
    - previous
      - abortion V23.2
      - hydatidiform mole V23.1
      - infertility V23.0
      - neonatal death V23.5
      - stillbirth V23.5
      - trophoblastic disease V23.1
      - vesicular mole V23.1
    - specified problem NEC V23.8❺
    - young
      - multigravida V23.84
      - primigravida V23.83
  - triplet NEC 651.1❺
    - with fetal loss and retention of one or more fetus(es) 651.4❺
    - affecting fetus or newborn 761.5
    - following (elective) fetal reduction 651.7
  - tubal (with rupture) 633.10
    - with intrauterine pregnancy 633.11
    - affecting fetus or newborn 761.4
  - twin NEC 651.0❺
    - with fetal loss and retention of one fetus 651.3❺
    - affecting fetus or newborn 761.5
    - following (elective) fetal reduction 651.7
  - unconfirmed V72.40
  - undelivered (no other diagnosis) V22.2
    - with false labor 644.1❺
    - high-risk V23.9
      - specified problem NEC V23.8❺
  - unwanted NEC V61.7
- **Pregnant uterus** – *see* condition
- **Preiser's disease** (osteoporosis) 733.09
- **Prekwashiorkor** 260
- **Preleukemia** 238.75
- **Preluxation of hip, congenital** (*see also* Subluxation, congenital, hip) 754.32
- **Premature** – *see also* condition
  - beats (nodal) 427.60
    - atrial 427.61
    - auricular 427.61
    - postoperative 997.1
    - specified type NEC 427.69
    - supraventricular 427.61
    - ventricular 427.69
  - birth NEC 765.1❺
  - closure
    - cranial suture 756.0
    - fontanel 756.0
    - foramen ovale 745.8
  - contractions 427.60
    - atrial 427.61
    - auricular 427.61
    - auriculoventricular 427.61
    - heart (extrasystole) 427.60
    - junctional 427.60
    - nodal 427.60
    - postoperative 997.1
    - ventricular 427.69
  - ejaculation 302.75
  - infant NEC 765.1❺
    - excessive 765.0❺
    - light-for-dates – *see* Light-for-dates
  - labor 644.2❺
    - threatened 644.0❺
  - lungs 770.4
  - menopause 256.31
  - puberty 259.1
  - rupture of membranes or amnion 658.1❺
    - affecting fetus or newborn 761.1
    - delayed delivery following 658.2❺
  - senility (syndrome) 259.8
  - separation, placenta (partial) – *see* Placenta, separation
  - ventricular systole 427.69
- **Prematurity** NEC 765.1❺
  - extreme 765.0❺
- **Premenstrual syndrome** 625.4

- **Premenstrual tension** 625.4
- **Premolarization, cuspids** 520.2
- **Premyeloma** 273.1
- **Prenatal**
  - care, normal pregnancy V22.1
    - first V22.0
  - death, cause unknown – *see* Death, fetus
  - screening – *see* Antenatal, screening
  - teeth 520.6
- **Prepartum** – *see* condition
- **Preponderance, left or right ventricular** 429.3
- **Prepuce** – *see* condition
- **PRES** (posterior reversible encephalopathy syndrome) 348.39
- **Presbycardia** 797
  - hypertensive (*see also* Hypertension, heart) 402.90
- **Presbycusis** 388.01
- **Presbyesophagus** 530.89
- **Presbyophrenia** 310.1
- **Presbyopia** 367.4
- **Prescription of contraceptives** NEC V25.02
  - diaphragm V25.02
  - oral (pill) V25.01
    - emergency V25.03
    - postcoital V25.03
    - repeat V25.41
  - repeat V25.40
    - oral (pill) V25.41
- **Presenile** – *see also* condition
  - aging 259.8
  - dementia (*see also* Dementia, presenile) 290.10
- **Presenility** 259.8
- **Presentation, fetal**
  - abnormal 652.9❺
    - with successful version 652.1❺
    - before labor, affecting fetus or newborn 761.7
    - causing obstructed labor 660.0❺
      - affecting fetus or newborn, any, except breech 763.1
    - in multiple gestation (one or more) 652.6❺
    - specified NEC 652.8❺
  - arm 652.7❺
    - causing obstructed labor 660.0❺
  - breech (buttocks) (complete) (frank) 652.2❺
    - with successful version 652.1❺
      - before labor, affecting fetus or newborn 761.7
    - before labor, affecting fetus or newborn 761.7
  - brow 652.4❺
    - causing obstructed labor 660.0❺
  - buttocks 652.2❺
  - chin 652.4❺
  - complete 652.2❺
  - compound 652.8❺
  - cord 663.0❺
  - extended head 652.4❺
  - face 652.4❺
    - to pubes 652.8❺
  - footling 652.8❺
  - frank 652.2❺
  - hand, leg, or foot NEC 652.8❺
  - incomplete 652.8❺
  - mentum 652.4❺
  - multiple gestation (one fetus or more) 652.6❺
  - oblique 652.3❺
    - with successful version 652.1❺
  - shoulder 652.8❺
    - affecting fetus or newborn 763.1
  - transverse 652.3❺
    - with successful version 652.1❺
  - umbilical cord 663.0❺
  - unstable 652.0❺
- **Prespondylolisthesis** (congenital) (lumbosacral) 756.11
- **Pressure**
  - area, skin ulcer (*see also* Decubitus) 707.00
  - atrophy, spine 733.99
  - birth, fetus or newborn NEC 767.9
  - brachial plexus 353.0
  - brain 348.4
    - injury at birth 767.0
  - cerebral – *see* Pressure, brain
  - chest 786.59
  - cone, tentorial 348.4
    - injury at birth 767.0
  - funis – *see* Compression, umbilical cord
  - hyposystolic (*see also* Hypotension) 458.9

Pressure – *continued*
  - increased
    - intracranial 781.99
      - due to
        - benign intracranial hypertension 348.2
        - hydrocephalus – *see* hydrocephalus
        - injury at birth 767.8
    - intraocular 365.00
  - lumbosacral plexus 353.1
  - mediastinum 519.3
  - necrosis (chronic) (skin) (*see also* Decubitus) 707.00
  - nerve – *see* Compression, nerve
  - paralysis (*see also* Neuropathy, entrapment) 355.9
  - sore (chronic) (*see also* Decubitus) 707.00
  - spinal cord 336.9
  - ulcer (chronic) (*see also* Decubitus) 707.00
  - umbilical cord – *see* Compression, umbilical cord
  - venous, increased 459.89
- **Pre-syncope** 780.2
- **Preterm infant** NEC 765.1❺
  - extreme 765.0❺
- **Priapism** (penis) 607.3
- **Prickling sensation** (*see also* Disturbance, sensation) 782.0
- **Prickly heat** 705.1
- **Primary** – *see* condition
- **Primigravida, elderly**
  - affecting
    - fetus or newborn 763.89
    - management of pregnancy, labor, and delivery 659.5❺
- **Primipara, old**
  - affecting
    - fetus or newborn 763.89
    - management of pregnancy, labor, and delivery 659.5❺
- **Primula dermatitis** 692.6
- **Primus varus** (bilateral) (metatarsus) 754.52
- ▶**PRIND** (prolonged reversible ischemic neurologic deficit)◀ 434.91 ▲
  - history of (personal) V12.54 ●
- **Pringle's disease** (tuberous sclerosis) 759.5
- **Prinzmetal's angina** 413.1
- **Prinzmetal-Massumi syndrome** (anterior chest wall) 786.52
- **Prizefighter ear** 738.7
- **Problem** (with) V49.9
  - academic V62.3
  - acculturation V62.4
  - adopted child V61.29
  - aged
    - in-law V61.3
    - parent V61.3
    - person NEC V61.8
  - alcoholism in family V61.41
  - anger reaction (*see also* Disturbance, conduct) 312.0❺
  - behavior, child 312.9
  - behavioral V40.9
    - specified NEC V40.3
  - betting V69.3
  - cardiorespiratory NEC V47.2
  - care of sick or handicapped person in family or household V61.49
  - career choice V62.2
  - communication V40.1
  - conscience regarding medical care V62.6
  - delinquency (juvenile) 312.9
  - diet, inappropriate V69.1
  - digestive NEC V47.3
  - ear NEC V41.3
  - eating habits, inappropriate V69.1
  - economic V60.2
    - affecting care V60.9
      - specified type NEC V60.8
  - educational V62.3
  - enuresis, child 307.6
  - exercise, lack of V69.0
  - eye NEC V41.1
  - family V61.9
    - specified circumstance NEC V61.8
  - fear reaction, child 313.0
  - feeding (elderly) (infant) 783.3
    - newborn 779.3
    - nonorganic 307.59

Problem – *continued*
  - fetal, affecting management of pregnancy 656.9❺
    - specified type NEC 656.8❺
  - financial V60.2
  - foster child V61.29
    - specified NEC V41.8
  - functional V41.9
    - specified type NEC V41.8
  - gambling V69.3
  - genital NEC V47.5
  - head V48.9
    - deficiency V48.0
    - disfigurement V48.6
    - mechanical V48.2
    - motor V48.2
    - movement of V48.2
    - sensory V48.4
    - specified condition NEC V48.8
  - hearing V41.2
  - high-risk sexual behavior V69.2
  - identity 313.82
  - influencing health status NEC V49.89
  - internal organ NEC V47.9
    - deficiency V47.0
    - mechanical or motor V47.1
  - interpersonal NEC V62.81
  - jealousy, child 313.3
  - learning V40.0
  - legal V62.5
  - life circumstance NEC V62.89
  - lifestyle V69.9
    - specified NEC V69.8
  - limb V49.9
    - deficiency V49.0
    - disfigurement V49.4
    - mechanical V49.1
    - motor V49.2
    - movement, involving
      - musculoskeletal system V49.1
      - nervous system V49.2
    - sensory V49.3
    - specified condition NEC V49.5
  - litigation V62.5
  - living alone V60.3
  - loneliness NEC V62.89
  - marital V61.10
    - involving
      - divorce V61.0
      - estrangement V61.0
      - psychosexual disorder 302.9
      - sexual function V41.7
    - relationship V61.10
  - mastication V41.6
  - medical care, within family V61.49
  - mental V40.9
    - specified NEC V40.2
  - mental hygiene, adult V40.9
  - multiparity V61.5
  - nail biting, child 307.9
  - neck V48.9
    - deficiency V48.1
    - disfigurement V48.7
    - mechanical V48.3
    - motor V48.3
    - movement V48.3
    - sensory V48.5
    - specified condition NEC V48.8
  - neurological NEC 781.99
  - none (feared complaint unfounded) V65.5
  - occupational V62.2
  - parent-child V61.20
    - relationship V61.20
  - partner V61.10
    - relationship V61.10
  - personal NEC V62.89
    - interpersonal conflict NEC V62.81
  - personality (*see also* Disorder, personality) 301.9
  - phase of life V62.89
  - placenta, affecting management of pregnancy 656.9❺
    - specified type NEC 656.8❺
  - poverty V60.2
  - presence of sick or handicapped person in family or household V61.49
  - psychiatric 300.9
  - psychosocial V62.9
    - specified type NEC V62.89
  - relational NEC V62.81
  - relationship, childhood 313.3
  - religious or spiritual belief
    - other than medical care V62.89

Premenstrual tension – Problem

- **Problem** – *continued*
  - religious or spiritual belief – *continued*
    - regarding medical care V62.6
  - self-damaging behavior V69.8
  - sexual
    - behavior, high-risk V69.2
    - function NEC V41.7
  - sibling
    - relational V61.8
    - relationship V61.8
  - sight V41.0
  - sleep disorder, child 307.40
  - sleep, lack of V69.4
  - smell V41.5
  - speech V40.1
  - spite reaction, child (*see also* Disturbance, conduct) 312.0❺
  - spoiled child reaction (*see also* Disturbance, conduct) 312.1❺
  - swallowing V41.6
  - tantrum, child (*see also* Disturbance, conduct) 312.1❺
  - taste V41.5
  - thumb sucking, child 307.9
  - tic (child) 307.21
  - trunk V48.9
    - deficiency V48.1
    - disfigurement V48.7
    - mechanical V48.3
    - motor V48.3
    - movement V48.3
    - sensory V48.5
    - specified condition NEC V48.8
  - unemployment V62.0
  - urinary NEC V47.4
  - voice production V41.4
- **Procedure** (surgical) **not done** NEC V64.3
  - because of
    - contraindication V64.1
    - patient's decision V64.2
      - for reasons of conscience or religion V62.6
    - specified reason NEC V64.3
- **Procidentia**
  - anus (sphincter) 569.1
  - rectum (sphincter) 569.1
  - stomach 537.89
  - uteri 618.1
- **Proctalgia** 569.42
  - fugax 564.6
  - spasmodic 564.6
    - psychogenic 307.89
- **Proctitis** 569.49
  - amebic 006.8
  - chlamydial 099.52
  - gonococcal 098.7
  - granulomatous 555.1
  - idiopathic 556.2
    - with ulcerative sigmoiditis 556.3
  - tuberculous (*see also* Tuberculosis) 014.8❺
  - ulcerative (chronic) (nonspecific) 556.2
    - with ulcerative sigmoiditis 556.3
- **Proctocele**
  - female (without uterine prolapse) 618.04
    - with uterine prolapse 618.4
      - complete 618.3
      - incomplete 618.2
  - male 569.49
- **Proctocolitis, idiopathic** 556.2
  - with ulcerative sigmoiditis 556.3
- **Proctoptosis** 569.1
- **Proctosigmoiditis** 569.89
  - ulcerative (chronic) 556.3
- **Proctospasm** 564.6
  - psychogenic 306.4
- **Prodromal-AIDS** – *see* Human immunodeficiency virus (disease) (illness) (infection)
- **Profichet's disease or syndrome** 729.9
- **Progeria** (adultorum) (syndrome) 259.8
- **Prognathism** (mandibular) (maxillary) 524.00
- **Progonoma** (melanotic) (M9363/0) – *see* Neoplasm, by site, benign
- **Progressive** – *see* condition
- **Prolapse, prolapsed**
  - anus, anal (canal) (sphincter) 569.1
  - arm or hand, complicating delivery 652.7❺
    - causing obstructed labor 660.0❺
      - affecting fetus or newborn 763.1
    - fetus or newborn 763.1
- **Prolapse, prolapsed** – *continued*
  - bladder (acquired) (mucosa) (sphincter)
    - congenital (female) (male) 756.71
    - female (*see also* Cystocele, female) 618.01
    - male 596.8
  - breast implant (prosthetic) 996.54
  - cecostomy 569.69
  - cecum 569.89
  - cervix, cervical (hypertrophied) 618.1
    - anterior lip, obstructing labor 660.2❺
      - affecting fetus or newborn 763.1
    - congenital 752.49
    - postpartal (old) 618.1
    - stump 618.84
  - ciliary body 871.1
  - colon (pedunculated) 569.89
  - colostomy 569.69
  - conjunctiva 372.73
  - cord – *see* Prolapse, umbilical cord
  - disc (intervertebral) – *see* Displacement, intervertebral disc
  - duodenum 537.89
  - eye implant (orbital) 996.59
    - lens (ocular) 996.53
  - fallopian tube 620.4
  - fetal extremity, complicating delivery 652.8❺
    - causing obstructed labor 660.0❺
    - fetus or newborn 763.1
  - funis – *see* Prolapse, umbilical cord
  - gastric (mucosa) 537.89
  - genital, female 618.9
    - specified NEC 618.89
  - globe 360.81
  - ileostomy bud 569.69
  - intervertebral disc – *see* Displacement, intervertebral disc
  - intestine (small) 569.89
  - iris 364.89 ▲
    - traumatic 871.1
  - kidney (*see also* Disease, renal) 593.0
    - congenital 753.3
  - laryngeal muscles or ventricle 478.79
  - leg, complicating delivery 652.8❺
    - causing obstructed labor 660.0❺
    - fetus or newborn 763.1
  - liver 573.8
  - meatus urinarius 599.5
  - mitral valve 424.0
  - ocular lens implant 996.53
  - organ or site, congenital NEC – *see* Malposition, congenital
  - ovary 620.4
  - pelvic (floor), female 618.89
  - perineum, female 618.89
  - pregnant uterus 654.4❺
  - rectum (mucosa) (sphincter) 569.1
    - due to Trichuris trichiuria 127.3
  - spleen 289.59
  - stomach 537.89
  - umbilical cord
    - affecting fetus or newborn 762.4
    - complicating delivery 663.0❺
  - ureter 593.89
    - with obstruction 593.4
  - ureterovesical orifice 593.89
  - urethra (acquired) (infected) (mucosa) 599.5
    - congenital 753.8
  - uterovaginal 618.4
    - complete 618.3
    - incomplete 618.2
    - specified NEC 618.89
  - uterus (first degree) (second degree) (third degree) (complete) (without vaginal wall prolapse) 618.1
    - with mention of vaginal wall prolapse – *see* Prolapse, uterovaginal
    - congenital 752.3
    - in pregnancy or childbirth 654.4❺
      - affecting fetus or newborn 763.1
      - causing obstructed labor 660.2❺
        - affecting fetus or newborn 763.1
    - postpartal (old) 618.1
  - uveal 871.1
  - vagina (anterior) (posterior) (vault) (wall) (without uterine prolapse) 618.00
    - with uterine prolapse 618.4
      - complete 618.3
      - incomplete 618.2
    - paravaginal 618.02
    - posthysterectomy 618.5
    - specified NEC 618.09
- **Prolapse, prolapsed** – *continued*
  - vitreous (humor) 379.26
    - traumatic 871.1
  - womb – *see* Prolapse, uterus
- **Prolapsus, female** 618.9
- **Proliferative** – *see* condition
- **Prolinemia** 270.8
- **Prolinuria** 270.8
- **Prolonged, prolongation**
  - bleeding time (*see also* Defect, coagulation) 790.92
    - "idiopathic" (in von Willebrand's disease) 286.4
  - coagulation time (*see also* Defect, coagulation) 790.92
  - gestation syndrome 766.22
  - labor 662.1❺
    - first stage 662.0❺
    - second stage 662.2❺
    - affecting fetus or newborn 763.89
  - PR interval 426.11
  - pregnancy 645.2❺
  - prothrombin time (*see also* Defect, coagulation) 790.92
  - QT interval 794.31
    - syndrome 426.82
  - rupture of membranes (24 hours or more prior to onset of labor) 658.2❺
  - uterine contractions in labor 661.4❺
    - affecting fetus or newborn 763.7
- **Prominauris** 744.29
- **Prominence**
  - auricle (ear) (congenital) 744.29
    - acquired 380.32
  - ischial spine or sacral promontory
    - with disproportion (fetopelvic) 653.3❺
      - affecting fetus or newborn 763.1
      - causing obstructed labor 660.1❺
        - affecting fetus or newborn 763.1
  - nose (congenital) 748.1
    - acquired 738.0
- **PROMM** (proximal myotonic myotonia) 359.21 ●
- **Pronation**
  - ankle 736.79
  - foot 736.79
    - congenital 755.67
- **Prophylactic**
  - administration of
    - antibiotics V07.39
    - antitoxin, any V07.2
    - antivenin V07.2
    - chemotherapeutic agent NEC V07.39
      - fluoride V07.31
    - diphtheria antitoxin V07.2
    - drug V07.39 ●
    - gamma globulin V07.2
    - immune sera (gamma globulin) V07.2
    - RhoGAM V07.2
    - tetanus antitoxin V07.2
  - chemotherapy NEC V07.39
    - fluoride V07.31
  - hormone replacement (postmenopausal) V07.4
  - immunotherapy V07.2
  - measure V07.9
    - specified type NEC V07.8
  - medication V07.39 ●
  - postmenopausal hormone replacement V07.4
  - sterilization V25.2
- **Proptosis** (ocular) (*see also* Exophthalmos) 376.30
  - thyroid 242.0❺
- **Propulsion**
  - eyeball 360.81
- **Prosecution, anxiety concerning** V62.5
- **Prostate, prostatic** – *see* condition
- **Prostatism** 600.90
  - with
    - other lower urinary tract symptoms (LUTS) 600.91
    - urinary
      - obstruction 600.91
      - retention 600.91
- **Prostatitis** (congestive) (suppurative) 601.9
  - acute 601.0
  - cavitary 601.8
  - chlamydial 099.54
  - chronic 601.1
  - diverticular 601.8
  - due to Trichomonas (vaginalis) 131.03

- **Prostatitis** – *continued*
  - fibrous 600.90
    - with
      - other lower urinary tract symptoms (LUTS) 600.91
      - urinary
        - obstruction 600.91
        - retention 600.91
  - gonococcal (acute) 098.12
    - chronic or duration of 2 months or over 098.32
  - granulomatous 601.8
  - hypertrophic 600.00
    - with
      - other lower urinary tract symptoms (LUTS) 600.01
      - urinary
        - obstruction 600.01
        - retention 600.01
  - specified type NEC 601.8
  - subacute 601.1
  - trichomonal 131.03
  - tuberculous (*see also* Tuberculosis) 016.5❺ *[601.4]*
- **Prostatocystitis** 601.3
- **Prostatorrhea** 602.8
- **Prostatoseminovesiculitis, trichomonal** 131.03
- **Prostration** 780.79
  - heat 992.5
    - anhydrotic 992.3
    - due to
      - salt (and water) depletion 992.4
      - water depletion 992.3
  - nervous 300.5
  - newborn 779.89
  - senile 797
- **Protanomaly** 368.51
- **Protanopia** (anomalous trichromat) (complete) (incomplete) 368.51
- **Protection** (against) (from) – *see* Prophylactic ●
- **Protein**
  - deficiency 260
  - malnutrition 260
  - sickness (prophylactic) (therapeutic) 999.5
- **Proteinemia** 790.99
- **Proteinosis**
  - alveolar, lung or pulmonary 516.0
  - lipid 272.8
  - lipoid (of Urbach) 272.8
- **Proteinuria** (*see also* Albuminuria) 791.0
  - Bence-Jones NEC 791.0
  - gestational 646.2❺
    - with hypertension – *see* Toxemia, of pregnancy
  - orthostatic 593.6
  - postural 593.6
- **Proteolysis, pathologic** 286.6
- **Protocoproporphyria** 277.1
- **Protoporphyria** (erythrohepatic) (erythropoietic) 277.1
- **Protrusio acetabuli** 718.65
- **Protrusion**
  - acetabulum (into pelvis) 718.65
  - device, implant, or graft – *see* Complications, mechanical
  - ear, congenital 744.29
  - intervertebral disc – *see* Displacement, intervertebral disc
  - nucleus pulposus – *see* Displacement, intervertebral disc
- **Proud flesh** 701.5
- **Prune belly** (syndrome) 756.71
- **Prurigo** (ferox) (gravis) (Hebra's) (hebrae) (mitis) (simplex) 698.2
  - agria 698.3
  - asthma syndrome 691.8
  - Besnier's (atopic dermatitis) (infantile eczema) 691.8
  - eczematodes allergicum 691.8
  - estivalis (Hutchinson's) 692.72
  - Hutchinson's 692.72
  - nodularis 698.3
  - psychogenic 306.3
- **Pruritus, pruritic** 698.9
  - ani 698.0
    - psychogenic 306.3
  - conditions NEC 698.9
    - psychogenic 306.3
  - due to Onchocerca volvulus 125.3
  - ear 698.9
  - essential 698.9
- **Pruritus, pruritic** – *continued*
  - genital organ(s) 698.1
    - psychogenic 306.3
  - gravidarum 646.8❺
  - hiemalis 698.8
  - neurogenic (any site) 306.3
  - perianal 698.0
  - psychogenic (any site) 306.3
  - scrotum 698.1
    - psychogenic 306.3
  - senile, senilis 698.8
  - Trichomonas 131.9
  - vulva, vulvae 698.1
    - psychogenic 306.3
- **Psammocarcinoma** (M8140/3) – *see* Neoplasm, by site, malignant
- **Pseudarthrosis, pseudoarthrosis** (bone) 733.82
  - joint following fusion V45.4
- **Pseudoacanthosis**
  - nigricans 701.8
- **Pseudoaneurysm** – *see* Aneurysm
- **Pseudoangina** (pectoris) – *see* Angina
- **Pseudoangioma** 452
- **Pseudo-Argyll-Robertson pupil** 379.45
- **Pseudoarteriosus** 747.89
- **Pseudoarthrosis** – *see* Pseudarthrosis
- **Pseudoataxia** 799.89
- **Pseudobulbar affect** (PBA) 310.8
- **Pseudobursa** 727.89
- **Pseudocholera** 025
- **Pseudochromidrosis** 705.89
- **Pseudocirrhosis, liver, pericardial** 423.2
- **Pseudocoarctation** 747.21
- **Pseudocowpox** 051.1
- **Pseudocoxalgia** 732.1
- **Pseudocroup** 478.75
- **Pseudocyesis** 300.11
- **Pseudocyst**
  - lung 518.89
  - pancreas 577.2
  - retina 361.19
- **Pseudodementia** 300.16
- **Pseudoelephantiasis neuroarthritica** 757.0
- **Pseudoemphysema** 518.89
- **Pseudoencephalitis**
  - superior (acute) hemorrhagic 265.1
- **Pseudoerosion cervix, congenital** 752.49
- **Pseudoexfoliation, lens capsule** 366.11
- **Pseudofracture** (idiopathic) (multiple) (spontaneous) (symmetrical) 268.2
- **Pseudoglanders** 025
- **Pseudoglioma** 360.44
- **Pseudogout** – *see* Chondrocalcinosis
- **Pseudohallucination** 780.1
- **Pseudohemianesthesia** 782.0
- **Pseudohemophilia** (Bernuth's) (hereditary) (type B) 286.4
  - type A 287.8
  - vascular 287.8
- **Pseudohermaphroditism** 752.7
  - with chromosomal anomaly – *see* Anomaly, chromosomal
  - adrenal 255.2
  - female (without adrenocortical disorder) 752.7
    - with adrenocortical disorder 255.2
    - adrenal 255.2
  - male (without gonadal disorder) 752.7
    - with
      - adrenocortical disorder 255.2
      - cleft scrotum 752.7
      - feminizing testis 259.5
      - gonadal disorder 257.9
    - adrenal 255.2
- **Pseudohole, macula** 362.54
- **Pseudo-Hurler's disease** (mucolipidosis III) 272.7
- **Pseudohydrocephalus** 348.2
- **Pseudohypertrophic muscular dystrophy** (Erb's) 359.1
- **Pseudohypertrophy, muscle** 359.1
- **Pseudohypoparathyroidism** 275.49
- **Pseudoinfluenza** 487.1
- **Pseudoinsomnia** 307.49
- **Pseudoleukemia** 288.8
  - infantile 285.8
- **Pseudomembranous** – *see* condition
- **Pseudomeningocele** (cerebral) (infective) 349.2
  - postprocedural 997.01
  - spinal 349.2
- **Pseudomenstruation** 626.8
- **Pseudomucinous**
  - cyst (ovary) (M8470/0) 220
  - peritoneum 568.89
- **Pseudomyeloma** 273.1
- **Pseudomyxoma peritonei** (M8480/6) 197.6
- **Pseudoneuritis optic** (nerve) 377.24
  - papilla 377.24
    - congenital 743.57
- **Pseudoneuroma** – *see* Injury, nerve, by site
- **Pseudo-obstruction**
  - intestine (chronic) (idiopathic) (intermittent secondary) (primary) 564.89
    - acute 560.89
- **Pseudopapilledema** 377.24
- **Pseudoparalysis**
  - arm or leg 781.4
  - atonic, congenital 358.8
- **Pseudopelade** 704.09
- **Pseudophakia** V43.1
- **Pseudopolycythemia** 289.0
- **Pseudopolyposis, colon** 556.4
- **Pseudoporencephaly** 348.0
- **Pseudopseudohypoparathyroidism** 275.49
- **Pseudopsychosis** 300.16
- **Pseudopterygium** 372.52
- **Pseudoptosis** (eyelid) 374.34
- **Pseudorabies** 078.89
- **Pseudoretinitis, pigmentosa** 362.65
- **Pseudorickets** 588.0
  - senile (Pozzi's) 731.0
- **Pseudorubella** 057.8
- **Pseudoscarlatina** 057.8
- **Pseudosclerema** 778.1
- **Pseudosclerosis** (brain)
  - Jakob's 046.1
  - of Westphal (-Strümpell) (hepatolenticular degeneration) 275.1
  - spastic 046.1
    - with dementia
      - with behavioral disturbance 046.1 *[294.11]*
      - without behavioral disturbance 046.1 *[294.10]*
- **Pseudoseizure** 780.39
  - non-psychiatric 780.39
  - psychiatric 300.11
- **Pseudotabes** 799.89
  - diabetic 250.6❺ *[337.1]*
- **Pseudotetanus** (*see also* Convulsions) 780.39
- **Pseudotetany** 781.7
  - hysterical 300.11
- **Pseudothalassemia** 285.0
- **Pseudotrichinosis** 710.3
- **Pseudotruncus arteriosus** 747.29
- **Pseudotuberculosis, pasteurella** (infection) 027.2
- **Pseudotumor**
  - cerebri 348.2
  - orbit (inflammatory) 376.11
- **Pseudo-Turner's syndrome** 759.89
- **Pseudoxanthoma elasticum** 757.39
- **Psilosis** (sprue) (tropical) 579.1
  - Monilia 112.89
  - nontropical 579.0
  - not sprue 704.00
- **Psittacosis** 073.9
- **Psoitis** 728.89
- **Psora** NEC 696.1
- **Psoriasis** 696.1
  - any type, except arthropathic 696.1
  - arthritic, arthropathic 696.0
  - buccal 528.6
  - flexural 696.1
  - follicularis 696.1
  - guttate 696.1
  - inverse 696.1
  - mouth 528.6
  - nummularis 696.1
  - psychogenic 316 *[696.1]*
  - punctata 696.1
  - pustular 696.1
  - rupioides 696.1

- **Psychosis** – *continued*
  - organic NEC 294.9
    - due to or associated with
      - addiction
        - alcohol (*see also* Psychosis, alcoholic) 291.9
        - drug (*see also* Psychosis, drug) 292.9
      - alcohol intoxication, acute (*see also* Psychosis, alcoholic) 291.9
      - alcoholism (*see also* Psychosis, alcoholic) 291.9
      - arteriosclerosis (cerebral) (*see also* Psychosis, arteriosclerotic) 290.40
      - cerebrovascular disease
        - acute (psychosis) 293.0
        - arteriosclerotic (*see also* Psychosis, arteriosclerotic) 290.40
      - childbirth – *see* Psychosis, puerperal
      - dependence
        - alcohol (*see also* Psychosis, alcoholic) 291.9
        - drug 292.9
      - disease
        - alcoholic liver (*see also* Psychosis, alcoholic) 291.9
        - brain
          - arteriosclerotic (*see also* Psychosis, arteriosclerotic) 290.40
        - cerebrovascular
          - acute (psychosis) 293.0
          - arteriosclerotic (*see also* Psychosis, arteriosclerotic) 290.40
        - endocrine or metabolic 293.9
          - acute (psychosis) 293.0
          - subacute (psychosis) 293.1
        - Jakob-Creutzfeldt (new variant)
          - with behavioral disturbance 046.1 *[294.11]*
          - without behavioral disturbance 046.1 *[294.10]*
        - liver, alcoholic (*see also* Psychosis, alcoholic) 291.9
      - disorder
        - cerebrovascular
          - acute (psychosis) 293.0
        - endocrine or metabolic 293.9
          - acute (psychosis) 293.0
          - subacute (psychosis) 293.1
      - epilepsy
        - with behavioral disturbance 345.9❺ *[294.11]*
        - without behavioral disturbance 345.9❺ *[294.10]*
        - transient (acute) 293.0
      - Huntington's chorea
        - with behavioral disturbance 333.4 *[294.11]*
        - without behavioral disturbance 333.4 *[294.10]*
      - infection
        - brain 293.9
          - acute (psychosis) 293.0
          - chronic 294.8
          - subacute (psychosis) 293.1
        - intracranial NEC 293.9
          - acute (psychosis) 293.0
          - chronic 294.8
          - subacute (psychosis) 293.1
      - intoxication
        - alcoholic (acute) (*see also* Psychosis, alcoholic) 291.9
          - pathological 291.4
        - drug (*see also* Psychosis, drug) 292.9
      - ischemia
        - cerebrovascular (generalized) (*see also* Psychosis, arteriosclerotic) 290.40
      - Jakob-Creutzfeldt disease (syndrome) (new variant)
        - with behavioral disturbance 046.1 *[294.11]*
        - without behavioral disturbance 046.1 *[294.10]*
      - multiple sclerosis
        - with behavioral disturbance 340 *[294.11]*
        - without behavioral disturbance 340 *[294.10]*
      - physical condition NEC 293.9
        - with
          - delusions 293.81
          - hallucinations 293.82
      - presenility 290.10
      - puerperium – *see* Psychosis, puerperal

- **Psychosis** – *continued*
  - organic – *continued*
    - due to or associated with – *continued*
      - sclerosis, multiple
        - with behavioral disturbance 340 *[294.11]*
        - without behavioral disturbance 340 *[294.10]*
      - senility 290.20
      - status epilepticus
        - with behavioral disturbance 345.3❺ *[294.11]*
        - without behavioral disturbance 345.3❺ *[294.10]*
      - trauma
        - brain (birth) (from electrical current) (surgical) 293.9
          - acute (psychosis) 293.0
          - chronic 294.8
          - subacute (psychosis) 293.1
      - unspecified physical condition 293.9
        - with
          - delusions 293.81
          - hallucinations 293.82
    - infective 293.9
      - acute (psychosis) 293.0
      - subacute 293.1
    - posttraumatic 293.9
      - acute 293.0
      - subacute 293.1
    - specified type NEC 294.8
    - transient 293.9
      - with
        - anxiety 293.84
        - delusions 293.81
        - depression 293.83
        - hallucinations 293.82
      - depressive type 293.83
      - hallucinatory type 293.82
      - paranoid type 293.81
      - specified type NEC 293.89
  - paranoic 297.1
  - paranoid (chronic) 297.9
    - alcoholic 291.5
    - chronic 297.1
    - climacteric 297.2
    - involutional 297.2
    - menopausal 297.2
    - protracted reactive 298.4
    - psychogenic 298.4
      - acute 298.3
    - schizophrenic (*see also* Schizophrenia) 295.3❺
    - senile 290.20
  - paroxysmal 298.9
    - senile 290.20
  - polyneuritic, alcoholic 291.1
  - postoperative 293.9
  - postpartum – *see* Psychosis, puerperal
  - prepsychotic (*see also* Schizophrenia) 295.5❺
  - presbyophrenic (type) 290.8
  - presenile (*see also* Dementia, presenile) 290.10
  - prison 300.16
  - psychogenic 298.8
    - depressive 298.0
    - paranoid 298.4
      - acute 298.3
  - puerperal
    - specified type – *see* categories 295-298❺
    - unspecified type 293.89
      - acute 293.0
      - chronic 293.89
      - subacute 293.1
  - reactive (emotional stress) (psychological trauma) 298.8
    - brief 298.8
    - confusion 298.2
    - depressive 298.0
    - excitation 298.1
  - schizo-affective (depressed) (excited) (*see also* Schizophrenia) 295.7❺
  - schizophrenia, schizophrenic (*see also* Schizophrenia) 295.9❺
    - borderline type 295.5❺
      - of childhood (*see also* Psychosis, childhood) 299.8❺
    - catatonic (excited) (withdrawn) 295.2❺
    - childhood type (*see also* Psychosis, childhood) 299.9❺
    - hebephrenic 295.1❺
    - incipient 295.5❺
    - latent 295.5❺
    - paranoid 295.3❺

- **Psychosis** – *continued*
  - schizophrenia, schizophrenic – *continued*
    - prepsychotic 295.5❺
    - prodromal 295.5❺
    - pseudoneurotic 295.5❺
    - pseudopsychopathic 295.5❺
    - schizophreniform 295.4❺
    - simple 295.0❺
    - undifferentiated type 295.9
  - schizophreniform 295.4❺
  - senile NEC 290.20
    - with
      - delusional features 290.20
      - depressive features 290.21
    - depressed type 290.21
    - paranoid type 290.20
    - simple deterioration 290.20
    - specified type – *see* categories 295-298❺
  - shared 297.3
  - situational (reactive) 298.8
  - symbiotic (childhood) (*see also* Psychosis, childhood) 299.1❺
  - toxic (acute) 293.9
- **Psychotic** (*see also* condition) 298.9
  - episode 298.9
    - due to or associated with physical conditions (*see also* Psychosis, organic) 293.9
- **Pterygium** (eye) 372.40
  - central 372.43
  - colli 744.5
  - double 372.44
  - peripheral (stationary) 372.41
    - progressive 372.42
  - recurrent 372.45
- **Ptilosis** 374.55
- **Ptomaine** (poisoning) (*see also* Poisoning, food) 005.9
- **Ptosis** (adiposa) 374.30
  - breast 611.8
  - cecum 569.89
  - colon 569.89
  - congenital (eyelid) 743.61
    - specified site NEC – *see* Anomaly, specified type NEC
  - epicanthus syndrome 270.2
  - eyelid 374.30
    - congenital 743.61
    - mechanical 374.33
    - myogenic 374.32
    - paralytic 374.31
  - gastric 537.5
  - intestine 569.89
  - kidney (*see also* Disease, renal) 593.0
    - congenital 753.3
  - liver 573.8
  - renal (*see also* Disease, renal) 593.0
    - congenital 753.3
  - splanchnic 569.89
  - spleen 289.59
  - stomach 537.5
  - viscera 569.89
- **PTSD** (Post-Traumatic Stress Disorder) 309.81
- **Ptyalism** 527.7
  - hysterical 300.11
  - periodic 527.2
  - pregnancy 646.8❺
  - psychogenic 306.4
- **Ptyalolithiasis** 527.5
- **Pubalgia** 848.8
- **Pubarche, precocious** 259.1
- **Pubertas praecox** 259.1
- **Puberty** V21.1
  - abnormal 259.9
  - bleeding 626.3
  - delayed 259.0
  - precocious (constitutional) (cryptogenic) (idiopathic) NEC 259.1
    - due to
      - adrenal
        - cortical hyperfunction 255.2
        - hyperplasia 255.2
      - cortical hyperfunction 255.2
      - ovarian hyperfunction 256.1
        - estrogen 256.0
      - pineal tumor 259.8
      - testicular hyperfunction 257.0
  - premature 259.1
    - due to
      - adrenal cortical hyperfunction 255.2
      - pineal tumor 259.8

- **Puberty** – *continued*
  - premature – *continued*
    - due to – *continued*
      - pituitary (anterior) hyperfunction 253.1
- **Puckering, macula** 362.56
- **Pudenda, pudendum** – *see* condition
- **Puente's disease** (simple glandular cheilitis) 528.5
- **Puerperal**
  - abscess
    - areola 675.1❺
    - Bartholin's gland 646.6❺
    - breast 675.1❺
    - cervix (uteri) 670❹
    - fallopian tube 670❹
    - genital organ 670❹
    - kidney 646.6❺
    - mammary 675.1❺
    - mesosalpinx 670❹
    - nabothian 646.6❺
    - nipple 675.0❺
    - ovary, ovarian 670❹
    - oviduct 670❹
    - parametric 670❹
    - para-uterine 670❹
    - pelvic 670❹
    - perimetric 670❹
    - periuterine 670❹
    - retro-uterine 670❹
    - subareolar 675.1❺
    - suprapelvic 670❹
    - tubal (ruptured) 670❹
    - tubo-ovarian 670❹
    - urinary tract NEC 646.6❺
    - uterine, uterus 670❹
    - vagina (wall) 646.6❺
    - vaginorectal 646.6❺
    - vulvovaginal gland 646.6❺
  - accident 674.9❺
  - adnexitis 670❹
  - afibrinogenemia, or other coagulation defect 666.3❺
  - albuminuria (acute) (subacute) 646.2❺
    - pre-eclamptic 642.4❺
  - anemia (conditions classifiable to 280-285) 648.2❺
  - anuria 669.3❺
  - apoplexy 674.0❺
  - asymptomatic bacteriuria 646.5❺
  - atrophy, breast 676.3❺
  - blood dyscrasia 666.3❺
  - caked breast 676.2❺
  - cardiomyopathy 674.5❺
  - cellulitis – *see* Puerperal, abscess
  - cerebrovascular disorder (conditions classifiable to 430-434, 436-437) 674.0❺
  - cervicitis (conditions classifiable to 616.0) 646.6❺
  - coagulopathy (any) 666.3❺
  - complications 674.9❺
    - specified type NEC 674.8❺
  - convulsions (eclamptic) (uremic) 642.6❺
    - with pre-existing hypertension 642.7❺
  - cracked nipple 676.1❺
  - cystitis 646.6❺
  - cystopyelitis 646.6❺
  - deciduitis (acute) 670❹
  - delirium NEC 293.9
  - diabetes (mellitus) (conditions classifiable to 250) 648.0❺
  - disease 674.9❺
    - breast NEC 676.3❺
    - cerebrovascular (acute) 674.0❺
    - nonobstetric NEC (*see also* Pregnancy, complicated, current disease or condition) 648.9❺
    - pelvis inflammatory 670❹
    - renal NEC 646.2❺
    - tubo-ovarian 670❹
    - Valsuani's (progressive pernicious anemia) 648.2❺
  - disorder
    - lactation 676.9❺
      - specified type NEC 676.8❺
    - nonobstetric NEC (*see also* Pregnancy, complicated, current disease or condition) 648.9❺
  - disruption
    - cesarean wound 674.1❺
    - episiotomy wound 674.2❺
    - perineal laceration wound 674.2❺
  - drug dependence (conditions classifiable to 304) 648.3❺
  - eclampsia 642.6❺
    - with pre-existing hypertension 642.7❺
  - embolism (pulmonary) 673.2❺
    - air 673.0❺
    - amniotic fluid 673.1❺
    - blood clot 673.2❺
    - brain or cerebral 674.0❺
    - cardiac 674.8❺
    - fat 673.8❺
    - intracranial sinus (venous) 671.5❺
    - pyemic 673.3❺
    - septic 673.3❺
    - spinal cord 671.5❺
  - endometritis (conditions classifiable to 615.0-615.9) 670❹
  - endophlebitis – *see* Puerperal, phlebitis
  - endotrachelitis 646.6❺
  - engorgement, breasts 676.2❺
  - erysipelas 670❹
  - failure
    - lactation 676.4❺
    - renal, acute 669.3❺
  - fever 670❹
    - meaning sepsis 670❹
    - meaning pyrexia (of unknown origin) 672❹
  - fissure, nipple 676.1❺
  - fistula
    - breast 675.1❺
    - mammary gland 675.1❺
    - nipple 675.0❺
  - galactophoritis 675.2❺
  - galactorrhea 676.6❺
  - gangrene
    - gas 670❹
    - uterus 670❹
  - gonorrhea (conditions classifiable to 098) 647.1❺
  - hematoma, subdural 674.0❺
  - hematosalpinx, infectional 670❹
  - hemiplegia, cerebral 674.0❺
  - hemorrhage 666.1❺
    - brain 674.0❺
    - bulbar 674.0❺
    - cerebellar 674.0❺
    - cerebral 674.0❺
    - cortical 674.0❺
    - delayed (after 24 hours) (uterine) 666.2❺
    - extradural 674.0❺
    - internal capsule 674.0❺
    - intracranial 674.0❺
    - intrapontine 674.0❺
    - meningeal 674.0❺
    - pontine 674.0❺
    - subarachnoid 674.0❺
    - subcortical 674.0❺
    - subdural 674.0❺
    - uterine, delayed 666.2❺
    - ventricular 674.0❺
  - hemorrhoids 671.8❺
  - hepatorenal syndrome 674.8❺
  - hypertrophy
    - breast 676.3❺
    - mammary gland 676.3❺
  - induration breast (fibrous) 676.3❺
  - infarction
    - lung – *see* Puerperal, embolism
    - pulmonary – *see* Puerperal, embolism
  - infection
    - Bartholin's gland 646.6❺
    - breast 675.2❺
      - with nipple 675.9❺
        - specified type NEC 675.8❺
    - cervix 646.6❺
    - endocervix 646.6❺
    - fallopian tube 670❹
    - generalized 670❹
    - genital tract (major) 670❹
      - minor or localized 646.6❺
    - kidney (bacillus coli) 646.6❺
    - mammary gland 675.2❺
    - mammary
      - with nipple 675.9❺
        - specified type NEC 675.8❺
    - nipple 675.0❺
      - with breast 675.9❺
        - specified type NEC 675.8❺
    - ovary 670❹
    - pelvic 670❹
    - peritoneum 670❹
    - renal 646.6❺
    - tubo-ovarian 670❹
    - urinary (tract) NEC 646.6❺
      - asymptomatic 646.5❺
    - uterus, uterine 670❹
    - vagina 646.6❺
  - inflammation – *see also* Puerperal, infection
    - areola 675.1❺
    - Bartholin's gland 646.6❺
    - breast 675.2❺
    - broad ligament 670❹
    - cervix (uteri) 646.6❺
    - fallopian tube 670❹
    - genital organs 670❹
      - localized 646.6❺
    - mammary gland 675.2❺
    - nipple 675.0❺
    - ovary 670❹
    - oviduct 670❹
    - pelvis 670❹
    - periuterine 670❹
    - tubal 670❹
    - vagina 646.6❺
    - vein – *see* Puerperal, phlebitis
  - inversion, nipple 676.3❺
  - ischemia, cerebral 674.0❺
  - lymphangitis 670❹
    - breast 675.2❺
  - malaria (conditions classifiable to 084) 647.4❺
  - malnutrition 648.9❺
  - mammillitis 675.0❺
  - mammitis 675.2❺
  - mania 296.0❺
    - recurrent episode 296.1❺
    - single episode 296.0❺
  - mastitis 675.2❺
    - purulent 675.1❺
    - retromammary 675.1❺
    - submammary 675.1❺
  - melancholia 296.2❺
    - recurrent episode 296.3❺
    - single episode 296.2❺
  - mental disorder (conditions classifiable to 290-303, 305.0, 305.2-305.9, 306-316, 317-319) 648.4❺
  - metritis (septic) (suppurative) 670❹
  - metroperitonitis 670❹
  - metrorrhagia 666.2❺
  - metrosalpingitis 670❹
  - metrovaginitis 670❹
  - milk leg 671.4❺
  - monoplegia, cerebral 674.0❺
  - necrosis
    - kidney, tubular 669.3❺
    - liver (acute) (subacute) (conditions classifiable to 570) 674.8❺
    - ovary 670❹
    - renal cortex 669.3❺
  - nephritis or nephrosis (conditions classifiable to 580-589) 646.2❺
    - with hypertension 642.1❺
  - nutritional deficiency (conditions classifiable to 260-269) 648.9❺
  - occlusion, precerebral artery 674.0❺
  - oliguria 669.3❺
  - oophoritis 670❹
  - ovaritis 670❹
  - paralysis
    - bladder (sphincter) 665.5❺
    - cerebral 674.0❺
  - paralytic stroke 674.0❺
  - parametritis 670❹
  - paravaginitis 646.6❺
  - pelviperitonitis 670❹
  - perimetritis 670❹
  - perimetrosalpingitis 670❹
  - perinephritis 646.6❺
  - perioophoritis 670❹
  - periphlebitis – *see* Puerperal, phlebitis
  - perisalpingitis 670❹
  - peritoneal infection 670❹
  - peritonitis (pelvic) 670❹
  - perivaginitis 646.6❺
  - phlebitis 671.9❺
    - deep 671.4❺
    - intracranial sinus (venous) 671.5❺
    - pelvic 671.4❺
    - specified site NEC 671.5❺
    - superficial 671.2❺
  - phlegmasia alba dolens 671.4❺

❹ Fourth-Digit Required ❺ Fifth-Digit Required *[code]* Manifestation Code ▶◀ Revised Text ● New Line ▲ Revised Code

Puerperal – *continued*
- placental polyp 674.4❺
- pneumonia, embolic – *see* Puerperal, embolism
- prediabetes 648.8❺
- pre-eclampsia (mild) 642.4❺
  - with pre-existing hypertension 642.7❺
  - severe 642.5❺
- psychosis, unspecified (*see also* Psychosis, puerperal) 293.89
- pyelitis 646.6❺
- pyelocystitis 646.6❺
- pyelohydronephrosis 646.6❺
- pyelonephritis 646.6❺
- pyelonephrosis 646.6❺
- pyemia 670❹
- pyocystitis 646.6❺
- pyohemia 670❹
- pyometra 670❹
- pyonephritis 646.6❺
- pyonephrosis 646.6❺
- pyo-oophoritis 670❹
- pyosalpingitis 670❹
- pyosalpinx 670❹
- pyrexia (of unknown origin) 672❹
- renal
  - disease NEC 646.2❺
  - failure, acute 669.3❺
- retention
  - decidua (fragments) (with delayed hemorrhage) 666.2❺
    - without hemorrhage 667.1❺
  - placenta (fragments) (with delayed hemorrhage) 666.2❺
    - without hemorrhage 667.1❺
  - secundines (fragments) (with delayed hemorrhage) 666.2❺
    - without hemorrhage 667.1❺
- retracted nipple 676.0❺
- rubella (conditions classifiable to 056) 647.5❺
- salpingitis 670❹
- salpingo-oophoritis 670❹
- salpingo-ovaritis 670❹
- salpingoperitonitis 670❹
- sapremia 670❹
- secondary perineal tear 674.2❺
- sepsis (pelvic) 670❹
- septicemia 670❹
- subinvolution (uterus) 674.8❺
- sudden death (cause unknown) 674.9❺
- suppuration – *see* Puerperal, abscess
- syphilis (conditions classifiable to 090-097) 647.0❺
- tetanus 670❹
- thelitis 675.0❺
- thrombocytopenia 666.3❺
- thrombophlebitis (superficial) 671.2❺
  - deep 671.4❺
  - pelvic 671.4❺
  - specified site NEC 671.5❺
- thrombosis (venous) – *see* Thrombosis, puerperal
- thyroid dysfunction (conditions classifiable to 240-246) 648.1❺
- toxemia (*see also* Toxemia, of pregnancy) 642.4❺
  - eclamptic 642.6❺
    - with pre-existing hypertension 642.7❺
  - pre-eclamptic (mild) 642.4❺
    - with
      - convulsions 642.6❺
      - pre-existing hypertension 642.7❺
    - severe 642.5❺
- tuberculosis (conditions classifiable to 010-018) 647.3❺
- uremia 669.3❺
- vaginitis (conditions classifiable to 616.1) 646.6❺
- varicose veins (legs) 671.0❺
  - vulva or perineum 671.1❺
- vulvitis (conditions classifiable to 616.1) 646.6❺
- vulvovaginitis (conditions classifiable to 616.1) 646.6❺
- white leg 671.4❺

Pulled muscle – *see* Sprain, by site

Pulmolithiasis 518.89

Pulmonary – *see* condition

Pulmonitis (unknown etiology) 486

Pulpitis (acute) (anachoretic) (chronic) (hyperplastic) (putrescent) (suppurative) (ulcerative) 522.0

Pulpless tooth 522.9

Pulse
- alternating 427.89
  - psychogenic 306.2
- bigeminal 427.89
- fast 785.0
- feeble, rapid, due to shock following injury 958.4
- rapid 785.0
- slow 427.89
- strong 785.9
- trigeminal 427.89
- water-hammer (*see also* Insufficiency, aortic) 424.1
- weak 785.9

Pulseless disease 446.7

Pulsus
- alternans or trigeminy 427.89
  - psychogenic 306.2

Punch drunk 310.2

Puncta lacrimalia occlusion 375.52

Punctiform hymen 752.49

Puncture (traumatic) – *see also* Wound, open, by site
- accidental, complicating surgery 998.2
- bladder, nontraumatic 596.6
- by
  - device, implant, or graft – *see* Complications, mechanical
  - foreign body
    - internal organs – *see also* Injury, internal, by site
      - by ingested object – *see* Foreign body
    - left accidentally in operation wound 998.4
  - instrument (any) during a procedure, accidental 998.2
- internal organs, abdomen, chest, or pelvis – *see* Injury, internal, by site
- kidney, nontraumatic 593.89

Pupil – *see* condition

Pupillary membrane 364.74
- persistent 743.46

Pupillotonia 379.46
- pseudotabetic 379.46

Purpura 287.2
- abdominal 287.0
- allergic 287.0
- anaphylactoid 287.0
- annularis telangiectodes 709.1
- arthritic 287.0
- autoerythrocyte sensitization 287.2
- autoimmune 287.0
- bacterial 287.0
- Bateman's (senile) 287.2
- capillary fragility (hereditary) (idiopathic) 287.8
- cryoglobulinemic 273.2
- devil's pinches 287.2
- fibrinolytic (*see also* Fibrinolysis) 286.6
- fulminans, fulminous 286.6
- gangrenous 287.0
- hemorrhagic (*see also* Purpura, thrombocytopenic) 287.39
  - nodular 272.7
  - nonthrombocytopenic 287.0
  - thrombocytopenic 287.39
- Henoch's (purpura nervosa) 287.0
- Henoch-Schönlein (allergic) 287.0
- hypergammaglobulinemic (benign primary) (Waldenström's) 273.0
- idiopathic 287.31
  - nonthrombocytopenic 287.0
  - thrombocytopenic 287.31
- immune thrombocytopenic 287.31
- infectious 287.0
- malignant 287.0
- neonatorum 772.6
- nervosa 287.0
- newborn NEC 772.6
- nonthrombocytopenic 287.2
  - hemorrhagic 287.0
  - idiopathic 287.0
- nonthrombopenic 287.2
- peliosis rheumatica 287.0
- pigmentaria, progressiva 709.09
- posttransfusion 287.4
- primary 287.0
- primitive 287.0
- red cell membrane sensitivity 287.2
- rheumatica 287.0
- Schönlein (-Henoch) (allergic) 287.0
- scorbutic 267
- senile 287.2
- simplex 287.2

Purpura – *continued*
- symptomatica 287.0
- telangiectasia annularis 709.1
- thrombocytopenic (*see also* Thrombocytopenia) 287.30
  - congenital 287.33
  - essential 287.30
  - hereditary 287.31
  - idiopathic 287.31
  - immune 287.31
  - neonatal, transitory (*see also* Thrombocytopenia, neonatal transitory) 776.1
  - primary 287.30
  - puerperal, postpartum 666.3❺
  - thrombotic 446.6
- thrombohemolytic (*see also* Fibrinolysis) 286.6
- thrombopenic (*see also* Thrombocytopenia) 287.30
  - congenital 287.33
  - essential 287.30
- thrombotic 446.6
  - thrombocytic 446.6
  - thrombocytopenic 446.6
- toxic 287.0
- variolosa 050.0
- vascular 287.0
- visceral symptoms 287.0
- Werlhof's (*see also* Purpura, thrombocytopenic) 287.39

Purpuric spots 782.7

Purulent – *see* condition

Pus
- absorption, general – *see* Septicemia
- in
  - stool 792.1
  - urine 791.9
- tube (rupture) (*see also* Salpingo-oophoritis) 614.2

Pustular rash 782.1

Pustule 686.9
- malignant 022.0
- nonmalignant 686.9

Putnam's disease (subacute combined sclerosis with pernicious anemia) 281.0 *[336.2]*

Putnam-Dana syndrome (subacute combined sclerosis with pernicious anemia) 281.0 *[336.2]*

Putrefaction, intestinal 569.89

Putrescent pulp (dental) 522.1

Pyarthritis – *see* Pyarthrosis

Pyarthrosis (*see also* Arthritis, pyogenic) 711.0❺
- tuberculous – *see* Tuberculosis, joint

Pycnoepilepsy, pycnolepsy (idiopathic) (*see also* Epilepsy) 345.0❺

Pyelectasia 593.89

Pyelectasis 593.89

Pyelitis (congenital) (uremic) 590.80
- with
  - abortion – *see* Abortion, by type, with specified complication NEC
  - contracted kidney 590.00
  - ectopic pregnancy (*see also* categories 633.0-633.9) 639.8
  - molar pregnancy (*see also* categories 630-632) 639.8
- acute 590.10
  - with renal medullary necrosis 590.11
- chronic 590.00
  - with
    - renal medullary necrosis 590.01
- complicating pregnancy, childbirth, or puerperium 646.6❺
  - affecting fetus or newborn 760.1
- cystica 590.3
- following
  - abortion 639.8
  - ectopic or molar pregnancy 639.8
- gonococcal 098.19
  - chronic or duration of 2 months or over 098.39
- tuberculous (*see also* Tuberculosis) 016.0❺ *[590.81]*

Pyelocaliectasis 593.89

Pyelocystitis (*see also* Pyelitis) 590.80

Pyelohydronephrosis 591

Pyelonephritis (*see also* Pyelitis) 590.80
- acute 590.10
  - with renal medullary necrosis 590.11
- chronic 590.00
- syphilitic (late) 095.4

Puerperal – Pyelonephritis

- **Pyelonephritis** – *continued*
  - tuberculous (*see also* Tuberculosis) 016.0❺ *[590.81]*
- **Pyelonephrosis** (*see also* Pyelitis) 590.80
  - chronic 590.00
- **Pyelophlebitis** 451.89
- **Pyelo-ureteritis cystica** 590.3
- **Pyemia, pyemic** (purulent) (*see also* Septicemia) 038.9
  - abscess – *see* Abscess
  - arthritis (*see also* Arthritis, pyogenic) 711.0❺
  - Bacillus coli 038.42
  - embolism ▶(*see also* Septicemia)◀ 415.12 ▲
  - fever 038.9
  - infection 038.9
  - joint (*see also* Arthritis, pyogenic) 711.0❺
  - liver 572.1
  - meningococcal 036.2
  - newborn 771.81
  - phlebitis – *see* Phlebitis
  - pneumococcal 038.2
  - portal 572.1
  - postvaccinal 999.39 ▲
  - specified organism NEC 038.8
  - staphylococcal 038.10
    - aureus 038.11
    - specified organism NEC 038.19
  - streptococcal 038.0
  - tuberculous – *see* Tuberculosis, miliary
- **Pygopagus** 759.4
- **Pykno-epilepsy, pyknolepsy** (idiopathic) (*see also* Epilepsy) 345.0❺
- **Pyle** (-Cohn) **disease** (craniometaphyseal dysplasia) 756.89
- **Pylephlebitis** (suppurative) 572.1
- **Pylethrombophlebitis** 572.1
- **Pylethrombosis** 572.1
- **Pyloritis** (*see also* Gastritis) 535.5❺
- **Pylorospasm** (reflex) 537.81
  - congenital or infantile 750.5
  - neurotic 306.4
  - newborn 750.5
  - psychogenic 306.4
- **Pylorus, pyloric** – *see* condition
- **Pyoarthrosis** – *see* Pyarthrosis
- **Pyocele**
  - mastoid 383.00
  - sinus (accessory) (nasal) (*see also* Sinusitis) 473.9
  - turbinate (bone) 473.9
  - urethra (*see also* Urethritis) 597.0
- **Pyococcal dermatitis** 686.00
- **Pyococcide, skin** 686.00
- **Pyocolpos** (*see also* Vaginitis) 616.10
- **Pyocyaneus dermatitis** 686.09
- **Pyocystitis** (*see also* Cystitis) 595.9
- **Pyoderma, pyodermia** 686.00
  - gangrenosum 686.01
  - specified type NEC 686.09
  - vegetans 686.8
- **Pyodermatitis** 686.00
  - vegetans 686.8
- **Pyogenic** – *see* condition
- **Pyohemia** – *see* Septicemia
- **Pyohydronephrosis** (*see also* Pyelitis) 590.80
- **Pyometra** 615.9
- **Pyometritis** (*see also* Endometritis) 615.9
- **Pyometrium** (*see also* Endometritis) 615.9
- **Pyomyositis** 728.0
  - ossificans 728.19
  - tropical (bungpagga) 040.81
- **Pyonephritis** (*see also* Pyelitis) 590.80
  - chronic 590.00
- **Pyonephrosis** (congenital) (*see also* Pyelitis) 590.80
  - acute 590.10
- **Pyo-oophoritis** (*see also* Salpingo-oophoritis) 614.2
- **Pyo-ovarium** (*see also* Salpingo-oophoritis) 614.2
- **Pyopericarditis** 420.99
- **Pyopericardium** 420.99
- **Pyophlebitis** – *see* Phlebitis
- **Pyopneumopericardium** 420.99
- **Pyopneumothorax** (infectional) 510.9
  - with fistula 510.0
  - subdiaphragmatic (*see also* Peritonitis) 567.29
  - subphrenic (*see also* Peritonitis) 567.29
- **Pyopneumothorax** – *continued*
  - tuberculous (*see also* Tuberculosis, pleura) 012.0❺
- **Pyorrhea** (alveolar) (alveolaris) 523.40
  - degenerative 523.5
- **Pyosalpingitis** (*see also* Salpingo-oophoritis) 614.2
- **Pyosalpinx** (*see also* Salpingo-oophoritis) 614.2
- **Pyosepticemia** – *see* Septicemia
- **Pyosis**
  - Corlett's (impetigo) 684
  - Manson's (pemphigus contagiosus) 684
- **Pyothorax** 510.9
  - with fistula 510.0
  - tuberculous (*see also* Tuberculosis, pleura) 012.0❺
- **Pyoureter** 593.89
  - tuberculous (*see also* Tuberculosis) 016.2❺
- **Pyramidopallidonigral syndrome** 332.0
- **Pyrexia** (of unknown origin) (P.U.O.) 780.6
  - atmospheric 992.0
  - during labor 659.2❺
  - environmentally-induced newborn 778.4
  - heat 992.0
  - newborn, environmentally-induced 778.4
  - puerperal 672❹
- **Pyroglobulinemia** 273.8
- **Pyromania** 312.33
- **Pyrosis** 787.1
- **Pyrroloporphyria** 277.1
- **Pyuria** (bacterial) 791.9

Q

- **Q fever** 083.0
  - with pneumonia 083.0 *[484.8]*
- **Quadricuspid aortic valve** 746.89
- **Quadrilateral fever** 083.0
- **Quadriparesis** – *see* Quadriplegia
  - meaning muscle weakness 728.87
- **Quadriplegia** 344.00
  - with fracture, vertebra (process) – *see* Fracture, vertebra, cervical, with spinal cord injury
  - brain (current episode) 437.8
  - C_1-C_4
    - complete 344.01
    - incomplete 344.02
  - C_5-C_7
    - complete 344.03
    - incomplete 344.04
  - cerebral (current episode) 437.8
  - congenital or infantile (cerebral) (spastic) (spinal) 343.2
  - cortical 437.8
  - embolic (current episode) (*see also* Embolism, brain) 434.1❺
  - infantile (cerebral) (spastic) (spinal) 343.2
  - newborn NEC 767.0
  - specified NEC 344.09
  - thrombotic (current episode) (*see also* Thrombosis, brain) 434.0❺
  - traumatic – *see* Injury, spinal, cervical
- **Quadruplet**
  - affected by maternal complications of pregnancy 761.5
  - healthy liveborn – *see* Newborn, multiple
  - pregnancy (complicating delivery) NEC 651.8❺
    - with fetal loss and retention of one or more fetus(es) 651.5❺
    - following (elective) fetal reduction 651.7
- **Quarrelsomeness** 301.3
- **Quartan**
  - fever 084.2
  - malaria (fever) 084.2
- **Queensland fever** 083.0
  - coastal 083.0
  - seven-day 100.89
- **Quervain's disease** 727.04
  - thyroid (subacute granulomatous thyroiditis) 245.1
- **Queyrat's erythroplasia** (M8080/2)
  - specified site – *see* Neoplasm, skin, in situ
  - unspecified site 233.5
- **Quincke's disease or edema** – *see* Edema, angioneurotic
- **Quinquaud's disease** (acne decalvans) 704.09
- **Quinsy** (gangrenous) 475
- **Quintan fever** 083.1
- **Quintuplet**
  - affected by maternal complications of pregnancy 761.5
  - healthy liveborn – *see* Newborn, multiple
  - pregnancy (complicating delivery) NEC 651.2❺
    - with fetal loss and retention of one or more fetus(es) 651.6❺
    - following (elective) fetal reduction 651.7
- **Quotidian**
  - fever 084.0
    - malaria (fever) 084.0

R

- **Rabbia** 071
- **Rabbit fever** (*see also* Tularemia) 021.9
- **Rabies** 071
  - contact V01.5
  - exposure to V01.5
  - inoculation V04.5
    - reaction – *see* Complications, vaccination
  - vaccination, prophylactic (against) V04.5
- **Rachischisis** (*see also* Spina bifida) 741.9❺
- **Rachitic** – *see also* condition
  - deformities of spine 268.1
  - pelvis 268.1
    - with disproportion (fetopelvic) 653.2❺
      - affecting fetus or newborn 763.1
      - causing obstructed labor 660.1❺
        - affecting fetus or newborn 763.1
- **Rachitis, rachitism** – *see also* Rickets
  - acute 268.0
  - fetalis 756.4
  - renalis 588.0
  - tarda 268.0
- **Racket nail** 757.5
- **Radial nerve** – *see* condition
- **Radiation effects or sickness** – *see also* Effect, adverse, radiation
  - cataract 366.46
  - dermatitis 692.82
    - sunburn (*see also* Sunburn) 692.71
- **Radiculitis** (pressure) (vertebrogenic) 729.2
  - accessory nerve 723.4
  - anterior crural 724.4
  - arm 723.4
  - brachial 723.4
  - cervical NEC 723.4
  - due to displacement of intervertebral disc – *see* Neuritis, due to, displacement intervertebral disc
  - leg 724.4
  - lumbar NEC 724.4
  - lumbosacral 724.4
  - rheumatic 729.2
  - syphilitic 094.89
  - thoracic (with visceral pain) 724.4
- **Radiculomyelitis** 357.0
  - toxic, due to
    - Clostridium tetani 037
    - Corynebacterium diphtheriae 032.89
- **Radiculopathy** (*see also* Radiculitis) 729.2
- **Radioactive substances, adverse effect** – *see* Effect, adverse, radioactive substance
- **Radiodermal burns** (acute) (chronic) (occupational) – *see* Burn, by site
- **Radiodermatitis** 692.82
- **Radionecrosis** – *see* Effect, adverse, radiation
- **Radiotherapy session** V58.0
- **Radium, adverse effect** – *see* Effect, adverse, radioactive substance
- **Raeder-Harbitz syndrome** (pulseless disease) 446.7
- **Rage** (*see also* Disturbance, conduct) 312.0❺
  - meaning rabies 071
- **Rag sorters' disease** 022.1
- **Raillietiniasis** 123.8
- **Railroad neurosis** 300.16
- **Railway spine** 300.16
- **Raised** – *see* Elevation
- **Raiva** 071
- **Rake teeth, tooth** 524.39
- **Rales** 786.7

❹ Fourth-Digit Required ❺ Fifth-Digit Required *[code]* Manifestation Code ▶◀ Revised Text ● New Line ▲ Revised Code

- **Ramifying renal pelvis** 753.3
- **Ramsay Hunt syndrome** (herpetic geniculate ganglionitis) 053.11
  - meaning dyssynergia cerebellaris myoclonica 334.2
- **Ranke's primary infiltration** (*see also* Tuberculosis) 010.0❺
- **Ranula** 527.6
  - congenital 750.26
- **Rape**
  - adult 995.83
  - alleged, observation or examination V71.5
  - child 995.53
- **Rapid**
  - feeble pulse, due to shock, following injury 958.4
  - heart (beat) 785.0
    - psychogenic 306.2
  - respiration 786.06
    - psychogenic 306.1
  - second stage (delivery) 661.3❺
    - affecting fetus or newborn 763.6
  - time-zone change syndrome 327.35
- **Rarefaction, bone** 733.99
- **Rash** 782.1
  - canker 034.1
  - diaper 691.0
  - drug (internal use) 693.0
    - contact 692.3
  - ECHO 9 virus 078.89
  - enema 692.89
  - food (*see also* Allergy, food) 693.1
  - heat 705.1
  - napkin 691.0
  - nettle 708.8
  - pustular 782.1
  - rose 782.1
    - epidemic 056.9
    - of infants 057.8
  - scarlet 034.1
  - serum (prophylactic) (therapeutic) 999.5
  - toxic 782.1
  - wandering tongue 529.1
- **Rasmussen's aneurysm** (*see also* Tuberculosis) 011.2❺
- **Rat-bite fever** 026.9
  - due to Streptobacillus moniliformis 026.1❺
  - spirochetal (morsus muris) 026.0❺
- **Rathke's pouch tumor** (M9350/1) 237.0
- **Raymond** (-Céstan) **syndrome** 433.8❺
- **Raynaud's**
  - disease or syndrome (paroxysmal digital cyanosis) 443.0
  - gangrene (symmetric) 443.0 *[785.4]*
  - phenomenon (paroxysmal digital cyanosis) (secondary) 443.0
- **RDS** 769
- **Reaction**
  - acute situational maladjustment (*see also* Reaction, adjustment) 309.9
  - adaptation (*see also* Reaction, adjustment) 309.9
  - adjustment 309.9
    - with
      - anxious mood 309.24
        - with depressed mood 309.28
      - conduct disturbance 309.3
        - combined with disturbance of emotions 309.4
      - depressed mood 309.0
        - brief 309.0
          - with anxious mood 309.28
        - prolonged 309.1
      - elective mutism 309.83
      - mixed emotions and conduct 309.4
      - mutism, elective 309.83
      - physical symptoms 309.82
      - predominant disturbance (of)
        - conduct 309.3
        - emotions NEC 309.29
          - mixed 309.28
        - mixed, emotions and conduct 309.4
        - specified type NEC 309.89
      - specific academic or work inhibition 309.23
      - withdrawal 309.83
    - depressive 309.0
      - with conduct disturbance 309.4
      - brief 309.0
      - prolonged 309.1
    - specified type NEC 309.89
  - adverse food NEC 995.7

Reaction – *continued*

- affective (*see also* Psychosis, affective) 296.90
  - specified type NEC 296.99
- aggressive 301.3
  - unsocialized (*see also* Disturbance, conduct) 312.0❺
- allergic (*see also* Allergy) 995.3
  - drug, medicinal substance, and biological – *see* Allergy, drug
  - food – *see* Allergy, food
  - serum 999.5
- anaphylactic – *see* Shock, anaphylactic
- anesthesia – *see* Anesthesia, complication
- anger 312.0❺
- antisocial 301.7
- antitoxin (prophylactic) (therapeutic) – *see* Complications, vaccination
- anxiety 300.00
- Arthus 995.21
- asthenic 300.5
- compulsive 300.3
- conversion (anesthetic) (autonomic) (hyperkinetic) (mixed paralytic) (paresthetic) 300.11
- deoxyribonuclease (DNA) (DNase) hypersensitivity NEC 287.2
- depressive 300.4
  - acute 309.0
  - affective (*see also* Psychosis, affective) 296.2❺
    - recurrent episode 296.3❺
    - single episode 296.2❺
  - brief 309.0
  - manic (*see also* Psychosis, affective) 296.80
  - neurotic 300.4
  - psychoneurotic 300.4
  - psychotic 298.0
- dissociative 300.15
- drug NEC (*see also* Table of Drugs and Chemicals) 995.20
  - allergic – *see also* Allergy, drug 995.27
  - correct substance properly administered 995.20
  - obstetric anesthetic or analgesic NEC 668.9❺
    - affecting fetus or newborn 763.5
    - specified drug – *see* Table of Drugs and Chemicals
  - overdose or poisoning 977.9
    - specified drug – *see* Table of Drugs and Chemicals
  - specific to newborn 779.4
  - transmitted via placenta or breast milk – *see* Absorption, drug, through placenta
  - withdrawal NEC 292.0
    - infant of dependent mother 779.5
  - wrong substance given or taken in error 977.9
    - specified drug – *see* Table of Drugs and Chemicals
- dyssocial 301.7
- dystonic, acute, due to drugs 333.72
- erysipeloid 027.1
- fear 300.20
  - child 313.0
- fluid loss, cerebrospinal 349.0
- food – *see also* Allergy, food
  - adverse NEC 995.7
  - anaphylactic shock – *see* Anaphylactic shock, due to, food
- foreign
  - body NEC 728.82
    - in operative wound (inadvertently left) 998.4
      - due to surgical material intentionally left – *see* Complications, due to (presence of) any device, implant, or graft classified to 996.0-996.5 NEC
  - substance accidentally left during a procedure (chemical) (powder) (talc) 998.7
    - body or object (instrument) (sponge) (swab) 998.4
- graft-versus-host (GVH) 996.85
- grief (acute) (brief) 309.0
  - prolonged 309.1
- gross stress (*see also* Reaction, stress, acute) 308.9
- group delinquent (*see also* Disturbance, conduct) 312.2❺
- Herxheimer's 995.0
- hyperkinetic (*see also* Hyperkinesia) 314.9
- hypochondriacal 300.7
- hypoglycemic, due to insulin 251.0
  - therapeutic misadventure 962.3

Reaction – *continued*

- hypomanic (*see also* Psychosis, affective) 296.0❺
  - recurrent episode 296.1❺
  - single episode 296.0❺
- hysterical 300.10
  - conversion type 300.11
  - dissociative 300.15
- id (bacterial cause) 692.89
- immaturity NEC 301.89
  - aggressive 301.3
  - emotional instability 301.59
- immunization – *see* Complications, vaccination
- incompatibility
  - blood group (ABO) (infusion) (transfusion) 999.6
  - Rh (factor) (infusion) (transfusion) 999.7
- inflammatory – *see* Infection
- infusion – *see* Complications, infusion
- inoculation (immune serum) – *see* Complications, vaccination
- insulin 995.23
- involutional
  - paranoid 297.2
  - psychotic (*see also* Psychosis, affective, depressive) 296.2❺
- leukemoid (basophilic) (lymphocytic) (monocytic) (myelocytic) (neutrophilic) 288.62
- LSD (*see also* Abuse, drugs, nondependent) 305.3❺
- lumbar puncture 349.0
- manic-depressive (*see also* Psychosis, affective) 296.80
  - depressed 296.2❺
    - recurrent episode 296.3❺
    - single episode 296.2❺
  - hypomanic 296.0❺
- neurasthenic 300.5
- neurogenic (*see also* Neurosis) 300.9
- neurotic NEC 300.9
- neurotic-depressive 300.4
- nitritoid – *see* Crisis, nitritoid
- obsessive-compulsive 300.3
- organic 293.9
  - acute 293.0
  - subacute 293.1
- overanxious, child or adolescent 313.0
- paranoid (chronic) 297.9
  - acute 298.3
  - climacteric 297.2
  - involutional 297.2
  - menopausal 297.2
  - senile 290.20
  - simple 297.0
- passive
  - aggressive 301.84
  - dependency 301.6
- personality (*see also* Disorder, personality) 301.9
- phobic 300.20
- postradiation – *see* Effect, adverse, radiation
- psychogenic NEC 300.9
- psychoneurotic (*see also* Neurosis) 300.9
  - anxiety 300.00
  - compulsive 300.3
  - conversion 300.11
  - depersonalization 300.6
  - depressive 300.4
  - dissociative 300.15
  - hypochondriacal 300.7
  - hysterical 300.10
    - conversion type 300.11
    - dissociative type 300.15
  - neurasthenic 300.5
  - obsessive 300.3
  - obsessive-compulsive 300.3
  - phobic 300.20
  - tension state 300.9
- psychophysiologic NEC (*see also* Disorder, psychosomatic) 306.9
  - cardiovascular 306.2
  - digestive 306.4
  - endocrine 306.6
  - gastrointestinal 306.4
  - genitourinary 306.50
  - heart 306.2
  - hemic 306.8
  - intestinal (large) (small) 306.4
  - laryngeal 306.1
  - lymphatic 306.8
  - musculoskeletal 306.0
  - pharyngeal 306.1
  - respiratory 306.1
  - skin 306.3

- **Reaction** – *continued*
  - psychophysiologic – *continued*
    - special sense organs 306.7
  - psychosomatic (*see also* Disorder, psychosomatic) 306.9
  - psychotic (*see also* Psychosis) 298.9
    - depressive 298.0
    - due to or associated with physical condition (*see also* Psychosis, organic) 293.9
    - involutional (*see also* Psychosis, affective) 296.2❺
      - recurrent episode 296.3❺
      - single episode 296.2❺
  - pupillary (myotonic) (tonic) 379.46
  - radiation – *see* Effect, adverse, radiation
  - runaway – *see also* Disturbance, conduct
    - socialized 312.2❺
    - undersocialized, unsocialized 312.1❺
  - scarlet fever toxin – *see* Complications, vaccination
  - schizophrenic (*see also* Schizophrenia) 295.9❺
    - latent 295.5❺
  - serological for syphilis – *see* Serology for syphilis
  - serum (prophylactic) (therapeutic) 999.5
    - immediate 999.4
  - situational (*see also* Reaction, adjustment) 309.9
    - acute, to stress 308.3
    - adjustment (*see also* Reaction, adjustment) 309.9
  - somatization (*see also* Disorder, psychosomatic) 306.9
  - spinal puncture 349.0
  - spite, child (*see also* Disturbance, conduct) 312.0❺
  - stress, acute 308.9
    - with predominant disturbance (of)
      - consciousness 308.1
      - emotions 308.0
      - mixed 308.4
      - psychomotor 308.2
      - specified type NEC 308.3
    - bone or cartilage – *see* Fracture, stress
  - surgical procedure – *see* Complications, surgical procedure
  - tetanus antitoxin – *see* Complications, vaccination
  - toxin-antitoxin – *see* Complications, vaccination
  - transfusion (blood) (bone marrow) (lymphocytes) (allergic) – *see* Complications, transfusion
  - tuberculin skin test, nonspecific (without active tuberculosis) 795.5
    - positive (without active tuberculosis) 795.5
  - ultraviolet – *see* Effect, adverse, ultraviolet
  - undersocialized, unsocialized – *see also* Disturbance, conduct
    - aggressive (type) 312.0❺
    - unaggressive (type) 312.1❺
  - vaccination (any) – *see* Complications, vaccination
  - white graft (skin) 996.52
  - withdrawing, child or adolescent 313.22
  - x-ray – *see* Effect, adverse, x-rays
- **Reactive depression** (*see also* Reaction, depressive) 300.4
  - neurotic 300.4
  - psychoneurotic 300.4
  - psychotic 298.0
- **Rebound tenderness** 789.6❺
- **Recalcitrant patient** V15.81
- **Recanalization, thrombus** – *see* Thrombosis
- **Recession, receding**
  - chamber angle (eye) 364.77
  - chin 524.06
  - gingival (postinfective) (postoperative) 523.20
    - generalized 523.25
    - localized 523.24
    - minimal 523.21
    - moderate 523.22
    - severe 523.23
- **Recklinghausen's disease** (M9540/1) 237.71
  - bones (osteitis fibrosa cystica) 252.01
- **Recklinghausen-Applebaum disease** (hemochromatosis) 275.0
- **Reclus' disease** (cystic) 610.1
- **Recrudescent typhus** (fever) 081.1
- **Recruitment, auditory** 388.44
- **Rectalgia** 569.42
- **Rectitis** 569.49
- **Rectocele**
  - female (without uterine prolapse) 618.04
    - with uterine prolapse 618.4
      - complete 618.3
- **Rectocele** – *continued*
  - female – *continued*
    - with uterine prolapse – *continued*
      - incomplete 618.2
  - in pregnancy or childbirth 654.4❺
    - causing obstructed labor 660.2❺
      - affecting fetus or newborn 763.1
  - male 569.49
  - vagina, vaginal (outlet) 618.04
- **Rectosigmoiditis** 569.89
  - ulcerative (chronic) 556.3
- **Rectosigmoid junction** – *see* condition
- **Rectourethral** – *see* condition
- **Rectovaginal** – *see* condition
- **Rectovesical** – *see* condition
- **Rectum, rectal** – *see* condition
- **Recurrent** – *see* condition
- **Red bugs** 133.8
- **Red cedar asthma** 495.8
- **Redness**
  - conjunctiva 379.93
  - eye 379.93
  - nose 478.19
- **Reduced ventilatory or vital capacity** 794.2
- **Reduction**
  - function
    - kidney (*see also* Disease, renal) 593.9
    - liver 573.8
  - ventilatory capacity 794.2
  - vital capacity 794.2
- **Redundant, redundancy**
  - abdomen 701.9
  - anus 751.5
  - cardia 537.89
  - clitoris 624.2
  - colon (congenital) 751.5
  - foreskin (congenital) 605
  - intestine 751.5
  - labia 624.3
  - organ or site, congenital NEC – *see* Accessory
  - panniculus (abdominal) 278.1
  - prepuce (congenital) 605
  - pylorus 537.89
  - rectum 751.5
  - scrotum 608.89
  - sigmoid 751.5
  - skin (of face) 701.9
    - eyelids 374.30
  - stomach 537.89
  - uvula 528.9
  - vagina 623.8
- **Reduplication** – *see* Duplication
- **Referral**
  - adoption (agency) V68.89
  - nursing care V63.8
  - patient without examination or treatment V68.81
  - social services V63.8
- **Reflex** – *see also* condition
  - blink, deficient 374.45
  - hyperactive gag 478.29
  - neurogenic bladder NEC 596.54
    - atonic 596.54
      - with cauda equina syndrome 344.61
  - vasoconstriction 443.9
  - vasovagal 780.2
- **Reflux**
  - esophageal 530.81
    - with esophagitis 530.11
  - esophagitis 530.11
  - gastroesophageal 530.81
  - mitral – *see* Insufficiency, mitral
  - ureteral – *see* Reflux, vesicoureteral
  - vesicoureteral 593.70
    - with
      - reflux nephropathy 593.73
        - bilateral 593.72
        - unilateral 593.71
- **Reformed gallbladder** 576.0
- **Reforming, artificial openings** (*see also* Attention to, artificial, opening) V55.9
- **Refractive error** (*see also* Error, refractive) 367.9
- **Refsum's disease or syndrome** (heredopathia atactica polyneuritiformis) 356.3
- **Refusal of**
  - food 307.59
    - hysterical 300.11
  - treatment because of, due to
    - patient's decision NEC V64.2
- **Refusal of** – *continued*
  - treatment because of, due to – *continued*
    - reason of conscience or religion V62.6
- **Regaud**
  - tumor (M8082/3) – *see* Neoplasm, nasopharynx, malignant
  - type carcinoma (M8082/3) – *see* Neoplasm, nasopharynx, malignant
- **Regional** – *see* condition
- **Regulation feeding** (elderly) (infant) 783.3
  - newborn 779.3
- **Regurgitated**
  - food, choked on 933.1
  - stomach contents, choked on 933.1
- **Regurgitation** 787.03 ▲
  - aortic (valve) (*see also* Insufficiency, aortic) 424.1
    - congenital 746.4
    - syphilitic 093.22
  - food – *see also* Vomiting
    - with reswallowing – *see* Rumination
    - newborn 779.3
  - gastric contents – *see* Vomiting
  - heart – *see* Endocarditis
  - mitral (valve) – *see also* Insufficiency, mitral
    - congenital 746.6
  - myocardial – *see* Endocarditis
  - pulmonary (heart) (valve) (*see also* Endocarditis, pulmonary) 424.3
  - stomach – *see* Vomiting
  - tricuspid – *see* Endocarditis, tricuspid
  - valve, valvular – *see* Endocarditis
  - vesicoureteral – *see* Reflux, vesicoureteral
- **Rehabilitation** V57.9
  - multiple types V57.89
  - occupational V57.21
  - specified type NEC V57.89
  - speech V57.3
  - vocational V57.22
- **Reichmann's disease or syndrome** (gastrosuccorrhea) 536.8
- **Reifenstein's syndrome** (hereditary familial hypogonadism, male) 259.5
- **Reilly's syndrome or phenomenon** (*see also* Neuropathy, peripheral, autonomic) 337.9
- **Reimann's periodic disease** 277.31
- **Reinsertion, contraceptive device** V25.42
- **Reiter's disease, syndrome, or urethritis** 099.3 *[711.1]*❺
- **Rejection**
  - food, hysterical 300.11
  - transplant 996.80
    - bone marrow 996.85
    - corneal 996.51
    - organ (immune or nonimmune cause) 996.80
      - bone marrow 996.85
      - heart 996.83
      - intestines 996.87
      - kidney 996.81
      - liver 996.82
      - lung 996.84
      - pancreas 996.86
      - specified NEC 996.89
    - skin 996.52
      - artificial 996.55
      - decellularized allodermis 996.55
- **Relapsing fever** 087.9
  - Carter's (Asiatic) 087.0
  - Dutton's (West African) 087.1
  - Koch's 087.9
  - louse-borne (epidemic) 087.0
  - Novy's (American) 087.1
  - Obermeyer's (European) 087.0
  - Spirillum 087.9
  - tick-borne (endemic) 087.1
- **Relaxation**
  - anus (sphincter) 569.49
    - due to hysteria 300.11
  - arch (foot) 734
    - congenital 754.61
  - back ligaments 728.4
  - bladder (sphincter) 596.59
  - cardio-esophageal 530.89
  - cervix (*see also* Incompetency, cervix) 622.5
  - diaphragm 519.4
  - inguinal rings – *see* Hernia, inguinal
  - joint (capsule) (ligament) (paralytic) (*see also* Derangement, joint) 718.90
    - congenital 755.8

❹ Fourth-Digit Required ❺ Fifth-Digit Required *[code]* Manifestation Code ▶◀ Revised Text ● New Line ▲ Revised Code

Relaxation – *continued*
- lumbosacral joint 724.6
- pelvic floor 618.89
- pelvis 618.89
- perineum 618.89
- posture 729.9
- rectum (sphincter) 569.49
- sacroiliac (joint) 724.6
- scrotum 608.89
- urethra (sphincter) 599.84
- uterus (outlet) 618.89
- vagina (outlet) 618.89
- vesical 596.59

Remains
- canal of Cloquet 743.51
- capsule (opaque) 743.51

Remittent fever (malarial) 084.6

Remnant
- canal of Cloquet 743.51
- capsule (opaque) 743.51
- cervix, cervical stump (acquired) (postoperative) 622.8
- cystic duct, postcholecystectomy 576.0
- fingernail 703.8
  - congenital 757.5
- meniscus, knee 717.5
- thyroglossal duct 759.2
- tonsil 474.8
  - infected 474.00
- urachus 753.7

Remote effect of cancer- *see* condition

Removal (of)
- catheter (urinary) (indwelling) V53.6
  - from artificial opening – *see* Attention to, artificial, opening
  - non-vascular V58.82
  - vascular V58.81
- cerebral ventricle (communicating) shunt V53.01
- device – *see also* Fitting (of)
  - contraceptive V25.42
  - fixation
    - external V54.89
    - internal V54.01
  - traction V54.89
- drains V58.49
- dressing
  - wound V58.30
    - nonsurgical V58.30
    - surgical V58.31
- ileostomy V55.2
- Kirschner wire V54.89
- non-vascular catheter V58.82
- pin V54.01
- plaster cast V54.89
- plate (fracture) V54.01
- rod V54.01
- screw V54.01
- splint, external V54.89
- staples V58.32
- subdermal implantable contraceptive V25.43
- sutures V58.32
- traction device, external V54.89
- vascular catheter V58.81
- wound packing V58.30
  - nonsurgical V58.30
  - surgical V58.31

Ren
- arcuatus 753.3
- mobile, mobilis (*see also* Disease, renal) 593.0
  - congenital 753.3
- unguliformis 753.3

Renal – *see also* condition
- glomerulohyalinosis-diabetic syndrome 250.4❺ *[581.81]*

Rendu-Osler-Weber disease or syndrome (familial hemorrhagic telangiectasia) 448.0

Reninoma (M8361/1) 236.91

Rénon-Delille syndrome 253.8

Repair
- pelvic floor, previous, in pregnancy or childbirth 654.4❺
  - affecting fetus or newborn 763.89
- scarred tissue V51

Replacement by artificial or mechanical device or prosthesis of (*see also* Fitting (of))
- artificial skin V43.83
- bladder V43.5
- blood vessel V43.4
- breast V43.82
- eye globe V43.0

Replacement by artificial or mechanical device or prosthesis of – *continued*
- heart
  - with
    - assist device V43.21
    - fully implantable artificial heart V43.22
  - valve V43.3
- intestine V43.89
- joint V43.60
  - ankle V43.66
  - elbow V43.62
  - finger V43.69
  - hip (partial) (total) V43.64
  - knee V43.65
  - shoulder V43.61
  - specified NEC V43.69
  - wrist V43.63
- kidney V43.89
- larynx V43.81
- lens V43.1
- limb(s) V43.7
- liver V43.89
- lung V43.89
- organ NEC V43.89
- pancreas V43.89
- skin (artificial) V43.83
- tissue NEC V43.89

Reprogramming
- cardiac pacemaker V53.31

Request for expert evidence V68.2

Reserve, decreased or low
- cardiac – *see* Disease, heart
  - kidney (*see also* Disease, renal) 593.9

Residual – *see also* condition
- bladder 596.8
- foreign body – *see* Retention, foreign body
- state, schizophrenic (*see also* Schizophrenia) 295.6❺
- urine 788.69

Resistance, resistant (to)
- activated protein C 289.81

Note – Use the following subclassification for categories V09.5, V09.7, V09.8, V09.9

0	*without mention of resistance to multiple drugs*	
1	*with resistance to multiple drugs*	
	V09.5	*quinolones and fluoroquinolones*
	V09.7	*antimycobacterial agents*
	V09.8	*specified drugs NEC*
	V09.9	*unspecified drugs*
9	*multiple sites*	

- drugs by microorganisms V09.9❺
  - Amikacin V09.4
  - aminoglycosides V09.4
  - Amodiaquine V09.5❺
  - Amoxicillin V09.0
  - Ampicillin V09.0
  - antimycobacterial agents V09.7❺
  - Azithromycin V09.2
  - Azlocillin V09.0
  - Aztreonam V09.1
  - B-lactam antibiotics V09.1
  - Bacampicillin V09.0
  - Bacitracin V09.8❺
  - Benznidazole V09.8❺
  - Capreomycin V09.7❺
  - Carbenicillin V09.0
  - Cefaclor V09.1
  - Cefadroxil V09.1
  - Cefamandole V09.1
  - Cefatetan V09.1
  - Cefazolin V09.1
  - Cefixime V09.1
  - Cefonicid V09.1
  - Cefoperazone V09.1
  - Ceforanide V09.1
  - Cefotaxime V09.1
  - Cefoxitin V09.1
  - Ceftazidine V09.1
  - Ceftizoxime V09.1
  - Ceftriaxone V09.1
  - Cefuroxime V09.1
  - Cephalexin V09.1
  - Cephaloglycin V09.1
  - Cephaloridine V09.1
  - cephalosporins V09.1
  - Cephalothin V09.1
  - Cephapirin V09.1
  - Cephradine V09.1

Resistance, resistant – *continued*
- drugs by microorganisms – *continued*
  - Chloramphenicol V09.8❺
  - Chloraquine V09.5❺
  - Chlorguanide V09.8❺
  - Chlorproguanil V09.8
  - Chlortetracyline V09.3
  - Cinoxacin V09.5❺
  - Ciprofloxacin V09.5❺
  - Clarithromycin V09.2
  - Clindamycin V09.8❺
  - Clioquinol V09.5❺
  - Clofazimine V09.7❺
  - Cloxacillin V09.0
  - Cyclacillin V09.0
  - Cycloserine V09.7❺
  - Dapsone [DZ] V09.7❺
  - Demeclocycline V09.3
  - Dicloxacillin V09.0
  - Doxycycline V09.3
  - Enoxacin V09.5❺
  - Erythromycin V09.2
  - Ethambutol [EMB] V09.7❺
  - Ethionamide [ETA] V09.7❺
  - fluoroquinolones NEC V09.5❺
  - Gentamicin V09.4
  - Halofantrine V09.8❺
  - Imipenem V09.1
  - Iodoquinol V09.5❺
  - Isoniazid [INH] V09.7❺
  - Kanamycin V09.4
  - macrolides V09.2
  - Mafenide V09.6
  - MDRO (multiple drug resistant organisms) NOS V09.91
  - Mefloquine V09.8❺
  - Melasoprol V09.8❺
  - Methicillin V09.0
  - Methacycline V09.3
  - Methenamine V09.8❺
  - Methicillin V09.0
  - Metronidazole V09.8❺
  - Mezlocillin V09.0
  - Minocycline V09.3
  - multiple drug resistant organisms NOS V09.91
  - Nafcillin V09.0
  - Nalidixic acid V09.5❺
  - Natamycin V09.2
  - Neomycin V09.4
  - Netilmicin V09.4
  - Nimorazole V09.8❺
  - Nitrofurantoin V09.8❺
  - Nitrofurtimox V09.8❺
  - Norfloxacin V09.5❺
  - Nystatin V09.2
  - Ofloxacin V09.5❺
  - Oleandomycin V09.2
  - Oxacillin V09.0
  - Oxytetracycline V09.3
  - Para-amino salicyclic acid [PAS] V09.7❺
  - Paromomycin V09.4
  - Penicillin (G) (V) (Vk) V09.0
  - penicillins V09.0
  - Pentamidine V09.8❺
  - Piperacillin V09.0
  - Primaquine V09.5❺
  - Proguanil V09.8❺
  - Pyrazinamide [PZA] V09.7❺
  - Pyrimethamine/Sulfalene V09.8❺
  - Pyrimethamine/Sulfodoxine V09.8❺
  - Quinacrine V09.5❺
  - Quinidine V09.8❺
  - Quinine V09.8❺
  - quinolones V09.5❺
  - Rifabutin V09.7❺
  - Rifampin [Rif] V09.7❺
  - Rifamycin V09.7❺
  - Rolitetracycline V09.3
  - specified drug(s) NEC V09.8❺
  - Spectinomycin V09.8❺
  - Spiramycin V09.2
  - Streptomycin [Sm] V09.4
  - Sulfacetamide V09.6
  - Sulfacytine V09.6
  - Sulfadiazine V09.6
  - Sulfadoxine V09.6
  - Sulfamethoxazole V09.6
  - Sulfapyridine V09.6
  - Sulfasalizine V09.6
  - Sulfasoxazole V09.6
  - sulfonamides V09.6
  - Sulfoxone V09.7❺

- **Resistance, resistant** – *continued*
  - drugs by microorganisms – *continued*
    - tetracycline V09.3
    - tetracyclines V09.3
    - Thiamphenicol V09.8❺
    - Ticarcillin V09.0
    - Tinidazole V09.8❺
    - Tobramycin V09.4
    - Triamphenicol V09.8❺
    - Trimethoprim V09.8❺
    - Vancomycin V09.8❺
  - insulin 277.7
  - thyroid hormone 246.8
- **Resorption**
  - biliary 576.8
    - purulent or putrid (*see also* Cholecystitis) 576.8
  - dental (roots) 521.40
    - alveoli 525.8
    - pathological
      - external 521.42
      - internal 521.41
      - specified NEC 521.49
  - septic – *see* Septicemia
  - teeth (roots) 521.40
    - pathological
      - external 521.42
      - internal 521.41
      - specified NEC 521.49
- **Respiration**
  - asymmetrical 786.09
  - bronchial 786.09
  - Cheyne-Stokes (periodic respiration) 786.04
  - decreased, due to shock following injury 958.4
  - disorder of 786.00
    - psychogenic 306.1
    - specified NEC 786.09
  - failure 518.81
    - acute 518.81
    - acute and chronic 518.84
    - chronic 518.83
    - newborn 770.84
  - insufficiency 786.09
    - acute 518.82
    - newborn NEC 770.89
  - Kussmaul (air hunger) 786.09
  - painful 786.52
  - periodic 786.09
    - high altitute 327.22
  - poor 786.09
    - newborn NEC 770.89
  - sighing 786.7
    - psychogenic 306.1
  - wheezing 786.07
- **Respiratory** – *see also* condition
  - distress 786.09
    - acute 518.82
    - fetus or newborn NEC 770.89
    - syndrome (newborn) 769
      - adult (following shock, surgery, or trauma) 518.5
        - specified NEC 518.82
  - failure 518.81
    - acute 518.81
    - acute and chronic 518.84
    - chronic 518.83
- **Respiratory syncytial virus** (RSV) 079.6
  - bronchiolitis 466.11
  - pneumonia 480.1
  - vaccination, prophylactic (against) V04.82
- **Response**
  - photoallergic 692.72
  - phototoxic 692.72
- **Rest, rests**
  - mesonephric duct 752.89
    - fallopian tube 752.11
  - ovarian, in fallopian tubes 752.19
  - wolffian duct 752.89
- **Restless legs syndrome** (RLS) 333.94
- **Restlessness** 799.2
- **Restoration of organ continuity from previous sterilization** (tuboplasty) (vasoplasty) V26.0
- **Restriction of housing space** V60.1
- **Restzustand, schizophrenic** (*see also* Schizophrenia) 295.6❺
- **Retained** – *see* Retention
- **Retardation**
  - development, developmental, specific (*see also* Disorder, development, specific) 315.9
    - learning, specific 315.2
      - arithmetical 315.1
      - language (skills) 315.31
        - expressive 315.31
        - mixed receptive-expressive 315.32
      - mathematics 315.1
      - reading 315.00
        - phonological 315.39
      - written expression 315.2
    - motor 315.4
  - endochondral bone growth 733.91
  - growth (physical) in childhood 783.43
    - due to malnutrition 263.2
    - fetal (intrauterine) 764.9❺
      - affecting management of pregnancy 656.5❺
  - intrauterine growth 764.9❺
    - affecting management of pregnancy 656.5❺
  - mental 319
    - borderline V62.89
    - mild, IQ 50-70 317
    - moderate, IQ 35-49 318.0
    - profound, IQ under 20 318.2
    - severe, IQ 20-34 318.1
  - motor, specific 315.4
  - physical 783.43
    - child 783.43
    - due to malnutrition 263.2
    - fetus (intrauterine) 764.9❺
      - affecting management of pregnancy 656.5❺
  - psychomotor NEC 307.9
  - reading 315.00
- **Retching** – *see* Vomiting
- **Retention, retained**
  - bladder (*see also* Retention, urine) 788.20
    - psychogenic 306.53
  - carbon dioxide 276.2
  - cyst – *see* Cyst
  - dead
    - fetus (after 22 completed weeks gestation) 656.4❺
      - early fetal death (before 22 completed weeks gestation) 632
    - ovum 631
  - decidua (following delivery) (fragments) (with hemorrhage) 666.2❺
    - without hemorrhage 667.1❺
  - deciduous tooth 520.6
  - dental root 525.3
  - fecal (*see also* Constipation) 564.00
  - fluid 276.6
  - foreign body – *see also* Foreign body, retained
    - bone 733.99
    - current trauma – *see* Foreign body, by site or type
    - middle ear 385.83
    - muscle 729.6
    - soft tissue NEC 729.6
  - gastric 536.8
  - membranes (following delivery) (with hemorrhage) 666.2❺
    - with abortion – *see* Abortion, by type
    - without hemorrhage 667.1❺
  - menses 626.8
  - milk (puerperal) 676.2❺
  - nitrogen, extrarenal 788.9
  - placenta (total) (with hemorrhage) 666.0❺
    - with abortion – *see* Abortion, by type
    - portions or fragments 666.2❺
      - without hemorrhage 667.1❺
    - without hemorrhage 667.0❺
  - products of conception
    - early pregnancy (fetal death before 22 completed weeks gestation) 632
    - following
      - abortion – *see* Abortion, by type
      - delivery 666.2❺
        - with hemorrhage 666.2❺
        - without hemorrhage 667.1❺
  - secundines (following delivery) (with hemorrhage) 666.2❺
    - with abortion – *see* Abortion, by type
    - complicating puerperium (delayed hemorrhage) 666.2❺
    - without hemorrhage 667.1❺
  - smegma, clitoris 624.8
- **Retention, retained** – *continued*
  - urine NEC 788.20
    - bladder, incomplete emptying 788.21
      - due to
        - benign prostatic hypertrophy (BPH) – *see* category 600
    - due to
      - benign prostatic hypertrophy (BPH) – *see* category 600
    - psychogenic 306.53
    - specified NEC 788.29
  - water (in tissue) (*see also* Edema) 782.3
- **Reticulation, dust** (occupational) 504
- **Reticulocytosis** NEC 790.99
- **Reticuloendotheliosis**
  - acute infantile (M9722/3) 202.5❺
  - leukemic (M9940/3) 202.4❺
  - malignant (M9720/3) 202.3❺
  - nonlipid (M9722/3) 202.5❺
- **Reticulohistiocytoma** (giant cell) 277.89
- **Reticulohistiocytosis, multicentric** 272.8
- **Reticulolymphosarcoma** (diffuse) (M9613/3) 200.8❺
  - follicular (M9691/3) 202.0❺
  - nodular (M9691/3) 202.0❺
- **Reticulosarcoma** (M9640/3) 200.0❺
  - nodular (M9642/3) 200.0❺
  - pleomorphic cell type (M9641/3) 200.0❺
- **Reticulosis** (skin)
  - acute of infancy (M9722/3) 202.5❺
  - familial hemophagocytic 288.4
  - histiocytic medullary (M9721/3) 202.3❺
  - lipomelanotic 695.89
  - malignant (M9720/3) 202.3❺
  - Sezary's (M9701/3) 202.2❺
- **Retina, retinal** – *see* condition
- **Retinitis** (*see also* Chorioretinitis) 363.20
  - albuminurica 585.9 *[363.10]*
  - arteriosclerotic 440.8 *[362.13]*
  - central angiospastic 362.41
  - Coat's 362.12
  - diabetic 250.5❺ *[362.01]*
  - disciformis 362.52
  - disseminated 363.10
    - metastatic 363.14
    - neurosyphilitic 094.83
    - pigment epitheliopathy 363.15
  - exudative 362.12
  - focal 363.00
    - in histoplasmosis 115.92
      - capsulatum 115.02
      - duboisii 115.12
    - juxtapapillary 363.05
    - macular 363.06
    - paramacular 363.06
    - peripheral 363.08
    - posterior pole NEC 363.07
  - gravidarum 646.8❺
  - hemorrhagica externa 362.12
  - juxtapapillary (Jensen's) 363.05
  - luetic – *see* Retinitis, syphilitic
  - metastatic 363.14
  - pigmentosa 362.74
  - proliferans 362.29
  - proliferating 362.29
  - punctata albescens 362.76
  - renal 585.9 *[363.13]*
  - syphilitic (secondary) 091.51
    - congenital 090.0 *[363.13]*
    - early 091.51
    - late 095.8 *[363.13]*
  - syphilitica, central, recurrent 095.8 *[363.13]*
  - tuberculous (*see also* Tuberculous) 017.3❺ *[363.13]*
- **Retinoblastoma** (M9510/3) 190.5
  - differentiated type (M9511/3) 190.5
  - undifferentiated type (M9512/3) 190.5
- **Retinochoroiditis** (*see also* Chorioretinitis) 363.20
  - central angiospastic 362.41
  - disseminated 363.10
    - metastatic 363.14
    - neurosyphilitic 094.83
    - pigment epitheliopathy 363.15
    - syphilitic 094.83
  - due to toxoplasmosis (acquired) (focal) 130.2
  - focal 363.00
    - in histoplasmosis 115.92
      - capsulatum 115.02
      - duboisii 115.12
    - juxtapapillary (Jensen's) 363.05

Retinochoroiditis – *continued*
- focal – *continued*
  - macular 363.06
  - paramacular 363.06
  - peripheral 363.08
  - posterior pole NEC 363.07
- juxtapapillaris 363.05
- syphilitic (disseminated) 094.83

Retinopathy (background) 362.10
- arteriosclerotic 440.8 *[362.13]*
- atherosclerotic 440.8 *[362.13]*
- central serous 362.41
- circinate 362.10
- Coat's 362.12
- diabetic 250.5❺ *[362.01]*
  - nonproliferative 250.5❺ *[362.03]*
    - mild 250.5❺ *[362.04]*
    - moderate 250.5❺ *[362.05]*
    - severe 250.5❺ *[362.06]*
  - proliferative 250.5❺ *[362.02]*
- exudative 362.12
- hypertensive 362.11
- nonproliferative
  - diabetic 250.5❺ *[362.03]*
    - mild 250.5❺ *[362.04]*
    - moderate 250.5❺ *[362.05]*
    - severe 250.5❺ *[362.06]*
- of prematurity 362.21
- pigmentary, congenital 362.74
- proliferative 362.29
  - diabetic 250.5 *[362.02]*
  - sickle-cell 282.60 *[362.29]*
- solar 363.31

Retinoschisis 361.10
- bullous 361.12
- congenital 743.56
- flat 361.11
- juvenile 362.73

Retractile testis 752.52

Retraction
- cervix – *see* Retraction, uterus
- drum (membrane) 384.82
- eyelid 374.41
- finger 736.29
- head 781.0
- lid 374.41
- lung 518.89
- mediastinum 519.3
- nipple 611.79
  - congenital 757.6
  - puerperal, postpartum 676.0❺
- palmar fascia 728.6
- pleura (*see also* Pleurisy) 511.0
- ring, uterus (Bandl's) (pathological) 661.4❺
  - affecting fetus or newborn 763.7
- sternum (congenital) 756.3
  - acquired 738.3
  - during respiration 786.9
- substernal 738.3
- supraclavicular 738.8
- syndrome (Duane's) 378.71
- uterus 621.6
- valve (heart) – *see* Endocarditis

Retrobulbar – *see* condition

Retrocaval ureter 753.4

Retrocecal – *see also* condition
- appendix (congenital) 751.5

Retrocession – *see* Retroversion

Retrodisplacement – *see* Retroversion

Retroflection, retroflexion – *see* Retroversion

Retrognathia, retrognathism (mandibular) (maxillary) 524.10

Retrograde
- ejaculation 608.87
- menstruation 626.8

Retroiliac ureter 753.4

Retroperineal – *see* condition

Retroperitoneal – *see* condition

Retroperitonitis 567.39

Retropharyngeal – *see* condition

Retroplacental – *see* condition

Retroposition – *see* Retroversion

Retrosternal thyroid (congenital) 759.2

Retroversion, retroverted
- cervix – *see* Retroversion, uterus
- female NEC (*see also* Retroversion, uterus) 621.6
- iris 364.70
- testis (congenital) 752.51

Retroversion, retroverted – *continued*
- uterus, uterine (acquired) (acute) (adherent) (any degree) (asymptomatic) (cervix) (postinfectional) (postpartal, old) 621.6
  - congenital 752.3
  - in pregnancy or childbirth 654.3❺
    - affecting fetus or newborn 763.89
    - causing obstructed labor 660.2❺
      - affecting fetus or newborn 763.1

Retrusion, premaxilla (developmental) 524.04

Rett's syndrome 330.8

Reverse, reversed
- peristalsis 787.4

Reye's syndrome 331.81

Reye-Sheehan syndrome (postpartum pituitary necrosis) 253.2

Rh (factor)
- hemolytic disease 773.0
- incompatibility, immunization, or sensitization
  - affecting management of pregnancy 656.1❺
  - fetus or newborn 773.0
  - transfusion reaction 999.7
- negative mother, affecting fetus or newborn 773.0
- titer elevated 999.7
- transfusion reaction 999.7

Rhabdomyolysis (idiopathic) 728.88

Rhabdomyoma (M8900/0) – *see also* Neoplasm, connective tissue, benign
- adult (M8904/0) – *see* Neoplasm, connective tissue, benign
- fetal (M8903/0) – *see* Neoplasm, connective tissue, benign
- glycogenic (M8904/0) – *see* Neoplasm, connective tissue, benign

Rhabdomyosarcoma (M8900/3) – *see also* Neoplasm connective tissue, malignant
- alveolar (M8920/3) – *see* Neoplasm, connective tissue, malignant
- embryonal (M8910/3) – *see* Neoplasm, connective tissue, malignant
- mixed type (M8902/3) – *see* Neoplasm, connective tissue, malignant
- pleomorphic (M8901/3) – *see* Neoplasm, connective tissue, malignant

Rhabdosarcoma (M8900/3) – *see* Rhabdomyosarcoma

Rhesus (factor) (Rh) incompatibility – *see* Rh, incompatibility

Rheumaticosis – *see* Rheumatism

Rheumatism, rheumatic (acute NEC) 729.0
- adherent pericardium 393
- arthritis
  - acute or subacute – *see* Fever, rheumatic
  - chronic 714.0
    - spine 720.0
- articular (chronic) NEC (*see also* Arthritis) 716.9❺
  - acute or subacute – *see* Fever, rheumatic
- back 724.9
- blennorrhagic 098.59
- carditis – *see* Disease, heart, rheumatic
- cerebral – *see* Fever, rheumatic
- chorea (acute) – *see* Chorea, rheumatic
- chronic NEC 729.0
- coronary arteritis 391.9
  - chronic 398.99
- degeneration, myocardium (*see also* Degeneration, myocardium, with rheumatic fever) 398.0
- desert 114.0
- febrile – *see* Fever, rheumatic
- fever – *see* Fever, rheumatic
- gonococcal 098.59
- gout 274.0
- heart
  - disease (*see also* Disease, heart, rheumatic) 398.90
  - failure (chronic) (congestive) (inactive) 398.91
- hemopericardium – *see* Rheumatic, pericarditis
- hydropericardium – *see* Rheumatic, pericarditis
- inflammatory (acute) (chronic) (subacute) – *see* Fever, rheumatic
- intercostal 729.0
  - meaning Tietze's disease 733.6
- joint (chronic) NEC (*see also* Arthritis) 716.9❺
  - acute – *see* Fever, rheumatic
- mediastinopericarditis – *see* Rheumatic, pericarditis

Rheumatism, rheumatic – *continued*
- muscular 729.0
- myocardial degeneration (*see also* Degeneration, myocardium, with rheumatic fever) 398.0
- myocarditis (chronic) (inactive) (with chorea) 398.0
  - active or acute 391.2
    - with chorea (acute) (rheumatic) (Sydenham's) 392.0
- myositis 729.1
- neck 724.9
- neuralgic 729.0
- neuritis (acute) (chronic) 729.2
- neuromuscular 729.0
- nodose – *see* Arthritis, nodosa
- nonarticular 729.0
- palindromic 719.30
  - ankle 719.37
  - elbow 719.32
  - foot 719.37
  - hand 719.34
  - hip 719.35
  - knee 719.36
  - multiple sites 719.39
  - pelvic region 719.35
  - shoulder (region) 719.31
  - specified site NEC 719.38
  - wrist 719.33
- pancarditis, acute 391.8
  - with chorea (acute) (rheumatic) (Sydenham's) 392.0
  - chronic or inactive 398.99
- pericarditis (active) (acute) (with effusion) (with pneumonia) 391.0
  - with chorea (acute) (rheumatic) (Sydenham's) 392.0
  - chronic or inactive 393
- pericardium – *see* Rheumatic, pericarditis
- pleuropericarditis – *see* Rheumatic, pericarditis
- pneumonia 390 *[517.1]*
- pneumonitis 390 *[517.1]*
- pneumopericarditis – *see* Rheumatic, pericarditis
- polyarthritis
  - acute or subacute – *see* Fever, rheumatic
  - chronic 714.0
- polyarticular NEC (*see also* Arthritis) 716.9❺
- psychogenic 306.0
- radiculitis 729.2
- sciatic 724.3
- septic – *see* Fever, rheumatic
- spine 724.9
- subacute NEC 729.0
- torticollis 723.5
- tuberculous NEC (*see also* Tuberculosis) 015.9❺
- typhoid fever 002.0

Rheumatoid – *see also* condition
- lungs 714.81

Rhinitis (atrophic) (catarrhal) (chronic) (croupous) (fibrinous) (hyperplastic) (hypertrophic) (membranous) (purulent) (suppurative) (ulcerative) 472.0
- with
  - hay fever (*see also* Fever, hay) 477.9
    - with asthma (bronchial) 493.0❺
  - sore throat – *see* Nasopharyngitis
- acute 460
- allergic (nonseasonal) (seasonal) (*see also* Fever, hay) 477.9
  - with asthma (*see also* Asthma) 493.0❺
  - due to food 477.1
- granulomatous 472.0
- infective 460
- obstructive 472.0
- pneumococcal 460
- syphilitic 095.8
  - congenital 090.0
- tuberculous (*see also* Tuberculosis) 012.8❺
- vasomotor (*see also* Fever, hay) 477.9

Rhinoantritis (chronic) 473.0
- acute 461.0

Rhinodacryolith 375.57

Rhinolalia (aperta) (clausa) (open) 784.49

Rhinolith 478.19
- nasal sinus (*see also* Sinusitis) 473.9

Rhinomegaly 478.19

Rhinopharyngitis (acute) (subacute) (*see also* Nasopharyngitis) 460
- chronic 472.2
- destructive ulcerating 102.5
- mutilans 102.5

Rhinophyma 695.3
Rhinorrhea 478.19
  cerebrospinal (fluid) 349.81
  paroxysmal (*see also* Fever, hay) 477.9
  spasmodic (*see also* Fever, hay) 477.9
Rhinosalpingitis 381.50
  acute 381.51
  chronic 381.52
Rhinoscleroma 040.1
Rhinosporidiosis 117.0
Rhinovirus infection 079.3
Rhizomelic chondrodysplasia punctata 277.86
Rhizomelique, pseudopolyarthritic 446.5
Rhoads and Bomford anemia (refractory) 238.72
Rhus
  diversiloba dermatitis 692.6
  radicans dermatitis 692.6
  toxicodendron dermatitis 692.6
  venenata dermatitis 692.6
  verniciflua dermatitis 692.6
Rhythm
  atrioventricular nodal 427.89
  disorder 427.9
    coronary sinus 427.89
    ectopic 427.89
    nodal 427.89
  escape 427.89
  heart, abnormal 427.9
    fetus or newborn – *see* Abnormal, heart rate
  idioventricular 426.89
    accelerated 427.89
  nodal 427.89
  sleep, inversion 327.39
    nonorganic origin 307.45
Rhytidosis facialis 701.8
Rib – *see also* condition
  cervical 756.2
Riboflavin deficiency 266.0
Rice bodies (*see also* Loose, body, joint) 718.1❺
  knee 717.6
Richter's hernia – *see* Hernia, Richter's
Ricinism 988.2
Rickets (active) (acute) (adolescent) (adult) (chest wall) (congenital) (current) (infantile) (intestinal) 268.0
  celiac 579.0
  fetal 756.4
  hemorrhagic 267
  hypophosphatemic with nephrotic-glycosuric dwarfism 270.0
  kidney 588.0
  late effect 268.1
  renal 588.0
  scurvy 267
  vitamin D-resistant 275.3
Rickettsial disease 083.9
  specified type NEC 083.8
Rickettsialpox 083.2
Rickettsiosis NEC 083.9
  specified type NEC 083.8
  tick-borne 082.9
    specified type NEC 082.8
  vesicular 083.2
Ricord's chancre 091.0
Riddoch's syndrome (visual disorientation) 368.16
Rider's
  bone 733.99
  chancre 091.0
Ridge, alveolus – *see also* condition
  edentulous
    atrophy 525.20
      mandible 525.20
        minimal 525.21
        moderate 525.22
        severe 525.23
      maxilla 525.20
        minimal 525.24
        moderate 525.25
        severe 525.26
  flabby 525.20
Ridged ear 744.29
Riedel's
  disease (ligneous thyroiditis) 245.3
  lobe, liver 751.69
  struma (ligneous thyroiditis) 245.3
  thyroiditis (ligneous) 245.3
Rieger's anomaly or syndrome (mesodermal dysgenesis, anterior ocular segment) 743.44
Riehl's melanosis 709.09
Rietti-Greppi-Micheli anemia or syndrome 282.49
Rieux's hernia – *see* Hernia, Rieux's
Rift Valley fever 066.3
Riga's disease (cachectic aphthae) 529.0
Riga-Fede disease (cachectic aphthae) 529.0
Riggs' disease (compound periodontitis) 523.40
Right middle lobe syndrome 518.0
Rigid, rigidity – *see also* condition
  abdominal 789.4❺
  articular, multiple congenital 754.89
  back 724.8
  cervix uteri
    in pregnancy or childbirth 654.6❺
      affecting fetus or newborn 763.89
      causing obstructed labor 660.2❺
        affecting fetus or newborn 763.1
  hymen (acquired) (congenital) 623.3
  nuchal 781.6
  pelvic floor
    in pregnancy or childbirth 654.4❺
      affecting fetus or newborn 763.89
      causing obstructed labor 660.2❺
        affecting fetus or newborn 763.1
  perineum or vulva
    in pregnancy or childbirth 654.8❺
      affecting fetus or newborn 763.89
      causing obstructed labor 660.2❺
        affecting fetus or newborn 763.1
  spine 724.8
  vagina
    in pregnancy or childbirth 654.7❺
      affecting fetus or newborn 763.89
      causing obstructed labor 660.2❺
        affecting fetus or newborn 763.1
Rigors 780.99
Riley-Day syndrome (familial dysautonomia) 742.8
RIND (reversible ischemic neurological deficit) 434.91 ●
  history of (personal) V12.54 ●
Ring(s)
  aorta 747.21
  Bandl's, complicating delivery 661.4❺
    affecting fetus or newborn 763.7
  contraction, complicating delivery 661.4❺
    affecting fetus or newborn 763.7
  esophageal (congenital) 750.3
  Fleischer (-Kayser) (cornea) 275.1 *[371.14]*
  hymenal, tight (acquired) (congenital) 623.3
  Kayser-Fleischer (cornea) 275.1 *[371.14]*
  retraction, uterus, pathological 661.4❺
    affecting fetus or newborn 763.7
  Schatzki's (esophagus) (congenital) (lower) 750.3
    acquired 530.3
  Soemmering's 366.51
  trachea, abnormal 748.3
  vascular (congenital) 747.21
  Vossius' 921.3
    late effect 366.21
Ringed hair (congenital) 757.4
Ringing in the ear (*see also* Tinnitus) 388.30
Ringworm 110.9
  beard 110.0
  body 110.5
  Burmese 110.9
  corporeal 110.5
  foot 110.4
  groin 110.3
  hand 110.2
  honeycomb 110.0
  nails 110.1
  perianal (area) 110.3
  scalp 110.0
  specified site NEC 110.8
  Tokelau 110.5
Rise, venous pressure 459.89
Risk
  factor – *see* Problem
  falling V15.88
  suicidal 300.9
Ritter's disease (dermatitis exfoliativa neonatorum) 695.81
Rivalry, sibling 313.3
Rivalta's disease (cervicofacial actinomycosis) 039.3
River blindness 125.3 *[360.13]*
Robert's pelvis 755.69
  with disproportion (fetopelvic) 653.0❺
    affecting fetus or newborn 763.1
    causing obstructed labor 660.1❺
      affecting fetus or newborn 763.1
Robin's syndrome 756.0
Robinson's (hidrotic) **ectodermal dysplasia** 757.31
Robles' disease (onchocerciasis) 125.3 *[360.13]*
Rochalimea- *see* Rickettsial disease
Rocky Mountain fever (spotted) 082.0
Rodent ulcer (M8090/3) – *see also* Neoplasm, skin, malignant
  cornea 370.07
Roentgen ray, adverse effect – *see* Effect, adverse, x-ray
Roetheln 056.9
Roger's disease (congenital interventricular septal defect) 745.4
Rokitansky's
  disease (*see also* Necrosis, liver) 570
  tumor 620.2
Rokitansky-Aschoff sinuses (mucosal outpouching of gallbladder) (*see also* Disease, gallbladder) 575.8
Rokitansky-Kuster-Hauser syndrome (congenital absence vagina) 752.49
Rollet's chancre (syphilitic) 091.0
Rolling of head 781.0
Romano-Ward syndrome (prolonged QT interval syndrome) 426.82
Romanus lesion 720.1
Romberg's disease or syndrome 349.89
Roof, mouth – *see* condition
Rosacea 695.3
  acne 695.3
  keratitis 695.3 *[370.49]*
Rosary, rachitic 268.0
Rose
  cold 477.0
  fever 477.0
  rash 782.1
    epidemic 056.9
    of infants 057.8
Rosen-Castleman-Liebow syndrome (pulmonary proteinosis) 516.0
Rosenbach's erysipelatoid or erysipeloid 027.1
Rosenthal's disease (factor XI deficiency) 286.2
Roseola 057.8
  infantum, infantilis ▶(*see also* Exanthem subitum)◀ 058.10 ▲
Rossbach's disease (hyperchlorhydria) 536.8
  psychogenic 306.4
Rossle-Urbach-Wiethe lipoproteinosis 272.8
Ross river fever 066.3
Rostan's asthma (cardiac) (*see also* Failure, ventricular, left) 428.1
Rot
  Barcoo (*see also* Ulcer, skin) 707.9
  knife-grinders' (*see also* Tuberculosis) 011.4❺
Rot-Bernhardt disease 355.1
Rotation
  anomalous, incomplete or insufficient – *see* Malrotation
  cecum (congenital) 751.4
  colon (congenital) 751.4
  manual, affecting fetus or newborn 763.89
  spine, incomplete or insufficient 737.8
  tooth, teeth 524.35
  vertebra, incomplete or insufficient 737.8
Röteln 056.9
Roth's disease or meralgia 355.1
Roth-Bernhardt disease or syndrome 355.1
Rothmund (-Thomson) **syndrome** 757.33
Rotor's disease or syndrome (idiopathic hyperbilirubinemia) 277.4
Rotundum ulcus – *see* Ulcer, stomach
Round
  back (with wedging of vertebrae) 737.10
    late effect of rickets 268.1
  hole, retina 361.31
    with detachment 361.01
  ulcer (stomach) – *see* Ulcer, stomach
  worms (infestation) (large) NEC 127.0
Roussy-Lévy syndrome 334.3

Routine postpartum follow-up V24.2
Roy (-Jutras) **syndrome** (acropachyderma) 757.39
Rubella (German measles) 056.9
  complicating pregnancy, childbirth, or puerperium 647.5❺
  complication 056.8
    neurological 056.00
      encephalomyelitis 056.01
      specified type NEC 056.09
    specified type NEC 056.79
  congenital 771.0
  contact V01.4
  exposure to V01.4
  maternal
    with suspected fetal damage affecting management of pregnancy 655.3❺
    affecting fetus or newborn 760.2
      manifest rubella in infant 771.0
  specified complications NEC 056.79
  vaccination, prophylactic (against) V04.3
Rubeola (measles) (*see also* Measles) 055.9
  complicated 055.8
  meaning rubella (*see also* Rubella) 056.9
  scarlatinosis 057.8
Rubeosis iridis 364.42
  diabetica 250.5❺ *[364.42]*
Rubinstein-Taybi's syndrome (brachydactylia, short stature and mental retardation) 759.89
Rud's syndrome (mental deficiency, epilepsy, and infantilism) 759.89
Rudimentary (congenital) – *see also* Agenesis
  arm 755.22
  bone 756.9
  cervix uteri 752.49
  eye (*see also* Microphthalmos) 743.10
  fallopian tube 752.19
  leg 755.32
  lobule of ear 744.21
  patella 755.64
  respiratory organs in thoracopagus 759.4
  tracheal bronchus 748.3
  uterine horn 752.3
  uterus 752.3
    in male 752.7
    solid or with cavity 752.3
  vagina 752.49
Ruiter-Pompen (-Wyers) **syndrome** (angiokeratoma corporis diffusum) 272.7
Ruled out condition (*see also* Observation, suspected) V71.9
Rumination – *see also* Vomiting
  disorder 307.53
  neurotic 300.3
  obsessional 300.3
  psychogenic 307.53
Runaway reaction – *see also* Disturbance, conduct
  socialized 312.2❺
  undersocialized, unsocialized 312.1❺
Runeberg's disease (progressive pernicious anemia) 281.0
Runge's syndrome (postmaturity) 766.22
Runny nose 784.99 ●
Rupia 091.3
  congenital 090.0
  tertiary 095.9
Rupture, ruptured 553.9
  abdominal viscera NEC 799.89
    obstetrical trauma 665.5❺
  abscess (spontaneous) – *see* Abscess, by site
  amnion – *see* Rupture, membranes
  aneurysm – *see* Aneurysm
  anus (sphincter) – *see* Laceration, anus
  aorta, aortic 441.5
    abdominal 441.3
    arch 441.1
    ascending 441.1
    descending 441.5
      abdominal 441.3
      thoracic 441.1
    syphilitic 093.0
    thoracoabdominal 441.6
    thorax, thoracic 441.1
    transverse 441.1
    traumatic (thoracic) 901.0
      abdominal 902.0
    valve or cusp (*see also* Endocarditis, aortic) 424.1
  appendix (with peritonitis) 540.0
    with peritoneal abscess 540.1

Rupture, ruptured – *continued*
  appendix – *continued*
    traumatic – *see* Injury, internal, gastrointestinal tract
  arteriovenous fistula, brain (congenital) 430
  artery 447.2
    brain (*see also* Hemorrhage, brain) 431
    coronary (*see also* Infarct, myocardium) 410.9❺
    heart (*see also* Infarct, myocardium) 410.9❺
    pulmonary 417.8
    traumatic (complication) (*see also* Injury, blood vessel, by site) 904.9
  bile duct, except cystic (*see also* Disease, biliary) 576.3
    cystic 575.4
    traumatic – *see* Injury, internal, intra-abdominal
  bladder (sphincter) 596.6
    with
      abortion – *see* Abortion, by type, with damage to pelvic organs
      ectopic pregnancy (*see also* categories 633.0-633.9) 639.2
      molar pregnancy (*see also* categories 630-632) 639.2
    following
      abortion 639.2
      ectopic or molar pregnancy 639.2
    nontraumatic 596.6
    obstetrical trauma 665.5❺
    spontaneous 596.6
    traumatic – *see* Injury, internal, bladder
  blood vessel (*see also* Hemorrhage) 459.0
    brain (*see also* Hemorrhage, brain) 431
    heart (*see also* Infarct, myocardium) 410.9❺
    traumatic (complication) (*see also* Injury, blood vessel, by site) 904.9
  bone – *see* Fracture, by site
  bowel 569.89
    traumatic – *see* Injury, internal, intestine
  Bowman's membrane 371.31
  brain
    aneurysm (congenital) (*see also* Hemorrhage, subarachnoid) 430
      late effect – *see* Late effect(s) (of) cerebrovascular disease
      syphilitic 094.87
    hemorrhagic (*see also* Hemorrhage, brain) 431
    injury at birth 767.0
    syphilitic 094.89
  capillaries 448.9
  cardiac (*see also* Infarct, myocardium) 410.9❺
  cartilage (articular) (current) – *see also* Sprain, by site
    knee – *see* Tear, meniscus
    semilunar – *see* Tear, meniscus
  cecum (with peritonitis) 540.0
    with peritoneal abscess 540.1
    traumatic 863.89
      with open wound into cavity 863.99
  cerebral aneurysm (congenital) (*see also* Hemorrhage, subarachnoid) 430
    late effect – *see* Late effect(s) (of) cerebrovascular disease
  cervix (uteri)
    with
      abortion – *see* Abortion, by type, with damage to pelvic organs
      ectopic pregnancy (*see also* categories 633.0-633.9) 639.2
      molar pregnancy (*see also* categories 630-632) 639.2
    following
      abortion 639.2
      ectopic or molar pregnancy 639.2
    obstetrical trauma 665.3❺
    traumatic – *see* Injury, internal, cervix
  chordae tendineae 429.5
  choroid (direct) (indirect) (traumatic) 363.63
  circle of Willis (*see also* Hemorrhage, subarachnoid) 430
    late effect – *see* Late effect(s) (of) cerebrovascular disease
  colon 569.89
    traumatic – *see* Injury, internal, colon
  cornea (traumatic) – *see also* Rupture, eye
    due to ulcer 370.00
  coronary (artery) (thrombotic) (*see also* Infarct, myocardium) 410.9❺
  corpus luteum (infected) (ovary) 620.1
  cyst – *see* Cyst
  cystic duct (*see also* Disease, gallbladder) 575.4

Rupture, ruptured – *continued*
  Descemet's membrane 371.33
    traumatic – *see* Rupture, eye
  diaphragm – *see also* Hernia, diaphragm
    traumatic – *see* Injury, internal, diaphragm
  diverticulum
    bladder 596.3
    intestine (large) (*see also* Diverticula) 562.10
      small 562.00
  duodenal stump 537.89
  duodenum (ulcer) – *see* Ulcer, duodenum, with perforation
  ear drum (*see also* Perforation, tympanum) 384.20
    with otitis media – *see* Otitis media
    traumatic – *see* Wound, open, ear
  esophagus 530.4
    traumatic 862.22
      with open wound into cavity 862.32
      cervical region – *see* Wound, open, esophagus
  eye (without prolapse of intraocular tissue) 871.0
    with
      exposure of intraocular tissue 871.1
      partial loss of intraocular tissue 871.2
      prolapse of intraocular tissue 871.1
    due to burn 940.5
  fallopian tube 620.8
    due to pregnancy – *see* Pregnancy, tubal
    traumatic – *see* Injury, internal, fallopian tube
  fontanel 767.3
  free wall (ventricle) (*see also* Infarct, myocardium) 410.9❺
  gallbladder or duct (*see also* Disease, gallbladder) 575.4
    traumatic – *see* Injury, internal, gallbladder
  gastric (*see also* Rupture, stomach) 537.89
    vessel 459.0
  globe (eye) (traumatic) – *see* Rupture, eye
  Graafian follicle (hematoma) 620.0
  heart (auricle) (ventricle) (*see also* Infarct, myocardium) 410.9❺
    infectional 422.90
    traumatic – *see* Rupture, myocardium, traumatic
  hymen 623.8
  internal
    organ, traumatic – *see also* Injury, internal, by site
      heart – *see* Rupture, myocardium, traumatic
      kidney – *see* Rupture, kidney
      liver – *see* Rupture, liver
      spleen – *see* Rupture, spleen, traumatic
    semilunar cartilage – *see* Tear, meniscus
  intervertebral disc – *see* Displacement, intervertebral disc
    traumatic (current) – *see* Dislocation, vertebra
  intestine 569.89
    traumatic – *see* Injury, internal, intestine
  intracranial, birth injury 767.0
  iris 364.76
    traumatic – *see* Rupture, eye
  joint capsule – *see* Sprain, by site
  kidney (traumatic) 866.03
    with open wound into cavity 866.13
    due to birth injury 767.8
    nontraumatic 593.89
  lacrimal apparatus (traumatic) 870.2
  lens (traumatic) 366.20
  ligament – *see also* Sprain, by site
    with open wound – *see* Wound, open, by site
    old (*see also* Disorder, cartilage, articular) 718.0❺
  liver (traumatic) 864.04
    with open wound into cavity 864.14
    due to birth injury 767.8
    nontraumatic 573.8
  lymphatic (node) (vessel) 457.8
  marginal sinus (placental) (with hemorrhage) 641.2❺
    affecting fetus or newborn 762.1
  meaning hernia – *see* Hernia
  membrana tympani (*see also* Perforation, tympanum) 384.20
    with otitis media – *see* Otitis media
    traumatic – *see* Wound, open, ear
  membranes (spontaneous)
    artificial
      delayed delivery following 658.3❺
        affecting fetus or newborn 761.1
      fetus or newborn 761.1
    delayed delivery following 658.2❺
      affecting fetus or newborn 761.1

Routine postpartum follow – Rupture, ruptured

- **Rupture, ruptured** – *continued*
  - membranes (spontaneous) – *continued*
    - premature (less than 24 hours prior to onset of labor) 658.1❺
      - affecting fetus or newborn 761.1
      - delayed delivery following 658.2❺
        - affecting fetus or newborn 761.1
  - meningeal artery (*see also* Hemorrhage, subarachnoid) 430
    - late effect – *see* Late effect(s) (of) cerebrovascular disease
  - meniscus (knee) – *see also* Tear, meniscus
    - old (*see also* Derangement, meniscus) 717.5
      - site other than knee – *see* Disorder, cartilage, articular
    - site other than knee – *see* Sprain, by site
  - mesentery 568.89
    - traumatic – *see* Injury, internal, mesentery
  - mitral – *see* Insufficiency, mitral
  - muscle (traumatic) NEC – *see also* Sprain, by site
    - with open wound – *see* Wound, open, by site
    - nontraumatic 728.83
  - musculotendinous cuff (nontraumatic) (shoulder) 840.4
  - mycotic aneurysm, causing cerebral hemorrhage (*see also* Hemorrhage, subarachnoid) 430
    - late effect – *see* Late effect(s) (of) cerebrovascular disease
  - myocardium, myocardial (*see also* Infarct, myocardium) 410.9❺
    - traumatic 861.03
      - with open wound into thorax 861.13
  - nontraumatic (meaning hernia) (*see also* Hernia, by site) 553.9
  - obstructed (*see also* Hernia, by site, with obstruction) 552.9
    - gangrenous (*see also* Hernia, by site, with gangrene) 551.9
  - operation wound 998.32
    - internal 998.31
  - ovary, ovarian 620.8
    - corpus luteum 620.1
    - follicle (graafian) 620.0
  - oviduct 620.8
    - due to pregnancy – *see* Pregnancy, tubal
  - pancreas 577.8
    - traumatic – *see* Injury, internal, pancreas
  - papillary muscle (ventricular) 429.6
  - pelvic
    - floor, complicating delivery 664.1❺
    - organ NEC – *see* Injury, pelvic, organs
  - penis (traumatic) – *see* Wound, open, penis
  - perineum 624.8
    - during delivery (*see also* Laceration, perineum, complicating delivery) 664.4❺
  - pharynx (nontraumatic) (spontaneous) 478.29
  - pregnant uterus (before onset of labor) 665.0❺
  - prostate (traumatic) – *see* Injury, internal, prostate
  - pulmonary
    - artery 417.8
    - valve (heart) (*see also* Endocarditis, pulmonary) 424.3
    - vein 417.8
    - vessel 417.8
  - pupil, sphincter 364.75
  - pus tube (*see also* Salpingo-oophoritis) 614.2
  - pyosalpinx (*see also* Salpingo-oophoritis) 614.2
  - rectum 569.49
    - traumatic – *see* Injury, internal, rectum
  - retina, retinal (traumatic) (without detachment) 361.30
    - with detachment (*see also* Detachment, retina, with retinal defect) 361.00
  - rotator cuff (capsule) (traumatic) 840.4
    - nontraumatic, complete 727.61
  - sclera 871.0
  - semilunar cartilage, knee (*see also* Tear, meniscus) 836.2
    - old (*see also* Derangement, meniscus) 717.5
  - septum (cardiac) 410.8❺
  - sigmoid 569.89
    - traumatic – *see* Injury, internal, colon, sigmoid
  - sinus of Valsalva 747.29
  - spinal cord – *see also* Injury, spinal, by site
    - due to injury at birth 767.4
    - fetus or newborn 767.4
    - syphilitic 094.89
    - traumatic – *see also* Injury, spinal, by site
      - with fracture – *see* Fracture, vertebra, by site, with spinal cord injury
  - spleen 289.59
    - congenital 767.8

- **Rupture, ruptured** – *continued*
  - spleen – *continued*
    - due to injury at birth 767.8
    - malarial 084.9
    - nontraumatic 289.59
    - spontaneous 289.59
    - traumatic 865.04
      - with open wound into cavity 865.14
  - splenic vein 459.0
  - stomach 537.89
    - due to injury at birth 767.8
    - traumatic – *see* Injury, internal, stomach
    - ulcer – *see* Ulcer, stomach, with perforation
  - synovium 727.50
    - specified site NEC 727.59
  - tendon (traumatic) – *see also* Sprain, by site
    - with open wound – *see* Wound, open, by site
    - Achilles 845.09
      - nontraumatic 727.67
    - ankle 845.09
      - nontraumatic 727.68
    - biceps (long bead) 840.8
      - nontraumatic 727.62
    - foot 845.10
      - interphalangeal (joint) 845.13
      - metatarsophalangeal (joint) 845.12
      - nontraumatic 727.68
      - specified site NEC 845.19
      - tarsometatarsal (joint) 845.11
    - hand 842.10
      - carpometacarpal (joint) 842.11
      - interphalangeal (joint) 842.13
      - metacarpophalangeal (joint) 842.12
      - nontraumatic 727.63
        - extensors 727.63
        - flexors 727.64
      - specified site NEC 842.19
    - nontraumatic 727.60
      - specified site NEC 727.69
    - patellar 844.8
      - nontraumatic 727.66
    - quadriceps 844.8
      - nontraumatic 727.65
    - rotator cuff (capsule) 840.4
      - nontraumatic, complete 727.61
    - wrist 842.00
      - carpal (joint) 842.01
      - nontraumatic 727.63
        - extensors 727.63
        - flexors 727.64
      - radiocarpal (joint) (ligament) 842.02
      - radioulnar (joint), distal 842.09
      - specified site NEC 842.09
  - testis (traumatic) 878.2
    - complicated 878.3
    - due to syphilis 095.8
  - thoracic duct 457.8
  - tonsil 474.8
  - traumatic
    - with open wound – *see* Wound, open, by site
    - aorta – *see* Rupture, aorta, traumatic
    - ear drum – *see* Wound, open, ear, drum
    - external site – *see* Wound, open, by site
    - eye 871.2
    - globe (eye) – *see* Wound, open, eyeball
    - internal organ (abdomen, chest, or pelvis) – *see also* Injury, internal, by site
      - heart – *see* Rupture, myocardium, traumatic
      - kidney – *see* Rupture, kidney
      - liver – *see* Rupture, liver
      - spleen – *see* Rupture, spleen, traumatic
    - ligament, muscle, or tendon – *see also* Sprain, by site
      - with open wound – *see* Wound, open, by site
    - meaning hernia – *see* Hernia
  - tricuspid (heart) (valve) – *see* Endocarditis, tricuspid
  - tube, tubal 620.8
    - abscess (*see also* Salpingo-oophoritis) 614.2
    - due to pregnancy – *see* Pregnancy, tubal
  - tympanum, tympanic (membrane) (*see also* Perforation, tympanum) 384.20
    - with otitis media – *see* Otitis media
    - traumatic – *see* Wound, open, ear, drum
  - umbilical cord 663.8❺
    - fetus or newborn 772.0
  - ureter (traumatic) (*see also* Injury, internal, ureter) 867.2
    - nontraumatic 593.89

- **Rupture, ruptured** – *continued*
  - urethra 599.84
    - with
      - abortion – *see* Abortion, by type, with damage to pelvic organs
      - ectopic pregnancy (*see also* categories 633.0-633.9) 639.2
      - molar pregnancy (*see also* categories 630-632) 639.2
    - following
      - abortion 639.2
      - ectopic or molar pregnancy 639.2
    - obstetrical trauma 665.5❺
    - traumatic – *see* Injury, internal urethra
  - uterosacral ligament 620.8
  - uterus (traumatic) – *see also* Injury, internal uterus
    - affecting fetus or newborn 763.89
    - during labor 665.1❺
    - nonpuerperal, nontraumatic 621.8
    - nontraumatic 621.8
    - pregnant (during labor) 665.1❺
      - before labor 665.0❺
  - vagina 878.6
    - complicated 878.7
    - complicating delivery – *see* Laceration, vagina, complicating delivery
  - valve, valvular (heart) – *see* Endocarditis
  - varicose vein – *see* Varicose vein
  - varix – *see* Varix
  - vena cava 459.0
  - ventricle (free wall) (left) (*see also* Infarct, myocardium) 410.9❺
  - vesical (urinary) 596.6
    - traumatic – *see* Injury, internal, bladder
  - vessel (blood) 459.0
    - pulmonary 417.8
  - viscus 799.89
  - vulva 878.4
    - complicated 878.5
    - complicating delivery 664.0❺
- **Russell's dwarf** (uterine dwarfism and craniofacial dysostosis) 759.89
- **Russell's dysentery** 004.8
- **Russell** (-Silver) **syndrome** (congenital hemihypertrophy and short stature) 759.89
- **Russian spring-summer type encephalitis** 063.0
- **Rust's disease** (tuberculous spondylitis) 015.0❺ *[720.81]*
- **Rustitskii's disease** (multiple myeloma) (M9730/3) 203.0❺
- **Ruysch's disease** (Hirschsprung's disease) 751.3
- **Rytand-Lipsitch syndrome** (complete atrioventricular block) 426.0

S

- **Saber**
  - shin 090.5
  - tibia 090.5
- **Sac, lacrimal** – *see* condition
- **Saccharomyces infection** (*see also* Candidiasis) 112.9
- **Saccharopinuria** 270.7
- **Saccular** – *see* condition
- **Sacculation**
  - aorta (nonsyphilitic) (*see also* Aneurysm, aorta) 441.9
    - ruptured 441.5
    - syphilitic 093.0
  - bladder 596.3
  - colon 569.89
  - intralaryngeal (congenital) (ventricular) 748.3
  - larynx (congenital) (ventricular) 748.3
  - organ or site, congenital – *see* Distortion
  - pregnant uterus, complicating delivery 654.4❺
    - affecting fetus or newborn 763.1
    - causing obstructed labor 660.2❺
      - affecting fetus or newborn 763.1
  - rectosigmoid 569.89
  - sigmoid 569.89
  - ureter 593.89
  - urethra 599.2
  - vesical 596.3
- **Sachs** (-Tay) **disease** (amaurotic familial idiocy) 330.1
- **Sacks-Libman disease** 710.0 *[424.91]*

Rupture, ruptured – Sacks-Libman disease

Sacralgia 724.6

Sacralization
- fifth lumbar vertebra 756.15
- incomplete (vertebra) 756.15

Sacrodynia 724.6

Sacroiliac joint – *see* condition

Sacroiliitis NEC 720.2

Sacrum – *see* condition

Saddle
- back 737.8
- embolus, aorta 444.0
- nose 738.0
  - congenital 754.0
  - due to syphilis 090.5

Sadism (sexual) 302.84

Saemisch's ulcer 370.04

Saenger's syndrome 379.46

Sago spleen 277.39

Sailors' skin 692.74

Saint
- Anthony's fire (*see also* Erysipelas) 035
- Guy's dance – *see* Chorea
- Louis-type encephalitis 062.3
- triad (*see also* Hernia, diaphragm) 553.3
- Vitus' dance – *see* Chorea

Salicylism
- correct substance properly administered 535.4❺
- overdose or wrong substance given or taken 965.1

Salivary duct or gland – *see also* condition
- virus disease 078.5

Salivation (excessive) (*see also* Ptyalism) 527.7

Salmonella (aertrycke) (choleraesuis) (enteritidis) (gallinarum) (suipestifer) (typhimurium) (*see also* Infection, Salmonella) 003.9
- arthritis 003.23
- carrier (suspected) of V02.3
- meningitis 003.21
- osteomyelitis 003.24
- pneumonia 003.22
- septicemia 003.1
- typhosa 002.0
  - carrier (suspected) of V02.1

Salmonellosis 003.0
- with pneumonia 003.22

Salpingitis (catarrhal) (fallopian tube) (nodular) (pseudofollicular) (purulent) (septic) (*see also* Salpingo-oophoritis) 614.2
- ear 381.50
  - acute 381.51
  - chronic 381.52
- Eustachian (tube) 381.50
  - acute 381.51
  - chronic 381.52
- follicularis 614.1
- gonococcal (chronic) 098.37
  - acute 098.17
- interstitial, chronic 614.1
- isthmica nodosa 614.1
- old – *see* Salpingo-oophoritis, chronic
- puerperal, postpartum, childbirth 670❹
- specific (chronic) 098.37
  - acute 098.17
- tuberculous (acute) (chronic) (*see also* Tuberculosis) 016.6❺
- venereal (chronic) 098.37
  - acute 098.17

Salpingocele 620.4

Salpingo-oophoritis (catarrhal) (purulent) (ruptured) (septic) (suppurative) 614.2
- acute 614.0
  - with
    - abortion – *see* Abortion, by type, with sepsis
    - ectopic pregnancy (*see also* categories 633.0-633.9) 639.0
    - molar pregnancy (*see also* categories 630-632) 639.0
  - following
    - abortion 639.0
    - ectopic or molar pregnancy 639.0
  - gonococcal 098.17
  - puerperal, postpartum, childbirth 670❹
  - tuberculous (*see also* Tuberculosis) 016.6❺
- chronic 614.1
  - gonococcal 098.37
  - tuberculous (*see also* Tuberculosis) 016.6❺
- complicating pregnancy 646.6❺
  - affecting fetus or newborn 760.8

Salpingo-oophoritis – *continued*
- gonococcal (chronic) 098.37
  - acute 098.17
- old – *see* Salpingo-oophoritis, chronic
- puerperal 670❹
- specific – *see* Salpingo-oophoritis, gonococcal
- subacute (*see also* Salpingo-oophoritis, acute) 614.0
- tuberculous (acute) (chronic) (*see also* Tuberculosis) 016.6❺
- venereal – *see* Salpingo-oophoritis, gonococcal

Salpingo-ovaritis (*see also* Salpingo-oophoritis) 614.2

Salpingoperitonitis (*see also* Salpingo-oophoritis) 614.2

Salt-losing
- nephritis (*see also* Disease, renal) 593.9
- syndrome (*see also* Disease, renal) 593.9

Salt-rheum (*see also* Eczema) 692.9

Salzmann's nodular dystrophy 371.46

Sampson's cyst or tumor 617.1

Sandblasters'
- asthma 502
- lung 502

Sander's disease (paranoia) 297.1

Sandfly fever 066.0

Sandhoff's disease 330.1

Sanfilippo's syndrome (mucopolysaccharidosis III) 277.5

Sanger-Brown's ataxia 334.2

San Joaquin Valley fever 114.0

Sao Paulo fever or typhus 082.0

Saponification, mesenteric 567.89

Sapremia – *see* Septicemia

Sarcocele (benign)
- syphilitic 095.8
  - congenital 090.5

Sarcoepiplocele (*see also* Hernia) 553.9

Sarcoepiplomphalocele (*see also* Hernia, umbilicus) 553.1

Sarcoid (any site) 135
- with lung involvement 135 *[517.8]*
- Boeck's 135
- Darier-Roussy 135
- Spiegler-Fendt 686.8

Sarcoidosis 135
- cardiac 135 *[425.8]*
- lung 135 *[517.8]*

Sarcoma (M8800/3) – *see also* Neoplasm, connective tissue, malignant
- alveolar soft part (M9581/3) – *see* Neoplasm, connective tissue, malignant
- ameloblastic (M9330/3) 170.1
  - upper jaw (bone) 170.0
- botryoid (M8910/3) – *see* Neoplasm, connective tissue, malignant
- botryoides (M8910/3) – *see* Neoplasm, connective tissue, malignant
- cerebellar (M9480/3) 191.6
  - circumscribed (arachnoidal) (M9471/3) 191.6
- circumscribed (arachnoidal) cerebellar (M9471/3) 191.6
- clear cell, of tendons and aponeuroses (M9044/3) – *see* Neoplasm, connective tissue, malignant
- embryonal (M8991/3) – *see* Neoplasm, connective tissue, malignant
- endometrial (stromal) (M8930/3) 182.0
  - isthmus 182.1
- endothelial (M9130/3) – *see also* Neoplasm, connective tissue, malignant
  - bone (M9260/3) – *see* Neoplasm, bone, malignant
- epithelioid cell (M8804/3) – *see* Neoplasm, connective tissue, malignant
- Ewing's (M9260/3) – *see* Neoplasm, bone, malignant
- follicular dendritic cell 202.9
- germinoblastic (diffuse) (M9632/3) 202.8❺
  - follicular (M9697/3) 202.0❺
- giant cell (M8802/3) – *see also* Neoplasm, connective tissue, malignant
  - bone (M9250/3) – *see* Neoplasm, bone, malignant
- glomoid (M8710/3) – *see* Neoplasm, connective tissue, malignant
- granulocytic (M9930/3) 205.3❺
- hemangioendothelial (M9130/3) – *see* Neoplasm, connective tissue, malignant

Sarcoma – *continued*
- hemorrhagic, multiple (M9140/3) – *see* Kaposi's, sarcoma
- Hodgkin's (M9662/3) 201.2❺
- immunoblastic (M9612/3) 200.8❺
- interdigitating dendritic cell 202.9
- Kaposi's (M9140/3) – *see* Kaposi's, sarcoma
- Kupffer cell (M9124/3) 155.0
- Langerhans cell 202.9❺
- leptomeningeal (M9530/3) – *see* Neoplasm, meninges, malignant
- lymphangioendothelial (M9170/3) – *see* Neoplasm, connective tissue, malignant
- lymphoblastic (M9630/3) 200.1❺
- lymphocytic (M9620/3) 200.1❺
- mast cell (M9740/3) 202.6❺
- melanotic (M8720/3) – *see* Melanoma
- meningeal (M9530/3) – *see* Neoplasm, meninges, malignant
- meningothelial (M9530/3) – *see* Neoplasm, meninges, malignant
- mesenchymal (M8800/3) – *see also* Neoplasm, connective tissue, malignant
  - mixed (M8990/3) – *see* Neoplasm, connective tissue, malignant
- mesothelial (M9050/3) – *see* Neoplasm, by site, malignant
- monstrocellular (M9481/3)
  - specified site – *see* Neoplasm, by site, malignant
  - unspecified site 191.9
- myeloid (M9930/3) 205.3❺
- neurogenic (M9540/3) – *see* Neoplasm, connective tissue, malignant
- odontogenic (M9270/3) 170.1
  - upper jaw (bone) 170.0
- osteoblastic (M9180/3) – *see* Neoplasm, bone, malignant
- osteogenic (M9180/3) – *see also* Neoplasm, bone, malignant
  - juxtacortical (M9190/3) – *see* Neoplasm, bone, malignant
  - periosteal (M9190/3) – *see* Neoplasm, bone, malignant
- periosteal (M8812/3) – *see also* Neoplasm, bone, malignant
  - osteogenic (M9190/3) – *see* Neoplasm, bone, malignant
- plasma cell (M9731/3) 203.8❺
- pleomorphic cell (M8802/3) – *see* Neoplasm, connective tissue, malignant
- reticuloendothelial (M9720/3) 202.3❺
- reticulum cell (M9640/3) 200.0❺
  - nodular (M9642/3) 200.0❺
  - pleomorphic cell type (M9641/3) 200.0❺
- round cell (M8803/3) – *see* Neoplasm, connective tissue, malignant
- small cell (M8803/3) – *see* Neoplasm, connective tissue, malignant
- spindle cell (M8801/3) – *see* Neoplasm, connective tissue, malignant
- stromal (endometrial) (M8930/3) 182.0
  - isthmus 182.1
- synovial (M9040/3) – *see also* Neoplasm, connective tissue, malignant
  - biphasic type (M9043/3) – *see* Neoplasm, connective tissue, malignant
  - epithelioid cell type (M9042/3) – *see* Neoplasm, connective tissue, malignant
  - spindle cell type (M9041/3) – *see* Neoplasm, connective tissue, malignant

Sarcomatosis
- meningeal (M9539/3) – *see* Neoplasm, meninges, malignant
- specified site NEC (M8800/3) – *see* Neoplasm, connective tissue, malignant
- unspecified site (M8800/6) 171.9

Sarcosinemia 270.8

Sarcosporidiosis 136.5

Satiety, early 780.94

Saturnine – *see* condition

Saturnism 984.9
- specified type of lead – *see* Table of Drugs and Chemicals

Satyriasis 302.89

Sauriasis – *see* Ichthyosis

Sauriderma 757.39

Sauriosis – *see* Ichthyosis

Savill's disease (epidemic exfoliative dermatitis) 695.89

- **SBE** (subacute bacterial endocarditis) 421.0
- **Scabies** (any site) 133.0
- **Scabs** 782.8
- **Scaglietti-Dagnini syndrome** (acromegalic macrospondylitis) 253.0
- **Scald, scalded** – *see also* Burn, by site
  - skin syndrome 695.1
- **Scalenus anticus** (anterior) **syndrome** 353.0
- **Scales** 782.8
- **Scalp** – *see* condition
- **Scaphocephaly** 756.0
- **Scaphoiditis, tarsal** 732.5
- **Scapulalgia** 733.90
- **Scapulohumeral myopathy** 359.1
- **Scar, scarring** (*see also* Cicatrix) 709.2
  - adherent 709.2
  - atrophic 709.2
  - cervix
    - in pregnancy or childbirth 654.6❺
      - affecting fetus or newborn 763.89
      - causing obstructed labor 660.2❺
        - affecting fetus or newborn 763.1
  - cheloid 701.4
  - chorioretinal 363.30
    - disseminated 363.35
    - macular 363.32
    - peripheral 363.34
    - posterior pole NEC 363.33
  - choroid (*see also* Scar, chorioretinal) 363.30
  - compression, pericardial 423.9
  - congenital 757.39
  - conjunctiva 372.64
  - cornea 371.00
    - xerophthalmic 264.6
  - due to previous cesarean delivery, complicating pregnancy or childbirth 654.2❺
    - affecting fetus or newborn 763.89
  - duodenal (bulb) (cap) 537.3
  - hypertrophic 701.4
  - keloid 701.4
  - labia 624.4
  - lung (base) 518.89
  - macula 363.32
    - disseminated 363.35
    - peripheral 363.34
  - muscle 728.89
  - myocardium, myocardial 412
  - painful 709.2
  - papillary muscle 429.81
  - posterior pole NEC 363.33
    - macular – *see* Scar, macula
  - postnecrotic (hepatic) (liver) 571.9
  - psychic V15.49
  - retina (*see also* Scar, chorioretinal) 363.30
  - trachea 478.9
  - uterus 621.8
    - in pregnancy or childbirth NEC 654.9❺
      - affecting fetus or newborn 763.89
      - from previous cesarean delivery 654.2❺
  - vulva 624.4
- **Scarabiasis** 134.1
- **Scarlatina** 034.1
  - anginosa 034.1
  - maligna 034.1
  - myocarditis, acute 034.1 *[422.0]*
    - old (*see also* Myocarditis) 429.0
  - otitis media 034.1 *[382.02]*
  - ulcerosa 034.1
- **Scarlatinella** 057.8
- **Scarlet fever** (albuminuria) (angina) (convulsions) (lesions of lid) (rash) 034.1
- **Schamberg's disease, dermatitis, or dermatosis** (progressive pigmentary dermatosis) 709.09
- **Schatzki's ring** (esophagus) (lower) (congenital) 750.3
  - acquired 530.3
- **Schaufenster krankheit** 413.9
- **Schaumann's**
  - benign lymphogranulomatosis 135
  - disease (sarcoidosis) 135
  - syndrome (sarcoidosis) 135
- **Scheie's syndrome** (mucopolysaccharidosis IS) 277.5
- **Schenck's disease** (sporotrichosis) 117.1
- **Scheuermann's disease or osteochondrosis** 732.0
- **Scheuthauer-Marie-Sainton syndrome** (cleidocranialis dysostosis) 755.59
- **Schilder** (-Flatau) **disease** 341.1
- **Schilling-type monocytic leukemia** (M9890/3) 206.9❺
- **Schimmelbusch's disease, cystic mastitis, or hyperplasia** 610.1
- **Schirmer's syndrome** (encephalocutaneous angiomatosis) 759.6
- **Schistocelia** 756.79
- **Schistoglossia** 750.13
- **Schistosoma infestation** – *see* Infestation, Schistosoma
- **Schistosomiasis** 120.9
  - Asiatic 120.2
  - bladder 120.0
  - chestermani 120.8
  - colon 120.1
  - cutaneous 120.3
  - due to
    - S. hematobium 120.0
    - S. japonicum 120.2
    - S. mansoni 120.1
    - S. mattheii 120.8
  - eastern 120.2
  - genitourinary tract 120.0
  - intestinal 120.1
  - lung 120.2
  - Manson's (intestinal) 120.1
  - Oriental 120.2
  - pulmonary 120.2
  - specified type NEC 120.8
  - vesical 120.0
- **Schizencephaly** 742.4
- **Schizo-affective psychosis** (*see also* Schizophrenia) 295.7❺
- **Schizodontia** 520.2
- **Schizoid personality** 301.20
  - introverted 301.21
  - schizotypal 301.22
- **Schizophrenia, schizophrenic** (reaction) 295.9❺

  Note – Use the following fifth-digit subclassification with category 295:

0	*unspecified*
1	*subchronic*
2	*chronic*
3	*subchronic with acute exacerbation*
4	*chronic with acute exacerbation*
5	*in remission*

  - acute (attack) NEC 295.8❺
    - episode 295.4❺
  - atypical form 295.8❺
  - borderline 295.5❺
  - catalepsy 295.2❺
  - catatonic (type) (acute) (excited) (withdrawn) 295.2❺
  - childhood (type) (*see also* Psychosis, childhood) 299.9❺
  - chronic NEC 295.6❺
  - coenesthesiopathic 295.8❺
  - cyclic (type) 295.7❺
  - disorganized (type) 295.1❺
  - flexibilitas cerea 295.2❺
  - hebephrenic (type) (acute) 295.1❺
  - incipient 295.5❺
  - latent 295.5❺
  - paranoid (type) (acute) 295.3❺
  - paraphrenic (acute) 295.3❺
  - prepsychotic 295.5❺
  - primary (acute) 295.0❺
  - prodromal 295.5❺
  - pseudoneurotic 295.5❺
  - pseudopsychopathic 295.5❺
  - reaction 295.9❺
  - residual type (state) 295.6❺
  - restzustand 295.6❺
  - schizo-affective (type) (depressed) (excited) 295.7❺
  - schizophreniform type 295.4❺
  - simple (type) (acute) 295.0❺
  - simplex (acute) 295.0❺
  - specified type NEC 295.8❺
  - syndrome of childhood NEC (*see also* Psychosis, childhood) 299.9❺
  - undifferentiated type 295.9❺
    - acute 295.8❺
    - chronic 295.6❺
- **Schizothymia** 301.20
  - introverted 301.21
  - schizotypal 301.22
- **Schlafkrankheit** 086.5
- **Schlatter's tibia** (osteochondrosis) 732.4
- **Schlatter-Osgood disease** (osteochondrosis, tibial tubercle) 732.4
- **Schloffer's tumor** (*see also* Peritonitis) 567.29
- **Schmidt's syndrome**
  - sphallo-pharyngo-laryngeal hemiplegia 352.6
  - thyroid-adrenocortical insufficiency 258.1
  - vagoaccessory 352.6
- **Schmincke**
  - carcinoma (M8082/3) – *see* Neoplasm, nasopharynx, malignant
  - tumor (M8082/3) – *see* Neoplasm, nasopharynx, malignant
- **Schmitz** (-Stutzer) **dysentery** 004.0
- **Schmorl's disease or nodes** 722.30
  - lumbar, lumbosacral 722.32
  - specified region NEC 722.39
  - thoracic, thoracolumbar 722.31
- **Schneider's syndrome** 047.9
- **Schneiderian**
  - carcinoma (M8121/3)
    - specified site – *see* Neoplasm, by site, malignant
    - unspecified site 160.0
  - papilloma (M8121/0)
    - specified site – *see* Neoplasm, by site, benign
    - unspecified site 212.0
- **Schnitzler syndrome** 273.1
- **Schoffer's tumor** (*see also* Peritonitis) 567.29
- **Scholte's syndrome** (malignant carcinoid) 259.2
- **Scholz's disease** 330.0
- **Scholz** (-Bielschowsky-Henneberg) **syndrome** 330.0
- **Schönlein** (-Henoch) **disease** (primary) (purpura) (rheumatic) 287.0
- **School examination** V70.3
- **Schottmüller's disease** (*see also* Fever, paratyphoid) 002.9
- **Schroeder's syndrome** (endocrine-hypertensive) 255.3
- **Schüller-Christian disease or syndrome** (chronic histiocytosis X) 277.89
- **Schultz's disease or syndrome** (agranulocytosis) 288.09
- **Schultze's acroparesthesia, simple** 443.89
- **Schwalbe-Ziehen-Oppenheimer disease** 333.6
- **Schwannoma** (M9560/0) – *see also* Neoplasm, connective tissues, benign
  - malignant (M9560/3) – *see* Neoplasm, connective tissue, malignant
- **Schwartz** (-Jampel) **syndrome** 359.23 ▲
- **Schwartz-Bartter syndrome** (inappropriate secretion of antidiuretic hormone) 253.6
- **Schweninger-Buzzi disease** (macular atrophy) 701.3
- **Sciatic** – *see* condition
- **Sciatica** (infectional) 724.3
  - due to
    - displacement of intervertebral disc 722.10
    - herniation, nucleus pulposus 722.10
  - wallet 724.3
- **Scimitar syndrome** (anomalous venous drainage, right lung to inferior vena cava) 747.49
- **Sclera** – *see* condition
- **Sclerectasia** 379.11
- **Scleredema**
  - adultorum 710.1
  - Buschke's 710.1
  - newborn 778.1
- **Sclerema**
  - adiposum (newborn) 778.1
  - adultorum 710.1
  - edematosum (newborn) 778.1
  - neonatorum 778.1
  - newborn 778.1
- **Scleriasis** – *see* Scleroderma
- **Scleritis** 379.00
  - with corneal involvement 379.05
  - anterior (annular) (localized) 379.03
  - brawny 379.06
  - granulomatous 379.09
  - posterior 379.07
  - specified NEC 379.09
  - suppurative 379.09
  - syphilitic 095.0
  - tuberculous (nodular) (*see also* Tuberculosis) 017.3❺ *[379.09]*
- **Sclerochoroiditis** (*see also* Scleritis) 379.00

Scleroconjunctivitis (*see also* Scleritis) 379.00
Sclerocystic ovary (syndrome) 256.4
Sclerodactylia 701.0
Scleroderma, sclerodermia (acrosclerotic) (diffuse) (generalized) (progressive) (pulmonary) 710.1
  circumscribed 701.0
  linear 701.0
  localized (linear) 701.0
  newborn 778.1
Sclerokeratitis 379.05
  meaning sclerosing keratitis 370.54
  tuberculous (*see also* Tuberculosis) 017.3❺ *[379.09]*
Scleroma, trachea 040.1
Scleromalacia
  multiple 731.0
  perforans 379.04
Scleromyxedema 701.8
Scleroperikeratitis 379.05
Sclerose en plaques 340
Sclerosis, sclerotic
  adrenal (gland) 255.8
  Alzheimer's 331.0
    with dementia – *see* Alzheimer's, dementia
  amyotrophic (lateral) 335.20
  annularis fibrosi
    aortic 424.1
    mitral 424.0
  aorta, aortic 440.0
    valve (*see also* Endocarditis, aortic) 424.1
  artery, arterial, arteriolar, arteriovascular – *see* Arteriosclerosis
  ascending multiple 340
  Baló's (concentric) 341.1
  basilar – *see* Sclerosis, brain
  bone (localized) NEC 733.99
  brain (general) (lobular) 341.9
    Alzheimer's – *see* Alzheimer's, dementia
    artery, arterial 437.0
    atrophic lobar 331.0
      with dementia
        with behavioral disturbance 331.0 *[294.11]*
        without behavioral disturbance 331.0 *[294.10]*
    diffuse 341.1
      familial (chronic) (infantile) 330.0
      infantile (chronic) (familial) 330.0
      Pelizaeus-Merzbacher type 330.0
    disseminated 340
    hereditary 334.2
    infantile (degenerative) (diffuse) 330.0
    insular 340
    Krabbe's 330.0
    miliary 340
    multiple 340
    Pelizaeus-Merzbacher 330.0
    progressive familial 330.0
    senile 437.0
    tuberous 759.5
  bulbar, progressive 340
  bundle of His 426.50
    left 426.3
    right 426.4
  cardiac – *see* Arteriosclerosis, coronary
  cardiorenal (*see also* Hypertension, cardiorenal) 404.90
  cardiovascular (*see also* Disease, cardiovascular) 429.2
    renal (*see also* Hypertension, cardiorenal) 404.90
  centrolobar, familial 330.0
  cerebellar – *see* Sclerosis, brain
  cerebral – *see* Sclerosis, brain
  cerebrospinal 340
    disseminated 340
    multiple 340
  cerebrovascular 437.0
  choroid 363.40
    diffuse 363.56
  combined (spinal cord) – *see also* Degeneration, combined
    multiple 340
  concentric, Balo's 341.1
  cornea 370.54
  coronary (artery) – *see* Arteriosclerosis, coronary
  corpus cavernosum
    female 624.8
    male 607.89

Sclerosis, sclerotic – *continued*
  Dewitzky's
    aortic 424.1
    mitral 424.0
  diffuse NEC 341.1
  disease, heart – *see* Arteriosclerosis, coronary
  disseminated 340
  dorsal 340
  dorsolateral (spinal cord) – *see* Degeneration, combined
  endometrium 621.8
  extrapyramidal 333.90
  eye, nuclear (senile) 366.16
  Friedreich's (spinal cord) 334.0
  funicular (spermatic cord) 608.89
  gastritis 535.4❺
  general (vascular) – *see* Arteriosclerosis
  gland (lymphatic) 457.8
  hepatic 571.9
  hereditary
    cerebellar 334.2
    spinal 334.0
  idiopathic cortical (Garre's) (*see also* Osteomyelitis) 730.1❺
  ilium, piriform 733.5
  insular 340
    pancreas 251.8
  islands of Langerhans 251.8
  kidney – *see* Sclerosis, renal
  larynx 478.79
  lateral 335.24
    amyotrophic 335.20
    descending 335.24
    primary 335.24
    spinal 335.24
  liver 571.9
  lobar, atrophic (of brain) 331.0
    with dementia
      with behavioral disturbance 331.0 *[294.11]*
      without behavioral disturbance 331.0 *[294.10]*
  lung (*see also* Fibrosis, lung) 515
  mastoid 383.1
  mitral – *see* Endocarditis, mitral
  Mönckeberg's (medial) (*see also* Arteriosclerosis, extremities) 440.20
  multiple (brain stem) (cerebral) (generalized) (spinal cord) 340
  myocardium, myocardial – *see* Arteriosclerosis, coronary
  nuclear (senile), eye 366.16
  ovary 620.8
  pancreas 577.8
  penis 607.89
  peripheral arteries (*see also* Arteriosclerosis, extremities) 440.20
  plaques 340
  pluriglandular 258.8
  polyglandular 258.8
  posterior (spinal cord) (syphilitic) 094.0
  posterolateral (spinal cord) – *see* Degeneration, combined
  prepuce 607.89
  primary lateral 335.24
  progressive systemic 710.1
  pulmonary (*see also* Fibrosis, lung) 515
    artery 416.0
    valve (heart) (*see also* Endocarditis, pulmonary) 424.3
  renal 587
    with
      cystine storage disease 270.0
      hypertension (*see also* Hypertension, kidney) 403.90
      hypertensive heart disease (conditions classifiable to 402) (*see also* Hypertension, cardiorenal) 404.90
    arteriolar (hyaline) (*see also* Hypertension, kidney) 403.90
    hyperplastic (*see also* Hypertension, kidney) 403.90
  retina (senile) (vascular) 362.17
  rheumatic
    aortic valve 395.9
    mitral valve 394.9
  Schilder's 341.1
  senile – *see* Arteriosclerosis
  spinal (cord) (general) (progressive) (transverse) 336.8
    ascending 357.0
    combined – *see also* Degeneration, combined
      multiple 340

Sclerosis, sclerotic – *continued*
  spinal – *continued*
    combined – *continued*
      syphilitic 094.89
    disseminated 340
    dorsolateral – *see* Degeneration, combined
    hereditary (Friedreich's) (mixed form) 334.0
    lateral (amyotrophic) 335.24
    multiple 340
    posterior (syphilitic) 094.0
  stomach 537.89
  subendocardial, congenital 425.3
  systemic (progressive) 710.1
    with lung involvement 710.1 *[517.2]*
  tricuspid (heart) (valve) – *see* Endocarditis, tricuspid
  tuberous (brain) 759.5
  tympanic membrane (*see also* Tympanosclerosis) 385.00
  valve, valvular (heart) – *see* Endocarditis
  vascular – *see* Arteriosclerosis
  vein 459.89
Sclerotenonitis 379.07
Sclerotitis (*see also* Scleritis) 379.00
  syphilitic 095.0
  tuberculous (*see also* Tuberculosis) 017.3❺ *[379.09]*
Scoliosis (acquired) (postural) 737.30
  congenital 754.2
  due to or associated with
    Charcôt-Marie-Tooth disease 356.1 *[737.43]*
    mucopolysaccharidosis 277.5 *[737.43]*
    neurofibromatosis 237.71 *[737.43]*
    osteitis
      deformans 731.0 *[737.43]*
      fibrosa cystica 252.01 *[737.43]*
    osteoporosis (*see also* Osteoporosis) 733.00 *[737.43]*
    poliomyelitis 138 *[737.43]*
    radiation 737.33
    tuberculosis (*see also* Tuberculosis) 015.0❺ *[737.43]*
  idiopathic 737.30
    infantile
      progressive 737.32
      resolving 737.31
  paralytic 737.39
  rachitic 268.1
  sciatic 724.3
  specified NEC 737.39
  thoracogenic 737.34
  tuberculous (*see also* Tuberculosis) 015.0❺ *[737.43]*
Scoliotic pelvis 738.6
  with disproportion (fetopelvic) 653.0❺
    affecting fetus or newborn 763.1
    causing obstructed labor 660.1❺
      affecting fetus or newborn 763.1
Scorbutus, scorbutic 267
  anemia 281.8
Scotoma (ring) 368.44
  arcuate 368.43
  Bjerrum 368.43
  blind spot area 368.42
  central 368.41
  centrocecal 368.41
  paracecal 368.42
  paracentral 368.41
  scintillating 368.12
  Seidel 368.43
Scratch – *see* Injury, superficial, by site
Scratchy throat 784.99 ●
Screening (for) V82.9
  alcoholism V79.1
  anemia, deficiency NEC V78.1
    iron V78.0
  anomaly, congenital V82.89
  antenatal , of mother V28.9
    alphafetoprotein levels, raised V28.1
    based on amniocentesis V28.2
      chromosomal anomalies V28.0
      raised alphafetoprotein levels V28.1
    fetal growth retardation using ultrasonics V28.4
    isoimmunization V28.5
    malformations using ultrasonics V28.3
    raised alphafetoprotein levels V28.1
    specified condition NEC V28.8
    Streptococcus B V28.6
  arterial hypertension V81.1
  arthropod-borne viral disease NEC V73.5

Screening (for) – *continued*
- asymptomatic bacteriuria V81.5
- bacterial
  - and spirochetal sexually transmitted diseases V74.5 ●
  - conjunctivitis V74.4
  - disease V74.9
    - sexually transmitted V74.5 ●
    - specified condition NEC V74.8
- bacteriuria, asymptomatic V81.5
- blood disorder NEC V78.9
  - specified type NEC V78.8
- bronchitis, chronic V81.3
- brucellosis V74.8
- cancer – *see* Screening, malignant neoplasm
- cardiovascular disease NEC V81.2
- cataract V80.2
- Chagas' disease V75.3
- chemical poisoning V82.5
- cholera V74.0
- cholesterol level V77.91
- chromosomal
  - anomalies
    - by amniocentesis, antenatal V28.0
    - maternal postnatal V82.4
  - athletes V70.3
- condition
  - cardiovascular NEC V81.2
  - eye NEC V80.2
  - genitourinary NEC V81.6
  - neurological V80.0
  - respiratory NEC V81.4
  - skin V82.0
  - specified NEC V82.89
- congenital
  - anomaly V82.89
    - eye V80.2
  - dislocation of hip V82.3
  - eye condition or disease V80.2
- conjunctivitis, bacterial V74.4
- contamination NEC (*see also* Poisoning) V82.5
- coronary artery disease V81.0
- cystic fibrosis V77.6
- deficiency anemia NEC V78.1
  - iron V78.0
- dengue fever V73.5
- depression V79.0
- developmental handicap V79.9
  - in early childhood V79.3
  - specified type NEC V79.8
- diabetes mellitus V77.1
- diphtheria V74.3
- disease or disorder V82.9
  - bacterial V74.9
    - specified NEC V74.8
  - blood V78.9
    - specified type NEC V78.8
  - blood-forming organ V78.9
    - specified type NEC V78.8 ❺
  - cardiovascular NEC V81.2
    - hypertensive V81.1
    - ischemic V81.0
  - Chagas' V75.3
  - chlamydial V73.98
    - specified NEC V73.88
  - ear NEC V80.3
  - endocrine NEC V77.99
  - eye NEC V80.2
  - genitourinary NEC V81.6
  - heart NEC V81.2
    - hypertensive V81.1
    - ischemic V81.0
  - HPV (human papillomavirus) V73.81 ●
  - human papillomavirus (HPV) V73.81 ●
  - immunity NEC V77.99
  - infectious NEC V75.9
  - lipoid NEC V77.91
  - mental V79.9
    - specified type NEC V79.8
  - metabolic NEC V77.99
    - inborn NEC V77.7
  - neurological V80.0
  - nutritional NEC V77.99
  - rheumatic NEC V82.2
  - rickettsial V75.0
  - sexually transmitted V74.5 ●
    - bacterial V74.5 ●
    - spirochetal V74.5 ●
  - sickle-cell V78.2
    - trait V78.2
  - specified type NEC V82.89
  - thyroid V77.0

Screening (for) – *continued*
- disease or disorder – *continued*
  - vascular NEC V81.2
    - ischemic V81.0
  - venereal V74.5
  - viral V73.99
    - arthropod-borne NEC V73.5
    - specified type NEC V73.89
- dislocation of hip, congenital V82.3
- drugs in athletes V70.3
- emphysema (chronic) V81.3
- encephalitis, viral (mosquito or tick borne) V73.5
- endocrine disorder NEC V77.99
- eye disorder NEC V80.2
  - congenital V80.2
- fever
  - dengue V73.5
  - hemorrhagic V73.5
  - yellow V73.4
- filariasis V75.6
- galactosemia V77.4
- genetic V82.79
  - disease carrier status V82.71
- genitourinary condition NEC V81.6
- glaucoma V80.1
- gonorrhea V74.5
- gout V77.5
- Hansen's disease V74.2
- heart disease NEC V81.2
  - hypertensive V81.1
  - ischemic V81.0
- heavy metal poisoning V82.5
- helminthiasis, intestinal V75.7
- hematopoietic malignancy V76.89
- hemoglobinopathies NEC V78.3
- hemorrhagic fever V73.5
- Hodgkin's disease V76.89
- hormones in athletes V70.3
- HPV (human papillomavirus) V73.81 ●
- human papillomavirus (HPV) V73.81 ●
- hypercholesterolemia V77.91
- hyperlipdemia V77.91
- hypertension V81.1
- immunity disorder NEC V77.99
- inborn errors of metabolism NEC V77.7
- infection
  - bacterial V74.9
    - specified type NEC V74.8
  - mycotic V75.4
  - parasitic NEC V75.8
- infectious disease V75.9
  - specified type NEC V75.8
- ingestion of radioactive substance V82.5
- intestinal helminthiasis V75.7
- iron deficiency anemia V78.0
- ischemic heart disease V81.0
- lead poisoning V82.5
- leishmaniasis V75.2
- leprosy V74.2
- leptospirosis V74.8
- leukemia V76.89
- lipoid disorder NEC V77.91
- lymphoma V76.89
- malaria V75.1
- malignant neoplasm (of) V76.9
  - bladder V76.3
  - blood V76.89
  - breast V76.10
    - mammogram NEC V76.12
      - for high-risk patient V76.11
    - specified type NEC V76.19
  - cervix V76.2
  - colon V76.51
  - colorectal V76.51
  - hematopoietic system V76.89
  - intestine V76.50
    - colon V76.51
    - small V76.52
  - lung V76.0
  - lymph (glands) V76.89
  - nervous system V76.81
  - oral cavity V76.42
  - other specified neoplasm NEC V76.89
  - ovary V76.46
  - prostate V76.44
  - rectum V76.41
  - respiratory organs V76.0
  - skin V76.43
  - specified sites NEC V76.49
  - testis V76.45

Screening (for) – *continued*
- malignant neoplasm (of) – *continued*
  - vagina V76.47
    - following hysterectomy for malignant condition V67.01
- malnutrition V77.2
- mammogram NEC V76.12
  - for high-risk patient V76.11
- maternal postnatal chromosomal anomalies V82.4
- measles V73.2
- mental
  - disorder V79.9
    - specified type NEC V79.8
  - retardation V79.2
- metabolic disorder NEC V77.99
- metabolic errors, inborn V77.7
- mucoviscidosis V77.6
- multiphasic V82.6
- mycosis V75.4
- mycotic infection V75.4
- nephropathy V81.5
- neurological condition V80.0
- nutritional disorder NEC V77.99
- obesity V77.8
- osteoporosis V82.81
- parasitic infection NEC V75.8
- phenylketonuria V77.3
- plague V74.8
- poisoning
  - chemical NEC V82.5
  - contaminated water supply V82.5
  - heavy metal V82.5
- poliomyelitis V73.0
- postnatal chromosomal anomalies, maternal V82.4
- prenatal – *see* Screening, antenatal
- pulmonary tuberculosis V74.1
- radiation exposure V82.5
- renal disease V81.5
- respiratory condition NEC V81.4
- rheumatic disorder NEC V82.2
- rheumatoid arthritis V82.1
- rickettsial disease V75.0
- rubella V73.3
- schistosomiasis V75.5
- senile macular lesions of eye V80.2
- sexually transmitted diseases V74.5 ●
  - bacterial V74.5 ●
  - spirochetal V74.5 ●
- sickle-cell anemia, disease, or trait V78.2
- skin condition V82.0
- sleeping sickness V75.3
- smallpox V73.1
- special V82.9
  - specified condition NEC V82.89
- specified type NEC V82.89
- spirochetal disease V74.9
  - sexually transmitted V74.5 ●
  - specified type NEC V74.8
- stimulants in athletes V70.3
- syphilis V74.5
- tetanus V74.8
- thyroid disorder V77.0
- trachoma V73.6
- trypanosomiasis V75.3
- tuberculosis, pulmonary V74.1
- venereal disease V74.5
- viral encephalitis
  - mosquito-borne V73.5
  - tick-borne V73.5
- whooping cough V74.8
- worms, intestinal V75.7
- yaws V74.6
- yellow fever V73.4

Scrofula (*see also* Tuberculosis) 017.2❺

Scrofulide (primary) (*see also* Tuberculosis) 017.0❺

Scrofuloderma, scrofulodermia (any site) (primary) (*see also* Tuberculosis) 017.0❺

Scrofulosis (universal) (*see also* Tuberculosis) 017.2❺

Scrofulosis lichen (primary) (*see also* Tuberculosis) 017.0❺

Scrofulous – *see* condition

Scrotal tongue 529.5
- congenital 750.13

Scrotum – *see* condition

Scurvy (gum) (infantile) (rickets) (scorbutic) 267

Sea-blue histiocyte syndrome 272.7

Seabright-Bantam syndrome
    (pseudohypoparathyroidism) 275.49
Seasickness 994.6
Seatworm 127.4
Sebaceous
  cyst (*see also* Cyst, sebaceous) 706.2
  gland disease NEC 706.9
Sebocystomatosis 706.2
Seborrhea, seborrheic 706.3
  adiposa 706.3
  capitis 690.11
  congestiva 695.4
  corporis 706.3
  dermatitis 690.10
    infantile 690.1❺
  diathesis in infants 695.89
  eczema 690.18
    infantile 690.12
  keratosis 702.19
    inflamed 702.11
  nigricans 759.89
  sicca 690.18
  wart 702.19
    inflamed 702.11
Seckel's syndrome 759.89
Seclusion pupil 364.74
Seclusiveness, child 313.22
Secondary – *see also* condition
  neoplasm – *see* Neoplasm, by site, malignant,
      secondary
Secretan's disease or syndrome (posttraumatic
    edema) 782.3
Secretion
  antidiuretic hormone, inappropriate (syndrome)
      253.6
  catecholamine, by pheochromocytoma 255.6
  hormone
    antidiuretic, inappropriate (syndrome) 253.6
    by
      carcinoid tumor 259.2
      pheochromocytoma 255.6
    ectopic NEC 259.3
  urinary
    excessive 788.42
    suppression 788.5
Section
  cesarean
    affecting fetus or newborn 763.4
    post mortem, affecting fetus or newborn 761.6
    previous, in pregnancy or childbirth 654.2❺
      affecting fetus or newborn 763.89
  nerve, traumatic – *see* Injury, nerve, by site
Seeligmann's syndrome (ichthyosis congenita) 757.1
Segmentation, incomplete (congenital) – *see also*
    Fusion
  bone NEC 756.9
  lumbosacral (joint) 756.15
  vertebra 756.15
    lumbosacral 756.15
▶**Seizure(s)**◀ 780.39
  akinetic (idiopathic) (*see also* Epilepsy) 345.0❺
    psychomotor 345.4❺
  apoplexy, apoplectic (*see also* Disease,
      cerebrovascular, acute) 436
  atonic (*see also* Epilepsy) 345.0❺
  autonomic 300.11
  brain or cerebral (*see also* Disease,
      cerebrovascular, acute) 436
  convulsive (*see also* Convulsions) 780.39
  cortical (focal) (motor) (*see also* Epilepsy)
      345.5❺
  due to stroke 438.89 ●
  epilepsy, epileptic (cryptogenic) (*see also*
      Epilepsy) 345.9❺
  epileptiform, epileptoid 780.39
    focal (*see also* Epilepsy) 345.5❺
  febrile (simple) 780.31
    with status epilepticus 345.3
    atypical 780.32
    complex 780.32
    complicated 780.32
  heart – *see* Disease, heart
  hysterical 300.11
  Jacksonian (focal) (*see also* Epilepsy) 345.5❺
    motor type 345.5❺
    sensory type 345.5❺
  newborn 779.0
  paralysis (*see also* Disease, cerebrovascular,
      acute) 436

Seizure(s) – *continued*
  recurrent 345.9
    epileptic – *see* Epilepsy
  repetitive 780.39
    epileptic – *see* Epilepsy
  salaam (*see also* Epilepsy) 345.6❺
  uncinate (*see also* Epilepsy) 345.4❺
Self-mutilation 300.9
Semicoma 780.09
Semiconsciousness 780.09
Seminal
  vesicle – *see* condition
  vesiculitis (*see also* Vesiculitis) 608.0
Seminoma (M9061/3)
  anaplastic type (M9062/3)
    specified site – *see* Neoplasm, by site,
        malignant
    unspecified site 186.9
  specified site – *see* Neoplasm, by site, malignant
  spermatocytic (M9063/3)
    specified site – *see* Neoplasm, by site,
        malignant
    unspecified site 186.9
  unspecified site 186.9
Semliki Forest encephalitis 062.8
Senear-Usher disease or syndrome (pemphigus
    erythematosus) 694.4
Senecio jacobae dermatitis 692.6
Senectus 797
Senescence 797
Senile (*see also* condition) 797
  cervix (atrophic) 622.8
  degenerative atrophy, skin 701.3
  endometrium (atrophic) 621.8
  fallopian tube (atrophic) 620.3
  heart (failure) 797
  lung 492.8
  ovary (atrophic) 620.3
  syndrome 259.8
  vagina, vaginitis (atrophic) 627.3
  wart 702.0
Senility 797
  with
    acute confusional state 290.3
    delirium 290.3
    mental changes 290.9
    psychosis NEC (*see also* Psychosis, senile)
        290.20
  premature (syndrome) 259.8
Sensation
  burning (*see also* Disturbance, sensation) 782.0
    tongue 529.6
  choking 784.99
  loss of (*see also* Disturbance, sensation) 782.0
  prickling (*see also* Disturbance, sensation) 782.0
  tingling (*see also* Disturbance, sensation) 782.0
Sense loss (touch) (*see also* Disturbance, sensation)
    782.0
  smell 781.1
  taste 781.1
Sensibility disturbance NEC (cortical) (deep)
    (vibratory) (*see also* Disturbance, sensation)
    782.0
Sensitive dentine 521.89
Sensitiver Beziehungswahn 297.8
Sensitivity, sensitization – *see also* Allergy
  autoerythrocyte 287.2
  carotid sinus 337.0
  child (excessive) 313.21
  cold, autoimmune 283.0
  methemoglobin 289.7
  suxamethonium 289.89
  tuberculin, without clinical or radiological
      symptoms 795.5
Sensory
  extinction 781.8
  neglect 781.8
Separation
  acromioclavicular – *see* Dislocation,
      acromioclavicular
  anxiety, abnormal 309.21
  apophysis, traumatic – *see* Fracture, by site
  choroid 363.70
    hemorrhagic 363.72
    serous 363.71
  costochondral (simple) (traumatic) – *see*
      Dislocation, costochondral

Separation – *continued*
  delayed
    umbilical cord 779.83
  epiphysis, epiphyseal
    nontraumatic 732.9
      upper femoral 732.2
    traumatic – *see* Fracture, by site
  fracture – *see* Fracture, by site
  infundibulum cardiac from right ventricle by a
      partition 746.83
  joint (current) (traumatic) – *see* Dislocation, by site
  placenta (normally implanted) – *see* Placenta,
      separation
  pubic bone, obstetrical trauma 665.6❺
  retina, retinal (*see also* Detachment, retina)
      361.9
    layers 362.40
      sensory (*see also* Retinoschisis) 361.10
    pigment epithelium (exudative) 362.42
      hemorrhagic 362.43
  sternoclavicular (traumatic) – *see* Dislocation,
      sternoclavicular
  symphysis pubis, obstetrical trauma 665.6❺
  tracheal ring, incomplete (congenital) 748.3
Sepsis (generalized) 995.91
  with
    abortion – *see* Abortion, by type, with sepsis
    acute organ dysfunction 995.92
    ectopic pregnancy (*see also* categories 633.0-
        633.9) 639.0
    molar pregnancy (*see also* categories 630-632)
        639.0
    multiple organ dysfunction (MOD) 995.92
  buccal 528.3
  complicating labor 659.3❺
  dental (pulpal origin) 522.4
  female genital organ NEC 614.9
  fetus (intrauterine) 771.81
  following
    abortion 639.0
    ectopic or molar pregnancy 639.0
    infusion, perfusion, or transfusion 999.39 ▲
  Friedländer's 038.49
  intraocular 360.00
  localized
    in operation wound 998.59
    skin (*see also* Abscess) 682.9
  malleus 024
  nadir 038.9
  newborn (organism unspecified) NEC 771.81
  oral 528.3
  puerperal, postpartum, childbirth (pelvic) 670❹
  resulting from infusion, injection, transfusion, or
      vaccination 999.39 ▲
  severe 995.92
  skin, localized (*see also* Abscess) 682.9
  umbilical (newborn) (organism unspecified)
      771.89
    tetanus 771.3
  urinary 599.0
    meaning sepsis 995.91
    meaning urinary tract infection 599.0
Septate – *see also* Septum
Septic – *see also* condition
  adenoids 474.01
    and tonsils 474.02
  arm (with lymphangitis) 682.3
  embolus – *see* Embolism
  finger (with lymphangitis) 681.00
  foot (with lymphangitis) 682.7
  gallbladder (*see also* Cholecystitis) 575.8
  hand (with lymphangitis) 682.4
  joint (*see also* Arthritis, septic) 711.0❺
  kidney (*see also* Infection, kidney) 590.9
  leg (with lymphangitis) 682.6
  mouth 528.3
  nail 681.9
    finger 681.02
    toe 681.11
  shock (endotoxic) 785.52
  sore (*see also* Abscess) 682.9
    throat 034.0
      milk-borne 034.0
      streptococcal 034.0
  spleen (acute) 289.59
  teeth (pulpal origin) 522.4
  throat 034.0
  thrombus – *see* Thrombosis
  toe (with lymphangitis) 681.1❺
  tonsils 474.00
    and adenoids 474.02

Septic – *continued*
- umbilical cord (newborn) (organism unspecified) 771.89
- uterus (*see also* Endometritis) 615.9

Septicemia, septicemic (generalized) (suppurative) 038.9
- with
  - abortion – *see* Abortion, by type, with sepsis
  - ectopic pregnancy (*see also* categories 633.0-633.9) 639.0
  - molar pregnancy (*see also* categories 630-632) 639.0
- Aerobacter aerogenes 038.49
- anaerobic 038.3
- anthrax 022.3
- Bacillus coli 038.42
- Bacteroides 038.3
- Clostridium 038.3
- complicating labor 659.3❺
- cryptogenic 038.9
- enteric gram-negative bacilli 038.40
- Enterobacter aerogenes 038.49
- Erysipelothrix (insidiosa) (rhusiopathiae) 027.1
- Escherichia coli 038.42
- following
  - abortion 639.0
  - ectopic or molar pregnancy 639.0
  - infusion, injection, transfusion, or vaccination 999.39 ▲
- Friedländer's (bacillus) 038.49
- gangrenous 038.9
- gonococcal 098.89
- gram-negative (organism) 038.40
  - anaerobic 038.3
- Hemophilus influenzae 038.41
- herpes (simplex) 054.5
- herpetic 054.5
- Listeria monocytogenes 027.0
- meningeal – *see* Meningitis
- meningococcal (chronic) (fulminating) 036.2
- navel, newborn (organism unspecified) 771.89
- newborn (organism unspecified) 771.81
- plague 020.2
- pneumococcal 038.2
- postabortal 639.0
- postoperative 998.59
- Proteus vulgaris 038.49
- Pseudomonas (aeruginosa) 038.43
- puerperal, postpartum 670❹
- Salmonella (aertrycke) (callinarum) (choleraesuis) (enteritidis) (suipestifer) 003.1
- Serratia 038.44
- Shigella (*see also* Dysentery, bacillary) 004.9
- specified organism NEC 038.8
- staphylococcal 038.10
  - aureus 038.11
  - specified organism NEC 038.19
- streptococcal (anaerobic) 038.0
- Streptococcus pneumoniae 038.2
- suipestifer 003.1
- umbilicus, newborn (organism unspecified) 771.89
- viral 079.99
- Yersinia enterocolitica 038.49

Septum, septate (congenital) – *see also* Anomaly, specified type NEC
- anal 751.2
- aqueduct of Sylvius 742.3
  - with spina bifida (*see also* Spina bifida) 741.0❺
- hymen 752.49
- uterus (*see also* Double, uterus) 752.2
- vagina 752.49
  - in pregnancy or childbirth 654.7❺
    - affecting fetus or newborn 763.89
    - causing obstructed labor 660.2❺
      - affecting fetus or newborn 763.1

Sequestration
- lung (congenital) (extralobar) (intralobar) 748.5
- orbit 376.10
- pulmonary artery (congenital) 747.3
- splenic 289.52

Sequestrum
- bone (*see also* Osteomyelitis) 730.1❺
  - jaw 526.4
- dental 525.8
- jaw bone 526.4
- sinus (accessory) (nasal) (*see also* Sinusitis) 473.9
  - maxillary 473.0

Sequoiosis asthma 495.8

Serology for syphilis
- doubtful
  - with signs or symptoms – *see* Syphilis, by site and stage
  - follow-up of latent syphilis – *see* Syphilis, latent
- false positive 795.6
- negative, with signs or symptoms – *see* Syphilis, by site and stage
- positive 097.1
  - with signs or symptoms – *see* Syphilis, by site and stage
  - false 795.6
  - follow-up of latent syphilis – *see* Syphilis, latent
  - only finding – *see* Syphilis, latent
- reactivated 097.1

Seroma - (postoperative) (non-infected) 998.13
- infected 998.51

Seropurulent – *see* condition

Serositis, multiple 569.89
- pericardial 423.2
- peritoneal 568.82
- pleural – *see* Pleurisy

Serotonin syndrome 333.99

Serous – *see* condition

Sertoli cell
- adenoma (M8640/0)
  - specified site – *see* Neoplasm, by site, benign
  - unspecified site
    - female 220
    - male 222.0
- carcinoma (M8640/3)
  - specified site – *see* Neoplasm, by site, malignant
  - unspecified site 186.9
- syndrome (germinal aplasia) 606.0
- tumor (M8640/0)
  - with lipid storage (M8641/0)
    - specified site – *see* Neoplasm, by site, benign
    - unspecified site
      - female 220
      - male 222.0
  - specified site – *see* Neoplasm, by site, benign
  - unspecified site
    - female 220
    - male 222.0

Sertoli-Leydig cell tumor (M8631/0)
- specified site – *see* Neoplasm, by site, benign
- unspecified site
  - female 220
  - male 222.0

Serum
- allergy, allergic reaction 999.5
  - shock 999.4
- arthritis 999.5 *[713.6]*
- complication or reaction NEC 999.5
- disease NEC 999.5
- hepatitis 070.3❺
- intoxication 999.5
- jaundice (homologous) – *see* Hepatitis, viral, type B
- neuritis 999.5
- poisoning NEC 999.5
- rash NEC 999.5
- reaction NEC 999.5
- sickness NEC 999.5

Sesamoiditis 733.99

Seven-day fever 061
- of
  - Japan 100.89
  - Queensland 100.89

Sever's disease or osteochondrosis (calcaneum) 732.5

Sex chromosome mosaics 758.81

Sex reassignment surgery status (*see also* Trans-sexualism) 302.50 ●

Sextuplet
- affected by maternal complication of pregnancy 761.5
- healthy liveborn – *see* Newborn, multiple
- pregnancy (complicating delivery) NEC 651.8❺
  - with fetal loss and retention of one or more fetus(es) 651.6❺
  - following (elective) fetal reduction 651.7

Sexual
- anesthesia 302.72
- deviation (*see also* Deviation, sexual) 302.9
- disorder (*see also* Deviation, sexual) 302.9
- frigidity (female) 302.72

Sexual – *continued*
- function, disorder of (psychogenic) 302.70
  - specified type NEC 302.79
- immaturity (female) (male) 259.0
- impotence 607.84
  - organic origin NEC 607.84
  - psychogenic 302.72
- precocity (constitutional) (cryptogenic) (female) (idiopathic) (male) NEC 259.1
  - with adrenal hyperplasia 255.2
- sadism 302.84

Sexuality, pathological (*see also* Deviation, sexual) 302.9

Sézary's disease, reticulosis, or syndrome (M9701/3) 202.2❺

Shadow, lung 793.1

Shaken infant syndrome 995.55

Shaking
- head (tremor) 781.0
- palsy or paralysis (*see also* Parkinsonism) 332.0

Shallowness, acetabulum 736.39

Shaver's disease or syndrome (bauxite pneumoconiosis) 503

Shearing
- artificial skin graft 996.55
- decellularized allodermis graft 996.55

Sheath (tendon) – *see* condition

Shedding
- nail 703.8
- teeth, premature, primary (deciduous) 520.6

Sheehan's disease or syndrome (postpartum pituitary necrosis) 253.2

Shelf, rectal 569.49

Shell
- shock (current) (*see also* Reaction, stress, acute) 308.9
  - lasting state 300.16
- teeth 520.5

Shield kidney 753.3

Shift, mediastinal 793.2

Shifting
- pacemaker 427.89
- sleep work schedule (affecting sleep) 327.36

Shiga's
- bacillus 004.0
- dysentery 004.0

Shigella (dysentery) (*see also* Dysentery, bacillary) 004.9
- carrier (suspected) of V02.3

Shigellosis (*see also* Dysentery, bacillary) 004.9

Shingles (*see also* Herpes, zoster) 053.9
- eye NEC 053.29

Shin splints 844.9

Shipyard eye or disease 077.1

Shirodkar suture, in pregnancy 654.5❺

Shock 785.50
- with
  - abortion – *see* Abortion, by type, with shock
  - ectopic pregnancy (*see also* categories 633.0-633.9) 639.5
  - molar pregnancy (*see also* categories 630-632) 639.5
- allergic – *see* Shock, anaphylactic
- anaclitic 309.21
- anaphylactic 995.0
  - chemical – *see* Table of Drugs and Chemicals
  - correct medicinal substance properly administered 995.0
  - drug or medicinal substance
    - correct substance properly administered 995.0
    - overdose or wrong substance given or taken 977.9
      - specified drug – *see* Table of Drugs and Chemicals
  - following sting(s) 989.5
  - food – *see* Anaphylactic shock, due to, food
  - immunization 999.4
  - serum 999.4
- anaphylactoid – *see* Shock, anaphylactic
- anesthetic
  - correct substance properly administered 995.4
  - overdose or wrong substance given 968.4
    - specified anesthetic – *see* Table of Drugs and Chemicals
- birth, fetus or newborn NEC 779.89
- cardiogenic 785.51

Shock – Siegal-Cattan-Mamou disease

- **Siemens' syndrome**
  - ectodermal dysplasia 757.31
  - keratosis follicularis spinulosa (decalvans) 757.39
- **Sighing respiration** 786.7
- **Sigmoid**
  - flexure – *see* condition
  - kidney 753.3
- **Sigmoiditis** – *see* Enteritis
- **Silfverskiöld's syndrome** 756.5❺
- **Silicosis, silicotic** (complicated) (occupational) (simple) 502
  - fibrosis, lung (confluent) (massive) (occupational) 502
  - non-nodular 503
  - pulmonum 502
- **Silicotuberculosis** (*see also* Tuberculosis) 011.4❺
- **Silo fillers' disease** 506.9
- **Silver's syndrome** (congenital hemihypertrophy and short stature) 759.89
- **Silver wire arteries, retina** 362.13
- **Silvestroni-Bianco syndrome** (thalassemia minima) 282.49
- **Simian crease** 757.2
- **Simmonds' cachexia or disease** (pituitary cachexia) 253.2
- **Simons' disease or syndrome** (progressive lipodystrophy) 272.6
- **Simple, simplex** – *see* condition
- **Sinding-Larsen disease** (juvenile osteopathia patellae) 732.4
- **Singapore hemorrhagic fever** 065.4
- **Singers' node or nodule** 478.5
- **Single**
  - atrium 745.69
  - coronary artery 746.85
  - umbilical artery 747.5
  - ventricle 745.3
- **Singultus** 786.8
  - epidemicus 078.89
- **Sinus** – *see also* Fistula
  - abdominal 569.81
  - arrest 426.6
  - arrhythmia 427.89
  - bradycardia 427.89
    - chronic 427.81
  - branchial cleft (external) (internal) 744.41
  - coccygeal (infected) 685.1
    - with abscess 685.0
  - dental 522.7
  - dermal (congenital) 685.1
    - with abscess 685.0
  - draining – *see* Fistula
  - infected, skin NEC 686.9
  - marginal, rupture or bleeding 641.2❺
    - affecting fetus or newborn 762.1
  - pause 426.6
  - pericranii 742.0
  - pilonidal (infected) (rectum) 685.1
    - with abscess 685.0
  - preauricular 744.46
  - rectovaginal 619.1
  - sacrococcygeal (dermoid) (infected) 685.1
    - with abscess 685.0
  - skin
    - infected NEC 686.9
    - noninfected- *see* Ulcer, skin
  - tachycardia 427.89
  - tarsi syndrome 726.79
  - testis 608.89
  - tract (postinfectional) – *see* Fistula
  - urachus 753.7
- **Sinuses, Rokitansky-Aschoff** (*see also* Disease, gallbladder) 575.8
- **Sinusitis** (accessory) (nasal) (hyperplastic) (nonpurulent) (purulent) (chronic) 473.9
  - with influenza, flu, or grippe 487.1
  - acute 461.9
    - ethmoidal 461.2
    - frontal 461.1
    - maxillary 461.0
    - specified type NEC 461.8
    - sphenoidal 461.3
  - allergic (*see also* Fever, hay) 477.9
  - antrum – *see* Sinusitis, maxillary
  - due to
    - fungus, any sinus 117.9
    - high altitude 993.1

- **Sinusitis** – *continued*
  - ethmoidal 473.2
    - acute 461.2
  - frontal 473.1
    - acute 461.1
  - influenzal 478.19
  - maxillary 473.0
    - acute 461.0
  - specified site NEC 473.8
  - sphenoidal 473.3
    - acute 461.3
  - syphilitic, any sinus 095.8
  - tuberculous, any sinus (*see also* Tuberculosis) 012.8❺
- **Sinusitis-bronchiectasis-situs inversus** (syndrome) (triad) 759.3
- **Sipple's syndrome** (medullary thyroid carcinoma-pheochromocytoma) 258.02 ▲
- **Sirenomelia** 759.89
- **Siriasis** 992.0
- **Sirkari's disease** 085.0
- **SIRS** (systemic inflammatory response syndrome) 995.90
  - due to
    - infectious process 995.91
      - with acute organ dysfunction 995.92
    - non-infectious process 995.93
      - with acute organ dysfunction 995.94
- **Siti** 104.0
- **Sitophobia** 300.29
- **Situation, psychiatric** 300.9
- **Situational**
  - disturbance (transient) (*see also* Reaction, adjustment) 309.9
    - acute 308.3
  - maladjustment, acute (*see also* Reaction, adjustment) 309.9
  - reaction (*see also* Reaction, adjustment) 309.9
    - acute 308.3
- **Situs inversus or transversus** 759.3
  - abdominalis 759.3
  - thoracis 759.3
- **Sixth disease**
  - due to ●
    - human herpesvirus 6 058.11 ●
    - human herpesvirus 7 058.12 ●
- **Sjögren** (-Gougerot) **syndrome or disease** (keratoconjunctivitis sicca) 710.2
  - with lung involvement 710.2 *[517.8]*
- **Sjögren-Larsson syndrome** (ichthyosis congenita) 757.1
- **Skeletal** – *see* condition
- **Skene's gland** – *see* condition
- **Skenitis** (*see also* Urethritis) 597.89
  - gonorrheal (acute) 098.0
    - chronic or duration of 2 months or over 098.2
- **Skerljevo** 104.0
- **Skevas-Zerfus disease** 989.5
- **Skin** – *see also* condition
  - donor V59.1
  - hidebound 710.9
- **SLAP lesion** (superior glenoid labrum) 840.7
- **Slate-dressers' lung** 502
- **Slate-miners' lung** 502
- **Sleep**
  - deprivation V69.4
  - disorder 780.50
    - with apnea – *see* Apnea, sleep
    - child 307.40
    - movement, unspecified 780.58
    - nonorganic origin 307.40
      - specified type NEC 307.49
  - disturbance 780.50
    - with apnea – *see* Apnea, sleep
    - nonorganic origin 307.40
      - specified type NEC 307.49
  - drunkenness 307.47
  - movement disorder, unspecified 780.58
  - paroxysmal (*see also* Narcolepsy) 347.00
  - related movement disorder, unspecified 780.58
  - rhythm inversion 327.39
    - nonorganic origin 307.45
  - walking 307.46
    - hysterical 300.13
- **Sleeping sickness** 086.5
  - late effect 139.8

- **Sleeplessness** (*see also* Insomnia) 780.52
  - menopausal 627.2
  - nonorganic origin 307.41
- **Slipped, slipping**
  - epiphysis (postinfectional) 732.9
    - traumatic (old) 732.9
      - current – *see* Fracture, by site
    - upper femoral (nontraumatic) 732.2
  - intervertebral disc – *see* Displacement, intervertebral disc
  - ligature, umbilical 772.3
  - patella 717.89
  - rib 733.99
  - sacroiliac joint 724.6
  - tendon 727.9
  - ulnar nerve, nontraumatic 354.2
  - vertebra NEC (*see also* Spondylolisthesis) 756.12
- **Slocumb's syndrome** 255.3
- **Sloughing** (multiple) (skin) 686.9
  - abscess – *see* Abscess, by site
  - appendix 543.9
  - bladder 596.8
  - fascia 728.9
  - graft – *see* Complications, graft
  - phagedena (*see also* Gangrene) 785.4
  - reattached extremity (*see also* Complications, reattached extremity) 996.90
  - rectum 569.49
  - scrotum 608.89
  - tendon 727.9
  - transplanted organ (*see also* Rejection, transplant, organ, by site) 996.80
  - ulcer (*see also* Ulcer, skin) 707.9
- **Slow**
  - feeding newborn 779.3
  - fetal, growth NEC 764.9❺
    - affecting management of pregnancy 656.5❺
- **Slowing**
  - heart 427.89
  - urinary stream 788.62
- **Sluder's neuralgia or syndrome** 337.0
- **Slurred, slurring, speech** 784.5
- **Small, smallness**
  - cardia reserve – *see* Disease, heart
  - for dates
    - fetus or newborn 764.0❺
      - with malnutrition 764.1❺
      - affecting management of pregnancy 656.5❺
  - infant, term 764.0❺
    - with malnutrition 764.1❺
    - affecting management of pregnancy 656.5❺
  - introitus, vagina 623.3
  - kidney, unknown cause 589.9
    - bilateral 589.1
    - unilateral 589.0
  - ovary 620.8
  - pelvis
    - with disproportion (fetopelvic) 653.1❺
      - affecting fetus or newborn 763.1
    - causing obstructed labor 660.1❺
      - affecting fetus or newborn 763.1
  - placenta – *see* Placenta, insufficiency
  - uterus 621.8
  - white kidney 582.9
- **Small-for-dates** (*see also* Light-for-dates) 764.0❺
  - affecting management of pregnancy 656.5❺
- **Smallpox** 050.9
  - contact V01.3
  - exposure to V01.3
  - hemorrhagic (pustular) 050.0
  - malignant 050.0
  - modified 050.2
  - vaccination
    - complications – *see* Complications, vaccination
    - prophylactic (against) V04.1
- **Smith's fracture** (separation) (closed) 813.41
  - open 813.51
- **Smith-Lemli-Opitz syndrome** (cerebrohepatorenal syndrome) 759.89
- **Smith-Magenis syndrome** 758.33
- **Smith-Strang disease** (oasthouse urine) 270.2
- **Smokers'**
  - bronchitis 491.0
  - cough 491.0
  - syndrome (*see also* Abuse, drugs, nondependent) 305.1
  - throat 472.1
  - tongue 528.6

- **Smoking complicating pregnancy, childbirth, or the puerperium** 649.0❺
- **Smothering spells** 786.09
- **Snaggle teeth, tooth** 524.39
- **Snapping**
  - finger 727.05
  - hip 719.65
  - jaw 524.69
    - temporomandibular joint sounds on opening or closing 524.64
  - knee 717.9
  - thumb 727.05
- **Sneddon-Wilkinson disease or syndrome** (subcorneal pustular dermatosis) 694.1
- **Sneezing** 784.99
  - intractable 478.19
- **Sniffing**
  - cocaine (*see also* Dependence) 304.2❺
  - either (*see also* Dependence) 304.6❺
  - glue (airplane) (*see also* Dependence) 304.6❺
- **Snoring** 786.09
- **Snow blindness** 370.24
- **Snuffles** (nonsyphilitic) 460
  - syphilitic (infant) 090.0
- **Social migrant** V60.0
- **Sodoku** 026.0
- **Soemmering's ring** 366.51
- **Soft** – *see also* condition
  - enlarged prostate 600.00
    - with
      - other lower urinary tract symptoms (LUTS) 600.01
      - urinary
        - obstruction 600.01
        - retention 600.01
  - nails 703.8
- **Softening**
  - bone 268.2
  - brain (necrotic) (progressive) 434.9❺
    - arteriosclerotic 437.0
    - congenital 742.4
    - embolic (*see also* Embolism, brain) 434.1❺
    - hemorrhagic (*see also* Hemorrhage, brain) 431
    - occlusive 434.9❺
    - thrombotic (*see also* Thrombosis, brain) 434.0❺
  - cartilage 733.92
  - cerebellar – *see* Softening, brain
  - cerebral – *see* Softening, brain
  - cerebrospinal – *see* Softening, brain
  - myocardial, heart (*see also* Degeneration, myocardial) 429.1
  - nails 703.8
  - spinal cord 336.8
  - stomach 537.89
- **Solar fever** 061
- **Soldier's**
  - heart 306.2
  - patches 423.1
- **Solitary**
  - cyst
    - bone 733.21
    - kidney 593.2
  - kidney (congenital) 753.0
  - tubercle, brain (*see also* Tuberculosis, brain) 013.2❺
  - ulcer, bladder 596.8
- **Somatization reaction, somatic reaction** (*see also* Disorder, psychosomatic) 306.9
  - disorder 300.81
- **Somatoform disorder** 300.82
  - atypical 300.82
  - severe 300.81
  - undifferentiated 300.82
- **Somnambulism** 307.46
  - hysterical 300.13
- **Somnolence** 780.09
  - nonorganic origin 307.43
  - periodic 349.89
- **Sonne dysentery** 004.3
- **Soor** 112.0
- **Sore**
  - Delhi 085.1
  - desert (*see also* Ulcer, skin) 707.9
  - eye 379.99
  - Lahore 085.1
  - mouth 528.9
    - canker 528.2
    - due to dentures 528.9
  - muscle 729.1
  - Naga (*see also* Ulcer, skin) 707.9
  - oriental 085.1
  - pressure (*see also* Decubitus) 707.00
    - with gangrene (*see also* Decubitus) 707.00 *[785.4]*
  - skin NEC 709.9
  - soft 099.0
  - throat 462
    - with influenza, flu, or grippe 487.1
    - acute 462
    - chronic 472.1
    - clergyman's 784.49
    - Coxsackie (virus) 074.0
    - diphtheritic 032.0
    - epidemic 034.0
    - gangrenous 462
    - herpetic 054.79
    - influenzal 487.1
    - malignant 462
    - purulent 462
    - putrid 462
    - septic 034.0
    - streptococcal (ulcerative) 034.0
    - ulcerated 462
    - viral NEC 462
      - Coxsackie 074.0
  - tropical (*see also* Ulcer, skin) 707.9
  - veldt (*see also* Ulcer, skin) 707.9
- **Sotos' syndrome** (cerebral gigantism) 253.0
- **Sounds**
  - friction, pleural 786.7
  - succussion, chest 786.7
  - temporomandibular joint
    - on opening or closing 524.64
- **South African cardiomyopathy syndrome** 425.2
- **South American**
  - blastomycosis 116.1
  - trypanosomiasis – *see* Trypanosomiasis
- **Southeast Asian hemorrhagic fever** 065.4
- **Spacing, teeth, abnormal** 524.30
  - excessive 524.32
- **Spade-like hand** (congenital) 754.89
- **Spading nail** 703.8
  - congenital 757.5
- **Spanemia** 285.9
- **Spanish collar** 605
- **Sparganosis** 123.5
- **Spasm, spastic, spasticity** (*see also* condition) 781.0
  - accommodation 367.53
  - ampulla of Vater (*see also* Disease, gallbladder) 576.8
  - anus, ani (sphincter) (reflex) 564.6
    - psychogenic 306.4
  - artery NEC 443.9
    - basilar 435.0
    - carotid 435.8
    - cerebral 435.9
      - specified artery NEC 435.8
    - retinal (*see also* Occlusion, retinal, artery) 362.30
    - vertebral 435.1
    - vertebrobasilar 435.3
  - Bell's 351.0
  - bladder (sphincter, external or internal) 596.8
  - bowel 564.9
    - psychogenic 306.4
  - bronchus, bronchiole 519.11
  - cardia 530.0
  - cardiac – *see* Angina
  - carpopedal (*see also* Tetany) 781.7
  - cecum 564.9
    - psychogenic 306.4
  - cerebral (arteries) (vascular) 435.9
    - specified artery NEC 435.8
  - cerebrovascular 435.9
  - cervix, complicating delivery 661.4❺
    - affecting fetus or newborn 763.7
  - ciliary body (of accommodation) 367.53
  - colon 564.1
    - psychogenic 306.4
  - common duct (*see also* Disease, biliary) 576.8
  - compulsive 307.22
  - conjugate 378.82
  - convergence 378.84
  - coronary (artery) – *see* Angina
  - diaphragm (reflex) 786.8
    - psychogenic 306.1
  - duodenum, duodenal (bulb) 564.89
  - esophagus (diffuse) 530.5
    - psychogenic 306.4
  - facial 351.8
  - fallopian tube 620.8
  - gait 781.2
  - gastrointestinal (tract) 536.8
    - psychogenic 306.4
  - glottis 478.75
    - hysterical 300.11
    - psychogenic 306.1
      - specified as conversion reaction 300.11
    - reflex through recurrent laryngeal nerve 478.75
  - habit 307.20
    - chronic 307.22
    - transient (of childhood) 307.21
  - heart – *see* Angina
  - hourglass – *see* Contraction, hourglass
  - hysterical 300.11
  - infantile (*see also* Epilepsy) 345.6❺
  - internal oblique, eye 378.51
  - intestinal 564.9
    - psychogenic 306.4
  - larynx, laryngeal 478.75
    - hysterical 300.11
    - psychogenic 306.1
      - specified as conversion reaction 300.11
  - levator palpebrae superioris 333.81
  - lightning (*see also* Epilepsy) 345.6❺
  - mobile 781.0
  - muscle 728.85
    - back 724.8
    - psychogenic 306.0
  - nerve, trigeminal 350.1
  - nervous 306.0
  - nodding 307.3
    - infantile (*see also* Epilepsy) 345.6❺
  - occupational 300.89
  - oculogyric 378.87
  - ophthalmic artery 362.30
  - orbicularis 781.0
  - perineal 625.8
  - peroneo-extensor (*see also* Flat, foot) 734
  - pharynx (reflex) 478.29
    - hysterical 300.11
    - psychogenic 306.1
      - specified as conversion reaction 300.11
  - pregnant uterus, complicating delivery 661.4❺
  - psychogenic 306.0
  - pylorus 537.81
    - adult hypertrophic 537.0
    - congenital or infantile 750.5
    - psychogenic 306.4
  - rectum (sphincter) 564.6
    - psychogenic 306.4
  - retinal artery NEC (*see also* Occlusion, retina, artery) 362.30
  - sacroiliac 724.6
  - salaam (infantile) (*see also* Epilepsy) 345.6❺
  - saltatory 781.0
  - sigmoid 564.9
    - psychogenic 306.4
  - sphincter of Oddi (*see also* Disease, gallbladder) 576.5
  - stomach 536.8
    - neurotic 306.4
  - throat 478.29
    - hysterical 300.11
    - psychogenic 306.1
      - specified as conversion reaction 300.11
  - tic 307.20
    - chronic 307.22
    - transient (of childhood) 307.21
  - tongue 529.8
  - torsion 333.6
  - trigeminal nerve 350.1
    - postherpetic 053.12
  - ureter 593.89
  - urethra (sphincter) 599.84
  - uterus 625.8
    - complicating labor 661.4❺
      - affecting fetus or newborn 763.7
  - vagina 625.1
    - psychogenic 306.51
  - vascular NEC 443.9
  - vasomotor NEC 443.9
  - vein NEC 459.89
  - vesical (sphincter, external or internal) 596.8
  - viscera 789.0❺

Spasmodic – *see* condition
Spasmophilia (*see also* Tetany) 781.7
Spasmus nutans 307.3
Spastic – *see also* Spasm
- child 343.9

Spasticity – *see also* Spasm
- cerebral, child 343.9

Speakers' throat 784.49
Specific, specified – *see* condition
Speech
- defect, disorder, disturbance, impediment NEC 784.5
  - psychogenic 307.9
- therapy V57.3

Spells 780.39
- breath-holding 786.9

Spencer's disease (epidemic vomiting) 078.82
Spens' syndrome (syncope with heart block) 426.9
Spermatic cord – *see* condition
Spermatocele 608.1
- congenital 752.89

Spermatocystitis 608.4
Spermatocytoma (M9063/3)
- specified site – *see* Neoplasm, by site, malignant
- unspecified site 186.9

Spermatorrhea 608.89
Sperm counts
- fertility testing V26.21
- following sterilization reversal V26.22
- postvasectomy V25.8

Sphacelus (*see also* Gangrene) 785.4
Sphenoidal – *see* condition
Sphenoiditis (chronic) (*see also* Sinusitis, sphenoidal) 473.3
Sphenopalatine ganglion neuralgia 337.0
Sphericity, increased, lens 743.36
Spherocytosis (congenital) (familial) (hereditary) 282.0
- hemoglobin disease 282.7
- sickle-cell (disease) 282.60

Spherophakia 743.36
Sphincter – *see* condition
Sphincteritis, sphincter of Oddi (*see also* Cholecystitis) 576.8
Sphingolipidosis 272.7
Sphingolipodystrophy 272.7
Sphingomyelinosis 272.7
Spicule tooth 520.2
Spider
- finger 755.59
- nevus 448.1
- vascular 448.1

Spiegler-Fendt sarcoid 686.8
Spielmeyer-Stock disease 330.1
Spielmeyer-Vogt disease 330.1
Spina bifida (aperta) 741.9❺

Note – Use the following fifth-digit subclassification with category 741:
0 unspecified region
1 cervical region
2 dorsal [thoracic] region
3 lumbar region

- with hydrocephalus 741.0❺
- fetal (suspected), affecting management of pregnancy 655.0❺
- occulta 756.17

Spindle, Krukenberg's 371.13
Spine, spinal – *see* condition
Spiradenoma (eccrine) (M8403/0) – *see* Neoplasm, skin, benign
Spirillosis NEC (*see also* Fever, relapsing) 087.9
Spirillum minus 026.0
Spirillum obermeieri infection 087.0
Spirochetal – *see* condition
Spirochetosis 104.9
- arthritic, arthritica 104.9 *[711.8]*❺
- bronchopulmonary 104.8
- icterohemorrhagica 100.0
- lung 104.8

Spitting blood (*see also* Hemoptysis) 786.3
Splanchnomegaly 569.89
Splanchnoptosis 569.89
Spleen, splenic – *see also* condition
- agenesis 759.0
- flexure syndrome 569.89
- neutropenia syndrome 289.53
- sequestration syndrome 289.52

Splenectasis (*see also* Splenomegaly) 789.2
Splenitis (interstitial) (malignant) (nonspecific) 289.59
- malarial (*see also* Malaria) 084.6
- tuberculous (*see also* Tuberculosis) 017.7❺

Splenocele 289.59
Splenomegalia – *see* Splenomegaly
Splenomegalic – *see* condition
Splenomegaly 789.2
- Bengal 789.2
- cirrhotic 289.51
- congenital 759.0
- congestive, chronic 289.51
- cryptogenic 789.2
- Egyptian 120.1
- Gaucher's (cerebroside lipidosis) 272.7
- idiopathic 789.2
- malarial (*see also* Malaria) 084.6
- neutropenic 289.53
- Niemann-Pick (lipid histiocytosis) 272.7
- siderotic 289.51
- syphilitic 095.8
  - congenital 090.0
- tropical (Bengal) (idiopathic) 789.2

Splenopathy 289.50
Splenopneumonia – *see* Pneumonia
Splenoptosis 289.59
Splinter – *see* Injury, superficial, by site
Split, splitting
- heart sounds 427.89
- lip, congenital (*see also* Cleft, lip) 749.10
- nails 703.8
- urinary stream 788.61

Spoiled child reaction (*see also* Disturbance, conduct) 312.1❺
Spondylarthritis (*see also* Spondylosis) 721.90
Spondylarthrosis (*see also* Spondylosis) 721.90
Spondylitis 720.9
- ankylopoietica 720.0
- ankylosing (chronic) 720.0
- atrophic 720.9
  - ligamentous 720.9
- chronic (traumatic) (*see also* Spondylosis) 721.90
- deformans (chronic) (*see also* Spondylosis) 721.90
- gonococcal 098.53
- gouty 274.0
- hypertrophic (*see also* Spondylosis) 721.90
- infectious NEC 720.9
- juvenile (adolescent) 720.0
- Kummell's 721.7
- Marie-Strümpell (ankylosing) 720.0
- muscularis 720.9
- ossificans ligamentosa 721.6
- osteoarthritica (*see also* Spondylosis) 721.90
- posttraumatic 721.7
- proliferative 720.0
- rheumatoid 720.0
- rhizomelica 720.0
- sacroiliac NEC 720.2
- senescent (*see also* Spondylosis) 721.90
- senile (*see also* Spondylosis) 721.90
- static (*see also* Spondylosis) 721.90
- traumatic (chronic) (*see also* Spondylosis) 721.90
- tuberculous (*see also* Tuberculosis) 015.0❺ *[720.81]*
- typhosa 002.0 *[720.81]*

Spondyloarthrosis (*see also* Spondylosis) 721.90
Spondylolisthesis (congenital) (lumbosacral) 756.12
- with disproportion (fetopelvic) 653.3❺
  - affecting fetus or newborn 763.1
  - causing obstructed labor 660.1❺
    - affecting fetus or newborn 763.1
- acquired 738.4
- degenerative 738.4
- traumatic 738.4
  - acute (lumbar) – *see* Fracture, vertebra, lumbar
  - site other than lumbosacral – *see* Fracture, vertebra, by site

Spondylolysis (congenital) 756.11
- acquired 738.4
- cervical 756.19

Spondylolysis – *continued*
- lumbosacral region 756.11
  - with disproportion (fetopelvic) 653.3❺
    - affecting fetus or newborn 763.1
    - causing obstructed labor 660.1❺
      - affecting fetus or newborn 763.1

Spondylopathy
- inflammatory 720.9
  - specified type NEC 720.89
- traumatic 721.7

Spondylose rhizomelique 720.0
Spondylosis 721.90
- with
  - disproportion 653.3❺
    - affecting fetus or newborn 763.1
    - causing obstructed labor 660.1❺
      - affecting fetus or newborn 763.1
  - myelopathy NEC 721.91
- cervical, cervicodorsal 721.0
  - with myelopathy 721.1
- inflammatory 720.9
- lumbar, lumbosacral 721.3
  - with myelopathy 721.42
- sacral 721.3
  - with myelopathy 721.42
- thoracic 721.2
  - with myelopathy 721.41
- traumatic 721.7

Sponge
- divers' disease 989.5
- inadvertently left in operation wound 998.4
- kidney (medullary) 753.17

Spongioblastoma (M9422/3)
- multiforme (M9440/3)
  - specified site – *see* Neoplasm, by site, malignant
  - unspecified site 191.9
- polare (M9423/3)
  - specified site – *see* Neoplasm, by site, malignant
  - unspecified site 191.9
- primitive polar (M9443/3)
  - specified site – *see* Neoplasm, by site, malignant
  - unspecified site 191.9
- specified site – *see* Neoplasm, by site, malignant
- unspecified site 191.9

Spongiocytoma (M9400/3)
- specified site – *see* Neoplasm, by site, malignant
- unspecified site 191.9

Spongioneuroblastoma (M9504/3) – *see* Neoplasm, by site, malignant
Spontaneous – *see also* condition
- fracture – *see* Fracture, pathologic

Spoon nail 703.8
- congenital 757.5

Sporadic – *see* condition
Sporotrichosis (bones) (cutaneous) (disseminated) (epidermal) (lymphatic) (lymphocutaneous) (mucous membranes) (pulmonary) (skeletal) (visceral) 117.1
Sporotrichum schenckii infection 117.1
Spots, spotting
- atrophic (skin) 701.3
- Bitôt's (in the young child) 264.1
- café au lait 709.09
- cayenne pepper 448.1
- complicating pregnancy 649.5❺
- cotton wool (retina) 362.83
- de Morgan's (senile angiomas) 448.1
- Fúchs' black (myopic) 360.21
- intermenstrual
  - irregular 626.6
  - regular 626.5
- interpalpebral 372.53
- Koplik's 055.9
- liver 709.09
- Mongolian (pigmented) 757.33
- of pregnancy 641.9❺
- purpuric 782.7
- ruby 448.1

Spotted fever – *see* Fever, spotted
Sprain, strain (joint) (ligament) (muscle) (tendon) 848.9
- abdominal wall (muscle) 848.8
- Achilles tendon 845.09
- acromioclavicular 840.0
- ankle 845.00
  - and foot 845.00

Sprain, strain – Sputum, abnormal

- **Squamous** – *see also* condition
  - cell metaplasia
    - bladder 596.8
    - cervix – *see* condition
  - epithelium in
    - cervical canal (congenital) 752.49
    - uterine mucosa (congenital) 752.3
  - metaplasia
    - bladder 596.8
    - cervix – *see* condition
- **Squashed nose** 738.0
  - congenital 754.0
- **Squeeze, divers'** 993.3
- **Squint** (*see also* Strabismus) 378.9
  - accommodative (*see also* Esotropia) 378.00
  - concomitant (*see also* Heterotropia) 378.30
- **Stab** – *see also* Wound, open, by site
  - internal organs – *see* Injury, internal, by site, with open wound
- **Staggering gait** 781.2
  - hysterical 300.11
- **Staghorn calculus** 592.0
- **Stähl's**
  - ear 744.29
  - pigment line (cornea) 371.11
- **Stahli's pigment lines** (cornea) 371.11
- **Stain, staining**
  - meconium 779.84
  - port wine 757.32
  - tooth, teeth (hard tissues) 521.7
    - due to
      - accretions 523.6
      - deposits (betel) (black) (green) (materia alba) (orange) (tobacco) 523.6
      - metals (copper) (silver) 521.7
      - nicotine 523.6
      - pulpal bleeding 521.7
      - tobacco 523.6
- **Stammering** 307.0
- **Standstill**
  - atrial 426.6
  - auricular 426.6
  - cardiac (*see also* Arrest, cardiac) 427.5
  - sinoatrial 426.6
  - sinus 426.6
  - ventricular (*see also* Arrest, cardiac) 427.5
- **Stannosis** 503
- **Stanton's disease** (melioidosis) 025
- **Staphylitis** (acute) (catarrhal) (chronic) (gangrenous) (membranous) (suppurative) (ulcerative) 528.3
- **Staphylococcemia** 038.10
  - aureus 038.11
  - specified organism NEC 038.19
- **Staphylococcus, staphylococcal** – *see* condition
- **Staphyloderma** (skin) 686.00
- **Staphyloma** 379.11
  - anterior, localized 379.14
  - ciliary 379.11
  - cornea 371.73
  - equatorial 379.13
  - posterior 379.12
  - posticum 379.12
  - ring 379.15
  - sclera NEC 379.11
- **Starch eating** 307.52
- **Stargardt's disease** 362.75
- **Starvation** (inanition) (due to lack of food) 994.2
  - edema 262
  - voluntary NEC 307.1
- **Stasis**
  - bile (duct) (*see also* Disease, biliary) 576.8
  - bronchus (*see also* Bronchitis) 490
  - cardiac (*see also* Failure, heart) 428.0
  - cecum 564.89
  - colon 564.89
  - dermatitis (*see also* Varix, with stasis dermatitis) 454.1
  - duodenal 536.8
  - eczema (*see also* Varix, with stasis dermatitis) 454.1
  - edema (*see also* Hypertension, venous) 459.30
  - foot 991.4
  - gastric 536.3
  - ileocecal coil 564.89
  - ileum 564.89
  - intestinal 564.89
  - jejunum 564.89
  - kidney 586

- **Stasis** – *continued*
  - liver 571.9
    - cirrhotic – *see* Cirrhosis, liver
  - lymphatic 457.8
  - pneumonia 514
  - portal 571.9
  - pulmonary 514
  - rectal 564.89
  - renal 586
    - tubular 584.5
  - stomach 536.3
  - ulcer
    - with varicose veins 454.0
    - without varicose veins 459.81
  - urine NEC (*see also* Retention, urine) 788.20
  - venous 459.81
- **State**
  - affective and paranoid, mixed, organic psychotic 294.8
  - agitated 307.9
    - acute reaction to stress 308.2
  - anxiety (neurotic) (*see also* Anxiety) 300.00
    - specified type NEC 300.09
  - apprehension (*see also* Anxiety) 300.00
    - specified type NEC 300.09
  - climacteric, female 627.2
    - following induced menopause 627.4
  - clouded
    - epileptic (*see also* Epilepsy) 345.9❺
    - paroxysmal (idiopathic) (*see also* Epilepsy) 345.9❺
  - compulsive (mixed) (with obsession) 300.3
  - confusional 298.9
    - acute 293.0
      - with
        - arteriosclerotic dementia 290.41
        - presenile brain disease 290.11
        - senility 290.3
      - alcoholic 291.0
      - drug-induced 292.81
    - epileptic 293.0
    - postoperative 293.9
    - reactive (emotional stress) (psychological trauma) 298.2
    - subacute 293.1
  - constitutional psychopathic 301.9
  - convulsive (*see also* Convulsions) 780.39
  - depressive NEC 311
    - induced by drug 292.84
    - neurotic 300.4
  - dissociative 300.15
  - hallucinatory 780.1
    - induced by drug 292.12
  - hypercoagulable (primary) 289.81
    - secondary 289.82
  - hyperdynamic beta-adrenergic circulatory 429.82
  - locked-in 344.81
  - menopausal 627.2
    - artificial 627.4
    - following induced menopause 627.4
  - neurotic NEC 300.9
    - with depersonalization episode 300.6
  - obsessional 300.3
  - oneiroid (*see also* Schizophrenia) 295.4❺
  - panic 300.01
  - paranoid 297.9
    - alcohol-induced 291.5
    - arteriosclerotic 290.42
    - climacteric 297.2
    - drug-induced 292.11
    - in
      - presenile brain disease 290.12
      - senile brain disease 290.20
    - involutional 297.2
    - menopausal 297.2
    - senile 290.20
    - simple 297.0
  - postleukotomy 310.0
  - pregnant (*see also* Pregnancy) V22.2
  - psychogenic, twilight 298.2
  - psychotic, organic (*see also* Psychosis, organic) 294.9
    - mixed paranoid and affective 294.8
    - senile or presenile NEC 290.9
    - transient NEC 293.9
      - with
        - anxiety 293.84
        - delusions 293.81
        - depression 293.83
        - hallucinations 293.82
  - residual schizophrenic (*see also* Schizophrenia) 295.6❺

- **State** – *continued*
  - tension (*see also* Anxiety) 300.9
  - transient organic psychotic 293.9
    - anxiety type 293.84
    - depressive type 293.83
    - hallucinatory type 293.83
    - paranoid type 293.81
    - specified type NEC 293.89
  - twilight
    - epileptic 293.0
    - psychogenic 298.2
  - vegetative (persistent) 780.03
- **Status** (post)
  - absence
    - epileptic (*see also* Epilepsy) 345.2
    - of organ, acquired (postsurgical) – *see* Absence, by site, acquired
  - anastomosis of intestine (for bypass) V45.3
  - anginosus 413.9
  - angioplasty, percutaneous transluminal coronary V45.82
  - ankle prosthesis V43.66
  - aortocoronary bypass or shunt V45.81
  - arthrodesis V45.4
  - artificially induced condition NEC V45.89
  - artificial opening (of) V44.9
    - gastrointestinal tract NEC V44.4
    - specified site NEC V44.8
    - urinary tract NEC V44.6
    - vagina V44.7
  - aspirator V46.0
  - asthmaticus (*see also* Asthma) 493.9❺
  - awaiting organ transplant V49.83
  - bariatric surgery V45.86
    - complicating pregnancy, childbirth, or the puerperium 649.2❺
  - bed confinement V49.84
  - breast implant removal V45.83
  - cardiac
    - device (in situ) V45.00
      - carotid sinus V45.09
        - fitting or adjustment V53.39
      - defibrillator, automatic implantable V45.02
      - pacemaker V45.01
        - fitting or adjustment V53.31
  - carotid sinus stimulator V45.09
  - cataract extraction V45.61
  - chemotherapy V66.2
    - current V58.69
  - circumcision, female 629.20
  - clitorectomy (female genital mutilation type I) 629.21
    - with excision of labia minora (female genital mutilation type II) 629.22
  - colostomy V44.3
  - contraceptive device V45.59
    - intrauterine V45.51
    - subdermal V45.52
  - convulsivus idiopathicus (*see also* Epilepsy) 345.3
  - coronary artery bypass or shunt V45.81
  - cutting
    - female genital 629.20
      - specified NEC 629.29
      - type I 629.21
      - type II 629.22
      - type III 629.23
      - type IV 629.29
  - cystostomy V44.50
    - appendico-vesicostomy V44.52
    - cutaneous-vesicostomy V44.51
    - specifed type NEC V44.59
  - defibrillator, automatic implantable cardiac V45.02
  - dental crowns V45.84
  - dental fillings V45.84
  - dental restoration V45.84
  - dental sealant V49.82
  - dialysis (hemo) (peritoneal) V45.1
  - donor V59.9
  - drug therapy or regimen V67.59
    - high-risk medication NEC V67.51
  - elbow prosthesis V43.62
  - enterostomy V44.4
  - epileptic, epilepticus (absence) (grand mal) (*see also* Epilepsy) 345.3
    - focal motor 345.7❺
    - partial 345.7❺
    - petit mal 345.2
    - psychomotor 345.7❺
    - temporal lobe 345.7❺

Status – *continued*
  estrogen receptor
    negative [ER-] V86.1
    positive [ER+] V86.0
  eye (adnexa) surgery V45.69
  female genital
    cutting 629.20
      specified NEC 629.29
      type I 629.21
      type II 629.22
      type III 629.23
      type IV 629.29
    mutilation 629.20
      type IV 629.29
    type I 629.21
    type II 629.22
    type III 629.23
  filtering bleb (eye) (postglaucoma) V45.69
    with rupture or complication 997.99
    postcataract extraction (complication) 997.99
  finger joint prosthesis V43.69
  gastric
    banding V45.86
      complicating pregnancy, childbirth, or the puerperium 649.2❺
    bypass for obesity V45.86
      complicating pregnancy, childbirth, or the puerperium 649.2❺
  gastrostomy V44.1
  grand mal 345.3
  heart valve prosthesis V43.3
  hemodialysis V45.1
  hip prosthesis (joint) (partial) (total) V43.64
  ileostomy V44.2
  infibulation (female genital mutilation type III) 629.23
  insulin pump V45.85
  intestinal bypass V45.3
  intrauterine contraceptive device V45.51
  jejunostomy V44.4
  knee joint prosthesis V43.65
  lacunaris 437.8
  lacunosis 437.8
  low birth weight V21.30
    less than 500 grams V21.31
    500-999 grams V21.32
    1000-1499 grams V21.33
    1500-1999 grams V21.34
    2000-2500 grams V21.35
  lymphaticus 254.8
  malignant neoplasm, ablated or excised – *see* History, malignant neoplasm
  marmoratus 333.79
  mutilation, female 629.20
    type I 629.21
    type II 629.22
    type III 629.23
    type IV 629.29
  nephrostomy V44.6
  neuropacemaker NEC V45.89
    brain V45.89
    carotid sinus V45.09
    neurologic NEC V45.89
  obesity surgery V45.86
    complicating pregnancy, childbirth, or the puerperium 649.2❺
  organ replacement
    by artificial or mechanical device or prosthesis of
      artery V43.4
      artificial skin V43.83
      bladder V43.5
      blood vessel V43.4
      breast V43.82
      eye globe V43.0
      heart
        assist device V43.21
        fully implantable artificial heart V43.22
        valve V43.3
      intestine V43.89
      joint V43.60
        ankle V43.66
        elbow V43.62
        finger V43.69
        hip (partial) (total) V43.64
        knee V43.65
        shoulder V43.61
        specified NEC V43.69
        wrist V43.63
      kidney V43.89
      larynx V43.81
      lens V43.1

Status – *continued*
  organ replacement – *continued*
    by artificial or mechanical device or prosthesis of – *continued*
      limb(s) V43.7
      liver V43.89
      lung V43.89
      organ NEC V43.89
      pancreas V43.89
      skin (artificial) V43.83
      tissue NEC V43.89
      vein V43.4
    by organ transplant (heterologous) (homologous) – *see* Status, transplant
  pacemaker
    brain V45.89
    cardiac V45.01
    carotid sinus V45.09
    neurologic NEC V45.89
    specified site NEC V45.89
  percutaneous transluminal coronary angioplasty V45.82
  peritoneal dialysis V45.1
  petit mal 345.2
  postcommotio cerebri 310.2
  postmenopausal (age related) (natural) V49.81
  postoperative NEC V45.89
  postpartum NEC V24.2
    care immediately following delivery V24.0
    routine follow-up V24.2
  postsurgical NEC V45.89
  renal dialysis V45.1
  respirator [ventilator] V46.11
    encounter
      during
        mechanical failure V46.14
        power failure V46.12
      for weaning V46.13
  reversed jejunal transposition (for bypass) V45.3
  sex reassignment surgery (*see also* Trans-sexualism) 302.50 ●
  shoulder prosthesis V43.61
  shunt
    aortocoronary bypass V45.81
    arteriovenous (for dialysis) V45.1
    cerebrospinal fluid V45.2
    vascular NEC V45.89
      aortocoronary (bypass) V45.81
    ventricular (communicating) (for drainage) V45.2
  sterilization
    tubal ligation V26.51
    vasectomy V26.52
  subdermal contraceptive device V45.52
  thymicolymphaticus 254.8
  thymicus 254.8
  thymolymphaticus 254.8
  tooth extraction 525.10
  tracheostomy V44.0
  transplant
    blood vessel V42.89
    bone V42.4
      marrow V42.81
    cornea V42.5
    heart V42.1
      valve V42.2
    intestine V42.84
    kidney V42.0
    liver V42.7
    lung V42.6
    organ V42.9
      specified site NEC V42.89
    pancreas V42.83
    peripheral stem cells V42.82
    skin V42.3
    stem cells, peripheral V42.82
    tissue V42.9
      specified type NEC V42.89
    vessel, blood V42.89
  tubal ligation V26.51
  ureterostomy V44.6
  urethrostomy V44.6
  vagina, artificial V44.7
  vascular shunt NEC V45.89
    aortocoronary (bypass) V45.81
  vasectomy V26.52
  ventilator [respirator] V46.11
    encounter
      during
        mechanical failure V46.14
        power failure V46.12
      for weaning V46.13
  wrist prosthesis V43.63

Stave fracture – *see* Fracture, metacarpus, metacarpal bone(s)

Steal
  subclavian artery 435.2
  vertebral artery 435.1

Stealing, solitary, child problem (*see also* Disturbance, conduct) 312.1❺

Steam burn – *see* Burn, by site

Steatocystoma multiplex 706.2

Steatoma (infected) 706.2
  eyelid (cystic) 374.84
    infected 373.13

Steatorrhea (chronic) 579.8
  with lacteal obstruction 579.2
  idiopathic 579.0
    adult 579.0
    infantile 579.0
  pancreatic 579.4
  primary 579.0
  secondary 579.8
  specified cause NEC 579.8
  tropical 579.1

Steatosis 272.8
  heart (*see also* Degeneration, myocardial) 429.1
  kidney 593.89
  liver 571.8

Steele-Richardson (-Olszewski) **Syndrome** 333.0

Stein's syndrome (polycystic ovary) 256.4

Stein-Leventhal syndrome (polycystic ovary) 256.4

Steinbrocker's syndrome (*see also* Neuropathy, peripheral, autonomic) 337.9

Steinert's disease 359.21 ▲

STEMI (ST elevation myocardial infarction) (*see also* Infarct, myocardium, ST elevation) 410.9❺

Stenocardia (*see also* Angina) 413.9

Stenocephaly 756.0

Stenosis (cicatricial) – *see also* Stricture
  ampulla of Vater 576.2
    with calculus, cholelithiasis, or stones – *see* Choledocholithiasis
  anus, anal (canal) (sphincter) 569.2
    congenital 751.2
  aorta (ascending) 747.22
    arch 747.10
    arteriosclerotic 440.0
    calcified 440.0
  aortic (valve) 424.1
    with
      mitral (valve)
        insufficiency or incompetence 396.2
        stenosis or obstruction 396.0
    atypical 396.0
    congenital 746.3
    rheumatic 395.0
      with
        insufficiency, incompetency or regurgitation 395.2
          with mitral (valve) disease 396.8
        mitral (valve)
          disease (stenosis) 396.0
          insufficiency or incompetence 396.2
          stenosis or obstruction 396.0
    specified cause, except rheumatic 424.1
    syphilitic 093.22
  aqueduct of Sylvius (congenital) 742.3
    with spina bifida (*see also* Spina bifida) 741.0❺
    acquired 331.4
  artery NEC ▶(*see also* Arteriosclerosis)◀ 447.1
    basilar – *see* Narrowing, artery, basilar
    carotid (common) (internal) – *see* Narrowing, artery, carotid
    celiac 447.4
    cerebral 437.0
      due to
        embolism (*see also* Embolism, brain) 434.1❺
        thrombus (*see also* Thrombosis, brain) 434.0❺
    extremities 440.20 ●
    precerebral – *see* Narrowing, artery, precerebral
    pulmonary (congenital) 747.3
      acquired 417.8
    renal 440.1
    vertebral – *see* Narrowing, artery, vertebral
  bile duct or biliary passage (*see also* Obstruction, biliary) 576.2
    congenital 751.61

Status – Stenosis

- **Stenosis** – *continued*
  - bladder neck (acquired) 596.0
    - congenital 753.6
  - brain 348.8
  - bronchus 519.19
    - syphilitic 095.8
  - cardia (stomach) 537.89
    - congenital 750.7
  - cardiovascular (*see also* Disease, cardiovascular) 429.2
  - carotid artery – *see* Narrowing, artery, carotid
  - cervix, cervical (canal) 622.4
    - congenital 752.49
    - in pregnancy or childbirth 654.6❺
      - affecting fetus or newborn 763.89
      - causing obstructed labor 660.2❺
        - affecting fetus or newborn 763.1
  - colon (*see also* Obstruction, intestine) 560.9
    - congenital 751.2
  - colostomy 569.62
  - common bile duct (*see also* Obstruction, biliary) 576.2
    - congenital 751.61
  - coronary (artery) – *see* Arteriosclerosis, coronary
  - cystic duct (*see also* Obstruction, gallbladder) 575.2
    - congenital 751.61
  - due to (presence of) any device, implant, or graft classifiable to 996.0-996.5 – *see* Complications, due to (presence of) any device, implant, or graft classified to 996.0-996.5 NEC
  - duodenum 537.3
    - congenital 751.1
  - ejaculatory duct NEC 608.89
  - endocervical os – *see* Stenosis, cervix
  - enterostomy 569.62
  - esophagostomy 530.87
  - esophagus 530.3
    - congenital 750.3
    - syphilitic 095.8
      - congenital 090.5
  - external ear canal 380.50
    - secondary to
      - inflammation 380.53
      - surgery 380.52
      - trauma 380.51
  - gallbladder (*see also* Obstruction, gallbladder) 575.2
  - glottis 478.74
  - heart valve (acquired) – *see also* Endocarditis
    - congenital NEC 746.89
      - aortic 746.3
      - mitral 746.5
      - pulmonary 746.02
      - tricuspid 746.1
  - hepatic duct (*see also* Obstruction, biliary) 576.2
  - hymen 623.3
  - hypertrophic subaortic (idiopathic) 425.1
  - infundibulum cardiac 746.83
  - intestine (*see also* Obstruction, intestine) 560.9
    - congenital (small) 751.1
      - large 751.2
  - lacrimal
    - canaliculi 375.53
    - duct 375.56
      - congenital 743.65
    - punctum 375.52
      - congenital 743.65
    - sac 375.54
      - congenital 743.65
  - lacrimonasal duct 375.56
    - congenital 743.65
    - neonatal 375.55
  - larynx 478.74
    - congenital 748.3
    - syphilitic 095.8
      - congenital 090.5
  - mitral (valve) (chronic) (inactive) 394.0
    - with
      - aortic (valve)
        - disease (insufficiency) 396.1
        - insufficiency or incompetence 396.1
        - stenosis or obstruction 396.0
      - incompetency, insufficiency or regurgitation 394.2
        - with aortic valve disease 396.8
    - active or acute 391.1
      - with chorea (acute) (rheumatic) (Sydenham's) 392.0
    - congenital 746.5
    - specified cause, except rheumatic 424.0

- **Stenosis** – *continued*
  - mitral – *continued*
    - syphilitic 093.21
  - myocardium, myocardial (*see also* Degeneration, myocardial) 429.1
    - hypertrophic subaortic (idiopathic) 425.1
  - nares (anterior) (posterior) 478.19
    - congenital 748.0
  - nasal duct 375.56
    - congenital 743.65
  - nasolacrimal duct 375.56
    - congenital 743.65
    - neonatal 375.55
  - organ or site, congenital NEC – *see* Atresia
  - papilla of Vater 576.2
    - with calculus, cholelithiasis, or stones – *see* Choledocholithiasis
  - pulmonary (artery) (congenital) 747.3
    - with ventricular septal defect, dextraposition of aorta and hypertrophy of right ventricle 745.2
    - acquired 417.8
    - infundibular 746.83
    - in tetralogy of Fallot 745.2
    - subvalvular 746.83
    - valve (*see also* Endocarditis, pulmonary) 424.3
      - congenital 746.02
    - vein 747.49
      - acquired 417.8
    - vessel NEC 417.8
  - pulmonic (congenital) 746.02
    - infundibular 746.83
    - subvalvular 746.83
  - pylorus (hypertrophic) 537.0
    - adult 537.0
    - congenital 750.5
    - infantile 750.5
  - rectum (sphincter) (*see also* Stricture, rectum) 569.2
  - renal artery 440.1
  - salivary duct (any) 527.8
  - sphincter of Oddi (*see also* Obstruction, biliary) 576.2
  - spinal 724.00
    - cervical 723.0
    - lumbar, lumbosacral 724.02
    - nerve (root) NEC 724.9
    - specified region NEC 724.09
    - thoracic, thoracolumbar 724.01
  - stomach, hourglass 537.6
  - subaortic 746.81
    - hypertrophic (idiopathic) 425.1
  - supra (valvular)-aortic 747.22
  - trachea 519.19
    - congenital 748.3
    - syphilitic 095.8
    - tuberculous (*see also* Tuberculosis) 012.8❺
  - tracheostomy 519.02
  - tricuspid (valve) (*see also* Endocarditis, tricuspid) 397.0
    - congenital 746.1
    - nonrheumatic 424.2
  - tubal 628.2
  - ureter (*see also* Stricture, ureter) 593.3
    - congenital 753.29
  - urethra (*see also* Stricture, urethra) 598.9
  - vagina 623.2
    - congenital 752.49
    - in pregnancy or childbirth 654.7❺
      - affecting fetus or newborn 763.89
      - causing obstructed labor 660.2❺
        - affecting fetus or newborn 763.1
  - valve (cardiac) (heart) (*see also* Endocarditis) 424.90
    - congenital NEC 746.89
      - aortic 746.3
      - mitral 746.5
      - pulmonary 746.02
      - tricuspid 746.1
      - urethra 753.6
  - valvular (*see also* Endocarditis) 424.90
    - congenital NEC 746.89
      - urethra 753.6
  - vascular graft or shunt 996.1
    - atherosclerosis – *see* Arteriosclerosis, extremities
    - embolism 996.74
    - occlusion NEC 996.74
    - thrombus 996.74
  - vena cava (inferior) (superior) 459.2
    - congenital 747.49
  - ventricular shunt 996.2

- **Stenosis** – *continued*
  - vulva 624.8
- **Stercolith** (*see also* Fecalith) 560.39
  - appendix 543.9
- **Stercoraceous, stercoral ulcer** 569.82
  - anus or rectum 569.41
- **Stereopsis, defective**
  - with fusion 368.33
  - without fusion 368.32
- **Stereotypies** NEC 307.3
- **Sterility**
  - female – *see* Infertility, female
  - male (*see also* Infertility, male) 606.9
- **Sterilization, admission for** V25.2
  - status
    - tubal ligation V26.51
    - vasectomy V26.52
- **Sternalgia** (*see also* Angina) 413.9
- **Sternopagus** 759.4
- **Sternum bifidum** 756.3
- **Sternutation** 784.99
- **Steroid**
  - effects (adverse) (iatrogenic)
    - cushingoid
      - correct substance properly administered 255.0
      - overdose or wrong substance given or taken 962.0
    - diabetes
      - correct substance properly administered 251.8
      - overdose or wrong substance given or taken 962.0
    - due to
      - correct substance properly administered 255.8
      - overdose or wrong substance given or taken 962.0
    - fever
      - correct substance properly administered 780.6
      - overdose or wrong substance given or taken 962.0
    - withdrawal
      - correct substance properly administered 255.41 ▲
      - overdose or wrong substance given or taken 962.0
  - responder 365.03
- **Stevens-Johnson disease or syndrome** (erythema multiforme exudativum) 695.1
- **Stewart-Morel syndrome** (hyperostosis frontalis interna) 733.3
- **Sticker's disease** (erythema infectiosum) 057.0
- **Stickler syndrome** 759.89
- **Sticky eye** 372.03
- **Stieda's disease** (calcification, knee joint) 726.62
- **Stiff**
  - back 724.8
  - neck (*see also* Torticollis) 723.5
- **Stiff-baby** 759.89
- **Stiff-man syndrome** 333.91
- **Stiffness, joint** NEC 719.50
  - ankle 719.57
  - back 724.8
  - elbow 719.52
  - finger 719.54
  - hip 719.55
  - knee 719.56
  - multiple sites 719.59
  - sacroiliac 724.6
  - shoulder 719.51
  - specified site NEC 719.58
  - spine 724.9
  - surgical fusion V45.4
  - wrist 719.53
- **Stigmata, congenital syphilis** 090.5
- **Still's disease or syndrome** 714.30
- **Still-Felty syndrome** (rheumatoid arthritis with splenomegaly and leukopenia) 714.1
- **Stillbirth, stillborn** NEC 779.9
- **Stiller's disease** (asthenia) 780.79
- **Stilling-Türk-Duane syndrome** (ocular retraction syndrome) 378.71
- **Stimulation, ovary** 256.1

- **Sting** (animal) (bee) (fish) (insect) (jellyfish) (Portuguese man-o-war) (wasp) (venomous) 989.5
  - anaphylactic shock or reaction 989.5
  - plant 692.6
- **Stippled epiphyses** 756.59
- **Stitch**
  - abscess 998.59
  - burst (in external operation wound) 998.32
    - internal 998.31
  - in back 724.5
- **Stojano's** (subcostal) **syndrome** 098.86
- **Stokes' disease** (exophthalmic goiter) 242.0❺
- **Stokes-Adams syndrome** (syncope with heart block) 426.9
- **Stokvis'** (-Talma) **disease** (enterogenous cyanosis) 289.7
- **Stomach** – *see* condition
- **Stoma malfunction**
  - colostomy 569.62
  - cystostomy 997.5
  - enterostomy 569.62
  - esophagostomy 530.87
  - gastrostomy 536.42
  - ileostomy 569.62
  - nephrostomy 997.5
  - tracheostomy 519.02
  - ureterostomy 997.5
- **Stomatitis** 528.00
  - angular 528.5
    - due to dietary or vitamin deficiency 266.0
  - aphthous 528.2
  - candidal 112.0
  - catarrhal 528.00
  - denture 528.9
  - diphtheritic (membranous) 032.0
  - due to
    - dietary deficiency 266.0
    - thrush 112.0
    - vitamin deficiency 266.0
  - epidemic 078.4
  - epizootic 078.4
  - follicular 528.00
  - gangrenous 528.1
  - herpetic 054.2
  - herpetiformis 528.2
  - malignant 528.00
  - membranous acute 528.00
  - monilial 112.0
  - mycotic 112.0
  - necrotic 528.1
    - ulcerative 101
  - necrotizing ulcerative 101
  - parasitic 112.0
  - septic 528.00
  - specified NEC 528.09
  - spirochetal 101
  - suppurative (acute) 528.00
  - ulcerative 528.00
    - necrotizing 101
  - ulceromembranous 101
  - vesicular 528.00
    - with exanthem 074.3
  - Vincent's 101
- **Stomatocytosis** 282.8
- **Stomatomycosis** 112.0
- **Stomatorrhagia** 528.9
- **Stone(s)** – *see also* Calculus
  - bladder 594.1
    - diverticulum 594.0
  - cystine 270.0
  - heart syndrome (*see also* Failure, ventricular, left) 428.1
  - kidney 592.0
  - prostate 602.0
  - pulp (dental) 522.2
  - renal 592.0
  - salivary duct or gland (any) 527.5
  - ureter 592.1
  - urethra (impacted) 594.2
  - urinary (duct) (impacted) (passage) 592.9
    - bladder 594.1
      - diverticulum 594.0
    - lower tract NEC 594.9
    - specified site 594.8
  - xanthine 277.2
- **Stonecutters' lung** 502
  - tuberculous (*see also* Tuberculosis) 011.4❺
- **Stonemasons'**
  - asthma, disease, or lung 502
    - tuberculous (*see also* Tuberculosis) 011.4❺
  - phthisis (*see also* Tuberculosis) 011.4❺
- **Stoppage**
  - bowel (*see also* Obstruction, intestine) 560.9
  - heart (*see also* Arrest, cardiac) 427.5
  - intestine (*see also* Obstruction, intestine) 560.9
  - urine NEC (*see also* Retention, urine) 788.20
- **Storm, thyroid** (apathetic) (*see also* Thyrotoxicosis) 242.9❺
- **Strabismus** (alternating) (congenital) (nonparalytic) 378.9
  - concomitant (*see also* Heterotropia) 378.30
    - convergent (*see also* Esotropia) 378.00
    - divergent (*see also* Exotropia) 378.10
  - convergent (*see also* Esotropia) 378.00
  - divergent (*see also* Exotropia) 378.10
  - due to adhesions, scars – *see* Strabismus, mechanical
  - in neuromuscular disorder NEC 378.73
    - intermittent 378.20
      - vertical 378.31
  - latent 378.40
    - convergent (esophoria) 378.41
    - divergent (exophoria) 378.42
    - vertical 378.43
  - mechanical 378.60
    - due to
      - Brown's tendon sheath syndrome 378.61
      - specified musculofascial disorder NEC 378.62
  - paralytic 378.50
    - third or oculomotor nerve (partial) 378.51
      - total 378.52
    - fourth or trochlear nerve 378.53
    - sixth or abducens nerve 378.54
  - specified type NEC 378.73
  - vertical (hypertropia) 378.31
- **Strain** – *see also* Sprain, by site
  - eye NEC 368.13
  - heart – *see* Disease, heart
  - meaning gonorrhea – *see* Gonorrhea
  - on urination 788.65
  - physical NEC V62.89
  - postural 729.9
  - psychological NEC V62.89
- **Strands**
  - conjunctiva 372.62
  - vitreous humor 379.25
- **Strangulation, strangulated** 994.7
  - appendix 543.9
  - asphyxiation or suffocation by 994.7
  - bladder neck 596.0
  - bowel – *see* Strangulation, intestine
  - colon – *see* Strangulation, intestine
  - cord (umbilical) – *see* Compression, umbilical cord
  - due to birth injury 767.8
  - food or foreign body (*see also* Asphyxia, food) 933.1
  - hemorrhoids 455.8
    - external 455.5
    - internal 455.2
  - hernia – *see also* Hernia, by site with obstruction
    - gangrenous – *see* Hernia, by site, with gangrene
  - intestine (large) (small) 560.2
    - with hernia – *see also* Hernia, by site, with obstruction
      - gangrenous – *see* Hernia, by site, with gangrene
    - congenital (small) 751.1
      - large 751.2
  - mesentery 560.2
  - mucus (*see also* Asphyxia, mucus) 933.1
    - newborn 770.18
  - omentum 560.2
  - organ or site, congenital NEC – *see* Atresia
  - ovary 620.8
    - due to hernia 620.4
  - penis 607.89
    - foreign body 939.3
  - rupture (*see also* Hernia, by site, with obstruction) 552.9
    - gangrenous (*see also* Hernia, by site, with gangrene) 551.9
  - stomach, due to hernia (*see also* Hernia, by site, with obstruction 552.9
    - with gangrene (*see also* Hernia, by site, with gangrene) 551.9
  - umbilical cord – *see* Compression, umbilical cord
  - vesicourethral orifice 596.0
- **Strangury** 788.1
- **Strawberry**
  - gallbladder (*see also* Disease, gallbladder) 575.6
  - mark 757.32
  - tongue (red) (white) 529.3
- **Straw itch** 133.8
- **Streak, ovarian** 752.0
- **Strephosymbolia** 315.01
  - secondary to organic lesion 784.69
- **Streptobacillary fever** 026.1
- **Streptobacillus moniliformis** 026.1
- **Streptococcemia** 038.0
- **Streptococcicosis** – *see* Infection, streptococcal
- **Streptococcus, streptococcal** – *see* condition
- **Streptoderma** 686.00
- **Streptomycosis** – *see* Actinomycosis
- **Streptothricosis** – *see* Actinomycosis
- **Streptothrix** – *see* Actinomycosis
- **Streptotrichosis** – *see* Actinomycosis
- **Stress** 308.9 ▲
  - fracture – *see* Fracture, stress
  - polycythemia 289.0
  - reaction (gross) (*see also* Reaction, stress, acute) 308.9
- **Stretching, nerve** – *see* Injury, nerve, by site
- **Striae** (albicantes) (atrophicae) (cutis distensae) (distensae) 701.3
- **Striations of nails** 703.8
- **Stricture** (*see also* Stenosis) 799.89
  - ampulla of Vater 576.2
    - with calculus, cholelithiasis, or stones – *see* Choledocholithiasis
  - anus (sphincter) 569.2
    - congenital 751.2
    - infantile 751.2
  - aorta (ascending) 747.22
    - arch 747.10
    - arteriosclerotic 440.0
    - calcified 440.0
  - aortic (valve) (*see also* Stenosis, aortic) 424.1
    - congenital 746.3
  - aqueduct of Sylvius (congenital) 742.3
    - with spina bifida (*see also* Spina bifida) 741.0❺
    - acquired 331.4
  - artery 447.1
    - basilar – *see* Narrowing, artery, basilar
    - carotid (common) (internal) – *see* Narrowing, artery, carotid
    - celiac 447.4
    - cerebral 437.0
      - congenital 747.81
      - due to
        - embolism (*see also* Embolism, brain) 434.1❺
        - thrombus (*see also* Thrombosis, brain) 434.0❺
    - congenital (peripheral) 747.60
      - cerebral 747.81
      - coronary 746.85
      - gastrointestinal 747.61
      - lower limb 747.64
      - renal 747.62
      - retinal 743.58
      - specified NEC 747.69
      - spinal 747.82
      - umbilical 747.5
      - upper limb 747.63
    - coronary – *see* Arteriosclerosis, coronary
      - congenital 746.85
    - precerebral – *see* Narrowing, artery, precerebral NEC
    - pulmonary (congenital) 747.3
      - acquired 417.8
    - renal 440.1
    - vertebral – *see* Narrowing, artery, vertebral
  - auditory canal (congenital) (external) 744.02
    - acquired (*see also* Stricture, ear canal, acquired) 380.50
  - bile duct or passage (any) (postoperative) (*see also* Obstruction, biliary) 576.2
    - congenital 751.61
  - bladder 596.8
    - congenital 753.6
    - neck 596.0
      - congenital 753.6
  - bowel (*see also* Obstruction, intestine) 560.9
  - brain 348.8

Sting – Stricture

Stricture – *continued*
bronchus 519.19
syphilitic 095.8
cardia (stomach) 537.89
congenital 750.7
cardiac – *see also* Disease, heart orifice (stomach) 537.89
cardiovascular (*see also* Disease, cardiovascular) 429.2
carotid artery – *see* Narrowing, artery, carotid
cecum (*see also* Obstruction, intestine) 560.9
cervix, cervical (canal) 622.4
congenital 752.49
in pregnancy or childbirth 654.6❺
affecting fetus or newborn 763.89
causing obstructed labor 660.2❺
affecting fetus or newborn 763.1
colon (*see also* Obstruction, intestine) 560.9
congenital 751.2
colostomy 569.62
common bile duct (*see also* Obstruction, biliary) 576.2
congenital 751.61
coronary (artery) – *see* Arteriosclerosis, coronary
congenital 746.85
cystic duct (*see also* Obstruction, gallbladder) 575.2
congenital 751.61
cystostomy 997.5
digestive organs NEC, congenital 751.8
duodenum 537.3
congenital 751.1
ear canal (external) (congenital) 744.02
acquired 380.50
secondary to
inflammation 380.53
surgery 380.52
trauma 380.51
ejaculatory duct 608.85
enterostomy 569.62
esophagostomy 530.87
esophagus (corrosive) (peptic) 530.3
congenital 750.3
syphilitic 095.8
congenital 090.5
Eustachian tube (*see also* Obstruction, Eustachian tube) 381.60
congenital 744.24
fallopian tube 628.2
gonococcal (chronic) 098.37
cute 098.17
tuberculous (*see also* Tuberculosis) 016.6❺
gallbladder (*see also* Obstruction, gallbladder) 575.2
congenital 751.69
glottis 478.74
heart – *see also* Disease, heart
congenital NEC 746.89
valve – *see also* Endocarditis
congenital NEC 746.89
aortic 746.3
mitral 746.5
pulmonary 746.02
tricuspid 746.1
hepatic duct (*see also* Obstruction, biliary) 576.2
hourglass, of stomach 537.6
hymen 623.3
hypopharynx 478.29
intestine (*see also* Obstruction, intestine) 560.9
congenital (small) 751.1
large 751.2
ischemic 557.1
lacrimal
canaliculi 375.53
congenital 743.65
punctum 375.52
congenital 743.65
sac 375.54
congenital 743.65
lacrimonasal duct 375.56
congenital 743.65
neonatal 375.55
larynx 478.79
congenital 748.3
syphilitic 095.8
congenital 090.5
lung 518.89
meatus
ear (congenital) 744.02
acquired (*see also* Stricture, ear canal, acquired) 380.50

Stricture – *continued*
meatus – *continued*
osseous (congenital) (ear) 744.03
acquired (*see also* Stricture, ear canal, acquired) 380.50
urinarius (*see also* Stricture, urethra) 598.9
congenital 753.6
mitral (valve) (*see also* Stenosis, mitral) 394.0
congenital 746.5
specified cause, except rheumatic 424.0
myocardium, myocardial (*see also* Degeneration, myocardial) 429.1
hypertrophic subaortic (idiopathic) 425.1
nares (anterior) (posterior) 478.19
congenital 748.0
nasal duct 375.56
congenital 743.65
neonatal 375.55
nasolacrimal duct 375.56
congenital 743.65
neonatal 375.55
nasopharynx 478.29
syphilitic 095.8
nephrostomy 997.5
nose 478.19
congenital 748.0
nostril (anterior) (posterior) 478.19
congenital 748.0
organ or site, congenital NEC – *see* Atresia
osseous meatus (congenital) (ear) 744.03
acquired (*see also* Stricture, ear canal, acquired) 380.50
os uteri (*see also* Stricture, cervix) 622.4
oviduct – *see* Stricture, fallopian tube
pelviureteric junction 593.3
pharynx (dilation) 478.29
prostate 602.8
pulmonary, pulmonic
artery (congenital) 747.3
acquired 417.8
noncongenital 417.8
infundibulum (congenital) 746.83
valve (*see also* Endocarditis, pulmonary) 424.3
congenital 746.02
vein (congenital) 747.49
acquired 417.8
vessel NEC 417.8
punctum lacrimale 375.52
congenital 743.65
pylorus (hypertrophic) 537.0
adult 537.0
congenital 750.5
infantile 750.5
rectosigmoid 569.89
rectum (sphincter) 569.2
congenital 751.2
due to
chemical burn 947.3
irradiation 569.2
lymphogranuloma venereum 099.1
gonococcal 098.7
inflammatory 099.1
syphilitic 095.8
tuberculous (*see also* Tuberculosis) 014.8❺
renal artery 440.1
salivary duct or gland (any) 527.8
sigmoid (flexure) (*see also* Obstruction, intestine) 560.9
spermatic cord 608.85
stoma (following) (of)
colostomy 569.62
cystostomy 997.5
enterostomy 569.62
esophagostomy 530.87
gastrostomy 536.42
ileostomy 569.62
nephrostomy 997.5
tracheostomy 519.02
ureterostomy 997.5
stomach 537.89
congenital 750.7
hourglass 537.6
subaortic 746.81
hypertrophic (acquired) (idiopathic) 425.1
subglottic 478.74
syphilitic NEC 095.8
tendon (sheath) 727.81
trachea 519.19
congenital 748.3
syphilitic 095.8
tuberculous (*see also* Tuberculosis) 012.8❺
tracheostomy 519.02

Stricture – *continued*
tricuspid (valve) (*see also* Endocarditis, tricuspid) 397.0
congenital 746.1
nonrheumatic 424.2
tunica vaginalis 608.85
ureter (postoperative) 593.3
congenital 753.29
tuberculous (*see also* Tuberculosis) 016.2❺
ureteropelvic junction 593.3
congenital 753.21
ureterovesical orifice 593.3
congenital 753.22
urethra (anterior) (meatal) (organic) (posterior) (spasmodic) 598.9
associated with schistosomiasis (*see also* Schistosomiasis) 120.9 *[598.01]*
congenital (valvular) 753.6
due to
infection 598.00
syphilis 095.8 *[598.01]*
trauma 598.1
gonococcal 098.2 *[598.01]*
gonorrheal 098.2 *[598.01]*
infective 598.00
late effect of injury 598.1
postcatheterization 598.2
postobstetric 598.1
postoperative 598.2
specified cause NEC 598.8
syphilitic 095.8 *[598.01]*
traumatic 598.1
valvular, congenital 753.6
urinary meatus (*see also* Stricture, urethra) 598.9
congenital 753.6
uterus, uterine 621.5
os (external) (internal) – *see* Stricture, cervix
vagina (outlet) 623.2
congenital 752.49
valve (cardiac) (heart) (*see also* Endocarditis) 424.90
congenital (cardiac) (heart) NEC 746.89
aortic 746.3
mitral 746.5
pulmonary 746.02
tricuspid 746.1
urethra 753.6
valvular (*see also* Endocarditis) 424.90
vascular graft or shunt 996.1
atherosclerosis – *see* Arteriosclerosis, extremities
embolism 996.74
occlusion NEC 996.74
thrombus 996.74
vas deferens 608.85
congenital 752.89
vein 459.2
vena cava (inferior) (superior) NEC 459.2
congenital 747.49
ventricular shunt 996.2
vesicourethral orifice 596.0
congenital 753.6
vulva (acquired) 624.8
Stridor 786.1
congenital (larynx) 748.3
Stridulous – *see* condition
Strippling of nails 703.8
Stroke 434.91
apoplectic (*see also* Disease, cerebrovascular, acute) 436
brain – *see* Infarct, brain
embolic 434.11
epileptic – *see* Epilepsy
healed or old V12.54 ▲
heart – *see* Disease, heart
heat 992.0
hemorrhagic – *see* Hemorrhage, brain
iatrogenic 997.02
in evolution 434.91 ▲
ischemic 434.91
late effect – *see* Late effect(s)) (of) cerebrovascular disease
lightning 994.0
paralytic – *see* Infarct, brain
postoperative 997.02
progressive 435.9
thrombotic 434.01
Stromatosis, endometrial (M8931/1) 236.0
Strong pulse 785.9
Strongyloides stercoralis infestation 127.2
Strongyloidiasis 127.2

- **Supervision** (of)
  - contraceptive method previously prescribed V25.40
    - intrauterine device V25.42
    - oral contraceptive (pill) V25.41
    - specified type NEC V25.49
    - subdermal implantable contraceptive V25.43
  - dietary (for) V65.3
    - allergy (food) V65.3
    - colitis V65.3
    - diabetes mellitus V65.3
    - food allergy intolerance V65.3
    - gastritis V65.3
    - hypercholesterolemia V65.3
    - hypoglycemia V65.3
    - intolerance (food) V65.3
    - obesity V65.3
    - specified NEC V65.3
  - lactation V24.1
  - pregnancy – *see* Pregnancy, supervision of
- **Supplemental teeth** 520.1
  - causing crowding 524.31
- **Suppression**
  - binocular vision 368.31
  - lactation 676.5❺
  - menstruation 626.8
  - ovarian secretion 256.39
  - renal 586
  - urinary secretion 788.5
  - urine 788.5
- **Suppuration, suppurative** – *see also* condition
  - accessory sinus (chronic) (*see also* Sinusitis) 473.9
  - adrenal gland 255.8
  - antrum (chronic) (*see also* Sinusitis, maxillary) 473.0
  - bladder (*see also* Cystitis) 595.89
  - bowel 569.89
  - brain 324.0
    - late effect 326
  - breast 611.0
    - puerperal, postpartum 675.1❺
  - dental periosteum 526.5
  - diffuse (skin) 686.00
  - ear (middle) (*see also* Otitis media) 382.4
    - external (*see also* Otitis, externa) 380.10
    - internal 386.33
  - ethmoidal (sinus) (chronic) (*see also* Sinusitis, ethmoidal) 473.2
  - fallopian tube (*see also* Salpingo-oophoritis) 614.2
  - frontal (sinus) (chronic) (*see also* Sinusitis, frontal) 473.1
  - gallbladder (*see also* Cholecystitis, acute) 575.0
  - gum 523.30
  - hernial sac – *see* Hernia, by site
  - intestine 569.89
  - joint (*see also* Arthritis, suppurative) 711.0❺
  - labyrinthine 386.33
  - lung 513.0
  - mammary gland 611.0
    - puerperal, postpartum 675.1❺
  - maxilla, maxillary 526.4
    - sinus (chronic) (*see also* Sinusitis, maxillary) 473.0
  - muscle 728.0
  - nasal sinus (chronic) (*see also* Sinusitis) 473.9
  - pancreas 577.0
  - parotid gland 527.2
  - pelvis, pelvic
    - female (*see also* Disease, pelvis, inflammatory) 614.4
      - acute 614.3
    - male (*see also* Peritonitis) 567.21
  - pericranial (*see also* Osteomyelitis) 730.2❺
  - salivary duct or gland (any) 527.2
  - sinus (nasal) (*see also* Sinusitis) 473.9
  - sphenoidal (sinus) (chronic) (*see also* Sinusitis, sphenoidal) 473.3
  - thymus (gland) 254.1
  - thyroid (gland) 245.0
  - tonsil 474.8
  - uterus (*see also* Endometritis) 615.9
  - vagina 616.10
  - wound – *see also* Wound, open, by site, complicated
    - dislocation – *see* Dislocation, by site, compound
    - fracture – *see* Fracture, by site, open
    - scratch or other superficial injury – *see* Injury, superficial, by site
- **Supraeruption, teeth** 524.34
- **Supraglottitis** 464.50
  - with obstruction 464.51
- **Suprapubic drainage** 596.8
- **Suprarenal** (gland) – *see* condition
- **Suprascapular nerve** – *see* condition
- **Suprasellar** – *see* condition
- **Supraspinatus syndrome** 726.10
- **Surfer knots** 919.8
  - infected 919.9
- **Surgery**
  - cosmetic NEC V50.1
    - following healed injury or operation V51
    - hair transplant V50.0
  - elective V50.9
    - breast augmentation or reduction V50.1
    - circumcision, ritual or routine (in absence of medical indication) V50.2
    - cosmetic NEC V50.1
    - ear piercing V50.3
    - face-lift V50.1
    - following healed injury or operation V51
    - hair transplant V50.0
  - not done because of
    - contraindication V64.1
    - patient's decision V64.2
    - specified reason NEC V64.3
  - plastic
    - breast augmentation or reduction V50.1
    - cosmetic V50.1
    - face-lift V50.1
    - following healed injury or operation V51
    - repair of scarred tissue (following healed injury or operation) V51
    - specified type NEC V50.8
  - previous, in pregnancy or childbirth
    - cervix 654.6❺
      - affecting fetus or newborn 763.89
      - causing obstructed labor 660.2❺
        - affecting fetus or newborn 763.1
    - pelvic soft tissues NEC 654.9❺
      - affecting fetus or newborn 763.89
      - causing obstructed labor 660.2❺
        - affecting fetus or newborn 763.1
    - perineum or vulva 654.8❺
    - uterus NEC 654.9❺
      - affecting fetus or newborn 763.89
      - causing obstructed labor 660.2❺
        - affecting fetus or newborn 763.1
      - from previous cesarean delivery 654.2❺
    - vagina 654.7❺
- **Surgical**
  - abortion – *see* Abortion, legal
  - emphysema 998.81
  - kidney (*see also* Pyelitis) 590.80
  - operation NEC 799.9
  - procedures, complication or misadventure – *see* Complications, surgical procedure
  - shock 998.0
- **Susceptibility**
  - genetic
    - to
      - MEN (multiple endocrine neoplasia) V84.81 ●
      - neoplasia ●
        - multiple endocrine [MEN] V84.81 ●
      - neoplasm
        - malignant, of
          - breast V84.01
          - endometrium V84.04
          - other V84.09
          - ovary V84.02
          - prostate V84.03
      - ▶specified◀ disease ▶NEC◀ V84.89 ▲
- **Suspected condition, ruled out** (*see also* Observation, suspected) V71.9
  - specified condition NEC V71.89
- **Suspended uterus, in pregnancy or childbirth** 654.4❺
  - affecting fetus or newborn 763.89
  - causing obstructed labor 660.2❺
    - affecting fetus or newborn 763.1
- **Sutton's disease** 709.09
- **Sutton and Gull's disease** (arteriolar nephrosclerosis) (*see also* Hypertension, kidney) 403.90
- **Suture**
  - burst (in external operation wound) 998.32
    - internal 998.31
  - inadvertently left in operation wound 998.4
  - removal V58.32
  - Shirodkar, in pregnancy (with or without cervical incompetence) 654.5❺
- **Swab inadvertently left in operation wound** 998.4
- **Swallowed, swallowing**
  - difficulty (*see also* Dysphagia) 787.20 ▲
  - foreign body NEC (*see also* Foreign body) 938
- **Swamp fever** 100.89
- **Swan neck hand** (intrinsic) 736.09
- **Sweat(s), sweating**
  - disease or sickness 078.2
  - excessive (*see also* Hyperhidrosis) 780.8
  - fetid 705.89
  - fever 078.2
  - gland disease 705.9
    - specified type NEC 705.89
  - miliary 078.2
  - night 780.8
- **Sweeley-Klionsky disease** (angiokeratoma corporis diffusum) 272.7
- **Sweet's syndrome** (acute febrile neutrophilic dermatosis) 695.89
- **Swelling** 782.3 ▲
  - abdominal (not referable to specific organ) 789.3❺
  - adrenal gland, cloudy 255.8
  - ankle 719.07
  - anus 787.99
  - arm 729.81
  - breast 611.72
  - Calabar 125.2
  - cervical gland 785.6
  - cheek 784.2
  - chest 786.6
  - ear 388.8
  - epigastric 789.3❺
  - extremity (lower) (upper) 729.81
  - eye 379.92
  - female genital organ 625.8
  - finger 729.81
  - foot 729.81
  - glands 785.6
  - gum 784.2
  - hand 729.81
  - head 784.2
  - inflammatory – *see* Inflammation
  - joint (*see also* Effusion, joint) 719.0❺
    - tuberculous – *see* Tuberculosis, joint
  - kidney, cloudy 593.89
  - leg 729.81
  - limb 729.81
  - liver 573.8
  - lung 786.6
  - lymph nodes 785.6
  - mediastinal 786.6
  - mouth 784.2
  - muscle (limb) 729.81
  - neck 784.2
  - nose or sinus 784.2
  - palate 784.2
  - pelvis 789.3❺
  - penis 607.83
  - perineum 625.8
  - rectum 787.99
  - scrotum 608.86
  - skin 782.2
  - splenic (*see also* Splenomegaly) 789.2
  - substernal 786.6
  - superficial, localized (skin) 782.2
  - testicle 608.86
  - throat 784.2
  - toe 729.81
  - tongue 784.2
  - tubular (*see also* Disease, renal) 593.9
  - umbilicus 789.3❺
  - uterus 625.8
  - vagina 625.8
  - vulva 625.8
  - wandering, due to Gnathostoma (spinigerum) 128.1
  - white – *see* Tuberculosis, arthritis
- **Swift's disease** 985.0
- **Swimmers'**
  - ear (acute) 380.12
  - itch 120.3
- **Swimming in the head** 780.4
- **Swollen** – *see also* Swelling
  - glands 785.6
- **Swyer-James syndrome** (unilateral hyperlucent lung) 492.8

Swyer's syndrome (XY pure gonadal dysgenesis) 752.7
Sycosis 704.8
barbae (not parasitic) 704.8
contagiosa 110.0
lupoid 704.8
mycotic 110.0
parasitic 110.0
vulgaris 704.8
Sydenham's chorea – *see* Chorea, Sydenham's
Sylvatic yellow fever 060.0
Sylvest's disease (epidemic pleurodynia) 074.1
Symblepharon 372.63
congenital 743.62
Symonds' syndrome 348.2
Sympathetic – *see* condition
Sympatheticotonia (*see also* Neuropathy, peripheral, autonomic) 337.9
Sympathicoblastoma (M9500/3)
specified site – *see* Neoplasm, by site, malignant
unspecified site 194.0
Sympathicogonioma (M9500/3) – *see* Sympathicoblastoma
Sympathoblastoma (M9500/3) – *see* Sympathicoblastoma
Sympathogonioma (M9500/3) – *see* Sympathicoblastoma
Symphalangy (*see also* Syndactylism) 755.10
Symptoms, specified (general) NEC 780.99
abdomen NEC 789.9
bone NEC 733.90
breast NEC 611.79
cardiac NEC 785.9
cardiovascular NEC 785.9
chest NEC 786.9
development NEC 783.9
digestive system NEC 787.99
eye NEC 379.99
gastrointestinal tract NEC 787.99
genital organs NEC
female 625.9
male 608.9
head and neck NEC 784.99
heart NEC 785.9
joint NEC 719.60
ankle 719.67
elbow 719.62
foot 719.67
hand 719.64
hip 719.65
knee 719.66
multiple sites 719.69
pelvic region 719.65
shoulder (region) 719.61
specified site NEC 719.68
wrist 719.63
larynx NEC 784.99
limbs NEC 729.89
lymphatic system NEC 785.9
menopausal 627.2
metabolism NEC 783.9
mouth NEC 528.9
muscle NEC 728.9
musculoskeletal NEC 781.99
limbs NEC 729.89
nervous system NEC 781.99
neurotic NEC 300.9
nutrition, metabolism, and development NEC 783.9
pelvis NEC 789.9
female 625.9
peritoneum NEC 789.9
respiratory system NEC 786.9
skin and integument NEC 782.9
subcutaneous tissue NEC 782.9
throat NEC 784.99
tonsil NEC 784.99
urinary system NEC 788.9
vascular NEC 785.9
Sympus 759.89
Synarthrosis 719.80
ankle 719.87
elbow 719.82
foot 719.87
hand 719.84
hip 719.85
knee 719.86
multiple sites 719.89
pelvic region 719.85

Synarthrosis – *continued*
shoulder (region) 719.81
specified site NEC 719.88
wrist 719.83
Syncephalus 759.4
Synchondrosis 756.9
abnormal (congenital) 756.9
ischiopubic (van Neck's) 732.1
Synchysis (senile) (vitreous humor) 379.21
scintillans 379.22
Syncope (near) (pre-) 780.2
anginosa 413.9
bradycardia 427.89
cardiac 780.2
carotid sinus 337.0
complicating delivery 669.2❺
due to lumbar puncture 349.0
fatal 798.1
heart 780.2
heat 992.1
laryngeal 786.2
tussive 786.2
vasoconstriction 780.2
vasodepressor 780.2
vasomotor 780.2
vasovagal 780.2
Syncytial infarct – *see* Placenta, abnormal
Syndactylism, syndactyly (multiple sites) 755.10
fingers (without fusion of bone) 755.11
with fusion of bone 755.12
toes (without fusion of bone) 755.13
with fusion of bone 755.14
Syndrome – *see also* Disease
5q minus 238.74
abdominal
acute 789.0❺
migraine 346.2❺
muscle deficiency 756.79
Abercrombie's (amyloid degeneration) 277.39
abnormal innervation 374.43
abstinence
alcohol 291.81
drug 292.0
Abt-Letterer-Siwe (acute histiocytosis X) (M9722/3) 202.5❺
Achard-Thiers (adrenogenital) 255.2
acid pulmonary aspiration 997.3
obstetric (Mendelson's) 668.0❺
acquired immune deficiency 042
acquired immunodeficiency 042
acrocephalosyndactylism 755.55
acute abdominal 789.0❺
acute chest 517.3
acute coronary 411.1
Adair-Dighton (brittle bones and blue sclera, deafness) 756.51
Adams-Stokes (-Morgagni) (syncope with heart block) 426.9
Addisonian 255.41 ▲
Adie (-Holmes) (pupil) 379.46
adiposogenital 253.8
adrenal
hemorrhage 036.3
meningococcic 036.3
adrenocortical 255.3
adrenogenital (acquired) (congenital) 255.2
feminizing 255.2
iatrogenic 760.79
virilism (acquired) (congenital) 255.2
affective organic NEC 293.89
drug-induced 292.84
afferent loop NEC 537.89
African macroglobulinemia 273.3
Ahumada-Del Castillo (nonpuerperal galactorrhea and amenorrhea) 253.1
air blast concussion – *see* Injury, internal, by site
Alagille 759.89
Albright (-Martin) (pseudohypoparathyroidism) 275.49
Albright-McCune-Sternberg (osteitis fibrosa disseminata) 756.59
alcohol withdrawal 291.81
Alder's (leukocyte granulation anomaly) 288.2
Aldrich (-Wiskott) (eczema-thrombocytopenia) 279.12
Alibert-Bazin (mycosis fungoides) (M9700/3) 202.1❺
Alice in Wonderland 293.89
Allen-Masters 620.6
Alligator baby (ichthyosis congenita) 757.1

Syndrome – *continued*
Alport's (hereditary hematuria-nephropathy-deafness) 759.89
Alvarez (transient cerebral ischemia) 435.9
alveolar capillary block 516.3
Alzheimer's 331.0
with dementia – *see* Alzheimer's, dementia
amnestic (confabulatory) 294.0
alcohol-induced persisting 291.1
drug-induced 292.83
posttraumatic 294.0
amotivational 292.89
amyostatic 275.1
amyotrophic lateral sclerosis 335.20
androgen insensitivity 259.5
Angelman 759.89
angina (*see also* Angina) 413.9
ankyloglossia superior 750.0
anterior
chest wall 786.52
compartment (tibial) 958.8
spinal artery 433.8❺
compression 721.1
tibial (compartment) 958.8
antibody deficiency 279.00
agammaglobulinemic 279.00
congenital 279.04
hypogammaglobulinemic 279.00
anticardiolipin antibody 795.79
antimongolism 758.39
antiphospholipid antibody 795.79
Anton (-Babinski) (hemiasomatognosia) 307.9
anxiety (*see also* Anxiety) 300.00
organic 293.84
aortic
arch 446.7
bifurcation (occlusion) 444.0
ring 747.21
Apert's (acrocephalosyndactyly) 755.55
Apert-Gallais (adrenogenital) 255.2
aphasia-apraxia-alexia 784.69
apical ballooning 429.83
"approximate answers" 300.16
arcuate ligament (-celiac axis) 447.4
arcus aortae 446.7
arc welders' 370.24
argentaffin, argintaffinoma 259.2
Argonz-Del Castillo (nonpuerperal galactorrhea and amenorrhea) 253.1
Argyll Robertson's (syphilitic) 094.89
nonsyphilitic 379.45
arm-shoulder (*see also* Neuropathy, peripheral, autonomic) 337.9
Armenian 277.31
Arnold-Chiari (*see also* Spina bifida) 741.0❺
type I 348.4
type II 741.0❺
type III 742.0
type IV 742.2
Arrillaga-Ayerza (pulmonary artery sclerosis with pulmonary hypertension) 416.0
arteriomesenteric duodenum occlusion 537.89
arteriovenous steal 996.73
arteritis, young female (obliterative brachiocephalic) 446.7
aseptic meningitis – *see* Meningitis, aseptic
Asherman's 621.5
Asperger's 299.8
asphyctic (*see also* Anxiety) 300.00
aspiration, of newborn, (massive) 770.18
meconium 770.12
ataxia-telangiectasia 334.8
Audry's (acropachyderma) 757.39
auriculotemporal 350.8
autosomal – *see also* Abnormal, autosomes NEC
deletion 758.39
5p 758.31
22q11.2 758.32
Avellis' 344.89
Axenfeld's 743.44
Ayerza (-Arrillaga) (pulmonary artery sclerosis with pulmonary hypertension) 416.0
Baader's (erythema multiforme exudativum) 695.1
Baastrup's 721.5
Babinski (-Vaquez) (cardiovascular syphilis) 093.89
Babinski-Fröhlich (adiposogenital dystrophy) 253.8
Babinski-Nageotte 344.89
Bagratuni's (temporal arteritis) 446.5
Bakwin-Krida (craniometaphyseal dysplasia) 756.89

Syndrome – Syndrome

④ Fourth-Digit Required ⑤ Fifth-Digit Required *[code]* Manifestation Code ▶◀ Revised Text ● New Line ▲ Revised Code

- **Syndrome** – *continued*
  - compartment(al) – *continued*
    - traumatic – *continued*
      - fingers 958.91
      - foot 958.92
      - forearm 958.91
      - hand 958.91
      - hip 958.92
      - leg 958.92
      - lower extremity 958.92
      - shoulder 958.91
      - specified site NEC 958.99
      - thigh 958.92
      - tibial 958.92
      - toes 958.92
      - upper extremity 958.91
      - wrist 958.91
  - compression 958.5
    - cauda equina 344.60
      - with neurogenic bladder 344.61
  - concussion 310.2
  - congenital
    - affecting more than one system 759.7
      - specified type NEC 759.89
    - central alveolar hypoventilation 327.25
    - facial diplegia 352.6
    - muscular hypertrophy-cerebral 759.89
  - congestion-fibrosis (pelvic) 625.5
  - conjunctivourethrosynovial 099.3
  - Conn (-Louis) (primary aldosteronism) 255.12
  - Conradi (-Hünermann) (chondrodysplasia calcificans congenita) 756.59
  - conus medullaris 336.8
  - Cooke-Apert-Gallais (adrenogenital) 255.2
  - Cornelia de Lange's (Amsterdam dwarf, mental retardation, and brachycephaly) 759.8❺
  - coronary insufficiency or intermediate 411.1
  - cor pulmonale 416.9
  - corticosexual 255.2
  - Costen's (complex) 524.60
  - costochondral junction 733.6
  - costoclavicular 353.0
  - costovertebral 253.0
  - Cotard's (paranoia) 297.1
  - Cowden 759.6
  - craniovertebral 723.2
  - Creutzfeldt-Jakob (new variant) 046.1
    - with dementia
      - with behavioral disturbance 046.1 *[294.11]*
      - without behavioral disturbance 046.1 *[294.10]*
  - crib death 798.0
  - cricopharyngeal 787.20 ▲
  - cri-du-chat 758.31
  - Crigler-Najjar (congenital hyperbilirubinemia) 277.4
  - crocodile tears 351.8
  - Cronkhite-Canada 211.3
  - croup 464.4
  - CRST (cutaneous systemic sclerosis) 710.1
  - crush 958.5
  - crushed lung (*see also* Injury, internal, lung) 861.20
  - Cruveilhier-Baumgarten (cirrhosis of liver) 571.5
  - cubital tunnel 354.2
  - Cuiffini-Pancoast (M8010/3) (carcinoma, pulmonary apex) 162.3
  - Curschmann (-Batten) (-Steinert) 359.21 ▲
  - Cushing's (iatrogenic) (idiopathic) (pituitary basophilism) (pituitary-dependent) 255.0
    - overdose or wrong substance given or taken 962.0
  - Cyriax's (slipping rib) 733.99
  - cystic duct stump 576.0
  - Da Costa's (neurocirculatory asthenia) 306.2
  - Dameshek's (erythroblastic anemia) 282.49
  - Dana-Putnam (subacute combined sclerosis with pernicious anemia) 281.0 *[336.2]*
  - Danbolt (-Closs) (acrodermatitis enteropathica) 686.8
  - Dandy-Walker (atresia, foramen of Magendie) 742.3
    - with spina bifida (*see also* Spina bifida) 741.0❺
  - Danlos' 756.83
  - Davies-Colley (slipping rib) 733.99
  - dead fetus 641.3❺
  - defeminization 255.2
  - defibrination (*see also* Fibrinolysis) 286.6
  - Degos' 447.8
  - Deiters' nucleus 386.19
  - Déjérine-Roussy 338.0
  - Déjérine-Thomas 333.0
- **Syndrome** – *continued*
  - de Lange's (Amsterdam dwarf, mental retardation, and brachycephaly) (Cornelia) 759.89
  - Del Castillo's (germinal aplasia) 606.0
  - deletion chromosomes 758.39
  - delusional
    - induced by drug 292.11
  - dementia-aphonia, of childhood (*see also* Psychosis, childhood) 299.1❺
  - demyelinating NEC 341.9
  - denial visual hallucination 307.9
  - depersonalization 300.6
  - Dercum's (adiposis dolorosa) 272.8
  - de Toni-Fanconi (-Debre) (cystinosis) 270.0
  - diabetes-dwarfism-obesity (juvenile) 258.1
  - diabetes mellitus-hypertension-nephrosis 250.4❺ *[581.81]*
  - diabetes mellitus in newborn infant 775.1
  - diabetes-nephrosis 250.4❺ *[581.81]*
  - diabetic amyotrophy 250.6❺ *[353.1]* ▲
  - Diamond-Blackfan (congenital hypoplastic anemia) 284.01
  - Diamond-Gardener (autoerythrocyte sensitization) 287.2
  - DIC (diffuse or disseminated intravascular coagulopathy) (*see also* Fibrinolysis) 286.6
  - diencephalohypophyseal NEC 253.8
  - diffuse cervicobrachial 723.3
  - diffuse obstructive pulmonary 496
  - DiGeorge's (thymic hypoplasia) 279.11
  - Dighton's 756.51
  - Di Guglielmo's (erythremic myelosis) (M9841/3) 207.0❺
  - disequilibrium 276.9
  - disseminated platelet thrombosis 446.6
  - Ditthomska 307.81
  - Doan-Wiseman (primary splenic neutropenia) 289.53
  - Döhle body-panmyelopathic 288.2
  - Donohue's (leprechaunism) 259.8
  - dorsolateral medullary (*see also* Disease, cerebrovascular, acute) 436
  - double athetosis 333.71
  - double whammy 360.81
  - Down's (mongolism) 758.0
  - Dresbach's (elliptocytosis) 282.1
  - Dressler's (postmyocardial infarction) 411.0
    - hemoglobinuria 283.2
    - postcardiotomy 429.4
  - drug withdrawal, infant, of dependent mother 779.5
  - dry skin 701.1
    - eye 375.15
  - DSAP (disseminated superficial actinic porokeratosis) 692.75
  - Duane's (retraction) 378.71
  - Duane-Stilling-Türk (ocular retraction syndrome) 378.71
  - Dubin-Johnson (constitutional hyperbilirubinemia) 277.4
  - Dubin-Sprinz (constitutional hyperbilirubinemia) 277.4
  - Duchenne's 335.22
  - due to abnormality
    - autosomal NEC (*see also* Abnormal, autosomes NEC) 758.5
      - 13 758.1
      - 18 758.2
      - 21 or 22 758.0
      - D_1 758.1
      - E_3 758.2
      - G 758.0
    - chromosomal 758.89
      - sex 758.81
  - dumping 564.2
    - nonsurgical 536.8
  - Duplay's 726.2
  - Dupré's (meningism) 781.6
  - Dyke-Young (acquired macrocytic hemolytic anemia) 283.9
  - dyspraxia 315.4
  - dystocia, dystrophia 654.9❺
  - Eagle-Barret 756.71
  - Eales' 362.18
  - Eaton-Lambert (*see also* Neoplasm, by site, malignant) 199.1 *[358.1]*
  - Ebstein's (downward displacement, tricuspid valve into right ventricle) 746.2
  - ectopic ACTH secretion 255.0
  - eczema-thrombocytopenia 279.12
  - Eddowes' (brittle bones and blue sclera) 756.51
- **Syndrome** – *continued*
  - Edwards' 758.2
  - efferent loop 537.89
  - effort (aviators') (psychogenic) 306.2
  - Ehlers-Danlos 756.83
  - Eisenmenger's (ventricular septal defect) 745.4
  - Ekbom's (restless legs) 333.94
  - Ekman's (brittle bones and blue sclera) 756.51
  - electric feet 266.2
  - Elephant man 237.71
  - Ellison-Zollinger (gastric hypersecretion with pancreatic islet cell tumor) 251.5
  - Ellis-van Creveld (chondroectodermal dysplasia) 756.55
  - embryonic fixation 270.2
  - empty sella (turcica) 253.8
  - endocrine-hypertensive 255.3
  - Engel-von Recklinghausen (osteitis fibrosa cystica) 252.01
  - enteroarticular 099.3
  - entrapment – *see* Neuropathy, entrapment
  - eosinophilia myalgia 710.5
  - epidemic vomiting 078.82
  - Epstein's – *see* Nephrosis
  - Erb (-Oppenheim)-Goldflam 358.00
  - Erdheim's (acromegalic macrospondylitis) 253.0
  - Erlacher-Blount (tibia vara) 732.4
  - erythrocyte fragmentation 283.19
  - euthyroid sick 790.94
  - Evans' (thrombocytopenic purpura) 287.32
  - excess cortisol, iatrogenic 255.0
  - exhaustion 300.5
  - extrapyramidal 333.90
  - eyelid-malar-mandible 756.0
  - eye retraction 378.71
  - Faber's (achlorhydric anemia) 280.9
  - Fabry (-Anderson) (angiokeratoma corporis diffusum) 272.7
  - facet 724.8
  - Fallot's 745.2
  - falx (*see also* Hemorrhage, brain) 431
  - familial eczema-thrombocytopenia 279.12
  - Fanconi's (anemia) (congenital pancytopenia) 284.09
  - Fanconi (-de Toni) (-Debré) (cystinosis) 270.0
  - Farber (-Uzman) (disseminated lipogranulomatosis) 272.8
  - fatigue NEC 300.5
    - chronic 780.71
  - faulty bowel habit (idiopathic megacolon) 564.7
  - FDH (focal dermal hypoplasia) 757.39
  - fecal reservoir 560.39
  - Feil-Klippel (brevicollis) 756.16
  - Felty's (rheumatoid arthritis with splenomegaly and leukopenia) 714.1
  - fertile eunuch 257.2
  - fetal alcohol 760.71
    - late effect 760.71
  - fibrillation-flutter 427.32
  - fibrositis (periarticular) 729.0
  - Fiedler's (acute isolated myocarditis) 422.91
  - Fiessinger-Leroy (-Reiter) 099.3
  - Fiessinger-Rendu (erythema multiforme exudativum) 695.1
  - first arch 756.0
  - fish odor 270.8
  - Fisher's 357.0
  - Fitz's (acute hemorrhagic pancreatitis) 577.0
  - Fitz-Hugh and Curtis 098.86
    - due to
      - Chlamydia trachomatis 099.56
      - Neisseria gonorrhoeae (gonoccocal peritonitis) 098.86
  - Flajani (-Basedow) (exophthalmic goiter) 242.0❺
  - floppy
    - infant 781.99
    - iris 364.81 ●
    - valve (mitral) 424.0
  - flush 259.2
  - Foix-Alajouanine 336.1
  - Fong's (hereditary osteo-onychodysplasia) 756.89
  - foramen magnum 348.4
  - Forbes-Albright (nonpuerperal amenorrhea and lactation associated with pituitary tumor) 253.1
  - Foster-Kennedy 377.04
  - Foville's (peduncular) 344.89
  - fragile X 759.83
  - Franceschetti's (mandibulofacial dysostosis) 756.0
  - Fraser's 759.89
  - Freeman-Sheldon 759.89

Syndrome – *continued*
- Frey's (auriculotemporal) 705.22
- Friderichsen-Waterhouse 036.3
- Friedrich-Erb-Arnold (acropachyderma) 757.39
- Fröhlich's (adiposogenital dystrophy) 253.8
- Froin's 336.8
- Frommel-Chiari 676.6 (5)
- frontal lobe 310.0
- Fukuhara 277.87
- Fuller Albright's (osteitis fibrosa disseminata) 756.59
- functional
  - bowel 564.9
  - prepubertal castrate 752.89
- Gaisböck's (polycythemia hypertonica) 289.0
- ganglion (basal, brain) 333.90
  - geniculi 351.1
- Ganser's, hysterical 300.16
- Gardner-Diamond (autoerythrocyte sensitization) 287.2
- gastroesophageal junction 530.0
- gastroesophageal laceration-hemorrhage 530.7
- gastrojejunal loop obstruction 537.89
- Gayet-Wernicke's (superior hemorrhagic polioencephalitis) 265.1
- Gee-Herter-Heubner (nontropical sprue) 579.0
- Gélineau's (*see also* Narcolepsy) 347.00
- genito-anorectal 099.1
- Gerhardt's (vocal cord paralysis) 478.30
- Gerstmann's (finger agnosia) 784.69
- Gianotti Crosti 057.8
  - due to known virus – *see* Infection, virus
  - due to unknown virus 057.8
- Gilbert's 277.4
- Gilford (-Hutchinson) (progeria) 259.8
- Gilles de la Tourette's 307.23
- Gillespie's (dysplasia oculodentodigitalis) 759.89
- Glénard's (enteroptosis) 569.89
- Glinski-Simmonds (pituitary cachexia) 253.2
- glucuronyl transferase 277.4
- glue ear 381.20
- Goldberg (-Maxwell) (-Morris) (testicular feminization) 259.5
- Goldenhar's (oculoauriculovertebral dysplasia) 756.0
- Goldflam-Erb 358.00
- Goltz-Gorlin (dermal hypoplasia) 757.39
- Goodpasture's (pneumorenal) 446.21
- Good's 279.06
- Gopalan's (burning feet) 266.2
- Gorlin-Chaudhry-Moss 759.89
- Gougerot (-Houwer)-Sjögren (keratoconjunctivitis sicca) 710.2
- Gougerot-Blum (pigmented purpuric lichenoid dermatitis) 709.1
- Gougerot-Carteaud (confluent reticulate papillomatosis) 701.8
- Gouley's (constrictive pericarditis) 423.2
- Gowers' (vasovagal attack) 780.2
- Gowers-Paton-Kennedy 377.04
- Gradenigo's 383.02
- Gray or grey (chloramphenicol) (newborn) 779.4
- Greig's (hypertelorism) 756.0
- Gubler-Millard 344.89
- Guérin-Stern (arthrogryposis multiplex congenita) 754.89
- Guillain-Barré (-Strohl) 357.0
- Gunn's (jaw-winking syndrome) 742.8
- Günther's (congenital erythropoietic porphyria) 277.1
- gustatory sweating 350.8
- H_3O 759.81
- Hadfield-Clarke (pancreatic infantilism) 577.8
- Haglund-Läwen-Fründ 717.89
- hair tourniquet – *see also* Injury, superficial, by site
  - finger 915.8
    - infected 915.9
  - penis 911.8
    - infected 911.9
  - toe 917.8
    - infected 917.9
- hairless women 257.8
- Hallermann-Strieff 756.0
- Hallervorden-Spatz 333.0
- Hamman's (spontaneous mediastinal emphysema) 518.1
- Hamman-Rich (diffuse interstitial pulmonary fibrosis) 516.3
- Hand-Schüller-Christian (chronic histiocytosis X) 277.89
- hand-foot 693.0 ▲

Syndrome – *continued*
- Hanot-Chauffard (-Troisier) (bronze diabetes) 275.0
- Harada's 363.22
- Hare's (M8010/3) (carcinoma, pulmonary apex) 162.3
- Harkavy's 446.0
- harlequin color change 779.89
- Harris' (organic hyperinsulinism) 251.1
- Hart's (pellagra-cerebellar ataxia-renal aminoaciduria) 270.0
- Hayem-Faber (achlorhydric anemia) 280.9
- Hayem-Widal (acquired hemolytic jaundice) 283.9
- Heberden's (angina pectoris) 413.9
- Hedinger's (malignant carcinoid) 259.2
- Hegglin's 288.2
- Heller's (infantile psychosis) (*see also* Psychosis, childhood) 299.1 (5)
- H.E.L.L.P 642.5 (5)
- hemolytic-uremic (adult) (child) 283.11
- hemophagocytic 288.4
  - infection-associated 288.4
- Hench-Rosenberg (palindromic arthritis) (*see also* Rheumatism, palindromic) 719.3 (5)
- Henoch-Schönlein (allergic purpura) 287.0
- hepatic flexure 569.89
- hepatorenal 572.4
  - due to a procedure 997.4
  - following delivery 674.8 (5)
- hepatourologic 572.4
- Herrick's (hemoglobin S disease) 282.61
- Herter (-Gee) (nontropical sprue) 579.0
- Heubner-Herter (nontropical sprue) 579.0
- Heyd's (hepatorenal) 572.4
- HHHO 759.81
- high grade myelodysplastic 238.73
  - with 5q deletion 238.73
- Hilger's 337.0
- histiocytic 288.4
- Hoffa (-Kastert) (liposynovitis prepatellaris) 272.8
- Hoffmann's 244.9 *[359.5]*
- Hoffmann-Bouveret (paroxysmal tachycardia) 427.2
- Hoffmann-Werdnig 335.0
- Holländer-Simons (progressive lipodystrophy) 272.6
- Holmes' (visual disorientation) 368.16
- Holmes-Adie 379.46
- Hoppe-Goldflam 358.00
- Horner's (*see also* Neuropathy, peripheral, autonomic) 337.9
  - traumatic – *see* Injury, nerve, cervical sympathetic
- hospital addiction 301.51
- Hunt's (herpetic geniculate ganglionitis) 053.11
  - dyssynergia cerebellaris myoclonica 334.2
- Hunter (-Hurler) (mucopolysaccharidosis II) 277.5
- hunterian glossitis 529.4
- Hurler (-Hunter) (mucopolysaccharidosis II) 277.5
- Hutchinson's incisors or teeth 090.5
- Hutchinson-Boeck (sarcoidosis) 135
- Hutchinson-Gilford (progeria) 259.8
- hydralazine
  - correct substance properly administered 695.4
  - overdose or wrong substance given or taken 972.6
- hydraulic concussion (abdomen) (*see also* Injury, internal, abdomen) 868.00
- hyperabduction 447.8
- hyperactive bowel 564.9
- hyperaldosteronism with hypokalemic alkalosis (Bartter's) 255.13
- hypercalcemic 275.42
- hypercoagulation NEC 289.89
- hypereosinophilic (idiopathic) 288.3
- hyperkalemic 276.7
- hyperkinetic – *see also* Hyperkinesia heart 429.82
- hyperlipemia-hemolytic anemia-icterus 571.1
- hypermobility 728.5
- hypernatremia 276.0
- hyperosmolarity 276.0
- hyperperfusion 997.01 ●
- hypersomnia-bulimia 349.89
- hypersplenic 289.4
- hypersympathetic (*see also* Neuropathy, peripheral, autonomic) 337.9
- hypertransfusion, newborn 776.4
- hyperventilation, psychogenic 306.1
- hyperviscosity (of serum) NEC 273.3
  - polycythemic 289.0
  - sclerothymic 282.8

Syndrome – *continued*
- hypoglycemic (familial) (neonatal) 251.2
  - functional 251.1
- hypokalemic 276.8
- hypophyseal 253.8
- hypophyseothalamic 253.8
- hypopituitarism 253.2
- hypoplastic left heart 746.7
- hypopotassemia 276.8
- hyposmolality 276.1
- hypotension, maternal 669.2 (5)
- hypothenar hammer 443.89 ●
- hypotonia-hypomentia-hypogonadism-obesity 759.81
- ICF (intravascular coagulation-fibrinolysis) (*see also* Fibrinolysis) 286.6
- idiopathic cardiorespiratory distress, newborn 769
- idiopathic nephrotic (infantile) 581.9
- iliotibial band 728.89
- Imerslund (-Gräsbeck) (anemia due to familial selective vitamin B12 malabsorption) 281.1
- immobility (paraplegic) 728.3
- immunity deficiency, combined 279.2
- impending coronary 411.1
- impingement
  - shoulder 726.2
  - vertebral bodies 724.4
- inappropriate secretion of antidiuretic hormone (ADH) 253.6
- incomplete
  - mandibulofacial 756.0
- infant
  - death, sudden (SIDS) 798.0
  - Hercules 255.2
  - of diabetic mother 775.0
  - shaken 995.55
- infantilism 253.3
- inferior vena cava 459.2
- influenza-like 487.1
- inspissated bile, newborn 774.4
- insufficient sleep 307.44
- intermediate coronary (artery) 411.1
- internal carotid artery (*see also* Occlusion, artery, carotid) 433.1 (5)
- interspinous ligament 724.8
- intestinal
  - carcinoid 259.2
  - gas 787.3
  - knot 560.2
- intraoperative floppy iris (IFIS) 364.81 ●
- intravascular
  - coagulation-fibrinolysis (ICF) (*see also* Fibrinolysis) 286.6
  - coagulopathy (*see also* Fibrinolysis) 286.6
- inverted Marfan's 759.89
- IRDS (idiopathic respiratory distress, newborn) 769
- irritable
  - bowel 564.1
  - heart 306.2
  - weakness 300.5
- ischemic bowel (transient) 557.9
  - chronic 557.1
  - due to mesenteric artery insufficiency 557.1
- Itsenko-Cushing (pituitary basophilism) 255.0
- IVC (intravascular coagulopathy) (*see also* Fibrinolysis) 286.6
- Ivemark's (asplenia with congenital heart disease) 759.0
- Jaccoud's 714.4
- Jackson's 344.89
- Jadassohn-Lewandowski (pachyonchia congenita) 757.5
- Jaffe-Lichtenstein (-Uehlinger) 252.01
- Jahnke's (encephalocutaneous angiomatosis) 759.6
- Jakob-Creutzfeldt (new variant) 046.1
  - with dementia
    - with behavioral disturbance 046.1 *[294.11]*
    - without behavioral disturbance 046.1 *[294.10]*
- Jaksch's (pseudoleukemia infantum) 285.8
- Jaksch-Hayem (-Luzet) (pseudoleukemia infantum) 285.8
- jaw-winking 742.8
- jejunal 564.2
- Jervell-Lange-Nielsen 426.82
- jet lag 327.35
- Jeune's (asphyxiating thoracic dystrophy of newborn) 756.4
- Job's (chronic granulomatous disease) 288.1

(4) Fourth-Digit Required (5) Fifth-Digit Required *[code]* Manifestation Code ►◄ Revised Text ● New Line ▲ Revised Code

④ Fourth-Digit Required ⑤ Fifth-Digit Required *[code]* Manifestation Code ▶◀ Revised Text ● New Line ▲ Revised Code

Syndrome – *continued*
- Sturge-Weber (-Dimitri) (encephalocutaneous angiomatosis) 759.6
- subclavian-carotid obstruction (chronic) 446.7
- subclavian steal 435.2
- subcoracoid-pectoralis minor 447.8
- subcostal 098.86
  - nerve compression 354.8
- subperiosteal hematoma 267
- subphrenic interposition 751.4
- sudden infant death (SIDS) 798.0
- Sudeck's 733.7
- Sudeck-Leriche 733.7
- superior
  - cerebellar artery (*see also* Disease, cerebrovascular, acute) 436
  - mesenteric artery 557.1
  - pulmonary sulcus (tumor) (M8010/3) 162.3
  - vena cava 459.2
- suprarenal cortical 255.3
- supraspinatus 726.10
- swallowed blood 777.3
- sweat retention 705.1
- Sweet's (acute febrile neutrophilic dermatosis) 695.89
- Swyer-James (unilateral hyperlucent lung) 492.8
- Swyer's (XY pure gonadal dysgenesis) 752.7
- Symonds' 348.2
- sympathetic
  - cervical paralysis 337.0
  - pelvic 625.5
- syndactylic oxycephaly 755.55
- syphilitic-cardiovascular 093.89
- systemic
  - fibrosclerosing 710.8
  - inflammatory response (SIRS) 995.90
    - due to
      - infectious process 995.91
        - with acute organ dysfunction 995.92
      - non-infectious process 995.93
        - with acute organ dysfunction 995.94
- systolic click (-murmur) 785.2
- Tabagism 305.1
- tachycardia-bradycardia 427.81
- Takayasu (-Onishi) (pulseless disease) 446.7
- Takotsubo 429.83
- Tapia's 352.6
- tarsal tunnel 355.5
- Taussig-Bing (transposition, aorta and overriding pulmonary artery) 745.11
- Taybi's (otopalatodigital) 759.89
- Taylor's 625.5
- teething 520.7
- tegmental 344.89
- telangiectasis-pigmentation-cataract 757.33
- temporal 383.02
  - lobectomy behavior 310.0
- temporomandibular joint-pain-dysfunction [TMJ] NEC 524.60
  - specified NEC 524.69
- Terry's 362.21
- testicular feminization 259.5
- testis, nonvirilizing 257.8
- tethered (spinal) cord 742.59
- thalamic 338.0
- Thibierge-Weissenbach (cutaneous systemic sclerosis) 710.1
- Thiele 724.6
- thoracic outlet (compression) 353.0
- thoracogenous rheumatic (hypertrophic pulmonary osteoarthropathy) 731.2
- Thorn's (*see also* Disease, renal) 593.9
- Thorson-Biörck (malignant carcinoid) 259.2
- thrombopenia-hemangioma 287.39
- thyroid-adrenocortical insufficiency 258.1
- Tietze's 733.6
- time-zone (rapid) 327.35
- Tobias' (carcinoma, pulmonary apex) (M8010/3) 162.3
- toilet seat 926.0
- Tolosa-Hunt 378.55
- Toni-Fanconi (cystinosis) 270.0
- Touraine's (hereditary osteo-onychodysplasia) 756.89
- Touraine-Solente-Golé (acropachyderma) 757.39
- toxic
  - oil 710.5
  - shock 040.82
- transfusion
  - fetal-maternal 772.0
  - twin
    - donor (infant) 772.0

Syndrome – *continued*
- transfusion – *continued*
  - twin – *continued*
    - recipient (infant) 776.4
- transient left ventricular apical ballooning 429.83
- Treacher Collins' (incomplete mandibulofacial dysostosis) 756.0
- trigeminal plate 259.8
- triplex X female 758.81
- trisomy NEC 758.5
  - 13 or D_1 758.1
  - 16-18 or E 758.2
  - 18 or E_3 758.2
  - 20 758.5
  - 21 or G (mongolism) 758.0
  - 22 or G (mongolism) 758.0
  - G 758.0
- Troisier-Hanot-Chauffard (bronze diabetes) 275.0
- tropical wet feet 991.4
- Trousseau's (thrombophlebitis migrans visceral cancer) 453.1
- Türk's (ocular retraction syndrome) 378.71
- Turner's 758.6
- Turner-Varny 758.6
- twin-to-twin transfusion 762.3
  - recipient twin 776.4
- Uehlinger's (acropachyderma) 757.39
- Ullrich (-Bonnevie) (-Turner) 758.6
- Ullrich-Feichtiger 759.89
- underwater blast injury (abdominal) (*see also* Injury, internal, abdomen) 868.00
- universal joint, cervix 620.6
- Unverricht (-Lundborg) 333.2
- Unverricht-Wagner (dermatomyositis) 710.3
- upward gaze 378.81
- Urbach-Oppenheim (necrobiosis lipoidica diabeticorum) 250.8❺ *[709.3]*
- Urbach-Wiethe (lipoid proteinosis) 272.8
- uremia, chronic 585.9
- urethral 597.81
- urethro-oculoarticular 099.3
- urethro-oculosynovial 099.3
- urohepatic 572.4
- uveocutaneous 364.24
- uveomeningeal, uveomeningitis 363.22
- vagohypoglossal 352.6
- vagovagal 780.2
- van Buchem's (hyperostosis corticalis) 733.3
- van der Hoeve's (brittle bones and blue sclera, deafness) 756.51
- van der Hoeve-Halbertsma-Waardenburg (ptosis-epicanthus) 270.2
- van der Hoeve-Waarderburg-Gualdi (ptosis-epicanthus) 270.2
- van Neck-Odelberg (juvenile osteochondrosis) 732.1
- vanishing twin 651.33
- vascular splanchnic 557.0
- vasomotor 443.9
- vasovagal 780.2
- VATER 759.89
- Velo-cardio-facial 758.32
- vena cava (inferior) (superior) (obstruction) 459.2
- Verbiest's (claudicatio intermittens spinalis) 435.1
- Vernet's 352.6
- vertebral
  - artery 435.1
    - compression 721.1
  - lumbar 724.4
  - steal 435.1
- vertebrogenic (pain) 724.5
- vertiginous NEC 386.9
- video display tube 723.8
- Villaret's 352.6
- Vinson-Plummer (sideropenic dysphagia) 280.8
- virilizing adrenocortical hyperplasia, congenital 255.2
- virus, viral 079.99
- visceral larval migrans 128.0
- visual disorientation 368.16
- vitamin B_6 deficiency 266.1
- vitreous touch 997.99
- Vogt's (corpus striatum) 333.71
- Vogt-Koyanagi 364.24
- Volkmann's 958.6
- von Bechterew-Stumpell (ankylosing spondylitis) 720.0
- von Graefe's 378.72
- von Hippel-Lindau (angiomatosis retinocerebellosa) 759.6

Syndrome – *continued*
- von Schroetter's (intermittent venous claudication) 453.8
- von Willebrand (-Jürgens) (angiohemophilia) 286.4
- Waardenburg-Klein (ptosis epicanthus) 270.2
- Wagner (-Unverricht) (dermatomyositis) 710.3
- Waldenström's (macroglobulinemia) 273.3
- Waldenström-Kjellberg (sideropenic dysphagia) 280.8
- Wallenberg's (posterior inferior cerebellar artery) (*see also* Disease, cerebrovascular, acute) 436
- Waterhouse (-Friderichsen) 036.3
- water retention 276.6
- Weber's 344.89
- Weber-Christian (nodular nonsuppurative panniculitis) 729.30
- Weber-Cockayne (epidermolysis bullosa) 757.39
- Weber-Dimitri (encephalocutaneous angiomatosis) 759.6
- Weber-Gubler 344.89
- Weber-Leyden 344.89
- Weber-Osler (familial hemorrhagic telangiectasia) 448.0
- Wegener's (necrotizing respiratory granulomatosis) 446.4
- Weill-Marchesani (brachymorphism and ectopia lentis) 759.89
- Weingarten's (tropical eosinophilia) 518.3
- Weiss-Baker (carotid sinus syncope) 337.0
- Weissenbach-Thibierge (cutaneous systemic sclerosis) 710.1
- Werdnig-Hoffmann 335.0
- Werlhof-Wichmann (*see also* Purpura, thrombocytopenic) 287.39
- Wermer's (polyendocrine adenomatosis) 258.01 ▲
- Werner's (progeria adultorum) 259.8
- Wernicke's (nonalcoholic) (superior hemorrhagic polioencephalitis) 265.1
- Wernicke-Korsakoff (nonalcoholic) 294.0
  - alcoholic 291.1
- Westphal-Strümpell (hepatolenticular degeneration) 275.1
- wet
  - brain (alcoholic) 303.9❺
  - feet (maceration) (tropical) 991.4
  - lung
    - adult 518.5
    - newborn 770.6
- whiplash 847.0
- Whipple's (intestinal lipodystrophy) 040.2
- "whistling face" (craniocarpotarsal dystrophy) 759.89
- Widal (-Abrami) (acquired hemolytic jaundice) 283.9
- Wilkie's 557.1
- Wilkinson-Sneddon (subcorneal pustular dermatosis) 694.1
- Willan-Plumbe (psoriasis) 696.1
- Willebrand (-Jürgens) (angiohemophilia) 286.4
- Willi-Prader (hypogenital dystrophy with diabetic tendency) 759.81
- Wilson's (hepatolenticular degeneration) 275.1
- Wilson-Mikity 770.7
- Wiskott-Aldrich (eczema-thrombocytopenia) 279.12
- withdrawal
  - alcohol 291.81
  - drug 292.0
    - infant of dependent mother 779.5
- Woakes' (ethmoiditis) 471.1
- Wolff-Parkinson-White (anomalous atrioventricular excitation) 426.7
- Wright's (hyperabduction) 447.8
- X
  - cardiac 413.9
  - dysmetabolic 277.7
- xiphoidalgia 733.99
- XO 758.6
- XXX 758.81
- XXXXY 758.81
- XXY 758.7
- yellow vernix (placental dysfunction) 762.2
- Zahorsky's 074.0
- Zellweger 277.86
- Zieve's (jaundice, hyperlipemia and hemolytic anemia) 571.1
- Zollinger-Ellison (gastric hypersecretion with pancreatic islet cell tumor) 251.5
- Zuelzer-Ogden (nutritional megaloblastic anemia) 281.2

Synechia (iris) (pupil) 364.70
anterior 364.72
peripheral 364.73
intrauterine (traumatic) 621.5
posterior 364.71
vulvae, congenital 752.49
Synesthesia (*see also* Disturbance, sensation) 782.0
Synodontia 520.2
Synophthalmus 759.89
Synorchidism 752.89
Synorchism 752.89
Synostosis (congenital) 756.59
astragaloscaphoid 755.67
radioulnar 755.53
talonavicular (bar) 755.67
tarsal 755.67
Synovial – *see* condition
Synovioma (M9040/3) – *see also* Neoplasm, connective tissue, malignant
benign (M9040/0) – *see* Neoplasm, connective tissue, benign
Synoviosarcoma (M9040/3) – *see* Neoplasm, connective tissue, malignant
Synovitis 727.00
chronic crepitant, wrist 727.2
due to crystals – *see* Arthritis, due to crystals
gonococcal 098.51
gouty 274.0
syphilitic 095.7
congenital 090.0
traumatic, current – *see* Sprain, by site
tuberculous – *see* Tuberculosis, synovitis
villonodular 719.20
ankle 719.27
elbow 719.22
foot 719.27
hand 719.24
hip 719.25
knee 719.26
multiple sites 719.29
pelvic region 719.25
shoulder (region) 719.21
specified site NEC 719.28
wrist 719.23
Syphilide 091.3
congenital 090.0
newborn 090.0
tubercular 095.8
congenital 090.0
Syphilis, syphilitic (acquired) 097.9
with lung involvement 095.1
abdomen (late) 095.2
acoustic nerve 094.86
adenopathy (secondary) 091.4
adrenal (gland) 095.8
with cortical hypofunction 095.8
age under 2 years NEC (*see also* Syphilis, congenital) 090.9 ⑤
acquired 097.9
alopecia (secondary) 091.82
anemia 095.8
aneurysm (artery) (ruptured) 093.89
aorta 093.0
central nervous system 094.89
congenital 090.5
anus 095.8
primary 091.1
secondary 091.3
aorta, aortic (arch) (abdominal) (insufficiency) (pulmonary) (regurgitation) (stenosis) (thoracic) 093.89
aneurysm 093.0
arachnoid (adhesive) 094.2
artery 093.89
cerebral 094.89
spinal 094.89
arthropathy (neurogenic) (tabetic) 094.0 *[713.5]*
asymptomatic – *see* Syphilis, latent
ataxia, locomotor (progressive) 094.0
atrophoderma maculatum 091.3
auricular fibrillation 093.89
Bell's palsy 094.89
bladder 095.8
bone 095.5
secondary 091.61
brain 094.89
breast 095.8
bronchus 095.8
bubo 091.0
bulbar palsy 094.89

Syphilis, syphilitic – *continued*
bursa (late) 095.7
cardiac decompensation 093.89
cardiovascular (early) (late) (primary) (secondary) (tertiary) 093.9
specified type and site NEC 093.89
causing death under 2 years of age (*see also* Syphilis, congenital) 090.9 ⑤
stated to be acquired NEC 097.9
central nervous system (any site) (early) (late) (latent) (primary) (recurrent) (relapse) (secondary) (tertiary) 094.9
with
ataxia 094.0
paralysis, general 094.1
juvenile 090.40
paresis (general) 094.1
juvenile 090.40
tabes (dorsalis) 094.0
juvenile 090.40
taboparesis 094.1
juvenile 090.40
aneurysm (ruptured) 094.87
congenital 090.40
juvenile 090.40
remission in (sustained) 094.9
serology doubtful, negative, or positive 094.9
specified nature or site NEC 094.89
vascular 094.89
cerebral 094.89
meningovascular 094.2
nerves 094.89
sclerosis 094.89
thrombosis 094.89
cerebrospinal 094.89
tabetic 094.0
cerebrovascular 094.89
cervix 095.8
chancre (multiple) 091.0
extragenital 091.2
Rollet's 091.2
Charcôt's joint 094.0 *[713.5]*
choked disc 094.89 *[377.00]*
chorioretinitis 091.51
congenital 090.0 *[363.13]*
late 094.83
choroiditis 091.51
congenital 090.0 *[363.13]*
late 094.83
prenatal 090.0 *[363.13]*
choroidoretinitis (secondary) 091.51
congenital 090.0 *[363.13]*
late 094.83
ciliary body (secondary) 091.52
late 095.8 *[364.11]*
colon (late) 095.8
combined sclerosis 094.89
complicating pregnancy, childbirth, or puerperium 647.0 ⑤
affecting fetus or newborn 760.2
condyloma (latum) 091.3
congenital 090.9 ⑤
with
encephalitis 090.41
paresis (general) 090.40
tabes (dorsalis) 090.40
taborparesis 090.40
chorioretinitis, choroiditis 090.0 *[363.13]*
early or less than 2 years after birth NEC 090.2
with manifestations 090.0
latent (without manifestations) 090.1
negative spinal fluid test 090.1
serology, positive 090.1
symptomatic 090.0
interstitial keratitis 090.3
juvenile neurosyphilis 090.40
late or 2 years or more after birth NEC 090.7 ⑤
chorioretinitis, choroiditis 090.5 *[363.13]*
interstitial keratitis 090.3
juvenile neurosyphilis NEC 090.40
latent (without manifestations) 090.6 ⑤
negative spinal fluid test 090.6 ⑤
serology, positive 090.6 ⑤
symptomatic or with manifestations NEC 090.5
interstitial keratitis 090.3
conjugal 097.9
tabes 094.0
conjunctiva 095.8 *[372.10]*
contact V01.6
cord, bladder 094.0

Syphilis, syphilitic – *continued*
cornea, late 095.8 *[370.59]*
coronary (artery) 093.89
sclerosis 093.89
coryza 095.8
congenital 090.0
cranial nerve 094.89
cutaneous – *see* Syphilis, skin
dacryocystitis 095.8
degeneration, spinal cord 094.89
d'emblée 095.8
dementia 094.1
paralytica 094.1
juvenilis 090.40
destruction of bone 095.5
dilatation, aorta 093.0
due to blood transfusion 097.9
dura mater 094.89
ear 095.8
inner 095.8
nerve (eighth) 094.86
neurorecurrence 094.86
early NEC 091.0
cardiovascular 093.9
central nervous system 094.9
paresis 094.1
tabes 094.0
latent (without manifestations) (less than 2 years after infection) 092.9
negative spinal fluid test 092.9
serological relapse following treatment 092.0
serology positive 092.9
paresis 094.1
relapse (treated, untreated) 091.7
skin 091.3
symptomatic NEC 091.89
extragenital chancre 091.2
primary, except extragenital chancre 091.0
secondary (*see also* Syphilis, secondary) 091.3
relapse (treated, untreated) 091.7
tabes 094.0
ulcer 091.3
eighth nerve 094.86
endemic, nonveneral 104.0
endocarditis 093.20
aortic 093.22
mitral 093.21
pulmonary 093.24
tricuspid 093.23
epididymis (late) 095.8
epiglottis 095.8
epiphysitis congenital) 090.0
esophagus 095.8
Eustachian tube 095.8
exposure to V01.6
eye 095.8 *[363.13]*
neuromuscular mechanism 094.85
eyelid 095.8 *[373.5]*
with gumma 095.8 *[373.5]*
ptosis 094.89
fallopian tube 095.8
fracture 095.5
gallbladder (late) 095.8
gastric 095.8
crisis 094.0
polyposis 095.8
general 097.9
paralysis 094.1
juvenile 090.40
genital (primary) 091.0
glaucoma 095.8
gumma (late) NEC 095.9
cardiovascular system 093.9
central nervous system 094.9
congenital 090.5
heart or artery 093.89
heart 093.89
block 093.89
decompensation 093.89
disease 093.89
failure 093.89
valve (*see also* Syphilis, endocarditis) 093.20
hemianesthesia 094.89
hemianopsia 095.8
hemiparesis 094.89
hemiplegia 094.89
hepatic artery 093.89
hepatitis 095.3
hepatomegaly 095.3
congenital 090.0

Syphilis, syphilitic – *continued*
- hereditaria tarda (*see also* Syphilis, congenital, late) 090.7❺
- hereditary (*see also* Syphilis, congenital) 090.9❺
  - interstitial keratitis 090.3
- Hutchinson's teeth 090.5
- hyalitis 095.8
- inactive – *see* Syphilis, latent
- infantum NEC (*see also* Syphilis, congenital) 090.9❺
- inherited – *see* Syphilis, congenital
- internal ear 095.8
- intestine (late) 095.8
- iris, iritis (secondary) 091.52
  - late 095.8 *[364.11]*
- joint (late) 095.8
- keratitis (congenital) (early) (interstitial) (late) (parenchymatous) (punctata profunda) 090.3
- kidney 095.4
- lacrimal apparatus 095.8
- laryngeal paralysis 095.8
- larynx 095.8
- late 097.0
  - cardiovascular 093.9
  - central nervous system 094.9
  - latent or 2 years or more after infection (without manifestation) 096
    - negative spinal fluid test 096
    - serology positive 096
  - paresis 094.1
  - specified site NEC 095.8
  - symptomatic or with symptoms 095.9
  - tabes 094.0
- latent 097.1
  - central nervous system 094.9
  - date of infection unspecified 097.1
  - early or less than 2 years after infection 092.9
  - late or 2 years or more after infection 096
  - serology
    - doubtful
      - follow-up of latent syphilis 097.1
        - central nervous system 094.9❹
        - date of infection unspecified 097.1
        - early or less than 2 years after infection 092.9❹
        - late or 2 years or more after infection 096
    - positive, only finding 097.1
      - date of infection unspecified 097.1
      - early or less than 2 years after infection 097.1
      - late or 2 years or more after infection 097.1
- lens 095.8
- leukoderma 091.3
  - late 095.8
- lienis 095.8
- lip 091.3
  - chancre 091.2
  - late 095.8
  - primary 091.2
- Lissauer's paralysis 094.1
- liver 095.3
  - secondary 091.62
- locomotor ataxia 094.0
- lung 095.1
- lymphadenitis (secondary) 091.4
- lymph gland (early) (secondary) 091.4
  - late 095.8
- macular atrophy of skin 091.3
  - striated 095.8
- maternal, affecting fetus or newborn 760.2
  - manifest syphilis in newborn – *see* Syphilis, congenital
- mediastinum (late) 095.8
- meninges (adhesive) (basilar) (brain) (spinal cord) 094.2
- meningitis 094.2
  - acute 091.81
  - congenital 090.42
- meningoencephalitis 094.2
- meningovascular 094.2
  - congenital 090.49
- mesarteritis 093.89
  - brain 094.89
  - spine 094.89
- middle ear 095.8
- mitral stenosis 093.21
- monoplegia 094.89
- mouth (secondary) 091.3
  - late 095.8

Syphilis, syphilitic – *continued*
- mucocutaneous 091.3
  - late 095.8
- mucous
  - membrane 091.3
    - late 095.8
  - patches 091.3
    - congenital 090.0
- mulberry molars 090.5
- muscle 095.6
- myocardium 093.82
- myositis 095.6
- nasal sinus 095.8
- neonatorum NEC (*see also* Syphilis, congenital) 090.9❺
- nerve palsy (any cranial nerve) 094.89
- nervous system, central 094.9
- neuritis 095.8
  - acoustic nerve 094.86
- neurorecidive of retina 094.83
- neuroretinitis 094.85
- newborn (*see also* Syphilis, congenital) 090.9❺
- nodular superficial 095.8
- nonvenereal, endemic 104.0
- nose 095.8
  - saddle back deformity 090.5
  - septum 095.8
    - perforated 095.8
- occlusive arterial disease 093.89
- ophthalmic 095.8 *[363.13]*
- ophthalmoplegia 094.89
- optic nerve (atrophy) (neuritis) (papilla) 094.84
- orbit (late) 095.8
- orchitis 095.8
- organic 097.9
- osseous (late) 095.5
- osteochondritis (congenital) 090.0
- osteoporosis 095.5
- ovary 095.8
- oviduct 095.8
- palate 095.8
  - gumma 095.8
  - perforated 090.5
- pancreas (late) 095.8
- pancreatitis 095.8
- paralysis 094.89
  - general 094.1
    - juvenile 090.40
- paraplegia 094.89
- paresis (general) 094.1
  - juvenile 090.40
- paresthesia 094.89
- Parkinson's disease or syndrome 094.82
- paroxysmal tachycardia 093.89
- pemphigus (congenital) 090.0
- penis 091.0
  - chancre 091.0
  - late 095.8
- pericardium 093.81
- perichondritis, larynx 095.8
- periosteum 095.5
  - congenital 090.0
  - early 091.61
  - secondary 091.61
- peripheral nerve 095.8
- petrous bone (late) 095.5
- pharynx 095.8
  - secondary 091.3
- pituitary (gland) 095.8
- placenta 095.8
- pleura (late) 095.8
- pneumonia, white 090.0
- pontine (lesion) 094.89
- portal vein 093.89
- primary NEC 091.2
  - anal 091.1
  - and secondary (*see also* Syphilis, secondary) 091.9
  - cardiovascular 093.9
  - central nervous system 094.9
  - extragenital chancre NEC 091.2
  - fingers 091.2
  - genital 091.0
  - lip 091.2
  - specified site NEC 091.2
  - tonsils 091.2
- prostate 095.8
- psychosis (intracranial gumma) 094.89
- ptosis (eyelid) 094.89
- pulmonary (late) 095.1
  - artery 093.89
- pulmonum 095.1

Syphilis, syphilitic – *continued*
- pyelonephritis 095.4
- recently acquired, symptomatic NEC 091.89
- rectum 095.8
- respiratory tract 095.8
- retina
  - late 094.83
  - neurorecidive 094.83
- retrobulbar neuritis 094.85
- salpingitis 095.8
- sclera (late) 095.0
- sclerosis
  - cerebral 094.89
  - coronary 093.89
  - multiple 094.89
  - subacute 094.89
- scotoma (central) 095.8
- scrotum 095.8
- secondary (and primary) 091.9
  - adenopathy 091.4
  - anus 091.3
  - bone 091.61
  - cardiovascular 093.9
  - central nervous system 094.9
  - chorioretinitis, choroiditis 091.51
  - hepatitis 091.62
  - liver 091.62
  - lymphadenitis 091.4
  - meningitis, acute 091.81
  - mouth 091.3
  - mucous membranes 091.3
  - periosteum 091.61
  - periostitis 091.61
  - pharynx 091.3
  - relapse (treated) (untreated) 091.7
  - skin 091.3
  - specified form NEC 091.89
  - tonsil 091.3
  - ulcer 091.3
  - viscera 091.69
  - vulva 091.3
- seminal vesicle (late) 095.8
- seronegative
  - with signs or symptoms – *see* Syphilis, by site and stage
- seropositive
  - with signs or symptoms – *see* Syphilis, by site or stage
  - follow-up of latent syphilis – *see* Syphilis, latent
  - only finding – *see* Syphilis, latent
- seventh nerve (paralysis) 094.89
- sinus 095.8
- sinusitis 095.8
- skeletal system 095.5
- skin (early) (secondary) (with ulceration) 091.3
  - late or tertiary 095.8
- small intestine 095.8
- spastic spinal paralysis 094.0
- spermatic cord (late) 095.8
- spinal (cord) 094.89
  - with
    - paresis 094.1
    - tabes 094.0
- spleen 095.8
- splenomegaly 095.8
- spondylitis 095.5
- staphyloma 095.8
- stigmata (congenital) 090.5
- stomach 095.8
- synovium (late) 095.7
- tabes dorsalis (early) (late) 094.0
  - juvenile 090.40
- tabetic type 094.0
  - juvenile 090.40
- taboparesis 094.1
  - juvenile 090.40
- tachycardia 093.89
- tendon (late) 095.7
- tertiary 097.0
  - with symptoms 095.8
  - cardiovascular 093.9
  - central nervous system 094.9
  - multiple NEC 095.8
  - specified site NEC 095.8
- testis 095.8
- thorax 095.8
- throat 095.8
- thymus (gland) 095.8
- thyroid (late) 095.8
- tongue 095.8
- tonsil (lingual) 095.8
  - primary 091.2

Syphilis, syphilitic – Taurodontism

❹ Fourth-Digit Required | ❺ Fifth-Digit Required | *[code]* Manifestation Code | ▶◀ Revised Text | ● New Line | ▲ Revised Code

- **Taussig-Bing defect, heart, or syndrome** (transposition, aorta and overriding pulmonary artery) 745.11
- **Tay's choroiditis** 363.41
- **Tay-Sachs**
  - amaurotic familial idiocy 330.1
  - disease 330.1
- **Taybi's syndrome** (otopalatodigital) 759.89
- **Taylor's**
  - disease (diffuse idiopathic cutaneous atrophy) 701.8
  - syndrome 625.5
- **Tear, torn** (traumatic) – *see also* Wound, open, by site
  - anus, anal (sphincter) 863.89
    - with open wound in cavity 863.99
    - complicating delivery ▶(healed) (old)◀ 654.8❺ ▲
      - with mucosa 664.3❺
      - not associated with third-degree perineal laceration 664.6❺ ●
    - nontraumatic, nonpuerperal ▶(healed) (old)◀ 569.43 ▲
  - articular cartilage, old (*see also* Disorder, cartilage, articular) 718.0❺
  - bladder
    - with
      - abortion – *see* Abortion, by type, with damage to pelvic organs
      - ectopic pregnancy (*see also* categories 633.0-633.9) 639.2
      - molar pregnancy (*see also* categories 630-632) 639.2
    - following
      - abortion 639.2
      - ectopic or molar pregnancy 639.2
    - obstetrical trauma 665.5❺
  - bowel
    - with
      - abortion – *see* Abortion, by type, with damage to pelvic organs
      - ectopic pregnancy (*see also* categories 633.0-633.9) 639.2
      - molar pregnancy (*see also* categories 630-632) 639.2
    - following
      - abortion 639.2
      - ectopic or molar pregnancy 639.2
    - obstetrical trauma 665.5❺
  - broad ligament
    - with
      - abortion – *see* Abortion, by type, with damage to pelvic organs
      - ectopic pregnancy (*see also* categories 633.0-633.9) 639.2
      - molar pregnancy (*see also* categories 630-632) 639.2
    - following
      - abortion 639.2
      - ectopic or molar pregnancy 639.2
    - obstetrical trauma 665.6❺
  - bucket handle (knee) (meniscus) – *see* Tear, meniscus
  - capsule
    - joint – *see* Sprain, by site
    - spleen – *see* Laceration, spleen, capsule
  - cartilage – *see also* Sprain, by site
    - articular, old (*see also* Disorder, cartilage, articular) 718.0❺
    - knee – *see* Tear, meniscus
    - semilunar (knee) (current injury) – *see* Tear, meniscus
  - cervix
    - with
      - abortion – *see* Abortion, by type, with damage to pelvic organs
      - ectopic pregnancy (*see also* categories 633.0-633.9) 639.2
      - molar pregnancy (*see also* categories 630-632) 639.2
    - following
      - abortion 639.2
      - ectopic or molar pregnancy 639.2
    - obstetrical trauma (current) 665.3❺
    - old 622.3
  - dural 998.2 ●
  - internal organ (abdomen, chest, or pelvis) – *see* Injury, internal, by site
  - ligament – *see also* Sprain, by site
    - with open wound – *see* Wound, open by site

Tear, torn – *continued*

  - meniscus (knee) (current injury) 836.2
    - bucket handle 836.0
      - old 717.0
    - lateral 836.1
      - anterior horn 836.1
        - old 717.42
      - bucket handle 836.1
        - old 717.41
      - old 717.40
      - posterior horn 836.1
        - old 717.43
      - specified site NEC 836.1
        - old 717.49
    - medial 836.0
      - anterior horn 836.0
        - old 717.1
      - bucket handle 836.0
        - old 717.0
      - old 717.3
      - posterior horn 836.0
        - old 717.2
    - old NEC 717.5
    - site other than knee – *see* Sprain, by site
  - muscle – *see also* Sprain, by site
    - with open wound – *see* Wound, open by site
  - pelvic
    - floor, complicating delivery 664.1❺
    - organ NEC
      - with
        - abortion – *see* Abortion, by type, with damage to pelvic organs
        - ectopic pregnancy (*see also* categories 633.0-633.9) 639.2
        - molar pregnancy (*see also* categories 630-632) 639.2
      - following
        - abortion 639.2
        - ectopic or molar pregnancy 639.2
      - obstetrical trauma 665.5❺
  - perineum – *see also* Laceration, perineum
    - obstetrical trauma 665.5❺
  - periurethral tissue
    - with
      - abortion – *see* Abortion, by type, with damage to pelvic organs
      - ectopic pregnancy (*see also* categories 633.0-633.9) 639.2
      - molar pregnancy (*see also* categories 630-632) 639.2
    - following
      - abortion 639.2
      - ectopic or molar pregnancy 639.2
    - obstetrical trauma 665.5❺
  - rectovaginal septum – *see* Laceration, rectovaginal septum
  - retina, retinal (recent) (with detachment) 361.00
    - without detachment 361.30
    - dialysis (juvenile) (with detachment) 361.04
    - giant (with detachment) 361.03
    - horseshoe (without detachment) 361.32
    - multiple (with detachment) 361.02
      - without detachment 361.33
    - old
      - delimited (partial) 361.06
      - partial 361.06
      - total or subtotal 361.07
    - partial (without detachment)
      - giant 361.03
      - multiple defects 361.02
      - old (delimited) 361.06
      - single defect 361.01
    - round hole (without detachment) 361.31
    - single defect (with detachment) 361.01
    - total or subtotal (recent) 361.05
      - old 361.07
  - rotator cuff (traumatic) 840.4
    - current injury 840.4
    - degenerative 726.10
    - nontraumatic 727.61
  - semilunar cartilage, knee (*see also* Tear, meniscus) 836.2
    - old 717.5
  - tendon – *see also* Sprain, by site
    - with open wound – *see* Wound, open by site
  - tentorial, at birth 767.0
  - umbilical cord
    - affecting fetus or newborn 772.0
    - complicating delivery 663.8❺

Tear, torn – *continued*

  - urethra
    - with
      - abortion – *see* Abortion, by type, with damage to pelvic organs
      - ectopic pregnancy (*see also* categories 633.0-633.9) 639.2
      - molar pregnancy (*see also* categories 630-632) 639.2
    - following
      - abortion 639.2
      - ectopic or molar pregnancy 639.2
    - obstetrical trauma 665.5❺
  - uterus – *see* Injury, internal, uterus
  - vagina – *see* Laceration, vagina
  - vessel, from catheter 998.2
  - vulva, complicating delivery 664.0❺
- **Tear stone** 375.57
- **Teeth, tooth** – *see also* condition
  - grinding 306.8
  - prenatal 520.6
- **Teething** 520.7
  - syndrome 520.7
- **Tegmental syndrome** 344.89
- **Telangiectasia, telangiectasis** (verrucous) 448.9
  - ataxic (cerebellar) 334.8
  - familial 448.0
  - hemorrhagic, hereditary (congenital) (senile) 448.0
  - hereditary hemorrhagic 448.0
  - retina 362.15
  - spider 448.1
- **Telecanthus** (congenital) 743.63
- **Telescoped bowel or intestine** (*see also* Intussusception) 560.0
- **Teletherapy, adverse effect** NEC 990
- **Telogen effluvium** 704.02
- **Temperature**
  - body, high (of unknown origin) (*see also* Pyrexia) 780.6
  - cold, trauma from 991.9
    - newborn 778.2
    - specified effect NEC 991.8
  - high
    - body (of unknown origin) (*see also* Pyrexia) 780.6
    - trauma from – *see* Heat
- **Temper tantrum** (childhood) (*see also* Disturbance, conduct) 312.1❺
- **Temple** – *see* condition
- **Temporal** – *see also* condition
  - lobe syndrome 310.0
- **Temporomandibular joint-pain-dysfunction syndrome** 524.60
- **Temporosphenoidal** – *see* condition
- **Tendency**
  - bleeding (*see also* Defect, coagulation) 286.9
  - homosexual, ego-dystonic 302.0
  - paranoid 301.0
  - suicide 300.9
- **Tenderness**
  - abdominal (generalized) (localized) 789.6❺
  - rebound 789.6❺
  - skin 782.0
- **Tendinitis, tendonitis** (*see also* Tenosynovitis) 726.90
  - Achilles 726.71
  - adhesive 726.90
    - shoulder 726.0
  - calcific 727.82
    - shoulder 726.11
  - gluteal 726.5
  - patellar 726.64
  - peroneal 726.79
  - pes anserinus 726.61
  - psoas 726.5
  - tibialis (anterior) (posterior) 726.72
  - trochanteric 726.5
- **Tendon** – *see* condition
- **Tendosynovitis** – *see* Tenosynovitis
- **Tendovaginitis** – *see* Tenosynovitis
- **Tenesmus** 787.99
  - rectal 787.99
  - vesical 788.9
- **Tenia** – *see* Taenia
- **Teniasis** – *see* Taeniasis
- **Tennis elbow** 726.32

- **Tenonitis** – *see also* Tenosynovitis
  - eye (capsule) 376.04
- **Tenontosynovitis** – *see* Tenosynovitis
- **Tenontothecitis** – *see* Tenosynovitis
- **Tenophyte** 727.9
- **Tenosynovitis** 727.00
  - adhesive 726.90
    - shoulder 726.0
  - ankle 727.06
  - bicipital (calcifying) 726.12
  - buttock 727.09
  - due to crystals – *see* Arthritis, due to crystals
  - elbow 727.09
  - finger 727.05
  - foot 727.06
  - gonococcal 098.51
  - hand 727.05
  - hip 727.09
  - knee 727.09
  - radial styloid 727.04
  - shoulder 726.10
    - adhesive 726.0
  - spine 720.1
  - supraspinatus 726.10
  - toe 727.06
  - tuberculous – *see* Tuberculosis, tenosynovitis
  - wrist 727.05
- **Tenovaginitis** – *see* Tenosynovitis
- **Tension**
  - arterial, high (*see also* Hypertension) 401.9
    - without diagnosis of hypertension 796.2
  - headache 307.81
  - intraocular (elevated) 365.00
  - nervous 799.2
  - ocular (elevated) 365.00
  - pneumothorax 512.0
    - iatrogenic 512.1
    - postoperative 512.1
    - spontaneous 512.0
  - premenstrual 625.4
  - state 300.9
- **Tentorium** – *see* condition
- **Teratencephalus** 759.89
- **Teratism** 759.7
- **Teratoblastoma** (malignant) (M9080/3) – *see* Neoplasm, by site, malignant
- **Teratocarcinoma** (M9081/3) – *see also* Neoplasm, by site, malignant
  - liver 155.0
- **Teratoma** (solid) (M9080/1) – *see also* Neoplasm, by site, uncertain behavior
  - adult (cystic) (M9080/0) – *see* Neoplasm, by site, benign
  - and embryonal carcinoma, mixed (M9081/3) – *see* Neoplasm, by site, malignant
  - benign (M9080/0) – *see* Neoplasm, by site, benign
  - combined with choriocarcinoma (M9101/3) – *see* Neoplasm, by site, malignant
  - cystic (adult) (M9080/0) – *see* Neoplasm, by site, benign
  - differentiated type (M9080/0) – *see* Neoplasm, by site, benign
  - embryonal (M9080/3) – *see also* Neoplasm, by site, malignant
    - liver 155.0
  - fetal
    - sacral, causing fetopelvic disproportion 653.7 ❺
  - immature (M9080/3) – *see* Neoplasm, by site, malignant
  - liver (M9080/3) 155.0
    - adult, benign, cystic, differentiated type, or mature (M9080/0) 211.5
  - malignant (M9080/3) – *see also* Neoplasm, by site, malignant
    - anaplastic type (M9082/3) – *see* Neoplasm, by site, malignant
    - intermediate type (M9083/3) – *see* Neoplasm, by site, malignant
    - liver (M9080/3) 155.0
    - trophoblastic (M9102/3)
      - specified site – *see* Neoplasm, by site, malignant
      - unspecified site 186.9
    - undifferentiated type (M9082/3) – *see* Neoplasm, by site, malignant
- **Teratoma** – *continued*
  - mature (M9080/0) – *see* Neoplasm, by site, benign
    - malignant (M9080/3) – *see* Neoplasm, by site, malignant ●
  - ovary (M9080/0) 220
    - embryonal, immature, or malignant (M9080/3) 183.0
  - suprasellar (M9080/3) – *see* Neoplasm, by site, malignant
  - testis (M9080/3) 186.9
    - adult, benign, cystic, differentiated type or mature (M9080/0) 222.0
    - undescended 186.0
- **Terminal care** V66.7
- **Termination**
  - anomalous – *see also* Malposition, congenital
    - portal vein 747.49
    - right pulmonary vein 747.42
  - pregnancy (legal) (therapeutic) (*see* Abortion, legal) 635.9 ❺
    - fetus NEC 779.6
    - illegal (*see also* Abortion, illegal) 636.9 ❺
- **Ternidens diminutus infestation** 127.7
- **Terrors, night** (child) 307.46
- **Terry's syndrome** 362.21
- **Tertiary** – *see* condition
- **Tessellated fundus, retina** (tigroid) 362.89
- **Test(s)**
  - adequacy
    - hemodialysis V56.31
    - peritoneal dialysis V56.32
  - AIDS virus V72.6
  - allergen V72.7
  - bacterial disease NEC (*see also* Screening, by name of disease) V74.9
  - basal metabolic rate V72.6
  - blood-alcohol V70.4
  - blood-drug V70.4
    - for therapeutic drug monitoring V58.83
  - blood typing V72.86
    - Rh typing V72.86
  - developmental, infant or child V20.2
  - Dick V74.8
  - fertility V26.21
  - genetic
    - female V26.32
    - for genetic disease carrier status
      - female V26.31
      - male V26.34
    - male V26.39
  - hearing V72.19
    - following failed hearing screening V72.11
  - HIV V72.6
  - human immunodeficiency virus V72.6
  - Kveim V82.89
  - laboratory V72.6
    - for medicolegal reason V70.4
  - male partner of habitual aborter V26.35
  - Mantoux (for tuberculosis) V74.1
  - mycotic organism V75.4
  - parasitic agent NEC V75.8
  - paternity V70.4
  - peritoneal equilibration V56.32
  - pregnancy
    - negative result V72.41
    - positive result V72.42
      - first pregnancy V72.42
    - unconfirmed V72.40
  - preoperative V72.84
    - cardiovascular V72.81
    - respiratory V72.82
    - specified NEC V72.83
  - procreative management NEC V26.29
    - genetic disease carrier status
      - female V26.31
      - male V26.34
  - Rh typing V72.86
  - sarcoidosis V82.89
  - Schick V74.3
  - Schultz-Charlton V74.8
  - skin, diagnostic
    - allergy V72.7
    - bacterial agent NEC (*see also* Screening, by name of disease) V74.9
    - Dick V74.8
    - hypersensitivity V72.7
    - Kveim V82.89
    - Mantoux V74.1
    - mycotic organism V75.4
    - parasitic agent NEC V75.8
- **Test(s)** – *continued*
  - skin, diagnostic – *continued*
    - sarcoidosis V82.89
    - Schick V74.3
    - Schultz-Charlton V74.8
    - tuberculin V74.1
  - specified type NEC V72.8 ❺
  - tuberculin V74.1
  - vision V72.0
  - Wassermann
    - positive (*see also* Serology for syphilis, positive) 097.1
      - false 795.6
- **Testicle, testicular, testis** – *see also* condition
  - feminization (syndrome) 259.5
- **Tetanus, tetanic** (cephalic) (convulsions) 037
  - with
    - abortion – *see* Abortion, by type, with sepsis
    - ectopic pregnancy (*see also* categories 633.0-633.9) 639.0
    - molar pregnancy (*see* categories 630-632) 639.0
  - following
    - abortion 639.0
    - ectopic or molar pregnancy 639.0
  - inoculation V03.7
    - reaction (due to serum) – *see* Complications, vaccination
  - neonatorum 771.3
  - puerperal, postpartum, childbirth 670 ❹
- **Tetany, tetanic** 781.7
  - alkalosis 276.3
  - associated with rickets 268.0
  - convulsions 781.7
    - hysterical 300.11
  - functional (hysterical) 300.11
  - hyperkinetic 781.7
    - hysterical 300.11
  - hyperpnea 786.01
    - hysterical 300.11
    - psychogenic 306.1
  - hyperventilation 786.01
    - hysterical 300.11
    - psychogenic 306.1
  - hypocalcemic, neonatal 775.4
  - hysterical 300.11
  - neonatal 775.4
  - parathyroid (gland) 252.1
  - parathyroprival 252.1
  - postoperative 252.1
  - postthyroidectomy 252.1
  - pseudotetany 781.7
    - hysterical 300.11
  - psychogenic 306.1
    - specified as conversion reaction 300.11
- **Tetralogy of Fallot** 745.2
- **Tetraplegia** – *see* Quadriplegia
- **Thailand hemorrhagic fever** 065.4
- **Thalassanemia** 282.49
- **Thalassemia** (alpha) (beta) (disease) (Hb-C) (Hb-D) (Hb-E) (Hb-H) (Hb-I) (high fetal gene) (high fetal hemoglobin) (intermedia) (major) (minima) (minor) (mixed) (trait) (with other hemoglobinopathy) 282.49
  - HB-S (without crisis) 282.41
    - with
      - crisis 282.42
      - vaso-occlusive pain 282.42
  - Sickle-cell (without crisis) 282.41
    - with
      - crisis 282.42
      - vaso-occlusive pain 282.42
- **Thalassemic variants** 282.49
- **Thaysen-Gee disease** (nontropical sprue) 579.0
- **Thecoma** (M8600/0) 220
  - malignant (M8600/3) 183.0
- **Thelarche, precocious** 259.1
- **Thelitis** 611.0
  - puerperal, postpartum 675.0 ❺
- **Therapeutic** – *see* condition
- **Therapy** V57.9
  - blood transfusion, without reported diagnosis V58.2
  - breathing V57.0
  - chemotherapy, antineoplastic V58.11
    - fluoride V07.31
    - prophylactic NEC V07.39
  - dialysis (intermittent) (treatment)
    - extracorporeal V56.0

Therapy – *continued*
- dialysis – *continued*
  - peritoneal V56.8
  - renal V56.0
  - specified type NEC V56.8
- exercise NEC V57.1
  - breathing V57.0
- extracorporeal dialysis (renal) V56.0
- fluoride prophylaxis V07.31
- hemodialysis V56.0
- hormone replacement (postmenopausal) V07.4
- immunotherapy antineoplastic V58.12
- long term oxygen therapy V46.2
- occupational V57.21
- orthoptic V57.4
- orthotic V57.81
- peritoneal dialysis V56.8
- physical NEC V57.1
- postmenopausal hormone replacement V07.4
- radiation V58.0
- speech V57.3
- vocational V57.22

Thermalgesia 782.0
Thermalgia 782.0
Thermanalgesia 782.0
Thermanesthesia 782.0
Thermic – *see* condition
Thermography (abnormal) 793.99
- breast 793.89

Thermoplegia 992.0
Thesaurismosis
- amyloid 277.39
- bilirubin 277.4
- calcium 275.40
- cystine 270.0
- glycogen (*see also* Disease, glycogen storage) 271.0
- kerasin 272.7
- lipoid 272.7
- melanin 255.41 ▲
- phosphatide 272.7
- urate 274.9

Thiaminic deficiency 265.1
- with beriberi 265.0

Thibierge-Weissenbach syndrome (cutaneous systemic sclerosis) 710.1
Thickened endometrium 793.5
Thickening
- bone 733.99
  - extremity 733.99
- breast 611.79
- hymen 623.3
- larynx 478.79
- nail 703.8
  - congenital 757.5
- periosteal 733.99
- pleura (*see also* Pleurisy) 511.0
- skin 782.8
- subepiglottic 478.79
- tongue 529.8
- valve, heart – *see* Endocarditis

Thiele syndrome 724.6
Thigh – *see* condition
Thinning vertebra (*see also* Osteoporosis) 733.00
Thirst, excessive 783.5
- due to deprivation of water 994.3

Thomsen's disease 359.22 ▲
Thomson's disease (congenital poikiloderma) 757.33
Thoracic – *see also* condition
- kidney 753.3
- outlet syndrome 353.0
- stomach – *see* Hernia, diaphragm

Thoracogastroschisis (congenital) 759.89
Thoracopagus 759.4
Thoracoschisis 756.3
Thoracoscopic surgical procedure converted to open procedure V64.42
Thorax – *see* condition
Thorn's syndrome (*see also* Disease, renal) 593.9
Thornwaldt's, Tornwaldt's
- bursitis (pharyngeal) 478.29
- cyst 478.26
- disease (pharyngeal bursitis) 478.29

Thorson-Biörck syndrome (malignant carcinoid) 259.2
Threadworm (infection) (infestation) 127.4
Threatened
- abortion or miscarriage 640.0❺
  - with subsequent abortion (*see also* Abortion, spontaneous) 634.9❺
  - affecting fetus 762.1
- labor 644.1❺
  - affecting fetus or newborn 761.8
  - premature 644.0❺
- miscarriage 640.0❺
  - affecting fetus 762.1
- premature
  - delivery 644.2❺
    - affecting fetus or newborn 761.8
  - labor 644.0❺
    - before 22 completed weeks gestation 640.0❺

Three-day fever 066.0
Threshers' lung 495.0
Thrix annulata (congenital) 757.4
Throat – *see* condition
Thrombasthenia (Glanzmann's) (hemorrhagic) (hereditary) 287.1
Thromboangiitis 443.1
- obliterans (general) 443.1
  - cerebral 437.1
  - vessels
    - brain 437.1
    - spinal cord 437.1

Thromboarteritis – *see* Arteritis
Thromboasthenia (Glanzmann's) (hemorrhagic) (hereditary) 287.1
Thrombocytasthenia (Glanzmann's) 287.1
Thrombocythemia (primary) (M9962/1) 238.71
- essential 238.71
- hemorrhagic 238.71
- idiopathic (hemorrhagic) (M9962/1) 238.71

Thrombocytopathy (dystrophic) (granulopenic) 287.1
Thrombocytopenia, thrombocytopenic 287.5
- with
  - absent radii (TAR) syndrome 287.33
  - giant hemangioma 287.39
- amegakaryocytic, congenital 287.33
- congenital 287.33
- cyclic 287.39
- dilutional 287.4
- due to
  - drugs 287.4
  - extracorporeal circulation of blood 287.4
  - massive blood transfusion 287.4
  - platelet alloimmunization 287.4
- essential 287.30
- hereditary 287.33
- Kasabach-Merritt 287.39
- neonatal, transitory 776.1
  - due to
    - exchange transfusion 776.1
    - idiopathic maternal thrombocytopenia 776.1
    - isoimmunization 776.1
- primary 287.30
- puerperal, postpartum 666.3❺
- purpura (*see also* Purpura, thrombocytopenic) 287.30
  - thrombotic 446.6
- secondary 287.4
- sex-linked 287.39

Thrombocytosis 238.71
- essential 238.71
- primary 238.71

Thromboembolism – *see* Embolism
Thrombopathy (Bernard-Soulier) 287.1
- constitutional 286.4
- Willebrand-Jürgens (angiohemophilia) 286.4

Thrombopenia (*see also* Thrombocytopenia) 287.5
Thrombophlebitis 451.9
- antecubital vein 451.82
- antepartum (superficial) 671.2❺
  - affecting fetus or newborn 760.3
  - deep 671.3❺
- arm 451.89
  - deep 451.83
  - superficial 451.82
- breast, superficial 451.89
- cavernous (venous) sinus – *see* Thrombophlebitis, intracranial venous sinus
- cephalic vein 451.82
- cerebral (sinus) (vein) 325
  - late effect – *see* category 326
  - nonpyogenic 437.6
    - in pregnancy or puerperium 671.5❺
    - late effect – *see* Late effect(s) (of) cerebrovascular disease
- due to implanted device – *see* Complications, due to (presence of) any device, implant, or graft classified to 996.0-996.5 NEC
- during or resulting from a procedure NEC 997.2
- femoral 451.11
- femoropopliteal 451.19
- following infusion, perfusion, or transfusion 999.2
- hepatic (vein) 451.89
- idiopathic, recurrent 453.1
- iliac vein 451.81
- iliofemoral 451.11
- intracranial venous sinus (any) 325
  - late effect – *see* category 326
  - nonpyogenic 437.6
    - in pregnancy or puerperium 671.5❺
    - late effect – *see* Late effect(s) (of) cerebrovascular disease
- jugular vein 451.89
- lateral (venous) sinus – *see* Thrombophlebitis, intracranial venous sinus
- leg 451.2
  - deep (vessels) 451.19
    - femoral vein 451.11
    - specified vessel NEC 451.19
  - superficial (vessels) 451.0
    - femoral vein 451.11
- longitudinal (venous) sinus – *see* Thrombophlebitis, intracranial venous sinus
- lower extremity 451.2
  - deep (vessels) 451.19
    - femoral vein 451.11
    - specified vessel NEC 451.19
  - superficial (vessels) 451.0
- migrans, migrating 453.1
- pelvic
  - with
    - abortion – *see* Abortion, by type, with sepsis
    - ectopic pregnancy (*see also* categories 633.0-633.9) 639.0
    - molar pregnancy (*see also* categories 630-632) 639.0
  - following
    - abortion 639.0
    - ectopic or molar pregnancy 639.0
  - puerperal 671.4❺
- popliteal vein 451.19
- portal (vein) 572.1
- postoperative 997.2
- pregnancy (superficial) 671.2❺
  - affecting fetus or newborn 760.3
  - deep 671.3❺
- puerperal, postpartum, childbirth (extremities) (superficial) 671.2❺
  - deep 671.4❺
  - pelvic 671.4❺
  - specified site NEC 671.5❺
- radial vein 451.82
- saphenous (greater) (lesser) 451.0
- sinus (intracranial) – *see* Thrombophlebitis, intracranial venous sinus
- specified site NEC 451.89
- tibial vein 451.19

Thrombosis, thrombotic (marantic) (multiple) (progressive) (vein) (vessel) 453.9
- with childbirth or during the puerperium – *see* Thrombosis, puerperal, postpartum
- antepartum – *see* Thrombosis, pregnancy
- aorta, aortic 444.1
  - abdominal 444.0
  - bifurcation 444.0
  - saddle 444.0
  - terminal 444.0
  - thoracic 444.1
  - valve – *see* Endocarditis, aortic
- apoplexy (*see also* Thrombosis, brain) 434.0❺
  - late effect – *see* Late effect(s) (of) cerebrovascular disease
- appendix, septic – *see* Appendicitis, acute
- arteriolar-capillary platelet, disseminated 446.6
- artery, arteries (postinfectional) 444.9
  - auditory, internal 433.8❺
  - basilar (*see also* Occlusion, artery, basilar) 433.0❺
  - carotid (common) (internal) (*see also* Occlusion, artery, carotid) 433.1❺
    - with other precerebral artery 433.3❺

Thrombosis, thrombotic – *continued*
- artery, arteries – *continued*
  - cerebellar (anterior inferior) (posterior inferior) (superior) 433.8❺
  - cerebral (*see also* Thrombosis, brain) 434.0❺
  - choroidal (anterior) 433.8❺
  - communicating posterior 433.8❺
  - coronary (*see also* Infarct, myocardium) 410.9❺
    - without myocardial infarction 411.81
    - due to syphilis 093.89
    - healed or specified as old 412
  - extremities 444.22
    - lower 444.22
    - upper 444.21
  - femoral 444.22
  - hepatic 444.89
  - hypophyseal 433.8❺
  - meningeal, anterior or posterior 433.8❺
  - mesenteric (with gangrene) 557.0
  - ophthalmic (*see also* Occlusion, retina) 362.30
  - pontine 433.8❺
  - popliteal 444.22
  - precerebral – *see* Occlusion, artery, precerebral NEC
  - pulmonary 415.19
    - iatrogenic 415.11
    - postoperative 415.11
    - septic 415.12 ●
  - renal 593.81
  - retinal (*see also* Occlusion, retina) 362.30
  - specified site NEC 444.89
  - spinal, anterior or posterior 433.8❺
  - traumatic (complication) (early) (*see also* Injury, blood vessel, by site) 904.9
  - vertebral (*see also* Occlusion, artery, vertebral) 433.2❺
    - with other precerebral artery 433.3❺
- atrial (endocardial) 424.90
  - without endocarditis 429.89
  - due to syphilis 093.89
- auricular (*see also* Infarct, myocardium) 410.9❺
- axillary (vein) 453.8
- basilar (artery) (*see also* Occlusion, artery, basilar) 433.0❺
- bland NEC 453.9
- brain (artery) (stem) 434.0❺
  - due to syphilis 094.89
  - iatrogenic 997.02
  - late effect – *see* Late effect(s) (of) cerebrovascular disease
  - postoperative 997.02
  - puerperal, postpartum, childbirth 674.0❺
  - sinus (*see also* Thrombosis, intracranial venous sinus) 325
- capillary 448.9
  - arteriolar, generalized 446.6
- cardiac (*see also* Infarct, myocardium) 410.9❺
  - due to syphilis 093.89
  - healed or specified as old 412
  - valve – *see* Endocarditis
- carotid (artery) (common) (internal) (*see also* Occlusion, artery, carotid) 433.1❺
  - with other precerebral artery 433.3❺
- cavernous sinus (venous) – *see* Thrombosis, intracranial venous sinus
- cerebellar artery (anterior inferior) (posterior inferior) (superior) 433.8❺
  - late effect – *see* Late effect(s) (of) cerebrovascular disease
- cerebral (arteries) (*see also* Thrombosis, brain) 434.0❺
  - late effect – *see* Late effect(s) (of) cerebrovascular disease
- coronary (artery) (*see also* Infarct, myocardium) 410.9❺
  - without myocardial infarction 411.81
  - due to syphilis 093.89
  - healed or specified as old 412
- corpus cavernosum 607.82
- cortical (*see also* Thrombosis, brain) 434.0❺
- due to (presence of) any device, implant, or graft classifiable to 996.0-996.5 – *see* Complications, due to (presence of) any device, implant, or graft classified to 996.0-996.5 NEC
- effort 453.8
- endocardial – *see* Infarct, myocardium
- eye (*see also* Occlusion, retina) 362.30
- femoral (vein) 453.8
  - with inflammation or phlebitis 451.11
  - artery 444.22

Thrombosis, thrombotic – *continued*
- femoral (vein) – *continued*
  - deep 453.41
- genital organ, male 608.83
- heart (chamber) (*see also* Infarct, myocardium) 410.9❺
- hepatic (vein) 453.0
  - artery 444.89
  - infectional or septic 572.1
- iliac (vein) 453.8
  - with inflammation or phlebitis 451.81
  - artery (common) (external) (internal) 444.81
- inflammation, vein – *see* Thrombophlebitis
- internal carotid artery (*see also* Occlusion, artery, carotid) 433.1❺
  - with other precerebral artery 433.3❺
- intestine (with gangrene) 557.0
- intracranial (*see also* Thrombosis, brain) 434.0❺
  - venous sinus (any) 325
    - nonpyogenic origin 437.6
      - in pregnancy or puerperium 671.5❺
- intramural (*see also* Infarct, myocardium) 410.9❺
  - without
    - cardiac condition 429.89
    - coronary artery disease 429.89
    - myocardial infarction 429.89
  - healed or specified as old 412
- jugular (bulb) 453.8
- kidney 593.81
  - artery 593.81
- lateral sinus (venous) – *see* Thrombosis, intracranial venous sinus
- leg 453.8
  - with inflammation or phlebitis – *see* Thrombophlebitis
  - deep (vessels) 453.40
    - lower (distal) 453.42
    - upper (proximal) 453.41
  - superficial (vessels) 453.8
- liver (venous) 453.0
  - artery 444.89
  - infectional or septic 572.1
  - portal vein 452
- longitudinal sinus (venous) – *see* Thrombosis, intracranial venous sinus
- lower extremity 453.8
  - deep vessels 453.40
    - calf 453.42
    - distal (lower leg) 453.42
    - femoral 453.41
    - iliac 453.41
    - lower leg 453.42
    - peroneal 453.42
    - popliteal 453.41
    - proximal (upper leg) 453.41
    - thigh 453.41
    - tibial 453.42
- lung 415.19
  - iatrogenic 415.11
  - postoperative 415.11
  - septic 415.12 ●
- marantic, dural sinus 437.6
- meninges (brain) (*see also* Thrombosis, brain) 434.0❺
- mesenteric (artery) (with gangrene) 557.0
  - vein (inferior) (superior) 557.0
- mitral – *see* Insufficiency, mitral
- mural (heart chamber) (*see also* Infarct, myocardium) 410.9❺
  - without
    - cardiac condition 429.89
    - coronary artery disease 429.89
    - myocardial infarction 429.89
  - due to syphilis 093.89
  - following myocardial infarction 429.79
  - healed or specified as old 412
- omentum (with gangrene) 557.0
- ophthalmic (artery) (*see also* Occlusion, retina) 362.30
- pampiniform plexus (male) 608.83
  - female 620.8
- parietal (*see also* Infarct, myocardium) 410.9❺
- penis, penile 607.82
- peripheral arteries 444.22
  - lower 444.22
  - upper 444.21
- platelet 446.6
- portal 452
  - due to syphilis 093.89
  - infectional or septic 572.1

Thrombosis, thrombotic – *continued*
- precerebral artery – *see also* Occlusion, artery, precerebral NEC
- pregnancy 671.9❺
  - deep (vein) 671.3❺
  - superficial (vein) 671.2❺
- puerperal, postpartum, childbirth 671.9❺
  - brain (artery) 674.0❺
    - venous 671.5❺
  - cardiac 674.8❺
  - cerebral (artery) 674.0❺
    - venous 671.5❺
  - deep (vein) 671.4❺
  - intracranial sinus (nonpyogenic) (venous) 671.5❺
  - pelvic 671.4❺
  - pulmonary (artery) 673.2❺
  - specified site NEC 671.5❺
  - superficial 671.2❺
- pulmonary (artery) (vein) 415.19
  - iatrogenic 415.11
  - postoperative 415.11
  - septic 415.12 ●
- renal (artery) 593.81
  - vein 453.3
- resulting from presence of shunt or other internal prosthetic device – *see* Complications, due to (presence of) any device, implant, or graft classifiable to 996.0-996.5 NEC
- retina, retinal (artery) 362.30
  - arterial branch 362.32
  - central 362.31
  - partial 362.33
  - vein
    - central 362.35
    - tributary (branch) 362.36
- scrotum 608.83
- seminal vesicle 608.83
- sigmoid (venous) sinus (*see* Thrombosis, intracranial venous sinus) 325
- silent NEC 453.9
- sinus, intracranial (venous) (any) (*see also* Thrombosis, intracranial venous sinus) 325
- softening, brain (*see also* Thrombosis, brain) 434.0❺
- specified site NEC 453.8
- spermatic cord 608.83
- spinal cord 336.1
  - due to syphilis 094.89
  - in pregnancy or puerperium 671.5❺
  - pyogenic origin 324.1
    - late effect – *see* category 326
- spleen, splenic 289.59
  - artery 444.89
- testis 608.83
- traumatic (complication) (early) (*see also* Injury, blood vessel, by site) 904.9
- tricuspid – *see* Endocarditis, tricuspid
- tumor – *see* Neoplasm, by site
- tunica vaginalis 608.83
- umbilical cord (vessels) 663.6❺
  - affecting fetus or newborn 762.6
- vas deferens 608.83
- vein
  - deep 453.40
  - lower extremity – *see* Thrombosis, lower extremity
- vena cava (inferior) (superior) 453.2

Thrombus – *see* Thrombosis

Thrush 112.0
- newborn 771.7

Thumb – *see also* condition
- gamekeeper's 842.12
- sucking (child problem) 307.9

Thygeson's superficial punctate keratitis 370.21

Thymergasia (*see also* Psychosis, affective) 296.80

Thymitis 254.8

Thymoma (benign) (M8580/0) 212.6
- malignant (M8580/3) 164.0

Thymus, thymic (gland) – *see* condition

Thyrocele (*see also* Goiter) 240.9

Thyroglossal – *see also* condition
- cyst 759.2
- duct, persistent 759.2

Thyroid (body) (gland) – *see also* condition
- hormone resistance 246.8
- lingual 759.2

Thyroiditis 245.9
- acute (pyogenic) (suppurative) 245.0
  - nonsuppurative 245.0

Thrombosis, thrombotic – Thyroiditis

Thyroiditis – *continued*
autoimmune 245.2
chronic (nonspecific) (sclerosing) 245.8
fibrous 245.3
lymphadenoid 245.2
lymphocytic 245.2
lymphoid 245.2
complicating pregnancy, childbirth, or puerperium 648.1❺
de Quervain's (subacute granulomatous) 245.1
fibrous (chronic) 245.3
giant (cell) (follicular) 245.1
granulomatous (de Quervain's) (subacute) 245.1
Hashimoto's (struma lymphomatosa) 245.2
iatrogenic 245.4
invasive (fibrous) 245.3
ligneous 245.3
lymphocytic (chronic) 245.2
lymphoid 245.2
lymphomatous 245.2
pseudotuberculous 245.1
pyogenic 245.0
radiation 245.4
Riedel's (ligneous) 245.3
subacute 245.1
suppurative 245.0
tuberculous (*see also* Tuberculosis) 017.5❺
viral 245.1
woody 245.3
Thyrolingual duct, persistent 759.2
Thyromegaly 240.9
Thyrotoxic
crisis or storm (*see also* Thyrotoxicosis) 242.9❺
heart failure (*see also* Thyrotoxicosis) 242.9❺ *[425.7]*
Thyrotoxicosis 242.9❺

Note – Use the following fifth-digit subclassification with category 242:
0 without mention of thyrotoxic crisis or storm
1 with mention of thyrotoxic crisis or storm

with
goiter (diffuse) 242.0❺
adenomatous 242.3❺
multinodular 242.2❺
uninodular 242.1❺
nodular 242.3❺
multinodular 242.2❺
uninodular 242.1❺
infiltrative
dermopathy 242.0❺
ophthalmopathy 242.0❺
thyroid acropachy 242.0❺
complicating pregnancy, childbirth, or puerperium 648.1❺
due to
ectopic thyroid nodule 242.4❺
ingestion of (excessive) thyroid material 242.8❺
specified cause NEC 242.8❺
factitia 242.8❺
heart 242.9❺ *[425.7]*
neonatal (transient) 775.3
TIA (transient ischemic attack) 435.9
with transient neurologic deficit 435.9
late effect – *see* Late effect(s) (of) cerebrovascular disease
Tibia vara 732.4
Tic 307.20
breathing 307.20
child problem 307.21
compulsive 307.22
convulsive 307.20
degenerative (generalized) (localized) 333.3
facial 351.8
douloureux (*see also* Neuralgia, trigeminal) 350.1
atypical 350.2
habit 307.20
chronic (motor or vocal) 307.22
transient (of childhood) 307.21
lid 307.20
transient (of childhood) 307.21
motor-verbal 307.23
occupational 300.89
orbicularis 307.20
transient (of childhood) 307.21
organic origin 333.3
postchoreic – *see* Chorea

Tic – *continued*
psychogenic 307.20
compulsive 307.22
salaam 781.0
spasm 307.20
chronic (motor or vocal) 307.22
transient (of childhood) 307.21
Tick (-borne) **fever** NEC 066.1
American mountain 066.1
Colorado 066.1
hemorrhagic NEC 065.3
Crimean 065.0
Kyasanur Forest 065.2
Omsk 065.1
mountain 066.1
nonexanthematous 066.1
Tick-bite fever NEC 066.1
African 087.1
Colorado (virus) 066.1
Rocky Mountain 082.0
Tick paralysis 989.5
Tics and spasms, compulsive 307.22
Tietze's disease or syndrome 733.6
Tight, tightness
anus 564.89
chest 786.59
fascia (lata) 728.9
foreskin (congenital) 605
hymen 623.3
introitus (acquired) (congenital) 623.3
rectal sphincter 564.89
tendon 727.81
Achilles (heel) 727.81
urethral sphincter 598.9
Tilting vertebra 737.9
Timidity, child 313.21
Tinea (intersecta) (tarsi) 110.9
amiantacea 110.0
asbestina 110.0
barbae 110.0
beard 110.0
black dot 110.0
blanca 111.2
capitis 110.0
corporis 110.5
cruris 110.3
decalvans 704.09
flava 111.0
foot 110.4
furfuracea 111.0
imbricata (Tokelau) 110.5
lepothrix 039.0
manuum 110.2
microsporic (*see also* Dermatophytosis) 110.9
nigra 111.1
nodosa 111.2
pedis 110.4
scalp 110.0
specified site NEC 110.8
sycosis 110.0
tonsurans 110.0
trichophytic (*see also* Dermatophytosis) 110.9
unguium 110.1
versicolor 111.0
Tingling sensation (*see also* Disturbance, sensation) 782.0
Tin-miners' lung 503
Tinnitus (aurium) 388.30
audible 388.32
objective 388.32
subjective 388.31
Tipped, teeth 524.33
Tipping
pelvis 738.6
with disproportion (fetopelvic) 653.0❺
affecting fetus or newborn 763.1
causing obstructed labor 660.1❺
affecting fetus or newborn 763.1
teeth 524.33
Tiredness 780.79
Tissue – *see* condition
Tobacco
abuse (affecting health) NEC (*see also* Abuse, drugs, nondependent) 305.1
heart 989.8❺
use disorder complicating pregnancy, childbirth, or the puerperium 649.0❺
Tobias' syndrome (carcinoma, pulmonary apex) (M8010/3) 162.3

Tocopherol deficiency 269.1
Todd's
cirrhosis – *see* Cirrhosis, biliary
paralysis (postepileptic transitory paralysis) 344.8❺
Toe – *see* condition
Toilet, artificial opening (*see also* Attention to, artificial, opening) V55.9
Tokelau ringworm 110.5
Tollwut 071
Tolosa-Hunt syndrome 378.55
Tommaselli's disease
correct substance properly administered 599.7
overdose or wrong substance given or taken 961.4
Tongue – *see also* condition
worms 134.1
Tongue tie 750.0
Toni-Fanconi syndrome (cystinosis) 270.0
Tonic pupil 379.46
Tonsil – *see* condition
Tonsillitis (acute) (catarrhal) (croupous) (follicular) (gangrenous) (infective) (lacunar) (lingual) (malignant) (membranous) (phlegmonous) (pneumococcal) (pseudomembranous) (purulent) (septic) (staphylococcal) (subacute) (suppurative) (toxic) (ulcerative) (vesicular) (viral) 463
with influenza, flu, or grippe 487.1
chronic 474.00
diphtheritic (membranous) 032.0
hypertrophic 474.00
influenzal 487.1
parenchymatous 475
streptococcal 034.0
tuberculous (*see also* Tuberculosis) 012.8❺
Vincent's 101
Tonsillopharyngitis 465.8
Tooth, teeth – *see* condition
Toothache 525.9
Topagnosis 782.0
Tophi (gouty) 274.0
ear 274.81
heart 274.82
specified site NEC 274.82
Torn – *see* Tear, torn
Tornwaldt's bursitis (disease) (pharyngeal bursitis) 478.29
cyst 478.26
Torpid liver 573.9
Torsion
accessory tube 620.5
adnexa (female) 620.5
aorta (congenital) 747.29
acquired 447.1
appendix
epididymis 608.24
testis 608.23
bile duct 576.8
with calculus, choledocholithiasis or stones – *see* Choledocholithiasis
congenital 751.69
bowel, colon, or intestine 560.2
cervix – *see* Malposition, uterus
duodenum 537.3
dystonia – *see* Dystonia, torsion
epididymis 608.24
appendix 608.24
fallopian tube 620.5
gallbladder (*see also* Disease, gallbladder) 575.8
congenital 751.69
gastric 537.89
hydatid of Morgagni (female) 620.5
kidney (pedicle) 593.89
Meckel's diverticulum (congenital) 751.0
mesentery 560.2
omentum 560.2
organ or site, congenital NEC – *see* Anomaly, specified type NEC
ovary (pedicle) 620.5
congenital 752.0
oviduct 620.5
penis 607.89
congenital 752.69
renal 593.89
spasm – *see* Dystonia, torsion
spermatic cord 608.22
extravaginal 608.21

Torsion – *continued*
- spermatic cord – *continued*
  - intravaginal 608.22
- spleen 289.59
- testicle, testis 608.20
  - appendix 608.23
- tibia 736.89
- umbilical cord – *see* Compression, umbilical cord
- uterus (*see also* Malposition, uterus) 621.6

Torticollis (intermittent) (spastic) 723.5
- congenital 754.1
  - sternomastoid 754.1
- due to birth injury 767.8
- hysterical 300.11
- ocular 781.93
- psychogenic 306.0
  - specified as conversion reaction 300.11
- rheumatic 723.5
- rheumatoid 714.0
- spasmodic 333.83
- traumatic, current NEC 847.0

Tortuous
- artery 447.1
- fallopian tube 752.19
- organ or site, congenital NEC – *see* Distortion
- renal vessel (congenital) 747.62
- retina vessel (congenital) 743.58
  - acquired 362.17
- ureter 593.4
- urethra 599.84
- vein – *see* Varicose, vein

Torula, torular (infection) 117.5
- histolytica 117.5
- lung 117.5

Torulosis 117.5

Torus
- fracture
  - fibula 823.41
    - with tibia 823.42
  - radius 813.45
  - tibia 823.40
    - with fibula 823.42
- mandibularis 526.81
- palatinus 526.81

Touch, vitreous 997.99

Touraine's syndrome (hereditary osteo-onychodysplasia) 756.89

Touraine-Solente-Golé syndrome (acropachyderma) 757.39

Tourette's disease (motor-verbal tic) 307.23

Tower skull 756.0
- with exophthalmos 756.0

Toxemia 799.89
- with
  - abortion – *see* Abortion, by type, with toxemia
- bacterial – *see* Septicemia
- biliary (*see also* Disease, biliary) 576.8
- burn – *see* Burn, by site
- congenital NEC 779.89
- eclamptic 642.6❺
  - with pre-existing hypertension 642.7❺
- erysipelatous (*see also* Erysipelas) 035
- fatigue 799.89
- fetus or newborn NEC 779.89
- food (*see also* Poisoning, food) 005.9
- gastric 537.89
- gastrointestinal 558.2
- intestinal 558.2
- kidney (*see also* Disease, renal) 593.9
- lung 518.89
- malarial NEC (*see also* Malaria) 084.6
- maternal (of pregnancy), affecting fetus or newborn 760.0
- myocardial – *see* Myocarditis, toxic
- of pregnancy (mild) (pre-eclamptic) 642.4❺
  - with
    - convulsions 642.6❺
    - pre-existing hypertension 642.7❺
  - affecting fetus or newborn 760.0
  - severe 642.5❺
- pre-eclamptic – *see* Toxemia, of pregnancy
- puerperal, postpartum – *see* Toxemia, of pregnancy
- pulmonary 518.89
- renal (*see also* Disease, renal) 593.9
- septic (*see also* Septicemia) 038.9
- small intestine 558.2
- staphylococcal 038.10
  - aureus 038.11
  - due to food 005.0

Toxemia – *continued*
- staphylococcal – *continued*
  - specified organism NEC 038.19
- stasis 799.89
- stomach 537.89
- uremic (*see also* Uremia) 586
- urinary 586

Toxemica cerebropathia psychica (nonalcoholic) 294.0
- alcoholic 291.1

Toxic (poisoning) – *see also* condition
- from drug or poison – *see* Table of Drugs and Chemicals
- oil syndrome 710.5
- shock syndrome 040.82
- thyroid (gland) (*see also* Thyrotoxicosis) 242.9❺

Toxicemia – *see* Toxemia

Toxicity
- dilantin
  - asymptomatic 796.0
  - symptomatic – *see* Table of Drugs and Chemicals
- drug
  - asymptomatic 796.0
  - symptomatic – *see* Table of Drugs and Chemicals
- fava bean 282.2
- from drug or poison
  - asymptomatic 796.0
  - symptomatic- *see* Table of Drugs and Chemicals

Toxicosis (*see also* Toxemia) 799.89
- capillary, hemorrhagic 287.0

Toxinfection 799.89
- gastrointestinal 558.2

Toxocariasis 128.0

Toxoplasma infection, generalized 130.9

Toxoplasmosis (acquired) 130.9
- with pneumonia 130.4
- congenital, active 771.2
- disseminated (multisystemic) 130.8
- maternal
  - with suspected damage to fetus affecting management of pregnancy 655.4❺
  - affecting fetus or newborn 760.2
    - manifest toxoplasmosis in fetus or newborn 771.2
- multiple sites 130.8
- multisystemic disseminated 130.8
- specified site NEC 130.7

Trabeculation, bladder 596.8

Trachea – *see* condition

Tracheitis (acute) (catarrhal) (infantile) (membranous) (plastic) (pneumococcal) (septic) (suppurative) (viral) 464.10
- with
  - bronchitis 490
    - acute or subacute 466.0
    - chronic 491.8
    - tuberculosis – *see* Tuberculosis, pulmonary
  - laryngitis (acute) 464.20
    - with obstruction 464.21
    - chronic 476.1
    - tuberculous (*see also* Tuberculosis, larynx) 012.3❺
  - obstruction 464.11
- chronic 491.8
  - with
    - bronchitis (chronic) 491.8
    - laryngitis (chronic) 476.1
  - due to external agent – *see* Condition, respiratory, chronic, due to
- diphtheritic (membranous) 032.3
  - due to external agent – *see* Inflammation, respiratory, upper, due to
- edematous 464.11
- influenzal 487.1
- streptococcal 034.0
- syphilitic 095.8
- tuberculous (*see also* Tuberculosis) 012.8❺

Trachelitis (nonvenereal) (*see also* Cervicitis) 616.0
- trichomonal 131.09

Tracheobronchial – *see* condition

Tracheobronchitis (*see also* Bronchitis) 490
- acute or subacute 466.0
  - with bronchospasm or obstruction 466.0
- chronic 491.8
- influenzal 487.1
- senile 491.8

Tracheobronchomegaly (congenital) 748.3
- with bronchiectasis 494.0
  - with (acute) exacerbation 494.1
- acquired 519.19
  - with bronchiectasis 494.0
    - with (acute) exacerbation 494.1

Tracheobronchopneumonitis – *see* Pneumonia, broncho

Tracheocele (external) (internal) 519.19
- congenital 748.3

Tracheomalacia 519.19
- congenital 748.3

Tracheopharyngitis (acute) 465.8
- chronic 478.9
  - due to external agent – *see* Condition, respiratory, chronic, due to
- due to external agent – *see* Inflammation, respiratory, upper, due to

Tracheostenosis 519.19
- congenital 748.3

Tracheostomy
- attention to V55.0
- complication 519.00
- granuloma 519.09
- hemorrhage 519.09
- infection 519.01
- malfunctioning 519.02
- obstruction 519.09
- sepsis 519.01
- status V44.0
- stenosis 519.02

Trachoma, trachomatous 076.9
- active (stage) 076.1
- contraction of conjunctiva 076.1
- dubium 076.0
- healed or late effect 139.1
- initial (stage) 076.0
- Türck's (chronic catarrhal laryngitis) 476.0

Trachyphonia 784.49

Training
- insulin pump V65.46
- orthoptic V57.4
- orthotic V57.81

Train sickness 994.6

Trait
- hemoglobin
  - abnormal NEC 282.7
    - with thalassemia 282.49
  - C (*see also* Disease, hemoglobin, C) 282.7
    - with elliptocytosis 282.7
  - S (Hb-S) 282.5
- Lepore 282.49
  - with other abnormal hemoglobin NEC 282.49
- paranoid 301.0
- sickle-cell 282.5
  - with
    - elliptocytosis 282.5
    - spherocytosis 282.5

Traits, paranoid 301.0

Tramp V60.0

Trance 780.09
- hysterical 300.13

Transaminasemia 790.4

Transfusion, blood
- donor V59.01
  - stem cells V59.02
- incompatible 999.6
- reaction or complication – *see* Complications, transfusion
- related acute lung injury (TRALI) 518.7
- syndrome
  - fetomaternal 772.0
  - twin-to-twin
    - blood loss (donor twin) 772.0
    - recipient twin 776.4
- without reported diagnosis V58.2

Transient – *see also* condition
- alteration of awareness 780.02
- blindness 368.12
- deafness (ischemic) 388.02
- global amnesia 437.7
- person (homeless) NEC V60.0

Transitional, lumbosacral joint of vertebra 756.19

Translocation
- autosomes NEC 758.5
  - 13-15 758.1
  - 16-18 758.2
  - 21 or 22 758.0
  - balanced in normal individual 758.4

- **Translocation** – *continued*
  - autosomes – *continued*
    - D_1 758.1
    - E_3 758.2
    - G 758.0
  - balanced autosomal in normal individual 758.4
  - chromosomes NEC 758.89
  - Down syndrome 758.0
- **Translucency, iris** 364.53
- **Transmission of chemical substances through the placenta** (affecting fetus or newborn) 760.70
  - alcohol 760.71
  - anticonvulsants 760.77
  - antifungals 760.74
  - anti-infective agents 760.74
  - antimetabolics 760.78
  - cocaine 760.75
  - "crack" 760.75
  - diethylstilbestrol [DES] 760.76
  - hallucinogenic agents 760.73
  - medicinal agents NEC 760.79
  - narcotics 760.72
  - obstetric anesthetic or analgesic drug 763.5
  - specified agent NEC 760.79
  - suspected, affecting management of pregnancy 655.5❺
- **Transplant(ed)**
  - bone V42.4
    - marrow V42.81
  - complication – *see also* Complications, due to (presence of) any device, implant, or graft classified to 996.0-996.5 NEC
    - bone marrow 996.85
    - corneal graft NEC 996.79
      - infection or inflammation 996.69
      - reaction 996.51
      - rejection 996.51
    - organ (failure) (immune or nonimmune cause) (infection) (rejection) 996.80
      - bone marrow 996.85
      - heart 996.83
      - intestines 996.87
      - kidney 996.81
      - liver 996.82
      - lung 996.84
      - pancreas 996.86
      - specified NEC 996.89
    - skin NEC 996.79
      - infection or inflammation 996.69
      - rejection 996.52
        - artificial 996.55
        - decellularized allodermis 996.55
  - cornea V42.5
  - hair V50.0
  - heart V42.1
    - valve V42.2
  - intestine V42.84
  - kidney V42.0
  - liver V42.7
  - lung V42.6
  - organ V42.9
    - specified NEC V42.89
  - pancreas V42.83
  - peripheral stem cells V42.82
  - skin V42.3
  - stem cells, peripheral V42.82
  - tissue V42.9
    - specified NEC V42.89
- **Transplants, ovarian, endometrial** 617.1
- **Transposed** – *see* Transposition
- **Transposition** (congenital) – *see also* Malposition, congenital
  - abdominal viscera 759.3
  - aorta (dextra) 745.11
  - appendix 751.5
  - arterial trunk 745.10
  - colon 751.5
  - great vessels (complete) 745.10
    - both originating from right ventricle 745.11
    - corrected 745.12
    - double outlet right ventricle 745.11
    - incomplete 745.11
    - partial 745.11
    - specified type NEC 745.19
  - heart 746.87
    - with complete transposition of viscera 759.3
  - intestine (large) (small) 751.5
  - pulmonary veins 747.49
  - reversed jejunal (for bypass) (status) V45.3
  - scrotal 752.81
- **Transposition** – *continued*
  - stomach 750.7
    - with general transposition of viscera 759.3
  - teeth, tooth 524.30
  - vessels (complete) 745.10
    - partial 745.11
  - viscera (abdominal) (thoracic) 759.3
- **Trans-sexualism** 302.50
  - with
    - asexual history 302.51
    - heterosexual history 302.53
    - homosexual history 302.52
- **Transverse** – *see also* condition
  - arrest (deep), in labor 660.3❺
    - affecting fetus or newborn 763.1
  - lie 652.3❺
    - before labor, affecting fetus or newborn 761.7
    - causing obstructed labor 660.0❺
      - affecting fetus or newborn 763.1
    - during labor, affecting fetus or newborn 763.1
- **Transvestism, transvestitism** (transvestic fetishism) 302.3
- **Trapped placenta** (with hemorrhage) 666.0❺
  - without hemorrhage 667.0❺
- **Trauma, traumatism** (*see also* Injury, by site) 959.9
  - birth – *see* Birth, injury NEC
  - causing hemorrhage of pregnancy or delivery 641.8❺
  - complicating
    - abortion – *see* Abortion, by type, with damage to pelvic organs
    - ectopic pregnancy (*see also* categories 633.0-633.9) 639.2
    - molar pregnancy (*see also* categories 630-632) 639.2
  - during delivery NEC 665.9❺
  - following
    - abortion 639.2
    - ectopic or molar pregnancy 639.2
  - maternal, during pregnancy, affecting fetus or newborn 760.5
  - neuroma – *see* Injury, nerve, by site
  - previous major, affecting management of pregnancy, childbirth, or puerperium V23.8❺
  - psychic (current) – *see also* Reaction, adjustment
    - previous (history) V15.49
  - psychologic, previous (affecting health) V15.49
  - transient paralysis – *see* Injury, nerve, by site
- **Traumatic** – *see* condition
- **Treacher Collins' syndrome** (incomplete facial dysostosis) 756.0
- **Treitz's hernia** – *see* Hernia, Treitz's
- **Trematode infestation** NEC 121.9
- **Trematodiasis** NEC 121.9
- **Trembles** 988.8
- **Trembling paralysis** (*see also* Parkinsonism) 332.0
- **Tremor** 781.0
  - essential (benign) 333.1
  - familial 333.1
  - flapping (liver) 572.8
  - hereditary 333.1
  - hysterical 300.11
  - intention 333.1
  - medication-induced postural 333.1
  - mercurial 985.0
  - muscle 728.85
  - Parkinson's (*see also* Parkinsonism) 332.0
  - psychogenic 306.0
    - specified as conversion reaction 300.11
  - senilis 797
  - specified type NEC 333.1
- **Trench**
  - fever 083.1
  - foot 991.4
  - mouth 101
  - nephritis – *see* Nephritis, acute
- **Treponema pallidum infection** (*see also* Syphilis) 097.9
- **Treponematosis** 102.9
  - due to
    - T. pallidum – *see* Syphilis
    - T. pertenue (yaws) (*see also* Yaws) 102.9
- **Triad**
  - Kartagener's 759.3
  - Reiter's (complete) (incomplete) 099.3
  - Saint's (*see also* Hernia, diaphragm) 553.3
- **Trichiasis** 704.2
  - cicatricial 704.2
- **Trichiasis** – *continued*
  - eyelid 374.05
    - with entropion (*see also* Entropion) 374.00
- **Trichinella spiralis** (infection) (infestation) 124
- **Trichinelliasis** 124
- **Trichinellosis** 124
- **Trichiniasis** 124
- **Trichinosis** 124
- **Trichobezoar** 938
  - intestine 936
  - stomach 935.2
- **Trichocephaliasis** 127.3
- **Trichocephalosis** 127.3
- **Trichocephalus infestation** 127.3
- **Trichoclasis** 704.2
- **Trichoepithelioma** (M8100/0) – *see also* Neoplasm, skin, benign
  - breast 217
  - genital organ NEC – *see* Neoplasm, by site, benign
  - malignant (M8100/3) – *see* Neoplasm, skin, malignant
- **Trichofolliculoma** (M8101/0) – *see* Neoplasm, skin, benign
- **Tricholemmoma** (M8102/0) – *see* Neoplasm, skin, benign
- **Trichomatosis** 704.2
- **Trichomoniasis** 131.9
  - bladder 131.09
  - cervix 131.09
  - intestinal 007.3
  - prostate 131.03
  - seminal vesicle 131.09
  - specified site NEC 131.8
  - urethra 131.02
  - urogenitalis 131.00
  - vagina 131.01
  - vulva 131.01
  - vulvovaginal 131.01
- **Trichomycosis** 039.0
  - axillaris 039.0
  - nodosa 111.2
  - nodularis 111.2
  - rubra 039.0
- **Trichonocardiosis** (axillaris) (palmellina) 039.0
- **Trichonodosis** 704.2
- **Trichophytid, trichophyton infection** (*see also* Dermatophytosis) 110.9
- **Trichophytide** – *see* Dermatophytosis
- **Trichophytobezoar** 938
  - intestine 936
  - stomach 935.2
- **Trichophytosis** – *see* Dermatophytosis
- **Trichoptilosis** 704.2
- **Trichorrhexis** (nodosa) 704.2
- **Trichosporosis nodosa** 111.2
- **Trichostasis spinulosa** (congenital) 757.4
- **Trichostrongyliasis** (small intestine) 127.6
- **Trichostrongylosis** 127.6
- **Trichostrongylus** (instabilis) infection 127.6
- **Trichotillomania** 312.39
- **Trichromat, anomalous** (congenital) 368.59
- **Trichromatopsia, anomalous** (congenital) 368.59
- **Trichuriasis** 127.3
- **Trichuris trichiuria** (any site) (infection) (infestation) 127.3
- **Tricuspid** (valve) – *see* condition
- **Trifid** – *see also* Accessory
  - kidney (pelvis) 753.3
  - tongue 750.13
- **Trigeminal neuralgia** (*see also* Neuralgia, trigeminal) 350.1
- **Trigeminoencephaloangiomatosis** 759.6
- **Trigeminy** 427.89
  - postoperative 997.1
- **Trigger finger** (acquired) 727.03
  - congenital 756.89
- **Trigonitis** (bladder) (chronic) (pseudomembranous) 595.3
  - tuberculous (*see also* Tuberculosis) 016.1❺
- **Trigonocephaly** 756.0
- **Trihexosidosis** 272.7
- **Trilobate placenta** – *see* Placenta, abnormal
- **Trilocular heart** 745.8

Translocation – Trilocular heart

Trimethylaminuria 270.8
Tripartita placenta – *see* Placenta, abnormal
Triple – *see also* Accessory
kidneys 753.3
uteri 752.2
X female 758.81
Triplegia 344.89
congenital or infantile 343.8
Triplet
affected by maternal complications of pregnancy 761.5
healthy liveborn – *see* Newborn, multiple
pregnancy (complicating delivery) NEC 651.1❺
with fetal loss and retention of one or more fetus(es) 651.4❺
following (elective) fetal reduction 651.7
Triplex placenta – *see* Placenta, abnormal
Triplication – *see* Accessory
Trismus 781.0
neonatorum 771.3
newborn 771.3
Trisomy (syndrome) NEC 758.5
13 (partial) 758.1
16-18 758.2
18 (partial) 758.2
21 (partial) 758.0
22 758.0
autosomes NEC 758.5
D_1 758.1
E_3 758.2
G (group) 758.0
group D1 758.1
group E 758.2
group G 758.0
Tritanomaly 368.53
Tritanopia 368.53
Troisier-Hanot-Chauffard syndrome (bronze diabetes) 275.0
Trombidiosis 133.8
Trophedema (hereditary) 757.0
congenital 757.0
Trophoblastic disease (*see also* Hydatidiform mole) 630
previous, affect. management of pregnancy V23.1
Tropholymphedema 757.0
Trophoneurosis NEC 356.9
arm NEC 354.9
disseminated 710.1
facial 349.89
leg NEC 355.8
lower extremity NEC 355.8
upper extremity NEC 354.9
Tropical – *see also* condition
maceration feet (syndrome) 991.4
wet foot (syndrome) 991.4
Trouble – *see also* Disease
bowel 569.9
heart – *see* Disease, heart
intestine 569.9
kidney (*see also* Disease, renal) 593.9
nervous 799.2
sinus (*see also* Sinusitis) 473.9
Trousseau's syndrome (thrombophlebitis migrans) 453.1
Truancy, childhood – *see also* Disturbance, conduct
socialized 312.2❺
undersocialized, unsocialized 312.1❺
Truncus
arteriosus (persistent) 745.0
common 745.0
communis 745.0
Trunk – *see* condition
Trychophytide – *see* Dermatophytosis
Trypanosoma infestation – *see* Trypanosomiasis
Trypanosomiasis 086.9
with meningoencephalitis 086.9 *[323.2]*
African 086.5
due to Trypanosoma 086.5
gambiense 086.3
rhodesiense 086.4
American 086.2
with
heart involvement 086.0
other organ involvement 086.1
without mention of organ involvement 086.2
Brazilian – *see* Trypanosomiasis, American
Chagas' – *see* Trypanosomiasis, American

Trypanosomiasis – *continued*
due to Trypanosoma
cruzi – *see* Trypanosomiasis, American
due to Trypanosoma – *continued*
gambiense 086.3
rhodesiense 086.4
gambiensis, Gambian 086.3
North American – *see* Trypanosomiasis, American
rhodesiensis, Rhodesian 086.4
South American – *see* Trypanosomiasis, American
T-shaped incisors 520.2
Tsutsugamushi fever 081.2
Tube, tubal, tubular – *see also* condition
ligation, admission for V25.2
Tubercle – *see also* Tuberculosis
brain, solitary 013.2❺
Darwin's 744.29
epithelioid noncaseating 135
Ghon, primary infection 010.0❺
Tuberculid, tuberculide (indurating) (lichenoid) (miliary) (papulonecrotic) (primary) (skin) (subcutaneous) (*see also* Tuberculosis) 017.0❺
Tuberculoma – *see also* Tuberculosis
brain (any part) 013.2❺
meninges (cerebral) (spinal) 013.1❺
spinal cord 013.4❺
Tuberculosis, tubercular, tuberculous (calcification) (calcified) (caseous) (chromogenic acid-fast bacilli) (congenital) (degeneration) (disease) (fibrocaseous) (fistula) (gangrene) (interstitial) (isolated circumscribed lesions) (necrosis) (parenchymatous) (ulcerative) 011.9

Note – Use the following fifth-digit subclassification with categories 010-018:

0 unspecified
1 bacteriological or histological examination not done
2 bacteriological or histological examination unknown (at present)
3 tubercle bacilli found (in sputum) by microscopy
4 tubercle bacilli not found (in sputum) by microscopy, but found by bacterial culture
5 tubercle bacilli not found by bacteriological examination, but tuberculosis confirmed histologically
6 tubercle bacilli not found by bacteriological or histological examination, but tuberculosis confirmed by other methods [inoculation of animals]

For tuberculous conditions specified as late effects or sequelae, see category 137.

abdomen 014.8❺
lymph gland 014.8❺
abscess 011.9❺
arm 017.9❺
bone (*see also* Osteomyelitis, due to, tuberculosis) 015.9❺ *[730.8]*❺
hip 015.1❺ *[730.85]*
knee 015.2❺ *[730.86]*
sacrum 015.0❺ *[730.88]*
specified site NEC 015.7❺ *[730.88]*
spinal 015.0❺ *[730.88]*
vertebra 015.0❺ *[730.88]*
brain 013.3❺
breast 017.9❺
Cowper's gland 016.5❺
dura (mater) 013.8❺
brain 013.3❺
spinal cord 013.5❺
epidural 013.8❺
brain 013.3❺
spinal cord 013.5❺
frontal sinus – *see* Tuberculosis, sinus
genital organs NEC 016.9❺
female 016.7❺
male 016.5❺
genitourinary NEC 016.9❺
gland (lymphatic) – *see* Tuberculosis, lymph gland
hip 015.1❺
iliopsoas 015.0❺ *[730.88]*
intestine 014.8❺
ischiorectal 014.8❺
joint 015.9❺
hip 015.1❺
knee 015.2❺
specified joint NEC 015.8❺

Tuberculosis, tubercular, tuberculous – *continued*
abscess – *continued*
joint – *continued*
vertebral 015.0❺ *[730.88]*
kidney 016.0❺ *[590.81]*
knee 015.2❺
lumbar 015.0❺ *[730.88]*
lung 011.2❺
primary, progressive 010.8❺
meninges (cerebral) (spinal) 013.0❺
pelvic 016.9❺
female 016.7❺
male 016.5❺
perianal 014.8❺
fistula 014.8❺
perinephritic 016.0❺ *[590.81]*
perineum 017.9❺
perirectal 014.8❺
psoas 015.0❺ *[730.88]*
rectum 014.8❺
retropharyngeal 012.8❺
sacrum 015.0❺ *[730.88]*
scrofulous 017.2❺
scrotum 016.5❺
skin 017.0❺
primary 017.0❺
spinal cord 013.5❺
spine or vertebra (column) 015.0❺ *[730.88]*
strumous 017.2❺
subdiaphragmatic 014.8❺
testis 016.5❺
thigh 017.9❺
urinary 016.3❺
kidney 016.0❺ *[590.81]*
uterus 016.7❺
accessory sinus – *see* Tuberculosis, sinus
Addison's disease 017.6❺
adenitis (*see also* Tuberculosis, lymph gland) 017.2❺
adenoids 012.8❺
adenopathy (*see also* Tuberculosis, lymph gland) 017.2❺
tracheobronchial 012.1❺
primary progressive 010.8❺
adherent pericardium 017.9❺ *[420.0]*
adnexa (uteri) 016.7❺
adrenal (capsule) (gland) 017.6❺
air passage NEC 012.8❺
alimentary canal 014.8❺
anemia 017.9❺
ankle (joint) 015.8❺
bone 015.5❺ *[730.87]*
anus 014.8❺
apex (*see also* Tuberculosis, pulmonary) 011.9❺
apical (*see also* Tuberculosis, pulmonary) 011.9❺
appendicitis 014.8❺
appendix 014.8❺
arachnoid 013.0❺
artery 017.9❺
arthritis (chronic) (synovial) 015.9❺ *[711.40]*
ankle 015.8❺ *[730.87]*
hip 015.1❺ *[711.45]*
knee 015.2❺ *[711.46]*
specified site NEC 015.8❺ *[711.48]*
spine or vertebra (column) 015.0❺ *[720.81]*
wrist 015.8❺ *[730.83]*
articular – *see* Tuberculosis, joint
ascites 014.0❺
asthma (*see also* Tuberculosis, pulmonary) 011.9❺
axilla, axillary 017.2❺
gland 017.2❺
bilateral (*see also* Tuberculosis, pulmonary) 011.9❺
bladder 016.1❺
bone (*see also* Osteomyelitis, due to, tuberculosis) 015.9❺ *[730.8]*
hip 015.1❺ *[730.85]*
knee 015.2❺ *[730.86]*
limb NEC 015.5❺ *[730.88]*
sacrum 015.0❺ *[730.88]*
specified site NEC 015.7❺ *[730.88]*
spinal or vertebral column 015.0❺ *[730.88]*
bowel 014.8❺
miliary 018.9❺
brain 013.2❺
breast 017.9❺
broad ligament 016.7❺
bronchi, bronchial, bronchus 011.3❺
ectasia, ectasis 011.5❺

Trimethylaminuria – Tuberculosis, tubercular, tuberculous

Tuberculosis, tubercular, tuberculous – *continued*
- bronchi, bronchial, bronchus – *continued*
  - fistula 011.3❺
    - primary, progressive 010.8❺
  - gland 012.1❺
    - primary, progressive 010.8❺
  - isolated 012.2❺
  - lymph gland or node 012.1❺
    - primary, progressive 010.8❺
- bronchiectasis 011.5❺
- bronchitis 011.3❺
- bronchopleural 012.0❺
- bronchopneumonia, bronchopneumonic 011.6❺
- bronchorrhagia 011.3❺
- bronchotracheal 011.3❺
  - isolated 012.2❺
- bronchus – *see* Tuberculosis, bronchi
- bronze disease (Addison's) 017.6❺
- buccal cavity 017.9❺
- bulbourethral gland 016.5❺
- bursa (*see also* Tuberculosis, joint) 015.9❺
- cachexia NEC (*see also* Tuberculosis, pulmonary) 011.9❺
- cardiomyopathy 017.9❺ *[425.8]*
- caries (*see also* Tuberculosis, bone) 015.9❺ *[730.8]*
- cartilage (*see also* Tuberculosis, bone) 015.9❺ *[730.8]*
  - intervertebral 015.0❺ *[730.88]*
- catarrhal (*see also* Tuberculosis, pulmonary) 011.9❺
- cecum 014.8❺
- cellular tissue (primary) 017.0❺
- cellulitis (primary) 017.0❺
- central nervous system 013.9❺
  - specified site NEC 013.8❺
- cerebellum (current) 013.2❺
- cerebral (current) 013.2❺
  - meninges 013.0❺
- cerebrospinal 013.6❺
  - meninges 013.0❺
- cerebrum (current) 013.2❺
- cervical 017.2❺
  - gland 017.2❺
  - lymph nodes 017.2❺
- cervicitis (uteri) 016.7❺
- cervix 016.7❺
- chest (*see also* Tuberculosis, pulmonary) 011.9❺
- childhood type or first infection 010.0❺
- choroid 017.3❺ *[363.13]*
- choroiditis 017.3❺ *[363.13]*
- ciliary body 017.3❺ *[364.11]*
- colitis 014.8❺
- colliers' 011.4❺
- colliquativa (primary) 017.0❺
- colon 014.8❺
  - ulceration 014.8❺
- complex, primary 010.0❺
- complicating pregnancy, childbirth, or puerperium 647.3❺
  - affecting fetus or newborn 760.2❺
- congenital 771.2❺
- conjunctiva 017.3❺ *[370.31]*
- connective tissue 017.9❺
  - bone – *see* Tuberculosis, bone
- contact V01.1
- converter (tuberculin skin test) (without disease) 795.5
- cornea (ulcer) 017.3❺ *[370.31]*
- Cowper's gland 016.5❺
- coxae 015.1❺ *[730.85]*
- coxalgia 015.1❺ *[730.85]*
- cul-de-sac of Douglas 014.8❺
- curvature, spine 015.0❺ *[737.40]*
- cutis (colliquativa) (primary) 017.0❺
- cyst, ovary 016.6❺
- cystitis 016.1❺
- dacryocystitis 017.3❺ *[375.32]*
- dactylitis 015.5❺
- diarrhea 014.8❺
- diffuse (*see also* Tuberculosis, miliary) 018.9❺
  - lung – *see* Tuberculosis, pulmonary
  - meninges 013.0❺
- digestive tract 014.8❺
- disseminated (*see also* Tuberculosis, miliary) 018.9❺
  - meninges 013.0❺
- duodenum 014.8❺
- dura (mater) 013.9❺
  - abscess 013.8❺
    - cerebral 013.3❺

Tuberculosis, tubercular, tuberculous – *continued*
- dura (mater) – *continued*
  - abscess – *continued*
    - spinal 013.5❺
- dysentery 014.8❺
- ear (inner) (middle) 017.4❺
  - bone 015.6❺
  - external (primary) 017.0❺
  - skin (primary) 017.0❺
- elbow 015.8❺
- emphysema – *see* Tuberculosis, pulmonary
- empyema 012.0❺
- encephalitis 013.6❺
- endarteritis 017.9❺
- endocarditis (any valve) 017.9❺ *[424.91]*
- endocardium (any valve) 017.9❺ *[424.91]*
- endocrine glands NEC 017.9❺
- endometrium 016.7❺
- enteric, enterica 014.8❺
- enteritis 014.8❺
- enterocolitis 014.8❺
- epididymis 016.4❺
- epididymitis 016.4❺
- epidural abscess 013.8❺
  - brain 013.3❺
  - spinal cord 013.5❺
- epiglottis 012.3❺
- episcleritis 017.3❺ *[379.00]*
- erythema (induratum) (nodosum) (primary) 017.1❺
- esophagus 017.8❺
- Eustachian tube 017.4❺
- exposure to V01.1❺
- exudative 012.0❺
  - primary, progressive 010.1❺
- eye 017.3❺
  - glaucoma 017.3❺ *[365.62]*
- eyelid (primary) 017.0❺
  - lupus 017.0❺ *[373.4]*
- fallopian tube 016.6❺
- fascia 017.9❺
- fauces 012.8❺
- finger 017.9❺
- first infection 010.0❺
- fistula, perirectal 014.8❺
- Florida 011.6❺
- foot 017.9❺
- funnel pelvis 137.3
- gallbladder 017.9❺
- galloping (*see also* Tuberculosis, pulmonary) 011.9❺
- ganglionic 015.9❺
- gastritis 017.9❺
- gastrocolic fistula 014.8❺
- gastroenteritis 014.8❺
- gastrointestinal tract 014.8❺
- general, generalized 018.9❺
  - acute 018.0❺
  - chronic 018.8❺
- genital organs NEC 016.9❺
  - female 016.7❺
  - male 016.5❺
- genitourinary NEC 016.9❺
- genu 015.2❺
- glandulae suprarenalis 017.6❺
- glandular, general 017.2❺
- glottis 012.3❺
- grinders' 011.4❺
- groin 017.2❺
- gum 017.9❺
- hand 017.9❺
- heart 017.9❺ *[425.8]*
- hematogenous – *see* Tuberculosis, miliary
- hemoptysis (*see also* Tuberculosis, pulmonary) 011.9❺
- hemorrhage NEC (*see also* Tuberculosis, pulmonary) 011.9❺
- hemothorax 012.0❺
- hepatitis 017.9❺
- hilar lymph nodes 012.1❺
  - primary, progressive 010.8❺
- hip (disease) (joint) 015.1❺
  - bone 015.1❺ *[730.85]*
- hydrocephalus 013.8❺
- hydropneumothorax 012.0❺
- hydrothorax 012.0❺
- hypoadrenalism 017.6❺
- hypopharynx 012.8❺
- ileocecal (hyperplastic) 014.8❺
- ileocolitis 014.8❺
- ileum 014.8❺
- iliac spine (superior) 015.0❺ *[730.88]*

Tuberculosis, tubercular, tuberculous – *continued*
- incipient NEC (*see also* Tuberculosis, pulmonary) 011.9❺
- indurativa (primary) 017.1❺
- infantile 010.0❺
- infection NEC 011.9❺
  - without clinical manifestation 010.0❺
- infraclavicular gland 017.2❺
- inguinal gland 017.2❺
- inguinalis 017.2❺
- intestine (any part) 014.8❺
- iris 017.3❺ *[364.11]*
- iritis 017.3❺ *[364.11]*
- ischiorectal 014.8❺
- jaw 015.7❺ *[730.88]*
- jejunum 014.8❺
- joint 015.9❺
  - hip 015.1❺
  - knee 015.2❺
  - specified site NEC 015.8❺
  - vertebral 015.0❺ *[730.88]*
- keratitis 017.3❺ *[370.31]*
  - interstitial 017.3❺ *[370.59]*
- keratoconjunctivitis 017.3❺ *[370.31]*
- kidney 016.0❺
- knee (joint) 015.2❺
- kyphoscoliosis 015.0❺ *[737.43]*
- kyphosis 015.0❺ *[737.41]*
- lacrimal apparatus, gland 017.3❺
- laryngitis 012.3❺
- larynx 012.3❺
- leptomeninges, leptomeningitis (cerebral) (spinal) 013.0❺
- lichenoides (primary) 017.0❺
- linguae 017.9❺
- lip 017.9❺
- liver 017.9❺
- lordosis 015.0❺ *[737.42]*
- lung – *see* Tuberculosis, pulmonary
- luposa 017.0❺
  - eyelid 017.0❺ *[373.4]*
- lymphadenitis – *see* Tuberculosis, lymph gland
- lymphangitis – *see* Tuberculosis, lymph gland
- lymphatic (gland) (vessel) – *see* Tuberculosis, lymph gland
- lymph gland or node (peripheral) 017.2❺
  - abdomen 014.8❺
  - bronchial 012.1❺
    - primary, progressive 010.8❺
  - cervical 017.2❺
  - hilar 012.1❺
    - primary, progressive 010.8❺
  - intrathoracic 012.1❺
    - primary, progressive 010.8❺
  - mediastinal 012.1❺
    - primary, progressive 010.8❺
  - mesenteric 014.8❺
  - peripheral 017.2❺
  - retroperitoneal 014.8❺
  - tracheobronchial 012.1❺
    - primary, progressive 010.8❺
- malignant NEC (*see also* Tuberculosis, pulmonary) 011.9❺
- mammary gland 017.9❺
- marasmus NEC (*see also* Tuberculosis, pulmonary) 011.9❺
- mastoiditis 015.6❺
- maternal, affecting fetus or newborn 760.2
- mediastinal (lymph) gland or node 012.1❺
  - primary, progressive 010.8❺
- mediastinitis 012.8❺
  - primary, progressive 010.8❺
- mediastinopericarditis 017.9❺ *[420.0]*
- mediastinum 012.8❺
  - primary, progressive 010.8❺
- medulla 013.9❺
  - brain 013.2❺
  - spinal cord 013.4❺
- melanosis, Addisonian 017.6❺
- membrane, brain 013.0❺
- meninges (cerebral) (spinal) 013.0❺
- meningitis (basilar) (brain) (cerebral) (cerebrospinal) (spinal) 013.0❺
- meningoencephalitis 013.0❺
- mesentery, mesenteric 014.8❺
  - lymph gland or node 014.8❺
- miliary (any site) 018.9❺
  - acute 018.0❺
  - chronic 018.8❺
  - specified type NEC 018.8❺
- millstone makers' 011.4❺
- miners' 011.4❺

Tuberculosis, tubercular, tuberculous – *continued*
- moulders' 011.4❺
- mouth 017.9❺
- multiple 018.9❺
  - acute 018.0❺
  - chronic 018.8❺
- muscle 017.9❺
- myelitis 013.6❺
- myocarditis 017.9❺ *[422.0]*
- myocardium 017.9❺ *[422.0]*
- nasal (passage) (sinus) 012.8❺
- nasopharynx 012.8❺
- neck gland 017.2❺
- nephritis 016.0❺ *[583.81]*
- nerve 017.9❺
- nose (septum) 012.8❺
- ocular 017.3❺
- old NEC 137.0❺
  - without residuals V12.01
- omentum 014.8❺
- oophoritis (acute) (chronic) 016.6❺
- optic 017.3❺ *[377.39]*
  - nerve trunk 017.3❺ *[377.39]*
  - papilla, papillae 017.3❺ *[377.39]*
- orbit 017.3❺
- orchitis 016.5❺ *[608.81]*
- organ, specified NEC 017.9❺
- orificialis (primary) 017.0❺
- osseous (*see also* Tuberculosis, bone) 015.9❺ *[730.8]*
- osteitis (*see also* Tuberculosis, bone) 015.9❺ *[730.8]*
- osteomyelitis (*see also* Tuberculosis, bone) 015.9❺ *[730.8]*
- otitis (media) 017.4❺
- ovaritis (acute) (chronic) 016.6❺
- ovary (acute) (chronic) 016.6❺
- oviducts (acute) (chronic) 016.6❺
- pachymeningitis 013.0❺
- palate (soft) 017.9❺
- pancreas 017.9❺
- papulonecrotic (primary) 017.0❺
- parathyroid glands 017.9❺
- paronychia (primary) 017.0❺
- parotid gland or region 017.9❺
- pelvic organ NEC 016.9❺
  - female 016.7❺
  - male 016.5❺
- pelvis (bony) 015.7❺ *[730.85]*
- penis 016.5❺
- peribronchitis 011.3❺
- pericarditis 017.9❺ *[420.0]*
- pericardium 017.9❺ *[420.0]*
- perichondritis, larynx 012.3❺
- perineum 017.9❺
- periostitis (*see also* Tuberculosis, bone) 015.9❺ *[730.8]*
- periphlebitis 017.9❺
  - eye vessel 017.3❺ *[362.18]*
  - retina 017.3❺ *[362.18]*
- perirectal fistula 014.8❺
- peritoneal gland 014.8❺
- peritoneum 014.0❺
- peritonitis 014.0❺
- pernicious NEC (*see also* Tuberculosis, pulmonary) 011.9❺
- pharyngitis 012.8❺
- pharynx 012.8❺
- phlyctenulosis (conjunctiva) 017.3❺ *[370.31]*
- phthisis NEC (*see also* Tuberculosis, pulmonary) 011.9❺
- pituitary gland 017.9❺
- placenta 016.7❺
- pleura, pleural, pleurisy, pleuritis (fibrinous) (obliterative) (purulent) (simple plastic) (with effusion) 012.0❺
  - primary, progressive 010.1❺
- pneumonia, pneumonic 011.6❺
- pneumothorax 011.7❺
- polyserositis 018.9❺
  - acute 018.0❺
  - chronic 018.8❺
- potters' 011.4❺
- prepuce 016.5❺
- primary 010.9❺
  - complex 010.0❺
  - complicated 010.8❺
    - with pleurisy or effusion 010.1❺
  - progressive 010.8❺
    - with pleurisy or effusion 010.1❺
  - skin 017.0❺
- proctitis 014.8❺

Tuberculosis, tubercular, tuberculous – *continued*
- prostate 016.5❺ *[601.4]*
- prostatitis 016.5❺ *[601.4]*
- pulmonaris (*see also* Tuberculosis, pulmonary) 011.9❺
- pulmonary (artery) (incipient) (malignant) (multiple round foci) (pernicious) (reinfection stage) 011.9❺
  - cavitated or with cavitation 011.2❺
    - primary, progressive 010.8❺
  - childhood type or first infection 010.0❺
  - chromogenic acid-fast bacilli 795.39
  - fibrosis or fibrotic 011.4❺
  - infiltrative 011.0❺
    - primary, progressive 010.9❺
  - nodular 011.1❺
  - specified NEC 011.8❺
  - sputum positive only 795.39
  - status following surgical collapse of lung NEC 011.9❺
- pyelitis 016.0❺ *[590.81]*
- pyelonephritis 016.0❺ *[590.81]*
- pyemia – *see* Tuberculosis, miliary
- pyonephrosis 016.0❺
- pyopneumothorax 012.0❺
- pyothorax 012.0❺
- rectum (with abscess) 014.8❺
  - fistula 014.8❺
- reinfection stage (*see also* Tuberculosis, pulmonary) 011.9❺
- renal 016.0❺
- renis 016.0❺
- reproductive organ 016.7❺
- respiratory NEC (*see also* Tuberculosis, pulmonary) 011.9❺
  - specified site NEC 012.8❺
- retina 017.3❺ *[363.13]*
- retroperitoneal (lymph gland or node) 014.8❺
  - gland 014.8❺
- retropharyngeal abscess 012.8❺
- rheumatism 015.9❺
- rhinitis 012.8❺
- sacroiliac (joint) 015.8❺
- sacrum 015.0❺ *[730.88]*
- salivary gland 017.9❺
- salpingitis (acute) (chronic) 016.6❺
- sandblasters' 011.4❺
- sclera 017.3❺ *[379.09]*
- scoliosis 015.0❺ *[737.43]*
- scrofulous 017.2❺
- scrotum 016.5❺
- seminal tract or vesicle 016.5❺ *[608.81]*
- senile NEC (*see also* Tuberculosis, pulmonary) 011.9❺
- septic NEC (*see also* Tuberculosis, miliary) 018.9❺
- shoulder 015.8❺
  - blade 015.7❺ *[730.8]*
- sigmoid 014.8❺
- sinus (accessory) (nasal) 012.8❺
  - bone 015.7❺ *[730.88]*
  - epididymis 016.4❺
- skeletal NEC (*see also* Osteomyelitis, due to tuberculosis) 015.9❺ *[730.8]*
- skin (any site) (primary) 017.0❺
- small intestine 014.8❺
- soft palate 017.9❺
- spermatic cord 016.5❺
- spinal
  - column 015.0❺ *[730.88]*
  - cord 013.4❺
  - disease 015.0❺ *[730.88]*
  - medulla 013.4❺
  - membrane 013.0❺
  - meninges 013.0❺
- spine 015.0❺ *[730.88]*
- spleen 017.7❺
- splenitis 017.7❺
- spondylitis 015.0❺ *[720.81]*
- spontaneous pneumothorax – *see* Tuberculosis, pulmonary
- sternoclavicular joint 015.8❺
- stomach 017.9❺
- stonemasons' 011.4❺
- struma 017.2❺
- subcutaneous tissue (cellular) (primary) 017.0❺
- subcutis (primary) 017.0❺
- subdeltoid bursa 017.9❺
- submaxillary 017.9❺
  - region 017.9❺
- supraclavicular gland 017.2❺
- suprarenal (capsule) (gland) 017.6❺

Tuberculosis, tubercular, tuberculous – *continued*
- swelling, joint (*see also* Tuberculosis, joint) 015.9❺
- symphysis pubis 015.7❺ *[730.88]*
- synovitis 015.9❺ *[727.01]*
  - hip 015.1❺ *[727.01]*
  - knee 015.2❺ *[727.01]*
  - specified site NEC 015.8❺ *[727.01]*
  - spine or vertebra 015.0❺ *[727.01]*
- systemic – *see* Tuberculosis, miliary
- tarsitis (eyelid) 017.0❺ *[373.4]*
  - ankle (bone) 015.5❺ *[730.87]*
- tendon (sheath) – *see* Tuberculosis, tenosynovitis
- tenosynovitis 015.9❺ *[727.01]*
  - hip 015.1❺ *[727.01]*
  - knee 015.2❺ *[727.01]*
  - specified site NEC 015.8❺ *[727.01]*
  - spine or vertebra 015.0❺ *[727.01]*
- testis 016.5❺ *[608.81]*
- throat 012.8❺
- thymus gland 017.9❺
- thyroid gland 017.5❺
- toe 017.9❺
- tongue 017.9❺
- tonsil (lingual) 012.8❺
- tonsillitis 012.8❺
- trachea, tracheal 012.8❺
  - gland 012.1❺
    - primary, progressive 010.8❺
  - isolated 012.2❺
- tracheobronchial 011.3❺
  - glandular 012.1❺
    - primary, progressive 010.8❺
  - isolated 012.2❺
  - lymph gland or node 012.1❺
    - primary, progressive 010.8❺
- tubal 016.6❺
- tunica vaginalis 016.5❺
- typhlitis 014.8❺
- ulcer (primary) (skin) 017.0❺
  - bowel or intestine 014.8❺
  - specified site NEC – *see* Tuberculosis, by site
- unspecified site – *see* Tuberculosis, pulmonary
- ureter 016.2❺
- urethra, urethral 016.3❺
- urinary organ or tract 016.3❺
  - kidney 016.0❺
- uterus 016.7❺
- uveal tract 017.3❺ *[363.13]*
- uvula 017.9❺
- vaccination, prophylactic (against) V03.2
- vagina 016.7❺
- vas deferens 016.5❺
- vein 017.9❺
- verruca (primary) 017.0❺
- verrucosa (cutis) (primary) 017.0❺
- vertebra (column) 015.0❺ *[730.88]*
- vesiculitis 016.5❺ *[608.81]*
- viscera NEC 014.8❺
- vulva 016.7❺ *[616.51]*
- wrist (joint)❺ 015.8
  - bone 015.5❺ *[730.83]*

Tuberculum
- auriculae 744.29
- occlusal 520.2
- paramolare 520.2

Tuberosity
- jaw, excessive 524.07
- maxillary, entire 524.07

Tuberous sclerosis (brain) 759.5

Tubo-ovarian – *see* condition

Tuboplasty, after previous sterilization V26.0

Tubotympanitis 381.10

Tularemia 021.9
- with
  - conjunctivitis 021.3
  - pneumonia 021.2
- bronchopneumonic 021.2
- conjunctivitis 021.3
- cryptogenic 021.1
- disseminated 021.8
- enteric 021.1
- generalized 021.8
- glandular 021.8
- intestinal 021.1
- oculoglandular 021.3
- ophthalmic 021.3
- pneumonia 021.2
- pulmonary 021.2
- specified NEC 021.8
- typhoidal 021.1

Tuberculosis, tubercular, tuberculous – Tularemia

Tularemia – *continued*
- ulceroglandular 021.0
- vaccination, prophylactic (against) V03.4

Tularensis conjunctivitis 021.3

Tumefaction – *see also* Swelling
- liver (*see also* Hypertrophy, liver) 789.1

Tumor (M8000/1) – *see also* Neoplasm, by site, unspecified nature
- Abrikossov's (M9580/0) – *see also* Neoplasm, connective tissue, benign
  - malignant (M9580/3) – *see* Neoplasm, connective tissue, malignant
- acinar cell (M8550/1) – *see* Neoplasm, by site, uncertain behavior
- acinic cell (M8550/1) – *see* Neoplasm, by site, uncertain behavior
- adenomatoid (M9054/0) – *see also* Neoplasm, by site, benign
  - odontogenic (M9300/0) 213.1
    - upper jaw (bone) 213.0
- adnexal (skin) (M8390/0) – *see* Neoplasm, skin, benign
- adrenal
  - cortical (benign) (M8370/0) 227.0
    - malignant (M8370/3) 194.0
  - rest (M8671/0) – *see* Neoplasm, by site, benign
- alpha cell (M8152/0)
  - malignant (M8152/3)
    - pancreas 157.4
    - specified site NEC – *see* Neoplasm, by site, malignant
    - unspecified site 157.4
  - pancreas 211.7
  - specified site NEC – *see* Neoplasm, by site, benign
  - unspecified site 211.7
- aneurysmal (*see also* Aneurysm) 442.9
- aortic body (M8691/1) 237.3
  - malignant (M8691/3) 194.6
- argentaffin (M8241/1) – *see* Neoplasm, by site, uncertain behavior
- basal cell (M8090/1) – *see also* Neoplasm, skin, uncertain behavior
- benign (M8000/0) – *see* Neoplasm, by site, benign
- beta cell (M8151/0)
  - malignant (M8151/3)
    - pancreas 157.4
    - specified site – *see* Neoplasm, by site, malignant
    - unspecified site 157.4
  - pancreas 211.7
  - specified site NEC – *see* Neoplasm, by site, benign
  - unspecified site 211.7
- blood – *see* Hematoma
- Brenner (M9000/0) 220
  - borderline malignancy (M9000/1) 236.2
  - malignant (M9000/3) 183.0
  - proliferating (M9000/1) 236.2
- Brooke's (M8100/0) – *see* Neoplasm, skin, benign
- brown fat (M8880/0) – *see* Lipoma, by site
- Burkitt's (M9750/3) 200.2❺
- calcifying epithelial odontogenic (M9340/0) 213.1
  - upper jaw (bone) 213.0
- carcinoid (M8240/1) – *see* Carcinoid
- carotid body (M8692/1) 237.3
  - malignant (M8692/3) 194.5
- Castleman's (mediastinal lymph node hyperplasia) 785.6
- cells (M8001/1) – *see also* Neoplasm, by site, unspecified nature
  - benign (M8001/0) – *see* Neoplasm, by site, benign
  - malignant (M8001/3) – *see* Neoplasm, by site, malignant
  - uncertain whether benign or malignant (M8001/1) – *see* Neoplasm, by site, uncertain nature
- cervix
  - in pregnancy or childbirth 654.6❺
    - affecting fetus or newborn 763.89
    - causing obstructed labor 660.2❺
      - affecting fetus or newborn 763.1
- chondromatous giant cell (M9230/0) – *see* Neoplasm, bone, benign

Tumor – *continued*
- chromaffin (M8700/0) – *see also* Neoplasm, by site, benign
  - malignant (M8700/3) – *see* Neoplasm, by site, malignant
- Cock's peculiar 706.2
- Codman's (benign chondroblastoma) (M9230/0) – *see* Neoplasm, bone, benign
- dentigerous, mixed (M9282/0) 213.1
  - upper jaw (bone) 213.0
- dermoid (M9084/0) – *see* Neoplasm, by site, benign
  - with malignant transformation (M9084/3) 183.0
- desmoid (extra-abdominal) (M8821/1) – *see also* Neoplasm, connective tissue, uncertain behavior
  - abdominal (M8822/1) – *see* Neoplasm, connective tissue, uncertain behavior
- embryonal (mixed) (M9080/1) – *see also* Neoplasm, by site, uncertain behavior
  - liver (M9080/3) 155.0
- endodermal sinus (M9071/3)
  - specified site – *see* Neoplasm, by site, malignant
  - unspecified site
    - female 183.0
    - male 186.9
- epithelial
  - benign (M8010/0) – *see* Neoplasm, by site, benign
  - malignant (M8010/3) – *see* Neoplasm, by site, malignant
- Ewing's (M9260/3) – *see* Neoplasm, bone, malignant
- fatty – *see* Lipoma
- fetal, causing disproportion 653.7❺
  - causing obstructed labor 660.1❺
- fibroid (M8890/0) – *see* Leiomyoma
- G cell (M8153/1)
  - malignant (M8153/3)
    - pancreas 157.4
    - specified site NEC – *see* Neoplasm, by site, malignant
    - unspecified site 157.4
  - specified site – *see* Neoplasm, by site, uncertain behavior
  - unspecified site 235.5
- giant cell (type) (M8003/1) – *see also* Neoplasm, by site, unspecified nature
  - bone (M9250/1) 238.0
    - malignant (M9250/3) – *see* Neoplasm, bone, malignant
  - chondromatous (M9230/0) – *see* Neoplasm, bone, benign
  - malignant (M8003/3) – *see* Neoplasm, by site, malignant
  - peripheral (gingiva) 523.8
  - soft parts (M9251/1) – *see also* Neoplasm, connective tissue, uncertain behavior
    - malignant (M9251/3) – *see* Neoplasm, connective tissue, malignant
  - tendon sheath 727.02
- glomus (M8711/0) – *see also* Hemangioma, by site
  - jugulare (M8690/1) 237.3
    - malignant (M8690/3) 194.6
- gonadal stromal (M8590/1) – *see* Neoplasm, by site, uncertain behavior
- granular cell (M9580/0) – *see also* Neoplasm, connective tissue, benign
  - malignant (M9580/3) – *see* Neoplasm, connective tissue, malignant
- granulosa cell (M8620/1) 236.2
  - malignant (M8620/3) 183.0
- granulosa cell-theca cell (M8621/1) 236.2
  - malignant (M8621/3) 183.0
- Grawitz's (hypernephroma) (M8312/3) 189.0
- hazard-crile (M8350/3) 193
- hemorrhoidal – *see* Hemorrhoids
- hilar cell (M8660/0) 220
- Hürthle cell (benign) (M8290/0) 226
  - malignant (M8290/3) 193
- hydatid (*see also* Echinococcus) 122.9
- hypernephroid (M8311/1) – *see also* Neoplasm, by site, uncertain behavior
- interstitial cell (M8650/1) – *see also* Neoplasm, by site, uncertain behavior
  - benign (M8650/0) – *see* Neoplasm, by site, benign
  - malignant (M8650/3) – *see* Neoplasm, by site, malignant

Tumor – *continued*
- islet cell (M8150/0)
  - malignant (M8150/3)
    - pancreas 157.4
    - specified site – *see* Neoplasm, by site, malignant
    - unspecified site 157.4
  - pancreas 211.7
  - specified site NEC – *see* Neoplasm, by site, benign
  - unspecified site 211.7
- juxtaglomerular (M8361/1) 236.91
- Krukenberg's (M8490/6) 198.6
- Leydig cell (M8650/1)
  - benign (M8650/0)
    - specified site – *see* Neoplasm, by site, benign
    - unspecified site
      - female 220
      - male 222.0
  - malignant (M8650/3)
    - specified site – *see* Neoplasm, by site, malignant
    - unspecified site
      - female 183.0
      - male 186.9
  - specified site – *see* Neoplasm, by site, uncertain behavior
  - unspecified site
    - female 236.2
    - male 236.4
- lipid cell, ovary (M8670/0) 220
- lipoid cell, ovary (M8670/0) 220
- lymphomatous, benign (M9590/0) – *see also* Neoplasm, by site, benign
- Malherbe's (M8110/0) – *see* Neoplasm, skin, benign
- malignant (M8000/3) – *see also* Neoplasm, by site, malignant
  - fusiform cell (type) (M8004/3) – *see* Neoplasm, by site, malignant
  - giant cell (type) (M8003/3) – *see* Neoplasm, by site, malignant
  - mixed NEC (M8940/3) – *see* Neoplasm, by site, malignant
  - small cell (type) (M8002/3) – *see* Neoplasm, by site, malignant
  - spindle cell (type) (M8004/3) – *see* Neoplasm, by site, malignant
- mast cell (M9740/1) 238.5
  - malignant (M9740/3) 202.6❺
- melanotic, neuroectodermal (M9363/0) – *see* Neoplasm, by site, benign
- Merkel cell – *see* Neoplasm, by site, malignant
- mesenchymal
  - malignant (M8800/3) – *see* Neoplasm, connective tissue, malignant
  - mixed (M8990/1) – *see* Neoplasm, connective tissue, uncertain behavior
- mesodermal, mixed (M8951/3) – *see also* Neoplasm, by site, malignant
  - liver 155.0
- mesonephric (M9110/1) – *see also* Neoplasm, by site, uncertain behavior
  - malignant (M9110/3) – *see* Neoplasm, by site, malignant
- metastatic
  - from specified site (M8000/3) – *see* Neoplasm, by site, malignant
  - to specified site (M8000/6) – *see* Neoplasm, by site, malignant, secondary
- mixed NEC (M8940/0) – *see also* Neoplasm, by site, benign
  - malignant (M8940/3) – *see* Neoplasm, by site, malignant
- mucocarcinoid, malignant (M8243/3) – *see* Neoplasm, by site, malignant
- mucoepidermoid (M8430/1) – *see* Neoplasm, by site, uncertain behavior
- Mullerian, mixed (M8950/3) – *see* Neoplasm, by site, malignant
- myoepithelial (M8982/0) – *see* Neoplasm, by site, benign
- neurogenic olfactory (M9520/3) 160.0
- nonencapsulated sclerosing (M8350/3) 193
- odontogenic (M9270/1) 238.0
  - adenomatoid (M9300/0) 213.1
    - upper jaw (bone) 213.0
  - benign (M9270/0) 213.1
    - upper jaw (bone) 213.0
  - calcifying epithelial (M9340/0) 213.1
    - upper jaw (bone) 213.0

Tumor – *continued*
  odontogenic – *continued*
    malignant (M9270/3) 170.1
      upper jaw (bone) 170.0
    squamous (M9312/0) 213.1
      upper jaw (bone) 213.0
  ovarian stromal (M8590/1) 236.2
  ovary
    in pregnancy or childbirth 654.4❺
      affecting fetus or newborn 763.89
      causing obstructed labor 660.2❺
        affecting fetus or newborn 763.1
  pacinian (M9507/0) – *see* Neoplasm, skin, benign
  Pancoast's (M8010/3) 162.3
  papillary – *see* Papilloma
  pelvic, in pregnancy or childbirth 654.9❺
    affecting fetus or newborn 763.89
    causing obstructed labor 660.2❺
      affecting fetus or newborn 763.1
  phantom 300.11
  plasma cell (M9731/1) 238.6
    benign (M9731/0) – *see* Neoplasm, by site, benign
    malignant (M9731/3) 203.8❺
  polyvesicular vitelline (M9071/3)
    specified site – *see* Neoplasm, by site, malignant
    unspecified site
      female 183.0
      male 186.9
  Pott's puffy (*see also* Osteomyelitis) 730.2❺
  Rathke's pouch (M9350/1) 237.0
  regaud's (M8082/3) – *see* Neoplasm, nasopharynx, malignant
  rete cell (M8140/0) 222.0
  retinal anlage (M9363/0) – *see* Neoplasm, by site, benign
  Rokitansky's 620.2
  salivary gland type, mixed (M8940/0) – *see also* Neoplasm, by site, benign
    malignant (M8940/3) – *see* Neoplasm, by site, malignant
  Sampson's 617.1
  Schloffer's (*see also* Peritonitis) 567.29
  Schmincke (M8082/3) – *see* Neoplasm, nasopharynx, malignant
  sebaceous (*see also* Cyst, sebaceous) 706.2
  secondary (M8000/6) – *see* Neoplasm, by site, secondary
  Sertoli cell (M8640/0)
    with lipid storage (M8641/0)
      specified site – *see* Neoplasm, by site, benign
      unspecified site
        female 220
        male 222.0
    specified site – *see* Neoplasm, by site, benign
    unspecified site
      female 220
      male 222.0
  Sertoli-Leydig cell (M8631/0)
    specified site, – *see* Neoplasm, by site, benign
    unspecified site
      female 220
      male 222.0
  sex cord (-stromal) (M8590/1) – *see* Neoplasm, by site, uncertain behavior
  skin appendage (M8390/0) – *see* Neoplasm, skin, benign
  soft tissue
    benign (M8800/0) – *see* Neoplasm, connective tissue, benign
    malignant (M8800/3) – *see* Neoplasm, connective tissue, malignant
  sternomastoid 754.1
  stromal
    abdomen
      benign 215.5
      malignant 171.5
      uncertain behavior 238.1
    digestive system 238.1
      benign 215.5
      malignant 171.5
      uncertain behavior 238.1
    gastric 238.1
      benign 215.5
      malignant 171.5
      uncertain behavior 238.1
    gastrointestinal 238.1
      benign 215.5
      malignant 171.5
      uncertain behavior 238.1

Tumor – *continued*
  stromal – *continued*
    intestine (small) (large) 238.1
      benign 215.5
      malignant 171.5
      uncertain behavior 238.1
    stomach 238.1
      benign 215.5
      malignant 171.5
      uncertain behavior 238.1
  superior sulcus (lung) (pulmonary) (syndrome) (M8010/3) 162.3
  suprasulcus (M8010/3) 162.3
  sweat gland (M8400/1) – *see also* Neoplasm, skin, uncertain behavior
    benign (M8400/0) – *see* Neoplasm, skin, benign
    malignant (M8400/3) – *see* Neoplasm, skin, malignant
  syphilitic brain 094.89
    congenital 090.49
  testicular stromal (M8590/1) 236.4
  theca cell (M8600/0) 220
  theca cell-granulosa cell (M8621/1) 236.2
  theca-lutein (M8610/0) 220
  turban (M8200/0) 216.4
  uterus
    in pregnancy or childbirth 654.1❺
      affecting fetus or newborn 763.89
      causing obstructed labor 660.2❺
        affecting fetus or newborn 763.1
  vagina
    in pregnancy or childbirth 654.7❺
      affecting fetus or newborn 763.89
      causing obstructed labor 660.2❺
        affecting fetus or newborn 763.1
  varicose (*see also* Varicose, vein) 454.9
  von Recklinghausen's (M9540/1) 237.71
  vulva
    in pregnancy or childbirth 654.8❺
      affecting fetus or newborn 763.89
      causing obstructed labor 660.2❺
        affecting fetus or newborn 763.1
  Warthin's (salivary gland) (M8561/0) 210.2
  white – *see also* Tuberculosis, arthritis
  White-Darier 757.39
  Wilms' (nephroblastoma) (M8960/3) 189.0
  yolk sac (M9071/3)
    specified site – *see* Neoplasm, by site, malignant
    unspecified site
      female 183.0
      male 186.9
Tumorlet (M8040/1) – *see* Neoplasm, by site, uncertain behavior
Tungiasis 134.1
Tunica vasculosa lentis 743.39
Tunnel vision 368.45
Turban tumor (M8200/0) 216.4
Türck's trachoma (chronic catarrhal laryngitis) 476.0
Türk's syndrome (ocular retraction syndrome) 378.71
Turner's
  hypoplasia (tooth) 520.4
  syndrome 758.6
  tooth 520.4
Turner-Kieser syndrome (hereditary osteo-onychodysplasia) 756.89
Turner-Varny syndrome 758.6
Turricephaly 756.0
Tussis convulsiva (*see also* Whooping cough) 033.9
Twin
  affected by maternal complications of pregnancy 761.5
  conjoined 759.4
  healthy liveborn – *see* Newborn, twin
  pregnancy (complicating delivery) NEC 651.0❺
    with fetal loss and retention of one fetus 651.3❺
    following (elective) fetal reduction 651.7
Twinning, teeth 520.2
Twist, twisted
  bowel, colon, or intestine 560.2
  hair (congenital) 757.4
  mesentery 560.2
  omentum 560.2
  organ or site, congenital NEC – *see* Anomaly, specified type NEC
  ovarian pedicle 620.5
    congenital 752.0

Twist, twisted – *continued*
  umbilical cord – *see* Compression, umbilical cord
Twitch 781.0
Tylosis 700
  buccalis 528.6
  gingiva 523.8
  linguae 528.6
  palmaris et plantaris 757.39
Tympanism 787.3
Tympanites (abdominal) (intestine) 787.3
Tympanitis – *see* Myringitis
Tympanosclerosis 385.00
  involving
    combined sites NEC 385.09
      with tympanic membrane 385.03
    tympanic membrane 385.01
      with ossicles 385.02
        and middle ear 385.03
Tympanum – *see* condition
Tympany
  abdomen 787.3
  chest 786.7
Typhlitis (*see also* Appendicitis) 541
Typhoenteritis 002.0
Typhogastric fever 002.0
Typhoid (abortive) (ambulant) (any site) (fever) (hemorrhagic) (infection) (intermittent) (malignant) (rheumatic) 002.0
  with pneumonia 002.0 *[484.8]*
  abdominal 002.0
  carrier (suspected) of V02.1
  cholecystitis (current) 002.0
  clinical (Widal and blood test negative) 002.0
  endocarditis 002.0 *[421.1]*
  inoculation reaction – *see* Complications, vaccination
  meningitis 002.0 *[320.7]*
  mesenteric lymph nodes 002.0
  myocarditis 002.0 *[422.0]*
  osteomyelitis (*see also* Osteomyelitis, due to, typhoid) 002.0 *[730.8]*❺
  perichondritis, larynx 002.0 *[478.71]*
  pneumonia 002.0 *[484.8]*
  spine 002.0 *[720.81]*
  ulcer (perforating) 002.0
  vaccination, prophylactic (against) V03.1
  Widal negative 002.0
Typhomalaria (fever) (*see also* Malaria) 084.6
Typhomania 002.0
Typhoperitonitis 002.0
Typhus (fever) 081.9
  abdominal, abdominalis 002.0
  African tick 082.1
  amarillic (*see also* Fever, Yellow) 060.9
  brain 081.9
  cerebral 081.9
  classical 080
  endemic (flea-borne) 081.0
  epidemic (louse-borne) 080
  exanthematic NEC 080
  exanthematicus SAI 080
    brillii SAI 081.1
    Mexicanus SAI 081.0
    pediculo vestimenti causa 080
    typhus murinus 081.0
  flea-borne 081.0
  Indian tick 082.1
  Kenya tick 082.1
  louse-borne 080
  Mexican 081.0
    flea-borne 081.0
    louse-borne 080
    tabardillo 080
  mite-borne 081.2
  murine 081.0
  North Asian tick-borne 082.2
  petechial 081.9
  Queensland tick 082.3
  rat 081.0
  recrudescent 081.1
  recurrent (*see also* Fever, relapsing) 087.9
  São Paulo 082.0
  scrub (China) (India) (Malaya) (New Guinea) 081.2
  shop (of Malaya) 081.0
  Siberian tick 082.2
  tick-borne NEC 082.9
  tropical 081.2
  vaccination, prophylactic (against) V05.8

Tyrosinemia 270.2
neonatal 775.89
Tyrosinosis (Medes) (Sakai) 270.2
Tyrosinuria 270.2
Tyrosyluria 270.2

U

Uehlinger's syndrome (acropachyderma) 757.39
Uhl's anomaly or disease (hypoplasia of myocardium, right ventricle) 746.84
Ulcer, ulcerated, ulcerating, ulceration, ulcerative 707.9
with gangrene 707.9 *[785.4]*
abdomen (wall) (*see also* Ulcer, skin) 707.8
ala, nose 478.19
alveolar process 526.5
amebic (intestine) 006.9
skin 006.6
anastomotic – *see* Ulcer, gastrojejunal
anorectal 569.41
antral – *see* Ulcer, stomach
anus (sphincter) (solitary) 569.41
varicose – *see* Varicose, ulcer, anus
aorta – *see* Aneurysm
aphthous (oral) (recurrent) 528.2
genital organ(s)
female 616.50 ▲
male 608.89
mouth 528.2
arm (*see also* Ulcer, skin) 707.8
arteriosclerotic plaque – *see* Arteriosclerosis, by site
artery NEC 447.2
without rupture 447.8
atrophic NEC – *see* Ulcer, skin
Barrett's (chronic peptic ulcer of esophagus) 530.85
bile duct 576.8
bladder (solitary) (sphincter) 596.8
bilharzial (*see also* Schistosomiasis) 120.9 *[595.4]*
submucosal (*see also* Cystitis) 595.1
tuberculous (*see also* Tuberculosis) 016.1❺
bleeding NEC – *see* Ulcer, peptic, with hemorrhage
bone 730.9❺
bowel (*see also* Ulcer, intestine) 569.82
breast 611.0
bronchitis 491.8
bronchus 519.19
buccal (cavity) (traumatic) 528.9
burn (acute) – *see* Ulcer, duodenum
Buruli 031.1
buttock (*see also* Ulcer, skin) 707.8
decubitus (*see also* Ulcer, decubitus) 707.00
cancerous (M8000/3) – *see* Neoplasm, by site, malignant
cardia – *see* Ulcer, stomach
cardio-esophageal (peptic) 530.20
with bleeding 530.21
cecum (*see also* Ulcer, intestine) 569.82
cervix (uteri) (trophic) 622.0
with mention of cervicitis 616.0
chancroidal 099.0
chest (wall) (*see also* Ulcer, skin) 707.8
Chiclero 085.4
chin (pyogenic) (*see also* Ulcer, skin) 707.8
chronic (cause unknown) – *see also* Ulcer, skin
penis 607.89
Cochin-China 085.1
colitis – *see* Colitis, ulcerative
colon (*see also* Ulcer, intestine) 569.82
conjunctiva (acute) (postinfectional) 372.00
cornea (infectional) 370.00
with perforation 370.06
annular 370.02
catarrhal 370.01
central 370.03
dendritic 054.42
marginal 370.01
mycotic 370.05
phlyctenular, tuberculous (*see also* Tuberculosis) 017.3❺ *[370.31]*
ring 370.02
rodent 370.07
serpent, serpiginous 370.04
superficial marginal 370.01

Ulcer, ulcerated, ulcerating, ulceration, ulcerative - *continued*
cornea – *continued*
tuberculous (*see also* Tuberculosis) 017.3❺ *[370.31]*
corpus cavernosum (chronic) 607.89
crural – *see* Ulcer, lower extremity
Curling's – *see* Ulcer, duodenum
Cushing's – *see* Ulcer, peptic
cystitis (interstitial) 595.1
decubitus (unspecified site) 707.00
with gangrene 707.00 *[785.4]*
ankle 707.06
back
lower 707.03
upper 707.02
buttock 707.05
elbow 707.01
head 707.09
heel 707.07
hip 707.04
other site 707.09
sacrum 707.03
shoulder blades 707.02
dendritic 054.42
diabetes, diabetic (mellitus) 250.8❺ *[707.9]*
lower limb 250.8❺ *[707.10]*
ankle 250.8❺ *[707.13]*
calf 250.8❺ *[707.12]*
foot 250.8❺ *[707.15]*
heel 250.8❺ *[707.14]*
knee 250.8❺ *[707.19]*
specified site NEC 250.8❺ *[707.19]*
thigh 250.8❺ *[707.11]*
toes 250.8❺ *[707.15]*
specified site NEC 250.8❺ *[707.8]*
Dieulafoy – *see* Lesion, Dieulafoy
due to
infection NEC – *see* Ulcer, skin
radiation, radium – *see* Ulcer, by site
trophic disturbance (any region) – *see* Ulcer, skin
x-ray – *see* Ulcer, by site
duodenum, duodenal (eroded) (peptic) 532.9❺

Note – Use the following fifth-digit subclassification with categories 531-534:
0 without mention of obstruction
1 with obstruction

with
hemorrhage (chronic) 532.4❺
and perforation 532.6❺
perforation (chronic) 532.5❺
and hemorrhage 532.6❺
acute 532.3❺
with
hemorrhage 532.0❺
and perforation 532.2❺
perforation 532.1❺
and hemorrhage 532.2❺
bleeding (recurrent) – *see* Ulcer, duodenum, with hemorrhage
chronic 532.7❺
with
hemorrhage 532.4❺
and perforation 532.6❺
perforation 532.5❺
and hemorrhage 532.6❺
penetrating – *see* Ulcer, duodenum, with perforation
perforating – *see* Ulcer, duodenum, with perforation
dysenteric NEC 009.0
elusive 595.1
endocarditis (any valve) (acute) (chronic) (subacute) 421.0
enteritis – *see* Colitis, ulcerative
enterocolitis 556.0
epiglottis 478.79
esophagus (peptic) 530.20
with bleeding 530.21
due to ingestion
aspirin 530.20
chemicals 530.20
medicinal agents 530.20
fungal 530.20
infectional 530.20
varicose (*see also* Varix, esophagus) 456.1
bleeding (*see also* Varix, esophagus, bleeding) 456.0
eye NEC 360.00
dendritic 054.42

Ulcer, ulcerated, ulcerating, ulceration, ulcerative - *continued*
eyelid (region) 373.01
face (*see also* Ulcer, skin) 707.8
fauces 478.29
Fenwick (-Hunner) (solitary) (*see also* Cystitis) 595.1
fistulous NEC – *see* Ulcer, skin
foot (indolent) (*see also* Ulcer, lower extremity) 707.15
perforating 707.15
leprous 030.1
syphilitic 094.0
trophic 707.15
varicose 454.0
inflamed or infected 454.2
frambesial, initial or primary 102.0
gallbladder or duct 575.8
gall duct 576.8
gangrenous (*see also* Gangrene) 785.4
gastric – *see* Ulcer, stomach
gastrocolic – *see* Ulcer, gastrojejunal
gastroduodenal – *see* Ulcer, peptic
gastroesophageal – *see* Ulcer, stomach
gastrohepatic – *see* Ulcer, stomach
gastrointestinal – *see* Ulcer, gastrojejunal
gastrojejunal (eroded) (peptic) 534.9

Note – Use the following fifth-digit subclassification with categories 531-534:
0 without mention of obstruction
1 with obstruction

with
hemorrhage (chronic) 534.4❺
and perforation 534.6❺
perforation 534.5❺
and hemorrhage 534.6❺
acute 534.3❺
with
hemorrhage 534.0❺
and perforation 534.2❺
perforation 534.1❺
and hemorrhage 534.2❺
bleeding (recurrent) – *see* Ulcer, gastrojejunal, with hemorrhage
chronic 534.7❺
with
hemorrhage 534.4❺
and perforation 534.6❺
perforation 534.5❺
and hemorrhage 534.6❺
penetrating – *see* Ulcer, gastrojejunal, with perforation
perforating – *see* Ulcer, gastrojejunal, with perforation
gastrojejunocolic – *see* Ulcer, gastrojejunal
genital organ
female 629.89
male 608.89
gingiva 523.8
gingivitis 523.10
glottis 478.79
granuloma of pudenda 099.2
groin (*see also* Ulcer, skin) 707.8
gum 523.8
gumma, due to yaws 102.4
hand (*see also* Ulcer, skin) 707.8
hard palate 528.9
heel (*see also* Ulcer, lower extremity) 707.14
decubitus (*see also* Ulcer, decubitus) 707.07
hemorrhoids 455.8
external 455.5
internal 455.2
hip (*see also* Ulcer, skin) 707.8
decubitus (*see also* Ulcer, decubitus) 707.04
Hunner's 595.1
hypopharynx 478.29
hypopyon (chronic) (subacute) 370.04
hypostaticum – *see* Ulcer, varicose
ileocolitis 556.1
ileum (*see also* Ulcer, intestine) 569.82
intestine, intestinal 569.82
with perforation 569.83
amebic 006.9
duodenal – *see* Ulcer, duodenum
granulocytopenic (with hemorrhage) 288.09
marginal 569.82
perforating 569.83
small, primary 569.82
stercoraceous 569.82
stercoral 569.82
tuberculous (*see also* Tuberculosis) 014.8❺

Tyrosinemia – Ulcer, ulcerated, ulcerating, ulceration, ulcerative

Ulcer, ulcerated, ulcerating, ulceration, ulcerative - *continued*
- intestine, intestinal – *continued*
  - typhoid (fever) 002.0
  - varicose 456.8
- ischemic 707.9
  - lower extremity (*see also* Ulcer, lower extremity) 707.10
    - ankle 707.13
    - calf 707.12
    - foot 707.15
    - heel 707.14
    - knee 707.19
    - specified site NEC 707.19
    - thigh 707.11
    - toes 707.15
- jejunum, jejunal – *see* Ulcer, gastrojejunal
- keratitis (*see also* Ulcer, cornea) 370.00
- knee – *see* Ulcer, lower extremity
- labium (majus) (minus) 616.50
- laryngitis (*see also* Laryngitis) 464.00
  - with obstruction 464.01
- larynx (aphthous) (contact) 478.79
  - diphtheritic 032.3
- leg – *see* Ulcer, lower extremity
- lip 528.5
- Lipschütz's 616.50
- lower extremity (atrophic) (chronic) (neurogenic) (perforating) (pyogenic) (trophic) (tropical) 707.10
  - with gangrene (*see also* Ulcer, lower extremity) 707.10 *[785.4]*
    - arteriosclerotic 440.24
  - ankle 707.13
  - arteriosclerotic 440.23
    - with gangrene 440.24
  - calf 707.12
  - decubitus 707.00
    - with gangrene 707.00 *[785.4]*
    - ankle 707.06
    - buttock 707.05
    - heel 707.07
    - hip 707.04
  - foot 707.15
  - heel 707.14
  - knee 707.19
  - specified site NEC 707.19
  - thigh 707.11
  - toes 707.15
  - varicose 454.0
    - inflamed or infected 454.2
- luetic – *see* Ulcer, syphilitic
- lung 518.89
  - tuberculous (*see also* Tuberculosis) 011.2❺
- malignant (M8000/3) – *see* Neoplasm, by site, malignant
- marginal NEC – *see* Ulcer, gastrojejunal
- meatus (urinarius) 597.89
- Meckel's diverticulum 751.0
- Meleney's (chronic undermining) 686.09
- Mooren's (cornea) 370.07
- mouth (traumatic) 528.9
- mycobacterial (skin) 031.1
- nasopharynx 478.29
- navel cord (newborn) 771.4
- neck (*see also* Ulcer, skin) 707.8
  - uterus 622.0
- neurogenic NEC – *see* Ulcer, skin
- nose, nasal (infectional) (passage) 478.19
  - septum 478.19
    - varicose 456.8
  - skin – *see* Ulcer, skin
  - spirochetal NEC 104.8
- oral mucosa (traumatic) 528.9
- palate (soft) 528.9
- penetrating NEC – *see* Ulcer, peptic, with perforation
- penis (chronic) 607.89
- peptic (site unspecified) 533.9

> *Note – Use the following fifth-digit subclassification with categories 531-534:*
> *0 without mention of obstruction*
> *1 with obstruction*

  - with
    - hemorrhage 533.4❺
      - and perforation 533.6❺
    - perforation (chronic) 533.5❺
      - and hemorrhage 533.6❺

Ulcer, ulcerated, ulcerating, ulceration, ulcerative - *continued*
- peptic – *continued*
  - acute 533.3❺
    - with
      - hemorrhage 533.0❺
        - and perforation 533.2❺
      - perforation 533.1❺
        - and hemorrhage 533.2❺
  - bleeding (recurrent) – *see* Ulcer, peptic, with hemorrhage
  - chronic 533.7❺
    - with
      - hemorrhage 533.4❺
        - and perforation 533.6❺
      - perforation 533.5❺
        - and hemorrhage 533.6❺
  - penetrating – *see* Ulcer, peptic, with perforation
- perforating NEC (*see also* Ulcer, peptic, with perforation) 533.5❺
  - skin 707.9
- perineum (*see also* Ulcer, skin) 707.8
- peritonsillar 474.8
- phagedenic (tropical) NEC – *see* Ulcer, skin
- pharynx 478.29
- phlebitis – *see* Phlebitis
- plaster (*see also* Ulcer, decubitus) 707.00
- popliteal space – *see* Ulcer, lower extremity
- postpyloric – *see* Ulcer, duodenum
- prepuce 607.89
- prepyloric – *see* Ulcer, stomach
- pressure (*see also* Ulcer, decubitus) 707.00
- primary of intestine 569.82
  - with perforation 569.83
- proctitis 556.2
  - with ulcerative sigmoiditis 556.3
- prostate 601.8
- pseudopeptic – *see* Ulcer, peptic
- pyloric – *see* Ulcer, stomach
- rectosigmoid 569.82
  - with perforation 569.83
- rectum (sphincter) (solitary) 569.41
  - stercoraceous, stercoral 569.41
  - varicose – *see* Varicose, ulcer, anus
- retina (*see also* Chorioretinitis) 363.20
- rodent (M8090/3) – *see also* Neoplasm, skin, malignant
  - cornea 370.07
- round – *see* Ulcer, stomach
- sacrum (region) (*see also* Ulcer, skin) 707.8
- Saemisch's 370.04
- scalp (*see also* Ulcer, skin) 707.8
- sclera 379.09
- scrofulous (*see also* Tuberculosis) 017.2❺
- scrotum 608.89
  - tuberculous (*see also* Tuberculosis) 016.5❺
  - varicose 456.4
- seminal vesicle 608.89
- sigmoid 569.82
  - with perforation 569.83
- skin (atrophic) (chronic) (neurogenic) (non-healing) (perforating) (pyogenic) (trophic) 707.9
  - with gangrene 707.9 *[785.4]*
  - amebic 006.6
  - decubitus (*see also* Ulcer, decubitus) 707.00
    - with gangrene 707.00 *[785.4]*
  - in granulocytopenia 288.09
  - lower extremity (*see also* Ulcer, lower extremity) 707.10
    - with gangrene 707.10 *[785.4]*
      - arteriosclerotic 440.24
    - ankle 707.13
    - arteriosclerotic 440.23
      - with gangrene 440.24
    - calf 707.12
    - foot 707.15
    - heel 707.14
    - knee 707.19
    - specified site NEC 707.19
    - thigh 707.11
    - toes 707.15
  - mycobacterial 031.1
  - syphilitic (early) (secondary) 091.3
  - tuberculous (primary) (*see also* Tuberculosis) 017.0❺
  - varicose – *see* Ulcer, varicose
- sloughing NEC – *see* Ulcer, skin
- soft palate 528.9
- solitary, anus or rectum (sphincter) 569.41
- sore throat 462
  - streptococcal 034.0
- spermatic cord 608.89

Ulcer, ulcerated, ulcerating, ulceration, ulcerative - *continued*
- spine (tuberculous) 015.0❺ *[730.88]*
- stasis (leg) (venous) 454.0
  - with varicose veins 454.0
  - without varicose veins 459.81
  - inflamed or infected 454.2
- stercoral, stercoraceous 569.82
  - with perforation 569.83
  - anus or rectum 569.41
- stoma, stomal – *see* Ulcer, gastrojejunal
- stomach (eroded) (peptic) (round) 531.9

> *Note – Use the following fifth-digit subclassification with categories 531-534:*
> *0 without mention of obstruction*
> *1 with obstruction*

  - with
    - hemorrhage 531.4❺
      - and perforation 531.6❺
    - perforation (chronic) 531.5❺
      - and hemorrhage 531.6❺
  - acute 531.3❺
    - with
      - hemorrhage 531.0❺
        - and perforation 531.2❺
      - perforation 531.1❺
        - and hemorrhage 531.2❺
  - bleeding (recurrent) – *see* Ulcer, stomach, with hemorrhage
  - chronic 531.7❺
    - with
      - hemorrhage 531.4❺
        - and perforation 531.6❺
      - perforation 531.5❺
        - and hemorrhage 531.6❺
  - penetrating – *see* Ulcer, stomach, with perforation
  - perforating – *see* Ulcer, stomach, with perforation
- stomatitis 528.00
- stress – *see* Ulcer, peptic
- strumous (tuberculous) (*see also* Tuberculosis) 017.2❺
- submental (*see also* Ulcer, skin) 707.8
- submucosal, bladder 595.1
- syphilitic (any site) (early) (secondary) 091.3
  - late 095.9
  - perforating 095.9
    - foot 094.0
- testis 608.89
- thigh – *see* Ulcer, lower extremity
- throat 478.29
  - diphtheritic 032.0
- toe – *see* Ulcer, lower extremity
- tongue (traumatic) 529.0
- tonsil 474.8
  - diphtheritic 032.0
- trachea 519.19
- trophic – *see* Ulcer, skin
- tropical NEC (*see also* Ulcer, skin) 707.9
- tuberculous – *see* Tuberculosis, ulcer
- tunica vaginalis 608.89
- turbinate 730.9❺
- typhoid (fever) 002.0
  - perforating 002.0
- umbilicus (newborn) 771.4
- unspecified site NEC – *see* Ulcer, skin
- urethra (meatus) (*see also* Urethritis) 597.89
- uterus 621.8
  - cervix 622.0
    - with mention of cervicitis 616.0
  - neck 622.0
    - with mention of cervicitis 616.0
- vagina 616.89
- valve, heart 421.0
- varicose (lower extremity, any part) 454.0
  - anus – *see* Varicose, ulcer, anus
  - broad ligament 456.5
  - esophagus (*see also* Varix, esophagus) 456.1
    - bleeding (*see also* Varix, esophagus, bleeding) 456.0
  - inflamed or infected 454.2
  - nasal septum 456.8
  - perineum 456.6
  - rectum – *see* Varicose, ulcer, anus
  - scrotum 456.4
  - specified site NEC 456.8
  - sublingual 456.3
  - vulva 456.6
- vas deferens 608.89
- vesical (*see also* Ulcer, bladder) 596.8

Ulcer, ulcerated, ulcerating, ulceration, ulcerative - *continued*
  vulva (acute) (infectional) 616.50
    Behçet's syndrome 136.1 *[616.51]*
    herpetic 054.12
    tuberculous 016.7❺ *[616.51]*
  vulvobuccal, recurring 616.50
  x-ray – *see* Ulcer, by site
  yaws 102.4
Ulcerosa scarlatina 034.1
Ulcus – *see also* Ulcer
  cutis tuberculosum (*see also* Tuberculosis) 017.0❺
  duodeni – *see* Ulcer, duodenum
  durum 091.0
    extragenital 091.2
  gastrojejunale – *see* Ulcer, gastrojejunal
  hypostaticum – *see* Ulcer, varicose
  molle (cutis) (skin) 099.0
  serpens corneae (pneumococcal) 370.04
  ventriculi – *see* Ulcer, stomach
Ulegyria 742.4
Ulerythema
  acneiforma 701.8
  centrifugum 695.4
  ophryogenes 757.4
Ullrich (-Bonnevie) (-Turner) **syndrome** 758.6
Ullrich-Feichtiger syndrome 759.89
Ulnar – *see* condition
Ulorrhagia 523.8
Ulorrhea 523.8
Umbilicus, umbilical – *see also* condition
  cord necrosis, affecting fetus or newborn 762.6
Unacceptable
  existing dental restoration
    contours 525.65
    morphology 525.65
Unavailability of medical facilities (at) V63.9
  due to
    investigation by social service agency V63.8
    lack of services at home V63.1
    remoteness from facility V63.0
    waiting list V63.2
  home V63.1
  outpatient clinic V63.0
  specified reason NEC V63.8
Uncinaria americana infestation 126.1
Uncinariasis (*see also* Ancylostomiasis) 126.9
Unconscious, unconsciousness 780.09
Underdevelopment – *see also* Undeveloped, sexual 259.0
Underfill, endodontic 526.63
Undernourishment 269.9
Undernutrition 269.9
Under observation – *see* Observation
Underweight 783.22
  for gestational age – *see* Light-for-dates
Underwood's disease (sclerema neonatorum) 778.1
Undescended – *see also* Malposition, congenital
  cecum 751.4
  colon 751.4
  testis 752.51
Undetermined diagnosis or cause 799.9
Undeveloped, undevelopment – *see also* Hypoplasia
  brain (congenital) 742.1
  cerebral (congenital) 742.1
  fetus or newborn 764.9❺
  heart 746.89
  lung 748.5
  testis 257.2
  uterus 259.0
Undiagnosed (disease) 799.9
Undulant fever (*see also* Brucellosis) 023.9
Unemployment, anxiety concerning V62.0
Unequal leg (acquired) (length) 736.81
  congenital 755.30
Unerupted teeth, tooth 520.6
Unextracted dental root 525.3
Unguis incarnatus 703.0
Unicornis uterus 752.3
Unicorporeus uterus 752.3
Uniformis uterus 752.3
Unilateral – *see also* condition
  development, breast 611.8
  organ or site, congenital NEC – *see* Agenesis
  vagina 752.49
Unilateralis uterus 752.3
Unilocular heart 745.8
Uninhibited bladder 596.54
  with cauda equina syndrome 344.61
  neurogenic (*see also* Neurogenic, bladder) 596.54
Union, abnormal – *see also* Fusion
  divided tendon 727.89
  larynx and trachea 748.3
Universal
  joint, cervix 620.6
  mesentery 751.4
Unknown
  cause of death 799.9
  diagnosis 799.9
Unna's disease (seborrheic dermatitis) 690.10
Unresponsiveness, adrenocorticotropin (ACTH) 255.41 ▲
Unsatisfactory
  restoration, tooth (existing) 525.60
    specified NEC 525.69
  smear 795.08
Unsoundness of mind (*see also* Psychosis) 298.9
Unspecified cause of death 799.9
Unstable
  back NEC 724.9
  colon 569.89
  joint – *see* Instability, joint
  lie 652.0❺
    affecting fetus or newborn (before labor) 761.7
    causing obstructed labor 660.0❺
      affecting fetus or newborn 763.1
  lumbosacral joint (congenital) 756.19
    acquired 724.6
  sacroiliac 724.6
  spine NEC 724.9
Untruthfulness, child problem (*see also* Disturbance, conduct) 312.0❺
Unverricht (-Lundborg) **disease, syndrome, or epilepsy** 333.2
Unverricht-Wagner syndrome (dermatomyositis) 710.3
Upper respiratory – *see* condition
Upset
  gastric 536.8
    psychogenic 306.4
  gastrointestinal 536.8
    psychogenic 306.4
    virus (*see also* Enteritis, viral) 008.8
  intestinal (large) (small) 564.9
    psychogenic 306.4
  menstruation 626.9
  mental 300.9
  stomach 536.8
    psychogenic 306.4
Urachus – *see also* condition
  patent 753.7
  persistent 753.7
Uratic arthritis 274.0
Urbach's lipoid proteinosis 272.8
Urbach-Oppenheim disease or syndrome (necrobiosis lipoidica diabeticorum) 250.8❺ *[709.3]*
Urbach-Wiethe disease or syndrome (lipoid proteinosis) 272.8
Urban yellow fever 060.1
Urea, blood, high – *see* Uremia
Uremia, uremic (absorption) (amaurosis) (amblyopia) (aphasia) (apoplexy) (coma) (delirium) (dementia) (dropsy) (dyspnea) (fever) (intoxication) (mania) (paralysis) (poisoning) (toxemia) (vomiting) 586
  with
    abortion – *see* Abortion, by type, with renal failure
    ectopic pregnancy (*see also* categories 633.0-633.9) 639.3
    hypertension (*see also* Hypertension, kidney) 403.91
    molar pregnancy (*see also* categories 630-632) 639.3
  chronic 585.9
  complicating
    abortion 639.3
    ectopic or molar pregnancy 639.3
    hypertension (*see also* Hypertension, kidney) 403.91
    labor and delivery 669.3❺
  congenital 779.89
Uremia, uremic – *continued*
  extrarenal 788.9
  hypertensive (chronic) (*see also* Hypertension, kidney) 403.91
  maternal NEC, affecting fetus or newborn 760.1
  neuropathy 585.9 *[357.4]*
  pericarditis 585.9 *[420.0]*
  prerenal 788.9
  pyelitic (*see also* Pyelitis) 590.80
Ureter, ureteral – *see* condition
Ureteralgia 788.0
Ureterectasis 593.89
Ureteritis 593.89
  cystica 590.3
  due to calculus 592.1
  gonococcal (acute) 098.19
    chronic or duration of 2 months or over 098.39
  nonspecific 593.89
Ureterocele (acquired) 593.89
  congenital 753.23
Ureterolith 592.1
Ureterolithiasis 592.1
Ureterostomy status V44.6
  with complication 997.5
Urethra, urethral – *see* condition
Urethralgia 788.9
Urethritis (abacterial) (acute) (allergic) (anterior) (chronic) (nonvenereal) (posterior) (recurrent) (simple) (subacute) (ulcerative) (undifferentiated) 597.80
  diplococcal (acute) 098.0
    chronic or duration of 2 months or over 098.2
  due to Trichomonas (vaginalis) 131.02
  gonococcal (acute) 098.0
    chronic or duration of 2 months or over 098.2
  nongonococcal (sexually transmitted) 099.40
    Chlamydia trachomatis 099.41
    Reiter's 099.3
    specified organism NEC 099.49
  nonspecific (sexually transmitted) (*see also* Urethritis, nongonococcal) 099.40
  not sexually transmitted 597.80
  Reiter's 099.3
  trichomonal or due to Trichomonas (vaginalis) 131.02
  tuberculous (*see also* Tuberculosis) 016.3❺
  venereal NEC (*see also* Urethritis, nongonococcal) 099.40
Urethrocele
  female 618.03
    with uterine prolapse 618.4
      complete 618.3
      incomplete 618.2
  male 599.5
Urethrolithiasis 594.2
Urethro-oculoarticular syndrome 099.3
Urethro-oculosynovial syndrome 099.3
Urethrorectal – *see* condition
Urethrorrhagia 599.84
Urethrorrhea 788.7
Urethrostomy status V44.6
  with complication 997.5
Urethrotrigonitis 595.3
Urethrovaginal – *see* condition
Urhidrosis, uridrosis 705.89
Uric acid
  diathesis 274.9
  in blood 790.6
Uricacidemia 790.6
Uricemia 790.6
Uricosuria 791.9
Urination
  frequent 788.41
  painful 788.1
  urgency 788.63
Urine, urinary – *see also* condition
  abnormality NEC 788.69
  blood in (*see also* Hematuria) 599.7
  discharge, excessive 788.42
  enuresis 788.30
    nonorganic origin 307.6
  extravasation 788.8
  frequency 788.41
  hesitancy 788.64
  incontinence 788.30
    active 788.30

Urine, urinary – *continued*
- incontinence – *continued*
  - female 788.30
    - stress 625.6
      - and urge 788.33
  - male 788.30
    - stress 788.32
      - and urge 788.33
  - mixed (stress and urge) 788.33
  - neurogenic 788.39
  - nonorganic origin 307.6
  - overflow 788.38
  - stress (female) 625.6
    - male NEC 788.32
- intermittent stream 788.61
- pus in 791.9
- retention or stasis NEC 788.20
  - bladder, incomplete emptying 788.21
  - psychogenic 306.53
  - specified NEC 788.29
- secretion
  - deficient 788.5
  - excessive 788.42
  - frequency 788.41
- strain 788.65
- stream
  - intermittent 788.61
  - slowing 788.62
  - splitting 788.61
  - weak 788.62
- urgency 788.63

Urinemia – *see* Uremia

Urinoma NEC 599.9
- bladder 596.8
- kidney 593.89
- renal 593.89
- ureter 593.89
- urethra 599.84

Uroarthritis, infectious 099.3

Urodialysis 788.5

Urolithiasis 592.9

Uronephrosis 593.89

Uropathy 599.9
- obstructive 599.60

Urosepsis 599.0
- meaning sepsis 995.91
- meaning urinary tract infection 599.0

Urticaria 708.9
- with angioneurotic edema 995.1
  - hereditary 277.6
- allergic 708.0
- cholinergic 708.5
- chronic 708.8
- cold, familial 708.2
- dermatographic 708.3
- due to
  - cold or heat 708.2
  - drugs 708.0
  - food 708.0
  - inhalants 708.0
  - plants 708.8
  - serum 999.5
- factitial 708.3
- giant 995.1
  - hereditary 277.6
- gigantea 995.1
  - hereditary 277.6
- idiopathic 708.1
- larynx 995.1
  - hereditary 277.6
- neonatorum 778.8
- nonallergic 708.1
- papulosa (Hebra) 698.2
- perstans hemorrhagica 757.39
- pigmentosa 757.33
- recurrent periodic 708.8
- serum 999.5
- solare 692.72
- specified type NEC 708.8
- thermal (cold) (heat) 708.2
- vibratory 708.4

Urticarioides acarodermatitis 133.9

Use of
- nonprescribed drugs (*see also* Abuse, drugs, nondependent) 305.9❺
- patent medicines (*see also* Abuse, drugs, nondependent) 305.9❺

Usher-Senear disease (pemphigus erythematosus) 694.4

Uta 085.5

Uterine size-date discrepancy 649.6❺

Uteromegaly 621.2

Uterovaginal – *see* condition

Uterovesical – *see* condition

Uterus – *see* condition

Utriculitis (utriculus prostaticus) 597.89

Uveal – *see* condition

Uveitis (anterior) (*see also* Iridocyclitis) 364.3
- acute or subacute 364.00
  - due to or associated with
    - gonococcal infection 098.41
    - herpes (simplex) 054.44
    - zoster 053.22
  - primary 364.01
  - recurrent 364.02
  - secondary (noninfectious) 364.04
    - infectious 364.03
- allergic 360.11
- chronic 364.10
  - due to or associated with
    - sarcoidosis 135 *[364.11]*
    - tuberculosis (*see also* Tuberculosis) 017.3❺ *[364.11]*
- due to
  - operation 360.11
  - toxoplasmosis (acquired) 130.2
    - congenital (active) 771.2
- granulomatous 364.10
- heterochromic 364.21
- lens-induced 364.23
- nongranulomatous 364.00
- posterior 363.20
  - disseminated – *see* Chorioretinitis, disseminated
  - focal – *see* Chorioretinitis, focal
- recurrent 364.02
- sympathetic 360.11
- syphilitic (secondary) 091.50
  - congenital 090.0 *[363.13]*
  - late 095.8 *[363.13]*
- tuberculous (*see also* Tuberculosis) 017.3❺ *[364.11]*

Uveoencephalitis 363.22

Uveokeratitis (*see also* Iridocyclitis) 364.3

Uveoparotid fever 135

Uveoparotitis 135

Uvula – *see* condition

Uvulitis (acute) (catarrhal) (chronic) (gangrenous) (membranous) (suppurative) (ulcerative) 528.3

V

Vaccination
- complication or reaction – *see* Complications, vaccination
- not carried out V64.00
  - because of
    - acute illness V64.01
    - allergy to vaccine or component V64.04
    - caregiver refusal V64.05
    - chronic illness V64.02
    - guardian refusal V64.05 ●
    - immune compromised state V64.03
    - parent refusal V64.05 ●
    - patient had disease being vaccinated against V64.08
    - patient refusal V64.06
    - reason NEC V64.09
    - religious reasons V64.07
- prophylactic (against) V05.9
  - arthropod-borne viral
    - disease NEC V05.1
    - encephalitis V05.0
  - chicken pox V05.4
  - cholera (alone) V03.0
    - with typhoid-paratyphoid (cholera + TAB) V06.0
  - common cold V04.7
  - diphtheria (alone) V03.5
    - with
      - poliomyelitis (DTP + polio) V06.3
      - tetanus V06.5
        - pertussis combined [DTP] (DTaP) V06.1
      - typhoid-paratyphoid (DTP + TAB) V06.2

Vaccination – *continued*
- prophylactic (against) – *continued*
  - disease (single) NEC V05.9
    - bacterial NEC V03.9
      - specified type NEC V03.89
    - combination NEC V06.9
      - specified type NEC V06.8
    - specified type NEC V05.8
  - encephalitis, viral, arthropod-borne V05.0
  - Hemophilus influenzae, type B [Hib] V03.81
  - hepatitis, viral V05.3
  - influenza V04.81
    - with
      - Streptococcus pneumoniae [pneumococcus] V06.6
  - leishmaniasis V05.2
  - measles (alone) V04.2
    - with mumps-rubella (MMR) V06.4
  - mumps (alone) V04.6
    - with measles and rubella (MMR) V06.4
  - pertussis alone V03.6
  - plague V03.3
  - poliomyelitis V04.0
    - with diphtheria-tetanus-pertussis (DTP polio) V06.3
  - rabies V04.5
  - respiratory syncytial virus (RSV) V04.82
  - rubella (alone) V04.3
    - with measles and mumps (MMR) V06.4
  - smallpox V04.1
  - Streptococcus pneumoniae [pneumococcus] V03.82
    - with
      - influenza V06.6
  - tetanus toxoid (alone) V03.7
    - with diphtheria [Td] [DT] V06.5
      - with
        - pertussis (DTP) (DTaP)V06.1
          - with poliomyelitis (DTP + polio) V06.3
  - tuberculosis (BCG) V03.2
  - tularemia V03.4
  - typhoid-paratyphoid (TAB) (alone) V03.1
    - with diphtheria-tetanus-pertussis (TAB + DTP) V06.2
  - varicella V05.4
  - viral
    - disease NEC V04.89
    - encephalitis, arthropod-borne V05.0
    - hepatitis V05.3
  - yellow fever V04.4

Vaccinia (generalized) 999.0
- congenital 771.2
- conjunctiva 999.39 ▲
- eyelids 999.0 *[373.5]*
- localized 999.39 ▲
- nose 999.39 ▲
- not from vaccination 051.0
  - eyelid 051.0 *[373.5]*
- sine vaccinatione 051.0
- without vaccination 051.0

Vacuum
- extraction of fetus or newborn 763.3
- in sinus (accessory) (nasal) (*see also* Sinusitis) 473.9

Vagabond V60.0

Vagabondage V60.0

Vagabonds' disease 132.1

Vagina, vaginal – *see* condition

Vaginalitis (tunica) 608.4

Vaginismus (reflex) 625.1
- functional 306.51
- hysterical 300.11
- psychogenic 306.51

Vaginitis (acute) (chronic) (circumscribed) (diffuse) (emphysematous) (Hemophilus vaginalis) (nonspecific) (nonvenereal) (ulcerative) 616.10
- with
  - abortion – *see* Abortion, by type, with sepsis
  - ectopic pregnancy (*see also* categories 633.0-633.9) 639.0
  - molar pregnancy (*see also* categories 630-632) 639.0
- adhesive, congenital 752.49
- atrophic, postmenopausal 627.3
- bacterial 616.10
- blennorrhagic (acute) 098.0
  - chronic or duration of 2 months or over 098.2
- candidal 112.1
- chlamydial 099.53

Vaginitis – *continued*
- complicating pregnancy or puerperium 646.6❺
  - affecting fetus or newborn 760.8
- congenital (adhesive) 752.49
- due to
  - C. albicans 112.1
  - Trichomonas (vaginalis) 131.01
- following
  - abortion 639.0
  - ectopic or molar pregnancy 639.0
- gonococcal (acute) 098.0
  - chronic or duration of 2 months or over 098.2
- granuloma 099.2
- Monilia 112.1
- mycotic 112.1
- pinworm 127.4 *[616.11]*
- postirradiation 616.10
- postmenopausal atrophic 627.3
- senile (atrophic) 627.3
- syphilitic (early) 091.0
  - late 095.8
- trichomonal 131.01
- tuberculous (*see also* Tuberculosis) 016.7❺
- venereal NEC 099.8

Vaginosis- *see* Vaginitis

Vagotonia 352.3

Vagrancy V60.0

VAIN I (vaginal intraepithelial neoplasia I) 623.0 ●

VAIN II (vaginal intraepithelial neoplasia II) 623.0 ●

VAIN III (vaginal intraepithelial neoplasia III) 233.31 ●

Vallecula – *see* condition

Valley fever 114.0

Valsuani's disease (progressive pernicious anemia, puerperal) 648.2❺

Valve, valvular (formation) – *see also* condition
- cerebral ventricle (communicating) in situ V45.2
- cervix, internal os 752.49
- colon 751.5
- congenital NEC – *see* Atresia
- formation congenital NEC – *see* Atresia
- heart defect – *see* Anomaly, heart, valve
- ureter 753.29
  - pelvic junction 753.21
  - vesical orifice 753.22
- urethra 753.6

Valvulitis (chronic) (*see also* Endocarditis) 424.90
- rheumatic (chronic) (inactive) (with chorea) 397.9
  - active or acute (aortic) (mitral) (pulmonary) (tricuspid) 391.1
- syphilitic NEC 093.20
  - aortic 093.22
  - mitral 093.21
  - pulmonary 093.24
  - tricuspid 093.23

Valvulopathy – *see* Endocarditis

van Bogaert's leukoencephalitis (sclerosing) (subacute) 046.2

van Bogaert-Nijssen (-Peiffer) **disease** 330.0

van Buchem's syndrome (hyperostosis corticalis) 733.3

Vancomycin (glycopeptide)
- intermediate staphylococcus aureus (VISA/GISA) V09.8
- resistant
  - enterococcus (VRE) V09.8
  - staphylococcus aureus (VRSA/GRSA) V09.8

van Creveld-von Gierke disease (glycogenosis I) 271.0

van den Bergh's disease (enterogenous cyanosis) 289.7

van der Hoeve's syndrome (brittle bones and blue sclera, deafness) 756.51

van der Hoeve-Halbertsma-Waardenburg syndrome (ptosis-epicanthus) 270.2

van der Hoeve-Waardenburg-Gualdi syndrome (ptosis-epicanthus) 270.2

Vanillism 692.89

Vanishing lung 492.0

Vanishing twin 651.33

van Neck (-Odelberg) **disease or syndrome** (juvenile osteochondrosis) 732.1

Vapor asphyxia or suffocation NEC 987.9
- specified agent – *see* Table of Drugs and Chemicals

Vaquez's disease (M9950/1) 238.4

Vaquez-Osler disease (polycythemia vera) (M9950/1) 238.4

Variance, lethal ball, prosthetic heart valve 996.02

Variants, thalassemic 282.49

Variations in hair color 704.3

Varicella 052.9
- with
  - complication 052.8
    - specified NEC 052.7
  - pneumonia 052.1
- exposure to V01.71
- vaccination and inoculation (against) (prophylactic) V05.4

Varices – *see* Varix

Varicocele (scrotum) (thrombosed) 456.4
- ovary 456.5
- perineum 456.6
- spermatic cord (ulcerated) 456.4

Varicose
- aneurysm (ruptured) (*see also* Aneurysm) 442.9
- dermatitis (lower extremity) – *see* Varicose, vein, inflamed or infected
- eczema – *see* Varicose, vein
- phlebitis – *see* Varicose, vein, inflamed or infected
- placental vessel – *see* Placenta, abnormal
- tumor – *see* Varicose, vein
- ulcer (lower extremity, any part) 454.0
  - anus 455.8
    - external 455.5
    - internal 455.2
  - esophagus (*see also* Varix, esophagus) 456.1
    - bleeding (*see also* Varix, esophagus, bleeding) 456.0
  - inflamed or infected 454.2
  - nasal septum 456.8
  - perineum 456.6
  - rectum – *see* Varicose, ulcer, anus
  - scrotum 456.4
  - specified site NEC 456.8
- vein (lower extremity) (ruptured) (*see also* Varix) 454.9
  - with
    - complications NEC 454.8
    - edema 454.8
    - inflammation or infection 454.1
      - ulcerated 454.2
    - pain 454.8
    - stasis dermatitis 454.1
      - with ulcer 454.2
    - swelling 454.8
    - ulcer 454.0
      - inflamed or infected 454.2
  - anus – *see* Hemorrhoids
  - broad ligament 456.5
  - congenital (peripheral) 747.60
    - gastrointestinal 747.61
    - lower limb 747.64
    - renal 747.62
    - specified NEC 747.69
    - upper limb 747.63
  - esophagus (ulcerated (*see also* Varix, esophagus) 456.1
    - bleeding (*see also* Varix, esophagus, bleeding) 456.0
  - inflamed or infected 454.1
    - with ulcer 454.2
  - in pregnancy or puerperium 671.0❺
    - vulva or perineum 671.1❺
  - nasal septum (with ulcer) 456.8
  - pelvis 456.5
  - perineum 456.6
    - in pregnancy, childbirth, or puerperium 671.1❺
  - rectum – *see* Hemorrhoids
  - scrotum (ulcerated) 456.4
  - specified site NEC 456.8
  - sublingual 456.3
  - ulcerated 454.0
    - inflamed or infected 454.2
  - umbilical cord, affecting fetus or newborn 762.6
  - urethra 456.8
  - vulva 456.6
    - in pregnancy, childbirth, or puerperium 671.1❺
- vessel – *see also* Varix
  - placenta – *see* Placenta, abnormal

Varicosis, varicosities, varicosity (*see also* Varix) 454.9

Variola 050.9
- hemorrhagic (pustular) 050.0
- major 050.0
- minor 050.1
- modified 050.2

Varioloid 050.2

Variolosa, purpura 050.0

Varix (lower extremity) (ruptured) 454.9
- with
  - complications NEC 454.8
  - edema 454.8
  - inflammation or infection 454.1
    - with ulcer 454.2
  - pain 454.8
  - stasis dermatitis 454.1
    - with ulcer 454.2
  - swelling 454.8
  - ulcer 454.0
    - with inflammation or infection 454.2
- aneurysmal (*see also* Aneurysm) 442.9
- anus – *see* Hemorrhoids
- arteriovenous (congenital) (peripheral) NEC 747.60
  - gastrointestinal 747.61
  - lower limb 747.64
  - renal 747.62
  - specified NEC 747.69
  - spinal 747.82
  - upper limb 747.63
- bladder 456.5
- broad ligament 456.5
- congenital (peripheral) 747.60
- esophagus (ulcerated) 456.1
  - bleeding 456.0
    - in
      - cirrhosis of liver 571.5 *[456.20]*
      - portal hypertension 572.3 *[456.20]*
  - congenital 747.69
  - in
    - cirrhosis of liver 571.5 *[456.21]*
      - with bleeding 571.5 *[456.20]*
    - portal hypertension 572.3 *[456.21]*
      - with bleeding 572.3 *[456.20]*
- gastric 456.8
- inflamed or infected 454.1
  - ulcerated 454.2
- in pregnancy or puerperium 671.0❺
  - perineum 671.1❺
  - vulva 671.1❺
- labia (majora) 456.6
- orbit 456.8
  - congenital 747.69
- ovary 456.5
- papillary 448.1
- pelvis 456.5
- perineum 456.6
  - in pregnancy or puerperium 671.1❺
- pharynx 456.8
- placenta – *see* Placenta, abnormal
- prostate 456.8
- rectum – *see* Hemorrhoids
- renal papilla 456.8
- retina 362.17
- scrotum (ulcerated) 456.4
- sigmoid colon 456.8
- specified site NEC 456.8
- spinal (cord) (vessels) 456.8
- spleen, splenic (vein) (with phlebolith) 456.8
- sublingual 456.3
- ulcerated 454.0
  - inflamed or infected 454.2
- umbilical cord, affecting fetus or newborn 762.6
- uterine ligament 456.5
- vocal cord 456.8
- vulva 456.6
  - in pregnancy, childbirth, or puerperium 671.1❺

Vasa previa 663.5❺
- affecting fetus or newborn 762.6
- hemorrhage from, affecting fetus or newborn 772.0

Vascular – *see also* condition
- loop on papilla (optic) 743.57
- sheathing, retina 362.13
- spasm 443.9
- spider 448.1

Vascularity, pulmonary, congenital 747.3

Vascularization
- choroid 362.16
- cornea 370.60
  - deep 370.63

Vascularization – *continued*
cornea – *continued*
localized 370.61
retina 362.16
subretinal 362.16
Vasculitis 447.6
allergic 287.0
cryoglobulinemic 273.2
disseminated 447.6
kidney 447.8
leukocytoclastic 446.29
nodular 695.2
retinal 362.18
rheumatic – *see* Fever, rheumatic
Vasculopathy
cardiac allograft 996.83
Vas deferens – *see* condition
Vas deferentitis 608.4
Vasectomy, admission for V25.2
Vasitis 608.4
nodosa 608.4
scrotum 608.4
spermatic cord 608.4
testis 608.4
tuberculous (*see also* Tuberculosis) 016.5❺
tunica vaginalis 608.4
vas deferens 608.4
Vasodilation 443.9
Vasomotor – *see* condition
Vasoplasty, after previous sterilization V26.0
Vasoplegia, splanchnic (*see also* Neuropathy, peripheral, autonomic) 337.9
Vasospasm 443.9
cerebral (artery) 435.9
with transient neurologic deficit 435.9
coronary 413.1
nerve
arm NEC 354.9
autonomic 337.9
brachial plexus 353.0
cervical plexus 353.2
leg NEC 355.8
lower extremity NEC 355.8
peripheral NEC 335.9
spinal NEC 355.9
sympathetic 337.9
upper extremity NEC 354.9
peripheral NEC 443.9
retina (artery) (*see also* Occlusion, retinal, artery) 362.30
Vasospastic – *see* condition
Vasovagal attack (paroxysmal) 780.2
psychogenic 306.2
Vater's ampulla – *see* condition
VATER syndrome 759.89
Vegetation, vegetative
adenoid (nasal fossa) 474.2
consciousness (persistent) 780.03
endocarditis (acute) (any valve) (chronic) (subacute) 421.0
heart (mycotic) (valve) 421.0
state (persistent) 780.03
Veil
Jackson's 751.4
over face (causing asphyxia) 768.9
Vein, venous – *see* condition
Veldt sore (*see also* Ulcer, skin) 707.9
Velo-cardio-facial syndrome 758.32
Velpeau's hernia – *see* Hernia, femoral
Venereal
balanitis NEC 099.8
bubo 099.1
disease 099.9
specified nature or type NEC 099.8
granuloma inguinale 099.2
lymphogranuloma (Durand-Nicolas-Favre), any site 099.1
salpingitis 098.37
urethritis (*see also* Urethritis, nongonococcal) 099.40
vaginitis NEC 099.8
warts 078.19
Vengefulness, in child (*see also* Disturbance, conduct) 312.0❺
Venofibrosis 459.89
Venom, venomous
bite or sting (animal or insect) 989.5
poisoning 989.5
Venous – *see* condition
Ventouse delivery NEC 669.5❺
affecting fetus or newborn 763.3
Ventral – *see* condition
Ventricle, ventricular – *see also* condition
escape 427.69
standstill (*see also* Arrest, cardiac) 427.5
Ventriculitis, cerebral (*see also* Meningitis) 322.9
Ventriculostomy status V45.2
Verbiest's syndrome (claudicatio intermittens spinalis) 435.1
Vernet's syndrome 352.6
Verneuil's disease (syphilitic bursitis) 095.7
Verruca (filiformis) 078.10
acuminata (any site) 078.11
necrogenica (primary) (*see also* Tuberculosis) 017.0❺
peruana 088.0
peruviana 088.0
plana (juvenilis) 078.19
plantaris 078.19
seborrheica 702.19
inflamed 702.11
senilis 702.0
tuberculosa (primary) (*see also* Tuberculosis) 017.0❺
venereal 078.19
viral NEC 078.10
Verrucosities (*see also* Verruca) 078.10
Verrucous endocarditis (acute) (any valve) (chronic) (subacute) 710.0 *[424.91]*
nonbacterial 710.0 *[424.91]*
Verruga
peruana 088.0
peruviana 088.0
Verse's disease (calcinosis intervertebralis) 275.49 *[722.90]*
Version
before labor, affecting fetus or newborn 761.7
cephalic (correcting previous malposition) 652.1❺
affecting fetus or newborn 763.1
cervix – *see* Version, uterus
uterus (postinfectional) (postpartal, old) (*see also* Malposition, uterus) 621.6
forward – *see* Anteversion, uterus
lateral – *see* Lateroversion, uterus
Vertebra, vertebral – *see* condition
Vertigo 780.4
auditory 386.19
aural 386.19
benign paroxysmal positional 386.11
central origin 386.2
cerebral 386.2
Dix and Hallpike (epidemic) 386.12
endemic paralytic 078.81
epidemic 078.81
Dix and Hallpike 386.12
Gerlier's 078.81
Pedersen's 386.12
vestibular neuronitis 386.12
epileptic – *see* Epilepsy
Gerlier's (epidemic) 078.81
hysterical 300.11
labyrinthine 386.10
laryngeal 786.2
malignant positional 386.2
Ménière's (*see also* Disease, Ménière's) 386.00
menopausal 627.2
otogenic 386.19
paralytic 078.81
paroxysmal positional, benign 386.11
Pedersen's (epidemic) 386.12
peripheral 386.10
specified type NEC 386.19
positional
benign paroxysmal 386.11
malignant 386.2
Verumontanitis (chronic) (*see also* Urethritis) 597.89
Vesania (*see also* Psychosis) 298.9
Vesical – *see* condition
Vesicle
cutaneous 709.8
seminal – *see* condition
skin 709.8
Vesicocolic – *see* condition
Vesicoperineal – *see* condition
Vesicorectal – *see* condition
Vesicourethrorectal – *see* condition
Vesicovaginal – *see* condition
Vesicular – *see* condition
Vesiculitis (seminal) 608.0
amebic 006.8
gonorrheal (acute) 098.14
chronic or duration of 2 months or over 098.34
trichomonal 131.09
tuberculous (*see also* Tuberculosis) 016.5❺ *[608.81]*
Vestibulitis (ear) (*see also* Labyrinthitis) 386.30
nose (external) 478.19
vulvar 616.10
Vestibulopathy, acute peripheral (recurrent) 386.12
Vestige, vestigial – *see also* Persistence
branchial 744.41
structures in vitreous 743.51
Vibriosis NEC 027.9
Vidal's disease (lichen simplex chronicus) 698.3
Video display tube syndrome 723.8
Vienna-type encephalitis 049.8
Villaret's syndrome 352.6
Villous – *see* condition
VIN I (vulvar intraepithelial neoplasia I) 624.01 ▲
VIN II (vulvar intraepithelial neoplasia II) 624.02 ▲
VIN III (vulvar intraepithelial neoplasia III) 233.32 ▲
Vincent's
angina 101
bronchitis 101
disease 101
gingivitis 101
infection (any site) 101
laryngitis 101
stomatitis 101
tonsillitis 101
Vinson-Plummer syndrome (sideropenic dysphagia) 280.8
Viosterol deficiency (*see also* Deficiency, calciferol) 268.9
Virchow's disease 733.99
Viremia 790.8
Virilism (adrenal) (female) NEC 255.2
with
3-beta-hydroxysteroid dehydrogenase defect 255.2
11-hydroxylase defect 255.2
21-hydroxylase defect 255.2
adrenal
hyperplasia 255.2
insufficiency (congenital) 255.2
cortical hyperfunction 255.2
Virilization (female) (suprarenal) (*see also* Virilism) 255.2
isosexual 256.4
Virulent bubo 099.0
Virus, viral – *see also* condition
infection NEC (*see also* Infection, viral) 079.99
septicemia 079.99
VISA (vancomycin intermediate staphylococcus aureus) V09.8
Viscera, visceral – *see* condition
Visceroptosis 569.89
Visible peristalsis 787.4
Vision, visual
binocular, suppression 368.31
blurred, blurring 368.8
hysterical 300.11
defect, defective (*see also* Impaired, vision) 369.9
disorientation (syndrome) 368.16
disturbance NEC (*see also* Disturbance, vision) 368.9
hysterical 300.11
examination V72.0
field, limitation 368.40
fusion, with defective steropsis 368.33
hallucinations 368.16
halos 368.16
loss 369.9
both eyes (*see also* Blindness, both eyes) 369.3
complete (*see also* Blindness, both eyes) 369.00
one eye 369.8
sudden 368.11

Vascularization – Vision, visual

❹ Fourth-Digit Required ❺ Fifth-Digit Required *[code]* Manifestation Code ▶◀ Revised Text ● New Line ▲ Revised Code

W

Vision, visual – Water-losing nephritis

Wound, open (by cutting or piercing instrument) (by firearms) (cut) (dissection) (incised) (laceration) (penetration) (perforating) (puncture) (with initial hemorrhage, not internal) 879.8

Note – For fracture with open wound, see Fracture.

For laceration, traumatic rupture, tear, or penetrating wound of internal organs, such as heart, lung, liver, kidney, pelvic organs, etc., whether or not accompanied by open wound or fracture in the same region, see Injury, internal.

For contused wound, see Contusion. For crush injury, see Crush. For abrasion, insect bite (nonvenomous), blister, or scratch, see Injury, superficial.

Complicated includes wounds with:
- *delayed healing*
- *delayed treatment*
- *foreign body*
- *primary infection*

For late effect of open wound, see Late, effect, wound, open, by site.

- abdomen, abdominal (external) (muscle) 879.2
  - complicated 879.3
  - wall (anterior) 879.2
    - complicated 879.3
    - lateral 879.4
      - complicated 879.5
- alveolar (process) 873.62
  - complicated 873.72
- ankle 891.0
  - with tendon involvement 891.2
  - complicated 891.1
- anterior chamber, eye (*see also* Wound, open, intraocular) 871.9
- anus 879.6
  - complicated 879.7
- arm 884.0
  - with tendon involvement 884.2
  - complicated 884.1
  - forearm 881.00
    - with tendon involvement 881.20
    - complicated 881.10
  - multiple sites – *see* Wound, open, multiple, upper limb
  - upper 880.03
    - with tendon involvement 880.23
    - complicated 880.13
    - multiple sites (with axillary or shoulder regions) 880.09
      - with tendon involvement 880.29
      - complicated 880.19
- artery – *see* Injury, blood vessel, by site
- auditory
  - canal (external) (meatus) 872.02
    - complicated 872.12
  - ossicles (incus) (malleus) (stapes) 872.62
    - complicated 872.72
- auricle, ear 872.01
  - complicated 872.11
- axilla 880.02
  - with tendon involvement 880.22
  - complicated 880.12
    - with tendon involvement 880.29
  - involving other sites of upper arm 880.09
    - complicated 880.19
- back 876.0
  - complicated 876.1
- bladder – *see* Injury, internal, bladder
- blood vessel – *see* Injury, blood vessel, by site
- brain – *see* Injury, intracranial, with open intracranial wound
- breast 879.0
  - complicated 879.1
- brow 873.42
  - complicated 873.52
- buccal mucosa 873.61
  - complicated 873.71
- buttock 877.0
  - complicated 877.1
- calf 891.0
  - with tendon involvement 891.2
  - complicated 891.1
- canaliculus lacrimalis 870.8
  - with laceration of eyelid 870.2
- canthus, eye 870.8
  - laceration – *see* Laceration, eyelid
- cavernous sinus – *see* Injury, intracranial
- cerebellum – *see* Injury, intracranial

Wound, open – *continued*
- cervical esophagus 874.4
  - complicated 874.5
- cervix – *see* Injury, internal, cervix
- cheek(s) (external) 873.41
  - complicated 873.51
  - internal 873.61
    - complicated 873.71
- chest (wall) (external) 875.0
  - complicated 875.1
- chin 873.44
  - complicated 873.54
- choroid 363.63
- ciliary body (eye) (*see also* Wound, open, intraocular) 871.9
- clitoris 878.8
  - complicated 878.9
- cochlea 872.64
  - complicated 872.74
- complicated 879.9
- conjunctiva – *see* Wound, open, intraocular
- cornea (nonpenetrating) (*see also* Wound, open, intraocular) 871.9
- costal region 875.0
  - complicated 875.1
- Descemet's membrane (*see also* Wound, open, intraocular) 871.9
- digit(s)
  - foot 893.0
    - with tendon involvement 893.2
    - complicated 893.1
  - hand 883.0
    - with tendon involvement 883.2
    - complicated 883.1
- drumhead, ear 872.61
  - complicated 872.71
- ear 872.8
  - canal 872.02
    - complicated 872.12
  - complicated 872.9
  - drum 872.61
    - complicated 872.71
  - external 872.00
    - complicated 872.10
  - multiple sites 872.69
    - complicated 872.79
  - ossicles (incus) (malleus) (stapes) 872.62
    - complicated 872.72
  - specified part NEC 872.69
    - complicated 872.79
- elbow 881.01
  - with tendon involvement 881.21
  - complicated 881.11
- epididymis 878.2
  - complicated 878.3
- epigastric region 879.2
  - complicated 879.3
- epiglottis 874.01
  - complicated 874.11
- esophagus (cervical) 874.4
  - complicated 874.5
  - thoracic – *see* Injury, internal, esophagus
- Eustachian tube 872.63
  - complicated 872.73
- extremity
  - lower (multiple) NEC 894.0
    - with tendon involvement 894.2
    - complicated 894.1
  - upper (multiple) NEC 884.0
    - with tendon involvement 884.2
    - complicated 884.1
- eye(s) (globe) – *see* Wound, open, intraocular
- eyeball NEC 871.9
  - laceration (*see also* Laceration, eyeball) 871.4
  - penetrating (*see also* Penetrating wound, eyeball) 871.7
- eyebrow 873.42
  - complicated 873.52
- eyelid NEC 870.8
  - laceration – *see* Laceration, eyelid
- face 873.40
  - complicated 873.50
  - multiple sites 873.49
    - complicated 873.59
  - specified part NEC 873.49
    - complicated 873.59
- fallopian tube – *see* Injury, internal, fallopian tube
- finger(s) (nail) (subungual) 883.0
  - with tendon involvement 883.2
  - complicated 883.1
- flank 879.4
  - complicated 879.5

Wound, open – *continued*
- foot (any part, except toe(s) alone) 892.0
  - with tendon involvement 892.2
  - complicated 892.1
- forearm 881.00
  - with tendon involvement 881.20
  - complicated 881.10
- forehead 873.42
  - complicated 873.52
- genital organs (external) NEC 878.8
  - complicated 878.9
  - internal – *see* Injury, internal, by site
- globe (eye) (*see also* Wound, open, eyeball) 871.9
- groin 879.4
  - complicated 879.5
- gum(s) 873.62
  - complicated 873.72
- hand (except finger(s) alone) 882.0
  - with tendon involvement 882.2
  - complicated 882.1
- head NEC 873.8
  - with intracranial injury – *see* Injury, intracranial
    - due to or associated with skull fracture – *see* Fracture, skull
  - complicated 873.9
  - scalp – *see* Wound, open, scalp
- heel 892.0
  - with tendon involvement 892.2
  - complicated 892.1
- high-velocity (grease gun) – *see* Wound, open, complicated, by site
- hip 890.0
  - with tendon involvement 890.2
  - complicated 890.1
- hymen 878.6
  - complicated 878.7
- hypochondrium 879.4
  - complicated 879.5
- hypogastric region 879.2
  - complicated 879.3
- iliac (region) 879.4
  - complicated 879.5
- incidental to
  - dislocation – *see* Dislocation, open, by site
  - fracture – *see* Fracture, open, by site
  - intracranial injury – *see* Injury, intracranial, with open intracranial wound
  - nerve injury – *see* Injury, nerve, by site
- inguinal region 879.4
  - complicated 879.5
- instep 892.0
  - with tendon involvement 892.2
  - complicated 892.1
- interscapular region 876.0
  - complicated 876.1
- intracranial – *see* Injury, intracranial, with open intracranial wound
- intraocular 871.9
  - with
    - partial loss (of intraocular tissue) 871.2
    - prolapse or exposure (of intraocular tissue) 871.1
  - laceration (*see also* Laceration, eyeball) 871.4
  - penetrating 871.7
    - with foreign body (nonmagnetic) 871.6
      - magnetic 871.5
  - without prolapse (of intraocular tissue) 871.0
- iris (*see also* Wound, open, eyeball) 871.9
- jaw (fracture not involved) 873.44
  - with fracture – *see* Fracture, jaw
  - complicated 873.54
- knee 891.0
  - with tendon involvement 891.2
  - complicated 891.1
- labium (majus) (minus) 878.4
  - complicated 878.5
- lacrimal apparatus, gland, or sac 870.8
  - with laceration of eyelid 870.2
- larynx 874.01
  - with trachea 874.00
    - complicated 874.10
  - complicated 874.11
- leg (multiple) 891.0
  - with tendon involvement 891.2
  - complicated 891.1
  - lower 891.0
    - with tendon involvement 891.2
    - complicated 891.1
  - thigh 890.0
    - with tendon involvement 890.2
    - complicated 890.1

Wound, open – *continued*
  leg – *continued*
    upper 890.0
      with tendon involvement 890.2
      complicated 890.1
  lens (eye) (alone) (*see also* Cataract, traumatic) 366.20
    with involvement of other eye structures – *see* Wound, open, eyeball
  limb
    lower (multiple) NEC 894.0
      with tendon involvement 894.2
      complicated 894.1
    upper (multiple) NEC 884.0
      with tendon involvement 884.2
      complicated 884.1
  lip 873.43
    complicated 873.53
  loin 876.0
    complicated 876.1
  lumbar region 876.0
    complicated 876.1
  malar region 873.41
    complicated 873.51
  mastoid region 873.49
    complicated 873.59
  mediastinum – *see* Injury, internal, mediastinum
  midthoracic region 875.0
    complicated 875.1
  mouth 873.60
    complicated 873.70
    floor 873.64
      complicated 873.74
    multiple sites 873.69
      complicated 873.79
    specified site NEC 873.69
      complicated 873.79
  multiple, unspecified site(s) 879.8

Note – Multiple open wounds of sites classifiable to the same four-digit category should be classified to that category unless they are in different limbs.

Multiple open wounds of sites classifiable to different four-digit categories, or to different limbs, should be coded separately.

    complicated 879.9
    lower limb(s) (one or both) (sites classifiable to more than one three-digit category in 890-893) 894.0
      with tendon involvement 894.2
      complicated 894.1
    upper limb(s) (one or both) (sites classifiable to more than one three-digit category in 880-883) 884.0
      with tendon involvement 884.2
      complicated 884.1
  muscle – *see* Sprain, by site
  nail
    finger(s) 883.0
      complicated 883.1
    thumb 883.0
      complicated 883.1
    toe(s) 893.0
      complicated 893.1
  nape (neck) 874.8
    complicated 874.9
    specified part NEC 874.8
      complicated 874.9
  nasal – *see also* Wound, open, nose
    cavity 873.22
      complicated 873.32
    septum 873.21
      complicated 873.31
    sinuses 873.23
      complicated 873.33
  nasopharynx 873.22
    complicated 873.32
  neck 874.8
    complicated 874.9
    nape 874.8
      complicated 874.9
    specified part NEC 874.8
      complicated 874.9
  nerve – *see* Injury, nerve, by site
  non-healing surgical 998.83
  nose 873.20
    complicated 873.30
    multiple sites 873.29
      complicated 873.39
    septum 873.21
      complicated 873.31

Wound, open – *continued*
  nose – *continued*
    sinuses 873.23
      complicated 873.33
  occipital region – *see* Wound, open, scalp
  ocular NEC 871.9
    adnexa 870.9
      specified region NEC 870.8
    laceration (*see also* Laceration, ocular) 871.4
    muscle (extraocular) 870.3
      with foreign body 870.4
      eyelid 870.1
      intraocular – *see* Wound, open, eyeball
    penetrating (*see also* Penetrating wound, ocular) 871.7
  orbit 870.8
    penetrating 870.3
      with foreign body 870.4
  orbital region 870.9
  ovary – *see* Injury, internal, pelvic organs
  palate 873.65
    complicated 873.75
  palm 882.0
    with tendon involvement 882.2
    complicated 882.1
  parathyroid (gland) 874.2
    complicated 874.3
  parietal region – *see* Wound, open, scalp
  pelvic floor or region 879.6
    complicated 879.7
  penis 878.0
    complicated 878.1
  perineum 879.6
    complicated 879.7
  periocular area 870.8
    laceration of skin 870.0
  pharynx 874.4
    complicated 874.5
  pinna 872.01
    complicated 872.11
  popliteal space 891.0
    with tendon involvement 891.2
    complicated 891.1
  prepuce 878.0
    complicated 878.1
  pubic region 879.2
    complicated 879.3
  pudenda 878.8
    complicated 878.9
  rectovaginal septum 878.8
    complicated 878.9
  sacral region 877.0
    complicated 877.1
  sacroiliac region 877.0
    complicated 877.1
  salivary (ducts) (glands) 873.69
    complicated 873.79
  scalp 873.0
    complicated 873.1
  scalpel, fetus or newborn 767.8
  scapular region 880.01
    with tendon involvement 880.21
    complicated 880.11
    involving other sites of upper arm 880.09
      with tendon involvement 880.29
      complicated 880.19
  sclera (*see also* Wound, open, intraocular) 871.9
  scrotum 878.2
    complicated 878.3
  seminal vesicle – *see* Injury, internal, pelvic organs
  shin 891.0
    with tendon involvement 891.2
    complicated 891.1
  shoulder 880.00
    with tendon involvement 880.20
    complicated 880.10
    involving other sites of upper arm 880.09
      with tendon involvement 880.29
      complicated 880.19
  skin NEC 879.8
    complicated 879.9
  skull – *see also* Injury, intracranial, with open intracranial wound
    with skull fracture – *see* Fracture, skull
  spermatic cord (scrotal) 878.2
    complicated 878.3
    pelvic region – *see* Injury, internal, spermatic cord
  spinal cord – *see* Injury, spinal
  sternal region 875.0
    complicated 875.1

Wound, open – *continued*
  subconjunctival – *see* Wound, open, intraocular
  subcutaneous NEC 879.8
    complicated 879.9
  submaxillary region 873.44
    complicated 873.54
  submental region 873.44
    complicated 873.54
  subungual
    finger(s) (thumb) – *see* Wound, open, finger
    toe(s) – *see* Wound, open, toe
  supraclavicular region 874.8
    complicated 874.9
  supraorbital 873.42
    complicated 873.52
  surgical, non-healing 998.83
  temple 873.49
    complicated 873.59
  temporal region 873.49
    complicated 873.59
  testis 878.2
    complicated 878.3
  thigh 890.0
    with tendon involvement 890.2
    complicated 890.1
  thorax, thoracic (external) 875.0
    complicated 875.1
  throat 874.8
    complicated 874.9
  thumb (nail) (subungual) 883.0
    with tendon involvement 883.2
    complicated 883.1
  thyroid (gland) 874.2
    complicated 874.3
  toe(s) (nail) (subungual) 893.0
    with tendon involvement 893.2
    complicated 893.1
  tongue 873.64
    complicated 873.74
  tonsil – *see* Wound, open, neck
  trachea (cervical region) 874.02
    with larynx 874.00
      complicated 874.10
    complicated 874.12
    intrathoracic – *see* Injury, internal, trachea
  trunk (multiple) NEC 879.6
    complicated 879.7
    specified site NEC 879.6
      complicated 879.7
  tunica vaginalis 878.2
    complicated 878.3
  tympanic membrane 872.61
    complicated 872.71
  tympanum 872.61
    complicated 872.71
  umbilical region 879.2
    complicated 879.3
  ureter – *see* Injury, internal, ureter
  urethra – *see* Injury, internal, urethra
  uterus – *see* Injury, internal, uterus
  uvula 873.69
    complicated 873.79
  vagina 878.6
    complicated 878.7
  vas deferens – *see* Injury, internal, vas deferens
  vitreous (humor) 871.2
  vulva 878.4
    complicated 878.5
  wrist 881.02
    with tendon involvement 881.22
    complicated 881.12
Wright's syndrome (hyperabduction) 447.8
  pneumonia 390 *[517.1]*
Wringer injury – *see* Crush injury, by site
Wrinkling of skin 701.8
Wrist – *see also* condition
  drop (acquired) 736.05
Wrong drug (given in error) NEC 977.9
  specified drug or substance – *see* Table of Drugs and Chemicals
Wry neck – *see also* Torticollis
  congenital 754.1
Wuchereria infestation 125.0
  bancrofti 125.0
  Brugia malayi 125.1
  malayi 125.1
Wuchereriasis 125.0
Wuchereriosis 125.0
Wuchernde struma langhans (M8332/3) 193

Wound, open – Wuchernde struma langhans

Volume 2

Section 2

Alphabetical Index to Poisoning and External Causes of Adverse Effects of Drugs and Other Chemical Substances

Table of Drugs and Chemicals

This table contains a classification of drugs and other chemical substances to identify poisoning states and external causes of adverse effects.

Each of the listed substances in the table is assigned a code according to the poisoning classification (960-989). These codes are used when there is a statement of poisoning, overdose, wrong substance given or taken, or intoxication.

The table also contains a listing of external causes of adverse effects. An adverse effect is a pathologic manifestation due to ingestion or exposure to drugs or other chemical substances (e.g., dermatitis, hypersensitivity reaction, aspirin gastritis). The adverse effect is to be identified by the appropriate code found in Section 1, Alphabetic Index to Diseases and Injuries. An external cause code can then be used to identify the circumstances involved. The table headings pertaining to external causes are defined below:

Accidental poisoning (E850–E869) — accidental overdose of drug, wrong substance given or taken, drug taken inadvertently, accidents in the usage of drugs and biologicals in medical and surgical procedures, and to show external causes of poisonings classifiable to 980-989.

Therapeutic use (E930–E949) — a correct substance properly administered in therapeutic or prophylactic dosage as the external cause of adverse effects.

Suicide attempt (E950–E952) — instances in which self-inflicted injuries or poisonings are involved.

Assault (E961-E962) – injury or poisoning inflicted by another person with the intent to injure or kill.

Undetermined (E980–E982) — to be used when the intent of the poisoning or injury cannot be determined whether it was intentional or accidental.

The American Hospital Formulary Service (AHFS) list numbers are included in the table to help classify new drugs not identified in the table by name. The AHFS list numbers are keyed to the continually revised AHFS (American Hospital Formulary Service, 2 vol. Washington, D.C.: American Society of Hospital Pharmacists, 1959). These listings are found in the table under the main term Drug.

Excluded from the table are radium and other radioactive substances. The classification of adverse effects and complications pertaining to these substances will be found in Index to Diseases and Injuries, and Index to External Causes of Injuries.

Although certain substances are indexed with one or more subentries, the majority are listed according to one use or state. It is recognized that many substances may be used in various ways, in medicine and in industry, and may cause adverse effects whatever the state of the agent (solid, liquid, or fumes arising from a liquid). In cases in which the reported data indicate a use or state not in the table, or which is clearly different from the one listed, an attempt should be made to classify the substance in the form which most nearly expresses the reported facts.

		External Cause (E-Code)				
Drug	**Poisoning**	**Accident**	**Therapeutic Use**	**Suicide Attempt**	**Assault**	**Undetermined**
1-propanol	980.3	E860.4	-	E950.9	E962.1	E980.9
2-propanol	980.2	E860.3	-	E950.9	E962.1	E980.9
2,4-D (dichlorophenoxyacetic acid)	989.4	E863.5	-	E950.6	E962.1	E980.7
2,4-toluene diisocyanate	983.0	E864.0	-	E950.7	E962.1	E980.6
2,4,5-T (trichlorophenoxyacetic acid)	989.2	E863.5	-	E950.6	E962.1	E980.7
14-hydroxydihydromorphinone	965.09	E850.2	E935.2	E950.0	E962.0	E980.0
ABOB	961.7	E857	E931.7	E950.4	E962.0	E980.4
Abrus (seed)	988.2	E865.3	-	E950.9	E962.1	E980.9
Absinthe	980.0	E860.1	-	E950.9	E962.1	E980.9
beverage	980.0	E860.0	-	E950.9	E962.1	E980.9
Acenocoumarin, acenocoumarol	964.2	E858.2	E934.2	E950.4	E962.0	E980.4
Acepromazine	969.1	E853.0	E939.1	E950.3	E962.0	E980.3
Acetal	982.8	E862.4	-	E950.9	E962.1	E980.9
Acetaldehyde (vapor)	987.8	E869.8	-	E952.8	E962.2	E982.8
liquid	989.89	E866.8	-	E950.9	E962.1	E980.9
Acetaminophen	965.4	E850.4	E935.4	E950.0	E962.0	E980.0
Acetaminosalol	965.1	E850.3	E935.3	E950.0	E962.0	E980.0
Acetanilid(e)	965.4	E850.4	E935.4	E950.0	E962.0	E980.0
Acetarsol, acetarsone	961.1	E857	E931.1	E950.4	E962.0	E980.4
Acetazolamide	974.2	E858.5	E944.2	E950.4	E962.0	E980.4
Acetic						
acid	983.1	E864.1	-	E950.7	E962.1	E980.6
with sodium acetate (ointment)	976.3	E858.7	E946.3	E950.4	E962.0	E980.4
irrigating solution	974.5	E858.5	E944.5	E950.4	E962.0	E980.4
lotion	976.2	E858.7	E946.2	E950.4	E962.0	E980.4
anhydride	983.1	E864.1	-	E950.7	E962.1	E980.6
ether (vapor)	982.8	E862.4	-	E950.9	E962.1	E980.9
Acetohexamide	962.3	E858.0	E932.3	E950.4	E962.0	E980.4
Acetomenaphihone	964.3	E858.2	E934.3	E950.4	E962.0	E980.4
Acetomorphine	965.01	E850.0	E935.0	E950.0	E962.0	E980.0
Acetone (oils) (vapor)	982.8	E862.4	-	E950.9	E962.1	E980.9
Acetophenazine (maleate)	969.1	E853.0	E939.1	E950.3	E962.0	E980.3
Acetophenetidin	965.4	E850.4	E935.4	E950.0	E962.0	E980.0
Acetophenone	982.0	E862.4	-	E950.9	E962.1	E980.9
Acetorphine	965.09	E850.2	E935.2	E950.0	E962.0	E980.0
Acetosulfone (sodium)	961.8	E857	E931.8	E950.4	E962.0	E980.4
Acetrizoate (sodium)	977.8	E858.8	E947.8	E950.4	E962.0	E980.4
Acetylcarbromal	967.3	E852.2	E937.3	E950.2	E962.0	E980.2
Acetylcholine (chloride)	971.0	E855.3	E941.0	E950.4	E962.0	E980.4
Acetylcysteine	975.5	E858.6	E945.5	E950.4	E962.0	E980.4
Acetyldigitoxin	972.1	E858.3	E942.1	E950.4	E962.0	E980.4
Acetyldihydrocodeine	965.09	E850.2	E935.2	E950.0	E962.0	E980.0
Acetyldihydrocodeinone	965.09	E850.2	E935.2	E950.0	E962.0	E980.0
Acetylene (gas) (industrial)	987.1	E868.1	-	E951.8	E962.2	E981.8
incomplete combustion of – *see* Carbon monoxide, fuel, utility						
tetrachloride (vapor)	982.3	E862.4	-	E950.9	E962.1	E980.9
Acetyliodosalicylic acid	965.1	E850.3	E935.3	E950.0	E962.0	E980.0
Acetylphenylhydrazine	965.8	E850.8	E935.8	E950.0	E962.0	E980.0
Acetylsalicylic acid	965.1	E850.3	E935.3	E950.0	E962.0	E980.0
Achromycin	960.4	E856	E930.4	E950.4	E962.0	E980.4
ophthalmic preparation	976.5	E858.7	E946.5	E950.4	E962.0	E980.4
topical NEC	976.0	E858.7	E946.0	E950.4	E962.0	E980.4
Acidifying agents	963.2	E858.1	E933.2	E950.4	E962.0	E980.4
Acids (corrosive) **NEC**	983.1	E864.1	-	E950.7	E962.1	E980.6
Aconite (wild)	988.2	E865.4	-	E950.9	E962.1	E980.9
Aconitine (liniment)	976.8	E858.7	E946.8	E950.4	E962.0	E980.4
Aconitum ferox	988.2	E865.4	-	E950.9	E962.1	E980.9
Acridine	983.0	E864.0	-	E950.7	E962.1	E980.6
vapor	987.8	E869.8	-	E952.8	E962.2	E982.8
Acriflavine	961.9	E857	E931.9	E950.4	E962.0	E980.4
Acrisorcin	976.0	E858.7	E946.0	E950.4	E962.0	E980.4
Acrolein (gas)	987.8	E869.8	-	E952.8	E962.2	E982.8
liquid	989.89	E866.8	-	E950.9	E962.1	E980.9
Actaea spicata	988.2	E865.4	-	E950.9	E962.1	E980.9
Acterol	961.5	E857	E931.5	E950.4	E962.0	E980.4
ACTH	962.4	E858.0	E932.4	E950.4	E962.0	E980.4
Acthar	962.4	E858.0	E932.4	E950.4	E962.0	E980.4
Actinomycin (C) (D)	960.7	E856	E930.7	E950.4	E962.0	E980.4
Adalin (acetyl)	967.3	E852.2	E937.3	E950.2	E962.0	E980.2
Adenosine (phosphate)	977.8	E858.8	E947.8	E950.4	E962.0	E980.4
Adhesives	989.89	E866.6	-	E950.9	E962.1	E980.9
ADH	962.5	E858.0	E932.5	E950.4	E962.0	E980.4
Adicillin	960.0	E856	E930.0	E950.4	E962.0	E980.4
Adiphenine	975.1	E855.6	E945.1	E950.4	E962.0	E980.4
Adjunct, pharmaceutical	977.4	E858.8	E947.4	E950.4	E962.0	E980.4
Adrenal (extract, cortex or medulla) (glucocorticoids) (hormones) (mineralocorticoids)	962.0	E858.0	E932.0	E950.4	E962.0	E980.4
ENT agent	976.6	E858.7	E946.6	E950.4	E962.0	E980.4
ophthalmic preparation	976.5	E858.7	E946.5	E950.4	E962.0	E980.4
topical NEC	976.0	E858.7	E946.0	E950.4	E962.0	E980.4
Adrenalin	971.2	E855.5	E941.2	E950.4	E962.0	E980.4
Adrenergic blocking agents	971.3	E855.6	E941.3	E950.4	E962.0	E980.4
Adrenergics	971.2	E855.5	E941.2	E950.4	E962.0	E980.4
Adrenochrome (derivatives)	972.8	E858.3	E942.8	E950.4	E962.0	E980.4
Adrenocorticotropic hormone	962.4	E858.0	E932.4	E950.4	E962.0	E980.4
Adrenocorticotropin	962.4	E858.0	E932.4	E950.4	E962.0	E980.4
Adriamycin	960.7	E856	E930.7	E950.4	E962.0	E980.4
Aerosol spray – *see* Sprays						
Aerosporin	960.8	E856	E930.8	E950.4	E962.0	E980.4
ENT agent	976.6	E858.7	E946.6	E950.4	E962.0	E980.4
ophthalmic preparation	976.5	E858.7	E946.5	E950.4	E962.0	E980.4
topical NEC	976.0	E858.7	E946.0	E950.4	E962.0	E980.4
Aethusa cynapium	988.2	E865.4	-	E950.9	E962.1	E980.9
Afghanistan black	969.6	E854.1	E939.6	E950.3	E962.0	E980.3
Aflatoxin	989.7	E865.9	-	E950.9	E962.1	E980.9
African boxwood	988.2	E865.4	-	E950.9	E962.1	E980.9
Agar (-agar)	973.3	E858.4	E943.3	E950.4	E962.0	E980.4
Agricultural agent NEC	989.89	E863.9	-	E950.6	E962.1	E980.7
Agrypnal	967.0	E851	E937.0	E950.1	E962.0	E980.1
Air contaminant(s), source or type not specified	987.9	E869.9	-	E952.9	E962.2	E982.9
specified type – *see* specific substance						
Akee	988.2	E865.4	-	E950.9	E962.1	E980.9
Akrinol	976.0	E858.7	E946.0	E950.4	E962.0	E980.4
Alantolactone	961.6	E857	E931.6	E950.4	E962.0	E980.4
Albamycin	960.8	E856	E930.8	E950.4	E962.0	E980.4
Albumin (normal human serum)	964.7	E858.2	E934.7	E950.4	E962.0	E980.4
Albuterol	975.7	E858.6	E945.7	E950.4	E962.0	E980.4
Alcohol	980.9	E860.9	-	E950.9	E962.1	E980.9
absolute	980.0	E860.1	-	E950.9	E962.1	E980.9
beverage	980.0	E860.0	E947.8	E950.9	E962.1	E980.9
amyl	980.3	E860.4	-	E950.9	E962.1	E980.9
antifreeze	980.1	E860.2	-	E950.9	E962.1	E980.9
butyl	980.3	E860.4	-	E950.9	E962.1	E980.9

● New Line ▲ Revised Code

		External Cause (E-Code)				
Drug	Poisoning	Accident	Therapeutic Use	Suicide Attempt	Assault	Undetermined
Alcohol – *continued*						
dehydrated	980.0	E860.1	-	E950.9	E862.1	E980.9
beverage	980.0	E860.0	E947.8	E950.9	E962.1	E980.9
denatured	980.0	E860.1	-	E950.9	E962.1	E980.9
deterrents	977.3	E858.8	E947.3	E950.4	E962.0	E980.4
diagnostic (gastric function)	977.8	E858.8	E947.8	E950.4	E962.0	E980.4
ethyl	980.0	E860.1	-	E950.9	E962.1	E980.9
beverage	980.0	E860.0	E947.8	E950.9	E962.1	E980.9
grain	980.0	E860.1	-	E950.9	E962.1	E980.9
beverage	980.0	E860.0	E947.8	E950.9	E962.1	E980.9
industrial	980.9	E860.9	-	E950.9	E962.1	E980.9
isopropyl	980.2	E860.3	-	E950.9	E962.1	E980.9
methyl	980.1	E860.2	-	E950.9	E962.1	E980.9
preparation for consumption	980.0	E860.0	E947.8	E950.9	E962.1	E980.9
propyl	980.3	E860.4	-	E950.9	E962.1	E980.9
secondary	980.2	E860.3	-	E950.9	E962.1	E980.9
radiator	980.1	E860.2	-	E950.9	E962.1	E980.9
rubbing	980.2	E860.3	-	E950.9	E962.1	E980.9
specified type NEC	980.8	E860.8	-	E950.9	E962.1	E980.9
surgical	980.9	E860.9	-	E950.9	E962.1	E980.9
vapor (from any type of alcohol)	987.8	E869.8	-	E952.8	E962.2	E982.8
wood	980.1	E860.2	-	E950.9	E962.1	E980.9
Alcuronium chloride	975.2	E858.6	E945.2	E950.4	E962.0	E980.4
Aldacione	974.4	E858.5	E944.4	E950.4	E962.0	E980.4
Aldicarb	989.3	E863.2	-	E950.6	E962.1	E980.7
Aldomet	972.6	E858.3	E942.6	E950.4	E962.0	E980.4
Aldosterone	962.0	E858.0	E932.0	E950.4	E962.0	E980.4
Aldrin (dust)	989.2	E863.0	-	E950.6	E962.1	E980.7
Algeldrate	973.0	E858.4	E943.0	E950.4	E962.0	E980.4
Alidase	963.4	E858.1	E933.4	E950.4	E962.0	E980.4
Aliphatic thiocyanates	989.0	E866.8	-	E950.9	E962.1	E980.9
Alkaline antiseptic solution (aromatic)	976.6	E858.7	E946.6	E950.4	E962.0	E980.4
Alkalinizing agents (medicinal)	963.3	E858.1	E933.3	E950.4	E962.0	E980.4
Alkalis, caustic	983.2	E864.2	-	E950.7	E962.1	E980.6
Alkalizing agents (medicinal)	963.3	E858.1	E933.3	E950.4	E962.0	E980.4
Alka-seltzer	965.1	E850.3	E935.3	E950.0	E962.0	E980.0
Alkavervir	972.6	E858.3	E942.6	E950.4	E962.0	E980.4
Allegron	969.0	E854.0	E939.0	E950.3	E962.0	E980.3
Alleve – *see* Naproxen						
Allobarbital, allobarbitone	967.0	E851	E937.0	E950.1	E962.0	E980.1
Allopurinol	974.7	E858.5	E944.7	E950.4	E962.0	E980.4
Allylestrenol	962.2	E858.0	E932.2	E950.4	E962.0	E980.4
Allylisopropylacetylurea	967.8	E852.8	E937.8	E950.2	E962.0	E980.2
Allylisopropylmalonylurea	967.0	E851	E937.0	E950.1	E962.0	E980.1
Allyltribromide	967.3	E852.2	E937.3	E950.2	E962.0	E980.2
Aloe, aloes, aloin	973.1	E858.4	E943.1	E950.4	E962.0	E980.4
Alosetron	973.8	E858.4	E943.8	E950.4	E962.0	E980.4
Aloxidone	966.0	E855.0	E936.0	E950.4	E962.0	E980.4
Aloxiprin	965.1	E850.3	E935.3	E950.0	E962.0	E980.0
Alpha amylase	963.4	E858.1	E933.4	E950.4	E962.0	E980.4
Alpha-1 blockers ●	971.3	E855.6	E941.3	E950.4	E962.0	E980.4
Alphaprodine (hydrochloride)	965.09	E850.2	E935.2	E950.0	E962.0	E980.0
Alpha tocopherol	963.5	E858.1	E933.5	E950.4	E962.0	E980.4
Alseroxylon	972.6	E858.3	E942.6	E950.4	E962.0	E980.4
Alum (ammonium) (potassium)	983.2	E864.2	-	E950.7	E962.1	E980.6
medicinal (astringent) NEC	976.2	E858.7	E946.2	E950.4	E962.0	E980.4
Aluminium, aluminum (gel) (hydroxide)	973.0	E858.4	E943.0	E950.4	E962.0	E980.4
acetate solution	976.2	E858.7	E946.2	E950.4	E962.0	E980.4
aspirin	965.1	E850.3	E935.3	E950.0	E962.0	E980.0
carbonate	973.0	E858.4	E943.0	E950.4	E962.0	E980.4
glycinate	973.0	E858.4	E943.0	E950.4	E962.0	E980.4
nicotinate	972.2	E858.3	E942.2	E950.4	E962.0	E980.4
ointment (surgical) (topical)	976.3	E858.7	E946.3	E950.4	E962.0	E980.4
phosphate	973.0	E858.4	E943.0	E950.4	E962.0	E980.4
subacetate	976.2	E858.7	E946.2	E950.4	E962.0	E980.4
topical NEC	976.3	E858.7	E946.3	E950.4	E962.0	E980.4
Alurate	967.0	E851	E937.0	E950.1	E962.0	E980.1
Alverine (citrate)	975.1	E858.6	E945.1	E950.4	E962.0	E980.4
Alvodine	965.09	E850.2	E935.2	E950.0	E962.0	E980.0
Amanita phalloides	988.1	E865.5	-	E950.9	E962.1	E980.9
Amantadine (hydrochloride)	966.4	E855.0	E936.4	E950.4	E962.0	E980.4
Ambazone	961.9	E857	E931.9	E950.4	E962.0	E980.4
Ambenonium	971.0	E855.3	E941.0	E950.4	E962.0	E980.4
Ambutonium bromide	971.1	E855.4	E941.1	E950.4	E962.0	E980.4
Ametazole	977.8	E858.8	E947.8	E950.4	E962.0	E980.4
Amethocaine (infiltration) (topical)	968.5	E855.2	E938.5	E950.4	E962.0	E980.4
nerve block (peripheral) (plexus)	968.6	E855.2	E938.6	E950.4	E962.0	E980.4
spinal	968.7	E855.2	E938.7	E950.4	E962.0	E980.4
Amethopterin	963.1	E858.1	E933.1	E950.4	E962.0	E980.4
Amfepramone	977.0	E858.8	E947.0	E950.4	E962.0	E980.4
Amidon	965.02	E850.1	E935.1	E950.0	E962.0	E980.0
Amidopyrine	965.5	E850.5	E935.5	E950.0	E962.0	E980.0
Aminacrine	976.0	E858.7	E946.0	E950.4	E962.0	E980.4
Aminitrozole	961.5	E857	E931.5	E950.4	E962.0	E980.4
Aminoacetic acid	974.5	E858.5	E944.5	E950.4	E962.0	E980.4
Amino acids	974.5	E858.5	E944.5	E950.4	E962.0	E980.4
Aminocaproic acid	964.4	E858.2	E934.4	E950.4	E962.0	E980.4
Aminoethylisothiourium	963.8	E858.1	E933.8	E950.4	E962.0	E980.4
Aminoglutethimide	966.3	E855.0	E936.3	E950.4	E962.0	E980.4
Aminometradine	974.3	E858.5	E944.3	E950.4	E962.0	E980.4
Aminopentamide	971.1	E855.4	E941.1	E950.4	E962.0	E980.4
Aminophenazone	965.5	E850.5	E935.5	E950.0	E962.0	E980.0
Aminophenol	983.0	E864.0	-	E950.7	E962.1	E980.6
Aminophenylpyridone	969.5	E853.8	E939.5	E950.3	E962.0	E980.3
Aminophyllin	975.7	E858.6	E945.7	E950.4	E962.0	E980.4
Aminopterin	963.1	E858.1	E933.1	E950.4	E962.0	E980.4
Aminopyrine	965.5	E850.5	E935.5	E950.0	E962.0	E980.0
Aminosalicylic acid	961.8	E857	E931.8	E950.4	E962.0	E980.4
Amiphenazole	970.1	E854.3	E940.1	E950.4	E962.0	E980.4
Amiquinsin	972.6	E858.3	E942.6	E950.4	E962.0	E980.4
Amisometradine	974.3	E858.5	E944.3	E950.4	E962.0	E980.4
Amitriptyline	969.0	E854.0	E939.0	E950.3	E962.0	E980.3
Ammonia (fumes) (gas) (vapor)	987.8	E869.8	-	E952.8	E962.2	E982.8
liquid (household) NEC	983.2	E861.4	-	E950.7	E962.1	E980.6
spirit, aromatic	970.8	E854.3	E940.8	E950.4	E962.0	E980.4
Ammoniated mercury	976.0	E858.7	E946.0	E950.4	E962.0	E980.4
Ammonium						
carbonate	983.2	E864.2	-	E950.7	E962.1	E980.6
chloride (acidifying agent)	963.2	E858.1	E933.2	E950.4	E962.0	E980.4
expectorant	975.5	E858.6	E945.5	E950.4	E962.0	E980.4
compounds (household) NEC	983.2	E861.4	-	E950.7	E962.1	E980.6
fumes (any usage)	987.8	E869.8	-	E952.8	E962.2	E982.8
industrial	983.2	E864.2	-	E950.7	E962.1	E980.6
ichthyosulronate	976.4	E858.7	E946.4	E950.4	E962.0	E980.4

Alcohol – Ammonium

● New Line ▲ Revised Code

		External Cause (E-Code)				
Drug	Poisoning	Accident	Therapeutic Use	Suicide Attempt	Assault	Undetermined
Ammonium – *continued*						
mandelate	961.9	E857	E931.9	E950.4	E962.0	E980.4
Amobarbital	967.0	E851	E937.0	E950.1	E962.0	E980.1
Amodiaquin(e)	961.4	E857	E931.4	E950.4	E962.0	E980.4
Amopyroquin(e)	961.4	E857	E931.4	E950.4	E962.0	E980.4
Amphenidone	969.5	E853.8	E939.5	E950.3	E962.0	E980.3
Amphetamine	969.7	E854.2	E939.7	E950.3	E962.0	E980.3
Amphomycin	960.8	E856	E930.8	E950.4	E962.0	E980.4
Amphotericin B	960.1	E856	E930.1	E950.4	E962.0	E980.4
topical	976.0	E858.7	E946.0	E950.4	E962.0	E980.4
Ampicillin	960.0	E856	E930.0	E950.4	E962.0	E980.4
Amprotropine	971.1	E855.4	E941.1	E950.4	E962.0	E980.4
Amygdalin	977.8	E858.8	E947.8	E950.4	E962.0	E980.4
Amyl						
acetate (vapor)	982.8	E862.4	-	E950.9	E962.1	E980.9
alcohol	980.3	E860.4	-	E950.9	E962.1	E980.9
nitrite (medicinal)	972.4	E858.3	E942.4	E950.4	E962.0	E980.4
Amylase (alpha)	963.4	E858.1	E933.4	E950.4	E962.0	E980.4
Amylene hydrate	980.8	E860.8	-	E950.9	E962.1	E980.9
Amylobarbitone	967.0	E851	E937.0	E950.1	E962.0	E980.1
Amylocaine	968.9	E855.2	E938.9	E950.4	E962.0	E980.4
infiltration (subcutaneous)	968.5	E855.2	E938.5	E950.4	E962.0	E980.4
nerve block (peripheral) (plexus)	968.6	E855.2	E938.6	E950.4	E962.0	E980.4
spinal	968.7	E855.2	E938.7	E950.4	E962.0	E980.4
topical (surface)	968.5	E855.2	E938.5	E950.4	E962.0	E980.4
Amytal (sodium)	967.0	E851	E937.0	E950.1	E962.0	E980.1
Analeptics	970.0	E854.3	E940.0	E950.4	E962.0	E980.4
Analgesics	965.9	E850.9	E935.9	E950.0	E962.0	E980.0
aromatic NEC	965.4	E850.4	E935.4	E950.0	E962.0	E980.0
non-narcotic NEC	965.7	E850.7	E935.7	E950.0	E962.0	E980.0
specified NEC	965.8	E850.8	E935.8	E950.0	E962.0	E980.0
Anamirta cocculus	988.2	E865.3	-	E950.9	E962.1	E980.9
Ancillin	960.0	E856	E930.0	E950.4	E962.0	E980.4
Androgens (anabolic congeners)	962.1	E858.0	E932.1	E950.4	E962.0	E980.4
Androstalone	962.1	E858.0	E932.1	E950.4	E962.0	E980.4
Androsterone	962.1	E858.0	E932.1	E950.4	E962.0	E980.4
Anemone pulsatilla	988.2	E865.4	-	E950.9	E962.1	E980.9
Anesthesia, anesthetic (general) NEC	968.4	E855.1	E938.4	E950.4	E962.0	E980.4
block (nerve) (plexus)	968.6	E855.2	E938.6	E950.4	E962.0	E980.4
gaseous NEC	968.2	E855.1	E938.2	E950.4	E962.0	E980.4
halogenated hydrocarbon derivatives NEC	968.2	E855.1	E938.2	E950.4	E962.0	E980.4
infiltration (intradermal) (subcutaneous) (submucosal)	968.5	E855.2	E938.5	E950.4	E962.0	E980.4
intravenous	968.3	E855.1	E938.3	E950.4	E962.0	E980.4
local NEC	968.9	E855.2	E938.9	E950.4	E962.0	E980.4
nerve blocking (peripheral) (plexus)	968.6	E855.2	E938.6	E950.4	E962.0	E980.4
rectal NEC	968.3	E855.1	E938.3	E950.4	E962.0	E980.4
spinal	968.7	E855.2	E938.7	E950.4	E962.0	E980.4
surface	968.5	E855.2	E938.5	E950.4	E962.0	E980.4
topical	968.5	E855.2	E938.5	E950.4	E962.0	E980.4
Aneurine	963.5	E858.1	E933.5	E950.4	E962.0	E980.4
Angio-Conray	977.8	E858.8	E947.8	E950.4	E962.0	E980.4
Angiotensin	971.2	E855.5	E941.2	E950.4	E962.0	E980.4
Anginine- *see* Glyceryl trinitrate	971.2	E855.5	E941.2	E950.4	E962.0	E980.4
Anhydrohydroxyprogesterone	962.2	E858.0	E932.2	E950.4	E962.0	E980.4
Anhydron	974.3	E858.5	E944.3	E950.4	E962.0	E980.4
Anileridine	965.09	E850.2	E935.2	E950.0	E962.0	E980.0
Aniline (dye) (liquid)	983.0	E864.0	-	E950.7	E962.1	E980.6
analgesic	965.4	E850.4	E935.4	E950.0	E962.0	E980.0
derivatives, therapeutic NEC	965.4	E850.4	E935.4	E950.0	E962.0	E980.0
vapor	987.8	E869.8	-	E952.8	E962.2	E982.8
Anisindione	964.2	E858.2	E934.2	E950.4	E962.0	E980.4
Aniscoropine	971.1	E855.4	E941.1	E950.4	E962.0	E980.4
Anorexic agents	977.0	E858.8	E947.0	E950.4	E962.0	E980.4
Ant (bite) (sting)	989.5	E905.5	-	E950.9	E962.1	E980.9
Antabuse	977.3	E858.8	E947.3	E950.4	E962.0	E980.4
Antacids	973.0	E858.4	E943.0	E950.4	E962.0	E980.4
Antazoline	963.0	E858.1	E933.0	E950.4	E962.0	E980.4
Anthelmintics	961.6	E857	E931.6	E950.4	E962.0	E980.4
Anthralin	976.4	E858.7	E946.4	E950.4	E962.0	E980.4
Anthramycin	960.7	E856	E930.7	E950.4	E962.0	E980.4
Antiadrenergics	971.3	E855.6	E941.3	E950.4	E962.0	E980.4
Antiallergic agents	963.0	E858.1	E933.0	E950.4	E962.0	E980.4
Antianemic agents NEC	964.1	E858.2	E934.1	E950.4	E962.0	E980.4
Antiaris toxicaria	988.2	E865.4	-	E950.9	E962.1	E980.9
Antiarteriesclerotic agents	972.2	E858.3	E942.2	E950.4	E962.0	E980.4
Antiasthmatics	975.7	E858.6	E945.7	E950.4	E962.0	E980.4
Antibiotics	960.9	E856	E930.9	E950.4	E962.0	E980.4
antifungal	960.1	E856	E930.1	E950.4	E962.0	E980.4
antimycobacterial	960.6	E856	E930.6	E950.4	E962.0	E980.4
antineoplastic	960.7	E856	E930.7	E950.4	E962.0	E980.4
cephalosporin (group)	960.5	E856	E930.5	E950.4	E962.0	E980.4
chloramphenicol (group)	960.2	E856	E930.2	E950.4	E962.0	E980.4
macrolides	960.3	E856	E930.3	E950.4	E962.0	E980.4
specified NEC	960.8	E856	E930.8	E950.4	E962.0	E980.4
tetracycline (group)	960.4	E856	E930.4	E950.4	E962.0	E980.4
Anticancer agents NEC	963.1	E858.1	E933.1	E950.4	E962.0	E980.4
antibiotics	960.7	E856	E930.7	E950.4	E962.0	E980.4
Anticholinergics	971.1	E855.4	E941.1	E950.4	E962.0	E980.4
Anticholinesterase (organophosphorus) (reversible)	971.0	E855.3	E941.0	E950.4	E962.0	E980.4
Anticoagulants	964.2	E858.2	E934.2	E950.4	E962.0	E980.4
antagonists	964.5	E858.2	E934.5	E950.4	E962.0	E980.4
Anti-common cold agents NEC	975.6	E858.6	E945.6	E950.4	E962.0	E980.4
Anticonvulsants NEC	966.3	E855.0	E936.3	E950.4	E962.0	E980.4
Antidepressants	969.0	E854.0	E939.0	E950.3	E962.0	E980.3
Antidiabetic agents	962.3	E858.0	E932.3	E950.4	E962.0	E980.4
Antidiarrheal agents	973.5	E858.4	E943.5	E950.4	E962.0	E980.4
Antidiuretic hormone	962.5	E858.0	E932.5	E950.4	E962.0	E980.4
Antidotes NEC	977.2	E858.8	E947.2	E950.4	E962.0	E980.4
Antiemetic agents	963.0	E858.1	E933.0	E950.4	E962.0	E980.4
Antiepilepsy agent NEC	966.3	E855.0	E936.3	E950.4	E962.0	E980.4
Antifertility pills	962.2	E858.0	E932.2	E950.4	E962.0	E980.4
Antiflatulents	973.8	E858.4	E943.8	E950.4	E962.0	E980.4
Antifreeze	989.89	E866.8	-	E950.9	E962.1	E980.9
alcohol	980.1	E860.2	-	E950.9	E962.1	E980.9
ethylene glycol	982.8	E862.4	-	E950.9	E962.1	E980.9
Antifungals (nonmedicinal) (sprays)	989.4	E863.6	-	E950.6	E962.1	E980.7
medicinal NEC	961.9	E857	E931.9	E950.4	E962.0	E980.4
antibiotic	960.1	E856	E930.1	E950.4	E962.0	E980.4
topical	976.0	E858.7	E946.0	E950.4	E962.0	E980.4
Antigastric secretion agents	973.0	E858.4	E943.0	E950.4	E962.0	E980.4
Antihelmintics	961.6	E857	E931.6	E950.4	E962.0	E980.4
Antihemophilic factor (human)	964.7	E858.2	E934.7	E950.4	E962.0	E980.4
Antihistamine	963.0	E858.1	E933.0	E950.4	E962.0	E980.4

● New Line ▲ Revised Code

		External Cause (E-Code)				
Drug	**Poisoning**	**Accident**	**Therapeutic Use**	**Suicide Attempt**	**Assault**	**Undetermined**
Antihypertensive agents NEC	972.6	E858.3	E942.6	E950.4	E962.0	E980.4
Anti-infectives NEC	961.9	E857	E931.9	E950.4	E962.0	E980.4
antibiotics	960.9	E856	E930.9	E950.4	E962.0	E980.4
specified NEC	960.8	E856	E930.8	E950.4	E962.0	E980.4
anthelmintic	961.6	E857	E931.6	E950.4	E962.0	E980.4
antimalarial	961.4	E857	E931.4	E950.4	E962.0	E980.4
antimycobacterial NEC	961.8	E857	E931.8	E950.4	E962.0	E980.4
antibiotics	960.6	E856	E930.6	E950.4	E962.0	E980.4
antiprotozoal NEC	961.5	E857	E931.5	E950.4	E962.0	E980.4
blood	961.4	E857	E931.4	E950.4	E962.0	E980.4
antiviral	961.7	E857	E931.7	E950.4	E962.0	E980.4
arsenical	961.1	E857	E931.1	E950.4	E962.0	E980.4
ENT agents	976.6	E858.7	E946.6	E950.4	E962.0	E980.4
heavy metals NEC	961.2	E857	E931.2	E950.4	E962.0	E980.4
local	976.0	E858.7	E946.0	E950.4	E962.0	E980.4
ophthalmic preparation	976.5	E858.7	E946.5	E950.4	E962.0	E980.4
topical NEC	976.0	E858.7	E946.0	E950.4	E962.0	E980.4
Anti-inflammatory agents (topical)	976.0	E858.7	E946.0	E950.4	E962.0	E980.4
Antiknock (tetraethyl lead)	984.1	E862.1	-	E950.9	E962.1	E980.9
Antilipemics	972.2	E858.3	E942.2	E950.4	E962.0	E980.4
Antimalarials	961.4	E857	E931.4	E950.4	E962.0	E980.4
Antimony (compounds) (vapor) NEC	985.4	E866.2	-	E950.9	E962.1	E980.9
anti-infectives	961.2	E857	E931.2	E950.4	E962.0	E980.4
pesticides (vapor)	985.4	E863.4	-	E950.6	E962.2	E980.7
potassium tartrate	961.2	E857	E931.2	E950.4	E962.0	E980.4
tartrated	961.2	E857	E931.2	E950.4	E962.0	E980.4
Antimuscarinic agents	971.1	E855.4	E941.1	E950.4	E962.0	E980.4
Antimycobacterials NEC	961.8	E857	E931.8	E950.4	E962.0	E980.4
antibiotics	960.6	E856	E930.6	E950.4	E962.0	E980.4
Antineoplastic agents	963.1	E858.1	E933.1	E950.4	E962.0	E980.4
antibiotics	960.7	E856	E930.7	E950.4	E962.0	E980.4
Anti-Parkinsonism agents	966.4	E855.0	E936.4	E950.4	E962.0	E980.4
Antiphlogistics	965.69	E850.6	E935.6	E950.0	E962.0	E980.0
Antiprotozoals NEC	961.5	E857	E931.5	E950.4	E962.0	E980.4
blood	961.4	E857	E931.4	E950.4	E962.0	E980.4
Antipruritics (local)	976.1	E858.7	E946.1	E950.4	E962.0	E980.4
Antipsychotic agents NEC	969.3	E853.8	E939.3	E950.3	E962.0	E980.3
Antipyretics	965.9	E850.9	E935.9	E950.0	E962.0	E980.0
specified NEC	965.8	E850.8	E935.8	E950.0	E962.0	E980.0
Antipyrine	965.5	E850.5	E935.5	E950.0	E962.0	E980.0
Antirabies serum (equine)	979.9	E858.8	E949.9	E950.4	E962.0	E980.4
Antirheumatics	965.69	E850.6	E935.6	E950.0	E962.0	E980.0
Antiseborrheics	976.4	E858.7	E946.4	E950.4	E962.0	E980.4
Antiseptics (external) (medicinal)	976.0	E858.7	E946.0	E950.4	E962.0	E980.4
Antistine	963.0	E858.1	E933.0	E950.4	E962.0	E980.4
Antithyroid agents	962.8	E858.0	E932.8	E950.4	E962.0	E980.4
Antitoxin, any	979.9	E858.8	E949.9	E950.4	E962.0	E980.4
Antituberculars	961.8	E857	E931.8	E950.4	E962.0	E980.4
antibiotics	960.6	E856	E930.6	E950.4	E962.0	E980.4
Antitussives	975.4	E858.6	E945.4	E950.4	E962.0	E980.4
Antivaricose agents (sclerosing)	972.7	E858.3	E942.7	E950.4	E962.0	E980.4
Antivenin (crotaline) (spider-bite)	979.9	E858.8	E949.9	E950.4	E962.0	E980.4
Antivert	963.0	E858.1	E933.0	E950.4	E962.0	E980.4
Antivirals NEC	961.7	E857	E931.7	E950.4	E962.0	E980.4
Ant poisons – *see* Pesticides						
Antrol	989.4	E863.4	-	E950.6	E962.1	E980.7
fungicide	989.4	E863.6	-	E950.6	E962.1	E980.7
Apomorphine hydrochloride (emetic)	973.6	E858.4	E943.6	E950.4	E962.0	E980.4
Appetite depressants, central	977.0	E858.8	E947.0	E950.4	E962.0	E980.4
Apresoline	972.6	E858.3	E942.6	E950.4	E962.0	E980.4
Aprobarbital, aprobarbitone	967.0	E851	E937.0	E950.1	E962.0	E980.1
Apronalide	967.8	E852.8	E937.8	E950.2	E962.0	E980.2
Aqua fortis	983.1	E864.1	-	E950.7	E962.1	E980.6
Arachis oil (topical)	976.3	E858.7	E946.3	E950.4	E962.0	E980.4
cathartic	973.2	E858.4	E943.2	E950.4	E962.0	E980.4
Aralen	961.4	E857	E931.4	E950.4	E962.0	E980.4
Arginine salts	974.5	E858.5	E944.5	E950.4	E962.0	E980.4
Argyrol	976.0	E858.7	E946.0	E950.4	E962.0	E980.4
ENT agent	976.6	E858.7	E946.6	E950.4	E962.0	E980.4
ophthalmic preparation	976.5	E858.7	E946.5	E950.4	E962.0	E980.4
Aristocort	962.0	E858.0	E932.0	E950.4	E962.0	E980.4
ENT agent	976.6	E858.7	E946.6	E950.4	E962.0	E980.4
ophthalmic preparation	976.5	E858.7	E946.5	E950.4	E962.0	E980.4
topical NEC	976.0	E858.7	E946.0	E950.4	E962.0	E980.4
Aromatics, corrosive	983.0	E864.0	-	E950.7	E962.1	E980.6
disinfectants	983.0	E861.4	-	E950.7	E962.1	E980.6
Arsenate of lead (insecticide)	985.1	E863.4	-	E950.8	E962.1	E980.8
herbicide	985.1	E863.5	-	E950.8	E962.1	E980.8
Arsenic, arsenicals (compounds) (dust) (fumes) (vapor) NEC	985.1	E866.3	-	E950.8	E962.1	E980.8
anti-infectives	961.1	E857	E931.1	E950.4	E962.0	E980.4
pesticide (dust) (fumes)	985.1	E863.4	-	E950.8	E962.1	E980.8
Arsine (gas)	985.1	E866.3	-	E950.8	E962.1	E980.8
Arsphenamine (silver)	961.1	E857	E931.1	E950.4	E962.0	E980.4
Arsthinol	961.1	E857	E931.1	E950.4	E962.0	E980.4
Artane	971.1	E855.4	E941.1	E950.4	E962.0	E980.4
Arthropod (venomous) **NEC**	989.5	E905.5	-	E950.9	E962.1	E980.9
Asbestos	989.81	E866.8	-	E950.9	E962.1	E980.9
Ascaridole	961.6	E857	E931.6	E950.4	E962.0	E980.4
Ascorbic acid	963.5	E858.1	E933.5	E950.4	E962.0	E980.4
Asiaticoside	976.0	E858.7	E946.0	E950.4	E962.0	E980.4
Aspidium (oleoresin)	961.6	E857	E931.6	E950.4	E962.0	E980.4
Aspirin	965.1	E850.3	E935.3	E950.0	E962.0	E980.0
Astringents (local)	976.2	E858.7	E946.2	E950.4	E962.0	E980.4
Atabrine	961.3	E857	E931.3	E950.4	E962.0	E980.4
Ataractics	969.5	E853.8	E939.5	E950.3	E962.0	E980.3
Atonia drug, intestinal	973.3	E858.4	E943.3	E950.4	E962.0	E980.4
Atophan	974.7	E858.5	E944.7	E950.4	E962.0	E980.4
Atropine	971.1	E855.4	E941.1	E950.4	E962.0	E980.4
Attapulgite	973.5	E858.4	E943.5	E950.4	E962.0	E980.4
Attenuvaxe	979.4	E858.8	E949.4	E950.4	E962.0	E980.4
Aureomycin	960.4	E856	E930.4	E950.4	E962.0	E980.4
ophthalmic preparation	976.5	E858.7	E946.5	E950.4	E962.0	E980.4
topical NEC	976.0	E858.7	E946.0	E950.4	E962.0	E980.4
Aurothioglucose	965.69	E850.6	E935.6	E950.0	E962.0	E980.0
Aurothioglycanide	965.69	E850.6	E935.6	E950.0	E962.0	E980.0
Aurothiomalate	965.69	E850.6	E935.6	E950.0	E962.0	E980.0
Automobile fuel	981	E862.1	-	E950.9	E962.1	E980.9
Autonomic nervous system agents NEC	971.9	E855.9	E941.9	E950.4	E962.0	E980.4
Aviosulfon	961.8	E857	E931.8	E950.4	E962.0	E980.4
Avomine	967.8	E852.8	E937.8	E950.2	E962.0	E980.2
Azacyclonol	969.5	E853.8	E939.5	E950.3	E962.0	E980.3
Azapetine	971.3	E855.6	E941.3	E950.4	E962.0	E980.4
Azaribine	963.1	E858.1	E933.1	E950.4	E962.0	E980.4
Azaserine	960.7	E856	E930.7	E950.4	E962.0	E980.4
Azathioprine	963.1	E858.1	E933.1	E950.4	E962.0	E980.4

● New Line ▲ Revised Code

Drug	Poisoning	External Cause (E-Code) Accident	Therapeutic Use	Suicide Attempt	Assault	Undetermined
Azosulfamide	961.0	E857	E931.0	E950.4	E962.0	E980.4
Azulfidine	961.0	E857	E931.0	E950.4	E962.0	E980.4
Azuresin	977.8	E858.8	E947.8	E950.4	E962.0	E980.4
Bacimycin	976.0	E858.7	E946.0	E950.4	E962.0	E980.4
ophthalmic preparation	976.5	E858.7	E946.5	E950.4	E962.0	E980.4
Bacitracin	960.8	E856	E930.8	E950.4	E962.0	E980.4
ENT agent	976.6	E858.7	E946.6	E950.4	E962.0	E980.4
ophthalmic preparation	976.5	E858.7	E946.5	E950.4	E962.0	E980.4
topical NEC	976.0	E858.7	E946.0	E950.4	E962.0	E980.4
Baking soda	963.3	E858.1	E933.3	E950.4	E962.0	E980.4
BAL	963.8	E858.1	E933.8	E950.4	E962.0	E980.4
Bamethan (sulfate)	972.5	E858.3	E942.5	E950.4	E962.0	E980.4
Bamipine	963.0	E858.1	E933.0	E950.4	E962.0	E980.4
Baneberry	988.2	E865.4	-	E950.9	E962.1	E980.9
Banewort	988.2	E865.4	-	E950.9	E962.1	E980.9
Barbenyl	967.0	E851	E937.0	E950.1	E962.0	E980.1
Barbital, barbitone	967.0	E851	E937.0	E950.1	E962.0	E980.1
Barbiturates, barbituric acid	967.0	E851	E937.0	E950.1	E962.0	E980.1
anesthetic (intravenous)	968.3	E855.1	E938.3	E950.4	E962.0	E980.4
Barium (carbonate) (chloride) (sulfate)	985.8	E866.4	-	E950.9	E962.1	E980.9
diagnostic agent	977.8	E858.8	E947.8	E950.4	E962.0	E980.4
pesticide	985.8	E863.4	-	E950.6	E962.1	E980.7
rodenticide	985.8	E863.7	-	E950.6	E962.1	E980.7
Barrier cream	976.3	E858.7	E946.3	E950.4	E962.0	E980.4
Battery acid or fluid	983.1	E864.1	-	E950.7	E962.1	E980.6
Bay rum	980.8	E860.8	-	E950.9	E962.1	E980.9
BCG vaccine	978.0	E858.8	E948.0	E950.4	E962.0	E980.4
Bearsfoot	988.2	E865.4	-	E950.9	E962.1	E980.9
Beclamide	966.3	E855.0	E936.3	E950.4	E962.0	E980.4
Bee (sting) (venom)	989.5	E905.3	-	E950.9	E962.1	E980.9
Belladonna (alkaloids)	971.1	E855.4	E941.1	E950.4	E962.0	E980.4
Bemegride	970.0	E854.3	E940.0	E950.4	E962.0	E980.4
Benactyzine	969.8	E855.8	E939.8	E950.3	E962.0	E980.3
Benadryl	963.0	E858.1	E933.0	E950.4	E962.0	E980.4
Bendrofluazide	974.3	E858.5	E944.3	E950.4	E962.0	E980.4
Bendroflumethiazide	974.3	E858.5	E944.3	E950.4	E962.0	E980.4
Benemid	974.7	E858.5	E944.7	E950.4	E962.0	E980.4
Benethamine penicillin G	960.0	E856	E930.0	E950.4	E962.0	E980.4
Benisone	976.0	E858.7	E946.0	E950.4	E962.0	E980.4
Benoquin	976.8	E858.7	E946.8	E950.4	E962.0	E980.4
Benoxinate	968.5	E855.2	E938.5	E950.4	E962.0	E980.4
Bentonite	976.3	E858.7	E946.3	E950.4	E962.0	E980.4
Benzalkonium (chloride)	976.0	E858.7	E946.0	E950.4	E962.0	E980.4
ophthalmic preparation	976.5	E858.7	E946.5	E950.4	E962.0	E980.4
Benzamidosalicylate (calcium)	961.8	E857	E931.8	E950.4	E962.0	E980.4
Benzathine penicillin	960.0	E856	E930.0	E950.4	E962.0	E980.4
Benzcarbimine	963.1	E858.1	E933.1	E950.4	E962.0	E980.4
Benzedrex	971.2	E855.5	E941.2	E950.4	E962.0	E980.4
Benzedrine (amphetamine)	969.7	E854.2	E939.7	E950.3	E962.0	E980.3
Benzene (acetyl) (dimethyl) (methyl) (solvent) (vapor)	982.0	E862.4	-	E950.9	E962.1	E980.9
hexachloride (gamma) (insecticide) (vapor)	989.2	E863.0	-	E950.6	E962.1	E980.7
Benzethonium	976.0	E858.7	E946.0	E950.4	E962.0	E980.4
Benzhexol (chloride)	966.4	E855.0	E936.4	E950.4	E962.0	E980.4
Benzilonium	971.1	E855.4	E941.1	E950.4	E962.0	E980.4
Benzin(e) – *see* Ligroin						
Benziodarone	972.4	E858.3	E942.4	E950.4	E962.0	E980.4
Benzocaine	968.5	E855.2	E938.5	E950.4	E962.0	E980.4
Benzodiapin	969.4	E853.2	E939.4	E950.3	E962.0	E980.3

Drug	Poisoning	External Cause (E-Code) Accident	Therapeutic Use	Suicide Attempt	Assault	Undetermined
Benzodiazepines (tranquilizers) **NEC**	969.4	E853.2	E939.4	E950.3	E962.0	E980.3
Benzoic acid (with salicylic acid) (anti-infective)	976.0	E858.7	E946.0	E950.4	E962.0	E980.4
Benzoin	976.3	E858.7	E946.3	E950.4	E962.0	E980.4
Benzol (vapor)	982.0	E862.4	-	E950.9	E962.1	E980.9
Benzomorphan	965.09	E850.2	E935.2	E950.0	E962.0	E980.0
Benzonatate	975.4	E858.6	E945.4	E950.4	E962.0	E980.4
Benzothiadiazides	974.3	E858.5	E944.3	E950.4	E962.0	E980.4
Benzoylpas	961.8	E857	E931.8	E950.4	E962.0	E980.4
Benzperidol	969.5	E853.8	E939.5	E950.3	E962.0	E980.3
Benzphetamine	977.0	E858.8	E947.0	E950.4	E962.0	E980.4
Benzpyrinium	971.0	E855.3	E941.0	E950.4	E962.0	E980.4
Benzquinamide	963.0	E858.1	E933.0	E950.4	E962.0	E980.4
Benzthiazide	974.3	E858.5	E944.3	E950.4	E962.0	E980.4
Benztropine	971.1	E855.4	E941.1	E950.4	E962.0	E980.4
Benzyl						
acetate	982.8	E862.4	-	E950.9	E962.1	E980.9
benzoate (anti-infective)	976.0	E858.7	E946.0	E950.4	E962.0	E980.4
morphine	965.09	E850.2	E935.2	E950.0	E962.0	E980.0
penicillin	960.0	E856	E930.0	E950.4	E962.0	E980.4
Bephenium hydroxynapthoate	961.6	E857	E931.6	E950.4	E962.0	E980.4
Bergamot oil	989.89	E866.8	-	E950.9	E962.1	E980.9
Berries, poisonous	988.2	E865.3	-	E950.9	E962.1	E980.9
Beryllium (compounds) (fumes)	985.3	E866.4	-	E950.9	E962.1	E980.9
Beta-carotene	976.3	E858.7	E946.3	E950.4	E962.0	E980.4
Beta-Chlor	967.1	E852.0	E937.1	E950.2	E962.0	E980.2
Betamethasone	962.0	E858.0	E932.0	E950.4	E962.0	E980.4
topical	976.0	E858.7	E946.0	E950.4	E962.0	E980.4
Betazole	977.8	E858.8	E947.8	E950.4	E962.0	E980.4
Bethanechol	971.0	E855.3	E941.0	E950.4	E962.0	E980.4
Bethanidine	972.6	E858.3	E942.6	E950.4	E962.0	E980.4
Betula oil	976.3	E858.7	E946.3	E950.4	E962.0	E980.4
Bhang	969.6	E854.1	E939.6	E950.3	E962.0	E980.3
Bialamicol	961.5	E857	E931.5	E950.4	E962.0	E980.4
Bichloride of mercury – *see* Mercury, chloride						
Bichromates (calcium) (crystals) (potassium) (sodium)	983.9	E864.3	-	E950.7	E962.1	E980.6
fumes	987.8	E869.8	-	E952.8	E962.2	E982.8
Biguanide derivatives, oral	962.3	E858.0	E932.3	E950.4	E962.0	E980.4
Biligrafin	977.8	E858.8	E947.8	E950.4	E962.0	E980.4
Bilopaque	977.8	E858.8	E947.8	E950.4	E962.0	E980.4
Bioflavonoids	972.8	E858.3	E942.8	E950.4	E962.0	E980.4
Biological substance NEC	979.9	E858.8	E949.9	E950.4	E962.0	E980.4
Biperiden	966.4	E855.0	E936.4	E950.4	E962.0	E980.4
Bisacodyl	973.1	E858.4	E943.1	E950.4	E962.0	E980.4
Bishydroxycoumarin	964.2	E858.2	E934.2	E950.4	E962.0	E980.4
Bismarsen	961.1	E857	E931.1	E950.4	E962.0	E980.4
Bismuth (compounds) NEC	985.8	E866.4	-	E950.9	E962.1	E980.9
anti-infectives	961.2	E857	E931.2	E950.4	E962.0	E980.4
subcarbonate	973.5	E858.4	E943.5	E950.4	E962.0	E980.4
sulfarsphenamine	961.1	E857	E931.1	E950.4	E962.0	E980.4
Bisphosphonates ●						
intravenous ●	963.1	E858.1	E933.7	E950.4	E962.0	E980.4
oral ●	963.1	E858.1	E933.6	E950.4	E962.0	E980.4
Bithionol	961.6	E857	E931.6	E950.4	E962.0	E980.4
Bitter almond oil	989.0	E866.8	-	E950.9	E962.1	E980.9
Bittersweet	988.2	E865.4	-	E950.9	E962.1	E930.9
Black						
flag	989.4	E863.4	-	E950.6	E962.1	E980.7

● New Line ▲ Revised Code

Drug	Poisoning	Accident	Therapeutic Use	Suicide Attempt	Assault	Undetermined
		External Cause (E-Code)				
Black – *continued*						
henbane	988.2	E865.4	-	E950.9	E962.1	E980.9
leaf (40)	989.4	E863.4	-	E950.6	E962.1	E980.7
widow spider (bite)	989.5	E905.1	-	E950.9	E962.1	E980.9
antivenin	979.9	E858.8	E949.9	E950.4	E962.0	E980.4
Blast furnace gas (carbon monoxide from)	986	E868.8	-	E952.1	E962.2	E982.1
Bleach NEC	983.9	E864.3	-	E950.7	E962.1	E980.6
Bleaching solutions	983.9	E864.3	-	E950.7	E962.1	E980.6
Bleomycin (sulfate)	960.7	E856	E930.7	E950.4	E962.0	E980.4
Blockain	968.9	E855.2	E938.9	E950.4	E962.0	E980.4
infiltration (subcutaneous)	968.5	E855.2	E938.5	E950.4	E962.0	E980.4
nerve block (peripheral) (plexus)	968.6	E855.2	E938.6	E950.4	E962.0	E980.4
topical (surface)	968.5	E855.2	E938.5	E950.4	E962.0	E980.4
Blood (derivatives) (natural) (plasma) (whole)	964.7	E858.2	E934.7	E950.4	E962.0	E980.4
affecting agent	964.9	E858.2	E934.9	E950.4	E962.0	E980.4
specified NEC	964.8	E858.2	E934.8	E950.4	E962.0	E980.4
substitute (macromolecular)	964.8	E858.2	E934.8	E950.4	E962.0	E980.4
Blue velvet	965.09	E850.2	E935.2	E950.0	E962.0	E980.0
Bone meal	989.89	E866.5	-	E950.9	E962.1	E980.9
Bonine	963.0	E858.1	E933.0	E950.4	E962.0	E980.4
Boracic acid	976.0	E858.7	E946.0	E950.4	E962.0	E980.4
ENT agent	976.6	E858.7	E946.6	E950.4	E962.0	E980.4
ophthalmic preparation	976.5	E858.7	E946.5	E950.4	E962.0	E980.4
Borate (cleanser) (sodium)	989.6	E861.3	-	E950.9	E962.1	E980.9
Borax (cleanser)	989.6	E861.3	-	E950.9	E962.1	E980.9
Boric acid	976.0	E858.7	E946.0	E950.4	E962.0	E980.4
ENT agent	976.6	E858.7	E946.6	E950.4	E962.0	E980.4
ophthalmic preparation	976.5	E858.7	E946.5	E950.4	E962.0	E980.4
Boron hydride NEC	989.89	E866.8	-	E950.9	E962.1	E980.9
fumes or gas	987.8	E869.8	-	E952.8	E962.2	E982.8
Botox	975.3	E858.6	E945.3	E950.4	E962.0	E980.4
Brake fluid vapor	987.8	E869.8	-	E952.8	E962.2	E982.8
Brass (compounds) (fumes)	985.8	E866.4	-	E950.9	E962.1	E980.9
Brasso	981	E861.3	-	E950.9	E962.1	E980.9
Bretylium (tosylate)	972.6	E858.3	E942.6	E950.4	E962.0	E980.4
Brevital (sodium)	968.3	E855.1	E938.3	E950.4	E962.0	E980.4
British antilewisite	963.8	E858.1	E933.8	E950.4	E962.0	E980.4
Bromal (hydrate)	967.3	E852.2	E937.3	E950.2	E962.0	E980.2
Bromelains	963.4	E858.1	E933.4	E950.4	E962.0	E980.4
Bromides NEC	967.3	E852.2	E937.3	E950.2	E962.0	E980.2
Bromine (vapor)	987.8	E869.8	-	E952.8	E962.2	E982.8
compounds (medicinal)	967.3	E852.2	E937.3	E950.2	E962.0	E980.2
Bromisovalum	967.3	E852.2	E937.3	E950.2	E962.0	E980.2
Bromobenzyl cyanide	987.5	E869.3	-	E952.8	E962.2	E982.8
Bromodiphenhydramine	963.0	E858.1	E933.0	E950.4	E962.0	E980.4
Bromoform	967.3	E852.2	E937.3	E950.2	E962.0	E980.2
Bromophenol blue reagent	977.8	E858.8	E947.8	E950.4	E962.0	E980.4
Bromosalicylhydroxamic acid	961.8	E857	E931.8	E950.4	E962.0	E980.4
Bromo-seltzer	965.4	E850.4	E935.4	E950.0	E962.0	E980.0
Brompheniramine	963.0	E858.1	E933.0	E950.4	E962.0	E980.4
Bromural	967.3	E852.2	E937.3	E950.2	E962.0	E980.2
Brown spider (bite) (venom)	989.5	E905.1	-	E950.9	E962.1	E980.9
Brucia	988.2	E865.3	-	E950.9	E962.1	E980.9
Brucine	989.1	E863.7	-	E950.6	E962.1	E980.7
Brunswick green – *see* Copper						
Bruten – *see* Ibuprofen						
Bryonia (alba) (dioica)	988.2	E865.4	-	E950.9	E962.1	E980.9
Buclizine	969.5	E853.8	E939.5	E950.3	E962.0	E980.3

Drug	Poisoning	Accident	Therapeutic Use	Suicide Attempt	Assault	Undetermined
		External Cause (E-Code)				
Bufferin	965.1	E850.3	E935.3	E950.0	E962.0	E980.0
Bufotenine	969.6	E854.1	E939.6	E950.3	E962.0	E980.3
Buphenine	971.2	E855.5	E941.2	E950.4	E962.0	E980.4
Bupivacaine	968.9	E855.2	E938.9	E950.4	E962.0	E980.4
infiltration (subcutaneous)	968.5	E855.2	E938.5	E950.4	E962.0	E980.4
nerve block (peripheral) (plexus)	968.6	E855.2	E938.6	E950.4	E962.0	E980.4
Busulfan	963.1	E858.1	E933.1	E950.4	E962.0	E980.4
Butabarbital (sodium)	967.0	E851	E937.0	E950.1	E962.0	E980.1
Butabarbitone	967.0	E851	E937.0	E950.1	E962.0	E980.1
Butabarpal	967.0	E851	E937.0	E950.1	E962.0	E980.1
Butacaine	968.5	E855.2	E938.5	E950.4	E962.0	E980.4
Butallylonal	967.0	E851	E937.0	E950.1	E962.0	E980.1
Butane (distributed in mobile container)	987.0	E868.0	-	E951.1	E962.2	E981.1
distributed through pipes	987.0	E867	-	E951.0	E962.2	E981.0
incomplete combustion of – *see* Carbon monoxide, butane						
Butanol	980.3	E860.4	-	E950.9	E962.1	E980.9
Butanone	982.8	E862.4	-	E950.9	E962.1	E980.9
Butaperazine	969.1	E853.0	E939.1	E950.3	E962.0	E980.3
Butazolidin	965.5	E850.5	E935.5	E950.0	E962.0	E980.0
Butethal	967.0	E851	E937.0	E950.1	E962.0	E980.1
Butethamate	971.1	E855.4	E941.1	E950.4	E962.0	E980.4
Buthalitone (sodium)	968.3	E855.1	E938.3	E950.4	E962.0	E980.4
Butisol (sodium)	967.0	E851	E937.0	E950.1	E962.0	E980.1
Butobarbital, butobarbitone	967.0	E851	E937.0	E950.1	E962.0	E980.1
Butriptyline	969.0	E854.0	E939.0	E950.3	E962.0	E980.3
Buttercups	988.2	E865.4	-	E950.9	E962.1	E980.9
Butter of antimony – *see* Antimony						
Butyl						
acetate (secondary)	982.8	E862.4	-	E950.9	E962.1	E980.9
alcohol	980.3	E860.4	-	E950.9	E962.1	E980.9
carbinol	980.8	E860.8	-	E950.9	E962.1	E980.9
carbitol	982.8	E862.4	-	E950.9	E962.1	E980.9
cellosolve	982.8	E862.4	-	E950.9	E962.1	E980.9
chloral (hydrate)	967.1	E852.0	E937.1	E950.2	E962.0	E980.2
formate	982.8	E862.4	-	E950.9	E962.1	E980.9
scopolammonium bromide	971.1	E855.4	E941.1	E950.4	E962.0	E980.4
Butyn	968.5	E855.2	E938.5	E950.4	E962.0	E980.4
Butyrophenone (-based tranquilizers)	969.2	E853.1	E939.2	E950.3	E962.0	E980.3
Cacodyl, cacodylic acid – *see* Arsenic						
Cactinomycin	960.7	E856	E930.7	E950.4	E962.0	E980.4
Cade oil	976.4	E858.7	E946.4	E950.4	E962.0	E980.4
Cadmium (chloride) (compounds) (dust) (fumes) (oxide)	985.5	E866.4	-	E950.9	E962.1	E980.9
sulfide (medicinal) NEC	976.4	E858.7	E946.4	E950.4	E962.0	E980.4
Caffeine	969.7	E854.2	E939.7	E950.3	E962.0	E980.3
Calabar bean	988.2	E865.4	-	E950.9	E962.1	E980.9
Caladium seguinium	988.2	E865.4	-	E950.9	E962.1	E980.9
Calamine (liniment) (lotion)	976.3	E858.7	E946.3	E950.4	E962.0	E980.4
Calciferol	963.5	E858.1	E933.5	E950.4	E962.0	E980.4
Calcium (salts) NEC	974.5	E858.5	E944.5	E950.4	E962.0	E980.4
acetylsalicylate	965.1	E850.3	E935.3	E950.0	E962.0	E980.0
benzamidosalicylate	961.8	E857	E931.8	E950.4	E962.0	E980.4
carbaspirin	965.1	E850.3	E935.3	E950.0	E962.0	E980.0
carbimide (citrated)	977.3	E858.8	E947.3	E950.4	E962.0	E980.4
carbonate (antacid)	973.0	E858.4	E943.0	E950.4	E962.0	E980.4
cyanide (citrated)	977.3	E858.8	E947.3	E950.4	E962.0	E980.4

● New Line ▲ Revised Code

Black – Calcium

		External Cause (E-Code)				
Drug	Poisoning	Accident	Therapeutic Use	Suicide Attempt	Assault	Undetermined
Calcium – *continued*						
dioctyl sulfosuccinate	973.2	E858.4	E943.2	E950.4	E962.0	E980.4
disodium edathamil	963.8	E858.1	E933.8	E950.4	E962.0	E980.4
disodium edetate	963.8	E858.1	E933.8	E950.4	E962.0	E980.4
EDTA	963.8	E858.1	E933.8	E950.4	E962.0	E980.4
hydrate, hydroxide	983.2	E864.2	-	E950.7	E962.1	E980.6
mandelate	961.9	E857	E931.9	E950.4	E962.0	E980.4
oxide	983.2	E864.2	-	E950.7	E962.1	E980.6
Calomel – *see* Mercury, chloride						
Caloric agents NEC	974.5	E858.5	E944.5	E950.4	E962.0	E980.4
Calusterone	963.1	E858.1	E933.1	E950.4	E962.0	E980.4
Camoquin	961.4	E857	E931.4	E950.4	E962.0	E980.4
Camphor (oil)	976.1	E858.7	E946.1	E950.4	E962.0	E980.4
Candeptin	976.0	E858.7	E946.0	E950.4	E962.0	E980.4
Candicidin	976.0	E858.7	E946.0	E950.4	E962.0	E980.4
Cannabinols	969.6	E854.1	E939.6	E950.3	E962.0	E980.3
Cannabis (derivatives) (indica) (sativa)	969.6	E854.1	E939.6	E950.3	E962.0	E980.3
Canned heat	980.1	E860.2	-	E950.9	E962.1	E980.9
Cantharides, cantharidin, cantharis	976.8	E858.7	E946.8	E950.4	E962.0	E980.4
Capillary agents	972.8	E858.3	E942.8	E950.4	E962.0	E980.4
Capreomycin	960.6	E856	E930.6	E950.4	E962.0	E980.4
Captodiame, captodiamine	969.5	E853.8	E939.5	E950.3	E962.0	E980.3
Caramiphen (hydrochloride)	971.1	E855.4	E941.1	E950.4	E962.0	E980.4
Carbachol	971.0	E855.3	E941.0	E950.4	E962.0	E980.4
Carbacrylamine resins	974.5	E858.5	E944.5	E950.4	E962.0	E980.4
Carbamate (sedative)	967.8	E852.8	E937.8	E950.2	E962.0	E980.2
herbicide	989.3	E863.5	-	E950.6	E962.1	E980.7
insecticide	989.3	E863.2	-	E950.6	E962.1	E980.7
Carbamazepine	966.3	E855.0	E936.3	E950.4	E962.0	E980.4
Carbamic esters	967.8	E852.8	E937.8	E950.2	E962.0	E980.2
Carbamide	974.4	E858.5	E944.4	E950.4	E962.0	E980.4
topical	976.8	E858.7	E946.8	E950.4	E962.0	E980.4
Carbamylcholine chloride	971.0	E855.3	E941.0	E950.4	E962.0	E980.4
Carbarsone	961.1	E857	E931.1	E950.4	E962.0	E980.4
Carbaryl	989.3	E863.2	-	E950.6	E962.1	E980.7
Carbaspirin	965.1	E850.3	E935.3	E950.0	E962.0	E980.0
Carbazochrome	972.8	E858.3	E942.8	E950.4	E962.0	E980.4
Carbenicillin	960.0	E856	E930.0	E950.4	E962.0	E980.4
Carbenoxolone	973.8	E858.4	E943.8	E950.4	E962.0	E980.4
Carbetapentane	975.4	E858.6	E945.4	E950.4	E962.0	E980.4
Carbimazole	962.8	E858.0	E932.8	E950.4	E962.0	E980.4
Carbinol	980.1	E860.2	-	E950.9	E962.1	E980.9
Carbinoxamine	963.0	E858.1	E933.0	E950.4	E962.0	E980.4
Carbitol	982.8	E862.4	-	E950.9	E962.1	E980.9
Carbocaine	968.9	E855.2	E938.9	E950.4	E962.0	E980.4
infiltration (subcutaneous)	968.5	E855.2	E938.5	E950.4	E962.0	E980.4
nerve block (peripheral) (plexus)	968.6	E855.2	E938.6	E950.4	E962.0	E980.4
topical (surface)	968.5	E855.2	E938.5	E950.4	E962.0	E980.4
Carbol-fuchsin solution	976.0	E858.7	E946.0	E950.4	E962.0	E980.4
Carbolic acid (*see also* Phenol)	983.0	E864.0	-	E950.7	E962.1	E980.6
Carbomycin	960.8	E856	E930.8	E950.4	E962.0	E980.4
Carbon						
bisulfide (liquid) (vapor)	982.2	E862.4	-	E950.9	E962.1	E980.9
dioxide (gas)	987.8	E869.8	-	E952.8	E962.2	E982.8
disulfide (liquid) (vapor)	982.2	E862.4	-	E950.9	E962.1	E980.9
monoxide (from incomplete combustion of) (in) NEC	986	E868.9	-	E952.1	E962.2	E982.1
blast furnace gas	986	E868.8	-	E952.1	E962.2	E982.1
Carbon – *continued*						
monoxide – *continued*						
butane (distributed in mobile container)	986	E868.0	-	E951.1	E962.2	E981.1
distributed through pipes	986	E867	-	E951.0	E962.2	E981.0
charcoal fumes	986	E868.3	-	E952.1	E962.2	E982.1
coal						
gas (piped)	986	E867	-	E951.0	E962.2	E981.0
solid (in domestic stoves, fireplaces)	986	E868.3	-	E952.1	E962.2	E982.1
coke (in domestic stoves, fireplaces)	986	E868.3	-	E952.1	E962.2	E982.1
exhaust gas (motor) not in transit	986	E868.2	-	E952.0	E962.2	E982.0
combustion engine, any not in watercraft	986	E868.2	-	E952.0	E962.2	E982.0
farm tractor, not in transit	986	E868.2	-	E952.0	E962.2	E982.0
gas engine	986	E868.2	-	E952.0	E962.2	E982.0
motor pump	986	E868.2	-	E952.0	E962.2	E982.0
motor vehicle, not in transit	986	E868.2	-	E952.0	E962.2	E982.0
fuel (in domestic use)	986	E868.3	-	E952.1	E962.2	E982.1
gas (piped)	986	E867	-	E951.0	E962.2	E981.0
in mobile container	986	E868.0	-	E951.1	E962.2	E981.1
utility	986	E868.1	-	E951.8	E962.2	E981.1
in mobile container	986	E868.0	-	E951.1	E962.2	E981.1
piped (natural)	986	E867	-	E951.0	E962.2	E981.0
illuminating gas	986	E868.1	-	E951.8	E962.2	E981.8
industrial fuels or gases, any	986	E868.8	-	E952.1	E962.2	E982.1
kerosene (in domestic stoves, fireplaces)	986	E868.3	-	E952.1	E962.2	E982.1
kiln gas or vapor	986	E868.8	-	E952.1	E962.2	E982.1
motor exhaust gas, not in transit	986	E868.2	-	E952.0	E962.2	E982.0
piped gas (manufactured) (natural)	986	E867	-	E951.0	E962.2	E981.0
producer gas	986	E868.8	-	E952.1	E962.2	E982.1
propane (distributed in mobile container)	986	E868.0	-	E951.1	E962.2	E981.1
distributed through pipes	986	E867	-	E951.0	E962.2	E981.0
specified source NEC	986	E868.8	-	E952.1	E962.2	E982.1
stove gas	986	E868.1	-	E951.8	E962.2	E981.8
piped	986	E867	-	E951.0	E962.2	E981.0
utility gas	986	E868.1	-	E951.8	E962.2	E981.8
piped	986	E867	-	E951.0	E962.2	E981.0
water gas	986	E868.1	-	E951.8	E962.2	E981.8
wood (in domestic stoves, fireplaces)	986	E868.3	-	E952.1	E962.2	E982.1
tetrachloride (vapor) NEC	987.8	E869.8	-	E952.8	E962.2	E982.8
liquid (cleansing agent) NEC	982.1	E861.3	-	E950.9	E962.1	E980.9
solvent	982.1	E862.4	-	E950.9	E962.1	E980.9
Carbonic acid (gas)	987.8	E869.8	-	E952.8	E962.2	E982.8
anhydrase inhibitors	974.2	E858.5	E944.2	E950.4	E962.0	E980.4
Carbowax	976.3	E858.7	E946.3	E950.4	E962.0	E980.4
Carbrital	967.0	E851	E937.0	E950.1	E962.0	E980.1
Carbromal (derivatives)	967.3	E852.2	E937.3	E950.2	E962.0	E980.2

● New Line ▲ Revised Code

Drug	Poisoning	External Cause (E-Code): Accident	Therapeutic Use	Suicide Attempt	Assault	Undetermined
Cardiac						
depressants	972.0	E858.3	E942.0	E950.4	E962.0	E980.4
rhythm regulators	972.0	E858.3	E942.0	E950.4	E962.0	E980.4
Cardiografin	977.8	E858.8	E947.8	E950.4	E962.0	E980.4
Cardio-green	977.8	E858.8	E947.8	E950.4	E962.0	E980.4
Cardiotonic glycosides	972.1	E858.3	E942.1	E950.4	E962.0	E980.4
Cardiovascular agents NEC	972.9	E858.3	E942.9	E950.4	E962.0	E980.4
Cardrase	974.2	E858.5	E944.2	E950.4	E962.0	E980.4
Carfusin	976.0	E858.7	E946.0	E950.4	E962.0	E980.4
Carisoprodol	968.0	E855.1	E938.0	E950.4	E962.0	E980.4
Carmustine	963.1	E858.1	E933.1	E950.4	E962.0	E980.4
Carotene	963.5	E858.1	E933.5	E950.4	E962.0	E980.4
Carphenazine (maleate)	969.1	E853.0	E939.1	E950.3	E962.0	E980.3
Carter's Little Pills	973.1	E858.4	E943.1	E950.4	E962.0	E980.4
Cascara (sagrada)	973.1	E858.4	E943.1	E950.4	E962.0	E980.4
Cassava	988.2	E865.4	-	E950.9	E962.1	E980.9
Castellani's paint	976.0	E858.7	E946.0	E950.4	E962.0	E980.4
Castor						
bean	988.2	E865.3	-	E950.9	E962.1	E980.9
oil	973.1	E858.4	E943.1	E950.4	E962.0	E980.4
Caterpillar (sting)	989.5	E905.5	-	E950.9	E962.1	E980.9
Catha (edulis)	970.8	E854.3	E940.8	E950.4	E962.0	E980.4
Cathartics NEC	973.3	E858.4	E943.3	E950.4	E962.0	E980.4
contact	973.1	E858.4	E943.1	E950.4	E962.0	E980.4
emollient	973.2	E858.4	E943.2	E950.4	E962.0	E980.4
intestinal irritants	973.1	E858.4	E943.1	E950.4	E962.0	E980.4
saline	973.3	E858.4	E943.3	E950.4	E962.0	E980.4
Cathomycin	960.8	E856	E930.8	E950.4	E962.0	E980.4
Caustic(s)	983.9	E864.4	-	E950.7	E962.1	E980.6
alkali	983.2	E864.2	-	E950.7	E962.1	E980.6
hydroxide	983.2	E864.2	-	E950.7	E962.1	E980.6
potash	983.2	E864.2	-	E950.7	E962.1	E980.6
soda	983.2	E864.2	-	E950.7	E962.1	E980.6
specified NEC	983.9	E864.3	-	E950.7	E962.1	E980.6
Ceepryn	976.0	E858.7	E946.0	E950.4	E962.0	E980.4
ENT agent	976.6	E858.7	E946.6	E950.4	E962.0	E980.4
lozenges	976.6	E858.7	E946.6	E950.4	E962.0	E980.4
Celestone	962.0	E858.0	E932.0	E950.4	E962.0	E980.4
topical	976.0	E858.7	E946.0	E950.4	E962.0	E980.4
Cellosolve	982.8	E862.4	-	E950.9	E962.1	E980.9
Cell stimulants and proliferants	976.8	E858.7	E946.8	E950.4	E962.0	E980.4
Cellulose derivatives, cathartic	973.3	E858.4	E943.3	E950.4	E962.0	E980.4
nitrates (topical)	976.3	E858.7	E946.3	E950.4	E962.0	E980.4
Centipede (bite)	989.5	E905.4	-	E950.9	E962.1	E980.9
Central nervous system						
depressants	968.4	E855.1	E938.4	E950.4	E962.0	E980.4
anesthetic (general) NEC	968.4	E855.1	E938.4	E950.4	E962.0	E980.4
gases NEC	968.2	E855.1	E938.2	E950.4	E962.0	E980.4
intravenous	968.3	E855.1	E938.3	E950.4	E962.0	E980.4
barbiturates	967.0	E851	E937.0	E950.1	E962.0	E980.1
bromides	967.3	E852.2	E937.3	E950.2	E962.0	E980.2
cannabis sativa	969.6	E854.1	E939.6	E950.3	E962.0	E980.3
chloral hydrate	967.1	E852.0	E937.1	E950.2	E962.0	E980.2
hallucinogenics	969.6	E854.1	E939.6	E950.3	E962.0	E980.3
hypnotics	967.9	E852.9	E937.9	E950.2	E962.0	E980.2
specified NEC	967.8	E852.8	E937.8	E950.2	E962.0	E980.2
muscle relaxants	968.0	E855.1	E938.0	E950.4	E962.0	E980.4
paraldehyde	967.2	E852.1	E937.2	E950.2	E962.0	E980.2
sedatives	967.9	E852.9	E937.9	E950.2	E962.0	E980.2
mixed NEC	967.6	E852.5	E937.6	E950.2	E962.0	E980.2

Drug	Poisoning	External Cause (E-Code): Accident	Therapeutic Use	Suicide Attempt	Assault	Undetermined
Central nervous system – *continued*						
depressants – *continued*						
sedatives – *continued*						
specified NEC	967.8	E852.8	E937.8	E950.2	E962.0	E980.2
muscle-tone depressants	968.0	E855.1	E938.0	E950.4	E962.0	E980.4
stimulants	970.9	E854.3	E940.9	E950.4	E962.0	E980.4
amphetamines	969.7	E854.2	E939.7	E950.3	E962.0	E980.3
analeptics	970.0	E854.3	E940.0	E950.4	E962.0	E980.4
antidepressants	969.0	E854.0	E939.0	E950.3	E962.0	E980.3
opiate antagonists	970.1	E854.3	E940.0	E950.4	E962.0	E980.4
specified NEC	970.8	E854.3	E940.8	E950.4	E962.0	E980.4
Cephalexin	960.5	E856	E930.5	E950.4	E962.0	E980.4
Cephaloglycin	960.5	E856	E930.5	E950.4	E962.0	E980.4
Cephaloridine	960.5	E856	E930.5	E950.4	E962.0	E980.4
Cephalosporins NEC	960.5	E856	E930.5	E950.4	E962.0	E980.4
N (adicillin)	960.0	E856	E930.0	E950.4	E962.0	E980.4
Cephalothin (sodium)	960.5	E856	E930.5	E950.4	E962.0	E980.4
Cerbera (odallam)	988.2	E865.4	-	E950.9	E962.1	E980.9
Cerberin	972.1	E858.3	E942.1	E950.4	E962.0	E980.4
Cerebral stimulants	970.9	E854.3	E940.9	E950.4	E962.0	E980.4
psychotherapeutic	969.7	E854.2	E939.7	E950.3	E962.0	E980.3
specified NEC	970.8	E854.3	E940.8	E950.4	E962.0	E980.4
Cetalkonium (chloride)	976.0	E858.7	E946.0	E950.4	E962.0	E980.4
Cetoxime	963.0	E858.1	E933.0	E950.4	E962.0	E980.4
Cetrimide	976.2	E858.7	E946.2	E950.4	E962.0	E980.4
Cetylpyridinium	976.0	E858.7	E946.0	E950.4	E962.0	E980.4
ENT agent	976.6	E858.7	E946.6	E950.4	E962.0	E980.4
lozenges	976.6	E858.7	E946.6	E950.4	E962.0	E980.4
Cevadilla – *see* Sabadilla						
Cevitamic acid	963.5	E858.1	E933.5	E950.4	E962.0	E980.4
Chalk, precipitated	973.0	E858.4	E943.0	E950.4	E962.0	E980.4
Charcoal						
fumes (carbon monoxide)	986	E868.3	-	E952.1	E962.2	E982.1
industrial	986	E868.8	-	E952.1	E962.2	E982.1
medicinal (activated)	973.0	E858.4	E943.0	E950.4	E962.0	E980.4
Chelating agents NEC	977.2	E858.8	E947.2	E950.4	E962.0	E980.4
Chelidonium majus	988.2	E865.4	-	E950.9	E962.1	E980.9
Chemical substance	989.9	E866.9	-	E950.9	E962.1	E980.9
specified NEC	989.89	E866.8	-	E950.9	E962.1	E980.9
Chemotherapy, antineoplastic	963.1	E858.1	E933.1	E950.4	E962.0	E980.4
Chenopodium (oil)	961.6	E857	E931.6	E950.4	E962.0	E980.4
Cherry laurel	988.2	E865.4	-	E950.9	E962.1	E980.9
Chiniofon	961.3	E857	E931.3	E950.4	E962.0	E980.4
Chlophedianol	975.4	E858.6	E945.4	E950.4	E962.0	E980.4
Chloral (betaine) (formamide) (hydrate)	967.1	E852.0	E937.1	E950.2	E962.0	E980.2
Chloralamide	967.1	E852.0	E937.1	E950.2	E962.0	E980.2
Chlorambucil	963.1	E858.1	E933.1	E950.4	E962.0	E980.4
Chloramphenicol	960.2	E856	E930.2	E950.4	E962.0	E980.4
ENT agent	976.6	E858.7	E946.6	E950.4	E962.0	E980.4
ophthalmic preparation	976.5	E858.7	E946.5	E950.4	E962.0	E980.4
topical NEC	976.0	E858.7	E946.0	E950.4	E962.0	E980.4
Chlorate(s) (potassium) (sodium) NEC	983.9	E864.3	-	E950.7	E962.1	E980.6
herbicides	989.4	E863.5	-	E950.6	E962.1	E980.7
Chlorcylizine	963.0	E858.1	E933.0	E950.4	E962.0	E980.4
Chlordan(e) (dust)	989.2	E863.0	-	E950.6	E962.1	E980.7
Chlordantoin	976.0	E858.7	E946.0	E950.4	E962.0	E980.4
Chlordiazepoxide	969.4	E853.2	E939.4	E950.3	E962.0	E980.3
Chloresium	976.8	E858.7	E946.8	E950.4	E962.0	E980.4
Chlorethiazol	967.1	E852.0	E937.1	E950.2	E962.0	E980.2

Drug	Poisoning	External Cause (E-Code) Accident	Therapeutic Use	Suicide Attempt	Assault	Undetermined
Chlorethyl – *see* Ethyl, chloride						
Chloretone	967.1	E852.0	E937.1	E950.2	E962.0	E980.2
Chlorex	982.3	E862.4	-	E950.9	E962.1	E980.9
Chlorhexadol	967.1	E852.0	E937.1	E950.2	E962.0	E980.2
Chlorhexidine (hydrochloride)	976.0	E858.7	E946.0	E950.4	E962.0	E980.4
Chlorhydroxyquinolin	976.0	E858.7	E946.0	E950.4	E962.0	E980.4
Chloride of lime (bleach)	983.9	E864.3	-	E950.7	E962.1	E980.6
Chlorinated						
camphene	989.2	E863.0	-	E950.6	E962.1	E980.7
diphenyl	989.89	E866.8	-	E950.9	E962.1	E980.9
hydrocarbons NEC	989.2	E863.0	-	E950.6	E962.1	E980.7
solvent	982.3	E862.4	-	E950.9	E962.1	E980.9
lime (bleach)	983.9	E864.3	-	E950.7	E962.1	E980.6
naphthalene – *see* Naphthalene						
pesticides NEC	989.2	E863.0	-	E950.6	E962.1	E980.7
soda – *see* Sodium, hypochlorite						
Chlorine (fumes) (gas)	987.6	E869.8	-	E952.8	E962.2	E982.8
bleach	983.9	E864.3	-	E950.7	E962.1	E980.6
compounds NEC	983.9	E864.3	-	E950.7	E962.1	E980.6
disinfectant	983.9	E861.4	-	E950.7	E962.1	E980.6
releasing agents NEC	983.9	E864.3	-	E950.7	E962.1	E980.6
Chlorisondamine	972.3	E858.3	E942.3	E950.4	E962.0	E980.4
Chlormadinone	962.2	E858.0	E932.2	E950.4	E962.0	E980.4
Chlormerodrin	974.0	E858.5	E944.0	E950.4	E962.0	E980.4
Chlormethiazole	967.1	E852.0	E937.1	E950.2	E962.0	E980.2
Chlormethylenecycline	960.4	E856	E930.4	E950.4	E962.0	E980.4
Chlormezanone	969.5	E853.8	E939.5	E950.3	E962.0	E980.3
Chloroacetophenone	987.5	E869.3	-	E952.8	E962.2	E982.8
Chloroaniline	983.0	E864.0	-	E950.7	E962.1	E980.6
Chlorobenzene, chlorobenzol	982.0	E862.4	-	E950.9	E962.1	E980.9
Chlorobutanol	967.1	E852.0	E937.1	E950.2	E962.0	E980.2
Chlorodinitrobenzene	983.0	E864.0	-	E950.7	E962.1	E980.6
dust or vapor	987.8	E869.8	-	E952.8	E962.2	E982.8
Chloroethane – *see* Ethyl, chloride						
Chloroform (fumes) (vapor)	987.8	E869.8	-	E952.8	E962.2	E932.8
anesthetic (gas)	968.2	E855.1	E938.2	E950.4	E962.0	E980.4
liquid NEC	968.4	E855.1	E938.4	E950.4	E962.0	E980.4
solvent	982.3	E862.4	-	E950.9	E962.1	E980.9
Chloroguanide	961.4	E857	E931.4	E950.4	E962.0	E980.4
Chloromycetin	960.2	E856	E930.2	E950.4	E962.0	E980.4
ENT agent	976.6	E858.7	E946.6	E950.4	E962.0	E980.4
ophthalmic preparation	976.5	E858.7	E946.5	E950.4	E962.0	E980.4
otic solution	976.6	E858.7	E946.6	E950.4	E962.0	E980.4
topical NEC	976.0	E858.7	E946.0	E950.4	E962.0	E980.4
Chloronitrobenzene	983.0	E864.0	-	E950.7	E962.1	E980.6
dust or vapor	987.8	E869.8	-	E952.8	E962.2	E982.8
Chlorophenol	983.0	E864.0	-	E950.7	E962.1	E980.6
Chlorophenothane	989.2	E863.0	-	E950.6	E962.1	E980.7
Chlorophyll (derivatives)	976.8	E858.7	E946.8	E950.4	E962.0	E980.4
Chloropicrin (fumes)	987.8	E869.8	-	E952.8	E962.2	E982.8
fumigant	989.4	E863.8	-	E950.6	E962.1	E980.7
fungicide	989.4	E863.6	-	E950.6	E962.1	E980.7
pesticide (fumes)	989.4	E863.4	-	E950.6	E962.1	E980.7
Chloroprocaine	968.9	E855.2	E938.9	E950.4	E962.0	E980.4
infiltration (subcutaneous)	968.5	E855.2	E938.5	E950.4	E962.0	E980.4
nerve block (peripheral) (plexus)	968.6	E855.2	E938.6	E950.4	E962.0	E980.4
Chloroptic	976.5	E858.7	E946.5	E950.4	E962.0	E980.4
Chloropurine	963.1	E858.1	E933.1	E950.4	E962.0	E980.4
Chloroquine (hydrochloride) (phosphate)	961.4	E857	E931.4	E950.4	E962.0	E980.4
Chlorothen	963.0	E858.1	E933.0	E950.4	E962.0	E980.4
Chlorothiazide	974.3	E858.5	E944.3	E950.4	E962.0	E980.4
Chlorotrianisene	962.2	E858.0	E932.2	E950.4	E962.0	E980.4
Chlorovinyldichloroarsine	985.1	E866.3	-	E950.8	E962.1	E980.8
Chloroxylenol	976.0	E858.7	E946.0	E950.4	E962.0	E980.4
Chlorphenesin (carbamate)	968.0	E855.1	E938.0	E950.4	E962.0	E980.4
topical (antifungal)	976.0	E858.7	E946.0	E950.4	E962.0	E980.4
Chlorpheniramine	963.0	E858.1	E933.0	E950.4	E962.0	E980.4
Chlorphenoxamine	966.4	E855.0	E936.4	E950.4	E962.0	E980.4
Chlorphentermine	977.0	E858.8	E947.0	E950.4	E962.0	E980.4
Chlorproguanil	961.4	E857	E931.4	E950.4	E962.0	E980.4
Chlorpromazine	969.1	E853.0	E939.1	E950.3	E962.0	E980.3
Chlorpropamide	962.3	E858.0	E932.3	E950.4	E962.0	E980.4
Chlorprothixene	969.3	E853.8	E939.3	E950.3	E962.0	E980.3
Chlorquinaldol	976.0	E858.7	E946.0	E950.4	E962.0	E980.4
Chlortetracycline	960.4	E856	E930.4	E950.4	E962.0	E980.4
Chlorthalidone	974.4	E858.5	E944.4	E950.4	E962.0	E980.4
Chlortrianisene	962.2	E858.0	E932.2	E950.4	E962.0	E980.4
Chlor-Trimeton	963.0	E858.1	E933.0	E950.4	E962.0	E980.4
Chlorzoxazone	968.0	E855.1	E938.0	E950.4	E962.0	E980.4
Choke damp	987.8	E869.8	-	E952.8	E962.2	E982.8
Cholebrine	977.8	E858.8	E947.8	E950.4	E962.0	E980.4
Cholera vaccine	978.2	E858.8	E948.2	E950.4	E962.0	E980.4
Cholesterol-lowering agents	972.2	E858.3	E942.2	E950.4	E962.0	E980.4
Cholestyramine (resin)	972.2	E858.3	E942.2	E950.4	E962.0	E980.4
Cholic acid	973.4	E858.4	E943.4	E950.4	E962.0	E980.4
Choline						
dihydrogen citrate	977.1	E858.8	E947.1	E950.4	E962.0	E980.4
salicylate	965.1	E850.3	E935.3	E950.0	E962.0	E980.0
theophyllinate	974.1	E858.5	E944.1	E950.4	E962.0	E980.4
Cholinergics	971.0	E855.3	E941.0	E950.4	E962.0	E980.4
Cholograrin	977.8	E858.8	E947.8	E950.4	E962.0	E980.4
Chorionic gonadoiropin	962.4	E858.0	E932.4	E950.4	E962.0	E980.4
Chromates	983.9	E864.3	-	E950.7	E962.1	E980.6
dust or mist	987.8	E869.8	-	E952.8	E962.2	E982.8
lead	984.0	E866.0	-	E950.9	E962.1	E980.9
paint	984.0	E861.5	-	E950.9	E962.1	E980.9
Chromic acid	983.9	E864.3	-	E950.7	E962.1	E980.6
dust or mist	987.8	E869.8	-	E952.8	E962.2	E982.8
Chromium	985.6	E866.4	-	E950.9	E962.1	E980.9
compounds – *see* Chromates						
Chromonar	972.4	E858.3	E942.4	E950.4	E962.0	E980.4
Chromyl chloride	983.9	E864.3	-	E950.7	E962.1	E980.6
Chrysarobin (ointment)	976.4	E858.7	E946.4	E950.4	E962.0	E980.4
Chrysazin	973.1	E858.4	E943.1	E950.4	E962.0	E980.4
Chymar	963.4	E858.1	E933.4	E950.4	E962.0	E980.4
ophthalmic preparation	976.5	E858.7	E946.5	E950.4	E962.0	E980.4
Chymotrypsin	963.4	E858.1	E933.4	E950.4	E962.0	E980.4
ophthalmic preparation	976.5	E858.7	E946.5	E950.4	E962.0	E980.4
Cicuta maculata or virosa	988.2	E865.4	-	E950.9	E962.1	E980.9
Cigarette lighter fluid	981	E862.1	-	E950.9	E962.1	E980.9
Cinchocaine (spinal)	968.7	E855.2	E938.7	E950.4	E962.0	E980.4
topical (surface)	968.5	E855.2	E938.5	E950.4	E962.0	E980.4
Cinchona	961.4	E857	E931.4	E950.4	E962.0	E980.4
Cinchonine alkaloids	961.4	E857	E931.4	E950.4	E962.0	E980.4
Cinchophen	974.7	E858.5	E944.7	E950.4	E962.0	E980.4
Cinnarizine	963.0	E858.1	E933.0	E950.4	E962.0	E980.4
Citanest	968.9	E855.2	E938.9	E950.4	E962.0	E980.4
infiltration (subcutaneous)	968.5	E855.2	E938.5	E950.4	E962.0	E980.4

● New Line ▲ Revised Code

Drug	Poisoning	External Cause (E-Code)				
		Accident	Therapeutic Use	Suicide Attempt	Assault	Undetermined
Citanest – *continued*						
nerve block (peripheral) (plexus)	968.6	E855.2	E938.6	E950.4	E962.0	E980.4
Citric acid	989.89	E866.8	-	E950.9	E962.1	E980.9
Citrovorum factor	964.1	E858.2	E934.1	E950.4	E962.0	E980.4
Claviceps purpurea	988.2	E865.4	-	E950.9	E962.1	E980.9
Cleaner, cleansing agent NEC	989.89	E861.3	-	E950.9	E962.1	E980.9
of paint or varnish	982.8	E862.9	-	E950.9	E962.1	E980.9
Clematis vitalba	988.2	E865.4	-	E950.9	E962.1	E980.9
Clemizole	963.0	E858.1	E933.0	E950.4	E962.0	E980.4
penicillin	960.0	E856	E930.0	E950.4	E962.0	E980.4
Clidinium	971.1	E855.4	E941.1	E950.4	E962.0	E980.4
Clindamycin	960.8	E856	E930.8	E950.4	E962.0	E980.4
Cliradon	965.09	E850.2	E935.2	E950.0	E962.0	E980.0
Clocortolone	962.0	E858.0	E932.0	E950.4	E962.0	E980.4
Clofedanol	975.4	E858.6	E945.4	E950.4	E962.0	E980.4
Clofibrate	972.2	E858.3	E942.2	E950.4	E962.0	E980.4
Clomethiazole	967.1	E852.0	E937.1	E950.2	E962.0	E980.2
Clomiphene	977.8	E858.8	E947.8	E950.4	E962.0	E980.4
Clonazepam	969.4	E853.2	E939.4	E950.3	E962.0	E980.3
Clonidine	972.6	E858.3	E942.6	E950.4	E962.0	E980.4
Clopamide	974.3	E858.5	E944.3	E950.4	E962.0	E980.4
Clorazepate	969.4	E853.2	E939.4	E950.3	E962.0	E980.3
Clorexolone	974.4	E858.5	E944.4	E950.4	E962.0	E980.4
Clorox (bleach)	983.9	E864.3	-	E950.7	E962.1	E980.6
Clortermine	977.0	E858.8	E947.0	E950.4	E962.0	E980.4
Clotrimazole	976.0	E858.7	E946.0	E950.4	E962.0	E980.4
Cloxacillin	960.0	E856	E930.0	E950.4	E962.0	E980.4
Coagulants NEC	964.5	E858.2	E934.5	E950.4	E962.0	E980.4
Coal (carbon monoxide from) – *see also* Carbon, monoxide, coal						
oil – *see* Kerosene						
tar NEC	983.0	E864.0	-	E950.7	E962.1	E980.6
fumes	987.8	E869.8	-	E952.8	E962.2	E982.8
medicinal (ointment)	976.4	E858.7	E946.4	E950.4	E962.0	E980.4
analgesics NEC	965.5	E850.5	E935.5	E950.0	E962.0	E980.0
naphtha (solvent)	981	E862.0	-	E950.9	E962.1	E980.9
Cobalt (fumes) (industrial)	985.8	E866.4	-	E950.9	E962.1	E980.9
Cobra (venom)	989.5	E905.0	-	E950.9	E962.1	E980.9
Coca (leaf)	970.8	E854.3	E940.8	E950.4	E962.0	E980.4
Cocaine (hydrochloride) (salt)	970.8	E854.3	E940.8	E950.4	E962.0	E980.4
topical anesthetic	968.5	E955.2	E938.5	E950.4	E962.0	E980.4
Coccidioidin	977.8	E858.8	E947.8	E950.4	E962.0	E980.4
Cocculus indicus	988.2	E865.3	-	E950.9	E962.1	E980.9
Cochineal	989.89	E866.8	-	E950.9	E962.1	E980.9
medicinal products	977.4	E858.8	E947.4	E950.4	E962.0	E980.4
Codeine	965.09	E850.2	E935.2	E950.0	E962.0	E980.0
Coffee	989.89	E866.8	-	E950.9	E962.1	E980.9
Cogentin	971.1	E855.4	E941.1	E950.4	E962.0	E980.4
Coke fumes or gas (carbon monoxide)	986	E868.3	-	E952.1	E962.2	E982.1
industrial use	986	E868.8	-	E952.1	E962.2	E982.1
Colace	973.2	E858.4	E943.2	E950.4	E962.0	E980.4
Colchicine	974.7	E858.5	E944.7	E950.4	E962.0	E980.4
Colchicum	988.2	E865.3	-	E950.9	E962.1	E980.9
Cold cream	976.3	E858.7	E946.3	E950.4	E962.0	E980.4
Colestipol	972.2	E858.3	E942.2	E950.4	E962.0	E980.4
Colistimethate	960.8	E856	E930.8	E950.4	E962.0	E980.4
Colistin	960.8	E856	E930.8	E950.4	E962.0	E980.4
Collagenase	976.8	E858.7	E946.8	E950.4	E962.0	E980.4
Collagen	977.8	E866.8	E947.8	E950.9	E962.1	E980.9
Collodion (flexible)	976.3	E858.7	E946.3	E950.4	E962.0	E980.4
Colocynth	973.1	E858.4	E943.1	E950.4	E962.0	E980.4
Coloring matter – *see* Dye(s)						
Combustion gas – *see* Carbon, monoxide						
Compazine	969.1	E853.0	E939.1	E950.3	E962.0	E980.3
Compound						
42 (warfarin)	989.4	E863.7	-	E950.6	E962.1	E980.7
269 (endrin)	989.2	E863.0	-	E950.6	E962.1	E980.7
497 (dieldrin)	989.2	E863.0	-	E950.6	E962.1	E980.7
1080 (sodium fluoroacetate)	989.4	E863.7	-	E950.6	E962.1	E980.7
3422 (parathion)	989.3	E863.1	-	E950.6	E962.1	E980.7
3911 (phorate)	989.3	E863.1	-	E950.6	E962.1	E980.7
3956 (toxaphene)	989.2	E863.0	-	E950.6	E962.1	E980.7
4049 (malathion)	989.3	E863.1	-	E950.6	E962.1	E980.7
4124 (dicapthon)	989.4	E863.4	-	E950.6	E962.1	E980.7
E (cortisone)	962.0	E858.0	E932.0	E950.4	E962.0	E980.4
F (hydrocortisone)	962.0	E858.0	E932.0	E950.4	E962.0	E980.4
Congo red	977.8	E858.8	E947.8	E950.4	E962.0	E980.4
Coniine, conine	965.7	E850.7	E935.7	E950.0	E962.0	E980.0
Conium (maculatum)	988.2	E865.4	-	E950.9	E962.1	E980.9
Conjugated estrogens (equine)	962.2	E858.0	E932.2	E950.4	E962.0	E980.4
Contac	975.6	E858.6	E945.6	E950.4	E962.0	E980.4
Contact lens solution	976.5	E858.7	E946.5	E950.4	E962.0	E980.4
Contraceptives (oral)	962.2	E858.0	E932.2	E950.4	E962.0	E980.4
vaginal	976.8	E858.7	E946.8	E950.4	E962.0	E980.4
Contrast media (roentgenographic)	977.8	E858.8	E947.8	E950.4	E962.0	E980.4
Convallaria majalis	988.2	E865.4	-	E950.9	E962.1	E980.9
Copper (dust) (fumes) (salts) NEC	985.8	E866.4	-	E950.9	E962.1	E980.9
arsenate, arsenite	985.1	E866.3	-	E950.8	E962.1	E980.8
insecticide	985.1	E863.4	-	E950.8	E962.1	E980.8
emetic	973.6	E858.4	E943.6	E950.4	E962.0	E980.4
fungicide	985.8	E863.6	-	E950.6	E962.1	E980.7
insecticide	985.8	E863.4	-	E950.6	E962.1	E980.7
oleate	976.0	E858.7	E946.0	E950.4	E962.0	E980.4
sulfate	983.9	E864.3	-	E950.7	E962.1	E980.6
fungicide	983.9	E863.6	-	E950.7	E962.1	E980.6
cupric	973.6	E858.4	E943.6	E950.4	E962.0	E980.4
cuprous	983.9	E864.3	-	E950.7	E962.1	E980.6
Copperhead snake (bite) (venom)	989.5	E905.0	-	E950.9	E962.1	E980.9
Coral (sting)	989.5	E905.6	-	E950.9	E962.1	E980.9
snake (bite) (venom)	989.5	E905.0	-	E950.9	E962.1	E980.9
Cordran	976.0	E858.7	E946.0	E950.4	E962.0	E980.4
Corn cures	976.4	E858.7	E946.4	E950.4	E962.0	E980.4
Cornhusker's lotion	976.3	E858.7	E946.3	E950.4	E962.0	E980.4
Corn starch	976.3	E858.7	E946.3	E950.4	E962.0	E980.4
Corrosive	983.9	E864.4	-	E950.7	E962.1	E980.6
acids NEC	983.1	E864.1	-	E950.7	E962.1	E980.6
aromatics	983.0	E864.0	-	E950.7	E962.1	E980.6
disinfectant	983.0	E861.4	-	E950.7	E962.1	E980.6
fumes NEC	987.9	E869.9	-	E952.9	E962.2	E982.9
specified NEC	983.9	E864.3	-	E950.7	E962.1	E980.6
sublimate – *see* Mercury, chloride						
Cortate	962.0	E858.0	E932.0	E950.4	E962.0	E980.4
Cort-Dome	962.0	E858.0	E932.0	E950.4	E962.0	E980.4
ENT agent	976.6	E858.7	E946.6	E950.4	E962.0	E980.4

● New Line ▲ Revised Code

Drug	Poisoning	External Cause (E-Code)				
		Accident	Therapeutic Use	Suicide Attempt	Assault	Undetermined
Cort-Dome – *continued*						
ophthalmic preparation	976.5	E858.7	E946.5	E950.4	E962.0	E980.4
topical NEC	976.0	E858.7	E946.0	E950.4	E962.0	E980.4
Cortef	962.0	E858.0	E932.0	E950.4	E962.0	E980.4
ENT agent	976.6	E858.7	E946.6	E950.4	E962.0	E980.4
ophthalmic preparation	976.5	E858.7	E946.5	E950.4	E962.0	E980.4
topical NEC	976.0	E858.7	E946.0	E950.4	E962.0	E980.4
Corticosteroids (fluorinated)	962.0	E858.0	E932.0	E950.4	E962.0	E980.4
ENT agent	976.6	E858.7	E946.6	E950.4	E962.0	E980.4
ophthalmic preparation	976.5	E858.7	E946.5	E950.4	E962.0	E980.4
topical NEC	976.0	E858.7	E946.0	E950.4	E962.0	E980.4
Corticotropin	962.4	E858.0	E932.4	E950.4	E962.0	E980.4
Cortisol	962.0	E858.0	E932.0	E950.4	E962.0	E980.4
ENT agent	976.6	E858.7	E946.6	E950.4	E962.0	E980.4
ophthalmic preparation	976.5	E858.7	E946.5	E950.4	E962.0	E980.4
topical NEC	976.0	E858.7	E946.0	E950.4	E962.0	E980.4
Cortisone derivatives (acetate)	962.0	E858.0	E932.0	E950.4	E962.0	E980.4
ENT agent	976.6	E858.7	E946.6	E950.4	E962.0	E980.4
ophthalmic preparation	976.5	E858.7	E946.5	E950.4	E962.0	E980.4
topical NEC	976.0	E858.7	E946.0	E950.4	E962.0	E980.4
Cortogen	962.0	E858.0	E932.0	E950.4	E962.0	E980.4
ENT agent	976.6	E858.7	E946.6	E950.4	E962.0	E980.4
ophthalmic preparation	976.5	E858.7	E946.5	E950.4	E962.0	E980.4
Corione	962.0	E858.0	E932.0	E950.4	E962.0	E980.4
ENT agent	976.6	E858.7	E946.6	E950.4	E962.0	E980.4
ophthalmic preparation	976.5	E858.7	E946.5	E950.4	E962.0	E980.4
Cortril	962.0	E858.0	E932.0	E950.4	E962.0	E980.4
ENT agent	976.6	E858.7	E946.6	E950.4	E962.0	E980.4
ophthalmic preparation	976.5	E858.7	E946.5	E950.4	E962.0	E980.4
topical NEC	976.0	E858.7	E946.0	E950.4	E962.0	E980.4
Cosmetics	989.89	E866.7	-	E950.9	E962.1	E980.9
Cosyntropin	977.8	E858.8	E947.8	E950.4	E962.0	E980.4
Cotarnine	964.5	E858.2	E934.5	E950.4	E962.0	E980.4
Cottonseed oil	976.3	E858.7	E946.3	E950.4	E962.0	E980.4
Cough mixtures (antitussives)	975.4	E858.6	E945.4	E950.4	E962.0	E980.4
containing opiates	965.09	E850.2	E935.2	E950.0	E962.0	E980.0
expectorants	975.5	E858.6	E945.5	E950.4	E962.0	E980.4
Coumadin	964.2	E858.2	E934.2	E950.4	E962.0	E980.4
rodenticide	989.4	E863.7	-	E950.6	E962.1	E980.7
Coumarin	964.2	E858.2	E934.2	E950.4	E962.0	E980.4
Coumetarol	964.2	E858.2	E934.2	E950.4	E962.0	E980.4
Cowbane	988.2	E865.4	-	E950.9	E962.1	E980.9
Cozyme	963.5	E858.1	E933.5	E950.4	E962.0	E980.4
Crack	970.8	E854.3	E940.8	E950.4	E962.0	E980.4
Creolin	983.0	E864.0	-	E950.7	E962.1	E980.6
disinfectant	983.0	E861.4	-	E950.7	E962.1	E980.6
Creosol (compound)	983.0	E864.0	-	E950.7	E962.1	E980.6
Creosote (beechwood) (coal tar)	983.0	E864.0	-	E950.7	E962.1	E980.6
medicinal (expectorant)	975.5	E858.6	E945.5	E950.4	E962.0	E980.4
syrup	975.5	E858.6	E945.5	E950.4	E962.0	E980.4
Cresol	983.0	E864.0	-	E950.7	E962.1	E980.6
disinfectant	983.0	E861.4	-	E950.7	E962.1	E980.6
Cresylic acid	983.0	E864.0	-	E950.7	E962.1	E980.6
Cropropamide	965.7	E850.7	E935.7	E950.0	E962.0	E980.0
with crotethamide	970.0	E854.3	E940.0	E950.4	E962.0	E980.4
Crotamiton	976.0	E858.7	E946.0	E950.4	E962.0	E980.4
Crotethamide	965.7	E850.7	E935.7	E950.0	E962.0	E980.0
with cropropamide	970.0	E854.3	E940.0	E950.4	E962.0	E980.4
Croton (oil)	973.1	E858.4	E943.1	E950.4	E962.0	E980.4
chloral	967.1	E852.0	E937.1	E950.2	E962.0	E980.2
Crude oil	981	E862.1	-	E950.9	E962.1	E980.9

Drug	Poisoning	External Cause (E-Code)				
		Accident	Therapeutic Use	Suicide Attempt	Assault	Undetermined
Cryogenine	965.8	E850.8	E935.8	E950.0	E962.0	E980.0
Cryolite (pesticide)	989.4	E863.4	-	E950.6	E962.1	E980.7
Cryptenamine	972.6	E858.3	E942.6	E950.4	E962.0	E980.4
Crystal violet	976.0	E858.7	E946.0	E950.4	E962.0	E980.4
Cuckoopint	988.2	E865.4	-	E950.9	E962.1	E980.9
Cumetharol	964.2	E858.2	E934.2	E950.4	E962.0	E980.4
Cupric sulfate	973.6	E858.4	E943.6	E950.4	E962.0	E980.4
Cuprous sulfate	983.9	E864.3	-	E950.7	E962.1	E980.6
Curare, curarine	975.2	E858.6	E945.2	E950.4	E962.0	E980.4
Cyanic acid – *see* Cyanide(s)						
Cyanide(s) (compounds) (hydrogen) (potassium) (sodium) NEC	989.0	E866.8	-	E950.9	E962.1	E980.9
dust or gas (inhalation) NEC	987.7	E869.8	-	E952.8	E962.2	E982.8
fumigant	989.0	E863.8	-	E950.6	E962.1	E980.7
mercuric – *see* Mercury						
pesticide (dust) (fumes)	989.0	E863.4	-	E950.6	E962.1	E980.7
Cyanocobalamin	964.1	E858.2	E934.1	E950.4	E962.0	E980.4
Cyanogen (chloride) (gas) **NEC**	987.8	E869.8	-	E952.8	E962.2	E982.8
Cyclaine	968.5	E855.2	E938.5	E950.4	E962.0	E980.4
Cyclamen europaeum	988.2	E865.4	-	E950.9	E962.1	E980.9
Cyclandelate	972.5	E858.3	E942.5	E950.4	E962.0	E980.4
Cyclazocine	965.09	E850.2	E935.2	E950.0	E962.0	E980.0
Cyclizine	963.0	E858.1	E933.0	E950.4	E962.0	E980.4
Cyclobarbital, cyclobarbitone	967.0	E851	E937.0	E950.1	E962.0	E980.1
Cycloguanil	961.4	E857	E931.4	E950.4	E962.0	E980.4
Cyclohexane	982.0	E862.4	-	E950.9	E962.1	E980.9
Cyclohexanol	980.8	E860.8	-	E950.9	E962.1	E980.9
Cyclohexanone	982.8	E862.4	-	E950.9	E962.1	E980.9
Cyclomethycaine	968.5	E855.2	E938.5	E950.4	E962.0	E980.4
Cyclopentamine	971.2	E855.5	E941.2	E950.4	E962.0	E980.4
Cyclopenthiazide	974.3	E858.5	E944.3	E950.4	E962.0	E980.4
Cyclopentolate	971.1	E855.4	E941.1	E950.4	E962.0	E980.4
Cyclophosphamide	963.1	E858.1	E933.1	E950.4	E962.0	E980.4
Cyclopropane	968.2	E855.1	E938.2	E950.4	E962.0	E980.4
Cycloserine	960.6	E856	E930.6	E950.4	E962.0	E980.4
Cyclothiazide	974.3	E858.5	E944.3	E950.4	E962.0	E980.4
Cycrimine	966.4	E855.0	E936.4	E950.4	E962.0	E980.4
Cymarin	972.1	E858.3	E942.1	E950.4	E962.0	E980.4
Cyproheptadine	963.0	E858.1	E933.0	E950.4	E962.0	E980.4
Cyprolidol	969.0	E854.0	E939.0	E950.3	E962.0	E980.3
Cytarabine	963.1	E858.1	E933.1	E950.4	E962.0	E980.4
Cytisus						
laburnum	988.2	E865.4	-	E950.9	E962.1	E980.9
scoparius	988.2	E865.4	-	E950.9	E962.1	E980.9
Cytomel	962.7	E858.0	E932.7	E950.4	E962.0	E980.4
Cytosine (antineoplastic)	963.1	E858.1	E933.1	E950.4	E962.0	E980.4
Cytoxan	963.1	E858.1	E933.1	E950.4	E962.0	E980.4
Dacarbazine	963.1	E858.1	E933.1	E950.4	E962.0	E980.4
Dactinomycin	960.7	E856	E930.7	E950.4	E962.0	E980.4
DADPS	961.8	E857	E931.8	E950.4	E962.0	E980.4
Dakin's solution (external)	976.0	E858.7	E946.0	E950.4	E962.0	E980.4
Dalmane	969.4	E853.2	E939.4	E950.3	E962.0	E980.3
DAM	977.2	E858.8	E947.2	E950.4	E962.0	E980.4
Danilone	964.2	E858.2	E934.2	E950.4	E962.0	E980.4
Danthron	973.1	E858.4	E943.1	E950.4	E962.0	E980.4
Dantrolene	975.2	E858.6	E945.2	E950.4	E962.0	E980.4
Daphne (gnidium) (mezereum)	988.2	E865.4	-	E950.9	E962.1	E980.9
berry	988.2	E865.3	-	E950.9	E962.1	E980.9

● New Line ▲ Revised Code

Drug	Poisoning	External Cause (E-Code)				
		Accident	Therapeutic Use	Suicide Attempt	Assault	Undetermined
Dapsone	961.8	E857	E931.8	E950.4	E962.0	E980.4
Daraprim	961.4	E857	E931.4	E950.4	E962.0	E980.4
Darnel	988.2	E865.3	-	E950.9	E962.1	E980.9
Darvon	965.8	E850.8	E935.8	E950.0	E962.0	E980.0
Daunorubicin	960.7	E856	E930.7	E950.4	E962.0	E980.4
DBI	962.3	E858.0	E932.3	E950.4	E962.0	E980.4
D-Con (rodenticide)	989.4	E863.7	-	E950.6	E962.1	E980.7
DDS	961.8	E857	E931.8	E950.4	E962.0	E980.4
DDT	989.2	E863.0	-	E950.6	E962.1	E980.7
Deadly nightshade	988.2	E865.4	-	E950.9	E962.1	E980.9
berry	988.2	E865.3	-	E950.9	E962.1	E980.9
Deanol	969.7	E854.2	E939.7	E950.3	E962.0	E980.3
Debrisoquine	972.6	E858.3	E942.6	E950.4	E962.0	E980.4
Decaborane	989.89	E866.8	-	E950.9	E962.1	E980.9
fumes	987.8	E869.8	-	E952.8	E962.2	E982.8
Decadron	962.0	E858.0	E932.0	E950.4	E962.0	E980.4
ENT agent	976.6	E858.7	E946.6	E950.4	E962.0	E980.4
ophthalmic preparation	976.5	E858.7	E946.5	E950.4	E962.0	E980.4
topical NEC	976.0	E858.7	E946.0	E950.4	E962.0	E980.4
Decahydronaphthalene	982.0	E862.4	-	E950.9	E962.1	E980.9
Decalin	982.0	E862.4	-	E950.9	E962.1	E980.9
Decamethonium	975.2	E858.6	E945.2	E950.4	E962.0	E980.4
Decholin	973.4	E858.4	E943.4	E950.4	E962.0	E980.4
sodium (diagnostic)	977.8	E858.8	E947.8	E950.4	E962.0	E980.4
Declomycin	960.4	E856	E930.4	E950.4	E962.0	E980.4
Deferoxamine	963.8	E858.1	E933.8	E950.4	E962.0	E980.4
Dehydrocholic acid	973.4	E858.4	E943.4	E950.4	E962.0	E980.4
DeKalin	982.0	E862.4	-	E950.9	E962.1	E980.9
Delalutin	962.2	E858.0	E932.2	E950.4	E962.0	E980.4
Delphinium	988.2	E865.3	-	E950.9	E962.1	E980.9
Deltasone	962.0	E858.0	E932.0	E950.4	E962.0	E980.4
Deltra	962.0	E858.0	E932.0	E950.4	E962.0	E980.4
Delvinal	967.0	E851	E937.0	E950.1	E962.0	E980.1
Demecarium (bromide)	971.0	E855.3	E941.0	E950.4	E962.0	E980.4
Demeclocycline	960.4	E856	E930.4	E950.4	E962.0	E980.4
Demecolcine	963.1	E858.1	E933.1	E950.4	E962.0	E980.4
Demelanizing agents	976.8	E858.7	E946.8	E950.4	E962.0	E980.4
Demerol	965.09	E850.2	E935.2	E950.0	E962.0	E980.0
Demethylchlortetracycline	960.4	E856	E930.4	E950.4	E962.0	E980.4
Demethyltetracycline	960.4	E856	E930.4	E950.4	E962.0	E980.4
Demeton	989.3	E863.1	-	E950.6	E962.1	E980.7
Demulcents	976.3	E858.7	E946.3	E950.4	E962.0	E980.4
Demulen	962.2	E858.0	E932.2	E950.4	E962.0	E980.4
Denatured alcohol	980.0	E860.1	-	E950.9	E962.1	E980.9
Dendrid	976.5	E858.7	E946.5	E950.4	E962.0	E980.4
Dental agents, topical	976.7	E858.7	E946.7	E950.4	E962.0	E980.4
Deodorant spray (feminine hygiene)	976.8	E858.7	E946.8	E950.4	E962.0	E980.4
Deoxyribonuclease	963.4	E858.1	E933.4	E950.4	E962.0	E980.4
Depressants						
appetite, central	977.0	E858.8	E947.0	E950.4	E962.0	E980.4
cardiac	972.0	E858.3	E942.0	E950.4	E962.0	E980.4
central nervous system (anesthetic)	968.4	E855.1	E938.4	E950.4	E962.0	E980.4
psychotherapeutic	969.5	E853.9	E939.5	E950.3	E962.0	E980.3
Dequalinium	976.0	E858.7	E946.0	E950.4	E962.0	E980.4
Dermolate	976.2	E858.7	E946.2	E950.4	E962.0	E980.4
DES	962.2	E858.0	E932.2	E950.4	E962.0	E980.4
Desenex	976.0	E858.7	E946.0	E950.4	E962.0	E980.4
Deserpidine	972.6	E858.3	E942.6	E950.4	E962.0	E980.4
Desipramine	969.0	E854.0	E939.0	E950.3	E962.0	E980.3
Deslanoside	972.1	E858.3	E942.1	E950.4	E962.0	E980.4
Desocodeine	965.09	E850.2	E935.2	E950.0	E962.0	E980.0
Desomorphine	965.09	E850.2	E935.2	E950.0	E962.0	E980.0
Desonide	976.0	E858.7	E946.0	E950.4	E962.0	E980.4
Desoxycorticosterone derivatives	962.0	E858.0	E932.0	E950.4	E962.0	E980.4
Desoxyephedrine	969.7	E854.2	E939.7	E950.3	E962.0	E980.3
DET	969.6	E854.1	E939.6	E950.3	E962.0	E980.3
Detergents (ingested) (synthetic)	989.6	E861.0	-	E950.9	E962.1	E980.9
external medication	976.2	E858.7	E946.2	E950.4	E962.0	E980.4
Deterrent, alcohol	977.3	E858.8	E947.3	E950.4	E962.0	E980.4
Detrothyronine	962.7	E858.0	E932.7	E950.4	E962.0	E980.4
Dettol (external medication)	976.0	E858.7	E946.0	E950.4	E962.0	E980.4
Dexamethasone	962.0	E858.0	E932.0	E950.4	E962.0	E980.4
ENT agent	976.6	E858.7	E946.6	E950.4	E962.0	E980.4
ophthalmic preparation	976.5	E858.7	E946.5	E950.4	E962.0	E980.4
topical NEC	976.0	E858.7	E946.0	E950.4	E962.0	E980.4
Dexamphetamine	969.7	E854.2	E939.7	E950.3	E962.0	E980.3
Dexedrine	969.7	E854.2	E939.7	E950.3	E962.0	E980.3
Dexpanthenol	963.5	E858.1	E933.5	E950.4	E962.0	E980.4
Dextran	964.8	E858.2	E934.8	E950.4	E962.0	E980.4
Dextriferron	964.0	E858.2	E934.0	E950.4	E962.0	E980.4
Dextroamphetamine	969.7	E854.2	E939.7	E950.3	E962.0	E980.3
Dextro calcium pantothenate	963.5	E858.1	E933.5	E950.4	E962.0	E980.4
Dextromethorphan	975.4	E858.6	E945.4	E950.4	E962.0	E980.4
Dextromoramide	965.09	E850.2	E935.2	E950.0	E962.0	E980.0
Dextro pantothenyl alcohol	963.5	E858.1	E933.5	E950.4	E962.0	E980.4
topical	976.8	E858.7	E946.8	E950.4	E962.0	E980.4
Dextropropoxyphene (hydrochloride)	965.8	E850.8	E935.8	E950.0	E962.0	E980.0
Dextrorphan	965.09	E850.2	E935.2	E950.0	E962.0	E980.0
Dextrose NEC	974.5	E858.5	E944.5	E950.4	E962.0	E980.4
Dextrothyroxin	962.7	E858.0	E932.7	E950.4	E962.0	E980.4
DFP	971.0	E855.3	E941.0	E950.4	E962.0	E980.4
DHE-45	972.9	E858.3	E942.9	E950.4	E962.0	E980.4
Diabinese	962.3	E858.0	E932.3	E950.4	E962.0	E980.4
Diacetyl monoxime	977.2	E858.8	E947.2	E950.4	E962.0	E980.4
Diacetylmorphine	965.01	E850.0	E935.0	E950.0	E962.0	E980.0
Diagnostic agents	977.8	E858.8	E947.8	E950.4	E962.0	E980.4
Dial (soap)	976.2	E858.7	E946.2	E950.4	E962.0	E980.4
sedative	967.0	E851	E937.0	E950.1	E962.0	E980.1
Diallylbarbituric acid	967.0	E851	E937.0	E950.1	E962.0	E980.1
Diaminodiphenylsulfone	961.8	E857	E931.8	E950.4	E962.0	E980.4
Diamorphine	965.01	E850.0	E935.0	E950.0	E962.0	E980.0
Diamox	974.2	E858.5	E944.2	E950.4	E962.0	E980.4
Diamthazole	976.0	E858.7	E946.0	E950.4	E962.0	E980.4
Diaphenylsulfone	961.8	E857	E931.8	E950.4	E962.0	E980.4
Diasone (sodium)	961.8	E857	E931.8	E950.4	E962.0	E980.4
Diazepam	969.4	E853.2	E939.4	E950.3	E962.0	E980.3
Diazinon	989.3	E863.1	-	E950.6	E962.1	E980.7
Diazomethane (gas)	987.8	E869.8	-	E952.8	E962.2	E982.8
Diazoxide	972.5	E858.3	E942.5	E950.4	E962.0	E980.4
Dibenamine	971.3	E855.6	E941.3	E950.4	E962.0	E980.4
Dibenzheptropine	963.0	E858.1	E933.0	E950.4	E962.0	E980.4
Dibenzyline	971.3	E855.6	E941.3	E950.4	E962.0	E980.4
Diborane (gas)	987.8	E869.8	-	E952.8	E962.2	E982.8
Dibromomannitol	963.1	E858.1	E933.1	E950.4	E962.0	E980.4
Dibucaine (spinal)	968.7	E855.2	E938.7	E950.4	E962.0	E980.4
topical (surface)	968.5	E855.2	E938.5	E950.4	E962.0	E980.4
Dibunate sodium	975.4	E858.6	E945.4	E950.4	E962.0	E980.4
Dibutoline	971.1	E855.4	E941.1	E950.4	E962.0	E980.4
Dicapthon	989.4	E863.4	-	E950.6	E962.1	E980.7
Dichloralphenazone	967.1	E852.0	E937.1	E950.2	E962.0	E980.2
Dichlorodifluoromethane	987.4	E869.2	-	E952.8	E962.2	E982.8

● New Line ▲ Revised Code

Drug	Poisoning	External Cause (E-Code)				
		Accident	Therapeutic Use	Suicide Attempt	Assault	Undetermined
Dichloroethane	982.3	E862.4	-	E950.9	E962.1	E980.9
Dichloroethylene	982.3	E862.4	-	E950.9	E962.1	E980.9
Dichloroethyl sulfide	987.8	E869.8	-	E952.8	E962.2	E982.8
Dichlorohydrin	982.3	E862.4	-	E950.9	E962.1	E980.9
Dichloromethane (solvent) (vapor)	982.3	E862.4	-	E950.9	E962.1	E980.9
Dichlorophen(e)	961.6	E857	E931.6	E950.4	E962.0	E980.4
Dichlorphenamide	974.2	E858.5	E944.2	E950.4	E962.0	E980.4
Dichlorvos	989.3	E863.1	-	E950.6	E962.1	E980.7
Diclofenac sodium	965.69	E850.6	E935.6	E950.0	E962.0	E980.0
Dicoumarin, dicumarol	964.2	E858.2	E934.2	E950.4	E962.0	E980.4
Dicyanogen (gas)	987.8	E869.8	-	E952.8	E962.2	E982.8
Dicyclomine	971.1	E855.4	E941.1	E950.4	E962.0	E980.4
Dieldrin (vapor)	989.2	E863.0		E950.6	E962.1	E980.1
Dienestrol	962.2	E858.0	E932.2	E950.4	E962.0	E980.4
Dietetics	977.0	E858.8	E947.0	E950.4	E962.0	E980.4
Diethazine	966.4	E855.0	E936.4	E950.4	E962.0	E980.4
Diethyl						
barbituric acid	967.0	E851	E937.0	E950.1	E962.0	E980.1
carbamazine	961.6	E857	E931.6	E950.4	E962.0	E980.4
carbinol	980.8	E860.8	-	E950.9	E962.1	E980.9
carbonate	982.8	E862.4	-	E950.9	E962.1	E980.9
ether (vapor) – *see* Ether(s)						
propion	977.0	E858.8	E947.0	E950.4	E962.0	E980.4
stilbestrol	962.2	E858.0	E932.2	E950.4	E962.0	E980.4
Diethylene						
dioxide	982.8	E862.4	-	E950.9	E962.1	E980.9
glycol (monoacetate) (monoethyl ether)	982.8	E862.4	-	E950.9	E962.1	E980.9
Diethylsulfone-diethylmethane	967.8	E852.8	E937.8	E950.2	E962.0	E980.2
Difencloxazine	965.09	E850.2	E935.2	E950.0	E962.0	E980.0
Diffusin	963.4	E858.1	E933.4	E950.4	E962.0	E980.4
Diflos	971.0	E855.3	E941.0	E950.4	E962.0	E980.4
Digestants	973.4	E858.4	E943.4	E950.4	E962.0	E980.4
Digitalin(e)	972.1	E858.3	E942.1	E950.4	E962.0	E980.4
Digitalis glycosides	972.1	E858.3	E942.1	E950.4	E962.0	E980.4
Digitoxin	972.1	E858.3	E942.1	E950.4	E962.0	E980.4
Digoxin	972.1	E858.3	E942.1	E950.4	E962.0	E980.4
Dihydrocodeine	965.09	E850.2	E935.2	E950.0	E962.0	E980.0
Dihydrocodeinone	965.09	E850.2	E935.2	E950.0	E962.0	E980.0
Dihydroergocristine	972.9	E858.3	E942.9	E950.4	E962.0	E980.4
Dihydroergotamine	972.9	E858.3	E942.9	E950.4	E962.0	E980.4
Dihydroergotoxine	972.9	E858.3	E942.9	E950.4	E962.0	E980.4
Dihydrohydroxycodeinone	965.09	E850.2	E935.2	E950.0	E962.0	E980.0
Dihydrohydroxymorphinone	965.09	E850.2	E935.2	E950.0	E962.0	E980.0
Dihydroisocodeine	965.09	E850.2	E935.2	E950.0	E962.0	E980.0
Dihydromorphine	965.09	E850.2	E935.2	E950.0	E962.0	E980.0
Dihydromorphinone	965.09	E850.2	E935.2	E950.0	E962.0	E980.0
Dihydrostreptomycin	960.6	E856	E930.6	E950.4	E962.0	E980.4
Dihydrotachysterol	962.6	E858.0	E932.6	E950.4	E962.0	E980.4
Dihydroxyanthraquinone	973.1	E858.4	E943.1	E950.4	E962.0	E980.4
Dihydroxycodeinone	965.09	E850.2	E935.2	E950.0	E962.0	E980.0
Diiodohydroxyquin	961.3	E857	E931.3	E950.4	E962.0	E980.4
topical	976.0	E858.7	E946.0	E950.4	E962.0	E980.4
Diiodohydroxyquinoline	961.3	E857	E931.3	E950.4	E962.0	E980.4
Dilantin	966.1	E855.0	E936.1	E950.4	E962.0	E980.4
Dilaudid	965.09	E850.2	E935.2	E950.0	E962.0	E980.0
Diloxanide	961.5	E857	E931.5	E950.4	E962.0	E980.4
Dimefline	970.0	E854.3	E940.0	E950.4	E962.0	E980.4
Dimenhydrinate	963.0	E858.1	E933.0	E950.4	E962.0	E980.4
Dimercaprol	963.8	E858.1	E933.8	E950.4	E962.0	E980.4
Dimercaptopropanol	963.8	E858.1	E933.8	E950.4	E962.0	E980.4

Drug	Poisoning	External Cause (E-Code)				
		Accident	Therapeutic Use	Suicide Attempt	Assault	Undetermined
Dimetane	963.0	E858.1	E933.0	E950.4	E962.0	E980.4
Dimethicone	976.3	E858.7	E946.3	E950.4	E962.0	E980.4
Dimethindene	963.0	E858.1	E933.0	E950.4	E962.0	E980.4
Dimethisoquin	968.5	E855.2	E938.5	E950.4	E962.0	E980.4
Dimethisterone	962.2	E858.0	E932.2	E950.4	E962.0	E980.4
Dimethoxanate	975.4	E858.6	E945.4	E950.4	E962.0	E980.4
Dimethyl						
arsine, arsinic acid – *see* Arsenic						
carbinol	980.2	E860.3	-	E950.9	E962.1	E980.9
diguanide	962.3	E858.0	E932.3	E950.4	E962.0	E980.4
ketone	982.8	E862.4	-	E950.9	E962.1	E980.9
vapor	987.8	E869.8	-	E952.8	E962.2	E982.8
meperidine	965.09	E850.2	E935.2	E950.0	E962.0	E980.0
parathion	989.3	E863.1	-	E950.6	E962.1	E980.7
polysiloxane	973.8	E858.4	E943.8	E950.4	E962.0	E980.4
sulfate (fumes)	987.8	E869.8	-	E952.8	E962.2	E982.8
liquid	983.9	E864.3	-	E950.7	E962.1	E980.6
sulfoxide NEC	982.8	E862.4	-	E950.9	E962.1	E980.9
medicinal	976.4	E858.7	E946.4	E950.4	E962.0	E980.4
triptamine	969.6	E854.1	E939.6	E950.3	E962.0	E980.3
tubocurarine	975.2	E858.6	E945.2	E950.4	E962.0	E980.4
Dindevan	964.2	E858.2	E934.2	E950.4	E962.0	E980.4
Dinitro (-ortho-) **cresol** (herbicide) (spray)	989.4	E863.5		E950.6	E962.1	E980.7
insecticide	989.4	E863.4	-	E950.6	E962.1	E980.7
Dinitrobenzene	983.0	E864.0	-	E950.7	E962.1	E980.6
vapor	987.8	E869.8	-	E952.8	E962.2	E982.8
Dinitro-orthocresol (herbicide)	989.4	E863.5	-	E950.6	E962.1	E980.7
insecticide	989.4	E863.4	-	E950.6	E962.1	E980.7
Dinitrophenol (herbicide) (spray)	989.4	E863.5	-	E950.6	E962.1	E980.7
insecticide	989.4	E863.4	-	E950.6	E962.1	E980.7
Dinoprost	975.0	E858.6	E945.0	E950.4	E962.0	E980.4
Dioctyl sulfosuccinate (calcium) (sodium)	973.2	E858.4	E943.2	E950.4	E962.0	E980.4
Diodoquin	961.3	E857	E931.3	E950.4	E962.0	E980.4
Dione derivatives NEC	966.3	E855.0	E936.3	E950.4	E962.0	E980.4
Dionin	965.09	E850.2	E935.2	E950.0	E962.0	E980.0
Dioxane	982.8	E862.4	-	E950.9	E962.1	E980.9
Dioxin – *see* Herbicides						
Dioxyline	972.5	E858.3	E942.5	E950.4	E962.0	E980.4
Dipentene	982.8	E862.4	-	E950.9	E962.1	E980.9
Diphemanil	971.1	E855.4	E941.1	E950.4	E962.0	E980.4
Diphenadione	964.2	E858.2	E934.2	E950.4	E962.0	E980.4
Diphenhydramine	963.0	E858.1	E933.0	E950.4	E962.0	E980.4
Diphenidol	963.0	E858.1	E933.0	E950.4	E962.0	E980.4
Diphenoxylate	973.5	E858.4	E943.5	E950.4	E962.0	E980.4
Diphenylchloroarsine	985.1	E866.3	-	E950.8	E962.1	E980.8
Diphenylhydantoin (sodium)	966.1	E855.0	E936.1	E950.4	E962.0	E980.4
Diphenylpyraline	963.0	E858.1	E933.0	E950.4	E962.0	E980.4
Diphtheria						
antitoxin	979.9	E858.8	E949.9	E950.4	E962.0	E980.4
toxoid	978.5	E858.8	E948.5	E950.4	E962.0	E980.4
with tetanus toxoid	978.9	E858.8	E948.9	E950.4	E962.0	E980.4
with pertussis component	978.6	E858.8	E948.6	E950.4	E962.0	E980.4
vaccine	978.5	E858.8	E948.5	E950.4	E962.0	E980.4
Dipipanone	965.09	E850.2	E935.2	E950.0	E962.0	E980.0
Diplovax	979.5	E858.8	E949.5	E950.4	E962.0	E980.4
Diprophylline	975.1	E858.6	E945.1	E950.4	E962.0	E980.4
Dipyridamole	972.4	E858.3	E942.4	E950.4	E962.0	E980.4
Dipyrone	965.5	E850.5	E935.5	E950.0	E962.0	E980.0

● New Line ▲ Revised Code

Drug	Poisoning	External Cause (E-Code) Accident	Therapeutic Use	Suicide Attempt	Assault	Undetermined
Diquat	989.4	E863.5	-	E950.6	E962.1	E980.7
Disinfectant NEC	983.9	E861.4	-	E950.7	E962.1	E980.6
alkaline	983.2	E861.4	-	E950.7	E962.1	E980.6
aromatic	983.0	E861.4	-	E950.7	E962.1	E980.6
Disipal	966.4	E855.0	E936.4	E950.4	E962.0	E980.4
Disodium edetate	963.8	E858.1	E933.8	E950.4	E962.0	E980.4
Disulfamide	974.4	E858.5	E944.4	E950.4	E962.0	E980.4
Disulfanilamide	961.0	E857	E931.0	E950.4	E962.0	E980.4
Disulfiram	977.3	E858.8	E947.3	E950.4	E962.0	E980.4
Dithiazanine	961.6	E857	E931.6	E950.4	E962.0	E980.4
Dithioglycerol	963.8	E858.1	E933.8	E950.4	E962.0	E980.4
Dithranot	976.4	E858.7	E946.4	E950.4	E962.0	E980.4
Diucardin	974.3	E858.5	E944.3	E950.4	E962.0	E980.4
Diupres	974.3	E858.5	E944.3	E950.4	E962.0	E980.4
Diuretics NEC	974.4	E858.5	E944.4	E950.4	E962.0	E980.4
carbonic acid anhydrase inhibitors	974.2	E858.5	E944.2	E950.4	E962.0	E980.4
mercurial	974.0	E858.5	E944.0	E950.4	E962.0	E980.4
osmotic	974.4	E858.5	E944.4	E950.4	E962.0	E980.4
purine derivatives	974.1	E858.5	E944.1	E950.4	E962.0	E980.4
saluretic	974.3	E858.5	E944.3	E950.4	E962.0	E980.4
Diuril	974.3	E858.5	E944.3	E950.4	E962.0	E980.4
Divinyl ether	968.2	E855.1	E938.2	E950.4	E962.0	E980.4
D-lysergic acid diethylamide	969.6	E854.1	E939.6	E950.3	E962.0	E980.3
DMCT	960.4	E856	E930.4	E950.4	E962.0	E980.4
DMSO	982.8	E862.4	-	E950.9	E962.1	E980.9
DMT	969.6	E854.1	E939.6	E950.3	E962.0	E980.3
DNOC	989.4	E863.5	-	E950.6	E962.1	E980.7
DOCA	962.0	E858.0	E932.0	E950.4	E962.0	E980.4
Dolophine	965.02	E850.1	E935.1	E950.0	E962.0	E980.0
Doloxene	965.8	E850.8	E935.8	E950.0	E962.0	E980.0
DOM	969.6	E854.1	E939.6	E950.3	E962.0	E980.3
Domestic gas – *see* Gas, utility						
Domiphen (bromide) (lozenges)	976.6	E858.7	E946.6	E950.4	E962.0	E980.4
Dopa (levo)	966.4	E855.0	E936.4	E950.4	E962.0	E980.4
Dopamine	971.2	E855.5	E941.2	E950.4	E962.0	E980.4
Doriden	967.5	E852.4	E937.5	E950.2	E962.0	E980.2
Dormiral	967.0	E851	E937.0	E950.1	E962.0	E980.1
Dormison	967.8	E852.8	E937.8	E950.2	E962.0	E980.2
Dornase	963.4	E858.1	E933.4	E950.4	E962.0	E980.4
Dorsacaine	968.5	E855.2	E938.5	E950.4	E962.0	E980.4
Dothiepin hydrochloride	969.0	E854.0	E939.0	E950.3	E962.0	E980.3
Doxapram	970.0	E854.3	E940.0	E950.4	E962.0	E980.4
Doxepin	969.0	E854.0	E939.0	E950.3	E962.0	E980.3
Doxorubicin	960.7	E856	E930.7	E950.4	E962.0	E980.4
Doxycycline	960.4	E856	E930.4	E950.4	E962.0	E980.4
Doxylamine	963.0	E858.1	E933.0	E950.4	E962.0	E980.4
Dramamine	963.0	E858.1	E933.0	E950.4	E962.0	E980.4
Drano (drain cleaner)	983.2	E864.2	-	E950.7	E962.1	E980.6
Dromoran	965.09	E850.2	E935.2	E950.0	E962.0	E980.0
Dromostanolone	962.1	E858.0	E932.1	E950.4	E962.0	E980.4
Droperidol	969.2	E853.1	E939.2	E950.3	E962.0	E980.3
Drotrecogin alfa	964.2	E858.2	E934.2	E950.4	E962.0	E980.4
Drug	977.9	E858.9	E947.9	E950.5	E962.0	E980.5
specified NEC	977.8	E858.8	E947.8	E950.4	E962.0	E980.4
AHFS List						
4:00 antihistamine drugs	963.0	E858.1	E933.0	E950.4	E962.0	E980.4
8:04 amebacides	961.5	E857	E931.5	E950.4	E962.0	E980.4
arsenical anti-infectives	961.1	E857	E931.1	E950.4	E962.0	E980.4
quinoline derivatives	961.3	E857	E931.3	E950.4	E962.0	E980.4

Drug	Poisoning	External Cause (E-Code) Accident	Therapeutic Use	Suicide Attempt	Assault	Undetermined
Drug – *continued*						
8:08 anthelmintics	961.6	E857	E931.6	E950.4	E962.0	E980.4
quinoline derivatives	961.3	E857	E931.3	E950.4	E962.0	E980.4
8:12.04 antifungal antibiotics	960.1	E856	E930.1	E950.4	E962.0	E980.4
8:12.06 cephalosporins	960.5	E856	E930.5	E950.4	E962.0	E980.4
8:12.08 chloramphenicol	960.2	E856	E930.2	E950.4	E962.0	E980.4
8:12.12 erythromycins	960.3	E856	E930.3	E950.4	E962.0	E980.4
8:12.16 penicillins	960.0	E856	E930.0	E950.4	E962.0	E980.4
8:12.20 streptomycins	960.6	E856	E930.6	E950.4	E962.0	E980.4
8:12.24 tetracyclines	960.4	E856	E930.4	E950.4	E962.0	E980.4
8:12.28 other antibiotics	960.8	E856	E930.8	E950.4	E962.0	E980.4
antimycobacterial	960.6	E856	E930.6	E950.4	E962.0	E980.4
macrolides	960.3	E856	E930.3	E950.4	E962.0	E980.4
8:16 antituberculars	961.8	E857	E931.8	E950.4	E962.0	E980.4
antibiotics	960.6	E856	E930.6	E950.4	E962.0	E980.4
8:18 antivirals	961.7	E857	E931.7	E950.4	E962.0	E980.4
8:20 plasmodicides (antimalarials)	961.4	E857	E931.4	E950.4	E962.0	E980.4
8:24 sulfonamides	961.0	E857	E931.0	E950.4	E962.0	E980.4
8:26 sulfones	961.8	E857	E931.8	E950.4	E962.0	E980.4
8:28 treponemicides	961.2	E857	E931.2	E950.4	E962.0	E980.4
8:32 trichomonacides	961.5	E857	E931.5	E950.4	E962.0	E980.4
nitrofuran derivatives	961.9	E857	E931.9	E950.4	E962.0	E980.4
quinoline derivatives	961.3	E857	E931.3	E950.4	E962.0	E980.4
8:36 urinary germicides	961.9	E857	E931.9	E950.4	E962.0	E980.4
quinoline derivatives	961.3	E857	E931.3	E950.4	E962.0	E980.4
8:40 other anti-infectives	961.9	E857	E931.9	E950.4	E962.0	E980.4
10:00 antineoplastic agents	963.1	E858.1	E933.1	E950.4	E962.0	E980.4
antibiotics	960.7	E856	E930.7	E950.4	E962.0	E980.4
progestogens	962.2	E858.0	E932.2	E950.4	E962.0	E980.4
12:04 parasympathomimetic (cholinergic) agents	971.0	E855.3	E941.0	E950.4	E962.0	E980.4
12:08 parasympatholytic (cholinergic-blocking) agents	971.1	E855.4	E941.1	E950.4	E962.0	E980.4
12:12 Sympathomimetic (adrenergic) agents	971.2	E855.5	E941.2	E950.4	E962.0	E980.4
12:16 sympatholytic (adrenergic-blocking) agents	971.3	E855.6	E941.3	E950.4	E962.0	E980.4
12:20 skeletal muscle relaxants						
central nervous system muscle-tone depressants	968.0	E855.1	E938.0	E950.4	E962.0	E980.4
myoneural blocking agents	975.2	E858.6	E945.2	E950.4	E962.0	E980.4
16:00 blood derivatives	964.7	E858.2	E934.7	E950.4	E962.0	E980.4
20:04 antianemia drugs	964.1	E858.2	E934.1	E950.4	E962.0	E980.4
20:04.04 iron preparations	964.0	E858.2	E934.0	E950.4	E962.0	E980.4
20:04.08 liver and stomach preparations	964.1	E858.2	E934.1	E950.4	E962.0	E980.4
20:12.04 anticoagulants	964.2	E858.2	E934.2	E950.4	E962.0	E980.4
20:12.08 antiheparin agents	964.5	E858.2	E934.5	E950.4	E962.0	E980.4
20:12.12 coagulants	964.5	E858.2	E934.5	E950.4	E962.0	E980.4
20:12.16 hemostatics NEC	964.5	E858.2	E934.5	E950.4	E962.0	E980.4
capillary active drugs	972.8	E858.3	E942.8	E950.4	E962.0	E980.4
24:04 cardiac drugs	972.9	E858.3	E942.9	E950.4	E962.0	E980.4
cardiotonic agents	972.1	E858.3	E942.1	E950.4	E962.0	E980.4
rhythm regulators	972.0	E858.3	E942.0	E950.4	E962.0	E980.4

● New Line ▲ Revised Code

Drug	Poisoning	External Cause (E-Code) Accident	Therapeutic Use	Suicide Attempt	Assault	Undetermined
Drug – *continued*						
24:06 antilipemic agents	972.2	E858.3	E942.2	E950.4	E962.0	E980.4
thyroid derivatives	962.7	E858.0	E932.7	E950.4	E962.0	E980.4
24:08 hypotensive agents	972.6	E858.3	E942.6	E950.4	E962.0	E980.4
adrenergic blocking agents	971.3	E855.6	E941.3	E950.4	E962.0	E980.4
ganglion blocking agents	972.3	E858.3	E942.3	E950.4	E962.0	E980.4
vasodilators	972.5	E858.3	E942.5	E950.4	E962.0	E980.4
24:12 vasodilating agents NEC	972.5	E858.3	E942.5	E950.4	E962.0	E980.4
coronary	972.4	E858.3	E942.4	E950.4	E962.0	E980.4
nicotinic acid derivatives	972.2	E858.3	E942.2	E950.4	E962.0	E980.4
24:16 sclerosing agents	972.7	E858.3	E942.7	E950.4	E962.0	E980.4
28:04 general anesthetics	968.4	E855.1	E938.4	E950.4	E962.0	E980.4
gaseous anesthetics	968.2	E855.1	E938.2	E950.4	E962.0	E980.4
halothane	968.1	E855.1	E938.1	E950.4	E962.0	E980.4
intravenous anesthetics	968.3	E855.1	E938.3	E950.4	E962.0	E980.4
28:08 analgesics and antipyretics	965.9	E850.9	E935.9	E950.0	E962.0	E980.0
antirheumatics	965.69	E850.6	E935.6	E950.0	E962.0	E980.0
aromatic analgesics	965.4	E850.4	E935.4	E950.0	E962.0	E980.0
non-narcotic NEC	965.7	E850.7	E935.7	E950.0	E962.0	E980.0
opium alkaloids	965.00	E850.2	E935.2	E950.0	E962.0	E980.0
heroin	965.01	E850.0	E935.0	E950.0	E962.0	E980.0
methadone	965.02	E850.1	E935.1	E950.0	E962.0	E980.0
specified type NEC	965.09	E850.2	E935.2	E950.0	E962.0	E980.0
pyrazole derivatives	965.5	E850.5	E935.5	E950.0	E962.0	E980.0
salicylates	965.1	E850.3	E935.3	E950.0	E962.0	E980.0
specified NEC	965.8	E850.8	E935.8	E950.0	E962.0	E980.0
28:10 narcotic antagonists	970.1	E854.3	E940.1	E950.4	E962.0	E980.4
28:12 anticonvulsants	966.3	E855.0	E936.3	E950.4	E962.0	E980.4
barbiturates	967.0	E851	E937.0	E950.1	E962.0	E980.1
benzodiazepine based tranquilizers	969.4	E853.2	E939.4	E950.3	E962.0	E980.3
bromides	967.3	E852.2	E937.3	E950.2	E962.0	E980.2
hydantoin derivatives	966.1	E855.0	E936.1	E950.4	E962.0	E980.4
oxazolidine (derivatives)	966.0	E855.0	E936.0	E950.4	E962.0	E980.4
succinimides	966.2	E855.0	E936.2	E950.4	E962.0	E980.4
28:16.04 antidepressants	969.0	E854.0	E939.0	E950.3	E962.0	E980.3
28:16.08 tranquilizers	969.5	E853.9	E939.5	E950.3	E962.0	E980.3
benzodiazepine based	969.4	E853.2	E939.4	E950.3	E962.0	E980.3
butyrophenone based	969.2	E853.1	E939.2	E950.3	E962.0	E980.3
major NEC	969.3	E853.8	E939.3	E950.3	E962.0	E980.3
phenothiazine-based	969.1	E853.0	E939.1	E950.3	E962.0	E980.3
28:16.12 other psychotherapeutic agents	969.8	E855.8	E939.8	E950.3	E962.0	E980.3
28:20 respiratory and cerebral stimulants	970.9	E854.3	E940.9	E950.4	E962.0	E980.4
analeplics	970.0	E854.3	E940.0	E950.4	E962.0	E980.4
anorexigenic agents	977.0	E858.8	E947.0	E950.4	E962.0	E980.4
psychostimulants	969.7	E854.2	E939.7	E950.3	E962.0	E980.3
specified NEC	970.8	E854.3	E940.8	E950.4	E962.0	E980.4
28:24 sedatives and hypnotics	967.9	E852.9	E937.9	E950.2	E962.0	E980.2
barbiturates	967.0	E851	E937.0	E950.1	E962.0	E980.1
benzodiazepine-based tranquilizers	969.4	E853.2	E939.4	E950.3	E962.0	E980.3
chloral hydrate (group)	967.1	E852.0	E937.1	E950.2	E962.0	E980.2

Drug	Poisoning	External Cause (E-Code) Accident	Therapeutic Use	Suicide Attempt	Assault	Undetermined
Drug – *continued*						
28:24 sedatives and hypnotics – *continued*						
glutethamide group	967.5	E852.4	E937.5	E950.2	E962.0	E980.2
intravenous anesthetics	968.3	E855.1	E938.3	E950.4	E962.0	E980.4
methaqualone (compounds)	967.4	E852.3	E937.4	E950.2	E962.0	E980.2
paraldehyde	967.2	E852.1	E937.2	E950.2	E962.0	E980.2
phenothiazine-based tranquilizers	969.1	E853.0	E939.1	E950.3	E962.0	E980.3
specified NEC	967.8	E852.8	E937.8	E950.2	E962.0	E980.2
thiobarbiturates	968.3	E855.1	E938.3	E950.4	E962.0	E980.4
tranquilizer NEC	969.5	E853.9	E939.5	E950.3	E962.0	E980.3
36:04 to 36:88 diagnostic agents	977.8	E858.8	E947.8	E950.4	E962.0	E980.4
40:00 electrolyte, caloric, and water balance agents NEC	974.5	E858.5	E944.5	E950.4	E962.0	E980.4
40:04 acidifying agents	963.2	E858.1	E933.2	E950.4	E962.0	E980.4
40:08 alkalinizing agents	963.3	E858.1	E933.3	E950.4	E962.0	E980.4
40:10 ammonia detoxicants	974.5	E858.5	E944.5	E950.4	E962.0	E980.4
40:12 replacement solutions	974.5	E858.5	E944.5	E950.4	E962.0	E980.4
plasma expanders	964.8	E858.2	E934.8	E950.4	E962.0	E980.4
40:16 sodium-removing resins	974.5	E858.5	E944.5	E950.4	E962.0	E980.4
40:18 potassium-removing resins	974.5	E858.5	E944.5	E950.4	E962.0	E980.4
40:20 caloric agents	974.5	E858.5	E944.5	E950.4	E962.0	E980.4
40:24 salt and sugar substitutes	974.5	E858.5	E944.5	E950.4	E962.0	E980.4
40:28 diuretics NEC	974.4	E858.5	E944.4	E950.4	E962.0	E980.4
carbonic acid anhydrase inhibitors	974.2	E858.5	E944.2	E950.4	E962.0	E980.4
mercurials	974.0	E858.5	E944.0	E950.4	E962.0	E980.4
purine derivatives	974.1	E858.5	E944.1	E950.4	E962.0	E980.4
saluretics	974.3	E858.5	E944.3	E950.4	E962.0	E980.4
thiazides	974.3	E858.5	E944.3	E950.4	E962.1	E980.4
40:36 irrigating solutions	974.5	E858.5	E944.5	E950.4	E962.0	E980.4
40:40 uricosuric agents	974.7	E858.5	E944.7	E950.4	E962.0	E980.4
44:00 enzymes	963.4	E858.1	E933.4	E950.4	E962.0	E980.4
fibrinolysis-affecting agents	964.4	E858.2	E934.4	E950.4	E962.0	E980.4
gastric agents	973.4	E858.4	E943.4	E950.4	E962.0	E980.4
48:00 expectorants and cough preparations						
antihistamine agents	963.0	E858.1	E933.0	E950.4	E962.0	E980.4
antitussives	975.4	E858.6	E945.4	E950.4	E962.0	E980.4
codeine derivatives	965.09	E850.2	E935.2	E950.0	E962.0	E980.0
expectorants	975.5	E858.6	E945.5	E950.4	E962.0	E980.4
narcotic agents NEC	965.09	E850.2	E935.2	E950.0	E962.0	E980.0
52:04 anti-infectives (EENT)						
ENT agent	976.6	E858.7	E946.6	E950.4	E962.0	E980.4
ophthalmic preparation	976.5	E858.7	E946.5	E950.4	E962.0	E980.4
52:04.04 antibiotics (EENT)						
ENT agent	976.6	E858.7	E946.6	E950.4	E962.0	E980.4
ophthalmic preparation	976.5	E858.7	E946.5	E950.4	E962.0	E980.4
52:04.06 antivirals (EENT)						
ENT agent	976.6	E858.7	E946.6	E950.4	E962.0	E980.4
ophthalmic preparation	976.5	E858.7	E946.5	E950.4	E962.0	E980.4

● New Line ▲ Revised Code

Drug	Poisoning	External Cause (E-Code) Accident	Therapeutic Use	Suicide Attempt	Assault	Undetermined
Drug – *continued*						
52:04.08 sulfonamides (EENT)						
ENT agent	976.6	E858.7	E946.6	E950.4	E962.0	E980.4
ophthalmic preparation	976.5	E858.7	E946.5	E950.4	E962.0	E980.4
52:04.12 miscellaneous anti-infectives (EENT)						
ENT agent	976.6	E858.7	E946.6	E950.4	E962.0	E980.4
ophthalmic preparation	976.5	E858.7	E946.5	E950.4	E962.0	E980.4
52:08 anti-inflammatory agents (EENT)						
ENT agent	976.6	E858.7	E946.6	E950.4	E962.0	E980.4
ophthalmic preparation	976.5	E858.7	E946.5	E950.4	E962.0	E980.4
52:10 carbonic anhydrase inhibitors	974.2	E858.5	E944.2	E950.4	E962.0	E980.4
52:12 contact lens solutions	976.5	E858.7	E946.5	E950.4	E962.0	E980.4
52:16 local anesthetics (EENT)	968.5	E855.2	E938.5	E950.4	E962.0	E980.4
52:20 miotics	971.0	E855.3	E941.0	E950.4	E962.0	E980.4
52:24 mydriatics						
adrenergics	971.2	E855.5	E941.2	E950.4	E962.0	E980.4
anticholinergics	971.1	E855.4	E941.1	E950.4	E962.0	E980.4
antimuscarinics	971.1	E855.4	E941.1	E950.4	E962.0	E980.4
parasympatholytics	971.1	E855.4	E941.1	E950.4	E962.0	E980.4
spasmolytics	971.1	E855.4	E941.1	E950.4	E962.0	E980.4
sympathomimetics	971.2	E855.5	E941.2	E950.4	E962.0	E980.4
52:28 mouth washes and gargles	976.6	E858.7	E946.6	E950.4	E962.0	E980.4
52:32 vasoconstrictors (EENT)	971.2	E855.5	E941.2	E950.4	E962.0	E980.4
52:36 unclassified agents (EENT)						
ENT agent	976.6	E858.7	E946.6	E950.4	E962.0	E980.4
ophthalmic preparation	976.5	E858.7	E946.5	E950.4	E962.0	E980.4
56:04 antacids and adsorbents	973.0	E858.4	E943.0	E950.4	E962.0	E980.4
56:08 antidiarrhea agents	973.5	E858.4	E943.5	E950.4	E962.0	E980.4
56:10 antiflatulents	973.8	E858.4	E943.8	E950.4	E962.0	E980.4
56:12 cathartics NEC	973.3	E858.4	E943.3	E950.4	E962.0	E980.4
emollients	973.2	E858.4	E943.2	E950.4	E962.0	E980.4
irritants	973.1	E858.4	E943.1	E950.4	E962.0	E980.4
56:16 digestants	973.4	E858.4	E943.4	E950.4	E962.0	E980.4
56:20 emetics and antiemetics						
antiemetics	963.0	E858.1	E933.0	E950.4	E962.0	E980.4
emetics	973.6	E858.4	E943.6	E950.4	E962.0	E980.4
56:24 lipotropic agents	977.1	E858.8	E947.1	E950.4	E962.0	E980.4
56:40 miscellaneous G.I. drugs	973.8	E858.4	E943.8	E950.4	E962.0	E980.4
60:00 gold compounds	965.69	E850.6	E935.6	E950.0	E962.0	E980.0
64:00 heavy metal antagonists	963.8	E858.1	E933.8	E950.4	E962.0	E980.4
68:04 adrenals	962.0	E858.0	E932.0	E950.4	E962.0	E980.4
68:08 androgens	962.1	E858.0	E932.1	E950.4	E962.0	E980.4
68:12 contraceptives, oral	962.2	E858.0	E932.2	E950.4	E962.0	E980.4
68:16 estrogens	962.2	E858.0	E932.2	E950.4	E962.0	E980.4
68:18 gonadotropins	962.4	E858.0	E932.4	E950.4	E962.0	E980.4
68:20 insulins and antidiabetic agents	962.3	E858.0	E932.3	E950.4	E962.0	E980.4
68:20.08 insulins	962.3	E858.0	E932.3	E950.4	E962.0	E980.4
68:24 parathyroid	962.6	E858.0	E932.6	E950.4	E962.0	E980.4
68:28 pituitary (posterior)	962.5	E858.0	E932.5	E950.4	E962.0	E980.4
anterior	962.4	E858.0	E932.4	E950.4	E962.0	E980.4
Drug – *continued*						
68:32 progestogens	962.2	E858.0	E932.2	E950.4	E962.0	E980.4
68:34 other corpus luteum						
hormones NEC	962.2	E858.0	E932.2	E950.4	E962.0	E980.4
68:36 thyroid and antithyroid						
antithyroid	962.8	E858.0	E932.8	E950.4	E962.0	E980.4
thyroid (derivatives)	962.7	E858.0	E932.7	E950.4	E962.0	E980.4
72:00 local anesthetics NEC	968.9	E855.2	E938.9	E950.4	E962.0	E980.4
infiltration (intradermal) (subcutaneous) (submucosal)	968.5	E855.2	E938.5	E950.4	E962.0	E980.4
nerve blocking (peripheral) (plexus) (regional)	968.6	E855.2	E938.6	E950.4	E962.0	E980.4
spinal	968.7	E855.2	E938.7	E950.4	E962.0	E980.4
topical (surface)	968.5	E855.2	E938.5	E950.4	E962.0	E980.4
76:00 oxytocics	975.0	E858.6	E945.0	E950.4	E962.0	E980.4
78:00 radioactive agents	990	-	-	-	-	-
80:04 serums NEC	979.9	E858.8	E949.9	E950.4	E962.0	E980.4
immune gamma globulin (human)	964.6	E858.2	E934.6	E950.4	E962.0	E980.4
80:08 toxoids NEC	978.8	E858.8	E948.8	E950.4	E962.0	E980.4
diphtheria	978.5	E858.8	E948.5	E950.4	E962.0	E980.4
and tetanus	978.9	E858.8	E948.9	E950.4	E962.0	E980.4
with pertussis component	978.6	E858.8	E948.6	E950.4	E962.0	E980.4
tetanus	978.4	E858.8	E948.4	E950.4	E962.0	E980.4
and diphtheria	978.9	E858.8	E948.9	E950.4	E962.0	E980.4
with pertussis component	978.6	E858.8	E948.6	E950.4	E962.0	E980.4
80:12 vaccines	979.9	E858.8	E949.9	E950.4	E962.0	E980.4
bacterial NEC	978.8	E858.8	E948.8	E950.4	E962.0	E980.4
with						
other bacterial components	978.9	E858.8	E948.9	E950.4	E962.0	E980.4
pertussis component	978.6	E858.8	E948.6	E950.4	E962.0	E980.4
viral and rickettsial components	979.7	E858.8	E949.7	E950.4	E962.0	E980.4
rickettsial NEC	979.6	E858.8	E949.6	E950.4	E962.0	E980.4
with						
bacterial component	979.7	E858.8	E949.7	E950.4	E962.0	E980.4
pertussis component	978.6	E858.8	E948.6	E950.4	E962.0	E980.4
viral component	979.7	E858.8	E949.7	E950.4	E962.0	E980.4
viral NEC	979.6	E858.8	E949.6	E950.4	E962.0	E980.4
with						
bacterial component	979.7	E858.8	E949.7	E950.4	E962.0	E980.4
pertussis component	978.6	E858.8	E948.6	E950.4	E962.0	E980.4
rickettsial component	979.7	E858.8	E949.7	E950.4	E962.0	E980.4
84:04.04 antibiotics (skin and mucous membrane)	976.0	E858.7	E946.0	E950.4	E962.0	E980.4
84:04.08 fungicides (skin and mucous membrane)	976.0	E858.7	E946.0	E950.4	E962.0	E980.4

Drug	Poisoning	External Cause (E-Code) Accident	Therapeutic Use	Suicide Attempt	Assault	Undetermined
Drug – *continued*						
84:04.12 scabicides and pediculicides (skin and mucous membrane)	976.0	E858.7	E946.0	E950.4	E962.0	E980.4
84:04.16 miscellaneous local anti-infectives (skin and mucous membrane)	976.0	E858.7	E946.0	E950.4	E962.0	E980.4
84:06 anti-inflammatory agents (skin and mucous membrane)	976.0	E858.7	E946.0	E950.4	E962.0	E980.4
84:08 antipruritics and local anesthetics						
antipruritics	976.1	E858.7	E946.1	E950.4	E962.0	E980.4
local anesthetics	968.5	E855.2	E938.5	E950.4	E962.0	E980.4
84:12 astringents	976.2	E858.7	E946.2	E950.4	E962.0	E980.4
84:16 cell stimulants and proliferants	976.8	E858.7	E946.8	E950.4	E962.0	E980.4
84:20 detergents	976.2	E858.7	E946.2	E950.4	E962.0	E980.4
84:24 emollients, demulcents, and protectants	976.3	E858.7	E946.3	E950.4	E962.0	E980.4
84:28 keratolytic agents	976.4	E858.7	E946.4	E950.4	E962.0	E980.4
84:32 keratoplastic agents	976.4	E858.7	E946.4	E950.4	E962.0	E980.4
84:36 miscellaneous agents (skin and mucous membrane)	976.8	E858.7	E946.8	E950.4	E962.0	E980.4
86:00 spasmolytic agents	975.1	E858.6	E945.1	E950.4	E962.0	E980.4
antiasthmatics	975.7	E858.6	E945.7	E950.4	E962.0	E980.4
papaverine	972.5	E858.3	E942.5	E950.4	E962.0	E980.4
theophylline	974.1	E858.5	E944.1	E950.4	E962.0	E980.4
88:04 vitamin A	963.5	E858.1	E933.5	E950.4	E962.0	E980.4
88:08 vitamin B complex	963.5	E858.1	E933.5	E950.4	E962.0	E980.4
hematopoietic vitamin	964.1	E858.2	E934.1	E950.4	E962.0	E980.4
nicotinic acid derivatives	972.2	E858.3	E942.2	E950.4	E962.0	E980.4
88:12 vitamin C	963.5	E858.1	E933.5	E950.4	E962.0	E980.4
88:16 vitamin D	963.5	E858.1	E933.5	E950.4	E962.0	E980.4
88:20 vitamin E	963.5	E858.1	E933.5	E950.4	E962.0	E980.4
88:24 vitamin K activity	964.3	E858.2	E934.3	E950.4	E962.0	E980.4
88:28 multivitamin preparations	963.5	E858.1	E933.5	E950.4	E962.0	E980.4
92:00 unclassified therapeutic agents	977.8	E858.8	E947.8	E950.4	E962.0	E980.4
Duboisine	971.1	E855.4	E941.1	E950.4	E962.0	E980.4
Dulcolax	973.1	E858.4	E943.1	E950.4	E962.0	E980.4
Duponol (C) (EP)	976.2	E858.7	E946.2	E950.4	E962.0	E980.4
Durabolin	962.1	E858.0	E932.1	E950.4	E962.0	E980.4
Dyclone	968.5	E855.2	E938.5	E950.4	E962.0	E980.4
Dyclonine	968.5	E855.2	E938.5	E950.4	E962.0	E980.4
Dydrogesterone	962.2	E858.0	E932.2	E950.4	E962.0	E980.4
Dyes NEC	989.89	E866.8	-	E950.9	E962.1	E980.9
diagnostic agents	977.8	E858.8	E947.8	E950.4	E962.0	E980.4
pharmaceutical NEC	977.4	E858.8	E947.4	E950.4	E962.0	E980.4
Dyfols	971.0	E855.3	E941.0	E950.4	E962.0	E980.4
Dymelor	962.3	E858.0	E932.3	E950.4	E962.0	E980.4
Dynamite	989.89	E866.8	-	E950.9	E962.1	E980.9
fumes	987.8	E869.8	-	E952.8	E962.2	E982.8
Dyphylline	975.1	E858.6	E945.1	E950.4	E962.0	E980.4
Ear preparations	976.6	E858.7	E946.6	E950.4	E962.0	E980.4
Echothiopate, ecothiopate	971.0	E855.3	E941.0	E950.4	E962.0	E980.4
Ecstacy	969.7	E854.2	E939.7	E950.3	E962.0	E980.3
Ectylurea	967.8	E852.8	E937.8	E950.2	E962.0	E980.2
Edathamil disodium	963.8	E858.1	E933.8	E950.4	E962.0	E980.4
Edecrin	974.4	E858.5	E944.4	E950.4	E962.0	E980.4
Edetate, disodium (calcium)	963.8	E858.1	E933.8	E950.4	E962.0	E980.4
Edrophonium	971.0	E855.3	E941.0	E950.4	E962.0	E980.4
Elase	976.8	E858.7	E946.8	E950.4	E962.0	E980.4
Elaterium	973.1	E858.4	E943.1	E950.4	E962.0	E980.4
Elder	988.2	E865.4	-	E950.9	E962.1	E980.9
berry, (unripe)	988.2	E865.3	-	E950.9	E962.1	E980.9
Electrolytes NEC	974.5	E858.5	E944.5	E950.4	E962.0	E980.4
Electrolytic agent NEC	974.5	E858.5	E944.5	E950.4	E962.0	E980.4
Embramine	963.0	E858.1	E933.0	E950.4	E962.0	E980.4
Emetics	973.6	E858.4	E943.6	E950.4	E962.0	E980.4
Emetine (hydrochloride)	961.5	E857	E931.5	E950.4	E962.0	E980.4
Emollients	976.3	E858.7	E946.3	E950.4	E962.0	E980.4
Emylcamate	969.5	E853.8	E939.5	E950.3	E962.0	E980.3
Encyprate	969.0	E854.0	E939.0	E950.3	E962.0	E980.3
Endocaine	968.5	E855.2	E938.5	E950.4	E962.0	E980.4
Endrin	989.2	E863.0	-	E950.6	E962.1	E980.7
Enflurane	968.2	E855.1	E938.2	E950.4	E962.0	E980.4
Enovid	962.2	E858.0	E932.2	E950.4	E962.0	E980.4
ENT preparations (anti-infectives)	976.6	E858.7	E946.6	E950.4	E962.0	E980.4
Enzodase	963.4	E858.1	E933.4	E950.4	E962.0	E980.4
Enzymes NEC	963.4	E858.1	E933.4	E950.4	E962.0	E980.4
Epanutin	966.1	E855.0	E936.1	E950.4	E962.0	E980.4
Ephedra (tincture)	971.2	E855.5	E941.2	E950.4	E962.0	E980.4
Ephedrine	971.2	E855.5	E941.2	E950.4	E962.0	E980.4
Epiestriol	962.2	E858.0	E932.2	E950.4	E962.0	E980.4
Epilim – *see* Sodium valproate						
Epinephrine	971.2	E855.5	E941.2	E950.4	E962.0	E980.4
Epsom salt	973.3	E858.4	E943.3	E950.4	E962.0	E980.4
Equanil	969.5	E853.8	E939.5	E950.3	E962.0	E980.3
Equisetum (diuretic)	974.4	E858.5	E944.4	E950.4	E962.0	E980.4
Ergometrine	975.0	E858.6	E945.0	E950.4	E962.0	E980.4
Ergonovine	975.0	E858.6	E945.0	E950.4	E962.0	E980.4
Ergot NEC	988.2	E865.4	-	E950.9	E962.1	E980.9
medicinal (alkaloids)	975.0	E858.6	E945.0	E950.4	E962.0	E980.4
Ergotamine (tartrate) (for migraine) **NEC**	972.9	E858.3	E942.9	E950.4	E962.0	E980.4
Ergotrate	975.0	E858.6	E945.0	E950.4	E962.0	E980.4
Erythrityl tetranitrate	972.4	E858.3	E942.4	E950.4	E962.0	E980.4
Erythrol tetranitrate	972.4	E858.3	E942.4	E950.4	E962.0	E980.4
Erythromycin	960.3	E856	E930.3	E950.4	E962.0	E980.4
ophthalmic preparation	976.5	E858.7	E946.5	E950.4	E962.0	E980.4
topical NEC	976.0	E858.7	E946.0	E950.4	E962.0	E980.4
Eserine	971.0	E855.3	E941.0	E950.4	E962.0	E980.4
Eskabarb	967.0	E851	E937.0	E950.1	E962.0	E980.1
Eskalith	969.8	E855.8	E939.8	E950.3	E962.0	E980.3
Estradiol (cypionate) (dipropionate) (valerate)	962.2	E858.0	E932.2	E950.4	E962.0	E980.4
Estriol	962.2	E858.0	E932.2	E950.4	E962.0	E980.4
Estrogens (with progestogens)	962.2	E858.0	E932.2	E950.4	E962.0	E980.4
Estrone	962.2	E858.0	E932.2	E950.4	E962.0	E980.4
Etafedrine	971.2	E855.5	E941.2	E950.4	E962.0	E980.4
Ethacrynate sodium	974.4	E858.5	E944.4	E950.4	E962.0	E980.4
Ethacrynic acid	974.4	E858.5	E944.4	E950.4	E962.0	E980.4
Ethambutol	961.8	E857	E931.8	E950.4	E962.0	E980.4
Ethamide	974.2	E858.5	E944.2	E950.4	E962.0	E980.4
Ethamivan	970.0	E854.3	E940.0	E950.4	E962.0	E980.4
Ethamsylate	964.5	E858.2	E934.5	E950.4	E962.0	E980.4
Ethanol	980.0	E860.1	-	E950.9	E962.1	E980.9
beverage	980.0	E860.0	-	E950.9	E962.1	E980.9
Ethchlorvynol	967.8	E852.8	E937.8	E950.2	E962.0	E980.2

● New Line ▲ Revised Code

		External Cause (E-Code)				
Drug	**Poisoning**	**Accident**	**Therapeutic Use**	**Suicide Attempt**	**Assault**	**Undetermined**
Ethebenecid	974.7	E858.5	E944.7	E950.4	E962.0	E980.4
Ether(s) (diethyl) (ethyl) (vapor)	987.8	E869.8	-	E952.8	E962.2	E982.8
anesthetic	968.2	E855.1	E938.2	E950.4	E962.0	E980.4
petroleum – *see* Ligroin solvent						
solvent	982.8	E862.4	-	E950.9	E962.1	E980.9
Ethidine chloride (vapor)	987.8	E869.8	-	E952.8	E962.2	E982.8
liquid (solvent)	982.3	E862.4	-	E950.9	E962.1	E980.9
Ethinamate	967.8	E852.8	E937.8	E950.2	E962.0	E980.2
Ethinylestradiol	962.2	E858.0	E932.2	E950.4	E962.0	E980.4
Ethionamide	961.8	E857	E931.8	E950.4	E962.0	E980.4
Ethisterone	962.2	E858.0	E932.2	E950.4	E962.0	E980.4
Ethobral	967.0	E851	E937.0	E950.1	E962.0	E980.1
Ethocaine (infiltration) (topical)	968.5	E855.2	E938.5	E950.4	E962.0	E980.4
nerve block (peripheral) (plexus)	968.6	E855.2	E938.6	E950.4	E962.0	E980.4
spinal	968.7	E855.2	E938.7	E950.4	E962.0	E980.4
Ethoheptazine (citrate)	965.7	E850.7	E935.7	E950.0	E962.0	E980.0
Ethopropazine	966.4	E855.0	E936.4	E950.4	E962.0	E980.4
Ethosuximide	966.2	E855.0	E936.2	E950.4	E962.0	E980.4
Ethotoin	966.1	E855.0	E936.1	E950.4	E962.0	E980.4
Ethoxazene	961.9	E857	E931.9	E950.4	E962.0	E980.4
Ethoxzolamide	974.2	E858.5	E944.2	E950.4	E962.0	E980.4
Ethyl						
acetate (vapor)	982.8	E862.4	-	E950.9	E962.1	E980.9
alcohol	980.0	E860.1	-	E950.9	E962.1	E980.9
beverage	980.0	E860.0	-	E950.9	E962.1	E980.9
aldehyde (vapor)	987.8	E869.8	-	E952.8	E962.2	E982.8
liquid	989.89	E866.8	-	E950.9	E962.1	E980.9
aminobenzoate	968.5	E855.2	E938.5	E950.4	E962.0	E980.4
biscoumacetate	964.2	E858.2	E934.2	E950.4	E962.0	E980.4
bromide (anesthetic)	968.2	E855.1	E938.2	E950.4	E962.0	E980.4
carbamate (antineoplastic)	963.1	E858.1	E933.1	E950.4	E962.0	E980.4
carbinol	980.3	E860.4	-	E950.9	E962.1	E980.9
chaulmoograte	961.8	E857	E931.8	E950.4	E962.0	E980.4
chloride (vapor)	987.8	E869.8	-	E952.8	E962.2	E982.8
anesthetic (local)	968.5	E855.2	E938.5	E950.4	E962.0	E980.4
inhaled	968.2	E855.1	E938.2	E950.4	E962.0	E980.4
solvent	982.3	E862.4	-	E950.9	E962.1	E980.9
estranol	962.1	E858.0	E932.1	E950.4	E962.0	E980.4
ether – *see* Ether(s)						
formate (solvent) NEC	982.8	E862.4	-	E950.9	E962.1	E980.9
iodoacetate	987.5	E869.3	-	E952.8	E962.2	E982.8
lactate (solvent) NEC	982.8	E862.4	-	E950.9	E962.1	E980.9
methylcarbinol	980.8	E860.8	-	E950.9	E962.1	E980.9
morphine	965.09	E850.2	E935.2	E950.0	E962.0	E980.0
Ethylene (gas)	987.1	E869.8	-	E952.8	E962.2	E982.8
anesthetic (general)	968.2	E855.1	E938.2	E950.4	E962.0	E980.4
chlorohydrin (vapor)	982.3	E862.4	-	E950.9	E962.1	E980.9
dichloride (vapor)	982.3	E862.4	-	E950.9	E962.1	E980.9
glycol(s) (any) (vapor)	982.8	E862.4	-	E950.9	E962.1	E980.9
Ethylidene						
chloride NEC	982.3	E862.4	-	E950.9	E962.1	E980.9
diethyl ether	982.8	-	E862.4	E950.9	E962.1	E980.9
Ethynodiol	962.2	E858.0	E932.2	E950.4	E962.0	E980.4
Etidocaine	968.9	E855.2	E938.9	E950.4	E962.0	E980.4
infiltration (subcutaneous)	968.5	E855.2	E938.5	E950.4	E962.0	E980.4
nerve (peripheral) (plexus)	968.6	E855.2	E938.6	E950.4	E962.0	E980.4
Etilfen	967.0	E851	E937.0	E950.1	E962.0	E980.1
Etomide	965.7	E850.7	E935.7	E950.0	E962.0	E980.0

		External Cause (E-Code)				
Drug	**Poisoning**	**Accident**	**Therapeutic Use**	**Suicide Attempt**	**Assault**	**Undetermined**
Etorphine	965.09	E850.2	E935.2	E950.0	E962.0	E980.0
Etoval	967.0	E851	E937.0	E950.1	E962.0	E980.1
Etrypiamine	969.0	E854.0	E939.0	E950.3	E962.0	E980.3
Eucaine	968.5	E855.2	E938.5	E950.4	E962.0	E980.4
Eucalyptus (oil) **NEC**	975.5	E858.6	E945.5	E950.4	E962.0	E980.4
Eucatropine	971.1	E855.4	E941.1	E950.4	E962.0	E980.4
Eucodal	965.09	E850.2	E935.2	E950.0	E962.0	E980.0
Euneryl	967.0	E851	E937.0	E950.1	E962.0	E980.1
Euphthalmine	971.1	E855.4	E941.1	E950.4	E962.0	E980.4
Eurax	976.0	E858.7	E946.0	E950.4	E962.0	E980.4
Euresol	976.4	E858.7	E946.4	E950.4	E962.0	E980.4
Euthroid	962.7	E858.0	E932.7	E950.4	E962.0	E980.4
Evans blue	977.8	E858.8	E947.8	E950.4	E962.0	E980.4
Evipal	967.0	E851	E937.0	E950.1	E962.0	E980.1
sodium	968.3	E855.1	E938.3	E950.4	E962.0	E980.4
Evipan	967.0	E851	E937.0	E950.1	E962.0	E980.1
sodium	968.3	E855.1	E938.3	E950.4	E962.0	E980.4
Exalgin	965.4	E850.4	E935.4	E950.0	E962.0	E980.0
Excipients, pharmaceutical	977.4	E858.8	E947.4	E950.4	E962.0	E980.4
Exhaust gas – *see* Carbon, monoxide						
Ex-Lax (phenolphthalein)	973.1	E858.4	E943.1	E950.4	E962.0	E980.4
Expectorants	975.5	E858.6	E945.5	E950.4	E962.0	E980.4
External medications (skin) (mucous membrane)	976.9	E858.7	E946.9	E950.4	E962.0	E980.4
dental agent	976.7	E858.7	E946.7	E950.4	E962.0	E980.4
ENT agent	976.6	E858.7	E946.6	E950.4	E962.0	E980.4
ophthalmic preparation	976.5	E858.7	E946.5	E950.4	E962.0	E980.4
specified NEC	976.8	E858.7	E946.8	E950.4	E962.0	E980.4
Eye agents (anti-infective)	976.5	E858.7	E946.5	E950.4	E962.0	E980.4
Factor IX complex (human)	964.5	E858.2	E934.5	E950.4	E962.0	E980.4
Fecal softeners	973.2	E858.4	E943.2	E950.4	E962.0	E980.4
Fenbutrazate	977.0	E858.8	E947.0	E950.4	E962.0	E980.4
Fencamfamin	970.8	E854.3	E940.8	E950.4	E962.0	E980.4
Fenfluramine	977.0	E858.8	E947.0	E950.4	E962.0	E980.4
Fenoprofen	965.61	E850.6	E935.6	E950.0	E962.0	E980.0
Fentanyl	965.09	E850.2	E935.2	E950.0	E962.0	E980.0
Fentazin	969.1	E853.0	E939.1	E930.3	E962.0	E980.3
Fenticlor, fentichlor	976.0	E858.7	E946.0	E950.4	E962.0	E980.4
Fer de lance (bite) (venom)	989.5	E905.0	-	E950.9	E962.1	E980.9
Ferric – *see* Iron						
Ferrocholinate	964.0	E858.2	E934.0	E950.4	E962.0	E980.4
Ferrous fumerate, gluconate, lactate, salt NEC, sulfate (medicinal)	964.0	E858.2	E934.0	E950.4	E962.0	E980.4
Ferrum – *see* Iron						
Fertilizers NEC	989.89	E866.5	-	E950.9	E962.1	E980.4
with herbicide mixture	989.4	E863.5	-	E950.6	E962.1	E980.7
Fibrinogen (human)	964.7	E858.2	E934.7	E950.4	E962.0	E980.4
Fibrinolysin	964.4	E858.2	E934.4	E950.4	E962.0	E980.4
Fibrinolysis-affecting agents	964.4	E858.2	E934.4	E950.4	E962.0	E980.4
Filix mas	961.6	E857	E931.6	E950.4	E962.0	E980.4
Fiorinal	965.1	E850.3	E935.3	E950.0	E962.0	E980.0
Fire damp	987.1	E869.8	-	E952.8	E962.2	E982.8
Fish, nonbacterial or noxious	988.0	E865.2	-	E950.9	E962.1	E980.9
shell	988.0	E865.1	-	E950.9	E962.1	E980.9
Flagyl	961.5	E857	E931.5	E950.4	E962.0	E980.4
Flavoxate	975.1	E858.6	E945.1	E950.4	E962.0	E980.4
Flaxedil	975.2	E858.6	E945.2	E950.4	E962.0	E980.4
Flaxseed (medicinal)	976.3	E858.7	E946.3	E950.4	E962.0	E980.4
Flomax ●	971.3	E855.6	E941.3	E950.4	E962.0	E980.4
Florantyrone	973.4	E858.4	E943.4	E950.4	E962.0	E980.4

		External Cause (E-Code)				
Drug	**Poisoning**	**Accident**	**Therapeutic Use**	**Suicide Attempt**	**Assault**	**Undetermined**
Floraquin	961.3	E857	E931.3	E950.4	E962.0	E980.4
Florinef	962.0	E858.0	E932.0	E950.4	E962.0	E980.4
ENT agent	976.6	E858.7	E946.6	E950.4	E962.0	E980.4
ophthalmic preparation	976.5	E858.7	E946.5	E950.4	E962.0	E980.4
topical NEC	976.0	E858.7	E946.0	E950.4	E962.0	E980.4
Flowers of sulfur	976.4	E858.7	E946.4	E950.4	E962.0	E980.4
Floxuridine	963.1	E858.1	E933.1	E950.4	E962.0	E980.4
Flucytosine	961.9	E857	E931.9	E950.4	E962.0	E980.4
Fludrocortisone	962.0	E858.0	E932.0	E950.4	E962.0	E980.4
ENT agent	976.6	E858.7	E946.6	E950.4	E962.0	E980.4
ophthalmic preparation	976.5	E858.7	E946.5	E950.4	E962.0	E980.4
topical NEC	976.0	E858.7	E946.0	E950.4	E962.0	E980.4
Flumethasone	976.0	E858.7	E946.0	E950.4	E962.0	E980.4
Flumethiazide	974.3	E858.5	E944.3	E950.4	E962.0	E980.4
Flumidin	961.7	E857	E931.7	E950.4	E962.0	E980.4
Flunitrazepam	969.4	E853.2	E939.4	E950.3	E962.0	E980.3
Fluocinolone	976.0	E858.7	E946.0	E950.4	E962.0	E980.4
Fluocortolone	962.0	E858.0	E932.0	E950.4	E962.0	E980.4
Fluohydrocortisone	962.0	E858.0	E932.0	E950.4	E962.0	E980.4
ENT agent	976.6	E858.7	E946.6	E950.4	E962.0	E980.4
ophthalmic preparation	976.5	E858.7	E946.5	E950.4	E962.0	E980.4
topical NEC	976.0	E858.7	E946.0	E950.4	E962.0	E980.4
Fluonid	976.0	E858.7	E946.0	E950.4	E962.0	E980.4
Fluopromazine	969.1	E853.0	E939.1	E950.3	E962.0	E980.3
Fluoracetate	989.4	E863.7	-	E950.6	E962.1	E980.7
Fluorescein (sodium)	977.8	E858.8	E947.8	E950.4	E962.0	E980.4
Fluoride(s) (pesticides) (sodium) NEC	989.4	E863.4	-	E950.6	E962.1	E980.7
hydrogen – *see* Hydrofluoric acid						
medicinal	976.7	E858.7	E946.7	E950.4	E962.0	E980.4
not pesticide NEC	983.9	E864.4	-	E950.7	E962.1	E980.6
stannous	976.7	E858.7	E946.7	E950.4	E962.0	E980.4
Fluorinated corticosteroids	962.0	E858.0	E932.0	E950.4	E962.0	E980.4
Fluorine (compounds) (gas)	987.8	E869.8	-	E952.8	E962.2	E982.8
salt – *see* Fluoride(s)						
Fluoristan	976.7	E858.7	E946.7	E950.4	E962.0	E980.4
Fluoroacetate	989.4	E863.7	-	E950.6	E962.1	E980.7
Fluorodeoxyuridine	963.1	E858.1	E933.1	E950.4	E962.0	E980.4
Fluorometholone (topical) NEC	976.0	E858.7	E946.0	E950.4	E962.0	E980.4
ophthalmic preparation	976.5	E858.7	E946.5	E950.4	E962.0	E980.4
Fluorouracil	963.1	E858.1	E933.1	E950.4	E962.0	E980.4
Fluothane	968.1	E855.1	E938.1	E950.4	E962.0	E980.4
Fluoxetine hydrochloride	969.0	E854.0	E939.0	E950.3	E962.0	E980.3
Fluoxymesterone	962.1	E858.0	E932.1	E950.4	E962.0	E980.4
Fluphenazine	969.1	E853.0	E939.1	E950.3	E962.0	E980.3
Fluprednisolone	962.0	E858.0	E932.0	E950.4	E962.0	E980.4
Flurandrenolide	976.0	E858.7	E946.0	E950.4	E962.0	E980.4
Flurazepam (hydrochloride)	969.4	E853.2	E939.4	E950.3	E962.0	E980.3
Flurbiprofen	965.61	E850.6	E935.6	E950.0	E962.0	E980.0
Flurobate	976.0	E858.7	E946.0	E950.4	E962.0	E980.4
Flurothyl	969.8	E855.8	E939.8	E950.3	E962.0	E980.3
Fluroxene	968.2	E855.1	E938.2	E950.4	E962.0	E980.4
Folacin	964.1	E858.2	E934.1	E950.4	E962.0	E980.4
Folic acid	964.1	E858.2	E934.1	E950.4	E962.0	E980.4
Follicle stimulating hormone	962.4	E858.0	E932.4	E950.4	E962.0	E980.4
Food, foodstuffs, nonbacterial or noxious	988.9	E865.9	-	E950.9	E962.1	E980.9
berries, seeds	988.2	E865.3	-	E950.9	E962.1	E980.9
fish	988.0	E865.2	-	E950.9	E962.1	E980.9
mushrooms	988.1	E865.5	-	E950.9	E962.1	E980.9

		External Cause (E-Code)				
Drug	**Poisoning**	**Accident**	**Therapeutic Use**	**Suicide Attempt**	**Assault**	**Undetermined**
Food, foodstuffs, nonbacterial or noxious – *continued*						
plants	988.2	E865.9	-	E950.9	E962.1	E980.9
specified type NEC	988.2	E865.4	-	E950.9	E962.1	E980.9
shellfish	988.0	E865.1	-	E950.9	E962.1	E980.9
specified NEC	988.8	E865.8	-	E950.9	E962.1	E980.9
Fool's parsley	988.2	E865.4	-	E950.9	E962.1	E980.9
Formaldehyde (solution)	989.89	E861.4	-	E950.9	E962.1	E980.9
fungicide	989.4	E863.6	-	E950.6	E962.1	E980.7
gas or vapor	987.8	E869.8	-	E952.8	E962.2	E982.8
Formalin	989.89	E861.4	-	E950.9	E962.1	E980.9
fungicide	989.4	E863.6	-	E950.6	E962.1	E980.7
vapor	987.8	E869.8	-	E952.8	E962.2	E982.8
Formic acid	983.1	E864.1	-	E950.7	E962.1	E980.6
vapor	987.8	E869.8	-	E952.8	E962.2	E982.8
Fowler's solution	985.1	E866.3	-	E950.8	E962.1	E980.8
Foxglove	988.2	E865.4	-	E950.9	E962.1	E980.9
Fox green	977.8	E858.8	E947.8	E950.4	E962.0	E980.4
Framycetin	960.8	E856	E930.8	E950.4	E962.0	E980.4
Frangula (extract)	973.1	E858.4	E943.1	E950.4	E962.0	E980.4
Frei antigen	977.8	E858.8	E947.8	E950.4	E962.0	E980.4
Freons	987.4	E869.2	-	E952.8	E962.2	E982.8
Fructose	974.5	E858.5	E944.5	E950.4	E962.0	E980.4
Frusemide	974.4	E858.5	E944.4	E950.4	E962.0	E980.4
FSH	962.4	E858.0	E932.4	E950.4	E962.0	E980.4
Fuel						
automobile	981	E862.1	-	E950.9	E962.1	E980.9
exhaust gas, not in transit	986	E868.2	-	E952.0	E962.2	E982.0
vapor NEC	987.1	E869.8	-	E952.8	E962.2	E982.8
gas (domestic use) – *see also* Carbon, monoxide, fuel						
utility	987.1	E868.1	-	E951.8	E962.2	E981.8
incomplete combustion of – *see* Carbon, monoxide, fuel, utility						
in mobile container	987.0	E868.0	-	E951.1	E962.2	E981.1
piped (natural)	987.1	E867	-	E951.0	E962.2	E981.0
industrial, incomplete combustion	986	E868.3	-	E952.1	E962.2	E982.1
Fugillin	960.8	E856	E930.8	E950.4	E962.0	E980.4
Fulminate of mercury	985.0	E866.1	-	E950.9	E962.1	E980.9
Fulvicin	960.1	E856	E930.1	E950.4	E962.0	E980.4
Fumadil	960.8	E856	E930.8	E950.4	E962.0	E980.4
Fumagillin	960.8	E856	E930.8	E950.4	E962.0	E980.4
Fumes (from)	987.9	E869.9	-	E952.9	E962.2	E982.9
carbon monoxide – *see* Carbon, monoxide						
charcoal (domestic use)	986	E868.3	-	E952.1	E962.2	E982.1
chloroform – *see* Chloroform						
coke (in domestic stoves, fireplaces)	986	E868.3	-	E952.1	E962.2	E982.1
corrosive NEC	987.8	E869.8	-	E952.8	E962.2	E982.8
ether – *see* Ether(s)						
freons	987.4	E869.2	-	E952.8	E962.2	E982.8
hydrocarbons	987.1	E869.8	-	E952.8	E962.2	E982.8
petroleum (liquefied)	987.0	E868.0	-	E951.1	E962.2	E981.1
distributed through pipes (pure or mixed with air)	987.0	E867	-	E951.0	E962.2	E981.0
lead – *see* Lead						

Drug	Poisoning	External Cause (E-Code) Accident	Therapeutic Use	Suicide Attempt	Assault	Undetermined
Fumes – *continued*						
metals – *see* specified metal						
nitrogen dioxide	987.2	E869.0	-	E952.8	E962.2	E982.8
pesticides – *see* Pesticides						
petroleum (liquefied)	987.0	E868.0	-	E951.1	E962.2	E981.1
distributed through pipes (pure or mixed with air)	987.0	E867	-	E951.0	E962.2	E981.0
polyester	987.8	E869.8	-	E952.8	E962.2	E982.8
specified source, other (*see also* substance specified)	987.8	E869.8	-	E952.8	E962.2	E982.8
sulfur dioxide	987.3	E869.1	-	E952.8	E962.2	E982.8
Fumigants	989.4	E863.8	-	E950.6	E962.1	E980.7
Fungi, noxious, used as food	988.1	E865.5	-	E950.9	E962.1	E980.9
Fungicides (*see also* Antifungals)	989.4	E863.6	-	E950.6	E962.1	E980.7
Fungizone	960.1	E856	E930.1	E950.4	E962.0	E980.4
topical	976.0	E858.7	E946.0	E950.4	E962.0	E980.4
Furacin	976.0	E858.7	E946.0	E950.4	E962.0	E980.4
Furadantin	961.9	E857	E931.9	E950.4	E962.0	E980.4
Furazolidone	961.9	E857	E931.9	E950.4	E962.0	E980.4
Furnace (coal burning) (domestic)**, gas from**	986	E868.3	-	E952.1	E962.2	E982.1
industrial	986	E868.8	-	E952.1	E962.2	E982.1
Furniture polish	989.89	E861.2	-	E950.9	E962.1	E980.9
Furosemide	974.4	E858.5	E944.4	E950.4	E962.0	E980.4
Furoxone	961.9	E857	E931.9	E950.4	E962.0	E980.4
Fusel oil (amyl) (butyl) (propyl)	980.3	E860.4	-	E950.9	E962.1	E980.9
Fusidic acid	960.8	E856	E930.8	E950.4	E962.0	E980.4
Gallamine	975.2	E858.6	E945.2	E950.4	E962.0	E980.4
Gallotannic acid	976.2	E858.7	E946.2	E950.4	E962.0	E980.4
Gamboge	973.1	E858.4	E943.1	E950.4	E962.0	E980.4
Gamimune	964.6	E858.2	E934.6	E950.4	E962.0	E980.4
Gamma-benzene hexachloride (vapor)	989.2	E863.0	-	E950.6	E962.1	E980.7
Gamma globulin	964.6	E858.2	E934.6	E950.4	E962.0	E980.4
Gamma Hydroxy Butyrate (GHB)	968.4	E855.1	E938.4	E950.4	E962.0	E980.4
Gamulin	964.6	E858.2	E934.6	E950.4	E962.0	E980.4
Ganglionic blocking agents	972.3	E858.3	E942.3	E950.4	E962.0	E980.4
Ganja	969.6	E854.1	E939.6	E950.3	E962.0	E980.3
Garamycin	960.8	E856	E930.8	E950.4	E962.0	E980.4
ophthalmic preparation	976.5	E858.7	E946.5	E950.4	E962.0	E980.4
topical NEC	976.0	E858.7	E946.0	E950.4	E962.0	E980.4
Gardenal	967.0	E851	E937.0	E950.1	E962.0	E980.1
Gardepanyl	967.0	E851	E937.0	E950.1	E962.0	E980.1
Gas	987.9	E869.9	-	E952.9	E962.2	E982.9
acetylene	987.1	E868.1	-	E951.8	E962.2	E981.8
incomplete combustion of – *see* Carbon, monoxide, fuel, utility						
air contaminants, source or type not specified	987.9	E869.9	-	E952.9	E962.2	E982.9
anesthetic (general) NEC	968.2	E855.1	E938.2	E950.4	E962.0	E980.4
blast furnace	986	E868.8	-	E952.1	E962.2	E982.1
butane – *see* Butane						
carbon monoxide – *see* Carbon, monoxide						
chlorine	987.6	E869.8	-	E952.8	E962.2	E982.8
coal – *see* Carbon, monoxide, coal						

Drug	Poisoning	External Cause (E-Code) Accident	Therapeutic Use	Suicide Attempt	Assault	Undetermined
Gas – *continued*						
cyanide	987.7	E869.8	-	E952.8	E962.2	E982.8
dicyanogen	987.8	E869.8	-	E952.8	E962.2	E982.8
domestic – *see* Gas, utility						
exhaust – *see* Carbon, monoxide, exhaust gas						
from wood- or coal-burning stove or fireplace	986	E868.3	-	E952.1	E962.2	E982.1
fuel (domestic use) – *see also* Carbon, monoxide, fuel						
industrial use	986	E868.8	-	E952.1	E962.2	E982.1
utility	987.1	E868.1	-	E951.8	E962.2	E981.8
incomplete combustion of – *see* Carbon, monoxide, fuel, utility						
in mobile container	987.0	E868.0	-	E951.1	E962.2	E981.1
piped (natural)	987.1	E867	-	E951.0	E962.2	E981.0
garage	986	E868.2	-	E952.0	E962.2	E982.0
hydrocarbon NEC	987.1	E869.8	-	E952.8	E962.2	E982.8
incomplete combustion of – *see* Carbon, monoxide, fuel, utility						
liquefied (mobile container)	987.0	E868.0	-	E951.1	E962.2	E981.1
piped	987.0	E867	-	E951.0	E962.2	E981.0
hydrocyanic acid	987.7	E869.8	-	E952.8	E962.2	E982.8
illuminating – *see* Gas, utility						
incomplete combustion, any – *see* Carbon, monoxide						
kiln	986	E868.8	-	E952.1	E962.2	E982.1
lacrimogenic	987.5	E869.3	-	E952.8	E962.2	E982.8
marsh	987.1	E869.8	-	E952.8	E962.2	E982.8
motor exhaust, not in transit	986	E868.8	-	E952.1	E962.2	E982.1
mustard – *see* Mustard, gas						
natural	987.1	E867	-	E951.0	E962.2	E981.0
nerve (war)	987.9	E869.9	-	E952.9	E962.2	E982.9
oils	981	E862.1	-	E950.9	E962.1	E980.9
petroleum (liquefied) (distributed in mobile containers)	987.0	E868.0	-	E951.1	E962.2	E981.1
piped (pure or mixed with air)	987.0	E867	-	E951.1	E962.2	E981.1
piped (manufactured) (natural) NEC	987.1	E867	-	E951.0	E962.2	E981.0
producer	986	E868.8	-	E952.1	E962.2	E982.1
propane – *see* Propane						
refrigerant (freon)	987.4	E869.2	-	E952.8	E962.2	E982.8
not freon	987.9	E869.9	-	E952.9	E962.2	E982.9
sewer	987.8	E869.8	-	E952.8	E962.2	E982.8
specified source NEC (*see also* substance specified)	987.8	E869.8	-	E952.8	E962.2	E982.8
stove – *see* Gas, utility						
tear	987.5	E869.3	-	E952.8	E962.2	E982.8

Fumes – Gas

● New Line ▲ Revised Code

Drug	Poisoning	External Cause (E-Code) Accident	Therapeutic Use	Suicide Attempt	Assault	Undetermined
Gas – *continued*						
utility (for cooking, heating, or lighting) (piped) NEC	987.1	E868.1	-	E951.8	E962.2	E981.8
incomplete combustion of – *see* Carbon, monoxide, fuel, utility						
in mobile container	987.0	E868.0	-	E951.1	E962.2	E981.1
piped (natural)	987.1	E867	-	E951.0	E962.2	E981.0
water	987.1	E868.1	-	E951.8	E962.2	E981.8
incomplete combustion of – *see* Carbon, monoxide, fuel, utility						
Gaseous substance – *see* Gas						
Gasoline, gasolene	981	E862.1	-	E950.9	E962.1	E980.9
vapor	987.1	E869.8	-	E952.8	E962.2	E982.8
Gastric enzymes	973.4	E858.4	E943.4	E950.4	E962.0	E980.4
Gastrograrin	977.8	E858.8	E947.8	E950.4	E962.0	E980.4
Gastrointestinal agents	973.9	E858.4	E943.9	E950.4	E962.0	E980.4
specified NEC	973.8	E858.4	E943.8	E950.4	E962.0	E980.4
Gaultheria procumbens	988.2	E865.4	-	E950.9	E962.1	E980.9
Gelatin (intravenous)	964.8	E858.2	E934.8	E950.4	E962.0	E980.4
absorbable (sponge)	964.5	E858.2	E934.5	E950.4	E962.0	E980.4
Gelfilm	976.8	E858.7	E946.8	E950.4	E962.0	E980.4
Gelfoam	964.5	E858.2	E934.5	E950.4	E962.0	E980.4
Gelsemine	970.8	E854.3	E940.8	E950.4	E962.0	E980.4
Gelsemium (sempervirens)	988.2	E865.4	-	E950.9	E962.1	E980.9
Gemonil	967.0	E851	E937.0	E950.1	E962.0	E980.1
Gentamicin	960.8	E856	E930.8	E950.4	E962.0	E980.4
ophthalmic preparation	976.5	E858.7	E946.5	E950.4	E962.0	E980.4
topical NEC	976.0	E858.7	E946.0	E950.4	E962.0	E980.4
Gentian violet	976.0	E858.7	E946.0	E950.4	E962.0	E980.4
Gexane	976.0	E858.7	E946.0	E950.4	E962.0	E980.4
Gila monster (venom)	989.5	E905.0	-	E950.9	E962.1	E980.9
Ginger, Jamaica	989.89	E866.8	-	E950.9	E962.1	E980.9
Gitalin	972.1	E858.3	E942.1	E950.4	E962.0	E980.4
Gitoxin	972.1	E858.3	E942.1	E950.4	E962.0	E980.4
Glandular extract (medicinal) **NEC**	977.9	E858.9	E947.9	E950.5	E962.0	E980.5
Glaucarubin	961.5	E857	E931.5	E950.4	E962.0	E980.4
Globin zinc insulin	962.3	E858.0	E932.3	E950.4	E962.0	E980.4
Glucagon	962.3	E858.0	E932.3	E950.4	E962.0	E980.4
Glucochloral	967.1	E852.0	E937.1	E950.2	E962.0	E980.2
Glucocorticoids	962.0	E858.0	E932.0	E950.4	E962.0	E980.4
Glucose	974.5	E858.5	E944.5	E950.4	E962.0	E980.4
oxidase reagent	977.8	E858.8	E947.8	E950.4	E962.0	E980.4
Glucosulfone sodium	961.8	E857	E931.8	E950.4	E962.0	E980.4
Glue(s)	989.89	E866.6	-	E950.9	E962.1	E980.9
Glutamic acid (hydrochloride)	973.4	E858.4	E943.4	E950.4	E962.0	E980.4
Glutalhione	963.8	E858.1	E933.8	E950.4	E962.0	E980.4
Glutaraldehyde	989.89	E861.4	-	E950.9	E962.1	E980.9
Glutethimide (group)	967.5	E852.4	E937.5	E950.2	E962.0	E980.2
Glycerin (lotion)	976.3	E858.7	E946.3	E950.4	E962.0	E980.4
Glycerol (topical)	976.3	E858.7	E946.3	E950.4	E962.0	E980.4
Glyceryl						
gualacolate	975.5	E858.6	E945.5	E950.4	E962.0	E980.4
triacetate (topical)	976.0	E858.7	E946.0	E950.4	E962.0	E980.4
trinitrate	972.4	E858.3	E942.4	E950.4	E962.0	E980.4
Glycine	974.5	E858.5	E944.5	E950.4	E962.0	E980.4
Glycobiarsol	961.1	E857	E931.1	E950.4	E962.0	E980.4
Glycols (ether)	982.8	E862.4	-	E950.9	E962.1	E980.9

Drug	Poisoning	External Cause (E-Code) Accident	Therapeutic Use	Suicide Attempt	Assault	Undetermined
Glycopyrrolate	971.1	E855.4	E941.1	E950.4	E962.0	E980.4
Glymidine	962.3	E858.0	E932.3	E950.4	E962.0	E980.4
Gold (compounds) (salts)	965.69	E850.6	E935.6	E950.0	E962.0	E980.0
Golden sulfide of antimony	985.4	E866.2	-	E950.9	E962.1	E980.9
Goldylocks	988.2	E865.4	-	E950.9	E962.1	E980.9
Gonadal tissue extract	962.9	E858.0	E932.9	E950.4	E962.0	E980.4
female	962.2	E858.0	E932.2	E950.4	E962.0	E980.4
male	962.1	E858.0	E932.1	E950.4	E962.0	E980.4
Gonadotropin	962.4	E858.0	E932.4	E950.4	E962.0	E980.4
Grain alcohol	980.0	E860.1	-	E950.9	E962.1	E980.9
beverage	980.0	E860.0	-	E950.9	E962.1	E980.9
Gramicidin	960.8	E856	E930.8	E950.4	E962.0	E980.4
Gratiola officinalis	988.2	E865.4	-	E950.9	E962.1	E980.9
Grease	989.89	E866.8	-	E950.9	E962.1	E980.9
Green hellebore	988.2	E865.4	-	E950.9	E962.1	E980.9
Green soap	976.2	E858.7	E946.2	E950.4	E962.0	E980.4
Grifulvin	960.1	E856	E930.1	E950.4	E962.0	E980.4
Griseofulvin	960.1	E856	E930.1	E950.4	E962.0	E980.4
Growth hormone	962.4	E858.0	E932.4	E950.4	E962.0	E980.4
Guaiacol	975.5	E858.6	E945.5	E950.4	E962.0	E980.4
Giuaiac reagent	977.8	E858.8	E947.8	E950.4	E962.0	E980.4
Guaifenesin	975.5	E858.6	E945.5	E950.4	E962.0	E980.4
Guaiphenesin	975.5	E858.6	E945.5	E950.4	E962.0	E980.4
Guanatol	961.4	E857	E931.4	E950.4	E962.0	E980.4
Guanethidine	972.6	E858.3	E942.6	E950.4	E962.0	E980.4
Guano	989.89	E866.5	-	E950.9	E962.1	E980.9
Guanochlor	972.6	E858.3	E942.6	E950.4	E962.0	E980.4
Guanoctine	972.6	E858.3	E942.6	E950.4	E962.0	E980.4
Guanoxan	972.6	E858.3	E942.6	E950.4	E962.0	E980.4
Hair treatment agent NEC	976.4	E858.7	E946.4	E950.4	E962.0	E980.4
Halcinonide	976.0	E858.7	E946.0	E950.4	E962.0	E980.4
Halethazole	976.0	E858.7	E946.0	E950.4	E962.0	E980.4
Hallucinogens	969.6	E854.1	E939.6	E950.3	E962.0	E980.3
Haloperidol	969.2	E853.1	E939.2	E950.3	E962.0	E980.3
Haloprogin	976.0	E858.7	E946.0	E950.4	E962.0	E980.4
Halotex	976.0	E858.7	E946.0	E950.4	E962.0	E980.4
Halothane	968.1	E855.1	E938.1	E950.4	E962.0	E980.4
Halquinols	976.0	E858.7	E946.0	E950.4	E962.0	E980.4
Harmonyl	972.6	E858.3	E942.6	E950.4	E962.0	E980.4
Hartmann's solution	974.5	E858.5	E944.5	E950.4	E962.0	E980.4
Hashish	969.6	E854.1	E939.6	E950.3	E962.0	E980.3
Hawaiian wood rose seeds	969.6	E854.1	E939.6	E950.3	E962.0	E980.3
Headache cures, drugs, powders NEC	977.9	E858.9	E947.9	E950.5	E962.0	E980.9
Heavenly Blue (morning glory)	969.6	E854.1	E939.6	E950.3	E962.0	E980.3
Heavy metal antagonists	963.8	E858.1	E933.8	E950.4	E962.0	E980.4
anti-infectives	961.2	E857	E931.2	E950.4	E962.0	E980.4
Hedaquinium	976.0	E858.7	E946.0	E950.4	E962.0	E980.4
Hedge hyssop	988.2	E865.4	-	E950.9	E962.1	E980.9
Heet	976.8	E858.7	E946.8	E950.4	E962.0	E980.4
Helenin	961.6	E857	E931.6	E950.4	E962.0	E980.4
Hellebore (black) (green) (white)	988.2	E865.4	-	E950.9	E962.1	E980.9
Hemlock	988.2	E865.4	-	E950.9	E962.1	E980.9
Hemostatics	964.5	E858.2	E934.5	E950.4	E962.0	E980.4
capillary active drugs	972.8	E858.3	E942.8	E950.4	E962.0	E980.4
Henbane	988.2	E865.4	-	E950.9	E962.1	E980.9
Heparin (sodium)	964.2	E858.2	E934.2	E950.4	E962.0	E980.4
Heptabarbital, heptabarbitone	967.0	E851	E937.0	E950.1	E962.0	E980.1
Heptachlor	989.2	E863.0	-	E950.6	E962.1	E980.7
Heptalgin	965.09	E850.2	E935.2	E950.0	E962.0	E980.0
Herbicides	989.4	E863.5	-	E950.6	E962.1	E980.7

● New Line ▲ Revised Code

		External Cause (E-Code)				
Drug	**Poisoning**	**Accident**	**Therapeutic Use**	**Suicide Attempt**	**Assault**	**Undetermined**
Heroin	965.01	E850.0	E935.0	E950.0	E962.0	E980.0
Herplex	976.5	E858.7	E946.5	E950.4	E962.0	E980.4
HES	964.8	E858.2	E934.8	E950.4	E962.0	E980.4
Hetastarch	964.8	E858.2	E934.8	E950.4	E962.0	E980.4
Hexachlorocyclohexane	989.2	E863.0	-	E950.6	E962.1	E980.7
Hexachlorophene	976.2	E858.7	E946.2	E950.4	E962.0	E980.4
Hexadimethrine (bromide)	964.5	E858.2	E934.5	E950.4	E962.0	E980.4
Hexanuorenium	975.2	E858.6	E945.2	E950.4	E962.0	E980.4
Hexa-germ	976.2	E858.7	E946.2	E950.4	E962.0	E980.4
Hexahydrophenol	980.8	E860.8	-	E950.9	E962.1	E980.9
Hexalin	980.8	E860.8	-	E950.9	E962.1	E980.9
Hexamethonium	972.3	E858.3	E942.3	E950.4	E962.0	E980.4
Hexamethyleneamine	961.9	E857	E931.9	E950.4	E962.0	E980.4
Hexamine	961.9	E857	E931.9	E950.4	E962.0	E980.4
Hexanone	982.8	E862.4	-	E950.9	E962.1	E980.9
Hexapropymate	967.8	E852.8	E937.8	E950.2	E962.0	E980.2
Hexestrol	962.2	E858.0	E932.2	E950.4	E962.0	E980.4
Hexethal (sodium)	967.0	E851	E937.0	E950.1	E962.0	E980.1
Hexetidine	976.0	E858.7	E946.0	E950.4	E962.0	E980.4
Hexobarbital, hexobarbitone	967.0	E851	E937.0	E950.1	E962.0	E980.1
sodium (anesthetic)	968.3	E855.1	E938.3	E950.4	E962.0	E980.4
soluble	968.3	E855.1	E938.3	E950.4	E962.0	E980.4
Hexocyclium	971.1	E855.4	E941.1	E950.4	E962.0	E980.4
Hexoestrol	962.2	E858.0	E932.2	E950.4	E962.0	E980.4
Hexone	982.8	E862.4	-	E950.9	E962.1	E980.9
Hexylcaine	968.5	E855.2	E938.5	E950.4	E962.0	E980.4
Hexylresorcinol	961.6	E857	E931.6	E950.4	E962.0	E980.4
Hinkle's pills	973.1	E858.4	E943.1	E950.4	E962.0	E980.4
Histalog	977.8	E858.8	E947.8	E950.4	E962.0	E980.4
Histamine (phosphate)	972.5	E858.3	E942.5	E950.4	E962.0	E980.4
Histoplasmin	977.8	E858.8	E947.8	E950.4	E962.0	E980.4
Holly berries	988.2	E865.3	-	E950.9	E962.1	E980.9
Homatropine	971.1	E855.4	E941.1	E950.4	E962.0	E980.4
Homo-tet	964.6	E858.2	E934.6	E950.4	E962.0	E980.4
Hormones (synthetic substitute) NEC	962.9	E858.0	E932.9	E950.4	E962.0	E980.4
adrenal cortical steroids	962.0	E858.0	E932.0	E950.4	E962.0	E980.4
antidiabetic agents	962.3	E858.0	E932.3	E950.4	E962.0	E980.4
follicle stimulating	962.4	E858.0	E932.4	E950.4	E962.0	E980.4
gonadotropic	962.4	E858.0	E932.4	E950.4	E962.0	E980.4
growth	962.4	E858.0	E932.4	E950.4	E962.0	E980.4
ovarian (substitutes)	962.2	E858.0	E932.2	E950.4	E962.0	E980.4
parathyroid (derivatives)	962.6	E858.0	E932.6	E950.4	E962.0	E980.4
pituitary (posterior)	962.5	E858.0	E932.5	E950.4	E962.0	E980.4
anterior	962.4	E858.0	E932.4	E950.4	E962.0	E980.4
thyroid (derivative)	962.7	E858.0	E932.7	E950.4	E962.0	E980.4
Hornet (sting)	989.5	E905.3	-	E950.9	E962.1	E980.9
Horticulture agent NEC	989.4	E863.9	-	E950.6	E962.1	E980.7
Hyaluronidase	963.4	E858.1	E933.4	E950.4	E962.0	E980.4
Hyazyme	963.4	E858.1	E933.4	E950.4	E962.0	E980.4
Hycodan	965.09	E850.2	E935.2	E950.0	E962.0	E980.0
Hydantoin derivatives	966.1	E855.0	E936.1	E950.4	E962.0	E980.4
Hydeltra	962.0	E858.0	E932.0	E950.4	E962.0	E980.4
Hydergine	971.3	E855.6	E941.3	E950.4	E962.0	E980.4
Hydrabamine penicillin	960.0	E856	E930.0	E950.4	E962.0	E980.4
Hydralazine, hydrallazine	972.6	E858.3	E942.6	E950.4	E962.0	E980.4
Hydrargaphen	976.0	E858.7	E946.0	E950.4	E962.0	E980.4
Hydrazine	983.9	E864.3	-	E950.7	E962.1	E980.6
Hydriodic acid	975.5	E858.6	E945.5	E950.4	E962.0	E980.4
Hydrocarbon gas	987.1	E869.8	-	E952.8	E962.2	E982.8
incomplete combustion of – *see* Carbon, monoxide, fuel, utility						
Hydrocarbon gas – *continued*						
liquefied (mobile container)	987.0	E868.0	-	E951.1	E962.2	E981.1
piped (natural)	987.0	E867	-	E951.0	E962.2	E981.0
Hydrochloric acid (liquid)	983.1	E864.1	-	E950.7	E962.1	E980.6
medicinal	973.4	E858.4	E943.4	E950.4	E962.0	E980.4
vapor	987.8	E869.8	-	E952.8	E962.2	E982.8
Hydrochlorothiazide	974.3	E858.5	E944.3	E950.4	E962.0	E980.4
Hydrocodone	965.09	E850.2	E935.2	E950.0	E962.0	E980.0
Hydrocortisone	962.0	E858.0	E932.0	E950.4	E962.0	E980.4
ENT agent	976.6	E858.7	E946.6	E950.4	E962.0	E980.4
ophthalmic preparation	976.5	E858.7	E946.5	E950.4	E962.0	E980.4
topical NEC	976.0	E858.7	E946.0	E950.4	E962.0	E980.4
Hydrocortone	962.0	E858.0	E932.0	E950.4	E962.0	E980.4
ENT agent	976.6	E858.7	E946.6	E950.4	E962.0	E980.4
ophthalmic preparation	976.5	E858.7	E946.5	E950.4	E962.0	E980.4
topical NEC	976.0	E858.7	E946.0	E950.4	E962.0	E980.4
Hydrocyanic acid – *see* Cyanide(s)						
Hydroflumethiazide	974.3	E858.5	E944.3	E950.4	E962.0	E980.4
Hydrofuoric acid (liquid)	983.1	E864.1	-	E950.7	E962.1	E980.6
vapor	987.8	E869.8	-	E952.8	E962.2	E982.8
Hydrogen	987.8	E869.8	-	E952.8	E962.2	E982.8
arsenide	985.1	E866.3	-	E950.8	E962.1	E980.8
arseniureted	985.1	E866.3	-	E950.8	E962.1	E980.8
cyanide (salts)	989.0	E866.8	-	E950.9	E962.1	E980.9
gas	987.7	E869.8	-	E952.8	E962.2	E982.8
fluoride (liquid)	983.1	E864.1	-	E950.7	E962.1	E980.6
vapor	987.8	E869.8	-	E952.8	E962.2	E982.8
peroxide (solution)	976.6	E858.7	E946.6	E950.4	E962.0	E980.4
phosphureted	987.8	E869.8	-	E952.8	E962.2	E982.8
sulfide (gas)	987.8	E869.8	-	E952.8	E962.2	E982.8
arseniureted	985.1	E866.3	-	E950.8	E962.1	E980.8
sulfureted	987.8	E869.8	-	E952.8	E962.2	E982.8
Hydromorphinol	965.09	E850.2	E935.2	E950.0	E962.0	E980.0
Hydromorphinone	965.09	E850.2	E935.2	E950.0	E962.0	E980.0
Hydromorphone	965.09	E850.2	E935.2	E950.0	E962.0	E980.0
Hydromox	974.3	E858.5	E944.3	E950.4	E962.0	E980.4
Hydrophilic lotion	976.3	E858.7	E946.3	E950.4	E962.0	E980.4
Hydroquinone	983.0	E864.0	-	E950.7	E962.1	E980.6
vapor	987.8	E869.8	-	E952.8	E962.2	E982.8
Hydrosulfuric acid (gas)	987.8	E869.8	-	E952.8	E962.2	E982.8
Hydrous wool fat (lotion)	976.3	E858.7	E946.3	E950.4	E962.0	E980.4
Hydroxide, caustic	983.2	E864.2	-	E950.7	E962.1	E980.6
Hydroxocobalamin	964.1	E858.2	E934.1	E950.4	E962.0	E980.4
Hydroxyamphetamine	971.2	E858.5	E941.2	E950.4	E962.0	E980.4
Hydroxychloroquine	961.4	E857	E931.4	E950.4	E962.0	E980.4
Hydroxydihydrocodeinone	965.09	E850.2	E935.2	E950.0	E962.0	E980.0
Hydroxyethyl starch	964.8	E858.2	E934.8	E950.4	E962.0	E980.4
Hydroxyphenamate	969.5	E853.8	E939.5	E950.3	E962.0	E980.3
Hydroxyphenylbutazone	965.5	E850.5	E935.5	E950.0	E962.0	E980.0
Hvdroxyprogesterone	962.2	E858.0	E932.2	E950.4	E962.0	E980.4
Hydroxyquinoline derivatives	961.3	E857	E931.3	E950.4	E962.0	E980.4
Hydroxystilbamidine	961.5	E857	E931.5	E950.4	E962.0	E980.4
Hydroxyurea	963.1	E858.1	E933.1	E950.4	E962.0	E980.4
Hydroxyzine	969.5	E853.8	E939.5	E950.3	E962.0	E980.3
Hyoscine (hydrobromide)	971.1	E855.4	E941.1	E950.4	E962.0	E980.4
Hyoscyamine	971.1	E855.4	E941.1	E950.4	E962.0	E980.4
Hyoscyamus (albus) (niger)	988.2	E865.4	-	E950.9	E962.1	E980.9
Hypaque	977.8	E858.8	E947.8	E950.4	E962.0	E980.4
Hypertussis	964.6	E858.2	E934.6	E950.4	E962.0	E980.4
Hypnotics NEC	967.9	E852.9	E937.9	E950.2	E962.0	E980.2

● New Line ▲ Revised Code

Drug	Poisoning	External Cause (E-Code) Accident	Therapeutic Use	Suicide Attempt	Assault	Undetermined
Hypochlorites – *see* Sodium, hypochlorite						
Hypotensive agents NEC	972.6	E858.3	E942.6	E950.4	E962.0	E980.4
Ibufenac	965.69	E850.6	E935.6	E950.0	E962.0	E980.0
Ibuprofen	965.61	E850.6	E935.6	E950.0	E962.0	E980.0
ICG	977.8	E858.8	E947.8	E950.4	E962.0	E980.4
Ichthammol	976.4	E858.7	E946.4	E950.4	E962.0	E980.4
Ichthyol	976.4	E858.7	E946.4	E950.4	E962.0	E980.4
Idoxuridine	976.5	E858.7	E946.5	E950.4	E962.0	E980.4
IDU	976.5	E858.7	E946.5	E950.4	E962.0	E980.4
Iletin	962.3	E858.0	E932.3	E950.4	E962.0	E980.4
Ilex	988.2	E865.4	-	E950.9	E962.1	E980.9
Illuminating gas – *see* Gas, utility						
Ilopan	963.5	E858.1	E933.5	E950.4	E962.0	E980.4
Ilotycin	960.3	E856	E930.3	E950.4	E962.0	E980.4
ophthalmic preparation	976.5	E858.7	E946.5	E950.4	E962.0	E980.4
topical NEC	976.0	E858.7	E946.0	E950.4	E962.0	E980.4
Imipramine	969.0	E854.0	E939.0	E950.3	E962.0	E980.3
Immu-G	964.6	E858.2	E934.6	E950.4	E962.0	E980.4
Immuglobin	964.6	E858.2	E934.6	E950.4	E962.0	E980.4
Immune serum globulin	964.6	E858.2	E934.6	E950.4	E962.0	E980.4
Immunosuppressive agents	963.1	E858.1	E933.1	E950.4	E962.0	E980.4
Immu-tetanus	964.6	E858.2	E934.6	E950.4	E962.0	E980.4
Indandione (derivatives)	964.2	E858.2	E934.2	E950.4	E962.0	E980.4
Inderal	972.0	E858.3	E942.0	E950.4	E962.0	E980.4
Indian						
hemp	969.6	E854.1	E939.6	E950.3	E962.0	E980.3
tobacco	988.2	E865.4	-	E950.9	E962.1	E980.9
Indigo carmine	977.8	E858.8	E947.8	E950.4	E962.0	E980.4
Indocin	965.69	E850.6	E935.6	E950.0	E962.0	E980.0
Indocyanine green	977.8	E858.8	E947.8	E950.4	E962.0	E980.4
Indomethacin	965.69	E850.6	E935.6	E950.0	E962.0	E980.0
Industrial						
alcohol	980.9	E860.9	-	E950.9	E962.1	E980.9
fumes	987.8	E869.8	-	E952.8	E962.2	E982.8
solvents (fumes) (vapors)	982.8	E862.9	-	E950.9	E962.1	E980.9
Influenza vaccine	979.6	E858.8	E949.6	E950.4	E962.0	E982.8
Ingested substances NEC	989.9	E866.9	-	E950.9	E962.1	E980.9
INH (isoniazid)	961.8	E857	E931.8	E950.4	E962.0	E980.4
Inhalation, gas (noxious) – *see* Gas						
Ink	989.89	E866.8	-	E950.9	E962.1	E980.9
Innovar	967.6	E852.5	E937.6	E950.2	E962.0	E980.2
Inositol niacinate	972.2	E858.3	E942.2	E950.4	E962.0	E980.4
Inproquone	963.1	E858.1	E933.1	E950.4	E962.0	E980.4
Insect (sting), **venomous**	989.5	E905.5	-	E950.9	E962.1	E980.9
Insecticides (*see also* Pesticides)	989.4	E863.4	-	E950.6	E962.1	E980.7
chlorinated	989.2	E863.0	-	E950.6	E962.1	E980.7
mixtures	989.4	E863.3	-	E950.6	E962.1	E980.7
organochlorine (compounds)	989.2	E863.0	-	E950.6	E962.1	E980.7
organophosphorus (compounds)	989.3	E863.1	-	E950.6	E962.1	E980.7
Insular tissue extract	962.3	E858.0	E932.3	E950.4	E962.0	E980.4
Insulin (amorphous) (globin) (isophane) (Lente) (NPH) (prolamine) (Semilente) (Ultralente) (zinc)	962.3	E858.0	E932.3	E950.4	E962.0	E980.4
Intranarcon	968.3	E855.1	E938.3	E950.4	E962.0	E980.4
Inulin	977.8	E858.8	E947.8	E950.4	E962.0	E980.4
Invert sugar	974.5	E858.5	E944.5	E950.4	E962.0	E980.4
Inza – *see* Naproxen						

Drug	Poisoning	External Cause (E-Code) Accident	Therapeutic Use	Suicide Attempt	Assault	Undetermined
Iodide NEC (*see also* Iodine)	976.0	E858.7	E946.0	E950.4	E962.0	E980.4
mercury (ointment)	976.0	E858.7	E946.0	E950.4	E962.0	E980.4
methylate	976.0	E858.7	E946.0	E950.4	E962.0	E980.4
potassium (expectorant) NEC	975.5	E858.6	E945.5	E950.4	E962.0	E980.4
Iodinated glycerol	975.5	E858.6	E945.5	E950.4	E962.0	E980.4
Iodine (antiseptic, external) (tincture) NEC	976.0	E858.7	E946.0	E950.4	E962.0	E980.4
diagnostic	977.8	E858.8	E947.8	E950.4	E962.0	E980.4
for thyroid conditions (antithyroid)	962.8	E858.0	E932.8	E950.4	E962.0	E980.4
vapor	987.8	E869.8	-	E952.8	E962.2	E982.8
Iodized oil	977.8	E858.8	E947.8	E950.4	E962.0	E980.4
Iodobismitol	961.2	E857	E931.2	E950.4	E962.0	E980.4
Iodochlorhydroxyquin	961.3	E857	E931.3	E950.4	E962.0	E980.4
topical	976.0	E858.7	E946.0	E950.4	E962.0	E980.4
Iodoform	976.0	E858.7	E946.0	E950.4	E962.0	E980.4
Iodopanoic acid	977.8	E858.8	E947.8	E950.4	E962.0	E980.4
Iodophthalein	977.8	E858.8	E947.8	E950.4	E962.0	E980.4
Ion exchange resins	974.5	E858.5	E944.5	E950.4	E962.0	E980.4
Iopanoic acid	977.8	E858.8	E947.8	E950.4	E962.0	E980.4
Iophendylate	977.8	E858.8	E947.8	E950.4	E962.0	E980.4
Iothiouracil	962.8	E858.0	E932.8	E950.4	E962.0	E980.4
Ipecac	973.6	E858.4	E943.6	E950.4	E962.0	E980.4
Ipecacuanha	973.6	E858.4	E943.6	E950.4	E962.0	E980.4
Ipodate	977.8	E858.8	E947.8	E950.4	E962.0	E980.4
Ipral	967.0	E851	E937.0	E950.1	E962.0	E980.1
Ipratropium	975.1	E858.6	E945.1	E950.4	E962.0	E980.4
Iproniazid	969.0	E854.0	E939.0	E950.3	E962.0	E980.3
Iron (compounds) (medicinal) (preparations)	964.0	E858.2	E934.0	E950.4	E962.0	E980.4
dextran	964.0	E858.2	E934.0	E950.4	E962.0	E980.4
nonmedicinal (dust) (fumes) NEC	985.8	E866.4	-	E950.9	E962.1	E980.9
Irritant drug	977.9	E858.9	E947.9	E950.5	E962.0	E980.5
Ismelin	972.6	E858.3	E942.6	E950.4	E962.0	E980.4
Isoamyl nitrite	972.4	E858.3	E942.4	E950.4	E962.0	E980.4
Isobutyl acetate	982.8	E862.4	-	E950.9	E962.1	E980.9
Isocarboxazid	969.0	E854.0	E939.0	E950.3	E962.0	E980.3
Isoephedrine	971.2	E855.5	E941.2	E950.4	E962.0	E980.4
Isoetharine	971.2	E855.5	E941.2	E950.4	E962.0	E980.4
Isofluorophate	971.0	E855.3	E941.0	E950.4	E962.0	E980.4
Isoniazid (INH)	961.8	E857	E931.8	E950.4	E962.0	E980.4
Isopentaquine	961.4	E857	E931.4	E950.4	E962.0	E980.4
Isophane insulin	962.3	E858.0	E932.3	E950.4	E962.0	E980.4
Isopregnenone	962.2	E858.0	E932.2	E950.4	E962.0	E980.4
Isoprenaline	971.2	E855.5	E941.2	E950.4	E962.0	E980.4
Isopropamide	971.1	E855.4	E941.1	E950.4	E962.0	E980.4
Isopropanol	980.2	E860.3	-	E950.9	E962.1	E980.9
topical (germicide)	976.0	E858.7	E946.0	E950.4	E962.0	E980.4
Isopropyl						
acetate	982.8	E862.4	-	E950.9	E962.1	E980.9
alcohol	980.2	E860.3	-	E950.9	E962.1	E980.9
topical (germicide)	976.0	E858.7	E946.0	E950.4	E962.0	E980.4
ether	982.8	E862.4	-	E950.9	E962.1	E980.9
Isoproterenol	971.2	E855.5	E941.2	E950.4	E962.0	E980.4
Isosorbide dinitrate	972.4	E858.3	E942.4	E950.4	E962.0	E980.4
Isothipendyl	963.0	E858.1	E933.0	E950.4	E962.0	E980.4
Isoxazolyl penicillin	960.0	E856	E930.0	E950.4	E962.0	E980.4
Isoxsuprine hydrochloride	972.5	E858.3	E942.5	E950.4	E962.0	E980.4
I-thyroxine sodium	962.7	E858.0	E932.7	E950.4	E962.0	E980.4
Jaborandi (pilocarpus) (extract)	971.0	E855.3	E941.0	E950.4	E962.0	E980.4

● New Line ▲ Revised Code

		External Cause (E-Code)				
Drug	**Poisoning**	**Accident**	**Therapeutic Use**	**Suicide Attempt**	**Assault**	**Undetermined**
Jalap	973.1	E858.4	E943.1	E950.4	E962.0	E980.4
Jamaica						
dogwood (bark)	965.7	E850.7	E935.7	E950.0	E962.0	E980.0
ginger	989.89	E866.8	-	E950.9	E962.1	E980.9
Jatropha	988.2	E865.4	-	E950.9	E962.1	E980.9
curcas	988.2	E865.3	-	E950.9	E962.1	E980.9
Jectofer	964.0	E858.2	E934.0	E950.4	E962.0	E980.4
Jellyfish (sting)	989.5	E905.6	-	E950.9	E962.1	E980.9
Jequirity (bean)	988.2	E865.3	-	E950.9	E962.1	E980.9
Jimson weed	988.2	E865.4	-	E950.9	E962.1	E980.9
seeds	988.2	E865.3	-	E950.9	E962.1	E980.9
Juniper tar (oil) (ointment)	976.4	E858.7	E946.4	E950.4	E962.0	E980.4
Kallikrein	972.5	E858.3	E942.5	E950.4	E962.0	E980.4
Kanamycin	960.6	E856	E930.6	E950.4	E962.0	E980.4
Kantrex	960.6	E856	E930.6	E950.4	E962.0	E980.4
Kaolin	973.5	E858.4	E943.5	E950.4	E962.0	E980.4
Karaya (gum)	973.3	E858.4	E943.3	E950.4	E962.0	E980.4
Kemithal	968.3	E855.1	E938.3	E950.4	E962.0	E980.4
Kenacort	962.0	E858.0	E932.0	E950.4	E962.0	E980.4
Keratolytics	976.4	E858.7	E946.4	E950.4	E962.0	E980.4
Keratoplastics	976.4	E858.7	E946.4	E950.4	E962.0	E980.4
Kerosene, kerosine (fuel) (solvent) NEC	981	E862.1	-	E950.9	E962.1	E980.9
insecticide	981	E863.4	-	E950.6	E962.1	E980.7
vapor	987.1	E869.8	-	E952.8	E962.2	E982.8
Ketamine	968.3	E855.1	E938.3	E950.4	E962.0	E980.4
Ketobemidone	965.09	E850.2	E935.2	E950.0	E962.0	E980.0
Ketols	982.8	E862.4	-	E950.9	E962.1	E980.9
Ketone oils	982.8	E862.4	-	E950.9	E962.1	E980.9
Ketoprofen	965.61	E850.6	E935.6	E950.0	E962.0	E980.0
Kiln gas or vapor (carbon monoxide)	986	E868.8	-	E952.1	E962.2	E982.1
Konsyl	973.3	E858.4	E943.3	E950.4	E962.0	E980.4
Kosam seed	988.2	E865.3	-	E950.9	E962.1	E980.9
Krait (venom)	989.5	E905.0	-	E950.9	E962.1	E980.9
Kwell (insecticide)	989.2	E863.0	-	E950.6	E962.1	E980.7
anti-infective (topical)	976.0	E858.7	E946.0	E950.4	E962.0	E980.4
Laburnum (flowers) (seeds)	988.2	E865.3	-	E950.9	E962.1	E980.9
leaves	988.2	E865.4	-	E950.9	E962.1	E980.9
Lacquers	989.89	E861.6	-	E950.9	E962.1	E980.9
Lacrimogenic gas	987.5	E869.3	-	E952.8	E962.2	E982.8
Lactic acid	983.1	E864.1	-	E950.7	E962.1	E980.6
Lactobacillus acidophilus	973.5	E858.4	E943.5	E950.4	E962.0	E980.4
Lactoflavin	963.5	E858.1	E933.5	E950.4	E962.0	E980.4
Lactuca (virosa) (extract)	967.8	E852.8	E937.8	E950.2	E962.0	E980.2
Lactucarium	967.8	E852.8	E937.8	E950.2	E962.0	E980.2
Laevulose	974.5	E858.5	E944.5	E950.4	E962.0	E980.4
Lanatoside (C)	972.1	E858.3	E942.1	E950.4	E962.0	E980.4
Lanolin (lotion)	976.3	E858.7	E946.3	E950.4	E962.0	E980.4
Largactil	969.1	E853.0	E939.1	E950.3	E962.0	E980.3
Larkspur	988.2	E865.3	-	E950.9	E962.1	E980.9
Laroxyl	969.0	E854.0	E939.0	E950.3	E962.0	E980.3
Lasix	974.4	E858.5	E944.4	E950.4	E962.0	E980.4
Latex	989.82	E866.8	-	E950.9	E962.1	E980.9
Lathyrus (seed)	988.2	E865.3	-	E950.9	E962.1	E980.9
Laudanum	965.09	E850.2	E935.2	E950.0	E962.0	E980.0
Laudexium	975.2	E858.6	E945.2	E950.4	E962.0	E980.4
Laurel, black or cherry	988.2	E865.4	-	E950.9	E962.1	E980.9
Laurolinium	976.0	E858.7	E946.0	E950.4	E962.0	E980.4
Lauryl sulfoacetate	976.2	E858.7	E946.2	E950.4	E962.0	E980.4
Laxatives NEC	973.3	E858.4	E943.3	E950.4	E962.0	E980.4
emollient	973.2	E858.4	E943.2	E950.4	E962.0	E980.4
L-dopa	966.4	E855.0	E936.4	E950.4	E962.0	E980.4

		External Cause (E-Code)				
Drug	**Poisoning**	**Accident**	**Therapeutic Use**	**Suicide Attempt**	**Assault**	**Undetermined**
L-Tryptophan – *see* amino acid						
Lead (dust) (fumes) (vapor) NEC	984.9	E866.0	-	E950.9	E962.1	E980.9
acetate (dust)	984.1	E866.0	-	E950.9	E962.1	E980.9
anti-infectives	961.2	E857	E931.2	E950.4	E962.0	E980.4
antiknock compound (tetraethyl)	984.1	E862.1	-	E950.9	E962.1	E980.9
arsenate, arsenite (dust) (insecticide) (vapor)	985.1	E863.4	-	E950.8	E962.1	E980.8
herbicide	985.1	E863.5	-	E950.8	E962.1	E980.8
carbonate	984.0	E866.0	-	E950.9	E962.1	E980.9
paint	984.0	E861.5	-	E950.9	E962.1	E980.9
chromate	984.0	E866.0	-	E950.9	E962.1	E980.9
paint	984.0	E861.5	-	E950.9	E962.1	E980.9
dioxide	984.0	E866.0	-	E950.9	E962.1	E980.9
inorganic (compound)	984.0	E866.0	-	E950.9	E962.1	E980.9
paint	984.0	E861.5	-	E950.9	E962.1	E980.9
iodide	984.0	E866.0	-	E950.9	E962.1	E980.9
pigment (paint)	984.0	E861.5	-	E950.9	E962.1	E980.9
monoxide (dust)	984.0	E866.0	-	E950.9	E962.1	E980.9
paint	984.0	E861.5	-	E950.9	E962.1	E980.9
organic	984.1	E866.0	-	E950.9	E962.1	E980.9
oxide	984.0	E866.0	-	E950.9	E962.1	E980.9
paint	984.0	E861.5	-	E950.9	E962.1	E980.9
paint	984.0	E861.5	-	E950.9	E962.1	E980.9
salts	984.0	E866.0	-	E950.9	E962.1	E980.9
specified compound NEC	984.8	E866.0	-	E950.9	E962.1	E980.9
tetra-ethyl	984.1	E862.1	-	E950.9	E962.1	E980.9
Lebanese red	969.6	E854.1	E939.6	E950.3	E962.0	E980.3
Lente Iletin (insulin)	962.3	E858.0	E932.3	E950.4	E962.0	E980.4
Leptazol	970.0	E854.3	E940.0	E950.4	E962.0	E980.4
Leritine	965.09	E850.2	E935.2	E950.0	E962.0	E980.0
Letter	962.7	E858.0	E932.7	E950.4	E962.0	E980.4
Lettuce opium	967.8	E852.8	E937.8	E950.2	E962.0	E980.2
Leucovorin (factor)	964.1	E858.2	E934.1	E950.4	E962.0	E980.4
Leukeran	963.1	E858.1	E933.1	E950.4	E962.0	E980.4
Levalbuterol	975.7	E858.6	E945.7	E950.4	E962.0	E980.4
Levallorphan	970.1	E854.3	E940.1	E950.4	E962.0	E980.4
Levanil	967.8	E852.8	E937.8	E950.2	E962.0	E980.2
Levarterenol	971.2	E855.5	E941.2	E950.4	E962.0	E980.4
Levodopa	966.4	E855.0	E936.4	E950.4	E962.0	E980.4
Levo-dromoran	965.09	E850.2	E935.2	E950.0	E962.0	E980.0
Levoid	962.7	E858.0	E932.7	E950.4	E962.0	E980.4
Levo-iso-methadone	965.02	E850.1	E935.1	E950.0	E962.0	E980.0
Levomepromazine	967.8	E852.8	E937.8	E950.2	E962.0	E980.2
Levoprome	967.8	E852.8	E937.8	E950.2	E962.0	E980.2
Levopropoxyphene	975.4	E858.6	E945.4	E950.4	E962.0	E980.4
Levorphan, levophanol	965.09	E850.2	E935.2	E950.0	E962.0	E980.0
Levothyroxine (sodium)	962.7	E858.0	E932.7	E950.4	E962.0	E980.4
Levsin	971.1	E855.4	E941.1	E950.4	E962.0	E980.4
Levulose	974.5	E858.5	E944.5	E950.4	E962.0	E980.4
Lewisite (gas)	985.1	E866.3	-	E950.8	E962.1	E980.8
Librium	969.4	E853.2	E939.4	E950.3	E962.0	E980.3
Lidex	976.0	E858.7	E946.0	E950.4	E962.0	E980.4
Lidocaine (infiltration) (topical)	968.5	E855.2	E938.5	E950.4	E962.0	E980.4
nerve block (peripheral) (plexus)	968.6	E855.2	E938.6	E950.4	E962.0	E980.4
spinal	968.7	E855.2	E938.7	E950.4	E962.0	E980.4
Lighter fluid	981	E862.1	-	E950.9	E962.1	E980.9

		External Cause (E-Code)				
Drug	Poisoning	Accident	Therapeutic Use	Suicide Attempt	Assault	Undetermined
Lignocaine (infiltration) (topical)	968.5	E855.2	E938.5	E950.4	E962.0	E980.4
nerve block (peripheral) (plexus)	968.6	E855.2	E938.6	E950.4	E962.0	E980.4
spinal	968.7	E855.2	E938.7	E950.4	E962.0	E980.4
Ligroin(e) (solvent)	981	E862.0	-	E950.9	E962.1	E980.9
vapor	987.1	E869.8	-	E952.8	E962.2	E982.8
Ligustrum vulgare	988.2	E865.3	-	E950.9	E962.1	E980.9
Lily of the valley	988.2	E865.4	-	E950.9	E962.1	E980.9
Lime (chloride)	983.2	E864.2	-	E950.7	E962.1	E980.6
solution, sulferated	976.4	E858.7	E946.4	E950.4	E962.0	E980.4
Limonene	982.8	E862.4	-	E950.9	E962.1	E980.9
Lincomycin	960.8	E856	E930.8	E950.4	E962.0	E980.4
Lindane (insecticide) (vapor)	989.2	E863.0	-	E950.6	E962.1	E980.7
anti-infective (topical)	976.0	E858.7	E946.0	E950.4	E962.0	E980.4
Liniments NEC	976.9	E858.7	E946.9	E950.4	E962.0	E980.4
Linoleic acid	972.2	E858.3	E942.2	E950.4	E962.0	E980.4
Liothyronine	962.7	E858.0	E932.7	E950.4	E962.0	E980.4
Liotrix	962.7	E858.0	E932.7	E950.4	E962.0	E980.4
Lipancreatin	973.4	E858.4	E943.4	E950.4	E962.0	E980.4
Lipo-Lutin	962.2	E858.0	E932.2	E950.4	E962.0	E980.4
Lipotropic agents	977.1	E858.8	E947.1	E950.4	E962.0	E980.4
Liquefied petroleum gases	987.0	E868.0	-	E951.1	E962.2	E981.1
piped (pure or mixed with air)	987.0	E867	-	E951.0	E962.2	E981.0
Liquid petrolatum	973.2	E858.4	E943.2	E950.4	E962.0	E980.4
substance	989.9	E866.9	-	E950.9	E962.1	E980.9
specified NEC	989.89	E866.8	-	E950.9	E962.1	E980.9
Lirugen	979.4	E858.8	E949.4	E950.4	E962.0	E980.4
Lithane	969.8	E855.8	E939.8	E950.3	E962.0	E980.3
Lithium	985.8	E866.4	-	E950.9	E962.1	E980.9
carbonate	969.8	E855.8	E939.8	E950.3	E962.0	E980.3
Lithonate	969.8	E855.8	E939.8	E950.3	E962.0	E980.3
Liver (extract) (injection) (preparations)	964.1	E858.2	E934.1	E950.4	E962.0	E980.4
Lizard (bite) (venom)	989.5	E905.0	-	E950.9	E962.1	E980.9
LMD	964.8	E858.2	E934.8	E950.4	E962.0	E980.4
Lobelia	988.2	E865.4	-	E950.9	E962.1	E980.9
Lobeline	970.0	E854.3	E940.0	E950.4	E962.0	E980.4
Locorten	976.0	E858.7	E946.0	E950.4	E962.0	E980.4
Lolium temulentum	988.2	E865.3	-	E950.9	E962.1	E980.9
Lomotil	973.5	E858.4	E943.5	E950.4	E962.0	E980.4
Lomustine	963.1	E858.1	E933.1	E950.4	E962.0	E980.4
Lophophora williamsii	969.6	E854.1	E939.6	E950.3	E962.0	E980.3
Lorazepam	969.4	E853.2	E939.4	E950.3	E962.0	E980.3
Lotions NEC	976.9	E858.7	E946.9	E950.4	E962.0	E980.4
Lotronexl	973.8	E858.4	E943.8	E950.4	E962.0	E980.4
Lotusate	967.0	E851	E937.0	E950.1	E962.0	E980.1
Lowila	976.2	E858.7	E946.2	E950.4	E962.0	E980.4
Loxapine	969.3	E853.8	E939.3	E950.3	E962.0	E980.3
Lozenges (throat)	976.6	E858.7	E946.6	E950.4	E962.0	E980.4
LSD (25)	969.6	E854.1	E939.6	E950.3	E962.0	E980.3
Lubricating oil NEC	981	E862.2	-	E950.9	E962.1	E980.9
Lucanthone	961.6	E857	E931.6	E950.4	E962.0	E980.4
Luminal	967.0	E851	E937.0	E950.1	E962.0	E980.1
Lung irritant (gas) **NEC**	987.9	E869.9	-	E952.9	E962.2	E982.9
Lutocylol	962.2	E858.0	E932.2	E950.4	E962.0	E980.4
Lutromone	962.2	E858.0	E932.2	E950.4	E962.0	E980.4
Lututrin	975.0	E858.6	E945.0	E950.4	E962.0	E980.4
Lye (concentrated)	983.2	E864.2	-	E950.7	E962.1	E980.6
Lygranum (skin test)	977.8	E858.8	E947.8	E950.4	E962.0	E980.4
Lymecycline	960.4	E856	E930.4	E950.4	E962.0	E980.4
Lymphogranuloma venereum antigen	977.8	E858.8	E947.8	E950.4	E962.0	E980.4
Lynestrenol	962.2	E858.0	E932.2	E950.4	E962.0	E980.4
Lyovac Sodium Edecrin	974.4	E858.5	E944.4	E950.4	E962.0	E980.4
Lypressin	962.5	E858.0	E932.5	E950.4	E962.0	E980.4
Lysergic acid (amide) (diethylamide)	969.6	E854.1	E939.6	E950.3	E962.0	E980.3
Lysergide	969.6	E854.1	E939.6	E950.3	E962.0	E980.3
Lysine vasopressin	962.5	E858.0	E932.5	E950.4	E962.0	E980.4
Lysol	983.0	E864.0	-	E950.7	E962.1	E980.6
Lytta (vitatta)	976.8	E858.7	E946.8	E950.4	E962.0	E980.4
Mace	987.5	E869.3	-	E952.8	E962.2	E982.8
Macrolides (antibiotics)	960.3	E856	E930.3	E950.4	E962.0	E980.4
Mafenide	976.0	E858.7	E946.0	E950.4	E962.0	E980.4
Magaldrate	973.0	E858.4	E943.0	E950.4	E962.0	E980.4
Magic mushroom	969.6	E854.1	E939.6	E950.3	E962.0	E980.3
Magnamycin	960.8	E856	E930.8	E950.4	E962.0	E980.4
Magnesia magma	973.0	E858.4	E943.0	E950.4	E962.0	E980.4
Magnesium (compounds) (fumes) NEC	985.8	E866.4	-	E950.9	E962.1	E980.9
antacid	973.0	E858.4	E943.0	E950.4	E962.0	E980.4
carbonate	973.0	E858.4	E943.0	E950.4	E962.0	E980.4
cathartic	973.3	E858.4	E943.3	E950.4	E962.0	E980.4
citrate	973.3	E858.4	E943.3	E950.4	E962.0	E980.4
hydroxide	973.0	E858.4	E943.0	E950.4	E962.0	E980.4
oxide	973.0	E858.4	E943.0	E950.4	E962.0	E980.4
sulfate (oral)	973.3	E858.4	E943.3	E950.4	E962.0	E980.4
intravenous	966.3	E855.0	E936.3	E950.4	E962.0	E980.4
trisilicate	973.0	E858.4	E943.0	E950.4	E962.0	E980.4
Malathion (insecticide)	989.3	E863.1	-	E950.6	E962.1	E980.7
Male fern (oleoresin)	961.6	E857	E931.6	E950.4	E962.0	E980.4
Mandelic acid	961.9	E857	E931.9	E950.4	E962.0	E980.4
Manganese compounds (fumes) **NEC**	985.2	E866.4	-	E950.9	E962.1	E980.9
Mannitol (diuretic) (medicinal) NEC	974.4	E858.5	E944.4	E950.4	E962.0	E980.4
hexanitrate	972.4	E858.3	E942.4	E950.4	E962.0	E980.4
mustard	963.1	E858.1	E933.1	E950.4	E962.0	E980.4
Mannomustine	963.1	E858.1	E933.1	E950.4	E962.0	E980.4
MAO inhibitors	969.0	E854.0	E939.0	E950.3	E962.0	E980.3
Mapharsen	961.1	E857	E931.1	E950.4	E962.0	E980.4
Marcaine	968.9	E855.2	E938.9	E950.4	E962.0	E980.4
infiltration (subcutaneous)	968.5	E855.2	E938.5	E950.4	E962.0	E980.4
nerve block (peripheral) (plexus)	968.6	E855.2	E938.6	E950.4	E962.0	E980.4
Marezine	963.0	E858.1	E933.0	E950.4	E962.0	E980.4
Marihuana, marijuana (derivatives)	969.6	E854.1	E939.6	E950.3	E962.0	E980.3
Marine animals or plants (sting)	989.5	E905.6	-	E950.9	E962.1	E980.9
Marplan	969.0	E854.0	E939.0	E950.3	E962.0	E980.3
Marsh gas	987.1	E869.8	-	E952.8	E962.2	E982.8
Marsilid	969.0	E854.0	E939.0	E950.3	E962.0	E980.3
Matulane	963.1	E858.1	E933.1	E950.4	E962.0	E980.4
Mazindol	977.0	E858.8	E947.0	E950.4	E962.0	E980.4
MDMA	969.7	E854.2	E939.7	E950.3	E962.0	E980.3
Meadow saffron	988.2	E865.3	-	E950.9	E962.1	E980.9
Measles vaccine	979.4	E858.8	E949.4	E950.4	E962.0	E980.4
Meat, noxious or nonbacterial	988.8	E865.0	-	E950.9	E962.1	E980.9
Mebanazine	969.0	E854.0	E939.0	E950.3	E962.0	E980.3
Mebaral	967.0	E851	E937.0	E950.1	E962.0	E980.1
Mebendazole	961.6	E857	E931.6	E950.4	E962.0	E980.4
Mebeverine	975.1	E858.6	E945.1	E950.4	E962.0	E980.4
Mebhydroline	963.0	E858.1	E933.0	E950.4	E962.0	E980.4
Mebrophenhydramine	963.0	E858.1	E933.0	E950.4	E962.0	E980.4

● New Line ▲ Revised Code

Drug	Poisoning	External Cause (E-Code)				
		Accident	Therapeutic Use	Suicide Attempt	Assault	Undetermined
Mebutamate	969.5	E853.8	E939.5	E950.3	E962.0	E980.3
Mecamylamine (chloride)	972.3	E858.3	E942.3	E950.4	E962.0	E980.4
Mechlorethamine hydrochloride	963.1	E858.1	E933.1	E950.4	E962.0	E980.4
Meclizene (hydrochloride)	963.0	E858.1	E933.0	E950.4	E962.0	E980.4
Meclofenoxate	970.0	E854.3	E940.0	E950.4	E962.0	E980.4
Meclozine (hydrochloride)	963.0	E858.1	E933.0	E950.4	E962.0	E980.4
Medazepam	969.4	E853.2	E939.4	E950.3	E962.0	E980.3
Medicine, medicinal substance	977.9	E858.9	E947.9	E950.5	E962.0	E980.5
specified NEC	977.8	E858.8	E947.8	E950.4	E962.0	E980.4
Medinal	967.0	E851	E937.0	E950.1	E962.0	E980.1
Medomin	967.0	E851	E937.0	E950.1	E962.0	E980.1
Medroxyprogesterone	962.2	E858.0	E932.2	E950.4	E962.0	E980.4
Medrysone	976.5	E858.7	E946.5	E950.4	E962.0	E980.4
Mefenamic acid	965.7	E850.7	E935.7	E950.0	E962.0	E980.0
Megahallucinogen	969.6	E854.1	E939.6	E950.3	E962.0	E980.3
Megestrol	962.2	E858.0	E932.2	E950.4	E962.0	E980.4
Meglumine	977.8	E858.8	E947.8	E950.4	E962.0	E980.4
Meladinin	976.3	E858.7	E946.3	E950.4	E962.0	E980.4
Melanizing agents	976.3	E858.7	E946.3	E950.4	E962.0	E980.4
Melarsoprol	961.1	E857	E931.1	E950.4	E962.0	E980.4
Melia azedarach	988.2	E865.3	-	E950.9	E962.1	E980.9
Mellaril	969.1	E853.0	E939.1	E950.3	E962.0	E980.3
Meloxine	976.3	E858.7	E946.3	E950.4	E962.0	E980.4
Melphalan	963.1	E858.1	E933.1	E950.4	E962.0	E980.4
Menadiol sodium diphosphate	964.3	E858.2	E934.3	E950.4	E962.0	E980.4
Menadione (sodium bisulfite)	964.3	E858.2	E934.3	E950.4	E962.0	E980.4
Menaphthone	964.3	E858.2	E934.3	E950.4	E962.0	E980.4
Meningococcal vaccine	978.8	E858.8	E948.8	E950.4	E962.0	E980.4
Menningovax-C	978.8	E858.8	E948.8	E950.4	E962.0	E980.4
Menotropins	962.4	E858.0	E932.4	E950.4	E962.0	E980.4
Menthol NEC	976.1	E858.7	E946.1	E950.4	E962.0	E980.4
Mepacrine	961.3	E857	E931.3	E950.4	E962.0	E980.4
Meparfynol	967.8	E852.8	E937.8	E950.2	E962.0	E980.2
Mepazine	969.1	E853.0	E939.1	E950.3	E962.0	E980.3
Mepenzolate	971.1	E855.4	E941.1	E950.4	E962.0	E980.4
Meperidine	965.09	E850.2	E935.2	E950.0	E962.0	E980.0
Mephenamin(e)	966.4	E855.0	E936.4	E950.4	E962.0	E980.4
Mephenesin (carbamate)	968.0	E855.1	E938.0	E950.4	E962.0	E980.4
Mephenoxalone	969.5	E853.8	E939.5	E950.3	E962.0	E980.3
Mephentermine	971.2	E855.5	E941.2	E950.4	E962.0	E980.4
Mephenytoin	966.1	E855.0	E936.1	E950.4	E962.0	E980.4
Mephobarbital	967.0	E851	E937.0	E950.1	E962.0	E980.1
Mepiperphenidol	971.1	E855.4	E941.1	E950.4	E962.0	E980.4
Mepivacaine	968.9	E855.2	E938.9	E950.4	E962.0	E980.4
infiltration (subcutaneous)	968.5	E855.2	E938.5	E950.4	E962.0	E980.4
nerve block (peripheral) (plexus)	968.6	E855.2	E938.6	E950.4	E962.0	E980.4
topical (surface)	968.5	E855.2	E938.5	E950.4	E962.0	E980.4
Meprednisone	962.0	E858.0	E932.0	E950.4	E962.0	E980.4
Meprobam	969.5	E853.8	E939.5	E950.3	E962.0	E980.3
Meprobamate	969.5	E853.8	E939.5	E950.3	E962.0	E980.3
Mepyramine (maleate)	963.0	E858.1	E933.0	E950.4	E962.0	E980.4
Meralluride	974.0	E858.5	E944.0	E950.4	E962.0	E980.4
Merbaphen	974.0	E858.5	E944.0	E950.4	E962.0	E980.4
Merbromin	976.0	E858.7	E946.0	E950.4	E962.0	E980.4
Mercaplomerin	974.0	E858.5	E944.0	E950.4	E962.0	E980.4
Mercaptopurine	963.1	E858.1	E933.1	E950.4	E962.0	E980.4
Mercumatilin	974.0	E858.5	E944.0	E950.4	E962.0	E980.4
Mercuramide	974.0	E858.5	E944.0	E950.4	E962.0	E980.4
Mercuranin	976.0	E858.7	E946.0	E950.4	E962.0	E980.4
Mercurochrome	976.0	E858.7	E946.0	E950.4	E962.0	E980.4
Mercury, mercuric, mercurous (compounds) (cyanide) (fumes) (nonmedicinal) (vapor) NEC	985.0	E866.1	-	E950.9	E962.1	E980.9
ammoniated	976.0	E858.7	E946.0	E950.4	E962.0	E980.4
anti-infective	961.2	E857	E931.2	E950.4	E962.0	E980.4
topical	976.0	E858.7	E946.0	E950.4	E962.0	E980.4
chloride (antiseptic) NEC	976.0	E858.7	E946.0	E950.4	E962.0	E980.4
fungicide	985.0	E863.6	-	E950.6	E962.1	E980.7
diuretic compounds	974.0	E858.5	E944.0	E950.4	E962.0	E980.4
fungicide	985.0	E863.6	-	E950.6	E962.1	E980.7
organic (fungicide)	985.0	E863.6	-	E950.6	E962.1	E980.7
Merethoxylline	974.0	E858.5	E944.0	E950.4	E962.0	E980.4
Mersalyl	974.0	E858.5	E944.0	E950.4	E962.0	E980.4
Merthiolate (topical)	976.0	E858.7	E946.0	E950.4	E962.0	E980.4
ophthalmic preparation	976.5	E858.7	E946.5	E950.4	E962.0	E980.4
Meruvax	979.4	E858.8	E949.4	E950.4	E962.0	E980.4
Mescal buttons	969.6	E854.1	E939.6	E950.3	E962.0	E980.3
Mescaline (salts)	969.6	E854.1	E939.6	E950.3	E962.0	E980.3
Mesoridazine besylate	969.1	E853.0	E939.1	E950.3	E962.0	E980.3
Mestanolone	962.1	E858.0	E932.1	E950.4	E962.0	E980.4
Mestranol	962.2	E858.0	E932.2	E950.4	E962.0	E980.4
Metactesylacetate	976.0	E858.7	E946.0	E950.4	E962.0	E980.4
Metaldehyde (snail killer) **NEC**	989.4	E863.4	-	E950.6	E962.1	E980.7
Metals (heavy) (nonmedicinal) NEC	985.9	E866.4	-	E950.9	E962.1	E980.9
dust, fumes, or vapor NEC	985.9	E866.4	-	E950.9	E962.1	E980.9
light NEC	985.9	E866.4	-	E950.9	E962.1	E980.9
dust, fumes, or vapor NEC	985.9	E866.4	-	E950.9	E962.1	E980.9
pesticides (dust) (vapor)	985.9	E863.4	-	E950.6	E962.1	E980.7
Metamucil	973.3	E858.4	E943.3	E950.4	E962.0	E980.4
Metaphen	976.0	E858.7	E946.0	E950.4	E962.0	E980.4
Metaproterenol	975.1	E858.6	E945.1	E950.4	E962.0	E980.4
Metaraminol	972.8	E858.3	E942.8	E950.4	E962.0	E980.4
Metaxalone	968.0	E855.1	E938.0	E950.4	E962.0	E980.4
Metformin	962.3	E858.0	E932.3	E950.4	E962.0	E980.4
Methacycline	960.4	E856	E930.4	E950.4	E962.0	E980.4
Methadone	965.02	E850.1	E935.1	E950.0	E962.0	E980.0
Methallenestril	962.2	E858.0	E932.2	E950.4	E962.0	E980.4
Methamphetamine	969.7	E854.2	E939.7	E950.3	E962.0	E980.3
Methandienone	962.1	E858.0	E932.1	E950.4	E962.0	E980.4
Methandriol	962.1	E858.0	E932.1	E950.4	E962.0	E980.4
Methandrostenolone	962.1	E858.0	E932.1	E950.4	E962.0	E980.4
Methane gas	987.1	E869.8	-	E952.8	E962.2	E982.8
Methanol	980.1	E860.2	-	E950.9	E962.1	E980.9
vapor	987.8	E869.8	-	E952.8	E962.2	E982.8
Methantheline	971.1	E855.4	E941.1	E950.4	E962.0	E980.4
Methaphenilene	963.0	E858.1	E933.0	E950.4	E962.0	E980.4
Methapyrilene	963.0	E858.1	E933.0	E950.4	E962.0	E980.4
Methaqualone (compounds)	967.4	E852.3	E937.4	E950.2	E962.0	E980.2
Metharbital, metharbitone	967.0	E851	E937.0	E950.1	E962.0	E980.1
Methazolamide	974.2	E858.5	E944.2	E950.4	E962.0	E980.4
Methdilazine	963.0	E858.1	E933.0	E950.4	E962.0	E980.4
Methedrine	969.7	E854.2	E939.7	E950.3	E962.0	E980.3
Methenamine (mandelate)	961.9	E857	E931.9	E950.4	E962.0	E980.4
Methenolone	962.1	E858.0	E932.1	E950.4	E962.0	E980.4
Methergine	975.0	E858.6	E945.0	E950.4	E962.0	E980.4
Methiacil	962.8	E858.0	E932.8	E950.4	E962.0	E980.4
Methicillin (sodium)	960.0	E856	E930.0	E950.4	E962.0	E980.4
Methimazole	962.8	E858.0	E932.8	E950.4	E962.0	E980.4

Mebutamate – Methimazole

● New Line ▲ Revised Code

		External Cause (E-Code)				
Drug	**Poisoning**	**Accident**	**Therapeutic Use**	**Suicide Attempt**	**Assault**	**Undetermined**
Methionine	977.1	E858.8	E947.1	E950.4	E962.0	E980.4
Methisazone	961.7	E857	E931.7	E950.4	E962.0	E980.4
Methitural	967.0	E851	E937.0	E950.1	E962.0	E980.1
Methixene	971.1	E855.4	E941.1	E950.4	E962.0	E980.4
Methobarbital, methobarbitone	967.0	E851	E937.0	E950.1	E962.0	E980.1
Methocarbamol	968.0	E855.1	E938.0	E950.4	E962.0	E980.4
Methohexital, methohexitone (sodium)	968.3	E855.1	E938.3	E950.4	E962.0	E980.4
Methoin	966.1	E855.0	E936.1	E950.4	E962.0	E980.4
Methopholine	965.7	E850.7	E935.7	E950.0	E962.0	E980.0
Methorate	975.4	E858.6	E945.4	E950.4	E962.0	E980.4
Methoserpidine	972.6	E858.3	E942.6	E950.4	E962.0	E980.4
Methotrexate	963.1	E858.1	E933.1	E950.4	E962.0	E980.4
Methotrimeprazine	967.8	E852.8	E937.8	E950.2	E962.0	E980.2
Methoxa-Dome	976.3	E858.7	E946.3	E950.4	E962.0	E980.4
Methoxamine	971.2	E855.5	E941.2	E950.4	E962.0	E980.4
Methoxsalen	976.3	E858.7	E946.3	E950.4	E962.0	E980.4
Methoxybenzyl penicillin	960.0	E856	E930.0	E950.4	E962.0	E980.4
Methoxychlor	989.2	E863.0	-	E950.6	E962.1	E980.7
Methoxyflurane	968.2	E855.1	E938.2	E950.4	E962.0	E980.4
Methoxyphenamine	971.2	E855.5	E941.2	E950.4	E962.0	E980.4
Methoxypromazine	969.1	E853.0	E939.1	E950.3	E962.0	E980.3
Methoxypsoralen	976.3	E858.7	E946.3	E950.4	E962.0	E980.4
Methscopolamine (bromide)	971.1	E855.4	E941.1	E950.4	E962.0	E980.4
Methsuximide	966.2	E855.0	E936.2	E950.4	E962.0	E980.4
Methyclothiazide	974.3	E858.5	E944.3	E950.4	E962.0	E980.4
Methyl						
acetate	982.8	E862.4	-	E950.9	E962.1	E980.9
acetone II	982.8	E862.4	-	E950.9	E962.1	E980.9
alcohol	980.1	E860.2	-	E950.9	E962.1	E980.9
amphetamine	969.7	E854.2	E939.7	E950.3	E962.0	E980.3
androstanolone	962.1	E858.0	E932.1	E950.4	E962.0	E980.4
atropine	971.1	E855.4	E941.1	E950.4	E962.0	E980.4
benzene	982.0	E862.4	-	E950.9	E962.1	E980.9
bromide (gas)	987.8	E869.8	-	E952.8	E962.2	E982.8
fumigant	987.8	E863.8	-	E950.6	E962.2	E980.7
butanol	980.8	E860.8	-	E950.9	E962.1	E980.9
carbinol	980.1	E860.2	-	E950.9	E962.1	E980.9
cellosolve	982.8	E862.4	-	E950.9	E962.1	E980.9
cellulose	973.3	E858.4	E943.3	E950.4	E962.0	E980.4
chloride (gas)	987.8	E869.8	-	E952.8	E962.2	E982.8
cyclohexane	982.8	E862.4	-	E950.9	E962.1	E980.9
cyclohexanone	982.8	E862.4	-	E950.9	E962.1	E980.9
dihydromorphinone	965.09	E850.2	E935.2	E950.0	E962.0	E980.0
ergometrine	975.0	E858.6	E945.0	E950.4	E962.0	E980.4
ergonovine	975.0	E858.6	E945.0	E950.4	E962.0	E980.4
ethyl ketone	982.8	E862.4	-	E950.9	E962.1	E980.9
hydrazine	983.9	E864.3	-	E950.7	E962.1	E980.6
isobutyl ketone	982.8	E862.4	-	E950.9	E962.1	E980.9
morphine NEC	965.09	E850.2	E935.2	E950.0	E962.0	E980.0
parafynol	967.8	E852.8	E937.8	E950.2	E962.0	E980.2
parathion	989.3	E863.1	-	E950.6	E962.1	E980.7
pentynol NEC	967.8	E852.8	E937.8	E950.2	E962.0	E980.2
peridol	969.2	E853.1	E939.2	E950.3	E962.0	E980.3
phenidate	969.7	E854.2	E939.7	E950.3	E962.0	E980.3
prednisolone	962.0	E858.0	E932.0	E950.4	E962.0	E980.4
ENT agent	976.6	E858.7	E946.6	E950.4	E962.0	E980.4
ophthalmic preparation	976.5	E858.7	E946.5	E950.4	E962.0	E980.4
topical NEC	976.0	E858.7	E946.0	E950.4	E962.0	E980.4
propylcarbinol	980.8	E860.8	-	E950.9	E962.1	E980.9
rosaniline NEC	976.0	E858.7	E946.0	E950.4	E962.0	E980.4
salicylate NEC	976.3	E858.7	E946.3	E950.4	E962.0	E980.4
Methyl – *continued*						
sulfate (fumes)	987.8	E869.8	-	E952.8	E962.2	E982.8
liquid	983.9	E864.3	-	E950.7	E962.1	E980.6
sulfonal	967.8	E852.8	E937.8	E950.2	E962.0	E980.2
testosterone	962.1	E858.0	E932.1	E950.4	E962.0	E980.4
thiouracil	962.8	E858.0	E932.8	E950.4	E962.0	E980.4
Methylated spirit	980.0	E860.1	-	E950.9	E962.1	E980.9
Methyldopa	972.6	E858.3	E942.6	E950.4	E962.0	E980.4
Methylene						
blue	961.9	E857	E931.9	E950.4	E962.0	E980.4
chloride or dichloride (solvent) NEC	982.3	E862.4	-	E950.9	E962.1	E980.9
Methylhexabital	967.0	E851	E937.0	E950.1	E962.0	E980.1
Methylparaben (ophthalmic)	976.5	E858.7	E946.5	E950.4	E962.0	E980.4
Methyprylon	967.5	E852.4	E937.5	E950.2	E962.0	E980.2
Methysergide	971.3	E855.6	E941.3	E950.4	E962.0	E980.4
Metoclopramide	963.0	E858.1	E933.0	E950.4	E962.0	E980.4
Metofoline	965.7	E850.7	E935.7	E950.0	E962.0	E980.0
Metopon	965.09	E850.2	E935.2	E950.0	E962.0	E980.0
Metronidazole	961.5	E857	E931.5	E950.4	E962.0	E980.4
Metycaine	968.9	E855.2	E938.9	E950.4	E962.0	E980.4
infiltration (subcutaneous)	968.5	E855.2	E938.5	E950.4	E962.0	E980.4
nerve block (peripheral) (plexus)	968.6	E855.2	E938.6	E950.4	E962.0	E980.4
topical (surface)	968.5	E855.2	E938.5	E950.4	E962.0	E980.4
Metyrapone	977.8	E858.8	E947.8	E950.4	E962.0	E980.4
Mevinphos	989.3	E863.1	-	E950.6	E962.1	E980.7
Mezereon (berries)	988.2	E865.3	-	E950.9	E962.1	E980.9
Micatin	976.0	E858.7	E946.0	E950.4	E962.0	E980.4
Miconazole	976.0	E858.7	E946.0	E950.4	E962.0	E980.4
Mifepristone	962.9	E858.0	E932.9	E950.4	E962.0	E980.4
Midol	965.1	E850.3	E935.3	E950.0	E962.0	E980.0
Milk of magnesia	973.0	E858.4	E943.0	E950.4	E962.0	E980.4
Millipede (tropical) (venomous)	989.5	E905.4	-	E950.9	E962.1	E980.9
Miltown	969.5	E853.8	E939.5	E950.3	E962.0	E980.3
Mineral						
oil (medicinal)	973.2	E858.4	E943.2	E950.4	E962.0	E980.4
nonmedicinal	981	E862.1	-	E950.9	E962.1	E980.9
topical	976.3	E858.7	E946.3	E950.4	E962.0	E980.4
salts NEC	974.6	E858.5	E944.6	E950.4	E962.0	E980.4
spirits	981	E862.0	-	E950.9	E962.1	E980.9
Minocycline	960.4	E856	E930.4	E950.4	E962.0	E980.4
Mithramycin (antineoplastic)	960.7	E856	E930.7	E950.4	E962.0	E980.4
Mitobronitol	963.1	E858.1	E933.1	E950.4	E962.0	E980.4
Mitomycin (antineoplastic)	960.7	E856	E930.7	E950.4	E962.0	E980.4
Mitotane	963.1	E858.1	E933.1	E950.4	E962.0	E980.4
Moderil	972.6	E858.3	E942.6	E950.4	E962.0	E980.4
Mogadon – *see* Nitrazepam						
Molindone	969.3	E853.8	E939.3	E950.3	E962.0	E980.3
Monistat	976.0	E858.7	E946.0	E950.4	E962.0	E980.4
Monkshood	988.2	E865.4	-	E950.9	E962.1	E980.9
Monoamine oxidase inhibitors	969.0	E854.0	E939.0	E950.3	E962.0	E980.3
Monochlorobenzene	982.0	E862.4	-	E950.9	E962.1	E980.9
Monosodium glutamate	989.89	E866.8	-	E950.9	E962.1	E980.9
Monoxide, carbon – *see* Carbon, monoxide						
Moperone	969.2	E853.1	E939.2	E950.3	E962.0	E980.3
Morning glory seeds	969.6	E854.1	E939.6	E950.3	E962.0	E980.3
Moroxydine (hydrochloride)	961.7	E857	E931.7	E950.4	E962.0	E980.4
Morphazinamide	961.8	E857	E931.8	E950.4	E962.0	E980.4
Morphinans	965.09	E850.2	E935.2	E950.0	E962.0	E980.0

● New Line ▲ Revised Code

Drug	Poisoning	External Cause (E-Code)				
		Accident	Therapeutic Use	Suicide Attempt	Assault	Undetermined
Morphine NEC	965.09	E850.2	E935.2	E950.0	E962.0	E980.0
antagonists	970.1	E854.3	E940.1	E950.4	E962.0	E980.4
Morpholinylethylmorphine	965.09	E850.2	E935.2	E950.0	E962.0	E980.0
Morrhuate sodium	972.7	E858.3	E942.7	E950.4	E962.0	E980.4
Moth balls (*see also* Pesticides)	989.4	E863.4	-	E950.6	E962.1	E980.7
naphthalene	983.0	E863.4	-	E950.7	E962.1	E980.6
Motor exhaust gas – *see* Carbon, monoxide, exhaust gas						
Mouth wash	976.6	E858.7	E946.6	E950.4	E962.0	E980.4
Mucolytic agent	975.5	E858.6	E945.5	E950.4	E962.0	E980.4
Mucomyst	975.5	E858.6	E945.5	E950.4	E962.0	E980.4
Mucous membrane agents (external)	976.9	E858.7	E946.9	E950.4	E962.0	E980.4
specified NEC	976.8	E858.7	E946.8	E950.4	E962.0	E980.4
Mumps						
immune globulin (human)	964.6	E858.2	E934.6	E950.4	E962.0	E980.4
skin test antigen	977.8	E858.8	E947.8	E950.4	E962.0	E980.4
vaccine	979.6	E858.8	E949.6	E950.4	E962.0	E980.4
Mumpsvax	979.6	E858.8	E949.6	E950.4	E962.0	E980.4
Muriatic acid – *see* Hydrochloric acid						
Muscarine	971.0	E855.3	E941.0	E950.4	E962.0	E980.4
Muscle affecting agents NEC	975.3	E858.6	E945.3	E950.4	E962.0	E980.4
oxytocic	975.0	E858.6	E945.0	E950.4	E962.0	E980.4
relaxants	975.3	E858.6	E945.3	E950.4	E962.0	E980.4
central nervous system	968.0	E855.1	E938.0	E950.4	E962.0	E980.4
skeletal	975.2	E858.6	E945.2	E950.4	E962.0	E980.4
smooth	975.1	E858.6	E945.1	E950.4	E962.0	E980.4
Mushrooms, noxious	988.1	E865.5	-	E950.9	E962.1	E980.9
Mussel, noxious	988.0	E865.1	-	E950.9	E962.1	E980.9
Mustard (emetic)	973.6	E858.4	E943.6	E950.4	E962.0	E980.4
gas	987.8	E869.8	-	E952.8	E962.2	E982.8
nitrogen	963.1	E858.1	E933.1	E950.4	E962.0	E980.4
Mustine	963.1	E858.1	E933.1	E950.4	E962.0	E980.4
M-vac	979.4	E858.8	E949.4	E950.4	E962.0	E980.4
Mycifradin	960.8	E856	E930.8	E950.4	E962.0	E980.4
topical	976.0	E858.7	E946.0	E950.4	E962.0	E980.4
Mycitracin	960.8	E856	E930.8	E950.4	E962.0	E980.4
ophthalmic preparation	976.5	E858.7	E946.5	E950.4	E962.0	E980.4
Mycostatin	960.1	E856	E930.1	E950.4	E962.0	E980.4
topical	976.0	E858.7	E946.0	E950.4	E962.0	E980.4
Mydriacyl	971.1	E855.4	E941.1	E950.4	E962.0	E980.4
Myelobromal	963.1	E858.1	E933.1	E950.4	E962.0	E980.4
Myleran	963.1	E858.1	E933.1	E950.4	E962.0	E980.4
Myochrysin(e)	965.69	E850.6	E935.6	E950.0	E962.0	E980.0
Myoneural blocking agents	975.2	E858.6	E945.2	E950.4	E962.0	E980.4
Myristica fragrans	988.2	E865.3	-	E950.9	E962.1	E980.9
Myristicin	988.2	E865.3	-	E950.9	E962.1	E980.9
Mysoline	966.3	E855.0	E936.3	E950.4	E962.0	E980.4
Nafcillin (sodium)	960.0	E856	E930.0	E950.4	E962.0	E980.4
Nail polish remover	982.8	E862.4	-	E950.9	E962.1	E908.9
Nalidixic acid	961.9	E857	E931.9	E950.4	E962.0	E980.4
Nalorphine	970.1	E854.3	E940.1	E950.4	E962.0	E980.4
Naloxone	970.1	E854.3	E940.1	E950.4	E962.0	E980.4
Nandrolone (decanoate) (phenproprioate)	962.1	E858.0	E932.1	E950.4	E962.0	E980.4
Naphazoline	971.2	E855.5	E941.2	E950.4	E962.0	E980.4
Naphtha (painter's) (petroleum)	981	E862.0	-	E950.9	E962.1	E980.9
solvent	981	E862.0	-	E950.9	E962.1	E980.9
vapor	987.1	E869.8	-	E952.8	E962.2	E982.8

Drug	Poisoning	External Cause (E-Code)				
		Accident	Therapeutic Use	Suicide Attempt	Assault	Undetermined
Naphthalene (chlorinated)	983.0	E864.0	-	E950.7	E962.1	E980.6
insecticide or moth repellent	983.0	E863.4	-	E950.7	E962.1	E980.6
vapor	987.8	E869.8	-	E952.8	E962.2	E982.8
Naphthol	983.0	E864.0	-	E950.7	E962.1	E980.6
Naphthylamine	983.0	E864.0	-	E950.7	E962.1	E980.6
Naprosyn – *see* Naproxen						
Naproxen	965.61	E850.6	E935.6	E950.0	E962.0	E980.0
Narcotic (drug)	967.9	E852.9	E937.9	E950.2	E962.0	E980.2
analgesic NEC	965.8	E850.8	E935.8	E950.0	E962.0	E980.0
antagonist	970.1	E854.3	E940.1	E950.4	E962.0	E980.4
specified NEC	967.8	E852.8	E937.8	E950.2	E962.0	E980.2
Narcotine	975.4	E858.6	E945.4	E950.4	E962.0	E980.4
Nardil	969.0	E854.0	E939.0	E950.3	E962.0	E980.3
Natrium cyanide – *see* Cyanide(s)						
Natural						
blood (product)	964.7	E858.2	E934.7	E950.4	E962.0	E980.4
gas (piped)	987.1	E867	-	E951.0	E962.2	E981.0
incomplete combustion	986	E867	-	E951.0	E962.2	E981.0
Nealbarbital, nealbarbitone	967.0	E851	E937.0	E950.1	E962.0	E980.1
Nectadon	975.4	E858.6	E945.4	E950.4	E962.0	E980.4
Nematocyst (sting)	989.5	E905.6	-	E950.9	E962.1	E980.9
Nembutal	967.0	E851	E937.0	E950.1	E962.0	E980.1
Neoarsphenamine	961.1	E857	E931.1	E950.4	E962.0	E980.4
Neocinchophen	974.7	E858.5	E944.7	E950.4	E962.0	E980.4
Neomycin	960.8	E856	E930.8	E950.4	E962.0	E980.4
ENT agent	976.6	E858.7	E946.6	E950.4	E962.0	E980.4
ophthalmic preparation	976.5	E858.7	E946.5	E950.4	E962.0	E980.4
topical NEC	976.0	E858.7	E946.0	E950.4	E962.0	E980.4
Neonal	967.0	E851	E937.0	E950.1	E962.0	E980.1
Neoprontosil	961.0	E857	E931.0	E950.4	E962.0	E980.4
Neosalvarsan	961.1	E857	E931.1	E950.4	E962.0	E980.4
Neosilversalvarsan	961.1	E857	E931.1	E950.4	E962.0	E980.4
Neosporin	960.8	E856	E930.8	E950.4	E962.0	E980.4
ENT agent	976.6	E858.7	E946.6	E950.4	E962.0	E980.4
opthalmic preparation	976.5	E858.7	E946.5	E950.4	E962.0	E980.4
topical NEC	976.0	E858.7	E946.0	E950.4	E962.0	E980.4
Neostigmine	971.0	E855.3	E941.0	E950.4	E962.0	E980.4
Neraval	967.0	E851	E937.0	E950.1	E962.0	E980.1
Neravan	967.0	E851	E937.0	E950.1	E962.0	E980.1
Nerium oleander	988.2	E865.4	-	E950.9	E962.1	E980.9
Nerve gases (war)	987.9	E869.9	-	E952.9	E962.2	E982.9
Nesacaine	968.9	E855.2	E938.9	E950.4	E962.0	E980.4
infiltration (subcutaneous)	968.5	E855.2	E938.5	E950.4	E962.0	E980.4
nerve block (peripheral) (plexus)	968.6	E855.2	E938.6	E950.4	E962.0	E980.4
Neurobarb	967.0	E851	E937.0	E950.1	E962.0	E980.1
Neuroleptics NEC	969.3	E853.8	E939.3	E950.3	E962.0	E980.3
Neuroprotective agent	977.8	E858.8	E947.8	E950.4	E962.0	E980.4
Neutral spirits	980.0	E860.1	-	E950.9	E962.1	E980.9
beverage	980.0	E860.0	-	E950.9	E962.1	E980.9
Niacin, niacinamide	972.2	E858.3	E942.2	E950.4	E962.0	E980.4
Nialamide	969.0	E854.0	E939.0	E950.3	E962.0	E980.3
Nickle (carbonyl) (compounds) (fumes) (tetracarbonyl) (vapor)	985.8	E866.4	-	E950.9	E962.1	E980.9
Niclosamide	961.6	E857	E931.6	E950.4	E962.0	E980.4
Nicomorphine	965.09	E850.2	E935.2	E950.0	E962.0	E980.0
Nicotinamide	972.2	E858.3	E942.2	E950.4	E962.0	E980.4
Nicotine (insecticide) (spray) (sulfate) NEC	989.4	E863.4	-	E950.6	E962.1	E980.7
not insecticide	989.89	E866.8	-	E950.9	E962.1	E980.9
Nicotinic acid (derivatives)	972.2	E858.3	E942.2	E950.4	E962.0	E980.4

● New Line ▲ Revised Code

Morphine – Nicotinic acid

Drug	Poisoning	External Cause (E-Code) Accident	Therapeutic Use	Suicide Attempt	Assault	Undetermined
Nicotinyl alcohol	972.2	E858.3	E942.2	E950.4	E962.0	E980.4
Nicoumalone	964.2	E858.2	E934.2	E950.4	E962.0	E980.4
Nifenazone	965.5	E850.5	E935.5	E950.0	E962.0	E980.0
Nifuraldezone	961.9	E857	E931.9	E950.4	E962.0	E980.4
Nightshade (deadly)	988.2	E865.4	-	E950.9	E962.1	E980.9
Nikethamide	970.0	E854.3	E940.0	E950.4	E962.0	E980.4
Nilstat	960.1	E856	E930.1	E950.4	E962.0	E980.4
topical	976.0	E858.7	E946.0	E950.4	E962.0	E980.4
Nimodipine	977.8	E858.8	E947.8	E950.4	E962.0	E980.4
Niridazole	961.6	E857	E931.6	E950.4	E962.0	E980.4
Nisentil	965.09	E850.2	E935.2	E950.0	E962.0	E980.0
Nitrates	972.4	E858.3	E942.4	E950.4	E962.0	E980.4
Nitrazepam	969.4	E853.2	E939.4	E950.3	E962.0	E980.3
Nitric						
acid (liquid)	983.1	E864.1	-	E950.7	E962.1	E980.6
vapor	987.8	E869.8	-	E952.8	E962.2	E982.8
oxide (gas)	987.2	E869.0	-	E952.8	E962.2	E982.8
Nitrite, amyl (medicinal) (vapor)	972.4	E858.3	E942.4	E950.4	E962.0	E980.4
Nitroaniline	983.0	E864.0	-	E950.7	E962.1	E980.6
vapor	987.8	E869.8	-	E952.8	E962.2	E982.8
Nitrobenzene, nitrobenzol	983.0	E864.0	-	E950.7	E962.1	E980.6
vapor	987.8	E869.8	-	E952.8	E962.2	E982.8
Nitrocellulose	976.3	E858.7	E946.3	E950.4	E962.0	E980.4
Nitrofuran derivatives	961.9	E857	E931.9	E950.4	E962.0	E980.4
Nitrofurantoin	961.9	E857	E931.9	E950.4	E962.0	E980.4
Nitrofurazone	976.0	E858.7	E946.0	E950.4	E962.0	E980.4
Nitrogen (dioxide) (gas) (oxide)	987.2	E869.0	-	E952.8	E962.2	E982.8
mustard (antineoplastic)	963.1	E858.1	E933.1	E950.4	E962.0	E980.4
Nitroglycerin, nitroglycerol (medicinal)	972.4	E858.3	E942.4	E950.4	E962.0	E980.4
nonmedicinal	989.89	E866.8	-	E950.9	E962.1	E980.9
fumes	987.8	E869.8	-	E952.8	E962.2	E982.8
Nitrohydrochloric acid	983.1	E864.1	-	E950.7	E962.1	E980.6
Nitromersol	976.0	E858.7	E946.0	E950.4	E962.0	E980.4
Nitronaphthalene	983.0	E864.0	-	E950.7	E962.2	E980.6
Nitrophenol	983.0	E864.0	-	E950.7	E962.2	E980.6
Nitrothiazol	961.6	E857	E931.6	E950.4	E962.0	E980.4
Nitrotoluene, nitrotoluol	983.0	E864.0	-	E950.7	E962.1	E980.6
vapor	987.8	E869.8	-	E952.8	E962.2	E982.8
Nitrous	968.2	E855.1	E938.2	E950.4	E962.0	E980.4
acid (liquid)	983.1	E864.1	-	E950.7	E962.1	E980.6
fumes	987.2	E869.0	-	E952.8	E962.2	E982.8
oxide (anesthetic) NEC	968.2	E855.1	E938.2	E950.4	E962.0	E980.4
Nitrozone	976.0	E858.7	E946.0	E950.4	E962.0	E980.4
Noctec	967.1	E852.0	E937.1	E950.2	E962.0	E980.2
Noludar	967.5	E852.4	E937.5	E950.2	E962.0	E980.2
Noptil	967.0	E851	E937.0	E950.1	E962.0	E980.1
Noradrenalin	971.2	E855.5	E941.2	E950.4	E962.0	E980.4
Noramidopyrine	965.5	E850.5	E935.5	E950.0	E962.0	E980.0
Norepinephrine	971.2	E855.5	E941.2	E950.4	E962.0	E980.4
Norethandrolone	962.1	E858.0	E932.1	E950.4	E962.0	E980.4
Norethindrone	962.2	E858.0	E932.2	E950.4	E962.0	E980.4
Norethisterone	962.2	E858.0	E932.2	E950.4	E962.0	E980.4
Norethynodrel	962.2	E858.0	E932.2	E950.4	E962.0	E980.4
Norlestrin	962.2	E858.0	E932.2	E950.4	E962.0	E980.4
Norlutin	962.2	E858.0	E932.2	E950.4	E962.0	E980.4
Normison – *see* Benzodiazepines						
Normorphine	965.09	E850.2	E935.2	E950.0	E962.0	E980.0
Nortriptyline	969.0	E854.0	E939.0	E950.3	E962.0	E980.3
Noscapine	975.4	E858.6	E945.4	E950.4	E962.0	E980.4

Drug	Poisoning	External Cause (E-Code) Accident	Therapeutic Use	Suicide Attempt	Assault	Undetermined
Nose preparations	976.6	E858.7	E946.6	E950.4	E962.0	E980.4
Novobiocin	960.8	E856	E930.8	E950.4	E962.0	E980.4
Novocain (infiltration) (topical)	968.5	E855.2	E938.5	E950.4	E962.0	E980.4
nerve block (peripheral) (plexus)	968.6	E855.2	E938.6	E950.4	E962.0	E980.4
spinal	968.7	E855.2	E938.7	E950.4	E962.0	E980.4
Noxythiolin	961.9	E857	E931.9	E950.4	E962.0	E980.4
NPH Iletin (insulin)	962.3	E858.0	E932.3	E950.4	E962.0	E980.4
Numorphan	965.09	E850.2	E935.2	E950.0	E962.0	E980.0
Nunol	967.0	E851	E937.0	E950.1	E962.0	E980.1
Nupercaine (spinal anesthetic)	968.7	E855.2	E938.7	E950.4	E962.0	E980.4
topical (surface)	968.5	E855.2	E938.5	E950.4	E962.0	E980.4
Nutmeg oil (liniment)	976.3	E858.7	E946.3	E950.4	E962.0	E980.4
Nux vomica	989.1	E863.7	-	E950.6	E962.1	E980.7
Nydrazid	961.8	E857	E931.8	E950.4	E962.0	E980.4
Nylidrin	971.2	E855.5	E941.2	E950.4	E962.0	E980.4
Nystatin	960.1	E856	E930.1	E950.4	E962.0	E980.4
topical	976.0	E858.7	E946.0	E950.4	E962.0	E980.4
Nytol	963.0	E858.1	E933.0	E950.4	E962.0	E980.4
Oblivion	967.8	E852.8	E937.8	E950.2	E962.0	E980.2
Octyl nitrite	972.4	E858.3	E942.4	E950.4	E962.0	E980.4
Oestradiol (cypionate) (dipropionate) (valerate)	962.2	E858.0	E932.2	E950.4	E962.0	E980.4
Oestriol	962.2	E858.0	E932.2	E950.4	E962.0	E980.4
Oestrone	962.2	E858.0	E932.2	E950.4	E962.0	E980.4
Oil (of) NEC	989.89	E866.8	-	E950.9	E962.1	E980.9
bitter almond	989.0	E866.8	-	E950.9	E962.1	E980.9
camphor	976.1	E858.7	E946.1	E950.4	E962.0	E980.4
colors	989.89	E861.6	-	E950.9	E962.1	E980.9
fumes	987.8	E869.8	-	E952.8	E962.2	E982.8
lubricating	981	E862.2	-	E950.9	E962.1	E980.9
specified source, other – *see* substance specified						
vitriol (liquid)	983.1	E864.1	-	E950.7	E962.1	E980.6
fumes	987.8	E869.8	-	E952.8	E962.2	E982.8
wintergreen (bitter) NEC	976.3	E858.7	E946.3	E950.4	E962.0	E980.4
Ointments NEC	976.9	E858.7	E946.9	E950.4	E962.0	E980.4
Oleander	988.2	E865.4	-	E950.9	E962.1	E980.9
Oleandomycin	960.3	E856	E930.3	E950.4	E962.0	E980.4
Oleovitamin A	963.5	E858.1	E933.5	E950.4	E962.0	E980.4
Oleum ricini	973.1	E858.4	E943.1	E950.4	E962.0	E980.4
Olive oil (medicinal) **NEC**	973.2	E858.4	E943.2	E950.4	E962.0	E980.4
OMPA	989.3	E863.1	-	E950.6	E962.1	E980.7
Oncovin	963.1	E858.1	E933.1	E950.4	E962.0	E980.4
Ophthaine	968.5	E855.2	E938.5	E950.4	E962.0	E980.4
Ophthetic	968.5	E855.2	E938.5	E950.4	E962.0	E980.4
Opiates, opioids, opium NEC	965.00	E850.2	E935.2	E950.0	E962.0	E980.0
antagonists	970.1	E854.3	E940.1	E950.4	E962.0	E980.4
Oracon	962.2	E858.0	E932.2	E950.4	E962.0	E980.4
Oragrafin	977.8	E858.8	E947.8	E950.4	E962.0	E980.4
Oral contraceptives	962.2	E858.0	E932.2	E950.4	E962.0	E980.4
Orciprenaline	975.1	E858.6	E945.1	E950.4	E962.0	E980.4
Organidin	975.5	E858.6	E945.5	E950.4	E962.0	E980.4
Organophosphates	989.3	E863.1	-	E950.6	E962.1	E980.7
Orimune	979.5	E858.8	E949.5	E950.4	E962.0	E980.4
Orinase	962.3	E858.0	E932.3	E950.4	E962.0	E980.4
Orphenadrine	966.4	E855.0	E936.4	E950.4	E962.0	E980.4
Ortal (sodium)	967.0	E851	E937.0	E950.1	E962.0	E980.1

● New Line ▲ Revised Code

Drug	Poisoning	External Cause (E-Code) Accident	Therapeutic Use	Suicide Attempt	Assault	Undetermined
Orthoboric acid	976.0	E858.7	E946.0	E950.4	E962.0	E980.4
ENT agent	976.6	E858.7	E946.6	E950.4	E962.0	E980.4
ophthalmic preparation	976.5	E858.7	E946.5	E950.4	E962.0	E980.4
Orthocaine	968.5	E855.2	E938.5	E950.4	E962.0	E980.4
Ortho-Novum	962.2	E858.0	E932.2	E950.4	E962.0	E980.4
Orthotolidine (reagent)	977.8	E858.8	E947.8	E950.4	E962.0	E980.4
Osmic acid (liquid)	983.1	E864.1	-	E950.7	E962.1	E980.6
fumes	987.8	E869.8	-	E952.8	E962.2	E982.8
Osmotic diuretics	974.4	E858.5	E944.4	E950.4	E962.0	E980.4
Ouabain	972.1	E858.3	E942.1	E950.4	E962.0	E980.4
Ovarian hormones (synthetic substitutes)	962.2	E858.0	E932.2	E950.4	E962.0	E980.4
Ovral	962.2	E858.0	E932.2	E950.4	E962.0	E980.4
Ovulation suppressants	962.2	E858.0	E932.2	E950.4	E962.0	E980.4
Ovulen	962.2	E858.0	E932.2	E950.4	E962.0	E980.4
Oxacillin (sodium)	960.0	E856	E930.0	E950.4	E962.0	E980.4
Oxalic acid	983.1	E864.1	-	E950.7	E962.1	E980.6
Oxanamide	969.5	E853.8	E939.5	E950.3	E962.0	E980.3
Oxandrolone	962.1	E858.0	E932.1	E950.4	E962.0	E980.4
Oxaprozin	965.61	E850.6	E935.6	E950.0	E962.0	E980.0
Oxazepam	969.4	E853.2	E939.4	E950.3	E962.0	E980.3
Oxazolidine derivatives	966.0	E855.0	E936.0	E950.4	E962.0	E980.4
Ox bile extract	973.4	E858.4	E943.4	E950.4	E962.0	E980.4
Oxedrine	971.2	E855.5	E941.2	E950.4	E962.0	E980.4
Oxeladin	975.4	E858.6	E945.4	E950.4	E962.0	E980.4
Oxethazaine NEC	968.5	E855.2	E938.5	E950.4	E962.0	E980.4
Oxidizing agents NEC	983.9	E864.3	-	E950.7	E962.1	E980.6
Oxolinic acid	961.3	E857	E931.3	E950.4	E962.0	E980.4
Oxophenarsine	961.1	E857	E931.1	E950.4	E962.0	E980.4
Oxsoralen	976.3	E858.7	E946.3	E950.4	E962.0	E980.4
Oxtriphylline	976.7	E858.6	E945.7	E950.4	E962.0	E980.4
Oxybuprocaine	968.5	E855.2	E938.5	E950.4	E962.0	E980.4
Oxybutynin	975.1	E858.6	E945.1	E950.4	E962.0	E980.4
Oxycodone	965.09	E850.2	E935.2	E950.0	E962.0	E980.0
Oxygen	987.8	E869.8	-	E952.8	E962.2	E982.8
Oxylone	976.0	E858.7	E946.0	E950.4	E962.0	E980.4
ophthalmic preparation	976.5	E858.7	E946.5	E950.4	E962.0	E980.4
Oxymesterone	962.1	E858.0	E932.1	E950.4	E962.0	E980.4
Oxymetazoline	971.2	E855.5	E941.2	E950.4	E962.0	E980.4
Oxymetholone	962.1	E858.0	E932.1	E950.4	E962.0	E980.4
Oxymorphone	965.09	E850.2	E935.2	E950.0	E962.0	E980.0
Oxypertine	969.0	E854.0	E939.0	E950.3	E962.0	E980.3
Oxyphenbutazone	965.5	E850.5	E935.5	E950.0	E962.0	E980.0
Oxyphencyclimine	971.1	E855.4	E941.1	E950.4	E962.0	E980.4
Oxyphenisatin	973.1	E858.4	E943.1	E950.4	E962.0	E980.4
Oxyphenonium	971.1	E855.4	E941.1	E950.4	E962.0	E980.4
Oxyquinoline	961.3	E857	E931.3	E950.4	E962.0	E980.4
Oxytetracycline	960.4	E856	E930.4	E950.4	E962.0	E980.4
Oxytocics	975.0	E858.6	E945.0	E950.4	E962.0	E980.4
Oxytocin	975.0	E858.6	E945.0	E950.4	E962.0	E980.4
Ozone	987.8	E869.8	-	E952.8	E962.2	E982.8
PABA	976.3	E858.7	E946.3	E950.4	E962.0	E980.4
Packed red cells	964.7	E858.2	E934.7	E950.4	E962.0	E980.4
Paint NEC	989.89	E861.6	-	E950.9	E962.1	E980.9
cleaner	982.8	E862.9	-	E950.9	E962.1	E980.9
fumes NEC	987.8	E869.8	-	E952.8	E962.1	E982.8
lead (fumes)	984.0	E861.5	-	E950.9	E962.1	E980.9
solvent NEC	982.8	E862.9	-	E950.9	E962.1	E980.9
stripper	982.8	E862.9	-	E950.9	E962.1	E980.9
Palfium	965.09	E850.2	E935.2	E950.0	E962.0	E980.0
Palivizumab	979.9	E858.8	E949.6	E950.4	E962.0	E980.4
Paludrine	961.4	E857	E931.4	E950.4	E962.0	E980.4
PAM	977.2	E855.8	E947.2	E950.4	E962.0	E980.4

Drug	Poisoning	External Cause (E-Code) Accident	Therapeutic Use	Suicide Attempt	Assault	Undetermined
Pamaquine (naphthoate)	961.4	E857	E931.4	E950.4	E962.0	E980.4
Pamprin	965.1	E850.3	E935.3	E950.0	E962.0	E980.0
Panadol	965.4	E850.4	E935.4	E950.0	E962.0	E980.0
Pancreatic dornase (mucolytic)	963.4	E858.1	E933.4	E950.4	E962.0	E980.4
Pancreatin	973.4	E858.4	E943.4	E950.4	E962.0	E980.4
Pancrelipase	973.4	E858.4	E943.4	E950.4	E962.0	E980.4
Pangamic acid	963.5	E858.1	E933.5	E950.4	E962.0	E980.4
Panthenol	963.5	E858.1	E933.5	E950.4	E962.0	E980.4
topical	976.8	E858.7	E946.8	E950.4	E962.0	E980.4
Pantopaque	977.8	E858.8	E947.8	E950.4	E962.0	E980.4
Pantopon	965.00	E850.2	E935.2	E950.0	E962.0	E980.0
Pantothenic acid	963.5	E858.1	E933.5	E950.4	E962.0	E980.4
Panwarfin	964.2	E858.2	E934.2	E950.4	E962.0	E980.4
Papain	973.4	E858.4	E943.4	E950.4	E962.0	E980.4
Papaverine	972.5	E858.3	E942.5	E950.4	E962.0	E980.4
Para-aminobenzoic acid	976.3	E858.7	E946.3	E950.4	E962.0	E980.4
Para-aminophenol derivatives	965.4	E850.4	E935.4	E950.0	E962.0	E980.0
Para-aminosalicylic acid (derivatives)	961.8	E857	E931.8	E950.4	E962.0	E980.4
Paracetaldehyde (medicinal)	967.2	E852.1	E937.2	E950.2	E962.0	E980.2
Paracetamol	965.4	E850.4	E935.4	E950.0	E962.0	E980.0
Paracodin	965.09	E850.2	E935.2	E950.0	E962.0	E980.0
Paradione	966.0	E855.0	E936.0	E950.4	E962.0	E980.4
Paraffin(s) (wax)	981	E862.3	-	E950.9	E962.1	E980.9
liquid (medicinal)	973.2	E858.4	E943.2	E950.4	E962.0	E980.4
nonmedicinal (oil)	981	E962.1	-	E950.9	E962.1	E980.9
Paraldehyde (medicinal)	967.2	E852.1	E937.2	E950.2	E962.0	E980.2
Paramethadione	966.0	E855.0	E936.0	E950.4	E962.0	E980.4
Paramethasone	962.0	E858.0	E932.0	E950.4	E962.0	E980.4
Paraquat	989.4	E863.5	-	E950.6	E962.1	E980.7
Parasympatholytics	971.1	E855.4	E941.1	E950.4	E962.0	E980.4
Parasympathomimetics	971.0	E855.3	E941.0	E950.4	E962.0	E980.4
Parathion	989.3	E863.1	-	E950.6	E962.1	E980.7
Parathormone	962.6	E858.0	E932.6	E950.4	E962.0	E980.4
Parathyroid (derivatives)	962.6	E858.0	E932.6	E950.4	E962.0	E980.4
Paratyphoid vaccine	978.1	E858.8	E948.1	E950.4	E962.0	E980.4
Paredrine	971.2	E855.5	E941.2	E950.4	E962.0	E980.4
Paregoric	965.00	E850.2	E935.2	E950.0	E962.0	E980.0
Pargyline	972.3	E858.3	E942.3	E950.4	E962.0	E980.4
Paris green	985.1	E866.3	-	E950.8	E962.1	E980.8
insecticide	985.1	E863.4	-	E950.8	E962.1	E980.8
Parnate	969.0	E854.0	E939.0	E950.3	E962.0	E980.3
Paromomycin	960.8	E856	E930.8	E950.4	E962.0	E980.4
Paroxypropione	963.1	E858.1	E933.1	E950.4	E962.0	E980.4
Parzone	965.09	E850.2	E935.2	E950.0	E962.0	E980.0
PAS	961.8	E857	E931.8	E950.4	E962.0	E980.4
PCBs	981	E862.3	-	E950.9	E962.1	E980.9
PCP (pentachlorophenol)	989.4	E863.6	-	E950.6	E962.1	E980.7
herbicide	989.4	E863.5	-	E950.6	E962.1	E980.7
insecticide	989.4	E863.4	-	E950.6	E962.1	E980.7
phencyclidine	968.3	E855.1	E938.3	E950.4	E962.0	E980.4
Peach kernel oil (emulsion)	973.2	E858.4	E943.2	E950.4	E962.0	E980.4
Peanut oil (emulsion) NEC	973.2	E858.4	E943.2	E950.4	E962.0	E980.4
topical	976.3	E858.7	E946.3	E950.4	E962.0	E980.4
Pearly Gates (morning glory seeds)	969.6	E854.1	E939.6	E950.3	E962.0	E980.3
Pecazine	969.1	E853.0	E939.1	E950.3	E962.0	E980.3
Pecilocin	960.1	E856	E930.1	E950.4	E962.0	E980.4
Pectin (with kaolin) **NEC**	973.5	E858.4	E943.5	E950.4	E962.0	E980.4
Pelletierine tannate	961.6	E857	E931.6	E950.4	E962.0	E980.4
Pemoline	969.7	E854.2	E939.7	E950.3	E962.0	E980.3

● New Line ▲ Revised Code

Orthoboric acid – Pemoline

Drug	Poisoning	External Cause (E-Code) Accident	Therapeutic Use	Suicide Attempt	Assault	Undetermined
Pempidine	972.3	E858.3	E942.3	E950.4	E962.0	E980.4
Penamecillin	960.0	E856	E930.0	E950.4	E962.0	E980.4
Penethamate hydriodide	960.0	E856	E930.0	E950.4	E962.0	E980.4
Penicillamine	963.8	E858.1	E933.8	E950.4	E962.0	E980.4
Penicillin (any type)	960.0	E856	E930.0	E950.4	E962.0	E980.4
Penicillinase	963.4	E858.1	E933.4	E950.4	E962.0	E980.4
Pentachlorophenol (fungicide)	989.4	E863.6	-	E950.6	E962.1	E980.7
herbicide	989.4	E863.5	-	E950.6	E962.1	E980.7
insecticide	989.4	E863.4	-	E950.6	E962.1	E980.7
Pentaerythritol	972.4	E858.3	E942.4	E950.4	E962.0	E980.4
chloral	967.1	E852.0	E937.1	E950.2	E962.0	E980.2
tetranitrate NEC	972.4	E858.3	E942.4	E950.4	E962.0	E980.4
Pentagastrin	977.8	E858.8	E947.8	E950.4	E962.0	E980.4
Pentalin	982.3	E862.4	-	E950.9	E962.1	E980.9
Pentamethonium (bromide)	972.3	E858.3	E942.3	E950.4	E962.0	E980.4
Pentamidine	961.5	E857	E931.5	E950.4	E962.0	E980.4
Pentanol	980.8	E860.8	-	E950.9	E962.1	E980.9
Pentaquine	961.4	E857	E931.4	E950.4	E962.0	E980.4
Peniazocine	965.8	E850.8	E935.8	E950.0	E962.0	E980.0
Penthienate	971.1	E855.4	E941.1	E950.4	E962.0	E980.4
Pentobarbital, pentobarbitone (sodium)	967.0	E851	E937.0	E950.1	E962.0	E980.1
Pentolinium (tartrate)	972.3	E858.3	E942.3	E950.4	E962.0	E980.4
Pentothal	968.3	E855.1	E938.3	E950.4	E962.0	E980.4
Pentyleneteirazol	970.0	E854.3	E940.0	E950.4	E962.0	E980.4
Pentylsalicylamide	961.8	E857	E931.8	E950.4	E962.0	E980.4
Pepsin	973.4	E858.4	E943.4	E950.4	E962.0	E980.4
Peptavlon	977.8	E858.8	E947.8	E950.4	E962.0	E980.4
Percaine (spinal)	968.7	E855.2	E938.7	E950.4	E962.0	E980.4
topical (surface)	968.5	E855.2	E938.5	E950.4	E962.0	E980.4
Perchloroethylene (vapor)	982.3	E862.4	-	E950.9	E962.1	E980.9
medicinal	961.6	E857	E931.6	E950.4	E962.0	E980.4
Percodan	965.09	E850.2	E935.2	E950.0	E962.0	E980.0
Percogesic	965.09	E850.2	E935.2	E950.0	E962.0	E980.0
Percorten	962.0	E858.0	E932.0	E950.4	E962.0	E980.4
Pergonal	962.4	E858.0	E932.4	E950.4	E962.0	E980.4
Perhexiline	972.4	E858.3	E942.4	E950.4	E962.0	E980.4
Periactin	963.0	E858.1	E933.0	E950.4	E962.0	E980.4
Periclor	967.1	E852.0	E937.1	E950.2	E962.0	E980.2
Pericyazine	969.1	E853.0	E939.1	E950.3	E962.0	E980.3
Peritrate	972.4	E858.3	E942.4	E950.4	E962.0	E980.4
Permanganates NEC	983.9	E864.3	-	E950.7	E962.1	E980.6
potassium (topical)	976.0	E858.7	E946.0	E950.4	E962.0	E980.4
Pernocton	967.0	E851	E937.0	E950.1	E962.0	E980.1
Pernoston	967.0	E851	E937.0	E950.1	E962.0	E980.1
Peronin(e)	965.09	E850.2	E935.2	E950.0	E962.0	E980.0
Perphenazine	969.1	E853.0	E939.1	E950.3	E962.0	E980.3
Pertofrane	969.0	E854.0	E939.0	E950.3	E962.0	E980.3
Pertussis						
immune serum (human)	964.6	E858.2	E934.6	E950.4	E962.0	E980.4
vaccine (with diphtheria toxoid) (with tetanus toxoid)	978.6	E858.8	E948.6	E950.4	E962.0	E980.4
Peruvian balsam	976.8	E858.7	E946.8	E950.4	E962.0	E980.4
Pesticides (dust) (fumes) (vapor)	989.4	E863.4	-	E950.6	E962.1	E980.7
arsenic	985.1	E863.4	-	E950.8	E962.1	E980.8
chlorinated	989.2	E863.0	-	E950.6	E962.1	E980.7
cyanide	989.0	E863.4	-	E950.6	E962.1	E980.7
kerosene	981	E863.4	-	E950.6	E962.1	E980.7
mixture (of compounds)	989.4	E863.3	-	E950.6	E962.1	E980.7
naphthalene	983.0	E863.4	-	E950.7	E962.1	E980.6

Drug	Poisoning	External Cause (E-Code) Accident	Therapeutic Use	Suicide Attempt	Assault	Undetermined
Pesticides – *continued*						
organochlorine (compounds)	989.2	E863.0	-	E950.6	E962.1	E980.7
petroleum (distillate) (products) NEC	981	E863.4	-	E950.6	E962.1	E980.7
specified ingredient NEC	989.4	E863.4	-	E950.6	E962.1	E980.7
strychnine	989.1	E863.4	-	E950.6	E962.1	E980.7
thallium	985.8	E863.7	-	E950.6	E962.1	E980.7
Pethidine (hydrochloride)	965.09	E850.2	E935.2	E950.0	E962.0	E980.0
Petrichloral	967.1	E852.0	E937.1	E950.2	E962.0	E980.2
Petrol	981	E862.1	-	E950.9	E962.1	E980.9
vapor	987.1	E869.8	-	E952.8	E962.2	E982.8
Petrolatum (jelly) (ointment)	976.3	E858.7	E946.3	E950.4	E962.0	E980.4
hydrophilic	976.3	E858.7	E946.3	E950.4	E962.0	E980.4
liquid	973.2	E858.4	E943.2	E950.4	E962.0	E980.4
topical	976.3	E858.7	E946.3	E950.4	E962.0	E980.4
nonmedicinal	981	E862.1	-	E950.9	E962.1	E980.9
Petroleum (cleaners) (fuels) (products) NEC	981	E862.1	-	E950.9	E962.1	E980.9
benzin(e) – *see* Ligroin(e)						
ether – *see* Ligroin(e)						
jelly – *see* Petrolatum						
naphtha – *see* Ligroin(e)						
pesticide	981	E863.4	-	E950.6	E962.1	E980.7
solids	981	E862.3	-	E950.9	E962.1	E980.9
solvents	981	E862.0	-	E950.9	E962.1	E980.9
vapor	987.1	E869.8	-	E952.8	E962.2	E982.8
Peyote	969.6	E854.1	E939.6	E950.3	E962.0	E980.3
Phanodorm, phanodorn	967.0	E851	E937.0	E950.1	E962.0	E980.1
Phanquinone, phanquone	961.5	E857	E931.5	E950.4	E962.0	E980.4
Pharmaceutical excipient or adjunct	977.4	E858.8	E947.4	E950.4	E962.0	E980.4
Phenacemide	966.3	E855.0	E936.3	E950.4	E962.0	E980.4
Phenacetin	965.4	E850.4	E935.4	E950.0	E962.0	E980.0
Phenadoxone	965.09	E850.2	E935.2	E950.0	E962.0	E980.0
Phenaglycodol	969.5	E853.8	E939.5	E950.3	E962.0	E980.3
Phenantoin	966.1	E855.0	E936.1	E950.4	E962.0	E980.4
Phenaphthazine reagent	977.8	E858.8	E947.8	E950.4	E962.0	E980.4
Phenazocine	965.09	E850.2	E935.2	E950.0	E962.0	E980.0
Phenazone	965.5	E850.5	E935.5	E950.0	E962.0	E980.0
Phenazopyridine	976.1	E858.7	E946.1	E950.4	E962.0	E980.4
Phenbenicillin	960.0	E856	E930.0	E950.4	E962.0	E980.4
Phenbutrazate	977.0	E858.8	E947.0	E950.4	E962.0	E980.4
Phencyclidine	968.3	E855.1	E938.3	E950.4	E962.0	E980.4
Phendimetrazine	977.0	E858.8	E947.0	E950.4	E962.0	E980.4
Phenelzine	969.0	E854.0	E939.0	E950.3	E962.0	E980.3
Phenergan	967.8	E852.8	E937.8	E950.2	E962.0	E980.2
Phenethicillin (potassium)	960.0	E856	E930.0	E950.4	E962.0	E980.4
Phenetsal	965.1	E850.3	E935.3	E950.0	E962.0	E980.0
Pheneturide	966.3	E855.0	E936.3	E950.4	E962.0	E980.4
Phenformin	962.3	E858.0	E932.3	E950.4	E962.0	E980.4
Phenglutarimide	971.1	E855.4	E941.1	E950.4	E962.0	E980.4
Phenicarbazide	965.8	E850.8	E935.8	E950.0	E962.0	E980.0
Phenindamine (tartrate)	963.0	E858.1	E933.0	E950.4	E962.0	E980.4
Phenindione	964.2	E858.2	E934.2	E950.4	E962.0	E980.4
Pheniprazine	969.0	E854.0	E939.0	E950.3	E962.0	E980.3
Pheniramine (maleate)	963.0	E858.1	E933.0	E950.4	E962.0	E980.4
Phenmetrazine	977.0	E858.8	E947.0	E950.4	E962.0	E980.4
Phenobal	967.0	E851	E937.0	E950.1	E962.0	E980.1
Phenobarbital	967.0	E851	E937.0	E950.1	E962.0	E980.1
Phenobarbitone	967.0	E851	E937.0	E950.1	E962.0	E980.1
Phenoctide	976.0	E858.7	E946.0	E950.4	E962.0	E980.4
Phenol (derivatives) NEC	983.0	E864.0	-	E950.7	E962.1	E980.6
disinfectant	983.0	E864.0	-	E950.7	E962.1	E980.6

● New Line ▲ Revised Code

		External Cause (E-Code)				
Drug	Poisoning	Accident	Therapeutic Use	Suicide Attempt	Assault	Undetermined
Phenol – *continued*						
pesticide	989.4	E863.4	-	E950.6	E962.1	E980.7
red	977.8	E858.8	E947.8	E950.4	E962.0	E980.4
Phenolphthalein	973.1	E858.4	E943.1	E950.4	E962.0	E980.4
Phenolsulfonphthalein	977.8	E858.8	E947.8	E950.4	E962.0	E980.4
Phenomorphan	965.09	E850.2	E935.2	E950.0	E962.0	E980.0
Phenonyl	967.0	E851	E937.0	E950.1	E962.0	E980.1
Phenoperidine	965.09	E850.2	E935.2	E950.0	E962.0	E980.0
Phenoquin	974.7	E858.5	E944.7	E950.4	E962.0	E980.4
Phenothiazines (tranquilizers) NEC	969.1	E853.0	E939.1	E950.3	E962.0	E980.3
insecticide	989.3	E863.4	-	E950.6	E962.1	E980.7
Phenoxybenzamiine	971.3	E855.6	E941.3	E950.4	E962.0	E980.4
Phenoxymethyl penicillin	960.0	E856	E930.0	E950.4	E962.0	E980.4
Phenprocoumon	964.2	E858.2	E934.2	E950.4	E962.0	E980.4
Phensuximide	966.2	E855.0	E936.2	E950.4	E962.0	E980.4
Phentermine	977.0	E858.8	E947.0	E950.4	E962.0	E980.4
Phentolamine	971.3	E855.6	E941.3	E950.4	E962.0	E980.4
Phenyl						
butazone	965.5	E850.5	E935.5	E950.0	E962.0	E980.0
enediamine	983.0	E864.0	-	E950.7	E962.1	E980.6
hydrazine	983.0	E864.0	E950.7	E962.1	E980.6	
antineoplastic	963.1	E858.1	E933.1	E950.4	E962.0	E980.4
mercuric compounds – *see* Mercury						
salicylaie	976.3	E858.7	E946.3	E950.4	E962.0	E980.4
Phenylephrin	971.2	E855.5	E941.2	E950.4	E962.0	E980.4
Phenylethylbiguanide	962.3	E858.0	E932.3	E950.4	E962.0	E980.4
Phenylpropanolamine	971.2	E855.5	E941.2	E950.4	E962.0	E980.4
Phenylsulfthion	989.3	E863.1	-	E950.6	E962.1	E980.7
Phenyramidol, phenyramidon	965.7	E850.7	E935.7	E950.0	E962.0	E980.0
Phenytoin	966.1	E855.0	E936.1	E950.4	E962.0	E980.4
pHisoHex	976.2	E858.7	E946.2	E950.4	E962.0	E980.4
Pholcodine	965.09	E850.2	E935.2	E950.0	E962.0	E980.0
Phorate	989.3	E863.1	-	E950.6	E962.1	E980.7
Phosdrin	989.3	E863.1	-	E950.6	E962.1	E980.7
Phosgene (gas)	987.8	E869.8	-	E952.8	E962.2	E982.8
Phosphate (tricresyl)	989.89	E866.8	-	E950.9	E962.1	E980.9
organic	989.3	E863.1	-	E950.6	E962.1	E980.7
solvent	982.8	E862.4	-	E950.9	E926.1	E980.9
Phosphine	987.8	E869.8	-	E952.8	E962.2	E982.8
fumigant	987.8	E863.8	-	E950.6	E962.2	E980.7
Phospholine	971.0	E855.3	E941.0	E950.4	E962.0	E980.4
Phosphoric acid	983.1	E864.1	-	E950.7	E962.1	E980.6
Phosphorus (compounds) NEC	983.9	E864.3	-	E950.7	E962.1	E980.6
rodenticide	983.9	E863.7	-	E950.7	E962.1	E980.6
Phthalimidoglutarimide	967.8	E852.8	E937.8	E950.2	E962.0	E980.2
Phthalylsulfathiazole	961.0	E857	E931.0	E950.4	E962.0	E980.4
Phylloquinone	964.3	E858.2	E934.3	E950.4	E962.0	E980.4
Physeptone	965.02	E850.1	E935.1	E950.0	E962.0	E980.0
Physostigma venenosum	988.2	E865.4	-	E950.9	E962.1	E980.9
Physostigmine	971.0	E855.3	E941.0	E950.4	E962.0	E980.4
Phytolacca decandra	988.2	E865.4	-	E950.9	E962.1	E980.9
Phytomenadione	964.3	E858.2	E934.3	E950.4	E962.0	E980.4
Phytonadione	964.3	E858.2	E934.3	E950.4	E962.0	E980.4
Picric (acid)	983.0	E864.0	-	E950.7	E962.1	E980.6
Picrotoxin	970.0	E854.3	E940.0	E950.4	E962.0	E980.4
Pilocarpine	971.0	E855.3	E941.0	E950.4	E962.0	E980.4
Pilocarpus (jaborandi) **extract**	971.0	E855.3	E941.0	E950.4	E962.0	E980.4
Pimaricin	960.1	E856	E930.1	E950.4	E962.0	E980.4
Piminodine	965.09	E850.2	E935.2	E950.0	E962.0	E980.0
Pine oil, pinesol (disinfectant)	983.9	E861.4	-	E950.7	E962.1	E980.6
Pinkroot	961.6	E857	E931.6	E950.4	E962.0	E980.4
Pipadone	965.09	E850.2	E935.2	E950.0	E962.0	E980.0
Pipamazine	963.0	E858.1	E933.0	E950.4	E962.0	E980.4
Pipazethate	975.4	E858.6	E945.4	E950.4	E962.0	E980.4
Pipenzolate	971.1	E855.4	E941.1	E950.4	E962.0	E980.4
Piperacetazine	969.1	E853.0	E939.1	E950.3	E962.0	E980.3
Piperazine NEC	961.6	E857	E931.6	E950.4	E962.0	E980.4
estrone sulfate	962.2	E858.0	E932.2	E950.4	E962.0	E980.4
Piper cubeba	988.2	E865.4	-	E950.9	E962.1	E980.9
Piperidione	975.4	E858.6	E945.4	E950.4	E962.0	E980.4
Piperidolate	971.1	E855.4	E941.1	E950.4	E962.0	E980.4
Piperocaine	968.9	E855.2	E938.9	E950.4	E962.0	E980.4
infiltration (subcutaneous)	968.5	E855.2	E938.5	E950.4	E962.0	E980.4
nerve block (peripheral) (plexus)	968.6	E855.2	E938.6	E950.4	E962.0	E980.4
topical (surface)	968.5	E855.2	E938.5	E950.4	E962.0	E980.4
Pipobroman	963.1	E858.1	E933.1	E950.4	E962.0	E980.4
Pipradrol	970.8	E854.3	E940.8	E950.4	E962.0	E980.4
Piscidia (bark) (erythrina)	965.7	E850.7	E935.7	E950.0	E962.0	E980.0
Pitch	983.0	E864.0	-	E950.7	E962.1	E980.6
Pitkin's solution	968.7	E855.2	E938.7	E950.4	E962.0	E980.4
Pitocin	975.0	E858.6	E945.0	E950.4	E962.0	E980.4
Pitressin (tannate)	962.5	E858.0	E932.5	E950.4	E962.0	E980.4
Pituitary extracts (posterior)	962.5	E858.0	E932.5	E950.4	E962.0	E980.4
anterior	962.4	E858.0	E932.4	E950.4	E962.0	E980.4
Pituitrin	962.5	E858.0	E932.5	E950.4	E962.0	E980.4
Placental extract	962.9	E858.0	E932.9	E950.4	E962.0	E980.4
Placidyl	967.8	E852.8	E937.8	E950.2	E962.0	E980.2
Plague vaccine	978.3	E858.8	E948.3	E950.4	E962.0	E980.4
Plant foods or fertilizers NEC	989.89	E866.5	-	E950.9	E962.1	E980.9
mixed with herbicides	989.4	E863.5	-	E950.6	E962.1	E930.7
Plants, noxious, used as food	988.2	E865.9	-	E950.9	E962.1	E980.9
berries and seeds	988.2	E865.3	-	E950.9	E962.1	E980.9
specified type NEC	988.2	E865.4	-	E950.9	E962.1	E980.9
Plasma (blood)	964.7	E858.2	E934.7	E950.4	E962.0	E980.4
expanders	964.8	E858.2	E934.8	E950.4	E962.0	E980.4
Plasmanate	964.7	E858.2	E934.7	E950.4	E962.0	E980.4
Plegicil	969.1	E853.0	E939.1	E950.3	E962.0	E980.3
Podophyllin	976.4	E858.7	E946.4	E950.4	E962.0	E980.4
Podophyllum resin	976.4	E858.7	E946.4	E950.4	E962.0	E980.4
Poison NEC	989.9	E866.9	-	E950.9	E962.1	E980.9
Poisonous berries	988.2	E865.3	-	E950.9	E962.1	E980.9
Pokeweed (any part)	988.2	E865.4	-	E950.9	E962.1	E980.9
Poldine	971.1	E855.4	E941.1	E950.4	E962.0	E980.4
Poliomyelitis vaccine	979.5	E858.8	E949.5	E950.4	E962.0	E980.4
Poliovirus vaccine	979.5	E858.8	E949.5	E950.4	E962.0	E980.4
Polish (car) (floor) (furniture) (metal) (silver)	989.89	E861.2	-	E950.9	E962.1	E980.9
abrasive	989.89	E861.3	-	E950.9	E962.1	E980.9
porcelain	989.89	E861.3	-	E950.9	E962.1	E980.9
Poloxalkol	973.2	E858.4	E943.2	E950.4	E962.0	E980.4
Polyaminostyrene resins	974.5	E858.5	E944.5	E950.4	E962.0	E980.4
Polychlorinated biphenyl – *see* PCBs						
Polycycline	960.4	E856	E930.4	E950.4	E962.0	E980.4
Polyester resin hardener	982.8	E862.4	-	E950.9	E962.1	E980.9
fumes	987.8	E869.8	-	E952.8	E962.2	E982.8
Polyestradiol (phosphate)	962.2	E858.0	E932.2	E950.4	E962.0	E980.4
Polyethanolamine alkyl sulfate	976.2	E858.7	E946.2	E950.4	E962.0	E980.4

● New Line ▲ Revised Code

Phenol – Polyethanolamine alkyl sulfate

		External Cause (E-Code)				
Drug	Poisoning	Accident	Therapeutic Use	Suicide Attempt	Assault	Undetermined
Polyethylene glycol	976.3	E858.7	E946.3	E950.4	E962.0	E980.4
Polyferose	964.0	E858.2	E934.0	E950.4	E962.0	E980.4
Polymyxin B	960.8	E856	E930.8	E950.4	E962.0	E980.4
ENT agent	976.6	E858.7	E946.6	E950.4	E962.0	E980.4
ophthalmic preparation	976.5	E858.7	E946.5	E950.4	E962.0	E980.4
topical NEC	976.0	E858.7	E946.0	E950.4	E962.0	E980.4
Polynoxylin(e)	976.0	E858.7	E946.0	E950.4	E962.0	E980.4
Polyoxymethyleneurea	976.0	E858.7	E946.0	E950.4	E962.0	E980.4
Polytetrafluoroethylene (inhaled)	987.8	E869.8	-	E952.8	E962.2	E982.8
Polythiazide	974.3	E858.5	E944.3	E950.4	E962.0	E980.4
Polyvinylpyrrolidone	964.8	E858.2	E934.8	E950.4	E962.0	E980.4
Pontocaine (hydrochloride) (infiltration) (topical)	968.5	E855.2	E938.5	E950.4	E962.0	E980.4
nerve block (peripheral) (plexus)	968.6	E855.2	E938.6	E950.4	E962.0	E980.4
spinal	968.7	E855.2	E938.7	E950.4	E962.0	E980.4
Pot	969.6	E854.1	E939.6	E950.3	E962.0	E980.3
Potash (caustic)	983.2	E864.2	-	E950.7	E962.1	E980.6
Potassic saline injection (lactated)	974.5	E858.5	E944.5	E950.4	E962.0	E980.4
Potassium (salts) NEC	974.5	E858.5	E944.5	E950.4	E962.0	E980.4
aminosalicylate	961.8	E857	E931.8	E950.4	E962.0	E980.4
arsenite (solution)	985.1	E866.3	-	E950.8	E962.1	E980.8
bichromate	983.9	E864.3	-	E950.7	E962.1	E980.6
bisulfate	983.9	E864.3	-	E950.7	E962.1	E980.6
bromide (medicinal) NEC	967.3	E852.2	E937.3	E950.2	E962.0	E980.2
carbonate	983.2	E864.2	-	E950.7	E962.1	E980.6
chlorate NEC	983.9	E864.3	-	E950.7	E962.1	E980.6
cyanide – *see* Cyanide						
hydroxide	983.2	E864.2	-	E950.7	E962.1	E980.6
iodide (expectorant) NEC	975.5	E858.6	E945.5	E950.4	E962.0	E980.4
nitrate	989.89	E866.8	-	E950.9	E962.1	E980.9
oxalate	983.9	E864.3	-	E950.7	E962.1	E980.6
perchlorate NEC	977.8	E858.8	E947.8	E950.4	E962.0	E980.4
antithyroid	962.8	E858.0	E932.8	E950.4	E962.0	E980.4
permanganate	976.0	E858.7	E946.0	E950.4	E962.0	E980.4
nonmedicinal	983.9	E864.3	-	E950.7	E962.1	E980.6
Povidone-iodine (anti-infective) **NEC**	976.0	E858.7	E946.0	E950.4	E962.0	E980.4
Practolol	972.0	E858.3	E942.0	E950.4	E962.0	E980.4
Pralidoxime (chloride)	977.2	E858.8	E947.2	E950.4	E962.0	E980.4
Pramoxine	968.5	E855.2	E938.5	E950.4	E962.0	E980.4
Prazosin	972.6	E858.3	E942.6	E950.4	E962.0	E980.4
Prednisolone	962.0	E858.0	E932.0	E950.4	E962.0	E980.4
ENT agent	976.6	E858.7	E946.6	E950.4	E962.0	E980.4
ophthalmic preparation	976.5	E858.7	E946.5	E950.4	E962.0	E980.4
topical NEC	976.0	E858.7	E946.0	E950.4	E962.0	E980.4
Prednisone	962.0	E858.0	E932.0	E950.4	E962.0	E980.4
Pregnanediol	962.2	E858.0	E932.2	E950.4	E962.0	E980.4
Pregneninolone	962.2	E858.0	E932.2	E950.4	E962.0	E980.4
Preludin	977.0	E858.8	E947.0	E950.4	E962.0	E980.4
Premarin	962.2	E858.0	E932.2	E950.4	E962.0	E980.4
Prenylamine	972.4	E858.3	E942.4	E950.4	E962.0	E980.4
Preparation H	976.8	E858.7	E946.8	E950.4	E962.0	E980.4
Preservatives	989.89	E866.8	-	E950.9	E962.1	E980.9
Pride of China	988.2	E865.3	-	E950.9	E962.1	E980.9
Prilocaine	968.9	E855.2	E938.9	E950.4	E962.0	E980.4
infiltration (subcutaneous)	968.5	E855.2	E938.5	E950.4	E962.0	E980.4
nerve block (peripheral) (plexus)	968.6	E855.2	E938.6	E950.4	E962.0	E980.4
Primaquine	961.4	E857	E931.4	E950.4	E962.0	E980.4
Primidone	966.3	E855.0	E936.3	E950.4	E962.0	E980.4
Primula (veris)	988.2	E865.4	-	E950.9	E962.1	E980.9

		External Cause (E-Code)				
Drug	Poisoning	Accident	Therapeutic Use	Suicide Attempt	Assault	Undetermined
Prinadol	965.09	E850.2	E935.2	E950.0	E962.0	E980.0
Priscol, Priscoline	971.3	E855.6	E941.3	E950.4	E962.0	E980.4
Privet	988.2	E865.4	-	E950.9	E962.1	E980.9
Privine	971.2	E855.5	E941.2	E950.4	E962.0	E980.4
Pro-Banthine	971.1	E855.4	E941.1	E950.4	E962.0	E980.4
Probarbital	967.0	E851	E937.0	E950.1	E962.0	E980.1
Probenecid	974.7	E858.5	E944.7	E950.4	E962.0	E980.4
Procainamide (hydrochloride)	972.0	E858.3	E942.0	E950.4	E962.0	E980.4
Procaine (hydrochloride) (infiltration) (topical)	968.5	E855.2	E938.5	E950.4	E962.0	E980.4
nerve block (periphreal) (plexus)	968.6	E855.2	E938.6	E950.4	E962.0	E980.4
penicillin G	960.0	E856	E930.0	E950.4	E962.0	E980.4
spinal	968.7	E855.2	E938.7	E950.4	E962.0	E980.4
Procalmidol	969.5	E853.8	E939.5	E950.3	E962.0	E980.3
Procarbazine	963.1	E858.1	E933.1	E950.4	E962.0	E980.4
Prochlorperazine	969.1	E853.0	E939.1	E950.3	E962.0	E980.3
Procyclidine	966.4	E855.0	E936.4	E950.4	E962.0	E980.4
Producer gas	986	E868.8	-	E952.1	E962.2	E982.1
Profenamine	966.4	E855.0	E936.4	E950.4	E962.0	E980.4
Profenil	975.1	E858.6	E945.1	E950.4	E962.0	E980.4
Progesterones	962.2	E858.0	E932.2	E950.4	E962.0	E980.4
Progestin	962.2	E858.0	E932.2	E950.4	E962.0	E980.4
Progestogens (with estrogens)	962.2	E858.0	E932.2	E950.4	E962.0	E980.4
Progestone	962.2	E858.0	E932.2	E950.4	E962.0	E980.4
Proguanil	961.4	E857	E931.4	E950.4	E962.0	E980.4
Prolactin	962.4	E858.0	E932.4	E950.4	E962.0	E980.4
Proloid	962.7	E858.0	E932.7	E950.4	E962.0	E980.4
Proluton	962.2	E858.0	E932.2	E950.4	E962.0	E980.4
Promacetin	961.8	E857	E931.8	E950.4	E962.0	E980.4
Promazine	969.1	E853.0	E939.1	E950.3	E962.0	E980.3
Promedol	965.09	E850.2	E935.2	E950.0	E962.0	E980.0
Promethazine	967.8	E852.8	E937.8	E950.2	E962.0	E980.2
Promin	961.8	E857	E931.8	E950.4	E962.0	E980.4
Pronestyl (hydrochloride)	972.0	E858.3	E942.0	E950.4	E962.0	E980.4
Pronetalol, pronethalol	972.0	E858.3	E942.0	E950.4	E962.0	E980.4
Prontosil	961.0	E857	E931.0	E950.4	E962.0	E980.4
Propamidine isethionate	961.5	E857	E931.5	E950.4	E962.0	E980.4
Propanal (medicinal)	967.8	E852.8	E937.8	E950.2	E962.0	E980.2
Propane (gas) (distributed in mobile container)	987.0	E868.0	-	E951.1	E962.2	E981.1
distributed through pipes	987.0	E867	-	E951.0	E962.2	E981.0
incomplete combustion of – *see* Carbon monoxide, Propane						
Propanidid	968.3	E855.1	E938.3	E950.4	E962.0	E980.4
Propanol	980.3	E860.4	-	E950.9	E962.1	E980.9
Propantheline	971.1	E855.4	E941.1	E950.4	E962.0	E980.4
Proparacaine	968.5	E855.2	E938.5	E950.4	E962.0	E980.4
Propatyl nitrate	972.4	E858.3	E942.4	E950.4	E962.0	E980.4
Propicillin	960.0	E856	E930.0	E950.4	E962.0	E980.4
Propiolactone (vapor)	987.8	E869.8	-	E952.8	E962.2	E982.8
Propiomazine	967.8	E852.8	E937.8	E950.2	E962.0	E980.2
Propionaidehyde (medicinal)	967.8	E852.8	E937.8	E950.2	E962.0	E980.2
Propionate compound	976.0	E858.7	E946.0	E950.4	E962.0	E980.4
Propion gel	976.0	E858.7	E946.0	E950.4	E962.0	E980.4
Propitocaine	968.9	E855.2	E938.9	E950.4	E962.0	E980.4
infiltration (subcutaneous)	968.5	E855.2	E938.5	E950.4	E962.0	E980.4
nerve block (peripheral) (plexus)	968.6	E855.2	E938.6	E950.4	E962.0	E980.4
Propoxur	989.3	E863.2	-	E950.6	E962.1	E980.7
Propoxycaine	968.9	E855.2	E938.9	E950.4	E962.0	E980.4
infiltration (subcutaneous)	968.5	E855.2	E938.5	E950.4	E962.0	E980.4

● New Line ▲ Revised Code

Drug	Poisoning	External Cause (E-Code) Accident	Therapeutic Use	Suicide Attempt	Assault	Undetermined
Propoxycaine – *continued*						
nerve block (peripheral) (plexus)	968.6	E855.2	E938.6	E950.4	E962.0	E980.4
topical (surface)	968.5	E855.2	E938.5	E950.4	E962.0	E980.4
Propoxyphene (hydrochloride)	965.8	E850.8	E935.8	E950.0	E962.0	E980.0
Propranolol	972.0	E858.3	E942.0	E950.4	E962.0	E980.4
Propyl						
alcohol	980.3	E860.4	-	E950.9	E962.1	E980.9
carbinol	980.3	E860.4	-	E950.9	E962.1	E980.9
hexadrine	971.2	E855.5	E941.2	E950.4	E962.0	E980.4
iodone	977.8	E858.8	E947.8	E950.4	E962.0	E980.4
thiouracil	962.8	E858.0	E932.8	E950.4	E962.0	E980.4
Propylene	987.1	E869.8	-	E952.8	E962.2	E982.8
Propylparaben (ophthalmic)	976.5	E858.7	E946.5	E950.4	E962.0	E980.4
Proscillaridin	972.1	E858.3	E942.1	E950.4	E962.0	E980.4
Prostaglandins	975.0	E858.6	E945.0	E950.4	E962.0	E980.4
Prostigmin	971.0	E855.3	E941.0	E950.4	E962.0	E980.4
Protamine (sulfate)	964.5	E858.2	E934.5	E950.4	E962.0	E980.4
zinc insulin	962.3	E858.0	E932.3	E950.4	E962.0	E980.4
Protectants (topical)	976.3	E858.7	E946.3	E950.4	E962.0	E980.4
Protein hydrolysate	974.5	E858.5	E944.5	E950.4	E962.0	E980.4
Prothiaden – *see* Dothiepin hydrochloride						
Prothionamide	961.8	E857	E931.8	E950.4	E962.0	E980.4
Prothipendyl	969.5	E853.8	E939.5	E950.3	E962.0	E980.3
Protokylol	971.2	E855.5	E941.2	E950.4	E962.0	E980.4
Protopam	977.2	E858.8	E947.2	E950.4	E962.0	E980.4
Protoveratrine(s) (A) (B)	972.6	E858.3	E942.6	E950.4	E962.0	E980.4
Protriptyline	969.0	E854.0	E939.0	E950.3	E962.0	E980.3
Provera	962.2	E858.0	E932.2	E950.4	E962.0	E980.4
Provitamin A	963.5	E858.1	E933.5	E950.4	E962.0	E980.4
Proxymetacaine	968.5	E855.2	E938.5	E950.4	E962.0	E980.4
Proxyphylline	975.1	E858.6	E945.1	E950.4	E962.0	E980.4
Prozac – *see* Fluoxetine hydrochloride						
Prunus						
laurocerasus	988.2	E865.4	-	E950.9	E962.1	E980.9
virginiana	988.2	E865.4	-	E950.9	E962.1	E980.9
Prussic acid	989.0	E866.8	-	E950.9	E962.1	E980.9
vapor	987.7	E869.8	-	E952.8	E962.2	E982.8
Pseudoephedrine	971.2	E855.5	E941.2	E950.4	E962.0	E980.4
Psilocin	969.6	E854.1	E939.6	E950.3	E962.0	E980.3
Psilocybin	969.6	E854.1	E939.6	E950.3	E962.0	E980.3
PSP	977.8	E858.8	E947.8	E950.4	E962.0	E980.4
Psychedelic agents	969.6	E854.1	E939.6	E950.3	E962.0	E980.3
Psychodysleptics	969.6	E854.1	E939.6	E950.3	E962.0	E980.3
Psychostimulants	969.7	E854.2	E939.7	E950.3	E962.0	E980.3
Psychotherapeutic agents	969.9	E855.9	E939.9	E950.3	E962.0	E980.3
antidepressants	969.0	E854.0	E939.0	E950.3	E962.0	E980.3
specified NEC	969.8	E855.8	E939.8	E950.3	E962.0	E980.3
tranquilizers NEC	969.5	E853.9	E939.5	E950.3	E962.0	E980.3
Psychotomimetic agents	969.6	E854.1	E939.6	E950.3	E962.0	E980.3
Psychotropic agents	969.9	E854.8	E939.9	E950.3	E962.0	E980.3
specified NEC	969.8	E854.8	E939.8	E950.3	E962.0	E980.3
Psyllium	973.3	E858.4	E943.3	E950.4	E962.0	E980.4
Pteroylglutamic acid	964.1	E858.2	E934.1	E950.4	E962.0	E980.4
Pteroyltriglutamate	963.1	E858.1	E933.1	E950.4	E962.0	E980.4
PTFE	987.8	E869.8	-	E952.8	E962.2	E982.8
Pulsatilla	988.2	E865.4	-	E950.9	E962.1	E980.9
Purex (bleach)	983.9	E864.3	-	E950.7	E962.1	E980.6
Purine diuretics	974.1	E858.5	E944.1	E950.4	E962.0	E980.4
Purinethol	963.1	E858.1	E933.1	E950.4	E962.0	E980.4
PVP	964.8	E858.2	E934.8	E950.4	E962.0	E980.4
Pyrabital	965.7	E850.7	E935.7	E950.0	E962.0	E980.0
Pyramidon	965.5	E850.5	E935.5	E950.0	E962.0	E980.0
Pyrantel (pamoate)	961.6	E857	E931.6	E950.4	E962.0	E980.4
Pyrathiazine	963.0	E858.1	E933.0	E950.4	E962.0	E980.4
Pyrazinamide	961.8	E857	E931.8	E950.4	E962.0	E980.4
Pyrazinoic acid (amide)	961.8	E857	E931.8	E950.4	E962.0	E980.4
Pyrazole (derivatives)	965.5	E850.5	E935.5	E950.0	E962.0	E980.0
Pyrazolone (analgesics)	965.5	E850.5	E935.5	E950.0	E962.0	E980.0
Pyrethrins, pyrethrum	989.4	E863.4	-	E950.6	E962.1	E980.7
Pyribenzamine	963.0	E858.1	E933.0	E950.4	E962.0	E980.4
Pyridine (liquid) (vapor)	982.0	E862.4	-	E950.9	E962.1	E980.9
aldoxime chloride	977.2	E858.8	E947.2	E950.4	E962.0	E980.4
Pyridium	976.1	E858.7	E946.1	E950.4	E962.0	E980.4
Pyridostigmine	971.0	E855.3	E941.0	E950.4	E962.0	E980.4
Pyridoxine	963.5	E858.1	E933.5	E950.4	E962.0	E980.4
Pyrilamine	963.0	E858.1	E933.0	E950.4	E962.0	E980.4
Pyrimethamine	961.4	E857	E931.4	E950.4	E962.0	E980.4
Pyrogallic acid	983.0	E864.0	-	E950.7	E962.1	E980.6
Pyroxylin	976.3	E858.7	E946.3	E950.4	E962.0	E980.4
Pyrrobutamine	963.0	E858.1	E933.0	E950.4	E962.0	E980.4
Pyrrocitine	968.5	E855.2	E938.5	E950.4	E962.0	E980.4
Pyrvinium (pamoate)	961.6	E857	E931.6	E950.4	E962.0	E980.4
PZI	962.3	E858.0	E932.3	E950.4	E962.0	E980.4
Quaalude	967.4	E852.3	E937.4	E950.2	E962.0	E980.2
Quaternary ammonia derivatives	971.1	E855.4	E941.1	E950.4	E962.0	E980.4
Quicklime	983.2	E864.2	-	E950.7	E962.1	E980.6
Quinacrine	961.3	E857	E931.3	E950.4	E962.0	E980.4
Quinaglute	972.0	E858.3	E942.0	E950.4	E962.0	E980.4
Quinalbarbitone	967.0	E851	E937.0	E950.1	E962.0	E980.1
Quinestradiol	962.2	E858.0	E932.2	E950.4	E962.0	E980.4
Quinethazone	974.3	E858.5	E944.3	E950.4	E962.0	E980.4
Quinidine (gluconate) (polygalacturonate) (salts) (sulfate)	972.0	E858.3	E942.0	E950.4	E962.0	E980.4
Quinine	961.4	E857	E931.4	E950.4	E962.0	E980.4
Quiniobine	961.3	E857	E931.3	E950.4	E962.0	E980.4
Quinolines	961.3	E857	E931.3	E950.4	E962.0	E980.4
Quotane	968.5	E855.2	E938.5	E950.4	E962.0	E980.4
Rabies						
immune globulin (human)	964.6	E858.2	E934.6	E950.4	E962.0	E980.4
vaccine	979.1	E858.8	E949.1	E950.4	E962.0	E980.4
Racemoramide	965.09	E850.2	E935.2	E950.0	E962.0	E980.0
Racemorphan	965.09	E850.2	E935.2	E950.0	E962.0	E980.0
Radiator alcohol	980.1	E860.2	-	E950.9	E962.1	E980.9
Radio-opaque (drugs) (materials)	977.8	E858.8	E947.8	E950.4	E962.0	E980.4
Ranunculus	988.2	E865.4	-	E950.9	E962.1	E980.9
Rat poison	989.4	E863.7	-	E950.6	E962.1	E980.7
Rattlesnake (venom)	989.5	E905.0	-	E950.9	E962.1	E980.9
Raudixin	972.6	E858.3	E942.6	E950.4	E962.0	E980.4
Rautensin	972.6	E858.3	E942.6	E950.4	E962.0	E980.4
Rautina	972.6	E858.3	E942.6	E950.4	E962.0	E980.4
Rautotal	972.6	E858.3	E942.6	E950.4	E962.0	E980.4
Rauwiloid	972.6	E858.3	E942.6	E950.4	E962.0	E980.4
Rauwoldin	972.6	E858.3	E942.6	E950.4	E962.0	E980.4
Rauwolfia (alkaloids)	972.6	E858.3	E942.6	E950.4	E962.0	E980.4
Realgar	985.1	E866.3	-	E950.8	E962.1	E980.8
Red cells, packed	964.7	E858.2	E934.7	E950.4	E962.0	E980.4
Reducing agents, industrial NEC	983.9	E864.3	-	E950.7	E962.1	E980.6
Refrigerant gas (freon)	987.4	E869.2	-	E952.8	E962.2	E982.8
not freon	987.9	E869.9	-	E952.9	E962.2	E982.9
Regroton	974.4	E858.5	E944.4	E950.4	E962.0	E980.4

● New Line ▲ Revised Code

Drug	Poisoning	External Cause (E-Code)				
		Accident	Therapeutic Use	Suicide Attempt	Assault	Undetermined
Rela	968.0	E855.1	E938.0	E950.4	E962.0	E980.4
Relaxants, skeletal muscle (autonomic)	975.2	E858.6	E945.2	E950.4	E962.0	E980.4
central nervous system	968.0	E855.1	E938.0	E950.4	E962.0	E980.4
Renese	974.3	E858.5	E944.3	E950.4	E962.0	E980.4
Renografin	977.8	E858.8	E947.8	E950.4	E962.0	E980.4
Replacement solutions	974.5	E858.5	E944.5	E950.4	E962.0	E980.4
Rescinnamine	972.6	E858.3	E942.6	E950.4	E962.0	E980.4
Reserpine	972.6	E858.3	E942.6	E950.4	E962.0	E980.4
Resorcin, resorcinol	976.4	E858.7	E946.4	E950.4	E962.0	E980.4
Respaire	975.5	E858.6	E945.5	E950.4	E962.0	E980.4
Respiratory agents NEC	975.8	E858.6	E945.8	E950.4	E962.0	E980.4
Retinoic acid	976.8	E858.7	E946.8	E950.4	E962.0	E980.4
Retinol	963.5	E858.1	E933.5	E950.4	E962.0	E980.4
Rh (D) immune globulin (human)	964.6	E858.2	E934.6	E950.4	E962.0	E980.4
Rhodine	965.1	E850.3	E935.3	E950.0	E962.0	E980.0
RhoGAM	964.6	E858.2	E934.6	E950.4	E962.0	E980.4
Riboflavin	963.5	E858.1	E933.5	E950.4	E962.0	E980.4
Ricin	989.89	E866.8	-	E950.9	E962.1	E980.9
Ricinus communis	988.2	E865.3	-	E950.9	E962.1	E980.9
Rickettsial vaccine NEC	979.6	E858.8	E949.6	E950.4	E962.0	E980.4
with viral and bacterial vaccine	979.7	E858.8	E949.7	E950.4	E962.0	E980.4
Rifampin	960.6	E856	E930.6	E950.4	E962.0	E980.4
Rimifon	961.8	E857	E931.8	E950.4	E962.0	E980.4
Ringer's injection (lactated)	974.5	E858.5	E944.5	E950.4	E962.0	E980.4
Ristocetin	960.8	E856	E930.8	E950.4	E962.0	E980.4
Ritalin	969.7	E854.2	E939.7	E950.3	E962.0	E980.3
Roach killers – *see* Pesticides						
Rocky Mountain spotted fever vaccine	979.6	E858.8	E949.6	E950.4	E962.0	E980.4
Rodenticides	989.4	E863.7	-	E950.6	E962.1	E980.7
Rohypnol	969.4	E853.2	E939.4	E950.3	E962.0	E980.3
Rolaids	973.0	E858.4	E943.0	E950.4	E962.0	E980.4
Rolitetracycline	960.4	E856	E930.4	E950.4	E962.0	E980.4
Romilar	975.4	E858.6	E945.4	E950.4	E962.0	E980.4
Rose water ointment	976.3	E858.7	E946.3	E950.4	E962.0	E980.4
Rotenone	989.4	E863.7	-	E950.6	E962.1	E980.7
Rotoxamine	963.0	E858.1	E933.0	E950.4	E962.0	E980.4
Rough-on-rats	989.4	E863.7	-	E950.6	E962.1	E980.7
RU486	962.9	E858.0	E932.9	E950.4	E962.0	E980.4
Rubbing alcohol	980.2	E860.3	-	E950.9	E962.1	E980.9
Rubella virus vaccine	979.4	E858.8	E949.4	E950.4	E962.0	E980.4
Rubelogen	979.4	E858.8	E949.4	E950.4	E962.0	E980.4
Rubeovax	979.4	E858.8	E949.4	E950.4	E962.0	E980.4
Rubidomycin	960.7	E856	E930.7	E950.4	E962.0	E980.4
Rue	988.2	E865.4	-	E950.9	E962.1	E980.9
Ruta	988.2	E865.4	-	E950.9	E962.1	E980.9
Sabadilla (medicinal)	976.0	E858.7	E946.0	E950.4	E962.0	E980.4
pesticide	989.4	E863.4	-	E950.6	E962.1	E980.7
Sabin oral vaccine	979.5	E858.8	E949.5	E950.4	E962.0	E980.4
Saccharated iron oxide	964.0	E858.2	E934.0	E950.4	E962.0	E980.4
Saccharin	974.5	E858.5	E944.5	E950.4	E962.0	E980.4
Safflower oil	972.2	E858.3	E942.2	E950.4	E962.0	E980.4
Salbutamol sulfate	975.7	E858.6	E945.7	E950.4	E962.0	E980.4
Salicylamide	965.1	E850.3	E935.3	E950.0	E962.0	E980.0
Salicylate(s)	965.1	E850.3	E935.3	E950.0	E962.0	E980.0
methyl	976.3	E858.7	E946.3	E950.4	E962.0	E980.4
theobromine calcium	974.1	E858.5	E944.1	E950.4	E962.0	E980.4
Salicylazosulfapyridine	961.0	E857	E931.0	E950.4	E962.0	E980.4
Salicylhydroxamic acid	976.0	E858.7	E946.0	E950.4	E962.0	E980.4

Drug	Poisoning	External Cause (E-Code)				
		Accident	Therapeutic Use	Suicide Attempt	Assault	Undetermined
Salicylic acid (keratolytic) NEC	976.4	E858.7	E946.4	E950.4	E962.0	E980.4
congeners	965.1	E850.3	E935.3	E950.0	E962.0	E980.0
salts	965.1	E850.3	E935.3	E950.0	E962.0	E980.0
Saliniazid	961.8	E857	E931.8	E950.4	E962.0	E980.4
Salol	976.3	E858.7	E946.3	E950.4	E962.0	E980.4
Salt (substitute) **NEC**	974.5	E858.5	E944.5	E950.4	E962.0	E980.4
Saluretics	974.3	E858.5	E944.3	E950.4	E962.0	E980.4
Saluron	974.3	E858.5	E944.3	E950.4	E962.0	E980.4
Salvarsan 606 (neosilver) (silver)	961.1	E857	E931.1	E950.4	E962.0	E980.4
Sambucus canadensis	988.2	E865.4	-	E950.9	E962.1	E980.9
berry	988.2	E865.3	-	E950.9	E962.1	E980.9
Sandril	972.6	E858.3	E942.6	E950.4	E962.0	E980.4
Sanguinaria canadensis	988.2	E865.4	-	E950.9	E962.1	E980.9
Saniflush (cleaner)	983.9	E861.3	-	E950.7	E962.1	E980.6
Santonin	961.6	E857	E931.6	E950.4	E962.0	E980.4
Santyl	976.8	E858.7	E946.8	E950.4	E962.0	E980.4
Sarkomycin	960.7	E856	E930.7	E950.4	E962.0	E980.4
Saroten	969.0	E854.0	E939.0	E950.3	E962.0	E980.3
Saturnine – *see* Lead						
Savin (oil)	976.4	E858.7	E946.4	E950.4	E962.0	E980.4
Scammony	973.1	E858.4	E943.1	E950.4	E962.0	E980.4
Scarlet red	976.8	E858.7	E946.8	E950.4	E962.0	E980.4
Scheele's green	985.1	E866.3	-	E950.8	E962.1	E980.8
insecticide	985.1	E863.4	-	E950.8	E962.1	E980.8
Schradan	989.3	E863.1	-	E950.6	E962.1	E980.7
Schweinfurt(h) green	985.1	E866.3	-	E950.8	E962.1	E980.8
insecticide	985.1	E863.4	-	E950.8	E962.1	E980.8
Scilla – *see* Squill						
Sclerosing agents	972.7	E858.3	E942.7	E950.4	E962.0	E980.4
Scopolamine	971.1	E855.4	E941.1	E950.4	E962.0	E980.4
Scouring powder	989.89	E861.3	-	E950.9	E962.1	E980.9
Sea						
anemone (sting)	989.5	E905.6	-	E950.9	E962.1	E980.9
cucumber (sting)	989.5	E905.6	-	E950.9	E962.1	E980.9
snake (bite) (venom)	989.5	E905.0	-	E950.9	E962.1	E980.9
urchin spine (puncture)	989.5	E905.6	-	E950.9	E962.1	E980.9
Secbutabarbital	967.0	E851	E937.0	E950.1	E962.0	E980.1
Secbutabarbitone	967.0	E851	E937.0	E950.1	E962.0	E980.1
Secobarbital	967.0	E851	E937.0	E950.1	E962.0	E980.1
Seconal	967.0	E851	E937.0	E950.1	E962.0	E980.1
Secretin	977.8	E858.8	E947.8	E950.4	E962.0	E980.4
Sedatives, nonbarbiturate	967.9	E852.9	E937.9	E950.2	E962.0	E980.2
specified NEC	967.8	E852.8	E937.8	E950.2	E962.0	E980.2
Sedormid	967.8	E852.8	E937.8	E950.2	E962.0	E980.2
Seed (plant)	988.2	E865.3	-	E950.9	E962.1	E980.9
disinfectant or dressing	989.89	E866.5	-	E950.9	E962.1	E980.9
Selenium (fumes) NEC	985.8	E866.4	-	E950.9	E962.1	E980.9
disulfide or sulfide	976.4	E858.7	E946.4	E950.4	E962.0	E980.4
Selsun	976.4	E858.7	E946.4	E950.4	E962.0	E980.4
Senna	973.1	E858.4	E943.1	E950.4	E962.0	E980.4
Septisol	976.2	E858.7	E946.2	E950.4	E962.0	E980.4
Serax	969.4	E853.2	E939.4	E950.3	E962.0	E980.3
Serenesil	967.8	E852.8	E937.8	E950.2	E962.0	E980.2
Serenium (hydrochloride)	961.9	E857	E931.9	E950.4	E962.0	E980.4
Serepax – *see* Oxazepam						
Sernyl	968.3	E855.1	E938.3	E950.4	E962.0	E980.4
Serotonin	977.8	E858.8	E947.8	E950.4	E962.0	E980.4
Serpasil	972.6	E858.3	E942.6	E950.4	E962.0	E980.4
Sewer gas	987.8	E869.8	-	E952.8	E962.2	E982.8
Shampoo	989.6	E861.0	-	E950.9	E962.1	E980.9
Shellfish, nonbacterial or noxious	988.0	E865.1	-	E950.9	E962.1	E980.9

Rela – Shellfish, nonbacterial or noxious

● New Line ▲ Revised Code

		External Cause (E-Code)				
Drug	Poisoning	Accident	Therapeutic Use	Suicide Attempt	Assault	Undetermined
Silicones NEC	989.83	E866.8	E947.8	E950.9	E962.1	E980.9
Silvadene	976.0	E858.7	E946.0	E950.4	E962.0	E980.4
Silver (compound) (medicinal) NEC	976.0	E858.7	E946.0	E950.4	E962.0	E980.4
anti-infectives	976.0	E858.7	E946.0	E950.4	E962.0	E980.4
arsphenamine	961.1	E857	E931.1	E950.4	E962.0	E980.4
nitrate	976.0	E858.7	E946.0	E950.4	E962.0	E980.4
ophthalmic preparation	976.5	E858.7	E946.5	E950.4	E962.0	E980.4
toughened (keratolytic)	976.4	E858.7	E946.4	E950.4	E962.0	E980.4
nonmedicinal (dust)	985.8	E866.4	-	E950.9	E962.1	E980.9
protein (mild) (strong)	976.0	E858.7	E946.0	E950.4	E962.0	E980.4
salvarsan	961.1	E857	E931.1	E950.4	E962.0	E980.4
Simethicone	973.8	E858.4	E943.8	E950.4	E962.0	E980.4
Sinequan	969.0	E854.0	E939.0	E950.3	E962.0	E980.3
Singoserp	972.6	E858.3	E942.6	E950.4	E962.0	E980.4
Sintrom	964.2	E858.2	E934.2	E950.4	E962.0	E980.4
Sitosterols	972.2	E858.3	E942.2	E950.4	E962.0	E980.4
Skeletal muscle relaxants	975.2	E858.6	E945.2	E950.4	E962.0	E980.4
Skin						
agents (external)	976.9	E858.7	E946.9	E950.4	E962.0	E980.4
specified NEC	976.8	E858.7	E946.8	E950.4	E962.0	E980.4
test antigen	977.8	E858.8	E947.8	E950.4	E962.0	E980.4
Sleep-eze	963.0	E858.1	E933.0	E950.4	E962.0	E980.4
Sleeping draught (drug) (pill) (tablet)	967.9	E852.9	E937.9	E950.2	E962.0	E980.2
Smallpox vaccine	979.0	E858.8	E949.0	E950.4	E962.0	E980.4
Smelter fumes NEC	985.9	E866.4	-	E950.9	E962.1	E980.9
Smog	987.3	E869.1	-	E952.8	E962.2	E982.8
Smoke NEC	987.9	E869.9	-	E952.9	E962.2	E982.9
Smooth muscle relaxant	975.1	E858.6	E945.1	E950.4	E962.0	E980.4
Snail killer	989.4	E863.4	-	E950.6	E962.1	E980.7
Snake (bite) (venom)	989.5	E905.0	-	E950.9	E962.1	E980.9
Snuff	989.89	E866.8	-	E950.9	E962.1	E980.9
Soap (powder) (product)	989.6	E861.1	-	E950.9	E962.1	E980.9
medicinal, soft	976.2	E858.7	E946.2	E950.4	E962.0	E980.4
Soda (caustic)	983.2	E864.2	-	E950.7	E962.1	E980.6
bicarb	963.3	E858.1	E933.3	E950.4	E962.0	E980.4
chlorinated – *see* Sodium, hypochlorite						
Sodium						
acetosulfone	961.8	E857	E931.8	E950.4	E962.0	E980.4
acetrizoate	977.8	E858.8	E947.8	E950.4	E962.0	E980.4
amytal	967.0	E851	E937.0	E950.1	E962.0	E980.1
arsenate – *see* Arsenic						
bicarbonate	963.3	E858.1	E933.3	E950.4	E962.0	E980.4
bichromate	983.9	E864.3	-	E950.7	E962.1	E980.6
biphosphate	963.2	E858.1	E933.2	E950.4	E962.0	E980.4
bisulfate	983.9	E864.3	-	E950.7	E962.1	E980.6
borate (cleanser)	989.6	E861.3	-	E950.9	E962.1	E980.9
bromide NEC	967.3	E852.2	E937.3	E950.2	E962.0	E980.2
cacodylate (nonmedicinal) NEC	978.8	E858.8	E948.8	E950.4	E962.0	E980.4
anti-infective	961.1	E857	E931.1	E950.4	E962.0	E980.4
herbicide	989.4	E863.5	-	E950.6	E962.1	E980.7
calcium edetate	963.8	E858.1	E933.8	E950.4	E962.0	E980.4
carbonate NEC	983.2	E864.2	-	E950.7	E962.1	E980.6
chlorate NEC	983.9	E864.3	-	E950.7	E962.1	E980.6
herbicide	983.9	E863.5	-	E950.7	E962.1	E980.6
chloride NEC	974.5	E858.5	E944.5	E950.4	E962.0	E980.4
chromate	983.9	E864.3	-	E950.7	E962.1	E980.6
citrate	963.3	E858.1	E933.3	E950.4	E962.0	E980.4
cyanide – *see* Cyanide(s)						
cyclamate	974.5	E858.5	E944.5	E950.4	E962.0	E980.4
diatrizoate	977.8	E858.8	E947.8	E950.4	E962.0	E980.4
Sodium – *continued*						
dibunate	975.4	E858.6	E945.4	E950.4	E962.0	E980.4
dioctyl sulfosuccinate	973.2	E858.4	E943.2	E950.4	E962.0	E980.4
edetate	963.8	E858.1	E933.8	E950.4	E962.0	E980.4
ethacrynate	974.4	E858.5	E944.4	E950.4	E962.0	E980.4
fluoracetate (dust) (rodenticide)	989.4	E863.7	-	E950.6	E962.1	E980.7
fluoride – *see* Fluoride(s)						
free salt	974.5	E858.5	E944.5	E950.4	E962.0	E980.4
glucosulfone	961.8	E857	E931.8	E950.4	E962.0	E980.4
hydroxide	983.2	E864.2	-	E950.7	E962.1	E980.6
hypochlorite (bleach) NEC	983.9	E864.3	-	E950.7	E962.1	E980.6
disinfectant	983.9	E861.4	-	E950.7	E962.1	E980.6
medicinal (anti-infective) (external)	976.0	E858.7	E946.0	E950.4	E962.0	E980.4
vapor	987.8	E869.8	-	E952.8	E962.2	E982.8
hyposulfite	976.0	E858.7	E946.0	E950.4	E962.0	E980.4
indigotindisulfonate	977.8	E858.8	E947.8	E950.4	E962.0	E980.4
iodide	977.8	E858.8	E947.8	E950.4	E962.0	E980.4
iothalamate	977.8	E858.8	E947.8	E950.4	E962.0	E980.4
iron edetate	964.0	E858.2	E934.0	E950.4	E962.0	E980.4
lactate	963.3	E858.1	E933.3	E950.4	E962.0	E980.4
lauryl sulfate	976.2	E858.7	E946.2	E950.4	E962.0	E980.4
L-triiodothyronine	962.7	E858.0	E932.7	E950.4	E962.0	E980.4
metrizoate	977.8	E858.8	E947.8	E950.4	E962.0	E980.4
monofluoracetate (dust) (rodenticide)	989.4	E863.7	-	E950.6	E962.1	E980.7
morrhuate	972.7	E858.3	E942.7	E950.4	E962.0	E980.4
nafcillin	960.0	E856	E930.0	E950.4	E962.0	E980.4
nitrate (oxidizing agent)	983.9	E864.3	-	E950.7	E962.1	E980.6
nitrite (medicinal)	972.4	E858.3	E942.4	E950.4	E962.0	E980.4
nitroferricyanide	972.6	E858.3	E942.6	E950.4	E962.0	E980.4
nitroprusside	972.6	E858.3	E942.6	E950.4	E962.0	E980.4
para-aminohippurate	977.8	E858.8	E947.8	E950.4	E962.0	E980.4
perborate (non-medicinal) NEC	989.89	E866.8	-	E950.9	E962.1	E980.9
medicinal	976.6	E858.7	E946.6	E950.4	E962.0	E980.4
soap	989.6	E861.1	-	E950.9	E962.1	E980.9
percarbonate – *see* Sodium, perborate						
phosphate	973.3	E858.4	E943.3	E950.4	E962.0	E980.4
polystyrene sulfonate	974.5	E858.5	E944.5	E950.4	E962.0	E980.4
propionate	976.0	E858.7	E946.0	E950.4	E962.0	E980.4
psylliate	972.7	E858.3	E942.7	E950.4	E962.0	E980.4
removing resins	974.5	E858.5	E944.5	E950.4	E962.0	E980.4
salicylate	965.1	E850.3	E935.3	E950.0	E962.0	E980.0
sulfate	973.3	E858.4	E943.3	E950.4	E962.0	E980.4
sulfoxone	961.8	E857	E931.8	E950.4	E962.0	E980.4
tetradecyl sulfate	972.7	E858.3	E942.7	E950.4	E962.0	E980.4
thiopental	968.3	E855.1	E938.3	E950.4	E962.0	E980.4
thiosalicylate	965.1	E850.3	E935.3	E950.0	E962.0	E980.0
thiosulfate	976.0	E858.7	E946.0	E950.4	E962.0	E980.4
tolbutdmide	977.8	E858.8	E947.8	E950.4	E962.0	E980.4
tyropanoate	977.8	E858.8	E947.8	E950.4	E962.0	E980.4
valproate	966.3	E855.0	E936.3	E950.4	E962.0	E980.4
Solanine	977.8	E858.8	E947.8	E950.4	E962.0	E980.4
Solanum dulcamara	988.2	E865.4	-	E950.9	E962.1	E980.9
Solapsone	961.8	E857	E931.8	E950.4	E962.0	E980.4
Solasulfone	961.8	E857	E931.8	E950.4	E962.0	E980.4
Soldering fluid	983.1	E864.1	-	E950.7	E962.1	E980.6
Solid substance	989.9	E866.9	-	E950.9	E962.1	E980.9
specified NEC	989.9	E866.8	-	E950.9	E962.1	E980.9
Solvents, industrial	982.8	E862.9	-	E950.9	E962.1	E980.9
naphtha	981	E862.0	-	E950.9	E962.1	E980.9

● New Line ▲ Revised Code

		External Cause (E-Code)				
Drug	**Poisoning**	**Accident**	**Therapeutic Use**	**Suicide Attempt**	**Assault**	**Undetermined**
Solvents, industrial – *continued*						
petroleum	981	E862.0	-	E950.9	E962.1	E980.9
specified NEC	982.8	E862.4	-	E950.9	E962.1	E980.9
Soma	968.0	E855.1	E938.0	E950.4	E962.0	E980.4
Somatotropin	962.4	E858.0	E932.4	E950.4	E962.0	E980.4
Sominex	963.0	E858.1	E933.0	E950.4	E962.0	E980.4
Somnos	967.1	E852.0	E937.1	E950.2	E962.0	E980.2
Somonal	967.0	E851	E937.0	E950.1	E962.0	E980.1
Soneryl	967.0	E851	E937.0	E950.1	E962.0	E980.1
Soothing syrup	977.9	E858.9	E947.9	E950.5	E962.0	E980.5
Sopor	967.4	E852.3	E937.4	E950.2	E962.0	E980.2
Soporific drug	967.9	E852.9	E937.9	E950.2	E962.0	E980.2
specified type NEC	967.8	E852.8	E937.8	E950.2	E962.0	E980.2
Sorbitol NEC	977.4	E858.8	E947.4	E950.4	E962.0	E980.4
Sotradecol	972.7	E858.3	E942.7	E950.4	E962.0	E980.4
Spacoline	975.1	E858.6	E945.1	E950.4	E962.0	E980.4
Spanish fly	976.8	E858.7	E946.8	E950.4	E962.0	E980.4
Sparine	969.1	E853.0	E939.1	E950.3	E962.0	E980.3
Sparteine	975.0	E858.6	E945.0	E950.4	E962.0	E980.4
Spasmolytics	975.1	E858.6	E945.1	E950.4	E962.0	E980.4
anticholinergics	971.1	E855.4	E941.1	E950.4	E962.0	E980.4
Spectinomycin	960.8	E856	E930.8	E950.4	E962.0	E980.4
Speed	969.7	E854.2	E939.7	E950.3	E962.0	E980.3
Spermicides	976.8	E858.7	E946.8	E950.4	E962.0	E980.4
Spider (bite) (venom)	989.5	E905.1	-	E950.9	E962.1	E980.9
antivenin	979.9	E858.8	E949.9	E950.4	E962.0	E980.4
Spigelia (root)	961.6	E857	E931.6	E950.4	E962.0	E980.4
Spiperone	969.2	E853.1	E939.2	E950.3	E962.0	E980.3
Spiramycin	960.3	E856	E930.3	E950.4	E962.0	E980.4
Spirilene	969.5	E853.8	E939.5	E950.3	E962.0	E980.3
Spirit(s) (neutral) NEC	980.0	E860.1	-	E950.9	E962.1	E980.9
beverage	980.0	E860.0	-	E950.9	E962.1	E980.9
industrial	980.9	E860.9	-	E950.9	E962.1	E980.9
mineral	981	E862.0	-	E950.9	E962.1	E980.9
of salt – *see* Hydrochloric acid						
surgical	980.9	E860.9	-	E950.9	E962.1	E980.9
Spironolactone	974.4	E858.5	E944.4	E950.4	E962.0	E980.4
Sponge, absorbable (gelatin)	964.5	E858.2	E934.5	E950.4	E962.0	E980.4
Sporostacin	976.0	E858.7	E946.0	E950.4	E962.0	E980.4
Sprays (aerosol)	989.89	E866.8	-	E950.9	E962.1	E980.9
cosmetic	989.89	E866.7	-	E950.9	E962.1	E980.9
medicinal NEC	977.9	E858.9	E947.9	E950.5	E962.0	E980.5
pesticides – *see* Pesticides						
specified content – *see* substance specified						
Spurge flax	988.2	E865.4	-	E950.9	E962.1	E980.9
Spurges	988.2	E865.4	-	E950.9	E962.1	E980.9
Squill (expectorant) NEC	975.5	E858.6	E945.5	E950.4	E962.0	E980.4
rat poison	989.4	E863.7	-	E950.6	E962.1	E980.7
Squirting cucumber (cathartic)	973.1	E858.4	E943.1	E950.4	E962.0	E980.4
Stains	989.89	E866.8	-	E950.9	E962.1	E980.9
Stannous – *see also* Tin						
fluoride	976.7	E858.7	E946.7	E950.4	E962.0	E980.4
Stanolone	962.1	E858.0	E932.1	E950.4	E962.0	E980.4
Stanozolol	962.1	E858.0	E932.1	E950.4	E962.0	E980.4
Staphisagria or stavesacre (pediculicide)	976.0	E858.7	E946.0	E950.4	E962.0	E980.4
Stelazine	969.1	E853.0	E939.1	E950.3	E962.0	E980.3
Stemetil	969.1	E853.0	E939.1	E950.3	E962.0	E980.3
Sterculia (cathartic) (gum)	973.3	E858.4	E943.3	E950.4	E962.0	E980.4

		External Cause (E-Code)				
Drug	**Poisoning**	**Accident**	**Therapeutic Use**	**Suicide Attempt**	**Assault**	**Undetermined**
Sternutator gas	987.8	E869.8	-	E952.8	E962.2	E982.8
Steroids NEC	962.0	E858.0	E932.0	E950.4	E962.0	E980.4
ENT agent	976.6	E858.7	E946.6	E950.4	E962.0	E980.4
ophthalmic preparation	976.5	E858.7	E946.5	E950.4	E962.0	E980.4
topical NEC	976.0	E858.7	E946.0	E950.4	E962.0	E980.4
Stibine	985.8	E866.4	-	E950.9	E962.1	E980.9
Stibophen	961.2	E857	E931.2	E950.4	E962.0	E980.4
Stilbamide, stilbamidine	961.5	E857	E931.5	E950.4	E962.0	E980.4
Stilbestrol	962.2	E858.0	E932.2	E950.4	E962.0	E980.4
Stimulants (central nervous system)	970.9	E854.3	E940.9	E950.4	E962.0	E980.4
analeptics	970.0	E854.3	E940.0	E950.4	E962.0	E980.4
opiate antagonist	970.1	E854.3	E940.1	E950.4	E962.0	E980.4
psychotherapeutic NEC	969.0	E854.0	E939.0	E950.3	E962.0	E980.3
specified NEC	970.8	E854.3	E940.8	E950.4	E962.0	E980.4
Storage batteries (acid) (cells)	983.1	E864.1	-	E950.7	E962.1	E980.6
Stovaine	968.9	E855.2	E938.9	E950.4	E962.0	E980.4
infiltration (subcutaneous)	968.5	E855.2	E938.5	E950.4	E962.0	E980.4
nerve block (peripheral) (plexus)	968.6	E855.2	E938.6	E950.4	E962.0	E980.4
spinal	968.7	E855.2	E938.7	E950.4	E962.0	E980.4
topical (surface)	968.5	E855.2	E938.5	E950.4	E962.0	E980.4
Stovarsal	961.1	E857	E931.1	E950.4	E962.0	E980.4
Stove gas – *see* Gas, utility						
Stoxil	976.5	E858.7	E946.5	E950.4	E962.0	E980.4
STP	969.6	E854.1	E939.6	E950.3	E962.0	E980.3
Stramonium (medicinal) NEC	971.1	E855.4	E941.1	E950.4	E962.0	E980.4
natural state	988.2	E865.4	-	E950.9	E962.1	E980.9
Streptodornase	964.4	E858.2	E934.4	E950.4	E962.0	E980.4
Streptoduocin	960.6	E856	E930.6	E950.4	E962.0	E980.4
Streptokinase	964.4	E858.2	E934.4	E950.4	E962.0	E980.4
Streptomycin	960.6	E856	E930.6	E950.4	E962.0	E980.4
Streptozocin	960.7	E856	E930.7	E950.4	E962.0	E980.4
Stripper (paint) (solvent)	982.8	E862.9	-	E950.9	E962.1	E980.9
Strobane	989.2	E863.0	-	E950.6	E962.1	E980.7
Strophanthin	972.1	E858.3	E942.1	E950.4	E962.0	E980.4
Strophanthus hispidus or kombe	988.2	E865.4	-	E950.9	E962.1	E980.9
Strychnine (rodenticide) (salts)	989.1	E863.7	-	E950.6	E962.1	E980.7
medicinal NEC	970.8	E854.3	E940.8	E950.4	E962.0	E980.4
Strychnos (ignatii) – *see* Strychnine						
Styramate	968.0	E855.1	E938.0	E950.4	E962.0	E980.4
Styrene	983.0	E864.0	-	E950.7	E962.1	E980.6
Succinimide (anticonvulsant)	966.2	E855.0	E936.2	E950.4	E962.0	E980.4
mercuric – *see* Mercury						
Succinylcholine	975.2	E858.6	E945.2	E950.4	E962.0	E980.4
Succinylsulfathiazole	961.0	E857	E931.0	E950.4	E962.0	E980.4
Sucrose	974.5	E858.5	E944.5	E950.4	E962.0	E980.4
Sulfacetamide	961.0	E857	E931.0	E950.4	E962.0	E980.4
ophthalmic preparation	976.5	E858.7	E946.5	E950.4	E962.0	E980.4
Sulfachlorpyridazine	961.0	E857	E931.0	E950.4	E962.0	E980.4
Sulfacytine	961.0	E857	E931.0	E950.4	E962.0	E980.4
Sulfadiazine	961.0	E857	E931.0	E950.4	E962.0	E980.4
silver (topical)	976.0	E858.7	E946.0	E950.4	E962.0	E980.4
Sulfadimethoxine	961.0	E857	E931.0	E950.4	E962.0	E980.4
Sulfadimidine	961.0	E857	E931.0	E950.4	E962.0	E980.4
Sulfaethidole	961.0	E857	E931.0	E950.4	E962.0	E980.4
Sulfafurazole	961.0	E857	E931.0	E950.4	E962.0	E980.4
Sulfaguanidine	961.0	E857	E931.0	E950.4	E962.0	E980.4
Sulfamerazine	961.0	E857	E931.0	E950.4	E962.0	E980.4
Sulfameter	961.0	E857	E931.0	E950.4	E962.0	E980.4

● New Line ▲ Revised Code

Drug	Poisoning	External Cause (E-Code)				
		Accident	Therapeutic Use	Suicide Attempt	Assault	Undetermined
Sulfamethizole	961.0	E857	E931.0	E950.4	E962.0	E980.4
Sulfamethoxazole	961.0	E857	E931.0	E950.4	E962.0	E980.4
Sulfamethoxydiazine	961.0	E857	E931.0	E950.4	E962.0	E980.4
Sulfamethoxypyridazine	961.0	E857	E931.0	E950.4	E962.0	E980.4
Sulfamethylthiazole	961.0	E857	E931.0	E950.4	E962.0	E980.4
Sulfamylon	976.0	E858.7	E946.0	E950.4	E962.0	E980.4
Sulfan blue (diagnostic dye)	977.8	E858.8	E947.8	E950.4	E962.0	E980.4
Sulfanilamide	961.0	E857	E931.0	E950.4	E962.0	E980.4
Sulfanilylguanidine	961.0	E857	E931.0	E950.4	E962.0	E980.4
Sulfaphenazole	961.0	E857	E931.0	E950.4	E962.0	E980.4
Sulfaphenylthiazole	961.0	E857	E931.0	E950.4	E962.0	E980.4
Sulfaproxyline	961.0	E857	E931.0	E950.4	E962.0	E980.4
Sulfapyridine	961.0	E857	E931.0	E950.4	E962.0	E980.4
Sulfapyrimidine	961.0	E857	E931.0	E950.4	E962.0	E980.4
Sulfarsphenamine	961.1	E857	E931.1	E950.4	E962.0	E980.4
Sulfasalazine	961.0	E857	E931.0	E950.4	E962.0	E980.4
Sulfasomizole	961.0	E857	E931.0	E950.4	E962.0	E980.4
Sulfasuxidine	961.0	E857	E931.0	E950.4	E962.0	E980.4
Sulfinpyrazone	974.7	E858.5	E944.7	E950.4	E962.0	E980.4
Sulfisoxazole	961.0	E857	E931.0	E950.4	E962.0	E980.4
ophthalmic preparation	976.5	E858.7	E946.5	E950.4	E962.0	E980.4
Sulfomyxin	960.8	E856	E930.8	E950.4	E962.0	E980.4
Sulfonal	967.8	E852.8	E937.8	E950.2	E962.0	E980.2
Sulfonamides (mixtures)	961.0	E857	E931.0	E950.4	E962.0	E980.4
Sulfones	961.8	E857	E931.8	E950.4	E962.0	E980.4
Sulfonethylmethane	967.8	E852.8	E937.8	E950.2	E962.0	E980.2
Sulfonmethane	967.8	E852.8	E937.8	E950.2	E962.0	E980.2
Sulfonphthal, sulfonphthol	977.8	E858.8	E947.8	E950.4	E962.0	E980.4
Sulfonylurea derivatives, oral	962.3	E858.0	E932.3	E950.4	E962.0	E980.4
Sulfoxone	961.8	E857	E931.8	E950.4	E962.0	E980.4
Sulfur, sulfureted, sulfuric, sulfurous, sulfuryl (compounds) NEC	989.89	E866.8	-	E950.9	E962.1	E980.9
acid	983.1	E864.1	-	E950.7	E962.1	E980.6
dioxide	987.3	E869.1	-	E952.8	E962.2	E982.8
ether – *see* Ether(s)						
hydrogen	987.8	E869.8	-	E952.8	E962.2	E982.8
medicinal (keratolytic) (ointment) NEC	976.4	E858.7	E946.4	E950.4	E962.0	E980.4
pesticide (vapor)	989.4	E863.4	-	E950.6	E962.1	E980.7
vapor NEC	987.8	E869.8	-	E952.8	E962.2	E982.8
Sulkowitch's reagent	977.8	E858.8	E947.8	E950.4	E962.0	E980.4
Sulph – *see also* Sulf-						
Sulphadione	961.8	E857	E931.8	E950.4	E962.0	E980.4
Sulthiame, sultiame	966.3	E855.0	E936.3	E950.4	E962.0	E980.4
Superinone	975.5	E858.6	E945.5	E950.4	E962.0	E980.4
Suramin	961.5	E857	E931.5	E950.4	E962.0	E980.4
Surfacaine	968.5	E855.2	E938.5	E950.4	E962.0	E980.4
Surital	968.3	E855.1	E938.3	E950.4	E962.0	E980.4
Sutilains	976.8	E858.7	E946.8	E950.4	E962.0	E980.4
Suxamethonium (bromide) (chloride) (iodide)	975.2	E858.6	E945.2	E950.4	E962.0	E980.4
Suxethonium (bromide)	975.2	E858.6	E945.2	E950.4	E962.0	E980.4
Sweet oil (birch)	976.3	E858.7	E946.3	E950.4	E962.0	E980.4
Sym-dichloroethyl ether	982.3	E862.4	-	E950.9	E962.1	E980.9
Sympatholytics	971.3	E855.6	E941.3	E950.4	E962.0	E980.4
Sympathomimetics	971.2	E855.5	E941.2	E950.4	E962.0	E980.4
Synagis	979.6	E858.8	E949.6	E950.4	E962.0	E980.4
Synalar	976.0	E858.7	E946.0	E950.4	E962.0	E980.4
Synthroid	962.7	E858.0	E932.7	E950.4	E962.0	E980.4
Syntocinon	975.0	E858.6	E945.0	E950.4	E962.0	E950.4
Syrosingopine	972.6	E858.3	E942.6	E950.4	E962.0	E980.4
Systemic agents (primarily)	963.9	E858.1	E933.9	E950.4	E962.0	E980.4
specified NEC	963.8	E858.1	E933.8	E950.4	E962.0	E980.4
Tablets (*see also* specified substance)	977.9	E858.9	E947.9	E950.5	E962.0	E980.5
Tace	962.2	E858.0	E932.2	E950.4	E962.0	E980.4
Tacrine	971.0	E855.3	E941.0	E950.4	E962.0	E980.4
Talbutal	967.0	E851	E937.0	E950.1	E962.0	E980.1
Talc	976.3	E858.7	E946.3	E950.4	E962.0	E980.4
Talcum	976.3	E858.7	E946.3	E950.4	E962.0	E980.4
Tamsulosin ●	971.3	E855.6	E941.3	E950.4	E962.0	E980.4
Tandearil, tanderil	965.5	E850.5	E935.5	E950.0	E962.0	E980.0
Tannic acid	983.1	E864.1	-	E950.7	E962.1	E980.6
medicinal (astringent)	976.2	E858.7	E946.2	E950.4	E962.0	E980.4
Tannin – *see* Tannic acid						
Tansy	988.2	E865.4	-	E950.9	E962.1	E980.9
TAO	960.3	E856	E930.3	E950.4	E962.0	E980.4
Tapazole	962.8	E858.0	E932.8	E950.4	E962.0	E980.4
Tar NEC	983.0	E864.0	-	E950.7	E962.1	E980.6
camphor – *see* Naphthalene						
fumes	987.8	E869.8	-	E952.8	E962.2	E982.8
Taractan	969.3	E853.8	E939.3	E950.3	E962.0	E980.3
Tarantula (venomous)	989.5	E905.1	-	E950.9	E962.1	E980.9
Tartar emetic (anti-infective)	961.2	E857	E931.2	E950.4	E962.0	E980.4
Tartaric acid	983.1	E864.1	-	E950.7	E962.1	E980.6
Tartrated antimony (anti-infective)	961.2	E857	E931.2	E950.4	E962.0	E980.4
TCA – *see* Trichloroacetic acid						
TDI	983.0	E864.0	-	E950.7	E962.1	E980.6
vapor	987.8	E869.8	-	E952.8	E962.2	E982.8
Tear gas	987.5	E869.3	-	E952.8	E962.2	E982.8
Teclothiazide	974.3	E858.5	E944.3	E950.4	E962.0	E980.4
Tegretol	966.3	E855.0	E936.3	E950.4	E962.0	E980.4
Telepaque	977.8	E858.8	E947.8	E950.4	E962.0	E980.4
Tellurium	985.8	E866.4	-	E950.9	E962.1	E980.9
fumes	985.8	E866.4	-	E950.9	E962.1	E980.9
TEM	963.1	E858.1	E933.1	E950.4	E962.0	E980.4
Temazepan – *see* Benzodiazepines						
TEPA	963.1	E858.1	E933.1	E950.4	E962.0	E980.4
TEPP	989.3	E863.1	-	E950.6	E962.1	E980.7
Terbutaline	971.2	E855.5	E941.2	E950.4	E962.0	E980.4
Teroxalene	961.6	E857	E931.6	E950.4	E962.0	E980.4
Terpin hydrate	975.5	E858.6	E945.5	E950.4	E962.0	E980.4
Terramycin	960.4	E856	E930.4	E950.4	E962.0	E980.4
Tessalon	975.4	E858.6	E945.4	E950.4	E962.0	E980.4
Testosterone	962.1	E858.0	E932.1	E950.4	E962.0	E980.4
Tetanus (vaccine)	978.4	E858.8	E948.4	E950.4	E962.0	E980.4
antitoxin	979.9	E858.8	E949.9	E950.4	E962.0	E980.4
immune globulin (human)	964.6	E858.2	E934.6	E950.4	E962.0	E980.4
toxoid	978.4	E858.8	E948.4	E950.4	E962.0	E980.4
with diphtheria toxoid	978.9	E858.8	E948.9	E950.4	E962.0	E980.4
with pertussis	978.6	E858.8	E948.6	E950.4	E962.0	E980.4
Tetrabenazine	969.5	E853.8	E939.5	E950.3	E962.0	E980.3
Tetracaine (infiltration) (topical)	968.5	E855.2	E938.5	E950.4	E962.0	E980.4
nerve block (peripheral) (plexus)	968.6	E855.2	E938.6	E950.4	E962.0	E980.4
spinal	968.7	E855.2	E938.7	E950.4	E962.0	E980.4
Tetrachlorethylene – *see* Tetrachloroethylene						
Tetrachlormethiazide	974.3	E858.5	E944.3	E950.4	E962.0	E980.4

		External Cause (E-Code)				
Drug	**Poisoning**	**Accident**	**Therapeutic Use**	**Suicide Attempt**	**Assault**	**Undetermined**
Tetrachloroethane (liquid) (vapor)	982.3	E862.4	-	E950.9	E962.1	E980.9
paint or varnish	982.3	E861.6	-	E950.9	E962.1	E980.9
Tetrachloroethylene (liquid) (vapor)	982.3	E862.4	-	E950.9	E962.1	E980.9
medicinal	961.6	E857	E931.6	E950.4	E962.0	E980.4
Tetrachloromethane – *see* Carbon, tetrachloride						
Tetracycline	960.4	E856	E930.4	E950.4	E962.0	E980.4
ophthalmic preparation	976.5	E858.7	E946.5	E950.4	E962.0	E980.4
topical NEC	976.0	E858.7	E946.0	E950.4	E962.0	E980.4
Tetraethylammonium chloride	972.3	E858.3	E942.3	E950.4	E962.0	E980.4
Tetraethyl lead (antiknock compound)	984.1	E862.1	-	E950.9	E962.1	E980.9
Tetraethyl pyrophosphate	989.3	E863.1	-	E950.6	E962.1	E980.7
Tetraethylthiuram disulfide	977.3	E858.8	E947.3	E950.4	E962.0	E980.4
Tetrahydroaminoacridine	971.0	E855.3	E941.0	E950.4	E962.0	E980.4
Tetrahydrocannabinol	969.6	E854.1	E939.6	E950.3	E962.0	E980.3
Tetrahydronaphthalene	982.0	E862.4	-	E950.9	E962.1	E980.9
Tetrahydrozoline	971.2	E855.5	E941.2	E950.4	E962.0	E980.4
Tetralin	982.0	E862.4	-	E950.9	E962.1	E980.9
Tetramethylthiuram (disulfide) NEC	989.4	E863.6	-	E950.6	E962.1	E980.7
medicinal	976.2	E858.7	E946.2	E950.4	E962.0	E980.4
Tetronal	967.8	E852.8	E937.8	E950.2	E962.0	E980.2
Tetryl	983.0	E864.0	-	E950.7	E962.1	E980.6
Thalidomide	967.8	E852.8	E937.8	E950.2	E962.0	E980.2
Thallium (compounds) (dust) NEC	985.8	E866.4	-	E950.9	E962.1	E980.9
pesticide (rodenticide)	985.8	E863.7	-	E950.6	E962.1	E980.7
THC	969.6	E854.1	E939.6	E950.3	E962.0	E980.3
Thebacon	965.09	E850.2	E935.2	E950.0	E962.0	E980.0
Thebaine	965.09	E850.2	E935.2	E950.0	E962.0	E980.0
Theobromine (calcium salicylate)	974.1	E858.5	E944.1	E950.4	E962.0	E980.4
Theophylline (diuretic)	974.1	E858.5	E944.1	E950.4	E962.0	E980.4
ethylenediamine	975.7	E858.6	E945.7	E950.4	E962.0	E980.4
Thiabendazole	961.6	E857	E931.6	E950.4	E962.0	E980.4
Thialbarbital, thialbarbitone	968.3	E855.1	E938.3	E950.4	E962.0	E980.4
Thiamine	963.5	E858.1	E933.5	E950.4	E962.0	E980.4
Thiamylal (sodium)	968.3	E855.1	E938.3	E950.4	E962.0	E980.4
Thiazesim	969.0	E854.0	E939.0	E950.3	E962.0	E980.3
Thiazides (diuretics)	974.3	E858.5	E944.3	E950.4	E962.0	E980.4
Thiethylperazine	963.0	E858.1	E933.0	E950.4	E962.0	E980.4
Thimerosal (topical)	976.0	E858.7	E946.0	E950.4	E962.0	E980.4
ophthalmic preparation	976.5	E858.7	E946.5	E950.4	E962.0	E980.4
Thioacetazone	961.8	E857	E931.8	E950.4	E962.0	E980.4
Thiobarbiturates	968.3	E855.1	E938.3	E950.4	E962.0	E980.4
Thiobismol	961.2	E857	E931.2	E950.4	E962.0	E980.4
Thiocarbamide	962.8	E858.0	E932.8	E950.4	E962.0	E980.4
Thiocarbarsone	961.1	E857	E931.1	E950.4	E962.0	E980.4
Thiocarlide	961.8	E857	E931.8	E950.4	E962.0	E980.4
Thioguanine	963.1	E858.1	E933.1	E950.4	E962.0	E980.4
Thiomercaptomerin	974.0	E858.5	E944.0	E950.4	E962.0	E980.4
Thiomerin	974.0	E858.5	E944.0	E950.4	E962.0	E980.4
Thiopental, thiopentone (sodium)	968.3	E855.1	E938.3	E950.4	E962.0	E980.4
Thiopropazate	969.1	E853.0	E939.1	E950.3	E962.0	E980.3
Thioproperazine	969.1	E853.0	E939.1	E950.3	E962.0	E980.3
Thioridazine	969.1	E853.0	E939.1	E950.3	E962.0	E980.3
Thio-TEPA, thiotepa	963.1	E858.1	E933.1	E950.4	E962.0	E980.4
Thiothixene	969.3	E853.8	E939.3	E950.3	E962.0	E980.3
Thiouracil	962.8	E858.0	E932.8	E950.4	E962.0	E980.4
Thiourea	962.8	E858.0	E932.8	E950.4	E962.0	E980.4

		External Cause (E-Code)				
Drug	**Poisoning**	**Accident**	**Therapeutic Use**	**Suicide Attempt**	**Assault**	**Undetermined**
Thiphenamil	971.1	E855.4	E941.1	E950.4	E962.0	E980.4
Thiram NEC	989.4	E863.6	-	E950.6	E962.1	E980.7
medicinal	976.2	E858.7	E946.2	E950.4	E962.0	E980.4
Thonzylamine	963.0	E858.1	E933.0	E950.4	E962.0	E980.4
Thorazine	969.1	E853.0	E939.1	E950.3	E962.0	E980.3
Thornapple	988.2	E865.4	-	E950.9	E962.1	E980.9
Throat preparation (lozenges) **NEC**	976.6	E858.7	E946.6	E950.4	E962.0	E980.4
Thrombin	964.5	E858.2	E934.5	E950.4	E962.0	E980.4
Thrombolysin	964.4	E858.2	E934.4	E950.4	E962.0	E980.4
Thymol	983.0	E864.0	-	E950.7	E962.1	E980.6
Thymus extract	962.9	E858.0	E932.9	E950.4	E962.0	E980.4
Thyroglobulin	962.7	E858.0	E932.7	E950.4	E962.0	E980.4
Thyroid (derivatives) (extract)	962.7	E858.0	E932.7	E950.4	E962.0	E980.4
Thyrolar	962.7	E858.0	E932.7	E950.4	E962.0	E980.4
Thyrothrophin, thyrotropin	977.8	E858.8	E947.8	E950.4	E962.0	E980.4
Thyroxin(e)	962.7	E858.0	E932.7	E950.4	E962.0	E980.4
Tigan	963.0	E858.1	E933.0	E950.4	E962.0	E980.4
Tigloidine	968.0	E855.1	E938.0	E950.4	E962.0	E980.4
Tin (chloride) (dust) (oxide) NEC	985.8	E866.4	-	E950.9	E962.1	E980.9
anti-infectives	961.2	E857	E931.2	E950.4	E962.0	E980.4
Tinactin	976.0	E858.7	E946.0	E950.4	E962.0	E980.4
Tincture, iodine – *see* Iodine						
Tindal	969.1	E853.0	E939.1	E950.3	E962.0	E980.3
Titanium (compounds) (vapor)	985.8	E866.4	-	E950.9	E962.1	E980.9
ointment	976.3	E858.7	E946.3	E950.4	E962.0	E980.4
Titroid	962.7	E858.0	E932.7	E950.4	E962.0	E980.4
TMTD – *see* Tetramethylthiuram disulfide						
TNT	989.89	E866.8	-	E950.9	E962.1	E980.9
fumes	987.8	E869.8	-	E952.8	E962.2	E982.8
Toadstool	988.1	E865.5	-	E950.9	E962.1	E980.9
Tobacco NEC	989.84	E866.8	-	E950.9	E962.1	E980.9
Indian	988.2	E865.4	-	E950.9	E962.1	E980.9
smoke, second-hand	987.8	E869.4	-	-	-	-
Tocopherol	963.5	E858.1	E933.5	E950.4	E962.0	E980.4
Tocosamine	975.0	E858.6	E945.0	E950.4	E962.0	E980.4
Tofranil	969.0	E854.0	E939.0	E950.3	E962.0	E980.3
Toilet deodorizer	989.89	E866.8	-	E950.9	E962.1	E980.9
Tolazamide	962.3	E858.0	E932.3	E950.4	E962.0	E980.4
Tolazoline	971.3	E855.6	E941.3	E950.4	E962.0	E980.4
Tolbutamide	962.3	E858.0	E932.3	E950.4	E962.0	E980.4
sodium	977.8	E858.8	E947.8	E950.4	E962.0	E980.4
Tolmetin	965.69	E850.6	E935.6	E950.0	E962.0	E980.0
Tolnaftate	976.0	E858.7	E946.0	E950.4	E962.0	E980.4
Tolpropamine	976.1	E858.7	E946.1	E950.4	E962.0	E980.4
Tolserol	968.0	E855.1	E938.0	E950.4	E962.0	E980.4
Toluene (liquid) (vapor)	982.0	E862.4	-	E950.9	E962.1	E980.9
diisocyanate	983.0	E864.0	-	E950.7	E962.1	E980.6
Toluidine	983.0	E864.0	-	E950.7	E962.1	E980.6
vapor	987.8	E869.8	-	E952.8	E962.2	E982.8
Toluol (liquid) (vapor)	982.0	E862.4	-	E950.9	E962.1	E980.9
Tolylene-2,4-diisocyanate	983.0	E864.0	-	E950.7	E962.1	E980.6
Tonics, cardiac	972.1	E858.3	E942.1	E950.4	E962.0	E980.4
Toxaphene (dust) (spray)	989.2	E863.0	-	E950.6	E962.1	E980.7
Toxoids NEC	978.8	E858.8	E948.8	E950.4	E962.0	E980.4
Tractor fuel NEC	981	E862.1	-	E950.9	E962.1	E980.9
Tragacanth	973.3	E858.4	E943.3	E950.4	E962.0	E980.4
Traniazoline	971.2	E855.5	E941.2	E950.4	E962.0	E980.4

		External Cause (E-Code)				
Drug	Poisoning	Accident	Therapeutic Use	Suicide Attempt	Assault	Undetermined
Tranquilizers	969.5	E853.9	E939.5	E950.3	E962.0	E980.3
benzodiazepine-based	969.4	E853.2	E939.4	E950.3	E962.0	E980.3
butyropherione-based	969.2	E853.1	E939.2	E950.3	E962.0	E980.3
major NEC	969.3	E853.8	E939.3	E950.3	E962.0	E980.3
phenothiazine-based	969.1	E853.0	E939.1	E950.3	E962.0	E980.3
specified NEC	969.5	E853.8	E939.5	E950.3	E962.0	E980.3
Trantoin	961.9	E857	E931.9	E950.4	E962.0	E980.4
Tranxene	969.4	E853.2	E939.4	E950.3	E962.0	E980.3
Tranylcypromine (sulfate)	969.0	E854.0	E939.0	E950.3	E962.0	E980.3
Trasentine	975.1	E858.6	E945.1	E950.4	E962.0	E980.4
Travert	974.5	E858.5	E944.5	E950.4	E962.0	E980.4
Trecator	961.8	E857	E931.8	E950.4	E962.0	E980.4
Tretinoin	976.8	E858.7	E946.8	E950.4	E962.0	E980.4
Triacetin	976.0	E858.7	E946.0	E950.4	E962.0	E980.4
Triacetyloleandomycin	960.3	E856	E930.3	E950.4	E962.0	E980.4
Triamcinolone	962.0	E858.0	E932.0	E950.4	E962.0	E980.4
ENT agent	976.6	E858.7	E946.6	E950.4	E962.0	E980.4
ophthalmic preparation	976.5	E858.7	E946.5	E950.4	E962.0	E980.4
topical NEC	976.0	E858.7	E946.0	E950.4	E962.0	E980.4
Triamterene	974.4	E858.5	E944.4	E950.4	E962.0	E980.4
Triaziquone	963.1	E858.1	E933.1	E950.4	E962.0	E980.4
Tribromacetaldehyde	967.3	E852.2	E937.3	E950.2	E962.0	E980.2
Tribromoethanol	968.2	E855.1	E938.2	E950.4	E962.0	E980.4
Tribromomethane	967.3	E852.2	E937.3	E950.2	E962.0	E980.2
Trichlorethane	982.3	E862.4	-	E950.9	E962.1	E980.9
Trichlormethiazide	974.3	E858.5	E944.3	E950.4	E962.0	E980.4
Trichloroacetic acid	983.1	E864.1	-	E950.7	E962.1	E980.6
medicinal (keratolytic)	976.4	E858.7	E946.4	E950.4	E962.0	E980.4
Trichloroethanol	967.1	E852.0	E937.1	E950.2	E962.0	E980.2
Trichloroethylene (liquid) (vapor)	982.3	E862.4	-	E950.9	E962.1	E980.9
anesthetic (gas)	968.2	E855.1	E938.2	E950.4	E962.0	E980.4
Trichloroethyl phosphate	967.1	E852.0	E937.1	E950.2	E962.0	E980.2
Trichlorofluoromethane NEC	987.4	E869.2	-	E952.8	E962.2	E982.8
Trichlorotriethylamine	963.1	E858.1	E933.1	E950.4	E962.0	E980.4
Trichomonacides NEC	961.5	E857	E931.5	E950.4	E962.0	E980.4
Trichomycin	960.1	E856	E930.1	E950.4	E962.0	E980.4
Triclofos	967.1	E852.0	E937.1	E950.2	E962.0	E980.2
Tricresyl phosphate	989.89	E866.8	-	E950.9	E962.1	E980.9
solvent	982.8	E862.4	-	E950.9	E962.1	E980.9
Tricyclamol	966.4	E855.0	E936.4	E950.4	E962.0	E980.4
Tridesilon	976.0	E858.7	E946.0	E950.4	E962.0	E980.4
Tridihexethyl	971.1	E855.4	E941.1	E950.4	E962.0	E980.4
Tridione	966.0	E855.0	E936.0	E950.4	E962.0	E980.4
Triethanolamine NEC	983.2	E864.2	-	E950.7	E962.1	E980.6
detergent	983.2	E861.0	-	E950.7	E962.1	E980.6
trinitrate	972.4	E858.3	E942.4	E950.4	E962.0	E980.4
Triethanomelamine	963.1	E858.1	E933.1	E950.4	E962.0	E980.4
Triethylene melamine	963.1	E858.1	E933.1	E950.4	E962.0	E980.4
Triethylenephosphoramide	963.1	E858.1	E933.1	E950.4	E962.0	E980.4
Triethylenethiophosphoramide	963.1	E858.1	E933.1	E950.4	E962.0	E980.4
Trifluoperazine	969.1	E853.0	E939.1	E950.3	E962.0	E980.3
Trifluperidol	969.2	E853.1	E939.2	E950.3	E962.0	E980.3
Triflupromazine	969.1	E853.0	E939.1	E950.3	E962.0	E980.3
Trihexyphenidyl	971.1	E855.4	E941.1	E950.4	E962.0	E980.4
Triiodothyronine	962.7	E858.0	E932.7	E950.4	E962.0	E980.4
Trilene	968.2	E855.1	E938.2	E950.4	E962.0	E980.4
Trimeprazine	963.0	E858.1	E933.0	E950.4	E962.0	E980.4
Trimetazidine	972.4	E858.3	E942.4	E950.4	E962.0	E980.4
Trimethadione	966.0	E855.0	E936.0	E950.4	E962.0	E980.4
Trimethaphan	972.3	E858.3	E942.3	E950.4	E962.0	E980.4
Trimethidinium	972.3	E858.3	E942.3	E950.4	E962.0	E980.4
Trimethobenzamide	963.0	E858.1	E933.0	E950.4	E962.0	E980.4

		External Cause (E-Code)				
Drug	Poisoning	Accident	Therapeutic Use	Suicide Attempt	Assault	Undetermined
Trimethylcarbinol	980.8	E860.8	-	E950.9	E962.1	E980.9
Trimethylpsoralen	976.3	E858.7	E946.3	E950.4	E962.0	E980.4
Trimeton	963.0	E858.1	E933.0	E950.4	E962.0	E980.4
Trimipramine	969.0	E854.0	E939.0	E950.3	E962.0	E980.3
Trimustine	963.1	E858.1	E933.1	E950.4	E962.0	E980.4
Trinitrin	972.4	E858.3	E942.4	E950.4	E962.0	E980.4
Trinitrophenol	983.0	E864.0	-	E950.7	E962.1	E980.6
Trinitrotoluene	989.89	E866.8	-	E950.9	E962.1	E980.9
fumes	987.8	E869.8	-	E952.8	E962.2	E982.8
Trional	967.8	E852.8	E937.8	E950.2	E962.0	E980.2
Trioxide of arsenic – *see* Arsenic						
Trioxsalen	976.3	E858.7	E946.3	E950.4	E962.0	E980.4
Tripelennamine	963.0	E858.1	E933.0	E950.4	E962.0	E980.4
Triperidol	969.2	E853.1	E939.2	E950.3	E962.0	E980.3
Triprolidine	963.0	E858.1	E933.0	E950.4	E962.0	E980.4
Trisoralen	976.3	E858.7	E946.3	E950.4	E962.0	E980.4
Troleandomycin	960.3	E856	E930.3	E950.4	E962.0	E980.4
Trolnitrate (phosphate)	972.4	E858.3	E942.4	E950.4	E962.0	E980.4
Trometamol	963.3	E858.1	E933.3	E950.4	E962.0	E980.4
Tromethamine	963.3	E858.1	E933.3	E950.4	E962.0	E980.4
Tronothane	968.5	E855.2	E938.5	E950.4	E962.0	E980.4
Tropicamide	971.1	E855.4	E941.1	E950.4	E962.0	E980.4
Troxidone	966.0	E855.0	E936.0	E950.4	E962.0	E980.4
Tryparsamide	961.1	E857	E931.1	E950.4	E962.0	E980.4
Trypsin	963.4	E858.1	E933.4	E950.4	E962.0	E980.4
Tryptizol	969.0	E854.0	E939.0	E950.3	E962.0	E980.3
Tuaminoheptane	971.2	E855.5	E941.2	E950.4	E962.0	E980.4
Tuberculin (old)	977.8	E858.8	E947.8	E950.4	E962.0	E980.4
Tubocurare	975.2	E858.6	E945.2	E950.4	E962.0	E980.4
Tubocurarine	975.2	E858.6	E945.2	E950.4	E962.0	E980.4
Turkish green	969.6	E854.1	E939.6	E950.3	E962.0	E980.3
Turpentine (spirits of) (liquid) (vapor)	982.8	E862.4	-	E950.9	E962.1	E980.9
Tybamate	969.5	E853.8	E939.5	E950.3	E962.0	E980.3
Tyloxapol	975.5	E858.6	E945.5	E950.4	E962.0	E980.4
Tymazoline	971.2	E855.5	E941.2	E950.4	E962.0	E980.4
Typhoid vaccine	978.1	E858.8	E948.1	E950.4	E962.0	E980.4
Typhus vaccine	979.2	E858.8	E949.2	E950.4	E962.0	E980.4
Tyrothricin	976.0	E858.7	E946.0	E950.4	E962.0	E980.4
ENT agent	976.6	E858.7	E946.6	E950.4	E962.0	E980.4
ophthalmic preparation	976.5	E858.7	E946.5	E950.4	E962.0	E980.4
Undecenoic acid	976.0	E858.7	E946.0	E950.4	E962.0	E980.4
Undecylenic acid	976.0	E858.7	E946.0	E950.4	E962.0	E980.4
Unna's boot	976.3	E858.7	E946.3	E950.4	E962.0	E980.4
Uracil mustard	963.1	E858.1	E933.1	E950.4	E962.0	E980.4
Uramustine	963.1	E858.1	E933.1	E950.4	E962.0	E980.4
Urari	975.2	E858.6	E945.2	E950.4	E962.0	E980.4
Urea	974.4	E858.5	E944.4	E950.4	E962.0	E980.4
topical	976.8	E858.7	E946.8	E950.4	E962.0	E980.4
Urethan(e) (antineoplastic)	963.1	E858.1	E933.1	E950.4	E962.0	E980.4
Urginea (maritima) (scilla) – *see* Squill						
Uric acid metabolism agents NEC	974.7	E858.5	E944.7	E950.4	E962.0	E980.4
Urokinase	964.4	E858.2	E934.4	E950.4	E962.0	E980.4
Urokon	977.8	E858.8	E947.8	E950.4	E962.0	E980.4
Urotropin	961.9	E857	E931.9	E950.4	E962.0	E980.4
Urtica	988.2	E865.4	-	E950.9	E962.1	E980.9
Utility gas – *see* Gas, utility						
Vaccine NEC	979.9	E858.8	E949.9	E950.4	E962.0	E980.4
bacterial NEC	978.8	E858.8	E948.8	E950.4	E962.0	E980.4

● New Line ▲ Revised Code

Drug	Poisoning	External Cause (E-Code) Accident	Therapeutic Use	Suicide Attempt	Assault	Undetermined
Vaccine – *continued*						
bacterial – *continued*						
with						
other bacterial component	978.9	E858.8	E948.9	E950.4	E962.0	E980.4
pertussis component	978.6	E858.8	E948.6	E950.4	E962.0	E980.4
viral-rickettsial component	979.7	E858.8	E949.7	E950.4	E962.0	E980.4
mixed NEC	978.9	E858.8	E948.9	E950.4	E962.0	E980.4
BCG	978.0	E858.8	E948.0	E950.4	E962.0	E980.4
cholera	978.2	E858.8	E948.2	E950.4	E962.0	E980.4
diphtheria	978.5	E858.8	E948.5	E950.4	E962.0	E980.4
influenza	979.6	E858.8	E949.6	E950.4	E962.0	E980.4
measles	979.4	E858.8	E949.4	E950.4	E962.0	E980.4
meningococcal	978.8	E858.8	E948.8	E950.4	E962.0	E980.4
mumps	979.6	E858.8	E949.6	E950.4	E962.0	E980.4
paratyphoid	978.1	E858.8	E948.1	E950.4	E962.0	E980.4
pertussis (with diphtheria toxoid) (with tetanus toxoid)	978.6	E858.8	E948.6	E950.4	E962.0	E980.4
plague	978.3	E858.8	E948.3	E950.4	E962.0	E980.4
poliomyelitis	979.5	E858.8	E949.5	E950.4	E962.0	E980.4
poliovirus	979.5	E858.8	E949.5	E950.4	E962.0	E980.4
rabies	979.1	E858.8	E949.1	E950.4	E962.0	E980.4
respiratory syncytial virus	979.6	E858.8	E949.6	E950.4	E962.0	E980.4
rickettsial NEC	979.6	E858.8	E949.6	E950.4	E962.0	E980.4
with						
bacterial component	979.7	E858.8	E949.7	E950.4	E962.0	E980.4
pertussis component	978.6	E858.8	E948.6	E950.4	E962.0	E980.4
viral component	979.7	E858.8	E949.7	E950.4	E962.0	E980.4
Rocky mountain spotted fever	979.6	E858.8	E949.6	E950.4	E962.0	E980.4
rotavirus	979.6	E858.8	E949.6	E950.4	E962.0	E980.4
rubella virus	979.4	E858.8	E949.4	E950.4	E962.0	E980.4
sabin oral	979.5	E858.8	E949.5	E950.4	E962.0	E980.4
smallpox	979.0	E858.8	E949.0	E950.4	E962.0	E980.4
tetanus	978.4	E858.8	E948.4	E950.4	E962.0	E980.4
typhoid	978.1	E858.8	E948.1	E950.4	E962.0	E980.4
typhus	979.2	E858.8	E949.2	E950.4	E962.0	E980.4
viral NEC	979.6	E858.8	E949.6	E950.4	E962.0	E980.4
with						
bacterial component	979.7	E858.8	E949.7	E950.4	E962.0	E980.4
pertussis component	978.6	E858.8	E948.6	E950.4	E962.0	E980.4
rickettsial component	979.7	E858.8	E949.7	E950.4	E962.0	E980.4
yellow fever	979.3	E858.8	E949.3	E950.4	E962.0	E980.4
Vaccinia immune globulin (human)	964.6	E858.2	E934.6	E950.4	E962.0	E980.4
Vaginal contraceptives	976.8	E858.7	E946.8	E950.4	E962.0	E980.4
Valethamate	971.1	E855.4	E941.1	E950.4	E962.0	E980.4
Valisone	976.0	E858.7	E946.0	E950.4	E962.0	E980.4
Valium	969.4	E853.2	E939.4	E950.3	E962.0	E980.3
Valmid	967.8	E852.8	E937.8	E950.2	E962.0	E980.2
Vanadium	985.8	E866.4	-	E950.9	E962.1	E980.9
Vancomycin	960.8	E856	E930.8	E950.4	E962.0	E980.4
Vapor (*see also* Gas)	987.9	E869.9	-	E952.9	E962.2	E982.9
kiln (carbon monoxide)	986	E868.8	-	E952.1	E962.2	E982.1
lead – *see* Lead						
specified source NEC - (*see also* specific substance)	987.8	E869.8	-	E952.8	E962.2	E982.8
Varidase	964.4	E858.2	E934.4	E950.4	E962.0	E980.4

Drug	Poisoning	External Cause (E-Code) Accident	Therapeutic Use	Suicide Attempt	Assault	Undetermined
Varnish	989.89	E861.6	-	E950.9	E962.1	E980.9
cleaner	982.8	E862.9	-	E950.9	E962.1	E980.9
Vaseline	976.3	E858.7	E946.3	E950.4	E962.0	E980.4
Vasodilan	972.5	E858.3	E942.5	E950.4	E962.0	E980.4
Vasodilators NEC	972.5	E858.3	E942.5	E950.4	E962.0	E980.4
coronary	972.4	E858.3	E942.4	E950.4	E962.0	E980.4
Vasopressin	962.5	E858.0	E932.5	E950.4	E962.0	E980.4
Vasopressor drugs	962.5	E858.0	E932.5	E950.4	E962.0	E980.4
Venom, venomous (bite) (sting)	989.5	E905.9	-	E950.9	E962.1	E980.9
arthropod NEC	989.5	E905.5	-	E950.9	E962.1	E980.9
bee	989.5	E905.3	-	E950.9	E962.1	E980.9
centipede	989.5	E905.4	-	E950.9	E962.1	E980.9
hornet	989.5	E905.3	-	E950.9	E962.1	E980.9
lizard	989.5	E905.0	-	E950.9	E962.1	E980.9
marine animals or plants	989.5	E905.6	-	E950.9	E962.1	E980.9
millipede (tropical)	989.5	E905.4	-	E950.9	E962.1	E980.9
plant NEC	989.5	E905.7	-	E950.9	E962.1	E980.9
marine	989.5	E905.6	-	E950.9	E962.1	E980.9
scorpion	989.5	E905.2	-	E950.9	E962.1	E980.9
snake	989.5	E905.0	-	E950.9	E962.1	E980.9
specified NEC	989.5	E905.8	-	E950.9	E962.1	E980.9
spider	989.5	E905.1	-	E950.9	E962.1	E980.9
wasp	989.5	E905.3	-	E950.9	E962.1	E980.9
Ventolin – *see* Salbutamol sulfate						
Veramon	967.0	E851	E937.0	E950.1	E962.0	E980.1
Veratrum						
album	988.2	E865.4	-	E950.9	E962.1	E980.9
alkaloids	972.6	E858.3	E942.6	E950.4	E962.0	E980.4
viride	988.2	E865.4	-	E950.9	E962.1	E980.9
Verdigris (*see also* Copper)	985.8	E866.4	-	E950.9	E962.1	E980.9
Veronal	967.0	E851	E937.0	E950.1	E962.0	E980.1
Veroxil	961.6	E857	E931.6	E950.4	E962.0	E980.4
Versidyne	965.7	E850.7	E935.7	E950.0	E962.0	E980.0
Viagra	972.5	E858.3	E942.5	E950.4	E962.0	E980.4
Vienna						
green	985.1	E866.3	-	E950.8	E962.1	E980.8
insecticide	985.1	E863.4	-	E950.6	E962.1	E980.7
red	989.89	E866.8	-	E950.9	E962.1	E980.9
pharmaceutical dye	977.4	E858.8	E947.4	E950.4	E962.0	E980.4
Vinbarbital, vinbarbitone	967.0	E851	E937.0	E950.1	E962.0	E980.1
Vinblastine	963.1	E858.1	E933.1	E950.4	E962.0	E980.4
Vincristine	963.1	E858.1	E933.1	E950.4	E962.0	E980.4
Vinesthene, vinethene	968.2	E855.1	E938.2	E950.4	E962.0	E980.4
Vinyl						
bital	967.0	E851	E937.0	E950.1	E962.0	E980.1
ether	968.2	E855.1	E938.2	E950.4	E962.0	E980.4
Vioform	961.3	E857	E931.3	E950.4	E962.0	E980.4
topical	976.0	E858.7	E946.0	E950.4	E962.0	E980.4
Viomycin	960.6	E856	E930.6	E950.4	E962.0	E980.4
Viosterol	963.5	E858.1	E933.5	E950.4	E962.0	E980.4
Viper (venom)	989.5	E905.0	-	E950.9	E962.1	E980.9
Viprynium (embonate)	961.6	E857	E931.6	E950.4	E962.0	E980.4
Virugon	961.7	E857	E931.7	E950.4	E962.0	E980.4
Visine	976.5	E858.7	E946.5	E950.4	E962.0	E980.4
Vitamins NEC	963.5	E858.1	E933.5	E950.4	E962.0	E980.4
B_{12}	964.1	E858.2	E934.1	E950.4	E962.0	E980.4
hematopoietic	964.1	E858.2	E934.1	E950.4	E962.0	E980.4
K	964.3	E858.2	E934.3	E950.4	E962.0	E980.4
Vleminckx's solution	976.4	E858.7	E946.4	E950.4	E962.0	E980.4
Voltaren – *see* Diclofenac sodium						

● New Line ▲ Revised Code

Drug	Poisoning	External Cause (E-Code): Accident	Therapeutic Use	Suicide Attempt	Assault	Undetermined
Warfarin (potassium) (sodium)	964.2	E858.2	E934.2	E950.4	E962.0	E980.4
rodenticide	989.4	E863.7	-	E950.6	E962.1	E980.7
Wasp (sting)	989.5	E905.3	-	E950.9	E962.1	E980.9
Water						
balance agents NEC	974.5	E858.5	E944.5	E950.4	E962.0	E980.4
gas	987.1	E868.1	-	E951.8	E962.2	E981.8
incomplete combustion of – *see* Carbon, monoxide, fuel, utility						
hemlock	988.2	E865.4	-	E950.9	E962.1	E980.9
moccasin (venom)	989.5	E905.0	-	E950.9	E962.1	E980.9
Wax (paraffin) (petroleum)	981	E862.3	-	E950.9	E962.1	E980.9
automobile	989.89	E861.2	-	E950.9	E962.1	E980.9
floor	981	E862.0	-	E950.9	E962.1	E980.9
Weed killers NEC	989.4	E863.5	-	E950.6	E962.1	E980.7
Welldorm	967.1	E852.0	E937.1	E950.2	E962.0	E980.2
White						
arsenic – *see* Arsenic						
hellebore	988.2	E865.4	-	E950.9	E962.1	E980.9
lotion (keratolytic)	976.4	E858.7	E946.4	E950.4	E962.0	E980.4
spirit	981	E862.0	-	E950.9	E962.1	E980.9
Whitewashes	989.89	E861.6	-	E950.9	E962.1	E980.9
Whole blood	964.7	E858.2	E934.7	E950.4	E962.0	E980.4
Wild						
black cherry	988.2	E865.4	-	E950.9	E962.1	E980.9
poisonous plants NEC	988.2	E865.4	-	E950.9	E962.1	E980.9
Window cleaning fluid	989.89	E861.3	-	E950.9	E962.1	E980.9
Wintergreen (oil)	976.3	E858.7	E946.3	E950.4	E962.0	E980.4
Witch hazel	976.2	E858.7	E946.2	E950.4	E962.0	E980.4
Wood						
alcohol	980.1	E860.2	-	E950.9	E962.1	E980.9
spirit	980.1	E860.2	-	E950.9	E962.1	E980.9
Woorali	975.2	E858.6	E945.2	E950.4	E962.0	E980.4
Wormseed, American	961.6	E857	E931.6	E950.4	E962.0	E980.4
Xanthine diuretics	974.1	E858.5	E944.1	E950.4	E962.0	E980.4
Xanthocillin	960.0	E856	E930.0	E950.4	E962.0	E980.4
Xanthotoxin	976.3	E858.7	E946.3	E950.4	E962.0	E980.4

Drug	Poisoning	External Cause (E-Code): Accident	Therapeutic Use	Suicide Attempt	Assault	Undetermined
Xigris	964.2	E858.2	E934.2	E950.4	E962.0	E980.4
Xylene (liquid) (vapor)	982.0	E862.4	-	E950.9	E962.1	E980.9
Xylocaine (infiltration) (topical)	968.5	E855.2	E938.5	E950.4	E962.0	E980.4
nerve block (peripheral) (plexus)	968.6	E855.2	E938.6	E950.4	E962.0	E980.4
spinal	968.7	E855.2	E938.7	E950.4	E962.0	E980.4
Xylol (liquid) (vapor)	982.0	E862.4	-	E950.9	E962.1	E980.9
Xylometazoline	971.2	E855.5	E941.2	E950.4	E962.0	E980.4
Yellow						
fever vaccine	979.3	E858.8	E949.3	E950.4	E962.0	E980.4
jasmine	988.2	E865.4	-	E950.9	E962.1	E980.9
Yew	988.2	E865.4	-	E950.9	E962.1	E980.9
Zactane	965.7	E850.7	E935.7	E950.0	E962.0	E980.0
Zaroxolyn	974.3	E858.5	E944.3	E950.4	E962.0	E980.4
Zephiran (topical)	976.0	E858.7	E946.0	E950.4	E962.0	E980.4
ophthalmic preparation	976.5	E858.7	E946.5	E950.4	E962.0	E980.4
Zerone	980.1	E860.2	-	E950.9	E962.1	E980.9
Zinc (compounds) (fumes) (salts) (vapor) NEC	985.8	E866.4	-	E950.9	E962.1	E980.9
anti-infectives	976.0	E858.7	E946.0	E950.4	E962.0	E980.4
antivaricose	972.7	E858.3	E942.7	E950.4	E962.0	E980.4
bacitracin	976.0	E858.7	E946.0	E950.4	E962.0	E980.4
chloride	976.2	E858.7	E946.2	E950.4	E962.0	E980.4
gelatin	976.3	E858.7	E946.3	E950.4	E962.0	E980.4
oxide	976.3	E858.7	E946.3	E950.4	E962.0	E980.4
peroxide	976.0	E858.7	E946.0	E950.4	E962.0	E980.4
pesticides	985.8	E863.4	-	E950.6	E962.1	E980.7
phosphide (rodenticide)	985.8	E863.7	-	E950.6	E962.1	E980.7
stearate	976.3	E858.7	E946.3	E950.4	E962.0	E980.4
sulfate (antivaricose)	972.7	E858.3	E942.7	E950.4	E962.0	E980.4
ENT agent	976.6	E858.7	E946.6	E950.4	E962.0	E980.4
ophthalmic solution	976.5	E858.7	E946.5	E950.4	E962.0	E980.4
topical NEC	976.0	E858.7	E946.0	E950.4	E962.0	E980.4
undecylenate	976.0	E858.7	E946.0	E950.4	E962.0	E980.4
Zovant	964.2	E858.2	E934.2	E950.4	E962.0	E980.4
Zoxazolamine	968.0	E855.1	E938.0	E950.4	E962.0	E980.4
Zygadenus (venenosus)	988.2	E865.4	-	E950.9	E962.1	E980.9

A

Abandonment
- causing exposure to weather conditions – *see* Exposure
- child, with intent to injure or kill E968.4
- helpless person, infant, newborn E904.0
  - with intent to injure or kill E968.4

Abortion, criminal, injury to child E968.8

Abuse (alleged) (suspected)
- adult
  - by
    - child E967.4
    - ex-partner E967.3
    - ex-spouse E967.3
    - father E967.0
    - grandchild E967.7
    - grandparent E967.6
    - mother E967.2
    - non-related caregiver E967.8
    - other relative E967.7
    - other specified person E967.1
    - partner E967.3
    - sibling E967.5
    - spouse E967.3
    - stepfather E967.0
    - stepmother E967.2
    - unspecified person E967.9
- child
  - by
    - boyfriend of parent or guardian E967.0
    - child E967.4
    - father E967.0
    - female partner of parent or guardian E967.2
    - girlfriend of parent or guardian E967.2
    - grandchild E967.7
    - grandparent E967.6
    - male partner of parent or guardian E967.0
    - mother E967.2
    - non-related caregiver E967.8
    - other relative E967.7
    - other specified person(s) E967.1
    - sibling E967.5
    - stepfather E967.0
    - stepmother E967.2
    - unspecified person E967.9

Accident (to) E928.9
- aircraft (in transit) (powered) E841❹
  - at landing, take-off E840❹
  - due to, caused by cataclysm – *see* categories E908❹, E909❹
  - late effect of E929.1
  - unpowered (*see also* Collision, aircraft, unpowered) E842❹
  - while alighting, boarding E843❹
- amphibious vehicle
  - on
    - land – *see* Accident, motor vehicle
    - water – *see* Accident, watercraft
- animal, ridden NEC E828❹
- animal-drawn vehicle NEC E827❹
- balloon (*see also* Collision, aircraft, unpowered) E842❹
- caused by, due to
  - abrasive wheel (metalworking) E919.3
  - animal NEC E906.9
    - being ridden (in sport or transport) E828
  - avalanche NEC E909.2
  - band saw E919.4
  - bench saw E919.4
  - bore, earth-drilling or mining (land) (seabed) E919.1
  - bulldozer E919.7
  - cataclysmic
    - earth surface movement or eruption E909.9
    - storm E908.9
  - chain
    - hoist E919.2
      - agricultural operations E919.0
      - mining operations E919.1
    - saw E920.1
  - circular saw E919.4
  - cold (excessive) (*see also* Cold, exposure to) E901.9
  - combine E919.0
    - conflagration – *see* Conflagration
  - corrosive liquid, substance NEC E924.1
  - cotton gin E919.8
  - crane E919.2
    - agricultural operations E919.0

Accident – *continued*
- caused by, due to – *continued*
  - crane – *continued*
    - mining operations E919.1
  - cutting or piercing instrument (*see also* Cut) E920.9
  - dairy equipment E919.8
  - derrick E919.2
    - agricultural operations E919.0
    - mining operations E919.1
  - drill E920.1
    - earth (land) (seabed) E919.1
    - hand (powered) E920.1
      - not powered E920.4
    - metalworking E919.3
    - woodworking E919.4
  - earth(-)
    - drilling machine E919.1
    - moving machine E919.7
    - scraping machine E919.7
  - electric
    - current (*see also* Electric shock) E925.9
    - motor – *see also* Accident, machine, by type of machine
      - current (of) – *see* Electric shock
  - elevator (building) (grain) E919.2
    - agricultural operations E919.0
    - mining operations E919.1
  - environmental factors NEC E928.9
  - excavating machine E919.7
  - explosive material (*see also* Explosion) E923.9
  - farm machine E919.0
  - fire, flames – *see also* Fire
    - conflagration – *see* Conflagration
  - firearm missile – *see* Shooting
  - forging (metalworking) machine E919.3
  - forklift (truck) E919.2
    - agricultural operations E919.0
    - mining operations E919.1
  - gas turbine E919.5
  - harvester E919.0
  - hay derrick, mower, or rake E919.0
  - heat (excessive) (*see also* Heat) E900.9
  - hoist (*see also* Accident, caused by, due to, lift) E919.2
    - chain – *see* Accident, caused by, due to, chain
    - shaft E919.1
  - hot
    - liquid E924.0
      - caustic or corrosive E924.1
    - object (not producing fire or flames) E924.8
    - substance E924.9
      - caustic or corrosive E924.1
      - liquid (metal) NEC E924.0
      - specified type NEC E924.8
  - human bite E928.3
  - ignition – *see* Ignition E919.4
  - internal combustion engine E919.5
  - landslide NEC E909.2
  - lathe (metalworking) E919.3
    - turnings E920.8
    - woodworking E919.4
  - lift, lifting (appliances) E919.2
    - agricultural operations E919.0
    - mining operations E919.1
    - shaft E919.1
  - lightning NEC E907
  - machine, machinery – *see also* Accident, machine
    - drilling, metal E919.3
    - manufacturing, for manufacture of steam
      - beverages E919.8
      - clothing E919.8
      - foodstuffs E919.8
      - paper E919.8
      - textiles E919.8
    - milling, metal E919.3
    - moulding E919.4
    - power press, metal E919.3
    - printing E919.8
    - rolling mill, metal E919.3
    - sawing, metal E919.3
    - specified type NEC E919.8
    - spinning E919.8
    - weaving E919.8
  - natural factor NEC E928.9
  - overhead plane E919.4
  - plane E920.4
    - overhead E919.4
  - powered
    - hand tool NEC E920.1

Accident – *continued*
- caused by, due to – *continued*
  - powered – *continued*
    - saw E919.4
      - hand E920.1
  - printing machine E919.8
  - pulley (block) E919.2
    - agricultural operations E919.0
    - mining operations E919.1
    - transmission E919.6
  - radial saw E919.4
  - radiation – *see* Radiation
  - reaper E919.0
  - road scraper E919.7
    - when in transport under its own power – *see* categories E810-E825❹
  - roller, coaster E919.8
  - sander E919.4
  - saw E920.4
    - band E919.4
    - bench E919.4
    - chain E920.1
    - circular E919.4
    - hand E920.4
      - powered E920.1
    - powered, except hand E919.4
    - radial E919.4
  - sawing machine, metal E919.3
  - shaft
    - hoist E919.1
    - lift E919.1
    - transmission E919.6
  - shears E920.4
    - hand E920.4
      - powered E920.1
    - mechanical E919.3
  - shovel E920.4
    - steam E919.7
  - spinning machine E919.8
  - steam – *see also* Burning, steam
    - engine E919.5
    - shovel E919.7
  - thresher E919.0
  - thunderbolt NEC E907
  - tractor E919.0
    - when in transport under its own power – *see* categories E810-E825❹
  - transmission belt, cable, chain, gear, pinion, pulley, shaft E919.6
  - turbine (gas) (water driven) E919.5
  - under-cutter E919.1
  - weaving machine E919.8
  - winch E919.2
    - agricultural operations E919.0
    - mining operations E919.1
- diving E883.0
  - with insufficient air supply E913.2
- glider (hang) (*see also* Collision, aircraft, unpowered) E842❹
- hovercraft
  - on
    - land – *see* Accident, motor vehicle
    - water – *see* Accident, watercraft
- ice yacht (*see also* Accident, vehicle NEC) E848
- in
  - medical, surgical procedure
    - as, or due to misadventure – *see* Misadventure
  - causing an abnormal reaction or later complication without mention of misadventure – *see* Reaction, abnormal
- kite carrying a person (*see also* Collision, involving aircraft, unpowered) E842❹
- land yacht (*see also* Accident, vehicle NEC) E848
- late effect of – *see* Late effect
- launching pad E845❹
- machine, machinery (*see also* Accident, caused by, due to, by specific type of machine) E919.9
  - agricultural including animal-powered premises E919.0
  - earth-drilling E919.1
  - earth moving or scraping E919.7
  - excavating E919.7
  - involving transport under own power on highway or transport vehicle – *see* categories E810-E825❹, E840-E845❹
  - lifting (appliances) E919.2
  - metalworking E919.3
  - mining E919.1

- **Accident** – *continued*
  - machine, machinery – *continued*
    - prime movers, except electric motors E919.5
      - electric motors – *see* Accident, machine, by specific type of machine
    - recreational E919.8
    - specified type NEC E919.8
    - transmission E919.6
    - watercraft (deck) (engine room) (galley) (laundry) (loading) E836❹
    - woodworking or forming E919.4
  - motor vehicle (on public highway) (traffic) E819❹
    - due to cataclysm – *see* categories E908❹, E909❹
    - involving
      - collision (*see also* Collision, motor vehicle) E812❹
    - nontraffic, not on public highway – *see* categories E820-E825❹
    - not involving collision – *see* categories E816-E819❹
  - nonmotor vehicle NEC E829❹
    - nonroad – *see* Accident, vehicle NEC
    - road, except pedal cycle, animal-drawn vehicle, or animal being ridden E829❹
  - nonroad vehicle NEC – *see* Accident, vehicle NEC
  - not elsewhere classifiable involving
    - cable car (not on rails) E847
      - on rails E829❹
    - coal car in mine E846
    - hand truck – *see* Accident, vehicle NEC
    - logging car E846
    - sled(ge), meaning snow or ice vehicle E848
    - tram, mine or quarry E846
    - truck
      - mine or quarry E846
      - self-propelled, industrial E846
      - station baggage E846
    - tub, mine or quarry E846
    - vehicle NEC E848
      - snow and ice E848
      - used only on industrial premises E846
    - wheelbarrow E848
  - occurring (at) (in)
    - apartment E849.0
    - baseball field, diamond E849.4
    - construction site, any E849.3
    - dock E849.8
      - yard E849.3
    - dormitory E849.7
    - factory (building) (premises) E849.3
    - farm E849.1
      - buildings E849.1
      - house E849.0
    - football field E849.4
    - forest E849.8
    - garage (place of work) E849.3
      - private (home) E849.0
    - gravel pit E849.2
    - gymnasium E849.4
    - highway E849.5
    - home (private) (residential) E849.0
      - institutional E849.7
    - hospital E849.7
    - hotel E849.6
    - house (private) (residential) E849.0
      - movie E849.6
      - public E849.6
    - institution, residential E849.7
    - jail E849.7
    - mine E849.2
    - motel E849.6
    - movie house E849.6
    - office (building) E849.6
    - orphanage E849.7
    - park (public) E849.4
      - mobile home E849.8
      - trailer E849.8
    - parking lot or place E849.8
    - place
      - industrial NEC E849.3
      - parking E849.8
      - public E849.8
        - specified place NEC E849.5
      - recreational NEC E849.4
      - sport NEC E849.4
    - playground (park) (school) E849.4
    - prison E849.6
    - public building NEC E849.6
    - quarry E849.2
    - railway
      - line NEC E849.8

- **Accident** – *continued*
  - occurring (at) (in) – *continued*
    - railway – *continued*
      - yard E849.3
    - residence
      - home (private) E849.0
    - resort (beach) (lake) (mountain) (seashore) (vacation) E849.4
    - restaurant E849.6
    - sand pit E849.2
    - school (building) (private) (public) (state) E849.6
      - reform E849.7
      - riding E849.4
    - seashore E849.8
      - resort E849.4
    - shop (place of work) E849.3
      - commercial E849.6
    - skating rink E849.4
    - sports palace E849.4
    - stadium E849.4
    - store E849.6
    - street E849.5
    - swimming pool (public) E849.4
      - private home or garden E849.0
    - tennis court E849.4
    - theatre, theater E849.6
    - trailer court E849.8
    - tunnel E849.8
      - under construction E849.2
    - warehouse E849.3
    - yard
      - dock E849.3
      - industrial E849.3
      - private (home) E849.0
      - railway E849.3
  - off-road type motor vehicle (not on public highway) NEC E821❹
    - on public highway – *see* categories E810-E819❹
  - pedal cycle E826❹
  - railway E807❹
    - due to cataclysm – *see* categories E908❹, E909❹
    - involving
      - avalanche E909.2
      - burning by engine, locomotive, train (*see also* Explosion, railway engine) E803❹
      - collision (*see also* collision, railway) E800❹
      - derailment (*see also* Derailment, railway) E802❹
      - explosion (*see also* Explosion, railway engine) E803❹
      - fall (*see also* Fall, from, railway rolling stock) E804❹
      - fire (*see also* Explosion, railway engine) E803❹
      - hitting by, being struck by
        - object falling in, on, from, rolling stock, train, vehicle E806❹
        - rolling stock, train, vehicle E805❹
      - overturning, railway rolling stock, train, vehicle (*see also* Derailment, railway) E802❹
      - running off rails, railway (*see also* Derailment, railway) E802❹
      - specified circumstances NEC E806❹
      - train or vehicle hit by
        - avalanche E909.2❹
        - failing object (earth, rock, tree) E806❹
          - due to cataclysm – *see* categories E908❹, E909❹
        - landslide E909.2❹
  - roller skate E885.1
  - scooter (nonmotorized) E885.0
  - skateboard E885.2
  - ski(ing) E885.3
    - jump E884.9
    - lift or tow (with chair or gondola) E847
  - snowboard E885.4
  - snow vehicle, motor driven (not on public highway) E820❹
    - on public highway – *see* categories E810-E819❹
  - spacecraft E845❹
  - specified cause NEC E928.8
  - street car E829❹
  - traffic NEC E819❹
  - vehicle NEC (with pedestrian) E848
    - battery powered
      - airport passenger vehicle E846
      - truck (baggage) (mail) E846

- **Accident** – *continued*
  - vehicle – *continued*
    - powered commercial or industrial (with other vehicle or object within commercial or industrial premises) E846
  - watercraft E838❹
    - with
      - drowning or submersion resulting from
        - accident other than to watercraft E832❹
        - accident to watercraft E830❹
      - injury, except drowning or submersion, resulting from
        - accident other than to watercraft – *see* categories E833-E838❹
        - accident to watercraft E831❹
    - due to, caused by cataclysm – *see* categories E908❹, E909❹
    - machinery E836❹
- **Acid throwing** E961
- **Acosta syndrome** E902.0
- **Aeroneurosis** E902.1
- **Aero-otitis media** – *see* Effects of, air pressure
- **Aerosinusitis** – *see* Effects of, air pressure
- **After-effect, late** – *see* Late effect
- **Air**
  - blast
    - in
      - terrorism E979.2
      - war operations E993
  - embolism (traumatic) NEC E928.9
    - in
      - infusion or transfusion E874.1
      - perfusion E874.2
  - sickness E903
- **Alpine sickness** E902.0
- **Altitude sickness** – *see* Effects of, air pressure
- **Anaphylactic shock, anaphylaxis** (*see also* Table of Drugs and Chemicals) E947.9
  - due to bite or sting (venomous) – *see* Bite, venomous
- **Andes disease** E902.0
- **Apoplexy**
  - heat – *see* Heat
- **Arachnidism** E905.1
- **Arson** E968.0
- **Asphyxia, asphyxiation**
  - by
    - chemical
      - in
        - terrorism E979.7
        - war operations E997.2
    - explosion – *see* Explosion E965.8
    - food (bone) (regurgitated food) (seed) E911
    - foreign object, except food E912
    - fumes
      - in
        - terrorism (chemical weapons) E979.7
        - war operations E997.2
    - gas – *see also* Table of Drugs and Chemicals
      - in
        - terrorism E979.7
        - war operations E997.2
      - legal
        - execution E978
        - intervention (tear) E972
      - tear E972
    - mechanical means (*see also* Suffocation) E913.9
  - from
    - conflagration – *see* Conflagration
    - fire – *see also* Fire E899
      - in
        - terrorism E979.3
        - war operations E990.9
    - ignition – *see* Ignition
- **Aspiration**
  - foreign body – *see* Foreign body, aspiration
  - mucus, not of newborn (with asphyxia, obstruction respiratory passage, suffocation) E912
  - phlegm (with asphyxia, obstruction respiratory passage, suffocation) E912
  - vomitus (with asphyxia, obstruction respiratory passage, suffocation) (*see also* Foreign body, aspiration, food) E911
- **Assassination** (attempt) (*see also* Assault) E968.9
- **Assault** (homicidal) (by) (in) E968.9
  - air gun E968.6
  - acid E961
    - swallowed E962.1
  - BB gun E968.6

Assault – *continued*
  bite NEC E968.8
    of human being E968.7
  bomb ((placed in) car or house) E965.8
    antipersonnel E965.5
    letter E965.7
    petrol E965.6
  brawl (hand) (fists) (foot) E960.0
  burning, burns (by fire) E968.0
    acid E961
      swallowed E962.1
    caustic, corrosive substance E961
      swallowed E962.1
    chemical from swallowing caustic, corrosive substance NEC E962.1
    hot liquid E968.3
    scalding E968.3
    vitriol E961
      swallowed E962.1
  caustic, corrosive substance E961
    swallowed E962.1
  cut, any part of body E966
  dagger E966
  drowning E964
  explosives) E965.9
    bomb (*see also* Assault, bomb) E965.8
    dynamite E965.8
  fight (hand) (fists) (foot) E960.0
    with weapon E968.9
      blunt or thrown E968.2
      cutting or piercing E966
      firearm – *see* Shooting, homicide
  fire E968.0
  firearm(s) – *see* Shooting, homicide
  garrotting E963
  gunshot (wound) – *see* Shooting, homicide
  hanging E963
  injury NEC E968.9
  knife E966
  late effect of E969
  ligature E963
  poisoning E962.9
    drugs or medicinals E962.0
    gas(es) or vapors, except drugs and medicinals E962.2
    solid or liquid substances, except drugs and medicinals E962.1
  puncture, any part of body E966
  pushing
    before moving object, train, vehicle E968.5
    from high place E968.1
  rape E960.1
  scalding E968.3
  shooting – *see* Shooting, homicide
  sodomy E960.1
  stab, any part of body E966
  strangulation E963
  submersion E964
  suffocation E963
  transport vehicle E968.5
  violence NEC E968.9
  vitriol E961
    swallowed E962.1
  weapon E968.9
    blunt or thrown E968.2
    cutting or piercing E966
    firearm – *see* Shooting, homicide
  wound E968.9
    cutting E966
    gunshot – *see* Shooting, homicide
    knife E966
    piercing E966
    puncture E966
    stab E966
Attack by animal NEC E906.9
Avalanche E909.2
  falling on or hitting
    motor vehicle (in motion) (on public highway) E909.2
    railway train E909.2
Aviators' disease E902.1

B

Barotitis, barodontalgia, berosinusitis, barotrauma (otitic) (sinus) – *see* Effects of, air pressure
Battered
  baby or child (syndrome) – *see* Abuse, child; category E967 ❹
  person other than baby or child – *see* Assault
Bayonet wound (*see also* Cut, by bayonet) E920.3
  in
    legal intervention E974
    terrorism E979.8
    war operations E995
Bean in nose E912
Bed set on fire NEC E898.0
Beheading (by guillotine)
  homicide E966
  legal execution E978
Bending, injury in E927
Bends E902.0
Bite
  animal (nonvenomous)NEC E906.5
  other specified (except arthropod) E906.3
    venomous NEC E905.9
  arthropod (nonvenomous) NEC E906.4
    venomous – *see* Sting
  black widow spider E905.1
  cat E906.3
  centipede E905.4
  cobra E905.0
  copperhead snake E905.0
  coral snake E905.0
  dog E906.0
  fer de lance E905.0
  gila monster E905.0
  human being
    accidental E928.3
    assault E968.7
  insect (nonvenomous) E906.4
    venomous – *see* Sting
  krait E905.0
  late effect of – *see* Late effect
  lizard E906.2
    venomous E905.0
  mamba E905.0
  marine animal
    nonvenomous E906.3
      snake E906.2
    venomous E905.6
      snake E905.0
  millipede E906.4
    venomous E905.4
  moray eel E906.3
  rat E906.1
  rattlesnake E905.0
  rodent, except rat E906.3
  serpent – *see* Bite, snake
  shark E906.3
  snake (venomous) E905.0
    nonvenomous E906.2
    sea E905.0
  spider E905.1
    nonvenomous E906.4
  tarantula (venomous) E905.1
  venomous NEC E905.9
    by specific animal – *see* category E905 ❹
  viper E905.0
  water moccasin E905.0
Blast (air)
  in
    terrorism E979.2
      from nuclear explosion E979.5
      underwater E979.0
    war operations E993
      from nuclear explosion E996
      underwater E992
Blizzard E908.3
Blow E928.9
  by law-enforcing agent, police (on duty) E975
    with blunt object (baton) (nightstick) (stave) (truncheon) E973
Blowing up (*see also* Explosion) E923.9
Brawl (hand) (fists) (foot) E960.0
Breakage (accidental)
  cable of cable car not on rails E847
  ladder (causing fall) E881.0
  part (any) of
    animal-drawn vehicle E827 ❹
    ladder (causing fall) E881.0
    motor vehicle
      in motion (on public highway) E818 ❹
        not on public highway E825 ❹
    nonmotor road vehicle, except animal-drawn vehicle or pedal cycle E829 ❹
    off-road type motor vehicle (not on public highway) NEC E821 ❹
      on public highway E818 ❹
    pedal cycle E826 ❹
Breakage – *continued*
  part (any) of – *continued*
    scaffolding (causing fall) E881.1
    snow vehicle, motor-driven (not on public highway) E820 ❹
      on public highway E818 ❹
    vehicle NEC – *see* Accident, vehicle
Broken
  glass
    fall on E888.0
    injury by E920.8
  power line (causing electric shock) E925.1
Bumping against, into (accidentally)
  object (moving) E917.9
    caused by crowd E917.1
      with subsequent fall E917.6
    furniture E917.3
      with subsequent fall E917.7
    in
      running water E917.2
      sports E917.0
        with subsequent fall E917.5
    stationary E917.4
      with subsequent fall E917.8
  person(s) E917.9
    with fall E886.9
      in sports E886.0
    as, or caused by, a crowd E917.1
      with subsequent fall E917.6
    in sports E917.0
      with fall E886.0
Burning, burns (accidental) (by) (from) (on) E899
  acid (any kind) E924.1
    swallowed – *see* Table of Drugs and Chemicals
  bedclothes (*see also* Fire, specified NEC) E898.0
  blowlamp (*see also* Fire, specified NEC) E898.1
  blowtorch (*see also* Fire, specified NEC) E898.1
  boat, ship, watercraft – *see* categories E830 ❹, E831 ❹, E837 ❹
  bonfire (controlled) E897
    uncontrolled E892
  candle (*see also* Fire, specified NEC) E898.1
  caustic liquid, substance E924.1
    swallowed – *see* Table of Drugs and Chemicals
  chemical E924.1
    from swallowing caustic, corrosive substance – *see* Table of Drugs and Chemicals
    in
      terrorism E979.7
      war operations E997.2
  cigar(s) or cigarette(s) (*see also* Fire, specified NEC) E898.1
  clothes, clothing, nightdress – *see* Ignition, clothes
    with conflagration – *see* Conflagration
  conflagration – *see* Conflagration
  corrosive liquid, substance E924.1
    swallowed – *see* Table of Drugs and Chemicals
  electric current (*see also* Electric shock) E925.9
  fire, flames (*see also* Fire) E899
  flare, Verey pistol E922.8
  heat
    from appliance (electrical) E924.8
    in local application, or packing during medical or surgical procedure E873.5
  homicide (attempt) (*see also* Assault, burning) E968.0
  hot
    liquid E924.0
      caustic or corrosive E924.1
    object (not producing fire or flames) E924.8
    substance E924.9
      caustic or corrosive E924.1
      liquid (metal) NEC E924.0
      specified type NEC E924.8
    tap water E924.2
  ignition – *see also* Ignition
    clothes, clothing, nightdress – *see also* Ignition, clothes
      with conflagration – *see* Conflagration
    highly inflammable material (benzine) (fat) (gasoline) (kerosine) (paraffin) (petrol) E894
  inflicted by other person
    stated as
      homicidal, intentional (*see also* Assault, burning) E968.0
      undetermined whether accidental or intentional (*see also* Burn, stated as undetermined whether accidental or intentional) E988.1

Burning, burns – *continued*
- internal, from swallowed caustic, corrosive liquid, substance – *see* Table of Drugs and Chemicals
- in
  - terrorism E979.3
    - from nuclear explosion E979.5
    - petrol bomb E979.3
  - war operations (from fire-producing device or conventional weapon) E990.9
    - from nuclear explosion E996
    - petrol bomb E990.0
- lamp (*see also* Fire, specified NEC) E898.1
- late effect of NEC E929.4
- lighter (cigar) (cigarette) (*see also* Fire, specified NEC) E898.1
- lightning E907
- liquid (boiling) (hot) (molten) E924.0
  - caustic, corrosive (external) E924.1
    - swallowed – *see* Table of Drugs and Chemicals
- local application of externally applied substance in medical or surgical care E873.5
- machinery – *see* Accident, machine
- matches (*see also* Fire, specified NEC) E898.1
- medicament, externally applied E873.5
- metal, molten E924.0
- object (hot) E924.8
  - producing fire or flames – *see* Fire
- oven (electric) (gas) E924.8
- pipe (smoking) (*see also* Fire, specified NEC) E898.1
- radiation – *see* Radiation
- railway engine, locomotive, train (*see also* Explosion, railway engine) E803❹
- self-inflicted (unspecified whether accidental or intentional) E988.1
  - caustic or corrosive substance NEC E988.7
  - stated as intentional, purposeful E958.1
    - caustic or corrosive substance NEC E958.7
- stated as undetermined whether accidental or intentional E988.1
  - caustic or corrosive substance NEC or E988.7
- steam E924.0
  - pipe E924.8
- substance (hot) E924.9
  - boiling or molten E924.0
  - caustic, corrosive (external) E924.1
    - swallowed – *see* Table of Drugs and Chemicals
- suicidal (attempt) NEC E958.1
  - caustic substance E958.7
  - late effect of E959
- tanning bed E926.2
- therapeutic misadventure
  - overdose of radiation E873.2
- torch, welding (*see also* Fire, specified NEC) E898.1
- trash fire (*see also* Burning, bonfire) E897
- vapor E924.0
- vitriol E924.1
- x-rays E926.3
  - in medical, surgical procedure – *see* Misadventure, failure, in dosage, radiation operations

Butted by animal E906.8

C

Cachexia, lead or saturnine E866.0
- from pesticide NEC (*see also* Table of Drugs and Chemicals) E863.4

Caisson disease E902.2

Capital punishment (any means) E978

Car sickness E903

Casualty (not due to war) NEC E928.9
- terrorism E979.8
- war (*see also* War operations) E995

Cat
- bite E906.3
- scratch E906.8

Cataclysmic (any injury)
- earth surface movement or eruption E909.9
  - specified type NEC E909.8
- storm or flood resulting from storm E908.9
  - specified type NEC E909.8

Catching fire – *see* Ignition

Caught
- between
  - objects (moving) (stationary and moving) E918
    - and machinery – *see* Accident, machine
- by cable car, not on rails E847
- in
  - machinery (moving parts of) – *see* Accident, machine
  - object E918

Cave-in (causing asphyxia, suffocation (by pressure)) (*see also* Suffocation, due to, cave-in) E913.3
- with injury other than asphyxia or suffocation E916
  - with asphyxia or suffocation (*see also* Suffocation, due to, cave-in) E913.3
- struck or crushed by E916
  - with asphyxia or suffocation (*see also* Suffocation, due to, cave-in) E913.3

Change(s) in air pressure – *see also* Effects of, air pressure
- sudden, in aircraft (ascent) (descent) (causing aeroneurosis or aviators' disease) E902.1

Chilblains E901.0
- due to manmade conditions E901.1

Choking (on) (any object except food or vomitus) E912
- apple E911
- bone E911
- food, any type (regurgitated) E911
- mucus or phlegm E912
- seed E911

Civil insurrection – *see* War operations

Cloudburst E908.8

Cold, exposure to (accidental) (excessive) (extreme) (place) E901.9
- causing chilblains or immersion foot E901.0
- due to
  - manmade conditions E901.1
  - specified cause NEC E901.8
  - weather (conditions) E901.0
- late effect of NEC E929.5
- self-inflicted (undetermined whether accidental or intentional) E988.3
  - suicidal E958.3
- suicide E958.3

Colic, lead, painters', or saturnine – *see* category E866❹

Collapse
- building (moveable) E916
  - burning (uncontrolled fire) E891.8
    - in terrorism E979.3
    - private E890.8
- dam E909.3
- due to heat – *see* Heat
- machinery – *see* Accident, machine or vehicle
- man-made structure E909.3
- postoperative NEC E878.9
- structure, burning NEC E891.8
  - burning (uncontrolled fire)
    - in terrorism E979.3

Collision (accidental)

Note – In the case of collisions between different types of vehicles, persons and objects, priority in classification is in the following order:

Aircraft
Watercraft
Motor vehicle
Railway vehicle
Pedal cycle
Animal-drawn vehicle
Animal being ridden
Streetcar or other
Nonmotor road vehicle
Other vehicle
Pedestrian or person using pedestrian conveyance
Object (except where falling from or set in motion by vehicle etc. listed above)

In the listing below, the combinations are listed only under the vehicle, etc., having priority. For definitions, see Supplementary Classification of External Causes of Injury and Poisoning (E800-E999).

- aircraft (with object or vehicle) (fixed) (movable) (moving) E841❹
  - with
    - person (while landing, taking off) (without accident to aircraft) E844❹

Collision – *continued*
- aircraft – *continued*
  - powered (in transit) (with unpowered aircraft) E841❹
    - while landing, taking off E840❹
  - unpowered E842❹
  - while landing, taking off E840❹
- animal being ridden (in sport or transport) E828❹
  - and
    - animal (being ridden) (herded) (unattended) E828❹
    - nonmotor road vehicle, except pedal cycle or animal-drawn vehicle E828❹
    - object (fallen) (fixed) (movable) (moving) not falling from or set in motion by vehicle of higher priority E828❹
    - pedestrian (conveyance or vehicle) E828❹
- animal-drawn vehicle E827❹
  - and
    - animal (being ridden) (herded) (unattended) E827❹
    - nonmotor road vehicle, except pedal cycle E827❹
    - object (fallen) (fixed) (movable) (moving) not falling from or set in motion by vehicle of higher priority E827❹
    - pedestrian (conveyance or vehicle) E827❹
    - streetcar E827❹
- motor vehicle (on public highway) (traffic accident) E812❹
  - after leaving, running off, public highway (without antecedent collision) (without re-entry) E816❹
    - with antecedent collision on public highway – *see* categories E810-E815❹
    - with re-entrance collision with another motor vehicle E811❹
  - and
    - abutment (bridge) (overpass) E815❹
    - animal (herded) (unattended) E815❹
      - carrying person, property E813❹
    - animal-drawn vehicle E813❹
    - another motor vehicle (abandoned) (disabled) (parked) (stalled) (stopped) E812❹
      - with, involving re-entrance (on same roadway) (across median strip) E811❹
    - any object, person, or vehicle off the public highway resulting from a noncollision motor vehicle nontraffic accident E816❹
    - avalanche, fallen or not moving E815❹
      - falling E909.2❹
    - boundary fence E815❹
    - culvert E815❹
    - fallen
      - stone E815❹
      - tree E815❹
    - guard post or guard rail E815❹
    - inter-highway divider E815❹
    - landslide, fallen or not moving E815❹
      - moving E909.2❹
    - machinery (road) E815❹
    - nonmotor road vehicle NEC E813❹
    - object (any object, person, or vehicle off the public highway resulting from a noncollision motor vehicle nontraffic accident) E815❹
      - off, normally not on, public highway resulting from a noncollision motor vehicle traffic accident E816❹
    - pedal cycle E813❹
    - pedestrian (conveyance) E814❹
    - person (using pedestrian conveyance) E814❹
    - post or pole (lamp) (light) (signal) (telephone) (utility) E815❹
    - railway rolling stock, train, vehicle E810❹
    - safety island E815❹
    - street car E813❹
    - traffic signal, sign, or marker (temporary) E815❹
    - tree E815❹
    - tricycle E813❹
    - wall of cut made for road E815❹
  - due to cataclysm – *see* categories E908❹, E909❹

Collision – *continued*
- motor vehicle – *continued*
  - not on public highway, nontraffic accident E822❹
    - and
      - animal (carrying person, property) (herded) (unattended) E822❹
      - animal-drawn vehicle E822❹
      - another motor vehicle (moving), except off-road motor vehicle E822❹
        - stationary E823❹
      - avalanche, fallen, not moving NEC E823❹
        - moving E909.2❹
      - landslide, fallen, not moving E823❹
        - moving E909.2❹
      - nonmotor vehicle (moving) E822❹
        - stationary E823❹
      - object (fallen) ((normally) (fixed) (movable but not in motion) (stationary) E823❹
        - moving, except when falling from, set in motion by, aircraft or cataclysm E822❹
      - pedal cycle (moving) E822❹
        - stationary E823❹
      - pedestrian (conveyance) E822❹
      - person (using pedestrian conveyance) E822❹
      - railway rolling stock, train, vehicle (moving) E822❹
        - stationary E823❹
      - road vehicle (any) (moving) E822❹
        - stationary E823❹
      - tricycle (moving) E822❹
        - stationary E823❹
- moving E909.2
- off-road type motor vehicle (not on public highway) E821❹
  - and
    - animal (being ridden) (-drawn vehicle) E821❹
    - another off-road motor vehicle, except snow vehicle E821❹
    - other motor vehicle, not on public highway E821❹
    - other object or vehicle NEC, fixed or movable, not set in motion by aircraft, motor vehicle on highway, or snow vehicle, motor-driven E821❹
    - pedal cycle E821❹
    - pedestrian (conveyance) E821❹
    - railway train E821❹
  - on public highway – *see* Collision, motor vehicle
- pedal cycle E826❹
  - and
    - animal (carrying person, property) (herded) (unherded) E826❹
    - animal-drawn vehicle E826❹
    - another pedal cycle E826❹
    - nonmotor road vehicle E826❹
    - object (fallen) (fixed) (movable) (moving) not falling from or set in motion by aircraft, motor vehicle, or railway train NEC E826❹
    - pedestrian (conveyance) E826❹
    - person (using pedestrian conveyance) E826❹
    - street car E826❹
- pedestrian(s) (conveyance) E917.9
  - with fall E886.9
    - in sports E886.0
  - and
    - crowd, human stampede E917.1
      - with subsequent fall E917.6
    - furniture E917.3
      - with subsequent fall E917.7
    - machinery – *see* Accident, machine
    - object (fallen) (moving) not falling from or set in motion by any vehicle classifiable to E800-E848, E917.9
      - caused by a crowd E917.1
        - with subsequent fall E917.6
      - furniture E917.3
        - with subsequent fall E917.7
      - in
        - running water E917.2
          - with drowning or submersion – *see* Submersion
        - sports E917.0
          - with subsequent fall E917.5
      - stationary E917.4
        - with subsequent fall E917.8
    - vehicle, nonmotor, nonroad E848

Collision – *continued*
- pedestrian(s) – *continued*
  - in
    - running water E917.2
      - with drowning or submersion – *see* Submersion
    - sports E917.0
      - with fall E886.0
- person(s) (using pedestrian conveyance) (*see also* Collision, pedestrian) E917.9
- railway (rolling stock) (train) (vehicle) (with (subsequent) derailment, explosion, fall or fire) E800❹
  - with antecedent derailment E802❹
  - and
    - animal (carrying person) (herded) (unattended) E801❹
    - another railway train or vehicle E800❹
    - buffers E801❹
    - fallen tree on railway E801❹
    - farm machinery, nonmotor (in transport) (stationary) E801❹
    - gates E801❹
    - nonmotor vehicle E801❹
    - object (fallen) (fixed) (movable) (movable) (moving) not falling from, set in motion by, aircraft or motor vehicle NEC E801❹
    - pedal cycle E801❹
    - pedestrian (conveyance) E805❹
    - person (using pedestrian conveyance) E805❹
    - platform E801❹
    - rock on railway E801❹
    - street car E801❹
- snow vehicle, motor-driven (not on public highway) E820❹
  - and
    - animal (being ridden) (-drawn vehicle) E820❹
    - another off-road motor vehicle E820❹
    - other motor vehicle, not on public highway E820❹
    - other object or vehicle NEC, fixed or movable, not set in motion by aircraft or motor vehicle on highway E820❹
    - pedal cycle E820❹
    - pedestrian (conveyance) E820❹
    - railway train E820❹
  - on public highway – *see* Collision, motor vehicle
- street car(s) E829❹
  - and
    - animal, herded, not being ridden, unattended E829❹
    - nonmotor road vehicle NEC E829❹
    - object (fallen) (fixed) (movable) (moving) not falling from or set in motion by aircraft, animal-drawn vehicle, animal being ridden, motor vehicle, pedal cycle, or railway train E829❹
    - pedestrian (conveyance) E829❹
    - person (using pedestrian conveyance) E829❹
- vehicle
  - animal-drawn – *see* Collision, animal-drawn vehicle
  - motor – *see* Collision, motor vehicle
  - nonmotor
    - nonroad E848
      - and
        - another nonmotor, nonroad vehicle E848
        - object (fallen) (fixed) (movable) (moving) not falling from or set in motion by aircraft, animal-drawn vehicle, animal being ridden, motor vehicle, nonmotor road vehicle, pedal cycle, railway train, or streetcar E848
    - road, except animal being ridden, animal-drawn vehicle, or pedal cycle E829❹
      - and
        - animal, herded, not being ridden, unattended E829❹
        - another nonmotor road vehicle, except animal being ridden, animal-drawn vehicle, or pedal cycle E829❹
        - object (fallen) (fixed) (movable) (moving) not falling from or set in motion by, aircraft, animal-drawn vehicle, animal being ridden, motor vehicle, pedal cycle, or railway train E829❹
        - pedestrian (conveyance) E829❹
        - person (using pedestrian conveyance) E829❹
        - vehicle, nonmotor, nonroad E829❹

Collision – *continued*
- watercraft E838❹
  - and
    - person swimming or water skiing E838❹
  - causing
    - drowning, submersion E830❹
    - injury except drowning, submersion E831❹

Combustion, spontaneous – *see* Ignition

Complication of medical or surgical procedure or treatment
- as an abnormal reaction – *see* Reaction, abnormal
- delayed, without mention of misadventure – *see* Reaction, abnormal
- due to misadventure – *see* Misadventure

Compression
- divers' squeeze E902.2
- trachea by
  - food E911
  - foreign body, except food E912

Conflagration
- building or structure, except private dwelling (barn) (church) (convalescent or residential home) (factory) (farm outbuilding) (hospital) (hotel) or (institution (educational) (dormitory) (residential)) (school) (shop) (store) (theatre) E891.9
  - with or causing (injury due to)
    - accident or injury NEC E891.9
      - specified circumstance NEC E891.8
    - burns, burning E891.3
    - carbon monoxide E891.2
    - fumes E891.2
      - polyvinylchloride (PVC) or similar material E891.1
    - smoke E891.2
  - causing explosion E891.0
  - in terrorism E979.3
- not in building or structure E892
- private dwelling (apartment) (boarding house) (camping place) (caravan) (farmhouse) (home (private)) (house) (lodging house) (private garage) (rooming house) (tenement) E890.9
  - with or causing (injury due to) accident or injury NEC E890.9
    - specified circumstance NEC E890.8
    - burns, burning E890.3
    - carbon monoxide E890.2
    - fumes E890.2
      - polyvinylchloride (PVC) or similar material E890.1
    - smoke E890.2
  - causing explosion E890.0

Constriction, external
- caused by
  - hair E928.4
  - other object E928.5

Contact with
- dry ice E901.1
- liquid air, hydrogen, nitrogen E901.1

Cramp(s)
- Heat – *see* Heat
- swimmers (*see also* category E910) E910.2❹
  - not in recreation or sport E910.3

Cranking (car) (truck) (bus) (engine), injury by E917.9

Crash
- aircraft (in transit) (powered) E841❹
  - at landing, take-off E840❹
  - in
    - terrorism E979.1
    - war operations E994
  - on runway NEC E840❹
  - stated as
    - homicidal E968.8
    - suicidal E958.6
    - undetermined whether accidental or intentional E988.6
  - unpowered E842❹
- glider E842❹
- motor vehicle – *see also* Accident, motor vehicle
  - homicidal E968.5
  - suicidal E958.5
  - undetermined whether accidental or intentional E988.5

Crushed (accidentally) E928.9
- between
  - boat(s), ship(s), watercraft (and dock or pier) (without accident to watercraft) E838❹
    - after accident to, or collision, watercraft E831❹
  - objects (moving) (stationary and moving) E918

Crushed – *continued*
by
avalanche NEC E909.2
boat, ship, watercraft after accident to, collision, watercraft E831❹
cave-in E916
with asphyxiation or suffocation (*see also* Suffocation, due to, cave-in) E913.3
crowd, human stampede E917.1
falling
aircraft (*see also* Accident, aircraft) E841❹
in
terrorism E979.1
war operations E994
earth, material E916
with asphyxiation or suffocation (*see also* Suffocation, due to, cave-in) E913.3
object E916
on ship, watercraft E838❹
while loading, unloading watercraft E838❹
landslide NEC E909.2
lifeboat after abandoning ship E831❹
machinery – *see* Accident, machine
railway rolling stock, train, vehicle (part of) E805❹
street car E829❹
vehicle NEC – *see* Accident, vehicle NEC
in
machinery – *see* Accident, machine
object E918
transport accident – *see* categories E800-E848❹
late effect of NEC E929.9

Cut, cutting (any part of body) (accidental) E920.9
by
arrow E920.8
axe E920.4
bayonet (*see also* Bayonet wound) E920.3
blender E920.2
broken glass E920.8
following fall E888.0
can opener E920.4
powered E920.2
chisel E920.4
circular saw E919.4
cutting or piercing instrument – *see also* category E920❹
following fall E888.0
late effect of E929.8
dagger E920.3
dart E920.8
drill – *see* Accident, caused by drill
edge of stiff paper E920 8
electric
beater E920.2
fan E920.2
knife E920.2
mixer E920.2
fork E920.4
garden fork E920.4
hand saw or tool (not powered) E920.4
powered E920.1
hedge clipper E920.4
powered E920.1
hoe E920.4
ice pick E920.4
knife E920.3
electric E920.2
lathe turnings E920.8
lawn mower E920.4
powered E920.0
riding E919.8
machine – *see* Accident, machine
meat
grinder E919.8
slicer E919.8
nails E920.8
needle E920.4
hypodermic E920.5
object, edged, pointed, sharp – *see* category E920❹
following fall E888.0
paper cutter E920.4
piercing instrument – *see also* category E920❹
late effect of E929.8
pitchfork E920.4
powered
can opener E920.2
garden cultivator E920.1
riding E919.8

Cut, cutting – *continued*
by – *continued*
powered – *continued*
hand saw E920.1
hand tool NEC E920.1
hedge clipper E920.1
household appliance or implement E920.2
lawn mower (hand) E920.0
riding E919.8
rivet gun E920.1
staple gun E920.1
rake E920.4
saw
circular E919.4
hand E920.4
scissors E920.4
screwdriver E920.4
sewing machine (electric) (powered) E920.2
not powered E920.4
shears E920.4
shovel E920.4
spade E920.4
splinters E920.8
sword E920.3
tin can lid E920.8
wood slivers E920.8
homicide (attempt) E966
inflicted by other person
stated as
intentional, homicidal E966
undetermined whether accidental or intentional E986
late effect of NEC E929.8
legal
execution E978
intervention E974
self-inflicted (unspecified whether accidental or intentional) E986
stated as intentional, purposeful E956
stated as undetermined whether accidental or intentional E986
suicidal (attempt) E956
terrorism E979.8
war operations E995

Cyclone E908.1

D

Death due to injury occurring one year or more previous – *see* Late effect

Decapitation (accidental circumstances) NEC E928.9
homicidal E966
legal execution (by guillotine) E978

Deprivation – *see also* Privation action E913.3
homicidal intent E968.4

Derailment (accidental)
railway (rolling stock) (train) (vehicle) (with subsequent collision) E802❹
with
collision (antecedent) (*see also* Collision, railway) E800❹
explosion (subsequent) (without antecedent collision) E802❹
antecedent collision E803❹ suffocation
fall (without collision (antecedent)) E802❹
fire (without collision (antecedent)) E802❹
street car E829❹

Descent
parachute (voluntary) (without accident to aircraft) E844❹
due to accident to aircraft – *see* categories E840-E842❹

Desertion
child, with intent to injure or kill E968.4
helpless person, infant, newborn E904.0
with intent to injure or kill E968.4

Destitution – *see* Privation

Disability, late effect or sequela of injury – *see* Late effect

Disease
Andes E902.0
aviators' E902.1
caisson E902.2
range E902.0

Divers' disease, palsy, paralysis, squeeze E902.0

Dog bite E906.0

Dragged by
cable car (not on rails) E847
on rails E829❹
motor vehicle (on highway) E814❹
not on highway, nontraffic accident E825❹
street car E829❹

Drinking poison (accidental) – *see* Table of Drugs and Chemicals

Drowning – *see* Submersion

Dust in eye E914

E

Earth falling (on) (with asphyxia or suffocation (by pressure)) (*see also* Suffocation, due to, cave-in) E913.3
as, or due to, a cataclysm (involving any transport vehicle) – *see* categories E908❹, E909❹
not due to cataclysmic action E913.3
motor vehicle (in motion) (on public highway) E813❹
not on public highway E825❹
nonmotor road vehicle NEC E829❹
pedal cycle E826❹
railway rolling stock, train, vehicle E806❹
street car E829❹
struck or crushed by E916
with asphyxiation or suffocation E913.3
with injury other than asphyxia, suffocation E916

Earthquake (any injury) E909.0

Effect(s) (adverse) of
air pressure E902.9
at high altitude E902.9
in aircraft E902.1
residence or prolonged visit (causing conditions classifiable to E902.0) E902.0
due to
diving E902.2
specified cause NEC E902.8
in aircraft E902.1
cold, excessive (exposure to) (*see also* Cold, exposure to) E901.9
heat (excessive) (*see also* Heat) E900.9
hot
place – *see* Heat
weather E900.0
insulation – *see* Heat
late – *see* Late effect of
motion E903
nuclear explosion or weapon
in
terrorism E979.5
war operations (blast) (fireball) (heat) (radiation) (direct) (secondary) E996
radiation – *see* Radiation
terrorism, secondary E979.9
travel E903

Electric shock, electrocution (accidental) (from exposed wire, faulty appliance, high voltage cable, live rail, open socket) (by) (in) E925.9
appliance or wiring
domestic E925.0
factory E925.2
farm (building) E925.8
house E925.0
home E925.0
industrial (conductor) (control apparatus) (transformer) E925.2
outdoors E925.8
public building E925.8
residential institution E925.8
school E925.8
specified place NEC E925.8
caused by other person
stated as
intentional, homicidal E968.8
undetermined whether accidental or intentional E988.4
electric power generating plant, distribution station E925.1
homicidal (attempt) E968.8
legal execution E978
lightning E907
machinery E925.9
domestic E925.0
factory E925.2
farm E925.8
home E925.0

Electric shock, electrocution – *continued*
  misadventure in medical or surgical procedure
    in electroshock therapy E873.4
  self-inflicted (undetermined whether accidental or intentional) E988.4
  stated as intentional E958.4
  stated as undetermined whether accidental or intentional E988.4
  suicidal (attempt) E958.4
  transmission line E925.1
Electrocution – *see* Electric shock
Embolism E921.1
  air (traumatic) NEC – *see* Air, embolism
Encephalitis
  lead or saturnine E866.0
    from pesticide NEC E863.4
Entanglement
  in
    bedclothes, causing suffocation E913.0
    wheel of pedal cycle E826❹
Entry of foreign body, material, any – *see* Foreign body
Execution, legal (any method) E978
Exhaustion
  cold – *see* Cold, exposure to
  due to excessive exertion E927
  heat – *see* Heat
Explosion (accidental) (in) (of) (on) E923.9
  acetylene E923.2
  aerosol can E921.8
  aircraft (in transit) (powered) E841❹
    at landing, take-off E840❹
    in
      terrorism E979.1
      war operations E994
    unpowered E842❹
  air tank (compressed) (in machinery) E921.1
  anesthetic gas in operating theatre E923.2
  automobile tire NEC E921.8
    causing transport accident – *see* categories E810-E825
  blasting (cap) (materials) E923.1
  boiler (machinery), not on transport vehicle E921.0
    steamship – *see* Explosion, watercraft
  bomb E923.8
    in
      terrorism E979.2
      war operations E993
        after cessation of hostilities E998
        atom, hydrogen or nuclear E996
        injury by fragments from E991.9
          antipersonnel bomb E991.3
  butane E923.2
  caused by
    other person
      stated as
        intentional. homicidal – *see* Assault, explosive
        undetermined whether accidental or homicidal E985.5
  coal gas E923.2
  detonator E923.1
  dynamite E923.1
  explosive (material) NEC E923.9
    gas(es) E923.2
    missile E923.8
      in
        terrorism E979.2
        war operations E993
          injury by fragments from E991.9
            antipersonnel bomb E991.3
    used in blasting operations E923.1
  fire-damp E923.2
  fireworks E923.0
  gas E923.2
    cylinder (in machinery) E921.1
    pressure tank (in machinery) E921.1
  gasoline (fumes) (tank) not in moving motor vehicle E923.2
  grain store (military) (munitions) E923.8
  grenade E923.8
    in
      terrorism E979.2
      war operations E993
        injury by fragments from E991.9
  homicide (attempt) – *see* Assault, explosive
  hot water heater, tank (in machinery) E921.0
  in mine (of explosive gases) NEC E923.2
  late effect of NEC E929.8

Explosion – *continued*
  machinery – *see also* Accident, machine
    pressure vessel – *see* Explosion, pressure vessel
  methane E923.2
  missile E923.8
    in
      terrorism E979.2
      war operations E993
        injury by fragments from E991.9
  motor vehicle (part of)
    in motion (on public highway) E818❹
      not on public highway E825❹
  munitions (dump) (factory) E923.8
    in
      terrorism E979.2
      war operations E993
  of mine E923.8
    in
      terrorism
        at sea or in harbor E979.0
        land E979.2
        marine E979.0
      war operations
        after cessation of hostilities E998
        at sea or in harbor E992
        land E993
          after cessation of hostilities E998
          injury by fragments from E991.9
        marine E992
  own weapons
    in
      terrorism (*see also* Suicide) E979.2
      war operations E993
        injury by fragments from E991.9
          antipersonnel bomb E991.3
  pressure
    cooker E921.8
    gas tank (in machinery) E921.1
    vessel (in machinery) E921.9
      on transport vehicle – *see* categories E800-E848❹
      specified type NEC E921.8
  propane E923.2
  railway engine, locomotive, train (boiler) (with subsequent collision, derailment, fall) E803❹
    with
      collision (antecedent) (*see also* Collision, railway) E800❹
      derailment (antecedent) E802❹
      fire (without antecedent collision or derailment) E803❹
  secondary fire resulting from – *see* Fire
  self-inflicted (unspecified whether accidental or intentional) E985.5
    stated as intentional, purposeful E955.5
  shell (artillery) E923.8
    in
      terrorism E979.2
      war operations E993
        injury by fragments from E991.9
  stated as undetermined whether caused accidentally or purposely inflicted E985.5
  steam or water lines (in machinery) E921.0
  suicide (attempted) E955.5
  terrorism – *see* Terrorism, explosion
  torpedo E923.8
    in
      terrorism E979.2
      war operations E992
  transport accident – *see* categories E800-E848❹
  war operations – *see* War operations, explosion
  watercraft (boiler) E837❹
    causing drowning, submersion (after jumping from watercraft) E830❹
Exposure (weather) (conditions) (rain) (wind) E904.3
  with homicidal intent E968.4
  environmental ●
    to ●
      algae bloom E928.6 ●
      blue-green algae bloom E928.6 ●
      brown tide E928.6 ●
      cyanobacteria bloom E928.6 ●
      Florida red tide E928.6 ●
      harmful algae ●
        and toxins E928.6 ●
        bloom E928.6 ●
      pfisteria piscicida E928.6 ●
      red tide E928.6 ●

Exposure – *continued*
  excessive E904.3
    cold (*see also* Cold, exposure to) E901.9
      self-inflicted – *see* Cold, exposure to, self-inflicted
    heat (*see also* Heat) E900.9
  fire – *see* Fire
  helpless person, infant, newborn due to abandonment or neglect E904.0
  noise E928.1
  prolonged in deep-freeze unit or refrigerator E901.1
  radiation – *see* Radiation
  resulting from transport accident – *see* categories E800-E848❹
  smoke from, due to
    fire – *see* Fire
    tobacco, second-hand E869.4
  vibration E928.2

F

Fall, falling (accidental) E888.9
  building E916
    burning E891.8
      private E890.8
  down
    escalator E880.0
    ladder E881.0
      in boat, ship, watercraft E833❹
    staircase E880.9
    stairs, steps – *see* Fall, from, stairs
  earth (with asphyxia or suffocation (by pressure)) (*see also* Earth, falling) E913.3
  from, off
    aircraft (at landing, take-off) (in-transit) (while alighting, boarding) E843❹
      resulting from accident to aircraft – *see* categories E840-E842❹
    animal (in sport or transport) E828❹
    animal-drawn vehicle E827❹
    balcony E882
    bed E884.4
    bicycle E826❹
    boat, ship, watercraft (into water) E832❹
      after accident to, collision, fire on E830❹
        and subsequently struck by (part of) boat E831❹
      and subsequently struck by (part of) while alighting, boat E838
      burning, crushed, sinking E830❹
        and subsequently struck by (part of) boat E831❹
    bridge E882
    building E882
      burning (uncontrolled fire) E891.8
        in terrorism E979.3
      private E890.8
    bunk in boat, ship, watercraft E834❹
      due to accident to watercraft E831❹
    cable car (not on rails) E847
      on rails E829❹
    car – *see* Fall from motor vehicle E884.9
    chair E884.2
    cliff E884.1
    commode E884.6
    curb (sidewalk) E880.1
    elevation aboard ship E834❹
      due to accident to ship E831❹
    embankment E884.9
    escalator E880.0
    fire escape E882
    flagpole E882
    furniture NEC E884.5
    gangplank (into water) (*see also* Fall, from, boat) E832❹
      to deck, dock E834❹
    hammock on ship E834❹
      due to accident to watercraft E831❹
    haystack E884.9
    high place NEC E884.9
      stated as undetermined whether accidental or intentional – *see* Jumping, from, high place
    horse (in sport or transport) E828❹
    in-line skates E885.1
    ladder E881.0
      in boat, ship, watercraft E833❹
        due to accident to watercraft E831❹

Fire – *continued*
- in, of, on, starting in – *continued*
  - tunnel (uncontrolled) E892
  - war operations (by fire-producing device or conventional weapon) E990.9
    - from nuclear explosion E996
    - petrol bomb E990.0
- late effect of NEC E929.4
- lumber (uncontrolled) E892
- mine (uncontrolled) E892
- prairie (uncontrolled) E892
- self-inflicted (unspecified whether accidental or intentional) E988.1
  - stated as intentional, purposeful E958.1
- specified NEC E898.1
  - with
    - conflagration – *see* Conflagration
    - ignition (of)
      - clothing – *see* Ignition, clothes
      - highly inflammable material (benzine) (fat) (gasoline) (kerosene) (paraffin) (petrol) E894
- started by other person
  - stated as
    - with intent to injure or kill E968.0
      - undetermined whether or not with intent to injure or kill E988.1
- suicide (attempted) E958.1
  - late effect of E959
- tunnel (uncontrolled) E892

Fireball effects from nuclear explosion
- in
  - terrorism E979.5
  - war operations E996

Fireworks (explosion) E923.0

Flash burns from explosion (*see also* Explosion) E923.9

Flood (any injury) (resulting from storm) E908.2
- caused by collapse of dam or manmade structure E909.3

Forced landing (aircraft) E840

Foreign body, object or material (entrance into (accidental))
- air passage (causing injury) E915
  - with asphyxia, obstruction, suffocation E912
    - food or vomitus E911
  - nose (with asphyxia, obstruction, suffocation) E912
    - causing injury without asphyxia, obstruction, suffocation E915
- alimentary canal (causing injury) (with obstruction) E915
  - with asphyxia, obstruction respiratory passage, suffocation E912
    - food E911
  - mouth E915
    - with asphyxia, obstruction, suffocation E912
      - food E911
  - pharynx E915
    - with asphyxia, obstruction, suffocation E912
      - food E911
- aspiration (with asphyxia, obstruction respiratory passage, suffocation) E912
  - causing injury without asphyxia, obstruction respiratory passage, suffocation E915
  - food (regurgitated) (vomited) E911
    - causing injury without asphyxia, obstruction respiratory passage, suffocation E915
  - mucus (not of newborn) E912
  - phlegm E912
- bladder (causing injury or obstruction) E915
- bronchus, bronchi – *see* Foreign body, air passages
- conjunctival sac E914
- digestive system – *see* Foreign body, alimentary canal
- ear (causing injury or obstruction) E915
- esophagus (causing injury or obstruction) (*see also* Foreign body, alimentary canal) E915
- eye (any part) E914
- eyelid E914
- hairball (stomach) (with obstruction) E915
- ingestion – *see* Foreign body, alimentary canal
- inhalation – *see* Foreign body, aspiration
- intestine (causing injury or obstruction) E915
- iris E914
- lacrimal apparatus E914
- larynx – *see* Foreign body, air passage
- late effect of NEC E929.8
- lung – *see* Foreign body, air passage

Foreign body, object or material – *continued*
- mouth – *see* Foreign body, alimentary canal, mouth
- nasal passage – *see* Foreign body, air passage, nose
- nose – *see* Foreign body, air passage, nose
- ocular muscle E914
- operation wound (left in) – *see* Misadventure, foreign object
- orbit E914
- pharynx – *see* Foreign body, alimentary canal, pharynx
- rectum (causing injury or obstruction) E915
- stomach (hairball) (causing injury or obstruction) E915
- tear ducts or glands E914
- trachea – *see* Foreign body, air passage
- urethra (causing injury or obstruction) E915
- vagina (causing injury or obstruction) E915

Found dead, injured
- from exposure (to) – *see* Exposure
- on
  - public highway E819❹
  - railway right of way E807❹

Fracture (circumstances unknown or unspecified) E887
- due to specified external means – *see* manner of accident
- late effect of NEC E929.3
- occurring in water transport NEC E835❹

Freezing – *see* Cold, exposure to

Frostbite E901.0
- due to manmade conditions E901.1

Frozen – *see* Cold, exposure to❹

G

Garrotting, homicidal (attempted) E963

Gored E906.8

Gunshot wound (*see also* Shooting) E922.9

H

Hailstones, injury by E904.3

Hairball (stomach) (with obstruction) E915

Hanged himself (*see also* Hanging, self-inflicted) E983.0

Hang gliding E842❹

Hanging (accidental) E913.8
- caused by other person
  - in accidental circumstances E913.8
  - stated as
    - intentional, homicidal E963
    - undetermined whether accidental or intentional E983.0
- homicide (attempt) E963
- in bed or cradle E913.0
- legal execution E978
- self-inflicted (unspecified whether accidental or intentional) E983.0
  - in accidental circumstances E913.8
  - stated as intentional, purposeful E953.0
- stated as undetermined whether accidental or intentional E983.0
- suicidal (attempt) E953.0

Heat (apoplexy) (collapse) (cramps) (effects of) (excessive) (exhaustion) (fever) (prostration) (stroke) E900.9
- due to
  - manmade conditions (as listed in E900.1, except boat, ship, watercraft) E900.1
  - weather (conditions) E900.0
- from
  - electric heating apparatus causing burning E924.8
  - nuclear explosion
    - in
      - terrorism E979.5
      - war operations E996
- generated in, boiler, engine, evaporator, fire room of boat, ship, watercraft E838❹
- inappropriate in local application or packing in medical or surgical procedure E873.5
- late effect of NEC E989

Hemorrhage
- delayed following medical or surgical treatment without mention of misadventure – *see* Reaction, abnormal
- during medical or surgical treatment as misadventure – *see* Misadventure, cut

High
- altitude, effects E902.9
- level of radioactivity, effects – *see* Radiation
- pressure effects – *see also* Effects of, air pressure
  - from rapid descent in water (causing caisson or divers' disease, palsy, or paralysis) E902.2
- temperature, effects – *see* Heat

Hit, hitting (accidental) by
- aircraft (propeller) (without accident to aircraft) E844❹
  - unpowered E842❹
- avalanche E909.2
- being thrown against object in or part of
  - motor vehicle (in motion) (on public highway) E818❹
    - not on public highway E825❹
  - nonmotor road vehicle NEC E829❹
  - street car E829❹
- boat, ship, watercraft
  - after fall from watercraft E838❹
    - damaged, involved in accident E831❹
  - while swimming, water skiing E838❹
- bullet (*see also* shooting) E922.9
  - from air gun E922.4
  - in
    - terrorism E979.4
    - war operations E991.2
      - rubber E991.0
- flare, Verey pistol (*see also* Shooting) E922.8
- hailstones E904.3
- landslide E909.2
- law-enforcing agent (on duty) E975
  - with blunt object (baton) (night stick) (stave) (truncheon) E973
- machine – *see* Accident, machine
- missile
  - firearm (*see also* shooting) E922.9
  - in
    - terrorism – *see* Terrorism, missle
    - war operations – *see* War operations, missle
- motor vehicle (on public highway) (traffic accident) E814❹
  - not on public highway, nontraffic accident E822❹
- nonmotor road vehicle NEC E829❹
- object
  - falling E916
    - from, in, on
      - aircraft E844❹
        - due to accident to aircraft – *see* categories E840-E842❹
        - unpowered E842❹
      - boat, ship, watercraft E838❹
        - due to accident to watercraft E831❹
      - building E916
        - burning E891.8
          - in terrorism E979.3
          - private E890.8
      - cataclysmic
        - earth surface movement or eruption E909.9
        - storm E908.9
      - cave-in E916
        - with asphyxiation or suffocation (*see also* Suffocation, due to, cave-in) E913.3
      - earthquake E909.0
      - motor vehicle (in motion) (on public highway) E818❹
        - not on public highway E825❹
        - stationary E916
      - nonmotor road vehicle NEC E829❹
      - pedal cycle E826❹
      - railway rolling stock, train, vehicle E806❹
      - street car E829❹
      - structure, burning NEC E891.8
      - vehicle, stationary E916
  - moving NEC – *see* Striking against, object
  - projected NEC – *see* Striking against, object
  - set in motion by
    - compressed air or gas, spring, striking, throwing – *see* Striking against, object
    - explosion – *see* Explosion

Fire – Hit, hitting

Hit, hitting – *continued*
- object – *continued*
  - thrown into, on, or towards
    - motor vehicle (in motion) (on public highway) E818❹
      - not on public highway E825❹
    - nonmotor road vehicle NEC E829❹
    - pedal cycle E826❹
    - street car E829❹
- off-road type motor vehicle (not on public highway) E821❹
  - on public highway E814❹
- other person(s) E917.9
  - with blunt or thrown object E917.9
    - in sports E917.0
      - with subsequent fall E917.5
    - intentionally, homicidal E968.2
  - as, or caused by, a crowd E917.1
    - with subsequent fall E917.6
  - in sports E917.0
- pedal cycle E826❹
- police (on duty) E975
  - with blunt object (baton) (nightstick) (stave) (truncheon) E973
- railway, rolling stock, train, vehicle (part of) E805❹
- shot – *see* Shooting
- snow vehicle, motor-driven (not on public highway) E820❹
  - on public highway E814❹
- street car E829❹
- vehicle NEC – *see* Accident, vehicle NEC

Homicide, homicidal (attempt) (justifiable) (*see also* Assault) E968.9

Hot
- liquid, object, substance, accident caused by – *see also* Accident, caused by, hot, by type of substance
  - late effect of E929.8
- place, effects – *see* Heat
- weather, effects E900.0

Humidity, causing problem E904.3

Hunger E904.1
- resulting from
  - abandonment or neglect E904.0
  - transport accident – *see* categories E800-E848

Hurricane (any injury) E908.0

Hypobarism, hypobaropethy – *see* Effects of, air pressure

Hypothermia – *see* Cold, exposure to

I

Ictus
- caloris – *see* Heat
- solaris E900.0

Ignition (accidental)
- anesthetic gas in operating theatre E923.2
- bedclothes
  - with
    - conflagration – *see* Conflagration
    - ignition (of)
      - clothing – *see* Ignition, clothes
      - highly inflammable material obstruction (benzine) (fat) (gasoline) (kerosene) (paraffin) (petrol) E894
- benzine E894
- clothes, clothing (from controlled fire) (in building) E893.9
  - with conflagration – *see* Conflagration
  - from
    - bonfire E893.2
    - highly inflammable material E894
    - sources or material as listed in E893.8
    - trash fire E893.2
    - uncontrolled fire – *see* Conflagration
  - in
    - private dwelling E893.0
    - specified building or structure, except of private dwelling E893.1
  - not in building or structure E893.2
- explosive material – *see* Explosion
- fat E894
- gasoline E894
- kerosene E894

Ignition – *continued*
- material
  - explosive – *see* Explosion
  - highly inflammable E894
    - with conflagration – *see* Conflagration
    - with explosion E923.2
- nightdress – *see* Ignition, clothes
- paraffin E894
- petrol E894

Immersion – *see* Submersion

Implantation of quills of porcupine E906.8

Inanition (from) E904.9
- hunger – *see* Lack of, food
- resulting from homicidal intent E968.4
- thirst – *see* Lack of, water

Inattention after, at birth E904.0
- homicidal, infanticidal intent E968.4

Infanticide (*see also* Assault)

Ingestion
- foreign body (causing injury) (with obstruction) – *see* Foreign body, alimentary canal
- poisonous substance NEC – *see* Table of Drugs and Chemicals

Inhalation
- excessively cold substance, manmade E901.1
- foreign body – *see* Foreign body, aspiration
- liquid air, hydrogen, nitrogen E901.1
- mucus, not of newborn (with asphyxia, obstruction respiratory passage, suffocation) E912
- phlegm (with asphyxia, obstruction respiratory passage, suffocation) E912
- poisonous gas – *see* Table of Drugs and Chemicals
- smoke from, due to
  - fire – *see* Fire
  - tobacco, second-hand E869.4
- vomitus (with asphyxia, obstruction respiratory passage, suffocation) E911

Injury, injured (accidental(ly)) NEC E928.9
- by, caused by, from
  - air rifle (B-B gun) E922.4
  - animal (not being ridden) NEC E906.9
    - being ridden (in sport or transport) E828❹
  - assault (*see also* Assault) E968.9
  - avalanche E909.2
  - bayonet (*see also* Bayonet wound) E920.3
  - being thrown against some part of, or object in
    - motor vehicle (in motion) (on public highway) E818❹
      - not on public highway E825❹
    - nonmotor road vehicle NEC E829❹
    - off-road motor vehicle NEC E821❹
    - railway train E806❹
    - snow vehicle, motor-driven E820❹
    - street car E829❹
  - bending E927
  - bite, human E928.3
  - broken glass E920.8
  - bullet – *see* Shooting
  - cave-in (*see also* Suffocation, due to, cave-in) E913.3
    - earth surface movement or eruption E909.9
    - storm E908.9
    - without asphyxiation or suffocation E916
  - cloudburst E908.8
  - cutting or piercing instrument (*see also* Cut) E920.9
  - cyclone E908.1
  - earth surface movement or eruption E909.9
  - earthquake E909.0❹
  - electric current (*see also* Electric shock) E925.9
  - explosion (*see also* Explosion) E923.9
  - fire – *see* Fire
  - flare, Verey pistol E922.8
  - flood E908.2
  - foreign body – *see* Foreign body
  - hailstones E904.3
  - hurricane E908.0
  - landslide E909.2❹
  - law-enforcing agent, police, in course of legal intervention – *see* Legal intervention
  - lightning E907
  - live rail or live wire – *see* Electric shock
  - machinery – *see also* Accident, machine
    - aircraft, without accident to aircraft E844❹
    - boat, ship, watercraft (deck) (engine room) (galley) (laundry) (loading) E836❹

Injury, injured – *continued*
- by, caused by, from – *continued*
  - missile
    - explosive E923.8
    - firearm – *see* Shooting
    - in
      - terrorism – *see* Terrorism, missle
      - war operations – *see* War operations, missle
  - moving part of motor vehicle (in motion) (on public highway) E818❹
    - not on public highway, nontraffic accident E825❹
    - while alighting, boarding, entering, leaving – *see* Fall, from, motor vehicle, while alighting, boarding
  - nail E920.8
  - needle (sewing) E920.4
    - hypodermic E920.5
  - noise E928.1
  - object
    - fallen on
      - motor vehicle (in motion) (on public highway) E818❹
        - not on public highway E825❹
    - falling – *see* Hit by, object, falling
  - paintball gun E922.5
  - radiation – *see* Radiation
  - railway rolling stock, train, vehicle (part of) E805❹
    - door or window E806❹
  - rotating propeller, aircraft E844❹
  - rough landing of off-road type motor vehicle (after leaving ground or rough terrain) E821❹
    - snow vehicle E820❹
  - saber (*see also* Wound, saber) E920.3
  - shot – *see* Shooting
  - sound waves E928.1
  - splinter or sliver, wood E920.8
  - straining E927
  - street car (door) E829❹
  - suicide (attempt) E958.9
  - sword E920.3
  - terrorism – *see* Terrorism
  - third rail – *see* Electric shock
  - thunderbolt E907
  - tidal wave E909.4
    - caused by storm E908.0
  - tornado E908.1
  - torrential rain E908.2
  - twisting E927
  - vehicle NEC – *see* Accident, vehicle NEC
  - vibration E928.2
  - volcanic eruption E909.1
  - weapon burst, in war operations E993
  - weightlessness (in spacecraft, real or simulated) E928.0
  - wood splinter or sliver E920.8
- due to
  - civil insurrection – *see* War operations
    - occurring after cessation of hostilities E998
  - terrorism – *see* Terrorism
  - war operations – *see* War operations
    - occurring after cessation of hostilities E998
- homicidal (*see also* Assault) E968.9
- in, on
  - civil insurrection – *see* War operations
  - fight E960.0
  - parachute descent (voluntary) (without accident to aircraft) E844❹
    - with accident to aircraft – *see* categories E840-E842❹
  - public highway E819❹
  - railway right of way E807❹
  - terrorism – *see* Terrorism
  - war operations – *see* War operations
- inflicted (by)
  - in course of arrest (attempted), suppression of disturbance, maintenance of order, by law enforcing agents – *see* Legal intervention
  - law-enforcing agent (on duty) – *see* Legal intervention
  - other person
    - stated as
      - accidental E928.9
      - homicidal, intentional – *see* Assault
      - undetermined whether accidental or intentional – *see* Injury, stated as undetermined
  - police (on duty) – *see* Legal intervention
- late effect of E929.9

Loss of control – *continued*
  off-road type motor vehicle (not on public highway) E821❹
    on public highway – *see* Loss of control, motor vehicle
  snow vehicle, motor-driven (not on public highway) E820❹
    on public highway – *see* Loss of control, motor vehicle
Lost at sea E832❹
  with accident to watercraft E830❹
  in war operations E995
Low
  pressure, effects – *see* Effects of, air pressure
  temperature, effects – *see* Cold exposure to
Lying before train, vehicle or other moving object (unspecified whether accidental or intentional) E988.0
  stated as intentional, purposeful, suicidal (attempt) E958.0
Lynching (*see also* Assault) E968.9

M

Malfunction, atomic power plant in water transport E838❹
Mangled (accidentally) NEC E928.9
Manhandling (in brawl, fight) E960.0
  legal intervention E975
Manslaughter (nonaccidental) – *see* Assault
Marble in nose E912
Mauled by animal E906.8
Medical procedure, complication of
  delayed or as an abnormal reaction without mention of misadventure – *see* Reaction, abnormal
  due to or as a result of misadventure – *see* Misadventure
Melting of fittings and furniture in burning
  in terrorism E979.3
Minamata disease E865.2
Misadventure(s) to patient(s) during surgical or medical care E876.9
  contaminated blood, fluid, drug or biological substance (presence of agents and toxins as listed in E875) E875.9
    administered (by) NEC E875.9
      infusion E875.0
      injection E875.1
      specified means NEC E875.2
      transfusion E875.0
      vaccination E875.1
  cut, cutting, puncture, perforation or hemorrhage (accidental) (inadvertent) (inappropriate) (during) E870.9
    aspiration of fluid or tissue (by puncture or catheterization, except heart) E870.5
    biopsy E870.8
      needle (aspirating) E870.5
    blood sampling E870.5
    catheterization E870.5
      heart E870.6
    dialysis (kidney) E870.2
    endoscopic examination E870.4
    enema E870.7
    infusion E870.1
    injection E870.3
    lumbar puncture E870.5
    needle biopsy E870.5
    paracentesis, abdominal E870.5
    perfusion E870.2
    specified procedure NEC E870.8
    surgical operation E870.0
    thoracentesis E870.5
    transfusion E870.1
    vaccination E870.3
  excessive amount of blood or other fluid during transfusion or infusion E873.0
  failure
    in dosage E873.9
      electroshock therapy E873.4
      inappropriate temperature (too hot or too cold) in local application and packing E873.5
      infusion
        excessive amount of fluid E873.0
        incorrect dilution of fluid E873.1

Misadventure(s) to patient(s) during surgical or medical care – *continued*
  failure – *continued*
      insulin-shock therapy E873.4
      nonadministration of necessary drug or medicinal E873.6
      overdose – *see also* Overdose
        radiation, in therapy E873.2
      radiation
        inadvertent exposure of patient (receiving radiation for test or therapy) E873.3
          not receiving radiation for test or therapy – *see* Radiation
        overdose E873.2
      specified procedure NEC E873.8
      transfusion
        excessive amount of blood E873.0
    mechanical, of instrument or apparatus (during procedure) E874.9
      aspiration of fluid or tissue (by puncture or catheterization, except of heart) E874.4
      biopsy E874.8
        needle (aspirating) E874.4
      blood sampling E874.4
      catheterization E874.4
        heart E874.5
      dialysis (kidney) E874.2
      endoscopic examination E874.3
      enema E874.8
      infusion E874.1
      injection E874.8
      lumbar puncture E874.4
      needle biopsy E874.4
      paracentesis, abdominal E874.4
      perfusion E874.2
      specified procedure NEC E874.8
      surgical operation E874.0
      thoracentesis E874.4
      transfusion E874.1
      vaccination E874.8
    sterile precautions (during procedure) E872.9
      aspiration of fluid or tissue (by puncture or catheterization, except heart) E872.5
      biopsy E872.8
        needle (aspirating) E872.5
      blood sampling E872.5
      catheterization E872.5
        heart E872.6
      dialysis (kidney) E872.2
      endoscopic examination E872.4
      enema E872.8
      infusion E872.1
      injection E872.3
      lumbar puncture E872.5
      needle biopsy E872.5
      paracentesis, abdominal E872.5
      perfusion E872.2
      removal of catheter or packing E872.8
    sterile precautions – *continued*
      specified procedure NEC E872.8
      surgical operation E872.0
      thoracentesis E872.5
      transfusion E872.1
      vaccination E872.3
    suture or ligature during surgical procedure E876.2
    to introduce or to remove tube or instrument E876.4
      foreign object left in body – *see* Misadventure, foreign object
  foreign object left in body (during procedure) E871.9
    aspiration of fluid or tissue (by puncture or catheterization, except heart) E871.5
    biopsy E871.8
      needle (aspirating) E871.5
    blood sampling E871.5
    catheterization E871.5
      heart E871.6
    dialysis (kidney) E871.2
    endoscopic examination E871.4
    enema E871.8
    infusion E871.1
    injection E871.3
    lumbar puncture E871.5
    needle biopsy E871.5
    paracentesis, abdominal E871.5
    perfusion E871.2
    removal of catheter or packing E871.7
    specified procedure NEC E871.8
    surgical operation E871.0
    thoracentesis E871.5

Misadventure(s) to patient(s) during surgical or medical care – *continued*
  foreign object left in body – *continued*
    transfusion E871.1
    vaccination E871.3
  hemorrhage – *see* Misadventure, cut
  inadvertent exposure of patient to radiation (being received for test or therapy) E873.3
  inappropriate
    operation performed E876.5
    temperature (too hot or too cold) in local application or packing E873.5
  infusion – *see also* Misadventure, by specific type, infusion
    excessive amount of fluid E873.0
    incorrect dilution of fluid E873.1
    wrong fluid E876.1
  mismatched blood in transfusion E876.0
  nonadministration of necessary drug or medicinal E873.6
  overdose – *see also* Overdose
    radiation, in therapy E873.2
  perforation – *see* Misadventure, cut
  performance of inappropriate operation E876.5
  puncture – *see* Misadventure, cut
  specified type NEC E876.8
    failure
      suture or ligature during surgical operation E876.2
      to introduce or to remove tube or instrument E876.4
        foreign object left in body E871.9
    infusion of wrong fluid E876.1
    performance of inappropriate operation E876.5
    transfusion of mismatched blood E876.0
    wrong
      fluid in infusion E876.1
      placement of endotracheal tube during anesthetic procedure E876.3
  transfusion – *see also* Misadventure, by specific type, transfusion
    excessive amount of blood E873.0
    mismatched blood E876.0
  wrong
    drug given in error – *see* Table of Drugs and Chemicals
    fluid in infusion E876.1
    placement of endotracheal tube during anesthetic procedure E876.3
Motion (effects) E903
  sickness E903
Mountain sickness E902.0
Mucus aspiration or inhalation, not of newborn (with asphyxia, obstruction respiratory passage, suffocation) E912
Mudslide of cataclysmic nature E909.2
Murder (attempt) (*see also* Assault) E968.9

N

Nail, injury by E920.8
Needlestick (sewing needle) E920.4
  hypodermic E920.5
Neglect – *see also* Privation
  criminal E968.4
  homicidal intent E968.4
Noise (causing injury) (pollution) E928.1

O

Object
  falling
    from, in, on, hitting
      aircraft E844❹
        due to accident to aircraft – *see* categories E840-E842❹
      machinery – *see also* Accident, machine
        not in operation E916
      motor vehicle (in motion) (on public highway) E818❹
        not on public highway E825❹
        stationary E916
        nonmotor road vehicle NEC E829❹
        pedal cycle E826❹
        person E916
        railway rolling stock, train, vehicle E806❹

Object – *continued*
- falling – *continued*
  - from, in, on, hitting – *continued*
    - motor vehicle – *continued*
      - street car E829❹
      - watercraft E838❹
        - due to accident to watercraft E831❹
- set in motion by
  - accidental explosion of pressure vessel – *see* category E921❹
  - firearm – *see* category E922❹
  - machine(ry) – *see* Accident, machine
  - transport vehicle – *see* categories E800-E848❹
- thrown from, in, on, towards
  - aircraft E844❹
  - cable car (not on rails) E847
    - on rails E829❹
  - motor vehicle (in motion) (on public highway) E818❹
    - not on public highway E825❹
  - nonmotor road vehicle NEC E829❹
  - pedal cycle E826❹
  - street car E829❹
  - vehicle NEC – *see* Accident, vehicle NEC

Obstruction
- air passages, larynx, respiratory passages
  - by
    - external means NEC – *see* Suffocation
    - food, any type (regurgitated) (vomited) E911
    - material or object, except food E912
    - mucus E912
    - phlegm E912
    - vomitus E911
- digestive tract, except mouth or pharynx
  - by
    - food, any type E915
    - foreign body (any) E915
- esophagus
  - food E911
  - foreign body, except food E912
  - without asphyxia or obstruction of respiratory passage E915
- mouth or pharynx
  - by
    - food, any type E911
    - material or object, except food E912
- respiration – *see* Obstruction, air passages

Oil in eye E914

Overdose
- anesthetic (drug) – *see* Table of Drugs and Chemicals
- drug – *see* Table of Drugs and Chemicals

Overexertion (lifting) (pulling) (pushing) E927

Overexposure (accidental) (to)
- cold (*see also* Cold, exposure to) E901.9
  - due to manmade conditions E901.1
- heat (*see also* Heat) E900.9
- radiation – *see* Radiation
- radioactivity – *see* Radiation
- sun, except sunburn E900.0
- weather – *see* Exposure

Overexposure – *continued*
- wind – *see* Exposure

Overheated (*see also* Heat) E900.9

Overlaid E913.0

Overturning (accidental)
- animal-drawn vehicle E827❹
- boat, ship, watercraft
  - causing
    - drowning, submersion E830❹
    - injury except drowning, submersion E831❹
- machinery – *see* Accident, machine
- motor vehicle (*see also* Loss of control, motor vehicle) E816❹
  - with antecedent collision on public highway – *see* Collision, motor vehicle
  - not on public highway, nontraffic accident E825❹
    - with antecedent collision – *see* Collision, motor vehicle, not on public highway
- nonmotor road vehicle NEC E829❹
- off-road type motor vehicle – *see* Loss of control, off-road type motor vehicle
- pedal cycle E826❹
- railway rolling stock, train, vehicle (*see also* Derailment, railway) E802❹
- street car E829❹
- vehicle NEC – *see* Accident, vehicle NEC

P

Palsy, divers' E902.2

Parachuting (voluntary) (without accident to aircraft) E844❹
- due to accident to aircraft – *see* categories E840-E842❹

Paralysis
- divers' E902.2
- lead or saturnine E866.0
  - from pesticide NEC E863.4

Pecked by bird E906.8

Phlegm aspiration or inhalation (with asphyxia, obstruction respirator), passage, suffocation) E912

Piercing (*see also* Cut) E920.9

Pinched
- between objects (moving) (stationary and moving) E918
- in object E918

Pinned under
- machine(ry) – *see* Accident, machine

Place of occurrence of accident – *see* Accident (to), occurring (at) (in)

Plumbism E866.0
- from insecticide NEC E863.4

Poisoning (accidental) (by) – *see also* Table of Drugs and Chemicals
- carbon monoxide
  - generated by
    - aircraft in transit E844❹
    - motor vehicle
      - in motion (on public highway) E818❹
        - not on public highway E825❹
    - watercraft (in transit) (not in transit) E838❹
- caused by injection of poisons or toxins into or through skin by plant thorns, spines, or other mechanism E905.7
  - marine or sea plants E905.6
- fumes or smoke due to
  - conflagration – *see* Conflagration
  - explosion or fire – *see* Fire
  - ignition – *see* Ignition
- gas
  - in legal intervention E972
  - legal execution, by E978
  - on watercraft E838❹
  - used as anesthetic – *see* Table of Drugs and Chemicals
- in
  - terrorism (chemical weapons) E979.7
  - war operations E997.2
- late effect of – *see* Late effect
- legal
  - execution E978
  - intervention
    - by gas E972

Pressure, external, causing asphyxia, suffocation (*see also* Suffocation) E913.9

Privation E904.9
- food (*see also* Lack of, food) E904.1
- helpless person, infant, newborn due to abandonment or neglect E904.0
- late effect of NEC E929.5
- resulting from transport accident – *see* categories E800-E848❹
- water (*see also* Lack of, water) E904.2

Projected objects, striking against or struck by – *see* Striking against, object

Prolonged stay in
- high attitude (causing conditions as listed in E902.0) E902.0
- weightless environment E928.0

Prostration
- heat – *see* Heat

Pulling, injury in E927

Puncture, puncturing (*see also* Cut) E920.9
- by
  - plant thorns or spines E920.8
    - toxic reaction E905.7
      - marine or sea plants E905.6
  - sea-urchin spine E905.6

Pushing (injury in) (overexertion) E927
- by other person(s) (accidental) E917.9
  - as, or caused by, a crowd, human stampede E917.1
    - with subsequent fall E917.6

Pushing – *continued*
- by other person(s) – *continued*
  - before moving vehicle or object
    - stated as
      - intentional, homicidal E968.5
      - undetermined whether accidental or intentional E988.8
  - from
    - high place
      - in accidental circumstances – *see* categories E880-E884❹
      - stated as
        - intentional, homicidal E968.1
        - undetermined whether accidental or intentional E987.9
          - man-made structure, except residential E987.1
          - natural site E987.2
          - residential E987.0
    - motor vehicle (*see also* Fall, from, motor vehicle) E818❹
      - stated as
        - intentional, homicidal E968.5
        - undetermined whether accidental or intentional E988.8
  - in sports E917.0
    - with fall E886.0
  - with fall E886.9
    - in sports E886.0

R

Radiation (exposure to) E926.9
- abnormal reaction to medical test or therapy E879.2
- arc lamps E926.2
- atomic power plant (malfunction) NEC E926.9
  - in water transport E838❹
- electromagnetic, ionizing E926.3
- gamma rays E926.3
- in
  - terrorism (from or following nuclear explosion) (direct) (secondary) E979.5
    - laser E979.8
  - war operations (from or following nuclear explosion) (direct) (secondary) E996
    - laser(s) E997.0
  - water transport E838❹
- inadvertent exposure of patient (receiving test or therapy) E873.3
- infrared (heaters and lamps) E926.1
  - excessive heat E900.1
- ionized, ionizing (particles, artificially accelerated) E926.8
  - electromagnetic E926.3
- isotopes, radioactive – *see* Radiation, radioactive isotopes
- laser(s) E926.4
  - in
    - terrorism E979.8
    - war operations E997.0
  - misadventure in medical care – *see* Misadventure, failure, in dosage, radiation
- late effect of NEC E929.8
  - excessive heat from – *see* Heat
- light sources (visible) (ultraviolet) E926.2
- misadventure in medical or surgical procedure – *see* Misadventure, failure, in dosage, radiation
- overdose (in medical or surgical pacemaker) procedure) E873.2
- radar E926.0
- radioactive isotopes E926.5
  - atomic power plant malfunction E926.5
    - in water transport E838❹
  - misadventure in medical or surgical treatment – *see* Misadventure, failure, in dosage, radiation
- radiobiologicals – *see* Radiation, radioactive isotopes
- radiofrequency E926.0
- radiopharmaceuticals – *see* Radiation, radioactive isotopes
- radium NEC E926.9
- sun E926.2
  - excessive heat from E900.0
- tanning bed E926.2
- welding arc or torch E926.2
  - excessive heat from E900.1

- **Radiation** – *continued*
  - x-rays (hard) (soft) E926.3
    - misadventure in medical or surgical treatment – *see* Misadventure, failure, in dosage, radiation
- **Rape** E960.1
- **Reaction, abnormal to or following** (medical or surgical procedure) E879.9
  - amputation (of limbs) E878.5
  - anastomosis (arteriovenous) (blood vessel) (gastrojejunal) (skin) (tendon) (natural, artificial material, tissue) E878.2
    - external stoma, creation of E878.3
  - aspiration (of fluid) E879.4
    - tissue E879.8
  - biopsy E879.8
  - blood
    - sampling E879.7
    - transfusion
      - procedure E879.8
  - bypass – *see* Reaction, abnormal, anastomosis
  - catheterization
    - cardiac E879.0
    - urinary E879.6
  - colostomy E878.3
  - cystostomy E878.3
  - dialysis (kidney) E879.1
  - drugs or biologicals – *see* Table of Drugs and Chemicals
  - duodenostomy E878.3
  - electroshock therapy E879.3
  - formation of external stoma E878.3
  - gastrostomy E878.3
  - graft – *see* Reaction, abnormal, anastomosis
  - hypothermia E879.8
  - implant, implantation (of)
    - artificial
      - internal device (cardiac pacemaker) (electrodes in brain) (heart valve prosthesis) (orthopedic) E878.1
      - material or tissue (for anastomosis or bypass) E878.2
        - with creation of external stoma E878.3
    - natural tissues (for anastomosis or bypass) E878.2
      - as transplantion – *see* Reaction, abnormal, transplant
      - with creation of external stoma E878.3
  - infusion
    - procedure E879.8
  - injection
    - procedure E879.8
  - insertion of gastric or duodenal sound E879.5
  - insulin-shock therapy E879.3
  - lumbar puncture E879.4
  - perfusion E879.1
  - procedures other than surgical operation (*see also* Reaction, abnormal, by specific type of procedure) E879.9
    - specified procedure NEC E879.8
  - radiological procedure or therapy E879.2
  - removal of organ (partial) (total) NEC E878.6
    - with
      - anastomosis, bypass or graft E878.2
      - formation of external stoma E878.3
      - implant of artificial internal device E878.1
      - transplant(ation)
        - partial organ E878.4
        - whole organ E878.0
  - sampling
    - blood E879.7
    - fluid NEC E879.4
    - tissue E879.8
  - shock therapy E879.3
  - surgical operation (*see also* Reaction, abnormal, by specified type of operation) E878.9
    - restorative NEC E878.4
      - with
        - anastomosis, bypass or graft E878.2
        - formation of external stoma E878.3
        - implant(ation) – *see* Reaction, abnormal, implant
        - transplantation) – *see* Reaction, abnormal, transplant
    - specified operation NEC E878.8
  - thoracentesis E879.4
  - transfusion
    - procedure E879.8
  - transplant, transplantation (heart) (kidney) (liver) E878.0
    - partial organ E878.4
- **Reaction, abnormal to or following** – *continued*
  - ureterostomy E878.3
  - vaccination E879.8
- **Reduction in**
  - atmospheric pressure – *see also* Effects of, air pressure
    - while surfacing from
      - deep water diving causing caisson or divers' disease, palsy or paralysis E902.2
      - underground E902.8
- **Residual** (effect) – *see* Late effect
- **Rock falling on or hitting** (accidentally)
  - motor vehicle (in motion) (on public highway) E818❹
    - not on public highway E825❹
  - nonmotor road vehicle NEC E829❹
  - pedal cycle E826❹
  - person E916
  - railway rolling stock, train, vehicle E806❹
- **Running off, away**
  - animal (being ridden) (in sport or transport) E828❹
    - not being ridden E906.8
  - animal-drawn vehicle E827❹
  - rails, railway (*see also* Derailment) E802❹
  - roadway
    - motor vehicle (without antecedent collision) E816❹
      - nontraffic accident E825❹
        - with antecedent collision – *see* categories Collision, motor vehicle, not on public highway
      - with
        - antecedent collision – *see* Collision motor vehicle
        - subsequent collision
          - involving any object, person or vehicle not on public of highway E816❹
          - on public highway E811❹
    - nonmotor road vehicle NEC E829❹
    - pedal cycle E826❹
- **Run over** (accidentally) (by)
  - animal (not being ridden) E906.8
    - being ridden (in sport or transport) E828❹
  - animal-drawn vehicle E827❹
  - machinery – *see* Accident, machine
  - motor vehicle (on public highway) – *see* Hit by, motor vehicle
  - nonmotor road vehicle NEC E829❹
  - railway train E805❹
  - street car E829❹
  - vehicle NEC E848

S

- **Saturnism** E866.0
  - from insecticide NEC E863.4
- **Scald, scalding** (accidental) (by) (from) (in) E924.0
  - acid – *see* Scald, caustic
  - boiling tap water E924.2
  - caustic or corrosive liquid, substance E924.1
    - swallowed – *see* Table of Drugs and Chemicals
  - homicide (attempt) – *see* Assault, burning
  - inflicted by other person
    - stated as
      - intentional or homicidal E968.3
      - undetermined whether accidental or intentional E988.2
  - late effect of NEC E929.8
  - liquid (boiling) (hot) E924.0
  - local application of externally applied substance in medical or surgical care E873.5
  - molten metal E924.0
  - self-inflicted (unspecified whether accidental or intentional) E988.2
    - stated as intentional, purposeful E958.2
  - stated as undetermined whether accidental or intentional E988.2
  - steam E924.0
  - tap water (boiling) E924.2
  - transport accident – *see* categories E800-E848
  - vapor E924.0
- **Scratch, cat** E906.8
- **Sea**
  - sickness E903
- **Self-mutilation** – *see* Suicide
- **Sequelae** (of)
  - in
    - terrorism E999.1
    - war operations E999.0
- **Shock**
  - anaphylactic (*see also* Table of Drugs and Chemicals) E947.9
    - due to
      - bite (venomous) – *see* Bite, venomous NEC
      - sting – *see* Sting
  - electric (*see also* Electric shock) E925.9
  - from electric appliance or current (*see also* Electric shock) E925.9
- **Shooting, shot** (accidental(ly)) E922.9
  - air gun E922.4
  - BB gun E922.4
  - hand gun (pistol) (revolver) E922.0
  - himself (*see also* Shooting, self-inflicted) E985.4
    - hand gun (pistol) (revolver) E985.0
    - military firearm, except hand gun E985.3
      - hand gun (pistol) (revolver) E985.0
    - rifle (hunting) E985.2
      - military E985.3
    - shotgun (automatic) E985.1
    - specified firearm NEC E985.4
    - Verey pistol E985.4
  - homicide (attempt) E965.4
    - air gun E968.6
    - BB gun E968.6
    - hand gun (pistol) (revolver) E965.0
    - military firearm, except hand gun E965.3
      - hand gun (pistol) (revolver) E965.0
    - paintball gun E965.4
    - rifle (hunting) E965.2
      - military E965.3
    - shotgun (automatic) E965.1
    - specified firearm NEC E965.4
    - Verey pistol E965.4
  - inflicted by other person
    - in accidental circumstances E922.9
      - hand gun (pistol) (revolver) E922.0
      - military firearm, except hand gun E922.3
        - hand gun (pistol) (revolver) E922.0
      - rifle (hunting) E922.2
        - military E922.3
      - shotgun (automatic) E922.1
      - specified firearm NEC E922.8
      - Verey pistol E922.8
    - stated as
      - intentional, homicidal E965.4
        - hand gun (pistol) (revolver) E955.4
        - military firearm, except hand gun E965.3
          - hand gun (pistol) (revolver) E965.0
        - paintball gun E965.4
        - rifle (hunting) E965.2
          - military E965.3
        - shotgun (automatic) E965.1
        - specified firearm E965.4
        - Verey pistol E965.4
      - undetermined whether accidental or intentional E985.4
        - air gun E985.6
        - BB gun E985.6
        - hand gun (pistol) (revolver) E985.0
        - military firearm, except hand gun E985.3
          - hand gun (pistol) (revolver) E985.0
        - paintball gun E985.7
        - rifle (hunting) E985.2
        - shotgun (automatic) E985.1
        - specified firearm NEC E985.4
        - Verey pistol E985.4
  - in
    - terrorism – *see* Terrorism, shooting
    - war operations – *see* War operations, shooting
  - legal
    - execution E978
    - intervention E970
  - military firearm, except hand gun E922.3
    - hand gun (pistol) (revolver) E922.0
  - paintball gun E922.5
  - rifle (hunting) E922.2
    - military E922.3
  - self-inflicted (unspecified whether accidental or intentional) E985.4
    - air gun E985.6
    - BB gun E985.6
    - hand gun (pistol) (revolver) E985.0
    - military firearm, except hand gun E985.3
      - hand gun (pistol) (revolver) E985.0
    - paintball gun E985.7
    - rifle (hunting) E985.2
      - military E985.3
    - shotgun (automatic) E985.1
    - specified firearm NEC E985.4

Shooting, shot – Submersion

Submersion – *continued*
- while – *continued*
  - snorkel diving E910.2
  - spear fishing underwater E910.1
  - surfboarding E910.2
  - swimming (swimming pool) E910.2
  - wading (in water) E910.2
  - water skiing E910.0

Sucked
- into
  - jet (aircraft) E844❹

Suffocation (accidental) (by external means) (by pressure) (mechanical) E913.9
- caused by other person
  - in accidental circumstances – *see* category E913❹
  - stated as
    - intentional, homicidal E963
    - undetermined whether accidental or intentional E983.9
      - by, in
        - hanging E983.0
        - plastic bag E983.1
        - specified means NEC E983.8
- due to, by
  - avalanche E909.2
  - bedclothes E913.0
  - bib E913.0
  - blanket E913.0
  - cave-in E913.3
    - caused by cataclysmic earth surface movement or eruption E909.9
  - conflagration – *see* Conflagration E983.8
  - explosion – *see* Explosion
  - falling earth, other substance E913.3 (attempted) (by) E958.9
  - fire – *see* Fire
  - food, any type (ingestion) (inhalation) (regurgitated) (vomited) E911
  - foreign body, except food (ingestion) (inhalation) E912
  - ignition – *see* Ignition
  - landslide E909.2
  - machine(ry) – *see* Accident, machine
  - material, object except food entering by nose or mouth, ingested, inhaled E912
  - mucus (aspiration) (inhalation), not of newborn E912
  - phlegm (aspiration) (inhalation) E912
  - pillow E913.0
  - plastic bag – *see* Suffocation, in, plastic bag
  - sheet (plastic) E913.0
  - specified means NEC E913.8
  - vomitus (aspiration) (inhalation) E911
- homicidal (attempt) E963
- in
  - airtight enclosed place E913.2
  - baby carriage E913.0
  - bed E913.0
  - closed place E913.2
  - cot, cradle E913.0
  - perambulator E913.0
  - plastic bag (in accidental circumstances) E913.1
    - homicidal, purposely inflicted by other person E963
    - self-inflicted (unspecified whether accidental or intentional) E983.1
      - in accidental circumstances E913.1
      - intentional, suicidal E953.1
    - stated as undetermined whether accidentally or purposely inflicted E983.1
    - suicidal, purposely self-inflicted E953.1
  - refrigerator E913.2
- self-inflicted – *see also* Suffocation, stated as undetermined whether accidental or intentional E953.9
  - in accidental circumstances – *see* category E913❹
  - stated as intentional, purposeful – *see* Suicide, suffocation
- stated as undetermined whether accidental or intentional E983.9
  - by, in
    - hanging E983.0
    - plastic bag E983.1
    - specified means NEC E983.8
- suicidal – *see* Suicide, suffocation

Suicide, suicidal (attempted) (by) E958.9
- burning, bums E958.1
- caustic substance E958.7
  - poisoning E950.7
  - swallowed E950.7
- cold, extreme E958.3
- cut (any part of body) E956
- cutting or piercing instrument (classifiable to E920) E956
- drowning E954
- electrocution E958.4
- explosive(s) (classifiable to E923) E955.5
- fire E958.1
- firearm (classifiable to E922) – *see* Shooting, suicidal
- hanging E953.0
- jumping
  - before moving object, train, vehicle E958.0
  - from high place – *see* Jumping, from, high place, stated as, suicidal
- knife E956
- late effect of E959
- motor vehicle, crashing of E958.5
- poisoning – *see* Table of Drugs and Chemicals
- puncture (any part of body) E956
- scald E958.2
- shooting – *see* Shooting, suicidal
- specified means NEC E958.8
- stab (any part of body) E956
- strangulation – *see* Suicide, suffocation
- submersion E954
- suffocation E953.9
  - by, in
    - hanging E953.0
    - plastic bag E953.1
    - specified means NEC E953.8
- wound NEC E958.9

Sunburn E926.2

Sunstroke E900.0

Supersonic waves (causing injury) E928.1

Surgical procedure, complication of
- delayed or as an abnormal reaction vehicle without mention of misadventure *see* Reaction, abnormal
- due to or as a result of misadventure – *see* Misadventure

Swallowed, swallowing
- foreign body – *see* Foreign body, alimentary canal
- poison – *see* Table of Drugs and Chemicals
- substance
  - caustic – *see* Table of Drugs and Chemicals drugs
  - corrosive – *see* Table of Drugs and Chemicals
  - poisonous – *see* Table of Drugs and Chemicals

Swimmers cramp (*see also* category E910) E910.2❹
- not in recreation or sport E910.3

Syndrome, battered
- baby or child – *see* Abuse, child
- wife – *see* Assault

T

Tackle in sport E886.0

Terrorism (injury) (by) (in) E979.8
- air blast E979.2
- aircraft burned, destroyed, exploded, shot down E979.1
  - used as a weapon E979.1
- anthrax E979.6
- asphyxia from
  - chemical (weapons) E979.7
  - fire, conflagration (caused by fire-producing device) E979.3
    - from nuclear explosion E979.5
  - gas or fumes E979.7
- bayonet E979.8
- biological agents E979.6
- blast (air) (effects) E979.2
  - from nuclear explosion E979.5
  - underwater E979.0
- bomb (antipersonnel) (mortar) (explosion) (fragments) E979.2
- bullet(s) (from carbine, machine gun, pistol, rifle, shotgun) E979.4

Terrorism – *continued*
- burn from
  - chemical E979.7
  - fire, conflagaration (caused by fire-producing device) E979.3
    - from nuclear explosion E979.5
  - gas E979.7
- burning aircraft E979.1
- chemical E979.7
- cholera E979.6
- conflagration E979.3
- crushed by falling aircraft E979.1
- depth-charge E979.0
- destruction of aircraft E979.1
- disability, as sequelae one year or more after injury E999.1
- drowning E979.8
- effect
  - of nuclear weapon (direct) (secondary) E979.5
  - secondary NEC E979.9
  - sequelae E999.1
- explosion (artillery shell) (breech-block) (cannon block) E979.2
  - aircraft E979.1
  - bomb (antipersonnel) (mortar) E979.2
    - nuclear (atom) (hydrogen) E979.5
  - depth-charge E979.0
  - grenade E979.2
  - injury by fragments from E979.2
  - land-mine E979.2
  - marine weapon E979.0
  - mine (land) E979.2
    - at sea or in harbor E979.0
    - marine E979.0
  - missle (explosive) NEC E979.2
  - munitions (dump) (factory) E979.2
  - nuclear (weapon) E979.5
    - other direct and secondary effects of E979.5
  - sea-based artillery shell E979.0
  - torpedo E979.0
- exposure to ionizing radiation from nuclear explosion E979.5
- falling aircraft E979.1
- fire or fire-producing device E979.3
- firearms E979.4
- fireball effects from nuclear explosion E979.5
- fragments from artillery shell, bomb NEC, grenade, guided missle, land-mine, rocket, shell, shrapnel E979.2
- gas or fumes E979.7
- grenade (explosion) (fragments) E979.2
- guided missle (explosion) (fragments) E979.2
  - nuclear E979.5
- heat from nuclear explosion E979.5
- hot substances E979.3
- hydrogen cyanide E979.7
- land mine (explosion) (fragments) E979.2
- laser(s) E979.8
- late effect of E999.1
- lewisite E979.7
- lung irritant (chemical) (fumes) (gas) E979.7
- marine mine E979.0
- mine E979.2
  - at sea E979.0
  - in harbor E979.0
  - land (explosion) (fragments) E979.2
  - marine E979.0
- missle (explosion) (fragments) (guided) E979.2
  - marine E979.0
  - nuclear E979.5
- mortar bomb (explosion) (fragments) E979.2
- mustard gas E979.7
- nerve gas E979.7
- nuclear weapons E979.5
- pellets (shotgun) E979.4
- petrol bomb E979.3
- phosgene E979.7
- piercing object E979.8
- poisoning (chemical) (fumes) (gas) E979.7
- radiation, ionizing from nuclear explosion E979.5
- rocket (explosion) (fragments) E979.2
- saber, sabre E979.8
- sarin E979.7
- screening smoke E979.7
- sequelae effect (of) E999.1
- shell (aircraft) (artillery) (cannon) (land-based) (explosion) (fragments) E979.2
  - sea-based E979.0
- shooting E979.4
  - bullet(s) E979.4
  - pellet(s) (rifle) (shotgun) E979.4
- shrapnel E979.2

Terrorism – *continued*
- smallpox E979.7
- stabbing object(s) E979.8
- submersion E979.8
- torpedo E979.0
- underwater blast E979.0
- vesicant (chemical) (fumes) (gas) E979.7
- weapon burst E979.2

Thermic fever E900.9

Thermoplegia E900.9

Thirst – *see also* Lack of water
- resulting from accident connected with transport – *see* categories E800-E848④

Thrown (accidentally)
- against object in or part of vehicle
  - by motion of vehicle
    - aircraft E844④
    - boat, ship, watercraft E838④
    - motor vehicle (on public highway) E818④
      - not on public highway E825
      - off-road type (not on public highway) E821④
        - on public highway E818④
        - snow vehicle E820④
          - on public highway E818④
  - nonmotor road vehicle NEC E829④
  - railway rolling stock, train, vehicle E806④
  - street car E829④
- from
  - animal (being ridden) (in sport or transport) E828④
  - high place, homicide (attempt) E968.1
  - machinery – *see* Accident, machine
  - vehicle NEC – *see* Accident, vehicle NEC
- off – *see* Thrown, from
- overboard (by motion of boat, ship, watercraft) E832④
  - by accident to boat, ship, watercraft E830④

Thunderbolt NEC E907

Tidal wave (any injury) E909.4
- caused by storm E908.0

Took
- overdose of drug – *see* Table of Drugs and Chemicals
- poison – *see* Table of Drugs and Chemicals

Tornado (any injury) E908.1

Torrential rain (any injury) E908.2

Traffic accident NEC E819④

Trampled by animal E906.8
- being ridden (in sport or transport) E828④

Trapped (accidentally)
- between
  - objects (moving) (stationary and moving) E918
- by
  - door of
    - elevator E918
    - motor vehicle (on public highway) (while alighting, boarding) – *see* Fall, from, motor vehicle, while alighting
    - railway train (underground) E806④
    - street car E829④
    - subway train E806④
- in object E918

Travel (effects) E903
- sickness E903

Tree
- falling on or hitting E916
  - motor vehicle (in motion) (on public highway) E818④
    - not on public highway E825④
  - nonmotor road vehicle NEC E829④
  - pedal cycle E826④
  - person E916
  - railway rolling stock, train, vehicle E806④
  - street car E829④

Trench foot E901.0

Tripping over animal, carpet, curb, rug, or small object (with fall) E885.9
- without fall – *see* Striking against, object

Tsunami E909.4

Twisting, Injury in E927

V

Violence, nonaccidental (*see also* Assault) E968.9

Volcanic eruption (any injury) E909.1

Vomitus in air passages (with asphyxia, obstruction or suffocation) E911

W

War operations (during hostilities) (injury) (by) (in) E995
- after cessation of hostilities, injury due to E998
- air blast E993
- aircraft burned, destroyed, exploded, shot down E991.9
- asphyxia from
  - chemical E997.2
  - fire, conflagration (caused by fire-producing device or conventional weapon) E990.9
    - from nuclear explosion E996
    - petrol bomb E990.0
  - fumes E997.2
  - gas E997.2
- battle wound NEC E995
- bayonet E995
- biological warfare agents E997.1
- blast (air) (effects) E993
  - from nuclear explosion E996
  - underwater E992
- bomb (mortar) (explosion) E993
  - after cessation of hostilities E998
  - fragments, injury by E991.9
    - antipersonnel E991.3
    - bullet(s) (from carbine, machine gun, pistol, rifle, shotgun) E991.2
  - rubber E991.0
- burn from
  - chemical E997.2
  - fire, conflagration (caused by fire-producing device or conventional weapon) E990.9
    - from nuclear explosion E996
    - petrol bomb E990.0
  - gas E997.2
- burning aircraft E994
- chemical E997.2
- chlorine E997.2
- conventional warfare, specified form NEC E995
- crushing by failing aircraft E994
- depth charge E992
- destruction of aircraft E994
- disability as sequela one year or more after injury E999.0
- drowning E995
- effect (direct) (secondary) nuclear weapon E996
- explosion (artillery shell) (breech block) (cannon shell) E993
  - after cessation of hostilities of bomb, mine placed in war E998
  - aircraft E994
  - bomb (mortar) E993
    - atom E996
    - hydrogen E996
    - injury by fragments from E991.9
      - antipersonnel E991.3
    - nuclear E996
  - depth charge E992
  - injury by fragments from E991.9
    - antipersonnel E991.3
  - marine weapon E992
  - mine
    - at sea or in harbor E992
    - land E993
      - injury by fragments from E991.9
    - marine E992
  - munitions (accidental) (being used in war) (dump) (factory) E993
  - nuclear (weapon) E996
  - own weapons (accidental) E993
    - injury by fragments from E991.9
      - antipersonnel E991.3
  - sea-based artillery shell E992
  - torpedo E992
- exposure to ionizing radiation from nuclear explosion E996
- failing aircraft E994
- fire or fire-producing device E990.9
  - petrol bomb E990.0
- fireball effects from nuclear explosion E996

War operations – *continued*
- fragments from
  - antipersonnel bomb E991.3
  - artillery shell, bomb NEC, grenade, guided missile, land mine, rocket, shell, shrapnel E991.9
- fumes E997.2
- gas E997.2
- grenade (explosion) E993
  - fragments, injury by E991.9
- guided missile (explosion) E993
  - fragments, injury by E991.9
  - nuclear E996
- heat from nuclear explosion E996
- injury due to, but occurring after cessation of hostilities E998
- lacrimator (gas) (chemical) E997.2
- land mine (explosion) E993
  - after cessation of hostilities E998
  - fragments, injury by E991.9
- laser(s) E997.0
- late effect of E999.0
- lewisite E997.2
- lung irritant (chemical) (fumes) (gas) E997.2
- marine mine E992
- mine
  - after cessation of hostilities E998
  - at sea E992
  - in harbor E992
  - land (explosion) E993
    - fragments, injury by E991.9
  - marine E992
- missile (guided) (explosion) E993
  - fragments, injury by E991.9
  - marine E992
  - nuclear E996
- mortar bomb (explosion) E993
  - fragments, injury by E991.9
- mustard gas E997.2
- nerve gas E997.2
- phosgene E997.2
- poisoning (chemical) (fumes) (gas) E997.2
- radiation , ionizing from nuclear explosion E996
- rocket (explosion) E993
  - fragments, injury by E991.9
- saber, sabre E995
- screening smoke E997.8
- shell (aircraft) (artillery) (cannon) (land based) (explosion) E993
  - fragments, injury by E991.9
  - sea-based E992
- shooting E991.2
  - after cessation of hostilities E998
  - bullet(s) E991.2
    - rubber E991.0
  - pellet(s) (rifle) E991.1
  - shrapnel E991.9
  - submersion E995
  - torpedo E992
  - unconventional warfare, except by nuclear weapon E997.9
  - biological (warfare) E997.1
  - gas, fumes, chemicals E997.2
  - laser(s) E997.0
  - specified type NEC E997.8
- underwater blast E992
- vesicant (chemical) (fumes) (gas) E997.2
- weapon burst E993

Washed
- away by flood – *see* Flood
- away by tidal wave – *see* Tidal wave
- off road by storm (transport vehicle) E908.9
- overboard E832

Weather exposure – *see also* Exposure
- cold E901.0
- hot E900.0

Weightlessness (causing injury) (effects of) (in spacecraft, real or simulated) E928.0

Wound (accidental) NEC (*see also* Injury) E928.9
- battle (*see also* War operations) E995
- bayonet E920.3
  - in
    - legal intervention E974
    - war operations E995
- gunshot – *see* Shooting
- incised – *see* Cut
- saber, sabre E920.3
  - in war operations E995

RAILWAY ACCIDENTS (E800-E807)

The following fourth-digit subdivisions are for use with categories E800-E807 to identify the injured person:

.0 Railway employee
Any person who by virtue of his employment in connection with a railway, whether by the railway company or not, is at increased risk of involvement in a railway accident, such as:
catering staff of train
driver
guard
porter
postal staff on train
railway fireman
shunter
sleeping car attendant

.1 Passenger on railway
Any authorized person traveling on a train, except a railway employee.
Excludes: intending passenger waiting at station (.8)
unauthorized rider on railway vehicle (.8)

.2 Pedestrian
See definition (r), Volume 1 page 297

.3 Pedal cyclist
See definition (p), Volume 1 page 297

.8 Other specified person
Intending passenger or bystander waiting at station
Unauthorized rider on railway vehicle

.9 Unspecified person

MOTOR VEHICLE TRAFFIC ACCIDENTS (E810-E819)

The following fourth-digit subdivisions are for use with categories E810-E819 to identify the injured person:

.0 Driver of motor vehicle other than motorcycle
See definition (l), Volume 1 pages 297-300

.1 Passenger in motor vehicle other than motorcycle
See definition (l), Volume 1 pages 297-300

.2 Motorcyclist
See definition (l), Volume 1 pages 297-300

.3 Passenger on motorcycle
See definition (l), Volume 1 pages 297-300

.4 Occupant of streetcar

.5 Rider of animal; occupant of animal-drawn vehicle

.6 Pedal cyclist
See definition (p), Volume 1 pages 297-300

.7 Pedestrian
See definition (r), Volume 1 pages 297-300

.8 Other specified person
Occupant of vehicle other than above
Person in railway train involved in accident
Unauthorized rider of motor vehicle

.9 Unspecified person

OTHER VEHICLE NONTRAFFIC ACCIDENTS (E820-E825)

The following fourth-digit subdivisions are for use with categories E820-E825 to identify the injured person:

.0 Driver of motor vehicle other than motorcycle
See definition (l), Volume 1 pages 297-301

.1 Passenger in motor vehicle other than motorcycle
See definition (l), Volume 1 pages 297-301

.2 Motorcyclist
See definition (l), Volume 1 pages 297-301

.3 Passenger on motorcycle
See definition (l), Volume 1 pages 297-301

.4 Occupant of streetcar

.5 Rider of animal; occupant of animal-drawn vehicle

.6 Pedal cyclist
See definition (p), Volume 1 pages 297-301

.7 Pedestrian
See definition (r), Volume 1 pages 297-301

.8 Other specified person
Occupant of vehicle other than above
Person in railway train involved in accident
Unauthorized rider of motor vehicle

.9 Unspecified person

OTHER ROAD VEHICLE ACCIDENTS (E826-E829)

The following fourth-digit subdivisions are for use with categories E826-E829 to identify the injured person:

.0 Pedestrian
See definition (r), Volume 1 pages 301-302

.1 Pedal cyclist
See definition (p), Volume 1 pages 301-302

.2 Rider of animal

.3 Occupant of animal-drawn vehicle

.4 Occupant of streetcar

.8 Other specified person

.9 Unspecified person

WATER TRANSPORT ACCIDENTS (E830-E838)

The following fourth-digit subdivisions are for use with categories E830-E838 to identify the injured person:

.0 Occupant of small boat, unpowered

.1 Occupant of small boat, powered
See definition (t), Volume 1 pages 302-303
Excludes: water skier (.4)

.2 Occupant of other watercraft crew
Persons:
engaged in operation of watercraft
providing passenger services [cabin attendants, ship's physician, catering personnel]
working on ship during voyage in other capacity [musician in band, operators of shops and beauty parlors]

.3 Occupant of other watercraft — other than crew
Passenger
Occupant of lifeboat, other than crew, after abandoning ship

.4 Water skier

.5 Swimmer

.6 Dockers, stevedores
Longshoreman employed on the dock in loading and unloading ships

.8 Other specified person
Immigration and custom officials on board ship
Person:
accompanying passenger or member of crew visiting boat
Pilot (guiding ship into port)

.9 Unspecified person

AIR AND SPACE TRANSPORT ACCIDENTS (E840-E845)

The following fourth-digit subdivisions are for use with categories E840-E845 to identify the injured person:

.0 Occupant of spacecraft

.1 Occupant of military aircraft, any
Crew in military aircraft [air force] [army] [national guard] [navy]
Passenger (civilian) (military) in military aircraft [air force] [army] [national guard] [navy]
Troops in military aircraft [air force] [army] [national guard] [navy]
Excludes: occupants of aircraft operated under jurisdiction of police departments (.5)
parachutist (.7)

.2 Crew of commercial aircraft (powered) in surface-to-surface transport

.3 Other occupant of commercial aircraft (powered) in surface-to-surface transport
Flight personnel:
not part of crew
on familiarization flight
Passenger on aircraft (powered) NOS

.4 Occupant of commercial aircraft (powered) in surface-to-air transport
Occupant [crew] [passenger] of aircraft (powered) engaged in activities, such as:
aerial spraying (crops) (fire retardants)
air drops of emergency supplies
air drops of parachutists, except from military craft
crop dusting
lowering of construction material [bridge or telephone pole]
sky writing

.5 Occupant of other powered aircraft
Occupant [crew] [passenger] of aircraft [powered] engaged in activities, such as:
aerobatic flying
aircraft racing
rescue operation
storm surveillance
traffic surveillance
Occupant of private plane NOS

.6 Occupant of unpowered aircraft, except parachutist
Occupant of aircraft classifiable to E842

.7 Parachutist (military) (other)
Person making voluntary descent
Excludes: person making descent after accident to aircraft (.1-.6)

.8 Ground crew, airline employee
Persons employed at airfields (civil) (military) or launching pads, not occupants of aircraft

.9 Other person

Tabular List

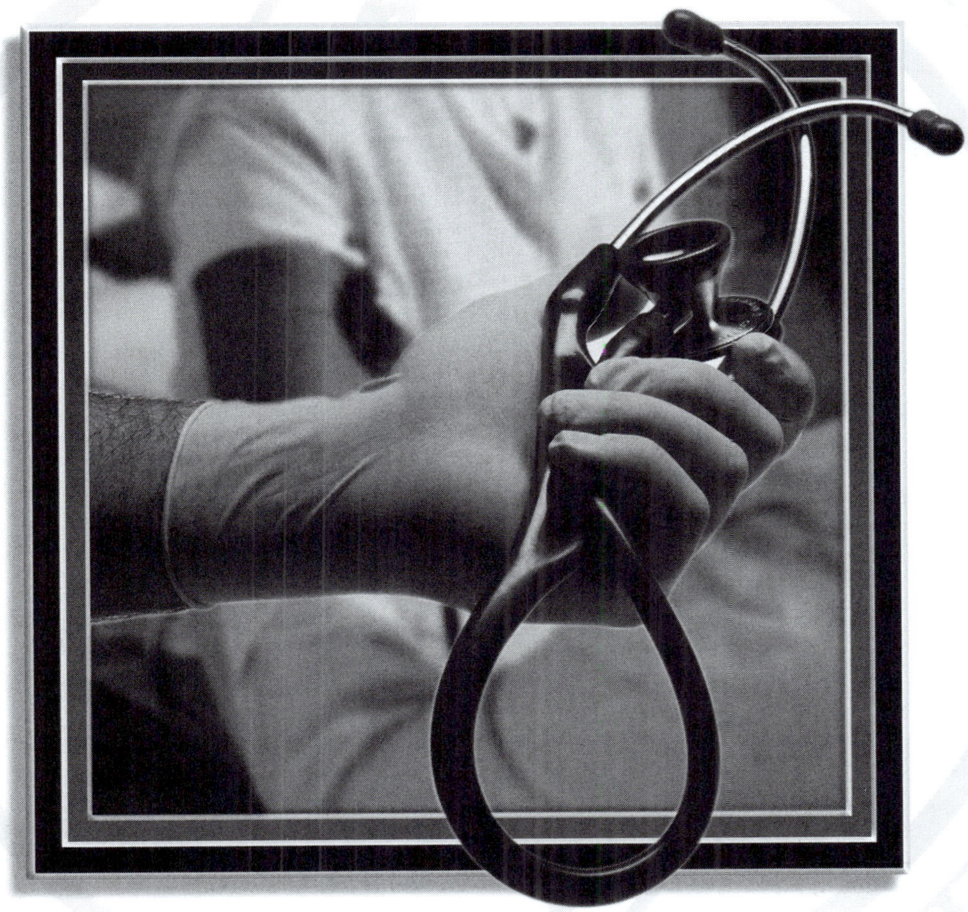

Volume 1 • Section 1

1. INFECTIOUS AND PARASITIC DISEASES (001-139)

Note: *Categories for "late effects" of infectious and parasitic diseases are to be found at 137-139.*

Includes diseases generally recognized as communicable or transmissible as well as a few diseases of unknown but possibly infectious origin

Excludes *acute respiratory infections (460-466)*
carrier or suspected carrier of infectious organism (V02.0-V02.9)
certain localized infections
influenza (487.0-487.8, ▶488◀)

INTESTINAL INFECTIOUS DISEASES (001-009)

Excludes *helminthiases (120.0-129)*

❹ **001 Cholera**
- **001.0 Due to Vibrio cholerae**
- **001.1 Due to Vibrio cholerae el tor**
- **001.9 Cholera, unspecified**

❹ **002 Typhoid and paratyphoid fevers**
- **002.0 Typhoid fever**
  Typhoid (fever) (infection) [any site]
- **002.1 Paratyphoid fever A**
- **002.2 Paratyphoid fever B**
- **002.3 Paratyphoid fever C**
- **002.9 Paratyphoid fever, unspecified**

❹ **003 Other salmonella infections**
Includes infection or food poisoning by Salmonella [any serotype]
- **003.0 Salmonella gastroenteritis**
  Salmonellosis
- **003.1 Salmonella septicemia**
  C&C Exclusions: 995.90, 995.91, 995.92, 995.93, 995.94
- ❺ **003.2 Localized salmonella infections**
  - ✖ **003.20 Localized salmonella infection, unspecified**
  - **003.21 Salmonella meningitis**
  - **003.22 Salmonella pneumonia**
  - **003.23 Salmonella arthritis**
  - **003.24 Salmonella osteomyelitis**
  - **003.29 Other**
- **003.8 Other specified salmonella infections**
- **003.9 Salmonella infection, unspecified**

❹ **004 Shigellosis**
Includes bacillary dysentery
- **004.0 Shigella dysenteriae**
  Infection by group A Shigella (Schmitz) (Shiga)
- **004.1 Shigella flexneri**
  Infection by group B Shigella
- **004.2 Shigella boydii**
  Infection by group C Shigella
- **004.3 Shigella sonnei**
  Infection by group D Shigella
- **004.8 Other specified shigella infections**
- **004.9 Shigellosis, unspecified**

❹ **005 Other food poisoning (bacterial)**
Excludes *salmonella infections (003.0-003.9)*
toxic effect of:
food contaminants (989.7)
noxious foodstuffs (988.0-988.9)
- **005.0 Staphylococcal food poisoning**
  Staphylococcal toxemia specified as due to food
- ▲ **005.1 Botulism food poisoning**
  ▶Botulism NOS◀
  Food poisoning due to Clostridium botulinum
  Excludes *▶infant botulism (040.41)◀*
  ▶wound botulism (040.42)◀

  DEF: Food poisoning caused by bacteria usually found in improperly canned or preserved foods. The botulinum neurotoxin affects the CNS and causes muscle paralysis.

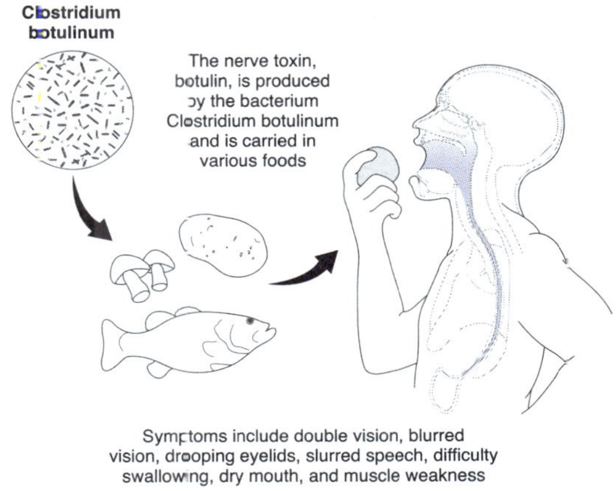

- **005.2 Food poisoning due to Clostridium perfringens [C. welchii]**
  Enteritis necroticans
- **005.3 Food poisoning due to other Clostridia**
- **005.4 Food poisoning due to Vibrio parahaemolyticus**
- ❺ **005.8 Other bacterial food poisoning**
  Excludes *salmonella food poisoning (003.0-003.9)*
  - **005.81 Food poisoning due to Vibrio vulnificus**
  - **005.89 Other bacterial food poisoning**
    Food poisoning due to Bacillus cereus
- **005.9 Food poisoning, unspecified**

❹ **006 Amebiasis**
Includes infection due to Entamoeba histolytica
Excludes *amebiasis due to organisms other than Entamoeba histolytica (007.8)*
- **006.0 Acute amebic dysentery without mention of abscess**
  Acute amebiasis

  DEF: Severe form of intestinal amebiasis causing stomach pain, bloody stools, and fever.
- **006.1 Chronic intestinal amebiasis without mention of abscess**
  Chronic:
  amebiasis
  amebic dysentery
- **006.2 Amebic nondysenteric colitis**
- **006.3 Amebic liver abscess**
  Hepatic amebiasis
- **006.4 Amebic lung abscess**
  Amebic abscess of lung (and liver)
- **006.5 Amebic brain abscess**
  Amebic abscess of brain (and liver) (and lung)
- **006.6 Amebic skin ulceration**
  Cutaneous amebiasis
- **006.8 Amebic infection of other sites**
  Amebic:
  appendicitis
  balanitis
  Ameboma
  Excludes *specific infections by free-living amebae (136.2)*
- **006.9 Amebiasis, unspecified**
  Amebiasis NOS

❹ 007 Other protozoal intestinal diseases

Includes protozoal:
colitis
diarrhea
dysentery

007.0 Balantidiasis
Infection by Balantidium coli

007.1 Giardiasis
Infection by Giardia lamblia
Lambliasis

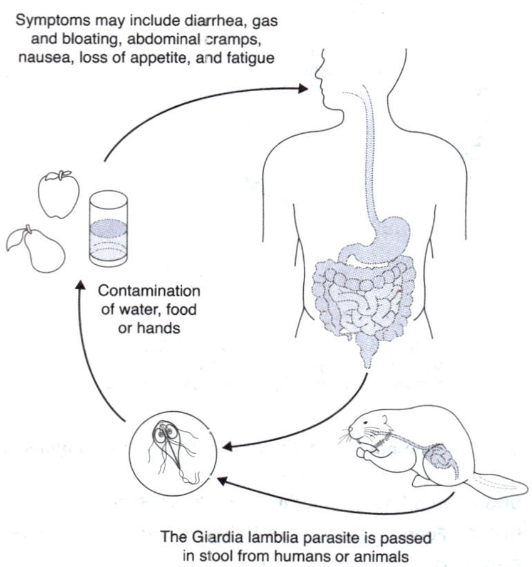

007.2 Coccidiosis
Infection by Isospora belli and Isospora hominis
Isosporiasis

007.3 Intestinal trichomoniasis

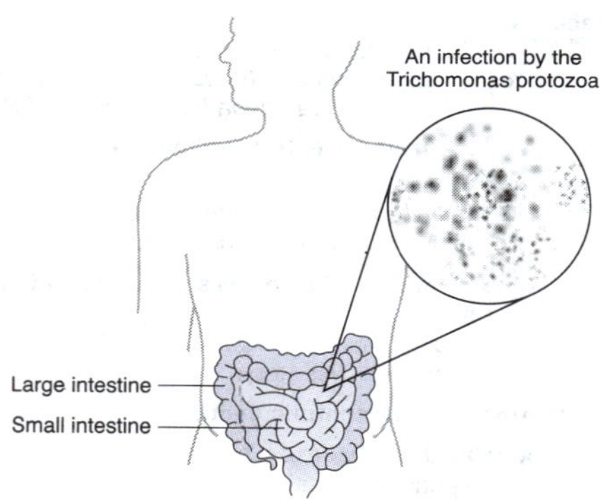

007.4 Cryptosporidiosis
AHA: 4Q 1997, 30

007.5 Cyclosporiasis
C&C Exclusions: 008.41, 008.42, 008.43, 008.44, 008.45, 008.46, 008.47, 008.49
AHA: 4Q 2000, 38

007.8 Other specified protozoal intestinal diseases
Amebiasis due to organisms other than Entamoeba histolytica

007.9 Unspecified protozoal intestinal disease
Flagellate diarrhea
Protozoal dysentery NOS

❹ 008 Intestinal infections due to other organisms

Includes any condition classifiable to 009.0-009.3 with mention of the responsible organisms

Excludes *food poisoning by these organisms (005.0-005.9)*

❺ 008.0 Escherichia coli [E. coli]
AHA: 4Q 1992, 17

008.00 E. coli, unspecified
E. coli enteritis NOS

Intestinal infections

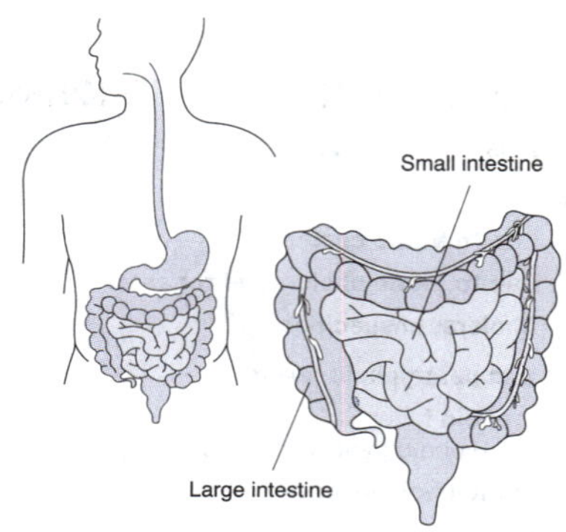

008.01 Enteropathogenic E. coli

008.02 Enterotoxigenic E. coli

008.03 Enteroinvasive E. coli

008.04 Enterohemorrhagic E. coli

008.09 Other intestinal E. coli infections

008.1 Arizona group of paracolon bacilli

008.2 Aerobacter aerogenes
Enterobacter aerogenes

008.3 Proteus (mirabilis) (morganii)

❺ 008.4 Other specified bacteria
AHA: 4Q 1992, 18

008.41 Staphylococcus
Staphylococcal enterocolitis
C&C Exclusions: 001.1, 002.0, 002.9, 003.0, 004.9, 005.0, 005.1, 005.2, 006.0, 006.1, 006.2, 006.9, 007.1, 007.2, 007.3, 007.4, 007.5, 007.8, 007.9, 008.00, 008.01, 008.02, 008.03, 008.04, 008.09, 008.1, 008.2, 008.3, 008.41, 008.42, 008.43, 008.44, 008.45, 008.46, 008.47, 008.49, 008.5, 008.61, 008.62, 008.63, 008.64, 008.65, 008.66, 008.67, 008.69, 008.8, 009.0, 014.80, 014.81, 014.82, 014.83, 014.84, 014.85, 014.86, 112.85, 129, 487.8, 536.3, 536.8, 555.0, 555.1, 555.2, 555.9, 556.0, 556.1, 556.2, 556.3, 556.4, 556.5, 556.6, 556.8, 556.9, 557.0, 557.1, 557.9, 558.2, 558.3, 558.9, 564.1, 775.0, 775.1, 775.2, 775.3, 775.4, 775.5, 775.6, 775.7, 775.8, 775.9, 777.5, 777.8

008.42 Pseudomonas
C&C Exclusions: See 008.41
AHA: 2Q 1989, 10

008.43 Campylobacter
C&C Exclusions: See 008.41

008.44 Yersinia enterocolitica
C&C Exclusions: See 008.41

008.45 Clostridium difficile
Pseudomembranous colitis
C&C Exclusions: See 008.41

008.46 Other anaerobes
Anaerobic enteritis NOS
Bacteroides (fragilis)
Gram-negative anaerobes
C&C Exclusions: See 008.41

008.47 Other gram-negative bacteria
Gram-negative enteritis NOS
Excludes *gram-negative anaerobes (008.46)*
C&C Exclusions: See 008.41

008.49 Other
C&C Exclusions: See 008.41
AHA: 2Q 1989, 10; 1Q 1988, 6

008.5 Bacterial enteritis, unspecified

5 **008.6 Enteritis due to specified virus**
AHA: 4Q 1992, 18

008.61 Rotavirus

008.62 Adenovirus

008.63 Norwalk virus
Norwalk-like agent

008.64 Other small round viruses [SRV's]
Small round virus NOS

008.65 Calicivirus

008.66 Astrovirus

008.67 Enterovirus NEC
Coxsackie virus
Echovirus
Excludes *poliovirus (045.0-045.9)*

008.69 Other viral enteritis
Torovirus
AHA: 1Q 2003, 10

008.8 Other organism, not elsewhere classified
Viral:
enteritis NOS
gastroenteritis
Excludes *influenza with involvement of gastrointestinal tract (487.8)*

4 **009 Ill-defined intestinal infections**
Excludes *diarrheal disease or intestinal infection due to specified organism (001.0-008.8)*
diarrhea following gastrointestinal surgery (564.4)
intestinal malabsorption (579.0-579.9)
ischemic enteritis (557.0-557.9)
other noninfectious gastroenteritis and colitis (558.1-558.9)
regional enteritis (555.0-555.9)
ulcerative colitis (556)

009.0 Infectious colitis, enteritis, and gastroenteritis
Colitis (septic)
Dysentery:
NOS
catarrhal
hemorrhagic
Enteritis (septic)
Gastroenteritis (septic)
AHA: 3Q 1999, 4

009.1 Colitis, enteritis, and gastroenteritis of presumed infectious origin
Excludes *colitis NOS (558.9)*
enteritis NOS (558.9)
gastroenteritis NOS (558.9)
AHA: 3Q 1999, 6

009.2 Infectious diarrhea
Diarrhea:
dysenteric
epidemic
Infectious diarrheal disease NOS

009.3 Diarrhea of presumed infectious origin
Excludes *diarrhea NOS (787.91)*
AHA: Nov-Dec 1987, 7

TUBERCULOSIS (010-018)

Includes infection by Mycobacterium tuberculosis (human) (bovine)
Excludes *congenital tuberculosis (771.2)*
late effects of tuberculosis (137.0-137.4)

The following fifth-digit subclassification is for use with categories 010-018:
0 **unspecified**
1 **bacteriological or histological examination not done**
2 **bacteriological or histological examination unknown (at present)**
3 **tubercle bacilli found (in sputum) by microscopy**
4 **tubercle bacilli not found (in sputum) by microscopy, but found by bacterial culture**
5 **tubercle bacilli not found by bacteriological examination, but tuberculosis confirmed histologically**
6 **tubercle bacilli not found by bacteriological or histological examination, but tuberculosis confirmed by other methods [inoculation of animals]**

4 **010 Primary tuberculous infection**
Requires fifth digit. See beginning of section 010-018 for codes and definitions.

5 **010.0 Primary tuberculous infection**
Excludes *nonspecific reaction to tuberculin skin test without active tuberculosis (795.5)*
positive PPD (795.5)
positive tuberculin skin test without active tuberculosis (795.5)

5 **010.1 Tuberculous pleurisy in primary progressive tuberculosis**

5 **010.8 Other primary progressive tuberculosis**
Excludes *tuberculous erythema nodosum (017.1)*

5 **010.9 Primary tuberculous infection, unspecified**

4 **011 Pulmonary tuberculosis**
Requires fifth digit. See beginning of section 010-018 for codes and definitions.
Use additional code to identify any associated silicosis (502)

5 **011.0 Tuberculosis of lung, infiltrative**
C&C Exclusions: 011.00, 011.01, 011.02, 011.03, 011.04, 011.05, 011.06, 011.10, 011.11, 011.12, 011.13, 011.14, 011.15, 011.16, 011.20, 011.21, 011.22, 011.23, 011.24, 011.25, 011.26, 011.30, 011.31, 011.32, 011.33, 011.34, 011.35, 011.36, 011.40, 011.41, 011.42, 011.43, 011.44, 011.45, 011.46, 011.50, 011.51, 011.52, 011.53, 011.54, 011.55, 011.56, 011.60, 011.61, 011.62, 011.63, 011.64, 011.65, 011.66, 011.70, 011.71, 011.72, 011.73, 011.74, 011.75, 011.76, 011.80, 011.81, 011.82, 011.83, 011.84, 011.85, 011.86, 011.90, 011.91, 011.92, 011.93, 011.94, 011.95, 011.96, 012.00, 012.01, 012.02, 012.03, 012.04, 012.05, 012.06, 012.10, 012.11, 012.12, 012.13, 012.14, 012.15, 012.16, 012.20, 012.21, 012.22, 012.23, 012.24, 012.25, 012.26, 012.30, 012.31, 012.32, 012.33, 012.34, 012.35, 012.36, 012.80, 012.81, 012.82, 012.83, 012.84, 012.85, 012.86, 017.90, 017.91, 017.92, 017.93, 017.94, 017.95, 017.96, 018.00, 018.01, 018.02, 018.03, 018.04, 018.05, 018.06, 018.80, 018.81, 018.82, 018.83, 018.84, 018.85, 018.86, 018.90, 018.91, 018.92, 018.93, 018.94, 018.95, 018.96, 031.0, 031.2, 031.8, 031.9, 041.81, 041.82, 041.83, 041.84, 041.85, 041.86, 041.89, 041.9, 079.82, 137.0, 139.8, 480.0, 480.1, 480.2, 480.3, 480.8, 480.9, 481, 482.0, 482.1, 482.2, 482.30, 482.31, 482.32, 482.39, 482.40, 482.41, 482.49, 482.81, 482.82, 482.83, 482.84, 482.89, 482.9, 483.0, 483.1, 483.8, 484.1, 484.3, 484.5, 484.6, 484.7, 484.8, 485, 486, 487.0, 487.1, 494.0, 494.1, 495.0, 495.1, 495.2, 495.3, 495.4, 495.5, 495.6, 495.7, 495.8, 495.9, 496, 500, 501, 502, 503, 504, 505, 506.0, 506.1, 506.2, 506.3, 506.4, 506.9, 507.0, 507.1, 507.8, 508.0, 508.1, 508.8, 508.9, 517.1, 518.89

5 **011.1 Tuberculosis of lung, nodular**
C&C Exclusions: See 011.0

5 **011.2 Tuberculosis of lung with cavitation**
C&C Exclusions: See 011.0

5 **011.3 Tuberculosis of bronchus**
Excludes *isolated bronchial tuberculosis (012.2)*
C&C Exclusions: See 011.0

A Adult (15+ years) M Maternity (12-55 years) N Newborn (0 years) P Pediatric (0-17 years) ♂ Male ♀ Female 2 Medicare Secondary Payer

❺ **011.4 Tuberculous fibrosis of lung**
C&C Exclusions: See 011.0

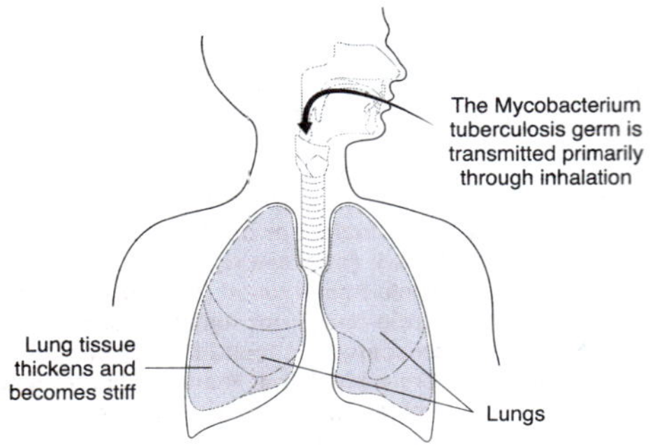

❺ **011.5 Tuberculous bronchiectasis**
C&C Exclusions: See 011.0

❺ **011.6 Tuberculous pneumonia [any form]**
C&C Exclusions: (for codes 011.60-011.65) See 011.0
C&C Exclusions: (for code 011.66) 011.66, 079.82, 139.8, 480.0, 480.1, 480.2, 480.3, 480.8, 480.9, 481, 482.0, 482.1, 482.2, 482.30, 482.31, 482.32, 482.39, 482.40, 482.41, 482.49, 482.81, 482.82, 482.83, 482.84, 482.89, 482.9, 483.0, 483.1, 483.8, 484.1, 484.3, 484.5, 484.6, 484.7, 484.8, 485, 486, 487.0, 487.1, 494.0, 494.1, 495.0, 495.1, 495.2, 495.3, 495.4, 495.5, 495.6, 495.7, 495.8, 495.9, 496, 500, 501, 502, 503, 504, 505, 506.0, 506.1, 506.2, 506.3, 506.4, 506.9, 507.0, 507.1, 507.8, 508.0, 508.1, 508.8, 508.9, 517.1, 518.89

❺ **011.7 Tuberculous pneumothorax**
C&C Exclusions: See 011.0

❺ **011.8 Other specified pulmonary tuberculosis**
C&C Exclusions: See 011.0

❺ **011.9 Pulmonary tuberculosis, unspecified**
Respiratory tuberculosis NOS
Tuberculosis of lung NOS
C&C Exclusions: See 011.0

❹ **012 Other respiratory tuberculosis**
Requires fifth digit. See beginning of section 010-018 for codes and definitions.
Excludes *respiratory tuberculosis, unspecified (011.9)*

❺ **012.0 Tuberculous pleurisy**
Tuberculosis of pleura
Tuberculous empyema
Tuberculous hydrothorax
Excludes *pleurisy with effusion without mention of cause (511.9)*
tuberculous pleurisy in primary progressive tuberculosis (010.1)
C&C Exclusions: See 011.0

❺ **012.1 Tuberculosis of intrathoracic lymph nodes**
Tuberculosis of lymph nodes:
- hilar
- mediastinal
- tracheobronchial

Tuberculous tracheobronchial adenopathy
Excludes *that specified as primary (010.0-010.9)*
C&C Exclusions: See 011.0

❺ **012.2 Isolated tracheal or bronchial tuberculosis**

❺ **012.3 Tuberculous laryngitis**
Tuberculosis of glottis

❺ **012.8 Other specified respiratory tuberculosis**
Tuberculosis of:
- mediastinum
- nasopharynx
- nose (septum)
- sinus [any nasal]

C&C Exclusions: See 011.0

❹ **013 Tuberculosis of meninges and central nervous system**
Requires fifth digit. See beginning of section 010-018 for codes and definitions.

❺ **013.0 Tuberculous meningitis**
Tuberculosis of meninges (cerebral) (spinal)
Tuberculous:
- leptomeningitis
- meningoencephalitis

Excludes *tuberculoma of meninges (013.1)*
C&C Exclusions: 003.21, 013.00, 013.01, 013.02, 013.03, 013.04, 013.05, 013.06, 013.10, 013.11, 013.12, 013.13, 013.14, 013.15, 013.16, 013.40, 013.41, 013.42, 013.43, 013.44, 013.45, 013.46, 013.50, 013.51, 013.52, 013.53, 013.54, 013.55, 013.56, 013.80, 013.81, 013.82, 013.83, 013.84, 013.85, 013.86, 013.90, 013.91, 013.92, 013.93, 013.94, 013.95, 013.96, 017.90, 017.91, 017.92, 017.93, 017.94, 017.95, 017.96, 031.2, 031.8, 031.9, 036.0, 041.81, 041.82, 041.83, 041.84, 041.85, 041.86, 041.89, 041.9, 047.0, 047.1, 047.8, 047.9, 049.0, 049.1, 053.0, 054.72, 072.1, 090.42, 091.81, 094.2, 098.89, 100.81, 112.83, 114.2, 115.01, 115.11, 115.91, 130.0, 137.1, 139.8, 320.0, 320.1, 320.2, 320.3, 320.7, 320.81, 320.82, 320.89, 320.9, 321.0, 321.1, 321.2, 321.3, 321.4, 321.8, 322.0, 322.1, 322.2, 322.9, 349.89, 349.9, 357.0

❺ **013.1 Tuberculoma of meninges**
C&C Exclusions: See 013.0

❺ **013.2 Tuberculoma of brain**
Tuberculosis of brain (current disease)
C&C Exclusions: 013.20, 013.21, 013.22, 013.23, 013.24, 013.25, 013.26, 013.30, 013.31, 013.32, 013.33, 013.34, 013.35, 013.36, 013.60, 013.61, 013.62, 013.63, 013.64, 013.65, 013.66, 013.80, 013.81, 013.82, 013.83, 013.84, 013.85, 013.86, 013.90, 013.91, 013.92, 013.93, 013.94, 013.95, 013.96, 017.90, 017.91, 017.92, 017.93, 017.94, 017.95, 017.96, 031.2, 031.8, 031.9, 041.81, 041.82, 041.83, 041.84, 041.85, 041.86, 041.89, 041.9, 137.1, 139.8

❺ **013.3 Tuberculous abscess of brain**
C&C Exclusions: See 013.2

❺ **013.4 Tuberculoma of spinal cord**
C&C Exclusions: 013.00, 013.01, 013.02, 013.03, 013.04, 013.05, 013.06, 013.10, 013.11, 013.12, 013.13, 013.14, 013.15, 013.16, 013.40, 013.41, 013.42, 013.43, 013.44, 013.45, 013.46, 013.50, 013.51, 013.52, 013.53, 013.54, 013.55, 013.56, 013.80, 013.81, 013.82, 013.83, 013.84, 013.85, 013.86, 013.90, 013.91, 013.92, 013.93, 013.94, 013.95, 013.96, 017.90, 017.91, 017.92, 017.93, 017.94, 017.95, 017.96, 031.2, 031.8, 031.9, 041.81, 041.82, 041.83, 041.84, 041.85, 041.86, 041.89, 041.9, 137.1, 139.8

❺ **013.5 Tuberculous abscess of spinal cord**
C&C Exclusions: See 013.4

❺ **013.6 Tuberculous encephalitis or myelitis**
C&C Exclusions: See 013.2

❺ **013.8 Other specified tuberculosis of central nervous system**
C&C Exclusions: 013.80, 013.81, 013.82, 013.83, 013.84, 013.85, 013.86, 013.90, 013.91, 013.92, 013.93, 013.94, 013.95, 013.96, 017.90, 017.91, 017.92, 017.93, 017.94, 017.95, 017.96, 031.2, 031.8, 031.9, 041.81, 041.82, 041.83, 041.84, 041.85, 041.86, 041.89, 041.9, 137.1, 139.8

❺ **013.9 Unspecified tuberculosis of central nervous system**
Tuberculosis of central nervous system NOS
C&C Exclusions: See 013.8

❹ **014 Tuberculosis of intestines, peritoneum, and mesenteric glands**
Requires fifth digit. See beginning of section 010-018 for codes and definitions.

❺ **014.0 Tuberculous peritonitis**
Tuberculous ascites
C&C Exclusions: 014.00, 014.01, 014.02, 014.03, 014.04, 014.05, 014.06, 014.80, 014.81, 014.82, 014.83, 014.84, 014.85, 014.86, 017.90, 017.91, 017.92, 017.93, 017.94, 017.95, 017.96, 031.2, 031.8, 031.9, 041.81, 041.82, 041.83, 041.84, 041.85, 041.86, 041.89, 041.9, 139.8

5 014.8 Other
Tuberculosis (of):
anus
intestine (large) (small)
mesenteric glands
rectum
retroperitoneal (lymph nodes)
Tuberculous enteritis
C&C Exclusions: (for codes 014.80, 014.82, and 014.83) See 014.0
C&C Exclusions: (for code 014.81) 014.81, 139.8

4 015 Tuberculosis of bones and joints
Requires fifth digit. See beginning of section 010-018 for codes and definitions.
Use additional code to identify manifestation, as:
tuberculous:
arthropathy (711.4)
necrosis of bone (730.8)
osteitis (730.8)
osteomyelitis (730.8)
synovitis (727.01)
tenosynovitis (727.01)

5 015.0 Vertebral column
Pott's disease
Use additional code to identify manifestation, as:
curvature of spine [Pott's] (737.4)
kyphosis (737.4)
spondylitis (720.81)

5 015.1 Hip

5 015.2 Knee

5 015.5 Limb bones
Tuberculous dactylitis

5 015.6 Mastoid
Tuberculous mastoiditis

5 015.7 Other specified bone

5 015.8 Other specified joint

5 015.9 Tuberculosis of unspecified bones and joints

4 016 Tuberculosis of genitourinary system
Requires fifth digit. See beginning of section 010-018 for codes and definitions.

5 016.0 Kidney
Renal tuberculosis
Use additional code to identify manifestation, as:
tuberculous:
nephropathy (583.81)
pyelitis (590.81)
pyelonephritis (590.81)
C&C Exclusions: 016.00, 016.01, 016.02, 016.03, 016.04, 016.05, 016.06, 016.10, 016.11, 016.12, 016.13, 016.14, 016.15, 016.16, 016.20, 016.21, 016.22, 016.23, 016.24, 016.25, 016.26, 016.30, 016.31, 016.32, 016.33, 016.34, 016.35, 016.36, 016.90, 016.91, 016.92, 016.93, 016.94, 016.95, 016.96, 017.90, 017.91, 017.92, 017.93, 017.94, 017.95, 017.96, 031.2, 031.8, 031.9, 041.81, 041.82, 041.83, 041.84, 041.85, 041.86, 041.89, 041.9, 137.2, 139.8

5 016.1 Bladder
C&C Exclusions: See 016.0

5 016.2 Ureter
C&C Exclusions: See 016.0

5 016.3 Other urinary organs
C&C Exclusions: See 016.0

5 016.4 Epididymis ♂
C&C Exclusions: 016.40, 016.41, 016.42, 016.43, 016.44, 016.45, 016.46, 016.50, 016.51, 016.52, 016.53, 016.54, 016.55, 016.56, 016.90, 016.91, 016.92, 016.93, 016.94, 016.95, 016.96, 017.90, 017.91, 017.92, 017.93, 017.94, 017.95, 017.96, 031.2, 031.8, 031.9, 041.81, 041.82, 041.83, 041.84, 041.85, 041.86, 041.89, 041.9, 137.2, 139.8

5 016.5 Other male genital organs ♂
Use additional code to identify manifestation, as:
tuberculosis of:
prostate (601.4)
seminal vesicle (608.81)
testis (608.81)
C&C Exclusions: See 016.4

5 016.6 Tuberculous oophoritis and salpingitis ♀
C&C Exclusions: 016.60, 016.61, 016.62, 016.63, 016.64, 016.65, 016.66, 016.70, 016.71, 016.72, 016.73, 016.74, 016.75, 016.76, 016.90, 016.91, 016.92, 016.93, 016.94, 016.95, 016.96, 017.90, 017.91, 017.92, 017.93, 017.94, 017.95, 017.96, 031.2, 031.8, 031.9, 041.81, 041.82, 041.83, 041.84, 041.85, 041.86, 041.89, 041.9, 137.2, 139.8

5 016.7 Other female genital organs ♀
Tuberculous:
cervicitis
endometritis
C&C Exclusions: See 016.6

5 016.9 Genitourinary tuberculosis, unspecified
C&C Exclusions: 016.90, 016.91, 016.92, 016.93, 016.94, 016.95, 016.96, 017.90, 017.91, 017.92, 017.93, 017.94, 017.95, 017.96, 031.2, 031.8, 031.9, 041.81, 041.82, 041.83, 041.84, 041.85, 041.86, 041.89, 041.9, 137.2, 139.8

4 017 Tuberculosis of other organs
Requires fifth digit. See beginning of section 010-018 for codes and definitions.

5 017.0 Skin and subcutaneous cellular tissue
Lupus:
exedens
vulgaris
Scrofuloderma
Tuberculosis:
colliquativa
cutis
lichenoides
papulonecrotica
verrucosa cutis
Excludes *lupus erythematosus (695.4)*
disseminated (710.0)
lupus NOS (710.0)
nonspecific reaction to tuberculin skin test without active tuberculosis (795.5)
positive PPD (795.5)
positive tuberculin skin test without active tuberculosis (795.5)

5 017.1 Erythema nodosum with hypersensitivity reaction in tuberculosis
Bazin's disease
Erythema:
induratum
nodosum, tuberculous
Tuberculosis indurativa
Excludes *erythema nodosum NOS (695.2)*

5 017.2 Peripheral lymph nodes
Scrofula
Scrofulous abscess
Tuberculous adenitis
Excludes *tuberculosis of lymph nodes:*
bronchial and mediastinal (012.1)
mesenteric and retroperitoneal (014.8)
tuberculous tracheobronchial adenopathy (012.1)
C&C Exclusions: 017.20, 017.21, 017.22, 017.23, 017.24, 017.25, 017.26, 017.90, 017.91, 017.92, 017.93, 017.94, 017.95, 017.96, 031.2, 031.8, 031.9, 041.81, 041.82, 041.83, 041.84, 041.85, 041.86, 041.89, 041.9, 139.8

❺ **017.3 Eye**

Use additional code to identify manifestation, as:
tuberculous:
episcleritis (379.09)
interstitial keratitis (370.59)
iridocyclitis, chronic (364.11)
keratoconjunctivitis (phlyctenular) (370.31)

C&C Exclusions: 017.30, 017.31, 017.32, 017.33, 017.34, 017.35, 017.36, 017.90, 017.91, 017.92, 017.93, 017.94, 017.95, 017.96, 031.2, 031.8, 031.9, 041.81, 041.82, 041.83, 041.84, 041.85, 041.86, 041.89, 041.9, 139.8

Tuberculosis of the eye

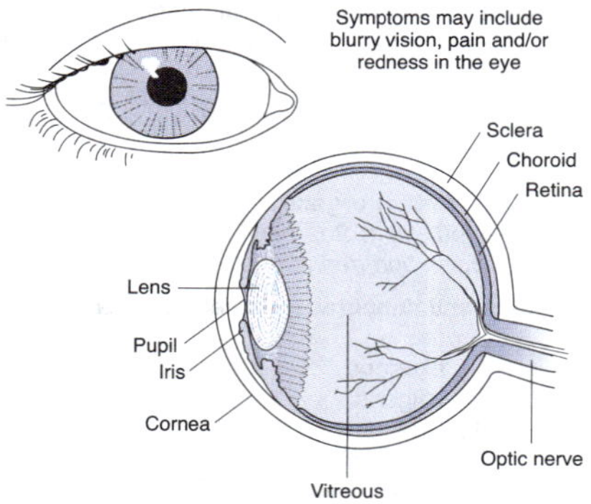

❺ **017.4 Ear**

Tuberculosis of ear
Tuberculous otitis media
Excludes *tuberculous mastoiditis (015.6)*

C&C Exclusions: 017.40, 017.41, 017.42, 017.43, 017.44, 017.45, 017.46, 017.90, 017.91, 017.92, 017.93, 017.94, 017.95, 017.96, 031.2, 031.8, 031.9, 041.81, 041.82, 041.83, 041.84, 041.85, 041.86, 041.89, 041.9, 139.8

❺ **017.5 Thyroid gland**

C&C Exclusions: 017.50, 017.51, 017.52, 017.53, 017.54, 017.55, 017.56, 017.90, 017.91, 017.92, 017.93, 017.94, 017.95, 017.96, 031.2, 031.8, 031.9, 041.81, 041.82, 041.83, 041.84, 041.85, 041.86, 041.89, 041.9, 139.8

❺ **017.6 Adrenal glands**

Addison's disease, tuberculous

C&C Exclusions: 017.60, 017.61, 017.62, 017.63, 017.64, 017.65, 017.66, 017.90, 017.91, 017.92, 017.93, 017.94, 017.95, 017.96, 031.2, 031.8, 031.9, 041.81, 041.82, 041.83, 041.84, 041.85, 041.86, 041.89, 041.9, 139.8

❺ **017.7 Spleen**

C&C Exclusions: 017.70, 017.71, 017.72, 017.73, 017.74, 017.75, 017.76, 017.90, 017.91, 017.92, 017.93, 017.94, 017.95, 017.96, 031.2, 031.8, 031.9, 041.81, 041.82, 041.83, 041.84, 041.85, 041.86, 041.89, 041.9, 139.8

❺ **017.8 Esophagus**

C&C Exclusions: 017.80, 017.81, 017.82, 017.83, 017.84, 017.85, 017.86, 017.90, 017.91, 017.92, 017.93, 017.94, 017.95, 017.96, 031.2, 031.8, 031.9, 041.81, 041.82, 041.83, 041.84, 041.85, 041.86, 041.89, 041.9, 139.8

❺ **017.9 Other specified organs**

Use additional code to identify manifestation, as:
tuberculosis of:
endocardium [any valve] (424.91)
myocardium (422.0)
pericardium (420.0)

C&C Exclusions: 017.90, 017.91, 017.92, 017.93, 017.94, 017.95, 017.96, 031.2, 031.8, 031.9, 041.81, 041.82, 041.83, 041.84, 041.85, 041.86, 041.89, 041.9, 079.82, 139.8, 480.3, 494.1

❹ **018 Miliary tuberculosis**

Requires fifth digit. See beginning of section 010-018 for codes and definitions.

Includes tuberculosis:
disseminated
generalized
miliary, whether of a single specified site, multiple sites, or unspecified site
polyserositis

❺ **018.0 Acute miliary tuberculosis**

C&C Exclusions: 017.90, 017.91, 017.92, 017.93, 017.94, 017.95, 017.96, 018.00, 018.01, 018.02, 018.03, 018.04, 018.05, 018.06, 018.80, 018.81, 018.82, 018.83, 018.84, 018.85, 018.86, 018.90, 018.91, 018.92, 018.93, 018.94, 018.95, 018.96, 031.2, 031.8, 031.9, 041.81, 041.82, 041.83, 041.84, 041.85, 041.86, 041.89, 041.9, 139.8

❺ **018.8 Other specified miliary tuberculosis**

C&C Exclusions: See 018.0

❺ **018.9 Miliary tuberculosis, unspecified**

C&C Exclusions: See 018.0

ZOONOTIC BACTERIAL DISEASES (020-027)

❹ **020 Plague**

Includes infection by Yersinia [Pasteurella] pestis

DEF: Infection with the *Yersinia pestis* bacillus, transmitted via flea, tick, and lice bites and by contact with infected persons or material.

020.0 Bubonic

020.1 Cellulocutaneous

020.2 Septicemic

C&C Exclusions: 995.90, 995.91, 995.92, 995.93, 995.94

DEF: High-density bloodstream infection in acute bubonic plague; may cause death before the appearance of buboes or pulmonary manifestations.

020.3 Primary pneumonic

DEF: Rapidly progressive, often fatal plague pneumonia caused by direct inhalation of bacteria with severe cough producing frothy, bloody, mucoid sputum.

020.4 Secondary pneumonic

020.5 Pneumonic, unspecified

020.8 Other specified types of plague

Abortive plague
Ambulatory plague
Pestis minor

020.9 Plague, unspecified

❹ **021 Tularemia**

Includes deerfly fever
infection by Francisella [Pasteurella] tularensis
rabbit fever

021.0 Ulceroglandular tularemia

021.1 Enteric tularemia

Tularemia:
cryptogenic
intestinal
typhoidal

021.2 Pulmonary tularemia

Bronchopneumonic tularemia

C&C Exclusions: 079.82, 480.3

021.3 Oculoglandular tularemia

021.8 Other specified tularemia

Tularemia:
generalized or disseminated
glandular

021.9 Unspecified tularemia

❹ **022 Anthrax**

AHA: 4Q 2002, 70

022.0 Cutaneous anthrax

Malignant pustule

022.1 Pulmonary anthrax

Respiratory anthrax
Wool-sorters' disease

022.2 Gastrointestinal anthrax

022.3 Anthrax septicemia

022.8 Other specified manifestations of anthrax

022.9 Anthrax, unspecified

❹ **023 Brucellosis**

Includes fever:
- Malta
- Mediterranean
- undulant

023.0 Brucella melitensis

023.1 Brucella abortus

023.2 Brucella suis

023.3 Brucella canis

023.8 Other brucellosis

Infection by more than one organism

023.9 Brucellosis, unspecified

024 Glanders

Infection by:
- Actinobacillus mallei
- Malleomyces mallei
- Pseudomonas mallei

Farcy
Malleus

025 Melioidosis

Infection by:
- Malleomyces pseudomallei
- Pseudomonas pseudomallei
- Whitmore's bacillus

Pseudoglanders

❹ **026 Rat-bite fever**

026.0 Spirillary fever

Rat-bite fever due to Spirillum minor [S. minus]
Sodoku

026.1 Streptobacillary fever

Epidemic arthritic erythema
Haverhill fever
Rat-bite fever due to Streptobacillus moniliformis

026.9 Unspecified rat-bite fever

❹ **027 Other zoonotic bacterial diseases**

027.0 Listeriosis

Infection by Listeria monocytogenes
Septicemia by Listeria monocytogenes
Use additional code to identify manifestations, as meningitis (320.7)

Excludes *congenital listeriosis (771.2)*

DEF: Infection with the gram-positive bacillus, *Listeria monocytogenes*, that may cause meningitis, eye infections, miscarriage, vomiting, and diarrhea.

027.1 Erysipelothrix infection

Erysipeloid (of Rosenbach)
Infection by Erysipelothrix insidiosa [E. rhusiopathiae]
Septicemia by Erysipelothrix insidiosa [E. rhusiopathiae]

027.2 Pasteurellosis

Mesenteric adenitis by Pasteurella multocida [P. septica]
Pasteurella pseudotuberculosis
Septic infection (cat bite) (dog bite) by Pasteurella multocida [P. septica]

Excludes *infection by:*
- *Francisella [Pasteurella] tularensis (021.0-021.9)*
- *Yersinia [Pasteurella] pestis (020.0-020.9)*

027.8 Other specified zoonotic bacterial diseases

027.9 Unspecified zoonotic bacterial disease

OTHER BACTERIAL DISEASES (030-041)

Excludes *bacterial venereal diseases (098.0-099.9)*
bartonellosis (088.0)

❹ **030 Leprosy**

Includes Hansen's disease
infection by Mycobacterium leprae

030.0 Lepromatous [type L]

Lepromatous leprosy (macular) (diffuse) (infiltrated) (nodular) (neuritic)

030.1 Tuberculoid [type T]

Tuberculoid leprosy (macular) (maculoanesthetic) (major) (minor) (neuritic)

030.2 Indeterminate [group I]

Indeterminate [uncharacteristic] leprosy (macular) (neuritic)

030.3 Borderline [group B]

Borderline or dimorphous leprosy (infiltrated) (neuritic)

030.8 Other specified leprosy

030.9 Leprosy, unspecified

❹ **031 Diseases due to other mycobacteria**

031.0 Pulmonary

Battey disease
Infection by Mycobacterium:
- avium
- intracellulare [Battey bacillus]
- kansasii

C&C Exclusions: 011.00, 011.01, 011.02, 011.03, 011.04, 011.05, 011.06, 011.10, 011.11, 011.12, 011.13, 011.14, 011.15, 011.16, 011.20, 011.21, 011.22, 011.23, 011.24, 011.25, 011.26, 011.30, 011.31, 011.32, 011.33, 011.34, 011.35, 011.36, 011.40, 011.41, 011.42, 011.43, 011.44, 011.45, 011.46, 011.50, 011.51, 011.52, 011.53, 011.54, 011.55, 011.56, 011.60, 011.61, 011.62, 011.63, 011.64, 011.65, 011.66, 011.70, 011.71, 011.72, 011.73, 011.74, 011.75, 011.76, 011.80, 011.81, 011.82, 011.83, 011.84, 011.85, 011.86, 011.90, 011.91, 011.92, 011.93, 011.94, 011.95, 011.96, 012.00, 012.01, 012.02, 012.03, 012.04, 012.05, 012.06, 012.10, 012.11, 012.12, 012.13, 012.14, 012.15, 012.16, 012.20, 012.21, 012.22, 012.23, 012.24, 012.25, 012.26, 012.30, 012.31, 012.32, 012.33, 012.34, 012.35, 012.36, 012.80, 012.81, 012.82, 012.83, 012.84, 012.85, 012.86, 017.90, 017.91, 017.92, 017.93, 017.94, 017.95, 017.96, 031.0, 031.2, 031.8, 031.9, 041.81, 041.82, 041.83, 041.84, 041.85, 041.86, 041.89, 041.9, 079.82, 137.0, 139.8, 480.0, 480.1, 480.2, 480.3, 480.8, 480.9, 481, 482.0, 482.1, 482.2, 482.30, 482.31, 482.32, 482.39, 482.40, 482.41, 482.49, 482.81, 482.82, 482.83, 482.84, 482.89, 482.9, 483.0, 483.1, 483.8, 484.1, 484.3, 484.5, 484.6, 484.7, 484.8, 485, 486, 487.0, 487.1, 494.0, 494.1, 495.0, 495.1, 495.2, 495.3, 495.4, 495.5, 495.6, 495.7, 495.8, 495.9, 496, 500, 501, 502, 503, 504, 505, 506.0, 506.1, 506.2, 506.3, 506.4, 506.9, 507.0, 507.1, 507.8, 508.0, 508.1, 508.8, 508.9, 517.1, 518.89

031.1 Cutaneous

Buruli ulcer
Infection by Mycobacterium:
- marinum [M. balnei]
- ulcerans

031.2 Disseminated

Disseminated mycobacterium avium-intracellulare complex (DMAC)
Mycobacterium avium-intracellulare complex (MAC) bacteremia

AHA: 4Q 1997, 31

031.8 Other specified mycobacterial diseases

031.9 Unspecified diseases due to mycobacteria

Atypical mycobacterium infection NOS

❹ **032 Diphtheria**

Includes infection by Corynebacterium diphtheriae

032.0 Faucial diphtheria

Membranous angina, diphtheritic

032.1 Nasopharyngeal diphtheria

032.2 Anterior nasal diphtheria

032.3 Laryngeal diphtheria

Laryngotracheitis, diphtheritic

A Adult (15+ years) M Maternity (12-55 years) N Newborn (0 years) P Pediatric (0-17 years) ♂ Male ♀ Female ❷ Medicare Secondary Payer

❺ **032.8 Other specified diphtheria**

032.81 Conjunctival diphtheria
Pseudomembranous diphtheritic conjunctivitis

032.82 Diphtheritic myocarditis

032.83 Diphtheritic peritonitis

032.84 Diphtheritic cystitis

032.85 Cutaneous diphtheria

032.89 Other

032.9 Diphtheria, unspecified

❹ **033 Whooping cough**
Includes pertussis
Use additional code to identify any associated pneumonia (484.3)

033.0 Bordetella pertussis [B. pertussis]

033.1 Bordetella parapertussis [B. parapertussis]

033.8 Whooping cough due to other specified organism
Bordetella bronchiseptica [B. bronchiseptica]

033.9 Whooping cough, unspecified organism

❹ **034 Streptococcal sore throat and scarlet fever**

034.0 Streptococcal sore throat
Septic:
angina
sore throat
Streptococcal:
angina
laryngitis
pharyngitis
tonsillitis

034.1 Scarlet fever
Scarlatina
Excludes *parascarlatina (057.8)*

DEF: Infection with group A beta-hemolytic streptococcal bacteria causing sore throat, fever, vomiting, and rough "sandpaper" rash on the trunk.

035 Erysipelas
Excludes *postpartum or puerperal erysipelas (670)*

DEF: Superficial cellulitis with dermal lymphatic involvement, commonly caused by group A beta-hemolytic streptococci; presents with shiny, raised, indurated, tender lesions with distinct margins, commonly on the legs and face.

❹ **036 Meningococcal infection**

036.0 Meningococcal meningitis
Cerebrospinal fever (meningococcal)
Meningitis:
cerebrospinal
epidemic
C&C Exclusions: 003.21, 013.00, 013.01, 013.02, 013.03, 013.04, 013.05, 013.06, 013.10, 013.11, 013.12, 013.13, 013.14, 013.15, 013.16, 036.0, 036.89, 036.9, 041.81, 041.82, 041.83, 041.84, 041.85, 041.86, 041.89, 041.9, 047.0, 047.1, 047.8, 047.9, 049.0, 049.1, 053.0, 054.72, 072.1, 090.42, 091.81, 094.2, 098.89, 100.81, 112.83, 114.2, 115.01, 115.11, 115.91, 130.0, 139.8, 320.0, 320.1, 320.2, 320.3, 320.7, 320.81, 320.82, 320.89, 320.9, 321.0, 321.1, 321.2, 321.3, 321.4, 321.8, 322.0, 322.1, 322.2, 322.9, 349.89, 349.9, 357.0

DEF: Inflammation of the membranes (meninges) around the brain or spinal cord causing fever, headache, stiff neck, muscle aches, and skin rashes.

036.1 Meningococcal encephalitis
C&C Exclusions: 036.1, 036.89, 036.9, 041.81, 041.82, 041.83, 041.84, 041.85, 041.86, 041.89, 041.9, 139.8

036.2 Meningococcemia
Meningococcal septicemia
C&C Exclusions: 003.1, 020.2, 036.2, 036.89, 036.9, 038.0, 038.10, 038.11, 038.19, 038.2, 038.3, 038.40, 038.41, 038.42, 038.43, 038.44, 038.49, 041.81, 041.82, 041.83, 041.84, 041.85, 041.86, 041.89, 041.9, 054.5, 139.8, 995.90, 995.91, 995.92, 995.93, 995.94

036.3 Waterhouse-Friderichsen syndrome, meningococcal
Meningococcal hemorrhagic adrenalitis
Meningococcic adrenal syndrome
Waterhouse-Friderichsen syndrome NOS
C&C Exclusions: 036.3, 036.89, 036.9, 041.81, 041.82, 041.83, 041.84, 041.85, 041.86, 041.89, 041.9, 139.8

❺ **036.4 Meningococcal carditis**

036.40 Meningococcal carditis, unspecified
C&C Exclusions: 036.40, 036.89, 036.9, 041.81, 041.82, 041.83, 041.84, 041.85, 041.86, 041.89, 041.9, 139.8

036.41 Meningococcal pericarditis
C&C Exclusions: 036.41, 036.89, 036.9, 041.81, 041.82, 041.83, 041.84, 041.85, 041.86, 041.89, 041.9, 139.8

036.42 Meningococcal endocarditis
C&C Exclusions: 036.42, 036.89, 036.9, 041.81, 041.82, 041.83, 041.84, 041.85, 041.86, 041.89, 041.9, 139.8

036.43 Meningococcal myocarditis
C&C Exclusions: 036.43, 041.81, 041.82, 041.83, 041.84, 041.85, 041.86, 041.89, 041.9, 139.8

❺ **036.8 Other specified meningococcal infections**

036.81 Meningococcal optic neuritis
C&C Exclusions: 036.81, 036.89, 036.9, 041.81, 041.82, 041.83, 041.84, 041.85, 041.86, 041.89, 041.9, 139.8

036.82 Meningococcal arthropathy
C&C Exclusions: 036.82, 036.89, 036.9, 041.81, 041.82, 041.83, 041.84, 041.85, 041.86, 041.89, 041.9, 139.8

036.89 Other
C&C Exclusions: 036.89, 036.9, 041.81, 041.82, 041.83, 041.84, 041.85, 041.86, 041.89, 041.9, 139.8

✖ **036.9 Meningococcal infection, unspecified**
Meningococcal infection NOS
C&C Exclusions: 036.89, 036.9, 041.81, 041.82, 041.83, 041.84, 041.85, 041.86, 041.89, 041.9, 139.8

037 Tetanus
Excludes *tetanus:*
complicating:
abortion (634-638 with .0, 639.0)
ectopic or molar pregnancy (639.0)
neonatorum (771.3)
puerperal (670)

DEF: Potentially fatal disease due to the neurotoxin of *Clostridium tetani*, entering the body through a contaminated wound, burn, or ulcer; causes muscular contractions, hyperreflexia, lockjaw, respiratory spasm, seizures, and paralysis.

C&C Exclusions: 037, 139.8

❹ **038 Septicemia**
Use additional code for systemic inflammatory response syndrome (SIRS) (995.91-995.92)
Excludes *bacteremia (790.7)*
septicemia (sepsis) of newborn (771.81)

AHA: 2Q 2004, 16; 4Q 1988, 10; 3Q 1988, 12

038.0 Streptococcal septicemia
C&C Exclusions: 003.1, 020.2, 036.2, 038.0, 038.10, 038.11, 038.19, 038.2, 038.3, 038.40, 038.41, 038.42, 038.43, 038.44, 038.49, 038.8, 038.9, 040.82, 040.89, 041.00, 041.01, 041.02, 041.03, 041.04, 041.05, 041.09, 041.10, 041.11, 041.19, 041.2, 041.3, 041.4, 041.5, 041.6, 041.7, 041.81, 041.82, 041.83, 041.84, 041.85, 041.86, 041.89, 041.9, 054.5, 139.8, 995.90, 995.91, 995.92, 995.93, 995.94

AHA: 4Q 2003, 79; 2Q 1996, 5

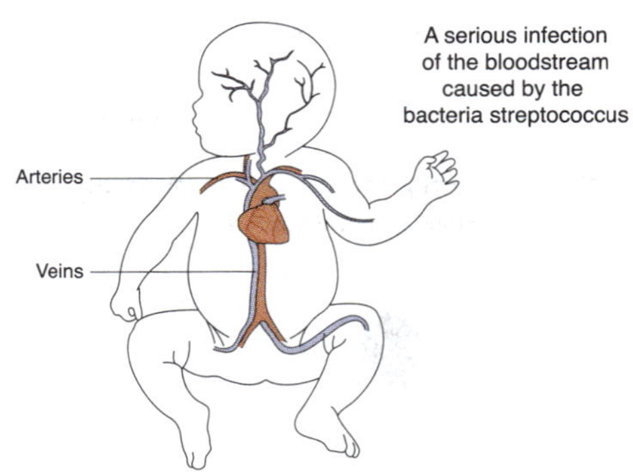

5 038.1 Staphylococcal septicemia
AHA: 4Q 1997, 32

038.10 Staphylococcal septicemia, unspecified
C&C Exclusions: See 038.0

038.11 Staphylococcus aureus septicemia
C&C Exclusions: See 038.0
AHA: 1Q 2005, 7; 2Q 2000, 5; 4Q 1998, 42

038.19 Other staphylococcal septicemia
C&C Exclusions: See 038.0
AHA: 2Q 2000, 5

038.2 Pneumococcal septicemia [Streptococcus pneumoniae septicemia]
C&C Exclusions: See 038.0
AHA: 2Q 1996, 5; 1Q 1991, 13

038.3 Septicemia due to anaerobes
Septicemia due to bacteroides
Excludes *gas gangrene (040.0)*
that due to anaerobic streptococci (038.0)
C&C Exclusions: See 038.0

5 038.4 Septicemia due to other gram-negative organisms

038.40 Gram-negative organism, unspecified
Gram-negative septicemia NOS
C&C Exclusions: See 038.0

038.41 Hemophilus influenzae [H. influenzae]
C&C Exclusions: See 038.0

038.42 Escherichia coli [E. coli]
C&C Exclusions: See 038.0
AHA: 4Q 2003, 73

038.43 Pseudomonas
C&C Exclusions: See 038.0

038.44 Serratia
C&C Exclusions: See 038.0

038.49 Other
C&C Exclusions: See 038.0

038.8 Other specified septicemias
Excludes *septicemia (due to):*
anthrax (022.3)
gonococcal (098.89)
herpetic (054.5)
meningococcal (036.2)
septicemic plague (020.2)
C&C Exclusions: See 038.0

038.9 Unspecified septicemia
Septicemia NOS
Excludes *bacteremia NOS (790.7)*
C&C Exclusions: See 038.0
AHA: 2Q 2005, 18-19; 2Q 2004, 16; 4Q 2003, 79; 2Q 2000, 3; 3Q 1999, 5, 9; 1Q 1998, 5; 3Q 1996, 16; 2Q 1996, 6

4 039 Actinomycotic infections
Includes actinomycotic mycetoma
infection by Actinomycetales, such as species of Actinomyces, Actinomadura, Nocardia, Streptomyces
maduromycosis (actinomycotic)
schizomycetoma (actinomycotic)

039.0 Cutaneous
Erythrasma
Trichomycosis axillaris

039.1 Pulmonary
Thoracic actinomycosis
C&C Exclusions: 079.82, 480.3

039.2 Abdominal

039.3 Cervicofacial

039.4 Madura foot
Excludes *madura foot due to mycotic infection (117.4)*

039.8 Of other specified sites

039.9 Of unspecified site
Actinomycosis NOS
Maduromycosis NOS
Nocardiosis NOS

4 040 Other bacterial diseases
Excludes *bacteremia NOS (790.7)*
bacterial infection NOS (041.9)

040.0 Gas gangrene
Gas bacillus infection or gangrene
Infection by Clostridium:
histolyticum
oedematiens
perfringens [welchii]
septicum
sordellii
Malignant edema
Myonecrosis, clostridial
Myositis, clostridial
C&C Exclusions: 040.0, 139.8
AHA: 1Q 1995, 11

040.1 Rhinoscleroma

040.2 Whipple's disease
Intestinal lipodystrophy

040.3 Necrobacillosis

● 5 040.4 Other specified botulism
Non-foodborne intoxication due to toxins of Clostridium botulinum [C. botulinum]
Excludes *botulism NOS (005.1)*
food poisoning due to toxins of Clostridium botulinum (005.1)

● 040.41 Infant botulism

● 040.42 Wound botulism
Non-foodborne botulism NOS
Use additional code to identify complicated open wound
DEF: Wound infection with *Clostridium botulinum* producing neurological effects of severe hypotonia and paralysis without gastrointestinal symptoms of food poisoning.

5 040.8 Other specified bacterial diseases

040.81 Tropical pyomyositis

040.82 Toxic shock syndrome
Use additional code to identify the organism
C&C Exclusions: 038.0, 038.10, 038.11, 038.19, 038.2, 038.3, 038.40, 038.41, 038.42, 038.43, 038.44, 038.49, 038.8, 038.9, 040.82, 680.0, 680.1, 680.2, 680.3, 680.4, 680.5, 680.6, 680.7, 680.8, 680.9, 682.0, 682.1, 682.2, 682.3, 682.5, 682.6, 682.7, 682.8, 682.9, 780.91, 780.92, 780.99, 785.50, 785.51, 785.59, 785.9, 799.8, 995.90, 995.91, 995.92, 995.93, 995.94
AHA: 4Q 2002, 44

040.89 Other
C&C Exclusions: 995.90, 995.91, 995.92, 995.93, 995.94
AHA: Nov-Dec 1986, 7

4 041 Bacterial infection in conditions classified elsewhere and of unspecified site
Note: *This category is provided to be used as an additional code to identify the bacterial agent in diseases classified elsewhere. This category will also be used to classify bacterial infections of unspecified nature or site.*
Excludes *bacteremia NOS (790.7)*
septicemia (038.0-038.9)
AHA: 2Q 2001, 12; Jul-Aug 1984, 19

5 041.0 Streptococcus
AHA: 1Q 2002, 3

041.00 Streptococcus, unspecified
C&C Exclusions: See 040.89

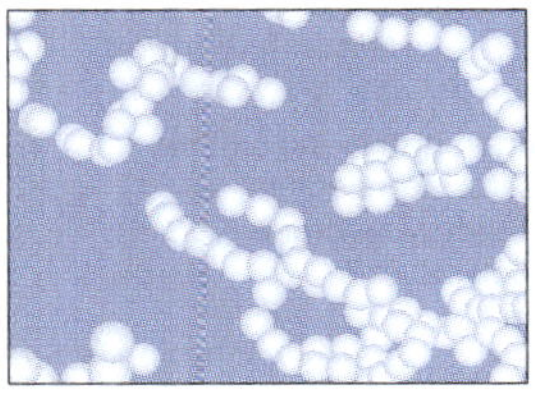

Streptococcus bacteria

Category 041 is used as a secondary code to a disease classified elsewhere in order to identify the bacterial agent involved in the infection.

041.01 Group A
C&C Exclusions: See 040.89

041.02 Group B
C&C Exclusions: See 040.89

041.03 Group C
C&C Exclusions: See 040.89

041.04 Group D [Enterococcus]
C&C Exclusions: See 040.89

041.05 Group G
C&C Exclusions: See 040.89

041.09 Other Streptococcus
C&C Exclusions: See 040.89

5 **041.1 Staphylococcus**
AHA: 4Q 2003, 104, 106; 2Q 2001, 11; 4Q 1998, 42, 54; 4Q 1997, 32

041.10 Staphylococcus, unspecified
C&C Exclusions: See 040.89
AHA: 2Q 2006, 15

041.11 Staphylococcus aureus
C&C Exclusions: See 040.89
AHA: 2Q 2006, 16

041.19 Other Staphylococcus
C&C Exclusions: See 040.89

041.2 Pneumococcus
C&C Exclusions: See 040.89

041.3 Friedländer's bacillus
Infection by Klebsiella pneumoniae
C&C Exclusions: See 040.89

041.4 Escherichia coli [E.coli]
C&C Exclusions: See 040.89

041.5 Hemophilus influenzae [H. influenzae]
C&C Exclusions: See 040.89

041.6 Proteus (mirabilis) (morganii)
C&C Exclusions: See 040.89

041.7 Pseudomonas
C&C Exclusions: See 040.89
AHA: 4Q 2002, 45

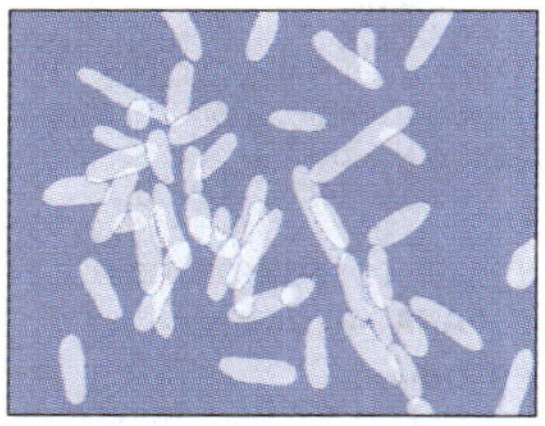

Pseudomonas is a common bacteria found in soil, water, and on the skins of humans and animals. It can cause minor skin infection or serious, life-threatening illness and can infect the blood, skin, bones, ears, eyes, urinary tract, heart valves, or lungs.

5 **041.8 Other specified bacterial infections**

041.81 Mycoplasma
Eaton's agent
Pleuropneumonia-like organisms [PPLO]
C&C Exclusions: See 040.89

041.82 Bacteroides fragilis
C&C Exclusions: See 040.89

041.83 Clostridium perfringens
C&C Exclusions: See 040.89

041.84 Other anaerobes
Gram-negative anaerobes
Excludes *Helicobacter pylori (041.86)*
C&C Exclusions: See 040.89

041.85 Other gram-negative organisms
Aerobacter aerogenes
Gram-negative bacteria NOS
Mima polymorpha
Serratia
Excludes *gram-negative anaerobes (041.84)*
AHA: 1Q 1995, 18
C&C Exclusions: See 040.89

041.86 Helicobacter pylori (H. pylori)
C&C Exclusions: See 040.89
DEF: Common gastric pathogen causing dyspepsia, gastritis, peptic ulcer disease, gastric adenocarcinoma, and gastric lymphoma.
AHA: 4Q 1995, 60

041.89 Other specified bacteria
C&C Exclusions: See 040.89
AHA: 2Q 2006, 7; 2Q 2003, 7

041.9 Bacterial infection, unspecified
C&C Exclusions: See 040.89
AHA: 2Q 1991, 9

HUMAN IMMUNODEFICIENCY VIRUS (HIV) INFECTION (042)

042 Human immunodeficiency virus [HIV] disease
Acquired immune deficiency syndrome
Acquired immunodeficiency syndrome
AIDS
AIDS-like syndrome
AIDS-related complex
ARC
HIV infection, symptomatic
Use additional code(s) to identify all manifestations of HIV
Use additional code to identify HIV-2 infection (079.53)
Excludes *asymptomatic HIV infection status (V08)*
exposure to HIV virus (V01.79)
nonspecific serologic evidence of HIV (795.71)
C&C Exclusions: 042, 139.8
AHA: 3Q 2006, 15; 1Q 2005, 7; 2Q 2004, 11; 1Q 2004, 5; 1Q 2003, 15; 1Q 1999, 14; 4Q 1997, 30-31; 1Q 1993, 21; 2Q 1992, 11; 3Q 1990, 17; Jul-Aug 1987, 8

POLIOMYELITIS AND OTHER NON-ARTHROPOD-BORNE VIRAL DISEASES OF CENTRAL NERVOUS SYSTEM (045-049)

4 **045 Acute poliomyelitis**
Excludes *late effects of acute poliomyelitis (138)*

The following fifth-digit subclassification is for use with category 045:
0 **poliovirus, unspecified type**
1 **poliovirus type I**
2 **poliovirus type II**
3 **poliovirus type III**

5 **045.0 Acute paralytic poliomyelitis specified as bulbar**
Infantile paralysis (acute) specified as bulbar
Poliomyelitis (acute) (anterior) specified as bulbar
Polioencephalitis (acute) (bulbar)
Polioencephalomyelitis (acute) (anterior) (bulbar)

5 **045.1 Acute poliomyelitis with other paralysis**
Paralysis:
acute atrophic, spinal
infantile, paralytic
Poliomyelitis (acute) with paralysis except bulbar
anterior
epidemic

5 **045.2 Acute nonparalytic poliomyelitis**
Poliomyelitis (acute) specified as nonparalytic
anterior
epidemic

5 **045.9 Acute poliomyelitis, unspecified**
Infantile paralysis unspecified whether paralytic or nonparalytic
Poliomyelitis (acute) unspecified whether paralytic or nonparalytic
anterior
epidemic

4 **046 Slow virus infection of central nervous system**

046.0 Kuru

046.1 Jakob-Creutzfeldt disease
Subacute spongiform encephalopathy

046.2 Subacute sclerosing panencephalitis
Dawson's inclusion body encephalitis
Van Bogaert's sclerosing leukoencephalitis
C&C Exclusions: 046.2, 139.8

046.3 Progressive multifocal leukoencephalopathy
Multifocal leukoencephalopathy NOS

046.8 Other specified slow virus infection of central nervous system

046.9 Unspecified slow virus infection of central nervous system

047 Meningitis due to enterovirus
Includes meningitis:
abacterial
aseptic
viral
Excludes *meningitis due to:*
adenovirus (049.1)
arthropod-borne virus (060.0-066.9)
leptospira (100.81)
virus of:
herpes simplex (054.72)
herpes zoster (053.0)
lymphocytic choriomeningitis (049.0)
mumps (072.1)
poliomyelitis (045.0-045.9)
any other infection specifically classified elsewhere

AHA: Jan-Feb 1987, 6

047.0 Coxsackie virus

047.1 ECHO virus
Meningo-eruptive syndrome

047.8 Other specified viral meningitis

047.9 Unspecified viral meningitis
Viral meningitis NOS

048 Other enterovirus diseases of central nervous system
Boston exanthem

049 Other non-arthropod-borne viral diseases of central nervous system
Excludes *late effects of viral encephalitis (139.0)*

049.0 Lymphocytic choriomeningitis
Lymphocytic:
meningitis (serous) (benign)
meningoencephalitis (serous) (benign)

049.1 Meningitis due to adenovirus

049.8 Other specified non-arthropod-borne viral diseases of central nervous system
Encephalitis:
acute:
inclusion body
necrotizing
epidemic
lethargica
Rio Bravo
von Economo's disease
Excludes ▶*human herpesvirus 6 encephalitis (058.21)*◀
▶*other human herpesvirus encephalitis (058.29)*◀

049.9 Unspecified non-arthropod-borne viral diseases of central nervous system
Viral encephalitis NOS

VIRAL DISEASES ACCOMPANIED BY EXANTHEM (050-057)

Excludes *arthropod-borne viral diseases (060.0-066.9)*
Boston exanthem (048)

050 Smallpox

050.0 Variola major
Hemorrhagic (pustular) smallpox
Malignant smallpox
Purpura variolosa

050.1 Alastrim
Variola minor

050.2 Modified smallpox
Varioloid

050.9 Smallpox, unspecified

051 Cowpox and paravaccinia

051.0 Cowpox
Vaccinia not from vaccination
Excludes *vaccinia (generalized) (from vaccination) (999.0)*

051.1 Pseudocowpox
Milkers' node

051.2 Contagious pustular dermatitis
Ecthyma contagiosum
Orf

051.9 Paravaccinia, unspecified
C&C Exclusions: 052.2

052 Chickenpox

052.0 Postvaricella encephalitis
Postchickenpox encephalitis
C&C Exclusions: 051.9, 052.0, 052.7, 052.8, 052.9, 078.88, 078.89, 079.81, 079.88, 079.89, 079.98, 079.99, 139.8

052.1 Varicella (hemorrhagic) pneumonitis
C&C Exclusions: 051.9, 052.1, 052.7, 052.8, 052.9, 078.88, 078.89, 079.81, 079.88, 079.89, 079.98, 079.99, 139.8

052.2 Postvaricella myelitis
Postchickenpox myelitis
C&C Exclusions: 052.0, 052.1, 052.2, 052.7, 052.8, 052.9, 053.14, 054.74

052.7 With other specified complications
C&C Exclusions: 051.9, 052.2, 052.7, 052.8, 052.9, 078.88, 078.89, 079.81, 079.88, 079.89, 079.98, 079.99, 139.8
AHA: 1Q 2002, 3

052.8 With unspecified complication
C&C Exclusions: See 052.7

052.9 Varicella without mention of complication
Chickenpox NOS
Varicella NOS
C&C Exclusions: See 052.7

053 Herpes zoster
Includes shingles
zona

053.0 With meningitis
C&C Exclusions: 003.21, 013.00, 013.01, 013.02, 013.03, 013.04 013.05, 013.06, 013.10, 013.11, 013.12, 013.13, 013.14 013.15, 013.16, 036.0, 047.0, 047.1, 047.8, 047.9, 049.0, 049.1, 053.0, 053.10, 053.11, 053.12, 053.13 053.14, 053.19, 053.79, 053.8, 053.9 054.72, 054.79 054.8, 054.9, 072.1, 078.88, 078.89, 079.81, 079.88 079.89, 079.98, 079.99, 090.42, 091.31, 094.2, 098.89 100.81, 112.83, 114.2, 115.01, 115.11, 115.91, 130.0, 139.8, 320.0, 320.1, 320.2, 320.3, 320.7, 320.81, 320.82 320.89, 320.9, 321.0, 321.1, 321.2, 321.3, 321.4, 321.8, 322.0, 322.1, 322.9, 349.89, 349.9, 357.0

053.1 With other nervous system complications

053.10 With unspecified nervous system complication
C&C Exclusions: 053.0, 053.10, 053.11, 053.12, 053.13, 053.14, 053.19, 053.79, 053.8, 053.9, 054.72, 054.79, 054.8, 054.9, 078.88, 078.89, 079.81, 079.88, 079.89, 079.98, 079.99, 139.8

053.11 Geniculate herpes zoster
Herpetic geniculate ganglionitis
C&C Exclusions: See 053.10

053.12 Postherpetic trigeminal neuralgia
C&C Exclusions: See 053.10

053.13 Postherpetic polyneuropathy
C&C Exclusions: See 053.10

053.14 Herpes zoster myelitis
C&C Exclusions: 052.2, 053.0, 053.10, 053.11, 053.12, 053.13, 053.14, 053.19, 053 79, 053.8, 054.74

053.19 Other
C&C Exclusions: See 053.10

⑤ **053.2 With ophthalmic complications**

Herpes zoster

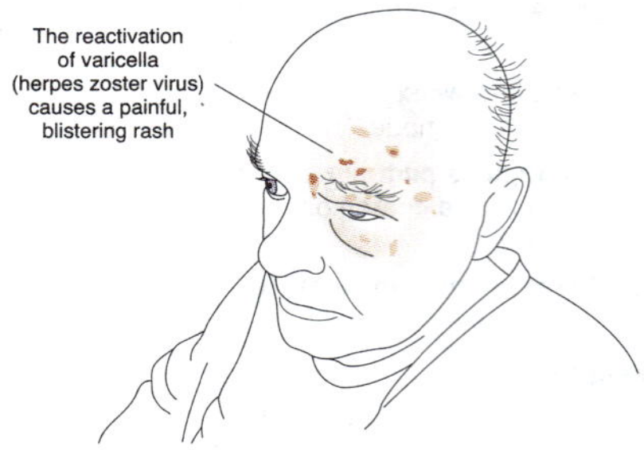

053.20 Herpes zoster dermatitis of eyelid
Herpes zoster ophthalmicus

053.21 Herpes zoster keratoconjunctivitis

053.22 Herpes zoster iridocyclitis

053.29 Other

⑤ **053.7 With other specified complications**

053.71 Otitis externa due to herpes zoster

053.79 Other
C&C Exclusions: 053.0, 053.10, 053.11, 053.12, 053.13, 053.14, 053.19, 053.20, 053.21, 053.22, 053.29, 053.71, 053.79, 053.8, 053.9, 054.0, 054.10, 054.11, 054.12, 054.13, 054.19, 054.2, 054.3, 054.40, 054.41, 054.42, 054.43, 054.44, 054.49, 054.5, 054.6, 054.71, 054.73, 054.79, 054.8, 054.9, 078.88, 078.89, 079.81, 079.88, 079.89, 079.98, 079.99, 139.8

✖ **053.8 With unspecified complication**
C&C Exclusions: See 053.7

053.9 Herpes zoster without mention of complication
Herpes zoster NOS
C&C Exclusions: 053.14

④ **054 Herpes simplex**
Excludes *congenital herpes simplex (771.2)*

054.0 Eczema herpeticum
Kaposi's varicelliform eruption
DEF: Infection with the herpes simplex virus at the site of an existing skin condition, often atopic dermatitis.

⑤ **054.1 Genital herpes**
AHA: Jan-Feb 1987, 15-16

054.10 Genital herpes, unspecified
Herpes progenitalis

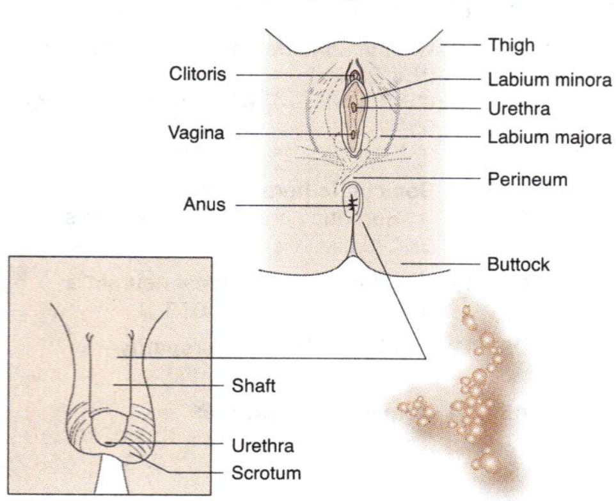

054.11 Herpetic vulvovaginitis ♀

054.12 Herpetic ulceration of vulva ♀

054.13 Herpetic infection of penis ♂

054.19 Other

054.2 Herpetic gingivostomatitis

054.3 Herpetic meningoencephalitis
Herpes encephalitis
Simian B disease
Excludes ▶*human herpesvirus 6 encephalitis (058.21)*◀
▶*other human herpesvirus encephalitis (058.29)*◀
C&C Exclusions: 054.3, 054.79, 054.8, 054.9, 139.8

⑤ **054.4 With ophthalmic complications**

✖ **054.40 With unspecified ophthalmic complication**

054.41 Herpes simplex dermatitis of eyelid

054.42 Dendritic keratitis

054.43 Herpes simplex disciform keratitis

054.44 Herpes simplex iridocyclitis

054.49 Other

054.5 Herpetic septicemia
C&C Exclusions: 003.1, 020.2, 036.2, 038.0, 038.10, 038.11, 038.19, 038.2, 038.3, 038.40, 038.41, 038.42, 038.43, 038.44, 038.49, 038.8, 038.9, 054.5, 054.79, 139.8, 995.90, 995.91, 995.92, 995.93, 995.94
AHA: 2Q 2000, 5

054.6 Herpetic whitlow
Herpetic felon

⑤ **054.7 With other specified complications**

054.71 Visceral herpes simplex
C&C Exclusions: 054.71, 054.72, 054.79, 054.8, 054.9, 139.8

054.72 Herpes simplex meningitis
C&C Exclusions: 003.21, 013.00, 013.01, 013.02, 013.03, 013.04, 013.05, 013.06, 013.10, 013.11, 013.12, 013.13, 013.14, 013.15, 013.16, 036.0, 047.0, 047.1, 047.8, 047.9, 049.0, 049.1, 053.0, 054.72, 054.79, 054.8, 054.9, 072.1, 090.42, 091.81, 094.2, 098.89, 100.81, 112.83, 114.2, 115.01, 115.11, 115.91, 130.0, 139.8, 320.0, 320.1, 320.2, 320.3, 320.7, 320.81, 320.82, 320.89, 320.9, 321.0, 321.1, 321.2, 321.3, 321.4, 321.8, 322.0, 322.1, 322.2, 322.9, 349.89, 349.9, 357.0

054.73 Herpes simplex otitis externa

054.74 Herpes simplex myelitis

054.79 Other
C&C Exclusions: 053.14, 054.74, 054.79, 054.8, 054.9, 078.88, 078.89, 079.81, 079.88, 079.89, 079.98, 079.99, 139.8

✖ **054.8 With unspecified complication**
C&C Exclusions: See 054.79

054.9 Herpes simplex without mention of complication
C&C Exclusions: 053.14, 054.74

④ **055 Measles**
Includes morbilli
rubeola

055.0 Postmeasles encephalitis
C&C Exclusions: 055.0, 055.79, 055.8, 055.9, 078.88, 078.89, 079.81, 079.88, 079.89, 079.98, 079.99, 139.8

055.1 Postmeasles pneumonia
C&C Exclusions: 055.1, 055.79, 055.8, 055.9, 078.88, 078.89, 079.81, 079.88, 079.89, 079.98, 079.99, 139.8

055.2 Postmeasles otitis media

⑤ **055.7 With other specified complications**

055.71 Measles keratoconjunctivitis
Measles keratitis
C&C Exclusions: 055.71, 055.79, 055.8, 055.9, 078.88, 078.89, 079.81, 079.88, 079.89, 079.98, 079.99, 139.8

055.79 Other
C&C Exclusions: 055.79, 055.79, 055.8, 055.9, 078.88, 078.89, 079.81, 079.88, 079.89, 079.98, 079.99, 139.8

✖ **055.8 With unspecified complication**
C&C Exclusions: 055.71, 055.79, 055.8, 055.9, 056.09, 078.88, 078.89, 079.81, 079.88, 079.89, 079.98, 079.99, 139.8

055.9 Measles without mention of complication

④ ⑤ Additional Digit Required ✖ Nonspecific PDx ⃠ Unacceptable PDx ✚ Manifestation Code ▶◀ Revised Text ● New Code ▲ Revised Code

056 Rubella
Includes German measles
Excludes *congenital rubella (771.0)*

056.0 With neurological complications

056.00 With unspecified neurological complication
C&C Exclusions: 056.00, 056.01, 056.09, 056.79, 056.8, 056.9, 078.88, 078.89, 079.81, 079.88, 079.89, 079.98, 079.99, 139.8

056.01 Encephalomyelitis due to rubella
Encephalitis due to rubella
Meningoencephalitis due to rubella
C&C Exclusions: See 056.00

056.09 Other
C&C Exclusions: See 056.00

056.7 With other specified complications

056.71 Arthritis due to rubella
C&C Exclusions: 056.71, 056.79, 056.8, 056.9, 078.88, 078.89, 079.81, 079.88, 079.89, 079.98, 079.99, 139.8

056.79 Other
C&C Exclusions: See 056.71

056.8 With unspecified complications
C&C Exclusions: 056.00, 056.01, 056.79, 056.8, 056.9, 078.88, 078.89, 079.81, 079.88, 079.89, 079.98, 079.99, 139.8

056.9 Rubella without mention of complication

057 Other viral exanthemata

057.0 Erythema infectiosum [fifth disease]

057.8 Other specified viral exanthemata
Dukes (-Filatow) disease
Fourth disease
Parascarlatina
Pseudoscarlatina
Excludes ►*exanthema subitum [sixth disease] (058.10-058.12)*◄
roseola infantum (058.10-058.12)

057.9 Viral exanthem, unspecified

OTHER HUMAN HERPESVIRUSES (058)

058 Other human herpesvirus
Excludes *congenital herpes (771.2)*
cytomegalovirus (078.5)
Epstein-Barr virus (075)
herpes NOS (054.0-054.9)
herpes simplex (054.0-054.9)
herpes zoster (053.0-053.9)
human herpesvirus NOS (054.0-054.9)
human herpesvirus 1 (054.0-054.9)
human herpesvirus 2 (054.0-054.9)
human herpesvirus 3 (052.0-053.9)
human herpesvirus 4 (075)
human herpesvirus 5 (078.5)
varicella (052.0-052.9)
varicella-zoster virus (052.0-053.9)

058.1 Roseola infantum
Exanthema subitum [sixth disease]
DEF: Common childhood herpes viral illness of mild upper respiratory symptoms, swollen glands, high fever lasting 3-7 days ending abruptly, followed by a rash.

058.10 Roseola infantum, unspecified
Exanthema subitum [sixth disease], unspecified

058.11 Roseola infantum due to human herpesvirus 6
Exanthema subitum [sixth disease] due to human herpesvirus 6

058.12 Roseola infantum due to human herpesvirus 7
Exanthema subitum [sixth disease] due to human herpesvirus 7

058.2 Other human herpesvirus encephalitis
Excludes *herpes encephalitis NOS (054.3)*
herpes simplex encephalitis (054.3)
human herpesvirus encephalitis NOS (054.3)
simian B herpesvirus encephalitis (054.3)

058.21 Human herpesvirus 6 encephalitis

058.29 Other human herpesvirus encephalitis
Human herpesvirus 7 encephalitis

058.8 Other human herpesvirus infections

058.81 Human herpesvirus 6 infection

058.82 Human herpesvirus 7 infection

058.89 Other human herpesvirus infection
Human herpesvirus 8 infection
Kaposi's sarcoma-associated herpesvirus infection

ARTHROPOD-BORNE VIRAL DISEASES (060-066)

Use additional code to identify any associated meningitis (321.2)
Excludes *late effects of viral encephalitis (139.0)*

060 Yellow fever

060.0 Sylvatic
Yellow fever:
jungle
sylvan

060.1 Urban

060.9 Yellow fever, unspecified

061 Dengue
Breakbone fever
Excludes *hemorrhagic fever caused by dengue virus (065.4)*

062 Mosquito-borne viral encephalitis

062.0 Japanese encephalitis
Japanese B encephalitis

062.1 Western equine encephalitis

062.2 Eastern equine encephalitis
Excludes *Venezuelan equine encephalitis (066.2)*

062.3 St. Louis encephalitis

062.4 Australian encephalitis
Australian arboencephalitis
Australian X disease
Murray Valley encephalitis

062.5 California virus encephalitis
Encephalitis:
California
La Crosse
Tahyna fever

062.8 Other specified mosquito-borne viral encephalitis
Encephalitis by Ilheus virus
Excludes *West Nile virus (066.40-066.49)*

062.9 Mosquito-borne viral encephalitis, unspecified

063 Tick-borne viral encephalitis
Includes diphasic meningoencephalitis

063.0 Russian spring-summer [taiga] encephalitis

063.1 Louping ill

063.2 Central European encephalitis

063.8 Other specified tick-borne viral encephalitis
Langat encephalitis
Powassan encephalitis

063.9 Tick-borne viral encephalitis, unspecified

064 Viral encephalitis transmitted by other and unspecified arthropods
Arthropod-borne viral encephalitis, vector unknown
Negishi virus encephalitis
Excludes *viral encephalitis NOS (049.9)*

065 Arthropod-borne hemorrhagic fever

065.0 Crimean hemorrhagic fever [CHF Congo virus]
Central Asian hemorrhagic fever

065.1 Omsk hemorrhagic fever

065.2 Kyasanur Forest disease

065.3 Other tick-borne hemorrhagic fever

065.4 Mosquito-borne hemorrhagic fever
Chikungunya hemorrhagic fever
Dengue hemorrhagic fever
Excludes *Chikungunya fever (066.3)*
dengue (061)
yellow fever (060.0-060.9)

065.8 Other specified arthropod-borne hemorrhagic fever
Mite-borne hemorrhagic fever

065.9 Arthropod-borne hemorrhagic fever, unspecified
Arbovirus hemorrhagic fever NOS

❹ **066 Other arthropod-borne viral diseases**

066.0 Phlebotomus fever
Changuinola fever
Sandfly fever

066.1 Tick-borne fever
Nairobi sheep disease
Tick fever:
American mountain
Colorado
Kemerovo
Quaranfil

066.2 Venezuelan equine fever
Venezuelan equine encephalitis

066.3 Other mosquito-borne fever
Fever (viral):
Bunyamwera
Bwamba
Chikungunya
Guama
Mayaro
Mucambo
O'Nyong-Nyong
Oropouche
Pixuna
Rift valley
Ross river
Wesselsbron
Zika
Excludes *dengue (061)*
yellow fever (060.0-060.9)

❺ **066.4 West Nile Fever**
AHA: 4Q 2002, 44

✖ **066.40 West Nile fever, unspecified**
West Nile fever NOS
West Nile fever without complications
West Nile virus NOS

066.41 West Nile fever with encephalitis
West Nile encephalitis
West Nile encephalomyelitis
AHA: 4Q 2004, 51

066.42 West Nile fever with other neurologic manifestation
Use additional code to specify the neurologic manifestation
AHA: 4Q 2004, 51

066.49 West Nile fever with other complications
Use additional code to specify the other conditions

066.8 Other specified arthropod-borne viral diseases
Chandipura fever
Piry fever

066.9 Arthropod-borne viral disease, unspecified
Arbovirus infection NOS

OTHER DISEASES DUE TO VIRUSES AND CHLAMYDIAE (070-079)

❹ **070 Viral hepatitis**
Includes viral hepatitis (acute) (chronic)
Excludes *cytomegalic inclusion virus hepatitis (078.5)*
AHA: 2Q, 2007, 6

070.0 Viral hepatitis A with hepatic coma

070.1 Viral hepatitis A without mention of hepatic coma
Infectious hepatitis

The following fifth-digit subclassification is for use with categories 070.2 and 070.3:
0 acute or unspecified, without mention of hepatitis delta
1 acute or unspecified, with hepatitis delta
2 chronic, without mention of hepatitis delta
3 chronic, with hepatitis delta

❺ **070.2 Viral hepatitis B with hepatic coma**
C&C Exclusions: 070.00, 070.01, 070.02, 070.03, 070.10, 070.11, 070.12, 070.13, 070.20, 070.21, 070.22, 070.23, 070.30, 070.31, 070.32, 070.33, 070.41, 070.42, 070.43, 070.44, 070.49, 070.51, 070.52, 070.53, 070.54, 070.59, 070.6, 070.9, 078.88, 078.89, 079.81, 079.88, 079.89, 079.98, 079.99, 139.8
AHA: 4Q 1991, 28

❺ **070.3 Viral hepatitis B without mention of hepatic coma**
Serum hepatitis
C&C Exclusions: See 070.2
AHA: 1Q 1993, 28; 4Q 1991, 28

❺ **070.4 Other specified viral hepatitis with hepatic coma**
AHA: 4Q 1991, 28

070.41 Acute hepatitis C with hepatic coma
C&C Exclusions: See 070.2

070.42 Hepatitis delta without mention of active hepatitis B disease with hepatic coma
Hepatitis delta with hepatitis B carrier state
C&C Exclusions: See 070.2

070.43 Hepatitis E with hepatic coma
C&C Exclusions: See 070.2

070.44 Chronic hepatitis C with hepatic coma
C&C Exclusions: See 070.2
AHA: 2Q, 2007, 7

070.49 Other specified viral hepatitis with hepatic coma
C&C Exclusions: See 070.2

❺ **070.5 Other specified viral hepatitis without mention of hepatic coma**
AHA: 4Q 1991, 28

070.51 Acute hepatitis C without mention of hepatic coma
C&C Exclusions: See 070.2

070.52 Hepatitis delta without mention of active hepatitis B disease or hepatic coma
C&C Exclusions: See 070.2

070.53 Hepatitis E without mention of hepatic coma
C&C Exclusions: See 070.2

070.54 Chronic hepatitis C without mention of hepatic coma
C&C Exclusions: See 070.2
AHA: 2Q 2006, 13

070.59 Other specified viral hepatitis without mention of hepatic coma
C&C Exclusions: See 070.2

070.6 Unspecified viral hepatitis with hepatic coma
Excludes *unspecified viral hepatitis C with hepatic coma (070.71)*
C&C Exclusions: See 070.2

❺ **070.7 Unspecified viral hepatitis C**

✖ **070.70 Unspecified viral hepatitis C without hepatic coma**
Unspecified viral hepatitis C NOS
C&C Exclusions: See 070.2
AHA: 4Q 2004, 52

✖ **070.71 Unspecified viral hepatitis C with hepatic coma**
C&C Exclusions: See 070.2
AHA: 4Q 2004, 52

070.9 Unspecified viral hepatitis without mention of hepatic coma
Viral hepatitis NOS
Excludes *unspecified viral hepatitis C without hepatic coma (070.70)*
C&C Exclusions: See 070.2

071 Rabies
Hydrophobia
Lyssa

❹ **072 Mumps**

072.0 Mumps orchitis ♂
C&C Exclusions: 072.0, 072.79, 072.8, 072.9, 078.88, 078.89, 079.81, 079.88, 079.89, 079.98, 079.99, 139.8

072.1 Mumps meningitis
C&C Exclusions: 003.21, 013.00, 013.01, 013.02, 013.03, 013.04, 013.05, 013.06, 013.10, 013.11, 013.12, 013.13, 013.14, 013.15, 013.16, 036.0, 047.0, 047.1, 047.8, 047.9, 049.0, 049.1, 053.0, 054.72, 072.1, 072.8, 072.9, 078.88, 078.89, 079.81, 079.88, 079.89, 079.98, 079.99, 090.42, 091.81, 094.2, 098.89, 100.81, 112.83, 114.2, 115.01, 115.11, 115.91, 130.0, 139.8, 320.0, 320.1, 320.2, 320.3, 320.7, 320.81, 320.82, 320.89, 320.9, 321.0, 321.1, 321.2, 321.3, 321.4, 321.8, 322.0, 322.1, 322.2, 322.9, 349.89, 349.9, 357.0

072.2 Mumps encephalitis
Mumps meningoencephalitis
C&C Exclusions: 072.2, 072.79, 072.8, 072.9, 078.88, 078.89, 079.81, 079.88, 079.89, 079.98, 079.99, 139.8

072.3 Mumps pancreatitis
C&C Exclusions: 072.3, 072.79, 072.8, 072.9, 078.88, 078.89, 079.81, 079.88, 079.89, 079.98, 079.99, 139.8

❺ **072.7 Mumps with other specified complications**

072.71 Mumps hepatitis
C&C Exclusions: 072.71, 072.79, 072.8, 072.9, 078.88, 078.89, 079.81, 079.88, 079.89, 079.98, 079.99, 139.8

072.72 Mumps polyneuropathy
C&C Exclusions: 072.72, 072.79, 072.8, 072.9, 078.88, 078.89, 079.81, 079.88, 079.89, 079.98, 079.99, 139.8

072.79 Other
C&C Exclusions: 072.79, 072.8, 072.9, 078.88, 078.89, 079.81, 079.88, 079.89, 079.98, 079.99, 139.8

✖ **072.8 Mumps with unspecified complication**
C&C Exclusions: 072.79, 072.8, 072.9, 078.88, 078.89, 079.81, 079.88, 079.89, 079.98, 079.99, 139.8

072.9 Mumps without mention of complication
Epidemic parotitis
Infectious parotitis

❹ **073 Ornithosis**
Includes parrot fever
psittacosis

073.0 With pneumonia
Lobular pneumonitis due to ornithosis

073.7 With other specified complications

✖ **073.8 With unspecified complication**

073.9 Ornithosis, unspecified

❹ **074 Specific diseases due to Coxsackie virus**
Excludes *Coxsackie virus:*
infection NOS (079.2)
meningitis (047.0)

074.0 Herpangina
Vesicular pharyngitis

074.1 Epidemic pleurodynia
Bornholm disease
Devil's grip
Epidemic:
myalgia
myositis

❺ **074.2 Coxsackie carditis**

✖ **074.20 Coxsackie carditis, unspecified**

074.21 Coxsackie pericarditis

074.22 Coxsackie endocarditis

074.23 Coxsackie myocarditis
Aseptic myocarditis of newborn

074.3 Hand, foot, and mouth disease
Vesicular stomatitis and exanthem

074.8 Other specified diseases due to Coxsackie virus
Acute lymphonodular pharyngitis

075 Infectious mononucleosis
Glandular fever
Monocytic angina
Pfeiffer's disease
AHA: 3Q 2001, 13; Mar-Apr 1987, 8

❹ **076 Trachoma**
Excludes *late effect of trachoma (139.1)*

076.0 Initial stage
Trachoma dubium

076.1 Active stage
Granular conjunctivitis (trachomatous)
Trachomatous:
follicular conjunctivitis
pannus

076.9 Trachoma, unspecified
Trachoma NOS

❹ **077 Other diseases of conjunctiva due to viruses and Chlamydiae**
Excludes *ophthalmic complications of viral diseases classified elsewhere*

077.0 Inclusion conjunctivitis
Paratrachoma
Swimming pool conjunctivitis
Excludes *inclusion blennorrhea (neonatal) (771.6)*

077.1 Epidemic keratoconjunctivitis
Shipyard eye

077.2 Pharyngoconjunctival fever
Viral pharyngoconjunctivitis

077.3 Other adenoviral conjunctivitis
Acute adenoviral follicular conjunctivitis

077.4 Epidemic hemorrhagic conjunctivitis
Apollo:
conjunctivitis
disease
Conjunctivitis due to enterovirus type 70
Hemorrhagic conjunctivitis (acute) (epidemic)

077.8 Other viral conjunctivitis
Newcastle conjunctivitis

❺ **077.9 Unspecified diseases of conjunctiva due to viruses and Chlamydiae**

077.98 Due to Chlamydiae

077.99 Due to viruses
Viral conjunctivitis NOS

❹ **078 Other diseases due to viruses and Chlamydiae**
Excludes *viral infection NOS (079.0-079.9)*
viremia NOS (790.8)

078.0 Molluscum contagiosum

❺ **078.1 Viral warts**
Viral warts due to human papillomavirus
AHA: 2Q 1997, 9; 4Q 1993, 22

078.10 Viral warts, unspecified
Condyloma NOS
Verruca NOS:
NOS
Vulgaris
Warts (infectious)

078.11 Condyloma acuminatum

078.19 Other specified viral warts
Genital warts NOS
Verruca:
plana
plantaris

078.2 Sweating fever
Miliary fever
Sweating disease

078.3 Cat-scratch disease
Benign lymphoreticulosis (of inoculation)
Cat-scratch fever

078.4 Foot and mouth disease
Aphthous fever
Epizootic:
aphthae
stomatitis

078.5 Cytomegaloviral disease
Cytomegalic inclusion disease
Salivary gland virus disease
Use additional code to identify manifestation, as:
cytomegalic inclusion virus:
hepatitis (573.1)
pneumonia (484.1)
Excludes *congenital cytomegalovirus infection (771.1)*
AHA: 1Q 2003, 10; 3Q 1998, 4; 2Q 1993, 11; 1Q 1989, 9

078.6 Hemorrhagic nephrosonephritis
Hemorrhagic fever:
epidemic
Korean
Russian
with renal syndrome

078.7 Arenaviral hemorrhagic fever
Hemorrhagic fever:
Argentine
Bolivian
Junin virus
Machupo virus

⑤ **078.8 Other specified diseases due to viruses and Chlamydiae**
Excludes *epidemic diarrhea (009.2)*
lymphogranuloma venereum (099.1)

078.81 Epidemic vertigo

078.82 Epidemic vomiting syndrome
Winter vomiting disease

078.88 Other specified diseases due to Chlamydiae
C&C Exclusions: 052.2, 053.14, 054.74
AHA: 4Q 1996, 22

078.89 Other specified diseases due to viruses
Epidemic cervical myalgia
Marburg disease
Tanapox
C&C Exclusions: See 078.88

④ **079 Viral and chlamydial infection in conditions classified elsewhere and of unspecified site**
Note: *This category is provided to be used as an additional code to identify the viral agent in diseases classifiable elsewhere. This category will also be used to classify virus infection of unspecified nature or site.*

079.0 Adenovirus
C&C Exclusions: See 078.88

079.1 ECHO virus
C&C Exclusions: See 078.88

079.2 Coxsackie virus
C&C Exclusions: See 078.88

079.3 Rhinovirus
C&C Exclusions: See 078.88

079.4 Human papillomavirus
C&C Exclusions: See 078.88
AHA: 2Q 1997, 9; 4Q 1993, 22

⑤ **079.5 Retrovirus**
Excludes *human immunodeficiency virus, type 1 [HIV-1] (042)*
human T-cell lymphotrophic virus, type III [HTLV-III] (042)
lymphadenopathy-associated virus [LAV] (042)
AHA: 4Q 1993, 22-23

079.50 Retrovirus, unspecified
C&C Exclusions: See 078.88

079.51 Human T-cell lymphotrophic virus, type I [HTLV-I]
C&C Exclusions: See 078.88

079.52 Human T-cell lymphotrophic virus, type II [HTLV-II]
C&C Exclusions: See 078.88

079.53 Human immunodeficiency virus, type 2 [HIV-2]
C&C Exclusions: See 078.88

079.59 Other specified retrovirus
C&C Exclusions: See 078.88

079.6 Respiratory syncytial virus (RSV)
C&C Exclusions: See 078.88
AHA: 4Q 1996, 27-28

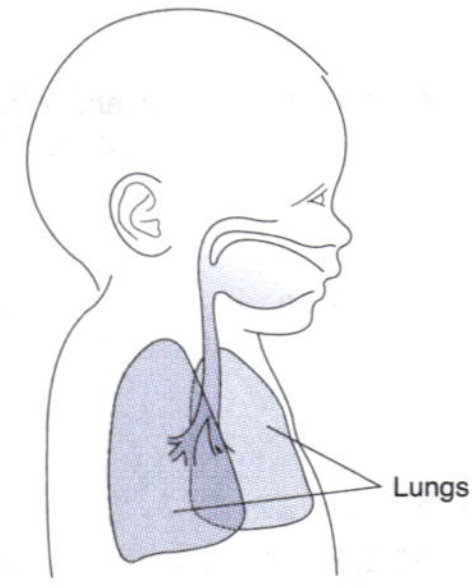

RSV is a common cause of many types of infections of the respiratory system, including bronchitis, bronchiolitis, pneumonia and croup. They occur most commonly and are most severe in infants, young children and the elderly.

⑤ **079.8 Other specified viral and chlamydial infections**
AHA: 1Q 1988, 12

079.81 Hantavirus
C&C Exclusions: See 078.88
AHA: 4Q 1995, 60

079.82 SARS-associated coronavirus
C&C Exclusions: 011.00, 011.01, 011.02, 011.03, 011.04, 011.05, 011.06, 011.10, 011.11, 011.12, 011.13, 011.14, 011.15, 011.16, 011.20, 011.21, 011.22, 011.23, 011.24, 011.25, 011.26, 011.30, 011.31, 011.32, 011.33, 011.34, 011.35, 011.36, 011.40, 011.41, 011.42, 011.43, 011.44, 011.45, 011.46, 011.50, 011.51, 011.52, 011.53, 011.54, 011.55, 011.56, 011.60, 011.61, 011.62, 011.63, 011.64, 011.65, 011.66, 011.70, 011.71, 011.72, 011.73, 011.74, 011.75, 011.76, 011.80, 011.81, 011.82, 011.83, 011.84, 011.85, 011.86, 011.90, 011.91, 011.92, 011.93, 011.94, 011.95, 011.96, 012.00, 012.01, 012.02, 012.03, 012.04, 012.05, 012.06, 012.10, 012.11, 012.12, 012.13, 012.14, 012.15, 012.16, 012.80, 012.81, 012.82, 012.83, 012.84, 012.85, 012.86, 017.90, 017.91, 017.92, 017.93, 017.94, 017.95, 017.96, 021.2, 031.0, 039.1, 079.82, 079.89, 115.05, 115.15, 115.95, 122.1, 130.4, 136.3, 480.0, 480.1, 480.2, 480.8, 480.9, 481, 482.0, 482.1, 482.2, 482.30, 482.31, 482.32, 482.39, 482.40, 482.41, 482.49, 482.81, 482.82, 482.83, 482.84, 482.89, 482.9, 483.0, 483.1, 483.8, 484.1, 484.3, 484.5, 484.6, 484.7, 484.8, 485, 486, 487.0, 487.1, 494.0, 494.1, 495.0, 495.1, 495.2, 495.3, 495.4, 495.5, 495.6, 495.7, 495.8, 495.9, 496, 500, 501, 502, 503, 504, 505, 506.0, 506.1, 506.2, 506.3, 506.4, 506.9, 507.0, 507.1, 507.8, 508.0, 508.1, 508.8, 508.9, 517.1, 517.8, 518.89, 519.8, 519.9
AHA: 4Q 2003, 46

● **079.83 Parvovirus B19**
Human parvovirus
Parvovirus NOS
Excludes *erythema infectiosum [fifth disease] (057.0)*

079.88 Other specified chlamydial infection
C&C Exclusions: 052.2, 053.14, 054.74

079.89 Other specified viral infection
C&C Exclusions: 052.2, 053.14, 054.74

⑤ **079.9 Unspecified viral and chlamydial infections**
Excludes *viremia NOS (790.8)*
AHA: 2Q 1991, 8

079.98 Unspecified chlamydial infection
Chlamydial infection NOS
C&C Exclusions: 052.2, 053.14, 054.74

079.99 Unspecified viral infection
Viral infection NOS
C&C Exclusions: 052.2, 053.14, 054.74

RICKETTSIOSES AND OTHER ARTHROPOD-BORNE DISEASES (080-088)

Excludes *arthropod-borne viral diseases (060.0-066.9)*

080 Louse-borne [epidemic] typhus
Typhus (fever):
classical
epidemic
exanthematic NOS
louse-borne

❹ **081 Other typhus**

081.0 Murine [endemic] typhus
Typhus (fever):
endemic
flea-borne

081.1 Brill's disease
Brill-Zinsser disease
Recrudescent typhus (fever)

081.2 Scrub typhus
Japanese river fever
Kedani fever
Mite-borne typhus
Tsutsugamushi

081.9 Typhus, unspecified
Typhus (fever) NOS

❹ **082 Tick-borne rickettsioses**

082.0 Spotted fevers
Rocky mountain spotted fever
Sao Paulo fever

082.1 Boutonneuse fever
African tick typhus
India tick typhus
Kenya tick typhus
Marseilles fever
Mediterranean tick fever

082.2 North Asian tick fever
Siberian tick typhus

082.3 Queensland tick typhus

❺ **082.4 Ehrlichiosis**
AHA: 4Q 2000, 38

✖ **082.40 Ehrlichiosis, unspecified**

082.41 Ehrlichiosis chaffeensis [E. chaffeensis]

082.49 Other ehrlichiosis

082.8 Other specified tick-borne rickettsioses
Lone star fever
AHA: 4Q 1999, 19

082.9 Tick-borne rickettsiosis, unspecified
Tick-borne typhus NOS

❹ **083 Other rickettsioses**

083.0 Q fever

083.1 Trench fever
Quintan fever
Wolhynian fever

083.2 Rickettsialpox
Vesicular rickettsiosis

083.8 Other specified rickettsioses

083.9 Rickettsiosis, unspecified

❹ **084 Malaria**
Note: Subcategories 084.0-084.6 exclude the listed conditions with mention of pernicious complications (084.8-084.9).
Excludes *congenital malaria (771.2)*

084.0 Falciparum malaria [malignant tertian]
Malaria (fever):
by Plasmodium falciparum
subtertian

084.1 Vivax malaria [benign tertian]
Malaria (fever) by Plasmodium vivax

084.2 Quartan malaria
Malaria (fever) by Plasmodium malariae
Malariae malaria

084.3 Ovale malaria
Malaria (fever) by Plasmodium ovale

084.4 Other malaria
Monkey malaria

084.5 Mixed malaria
Malaria (fever) by more than one parasite

084.6 Malaria, unspecified
Malaria (fever) NOS

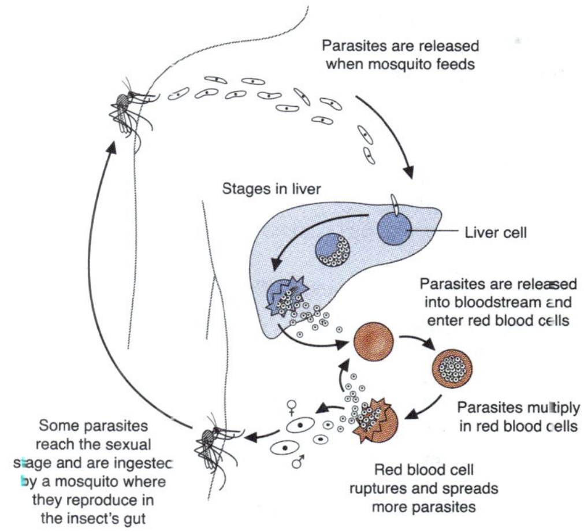

084.7 Induced malaria
Therapeutically induced malaria
Excludes *accidental infection from syringe, blood transfusion, etc. (084.0-084.6, above, according to parasite species)*
transmission from mother to child during delivery (771.2)

084.8 Blackwater fever
Hemoglobinuric:
fever (bilious)
malaria
Malarial hemoglobinuria

084.9 Other pernicious complications of malaria
Algid malaria
Cerebral malaria
Use additional code to identify complication, as:
malarial:
hepatitis (573.2)
nephrosis (581.81)

❹ **085 Leishmaniasis**

085.0 Visceral [kala-azar]
Dumdum fever
Infection by Leishmania:
donovani
infantum
Leishmaniasis:
dermal, post-kala-azar
Mediterranean
visceral (Indian)

085.1 Cutaneous, urban
Aleppo boil
Baghdad boil
Delhi boil
Infection by Leishmania tropica (minor)
Leishmaniasis, cutaneous:
dry form
late
recurrent
ulcerating
Oriental sore

085.2 Cutaneous, Asian desert
Infection by Leishmania tropica major
Leishmaniasis, cutaneous:
acute necrotizing
rural
wet form
zoonotic form

085.3 Cutaneous, Ethiopian
Infection by Leishmania ethiopica
Leishmaniasis, cutaneous:
diffuse
lepromatous

085.4 Cutaneous, American
Chiclero ulcer
Infection by Leishmania mexicana
Leishmaniasis tegumentaria diffusa

085.5 Mucocutaneous (American)
Espundia
Infection by Leishmania braziliensis
Uta

085.9 Leishmaniasis, unspecified

4 086 Trypanosomiasis
Use additional code to identify manifestations, as:
trypanosomiasis:
encephalitis (323.2)
meningitis (321.3)

086.0 Chagas' disease with heart involvement
American trypanosomiasis with heart involvement
Infection by Trypanosoma cruzi with heart involvement
Any condition classifiable to 086.2 with heart involvement
C&C Exclusions: 086.0, 139.8

086.1 Chagas' disease with other organ involvement
American trypanosomiasis with involvement of organ other than heart
Infection by Trypanosoma cruzi with involvement of organ other than heart
Any condition classifiable to 086.2 with involvement of organ other than heart

086.2 Chagas' disease without mention of organ involvement
American trypanosomiasis
Infection by Trypanosoma cruzi

086.3 Gambian trypanosomiasis
Gambian sleeping sickness
Infection by Trypanosoma gambiense

086.4 Rhodesian trypanosomiasis
Infection by Trypanosoma rhodesiense
Rhodesian sleeping sickness

086.5 African trypanosomiasis, unspecified
Sleeping sickness NOS

086.9 Trypanosomiasis, unspecified

4 087 Relapsing fever
Includes recurrent fever

087.0 Louse-borne

087.1 Tick-borne

087.9 Relapsing fever, unspecified

4 088 Other arthropod-borne diseases

088.0 Bartonellosis
Carrión's disease
Oroya fever
Verruga peruana

5 088.8 Other specified arthropod-borne diseases
AHA: 4Q 1991, 15; 3Q 1990, 14; 2Q 1989, 10

088.81 Lyme disease
Erythema chronicum migrans
DEF: Tick-transmitted infection caused by *Borrelia burgdorferi*, manifesting with erythema chronicum migrans, myalgia, arthritis of the large joints, and nervous and cardiovascular system involvement.

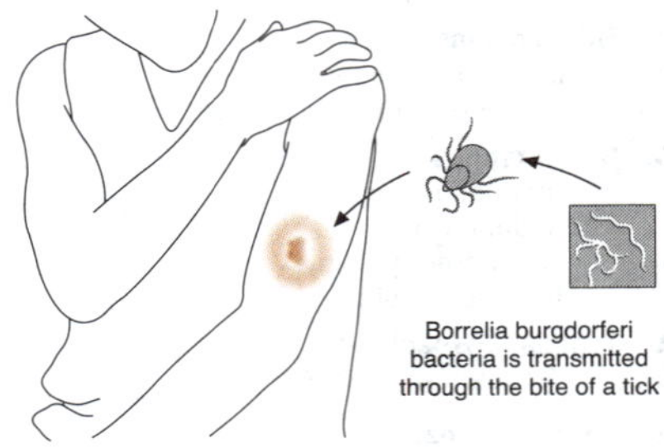

088.82 Babesiosis
Babesiasis
AHA: 4Q 1993, 23

088.89 Other

088.9 Arthropod-borne disease, unspecified

SYPHILIS AND OTHER VENEREAL DISEASES (090-099)

Excludes *nonvenereal endemic syphilis (104.0)*
urogenital trichomoniasis (131.0)

4 090 Congenital syphilis

090.0 Early congenital syphilis, symptomatic
Congenital syphilitic:
choroiditis
coryza (chronic)
hepatomegaly
mucous patches
periostitis
splenomegaly
Syphilitic (congenital):
epiphysitis
osteochondritis
pemphigus
Any congenital syphilitic condition specified as early or manifest less than two years after birth

090.1 Early congenital syphilis, latent
Congenital syphilis without clinical manifestations, with positive serological reaction and negative spinal fluid test, less than two years after birth

090.2 Early congenital syphilis, unspecified
Congenital syphilis NOS, less than two years after birth

090.3 Syphilitic interstitial keratitis
Syphilitic keratitis:
parenchymatous
punctata profunda
Excludes *interstitial keratitis NOS (370.50)*

5 **090.4 Juvenile neurosyphilis**
Use additional code to identify any associated mental disorder

090.40 Juvenile neurosyphilis, unspecified
Congenital neurosyphilis
Dementia paralytica juvenilis
Juvenile:
general paresis
tabes
taboparesis
C&C Exclusions: 090.0, 090.1, 090.2, 090.3, 090.40, 090.41, 090.42, 090.49, 090.5, 090.6, 090.7, 090.9, 091.0, 091.1, 091.2, 091.3, 091.4, 091.50, 091.51, 091.52, 091.61, 091.62, 091.69, 091.7, 091.81, 091.82, 091.89, 091.9, 092.0, 092.9, 093.0, 093.1, 093.20, 093.21, 093.22, 093.23, 093.24, 093.81, 093.82, 093.89, 093.9, 094.0, 094.1, 094.2, 094.3, 094.81, 094.82, 094.83, 094.84, 094.85, 094.86, 094.87, 094.89, 095.0, 095.1, 095.2, 095.3, 095.4, 095.5, 095.6, 095.7, 095.8, 095.9, 096, 097.0, 097.1, 097.9, 099.40, 099.41, 099.49, 099.50, 099.51, 099.52, 099.53, 099.54, 099.55, 099.56, 099.59, 099.8, 099.9, 139.8

090.41 Congenital syphilitic encephalitis
C&C Exclusions: See 090.40

090.42 Congenital syphilitic meningitis
C&C Exclusions: 003.21, 013.00, 013.01, 013.02, 013.03, 013.04, 013.05, 013.06, 013.10, 013.11, 013.12, 013.13, 013.14, 013.15, 013.16, 036.0, 047.0, 047.1, 047.8, 047.9, 049.0, 049.1, 053.0, 054.72, 072.1, 090.0, 090.1, 090.2, 090.3, 090.40, 090.41, 090.42, 090.49, 090.5, 090.6, 090.7, 090.9, 091.0, 091.1, 091.2, 091.3, 091.4, 091.50, 091.51, 091.52, 091.61, 091.62, 091.69, 091.7, 091.81, 091.82, 091.89, 091.9, 092.0, 092.9, 093.0, 093.1, 093.20, 093.21, 093.22, 093.23, 093.24, 093.81, 093.82, 093.89, 093.9, 094.0, 094.1, 094.2, 094.3, 094.81, 094.82, 094.83, 094.84, 094.85, 094.86, 094.87, 094.89, 095.0, 095.1, 095.2, 095.3, 095.4, 095.5, 095.6, 095.7, 095.8, 095.9, 096, 097.0, 097.1, 097.9, 099.40, 099.41, 099.49, 099.50, 099.51, 099.52, 099.53, 099.54, 099.55, 099.56, 099.59, 099.8, 099.9, 100.81, 112.83, 114.2, 115.01, 115.11, 115.91, 130.0, 139.8, 320.0, 320.1, 320.2, 320.3, 320.7, 320.81, 320.82, 320.89, 320.9, 321.0, 321.1, 321.2, 321.3, 321.4, 321.8, 322.0, 322.1, 322.2, 322.9, 349.89, 349.9, 357.0

090.49 Other
C&C Exclusions: See 090.40

090.5 Other late congenital syphilis, symptomatic
Gumma due to congenital syphilis
Hutchinson's teeth
Syphilitic saddle nose
Any congenital syphilitic condition specified as late or manifest two years or more after birth

090.6 Late congenital syphilis, latent
Congenital syphilis without clinical manifestations, with positive serological reaction and negative spinal fluid test, two years or more after birth

090.7 Late congenital syphilis, unspecified
Congenital syphilis NOS, two years or more after birth

090.9 Congenital syphilis, unspecified

4 **091 Early syphilis, symptomatic**
Excludes *early cardiovascular syphilis (093.0-093.9)*
early neurosyphilis (094.0-094.9)

091.0 Genital syphilis (primary)
Genital chancre

091.1 Primary anal syphilis

091.2 Other primary syphilis
Primary syphilis of:
breast
fingers
lip
tonsils

091.3 Secondary syphilis of skin or mucous membranes
Condyloma latum
Secondary syphilis of:
anus
mouth
pharynx
skin
tonsils
vulva

091.4 Adenopathy due to secondary syphilis
Syphilitic adenopathy (secondary)
Syphilitic lymphadenitis (secondary)

5 **091.5 Uveitis due to secondary syphilis**

091.50 Syphilitic uveitis, unspecified

091.51 Syphilitic chorioretinitis (secondary)

091.52 Syphilitic iridocyclitis (secondary)

5 **091.6 Secondary syphilis of viscera and bone**

091.61 Secondary syphilitic periostitis

091.62 Secondary syphilitic hepatitis
Secondary syphilis of liver

091.69 Other viscera

091.7 Secondary syphilis, relapse
Secondary syphilis, relapse (treated) (untreated)

5 **091.8 Other forms of secondary syphilis**

091.81 Acute syphilitic meningitis (secondary)

091.82 Syphilitic alopecia

091.89 Other

091.9 Unspecified secondary syphilis

4 **092 Early syphilis, latent**
Includes syphilis (acquired) without clinical manifestations, with positive serological reaction and negative spinal fluid test, less than two years after infection

092.0 Early syphilis, latent, serological relapse after treatment

092.9 Early syphilis, latent, unspecified

4 **093 Cardiovascular syphilis**

093.0 Aneurysm of aorta, specified as syphilitic
Dilatation of aorta, specified as syphilitic

093.1 Syphilitic aortitis

5 **093.2 Syphilitic endocarditis**

093.20 Valve, unspecified
Syphilitic ostial coronary disease
C&C Exclusions: See 090.40

093.21 Mitral valve
C&C Exclusions: See 090.40

093.22 Aortic valve
Syphilitic aortic incompetence or stenosis
C&C Exclusions: See 090.40

093.23 Tricuspid valve
C&C Exclusions: See 090.40

093.24 Pulmonary valve
C&C Exclusions: See 090.40

5 **093.8 Other specified cardiovascular syphilis**

093.81 Syphilitic pericarditis
C&C Exclusions: See 090.40

093.82 Syphilitic myocarditis
C&C Exclusions: See 090.40

093.89 Other
C&C Exclusions: See 090.40

093.9 Cardiovascular syphilis, unspecified
C&C Exclusions: See 090.40

094 Neurosyphilis
Use additional code to identify any associated mental disorder

094.0 Tabes dorsalis
Locomotor ataxia (progressive)
Posterior spinal sclerosis (syphilitic)
Tabetic neurosyphilis
Use additional code to identify manifestation, as:
neurogenic arthropathy [Charcot's joint disease] (713.5)
C&C Exclusions: See 090.40

094.1 General paresis
Dementia paralytica
General paralysis (of the insane) (progressive)
Paretic neurosyphilis
Taboparesis
C&C Exclusions: See 090.40

094.2 Syphilitic meningitis
Meningovascular syphilis
Excludes *acute syphilitic meningitis (secondary) (091.81)*
C&C Exclusions: See 090.42

094.3 Asymptomatic neurosyphilis
C&C Exclusions: See 090.40

094.8 Other specified neurosyphilis

094.81 Syphilitic encephalitis
C&C Exclusions: See 090.40

094.82 Syphilitic Parkinsonism

094.83 Syphilitic disseminated retinochoroiditis

094.84 Syphilitic optic atrophy

094.85 Syphilitic retrobulbar neuritis

094.86 Syphilitic acoustic neuritis

094.87 Syphilitic ruptured cerebral aneurysm
C&C Exclusions: See 090.40

094.89 Other
C&C Exclusions: See 090.40

094.9 Neurosyphilis, unspecified
Gumma (syphilitic) of central nervous system NOS
Syphilis (early) (late) of central nervous system NOS
Syphiloma of central nervous system NOS
C&C Exclusions: See 090.40

095 Other forms of late syphilis, with symptoms
Includes gumma (syphilitic)
tertiary, or unspecified stage

095.0 Syphilitic episcleritis

095.1 Syphilis of lung

095.2 Syphilitic peritonitis

095.3 Syphilis of liver

095.4 Syphilis of kidney

095.5 Syphilis of bone

095.6 Syphilis of muscle
Syphilitic myositis

095.7 Syphilis of synovium, tendon, and bursa
Syphilitic:
bursitis
synovitis

095.8 Other specified forms of late symptomatic syphilis
Excludes *cardiovascular syphilis (093.0-093.9)*
neurosyphilis (094.0-094.9)

095.9 Late symptomatic syphilis, unspecified

096 Late syphilis, latent
Syphilis (acquired) without clinical manifestations, with positive serological reaction and negative spinal fluid test, two years or more after infection

097 Other and unspecified syphilis

097.0 Late syphilis, unspecified

097.1 Latent syphilis, unspecified
Positive serological reaction for syphilis

097.9 Syphilis, unspecified
Syphilis (acquired) NOS
Excludes *syphilis NOS causing death under two years of age (090.9)*

098 Gonococcal infections

098.0 Acute, of lower genitourinary tract
Gonococcal:
Bartholinitis (acute)
urethritis (acute)
vulvovaginitis (acute)
Gonorrhea (acute):
NOS
genitourinary (tract) NOS
C&C Exclusions: 098.0, 098.10, 098.11, 098.12, 098.13, 098.14, 098.15, 098.16, 098.17, 098.19, 098.2, 098.30, 098.31, 098.32, 098.33, 098.34, 098.35, 098.36, 098.37, 098.39, 098.89, 099.40, 099.41, 099.49, 099.50, 099.51, 099.52, 099.53, 099.54, 099.55, 099.56, 099.59, 099.8, 099.9, 139.8

098.1 Acute, of upper genitourinary tract

098.10 Gonococcal infection (acute) of upper genitourinary tract, site unspecified
C&C Exclusions: See 098.0

098.11 Gonococcal cystitis (acute)
Gonorrhea (acute) of bladder
C&C Exclusions: See 098.0

098.12 Gonococcal prostatitis (acute) ♂
C&C Exclusions: See 098.0

098.13 Gonococcal epididymo-orchitis (acute) ♂
Gonococcal orchitis (acute)
C&C Exclusions: See 098.0

098.14 Gonococcal seminal vesiculitis (acute) ♂
Gonorrhea (acute) of seminal vesicle
C&C Exclusions: See 098.0

098.15 Gonococcal cervicitis (acute) ♀
Gonorrhea (acute) of cervix
C&C Exclusions: See 098.0

098.16 Gonococcal endometritis (acute) ♀
Gonorrhea (acute) of uterus
C&C Exclusions: See 098.0

098.17 Gonococcal salpingitis, specified as acute ♀
C&C Exclusions: See 098.0

098.19 Other
C&C Exclusions: See 098.0

098.2 Chronic, of lower genitourinary tract
Gonococcal specified as chronic or with duration of two months or more:
Bartholinitis specified as chronic or with duration of two months or more
urethritis specified as chronic or with duration of two months or more
vulvovaginitis specified as chronic or with duration of two months or more
Gonorrhea specified as chronic or with duration of two months or more:
NOS specified as chronic or with duration of two months or more
genitourinary (tract) specified as chronic or with duration of two months or more
Any condition classifiable to 098.0 specified as chronic or with duration of two months or more

098.3 Chronic, of upper genitourinary tract
Any condition classifiable to 098.1 stated as chronic or with a duration of two months or more

098.30 Chronic gonococcal infection of upper genitourinary tract, site unspecified

098.31 Gonococcal cystitis, chronic
Any condition classifiable to 098.11, specified as chronic
Gonorrhea of bladder, chronic

098.32 Gonococcal prostatitis, chronic ♂
Any condition classifiable to 098.12, specified as chronic

098.33 Gonococcal epididymo-orchitis, chronic ♂
Any condition classifiable to 098.13, specified as chronic
Chronic gonococcal orchitis

Additional Digit Required · Nonspecific PDx · Unacceptable PDx · Manifestation Code · Revised Text · New Code · Revised Code

098.34 Gonococcal seminal vesiculitis, chronic ♂
Any condition classifiable to 098.14, specified as chronic
Gonorrhea of seminal vesicle, chronic

098.35 Gonococcal cervicitis, chronic ♀
Any condition classifiable to 098.15, specified as chronic
Gonorrhea of cervix, chronic

098.36 Gonococcal endometritis, chronic ♀
Any condition classifiable to 098.16, specified as chronic

098.37 Gonococcal salpingitis (chronic) ♀

098.39 Other

5 **098.4 Gonococcal infection of eye**

098.40 Gonococcal conjunctivitis (neonatorum)
Gonococcal ophthalmia (neonatorum)

098.41 Gonococcal iridocyclitis

098.42 Gonococcal endophthalmia

098.43 Gonococcal keratitis

098.49 Other

5 **098.5 Gonococcal infection of joint**

098.50 Gonococcal arthritis
Gonococcal infection of joint NOS

098.51 Gonococcal synovitis and tenosynovitis

098.52 Gonococcal bursitis

098.53 Gonococcal spondylitis

098.59 Other
Gonococcal rheumatism

098.6 Gonococcal infection of pharynx

098.7 Gonococcal infection of anus and rectum
Gonococcal proctitis

5 **098.8 Gonococcal infection of other specified sites**

098.81 Gonococcal keratosis (blennorrhagica)

098.82 Gonococcal meningitis

098.83 Gonococcal pericarditis

098.84 Gonococcal endocarditis

098.85 Other gonococcal heart disease

098.86 Gonococcal peritonitis

098.89 Other
Gonococcemia

4 **099 Other venereal diseases**

099.0 Chancroid
Bubo (inguinal):
- chancroidal
- due to Hemophilus ducreyi

Chancre:
- Ducrey's
- simple
- soft

Ulcus molle (cutis) (skin)

099.1 Lymphogranuloma venereum
Climatic or tropical bubo
(Durand-) Nicolas-Favre disease
Esthiomene
Lymphogranuloma inguinale

DEF: Sexually transmitted infection by *Chlamydia trachomatis*, seen in warm climates; presents with primary cutaneous or mucosal lesion at infection site and acute unilateral or bilateral lymphadenopathy.

099.2 Granuloma inguinale
Donovanosis
Granuloma pudendi (ulcerating)
Granuloma venereum
Pudendal ulcer

099.3 Reiter's disease
Reiter's syndrome
Use additional code for associated:
- arthropathy (711.1)
- conjunctivitis (372.33)

5 **099.4 Other nongonococcal urethritis [NGU]**

099.40 Unspecified
Nonspecific urethritis

099.41 Chlamydia trachomatis

099.49 Other specified organism

5 **099.5 Other venereal diseases due to Chlamydia trachomatis**
Excludes *Chlamydia trachomatis infection of conjunctiva (076.0-076.9, 077.0, 077.9)*
Lymphogranuloma venereum (099.1)

✖ **099.50 Unspecified site**

099.51 Pharynx

099.52 Anus and rectum

099.53 Lower genitourinary sites
Excludes *urethra (099.41)*
Use additional code to specify site of infection, such as:
- bladder (595.4)
- cervix (616.0)
- vagina and vulva (616.11)

099.54 Other genitourinary sites
Use additional code to specify site of infection, such as:
- pelvic inflammatory disease NOS (614.9)
- testis and epididymis (604.91)

099.55 Unspecified genitourinary site

099.56 Peritoneum
Perihepatitis

099.59 Other specified site

099.8 Other specified venereal diseases

✖ **099.9 Venereal disease, unspecified**

OTHER SPIROCHETAL DISEASES (100-104)

4 **100 Leptospirosis**

100.0 Leptospirosis icterohemorrhagica
Leptospiral or spirochetal jaundice (hemorrhagic)
Weil's disease

5 **100.8 Other specified leptospiral infections**

100.81 Leptospiral meningitis (aseptic)

100.89 Other
Fever:
- Fort Bragg
- pretibial
- swamp

Infection by Leptospira:
- australis
- bataviae
- pyrogenes

✖ **100.9 Leptospirosis, unspecified**

101 Vincent's angina
Acute necrotizing ulcerative:
- gingivitis
- stomatitis

Fusospirochetal pharyngitis
Spirochetal stomatitis
Trench mouth
Vincent's:
- gingivitis
- infection [any site]

4 **102 Yaws**
Includes frambesia
pian

102.0 Initial lesions
Chancre of yaws
Frambesia, initial or primary
Initial frambesial ulcer
Mother yaw

102.1 Multiple papillomata and wet crab yaws
Butter yaws
Frambesioma
Pianoma
Plantar or palmar papilloma of yaws

102.2 Other early skin lesions
Early yaws (cutaneous) (macular) (papular) (maculopapular) (micropapular)
Frambeside of early yaws
Cutaneous yaws, less than five years after infection

102.3 Hyperkeratosis
Ghoul hand
Hyperkeratosis, palmar or plantar (early) (late) due to yaws
Worm-eaten soles

102.4 Gummata and ulcers
Gummatous frambeside
Nodular late yaws (ulcerated)

102.5 Gangosa
Rhinopharyngitis mutilans

102.6 Bone and joint lesions
Goundou of yaws (late)
Gumma, bone of yaws (late)
Gummatous osteitis or periostitis of yaws (late)
Hydrarthrosis of yaws (early) (late)
Osteitis of yaws (early) (late)
Periostitis (hypertrophic) of yaws (early) (late)

102.7 Other manifestations
Juxta-articular nodules of yaws
Mucosal yaws

102.8 Latent yaws
Yaws without clinical manifestations, with positive serology

102.9 Yaws, unspecified

4 **103 Pinta**

103.0 Primary lesions
Chancre (primary) of pinta [carate]
Papule (primary) of pinta [carate]
Pintid of pinta [carate]

103.1 Intermediate lesions
Erythematous plaques of pinta [carate]
Hyperchromic lesions of pinta [carate]
Hyperkeratosis of pinta [carate]

103.2 Late lesions
Cardiovascular lesions of pinta [carate]
Skin lesions of pinta [carate]:
achromic of pinta [carate]
cicatricial of pinta [carate]
dyschromic of pinta [carate]
Vitiligo of pinta [carate]

103.3 Mixed lesions
Achromic and hyperchromic skin lesions of pinta [carate]

103.9 Pinta, unspecified

4 **104 Other spirochetal infection**

104.0 Nonvenereal endemic syphilis
Bejel
Njovera

104.8 Other specified spirochetal infections
Excludes *relapsing fever (087.0-087.9)*
syphilis (090.0-097.9)

104.9 Spirochetal infection, unspecified

MYCOSES (110-118)

Use additional code to identify manifestation, as:
arthropathy (711.6)
meningitis (321.0-321.1)
otitis externa (380.15)
Excludes *infection by Actinomycetales, such as species of Actinomyces, Actinomadura, Nocardia, Streptomyces (039.0-039.9)*

4 **110 Dermatophytosis**
Includes infection by species of Epidermophyton, Microsporum, and Trichophyton
tinea, any type except those in 111

110.0 Of scalp and beard
Kerion
Sycosis, mycotic
Trichophytic tinea [black dot tinea], scalp

110.1 Of nail
Dermatophytic onychia
Onychomycosis
Tinea unguium

Dermatophytosis of the nail
A fungal infection of the skin caused by a parasitic fungus occuring under a finger or toe nail

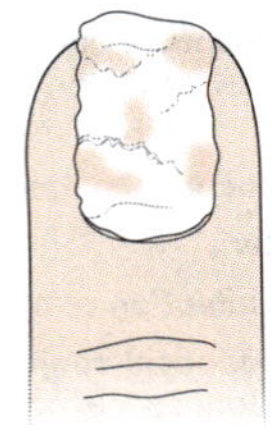

110.2 Of hand
Tinea manuum

110.3 Of groin and perianal area
Dhobie itch
Eczema marginatum
Tinea cruris

DEF: Fungal infection of the groin commonly known as jock itch.

110.4 Of foot
Athlete's foot
Tinea pedis

110.5 Of the body
Herpes circinatus
Tinea imbricata [Tokelau]

110.6 Deep seated dermatophytosis
Granuloma trichophyticum
Majocchi's granuloma

110.8 Of other specified sites

✖ **110.9 Of unspecified site**
Favus NOS
Microsporic tinea NOS
Ringworm NOS

4 **111 Dermatomycosis, other and unspecified**

111.0 Pityriasis versicolor
Infection by Malassezia [Pityrosporum] furfur
Tinea flava
Tinea versicolor

111.1 Tinea nigra
Infection by Cladosporium species
Keratomycosis nigricans
Microsporosis nigra
Pityriasis nigra
Tinea palmaris nigra

111.2 Tinea blanca
Infection by Trichosporon (beigelii) cutaneum
White piedra

111.3 Black piedra
Infection by Piedraia hortai

111.8 Other specified dermatomycoses

111.9 Dermatomycosis, unspecified

❹ 112 Candidiasis

Includes infection by Candida species
moniliasis

Excludes *neonatal monilial infection (771.7)*

112.0 Of mouth
Thrush (oral)
C&C Exclusions: 112.0, 112.1, 112.2, 112.3, 112.4, 112.5, 112.81, 112.82, 112.83, 112.84, 112.85, 112.89, 117.9, 139.8

Candidiasis of the mouth (thrush)

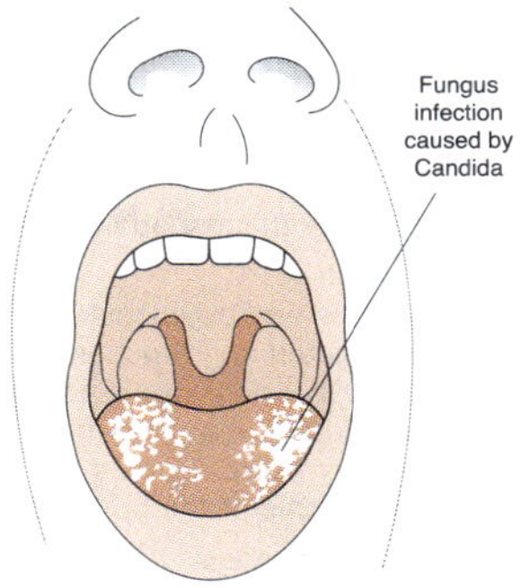

112.1 Of vulva and vagina ♀
Candidal vulvovaginitis
Monilial vulvovaginitis

112.2 Of other urogenital sites
Candidal balanitis
AHA: 4Q 2003, 105; 4Q 1996, 33

112.3 Of skin and nails
Candidal intertrigo
Candidal onychia
Candidal perionyxis [paronychia]

112.4 Of lung
Candidal pneumonia
C&C Exclusions: See 112.0
AHA: 2Q 1998, 7

112.5 Disseminated
Systemic candidiasis
C&C Exclusions: See 112.0
AHA: 2Q 2000, 5; 2Q 1989, 10

❺ 112.8 Of other specified sites

112.81 Candidal endocarditis
C&C Exclusions: See 112.0

112.82 Candidal otitis externa
Otomycosis in moniliasis
C&C Exclusions: See 112.0

112.83 Candidal meningitis
C&C Exclusions: 003.21, 013.00, 013.01, 013.02, 013.03, 013.04, 013.05, 013.06, 013.10, 013.11, 013.12, 013.13, 013.14, 013.15, 013.16, 036.0, 047.0, 047.1, 047.8, 047.9, 049.0, 049.1, 053.0, 054.72, 072.1, 090.42, 091.81, 094.2, 098.89, 100.81, 112.0, 112.1, 112.2, 112.3, 112.4, 112.5, 112.81, 112.82, 112.83, 112.84, 112.85, 112.89, 114.2, 115.01, 115.11, 115.91, 117.9, 130.0, 139.8, 320.0, 320.1, 320.2, 320.3, 320.7, 320.81, 320.82, 320.89, 320.9, 321.0, 321.1, 321.2, 321.3, 321.4, 321.8, 322.0, 322.1, 322.2, 322.9, 349.89, 349.9, 357.0

112.84 Candidal esophagitis
C&C Exclusions: See 112.0
AHA: 4Q 1992, 19

112.85 Candidal enteritis
C&C Exclusions: See 112.0
AHA: 4Q 1992, 19

112.89 Other
AHA: 1Q 1992, 17; 3Q 1991, 20

✖ **112.9 Of unspecified site**

❹ 114 Coccidioidomycosis

Includes infection by Coccidioides (immitis)
Posada-Wernicke disease

AHA: 4Q 1993, 23

114.0 Primary coccidioidomycosis (pulmonary)
Acute pulmonary coccidioidomycosis
Coccidioidomycotic pneumonitis
Desert rheumatism
Pulmonary coccidioidomycosis
San Joaquin Valley fever
C&C Exclusions: 114.0, 114.3, 114.4, 114.5, 114.9, 117.9, 139.8

A respiratory disease caused by inhaling the fungus Coccidioides immitis

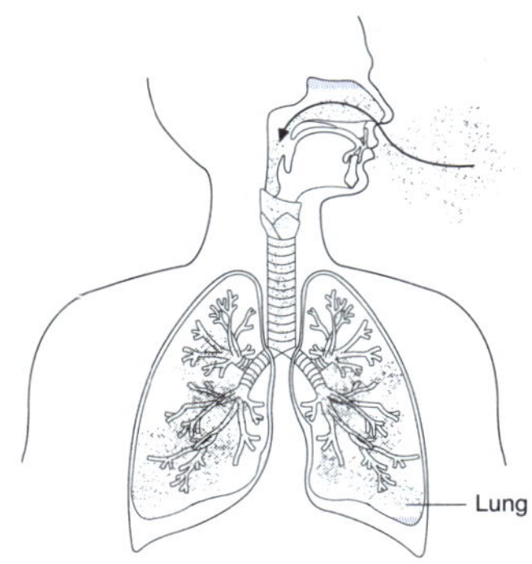

114.1 Primary extrapulmonary coccidioidomycosis
Chancriform syndrome
Primary cutaneous coccidioidomycosis

114.2 Coccidioidal meningitis
C&C Exclusions: 003.21, 013.00, 013.01, 013.02, 013.03, 013.04, 013.05, 013.06, 013.10, 013.11, 013.12, 013.13, 013.14, 013.15, 013.16, 036.0, 047.0, 047.1, 047.8, 047.9, 049.0, 049.1, 053.0, 054.72, 072.1, 090.42, 091.81, 094.2, 098.89, 100.81, 112.83, 114.2, 114.3, 114.4, 114.5, 114.9, 115.01, 115.11, 115.91, 117.9, 130.0, 139.8, 320.0, 320.1, 320.2, 320.3, 320.7, 320.81, 320.82, 320.89, 320.9, 321.0, 321.1, 321.2, 321.3, 321.4, 321.8, 322.0, 322.1, 322.2, 322.9, 349.89, 349.9, 357.0

114.3 Other forms of progressive coccidioidomycosis
Coccidioidal granuloma
Disseminated coccidioidomycosis
C&C Exclusions: 114.3, 114.9, 117.9, 139.8

114.4 Chronic pulmonary coccidioidomycosis

114.5 Pulmonary coccidioidomycosis, unspecified

✖ **114.9 Coccidioidomycosis, unspecified**
C&C Exclusions: See 114.3

❹ 115 Histoplasmosis

The following fifth-digit subclassification is for use with category 115:

- **0** **without mention of manifestation**
- **1** **meningitis**
- **2** **retinitis**
- **3** **pericarditis**
- **4** **endocarditis**
- **5** **pneumonia**
- **9** **other**

❺ 115.0 Infection by Histoplasma capsulatum
American histoplasmosis
Darling's disease
Reticuloendothelial cytomycosis
Small form histoplasmosis
C&C Exclusions: (for code 115.00) 115.00, 115.09, 115.90, 115.99, 117.9, 139.8
C&C Exclusions: (for code 115.01) 003.21, 013.00, 013.01, 013.02, 013.03, 013.04, 013.05, 013.06, 013.10, 013.11, 013.12, 013.13, 013.14, 013.15, 013.16, 036.0, 047.0, 047.1, 047.8, 047.9, 049.0, 049.1, 053.0, 054.72, 072.1, 090.42, 091.81, 094.2, 098.89, 100.81, 112.83, 114.2, 115.00, 115.01, 115.11, 115.90, 115.91, 115.99, 117.9, 130.0, 137.1, 139.8, 320.0, 320.1, 320.2, 320.3, 320.7, 320.81, 320.82, 320.89, 320.9, 321.0, 321.1, 321.2, 321.3, 321.4, 321.8, 322.0, 322.1, 322.2, 322.9, 349.89, 349.9, 357.0

C&C Exclusions: (for code 115.02) 115.00, 115.02, 115.09, 115.90, 115.92, 115.99, 117.9, 139.8
C&C Exclusions: (for code 115.03) 115.00, 115.03, 115.09, 115.90, 115.93, 115.99, 117.9, 139.8
C&C Exclusions: (for code 115.04) 115.00, 115.04, 115.09, 115.90, 115.94, 115.99, 117.9, 139.8
C&C Exclusions: (for code 115.05) 079.82, 115.00, 115.05, 115.09, 115.90, 115.95, 115.99, 117.9, 139.8, 480.0, 480.1, 480.2, 480.3, 480.8, 480.9, 481, 482.0, 482.1, 482.2, 482.30, 482.31, 482.32, 482.39, 482.40, 482.41, 482.49, 482.81, 482.82, 482.83, 482.84, 482.89, 482.9, 483.0, 483.1, 483.8, 484.1, 484.3, 484.5, 484.6, 484.7, 484.8, 485, 486, 487.0, 487.1, 494.0, 494.1, 495.0, 495.1, 495.2, 495.3, 495.4, 495.5, 495.6, 495.7, 495.8, 495.9, 496, 500, 501, 502, 503, 504, 505, 506.0, 506.1, 506.2, 506.3, 506.4, 506.9, 507.0, 507.1, 507.8, 508.0, 508.1, 508.8, 508.9, 517.1, 518.89

5 **115.1 Infection by Histoplasma duboisii**
African histoplasmosis
Large form histoplasmosis
C&C Exclusions: (for code 115.10) 115.10, 115.19, 115.90, 115.99, 117.9, 139.8
C&C Exclusions: (for code 115.11) 003.21, 013.00, 013.01, 013.02, 013.03, 013.04, 013.05, 013.06, 013.10, 013.11, 013.12, 013.13, 013.14, 013.15, 013.16, 036.0, 047.0, 047.1, 047.8, 047.9, 049.0, 049.1, 053.0, 054.72, 072.1, 090.42, 091.81, 094.2, 098.89, 100.81, 112.83, 114.2, 115.01, 115.10, 115.11, 115.19, 115.90, 115.91, 115.99, 117.9, 130.0, 137.1, 139.8, 320.0, 320.1, 320.2, 320.3, 320.7, 320.81, 320.82, 320.89, 320.9, 321.0, 321.1, 321.2, 321.3, 321.4, 321.8, 322.0, 322.1, 322.2, 322.9, 349.89, 349.9, 357.0
C&C Exclusions: (for code 115.12) 115.10, 115.12, 115.19, 115.90, 115.92, 115.99, 117.9, 139.8
C&C Exclusions: (for code 115.13) 115.10, 115.13, 115.19, 115.90, 115.93, 115.99, 117.9, 139.8
C&C Exclusions: (for code 115.14) 115.10, 115.14, 115.19, 115.90, 115.94, 115.99, 117.9, 139.8
C&C Exclusions: (for code 115.15) 079.82, 115.05, 115.10, 115.15, 115.19, 115.90, 115.95, 115.99, 117.9, 139.8, 480.0, 480.1, 480.2, 480.3, 480.8, 480.9, 481, 482.0, 482.1, 482.2, 482.30, 482.31, 482.32, 482.39, 482.40, 482.41, 482.49, 482.81, 482.82, 482.83, 482.84, 482.89, 482.9, 483.0, 483.1, 483.8, 484.1, 484.3, 484.5, 484.6, 484.7, 484.8, 485, 486, 487.0, 487.1, 494.0, 494.1, 495.0, 495.1, 495.2, 495.3, 495.4, 495.5, 495.6, 495.7, 495.8, 495.9, 496, 500, 501, 502, 503, 504, 505, 506.0, 506.1, 506.2, 506.3, 506.4, 506.9, 507.0, 507.1, 507.8, 508.0, 508.1, 508.8, 508.9, 517.1, 518.89

5 **115.9 Histoplasmosis, unspecified**
Histoplasmosis NOS
C&C Exclusions: (for code 115.90) 115.90, 115.99, 117.9, 139.8
C&C Exclusions: (for code 115.91) 003.21, 013.00, 013.01, 013.02, 013.03, 013.04, 013.05, 013.06, 013.10, 013.11, 013.12, 013.13, 013.14, 013.15, 013.16, 036.0, 047.0, 047.1, 047.8, 047.9, 049.0, 049.1, 053.0, 054.72, 072.1, 090.42, 091.81, 094.2, 098.89, 100.81, 112.83, 114.2, 115.01, 115.11, 115.91, 115.99, 117.9, 130.0, 137.1, 139.8, 320.0, 320.1, 320.2, 320.3, 320.7, 320.81, 320.82, 320.89, 320.9, 321.0, 321.1, 321.2, 321.3, 321.4, 321.8, 322.0, 322.1, 322.2, 322.9, 349.89, 349.9, 357.0
C&C Exclusions: (for code 115.92) 115.92, 115.99, 117.9, 139.8
C&C Exclusions: (for code 115.93) 115.93, 115.99, 117.9, 139.8
C&C Exclusions: (for code 115.94) 115.94, 115.99, 117.9, 139.8
C&C Exclusions: (for code 115.95) 079.82, 115.05, 115.15, 115.95, 115.99, 117.9, 139.8, 480.3
C&C Exclusions: (for code 115.99) 115.99, 117.9, 139.8

4 **116 Blastomycotic infection**

116.0 Blastomycosis
Blastomycotic dermatitis
Chicago disease
Cutaneous blastomycosis
Disseminated blastomycosis
Gilchrist's disease
Infection by Blastomyces [Ajellomyces] dermatitidis
North American blastomycosis
Primary pulmonary blastomycosis
C&C Exclusions: 116.0, 117.9, 139.8

116.1 Paracoccidioidomycosis
Brazilian blastomycosis
Infection by Paracoccidioides [Blastomyces] brasiliensis
Lutz-Splendore-Almeida disease
Mucocutaneous-lymphangitic paracoccidioidomycosis
Pulmonary paracoccidioidomycosis
South American blastomycosis
Visceral paracoccidioidomycosis
C&C Exclusions: 116.1, 117.9, 139.8

116.2 Lobomycosis
Infections by Loboa [Blastomyces] loboi
Keloidal blastomycosis
Lobo's disease

4 **117 Other mycoses**

117.0 Rhinosporidiosis
Infection by Rhinosporidium seeberi

117.1 Sporotrichosis
Cutaneous sporotrichosis
Disseminated sporotrichosis
Infection by Sporothrix [Sporotrichum] schenckii
Lymphocutaneous sporotrichosis
Pulmonary sporotrichosis
Sporotrichosis of the bones

117.2 Chromoblastomycosis
Chromomycosis
Infection by Cladosporidium carrionii, Fonsecaea compactum, Fonsecaea pedrosoi, Phialophora verrucosa

117.3 Aspergillosis
Infection by Aspergillus species, mainly A. fumigatus, A. flavus group, A. terreus group
C&C Exclusions: 117.3, 117.9, 139.8
AHA: 4Q 1997, 40

117.4 Mycotic mycetomas
Infection by various genera and species of Ascomycetes and Deuteromycetes, such as Acremonium [Cephalosporium] falciforme, Neotestudina rosatii, Madurella grisea, Madurella mycetomii, Pyrenochaeta romeroi, Zopfia [Leptosphaeria] senegalensis
Madura foot, mycotic
Maduromycosis, mycotic
Excludes *actinomycotic mycetomas (039.0-039.9)*
C&C Exclusions: 117.4, 117.9, 139.8

117.5 Cryptococcosis
Busse-Buschke's disease
European cryptococcosis
Infection by Cryptococcus neoformans
Pulmonary cryptococcosis
Systemic cryptococcosis
Torula
C&C Exclusions: 117.5, 117.9, 139.8

117.6 Allescheriosis [Petriellidosis]
Infections by Allescheria [Petriellidium] boydii [Monosporium apiospermum]
Excludes *mycotic mycetoma (117.4)*
C&C Exclusions: 117.6, 117.9, 139.8

117.7 Zygomycosis [Phycomycosis or Mucormycosis]
Infection by species of Absidia, Basidiobolus, Conidiobolus, Cunninghamella, Entomophthora, Mucor, Rhizopus, Saksenaea
C&C Exclusions: 117.7, 117.9, 139.8

117.8 Infection by dematiacious fungi [Phaehyphomycosis]
Infection by dematiacious fungi, such as Cladosporium trichoides [bantianum], Dreschlera hawaiiensis, Phialophora gougerotii, Phialophora jeanselmi

117.9 Other and unspecified mycoses

118 Opportunistic mycoses
Infection of skin, subcutaneous tissues, and/or organs by a wide variety of fungi generally considered to be pathogenic to compromised hosts only (e.g., infection by species of Alternaria, Dreschlera, Fusarium)
C&C Exclusions: 117.9, 118, 139.8

HELMINTHIASES (120-129)

❹ **120 Schistosomiasis [bilharziasis]**

120.0 Schistosoma haematobium
Vesical schistosomiasis NOS

120.1 Schistosoma mansoni
Intestinal schistosomiasis NOS

120.2 Schistosoma japonicum
Asiatic schistosomiasis NOS
Katayama disease or fever

120.3 Cutaneous
Cercarial dermatitis
Infection by cercariae of Schistosoma
Schistosome dermatitis
Swimmers' itch

120.8 Other specified schistosomiasis
Infection by Schistosoma:
- bovis
- intercalatum
- mattheii
- spindale

Schistosomiasis chestermani

120.9 Schistosomiasis, unspecified
Blood flukes NOS
Hemic distomiasis

❹ **121 Other trematode infections**

121.0 Opisthorchiasis
Infection by:
- cat liver fluke
- Opisthorchis (felineus) (tenuicollis) (viverrini)

121.1 Clonorchiasis
Biliary cirrhosis due to clonorchiasis
Chinese liver fluke disease
Hepatic distomiasis due to Clonorchis sinensis
Oriental liver fluke disease

121.2 Paragonimiasis
Infection by Paragonimus
Lung fluke disease (oriental)
Pulmonary distomiasis

121.3 Fascioliasis
Infection by Fasciola:
- gigantica
- hepatica

Liver flukes NOS
Sheep liver fluke infection

121.4 Fasciolopsiasis
Infection by Fasciolopsis (buski)
Intestinal distomiasis

121.5 Metagonimiasis
Infection by Metagonimus yokogawai

121.6 Heterophyiasis
Infection by:
- Heterophyes heterophyes
- Stellantchasmus falcatus

121.8 Other specified trematode infections
Infection by:
- Dicrocoelium dendriticum
- Echinostoma ilocanum
- Gastrodiscoides hominis

121.9 Trematode infection, unspecified
Distomiasis NOS
Fluke disease NOS

❹ **122 Echinococcosis**
Includes echinococciasis
hydatid disease
hydatidosis

122.0 Echinococcus granulosus infection of liver

122.1 Echinococcus granulosus infection of lung
C&C Exclusions: 079.82, 480.3

122.2 Echinococcus granulosus infection of thyroid

122.3 Echinococcus granulosus infection, other

122.4 Echinococcus granulosus infection, unspecified

122.5 Echinococcus multilocularis infection of liver

122.6 Echinococcus multilocularis infection, other

122.7 Echinococcus multilocularis infection, unspecified

122.8 Echinococcosis, unspecified, of liver

122.9 Echinococcosis, other and unspecified

❹ **123 Other cestode infection**

123.0 Taenia solium infection, intestinal form
Pork tapeworm (adult) (infection)

123.1 Cysticercosis
Cysticerciasis
Infection by Cysticercus cellulosae [larval form of Taenia solium]
AHA: 2Q 1997, 8

123.2 Taenia saginata infection
Beef tapeworm (infection)
Infection by Taeniarhynchus saginatus

123.3 Taeniasis, unspecified

123.4 Diphyllobothriasis, intestinal
Diphyllobothrium (adult) (latum) (pacificum) infection
Fish tapeworm (infection)

123.5 Sparganosis [larval diphyllobothriasis]
Infection by:
- Diphyllobothrium larvae
- Sparganum (mansoni) (proliferum)
- Spirometra larvae

123.6 Hymenolepiasis
Dwarf tapeworm (infection)
Hymenolepis (diminuta) (nana) infection
Rat tapeworm (infection)

123.8 Other specified cestode infection
Diplogonoporus (grandis) infection
Dipylidium (caninum) infection
Dog tapeworm (infection)

123.9 Cestode infection, unspecified
Tapeworm (infection) NOS

124 Trichinosis
Trichinella spiralis infection
Trichinellosis
Trichiniasis

❹ **125 Filarial infection and dracontiasis**

125.0 Bancroftian filariasis
Chyluria due to Wuchereria bancrofti
Elephantiasis due to Wuchereria bancrofti
Infection due to Wuchereria bancrofti
Lymphadenitis due to Wuchereria bancrofti
Lymphangitis due to Wuchereria bancrofti
Wuchereriasis

125.1 Malayan filariasis
Brugia filariasis due to Brugia [Wuchereria] malayi
Chyluria due to Brugia [Wuchereria] malayi
Elephantiasis due to Brugia [Wuchereria] malayi
Infection due to Brugia [Wuchereria] malayi
Lymphadenitis due to Brugia [Wuchereria] malayi
Lymphangitis due to Brugia [Wuchereria] malayi

125.2 Loiasis
Eyeworm disease of Africa
Loa loa infection

125.3 Onchocerciasis
Onchocerca volvulus infection
Onchocercosis

125.4 Dipetalonemiasis
Infection by:
- Acanthocheilonema perstans
- Dipetalonema perstans

125.5 Mansonella ozzardi infection
Filariasis ozzardi

125.6 Other specified filariasis
Dirofilaria infection
Infection by:
- Acanthocheilonema streptocerca
- Dipetalonema streptocerca

125.7 Dracontiasis
Guinea-worm infection
Infection by Dracunculus medinensis

125.9 Unspecified filariasis

❹ **126 Ancylostomiasis and necatoriasis**
Includes cutaneous larva migrans due to Ancylostoma
hookworm (disease) (infection)
uncinariasis

126.0 Ancylostoma duodenale

126.1 Necator americanus

126.2 Ancylostoma braziliense

126.3 Ancylostoma ceylanicum

126.8 Other specified Ancylostoma

126.9 Ancylostomiasis and necatoriasis, unspecified
Creeping eruption NOS
Cutaneous larva migrans NOS

❹ **127 Other intestinal helminthiases**

127.0 Ascariasis
Ascaridiasis
Infection by Ascaris lumbricoides
Roundworm infection

127.1 Anisakiasis
Infection by Anisakis larva

127.2 Strongyloidiasis
Infection by Strongyloides stercoralis
Excludes *trichostrongyliasis (127.6)*

127.3 Trichuriasis
Infection by Trichuris trichiuria
Trichocephaliasis
Whipworm (disease) (infection)

127.4 Enterobiasis
Infection by Enterobius vermicularis
Oxyuriasis
Oxyuris vermicularis infection
Pinworm (disease) (infection)
Threadworm infection

127.5 Capillariasis
Infection by Capillaria philippinensis
Excludes *infection by Capillaria hepatica (128.8)*

127.6 Trichostrongyliasis
Infection by Trichostrongylus species

127.7 Other specified intestinal helminthiasis
Infection by:
Oesophagostomum apiostomum and related species
Ternidens diminutus
Other specified intestinal helminth
Physalopteriasis

127.8 Mixed intestinal helminthiasis
Infection by intestinal helminths classified to more than one of the categories 120.0-127.7
Mixed helminthiasis NOS

✖ **127.9 Intestinal helminthiasis, unspecified**

❹ **128 Other and unspecified helminthiases**

128.0 Toxocariasis
Larva migrans visceralis
Toxocara (canis) (cati) infection
Visceral larva migrans syndrome

128.1 Gnathostomiasis
Infection by Gnathostoma spinigerum and related species

128.8 Other specified helminthiasis
Infection by:
Angiostrongylus cantonensis
Capillaria hepatica
other specified helminth

128.9 Helminth infection, unspecified
Helminthiasis NOS
Worms NOS

✖ **129 Intestinal parasitism, unspecified**

OTHER INFECTIOUS AND PARASITIC DISEASES (130-136)

❹ **130 Toxoplasmosis**
Includes infection by toxoplasma gondii
toxoplasmosis (acquired)
Excludes *congenital toxoplasmosis (771.2)*

130.0 Meningoencephalitis due to toxoplasmosis
Encephalitis due to acquired toxoplasmosis
C&C Exclusions: 130.0, 130.7, 130.8, 139.8

130.1 Conjunctivitis due to toxoplasmosis
C&C Exclusions: 130.1, 130.7, 130.8, 139.8

130.2 Chorioretinitis due to toxoplasmosis
Focal retinochoroiditis due to acquired toxoplasmosis
C&C Exclusions: 130.2, 130.7, 130.8, 139.8

130.3 Myocarditis due to toxoplasmosis
C&C Exclusions: 130.3, 130.7, 130.8, 139.8

130.4 Pneumonitis due to toxoplasmosis
C&C Exclusions: 079.82, 130.4, 130.7, 130.8, 130.9, 139.8, 480.0, 480.1, 480.2, 480.3, 480.8, 480.9, 481, 482.0, 482.1, 482.2, 482.30, 482.31, 482.32, 482.39, 482.40, 482.41, 482.49, 482.81, 482.82, 482.83, 482.84, 482.89, 482.9, 483.0, 483.1, 483.8, 484.1, 484.3, 484.5, 484.6, 484.7, 484.8, 485, 486, 487.0, 487.1, 494.0, 494.1, 495.0, 495.1, 495.2, 495.3, 495.4, 495.5, 495.6, 495.7, 495.8, 495.9, 496, 500, 501, 502, 503, 504, 505, 506.0, 506.1, 506.2, 506.3, 506.4, 506.9, 507.0, 507.1, 507.8, 508.0, 508.1, 508.8, 508.9, 517.1, 518.89

130.5 Hepatitis due to toxoplasmosis
C&C Exclusions: 130.5, 130.7, 130.8, 139.8

130.7 Toxoplasmosis of other specified sites
C&C Exclusions: 130.7, 130.8, 139.8

130.8 Multisystemic disseminated toxoplasmosis
Toxoplasmosis of multiple sites
C&C Exclusions: See 130.7

✖ **130.9 Toxoplasmosis, unspecified**

❹ **131 Trichomoniasis**
Includes infection due to Trichomonas (vaginalis)

❺ **131.0 Urogenital trichomoniasis**

✖ **131.00 Urogenital trichomoniasis, unspecified**
Fluor (vaginalis) trichomonal or due to Trichomonas (vaginalis)
Leukorrhea (vaginalis) trichomonal or due to Trichomonas (vaginalis)

131.01 Trichomonal vulvovaginitis ♀
Vaginitis, trichomonal or due to Trichomonas (vaginalis)

131.02 Trichomonal urethritis

A sexually transmitted diesease caused by the protozoan Trichomonas vaginalis infecting the urethra

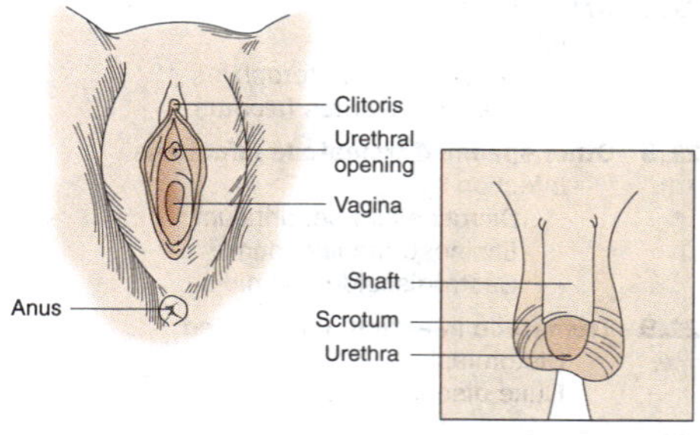

131.03 Trichomonal prostatitis ♂

131.09 Other

131.8 Other specified sites
Excludes *intestinal (007.3)*

✖ **131.9 Trichomoniasis, unspecified**

❹ **132 Pediculosis and phthirus infestation**

132.0 Pediculus capitis [head louse]

132.1 Pediculus corporis [body louse]

132.2 Phthirus pubis [pubic louse]
Pediculus pubis

❹ ❺ Additional Digit Required ✖ Nonspecific PDx ⊘ Unacceptable PDx ✚ Manifestation Code ▶◀ Revised Text ● New Code ▲ Revised Code

132.3 Mixed infestation
Infestation classifiable to more than one of the categories 132.0-132.2

✖ **132.9 Pediculosis, unspecified**

❹ **133 Acariasis**

133.0 Scabies
Infestation by Sarcoptes scabiei
Norwegian scabies
Sarcoptic itch

133.8 Other acariasis
Chiggers
Infestation by:
Demodex folliculorum
Trombicula

133.9 Acariasis, unspecified
Infestation by mites NOS

❹ **134 Other infestation**

134.0 Myiasis
Infestation by:
Dermatobia (hominis)
fly larvae
Gasterophilus (intestinalis)
maggots
Oestrus ovis

134.1 Other arthropod infestation
Infestation by:
chigoe
sand flea
Tunga penetrans
Jigger disease
Scarabiasis
Tungiasis

134.2 Hirudiniasis
Hirudiniasis (external) (internal)
Leeches (aquatic) (land)

134.8 Other specified infestations

134.9 Infestation, unspecified
Infestation (skin) NOS
Skin parasites NOS

135 Sarcoidosis
Besnier-Boeck-Schaumann disease
Lupoid (miliary) of Boeck
Lupus pernio (Besnier)
Lymphogranulomatosis, benign (Schaumann's)
Sarcoid (any site):
NOS
Boeck
Darier-Roussy
Uveoparotid fever
C&C Exclusions: 135, 139.8

❹ **136 Other and unspecified infectious and parasitic diseases**

136.0 Ainhum
Dactylolysis spontanea

136.1 Behçet's syndrome
DEF: Relapsing inflammatory disorder with recurring painful sores of the mouth, skin, and genitals; swollen joints; severe uveitis, retinal vasculitis, optic atrophy; and digestive system involvement.

136.2 Specific infections by free-living amebae
Meningoencephalitis due to Naegleria

136.3 Pneumocystosis
Pneumonia due to Pneumocystis carinii
Pneumonia due to Pneumocystis jiroveci
C&C Exclusions: 079.82, 136.3, 480.0, 480.1, 480.2, 480.3, 480.8, 480.9, 481, 482.0, 482.1, 482.2, 482.30, 482.31, 482.32, 482.39, 482.40, 482.41, 482.49, 482.81, 482.82, 482.83, 482.84, 482.89, 482.9, 483.0, 483.1, 483.8, 484.1, 484.3, 484.5, 484.6, 484.7, 484.8, 485, 486, 487.0, 487.1, 494.0, 494.1, 495.0, 495.1, 495.2, 495.3, 495.4, 495.5, 495.6, 495.7, 495.8, 495.9, 496, 500, 501, 502, 503, 504, 505, 506.0, 506.1, 506.2, 506.3, 506.4, 506.9, 507.0, 507.1, 507.8, 508.0, 508.1, 508.8, 508.9, 517.1, 518.89
AHA: 1Q 2005, 7; 1Q 2003, 15; Nov-Dec 1987, 5-6

136.4 Psorospermiasis

136.5 Sarcosporidiosis
Infection by Sarcocystis lindemanni

136.8 Other specified infectious and parasitic diseases
Candiru infestation

✖ **136.9 Unspecified infectious and parasitic diseases**
Infectious disease NOS
Parasitic disease NOS
AHA: 2Q 1991, 8

LATE EFFECTS OF INFECTIOUS AND PARASITIC DISEASES (137-139)

❹ **137 Late effects of tuberculosis**
Note: *This category is to be used to indicate conditions classifiable to 010-018 as the cause of late effects, which are themselves classified elsewhere. The "late effects" include those specified as such, as sequelae, or as due to old or inactive tuberculosis, without evidence of active disease.*

✖ **137.0 Late effects of respiratory or unspecified tuberculosis**
C&C Exclusions: 137.0, 139.8

✖ **137.1 Late effects of central nervous system tuberculosis**
C&C Exclusions: 137.1, 139.8

✖ **137.2 Late effects of genitourinary tuberculosis**
C&C Exclusions: 137.2, 139.8

✖ **137.3 Late effects of tuberculosis of bones and joints**

✖ **137.4 Late effects of tuberculosis of other specified organs**

✖ **138 Late effects of acute poliomyelitis**
Note: *This category is to be used to indicate conditions classifiable to 045 as the cause of late effects, which are themselves classified elsewhere. The "late effects" include conditions specified as such, or as sequelae, or as due to old or inactive poliomyelitis, without evidence of active disease.*
C&C Exclusions: 138, 139.8

❹ **139 Late effects of other infectious and parasitic diseases**
Note: *This category is to be used to indicate conditions classifiable to categories 001-009, 020-041, 046-136 as the cause of late effects, which are themselves classified elsewhere. The "late effects" include conditions specified as such; they also include sequela of diseases classifiable to the above categories if there is evidence that the disease itself is no longer present.*

✖ **139.0 Late effects of viral encephalitis**
Late effects of conditions classifiable to 049.8-049.9, 062-064

✖ **139.1 Late effects of trachoma**
Late effects of conditions classifiable to 076

✖ **139.8 Late effects of other and unspecified infectious and parasitic diseases**
C&C Exclusions: 052.2, 053.14, 054.74, 995.90, 995.91, 995.92, 995.93, 995.94
AHA: 2Q 2006, 18; 4Q 1991, 15; 3Q 1990, 14; Mar-Apr 1987, 8

2. NEOPLASMS (140-239)

DEF: A neoplasm is abnormal tissue that grows more rapidly than normal and lacks the organization and functionality of the tissue around it. Ordinary cells receive feedback limiting the creation of new cells after a certain number of divisions so that new cells are generated properly for tissue repair and growth. Tumors develop when cells cease responding to the feedback and grow without control, causing damage to the surrounding cells, and disrupting the normal function of the body. A neoplasm can be classified as either malignant, benign, or carcinoma in situ. A malignant tumor is one that grows quickly and destructively invades surrounding tissue. A benign neoplasm is one that is neither growing excessively nor destroying surrounding cells, but may cause damage or dysfunction due to its size or effect on adjacent tissue. A carcinoma in situ is a neoplasm undergoing malignant changes but still contained within its originating site and has not invaded surrounding tissue. The primary neoplasm is the site where the cancerous cells are believed to have originated. A secondary neoplasm is one at another location where malignant cells from a primary site were transported through the lymphatic or circulatory system. In some cases, a primary site other than the known neoplasm cannot be found, but the presenting tumor is ruled as a secondary one because its characteristics are inconsistent with a primary tumor at that site. Neoplasms are organized by the level of malignancy, whether the tumor in question is a primary or a secondary one, and by location.

1. Content:
   This chapter contains the following broad groups:
   - 140-195 Malignant neoplasms, stated or presumed to be primary, of specified sites, except of lymphatic and hematopoietic tissue
   - 196-198 Malignant neoplasms, stated or presumed to be secondary, of specified sites
   - 199 Malignant neoplasms, without specification of site
   - 200-208 Malignant neoplasms, stated or presumed to be primary, of lymphatic and hematopoietic tissue
   - 210-229 Benign neoplasms
   - 230-234 Carcinoma in situ
   - 235-238 Neoplasms of uncertain behavior [see Note, at beginning of section 235-238]
   - 239 Neoplasms of unspecified nature
2. Functional activity
   All neoplasms are classified in this chapter, whether or not functionally active. An additional code from Chapter 3 may be used to identify such functional activity associated with any neoplasm, e.g.:
   - catecholamine-producing malignant pheochromocytoma of adrenal:
     code 194.0, additional code 255.6
   - basophil adenoma of pituitary with Cushing's syndrome:
     code 227.3, additional code 255.0
3. Morphology [Histology]
   For those wishing to identify the histological type of neoplasms, a comprehensive coded nomenclature, which comprises the morphology rubrics of the ICD-Oncology, is found in appendix A.
4. Malignant neoplasms overlapping site boundaries
   Categories 140-195 are for the classification of primary malignant neoplasms according to their point of origin. A malignant neoplasm that overlaps two or more subcategories within a three-digit rubric and whose point of origin cannot be determined should be classified to the subcategory .8 "Other."
   For example, "carcinoma involving tip and ventral surface of tongue" should be assigned to 141.8. On the other hand, "carcinoma of tip of tongue, extending to involve the ventral surface" should be coded to 141.2, as the point of origin, the tip, is known. Three subcategories (149.8, 159.8, 165.8) have been provided for malignant neoplasms that overlap the boundaries of three-digit rubrics within certain systems.
   Overlapping malignant neoplasms that cannot be classified as indicated above should be assigned to the appropriate subdivision of category 195 (Malignant neoplasm of other and ill-defined sites).

AHA: 2Q 1990, 7

MALIGNANT NEOPLASM OF LIP, ORAL CAVITY, AND PHARYNX (140-149)

Excludes carcinoma in situ (230.0)

④ **140 Malignant neoplasm of lip**
Excludes skin of lip (173.0)

140.0 Upper lip, vermilion border
Upper lip:
NOS
external
lipstick area

140.1 Lower lip, vermilion border
Lower lip:
NOS
external
lipstick area

140.3 Upper lip, inner aspect
Upper lip:
buccal aspect
frenulum
mucosa
oral aspect

140.4 Lower lip, inner aspect
Lower lip:
buccal aspect
frenulum
mucosa
oral aspect

140.5 Lip, unspecified, inner aspect
Lip, not specified whether upper or lower:
buccal aspect
frenulum
mucosa
oral aspect

140.6 Commissure of lip
Labial commissure

140.8 Other sites of lip
Malignant neoplasm of contiguous or overlapping sites of lip whose point of origin cannot be determined

✖ **140.9 Lip, unspecified, vermilion border**
Lip, not specified as upper or lower:
NOS
external
lipstick area

④ **141 Malignant neoplasm of tongue**

141.0 Base of tongue
Dorsal surface of base of tongue
Fixed part of tongue NOS
AHA: 4Q 2006, 90-91

141.1 Dorsal surface of tongue
Anterior two-thirds of tongue, dorsal surface
Dorsal tongue NOS
Midline of tongue
Excludes dorsal surface of base of tongue (141.0)

141.2 Tip and lateral border of tongue

141.3 Ventral surface of tongue
Anterior two-thirds of tongue, ventral surface
Frenulum linguae

141.4 Anterior two-thirds of tongue, part unspecified
Mobile part of tongue NOS

141.5 Junctional zone
Border of tongue at junction of fixed and mobile parts at insertion of anterior tonsillar pillar

141.6 Lingual tonsil

141.8 Other sites of tongue
Malignant neoplasm of contiguous or overlapping sites of tongue whose point of origin cannot be determined

✖ **141.9 Tongue, unspecified**
Tongue NOS

Malignant neoplasm of tongue

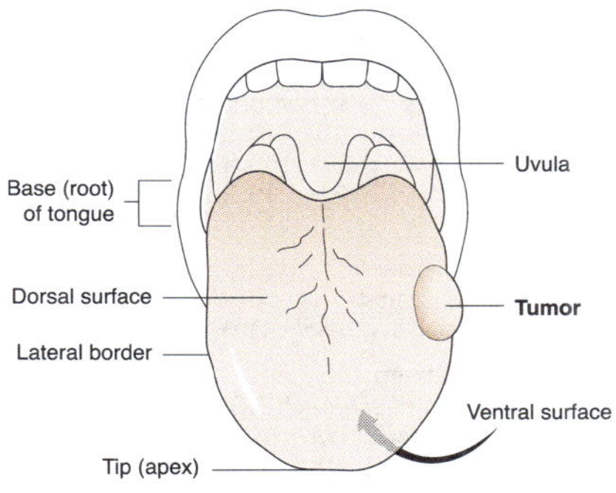

❹ **142 Malignant neoplasm of major salivary glands**
Includes salivary ducts
Excludes *malignant neoplasm of minor salivary glands:*
NOS (145.9)
buccal mucosa (145.0)
soft palate (145.3)
tongue (141.0-141.9)
tonsil, palatine (146.0)

142.0 Parotid gland

142.1 Submandibular gland
Submaxillary gland

142.2 Sublingual gland

142.8 Other major salivary glands
Malignant neoplasm of contiguous or overlapping sites of salivary glands and ducts whose point of origin cannot be determined

✖ **142.9 Salivary gland, unspecified**
Salivary gland (major) NOS

❹ **143 Malignant neoplasm of gum**
Includes alveolar (ridge) mucosa
gingiva (alveolar) (marginal)
interdental papillae
Excludes *malignant odontogenic neoplasms (170.0-170.1)*

143.0 Upper gum

143.1 Lower gum

143.8 Other sites of gum
Malignant neoplasm of contiguous or overlapping sites of gum whose point of origin cannot be determined

✖ **143.9 Gum, unspecified**

❹ **144 Malignant neoplasm of floor of mouth**

144.0 Anterior portion
Anterior to the premolar-canine junction

144.1 Lateral portion

144.8 Other sites of floor of mouth
Malignant neoplasm of contiguous or overlapping sites of floor of mouth whose point of origin cannot be determined

✖ **144.9 Floor of mouth, part unspecified**

❹ **145 Malignant neoplasm of other and unspecified parts of mouth**
Excludes *mucosa of lips (140.0-140.9)*

145.0 Cheek mucosa
Buccal mucosa
Cheek, inner aspect

145.1 Vestibule of mouth
Buccal sulcus (upper) (lower)
Labial sulcus (upper) (lower)

145.2 Hard palate

145.3 Soft palate
Excludes *nasopharyngeal [posterior] [superior] surface of soft palate (147.3)*

145.4 Uvula

145.5 Palate, unspecified
Junction of hard and soft palate
Roof of mouth

145.6 Retromolar area

145.8 Other specified parts of mouth
Malignant neoplasm of contiguous or overlapping sites of mouth whose point of origin cannot be determined

145.9 Mouth, unspecified
Buccal cavity NOS
Minor salivary gland, unspecified site
Oral cavity NOS

❹ **146 Malignant neoplasm of oropharynx**

146.0 Tonsil
Tonsil:
NOS
faucial
palatine
Excludes *lingual tonsil (141.6)*
pharyngeal tonsil (147.1)
AHA: Sep-Oct 1987, 8

146.1 Tonsillar fossa

146.2 Tonsillar pillars (anterior) (posterior)
Faucial pillar
Glossopalatine fold
Palatoglossal arch
Palatopharyngeal arch

146.3 Vallecula
Anterior and medial surface of the pharyngoepiglottic fold

146.4 Anterior aspect of epiglottis
Epiglottis, free border [margin]
Glossoepiglottic fold(s)
Excludes *epiglottis:*
NOS (161.1)
suprahyoid portion (161.1)

146.5 Junctional region
Junction of the free margin of the epiglottis, the aryepiglottic fold, and the pharyngoepiglottic fold

146.6 Lateral wall of oropharynx

146.7 Posterior wall of oropharynx

146.8 Other specified sites of oropharynx
Branchial cleft
Malignant neoplasm of contiguous or overlapping sites of oropharynx whose point of origin cannot be determined

✖ **146.9 Oropharynx, unspecified**
AHA: 2Q 2002, 6

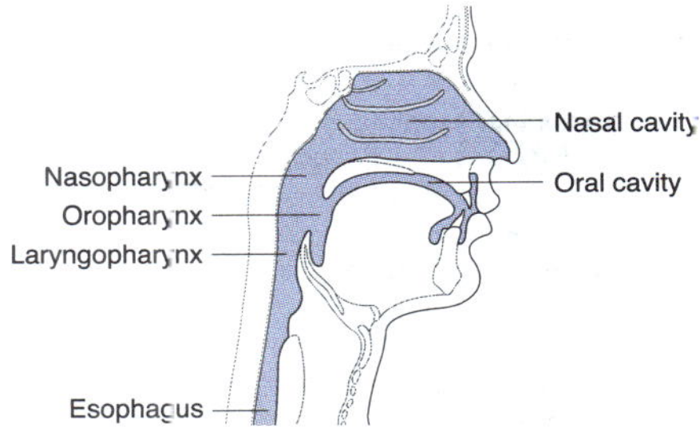

❹ **147 Malignant neoplasm of nasopharynx**

147.0 Superior wall
Roof of nasopharynx

147.1 Posterior wall
Adenoid
Pharyngeal tonsil

147.2 Lateral wall
Fossa of Rosenmüller
Opening of auditory tube
Pharyngeal recess

147.3 Anterior wall
Floor of nasopharynx
Nasopharyngeal [posterior] [superior] surface of soft palate
Posterior margin of nasal septum and choanae

147.8 Other specified sites of nasopharynx
Malignant neoplasm of contiguous or overlapping sites of nasopharynx whose point of origin cannot be determined

✖ **147.9 Nasopharynx, unspecified**
Nasopharyngeal wall NOS

❹ **148 Malignant neoplasm of hypopharynx**

148.0 Postcricoid region

148.1 Pyriform sinus
Pyriform fossa

148.2 Aryepiglottic fold, hypopharyngeal aspect
Aryepiglottic fold or interarytenoid fold:
NOS
marginal zone
Excludes *aryepiglottic fold or interarytenoid fold, laryngeal aspect (161.1)*

148.3 Posterior hypopharyngeal wall

148.8 Other specified sites of hypopharynx
Malignant neoplasm of contiguous or overlapping sites of hypopharynx whose point of origin cannot be determined

148.9 Hypopharynx, unspecified
Hypopharyngeal wall NOS
Hypopharynx NOS

❹ **149 Malignant neoplasm of other and ill-defined sites within the lip, oral cavity, and pharynx**

149.0 Pharynx, unspecified

149.1 Waldeyer's ring

149.8 Other
Malignant neoplasms of lip, oral cavity, and pharynx whose point of origin cannot be assigned to any one of the categories 140-148
Excludes *"book leaf" neoplasm [ventral surface of tongue and floor of mouth] (145.8)*

149.9 Ill-defined

MALIGNANT NEOPLASM OF DIGESTIVE ORGANS AND PERITONEUM (150-159)

Excludes *carcinoma in situ (230.1-230.9)*

❹ **150 Malignant neoplasm of esophagus**

150.0 Cervical esophagus
C&C Exclusions: 150.0, 150.1, 150.2, 150.3, 150.4, 150.5, 150.8, 150.9, 159.0, 159.8, 159.9, 176.3, 195.8, 199.0, 199.1, 239.0, 239.8, 239.9

150.1 Thoracic esophagus
C&C Exclusions: See 150.0

150.2 Abdominal esophagus
Excludes *adenocarcinoma (151.0)*
cardio-esophageal junction (151.0)
C&C Exclusions: See 150.0

150.3 Upper third of esophagus
Proximal third of esophagus
C&C Exclusions: See 150.0

150.4 Middle third of esophagus
C&C Exclusions: See 150.0

150.5 Lower third of esophagus
Distal third of esophagus
Excludes *adenocarcinoma (151.0)*
cardio-esophageal junction (151.0)
C&C Exclusions: See 150.0

150.8 Other specified part
Malignant neoplasm of contiguous or overlapping sites of esophagus whose point of origin cannot be determined
C&C Exclusions: See 150.0

✖ **150.9 Esophagus, unspecified**
C&C Exclusions: See 150.0

❹ **151 Malignant neoplasm of stomach**
Excludes *malignant stromal tumor of stomach (171.5)*

151.0 Cardia
Cardiac orifice
Cardio-esophageal junction
Excludes *squamous cell carcinoma (150.2, 150.5)*
C&C Exclusions: 151.0, 151.1, 151.2, 151.3, 151.4, 151.5, 151.8, 151.9, 159.0, 159.8, 159.9, 176.3, 195.8, 199.0, 199.1, 239.0, 239.8, 239.9

151.1 Pylorus
Prepylorus
Pyloric canal
C&C Exclusions: See 151.0

151.2 Pyloric antrum
Antrum of stomach NOS
C&C Exclusions: See 151.0

151.3 Fundus of stomach
C&C Exclusions: See 151.0

151.4 Body of stomach
C&C Exclusions: See 151.0

151.5 Lesser curvature, unspecified
Lesser curvature, not classifiable to 151.1-151.4
C&C Exclusions: See 151.0

151.6 Greater curvature, unspecified
Greater curvature, not classifiable to 151.0-151.4
C&C Exclusions: See 151.0

151.8 Other specified sites of stomach
Anterior wall, not classifiable to 151.0-151.4
Posterior wall, not classifiable to 151.0-151.4
Malignant neoplasm of contiguous or overlapping sites of stomach whose point of origin cannot be determined
C&C Exclusions: See 151.0

✖ **151.9 Stomach, unspecified**
Carcinoma ventriculi
Gastric cancer
C&C Exclusions: See 151.0
AHA: 2Q 2001, 17

❹ **152 Malignant neoplasm of small intestine, including duodenum**
Excludes *malignant stromal tumor of small intestine (171.5)*

152.0 Duodenum
C&C Exclusions: 152.0, 152.8, 152.9, 159.0, 159.8, 159.9, 176.3, 195.8, 199.0, 199.1, 239.0, 239.8, 239.9

152.1 Jejunum
C&C Exclusions: 152.1, 152.8, 152.9, 159.0, 159.8, 159.9, 176.3, 195.8, 199.0, 199.1, 239.0, 239.8, 239.9

152.2 Ileum
Excludes *ileocecal valve (153.4)*
C&C Exclusions: 152.2, 152.8, 152.9, 159.0, 159.8, 159.9, 176.3, 195.8, 199.0, 199.1, 239.0, 239.8, 239.9

152.3 Meckel's diverticulum
C&C Exclusions: 152.3, 152.8, 152.9, 159.0, 159.8, 159.9, 176.3, 195.8, 199.0, 199.1, 239.0, 239.8, 239.9

152.8 Other specified sites of small intestine
Duodenojejunal junction
Malignant neoplasm of contiguous or overlapping sites of small intestine whose point of origin cannot be determined
C&C Exclusions: 152.8, 152.9, 159.0, 159.8, 159.9, 176.3, 195.8, 199.0, 199.1, 239.0, 239.8, 239.9

✖ **152.9 Small intestine, unspecified**
C&C Exclusions: See 152.8

❹ **153 Malignant neoplasm of colon**

153.0 Hepatic flexure
C&C Exclusions: 153.0, 153.8, 153.9, 159.0, 159.8, 159.9, 176.3, 195.8, 199.0, 199.1, 239.0, 239.8, 239.9

153.1 Transverse colon
C&C Exclusions: 153.1, 153.8, 153.9, 159.0, 159.8, 159.9, 176.3, 195.8, 199.0, 199.1, 239.0, 239.8, 239.9

153.2 Descending colon
Left colon
C&C Exclusions: 153.2, 153.8, 153.9, 159.0, 159.8, 159.9, 176.3, 195.8, 199.0, 199.1, 239.0, 239.8, 239.9

153.3 Sigmoid colon
Sigmoid (flexure)
Excludes *rectosigmoid junction (154.0)*
C&C Exclusions: 153.3, 153.8, 153.9, 159.0, 159.8, 159.9, 176.3, 195.8, 199.0, 199.1, 239.0, 239.8, 239.9

153.4 Cecum
Ileocecal valve
C&C Exclusions: 153.4, 153.8, 153.9, 159.0, 159.8, 159.9, 176.3, 195.8, 199.0, 199.1, 239.0, 239.8, 239.9

153.5 Appendix
C&C Exclusions: 153.5, 153.8, 153.9, 159.0, 159.8, 159.9, 176.3, 195.8, 199.0, 199.1, 239.0, 239.8, 239.9

153.6 Ascending colon
Right colon
C&C Exclusions: 153.6, 153.8, 153.9, 159.0, 159.8, 159.9, 176.3, 195.8, 199.0, 199.1, 239.0, 239.8, 239.9

Malignant neoplasm of colon

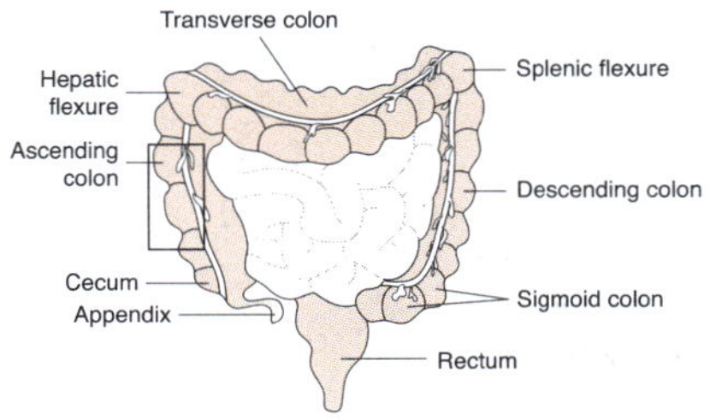

Colon cancer stages

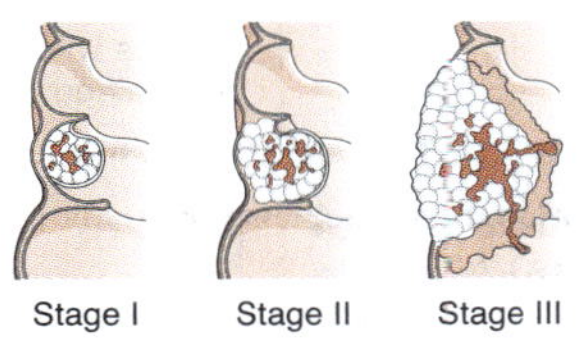

153.7 Splenic flexure
C&C Exclusions: 153.7, 153.8, 153.9, 159.0, 159.8, 159.9, 176.3, 195.8, 199.0, 199.1, 239.0, 239.8, 239.9

153.8 Other specified sites of large intestine
Malignant neoplasm of contiguous or overlapping sites of colon whose point of origin cannot be determined
Excludes *ileocecal valve (153.4)*
rectosigmoid junction (154.0)
C&C Exclusions: 153.8, 153.9, 159.0, 159.8, 159.9, 176.3, 195.8, 199.0, 199.1, 239.0, 239.8, 239.9

✖ **153.9 Colon, unspecified**
Large intestine NOS
C&C Exclusions: See 153.8

❹ **154 Malignant neoplasm of rectum, rectosigmoid junction, and anus**

154.0 Rectosigmoid junction
Colon with rectum
Rectosigmoid (colon)
C&C Exclusions: 154.0, 154.8, 159.0, 159.8, 159.9, 176.3, 195.8, 199.0, 199.1, 239.0, 239.8, 239.9

154.1 Rectum
Rectal ampulla
C&C Exclusions: 154.1, 154.8, 159.0, 159.8, 159.9, 176.3, 195.8, 199.0, 199.1, 239.0, 239.8, 239.9

154.2 Anal canal
Anal sphincter
Excludes *skin of anus (172.5, 173.5)*
C&C Exclusions: 154.2, 154.3, 154.8, 159.0, 159.8, 159.9, 176.3, 195.8, 199.0, 199.1, 239.0, 239.8, 239.9
AHA: 1Q 2001, 8

✖ **154.3 Anus, unspecified**
Excludes *anus:*
margin (172.5, 173.5)
skin (172.5, 173.5)
perianal skin (172.5, 173.5)
C&C Exclusions: See 154.2

154.8 Other
Anorectum
Cloacogenic zone
Malignant neoplasm of contiguous or overlapping sites of rectum, rectosigmoid junction, and anus whose point of origin cannot be determined
C&C Exclusions: 154.8, 159.0, 159.8, 159.9, 176.3, 195.8, 199.0, 199.1, 239.0, 239.8, 239.9

❹ **155 Malignant neoplasm of liver and intrahepatic bile ducts**

155.0 Liver, primary
Carcinoma:
liver, specified as primary
hepatocellular
liver cell
Hepatoblastoma
C&C Exclusions: 155.0, 155.1, 155.2, 159.0, 159.8, 159.9, 176.3, 195.8, 199.0, 199.1, 239.0, 239.8, 239.9

155.1 Intrahepatic bile ducts
Canaliculi biliferi
Interlobular:
bile ducts
biliary canals
Intrahepatic:
biliary passages
canaliculi
gall duct
Excludes *hepatic duct (156.1)*
C&C Exclusions: See 155.0

155.2 Liver, not specified as primary or secondary
C&C Exclusions: See 155.0

❹ **156 Malignant neoplasm of gallbladder and extrahepatic bile ducts**

156.0 Gallbladder
C&C Exclusions: 156.0, 156.8, 156.9, 159.0, 159.8, 159.9, 176.3, 195.8, 199.0, 199.1, 239.0, 239.8, 239.9

156.1 Extrahepatic bile ducts
Biliary duct or passage NOS
Common bile duct
Cystic duct
Hepatic duct
Sphincter of Oddi
C&C Exclusions: 156.1, 156.8, 156.9, 159.0, 159.8, 159.9, 176.3, 195.8, 199.0, 199.1, 239.0, 239.8, 239.9

156.2 Ampulla of Vater
C&C Exclusions: 156.2, 156.8, 156.9, 159.0, 159.8, 159.9, 176.3, 195.8, 199.0, 199.1, 239.0, 239.8, 239.9

156.8 Other specified sites of gallbladder and extrahepatic bile ducts
Malignant neoplasm of contiguous or overlapping sites of gallbladder and extrahepatic bile ducts whose point of origin cannot be determined
C&C Exclusions: 156.8, 156.9, 159.0, 159.8, 159.9, 176.3, 195.8, 199.0, 199.1, 239.0, 239.8, 239.9

156.9 Biliary tract, part unspecified
Malignant neoplasm involving both intrahepatic and extrahepatic bile ducts
C&C Exclusions: See 156.8

❹ **157 Malignant neoplasm of pancreas**

157.0 Head of pancreas
C&C Exclusions: 157.0, 157.1, 157.2, 157.3, 157.4, 157.8, 157.9, 159.0, 159.8, 159.9, 176.3, 195.8, 199.0, 199.1, 239.0, 239.8, 239.9
AHA: 2Q 2005, 9; 4Q 2000, 40

157.1 Body of pancreas
C&C Exclusions: See 157.0

157.2 Tail of pancreas
C&C Exclusions: See 157.0

157.3 Pancreatic duct
Duct of:
Santorini
Wirsung
C&C Exclusions: See 157.0

157.4 Islets of Langerhans
Islets of Langerhans, any part of pancreas
Use additional code to identify any functional activity
C&C Exclusions: See 157.0

157.8 Other specified sites of pancreas
Ectopic pancreatic tissue
Malignant neoplasm of contiguous or overlapping sites of pancreas whose point of origin cannot be determined
C&C Exclusions: See 157.0

✖ **157.9 Pancreas, part unspecified**
C&C Exclusions: See 157.0
AHA: 4Q 1989, 11

❹ **158 Malignant neoplasm of retroperitoneum and peritoneum**

158.0 Retroperitoneum
Periadrenal tissue
Perinephric tissue
Perirenal tissue
Retrocecal tissue

158.8 Specified parts of peritoneum
Cul-de-sac (of Douglas)
Mesentery
Mesocolon
Omentum
Peritoneum:
  parietal
  pelvic
Rectouterine pouch
Malignant neoplasm of contiguous or overlapping sites of retroperitoneum and peritoneum whose point of origin cannot be determined

✖ **158.9 Peritoneum, unspecified**

❹ **159 Malignant neoplasm of other and ill-defined sites within the digestive organs and peritoneum**

✖ **159.0 Intestinal tract, part unspecified**
Intestine NOS

159.1 Spleen, not elsewhere classified
Angiosarcoma of spleen
Fibrosarcoma of spleen
Excludes *Hodgkin's disease (201.0-201.9)*
lymphosarcoma (200.1)
reticulosarcoma (200.0)

159.8 Other sites of digestive system and intra-abdominal organs
Malignant neoplasm of digestive organs and peritoneum whose point of origin cannot be assigned to any one of the categories 150-158
Excludes *anus and rectum (154.8)*
cardio-esophageal junction (151.0)
colon and rectum (154.0)

159.9 Ill-defined
Alimentary canal or tract NOS
Gastrointestinal tract NOS
Excludes *abdominal NOS (195.2)*
intra-abdominal NOS (195.2)

MALIGNANT NEOPLASM OF RESPIRATORY AND INTRATHORACIC ORGANS (160-165)

Excludes *carcinoma in situ (231.0-231.9)*

❹ **160 Malignant neoplasm of nasal cavities, middle ear, and accessory sinuses**

160.0 Nasal cavities
Cartilage of nose
Conchae, nasal
Internal nose
Septum of nose
Vestibule of nose
Excludes *nasal bone (170.0)*
nose NOS (195.0)
olfactory bulb (192.0)
posterior margin of septum and choanae (147.3)
skin of nose (172.3, 173.3)
turbinates (170.0)

160.1 Auditory tube, middle ear, and mastoid air cells
Antrum tympanicum
Eustachian tube
Tympanic cavity
Excludes *auditory canal (external) (172.2, 173.2)*
bone of ear (meatus) (170.0)
cartilage of ear (171.0)
ear (external) (skin) (172.2, 173.2)

Malignant neoplasm of auditory tube, middle ear, or mastoid air cells

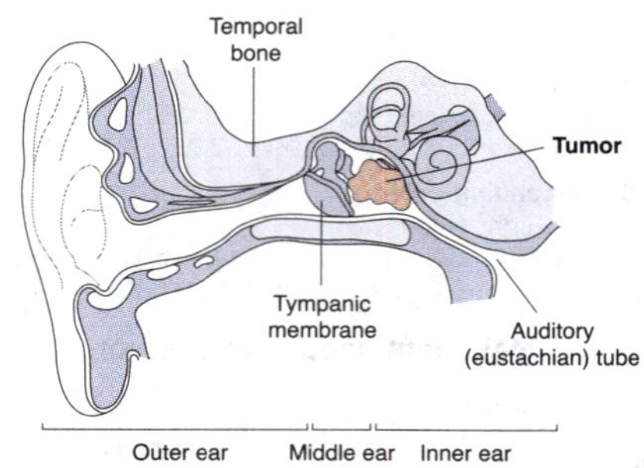

160.2 Maxillary sinus
Antrum (Highmore) (maxillary)

160.3 Ethmoidal sinus

160.4 Frontal sinus

160.5 Sphenoidal sinus

160.8 Other
Malignant neoplasm of contiguous or overlapping sites of nasal cavities, middle ear, and accessory sinuses whose point of origin cannot be determined

✖ **160.9 Accessory sinus, unspecified**

❹ **161 Malignant neoplasm of larynx**

161.0 Glottis
Intrinsic larynx
Laryngeal commissure (anterior) (posterior)
True vocal cord
Vocal cord NOS

161.1 Supraglottis
Aryepiglottic fold or interarytenoid fold, laryngeal aspect
Epiglottis (suprahyoid portion) NOS
Extrinsic larynx
False vocal cords
Posterior (laryngeal) surface of epiglottis
Ventricular bands
Excludes *anterior aspect of epiglottis (146.4)*
aryepiglottic fold or interarytenoid fold:
  NOS (148.2)
  hypopharyngeal aspect (148.2)
  marginal zone (148.2)

161.2 Subglottis

161.3 Laryngeal cartilages
Cartilage:
  arytenoid
  cricoid
  cuneiform
  thyroid

161.8 Other specified sites of larynx
Malignant neoplasm of contiguous or overlapping sites of larynx whose point of origin cannot be determined

✖ **161.9 Larynx, unspecified**

❹ **162 Malignant neoplasm of trachea, bronchus, and lung**

162.0 Trachea
Cartilage of trachea
Mucosa of trachea

162.2 Main bronchus
Carina
Hilus of lung
C&C Exclusions: 162.2, 162.8, 162.9, 165.8, 165.9, 176.4, 195.8, 199.0, 199.1, 239.1, 239.8, 239.9

162.3 Upper lobe, bronchus or lung
C&C Exclusions: 162.3, 162.8, 162.9, 165.8, 165.9, 176.4, 195.8, 199.0, 199.1, 239.1, 239.8, 239.9
AHA: 1Q 2004, 4

162.4 Middle lobe, bronchus or lung
C&C Exclusions: 162.4, 162.8, 162.9, 165.8, 165.9, 176.4, 195.8, 199.0, 199.1, 239.1, 239.8, 239.9

162.5 Lower lobe, bronchus or lung
C&C Exclusions: 162.5, 162.8, 162.9, 165.8, 165.9, 176.4, 195.8, 199.0, 199.1, 239.1, 239.8, 239.9

162.8 Other parts of bronchus or lung
Malignant neoplasm of contiguous or overlapping sites of bronchus or lung whose point of origin cannot be determined
C&C Exclusions: 162.8, 162.9, 165.8, 165.9, 176.4, 195.8, 199.0, 199.1, 239.1, 239.8, 239.9
AHA: 3Q 2006, 8

✖ **162.9 Bronchus and lung, unspecified**
C&C Exclusions: See 162.8
AHA: 3Q 2006, 14-15; 2Q 1997, 3; 4Q 1996, 48

❹ **163 Malignant neoplasm of pleura**

163.0 Parietal pleura
C&C Exclusions: 163.0, 163.1, 163.8, 163.9, 165.8, 165.9, 195.8, 199.0, 199.1, 239.1, 239.8, 239.9

163.1 Visceral pleura
C&C Exclusions: See 163.0

163.8 Other specified sites of pleura
Malignant neoplasm of contiguous or overlapping sites of pleura whose point of origin cannot be determined
C&C Exclusions: See 163.0

✖ **163.9 Pleura, unspecified**
C&C Exclusions: See 163.0

❹ **164 Malignant neoplasm of thymus, heart, and mediastinum**

164.0 Thymus
C&C Exclusions: 164.0

164.1 Heart
Endocardium
Epicardium
Myocardium
Pericardium
Excludes *great vessels (171.4)*
C&C Exclusions: 164.1

164.2 Anterior mediastinum
C&C Exclusions: 164.2, 164.3, 164.8, 164.9, 165.8, 165.9, 195.8, 199.0, 199.1, 239.1, 239.8, 239.9

164.3 Posterior mediastinum
C&C Exclusions: See 164.2

164.8 Other
Malignant neoplasm of contiguous or overlapping sites of thymus, heart, and mediastinum whose point of origin cannot be determined
C&C Exclusions: See 164.2

✖ **164.9 Mediastinum, part unspecified**
C&C Exclusions: See 164.2

❹ **165 Malignant neoplasm of other and ill-defined sites within the respiratory system and intrathoracic organs**

165.0 Upper respiratory tract, part unspecified

165.8 Other
Malignant neoplasm of respiratory and intrathoracic organs whose point of origin cannot be assigned to any one of the categories 160-164

165.9 Ill-defined sites within the respiratory system
Respiratory tract NOS
Excludes *intrathoracic NOS (195.1)*
thoracic NOS (195.1)

MALIGNANT NEOPLASM OF BONE, CONNECTIVE TISSUE, SKIN, AND BREAST (170-176)

Excludes *carcinoma in situ:*
breast (233.0)
skin (232.0-232.9)

❹ **170 Malignant neoplasm of bone and articular cartilage**
Includes cartilage (articular) (joint)
periosteum
Excludes *bone marrow NOS (202.9)*
cartilage:
ear (171.0)
eyelid (171.0)
larynx (161.3)
nose (160.0)
synovia (171.0-171.9)

170.0 Bones of skull and face, except mandible
Bone:
ethmoid
frontal
malar
nasal
occipital
orbital
parietal
sphenoid
temporal
zygomatic
Maxilla (superior)
Turbinate
Upper jaw bone
Vomer
Excludes *carcinoma, any type except intraosseous or odontogenic:*
maxilla, maxillary (sinus) (160.2)
upper jaw bone (143.0)
jaw bone (lower) (170.1)

170.1 Mandible
Inferior maxilla
Jaw bone NOS
Lower jaw bone
Excludes *carcinoma, any type except intraosseous or odontogenic:*
jaw bone NOS (143.9)
lower (143.1)
upper jaw bone (170.0)

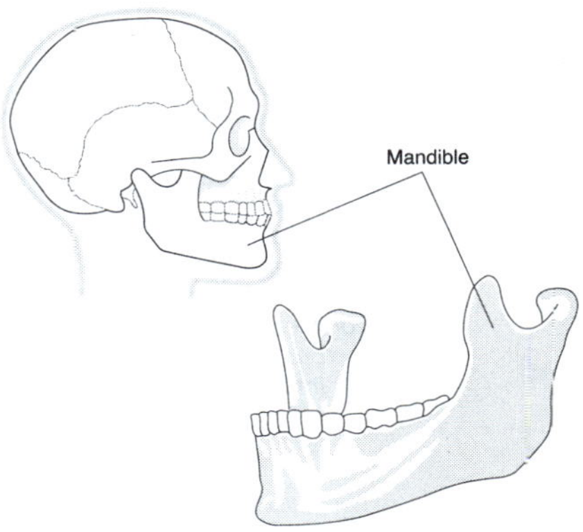

170.2 Vertebral column, excluding sacrum and coccyx
Spinal column
Spine
Vertebra
Excludes *sacrum and coccyx (170.6)*

170.3 Ribs, sternum, and clavicle
Costal cartilage
Costovertebral joint
Xiphoid process

170.4 Scapula and long bones of upper limb
Acromion
Bones NOS of upper limb
Humerus
Radius
Ulna
AHA: 2Q 1999, 9

170.5 Short bones of upper limb
Carpal
Cuneiform, wrist
Metacarpal
Navicular, of hand
Phalanges of hand
Pisiform
Scaphoid (of hand)
Semilunar or lunate
Trapezium
Trapezoid
Unciform

170.6 Pelvic bones, sacrum, and coccyx
Coccygeal vertebra
Ilium
Ischium
Pubic bone
Sacral vertebra

170.7 Long bones of lower limb
Bones NOS of lower limb
Femur
Fibula
Tibia

170.8 Short bones of lower limb
Astragalus [talus]
Calcaneus
Cuboid
Cuneiform, ankle
Metatarsal
Navicular (of ankle)
Patella
Phalanges of foot
Tarsal

✖ **170.9 Bone and articular cartilage, site unspecified**

❹ **171 Malignant neoplasm of connective and other soft tissue**
Includes blood vessel
bursa
fascia
fat
ligament, except uterine
malignant stromal tumors
muscle
peripheral, sympathetic, and parasympathetic nerves and ganglia
synovia
tendon (sheath)
Excludes *cartilage (of):*
articular (170.0-170.9)
larynx (161.3)
nose (160.0)
connective tissue:
breast (174.0-175.9)
internal organs (except stromal tumors) - code to malignant neoplasm of the site [e.g., leiomyosarcoma of stomach, 151.9]
heart (164.1)
uterine ligament (183.4)

171.0 Head, face, and neck
Cartilage of:
ear
eyelid
AHA: 2Q 1999, 6

171.2 Upper limb, including shoulder
Arm
Finger
Forearm
Hand

171.3 Lower limb, including hip
Foot
Leg
Popliteal space
Thigh
Toe

171.4 Thorax
Axilla
Diaphragm
Great vessels
Excludes *heart (164.1)*
mediastinum (164.2-164.9)
thymus (164.0)

171.5 Abdomen
Abdominal wall
Hypochondrium
Excludes *peritoneum (158.8)*
retroperitoneum (158.0)

171.6 Pelvis
Buttock
Groin
Inguinal region
Perineum
Excludes *pelvic peritoneum (158.8)*
retroperitoneum (158.0)
uterine ligament, any (183.3-183.5)

171.7 Trunk, unspecified
Back NOS
Flank NOS

171.8 Other specified sites of connective and other soft tissue
Malignant neoplasm of contiguous or overlapping sites of connective tissue whose point of origin cannot be determined

✖ **171.9 Connective and other soft tissue, site unspecified**

❹ **172 Malignant melanoma of skin**
Includes melanocarcinoma
melanoma (skin) NOS
Excludes *skin of genital organs (184.0-184.9, 187.1-187.9)*
sites other than skin - code to malignant neoplasm of the site

172.0 Lip
Excludes *vermilion border of lip (140.0-140.1, 140.9)*

172.1 Eyelid, including canthus

172.2 Ear and external auditory canal
Auricle (ear)
Auricular canal, external
External [acoustic] meatus
Pinna

172.3 Other and unspecified parts of face
Cheek (external)
Chin
Eyebrow
Forehead
Nose, external
Temple

Malignant melanoma of skin

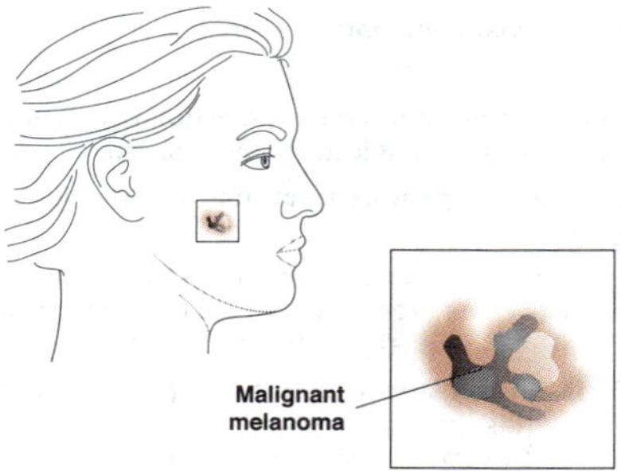

172.4 Scalp and neck

172.5 Trunk, except scrotum
Axilla
Breast
Buttock
Groin
Perianal skin
Perineum
Umbilicus
Excludes *anal canal (154.2)*
anus NOS (154.3)
scrotum (187.7)

172.6 Upper limb, including shoulder
Arm
Finger
Forearm
Hand

172.7 Lower limb, including hip
Ankle
Foot
Heel
Knee
Leg
Popliteal area
Thigh
Toe

172.8 Other specified sites of skin
Malignant melanoma of contiguous or overlapping sites of skin whose point of origin cannot be determined

✖ **172.9 Melanoma of skin, site unspecified**

❹ **173 Other malignant neoplasm of skin**
Includes malignant neoplasm of:
sebaceous glands
sudoriferous, sudoriparous glands
sweat glands
Excludes *Kaposi's sarcoma (176.0-176.9)*
malignant melanoma of skin (172.0-172.9)
skin of genital organs (184.0-184.9, 187.1-187.9)
AHA: 1Q 2000, 18; 2Q 1996, 12

173.0 Skin of lip
Excludes *vermilion border of lip (140.0-140.1, 140.9)*

173.1 Eyelid, including canthus
Excludes *cartilage of eyelid (171.0)*

173.2 Skin of ear and external auditory canal
Auricle (ear)
Auricular canal, external
External meatus
Pinna
Excludes *cartilage of ear (171.0)*

173.3 Skin of other and unspecified parts of face
Cheek, external
Chin
Eyebrow
Forehead
Nose, external
Temple
AHA: 1Q 2000, 3

173.4 Scalp and skin of neck

173.5 Skin of trunk, except scrotum
Axillary fold
Perianal skin
Skin of:
abdominal wall
anus
back
breast
buttock
chest wall
groin
perineum
Umbilicus
Excludes *anal canal (154.2)*
anus NOS (154.3)
skin of scrotum (187.7)
AHA: 1Q 2001, 8

173.6 Skin of upper limb, including shoulder
Arm
Finger
Forearm
Hand

Malignant neoplasm of skin of upper limb

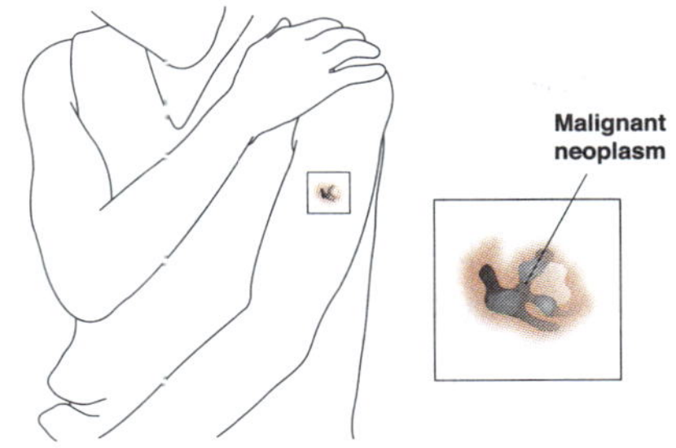

173.7 Skin of lower limb, including hip
Ankle
Foot
Heel
Knee
Leg
Popliteal area
Thigh
Toe

173.8 Other specified sites of skin
Malignant neoplasm of contiguous or overlapping sites of skin whose point of origin cannot be determined

✖ **173.9 Skin, site unspecified**

❹ **174 Malignant neoplasm of female breast**
Use additional code to identify estrogen receptor status (V86.0-V86.1)
Includes breast (female)
connective tissue
soft parts
Paget's disease of:
breast
nipple
Excludes *skin of breast (172.5, 173.5)*
AHA: 3Q 1997, 8; 4Q 1989, 11

174.0 Nipple and areola ♀

174.1 Central portion ♀

174.2 Upper-inner quadrant ♀

174.3 Lower-inner quadrant ♀

174.4 Upper-outer quadrant ♀
AHA: 1Q 2004, 3

174.5 Lower-outer quadrant ♀

174.6 Axillary tail ♀

174.8 Other specified sites of female breast ♀
Ectopic sites
Inner breast
Lower breast
Midline of breast
Outer breast
Upper breast
Malignant neoplasm of contiguous or overlapping sites of breast whose point of origin cannot be determined

✖ **174.9 Breast (female), unspecified** ♀
AHA: 3Q 2005, 11

❹ **175 Malignant neoplasm of male breast**
Use additional code to identify estrogen receptor status (V86.0-V86.1)
Excludes *skin of breast (172.5, 173.5)*

175.0 Nipple and areola ♂

175.9 Other and unspecified sites of male breast ♂
Ectopic breast tissue, male

④ **176 Kaposi's sarcoma**
AHA: 4Q 1991, 24

176.0 Skin

Kaposi's sarcoma; skin

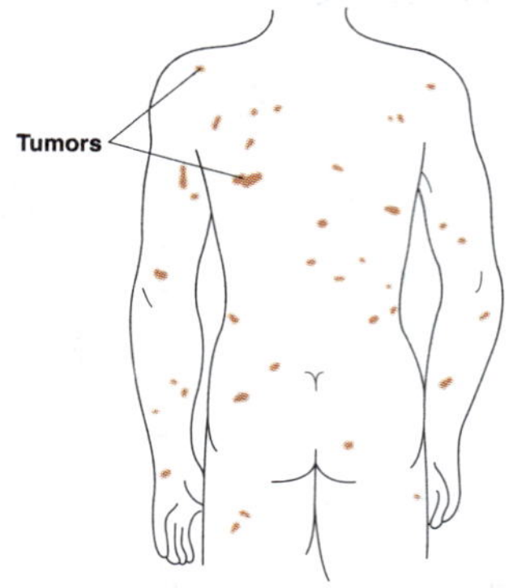

176.1 Soft tissue
Includes blood vessel
connective tissue
fascial
ligament
lymphatic(s) NEC
muscle
Excludes *lymph glands and nodes (176.5)*

176.2 Palate

176.3 Gastrointestinal sites

176.4 Lung
C&C Exclusions: 162.8, 162.9, 165.8, 165.9, 176.4, 195.8, 199.0, 199.1, 239.1, 239.8, 239.9

176.5 Lymph nodes
C&C Exclusions: 176.5, 195.8, 196.0, 196.1, 196.2, 196.3, 196.4, 196.5, 196.6, 196.8, 196.9, 199.0, 199.1, 239.8, 239.9

176.8 Other specified sites
Oral cavity NEC

✖ **176.9 Unspecified**
Viscera NOS

MALIGNANT NEOPLASM OF GENITOURINARY ORGANS (179-189)

Excludes *carcinoma in situ (233.1-233.9)*

✖ **179 Malignant neoplasm of uterus, part unspecified** ♀

④ **180 Malignant neoplasm of cervix uteri**
Includes invasive malignancy [carcinoma]
Excludes *carcinoma in situ (233.1)*

180.0 Endocervix ♀
Cervical canal NOS
Endocervical canal
Endocervical gland

180.1 Exocervix ♀

180.8 Other specified sites of cervix ♀
Cervical stump
Squamocolumnar junction of cervix
Malignant neoplasm of contiguous or overlapping sites of cervix uteri whose point of origin cannot be determined

✖ **180.9 Cervix uteri, unspecified** ♀

181 Malignant neoplasm of placenta ♀
Choriocarcinoma NOS
Chorioepithelioma NOS
Excludes *chorioadenoma (destruens) (236.1)*
hydatidiform mole (630)
malignant (236.1)
invasive mole (236.1)
male choriocarcinoma NOS (186.0-186.9)

④ **182 Malignant neoplasm of body of uterus**
Excludes *carcinoma in situ (233.2)*

182.0 Corpus uteri, except isthmus ♀
Cornu
Endometrium
Fundus
Myometrium

182.1 Isthmus ♀
Lower uterine segment

182.8 Other specified sites of body of uterus ♀
Malignant neoplasm of contiguous or overlapping sites of body of uterus whose point of origin cannot be determined
Excludes *uterus NOS (179)*

④ **183 Malignant neoplasm of ovary and other uterine adnexa**
Excludes *Douglas' cul-de-sac (158.8)*

183.0 Ovary ♀
Use additional code to identify any functional activity

183.2 Fallopian tube ♀
Oviduct
Uterine tube

183.3 Broad ligament ♀
Mesovarium
Parovarian region

183.4 Parametrium ♀
Uterine ligament NOS
Uterosacral ligament

183.5 Round ligament ♀
AHA: 3Q 1999, 5

183.8 Other specified sites of uterine adnexa ♀
Tubo-ovarian
Utero-ovarian
Malignant neoplasm of contiguous or overlapping sites of ovary and other uterine adnexa whose point of origin cannot be determined

✖ **183.9 Uterine adnexa, unspecified** ♀

④ **184 Malignant neoplasm of other and unspecified female genital organs**
Excludes *carcinoma in situ (▶233.30–233.39◀)*

184.0 Vagina ♀
Gartner's duct
Vaginal vault

184.1 Labia majora ♀
Greater vestibular [Bartholin's] gland

184.2 Labia minora ♀

184.3 Clitoris ♀

184.4 Vulva, unspecified ♀
External female genitalia NOS
Pudendum

184.8 Other specified sites of female genital organs ♀
Malignant neoplasm of contiguous or overlapping sites of female genital organs whose point of origin cannot be determined

184.9 Female genital organ, site unspecified ♀
Female genitourinary tract NOS

185 Malignant neoplasm of prostate ♂
Excludes *seminal vesicles (187.8)*
C&C Exclusions: 599.60, 599.69
AHA: 3Q 2003, 13; 3Q 1999, 5; 3Q 1992, 7

④ **186 Malignant neoplasm of testis**
Use additional code to identify any functional activity

186.0 Undescended testis ♂
Ectopic testis
Retained testis

186.9 Other and unspecified testis ♂
Testis:
NOS
descended
scrotal

187 Malignant neoplasm of penis and other male genital organs

187.1 Prepuce ♂
Foreskin

187.2 Glans penis ♂

187.3 Body of penis ♂
Corpus cavernosum

187.4 Penis, part unspecified ♂
Skin of penis NOS

187.5 Epididymis ♂

187.6 Spermatic cord ♂
Vas deferens

187.7 Scrotum ♂
Skin of scrotum

187.8 Other specified sites of male genital organs ♂
Seminal vesicle
Tunica vaginalis
Malignant neoplasm of contiguous or overlapping sites of penis and other male genital organs whose point of origin cannot be determined

187.9 Male genital organ, site unspecified ♂
Male genital organ or tract NOS

188 Malignant neoplasm of bladder
Excludes *carcinoma in situ (233.7)*

188.0 Trigone of urinary bladder
C&C Exclusions: 599.60, 599.69

188.1 Dome of urinary bladder
C&C Exclusions: See 188.0

188.2 Lateral wall of urinary bladder
C&C Exclusions: See 188.0

188.3 Anterior wall of urinary bladder
C&C Exclusions: See 188.0

188.4 Posterior wall of urinary bladder
C&C Exclusions: See 188.0

188.5 Bladder neck
Internal urethral orifice
C&C Exclusions: See 188.0

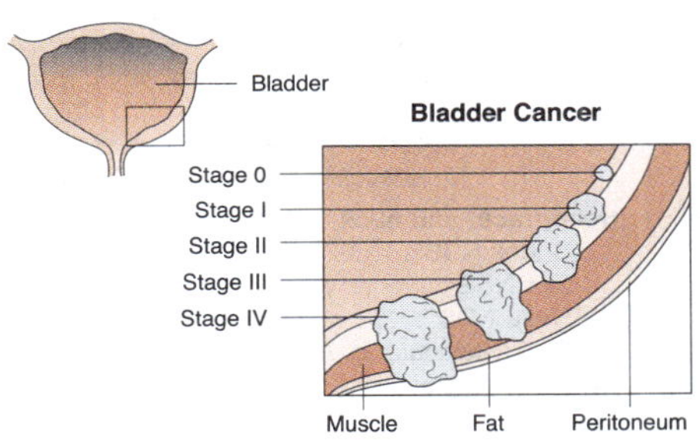

188.6 Ureteric orifice
C&C Exclusions: See 188.0

188.7 Urachus
C&C Exclusions: See 188.0

188.8 Other specified sites of bladder
Malignant neoplasm of contiguous or overlapping sites of bladder whose point of origin cannot be determined
C&C Exclusions: See 188.0

188.9 Bladder, part unspecified
Bladder wall NOS
C&C Exclusions: See 188.0
AHA: 1Q 2000, 5

189 Malignant neoplasm of kidney and other and unspecified urinary organs

189.0 Kidney, except pelvis
Kidney NOS
Kidney parenchyma
C&C Exclusions: 189.0, 189.1, 189.8, 189.9, 195.8, 199.0, 199.1, 239.5, 239.8, 239.9
AHA: 2Q 2005, 4; 2Q 2004, 4

189.1 Renal pelvis
Renal calyces
Ureteropelvic junction
C&C Exclusions: See 189.0

189.2 Ureter
Excludes *ureteric orifice of bladder (188.6)*
C&C Exclusions: 189.2, 189.8, 189.9, 195.8, 199.0, 199.1, 239.5, 239.8, 239.9, 599.60, 599.69

189.3 Urethra
Excludes *urethral orifice of bladder (188.5)*
C&C Exclusions: 599.60, 599.69

189.4 Paraurethral glands
C&C Exclusions: See 189.3

189.8 Other specified sites of urinary organs
Malignant neoplasm of contiguous or overlapping sites of kidney and other urinary organs whose point of origin cannot be determined
C&C Exclusions: See 189.3

189.9 Urinary organ, site unspecified
Urinary system NOS
C&C Exclusions: See 189.3

MALIGNANT NEOPLASM OF OTHER AND UNSPECIFIED SITES (190-199)

Excludes *carcinoma in situ (234.0-234.9)*

190 Malignant neoplasm of eye
Excludes *carcinoma in situ (234.0)*
eyelid (skin) (172.1, 173.1)
cartilage (171.0)
optic nerve (192.0)
orbital bone (170.0)

190.0 Eyeball, except conjunctiva, cornea, retina, and choroid
Ciliary body
Crystalline lens
Iris
Sclera
Uveal tract

190.1 Orbit
Connective tissue of orbit
Extraocular muscle
Retrobulbar
Excludes *bone of orbit (170.0)*

190.2 Lacrimal gland

190.3 Conjunctiva

190.4 Cornea

190.5 Retina

190.6 Choroid

190.7 Lacrimal duct
Lacrimal sac
Nasolacrimal duct

190.8 Other specified sites of eye
Malignant neoplasm of contiguous or overlapping sites of eye whose point of origin cannot be determined

190.9 Eye, part unspecified

191 Malignant neoplasm of brain
Excludes *cranial nerves (192.0)*
retrobulbar area (190.1)

191.0 Cerebrum, except lobes and ventricles
Basal ganglia
Cerebral cortex
Corpus striatum
Globus pallidus
Hypothalamus
Thalamus
C&C Exclusions: 191.0, 191.1, 191.2, 191.3, 191.4, 191.5, 191.6, 191.7, 191.8, 191.9, 192.0, 192.1, 192.8, 192.9, 195.8, 199.0, 199.1, 239.6, 239.7, 239.8, 239.9

191.1 Frontal lobe
C&C Exclusions: See 191.0
AHA: 4Q 2005, 118

191.2 Temporal lobe
Hippocampus
Uncus
C&C Exclusions: See 191.0

191.3 Parietal lobe
C&C Exclusions: See 191.0

191.4 Occipital lobe
C&C Exclusions: See 191.0

191.5 Ventricles
Choroid plexus
Floor of ventricle
C&C Exclusions: See 191.0

191.6 Cerebellum NOS
Cerebellopontine angle
C&C Exclusions: See 191.0

191.7 Brain stem
Cerebral peduncle
Medulla oblongata
Midbrain
Pons
C&C Exclusions: See 191.0

191.8 Other parts of brain
Corpus callosum
Tapetum
Malignant neoplasm of contiguous or overlapping sites of brain whose point of origin cannot be determined
C&C Exclusions: See 191.0

191.9 Brain, unspecified
Cranial fossa NOS
C&C Exclusions: See 191.0

❹ **192 Malignant neoplasm of other and unspecified parts of nervous system**
Excludes *peripheral, sympathetic, and parasympathetic nerves and ganglia (171.0-171.9)*

192.0 Cranial nerves
Olfactory bulb
C&C Exclusions: 192.0, 192.8, 192.9, 195.8, 199.0, 199.1, 239.6, 239.7, 239.8, 239.9

192.1 Cerebral meninges
Dura (mater)
Falx (cerebelli) (cerebri)
Meninges NOS
Tentorium
C&C Exclusions: 192.1, 192.8, 192.9, 195.8, 199.0, 199.1, 239.6, 239.7, 239.8, 239.9

192.2 Spinal cord
Cauda equina
C&C Exclusions: 192.2, 192.8, 192.9, 195.8, 199.0, 199.1, 239.6, 239.7, 239.8, 239.9

Malignant neoplasm; spinal cord

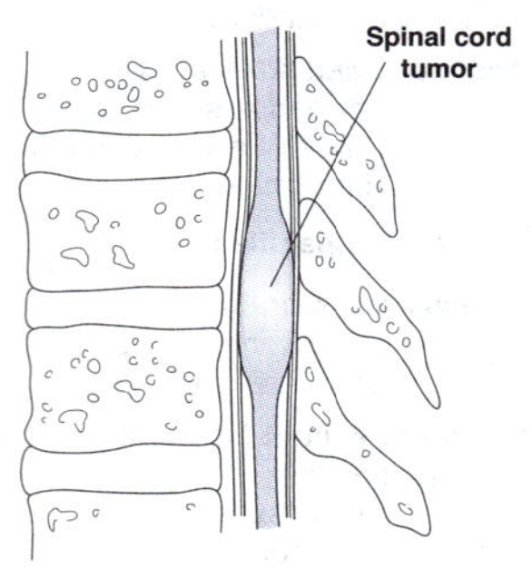

192.3 Spinal meninges
C&C Exclusions: 192.3, 192.8, 192.9, 195.8, 199.0, 199.1, 239.6, 239.7, 239.8, 239.9

192.8 Other specified sites of nervous system
Malignant neoplasm of contiguous or overlapping sites of other parts of nervous system whose point of origin cannot be determined
C&C Exclusions: 191.0, 191.1, 191.2, 191.3, 191.4, 191.5, 191.6, 191.7, 191.8, 191.9, 192.0, 192.1, 192.8, 192.9, 195.8, 199.0, 199.1, 239.6, 239.7, 239.8, 239.9

✖ **192.9 Nervous system, part unspecified**
Nervous system (central) NOS
Excludes *meninges NOS (192.1)*

193 Malignant neoplasm of thyroid gland
Thyroglossal duct
Use additional code to identify any functional activity

❹ **194 Malignant neoplasm of other endocrine glands and related structures**
Use additional code to identify any functional activity
Excludes *islets of Langerhans (157.4)*
ovary (183.0)
testis (186.0-186.9)
thymus (164.0)

194.0 Adrenal gland
Adrenal cortex
Adrenal medulla
Suprarenal gland

194.1 Parathyroid gland

194.3 Pituitary gland and craniopharyngeal duct
Craniobuccal pouch
Hypophysis
Rathke's pouch
Sella turcica
AHA: Jul-Aug 1985, 9

194.4 Pineal gland

194.5 Carotid body

194.6 Aortic body and other paraganglia
Coccygeal body
Glomus jugulare
Para-aortic body

194.8 Other
Pluriglandular involvement NOS
Note: *If the sites of multiple involvements are known, they should be coded separately.*

✖ **194.9 Endocrine gland, site unspecified**

❹ **195 Malignant neoplasm of other and ill-defined sites**
Includes malignant neoplasms of contiguous sites, not elsewhere classified, whose point of origin cannot be determined
Excludes *malignant neoplasm:*
lymphatic and hematopoietic tissue (200.0-208.9)
secondary sites (196.0-198.8)
unspecified site (199.0-199.1)

195.0 Head, face, and neck
Cheek NOS
Jaw NOS
Nose NOS
Supraclavicular region NOS
AHA: 4Q 2003, 107

195.1 Thorax
Axilla
Chest (wall) NOS
Intrathoracic NOS

195.2 Abdomen
Intra-abdominal NOS
AHA: 2Q 1997, 3

195.3 Pelvis
Groin
Inguinal region NOS
Presacral region
Sacrococcygeal region
Sites overlapping systems within pelvis, as:
rectovaginal (septum)
rectovesical (septum)

195.4 Upper limb

195.5 Lower limb

195.8 Other specified sites
Back NOS
Flank NOS
Trunk NOS

4 196 Secondary and unspecified malignant neoplasm of lymph nodes

Excludes *any malignant neoplasm of lymph nodes, specified as primary (200.0-202.9)*
Hodgkin's disease (201.0-201.9)
lymphosarcoma (200.1)
reticulosarcoma (200.0)
other forms of lymphoma (202.0-202.9)

AHA: 2Q 1992, 3; May-Jun 1985, 3

196.0 Lymph nodes of head, face, and neck
Cervical
Cervicofacial
Scalene
Supraclavicular
C&C Exclusions: 176.5, 195.8, 196.0, 196.1, 196.2, 196.3, 196.4, 196.5, 196.6, 196.8, 196.9, 199.0, 199.1, 239.8, 239.9

196.1 Intrathoracic lymph nodes
Bronchopulmonary
Intercostal
Mediastinal
Tracheobronchial
C&C Exclusions: See 196.0
AHA: 3Q 2006, 8

196.2 Intra-abdominal lymph nodes
Intestinal
Mesenteric
Retroperitoneal
C&C Exclusions: See 196.0
AHA: 4Q 2003, 111

196.3 Lymph nodes of axilla and upper limb
Brachial
Epitrochlear
Infraclavicular
Pectoral
C&C Exclusions: See 196.0

196.5 Lymph nodes of inguinal region and lower limb
Femoral
Groin
Popliteal
Tibial
C&C Exclusions: See 196.0

196.6 Intrapelvic lymph nodes
Hypogastric
Iliac
Obturator
Parametrial
C&C Exclusions: See 196.0

196.8 Lymph nodes of multiple sites
C&C Exclusions: See 196.0

✖ 196.9 Site unspecified
Lymph nodes NOS
C&C Exclusions: See 196.0

4 197 Secondary malignant neoplasm of respiratory and digestive systems

Excludes *lymph node metastasis (196.0-196.9)*

AHA: May-Jun 1985, 3

197.0 Lung
Bronchus
C&C Exclusions: 195.8, 197.0, 197.3, 198.89, 199.0, 199.1, 239.8, 239.9
AHA: 1Q 2006, 5; 2Q 1999, 9

197.1 Mediastinum
C&C Exclusions: 195.8, 197.1, 197.3, 198.89, 199.0, 199.1, 239.8, 239.9
AHA: 3Q 2006, 8

197.2 Pleura
C&C Exclusions: 195.8, 197.2, 197.3, 198.89, 199.0, 199.1, 239.8, 239.9
AHA: 4Q 2003, 110; 4Q 1989, 11

197.3 Other respiratory organs
Trachea
C&C Exclusions: 195.8, 197.0, 197.1, 197.2, 197.3, 198.89, 199.0, 199.1, 239.8, 239.9

197.4 Small intestine, including duodenum
C&C Exclusions: 195.8, 197.4, 197.8, 198.89, 199.0, 199.1, 239.8, 239.9

197.5 Large intestine and rectum
C&C Exclusions: 195.8, 197.5, 197.8, 198.89, 199.0, 199.1, 239.8, 239.9

197.6 Retroperitoneum and peritoneum
C&C Exclusions: 195.8, 197.6, 197.8, 198.89, 199.0, 199.1, 239.8, 239.9
AHA: 2Q 2004, 4; 4Q 1989, 11

197.7 Liver, specified as secondary
C&C Exclusions: 195.8, 197.7, 197.8, 198.89, 199.0, 199.1, 239.8, 239.9
AHA: 1Q 2006, 5; 2Q 2005, 9

197.8 Other digestive organs and spleen
C&C Exclusions: 195.8, 197.4, 197.5, 197.6, 197.7, 197.8, 198.89, 199.0, 199.1, 239.8, 239.9
AHA: 2Q 1997, 3; 2Q 1992, 3

4 198 Secondary malignant neoplasm of other specified sites

Excludes *lymph node metastasis (196.0-196.9)*

AHA: May-Jun 1985, 3

198.0 Kidney
C&C Exclusions: 195.8, 198.0, 198.1, 198.89, 199.0, 199.1, 239.8, 239.9

198.1 Other urinary organs
C&C Exclusions: See 198.0

198.2 Skin
Skin of breast
C&C Exclusions: 195.8, 198.2, 198.89, 199.0, 199.1, 239.8 239.9

198.3 Brain and spinal cord
C&C Exclusions: 195.8, 198.3, 198.89, 199.0, 199.1, 239.8, 239.9
AHA: 3Q 1999, 7

198.4 Other parts of nervous system
Meninges (cerebral) (spinal)
C&C Exclusions: 195.8, 198.4, 198.89, 199.0, 199.1, 239.8, 239.9
AHA: Jan-Feb 1987, 7

198.5 Bone and bone marrow
C&C Exclusions: 195.8, 198.5, 198.89, 199.0, 199.1, 239.8, 239.9
AHA: 1Q 2007, 6; 4Q 2003, 110; 3Q 1999, 5; 2Q 1992, 3; 1Q 1991, 16; 4Q 1989, 10

198.6 Ovary ♀
C&C Exclusions: 195.8, 198.6, 198.89, 199.0, 199.1, 239.8, 239.9

198.7 Adrenal gland
Suprarenal gland
C&C Exclusions: 195.8, 198.7, 198.89, 199.0, 199.1, 239.8, 239.9

5 198.8 Other specified sites

198.81 Breast
Excludes *skin of breast (198.2)*
C&C Exclusions: 195.8, 198.81, 198.89, 199.0, 199.1, 239.8, 239.9

198.82 Genital organs
C&C Exclusions: 195.8, 198.82, 198.89, 199.0, 199.1, 239.8, 239.9

198.89 Other
Excludes *retroperitoneal lymph nodes (196.2)*
C&C Exclusions: 195.8, 198.89, 199.0, 199.1, 239.8, 239.9
AHA: 2Q 2005, 4; 2Q 1997, 4

4 199 Malignant neoplasm without specification of site

199.0 Disseminated
Carcinomatosis unspecified site (primary) (secondary)
Generalized:
cancer unspecified site (primary) (secondary)
malignancy unspecified site (primary) (secondary)
Multiple cancer unspecified site (primary) (secondary)
C&C Exclusions: See 198.89
AHA: 4Q 1989, 10

✖ 199.1 Other
Cancer unspecified site (primary) (secondary)
Carcinoma unspecified site (primary) (secondary)
Malignancy unspecified site (primary) (secondary)
AHA: 3Q 2006, 15; 1Q 2006, 5

A Adult (15+ years) M Maternity (12-55 years) N Newborn (0 years) P Pediatric (0-17 years) ♂ Male ♀ Female ② Medicare Secondary Payer

MALIGNANT NEOPLASM OF LYMPHATIC AND HEMATOPOIETIC TISSUE (200-208)

Excludes *secondary neoplasm of:*
bone marrow (198.5)
spleen (197.8)
secondary and unspecified neoplasm of lymph nodes (196.0-196.9)

The following fifth-digit subclassification is for use with categories 200-202:

0 unspecified site, extranodal and solid organ sites
1 lymph nodes of head, face, and neck
2 intrathoracic lymph nodes
3 intra-abdominal lymph nodes
4 lymph nodes of axilla and upper limb
5 lymph nodes of inguinal region and lower limb
6 intrapelvic lymph nodes
7 spleen
8 lymph nodes of multiple sites

▲4 **200 Lymphosarcoma and reticulosarcoma and other specified malignant tumors of lymphatic tissue**
Requires fifth digit. See note before section 200 for codes and definitions.
AHA: 2Q 1992, 3; Nov-Dec 1986, 5

5 **200.0 Reticulosarcoma**
Lymphoma (malignant):
histiocytic (diffuse):
nodular
pleomorphic cell type
reticulum cell type
Reticulum cell sarcoma:
NOS
pleomorphic cell type
C&C Exclusions: (for codes 200.00, 200.08) 200.00, 200.01, 200.02, 200.03, 200.04, 200.05, 200.06, 200.07, 200.08, 239.8, 239.9
C&C Exclusions: (for code 200.01) 200.00, 200.01, 200.08, 239.8, 239.9
C&C Exclusions: (for code 200.02) 200.00, 200.02, 200.08, 239.8, 239.9
C&C Exclusions: (for code 200.03) 200.00, 200.03, 200.08, 239.8, 239.9
C&C Exclusions: (for code 200.04) 200.00, 200.04, 200.08, 239.8, 239.9
C&C Exclusions: (for code 200.05) 200.00, 200.05, 200.08, 239.8, 239.9
C&C Exclusions: (for code 200.06) 200.00, 200.06, 200.08, 239.8, 239.9
C&C Exclusions: (for code 200.07) 200.00, 200.07, 200.08, 239.8, 239.9
AHA: For Code 200.03: 3Q 2001, 12

5 **200.1 Lymphosarcoma**
Lymphoblastoma (diffuse)
Lymphoma (malignant):
lymphoblastic (diffuse)
lymphocytic (cell type) (diffuse)
lymphosarcoma type
Lymphosarcoma:
NOS
diffuse NOS
lymphoblastic (diffuse)
lymphocytic (diffuse)
prolymphocytic
Excludes *lymphosarcoma:*
follicular or nodular (202.0)
mixed cell type (200.8)
lymphosarcoma cell leukemia (207.8)
C&C Exclusions: (for codes 200.10, 200.18) 200.10, 200.11, 200.12, 200.13, 200.14, 200.15, 200.16, 200.17, 200.18, 239.8, 239.9
C&C Exclusions: (for code 200.11) 200.10, 200.11, 200.18, 239.8, 239.9
C&C Exclusions: (for code 200.12) 200.10, 200.12, 200.18, 239.8, 239.9
C&C Exclusions: (for code 200.13) 200.10, 200.13, 200.18, 239.8, 239.9
C&C Exclusions: (for code 200.14) 200.10, 200.14, 200.18, 239.8, 239.9
C&C Exclusions: (for code 200.15) 200.10, 200.15, 200.18, 239.8, 239.9
C&C Exclusions: (for code 200.16) 200.10, 200.16, 200.18, 239.8, 239.9
C&C Exclusions: (for code 200.17) 200.10, 200.17, 200.18, 239.8, 239.9

5 **200.2 Burkitt's tumor or lymphoma**
Malignant lymphoma, Burkitt's type
C&C Exclusions: (for codes 200.20, 200.28) 200.20, 200.21, 200.22, 200.23, 200.24, 200.25, 200.26, 200.27, 200.28, 239.8, 239.9
C&C Exclusions: (for code 200.21) 200.20, 200.21, 200.28, 239.8, 239.9
C&C Exclusions: (for code 200.22) 200.20, 200.22, 200.28, 239.8, 239.9
C&C Exclusions: (for code 200.23) 200.20, 200.23, 200.28, 239.8, 239.9
C&C Exclusions: (for code 200.24) 200.20, 200.24, 200.28, 239.8, 239.9
C&C Exclusions: (for code 200.25) 200.20, 200.25, 200.28, 239.8, 239.9
C&C Exclusions: (for code 200.26) 200.20, 200.26, 200.28, 239.8, 239.9
C&C Exclusions: (for code 200.27) 200.20, 200.27, 200.28, 239.8, 239.9

●5 **200.3 Marginal zone lymphoma**
Extranodal marginal zone B-cell lymphoma
Mucosa associated lymphoid tissue [MALT]
Nodal marginal zone B-cell lymphoma
Splenic marginal zone B-cell lymphoma
DEF: Uncommon, low-grade, slow-growing B-cell non-Hodgkin's lymphoma involving the marginal, patchy area of the lymph node outside the mantle zone; not very responsive to traditional therapy.

●5 **200.4 Mantle cell lymphoma**

●5 **200.5 Primary central nervous system lymphoma**
DEF: Rare lymphoma of the brain, spinal cord, eyes, and/or meningeal coverings, causing personality change, headache, memory and progressive vision loss.

●5 **200.6 Anaplastic large cell lymphoma**
DEF: Rare lymphoma, usually of cancerous T-cells; presents as high-grade, aggressive, systemic form associated with chromosome abnormality or slow-growing, limited cutaneous form.

●5 **200.7 Large cell lymphoma**
DEF: Common, aggressive B- or T-cell lymphomas that tend to metastasize with extranodal, infiltrating tumors that obstruct organs, causing site-related symptoms.

5 200.8 Other named variants
Lymphoma (malignant):
lymphoplasmacytoid type
mixed lymphocytic-histiocytic (diffuse)
Lymphosarcoma, mixed cell type (diffuse)
Reticulolymphosarcoma (diffuse)
C&C Exclusions: (for codes 200.80, 200.88) 200.80, 200.81, 200.82, 200.83, 200.84, 200.85, 200.86, 200.87, 200.88, 239.8, 239.9
C&C Exclusions: (for code 200.81) 200.80, 200.81, 200.88, 239.8, 239.9
C&C Exclusions: (for code 200.82) 200.80, 200.82, 200.88, 239.8, 239.9
C&C Exclusions: (for code 200.83) 200.80, 200.83, 200.88, 239.8, 239.9
C&C Exclusions: (for code 200.84) 200.80, 200.84, 200.88, 239.8, 239.9
C&C Exclusions: (for code 200.85) 200.80, 200.85, 200.88, 239.8, 239.9
C&C Exclusions: (for code 200.86) 200.80, 200.86, 200.88, 239.8, 239.9
C&C Exclusions: (for code 200.87) 200.80, 200.87, 200.88, 239.8, 239.9

4 201 Hodgkin's disease
Requires fifth digit. See note before section 200 for codes and definitions.
AHA: 2Q 1992, 3; Nov-Dec 1986, 5

5 201.0 Hodgkin's paragranuloma
C&C Exclusions: (for codes 201.00, 201.08) 201.00, 201.01, 201.02, 201.03, 201.04, 201.05, 201.06, 201.07, 201.08, 201.90, 201.98, 239.8, 239.9
C&C Exclusions: (for code 201.01) 201.00, 201.01, 201.08, 201.90, 201.91, 239.8, 239.9
C&C Exclusions: (for code 201.02) 201.00, 201.02, 201.08, 201.90, 201.92, 239.8, 239.9
C&C Exclusions: (for code 201.03) 201.00, 201.03, 201.08, 201.90, 201.93, 239.8, 239.9
C&C Exclusions: (for code 201.04) 201.00, 201.04, 201.08, 201.90, 201.94, 239.8, 239.9
C&C Exclusions: (for code 201.05) 201.00, 201.05, 201.08, 201.90, 201.95, 239.8, 239.9
C&C Exclusions: (for code 201.06) 201.00, 201.06, 201.08, 201.90, 201.96, 239.8, 239.9
C&C Exclusions: (for code 201.07) 201.00, 201.07, 201.08, 201.90, 201.97, 239.8, 239.9

5 201.1 Hodgkin's granuloma
C&C Exclusions: (for codes 201.10, 201.18) 201.10, 201.11, 201.12, 201.13, 201.14, 201.15, 201.16, 201.17, 201.18, 201.90, 201.98, 239.8, 239.9
C&C Exclusions: (for code 201.11) 201.10, 201.11, 201.18, 201.90, 201.91, 201.98, 239.8, 239.9
C&C Exclusions: (for code 201.12) 201.10, 201.12, 201.18, 201.90, 201.92, 201.98, 239.8, 239.9
C&C Exclusions: (for code 201.13) 201.10, 201.13, 201.18, 201.90, 201.93, 201.98, 239.8, 239.9
C&C Exclusions: (for code 201.14) 201.10, 201.14, 201.18, 201.90, 201.94, 201.98, 239.8, 239.9
C&C Exclusions: (for code 201.15) 201.10, 201.15, 201.18, 201.90, 201.95, 201.98, 239.8, 239.9
C&C Exclusions: (for code 201.16) 201.10, 201.16, 201.18, 201.90, 201.96, 201.98, 239.8, 239.9
C&C Exclusions: (for code 201.17) 201.10, 201.17, 201.18, 201.90, 201.97, 201.98, 239.8, 239.9
AHA: 2Q 1999, 7

5 201.2 Hodgkin's sarcoma
C&C Exclusions: (for codes 201.20, 201.28) 201.20, 201.21, 201.22, 201.23, 201.24, 201.25, 201.26, 201.27, 201.28, 201.90, 201.98, 239.8, 239.9
C&C Exclusions: (for code 201.21) 201.20, 201.21, 201.28, 201.90, 201.91, 201.98, 239.8, 239.9
C&C Exclusions: (for code 201.22) 201.20, 201.22, 201.28, 201.90, 201.92, 201.98, 239.8, 239.9
C&C Exclusions: (for code 201.23) 201.20, 201.23, 201.28, 201.90, 201.93, 201.98, 239.8, 239.9
C&C Exclusions: (for code 201.24) 201.20, 201.24, 201.28, 201.90, 201.94, 201.98, 239.8, 239.9
C&C Exclusions: (for code 201.25) 201.20, 201.25, 201.28, 201.90, 201.95, 201.98, 239.8, 239.9
C&C Exclusions: (for code 201.26) 201.20, 201.26, 201.28, 201.90, 201.96, 201.98, 239.8, 239.9
C&C Exclusions: (for code 201.27) 201.20, 201.27, 201.28, 201.90, 201.97, 201.98, 239.8, 239.9

5 201.4 Lymphocytic-histiocytic predominance
C&C Exclusions: (for codes 201.40, 201.48) 201.40, 201.41, 201.42, 201.43, 201.44, 201.45, 201.46, 201.47, 201.48, 201.90, 201.98, 239.8, 239.9
C&C Exclusions: (for code 201.41) 201.40, 201.41, 201.48, 201.90, 201.91, 201.98, 239.8, 239.9
C&C Exclusions: (for code 201.42) 201.40, 201.42, 201.48, 201.90, 201.92, 201.98, 239.8, 239.9
C&C Exclusions: (for code 201.43) 201.40, 201.43, 201.48, 201.90, 201.93, 201.98, 239.8, 239.9
C&C Exclusions: (for code 201.44) 201.40, 201.44, 201.48, 201.90, 201.94, 201.98, 239.8, 239.9
C&C Exclusions: (for code 201.45) 201.40, 201.45, 201.48, 201.90, 201.95, 201.98, 239.8, 239.9
C&C Exclusions: (for code 201.46) 201.40, 201.46, 201.48, 201.90, 201.96, 201.98, 239.8, 239.9
C&C Exclusions: (for code 201.47) 201.40, 201.47, 201.48, 201.90, 201.97, 201.98, 239.8, 239.9

5 201.5 Nodular sclerosis
Hodgkin's disease, nodular sclerosis:
NOS
cellular phase
C&C Exclusions: (for codes 201.50, 201.58) 201.50, 201.51, 201.52, 201.53, 201.54, 201.55, 201.56, 201.57, 201.58, 201.90, 201.98, 239.8, 239.9
C&C Exclusions: (for code 201.51) 201.50, 201.51, 201.58, 201.90, 201.91, 201.98, 239.8, 239.9
C&C Exclusions: (for code 201.52) 201.50, 201.52, 201.58, 201.90, 201.92, 201.98, 239.8, 239.9
C&C Exclusions: (for code 201.53) 201.50, 201.53, 201.58, 201.90, 201.93, 201.98, 239.8, 239.9
C&C Exclusions: (for code 201.54) 201.50, 201.54, 201.58, 201.90, 201.94, 201.98, 239.8, 239.9
C&C Exclusions: (for code 201.55) 201.50, 201.55, 201.58, 201.90, 201.95, 201.98, 239.8, 239.9
C&C Exclusions: (for code 201.56) 201.50, 201.56, 201.58, 201.90, 201.96, 201.98, 239.8, 239.9
C&C Exclusions: (for code 201.57) 201.50, 201.57, 201.58, 201.90, 201.97, 201.98, 239.8, 239.9

5 201.6 Mixed cellularity
C&C Exclusions: (for codes 201.60, 201.68) 201.60, 201.61, 201.62, 201.63, 201.64, 201.65, 201.66, 201.67, 201.68, 201.90, 201.98, 239.8, 239.9
C&C Exclusions: (for code 201.61) 201.60, 201.61, 201.68, 201.90, 201.91, 201.98, 239.8, 239.9
C&C Exclusions: (for code 201.62) 201.60, 201.62, 201.68, 201.90, 201.92, 201.98, 239.8, 239.9
C&C Exclusions: (for code 201.63) 201.60, 201.63, 201.68, 201.90, 201.93, 201.98, 239.8, 239.9
C&C Exclusions: (for code 201.64) 201.60, 201.64, 201.68, 201.90, 201.94, 201.98, 239.8, 239.9
C&C Exclusions: (for code 201.65) 201.60, 201.65, 201.68, 201.90, 201.95, 201.98, 239.8, 239.9
C&C Exclusions: (for code 201.66) 201.60, 201.66, 201.68, 201.90, 201.96, 201.98, 239.8, 239.9
C&C Exclusions: (for code 201.67) 201.60, 201.67, 201.68, 201.90, 201.97, 201.98, 239.8, 239.9

5 201.7 Lymphocytic depletion
Hodgkin's disease, lymphocytic depletion:
NOS
diffuse fibrosis
reticular type
C&C Exclusions: (for codes 201.70, 201.78) 201.70, 201.71, 201.72, 201.73, 201.74, 201.75, 201.76, 201.77, 201.78, 201.90, 201.98, 239.8, 239.9
C&C Exclusions: (for code 201.71) 201.70, 201.71, 201.78, 201.90, 201.91, 201.98, 239.8, 239.9
C&C Exclusions: (for code 201.72) 201.70, 201.72, 201.78, 201.90, 201.92, 201.98, 239.8, 239.9
C&C Exclusions: (for code 201.73) 201.70, 201.73, 201.78, 201.90, 201.93, 201.98, 239.8, 239.9
C&C Exclusions: (for code 201.74) 201.70, 201.74, 201.78, 201.90, 201.94, 201.98, 239.8, 239.9
C&C Exclusions: (for code 201.75) 201.70, 201.75, 201.78, 201.90, 201.95, 201.98, 239.8, 239.9
C&C Exclusions: (for code 201.76) 201.70, 201.76, 201.78, 201.90, 201.96, 201.98, 239.8, 239.9
C&C Exclusions: (for code 201.77) 201.70, 201.77, 201.78, 201.90, 201.97, 201.98, 239.8, 239.9

❺ **201.9 Hodgkin's disease, unspecified**

Hodgkin's:
- disease NOS
- lymphoma NOS

Malignant:
- lymphogranuloma
- lymphogranulomatosis

C&C Exclusions: (for codes 201.90, 201.98) 201.90, 201.91, 201.92, 201.93, 201.94, 201.95, 201.96, 201.97, 201.98, 239.8, 239.9
C&C Exclusions: (for code 201.91) 201.90, 201.91, 201.98, 239.8, 239.9
C&C Exclusions: (for code 201.92) 201.90, 201.92, 201.98, 239.8, 239.9
C&C Exclusions: (for code 201.93) 201.90, 201.93, 201.98, 239.8, 239.9
C&C Exclusions: (for code 201.94) 201.90, 201.94, 201.98, 239.8, 239.9
C&C Exclusions: (for code 201.95) 201.90, 201.95, 201.98, 239.8, 239.9
C&C Exclusions: (for code 201.96) 201.90, 201.96, 201.98, 239.8, 239.9
C&C Exclusions: (for code 201.97) 201.90, 201.97, 201.98, 239.8, 239.9

Hodgkin's disease

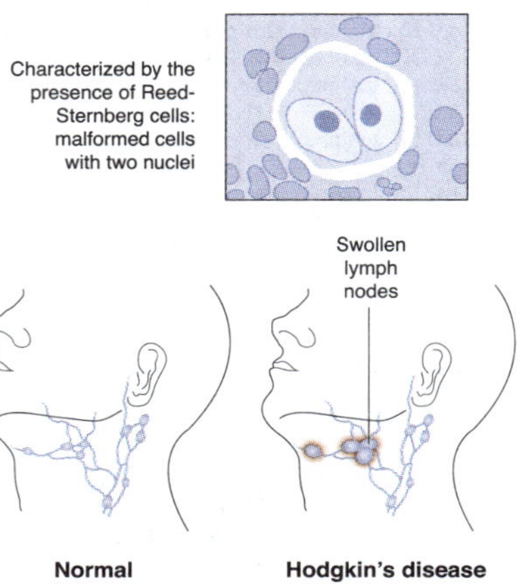

❹ **202 Other malignant neoplasms of lymphoid and histiocytic tissue**

Requires fifth digit. See note before section 200 for codes and definitions.

AHA: 2Q 1992, 3; Nov-Dec 1986, 5

❺ **202.0 Nodular lymphoma**

Brill-Symmers disease

Lymphoma:
- follicular (giant)
- lymphocytic, nodular

Lymphosarcoma:
- follicular (giant)
- nodular

C&C Exclusions: (for codes 202.00, 202.08) 202.00, 202.01, 202.02, 202.03, 202.04, 202.05, 202.06, 202.08, 202.80, 202.90, 239.8, 239.9
C&C Exclusions: (for code 202.01) 202.00, 202.01, 202.08, 202.81, 202.91, 239.8, 239.9
C&C Exclusions: (for code 202.02) 202.00, 202.02, 202.08, 202.82, 202.92, 239.8, 239.9
C&C Exclusions: (for code 202.03) 202.00, 202.03, 202.08, 202.83, 202.93, 239.8, 239.9
C&C Exclusions: (for code 202.04) 202.00, 202.04, 202.08, 202.84, 202.94, 239.8, 239.9
C&C Exclusions: (for code 202.05) 202.00, 202.05, 202.08, 202.85, 202.95, 239.8, 239.9
C&C Exclusions: (for code 202.06) 202.00, 202.06, 202.08, 202.86, 202.96, 239.8, 239.9
C&C Exclusions: (for code 202.07) 202.00, 202.07, 202.08, 202.87, 202.97, 239.8, 239.9

❺ **202.1 Mycosis fungoides**

C&C Exclusions: (for codes 202.10, 202.18) 202.10, 202.11, 202.12, 202.13, 202.14, 202.15, 202.16, 202.08, 202.80, 202.90, 239.8, 239.9
C&C Exclusions: (for code 202.11) 202.10, 202.11, 202.18, 202.81, 202.91, 239.8, 239.9
C&C Exclusions: (for code 202.12) 202.10, 202.12, 202.18, 202.82, 202.92, 239.8, 239.9
C&C Exclusions: (for code 202.13) 202.10, 202.13, 202.18, 202.83, 202.93, 239.8, 239.9
C&C Exclusions: (for code 202.14) 202.10, 202.14, 202.18, 202.84, 202.94, 239.8, 239.9
C&C Exclusions: (for code 202.15) 202.10, 202.15, 202.18, 202.85, 202.95, 239.8, 239.9
C&C Exclusions: (for code 202.16) 202.10, 202.16, 202.18, 202.86, 202.96, 239.8, 239.9
C&C Exclusions: (for code 202.17) 202.10, 202.17, 202.18, 202.87, 202.97, 239.8, 239.9

AHA: 2Q 1992, 4

❺ **202.2 Sézary's disease**

C&C Exclusions: (for codes 202.20, 202.28) 202.20, 202.21, 202.22, 202.23, 202.24, 202.25, 202.26, 202.08, 202.80, 202.90, 239.8, 239.9
C&C Exclusions: (for code 202.21) 202.20, 202.21, 202.28, 202.81, 202.91, 239.8, 239.9
C&C Exclusions: (for code 202.22) 202.20, 202.22, 202.28, 202.82, 202.92, 239.8, 239.9
C&C Exclusions: (for code 202.23) 202.20, 202.23, 202.28, 202.83, 202.93, 239.8, 239.9
C&C Exclusions: (for code 202.24) 202.20, 202.24, 202.28, 202.84, 202.94, 239.8, 239.9
C&C Exclusions: (for code 202.25) 202.20, 202.25, 202.28, 202.85, 202.95, 239.8, 239.9
C&C Exclusions: (for code 202.26) 202.20, 202.26, 202.28, 202.86, 202.96, 239.8, 239.9
C&C Exclusions: (for code 202.27) 202.20, 202.27, 202.28, 202.87, 202.97, 239.8, 239.9

AHA: 2Q 1999, 7

❺ **202.3 Malignant histiocytosis**

Histiocytic medullary reticulosis

Malignant:
- reticuloendotheliosis
- reticulosis

C&C Exclusions: (for codes 202.30, 202.38) 202.30, 202.31, 202.32, 202.33, 202.34, 202.35, 202.36, 202.38, 202.80, 202.90, 239.8, 239.9
C&C Exclusions: (for code 202.31) 202.30, 202.31, 202.38, 202.81, 202.91, 239.8, 239.9
C&C Exclusions: (for code 202.32) 202.30, 202.32, 202.38, 202.82, 202.92, 239.8, 239.9
C&C Exclusions: (for code 202.33) 202.30, 202.33, 202.38, 202.83, 202.93, 239.8, 239.9
C&C Exclusions: (for code 202.34) 202.30, 202.34, 202.38, 202.84, 202.94, 239.8, 239.9
C&C Exclusions: (for code 202.35) 202.30, 202.35, 202.38, 202.85, 202.95, 239.8, 239.9
C&C Exclusions: (for code 202.36) 202.30, 202.36, 202.38, 202.86, 202.96, 239.8, 239.9
C&C Exclusions: (for code 202.37) 202.30, 202.37, 202.38, 202.87, 202.97, 239.8, 239.9

❺ **202.4 Leukemic reticuloendotheliosis**

Hairy-cell leukemia

C&C Exclusions: (for codes 202.40, 202.48) 202.40, 202.41, 202.42, 202.43, 202.44, 202.45, 202.46, 202.48, 202.80, 202.90, 239.8, 239.9
C&C Exclusions: (for code 202.41) 202.40, 202.41, 202.48, 202.81, 202.91, 239.8, 239.9
C&C Exclusions: (for code 202.42) 202.40, 202.42, 202.48, 202.82, 202.92, 239.8, 239.9
C&C Exclusions: (for code 202.43) 202.40, 202.43, 202.48, 202.83, 202.93, 239.8, 239.9
C&C Exclusions: (for code 202.44) 202.40, 202.44, 202.48, 202.84, 202.94, 239.8, 239.9
C&C Exclusions: (for code 202.45) 202.40, 202.45, 202.48, 202.85, 202.95, 239.8, 239.9
C&C Exclusions: (for code 202.46) 202.40, 202.46, 202.48, 202.86, 202.96, 239.8, 239.9
C&C Exclusions: (for code 202.47) 202.40, 202.47, 202.48, 202.87, 202.97, 239.8, 239.9

202.5 Letterer-Siwe disease
Acute:
differentiated progressive histiocytosis
histiocytosis X (progressive)
infantile reticuloendotheliosis
reticulosis of infancy
Excludes *Hand-Schüller-Christian disease (277.89)*
histiocytosis (acute) (chronic) (277.89)
histiocytosis X (chronic) (277.89)
C&C Exclusions: (for codes 202.50, 202.58) 202.50, 202.51, 202.52, 202.53, 202.54, 202.55, 202.56, 202.58, 202.80, 202.90, 239.8, 239.9
C&C Exclusions: (for code 202.51) 202.50, 202.51, 202.58, 202.81, 202.91, 239.8, 239.9
C&C Exclusions: (for code 202.52) 202.50, 202.52, 202.58, 202.82, 202.92, 239.8, 239.9
C&C Exclusions: (for code 202.53) 202.50, 202.53, 202.58, 202.83, 202.93, 239.8, 239.9
C&C Exclusions: (for code 202.54) 202.50, 202.54, 202.58, 202.84, 202.94, 239.8, 239.9
C&C Exclusions: (for code 202.55) 202.50, 202.55, 202.58, 202.85, 202.95, 239.8, 239.9
C&C Exclusions: (for code 202.56) 202.50, 202.56, 202.58, 202.86, 202.96, 239.8, 239.9
C&C Exclusions: (for code 202.57) 202.50, 202.57, 202.58, 202.87, 202.97, 239.8, 239.9

202.6 Malignant mast cell tumors
Malignant:
mastocytoma
mastocytosis
Mast cell sarcoma
Systemic tissue mast cell disease
Excludes *mast cell leukemia (207.8)*
C&C Exclusions: (for codes 202.60, 202.68) 202.60, 202.61, 202.62, 202.63, 202.64, 202.65, 202.66, 202.68, 202.80, 202.90, 239.8, 239.9
C&C Exclusions: (for code 202.61) 202.60, 202.61, 202.68, 202.81, 202.91, 239.8, 239.9
C&C Exclusions: (for code 202.62) 202.60, 202.62, 202.68, 202.82, 202.92, 239.8, 239.9
C&C Exclusions: (for code 202.63) 202.60, 202.63, 202.68, 202.83, 202.93, 239.8, 239.9
C&C Exclusions: (for code 202.64) 202.60, 202.64, 202.68, 202.84, 202.94, 239.8, 239.9
C&C Exclusions: (for code 202.65) 202.60, 202.65, 202.68, 202.85, 202.95, 239.8, 239.9
C&C Exclusions: (for code 202.66) 202.60, 202.66, 202.68, 202.86, 202.96, 239.8, 239.9
C&C Exclusions: (for code 202.67) 202.60, 202.67, 202.68, 202.87, 202.97, 239.8, 239.9

● **202.7 Peripheral T-cell lymphoma**
DEF: Aggressive, non-Hodgkin's lymphoma derived from mature neoplastic T-cell lymphocytes that have moved to other tissue, causing site-related symptoms and generalized lymphadenopathy.

202.8 Other lymphomas
Lymphoma (malignant):
NOS
diffuse
Excludes *benign lymphoma (229.0)*
C&C Exclusions: (for codes 202.80, 202.88) 202.80, 202.81, 202.82, 202.83, 202.84, 202.85, 202.86, 202.87, 202.88, 202.90, 239.8, 239.9
C&C Exclusions: (for code 202.81) 202.80, 202.81, 202.88, 202.91, 239.8, 239.9
C&C Exclusions: (for code 202.82) 202.80, 202.82, 202.88, 202.92, 239.8, 239.9
C&C Exclusions: (for code 202.83) 202.80, 202.83, 202.88, 202.93, 239.8, 239.9
C&C Exclusions: (for code 202.84) 202.80, 202.84, 202.88, 202.94, 239.8, 239.9
C&C Exclusions: (for code 202.85) 202.80, 202.85, 202.88, 202.95, 239.8, 239.9
C&C Exclusions: (for code 202.86) 202.80, 202.86, 202.88, 202.96, 239.8, 239.9
C&C Exclusions: (for code 202.87) 202.80, 202.87, 202.88, 202.97, 239.8, 239.9
AHA: 4Q 2006, 135-136; 2Q 1992, 4; For Code 202.80: 2Q 2006, 21

202.9 Other and unspecified malignant neoplasms of lymphoid and histiocytic tissue
Follicular dendritic cell sarcoma
Interdigitating dendritic cell sarcoma
Langerhans cell sarcoma
Malignant neoplasm of bone marrow NOS
C&C Exclusions: (for codes 202.90, 202.98) 202.90, 202.91, 202.92, 202.93, 202.94, 202.95, 202.96, 202.97, 202.98, 239.8, 239.9
C&C Exclusions: (for code 202.91) 202.90, 202.91, 202.98, 239.8, 239.9
C&C Exclusions: (for code 202.92) 202.90, 202.92, 202.98, 239.8, 239.9
C&C Exclusions: (for code 202.93) 202.90, 202.93, 202.98, 239.8, 239.9
C&C Exclusions: (for code 202.94) 202.90, 202.94, 202.98, 239.8, 239.9
C&C Exclusions: (for code 202.95) 202.90, 202.95, 202.98, 239.8, 239.9
C&C Exclusions: (for code 202.96) 202.90, 202.96, 202.98, 239.8, 239.9
C&C Exclusions: (for code 202.97) 202.90, 202.97, 202.98, 239.8, 239.9

203 Multiple myeloma and immunoproliferative neoplasms

The following fifth-digit subclassification is for use with category 203:
0 without mention of remission
1 in remission

203.0 Multiple myeloma
Kahler's disease
Myelomatosis
Excludes *solitary myeloma (238.6)*
C&C Exclusions: 203.00, 203.01, 203.10, 203.11, 203.80, 203.81, 204.00, 204.01, 204.10, 204.11, 204.20, 204.21, 204.80, 204.81, 204.90, 204.91, 205.00, 205.01, 205.10, 205.11, 205.20, 205.21, 205.30, 205.31, 205.80, 205.81, 205.90, 205.91, 206.00, 206.01, 206.10, 206.11, 206.20, 206.21, 206.80, 206.81, 206.90, 206.91, 207.00, 207.01, 207.10, 207.11, 207.20, 207.21, 207.80, 207.81, 208.00, 208.01, 208.10, 208.11, 208.20, 208.21, 208.80, 208.81, 208.90, 208.91, 239.8, 239.9
AHA: 1Q 1996, 16; 4Q 1991, 26

Multiple myeloma

A type of cancer characterized by excessive numbers of malignant plasma cells in the bone marrow

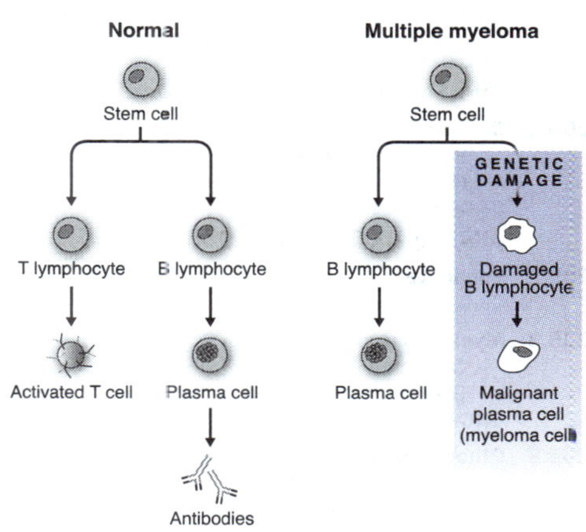

203.1 Plasma cell leukemia
Plasmacytic leukemia
C&C Exclusions: See 203.0
AHA: 4Q 1990, 26; Sep-Oct 1986, 12

203.8 Other immunoproliferative neoplasms
C&C Exclusions: See 203.0
AHA: 4Q 1990, 26; Sep-Oct 1986, 12

❹ **204 Lymphoid leukemia**

Includes leukemia:
- lymphatic
- lymphoblastic
- lymphocytic
- lymphogenous

The following fifth-digit subclassification is for use with category 204:
- **0 without mention of remission**
- **1 in remission**

❺ **204.0 Acute**

Excludes *acute exacerbation of chronic lymphoid leukemia (204.1)*

C&C Exclusions: See 203.0

AHA: 3Q 1999, 6

❺ **204.1 Chronic**

C&C Exclusions: See 203.0

❺ **204.2 Subacute**

C&C Exclusions: See 203.0

❺ **204.8 Other lymphoid leukemia**

Aleukemic leukemia:
- lymphatic
- lymphocytic
- lymphoid

C&C Exclusions: See 203.0

✖❺ **204.9 Unspecified lymphoid leukemia**

C&C Exclusions: See 203.0

❹ **205 Myeloid leukemia**

Includes leukemia:
- granulocytic
- myeloblastic
- myelocytic
- myelogenous
- myelomonocytic
- myelosclerotic
- myelosis

AHA: 3Q 1993, 3; 4Q 1991, 26; 4Q 1990, 3; May-Jun 1985, 18

The following fifth-digit subclassification is for use with category 205:
- **0 without mention of remission**
- **1 in remission**

❺ **205.0 Acute**

Acute promyelocytic leukemia

Excludes *acute exacerbation of chronic myeloid leukemia (205.1)*

C&C Exclusions: See 203.0

AHA: For Code 205.00: 2Q 2006, 21

❺ **205.1 Chronic**

Eosinophilic leukemia
Neutrophilic leukemia

C&C Exclusions: See 203.0

AHA: 1Q 2000, 6; Jul-Aug 1985, 13

❺ **205.2 Subacute**

C&C Exclusions: See 203.0

❺ **205.3 Myeloid sarcoma**

Chloroma
Granulocytic sarcoma

C&C Exclusions: See 203.0

❺ **205.8 Other myeloid leukemia**

Aleukemic leukemia:
- granulocytic
- myelogenous
- myeloid

Aleukemic myelosis

C&C Exclusions: See 203.0

✖❺ **205.9 Unspecified myeloid leukemia**

C&C Exclusions: See 203.0

❹ **206 Monocytic leukemia**

Includes leukemia:
- histiocytic
- monoblastic
- monocytoid

The following fifth-digit subclassification is for use with category 206:
- **0 without mention of remission**
- **1 in remission**

❺ **206.0 Acute**

Excludes *acute exacerbation of chronic monocytic leukemia (206.1)*

C&C Exclusions: See 203.0

❺ **206.1 Chronic**

C&C Exclusions: See 203.0

❺ **206.2 Subacute**

C&C Exclusions: See 203.0

❺ **206.8 Other monocytic leukemia**

Aleukemic:
- monocytic leukemia
- monocytoid leukemia

C&C Exclusions: See 203.0

✖❺ **206.9 Unspecified monocytic leukemia**

C&C Exclusions: See 203.0

❹ **207 Other specified leukemia**

Excludes *leukemic reticuloendotheliosis (202.4)*
plasma cell leukemia (203.1)

The following fifth-digit subclassification is for use with category 207:
- **0 without mention of remission**
- **1 in remission**

❺ **207.0 Acute erythremia and erythroleukemia**

Acute erythremic myelosis
Di Guglielmo's disease
Erythremic myelosis

C&C Exclusions: See 203.0

❺ **207.1 Chronic erythremia**

Heilmeyer-Schöner disease

C&C Exclusions: See 203.0

❺ **207.2 Megakaryocytic leukemia**

Megakaryocytic myelosis
Thrombocytic leukemia

C&C Exclusions: See 203.0

❺ **207.8 Other specified leukemia**

Lymphosarcoma cell leukemia

C&C Exclusions: See 203.0

Leukemia begins in a cell in the bone marrow. The cell undergoes a leukemic change and it multiplies into many cells. The leukemia cells grow and survive better than normal cells and eventually crowd out the normal cells.

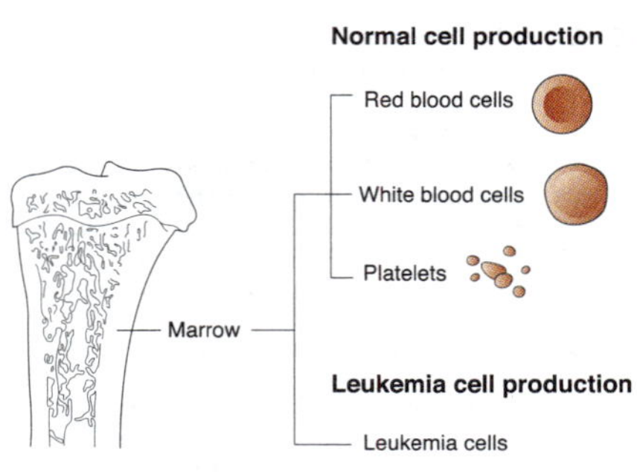

❹ **208 Leukemia of unspecified cell type**

The following fifth-digit subclassification is for use with category 208:
- **0 without mention of remission**
- **1 in remission**

❺ **208.0 Acute**

Acute leukemia NOS
Blast cell leukemia
Stem cell leukemia

Excludes *acute exacerbation of chronic unspecified leukemia (208.1)*

C&C Exclusions: See 203.0

5 **208.1 Chronic**
Chronic leukemia NOS
C&C Exclusions: See 203.0

5 **208.2 Subacute**
Subacute leukemia NOS
C&C Exclusions: See 203.0

5 **208.8 Other leukemia of unspecified cell type**
C&C Exclusions: See 203.0

✖ 5 **208.9 Unspecified leukemia**
Leukemia NOS
C&C Exclusions: See 203.0

BENIGN NEOPLASMS (210-229)

4 **210 Benign neoplasm of lip, oral cavity, and pharynx**
Excludes *cyst (of):*
jaw (526.0-526.2, 526.89)
oral soft tissue (528.4)
radicular (522.8)

210.0 Lip
Frenulum labii
Lip (inner aspect) (mucosa) (vermilion border)
Excludes *labial commissure (210.4)*
skin of lip (216.0)

210.1 Tongue
Lingual tonsil

210.2 Major salivary glands
Gland:
parotid
sublingual
submandibular
Excludes *benign neoplasms of minor salivary glands:*
NOS (210.4)
buccal mucosa (210.4)
lips (210.0)
palate (hard) (soft) (210.4)
tongue (210.1)
tonsil, palatine (210.5)

210.3 Floor of mouth

210.4 Other and unspecified parts of mouth
Gingiva
Gum (upper) (lower)
Labial commissure
Oral cavity NOS
Oral mucosa
Palate (hard) (soft)
Uvula
Excludes *benign odontogenic neoplasms of bone (213.0-213.1)*
developmental odontogenic cysts (526.0)
mucosa of lips (210.0)
nasopharyngeal [posterior] [superior] surface of soft palate (210.7)

210.5 Tonsil
Tonsil (faucial) (palatine)
Excludes *lingual tonsil (210.1)*
pharyngeal tonsil (210.7)
tonsillar:
fossa (210.6)
pillars (210.6)

210.6 Other parts of oropharynx
Branchial cleft or vestiges
Epiglottis, anterior aspect
Fauces NOS
Mesopharynx NOS
Tonsillar:
fossa
pillars
Vallecula
Excludes *epiglottis:*
NOS (212.1)
suprahyoid portion (212.1)

210.7 Nasopharynx
Adenoid tissue
Lymphadenoid tissue
Pharyngeal tonsil
Posterior nasal septum

210.8 Hypopharynx
Arytenoid fold
Laryngopharynx
Postcricoid region
Pyriform fossa

210.9 Pharynx, unspecified
Throat NOS

4 **211 Benign neoplasm of other parts of digestive system**
Excludes *benign stromal tumors of digestive system (215.5)*

211.0 Esophagus

211.1 Stomach
Body of stomach
Cardia of stomach
Cardiac orifice
Fundus of stomach
Pylorus

211.2 Duodenum, jejunum, and ileum
Small intestine NOS
Excludes *ampulla of Vater (211.5)*
ileocecal valve (211.3)

211.3 Colon
Appendix
Cecum
Ileocecal valve
Large intestine NOS
Excludes *rectosigmoid junction (211.4)*
AHA: 3Q 2005, 17; 2Q 2005, 16; 4Q 2001, 56

211.4 Rectum and anal canal
Anal canal or sphincter
Anus NOS
Rectosigmoid junction
Excludes *anus:*
margin (216.5)
skin (216.5)
perianal skin (216.5)

211.5 Liver and biliary passages
Ampulla of Vater
Common bile duct
Cystic duct
Gallbladder
Hepatic duct
Sphincter of Oddi

211.6 Pancreas, except islets of Langerhans

211.7 Islets of Langerhans
Islet cell tumor
Use additional code to identify any functional activity

211.8 Retroperitoneum and peritoneum
Mesentery
Mesocolon
Omentum
Retroperitoneal tissue

211.9 Other and unspecified site
Alimentary tract NOS
Digestive system NOS
Gastrointestinal tract NOS
Intestinal tract NOS
Intestine NOS
Spleen, not elsewhere classified

❹ 212 Benign neoplasm of respiratory and intrathoracic organs

212.0 Nasal cavities, middle ear, and accessory sinuses

Cartilage of nose
Eustachian tube
Nares
Septum of nose
Sinus:
  ethmoidal
  frontal
  maxillary
  sphenoidal

Excludes *auditory canal (external) (216.2)*
bone of:
  ear (213.0)
  nose [turbinates] (213.0)
cartilage of ear (215.0)
ear (external) (skin) (216.2)
nose NOS (229.8)
  skin (216.3)
olfactory bulb (225.1)
polyp of:
  accessory sinus (471.8)
  ear (385.30-385.35)
  nasal cavity (471.0)
posterior margin of septum and choanae (210.7)

212.1 Larynx

Cartilage:
  arytenoid
  cricoid
  cuneiform
  thyroid
Epiglottis (suprahyoid portion) NOS
Glottis
Vocal cords (false) (true)

Excludes *epiglottis, anterior aspect (210.6)*
polyp of vocal cord or larynx (478.4)

212.2 Trachea

212.3 Bronchus and lung

Carina
Hilus of lung

212.4 Pleura

212.5 Mediastinum

212.6 Thymus

212.7 Heart

Excludes *great vessels (215.4)*

212.8 Other specified sites

✖ **212.9 Site unspecified**

Respiratory organ NOS
Upper respiratory tract NOS

Excludes *intrathoracic NOS (229.8)*
thoracic NOS (229.8)

❹ 213 Benign neoplasm of bone and articular cartilage

Includes cartilage (articular) (joint)
periosteum

Excludes *cartilage of:*
  ear (215.0)
  eyelid (215.0)
  larynx (212.1)
  nose (212.0)
exostosis NOS (726.91)
synovia (215.0-215.9)

213.0 Bones of skull and face

Excludes *lower jaw bone (213.1)*

213.1 Lower jaw bone

213.2 Vertebral column, excluding sacrum and coccyx

213.3 Ribs, sternum, and clavicle

213.4 Scapula and long bones of upper limb

213.5 Short bones of upper limb

213.6 Pelvic bones, sacrum, and coccyx

213.7 Long bones of lower limb

213.8 Short bones of lower limb

✖ **213.9 Bone and articular cartilage, site unspecified**

❹ 214 Lipoma

Includes angiolipoma
fibrolipoma
hibernoma
lipoma (fetal) (infiltrating) (intramuscular)
myelolipoma
myxolipoma

214.0 Skin and subcutaneous tissue of face

214.1 Other skin and subcutaneous tissue

214.2 Intrathoracic organs

214.3 Intra-abdominal organs

214.4 Spermatic cord ♂

214.8 Other specified sites

AHA: 3Q 1994, 7

✖ **214.9 Lipoma, unspecified site**

❹ 215 Other benign neoplasm of connective and other soft tissue

Includes blood vessel
bursa
fascia
ligament
muscle
peripheral, sympathetic, and parasympathetic nerves and ganglia
synovia
tendon (sheath)

Excludes *cartilage:*
  articular (213.0-213.9)
  larynx (212.1)
  nose (212.0)
connective tissue of:
  breast (217)
  internal organ, except lipoma and hemangioma - code to benign neoplasm of the site
lipoma (214.0-214.9)

215.0 Head, face, and neck

215.2 Upper limb, including shoulder

215.3 Lower limb, including hip

215.4 Thorax

Excludes *heart (212.7)*
mediastinum (212.5)
thymus (212.6)

215.5 Abdomen

Abdominal wall
Benign stromal tumors of abdomen
Hypochondrium

215.6 Pelvis

Buttock
Groin
Inguinal region
Perineum

Excludes *uterine:*
  leiomyoma (218.0-218.9)
  ligament, any (221.0)

215.7 Trunk, unspecified

Back NOS
Flank NOS

215.8 Other specified sites

✖ **215.9 Site unspecified**

❹ 216 Benign neoplasm of skin

Includes blue nevus
dermatofibroma
hydrocystoma
pigmented nevus
syringoadenoma
syringoma

Excludes *skin of genital organs (221.0-222.9)*

AHA: 1Q 2000, 21

216.0 Skin of lip

Excludes *vermilion border of lip (210.0)*

216.1 Eyelid, including canthus

Excludes *cartilage of eyelid (215.0)*

216.2 Ear and external auditory canal
Auricle (ear)
Auricular canal, external
External meatus
Pinna
Excludes *cartilage of ear (215.0)*

216.3 Skin of other and unspecified parts of face
Cheek, external
Eyebrow
Nose, external
Temple

216.4 Scalp and skin of neck
AHA: 3Q 1991, 12

216.5 Skin of trunk, except scrotum
Axillary fold
Perianal skin
Skin of:
- abdominal wall
- anus
- back
- breast
- buttock
- chest wall
- groin
- perineum

Umbilicus
Excludes *anal canal (211.4)*
anus NOS (211.4)
skin of scrotum (222.4)

216.6 Skin of upper limb, including shoulder

216.7 Skin of lower limb, including hip

216.8 Other specified sites of skin

216.9 Skin, site unspecified

217 Benign neoplasm of breast
Breast (male) (female)
- connective tissue
- glandular tissue
- soft parts

Excludes *adenofibrosis (610.2)*
benign cyst of breast (610.0)
fibrocystic disease (610.1)
skin of breast (216.5)
AHA: 1Q 2000, 4

218 Uterine leiomyoma
Includes fibroid (bleeding) (uterine)
uterine:
- fibromyoma
- myoma

218.0 Submucous leiomyoma of uterus ♀

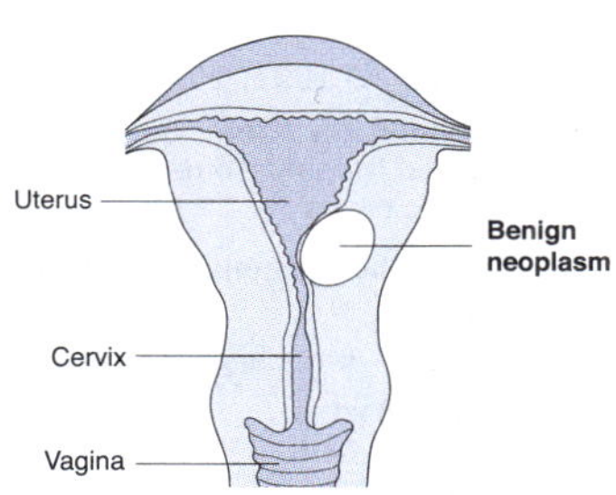

218.1 Intramural leiomyoma of uterus ♀
Interstitial leiomyoma of uterus

218.2 Subserous leiomyoma of uterus ♀
Subperitoneal leiomyoma of uterus

218.9 Leiomyoma of uterus, unspecified ♀
AHA: 1Q 2003, 4

219 Other benign neoplasm of uterus

219.0 Cervix uteri ♀

219.1 Corpus uteri ♀
Endometrium
Fundus
Myometrium

219.8 Other specified parts of uterus ♀

219.9 Uterus, part unspecified ♀

220 Benign neoplasm of ovary ♀
Use additional code to identify any functional activity (256.0-256.1)
Excludes *cyst:*
- *corpus albicans (620.2)*
- *corpus luteum (620.1)*
- *endometrial (617.1)*
- *follicular (atretic) (620.0)*
- *graafian follicle (620.0)*
- *ovarian NOS (620.2)*
- *retention (620.2)*

221 Benign neoplasm of other female genital organs
Includes adenomatous polyp
benign teratoma
Excludes *cyst:*
- *epoophoron (752.11)*
- *fimbrial (752.11)*
- *Gartner's duct (752.11)*
- *parovarian (752.11)*

221.0 Fallopian tube and uterine ligaments ♀
Oviduct
Parametrium
Uterine ligament (broad) (round) (uterosacral)
Uterine tube

221.1 Vagina ♀

221.2 Vulva ♀
Clitoris
External female genitalia NOS
Greater vestibular [Bartholin's] gland
Labia (majora) (minora)
Pudendum
Excludes *Bartholin's (duct) (gland) cyst (616.2)*

221.8 Other specified sites of female genital organs ♀

221.9 Female genital organ, site unspecified ♀
Female genitourinary tract NOS

222 Benign neoplasm of male genital organs

222.0 Testis ♂
Use additional code to identify any functional activity

222.1 Penis ♂
Corpus cavernosum
Glans penis
Prepuce

222.2 Prostate ♂
Excludes *adenomatous hyperplasia of prostate (600.20-600.21)*
prostatic:
- *adenoma (600.20-600.21)*
- *enlargement (600.00-600.01)*
- *hypertrophy (600.00-600.01)*

222.3 Epididymis ♂

222.4 Scrotum ♂
Skin of scrotum

222.8 Other specified sites of male genital organs ♂
Seminal vesicle
Spermatic cord

222.9 Male genital organ, site unspecified ♂
Male genitourinary tract NOS

223 Benign neoplasm of kidney and other urinary organs

223.0 Kidney, except pelvis
Kidney NOS
Excludes *renal:*
- *calyces (223.1)*
- *pelvis (223.1)*

223.1 Renal pelvis

223.2 Ureter
Excludes *ureteric orifice of bladder (223.3)*

223.3 Bladder

223.8 Other specified sites of urinary organs

223.81 Urethra
Excludes *urethral orifice of bladder (223.3)*

223.89 Other
Paraurethral glands

✖ **223.9 Urinary organ, site unspecified**
Urinary system NOS

❹ **224 Benign neoplasm of eye**
Excludes *cartilage of eyelid (215.0)*
eyelid (skin) (216.1)
optic nerve (225.1)
orbital bone (213.0)

224.0 Eyeball, except conjunctiva, cornea, retina, and choroid
Ciliary body
Iris
Sclera
Uveal tract

224.1 Orbit
Excludes *bone of orbit (213.0)*

224.2 Lacrimal gland

224.3 Conjunctiva

224.4 Cornea

224.5 Retina
Excludes *hemangioma of retina (228.03)*

224.6 Choroid

224.7 Lacrimal duct
Lacrimal sac
Nasolacrimal duct

224.8 Other specified parts of eye

✖ **224.9 Eye, part unspecified**

❹ **225 Benign neoplasm of brain and other parts of nervous system**
Excludes *hemangioma (228.02)*
neurofibromatosis (237.7)
peripheral, sympathetic, and parasympathetic nerves and ganglia (215.0-215.9)
retrobulbar (224.1)

225.0 Brain

225.1 Cranial nerves
AHA: 4Q 2004, 113

225.2 Cerebral meninges
Meninges NOS
Meningioma (cerebral)

225.3 Spinal cord
Cauda equina

225.4 Spinal meninges
Spinal meningioma

225.8 Other specified sites of nervous system

✖ **225.9 Nervous system, part unspecified**
Nervous system (central) NOS
Excludes *meninges NOS (225.2)*

226 Benign neoplasm of thyroid glands
Use additional code to identify any functional activity

❹ **227 Benign neoplasm of other endocrine glands and related structures**
Use additional code to identify any functional activity
Excludes *ovary (220)*
pancreas (211.6)
testis (222.0)

227.0 Adrenal gland
Suprarenal gland

227.1 Parathyroid gland

227.3 Pituitary gland and craniopharyngeal duct (pouch)
Craniobuccal pouch
Hypophysis
Rathke's pouch
Sella turcica

227.4 Pineal gland
Pineal body

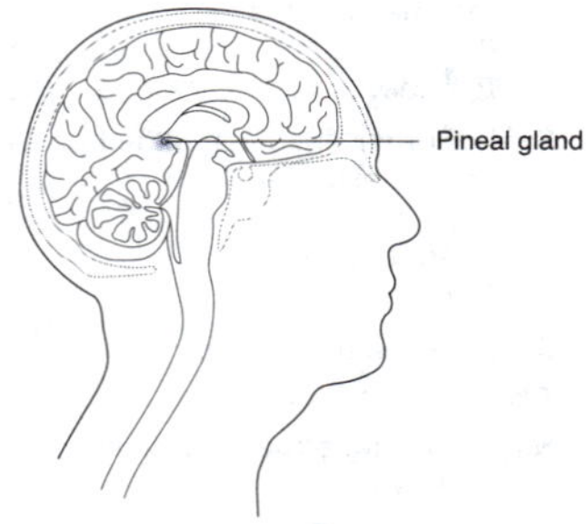

227.5 Carotid body

227.6 Aortic body and other paraganglia
Coccygeal body
Glomus jugulare
Para-aortic body
AHA: Nov-Dec 1984, 17

227.8 Other

✖ **227.9 Endocrine gland, site unspecified**

❹ **228 Hemangioma and lymphangioma, any site**
Includes angioma (benign) (cavernous) (congenital) NOS
cavernous nevus
glomus tumor
hemangioma (benign) (congenital)
Excludes *benign neoplasm of spleen, except hemangioma and lymphangioma (211.9)*
glomus jugulare (227.6)
nevus:
NOS (216.0-216.9)
blue or pigmented (216.0-216.9)
vascular (757.32)
AHA: 1Q 2000, 21

❺ **228.0 Hemangioma, any site**
AHA: Jan-Feb 1985, 19

✖ **228.00 Of unspecified site**

228.01 Of skin and subcutaneous tissue

228.02 Of intracranial structures

228.03 Of retina

228.04 Of intra-abdominal structures
Peritoneum
Retroperitoneal tissue

228.09 Of other sites
Systemic angiomatosis
AHA: 3Q 1991, 20

228.1 Lymphangioma, any site
Congenital lymphangioma
Lymphatic nevus

❹ **229 Benign neoplasm of other and unspecified sites**

229.0 Lymph nodes
Excludes *lymphangioma (228.1)*

229.8 Other specified sites
Intrathoracic NOS
Thoracic NOS

✖ **229.9 Site unspecified**

CARCINOMA IN SITU (230-234)

Includes Bowen's disease
erythroplasia
Queyrat's erythroplasia
Excludes *leukoplakia - see Alphabetic Index*

4 230 Carcinoma in situ of digestive organs

230.0 Lip, oral cavity, and pharynx
Gingiva
Hypopharynx
Mouth [any part]
Nasopharynx
Oropharynx
Salivary gland or duct
Tongue
Excludes *aryepiglottic fold or interarytenoid fold, laryngeal aspect (231.0)*
epiglottis:
NOS (231.0)
suprahyoid portion (231.0)
skin of lip (232.0)

230.1 Esophagus

230.2 Stomach
Body of stomach
Cardia of stomach
Cardiac orifice
Fundus of stomach
Pylorus

230.3 Colon
Appendix
Cecum
Ileocecal valve
Large intestine NOS
Excludes *rectosigmoid junction (230.4)*

230.4 Rectum
Rectosigmoid junction

230.5 Anal canal
Anal sphincter

✖ **230.6 Anus, unspecified**
Excludes *anus:*
margin (232.5)
skin (232.5)
perianal skin (232.5)

230.7 Other and unspecified parts of intestine
Duodenum
Ileum
Jejunum
Small intestine NOS
Excludes *ampulla of Vater (230.8)*

230.8 Liver and biliary system
Ampulla of Vater
Common bile duct
Cystic duct
Gallbladder
Hepatic duct
Sphincter of Oddi

230.9 Other and unspecified digestive organs
Digestive organ NOS
Gastrointestinal tract NOS
Pancreas
Spleen

4 231 Carcinoma in situ of respiratory system

231.0 Larynx
Cartilage:
arytenoid
cricoid
cuneiform
thyroid
Epiglottis:
NOS
posterior surface
suprahyoid portion
Vocal cords (false) (true)
Excludes *aryepiglottic fold or interarytenoid fold:*
NOS (230.0)
hypopharyngeal aspect (230.0)
marginal zone (230.0)

231.1 Trachea

231.2 Bronchus and lung
Carina
Hilus of lung

231.8 Other specified parts of respiratory system
Accessory sinuses
Middle ear
Nasal cavities
Pleura
Excludes *ear (external) (skin) (232.2)*
nose NOS (234.8)
skin (232.3)

✖ **231.9 Respiratory system, part unspecified**
Respiratory organ NOS

4 232 Carcinoma in situ of skin
Includes pigment cells

232.0 Skin of lip
Excludes *vermilion border of lip (230.0)*

232.1 Eyelid, including canthus

A tumor that has been detected and has the characteristics of malignancy but has not invaded other tissues

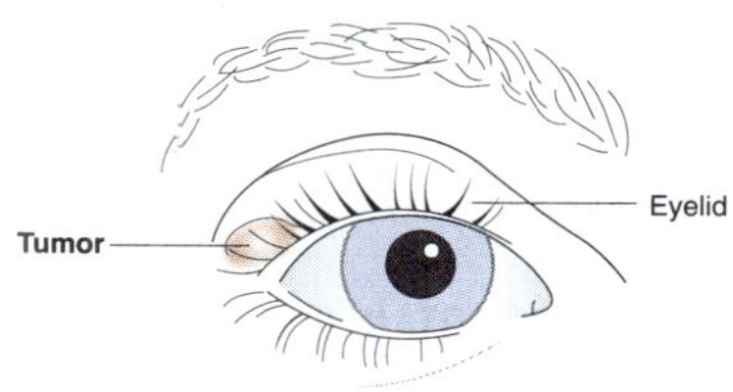

232.2 Ear and external auditory canal

232.3 Skin of other and unspecified parts of face

232.4 Scalp and skin of neck

232.5 Skin of trunk, except scrotum
Anus, margin
Axillary fold
Perianal skin
Skin of:
abdominal wall
anus
back
breast
buttock
chest wall
groin
perineum
Umbilicus
Excludes *anal canal (230.5)*
anus NOS (230.6)
skin of genital organs (▶233.30-233.39◀, 233.5-233.6)

232.6 Skin of upper limb, including shoulder

232.7 Skin of lower limb, including hip

232.8 Other specified sites of skin

✖ **232.9 Skin, site unspecified**

4 233 Carcinoma in situ of breast and genitourinary system

233.0 Breast
Excludes *Paget's disease (174.0-174.9)*
skin of breast (232.5)

233.1 Cervix uteri ♀
▶ Adenocarcinoma in situ of cervix◀
Cervical intraepithelial glandular neoplasia
Cervical intraepithelial neoplasia III [CIN III]
Severe dysplasia of cervix
Excludes *cervical intraepithelial neoplasia II [CIN II] (622.12)*
cytologic evidence of malignancy without histologic confirmation (795.06)
high grade squamous intraepithelial lesion (HGSIL) (795.04)
moderate dysplasia of cervix (622.12)
AHA: 3Q 1992, 7; 3Q 1992, 8; 1Q 1991, 11

233.2 Other and unspecified parts of uterus ♀

❺ **233.3 Other and unspecified female genital organs**

● ✖ **233.30 Unspecified female genital organ** ♀

● **233.31 Vagina** ♀
Severe dysplasia of vagina
Vaginal intraepithelial neoplasia III [VAIN III]

● **233.32 Vulva** ♀
Severe dysplasia of vulva
Vulvar intraepithelial neoplasia III [VIN III]

● **233.39 Other female genital organ** ♀

233.4 Prostate ♂

233.5 Penis ♂

233.6 Other and unspecified male genital organs ♂

233.7 Bladder

233.9 Other and unspecified urinary organs

❹ **234 Carcinoma in situ of other and unspecified sites**

234.0 Eye
Excludes *cartilage of eyelid (234.8)*
eyelid (skin) (232.1)
optic nerve (234.8)
orbital bone (234.8)

234.8 Other specified sites
Endocrine gland [any]

✖ **234.9 Site unspecified**
Carcinoma in situ NOS

NEOPLASMS OF UNCERTAIN BEHAVIOR (235-238)

Note: *Categories 235-238 classify by site certain histomorphologically well-defined neoplasms, the subsequent behavior of which cannot be predicted from the present appearance.*

❹ **235 Neoplasm of uncertain behavior of digestive and respiratory systems**
Excludes *stromal tumors of uncertain behavior of digestive system (238.1)*

235.0 Major salivary glands
Gland:
parotid
sublingual
submandibular
Excludes *minor salivary glands (235.1)*

235.1 Lip, oral cavity, and pharynx
Gingiva
Hypopharynx
Minor salivary glands
Mouth
Nasopharynx
Oropharynx
Tongue
Excludes *aryepiglottic fold or interarytenoid fold, laryngeal aspect (235.6)*
epiglottis:
NOS (235.6)
suprahyoid portion (235.6)
skin of lip (238.2)

235.2 Stomach, intestines, and rectum

235.3 Liver and biliary passages
Ampulla of Vater
Bile ducts [any]
Gallbladder
Liver

235.4 Retroperitoneum and peritoneum

235.5 Other and unspecified digestive organs
Anal:
canal
sphincter
Anus NOS
Esophagus
Pancreas
Spleen
Excludes *anus:*
margin (238.2)
skin (238.2)
perianal skin (238.2)

235.6 Larynx
Excludes *aryepiglottic fold or interarytenoid fold:*
NOS (235.1)
hypopharyngeal aspect (235.1)
marginal zone (235.1)

235.7 Trachea, bronchus, and lung

235.8 Pleura, thymus, and mediastinum

235.9 Other and unspecified respiratory organs
Accessory sinuses
Middle ear
Nasal cavities
Respiratory organ NOS
Excludes *ear (external) (skin) (238.2)*
nose (238.8)
skin (238.2)

❹ **236 Neoplasm of uncertain behavior of genitourinary organs**

236.0 Uterus ♀

236.1 Placenta ♀
Chorioadenoma (destruens)
Invasive mole
Malignant hydatid(iform) mole

236.2 Ovary ♀
Use additional code to identify any functional activity

236.3 Other and unspecified female genital organs ♀

236.4 Testis ♂
Use additional code to identify any functional activity

236.5 Prostate ♂

236.6 Other and unspecified male genital organs ♂

236.7 Bladder

❺ **236.9 Other and unspecified urinary organs**

✖ **236.90 Urinary organ, unspecified**

236.91 Kidney and ureter

236.99 Other

❹ **237 Neoplasm of uncertain behavior of endocrine glands and nervous system**

237.0 Pituitary gland and craniopharyngeal duct
Use additional code to identify any functional activity

237.1 Pineal gland

237.2 Adrenal gland
Suprarenal gland
Use additional code to identify any functional activity

237.3 Paraganglia
Aortic body
Carotid body
Coccygeal body
Glomus jugulare
AHA: Nov-Dec 1984, 17

237.4 Other and unspecified endocrine glands
Parathyroid gland
Thyroid gland

237.5 Brain and spinal cord

237.6 Meninges
Meninges:
NOS
cerebral
spinal

❺ **237.7 Neurofibromatosis**
von Recklinghausen's disease

✖ **237.70 Neurofibromatosis, unspecified**

237.71 Neurofibromatosis, type 1 [von Recklinghausen's disease]

237.72 Neurofibromatosis, type 2 [acoustic neurofibromatosis]

237.9 Other and unspecified parts of nervous system
Cranial nerves
Excludes *peripheral, sympathetic, and parasympathetic nerves and ganglia (238.1)*

❹ **238 Neoplasm of uncertain behavior of other and unspecified sites and tissues**

238.0 Bone and articular cartilage
Excludes *cartilage:*
ear (238.1)
eyelid (238.1)
larynx (235.6)
nose (235.9)
synovia (238.1)

238.1 Connective and other soft tissue
Peripheral, sympathetic, and parasympathetic nerves and ganglia
Stromal tumors of digestive system
Excludes *cartilage (of):*
articular (238.0)
larynx (235.6)
nose (235.9)
connective tissue of breast (238.3)

238.2 Skin
Excludes *anus NOS (235.5)*
skin of genital organs (236.3, 236.6)
vermilion border of lip (235.1)

238.3 Breast
Excludes *skin of breast (238.2)*

238.4 Polycythemia vera

238.5 Histiocytic and mast cells
Mast cell tumor NOS
Mastocytoma NOS

238.6 Plasma cells
Plasmacytoma NOS
Solitary myeloma

❺ **238.7 Other lymphatic and hematopoietic tissues**
Excludes *acute myelogenous leukemia (205.0)*
chronic myelomonocytic leukemia (205.1)
myelofibrosis (289.83)
myelosclerosis NOS (289.89)
myelosis:
NOS (205.9)
megakaryocytic (207.2)

AHA: 3Q 2001, 13; 1Q 1997, 5; 2Q 1989, 8

238.71 Essential thrombocythemia
Essential hemorrhagic thrombocythemia
Essential thrombocytosis
Idiopathic (hemorrhagic) thrombocythemia
Primary thrombocytosis

238.72 Low grade myelodysplastic syndrome lesions
Refractory anemia (RA)
Refractory anemia with ringed sideroblasts (RARS)
Refractory cytopenia with multilineage dysplasia (RCMD)
Refractory cytopenia with multilineage dysplasia and ringed sideroblasts (RCMD-RS)

238.73 High grade myelodysplastic syndrome lesions
Refractory anemia with excess blasts-1 (RAEB-1)
Refractory anemia with excess blasts-2 (RAEB-2)

238.74 Myelodysplastic syndrome with 5q deletion
5q minus syndrome NOS
Excludes *constitutional 5q deletion (758.39)*
high grade myelodysplastic syndrome with 5q deletion (238.73)

✖ **238.75 Myelodysplastic syndrome, unspecified**

238.76 Myelofibrosis with myeloid metaplasia
Agnogenic myeloid metaplasia
Idiopathic myelofibrosis (chronic)
Myelosclerosis with myeloid metaplasia
Primary myelofibrosis
Excludes *myelofibrosis NOS (289.83)*
myelophthisic anemia (284.2)
myelophthisis (284.2)
secondary myelofibrosis (289.83)

238.79 Other lymphatic and hematopoietic tissues
Lymphoproliferative disease (chronic) NOS
Megakaryocytic myelosclerosis
Myeloproliferative disease (chronic) NOS
Panmyelosis (acute)

238.8 Other specified sites
Eye
Heart
Excludes *eyelid (skin) (238.2)*
cartilage (238.1)

238.9 Site unspecified

NEOPLASMS OF UNSPECIFIED NATURE (239)

❹ **239 Neoplasms of unspecified nature**
Note: *Category 239 classifies by site neoplasms of unspecified morphology and behavior. The term "mass," unless otherwise stated, is not to be regarded as a neoplastic growth.*
Includes "growth" NOS
neoplasm NOS
new growth NOS
tumor NOS

✖ **239.0 Digestive system**
Excludes *anus:*
margin (239.2)
skin (239.2)
perianal skin (239.2)

✖ **239.1 Respiratory system**

✖ **239.2 Bone, soft tissue, and skin**
Excludes *anal canal (239.0)*
anus NOS (239.0)
bone marrow (202.9)
cartilage:
larynx (239.1)
nose (239.1)
connective tissue of breast (239.3)
skin of genital organs (239.5)
vermilion border of lip (239.0)

✖ **239.3 Breast**
Excludes *skin of breast (239.2)*

✖ **239.4 Bladder**

239.5 Other genitourinary organs

✖ **239.6 Brain**
Excludes *cerebral meninges (239.7)*
cranial nerves (239.7)

✖ **239.7 Endocrine glands and other parts of nervous system**
Excludes *peripheral, sympathetic, and parasympathetic nerves and ganglia (239.2)*

✖ **239.8 Other specified sites**
Excludes *eyelid (skin) (239.2)*
cartilage (239.2)
great vessels (239.2)
optic nerve (239.7)

✖ **239.9 Site unspecified**

A Adult (15+ years) M Maternity (12-55 years) N Newborn (0 years) P Pediatric (0-17 years) ♂ Male ♀ Female ❷ Medicare Secondary Payer

3. ENDOCRINE, NUTRITIONAL AND METABOLIC DISEASES, AND IMMUNITY DISORDERS (240-279)

Note: *All neoplasms, whether functionally active or not, are classified in Chapter 2. Codes in Chapter 3 (i.e., 242.8, 246.0, 251-253, 255-259) may be used to identify such functional activity associated with any neoplasm, or by ectopic endocrine tissue.*

Excludes *endocrine and metabolic disturbances specific to the fetus and newborn (775.0-775.9)*

DISORDERS OF THYROID GLAND (240-246)

❹ **240 Simple and unspecified goiter**

DEF: Thyroid gland enlargement presenting as a swelling in the neck, usually due to thyroid-stimulating hormone (TSH) overload.

240.0 Goiter, specified as simple

Any condition classifiable to 240.9, specified as simple

DEF: Enlarged thyroid that functions normally.

240.9 Goiter, unspecified

Enlargement of thyroid
Goiter or struma:
- NOS
- diffuse colloid
- endemic
- hyperplastic
- nontoxic (diffuse)
- parenchymatous
- sporadic

Excludes *congenital (dyshormonogenic) goiter (246.1)*

❹ **241 Nontoxic nodular goiter**

Excludes *adenoma of thyroid (226)*
cystadenoma of thyroid (226)

DEF: One or more nodules (hard knobs) on the thyroid that do not impair its normal function.

241.0 Nontoxic uninodular goiter

Thyroid nodule
Uninodular goiter (nontoxic)

241.1 Nontoxic multinodular goiter

Multinodular goiter (nontoxic)

241.9 Unspecified nontoxic nodular goiter

Adenomatous goiter
Nodular goiter (nontoxic) NOS
Struma nodosa (simplex)

❹ **242 Thyrotoxicosis with or without goiter**

Excludes *neonatal thyrotoxicosis (775.3)*

DEF: Hyperthyroid conditions with excessive hormone production and speeding up of body functions: increased heart rate and blood pressure, excessive sweating, hand tremors, nervousness and anxiety, insomnia, and weight loss with increased appetite.

The following fifth-digit subclassification is for use with category 242:
- **0 without mention of thyrotoxic crisis or storm**
- **1 with mention of thyrotoxic crisis or storm**

❺ **242.0 Toxic diffuse goiter**

Basedow's disease
Exophthalmic or toxic goiter NOS
Graves' disease
Primary thyroid hyperplasia

C&C Exclusions: 017.50, 017.51, 017.52, 017.53, 017.54, 017.55, 017.56, 017.90, 017.91, 017.92, 017.93, 017.94, 017.95, 017.96, 240.0, 240.9, 241.0, 241.1, 241.9, 242.00, 242.01, 242.10, 242.11, 242.20, 242.21, 242.30, 242.31, 242.40, 242.41, 242.80, 242.81, 242.90, 242.91, 243, 244.0, 244.1, 244.2, 244.3, 244.8, 244.9, 245.0, 245.1, 245.2, 245.3, 245.4, 245.8, 245.9, 246.0, 246.1, 246.2, 246.3, 246.8, 246.9, 259.8, 259.9

❺ **242.1 Toxic uninodular goiter**

Thyroid nodule, toxic or with hyperthyroidism
Uninodular goiter, toxic or with hyperthyroidism

C&C Exclusions: See 242.0

❺ **242.2 Toxic multinodular goiter**

Secondary thyroid hyperplasia

C&C Exclusions: See 242.0

❺ **242.3 Toxic nodular goiter, unspecified**

Adenomatous goiter, toxic or with hyperthyroidism
Nodular goiter, toxic or with hyperthyroidism
Struma nodosa, toxic or with hyperthyroidism
Any condition classifiable to 241.9 specified as toxic or with hyperthyroidism

C&C Exclusions: See 242.0

❺ **242.4 Thyrotoxicosis from ectopic thyroid nodule**

C&C Exclusions: See 242.0

❺ **242.8 Thyrotoxicosis of other specified origin**

Overproduction of thyroid-stimulating hormone [TSH]
Thyrotoxicosis:
- factitia from ingestion of excessive thyroid material

Use additional E code to identify cause, if drug-induced

C&C Exclusions: See 242.0

❺ **242.9 Thyrotoxicosis without mention of goiter or other cause**

Hyperthyroidism NOS
Thyrotoxicosis NOS

C&C Exclusions: See 242.0

243 Congenital hypothyroidism

Congenital thyroid insufficiency
Cretinism (athyrotic) (endemic)
Use additional code to identify associated mental retardation

Excludes *congenital (dyshormonogenic) goiter (246.1)*

DEF: Underactive thyroid gland present at birth with inadequate hormone production and slowed metabolic processes. Untreated, it can cause brain damage, mental retardation, and developmental delays.

❹ **244 Acquired hypothyroidism**

Includes athyroidism (acquired)
hypothyroidism (acquired)
myxedema (adult) (juvenile)
thyroid (gland) insufficiency (acquired)

DEF: Underactive thyroid gland due to outside influences, causing an inadequate production of thyroid hormone and a slowing of metabolic processes.

Normal **Hypothyroidism**

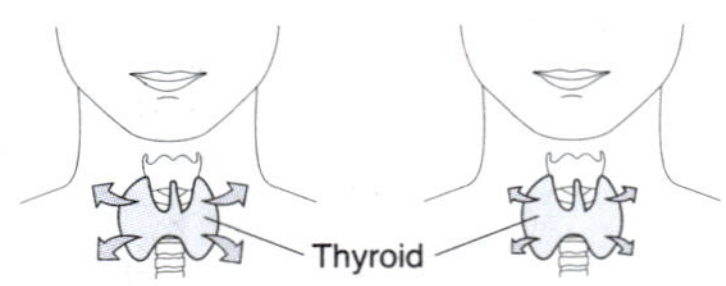

Normal thyroid hormone production — Insufficient thyroid hormone production

244.0 Postsurgical hypothyroidism

244.1 Other postablative hypothyroidism

Hypothyroidism following therapy, such as irradiation

244.2 Iodine hypothyroidism

Hypothyroidism resulting from administration or ingestion of iodide
Use additional E code to identify drug

244.3 Other iatrogenic hypothyroidism

Hypothyroidism resulting from:
- P-aminosalicylic acid [PAS]
- Phenylbutazone
- Resorcinol

Iatrogenic hypothyroidism NOS
Use additional E code to identify drug

244.8 Other specified acquired hypothyroidism

Secondary hypothyroidism NEC

AHA: Jul-Aug 1985, 9

244.9 Unspecified hypothyroidism

Hypothyroidism, primary or NOS
Myxedema, primary or NOS

AHA: 3Q 1999, 19; 4Q 1996, 29

❹ 245 Thyroiditis

245.0 Acute thyroiditis
Abscess of thyroid
Thyroiditis:
  nonsuppurative, acute
  pyogenic
  suppurative
Use additional code to identify organism

DEF: Painful infection of the thyroid gland, often with abscess and pus formation.

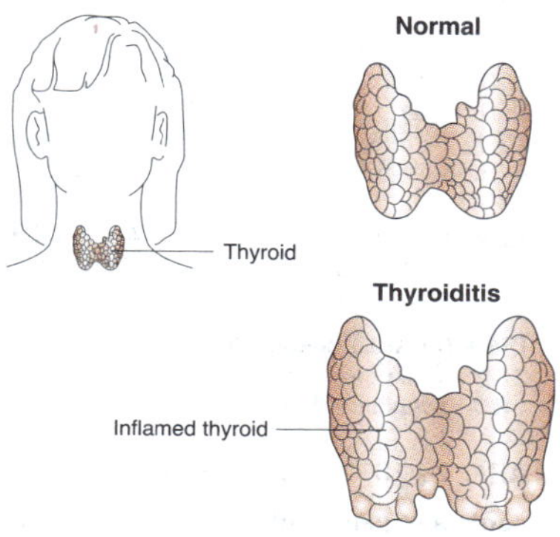

245.1 Subacute thyroiditis
Thyroiditis:
  de Quervain's
  giant cell
  granulomatous
  viral

245.2 Chronic lymphocytic thyroiditis
Hashimoto's disease
Struma lymphomatosa
Thyroiditis:
  autoimmune
  lymphocytic (chronic)

DEF: Autoimmune inflammation of the thyroid with lymphocyte infiltration that presents with painless thyroid enlargement and hypothyroid symptoms.

245.3 Chronic fibrous thyroiditis
Struma fibrosa
Thyroiditis:
  invasive (fibrous)
  ligneous
  Riedel's

245.4 Iatrogenic thyroiditis
Use additional E code to identify cause

245.8 Other and unspecified chronic thyroiditis
Chronic thyroiditis:
  NOS
  nonspecific

245.9 Thyroiditis, unspecified
Thyroiditis NOS

❹ 246 Other disorders of thyroid

246.0 Disorders of thyrocalcitonin secretion
Hypersecretion of calcitonin or thyrocalcitonin

246.1 Dyshormonogenic goiter
Congenital (dyshormonogenic) goiter
Goiter due to enzyme defect in synthesis of thyroid hormone
Goitrous cretinism (sporadic)

246.2 Cyst of thyroid
Excludes *cystadenoma of thyroid (226)*

246.3 Hemorrhage and infarction of thyroid

246.8 Other specified disorders of thyroid
Abnormality of thyroid-binding globulin
Atrophy of thyroid
Hyper-TBG-nemia
Hypo-TBG-nemia

AHA: 2Q 2006, 5

✖ 246.9 Unspecified disorder of thyroid

DISEASES OF OTHER ENDOCRINE GLANDS (250-259)

❹ 250 Diabetes mellitus
Excludes *gestational diabetes (648.8)*
hyperglycemia NOS (▶790.29◀)
neonatal diabetes mellitus (775.1)
nonclinical diabetes (790.29)

DEF: Underproduction or underutilization of insulin; presents with abnormally high blood sugar (glucose) levels, resulting in impaired carbohydrate and fat metabolism.

AHA: 4Q 2004, 56; 2Q 2004, 17; 2Q 2002, 13; 2Q 2001, 16; 2Q 1998, 15; 4Q 1997, 32; 2Q 1997, 14; 3Q 1996, 5; 4Q 1993, 19; 2Q 1992, 5; 3Q 1991, 3; 2Q 1990, 22; Nov-Dec 1985, 11

The following fifth-digit subclassification is for use with category 250:
0 type II or unspecified type, not stated as uncontrolled
  Fifth-digit 0 is for use for type II patients, even if the patient requires insulin
  Use additional code, if applicable, for associated long-term (current) insulin use V58.67
1 type I [juvenile type], not stated as uncontrolled
2 type II or unspecified type, uncontrolled
  Fifth-digit 2 is for use for type II patients, even if the patient requires insulin
  Use additional code, if applicable, for associated long-term (current) insulin use V58.67
3 type I [juvenile type], uncontrolled

❺ 250.0 Diabetes mellitus without mention of complication
Diabetes mellitus without mention of complication or manifestation classifiable to 250.1-250.9
Diabetes (mellitus) NOS

C&C Exclusions: (for codes 250.01-250.03) 250.00, 250.01, 250.02, 250.03, 250.10, 250.11, 250.12, 250.13, 250.20, 250.21, 250.22, 250.23, 250.30, 250.31, 250.32, 250.33, 250.40, 250.41, 250.42, 250.43, 250.50, 250.51, 250.52, 250.53, 250.60, 250.61, 250.62, 250.63, 250.70, 250.71, 250.72, 250.73, 250.80, 250.81, 250.82, 250.83, 250.90, 250.91, 250.92, 250.93, 251.0, 251.1, 251.2, 251.3, 259.8, 259.9

AHA: 1Q 2006, 14; 4Q 1997, 32; 3Q 1991, 3, 12; Nov-Dec 1985, 11; For Code 250.00: 1Q 2005, 15; 4Q 2004, 55; 4Q 2003, 105, 108; 2Q 2003, 16; 1Q 2002, 7, 11; For Code 250.01: 4Q 2004, 55; 4Q 2003, 110; 2Q 2003, 6; For Code 250.02: 1Q 2003, 5

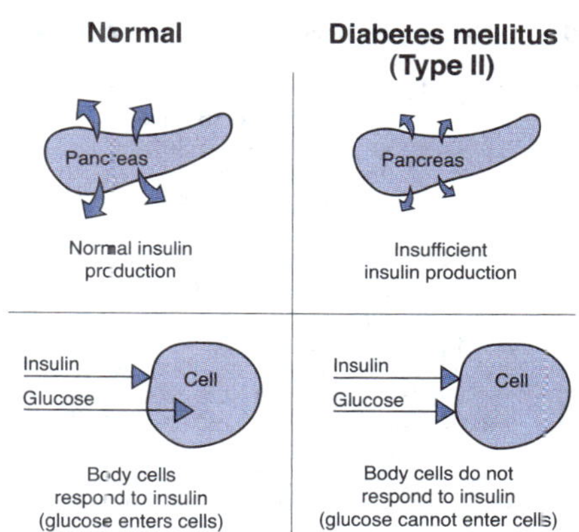

❺ 250.1 Diabetes with ketoacidosis
Diabetic:
  acidosis without mention of coma
  ketosis without mention of coma

DEF: Diabetic complication characterized by hyperglycemia, hyperketonemia, and metabolic acidosis; often presents with nausea, vomiting, and abdominal pain; may progress to cerebral edema or lead to coma and/or death.

C&C Exclusions: (for codes 250.11-250.13) See 250.0

AHA: For Code 250.11: 4Q 2003, 82; For Code 250.13: 2Q 2006, 19

5 250.2 Diabetes with hyperosmolarity
Hyperosmolar (nonketotic) coma

DEF: Metabolic diabetic complication presenting with altered consciousness varying from confusion or disorientation to coma, usually resulting from extreme dehydration.

C&C Exclusions: (for codes 250.21-250.23) See 250.0

AHA: 4Q 1993, 19; 3Q 1991, 7

5 250.3 Diabetes with other coma
Diabetic coma (with ketoacidosis)
Diabetic hypoglycemic coma
Insulin coma NOS

Excludes *diabetes with hyperosmolar coma (250.2)*

C&C Exclusions: (for codes 250.31-250.33) See 250.0

AHA: 3Q 1991, 7, 12

5 250.4 Diabetes with renal manifestations
Use additional code to identify manifestation, as:
chronic kidney disease (585.1-585.9)
diabetic:
nephropathy NOS (583.81)
nephrosis (581.81)
intercapillary glomerulosclerosis (581.81)
Kimmelstiel-Wilson syndrome (581.81)

C&C Exclusions: (for code 250.40) 585.1, 585.2, 585.3, 585.4, 585.5, 585.6, 585.9

C&C Exclusions: (for codes 250.41-250.43) 250.00, 250.01, 250.02, 250.03, 250.10, 250.11, 250.12, 250.13, 250.20, 250.21, 250.22, 250.23, 250.30, 250.31, 250.32, 250.33, 250.40, 250.41, 250.42, 250.43, 250.50, 250.51, 250.52, 250.53, 250.60, 250.61, 250.62, 250.63, 250.70, 250.71, 250.72, 250.73, 250.80, 250.81, 250.82, 250.83, 250.90, 250.91, 250.92, 250.93, 251.0, 251.1, 251.2, 251.3, 259.8, 259.9, 585.1, 585.2, 585.3, 585.4, 585.5, 585.6, 585.9

AHA: 3Q 1991, 8, 12; Sep-Oct 1987, 9; Sep-Oct 1984, 3; For Code 250.40: 1Q 2003, 20

5 250.5 Diabetes with ophthalmic manifestations
Use additional code to identify manifestation, as:
diabetic:
blindness (369.00-369.9)
cataract (366.41)
glaucoma (365.44)
macular edema (362.07)
retinal edema (362.07)
retinopathy (362.01-362.07)

C&C Exclusions: (for codes 250.51-250.53) See 250.0

AHA: 4Q 2005, 65; 3Q 1991, 8; Sep-Oct 1985, 11; For Code 250.50: 4Q 2005, 67

5 250.6 Diabetes with neurological manifestations
Use additional code to identify manifestation, as:
diabetic:
amyotrophy (▶353.1◀)
gastroparalysis (536.3)
gastroparesis (536.3)
mononeuropathy (354.0-355.9)
neurogenic arthropathy (713.5)
peripheral autonomic neuropathy (337.1)
polyneuropathy (357.2)

C&C Exclusions: 250.00, 250.01, 250.02, 250.03, 250.10, 250.11, 250.12, 250.13, 250.20, 250.21, 250.22, 250.23, 250.30, 250.31, 250.32, 250.33, 250.40, 250.41, 250.42, 250.43, 250.50, 250.51, 250.52, 250.53, 250.60, 250.61, 250.62, 250.63, 250.70, 250.71, 250.72, 250.73, 250.80, 250.81, 250.82, 250.83, 250.90, 250.91, 250.92, 250.93, 251.0, 251.1, 251.2, 251.3, 259.8, 259.9, 358.00, 358.01

AHA: 2Q 1993, 6; 2Q 1992, 15; 3Q 1991, 9; Nov-Dec 1984, 9; For Code 250.60: 4Q 2003, 105; For Code 250.61: 2Q 2004, 7

5 250.7 Diabetes with peripheral circulatory disorders
Use additional code to identify manifestation, as:
diabetic:
gangrene (785.4)
peripheral angiopathy (443.81)

C&C Exclusions: (for code 250.70) 445.01, 445.02, 445.81, 445.89

C&C Exclusions: (for codes 250.71-250.73) See 250.0

AHA: 1Q 1996, 10; 3Q 1994, 5; 2Q 1994, 17; 3Q 1991, 10, 12; 3Q 1990, 15; For Code 250.70: 1Q 2004, 14

5 250.8 Diabetes with other specified manifestations
Diabetic hypoglycemia
Hypoglycemic shock
Use additional code to identify manifestation, as:
any associated ulceration (707.10-707.9)
diabetic bone changes (731.8)
Use additional E code to identify cause, if drug-induced

C&C Exclusions: (for code 250.80) 585.1, 585.2, 585.3, 585.4, 585.5, 585.6, 585.9

C&C Exclusions: (for codes 250.81-250.83) 250.00, 250.01, 250.02, 250.03, 250.10, 250.11, 250.12, 250.13, 250.20, 250.21, 250.22, 250.23, 250.30, 250.31, 250.32, 250.33, 250.40, 250.41, 250.42, 250.43, 250.50, 250.51, 250.52, 250.53, 250.60, 250.61, 250.62, 250.63, 250.70, 250.71, 250.72, 250.73, 250.80, 250.81, 250.82, 250.83, 250.90, 250.91, 250.92, 250.93, 251.0, 251.1, 251.2, 251.3, 259.8, 259.9, 358.00, 358.01, 445.01, 445.02, 445.81, 445.89, 585.1, 585.2, 585.3, 585.4, 585.5, 585.6, 585.9

AHA: 4Q 2000, 44; 4Q 1997, 43; 2Q 1997, 16; 4Q 1993, 20; 3Q 1991, 10; For Code 250.80: 1Q 2004, 14

5 250.9 Diabetes with unspecified complication

C&C Exclusions: (for code 250.90) See 250.80

C&C Exclusions: (for codes 250.91-250.93) See 250.81-250.83

AHA: 2Q 1992, 15; 3Q 1991, 7, 12

4 251 Other disorders of pancreatic internal secretion

251.0 Hypoglycemic coma
Iatrogenic hyperinsulinism
Non-diabetic insulin coma
Use additional E code to identify cause, if drug-induced

Excludes *hypoglycemic coma in diabetes mellitus (250.3)*

C&C Exclusions: See 250.0

AHA: Mar-Apr 1985, 8

251.1 Other specified hypoglycemia
Hyperinsulinism:
NOS
ectopic
functional
Hyperplasia of pancreatic islet beta cells NOS

Excludes *hypoglycemia in diabetes mellitus (250.8)*
hypoglycemia in infant of diabetic mother (775.0)
hypoglycemic coma (251.0)
neonatal hypoglycemia (775.6)

Use additional E code to identify cause, if drug-induced

AHA: 1Q 2003, 10

251.2 Hypoglycemia, unspecified
Hypoglycemia:
NOS
reactive
spontaneous

Excludes *hypoglycemia:*
with coma (251.0)
in diabetes mellitus (250.8)
leucine-induced (270.3)

AHA: Mar-Apr 1985, 8

251.3 Postsurgical hypoinsulinemia
Hypoinsulinemia following complete or partial pancreatectomy
Postpancreatectomy hyperglycemia

C&C Exclusions: See 250.0

AHA: 3Q 1991, 6

251.4 Abnormality of secretion of glucagon
Hyperplasia of pancreatic islet alpha cells with glucagon excess

251.5 Abnormality of secretion of gastrin
Hyperplasia of pancreatic alpha cells with gastrin excess
Zollinger-Ellison syndrome

C&C Exclusions: 530.21, 537.84, 569.86

251.8 Other specified disorders of pancreatic internal secretion

AHA: 2Q 1998, 15; 3Q 1991, 6

✖ 251.9 Unspecified disorder of pancreatic internal secretion
Islet cell hyperplasia NOS

4 252 Disorders of parathyroid gland

5 252.0 Hyperparathyroidism

Excludes *ectopic hyperparathyroidism (259.3)*

✖ 252.00 Hyperparathyroidism, unspecified

252.01 Primary hyperparathyroidism

Hyperplasia of parathyroid

DEF: Excessive production of parathyroid hormone, usually caused by hyperplasia of the gland itself.

252.02 Secondary hyperparathyroidism, non-renal

Excludes *secondary hyperparathyroidism (of renal origin) (588.81)*

AHA: 4Q 2004, 57-59

252.08 Other hyperparathyroidism

Tertiary hyperparathyroidism

252.1 Hypoparathyroidism

Parathyroiditis (autoimmune)
Tetany:
parathyroid
parathyroprival

Excludes *pseudohypoparathyroidism (275.49)*
pseudopseudohypoparathyroidism (275.49)
tetany NOS (781.7)
transitory neonatal hypoparathyroidism (775.4)

DEF: Reduced production of parathyroid hormone due to autoimmune disease, genetic factors, or gland removal.

C&C Exclusions: 252.0, 252.1, 252.8, 252.9, 259.8, 259.9

252.8 Other specified disorders of parathyroid gland

Cyst of parathyroid gland
Hemorrhage of parathyroid gland

✖ 252.9 Unspecified disorder of parathyroid gland

4 253 Disorders of the pituitary gland and its hypothalamic control

Includes the listed conditions whether the disorder is in the pituitary or the hypothalamus

Excludes *Cushing's syndrome (255.0)*

253.0 Acromegaly and gigantism

Overproduction of growth hormone

253.1 Other and unspecified anterior pituitary hyperfunction

Forbes-Albright syndrome

Excludes *overproduction of:*
ACTH (255.3)
thyroid-stimulating hormone [TSH] (242.8)

AHA: Jul-Aug 1985, 9

253.2 Panhypopituitarism

Cachexia, pituitary
Necrosis of pituitary (postpartum)
Pituitary insufficiency NOS
Sheehan's syndrome
Simmonds' disease

Excludes *iatrogenic hypopituitarism (253.7)*

C&C Exclusions: 253.0, 253.1, 253.2, 253.3, 253.4, 253.5, 253.6, 253.7, 253.8, 253.9, 259.8, 259.9

253.3 Pituitary dwarfism

Isolated deficiency of (human) growth hormone [HGH]
Lorain-Levi dwarfism

253.4 Other anterior pituitary disorders

Isolated or partial deficiency of an anterior pituitary hormone, other than growth hormone
Prolactin deficiency

AHA: Jul-Aug 1985, 9

253.5 Diabetes insipidus

Vasopressin deficiency

Excludes *nephrogenic diabetes insipidus (588.1)*

DEF: Insufficient vasopressin characterized by intense thirst and excretion of large amounts of urine.

C&C Exclusions: 253.0, 253.1, 253.2, 253.4, 253.5, 253.6, 253.7, 253.8, 253.9, 259.8, 259.9

253.6 Other disorders of neurohypophysis

Syndrome of inappropriate secretion of antidiuretic hormone [ADH]

Excludes *ectopic antidiuretic hormone secretion (259.3)*

253.7 Iatrogenic pituitary disorders

Hypopituitarism:
hormone-induced
hypophysectomy-induced
postablative
radiotherapy-induced
Use additional E code to identify cause

253.8 Other disorders of the pituitary and other syndromes of diencephalohypophyseal origin

Abscess of pituitary
Adiposogenital dystrophy
Cyst of Rathke's pouch
Fröhlich's syndrome

Excludes *craniopharyngioma (237.0)*

✖ 253.9 Unspecified

Dyspituitarism

4 254 Diseases of thymus gland

Excludes *aplasia or dysplasia with immunodeficiency (279.2)*
hypoplasia with immunodeficiency (279.2)
myasthenia gravis (358.00-358.01)

254.0 Persistent hyperplasia of thymus

Hypertrophy of thymus

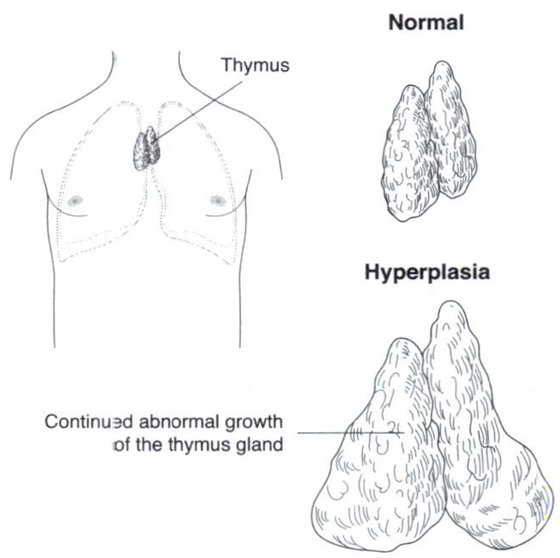

254.1 Abscess of thymus

254.8 Other specified diseases of thymus gland

Atrophy of thymus
Cyst of thymus

Excludes *thymoma (212.6)*

✖ 254.9 Unspecified disease of thymus gland

4 255 Disorders of adrenal glands

Includes the listed conditions whether the basic disorder is in the adrenals or is pituitary-induced

255.0 Cushing's syndrome

Adrenal hyperplasia due to excess ACTH
Cushing's syndrome:
NOS
iatrogenic
idiopathic
pituitary-dependent
Ectopic ACTH syndrome
Iatrogenic syndrome of excess cortisol
Overproduction of cortisol
Use additional E code to identify cause, if drug-induced

Excludes *congenital adrenal hyperplasia (255.2)*

C&C Exclusions: 255.0, 255.1, 255.2, 259.8, 259.9

5 255.1 Hyperaldosteronism

DEF: Excessive aldosterone production; typically presents with loss of potassium, muscular weakness, and elevated blood pressure.

AHA: 4Q 2003, 48

✖ 255.10 Hyperaldosteronism, unspecified

Aldosteronism NOS
Primary aldosteronism, unspecified

Excludes *Conn's syndrome (255.12)*

C&C Exclusions: 255.0, 258.0, 258.1, 258.8, 258.9

A Adult (15+ years) M Maternity (12-55 years) N Newborn (0 years) P Pediatric (0-17 years) ♂ Male ♀ Female ❷ Medicare Secondary Payer

255.11 Glucocorticoid-remediable aldosteronism
Familial aldosteronism type I
Excludes *Conn's syndrome (255.12)*
C&C Exclusions: See 255.10

255.12 Conn's syndrome
DEF: Excess secretion of aldosterone due to an adrenocortical adenoma, causing hypokalemia, alkalosis, muscular weakness, polyuria, polydipsia, and hypertension.
C&C Exclusions: See 255.10

255.13 Bartter's syndrome
C&C Exclusions: See 255.10

255.14 Other secondary aldosteronism
C&C Exclusions: See 255.10

255.2 Adrenogenital disorders
Achard-Thiers syndrome
Adrenogenital syndromes, virilizing or feminizing, whether acquired or associated with congenital adrenal hyperplasia consequent on inborn enzyme defects in hormone synthesis
Congenital adrenal hyperplasia
Female adrenal pseudohermaphroditism
Male:
macrogenitosomia praecox
sexual precocity with adrenal hyperplasia
Virilization (female) (suprarenal)
Excludes *adrenal hyperplasia due to excess ACTH (255.0)*
isosexual virilization (256.4)

255.3 Other corticoadrenal overactivity
Acquired benign adrenal androgenic overactivity
Overproduction of ACTH
C&C Exclusions: 017.60, 017.61, 017.62, 017.63, 017.64, 017.65, 017.66, 017.90, 017.91, 017.92, 017.93, 017.94, 017.95, 017.96, 255.3, 255.4, 255.5, 255.6, 255.8, 255.9, 259.8, 259.9

❺ **255.4 Corticoadrenal insufficiency**
Excludes *tuberculous Addison's disease (017.6)*
C&C Exclusions: See 255.3
AHA: 3Q 2006, 24

● **255.41 Glucocorticoid deficiency**
Addisonian crisis
Addison's disease NOS
Adrenal:
atrophy (autoimmune)
calcification
crisis
hemorrhage
infarction
insufficiency NOS
Combined glucocorticoid and mineralocorticoid deficiency
Corticoadrenal insufficiency NOS
DEF: Low levels of the glucocorticoid hormone, cortisol, secreted by the adrenal glands and responsible for regulating blood pressure, cardiovascular function, inflammatory response, insulin effects, and metabolism.

● **255.42 Mineralocorticoid deficiency**
Hypoaldosteronism
Excludes *combined glucocorticoid and mineralocorticoid deficiency (255.41)*

255.5 Other adrenal hypofunction
Adrenal medullary insufficiency
Excludes *Waterhouse-Friderichsen syndrome (meningococcal) (036.3)*
C&C Exclusions: See 255.3

255.6 Medulloadrenal hyperfunction
Catecholamine secretion by pheochromocytoma
DEF: Overproduction of adrenaline hormones by the adrenal medulla, causing heart disease, high blood pressure, and related problems.
C&C Exclusions: See 255.3

255.8 Other specified disorders of adrenal glands
Abnormality of cortisol-binding globulin

255.9 Unspecified disorder of adrenal glands

❹ **256 Ovarian dysfunction**
AHA: 4Q 2000, 51

256.0 Hyperestrogenism ♀

256.1 Other ovarian hyperfunction ♀
Hypersecretion of ovarian androgens
AHA: 2Q 1995, 15

256.2 Postablative ovarian failure ♀
Ovarian failure:
iatrogenic
postirradiation
postsurgical
Use additional code for states associated with artificial menopause (627.4)
Excludes *acquired absence of ovary (V45.77)*
asymptomatic age-related (natural) postmenopausal status (V49.81)
AHA: 2Q 2002, 12

❺ **256.3 Other ovarian failure**
Use additional code for states associated with natural menopause (627.2)
Excludes *asymptomatic age-related (natural) postmenopausal status (V49.81)*
AHA: 4Q 2001, 41

256.31 Premature menopause ♀ [A]
C&C Exclusions: 258.0, 258.1, 258.8, 258.9

256.39 Other ovarian failure ♀
Delayed menarche
Ovarian hypofunction
Primary ovarian failure NOS
C&C Exclusions: See 256.31

256.4 Polycystic ovaries ♀
Isosexual virilization
Stein-Leventhal syndrome
DEF: Ovaries containing multiple, small follicular cysts filled with yellow or blood-stained, thin serous fluid.

256.8 Other ovarian dysfunction ♀

✖ **256.9 Unspecified ovarian dysfunction** ♀

❹ **257 Testicular dysfunction**

257.0 Testicular hyperfunction ♂
Hypersecretion of testicular hormones
DEF: Excessive testosterone production, often due to an active tumor on the testicle. Commonly presents with increased muscle and bone growth in children and increased secondary sex characteristics.

The secretion of too much testosterone into the body

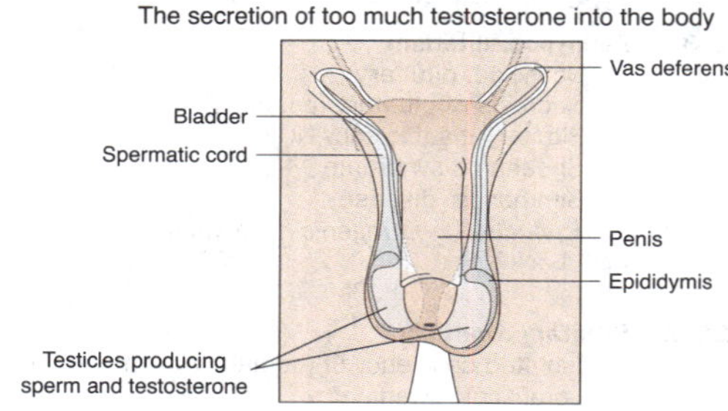

257.1 Postablative testicular hypofunction ♂
Testicular hypofunction:
iatrogenic
postirradiation
postsurgical

257.2 Other testicular hypofunction ♂
Defective biosynthesis of testicular androgen
Eunuchoidism:
NOS
hypogonadotropic
Failure:
Leydig's cell, adult
seminiferous tubule, adult
Testicular hypogonadism
Excludes *azoospermia (606.0)*

257.8 Other testicular dysfunction ♂
Excludes *androgen insensitivity syndrome (259.5)*

✖ **257.9 Unspecified testicular dysfunction** ♂

❹ **258 Polyglandular dysfunction and related disorders**

❺ **258.0 Polyglandular activity in multiple endocrine adenomatosis**
▶ Multiple endocrine neoplasia [MEN] syndromes◀
▶ Use additional codes to identify any malignancies and other conditions associated with the syndromes◀
C&C Exclusions: 240.0, 240.9, 241.0, 241.1, 241.9, 242.00, 242.01, 242.10, 242.11, 242.20, 242.21, 242.30, 242.31, 242.40, 242.41, 242.80, 242.81, 242.90, 242.91, 243, 244.0, 244.1, 244.2, 244.3, 244.8, 244.9, 245.0, 245.1, 245.2, 245.3, 245.4, 245.8, 245.9, 246.0, 246.1, 246.2, 246.3, 246.8, 246.9, 250.00, 250.01, 250.02, 250.03, 250.10, 250.11, 250.12, 250.13, 250.20, 250.21, 250.22, 250.23, 250.30, 250.31, 250.32, 250.33, 250.40, 250.41, 250.42, 250.43, 250.50, 250.51, 250.52, 250.53, 250.60, 250.61, 250.62, 250.63, 250.70, 250.71, 250.72, 250.73, 250.80, 250.81, 250.82, 250.83, 250.90, 250.91, 250.92, 250.93, 251.0, 251.1, 251.2, 251.3, 251.4, 251.5, 252.0, 252.1, 252.8, 252.9, 253.0, 253.1, 253.2, 253.3, 253.4, 253.5, 253.6, 253.7, 253.8, 253.9, 254.0, 254.1, 254.8, 254.9, 255.0, 255.1, 255.2, 255.3, 255.4, 255.5, 255.6, 255.8, 255.9, 256.0, 256.1, 256.2, 256.31, 256.39, 256.4, 256.8, 256.9, 257.0, 257.1, 257.2, 257.8, 257.9, 258.0, 258.1, 258.8, 258.9, 259.0, 259.1, 259.2, 259.3, 259.4, 259.8, 259.9

● **258.01 Multiple endocrine neoplasia [MEN] type I**
Wermer's syndrome
DEF: Hyperplasia or tumors of the parathyroid, pancreatic islet cells, and pituitary gland; causes oversecretion of hormones, kidney stones, infertility, and severe peptic ulcers.

● **258.02 Multiple endocrine neoplasia [MEN] type IIA**
Sipple's syndrome
DEF: Triad of thyroid medullary carcinoma, adrenal gland tumor, and parathyroid hyperplasia.

● **258.03 Multiple endocrine neoplasia [MEN] type IIB**

258.1 Other combinations of endocrine dysfunction
Lloyd's syndrome
Schmidt's syndrome
DEF: Schmidt's syndrome: hypofunction of more than one endocrine gland in different combinations, including the thyroid, adrenals, gonads, parathyroids, and pancreas; occurs primarily in adult females.
C&C Exclusions: See 258.0

258.8 Other specified polyglandular dysfunction
C&C Exclusions: See 258.0

✖ **258.9 Polyglandular dysfunction, unspecified**
C&C Exclusions: See 258.0

❹ **259 Other endocrine disorders**

259.0 Delay in sexual development and puberty, not elsewhere classified
Delayed puberty

259.1 Precocious sexual development and puberty, not elsewhere classified P
Sexual precocity:
NOS
constitutional
cryptogenic
idiopathic

259.2 Carcinoid syndrome
Hormone secretion by carcinoid tumors
C&C Exclusions: 259.2, 259.3, 259.8, 259.9

259.3 Ectopic hormone secretion, not elsewhere classified
Ectopic:
antidiuretic hormone secretion [ADH]
hyperparathyroidism
Excludes *ectopic ACTH syndrome (255.0)*
AHA: Nov-Dec 1985, 4

259.4 Dwarfism, not elsewhere classified
Dwarfism:
NOS
constitutional
Excludes *dwarfism:*
achondroplastic (756.4)
intrauterine (759.7)
nutritional (263.2)
pituitary (253.3)
renal (588.0)
progeria (259.8)

259.5 Androgen insensitivity syndrome
Partial androgen insensitivity
Reifenstein syndrome
C&C Exclusions: 242.00, 242.01, 242.10, 242.11, 242.20, 242.21, 242.30, 242.31, 242.40, 242.41, 242.80, 242.81, 242.90, 242.91, 250.01, 250.02, 250.03, 250.11, 250.12, 250.13, 250.21, 250.22, 250.23, 250.31, 250.32, 250.33, 250.41, 250.42, 250.43, 250.51, 250.52, 250.53, 250.61, 250.62, 250.63, 250.71, 250.72, 250.73, 250.81, 250.82, 250.83, 250.91, 250.92, 250.93, 251.0, 251.3, 252.1, 253.2, 253.5, 254.1, 255.0, 255.3, 255.4, 255.5, 255.6, 258.0, 258.1, 258.8, 258.9, 259.2
AHA: 4Q 2005, 53

259.8 Other specified endocrine disorders
Pineal gland dysfunction
Progeria
Werner's syndrome

259.9 Unspecified endocrine disorder
Disturbance:
endocrine NOS
hormone NOS
Infantilism NOS

NUTRITIONAL DEFICIENCIES (260-269)

Excludes *deficiency anemias (280.0-281.9)*

260 Kwashiorkor
Nutritional edema with dyspigmentation of skin and hair
C&C Exclusions: 260, 262, 263.0, 263.1, 263.2, 263.8, 263.9

261 Nutritional marasmus
Nutritional atrophy
Severe calorie deficiency
Severe malnutrition NOS
C&C Exclusions: See 260
AHA: 2Q 2006, 12

262 Other severe protein-calorie malnutrition
Nutritional edema without mention of dyspigmentation of skin and hair
C&C Exclusions: See 260
AHA: 4Q 1992, 24; Jul-Aug 1985, 12

❹ **263 Other and unspecified protein-calorie malnutrition**
AHA: 4Q 1992, 24

263.0 Malnutrition of moderate degree
C&C Exclusions: See 260
AHA: Jul-Aug 1985, 1

263.1 Malnutrition of mild degree
C&C Exclusions: See 260
AHA: Jul-Aug 1985, 1

263.2 Arrested development following protein-calorie malnutrition
Nutritional dwarfism
Physical retardation due to malnutrition
C&C Exclusions: See 260

263.8 Other protein-calorie malnutrition
C&C Exclusions: See 260

263.9 Unspecified protein-calorie malnutrition
Dystrophy due to malnutrition
Malnutrition (calorie) NOS
Excludes *nutritional deficiency NOS (269.9)*
C&C Exclusions: See 260
AHA: 4Q 2003, 109; Nov-Dec 1984, 19

Protein-calorie malnutrition

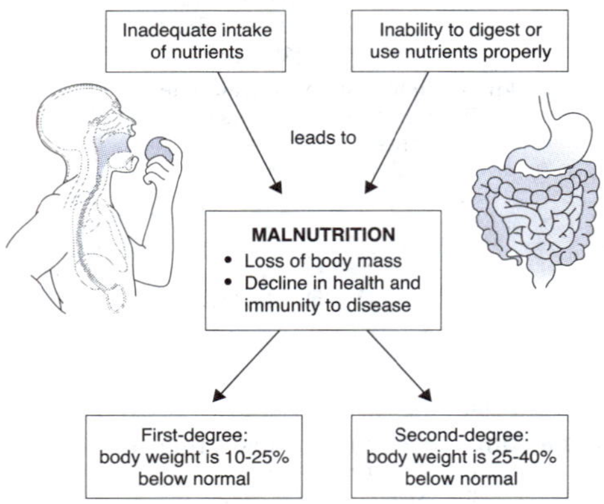

❹ **264 Vitamin A deficiency**
DEF: Vitamin A plays an important role in vision, bone growth, reproduction, and cell division and is stored in the liver.

264.0 With conjunctival xerosis
DEF: Vitamin A deficiency with dryness of the membrane that lines the eyelids and covers the exposed surface of the sclera.

264.1 With conjunctival xerosis and Bitot's spot
Bitot's spot in the young child
DEF: Vitamin A deficiency with superficial spots of keratinized epithelium on the conjunctiva, accompanied by dryness.

264.2 With corneal xerosis

264.3 With corneal ulceration and xerosis

264.4 With keratomalacia
DEF: Vitamin A deficiency with softening of the corneas that may lead to corneal infection or rupture.

264.5 With night blindness

264.6 With xerophthalmic scars of cornea

264.7 Other ocular manifestations of vitamin A deficiency
Xerophthalmia due to vitamin A deficiency

264.8 Other manifestations of vitamin A deficiency
Follicular keratosis due to vitamin A deficiency
Xeroderma due to vitamin A deficiency

264.9 Unspecified vitamin A deficiency
Hypovitaminosis A NOS

Body does not take in a sufficient amount of Vitamin A or does not absorb Vitamin A properly. The most common symptoms include dry eyes and eye inflammation.

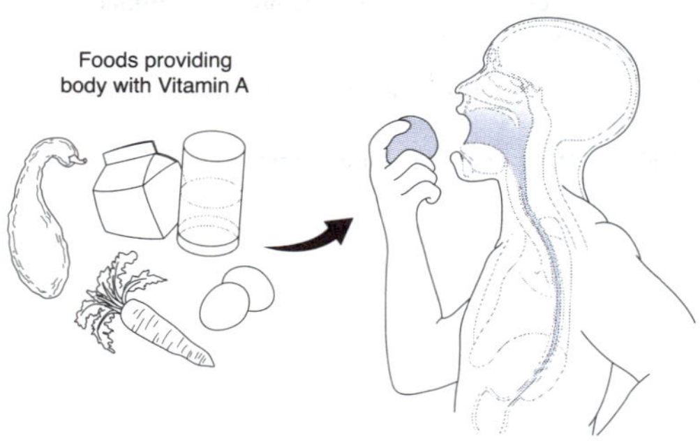

❹ **265 Thiamine and niacin deficiency states**

265.0 Beriberi
DEF: Severe vitamin B_1 deficiency causing nerve, heart, and/or brain abnormalities.

265.1 Other and unspecified manifestations of thiamine deficiency
Other vitamin B_1 deficiency states

265.2 Pellagra
Deficiency:
niacin (-tryptophan)
nicotinamide
nicotinic acid
vitamin PP
Pellagra (alcoholic)
DEF: Niacin and amino acid tryptophan deficiency affecting the skin, digestive tract, and brain.

❹ **266 Deficiency of B-complex components**

266.0 Ariboflavinosis
Riboflavin [vitamin B_2] deficiency
DEF: Riboflavin deficiency causing dry throat and nasal passages, mouth sores, magenta-colored tongue, and overproduction of oil on the skin.
AHA: Sep-Oct 1986, 10

266.1 Vitamin B_6 deficiency
Deficiency:
pyridoxal
pyridoxamine
pyridoxine
Vitamin B_6 deficiency syndrome
Excludes *vitamin B_6-responsive sideroblastic anemia (285.0)*

266.2 Other B-complex deficiencies
Deficiency:
cyanocobalamin
folic acid
vitamin B_{12}
Excludes *combined system disease with anemia (281.0-281.1)*
deficiency anemias (281.0-281.9)
subacute degeneration of spinal cord with anemia (281.0-281.1)

266.9 Unspecified vitamin B deficiency

267 Ascorbic acid deficiency
Deficiency of vitamin C
Scurvy
Excludes *scorbutic anemia (281.8)*
DEF: Condition known as scurvy caused by deficiency of ascorbic acid (vitamin C) and marked by weakness, anemia, spongy gums, and mucocutaneous hemorrhages.

❹ **268 Vitamin D deficiency**
Excludes *vitamin D-resistant:*
osteomalacia (275.3)
rickets (275.3)

268.0 Rickets, active
Excludes *celiac rickets (579.0)*
renal rickets (588.0)
DEF: Childhood disease caused by a lack of vitamin D, resulting in soft, spongy bones and causing bone pain as well as skeletal deformities (e.g., bowlegs, scoliosis), distortion of the rib cage, and oddly-shaped skull.

✖ **268.1 Rickets, late effect**
Any condition specified as due to rickets and stated to be a late effect or sequela of rickets
► *Code first*◄ *the nature of late effect*

268.2 Osteomalacia, unspecified
DEF: Deficient levels of calcium in the bone, resulting in bone softening.

268.9 Unspecified vitamin D deficiency
Avitaminosis D

❹ ❺ Additional Digit Required ✖ Nonspecific PDx ⃠ Unacceptable PDx ✚ Manifestation Code ►◄ Revised Text ● New Code ▲ Revised Code

4 269 Other nutritional deficiencies

269.0 Deficiency of vitamin K

Excludes *deficiency of coagulation factor due to vitamin K deficiency (286.7)*
vitamin K deficiency of newborn (776.0)

C&C Exclusions: 269.0

269.1 Deficiency of other vitamins

Deficiency:
vitamin E
vitamin P

269.2 Unspecified vitamin deficiency

Multiple vitamin deficiency NOS

269.3 Mineral deficiency, not elsewhere classified

Deficiency:
calcium, dietary
iodine

Excludes *deficiency:*
calcium NOS (275.40)
potassium (276.8)
sodium (276.1)

269.8 Other nutritional deficiency

Excludes *adult failure to thrive (783.7)*
failure to thrive in childhood (783.41)
feeding problems (783.3)
newborn (779.3)

269.9 Unspecified nutritional deficiency

OTHER METABOLIC AND IMMUNITY DISORDERS (270-279)

Use additional code to identify any associated mental retardation

4 270 Disorders of amino-acid transport and metabolism

Excludes *abnormal findings without manifest disease (790.0-796.9)*
disorders of purine and pyrimidine metabolism (277.1-277.2)
gout (274.0-274.9)

270.0 Disturbances of amino-acid transport

Cystinosis
Cystinuria
Fanconi (-de Toni) (-Debré) syndrome
Glycinuria (renal)
Hartnup disease

270.1 Phenylketonuria [PKU]

Hyperphenylalaninemia

DEF: Inherited metabolic disorder caused by an enzyme deficiency resulting in accumulation of phenylalanine and its metabolites in the blood with excess excretion in the urine; causes mental retardation, seizures, eczema, and abnormal body odor.

270.2 Other disturbances of aromatic amino-acid metabolism

Albinism
Alkaptonuria
Alkaptonuric ochronosis
Disturbances of metabolism of tyrosine and tryptophan
Homogentisic acid defects
Hydroxykynureninuria
Hypertyrosinemia
Indicanuria
Kynureninase defects
Oasthouse urine disease
Ochronosis
Tyrosinosis
Tyrosinuria
Waardenburg syndrome

Excludes *vitamin B_6-deficiency syndrome (266.1)*

AHA: 3Q 1999, 20

270.3 Disturbances of branched-chain amino-acid metabolism

Disturbances of metabolism of leucine, isoleucine, and valine
Hypervalinemia
Intermittent branched-chain ketonuria
Leucine-induced hypoglycemia
Leucinosis
Maple syrup urine disease

AHA: 3Q 2000, 8

270.4 Disturbances of sulphur-bearing amino-acid metabolism

Cystathioninemia
Cystathioninuria
Disturbances of metabolism of methionine, homocystine, and cystathionine
Homocystinuria
Hypermethioninemia
Methioninemia

AHA: 2Q, 2007, 9 ; 1Q 2004, 6

270.5 Disturbances of histidine metabolism

Carnosinemia
Histidinemia
Hyperhistidinemia
Imidazole aminoaciduria

270.6 Disorders of urea cycle metabolism

Argininosuccinic aciduria
Citrullinemia
Disorders of metabolism of ornithine, citrulline, argininosuccinic acid, arginine, and ammonia
Hyperammonemia
Hyperornithinemia

270.7 Other disturbances of straight-chain amino-acid metabolism

Glucoglycinuria
Glycinemia (with methylmalonic acidemia)
Hyperglycinemia
Hyperlysinemia
Other disturbances of metabolism of glycine, threonine, serine, glutamine, and lysine
Pipecolic acidemia
Saccharopinuria

AHA: 3Q 2000, 8

270.8 Other specified disorders of amino-acid metabolism

Alaninemia
Ethanolaminuria
Glycoprolinuria
Hydroxyprolinemia
Hyperprolinemia
Iminoacidopathy
Prolinemia
Prolinuria
Sarcosinemia

✖ **270.9 Unspecified disorder of amino-acid metabolism**

4 271 Disorders of carbohydrate transport and metabolism

Excludes *abnormality of secretion of glucagon (251.4)*
diabetes mellitus (250.0-250.9)
hypoglycemia NOS (251.2)
mucopolysaccharidosis (277.5)

271.0 Glycogenosis

Amylopectinosis
Glucose-6-phosphatase deficiency
Glycogen storage disease
McArdle's disease
Pompe's disease
von Gierke's disease

AHA: 1Q 1998, 5

271.1 Galactosemia

Galactose-1-phosphate uridyl transferase deficiency
Galactosuria

271.2 Hereditary fructose intolerance

Essential benign fructosuria
Fructosemia

271.3 Intestinal disaccharidase deficiencies and disaccharide malabsorption

Intolerance or malabsorption (congenital) (of):
glucose-galactose
lactose
sucrose-isomaltose

271.4 Renal glycosuria

Renal diabetes

DEF: Excess glucose in the urine with normal levels in the blood, due to renal tubules' inability to reabsorb glucose completely.

271.8 Other specified disorders of carbohydrate transport and metabolism
Essential benign pentosuria
Fucosidosis
Glycolic aciduria
Hyperoxaluria (primary)
Mannosidosis
Oxalosis
Xylosuria
Xylulosuria

✖ **271.9 Unspecified disorder of carbohydrate transport and metabolism**

❹ **272 Disorders of lipoid metabolism**
Excludes *localized cerebral lipidoses (330.1)*

272.0 Pure hypercholesterolemia
Familial hypercholesterolemia
Fredrickson Type IIa hyperlipoproteinemia
Hyperbetalipoproteinemia
Hyperlipidemia, Group A
Low-density-lipoid-type [LDL] hyperlipoproteinemia
AHA: 4Q 2005, 71

272.1 Pure hyperglyceridemia
Endogenous hyperglyceridemia
Fredrickson Type IV hyperlipoproteinemia
Hyperlipidemia, Group B
Hyperprebetalipoproteinemia
Hypertriglyceridemia, essential
Very-low-density-lipoid-type [VLDL] hyperlipoproteinemia

272.2 Mixed hyperlipidemia
Broad- or floating-betalipoproteinemia
Fredrickson Type IIb or III hyperlipoproteinemia
Hyperbetalipoproteinemia with prebetalipoproteinemia
Hypercholesterolemia with endogenous hyperglyceridemia
Tubo-eruptive xanthoma
Xanthoma tuberosum

272.3 Hyperchylomicronemia
Bürger-Grütz syndrome
Fredrickson type I or V hyperlipoproteinemia
Hyperlipidemia, Group D
Mixed hyperglyceridemia

272.4 Other and unspecified hyperlipidemia
Alpha-lipoproteinemia
Combined hyperlipidemia
Hyperlipidemia NOS
Hyperlipoproteinemia NOS
AHA: 1Q 2005, 17

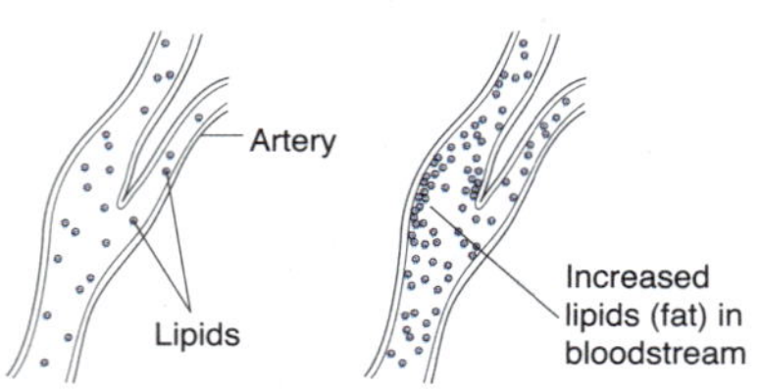

272.5 Lipoprotein deficiencies
Abetalipoproteinemia
Bassen-Kornzweig syndrome
High-density lipoid deficiency
Hypoalphalipoproteinemia
Hypobetalipoproteinemia (familial)

272.6 Lipodystrophy
Barraquer-Simons disease
Progressive lipodystrophy
Use additional E code to identify cause, if iatrogenic
Excludes *intestinal lipodystrophy (040.2)*
DEF: Defective fat metabolism resulting in abnormal or degenerative subcutaneous fat deposits that appear as lumps or dents under the skin.

272.7 Lipidoses
Chemically induced lipidosis
Disease:
- Anderson's
- Fabry's
- Gaucher's
- I cell [mucolipidosis I]
- lipoid storage NOS
- Niemann-Pick
- pseudo-Hurler's or mucolipidosis III
- triglyceride storage, Type I or II
- Wolman's or triglyceride storage, Type III

Mucolipidosis II
Primary familial xanthomatosis
Excludes *cerebral lipidoses (330.1)*
Tay-Sachs disease (330.1)

272.8 Other disorders of lipoid metabolism
Hoffa's disease or liposynovitis prepatellaris
Launois-Bensaude's lipomatosis
Lipoid dermatoarthritis

✖ **272.9 Unspecified disorder of lipoid metabolism**

❹ **273 Disorders of plasma protein metabolism**
Excludes *agammaglobulinemia and hypogammaglobulinemia (279.0-279.2)*
coagulation defects (286.0-286.9)
hereditary hemolytic anemias (282.0-282.9)

273.0 Polyclonal hypergammaglobulinemia
Hypergammaglobulinemic purpura:
- benign primary
- Waldenström's

273.1 Monoclonal paraproteinemia
Benign monoclonal hypergammaglobulinemia [BMH]
Monoclonal gammopathy:
- NOS
- associated with lymphoplasmacytic dyscrasias
- benign

Paraproteinemia:
- benign (familial)
- secondary to malignant or inflammatory disease

273.2 Other paraproteinemias
Cryoglobulinemic:
- purpura
- vasculitis

Mixed cryoglobulinemia

273.3 Macroglobulinemia
Macroglobulinemia (idiopathic) (primary)
Waldenström's macroglobulinemia

273.4 Alpha-1-antitrypsin deficiency
AAT deficiency

273.8 Other disorders of plasma protein metabolism
Abnormality of transport protein
Bisalbuminemia
AHA: 2Q 1998, 11

✖ **273.9 Unspecified disorder of plasma protein metabolism**

❹ **274 Gout**
Excludes *lead gout (984.0-984.9)*
AHA: 2Q 1995, 4

274.0 Gouty arthropathy

Inflammation of one or more joints due to gout

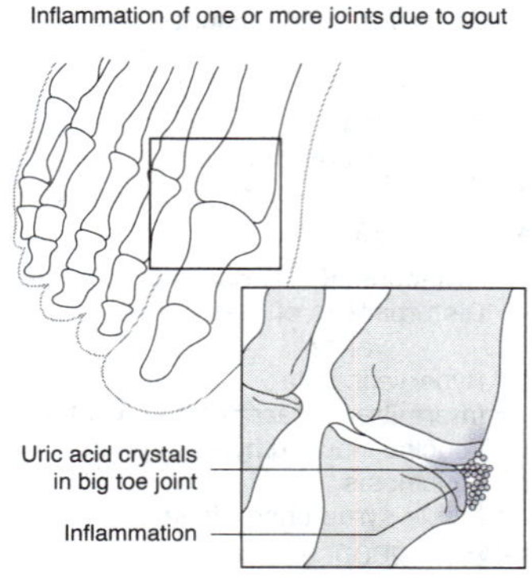

5 **274.1 Gouty nephropathy**

274.10 Gouty nephropathy, unspecified
C&C Exclusions: 585.1, 585.2, 585.3, 585.4, 585.5, 585.6, 585.9
AHA: Nov-Dec 1985, 15

274.11 Uric acid nephrolithiasis
C&C Exclusions: 599.60, 599.69

274.19 Other
C&C Exclusions: See 274.10

5 **274.8 Gout with other specified manifestations**

274.81 Gouty tophi of ear

274.82 Gouty tophi of other sites
Gouty tophi of heart

274.89 Other
Use additional code to identify manifestations, as:
gouty:
iritis (364.11)
neuritis (357.4)

274.9 Gout, unspecified

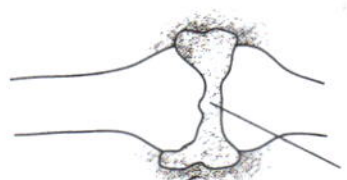

4 **275 Disorders of mineral metabolism**
Excludes *abnormal findings without manifest disease (790.0-796.9)*

275.0 Disorders of iron metabolism
Bronzed diabetes
Hemochromatosis
Pigmentary cirrhosis (of liver)
Excludes *anemia:*
iron deficiency (280.0-280.9)
sideroblastic (285.0)
AHA: 2Q 1997, 11

275.1 Disorders of copper metabolism
Hepatolenticular degeneration
Wilson's disease

275.2 Disorders of magnesium metabolism
Hypermagnesemia
Hypomagnesemia

275.3 Disorders of phosphorus metabolism
Familial hypophosphatemia
Hypophosphatasia
Vitamin D-resistant:
osteomalacia
rickets

5 **275.4 Disorders of calcium metabolism**
Excludes *parathyroid disorders (252.00-252.9)*
vitamin D deficiency (268.0-268.9)
AHA: 4Q 1997, 33

✖ **275.40 Unspecified disorder of calcium metabolism**

275.41 Hypocalcemia
DEF: Reduced calcium levels in the blood causing hyperactive deep tendon reflexes, Chvostek's sign, muscle and abdominal cramps, and carpopedal spasm.

275.42 Hypercalcemia
DEF: Excess calcium levels in the blood causing fatigue, muscle weakness, depression, anorexia, nausea, and constipation.
AHA: 4Q 2003, 110

275.49 Other disorders of calcium metabolism
Nephrocalcinosis
Pseudohypoparathyroidism
Pseudopseudohypoparathyroidism

275.8 Other specified disorders of mineral metabolism

✖ **275.9 Unspecified disorder of mineral metabolism**

4 **276 Disorders of fluid, electrolyte, and acid-base balance**
Excludes *diabetes insipidus (253.5)*
familial periodic paralysis (359.3)

276.0 Hyperosmolality and/or hypernatremia
Sodium [Na] excess
Sodium [Na] overload
C&C Exclusions: 276.0, 276.1, 276.2, 276.3, 276.4, 276.50, 276.51, 276.52, 276.6, 276.7, 276.8, 276.9

276.1 Hyposmolality and/or hyponatremia
Sodium [Na] deficiency
C&C Exclusions: See 276.0

276.2 Acidosis
Acidosis:
NOS
lactic
metabolic
respiratory
Excludes *diabetic acidosis (250.1)*
C&C Exclusions: See 276.0
AHA: Jan-Feb 1987, 15

276.3 Alkalosis
Alkalosis:
NOS
metabolic
respiratory
C&C Exclusions: See 276.0

276.4 Mixed acid-base balance disorder
Hypercapnia with mixed acid-base disorder
C&C Exclusions: See 276.0

5 **276.5 Volume depletion**
Excludes *hypovolemic shock:*
postoperative (998.0)
traumatic (958.4)
AHA: 4Q 2005, 54; 2Q 2005, 9; 1Q 2003, 5, 22; 3Q 2002, 21; 4Q 1997, 30; 2Q 1988, 9

✖ **276.50 Volume depletion, unspecified**
C&C Exclusions: See 276.0

276.51 Dehydration
C&C Exclusions: See 276.0

276.52 Hypovolemia
Depletion of volume of plasma
DEF: Abnormal decrease in the total volume of circulating blood with a corresponding loss of sodium electrolytes.
C&C Exclusions: See 276.0

276.6 Fluid overload
Fluid retention
Excludes *ascites (▶789.51-789.59◀)*
localized edema (782.3)
C&C Exclusions: See 276.0
AHA: 4Q 2006, 136

276.7 Hyperpotassemia
Hyperkalemia
Potassium [K]:
excess
intoxication
overload
C&C Exclusions: See 276.0
AHA: 1Q 2005, 9; 2Q 2001, 12

276.8 Hypopotassemia
Hypokalemia
Potassium [K] deficiency
DEF: Low potassium level in the blood causing neuromuscular disorders ranging from weakness to paralysis, electrocardiographic abnormalities, renal disease, and gastrointestinal disorders.
C&C Exclusions: See 276.0

276.9 Electrolyte and fluid disorders not elsewhere classified
Electrolyte imbalance
Hyperchloremia
Hypochloremia
Excludes *electrolyte imbalance:*
associated with hyperemesis gravidarum (643.1)
complicating labor and delivery (669.0)
following abortion and ectopic or molar pregnancy (634-638 with .4, 639.4)
C&C Exclusions: See 276.0
AHA: Jan-Feb 1987, 15

④ **277 Other and unspecified disorders of metabolism**

⑤ **277.0 Cystic fibrosis**
Fibrocystic disease of the pancreas
Mucoviscidosis
DEF: Defective gene causing overproduction of mucous that builds up in lung passages, resulting in life-threatening respiratory problems.
AHA: 4Q 1990, 16; 3Q 1990, 18

277.00 Without mention of meconium ileus
Cystic fibrosis NOS
C&C Exclusions: 277.00, 277.01, 277.02, 277.03, 277.09
AHA: 2Q 2003, 12

277.01 With meconium ileus N
Meconium:
ileus (of newborn)
obstruction of intestine in mucoviscidosis
C&C Exclusions: See 277.00

277.02 With pulmonary manifestations
Cystic fibrosis with pulmonary exacerbation
Use additional code to identify any infectious organism present, such as:
psuedomonas (041.7)
C&C Exclusions: See 277.00
AHA: 4Q 2002, 45-46

277.03 With gastrointestinal manifestations
Excludes *with meconium ileus (277.01)*
C&C Exclusions: See 277.00
AHA: 4Q 2002, 45

277.09 With other manifestations
C&C Exclusions: See 277.00

277.1 Disorders of porphyrin metabolism
Hematoporphyria
Hematoporphyrinuria
Hereditary coproporphyria
Porphyria
Porphyrinuria
Protocoproporphyria
Protoporphyria
Pyrroloporphyria

277.2 Other disorders of purine and pyrimidine metabolism
Hypoxanthine-guanine-phosphoribosyltransferase deficiency [HG-PRT deficiency]
Lesch-Nyhan syndrome
Xanthinuria
Excludes *gout (274.0-274.9)*
orotic aciduric anemia (281.4)

⑤ **277.3 Amyloidosis**
AHA: 1Q 1996, 16

✖ **277.30 Amyloidosis, unspecified**
Amyloidosis NOS

277.31 Familial Mediterranean fever
Benign paroxysmal peritonitis
Hereditary amyloid nephropathy
Periodic familial polyserositis
Recurrent polyserositis

277.39 Other amyloidosis
Hereditary cardiac amyloidosis
Inherited systemic amyloidosis
Neuropathic (Portuguese) (Swiss) amyloidosis
Secondary amyloidosis

277.4 Disorders of bilirubin excretion
Hyperbilirubinemia:
congenital
constitutional
Syndrome:
Crigler-Najjar
Dubin-Johnson
Gilbert's
Rotor's
Excludes *hyperbilirubinemias specific to the perinatal period (774.0-774.7)*
DEF: Gilbert's syndrome: an inborn error of bilirubin metabolism causing a benign elevation of unconjugated bilirubin with no liver damage or hematologic abnormalities.

277.5 Mucopolysaccharidosis
Gargoylism
Hunter's syndrome
Hurler's syndrome
Lipochondrodystrophy
Maroteaux-Lamy syndrome
Morquio-Brailsford disease
Osteochondrodystrophy
Sanfilippo's syndrome
Scheie's syndrome

277.6 Other deficiencies of circulating enzymes
Hereditary angioedema

277.7 Dysmetabolic syndrome X
Use additional code for associated manifestation, such as:
cardiovascular disease (414.00-414.07)
obesity (278.00-278.01)
AHA: 4Q 2001, 42

⑤ **277.8 Other specified disorders of metabolism**
AHA: 4Q 2003, 50; 2Q 2001, 18; Sep-Oct 1987, 9

277.81 Primary carnitine deficiency

277.82 Carnitine deficiency due to inborn errors of metabolism

277.83 Iatrogenic carnitine deficiency
Carnitine deficiency due to:
hemodialysis
valproic acid therapy

277.84 Other secondary carnitine deficiency

277.85 Disorders of fatty acid oxidation
Carnitine palmitoyltransferase deficiencies (CPT1, CPT2)
Glutaric aciduria type II (type IIA, IIB, IIC)
Long chain 3-hydroxyacyl CoA dehydrogenase deficiency (LCHAD)
Long chain/very long chain acyl CoA dehydrogenase deficiency (LCAD, VLCAD)
Medium chain acyl CoA dehydrogenase deficiency (MCAD)
Short chain acyl CoA dehydrogenase deficiency (SCAD)
Excludes *primary carnitine deficiency (277.81)*

277.86 Peroxisomal disorders
Adrenomyeloneuropathy
Neonatal adrenoleukodystrophy
Rhizomelic chondrodysplasia punctata
X-linked adrenoleukodystrophy
Zellweger syndrome
Excludes *infantile Refsum disease (356.3)*

277.87 Disorders of mitochondrial metabolism
Kearns-Sayre syndrome
Mitochondrial Encephalopathy, Lactic Acidosis and Stroke-like episodes (MELAS syndrome)
Mitochondrial Neurogastrointestinal Encephalopathy syndrome (MNGIE)
Myoclonus with Epilepsy and with Ragged Red Fibers (MERRF syndrome)
Neuropathy, Ataxia and Retinitis Pigmentosa (NARP syndrome)
Use additional code for associated conditions
Excludes *disorders of pyruvate metabolism (271.8)*
Leber's optic atrophy (377.16)
Leigh's subacute necrotizing encephalopathy (330.8)
Reye's syndrome (331.81)
AHA: 4Q 2004, 62

277.89 Other specified disorders of metabolism
Hand-Schüller-Christian disease
Histiocytosis (acute) (chronic)
Histiocytosis X (chronic)
Excludes *histiocytosis:*
acute differentiated progressive (202.5)
X, acute (progressive) (202.5)

277.9 Unspecified disorder of metabolism
Enzymopathy NOS

278 Overweight, obesity and other hyperalimentation
Excludes *hyperalimentation NOS (783.6)*
poisoning by vitamins NOS (963.5)
polyphagia (783.6)

278.0 Overweight and obesity
Use additional code to identify Body Mass Index (BMI), if known (V85.0-V85.54)
Excludes *adiposogenital dystrophy (253.8)*
obesity of endocrine origin NOS (259.9)
AHA: 4Q 2005, 97

278.00 Obesity, unspecified
Obesity NOS
AHA: 4Q 2001, 42; 1Q 1999, 5-6

278.01 Morbid obesity
Severe obesity
AHA: 2Q 2006, 6; 3Q 2003, 6-8

278.02 Overweight
AHA: 4Q 2005, 55

278.1 Localized adiposity
Fat pad
AHA: 2Q 2006, 11

278.2 Hypervitaminosis A

278.3 Hypercarotinemia
DEF: Elevated carotene levels in the blood from excessive ingestion of carotenoids or the inability to convert carotenoids to vitamin A; often presents with yellowing of the skin.

278.4 Hypervitaminosis D

278.8 Other hyperalimentation

279 Disorders involving the immune mechanism

279.0 Deficiency of humoral immunity

279.00 Hypogammaglobulinemia, unspecified
Agammaglobulinemia NOS

279.01 Selective IgA immunodeficiency

279.02 Selective IgM immunodeficiency
C&C Exclusions: 279.02, 279.03, 279.04, 279.05, 279.06, 279.09, 279.10, 279.11, 279.12, 279.13, 279.19, 279.2, 279.3, 279.4, 279.8, 279.9

279.03 Other selective immunoglobulin deficiencies
Selective deficiency of IgG
C&C Exclusions: See 279.02

279.04 Congenital hypogammaglobulinemia
Agammaglobulinemia:
Bruton's type
X-linked
C&C Exclusions: See 279.02

279.05 Immunodeficiency with increased IgM
Immunodeficiency with hyper-IgM:
autosomal recessive
X-linked
C&C Exclusions: See 279.02

279.06 Common variable immunodeficiency
Dysgammaglobulinemia (acquired) (congenital) (primary)
Hypogammaglobulinemia:
acquired primary
congenital non-sex-linked
sporadic
C&C Exclusions: See 279.02

279.09 Other
Transient hypogammaglobulinemia of infancy

279.1 Deficiency of cell-mediated immunity

279.10 Immunodeficiency with predominant T-cell defect, unspecified
C&C Exclusions: See 279.02
AHA: Sep-Oct 1987, 10

279.11 DiGeorge's syndrome
Pharyngeal pouch syndrome
Thymic hypoplasia
DEF: Congenital disorder with hypoplasia or aplasia of the thymus and parathyroid glands; associated with congenital heart defects, great vessel anomalies, esophageal atresia, and abnormal facial structure.
C&C Exclusions: See 279.02

279.12 Wiskott-Aldrich syndrome
DEF: X-linked immunodeficiency syndrome presenting with eczema, thrombocytopenia, and recurrent pyogenic infection.
C&C Exclusions: See 279.02

279.13 Nezelof's syndrome
Cellular immunodeficiency with abnormal immunoglobulin deficiency
C&C Exclusions: See 279.02

279.19 Other
Excludes *ataxia-telangiectasia (334.8)*
C&C Exclusions: See 279.02

279.2 Combined immunity deficiency
Agammaglobulinemia:
autosomal recessive
Swiss-type
X-linked recessive
Severe combined immunodeficiency [SCID]
Thymic:
alymphoplasia
aplasia or dysplasia with immunodeficiency
Excludes *thymic hypoplasia (279.11)*
C&C Exclusions: See 279.02

279.3 Unspecified immunity deficiency
C&C Exclusions: See 279.02

279.4 Autoimmune disease, not elsewhere classified
Autoimmune disease NOS
Excludes *transplant failure or rejection (996.80-996.89)*
C&C Exclusions: See 279.02

279.8 Other specified disorders involving the immune mechanism
Single complement [C_1-C_9] deficiency or dysfunction
C&C Exclusions: See 279.02

279.9 Unspecified disorder of immune mechanism
C&C Exclusions: See 279.02
AHA: 3Q 1992, 13

A Adult (15+ years) M Maternity (12-55 years) N Newborn (0 years) P Pediatric (0-17 years) ♂ Male ♀ Female ❷ Medicare Secondary Payer

4. DISEASES OF THE BLOOD AND BLOOD-FORMING ORGANS (280-289)

4 280 Iron deficiency anemias

Includes anemia:
- asiderotic
- hypochromic-microcytic
- sideropenic

Excludes familial microcytic anemia (282.49)

280.0 Secondary to blood loss (chronic)

Normocytic anemia due to blood loss

Excludes acute posthemorrhagic anemia (285.1)

C&C Exclusions: 280.0, 280.1, 280.8, 280.9, 281.0, 281.1, 281.2, 281.3, 281.4, 281.8, 281.9, 282.0, 282.1, 282.2, 282.3, 282.41, 282.42, 282.49, 282.5, 282.60, 282.61, 282.62, 282.63, 282.64, 282.68, 282.69, 282.7, 282.8, 282.9, 283.0, 283.10, 283.11, 283.19, 283.2, 283.9, 284.0, 284.8, 284.9, 285.0, 285.1, 285.21, 285.22, 285.29, 285.8, 285.9, 289.8, 289.9

AHA: 4Q 1993, 34

280.1 Secondary to inadequate dietary iron intake

280.8 Other specified iron deficiency anemias

Paterson-Kelly syndrome
Plummer-Vinson syndrome
Sideropenic dysphagia

280.9 Iron deficiency anemia, unspecified

Anemia:
- achlorhydric
- chlorotic
- idiopathic hypochromic
- iron [Fe] deficiency NOS

4 281 Other deficiency anemias

281.0 Pernicious anemia

Anemia:
- Addison's
- Biermer's
- congenital pernicious

Congenital intrinsic factor [Castle's] deficiency

Excludes combined system disease without mention of anemia (266.2)
subacute degeneration of spinal cord without mention of anemia (266.2)

DEF: Anemia due to underlying Vitamin B_{12} malabsorption caused by inadequate production of intrinsic factor in the gastric mucosa.

AHA: Nov-Dec 1984, 1; Sep-Oct 1984, 16

281.1 Other vitamin B_{12} deficiency anemia

Anemia:
- vegan's
- vitamin B_{12} deficiency (dietary)
- due to selective vitamin B_{12} malabsorption with proteinuria

Syndrome:
- Imerslund's
- Imerslund-Gräsbeck

Excludes combined system disease without mention of anemia (266.2)
subacute degeneration of spinal cord without mention of anemia (266.2)

DEF: Deficiency of Vitamin B_{12} in diet. Symptoms include loss of appetite, diarrhea, numbness and tingling in the hands and/or feet, pale skin color, and a soreness in the mouth and/or tongue

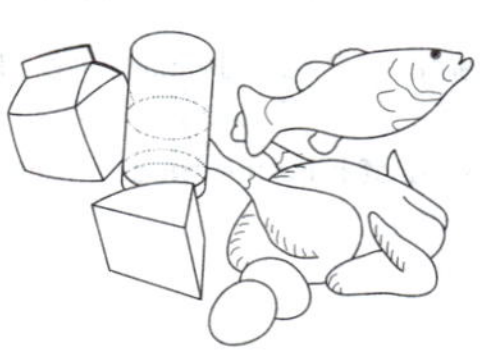

Meat, fish, dairy products, and eggs are the best sources of Vitamin B_{12}

281.2 Folate-deficiency anemia

Congenital folate malabsorption
Folate or folic acid deficiency anemia:
- NOS
- dietary
- drug-induced

Goat's milk anemia
Nutritional megaloblastic anemia (of infancy)
Use additional E code to identify drug

281.3 Other specified megaloblastic anemias, not elsewhere classified

Combined B_{12} and folate-deficiency anemia

281.4 Protein-deficiency anemia

Amino-acid-deficiency anemia

C&C Exclusions: See 280.0

281.8 Anemia associated with other specified nutritional deficiency

Scorbutic anemia

C&C Exclusions: See 280.0

281.9 Unspecified deficiency anemia

Anemia:
- dimorphic
- macrocytic
- megaloblastic NOS
- nutritional NOS
- simple chronic

4 282 Hereditary hemolytic anemias

282.0 Hereditary spherocytosis

Acholuric (familial) jaundice
Congenital hemolytic anemia (spherocytic)
Congenital spherocytosis
Minkowski-Chauffard syndrome
Spherocytosis (familial)

Excludes hemolytic anemia of newborn (773.0-773.5)

DEF: Congenital form of spherocytosis with hemolytic anemia, abnormal fragility of erythrocytes, jaundice, and splenomegaly.

282.1 Hereditary elliptocytosis

Elliptocytosis (congenital)
Ovalocytosis (congenital) (hereditary)

282.2 Anemias due to disorders of glutathione metabolism

Anemia:
- 6-phosphogluconic dehydrogenase deficiency
- enzyme deficiency, drug-induced
- erythrocytic glutathione deficiency
- glucose-6-phosphate dehydrogenase [G-6-PD] deficiency
- glutathione-reductase deficiency
- hemolytic nonspherocytic (hereditary), type I

Disorder of pentose phosphate pathway
Favism

282.3 Other hemolytic anemias due to enzyme deficiency

Anemia:
- hemolytic nonspherocytic (hereditary), type II
- hexokinase deficiency
- pyruvate kinase [PK] deficiency
- triosephosphate isomerase deficiency

5 282.4 Thalassemias

Excludes sickle-cell:
disease (282.60-282.69)
trait (282.5)

AHA: 4Q 2003, 51

282.41 Sickle-cell thalassemia without crisis

Sickle-cell thalassemia NOS
Thalassemia Hb-S disease without crisis

C&C Exclusions: 280.0, 281.4, 281.8, 282.41, 282.42, 282.49, 282.60, 282.61, 282.62, 282.63, 282.64, 282.68, 282.69, 283.0, 283.10, 283.11, 283.19, 283.2, 283.9, 284.8, 284.9, 285.0, 285.1

282.42 Sickle-cell thalassemia with crisis

Sickle-cell thalassemia with vaso-occlusive pain
Thalassemia Hb-S disease with crisis
Use additional code for types of crisis, such as:
- acute chest syndrome (517.3)
- splenic sequestration (289.52)

C&C Exclusions: See 282.41

282.49 Other thalassemia
Cooley's anemia
Hb-Bart's disease
Hereditary leptocytosis
Mediterranean anemia (with other hemoglobinopathy)
Microdrepanocytosis
Thalassemia (alpha) (beta) (intermedia) (major) (minima) (minor) (mixed) (trait) (with other hemoglobinopathy)
Thalassemia NOS
C&C Exclusions: See 282.41

282.5 Sickle-cell trait
Hb-AS genotype
Hemoglobin S [Hb-S] trait
Heterozygous:
 hemoglobin S
 Hb-S
Excludes *that with other hemoglobinopathy (282.60-282.69)*
that with thalassemia (282.49)

❺ **282.6 Sickle-cell disease**
Sickle cell anemia
Excludes *sickle-cell thalassemia (282.41-282.42)*
sickle-cell trait (282.5)
DEF: Chronic, hereditary disease in which red blood cells contain abnormal hemoglobin S and are stiff and misshapen like a crescent, inhibiting blood flow through small blood vessels.

282.60 Sickle-cell disease, unspecified
Sickle-cell anemia NOS
C&C Exclusions: See 280.0
AHA: 2Q 1997, 11

Normal red blood cells
Cells are compact and flexible, enabling them to squeeze through small capillaries

Sickled red blood cells
Cells are stiff and angular, causing them to become stuck in small capillaries

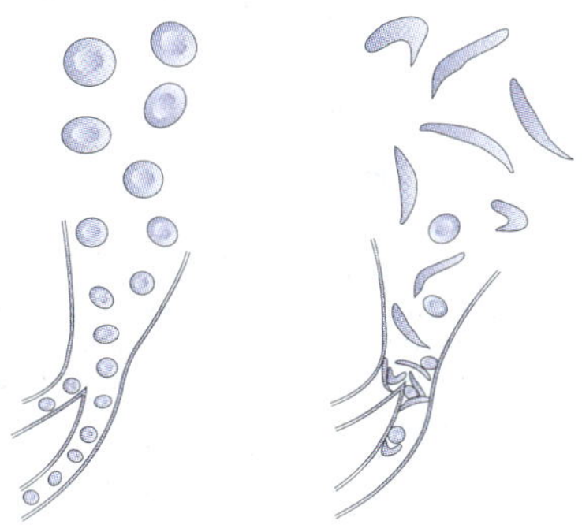

282.61 Hb-SS disease without crisis
C&C Exclusions: See 280.0
AHA: 2Q, 2007, 10

282.62 Hb-SS disease with crisis
Hb-SS disease with vaso-occlusive pain
Sickle-cell crisis NOS
Use additional code for types of crisis, such as:
 acute chest syndrome (517.3)
 splenic sequestration (289.52)
C&C Exclusions: See 280.0
AHA: 4Q 2003, 56; 2Q 1998, 8; 2Q 1991, 15

282.63 Sickle-cell/Hb-C disease without crisis
Hb-S/Hb-C disease without crisis
C&C Exclusions: See 280.0

282.64 Sickle-cell/Hb-C disease with crisis
Hb-S/Hb-C disease with crisis
Sickle-cell/Hb-C disease with vaso-occlusive disease
Use additional code for type of crisis, such as:
 acute chest syndrome (517.3)
 splenic sequestration (289.52)
C&C Exclusions: See 282.41
AHA: 4Q 2003, 51

282.68 Other sickle-cell disease without crisis
Hb-S/Hb-D disease without crisis
Hb-S/Hb-E disease without crisis
Sickle-cell/Hb-D disease without crisis
Sickle-cell/Hb-E disease without crisis
C&C Exclusions: See 282.41
AHA: 4Q 2003, 51

282.69 Other sickle-cell disease with crisis
Hb-S/Hb-D disease with crisis
Hb-S/Hb-E disease with crisis
Other sickle-cell disease with vaso-occlusive pain
Sickle-cell/Hb-D disease with crisis
Sickle-cell/Hb-E disease with crisis
Use additional code for types of crisis, such as:
 acute chest syndrome (517.3)
 splenic sequestration (289.52)
C&C Exclusions: See 280.0

282.7 Other hemoglobinopathies
Abnormal hemoglobin NOS
Congenital Heinz-body anemia
Disease:
 hemoglobin C [Hb-C]
 hemoglobin D [Hb-D]
 hemoglobin E [Hb-E]
 hemoglobin Zurich [Hb-Zurich]
Hemoglobinopathy NOS
Hereditary persistence of fetal hemoglobin [HPFH]
Unstable hemoglobin hemolytic disease
Excludes *familial polycythemia (289.6)*
hemoglobin M [Hb-M] disease (289.7)
high-oxygen-affinity hemoglobin (289.0)
C&C Exclusions: 282.41, 282.42, 282.49, 282.64, 282.68

282.8 Other specified hereditary hemolytic anemias
Stomatocytosis
C&C Exclusions: See 282.7

282.9 Hereditary hemolytic anemia, unspecified
Hereditary hemolytic anemia NOS
C&C Exclusions: See 282.7

❹ **283 Acquired hemolytic anemias**
AHA: Nov-Dec 1984, 1

283.0 Autoimmune hemolytic anemias
Autoimmune hemolytic disease (cold type) (warm type)
Chronic cold hemagglutinin disease
Cold agglutinin disease or hemoglobinuria
Hemolytic anemia:
 cold type (secondary) (symptomatic)
 drug-induced
 warm type (secondary) (symptomatic)
Use additional E code to identify cause, if drug-induced
Excludes *Evans' syndrome (287.32)*
hemolytic disease of newborn (773.0-773.5)
C&C Exclusions: See 280.0

❺ **283.1 Non-autoimmune hemolytic anemias**
AHA: 4Q 1993, 25

283.10 Non-autoimmune hemolytic anemia, unspecified
C&C Exclusions: See 280.0

283.11 Hemolytic-uremic syndrome
DEF: Condition in which platelets become clogged in narrow renal blood vessels, leading to the destruction of red blood cells and kidney failure. Symptoms include severe abdominal pain, diarrhea, nausea, and vomiting.
C&C Exclusions: See 280.0

283.19 Other non-autoimmune hemolytic anemias
Hemolytic anemia:
 mechanical
 microangiopathic
 toxic
Use additional E code to identify cause
C&C Exclusions: See 280.0

283.2 Hemoglobinuria due to hemolysis from external causes
Acute intravascular hemolysis
Hemoglobinuria:
from exertion
march
paroxysmal (cold) (nocturnal)
due to other hemolysis
Marchiafava-Micheli syndrome
Use additional E code to identify cause
C&C Exclusions: See 280.0

283.9 Acquired hemolytic anemia, unspecified
Acquired hemolytic anemia NOS
Chronic idiopathic hemolytic anemia
C&C Exclusions: See 280.0

④ 284 Aplastic anemia and other bone marrow failure syndromes
AHA: 1Q 1991, 14; Nov-Dec 1984, 1; Sep-Oct 1984, 16

⑤ 284.0 Constitutional aplastic anemia
AHA: 1Q 1991, 14

284.01 Constitutional red blood cell aplasia
Aplasia, (pure) red cell:
congenital
of infants
primary
Blackfan-Diamond syndrome
Familial hypoplastic anemia
C&C Exclusions: 280.0, 281.4, 281.8, 282.41, 282.42, 282.49, 282.80, 282.81, 282.82, 282.83, 282.84, 282.88, 282.89, 283.0, 283.10, 283.11, 283.19, 283.2, 283.9, 284.8, 284.9, 285.0, 285.1

284.09 Other constitutional aplastic anemia
Fanconi's anemia
Pancytopenia with malformations
C&C Exclusions: See 284.01

284.1 Pancytopenia
Excludes *pancytopenia (due to) (with):*
aplastic anemia NOS (284.9)
bone marrow infiltration (284.2)
constitutional red blood cell aplasia (284.01)
drug induced (▶284.89◀)
hairy cell leukemia (202.4)
human immunodeficiency virus disease (042)
leukoerythroblastic anemia (284.2)
malformations (284.09)
myelodysplastic syndromes (238.72-238.75)
myeloproliferative disease (238.79)
other constitutional aplastic anemia (284.09)
DEF: Decreased count of all elements in the blood: red blood cells, white blood cells, and platelets.
C&C Exclusions: See 284.01

+ *284.2 Myelophthisis*
Leukoerythroblastic anemia
Myelophthisic anemia
Code first the underlying disorder, such as:
malignant neoplasm of breast (174.0-174.9, 175.0-175.9)
tuberculosis (015.0-015.9)
Excludes *idiopathic myelofibrosis (238.76)*
myelofibrosis NOS (289.83)
myelofibrosis with myeloid metaplasia (238.76)
primary myelofibrosis (238.76)
secondary myelofibrosis (289.83)
C&C Exclusions: See 284.01

⑤ 284.8 Other specified aplastic anemias
C&C Exclusions: 280.0, 280.1, 280.8, 280.9, 281.0, 281.1, 281.2, 281.3, 281.4, 281.8, 281.9, 282.0, 282.1, 282.2, 282.3, 282.41, 282.42, 282.49, 282.5, 282.60, 282.61, 282.62, 282.63, 282.64, 282.68, 282.69, 282.7, 282.8, 282.9, 283.0, 283.10, 283.11, 283.19, 283.2, 283.9, 284.8, 284.9, 285.0, 285.1, 285.21, 285.22, 285.29, 285.8, 285.9, 289.8, 289.9
AHA: 3Q 2005, 11; 1Q 1997, 5; 1Q 1992, 15; 1Q 1991, 14

● 284.81 Red cell aplasia (acquired) (adult) (with thymoma)
Red cell aplasia NOS
DEF: Decline of RBC precursor cells in the bone marrow until nearly absent while WBC precursors are present at normal levels; causes normochromic, normoblastic anemia.

● 284.89 Other specified aplastic anemias
Aplastic anemia (due to):
chronic systemic disease
drugs
infection
radiation
toxic (paralytic)
Use additional E code to identify cause

284.9 Aplastic anemia, unspecified
Anemia:
aplastic (idiopathic) NOS
aregenerative
hypoplastic NOS
nonregenerative
Medullary hypoplasia
Excludes *refractory anemia (238.72)*
C&C Exclusions: See 284.8

④ 285 Other and unspecified anemias
AHA: 1Q 1991, 14; Nov-Dec 1984, 1

285.0 Sideroblastic anemia
Anemia:
hypochromic with iron loading
sideroachrestic
sideroblastic:
acquired
congenital
hereditary
primary
secondary (drug-induced) (due to disease)
sex-linked hypochromic
vitamin B_6-responsive
Pyridoxine-responsive (hypochromic) anemia
Use additional E code to identify cause, if drug-induced
Excludes *refractory sideroblastic anemia (238.72)*
DEF: Group of blood disorders in which the bone marrow's ability to produce normal red blood cells is impaired and sideroblasts, or deformed red blood cells, are present in the bloodstream.
C&C Exclusions: See 284.8

285.1 Acute posthemorrhagic anemia
Anemia due to acute blood loss
Excludes *anemia due to chronic blood loss (280.0)*
blood loss anemia NOS (280.0)
C&C Exclusions: See 284.8
AHA: 1Q 2007, 19; 2Q 1992, 15

⑤ 285.2 Anemia of chronic disease
Anemia in chronic illness
AHA: 4Q 2000, 39

285.21 Anemia in chronic kidney disease
Anemia in end stage renal disease
Erythropoietin-resistant anemia (EPO resistant anemia)
C&C Exclusions: See 284.8

285.22 Anemia in neoplastic disease
C&C Exclusions: See 284.8

285.29 Anemia of other chronic disease
Anemia in other chronic illness
C&C Exclusions: See 284.8

285.8 Other specified anemias
Anemia:
- dyserythropoietic (congenital)
- dyshematopoietic (congenital)
- von Jaksch's

Infantile pseudoleukemia

C&C Exclusions: See 284.8

AHA: 1Q 1991, 16

285.9 Anemia, unspecified
Anemia:
- NOS
- essential
- normocytic, not due to blood loss
- profound
- progressive
- secondary

Oligocythemia

Excludes *anemia (due to):*
- *blood loss:*
  - *acute (285.1)*
  - *chronic or unspecified (280.0)*
- *iron deficiency (280.0-280.9)*

C&C Exclusions: See 284.8

AHA: 1Q 2007, 19; 1Q 2002, 14; 2Q 1992, 16; Mar-Apr 1985, 13; Nov-Dec 1984, 1

4 286 Coagulation defects

286.0 Congenital factor VIII disorder
Antihemophilic globulin [AHG] deficiency
Factor VIII (functional) deficiency
Hemophilia:
- NOS
- A
- classical
- familial
- hereditary

Subhemophilia

Excludes *factor VIII deficiency with vascular defect (286.4)*

DEF: Most common form of hemophilia, referred to as classic hemophilia or hemophilia A; characterized by profuse bleeding from injuries, as well as bleeding from the joints, muscles, digestive tract, and brain.

C&C Exclusions: 286.0, 286.1, 286.2, 286.3, 286.4, 286.5, 286.6, 286.7, 286.9, 287.0, 287.1, 287.2, 287.30, 287.31, 287.32, 287.33, 287.39, 287.4, 287.5, 287.8, 287.9, 289.8, 289.9

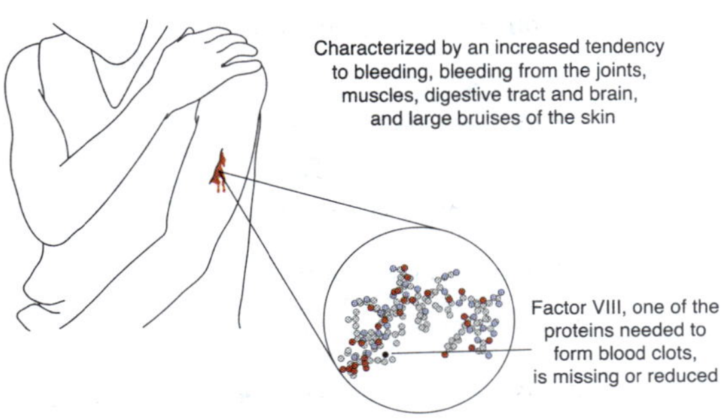

286.1 Congenital factor IX disorder
Christmas disease
Deficiency:
- factor IX (functional)
- plasma thromboplastin component [PTC]

Hemophilia B

C&C Exclusions: See 286.0

286.2 Congenital factor XI deficiency
Hemophilia C
Plasma thromboplastin antecedent [PTA] deficiency
Rosenthal's disease

C&C Exclusions: See 286.0

286.3 Congenital deficiency of other clotting factors
Congenital afibrinogenemia
Deficiency:
- AC globulin
- factor:
  - I [fibrinogen]
  - II [prothrombin]
  - V [labile]
  - VII [stable]
  - X [Stuart-Prower]
  - XII [Hageman]
  - XIII [fibrin stabilizing]
- Laki-Lorand factor
- proaccelerin

Disease:
- Owren's
- Stuart-Prower

Dysfibrinogenemia (congenital)
Dysprothrombinemia (constitutional)
Hypoproconvertinemia
Hypoprothrombinemia (hereditary)
Parahemophilia

C&C Exclusions: See 286.0

286.4 von Willebrand's disease
Angiohemophilia (A) (B)
Constitutional thrombopathy
Factor VIII deficiency with vascular defect
Pseudohemophilia type B
Vascular hemophilia
von Willebrand's (-Jürgens') disease

Excludes *factor VIII deficiency:*
- *NOS (286.0)*
- *with functional defect (286.0)*

hereditary capillary fragility (287.8)

C&C Exclusions: See 286.0

286.5 Hemorrhagic disorder due to intrinsic circulating anticoagulants
Antithrombinemia
Antithromboplastinemia
Antithromboplastino-genemia
Hyperheparinemia
Increase in:
- anti-VIIIa
- anti-IXa
- anti-Xa
- anti-XIa
- antithrombin

Secondary hemophilia
Systemic lupus erythematosus [SLE] inhibitor

C&C Exclusions: See 286.0

AHA: 3Q 1992, 15; 3Q 1990, 14

286.6 Defibrination syndrome
Afibrinogenemia, acquired
Consumption coagulopathy
Diffuse or disseminated intravascular coagulation [DIC syndrome]
Fibrinolytic hemorrhage, acquired
Hemorrhagic fibrinogenolysis
Pathologic fibrinolysis
Purpura:
- fibrinolytic
- fulminans

Excludes *that complicating:*
- *abortion (634-638 with .1, 639.1)*
- *pregnancy or the puerperium (641.3, 666.3)*

disseminated intravascular coagulation in newborn (776.2)

DEF: Bleeding disorder characterized by an abnormal reduction in the elements involved in blood clotting; marked by profuse hemorrhaging in the late stages.

C&C Exclusions: See 286.0

AHA: 4Q 1993, 29

286.7 Acquired coagulation factor deficiency
Deficiency of coagulation factor due to:
liver disease
vitamin K deficiency
Hypoprothrombinemia, acquired
Use additional E-code to identify cause, if drug-induced
Excludes *vitamin K deficiency of newborn (776.0)*
C&C Exclusions: See 286.0
AHA: 4Q 1993, 29

286.9 Other and unspecified coagulation defects
Defective coagulation NOS
Deficiency, coagulation factor NOS
Delay, coagulation
Disorder:
coagulation
hemostasis
Excludes *abnormal coagulation profile (790.92)*
hemorrhagic disease of newborn (776.0)
that complicating:
abortion (634-638 with .1, 639.1)
pregnancy or the puerperium (641.3, 666.3)
C&C Exclusions: See 286.0

❹ 287 Purpura and other hemorrhagic conditions
Excludes *hemorrhagic thrombocythemia (238.79)*
purpura fulminans (286.6)
AHA: 1Q 1991, 14

287.0 Allergic purpura
Peliosis rheumatica
Purpura:
anaphylactoid
autoimmune
Henoch's
nonthrombocytopenic:
hemorrhagic
idiopathic
rheumatica
Schönlein-Henoch
vascular
Vasculitis, allergic
Excludes *hemorrhagic purpura (287.39)*
purpura annularis telangiectodes (709.1)
DEF: Allergic reaction causing hemorrhaging of the skin and mucous membranes; produces purple discolorations on the skin surface.
C&C Exclusions: See 286.0

287.1 Qualitative platelet defects
Thrombasthenia (hemorrhagic) (hereditary)
Thrombocytasthenia
Thrombocytopathy (dystrophic)
Thrombopathy (Bernard-Soulier)
Excludes *von Willebrand's disease (286.4)*
C&C Exclusions: See 286.0

287.2 Other nonthrombocytopenic purpuras
Purpura:
NOS
senile
simplex
C&C Exclusions: See 286.0

❺ 287.3 Primary thrombocytopenia
Excludes *thrombotic thrombocytopenic purpura (446.6)*
transient thrombocytopenia of newborn (776.1)
AHA: 4Q 2005, 56

✖ 287.30 Primary thrombocytopenia, unspecified
Megakaryocytic hypoplasia
C&C Exclusions: See 286.0

287.31 Immune thrombocytopenic purpura
Idiopathic thrombocytopenic purpura
Tidal platelet dysgenesis
C&C Exclusions: See 286.0
AHA: 4Q 2005, 57

287.32 Evans' syndrome
C&C Exclusions: See 286.0

287.33 Congenital and hereditary thrombocytopenic purpura
Congenital and hereditary thrombocytopenia
Thrombocytopenia with absent radii (TAR) syndrome
Excludes *Wiskott-Aldrich syndrome (279.12)*
C&C Exclusions: See 286.0

287.39 Other primary thrombocytopenia
C&C Exclusions: See 286.0

287.4 Secondary thrombocytopenia
Posttransfusion purpura
Thrombocytopenia (due to):
dilutional
drugs
extracorporeal circulation of blood
massive blood transfusion
platelet alloimmunization
Use additional E code to identify cause
Excludes *transient thrombocytopenia of newborn (776.1)*
C&C Exclusions: See 286.0
AHA: 4Q 1999, 22; 4Q 1993, 29

287.5 Thrombocytopenia, unspecified
C&C Exclusions: See 286.0

287.8 Other specified hemorrhagic conditions
Capillary fragility (hereditary)
Vascular pseudohemophilia
C&C Exclusions: See 286.0

287.9 Unspecified hemorrhagic conditions
Hemorrhagic diathesis (familial)
C&C Exclusions: See 286.0

❹ 288 Diseases of white blood cells
Excludes *leukemia (204.0-208.9)*
AHA: 1Q 1991, 14

❺ 288.0 Neutropenia
Decreased absolute neutrophil count (ANC)
Use additional code for any associated:
▶fever (780.6)◀
▶mucositis (478.11, 528.00-528.09, 538, 616.81)◀
Excludes *neutropenic splenomegaly (289.53)*
transitory neonatal neutropenia (776.7)
AHA: 3Q 2005, 11; 3Q 1999, 6; 2Q 1999, 9; 3Q 1996, 16; 2Q 1996, 6

✖ 288.00 Neutropenia, unspecified
C&C Exclusions: 288.1, 288.2, 288.3, 288.8, 288.9, 289.81, 289.82, 289.9

288.01 Congenital neutropenia
Congenital agranulocytosis
Infantile genetic agranulocytosis
Kostmann's syndrome
C&C Exclusions: See 288.00

288.02 Cyclic neutropenia
Cyclic hematopoiesis
Periodic neutropenia
C&C Exclusions: See 288.00

288.03 Drug induced neutropenia
Use additional E code to identify drug
C&C Exclusions: See 288.00
AHA: 4Q 2006, 73

288.04 Neutropenia due to infection
C&C Exclusions: See 288.00

288.09 Other neutropenia
Agranulocytosis
Neutropenia:
immune
toxic
C&C Exclusions: See 288.00

Agranulocytosis

A sudden, severe condition characterized by high fever and a steep drop in the number of white blood cells in the bloodstream

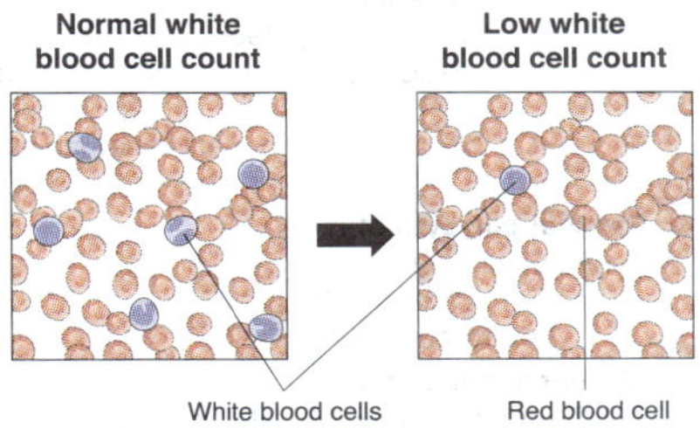

288.1 Functional disorders of polymorphonuclear neutrophils
Chronic (childhood) granulomatous disease
Congenital dysphagocytosis
Job's syndrome
Lipochrome histiocytosis (familial)
Progressive septic granulomatosis
C&C Exclusions: 288.0, 288.1, 288.2, 288.3, 288.8, 288.9, 289.81, 289.82, 289.8, 289.9

288.2 Genetic anomalies of leukocytes
Anomaly (granulation) (granulocyte) or syndrome:
Alder's (-Reilly)
Chédiak-Steinbrinck (-Higashi)
Jordan's
May-Hegglin
Pelger-Huet
Hereditary:
hypersegmentation
hyposegmentation
leukomelanopathy
C&C Exclusions: See 288.1

288.3 Eosinophilia
Eosinophilia:
allergic
hereditary
idiopathic
secondary
Eosinophilic leukocytosis
Excludes *Löffler's syndrome (518.3)*
pulmonary eosinophilia (518.3)
C&C Exclusions: See 288.1
DEF: Elevated number of eosinophils in the bloodstream.
AHA: 3Q 2000, 11

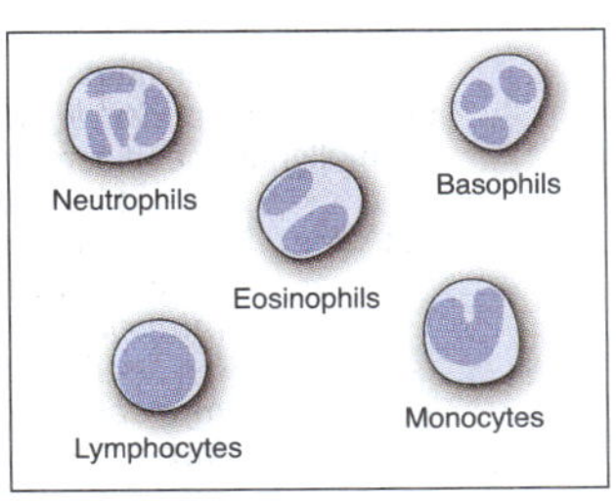

White blood cells

288.4 Hemophagocytic syndromes
Familial hemophagocytic lymphohistiocytosis
Familial hemophagocytic reticulosis
Hemophagocytic syndrome, infection-associated
Histiocytic syndromes
Macrophage activation syndrome
C&C Exclusions: 288.1, 289.81, 289.82

288.5 Decreased white blood cell count
Excludes *neutropenia (288.01-288.09)*

288.50 Leukocytopenia, unspecified
Decreased leukocytes, unspecified
Decreased white blood cell count, unspecified
Leukopenia NOS
C&C Exclusions: See 288.4

288.51 Lymphocytopenia
Decreased lymphocytes
C&C Exclusions: See 288.4

288.59 Other decreased white blood cell count
Basophilic leukopenia
Eosinophilic leukopenia
Monocytopenia
Plasmacytopenia
C&C Exclusions: See 288.4

288.6 Elevated white blood cell count
Excludes *eosinophilia (288.3)*

288.60 Leukocytosis, unspecified
Elevated leukocytes, unspecified
Elevated white blood cell count, unspecified
C&C Exclusions: See 288.4

288.61 Lymphocytosis (symptomatic)
Elevated lymphocytes
C&C Exclusions: See 288.4

288.62 Leukemoid reaction
Basophilic leukemoid reaction
Lymphocytic leukemoid reaction
Monocytic leukemoid reaction
Myelocytic leukemoid reaction
Neutrophilic leukemoid reaction
C&C Exclusions: See 288.4

288.63 Monocytosis (symptomatic)
Excludes *infectious mononucleosis (075)*
C&C Exclusions: See 288.4

288.64 Plasmacytosis
C&C Exclusions: See 288.4

288.65 Basophilia
C&C Exclusions: See 288.4

● **288.66 Bandemia**
Bandemia without diagnosis of specific infection
Excludes *confirmed infection – code to infection*
leukemia (204.00-208.9)
DEF: Nonspecific elevated count of immature white blood cells even when other white blood cell counts are normal.

288.69 Other elevated white blood cell count
C&C Exclusions: See 288.4

288.8 Other specified disease of white blood cells
Excludes *decreased white blood cell counts (288.50-288.59)*
elevated white blood cell counts (288.60-288.69)
immunity disorders (279.0-279.9)
C&C Exclusions: See 288.1
AHA: Mar-Apr 1987, 12

288.9 Unspecified disease of white blood cells
C&C Exclusions: See 288.1

❹ 289 Other diseases of blood and blood-forming organs

289.0 Polycythemia, secondary

High-oxygen-affinity hemoglobin
Polycythemia:
acquired
benign
due to:
fall in plasma volume
high altitude
emotional
erythropoietin
hypoxemic
nephrogenous
relative
spurious
stress

Excludes *polycythemia:*
neonatal (776.4)
primary (238.4)
vera (238.4)

289.1 Chronic lymphadenitis

Chronic:
adenitis any lymph node, except mesenteric
lymphadenitis any lymph node, except mesenteric

Excludes *acute lymphadenitis (683)*
mesenteric (289.2)
enlarged glands NOS (785.6)

289.2 Nonspecific mesenteric lymphadenitis

Mesenteric lymphadenitis (acute) (chronic)

289.3 Lymphadenitis, unspecified, except mesenteric

AHA: 2Q 1992, 8

Inflammation of one or more lymph nodes

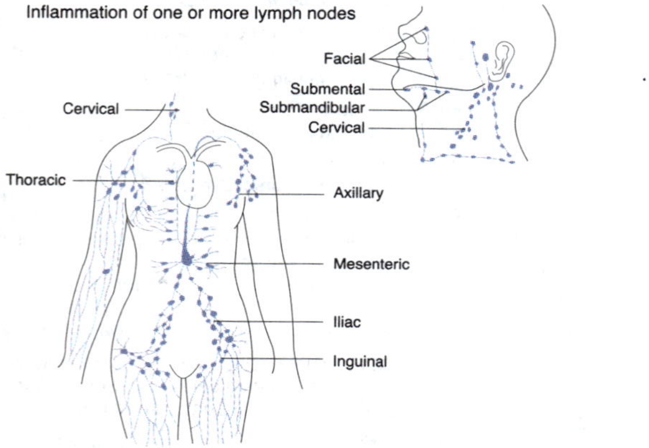

289.4 Hypersplenism

"Big spleen" syndrome
Dyssplenism
Hypersplenia

Excludes *primary splenic neutropenia (289.53)*

❺ 289.5 Other diseases of spleen

✖ 289.50 Disease of spleen, unspecified

289.51 Chronic congestive splenomegaly

✚ *289.52 Splenic sequestration*

Code first sickle-cell disease in crisis (282.42, 282.62, 282.64, 282.69)

DEF: Red blood cells trapped within the spleen due to Hb SS sickle cell disease, causing a dangerous fall in hemoglobin and potential hypovolemic shock or death; manifests with sudden weakness, tachycardia, tachypnea, pallor, and abdominal fullness.

AHA: 4Q 2003, 51

289.53 Neutropenic splenomegaly

289.59 Other

Lien migrans
Perisplenitis
Splenic:
abscess
atrophy
cyst
fibrosis
infarction
rupture, nontraumatic
Splenitis
Wandering spleen

Excludes *bilharzial splenic fibrosis (120.0-120.9)*
hepatolienal fibrosis (571.5)
splenomegaly NOS (789.2)

289.6 Familial polycythemia

Familial:
benign polycythemia
erythrocytosis

289.7 Methemoglobinemia

Congenital NADH [DPNH]-methemoglobin-reductase deficiency
Hemoglobin M [Hb-M] disease
Methemoglobinemia:
NOS
acquired (with sulfhemoglobinemia)
hereditary
toxic
Stokvis' disease
Sulfhemoglobinemia
Use additional E code to identify cause

❺ 289.8 Other specified diseases of blood and blood-forming organs

AHA: 4Q 2003, 56; 1Q 2002, 16; 2Q 1989, 8; Mar-Apr 1987, 12

289.81 Primary hypercoagulable state

Activated protein C resistance
Antithrombin III deficiency
Factor V Leiden mutation
Lupus anticoagulant
Protein C deficiency
Protein S deficiency
Prothrombin gene mutation

DEF: Abnormal development of blood clots in arteries or veins.

C&C Exclusions: 280.0, 281.4, 281.8, 282.41, 282.42, 282.49, 282.60, 282.61, 282.62, 282.63, 282.64, 282.68, 282.69, 283.0, 283.10, 283.11, 283.19, 283.2, 283.9, 284.8, 284.9, 285.0, 285.1, 286.0, 286.1, 286.2, 286.3, 286.4, 286.5, 286.6, 286.7, 286.9, 287.0, 287.1, 287.2, 287.30, 287.31, 287.32, 287.33, 287.39, 287.4, 287.5, 287.8, 287.9, 288.1, 289.81, 289.82

289.82 Secondary hypercoagulable state

C&C Exclusions: See 289.81

✚ *289.83 Myelofibrosis*

Myelofibrosis NOS
Secondary myelofibrosis
Code first the underlying disorder, such as:
malignant neoplasm of breast (174.0-174.9, 175.0-175.9)

Excludes *idiopathic myelofibrosis (238.76)*
leukoerythroblastic anemia (284.2)
myelofibrosis with myeloid metaplasia (238.76)
myelophthisic anemia (284.2)
myelophthisis (284.2)
primary myelofibrosis (238.76)

C&C Exclusions: See 289.81

289.89 Other specified diseases of blood and blood-forming organs

Hypergammaglobulinemia
Pseudocholinesterase deficiency

C&C Exclusions: See 289.81

289.9 Unspecified diseases of blood and blood-forming organs

Blood dyscrasia NOS
Erythroid hyperplasia

C&C Exclusions: 282.41, 282.42, 282.49, 282.64, 282.68, 287.30, 287.31, 287.32, 287.33, 287.39, 289.81, 289.82

AHA: Mar-Apr 1985, 14

5. MENTAL DISORDERS (290-319)

PSYCHOSES (290-299)

Excludes *mental retardation (317-319)*

ORGANIC PSYCHOTIC CONDITIONS (290-294)

Includes psychotic organic brain syndrome

Excludes *nonpsychotic syndromes of organic etiology (310.0-310.9)*
psychoses classifiable to 295-298 and without impairment of orientation, comprehension, calculation, learning capacity, and judgement, but associated with physical disease, injury, or condition affecting the brain [e.g., following childbirth] (295.0-298.8)

❹ **290 Dementias**

Code first the associated neurological condition

Excludes *dementia due to alcohol (291.0-291.2)*
dementia due to drugs (292.82)
dementia not classified as senile, presenile, or arteriosclerotic (294.10-294.11)
psychoses classifiable to 295-298 occurring in the senium without dementia or delirium (295.0-298.8)
senility with mental changes of nonpsychotic severity (310.1)
transient organic psychotic conditions (293.0-293.9)

290.0 Senile dementia, uncomplicated A

Senile dementia:
NOS
simple type

Excludes *mild memory disturbances, not amounting to dementia, associated with senile brain disease (310.1)*
senile dementia with:
delirium or confusion (290.3)
delusional [paranoid] features (290.20)
depressive features (290.21)

AHA: 4Q 1999, 4

❺ **290.1 Presenile dementia**

Brain syndrome with presenile brain disease

Excludes *arteriosclerotic dementia (290.40-290.43)*
dementia associated with other cerebral conditions (294.10-294.11)

AHA: Nov-Dec 1984, 20

290.10 Presenile dementia, uncomplicated A

Presenile dementia:
NOS
simple type

DEF: Loss of cognitive and intellectual functions, such as impaired memory, judgment, and intellect, without impaired perception or consciousness, in patients younger than 65.

290.11 Presenile dementia with delirium A

Presenile dementia with acute confusional state

AHA: 1Q 1988, 3

290.12 Presenile dementia with delusional features A

Presenile dementia, paranoid type

290.13 Presenile dementia with depressive features A

Presenile dementia, depressed type

❺ **290.2 Senile dementia with delusional or depressive features**

Excludes *senile dementia:*
NOS (290.0)
with delirium and/or confusion (290.3)

290.20 Senile dementia with delusional features A

Senile dementia, paranoid type
Senile psychosis NOS

290.21 Senile dementia with depressive features A

290.3 Senile dementia with delirium A

Senile dementia with acute confusional state

Excludes *senile:*
dementia NOS (290.0)
psychosis NOS (290.20)

❺ **290.4 Vascular dementia**

Multi-infarct dementia or psychosis
Use additional code to identify cerebral atherosclerosis (437.0)

Excludes *suspected cases with no clear evidence of arteriosclerosis (290.9)*

AHA: 1Q 1988, 3

290.40 Vascular dementia, uncomplicated A

Arteriosclerotic dementia:
NOS
simple type

290.41 Vascular dementia with delirium A

Arteriosclerotic dementia with acute confusional state

290.42 Vascular dementia with delusions A

Arteriosclerotic dementia, paranoid type

290.43 Vascular dementia with depressed mood A

Arteriosclerotic dementia, depressed type

290.8 Other specified senile psychotic conditions

Presbyophrenic psychosis

290.9 Unspecified senile psychotic condition A

❹ **291 Alcohol-induced mental disorders**

Excludes *alcoholism without psychosis (303.0-303.9)*

AHA: 1Q 1988, 3; Sep-Oct 1986, 3

291.0 Alcohol withdrawal delirium

Alcoholic delirium
Delirium tremens

Excludes *alcohol withdrawal (291.81)*

DEF: Delirium occuring when an alcoholic is denied alcohol for a significant period of time.

C&C Exclusions: 291.0, 291.1, 291.2, 291.3, 291.4, 291.5, 291.81, 291.89, 291.9, 292.0, 292.1, 292.2, 292.81, 292.82, 292.83, 292.84, 292.89, 292.9, 293.0, 293.1, 293.81, 293.82, 293.83, 293.84, 293.89, 293.9, 294.0, 294.10, 294.11, 294.8, 294.9, 303.00, 303.01, 303.02, 303.03, 303.90, 303.91, 303.92, 303.93, 304.00, 304.01, 304.02, 304.03, 304.10, 304.11, 304.12, 304.13, 304.20, 304.21, 304.22, 304.23, 304.30, 304.31, 304.32, 304.33, 304.40, 304.41, 304.42, 304.43, 304.50, 304.51, 304.52, 304.53, 304.60, 304.61, 304.62, 304.63, 304.70, 304.71, 304.72, 304.73, 304.80, 304.81, 304.82, 304.83, 304.90, 304.91, 305.00, 305.01, 305.02, 305.03, 305.20, 305.21, 305.22, 305.23, 305.30, 305.31, 305.32, 305.33, 305.40, 305.41, 305.42, 305.43, 305.50, 305.51, 305.52, 305.53, 305.60, 305.61, 305.62, 305.63, 305.70, 305.71, 305.72, 305.73, 305.80, 305.81, 305.82, 305.83, 305.90, 305.91, 305.92, 305.93, 790.3

AHA: 2Q 1991, 11

291.1 Alcohol-induced persisting amnestic disorder

Alcoholic polyneuritic psychosis
Korsakoff's psychosis, alcoholic
Wernicke-Korsakoff syndrome (alcoholic)

C&C Exclusions: See 291.0

291.2 Alcohol-induced persisting dementia

Alcoholic dementia NOS
Alcoholism associated with dementia NOS
Chronic alcoholic brain syndrome

DEF: Lasting state of dementia due to chronic alcoholism.

C&C Exclusions: See 291.0

291.3 Alcohol-induced psychotic disorder with hallucinations

Alcoholic:
hallucinosis (acute)
psychosis with hallucinosis

Excludes *alcohol withdrawal with delirium (291.0)*
schizophrenia (295.0-295.9) and paranoid states (297.0-297.9) taking the form of chronic hallucinosis with clear consciousness in an alcoholic

C&C Exclusions: See 291.0

AHA: 2Q 1991, 11

A Adult (15+ years) | M Maternity (12-55 years) | N Newborn (0 years) | P Pediatric (0-17 years) | ♂ Male | ♀ Female | ❷ Medicare Secondary Payer

291.4 Idiosyncratic alcohol intoxication
Pathologic:
alcohol intoxication
drunkenness
Excludes *acute alcohol intoxication (305.0)*
in alcoholism (303.0)
simple drunkenness (305.0)
C&C Exclusions: See 291.0

291.5 Alcohol-induced psychotic disorder with delusions
Alcoholic:
paranoia
psychosis, paranoid type
Excludes *nonalcoholic paranoid states (297.0-297.9)*
schizophrenia, paranoid type (295.3)

❺ **291.8 Other specified alcohol-induced mental disorders**
AHA: 3Q 1994, 13; Jul-Aug 1985, 10

291.81 Alcohol withdrawal
Alcohol:
abstinence syndrome or symptoms
withdrawal syndrome or symptoms
Excludes *alcohol withdrawal:*
delirium (291.0)
hallucinosis (291.3)
delirium tremens (291.0)
C&C Exclusions: 291.0, 291.1, 291.2, 291.3, 291.4, 291.5, 291.81, 291.89, 291.9, 292.0, 292.11, 292.12, 292.2, 292.81, 292.82, 292.83, 292.84, 292.89, 292.9, 293.0, 293.1, 293.81, 293.82, 293.83, 293.84, 293.89, 293.9, 294.0, 294.10, 294.11, 294.8, 294.9, 303.00, 303.01, 303.02, 303.03, 303.90, 303.91, 303.92, 303.93, 304.00, 304.01, 304.02, 304.03, 304.10, 304.11, 304.12, 304.13, 304.20, 304.21, 304.22, 304.23, 304.30, 304.31, 304.32, 304.33, 304.40, 304.41, 304.42, 304.43, 304.50, 304.51, 304.52, 304.53, 304.60, 304.61, 304.62, 304.63, 304.70, 304.71, 304.72, 304.73, 304.80, 304.81, 304.82, 304.83, 304.90, 304.91, 304.92, 304.93, 305.00, 305.01, 305.02, 305.03, 305.20, 305.21, 305.22, 305.23, 305.30, 305.31, 305.32, 305.33, 305.40, 305.41, 305.42, 305.43, 305.50, 305.51, 305.52, 305.53, 305.60, 305.61, 305.62, 305.63, 305.70, 305.71, 305.72, 305.73, 305.80, 305.81, 305.82, 305.83, 305.90, 305.91, 305.92, 305.93, 790.3
AHA: 4Q 1996, 28; 2Q 1991, 11

291.82 Alcohol-induced sleep disorders
Alcohol-induced circadian rhythm sleep disorders
Alcohol-induced hypersomnia
Alcohol-induced insomnia
Alcohol-induced parasomnia
DEF: Disruption of normal sleep patterns due to the consumption of alcohol.
C&C Exclusions: See 291.81

291.89 Other
Alcohol-induced anxiety disorder
Alcohol-induced mood disorder
Alcohol-induced sexual dysfunction
C&C Exclusions: See 291.81

291.9 Unspecified alcohol-induced mental disorders
Alcoholic:
mania NOS
psychosis NOS
Alcoholism (chronic) with psychosis
Alcohol-related disorder NOS
C&C Exclusions: See 291.0

❹ **292 Drug-induced mental disorders**
Includes organic brain syndrome associated with consumption of drugs
Use additional code for any associated drug dependence (304.0-304.9)
Use additional E code to identify drug
AHA: 3Q 2004, 8; 2Q 1991, 11; Sep-Oct 1986, 3

292.0 Drug withdrawal
Drug:
abstinence syndrome or symptoms
withdrawal syndrome or symptoms
DEF: Curtailed drug use, resulting in physical or psychological symptoms lasting hours to weeks, commonly featuring headache, anxiety, depression, chills, sweats, and tremors.
C&C Exclusions: See 291.0
AHA: 1Q 1997, 12; 1Q 1988, 3

❺ **292.1 Drug-induced psychotic disorders**

292.11 Drug-induced psychotic disorder with delusions
Paranoid state induced by drugs
C&C Exclusions: See 291.0

292.12 Drug-induced psychotic disorder with hallucinations
Hallucinatory state induced by drugs
Excludes *states following LSD or other hallucinogens, lasting only a few days or less ["bad trips"] (305.3)*
C&C Exclusions: See 291.0

292.2 Pathological drug intoxication
Drug reaction resulting in brief psychotic states:
NOS
idiosyncratic
pathologic
Excludes *expected brief psychotic reactions to hallucinogens ["bad trips"] (305.3)*
physiological side-effects of drugs (e.g., dystonias)
C&C Exclusions: See 291.0

❺ **292.8 Other specified drug-induced mental disorders**
AHA: 1Q 1988, 3

292.81 Drug-induced delirium
C&C Exclusions: See 291.0

292.82 Drug-induced persisting dementia
C&C Exclusions: See 291.0

292.83 Drug-induced persisting amnestic disorder
C&C Exclusions: See 291.0

292.84 Drug-induced mood disorder
Depressive state induced by drugs
C&C Exclusions: See 291.0

292.85 Drug-induced sleep disorders
Drug-induced circadian rhythm sleep disorders
Drug-induced hypersomnia
Drug-induced insomnia
Drug-induced parasomnia
C&C Exclusions: 291.0, 291.1, 291.2, 291.3, 291.4, 291.81, 291.89, 291.9, 292.0, 292.11, 292.12, 292.2, 292.81, 292.82, 292.83, 292.84, 292.89, 292.9, 293.81, 293.82, 293.83, 293.84, 303.00, 303.01, 303.02, 303.90, 303.91, 303.92, 304.00, 304.01, 304.02, 304.10, 304.11, 304.12, 304.20, 304.21, 304.22, 304.40, 304.41, 304.42, 304.50, 304.51, 304.52, 304.60, 304.61, 304.62, 304.70, 304.71, 304.72, 304.80, 304.81, 304.82, 304.90, 304.91, 304.92, 304.50, 304.51, 304.52, 304.60, 304.61, 304.62, 304.70, 304.71, 304.72, 304.80, 304.81, 304.82, 304.90, 304.91, 304.92, 305.00, 305.01, 305.02, 305.30, 305.31, 305.32, 305.40, 305.41, 305.42, 305.50, 305.51, 305.52, 305.60, 305.61, 305.62, 305.70, 305.71, 305.72, 305.90, 305.91, 305.92, 710.5

292.89 Other
Drug-induced anxiety disorder
Drug-induced organic personality syndrome
Drug-induced sexual dysfunction
Drug intoxication
C&C Exclusions: See 291.0

❹ ❺ Additional Digit Required ✖ Nonspecific PDx ⊘ Unacceptable PDx ✚ Manifestation Code ▶◀ Revised Text ● New Code ▲ Revised Code

292.9 Unspecified drug-induced mental disorder
Drug-related disorder NOS
Organic psychosis NOS due to or associated with drugs
C&C Exclusions: See 291.0

❹ **293 Transient mental disorders due to conditions classified elsewhere**
Includes transient organic mental disorders not associated with alcohol or drugs
Code first the associated physical or neurological condition
Excludes confusional state or delirium superimposed on senile dementia (290.3)
dementia due to:
alcohol (291.0-291.9)
arteriosclerosis (290.40-290.43)
drugs (292.82)
senility (290.0)

293.0 Delirium due to conditions classified elsewhere
Acute:
confusional state
infective psychosis
organic reaction
posttraumatic organic psychosis
psycho-organic syndrome
Acute psychosis associated with endocrine, metabolic, or cerebrovascular disorder
Epileptic:
confusional state
twilight state
AHA: 1Q 1988, 3

293.1 Subacute delirium
Subacute:
confusional state
infective psychosis
organic reaction
posttraumatic organic psychosis
psycho-organic syndrome
psychosis associated with endocrine or metabolic disorder

❺ **293.8 Other specified transient mental disorders due to conditions classified elsewhere**

293.81 Psychotic disorder with delusions in conditions classified elsewhere
Transient organic psychotic condition, paranoid type
C&C Exclusions: 291.0, 291.1, 291.2, 291.3, 291.4, 291.5, 291.81, 291.89, 291.9, 292.0, 292.11, 292.12, 292.2, 292.81, 292.82, 292.83, 292.84, 292.89, 292.9, 293.0, 293.9, 294.0, 294.10, 294.11, 294.8, 294.9, 303.00, 303.01, 303.02, 303.03, 303.90, 303.91, 303.92, 303.93, 304.00, 304.01, 304.02, 304.03, 304.10, 304.11, 304.12, 304.13, 304.20, 304.21, 304.22, 304.23, 304.30, 304.31, 304.32, 304.33, 304.40, 304.41, 304.42, 304.43, 304.50, 304.51, 304.52, 304.53, 304.60, 304.61, 304.62, 304.63, 304.70, 304.71, 304.72, 304.73, 304.80, 304.81, 304.82, 304.83, 304.90, 304.91, 304.92, 304.93, 305.00, 305.01, 305.02, 305.03, 305.20, 305.21, 305.22, 305.23, 305.30, 305.31, 305.32, 305.33, 305.40, 305.41, 305.42, 305.43, 305.50, 305.51, 305.52, 305.53, 305.60, 305.61, 305.62, 305.63, 305.70, 305.71, 305.72, 305.73, 305.80, 305.81, 305.82, 305.83, 305.90, 305.91, 305.92, 305.93, 790.3

293.82 Psychotic disorder with hallucinations in conditions classified elsewhere
Transient organic psychotic condition, hallucinatory type
C&C Exclusions: See 293.81

293.83 Mood disorder in conditions classified elsewhere
Transient organic psychotic condition, depressive type
C&C Exclusions: See 293.81

293.84 Anxiety disorder in conditions classified elsewhere
C&C Exclusions: See 293.81
AHA: 4Q 1996, 29

293.89 Other
Catatonic disorder in conditions classified elsewhere

293.9 Unspecified transient mental disorder in conditions classified elsewhere
Organic psychosis:
infective NOS
posttraumatic NOS
transient NOS
Psycho-organic syndrome

❹ **294 Persistent mental disorders due to conditions classified elsewhere**
Includes organic psychotic brain syndromes (chronic), not elsewhere classified
AHA: Mar-Apr 1985, 12

294.0 Amnestic disorder in conditions classified elsewhere
Korsakoff's psychosis or syndrome (nonalcoholic)
Code first underlying condition
Excludes alcoholic:
amnestic syndrome (291.1)
Korsakoff's psychosis (291.1)

❺ **294.1 Dementia in conditions classified elsewhere**
Dementia of the Alzheimer's type
Code first any underlying physical condition, as:
dementia in:
Alzheimer's disease (331.0)
cerebral lipidoses (330.1)
dementia with Lewy bodies (331.82)
dementia with Parkinsonism (331.82)
epilepsy (345.0-345.9)
frontal dementia (331.19)
frontotemporal dementia (331.19)
general paresis [syphilis] (094.1)
hepatolenticular degeneration (275.1)
Huntington's chorea (333.4)
Jakob-Creutzfeldt disease (046.1)
multiple sclerosis (340)
Pick's disease of the brain (331.11)
polyarteritis nodosa (446.0)
syphilis (094.1)
Excludes dementia:
arteriosclerotic (290.40-290.43)
presenile (290.10-290.13)
senile (290.0)
epileptic psychosis NOS (294.8)
AHA: 4Q 2000, 40; 1Q 1999, 14; Nov-Dec 1985, 5

✚ ***294.10 Dementia in conditions classified elsewhere without behavioral disturbance***
Dementia in conditions classified elsewhere NOS
C&C Exclusions: 291.0, 291.1, 291.2, 291.3, 291.4, 291.81, 291.89, 291.9, 292.0, 292.11, 292.12, 292.2, 292.81, 292.82, 292.83, 292.84, 292.89, 292.9, 293.81, 293.82, 293.83, 293.84

✚ ***294.11 Dementia in conditions classified elsewhere with behavioral disturbance***
Aggressive behavior
Combative behavior
Violent behavior
Wandering off
C&C Exclusions: See 294.10
AHA: 4Q 2000, 41

294.8 Other persistent mental disorders due to conditions classified elsewhere
Amnestic disorder NOS
Dementia NOS
Epileptic psychosis NOS
Mixed paranoid and affective organic psychotic states
Use additional code for associated epilepsy (345.0-345.9)
Excludes mild memory disturbances, not amounting to dementia (310.1)
AHA: 3Q 2003, 14; 1Q 1988, 5

294.9 Unspecified persistent mental disorders due to conditions classified elsewhere
Cognitive disorder NOS
Organic psychosis (chronic)
AHA: 2Q, 2007, 5

OTHER PSYCHOSES (295-299)

Use additional code to identify any associated physical disease, injury, or condition affecting the brain with psychoses classifiable to 295-298

4 295 Schizophrenic disorders

Includes schizophrenia of the types described in 295.0-295.9 occurring in children

Excludes *childhood type schizophrenia (299.9)*
infantile autism (299.0)

DEF: Chronic, severe, and disabling mental disorders appearing in early adulthood and affecting behavior and thought patterns with unknown cause. Patients hear voices and experience cognitive deficits, hallucinations, delusions, and disordered thoughts out of contact with reality, causing fearfulness, withdrawal, and extreme agitation.

The following fifth-digit subclassification is for use with category 295:

- **0 unspecified**
- **1 subchronic**
- **2 chronic**
- **3 subchronic with acute exacerbation**
- **4 chronic with acute exacerbation**
- **5 in remission**

5 295.0 Simple type

Schizophrenia simplex

Excludes *latent schizophrenia (295.5)*

DEF: Least severe type of schizophrenia; symptoms include a gradual withdrawal from contact with others, as well as mild hallucinations and delusions.

C&C Exclusions: (for codes 295.00-295.04) 295.00, 295.01, 295.02, 295.03, 295.04, 295.05, 295.10, 295.11, 295.12, 295.13, 295.14, 295.15, 295.20, 295.21, 295.22, 295.23, 295.24, 295.25, 295.30, 295.31, 295.32, 295.33, 295.34, 295.35, 295.40, 295.41, 295.42, 295.43, 295.44, 295.45, 295.50, 295.51, 295.52, 295.53, 295.54, 295.55, 295.60, 295.61, 295.62, 295.63, 295.64, 295.65, 295.70, 295.71, 295.72, 295.73, 295.74, 295.75, 295.80, 295.81, 295.82, 295.83, 295.84, 295.85, 295.90, 295.91, 295.92, 295.93, 295.94, 295.95, 300.00, 300.01, 300.02, 300.09, 300.10, 300.12, 300.13, 300.14, 300.15, 300.16, 300.19, 300.20, 300.21, 300.22, 300.23, 300.29, 300.3, 300.4, 300.5, 300.6, 300.7, 300.81, 300.82, 300.89, 300.9, 301.0, 301.10, 301.11, 301.12, 301.13, 301.20, 301.21, 301.22, 301.3, 301.4, 301.50, 301.51, 301.59, 301.6, 301.7, 301.81, 301.82, 301.83, 301.84, 301.89, 301.9, 306.0, 306.1, 306.2, 306.3, 306.4, 306.50, 306.51, 306.52, 306.53, 306.59, 306.6, 306.7, 306.8, 306.9, 307.0, 307.1, 307.20, 307.21, 307.22, 307.23, 307.3, 307.40, 307.41, 307.42, 307.43, 307.44, 307.45, 307.46, 307.47, 307.48, 307.49, 307.50, 307.51, 307.52, 307.53, 307.54, 307.59, 307.6, 307.7, 307.80, 307.81, 307.89, 307.9, 308.0, 308.1, 308.2, 308.3, 308.4, 308.9, 309.0, 309.1, 309.21, 309.22, 309.23, 309.24, 309.28, 309.29, 309.3, 309.4, 309.81, 309.82, 309.83, 309.89, 309.9, 310.0, 310.1, 310.2, 310.8, 310.9, 311, 312.00, 312.01, 312.02, 312.03, 312.10, 312.11, 312.12, 312.13, 312.20, 312.21, 312.22, 312.23, 312.30, 312.31, 312.32, 312.33, 312.34, 312.35, 312.39, 312.4, 312.81, 312.82, 312.89, 312.9, 313.0, 313.1, 313.21, 313.22, 313.23, 313.3, 313.81, 313.82, 313.83, 313.89, 313.9, 314.00, 314.01, 314.1, 314.2, 314.8, 314.9, 315.00, 315.01, 315.02, 315.09, 315.1, 315.2, 315.31, 315.32, 315.39, 315.4, 315.5, 315.8, 315.9, 316, 317, 318.0, 318.1, 318.2, 319

5 295.1 Disorganized type

Hebephrenia
Hebephrenic type schizophrenia

DEF: Schizophrenia characterized by inappropriate, disinhibited behavior, and displays of strange emotional responses and agitation.

C&C Exclusions: (for codes 295.10-295.14) See 295.0

5 295.2 Catatonic type

Catatonic (schizophrenia):
- agitation
- excitation
- excited type
- stupor
- withdrawn type

Schizophrenic:
- catalepsy
- catatonia
- flexibilitas cerea

C&C Exclusions: (for codes 295.21-295.24) See 295.0

5 295.3 Paranoid type

Paraphrenic schizophrenia

Excludes *involutional paranoid state (297.2)*
paranoia (297.1)
paraphrenia (297.2)

DEF: Schizophrenia marked by displays of megalomania, delusions of persecution and/or grandeur, hallucinations, and aggressive behavior.

C&C Exclusions: (for codes 295.30-295.34) See 295.0

5 295.4 Schizophreniform disorder

Oneirophrenia
Schizophreniform:
- attack
- psychosis, confusional type

Excludes *acute forms of schizophrenia of:*
catatonic type (295.2)
hebephrenic type (295.1)
paranoid type (295.3)
simple type (295.0)
undifferentiated type (295.8)

C&C Exclusions: (for codes 295.40-295.44) See 295.0

5 295.5 Latent schizophrenia

Latent schizophrenic reaction
Schizophrenia:
- borderline
- incipient
- prepsychotic
- prodromal
- pseudoneurotic
- pseudopsychopathic

Excludes *schizoid personality (301.20-301.22)*

5 295.6 Residual type

Chronic undifferentiated schizophrenia
Restzustand (schizophrenic)
Schizophrenic residual state

C&C Exclusions: (for codes 295.60-295.64) See 295.0

AHA: For Code 295.62: 4Q 2006, 78

5 295.7 Schizoaffective disorder

Cyclic schizophrenia
Mixed schizophrenic and affective psychosis
Schizo-affective psychosis
Schizophreniform psychosis, affective type

C&C Exclusions: (for codes 295.70-295.74) See 295.0

5 295.8 Other specified types of schizophrenia

Acute (undifferentiated) schizophrenia
Atypical schizophrenia
Cenesthopathic schizophrenia

Excludes *infantile autism (299.0)*

C&C Exclusions: (for codes 295.80-295.84) See 295.0

5 295.9 Unspecified schizophrenia

Schizophrenia:
- NOS
- mixed NOS
- undifferentiated NOS
- undifferentiated type

Schizophrenic reaction NOS
Schizophreniform psychosis NOS

C&C Exclusions: (for codes 295.90-295.94) See 295.0

AHA: 3Q 1995, 6

4 296 Episodic mood disorders

Includes episodic affective disorders

Excludes *neurotic depression (300.4)*
reactive depressive psychosis (298.0)
reactive excitation (298.1)

AHA: Mar-Apr 1985, 14

The following fifth-digit subclassification is for use with categories 296.0-296.6:

- **0 unspecified**
- **1 mild**
- **2 moderate**
- **3 severe, without mention of psychotic behavior**
- **4 severe, specified as with psychotic behavior**
- **5 in partial or unspecified remission**
- **6 in full remission**

5 296.0 Bipolar I disorder, single manic episode
Hypomania (mild) NOS single episode or unspecified
Hypomanic psychosis single episode or unspecified
Mania (monopolar) NOS single episode or unspecified
Manic-depressive psychosis or reaction, single episode or unspecified:
hypomanic, single episode or unspecified
manic, single episode or unspecified
Excludes *circular type, if there was a previous attack of depression (296.4)*
C&C Exclusions: (for code 296.04) See 295.0

5 296.1 Manic disorder, recurrent episode
Any condition classifiable to 296.0, stated to be recurrent
Excludes *circular type, if there was a previous attack of depression (296.4)*
C&C Exclusions: (for code 296.14) See 295.0

5 296.2 Major depressive disorder, single episode
Depressive psychosis, single episode or unspecified
Endogenous depression, single episode or unspecified
Involutional melancholia, single episode or unspecified
Manic-depressive psychosis or reaction, depressed type, single episode or unspecified
Monopolar depression, single episode or unspecified
Psychotic depression, single episode or unspecified
Excludes *circular type, if previous attack was of manic type (296.5)*
depression NOS (311)
reactive depression (neurotic) (300.4)
psychotic (298.0)

5 296.3 Major depressive disorder, recurrent episode
Any condition classifiable to 296.2, stated to be recurrent
Excludes *circular type, if previous attack was of manic type (296.5)*
depression NOS (311)
reactive depression (neurotic) (300.4)
psychotic (298.0)
C&C Exclusions: (for code 296.34) See 295.0

5 296.4 Bipolar I disorder, most recent episode (or current) manic
Bipolar disorder, now manic
Manic-depressive psychosis, circular type but currently manic
Excludes *brief compensatory or rebound mood swings (296.99)*
C&C Exclusions: (for code 296.44) See 295.0

5 296.5 Bipolar I disorder, most recent episode (or current) depressed
Bipolar disorder, now depressed
Manic-depressive psychosis, circular type but currently depressed
Excludes *brief compensatory or rebound mood swings (296.99)*
C&C Exclusions: (for code 296.54) See 295.0

5 296.6 Bipolar I disorder, most recent episode (or current) mixed
Manic-depressive psychosis, circular type, mixed
C&C Exclusions: (for code 296.64) See 295.0

296.7 Bipolar I disorder, most recent episode (or current) unspecified
Atypical bipolar affective disorder NOS
Manic-depressive psychosis, circular type, current condition not specified as either manic or depressive

5 296.8 Other and unspecified bipolar disorders

296.80 Bipolar disorder, unspecified
Bipolar disorder, NOS
Manic-depressive:
reaction NOS
syndrome NOS

296.81 Atypical manic disorder

296.82 Atypical depressive disorder

296.89 Other
Bipolar II disorder
Manic-depressive psychosis, mixed type

5 296.9 Other and unspecified episodic mood disorder
Excludes *psychogenic affective psychoses (298.0-298.8)*

296.90 Unspecified episodic mood disorder
Affective psychosis NOS
Melancholia NOS
Mood disorder, NOS
AHA: Mar-Apr 1985, 14

296.99 Other specified episodic mood disorder
Mood swings:
brief compensatory
rebound

4 297 Delusional disorders
Includes paranoid disorders
Excludes *acute paranoid reaction (298.3)*
alcoholic jealousy or paranoid state (291.5)
paranoid schizophrenia (295.3)

297.0 Paranoid state, simple

297.1 Delusional disorder
Chronic paranoid psychosis
Sander's disease
Systematized delusions
Excludes *paranoid personality disorder (301.0)*

297.2 Paraphrenia
Involutional paranoid state
Late paraphrenia
Paraphrenia (involutional)

297.3 Shared psychotic disorder
Folie à deux
Induced psychosis or paranoid disorder

297.8 Other specified paranoid states
Paranoia querulans
Sensitiver Beziehungswahn
Excludes *acute paranoid reaction or state (298.3)*
senile paranoid state (290.20)

297.9 Unspecified paranoid state
Paranoid:
disorder NOS
psychosis NOS
reaction NOS
state NOS
AHA: Jul-Aug 1985, 9

4 298 Other nonorganic psychoses
Includes psychotic conditions due to or provoked by:
emotional stress
environmental factors as major part of etiology

DEF: Severe emotional disorders featuring personality derangement, loss of contact with reality, and impairment of social functioning.

298.0 Depressive type psychosis
Psychogenic depressive psychosis
Psychotic reactive depression
Reactive depressive psychosis
Excludes *manic-depressive psychosis, depressed type (296.2-296.3)*
neurotic depression (300.4)
reactive depression NOS (300.4)
C&C Exclusions: See 295.0

298.1 Excitative type psychosis
Acute hysterical psychosis
Psychogenic excitation
Reactive excitation
Excludes *manic-depressive psychosis, manic type (296.0-296.1)*

298.2 Reactive confusion
Psychogenic confusion
Psychogenic twilight state
Excludes *acute confusional state (293.0)*

298.3 Acute paranoid reaction
Acute psychogenic paranoid psychosis
Bouffée délirante
Excludes *paranoid states (297.0-297.9)*
C&C Exclusions: See 295.0

298.4 Psychogenic paranoid psychosis
Protracted reactive paranoid psychosis
C&C Exclusions: See 295.0

298.8 Other and unspecified reactive psychosis
Brief psychotic disorder
Brief reactive psychosis NOS
Hysterical psychosis
Psychogenic psychosis NOS
Psychogenic stupor
Excludes *acute hysterical psychosis (298.1)*

298.9 Unspecified psychosis
Atypical psychosis
Psychosis NOS
Psychotic disorder NOS

❹ **299 Pervasive developmental disorders**
Excludes *adult type psychoses occurring in childhood, as:*
affective disorders (296.0-296.9)
manic-depressive disorders (296.0-296.9)
schizophrenia (295.0-295.9)

The following fifth-digit subclassification is for use with category 299:
0 current or active state
1 residual state

❺ **299.0 Autistic disorder**
Childhood autism
Infantile psychosis
Kanner's syndrome
Excludes *disintegrative psychosis (299.1)*
Heller's syndrome (299.1)
schizophrenic syndrome of childhood (299.9)
C&C Exclusions: (for code 299.00) See 295.0

❺ **299.1 Childhood disintegrative disorder**
Heller's syndrome
Use additional code to identify any associated neurological disorder
Excludes *infantile autism (299.0)*
schizophrenic syndrome of childhood (299.9)
DEF: Neurological disorder appearing at a young age that impairs social development and communication skills, and resulting in abnormal behavior that varies in degree of severity and ability to function.
C&C Exclusions: (for code 299.10) See 295.0

❺ **299.8 Other specified pervasive developmental disorders**
Asperger's disorder
Atypical childhood psychosis
Borderline psychosis of childhood
Excludes *simple stereotypes without psychotic disturbance (307.3)*
C&C Exclusions: (for code 299.80) See 295.0

❺ **299.9 Unspecified pervasive developmental disorder**
Child psychosis NOS
Pervasive developmental disorder NOS
Schizophrenia, childhood type NOS
Schizophrenic syndrome of childhood NOS
Excludes *schizophrenia of adult type occurring in childhood (295.0-295.9)*
C&C Exclusions: (for code 299.90) See 295.0

NEUROTIC DISORDERS, PERSONALITY DISORDERS, AND OTHER NONPSYCHOTIC MENTAL DISORDERS (300-316)

❹ **300 Anxiety, dissociative and somatoform disorders**

❺ **300.0 Anxiety states**
Excludes *anxiety in:*
acute stress reaction (308.0)
transient adjustment reaction (309.24)
neurasthenia (300.5)
psychophysiological disorders (306.0-306.9)
separation anxiety (309.21)

300.00 Anxiety state, unspecified
Anxiety:
neurosis
reaction
state (neurotic)
Atypical anxiety disorder
AHA: 1Q 2002, 6

300.01 Panic disorder without agoraphobia
Panic:
attack
state
Excludes *panic disorder with agoraphobia (300.21)*
DEF: Unexplained bouts of intense fear or anxiety, accompanied by physiological symptoms of elevated heart rate, sweating, trembling, dizziness, and dyspnea.

300.02 Generalized anxiety disorder
DEF: Persistent, uncontrollable worry about aspects of a person's life; diagnosed when symptoms last longer than six months, with anxiety present on the majority of days in that time.

300.09 Other

❺ **300.1 Dissociative, conversion and factitious disorders**
Excludes *adjustment reaction (309.0-309.9)*
anorexia nervosa (307.1)
gross stress reaction (308.0-308.9)
hysterical personality (301.50-301.59)
psychophysiologic disorders (306.0-306.9)

300.10 Hysteria, unspecified

300.11 Conversion disorder
Astasia-abasia, hysterical
Conversion hysteria or reaction
Hysterical:
blindness
deafness
paralysis
AHA: Nov-Dec 1985, 15

300.12 Dissociative amnesia
Hysterical amnesia
DEF: Psychological trauma causing temporary forgetting of personal information and inability to perform complex tasks, like driving or cooking.

300.13 Dissociative fugue
Hysterical fugue
DEF: Disorder occurring in response to a severe, recent stressor, in which the patient invents a new personality and becomes unable to remember his/her previous identity, lasting days or months.

300.14 Dissociative identity disorder

300.15 Dissociative disorder or reaction, unspecified

300.16 Factitious disorder with predominantly psychological signs and symptoms
Compensation neurosis
Ganser's syndrome, hysterical

300.19 Other and unspecified factitious illness
Factitious disorder (with combined psychological and physical signs and symptoms)(with predominantly physical signs and symptoms) NOS
Excludes *multiple operations or hospital addiction syndrome (301.51)*

❺ **300.2 Phobic disorders**
Excludes *anxiety state not associated with a specific situation or object (300.00-300.09)*
obsessional phobias (300.3)

300.20 Phobia, unspecified
Anxiety-hysteria NOS
Phobia NOS

300.21 Agoraphobia with panic disorder
Fear of:
open spaces with panic attacks
streets with panic attacks
travel with panic attacks
Panic disorder with agoraphobia
Excludes *agoraphobia without panic disorder (300.22)*
panic disorder without agoraphobia (300.01)
DEF: Fear of open spaces or crowds, traveling, or leaving a safe place, accompanied by panic attacks.

300.22 Agoraphobia without mention of panic attacks
Any condition classifiable to 300.21 without mention of panic attacks

300.23 Social phobia
Fear of:
- eating in public
- public speaking
- washing in public

DEF: Intense fear of appearing in public, especially in situations where one is the center of attention.

300.29 Other isolated or specific phobias
Acrophobia
Animal phobias
Claustrophobia
Fear of crowds

300.3 Obsessive-compulsive disorders
Anancastic neurosis
Compulsive neurosis
Obsessional phobia [any]
Excludes *obsessive-compulsive symptoms occurring in:*
- *endogenous depression (296.2-296.3)*
- *organic states (e.g., encephalitis)*
- *schizophrenia (295.0-295.9)*

DEF: Recurrent obsessions of thought or action that are time-consuming or disruptive to daily life and can produce anxiety or distress.

300.4 Dysthymic disorder
Anxiety depression
Depression with anxiety
Depressive reaction
Neurotic depressive state
Reactive depression
Excludes *adjustment reaction with depressive symptoms (309.0-309.1)*
depression NOS (311)
manic-depressive psychosis, depressed type (296.2-296.3)
reactive depressive psychosis (298.0)

DEF: Type of reactive depression brought about by changes or events in the patient's life; may be accompanied by anxiety.

300.5 Neurasthenia
Fatigue neurosis
Nervous debility
Psychogenic:
- asthenia
- general fatigue

Use additional code to identify any associated physical disorder
Excludes *anxiety state (300.00-300.09)*
neurotic depression (300.4)
psychophysiological disorders (306.0-306.9)
specific nonpsychotic mental disorders following organic brain damage (310.0-310.9)

300.6 Depersonalization disorder
Derealization (neurotic)
Neurotic state with depersonalization episode
Excludes *depersonalization associated with:*
- *anxiety (300.00-300.09)*
- *depression (300.4)*
- *manic-depressive disorder or psychosis (296.0-296.9)*
- *schizophrenia (295.0-295.9)*

300.7 Hypochondriasis
Body dysmorphic disorder
Excludes *hypochondriasis in:*
- *hysteria (300.10-300.19)*
- *manic-depressive psychosis, depressed type (296.2-296.3)*
- *neurasthenia (300.5)*
- *obsessional disorder (300.3)*
- *schizophrenia (295.0-295.9)*

DEF: Chronic worry about nonexistent illnesses that one believes one may have.

5 **300.8 Somatoform disorders**

300.81 Somatization disorder
Briquet's disorder
Severe somatoform disorder

300.82 Undifferentiated somatoform disorder
Atypical somatoform disorder
Somatoform disorder NOS
AHA: 4Q 1996, 29

300.89 Other somatoform disorders
Occupational neurosis, including writers' cramp
Psychasthenia
Psychasthenic neurosis

300.9 Unspecified nonpsychotic mental disorder
Psychoneurosis NOS

4 **301 Personality disorders**
Includes character neurosis
Use additional code to identify any associated neurosis or psychosis, or physical condition
Excludes *nonpsychotic personality disorder associated with organic brain syndromes (310.0-310.9)*

301.0 Paranoid personality disorder
Fanatic personality
Paranoid personality (disorder)
Paranoid traits
Excludes *acute paranoid reaction (298.3)*
alcoholic paranoia (291.5)
paranoid schizophrenia (295.3)
paranoid states (297.0-297.9)
AHA: Jul-Aug 1985, 9

5 **301.1 Affective personality disorder**
Excludes *affective psychotic disorders (296.0-296.9)*
neurasthenia (300.5)
neurotic depression (300.4)

301.10 Affective personality disorder, unspecified

301.11 Chronic hypomanic personality disorder
Chronic hypomanic disorder
Hypomanic personality
DEF: Mild hyperactivity and euphoria to an extent that it interferes with daily life.

301.12 Chronic depressive personality disorder
Chronic depressive disorder
Depressive character or personality

301.13 Cyclothymic disorder
Cycloid personality
Cyclothymia
Cyclothymic personality
DEF: Mild mood swings between elevated mood and mild depression.

5 **301.2 Schizoid personality disorder**
Excludes *schizophrenia (295.0-295.9)*

301.20 Schizoid personality disorder, unspecified

301.21 Introverted personality

301.22 Schizotypal personality disorder

301.3 Explosive personality disorder
Aggressive:
- personality
- reaction

Aggressiveness
Emotional instability (excessive)
Pathological emotionality
Quarrelsomeness
Excludes *dyssocial personality (301.7)*
hysterical neurosis (300.10-300.19)

DEF: Disorder in which a person is quick to anger, aggressive, abnormally emotional, and argumentative.

301.4 Obsessive-compulsive personality disorder
Anancastic personality
Obsessional personality
Excludes *obsessive-compulsive disorder (300.3)*
phobic state (300.20-300.29)

A Adult (15+ years) M Maternity (12-55 years) N Newborn (0 years) P Pediatric (0-17 years) ♂ Male ♀ Female ② Medicare Secondary Payer

⑤ **301.5 Histrionic personality disorder**
Excludes *hysterical neurosis (300.10-300.19)*

301.50 Histrionic personality disorder, unspecified
Hysterical personality NOS

301.51 Chronic factitious illness with physical symptoms
Hospital addiction syndrome
Multiple operations syndrome
Munchausen syndrome

301.59 Other histrionic personality disorder
Personality:
emotionally unstable
labile
psychoinfantile

301.6 Dependent personality disorder
Asthenic personality
Inadequate personality
Passive personality
Excludes *neurasthenia (300.5)*
passive-aggressive personality (301.84)

301.7 Antisocial personality disorder
Amoral personality
Asocial personality
Dyssocial personality
Personality disorder with predominantly sociopathic or asocial manifestation
Excludes *disturbance of conduct without specifiable personality disorder (312.0-312.9)*
explosive personality (301.3)

AHA: Sep-Oct 1984, 16

⑤ **301.8 Other personality disorders**

301.81 Narcissistic personality disorder
DEF: Exaggerated sense of self-importance, lack of social inhibition, lying, lack of empathy for others, and a sense of entitlement.

301.82 Avoidant personality disorder

301.83 Borderline personality disorder

301.84 Passive-aggressive personality

301.89 Other
Personality:
eccentric
"haltlose" type
immature
masochistic
psychoneurotic
Excludes *psychoinfantile personality (301.59)*

301.9 Unspecified personality disorder
Pathological personality NOS
Personality disorder NOS
Psychopathic:
constitutional state
personality (disorder)

④ **302 Sexual and gender identity disorders**
Excludes *sexual disorder manifest in:*
organic brain syndrome (290.0-294.9, 310.0-310.9)
psychosis (295.0-298.9)

302.0 Ego-dystonic sexual orientation
Ego-dystonic lesbianism
Sexual orientation conflict disorder
Excludes *homosexual pedophilia (302.2)*

302.1 Zoophilia
Bestiality
DEF: Sexual attraction to animals.

302.2 Pedophilia

302.3 Transvestic fetishism
Excludes *trans-sexualism (302.5)*

302.4 Exhibitionism
DEF: Compulsion to expose genitals in public.

⑤ **302.5 Trans-sexualism**
▶ Sex reassignment surgery status◀
Excludes *transvestism (302.3)*

302.50 With unspecified sexual history

302.51 With asexual history

302.52 With homosexual history

302.53 With heterosexual history

302.6 Gender identity disorder in children
Feminism in boys
Gender identity disorder NOS
Excludes *gender identity disorder in adult (302.85)*
trans-sexualism (302.50-302.53)
transvestism (302.3)

⑤ **302.7 Psychosexual dysfunction**
Excludes *impotence of organic origin (607.84)*
normal transient symptoms from ruptured hymen
transient or occasional failures of erection due to fatigue, anxiety, alcohol, or drugs

DEF: Psychological problems interfering with normal sexual activities.

302.70 Psychosexual dysfunction, unspecified
Sexual dysfunction NOS

302.71 Hypoactive sexual desire disorder
Excludes *decreased sexual desire (799.81)*
DEF: Markedly decreased sexual desire.

302.72 With inhibited sexual excitement
Female sexual arousal disorder
Frigidity
Impotence
Male erectile disorder

302.73 Female orgasmic disorder ♀

302.74 Male orgasmic disorder ♂

302.75 Premature ejaculation ♂

302.76 Dyspareunia, psychogenic ♀

302.79 With other specified psychosexual dysfunctions
Sexual aversion disorder

⑤ **302.8 Other specified psychosexual disorders**

302.81 Fetishism

302.82 Voyeurism
DEF: Uncontrollable compulsion to covertly observe others who are nude or engaged in sexual activity.

302.83 Sexual masochism
DEF: Psychosexual disorder marked by the need to be humiliated or hurt to achieve sexual gratification.

302.84 Sexual sadism
DEF: Psychosexual disorder marked by the need to humiliate or injure others to achieve sexual gratification.

302.85 Gender identity disorder in adolescents or adults
▶ Use additional code to identify sex reassignment surgery status (302.5)◀
Excludes *gender identity disorder NOS (302.6)*
gender identity disorder in children (302.6)

302.89 Other
Frotteurism
Nymphomania
Satyriasis

302.9 Unspecified psychosexual disorder
Paraphilia NOS
Pathologic sexuality NOS
Sexual deviation NOS
Sexual disorder NOS

303 Alcohol dependence syndrome

Use additional code to identify any associated condition, as:
- alcoholic psychoses (291.0-291.9)
- drug dependence (304.0-304.9)
- physical complications of alcohol, such as:
  - cerebral degeneration (331.7)
  - cirrhosis of liver (571.2)
  - epilepsy (345.0-345.9)
  - gastritis (535.3)
  - hepatitis (571.1)
  - liver damage NOS (571.3)

Excludes *drunkenness NOS (305.0)*

AHA: 3Q 1995, 6; 2Q 1991, 9; 4Q 1988, 8; Sep-Oct 1986, 3

The following fifth-digit subclassification is for use with category 303:
- **0 unspecified**
- **1 continuous**
- **2 episodic**
- **3 in remission**

303.0 Acute alcoholic intoxication
Acute drunkenness in alcoholism
C&C Exclusions: (for codes 303.00-303.02) 291.0, 291.1, 291.2, 291.3, 291.4, 291.5, 291.81, 291.89, 291.9, 292.0, 292.1, 292.2, 292.81, 292.82, 292.83, 292.84, 292.89, 292.9, 303.00, 303.01, 303.02, 303.03, 303.90, 303.91, 303.92, 303.93, 304.00, 304.01, 304.02, 304.03, 304.10, 304.11, 304.12, 304.13, 304.20, 304.21, 304.22, 304.23, 304.30, 304.31, 304.32, 304.33, 304.40, 304.41, 304.42, 304.43, 304.50, 304.51, 304.52, 304.53, 304.60, 304.61, 304.62, 304.63, 304.70, 304.71, 304.72, 304.73, 304.80, 304.81, 304.82, 304.83, 304.90, 304.91, 305.00, 305.01, 305.02, 305.03, 305.20, 305.21, 305.22, 305.23, 305.30, 305.31, 305.32, 305.33, 305.40, 305.41, 305.42, 305.43, 305.50, 305.51, 305.52, 305.53, 305.60, 305.61, 305.62, 305.63, 305.70, 305.71, 305.72, 305.73, 305.80, 305.81, 305.82, 305.83, 305.90, 305.91, 305.92, 305.93, 790.3

303.9 Other and unspecified alcohol dependence
Chronic alcoholism
Dipsomania
C&C Exclusions: (for codes 303.90-303.92) See 303.0
AHA: 2Q 2002, 4; 2Q 1989, 9

304 Drug dependence

Excludes *nondependent abuse of drugs (305.1-305.9)*

AHA: 2Q 1991, 10; 4Q 1988, 8; Sep-Oct 1986, 3

The following fifth-digit subclassification is for use with category 304:
- **0 unspecified**
- **1 continuous**
- **2 episodic**
- **3 in remission**

304.0 Opioid type dependence
Heroin
Meperidine
Methadone
Morphine
Opium
Opium alkaloids and their derivatives
Synthetics with morphine-like effects
C&C Exclusions: (for codes 304.00-304.02) See 303.0
AHA: For code 304.00: 2Q 2006, 7

304.1 Sedative, hypnotic or anxiolytic dependence
Barbiturates
Nonbarbiturate sedatives and tranquilizers with a similar effect:
- chlordiazepoxide
- diazepam
- glutethimide
- meprobamate
- methaqualone

C&C Exclusions: (for codes 304.10-304.12) See 303.0

304.2 Cocaine dependence
Coca leaves and derivatives
C&C Exclusions: (for codes 304.20-304.22) See 303.0

304.3 Cannabis dependence
Hashish
Hemp
Marihuana

304.4 Amphetamine and other psychostimulant dependence
Methylphenidate
Phenmetrazine
C&C Exclusions: (for codes 304.40-304.42) See 303.0

304.5 Hallucinogen dependence
Dimethyltryptamine [DMT]
Lysergic acid diethylamide [LSD] and derivatives
Mescaline
Psilocybin
C&C Exclusions: (for codes 304.50-304.52) See 303.0

304.6 Other specified drug dependence
Absinthe addiction
Glue sniffing
Inhalant dependence
Phencyclidine dependence

Excludes *tobacco dependence (305.1)*

C&C Exclusions: (for codes 304.60-304.62) See 303.0

304.7 Combinations of opioid type drug with any other
C&C Exclusions: (for codes 304.70-304.72) See 303.0
AHA: Mar-Apr 1986, 12

304.8 Combinations of drug dependence excluding opioid type drug
C&C Exclusions: (for codes 304.80-304.82) See 303.0
AHA: Mar-Apr 1986, 12

304.9 Unspecified drug dependence
Drug addiction NOS
Drug dependence NOS
C&C Exclusions: (for codes 304.90-304.92) See 303.0
AHA: For Code: 304.90: 4Q 2003, 103

305 Nondependent abuse of drugs

Note: *Includes cases where a person, for whom no other diagnosis is possible, has come under medical care because of the maladaptive effect of a drug on which he is not dependent and that he has taken on his own initiative to the detriment of his health or social functioning.*

Excludes *alcohol dependence syndrome (303.0-303.9)*
drug dependence (304.0-304.9)
drug withdrawal syndrome (292.0)
poisoning by drugs or medicinal substances (960.0-979.9)

AHA: 2Q 1991, 10; 4Q 1988, 8; Sep-Oct 1986, 3

The following fifth-digit subclassification is for use with codes 305.0, 305.2-305.9
- **0 unspecified**
- **1 continuous**
- **2 episodic**
- **3 in remission**

305.0 Alcohol abuse
Drunkenness NOS
Excessive drinking of alcohol NOS
"Hangover" (alcohol)
Inebriety NOS

Excludes *acute alcohol intoxication in alcoholism (303.0)*
alcoholic psychoses (291.0-291.9)

C&C Exclusions: (for codes 305.00-305.02) See 303.0
AHA: 3Q 1996, 16

305.1 Tobacco use disorder
Tobacco dependence

Excludes *history of tobacco use (V15.82)*
smoking complicating pregnancy (649.0)
tobacco use disorder complicating pregnancy (649.0)

AHA: 2Q 1996, 10; Nov-Dec 1984, 12

305.2 Cannabis abuse

305.3 Hallucinogen abuse
Acute intoxication from hallucinogens ["bad trips"]
LSD reaction
C&C Exclusions: (for codes 305.30-305.32) See 303.0

305.4 Sedative, hypnotic or anxiolytic abuse
C&C Exclusions: (for codes 305.40-305.42) See 303.0

305.5 Opioid abuse
C&C Exclusions: (for codes 305.50-305.52) See 303.0

5 **305.6 Cocaine abuse**
C&C Exclusions: (for codes 305.60-305.62) See 303.0
AHA: 1Q 1993, 25; For Code 305.60: 1Q 2005, 6

5 **305.7 Amphetamine or related acting sympathomimetic abuse**
C&C Exclusions: (for codes 305.70-305.72) See 303.0

5 **305.8 Antidepressant type abuse**

5 **305.9 Other, mixed, or unspecified drug abuse**
Caffeine intoxication
Inhalant abuse
"Laxative habit"
Misuse of drugs NOS
Nonprescribed use of drugs or patent medicinals
Phencyclidine abuse
C&C Exclusions: (for codes 305.90-305.92) See 303.0
AHA: 3Q 1999, 20

4 **306 Physiological malfunction arising from mental factors**
Includes psychogenic:
physical symptoms not involving tissue damage
physiological manifestations not involving tissue damage
Excludes *hysteria (300.11-300.19)*
physical symptoms secondary to a psychiatric disorder classified elsewhere
psychic factors associated with physical conditions involving tissue damage classified elsewhere (316)
specific nonpsychotic mental disorders following organic brain damage (310.0-310.9)

306.0 Musculoskeletal
Psychogenic paralysis
Psychogenic torticollis
Excludes *Gilles de la Tourette's syndrome (307.23)*
paralysis as hysterical or conversion reaction (300.11)
tics (307.20-307.22)

306.1 Respiratory
Psychogenic:
air hunger
cough
hiccough
hyperventilation
yawning
Excludes *psychogenic asthma (316 and 493.9)*

306.2 Cardiovascular
Cardiac neurosis
Cardiovascular neurosis
Neurocirculatory asthenia
Psychogenic cardiovascular disorder
Excludes *psychogenic paroxysmal tachycardia (316 and 427.2)*
AHA: Jul-Aug 1985, 14

306.3 Skin
Psychogenic pruritus
Excludes *psychogenic:*
alopecia (316 and 704.00)
dermatitis (316 and 692.9)
eczema (316 and 691.8 or 692.9)
urticaria (316 and 708.0-708.9)

306.4 Gastrointestinal
Aerophagy
Cyclical vomiting, psychogenic
Diarrhea, psychogenic
Nervous gastritis
Psychogenic dyspepsia
Excludes *cyclical vomiting NOS (536.2)*
globus hystericus (300.11)
mucous colitis (316 and 564.9)
psychogenic:
cardiospasm (316 and 530.0)
duodenal ulcer (316 and 532.0-532.9)
gastric ulcer (316 and 531.0-531.9)
peptic ulcer NOS (316 and 533.0-533.9)
vomiting NOS (307.54)
AHA: 2Q 1989, 11

5 **306.5 Genitourinary**
Excludes *enuresis, psychogenic (307.6)*
frigidity (302.72)
impotence (302.72)
psychogenic dyspareunia (302.76)

306.50 Psychogenic genitourinary malfunction, unspecified

306.51 Psychogenic vaginismus ♀
Functional vaginismus

306.52 Psychogenic dysmenorrhea ♀
DEF: Mental factors causing a woman to experience painful menstruation.

306.53 Psychogenic dysuria
DEF: Mental factors causing the patient to experience painful urination.

306.59 Other
AHA: Mar-Apr 1987, 11

306.6 Endocrine

306.7 Organs of special sense
Excludes *hysterical blindness or deafness (300.11)*
psychophysical visual disturbances (368.16)

306.8 Other specified psychophysiological malfunction
Bruxism
Teeth grinding

306.9 Unspecified psychophysiological malfunction
Psychophysiologic disorder NOS
Psychosomatic disorder NOS

4 **307 Special symptoms or syndromes, not elsewhere classified**
Note: This category is intended for use if the psychopathology is manifested by a single specific symptom or group of symptoms which is not part of an organic illness or other mental disorder classifiable elsewhere.
Excludes *those due to mental disorders classified elsewhere*
those of organic origin

307.0 Stuttering
Excludes *dysphasia (784.5)*
lisping or lalling (307.9)
retarded development of speech (315.31-315.39)
DEF: Normal flow of speech disrupted by repeated sounds or pauses.

307.1 Anorexia nervosa
Excludes *eating disturbance NOS (307.50)*
feeding problem (783.3)
of nonorganic origin (307.59)
loss of appetite (783.0)
of nonorganic origin (307.59)
C&C Exclusions: 306.4, 306.8, 306.9, 307.1, 307.50, 307.51, 307.52, 307.53, 307.54, 307.59, 309.22
AHA: 2Q 2006, 12; 4Q 1989, 11

5 **307.2 Tics**
Excludes *nail-biting or thumb-sucking (307.9)*
stereotypes occurring in isolation (307.3)
tics of organic origin (333.3)

307.20 Tic disorder, unspecified
Tic disorder NOS

307.21 Transient tic disorder

307.22 Chronic motor or vocal tic disorder

307.23 Tourette's disorder
Motor-verbal tic disorder

307.3 Stereotypic movement disorder
Body-rocking
Head banging
Spasmus nutans
Stereotypes NOS
Excludes *tics (307.20-307.23)*
of organic origin (333.3)

5 307.4 Specific disorders of sleep of nonorganic origin

Excludes *narcolepsy (347.00-347.11)*
organic hypersomnia (327.10-327.19)
organic insomnia (327.00-327.09)
those of unspecified cause (780.50-780.59)

307.40 Nonorganic sleep disorder, unspecified

307.41 Transient disorder of initiating or maintaining sleep

Adjustment insomnia
Hyposomnia associated with acute or intermittent emotional reactions or conflicts
Insomnia associated with acute or intermittent emotional reactions or conflicts
Sleeplessness associated with acute or intermittent emotional reactions or conflicts

307.42 Persistent disorder of initiating or maintaining sleep

Hyposomnia, insomnia, or sleeplessness associated with:
anxiety
conditioned arousal
depression (major) (minor)
psychosis
Idiopathic insomnia
Paradoxical insomnia
Primary insomnia
Psychophysiological insomnia

307.43 Transient disorder of initiating or maintaining wakefulness

Hypersomnia associated with acute or intermittent emotional reactions or conflicts

307.44 Persistent disorder of initiating or maintaining wakefulness

Hypersomnia associated with depression (major) (minor)
Insufficient sleep syndrome
Primary hypersomnia
Excludes *sleep deprivation (V69.4)*

307.45 Circadian rhythm sleep disorder of nonorganic origin

307.46 Sleep arousal disorder

Night terror disorder
Night terrors
Sleep terror disorder
Sleepwalking
Somnambulism

307.47 Other dysfunctions of sleep stages or arousal from sleep

Nightmare disorder
Nightmares:
NOS
REM-sleep type
Sleep drunkenness

307.48 Repetitive intrusions of sleep

Repetitive intrusion of sleep with:
atypical polysomnographic features
environmental disturbances
repeated REM-sleep interruptions

307.49 Other

"Short-sleeper"
Subjective insomnia complaint

5 307.5 Other and unspecified disorders of eating

Excludes *anorexia:*
nervosa (307.1)
of unspecified cause (783.0)
overeating, of unspecified cause (783.6)
vomiting:
NOS (787.0)
cyclical (536.2)
psychogenic (306.4)

307.50 Eating disorder, unspecified

Eating disorder NOS

307.51 Bulimia nervosa

Overeating of nonorganic origin

DEF: Binge eating followed by self-induced vomiting.

307.52 Pica

Perverted appetite of nonorganic origin

DEF: Compulsion to eat inedible substances, such as dirt or rocks.

307.53 Rumination disorder

Regurgitation, of nonorganic origin, of food with reswallowing
Excludes *obsessional rumination (300.3)*

307.54 Psychogenic vomiting

307.59 Other

Feeding disorder of infancy or early childhood of nonorganic origin
Infantile feeding disturbances of nonorganic origin
Loss of appetite of nonorganic origin

307.6 Enuresis

Enuresis (primary) (secondary) of nonorganic origin
Excludes *enuresis of unspecified cause (788.3)*

307.7 Encopresis

Encopresis (continuous) (discontinuous) of nonorganic origin
Excludes *encopresis of unspecified cause (787.6)*

5 307.8 Pain disorders related to psychological factors

307.80 Psychogenic pain, site unspecified

307.81 Tension headache

Excludes *headache:*
NOS (784.0)
migraine (346.0-346.9)

AHA: Nov-Dec 1985, 16

307.89 Other

Code first to type or site of pain
Excludes *pain disorder exclusively attributed to psychological factors (307.80)*
psychogenic pain (307.80)

307.9 Other and unspecified special symptoms or syndromes, not elsewhere classified

Communication disorder NOS
Hair plucking
Lalling
Lisping
Masturbation
Nail-biting
Thumb-sucking

4 308 Acute reaction to stress

Includes catastrophic stress
combat fatigue
gross stress reaction (acute)
transient disorders in response to exceptional physical or mental stress which usually subside within hours or days
Excludes *adjustment reaction or disorder (309.0-309.9)*
chronic stress reaction (309.1-309.9)

308.0 Predominant disturbance of emotions

Anxiety as acute reaction to exceptional [gross] stress
Emotional crisis as acute reaction to exceptional [gross] stress
Panic state as acute reaction to exceptional [gross] stress

308.1 Predominant disturbance of consciousness

Fugues as acute reaction to exceptional [gross] stress

308.2 Predominant psychomotor disturbance

Agitation states as acute reaction to exceptional [gross] stress
Stupor as acute reaction to exceptional [gross] stress

308.3 Other acute reactions to stress

Acute situational disturbance
Acute stress disorder
Excludes *prolonged posttraumatic emotional disturbance (309.81)*

308.4 Mixed disorders as reaction to stress

308.9 Unspecified acute reaction to stress

④ 309 Adjustment reaction

Includes adjustment disorders
reaction (adjustment) to chronic stress

Excludes *acute reaction to major stress (308.0-308.9)*
neurotic disorders (300.0-300.9)

309.0 Adjustment disorder with depressed mood

Grief reaction

Excludes *affective psychoses (296.0-296.9)*
neurotic depression (300.4)
prolonged depressive reaction (309.1)
psychogenic depressive psychosis (298.0)

309.1 Prolonged depressive reaction

Excludes *affective psychoses (296.0-296.9)*
brief depressive reaction (309.0)
neurotic depression (300.4)
psychogenic depressive psychosis (298.0)

DEF: Prolonged depressive state as a reaction to an event or change in the patient's life.

⑤ 309.2 With predominant disturbance of other emotions

309.21 Separation anxiety disorder

DEF: Abnormal anxiety when separated from a parent, guardian, or usual environment.

309.22 Emancipation disorder of adolescence and early adult life

309.23 Specific academic or work inhibition

309.24 Adjustment disorder with anxiety

309.28 Adjustment disorder with mixed anxiety and depressed mood

Adjustment reaction with anxiety and depression

309.29 Other

Culture shock

309.3 Adjustment disorder with disturbance of conduct

Conduct disturbance as adjustment reaction
Destructiveness as adjustment reaction

Excludes *destructiveness in child (312.9)*
disturbance of conduct NOS (312.9)
dyssocial behavior without manifest psychiatric disorder (V71.01-V71.02)
personality disorder with predominantly sociopathic or asocial manifestations (301.7)

309.4 Adjustment disorder with mixed disturbance of emotions and conduct

⑤ 309.8 Other specified adjustment reactions

309.81 Posttraumatic stress disorder

Chronic posttraumatic stress disorder
Concentration camp syndrome
Posttraumatic stress disorder NOS
Post-traumatic stress disorder (PTSD)

Excludes *acute stress disorder (308.3)*
posttraumatic brain syndrome:
nonpsychotic (310.2)
psychotic (293.0-293.9)

DEF: Chronic stressful response to traumatic events such as combat, rape, physical assault, and natural disasters with sudden, powerful memories (flashbacks) of the event, anxiety, and panic.

309.82 Adjustment reaction with physical symptoms

309.83 Adjustment reaction with withdrawal

Elective mutism as adjustment reaction
Hospitalism (in children) NOS

309.89 Other

309.9 Unspecified adjustment reaction

Adaptation reaction NOS
Adjustment reaction NOS

④ 310 Specific nonpsychotic mental disorders due to brain damage

Excludes *neuroses, personality disorders, or other nonpsychotic conditions occurring in a form similar to that seen with functional disorders but in association with a physical condition (300.0-300.9, 301.0-301.9)*

310.0 Frontal lobe syndrome

Lobotomy syndrome
Postleucotomy syndrome [state]

Excludes *postcontusion syndrome (310.2)*

DEF: Damage to the frontal lobe of the brain, typically manifesting as apathy, a lack of planning, emotional bluntness, and the absence of abstract thought.

310.1 Personality change due to conditions classified elsewhere

Cognitive or personality change of other type, of nonpsychotic severity
Organic psychosyndrome of nonpsychotic severity
Presbyophrenia NOS
Senility with mental changes of nonpsychotic severity

Excludes *memory loss of unknown cause (780.93)*

AHA: 2Q 2005, 6

310.2 Postconcussion syndrome

Postcontusion syndrome or encephalopathy
Posttraumatic brain syndrome, nonpsychotic
Status postcommotio cerebri

Excludes *any organic psychotic conditions following head injury (293.0-294.0)*
frontal lobe syndrome (310.0)
postencephalitic syndrome (310.8)

DEF: Symptoms such as headache, amnesia, and lack of concentration due to a severe blow to the skull.

AHA: 4Q 1990, 24

310.8 Other specified nonpsychotic mental disorders following organic brain damage

Mild memory disturbance
Postencephalitic syndrome
Other focal (partial) organic psychosyndromes

310.9 Unspecified nonpsychotic mental disorder following organic brain damage

AHA: 4Q 2003, 103

311 Depressive disorder, not elsewhere classified

Depressive disorder NOS
Depressive state NOS
Depression NOS

Excludes *acute reaction to major stress with depressive symptoms (308.0)*
affective personality disorder (301.10-301.13)
affective psychoses (296.0-296.9)
brief depressive reaction (309.0)
depressive states associated with stressful events (309.0-309.1)
disturbance of emotions specific to childhood and adolescence, with misery and unhappiness (313.1)
mixed adjustment reaction with depressive symptoms (309.4)
neurotic depression (300.4)
prolonged depressive adjustment reaction (309.1)
psychogenic depressive psychosis (298.0)

AHA: 4Q 2003, 75

4 312 Disturbance of conduct, not elsewhere classified
Excludes *adjustment reaction with disturbance of conduct (309.3)*
drug dependence (304.0-304.9)
dyssocial behavior without manifest psychiatric disorder (V71.01-V71.02)
personality disorder with predominantly sociopathic or asocial manifestations (301.7)
sexual deviations (302.0-302.9)

The following fifth-digit subclassification is for use with categories 312.0-312.2:
0 **unspecified**
1 **mild**
2 **moderate**
3 **severe**

5 312.0 Undersocialized conduct disorder, aggressive type
Aggressive outburst
Anger reaction
Unsocialized aggressive disorder

5 312.1 Undersocialized conduct disorder, unaggressive type
Childhood truancy, unsocialized
Solitary stealing
Tantrums

5 312.2 Socialized conduct disorder
Childhood truancy, socialized
Group delinquency
Excludes *gang activity without manifest psychiatric disorder (V71.01)*

5 312.3 Disorders of impulse control, not elsewhere classified

312.30 Impulse control disorder, unspecified

312.31 Pathological gambling

312.32 Kleptomania
DEF: Irresistible impulse to steal.

312.33 Pyromania
DEF: Uncontrollable impulse to set fires.

312.34 Intermittent explosive disorder

312.35 Isolated explosive disorder

312.39 Other
Trichotillomania

312.4 Mixed disturbance of conduct and emotions
Neurotic delinquency
Excludes *compulsive conduct disorder (312.3)*

5 312.8 Other specified disturbances of conduct, not elsewhere classified

312.81 Conduct disorder, childhood onset type

312.82 Conduct disorder, adolescent onset type

312.89 Other conduct disorder
Conduct disorder of unspecified onset

312.9 Unspecified disturbance of conduct
Delinquency (juvenile)
Disruptive behavior disorder NOS

4 313 Disturbance of emotions specific to childhood and adolescence
Excludes *adjustment reaction (309.0-309.9)*
emotional disorder of neurotic type (300.0-300.9)
masturbation, nail-biting, thumb-sucking, and other isolated symptoms (307.0-307.9)

313.0 Overanxious disorder
Anxiety and fearfulness of childhood and adolescence
Overanxious disorder of childhood and adolescence
Excludes *abnormal separation anxiety (309.21)*
anxiety states (300.00-300.09)
hospitalism in children (309.83)
phobic state (300.20-300.29)

313.1 Misery and unhappiness disorder
Excludes *depressive neurosis (300.4)*

5 313.2 Sensitivity, shyness, and social withdrawal disorder
Excludes *infantile autism (299.0)*
schizoid personality (301.20-301.22)
schizophrenia (295.0-295.9)

313.21 Shyness disorder of childhood
Sensitivity reaction of childhood or adolescence

313.22 Introverted disorder of childhood
Social withdrawal of childhood or adolescence
Withdrawal reaction of childhood or adolescence

313.23 Selective mutism
Excludes *elective mutism as adjustment reaction (309.83)*

313.3 Relationship problems
Sibling jealousy
Excludes *relationship problems associated with aggression, destruction, or other forms of conduct disturbance (312.0-312.9)*

5 313.8 Other or mixed emotional disturbances of childhood or adolescence

313.81 Oppositional defiant disorder

313.82 Identity disorder
Identity problem

313.83 Academic underachievement disorder

313.89 Other P
Reactive attachment disorder of infancy or early childhood

313.9 Unspecified emotional disturbance of childhood or adolescence P
Mental disorder of infancy, childhood or adolescence NOS

4 314 Hyperkinetic syndrome of childhood
Excludes *hyperkinesis as symptom of underlying disorder - code the underlying disorder*

5 314.0 Attention deficit disorder
Adult
Child

314.00 Without mention of hyperactivity
Predominantly inattentive type
AHA: 1Q 1997, 8

314.01 With hyperactivity
Combined type
Overactivity NOS
Predominantly hyperactive/impulsive type
Simple disturbance of attention with overactivity
AHA: 1Q 1997, 8

314.1 Hyperkinesis with developmental delay
Developmental disorder of hyperkinesis
Use additional code to identify any associated neurological disorder

314.2 Hyperkinetic conduct disorder
Hyperkinetic conduct disorder without developmental delay
Excludes *hyperkinesis with significant delays in specific skills (314.1)*

314.8 Other specified manifestations of hyperkinetic syndrome

314.9 Unspecified hyperkinetic syndrome
Hyperkinetic reaction of childhood or adolescence NOS
Hyperkinetic syndrome NOS

4 315 Specific delays in development
Excludes *that due to a neurological disorder (320.0-389.9)*

5 315.0 Specific reading disorder

315.00 Reading disorder, unspecified

315.01 Alexia

315.02 Developmental dyslexia

315.09 Other
Specific spelling difficulty

315.1 Mathematics disorder
Dyscalculia

315.2 Other specific learning difficulties
Disorder of written expression
Excludes *specific arithmetical disorder (315.1)*
specific reading disorder (315.00-315.09)

5 **315.3 Developmental speech or language disorder**

315.31 Expressive language disorder
Developmental aphasia
Word deafness
Excludes *acquired aphasia (784.3)*
elective mutism (309.83, 313.0, 313.23)

315.32 Mixed receptive-expressive language disorder
▶ Central auditory processing disorder◀
Excludes ▶*acquired auditory processing disorder (388.45)*◀

DEF: Problems comprehending as well as expressing verbal language.

AHA: 2Q 2005, 5; 4Q 1996, 30

● **315.34 Speech and language developmental delay due to hearing loss**
Use additional code to identify type of hearing loss (389.00-389.9)

315.39 Other
Developmental articulation disorder
Dyslalia
Phonological disorder
Excludes *lisping and lalling (307.9)*
stammering and stuttering (307.0)

315.4 Developmental coordination disorder
Clumsiness syndrome
Dyspraxia syndrome
Specific motor development disorder

315.5 Mixed development disorder
AHA: 2Q 2002, 11

315.8 Other specified delays in development

315.9 Unspecified delay in development
Developmental disorder NOS
Learning disorder NOS

316 Psychic factors associated with diseases classified elsewhere
Psychologic factors in physical conditions classified elsewhere
Use additional code to identify the associated physical condition, as:
psychogenic:
asthma (493.9)
dermatitis (692.9)
duodenal ulcer (532.0-532.9)
eczema (691.8, 692.9)
gastric ulcer (531.0-531.9)
mucous colitis (564.9)
paroxysmal tachycardia (427.2)
ulcerative colitis (556)
urticaria (708.0-708.9)
psychosocial dwarfism (259.4)
Excludes *physical symptoms and physiological malfunctions, not involving tissue damage, of mental origin (306.0-306.9)*

MENTAL RETARDATION (317-319)

Use additional code(s) to identify any associated psychiatric or physical condition(s)

317 Mild mental retardation
High-grade defect
IQ 50-70
Mild mental subnormality

4 **318 Other specified mental retardation**

318.0 Moderate mental retardation
IQ 35-49
Moderate mental subnormality

318.1 Severe mental retardation
IQ 20-34
Severe mental subnormality

318.2 Profound mental retardation
IQ under 20
Profound mental subnormality

319 Unspecified mental retardation
Mental deficiency NOS
Mental subnormality NOS

6. DISEASES OF THE NERVOUS SYSTEM AND SENSE ORGANS (320-389)

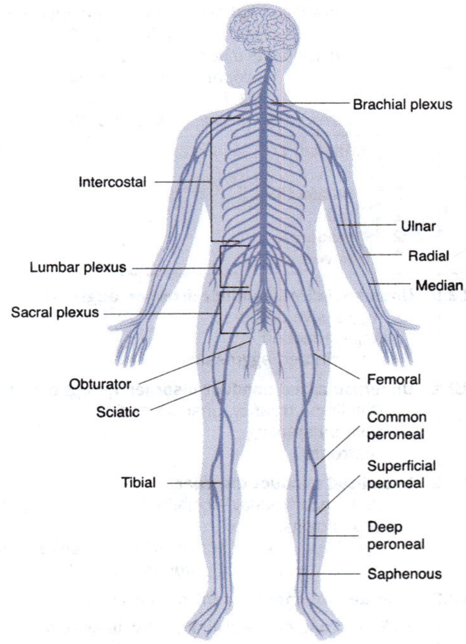

INFLAMMATORY DISEASES OF THE CENTRAL NERVOUS SYSTEM (320-326)

4 **320 Bacterial meningitis**
Includes arachnoiditis bacterial
leptomeningitis bacterial
meningitis bacterial
meningoencephalitis bacterial
meningomyelitis bacterial
pachymeningitis bacterial

DEF: Bacterial infection of the tissues (meninges) surrounding the brain and spinal cord, causing fever, headache, vomiting, malaise, and stiff neck and may progress to confusion, stupor, convulsions, coma, and death.

AHA: Jan-Feb 1987, 6

320.0 Hemophilus meningitis
Meningitis due to Hemophilus influenzae [H. influenzae]
C&C Exclusions: 003.21, 013.00, 013.01, 013.02, 013.03, 013.04, 013.05, 013.06, 013.10, 013.11, 013.12, 013.13, 013.14, 013.15, 013.16, 036.0, 047.0, 047.1, 047.8, 047.9, 049.0, 049.1, 053.0, 054.72, 072.1, 090.42, 091.81, 094.2, 098.89, 100.81, 112.83, 114.2, 115.01, 115.11, 115.91, 130.0, 250.60, 250.61, 250.62, 250.63, 250.80, 250.81, 250.82, 250.83, 250.90, 250.91, 250.92, 250.93, 320.0, 320.1, 320.2, 320.3, 320.7, 320.81, 320.82, 320.89, 320.9, 321.0, 321.1, 321.2, 321.3, 321.4, 321.8, 322.0, 322.1, 322.2, 322.9, 349.89, 349.9, 357.0

320.1 Pneumococcal meningitis
C&C Exclusions: See 320.0

320.2 Streptococcal meningitis
C&C Exclusions: See 320.0

320.3 Staphylococcal meningitis
C&C Exclusions: See 320.0

Meningitis, an infection of the lining of the brain and spinal cord, caused by the bacteria staphylococcus

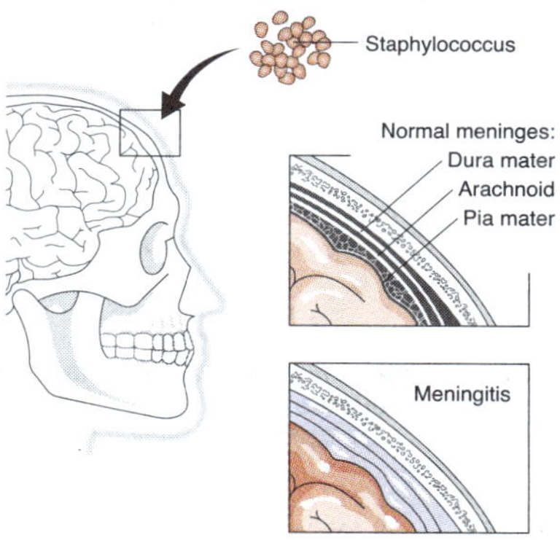

+ ***320.7 Meningitis in other bacterial diseases classified elsewhere***
Code first underlying disease as:
actinomycosis (039.8)
listeriosis (027.0)
typhoid fever (002.0)
whooping cough (033.0-033.9)
Excludes *meningitis (in):*
epidemic (036.0)
gonococcal (098.82)
meningococcal (036.0)
salmonellosis (003.21)
syphilis:
NOS (094.2)
congenital (090.42)
meningovascular (094.2)
secondary (091.81)
tuberculosis (013.0)
C&C Exclusions: See 320.0

5 **320.8 Meningitis due to other specified bacteria**

320.81 Anaerobic meningitis
Bacteroides (fragilis)
Gram-negative anaerobes
C&C Exclusions: See 320.0

320.82 Meningitis due to gram-negative bacteria, not elsewhere classified
Aerobacter aerogenes
Escherichia coli [E. coli]
Friedlander bacillus
Klebsiella pneumoniae
Proteus morganii
Pseudomonas
Excludes *gram-negative anaerobes (320.81)*
C&C Exclusions: See 320.0

320.89 Meningitis due to other specified bacteria
Bacillus pyocyaneus
C&C Exclusions: See 320.0

320.9 Meningitis due to unspecified bacterium
Meningitis:
bacterial NOS
purulent NOS
pyogenic NOS
suppurative NOS
C&C Exclusions: See 320.0

4 **321 Meningitis due to other organisms**
Includes arachnoiditis due to organisms other than bacteria
leptomeningitis due to organisms other than bacteria
meningitis due to organisms other than bacteria
pachymeningitis due to organisms other than bacteria

DEF: Infection of the tissues (meninges) surrounding the brain and spinal cord due to non-bacterial organisms.

AHA: Jan-Feb 1987, 6

+ ***321.0 Cryptococcal meningitis***
Code first underlying disease (117.5)
C&C Exclusions: See 320.0

+ ***321.1 Meningitis in other fungal diseases***
Code first underlying disease (110.0-118)
Excludes *meningitis in:*
candidiasis (112.83)
coccidioidomycosis (114.2)
histoplasmosis (115.01, 115.11, 115.91)
C&C Exclusions: See 320.0

+ ***321.2 Meningitis due to viruses not elsewhere classified***
Code first underlying disease, as:
meningitis due to arbovirus (060.0-066.9)
Excludes *meningitis (due to):*
abacterial (047.0-047.9)
adenovirus (049.1)
aseptic NOS (047.9)
Coxsackie (virus) (047.0)
ECHO virus (047.1)
enterovirus (047.0-047.9)
herpes simplex virus (054.72)
herpes zoster virus (053.0)
lymphocytic choriomeningitis virus (049.0)
mumps (072.1)
viral NOS (047.9)
meningo-eruptive syndrome (047.1)
C&C Exclusions: 003.21, 013.00, 013.01, 013.02, 013.03, 013.04, 013.05, 013.06, 013.10, 013.11, 013.12, 013.13, 013.14, 013.15, 013.16, 036.0, 047.0, 047.1, 047.8, 047.9, 049.0, 049.1, 053.0, 054.72, 072.1, 090.42, 091.81, 094.2, 098.89, 100.81, 112.83, 114.2, 115.01, 115.11, 115.91, 130.0, 320.0, 320.1, 320.2, 320.3, 320.7, 320.81, 320.82, 320.89, 320.9, 321.0, 321.1, 321.2, 321.3, 321.4, 321.8, 322.0, 322.1, 322.2, 322.9, 349.89, 349.9, 357.0
AHA: 4Q 2004, 51

+ ***321.3 Meningitis due to trypanosomiasis***
Code first underlying disease (086.0-086.9)
C&C Exclusions: See 320.0

+ ***321.4 Meningitis in sarcoidosis***
Code first underlying disease (135)
C&C Exclusions: See 320.0

+ ***321.8 Meningitis due to other nonbacterial organisms classified elsewhere***
Code first underlying disease
Excludes *leptospiral meningitis (100.81)*
C&C Exclusions: See 320.0

4 **322 Meningitis of unspecified cause**
Includes arachnoiditis with no organism specified as cause
leptomeningitis with no organism specified as cause
meningitis with no organism specified as cause
pachymeningitis with no organism specified as cause

AHA: Jan-Feb 1987, 6

322.0 Nonpyogenic meningitis
Meningitis with clear cerebrospinal fluid
C&C Exclusions: See 320.0

322.1 Eosinophilic meningitis
C&C Exclusions: See 320.0

322.2 Chronic meningitis
C&C Exclusions: See 320.0

322.9 Meningitis, unspecified
C&C Exclusions: See 320.0

4 323 Encephalitis, myelitis, and encephalomyelitis

Includes acute disseminated encephalomyelitis
meningoencephalitis, except bacterial
meningomyelitis, except bacterial
myelitis:
ascending
transverse

Excludes *acute transverse myelitis NOS (341.20)*
acute transverse myelitis in conditions classified elsewhere (341.21)
bacterial:
meningoencephalitis (320.0-320.9)
meningomyelitis (320.0-320.9)
idiopathic transverse myelitis (341.22)

DEF: Encephalitis: Inflammation of the brain.

DEF: Myelitis: Inflammation of the spinal cord.

DEF: Encephalomyelitis: Inflammation of both the brain and the spinal cord.

5 323.0 Encephalitis, myelitis, and encephalomyelitis in viral diseases classified elsewhere
Code first underlying disease, as:
cat-scratch disease (078.3)
infectious mononucleosis (075)
ornithosis (073.7)

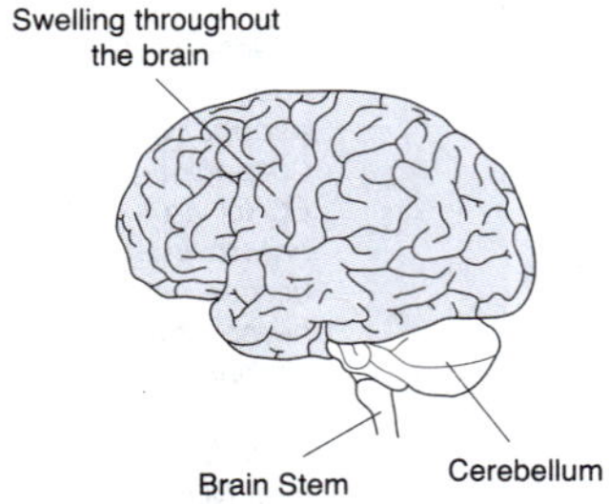

+ *323.01 Encephalitis and encephalomyelitis in viral diseases classified elsewhere*
Excludes *encephalitis (in):*
arthropod-borne viral (062.0-064)
herpes simplex (054.3)
mumps (072.2)
other viral diseases of central nervous system (049.8-049.9)
poliomyelitis (045.0-045.9)
rubella (056.01)
slow virus infections of central nervous system (046.0-046.9)
viral NOS (049.9)
West Nile (066.41)
C&C Exclusions: 052.2, 053.14, 054.74

+ *323.02 Myelitis in viral diseases classified elsewhere*
Excludes *myelitis (in):*
herpes simplex (054.74)
herpes zoster (053.14)
other viral diseases of central nervous system (049.8-049.9)
poliomyelitis (045.0-045.9)
rubella (056.01)
C&C Exclusions: See 323.01

+ *323.1 Encephalitis, myelitis, and encephalomyelitis in rickettsial diseases classified elsewhere*
Code first underlying disease (080-083.9)

+ *323.2 Encephalitis, myelitis, and encephalomyelitis in protozoal diseases classified elsewhere*
Code first underlying disease, as:
malaria (084.0-084.9)
trypanosomiasis (086.0-086.9)

5 323.4 Other encephalitis, myelitis, and encephalomyelitis due to infection classified elsewhere
Code first underlying disease

+ *323.41 Other encephalitis and encephalomyelitis due to infection classified elsewhere*
Excludes *encephalitis (in):*
meningococcal (036.1)
syphilis:
NOS (094.81)
congenital (090.41)
toxoplasmosis (130.0)
tuberculosis (013.6)
meningoencephalitis due to free-living amebae [Naegleria] (136.2)
C&C Exclusions: See 323.01

+ *323.42 Other myelitis due to infection classified elsewhere*
Excludes *myelitis (in):*
syphilis (094.89)
tuberculosis (013.6)
C&C Exclusions: See 323.01

5 323.5 Encephalitis, myelitis, and encephalomyelitis following immunization procedures
Use additional E code to identify vaccine

323.51 Encephalitis and encephalomyelitis following immunization procedures
Encephalitis postimmunization or postvaccinal
Encephalomyelitis postimmunization or postvaccinal
C&C Exclusions: See 323.01

323.52 Myelitis following immunization procedures
Myelitis postimmunization or postvaccinal
C&C Exclusions: See 323.01

5 323.6 Postinfectious encephalitis, myelitis, and encephalomyelitis
Code first underlying disease

+ *323.61 Infectious acute disseminated encephalomyelitis (ADEM)*
Acute necrotizing hemorrhagic encephalopathy
Excludes *noninfectious acute disseminated encephalomyelitis (ADEM) (323.81)*
C&C Exclusions: See 323.01

+ *323.62 Other postinfectious encephalitis and encephalomyelitis*
Excludes *encephalitis:*
postchickenpox (052.0)
postmeasles (055.0)
C&C Exclusions: See 323.01

+ *323.63 Postinfectious myelitis*
Excludes *herpes simplex myelitis (054.74)*
herpes zoster myelitis (053.14)
postchickenpox myelitis (052.2)
C&C Exclusions: See 323.01

5 323.7 Toxic encephalitis, myelitis, and encephalomyelitis
Code first underlying cause, as:
carbon tetrachloride (982.1)
hydroxyquinoline derivatives (961.3)
lead (984.0-984.9)
mercury (985.0)
thallium (985.8)
AHA: 2Q 1997, 8

+ *323.71 Toxic encephalitis and encephalomyelitis*
C&C Exclusions: See 323.01

+ *323.72 Toxic myelitis*
C&C Exclusions: See 323.01

5 323.8 Other causes of encephalitis, myelitis, and encephalomyelitis

323.81 Other causes of encephalitis and encephalomyelitis
Noninfectious acute disseminated encephalomyelitis (ADEM)
C&C Exclusions: See 323.01

323.82 Other causes of myelitis
Transverse myelitis NOS
C&C Exclusions: See 323.01

323.9 Unspecified cause of encephalitis, myelitis, and encephalomyelitis
AHA: 1Q 2006, 8

324 Intracranial and intraspinal abscess

324.0 Intracranial abscess
Abscess (embolic):
cerebellar
cerebral
Abscess (embolic) of brain [any part]:
epidural
extradural
otogenic
subdural
Excludes *tuberculous (013.3)*
C&C Exclusions: 006.5, 013.20, 013.21, 013.22, 013.23, 013.24, 013.25, 013.26, 013.30, 013.31, 013.32, 013.33, 013.34, 013.35, 013.36, 250.60, 250.61, 250.62, 250.63, 250.80, 250.81, 250.82, 250.83, 250.90, 250.91, 250.92, 250.93, 324.0, 324.1, 324.9, 325, 348.8, 348.9

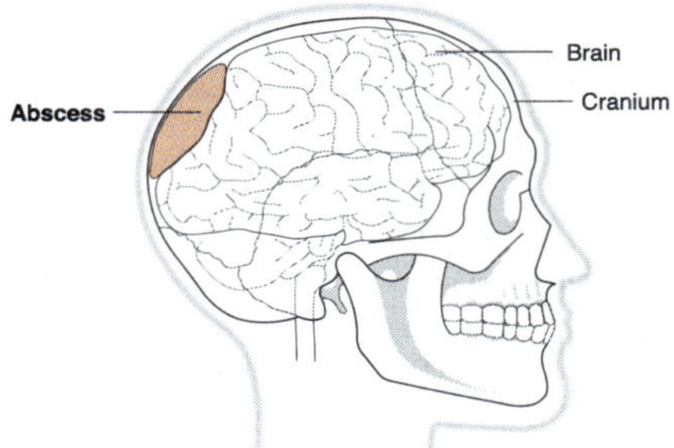

324.1 Intraspinal abscess
Abscess (embolic) of spinal cord [any part]:
epidural
extradural
subdural
Excludes *tuberculous (013.5)*
C&C Exclusions: 006.5, 013.20, 013.21, 013.22, 013.23, 013.24, 013.25, 013.26, 013.30, 013.31, 013.32, 013.33, 013.34, 013.35, 013.36, 250.60, 250.61, 250.62, 250.63, 250.80, 250.81, 250.82, 250.83, 250.90, 250.91, 250.92, 250.93, 324.1

324.9 Of unspecified site
Extradural or subdural abscess NOS
C&C Exclusions: 006.5, 013.20, 013.21, 013.22, 013.23, 013.24, 013.25, 013.26, 013.30, 013.31, 013.32, 013.33, 013.34, 013.35, 013.36, 250.60, 250.61, 250.62, 250.63, 250.80, 250.81, 250.82, 250.83, 250.90, 250.91, 250.92, 250.93, 324.0, 324.1, 324.9, 325

325 Phlebitis and thrombophlebitis of intracranial venous sinuses
Embolism of cavernous, lateral, or other intracranial or unspecified intracranial venous sinus
Endophlebitis of cavernous, lateral, or other intracranial or unspecified intracranial venous sinus
Phlebitis, septic or suppurative of cavernous, lateral, or other intracranial or unspecified intracranial venous sinus
Thrombophlebitis of cavernous, lateral, or other intracranial or unspecified intracranial venous sinus
Thrombosis of cavernous, lateral, or other intracranial or unspecified intracranial venous sinus
Excludes *that specified as:*
complicating pregnancy, childbirth, or the puerperium (671.5)
of nonpyogenic origin (437.6)
DEF: Inflammation and/or blood clot formation in a large vein or channel for venous blood circulation in the brain.

326 Late effects of intracranial abscess or pyogenic infection
Note: *This category is to be used to indicate conditions whose primary classification is to 320-325 [excluding 320.7, 321.0-321.8, 323.01-323.42, 323.61-323.72] as the cause of late effects, themselves classifiable elsewhere. The "late effects" include conditions specified as such, or as sequelae, which may occur at any time after the resolution of the causal condition.*
Use additional code to identify condition, as:
hydrocephalus (331.4)
paralysis (342.0-342.9, 344.0-344.9)

ORGANIC SLEEP DISORDERS (327)

327 Organic sleep disorders
AHA: 4Q 2005, 59-64

327.0 Organic disorders of initiating and maintaining sleep [Organic insomnia]
Excludes *insomnia NOS (780.52)*
insomnia not due to a substance or known physiological condition (307.41-307.42)
insomnia with sleep apnea NOS (780.51)

327.00 Organic insomnia, unspecified

327.01 Insomnia due to medical condition classified elsewhere
Code first underlying condition
Excludes *insomnia due to mental disorder (327.02)*

327.02 Insomnia due to mental disorder
Code first mental disorder
Excludes *alcohol-induced insomnia (291.82)*
drug-induced insomnia (292.85)

327.09 Other organic insomnia

327.1 Organic disorders of excessive somnolence [Organic hypersomnia]
Excludes *hypersomnia NOS (780.54)*
hypersomnia not due to a substance or known physiological condition (307.43-307.44)
hypersomnia with sleep apnea NOS (780.53)

327.10 Organic hypersomnia, unspecified

327.11 Idiopathic hypersomnia with long sleep time

327.12 Idiopathic hypersomnia without long sleep time

327.13 Recurrent hypersomnia
Kleine-Levin syndrome
Menstrual related hypersomnia

327.14 Hypersomnia due to medical condition classified elsewhere
Code first underlying condition
Excludes *hypersomnia due to mental disorder (327.15)*

327.15 Hypersomnia due to mental disorder
Code first mental disorder
Excludes *alcohol-induced hypersomnia (291.82)*
drug-induced hypersomnia (292.85)

327.19 Other organic hypersomnia

327.2 Organic sleep apnea
Excludes *Cheyne-Stokes breathing (786.04)*
hypersomnia with sleep apnea NOS (780.53)
insomnia with sleep apnea NOS (780.51)
sleep apnea in newborn (770.81-770.82)
sleep apnea NOS (780.57)

327.20 Organic sleep apnea, unspecified

327.21 Primary central sleep apnea

327.22 High altitude periodic breathing

327.23 Obstructive sleep apnea (adult) (pediatric)

327.24 Idiopathic sleep related nonobstructive alveolar hypoventilation
Sleep related hypoxia

327.25 Congenital central alveolar hypoventilation syndrome

327.26 Sleep related hypoventilation/hypoxemia in conditions classified elsewhere
Code first underlying condition

327.27 Central sleep apnea in conditions classified elsewhere
Code first underlying condition

327.29 Other organic sleep apnea

Nervous System and Sense Organs
323.9 – 327.29

327.3 Circadian rhythm sleep disorder
Organic disorder of sleep-wake cycle
Organic disorder of sleep-wake schedule
Excludes *alcohol-induced circadian rhythm sleep disorder (291.82)*
circadian rhythm sleep disorder of nonorganic origin (307.45)
disruption of 24 hour sleep wake cycle NOS (780.55)
drug-induced circadian rhythm sleep disorder (292.85)

327.30 Circadian rhythm sleep disorder, unspecified

327.31 Circadian rhythm sleep disorder, delayed sleep phase type

327.32 Circadian rhythm sleep disorder, advanced sleep phase type

327.33 Circadian rhythm sleep disorder, irregular sleep-wake type

327.34 Circadian rhythm sleep disorder, free-running type

327.35 Circadian rhythm sleep disorder, jet lag type

327.36 Circadian rhythm sleep disorder, shift work type

+ ***327.37 Circadian rhythm sleep disorder in conditions classified elsewhere***
Code first underlying condition

327.39 Other circadian rhythm sleep disorder

327.4 Organic parasomnia
Excludes *alcohol-induced parasomnia (291.82)*
drug-induced parasomnia (292.85)
parasomnia not due to a known physiological condition (307.47)

327.40 Organic parasomnia, unspecified

327.41 Confusional arousals

327.42 REM sleep behavior disorder

327.43 Recurrent isolated sleep paralysis

+ ***327.44 Parasomnia in conditions classified elsewhere***
Code first underlying condition

327.49 Other organic parasomnia

327.5 Organic sleep related movement disorders
Excludes *restless legs syndrome (333.94)*
sleep related movement disorder NOS (780.58)

327.51 Periodic limb movement disorder
Periodic limb movement sleep disorder
DEF: Involuntary limb movement or jerking during or just before sleep.

327.52 Sleep related leg cramps

327.53 Sleep related bruxism
DEF: Grinding the teeth during sleep.

327.59 Other organic sleep related movement disorders

327.8 Other organic sleep disorders

HEREDITARY AND DEGENERATIVE DISEASES OF THE CENTRAL NERVOUS SYSTEM (330-337)

Excludes *hepatolenticular degeneration (275.1)*
multiple sclerosis (340)
other demyelinating diseases of central nervous system (341.0-341.9)

330 Cerebral degenerations usually manifest in childhood
Use additional code to identify associated mental retardation

330.0 Leukodystrophy
Krabbe's disease
Leukodystrophy:
NOS
globoid cell
metachromatic
sudanophilic
Pelizaeus-Merzbacher disease
Sulfatide lipidosis

330.1 Cerebral lipidoses
Amaurotic (familial) idiocy
Disease:
Batten
Jansky-Bielschowsky
Kufs'
Spielmeyer-Vogt
Tay-Sachs
Gangliosidosis

+ ***330.2 Cerebral degeneration in generalized lipidoses***
Code first underlying disease, as:
Fabry's disease (272.7)
Gaucher's disease (272.7)
Niemann-Pick disease (272.7)
sphingolipidosis (272.7)

+ ***330.3 Cerebral degeneration of childhood in other diseases classified elsewhere***
Code first underlying disease, as:
Hunter's disease (277.5)
mucopolysaccharidosis (277.5)

330.8 Other specified cerebral degenerations in childhood
Alpers' disease or gray-matter degeneration
Infantile necrotizing encephalomyelopathy
Leigh's disease
Subacute necrotizing encephalopathy or encephalomyelopathy
AHA: Nov-Dec 1985, 5

330.9 Unspecified cerebral degeneration in childhood

331 Other cerebral degenerations
▶ Use additional code, where applicable, to identify:◀
▶ with behavioral disturbance (294.11)◀
▶ without behavioral disturbance (294.10)◀

331.0 Alzheimer's disease
DEF: Progressive degenerative disease of the brain of unknown cause with diffuse atrophy throughout the cerebral cortex; it initially presents with slight memory disturbance or personality changes that progressively deteriorate to profound memory loss and dementia.
AHA: 4Q 2000, 41; 4Q 1999, 7; Nov-Dec 1984, 20

331.1 Frontotemporal dementia
Use additional code for associated behavioral disturbances (294.10-294.11)
AHA: 4Q 2003, 57

331.11 Pick's disease
DEF: Rare, progressive, degenerative disease of the brain, similar to Alzheimer's disease but with cortical atrophy confined to the frontal and temporal lobes.

331.19 Other frontotemporal dementia
Frontal dementia

331.2 Senile degeneration of brain
Excludes *senility NOS (797)*

331.3 Communicating hydrocephalus
▶ Secondary normal pressure hydrocephalus◀
Excludes *congenital hydrocephalus (742.3)*
▶ *idiopathic normal pressure hydrocephalus (331.5)*◀
▶ *normal pressure hydrocephalus (331.5)*◀
▶ *spina bifida with hydrocephalus (741.0)*◀
AHA: Sep-Oct 1985, 12

331.4 Obstructive hydrocephalus
Acquired hydrocephalus NOS
Excludes *congenital hydrocephalus (742.3)*
▶ *idiopathic normal pressure hydrocephalus (331.5)*◀
▶ *normal pressure hydrocephalus (331.5)*◀
▶ *spina bifida with hydrocephalus (741.0)*◀
C&C Exclusions: 250.60, 250.61, 250.62, 250.63, 250.80, 250.81, 250.82, 250.83, 250.90, 250.91, 250.92, 250.93, 331.3, 331.4, 331.7, 331.89, 331.9, 348.8, 348.9, 741.00, 741.01, 741.02, 741.03, 742.3, 742.4, 742.59, 742.8, 742.9
AHA: 4Q 2003, 106; 1Q 1999, 9

● **331.5 Idiopathic normal pressure hydrocephalus (INPH)**
Normal pressure hydrocephalus NOS
Excludes *congenital hydrocephalus (742.3)*
secondary normal pressure hydrocephalus (331.3)
spina bifida with hydrocephalus (741.0)

DEF: Disruption of normal cerebrospinal fluid circulation and gradual ventricular enlargement without known cause resulting in abnormal gait, cognitive impairment, and urinary incontinence.

+ ***331.7 Cerebral degeneration in diseases classified elsewhere***
Code first underlying disease, as:
alcoholism (303.0-303.9)
beriberi (265.0)
cerebrovascular disease (430-438)
congenital hydrocephalus (741.0, 742.3)
neoplastic disease (140.0-239.9)
myxedema (244.0-244.9)
vitamin B_{12} deficiency (266.2)
Excludes *cerebral degeneration in:*
Jakob-Creutzfeldt disease (046.1)
progressive multifocal leukoencephalopathy (046.3)
subacute spongiform encephalopathy (046.1)

5 **331.8 Other cerebral degeneration**

331.81 Reye's syndrome P
DEF: Rare, acute, sometimes fatal disease of childhood with recurrent vomiting, elevated serum transaminase levels, and liver changes, followed by acute brain swelling, disturbances of consciousness, and seizures.

331.82 Dementia with Lewy bodies
Dementia with Parkinsonism
Lewy body dementia
Lewy body disease
Use additional code for associated behavioral disturbances (294.10-294.11)
C&C Exclusions: 331.4
AHA: 4Q 2003, 57

331.83 Mild cognitive impairment, so stated
Excludes *altered mental status (780.97)*
cerebral degeneration (331.0-331.9)
change in mental status (780.97)
cognitive deficits following (late effects of) cerebral hemorrhage or infarction (438.0)
cognitive impairment due to intracranial or head injury (850-854, 959.01)
cognitive impairment due to late effect of intracranial injury (907.0)
dementia (290.0-290.43, 294.8)
mild memory disturbance (310.8)
neurologic neglect syndrome (781.8)
personality change, nonpsychotic (310.1)
DEF: Impairment in memory or other specific cognitive function, beyond what is normally seen at a given age, but with function remaining relatively intact in the other cognitive domains.
C&C Exclusions: See 331.82

331.89 Other
Cerebral ataxia

✖ **331.9 Cerebral degeneration, unspecified**

4 **332 Parkinson's disease**
Excludes *dementia with Parkinsonism (331.82)*

332.0 Paralysis agitans
Parkinsonism or Parkinson's disease:
NOS
idiopathic
primary
AHA: Mar-Apr 1987, 7

332.1 Secondary Parkinsonism
Neuroleptic-induced Parkinsonism
Parkinsonism due to drugs
Use additional E code to identify drug, if drug-induced
Excludes *Parkinsonism (in):*
Huntington's disease (333.4)
progressive supranuclear palsy (333.0)
Shy-Drager syndrome (333.0)
syphilitic (094.82)

4 **333 Other extrapyramidal disease and abnormal movement disorders**
Includes other forms of extrapyramidal, basal ganglia, or striatopallidal disease
Excludes *abnormal movements of head NOS (781.0)*
sleep related movement disorders (327.51-327.59)

333.0 Other degenerative diseases of the basal ganglia
Atrophy or degeneration:
olivopontocerebellar [Déjérine-Thomas syndrome]
pigmentary pallidal [Hallervorden-Spatz disease]
striatonigral
Parkinsonian syndrome associated with:
idiopathic orthostatic hypotension
symptomatic orthostatic hypotension
Progressive supranuclear ophthalmoplegia
Shy-Drager syndrome
AHA: 3Q 1996, 8

333.1 Essential and other specified forms of tremor
Benign essential tremor
Familial tremor
Medication-induced postural tremor
Use additional E code to identify drug, if drug-induced
Excludes *tremor NOS (781.0)*

333.2 Myoclonus
Familial essential myoclonus
Progressive myoclonic epilepsy
Unverricht-Lundborg disease
Use additional E code to identify drug, if drug-induced
DEF: Spontaneous contractions of a muscle or group of muscles as part of a disease process, drug side effect, or normal physiological response.
AHA: 3Q 1997, 4; Mar-Apr 1987, 12

333.3 Tics of organic origin
Use additional E code to identify drug, if drug-induced
Excludes *Gilles de la Tourette's syndrome (307.23)*
habit spasm (307.22)
tic NOS (307.20)

333.4 Huntington's chorea

333.5 Other choreas
Hemiballism(us)
Paroxysmal choreo-athetosis
Use additional E code to identify drug, if drug-induced
Excludes *Sydenham's or rheumatic chorea (392.0-392.9)*

333.6 Genetic torsion dystonia
Dystonia:
deformans progressiva
musculorum deformans
(Schwalbe-) Ziehen-Oppenheim disease

5 **333.7 Acquired torsion dystonia**

333.71 Athetoid cerebral palsy
Double athetosis (syndrome)
Vogt's disease
Excludes *infantile cerebral palsy (343.0-343.9)*
DEF: Permanent, nonprogressive, motor disorder caused by brain damage from birth trauma or intrauterine pathology and characterized by uncontrolled, writhing movements of the hands, feet, arms, or legs.
C&C Exclusions: 781.7

333.72 Acute dystonia due to drugs
Acute dystonic reaction due to drugs
Neuroleptic induced acute dystonia
Use additional E code to identify drug
Excludes *blepharospasm due to drugs (333.85)*
orofacial dyskinesia due to drugs (333.85)
secondary Parkinsonism (332.1)
subacute dyskinesia due to drugs (333.85)
tardive dyskinesia (333.85)
C&C Exclusions: See 333.71

333.79 Other acquired torsion dystonia
C&C Exclusions: See 333.71

5 **333.8 Fragments of torsion dystonia**
Use additional E code to identify drug, if drug-induced

333.81 Blepharospasm
Excludes *blepharospasm due to drugs (333.85)*
DEF: Spasm of the orbicularis oculi muscle, causing uncontrolled winking or blinking.

333.82 Orofacial dyskinesia
Excludes *orofacial dyskinesia due to drugs (333.85)*

333.83 Spasmodic torticollis
Excludes *torticollis:*
NOS (723.5)
hysterical (300.11)
psychogenic (306.0)
DEF: Contractions of the neck muscles causing uncontrolled head movements.

333.84 Organic writers' cramp
Excludes *psychogenic (300.89)*

333.85 Subacute dyskinesia due to drugs
Blepharospasm due to drugs
Orofacial dyskinesia due to drugs
Tardive dyskinesia
Use additional E code to identify drug
Excludes *acute dystonia due to drugs (333.72)*
acute dystonic reaction due to drugs (333.72)
secondary Parkinsonism (332.1)
C&C Exclusions: See 333.71
AHA: 4Q 2006, 78

333.89 Other

5 **333.9 Other and unspecified extrapyramidal diseases and abnormal movement disorders**

333.90 Unspecified extrapyramidal disease and abnormal movement disorder
Medication-induced movement disorders NOS
Use additional E code to identify drug, if drug-induced

333.91 Stiff-man syndrome
DEF: Progressive fluctuating rigidity of axial and limb muscles in the absence of any signs of cerebral and/or spinal cord disease.

333.92 Neuroleptic malignant syndrome
Use additional E code to identify drug
Excludes *neuroleptic induced Parkinsonism (332.1)*
AHA: 4Q 1994, 37

333.93 Benign shuddering attacks
DEF: Mild, non-disabling, non-dangerous, epileptic-like muscle spasms which last 5-15 seconds.
AHA: 4Q 1994, 37

333.94 Restless legs syndrome (RLS)
DEF: Irresistible urge to move the legs, particularly when sitting or lying down, with leg sensations such as creeping, crawling, itching, tugging, tightening, or pulling alleviated upon movement.

333.99 Other
Neuroleptic-induced acute akathisia
Use additional E code to identify drug, if drug-induced
AHA: 4Q 2004, 95; 2Q 2004, 12; 4Q 1994, 37

4 **334 Spinocerebellar disease**
Excludes *olivopontocerebellar degeneration (333.0)*
peroneal muscular atrophy (356.1)

334.0 Friedreich's ataxia

334.1 Hereditary spastic paraplegia
DEF: Hereditary disorder characterized by lower-limb spasticity and near total loss of joint flexibility while the upper limbs remain unaffected.

334.2 Primary cerebellar degeneration
Cerebellar ataxia:
Marie's
Sanger-Brown
Dyssynergia cerebellaris myoclonica
Primary cerebellar degeneration:
NOS
hereditary
sporadic
AHA: Mar-Apr 1987, 9

334.3 Other cerebellar ataxia
Cerebellar ataxia NOS
Use additional E code to identify drug, if drug-induced

+ ***334.4 Cerebellar ataxia in diseases classified elsewhere***
Code first underlying disease, as:
alcoholism (303.0-303.9)
myxedema (244.0-244.9)
neoplastic disease (140.0-239.9)

334.8 Other spinocerebellar diseases
Ataxia-telangiectasia [Louis-Bar syndrome]
Corticostriatal-spinal degeneration

✖ **334.9 Spinocerebellar disease, unspecified**

4 **335 Anterior horn cell disease**

335.0 Werdnig-Hoffmann disease
Infantile spinal muscular atrophy
Progressive muscular atrophy of infancy
C&C Exclusions: 250.60, 250.61, 250.62, 250.63, 250.80, 250.81, 250.82, 250.83, 250.90, 250.91, 250.92, 250.93, 334.8, 334.9, 335.0, 335.10, 335.11, 335.19, 335.20, 335.21, 335.22, 335.23, 335.24, 335.29, 335.8, 335.9, 336.0, 336.1, 336.2, 336.3, 336.8, 336.9, 337.0, 337.1, 337.20, 337.21, 337.22, 337.29, 337.3, 337.9, 349.89, 349.9

5 **335.1 Spinal muscular atrophy**

335.10 Spinal muscular atrophy, unspecified
C&C Exclusions: See 335.0

335.11 Kugelberg-Welander disease
Spinal muscular atrophy:
familial
juvenile
C&C Exclusions: See 335.0

335.19 Other
Adult spinal muscular atrophy
C&C Exclusions: See 335.0

335.2 Motor neuron disease

335.20 Amyotrophic lateral sclerosis A

Motor neuron disease (bulbar) (mixed type)

C&C Exclusions: See 335.0

AHA: 4Q 1995, 81

Amyotrophic lateral sclerosis (ALS)

Also known as Lou Gehrig's Disease, ALS is caused by the degeneration and death of motor neurons in the spinal cord and brain

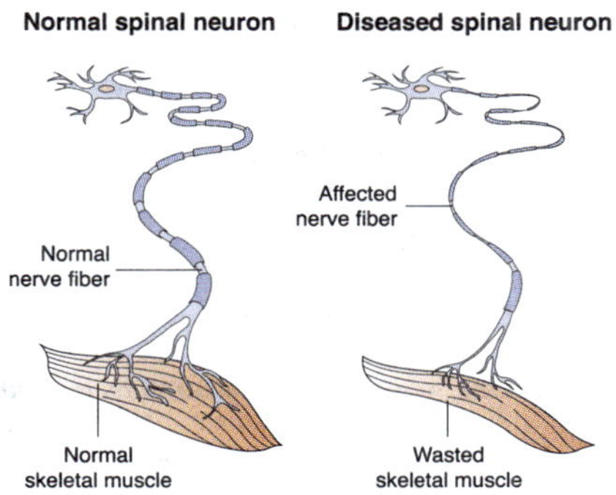

335.21 Progressive muscular atrophy

Duchenne-Aran muscular atrophy
Progressive muscular atrophy (pure)

C&C Exclusions: See 335.0

335.22 Progressive bulbar palsy

C&C Exclusions: See 335.0

335.23 Pseudobulbar palsy

DEF: Spastic weakness of the muscles associated with the cranial nerves (e.g., muscles of the face, pharynx, and tongue) due to lesions of the corticospinal tract.

C&C Exclusions: See 335.0

335.24 Primary lateral sclerosis

C&C Exclusions: See 335.0

335.29 Other

C&C Exclusions: See 335.0

335.8 Other anterior horn cell diseases

C&C Exclusions: See 335.0

335.9 Anterior horn cell disease, unspecified

C&C Exclusions: See 335.0

336 Other diseases of spinal cord

336.0 Syringomyelia and syringobulbia

DEF: Cyst formation within the spinal cord resulting from trauma, hemorrhage, meningitis, tumor, or Chiari I malformation. The cyst grows, destroying the cord's center and causing neurologic deficits that progress to greater degrees when not treated surgically.

AHA: 1Q 1989, 10

336.1 Vascular myelopathies

Acute infarction of spinal cord (embolic) (nonembolic)
Arterial thrombosis of spinal cord
Edema of spinal cord
Hematomyelia
Subacute necrotic myelopathy

+ ***336.2 Subacute combined degeneration of spinal cord in diseases classified elsewhere***

Code first underlying disease, as:
other vitamin B_{12} deficiency anemia (281.1)
pernicious anemia (281.0)
vitamin B_{12} deficiency (266.2)

+ ***336.3 Myelopathy in other diseases classified elsewhere***

Code first underlying disease, as:
myelopathy in neoplastic disease (140.0-239.9)

Excludes *myelopathy in:*
intervertebral disc disorder (722.70-722.73)
spondylosis (721.1, 721.41-721.42, 721.91)

AHA: 3Q 1999, 5

336.8 Other myelopathy

Myelopathy:
drug-induced
radiation-induced
Use additional E code to identify cause

336.9 Unspecified disease of spinal cord

Cord compression NOS
Myelopathy NOS

Excludes *myelitis (323.02, 323.1, 323.2, 323.42, 323.52, 323.63, 323.72, 323.82, 323.9)*
spinal (canal) stenosis (723.0, 724.00-724.09)

337 Disorders of the autonomic nervous system

Includes disorders of peripheral autonomic, sympathetic, parasympathetic, or vegetative system

Excludes *familial dysautonomia [Riley-Day syndrome] (742.8)*

337.0 Idiopathic peripheral autonomic neuropathy

Carotid sinus syncope or syndrome
Cervical sympathetic dystrophy or paralysis

DEF: Carotid sinus syncope: spontaneous syncope due to overactivity of the carotid sinus reflex or syncope produced by pressure applied to one or both carotid sinuses.

+ ***337.1 Peripheral autonomic neuropathy in disorders classified elsewhere***

Code first underlying disease, as:
amyloidosis (277.30-277.39)
diabetes (250.6)

AHA: 2Q 1993, 6; 3Q 1991, 9; Nov-Dec 1984, 9

337.2 Reflex sympathetic dystrophy

AHA: 4Q 1993, 24

337.20 Reflex sympathetic dystrophy, unspecified

337.21 Reflex sympathetic dystrophy of the upper limb

337.22 Reflex sympathetic dystrophy of the lower limb

337.29 Reflex sympathetic dystrophy of other specified site

337.3 Autonomic dysreflexia

Use additional code to identify the cause, such as:
decubitus ulcer (707.00-707.09)
fecal impaction (560.39)
urinary tract infection (599.0)

AHA: 4Q 1998, 37

337.9 Unspecified disorder of autonomic nervous system

PAIN (338)

338 Pain, not elsewhere classified

Use additional code to identify:
pain associated with psychological factors (307.89)

Excludes *generalized pain (780.96)*
localized pain, unspecified type - code to pain by site
pain disorder exclusively attributed to psychological factors (307.80)

AHA: 2Q, 2007, 15

338.0 Central pain syndrome

Déjérine-Roussy syndrome
Myelopathic pain syndrome
Thalamic pain syndrome (hyperesthetic)

C&C Exclusions: 040.82, 440.24, 780.01, 780.03, 780.1, 780.31, 780.32, 780.39, 781.7, 785.4, 785.50, 785.51, 785.52, 785.59, 786.3, 788.20, 788.29, 789.5, 790.7, 791.1, 791.3, 799.01, 799.02, 799.1, 799.4

338.1 Acute pain

338.11 Acute pain due to trauma

C&C Exclusions: See 338.0

338.12 Acute post-thoracotomy pain

Post-thoracotomy pain NOS

C&C Exclusions: See 338.0

338.18 Other acute postoperative pain

Postoperative pain NOS

C&C Exclusions: See 338.0

338.19 Other acute pain
Excludes neoplasm related acute pain (338.3)
C&C Exclusions: See 338.0
AHA: 2Q, 2007, 14

❺ **338.2 Chronic pain**
Excludes causalgia (355.9):
lower limb (355.71)
upper limb (354.4)
chronic pain syndrome (338.4)
myofascial pain syndrome (729.1)
neoplasm related chronic pain (338.3)
reflex sympathetic dystrophy (337.20-337.29)

338.21 Chronic pain due to trauma
C&C Exclusions: See 338.0

338.22 Chronic post-thoracotomy pain
C&C Exclusions: See 338.0

338.28 Other chronic postoperative pain
C&C Exclusions: See 338.0

338.29 Other chronic pain
C&C Exclusions: See 338.0

338.3 Neoplasm related pain (acute) (chronic)
Cancer associated pain
Pain due to malignancy (primary) (secondary)
Tumor associated pain
C&C Exclusions: See 338.0
AHA: 2Q, 2007, 14

338.4 Chronic pain syndrome
Chronic pain associated with significant psychosocial dysfunction
C&C Exclusions: See 338.0
AHA: 2Q, 2007, 14

OTHER DISORDERS OF THE CENTRAL NERVOUS SYSTEM (340-349)

340 Multiple sclerosis
Disseminated or multiple sclerosis:
NOS
brain stem
cord
generalized
C&C Exclusions: 250.60, 250.61, 250.62, 250.63, 250.80, 250.81, 250.82, 250.83, 250.90, 250.91, 250.92, 250.93, 340, 341.8, 341.9

Multiple sclerosis (MS)

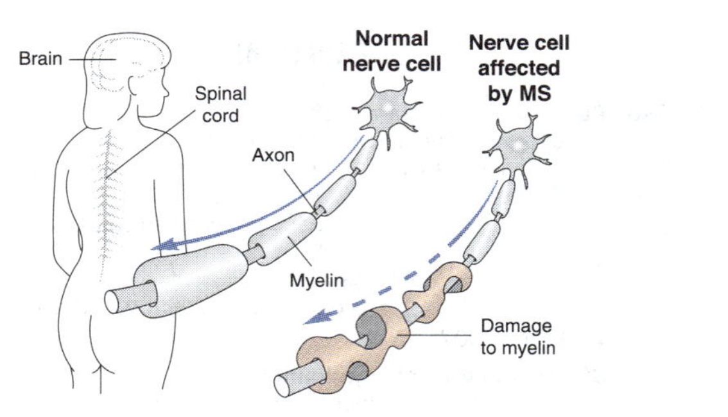

❹ **341 Other demyelinating diseases of central nervous system**

341.0 Neuromyelitis optica

341.1 Schilder's disease
Balo's concentric sclerosis
Encephalitis periaxialis:
concentrica [Balo's]
diffusa [Schilder's]
DEF: Leukoencephalopathy with massive destruction of the brain's white matter, cavity formation, and glial scarring, causing blindness, deafness, spasticity, and progressive mental deterioration.

❺ **341.2 Acute (transverse) myelitis**
Excludes acute (transverse) myelitis (in) (due to):
following immunization procedures (323.52)
infection classified elsewhere (323.42)
postinfectious (323.63)
protozoal diseases classified elsewhere (323.2)
rickettsial diseases classified elsewhere (323.1)
toxic (323.72)
viral diseases classified elsewhere (323.02)
transverse myelitis NOS (323.82)
DEF: Spinal cord disorder with inflammatory lesions across the entire width of one level; numbness, back pain, weakness, sensory loss, motor and sphincter deficits, loss of bladder and bowel control appear quickly and progress to paraplegia.

✖ **341.20 Acute (transverse) myelitis NOS**
C&C Exclusions: 052.2, 053.14, 054.74, 349.82

✚ ***341.21 Acute (transverse) myelitis in conditions classified elsewhere***
Code first underlying condition
C&C Exclusions: See 341.20

341.22 Idiopathic transverse myelitis
C&C Exclusions: See 341.20

341.8 Other demyelinating diseases of central nervous system
Central demyelination of corpus callosum
Central pontine myelinosis
Marchiafava (-Bignami) disease
AHA: Nov-Dec 1987, 6

✖ **341.9 Demyelinating disease of central nervous system, unspecified**

❹ **342 Hemiplegia and hemiparesis**
Note: This category is to be used when hemiplegia (complete) (incomplete) is reported without further specification, or is stated to be old or long-standing but of unspecified cause. The category is also for use in multiple coding to identify these types of hemiplegia resulting from any cause.
Excludes congenital (343.1)
hemiplegia due to late effect of cerebrovascular accident (438.20-438.22)
infantile NOS (343.4)
AHA: 4Q 1994, 38

The following fifth-digits are for use with codes 342.0-342.9
0 affecting unspecified side
1 affecting dominant side
2 affecting nondominant side

❺ **342.0 Flaccid hemiplegia**

❺ **342.1 Spastic hemiplegia**

❺ **342.8 Other specified hemiplegia**

❺ **342.9 Hemiplegia, unspecified**
AHA: 4Q 1998, 87

4 343 Infantile cerebral palsy

Includes
cerebral:
palsy NOS
spastic infantile paralysis
congenital spastic paralysis (cerebral)
Little's disease
paralysis (spastic) due to birth injury:
intracranial
spinal

Excludes
athetoid cerebral palsy (333.71)
hereditary cerebral paralysis, such as:
hereditary spastic paraplegia (334.1)
Vogt's disease (333.71)
spastic paralysis specified as noncongenital or noninfantile (344.0-344.9)

DEF: Group of persisting, nonprogressive motor disorders, sometimes with cognitive defects, appearing in young children as a result of brain damage from birth trauma or intrauterine pathology.

343.0 Diplegic
Congenital diplegia
Congenital paraplegia
DEF: Palsy affecting one set of limbs on both sides of the body (e.g., both arms or both legs).

343.1 Hemiplegic
Congenital hemiplegia
Excludes *infantile hemiplegia NOS (343.4)*
DEF: Palsy affecting the limbs on either the left or right side (e.g., the right arm and right leg).

343.2 Quadriplegic
Tetraplegic
DEF: Palsy presenting with paralysis of all four limbs.
C&C Exclusions: 250.60, 250.61, 250.62, 250.63, 250.80, 250.81, 250.82, 250.83, 250.90, 250.91, 250.92, 250.93, 342.00, 342.01, 342.02, 342.10, 342.11, 342.12, 342.80, 342.81, 342.82, 342.90, 342.91, 342.92, 343.0, 343.1, 343.2, 343.3, 343.4, 343.8, 343.9, 344.00, 344.01, 344.02, 344.03, 344.04, 344.09, 344.1, 344.2, 344.30, 344.31, 344.32, 344.40, 344.41, 344.42, 344.5, 344.6, 344.60, 344.61, 344.9, 348.8, 348.9, 349.89, 742.59, 742.8, 742.9

343.3 Monoplegic

343.4 Infantile hemiplegia
Infantile hemiplegia (postnatal) NOS

343.8 Other specified infantile cerebral palsy

✖ **343.9 Infantile cerebral palsy, unspecified**
Cerebral palsy NOS
AHA: 4Q 2005, 1989

4 344 Other paralytic syndromes

Note: *This category is to be used when the listed conditions are reported without further specification or are stated to be old or long-standing but of unspecified cause. The category is also for use in multiple coding to identify these conditions resulting from any cause.*

Includes
paralysis (complete) (incomplete), except as classifiable to 342 and 343

Excludes
congenital or infantile cerebral palsy (343.0-343.9)
hemiplegia (342.0-342.9)
congenital or infantile (343.1, 343.4)

5 344.0 Quadriplegia and quadriparesis

344.00 Quadriplegia, unspecified
C&C Exclusions: See 343.2
AHA: 4Q 2003, 103; 4Q 1998, 38

344.01 C_1-C_4, complete
C&C Exclusions: See 343.2

344.02 C_1-C_4, incomplete
C&C Exclusions: See 343.2

344.03 C_5-C_7, complete
C&C Exclusions: See 343.2

344.04 C_5-C_7, incomplete
C&C Exclusions: See 343.2

344.09 Other
C&C Exclusions: See 343.2
AHA: 1Q 2001, 12; 4Q 1998, 39

344.1 Paraplegia
Paralysis of both lower limbs
Paraplegia (lower)
AHA: 4Q 2003, 110; Mar-Apr 1987, 10

344.2 Diplegia of upper limbs
Diplegia (upper)
Paralysis of both upper limbs

5 344.3 Monoplegia of lower limb
Paralysis of lower limb
Excludes *monoplegia of lower limb due to late effect of cerebrovascular accident (438.40-438.42)*

344.30 Affecting unspecified side

344.31 Affecting dominant side

344.32 Affecting nondominant side

5 344.4 Monoplegia of upper limb
Paralysis of upper limb
Excludes *monoplegia of upper limb due to late effect of cerebrovascular accident (438.30-438.32)*

344.40 Affecting unspecified side

344.41 Affecting dominant side

344.42 Affecting nondominant side

344.5 Unspecified monoplegia

5 344.6 Cauda equina syndrome
DEF: Compression of spinal nerve roots causing dull aching pain in the perineum, bladder, and sacrum with associated paresthesias and/or paralysis.

344.60 Without mention of neurogenic bladder

344.61 With neurogenic bladder
Acontractile bladder
Autonomic hyperreflexia of bladder
Cord bladder
Detrusor hyperreflexia
C&C Exclusions: 599.60, 599.69
AHA: May-Jun 1987, 12; Mar-Apr 1987, 10

5 344.8 Other specified paralytic syndromes

344.81 Locked-in state
DEF: Condition in which a person remains conscious and retains normal cognitive function, but loses all power of movement, except for the eyes.
AHA: 4Q 1993, 24

344.89 Other specified paralytic syndrome
AHA: 2Q 1999, 4

✖ **344.9 Paralysis, unspecified**

4 345 Epilepsy and recurrent seizures
Excludes *progressive myoclonic epilepsy (333.2)*
AHA: 1Q 1993 24; 2Q 1992, 8; 4Q 1992, 23

The following fifth-digit subclassification is for use with categories 345.0, 345.1, 345.4-345.9:
0 without mention of intractable epilepsy
1 with intractable epilepsy

5 345.0 Generalized nonconvulsive epilepsy
Absences:
atonic
typical
Minor epilepsy
Petit mal
Pykno-epilepsy
Seizures:
akinetic
atonic
C&C Exclusions: (for code 345.00) 780.32
C&C Exclusions: (for code 345.01) 250.60, 250.61, 250.62, 250.63, 345.00, 345.01, 345.10, 345.11, 345.2, 345.3, 345.40, 345.41, 345.50, 345.51, 345.60, 345.61, 345.70, 345.71, 345.80, 345.81, 345.90, 345.91, 348.8, 348.9, 349.89, 349.9, 780.32
AHA: For Code 345.00: 1Q 2004, 18

Nervous System and Sense Organs 343 – 345.0

345.1 Generalized convulsive epilepsy
Epileptic seizures:
clonic
myoclonic
tonic
tonic-clonic
Grand mal
Major epilepsy
Excludes convulsions:
NOS (780.39)
infantile (780.39)
newborn (779.0)
infantile spasms (345.6)
C&C Exclusions: (for code 345.10) See 345.0
AHA: 3Q 1997, 4

345.2 Petit mal status
Epileptic absence status
C&C Exclusions: See 345.0

345.3 Grand mal status
Status epilepticus NOS
Excludes *epilepsia partialis continua (345.7)*
status:
psychomotor (345.7)
temporal lobe (345.7)
C&C Exclusions: See 345.0
AHA: 3Q 2005, 12

345.4 Localization-related (focal) (partial) epilepsy and epileptic syndromes with complex partial seizures
Epilepsy:
limbic system
partial:
secondarily generalized
with impairment of consciousness
with memory and ideational disturbances
psychomotor
psychosensory
temporal lobe
Epileptic automatism
C&C Exclusions: (for code 345.40) See 345.00
C&C Exclusions: (for code 345.41) See 345.01

345.5 Localization-related (focal) (partial) epilepsy and epileptic syndromes with simple partial seizures
Epilepsy:
Bravais-Jacksonian NOS
focal (motor) NOS
Jacksonian NOS
motor partial
partial NOS:
without impairment of consciousness
sensory-induced
somatomotor
somatosensory
visceral
visual
C&C Exclusions: (for code 345.50) See 345.00
C&C Exclusions: (for code 345.51) See 345.01

345.6 Infantile spasms
Hypsarrhythmia
Lightning spasms
Salaam attacks
Excludes *salaam tic (781.0)*
C&C Exclusions: (for code 345.60) See 345.00
C&C Exclusions: (for code 345.61) See 345.01
AHA: Nov-Dec 1984, 12

345.7 Epilepsia partialis continua
Kojevnikov's epilepsy
C&C Exclusions: (for code 345.70) See 345.00
C&C Exclusions: (for code 345.71) See 345.01

345.8 Other forms of epilepsy and recurrent seizures
Epilepsy:
cursive [running]
gelastic
C&C Exclusions: (for code 345.80) See 345.00
C&C Exclusions: (for code 345.81) See 345.01

345.9 Epilepsy, unspecified
Epileptic convulsions, fits, or seizures NOS
Recurrent seizures NOS
Seizure disorder NOS
Excludes *convulsion (convulsive) disorder (780.39)*
convulsive seizure or fit NOS (780.39)
recurrent convulsions (780.39)
C&C Exclusions: (for code 345.90) See 345.00
C&C Exclusions: (for code 345.91) See 345.01
AHA: Nov-Dec 1987, 12

346 Migraine
DEF: Periodic severe headaches, usually temporal and unilateral at onset, that present with aura, irritability, nausea, vomiting, constipation or diarrhea, and commonly photophobia.

The following fifth-digit subclassification is for use with category 346:
0 without mention of intractable migraine
1 with intractable migraine, so stated

346.0 Classical migraine
Migraine preceded or accompanied by transient focal neurological phenomena
Migraine with aura
DEF: Migraine with neurological symptoms such as blind spots, flashing lights, zigzag visual patterns, or a tingling, pins-and-needles sensation in the head before migraine onset.

346.1 Common migraine
Atypical migraine
Sick headache

346.2 Variants of migraine
Cluster headache
Histamine cephalgia
Horton's neuralgia
Migraine:
abdominal
basilar
lower half
retinal
Neuralgia:
ciliary
migrainous

346.8 Other forms of migraine
Migraine:
hemiplegic
ophthalmoplegic

346.9 Migraine, unspecified
AHA: Nov-Dec 1985, 16

347 Cataplexy and narcolepsy
DEF: Cataplexy: abrupt attacks of muscular weakness and loss of muscle tone triggered by an emotional stimulus.
DEF: Narcolepsy: recurrent, uncontrollable episodes of falling into a deep sleep.

347.0 Narcolepsy
347.00 Without cataplexy
Narcolepsy NOS
347.01 With cataplexy

347.1 Narcolepsy in conditions classified elsewhere
Code first underlying condition
347.10 Without cataplexy
347.11 With cataplexy

348 Other conditions of brain
348.0 Cerebral cysts
Arachnoid cyst
Porencephalic cyst
Porencephaly, acquired
Pseudoporencephaly
Excludes *porencephaly (congenital) (742.4)*

348.1 Anoxic brain damage
Excludes *that occurring in:*
abortion (634-638 with .7, 639.8)
ectopic or molar pregnancy (639.8)
labor or delivery (668.2, 669.4)
that of newborn (767.0, 768.0-768.9, 772.1-772.2)
Use additional E code to identify cause
C&C Exclusions: 250.60, 250.61, 250.62, 250.63, 250.80, 250.81, 250.82, 250.83, 250.90, 250.91, 250.92, 250.93, 348.1, 348.2, 349.89, 349.9

348.2 Benign intracranial hypertension
Pseudotumor cerebri
Excludes *hypertensive encephalopathy (437.2)*

❺ **348.3 Encephalopathy, not elsewhere classified**
AHA: 4Q 2003, 58; 3Q 1997, 4

348.30 Encephalopathy, unspecified
C&C Exclusions: 349.82

Any disease or disorder of the brain that alters brain function or structure

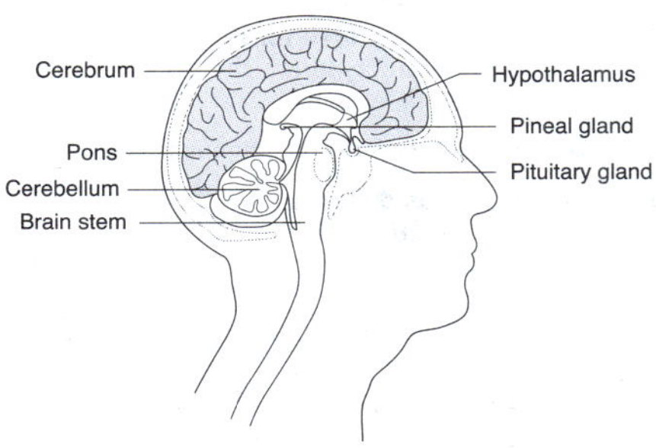

348.31 Metabolic encephalopathy
Septic encephalopathy
Excludes *toxic metabolic encephalopathy (349.82)*
DEF: Neuropsychiatric disturbances due to metabolic brain disease, commonly caused by hypoxia, ischemia, hypoglycemia, or diseases of other organs.
C&C Exclusions: See 348.30

348.39 Other encephalopathy
Excludes *encephalopathy:*
alcoholic (291.2)
hepatic (572.2)
hypertensive (437.2)
toxic (349.82)
C&C Exclusions: See 348.30

348.4 Compression of brain
Compression brain (stem)
Herniation brain (stem)
Posterior fossa compression syndrome
AHA: 4Q 1994, 37

348.5 Cerebral edema

348.8 Other conditions of brain
Cerebral:
calcification
fungus
C&C Exclusions: 780.32
AHA: Sep-Oct 1987, 9

✖ **348.9 Unspecified condition of brain**
C&C Exclusions: 348.8

❹ **349 Other and unspecified disorders of the nervous system**

349.0 Reaction to spinal or lumbar puncture
Headache following lumbar puncture
AHA: 2Q 1999, 9; 3Q 1990, 18

349.1 Nervous system complications from surgically implanted device
Excludes *immediate postoperative complications (997.00-997.09)*
mechanical complications of nervous system device (996.2)
C&C Exclusions: 250.60, 250.61, 250.62, 250.63, 250.80, 250.81, 250.82, 250.83, 250.90, 250.91, 250.92, 250.93, 349.1, 349.89, 349.9

349.2 Disorders of meninges, not elsewhere classified
Adhesions, meningeal (cerebral) (spinal)
Cyst, spinal meninges
Meningocele, acquired
Pseudomeningocele, acquired
AHA: 1Q 2006, 15; 2Q 1998, 18; 3Q 1994, 4

❺ **349.8 Other specified disorders of nervous system**

349.81 Cerebrospinal fluid rhinorrhea
Excludes *cerebrospinal fluid otorrhea (388.61)*
DEF: Discharge of cerebrospinal fluid through the nose.
C&C Exclusions: 250.60, 250.61, 250.62, 250.63, 250.80, 250.81, 250.82, 250.83, 250.90, 250.91, 250.92, 250.93, 349.81, 349.89, 349.9

349.82 Toxic encephalopathy
Toxic metabolic encephalopathy
Use additional E code to identify cause
C&C Exclusions: 013.60, 013.61, 013.62, 013.63, 013.64, 013.65, 013.66, 017.90, 017.91, 017.92, 017.93, 017.94, 017.95, 017.96, 036.1, 049.8, 049.9, 052.0, 054.3, 062.0, 062.1, 062.2, 062.3, 062.4, 062.5, 062.8, 062.9, 063.0, 063.1, 063.2, 063.8, 063.9, 072.2, 090.41, 094.81, 130.0, 250.60, 250.61, 250.62, 250.63, 250.80, 250.81, 250.82, 250.83, 250.90, 250.91, 250.92, 250.93, 323.0, 323.1, 323.2, 323.3, 323.4, 323.5, 323.6, 323.7, 323.8, 323.9, 348.3, 348.8, 348.9, 349,82, 349.89, 349.9
AHA: 4Q 1993, 29

Brain tissue degeneration due to toxic substance

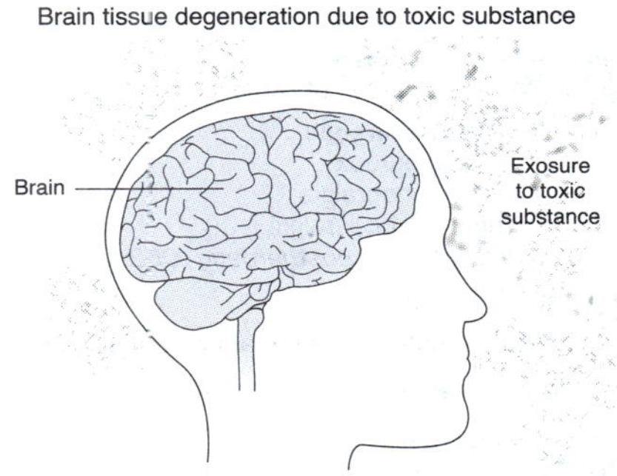

349.89 Other
C&C Exclusions: 358.00, 358.01, 780.32

✖ **349.9 Unspecified disorders of nervous system**
Disorder of nervous system (central) NOS
C&C Exclusions: See 349.89

DISORDERS OF THE PERIPHERAL NERVOUS SYSTEM (350-359)

Excludes *diseases of:*
acoustic [8th] nerve (388.5)
oculomotor [3rd, 4th, 6th] nerves (378.0-378.9)
optic [2nd] nerve (377.0-377.9)
peripheral autonomic nerves (337.0-337.9)
neuralgia NOS or "rheumatic" (729.2)
neuritis NOS or "rheumatic" (729.2)
peripheral neuritis in pregnancy (646.4)
radiculitis NOS or "rheumatic" (729.2)

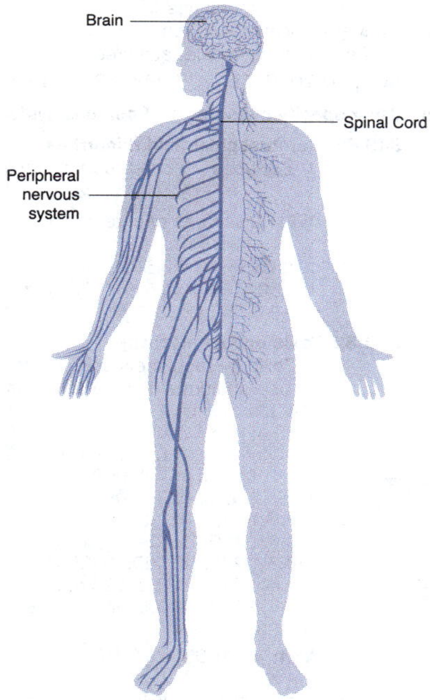

❹ **350 Trigeminal nerve disorders**
Includes disorders of 5th cranial nerve

350.1 Trigeminal neuralgia
Tic douloureux
Trifacial neuralgia
Trigeminal neuralgia NOS
Excludes *postherpetic (053.12)*

350.2 Atypical face pain

350.8 Other specified trigeminal nerve disorders

✖ **350.9 Trigeminal nerve disorder, unspecified**

❹ **351 Facial nerve disorders**
Includes disorders of 7th cranial nerve
Excludes *that in newborn (767.5)*

351.0 Bell's palsy
Facial palsy
DEF: Temporary, unilateral facial muscle weakness or paralysis resulting from damage or trauma to one of the paired facial nerves.

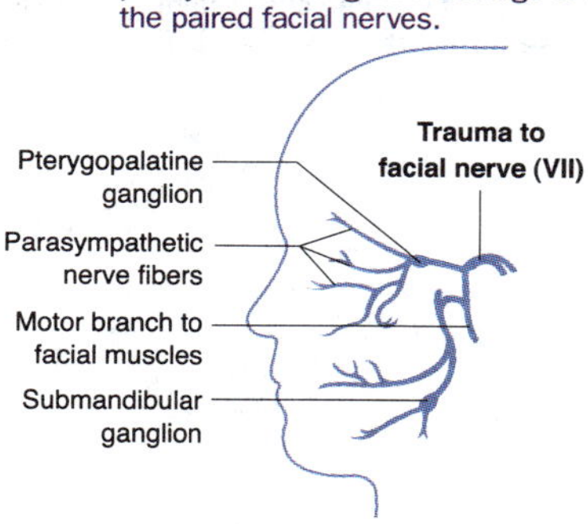

351.1 Geniculate ganglionitis
Geniculate ganglionitis NOS
Excludes *herpetic (053.11)*
DEF: Inflammation of the facial nerve ganglion.

351.8 Other facial nerve disorders
Facial myokymia
Melkersson's syndrome
DEF: Melkersson's syndrome: chronic, noninflammatory facial swelling, usually confined to the lips, with recurrent facial palsy and sometimes a fissured tongue.
AHA: 3Q 2002, 13

✖ **351.9 Facial nerve disorder, unspecified**

❹ **352 Disorders of other cranial nerves**

352.0 Disorders of olfactory [1st] nerve

352.1 Glossopharyngeal neuralgia
AHA: 2Q 2002, 8

352.2 Other disorders of glossopharyngeal [9th] nerve

352.3 Disorders of pneumogastric [10th] nerve
Disorders of vagal nerve
Excludes *paralysis of vocal cords or larynx (478.30-478.34)*

352.4 Disorders of accessory [11th] nerve

352.5 Disorders of hypoglossal [12th] nerve

352.6 Multiple cranial nerve palsies
Collet-Sicard syndrome
Polyneuritis cranialis

✖ **352.9 Unspecified disorder of cranial nerves**

❹ **353 Nerve root and plexus disorders**
Excludes *conditions due to:*
intervertebral disc disorders (722.0-722.9)
spondylosis (720.0-721.9)
vertebrogenic disorders (723.0-724.9)

353.0 Brachial plexus lesions
Cervical rib syndrome
Costoclavicular syndrome
Scalenus anticus syndrome
Thoracic outlet syndrome
Excludes *brachial neuritis or radiculitis NOS (723.4)*
that in newborn (767.6)
AHA: 3Q 2006, 12

353.1 Lumbosacral plexus lesions
▶*Code first, if applicable, associated diabetes mellitus (250.6)*◀

353.2 Cervical root lesions, not elsewhere classified

353.3 Thoracic root lesions, not elsewhere classified

353.4 Lumbosacral root lesions, not elsewhere classified

353.5 Neuralgic amyotrophy
Parsonage-Aldren-Turner syndrome

353.6 Phantom limb (syndrome)

353.8 Other nerve root and plexus disorders

✖ **353.9 Unspecified nerve root and plexus disorder**

❹ **354 Mononeuritis of upper limb and mononeuritis multiplex**

354.0 Carpal tunnel syndrome
Median nerve entrapment
Partial thenar atrophy
DEF: Pain, burning, tingling and/or numbness in the fingers and hand, often extending to the elbow, due to compression of the median nerve within the carpal tunnel.

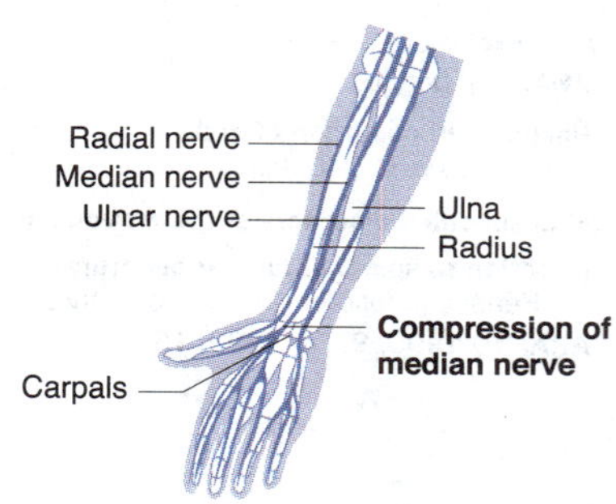

354.1 Other lesion of median nerve
Median nerve neuritis

354.2 Lesion of ulnar nerve
Cubital tunnel syndrome
Tardy ulnar nerve palsy

354.3 Lesion of radial nerve
Acute radial nerve palsy
AHA: Nov-Dec 1987, 6

354.4 Causalgia of upper limb
Excludes *causalgia:*
NOS (355.9)
lower limb (355.71)

354.5 Mononeuritis multiplex
Combinations of single conditions classifiable to 354 or 355

354.8 Other mononeuritis of upper limb

354.9 Mononeuritis of upper limb, unspecified

4 **355 Mononeuritis of lower limb**

355.0 Lesion of sciatic nerve
Excludes *sciatica NOS (724.3)*
AHA: 2Q 1989, 12

355.1 Meralgia paresthetica
Lateral cutaneous femoral nerve of thigh compression or syndrome

355.2 Other lesion of femoral nerve

355.3 Lesion of lateral popliteal nerve
Lesion of common peroneal nerve

Injury to the popliteal nerve affects the ability of the patient to flex their foot upward at the ankle

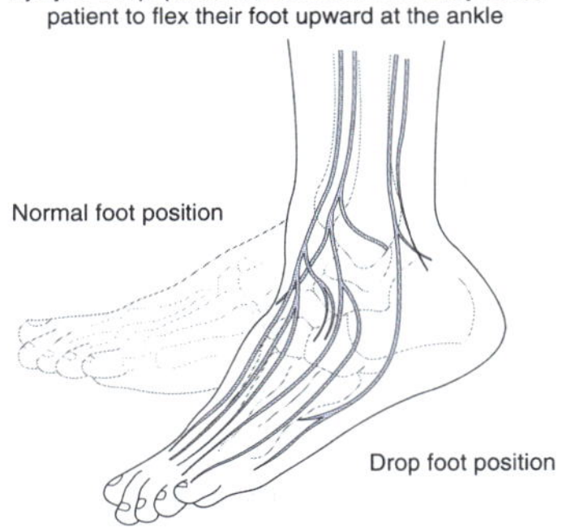

355.4 Lesion of medial popliteal nerve

355.5 Tarsal tunnel syndrome
DEF: Pain, burning, tingling and/or numbness of the sole of the foot, often extending to the ankle, due to compression of the posterior tibial nerve or plantar nerves within the tarsal tunnel.

355.6 Lesion of plantar nerve
Morton's metatarsalgia, neuralgia, or neuroma

5 **355.7 Other mononeuritis of lower limb**

355.71 Causalgia of lower limb
Excludes *causalgia:*
NOS (355.9)
upper limb (354.4)

355.79 Other mononeuritis of lower limb

355.8 Mononeuritis of lower limb, unspecified

355.9 Mononeuritis of unspecified site
Causalgia NOS
Excludes *causalgia:*
lower limb (355.71)
upper limb (354.4)

4 **356 Hereditary and idiopathic peripheral neuropathy**

356.0 Hereditary peripheral neuropathy
Déjérine-Sottas disease

356.1 Peroneal muscular atrophy
Charcôt-Marie-Tooth disease
Neuropathic muscular atrophy

356.2 Hereditary sensory neuropathy

356.3 Refsum's disease
Heredopathia atactica polyneuritiformis

356.4 Idiopathic progressive polyneuropathy

356.8 Other specified idiopathic peripheral neuropathy
Supranuclear paralysis

✖ **356.9 Unspecified**

4 **357 Inflammatory and toxic neuropathy**

357.0 Acute infective polyneuritis
Guillain-Barre syndrome
Postinfectious polyneuritis
C&C Exclusions: 003.21, 013.00, 013.01, 013.02, 013.03, 013.04, 013.05, 013.06, 013.10, 013.11, 013.12, 013.13, 013.14, 013.15, 013.16, 036.0, 036.89, 041.81, 041.82, 041.83, 041.84, 041.85, 041.86, 041.89, 041.9, 047.0, 047.1, 047.8, 047.9, 049.0, 049.1, 053.0, 054.72, 072.1, 090.42, 091.81, 094.2, 098.89, 100.81, 112.83, 114.2, 115.01, 115.11, 115.91, 130.0, 139.8, 320.0, 320.1, 320.2, 320.3, 320.7, 320.81, 320.82, 320.89, 320.9, 321.0, 321.1, 321.2, 321.3, 321.4, 321.8, 322.0, 322.1, 322.2, 322.9, 349.89, 349.9, 357.0
AHA: 2Q 1998, 12

+ ***357.1 Polyneuropathy in collagen vascular disease***
Code first underlying disease, as:
disseminated lupus erythematosus (710.0)
polyarteritis nodosa (446.0)
rheumatoid arthritis (714.0)

+ ***357.2 Polyneuropathy in diabetes***
Code first underlying disease (250.6)
AHA: 4Q 2003, 105; 2Q 1992, 15; 3Q 1991, 9

+ ***357.3 Polyneuropathy in malignant disease***
Code first underlying disease (140.0-208.9)

+ ***357.4 Polyneuropathy in other diseases classified elsewhere***
Code first underlying disease, as:
amyloidosis (277.30-277.39)
beriberi (265.0)
chronic uremia (585.9)
deficiency of B vitamins (266.0-266.9)
diphtheria (032.0-032.9)
hypoglycemia (251.2)
pellagra (265.2)
porphyria (277.1)
sarcoidosis (135)
uremia NOS (586)
Excludes *polyneuropathy in:*
herpes zoster (053.13)
mumps (072.72)
AHA: 2Q 1998, 15

357.5 Alcoholic polyneuropathy
DEF: Loss of nerve function due to damage from prolonged, excessive alcohol consumption; commonly presents with numbness, weakness, and burning in the feet.

357.6 Polyneuropathy due to drugs
Use additional E code to identify drug

357.7 Polyneuropathy due to other toxic agents
Use additional E code to identify toxic agent

5 **357.8 Other**
AHA: 4Q 2002, 47; 2Q 1998, 12

357.81 Chronic inflammatory demyelinating polyneuritis

357.82 Critical illness polyneuropathy
Acute motor neuropathy
AHA: 4Q 2003, 111

357.89 Other inflammatory and toxic neuropathy

✖ **357.9 Unspecified**

4 **358 Myoneural disorders**

5 **358.0 Myasthenia gravis**
AHA: 4Q 2003, 59

358.00 Myasthenia gravis without (acute) exacerbation
Myasthenia gravis NOS
C&C Exclusions: 250.60, 250.61, 250.62, 250.63, 250.80, 250.81, 250.82, 250.83, 250.90, 250.91, 250.92, 250.93, 349.89, 349.9, 358.00, 358.01, 358.1

358.01 Myasthenia gravis with (acute) exacerbation
Myasthenia gravis in crisis
C&C Exclusions: See 358.00
AHA: 1Q 2005, 4; 4Q 2004, 139

+ ***358.1 Myasthenic syndromes in diseases classified elsewhere***
Amotrophy from stated cause classified elsewhere
Eaton-Lambert syndrome from stated cause classified elsewhere
Code first underlying disease, as:
botulism (005.1)
hypothyroidism (244.0-244.9)
malignant neoplasm (140.0-208.9)
pernicious anemia (281.0)
thyrotoxicosis (242.0-242.9)
C&C Exclusions: 250.60, 250.61, 250.62, 250.63, 250.80, 250.81, 250.82, 250.83, 250.90, 250.91, 250.92, 250.93, 349.89, 349.9, 358.00, 358.01, 358.1

358.2 Toxic myoneural disorders
Use additional E code to identify toxic agent

358.8 Other specified myoneural disorders

✖ **358.9 Myoneural disorders, unspecified**
AHA: 2Q 2002, 16

❹ **359 Muscular dystrophies and other myopathies**
Excludes *idiopathic polymyositis (710.4)*

359.0 Congenital hereditary muscular dystrophy
Benign congenital myopathy
Central core disease
Centronuclear myopathy
Myotubular myopathy
Nemaline body disease
Excludes *arthrogryposis multiplex congenita (754.89)*
C&C Exclusions: 250.60, 250.61, 250.62, 250.63, 250.80, 250.81, 250.82, 250.83, 250.90, 250.91, 250.92, 250.93, 349.89, 349.9, 359.0, 359.1

359.1 Hereditary progressive muscular dystrophy
Muscular dystrophy:
- NOS
- distal
- Duchenne
- Erb's
- fascioscapulohumeral
- Gower's
- Landouzy-Déjérine
- limb-girdle
- ocular
- oculopharyngeal

C&C Exclusions: See 358.00

❺ **359.2 Myotonic disorders**
Excludes ▶*periodic paralysis (359.3)*◀

● **359.21 Myotonic muscular dystrophy**
Dystrophia myotonica
Myotonia atrophica
Myotonic dystrophy
Proximal myotonic myopathy (PROMM)
Steinert's disease

● **359.22 Myotonia congenita**
Acetazolamide responsive myotonia congenita
Dominant form (Thomsen's disease)
Recessive form (Becker's disease)
DEF: Inability to quickly relax muscles after voluntary contraction, particularly with sudden activity after rest.

● **359.23 Myotonic chondrodystrophy**
Congenital myotonic chondrodystrophy
Schwartz-Jampel disease

● **359.24 Drug induced myotonia**
Use additional E code to identify drug

● ✖ **359.29 Other specified myotonic disorder**
Myotonia fluctuans
Myotonia levior
Myotonia permanens
Paramyotonia congenita (of von Eulenburg)

▲ **359.3 Periodic paralysis**
▶ Familial periodic paralysis◀
▶ Hyperkalemic periodic paralysis◀
Hypokalemic familial periodic paralysis
▶ Hypokalemic periodic paralysis◀
▶ Potassium sensitive periodic paralysis◀
Excludes ▶*paramyotonia congenita (of von Eulenburg) (359.29)*◀

359.4 Toxic myopathy
Use additional E code to identify toxic agent
AHA: 1Q 1988, 5

+ ***359.5 Myopathy in endocrine diseases classified elsewhere***
Code first underlying disease, as:
Addison's disease (▶255.41◀)
Cushing's syndrome (255.0)
hypopituitarism (253.2)
myxedema (244.0-244.9)
thyrotoxicosis (242.0-242.9)

+ ***359.6 Symptomatic inflammatory myopathy in diseases classified elsewhere***
Code first underlying disease, as:
amyloidosis (277.30-277.39)
disseminated lupus erythematosus (710.0)
malignant neoplasm (140.0-208.9)
polyarteritis nodosa (446.0)
rheumatoid arthritis (714.0)
sarcoidosis (135)
scleroderma (710.1)
Sjögren's disease (710.2)

❺ **359.8 Other myopathies**
AHA: 4Q 2002, 47; 3Q 1990, 17

359.81 Critical illness myopathy
Acute necrotizing myopathy
Acute quadriplegic myopathy
Intensive care (ICU) myopathy
Myopathy of critical illness

359.89 Other myopathies

✖ **359.9 Myopathy, unspecified**

DISORDERS OF THE EYE AND ADNEXA (360-379)

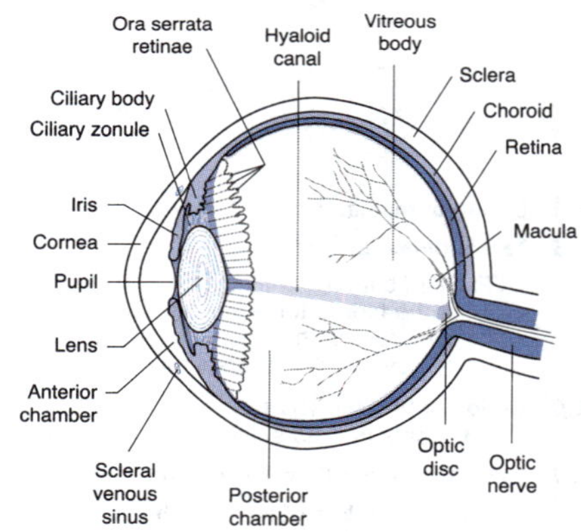

❹ **360 Disorders of the globe**
Includes disorders affecting multiple structures of eye

❺ **360.0 Purulent endophthalmitis**
Excludes *bleb associated endophthalmitis (379.63)*

360.00 Purulent endophthalmitis, unspecified

An inflammation of the tissues of the eye resulting in the formation of pus

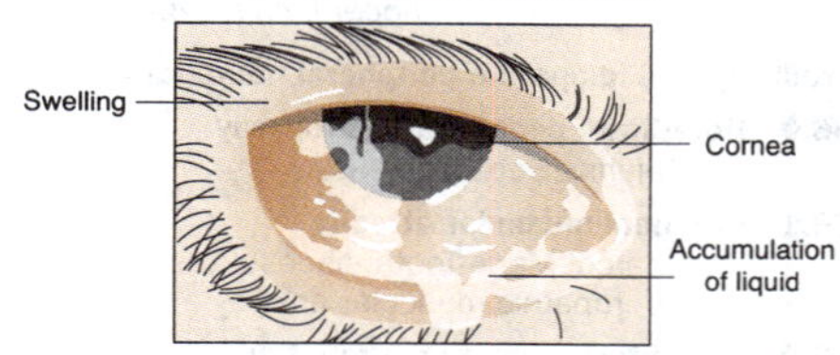

360.01 Acute endophthalmitis

360.02 Panophthalmitis

DEF: Inflammation affecting all the structures or tissues of the eye.

360.03 Chronic endophthalmitis

360.04 Vitreous abscess

❺ **360.1 Other endophthalmitis**

Excludes *bleb associated endophthalmitis (379.63)*

360.11 Sympathetic uveitis

360.12 Panuveitis

360.13 Parasitic endophthalmitis NOS

360.14 Ophthalmia nodosa

360.19 Other

Phacoanaphylactic endophthalmitis

❺ **360.2 Degenerative disorders of globe**

AHA: 3Q 1991, 3

360.20 Degenerative disorder of globe, unspecified

360.21 Progressive high (degenerative) myopia

Malignant myopia

360.23 Siderosis

360.24 Other metallosis

Chalcosis

360.29 Other

Excludes *xerophthalmia (264.7)*

❺ **360.3 Hypotony of eye**

360.30 Hypotony, unspecified

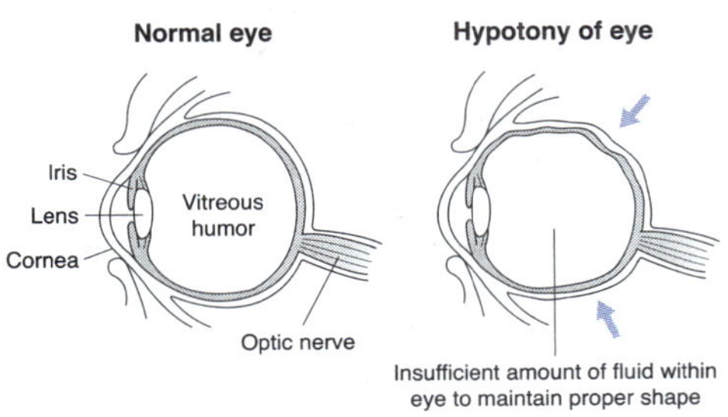

360.31 Primary hypotony

360.32 Ocular fistula causing hypotony

360.33 Hypotony associated with other ocular disorders

360.34 Flat anterior chamber

❺ **360.4 Degenerated conditions of globe**

360.40 Degenerated globe or eye, unspecified

360.41 Blind hypotensive eye

Atrophy of globe
Phthisis bulbi

DEF: Loss of vision due to extremely low intraocular fluid causing the eye to lose its shape.

360.42 Blind hypertensive eye

Absolute glaucoma

360.43 Hemophthalmos, except current injury

Excludes *traumatic (871.0-871.9, 921.0-921.9)*

DEF: Accumulation of blood within the eyeball that is not due to a current injury.

360.44 Leucocoria

❺ **360.5 Retained (old) intraocular foreign body, magnetic**

Excludes *current penetrating injury with magnetic foreign body (871.5)*
retained (old) foreign body of orbit (376.6)

360.50 Foreign body, magnetic, intraocular, unspecified

360.51 Foreign body, magnetic, in anterior chamber

360.52 Foreign body, magnetic, in iris or ciliary body

360.53 Foreign body, magnetic, in lens

360.54 Foreign body, magnetic, in vitreous

360.55 Foreign body, magnetic, in posterior wall

360.59 Foreign body, magnetic, in other or multiple sites

❺ **360.6 Retained (old) intraocular foreign body, nonmagnetic**

Retained (old) foreign body:
NOS
nonmagnetic

Excludes *current penetrating injury with (nonmagnetic) foreign body (871.6)*
retained (old) foreign body in orbit (376.6)

360.60 Foreign body, intraocular, unspecified

360.61 Foreign body in anterior chamber

360.62 Foreign body in iris or ciliary body

360.63 Foreign body in lens

360.64 Foreign body in vitreous

360.65 Foreign body in posterior wall

360.69 Foreign body in other or multiple sites

❺ **360.8 Other disorders of globe**

360.81 Luxation of globe

360.89 Other

✖ **360.9 Unspecified disorder of globe**

❹ **361 Retinal detachments and defects**

❺ **361.0 Retinal detachment with retinal defect**

Rhegmatogenous retinal detachment

Excludes *detachment of retinal pigment epithelium (362.42-362.43)*
retinal detachment (serous) (without defect) (361.2)

361.00 Retinal detachment with retinal defect, unspecified

361.01 Recent detachment, partial, with single defect

361.02 Recent detachment, partial, with multiple defects

361.03 Recent detachment, partial, with giant tear

361.04 Recent detachment, partial, with retinal dialysis

Dialysis (juvenile) of retina (with detachment)

361.05 Recent detachment, total or subtotal

361.06 Old detachment, partial

Delimited old retinal detachment

361.07 Old detachment, total or subtotal

❺ **361.1 Retinoschisis and retinal cysts**

Excludes *juvenile retinoschisis (362.73)*
microcystoid degeneration of retina (362.62)
parasitic cyst of retina (360.13)

361.10 Retinoschisis, unspecified

361.11 Flat retinoschisis

361.12 Bullous retinoschisis

361.13 Primary retinal cysts

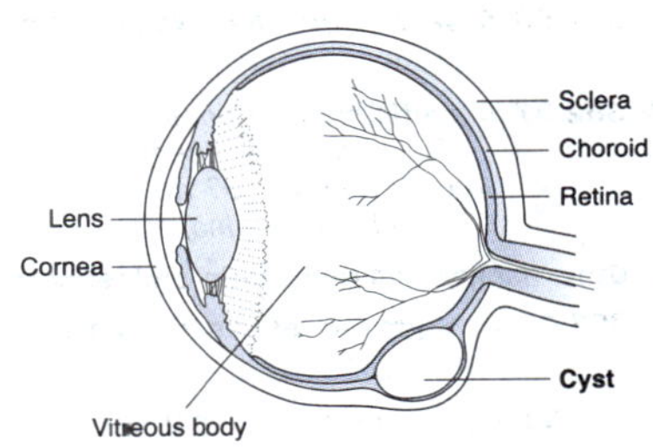

361.14 Secondary retinal cysts

361.19 Other

Pseudocyst of retina

361.2 Serous retinal detachment

Retinal detachment without retinal defect

Excludes *central serous retinopathy (362.41)*
retinal pigment epithelium detachment (362.42-362.43)

5 361.3 Retinal defects without detachment
Excludes *chorioretinal scars after surgery for detachment (363.30-363.35)*
peripheral retinal degeneration without defect (362.60-362.66)

361.30 Retinal defect, unspecified
Retinal break(s) NOS

361.31 Round hole of retina without detachment

361.32 Horseshoe tear of retina without detachment
Operculum of retina without mention of detachment

361.33 Multiple defects of retina without detachment

5 361.8 Other forms of retinal detachment

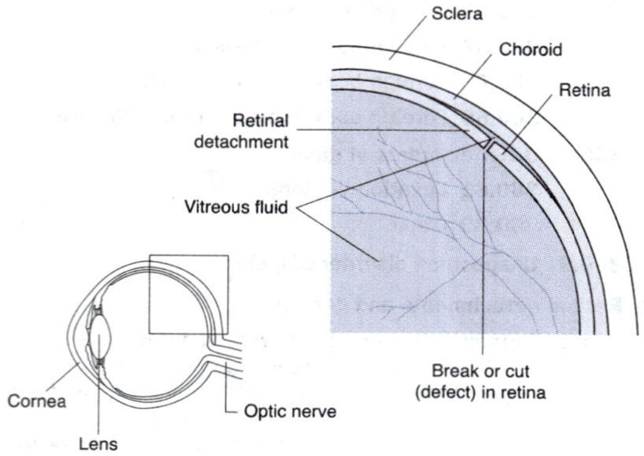

361.81 Traction detachment of retina
Traction detachment with vitreoretinal organization

361.89 Other
AHA: 3Q 1999, 12

✖ **361.9 Unspecified retinal detachment**
AHA: Nov-Dec 1987, 10

4 362 Other retinal disorders
Excludes *chorioretinal scars (363.30-363.35)*
chorioretinitis (363.0-363.2)

5 362.0 Diabetic retinopathy
Code first diabetes (250.5)
AHA: 4Q 2005, 65; 3Q 1991, 8

+ ***362.01 Background diabetic retinopathy***
Diabetic retinal microaneurysms
Diabetic retinopathy NOS

+ ***362.02 Proliferative diabetic retinopathy***
AHA: 3Q 1996, 5

+ ***362.03 Nonproliferative diabetic retinopathy NOS***

+ ***362.04 Mild nonproliferative diabetic retinopathy***

+ ***362.05 Moderate nonproliferative diabetic retinopathy***

+ ***362.06 Severe nonproliferative diabetic retinopathy***
AHA: 4Q 2005, 67

+ ***362.07 Diabetic macular edema***
Diabetic retinal edema
Note: *Code 362.07 must be used with a code for diabetic retinopathy (362.01-362.06)*

5 362.1 Other background retinopathy and retinal vascular changes

362.10 Background retinopathy, unspecified
AHA: 1Q 2006, 12

362.11 Hypertensive retinopathy
AHA: 3Q 1990, 3

362.12 Exudative retinopathy
Coats' syndrome
AHA: 3Q 1999, 12

362.13 Changes in vascular appearance
Vascular sheathing of retina
Use additional code for any associated atherosclerosis (440.8)

362.14 Retinal microaneurysms NOS

362.15 Retinal telangiectasia

362.16 Retinal neovascularization NOS
Neovascularization:
choroidal
subretinal

362.17 Other intraretinal microvascular abnormalities
Retinal varices

362.18 Retinal vasculitis
Eales' disease
Retinal:
arteritis
endarteritis
perivasculitis
phlebitis

5 362.2 Other proliferative retinopathy

362.21 Retrolental fibroplasia
DEF: Abnormal development of retinal blood vessels into the clear gel at the back of the eye in premature infants, causing scar tissue formation and retinal loosening or detachment.

362.29 Other nondiabetic proliferative retinopathy
AHA: 3Q 1996, 5

5 362.3 Retinal vascular occlusion

362.30 Retinal vascular occlusion, unspecified

362.31 Central retinal artery occlusion

362.32 Arterial branch occlusion

362.33 Partial arterial occlusion
Hollenhorst plaque
Retinal microembolism

362.34 Transient arterial occlusion
Amaurosis fugax
AHA: 1Q 2000, 16

362.35 Central retinal vein occlusion
AHA: 2Q 1993, 6

362.36 Venous tributary (branch) occlusion

362.37 Venous engorgement
Occlusion:
of retinal vein
incipient of retinal vein
partial of retinal vein

5 362.4 Separation of retinal layers
Excludes *retinal detachment (serous) (361.2)*
rhegmatogenous (361.00-361.07)

362.40 Retinal layer separation, unspecified

362.41 Central serous retinopathy
DEF: Fluid seepage from the choroid into the retina, causing the retinal layers to fill and separate from each other.

362.42 Serous detachment of retinal pigment epithelium
Exudative detachment of retinal pigment epithelium

362.43 Hemorrhagic detachment of retinal pigment epithelium

❺ 362.5 Degeneration of macula and posterior pole
Excludes *degeneration of optic disc (377.21-377.24)*
hereditary retinal degeneration [dystrophy] (362.70-362.77)

362.50 Macular degeneration (senile), unspecified

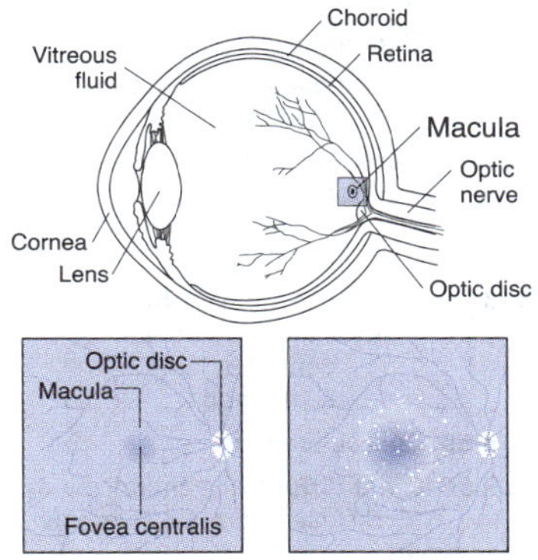

Normal Macular degeneration

362.51 Nonexudative senile macular degeneration
Senile macular degeneration:
atrophic
dry

362.52 Exudative senile macular degeneration
Kuhnt-Junius degeneration
Senile macular degeneration:
disciform
wet

362.53 Cystoid macular degeneration
Cystoid macular edema

362.54 Macular cyst, hole, or pseudohole

362.55 Toxic maculopathy
Use additional E code to identify drug, if drug induced

362.56 Macular puckering
Preretinal fibrosis

362.57 Drusen (degenerative)

❺ 362.6 Peripheral retinal degenerations
Excludes *hereditary retinal degeneration [dystrophy] (362.70-362.77)*
retinal degeneration with retinal defect (361.00-361.07)

362.60 Peripheral retinal degeneration, unspecified

362.61 Paving stone degeneration

362.62 Microcystoid degeneration
Blessig's cysts
Iwanoff's cysts

362.63 Lattice degeneration
Palisade degeneration of retina

362.64 Senile reticular degeneration

362.65 Secondary pigmentary degeneration
Pseudoretinitis pigmentosa

362.66 Secondary vitreoretinal degenerations

❺ 362.7 Hereditary retinal dystrophies

362.70 Hereditary retinal dystrophy, unspecified

+ ***362.71 Retinal dystrophy in systemic or cerebroretinal lipidoses***
Code first underlying disease, as:
cerebroretinal lipidoses (330.1)
systemic lipidoses (272.7)

+ ***362.72 Retinal dystrophy in other systemic disorders and syndromes***
Code first underlying disease, as:
Bassen-Kornzweig syndrome (272.5)
Refsum's disease (356.3)

362.73 Vitreoretinal dystrophies
Juvenile retinoschisis

362.74 Pigmentary retinal dystrophy
Retinal dystrophy, albipunctate
Retinitis pigmentosa

362.75 Other dystrophies primarily involving the sensory retina
Progressive cone (-rod) dystrophy
Stargardt's disease

DEF: Stargardt's disease: genetic condition causing degeneration of the macula, occurring by age 20, with rapid loss of visual acuity and abnormal pigmentation of the macula.

362.76 Dystrophies primarily involving the retinal pigment epithelium
Fundus flavimaculatus
Vitelliform dystrophy

362.77 Dystrophies primarily involving Bruch's membrane
Dystrophy:
hyaline
pseudoinflammatory foveal
Hereditary drusen

❺ 362.8 Other retinal disorders
Excludes *chorioretinal inflammations (363.0-363.2)*
chorioretinal scars (363.30-363.35)

362.81 Retinal hemorrhage
Hemorrhage:
preretinal
retinal (deep) (superficial)
subretinal

AHA: 4Q 1996, 43

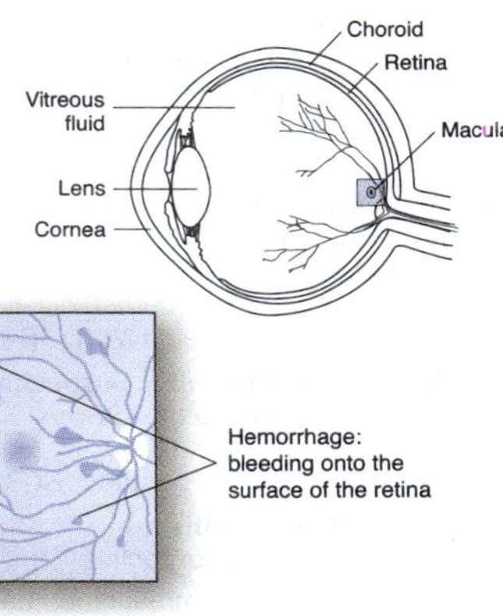

362.82 Retinal exudates and deposits

362.83 Retinal edema
Retinal:
cotton wool spots
edema (localized) (macular) (peripheral)

362.84 Retinal ischemia

362.85 Retinal nerve fiber bundle defects

362.89 Other retinal disorders

✖ **362.9 Unspecified retinal disorder**

❹ 363 Chorioretinal inflammations, scars, and other disorders of choroid

❺ 363.0 Focal chorioretinitis and focal retinochoroiditis
Excludes *focal chorioretinitis or retinochoroiditis in:*
histoplasmosis (115.02, 115.12, 115.92)
toxoplasmosis (130.2)
congenital infection (771.2)

363.00 Focal chorioretinitis, unspecified
Focal:
choroiditis or chorioretinitis NOS
retinitis or retinochoroiditis NOS

363.01 Focal choroiditis and chorioretinitis, juxtapapillary

363.03 Focal choroiditis and chorioretinitis of other posterior pole

A Adult (15+ years) M Maternity (12-55 years) N Newborn (0 years) P Pediatric (0-17 years) ♂ Male ♀ Female ❷ Medicare Secondary Payer

363.04 Focal choroiditis and chorioretinitis, peripheral

363.05 Focal retinitis and retinochoroiditis, juxtapapillary
Neuroretinitis

363.06 Focal retinitis and retinochoroiditis, macular or paramacular

363.07 Focal retinitis and retinochoroiditis of other posterior pole

363.08 Focal retinitis and retinochoroiditis, peripheral

5 **363.1 Disseminated chorioretinitis and disseminated retinochoroiditis**
Excludes *disseminated choroiditis or chorioretinitis in secondary syphilis (091.51)*
neurosyphilitic disseminated retinitis or retinochoroiditis (094.83)
retinal (peri)vasculitis (362.18)

363.10 Disseminated chorioretinitis, unspecified
Disseminated:
choroiditis or chorioretinitis NOS
retinitis or retinochoroiditis NOS

363.11 Disseminated choroiditis and chorioretinitis, posterior pole

363.12 Disseminated choroiditis and chorioretinitis, peripheral

363.13 Disseminated choroiditis and chorioretinitis, generalized
Code first any underlying disease, as:
tuberculosis (017.3)

363.14 Disseminated retinitis and retinochoroiditis, metastatic

363.15 Disseminated retinitis and retinochoroiditis, pigment epitheliopathy
Acute posterior multifocal placoid pigment epitheliopathy

5 **363.2 Other and unspecified forms of chorioretinitis and retinochoroiditis**
Excludes *panophthalmitis (360.02)*
sympathetic uveitis (360.11)
uveitis NOS (364.3)

363.20 Chorioretinitis, unspecified
Choroiditis NOS
Retinitis NOS
Uveitis, posterior NOS

363.21 Pars planitis
Posterior cyclitis

DEF: Inflammation of the peripheral retina and the ciliary body, the hair-like structures that hold the lens of the eye in place.

363.22 Harada's disease

5 **363.3 Chorioretinal scars**
Scar (postinflammatory) (postsurgical) (posttraumatic):
choroid
retina

363.30 Chorioretinal scar, unspecified

363.31 Solar retinopathy

DEF: Scar on the retina resulting from solar radiation.

363.32 Other macular scars

363.33 Other scars of posterior pole

363.34 Peripheral scars

363.35 Disseminated scars

5 **363.4 Choroidal degenerations**

363.40 Choroidal degeneration, unspecified
Choroidal sclerosis NOS

363.41 Senile atrophy of choroid

363.42 Diffuse secondary atrophy of choroid

363.43 Angioid streaks of choroid

5 **363.5 Hereditary choroidal dystrophies**
Hereditary choroidal atrophy:
partial [choriocapillaris]
total [all vessels]

363.50 Hereditary choroidal dystrophy or atrophy, unspecified

363.51 Circumpapillary dystrophy of choroid, partial

363.52 Circumpapillary dystrophy of choroid, total
Helicoid dystrophy of choroid

363.53 Central dystrophy of choroid, partial
Dystrophy, choroidal:
central areolar
circinate

363.54 Central choroidal atrophy, total
Dystrophy, choroidal:
central gyrate
serpiginous

363.55 Choroideremia

363.56 Other diffuse or generalized dystrophy, partial
Diffuse choroidal sclerosis

363.57 Other diffuse or generalized dystrophy, total
Generalized gyrate atrophy, choroid

5 **363.6 Choroidal hemorrhage and rupture**

363.61 Choroidal hemorrhage, unspecified

363.62 Expulsive choroidal hemorrhage

363.63 Choroidal rupture

5 **363.7 Choroidal detachment**

363.70 Choroidal detachment, unspecified

363.71 Serous choroidal detachment

363.72 Hemorrhagic choroidal detachment

363.8 Other disorders of choroid
AHA: 1Q 2006, 12

✖ **363.9 Unspecified disorder of choroid**

4 **364 Disorders of iris and ciliary body**

5 **364.0 Acute and subacute iridocyclitis**
Anterior uveitis, acute, subacute
Cyclitis, acute, subacute
Iridocyclitis, acute, subacute
Iritis, acute, subacute
Excludes *gonococcal (098.41)*
herpes simplex (054.44)
herpes zoster (053.22)

364.00 Acute and subacute iridocyclitis, unspecified

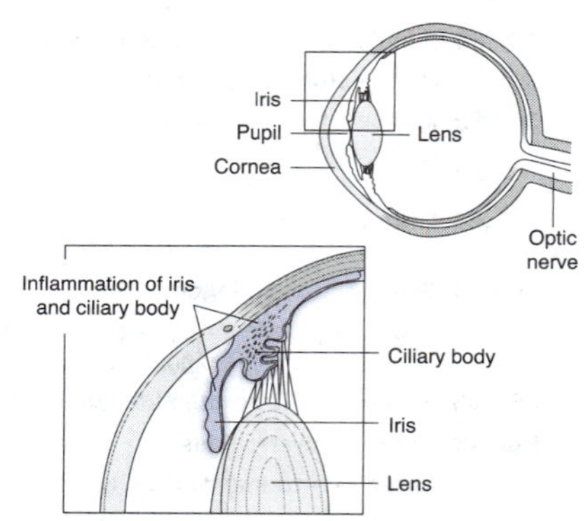

364.01 Primary iridocyclitis

364.02 Recurrent iridocyclitis

364.03 Secondary iridocyclitis, infectious

364.04 Secondary iridocyclitis, noninfectious
Aqueous:
cells
fibrin
flare

364.05 Hypopyon

DEF: Accumulation of pus in the anterior chamber of the eye.

5 364.1 Chronic iridocyclitis
Excludes *posterior cyclitis (363.21)*

364.10 Chronic iridocyclitis, unspecified

+ *364.11 Chronic iridocyclitis in diseases classified elsewhere*
Code first underlying disease, as:
sarcoidosis (135)
tuberculosis (017.3)
Excludes *syphilitic iridocyclitis (091.52)*

5 364.2 Certain types of iridocyclitis
Excludes *posterior cyclitis (363.21)*
sympathetic uveitis (360.11)

364.21 Fuchs' heterochromic cyclitis

364.22 Glaucomatocyclitic crises

364.23 Lens-induced iridocyclitis

364.24 Vogt-Koyanagi syndrome

364.3 Unspecified iridocyclitis
Uveitis NOS

5 364.4 Vascular disorders of iris and ciliary body

364.41 Hyphema
Hemorrhage of iris or ciliary body
DEF: Bleeding in the iris, usually as a result of trauma, and pools in the bottom of the cornea causing vision to be extremely blurred.

364.42 Rubeosis iridis
Neovascularization of iris or ciliary body

5 364.5 Degenerations of iris and ciliary body

364.51 Essential or progressive iris atrophy

364.52 Iridoschisis

364.53 Pigmentary iris degeneration
Acquired heterochromia of iris
Pigment dispersion syndrome of iris
Translucency of iris
DEF: Fading of the pigmentation (color) of the iris, allowing light to seep in rather than being blocked; presents with light-sensitivity and blurred vision.

364.54 Degeneration of pupillary margin
Atrophy of sphincter of iris
Ectropion of pigment epithelium of iris

364.55 Miotic cysts of pupillary margin
DEF: Fluid-filled pockets in the iris at the pupil's edge, causing the iris to contract and interfering with vision when light is less than optimal.

364.56 Degenerative changes of chamber angle

364.57 Degenerative changes of ciliary body

364.59 Other iris atrophy
Iris atrophy (generalized) (sector shaped)

5 364.6 Cysts of iris, ciliary body, and anterior chamber
Excludes *miotic pupillary cyst (364.55)*
parasitic cyst (360.13)

364.60 Idiopathic cysts

364.61 Implantation cysts
Epithelial down-growth, anterior chamber
Implantation cysts (surgical) (traumatic)

364.62 Exudative cysts of iris or anterior chamber

364.63 Primary cyst of pars plana

364.64 Exudative cyst of pars plana

5 364.7 Adhesions and disruptions of iris and ciliary body
Excludes *flat anterior chamber (360.34)*

364.70 Adhesions of iris, unspecified
Synechiae (iris) NOS

364.71 Posterior synechiae
DEF: Adhesion where the lens and the iris grow together, preventing the iris from dilating and contracting properly.

364.72 Anterior synechiae

364.73 Goniosynechiae
Peripheral anterior synechiae

364.74 Pupillary membranes
Iris bombé
Pupillary:
occlusion
seclusion

364.75 Pupillary abnormalities
Deformed pupil
Ectopic pupil
Rupture of sphincter, pupil

364.76 Iridodialysis
DEF: Separation or loosening of the iris from its root at the ciliary body, usually from trauma or surgical accident.

364.77 Recession of chamber angle

5 364.8 Other disorders of iris and ciliary body

● 364.81 Floppy iris syndrome
Intraoperative floppy iris syndrome (IFIS)
Use additional E code to identify cause, such as:
sympatholytics [antiadrenergics] causing adverse effect in therapeutic use (E941.3)
DEF: Syndrome occurring in one who has taken alpha-blockers; a dilated iris does not stay dilated, causing potentially injurious surgical complications.

● 364.89 Other disorders of iris and ciliary body
Prolapse of iris NOS
Excludes *prolapse of iris in recent wound (871.1)*

✖ 364.9 Unspecified disorder of iris and ciliary body

4 365 Glaucoma
Excludes *blind hypertensive eye [absolute glaucoma] (360.42)*
congenital glaucoma (743.20-743.22)
DEF: Increase in intraocular pressure causing pathologic changes in the optic disk and defects in the field of vision.

5 365.0 Borderline glaucoma [glaucoma suspect]
AHA: 1Q 1990, 8

365.00 Preglaucoma, unspecified

365.01 Open angle with borderline findings
Open angle with:
borderline intraocular pressure
cupping of optic discs

365.02 Anatomical narrow angle

365.03 Steroid responders

365.04 Ocular hypertension

5 365.1 Open-angle glaucoma

365.10 Open-angle glaucoma, unspecified
Wide-angle glaucoma NOS

An increase in fluid pressure in the eye resulting from the outflow of ocular fluid being blocked

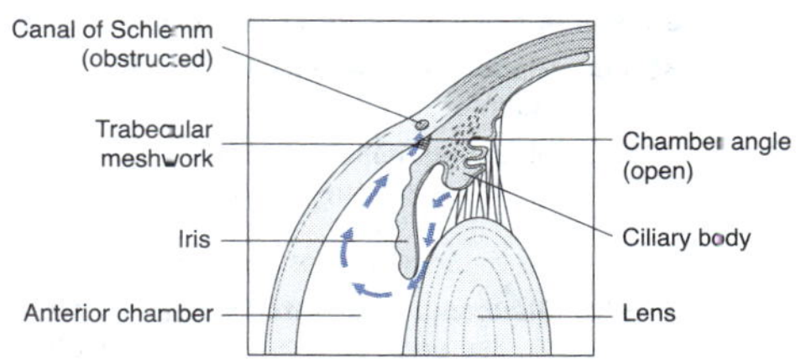

365.11 Primary open angle glaucoma
Chronic simple glaucoma

365.12 Low tension glaucoma

365.13 Pigmentary glaucoma
DEF: Granules of pigment coloring the eye break off and block drainage canals, increasing intraocular pressure.

365.14 Glaucoma of childhood
Infantile or juvenile glaucoma

365.15 Residual stage of open angle glaucoma

5 **365.2 Primary angle-closure glaucoma**

365.20 Primary angle-closure glaucoma, unspecified

365.21 Intermittent angle-closure glaucoma

Angle-closure glaucoma:
interval
subacute

365.22 Acute angle-closure glaucoma

DEF: Severe, sudden increase in intraocular pressure due to a blockage of the chamber angle at the junction of the iris and cornea, preventing normal aqueous fluid drainage and causing rapid loss of vision.

365.23 Chronic angle-closure glaucoma

AHA: 2Q 1998, 16

365.24 Residual stage of angle-closure glaucoma

5 **365.3 Corticosteroid-induced glaucoma**

365.31 Glaucomatous stage

365.32 Residual stage

5 **365.4 Glaucoma associated with congenital anomalies, dystrophies, and systemic syndromes**

+ ***365.41 Glaucoma associated with chamber angle anomalies***

Code first associated disorder, as:
Axenfeld's anomaly (743.44)
Rieger's anomaly or syndrome (743.44)

+ ***365.42 Glaucoma associated with anomalies of iris***

Code first associated disorder, as:
aniridia (743.45)
essential iris atrophy (364.51)

+ ***365.43 Glaucoma associated with other anterior segment anomalies***

Code first associated disorder, as:
microcornea (743.41)

+ ***365.44 Glaucoma associated with systemic syndromes***

Code first associated disease, as:
neurofibromatosis (237.7)
Sturge-Weber (-Dimitri) syndrome (759.6)

5 **365.5 Glaucoma associated with disorders of the lens**

365.51 Phacolytic glaucoma

Use additional code for associated hypermature cataract (366.18)

DEF: Leakage of lens protein from a mature cataract into the aqueous fluid, blocking fluid outflow and causing pressure buildup.

365.52 Pseudoexfoliation glaucoma

Use additional code for associated pseudoexfoliation of capsule (366.11)

365.59 Glaucoma associated with other lens disorders

Use additional code for associated disorder, as:
dislocation of lens (379.33-379.34)
spherophakia (743.36)

5 **365.6 Glaucoma associated with other ocular disorders**

365.60 Glaucoma associated with unspecified ocular disorder

365.61 Glaucoma associated with pupillary block

Use additional code for associated disorder, as:
seclusion of pupil [iris bombé] (364.74)

365.62 Glaucoma associated with ocular inflammations

Use additional code for associated disorder, as:
glaucomatocyclitic crises (364.22)
iridocyclitis (364.0-364.3)

365.63 Glaucoma associated with vascular disorders

Use additional code for associated disorder, as:
central retinal vein occlusion (362.35)
hyphema (364.41)

365.64 Glaucoma associated with tumors or cysts

Use additional code for associated disorder, as:
benign neoplasm (224.0-224.9)
epithelial down-growth (364.61)
malignant neoplasm (190.0-190.9)

365.65 Glaucoma associated with ocular trauma

Use additional code for associated condition, as:
contusion of globe (921.3)
recession of chamber angle (364.77)

5 **365.8 Other specified forms of glaucoma**

365.81 Hypersecretion glaucoma

DEF: Overproduction of ocular fluid rather than insufficient drainage that causes increased intraocular pressure.

365.82 Glaucoma with increased episcleral venous pressure

DEF: Blood pressure of the veins in the white of the eye increases as the pressure of intraocular fluid increases.

365.83 Aqueous misdirection

Malignant glaucoma

AHA: 4Q 2002, 48

365.89 Other specified glaucoma

AHA: 2Q 1998, 16

✖ **365.9 Unspecified glaucoma**

AHA: 3Q 2003, 14; 2Q 2001, 16

4 **366 Cataract**

Excludes *congenital cataract (743.30-743.34)*

DEF: Partial or complete clouding on or in the lens or lens capsule of the eye, obscuring vision.

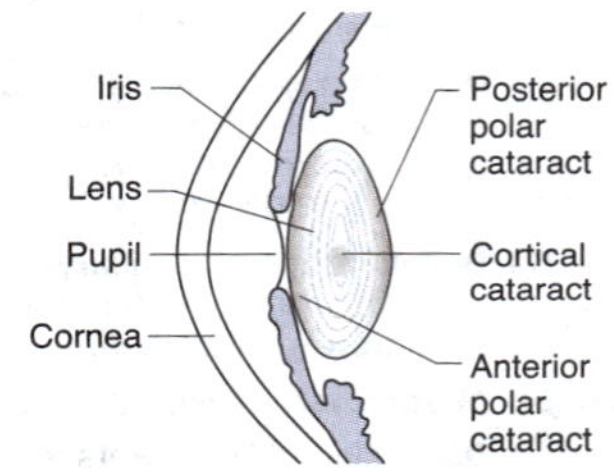

5 **366.0 Infantile, juvenile, and presenile cataract**

366.00 Nonsenile cataract, unspecified

366.01 Anterior subcapsular polar cataract

366.02 Posterior subcapsular polar cataract

366.03 Cortical, lamellar, or zonular cataract

366.04 Nuclear cataract

366.09 Other and combined forms of nonsenile cataract

5 **366.1 Senile cataract**

AHA: 3Q 1991, 9; Sep-Oct 1985, 10

366.10 Senile cataract, unspecified A

AHA: 1Q 2003, 5

366.11 Pseudoexfoliation of lens capsule A

366.12 Incipient cataract A

Cataract:
coronary
immature NOS
punctate
Water clefts

366.13 Anterior subcapsular polar senile cataract A

366.14 Posterior subcapsular polar senile cataract A

366.15 Cortical senile cataract A

366.16 Nuclear sclerosis A

Cataracta brunescens
Nuclear cataract

366.17 Total or mature cataract A

366.18 Hypermature cataract A
Morgagni cataract

366.19 Other and combined forms of senile cataract A

⑤ **366.2 Traumatic cataract**

366.20 Traumatic cataract, unspecified

366.21 Localized traumatic opacities
Vossius' ring

366.22 Total traumatic cataract

366.23 Partially resolved traumatic cataract

⑤ **366.3 Cataract secondary to ocular disorders**

366.30 Cataracta complicata, unspecified

366.31 Glaucomatous flecks (subcapsular)
Code first underlying glaucoma (365.0-365.9)

366.32 Cataract in inflammatory disorders
Code first underlying condition, as:
chronic choroiditis (363.0-363.2)

366.33 Cataract with neovascularization
Code first underlying condition, as:
chronic iridocyclitis (364.10)

366.34 Cataract in degenerative disorders
Sunflower cataract
Code first underlying condition, as:
chalcosis (360.24)
degenerative myopia (360.21)
pigmentary retinal dystrophy (362.74)

⑤ **366.4 Cataract associated with other disorders**

+ ***366.41 Diabetic cataract***
Code first diabetes (250.5)
AHA: 3Q 1991, 9; Sep-Oct 1985, 11

+ ***366.42 Tetanic cataract***
Code first underlying disease as:
calcinosis (275.40)
hypoparathyroidism (252.1)

+ ***366.43 Myotonic cataract***
Code first underlying disorder (▶359.21-359.29◀)

+ ***366.44 Cataract associated with other syndromes***
Code first underlying condition, as:
craniofacial dysostosis (756.0)
galactosemia (271.1)

366.45 Toxic cataract
Drug-induced cataract
Use additional E code to identify drug or other toxic substance

DEF: Cataract caused by exposure to a drug or other toxic substance, such as a miotic, antimiotic, corticosteroid, metal, nitro compound, or substituted hydrocarbon.

366.46 Cataract associated with radiation and other physical influences
Use additional E code to identify cause

⑤ **366.5 After-cataract**

366.50 After-cataract, unspecified
Secondary cataract NOS

366.51 Soemmering's ring

DEF: Doughnut-shaped remnant of lens behind the pupil, occurring after cataract surgery or secondary to trauma.

366.52 Other after-cataract, not obscuring vision

366.53 After-cataract, obscuring vision

366.8 Other cataract
Calcification of lens

✖ **366.9 Unspecified cataract**

④ **367 Disorders of refraction and accommodation**

367.0 Hypermetropia
Far-sightedness
Hyperopia

367.1 Myopia
Near-sightedness

⑤ **367.2 Astigmatism**

DEF: Condition in which the cornea is not shaped perfectly round, causing light to focus on more than one point of the retina and resulting in blurred vision.

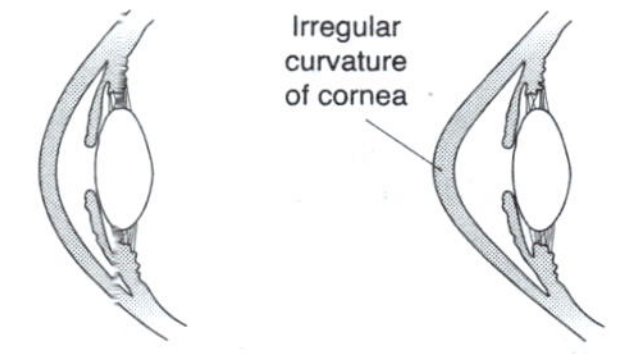

367.20 Astigmatism, unspecified

367.21 Regular astigmatism

367.22 Irregular astigmatism

⑤ **367.3 Anisometropia and aniseikonia**

367.31 Anisometropia

367.32 Aniseikonia

367.4 Presbyopia

DEF: Lens of the eye loses its elasticity due to age, making it more difficult to focus on near points.

⑤ **367.5 Disorders of accommodation**

367.51 Paresis of accommodation
Cycloplegia

367.52 Total or complete internal ophthalmoplegia

367.53 Spasm of accommodation

DEF: Abnormal, uncontrolled contraction of the ciliary muscle, usually initially presenting as near-sightedness.

⑤ **367.8 Other disorders of refraction and accommodation**

367.81 Transient refractive change

367.89 Other
Drug-induced disorders of refraction and accommodation
Toxic disorders of refraction and accommodation

✖ **367.9 Unspecified disorder of refraction and accommodation**

④ **368 Visual disturbances**

Excludes *electrophysiological disturbances (794.11-794.14)*

⑤ **368.0 Amblyopia ex anopsia**

The loss of visual acuity in the absence of a detectable organic disease

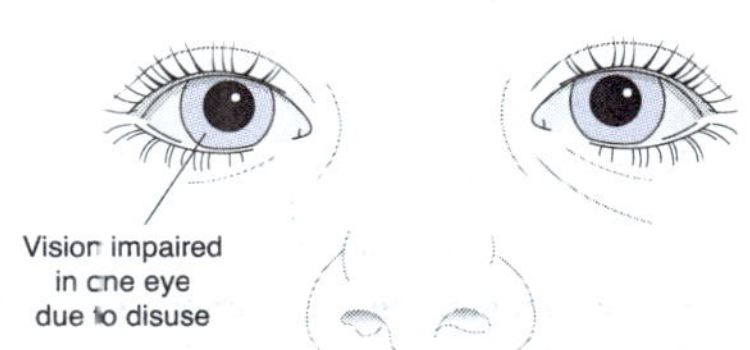

368.00 Amblyopia, unspecified

368.01 Strabismic amblyopia
Suppression amblyopia

368.02 Deprivation amblyopia

368.03 Refractive amblyopia

⑤ **368.1 Subjective visual disturbances**

368.10 Subjective visual disturbance, unspecified

368.11 Sudden visual loss

368.12 Transient visual loss
Concentric fading
Scintillating scotoma

368.13 Visual discomfort
Asthenopia
Eye strain
Photophobia

368.14 Visual distortions of shape and size
Macropsia
Metamorphopsia
Micropsia

368.15 Other visual distortions and entoptic phenomena
Photopsia
Refractive:
diplopia
polyopia
Visual halos

DEF: Photopsia: sparks or flashes in the field of vision, due to retinal irritation.

368.16 Psychophysical visual disturbances
Visual:
agnosia
disorientation syndrome
hallucinations

368.2 Diplopia
Double vision

❺ **368.3 Other disorders of binocular vision**

368.30 Binocular vision disorder, unspecified

368.31 Suppression of binocular vision

368.32 Simultaneous visual perception without fusion

DEF: Imaging from both eyes reaches the brain and are both processed, but without being merged into a single image; the patient sees two side-by-side images instead of one.

368.33 Fusion with defective stereopsis

368.34 Abnormal retinal correspondence

❺ **368.4 Visual field defects**

368.40 Visual field defect, unspecified

368.41 Scotoma involving central area
Scotoma:
central
centrocecal
paracentral

DEF: Blind spot (scotoma) in the central five degrees of the patient's vision.

368.42 Scotoma of blind spot area
Enlarged:
angioscotoma
blind spot
Paracecal scotoma

368.43 Sector or arcuate defects
Scotoma:
arcuate
Bjerrum
Seidel

368.44 Other localized visual field defect
Scotoma:
NOS
ring
Visual field defect:
nasal step
peripheral

368.45 Generalized contraction or constriction

368.46 Homonymous bilateral field defects
Hemianopsia (altitudinal) (homonymous)
Quadrant anopia

368.47 Heteronymous bilateral field defects
Hemianopsia:
binasal
bitemporal

❺ **368.5 Color vision deficiencies**
Color blindness

368.51 Protan defect
Protanomaly
Protanopia

368.52 Deutan defect
Deuteranomaly
Deuteranopia

368.53 Tritan defect
Tritanomaly
Tritanopia

368.54 Achromatopsia
Monochromatism (cone) (rod)

368.55 Acquired color vision deficiencies

368.59 Other color vision deficiencies

❺ **368.6 Night blindness**
Nyctalopia

368.60 Night blindness, unspecified

368.61 Congenital night blindness
Hereditary night blindness
Oguchi's disease

368.62 Acquired night blindness
Excludes that due to vitamin A deficiency (264.5)

368.63 Abnormal dark adaptation curve
Abnormal threshold of cones or rods
Delayed adaptation of cones or rods

368.69 Other night blindness

368.8 Other specified visual disturbances
Blurred vision NOS
AHA: 4Q 2002, 56

✖ **368.9 Unspecified visual disturbance**
AHA: 1Q 2004, 15

❹ **369 Blindness and low vision**

Note: Visual impairment refers to a functional limitation of the eye (e.g., limited visual acuity or visual field). It should be distinguished from visual disability, indicating a limitation of the abilities of the individual (e.g., limited reading skills, vocational skills), and from visual handicap, indicating a limitation of personal and socioeconomic independence (e.g., limited mobility, limited employability).

The levels of impairment defined in the table after 369.08 are based on the recommendations of the WHO Study Group on Prevention of Blindness (Geneva, November 6-10, 1972; WHO Technical Report Series 518), and of the International Council of Ophthalmology (1976).
Note that definitions of blindness vary in different settings. For international reporting, WHO defines blindness as profound impairment. This definition can be applied to blindness of one eye (369.1, 369.6) and to blindness of the individual (369.0).

For determination of benefits in the U.S.A., the definition of legal blindness as severe impairment is often used. This definition applies to blindness of the individual only.

Excludes correctable impaired vision due to refractive errors (367.0-367.9)

❺ **369.0 Profound impairment, both eyes**

✖ **369.00 Impairment level not further specified**
Blindness:
NOS according to WHO definition
both eyes

✖ **369.01 Better eye: total impairment; lesser eye: total impairment**

✖ **369.02 Better eye: near-total impairment; lesser eye: not further specified**

✖ **369.03 Better eye: near-total impairment; lesser eye: total impairment**

✖ **369.04 Better eye: near-total impairment; lesser eye: near-total impairment**

✖ **369.05 Better eye: profound impairment; lesser eye: not further specified**

✖ **369.06 Better eye: profound impairment; lesser eye: total impairment**

✖ **369.07 Better eye: profound impairment; lesser eye: near-total impairment**

✖ **369.08 Better eye: profound impairment; lesser eye: profound impairment**

<table>
<tr><td colspan="2">Classification</td><td>Levels of Visual Impairment</td><td rowspan="2">Additional descriptors which may be encountered</td></tr>
<tr><td>"legal"</td><td>WHO</td><td>Visual acuity and/or visual field limitation (whichever is worse)</td></tr>
<tr><td rowspan="3"></td><td rowspan="2">(Near-) Normal Vision</td><td>Range of Normal Vision
20/10 20/13 20/16 20/20 20/25
2.0 1.6 1.25 1.0 0.8</td><td></td></tr>
<tr><td>Near-Normal Vision
20/30 20/40 20/50 20/60
0.7 0.6 0.5 0.4 0.3</td><td></td></tr>
<tr><td rowspan="2">Low Vision</td><td>Moderate Visual Impairment
20/70 20/80 20/100 20/125 20/160
0.25 0.20 0.16 0.12</td><td>Moderate low vision</td></tr>
<tr><td rowspan="4">Legal Blindness (USA) both eyes</td><td>Severe Visual Impairment
20/200 20/250 20/320 20/400
0.10 0.08 0.06 0.05
Visual field: 20 degrees or less</td><td>Severe low vision, "Legal" blindness</td></tr>
<tr><td rowspan="3">Blindness (WHO) one or both eyes</td><td>Profound Visual Impairment
20/500 20/630 20/800 20/1000
0.04 0.03 0.025 0.02
Count fingers at: less than 3m (10 ft.)
Visual field: 10 degrees or less</td><td>Profound low vision, Moderate blindness</td></tr>
<tr><td>Near-Total Visual Impairment
Visual acuity: less than 0.02 (20/1000)
Count fingers at: 1m (3ft.) or less
Hand movements: 5m (15ft.) or less
Light projection, light perception
Visual field: 5 degrees or less</td><td>Severe blindness, Near-total blindness</td></tr>
<tr><td>Total Visual Impairment
No light perception (NLP)</td><td>Total blindness</td></tr>
<tr><td colspan="4">Visual acuity refers to best achievable acuity with correction.
Non-listed Snellen fractions may be classified by converting to the nearest decimal equivalent, e.g. 10/200 = .05, 6/30 = .20.
CF (count fingers) without designation of distance, may be classified to profound impairment.
HM (hand motion) without designation of distance, may be classified to near-total impairment.
Visual field measurements refer to the largest field diameter for a 1/100 white test object.</td></tr>
</table>

⑤ **369.1 Moderate or severe impairment, better eye, profound impairment lesser eye**

✖ **369.10 Impairment level not further specified**
Blindness, one eye, low vision other eye

✖ **369.11 Better eye: severe impairment; lesser eye: blind, not further specified**

✖ **369.12 Better eye: severe impairment; lesser eye: total impairment**

✖ **369.13 Better eye: severe impairment; lesser eye: near-total impairment**

✖ **369.14 Better eye: severe impairment; lesser eye: profound impairment**

✖ **369.15 Better eye: moderate impairment; lesser eye: blind, not further specified**

✖ **369.16 Better eye: moderate impairment; lesser eye: total impairment**

✖ **369.17 Better eye: moderate impairment; lesser eye: near-total impairment**

✖ **369.18 Better eye: moderate impairment; lesser eye: profound impairment**

⑤ **369.2 Moderate or severe impairment, both eyes**

✖ **369.20 Impairment level not further specified**
Low vision, both eyes NOS

✖ **369.21 Better eye: severe impairment; lesser eye: not further specified**

✖ **369.22 Better eye: severe impairment; lesser eye: severe impairment**

✖ **369.23 Better eye: moderate impairment; lesser eye: not further specified**

✖ **369.24 Better eye: moderate impairment; lesser eye: severe impairment**

✖ **369.25 Better eye: moderate impairment; lesser eye: moderate impairment**

✖ **369.3 Unqualified visual loss, both eyes**
Excludes *blindness NOS:*
legal [U.S.A. definition] (369.4)
WHO definition (369.00)

✖ **369.4 Legal blindness, as defined in U.S.A.**
Blindness NOS according to U.S.A. definition
Excludes *legal blindness with specification of impairment level (369.01-369.08, 369.11-369.14, 369.21-369.22)*

⑤ **369.6 Profound impairment, one eye**

✖ **369.60 Impairment level not further specified**
Blindness, one eye

✖ **369.61 One eye: total impairment; other eye: not specified**

✖ **369.62 One eye: total impairment; other eye: near-normal vision**

✖ **369.63 One eye: total impairment; other eye: normal vision**

✖ **369.64 One eye: near-total impairment; other eye: not specified**

✖ **369.65 One eye: near-total impairment; other eye: near-normal vision**

✖ **369.66 One eye: near-total impairment; other eye: normal vision**

✖ **369.67 One eye: profound impairment; other eye: not specified**

✖ **369.68 One eye: profound impairment; other eye: near-normal vision**

✖ **369.69 One eye: profound impairment; other eye: normal vision**

⑤ **369.7 Moderate or severe impairment, one eye**

✖ **369.70 Impairment level not further specified**
Low vision, one eye

✖ **369.71 One eye: severe impairment; other eye: not specified**

✖ **369.72 One eye: severe impairment; other eye: near-normal vision**

✖ **369.73 One eye: severe impairment; other eye: normal vision**

✖ **369.74 One eye: moderate impairment; other eye: not specified**

✖ **369.75 One eye: moderate impairment; other eye: near-normal vision**

✖ **369.76 One eye: moderate impairment; other eye: normal vision**

✖ **369.8 Unqualified visual loss, one eye**

✖ **369.9 Unspecified visual loss**
AHA: 4Q 2002, 114; 3Q 2002, 20

④ **370 Keratitis**

⑤ **370.0 Corneal ulcer**
Excludes *that due to vitamin A deficiency (264.3)*

370.00 Corneal ulcer, unspecified

370.01 Marginal corneal ulcer

370.02 Ring corneal ulcer
DEF: Ring of ulceration encircling the entire edge of the cornea.

370.03 Central corneal ulcer

370.04 Hypopyon ulcer
Serpiginous ulcer

370.05 Mycotic corneal ulcer
DEF: Corneal ulcer caused by a fungal infection.

370.06 Perforated corneal ulcer

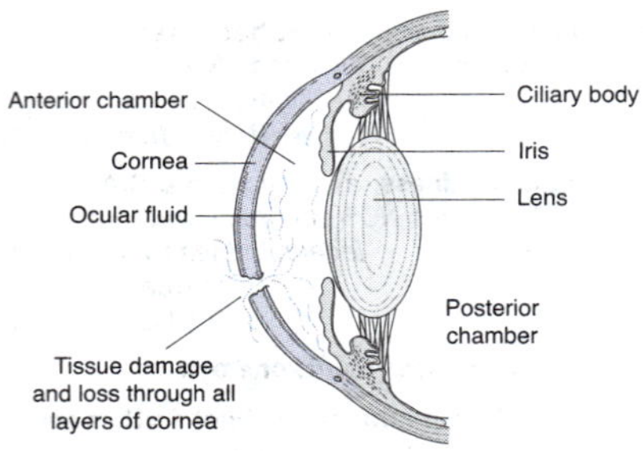

370.07 Mooren's ulcer

⑤ **370.2 Superficial keratitis without conjunctivitis**
Excludes *dendritic [herpes simplex] keratitis (054.42)*

370.20 Superficial keratitis, unspecified

370.21 Punctate keratitis
Thygeson's superficial punctate keratitis

370.22 Macular keratitis
Keratitis:
areolar
nummular
stellate
striate

370.23 Filamentary keratitis
DEF: Keratitis with twisted filaments of mucoid material on the surface of the cornea.

370.24 Photokeratitis
Snow blindness
Welders' keratitis
DEF: Painful, inflamed cornea that develops due to over-exposure to ultraviolet light.
AHA: 3Q 1996, 6

⑤ **370.3 Certain types of keratoconjunctivitis**
DEF: Inflammation of both the cornea and conjunctiva; presents with burning, bloodshot, watery eyes sensitive to bright light, blurred vision, and a sensation of something in the eye.

370.31 Phlyctenular keratoconjunctivitis
Phlyctenulosis
Use additional code for any associated tuberculosis (017.3)

370.32 Limbar and corneal involvement in vernal conjunctivitis
Use additional code for vernal conjunctivitis (372.13)

370.33 Keratoconjunctivitis sicca, not specified as Sjögren's
Excludes *Sjögren's syndrome (710.2)*

370.34 Exposure keratoconjunctivitis
DEF: Dryness and inflammation of the cornea and conjunctiva caused by the failure of the eyelid to completely close during sleep and/or blinking.
AHA: 3Q 1996, 6

370.35 Neurotrophic keratoconjunctivitis

⑤ **370.4 Other and unspecified keratoconjunctivitis**

370.40 Keratoconjunctivitis, unspecified
Superficial keratitis with conjunctivitis NOS

+ ***370.44 Keratitis or keratoconjunctivitis in exanthema***
Code first underlying condition (050.0-052.9)
Excludes *herpes simplex (054.43)*
herpes zoster (053.21)
measles (055.71)

370.49 Other
Excludes *epidemic keratoconjunctivitis (077.1)*

⑤ **370.5 Interstitial and deep keratitis**

370.50 Interstitial keratitis, unspecified

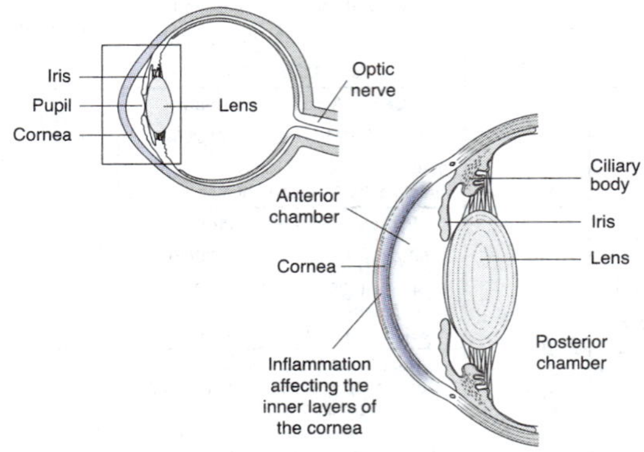

370.52 Diffuse interstitial keratitis
Cogan's syndrome

370.54 Sclerosing keratitis

370.55 Corneal abscess

370.59 Other
Excludes *disciform herpes simplex keratitis (054.43)*
syphilitic keratitis (090.3)

⑤ **370.6 Corneal neovascularization**

370.60 Corneal neovascularization, unspecified

370.61 Localized vascularization of cornea

370.62 Pannus (corneal)
AHA: 3Q 2002, 20

370.63 Deep vascularization of cornea

370.64 Ghost vessels (corneal)

370.8 Other forms of keratitis
AHA: 3Q 1994, 5

✖ **370.9 Unspecified keratitis**

④ **371 Corneal opacity and other disorders of cornea**

⑤ **371.0 Corneal scars and opacities**
Excludes *that due to vitamin A deficiency (264.6)*

371.00 Corneal opacity, unspecified
Corneal scar NOS

371.01 Minor opacity of cornea
Corneal nebula

371.02 Peripheral opacity of cornea
Corneal macula not interfering with central vision

371.03 Central opacity of cornea
Corneal:
leucoma interfering with central vision
macula interfering with central vision

371.04 Adherent leucoma
DEF: Thick, opaque overgrowth of the cornea onto the iris.

+ ***371.05 Phthisical cornea***
Code first underlying tuberculosis (017.3)
DEF: Wasting and corresponding opacity of the cornea due to tuberculosis.

⑤ **371.1 Corneal pigmentations and deposits**

371.10 Corneal deposit, unspecified

371.11 Anterior pigmentations
Stähli's lines

371.12 Stromal pigmentations
Hematocornea

371.13 Posterior pigmentations
Krukenberg spindle

371.14 Kayser-Fleischer ring
DEF: Gray-green or brownish ring of copper deposits on the exterior of the cornea that slowly grow inward; often seen with liver disorders.

371.15 Other deposits associated with metabolic disorders

371.16 Argentous deposits

❺ **371.2 Corneal edema**

371.20 Corneal edema, unspecified

371.21 Idiopathic corneal edema

371.22 Secondary corneal edema

371.23 Bullous keratopathy

371.24 Corneal edema due to wearing of contact lenses

❺ **371.3 Changes of corneal membranes**

371.30 Corneal membrane change, unspecified

371.31 Folds and rupture of Bowman's membrane

371.32 Folds in Descemet's membrane
DEF: Fold in the membrane between the innermost layer of the cornea and the stroma (strong, supportive layer), affecting vision and preventing the flow of nutrients out to the cornea.

371.33 Rupture in Descemet's membrane

❺ **371.4 Corneal degenerations**

371.40 Corneal degeneration, unspecified

371.41 Senile corneal changes
Arcus senilis
Hassall-Henle bodies

371.42 Recurrent erosion of cornea
Excludes *Mooren's ulcer (370.07)*

371.43 Band-shaped keratopathy
DEF: Degeneration of the cornea in which calcium deposits are laid in horizontal band-like layers, obscuring the patient's vision.

371.44 Other calcerous degenerations of cornea

371.45 Keratomalacia NOS
Excludes *that due to vitamin A deficiency (264.4)*

371.46 Nodular degeneration of cornea
Salzmann's nodular dystrophy

371.48 Peripheral degenerations of cornea
Marginal degeneration of cornea [Terrien's]

371.49 Other
Discrete colliquative keratopathy

❺ **371.5 Hereditary corneal dystrophies**

371.50 Corneal dystrophy, unspecified

A genetic condition that causes the cornea to weaken and degenerate so as to become opaque, retain fluid (edema), or develop other lesions

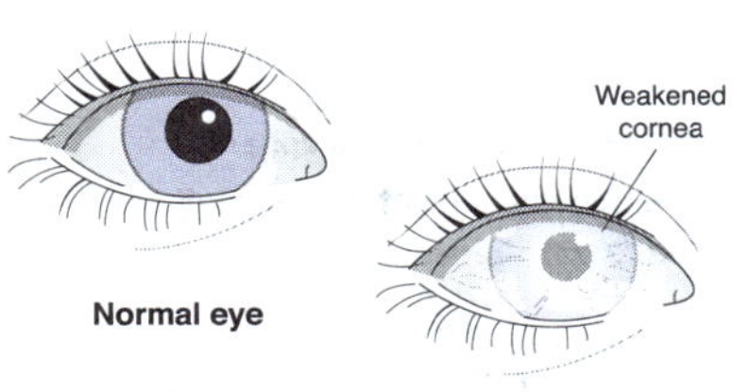

371.51 Juvenile epithelial corneal dystrophy
DEF: Multiple lesions on the outermost layer of the cornea occurring in the early years, which gradually grow together and obscure vision.

371.52 Other anterior corneal dystrophies
Corneal dystrophy:
microscopic cystic
ring-like

371.53 Granular corneal dystrophy

371.54 Lattice corneal dystrophy

371.55 Macular corneal dystrophy

371.56 Other stromal corneal dystrophies
Crystalline corneal dystrophy

371.57 Endothelial corneal dystrophy
Combined corneal dystrophy
Cornea guttata
Fuchs' endothelial dystrophy

371.58 Other posterior corneal dystrophies
Polymorphous corneal dystrophy

❺ **371.6 Keratoconus**

371.60 Keratoconus, unspecified

371.61 Keratoconus, stable condition

371.62 Keratoconus, acute hydrops

❺ **371.7 Other corneal deformities**

371.70 Corneal deformity, unspecified

371.71 Corneal ectasia

371.72 Descemetocele

371.73 Corneal staphyloma

❺ **371.8 Other corneal disorders**

371.81 Corneal anesthesia and hypoesthesia
DEF: Decreased or complete loss of corneal sensitivity to pain and irritation.

371.82 Corneal disorder due to contact lens
Excludes *corneal edema due to contact lens (371.24)*

371.89 Other
AHA: 3Q 1999, 12

✖ **371.9 Unspecified corneal disorder**

❹ **372 Disorders of conjunctiva**
Excludes *keratoconjunctivitis (370.3-370.4)*

❺ **372.0 Acute conjunctivitis**

372.00 Acute conjunctivitis, unspecified

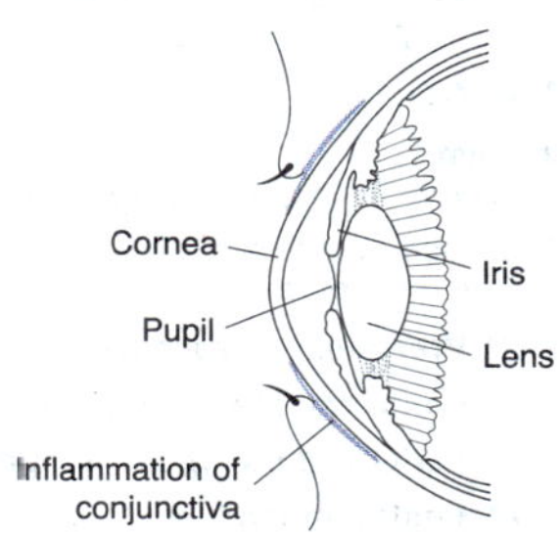

372.01 Serous conjunctivitis, except viral
Excludes *viral conjunctivitis NOS (077.9)*

372.02 Acute follicular conjunctivitis
Conjunctival folliculosis NOS
Excludes *conjunctivitis:*
adenoviral (acute follicular) (077.3)
epidemic hemorrhagic (077.4)
inclusion (077.0)
Newcastle (077.8)
epidemic keratoconjunctivitis (077.1)
pharyngoconjunctival fever (077.2)

372.03 Other mucopurulent conjunctivitis
Catarrhal conjunctivitis
Excludes *blennorrhea neonatorum (gonococcal) (098.40)*
neonatal conjunctivitis (771.6)
ophthalmia neonatorum NOS (771.6)
DEF: Inflammation of the conjunctiva with the production of mucous and pus.

372.04 Pseudomembranous conjunctivitis
Membranous conjunctivitis
Excludes *diphtheritic conjunctivitis (032.81)*

372.05 Acute atopic conjunctivitis
DEF: Sudden, severe case of conjunctivitis caused by allergies.

5 **372.1 Chronic conjunctivitis**
372.10 Chronic conjunctivitis, unspecified
372.11 Simple chronic conjunctivitis
372.12 Chronic follicular conjunctivitis
372.13 Vernal conjunctivitis
DEF: Seasonal inflammation of the conjunctiva due to an allergic reaction to pollen, mold, or another seasonal factor.
AHA: 3Q 1996, 8
372.14 Other chronic allergic conjunctivitis
AHA: 3Q 1996, 8
+ ***372.15 Parasitic conjunctivitis***
Code first underlying disease as:
filariasis (125.0-125.9)
mucocutaneous leishmaniasis (085.5)

5 **372.2 Blepharoconjunctivitis**
372.20 Blepharoconjunctivitis, unspecified
372.21 Angular blepharoconjunctivitis
372.22 Contact blepharoconjunctivitis
DEF: Inflammation of the conjunctiva and eyelid due to wearing contact lenses.

5 **372.3 Other and unspecified conjunctivitis**
372.30 Conjunctivitis, unspecified
+ ***372.31 Rosacea conjunctivitis***
Code first underlying rosacea dermatitis (695.3)
+ ***372.33 Conjunctivitis in mucocutaneous disease***
Code first underlying disease as:
erythema multiforme (695.1)
Reiter's disease (099.3)
Excludes *ocular pemphigoid (694.61)*
372.39 Other

5 **372.4 Pterygium**
Excludes *pseudopterygium (372.52)*
DEF: Raised, wedge-shaped overgrowth of the conjunctiva onto the cornea of the eye.
372.40 Pterygium, unspecified
372.41 Peripheral pterygium, stationary
372.42 Peripheral pterygium, progressive
372.43 Central pterygium
DEF: Pterygium which has grown into the center of the cornea, entering the patient's visual field.
372.44 Double pterygium
372.45 Recurrent pterygium

5 **372.5 Conjunctival degenerations and deposits**
372.50 Conjunctival degeneration, unspecified
372.51 Pinguecula
DEF: Small, nonmalignant, yellowish growth on the conjunctiva often asymptomatic and requiring no treatment but may cause irritation.
372.52 Pseudopterygium
372.53 Conjunctival xerosis
Excludes *conjunctival xerosis due to vitamin A deficiency (264.0, 264.1, 264.7)*
372.54 Conjunctival concretions
DEF: Yellow-white granules or cysts which form just beneath the conjunctiva, wearing it away and causing the sensation of a foreign body in the eye.
372.55 Conjunctival pigmentations
Conjunctival argyrosis
372.56 Conjunctival deposits

5 **372.6 Conjunctival scars**
372.61 Granuloma of conjunctiva
372.62 Localized adhesions and strands of conjunctiva
372.63 Symblepharon
Extensive adhesions of conjunctiva
DEF: Conjunctiva of the eyelid that has adhered to the eye, sometimes over the cornea, requiring surgical removal.
372.64 Scarring of conjunctiva
Contraction of eye socket (after enucleation)

5 **372.7 Conjunctival vascular disorders and cysts**
372.71 Hyperemia of conjunctiva
372.72 Conjunctival hemorrhage
Hyposphagma
Subconjunctival hemorrhage
372.73 Conjunctival edema
Chemosis of conjunctiva
Subconjunctival edema
372.74 Vascular abnormalities of conjunctiva
Aneurysm(ata) of conjunctiva
372.75 Conjunctival cysts

5 **372.8 Other disorders of conjunctiva**
372.81 Conjunctivochalasis
DEF: Loosening of the conjunctiva's attachment to the eye, causing wrinkling, dryness, and a tendency to trap particles in the folds, causing chronic inflammation.
AHA: 4Q 2000, 41
372.89 Other disorders of conjunctiva

✖ **372.9 Unspecified disorder of conjunctiva**

4 **373 Inflammation of eyelids**
5 **373.0 Blepharitis**
Excludes *blepharoconjunctivitis (372.20-372.22)*
373.00 Blepharitis, unspecified
373.01 Ulcerative blepharitis

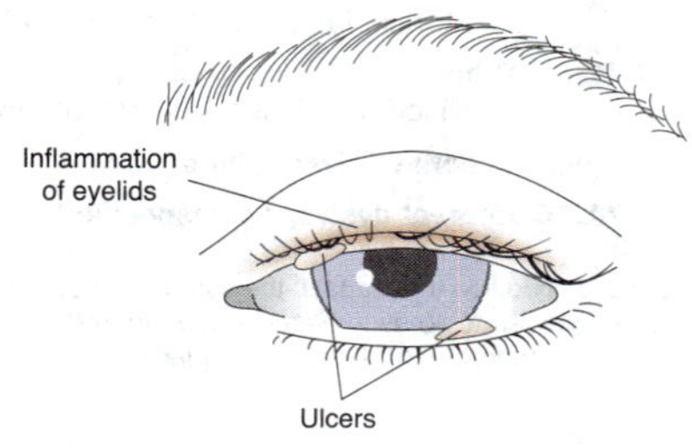

373.02 Squamous blepharitis

5 **373.1 Hordeolum and other deep inflammation of eyelid**
373.11 Hordeolum externum
Hordeolum NOS
Stye
DEF: Infection of an oil gland in an eyelash follicle.
373.12 Hordeolum internum
Infection of meibomian gland
373.13 Abscess of eyelid
Furuncle of eyelid

373.2 Chalazion
Meibomian (gland) cyst
Excludes *infected meibomian gland (373.12)*

❺ **373.3 Noninfectious dermatoses of eyelid**

373.31 Eczematous dermatitis of eyelid

373.32 Contact and allergic dermatitis of eyelid

373.33 Xeroderma of eyelid

373.34 Discoid lupus erythematosus of eyelid

+ ***373.4 Infective dermatitis of eyelid of types resulting in deformity***
Code first underlying disease, as:
leprosy (030.0-030.9)
lupus vulgaris (tuberculous) (017.0)
yaws (102.0-102.9)

+ ***373.5 Other infective dermatitis of eyelid***
Code first underlying disease, as:
actinomycosis (039.3)
impetigo (684)
mycotic dermatitis (110.0-111.9)
vaccinia (051.0)
postvaccination (999.0)
Excludes *herpes:*
simplex (054.41)
zoster (053.20)

+ ***373.6 Parasitic infestation of eyelid***
Code first underlying disease, as:
leishmaniasis (085.0-085.9)
loiasis (125.2)
onchocerciasis (125.3)
pediculosis (132.0)

373.8 Other inflammations of eyelids

✖ **373.9 Unspecified inflammation of eyelid**

❹ **374 Other disorders of eyelids**

❺ **374.0 Entropion and trichiasis of eyelid**
DEF: Entropion: inward curling of the eyelid margin, usually the bottom, so the lashes irritate the surface of the eyeball.

374.00 Entropion, unspecified

374.01 Senile entropion A

374.02 Mechanical entropion

374.03 Spastic entropion

374.04 Cicatricial entropion

374.05 Trichiasis without entropion
DEF: Trichiasis: ingrowing eyelashes

❺ **374.1 Ectropion**
DEF: Outward curling of the eyelid away from the eye, usually the lower, exposing the inner surface and causing irritation, dryness, and possible damage.

374.10 Ectropion, unspecified

374.11 Senile ectropion A

374.12 Mechanical ectropion

374.13 Spastic ectropion

374.14 Cicatricial ectropion

❺ **374.2 Lagophthalmos**

374.20 Lagophthalmos, unspecified

374.21 Paralytic lagophthalmos

374.22 Mechanical lagophthalmos

374.23 Cicatricial lagophthalmos
DEF: Inability to completely close the eye due to the presence of scar tissue.

❺ **374.3 Ptosis of eyelid**

374.30 Ptosis of eyelid, unspecified
AHA: 2Q 1996, 11

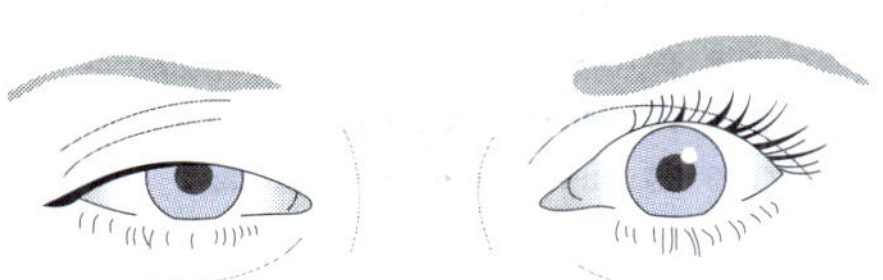

374.31 Paralytic ptosis

374.32 Myogenic ptosis

374.33 Mechanical ptosis

374.34 Blepharochalasis
Pseudoptosis

❺ **374.4 Other disorders affecting eyelid function**
Excludes *blepharoclonus (333.81)*
blepharospasm (333.81)
facial nerve palsy (351.0)
third nerve palsy or paralysis (378.51-378.52)
tic (psychogenic) (307.20-307.23)
organic (333.3)

374.41 Lid retraction or lag

374.43 Abnormal innervation syndrome
Jaw-blinking
Paradoxical facial movements
DEF: Sagging of the skin of the upper eyelid over the eye, obstructing vision; usually due to changes in elastin and collagen, affecting the skin's elasticity.

374.44 Sensory disorders

374.45 Other sensorimotor disorders
Deficient blink reflex

374.46 Blepharophimosis
Ankyloblepharon
DEF: Hereditary disorder in which the palpebral fissures (space between the eyelids) is narrowed, giving the appearance of continually squinting.

❺ **374.5 Degenerative disorders of eyelid and periocular area**

374.50 Degenerative disorder of eyelid, unspecified

+ ***374.51 Xanthelasma***
Xanthoma (planum) (tuberosum) of eyelid
Code first underlying condition (272.0-272.9)

374.52 Hyperpigmentation of eyelid
Chloasma
Dyspigmentation

374.53 Hypopigmentation of eyelid
Vitiligo of eyelid

374.54 Hypertrichosis of eyelid

374.55 Hypotrichosis of eyelid
Madarosis of eyelid

374.56 Other degenerative disorders of skin affecting eyelid

❺ **374.8 Other disorders of eyelid**

374.81 Hemorrhage of eyelid
Excludes *black eye (921.0)*

374.82 Edema of eyelid
Hyperemia of eyelid

374.83 Elephantiasis of eyelid

374.84 Cysts of eyelids
Sebaceous cyst of eyelid

374.85 Vascular anomalies of eyelid

374.86 Retained foreign body of eyelid

374.87 Dermatochalasis

374.89 Other disorders of eyelid

✖ **374.9 Unspecified disorder of eyelid**

❹ **375 Disorders of lacrimal system**

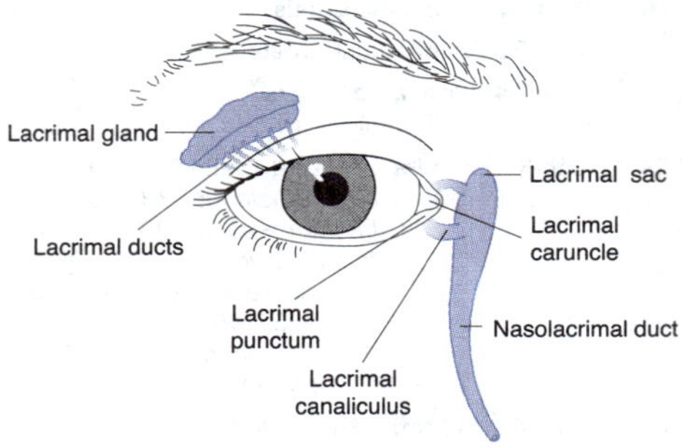

❺ **375.0 Dacryoadenitis**

DEF: Inflammation of the lacrimal gland.

375.00 Dacryoadenitis, unspecified

375.01 Acute dacryoadenitis

375.02 Chronic dacryoadenitis

375.03 Chronic enlargement of lacrimal gland

❺ **375.1 Other disorders of lacrimal gland**

375.11 Dacryops

DEF: Overproduction of tears causing constant tearing.

375.12 Other lacrimal cysts and cystic degeneration

375.13 Primary lacrimal atrophy

DEF: Wasting of the lacrimal glands causing severe dryness with decreased tear production.

375.14 Secondary lacrimal atrophy

375.15 Tear film insufficiency, unspecified

Dry eye syndrome

AHA: 3Q 1996, 6

375.16 Dislocation of lacrimal gland

DEF: Lacrimal gland separated from the tear ducts, preventing tears from passing normally to the eye.

❺ **375.2 Epiphora**

375.20 Epiphora, unspecified as to cause

Tear overflow caused by overproduction or blockage of lacrimal passages

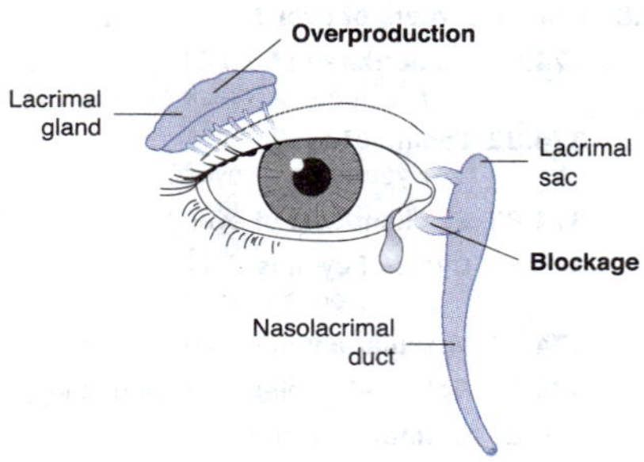

375.21 Epiphora due to excess lacrimation

375.22 Epiphora due to insufficient drainage

❺ **375.3 Acute and unspecified inflammation of lacrimal passages**

Excludes *neonatal dacryocystitis (771.6)*

375.30 Dacryocystitis, unspecified

375.31 Acute canaliculitis, lacrimal

DEF: Severe, sudden inflammation of the lacrimal passages or tear ducts.

375.32 Acute dacryocystitis

Acute peridacryocystitis

DEF: Sudden, severe inflammation of the tear sac, usually due to blockage of the tear ducts.

375.33 Phlegmonous dacryocystitis

❺ **375.4 Chronic inflammation of lacrimal passages**

375.41 Chronic canaliculitis

375.42 Chronic dacryocystitis

375.43 Lacrimal mucocele

DEF: Inflammation of the lacrimal system in which the tear ducts, and then the eyes, become filled with mucous.

❺ **375.5 Stenosis and insufficiency of lacrimal passages**

375.51 Eversion of lacrimal punctum

DEF: Tear duct exit turned away from the eye, causing tears to flow directly onto the face instead of moistening the eyeball.

375.52 Stenosis of lacrimal punctum

375.53 Stenosis of lacrimal canaliculi

375.54 Stenosis of lacrimal sac

375.55 Obstruction of nasolacrimal duct, neonatal

Excludes *congenital anomaly of nasolacrimal duct (743.65)*

375.56 Stenosis of nasolacrimal duct, acquired

375.57 Dacryolith

❺ **375.6 Other changes of lacrimal passages**

375.61 Lacrimal fistula

375.69 Other

❺ **375.8 Other disorders of lacrimal system**

375.81 Granuloma of lacrimal passages

375.89 Other

✖ **375.9 Unspecified disorder of lacrimal system**

❹ **376 Disorders of the orbit**

❺ **376.0 Acute inflammation of orbit**

376.00 Acute inflammation of orbit, unspecified

376.01 Orbital cellulitis

Abscess of orbit

376.02 Orbital periostitis

376.03 Orbital osteomyelitis

376.04 Tenonitis

❺ **376.1 Chronic inflammatory disorders of orbit**

376.10 Chronic inflammation of orbit, unspecified

376.11 Orbital granuloma

Pseudotumor (inflammatory) of orbit

376.12 Orbital myositis

DEF: Inflammation of one of the muscles that moves the eyeball.

+ ***376.13 Parasitic infestation of orbit***

Code first underlying disease, as:

hydatid infestation of orbit (122.3, 122.6, 122.9)

myiasis of orbit (134.0)

❺ **376.2 Endocrine exophthalmos**

Code first underlying thyroid disorder (242.0-242.9)

+ ***376.21 Thyrotoxic exophthalmos***

DEF: Excess production of thyroid hormones causing painful inflammation of the eye muscles, and protrusion of the eye from the socket.

+ ***376.22 Exophthalmic ophthalmoplegia***

❺ **376.3 Other exophthalmic conditions**

376.30 Exophthalmos, unspecified

376.31 Constant exophthalmos

376.32 Orbital hemorrhage

376.33 Orbital edema or congestion

376.34 Intermittent exophthalmos

376.35 Pulsating exophthalmos

376.36 Lateral displacement of globe
DEF: Condition in which the eyeball is situated towards the side of the head, away from the nose.

376.4 Deformity of orbit
376.40 Deformity of orbit, unspecified
376.41 Hypertelorism of orbit
376.42 Exostosis of orbit
DEF: Abnormal bone growth of the eye socket; can impair vision and prevent the eye from moving properly.
376.43 Local deformities due to bone disease
376.44 Orbital deformities associated with craniofacial deformities
376.45 Atrophy of orbit
376.46 Enlargement of orbit
376.47 Deformity due to trauma or surgery

376.5 Enophthalmos
DEF: Condition in which the eye is recessed abnormally deep within the eye socket.
376.50 Enophthalmos, unspecified as to cause
376.51 Enophthalmos due to atrophy of orbital tissue
376.52 Enophthalmos due to trauma or surgery

376.6 Retained (old) foreign body following penetrating wound of orbit
Retrobulbar foreign body

376.8 Other orbital disorders
376.81 Orbital cysts
Encephalocele of orbit
AHA: 3Q 1999, 13
376.82 Myopathy of extraocular muscles
376.89 Other

376.9 Unspecified disorder of orbit

377 Disorders of optic nerve and visual pathways

377.0 Papilledema
DEF: Swelling of the optic disk (the part of the retina that connects to the optic nerve) caused by increased intracranial pressure.
377.00 Papilledema, unspecified
C&C Exclusions: 017.30, 017.31, 017.32, 017.33, 017.34, 0173.5, 017.36, 017.90, 017.91, 017.92, 017.93, 017.94, 017.95, 017.96, 036.81, 250.50, 250.51, 250.52, 250.53, 250.80, 250.81, 250.82, 250.83, 250.90, 250.91, 250.92, 250.93, 377.00, 377.01, 377.02, 377.03, 377.14, 377.24, 379.8, 379.90, 379.99, 743.8, 743.9
377.01 Papilledema associated with increased intracranial pressure
C&C Exclusions: See 377.00
377.02 Papilledema associated with decreased ocular pressure
C&C Exclusions: See 377.00
377.03 Papilledema associated with retinal disorder
377.04 Foster-Kennedy syndrome
DEF: Disease that presents with papilledema in one eye and atrophy of the optic nerve of the other; caused by increased intracranial pressure from a tumor.

377.1 Optic atrophy
377.10 Optic atrophy, unspecified
377.11 Primary optic atrophy
Excludes *neurosyphilitic optic atrophy (094.84)*
377.12 Postinflammatory optic atrophy
377.13 Optic atrophy associated with retinal dystrophies
377.14 Glaucomatous atrophy [cupping] of optic disc
377.15 Partial optic atrophy
Temporal pallor of optic disc
377.16 Hereditary optic atrophy
Optic atrophy:
dominant hereditary
Leber's

377.2 Other disorders of optic disc
377.21 Drusen of optic disc
377.22 Crater-like holes of optic disc
377.23 Coloboma of optic disc
DEF: Congenital defect of the iris in which there is a gap, hole, or cleft that failed to close; may cause ghost images, blurred or decreased visual acuity.
377.24 Pseudopapilledema

377.3 Optic neuritis
Excludes *meningococcal optic neuritis (036.81)*
377.30 Optic neuritis, unspecified
377.31 Optic papillitis
DEF: Swelling of the optic disc where the optic nerve connects to the retina.
377.32 Retrobulbar neuritis (acute)
Excludes *syphilitic retrobulbar neuritis (094.85)*
DEF: Inflammation of the optic nerve directly behind the eye.
377.33 Nutritional optic neuropathy
377.34 Toxic optic neuropathy
Toxic amblyopia
377.39 Other
Excludes *ischemic optic neuropathy (377.41)*

377.4 Other disorders of optic nerve
377.41 Ischemic optic neuropathy
377.42 Hemorrhage in optic nerve sheaths
377.43 Optic nerve hypoplasia
AHA: 4Q 2006, 82
377.49 Other
Compression of optic nerve

377.5 Disorders of optic chiasm
377.51 Associated with pituitary neoplasms and disorders
DEF: Interruption of neural impulses from the eye to the brain due to a tumor or other disorder of the pituitary gland.
377.52 Associated with other neoplasms
377.53 Associated with vascular disorders
377.54 Associated with inflammatory disorders

377.6 Disorders of other visual pathways
377.61 Associated with neoplasms
377.62 Associated with vascular disorders
377.63 Associated with inflammatory disorders

377.7 Disorders of visual cortex
Excludes *visual:*
agnosia (368.16)
hallucinations (368.16)
halos (368.15)
377.71 Associated with neoplasms
377.72 Associated with vascular disorders
377.73 Associated with inflammatory disorders
377.75 Cortical blindness
DEF: Blindness caused by a defect of the brain and not the eyes.

377.9 Unspecified disorder of optic nerve and visual pathways

❹ **378 Strabismus and other disorders of binocular eye movements**
Excludes *nystagmus and other irregular eye movements (379.50-379.59)*

❺ **378.0 Esotropia**
Convergent concomitant strabismus
Excludes *intermittent esotropia (378.20-378.22)*

378.00 Esotropia, unspecified

A type of strabismus in which one or both eyes turn inwards

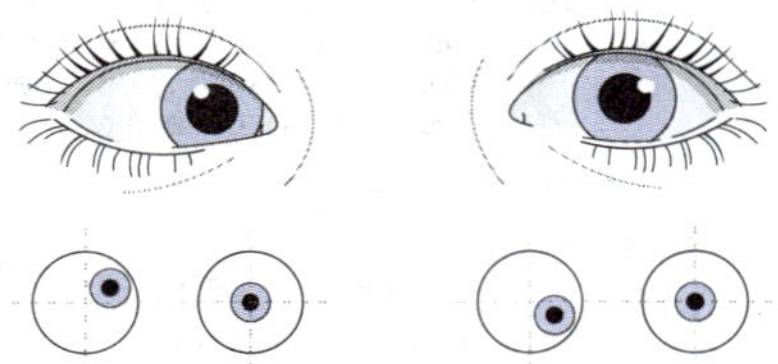

Esotropia with A pattern: eye deviates upwards and inwards

Esotropia with V pattern: eye deviates downwards and inwards

378.01 Monocular esotropia

378.02 Monocular esotropia with A pattern

378.03 Monocular esotropia with V pattern

378.04 Monocular esotropia with other noncomitancies
Monocular esotropia with X or Y pattern

378.05 Alternating esotropia

378.06 Alternating esotropia with A pattern

378.07 Alternating esotropia with V pattern

378.08 Alternating esotropia with other noncomitancies
Alternating esotropia with X or Y pattern

❺ **378.1 Exotropia**
Divergent concomitant strabismus
Excludes *intermittent exotropia (378.20, 378.23-378.24)*

378.10 Exotropia, unspecified

A type of strabismus in which one or both eyes turn outwards

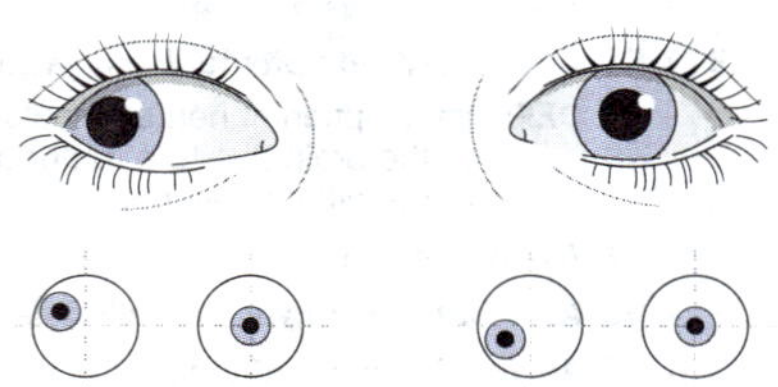

Exotropia with V pattern: eye deviates downwards and outwards

Exotropia with A pattern: eye deviates upwards and outwards

378.11 Monocular exotropia

378.12 Monocular exotropia with A pattern

378.13 Monocular exotropia with V pattern

378.14 Monocular exotropia with other noncomitancies
Monocular exotropia with X or Y pattern

378.15 Alternating exotropia

378.16 Alternating exotropia with A pattern

378.17 Alternating exotropia with V pattern

378.18 Alternating exotropia with other noncomitancies
Alternating exotropia with X or Y pattern

❺ **378.2 Intermittent heterotropia**
Excludes *vertical heterotropia (intermittent) (378.31)*

378.20 Intermittent heterotropia, unspecified
Intermittent:
esotropia NOS
exotropia NOS

378.21 Intermittent esotropia, monocular

378.22 Intermittent esotropia, alternating

378.23 Intermittent exotropia, monocular

378.24 Intermittent exotropia, alternating

❺ **378.3 Other and unspecified heterotropia**

378.30 Heterotropia, unspecified

378.31 Hypertropia
Vertical heterotropia (constant) (intermittent)

378.32 Hypotropia

378.33 Cyclotropia

378.34 Monofixation syndrome
Microtropia

378.35 Accommodative component in esotropia

❺ **378.4 Heterophoria**

378.40 Heterophoria, unspecified

378.41 Esophoria

378.42 Exophoria

378.43 Vertical heterophoria

378.44 Cyclophoria

378.45 Alternating hyperphoria

❺ **378.5 Paralytic strabismus**

378.50 Paralytic strabismus, unspecified

378.51 Third or oculomotor nerve palsy, partial
AHA: 3Q 1991, 9

378.52 Third or oculomotor nerve palsy, total
AHA: 2Q 1989, 12

378.53 Fourth or trochlear nerve palsy
AHA: 2Q 2001, 21

378.54 Sixth or abducens nerve palsy
AHA: 2Q 1989, 12

378.55 External ophthalmoplegia

378.56 Total ophthalmoplegia
DEF: Paralysis of all of the muscles that move the eye as well as the muscles controlling the diameter of the pupil and shape of the lens.

❺ **378.6 Mechanical strabismus**

378.60 Mechanical strabismus, unspecified

378.61 Brown's (tendon) sheath syndrome
DEF: Condition in which the muscle that moves the eye upward and inward is too short, impairing eye movement.

378.62 Mechanical strabismus from other musculofascial disorders

378.63 Limited duction associated with other conditions

❺ **378.7 Other specified strabismus**

378.71 Duane's syndrome
DEF: Abnormal fibrous tissue attached to the muscles that move one of the eyes, inhibiting proper movement.

378.72 Progressive external ophthalmoplegia

378.73 Strabismus in other neuromuscular disorders

❺ **378.8 Other disorders of binocular eye movements**
Excludes *nystagmus (379.50-379.56)*

378.81 Palsy of conjugate gaze

378.82 Spasm of conjugate gaze

378.83 Convergence insufficiency or palsy

378.84 Convergence excess or spasm
DEF: Eyes fail to move in a coordinated fashion when viewing objects up close.

378.85 Anomalies of divergence

378.86 Internuclear ophthalmoplegia

378.87 Other dissociated deviation of eye movements
Skew deviation

✖ **378.9 Unspecified disorder of eye movements**
Ophthalmoplegia NOS
Strabismus NOS
AHA: 2Q 2001, 21

❹ **379 Other disorders of eye**

❺ **379.0 Scleritis and episcleritis**

Excludes *syphilitic episcleritis (095.0)*

379.00 Scleritis, unspecified
Episcleritis NOS

379.01 Episcleritis periodica fugax

DEF: Periodic attacks of inflammation of the sclera; typically of rapid onset and short duration.

379.02 Nodular episcleritis

379.03 Anterior scleritis

379.04 Scleromalacia perforans

379.05 Scleritis with corneal involvement
Scleroperikeratitis

379.06 Brawny scleritis

DEF: Severe inflammation of the sclera affecting the border between the sclera and the cornea.

379.07 Posterior scleritis
Sclerotenonitis

379.09 Other
Scleral abscess

❺ **379.1 Other disorders of sclera**

Excludes *blue sclera (743.47)*

379.11 Scleral ectasia
Scleral staphyloma NOS

DEF: Contents of the eyeball protrude through an abnormally thin section of the sclera.

379.12 Staphyloma posticum

379.13 Equatorial staphyloma

379.14 Anterior staphyloma, localized

379.15 Ring staphyloma

379.16 Other degenerative disorders of sclera

379.19 Other

❺ **379.2 Disorders of vitreous body**

379.21 Vitreous degeneration
Vitreous:
cavitation
detachment
liquefaction

379.22 Crystalline deposits in vitreous
Asteroid hyalitis
Synchysis scintillans

379.23 Vitreous hemorrhage

AHA: 3Q 1991, 15

Blood is found mixing with the vitreous matter

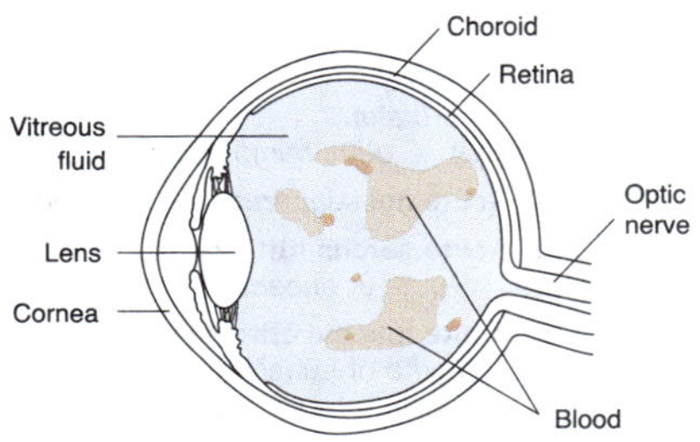

379.24 Other vitreous opacities
Vitreous floaters

379.25 Vitreous membranes and strands

379.26 Vitreous prolapse

379.29 Other disorders of vitreous

Excludes *vitreous abscess (360.04)*

AHA: 1Q 1999, 11

❺ **379.3 Aphakia and other disorders of lens**

Excludes *after-cataract (366.50-366.53)*

379.31 Aphakia

Excludes *cataract extraction status (V45.61)*

DEF: Absence of the crystalline lens of the eye: usually occurs following the surgical removal of cataracts.

379.32 Subluxation of lens

379.33 Anterior dislocation of lens

379.34 Posterior dislocation of lens

379.39 Other disorders of lens

❺ **379.4 Anomalies of pupillary function**

379.40 Abnormal pupillary function, unspecified

379.41 Anisocoria

DEF: Pupils of unequal size.

379.42 Miosis (persistent), not due to miotics

379.43 Mydriasis (persistent), not due to mydriatics

379.45 Argyll Robertson pupil, atypical
Argyll Robertson phenomenon or pupil, nonsyphilitic

Excludes *Argyll Robertson pupil (syphilitic) (094.89)*

379.46 Tonic pupillary reaction
Adie's pupil or syndrome

379.49 Other
Hippus
Pupillary paralysis

❺ **379.5 Nystagmus and other irregular eye movements**

379.50 Nystagmus, unspecified

AHA: 4Q 2002, 68; 2Q 2001, 21

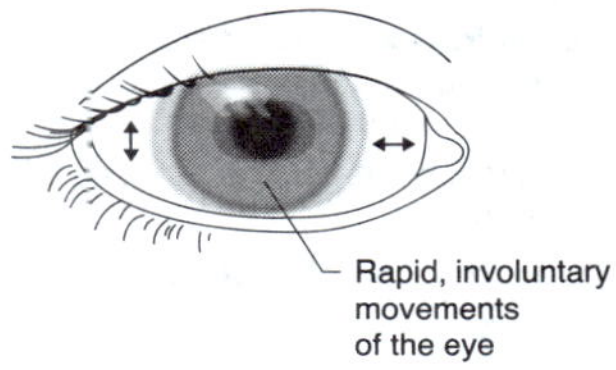

379.51 Congenital nystagmus

379.52 Latent nystagmus

379.53 Visual deprivation nystagmus

379.54 Nystagmus associated with disorders of the vestibular system

379.55 Dissociated nystagmus

379.56 Other forms of nystagmus

379.57 Deficiencies of saccadic eye movements
Abnormal optokinetic response

DEF: Rapid and involuntary eye movement while changing focus on stationary objects.

379.58 Deficiencies of smooth pursuit movements

DEF: Jerking eye movement while tracking a moving object.

379.59 Other irregularities of eye movements
Opsoclonus

❺ **379.6 Inflammation (infection) of postprocedural bleb**
Postprocedural blebitis

✖ **379.60 Inflammation (infection) of postprocedural bleb, unspecified**

C&C Exclusions: 377.00, 377.01, 377.02

379.61 Inflammation (infection) of postprocedural bleb, stage 1

C&C Exclusions: See 379.60

379.62 Inflammation (infection) of postprocedural bleb, stage 2

C&C Exclusions: See 379.60

AHA: 4Q 2006, 83

379.63 Inflammation (infection) of postprocedural bleb, stage 3
Bleb associated endophthalmitis
C&C Exclusions: See 379.60

379.8 Other specified disorders of eye and adnexa

❺ **379.9 Unspecified disorder of eye and adnexa**

379.90 Disorder of eye, unspecified

379.91 Pain in or around eye

379.92 Swelling or mass of eye

379.93 Redness or discharge of eye

379.99 Other ill-defined disorders of eye
Excludes *blurred vision NOS (368.8)*

DISEASES OF THE EAR AND MASTOID PROCESS (380-389)

Ear anatomy

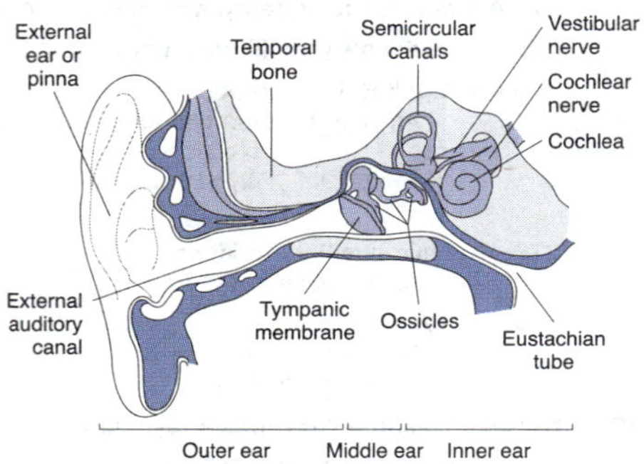

❹ **380 Disorders of external ear**

❺ **380.0 Perichondritis and chondritis of pinna**
Chondritis of auricle
Perichondritis of auricle
DEF: Inflammation of the cartilage of the outer, visible part of the ear.

380.00 Perichondritis of pinna, unspecified

380.01 Acute perichondritis of pinna

380.02 Chronic perichondritis of pinna

380.03 Chondritis of pinna
AHA: 4Q 2004, 76

❺ **380.1 Infective otitis externa**
DEF: Infection of the outer ear canal.

380.10 Infective otitis externa, unspecified
Otitis externa (acute):
NOS
circumscribed
diffuse
hemorrhagica
infective NOS

380.11 Acute infection of pinna
Excludes *furuncular otitis externa (680.0)*

380.12 Acute swimmers' ear
Beach ear
Tank ear

✚ ***380.13 Other acute infections of external ear***
Code first underlying disease, as:
erysipelas (035)
impetigo (684)
seborrheic dermatitis (690.10-690.18)
Excludes *herpes simplex (054.73)*
herpes zoster (053.71)

380.14 Malignant otitis externa

✚ ***380.15 Chronic mycotic otitis externa***
Code first underlying disease, as:
aspergillosis (117.3)
otomycosis NOS (111.9)
Excludes *candidal otitis externa (112.82)*
DEF: Fungal infection of the outer ear lasting for an extended period of time.

380.16 Other chronic infective otitis externa
Chronic infective otitis externa NOS

❺ **380.2 Other otitis externa**

380.21 Cholesteatoma of external ear
Keratosis obturans of external ear (canal)
Excludes *cholesteatoma NOS (385.30-385.35)*
postmastoidectomy (383.32)

380.22 Other acute otitis externa
Acute otitis externa:
actinic
chemical
contact
eczematoid
reactive

380.23 Other chronic otitis externa
Chronic otitis externa NOS

❺ **380.3 Noninfectious disorders of pinna**

380.30 Disorder of pinna, unspecified

380.31 Hematoma of auricle or pinna
DEF: Swelling filled with blood on the outer ear.

380.32 Acquired deformities of auricle or pinna
Excludes *cauliflower ear (738.7)*
AHA: 3Q 2003, 12

380.39 Other
Excludes *gouty tophi of ear (274.81)*

380.4 Impacted cerumen
Wax in ear
DEF: Ear wax blocking the external ear canal.

❺ **380.5 Acquired stenosis of external ear canal**
Collapse of external ear canal

380.50 Acquired stenosis of external ear canal, unspecified as to cause

380.51 Secondary to trauma

380.52 Secondary to surgery

380.53 Secondary to inflammation

❺ **380.8 Other disorders of external ear**

380.81 Exostosis of external ear canal
DEF: A bony growth covered with cartilage on the outer ear.

380.89 Other

✖ **380.9 Unspecified disorder of external ear**

❹ **381 Nonsuppurative otitis media and Eustachian tube disorders**

❺ **381.0 Acute nonsuppurative otitis media**
Acute tubotympanic catarrh
Otitis media, acute or subacute:
catarrhal
exudative
transudative
with effusion
Excludes *otitic barotrauma (993.0)*

381.00 Acute nonsuppurative otitis media, unspecified

381.01 Acute serous otitis media
Acute or subacute secretory otitis media

381.02 Acute mucoid otitis media
Acute or subacute seromucinous otitis media
Blue drum syndrome

381.03 Acute sanguinous otitis media
DEF: Middle ear infection accompanied by bleeding from the ear's structures or membranes.

381.04 Acute allergic serous otitis media

381.05 Acute allergic mucoid otitis media

381.06 Acute allergic sanguinous otitis media

❺ **381.1 Chronic serous otitis media**
Chronic tubotympanic catarrh

381.10 Chronic serous otitis media, simple or unspecified

381.19 **Other**
Serosanguinous chronic otitis media

5 381.2 **Chronic mucoid otitis media**
Glue ear
Excludes *adhesive middle ear disease (385.10-385.19)*

DEF: Long-term middle ear infection causing mucous to become trapped in the middle ear.

381.20 **Chronic mucoid otitis media, simple or unspecified**

381.29 **Other**
Mucosanguinous chronic otitis media

381.3 **Other and unspecified chronic nonsuppurative otitis media**
Otitis media, chronic:
- allergic
- exudative
- secretory
- seromucinous
- transudative
- with effusion

381.4 **Nonsuppurative otitis media, not specified as acute or chronic**
Otitis media:
- allergic
- catarrhal
- exudative
- mucoid
- secretory
- seromucinous
- serous
- transudative
- with effusion

Middle ear

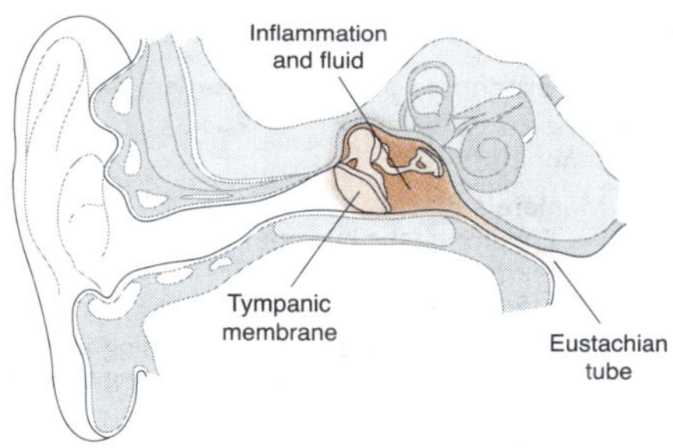

5 381.5 **Eustachian salpingitis**

381.50 **Eustachian salpingitis, unspecified**

381.51 **Acute Eustachian salpingitis**

381.52 **Chronic Eustachian salpingitis**

5 381.6 **Obstruction of Eustachian tube**
Stenosis of Eustachian tube
Stricture of Eustachian tube

381.60 **Obstruction of Eustachian tube, unspecified**

381.61 **Osseous obstruction of Eustachian tube**
Obstruction of Eustachian tube from cholesteatoma, polyp, or other osseous lesion

381.62 **Intrinsic cartilagenous obstruction of Eustachian tube**

381.63 **Extrinsic cartilagenous obstruction of Eustachian tube**
Compression of Eustachian tube

381.7 **Patulous Eustachian tube**

5 381.8 **Other disorders of Eustachian tube**

381.81 **Dysfunction of Eustachian tube**

381.89 **Other**

✖ 381.9 **Unspecified Eustachian tube disorder**

4 382 **Suppurative and unspecified otitis media**

5 382.0 **Acute suppurative otitis media**
Otitis media, acute:
- necrotizing NOS
- purulent

382.00 **Acute suppurative otitis media without spontaneous rupture of ear drum**

382.01 **Acute suppurative otitis media with spontaneous rupture of ear drum**

+ *382.02* ***Acute suppurative otitis media in diseases classified elsewhere***
Code first underlying disease, as:
- influenza (487.8)
- scarlet fever (034.1)

Excludes *postmeasles otitis (055.2)*

382.1 **Chronic tubotympanic suppurative otitis media**
Benign chronic suppurative otitis media (with anterior perforation of ear drum)
Chronic tubotympanic disease (with anterior perforation of ear drum)

382.2 **Chronic atticoantral suppurative otitis media**
Chronic atticoantral disease (with posterior or superior marginal perforation of ear drum)
Persistent mucosal disease (with posterior or superior marginal perforation of ear drum)

382.3 **Unspecified chronic suppurative otitis media**
Chronic purulent otitis media
Excludes *tuberculous otitis media (017.4)*

382.4 **Unspecified suppurative otitis media**
Purulent otitis media NOS

✖ 382.9 **Unspecified otitis media**
Otitis media:
- NOS
- acute NOS
- chronic NOS

AHA: Nov-Dec 1984, 16

4 383 **Mastoiditis and related conditions**

5 383.0 **Acute mastoiditis**
Abscess of mastoid
Empyema of mastoid

383.00 **Acute mastoiditis without complications**

383.01 **Subperiosteal abscess of mastoid**
C&C Exclusions: 015.60, 015.61, 015.62, 015.63, 015.64, 015.65, 015.66, 017.40, 017.41, 017.42, 017.43, 017.44, 017.45, 017.46, 017.90, 017.91, 017.92, 017.93, 017.94, 017.95, 017.96, 383.00, 383.01, 383.02, 383.1, 383.20, 383.21, 383.22, 383.30, 383.31, 383.32, 383.33, 383.81, 383.89, 383.9, 388.71, 388.72, 388.8, 388.9, 744.00, 744.02, 744.09, 744.29, 744.3

383.02 **Acute mastoiditis with other complications**
Gradenigo's syndrome

383.1 **Chronic mastoiditis**
Caries of mastoid
Fistula of mastoid
Excludes *tuberculous mastoiditis (015.6)*

5 383.2 **Petrositis**
Coalescing osteitis of petrous bone
Inflammation of petrous bone
Osteomyelitis of petrous bone

DEF: Inflammation of the dense, hard bone behind the temple protecting the inner ear.

383.20 **Petrositis, unspecified**

383.21 **Acute petrositis**

383.22 **Chronic petrositis**

5 383.3 **Complications following mastoidectomy**

383.30 **Postmastoidectomy complication, unspecified**
C&C Exclusions: See 383.1

383.31 **Mucosal cyst of postmastoidectomy cavity**

383.32 **Recurrent cholesteatoma of postmastoidectomy cavity**

A Adult (15+ years) M Maternity (12-55 years) N Newborn (0 years) P Pediatric (0-17 years) ♂ Male ♀ Female 2 Medicare Secondary Payer

383.33 Granulations of postmastoidectomy cavity
Chronic inflammation of postmastoidectomy cavity

❺ **383.8 Other disorders of mastoid**

383.81 Postauricular fistula
C&C Exclusions: See 383.1

383.89 Other

✖ **383.9 Unspecified mastoiditis**

❹ **384 Other disorders of tympanic membrane**

❺ **384.0 Acute myringitis without mention of otitis media**

384.00 Acute myringitis, unspecified
Acute tympanitis NOS

384.01 Bullous myringitis
Myringitis bullosa hemorrhagica
DEF: Inflammation of the eardrum caused by a virus and characterized by blood-filled blisters.

384.09 Other

384.1 Chronic myringitis without mention of otitis media
Chronic tympanitis

❺ **384.2 Perforation of tympanic membrane**
Perforation of ear drum:
NOS
persistent posttraumatic
postinflammatory
Excludes *otitis media with perforation of tympanic membrane (382.00-382.9)*
traumatic perforation [current injury] (872.61)

384.20 Perforation of tympanic membrane, unspecified

384.21 Central perforation of tympanic membrane

384.22 Attic perforation of tympanic membrane
Pars flaccida

384.23 Other marginal perforation of tympanic membrane

384.24 Multiple perforations of tympanic membrane

384.25 Total perforation of tympanic membrane

❺ **384.8 Other specified disorders of tympanic membrane**

384.81 Atrophic flaccid tympanic membrane
Healed perforation of ear drum
DEF: Eardrum that has wasted away and lost its tension, resulting in severe hearing loss.

384.82 Atrophic nonflaccid tympanic membrane

✖ **384.9 Unspecified disorder of tympanic membrane**

❹ **385 Other disorders of middle ear and mastoid**
Excludes *mastoiditis (383.0-383.9)*

❺ **385.0 Tympanosclerosis**
DEF: Thickening and hardening of the eardrum, reducing its ability to vibrate and transmit sound.

385.00 Tympanosclerosis, unspecified as to involvement

385.01 Tympanosclerosis involving tympanic membrane only

385.02 Tympanosclerosis involving tympanic membrane and ear ossicles

385.03 Tympanosclerosis involving tympanic membrane, ear ossicles, and middle ear

385.09 Tympanosclerosis involving other combination of structures

❺ **385.1 Adhesive middle ear disease**
Adhesive otitis
Otitis media:
chronic adhesive
fibrotic
Excludes *glue ear (381.20-381.29)*

385.10 Adhesive middle ear disease, unspecified as to involvement

385.11 Adhesions of drum head to incus

385.12 Adhesions of drum head to stapes

385.13 Adhesions of drum head to promontorium

385.19 Other adhesions and combinations

❺ **385.2 Other acquired abnormality of ear ossicles**

385.21 Impaired mobility of malleus
Ankylosis of malleus

385.22 Impaired mobility of other ear ossicles
Ankylosis of ear ossicles, except malleus

385.23 Discontinuity or dislocation of ear ossicles

385.24 Partial loss or necrosis of ear ossicles

❺ **385.3 Cholesteatoma of middle ear and mastoid**
Cholesterosis of (middle) ear
Epidermosis of (middle) ear
Keratosis of (middle) ear
Polyp of (middle) ear
Excludes *cholesteatoma:*
external ear canal (380.21)
recurrent of postmastoidectomy cavity (383.32)
DEF: Cyst-like mass filled with cell debris and cholesterol crystals in the middle ear and/or mastoid process that can damage the ossicles, causing deafness, vertigo, and nerve deterioration.

385.30 Cholesteatoma, unspecified

385.31 Cholesteatoma of attic

385.32 Cholesteatoma of middle ear

385.33 Cholesteatoma of middle ear and mastoid
AHA: 3Q 2000, 10

385.35 Diffuse cholesteatosis

❺ **385.8 Other disorders of middle ear and mastoid**

385.82 Cholesterin granuloma

385.83 Retained foreign body of middle ear
AHA: 3Q 1994, 7; Nov-Dec 1987, 9

385.89 Other

✖ **385.9 Unspecified disorder of middle ear and mastoid**

❹ **386 Vertiginous syndromes and other disorders of vestibular system**
Excludes *vertigo NOS (780.4)*
AHA: Mar-Apr 1985, 12

❺ **386.0 Méniére's disease**
Endolymphatic hydrops
Lermoyez's syndrome
Méniére's syndrome or vertigo
DEF: Disorder of the inner ear causing attacks of vertigo, tinnitus, and progressive hearing loss involving all tones.

386.00 Méniére's disease, unspecified
Méniére's disease (active)

386.01 Active Méniére's disease, cochleovestibular

386.02 Active Méniére's disease, cochlear

386.03 Active Méniére's disease, vestibular

386.04 Inactive Méniére's disease
Méniére's disease in remission

❺ **386.1 Other and unspecified peripheral vertigo**
Excludes *epidemic vertigo (078.81)*

386.10 Peripheral vertigo, unspecified

386.11 Benign paroxysmal positional vertigo
Benign paroxysmal positional nystagmus
DEF: Severe vertigo and nystagmus caused by calcified debris within the inner ear that migrates to the semicircular canal and causes endolymph displacement when the head is turned in the direction of the affected ear.

386.12 Vestibular neuronitis
Acute (and recurrent) peripheral vestibulopathy

386.19 Other
Aural vertigo
Otogenic vertigo

386.2 Vertigo of central origin
Central positional nystagmus
Malignant positional vertigo

5 386.3 Labyrinthitis

386.30 Labyrinthitis, unspecified

386.31 Serous labyrinthitis
Diffuse labyrinthitis
DEF: Inflammation of the inner ear, accompanied by fluid buildup.

386.32 Circumscribed labyrinthitis
Focal labyrinthitis

386.33 Suppurative labyrinthitis
Purulent labyrinthitis
DEF: Inflammation of the inner ear, accompanied by a discharge of pus.

386.34 Toxic labyrinthitis

386.35 Viral labyrinthitis

5 386.4 Labyrinthine fistula

386.40 Labyrinthine fistula, unspecified

386.41 Round window fistula

386.42 Oval window fistula

386.43 Semicircular canal fistula

386.48 Labyrinthine fistula of combined sites

5 386.5 Labyrinthine dysfunction

386.50 Labyrinthine dysfunction, unspecified

386.51 Hyperactive labyrinth, unilateral
DEF: Labyrinth of one ear is extra sensitive to sound, gravitation, and pressure changes, causing ear pain, tinnitus, and vertigo.

386.52 Hyperactive labyrinth, bilateral

386.53 Hypoactive labyrinth, unilateral

386.54 Hypoactive labyrinth, bilateral

386.55 Loss of labyrinthine reactivity, unilateral
DEF: Complete loss of inner ear sensitivity to sound, gravitation, and pressure on one side.

386.56 Loss of labyrinthine reactivity, bilateral

386.58 Other forms and combinations

386.8 Other disorders of labyrinth

386.9 Unspecified vertiginous syndromes and labyrinthine disorders

4 387 Otosclerosis
Includes otospongiosis

387.0 Otosclerosis involving oval window, nonobliterative

387.1 Otosclerosis involving oval window, obliterative

387.2 Cochlear otosclerosis
Otosclerosis involving:
otic capsule
round window

387.8 Other otosclerosis

✖ 387.9 Otosclerosis, unspecified

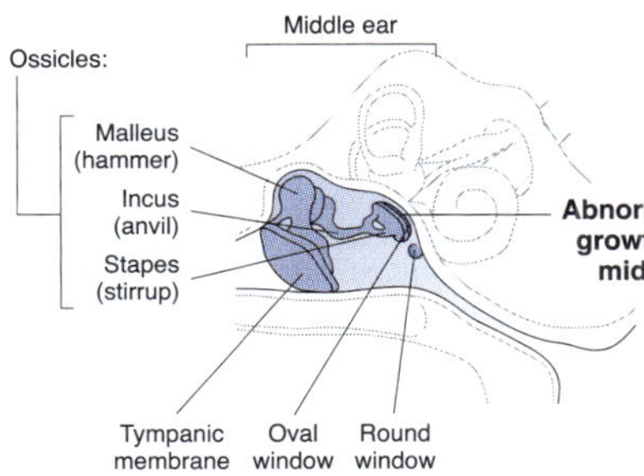

4 388 Other disorders of ear

5 388.0 Degenerative and vascular disorders of ear

✖ 388.00 Degenerative and vascular disorders, unspecified

388.01 Presbyacusis
DEF: Gradual hearing loss that normally occurs with age.

388.02 Transient ischemic deafness
DEF: A passing hearing loss that occurs when blood flow to the auditory organs is decreased due to injury or disease.

5 388.1 Noise effects on inner ear

✖ 388.10 Noise effects on inner ear, unspecified

388.11 Acoustic trauma (explosive) to ear
Otitic blast injury

388.12 Noise-induced hearing loss

388.2 Sudden hearing loss, unspecified

5 388.3 Tinnitus
DEF: Ringing, hissing, roaring, or other sound in the ear in the absence of any apparent stimulus.

✖ 388.30 Tinnitus, unspecified

388.31 Subjective tinnitus

388.32 Objective tinnitus

5 388.4 Other abnormal auditory perception

✖ 388.40 Abnormal auditory perception, unspecified

388.41 Diplacusis
DEF: One sound is heard as two separate sounds at different tones or pitches.

388.42 Hyperacusis
DEF: Hearing is abnormally heightened; normal sounds seem amplified, even cause ear pain.

388.43 Impairment of auditory discrimination

388.44 Recruitment

● 388.45 Acquired auditory processing disorder
Auditory processing disorder NOS
Excludes *central auditory processing disorder (315.32)*

388.5 Disorders of acoustic nerve
Acoustic neuritis
Degeneration of acoustic or eighth nerve
Disorder of acoustic or eighth nerve
Excludes *acoustic neuroma (225.1)*
syphilitic acoustic neuritis (094.86)
AHA: Mar-Apr 1987, 8

5 388.6 Otorrhea
DEF: Fluid leaking from the ear.

✖ 388.60 Otorrhea, unspecified
Discharging ear NOS

388.61 Cerebrospinal fluid otorrhea
Excludes *cerebrospinal fluid rhinorrhea (349.81)*

388.69 Other
Otorrhagia

5 388.7 Otalgia

✖ 388.70 Otalgia, unspecified
Earache NOS

388.71 Otogenic pain

388.72 Referred pain

388.8 Other disorders of ear

✖ 388.9 Unspecified disorder of ear

4 389 Hearing loss

5 389.0 Conductive hearing loss
Conductive deafness
▶ Excludes *mixed conductive and sensorineural hearing loss (389.20-389.22)*◀
DEF: Loss of audio acuity caused by transmission interference of sound waves before they can reach the inner ear and the auditory nerve.
AHA: 4Q 1989, 5

✖ 389.00 Conductive hearing loss, unspecified

389.01 Conductive hearing loss, external ear

389.02 Conductive hearing loss, tympanic membrane

389.03 Conductive hearing loss, middle ear

389.04 Conductive hearing loss, inner ear

● **389.05 Conductive hearing loss, unilateral**

● **389.06 Conductive hearing loss, bilateral**

389.08 Conductive hearing loss of combined types

5 **389.1 Sensorineural hearing loss**

Perceptive hearing loss or deafness

Excludes *abnormal auditory perception (388.40-388.44)*
▶ mixed conductive and sensorineural hearing loss (389.20-389.22)◀
psychogenic deafness (306.7)

AHA: 4Q 1989, 5

✖ **389.10 Sensorineural hearing loss, unspecified**

AHA: 1Q 1993, 29

389.11 Sensory hearing loss, bilateral

DEF: Hearing loss from damage or dysfunction of the hair-like cells of the cochlea in the inner ear.

389.12 Neural hearing loss, bilateral

DEF: Hearing loss stemming from damage to the eighth cranial (auditory) nerve, caused by neurological damage and neuromas.

● **389.13 Neural hearing loss, unilateral**

▲ **389.14 Central hearing loss**

DEF: Hearing loss caused by a disorder of the brain affecting the auditory pathway or the processing of information from the acoustic nerve.

389.15 Sensorineural hearing loss, unilateral

389.16 Sensorineural hearing loss, asymmetrical

● **389.17 Sensory hearing loss, unilateral**

▲ **389.18 Sensorineural hearing loss, bilateral**

5 **389.2 Mixed conductive and sensorineural hearing loss**

Deafness or hearing loss of type classifiable to ▶389.00-389.08◀ with type classifiable to ▶389.10-389.18◀

● **389.20 Mixed hearing loss, unspecified**

● **389.21 Mixed hearing loss, unilateral**

● **389.22 Mixed hearing loss, bilateral**

▲✖ **389.7 Deaf nonspeaking, not elsewhere classifiable**

389.8 Other specified forms of hearing loss

✖ **389.9 Unspecified hearing loss**

Deafness NOS

AHA: 1Q 2004, 15

7. DISEASES OF THE CIRCULATORY SYSTEM (390-459)

Circulatory system

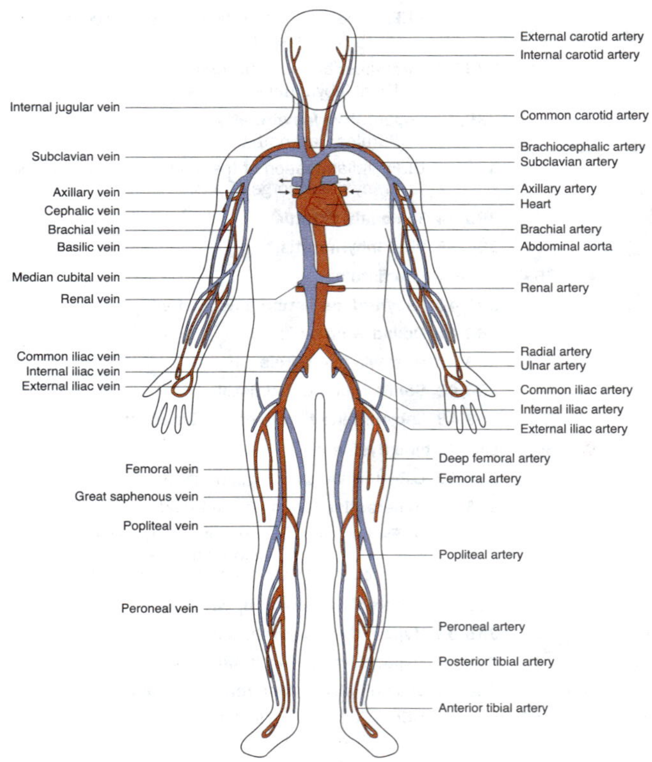

ACUTE RHEUMATIC FEVER (390-392)

390 Rheumatic fever without mention of heart involvement

Arthritis, rheumatic, acute or subacute
Rheumatic fever (active) (acute)
Rheumatism, articular, acute or subacute

Excludes *that with heart involvement (391.0-391.9)*

DEF: Delayed, febrile, inflammatory disease resulting about 20 days after streptococcal infection; presents with joint pain, migratory arthritis, skin rash on the trunk and proximal extremities, nosebleeds; can cause cardiac damage.

4 **391 Rheumatic fever with heart involvement**

Excludes *chronic heart diseases of rheumatic origin (393.0-398.9) unless rheumatic fever is also present or there is evidence of recrudescence or activity of the rheumatic process*

391.0 Acute rheumatic pericarditis

Rheumatic:
fever (active) (acute) with pericarditis
pericarditis (acute)

Any condition classifiable to 390 with pericarditis

Excludes *that not specified as rheumatic (420.0-420.9)*

391.1 Acute rheumatic endocarditis
Rheumatic:
endocarditis, acute
fever (active) (acute) with endocarditis or valvulitis
valvulitis acute
Any condition classifiable to 390 with endocarditis or valvulitis

Endocarditis

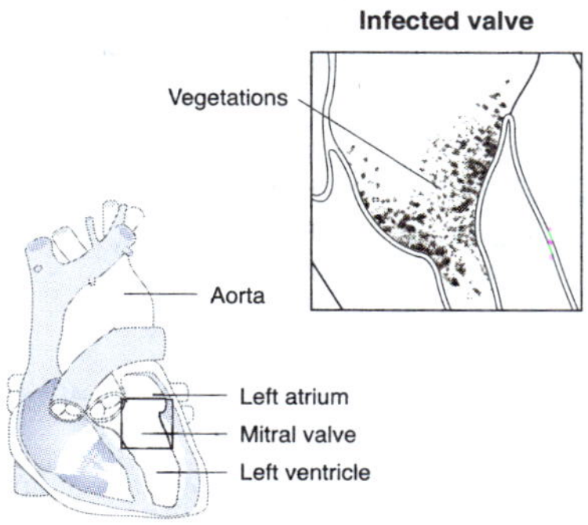

391.2 Acute rheumatic myocarditis
Rheumatic fever (active) (acute) with myocarditis
Any condition classifiable to 390 with myocarditis

391.8 Other acute rheumatic heart disease
Rheumatic:
fever (active) (acute) with other or multiple types of heart involvement
pancarditis, acute
Any condition classifiable to 390 with other or multiple types of heart involvement

391.9 Acute rheumatic heart disease, unspecified
Rheumatic:
carditis, acute
fever (active) (acute) with unspecified type of heart involvement
heart disease, active or acute
Any condition classifiable to 390 with unspecified type of heart involvement

❹ **392 Rheumatic chorea**
Includes Sydenham's chorea
Excludes *chorea:*
NOS (333.5)
Huntington's (333.4)

392.0 With heart involvement
Rheumatic chorea with heart involvement of any type classifiable to 391

392.9 Without mention of heart involvement

CHRONIC RHEUMATIC HEART DISEASE (393-398)

393 Chronic rheumatic pericarditis
Adherent pericardium, rheumatic
Chronic rheumatic:
mediastinopericarditis
myopericarditis
Excludes *pericarditis NOS or not specified as rheumatic (423.0-423.9)*

❹ **394 Diseases of mitral valve**
Excludes *that with aortic valve involvement (396.0-396.9)*

394.0 Mitral stenosis
Mitral (valve):
obstruction (rheumatic)
stenosis NOS
C&C Exclusions: 390, 391.8, 391.9, 394.0, 394.1, 394.2, 394.9, 396.0, 396.1, 396.2, 396.3, 396.8, 396.9, 397.9, 398.90, 398.99, 424.0, 459.89, 459.9

394.1 Rheumatic mitral insufficiency
Rheumatic mitral:
incompetence
regurgitation
Excludes *that not specified as rheumatic (424.0)*
C&C Exclusions: See 394.0
AHA: 2Q 2005, 14

394.2 Mitral stenosis with insufficiency
Mitral stenosis with incompetence or regurgitation
C&C Exclusions: See 394.0
AHA: 1Q 2007, 11-12

394.9 Other and unspecified mitral valve diseases
Mitral (valve):
disease (chronic)
failure
C&C Exclusions: See 394.0

❹ **395 Diseases of aortic valve**
Excludes *that not specified as rheumatic (424.1)*
that with mitral valve involvement (396.0-396.9)

395.0 Rheumatic aortic stenosis
Rheumatic aortic (valve) obstruction
C&C Exclusions: 390, 391.8, 391.9, 395.0, 395.1, 395.2, 395.9, 396.0, 396.1, 396.2, 396.3, 396.8, 396.9, 397.9, 398.90, 398.99, 424.0, 459.89, 459.9
AHA: 4Q 1988, 8

395.1 Rheumatic aortic insufficiency
Rheumatic aortic:
incompetence
regurgitation
C&C Exclusions: See 395.0

395.2 Rheumatic aortic stenosis with insufficiency
Rheumatic aortic stenosis with incompetence or regurgitation
C&C Exclusions: See 395.0

395.9 Other and unspecified rheumatic aortic diseases
Rheumatic aortic (valve) disease
C&C Exclusions: See 395.0

❹ **396 Diseases of mitral and aortic valves**
Includes involvement of both mitral and aortic valves, whether specified as rheumatic or not
AHA: Nov-Dec 1987, 8

396.0 Mitral valve stenosis and aortic valve stenosis
Atypical aortic (valve) stenosis
Mitral and aortic (valve) obstruction (rheumatic)
C&C Exclusions: 390, 391.8, 391.9, 394.0, 394.1, 394.2, 394.9, 396.0, 396.1, 396.2, 396.3, 396.8, 396.9, 397.9, 398.90, 398.99, 424.0, 424.1, 459.89, 459.9

396.1 Mitral valve stenosis and aortic valve insufficiency
C&C Exclusions: See 396.0

396.2 Mitral valve insufficiency and aortic valve stenosis
C&C Exclusions: See 396.0
AHA: 2Q 2000, 16

396.3 Mitral valve insufficiency and aortic valve insufficiency
Mitral and aortic (valve):
incompetence
regurgitation
C&C Exclusions: See 396.0

396.8 Multiple involvement of mitral and aortic valves
Stenosis and insufficiency of mitral or aortic valve with stenosis or insufficiency, or both, of the other valve
C&C Exclusions: See 396.0

396.9 Mitral and aortic valve diseases, unspecified
C&C Exclusions: See 396.0

❹ **397 Diseases of other endocardial structures**

397.0 Diseases of tricuspid valve
Tricuspid (valve) (rheumatic):
disease
insufficiency
obstruction
regurgitation
stenosis
C&C Exclusions: 397.0, 398.90, 398.99, 424.0, 424.1, 459.89, 459.9
AHA: 3Q 2006, 7; 2Q 2000,16

397.1 Rheumatic diseases of pulmonary valve
Excludes *that not specified as rheumatic (424.3)*
C&C Exclusions: 397.1, 398.90, 398.99, 424.0, 424.1, 459.89, 459.9

397.9 Rheumatic diseases of endocardium, valve unspecified
Rheumatic:
endocarditis (chronic)
valvulitis (chronic)
Excludes *that not specified as rheumatic (424.90-424.99)*
C&C Exclusions: 390, 391.1, 391.8, 391.9, 394.0, 394.1, 394.2, 394.9, 395.0, 395.1, 395.2, 395.9, 397.1, 397.9, 398.90, 398.99, 421.0, 421.1, 421.9, 424.0, 424.1, 424.2, 424.3, 424.90, 424.91, 424.99, 459.89, 459.9

❹ **398 Other rheumatic heart disease**

398.0 Rheumatic myocarditis
Rheumatic degeneration of myocardium
Excludes *myocarditis not specified as rheumatic (429.0)*
DEF: Chronic inflammation and degeneration of heart muscle due to rheumatic heart disease.
C&C Exclusions: 390, 391.2, 391.8, 391.9, 398.0, 398.90, 398.99, 422.0, 422.90, 422.91, 422.92, 422.93, 422.99, 429.0, 429.71, 429.79, 459.89, 459.9

❺ **398.9 Other and unspecified rheumatic heart diseases**

398.90 Rheumatic heart disease, unspecified
Rheumatic:
carditis
heart disease NOS
Excludes *carditis not specified as rheumatic (429.89)*
heart disease NOS not specified as rheumatic (429.9)

398.91 Rheumatic heart failure (congestive)
Rheumatic left ventricular failure
DEF: Severe rheumatic damage to heart valves causing heart failure.
C&C Exclusions: 398.90, 398.91, 398.99, 402.01, 402.11, 402.91, 428.0, 428.1, 428.20, 428.21, 428.22, 428.23, 428.30, 428.31, 428.32, 428.33, 428.40, 428.41, 428.42, 428.43, 428.9, 459.89, 459.9
AHA: 2Q 2005, 14; 1Q 1995, 6; 3Q 1988, 3

398.99 Other

HYPERTENSIVE DISEASE (401-405)

Excludes *that complicating pregnancy, childbirth, or the puerperium (642.0-642.9)*
that involving coronary vessels (410.00-414.9)
AHA: 3Q 1990, 3; 2Q 1989, 12; Sep-Oct 1987, 9; Jul-Aug 1984, 11

❹ **401 Essential hypertension**
Includes high blood pressure
hyperpiesia
hyperpiesis
hypertension (arterial) (essential) (primary) (systemic)
hypertensive vascular:
degeneration
disease
Excludes *elevated blood pressure without diagnosis of hypertension (796.2)*
pulmonary hypertension (416.0-416.9)
that involving vessels of:
brain (430-438)
eye (362.11)
AHA: 2Q 1992, 5

401.0 Malignant
C&C Exclusions: 401.0, 401.1, 401.9, 402.00, 402.01, 402.10, 402.11, 402.90, 402.91, 403.00, 403.01, 403.10, 403.11, 403.90, 403.91, 404.00, 404.01, 404.02, 404.03, 404.10, 404.11, 404.12, 404.13, 404.90, 404.91, 404.92, 404.93, 405.01, 405.09, 405.11, 405.19, 405.91, 405.99, 459.89, 459.9
AHA: May-Jun 1985, 19

401.1 Benign

401.9 Unspecified
AHA: 4Q 2005, 71; 3Q 2005, 8; 4Q 2004, 78; 4Q 2003, 105, 108, 111; 3Q 2003, 14; 2Q 2003, 16; 4Q 1997, 37

❹ **402 Hypertensive heart disease**
Use additional code to specify type of heart failure (428.0-428.43), if known
Includes hypertensive:
cardiomegaly
cardiopathy
cardiovascular disease
heart (disease) (failure)
any condition classifiable to 429.0-429.3, 429.8, 429.9 due to hypertension
AHA: 4Q 2002, 49; 2Q 1993, 9; Nov-Dec 1984, 18

❺ **402.0 Malignant**

402.00 Without heart failure
C&C Exclusions: See 401.0

402.01 With heart failure
C&C Exclusions: 398.91, 401.0, 401.1, 401.9, 402.00, 402.01, 402.10, 402.11, 402.90, 402.91, 403.00, 403.01, 403.10, 403.11, 403.90, 403.91, 404.00, 404.01, 404.02, 404.03, 404.10, 404.11, 404.12, 404.13, 404.90, 404.91, 404.92, 404.93, 405.01, 405.09, 405.11, 405.19, 405.91, 405.99, 428.0, 428.1, 428.20, 428.21, 428.22, 428.23, 428.30, 428.31, 428.32, 428.33, 428.40, 428.41, 428.42, 428.43, 428.9, 459.89, 459.9

❺ **402.1 Benign**

402.10 Without heart failure

402.11 With heart failure
C&C Exclusions: See 402.01

❺ **402.9 Unspecified**

402.90 Without heart failure

402.91 With heart failure
C&C Exclusions: See 402.01
AHA: 4Q 2002, 52; 1Q 1993, 19; 2Q 1989, 12

❹ **403 Hypertensive chronic kidney disease**
Includes arteriolar nephritis
arteriosclerosis of:
kidney
renal arterioles
arteriosclerotic nephritis (chronic) (interstitial)
hypertensive:
nephropathy
renal failure
uremia (chronic)
nephrosclerosis
renal sclerosis with hypertension
any condition classifiable to 585, 586, or 587 with any condition classifiable to 401
Excludes *acute renal failure (584.5-584.9)*
renal disease stated as not due to hypertension
renovascular hypertension (405.0-405.9 with fifth-digit 1)
AHA: 4Q 2005, 68; 4Q 1992, 22; 2Q 1992, 5

The following fifth-digit subclassification is for use with category 403:
0 **with chronic kidney disease stage I through stage IV, or unspecified**
Use additional code to identify the stage of chronic kidney disease (585.1-585.4, 585.9)
1 **with chronic kidney disease stage V or end stage renal disease**
Use additional code to identify the stage of chronic kidney disease (585.5-585.6)

❺ **403.0 Malignant**
C&C Exclusions: 401.0, 401.1, 401.9, 402.00, 402.01, 402.10, 402.11, 402.90, 402.91, 403.00, 403.01, 403.10, 403.11, 403.90, 403.91, 404.00, 404.01, 404.02, 404.03, 404.10, 404.11, 404.12, 404.13, 404.90, 404.91, 404.92, 404.93, 405.01, 405.09, 405.11, 405.19, 405.91, 405.99, 459.89, 459.9

❺ **403.1 Benign**
C&C Exclusions: **(for code 403.11)** See 403.0

❹ ❺ Additional Digit Required ✖ Nonspecific PDx ⊘ Unacceptable PDx ✚ Manifestation Code ►◄ Revised Text ● New Code ▲ Revised Code

❺ **403.9 Unspecified**
C&C Exclusions: (for code 403.91) See 403.0
AHA: For Code 403.90: 4Q 2006, 86; For Code: 403.91: 4Q 2005, 69; 1Q 2004, 14; 1Q 2003, 20; 2Q 2001, 11; 3Q 1991, 8

❹ **404 Hypertensive heart and chronic kidney disease**
Use additional code to specify type of heart failure (428.0-428.43), if known
Includes disease:
cardiorenal
cardiovascular renal
any condition classifiable to 402 with any condition classifiable to 403

DEF: Simultaneous disease of the heart and kidneys caused by high blood pressure.

AHA: 4Q 2005, 68; 4Q 2002, 49; 3Q 1990, 3; Jul-Aug 1984, 14

The following fifth-digit subclassification is for use with category 404:
0 without heart failure and with chronic kidney disease stage I through stage IV, or unspecified
Use additional code to identify the stage of chronic kidney disease (585.1-585.4, 585.9)
1 with heart failure and with chronic kidney disease stage I through stage IV, or unspecified
Use additional code to identify the stage of chronic kidney disease (585.1-585.4, 585.9)
2 without heart failure and with chronic kidney disease stage V or end stage renal disease
Use additional code to identify the stage of chronic kidney disease (585.5-585.6)
3 with heart failure and chronic kidney disease stage V or end stage renal disease
Use additional code to identify the stage of chronic kidney disease (585.5-585.6)

❺ **404.0 Malignant**
C&C Exclusions: See 403.0

❺ **404.1 Benign**
C&C Exclusions: (for codes 404.11-404.13) See 403.0

❺ **404.9 Unspecified**
C&C Exclusions: (for codes 404.91-404.93) See 403.0

❹ **405 Secondary hypertension**
AHA: 3Q 1990, 3; Sep-Oct 1987, 9, 11; Jul-Aug 1984, 14

❺ **405.0 Malignant**
405.01 Renovascular
C&C Exclusions: See 403.0
405.09 Other
C&C Exclusions: See 403.0

❺ **405.1 Benign**
405.11 Renovascular
405.19 Other

❺ **405.9 Unspecified**
405.91 Renovascular
405.99 Other
AHA: 3Q 2000, 4

ISCHEMIC HEART DISEASE (410-414)

Includes that with mention of hypertension
Use additional code to identify presence of hypertension (401.0-405.9)

AHA: 3Q 1991, 10; Jul-Aug 1984, 5

❹ **410 Acute myocardial infarction**
Includes cardiac infarction
coronary (artery):
embolism
occlusion
rupture
thrombosis
infarction of heart, myocardium, or ventricle
rupture of heart, myocardium, or ventricle
ST elevation (STEMI) and non-ST elevation (NSTEMI) myocardial infarction
any condition classifiable to 414.1-414.9 specified as acute or with a stated duration of 8 weeks or less

DEF: An area of heart muscle begins to die or suffer permanent damage from lack of oxygen.

AHA: 2Q 2006, 9; 4Q 2005, 69; 3Q 2001, 21; 3Q 1998, 15; 4Q 1997, 37; 3Q 1995, 9; 4Q 1992, 24; 1Q 1992, 10; 3Q 1991, 18; 1Q 1991, 14; 3Q 1989, 3

The following fifth-digit subclassification is for use with category 410:
0 episode of care unspecified
Use when the source document does not contain sufficient information for the assignment of fifth-digit 1 or 2.
1 initial episode of care
Use fifth-digit 1 to designate the first episode of care (regardless of facility site) for a newly diagnosed myocardial infarction. The fifth-digit 1 is assigned regardless of the number of times a patient may be transferred during the initial episode of care.
2 subsequent episode of care
Use fifth-digit 2 to designate an episode of care following the initial episode when the patient is admitted for further observation, evaluation or treatment for a myocardial infarction that has received initial treatment, but is still less than 8 weeks old.

❺ **410.0 Of anterolateral wall**
ST elevation myocardial infarction (STEMI) of anterolateral wall
C&C Exclusions: (for code 410.01) 410.00, 410.01, 410.02, 410.10, 410.11, 410.12, 410.20, 410.21, 410.22, 410.30, 410.31, 410.32, 410.40, 410.41, 410.42, 410.50, 410.51, 410.52, 410.60, 410.61, 410.62, 410.70, 410.71, 410.72, 410.80, 410.81, 410.82, 410.90, 410.91, 410.92, 459.89, 459.9

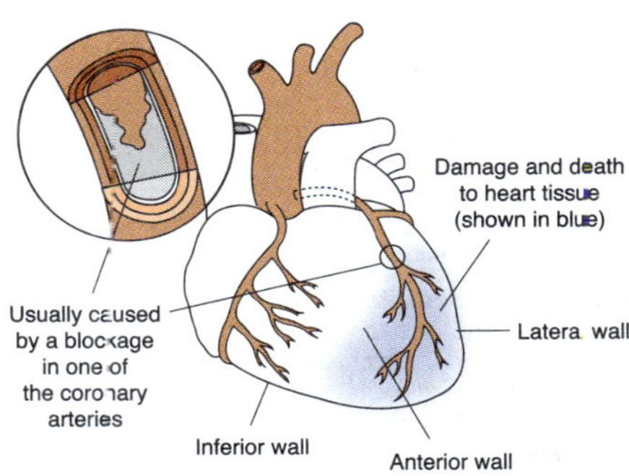

⑤ **410.1 Of other anterior wall**

Infarction:
- anterior (wall) NOS (with contiguous portion of intraventricular septum)
- anteroapical (with contiguous portion of intraventricular septum)
- anteroseptal (with contiguous portion of intraventricular septum)

ST elevation myocardial infarction (STEMI) of other anterior wall

C&C Exclusions: (for code 410.11) See 410.0

AHA: For Code 410.11: 3Q 2003, 10

⑤ **410.2 Of inferolateral wall**

ST elevation myocardial infarction (STEMI) of inferolateral wall

C&C Exclusions: (for code 410.21) See 410.0

⑤ **410.3 Of inferoposterior wall**

ST elevation myocardial infarction (STEMI) of inferoposterior wall

C&C Exclusions: (for code 410.31) See 410.0

⑤ **410.4 Of other inferior wall**

Infarction:
- diaphragmatic wall NOS (with contiguous portion of intraventricular septum)
- inferior (wall) NOS (with contiguous portion of intraventricular septum)

ST elevation myocardial infarction (STEMI) of other inferior wall

C&C Exclusions: (for code 410.41) See 410.0

AHA: 1Q 2000, 7, 26; 4Q 1999, 9; 3Q 1997, 10; For Code 410.41: 3Q 2006, 8-9; 2Q 2001, 8-9

⑤ **410.5 Of other lateral wall**

Infarction:
- apical-lateral
- basal-lateral
- high lateral
- posterolateral

ST elevation myocardial infarction (STEMI) of other lateral wall

C&C Exclusions: (for code 410.51) See 410.0

⑤ **410.6 True posterior wall infarction**

Infarction:
- posterobasal
- strictly posterior

ST elevation myocardial infarction (STEMI) of true posterior wall

C&C Exclusions: (for code 410.61) See 410.0

⑤ **410.7 Subendocardial infarction**

Non-ST elevation myocardial infarction (NSTEMI)
Nontransmural infarction

C&C Exclusions: (for code 410.71) See 410.0

AHA: 1Q 2000, 7; For Code 410.71: 4Q 2005, 71; 2Q 2005, 19

⑤ **410.8 Of other specified sites**

Infarction of:
- atrium
- papillary muscle
- septum alone

ST elevation myocardial infarction (STEMI) of other specified sites

C&C Exclusions: (for code 410.81) See 410.0

✖⑤ **410.9 Unspecified site**

Acute myocardial infarction NOS
Coronary occlusion NOS
Myocardial infarction NOS

C&C Exclusions: (for code 410.91) See 410.0

AHA: 1Q 1996, 17; 1Q 1992, 9; For Code 410.91: 2Q 2005, 18; 3Q 2002, 5

④ **411 Other acute and subacute forms of ischemic heart disease**

AHA: 4Q 1994, 55; 3Q 1991, 24

411.0 Postmyocardial infarction syndrome

Dressler's syndrome

DEF: Fever, chest pain, pleuritis, and pericarditis weeks or months after heart injury caused by surgery or myocardial infarction.

C&C Exclusions: 411.0, 411.81, 411.89, 459.89, 459.9

411.1 Intermediate coronary syndrome

Impending infarction
Preinfarction angina
Preinfarction syndrome
Unstable angina

Excludes *angina (pectoris) (413.9)*
decubitus (413.0)

C&C Exclusions: 410.00, 410.01, 410.02, 410.10, 410.11, 410.12, 410.20, 410.21, 410.22, 410.30, 410.31, 410.32, 410.40, 410.41, 410.42, 410.50, 410.51, 410.52, 410.60, 410.61, 410.62, 410.70, 410.71, 410.72, 410.80, 410.81, 410.82, 410.90, 410.91, 410.92, 411.1, 411.81, 411.89, 413.0, 413.1, 413.9, 414.8, 414.9, 459.89, 459.9

AHA: 4Q 2005, 105; 2Q 2004, 3; 1Q 2003, 12; 3Q 2001, 15; 2Q 2001, 7, 9; 4Q 1998, 86; 2Q 1996, 10; 3Q 1991, 24; 1Q 1991, 14; 3Q 1990, 6; 4Q 1989, 10

⑤ **411.8 Other**

AHA: 3Q 1991, 18; 3Q 1989, 4

411.81 Acute coronary occlusion without myocardial infarction

Acute coronary (artery):
- embolism without or not resulting in myocardial infarction
- obstruction without or not resulting in myocardial infarction
- occlusion without or not resulting in myocardial infarction
- thrombosis without or not resulting in myocardial infarction

Excludes *obstruction without infarction due to atherosclerosis (414.00-414.07)*
occlusion without infarction due to atherosclerosis (414.00-414.07)

DEF: An area of the heart is deprived of oxygen without suffering permanent tissue damage.

C&C Exclusions: 410.00, 410.01, 410.02, 410.10, 410.11, 410.12, 410.20, 410.21, 410.22, 410.30, 410.31, 410.32, 410.40, 410.41, 410.42, 410.50, 410.51, 410.52, 410.60, 410.61, 410.62, 410.70, 410.71, 410.72, 410.80, 410.81, 410.82, 410.90, 410.91, 410.92, 411.0, 411.1, 411.81, 411.89, 413.0, 413.1, 413.9, 414.8, 414.9, 459.89, 459.9

AHA: 3Q 1991, 24; 1Q 1991, 14

411.89 Other

Coronary insufficiency (acute)
Subendocardial ischemia

C&C Exclusions: See 411.81

AHA: 3Q 2001, 14; 1Q 1992, 9

✖ **412 Old myocardial infarction**

Healed myocardial infarction
Past myocardial infarction diagnosed on ECG [EKG] or other special investigation, but currently presenting no symptoms

AHA: 2Q 2003, 10; 2Q 2001, 9; 3Q 1998, 15; 2Q 1991, 22; 3Q 1990, 7

④ **413 Angina pectoris**

413.0 Angina decubitus

Nocturnal angina

DEF: Severe chest pain occuring when the patient is lying down.

C&C Exclusions: 410.00, 410.01, 410.02, 410.10, 410.11, 410.12, 410.20, 410.21, 410.22, 410.30, 410.31, 410.32, 410.40, 410.41, 410.42, 410.50, 410.51, 410.52, 410.60, 410.61, 410.62, 410.70, 410.71, 410.72, 410.80, 410.81, 410.82, 410.90, 410.91, 410.92, 411.1, 411.81, 411.89, 413.0, 413.1, 413.9, 414.8, 414.9, 459.89, 459.9

413.1 Prinzmetal angina

Variant angina pectoris

C&C Exclusions: See 413.0

AHA: 3Q 2006, 23

413.9 Other and unspecified angina pectoris
Angina:
NOS
cardiac
of effort
Anginal syndrome
Status anginosus
Stenocardia
Syncope anginosa
Excludes *preinfarction angina (411.1)*
C&C Exclusions: See 413.0
AHA: 3Q 2002, 4; 3Q 1991, 16; 3Q 1990, 6

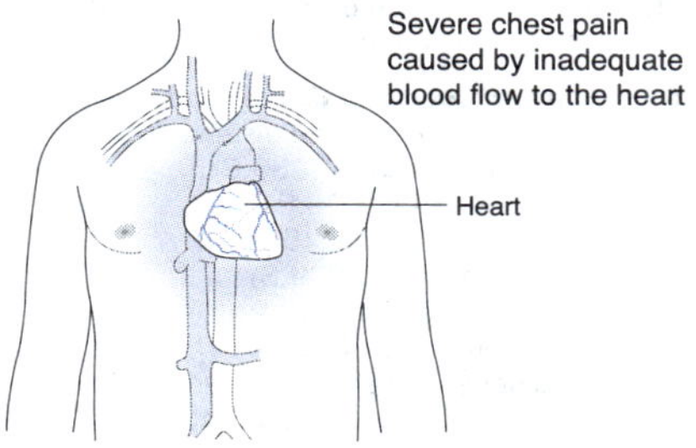

❹ 414 Other forms of chronic ischemic heart disease
Excludes *arteriosclerotic cardiovascular disease [ASCVD] (429.2)*
cardiovascular:
arteriosclerosis or sclerosis (429.2)
degeneration or disease (429.2)

❺ 414.0 Coronary atherosclerosis
Arteriosclerotic heart disease [ASHD]
Atherosclerotic heart disease
Coronary (artery):
arteriosclerosis
arteritis or endarteritis
atheroma
sclerosis
stricture
Excludes *embolism of graft (996.72)*
occlusion NOS of graft (996.72)
thrombus of graft (996.72)
▶ Use additional code, if applicable, to identify chronic total occlusion of coronary artery (414.2)◀
DEF: Clogging of coronary arteries with fatty plaque build-up, restricting blood flow and hardening the arteries.
AHA: 2Q 1997, 13; 2Q 1995, 17; 4Q 1994, 49; 2Q 1994, 13; 1Q 1994, 6; 3Q 1990, 7

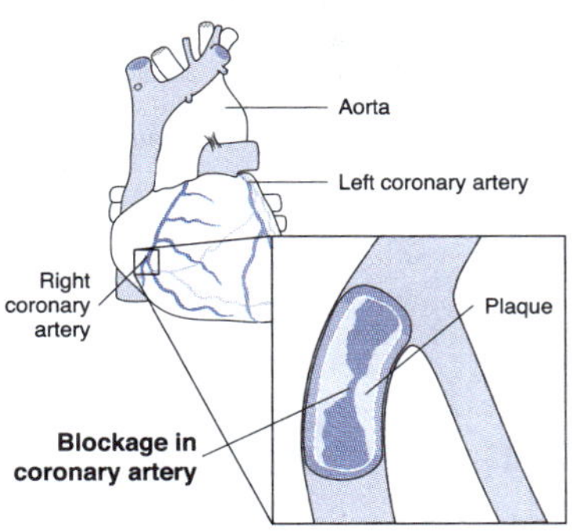

414.00 Of unspecified type of vessel, native or graft A
AHA: 1Q 2004, 24; 2Q 2003, 16; 3Q 2001, 15; 4Q 1999, 4; 3Q 1997, 15; 4Q 1996, 31

414.01 Of native coronary artery A
AHA: 4Q 2005, 71; 2Q 2004, 3; 4Q 2003, 108; 3Q 2003.9, 14; 3Q 2002, 4-9; 3Q 2001, 15; 2Q 2001, 8-9; 3Q 1997, 15; 4Q 1996, 31; 2Q 1996, 10

414.02 Of autologous vein bypass graft A

414.03 Of nonautologous biological bypass graft A

414.04 Of artery bypass graft A
Internal mammary artery
AHA: 4Q 1996, 31

414.05 Of unspecified type of bypass graft A
Bypass graft NOS
AHA: 3Q 1997, 15; 4Q 1996, 31

414.06 Of native coronary artery of transplanted heart
AHA: 4Q 2003, 60

414.07 Of bypass graft (artery) (vein) of transplanted heart A

❺ 414.1 Aneurysm and dissection of heart
AHA: 4Q 2002, 54

414.10 Aneurysm of heart (wall)
Aneurysm (arteriovenous):
mural
ventricular

414.11 Aneurysm of coronary vessels
Aneurysm (arteriovenous) of coronary vessels
AHA: 3Q 2003, 10; 1Q 1999, 17

414.12 Dissection of coronary artery

A tear in the intimal arterial wall of a coronary artery resulting in the sudden intrusion of blood within the layers of the wall

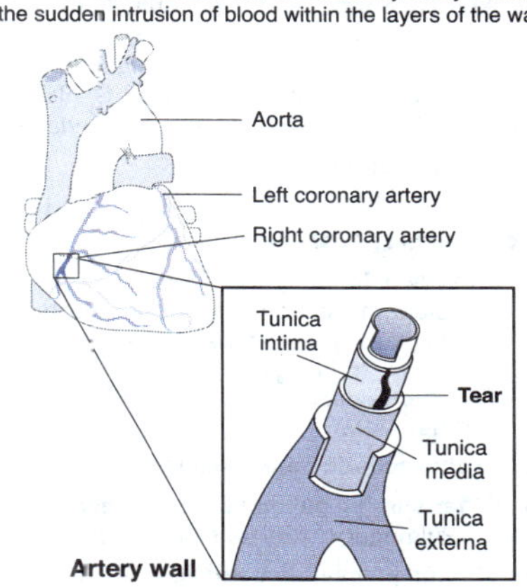

414.19 Other aneurysm of heart
Arteriovenous fistula, acquired, of heart

●✚ ***414.2 Chronic total occlusion of coronary artery***
Complete occlusion of coronary artery
Total occlusion of coronary artery
Code first coronary atherosclerosis (414.00-414.07)
Excludes acute coronary occlusion with myocardial infarction (410.00-410.92)
acute coronary occlusion without myocardial infarction (411.81)

414.8 Other specified forms of chronic ischemic heart disease
Chronic coronary insufficiency
Ischemia, myocardial (chronic)
Any condition classifiable to 410 specified as chronic, or presenting with symptoms after 8 weeks from date of infarction
Excludes *coronary insufficiency (acute) (411.89)*
AHA: 3Q 2001, 15; 1Q 1992, 10; 3Q 1990, 7, 15; 2Q 1990, 19

✖ **414.9 Chronic ischemic heart disease, unspecified**
Ischemic heart disease NOS

DISEASES OF PULMONARY CIRCULATION (415-417)

❹ 415 Acute pulmonary heart disease

415.0 Acute cor pulmonale
Excludes *cor pulmonale NOS (416.9)*
DEF: Enlarged right heart ventricle due to obstruction of the pulmonary artery.
C&C Exclusions: 415.0, 416.8, 416.9, 459.89, 459.9

❺ 415.1 Pulmonary embolism and infarction
Pulmonary (artery) (vein):
- apoplexy
- embolism
- infarction (hemorrhagic)
- thrombosis

Excludes *that complicating:*
- *abortion (634-638 with .6, 639.6)*
- *ectopic or molar pregnancy (639.6)*
- *pregnancy, childbirth, or the puerperium (673.0-673.8)*

AHA: 4Q 1990, 25

415.11 Iatrogenic pulmonary embolism and infarction
C&C Exclusions: 415.11, 415.19, 459.89, 459.9
AHA: 4Q 1995, 58

● 415.12 Septic pulmonary embolism
Septic embolism NOS
Code first underlying infection, such as:
septicemia (038.0-038.9)
Excludes *septic arterial embolism (449)*

415.19 Other
C&C Exclusions: See 415.11

❹ 416 Chronic pulmonary heart disease

416.0 Primary pulmonary hypertension
Idiopathic pulmonary arteriosclerosis
Pulmonary hypertension (essential) (idiopathic) (primary)
C&C Exclusions: 416.0, 416.8, 416.9, 417.8, 417.9, 459.89, 459.9

416.1 Kyphoscoliotic heart disease

416.8 Other chronic pulmonary heart diseases
Pulmonary hypertension, secondary

416.9 Chronic pulmonary heart disease, unspecified
Chronic cardiopulmonary disease
Cor pulmonale (chronic) NOS

❹ 417 Other diseases of pulmonary circulation

417.0 Arteriovenous fistula of pulmonary vessels
Excludes *congenital arteriovenous fistula (747.3)*

417.1 Aneurysm of pulmonary artery
Excludes *congenital aneurysm (747.3)*
DEF: Bulging in one portion of the artery's wall that brings blood to the lungs, forming a pouch or sac with the potential for rupture.

417.8 Other specified diseases of pulmonary circulation
Pulmonary:
- arteritis
- endarteritis

Rupture of pulmonary vessel
Stricture of pulmonary vessel

✖ 417.9 Unspecified disease of pulmonary circulation

OTHER FORMS OF HEART DISEASE (420-429)

❹ 420 Acute pericarditis
Includes acute:
- mediastinopericarditis
- myopericarditis
- pericardial effusion
- pleuropericarditis
- pneumopericarditis

Excludes *acute rheumatic pericarditis (391.0)*
postmyocardial infarction syndrome [Dressler's] (411.0)
DEF: Serious inflammation of the membranous sac around the heart causing chest pain, coughing, fatigue, and fever.

✚ *420.0 Acute pericarditis in diseases classified elsewhere*
Code first underlying disease, as:
- actinomycosis (039.8)
- amebiasis (006.8)
- chronic uremia (585.9)
- nocardiosis (039.8)
- tuberculosis (017.9)
- uremia NOS (586)

Excludes *pericarditis (acute) (in):*
- *Coxsackie (virus) (074.21)*
- *gonococcal (098.83)*
- *histoplasmosis (115.0-115.9 with fifth-digit 3)*
- *meningococcal infection (036.41)*
- *syphilitic (093.81)*

C&C Exclusions: 391.0, 393, 420.0, 420.90, 420.91, 420.99, 423.8, 423.9, 459.89, 459.9

❺ 420.9 Other and unspecified acute pericarditis

420.90 Acute pericarditis, unspecified
Pericarditis (acute):
- NOS
- infective NOS
- sicca

C&C Exclusions: See 420.0
AHA: 2Q 1989, 12

420.91 Acute idiopathic pericarditis
Pericarditis, acute:
- benign
- nonspecific
- viral

C&C Exclusions: See 420.0

420.99 Other
Pericarditis (acute):
- pneumococcal
- purulent
- staphylococcal
- streptococcal
- suppurative

Pneumopyopericardium
Pyopericardium
Excludes *pericarditis in diseases classified elsewhere (420.0)*
C&C Exclusions: See 420.0

❹ 421 Acute and subacute endocarditis

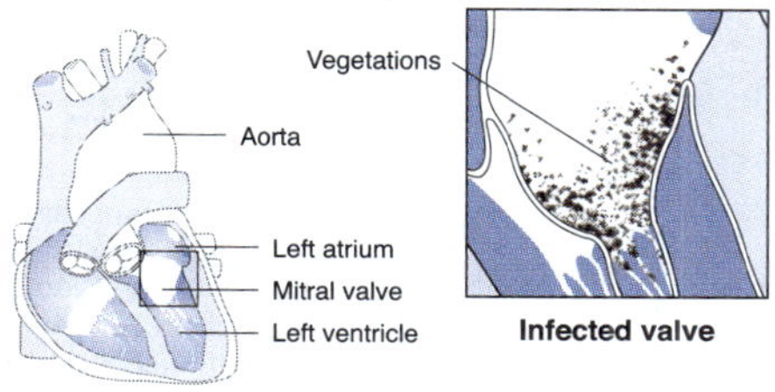

421.0 Acute and subacute bacterial endocarditis
Endocarditis (acute) (chronic) (subacute):
bacterial
infective NOS
lenta
malignant
purulent
septic
ulcerative
vegetative
Infective aneurysm
Subacute bacterial endocarditis [SBE]
Use additional code, if desired, to identify infectious organism [e.g., Streptococcus 041.0, Staphylococcus 041.1]
C&C Exclusions: 391.1, 397.9, 421.0, 421.1, 421.9, 424.90, 424.91, 424.99, 459.89, 459.9
AHA: 1Q 1999, 12; 1Q 1991, 15

✚ *421.1 Acute and subacute infective endocarditis in diseases classified elsewhere*
Code first underlying disease, as:
blastomycosis (116.0)
Q fever (083.0)
typhoid (fever) (002.0)
Excludes *endocarditis (in):*
Coxsackie (virus) (074.22)
gonococcal (098.84)
histoplasmosis (115.0-115.9 with fifth-digit 4)
meningococcal infection (036.42)
monilial (112.81)
C&C Exclusions: See 421.0

421.9 Acute endocarditis, unspecified
Endocarditis, acute or subacute
Myoendocarditis, acute or subacute
Periendocarditis, acute or subacute
Excludes *acute rheumatic endocarditis (391.1)*
C&C Exclusions: See 421.0

❹ 422 Acute myocarditis
Excludes *acute rheumatic myocarditis (391.2)*
DEF: Severe inflammation of heart muscle tissue.

✚ *422.0 Acute myocarditis in diseases classified elsewhere*
Code first underlying disease, as:
myocarditis (acute):
influenzal (487.8)
tuberculous (017.9)
Excludes *myocarditis (acute) (due to):*
aseptic, of newborn (074.23)
Coxsackie (virus) (074.23)
diphtheritic (032.82)
meningococcal infection (036.43)
syphilitic (093.82)
toxoplasmosis (130.3)
C&C Exclusions: 391.2, 398.0, 422.0, 422.90, 422.91, 422.92, 422.93, 422.99, 429.0, 429.71, 429.79, 459.89, 459.9

❺ 422.9 Other and unspecified acute myocarditis

422.90 Acute myocarditis, unspecified
Acute or subacute (interstitial) myocarditis
C&C Exclusions: See 422.0

422.91 Idiopathic myocarditis
Myocarditis (acute or subacute):
Fiedler's
giant cell
isolated (diffuse) (granulomatous)
nonspecific granulomatous
C&C Exclusions: See 422.0

422.92 Septic myocarditis
Myocarditis, acute or subacute:
pneumococcal
staphylococcal
Use additional code to identify infectious organism [e.g., Staphylococcus 041.1]
Excludes *myocarditis, acute or subacute:*
in bacterial diseases classified elsewhere (422.0)
streptococcal (391.2)
C&C Exclusions: See 422.0

422.93 Toxic myocarditis
DEF: Inflammation of heart muscle as a result of noxious drugs or substances in the body.
C&C Exclusions: See 422.0

422.99 Other
C&C Exclusions: See 422.0

❹ 423 Other diseases of pericardium
Excludes *that specified as rheumatic (393)*

423.0 Hemopericardium
DEF: Bleeding causing the sac around the heart to fill with blood.
C&C Exclusions: 423.0, 423.1, 423.2, 423.8, 423.9, 459.89, 459.9

423.1 Adhesive pericarditis
Adherent pericardium
Fibrosis of pericardium
Milk spots
Pericarditis:
adhesive
obliterative
Soldiers' patches
DEF: Pericardial inflammation with adhesion between the two pericardial layers or between the pericardium and the heart or neighboring structures.
C&C Exclusions: See 423.0

423.2 Constrictive pericarditis
Concato's disease
Pick's disease of heart (and liver)
C&C Exclusions: See 423.0

● 423.3 Cardiac tamponade
Code first the underlying cause
DEF: Increased pressure on the heart due to fluid in the pericardial sac, impairing the ventricles' filling action and causing decreased cardiac output.

423.8 Other specified diseases of pericardium
Calcification of pericardium
Fistula of pericardium
AHA: 2Q 1989, 12

423.9 Unspecified disease of pericardium
AHA: 1Q 2007, 11-12

❹ 424 Other diseases of endocardium

Excludes *bacterial endocarditis (421.0-421.9)*
rheumatic endocarditis (391.1, 394.0-397.9)
syphilitic endocarditis (093.20-093.24)

424.0 Mitral valve disorders

Mitral (valve):
- incompetence NOS of specified cause, except rheumatic
- insufficiency NOS of specified cause, except rheumatic
- regurgitation NOS of specified cause, except rheumatic

Excludes *mitral (valve):*
disease (394.9)
failure (394.9)
stenosis (394.0)
the listed conditions:
specified as rheumatic (394.1)
unspecified as to cause but with mention of:
diseases of aortic valve (396.0-396.9)
mitral stenosis or obstruction (394.2)

C&C Exclusions: 394.0, 394.1, 394.2, 394.9, 396.0, 396.1, 396.2, 396.3, 396.8, 396.9, 424.0, 459.89, 459.9

AHA: 3Q 2006, 7; 2Q 2000, 16; 3Q 1998, 11; Nov-Dec 1987, 8; Nov-Dec 1984, 8

424.1 Aortic valve disorders

Aortic (valve):
- incompetence NOS of specified cause, except rheumatic
- insufficiency NOS of specified cause, except rheumatic
- regurgitation NOS of specified cause, except rheumatic
- stenosis NOS of specified cause, except rheumatic

Excludes *hypertrophic subaortic stenosis (425.1)*
that specified as rheumatic (395.0-395.9)
that of unspecified cause but with mention of diseases of mitral valve (396.0-396.9)

C&C Exclusions: 395.0, 395.1, 395.2, 395.9, 396.0, 396.1, 396.2, 396.3, 396.8, 396.9, 424.1, 459.89, 459.9

AHA: 4Q 1988, 8; Nov-Dec 1987, 8

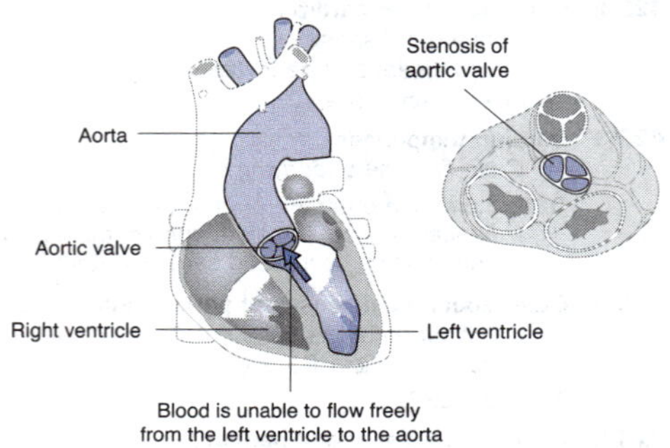

424.2 Tricuspid valve disorders, specified as nonrheumatic

Tricuspid valve:
- incompetence of specified cause, except rheumatic
- insufficiency of specified cause, except rheumatic
- regurgitation of specified cause, except rheumatic
- stenosis of specified cause, except rheumatic

Excludes *rheumatic or of unspecified cause (397.0)*

C&C Exclusions: 397.0, 424.2, 459.89, 459.9

424.3 Pulmonary valve disorders

Pulmonic:
- incompetence NOS
- insufficiency NOS
- regurgitation NOS
- stenosis NOS

Excludes *that specified as rheumatic (397.1)*

C&C Exclusions: 397.1, 424.3, 459.89, 459.9

❺ 424.9 Endocarditis, valve unspecified

424.90 Endocarditis, valve unspecified, unspecified cause

Endocarditis (chronic):
- NOS
- nonbacterial thrombotic

Valvular:
- incompetence of unspecified valve, unspecified cause
- insufficiency of unspecified valve, unspecified cause
- regurgitation of unspecified valve, unspecified cause
- stenosis of unspecified valve, unspecified cause

Valvulitis (chronic)

C&C Exclusions: 424.90, 424.91, 424.99, 459.89, 459.9

+ *424.91 Endocarditis in diseases classified elsewhere*

Code first underlying disease, as:
- atypical verrucous endocarditis [Libman-Sacks] (710.0)
- disseminated lupus erythematosus (710.0)
- tuberculosis (017.9)

Excludes *syphilitic (093.20-093.24)*

C&C Exclusions: See 424.90

424.99 Other

Any condition classifiable to 424.90 with specified cause, except rheumatic

Excludes *endocardial fibroelastosis (425.3)*
that specified as rheumatic (397.9)

C&C Exclusions: See 424.90

❹ 425 Cardiomyopathy

Includes myocardiopathy

AHA: Jul-Aug 1985, 15

425.0 Endomyocardial fibrosis

C&C Exclusions: 425.0, 425.1, 425.2, 425.3, 425.4, 425.5, 425.6, 425.7, 425.8, 425.9, 459.89, 459.9

425.1 Hypertrophic obstructive cardiomyopathy

Hypertrophic subaortic stenosis (idiopathic)

DEF: Abnormal thickening of the heart muscle obstructing blood flow through the left ventricle.

C&C Exclusions: See 425.0

425.2 Obscure cardiomyopathy of Africa

Becker's disease
Idiopathic mural endomyocardial disease

C&C Exclusions: See 425.0

425.3 Endocardial fibroelastosis

Elastomyofibrosis

C&C Exclusions: See 425.0

425.4 Other primary cardiomyopathies

Cardiomyopathy:
- NOS
- congestive
- constrictive
- familial
- hypertrophic
- idiopathic
- nonobstructive
- obstructive
- restrictive

Cardiovascular collagenosis

C&C Exclusions: See 425.0

AHA: 1Q 2007, 20; 2Q 2005, 14; 1Q 2000, 22; 4Q 1997, 55; 2Q 1990, 19

425.5 Alcoholic cardiomyopathy

C&C Exclusions: See 425.0

AHA: Sep-Oct 1985, 15

+ *425.7 Nutritional and metabolic cardiomyopathy*

Code first underlying disease, as:
- amyloidosis (277.30-277.39)
- beriberi (265.0)
- cardiac glycogenosis (271.0)
- mucopolysaccharidosis (277.5)
- thyrotoxicosis (242.0-242.9)

Excludes *gouty tophi of heart (274.82)*

C&C Exclusions: See 425.0

+ **_425.8 Cardiomyopathy in other diseases classified elsewhere_**
 Code first underlying disease, as:
 Friedreich's ataxia (334.0)
 myotonia atrophica (▶359.21◀)
 progressive muscular dystrophy (359.1)
 sarcoidosis (135)
 Excludes *cardiomyopathy in Chagas' disease (086.0)*
 C&C Exclusions: See 425.0
 AHA: 2Q 1993, 9

425.9 Secondary cardiomyopathy, unspecified
 C&C Exclusions: See 425.0

❹ **426 Conduction disorders**

426.0 Atrioventricular block, complete
 Third degree atrioventricular block
 DEF: No conduction of electrical impulses occurs between the atria and ventricles, requiring a pacemaker to maintain rhythm.
 C&C Exclusions: 426.0, 426.10, 426.11, 426.12, 426.13, 426.2, 426.3, 426.4, 426.50, 426.51, 426.52, 426.53, 426.54, 426.6, 426.7, 426.81, 426.89, 426.9, 427.0, 427.1, 427.2, 427.31, 427.32, 427.41, 427.42, 427.5, 427.89, 459.89, 459.9
 AHA: 2Q 2006, 14

❺ **426.1 Atrioventricular block, other and unspecified**

426.10 Atrioventricular block, unspecified
 Atrioventricular [AV] block (incomplete) (partial)

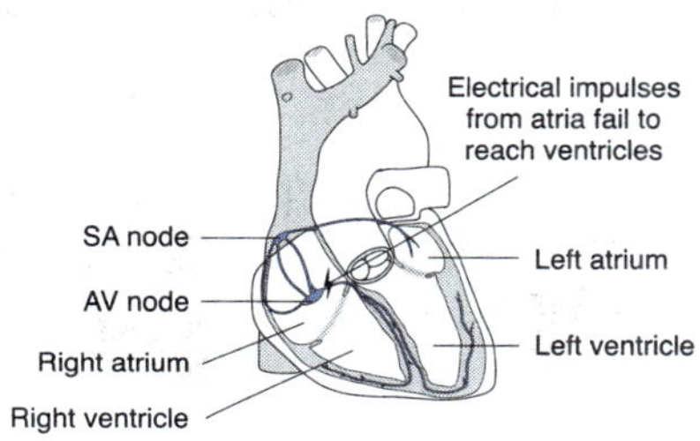

426.11 First degree atrioventricular block
 Incomplete atrioventricular block, first degree
 Prolonged P-R interval NOS
 AHA: 2Q 2006, 14

426.12 Mobitz (type) II atrioventricular block
 Incomplete atrioventricular block:
 Mobitz (type) II
 second degree, Mobitz (type) II
 C&C Exclusions: See 426.0
 AHA: 2Q 2006, 14

426.13 Other second degree atrioventricular block
 Incomplete atrioventricular block:
 Mobitz (type) I [Wenckebach's]
 second degree:
 NOS
 Mobitz (type) I
 with 2:1 atrioventricular response [block]
 Wenckebach's phenomenon
 C&C Exclusions: See 426.0

426.2 Left bundle branch hemiblock
 Block:
 left anterior fascicular
 left posterior fascicular

426.3 Other left bundle branch block
 Left bundle branch block:
 NOS
 anterior fascicular with posterior fascicular
 complete
 main stem

426.4 Right bundle branch block
 AHA: 3Q 2000, 3

❺ **426.5 Bundle branch block, other and unspecified**

✖ **426.50 Bundle branch block, unspecified**

426.51 Right bundle branch block and left posterior fascicular block

426.52 Right bundle branch block and left anterior fascicular block

426.53 Other bilateral bundle branch block
 Bifascicular block NOS
 Bilateral bundle branch block NOS
 Right bundle branch with left bundle branch block (incomplete) (main stem)
 C&C Exclusions: See 426.0

426.54 Trifascicular block
 C&C Exclusions: See 426.0

426.6 Other heart block
 Intraventricular block:
 NOS
 diffuse
 myofibrillar
 Sinoatrial block
 Sinoauricular block
 C&C Exclusions: See 426.0

426.7 Anomalous atrioventricular excitation
 Atrioventricular conduction:
 accelerated
 accessory
 pre-excitation
 Ventricular pre-excitation
 Wolff-Parkinson-White syndrome
 C&C Exclusions: See 426.0

❺ **426.8 Other specified conduction disorders**

426.81 Lown-Ganong-Levine syndrome
 Syndrome of short P-R interval, normal QRS complexes, and supraventricular tachycardias
 C&C Exclusions: See 426.0

426.82 Long QT syndrome
 DEF: Hereditary defect of the heart's electrical conduction system with an abnormally long gap in the time it takes for the ventricles to contract.
 C&C Exclusions: See 426.0
 AHA: 4Q 2005, 72

426.89 Other
 Dissociation:
 atrioventricular [AV]
 interference
 isorhythmic
 Nonparoxysmal AV nodal tachycardia
 C&C Exclusions: See 426.0

426.9 Conduction disorder, unspecified
 Heart block NOS
 Stokes-Adams syndrome

❹ **427 Cardiac dysrhythmias**
 Excludes *that complicating:*
 abortion (634-638 with .7, 639.8)
 ectopic or molar pregnancy (639.8)
 labor or delivery (668.1, 669.4)
 AHA: Jul-Aug 1985, 15

427.0 Paroxysmal supraventricular tachycardia
 Paroxysmal tachycardia:
 atrial [PAT]
 atrioventricular [AV]
 junctional
 nodal
 DEF: Abnormally rapid atrial rhythm occurring from time to time, most often in the young.
 C&C Exclusions: See 426.0

427.1 Paroxysmal ventricular tachycardia
 Ventricular tachycardia (paroxysmal)
 DEF: Potentially lethal rapid heart beat initiating in the ventricles marked by three or more consecutive premature beats.
 C&C Exclusions: See 426.0
 AHA: 2Q 2006, 16; 3Q 1995, 9; Mar-Apr 1986, 11

427.2 Paroxysmal tachycardia, unspecified
 Bouveret-Hoffmann syndrome
 Paroxysmal tachycardia:
 NOS
 essential
 C&C Exclusions: See 426.0

⑤ 427.3 Atrial fibrillation and flutter

427.31 Atrial fibrillation

C&C Exclusions: See 426.0

AHA: 3Q 2005, 8; 4Q 2004, 78, 121; 3Q 2004, 7; 4Q 2003, 95, 105; 1Q 2003, 8; 2Q 1999, 17; 3Q 1995, 8

Irregular, rapid atrial contractions

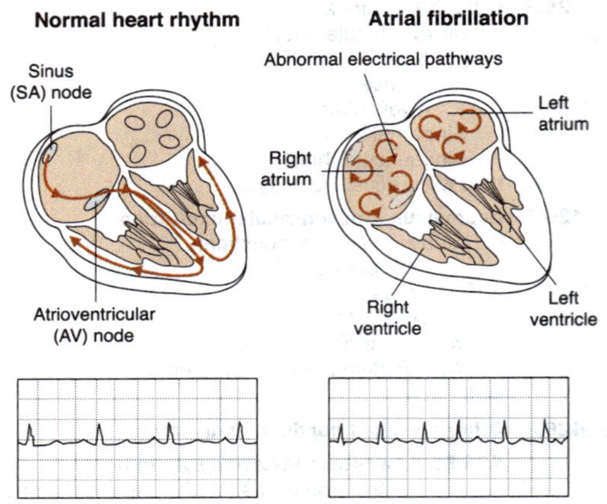

427.32 Atrial flutter

C&C Exclusions: See 426.0

AHA: 4Q 2003, 94

⑤ 427.4 Ventricular fibrillation and flutter

427.41 Ventricular fibrillation

C&C Exclusions: See 426.0

AHA: 3Q 2002, 5

427.42 Ventricular flutter

C&C Exclusions: See 426.0

✖ 427.5 Cardiac arrest

Cardiorespiratory arrest

C&C Exclusions: 427.0, 427.1, 427.2, 427.31, 427.32, 427.41, 427.42, 427.5, 459.89, 459.9

AHA: 3Q 2002, 5; 2Q 2000, 12; 3Q 1995, 8; 2Q 1988, 8

⑤ 427.6 Premature beats

427.60 Premature beats, unspecified

Ectopic beats
Extrasystoles
Extrasystolic arrhythmia
Premature contractions or systoles NOS

427.61 Supraventricular premature beats

Atrial premature beats, contractions, or systoles

427.69 Other

Ventricular premature beats, contractions, or systoles

AHA: 4Q 1993, 42

⑤ 427.8 Other specified cardiac dysrhythmias

427.81 Sinoatrial node dysfunction

Sinus bradycardia:
- persistent
- severe

Syndrome:
- sick sinus
- tachycardia-bradycardia

Excludes *sinus bradycardia NOS (427.89)*

AHA: 3Q 2000, 8

427.89 Other

Rhythm disorder:
- coronary sinus
- ectopic
- nodal

Wandering (atrial) pacemaker

Excludes *carotid sinus syncope (337.0)*
neonatal bradycardia (779.81)
neonatal tachycardia (779.82)
reflex bradycardia (337.0)
tachycardia NOS (785.0)

✖ 427.9 Cardiac dysrhythmia, unspecified

Arrhythmia (cardiac) NOS

AHA: 2Q 1989, 10

④ 428 Heart failure

Code, if applicable, heart failure due to hypertension first (402.0-402.9, with fifth-digit 1 or 404.0-404.9 with fifth-digit 1 or 3)

Excludes *rheumatic (398.91)*
that complicating:
abortion (634-638 with .7, 639.8)
ectopic or molar pregnancy (639.8)
labor or delivery (668.1, 669.4)

AHA: 4Q 2002, 49; 3Q 1998, 5; 2Q 1990, 16; 2Q 1990, 19; 2Q 1989, 10; 3Q 1988, 3

428.0 Congestive heart failure, unspecified

Congestive heart disease
Right heart failure (secondary to left heart failure)

Excludes *fluid overload NOS (276.6)*

C&C Exclusions: 398.91, 402.01, 402.11, 402.91, 428.0, 428.1, 428.20, 428.21, 428.22, 428.23, 428.30, 428.31, 428.32, 428.33, 428.40, 428.41, 428.42, 428.43, 428.9, 459.89, 459.9, 518.4

AHA: 1Q 2007, 20; 3Q 2006, 7; 4Q 2005, 120; 3Q 2005, 8; 1Q 2005, 5, 9; 4Q 2004, 140; 3Q 2004, 7; 4Q 2003, 109; 1Q 2003, 9; 4Q 2002, 52; 2Q 2001, 13; 4Q 2000, 48; 2Q 2000, 16; 1Q 2000, 22; 4Q 1999, 4; 1Q 1999, 11; 4Q 1997, 55; 3Q 1997, 10; 3Q 1996, 9; 3Q 1991, 18-19; 2Q 1989, 12

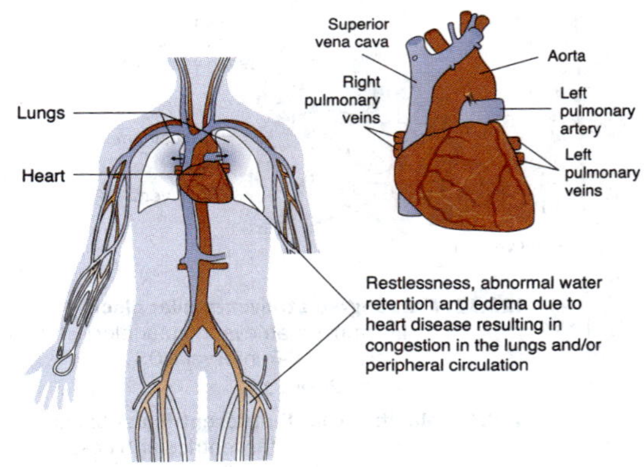

428.1 Left heart failure

Acute edema of lung with heart disease NOS or heart failure
Acute pulmonary edema with heart disease NOS or heart failure
Cardiac asthma
Left ventricular failure

C&C Exclusions: See 428.0

⑤ 428.2 Systolic heart failure

Excludes *combined systolic and diastolic heart failure (428.40-428.43)*

DEF: Heart muscle fails to contract with adequate force and not enough oxygen-rich blood is pumped to the body.

✖ 428.20 Unspecified

C&C Exclusions: See 428.0

428.21 Acute

C&C Exclusions: See 428.0

428.22 Chronic

C&C Exclusions: See 428.0

AHA: 4Q 2005, 120

428.23 Acute on chronic

C&C Exclusions: See 428.0

AHA: 1Q 2003, 9

❺ **428.3 Diastolic heart failure**

Excludes *combined systolic and diastolic heart failure (428.40-428.43)*

DEF: Heart muscle contracts normally but ventricles fail to relax properly after contraction, resulting in less blood entering the heart.

✖ **428.30 Unspecified**
C&C Exclusions: See 428.0
AHA: 4Q 2002, 52

428.31 Acute
C&C Exclusions: See 428.0

428.32 Chronic
C&C Exclusions: See 428.0

428.33 Acute on chronic
C&C Exclusions: See 428.0
AHA: 1Q 2007, 20

❺ **428.4 Combined systolic and diastolic heart failure**

DEF: Heart fails both to contract and relax properly, resulting in an insufficient amount of blood moving through the circulatory system.

✖ **428.40 Unspecified**
C&C Exclusions: See 428.0

428.41 Acute
C&C Exclusions: See 428.0
AHA: 4Q 2004, 140

428.42 Chronic
C&C Exclusions: See 428.0

428.43 Acute on chronic
C&C Exclusions: See 428.0
AHA: 3Q 2006, 7; 4Q 2002, 52

✖ **428.9 Heart failure, unspecified**
Cardiac failure NOS
Heart failure NOS
Myocardial failure NOS
Weak heart
C&C Exclusions: See 428.0
AHA: 2Q 1989, 10; Nov-Dec 1985, 14

❹ **429 Ill-defined descriptions and complications of heart disease**

429.0 Myocarditis, unspecified
Myocarditis (with mention of arteriosclerosis):
NOS (with mention of arteriosclerosis)
chronic (interstitial) (with mention of arteriosclerosis)
fibroid (with mention of arteriosclerosis)
senile (with mention of arteriosclerosis)
Use additional code to identify presence of arteriosclerosis

Excludes *acute or subacute (422.0-422.9)*
rheumatic (398.0)
acute (391.2)
that due to hypertension (402.0-402.9)

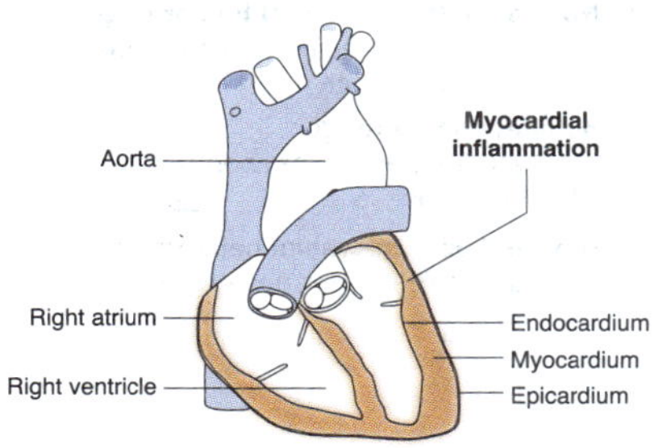

429.1 Myocardial degeneration
Degeneration of heart or myocardium (with mention of arteriosclerosis):
fatty (with mention of arteriosclerosis)
mural (with mention of arteriosclerosis)
muscular (with mention of arteriosclerosis)
Myocardial (with mention of arteriosclerosis):
degeneration (with mention of arteriosclerosis)
disease (with mention of arteriosclerosis)
Use additional code to identify presence of arteriosclerosis

Excludes *that due to hypertension (402.0-402.9)*

429.2 Cardiovascular disease, unspecified
Arteriosclerotic cardiovascular disease [ASCVD]
Cardiovascular arteriosclerosis
Cardiovascular:
degeneration (with mention of arteriosclerosis)
disease (with mention of arteriosclerosis)
sclerosis (with mention of arteriosclerosis)
Use additional code to identify presence of arteriosclerosis

Excludes *that due to hypertension (402.0-402.9)*

429.3 Cardiomegaly
Cardiac:
dilatation
hypertrophy
Ventricular dilatation

Excludes *that due to hypertension (402.0-402.9)*

DEF: Abnormal enlargement of the heart.

429.4 Functional disturbances following cardiac surgery
Cardiac insufficiency following cardiac surgery or due to prosthesis
Heart failure following cardiac surgery or due to prosthesis
Postcardiotomy syndrome
Postvalvulotomy syndrome

Excludes *cardiac failure in the immediate postoperative period (997.1)*

C&C Exclusions: 429.4, 429.71, 429.79, 459.89, 459.9
AHA: 2Q 2002, 12; Nov-Dec 1985, 6

429.5 Rupture of chordae tendineae

DEF: Tear in the fibrous, cord-like tissue connecting the papillary muscles to the valves, holding the valve flaps in place to prevent their eversion.

C&C Exclusions: 429.5, 429.71, 429.79, 459.89, 459.9

429.6 Rupture of papillary muscle
C&C Exclusions: 429.6, 429.71, 429.79, 429.81, 459.89, 459.9

❺ **429.7 Certain sequelae of myocardial infarction, not elsewhere classified**
Use additional code to identify the associated myocardial infarction:
with onset of 8 weeks or less (410.00-410.92)
with onset of more than 8 weeks (414.8)

Excludes *congenital defects of heart (745, 746)*
coronary aneurysm (414.11)
disorders of papillary muscle (429.6, 429.81)
postmyocardial infarction syndrome (411.0)
rupture of chordae tendineae (429.5)

AHA: 3Q 1989, 5

429.71 Acquired cardiac septal defect A

Excludes *acute septal infarction (410.00-410.92)*

C&C Exclusions: 422.0, 422.90, 422.91, 422.92, 422.93, 422.99, 429.0, 429.4, 429.5, 429.6, 429.71, 429.79, 429.81, 429.82, 459.89, 459.9, 745.0, 745.10, 745.11, 745.12, 745.19, 745.2, 745.3, 745.4, 745.5, 745.60, 745.61, 745.69, 745.7, 745.8, 745.9, 746.89, 746.9, 747.83, 747.89, 747.9, 759.7, 759.81, 759.82, 759.83, 759.89

429.79 Other A
Mural thrombus (atrial) (ventricular) acquired, following myocardial infarction
C&C Exclusions: See 429.71
AHA: 1Q 1992, 10

5 429.8 Other ill-defined heart diseases

429.81 Other disorders of papillary muscle

Papillary muscle:
- atrophy
- degeneration
- dysfunction
- incompetence
- incoordination
- scarring

C&C Exclusions: 429.6, 429.71, 429.79, 429.81, 459.89, 459.9

429.82 Hyperkinetic heart disease

C&C Exclusions: 429.71, 429.79, 429.82, 459.89, 459.9

429.83 Takotsubo syndrome

Broken heart syndrome
Reversible left ventricular dysfunction following sudden emotional stress
Stress induced cardiomyopathy
Transient left ventricular apical ballooning syndrome

AHA: 4Q 2006, 87

429.89 Other

Carditis

Excludes *that due to hypertension (402.0-402.9)*

AHA: 2Q 2006, 19; 3Q 2005, 14; 1Q 1992, 10

✖ 429.9 Heart disease, unspecified

Heart disease (organic) NOS
Morbus cordis NOS

Excludes *that due to hypertension (402.0-402.9)*

AHA: 1Q 1993, 19

CEREBROVASCULAR DISEASE (430-438)

Includes with mention of hypertension (conditions classifiable to 401-405)

Use additional code to identify presence of hypertension

Excludes *any condition classifiable to 430-434, 436, 437 occurring during pregnancy, childbirth, or the puerperium, or specified as puerperal (674.0)*
iatrogenic cerebrovascular infarction or hemorrhage (997.02)

AHA: 1Q 1993, 27; 3Q 1991, 10; 3Q 1990, 3; 2Q 1989, 8; Mar-Apr 1985, 6

430 Subarachnoid hemorrhage

Meningeal hemorrhage
Ruptured:
- berry aneurysm
- (congenital) cerebral aneurysm NOS

Excludes *syphilitic ruptured cerebral aneurysm (094.87)*

DEF: Bleeding between the brain and the middle membrane covering the brain within the cerebrospinal fluid filled spaces.

C&C Exclusions: 430, 431, 432.0, 432.1, 432.9, 459.89, 459.9, 780.01, 780.02, 780.03, 780.09, 800.00, 800.01, 800.02, 800.03, 800.04, 800.05, 800.06, 800.09, 800.10, 800.11, 800.12, 800.13, 800.14, 800.15, 800.16, 800.19, 800.20, 800.21, 800.22, 800.23, 800.24, 800.25, 800.26, 800.29, 800.30, 800.31, 800.32, 800.33, 800.34, 800.35, 800.36, 800.39, 800.40, 800.41, 800.42, 800.43, 800.44, 800.45, 800.46, 800.49, 800.50, 800.51, 800.52, 800.53, 800.54, 800.55, 800.56, 800.59, 800.60, 800.61, 800.62, 800.63, 800.64, 800.65, 800.66, 800.69, 800.70, 800.71, 800.72, 800.73, 800.74, 800.75, 800.76, 800.79, 800.80, 800.81, 800.82, 800.83, 800.84, 800.85, 800.86, 800.89, 800.90, 800.91, 800.92, 800.93, 800.94, 800.95, 800.96, 800.99, 801.00, 801.01, 801.02, 801.03, 801.04, 801.05, 801.06, 801.09, 801.10, 801.11, 801.12, 801.13, 801.14, 801.15, 801.16, 801.19, 801.20, 801.21, 801.22, 801.23, 801.24, 801.25, 801.26, 801.29, 801.30, 801.31, 801.32, 801.33, 801.34, 801.35, 801.36, 801.39, 801.40, 801.41, 801.42, 801.43, 801.44, 801.45, 801.46, 801.49, 801.50, 801.51, 801.52, 801.53, 801.54, 801.55, 801.56, 801.59, 801.60, 801.61, 801.62, 801.63, 801.64, 801.65, 801.66, 801.69, 801.70, 801.71, 801.72, 801.73, 801.74, 801.75, 801.76, 801.79, 801.80, 801.81, 801.82, 801.83, 801.84, 801.85, 801.86, 801.89, 801.90, 801.91, 801.92, 801.93, 801.94, 801.95, 801.96, 801.99, 803.00, 803.01, 803.02, 803.03, 803.04, 803.05, 803.06, 803.09, 803.10, 803.11, 803.12, 803.13, 803.14, 803.15, 803.16, 803.19, 803.20, 803.21, 803.22, 803.23, 803.24, 803.25, 803.26, 803.29, 803.30, 803.31, 803.32, 803.33, 803.34, 803.35, 803.36, 803.39, 803.40, 803.41, 803.42, 803.43, 803.44, 803.45, 803.46, 803.49, 803.50, 803.51, 803.52, 803.53, 803.54, 803.55, 803.56, 803.59, 803.60, 803.61, 803.62, 803.63, 803.64, 803.65, 803.66, 803.69, 803.70, 803.71, 803.72, 803.73, 803.74, 803.75, 803.76, 803.79, 803.80, 803.81, 803.82, 803.83, 803.84, 803.85, 803.86, 803.89, 803.90, 803.91, 803.92, 803.93, 803.94, 803.95, 803.96, 803.99, 804.00, 804.01, 804.02, 804.03, 804.04, 804.05, 804.06, 804.09, 804.10, 804.11, 804.12, 804.13, 804.14, 804.15, 804.16, 804.19, 804.20, 804.21, 804.22, 804.23, 804.24, 804.25, 804.26, 804.29, 804.30, 804.31, 804.32, 804.33, 804.34, 804.35, 804.36, 804.39, 804.40, 804.41, 804.42, 804.43, 804.44, 804.45, 804.46, 804.49, 804.50, 804.51, 804.52, 804.53, 804.54, 804.55, 804.56, 804.59, 804.60, 804.61, 804.62, 804.63, 804.64, 804.65, 804.66, 804.69, 804.70, 804.71, 804.72, 804.73, 804.74, 804.75, 804.76, 804.79, 804.80, 804.81, 804.82, 804.83, 804.84, 804.85, 804.86, 804.89, 804.90, 804.91, 804.92, 804.93, 804.94, 804.95, 804.96, 850.0, 850.1, 850.2, 850.3, 850.5, 850.9, 851.00, 851.01, 851.02, 851.03, 851.04, 851.05, 851.06, 851.09, 851.10, 851.11, 851.12, 851.13, 851.14, 851.15, 851.16, 851.19, 851.20, 851.21, 851.22, 851.23, 851.24, 851.25, 851.26, 851.29, 851.30, 851.31, 851.32, 851.33, 851.34, 851.35, 851.36, 851.39, 851.40, 851.41, 851.42, 851.43, 851.44, 851.45, 851.46, 851.49, 851.50, 851.51, 851.52, 851.53, 851.54, 851.55, 851.56, 851.59, 851.60, 851.61, 851.62, 851.63, 851.64, 851.65, 851.66, 851.69, 851.70, 851.71, 851.72, 851.73, 851.74, 851.75, 851.76, 851.79, 851.80, 851.81, 851.82, 851.83, 851.84, 851.85, 851.86, 851.89, 851.90, 851.91, 851.92, 851.93, 851.94, 851.95, 851.96, 851.99, 852.00, 852.01, 852.02, 852.03, 852.04, 852.05, 852.06, 852.09, 852.10, 852.11, 852.12, 852.13, 852.14, 852.15, 852.16, 852.19, 852.21, 852.22, 852.23, 852.24, 852.25, 852.26, 852.29, 852.30, 852.31, 852.32, 852.33, 852.34, 852.35, 852.36, 852.39, 852.40, 852.41, 852.42, 852.43, 852.44, 852.45, 852.46, 852.49, 852.50, 852.51, 852.52, 852.53, 852.54, 852.55, 852.56, 852.59, 853.00, 853.01, 853.02, 853.03, 853.04, 853.05, 853.06, 853.09, 853.10, 853.11, 853.12, 853.13, 853.14, 853.15, 853.16, 853.19, 854.00, 854.01, 854.02, 854.03, 854.04, 854.05, 854.06, 854.09, 854.10, 854.11, 854.12, 854.13, 854.14, 854.15, 854.16, 854.19

AHA: 4Q 2004, 77

431 Intracerebral hemorrhage

Hemorrhage (of):
- basilar
- bulbar
- cerebellar
- cerebral
- cerebromeningeal
- cortical
- internal capsule
- intrapontine
- pontine
- subcortical
- ventricular

Rupture of blood vessel in brain

DEF: Bleeding inside the brain.

C&C Exclusions: See 430

AHA: 4Q 2004, 77

4 432 Other and unspecified intracranial hemorrhage

AHA: 4Q 2004, 77

432.0 Nontraumatic extradural hemorrhage

Nontraumatic epidural hemorrhage

C&C Exclusions: See 430

432.1 Subdural hemorrhage

Subdural hematoma, nontraumatic

C&C Exclusions: See 430

✖ 432.9 Unspecified intracranial hemorrhage

Intracranial hemorrhage NOS

❹ **433 Occlusion and stenosis of precerebral arteries**

Includes embolism of basilar, carotid, and vertebral arteries
narrowing of basilar, carotid, and vertebral arteries
obstruction of basilar, carotid, and vertebral arteries
thrombosis of basilar, carotid, and vertebral arteries

Excludes *insufficiency NOS of precerebral arteries (435.0-435.9)*

AHA: 2Q 1995, 14; 3Q 1990, 16

The following fifth-digit subclassification is for use with category 433:
0 without mention of cerebral infarction
1 with cerebral infarction

❺ **433.0 Basilar artery**
C&C Exclusions: (for code 433.01) 250.70, 250.71, 250.72, 250.73, 250.80, 250.81, 250.82, 250.83, 250.90, 250.91, 250.92, 250.93, 433.00, 433.01, 433.10, 433.11, 433.20, 433.21, 433.30, 433.31, 433.80, 433.81, 433.90, 433.91, 435.0, 459.89, 459.9

Basilar artery occlusion and stenosis
With cerebral infarction

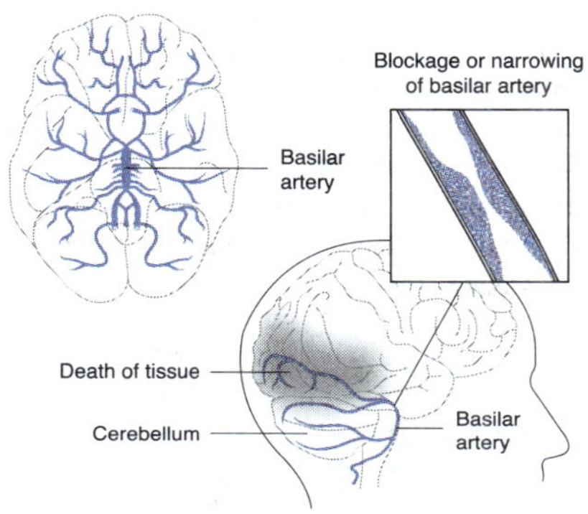

❺ **433.1 Carotid artery**
C&C Exclusions: (for code 433.11) 250.70, 250.71, 250.72, 250.73, 250.80, 250.81, 250.82, 250.83, 250.90, 250.91, 250.92, 250.93, 433.00, 433.01, 433.10, 433.11, 433.20, 433.21, 433.30, 433.31, 433.80, 433.81, 433.90, 433.91, 459.89, 459.9
AHA: 1Q 2000, 16; For Code 433.10: 1Q 2006, 17; 1Q 2002, 7, 10

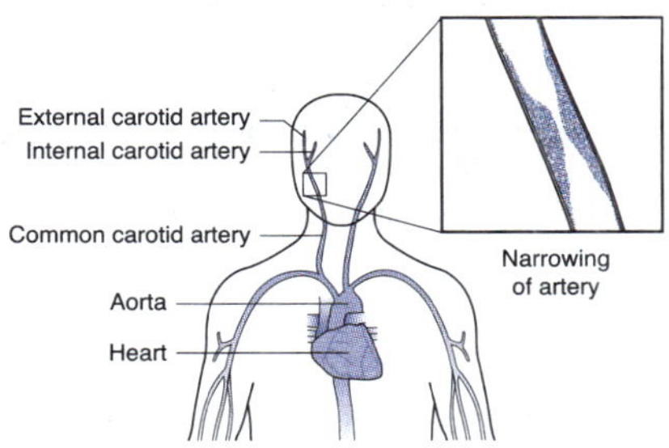

❺ **433.2 Vertebral artery**
C&C Exclusions: (for code 433.21) 250.70, 250.71, 250.72, 250.73, 250.80, 250.81, 250.82, 250.83, 250.90, 250.91, 250.92, 250.93, 433.00, 433.01, 433.10, 433.11, 433.20, 433.21, 433.30, 433.31, 433.80, 433.81, 433.90, 433.91, 435.1, 459.89, 459.9

❺ **433.3 Multiple and bilateral**
C&C Exclusions: (for code 433.31) See 433.1
AHA: 2Q 2002, 19; For Code 433.30: 1Q 2006, 17

❺ **433.8 Other specified precerebral artery**
C&C Exclusions: (for code 433.81) See 433.0

❺ **433.9 Unspecified precerebral artery**
(✖ is only valid for fifth-digit "0")
Precerebral artery NOS
C&C Exclusions: (for code 433.91) See 433.0

❹ **434 Occlusion of cerebral arteries**
AHA: 2Q 1995, 14

The following fifth-digit subclassification is for use with category 434:
0 without mention of cerebral infarction
1 with cerebral infarction

❺ **434.0 Cerebral thrombosis**
Thrombosis of cerebral arteries
DEF: Obstruction of an artery supplying blood to the brain by a blood clot.
C&C Exclusions: (for code 434.01) 250.70, 250.71, 250.72, 250.73, 250.80, 250.81, 250.82, 250.83, 250.90, 250.91, 250.92, 250.93, 434.00, 434.01, 434.10, 434.11, 434.90, 434.91, 436, 459.89, 459.9
AHA: For Code 434.01: 4Q 2004, 77

❺ **434.1 Cerebral embolism**
DEF: Artery to the brain blocked by an air bubble, foreign object, or piece of thrombus that has traveled until it becomes lodged.
C&C Exclusions: (for code 434.11) See 434.0
AHA: 3Q 1997, 11; For Code 434.11: 4Q 2004, 77

❺ **434.9 Cerebral artery occlusion, unspecified**
(✖ is only valid for fifth-digit "0")
C&C Exclusions: (for code 434.91) See 434.0
AHA: 4Q 1998, 87; For Code 434.91: 1Q 2007, 23-24; 4Q 2004, 77-78

❹ **435 Transient cerebral ischemia**

Includes cerebrovascular insufficiency (acute) with transient focal neurological signs and symptoms
insufficiency of basilar, carotid, and vertebral arteries
spasm of cerebral arteries

Excludes *acute cerebrovascular insufficiency NOS (437.1)*
that due to any condition classifiable to 433 (433.0-433.9)

435.0 Basilar artery syndrome

435.1 Vertebral artery syndrome

435.2 Subclavian steal syndrome

435.3 Vertebrobasilar artery syndrome
AHA: 4Q 1995, 60

435.8 Other specified transient cerebral ischemias

435.9 Unspecified transient cerebral ischemia
Impending cerebrovascular accident
Intermittent cerebral ischemia
Transient ischemic attack [TIA]
AHA: Nov-Dec 1985, 12

436 Acute, but ill-defined, cerebrovascular disease
Apoplexy, apoplectic:
NOS
attack
cerebral
seizure
Cerebral seizure

Excludes *any condition classifiable to categories 430-435*
cerebrovascular accident (434.91)
CVA (ischemic) (434.91)
embolic (434.11)
hemorrhagic (430, 431, 432.0-432.9)
thrombotic (434.01)
postoperative cerebrovascular accident (997.02)
stroke (ischmic) (434.91)
embolic (434.11)
hemorrhagic (430, 431, 432.0-432.9)
thrombotic (434.01)

C&C Exclusions: 250.70, 250.71, 250.72, 250.73, 250.80, 250.81, 250.82, 250.83, 250.90, 250.91, 250.92, 250.93, 430, 431, 432.0, 432.1, 432.9, 434.00, 434.01, 434.10, 434.11, 434.90, 434.91, 436, 459.89, 459.9, 780.01, 780.02, 780.03, 780.09, 800.00, 800.01, 800.02, 800.03, 800.04, 800.05, 800.06, 800.09, 800.10, 800.11, 800.12, 800.13, 800.14, 800.15, 800.16, 800.19, 800.20, 800.21, 800.22, 800.23, 800.24, 800.25, 800.26, 800.29, 800.30, 800.31, 800.32, 800.33, 800.34, 800.35, 800.36, 800.39, 800.40, 800.41, 800.42, 800.43, 800.44, 800.45, 800.46, 800.49, 800.50, 800.51, 800.52, 800.53, 800.54, 800.55, 800.56, 800.59, 800.60, 800.61, 800.62, 800.63, 800.64, 800.65, 800.66, 800.69, 800.70, 800.71, 800.72, 800.73, 800.74, 800.75, 800.76, 800.79, 800.80, 800.81, 800.82, 800.83, 800.84, 800.85, 800.86, 800.89, 800.90, 800.91, 800.92, 800.93, 800.94, 800.95, 800.96, 800.99, 801.00,

801.01, 801.02, 801.03, 801.04, 801.05, 801.06, 801.09, 801.10, 801.11, 801.12, 801.13, 801.14, 801.15, 801.16, 801.19, 801.20, 801.21, 801.22, 801.23, 801.24, 801.25, 801.26, 801.29, 801.30, 801.31, 801.32, 801.33, 801.34, 801.35, 801.36, 801.39, 801.40, 801.41, 801.42, 801.43, 801.44, 801.45, 801.46, 801.49, 801.50, 801.51, 801.52, 801.53, 801.54, 801.55, 801.56, 801.59, 801.60, 801.61, 801.62, 801.63, 801.64, 801.65, 801.66, 801.69, 801.70, 801.71, 801.72, 801.73, 801.74, 801.75, 801.76, 801.79, 801.80, 801.81, 801.82, 801.83, 801.84, 801.85, 801.86, 801.89, 801.90, 801.91, 801.92, 801.93, 801.94, 801.95, 801.96, 801.99, 803.00, 803.01, 803.02, 803.03, 803.04, 803.05, 803.06, 803.09, 803.10, 803.11, 803.12, 803.13, 803.14, 803.15, 803.16, 803.19, 803.20, 803.21, 803.22, 803.23, 803.24, 803.25, 803.26, 803.29, 803.30, 803.31, 803.32, 803.33, 803.34, 803.35, 803.36, 803.39, 803.40, 803.41, 803.42, 803.43, 803.44, 803.45, 803.46, 803.49, 803.50, 803.51, 803.52, 803.53, 803.54, 803.55, 803.56, 803.59, 803.60, 803.61, 803.62, 803.63, 803.64, 803.65, 803.66, 803.69, 803.70, 803.71, 803.72, 803.73, 803.74, 803.75, 803.76, 803.79, 803.80, 803.81, 803.82, 803.83, 803.84, 803.85, 803.86, 803.89, 803.90, 803.91, 803.92, 803.93, 803.94, 803.95, 803.96, 803.99, 804.00, 804.01, 804.02, 804.03, 804.04, 804.05, 804.06, 804.09, 804.10, 804.11, 804.12, 804.13, 804.14, 804.15, 804.16, 804.19, 804.20, 804.21, 804.22, 804.23, 804.24, 804.25, 804.26, 804.29, 804.30, 804.31, 804.32, 804.33, 804.34, 804.35, 804.36, 804.39, 804.40, 804.41, 804.42, 804.43, 804.44, 804.45, 804.46, 804.49, 804.50, 804.51, 804.52, 804.53, 804.54, 804.55, 804.56, 804.59, 804.60, 804.61, 804.62, 804.63, 804.64, 804.65, 804.66, 804.69, 804.70, 804.71, 804.72, 804.73, 804.74, 804.75, 804.76, 804.79, 804.80, 804.81, 804.82, 804.83, 804.84, 804.85, 804.86, 804.89, 804.90, 804.91, 804.92, 804.93, 804.94, 804.95, 804.96, 850.0, 850.1, 850.2, 850.3, 850.5, 850.9, 851.00, 851.01, 851.02, 851.03, 851.04, 851.05, 851.06, 851.09, 851.10, 851.11, 851.12, 851.13, 851.14, 851.15, 851.16, 851.19, 851.20, 851.21, 851.22, 851.23, 851.24, 851.25, 851.26, 851.29, 851.30, 851.31, 851.32, 851.33, 851.34, 851.35, 851.36, 851.39, 851.40, 851.41, 851.42, 851.43, 851.44, 851.45, 851.46, 851.49, 851.50, 851.51, 851.52, 851.53, 851.54, 851.55, 851.56, 851.59, 851.60, 851.61, 851.62, 851.63, 851.64, 851.65, 851.66, 851.69, 851.70, 851.71, 851.72, 851.73, 851.74, 851.75, 851.76, 851.79, 851.80, 851.81, 851.82, 851.83, 851.84, 851.85, 851.86, 851.89, 851.90, 851.91, 851.92, 851.93, 851.94, 851.95, 851.96, 851.99, 852.00, 852.01, 852.02, 852.03, 852.04, 852.05, 852.06, 852.09, 852.10, 852.11, 852.12, 852.13, 852.14, 852.15, 852.16, 852.19, 852.21, 852.22, 852.23, 852.24, 852.25, 852.26, 852.29, 852.30, 852.31, 852.32, 852.33, 852.34, 852.35, 852.36, 852.39, 852.40, 852.41, 852.42, 852.43, 852.44, 852.45, 852.46, 852.49, 852.50, 852.51, 852.52, 852.53, 852.54, 852.55, 852.56, 852.59, 853.00, 853.01, 853.02, 853.03, 853.04, 853.05, 853.06, 853.09, 853.10, 853.11, 853.12, 853.13, 853.14, 853.15, 853.16, 853.19, 854.00, 854.01, 854.02, 854.03, 854.04, 854.05, 854.06, 854.09, 854.10, 854.11, 854.12, 854.13, 854.14, 854.15, 854.16, 854.19

AHA: 4Q 2004, 77; 4Q 1999, 3

❹ **437 Other and ill-defined cerebrovascular disease**

437.0 Cerebral atherosclerosis A

Atheroma of cerebral arteries
Cerebral arteriosclerosis

437.1 Other generalized ischemic cerebrovascular disease

Acute cerebrovascular insufficiency NOS
Cerebral ischemia (chronic)

437.2 Hypertensive encephalopathy

C&C Exclusions: 250.70, 250.71, 250.72, 250.73, 250.80, 250.81, 250.82, 250.83, 250.90, 250.91, 250.92, 250.93, 437.2, 459.89, 459.9

AHA: Jul-Aug 1984, 14

437.3 Cerebral aneurysm, nonruptured

Internal carotid artery, intracranial portion
Internal carotid artery NOS

Excludes *congenital cerebral aneurysm, nonruptured (747.81)*
internal carotid artery, extracranial portion (442.81)

DEF: Temporary loss of short-term memory due to interrupted blood flow to certain areas of the brain.

437.4 Cerebral arteritis

C&C Exclusions: 250.70, 250.71, 250.72, 250.73, 250.80, 250.81, 250.82, 250.83, 250.90, 250.91, 250.92, 250.93, 437.4, 459.89, 459.9

AHA: 4Q 1999, 21

437.5 Moyamoya disease

C&C Exclusions: 250.70, 250.71, 250.72, 250.73, 250.80, 250.81, 250.82, 250.83, 250.90, 250.91, 250.92, 250.93, 437.5, 459.89, 459.9

437.6 Nonpyogenic thrombosis of intracranial venous sinus

Excludes *pyogenic (325)*

C&C Exclusions: 250.70, 250.71, 250.72, 250.73, 250.80, 250.81, 250.82, 250.83, 250.90, 250.91, 250.92, 250.93, 437.6, 459.89, 459.9

437.7 Transient global amnesia

AHA: 4Q 1992, 20

437.8 Other

✖ **437.9 Unspecified**

Cerebrovascular disease or lesion NOS

❹ **438 Late effects of cerebrovascular disease**

Note: *This category is to be used to indicate conditions in 430-437 as the cause of late effects. The "late effects" include conditions specified as such, or as sequelae, which may occur at any time after the onset of the causal condition.*

Excludes ▶ *personal history of:*◀
▶ *cerebral infarction without residual deficits (V12.54)*◀
▶ *PRIND (Prolonged reversible ischemic neurologic deficit) (V12.54)*◀
▶ *RIND (Reversible ischemic neurological deficit) (V12.54)*◀
▶ *transient ischemic attack (TIA) (V12.54)*◀

AHA: 3Q 2006, 4, 6; 4Q 1999, 4, 6-7; 4Q 1998, 39, 88; 4Q 1997, 35, 37; 4Q 1992, 21; Nov-Dec 1986, 12; Mar-Apr 1986, 7

438.0 Cognitive deficits

❺ **438.1 Speech and language deficits**

438.10 Speech and language deficit, unspecified

438.11 Aphasia

DEF: Impaired or complete loss of the ability to communicate with language or symbols.

AHA: 4Q 2003, 105; 4Q 1997, 36

438.12 Dysphasia

DEF: Speech impairment resulting from brain damage or illness.

AHA: 4Q 1999, 3, 9

438.19 Other speech and language deficits

❺ **438.2 Hemiplegia/hemiparesis**

DEF: Paralysis affecting one side of the body.

438.20 Hemiplegia affecting unspecified side

AHA: 4Q 2003, 105; 4Q 1999, 3, 9

438.21 Hemiplegia affecting dominant side

438.22 Hemiplegia affecting nondominant side

AHA: 4Q 2003, 105; 1Q 2002, 16

❺ **438.3 Monoplegia of upper limb**

438.30 Monoplegia of upper limb affecting unspecified side

438.31 Monoplegia of upper limb affecting dominant side

438.32 Monoplegia of upper limb affecting nondominant side

❺ **438.4 Monoplegia of lower limb**

438.40 Monoplegia of lower limb affecting unspecified side

438.41 Monoplegia of lower limb affecting dominant side

438.42 Monoplegia of lower limb affecting nondominant side

438.5 Other paralytic syndrome

Use additional code to identify type of paralytic syndrome, such as:
locked-in state (344.81)
quadriplegia (344.00-344.09)

Excludes *late effects of cerebrovascular accident with:*
hemiplegia/hemiparesis (438.20-438.22)
monoplegia of lower limb (438.40-438.42)
monoplegia of upper limb (438.40-438.42)

438.50 Other paralytic syndrome affecting unspecified side

438.51 Other paralytic syndrome affecting dominant side

438.52 Other paralytic syndrome affecting nondominant side

438.53 Other paralytic syndrome, bilateral
AHA: 4Q 1998, 39

438.6 Alterations of sensations
Use additional code to identify the altered sensation

438.7 Disturbance of vision
Use additional code to identify the visual disturbance
AHA: 4Q 2002, 56

438.8 Other late effects of cerebrovascular disease

438.81 Apraxia

438.82 Dysphagia
▶ Use additional code to identify the type of dysphagia, if known (787.20-787.29)◀

438.83 Facial weakness
Facial droop

438.84 Ataxia
DEF: Inability to coordinate muscle movement.
AHA: 4Q 2002, 56

438.85 Vertigo
DEF: Sensation of dizziness or falling off balance.

438.89 Other late effects of cerebrovascular disease
Use additional code to identify the late effect
AHA: 1Q 2005, 13; 4Q 1998, 39

438.9 Unspecified late effects of cerebrovascular disease

DISEASES OF ARTERIES, ARTERIOLES, AND CAPILLARIES (440-▶449◀)

440 Atherosclerosis

Includes arteriolosclerosis
arteriosclerosis (obliterans) (senile)
arteriosclerotic vascular disease
atheroma
degeneration:
arterial
arteriovascular
vascular
endarteritis deformans or obliterans
senile:
arteritis
endarteritis

Excludes *atheroembolism (445.01-445.89)*
atherosclerosis of bypass graft of the extremities (440.30-440.32)

DEF: Fatty plague deposits that reduce the diameter and elasticity of an artery.

440.0 Of aorta A
AHA: 2Q 1993, 7; 2Q 1993, 8; 4Q 1988, 8

440.1 Of renal artery A
Excludes *atherosclerosis of renal arterioles (403.00-403.91)*

440.2 Of native arteries of the extremities
▶ Use additional code, if applicable, to identify chronic total occlusion of artery of the extremities (440.4)◀
Excludes *atherosclerosis of bypass graft of the extremities (440.30-440.32)*
AHA: 4Q 1994, 49; 4Q 1993, 27; 4Q 1992, 25; 3Q 1990, 15; Mar-Apr 1987, 6

440.20 Atherosclerosis of the extremities, unspecified A

440.21 Atherosclerosis of the extremities with intermittent claudication A

440.22 Atherosclerosis of the extremities with rest pain A
Any condition classifiable to 440.21

440.23 Atherosclerosis of the extremities with ulceration A
Any condition classifiable to 440.21-440.22
Use additional code for any associated ulceration (707.10-707.9)
C&C Exclusions: 707.10, 707.11, 707.12, 707.13, 707.14, 707.15, 707.19
AHA: 4Q 2000, 44

440.24 Atherosclerosis of the extremities with gangrene
Any condition classifiable to 440.21, 440.22, and 440.23 with ischemic gangrene 785.4
Use additional code for any associated ulceration (707.10-707.9)
Excludes *gas gangrene 040.0*
C&C Exclusions: 440.24, 780.91, 780.92, 780.99, 785.4, 799.8
AHA: 4Q 2003, 109; 3Q 2003, 14; 4Q 1995, 54; 1Q 1995, 11

440.29 Other A

440.3 Of bypass graft of the extremities
Excludes *atherosclerosis of native artery of the extremity (440.21-440.24)*
embolism [occlusion NOS] [thrombus] of graft (996.74)
AHA: 4Q 1994, 49

440.30 Of unspecified graft A

440.31 Of autologous vein bypass graft A

440.32 Of nonautologous vein bypass graft A

●+ ***440.4 Chronic total occlusion of artery of the extremities***
Complete occlusion of artery of the extremities
Total occlusion of artery of the extremities
Code first atherosclerosis of arteries of the extremities (440.20-440.29, 440.30-440.32)
Excludes *acute occlusion of artery of extremity (444.21-444.22)*

440.8 Of other specified arteries A
Excludes *basilar (433.0)*
carotid (433.1)
cerebral (437.0)
coronary (414.00-414.07)
mesenteric (557.1)
precerebral (433.0-433.9)
pulmonary (416.0)
vertebral (433.2)

440.9 Generalized and unspecified atherosclerosis A
Arteriosclerotic vascular disease NOS
Excludes *arteriosclerotic cardiovascular disease [ASCVD] (429.2)*

441 Aortic aneurysm and dissection
Excludes *syphilitic aortic aneurysm (093.0)*
traumatic aortic aneurysm (901.0, 902.0)

441.0 Dissection of aorta
AHA: 4Q 1989, 10

441.00 Unspecified site
C&C Exclusions: 250.70, 250.71, 250.72, 250.73, 250.80, 250.81, 250.82, 250.83, 250.90, 250.91, 250.92, 250.93, 441.00, 441.01, 441.02, 441.03, 441.1, 441.2, 441.3, 441.4, 441.5, 441.6, 441.7, 441.9, 459.89, 459.9

441.01 Thoracic
C&C Exclusions: See 441.00

441.02 Abdominal
C&C Exclusions: See 441.00

441.03 Thoracoabdominal
C&C Exclusions: See 441.00

441.1 Thoracic aneurysm, ruptured
C&C Exclusions: See 441.00

441.2 Thoracic aneurysm without mention of rupture
AHA: 3Q 1992, 10

441.3 Abdominal aneurysm, ruptured
C&C Exclusions: See 441.00

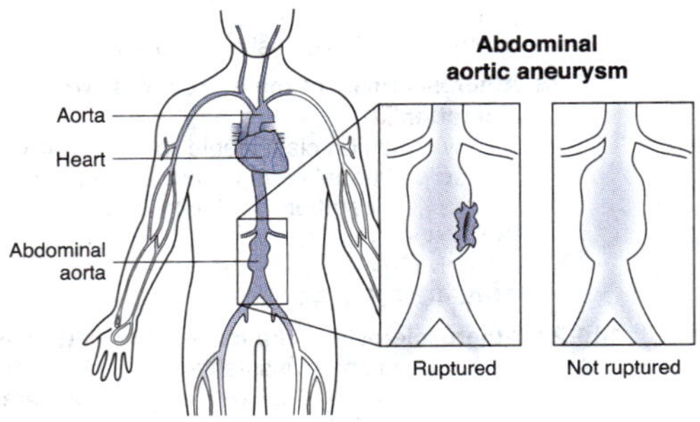

441.4 Abdominal aneurysm without mention of rupture

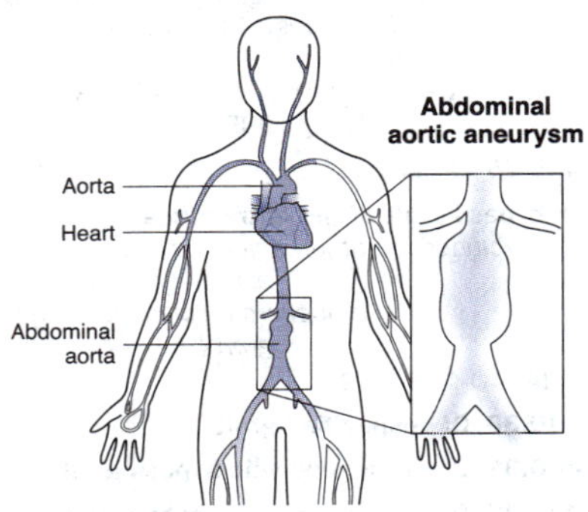

AHA: 4Q 2000, 64; 1Q 1999, 15-17; 3Q 1992, 10

441.5 Aortic aneurysm of unspecified site, ruptured
Rupture of aorta NOS
C&C Exclusions: See 441.00

441.6 Thoracoabdominal aneurysm, ruptured
C&C Exclusions: See 441.00

441.7 Thoracoabdominal aneurysm, without mention of rupture
AHA: 2Q 2006, 16

✖ **441.9 Aortic aneurysm of unspecified site without mention of rupture**
Aneurysm
Dilatation of aorta
Hyaline necrosis of aorta

❹ **442 Other aneurysm**
Includes aneurysm (ruptured) (cirsoid) (false) (varicose)
aneurysmal varix
Excludes *arteriovenous aneurysm or fistula:*
acquired (447.0)
congenital (747.60-747.69)
traumatic (900.0-904.9)

442.0 Of artery of upper extremity

442.1 Of renal artery

442.2 Of iliac artery
AHA: 1Q 1999, 16-17

442.3 Of artery of lower extremity
Aneurysm:
femoral artery
popliteal artery
AHA: 3Q 2002, 24-26; 1Q 1999, 16

❺ **442.8 Of other specified artery**

442.81 Artery of neck
Aneurysm of carotid artery (common) (external) (internal, extracranial portion)
Excludes *internal carotid artery, intracranial portion (437.3)*

442.82 Subclavian artery

442.83 Splenic artery

442.84 Other visceral artery
Aneurysm:
celiac artery
gastroduodenal artery
gastroepiploic artery
hepatic artery
pancreaticoduodenal artery
superior mesenteric artery

442.89 Other
Aneurysm:
mediastinal artery
spinal artery
Excludes *cerebral (nonruptured) (437.3)*
congenital (747.81)
ruptured (430)
coronary (414.11)
heart (414.10)
pulmonary (417.1)

✖ **442.9 Of unspecified site**

❹ **443 Other peripheral vascular disease**

443.0 Raynaud's syndrome
Raynaud's:
disease
phenomenon (secondary)
Use additional code to identify gangrene (785.4)

443.1 Thromboangiitis obliterans [Buerger's disease]
Presenile gangrene
DEF: Medium-sized blood vessels of the hands and feet become inflamed and blocked by blood clots, causing gangrene of the extremities.

❺ **443.2 Other arterial dissection**
Excludes *dissection of aorta (441.00-441.03)*
dissection of coronary arteries (414.12)
AHA: 4Q 2002, 54

443.21 Dissection of carotid artery

443.22 Dissection of iliac artery

443.23 Dissection of renal artery

443.24 Dissection of vertebral artery

443.29 Dissection of other artery

❺ **443.8 Other specified peripheral vascular diseases**

✚ ***443.81 Peripheral angiopathy in diseases classified elsewhere***
Code first underlying disease, as:
diabetes mellitus (250.7)
AHA: 1Q 2004, 14; 3Q 1991, 10

443.82 Erythromelalgia
DEF: Abnormal dilation of extremity blood vessels, especially in the feet, causing a painful, burning sensation, and redness.
AHA: 4Q 2005, 73

443.89 Other
Acrocyanosis
Acroparesthesia:
simple [Schultze's type]
vasomotor [Nothnagel's type]
Erythrocyanosis
Excludes *chilblains (991.5)*
frostbite (991.0-991.3)
immersion foot (991.4)

443.9 Peripheral vascular disease, unspecified
Intermittent claudication NOS
Peripheral:
angiopathy NOS
vascular disease NOS
Spasm of artery
Excludes *atherosclerosis of the arteries of the extremities (440.20-440.22)*
spasm of cerebral artery (435.0-435.9)
AHA: 4Q 1992, 25; 3Q 1991, 10

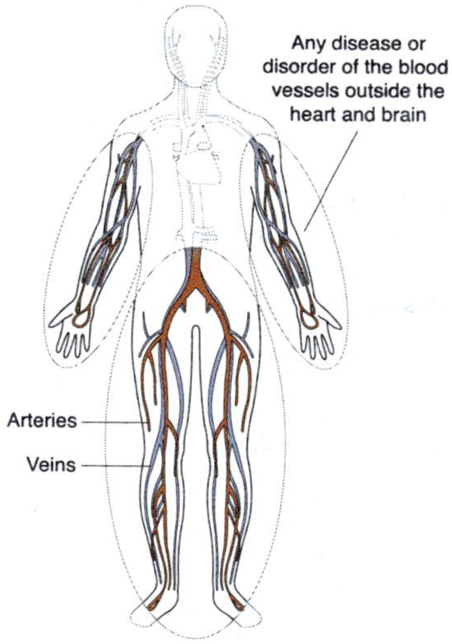

❹ **444 Arterial embolism and thrombosis**
Includes infarction:
embolic
thrombotic
occlusion
Excludes *atheroembolism (445.01-445.89)*
▶ *septic arterial embolism (449)*◀
that complicating:
abortion (634-638 with .6, 639.6)
ectopic or molar pregnancy (639.6)
pregnancy, childbirth, or the puerperium (673.0-673.8)
AHA: 2Q 1992, 11; 4Q 1990, 27

444.0 Of abdominal aorta
Aortic bifurcation syndrome
Aortoiliac obstruction
Leriche's syndrome
Saddle embolus
C&C Exclusions: 250.70, 250.71, 250.72, 250.73, 250.80, 250.81, 250.82, 250.83, 250.90, 250.91, 250.92, 250.93, 444.0, 444.89, 444.9, 459.89, 459.9
AHA: 2Q 1993, 7; 4Q 1990, 27

444.1 Of thoracic aorta
Embolism or thrombosis of aorta (thoracic)
C&C Exclusions: 250.70, 250.71, 250.72, 250.73, 250.80, 250.81, 250.82, 250.83, 250.90, 250.91, 250.92, 250.93, 444.1, 444.89, 444.9, 459.89, 459.9

❺ **444.2 Of arteries of the extremities**
AHA: Mar-Apr 1987, 6

444.21 Upper extremity
C&C Exclusions: 250.70, 250.71, 250.72, 250.73, 250.80, 250.81, 250.82, 250.83, 250.90, 250.91, 250.92, 250.93, 444.21, 444.89, 444.9, 459.89, 459.9

444.22 Lower extremity
Arterial embolism or thrombosis:
femoral
peripheral NOS
popliteal
Excludes *iliofemoral (444.81)*
C&C Exclusions: 250.70, 250.71, 250.72, 250.73, 250.80, 250.81, 250.82, 250.83, 250.90, 250.91, 250.92, 250.93, 444.22, 444.89, 444.9, 459.89, 459.9
AHA: 3Q 2003, 10; 1Q 2003, 17; 3Q 1990, 16

❺ **444.8 Of other specified artery**

444.81 Iliac artery
C&C Exclusions: 250.70, 250.71, 250.72, 250.73, 250.80, 250.81, 250.82, 250.83, 250.90, 250.91, 250.92, 250.93, 444.81, 444.89, 444.9, 459.89, 459.9
AHA: 1Q 2003, 16

444.89 Other
Excludes *basilar (433.0)*
carotid (433.1)
cerebral (434.0-434.9)
coronary (410.00-410.92)
mesenteric (557.0)
ophthalmic (362.30-362.34)
precerebral (433.0-433.9)
pulmonary (415.19)
renal (593.81)
retinal (362.30-362.34)
vertebral (433.2)
C&C Exclusions: 250.70, 250.71, 250.72, 250.73, 250.80, 250.81, 250.82, 250.83, 250.90, 250.91, 250.92, 250.93, 444.89, 444.9, 445.01, 445.02, 445.81, 445.89, 459.89, 459.9

✖ **444.9 Of unspecified artery**
C&C Exclusions: See 444.89

❹ **445 Atheroembolism**
Includes Atherothrombotic microembolism
Cholesterol embolism
DEF: Obstruction of an artery by a traveling fat deposit that has become lodged.
AHA: 4Q 2002, 57

❺ **445.0 Of extremities**

445.01 Upper extremity
C&C Exclusions: 250.70, 250.71, 250.72, 250.73, 250.80, 250.81, 250.82, 250.83, 250.90, 250.91, 250.92, 250.93, 444.89, 444.9, 445.01, 459.89, 459.9

445.02 Lower extremity
C&C Exclusions: 250.70, 250.71, 250.72, 250.73, 250.80, 250.81, 250.82, 250.83, 250.90, 250.91, 250.92, 250.93, 444.89, 444.9, 445.02, 459.89, 459.9

❺ **445.8 Of other sites**

445.81 Kidney
Use additional code for any associated acute renal failure or chronic kidney disease (584, 585)
C&C Exclusions: 250.70, 250.71, 250.72, 250.73, 250.80, 250.81, 250.82, 250.83, 250.90, 250.91, 250.92, 250.93, 444.89, 444.9, 445.81, 459.89, 459.9

445.89 Other site
C&C Exclusions: 250.70, 250.71, 250.72, 250.73, 250.80, 250.81, 250.82, 250.83, 250.90, 250.91, 250.92, 250.93, 444.89, 444.9, 445.89, 459.89, 459.9

④ **446 Polyarteritis nodosa and allied conditions**

446.0 Polyarteritis nodosa
Disseminated necrotizing periarteritis
Necrotizing angiitis
Panarteritis (nodosa)
Periarteritis (nodosa)

DEF: The body's immune system mistakenly attacks small and medium-sized blood vessels, resulting in tissue death.

C&C Exclusions: 250.70, 250.71, 250.72, 250.73, 250.80, 250.81, 250.82, 250.83, 250.90, 250.91, 250.92, 250.93, 446.0, 446.1, 446.20, 446.21, 446.29, 446.3, 446.4, 446.5, 446.6, 446.7, 459.89, 459.9

446.1 Acute febrile mucocutaneous lymph node syndrome [MCLS]
Kawasaki disease

⑤ **446.2 Hypersensitivity angiitis**
Excludes *antiglomerular basement membrane disease without pulmonary hemorrhage (583.89)*

✖ **446.20 Hypersensitivity angiitis, unspecified**
C&C Exclusions: See 446.0

446.21 Goodpasture's syndrome
Antiglomerular basement membrane antibody-mediated nephritis with pulmonary hemorrhage
Use additional code to identify renal disease (583.81)
C&C Exclusions: See 446.0

446.29 Other specified hypersensitivity angiitis
C&C Exclusions: See 446.0
AHA: 1Q 1995, 3

446.3 Lethal midline granuloma
Malignant granuloma of face

DEF: Severe tumor associated with infection that appears in the nose or sinuses and results in death.

C&C Exclusions: See 446.0
AHA: 3Q 2000, 11

446.4 Wegener's granulomatosis
Necrotizing respiratory granulomatosis
Wegener's syndrome
C&C Exclusions: See 446.0
AHA: 3Q 2000, 11

446.5 Giant cell arteritis
Cranial arteritis
Horton's disease
Temporal arteritis
C&C Exclusions: See 446.0

446.6 Thrombotic microangiopathy
Moschcowitz's syndrome
Thrombotic thrombocytopenic purpura
C&C Exclusions: See 446.0

446.7 Takayasu's disease
Aortic arch arteritis
Pulseless disease
C&C Exclusions: See 446.0

④ **447 Other disorders of arteries and arterioles**

447.0 Arteriovenous fistula, acquired
Arteriovenous aneurysm, acquired
Excludes *cerebrovascular (437.3)*
coronary (414.19)
pulmonary (417.0)
surgically created arteriovenous shunt or fistula:
complication (996.1, 996.61-996.62)
status or presence (V45.1)
traumatic (900.0-904.9)

447.1 Stricture of artery
AHA: 2Q 1993, 8; Mar-Apr 1987, 6

447.2 Rupture of artery
Erosion of artery
Fistula, except arteriovenous of artery
Ulcer of artery
Excludes *traumatic rupture of artery (900.0-904.9)*

447.3 Hyperplasia of renal artery
Fibromuscular hyperplasia of renal artery

447.4 Celiac artery compression syndrome
Celiac axis syndrome
Marable's syndrome

447.5 Necrosis of artery

447.6 Arteritis, unspecified
Aortitis NOS
Endarteritis NOS
Excludes *arteritis, endarteritis:*
aortic arch (446.7)
cerebral (437.4)
coronary (414.00-414.07)
deformans (440.0-440.9)
obliterans (440.0-440.9)
pulmonary (417.8)
senile (440.0-440.9)
polyarteritis NOS (446.0)
syphilitic aortitis (093.1)
AHA: 1Q 1995, 3

447.8 Other specified disorders of arteries and arterioles
Fibromuscular hyperplasia of arteries, except renal

✖ **447.9 Unspecified disorders of arteries and arterioles**

④ **448 Disease of capillaries**

448.0 Hereditary hemorrhagic telangiectasia
Rendu-Osler-Weber disease

448.1 Nevus, non-neoplastic
Nevus:
araneus
senile
spider
stellar
Excludes *neoplastic (216.0-216.9)*
port wine (757.32)
strawberry (757.32)

448.9 Other and unspecified capillary diseases
Capillary:
hemorrhage
hyperpermeability
thrombosis
Excludes *capillary fragility (hereditary) (287.8)*

● **449 Septic arterial embolism**
Code first underlying infection, such as:
infective endocarditis (421.0)
lung abscess (513.0)
Use additional code to identify the site of the embolism (433.0-433.9, 444.0-444.9)
Excludes *septic pulmonary embolism (415.12)*

DEF: Dislodged material from a centralized infection lodged in a small arteriole, causing tissue death due to bacteria and lack of blood supply.

DISEASES OF VEINS AND LYMPHATICS, AND OTHER DISEASES OF CIRCULATORY SYSTEM (451-459)

④ **451 Phlebitis and thrombophlebitis**
Includes endophlebitis
inflammation, vein
periphlebitis
suppurative phlebitis
Use additional E code to identify drug if drug-induced
Excludes *that complicating:*
abortion (634-638 with .7, 639.8)
ectopic or molar pregnancy (639.8)
pregnancy, childbirth, or the puerperium (671.0-671.9)
that due to or following:
implant or catheter device (996.61-996.62)
infusion, perfusion, or transfusion (999.2)
AHA: 1Q 1992, 16

451.0 Of superficial vessels of lower extremities
Saphenous vein (greater) (lesser)
C&C Exclusions: 250.70, 250.71, 250.72, 250.73, 250.80, 250.81, 250.82, 250.83, 250.90, 250.91, 250.92, 250.93, 451.0, 451.11, 451.19, 451.2, 451.81, 451.82, 451.83, 451.84, 451.89, 451.9, 459.89, 459.9
AHA: 3Q 1991, 16

451.1 Of deep vessels of lower extremities
AHA: 3Q 1991, 16

451.11 Femoral vein (deep) (superficial)
C&C Exclusions: See 451.0

451.19 Other
Femoropopliteal vein
Popliteal vein
Tibial vein
C&C Exclusions: See 451.0

451.2 Of lower extremities, unspecified
C&C Exclusions: See 451.0
AHA: 4Q 2004, 80

451.8 Of other sites
Excludes *intracranial venous sinus (325)*
nonpyogenic (437.6)
portal (vein) (572.1)

451.81 Iliac vein
C&C Exclusions: See 451.0

451.82 Of superficial veins of upper extremities
Antecubital vein
Basilic vein
Cephalic vein

451.83 Of deep veins of upper extremities
Brachial vein
Radial vein
Ulnar vein

451.84 Of upper extremities, unspecified

451.89 Other
Axillary vein
Jugular vein
Subclavian vein
Thrombophlebitis of breast (Mondor's disease)

451.9 Of unspecified site

452 Portal vein thrombosis
Portal (vein) obstruction
Excludes *hepatic vein thrombosis (453.0)*
phlebitis of portal vein (572.1)
C&C Exclusions: 250.70, 250.71, 250.72, 250.73, 250.80, 250.81, 250.82, 250.83, 250.90, 250.91, 250.92, 250.93, 452, 453.8, 453.9, 459.89, 459.9

453 Other venous embolism and thrombosis
Excludes *that complicating:*
abortion (634-638 with .7, 639.8)
ectopic or molar pregnancy (639.8)
pregnancy, childbirth, or the puerperium (671.0-671.9)
that with inflammation, phlebitis, and thrombophlebitis (451.0-451.9)
AHA: 1Q 1992, 16

453.0 Budd-Chiari syndrome
Hepatic vein thrombosis
DEF: Obstruction or occlusion of the hepatic veins, causing an enlarged liver, abdominal pain/ tenderness, intractable ascites, mild jaundice, portal hypertension, and liver failure.
C&C Exclusions: 250.70, 250.71, 250.72, 250.73, 250.80, 250.81, 250.82, 250.83, 250.90, 250.91, 250.92, 250.93, 453.0, 453.8, 453.9, 459.89, 459.9

453.1 Thrombophlebitis migrans
C&C Exclusions: 250.70, 250.71, 250.72, 250.73, 250.80, 250.81, 250.82, 250.83, 250.90, 250.91, 250.92, 250.93, 453.1, 453.8, 453.9, 459.89, 459.9

453.2 Of vena cava
C&C Exclusions: 250.70, 250.71, 250.72, 250.73, 250.80, 250.81, 250.82, 250.83, 250.90, 250.91, 250.92, 250.93, 453.2, 453.8, 453.9, 459.89, 459.9

453.3 Of renal vein
C&C Exclusions: 250.70, 250.71, 250.72, 250.73, 250.80, 250.81, 250.82, 250.83, 250.90, 250.91, 250.92, 250.93, 453.3, 453.8, 453.9, 459.89, 459.9

453.4 Venous embolism and thrombosis of deep vessels of lower extremity

453.40 Venous embolism and thrombosis of unspecified deep vessels of lower extremity
Deep vein thrombosis NOS
DVT NOS

453.41 Venous embolism and thrombosis of deep vessels of proximal lower extremity
Femoral
Iliac
Popliteal
Thigh
Upper leg NOS
AHA: 4Q 2004, 79

453.42 Venous embolism and thrombosis of deep vessels of distal lower extremity
Calf
Lower leg NOS
Peroneal
Tibial

453.8 Of other specified veins
Excludes *cerebral (434.0-434.9)*
coronary (410.00-410.92)
intracranial venous sinus (325)
nonpyogenic (437.6)
mesenteric (557.0)
portal (452)
precerebral (433.0-433.9)
pulmonary (415.19)
C&C Exclusions: 250.70, 250.71, 250.72, 250.73, 250.80, 250.81, 250.82, 250.83, 250.90, 250.91, 250.92, 250.93, 453.8, 453.9, 459.89, 459.9
AHA: 3Q 1991, 16; Mar-Apr 1987, 6

453.9 Of unspecified site
Embolism of vein
Thrombosis (vein)
C&C Exclusions: See 453.8

454 Varicose veins of lower extremities
Excludes *that complicating pregnancy, childbirth, or the puerperium (671.0)*
DEF: Swollen, dilated veins in the legs.
AHA: 2Q 1991, 20

454.0 With ulcer A
Varicose ulcer (lower extremity, any part)
Varicose veins with ulcer of lower extremity [any part] or of unspecified site
Any condition classifiable to 454.9 with ulcer or specified as ulcerated
AHA: 4Q 1999, 18

454.1 With inflammation A
Stasis dermatitis
Varicose veins with inflammation of lower extremity [any part] or of unspecified site
Any condition classifiable to 454.9 with inflammation or specified as inflamed

454.2 With ulcer and inflammation A
Varicose veins with ulcer and inflammation of lower extremity [any part] or of unspecified site
Any condition classifiable to 454.9 with ulcer and inflammation

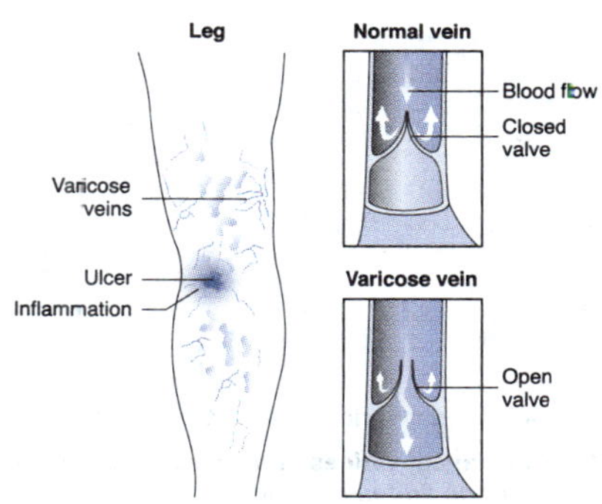

454.8 With other complications
Edema
Pain
Swelling
AHA: 4Q 2002, 58

A Adult (15+ years) M Maternity (12-55 years) N Newborn (0 years) P Pediatric (0-17 years) ♂ Male ♀ Female ❷ Medicare Secondary Payer

454.9 Asymptomatic varicose veins A
Phlebectasia of lower extremity [any part] or of unspecified site
Varicose veins NOS
Varicose veins of lower extremity [any part] or of unspecified site
Varix of lower extremity [any part] or of unspecified site
AHA: 4Q 2002, 58

④ **455 Hemorrhoids**
Includes hemorrhoids (anus) (rectum)
piles
varicose veins, anus or rectum
Excludes *that complicating pregnancy, childbirth, or the puerperium (671.8)*

DEF: Dilated, swollen, painful veins in the anus or rectum.

455.0 Internal hemorrhoids without mention of complication
AHA: 3Q 2005, 17

455.1 Internal thrombosed hemorrhoids

455.2 Internal hemorrhoids with other complication
Internal hemorrhoids:
- bleeding
- prolapsed
- strangulated
- ulcerated

AHA: 3Q 2005, 17; 1Q 2003, 8

455.3 External hemorrhoids without mention of complication
AHA: 1Q 2007, 13; 3Q 2005, 17

455.4 External thrombosed hemorrhoids

455.5 External hemorrhoids with other complication
External hemorrhoids:
- bleeding
- prolapsed
- strangulated
- ulcerated

AHA: 3Q 2005, 17; 1Q 2003, 8

455.6 Unspecified hemorrhoids without mention of complication
Hemorrhoids NOS

455.7 Unspecified thrombosed hemorrhoids
Thrombosed hemorrhoids, unspecified whether internal or external

455.8 Unspecified hemorrhoids with other complication
Hemorrhoids, unspecified whether internal or external:
- bleeding
- prolapsed
- strangulated
- ulcerated

455.9 Residual hemorrhoidal skin tags
Skin tags, anus or rectum

④ **456 Varicose veins of other sites**

456.0 Esophageal varices with bleeding
C&C Exclusions: 251.5, 456.0, 456.20, 459.89, 459.9, 530.21, 530.7, 530.82, 531.00, 531.01, 531.10, 531.11, 531.20, 531.21, 531.30, 531.31, 531.40, 531.41, 531.50, 531.51, 531.60, 531.61, 531.70, 531.71, 531.90, 531.91, 532.00, 532.01, 532.10, 532.11, 532.20, 532.21, 532.30, 532.31, 532.40, 532.41, 532.50, 532.51, 532.60, 532.61, 532.70, 532.71, 532.90, 532.91, 533.00, 533.01, 533.10, 533.11, 533.20, 533.21, 533.30, 533.31, 533.40, 533.41, 533.50, 533.51, 533.60, 533.61, 533.70, 533.71, 533.90, 533.91, 534.00, 534.01, 534.10, 534.11, 534.20, 534.21, 534.30, 534.31, 534.40, 534.41, 534.50, 534.51, 534.60, 534.61, 534.70, 534.71, 534.90, 534.91, 535.01, 535.11, 535.21, 535.31, 535.41, 535.51, 535.61, 537.83, 537.84, 562.02, 562.03, 562.12, 562.13, 569.3, 569.85, 569.86, 578.0, 578.1, 578.9

456.1 Esophageal varices without mention of bleeding

⑤ **456.2 Esophageal varices in diseases classified elsewhere**
Code first underlying disease, as:
- cirrhosis of liver (571.0-571.9)
- portal hypertension (572.3)

✚ ***456.20 With bleeding***
C&C Exclusions: 456.0, 456.20, 459.89, 459.9, 530.82
AHA: Nov-Dec 1985, 14

✚ ***456.21 Without mention of bleeding***
AHA: 3Q 2005, 15; 2Q 2002, 4

456.3 Sublingual varices

456.4 Scrotal varices ♂
Varicocele

456.5 Pelvic varices
Varices of broad ligament

Varicose veins on structures in the pelvis

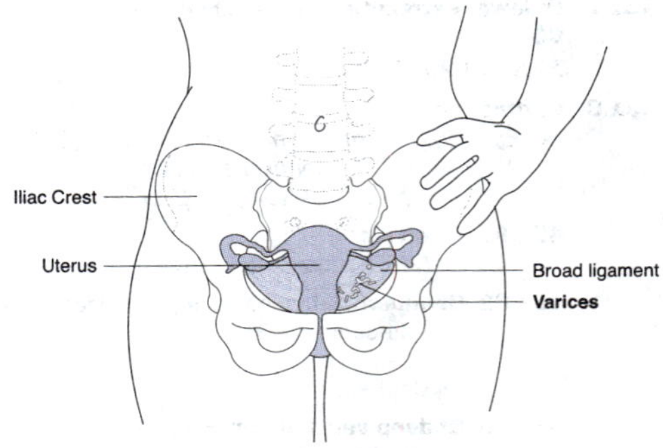

456.6 Vulval varices ♀
Varices of perineum
Excludes *that complicating pregnancy, childbirth, or the puerperium (671.1)*

456.8 Varices of other sites
Varicose veins of nasal septum (with ulcer)
Excludes *placental varices (656.7)*
retinal varices (362.17)
varicose ulcer of unspecified site (454.0)
varicose veins of unspecified site (454.9)

AHA: 2Q 2002, 4

④ **457 Noninfectious disorders of lymphatic channels**

457.0 Postmastectomy lymphedema syndrome A
Elephantiasis due to mastectomy
Obliteration of lymphatic vessel due to mastectomy

DEF: Localized edema in the upper arm following breast and lymph node removal due to lack of lymph circulation through the chest area.

AHA: 2Q 2002, 12

457.1 Other lymphedema
Elephantiasis (nonfilarial) NOS
Lymphangiectasis
Lymphedema:
- acquired (chronic)
- praecox
- secondary

Obliteration, lymphatic vessel
Excludes *elephantiasis (nonfilarial):*
congenital (757.0)
eyelid (374.83)
vulva (624.8)

AHA: 3Q 2004, 5

457.2 Lymphangitis
Lymphangitis:
- NOS
- chronic
- subacute

Excludes *acute lymphangitis (682.0-682.9)*

457.8 Other noninfectious disorders of lymphatic channels
Chylocele (nonfilarial)
Chylous:
- ascites
- cyst

Lymph node or vessel:
- fistula
- infarction
- rupture

Excludes *chylocele:*
filarial (125.0-125.9)
tunica vaginalis (nonfilarial) (608.84)

AHA: 1Q 2004, 5; 3Q 2003, 17

✖ **457.9 Unspecified noninfectious disorder of lymphatic channels**

❹ **458 Hypotension**

Includes hypopiesis

Excludes *cardiovascular collapse (785.50)*
maternal hypotension syndrome (669.2)
shock (785.50-785.59)
Shy-Drager syndrome (333.0)

458.0 Orthostatic hypotension

Hypotension:
orthostatic (chronic)
postural

DEF: Abnormally low blood pressure that occurs when the patient moves to a standing or upright position.

AHA: 3Q 2000, 8; 3Q 1991, 9

458.1 Chronic hypotension

Permanent idiopathic hypotension

❺ **458.2 Iatrogenic hypotension**

AHA: 4Q 2003, 60; 3Q 2002, 12; 4Q 1995, 57

458.21 Hypotension of hemodialysis

Intra-dialytic hypotension

AHA: 4Q 2003, 61

458.29 Other iatrogenic hypotension

Postoperative hypotension

458.8 Other specified hypotension

AHA: 4Q 1997, 37

458.9 Hypotension, unspecified

Hypotension (arterial) NOS

❹ **459 Other disorders of circulatory system**

459.0 Hemorrhage, unspecified

Rupture of blood vessel NOS
Spontaneous hemorrhage NEC

Excludes *hemorrhage:*
gastrointestinal NOS (578.9)
in newborn NOS (772.9)
secondary or recurrent following trauma (958.2)
traumatic rupture of blood vessel (900.0-904.9)

C&C Exclusions: 459.0, 459.89, 459.9

AHA: 4Q 1990, 26

❺ **459.1 Postphlebitic syndrome**

Chronic venous hypertension due to deep vein thrombosis

Excludes *chronic venous hypertension without deep vein thrombosis (459.30-459.39)*

AHA: 4Q 2002, 58; 2Q 1991, 20

459.10 Postphlebitic syndrome without complications

Asymptomatic postphlebitic syndrome
Postphlebitic syndrome NOS

459.11 Postphlebitic syndrome with ulcer

459.12 Postphlebitic syndrome with inflammation

459.13 Postphlebitic syndrome with ulcer and inflammation

459.19 Postphlebitic syndrome with other complication

459.2 Compression of vein

Stricture of vein
Vena cava syndrome (inferior) (superior)

❺ **459.3 Chronic venous hypertension (idiopathic)**

Stasis edema

Excludes *chronic venous hypertension due to deep vein thrombosis (459.10-459.19)*
varicose veins (454.0-454.9)

AHA: 4Q 2002, 59

459.30 Chronic venous hypertension without complications

Asymptomatic chronic venous hypertension
Chronic venous hypertension NOS

459.31 Chronic venous hypertension with ulcer

AHA: 4Q 2002, 43

459.32 Chronic venous hypertension with inflammation

459.33 Chronic venous hypertension with ulcer and inflammation

459.39 Chronic venous hypertension with other complication

❺ **459.8 Other specified disorders of circulatory system**

AHA: 3Q 2004, 5; 2Q 1991, 20; Mar-Apr 1987, 6

459.81 Venous (peripheral) insufficiency, unspecified

Chronic venous insufficiency NOS
Use additional code for any associated ulceration (707.10-707.9)

459.89 Other

Collateral circulation (venous), any site
Phlebosclerosis
Venofibrosis

C&C Exclusions: 428.20, 428.21, 428.22, 428.23, 428.30, 428.31, 428.32, 428.33, 428.40, 428.41, 428.42, 428.43, 428.9, 445.01, 445.02, 445.81, 445.89

✖ **459.9 Unspecified circulatory system disorder**

C&C Exclusions: See 459.89

8. DISEASES OF THE RESPIRATORY SYSTEM (460-519)

Use additional code to identify infectious organism

ACUTE RESPIRATORY INFECTIONS (460-466)

Excludes *pneumonia and influenza (480.0-▶488◀)*

460 Acute nasopharyngitis [common cold]
Coryza (acute)
Nasal catarrh, acute
Nasopharyngitis:
  NOS
  acute
  infective NOS
Rhinitis:
  acute
  infective
Excludes *nasopharyngitis, chronic (472.2)*
pharyngitis:
  acute or unspecified (462)
  chronic (472.1)
rhinitis:
  allergic (477.0-477.9)
  chronic or unspecified (472.0)
sore throat:
  acute or unspecified (462)
  chronic (472.1)
AHA: 1Q 1988, 12

❹ **461 Acute sinusitis**
Includes abscess, acute, of sinus (accessory) (nasal)
empyema, acute, of sinus (accessory) (nasal)
infection, acute, of sinus (accessory) (nasal)
inflammation, acute, of sinus (accessory) (nasal)
suppuration, acute, of sinus (accessory) (nasal)
Excludes *chronic or unspecified sinusitis (473.0-473.9)*

An infection of a maxillary sinus

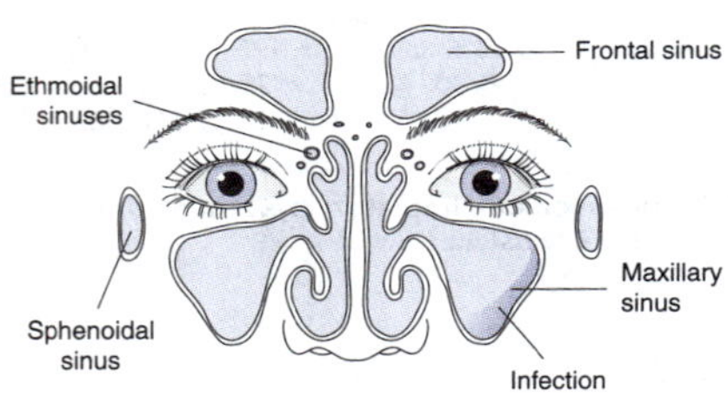

461.0 Maxillary
Acute antritis

461.1 Frontal

461.2 Ethmoidal

461.3 Sphenoidal

461.8 Other acute sinusitis
Acute pansinusitis

✖ **461.9 Acute sinusitis, unspecified**
Acute sinusitis NOS

462 Acute pharyngitis
Acute sore throat NOS
Pharyngitis (acute):
  NOS
  gangrenous
  infective
  phlegmonous
  pneumococcal
  staphylococcal
  suppurative
  ulcerative
Sore throat (viral) NOS
Viral pharyngitis
Excludes *abscess:*
  peritonsillar [quinsy] (475)
  pharyngeal NOS (478.29)
  retropharyngeal (478.24)
chronic pharyngitis (472.1)
infectious mononucleosis (075)
that specified as (due to):
  Coxsackie (virus) (074.0)
  gonococcus (098.6)
  herpes simplex (054.79)
  influenza (487.1)
  septic (034.0)
  streptococcal (034.0)
AHA: 4Q 1999, 26; Sep-Oct 1985, 8

463 Acute tonsillitis
Tonsillitis (acute):
  NOS
  follicular
  gangrenous
  infective
  pneumococcal
  septic
  staphylococcal
  suppurative
  ulcerative
  viral
Excludes *chronic tonsillitis (474.0)*
hypertrophy of tonsils (474.1)
peritonsillar abscess [quinsy] (475)
sore throat:
  acute or NOS (462)
  septic (034.0)
streptococcal tonsillitis (034.0)
AHA: Nov-Dec 1984, 16

❹ **464 Acute laryngitis and tracheitis**
Excludes *that associated with influenza (487.1)*
that due to Streptococcus (034.0)

❺ **464.0 Acute laryngitis**
Laryngitis (acute):
  NOS
  edematous
  Hemophilus influenzae [H. influenzae]
  pneumococcal
  septic
  suppurative
  ulcerative
Excludes *chronic laryngitis (476.0-476.1)*
influenzal laryngitis (487.1)
AHA: 4Q 2001, 42

464.00 Without mention of obstruction

464.01 With obstruction

❺ **464.1 Acute tracheitis**
Tracheitis (acute):
  NOS
  catarrhal
  viral
Excludes *chronic tracheitis (491.8)*

464.10 Without mention of obstruction

464.11 With obstruction
C&C Exclusions: 012.20, 012.21, 012.22, 012.23, 012.24, 012.25, 012.26, 012.30, 012.31, 012.32, 012.33, 012.34, 012.35, 012.36, 012.80, 012.81, 012.82, 012.83, 012.84, 012.85, 012.86, 017.90, 017.91, 017.92, 017.93, 017.94, 017.95, 017.96, 464.10, 464.11, 464.20, 464.21, 464.30, 464.31, 519.8, 519.9

464.2 Acute laryngotracheitis
Laryngotracheitis (acute)
Tracheitis (acute) with laryngitis (acute)
Excludes *chronic laryngotracheitis (476.1)*

464.20 Without mention of obstruction

464.21 With obstruction
C&C Exclusions: See 464.11

464.3 Acute epiglottitis
Viral epiglottitis
Excludes *epiglottitis, chronic (476.1)*

464.30 Without mention of obstruction

464.31 With obstruction
C&C Exclusions: See 464.11

464.4 Croup
Croup syndrome

464.5 Supraglottitis, unspecified
AHA: 4Q 2001, 42

464.50 Without mention of obstruction
AHA: 4Q 2001, 43

464.51 With obstruction

465 Acute upper respiratory infections of multiple or unspecified sites
Excludes *upper respiratory infection due to:*
influenza (487.1)
Streptococcus (034.0)

465.0 Acute laryngopharyngitis

465.8 Other multiple sites
Multiple URI

465.9 Unspecified site
Acute URI NOS
Upper respiratory infection (acute)

466 Acute bronchitis and bronchiolitis
Includes that with:
bronchospasm
obstruction

466.0 Acute bronchitis
Bronchitis, acute or subacute:
fibrinous
membranous
pneumococcal
purulent
septic
viral
with tracheitis
Croupous bronchitis
Tracheobronchitis, acute
Excludes *acute bronchitis with chronic obstructive pulmonary disease (491.22)*
AHA: 4Q 2004, 137; 1Q 2004, 3; 4Q 2002, 46; 4Q 1996, 28; 4Q 1991, 24; 1Q 1988, 12

466.1 Acute bronchiolitis
Bronchiolitis (acute)
Capillary pneumonia

466.11 Acute bronchiolitis due to respiratory syncytial virus (RSV)
AHA: 1Q 2005, 10; 4Q 1996, 27

466.19 Acute bronchiolitis due to other infectious organisms
Use additional code to identify organism

OTHER DISEASES OF THE UPPER RESPIRATORY TRACT (470-478)

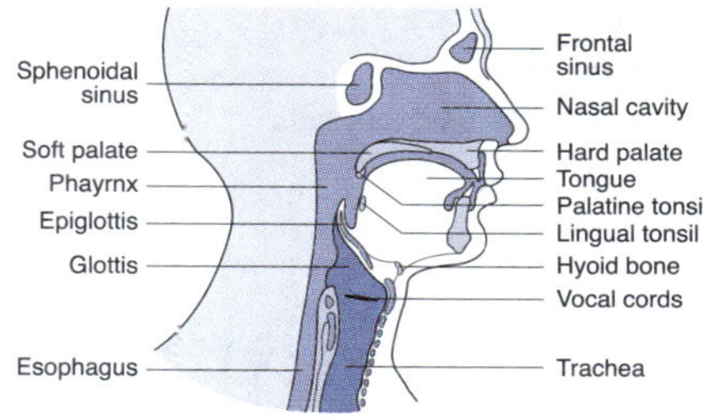

470 Deviated nasal septum
Deflected septum (nasal) (acquired)
Excludes *congenital (754.0)*
DEF: Cartilage separating the nostrils is shifted out of position, usually due to trauma.

471 Nasal polyps
Excludes *adenomatous polyps (212.0)*

471.0 Polyp of nasal cavity
Polyp:
choanal
nasopharyngeal

471.1 Polypoid sinus degeneration
Woakes' syndrome or ethmoiditis

471.8 Other polyp of sinus
Polyp of sinus:
accessory
ethmoidal
maxillary
sphenoidal

471.9 Unspecified nasal polyp
Nasal polyp NOS

472 Chronic pharyngitis and nasopharyngitis

472.0 Chronic rhinitis
Ozena
Rhinitis:
NOS
atrophic
granulomatous
hypertrophic
obstructive
purulent
ulcerative
Excludes *allergic rhinitis (477.0-477.9)*

472.1 Chronic pharyngitis
Chronic sore throat
Pharyngitis:
atrophic
granular (chronic)
hypertrophic

472.2 Chronic nasopharyngitis
Excludes *acute or unspecified nasopharyngitis (460)*

473 Chronic sinusitis
Includes abscess (chronic) of sinus (accessory) (nasal)
empyema (chronic) of sinus (accessory) (nasal)
infection (chronic) of sinus (accessory) (nasal)
suppuration (chronic) of sinus (accessory) (nasal)
Excludes *acute sinusitis (461.0-461.9)*

473.0 Maxillary
Antritis (chronic)

473.1 Frontal

473.2 Ethmoidal
Excludes *Woakes' ethmoiditis (471.1)*

473.3 Sphenoidal

473.8 Other chronic sinusitis
Pansinusitis (chronic)

473.9 Unspecified sinusitis (chronic)
Sinusitis (chronic) NOS

④ **474 Chronic disease of tonsils and adenoids**

⑤ **474.0 Chronic tonsillitis and adenoiditis**
Excludes *acute or unspecified tonsillitis (463)*
AHA: 4Q 1997, 38

474.00 Chronic tonsillitis

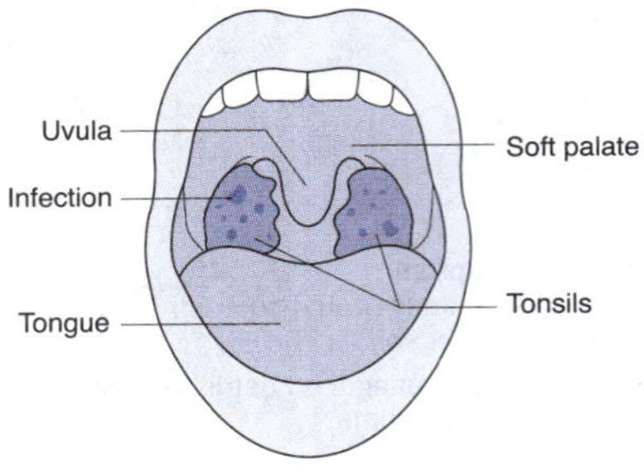

474.01 Chronic adenoiditis

474.02 Chronic tonsillitis and adenoiditis

⑤ **474.1 Hypertrophy of tonsils and adenoids**
Enlargement of tonsils or adenoids
Hyperplasia of tonsils or adenoids
Hypertrophy of tonsils or adenoids
Excludes *that with:*
adenoiditis (474.01)
adenoiditis and tonsillitis (474.02)
tonsillitis (474.00)

474.10 Tonsils with adenoids
AHA: 2Q 2005, 16

474.11 Tonsils alone

474.12 Adenoids alone

474.2 Adenoid vegetations
DEF: Fungal growths around the adenoids at the top of the throat.

474.8 Other chronic disease of tonsils and adenoids
Amygdalolith
Calculus, tonsil
Cicatrix of tonsil (and adenoid)
Tonsillar tag
Ulcer, tonsil

✖ **474.9 Unspecified chronic disease of tonsils and adenoids**
Disease (chronic) of tonsils (and adenoids)

475 Peritonsillar abscess
Abscess of tonsil
Peritonsillar cellulitis
Quinsy
Excludes *tonsillitis:*
acute or NOS (463)
chronic (474.0)

④ **476 Chronic laryngitis and laryngotracheitis**

476.0 Chronic laryngitis
Laryngitis:
catarrhal
hypertrophic
sicca

476.1 Chronic laryngotracheitis
Laryngitis, chronic, with tracheitis (chronic)
Tracheitis, chronic, with laryngitis
Excludes *chronic tracheitis (491.8)*
laryngitis and tracheitis, acute or unspecified (464.00-464.51)
DEF: Long-term inflammation extending past the vocal cords and into the trachea.

④ **477 Allergic rhinitis**
Includes allergic rhinitis (nonseasonal) (seasonal)
hay fever
spasmodic rhinorrhea
Excludes *allergic rhinitis with asthma (bronchial) (493.0)*

477.0 Due to pollen
Pollinosis

477.1 Due to food
AHA: 4Q 2000, 42

477.2 Due to animal (cat) (dog) hair and dander

477.8 Due to other allergen

477.9 Cause unspecified
AHA: 2Q 1997, 9

④ **478 Other diseases of upper respiratory tract**

478.0 Hypertrophy of nasal turbinates

⑤ **478.1 Other diseases of nasal cavity and sinuses**
Excludes *varicose ulcer of nasal septum (456.8)*

478.11 Nasal mucositis (ulcerative)
Use additional E code to identify adverse effects of therapy, such as:
antineoplastic and immunosuppressive drugs (E930.7, E933.1)
radiation therapy (E879.2)

478.19 Other diseases of nasal cavity and sinuses
Abscess of nose (septum)
Cyst or mucocele of sinus (nasal)
Necrosis of nose (septum)
Rhinolith
Ulcer of nose (septum)

⑤ **478.2 Other diseases of pharynx, not elsewhere classified**

478.20 Unspecified disease of pharynx

478.21 Cellulitis of pharynx or nasopharynx
C&C Exclusions: 478.20, 478.21, 478.22, 478.23, 478.24, 519.8, 519.9

478.22 Parapharyngeal abscess
DEF: Pus-filled sore at the back of the throat.
C&C Exclusions: See 478.21

478.24 Retropharyngeal abscess
C&C Exclusions: See 478.21

478.25 Edema of pharynx or nasopharynx

478.26 Cyst of pharynx or nasopharynx

478.29 Other
Abscess of pharynx or nasopharynx
Excludes *ulcerative pharyngitis (462)*

⑤ **478.3 Paralysis of vocal cords or larynx**

478.30 Paralysis, unspecified
Laryngoplegia
Paralysis of glottis
C&C Exclusions: 478.30, 478.31, 478.32, 478.33, 478.34, 478.5, 478.70, 519.8, 519.9

478.31 Unilateral, partial
C&C Exclusions: See 478.30

478.32 Unilateral, complete
C&C Exclusions: See 478.30

478.33 Bilateral, partial
C&C Exclusions: See 478.30

478.34 Bilateral, complete
C&C Exclusions: See 478.30

478.4 Polyp of vocal cord or larynx
Excludes *adenomatous polyps (212.1)*

478.5 Other diseases of vocal cords
Abscess of vocal cords
Cellulitis of vocal cords
Chorditis (fibrinous) (nodosa) (tuberosa)
Granuloma of vocal cords
Leukoplakia of vocal cords
Singers' nodes

478.6 Edema of larynx
Edema (of):
glottis
subglottic
supraglottic

⑤ **478.7 Other diseases of larynx, not elsewhere classified**

478.70 Unspecified disease of larynx

478.71 Cellulitis and perichondritis of larynx

478.74 Stenosis of larynx

Abnormal narrowing or constriction of larynx

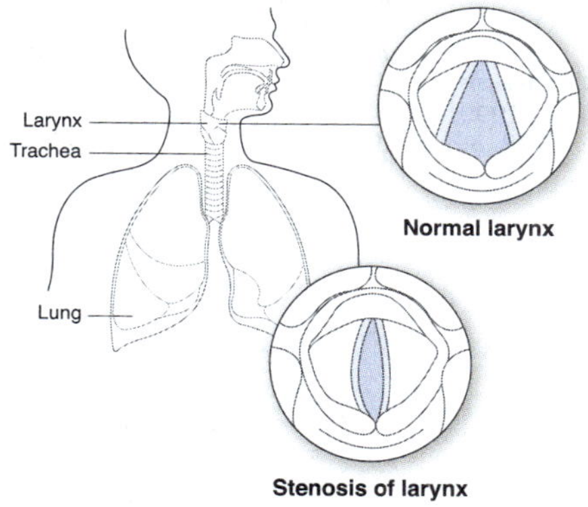

478.75 Laryngeal spasm
Laryngismus (stridulus)

478.79 Other
Abscess of larynx
Necrosis of larynx
Obstruction of larynx
Pachyderma of larynx
Ulcer of larynx
Excludes *ulcerative laryngitis (464.00-464.01)*

AHA: 3Q 1991, 20

478.8 Upper respiratory tract hypersensitivity reaction, site unspecified
Excludes *hypersensitivity reaction of lower respiratory tract, as:*
extrinsic allergic alveolitis (495.0-495.9)
pneumoconiosis (500-505)

478.9 Other and unspecified diseases of upper respiratory tract
Abscess of trachea
Cicatrix of trachea

PNEUMONIA AND INFLUENZA (480-►488◄)

Excludes *pneumonia:*
allergic or eosinophilic (518.3)
aspiration:
NOS (507.0)
newborn (770.18)
solids and liquids (507.0-507.8)
congenital (770.0)
lipoid (507.1)
passive (514)
rheumatic (390)

❹ **480 Viral pneumonia**

480.0 Pneumonia due to adenovirus
C&C Exclusions: 079.82, 480.3

480.1 Pneumonia due to respiratory syncytial virus
C&C Exclusions: See 480.0
AHA: 4Q 1996, 28; 1Q 1988, 12

480.2 Pneumonia due to parainfluenza virus
C&C Exclusions: See 480.0

480.3 Pneumonia due to SARS-associated coronavirus
C&C Exclusions: See 480.0
AHA: 4Q 2003, 46-47

480.8 Pneumonia due to other virus not elsewhere classified
Excludes *congenital rubella pneumonitis (771.0)*
influenza with pneumonia, any form (487.0)
pneumonia complicating viral diseases classified elsewhere (484.1-484.8)
C&C Exclusions: See 480.0

480.9 Viral pneumonia, unspecified
C&C Exclusions: See 480.0
AHA: 3Q 1998, 5

481 Pneumococcal pneumonia [Streptococcus pneumoniae pneumonia]
Lobar pneumonia, organism unspecified
C&C Exclusions: 011.00, 011.01, 011.02, 011.03, 011.04, 011.05, 011.06, 011.10, 011.11, 011.12, 011.13, 011.14, 011.15, 011.16, 011.20, 011.21, 011.22, 011.23, 011.24, 011.25, 011.26, 011.30, 011.31, 011.32, 011.33, 011.34, 011.35, 011.36, 011.40, 011.41, 011.42, 011.43, 011.44, 011.45, 011.46, 011.50, 011.51, 011.52, 011.53, 011.54, 011.55, 011.56, 011.60, 011.61, 011.62, 011.63, 011.64, 011.65, 011.66, 011.70, 011.71, 011.72, 011.73, 011.74, 011.75, 011.76, 011.80, 011.81, 011.82, 011.83, 011.84, 011.85, 011.86, 011.90, 011.91, 011.92, 011.93, 011.94, 011.95, 011.96, 012.00, 012.01, 012.02, 012.03, 012.04, 012.05, 012.06, 012.10, 012.11, 012.12, 012.13, 012.14, 012.15, 012.16, 012.80, 012.81, 012.82, 012.83, 012.84, 012.85, 012.86, 017.90, 017.91, 017.92, 017.93, 017.94, 017.95, 017.96, 021.2, 031.0, 039.1, 079.82, 115.05, 115.15, 115.95, 122.1, 130.4, 136.3, 480.0, 480.1, 480.2, 480.3, 480.8, 480.9, 481, 482.0, 482.1, 482.2, 482.30, 482.31, 482.32, 482.39, 482.40, 482.41, 482.49, 482.81, 482.82, 482.83, 482.84, 482.89, 482.9, 483.0, 483.1, 483.8, 484.1, 484.3, 484.5, 484.6, 484.7 484.8, 485, 486, 487.0, 487.1, 494.0, 494.1, 495.0, 495.1, 495.2, 495.3, 495.4, 495.5, 495.6, 495.7, 495.8, 495.9, 496, 500, 501, 502, 503, 504, 505, 506.0, 506.1, 506.2, 506.3, 506.4, 506.9, 507.0, 507.1, 507.8, 508.0, 508.1, 508.8, 508.9, 517.1, 517.2, 517.8, 518.89, 519.8, 519.9, 748.61
AHA: 2Q 1998, 7; 4Q 1992, 19; 1Q 1992, 18; 1Q 1991, 13; 1Q 1988, 13; Mar-Apr 1985, 6

❹ **482 Other bacterial pneumonia**

482.0 Pneumonia due to Klebsiella pneumoniae
C&C Exclusions: See 481

482.1 Pneumonia due to Pseudomonas
C&C Exclusions: See 481

482.2 Pneumonia due to Hemophilus influenzae [H. influenzae]
C&C Exclusions: See 481
AHA: 2Q 2005, 19

❺ **482.3 Pneumonia due to Streptococcus**
Excludes *Streptococcus pneumoniae pneumonia (481)*
AHA: 1Q 1988, 13

482.30 Streptococcus, unspecified
C&C Exclusions: See 481

482.31 Group A
C&C Exclusions: See 481

482.32 Group B
C&C Exclusions: See 481

482.39 Other Streptococcus
C&C Exclusions: See 481

❺ **482.4 Pneumonia due to Staphylococcus**
AHA: 3Q 1991, 16

482.40 Pneumonia due to Staphylococcus, unspecified
C&C Exclusions: See 481

482.41 Pneumonia due to Staphylococcus aureus
C&C Exclusions: See 481

482.49 Other Staphylococcus pneumonia
C&C Exclusions: See 481

❺ **482.8 Pneumonia due to other specified bacteria**
Excludes *pneumonia complicating infectious disease classified elsewhere (484.1-484.8)*
AHA: 3Q 1988, 11

482.81 Anaerobes
Bacteroides (melaninogenicus)
Gram-negative anaerobes
C&C Exclusions: See 481

482.82 Escherichia coli [E. coli]
C&C Exclusions: See 481

482.83 Other gram-negative bacteria
Gram-negative pneumonia NOS
Proteus
Serratia marcescens
Excludes *gram-negative anaerobes (482.81)*
Legionnaires' disease (482.84)
AHA: 2Q 1998, 5; 3Q 1994, 9
C&C Exclusions: See 481

482.84 Legionnaires' disease
C&C Exclusions: See 481
AHA: 4Q 1997, 38

482.89 Other specified bacteria
C&C Exclusions: See 481
AHA: 2Q 1997, 6

482.9 Bacterial pneumonia unspecified
C&C Exclusions: See 481
AHA: 2Q 1998, 6; 2Q 1997, 6; 1Q 1994, 17

❹ **483 Pneumonia due to other specified organism**
AHA: Nov-Dec 1987, 5

483.0 Mycoplasma pneumoniae
Eaton's agent
Pleuropneumonia-like organisms [PPLO]
C&C Exclusions: See 481

483.1 Chlamydia
C&C Exclusions: See 481
AHA: 4Q 1996, 31

483.8 Other specified organism
C&C Exclusions: See 481

❹ **484 Pneumonia in infectious diseases classified elsewhere**
Excludes *influenza with pneumonia, any form (487.0)*

+ ***484.1 Pneumonia in cytomegalic inclusion disease***
Code first underlying disease, as: (078.5)
C&C Exclusions: See 481

+ ***484.3 Pneumonia in whooping cough***
Code first underlying disease, as: (033.0-033.9)
C&C Exclusions: See 481

+ ***484.5 Pneumonia in anthrax***
Code first underlying disease (022.1)
C&C Exclusions: See 481

+ ***484.6 Pneumonia in aspergillosis***
Code first underlying disease (117.3)
C&C Exclusions: See 481
AHA: 4Q 1997, 40

+ ***484.7 Pneumonia in other systemic mycoses***
Code first underlying disease
Excludes *pneumonia in:*
candidiasis (112.4)
coccidioidomycosis (114.0)
histoplasmosis (115.0-115.9 with fifth-digit 5)
C&C Exclusions: See 481

+ ***484.8 Pneumonia in other infectious diseases classified elsewhere***
Code first underlying disease, as:
Q fever (083.0)
typhoid fever (002.0)
Excludes *pneumonia in:*
actinomycosis (039.1)
measles (055.1)
nocardiosis (039.1)
ornithosis (073.0)
Pneumocystis carinii (136.3)
salmonellosis (003.22)
toxoplasmosis (130.4)
tuberculosis (011.6)
tularemia (021.2)
varicella (052.1)
C&C Exclusions: See 481

485 Bronchopneumonia, organism unspecified
Bronchopneumonia:
hemorrhagic
terminal
Pleurobronchopneumonia
Pneumonia:
lobular
segmental
Excludes *bronchiolitis (acute) (466.11- 466.19)*
chronic (491.8)
lipoid pneumonia (507.1)
C&C Exclusions: See 481

486 Pneumonia, organism unspecified
Excludes *hypostatic or passive pneumonia (514)*
influenza with pneumonia, any form (487.0)
inhalation or aspiration pneumonia due to foreign materials (507.0-507.8)
pneumonitis due to fumes and vapors (506.0)
C&C Exclusions: See 481
AHA: 4Q 1999, 6; 3Q 1999, 9; 3Q 1998, 7; 2Q 1998, 4-5; 1Q 1998, 8; 3Q 1997, 9; 3Q 1994, 10; 3Q 1988, 11

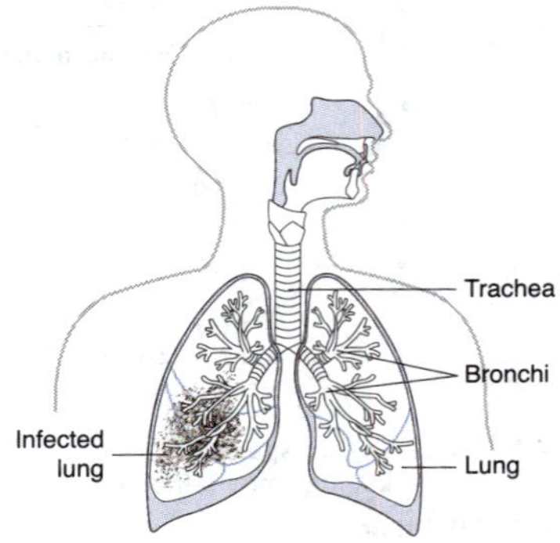

❹ **487 Influenza**
Excludes *Hemophilus influenzae [H. influenzae]:*
infection NOS (041.5)
laryngitis (464.00-464.01)
meningitis (320.0)
▶*influenza due to identified avian influenza virus (488)*◀

487.0 With pneumonia
Influenza with pneumonia, any form
Influenzal:
bronchopneumonia
pneumonia
Use additional code to identify the type of pneumonia (480.0-480.9, 481, 482.0-482.9, 483.0-483.8, 485)
C&C Exclusions: See 481
AHA: 1Q 2006, 18

487.1 With other respiratory manifestations
Influenza NOS
Influenzal:
laryngitis
pharyngitis
respiratory infection (upper) (acute)
C&C Exclusions: 079.82, 480.3, 494.1
AHA: 1Q 2006, 18; 2Q 2005, 18; 4Q 1999, 26

487.8 With other manifestations
Encephalopathy due to influenza
Influenza with involvement of gastrointestinal tract
Excludes *"intestinal flu" [viral gastroenteritis] (008.8)*

● **488 Influenza due to identified avian influenza virus**
Note: *Influenza caused by influenza viruses that normally infect only birds and, less commonly, other animals*
Excludes *influenza caused by other influenza viruses (487)*

CHRONIC OBSTRUCTIVE PULMONARY DISEASE AND ALLIED CONDITIONS (490-496)

AHA: 3Q 1988, 5

490 Bronchitis, not specified as acute or chronic
Bronchitis NOS:
catarrhal
with tracheitis NOS
Tracheobronchitis NOS
Excludes *bronchitis:*
allergic NOS (493.9)
asthmatic NOS (493.9)
due to fumes and vapors (506.0)

Bronchitis

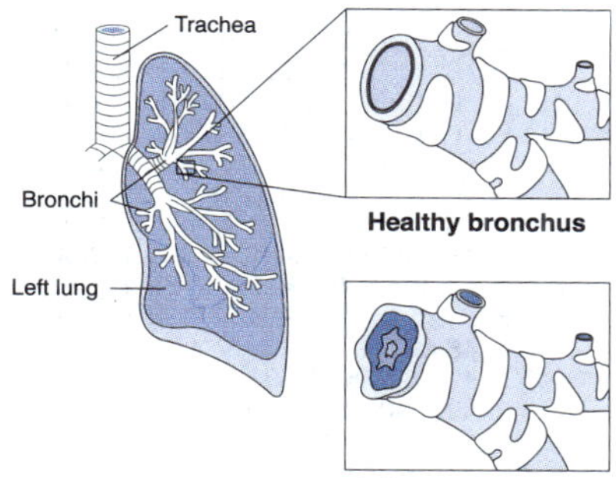

491 Chronic bronchitis
Excludes *chronic obstructive asthma (493.2)*

491.0 Simple chronic bronchitis
Catarrhal bronchitis, chronic
Smokers' cough

491.1 Mucopurulent chronic bronchitis
Bronchitis (chronic) (recurrent):
fetid
mucopurulent
purulent
C&C Exclusions: 491.1, 491.20, 491.21, 491.8, 491.9
AHA: 3Q 1988, 12

491.2 Obstructive chronic bronchitis
Bronchitis:
emphysematous
obstructive (chronic) (diffuse)
Bronchitis with:
chronic airway obstruction
emphysema
Excludes *asthmatic bronchitis (acute) (NOS) 493.9*
chronic obstructive asthma 493.2
AHA: 3Q 1997, 9; 4Q 1991, 25; 2Q 1991, 21

491.20 Without exacerbation
Emphysema with chronic bronchitis
C&C Exclusions: See 491.1
AHA: 3Q 1997, 9

491.21 With (acute) exacerbation
Acute exacerbation of chronic obstructive pulmonary disease [COPD]
Decompensated chronic obstructive pulmonary disease [COPD]
Decompensated chronic obstructive pulmonary disease [COPD] with exacerbation
Exludes: *chronic obstructive asthma with acute exacerbation 493.22*
C&C Exclusions: See 491.1
AHA: 1Q 2004, 3; 3Q 2002, 18-19; 4Q 2001, 43; 2Q 1996, 10

491.22 With acute bronchitis
C&C Exclusions: See 491.1
AHA: 3Q 2006, 20; 4Q 2004, 82

491.8 Other chronic bronchitis
Chronic:
tracheitis
tracheobronchitis
C&C Exclusions: See 491.1

491.9 Unspecified chronic bronchitis
C&C Exclusions: See 491.1

492 Emphysema
DEF: Abnormal enlargement of the air sacs in the lungs, which lose their elasticity, making breathing increasingly difficult.
AHA: 2Q 1991, 21

492.0 Emphysematous bleb
Giant bullous emphysema
Ruptured emphysematous bleb
Tension pneumatocele
Vanishing lung
AHA: 2Q 1993, 3

492.8 Other emphysema
Emphysema (lung or pulmonary):
NOS
centriacinar
centrilobular
obstructive
panacinar
panlobular
unilateral
vesicular
MacLeod's syndrome
Swyer-James syndrome
Unilateral hyperlucent lung
Excludes *emphysema:*
with chronic bronchitis (491.20-491.22)
compensatory (518.2)
due to fumes and vapors (506.4)
interstitial (518.1)
newborn (770.2)
mediastinal (518.1)
surgical (subcutaneous) (998.81)
traumatic (958.7)
C&C Exclusions: 492.0, 492.8, 493.20, 493.21
AHA: 1Q 2005, 4; 4Q 1993, 41; Jul-Aug 1984, 17

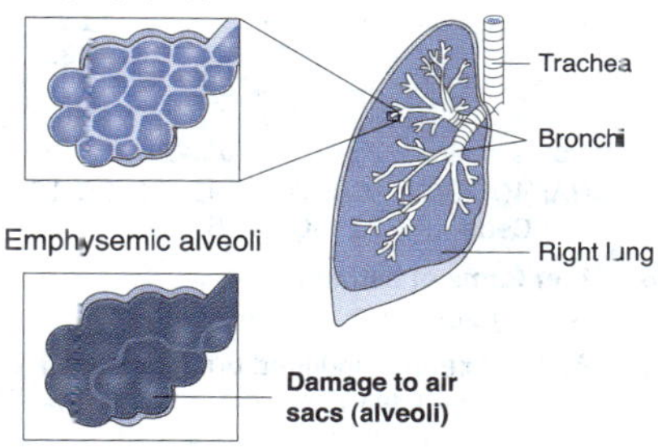

Respiratory System

❹ **493 Asthma**

Excludes *wheezing NOS (786.07)*

DEF: Condition in which the bronchial tubes spasm and constrict acutely in response to a specific trigger like an allergen, exercise, or emotional stress.

AHA: 4Q 2004, 137; 4Q 2003, 62; 4Q 2001, 43; 4Q 2000, 42; 1Q 1991, 13; 3Q 1988, 9; Jul-Aug 1985, 8; Nov-Dec 1984, 17

The following fifth-digit subclassification is for use with codes 493.0-493.2, 493.9:

- **0 unspecified**
- **1 with status asthmaticus**
- **2 with (acute) exacerbation**

❺ **493.0 Extrinsic asthma**

Asthma:
- allergic with stated cause
- atopic
- childhood
- hay
- platinum

Hay fever with asthma

Excludes *asthma:*
- *allergic NOS (493.9)*
- *detergent (507.8)*
- *miners' (500)*
- *wood (495.8)*

DEF: Bronchial spasming attacks brought on by factors outside the body, such as pollution, allergens, or cigarette smoke.

C&C Exclusions: (for codes 493.01-493.02) 493.00, 493.01, 493.02, 493.10, 493.11, 493.12, 493.20, 493.21, 493.22, 493.90, 493.91, 493.92, 517.8, 518.89, 519.8, 519.9

❺ **493.1 Intrinsic asthma**

Late-onset asthma

C&C Exclusions: See 493.0

AHA: 3Q 1988, 9; Mar-Apr 1985, 7

❺ **493.2 Chronic obstructive asthma**

Asthma with chronic obstructive pulmonary disease (COPD)

Chronic asthmatic bronchitis

Excludes *acute bronchitis (466.0)*
chronic obstructive bronchitis (491.20-491.22)

C&C Exclusions: (for codes 493.20-493.21) 491.1, 491.20, 491.21, 491.8, 491.9, 492.0, 492.8, 493.00, 493.01, 493.02, 493.10, 493.11, 493.12, 493.20, 493.21, 493.22, 493.90, 493.91, 493.92, 517.8, 518.89, 519.8, 519.9

C&C Exclusions: (for code 493.22) See 493.0

AHA: 4Q 2003, 108; 2Q 1991, 21; 2Q 1990, 20; For Code 493.22: 3Q 2006, 20

❺ **493.8 Other forms of asthma**

AHA: 4Q 2003, 62

493.81 Exercise induced bronchospasm

C&C Exclusions: 493.01, 493.02, 493.11, 493.12, 493.20, 493.21, 493.22, 493.90, 493.91, 493.92

493.82 Cough variant asthma

C&C Exclusions: See 493.81

❺ **493.9 Asthma, unspecified**

Asthma (bronchial) (allergic NOS)

Bronchitis:
- allergic
- asthmatic

C&C Exclusions: (for code 493.90-493.92) See 493.0

AHA: 4Q 1997, 40; For Code 493.90: 4Q 2004, 137; 4Q 2003, 108; 4Q 1999, 25; 1Q 1997, 7; For code 493.91: 1Q 2005, 5; For Code 493.92: 1Q 2003, 9

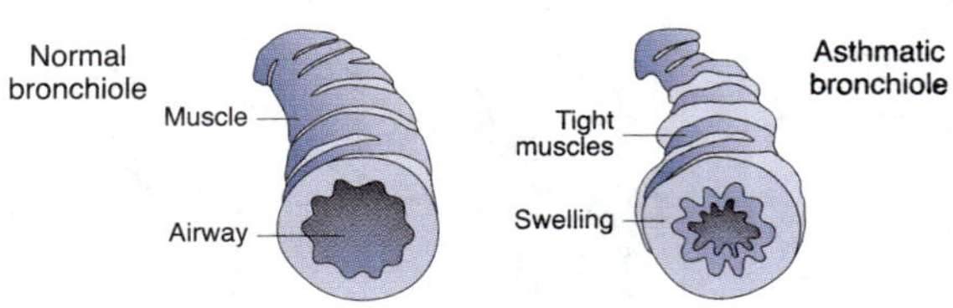

❹ **494 Bronchiectasis**

Bronchiectasis (fusiform) (postinfectious) (recurrent)

Bronchiolectasis

Excludes *congenital (748.61)*
tuberculous bronchiectasis (current disease) (011.5)

DEF: Destruction and widening of the large airways, often due to recurrent, severe infection or inflammation, or following foreign body obstruction.

AHA: 4Q 2000, 42

494.0 Bronchiectasis without acute exacerbation

C&C Exclusions: 011.00, 011.01, 011.02, 011.03, 011.04, 011.05, 011.06, 011.10, 011.11, 011.12, 011.13, 011.14, 011.15, 011.16, 011.20, 011.21, 011.22, 011.23, 011.24, 011.25, 011.26, 011.30, 011.31, 011.32, 011.33, 011.34, 011.35, 011.36, 011.40, 011.41, 011.42, 011.43, 011.44, 011.45, 011.46, 011.50, 011.51, 011.52, 011.53, 011.54, 011.55, 011.56, 011.60, 011.61, 011.62, 011.63, 011.64, 011.65, 011.66, 011.70, 011.71, 011.72, 011.73, 011.74, 011.75, 011.76, 011.80, 011.81, 011.82, 011.83, 011.84, 011.85, 011.86, 011.90, 011.91, 011.92, 011.93, 011.94, 011.95, 011.96, 012.00, 012.01, 012.02, 012.03, 012.04, 012.05, 012.06, 012.10, 012.11, 012.12, 012.13, 012.14, 012.15, 012.16, 031.0, 079.82, 115.05, 115.15, 130.4, 136.3, 137.0, 139.8, 480.0, 480.1, 480.2, 480.3, 480.8, 480.9, 481, 482.0, 482.1, 482.2, 482.30, 482.31, 482.32, 482.39, 482.40, 482.41, 482.49, 482.81, 482.82, 482.83, 482.84, 482.89, 482.9, 483.0, 483.1, 483.8, 484.1, 484.3, 484.5, 484.6, 484.7, 484.8, 485, 486, 487.0, 495.0, 495.1, 495.2, 495.3, 495.4, 495.5, 495.6, 495.7, 495.8, 495.9, 496, 506.0, 506.1, 507.0, 507.1, 507.8, 508.0, 508.1, 515, 516.0, 516.1, 516.2, 516.3, 516.8, 516.9, 517.1, 517.2, 517.8, 748.61

494.1 Bronchiectasis with acute exacerbation

C&C Exclusions: 011.00, 011.01, 011.02, 011.03, 011.04, 011.05, 011.06, 011.10, 011.11, 011.12, 011.13, 011.14, 011.15, 011.16, 011.20, 011.21, 011.22, 011.23, 011.24, 011.25, 011.26, 011.30, 011.31, 011.32, 011.33, 011.34, 011.35, 011.36, 011.40, 011.41, 011.42, 011.43, 011.44, 011.45, 011.46, 011.50, 011.51, 011.52, 011.53, 011.54, 011.55, 011.56, 011.60, 011.61, 011.62, 011.63, 011.64, 011.65, 011.66, 011.70, 011.71, 011.72, 011.73, 011.74, 011.75, 011.76, 011.80, 011.81, 011.82, 011.83, 011.84, 011.85, 011.86, 011.90, 011.91, 011.92, 011.93, 011.94, 011.95, 011.96, 012.00, 012.01, 012.02, 012.03, 012.04, 012.05, 012.06, 012.10, 012.11, 012.12, 012.13, 012.14, 012.15, 012.16, 017.90, 017.91, 017.92, 017.93, 017.94, 017.95, 017.96, 031.0, 079.82, 115.05, 115.15, 130.4, 136.3, 480.3, 481, 482.0, 482.1, 482.2, 482.30, 482.31, 482.32, 482.39, 482.40, 482.41, 482.49, 482.81, 482.82, 482.83, 482.84, 482.89, 482.9, 483.0, 483.1, 483.8, 484.1, 484.3, 484.5, 484.6, 484.7, 484.8, 485, 486, 487.0, 487.1, 494.1, 495.0, 495.1, 495.2, 495.3, 495.4,495.5, 495.6, 495.7, 495.8, 495.9, 496, 506.0, 506.1, 506.4, 506.9, 507.0, 507.1, 507.8, 508.0, 508.1, 515, 516.0, 516.1, 516.2, 516.3, 516.8, 516.9, 517.1, 517.2, 517.8, 748.61

④ 495 Extrinsic allergic alveolitis

Includes allergic alveolitis and pneumonitis due to inhaled organic dust particles of fungal, thermophilic actinomycete, or other origin

DEF: Inflammation of the small, inner air sacs in the lungs, due to an allergic reaction triggered by inhaled organic substances or microorganisms.

495.0 Farmers' lung

C&C Exclusions: 011.00, 011.01, 011.02, 011.03, 011.04, 011.05, 011.06, 011.10, 011.11, 011.12, 011.13, 011.14, 011.15, 011.16, 011.20, 011.21, 011.22, 011.23, 011.24, 011.25, 011.26, 011.30, 011.31, 011.32, 011.33, 011.34, 011.35, 011.36, 011.40, 011.41, 011.42, 011.43, 011.44, 011.45, 011.46, 011.50, 011.51, 011.52, 011.53, 011.54, 011.55, 011.56, 011.60, 011.61, 011.62, 011.63, 011.64, 011.65, 011.66, 011.70, 011.71, 011.72, 011.73, 011.74, 011.75, 011.76, 011.80, 011.81, 011.82, 011.83, 011.84, 011.85, 011.86, 011.90, 011.91, 011.92, 011.93, 011.94, 011.95, 011.96, 012.00, 012.01, 012.02, 012.03, 012.04, 012.05, 012.06, 012.10, 012.11, 012.12, 012.13, 012.14, 012.15, 012.16, 012.80, 012.81, 012.82, 012.83, 012.84, 012.85, 012.86, 017.90, 017.91, 017.92, 017.93, 017.94, 017.95, 017.96, 021.2, 031.0, 039.1, 079.82, 115.05, 115.15, 115.95, 122.1, 130.4, 136.3, 480.0, 480.1, 480.2, 480.3, 480.8, 480.9, 481, 482.0, 482.1, 482.2, 482.30, 482.31, 482.32, 482.39, 482.40, 482.41, 482.49, 482.81, 482.82, 482.83, 482.84, 482.89, 482.9, 483.0, 483.1, 483.8, 484.1, 484.3, 484.5, 484.6, 484.7, 484.8, 485, 486, 487.0, 487.1, 494.0, 494.1, 495.0, 495.1, 495.2, 495.3, 495.4, 495.5, 495.6, 495.7, 495.8, 495.9, 496, 500, 501, 502, 503, 504, 505, 506.0, 506.1, 506.2, 506.3, 506.4, 506.9, 507.0, 507.1, 507.8, 508.0, 508.1, 508.8, 508.9, 517.1, 517.8, 518.89, 519.8, 519.9, 748.61

495.1 Bagassosis

C&C Exclusions: See 495.0

495.2 Bird-fanciers' lung

Budgerigar-fanciers' disease or lung
Pigeon-fanciers' disease or lung

C&C Exclusions: See 495.0

495.3 Suberosis

Cork-handlers' disease or lung

C&C Exclusions: See 495.0

495.4 Malt workers' lung

Alveolitis due to Aspergillus clavatus

C&C Exclusions: See 495.0

495.5 Mushroom workers' lung

C&C Exclusions: See 495.0

495.6 Maple bark-strippers' lung

Alveolitis due to Cryptostroma corticale

C&C Exclusions: See 495.0

495.7 "Ventilation" pneumonitis

Allergic alveolitis due to fungal, thermophilic actinomycete, and other organisms growing in ventilation [air conditioning] systems

C&C Exclusions: See 495.0

495.8 Other specified allergic alveolitis and pneumonitis

Cheese-washers' lung
Coffee workers' lung
Fish-meal workers' lung
Furriers' lung
Grain-handlers' disease or lung
Pituitary snuff-takers' disease
Sequoiosis or red-cedar asthma
Wood asthma

C&C Exclusions: See 495.0

495.9 Unspecified allergic alveolitis and pneumonitis

Alveolitis, allergic (extrinsic)
Hypersensitivity pneumonitis

C&C Exclusions: See 495.0

496 Chronic airway obstruction, not elsewhere classified

Chronic:
- nonspecific lung disease
- obstructive lung disease
- obstructive pulmonary disease [COPD] NOS

Note: This code is not to be used with any code from categories 491-493

Excludes *chronic obstructive lung disease [COPD] specified (as) (with):*
- *allergic alveolitis (495.0-495.9)*
- *asthma (493.2)*
- *bronchiectasis (494.0-494.1)*
- *bronchitis (491.20-491.22)*
  - *with emphysema (491.20-491.22)*
- *decompensated (491.21)*

emphysema (492.0-492.8)

C&C Exclusions: 017.90, 017.91, 017.92, 017.93, 017.94, 017.95, 017.96, 079.82, 480.3, 487.1, 494.0, 494.1, 496, 506.1, 506.4, 506.9, 748.61

AHA: 4Q 2003, 109; 2Q 2000, 15; 2Q 1992, 16; 2Q 1991, 21; 3Q 1988, 56

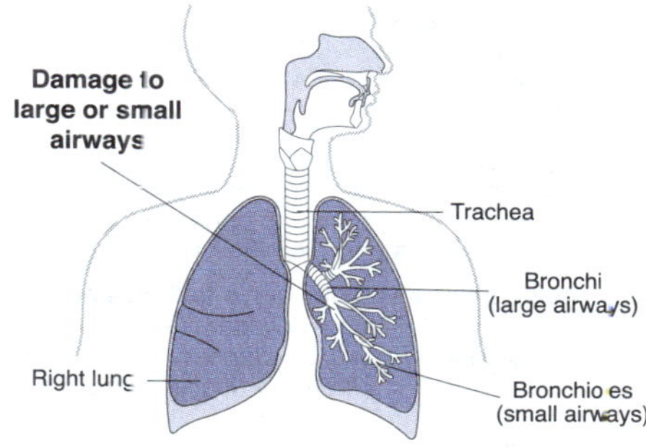

PNEUMOCONIOSES AND OTHER LUNG DISEASES DUE TO EXTERNAL AGENTS (500-508)

500 Coal workers' pneumoconiosis A

Anthracosilicosis
Anthracosis
Black lung disease
Coal workers' lung
Miners' asthma

DEF: Silicotic nodules and scar-tissue formation in the lungs due to prolonged inhalation and collection of coal dust particles in the bronchioles.

C&C Exclusions: 079.82, 480.3

501 Asbestosis A

DEF: Chronic lung disease caused by inhaling asbestos particles over a prolonged period.

C&C Exclusions: See 500

502 Pneumoconiosis due to other silica or silicates

Pneumoconiosis due to talc
Silicotic fibrosis (massive) of lung
Silicosis (simple) (complicated)

C&C Exclusions: See 500

503 Pneumoconiosis due to other inorganic dust

Aluminosis (of lung)
Bauxite fibrosis (of lung)
Berylliosis
Graphite fibrosis (of lung)
Siderosis
Stannosis

C&C Exclusions: See 500

504 Pneumonopathy due to inhalation of other dust

Byssinosis
Cannabinosis
Flax-dressers' disease

Excludes *allergic alveolitis (495.0-495.9)*
asbestosis (501)
bagassosis (495.1)
farmers' lung (495.0)

505 Pneumoconiosis, unspecified
C&C Exclusions: See 500

506 Respiratory conditions due to chemical fumes and vapors
Use additional E code to identify cause

506.0 Bronchitis and pneumonitis due to fumes and vapors
Chemical bronchitis (acute)
C&C Exclusions: 011.00, 011.01, 011.02, 011.03, 011.04, 011.05, 011.06, 011.10, 011.11, 011.12, 011.13, 011.14, 011.15, 011.16, 011.20, 011.21, 011.22, 011.23, 011.24, 011.25, 011.26, 011.30, 011.31, 011.32, 011.33, 011.34, 011.35, 011.36, 011.40, 011.41, 011.42, 011.43, 011.44, 011.45, 011.46, 011.50, 011.51, 011.52, 011.53, 011.54, 011.55, 011.56, 011.60, 011.61, 011.62, 011.63, 011.64, 011.65, 011.66, 011.70, 011.71, 011.72, 011.73, 011.74, 011.75, 011.76, 011.80, 011.81, 011.82, 011.83, 011.84, 011.85, 011.86, 011.90, 011.91, 011.92, 011.93, 011.94, 011.95, 011.96, 012.00, 012.01, 012.02, 012.03, 012.04, 012.05, 012.06, 012.10, 012.11, 012.12, 012.13, 012.14, 012.15, 012.16, 012.80, 012.81, 012.82, 012.83, 012.84, 012.85, 012.86, 017.90, 017.91, 017.92, 017.93, 017.94, 017.95, 017.96, 021.2, 031.0, 039.1, 079.82, 115.05, 115.15, 115.95, 122.1, 130.4, 136.3, 480.0, 480.1, 480.2, 480.3, 480.8, 480.9, 481, 482.0, 482.1, 482.2, 482.30, 482.31, 482.32, 482.39, 482.40, 482.41, 482.49, 482.81, 482.82, 482.83, 482.84, 482.89, 482.9, 483.0, 483.1, 483.8, 484.1, 484.3, 484.5, 484.6, 484.7, 484.8, 485, 486, 487.0, 487.1, 494.0, 494.1, 495.0, 495.1, 495.2, 495.3, 495.4, 495.5, 495.6, 495.7, 495.8, 495.9, 496, 500, 501, 502, 503, 504, 505, 506.0, 506.1, 506.2, 506.3, 506.4, 506.9, 507.0, 507.1, 507.8, 508.0, 508.1, 508.8, 508.9, 517.1, 517.8, 518.89, 519.8, 519.9, 748.61

506.1 Acute pulmonary edema due to fumes and vapors
Chemical pulmonary edema (acute)
Excludes *acute pulmonary edema NOS (518.4)*
chronic or unspecified pulmonary edema (514)
C&C Exclusions: See 506.0
AHA: 3Q 1988, 4

506.2 Upper respiratory inflammation due to fumes and vapors
C&C Exclusions: 079.82, 480.3
AHA: 3Q 2005, 10

506.3 Other acute and subacute respiratory conditions due to fumes and vapors
C&C Exclusions: See 506.2

506.4 Chronic respiratory conditions due to fumes and vapors
Emphysema (diffuse) (chronic) due to inhalation of chemical fumes and vapors
Obliterative bronchiolitis (chronic) (subacute) due to inhalation of chemical fumes and vapors
Pulmonary fibrosis (chronic) due to inhalation of chemical fumes and vapors
C&C Exclusions: See 506.0

506.9 Unspecified respiratory conditions due to fumes and vapors
Silo-fillers' disease
C&C Exclusions: See 506.0

507 Pneumonitis due to solids and liquids
Excludes *fetal aspiration pneumonitis (770.18)*
AHA: 3Q 1991, 16

507.0 Due to inhalation of food or vomitus
Aspiration pneumonia (due to):
- NOS
- food (regurgitated)
- gastric secretions
- milk
- saliva
- vomitus

C&C Exclusions: See 506.0
AHA: 1Q 1989, 10

507.1 Due to inhalation of oils and essences
Lipoid pneumonia (exogenous)
Excludes *endogenous lipoid pneumonia (516.8)*
C&C Exclusions: See 506.0

507.8 Due to other solids and liquids
Detergent asthma
C&C Exclusions: See 506.0

508 Respiratory conditions due to other and unspecified external agents
Use additional E code to identify cause

508.0 Acute pulmonary manifestations due to radiation
Radiation pneumonitis
C&C Exclusions: See 506.0
AHA: 2Q 1988, 4

508.1 Chronic and other pulmonary manifestations due to radiation
Fibrosis of lung following radiation
C&C Exclusions: See 506.0

508.8 Respiratory conditions due to other specified external agents
C&C Exclusions: See 506.2

508.9 Respiratory conditions due to unspecified external agent
C&C Exclusions: See 506.2

OTHER DISEASES OF RESPIRATORY SYSTEM (510-519)

510 Empyema
Use additional code to identify infectious organism (041.0-041.9)
Excludes *abscess of lung (513.0)*
DEF: Pus discharges into the space between the lungs and the chest wall, usually due to an infection of the lungs.

510.0 With fistula
Fistula:
- bronchocutaneous
- bronchopleural
- hepatopleural
- mediastinal
- pleural
- thoracic

Any condition classifiable to 510.9 with fistula
C&C Exclusions: 510.0, 510.9, 517.8, 518.89, 519.8, 519.9

510.9 Without mention of fistula
Abscess:
- pleura
- thorax

Empyema (chest) (lung) (pleura)
Fibrinopurulent pleurisy
Pleurisy:
- purulent
- septic
- seropurulent
- suppurative

Pyopneumothorax
Pyothorax
C&C Exclusions: See 510.0
AHA: 3Q 1994, 6

511 Pleurisy
Excludes *malignant pleural effusion (197.2)*
pleurisy with mention of tuberculosis, current disease (012.0)

511.0 Without mention of effusion or current tuberculosis
Adhesion, lung or pleura
Calcification of pleura
Pleurisy (acute) (sterile):
- diaphragmatic
- fibrinous
- interlobar

Pleurisy:
- NOS
- pneumococcal
- staphylococcal
- streptococcal

Thickening of pleura
AHA: 3Q 1994, 5

511.1 With effusion, with mention of a bacterial cause other than tuberculosis

Pleurisy with effusion (exudative) (serous):
- pneumococcal
- staphylococcal
- streptococcal
- other specified nontuberculous bacterial cause

C&C Exclusions: 011.00, 011.01, 011.02, 011.03, 011.04, 011.05, 011.06, 011.10, 011.11, 011.12, 011.13, 011.14, 011.15, 011.16, 011.20, 011.21, 011.22, 011.23, 011.24, 011.25, 011.26, 011.30, 011.31, 011.32, 011.33, 011.34, 011.35, 011.36, 011.40, 011.41, 011.42, 011.43, 011.44, 011.45, 011.46, 011.50, 011.51, 011.52, 011.53, 011.54, 011.55, 011.56, 011.60, 011.61, 011.62, 011.63, 011.64, 011.65, 011.66, 011.70, 011.71, 011.72, 011.73, 011.74, 011.75, 011.76, 011.80, 011.81, 011.82, 011.83, 011.84, 011.85, 011.86, 011.90, 011.91, 011.92, 011.93, 011.94, 011.95, 011.96, 012.00, 012.01, 012.02, 012.03, 012.04, 012.05, 012.06, 012.10, 012.11, 012.12, 012.13, 012.14, 012.15, 012.16, 012.80, 012.81, 012.82, 012.83, 012.84, 012.85, 012.86, 017.90, 017.91, 017.92, 017.93, 017.94, 017.95, 017.96, 511.0, 511.1, 511.8, 511.9, 517.8, 518.89, 519.8, 519.9

511.8 Other specified forms of effusion, except tuberculous

Encysted pleurisy
Hemopneumothorax
Hemothorax
Hydropneumothorax
Hydrothorax

Excludes *traumatic (860.2-860.5, 862.29, 862.39)*

C&C Exclusions: See 511.1

AHA: 1Q 1997, 10

511.9 Unspecified pleural effusion

Pleural effusion NOS
Pleurisy:
- exudative
- serofibrinous
- serous
- with effusion NOS

C&C Exclusions: See 511.1

AHA: 2Q 2003, 7; 3Q 1991, 19; 4Q 1989, 11

❹ 512 Pneumothorax

512.0 Spontaneous tension pneumothorax

C&C Exclusions: 512.0, 512.1, 512.8, 517.8, 518.89, 519.8, 519.9

AHA: 3Q 1994, 5

512.1 Iatrogenic pneumothorax

Postoperative pneumothorax

C&C Exclusions: See 512.0

AHA: 4Q 1994, 40

512.8 Other spontaneous pneumothorax

Pneumothorax:
- NOS
- acute
- chronic

Excludes *pneumothorax:*
- *congenital (770.2)*
- *traumatic (860.0-860.1, 860.4-860.5)*
- *tuberculous, current disease (011.7)*

C&C Exclusions: See 512.0

AHA: 2Q 1993, 3

A lung collapses due to an accumulation of air or gas in the chest cavity

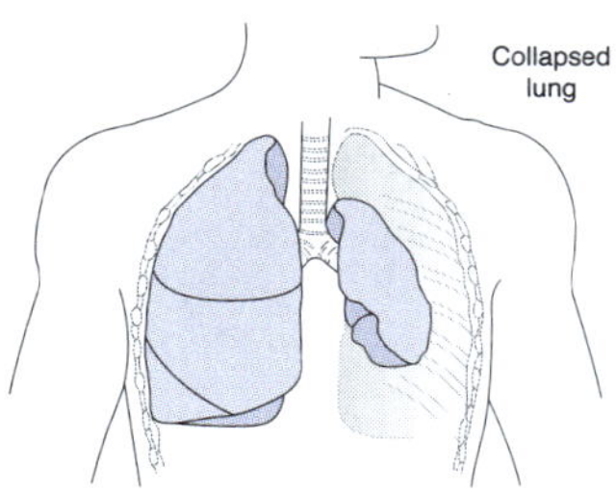

❹ 513 Abscess of lung and mediastinum

513.0 Abscess of lung

Abscess (multiple) of lung
Gangrenous or necrotic pneumonia
Pulmonary gangrene or necrosis

C&C Exclusions: 006.4, 011.00, 011.01, 011.02, 011.03, 011.04, 011.05, 011.06, 011.10, 011.11, 011.12, 011.13, 011.14, 011.15, 011.16, 011.20, 011.21, 011.22, 011.23, 011.24, 011.25, 011.26, 011.30, 011.31, 011.32, 011.33, 011.34, 011.35, 011.36, 011.40, 011.41, 011.42, 011.43, 011.44, 011.45, 011.46, 011.50, 011.51, 011.52, 011.53, 011.54, 011.55, 011.56, 011.60, 011.61, 011.62, 011.63, 011.64, 011.65, 011.66, 011.70, 011.71, 011.72, 011.73, 011.74, 011.75, 011.76, 011.80, 011.81, 011.82, 011.83, 011.84, 011.85, 011.86, 011.90, 011.91, 011.92, 011.93, 011.94, 011.95, 011.96, 012.00, 012.01, 012.02, 012.03, 012.04, 012.05, 012.06, 012.10, 012.11, 012.12, 012.13, 012.14, 012.15, 012.16, 012.80, 012.81, 012.82, 012.83, 012.84, 012.85, 012.86, 017.90, 017.91, 017.92, 017.93, 017.94, 017.95, 017.96, 513.0, 519.8, 519.9

AHA: 2Q 1998, 7

513.1 Abscess of mediastinum

C&C Exclusions: 513.1, 519.8, 519.9

514 Pulmonary congestion and hypostasis

Hypostatic:
- bronchopneumonia
- pneumonia

Passive pneumonia
Pulmonary congestion (chronic) (passive)
Pulmonary edema:
- NOS
- chronic

Excludes *acute pulmonary edema:*
- *NOS (518.4)*
- *with mention of heart disease or failure (428.1)*

hypostatic pneumonia due to or specified as a specific type of pneumonia - code to the type of pneumonia (480.0-480.9, 481, 482.0-482.49, 483.0-483.8, 485, 486, 487.0)

AHA: 2Q 1998, 6; 3Q 1988, 5

515 Postinflammatory pulmonary fibrosis

Cirrhosis of lung chronic or unspecified
Fibrosis of lung (atrophic) (confluent) (massive) (perialveolar) (peribronchial) chronic or unspecified
Induration of lung chronic or unspecified

DEF: Formation of fibrous tissue and scarring in the lungs after the lungs have been inflamed for a significant period of time.

C&C Exclusions: 011.00, 011.01, 011.02, 011.03, 011.04, 011.05, 011.06, 011.10, 011.11, 011.12, 011.13, 011.14, 011.15, 011.16, 011.20, 011.21, 011.22, 011.23, 011.24, 011.25, 011.26, 011.30, 011.31, 011.32, 011.33, 011.34, 011.35, 011.36, 011.40, 011.41, 011.42, 011.43, 011.44, 011.45, 011.46, 011.50, 011.51, 011.52, 011.53, 011.54, 011.55, 011.56, 011.60, 011.61, 011.62, 011.63, 011.64, 011.65, 011.66, 011.70, 011.71, 011.72, 011.73, 011.74, 011.75, 011.76, 011.80, 011.81, 011.82, 011.83, 011.84, 011.85, 011.86, 011.90, 011.91, 011.92, 011.93, 011.94, 011.95, 011.96, 012.00, 012.01, 012.02, 012.03, 012.04, 012.05, 012.06, 012.10, 012.11, 012.12, 012.13, 012.14, 012.15, 012.16, 012.80, 012.81, 012.82, 012.83, 012.84, 012.85, 012.86, 017.90, 017.91, 017.92, 017.93, 017.94, 017.95, 017.96, 494.0, 494.1, 495.0, 495.1, 495.2, 495.3, 495.4, 495.5, 495.6, 495.7, 495.8, 495.9, 496, 500, 501, 502, 503, 504, 505, 506.0, 506.1, 506.2, 506.3, 506.4, 506.9, 507.0, 507.1, 507.8, 508.0, 508.1, 508.8, 508.9, 515, 516.0, 516.1, 516.2, 516.3, 516.8, 516.9, 517.2, 517.8, 518.89, 519.8, 519.9, 748.61

❹ 516 Other alveolar and parietoalveolar pneumonopathy

516.0 Pulmonary alveolar proteinosis

DEF: The production of abnormally high amounts of surfactant, the substance secreted by the lungs to keep alveoli open.

C&C Exclusions: See 515

+ *516.1 Idiopathic pulmonary hemosiderosis*

Essential brown induration of lung
Code first underlying disease (275.0)

C&C Exclusions: See 515

516.2 Pulmonary alveolar microlithiasis

DEF: Rare disease in which small calcium deposits form in the alveoli of the lungs.

C&C Exclusions: See 515

516.3 Idiopathic fibrosing alveolitis
Alveolar capillary block
Diffuse (idiopathic) (interstitial) pulmonary fibrosis
Hamman-Rich syndrome
C&C Exclusions: See 515

516.8 Other specified alveolar and parietoalveolar pneumonopathies
Endogenous lipoid pneumonia
Interstitial pneumonia (desquamative) (lymphoid)
Excludes *lipoid pneumonia, exogenous or unspecified (507.1)*
C&C Exclusions: See 515
AHA: 2Q 2006, 20; 1Q 1992, 12

✖ **516.9 Unspecified alveolar and parietoalveolar pneumonopathy**
C&C Exclusions: See 515

❹ **517 Lung involvement in conditions classified elsewhere**
Excludes *rheumatoid lung (714.81)*

✚ ***517.1 Rheumatic pneumonia***
Code first underlying disease (390)
C&C Exclusions: 011.00, 011.01, 011.02, 011.03, 011.04, 011.05, 011.06, 011.10, 011.11, 011.12, 011.13, 011.14, 011.15, 011.16, 011.20, 011.21, 011.22, 011.23, 011.24, 011.25, 011.26, 011.30, 011.31, 011.32, 011.33, 011.34, 011.35, 011.36, 011.40, 011.41, 011.42, 011.43, 011.44, 011.45, 011.46, 011.50, 011.51, 011.52, 011.53, 011.54, 011.55, 011.56, 011.60, 011.61, 011.62, 011.63, 011.64, 011.65, 011.66, 011.70, 011.71, 011.72, 011.73, 011.74, 011.75, 011.76, 011.80, 011.81, 011.82, 011.83, 011.84, 011.85, 011.86, 011.90, 011.91, 011.92, 011.93, 011.94, 011.95, 011.96, 012.00, 012.01, 012.02, 012.03, 012.04, 012.05, 012.06, 012.10, 012.11, 012.12, 012.13, 012.14, 012.15, 012.16, 012.80, 012.81, 012.82, 012.83, 012.84, 012.85, 012.86, 017.90, 017.91, 017.92, 017.93, 017.94, 017.95, 017.96, 079.82, 480.0, 480.1, 480.2, 480.3, 480.8, 480.9, 481, 482.0, 482.1, 482.2, 482.30, 482.31, 482.32, 482.39, 482.40, 482.41, 482.49, 482.81, 482.82, 482.83, 482.84, 482.89, 482.9, 483.0, 483.1, 483.8, 484.1, 484.3, 484.5, 484.6, 484.7, 484.8, 485, 486, 487.0, 487.1, 494.0, 494.1, 495.0, 495.1, 495.2, 495.3, 495.4, 495.5, 495.6, 495.7, 495.8, 495.9, 496, 500, 501, 502, 503, 504, 505, 506.0, 506.1, 506.2, 506.3, 506.4, 506.9, 507.0, 507.1, 507.8, 508.0, 508.1, 508.8, 508.9, 515, 516.0, 516.1, 516.2, 516.3, 516.8, 516.9, 517.1, 517.2, 517.8, 518.89, 519.8, 519.9, 748.61

✚ ***517.2 Lung involvement in systemic sclerosis***
Code first underlying disease (710.1)
C&C Exclusions: 011.00, 011.01, 011.02, 011.03, 011.04, 011.05, 011.06, 011.10, 011.11, 011.12, 011.13, 011.14, 011.15, 011.16, 011.20, 011.21, 011.22, 011.23, 011.24, 011.25, 011.26, 011.30, 011.31, 011.32, 011.33, 011.34, 011.35, 011.36, 011.40, 011.41, 011.42, 011.43, 011.44, 011.45, 011.46, 011.50, 011.51, 011.52, 011.53, 011.54, 011.55, 011.56, 011.60, 011.61, 011.62, 011.63, 011.64, 011.65, 011.66, 011.70, 011.71, 011.72, 011.73, 011.74, 011.75, 011.76, 011.80, 011.81, 011.82, 011.83, 011.84, 011.85, 011.86, 011.90, 011.91, 011.92, 011.93, 011.94, 011.95, 011.96, 012.00, 012.01, 012.02, 012.03, 012.04, 012.05, 012.06, 012.10, 012.11, 012.12, 012.13, 012.14, 012.15, 012.16, 012.80, 012.81, 012.82, 012.83, 012.84, 012.85, 012.86, 017.90, 017.91, 017.92, 017.93, 017.94, 017.95, 017.96, 494.0, 494.1, 495.0, 495.1, 495.2, 495.3, 495.4, 495.5, 495.6, 495.7, 495.8, 495.9, 496, 500, 501, 502, 503, 504, 505, 506.0, 506.1, 506.2, 506.3, 506.4, 506.9, 507.0, 507.1, 507.8, 508.0, 508.1, 508.8, 508.9, 515, 516.0, 516.1, 516.2, 516.3, 516.8, 516.9, 517.2, 518.89, 519.8, 519.9, 748.61

✚ ***517.3 Acute chest syndrome***
Code first sickle-cell disease in crisis (282.42, 282.62, 282.64, 282.69)
C&C Exclusions: 280.0, 281.4, 281.8, 282.41, 282.42, 282.49, 282.60, 282.61, 282.62, 282.63, 282.64, 282.68, 282.69, 283.0, 283.10, 283.11, 283.19, 283.2, 283.9, 284.8, 284.9, 285.0, 285.1
AHA: 4Q 2003, 51, 56

✚ ***517.8 Lung involvement in other diseases classified elsewhere***
Code first underlying disease, as:
amyloidosis (277.30-277.39)
polymyositis (710.4)
sarcoidosis (135)
Sjögren's disease (710.2)
systemic lupus erythematosus (710.0)
Excludes *syphilis (095.1)*
C&C Exclusions: 011.00, 011.01, 011.02, 011.03, 011.04, 011.05, 011.06, 011.10, 011.11, 011.12, 011.13, 011.14, 011.15, 011.16, 011.20, 011.21, 011.22, 011.23, 011.24, 011.25, 011.26, 011.30, 011.31, 011.32, 011.33, 011.34, 011.35, 011.36, 011.40, 011.41, 011.42, 011.43, 011.44, 011.45, 011.46, 011.50, 011.51, 011.52, 011.53, 011.54, 011.55, 011.56, 011.60, 011.61, 011.62, 011.63, 011.64, 011.65, 011.66, 011.70, 011.71, 011.72, 011.73, 011.74, 011.75, 011.76, 011.80, 011.81, 011.82, 011.83, 011.84, 011.85, 011.86, 011.90, 011.91, 011.92, 011.93, 011.94, 011.95, 011.96, 012.00, 012.01, 012.02, 012.03, 012.04, 012.05, 012.06, 012.10, 012.11, 012.12, 012.13, 012.14, 012.15, 012.16, 012.80, 012.81, 012.82, 012.83, 012.84, 012.85, 012.86, 017.90, 017.91, 017.92, 017.93, 017.94, 017.95, 017.96, 079.82, 480.3, 493.02, 493.12, 493.22, 493.92, 494.0, 494.1, 495.0, 495.1, 495.2, 495.3, 495.4, 495.5, 495.6, 495.7, 495.8, 495.9, 496, 500, 501, 502, 503, 504, 505, 506.0, 506.1, 506.2, 506.3, 506.4, 506.9, 507.0, 507.1, 507.8, 508.0, 508.1, 508.8, 508.9, 515, 516.0, 516.1, 516.2, 516.3, 516.8, 516.9, 517.2, 518.89, 519.8, 519.9, 748.61
AHA: 2Q 2003, 7

❹ **518 Other diseases of lung**

518.0 Pulmonary collapse
Atelectasis
Collapse of lung
Middle lobe syndrome
Excludes *atelectasis:*
congenital (partial) (770.5)
primary (770.4)
tuberculous, current disease (011.8)
C&C Exclusions: 518.0, 519.8, 519.9
AHA: 4Q 1990, 25

518.1 Interstitial emphysema
Mediastinal emphysema
Excludes *surgical (subcutaneous) emphysema (998.81)*
that in fetus or newborn (770.2)
traumatic emphysema (958.7)
C&C Exclusions: 518.1, 519.8, 519.9

518.2 Compensatory emphysema

518.3 Pulmonary eosinophilia
Eosinophilic asthma
Löffler's syndrome
Pneumonia:
allergic
eosinophilic
Tropical eosinophilia

518.4 Acute edema of lung, unspecified
Acute pulmonary edema NOS
Pulmonary edema, postoperative
Excludes *pulmonary edema:*
acute, with mention of heart disease or failure (428.1)
chronic or unspecified (514)
due to external agents (506.0-508.9)
DEF: Sudden, severe accumulation of fluid in the lungs.
C&C Exclusions: 398.91, 428.0, 428.1, 428.20, 428.21, 428.22, 428.23, 428.30, 428.31, 428.32, 428.33, 428.40, 428.41, 428.42, 428.43, 428.9, 518.4, 519.8, 519.9

518.5 Pulmonary insufficiency following trauma and surgery
Adult respiratory distress syndrome
Pulmonary insufficiency following:
shock
surgery
trauma
Shock lung
Excludes *adult respiratory distress syndrome associated with other conditions (518.82)*
pneumonia:
aspiration (507.0)
hypostatic (514)
respiratory failure in other conditions (518.81, 518.83-518.84)
C&C Exclusions: 518.5, 519.8, 519.9
AHA: 4Q 2004, 139; 3Q 1988, 3, 7; Sep-Oct 1987, 1

518.6 Allergic bronchopulmonary aspergillosis
C&C Exclusions: 518.6, 519.8, 519.9
AHA: 4Q 1997, 39

518.7 Transfusion related acute lung injury (TRALI)
C&C Exclusions: 518.7, 997.3
AHA: 4Q 2006, 91

❺ **518.8 Other diseases of lung**

518.81 Acute respiratory failure
Respiratory failure NOS
Excludes *acute and chronic respiratory failure (518.84)*
acute respiratory distress (518.82)
chronic respiratory failure (518.83)
respiratory arrest (799.1)
respiratory failure, newborn (770.84)
C&C Exclusions: 518.81, 518.82, 518.83, 518.84, 518.89, 519.8, 519.9, 799.01, 799.02, 799.1
AHA: 4Q 2005, 96; 2Q 2005, 19; 1Q 2005, 3-8; 4Q 2004, 139; 1Q 2003; 15; 4Q 1998, 41; 3Q 1991, 14; 2Q 1991, 3; 4Q 1990, 25; 2Q 1990; 20; 3Q 1988, 7, 10; Sep-Oct 1987, 1

518.82 Other pulmonary insufficiency, not elsewhere classified
Acute respiratory distress
Acute respiratory insufficiency
Adult respiratory distress syndrome NEC
Excludes *adult respiratory distress syndrome associated with trauma or surgery (518.5)*
pulmonary insufficiency following trauma or surgery (518.5)
respiratory distress:
NOS (786.09)
newborn (770.89)
syndrome, newborn (769)
shock lung (518.5)
C&C Exclusions: See 518.81
AHA: 4Q 2003, 105; 2Q 1991, 21; 3Q 1988, 7

518.83 Chronic respiratory failure
C&C Exclusions: See 518.81
AHA: 4Q 2005, 96; 4Q 2003, 111

518.84 Acute and chronic respiratory failure
Acute on chronic respiratory failure
C&C Exclusions: See 518.81

518.89 Other diseases of lung, not elsewhere classified
Broncholithiasis
Calcification of lung
Lung disease NOS
Pulmolithiasis
C&C Exclusions: 079.82, 480.3, 493.02, 493.12, 493.22, 493.92
AHA: 3Q 1990, 18; 4Q 1988, 6

❹ **519 Other diseases of respiratory system**

❺ **519.0 Tracheostomy complications**

✖ **519.00 Tracheostomy complication, unspecified**
C&C Exclusions: 519.00, 519.01, 519.02, 519.09, 519.1, 519.8, 519.9

519.01 Infection of tracheostomy
Use additional code to identify type of infection, such as:
abscess or cellulitis of neck (682.1)
septicemia (038.0-038.9)
Use additional code to identify organism (041.00-041.9)
C&C Exclusions: See 519.00
AHA: 4Q 1998, 41

519.02 Mechanical complication of tracheostomy
Tracheal stenosis due to tracheostomy
C&C Exclusions: See 519.00

519.09 Other tracheostomy complications
Hemorrhage due to tracheostomy
Tracheoesophageal fistula due to tracheostomy
C&C Exclusions: See 519.00

❺ **519.1 Other diseases of trachea and bronchus, not elsewhere classified**
AHA: 3Q 2002, 18; 3Q 1988, 6

519.11 Acute bronchospasm
Bronchospasm NOS
Excludes *acute bronchitis with bronchospasm (466.0)*
asthma (493.00-493.92)
exercise induced bronchospasm (493.81)
DEF: Constriction or contraction of the smooth muscle in the large air passages, severely limiting airflow.
C&C Exclusions: 519.00, 519.01, 519.02, 519.09

519.19 Other diseases of trachea and bronchus
Calcification of bronchus or trachea
Stenosis of bronchus or trachea
Ulcer of bronchus or trachea
C&C Exclusions: See 519.11

519.2 Mediastinitis
C&C Exclusions: 519.2, 519.3, 519.8, 519.9

519.3 Other diseases of mediastinum, not elsewhere classified
Fibrosis of mediastinum
Hernia of mediastinum
Retraction of mediastinum

519.4 Disorders of diaphragm
Diaphragmitis
Paralysis of diaphragm
Relaxation of diaphragm
Excludes *congenital defect of diaphragm (756.6)*
diaphragmatic hernia (551-553 with .3)
congenital (756.6)

519.8 Other diseases of respiratory system, not elsewhere classified
C&C Exclusions: 079.82, 480.3, 493.02, 493.12, 493.22, 493.92
AHA: 4Q 1989, 12

✖ **519.9 Unspecified disease of respiratory system**
Respiratory disease (chronic) NOS
C&C Exclusions: See 519.8

9. DISEASES OF THE DIGESTIVE SYSTEM (520-579)

Digestive system

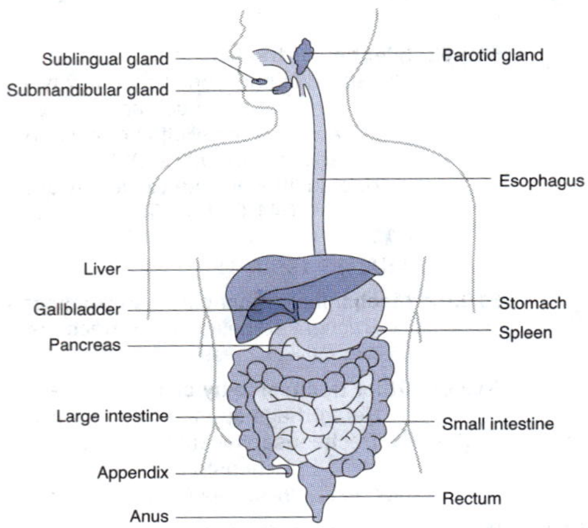

DISEASES OF ORAL CAVITY, SALIVARY GLANDS, AND JAWS (520-529)

Oral cavity anatomy

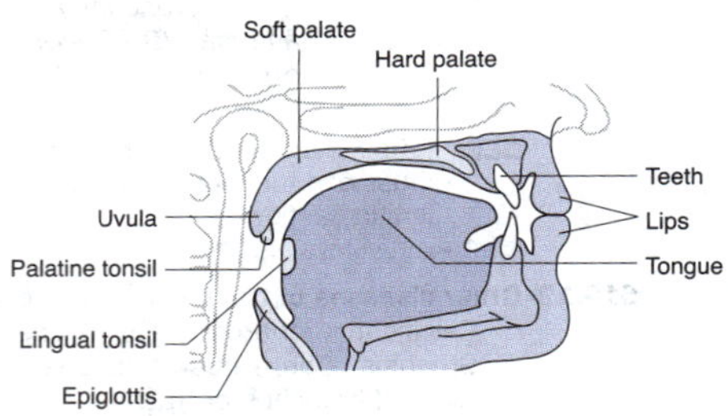

❹ **520 Disorders of tooth development and eruption**

520.0 Anodontia
Absence of teeth (complete) (congenital) (partial)
Hypodontia
Oligodontia
Excludes *acquired absence of teeth (525.10-525.19)*

DEF: Defect in which many or all of the teeth do not develop and are absent from the mouth.

520.1 Supernumerary teeth
Distomolar
Fourth molar
Mesiodens
Paramolar
Supplemental teeth
Excludes *supernumerary roots (520.2)*

520.2 Abnormalities of size and form
Concrescence of teeth
Dens evaginatus
Dens in dente
Dens invaginatus
Enamel pearls
Fusion of teeth
Gemination of teeth
Macrodontia
Microdontia
Peg-shaped [conical] teeth
Supernumerary roots
Taurodontism
Tuberculum paramolare
Excludes *that due to congenital syphilis (090.5)*
tuberculum Carabelli, which is regarded as a normal variation

520.3 Mottled teeth
Dental fluorosis
Mottling of enamel
Nonfluoride enamel opacities

520.4 Disturbances of tooth formation
Aplasia and hypoplasia of cementum
Dilaceration of tooth
Enamel hypoplasia (neonatal) (postnatal) (prenatal)
Horner's teeth
Hypocalcification of teeth
Regional odontodysplasia
Turner's tooth
Excludes *Hutchinson's teeth and mulberry molars in congenital syphilis (090.5)*
mottled teeth (520.3)

520.5 Hereditary disturbances in tooth structure, not elsewhere classified
Amelogenesis imperfecta
Dentinal dysplasia
Dentinogenesis imperfecta
Odontogenesis imperfecta
Shell teeth

520.6 Disturbances in tooth eruption
Teeth:
- embedded
- impacted
- natal
- neonatal
- prenatal
- primary [deciduous]:
  - persistent
  - shedding, premature

Tooth eruption:
- late
- obstructed
- premature

Excludes *exfoliation of teeth (attributable to disease of surrounding tissues) (525.0-525.19)*

AHA: 1Q 2006, 18; 2Q 2005, 15

520.7 Teething syndrome

520.8 Other specified disorders of tooth development and eruption
Color changes during tooth formation
Pre-eruptive color changes
Excludes *posteruptive color changes (521.7)*

✖ **520.9 Unspecified disorder of tooth development and eruption**

❹ **521 Diseases of hard tissues of teeth**

❺ **521.0 Dental caries**
AHA: 4Q 2001, 44

✖ **521.00 Dental caries, unspecified**

521.01 Dental caries limited to enamel
Initial caries
White spot lesion

521.02 Dental caries extending into dentine

521.03 Dental caries extending into pulp

521.04 Arrested dental caries

521.05 Odontoclasia
Infantile melanodontia
Melanodontoclasia
Excludes *internal and external resorption of teeth (521.40-521.49)*

521.06 Dental caries pit and fissure
Primary dental caries, pit and fissure origin

521.07 Dental caries of smooth surface
Primary dental caries, smooth surface origin

521.08 Dental caries of root surface
Primary dental caries, root surface

521.09 Other dental caries
AHA: 3Q 2002, 14

❺ **521.1 Excessive attrition (approximal wear) (occlusal wear)**

DEF: Teeth exhibit excessive wear and tear as a result of tooth-to-tooth contact, often due to grinding the teeth.

✖ **521.10 Excessive attrition, unspecified**

521.11 Excessive attrition, limited to enamel

521.12 Excessive attrition, extending into dentine

521.13 Excessive attrition, extending into pulp

521.14 Excessive attrition, localized

521.15 Excessive attrition, generalized

⑤ **521.2 Abrasion**

Abrasion of teeth:
- dentifrice
- habitual
- occupational
- ritual
- traditional

Wedge defect NOS of teeth

DEF: Teeth exhibit specific wear and tear as a result of tooth contact with another object.

✖ **521.20 Abrasion, unspecified**

521.21 Abrasion, limited to enamel

521.22 Abrasion, extending into dentine

521.23 Abrasion, extending into pulp

521.24 Abrasion, localized

521.25 Abrasion, generalized

⑤ **521.3 Erosion**

Erosion of teeth:
- NOS
- due to:
  - medicine
  - persistent vomiting
- idiopathic
- occupational

✖ **521.30 Erosion, unspecified**

521.31 Erosion, limited to enamel

521.32 Erosion, extending into dentine

521.33 Erosion, extending into pulp

521.34 Erosion, localized

521.35 Erosion, generalized

⑤ **521.4 Pathological resorption**

✖ **521.40 Pathological resorption, unspecified**

521.41 Pathological resorption, internal

521.42 Pathological resorption, external

521.49 Other pathological resorption

Internal granuloma of pulp

521.5 Hypercementosis

Cementation hyperplasia

521.6 Ankylosis of teeth

DEF: Roots of the teeth grow into and merge with the bone of the jaw; most often occurring during development of baby teeth.

521.7 Intrinsic posteruptive color changes

Staining [discoloration] of teeth:
- NOS
- due to:
  - drugs
  - metals
  - pulpal bleeding

Excludes *accretions [deposits] on teeth (523.6)*
extrinsic color changes (523.6)
pre-eruptive color changes (520.8)

⑤ **521.8 Other specified diseases of hard tissues of teeth**

521.81 Cracked tooth

Excludes *asymptomatic craze lines in enamel - omit code*
broken tooth due to trauma (873.63, 873.73)
fractured tooth due to trauma (873.63, 873.73)

521.89 Other specified diseases of hard tissues of teeth

Irradiated enamel
Sensitive dentin

✖ **521.9 Unspecified disease of hard tissues of teeth**

④ **522 Diseases of pulp and periapical tissues**

522.0 Pulpitis

Pulpal:
- abscess
- polyp

Pulpitis:
- acute
- chronic (hyperplastic) (ulcerative)
- suppurative

DEF: Painful inflammation of the soft living tissue containing nerves within the center of the tooth.

522.1 Necrosis of the pulp

Pulp gangrene

522.2 Pulp degeneration

Denticles
Pulp calcifications
Pulp stones

522.3 Abnormal hard tissue formation in pulp

Secondary or irregular dentin

522.4 Acute apical periodontitis of pulpal origin

DEF: Severe inflammation of the periodontal ligament connecting the tooth to the jawbone due to infection or necrosis of the soft, living tissue in the center of the tooth.

522.5 Periapical abscess without sinus

Abscess:
- dental
- dentoalveolar

Excludes *periapical abscess with sinus (522.7)*

522.6 Chronic apical periodontitis

Apical or periapical granuloma
Apical periodontitis NOS

522.7 Periapical abscess with sinus

Fistula:
- alveolar process
- dental

522.8 Radicular cyst

Cyst:
- apical (periodontal)
- periapical
- radiculodental
- residual radicular

Excludes *lateral developmental or lateral periodontal cyst (526.0)*

522.9 Other and unspecified diseases of pulp and periapical tissues

④ **523 Gingival and periodontal diseases**

⑤ **523.0 Acute gingivitis**

Excludes *acute necrotizing ulcerative gingivitis (101)*
herpetic gingivostomatitis (054.2)

An inflammation of the gums caused by a bacterial infection

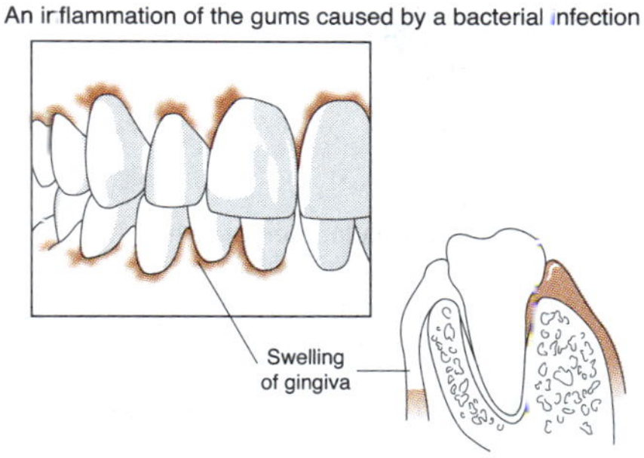

523.00 Acute gingivitis, plaque induced

Acute gingivitis NOS

523.01 Acute gingivitis, non-plaque induced

523.1 Chronic gingivitis
Gingivitis (chronic):
desquamative
hyperplastic
simple marginal
ulcerative
Excludes *herpetic gingivostomatitis (054.2)*

523.10 Chronic gingivitis, plaque induced
Chronic gingivitis NOS
Gingivitis NOS

523.11 Chronic gingivitis, non-plaque induced

523.2 Gingival recession
Gingival recession (postinfective) (postoperative)
DEF: Gums that have receded, exposing more tooth.

523.20 Gingival recession, unspecified
523.21 Gingival recession, minimal
523.22 Gingival recession, moderate
523.23 Gingival recession, severe
523.24 Gingival recession, localized
523.25 Gingival recession, generalized

523.3 Aggressive and acute periodontitis
Acute:
pericementitis
pericoronitis
Excludes *acute apical periodontitis (522.4)*
periapical abscess (522.5, 522.7)

523.30 Aggressive periodontitis, unspecified
523.31 Aggressive periodontitis, localized
Periodontal abscess
523.32 Aggressive periodontitis, generalized
523.33 Acute periodontitis

523.4 Chronic periodontitis
Chronic pericoronitis
Pericementitis (chronic)
Periodontitis:
NOS
complex
simplex
Excludes *chronic apical periodontitis (522.6)*

523.40 Chronic periodontitis, unspecified
523.41 Chronic periodontitis, localized
523.42 Chronic periodontitis, generalized

523.5 Periodontosis
DEF: Serious inflammation and infection of the ligaments and bones supporting the tooth and leading to tooth loss.

523.6 Accretions on teeth
Dental calculus:
subgingival
supragingival
Deposits on teeth:
betel
materia alba
soft
tartar
tobacco
Extrinsic discoloration of teeth
Excludes *intrinsic discoloration of teeth (521.7)*
DEF: Calculous deposits or tartar build-up that resists removal by normal brushing and requires profession cleaning.

523.8 Other specified periodontal diseases
Giant cell:
epulis
peripheral granuloma
Gingival:
cysts
enlargement NOS
fibromatosis
Gingival polyp
Periodontal lesions due to traumatic occlusion
Peripheral giant cell granuloma
Excludes *leukoplakia of gingiva (528.6)*

523.9 Unspecified gingival and periodontal disease
AHA: 3Q 2002, 14

524 Dentofacial anomalies, including malocclusion

524.0 Major anomalies of jaw size
Excludes *hemifacial atrophy or hypertrophy (754.0)*
unilateral condylar hyperplasia or hypoplasia of mandible (526.89)

524.00 Unspecified anomaly
524.01 Maxillary hyperplasia
524.02 Mandibular hyperplasia
524.03 Maxillary hypoplasia
524.04 Mandibular hypoplasia
524.05 Macrogenia
DEF: Abnormally large chin.
524.06 Microgenia
524.07 Excessive tuberosity of jaw
Entire maxillary tuberosity
524.09 Other specified anomaly

524.1 Anomalies of relationship of jaw to cranial base
524.10 Unspecified anomaly
Prognathism
Retrognathism
524.11 Maxillary asymmetry
524.12 Other jaw asymmetry
524.19 Other specified anomaly

524.2 Anomalies of dental arch relationship
Anomaly of dental arch
Excludes *hemifacial atrophy or hypertrophy (754.0)*
soft tissue impingement (524.81-524.82)
unilateral condylar hyperplasia or hypoplasia of mandible (526.89)

524.20 Unspecified anomaly of dental arch relationship
524.21 Malocclusion, Angle's class I
Neutro-occlusion

Angle's Classification of Malocclusion

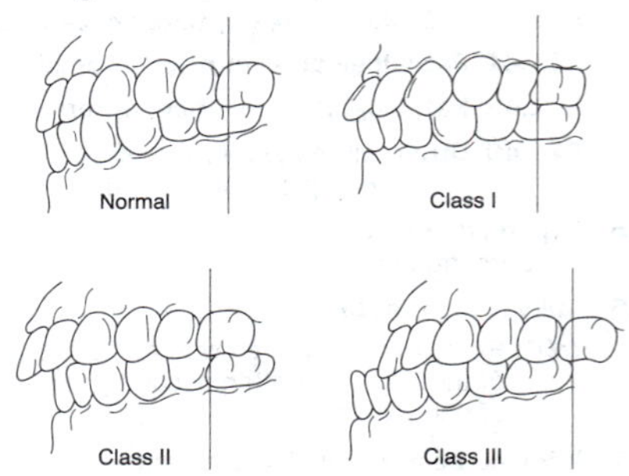

524.22 Malocclusion, Angle's class II
Disto-occlusion Division I
Disto-occlusion Division II
524.23 Malocclusion, Angle's class III
Mesio-occlusion
524.24 Open anterior occlusal relationship
Anterior open bite
524.25 Open posterior occlusal relationship
Posterior open bite
524.26 Excessive horizontal overlap
Excessive horizontal overjet
524.27 Reverse articulation
Anterior articulation
Crossbite
Posterior articulation
524.28 Anomalies of interarch distance
Excessive interarch distance
Inadequate interarch distance
524.29 Other anomalies of dental arch relationship
Other anomalies of dental arch

5 524.3 Anomalies of tooth position of fully erupted teeth
Excludes *impacted or embedded teeth with abnormal position of such teeth or adjacent teeth (520.6)*

✖ **524.30 Unspecified anomaly of tooth position**
Diastema of teeth NOS
Displacement of teeth NOS
Transposition of teeth NOS

524.31 Crowding of teeth

524.32 Excessive spacing of teeth

524.33 Horizontal displacement of teeth
Tipped teeth
Tipping of teeth

524.34 Vertical displacement of teeth
Extruded tooth
Infraeruption of teeth
Intruded tooth
Supraeruption of teeth

524.35 Rotation of tooth/teeth

524.36 Insufficient interocclusal distance of teeth (ridge)
Lack of adequate intermaxillary vertical dimension

524.37 Excessive interocclusal distance of teeth
Excessive intermaxillary vertical dimension
Loss of occlusal vertical dimension

524.39 Other anomalies of tooth position

524.4 Malocclusion, unspecified

5 524.5 Dentofacial functional abnormalities

✖ **524.50 Dentofacial functional abnormality, unspecified**

524.51 Abnormal jaw closure

524.52 Limited mandibular range of motion

524.53 Deviation in opening and closing of the mandible

524.54 Insufficient anterior guidance
Insufficient anterior occlusal guidance

524.55 Centric occlusion maximum intercuspation discrepancy
Centric occlusion of teeth discrepancy

524.56 Non-working side interference
Balancing side interference

524.57 Lack of posterior occlusal support

524.59 Other dentofacial functional abnormalities
Abnormal swallowing
Mouth breathing
Sleep postures
Tongue, lip, or finger habits

5 524.6 Temporomandibular joint disorders
Excludes *current temporomandibular joint:*
dislocation (830.0-830.1)
strain (848.1)

✖ **524.60 Temporomandibular joint disorders, unspecified**
Temporomandibular joint-pain-dysfunction syndrome [TMJ]

524.61 Adhesions and ankylosis (bony or fibrous)

524.62 Arthralgia of temporomandibular joint

524.63 Articular disc disorder (reducing or nonreducing)

524.64 Temporomandibular joint sounds on opening and/or closing the jaw

524.69 Other specified temporomandibular joint disorders

5 524.7 Dental alveolar anomalies

✖ **524.70 Unspecified alveolar anomaly**

524.71 Alveolar maxillary hyperplasia

524.72 Alveolar mandibular hyperplasia

524.73 Alveolar maxillary hypoplasia

524.74 Alveolar mandibular hypoplasia

524.75 Vertical displacement of alvoelus and teeth
Extrusion of alveolus and teeth

524.76 Occlusal plane deviation

524.79 Other specified alveolar anomaly

5 524.8 Other specified dentofacial anomalies

524.81 Anterior soft tissue impingement

524.82 Posterior soft tissue impingement

524.89 Other specified dentofacial anomalies

✖ **524.9 Unspecified dentofacial anomalies**

4 525 Other diseases and conditions of the teeth and supporting structures

525.0 Exfoliation of teeth due to systemic causes

5 525.1 Loss of teeth due to trauma, extraction, or periodontal disease
Code first class of edentulism (525.40-525.44, 525.50-525.54)
AHA: 4Q 2005, 74; 4Q 2001, 44

+ ***525.10 Acquired absence of teeth, unspecified***
Tooth extraction status, NOS

+ ***525.11 Loss of teeth due to trauma***

+ ***525.12 Loss of teeth due to periodontal disease***

+ ***525.13 Loss of teeth due to caries***

+ ***525.19 Other loss of teeth***

5 525.2 Atrophy of edentulous alveolar ridge

✖ **525.20 Unspecified atrophy of edentulous alveolar ridge**
Atrophy of the mandible NOS
Atrophy of the maxilla NOS

525.21 Minimal atrophy of the mandible

525.22 Moderate atrophy of the mandible

525.23 Severe atrophy of the mandible

525.24 Minimal atrophy of the maxilla

525.25 Moderate atrophy of the maxilla

525.26 Severe atrophy of the maxilla

525.3 Retained dental root
DEF: Part or all of the root structure of a tooth remains in the jaw after the tooth is extracted or otherwise lost.

5 525.4 Complete edentulism
Use additional code to identify cause of edentulism (525.10-525.19)
AHA: 4Q 2005, 74

✖ **525.40 Complete edentulism, unspecified**
Edentulism NOS

525.41 Complete edentulism, class I

525.42 Complete edentulism, class II

525.43 Complete edentulism, class III

525.44 Complete edentulism, class IV

5 525.5 Partial edentulism
Use additional code to identify cause of edentulism (525.10-525.19)
AHA: 4Q 2005, 74

✖ **525.50 Partial edentulism, unspecified**

525.51 Partial edentulism, class I

525.52 Partial edentulism, class II

525.53 Partial edentulism, class III

525.54 Partial edentulism, class IV

5 525.6 Unsatisfactory restoration of tooth
Defective bridge, crown, fillings
Defective dental restoration
Excludes *dental restoration status (V45.84)*
unsatisfactory endodontic treatment (526.61-526.69)

✖ **525.60 Unspecified unsatisfactory restoration of tooth**
Unspecified defective dental restoration

525.61 Open restoration margins
Dental restoration failure of marginal integrity
Open margin on tooth restoration

525.62 Unrepairable overhanging of dental restorative materials
Overhanging of tooth restoration

525.63 Fractured dental restorative material without loss of material
Excludes *cracked tooth (521.81)*
fractured tooth (873.63, 873.73)

525.64 Fractured dental restorative material with loss of material
Excludes *cracked tooth (521.81)*
fractured tooth (873.63, 873.73)

525.65 Contour of existing restoration of tooth biologically incompatible with oral health
Dental restoration failure of periodontal anatomical integrity
Unacceptable contours of existing restoration
Unacceptable morphology of existing restoration

525.66 Allergy to existing dental restorative material
Use additional code to identify the specific type of allergy

525.67 Poor aesthetics of existing restoration
Dental restoration aesthetically inadequate or displeasing

525.69 Other unsatisfactory restoration of existing tooth

● ❺ **525.7 Endosseous dental implant failure**

● **525.71 Osseointegration failure of dental implant**
Hemorrhagic complications of dental implant placement
Iatrogenic osseointegration failure of dental implant
Osseointegration failure of dental implant due to:
complications of systemic disease
poor bone quality
Pre-integration failure of dental implant NOS
Pre-osseointegration failure of dental implant

● **525.72 Post-osseointegration biological failure of dental implant**
Failure of dental implant due to:
lack of attached gingiva
occlusal trauma (caused by poor prosthetic design)
parafunctional habits
periodontal infection (peri-implantitis)
poor oral hygiene
Iatrogenic post-osseointegration failure of dental implant
Post-osseointegration failure of dental implant due to complications of systemic disease

● **525.73 Post-osseointegration mechanical failure of dental implant**
Excludes *cracked tooth (521.81)*
fractured dental restorative material with loss of material (525.64)
fractured dental restorative material without loss of material (525.63)
fractured tooth (873.63, 873.73)

● **525.79 Other endosseous dental implant failure**
Dental implant failure NOS

525.8 Other specified disorders of the teeth and supporting structures
Enlargement of alveolar ridge NOS
Irregular alveolar process

✖ **525.9 Unspecified disorder of the teeth and supporting structures**

❹ **526 Diseases of the jaws**

526.0 Developmental odontogenic cysts
Cyst:
dentigerous
eruption
follicular
lateral developmental
lateral periodontal
primordial
Keratocyst
Excludes *radicular cyst (522.8)*

526.1 Fissural cysts of jaw
Cyst:
globulomaxillary
incisor canal
median anterior maxillary
median palatal
nasopalatine
palatine of papilla
Excludes *cysts of oral soft tissues (528.4)*

526.2 Other cysts of jaws
Cyst of jaw:
NOS
aneurysmal
hemorrhagic
traumatic

526.3 Central giant cell (reparative) granuloma
Excludes *peripheral giant cell granuloma (523.8)*

526.4 Inflammatory conditions
Abscess of jaw (acute) (chronic) (suppurative)
Osteitis of jaw (acute) (chronic) (suppurative)
Osteomyelitis (neonatal) of jaw (acute) (chronic) (suppurative)
Periostitis of jaw (acute) (chronic) (suppurative)
Sequestrum of jaw bone
Excludes *alveolar osteitis (526.5)*
▶ *osteonecrosis of jaw (733.45)*◀

526.5 Alveolitis of jaw
Alveolar osteitis
Dry socket
DEF: Inflammation of the tooth sockets.

❺ **526.6 Periradicular pathology associated with previous endodontic treatment**

526.61 Perforation of root canal space

526.62 Endodontic overfill

526.63 Endodontic underfill

526.69 Other periradicular pathology associated with previous endodontic treatment

❺ **526.8 Other specified diseases of the jaws**

526.81 Exostosis of jaw
Torus mandibularis
Torus palatinus

526.89 Other
Cherubism
Fibrous dysplasia of jaw(s)
Latent bone cyst of jaw(s)
Osteoradionecrosis of jaw(s)
Unilateral condylar hyperplasia or hypoplasia of mandible

✖ **526.9 Unspecified disease of the jaws**

❹ **527 Diseases of the salivary glands**

527.0 Atrophy
DEF: Wasting of the saliva glands, resulting in insufficient saliva production.

527.1 Hypertrophy

527.2 Sialoadenitis
Parotitis:
NOS
allergic
toxic
Sialoangitis
Sialodochitis
Excludes *epidemic or infectious parotitis (072.0-072.9)*
uveoparotid fever (135)

527.3 Abscess
C&C Exclusions: 527.0, 527.1, 527.2, 527.3, 527.4, 527.5, 527.6, 527.7, 527.8, 527.9, 537.89, 537.9

527.4 Fistula
Excludes *congenital fistula of salivary gland (750.24)*
C&C Exclusions: See 527.3

527.5 Sialolithiasis
Calculus of salivary gland or duct
Stone of salivary gland or duct
Sialodocholithiasis
DEF: Calculus or stone formation in the salivary gland.

527.6 Mucocele
Mucous:
  extravasation cyst of salivary gland
  retention cyst of salivary gland
Ranula

A type of cyst filled with mucous caused by the rupturing of a salivary gland duct

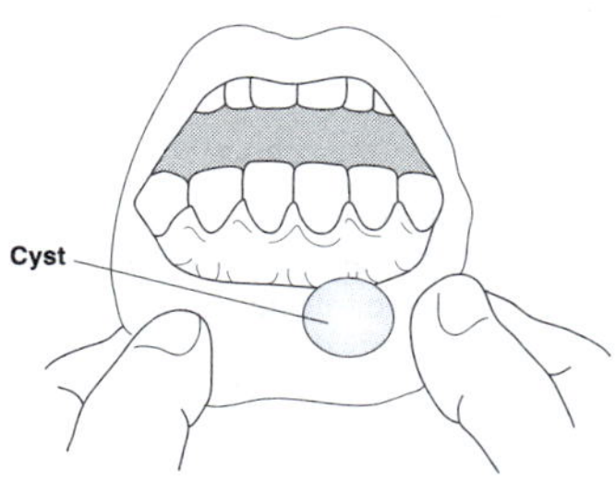

527.7 Disturbance of salivary secretion
Hyposecretion
Ptyalism
Sialorrhea
Xerostomia

527.8 Other specified diseases of the salivary glands
Benign lymphoepithelial lesion of salivary gland
Sialectasia
Sialosis
Stenosis of salivary duct
Stricture of salivary duct

✖ **527.9 Unspecified disease of the salivary glands**

❹ **528 Diseases of the oral soft tissues, excluding lesions specific for gingiva and tongue**

❺ **528.0 Stomatitis and mucositis (ulcerative)**
Excludes *cellulitis and abscess of mouth (528.3)*
diphtheritic stomatitis (032.0)
epizootic stomatitis (078.4)
gingivitis (523.0-523.1)
oral thrush (112.0)
Stevens-Johnson syndrome (695.1)
stomatitis:
  acute necrotizing ulcerative (101)
  aphthous (528.2)
  gangrenous (528.1)
  herpetic (054.2)
  Vincent's (101)
AHA: 2Q 1999, 9

✖ **528.00 Stomatitis and mucositis, unspecified**
Mucositis NOS
Ulcerative mucositis NOS
Ulcerative stomatitis NOS
Vesicular stomatitis NOS
DEF: Stomatitis: Painful inflammation of the soft tissues of the mouth, usually from a viral infection.
C&C Exclusions: 528.3

528.01 Mucositis (ulcerative) due to antineoplastic therapy
Use additional E code to identify adverse effects of therapy, such as:
  antineoplastic and immunosuppressive drugs (E930.7, E933.1)
  radiation therapy (E879.2)
DEF: Mucositis: Painful inflammation and ulcerative sores of mucous membranes, such as those lining the alimentary tract, resulting from chemotherapy or radiation.
C&C Exclusions: See 528.00
AHA: 4Q 2006, 90

528.02 Mucositis (ulcerative) due to other drugs
Use additional E code to identify drug
C&C Exclusions: See 528.00

528.09 Other stomatitis and mucositis (ulcerative)
C&C Exclusions: See 528.00

528.1 Cancrum oris
Gangrenous stomatitis
Noma

528.2 Oral aphthae
Aphthous stomatitis
Canker sore
Periadenitis mucosa necrotica recurrens
Recurrent aphthous ulcer
Stomatitis herpetiformis
Excludes *herpetic stomatitis (054.2)*

528.3 Cellulitis and abscess
Cellulitis of mouth (floor)
Ludwig's angina
Oral fistula
Excludes *abscess of tongue (529.0)*
cellulitis or abscess of lip (528.5)
fistula (of):
  dental (522.7)
  lip (528.5)
gingivitis (523.00-523.11)
C&C Exclusions: 528.0, 528.3, 529.0, 529.2

528.4 Cysts
Dermoid cyst of mouth
Epidermoid cyst of mouth
Epstein's pearl of mouth
Lymphoepithelial cyst of mouth
Nasoalveolar cyst of mouth
Nasolabial cyst of mouth
Excludes *cyst:*
  gingiva (523.8)
  tongue (529.8)

528.5 Diseases of lips
Abscess of lip(s)
Cellulitis of lip(s)
Cheilitis:
  NOS
  angular
Cheilodynia
Cheilosis
Fistula of lip(s)
Hypertrophy of lip(s)
Excludes *actinic cheilitis (692.79)*
congenital fistula of lip (750.25)
leukoplakia of lips (528.6)
AHA: Sep-Oct 1986, 10

528.6 Leukoplakia of oral mucosa, including tongue
Leukokeratosis of oral mucosa
Leukoplakia of:
  gingiva
  lips
  tongue
Excludes *carcinoma in situ (230.0, 232.0)*
leukokeratosis nicotina palati (528.79)

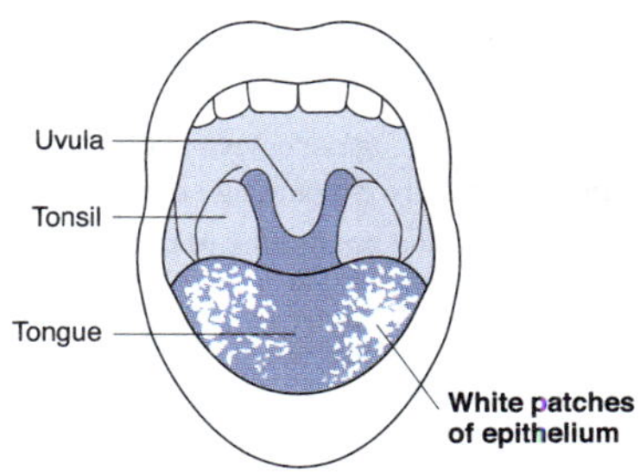

❺ **528.7 Other disturbances of oral epithelium, including tongue**
Excludes *carcinoma in situ (230.0, 232.0)*
leukokeratosis NOS (▶702.8◀)

528.71 Minimal keratinized residual ridge mucosa
Minimal keratinization of alveolar ridge mucosa

528.72 Excessive keratinized residual ridge mucosa
Excessive keratinization of alveolar ridge mucosa

528.79 Other disturbances of oral epithelium, including tongue
Erythroplakia of mouth or tongue
Focal epithelial hyperplasia of mouth or tongue
Leukoedema of mouth or tongue
Leukokeratosis nicotina palati
Other oral epithelium disturbances

528.8 Oral submucosal fibrosis, including of tongue
DEF: Buildup of fibrous (scar-like) tissue within the soft tissues of the mouth, causing rigidity and inability to open the mouth.

528.9 Other and unspecified diseases of the oral soft tissues
Cheek and lip biting
Denture sore mouth
Denture stomatitis
Eosinophilic granuloma of oral mucosa
Irritative hyperplasia of oral mucosa
Melanoplakia
Papillary hyperplasia of palate
Pyogenic granuloma of oral mucosa
Ulcer (traumatic) of oral mucosa

❹ **529 Diseases and other conditions of the tongue**

529.0 Glossitis
Abscess of tongue
Ulceration (traumatic) of tongue
Excludes *glossitis:*
benign migratory (529.1)
Hunter's (529.4)
median rhomboid (529.2)
Moeller's (529.4)
DEF: Changes in the appearance of the tongue due to inflammation.

529.1 Geographic tongue
Benign migratory glossitis
Glossitis areata exfoliativa

529.2 Median rhomboid glossitis

529.3 Hypertrophy of tongue papillae
Black hairy tongue
Coated tongue
Hypertrophy of foliate papillae
Lingua villosa nigra

529.4 Atrophy of tongue papillae
Bald tongue
Glazed tongue
Glossitis:
Hunter's
Moeller's
Glossodynia exfoliativa
Smooth atrophic tongue

529.5 Plicated tongue
Fissured tongue
Furrowed tongue
Scrotal tongue
Excludes *fissure of tongue, congenital (750.13)*

529.6 Glossodynia
Glossopyrosis
Painful tongue
Excludes *glossodynia exfoliativa (529.4)*
DEF: Pain and/or a burning sensation in the tongue.

529.8 Other specified conditions of the tongue
Atrophy (of) tongue
Crenated (of) tongue
Enlargement (of) tongue
Glossocele
Glossoptosis
Hypertrophy (of) tongue
Excludes *erythroplasia of tongue (528.79)*
leukoplakia of tongue (528.6)
macroglossia (congenital) (750.15)
microglossia (congenital) (750.16)
oral submucosal fibrosis (528.8)

✖ **529.9 Unspecified condition of the tongue**

DISEASES OF ESOPHAGUS, STOMACH, AND DUODENUM (530-538)

Esophageal anatomy

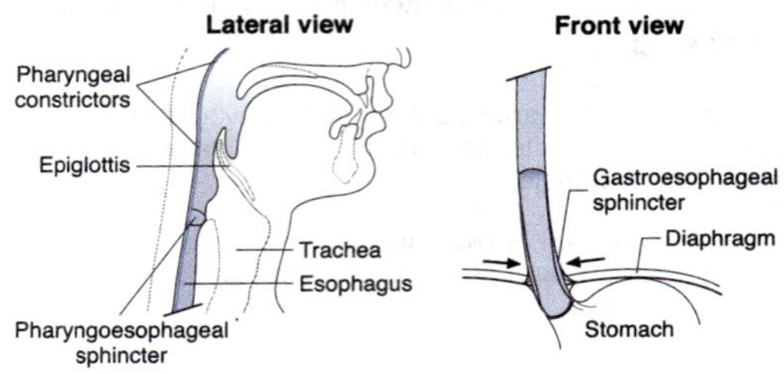

❹ **530 Diseases of esophagus**
Excludes *esophageal varices (456.0-456.2)*

530.0 Achalasia and cardiospasm
Achalasia (of cardia)
Aperistalsis of esophagus
Megaesophagus
Excludes *congenital cardiospasm (750.7)*

❺ **530.1 Esophagitis**
Abscess of esophagus
Esophagitis:
NOS
chemical
peptic
postoperative
regurgitant
Use additional E code to identify cause, if induced by chemical
Excludes *tuberculous esophagitis (017.8)*
AHA: 4Q 1993, 27; 1Q 1992, 17; 3Q 1991, 20

530.10 Esophagitis, unspecified
AHA: 3Q 2005, 17

530.11 Reflux esophagitis
DEF: Esophageal inflammation due to reflux of gastric acid from the stomach back up into the esophagus.
AHA: 4Q 1995, 82

530.12 Acute esophagitis
AHA: 4Q 2001, 45

530.19 Other esophagitis
AHA: 3Q 2001, 10

❺ **530.2 Ulcer of esophagus**
Ulcer of esophagus:
fungal
peptic
Ulcer of esophagus due to ingestion of:
aspirin
chemicals
medicines
Use additional E code to identify cause, if induced by chemical or drug
AHA: 4Q 2003, 63

530.20 Ulcer of esophagus without bleeding
Ulcer of esophagus NOS
C&C Exclusions: 456.0, 530.21, 530.7, 530.82, 531.00, 531.01, 531.10, 531.11, 531.20, 531.21, 531.31, 531.40, 531.41, 531.50, 531.51, 531.60, 531.61, 531.71, 531.91, 532.00, 532.01, 532.10, 532.11, 532.20, 532.21, 532.31, 532.40, 532.41, 532.50, 532.51, 532.60, 532.61, 532.71, 532.91, 533.00, 533.01, 533.10, 533.11, 533.20, 533.21, 533.31, 533.40, 533.41, 533.50, 533.51, 533.60, 533.61, 533.71, 533.91, 534.00, 534.01, 534.10, 534.11, 534.20, 534.21, 534.31, 534.40, 534.41, 534.50, 534.51, 534.60, 534.61, 534.71, 534.91, 535.01, 535.11, 535.21, 535.31, 535.41, 535.51, 535.61, 537.83, 537.84, 562.02, 562.03, 562.12, 562.13, 569.3, 569.85, 569.86, 578.0, 578.1, 578.9

530.21 Ulcer of esophagus with bleeding
Excludes *bleeding esophageal varices (456.0, 456.20)*
C&C Exclusions: See 530.20

A lesion that develops on the interior wall of the esophagus

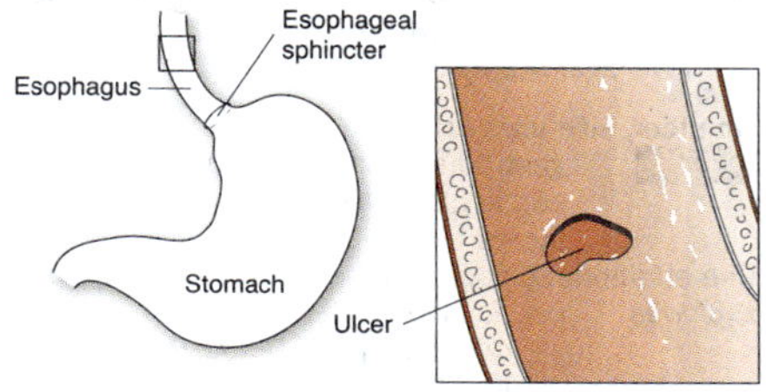

530.3 Stricture and stenosis of esophagus
Compression of esophagus
Obstruction of esophagus
Excludes *congenital stricture of esophagus (750.3)*
AHA: 2Q 2001, 4; 2Q 1997, 3; 1Q 1988, 13

530.4 Perforation of esophagus
Rupture of esophagus
Excludes *traumatic perforation of esophagus (862.22, 862.32, 874.4-874.5)*
C&C Exclusions: 530.4, 530.7, 530.81, 530.83, 530.84, 530.89, 530.9

530.5 Dyskinesia of esophagus
Corkscrew esophagus
Curling esophagus
Esophagospasm
Spasm of esophagus
Excludes *cardiospasm (530.0)*
DEF: Weakened, paralyzed, or uncoordinated movement of esophageal muscles, causing difficulty swallowing.
AHA: 1Q 1988, 13; Nov-Dec 1984, 19

530.6 Diverticulum of esophagus, acquired
Diverticulum, acquired:
- epiphrenic
- pharyngoesophageal
- pulsion
- subdiaphragmatic
- traction
- Zenker's (hypopharyngeal)

Esophageal pouch, acquired
Esophagocele, acquired
Excludes *congenital diverticulum of esophagus (750.4)*
AHA: Jan-Feb 1985, 3

530.7 Gastroesophageal laceration-hemorrhage syndrome
Mallory-Weiss syndrome
DEF: Esophagus becomes torn and bleeds near its connection to the stomach due to prolonged vomiting, hiccuping, or other spasmodic activity.
C&C Exclusions: 251.5, 456.0, 530.21, 530.4, 530.7, 530.81, 530.82, 530.83, 530.84, 530.89, 530.9, 531.00, 531.01, 531.10, 531.11, 531.20, 531.21, 531.30, 531.31, 531.40, 531.41, 531.50, 531.51, 531.60, 531.61, 531.70, 531.71, 531.90, 531.91, 532.00, 532.01, 532.10, 532.11, 532.20, 532.21, 532.30, 532.31, 532.40, 532.41, 532.50, 532.51, 532.60, 532.61, 532.70, 532.71, 532.90, 532.91, 533.00, 533.01, 533.10, 533.11, 533.20, 533.21, 533.30, 533.31, 533.40, 533.41, 533.50, 533.51, 533.60, 533.61, 533.70, 533.71, 533.90, 533.91, 534.00, 534.01, 534.10, 534.11, 534.20, 534.21, 534.30, 534.31, 534.40, 534.41, 534.50, 534.51, 534.60, 534.61, 534.70, 534.71, 534.90, 534.91, 535.01, 535.11, 535.21, 535.31, 535.41, 535.51, 535.61, 537.83, 537.84, 562.02, 562.03, 562.12, 562.13, 569.3, 569.85, 569.86, 578.0, 578.1, 578.9

5 **530.8 Other specified disorders of esophagus**

530.81 Esophageal reflux
Gastroesophageal reflux
Excludes *reflux esophagitis (530.11)*
AHA: 2Q 2001, 4; 1Q 1995, 7; 4Q 1992, 27

530.82 Esophageal hemorrhage
Excludes *hemorrhage due to esophageal varices (456.0-456.2)*
C&C Exclusions: 251.5, 456.0, 456.20, 459.89, 459.9, 530.21, 530.7, 530.82, 531.00, 531.01, 531.10, 531.11, 531.20, 531.21, 531.30, 531.31, 531.40, 531.41, 531.50, 531.51, 531.60, 531.61, 531.70, 531.71, 531.90, 531.91, 532.00, 532.01, 532.10, 532.11, 532.20, 532.21, 532.30, 532.31, 532.40, 532.41, 532.50, 532.51, 532.60, 532.61, 532.70, 532.71, 532.90, 532.91, 533.00, 533.01, 533.10, 533.11, 533.20, 533.21, 533.30, 533.31, 533.40, 533.41, 533.50, 533.51, 533.60, 533.61, 533.70, 533.71, 533.90, 533.91, 534.00, 534.01, 534.10, 534.11, 534.20, 534.21, 534.30, 534.31, 534.40, 534.41, 534.50, 534.51, 534.61, 534.70, 534.71, 534.90, 534.91, 535.01, 535.10, 535.11, 535.21, 535.31, 535.41, 535.51, 535.61, 537.83, 537.84, 562.02, 562.03, 562.12, 562.13, 569.3, 569.85, 569.86, 578.0, 578.1, 578.9
AHA: 1Q 2005, 17

530.83 Esophageal leukoplakia

530.84 Tracheoesophageal fistula
Excludes *congenital tracheoesophageal fistula (750.3)*
C&C Exclusions: 530.4, 530.7, 530.81, 530.83, 530.84, 530.89, 530.9

530.85 Barrett's esophagus
C&C Exclusions: See 530.20
AHA: 4Q 2003, 63

530.86 Infection of esophagostomy
Use additional code to specify infection

530.87 Mechanical complication of esophagostomy
Malfunction of esophagostomy

530.89 Other
Excludes *Paterson-Kelly syndrome (280.8)*

✖ **530.9 Unspecified disorder of esophagus**

4 **531 Gastric ulcer**
Includes ulcer (peptic):
- prepyloric
- pylorus
- stomach

Use additional E code to identify drug, if drug-induced
Excludes *peptic ulcer NOS (533.0-533.9)*
AHA: 1Q 1991, 15; 4Q 1990, 27

The following fifth-digit subclassification is for use with category 531:
0 without mention of obstruction
1 with obstruction

5 **531.0 Acute with hemorrhage**
C&C Exclusions: 251.5, 456.0, 530.21, 530.7, 530.82, 531.00, 531.01, 531.10, 531.11, 531.20, 531.21, 531.30, 531.31, 531.40, 531.41, 531.50, 531.51, 531.60, 531.61, 531.70, 531.71, 531.90, 531.91, 532.00, 532.01, 532.10, 532.11, 532.20, 532.21, 532.30, 532.31, 532.40, 532.41, 532.50, 532.51, 532.60, 532.61, 532.70, 532.71, 532.90, 532.91, 533.00, 533.01, 533.10, 533.11, 533.20, 533.21, 533.30, 533.31, 533.40, 533.41, 533.50, 533.51, 533.60, 533.61, 533.70, 533.71, 533.90, 533.91, 534.00, 534.01, 534.10, 534.11, 534.20, 534.21, 534.30, 534.31, 534.40, 534.41, 534.50, 534.51, 534.60, 534.61, 534.70, 534.71, 534.90, 534.91, 535.01, 535.11, 535.21, 535.31, 535.41, 535.51, 535.61, 537.83, 537.84, 537.89, 537.9, 562.02, 562.03, 562.12, 562.13, 569.3, 569.85, 569.86, 578.0, 578.1, 578.9
AHA: Nov-Dec 1984, 15

5 **531.1 Acute with perforation**
C&C Exclusions: See 531.0

5 **531.2 Acute with hemorrhage and perforation**
C&C Exclusions: See 531.0

5 **531.3 Acute without mention of hemorrhage or perforation**
C&C Exclusions: See 531.0

Digestive System

530.21 – 531.3

A Adult (15+ years) M Maternity (12-55 years) N Newborn (0 years) P Pediatric (0-17 years) ♂ Male ♀ Female 2 Medicare Secondary Payer

531.4 Chronic or unspecified with hemorrhage
C&C Exclusions: See 531.0
AHA: 4Q 1990, 22

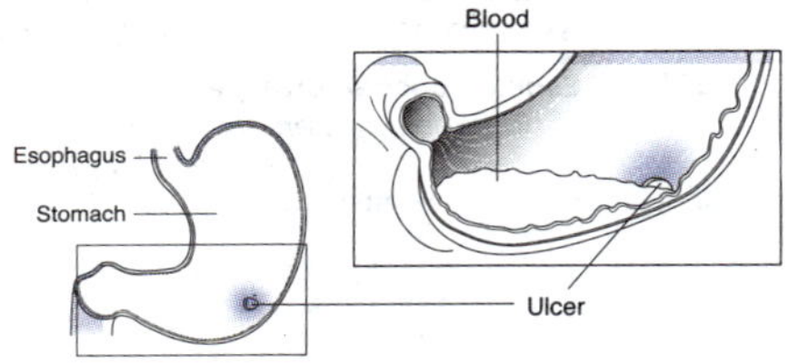

531.5 Chronic or unspecified with perforation
C&C Exclusions: See 531.0

531.6 Chronic or unspecified with hemorrhage and perforation
C&C Exclusions: See 531.0

531.7 Chronic without mention of hemorrhage or perforation
C&C Exclusions: See 531.0

531.9 Unspecified as acute or chronic, without mention of hemorrhage or perforation
C&C Exclusions: See 531.0

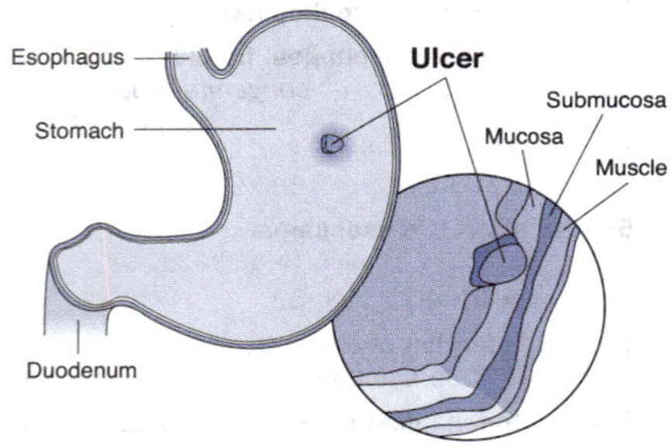

532 Duodenal ulcer
Includes erosion (acute) of duodenum
ulcer (peptic):
duodenum
postpyloric
Use additional E code to identify drug, if drug-induced
Excludes *peptic ulcer NOS (533.0-533.9)*
AHA: 4Q 1990, 27; 1Q 1991, 15

The following fifth-digit subclassification is for use with category 532:
0 without mention of obstruction
1 with obstruction

532.0 Acute with hemorrhage
C&C Exclusions: 251.5, 456.0, 530.21, 530.7, 530.82, 531.00, 531.01, 531.10, 531.11, 531.20, 531.21, 531.30, 531.31, 531.40, 531.41, 531.50, 531.51, 531.60, 531.61, 531.70, 531.71, 531.90, 531.91, 532.00, 532.01, 532.10, 532.11, 532.20, 532.21, 532.30, 532.31, 532.40, 532.41, 532.50, 532.51, 532.60, 532.61, 532.70, 532.71, 532.90, 532.91, 533.00, 533.01, 533.10, 533.11, 533.20, 533.21, 533.30, 533.31, 533.40, 533.41, 533.50, 533.51, 533.60, 533.61, 533.70, 533.71, 533.90, 533.91, 534.00, 534.01, 534.10, 534.11, 534.20, 534.21, 534.30, 534.31, 534.40, 534.41, 534.50, 534.51, 534.60, 534.61, 534.70, 534.71, 534.90, 534.91, 535.01, 535.11, 535.21, 535.31, 535.41, 535.51, 535.61, 537.3, 537.83, 537.84, 537.89, 537.9, 562.02, 562.03, 562.12, 562.13, 569.3, 569.85, 569.86, 578.0, 578.1, 578.9
AHA: 4Q 1990, 22

532.1 Acute with perforation
C&C Exclusions: See 532.0

532.2 Acute with hemorrhage and perforation
C&C Exclusions: See 532.0

532.3 Acute without mention of hemorrhage or perforation
C&C Exclusions: See 532.0

532.4 Chronic or unspecified with hemorrhage
C&C Exclusions: See 532.0

532.5 Chronic or unspecified with perforation
C&C Exclusions: See 532.0

532.6 Chronic or unspecified with hemorrhage and perforation
C&C Exclusions: See 532.0

532.7 Chronic without mention of hemorrhage or perforation
C&C Exclusions: See 532.0

532.9 Unspecified as acute or chronic, without mention of hemorrhage or perforation
C&C Exclusions: See 532.0

533 Peptic ulcer, site unspecified
Includes gastroduodenal ulcer NOS
peptic ulcer NOS
stress ulcer NOS
Use additional E code to identify drug, if drug-induced
Excludes *peptic ulcer:*
duodenal (532.0-532.9)
gastric (531.0-531.9)
AHA: 1Q 1991, 15; 4Q 1990, 27

The following fifth-digit subclassification is for use with category 533:
0 without mention of obstruction
1 with obstruction

533.0 Acute with hemorrhage
C&C Exclusions: 251.5, 456.0, 530.21, 530.7, 530.82, 531.00, 531.01, 531.10, 531.11, 531.20, 531.21, 531.30, 531.31, 531.40, 531.41, 531.50, 531.51, 531.60, 531.61, 531.70, 531.71, 531.90, 531.91, 532.00, 532.01, 532.10, 532.11, 532.20, 532.21, 532.30, 532.31, 532.40, 532.41, 532.50, 532.51, 532.60, 532.61, 532.70, 532.71, 532.90, 532.91, 533.00, 533.01, 533.10, 533.11, 533.20, 533.21, 533.30, 533.31, 533.40, 533.41, 533.50, 533.51, 533.60, 533.61, 533.70, 533.71, 533.90, 533.91, 534.00, 534.01, 534.10, 534.11, 534.20, 534.21, 534.30, 534.31, 534.40, 534.41, 534.50, 534.51, 534.60, 534.61, 534.70, 534.71, 534.90, 534.91, 535.01, 535.11, 535.21, 535.31, 535.41, 535.51, 535.61, 537.83, 537.84, 537.89, 537.9, 562.02, 562.03, 562.12, 562.13, 569.3, 569.85, 569.86, 578.0, 578.1, 578.9

533.1 Acute with perforation
C&C Exclusions: See 533.0

533.2 Acute with hemorrhage and perforation
C&C Exclusions: See 533.0

533.3 Acute without mention of hemorrhage and perforation
C&C Exclusions: See 533.0

533.4 Chronic or unspecified with hemorrhage
C&C Exclusions: See 533.0

533.5 Chronic or unspecified with perforation
C&C Exclusions: See 533.0

533.6 Chronic or unspecified with hemorrhage and perforation
C&C Exclusions: See 533.0

533.7 Chronic without mention of hemorrhage or perforation
C&C Exclusions: See 533.0
AHA: 2Q 1989, 16

533.9 Unspecified as acute or chronic, without mention of hemorrhage or perforation
C&C Exclusions: See 533.0

534 Gastrojejunal ulcer

Includes ulcer (peptic) or erosion:
anastomotic
gastrocolic
gastrointestinal
gastrojejunal
jejunal
marginal
stomal

Excludes *primary ulcer of small intestine (569.82)*

AHA: 1Q 1991, 15; 4Q 1990, 27

The following fifth-digit subclassification is for use with category 534:
0 without mention of obstruction
1 with obstruction

534.0 Acute with hemorrhage
C&C Exclusions: 251.5, 456.0, 530.21, 530.7, 530.82, 531.00, 531.01, 531.10, 531.11, 531.20, 531.21, 531.30, 531.31, 531.40, 531.41, 531.50, 531.51, 531.60, 531.61, 531.70, 531.71, 531.90, 531.91, 532.00, 532.01, 532.10, 532.11, 532.20, 532.21, 532.30, 532.31, 532.40, 532.41, 532.50, 532.51, 532.60, 532.61, 532.70, 532.71, 532.90, 532.91, 533.00, 533.01, 533.10, 533.11, 533.20, 533.21, 533.30, 533.31, 533.40, 533.41, 533.50, 533.51, 533.60, 533.61, 533.70, 533.71, 533.90, 533.91, 534.00, 534.01, 534.10, 534.11, 534.20, 534.21, 534.30, 534.31, 534.40, 534.41, 534.50, 534.51, 534.60, 534.61, 534.70, 534.71, 534.90, 534.91, 535.01, 535.11, 535.21, 535.31, 535.41, 535.51, 535.61, 537.83, 537.84, 537.89, 537.9, 562.02, 562.03, 562.12, 562.13, 569.3, 569.85, 569.86 578.0, 578.1, 578.9

534.1 Acute with perforation
C&C Exclusions: See 534.0

534.2 Acute with hemorrhage and perforation
C&C Exclusions: See 534.0

534.3 Acute without mention of hemorrhage or perforation
C&C Exclusions: See 534.0

534.4 Chronic or unspecified with hemorrhage
C&C Exclusions: See 534.0

534.5 Chronic or unspecified with perforation
C&C Exclusions: See 534.0

534.6 Chronic or unspecified with hemorrhage and perforation
C&C Exclusions: See 534.0

534.7 Chronic without mention of hemorrhage or perforation
C&C Exclusions: See 534.0

534.9 Unspecified as acute or chronic, without mention of hemorrhage or perforation
C&C Exclusions: See 534.0

535 Gastritis and duodenitis
AHA: 2Q 1992, 9; 4Q 1991, 25

The following fifth-digit subclassification is for use with category 535:
0 without mention of hemorrhage
1 with hemorrhage

535.0 Acute gastritis
C&C Exclusions: (for code 535.01) 251.5, 456.0, 530.21, 530.7, 530.82, 531.00, 531.01, 531.10, 531.11, 531.20, 531.21, 531.30, 531.31, 531.40, 531.41, 531.50, 531.51, 531.60, 531.61, 531.70, 531.71, 531.90, 531.91, 532.00, 532.01, 532.10, 532.11, 532.20, 532.21, 532.30, 532.31, 532.40, 532.41, 532.50, 532.51, 532.60, 532.61, 532.70, 532.71, 532.90, 532.91, 533.00, 533.01, 533.10, 533.11, 533.20, 533.21, 533.30, 533.31, 533.40, 533.41, 533.50, 533.51, 533.60, 533.61, 533.70, 533.71, 533.90, 533.91, 534.00, 534.01, 534.10, 534.11, 534.20, 534.21, 534.30, 534.31, 534.40, 534.41, 534.50, 534.51, 534.60, 534.61, 534.70, 534.71, 534.90, 534.91, 535.01, 535.11, 535.21, 535.31, 535.41, 535.51, 535.61, 537.83, 537.84, 562.02, 562.03, 562.12, 562.13, 569.3, 569.85, 569.86, 578.0, 578.1, 578.9
AHA: 2Q 1992, 8; Nov-Dec 1986, 9

535.1 Atrophic gastritis
Gastritis:
atrophic-hyperplastic
chronic (atrophic)
C&C Exclusions: (for code 535.11) See 535.0
AHA: 1Q 1994, 18

535.2 Gastric mucosal hypertrophy
Hypertrophic gastritis
DEF: Overgrowth of the lining of the stomach, causing nausea and vomiting, pain and swelling, loss of appetite and weight.
C&C Exclusions: (for code 535.21) See 535.0

535.3 Alcoholic gastritis
C&C Exclusions: (for code 535.31) See 535.0

535.4 Other specified gastritis
Gastritis:
allergic
bile induced
irritant
superficial
toxic
C&C Exclusions: (for code 535.41) See 535.0
AHA: 4Q 1990, 27

535.5 Unspecified gastritis and gastroduodenitis
C&C Exclusions: (for code 535.51) See 535.0
AHA: For Code 535.50: 3Q 2005, 17; 4Q 1999, 25

535.6 Duodenitis
C&C Exclusions: (for code 535.61) See 535.0
AHA: For Code 535.60: 3Q 2005, 17

536 Disorders of function of stomach
Excludes *functional disorders of stomach specified as psychogenic (306.4)*

536.0 Achlorhydria
DEF: Absence of hydrochloric acid in the stomach's gastric secretions, most often from antibodies against cells producing gastric acid, or a symptom of *H. pylori* infection, atrophic gastritis, or cancer.

536.1 Acute dilatation of stomach
Acute distention of stomach
DEF: Distention of the stomach due to excessive gas build-up or bowel obstruction, preventing passage of food.
C&C Exclusions: 536.1

536.2 Persistent vomiting
Habit vomiting
Persistent vomiting [not of pregnancy]
Uncontrollable vomiting
Excludes *excessive vomiting in pregnancy (643.0-643.9)*
vomiting NOS (787.0)

+ ***536.3 Gastroparesis***
Gastroparalysis
▶ *Code first underlying disease, such as:*◀
▶ diabetes mellitus (250.6)◀
AHA: 2Q 2004, 7; 2Q 2001, 4; 4Q 1994, 42

536.4 Gastrostomy complications
AHA: 4Q 1998, 42

536.40 Gastrostomy complication, unspecified
C&C Exclusions: 536.40, 536.41, 536.42, 536.49, 997.4, 997.71, 997.91, 997.99, 998.81, 998.83, 998.9

536.41 Infection of gastrostomy
Use additional code to identify type of infection, such as:
abscess or cellulitis of abdomen (682.2)
septicemia (038.0-038.9)
Use additional code to identify organism (041.00-041.9)
C&C Exclusions: See 536.40
AHA: 4Q 1998, 42

536.42 Mechanical complication of gastrostomy
C&C Exclusions: See 536.40

536.49 Other gastrostomy complications
C&C Exclusions: See 536.40
AHA: 4Q 1998, 42

Digestive System

534 – 536.49

A Adult (15+ years) M Maternity (12-55 years) N Newborn (0 years) P Pediatric (0-17 years) ♂ Male ♀ Female ❷ Medicare Secondary Payer

536.8 Dyspepsia and other specified disorders of function of stomach
Achylia gastrica
Hourglass contraction of stomach
Hyperacidity
Hyperchlorhydria
Hypochlorhydria
Indigestion
Tachygastria
Excludes *achlorhydria (536.0)*
heartburn (787.1)
AHA: 2Q 1993, 6; 2Q 1989, 16; Nov-Dec 1984, 9

536.9 Unspecified functional disorder of stomach
Functional gastrointestinal:
disorder
disturbance
irritation

④ 537 Other disorders of stomach and duodenum

537.0 Acquired hypertrophic pyloric stenosis
Constriction of pylorus, acquired or adult
Obstruction of pylorus, acquired or adult
Stricture of pylorus, acquired or adult
Excludes *congenital or infantile pyloric stenosis (750.5)*
C&C Exclusions: 536.3, 536.8, 536.9, 537.0, 537.3, 750.5, 750.8, 750.9, 751.1, 751.5
AHA: 2Q 2001, 4; Jan-Feb 1985, 14

537.1 Gastric diverticulum
Excludes *congenital diverticulum of stomach (750.7)*
AHA: Jan-Feb 1985, 4

537.2 Chronic duodenal ileus

537.3 Other obstruction of duodenum
Cicatrix of duodenum
Stenosis of duodenum
Stricture of duodenum
Volvulus of duodenum
Excludes *congenital obstruction of duodenum (751.1)*
C&C Exclusions: 537.3, 750.8, 750.9, 751.1, 751.5

537.4 Fistula of stomach or duodenum
Gastrocolic fistula
Gastrojejunocolic fistula
C&C Exclusions: 537.4, 750.8, 750.9, 751.5

537.5 Gastroptosis
DEF: Abnormal downward displacement of the stomach from its normal position below the diaphragm into the lower abdomen.

537.6 Hourglass stricture or stenosis of stomach
Cascade stomach
Excludes *congenital hourglass stomach (750.7)*
hourglass contraction of stomach (536.8)

⑤ 537.8 Other specified disorders of stomach and duodenum
AHA: 4Q 1991, 25

537.81 Pylorospasm
Excludes *congenital pylorospasm (750.5)*

537.82 Angiodysplasia of stomach and duodenum without mention of hemorrhage
AHA: 3Q 1996, 10; 4Q 1990, 4

537.83 Angiodysplasia of stomach and duodenum with hemorrhage
C&C Exclusions: 251.5, 456.0, 530.21, 530.7, 530.82, 531.00, 531.01, 531.10, 531.11, 531.20, 531.21, 531.30, 531.31, 531.40, 531.41, 531.50, 531.51, 531.60, 531.61, 531.70, 531.71, 531.90, 531.91, 532.00, 532.01, 532.10, 532.11, 532.20, 532.21, 532.30, 532.31, 532.40, 532.41, 532.50, 532.51, 532.60, 532.61, 532.70, 532.71, 532.90, 532.91, 533.00, 533.01, 533.10, 533.11, 533.20, 533.21, 533.30, 533.31, 533.40, 533.41, 533.50, 533.51, 533.60, 533.61, 533.70, 533.71, 533.90, 533.91, 534.00, 534.01, 534.10, 534.11, 534.20, 534.21, 534.30, 534.31, 534.40, 534.41, 534.50, 534.51, 534.60, 534.61, 534.70, 534.71, 534.90, 534.91, 535.01, 535.11, 535.21, 535.31, 535.41, 535.51, 535.61, 537.83, 537.84, 562.02, 562.03, 562.12, 562.13, 569.3, 569.85, 569.86, 578.0, 578.1, 578.9

537.84 Dieulafoy lesion (hemorrhagic) of stomach and duodenum
DEF: Abnormality of arteriole within the digestive tract protruding through a tiny mucosal defect, usually near the gastroesophageal junction, that can cause massive gastrointestinal bleeding.
C&C Exclusions: 251.5, 530.21, 530.7, 530.82, 531.00, 531.01, 531.10, 531.11, 531.20, 531.21, 531.30, 531.31, 531.40, 531.41, 531.50, 531.51, 531.60, 531.61, 531.70, 531.71, 531.90, 531.91, 532.00, 532.01, 532.10, 532.11, 532.20, 532.21, 532.30, 532.31, 532.40, 532.41, 532.50, 532.51, 532.60, 532.61, 532.70, 532.71, 532.90, 532.91, 533.00, 533.01, 533.10, 533.11, 533.20, 533.21, 533.30, 533.31, 533.40, 533.41, 533.50, 533.51, 533.60, 533.61, 533.70, 533.71, 533.90, 533.91, 534.00, 534.01, 534.10, 534.11, 534.20, 534.21, 534.30, 534.31, 534.40, 534.41, 534.50, 534.51, 534.60, 534.61, 534.70, 534.71, 534.90, 534.91, 535.01, 535.11, 535.21, 535.31, 535.41, 535.51, 535.61, 537.83, 537.84, 562.02, 562.03, 562.12, 562.13, 569.3, 569.85, 569.86, 578.0, 578.1, 578.9
AHA: 4Q 2002, 60

537.89 Other
Gastric or duodenal:
prolapse
rupture
Intestinal metaplasia of gastric mucosa
Passive congestion of stomach
Excludes *diverticula of duodenum (562.00-562.01)*
gastrointestinal hemorrhage (578.0-578.9)
C&C Exclusions: 530.21
AHA: 3Q 2005, 15; Nov-Dec 1984, 7

✖ 537.9 Unspecified disorder of stomach and duodenum
C&C Exclusions: See 537.89

538 Gastrointestinal mucositis (ulcerative)
Use additional E code to identify adverse effects of therapy, such as:
antineoplastic and immunosuppressive drugs (E930.7, E933.1)
radiation therapy (E879.2)
Excludes *mucositis (ulcerative) of mouth and oral soft tissue (528.00-528.09)*
C&C Exclusions: 527.3, 527.4, 530.21, 531.00, 531.01, 531.10, 531.11, 531.20, 531.21, 531.30, 531.31, 531.40, 531.41, 531.50, 531.51, 531.60, 531.61, 531.71, 531.91, 532.00, 532.01, 532.10, 532.11, 532.20, 532.21, 532.30, 532.31, 532.40, 532.41, 532.50, 532.51, 532.60, 532.61, 532.71, 532.91, 533.00, 533.01, 533.10, 533.11, 533.20, 533.21, 533.31, 533.40, 533.41, 533.50, 533.51, 533.60, 533.61, 533.71, 533.91, 534.00, 534.01, 534.10, 534.11, 534.20, 534.21, 534.31, 534.40, 534.41, 534.50, 534.51, 534.60, 534.61, 534.71, 534.91, 540.0, 540.1, 540.9, 550.00, 550.01, 550.02, 550.03, 550.10, 550.11, 550.12, 550.13, 551.00, 551.01, 551.02, 551.03, 551.1, 551.20, 551.21, 551.29, 551.8, 551.9, 552.00, 552.01, 552.02, 552.03

APPENDICITIS (540-543)

❹ **540 Acute appendicitis**
AHA: Nov-Dec 1984, 19

540.0 With generalized peritonitis
Appendicitis (acute) with: perforation, peritonitis (generalized), rupture:
- fulminating
- gangrenous
- obstructive

Cecitis (acute) with: perforation, peritonitis (generalized), rupture
Rupture of appendix
Excludes *acute appendicitis with peritoneal abscess (540.1)*
C&C Exclusions: 537.89, 537.9, 540.0, 540.1, 540.9, 541, 542, 543.0, 543.9

540.1 With peritoneal abscess
Abscess of appendix
With generalized peritonitis
C&C Exclusions: See 540.0
AHA: Nov-Dec 1984, 19

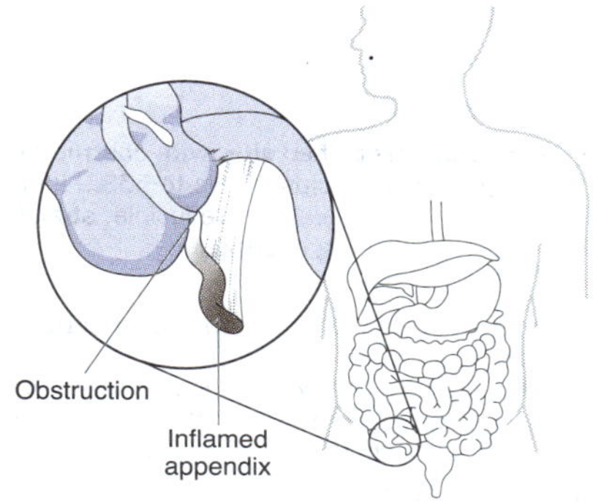

540.9 Without mention of peritonitis
Acute:
appendicitis without mention of perforation, peritonitis, or rupture:
- fulminating
- gangrenous
- inflamed
- obstructive

cecitis without mention of perforation, peritonitis, or rupture
C&C Exclusions: See 540.0
AHA: 1Q 2001, 15; 4Q 1997, 52

541 Appendicitis, unqualified
AHA: 2Q 1990, 26

542 Other appendicitis
Appendicitis:
- chronic
- recurrent
- relapsing
- subacute

Excludes *hyperplasia (lymphoid) of appendix (543.0)*
AHA: 1Q 2001, 15

❹ **543 Other diseases of appendix**

543.0 Hyperplasia of appendix (lymphoid)

543.9 Other and unspecified diseases of appendix
Appendicular or appendiceal:
- colic
- concretion
- fistula

Diverticulum of appendix
Fecalith of appendix
Intussusception of appendix
Mucocele of appendix
Stercolith of appendix

HERNIA OF ABDOMINAL CAVITY (550-553)

Includes hernia:
- acquired
- congenital, except diaphragmatic or hiatal

❹ **550 Inguinal hernia**
Includes bubonocele
inguinal hernia (direct) (double) (indirect) (oblique) (sliding)
scrotal hernia
DEF: Weakness in the muscles in the groin area between the abdomen and thigh, allowing part of the intestine to bulge through the muscle wall.
AHA: Nov-Dec 1985, 12

The following fifth-digit subclassification is for use with category 550:
- **0 unilateral or unspecified (not specified as recurrent)**
  Unilateral NOS
- **1 unilateral or unspecified, recurrent**
- **2 bilateral (not specified as recurrent)**
  Bilateral NOS
- **3 bilateral, recurrent**

❺ **550.0 Inguinal hernia, with gangrene**
Inguinal hernia with gangrene (and obstruction)
C&C Exclusions: 537.89, 537.9, 550.00, 550.01, 550.02, 550.03, 550.10, 550.11, 550.12, 550.13, 550.90, 550.91, 550.92, 550.93, 552.8, 552.9, 553.8, 553.9

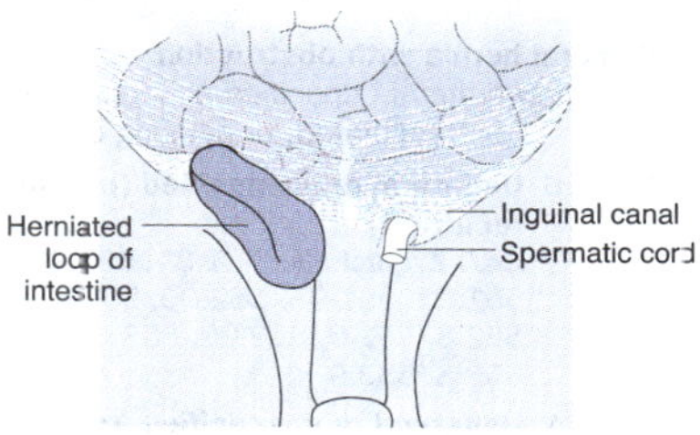

❺ **550.1 Inguinal hernia, with obstruction, without mention of gangrene**
Inguinal hernia with mention of incarceration, irreducibility, or strangulation
C&C Exclusions: See 550.0

❺ **550.9 Inguinal hernia, without mention of obstruction or gangrene**
Inguinal hernia NOS
AHA: For Code 550.91: 3Q 2003, 10; 1Q 2003, 4

❹ **551 Other hernia of abdominal cavity, with gangrene**
Includes that with gangrene (and obstruction)

❺ **551.0 Femoral hernia with gangrene**

551.00 Unilateral or unspecified (not specified as recurrent)
Femoral hernia NOS with gangrene
C&C Exclusions: 537.89, 537.9, 551.00, 551.01, 551.02, 551.03, 552.8, 552.9, 553.00, 553.01, 553.02, 553.03, 553.8, 553.9

551.01 Unilateral or unspecified, recurrent
C&C Exclusions: See 551.00

551.02 Bilateral (not specified as recurrent)
C&C Exclusions: See 551.00

551.03 Bilateral, recurrent
C&C Exclusions: See 551.00

551.1 Umbilical hernia with gangrene
Parumbilical hernia specified as gangrenous
C&C Exclusions: 537.89, 537.9, 551.1, 551.20, 551.21, 551.29, 552.1, 552.20, 552.21, 552.29, 552.8, 552.9, 553.1, 553.20, 553.21, 553.29, 553.8, 553.9

❺ **551.2 Ventral hernia with gangrene**

551.20 Ventral, unspecified, with gangrene
C&C Exclusions: See 551.1

551.21 Incisional, with gangrene
Hernia:
- postoperative specified as gangrenous
- recurrent, ventral specified as gangrenous

C&C Exclusions: See 551.1

551.29 Other
Epigastric hernia specified as gangrenous
C&C Exclusions: See 551.1

551.3 Diaphragmatic hernia with gangrene
Hernia:
hiatal (esophageal) (sliding) specified as gangrenous
paraesophageal specified as gangrenous
Thoracic stomach specified as gangrenous
Excludes *congenital diaphragmatic hernia (756.6)*
C&C Exclusions: 551.3, 552.3, 552.8, 552.9, 553.3, 553.8, 553.9

551.8 Hernia of other specified sites, with gangrene
Any condition classifiable to 553.8 if specified as gangrenous
C&C Exclusions: 537.89, 537.9, 550.00, 550.01, 550.02, 550.03, 550.10, 550.11, 550.12, 550.13, 550.90, 550.91, 550.92, 550.93, 551.00, 551.01, 551.02, 551.03, 551.1, 551.20, 551.21, 551.29, 551.3, 551.8, 551.9, 552.00, 552.01, 552.02, 552.03, 552.1, 552.20, 552.21, 552.29, 552.3, 552.8, 552.9, 553.00, 553.01, 553.02, 553.03, 553.1, 553.20, 553.21, 553.29, 553.3, 553.8, 553.9

551.9 Hernia of unspecified site, with gangrene
Any condition classifiable to 553.9 if specified as gangrenous
C&C Exclusions: See 551.8

❹ **552 Other hernia of abdominal cavity, with obstruction, but without mention of gangrene**
Excludes *that with mention of gangrene (551.0-551.9)*

❺ **552.0 Femoral hernia with obstruction**
Femoral hernia specified as incarcerated, irreducible, strangulated, or causing obstruction

552.00 Unilateral or unspecified (not specified as recurrent)
C&C Exclusions: 537.89, 537.9, 551.00, 551.01, 551.02, 551.03, 552.00, 552.01, 552.02, 552.03, 552.8, 552.9, 553.00, 553.01, 553.02, 553.03, 553.8, 553.9

552.01 Unilateral or unspecified, recurrent
C&C Exclusions: See 552.00

552.02 Bilateral (not specified as recurrent)
C&C Exclusions: See 552.00

552.03 Bilateral, recurrent
C&C Exclusions: See 552.00

552.1 Umbilical hernia with obstruction
Parumbilical hernia specified as incarcerated, irreducible, strangulated, or causing obstruction
C&C Exclusions: 551.1, 551.20, 551.21, 551.29, 552.1, 552.20, 552.21, 552.29, 552.8, 552.9, 553.8, 553.9

❺ **552.2 Ventral hernia with obstruction**
Ventral hernia specified as incarcerated, irreducible, strangulated, or causing obstruction

552.20 Ventral, unspecified, with obstruction
C&C Exclusions: See 552.1

552.21 Incisional, with obstruction
Hernia:
postoperative specified as incarcerated, irreducible, strangulated, or causing obstruction
recurrent, ventral specified as incarcerated, irreducible, strangulated, or causing obstruction
C&C Exclusions: See 552.1
AHA: 3Q 2003, 11

552.29 Other
Epigastric hernia specified as incarcerated, irreducible, strangulated, or causing obstruction
C&C Exclusions: See 552.1

552.3 Diaphragmatic hernia with obstruction
Hernia:
hiatal (esophageal) (sliding) specified as incarcerated, irreducible, strangulated, or causing obstruction
paraesophageal specified as incarcerated, irreducible, strangulated, or causing obstruction
Thoracic stomach specified as incarcerated, irreducible, strangulated, or causing obstruction
Excludes *congenital diaphragmatic hernia (756.6)*
C&C Exclusions: 551.3, 552.3, 552.8, 552.9, 553.3, 553.8, 553.9

552.8 Hernia of other specified sites, with obstruction
Any condition classifiable to 553.8 if specified as incarcerated, irreducible, strangulated, or causing obstruction
Excludes *hernia due to adhesion with obstruction (560.81)*
C&C Exclusions: 550.00, 550.01, 550.02, 550.03, 550.10, 550.11, 550.12, 550.13, 550.90, 550.91, 550.92, 550.93, 551.00, 551.01, 551.02, 551.03, 551.1, 551.20, 551.21, 551.29, 551.3, 551.8, 551.9, 552.00, 552.01, 552.02, 552.03, 552.1, 552.20, 552.21, 552.29, 552.3, 552.8, 552.9, 553.00, 553.01, 553.02, 553.03, 553.1, 553.20, 553.21, 553.29, 553.3, 553.8, 553.9
AHA: 1Q 2004, 10

552.9 Hernia of unspecified site, with obstruction
Any condition classifiable to 553.9 if specified as incarcerated, irreducible, strangulated, or causing obstruction
C&C Exclusions: See 552.9

❹ **553 Other hernia of abdominal cavity without mention of obstruction or gangrene**
Excludes *the listed conditions with mention of:*
gangrene (and obstruction) (551.0-551.9)
obstruction (552.0-552.9)

❺ **553.0 Femoral hernia**

553.00 Unilateral or unspecified (not specified as recurrent)
Femoral hernia NOS

553.01 Unilateral or unspecified, recurrent

553.02 Bilateral (not specified as recurrent)

553.03 Bilateral, recurrent

553.1 Umbilical hernia
Parumbilical hernia

❺ **553.2 Ventral hernia**

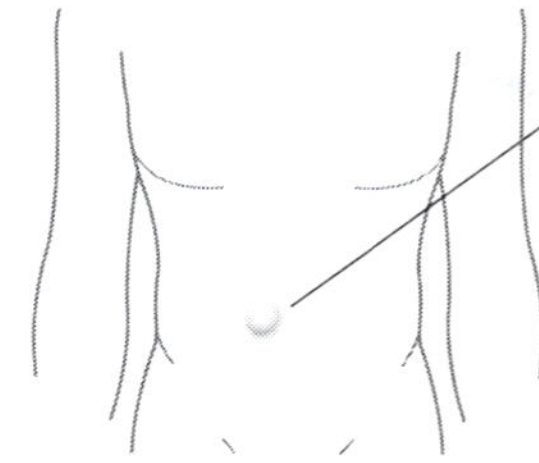

553.20 Ventral, unspecified
AHA: 2Q 2006, 11; 3Q 2003,6

553.21 Incisional
Hernia:
postoperative
recurrent, ventral
AHA: 3Q 2003, 6

553.29 Other
Hernia:
epigastric
spigelian

553.3 Diaphragmatic hernia
Hernia:
hiatal (esophageal) (sliding)
paraesophageal
Thoracic stomach
Excludes *congenital:*
diaphragmatic hernia (756.6)
hiatal hernia (750.6)
esophagocele (530.6)
AHA: 2Q 2001, 6; 1Q 2000, 6

553.8 Hernia of other specified sites
Hernia:
ischiatic
ischiorectal
lumbar
obturator
pudendal
retroperitoneal
sciatic
Other abdominal hernia of specified site
Excludes *vaginal enterocele (618.6)*

✖ **553.9 Hernia of unspecified site**
Enterocele
Epiplocele
Hernia:
NOS
interstitial
intestinal
intra-abdominal
Rupture (nontraumatic)
Sarcoepiplocele

NONINFECTIOUS ENTERITIS AND COLITIS (555-558)

❹ **555 Regional enteritis**
Includes Crohn's disease
Granulomatous enteritis
Excludes *ulcerative colitis (556)*

Regional enteritis
Inflammation of the intestinal tract

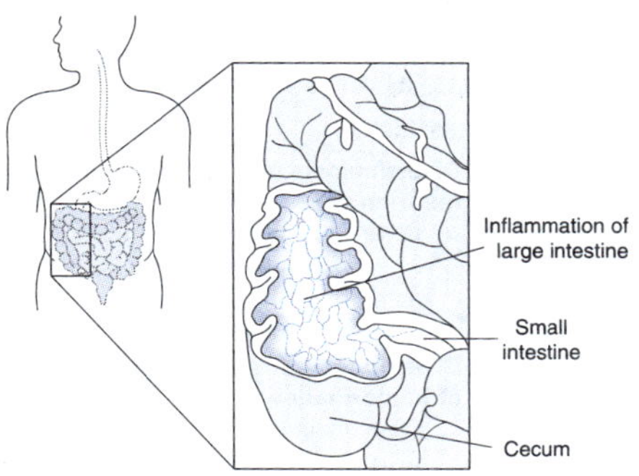

555.0 Small intestine
Ileitis:
regional
segmental
terminal
Regional enteritis or Crohn's disease of:
duodenum
ileum
jejunum

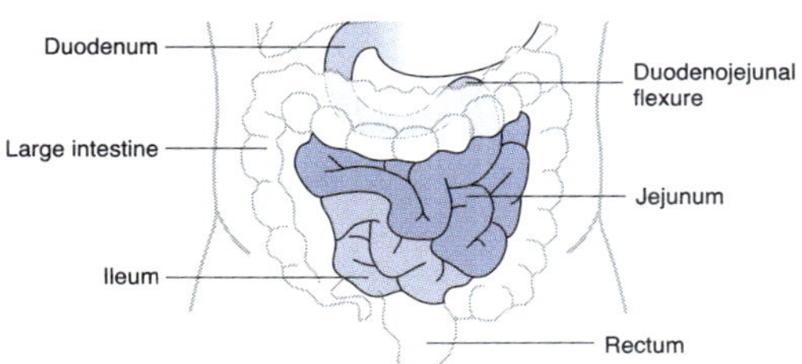

555.1 Large intestine
Colitis:
granulomatous
regional
transmural
Regional enteritis or Crohn's disease of:
colon
large bowel
rectum
AHA: 3Q 1999, 8

555.2 Small intestine with large intestine
Regional ileocolitis
AHA: 1Q 2003, 18

555.9 Unspecified site
Crohn's disease NOS
Regional enteritis NOS
AHA: 2Q 2005, 11; 3Q 1999, 8; 4Q 1997, 42; 2Q 1997, 3

❹ **556 Ulcerative colitis**
DEF: Inflammation of the intestinal lining with ulcer formation, causing diarrhea as the colon empties frequently.

556.0 Ulcerative (chronic) enterocolitis

556.1 Ulcerative (chronic) ileocolitis

556.2 Ulcerative (chronic) proctitis

556.3 Ulcerative (chronic) proctosigmoiditis

556.4 Pseudopolyposis of colon
DEF: Polyp-like localized inflammations of the colon.

556.5 Left-sided ulcerative (chronic) colitis

556.6 Universal ulcerative (chronic) colitis
Pancolitis

556.8 Other ulcerative colitis

556.9 Ulcerative colitis, unspecified
Ulcerative enteritis NOS
AHA: 1Q 2003, 10

❹ **557 Vascular insufficiency of intestine**
Excludes *necrotizing enterocolitis of the newborn (777.5)*

557.0 Acute vascular insufficiency of intestine
Acute:
hemorrhagic enterocolitis
ischemic colitis, enteritis, or enterocolitis
massive necrosis of intestine
Bowel infarction
Embolism of mesenteric artery
Fulminant enterocolitis
Hemorrhagic necrosis of intestine
Infarction of appendices epiploicae
Intestinal gangrene
Intestinal infarction (acute) (agnogenic) (hemorrhagic) (nonocclusive)
Mesenteric infarction (embolic) (thrombotic)
Necrosis of intestine
Terminal hemorrhagic enteropathy
Thrombosis of mesenteric artery
C&C Exclusions: 557.0, 557.1
AHA: 4Q 2001, 53

557.1 Chronic vascular insufficiency of intestine
Angina, abdominal
Chronic ischemic colitis, enteritis, or enterocolitis
Ischemic stricture of intestine
Mesenteric:
angina
artery syndrome (superior)
vascular insufficiency
AHA: 3Q 1996, 9; 4Q 1990, 4; Nov-Dec 1986, 11; Nov-Dec 1984, 7

557.9 Unspecified vascular insufficiency of intestine
Alimentary pain due to vascular insufficiency
Ischemic colitis, enteritis, or enterocolitis NOS

❹ **558 Other and unspecified noninfectious gastroenteritis and colitis**
Excludes *infectious:*
colitis, enteritis, or gastroenteritis (009.0-009.1)
diarrhea (009.2-009.3)

558.1 Gastroenteritis and colitis due to radiation
Radiation enterocolitis
C&C Exclusions: 558.1

558.2 Toxic gastroenteritis and colitis
Use additional E code to identify cause
C&C Exclusions: 558.2

558.3 Allergic gastroenteritis and colitis
Use additional code to identify type of food allergy (V15.01-V15.05)
C&C Exclusions: 008.41, 008.42, 008.43, 008.44, 008.45, 008.46, 008.47, 008.49
AHA: 1Q 2003, 12; 4Q 2000, 42

558.9 Other and unspecified noninfectious gastroenteritis and colitis
Colitis, NOS, dietetic, or noninfectious
Enteritis, NOS, dietetic, or noninfectious
Gastroenteritis, NOS, dietetic, or noninfectious
Ileitis, NOS, dietetic, or noninfectious
Jejunitis, NOS, dietetic, or noninfectious
Sigmoiditis, NOS, dietetic, or noninfectious
AHA: 3Q 1999, 4, 6; Nov-Dec 1987, 7

OTHER DISEASES OF INTESTINES AND PERITONEUM (560-569)

❹ **560 Intestinal obstruction without mention of hernia**
Excludes *duodenum (537.2-537.3)*
inguinal hernia with obstruction (550.1)
intestinal obstruction complicating hernia (552.0-552.9)
mesenteric:
embolism (557.0)
infarction (557.0)
thrombosis (557.0)
neonatal intestinal obstruction (277.01, 777.1-777.2, 777.4)

560.0 Intussusception
Intussusception (colon) (intestine) (rectum)
Invagination of intestine or colon
Excludes *intussusception of appendix (543.9)*
C&C Exclusions: 560.0, 560.1, 560.2, 560.30, 560.31, 560.39, 560.81, 560.89, 560.9, 569.89, 569.9
AHA: 4Q 1998, 82

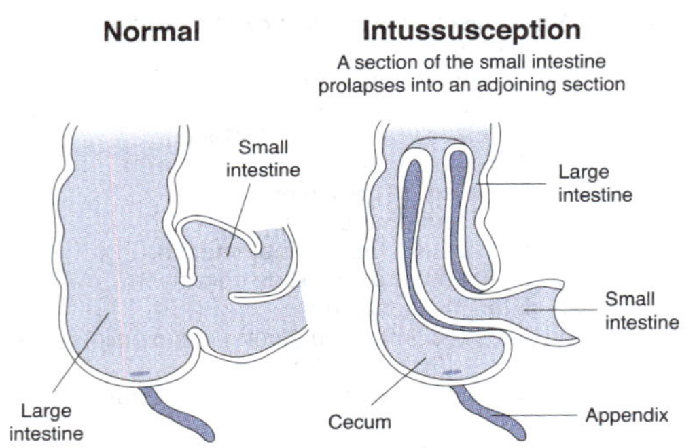

560.1 Paralytic ileus
Adynamic ileus
Ileus (of intestine) (of bowel) (of colon)
Paralysis of intestine or colon
Excludes *gallstone ileus (560.31)*
DEF: Blockage between the small and large intestine due to nonfunctioning muscle wall; may occur due to fluid imbalance, nerve damage, decreased blood supply, or toxins.
C&C Exclusions: See 560.0
AHA: Jan-Feb 1987, 13

560.2 Volvulus
Knotting of intestine, bowel, or colon
Strangulation of intestine, bowel, or colon
Torsion of intestine, bowel, or colon
Twist of intestine, bowel, or colon
DEF: Twisting of the intestine, constricting the passageway and cutting off blood supply to the area; presents with sudden, severe abdominal pain, vomiting, and abdominal distention.
C&C Exclusions: See 560.0

❺ **560.3 Impaction of intestine**

560.30 Impaction of intestine, unspecified
Impaction of colon
C&C Exclusions: See 560.0

560.31 Gallstone ileus
Obstruction of intestine by gallstone
C&C Exclusions: See 560.0

560.39 Other
Concretion of intestine
Enterolith
Fecal impaction
C&C Exclusions: See 560.0
AHA: 4Q 1998, 38

❺ **560.8 Other specified intestinal obstruction**

560.81 Intestinal or peritoneal adhesions with obstruction (postoperative) (postinfection)
Excludes *adhesions without obstruction (568.0)*
C&C Exclusions: See 560.0
AHA: 4Q 1995, 55; 3Q 1995, 6; Nov-Dec 1987, 9

560.89 Other
Acute pseudo-obstruction of intestine
Mural thickening causing obstruction
Excludes *ischemic stricture of intestine (557.1)*
C&C Exclusions: See 560.0
AHA: 2Q 1997, 3; 1Q 1988, 6

560.9 Unspecified intestinal obstruction
Enterostenosis
Obstruction of intestine or colon
Occlusion of intestine or colon
Stenosis of intestine or colon
Stricture of intestine or colon
Excludes *congenital stricture or stenosis of intestine (751.1-751.2)*
C&C Exclusions: See 560.0

❹ **562 Diverticula of intestine**
Use additional code to identify any associated:
peritonitis (567.0-567.9)
Excludes *congenital diverticulum of colon (751.5)*
diverticulum of appendix (543.9)
Meckel's diverticulum (751.0)
AHA: 4Q 1991, 25; Jan-Feb 1985, 1

❺ **562.0 Small intestine**

562.00 Diverticulosis of small intestine (without mention of hemorrhage)
Diverticulosis:
duodenum without mention of diverticulitis
ileum without mention of diverticulitis
jejunum without mention of diverticulitis

562.01 Diverticulitis of small intestine (without mention of hemorrhage)
Diverticulitis (with diverticulosis):
duodenum
ileum
jejunum
small intestine

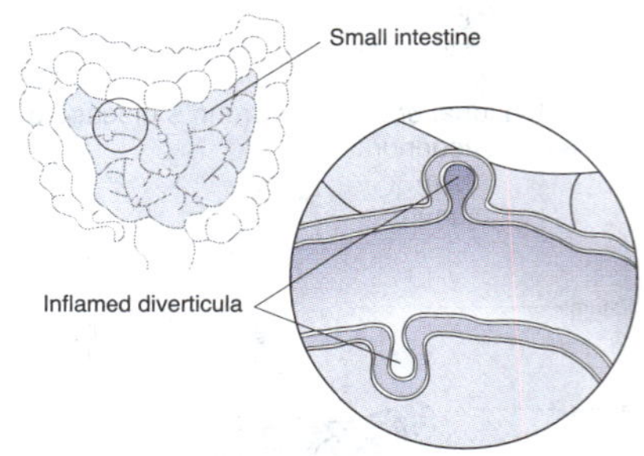

562.02 Diverticulosis of small intestine with hemorrhage
C&C Exclusions: 251.5, 456.0, 530.21, 530.7, 530.82, 531.00, 531.01, 531.10, 531.11, 531.20, 531.21, 531.30, 531.31, 531.40, 531.41, 531.50, 531.51, 531.60, 531.61, 531.70, 531.71, 531.90, 531.91, 532.00, 532.01, 532.10, 532.11, 532.20, 532.21, 532.30, 532.31, 532.40, 532.41, 532.50, 532.51, 532.60, 532.61, 532.70, 532.71, 532.90, 532.91, 533.00, 533.01, 533.10, 533.11, 533.20, 533.21, 533.30, 533.31, 533.40, 533.41, 533.50, 533.51, 533.60, 533.61, 533.70, 533.71, 533.90, 533.91, 534.00, 534.01, 534.10, 534.11, 534.20, 534.21, 534.30, 534.31, 534.40, 534.41, 534.50, 534.51, 534.60, 534.61, 534.70, 534.71, 534.90, 534.91, 535.01, 535.11, 535.21, 535.31, 535.41, 535.51, 535.61, 537.83, 537.84, 562.02, 562.03, 562.12, 562.13, 569.3, 569.85, 569.86, 578.0, 578.1, 578.9

562.03 Diverticulitis of small intestine with hemorrhage
C&C Exclusions: See 562.02

5 **562.1 Colon**
AHA: 3Q 2005, 17; 3Q 2002, 15; 4Q 1990, 21; Jan-Feb 1985, 5

562.10 Diverticulosis of colon (without mention of hemorrhage)
Diverticulosis without mention of diverticulitis:
NOS
intestine (large) without mention of diverticulitis
Diverticular disease (colon) without mention of diverticulitis

562.11 Diverticulitis of colon without mention of hemorrhage
Diverticulitis (with diverticulosis):
NOS
colon
intestine (large)
AHA: 1Q 1996, 14; Jan-Feb 1985, 5

562.12 Diverticulosis of colon with hemorrhage
C&C Exclusions: See 562.02

562.13 Diverticulitis of colon with hemorrhage
C&C Exclusions: See 562.02

4 **564 Functional digestive disorders, not elsewhere classified**
Excludes *functional disorders of stomach (536.0-536.9)*
those specified as psychogenic (306.4)

5 **564.0 Constipation**
Excludes *psychogenic constipation (306.4)*
AHA: 4Q 2001, 45

✖ **564.00 Constipation, unspecified**

564.01 Slow transit constipation
DEF: Dysfunction of intestinal smooth muscles that move matter, causing slow stool movement.

564.02 Outlet dysfunction constipation

564.09 Other constipation

564.1 Irritable bowel syndrome
Irritable colon
Spastic colon
DEF: Functional disorder of hypersensitive nerves and muscles in the colon, causing cramping, pain, diarrhea, and/or constipation.
AHA: 1Q 1988, 6

564.2 Postgastric surgery syndromes
Dumping syndrome
Jejunal syndrome
Postgastrectomy syndrome
Postvagotomy syndrome
Excludes *malnutrition following gastrointestinal surgery (579.3)*
postgastrojejunostomy ulcer (534.0-534.9)
AHA: 1Q 1995, 11

564.3 Vomiting following gastrointestinal surgery
Vomiting (bilious) following gastrointestinal surgery

564.4 Other postoperative functional disorders
Diarrhea following gastrointestinal surgery
Excludes *colostomy and enterostomy complications (569.60-569.69)*

564.5 Functional diarrhea
Excludes *diarrhea:*
NOS (787.91)
psychogenic (306.4)

564.6 Anal spasm
Proctalgia fugax

564.7 Megacolon, other than Hirschsprung's
Dilatation of colon
Excludes *megacolon:*
congenital [Hirschsprung's] (751.3)
toxic (556)

5 **564.8 Other specified functional disorders of intestine**
Excludes *malabsorption (579.0-579.9)*
AHA: 1Q 1988, 6

564.81 Neurogenic bowel
DEF: Intestinal dysfunction due to spinal cord damage.
AHA: 1Q 2001, 12; 4Q 1998, 45

564.89 Other functional disorders of intestine
Atony of colon

✖ **564.9 Unspecified functional disorder of intestine**

4 **565 Anal fissure and fistula**

565.0 Anal fissure
Excludes ▶ *anal sphincter tear (healed) (non-traumatic) (old) (569.43)*◀
traumatic (863.89, 863.99)
DEF: Cut or tear in the tissue lining the anus, causing painful defecation and red blood streaks in stool, especially when passing hard, dry stool.

565.1 Anal fistula
Fistula:
anorectal
rectal
rectum to skin
Excludes *fistula of rectum to internal organs - see Alphabetic Index*
ischiorectal fistula (566)
rectovaginal fistula (619.1)
AHA: 1Q 2007, 13

566 Abscess of anal and rectal regions
Abscess:
ischiorectal
perianal
perirectal
Cellulitis:
anal
perirectal
rectal
Ischiorectal fistula
C&C Exclusions: 566

4 **567 Peritonitis and retroperitoneal infections**
Excludes *peritonitis:*
benign paroxysmal (277.31)
pelvic, female (614.5, 614.7)
periodic familial (277.31)
puerperal (670)
with or following:
abortion (634-638 with .0, 639.0)
appendicitis (540.0-540.1)
ectopic or molar pregnancy (639.0)

+ ***567.0 Peritonitis in infectious diseases classified elsewhere***
Code first underlying disease
Excludes *peritonitis:*
gonococcal (098.86)
syphilitic (095.2)
tuberculous (014.0)
C&C Exclusions: 567.0, 567.1, 567.21, 567.22, 567.23, 567.29, 567.38, 567.39, 567.81, 567.82, 567.89, 567.9, 569.89, 569.9

567.1 Pneumococcal peritonitis
C&C Exclusions: See 567.0

567.2 Other suppurative peritonitis
AHA: 4Q 2005, 74; 2Q 2001, 11-12; 3Q 1999, 9; 2Q 1998, 19

567.21 Peritonitis (acute) generalized
Pelvic peritonitis, male
C&C Exclusions: See 567.0

567.22 Peritoneal abscess
Abscess (of):
- abdominopelvic
- mesenteric
- omentum
- peritoneum
- retrocecal
- subdiaphragmatic
- subhepatic
- subphrenic

C&C Exclusions: See 567.0

567.23 Spontaneous bacterial peritonitis
Excludes *bacterial peritonitis NOS (567.29)*
C&C Exclusions: See 567.0

567.29 Other suppurative peritonitis
Subphrenic peritonitis
C&C Exclusions: See 567.0

567.3 Retroperitoneal infections
AHA: 4Q 2005, 74

567.31 Psoas muscle abscess
C&C Exclusions: 567.31, 728.0, 728.86, 728.88

567.38 Other retroperitoneal abscess
C&C Exclusions: See 567.0
AHA: 4Q 2005, 77

567.39 Other retroperitoneal infections
C&C Exclusions: See 567.0

567.8 Other specified peritonitis
AHA: 4Q 2005, 74

567.81 Choleperitonitis
Peritonitis due to bile
C&C Exclusions: See 567.0

567.82 Sclerosing mesenteritis
Fat necrosis of peritoneum
(Idiopathic) sclerosing mesenteric fibrosis
Mesenteric lipodystrophy
Mesenteric panniculitis
Retractile mesenteritis
DEF: Rare, idiopathic lesions of fat necrosis, fibrosis, and chronic inflammation causing single or multiple lesions, or diffuse thickening of the mesentery.
C&C Exclusions: See 567.0
AHA: 4Q 2005, 77

567.89 Other specified peritonitis
Chronic proliferative peritonitis
Mesenteric saponification
Peritonitis due to urine
C&C Exclusions: See 567.0

567.9 Unspecified peritonitis
Peritonitis:
- NOS
- of unspecified cause

C&C Exclusions: 567.21, 567.22, 567.23, 567.29, 567.38, 567.39, 567.81, 567.82, 567.89
AHA: 1Q 2004, 10

568 Other disorders of peritoneum

568.0 Peritoneal adhesions (postoperative) (postinfection)
Adhesions (of):
- abdominal (wall)
- diaphragm
- intestine
- male pelvis
- mesenteric
- omentum
- stomach

Adhesive bands
Excludes *adhesions:*
pelvic, female (614.6)
with obstruction:
duodenum (537.3)
intestine (560.81)
AHA: 3Q 2003, 7, 11; 4Q 1995, 55; 3Q 1995, 7; Sep-Oct 1985, 11

Peritoneal adhesions

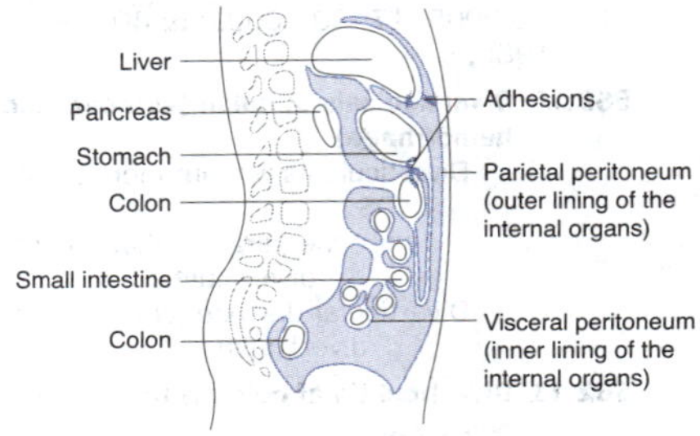

568.8 Other specified disorders of peritoneum

568.81 Hemoperitoneum (nontraumatic)
C&C Exclusions: 568.81

568.82 Peritoneal effusion (chronic)
Excludes *ascites NOS (►789.51-789.59◄)*
DEF: Seepage of fluid other than blood into the peritoneal cavity.

568.89 Other
Peritoneal:
- cyst
- granuloma

568.9 Unspecified disorder of peritoneum

569 Other disorders of intestine

569.0 Anal and rectal polyp
Anal and rectal polyp NOS
Excludes *adenomatous anal and rectal polyp (211.4)*

569.1 Rectal prolapse
Procidentia:
- anus (sphincter)
- rectum (sphincter)

Proctoptosis
Prolapse:
- anal canal
- rectal mucosa

Excludes *prolapsed hemorrhoids (455.2, 455.5)*
DEF: Rectal tissue falls from its usual position, turning itself inside out and protruding from the body in late stages.

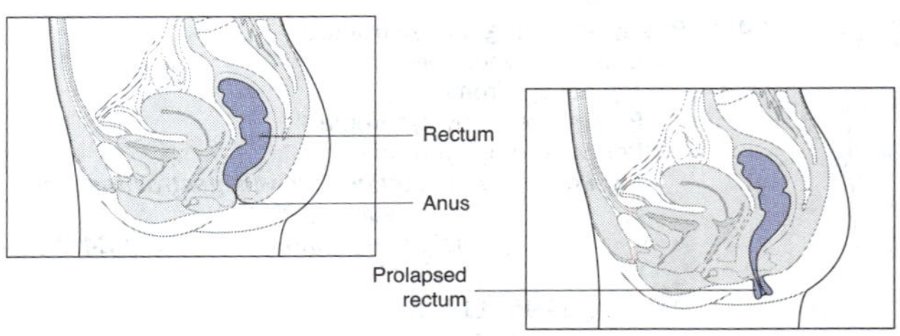

569.2 Stenosis of rectum and anus
Stricture of anus (sphincter)

569.3 Hemorrhage of rectum and anus

Excludes *gastrointestinal bleeding NOS (578.9)*
melena (578.1)

C&C Exclusions: 251.5, 456.0, 530.21, 530.7, 530.82, 531.00, 531.01, 531.10, 531.11, 531.20, 531.21, 531.30, 531.31, 531.40, 531.41, 531.50, 531.51, 531.60, 531.61, 531.70, 531.71, 531.90, 531.91, 532.00, 532.01, 532.10, 532.11, 532.20, 532.21, 532.30, 532.31, 532.40, 532.41, 532.50, 532.51, 532.60, 532.61, 532.70, 532.71, 532.90, 532.91, 533.00, 533.01, 533.10, 533.11, 533.20, 533.21, 533.30, 533.31, 533.40, 533.41, 533.50, 533.51, 533.60, 533.61, 533.70, 533.71, 533.90, 533.91, 534.00, 534.01, 534.10, 534.11, 534.20, 534.21, 534.30, 534.31, 534.40, 534.41, 534.50, 534.51, 534.60, 534.61, 534.70, 534.71, 534.90, 534.91, 535.01, 535.11, 535.21, 535.31, 535.41, 535.51, 535.61, 537.83, 537.84, 562.02, 562.03, 562.12, 562.13, 569.3, 569.85, 569.86, 578.0, 578.1, 578.9

AHA: 3Q 2005, 17

5 **569.4 Other specified disorders of rectum and anus**

569.41 Ulcer of anus and rectum

Solitary ulcer of anus (sphincter) or rectum (sphincter)
Stercoral ulcer of anus (sphincter) or rectum (sphincter)

DEF: Open sore in the rectum and/or causing pain that worsens during defecation and blood or mucous in the stool.

569.42 Anal or rectal pain

AHA: 1Q 2003, 8; 1Q 1996, 13

Tear of anus, nontraumatic
Use additional code for any associated fecal incontinence (787.6)

Excludes *anal fissure (565.0)*
anal sphincter tear (healed) (old) complicating delivery (654.8)

● **569.43 Anal sphincter tear (healed) (old)**

Tear of anus, nontraumatic
Use additional code for any associated fecal incontinence (787.6)

Excludes *anal fissure (565.0)*
anal sphincter tear (healed) (old) complicating delivery (654.8)

569.49 Other

Granuloma of rectum (sphincter)
Hypertrophy of anal papillae
Proctitis NOS
Rupture of rectum (sphincter)

Excludes *fistula of rectum to:*
internal organs - see Alphabetic Index
skin (565.1)
hemorrhoids (455.0-455.9)
incontinence of sphincter ani (787.6)

569.5 Abscess of intestine

Excludes *appendiceal abscess (540.1)*

C&C Exclusions: 569.5

5 **569.6 Colostomy and enterostomy complications**

AHA: 4Q 1995, 58

✖ **569.60 Colostomy and enterostomy complication, unspecified**

C&C Exclusions: 569.60, 569.61, 569.62, 569.69

569.61 Infection of colostomy and enterostomy

Use additional code to specify type of infection, such as:
abscess or cellulitis of abdomen (682.2)
septicemia (038.0-038.9)
Use additional code to identify organism (041.00-041.9)

C&C Exclusions: See 569.60

569.62 Mechanical complication of colostomy and enterostomy

Malfunction of colostomy and enterostomy

C&C Exclusions: 536.40, 536.41, 536.42, 536.49, 569.60, 569.61, 569.62, 569.69, 997.4, 997.71, 997.91, 997.99, 998.81, 998.83, 998.9

AHA: 2Q 2005, 11; 1Q 2003, 10; 4Q 1998, 44

569.69 Other complication

Fistula
Hernia
Prolapse

C&C Exclusions: See 569.60

AHA: 3Q 1998, 16

5 **569.8 Other specified disorders of intestine**

AHA: 4Q 1991, 25

569.81 Fistula of intestine, excluding rectum and anus

Fistula:
abdominal wall
enterocolic
enteroenteric
ileorectal

Excludes *fistula of intestine to internal organs – see Alphabetic Index*
persistent postoperative fistula (998.6)

DEF: Abnormal passageway between loops of the intestine or the intestine and another organ or the abdominal wall.

AHA: 3Q 1999, 8

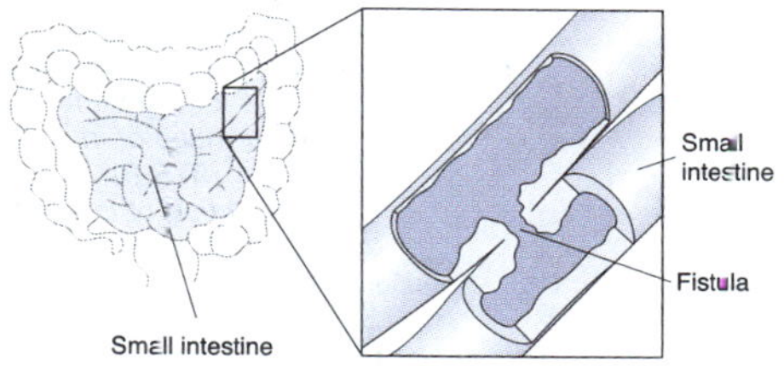

569.82 Ulceration of intestine

Primary ulcer of intestine
Ulceration of colon

Excludes *that with perforation (569.83)*

569.83 Perforation of intestine

DEF: Hole in the intestinal wall allowing food and/or fecal matter to leak into the abdominal cavity.

C&C Exclusions: 569.83

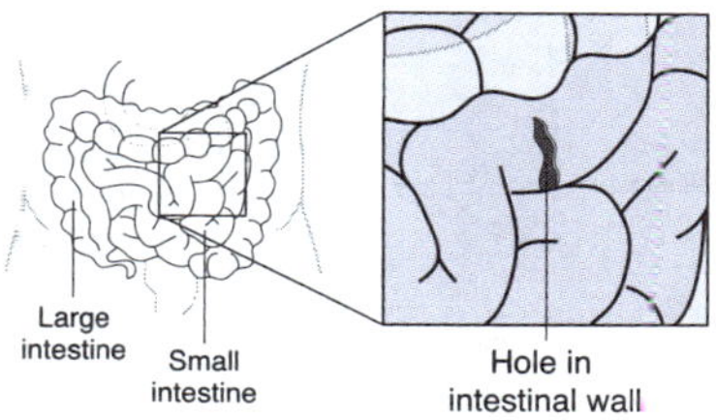

569.84 Angiodysplasia of intestine (without mention of hemorrhage)

AHA: 3Q 1996, 10; 4Q 1990, 4, 21

569.85 Angiodysplasia of intestine with hemorrhage

DEF: Dilated intestinal blood vessels with corresponding thinning and weakening of vessel walls and bleeding into the intestinal tract.

C&C Exclusions: 251.5, 456.0, 530.21, 530.7, 530.82, 531.00, 531.01, 531.10, 531.11, 531.20, 531.21, 531.30, 531.31, 531.40, 531.41, 531.50, 531.51, 531.60, 531.61, 531.70, 531.71, 531.90, 531.91, 532.00, 532.01, 532.10, 532.11, 532.20, 532.21, 532.30, 532.31, 532.40, 532.41, 532.50, 532.51, 532.60, 532.61, 532.70, 532.71, 532.90, 532.91, 533.00, 533.01, 533.10, 533.11, 533.20, 533.21, 533.30, 533.31, 533.40, 533.41, 533.50, 533.51, 533.60, 533.61, 533.70, 533.71, 533.90, 533.91, 534.00, 534.01, 534.10, 534.11, 534.20, 534.21, 534.30, 534.31, 534.40, 534.41, 534.50, 534.51, 534.60, 534.61, 534.70, 534.71, 534.90, 534.91, 535.01, 535.11, 535.21, 535.31, 535.41, 535.51, 535.61, 537.83, 537.84, 562.02, 562.03, 562.12, 562.13, 569.3, 569.85, 569.86, 578.0, 578.1, 578.9

AHA: 3Q 1996, 9

Skin and Subcutaneous Tissue

569.3 – 569.85

A Adult (15+ years) M Maternity (12-55 years) N Newborn (0 years) P Pediatric (0-17 years) ♂ Male ♀ Female 2 Medicare Secondary Payer

569.86 Dieulafoy lesion (hemorrhagic) of intestine
C&C Exclusions: 251.1, 530.2, 530.7, 530.82, 531.00, 531.01, 531.10, 531.11, 531.20, 531.21, 531.30, 531.31, 531.40, 531.41, 531.50, 531.51, 531.60, 531.61, 531.70, 531.71, 531.90, 531.91, 532.00, 532.01, 532.10, 532.11, 532.20, 532.21, 532.30, 532.31, 532.40, 532.41, 532.50, 532.51, 532.60, 532.61, 532.70, 532.71, 532.90, 532.91, 533.00, 533.01, 533.10, 533.11, 533.20, 533.21, 533.30, 533.31, 533.40, 533.41, 533.50, 533.51, 533.60, 533.61, 533.70, 533.71, 533.90, 533.91, 534.00, 534.01, 534.10, 534.11, 534.20, 534.21, 534.30, 534.31, 534.40, 534.41, 534.50, 534.51, 534.60, 534.61, 534.70, 534.71, 534.90, 534.91, 535.01, 535.11, 535.21, 535.31, 535.41, 535.51, 535.61, 537.83, 537.84, 562.02, 562.03, 562.12, 562.13, 569.3, 569.85, 569.86, 578.0, 578.1, 578.9
AHA: 4Q 2002, 60-61

569.89 Other
Enteroptosis
Granuloma of intestine
Pericolitis
Perisigmoiditis
Prolapse of intestine
Visceroptosis
Excludes *gangrene of intestine, mesentery, or omentum (557.0)*
hemorrhage of intestine NOS (578.9)
obstruction of intestine (560.0-560.9)
C&C Exclusions: 567.21, 567.22, 567.23, 567.29, 567.38, 567.39, 567.81, 567.82, 567.89
AHA: 3Q 1996, 3

✖ **569.9 Unspecified disorder of intestine**
C&C Exclusions: See 569.89

OTHER DISEASES OF DIGESTIVE SYSTEM (570-579)

Liver

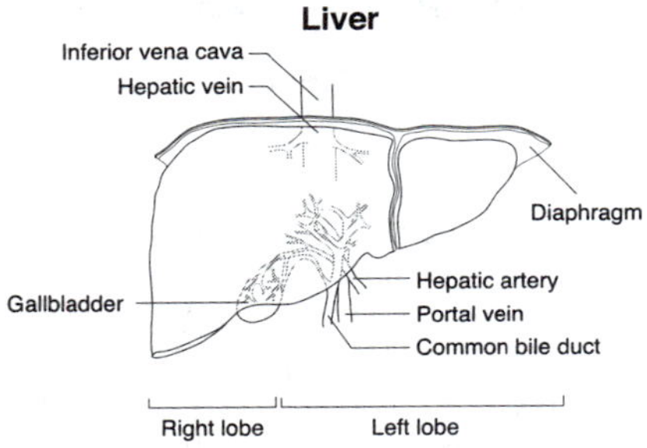

570 Acute and subacute necrosis of liver
Acute hepatic failure
Acute or subacute hepatitis, not specified as infective
Necrosis of liver (acute) (diffuse) (massive) (subacute)
Parenchymatous degeneration of liver
Yellow atrophy (liver) (acute) (subacute)
Excludes *icterus gravis of newborn (773.0-773.2)*
serum hepatitis (070.2-070.3)
that with:
abortion (634-638 with .7, 639.8)
ectopic or molar pregnancy (639.8)
pregnancy, childbirth, or the puerperium (646.7)
viral hepatitis (070.0-070.9)
C&C Exclusions: 570, 573.4, 573.8, 573.9
AHA: 2Q 2005, 9; 1Q 2000, 22

❹ **571 Chronic liver disease and cirrhosis**

571.0 Alcoholic fatty liver [A]
DEF: Accumulation of fats and fatty acids in the liver caused by excessive alcohol consumption.

571.1 Acute alcoholic hepatitis [A]
Acute alcoholic liver disease
AHA: 2Q 2002, 4

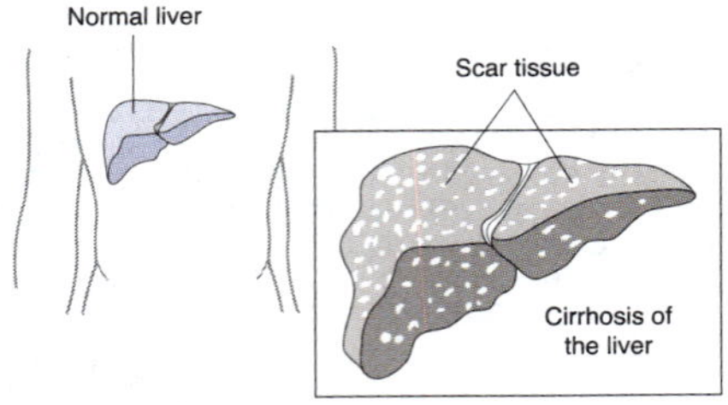

571.2 Alcoholic cirrhosis of liver [A]
Florid cirrhosis
Laennec's cirrhosis (alcoholic)
DEF: Normal, healthy tissue of the liver is replaced by debilitating scar tissue due to long-term, excessive alcohol consumption.
C&C Exclusions: 571.2, 573.8, 573.9
AHA: 2Q 2002, 4; 1Q 2002, 3; Nov-Dec 1985, 14

571.3 Alcoholic liver damage, unspecified [A]

❺ **571.4 Chronic hepatitis**
Excludes *viral hepatitis (acute) (chronic) (070.0-070.9)*

571.40 Chronic hepatitis, unspecified

571.41 Chronic persistent hepatitis

571.49 Other
Chronic hepatitis:
active
aggressive
Recurrent hepatitis
C&C Exclusions: 571.49, 571.5, 571.6, 571.8, 571.9, 573.8, 573.9
AHA: 3Q 1999, 19; Nov-Dec 1985, 14

571.5 Cirrhosis of liver without mention of alcohol
Cirrhosis of liver:
NOS
cryptogenic
macronodular
micronodular
posthepatitic
postnecrotic
Healed yellow atrophy (liver)
Portal cirrhosis
C&C Exclusions: See 571.49

571.6 Biliary cirrhosis
Chronic nonsuppurative destructive cholangitis
Cirrhosis:
cholangitic
cholestatic
DEF: Scar tissue formation of the ducts carrying bile from the liver to the small intestine, resulting in bile build-up and liver damage leading to cirrhosis.
C&C Exclusions: See 571.49

571.8 Other chronic nonalcoholic liver disease
Chronic yellow atrophy (liver)
Fatty liver, without mention of alcohol
AHA: 2Q 1996, 12

571.9 Unspecified chronic liver disease without mention of alcohol

❹ **572 Liver abscess and sequelae of chronic liver disease**

572.0 Abscess of liver
Excludes *amebic liver abscess (006.3)*
C&C Exclusions: 006.3, 572.0, 572.1, 573.8, 573.9

572.1 Portal pyemia
Phlebitis of portal vein
Portal thrombophlebitis
Pylephlebitis
Pylethrombophlebitis
C&C Exclusions: See 572.0

572.2 Hepatic coma
Hepatic encephalopathy
Hepatocerebral intoxication
Portal-systemic encephalopathy
► *Excludes* *hepatic coma associated with viral hepatitis – see category 070*◄
C&C Exclusions: 572.2, 573.8, 573.9
AHA: 2Q 2005, 9; 1Q 2002, 3; 3Q 1995, 14

572.3 Portal hypertension
AHA: 3Q 2005, 15

572.4 Hepatorenal syndrome
Excludes *that following delivery (674.8)*
C&C Exclusions: 572.4, 573.8, 573.9
AHA: 3Q 1993, 15

572.8 Other sequelae of chronic liver disease

④ **573 Other disorders of liver**
Excludes *amyloid or lardaceous degeneration of liver (277.39)*
congenital cystic disease of liver (751.62)
glycogen infiltration of liver (271.0)
hepatomegaly NOS (789.1)
portal vein obstruction (452)

573.0 Chronic passive congestion of liver
DEF: Overly full, distended gallbladder due to accumulation of mucous and watery material rather than stone formation.

+ ***573.1 Hepatitis in viral diseases classified elsewhere***
Code first underlying disease, as:
Coxsackie virus disease (074.8)
cytomegalic inclusion virus disease (078.5)
infectious mononucleosis (075)
Excludes *hepatitis (in):*
mumps (072.71)
viral (070.0-070.9)
yellow fever (060.0-060.9)
C&C Exclusions: 573.1, 573.2, 573.3, 573.8, 573.9

+ ***573.2 Hepatitis in other infectious diseases classified elsewhere***
Code first underlying disease, as:
malaria (084.9)
Excludes *hepatitis in:*
late syphilis (095.3)
secondary syphilis (091.62)
toxoplasmosis (130.5)
C&C Exclusions: See 573.1

573.3 Hepatitis, unspecified
Toxic (noninfectious) hepatitis
Use additional E code to identify cause
C&C Exclusions: See 573.1
AHA: 3Q 1998, 3-4; 4Q 1990, 26

573.4 Hepatic infarction
C&C Exclusions: 570, 573.4, 573.8, 573.9

573.8 Other specified disorders of liver
Hepatoptosis

✖ **573.9 Unspecified disorder of liver**

④ **574 Cholelithiasis**
The following fifth-digit subclassification is for use with category 574:
0 without mention of obstruction
1 with obstruction

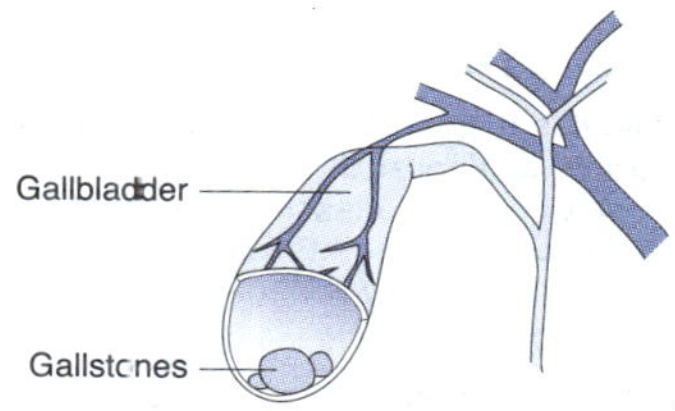

⑤ **574.0 Calculus of gallbladder with acute cholecystitis**
Biliary calculus with acute cholecystitis
Calculus of cystic duct with acute cholecystitis
Cholelithiasis with acute cholecystitis
Any condition classifiable to 574.2 with acute cholecystitis
C&C Exclusions: (for code 574.00) 574.00, 574.01, 574.10, 574.11, 574.20, 574.21, 574.40, 574.60, 574.61, 574.80, 574.81, 575.0, 575.10, 575.11, 575.12, 575.9, 576.8, 576.9
C&C Exclusions: (for code 574.01) 574.00, 574.01, 574.10, 574.11, 574.20, 574.21, 574.60, 574.61, 574.80, 574.81, 575.0, 575.10, 575.11, 575.12, 575.9, 576.8, 576.9
AHA: 4Q 1996, 32

⑤ **574.1 Calculus of gallbladder with other cholecystitis**
Biliary calculus with cholecystitis
Calculus of cystic duct with cholecystitis
Cholelithiasis with cholecystitis
Cholecystitis with cholelithiasis NOS
Any condition classifiable to 574.2 with cholecystitis (chronic)
C&C Exclusions: See 574.0
AHA: 3Q 1999, 9; 4Q 1996, 32, 69; 2Q 1996, 13; For Code 574.10: 1Q 2003, 5

⑤ **574.2 Calculus of gallbladder without mention of cholecystitis**
Biliary:
calculus NOS
colic NOS
Calculus of cystic duct
Cholelithiasis NOS
Colic (recurrent) of gallbladder
Gallstone (impacted)
C&C Exclusions: (for code 574.21) See 574.0
AHA: For Code 574.20: 1Q 1988, 14

⑤ **574.3 Calculus of bile duct with acute cholecystitis**
Calculus of bile duct [any] with acute cholecystitis
Choledocholithiasis with acute cholecystitis
Any condition classifiable to 574.5 with acute cholecystitis
C&C Exclusions: 574.30, 574.31, 574.40, 574.41, 574.50, 574.51, 574.60, 574.61, 574.70, 574.71, 574.80, 574.81, 574.90, 574.91, 575.0, 575.10, 575.11, 575.12, 576.8, 576.9

⑤ **574.4 Calculus of bile duct with other cholecystitis**
Calculus of bile duct [any] with cholecystitis (chronic)
Choledocholithiasis with cholecystitis (chronic)
Any condition classifiable to 574.5 with cholecystitis (chronic)
C&C Exclusions: See 574.3

⑤ **574.5 Calculus of bile duct without mention of cholecystitis**
Calculus of:
bile duct [any]
common duct
hepatic duct
Choledocholithiasis
Hepatic:
colic (recurrent)
lithiasis
C&C Exclusions: See 574.3
AHA: 3Q 1994, 11

⑤ **574.6 Calculus of gallbladder and bile duct with acute cholecystitis**
Any condition classifiable to 574.0 and 574.3
C&C Exclusions: 574.60, 574.61, 575.0, 575.10, 575.11, 575.12, 575.9, 576.8, 576.9
AHA: 4Q 1996, 32

5 **574.7 Calculus of gallbladder and bile duct with other cholecystitis**
Any condition classifiable to 574.1 and 574.4
C&C Exclusions: 574.30, 574.31, 574.40, 574.41, 574.50, 574.51, 574.60, 574.61, 574.70, 574.71, 574.80, 574.81, 574.90, 574.91, 575.0, 575.10, 575.11, 575.12, 576.8, 576.9
AHA: 4Q 1996, 32

5 **574.8 Calculus of gallbladder and bile duct with acute and chronic cholecystitis**
Any condition classifiable to 574.6 and 574.7
C&C Exclusions: 574.80, 574.81, 574.90, 574.91, 575.0, 575.10, 575.11, 575.12, 576.8, 576.9
AHA: 4Q 1996, 32

5 **574.9 Calculus of gallbladder and bile duct without cholecystitis**
Any condition classifiable to 574.2 and 574.5
C&C Exclusions: See 574.7
AHA: 4Q 1996, 32

4 **575 Other disorders of gallbladder**

575.0 Acute cholecystitis
Abscess of gallbladder without mention of calculus
Angiocholecystitis without mention of calculus
Cholecystitis without mention of calculus:
- emphysematous (acute)
- gangrenous
- suppurative

Empyema of gallbladder without mention of calculus
Gangrene of gallbladder without mention of calculus
Excludes *that with:*
- *acute and chronic cholecystitis (575.12)*
- *choledocholithiasis (574.3)*
- *choledocholithiasis and cholelithiasis (574.6)*
- *cholelithiasis (574.0)*

C&C Exclusions: 574.60, 574.61, 574.80, 574.81, 575.0, 575.10, 575.11, 575.12, 575.9, 576.8, 576.9
AHA: 3Q 1991, 17

5 **575.1 Other cholecystitis**
Cholecystitis without mention of calculus:
- NOS without mention of calculus
- chronic without mention of calculus

Excludes *that with:*
- *choledocholithiasis (574.4)*
- *choledocholithiasis and cholelithiasis (574.8)*
- *cholelithiasis (574.1)*

AHA: 4Q 1996, 32

✖ **575.10 Cholecystitis, unspecified**
Cholecystitis NOS

575.11 Chronic cholecystitis

575.12 Acute and chronic cholecystitis
C&C Exclusions: 575.0, 575.10, 575.11, 575.12, 575.9, 576.8, 576.9
AHA: 4Q 1997, 52; 4Q 1996, 32

575.2 Obstruction of gallbladder
Occlusion of cystic duct or gallbladder without mention of calculus
Stenosis of cystic duct or gallbladder without mention of calculus
Stricture of cystic duct or gallbladder without mention of calculus
Excludes *that with calculus (574.0-574.2 with fifth digit 1)*
C&C Exclusions: 575.2, 575.3, 575.4, 575.5, 575.6, 575.8, 575.9, 576.8, 576.9

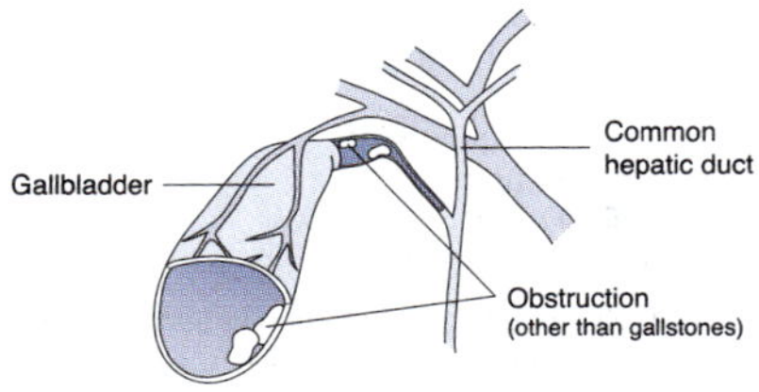

575.3 Hydrops of gallbladder
Mucocele of gallbladder
C&C Exclusions: See 575.2
AHA: 2Q 1989, 13

575.4 Perforation of gallbladder
Rupture of cystic duct or gallbladder
C&C Exclusions: See 575.2

575.5 Fistula of gallbladder
Fistula:
- cholecystoduodenal
- cholecystoenteric

C&C Exclusions: See 575.2

575.6 Cholesterolosis of gallbladder
Strawberry gallbladder
DEF: Build-up of cholesterol deposits on the surface of the gallbladder, giving it a "strawberry" appearance.
AHA: 4Q 1990, 17

575.8 Other specified disorders of gallbladder
Adhesions (of) cystic duct or gallbladder
Atrophy (of) cystic duct or gallbladder
Biliary dyskinesia
Cyst (of) cystic duct or gallbladder
Hypertrophy (of) cystic duct or gallbladder
Nonfunctioning (of) cystic duct or gallbladder
Ulcer (of) cystic duct or gallbladder
Excludes *Hartmann's pouch of intestine (V44.3)*
nonvisualization of gallbladder (793.3)
AHA: 4Q 1990, 26; 2Q 1989, 13

✖ **575.9 Unspecified disorder of gallbladder**

4 **576 Other disorders of biliary tract**
Excludes *that involving the:*
- *cystic duct (575.0-575.9)*
- *gallbladder (575.0-575.9)*

576.0 Postcholecystectomy syndrome
AHA: 1Q 1988, 10

576.1 Cholangitis
Cholangitis:
- NOS
- acute
- ascending
- chronic
- primary
- recurrent
- sclerosing
- secondary
- stenosing
- suppurative

DEF: Infection of the biliary tract; presents with pain in the upper-right abdomen which may grow worse after a fatty meal, fever, nausea, vomiting, flatulence, pale-colored stool, and jaundice (yellowing of the eyes and skin).
C&C Exclusions: 576.1, 576.8, 576.9
AHA: 2Q 1999, 13

576.2 Obstruction of bile duct
Occlusion of bile duct, except cystic duct, without mention of calculus
Stenosis of bile duct, except cystic duct, without mention of calculus
Stricture of bile duct, except cystic duct, without mention of calculus
Excludes *congenital (751.61)*
that with calculus (574.3-574.5 with fifth-digit 1)
AHA: 3Q 2003, 17-18; 1Q 2001, 8; 2Q 1999, 13

576.3 Perforation of bile duct
Rupture of bile duct, except cystic duct
C&C Exclusions: 576.3, 576.4, 576.8, 576.9

576.4 Fistula of bile duct
Choledochoduodenal fistula
C&C Exclusions: See 576.3

576.5 Spasm of sphincter of Oddi

576.8 Other specified disorders of biliary tract
Adhesions of bile duct [any]
Atrophy of bile duct [any]
Cyst of bile duct [any]
Hypertrophy of bile duct [any]
Stasis of bile duct [any]
Ulcer of bile duct [any]
Excludes *congenital choledochal cyst (751.69)*
AHA: 3Q 2003, 17; 2Q 1999, 14

576.9 Unspecified disorder of biliary tract

577 Diseases of pancreas

577.0 Acute pancreatitis
Abscess of pancreas
Necrosis of pancreas:
acute
infective
Pancreatitis:
NOS
acute (recurrent)
apoplectic
hemorrhagic
subacute
suppurative
Excludes *mumps pancreatitis (072.3)*
C&C Exclusions: 577.0, 577.1, 577.8, 577.9
AHA: 3Q 1999, 9; 2Q 1998, 19; 2Q 1996, 13; 2Q 1989, 9

577.1 Chronic pancreatitis
Chronic pancreatitis:
NOS
infectious
interstitial
Pancreatitis:
painless
recurrent
relapsing
AHA: 1Q 2001, 8; 2Q 1996, 13; 3Q 1994, 11

577.2 Cyst and pseudocyst of pancreas
C&C Exclusions: 577.2, 577.8, 577.9

577.8 Other specified diseases of pancreas
Atrophy of pancreas
Calculus of pancreas
Cirrhosis of pancreas
Fibrosis of pancreas
Pancreatic:
infantilism
necrosis:
NOS
aseptic
fat
Pancreatolithiasis
Excludes *fibrocystic disease of pancreas (277.00-277.09)*
islet cell tumor of pancreas (211.7)
pancreatic steatorrhea (579.4)
AHA: 1Q 2001, 8

577.9 Unspecified disease of pancreas

578 Gastrointestinal hemorrhage
Excludes *that with mention of:*
angiodysplasia of stomach and duodenum (537.83)
angiodysplasia of intestine (569.85)
diverticulitis, intestine:
large (562.13)
small (562.03)
diverticulosis, intestine:
large (562.12)
small (562.02)
gastritis and duodenitis (535.0-535.6)
ulcer:
duodenal, gastric, gastrojejunal, or peptic (531.00-534.91)
AHA: 2Q 1992, 9; 4Q 1990, 20

578.0 Hematemesis
Vomiting of blood
C&C Exclusions: 251.5, 456.0, 530.21, 530.7, 530.82, 531.00, 531.01, 531.10, 531.11, 531.20, 531.21, 531.30, 531.31, 531.40, 531.41, 531.50, 531.51, 531.60, 531.61, 531.70, 531.71, 531.90, 531.91, 532.00, 532.01, 532.10, 532.11, 532.20, 532.21, 532.30, 532.31, 532.40, 532.41, 532.50, 532.51, 532.60, 532.61, 532.70, 532.71, 532.90, 532.91, 533.00, 533.01, 533.10, 533.11, 533.20, 533.21, 533.30, 533.31, 533.40, 533.41, 533.50, 533.51, 533.60, 533.61, 533.70, 533.71, 533.90, 533.91, 534.00, 534.01, 534.10, 534.11, 534.20, 534.21, 534.30, 534.31, 534.40, 534.41, 534.50, 534.51, 534.60, 534.61, 534.70, 534.71, 534.90, 534.91, 535.01, 535.11, 535.21, 535.31, 535.41, 535.51, 535.61, 537.83, 537.84, 562.02, 562.03, 562.12, 562.13, 569.3, 569.85, 569.86, 578.0, 578.1, 578.9
AHA: 2Q 2002, 4

578.1 Blood in stool
Melena
Excludes *melena of the newborn (772.4, 777.3)*
occult blood (792.1)
C&C Exclusions: See 578.0
AHA: 2Q 2006, 17; 2Q 1992, 8

578.9 Hemorrhage of gastrointestinal tract, unspecified
Gastric hemorrhage
Intestinal hemorrhage
C&C Exclusions: See 578.0
AHA: 4Q 2006, 91; 3Q 2005, 17; Nov-Dec 1986, 9

579 Intestinal malabsorption

579.0 Celiac disease
Celiac:
crisis
infantilism
rickets
Gee (-Herter) disease
Gluten enteropathy
Idiopathic steatorrhea
Nontropical sprue

579.1 Tropical sprue
Sprue:
NOS
tropical
Tropical steatorrhea

579.2 Blind loop syndrome
Postoperative blind loop syndrome

579.3 Other and unspecified postsurgical nonabsorption
Hypoglycemia following gastrointestinal surgery
Malnutrition following gastrointestinal surgery
C&C Exclusions: 579.3, 579.4, 579.8, 579.9
AHA: 4Q 2003, 104

579.4 Pancreatic steatorrhea
DEF: Insufficient pancreatic enzyme excretions causing severe malabsorption and nutrient deficiencies with loose stools containing unabsorbed fat.

579.8 Other specified intestinal malabsorption
Enteropathy:
exudative
protein-losing
Steatorrhea (chronic)
AHA: 1Q 1988, 6

579.9 Unspecified intestinal malabsorption
Malabsorption syndrome NOS
AHA: 4Q 2004, 59

Digestive System

576.8 – 579.9

10. DISEASES OF THE GENITOURINARY SYSTEM (580-629)

NEPHRITIS, NEPHROTIC SYNDROME, AND NEPHROSIS (580-589)

Excludes hypertensive chronic kidney disease (403.00-403.91, 404.00-404.93)

④ **580 Acute glomerulonephritis**

Includes acute nephritis

580.0 With lesion of proliferative glomerulonephritis

Acute (diffuse) proliferative glomerulonephritis
Acute poststreptococcal glomerulonephritis

C&C Exclusions: 016.00, 016.01, 016.02, 016.03, 016.04, 016.05, 016.06, 016.30, 016.31, 016.32, 016.33, 016.34, 016.35, 016.36, 016.90, 016.91, 016.92, 016.93, 016.94, 016.95, 016.96, 017.90, 017.91, 017.92, 017.93, 017.94, 017.95, 017.96, 098.10, 098.19, 098.30, 098.31, 098.89, 112.2, 131.00, 131.8, 131.9, 250.40, 250.41, 250.42, 250.43, 250.80, 250.81, 250.82, 250.83, 250.90, 250.91, 250.92, 250.93, 274.10, 274.19, 580.0, 580.4, 580.81, 580.89, 580.9, 581.0, 581.1, 581.2, 581.3, 581.81, 581.89, 581.9, 582.0, 582.1, 582.2, 582.4, 582.81, 582.89, 582.9, 583.0, 583.1, 583.2, 583.4, 583.6, 583.7, 583.81, 583.89, 583.9, 584.5, 584.6, 584.7, 584.8, 584.9, 585.1, 585.2, 585.3, 585.4, 585.5, 585.6, 585.9, 586, 587, 588.0, 588.1, 588.8, 588.9, 589.0, 589.1, 589.9, 590.00, 590.01, 590.10, 590.11, 590.2, 590.3, 590.80, 590.81, 590.9, 591, 593.0, 593.1, 593.2, 593.89, 593.9, 599.7, 599.81, 599.82, 599.83, 599.84, 599.89, 599.9

580.4 With lesion of rapidly progressive glomerulonephritis

Acute nephritis with lesion of necrotizing glomerulitis

C&C Exclusions: See 580.0

⑤ **580.8 With other specified pathological lesion in kidney**

✚ ***580.81 Acute glomerulonephritis in diseases classified elsewhere***

Code first underlying disease, as:
infectious hepatitis (070.0-070.9)
mumps (072.79)
subacute bacterial endocarditis (421.0)
typhoid fever (002.0)

C&C Exclusions: See 580.0

580.89 Other

Glomerulonephritis, acute, with lesion of:
exudative nephritis
interstitial (diffuse) (focal) nephritis

C&C Exclusions: 016.00, 016.01, 016.02, 016.03, 016.04, 016.05, 016.06, 016.30, 016.31, 016.32, 016.33, 016.34, 016.35, 016.36, 016.90, 016.91, 016.92, 016.93, 016.94, 016.95, 016.96, 017.90, 017.91, 017.92, 017.93, 017.94, 017.95, 017.96, 098.10, 098.19, 098.30, 098.31, 098.89, 112.2, 131.00, 131.8, 131.9, 274.10, 274.19, 580.0, 580.4, 580.81, 580.89, 580.9, 581.0, 581.1, 581.2, 581.3, 581.81, 581.89, 581.9, 582.0, 582.1, 582.2, 582.4, 582.81, 582.89, 582.9, 583.0, 583.1, 583.2, 583.4, 583.6, 583.7, 583.81, 583.89, 583.9, 584.5, 584.6, 584.7, 584.8, 584.9, 585.1, 585.2, 585.3, 585.4, 585.5, 585.6, 585.9, 586, 587, 588.0, 588.1, 588.8, 588.9, 589.0, 589.1, 589.9, 590.00, 590.01, 590.10, 590.11, 590.2, 590.3, 590.80, 590.81, 590.9, 591, 593.0, 593.1, 593.2, 593.89, 593.9, 599.7, 599.81, 599.82, 599.83, 599.84, 599.89, 599.9

580.9 Acute glomerulonephritis with unspecified pathological lesion in kidney

Glomerulonephritis:
NOS specified as acute
hemorrhagic specified as acute
Nephritis specified as acute
Nephropathy specified as acute

C&C Exclusions: 016.00, 016.01, 016.02, 016.03, 016.04, 016.05, 016.06, 016.30, 016.31, 016.32, 016.33, 016.34, 016.35, 016.36, 016.90, 016.91, 016.92, 016.93, 016.94, 016.95, 016.96, 017.90, 017.91, 017.92, 017.93, 017.94, 017.95, 017.96, 098.10, 098.19, 098.30, 098.31, 098.89, 112.2, 131.00, 131.8, 131.9, 250.40, 250.41, 250.42, 250.43, 250.80, 250.81, 250.82, 250.83, 250.90, 250.91, 250.92, 250.93, 274.10, 274.19, 580.0, 580.4, 580.81, 580.89, 580.9, 581.0, 581.1, 581.2, 581.3, 581.81, 581.89, 581.9, 582.0, 582.1, 582.2, 582.4, 582.81, 582.89, 582.9, 583.0, 583.1, 583.2, 583.4, 583.6, 583.7, 583.81, 583.89, 583.9, 584.5, 584.6, 584.7, 584.8, 584.9, 585.1, 585.2, 585.3, 585.4, 585.5, 585.6, 585.9, 586, 587, 588.0, 588.1, 588.8, 588.9, 589.0, 589.1, 589.9, 590.00, 590.01, 590.10, 590.11, 590.2, 590.3, 590.80, 590.81, 590.9, 591, 593.0, 593.1, 593.2, 593.89, 593.9, 599.7, 599.81, 599.82, 599.83, 599.84, 599.89, 599.9

④ **581 Nephrotic syndrome**

581.0 With lesion of proliferative glomerulonephritis

C&C Exclusions: See 580.9

581.1 With lesion of membranous glomerulonephritis

Epimembranous nephritis
Idiopathic membranous glomerular disease
Nephrotic syndrome with lesion of:
focal glomerulosclerosis
sclerosing membranous glomerulonephritis
segmental hyalinosis

C&C Exclusions: See 580.9

581.2 With lesion of membranoproliferative glomerulonephritis

Nephrotic syndrome with lesion (of):
endothelial glomerulonephritis
hypocomplementemic persistent glomerulonephritis
lobular glomerulonephritis
mesangiocapillary glomerulonephritis
mixed membranous and proliferative glomerulonephritis

C&C Exclusions: See 580.9

581.3 With lesion of minimal change glomerulonephritis

Foot process disease
Lipoid nephrosis
Minimal change:
glomerular disease
glomerulitis
nephrotic syndrome

C&C Exclusions: See 580.9

AHA: 1Q 2007, 23

⑤ **581.8 With other specified pathological lesion in kidney**

✚ ***581.81 Nephrotic syndrome in diseases classified elsewhere***

Code first underlying disease, as:
amyloidosis (277.30-277.39)
diabetes mellitus (250.4)
malaria (084.9)
polyarteritis (446.0)
systemic lupus erythematosus (710.0)

Excludes *nephrosis in epidemic hemorrhagic fever (078.6)*

C&C Exclusions: See 580.9

AHA: 3Q 1991, 8, 12; Sep-Oct 1985, 3

581.89 Other

Glomerulonephritis with edema and lesion of:
exudative nephritis
interstitial (diffuse) (focal) nephritis

C&C Exclusions: See 580.9

581.9 Nephrotic syndrome with unspecified pathological lesion in kidney
Glomerulonephritis with edema NOS
Nephritis:
nephrotic NOS
with edema NOS
Nephrosis NOS
Renal disease with edema NOS
C&C Exclusions: See 580.9

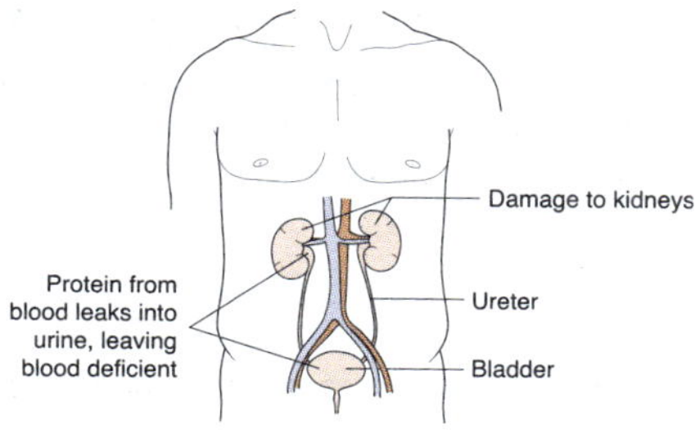

❹ **582 Chronic glomerulonephritis**
Includes chronic nephritis

582.0 With lesion of proliferative glomerulonephritis
Chronic (diffuse) proliferative glomerulonephritis
C&C Exclusions: 585.1, 585.2, 585.3, 585.4, 585.5, 585.6, 585.9

582.1 With lesion of membranous glomerulonephritis
Chronic glomerulonephritis:
membranous
sclerosing
Focal glomerulosclerosis
Segmental hyalinosis
C&C Exclusions: See 582.0
AHA: Sep-Oct 1984, 16

582.2 With lesion of membranoproliferative glomerulonephritis
Chronic glomerulonephritis:
endothelial
hypocomplementemic persistent
lobular
membranoproliferative
mesangiocapillary
mixed membranous and proliferative
C&C Exclusions: See 582.0

582.4 With lesion of rapidly progressive glomerulonephritis
Chronic nephritis with lesion of necrotizing glomerulitis
C&C Exclusions: See 582.0

❺ **582.8 With other specified pathological lesion in kidney**

+ ***582.81 Chronic glomerulonephritis in diseases classified elsewhere***
Code first underlying disease, as:
amyloidosis (277.30-277.39)
systemic lupus erythematosus (710.0)
C&C Exclusions: See 582.0

582.89 Other
Chronic glomerulonephritis with lesion of:
exudative nephritis
interstitial (diffuse) (focal) nephritis
C&C Exclusions: See 582.0

582.9 Chronic glomerulonephritis with unspecified pathological lesion in kidney
Glomerulonephritis: specified as chronic
NOS specified as chronic
hemorrhagic specified as chronic
Nephritis specified as chronic
Nephropathy specified as chronic
C&C Exclusions: See 582.0
AHA: 2Q 2001, 12

❹ **583 Nephritis and nephropathy, not specified as acute or chronic**
Includes "renal disease" so stated, not specified as acute or chronic but with stated pathology or cause

583.0 With lesion of proliferative glomerulonephritis
Proliferative:
glomerulonephritis (diffuse) NOS
nephritis NOS
nephropathy NOS
C&C Exclusions: See 582.0

583.1 With lesion of membranous glomerulonephritis
Membranous:
glomerulonephritis NOS
nephritis NOS
Membranous nephropathy NOS
C&C Exclusions: See 582.0

583.2 With lesion of membranoproliferative glomerulonephritis
Membranoproliferative:
glomerulonephritis NOS
nephritis NOS
nephropathy NOS
Nephritis NOS, with lesion of:
hypocomplementemic persistent glomerulonephritis
lobular glomerulonephritis
mesangiocapillary glomerulonephritis
mixed membranous and proliferative glomerulonephritis
C&C Exclusions: See 582.0

583.4 With lesion of rapidly progressive glomerulonephritis
Necrotizing or rapidly progressive:
glomerulitis NOS
glomerulonephritis NOS
nephritis NOS
nephropathy NOS
Nephritis, unspecified, with lesion of necrotizing glomerulitis
C&C Exclusions: See 580.9

583.6 With lesion of renal cortical necrosis
Nephritis NOS with (renal) cortical necrosis
Nephropathy NOS with (renal) cortical necrosis
Renal cortical necrosis NOS
C&C Exclusions: See 582.0

583.7 With lesion of renal medullary necrosis
Nephritis NOS with (renal) medullary [papillary] necrosis
Nephropathy NOS with (renal) medullary [papillary] necrosis
C&C Exclusions: See 582.0

❺ **583.8 With other specified pathological lesion in kidney**

+ ***583.81 Nephritis and nephropathy, not specified as acute or chronic, in diseases classified elsewhere***
Code first underlying disease, as:
amyloidosis (277.30-277.39)
diabetes mellitus (250.4)
gonococcal infection (098.19)
Goodpasture's syndrome (446.21)
systemic lupus erythematosus (710.0)
tuberculosis (016.0)
Excludes gouty nephropathy (274.10)
syphilitic nephritis (095.4)
C&C Exclusions: See 582.0
AHA: 2Q 2003, 7; 3Q 1991, 8; Sep-Oct 1985, 3

583.89 Other
Glomerulitis with lesion of:
exudative nephritis
interstitial nephritis
Glomerulonephritis with lesion of:
exudative nephritis
interstitial nephritis
Nephritis with lesion of:
exudative nephritis
interstitial nephritis
Nephropathy with lesion of:
exudative nephritis
interstitial nephritis
Renal disease with lesion of:
exudative nephritis
interstitial nephritis
C&C Exclusions: See 582.0

583.9 With unspecified pathological lesion in kidney
Glomerulitis NOS
Glomerulonephritis NOS
Nephritis NOS
Nephropathy NOS
Excludes *nephropathy complicating pregnancy, labor, or the puerperium (642.0-642.9, 646.2)*
renal disease NOS with no stated cause (593.9)
C&C Exclusions: See 582.0

4 584 Acute renal failure
Excludes *following labor and delivery (669.3)*
posttraumatic (958.5)
that complicating:
abortion (634-638 with .3, 639.3)
ectopic or molar pregnancy (639.3)
AHA: 1Q 1993, 18; 2Q 1992, 5; 4Q 1992, 22

584.5 With lesion of tubular necrosis
Lower nephron nephrosis
Renal failure with (acute) tubular necrosis
Tubular necrosis:
NOS
acute
C&C Exclusions: 250.40, 250.41, 250.42, 250.43, 250.80, 250.81, 250.82, 250.83, 250.90, 250.91, 250.92, 250.93, 274.10, 274.19, 580.0, 580.4, 580.81, 580.89, 580.9, 581.0, 581.1, 581.2, 581.3, 581.81, 581.89, 581.9, 582.0, 582.1, 582.2, 582.4, 582.81, 582.89, 582.9, 583.0, 583.1, 583.2, 583.4, 583.6, 583.7, 583.81, 583.89, 583.9, 584.5, 584.6, 584.7, 584.8, 584.9, 585.1, 585.2, 585.3, 585.4, 585.5, 585.6, 585.9, 586, 587, 588.0, 588.1, 588.8, 588.9, 589.0, 589.1, 589.9, 590.00, 590.01, 590.10, 590.11, 590.2, 590.3, 590.80, 590.81, 590.9, 591, 593.0, 593.1, 593.2, 593.89, 593.9, 599.7, 599.81, 599.82, 599.83, 599.84, 599.89, 599.9, 753.0, 753.20, 753.21, 753.22, 753.23, 753.29, 753.3, 753.9

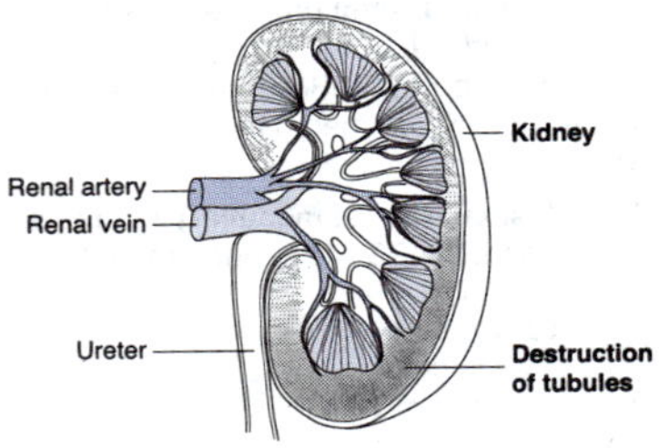

584.6 With lesion of renal cortical necrosis
C&C Exclusions: See 584.5

584.7 With lesion of renal medullary [papillary] necrosis
Necrotizing renal papillitis
C&C Exclusions: See 584.5

584.8 With other specified pathological lesion in kidney
C&C Exclusions: 250.40, 250.41, 250.42, 250.43, 250.80, 250.81, 250.82, 250.83, 250.90, 250.91, 250.92, 250.93, 274.10, 274.19, 580.0, 580.4, 580.81, 580.89, 580.9, 581.0, 581.1, 581.2, 581.3, 581.81, 581.89, 581.9, 582.0, 582.1, 582.2, 582.4, 582.81, 582.89, 582.9, 583.0, 583.1, 583.2, 583.4, 583.6, 583.7, 583.81, 583.89, 583.9, 584.5, 584.6, 584.7, 584.8, 584.9, 585.1, 585.2, 585.3, 585.4, 585.5, 585.6, 585.9, 586, 587, 588.0, 588.1, 588.8, 588.9, 589.0, 589.1, 589.9, 590.00, 590.01, 590.10, 590.11, 590.2, 590.3, 590.80, 590.81, 590.9, 591, 593.0, 593.1, 593.2, 593.89, 593.9, 599.7, 599.81, 599.82, 599.83, 599.84, 599.89, 599.9

584.9 Acute renal failure, unspecified
C&C Exclusions: See 584.5
AHA: 2Q 2005, 18; 2Q 2003, 7; 1Q 2003, 22; 3Q 2002, 21, 28; 2Q 2001, 14; 1Q 2000, 22; 3Q 1996, 9; 4Q 1988, 1

4 585 Chronic kidney disease (CKD)
Chronic uremia
Code first hypertensive chronic kidney disease, if applicable, (403.00-403.91, 404.00▶404.93◀)
Use additional code to identify kidney transplant status, if applicable (V42.0)
Use additional code to identify manifestation as:
uremic:
neuropathy (357.4)
pericarditis (420.0)
AHA: 4Q 2005, 68, 77; 1Q 2004, 5; 4Q 2003, 61, 111; 2Q 2003, 7; 2Q 2001, 12-13; 1Q 2001, 3; 4Q 1998, 55; 3Q 1998, 6-7; 2Q 1998, 20; 3Q 1996, 9; 1Q 1993, 18; 3Q 1991, 8; 4Q 1989, 1; Nov-Dec 1985, 15; Sep-Oct 1984, 3

585.1 Chronic kidney disease, Stage I
C&C Exclusions: 580.0, 580.4, 580.81, 580.89, 580.9, 581.0, 581.1, 581.2, 581.3, 581.81, 581.89, 581.9, 583.4, 584.5, 584.6, 584.7, 584.8, 584.9, 585.1, 585.2, 585.3, 585.4, 585.5, 585.6, 585.9, 590.10, 590.11, 590.2, 590.3, 590.80, 590.81, 590.9, 591

585.2 Chronic kidney disease, Stage II (mild)
C&C Exclusions: See 585.1

585.3 Chronic kidney disease, Stage III (moderate)
C&C Exclusions: See 585.1
AHA: 4Q 2005, 69

585.4 Chronic kidney disease, Stage IV (severe)
C&C Exclusions: See 585.1

585.5 Chronic kidney disease, Stage V
Excludes *chronic kidney disease, Stage V requiring chronic dialysis (585.6)*
C&C Exclusions: See 585.1

585.6 End stage renal disease
Chronic kidney disease requiring chronic dialysis
C&C Exclusions: See 585.1
AHA: 4Q 2006, 136; 4Q 2005, 79

✖ 585.9 Chronic kidney disease, unspecified
Chronic renal disease
Chronic renal failure NOS
Chronic renal insufficiency
C&C Exclusions: See 585.1
AHA: 4Q 2006, 86; 4Q 2005, 79

586 Renal failure, unspecified
Uremia NOS
Excludes *following labor and delivery (669.3)*
posttraumatic renal failure (958.5)
that complicating:
abortion (634-638 with .3, 639.3)
ectopic or molar pregnancy (639.3)
uremia:
extrarenal (788.9)
prerenal (788.9)
with any condition classifiable to 401 (403.0-403.9 with fifth-digit 1)
C&C Exclusions: 585.1, 585.2, 585.3, 585.4, 585.5, 585.6, 585.9
AHA: 3Q 1998, 6; 1Q 1993, 18

587 Renal sclerosis, unspecified
Atrophy of kidney
Contracted kidney
Renal:
cirrhosis
fibrosis
Excludes *nephrosclerosis (arteriolar) (arteriosclerotic) (403.00-403.92)*
with hypertension (403.00-403.92)
C&C Exclusions: See 586

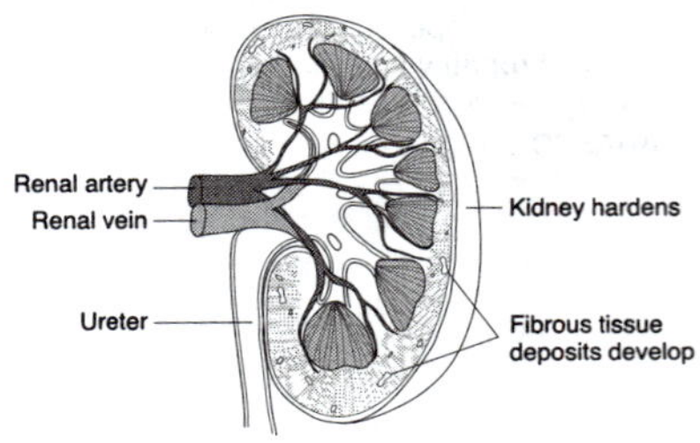

④ **588 Disorders resulting from impaired renal function**

588.0 Renal osteodystrophy
Azotemic osteodystrophy
Phosphate-losing tubular disorders
Renal:
dwarfism
infantilism
rickets
C&C Exclusions: See 586

588.1 Nephrogenic diabetes insipidus
Excludes *diabetes insipidus NOS (253.5)*
C&C Exclusions: See 586

⑤ **588.8 Other specified disorders resulting from impaired renal function**
Excludes *secondary hypertension (405.0-405.9)*

588.81 Secondary hyperparathyroidism (of renal origin)
Secondary hyperparathyroidism NOS
C&C Exclusions: See 586
AHA: 4Q 2004, 58-59

588.89 Other specified disorders resulting from impaired renal function
Hypokalemic nephropathy
C&C Exclusions: See 586

✖ **588.9 Unspecified disorder resulting from impaired renal function**
C&C Exclusions: See 586

④ **589 Small kidney of unknown cause**

✖ **589.0 Unilateral small kidney**
C&C Exclusions: See 586

✖ **589.1 Bilateral small kidneys**
C&C Exclusions: See 586

✖ **589.9 Small kidney, unspecified**
C&C Exclusions: See 586

OTHER DISEASES OF URINARY SYSTEM (590-599)

④ **590 Infections of kidney**
Use additional code to identify organism, such as Escherichia coli [E. coli] (041.4)

⑤ **590.0 Chronic pyelonephritis**
Chronic pyelitis
Chronic pyonephrosis
Code, if applicable, any causal condition first

590.00 Without lesion of renal medullary necrosis
C&C Exclusions: See 586

590.01 With lesion of renal medullary necrosis
C&C Exclusions: See 586

⑤ **590.1 Acute pyelonephritis**
Acute pyelitis
Acute pyonephrosis

590.10 Without lesion of renal medullary necrosis
C&C Exclusions: 016.00, 016.01, 016.02, 016.03, 016.04, 016.05, 016.06, 016.30, 016.31, 016.32, 016.33, 016.34, 016.35, 016.36, 016.90, 016.91, 016.92, 016.93, 016.94, 016.95, 016.96, 017.90, 017.91, 017.92, 017.93, 017.94, 017.95, 017.96, 098.10, 098.19, 098.30, 098.31, 098.89, 112.2, 131.00, 131.8, 131.9, 250.40, 250.41, 250.42, 250.43, 250.80, 250.81, 250.82, 250.83, 250.90, 250.91, 250.92, 250.93, 274.10, 274.19, 580.0, 580.4, 580.81, 580.89, 580.9, 581.0, 581.1, 581.2, 581.3, 581.81, 581.89, 581.9, 582.0, 582.1, 582.2, 582.4, 582.81, 582.89, 582.9, 583.0, 583.1, 583.2, 583.4, 583.6, 583.7, 583.81, 583.89, 583.9, 584.5, 584.6, 584.7, 584.8, 584.9, 585.1, 585.2, 585.3, 585.4, 585.5, 585.6, 585.9, 586, 587, 588.0, 588.1, 588.8, 588.9, 589.0, 589.1, 589.9, 590.00, 590.01, 590.10, 590.11, 590.2, 590.3, 590.80, 590.81, 590.9, 591, 593.0, 593.1, 593.2, 593.89, 593.9, 599.7, 599.81, 599.82, 599.83, 599.84, 599.89, 599.9

590.11 With lesion of renal medullary necrosis
C&C Exclusions: See 590.10

590.2 Renal and perinephric abscess
Abscess:
kidney
nephritic
perirenal
Carbuncle of kidney
C&C Exclusions: See 590.10

590.3 Pyeloureteritis cystica
Infection of renal pelvis and ureter
Ureteritis cystica
DEF: Infection of renal pelvis and ureter with development of small cysts in the kidney and ureter.
C&C Exclusions: 016.00, 016.01, 016.02, 016.03, 016.04, 016.05, 016.06, 016.30, 016.31, 016.32, 016.33, 016.34, 016.35, 016.36, 016.90, 016.91, 016.92, 016.93, 016.94, 016.95, 016.96, 017.90, 017.91, 017.92, 017.93, 017.94, 017.95, 017.96, 098.10, 098.19, 098.30, 098.31, 098.89, 112.2, 131.00, 131.8, 131.9, 274.10, 274.19, 580.0, 580.4, 580.81, 580.89, 580.9, 581.0, 581.1, 581.2, 581.3, 581.81, 581.89, 581.9, 582.0, 582.1, 582.2, 582.4, 582.81, 582.89, 582.9, 583.0, 583.1, 583.2, 583.4, 583.6, 583.7, 583.81, 583.89, 583.9, 584.5, 584.6, 584.7, 584.8, 584.9, 585.1, 585.2, 585.3, 585.4, 585.5, 585.6, 585.9, 586, 587, 588.0, 588.1, 588.8, 588.9, 589.0, 589.1, 589.9, 590.00, 590.01, 590.10, 590.11, 590.2, 590.3, 590.80, 590.81, 590.9, 591, 593.0, 593.1, 593.2, 593.89, 593.9, 599.7, 599.81, 599.82, 599.83, 599.84, 599.89, 599.9

⑤ **590.8 Other pyelonephritis or pyonephrosis, not specified as acute or chronic**

590.80 Pyelonephritis, unspecified
Pyelitis NOS
Pyelonephritis NOS
C&C Exclusions: See 590.3
AHA: 1Q 1998, 10; 4Q 1997, 40

+ ***590.81 Pyelitis or pyelonephritis in diseases classified elsewhere***
Code first underlying disease, as:
tuberculosis (016.0)
C&C Exclusions: See 590.3

✖ **590.9 Infection of kidney, unspecified**
Excludes *urinary tract infection NOS (599.0)*
C&C Exclusions: See 590.3

591 Hydronephrosis
Hydrocalycosis
Hydronephrosis
Hydroureteronephrosis
Excludes *congenital hydronephrosis (753.29)*
hydroureter (593.5)
DEF: Stretching or dilation of kidneys where urine collects because of an outflow obstruction.
C&C Exclusions: See 590.3

④ **592 Calculus of kidney and ureter**
Excludes *nephrocalcinosis (275.49)*

592.0 Calculus of kidney
Nephrolithiasis NOS
Renal calculus or stone
Staghorn calculus
Stone in kidney
Excludes *uric acid nephrolithiasis (274.11)*
AHA: 1Q 2000, 4

592.1 Calculus of ureter
Ureteric stone
Ureterolithiasis
C&C Exclusions: 592.0, 592.1, 592.9, 593.3, 593.4, 593.5, 593.89, 593.9, 594.0, 594.1, 594.2, 594.8, 594.9, 599.60, 599.69, 599.7, 599.81, 599.82, 599.83 599.84, 599.89, 599.9
AHA: 2Q 1998, 9; 1Q 1998, 10; 1Q 1991, 11

592.9 Urinary calculus, unspecified
C&C Exclusions: 599.60, 599.69
AHA: 1Q 1998, 10; 4Q 1997, 40

④ **593 Other disorders of kidney and ureter**

593.0 Nephroptosis
Floating kidney
Mobile kidney
C&C Exclusions: 585.1, 585.2, 585.3, 585.4, 585.5, 585.6, 585.9

593.1 Hypertrophy of kidney
C&C Exclusions: See 593.0

593.2 Cyst of kidney, acquired
Cyst (multiple) (solitary) of kidney, not congenital
Peripelvic (lymphatic) cyst
Excludes *calyceal or pyelogenic cyst of kidney (591)*
congenital cyst of kidney (753.1)
polycystic (disease of) kidney (753.1)
C&C Exclusions: See 593.0
AHA: 4Q 1990, 3

593.3 Stricture or kinking of ureter
Angulation of ureter (postoperative)
Constriction of ureter (postoperative)
Stricture of pelviureteric junction
C&C Exclusions: See 592.9
AHA: 2Q 1998, 9

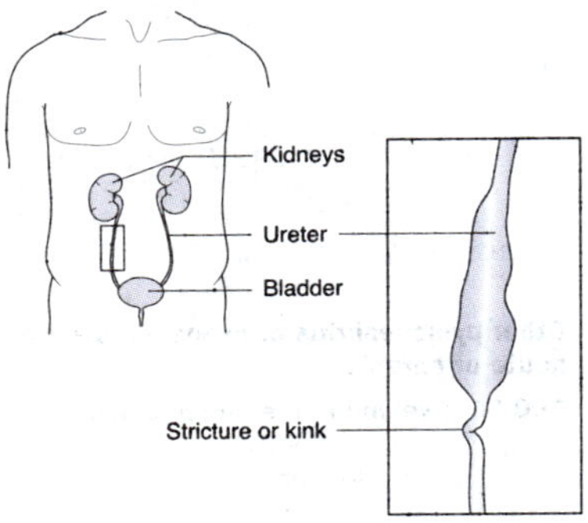

593.4 Other ureteric obstruction
Idiopathic retroperitoneal fibrosis
Occlusion NOS of ureter
Excludes *that due to calculus (592.1)*
C&C Exclusions: See 592.9
AHA: 2Q 1997, 4

593.5 Hydroureter
Excludes *congenital hydroureter (753.22)*
hydroureteronephrosis (591)
C&C Exclusions: 593.3, 593.4, 593.5, 593.89, 593.9, 595.0, 595.1, 595.2, 595.3, 595.4, 595.81, 595.82, 595.89, 595.9, 596.8, 596.9, 599.0, 599.60, 599.69, 599.7, 599.81, 599.82, 599.83, 599.84, 599.89, 599.9, 753.4, 753.5, 753.9

593.6 Postural proteinuria
Benign postural proteinuria
Orthostatic proteinuria
Excludes *proteinuria NOS (791.0)*

5 **593.7 Vesicoureteral reflux**
DEF: Abnormal retrograde flow of urine from bladder back into the ureter and kidney; may cause prorgressive, long-term damage.
AHA: 4Q 1994, 42

593.70 Unspecified or without reflux nephropathy

593.71 With reflux nephropathy, unilateral

593.72 With reflux nephropathy, bilateral

593.73 With reflux nephropathy NOS

5 **593.8 Other specified disorders of kidney and ureter**

593.81 Vascular disorders of kidney
Renal (artery):
embolism
hemorrhage
thrombosis
Renal infarction

593.82 Ureteral fistula
Intestinoureteral fistula
Excludes *fistula between ureter and female genital tract (619.0)*

593.89 Other
Adhesions, kidney or ureter
Periureteritis
Polyp of ureter
Pyelectasia
Ureterocele
Excludes *tuberculosis of ureter (016.2)*
ureteritis cystica (590.3)
C&C Exclusions: 585.1, 585.2, 585.3, 585.4, 585.5, 585.6, 585.9

593.9 Unspecified disorder of kidney and ureter
Acute renal disease
Acute renal insufficiency
Renal disease NOS
Salt-losing nephritis or syndrome
Excludes *chronic renal insufficiency (585.9)*
cystic kidney disease (753.1)
nephropathy, so stated (583.0-583.9)
renal disease:
arising in pregnancy or the puerperium (642.1-642.2, 642.4-642.7, 646.2)
not specified as acute or chronic, but with stated pathology or cause (583.0-583.9)
C&C Exclusions: See 593.89
AHA: 4Q 2005, 79; 1Q 1993, 17

4 **594 Calculus of lower urinary tract**

594.0 Calculus in diverticulum of bladder
C&C Exclusions: See 592.9

594.1 Other calculus in bladder
Urinary bladder stone
Excludes *staghorn calculus (592.0)*
C&C Exclusions: See 592.9

594.2 Calculus in urethra
C&C Exclusions: See 592.9

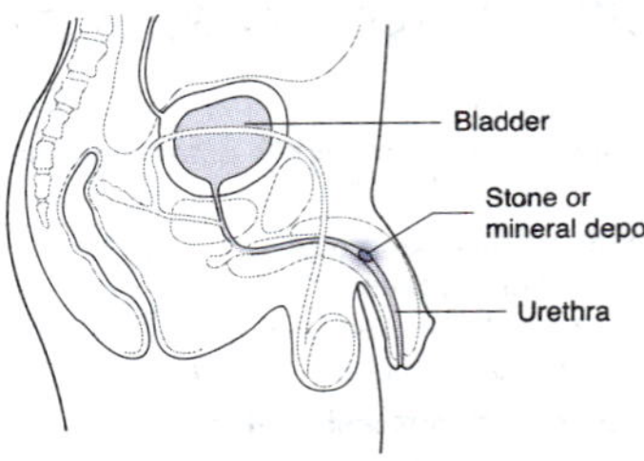

594.8 Other lower urinary tract calculus
C&C Exclusions: See 592.9
AHA: Jan-Feb 1985, 16

594.9 Calculus of lower urinary tract, unspecified
Excludes *calculus of urinary tract NOS (592.9)*
C&C Exclusions: See 592.9

4 **595 Cystitis**
Use additional code to identify organism, such as Escherichia coli [E. coli] (041.4)
Excludes *prostatocystitis (601.3)*

595.0 Acute cystitis
Excludes *trigonitis (595.3)*
C&C Exclusions: 016.10, 016.11, 016.12, 016.13, 016.14, 016.15, 016.16, 016.30, 016.31, 016.32, 016.33, 016.34, 016.35, 016.36, 016.90, 016.91, 016.92, 016.93, 016.94, 016.95, 016.96, 017.90, 017.91, 017.92, 017.93, 017.94, 017.95, 017.96, 098.0, 098.11, 098.2, 098.39, 098.89, 112.2, 131.00, 131.8, 131.9, 593.3, 593.4, 593.5, 593.89, 593.9, 595.0, 595.1, 595.2, 595.3, 595.4, 595.81, 595.82, 595.89, 595.9, 596.8, 596.9, 599.0, 599.60, 599.69, 599.7, 599.81, 599.82, 599.83, 599.84, 599.89, 599.9
AHA: 2Q 1999, 15

595.1 Chronic interstitial cystitis
Hunner's ulcer
Panmural fibrosis of bladder
Submucous cystitis
C&C Exclusions: See 595.0

595.2 Other chronic cystitis
Chronic cystitis NOS
Subacute cystitis
Excludes *trigonitis (595.3)*
C&C Exclusions: See 595.0

595.3 Trigonitis
Follicular cystitis
Trigonitis (acute) (chronic)
Urethrotrigonitis
DEF: Inflammation of the mouth of the bladder where it drains into the urethra.
C&C Exclusions: See 592.9

+ *595.4 Cystitis in diseases classified elsewhere*
Code first underlying disease, as:
actinomycosis (039.8)
amebiasis (006.8)
bilharziasis (120.0-120.9)
Echinococcus infestation (122.3, 122.6)
Excludes *cystitis:*
diphtheritic (032.84)
gonococcal (098.11, 098.31)
monilial (112.2)
trichomonal (131.09)
tuberculous (016.1)
C&C Exclusions: See 595.0

⑤ 595.8 Other specified types of cystitis

595.81 Cystitis cystica
DEF: Inflammation of the bladder with formation of cysts on the interior bladder wall.
C&C Exclusions: See 595.0

595.82 Irradiation cystitis
Use additional E code to identify cause
C&C Exclusions: See 595.0

595.89 Other
Abscess of bladder
Cystitis:
bullous
emphysematous
glandularis
C&C Exclusions: See 595.0

✖ 595.9 Cystitis, unspecified
C&C Exclusions: See 595.0

④ 596 Other disorders of bladder
Use additional code to identify urinary incontinence (625.6, 788.30-788.39)
AHA: Mar-Apr 1987, 10

596.0 Bladder neck obstruction
Contracture (acquired) of bladder neck or vesicourethral orifice
Obstruction (acquired) of bladder neck or vesicourethral orifice
Stenosis (acquired) of bladder neck or vesicourethral orifice
Excludes *congenital (753.6)*
DEF: Blockage in the opening between the bladder and the urethra, causing distention and decreased urine output.
C&C Exclusions: 185, 188.0, 188.1, 188.2, 188.3, 188.4, 188.5, 188.6, 188.7, 188.8, 188.9, 189.3, 189.4, 189.8, 189.9, 596.0, 596.4, 596.51, 596.52, 596.53, 596.54, 596.55, 596.59, 596.8, 596.9, 599.60, 599.69, 600.0, 600.1, 600.2, 600.3, 600.9, 601.1, 601.2, 601.3, 601.4, 601.8, 601.9, 602.0, 602.1, 602.2, 602.3, 602.8, 602.9
AHA: 3Q 2002, 28; 2Q 2001, 14; Nov-Dec 1986, 10

596.1 Intestinovesical fistula
Fistula:
enterovesical
vesicocolic
vesicoenteric
vesicorectal
DEF: Abnormal passage between the bladder and the intestines.
C&C Exclusions: 098.0, 098.2, 098.39, 098.89, 596.1, 596.2, 596.8, 596.9, 599.7, 599.81, 599.82, 599.83, 599.84, 599.89, 599.9, 788.1

596.2 Vesical fistula, not elsewhere classified
Fistula:
bladder NOS
urethrovesical
vesicocutaneous
vesicoperineal
Excludes *fistula between bladder and female genital tract (619.0)*
C&C Exclusions: See 596.1

596.3 Diverticulum of bladder
Diverticulitis of bladder
Diverticulum (acquired) (false) of bladder
Excludes *that with calculus in diverticulum of bladder (594.0)*

596.4 Atony of bladder
High compliance bladder
Hypotonicity of bladder
Inertia of bladder
Excludes *neurogenic bladder (596.54)*
C&C Exclusions: 596.4, 596.51, 596.52, 596.53, 596.54, 596.55, 596.59, 596.8, 596.9, 599.7, 599.81, 599.82, 599.83, 599.84, 599.89, 599.9, 788.1

⑤ 596.5 Other functional disorders of bladder
Excludes *cauda equina syndrome with neurogenic bladder (344.61)*

596.51 Hypertonicity of bladder
Hyperactivity
Overactive bladder
C&C Exclusions: See 592.9

596.52 Low bladder compliance
DEF: Bladder has high pressures with low volume and detrusor instability; the muscle is not able to stretch to accommodate filling completely to hold urine, causing frequent urination.
C&C Exclusions: See 592.9

596.53 Paralysis of bladder
C&C Exclusions: See 592.9

596.54 Neurogenic bladder NOS
C&C Exclusions: See 592.9
AHA: 1Q 2001, 12

596.55 Detrusor sphincter dyssynergia
C&C Exclusions: See 592.9

596.59 Other functional disorder of bladder
Detrusor instability
C&C Exclusions: See 592.9

596.6 Rupture of bladder, nontraumatic
C&C Exclusions: 599.60, 599.69

596.7 Hemorrhage into bladder wall
Hyperemia of bladder
Excludes *acute hemorrhagic cystitis (595.0)*
C&C Exclusions: See 596.6

596.8 Other specified disorders of bladder
Bladder:
calcified
contracted
hemorrhage
hypertrophy
Excludes *cystocele, female (618.01-618.02, 618.09, 618.2-618.4)*
hernia or prolapse of bladder, female (618.01-618.02, 618.09, 618.2-618.4)
C&C Exclusions: See 592.9
AHA: Jan-Feb 1985, 8

✖ 596.9 Unspecified disorder of bladder
C&C Exclusions: See 592.9
AHA: Jan-Feb 1985, 8

④ 597 Urethritis, not sexually transmitted, and urethral syndrome

Excludes *nonspecific urethritis, so stated (099.4)*

597.0 Urethral abscess

Abscess:
- periurethral
- urethral (gland)

Abscess of:
- bulbourethral gland
- Cowper's gland
- Littré's gland

Periurethral cellulitis

Excludes *urethral caruncle (599.3)*

C&C Exclusions: 098.0, 098.2, 098.39, 098.89, 099.40, 099.41, 099.49, 112.2, 131.00, 131.02, 131.8, 131.9, 597.0, 597.80, 597.81, 597.89, 598.00, 598.01, 598.8, 598.9, 599.0, 599.60, 599.69, 599.7, 599.81, 599.82, 599.83, 599.84, 599.89, 599.9, 607.1, 607.2, 607.3, 607.81, 607.82, 607.83, 607.89, 607.9, 608.4, 608.81, 608.85, 608.87, 608.89, 752.61, 752.62, 752.63, 752.64, 752.65, 752.69, 752.8, 752.9, 753.6, 753.7, 753.8, 753.9, 788.1

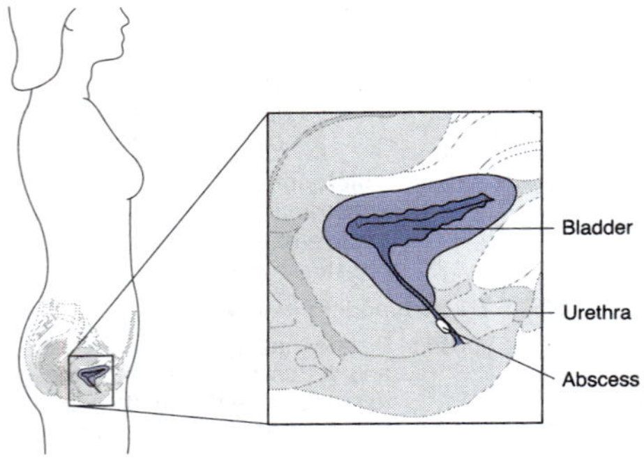

⑤ 597.8 Other urethritis

597.80 Urethritis, unspecified

597.81 Urethral syndrome NOS

597.89 Other

Adenitis, Skene's glands
Cowperitis
Meatitis, urethral
Ulcer, urethra (meatus)
Verumontanitis

Excludes *trichomonal (131.02)*

④ 598 Urethral stricture

Includes pinhole meatus
stricture of urinary meatus

Use additional code to identify urinary incontinence (625.6, 788.30-788.39)

Excludes *congenital stricture of urethra and urinary meatus (753.6)*

⑤ 598.0 Urethral stricture due to infection

598.00 Due to unspecified infection

C&C Exclusions: 599.60, 599.69

+ *598.01 Due to infective diseases classified elsewhere*

Code first underlying disease, as:
- gonococcal infection (098.2)
- schistosomiasis (120.0-120.9)
- syphilis (095.8)

C&C Exclusions: See 598.00

598.1 Traumatic urethral stricture

Stricture of urethra:
- late effect of injury
- postobstetric

Excludes *postoperative following surgery on genitourinary tract (598.2)*

C&C Exclusions: 098.0, 098.2, 098.39, 098.89, 131.02, 598.1, 598.2, 598.8, 598.9, 599.60, 599.69, 599.7, 599.81, 599.82, 599.83, 599.84, 599.89, 599.9, 752.61, 752.62, 752.63, 752.64, 752.65, 752.69, 753.6, 753.7, 753.8, 753.9, 788.1

598.2 Postoperative urethral stricture

Postcatheterization stricture of urethra

C&C Exclusions: See 598.2

AHA: 3Q 1997, 6

598.8 Other specified causes of urethral stricture

C&C Exclusions: See 592.9

AHA: Nov-Dec 1984, 9

✖ 598.9 Urethral stricture, unspecified

C&C Exclusions: See 592.9

④ 599 Other disorders of urethra and urinary tract

599.0 Urinary tract infection, site not specified

Use additional code to identify organism, such as Escherichia coli [E. coli] (041.4)

Excludes *Candidiasis of urinary tract (112.2)*
urinary tract infection of newborn (771.82)

C&C Exclusions: 098.2, 098.39, 098.89, 099.40, 099.41, 099.49, 112.2, 131.00, 131.8, 131.9, 590.10, 590.11, 590.2, 590.3, 590.80, 590.81, 590.9, 591, 593.89, 593.9, 599.60, 599.69, 599.7, 599.81, 599.82, 599.83, 599.84, 599.89, 599.9, 788.1, 996.64

AHA: 3Q 2005, 12; 2Q 2004, 13; 4Q 2003, 79; 4Q 1999, 6; 2Q 1999, 15; 1Q 1998, 5; 2Q 1996, 7; 4Q 1996, 33; 2Q 1995, 7; 1Q 1992, 13

599.1 Urethral fistula

Fistula:
- urethroperineal
- urethrorectal

Urinary fistula NOS

Excludes *fistula:*
- *urethroscrotal (608.89)*
- *urethrovaginal (619.0)*
- *urethrovesicovaginal (619.0)*

C&C Exclusions: See 592.9

599.2 Urethral diverticulum

C&C Exclusions: See 592.9

599.3 Urethral caruncle

Polyp of urethra

C&C Exclusions: See 592.9

599.4 Urethral false passage

C&C Exclusions: 597.0, 597.80, 597.81, 597.89, 598.00, 598.01, 598.8, 598.9, 599.0, 599.60, 599.69, 599.7, 599.81, 599.82, 599.83, 599.84, 599.89, 599.9, 607.1, 607.2, 607.3, 607.81, 607.82, 607.83, 607.89, 607.9, 608.4, 608.81, 608.85, 608.87, 608.89, 752.61, 752.62, 752.63, 752.64, 752.65, 752.69, 752.8, 752.9, 753.9, 788.1

599.5 Prolapsed urethral mucosa

Prolapse of urethra
Urethrocele

Excludes *urethrocele, female (618.03, 618.09, 618.2-618.4)*

C&C Exclusions: See 592.9

❺ **599.6 Urinary obstruction**
Use additional code to identify urinary incontinence (625.6, 788.30-788.39)
Excludes *obstructive nephropathy NOS (593.89)*
AHA: 4Q 2005, 80

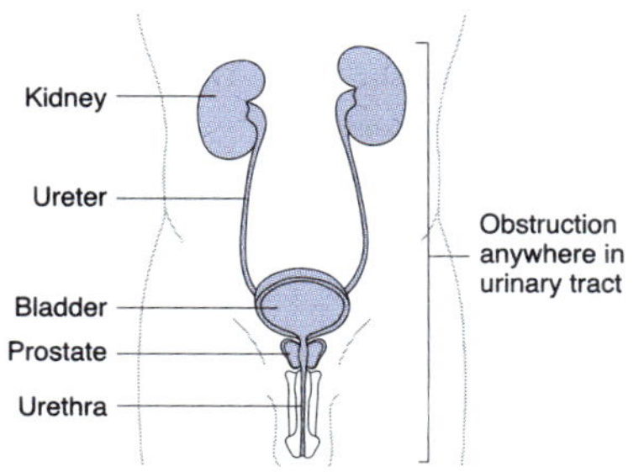

✖ **599.60 Urinary obstruction, unspecified**
Obstructive uropathy NOS
Urinary (tract) obstruction NOS
C&C Exclusions: 185, 188.0, 188.1, 188.2, 188.3, 188.4, 188.5, 188.6, 188.7, 188.8, 188.9, 189.2, 189.3, 189.4, 189.8, 189.9, 274.11, 344.61, 592.1, 592.9, 593.3, 593.4, 593.5, 593.89, 593.9, 594.0, 594.1, 594.2, 594.8, 594.9, 595.0, 595.1, 595.2, 595.3, 595.4, 595.81, 595.82, 595.89, 595.9, 596.0, 596.51, 596.52, 596.53, 596.54, 596.55, 596.59, 596.8, 596.9, 597.0, 597.80, 597.81, 597.89, 598.00, 598.01, 598.1, 598.2, 598.8, 598.9, 599.0, 599.4, 599.60, 599.69, 599.7, 599.81, 599.82, 599.83, 599.84, 599.89, 599.9, 600.0, 600.1, 600.2, 600.3, 600.9, 601.1, 601.2, 601.3, 601.4, 601.8, 601.9, 602.0, 602.1, 602.2, 602.3, 602.8, 602.9, 753.0, 753.10, 753.11, 753.12, 753.13, 753.14, 753.15, 753.16, 753.17, 753.19, 753.20, 753.21, 753.22, 753.23, 753.29, 753.3, 753.9, 788.1, 788.20, 788.29

599.69 Urinary obstruction, not elsewhere classified
Code, if applicable, any causal condition first, such as:
hyperplasia of prostate (600.0-600.9 with fifth digit 1)
C&C Exclusions: See 599.60

599.7 Hematuria
Hematuria (benign) (essential)
Excludes *hemoglobinuria (791.2)*
DEF: Presence of blood in the urine.
C&C Exclusions: 585.1, 585.2, 585.3, 585.4, 585.5, 585.6, 585.9, 592.0, 592.1, 592.9, 593.89, 593.9, 594.0, 594.1, 594.2, 594.8, 594.9, 596.6, 596.7, 599.60, 599.69, 599.7, 599.81, 599.82, 599.83, 599.84, 599.89, 599.9
AHA: 1Q 2000, 5; 3Q 1995, 8

❺ **599.8 Other specified disorders of urethra and urinary tract**
Use additional code to identify urinary incontinence (625.6, 788.30-788.39)
Excludes *symptoms and other conditions classifiable to 788.0-788.2, 788.4-788.9, 791.0-791.9*

599.81 Urethral hypermobility
C&C Exclusions: 585.1, 585.2, 585.3, 585.4, 585.5, 585.6, 585.9, 599.60, 599.69

599.82 Intrinsic (urethral) sphincter deficiency [ISD]
C&C Exclusions: See 599.81
AHA: 2Q 1996, 15

599.83 Urethral instability
C&C Exclusions: See 599.81

599.84 Other specified disorders of urethra
Rupture of urethra (nontraumatic)
Urethral:
cyst
granuloma
C&C Exclusions: See 599.81

599.89 Other specified disorders of urinary tract
C&C Exclusions: See 599.81

✖ **599.9 Unspecified disorder of urethra and urinary tract**

DISEASES OF MALE GENITAL ORGANS (600-608)

❹ **600 Hyperplasia of prostate**
Includes enlarged prostate
AHA: 3Q 2005, 20; 4Q 2000, 43; 3Q 1994, 12; 3Q 1992, 7; Nov-Dec 1986, 10

❺ **600.0 Hypertrophy (benign) of prostate**
Benign prostatic hypertrophy
Enlargement of prostate
Smooth enlarged prostate
Soft enlarged prostate
AHA: 4Q 2003, 63; 1Q 2003, 6; 3Q 2002, 28; 2Q 2001, 14

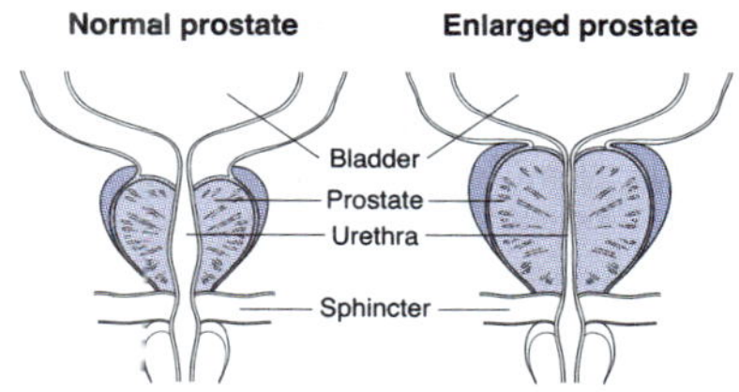

600.00 Hypertrophy (benign) of prostate without urinary obstruction and other lower urinary tract symptoms (LUTS) ♂A
Hypertrophy (benign) of prostate NOS
C&C Exclusions: 596.0, 599.60, 599.69, 601.0, 601.2, 601.3, 602.1, 788.20, 788.29

600.01 Hypertrophy (benign) of prostate with urinary obstruction and other lower urinary tract symptoms (LUTS) ♂A
Hypertrophy (benign) of prostate with urinary retention
Use additional code to identify symptoms:
incomplete bladder emptying (788.21)
nocturia (788.43)
straining on urination (788.65)
urinary frequency (788.41)
urinary hesitancy (788.64)
urinary incontinence (788.30-788.39)
urinary obstruction (599.69)
urinary retention (788.20)
urinary urgency (788.63)
weak urinary stream (788.62)
C&C Exclusions: See 600.00
AHA: 4Q 2006, 95; 4Q 2003, 64

❺ **600.1 Nodular prostate**
Hard, firm prostate
Multinodular prostate
Excludes *malignant neoplasm of prostate (185)*
AHA: 4Q 2003, 63

600.10 Nodular prostate without urinary obstruction ♂A
Nodular prostate NOS
C&C Exclusions: See 600.00

600.11 Nodular prostate with urinary obstruction ♂A
Nodular prostate with urinary retention
C&C Exclusions: See 600.00

❺ **600.2 Benign localized hyperplasia of prostate**
Adenofibromatous hypertrophy of prostate
Adenoma of prostate
Fibroadenoma of prostate
Fibroma of prostate
Myoma of prostate
Polyp of prostate
Excludes *benign neoplasms of prostate (222.2)*
hypertrophy of prostate (600.00-600.01)
malignant neoplasm of prostate (185)
AHA: 4Q 2003, 63

600.20 Benign localized hyperplasia of prostate without urinary obstruction and other lower urinary tract symptoms (LUTS) ♂A
Benign localized hyperplasia of prostate NOS
C&C Exclusions: See 600.00

600.21 Benign localized hyperplasia of prostate with urinary obstruction and other lower urinary tract symptoms (LUTS) ♂ A
Benign localized hyperplasia of prostate with urinary retention
Use additional code to identify symptoms:
incomplete bladder emptying (788.21)
nocturia (788.43)
straining on urination (788.65)
urinary frequency (788.41)
urinary hesitancy (788.64)
urinary incontinence (788.30-788.39)
urinary obstruction (599.69)
urinary retention (788.20)
urinary urgency (788.63)
weak urinary stream (788.62)
C&C Exclusions: See 600.00

600.3 Cyst of prostate ♂ A
C&C Exclusions: See 600.00

5 **600.9 Hyperplasia of prostate, unspecified**
Median bar
Prostatic obstruction NOS
AHA: 4Q 2003, 63

✖ **600.90 Hyperplasia of prostate, unspecified, without urinary obstruction and other lower urinary tract symptoms (LUTS)** ♂ A
Hyperplasia of prostate NOS
C&C Exclusions: See 600.00

✖ **600.91 Hyperplasia of prostate, unspecified, with urinary obstruction and other lower urinary tract symptoms (LUTS)** ♂ A
Hyperplasia of prostate, unspecified, with urinary retention
Use additional code to identify symptoms:
incomplete bladder emptying (788.21)
nocturia (788.43)
straining on urination (788.65)
urinary frequency (788.41)
urinary hesitancy (788.64)
urinary incontinence (788.30-788.39)
urinary obstruction (599.69)
urinary retention (788.20)
urinary urgency (788.63)
weak urinary stream (788.62)
C&C Exclusions: See 600.00

4 **601 Inflammatory diseases of prostate**
Use additional code to identify organism, such as Staphylococcus (041.1), or Streptococcus (041.0)

601.0 Acute prostatitis ♂ A
C&C Exclusions: 098.12, 098.32, 098.89, 112.2, 131.00, 131.03, 131.8, 131.9, 599.60, 599.69, 600.0, 600.1, 600.2, 600.3, 600.9, 601.1, 601.2, 601.3, 601.4, 601.8, 601.9, 602.0, 602.1, 602.2, 602.3, 602.8, 602.9

601.1 Chronic prostatitis ♂ A
C&C Exclusions: 599.60, 599.69

601.2 Abscess of prostate ♂ A
C&C Exclusions: See 601.0

601.3 Prostatocystitis ♂ A
C&C Exclusions: See 601.0

+ ***601.4 Prostatitis in diseases classified elsewhere*** ♂ A
Code first underlying disease, as:
actinomycosis (039.8)
blastomycosis (116.0)
syphilis (095.8)
tuberculosis (016.5)
Excludes *prostatitis:*
gonococcal (098.12, 098.32)
monilial (112.2)
trichomonal (131.03)

601.8 Other specified inflammatory diseases of prostate ♂ A
Prostatitis:
cavitary
diverticular
granulomatous

✖ **601.9 Prostatitis, unspecified** ♂ A
Prostatitis NOS
C&C Exclusions: See 601.1

4 **602 Other disorders of prostate**

602.0 Calculus of prostate ♂ A
Prostatic stone
C&C Exclusions: See 601.1

602.1 Congestion or hemorrhage of prostate ♂ A
C&C Exclusions: See 601.0

602.2 Atrophy of prostate ♂ A
C&C Exclusions: See 601.1

602.3 Dysplasia of prostate ♂
Prostatic intraepithelial neoplasia I (PIN I)
Prostatic intraepithelial neoplasia II (PIN II)
Excludes *prostatic intraepithelial neoplasia III (PIN III) (233.4)*
C&C Exclusions: 596.0, 599.60, 599.69, 601.0, 601.2, 601.3, 602.1, 788.20, 788.29
AHA: 4Q 2001, 46

602.8 Other specified disorders of prostate ♂ A
Fistula of prostate
Infarction of prostate
Stricture of prostate
Periprostatic adhesions
C&C Exclusions: See 601.1

✖ **602.9 Unspecified disorder of prostate** ♂ A
C&C Exclusions: See 601.1

4 **603 Hydrocele**
Includes hydrocele of spermatic cord, testis, or tunica vaginalis
Excludes *congenital (778.6)*
DEF: Collection of serous fluid on the tunica vaginalis, spermatic cord, or testicle from acute local injury, infection, radiotherapy, or gradual fluid accumulation.

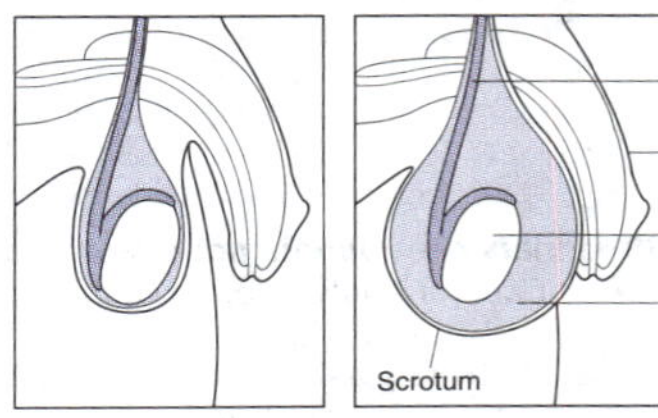

603.0 Encysted hydrocele

603.1 Infected hydrocele
Use additional code to identify organism
C&C Exclusions: 112.2, 131.00, 131.8, 131.9, 603.0, 603.1, 603.8, 603.9

603.8 Other specified types of hydrocele

603.9 Hydrocele, unspecified

4 **604 Orchitis and epididymitis**
Use additional code to identify organism such as Escherichia coli [E. coli] (041.4), Staphylococcus (041.1), or Streptococcus (041.0)

604.0 Orchitis, epididymitis, and epididymo-orchitis, with abscess ♂
Abscess of epididymis or testis
C&C Exclusions: 072.0, 098.13, 098.14, 098.33, 098.34, 098.89, 112.2, 131.00, 131.8, 131.9, 604.0, 604.90, 604.91, 604.99

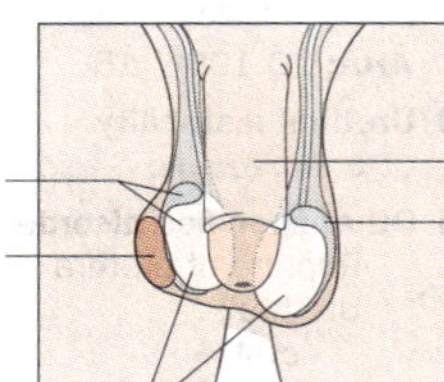

⑤ **604.9 Other orchitis, epididymitis, and epididymo-orchitis, without mention of abscess**

604.90 Orchitis and epididymitis, unspecified ♂

\+ ***604.91 Orchitis and epididymitis in diseases classified elsewhere*** ♂

Code first underlying disease, as:
- diphtheria (032.89)
- filariasis (125.0-125.9)
- syphilis (095.8)

Excludes *orchitis:*
- *gonococcal (098.13, 098.33)*
- *mumps (072.0)*
- *tuberculous (016.5)*

tuberculous epididymitis (016.4)

604.99 Other ♂

605 Redundant prepuce and phimosis ♂
- Adherent prepuce
- Paraphimosis
- Phimosis (congenital)
- Tight foreskin

④ **606 Infertility, male**

AHA: 2Q 1996, 9

606.0 Azoospermia ♂ A
- Absolute infertility
- Infertility due to:
  - germinal (cell) aplasia
  - spermatogenic arrest (complete)

606.1 Oligospermia ♂ A
- Infertility due to:
  - germinal cell desquamation
  - hypospermatogenesis
  - incomplete spermatogenic arrest

606.8 Infertility due to extratesticular causes ♂ A
- Infertility due to:
  - drug therapy
  - infection
  - obstruction of efferent ducts
  - radiation
  - systemic disease

606.9 Male infertility, unspecified ♂ A

④ **607 Disorders of penis**

Excludes *phimosis (605)*

607.0 Leukoplakia of penis ♂
- Kraurosis of penis

Excludes *carcinoma in situ of penis (233.5)*
erythroplasia of Queyrat (233.5)

607.1 Balanoposthitis ♂
- Balanitis
- Use additional code to identify organism

607.2 Other inflammatory disorders of penis ♂
- Abscess of corpus cavernosum or penis
- Boil of corpus cavernosum or penis
- Carbuncle of corpus cavernosum or penis
- Cellulitis of corpus cavernosum or penis
- Cavernitis (penis)
- Use additional code to identify organism

Excludes *herpetic infection (054.13)*

607.3 Priapism ♂
- Painful erection

⑤ **607.8 Other specified disorders of penis**

607.81 Balanitis xerotica obliterans ♂
- Induratio penis plastica

DEF: Chronic skin condition of the penis causing atrophic, white, patches on the foreskin and glans with hardened, indurated tissue near the meatus.

607.82 Vascular disorders of penis ♂
- Embolism of corpus cavernosum or penis
- Hematoma (nontraumatic) of corpus cavernosum or penis
- Hemorrhage of corpus cavernosum or penis
- Thrombosis of corpus cavernosum or penis

607.83 Edema of penis ♂

607.84 Impotence of organic origin ♂ A

Excludes *nonorganic (302.72)*

AHA: 3Q 1991, 11

607.85 Peyronie's disease ♂

C&C Exclusions: 597.0, 599.4

AHA: 4Q 2003, 64

607.89 Other ♂
- Atrophy of corpus cavernosum or penis
- Fibrosis of corpus cavernosum or penis
- Hypertrophy of corpus cavernosum or penis
- Ulcer (chronic) of corpus cavernosum or penis

607.9 Unspecified disorder of penis ♂

④ **608 Other disorders of male genital organs**

608.0 Seminal vesiculitis ♂
- Abscess of seminal vesicle
- Cellulitis of seminal vesicle
- Vesiculitis (seminal)
- Use additional code to identify organism

Excludes *gonococcal infection (098.14, 098.34)*

608.1 Spermatocele ♂

DEF: Cyst on the epididymis or testicle containing sperm.

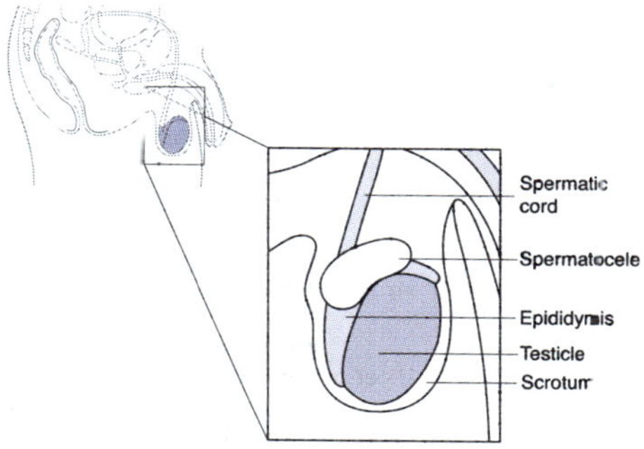

⑤ **608.2 Torsion of testis**

DEF: Testicle becomes twisted inside the scrotum, cutting off the blood supply.

✖ **608.20 Torsion of testis, unspecified** ♂

608.21 Extravaginal torsion of spermatic cord ♂

608.22 Intravaginal torsion of spermatic cord ♂
- ▶ Torsion of spermatic cord NOS◀

608.23 Torsion of appendix testis ♂

608.24 Torsion of appendix epididymis ♂

608.3 Atrophy of testis ♂

608.4 Other inflammatory disorders of male genital organs ♂
- Abscess of scrotum, spermatic cord, testis [except abscess], tunica vaginalis, or vas deferens
- Boil of scrotum, spermatic cord, testis [except abscess], tunica vaginalis, or vas deferens
- Carbuncle of scrotum, spermatic cord, testis [except abscess], tunica vaginalis, or vas deferens
- Cellulitis of scrotum, spermatic cord, testis [except abscess], tunica vaginalis, or vas deferens
- Vasitis
- Use additional code to identify organism

Excludes *abscess of testis (604.0)*

⑤ **608.8 Other specified disorders of male genital organs**

\+ ***608.81 Disorders of male genital organs in diseases classified elsewhere*** ♂

Code first underlying disease, as:
- filariasis (125.0-125.9)
- tuberculosis (016.5)

608.82 Hematospermia ♂

AHA: 4Q 2001, 46

A Adult (15+ years) M Maternity (12-55 years) N Newborn (0 years) P Pediatric (0-17 years) ♂ Male ♀ Female ② Medicare Secondary Payer

608.83 Vascular disorders ♂
Hematocele NOS, male
Hematoma (nontraumatic) of seminal vesicle, spermatic cord, testis, scrotum, tunica vaginalis, or vas deferens
Hemorrhage of seminal vesicle, spermatic cord, testis, scrotum, tunica vaginalis, or vas deferens
Thrombosis of seminal vesicle, spermatic cord, testis, scrotum, tunica vaginalis, or vas deferens
AHA: 4Q 2003, 110

608.84 Chylocele of tunica vaginalis ♂

608.85 Stricture ♂
Stricture of:
spermatic cord
tunica vaginalis
vas deferens

608.86 Edema ♂

608.87 Retrograde ejaculation ♂
DEF: Bladder neck remains open during ejaculation, causing semen to flow backwards into the bladder.
C&C Exclusions: See 607.85
AHA: 4Q 2001, 46

608.89 Other ♂
Atrophy of seminal vesicle, spermatic cord, testis, scrotum tunica vaginalis, or vas deferens
Fibrosis of seminal vesicle, spermatic cord, testis, scrotum tunica vaginalis, or vas deferens
Hypertrophy of seminal vesicle, spermatic cord, testis, scrotum tunica vaginalis, or vas deferens
Ulcer of seminal vesicle, spermatic cord, testis, scrotum tunica vaginalis, or vas deferens
Excludes *atrophy of testis (608.3)*

✖ **608.9 Unspecified disorder of male genital organs ♂**

DISORDERS OF BREAST (610-611)

❹ **610 Benign mammary dysplasias**

610.0 Solitary cyst of breast
Cyst (solitary) of breast

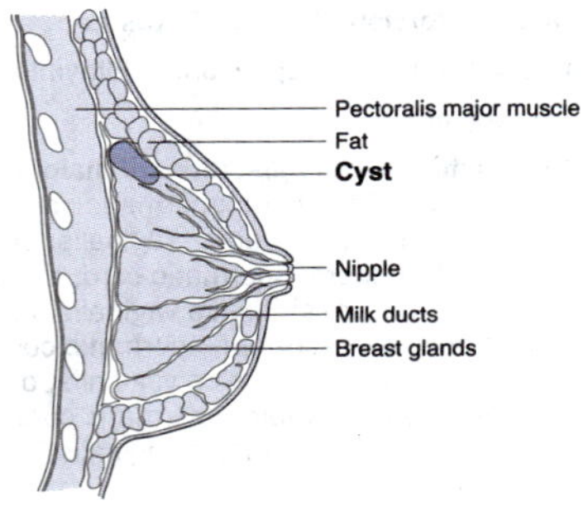

610.1 Diffuse cystic mastopathy A
Chronic cystic mastitis
Cystic breast
Fibrocystic disease of breast
AHA: 2Q 2006, 10

610.2 Fibroadenosis of breast
Fibroadenosis of breast:
NOS
chronic
cystic
diffuse
periodic
segmental

610.3 Fibrosclerosis of breast

610.4 Mammary duct ectasia
Comedomastitis
Duct ectasia
Mastitis:
periductal
plasma cell
DEF: Dilated milk duct filled with fluid; becomes inflamed and clogged with a thick, sticky substance, causing discharge and tenderness.

610.8 Other specified benign mammary dysplasias
Mazoplasia
Sebaceous cyst of breast

✖ **610.9 Benign mammary dysplasia, unspecified**

❹ **611 Other disorders of breast**
Excludes *that associated with lactation or the puerperium (675.0-676.9)*

611.0 Inflammatory disease of breast
Abscess (acute) (chronic) (nonpuerperal) of:
areola
breast
Mammillary fistula
Mastitis (acute) (subacute) (nonpuerperal):
NOS
infective
retromammary
submammary
Excludes *carbuncle of breast (680.2)*
chronic cystic mastitis (610.1)
neonatal infective mastitis (771.5)
thrombophlebitis of breast [Mondor's disease] (451.89)

611.1 Hypertrophy of breast
Gynecomastia
Hypertrophy of breast:
NOS
massive pubertal

611.2 Fissure of nipple

611.3 Fat necrosis of breast
Fat necrosis (segmental) of breast

611.4 Atrophy of breast

611.5 Galactocele
DEF: Cyst in the breast containing milk.

611.6 Galactorrhea not associated with childbirth
DEF: Inappropriate discharge of milk from the breast.

❺ **611.7 Signs and symptoms in breast**

611.71 Mastodynia
Pain in breast

611.72 Lump or mass in breast
C&C Exclusions: 610.0, 610.1, 610.2, 610.3, 610.4, 610.8, 610.9, 611.0, 611.1, 611.2, 611.3, 611.4, 611.5, 611.6, 611.71, 611.72, 611.79, 611.8, 611.9
AHA: 2Q 2003, 4-5

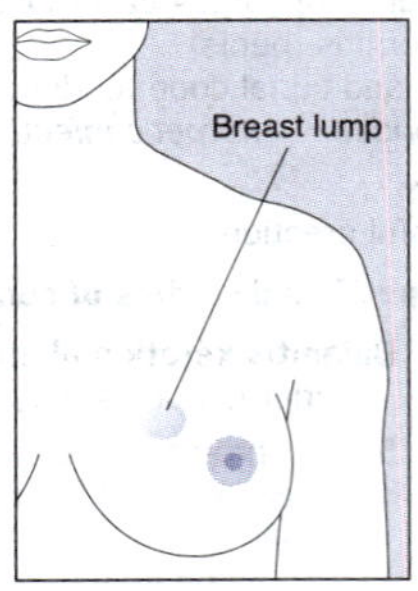

611.79 Other
Induration of breast
Inversion of nipple
Nipple discharge
Retraction of nipple

611.8 Other specified disorders of breast
Hematoma (nontraumatic) of breast
Infarction of breast
Occlusion of breast duct
Subinvolution of breast (postlactational) (postpartum)

611.9 Unspecified breast disorder

INFLAMMATORY DISEASE OF FEMALE PELVIC ORGANS (614-616)

Use additional code to identify organism, such as Staphylococcus (041.1), or Streptococcus (041.0)
Excludes *that associated with pregnancy, abortion, childbirth, or the puerperium (630-676.9)*

④ 614 Inflammatory disease of ovary, fallopian tube, pelvic cellular tissue, and peritoneum
Excludes *endometritis (615.0-615.9)*
major infection following delivery (670)
that complicating:
abortion (634-638 with .0, 639.0)
ectopic or molar pregnancy (639.0)
pregnancy or labor (646.6)

614.0 Acute salpingitis and oophoritis ♀
Any condition classifiable to 614.2, specified as acute or subacute
C&C Exclusions: 016.60, 016.61, 016.62, 016.63, 016.64, 016.65, 016.66, 016.70, 016.71, 016.72, 016.73, 016.74, 016.75, 016.76, 016.90, 016.91, 016.92, 016.93, 016.94, 016.95, 016.96, 017.90, 017.91, 017.92, 017.93, 017.94, 017.95, 017.96, 098.15, 098.16, 098.17, 098.35, 098.36, 098.37, 098.89, 112.2, 131.00, 131.8, 131.9, 614.0, 614.1, 614.2, 614.3, 614.4, 614.5, 614.6, 614.7, 614.8, 614.9, 615.0, 615.1, 615.9, 616.8, 616.9, 625.8, 625.9, 629.8, 629.9, 752.8, 752.9

614.1 Chronic salpingitis and oophoritis ♀
Hydrosalpinx
Salpingitis:
follicularis
isthmica nodosa
Any condition classifiable to 614.2, specified as chronic

614.2 Salpingitis and oophoritis not specified as acute, subacute, or chronic ♀
Abscess (of):
fallopian tube
ovary
tubo-ovarian
Oophoritis
Perioophoritis
Perisalpingitis
Pyosalpinx
Salpingitis
Salpingo-oophoritis
Tubo-ovarian inflammatory disease
Excludes *gonococcal infection (chronic) (098.37)*
acute (098.17)
tuberculous (016.6)
AHA: 2Q 1991, 5

614.3 Acute parametritis and pelvic cellulitis ♀
Acute inflammatory pelvic disease
Any condition classifiable to 614.4, specified as acute
C&C Exclusions: See 614.0

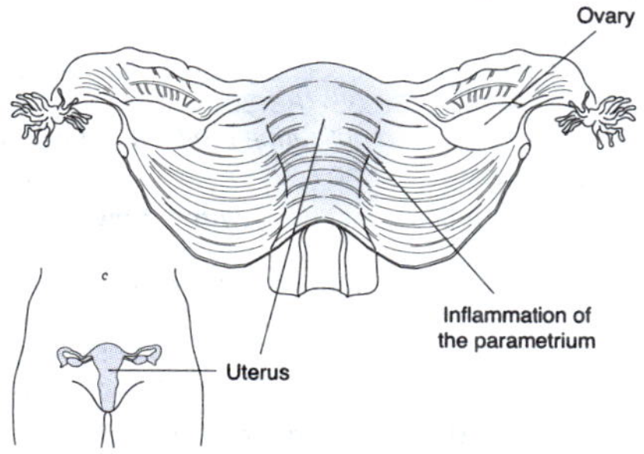

614.4 Chronic or unspecified parametritis and pelvic cellulitis ♀
Abscess (of):
broad ligament chronic or NOS
parametrium chronic or NOS
pelvis, female chronic or NOS
pouch of Douglas chronic or NOS
Chronic inflammatory pelvic disease
Pelvic cellulitis, female
Excludes *tuberculous (016.7)*

614.5 Acute or unspecified pelvic peritonitis, female ♀
C&C Exclusions: See 614.0
AHA: 4Q 2005, 74

614.6 Pelvic peritoneal adhesions, female (postoperative) (postinfection) ♀
Adhesions:
peritubal
tubo-ovarian
Use additional code to identify any associated infertility (628.2)
AHA: 3Q 2003, 6; 1Q 2003, 4; 3Q 1995, 7 3Q 1994, 12

614.7 Other chronic pelvic peritonitis, female ♀
Excludes *tuberculous (016.7)*

614.8 Other specified inflammatory disease of female pelvic organs and tissues ♀

614.9 Unspecified inflammatory disease of female pelvic organs and tissues ♀
Pelvic infection or inflammation, female NOS
Pelvic inflammatory disease [PID]

④ 615 Inflammatory diseases of uterus, except cervix
Excludes *following delivery (670)*
hyperplastic endometritis (621.30-621.33)
that complicating:
abortion (634-638 with .0, 639.0)
ectopic or molar pregnancy (639.0)
pregnancy or labor (646.6)

615.0 Acute ♀
Any condition classifiable to 615.9, specified as acute or subacute
C&C Exclusions: 016.60, 016.61, 016.62, 016.63, 016.64, 016.65, 016.66, 016.70, 016.71, 016.72, 016.73, 016.74, 016.75, 016.76, 016.90, 016.91, 016.92, 016.93, 016.94, 016.95, 016.96, 017.90, 017.91, 017.92, 017.93, 017.94, 017.95, 017.96, 098.15, 098.16, 098.17, 098.35, 098.36, 098.37, 098.89, 112.2, 131.00, 131.8, 131.9, 614.0, 614.1, 614.2, 614.3, 614.4, 614.5, 614.6, 614.7, 614.8, 614.9, 615.0, 615.1, 615.9, 616.0, 616.8, 616.9, 621.8, 621.9, 625.8, 625.9, 629.8, 629.9, 752.8, 752.9

615.1 Chronic ♀
Any condition classifiable to 615.9, specified as chronic

615.9 Unspecified inflammatory disease of uterus ♀
Endometritis
Endomyometritis
Metritis
Myometritis
Perimetritis
Pyometra
Uterine abscess

④ 616 Inflammatory disease of cervix, vagina, and vulva
Excludes *that complicating:*
abortion (634-638 with .0, 639.0)
ectopic or molar pregnancy (639.0)
pregnancy, childbirth, or the puerperium (646.6)

616.0 Cervicitis and endocervicitis ♀
Cervicitis with or without mention of erosion or ectropion
Endocervicitis with or without mention of erosion or ectropion
Nabothian (gland) cyst or follicle
Excludes *erosion or ectropion without mention of cervicitis (622.0)*

Genitourinary System

611.8 – 616.0

❺ **616.1 Vaginitis and vulvovaginitis**

616.10 Vaginitis and vulvovaginitis, unspecified ♀
Vaginitis:
NOS
postirradiation
Vulvitis NOS
Vulvovaginitis NOS
Use additional code to identify organism, such as Escherichia coli [E. coli] (041.4), Staphylococcus (041.1), or Streptococcus (041.0)
Excludes *noninfective leukorrhea (623.5)*
postmenopausal or senile vaginitis (627.3)

+ ***616.11 Vaginitis and vulvovaginitis in diseases classified elsewhere*** ♀
Code first underlying disease, as:
pinworm vaginitis (127.4)
Excludes *herpetic vulvovaginitis (054.11)*
monilial vulvovaginitis (112.1)
trichomonal vaginitis or vulvovaginitis (131.01)

616.2 Cyst of Bartholin's gland ♀
Bartholin's duct cyst

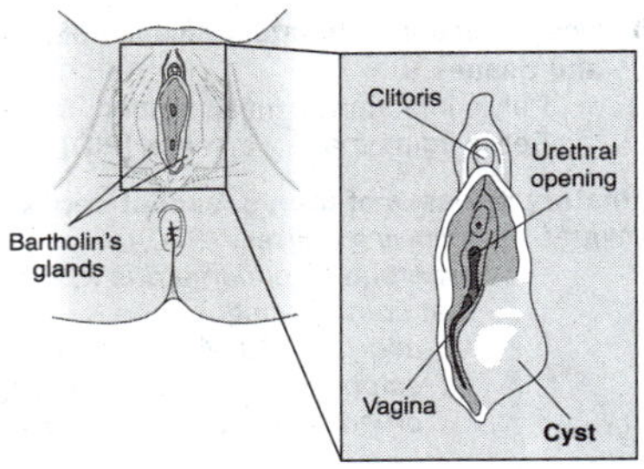

616.3 Abscess of Bartholin's gland ♀
Vulvovaginal gland abscess
C&C Exclusions: 016.70, 016.71, 016.72, 016.73, 016.74, 016.75, 016.76, 016.90, 016.91, 016.92, 016.93, 016.94, 016.95, 016.96, 017.90, 017.91, 017.92, 017.93, 017.94, 017.95, 017.96, 112.1, 112.2, 131.00, 131.01, 131.8, 131.9, 616.0, 616.8, 616.9, 624.3, 624.4, 624.5, 624.6, 624.8, 624.9, 625.8, 625.9, 629.8, 629.9, 752.8, 752.9

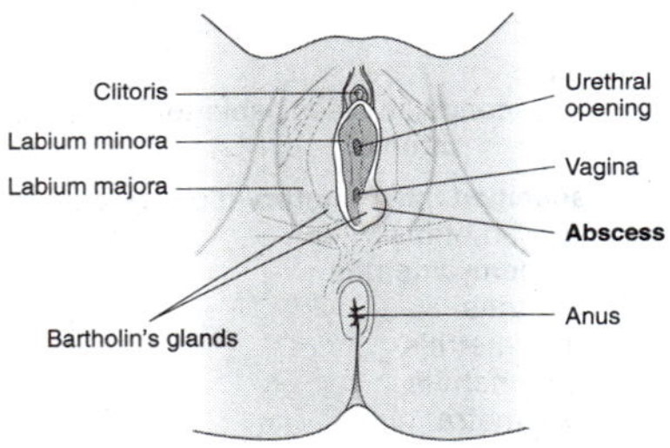

616.4 Other abscess of vulva ♀
Abscess of vulva
Carbuncle of vulva
Furuncle of vulva
C&C Exclusions: See 616.3

❺ **616.5 Ulceration of vulva**

616.50 Ulceration of vulva, unspecified ♀
Ulcer NOS of vulva

+ ***616.51 Ulceration of vulva in diseases classified elsewhere*** ♀
Code first underlying disease, as:
Behçet's syndrome (136.1)
tuberculosis (016.7)
Excludes *vulvar ulcer (in):*
gonococcal (098.0)
herpes simplex (054.12)
syphilitic (091.0)

❺ **616.8 Other specified inflammatory diseases of cervix, vagina, and vulva**
Excludes *noninflammatory disorders of:*
cervix (622.0-622.9)
vagina (623.0-623.9)
vulva (624.0-624.9)

616.81 Mucositis (ulcerative) of cervix, vagina, and vulva ♀
Use additional E code to identify adverse effects of therapy, such as:
antineoplastic and immunosuppressive drugs (E930.7, E933.1)
radiation therapy (E879.2)

616.89 Other inflammatory disease of cervix, vagina, and vulva ♀
Caruncle, vagina or labium
Ulcer, vagina

✖ **616.9 Unspecified inflammatory disease of cervix, vagina, and vulva** ♀

OTHER DISORDERS OF FEMALE GENITAL TRACT (617-629)

❹ **617 Endometriosis**
DEF: Tissue like that lining the uterus grows outside the uterus in the pelvis, abdomen, and on other organs; causes pain and infertility.

617.0 Endometriosis of uterus ♀
Adenomyosis
Endometriosis:
cervix
internal
myometrium
Excludes *stromal endometriosis (236.0)*
AHA: 3Q 1992, 7

617.1 Endometriosis of ovary ♀
Chocolate cyst of ovary
Endometrial cystoma of ovary

617.2 Endometriosis of fallopian tube ♀

617.3 Endometriosis of pelvic peritoneum ♀
Endometriosis:
broad ligament
cul-de-sac (Douglas')
parametrium
round ligament

617.4 Endometriosis of rectovaginal septum and vagina ♀

617.5 Endometriosis of intestine ♀
Endometriosis:
appendix
colon
rectum

617.6 Endometriosis in scar of skin ♀

617.8 Endometriosis of other specified sites ♀
Endometriosis:
bladder
lung
umbilicus
vulva

✖ **617.9 Endometriosis, site unspecified** ♀

❹ **618 Genital prolapse**
Use additional code to identify urinary incontinence (625.6, 788.31, 788.33-788.39)
Excludes *that complicating pregnancy, labor, or delivery (654.4)*

❺ **618.0 Prolapse of vaginal walls without mention of uterine prolapse**
Excludes *that with uterine prolapse (618.2-618.4)*
enterocele (618.6)
vaginal vault prolapse following hysterectomy (618.5)

✖ **618.00 Unspecified prolapse of vaginal walls** ♀
Vaginal prolapse NOS

618.01 Cystocele, midline ♀
Cystocele NOS

618.02 Cystocele, lateral ♀
Paravaginal
DEF: Bladder bulges through the side wall of the vagina.

618.03 Urethrocele ♀

618.04 Rectocele ♀
Proctocele

618.05 Perineocele ♀

618.09 Other prolapse of vaginal walls without mention of uterine prolapse ♀
Cystourethrocele

618.1 Uterine prolapse without mention of vaginal wall prolapse ♀
Descensus uteri
Uterine prolapse:
NOS
complete
first degree
second degree
third degree
Excludes *that with mention of cystocele, urethrocele, or rectocele (618.2-618.4)*

DEF: Uterine displacement downwards into the vaginal canal.

618.2 Uterovaginal prolapse, incomplete ♀

618.3 Uterovaginal prolapse, complete ♀

618.4 Uterovaginal prolapse, unspecified ♀

618.5 Prolapse of vaginal vault after hysterectomy ♀

618.6 Vaginal enterocele, congenital or acquired ♀
Pelvic enterocele, congenital or acquired

618.7 Old laceration of muscles of pelvic floor ♀

5 618.8 Other specified genital prolapse

618.81 Incompetence or weakening of pubocervical tissue ♀

618.82 Incompetence or weakening of rectovaginal tissue ♀

618.83 Pelvic muscle wasting ♀
Disuse atrophy of pelvic muscle and anal sphincter

618.84 Cervical stump prolapse ♀

618.89 Other specified genital prolapse ♀

618.9 Unspecified genital prolapse ♀

4 619 Fistula involving female genital tract
Excludes *vesicorectal and intestinovesical fistula (596.1)*

619.0 Urinary-genital tract fistula, female ♀
Fistula:
cervicovesical
ureterovaginal
urethrovaginal
urethrovesicovaginal
uteroureteric
uterovesical
vesicocervicovaginal
vesicovaginal

619.1 Digestive-genital tract fistula, female ♀
Fistula:
intestinouterine
intestinovaginal
rectovaginal
rectovulval
sigmoidovaginal
uterorectal

619.2 Genital tract-skin fistula, female ♀
Fistula:
uterus to abdominal wall
vaginoperineal

An abnormal tube-like passage connecting the genital tract to the skin surface

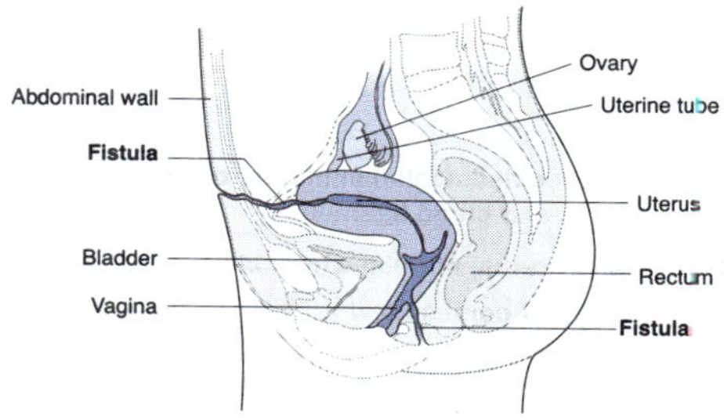

619.8 Other specified fistulas involving female genital tract ♀
Fistula:
cervix
cul-de-sac (Douglas')
uterus
vagina

619.9 Unspecified fistula involving female genital tract ♀

4 620 Noninflammatory disorders of ovary, fallopian tube, and broad ligament
Excludes *hydrosalpinx (614.1)*

620.0 Follicular cyst of ovary ♀
Cyst of graafian follicle
DEF: Fluid-filled sac on the ovary caused by larger than normal growth of a follicle that does not rupture to release the egg.

620.1 Corpus luteum cyst or hematoma ♀
Corpus luteum hemorrhage or rupture
Lutein cyst

620.2 Other and unspecified ovarian cyst ♀
Cyst of ovary:
NOS
corpus albicans
retention NOS
serous
theca-lutein
Simple cystoma of ovary
Excludes *cystadenoma (benign) (serous) (220)*
developmental cysts (752.0)
neoplastic cysts (220)
polycystic ovaries (256.4)
Stein-Leventhal syndrome (256.4)

620.3 Acquired atrophy of ovary and fallopian tube ♀
Senile involution of ovary

620.4 Prolapse or hernia of ovary and fallopian tube ♀
Displacement of ovary and fallopian tube
Salpingocele

620.5 Torsion of ovary, ovarian pedicle, or fallopian tube ♀
Torsion:
accessory tube
hydatid of Morgagni

620.6 Broad ligament laceration syndrome ♀
Masters-Allen syndrome

620.7 Hematoma of broad ligament ♀
Hematocele, broad ligament
C&C Exclusions: 620.6, 620.7, 620.8, 620.9, 625.8, 625.9, 629.8, 629.9, 752.8, 752.9

620.8 Other noninflammatory disorders of ovary, fallopian tube, and broad ligament ♀
Cyst of broad ligament or fallopian tube
Hematosalpinx of ovary or fallopian tube
Infarction of ovary or fallopian tube
Polyp of broad ligament or fallopian tube
Rupture of ovary or fallopian tube
Excludes *hematosalpinx in ectopic pregnancy (639.2)*
peritubal adhesions (614.6)
torsion of ovary, ovarian pedicle, or fallopian tube (620.5)

✖ **620.9 Unspecified noninflammatory disorder of ovary, fallopian tube, and broad ligament** ♀

❹ **621 Disorders of uterus, not elsewhere classified**

621.0 Polyp of corpus uteri ♀
Polyp:
endometrium
uterus NOS
Excludes *cervical polyp NOS (622.7)*

621.1 Chronic subinvolution of uterus ♀
Excludes *puerperal (674.8)*
AHA: 1Q 1991, 11

621.2 Hypertrophy of uterus ♀
Bulky or enlarged uterus
Excludes *puerperal (674.8)*

❺ **621.3 Endometrial hyperplasia**
Hyperplasia (adenomatous) (cystic) (glandular) of endometrium
Hyperplastic endometritis
DEF: Overgrowth of cells lining the uterus.

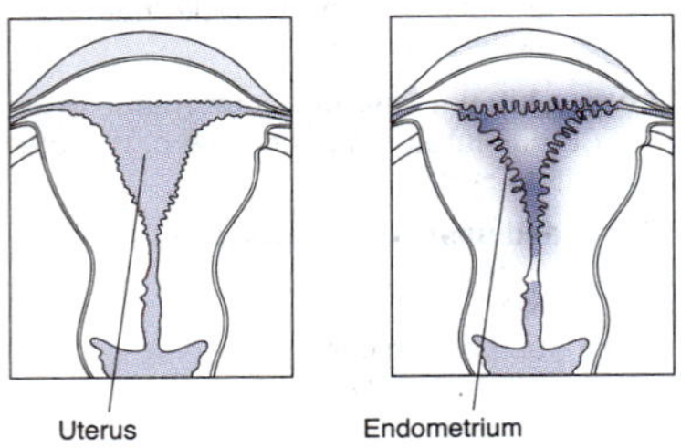

✖ **621.30 Endometrial hyperplasia, unspecified** ♀
Endometrial hyperplasia NOS

621.31 Simple endometrial hyperplasia without atypia ♀

621.32 Complex endometrial hyperplasia without atypia ♀

621.33 Endometrial hyperplasia with atypia ♀

621.4 Hematometra ♀
Hemometra
Excludes *that in congenital anomaly (752.2-752.3)*
DEF: Blood accumulated in the uterus.

621.5 Intrauterine synechiae ♀
Adhesions of uterus
Band(s) of uterus

621.6 Malposition of uterus ♀
Anteversion of uterus
Retroflexion of uterus
Retroversion of uterus
Excludes *malposition complicating pregnancy, labor, or delivery (654.3-654.4)*
prolapse of uterus (618.1-618.4)

621.7 Chronic inversion of uterus ♀
Excludes *current obstetrical trauma (665.2)*
prolapse of uterus (618.1-618.4)

621.8 Other specified disorders of uterus, not elsewhere classified ♀
Atrophy, acquired of uterus
Cyst of uterus
Fibrosis NOS of uterus
Old laceration (postpartum) of uterus
Ulcer of uterus
Excludes *bilharzial fibrosis (120.0-120.9)*
endometriosis (617.0)
fistulas (619.0-619.8)
inflammatory diseases (615.0-615.9)

✖ **621.9 Unspecified disorder of uterus** ♀

❹ **622 Noninflammatory disorders of cervix**
Excludes *abnormality of cervix complicating pregnancy, labor, or delivery (654.5-654.6)*
fistula (619.0-619.8)

622.0 Erosion and ectropion of cervix ♀
Eversion of cervix
Ulcer of cervix
Excludes *that in chronic cervicitis (616.0)*

❺ **622.1 Dysplasia of cervix (uteri)**
Excludes *abnormal results from cervical cytologic examination ▶without histologic confirmation (795.00-795.09)◀*
carcinoma in situ of cervix (233.1)
cervical intraepithelial neoplasia III [CIN III] (233.1)
AHA: 1Q 1991, 11

✖ **622.10 Dysplasia of cervix, unspecified** ♀
Anaplasia of cervix
Cervical atypism
Cervical dysplasia NOS

622.11 Mild dysplasia of cervix ♀
Cervical intraepithelial neoplasia I [CIN I]

622.12 Moderate dysplasia of cervix ♀
Cervical intraepithelial neoplasia II [CIN II]
Excludes *carcinoma in situ of cervix (233.1)*
cervical intraepithelial neoplasia III [CIN III] (233.1)
severe dysplasia (233.1)

622.2 Leukoplakia of cervix (uteri) ♀
Excludes *carcinoma in situ of cervix (233.1)*

622.3 Old laceration of cervix ♀
Adhesions of cervix
Band(s) of cervix
Cicatrix (postpartum) of cervix
Excludes *current obstetrical trauma (665.3)*

622.4 Stricture and stenosis of cervix ♀
Atresia (acquired) of cervix
Contracture of cervix
Occlusion of cervix
Pinpoint os uteri
Excludes *congenital (752.49)*
that complicating labor (654.6)

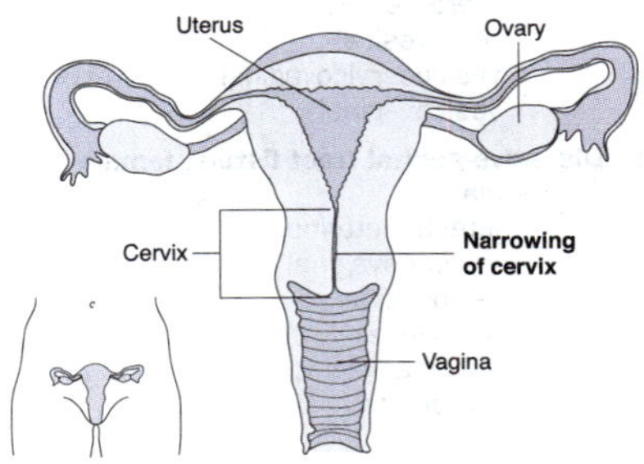

622.5 Incompetence of cervix ♀
Excludes *complicating pregnancy (654.5)*
that affecting fetus or newborn (761.0)

622.6 Hypertrophic elongation of cervix ♀

622.7 Mucous polyp of cervix ♀
Polyp NOS of cervix
Excludes *adenomatous polyp of cervix (219.0)*

622.8 Other specified noninflammatory disorders of cervix ♀
Atrophy (senile) of cervix
Cyst of cervix
Fibrosis of cervix
Hemorrhage of cervix
Excludes *endometriosis (617.0)*
fistula (619.0-619.8)
inflammatory diseases (616.0)

✖ **622.9 Unspecified noninflammatory disorder of cervix ♀**

④ **623 Noninflammatory disorders of vagina**
Excludes *abnormality of vagina complicating pregnancy, labor, or delivery (654.7)*
congenital absence of vagina (752.49)
congenital diaphragm or bands (752.49)
fistulas involving vagina (619.0-619.8)

623.0 Dysplasia of vagina ♀
▶ Vaginal intraepithelial neoplasia I and II [VAIN I and II]◀
Excludes *carcinoma in situ of vagina (▶233.31◀)*
▶ *severe dysplasia of vagina (233.31)*◀
▶ *vaginal intraepithelial neoplasia III [VAIN III] (233.31)*◀

623.1 Leukoplakia of vagina ♀
DEF: White plaque on the mucosal surface of vagina that develops into thickened, rough-textured grayish white lesions.

623.2 Stricture or atresia of vagina ♀
Adhesions (postoperative) (postradiation) of vagina
Occlusion of vagina
Stenosis, vagina
Use additional E code to identify any external cause
Excludes *congenital atresia or stricture (752.49)*

623.3 Tight hymenal ring ♀
Rigid hymen acquired or congenital
Tight hymenal ring acquired or congenital
Tight introitus acquired or congenital
Excludes *imperforate hymen (752.42)*

623.4 Old vaginal laceration ♀
Excludes *old laceration involving muscles of pelvic floor (618.7)*

623.5 Leukorrhea, not specified as infective ♀
Leukorrhea NOS of vagina
Vaginal discharge NOS
Excludes *trichomonal (131.00)*

623.6 Vaginal hematoma ♀
Excludes *current obstetrical trauma (665.7)*

623.7 Polyp of vagina ♀

623.8 Other specified noninflammatory disorders of vagina ♀
Cyst of vagina
Hemorrhage of vagina

✖ **623.9 Unspecified noninflammatory disorder of vagina ♀**

④ **624 Noninflammatory disorders of vulva and perineum**
Excludes *abnormality of vulva and perineum complicating pregnancy, labor, or delivery (654.8)*
condyloma acuminatum (078.1)
fistulas involving:
perineum - see Alphabetic Index
vulva (619.0-619.8)
vulval varices (456.6)
vulvar involvement in skin conditions (690-709.9)

⑤ **624.0 Dystrophy of vulva**
Excludes *carcinoma in situ of vulva (▶233.32◀)*
▶ *severe dysplasia of vulva (233.32)*◀
▶ *vulvar intraepithelial neoplasia III [VIN III] (233.32)* ◀

● **624.01 Vulvar intraepithelial neoplasia I [VIN I] ♀**
Mild dysplasia of vulva

● **624.02 Vulvar intraepithelial neoplasia II [VIN II] ♀**
Moderate dysplasia of vulva

● **624.09 Other dystrophy of vulva ♀**
Kraurosis of vulva
Leukoplakia of vulva

624.1 Atrophy of vulva ♀

A partial or complete wasting away of the vulva

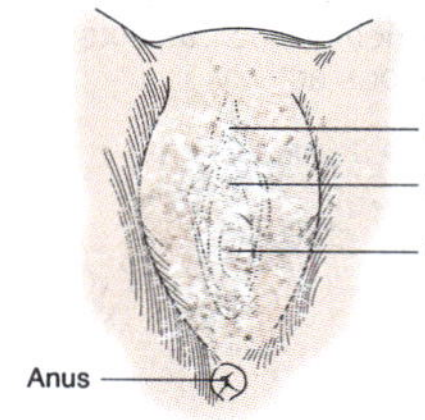

624.2 Hypertrophy of clitoris ♀
Excludes *that in endocrine disorders (255.2, 256.1)*

624.3 Hypertrophy of labia ♀
Hypertrophy of vulva NOS

624.4 Old laceration or scarring of vulva ♀

624.5 Hematoma of vulva ♀
Excludes *that complicating delivery (664.5)*

624.6 Polyp of labia and vulva ♀

624.8 Other specified noninflammatory disorders of vulva and perineum ♀
Cyst of vulva
Edema of vulva
Stricture of vulva
AHA: 1Q 2003, 13; 1Q 1995, 8

✖ **624.9 Unspecified noninflammatory disorder of vulva and perineum ♀**

④ **625 Pain and other symptoms associated with female genital organs**

625.0 Dyspareunia ♀
Excludes *psychogenic dyspareunia (302.76)*
DEF: Pain during sexual intercourse.

625.1 Vaginismus ♀
Colpospasm
Vulvismus
Excludes *psychogenic vaginismus (306.51)*
DEF: Severe, painful spasms of the vaginal muscles that prevent sexual intercourse.

625.2 Mittelschmerz ♀
Intermenstrual pain
Ovulation pain

625.3 Dysmenorrhea ♀
Painful menstruation
Excludes *psychogenic dysmenorrhea (306.52)*
AHA: 2Q 1994, 12

625.4 Premenstrual tension syndromes ♀
Menstrual:
migraine
molimen
Premenstrual dysphoric disorder
Premenstrual syndrome
Premenstrual tension NOS
AHA: 4Q 2003, 116

625.5 Pelvic congestion syndrome ♀
Congestion-fibrosis syndrome
Taylor's syndrome
DEF: Varicose veins in the pelvis causing pressure build-up, bulging, and congestion with painful symptoms.

625.6 Stress incontinence, female ♀
Excludes *mixed incontinence (788.33)*
stress incontinence, male (788.32)

DEF: Involuntary loss of bladder control during physical movements, such as coughing, sneezing, or other strenuous activity.

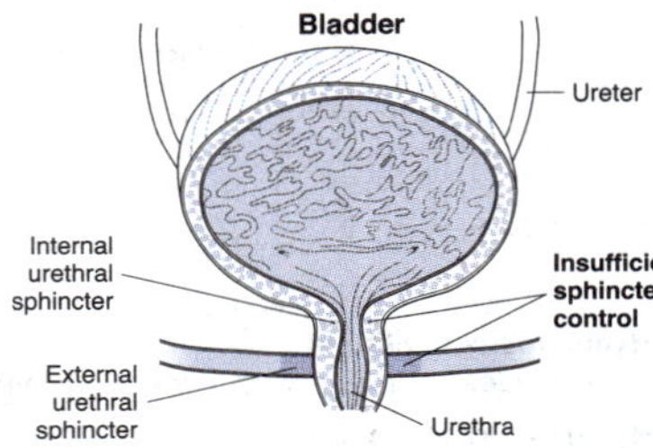

625.8 Other specified symptoms associated with female genital organs ♀
AHA: Nov-Dec 1985, 16

625.9 Unspecified symptom associated with female genital organs ♀
AHA: 4Q 2006, 110

❹ **626 Disorders of menstruation and other abnormal bleeding from female genital tract**
Excludes *menopausal and premenopausal bleeding (627.0)*
pain and other symptoms associated with menstrual cycle (625.2-625.4)
postmenopausal bleeding (627.1)

626.0 Absence of menstruation ♀
Amenorrhea (primary) (secondary)

626.1 Scanty or infrequent menstruation ♀
Hypomenorrhea
Oligomenorrhea

626.2 Excessive or frequent menstruation ♀
Heavy periods
Menometrorrhagia
Menorrhagia
Polymenorrhea
Excludes *premenopausal (627.0)*
that in puberty (626.3)

626.3 Puberty bleeding ♀
Excessive bleeding associated with onset of menstrual periods
Pubertal menorrhagia

626.4 Irregular menstrual cycle ♀
Irregular:
bleeding NOS
menstruation
periods

626.5 Ovulation bleeding ♀
Regular intermenstrual bleeding

626.6 Metrorrhagia ♀
Bleeding unrelated to menstrual cycle
Irregular intermenstrual bleeding

626.7 Postcoital bleeding ♀
DEF: Bleeding after sexual intercourse.

626.8 Other ♀
Dysfunctional or functional uterine hemorrhage NOS
Menstruation:
retained
suppression of

✖ **626.9 Unspecified** ♀

❹ **627 Menopausal and postmenopausal disorders**
Excludes *asymptomatic age-related (natural) postmenopausal status (V49.81)*

627.0 Premenopausal menorrhagia ♀
Excessive bleeding associated with onset of menopause
Menorrhagia:
climacteric
menopausal
preclimacteric

627.1 Postmenopausal bleeding ♀

627.2 Symptomatic menopausal or female climacteric states ♀
Symptoms, such as flushing, sleeplessness, headache, lack of concentration, associated with the menopause

627.3 Postmenopausal atrophic vaginitis ♀
Senile (atrophic) vaginitis

627.4 Symptomatic states associated with artificial menopause ♀
Postartificial menopause syndromes
Any condition classifiable to 627.1, 627.2, or 627.3 which follows induced menopause

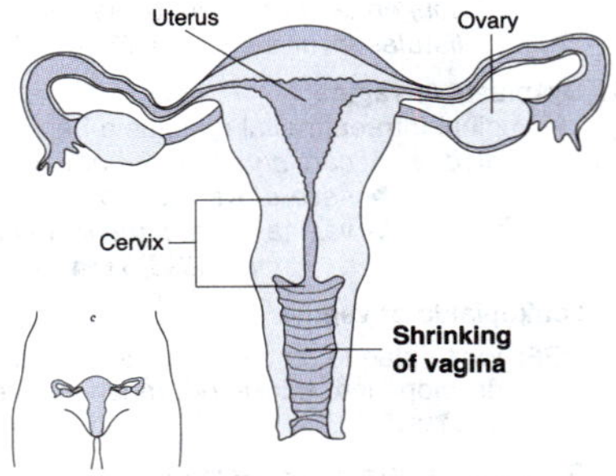

627.8 Other specified menopausal and postmenopausal disorders ♀
Excludes *premature menopause NOS (256.31)*

✖ **627.9 Unspecified menopausal and postmenopausal disorder** ♀

❹ **628 Infertility, female**
Includes primary and secondary sterility
AHA: 2Q 1996, 9; 1Q 1995, 7

628.0 Associated with anovulation ♀
Anovulatory cycle
Use additional code for any associated Stein-Leventhal syndrome (256.4)

✚ ***628.1 Of pituitary-hypothalamic origin*** ♀
Code first underlying disease, as:
adiposogenital dystrophy (253.8)
anterior pituitary disorder (253.0-253.4)

628.2 Of tubal origin ♀
Infertility associated with congenital anomaly of tube
Tubal:
block
occlusion
stenosis
Use additional code for any associated peritubal adhesions (614.6)

628.3 Of uterine origin ♀
Infertility associated with congenital anomaly of uterus
Nonimplantation
Use additional code for any associated tuberculous endometritis (016.7)

628.4 Of cervical or vaginal origin ♀
Infertility associated with:
anomaly or cervical mucus
congenital structural anomaly
dysmucorrhea

628.8 Of other specified origin ♀

628.9 Of unspecified origin ♀

❹ **629 Other disorders of female genital organs**

629.0 Hematocele, female, not elsewhere classified ♀
Excludes *hematocele or hematoma:*
broad ligament (620.7)
fallopian tube (620.8)
that associated with ectopic pregnancy (633.00-633.91)
uterus (621.4)
vagina (623.6)
vulva (624.5)

629.1 Hydrocele, canal of Nuck ♀
Cyst of canal of Nuck (acquired)
Excludes *congenital (752.41)*
DEF: Fluid filled sac in the canal of Nuck, the narrow cavity between the vaginal canal and the uterus.

❺ **629.2 Female genital mutilation status**
Female circumcision status
Female genital cutting
AHA: 4Q 2004, 88

✖ **629.20 Female genital mutilation status, unspecified** ♀
Female genital cutting status, unspecified
Female genital mutilation NOS

629.21 Female genital mutilation Type I status ♀
Clitorectomy status
Female genital cutting Type I status

629.22 Female genital mutilation Type II status ♀
Clitorectomy with excision of labia minora status
Female genital cutting Type II status
AHA: 4Q 2004, 90

629.23 Female genital mutilation Type III status ♀
Female genital cutting Type III status
Infibulation status
AHA: 4Q 2004, 90

629.29 Other female genital mutilation status ♀
Female genital cutting Type IV status
Female genital mutilation Type IV status
Other female genital cutting status

❺ **629.8 Other specified disorders of female genital organs**

629.81 Habitual aborter without current pregnancy ♀
Excludes *habitual aborter with current pregnancy (646.3)*

629.89 Other specified disorders of female genital organs ♀

629.9 Unspecified disorder of female genital organs ♀

11. COMPLICATIONS OF PREGNANCY, CHILDBIRTH, AND THE PUERPERIUM (630-677)

ECTOPIC AND MOLAR PREGNANCY (630-633)

Use additional code from category 639 to identify any complications

630 Hydatidiform mole ♀M
Trophoblastic disease NOS
Vesicular mole
Excludes *chorioadenoma (destruens) (236.1)*
chorionepithelioma (181)
malignant hydatidiform mole (236.1)
DEF: Fertilized egg tissue develops into an abnormal, potentially cancerous, grape-like cluster of cells instead of a normal embyro and placenta.

631 Other abnormal product of conception ♀M
Blighted ovum
Mole:
NOS
carneous
fleshy
stone

632 Missed abortion ♀M
Early fetal death before completion of 22 weeks' gestation with retention of dead fetus
Retained products of conception, not following spontaneous or induced abortion or delivery
Excludes *failed induced abortion (638.0-638.9)*
fetal death (intrauterine) (late) (656.4)
missed delivery (656.4)
that with abnormal product of conception (630, 631)
AHA: 1Q 2001, 5

❹ **633 Ectopic pregnancy**
Includes ruptured ectopic pregnancy
AHA: 4Q 2002, 61

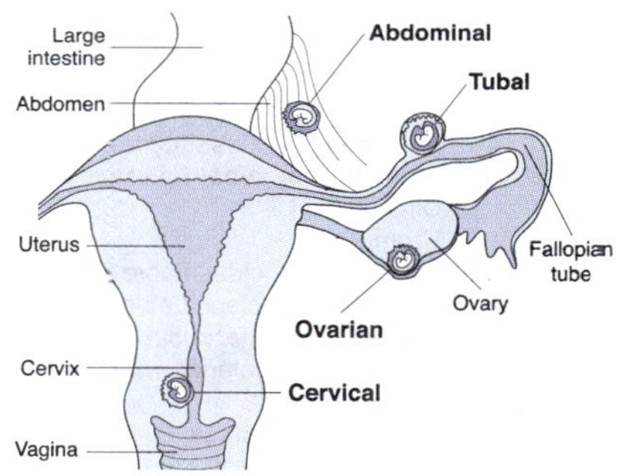

❺ **633.0 Abdominal pregnancy**
Intraperitoneal pregnancy

633.00 Abdominal pregnancy without intrauterine pregnancy ♀M

633.01 Abdominal pregnancy with intrauterine pregnancy ♀M

❺ **633.1 Tubal pregnancy**
Fallopian pregnancy
Rupture of (fallopian) tube due to pregnancy
Tubal abortion
DEF: Fertilized egg implants itself within the fallopian tube where the embryo grows and may rupture the tube.
AHA: 2Q 1990, 27

633.10 Tubal pregnancy without intrauterine pregnancy ♀M

633.11 Tubal pregnancy with intrauterine pregnancy ♀M

❺ **633.2 Ovarian pregnancy**

633.20 Ovarian pregnancy without intrauterine pregnancy ♀M

633.21 Ovarian pregnancy with intrauterine pregnancy ♀M

❺ **633.8 Other ectopic pregnancy**
Pregnancy:
cervical
combined
cornual
intraligamentous
mesometric
mural

633.80 Other ectopic pregnancy without intrauterine pregnancy ♀M

633.81 Other ectopic pregnancy with intrauterine pregnancy ♀M

❺ **633.9 Unspecified ectopic pregnancy**

✖ **633.90 Unspecified ectopic pregnancy without intrauterine pregnancy** ♀M

✖ **633.91 Unspecified ectopic pregnancy with intrauterine pregnancy** ♀M

OTHER PREGNANCY WITH ABORTIVE OUTCOME (634-639)

The following fourth-digit subdivisions are for use with categories 634-638:

.0 Complicated by genital tract and pelvic infection
Endometritis
Salpingo-oophoritis
Sepsis NOS
Septicemia NOS
Any condition classifiable to 639.0, with condition classifiable to 634-638
Excludes *urinary tract infection (634-638 with .7)*

.1 Complicated by delayed or excessive hemorrhage
Afibrinogenemia
Defibrination syndrome
Intravascular hemolysis
Any condition classifiable to 639.1, with condition classifiable to 634-638

.2 Complicated by damage to pelvic organs and tissues
Laceration, perforation, or tear of:
bladder
uterus
Any condition classifiable to 639.2, with condition classifiable to 634-638

.3 Complicated by renal failure
Oliguria
Uremia
Any condition classifiable to 639.3, with condition classifiable to 634-638

.4 Complicated by metabolic disorder
Electrolyte imbalance with conditions classifiable to 634-638

.5 Complicated by shock
Circulatory collapse
Shock (postoperative) (septic)
Any condition classifiable to 639.5, with condition classifiable to 634-638

.6 Complicated by embolism
Embolism:
NOS
amniotic fluid
pulmonary
Any condition classifiable to 639.6, with condition classifiable to 634-638

.7 With other specified complications
Cardiac arrest or failure
Urinary tract infection
Any condition classifiable to 639.8, with condition classifiable to 634-638

.8 With unspecified complications

.9 Without mention of complication

❹ **634 Spontaneous abortion**
Includes miscarriage
spontaneous abortion
AHA: 2Q 1991, 16

Requires fifth digit to identify stage:
0 unspecified
1 incomplete
2 complete

❺ **634.0 Complicated by genital tract and pelvic infection** ♀M
C&C Exclusions: (for code 634.00) 634.00, 634.01, 634.02, 634.10, 634.11, 634.12, 634.20, 634.21, 634.22, 634.30, 634.31, 634.32, 634.40, 634.41, 634.42, 634.50, 634.51, 634.52, 634.60, 634.61, 634.62, 634.70, 634.71, 634.72, 634.80, 634.81, 634.82, 634.90, 634.91, 634.92, 635.00, 635.01, 635.02, 635.10, 635.11, 635.12, 635.20, 635.21, 635.22, 635.30, 635.31, 635.32, 635.40, 635.41, 635.42, 635.50, 635.51, 635.52, 635.60, 635.61, 635.62, 635.70, 635.71, 635.72, 635.80, 635.81, 635.82, 635.90, 635.91, 635.92, 636.00, 636.01, 636.02, 636.10, 636.11, 636.12, 636.20, 636.21, 636.22, 636.30, 636.31, 636.32, 636.40, 636.41, 636.42, 636.50, 636.51, 636.52, 636.60, 636.61, 636.62, 636.70, 636.71, 636.72, 636.80, 636.81, 636.82, 636.90, 636.91, 636.92, 637.00, 637.01, 637.02, 637.10, 637.11, 637.12, 637.20, 637.21, 637.22, 637.30, 637.31, 637.32, 637.40, 637.41, 637.42, 637.50, 637.51, 637.52, 637.60, 637.61, 637.62, 637.70, 637.71, 637.72, 637.80, 637.81, 637.82, 637.90, 637.91, 637.92, 638.0, 638.1, 638.2, 638.3, 638.4, 638.5, 638.6, 638.7, 638.8, 638.9, 640.00, 640.01, 640.03, 640.80, 640.81, 640.83, 640.90, 640.91, 640.93, 641.00, 641.01, 641.03, 641.10, 641.11, 641.13, 641.20, 641.21, 641.23, 646.80, 646.81, 646.82, 646.83, 646.84, 646.90, 646.91, 646.93, 648.90, 648.91, 648.92, 648.93, 648.94, 650, 669.40, 669.41, 669.42, 669.43, 669.44, 669.80, 669.81, 669.82, 669.83, 669.84, 669.90, 669.91, 669.92, 669.93, 669.94

❺ **634.1 Complicated by delayed or excessive hemorrhage** ♀M

❺ **634.2 Complicated by damage to pelvic organs or tissues** ♀M

❺ **634.3 Complicated by renal failure** ♀M

❺ **634.4 Complicated by metabolic disorder** ♀M

❺ **634.5 Complicated by shock** ♀M

❺ **634.6 Complicated by embolism** ♀M

❺ **634.7 With other specified complications** ♀M

❺ **634.8 With unspecified complication** ♀M

❺ **634.9 Without mention of complication** ♀M

❹ **635 Legally induced abortion**
Includes abortion or termination of pregnancy:
elective
legal
therapeutic
Excludes *menstrual extraction or regulation (V25.3)*
AHA: 2Q 1994, 14

Requires fifth digit to identify stage:
0 unspecified
1 incomplete
2 complete

❺ **635.0 Complicated by genital tract and pelvic infection** ♀M

❺ **635.1 Complicated by delayed or excessive hemorrhage** ♀M

❺ **635.2 Complicated by damage to pelvic organs or tissues** ♀M

❺ **635.3 Complicated by renal failure** ♀M

❺ **635.4 Complicated by metabolic disorder** ♀M

❺ **635.5 Complicated by shock** ♀M

❺ **635.6 Complicated by embolism** ♀M

❺ **635.7 With other specified complications** ♀M

❺ **635.8 With unspecified complication** ♀M

❺ **635.9 Without mention of complication** ♀M

4 636 Illegally induced abortion
Includes abortion:
criminal
illegal
self-induced

Requires fifth digit to identify stage:
0 **unspecified**
1 **incomplete**
2 **complete**

5 **636.0 Complicated by genital tract and pelvic infection** ♀M
5 **636.1 Complicated by delayed or excessive hemorrhage** ♀M
5 **636.2 Complicated by damage to pelvic organs or tissues** ♀M
5 **636.3 Complicated by renal failure** ♀M
5 **636.4 Complicated by metabolic disorder** ♀M
5 **636.5 Complicated by shock** ♀M
5 **636.6 Complicated by embolism** ♀M
5 **636.7 With other specified complications** ♀M
5 **636.8 With unspecified complication** ♀M
5 **636.9 Without mention of complication** ♀M

4 637 Unspecified abortion
Includes abortion NOS
retained products of conception following abortion, not classifiable elsewhere

Requires fifth digit to identify stage:
0 **unspecified**
1 **incomplete**
2 **complete**

5 **637.0 Complicated by genital tract and pelvic infection** ♀M
5 **637.1 Complicated by delayed or excessive hemorrhage** ♀M
5 **637.2 Complicated by damage to pelvic organs or tissues** ♀M
5 **637.3 Complicated by renal failure** ♀M
5 **637.4 Complicated by metabolic disorder** ♀M
5 **637.5 Complicated by shock** ♀M
5 **637.6 Complicated by embolism** ♀M
5 **637.7 With other specified complications** ♀M
5 **637.8 With unspecified complication** ♀M
5 **637.9 Without mention of complication** ♀M

4 638 Failed attempted abortion
Includes failure of attempted induction of (legal) abortion
Excludes incomplete abortion (634.0-637.9)

638.0 Complicated by genital tract and pelvic infection ♀M
638.1 Complicated by delayed or excessive hemorrhage ♀M
638.2 Complicated by damage to pelvic organs or tissues ♀M
638.3 Complicated by renal failure ♀M
638.4 Complicated by metabolic disorder ♀M
638.5 Complicated by shock ♀M
638.6 Complicated by embolism ♀M
638.7 With other specified complications ♀M
638.8 With unspecified complication ♀M
638.9 Without mention of complication ♀M

4 639 Complications following abortion and ectopic and molar pregnancies
Note: This category is provided for use when it is required to classify separately the complications classifiable to the fourth digit level in categories 634-638; for example:
a) when the complication itself was responsible for an episode of medical care, the abortion, ectopic or molar pregnancy itself having been dealt with at a previous episode
b) when these conditions are immediate complications of ectopic or molar pregnancies classifiable to 630-633 where they cannot be identified at fourth digit level.

639.0 Genital tract and pelvic infection ♀M
Endometritis following conditions classifiable to 630-638
Parametritis following conditions classifiable to 630-638
Pelvic peritonitis following conditions classifiable to 630-638
Salpingitis following conditions classifiable to 630-638
Salpingo-oophoritis following conditions classifiable to 630-638
Sepsis NOS following conditions classifiable to 630-638
Septicemia NOS following conditions classifiable to 630-638
Excludes urinary tract infection (639.8)
C&C Exclusions: 639.0, 639.2, 639.3, 639.4, 639.5, 639.6, 639.8, 639.9, 640.00, 640.01, 640.03, 640.80, 640.81, 640.83, 640.90, 640.91, 640.93, 641.00, 641.01, 641.03, 641.10, 641.11, 641.13, 641.20, 641.21, 641.23, 646.80, 646.81, 646.82, 646.83, 646.84, 646.90, 646.91, 646.93, 648.90, 648.91, 648.92, 648.93, 648.94, 650, 669.40, 669.41, 669.42, 669.43, 669.44, 669.80, 669.81, 669.82, 669.83, 669.84, 669.90, 669.91, 669.92, 669.93, 669.94

639.1 Delayed or excessive hemorrhage ♀M
Afibrinogenemia following conditions classifiable to 630-638
Defibrination syndrome following conditions classifiable to 630-638
Intravascular hemolysis following conditions classifiable to 630-638
C&C Exclusions: 639.1, 639.2, 639.3, 639.4, 639.5, 639.6, 639.8, 639.9, 640.00, 640.01, 640.03, 640.80, 640.81, 640.83, 640.90, 640.91, 640.93, 641.00, 641.01, 641.03, 641.10, 641.11, 641.13, 641.20, 641.21, 641.23, 646.80, 646.81, 646.82, 646.83, 646.84, 646.90, 646.91, 646.93, 648.90, 648.91, 648.92, 648.93, 648.94, 650, 669.40, 669.41, 669.42, 669.43, 669.44, 669.80, 669.81, 669.82, 669.83, 669.84, 669.90, 669.91, 669.92, 669.93, 669.94

639.2 Damage to pelvic organs and tissues ♀M
Laceration, perforation, or tear of:
bladder following conditions classifiable to 630-638
bowel following conditions classifiable to 630-638
broad ligament following conditions classifiable to 630-638
cervix following conditions classifiable to 630-638
periurethral tissue following conditions classifiable to 630-638
uterus following conditions classifiable to 630-638
vagina following conditions classifiable to 630-638
C&C Exclusions: 639.2, 639.3, 639.4, 639.5, 639.6, 639.8, 639.9, 640.00, 640.01, 640.03, 640.80, 640.81, 640.83, 640.90, 640.91, 640.93, 641.00, 641.01, 641.03, 641.10, 641.11, 641.13, 641.20, 641.21, 641.23, 646.80, 646.81, 646.82, 646.83, 646.84, 646.90, 646.91, 646.93, 648.90, 648.91, 648.92, 648.93, 648.94, 650, 669.40, 669.41, 669.42, 669.43, 669.44, 669.80, 669.81, 669.82, 669.83, 669.84, 669.90, 669.91, 669.92, 669.93, 669.94

639.3 Renal failure ♀M
Oliguria following conditions classifiable to 630-638
Renal:
failure (acute) following conditions classifiable to 630-638
shutdown following conditions classifiable to 630-638
tubular necrosis following conditions classifiable to 630-638
Uremia following conditions classifiable to 630-638
C&C Exclusions: See 639.2

639.4 Metabolic disorders ♀M
Electrolyte imbalance following conditions classifiable to 630-638
C&C Exclusions: See 639.2

Complications of Pregnancy, Childbirth, and the Puerperium 636 – 639.4

A Adult (15+ years) M Maternity (12-55 years) N Newborn (0 years) P Pediatric (0-17 years) ♂Male ♀Female 2 Medicare Secondary Payer

639.5 Shock ♀M
Circulatory collapse following conditions classifiable to 630-638
Shock (postoperative) (septic) following conditions classifiable to 630-638
C&C Exclusions: See 639.2

639.6 Embolism ♀M
Embolism:
NOS following conditions classifiable to 630-638
air following conditions classifiable to 630-638
amniotic fluid following conditions classifiable to 630-638
blood-clot following conditions classifiable to 630-638
fat following conditions classifiable to 630-638
pulmonary following conditions classifiable to 630-638
pyemic following conditions classifiable to 630-638
septic following conditions classifiable to 630-638
soap following conditions classifiable to 630-638
C&C Exclusions: See 639.2

639.8 Other specified complications following abortion or ectopic and molar pregnancy ♀M
Acute yellow atrophy or necrosis of liver following conditions classifiable to 630-638
Cardiac arrest or failure following conditions classifiable to 630-638
Cerebral anoxia following conditions classifiable to 630-638
Urinary tract infection following conditions classifiable to 630-638
C&C Exclusions: See 639.2

639.9 Unspecified complication following abortion or ectopic and molar pregnancy ♀M
Complication(s) not further specified following conditions classifiable to 630-638
C&C Exclusions: See 639.2

COMPLICATIONS MAINLY RELATED TO PREGNANCY (640-649)

Includes the listed conditions even if they arose or were present during labor, delivery, or the puerperium

AHA: 2Q 1990, 11

The following fifth-digit subclassification is for use with categories 640-649 to denote the current episode of care:

0 **unspecified as to episode of care or not applicable**
1 **delivered, with or without mention of antepartum condition**
Antepartum condition with delivery
Delivery NOS (with mention of antepartum complication during current episode of care)
Intrapartum obstetric condition (with mention of antepartum complication during current episode of care)
Pregnancy, delivered (with mention of antepartum complication during current episode of care)
2 **delivered, with mention of postpartum complication**
Delivery with mention of puerperal complication during current episode of care
3 **antepartum condition or complication**
Antepartum obstetric condition, not delivered during the current episode of care
4 **postpartum condition or complication**
Postpartum or puerperal obstetric condition or complication following delivery that occurred:
during previous episode of care
outside hospital, with subsequent admission for observation or care

④ **640 Hemorrhage in early pregnancy**
Requires fifth digit; valid digits are in [brackets] under each code. See beginning of section 640-649 for definitions.
Includes hemorrhage before completion of 22 weeks' gestation

⑤ **640.0 Threatened abortion** ♀M
[0,1,3]
C&C Exclusions: 640.00, 640.01, 640.03, 640.80, 640.81, 640.83, 640.90, 640.91, 640.93, 641.00, 641.01, 641.03, 641.10, 641.11, 641.13, 646.80, 646.81, 646.82, 646.83, 646.84, 646.90, 646.91, 646.93, 648.90, 648.91, 648.92, 648.93, 648.94, 650, 669.40, 669.41, 669.42, 669.43, 669.44, 669.80, 669.81, 669.82, 669.83, 669.84, 669.90, 669.91, 669.92, 669.93, 669.94

⑤ **640.8 Other specified hemorrhage in early pregnancy** ♀M
[0,1,3]
C&C Exclusions: See 640.0

✖⑤ **640.9 Unspecified hemorrhage in early pregnancy** ♀M
[0,1,3]
C&C Exclusions: See 640.0

④ **641 Antepartum hemorrhage, abruptio placentae, and placenta previa**
Requires fifth digit; valid digits are in [brackets] under each code. See beginning of section 640-649 for definitions.

⑤ **641.0 Placenta previa without hemorrhage** ♀M
[0,1,3]
(✖ is only valid for fifth-digit "0")
Low implantation of placenta without hemorrhage
Placenta previa noted:
during pregnancy without hemorrhage
before labor (and delivered by cesarean delivery) without hemorrhage
DEF: Placenta situated at the bottom of the uterus, over the opening of the cervix.
C&C Exclusions: See 640.0

⑤ **641.1 Hemorrhage from placenta previa** ♀M
[0,1,3]
(✖ is only valid for fifth-digit "0")
Low-lying placenta NOS or with hemorrhage (intrapartum)
Placenta previa:
incomplete NOS or with hemorrhage (intrapartum)
marginal NOS or with hemorrhage (intrapartum)
partial NOS or with hemorrhage (intrapartum)
total NOS or with hemorrhage (intrapartum)
Excludes *hemorrhage from vasa previa (663.5)*
C&C Exclusions: See 640.0

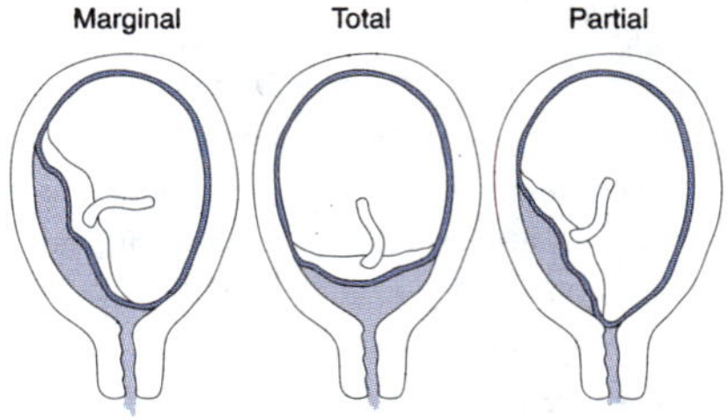

⑤ **641.2 Premature separation of placenta** ♀M
[0,1,3]
(✖ is only valid for fifth-digit "0")
Ablatio placentae
Abruptio placentae
Accidental antepartum hemorrhage
Couvelaire uterus
Detachment of placenta (premature)
Premature separation of normally implanted placenta

❺ 641.3 Antepartum hemorrhage associated with coagulation defects ♀ M

[0,1,3] (✖ is only valid for fifth-digit "0")

Antepartum or intrapartum hemorrhage associated with:
- afibrinogenemia
- hyperfibrinolysis
- hypofibrinogenemia

Excludes *coagulation defects not associated with antepartum hemorrhage (649.3)*

C&C Exclusions: 641.30, 641.31, 641.33, 641.80, 641.81, 641.83, 641.90, 641.91, 641.93, 646.80, 646.81, 646.82, 646.83, 646.84, 646.90, 646.91, 646.93, 648.90, 648.91, 648.92, 648.93, 648.94, 650, 669.40, 669.41, 669.42, 669.43, 669.44, 669.80, 669.81, 669.82, 669.83, 669.84, 669.90, 669.91, 669.92, 669.93, 669.94

❺ 641.8 Other antepartum hemorrhage ♀ M

[0,1,3] (✖ is only valid for fifth-digit "0")

Antepartum or intrapartum hemorrhage associated with:
- trauma
- uterine leiomyoma

C&C Exclusions: See 641.3

✖❺ 641.9 Unspecified antepartum hemorrhage ♀ M

[0,1,3]

Hemorrhage:
- antepartum NOS
- intrapartum NOS
- of pregnancy NOS

C&C Exclusions: See 641.3

❹ 642 Hypertension complicating pregnancy, childbirth, and the puerperium

Requires fifth digit; valid digits are in [brackets] under each code. See beginning of section 640-649 for definitions.

❺ 642.0 Benign essential hypertension complicating pregnancy, childbirth, and the puerperium ♀ M

[0-4] (✖ is only valid for fifth-digit "0")

Hypertension:
- benign essential specified as complicating, or as a reason for obstetric care during pregnancy, childbirth, or the puerperium
- chronic NOS specified as complicating, or as a reason for obstetric care during pregnancy, childbirth, or the puerperium
- essential specified as complicating, or as a reason for obstetric care during pregnancy, childbirth, or the puerperium
- pre-existing NOS specified as complicating, or as a reason for obstetric care during pregnancy, childbirth, or the puerperium

❺ 642.1 Hypertension secondary to renal disease, complicating pregnancy, childbirth, and the puerperium ♀ M

[0-4] (✖ is only valid for fifth-digit "0")

Hypertension secondary to renal disease, specified as complicating, or as a reason for obstetric care during pregnancy, childbirth, or the puerperium

❺ 642.2 Other pre-existing hypertension complicating pregnancy, childbirth, and the puerperium ♀ M

[0-4] (✖ is only valid for fifth-digit "0")

Hypertensive:
- chronic kidney disease specified as complicating, or as a reason for obstetric care during pregnancy, childbirth, or the puerperium
- heart and chronic kidney disease specified as complicating, or as a reason for obstetric care during pregnancy, childbirth, or the puerperium
- heart disease specified as complicating, or as a reason for obstetric care during pregnancy, childbirth, or the puerperium

Malignant hypertension specified as complicating, or as a reason for obstetric care during pregnancy, childbirth, or the puerperium

❺ 642.3 Transient hypertension of pregnancy ♀ M

[0-4] (✖ is only valid for fifth-digit "0")

Gestational hypertension

Transient hypertension, so described, in pregnancy, childbirth, or the puerperium

AHA: 3Q 1990, 4

❺ 642.4 Mild or unspecified pre-eclampsia ♀ M

[0-4] (✖ is only valid for fifth-digit "0")

Hypertension in pregnancy, childbirth, or the puerperium, not specified as pre-existing, with either albuminuria or edema, or both; mild or unspecified

Pre-eclampsia:
- NOS
- mild

Toxemia (pre-eclamptic):
- NOS
- mild

Excludes *albuminuria in pregnancy, without mention of hypertension (646.2)*
edema in pregnancy, without mention of hypertension (646.1)

C&C Exclusions: 642.00, 642.01, 642.02, 642.03, 642.04, 642.10, 642.11, 642.12, 642.13, 642.14, 642.20, 642.21, 642.22, 642.23, 642.24, 642.30, 642.31, 642.32, 642.33, 642.34, 642.40, 642.41, 642.42, 642.43, 642.44, 642.50, 642.51, 642.52, 642.53, 642.54, 642.60, 642.61, 642.62, 642.63, 642.64, 642.70, 642.71, 642.72, 642.73, 642.74, 642.90, 642.91, 642.92, 642.93, 642.94, 646.10, 646.11, 646.12, 646.13, 646.14, 646.80, 646.81, 646.82, 646.83, 646.84, 646.90, 646.91, 646.93, 648.90, 648.91, 648.92, 648.93, 648.94, 650, 669.40, 669.41, 669.42, 669.43, 669.44, 669.80, 669.81, 669.82, 669.83, 669.84, 669.90, 669.91, 669.92, 669.93, 669.94

❺ 642.5 Severe pre-eclampsia ♀ M

[0-4] (✖ is only valid for fifth-digit "0")

Hypertension in pregnancy, childbirth, or the puerperium, not specified as pre-existing, with either albuminuria or edema, or both; specified as severe

Pre-eclampsia, severe

Toxemia (pre-eclamptic), severe

C&C Exclusions: See 642.4

AHA: Nov-Dec 1985, 3

❺ 642.6 Eclampsia ♀ M

[0-4] (✖ is only valid for fifth-digit "0")

Toxemia:
- eclamptic
- with convulsions

C&C Exclusions: See 642.4

❺ 642.7 Pre-eclampsia or eclampsia superimposed on pre-existing hypertension ♀ M

[0-4] (✖ is only valid for fifth-digit "0")

Conditions classifiable to 642.4-642.6, with conditions classifiable to 642.0-642.2

C&C Exclusions: See 642.4

Pre-eclampsia

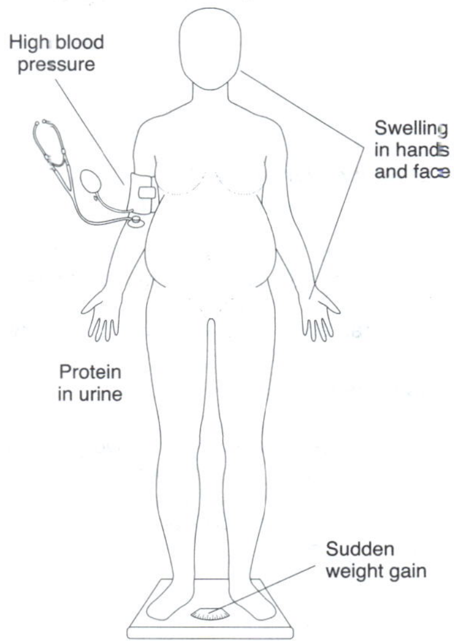

642.9 Unspecified hypertension complicating pregnancy, childbirth, or the puerperium
[0-4] (✖ is only valid for fifth-digit "0")
Hypertension NOS, without mention of albuminuria or edema, complicating pregnancy, childbirth, or the puerperium

643 Excessive vomiting in pregnancy
Requires fifth digit; valid digits are in [brackets] under each code. See beginning of section 640-649 for definitions.
Includes hyperemesis arising during pregnancy
hyperemesis gravidarum
vomiting:
persistent arising during pregnancy
vicious arising during pregnancy

643.0 Mild hyperemesis gravidarum
[0,1,3] (✖ is only valid for fifth-digit "0")
Hyperemesis gravidarum, mild or unspecified, starting before the end of the 22nd week of gestation

643.1 Hyperemesis gravidarum with metabolic disturbance
[0,1,3] (✖ is only valid for fifth-digit "0")
Hyperemesis gravidarum, starting before the end of the 22nd week of gestation, with metabolic disturbance, such as:
carbohydrate depletion
dehydration
electrolyte imbalance

643.2 Late vomiting of pregnancy
[0,1,3] (✖ is only valid for fifth-digit "0")
Excessive vomiting starting after 22 completed weeks of gestation

643.8 Other vomiting complicating pregnancy
[0,1,3] (✖ is only valid for fifth-digit "0")
Vomiting due to organic disease or other cause, specified as complicating pregnancy, or as a reason for obstetric care during pregnancy
Use additional code to specify cause

643.9 Unspecified vomiting of pregnancy
[0,1,3] (✖ is only valid for fifth-digit "0")
Vomiting as a reason for care during pregnancy, length of gestation unspecified

644 Early or threatened labor
Requires fifth digit; valid digits are in [brackets] under each code. See beginning of section 640-649 for definitions.

644.0 Threatened premature labor
[0,3] (✖ is only valid for fifth-digit "0")
Premature labor after 22 weeks, but before 37 completed weeks of gestation without delivery
Excludes *that occurring before 22 completed weeks of gestation (640.0)*
C&C Exclusions: 644.00, 644.03, 644.10, 644.13, 644.20, 644.21, 646.80, 646.81, 646.82, 646.83, 646.84, 646.90, 646.91, 646.93, 648.90, 648.91, 648.92, 648.93, 648.94, 650, 669.40, 669.41, 669.42, 669.43, 669.44, 669.80, 669.81, 669.82, 669.83, 669.84, 669.90, 669.91, 669.92, 669.93, 669.94

644.1 Other threatened labor
[0,3] (✖ is only valid for fifth-digit "0")
False labor:
NOS without delivery
after 37 completed weeks of gestation without delivery
Threatened labor NOS without delivery
C&C Exclusions: See 644.0

644.2 Early onset of delivery
[0-1] (✖ is only valid for fifth-digit "0")
Onset (spontaneous) of delivery before 37 completed weeks of gestation
Premature labor with onset of delivery before 37 completed weeks of gestation
AHA: 2Q 1991, 16

645 Late pregnancy
Requires fifth digit; valid digits are in [brackets] under each code. See beginning of section 640-649 for definitions.
AHA: 4Q 2000, 43; 4Q 1991, 26

645.1 Post term pregnancy
[0,1,3]
Pregnancy over 40 completed weeks to 42 completed weeks gestation

645.2 Prolonged pregnancy
[0,1,3]
Pregnancy which has advanced beyond 42 completed weeks of gestation

646 Other complications of pregnancy, not elsewhere classified
Use additional code(s) to further specify complication
Requires fifth digit; valid digits are in [brackets] under each code. See beginning of section 640-649 for definitions.
AHA: 4Q 1995, 59

646.0 Papyraceous fetus
[0,1,3] (✖ is only valid for fifth-digit "0")

646.1 Edema or excessive weight gain in pregnancy, without mention of hypertension
[0-4] (✖ is only valid for fifth-digit "0")
Gestational edema
Maternal obesity syndrome
Excludes *that with mention of hypertension (642.0-642.9)*

646.2 Unspecified renal disease in pregnancy, without mention of hypertension
[0-4] (✖ is only valid for fifth-digit "0")
Albuminuria in pregnancy or the puerperium, without mention of hypertension
Gestational proteinuria in pregnancy or the puerperium, without mention of hypertension
Nephropathy NOS in pregnancy or the puerperium, without mention of hypertension
Renal disease NOS in pregnancy or the puerperium, without mention of hypertension
Uremia in pregnancy or the puerperium, without mention of hypertension
Excludes *that with mention of hypertension (642.0-642.9)*

646.3 Habitual aborter
[0-1,3] (✖ is only valid for fifth-digit "0")
Excludes *with current abortion (634.0-634.9)*
without current pregnancy (▶629.81◀)

646.4 Peripheral neuritis in pregnancy
[0-4] (✖ is only valid for fifth-digit "0")

646.5 Asymptomatic bacteriuria in pregnancy
[0-4] (✖ is only valid for fifth-digit "0")

646.6 Infections of genitourinary tract in pregnancy
[0-4] (✖ is only valid for fifth-digit "0")
Conditions classifiable to 590, 595, 597, 599.0, 616 complicating pregnancy, childbirth, or the puerperium
Conditions classifiable to 614.0-614.5, 614.7-614.9, 615 complicating pregnancy or labor
Excludes *major puerperal infection (670)*
C&C Exclusions: 646.60, 646.61, 646.62, 646.63, 646.64, 646.80, 646.81, 646.82, 646.83, 646.84, 646.90, 646.91, 646.93, 648.90, 648.91, 648.92, 648.93, 648.94, 650, 669.40, 669.41, 669.42, 669.43, 669.44, 669.80, 669.81, 669.82, 669.83, 669.84, 669.90, 669.91, 669.92, 669.93, 669.94
AHA: For Code 646.63: 4Q 2004, 90

5 **646.7 Liver disorders in pregnancy** ♀M
[0,1,3]
(✖ is only valid for fifth-digit "0")
Acute yellow atrophy of liver (obstetric) (true) of pregnancy
Icterus gravis of pregnancy
Necrosis of liver of pregnancy
Excludes *hepatorenal syndrome following delivery (674.8)*
viral hepatitis (647.6)
C&C Exclusions: 646.70, 646.71, 646.73, 646.80, 646.81, 646.82, 646.83, 646.84, 646.90, 646.91, 646.93, 648.90, 648.91, 648.92, 648.93, 648.94, 650, 669.40, 669.41, 669.42, 669.43, 669.44, 669.80, 669.81, 669.82, 669.83, 669.84, 669.90, 669.91, 669.92, 669.93, 669.94

5 **646.8 Other specified complications of pregnancy** ♀M
[0-4]
(✖ is only valid for fifth-digit "0")
Fatigue during pregnancy
Herpes gestationis
Insufficient weight gain of pregnancy
C&C Exclusions: 646.50, 646.51, 646.52, 646.53, 646.54
AHA: 3Q 1998, 16; Jan-Feb 1985, 19

5 **646.9 Unspecified complication of pregnancy** ♀M
[0,1,3]
(✖ is only valid for fifth-digit "0")
C&C Exclusions: See 646.8

4 **647 Infectious and parasitic conditions in the mother classifiable elsewhere, but complicating pregnancy, childbirth, or the puerperium**
Use additional code(s) to further specify complication
Requires fifth digit; valid digits are in [brackets] under each code. See beginning of section 640-649 for definitions.
Includes the listed conditions when complicating the pregnant state, aggravated by the pregnancy, or when a main reason for obstetric care
Excludes *those conditions in the mother known or suspected to have affected the fetus (655.0-655.9)*

5 **647.0 Syphilis** ♀M
[0-4]
(✖ is only valid for fifth-digit "0")
Conditions classifiable to 090-097

5 **647.1 Gonorrhea** ♀M
[0-4]
(✖ is only valid for fifth-digit "0")
Conditions classifiable to 098

5 **647.2 Other venereal diseases** ♀M
[0-4]
(✖ is only valid for fifth-digit "0")
Conditions classifiable to 099

5 **647.3 Tuberculosis** ♀M
[0-4]
(✖ is only valid for fifth-digit "0")
Conditions classifiable to 010-018
C&C Exclusions: 646.80, 646.81, 646.82, 646.83, 646.84, 646.90, 646.91, 646.93, 647.30, 647.31, 647.32, 647.33, 647.34, 648.90, 648.91, 648.92, 648.93, 648.94, 650, 669.40, 669.41, 669.42, 669.43, 669.44, 669.80, 669.81, 669.82, 669.83, 669.84, 669.90, 669.91, 669.92, 669.93, 669.94

5 **647.4 Malaria** ♀M
[0-4]
(✖ is only valid for fifth-digit "0")
Conditions classifiable to 084
C&C Exclusions: 646.80, 646.81, 646.82, 646.83, 646.84, 646.90, 646.91, 646.93, 647.40, 647.41, 647.42, 647.43, 647.44, 648.90, 648.91, 648.92, 648.93, 648.94, 650, 669.40, 669.41, 669.42, 669.43, 669.44, 669.80, 669.81, 669.82, 669.83, 669.84, 669.90, 669.91, 669.92, 669.93, 669.94

5 **647.5 Rubella** ♀M
[0-4]
(✖ is only valid for fifth-digit "0")
Conditions classifiable to 056

5 **647.6 Other viral diseases** ♀M
[0-4]
(✖ is only valid for fifth-digit "0")
Conditions classifiable to 042 and 050-079, except 056
AHA: Jan-Feb 1985, 15

5 **647.8 Other specified infectious and parasitic diseases** ♀M
[0-4]
(✖ is only valid for fifth-digit "0")

✖5 **647.9 Unspecified infection or infestation** ♀M
[0-4]

4 **648 Other current conditions in the mother classifiable elsewhere, but complicating pregnancy, childbirth, or the puerperium**
Use additional code(s) to identify the condition
Requires fifth digit; valid digits are in [brackets] under each code. See beginning of section 640-649 for definitions.
Includes the listed conditions when complicating the pregnant state, aggravated by the pregnancy, or when a main reason for obstetric care
Excludes *those conditions in the mother known or suspected to have affected the fetus (655.0-665.9)*

5 **648.0 Diabetes mellitus** ♀M
[0-4]
(✖ is only valid for fifth-digit "0")
Conditions classifiable to 250
Excludes *gestational diabetes (648.8)*
C&C Exclusions: 646.80, 646.81, 646.82, 646.83, 646.84, 646.90, 646.91, 646.93, 648.00, 648.01, 648.02, 648.03, 648.04, 648.90, 648.91, 648.92, 648.93, 648.94, 650, 669.40, 669.41, 669.42, 669.43, 669.44, 669.80, 669.81, 669.82, 669.83, 669.84, 669.90, 669.91, 669.92, 669.93, 669.94
AHA: 3Q 1991, 5, 11

5 **648.1 Thyroid dysfunction** ♀M
[0-4]
(✖ is only valid for fifth-digit "0")
Conditions classifiable to 240-246

5 **648.2 Anemia** ♀M
[0-4]
(✖ is only valid for fifth-digit "0")
Conditions classifiable to 280-285
C&C Exclusions: 646.80, 646.81, 646.82, 646.83, 646.84, 646.90, 646.91, 646.93, 648.20, 648.21, 648.22, 648.23, 648.24, 648.90, 648.91, 648.92, 648.93, 648.94, 650, 669.40, 669.41, 669.42, 669.43, 669.44, 669.80, 669.81, 669.82, 669.83, 669.84, 669.90, 669.91, 669.92, 669.93, 669.94
AHA: For Code 648.22: 1Q 2002, 14

5 **648.3 Drug dependence** ♀M
[0-4]
(✖ is only valid for fifth-digit "0")
Conditions classifiable to 304
C&C Exclusions: 646.80, 646.81, 646.82, 646.83, 646.84, 646.90, 646.91, 646.93, 648.30, 648.31, 648.32, 648.33, 648.34, 648.90, 648.91, 648.92, 648.93, 648.94, 650, 669.40, 669.41, 669.42, 669.43, 669.44, 669.80, 669.81, 669.82, 669.83, 669.84, 669.90, 669.91, 669.92, 669.93, 669.94
AHA: 2Q 1998, 13; 4Q 1988, 8

5 **648.4 Mental disorders** ♀M
[0-4]
(✖ is only valid for fifth-digit "0")
Conditions classifiable to 290-303, 305.0, 305.2-305.9, 306-316, 317-319
AHA: 2Q 1998, 13; 4Q 1995, 63

5 **648.5 Congenital cardiovascular disorders** ♀M
[0-4]
(✖ is only valid for fifth-digit "0")
Conditions classifiable to 745-747
C&C Exclusions: 646.80, 646.81, 646.82, 646.83, 646.84, 646.90, 646.91, 646.93, 648.50, 648.51, 648.52, 648.53, 648.54, 648.60, 648.61, 648.62, 648.63, 648.64, 648.90, 648.91, 648.92, 648.93, 648.94, 650, 669.40, 669.41, 669.42, 669.43, 669.44, 669.80, 669.81, 669.82, 669.83, 669.84, 669.90, 669.91, 669.92, 669.93, 669.94

5 **648.6 Other cardiovascular diseases** ♀M
[0-4]
(✖ is only valid for fifth-digit "0")
Conditions classifiable to 390-398, 410-429
Excludes *cerebrovascular disorders in the puerperium (674.0)*
peripartum cardiomyopathy (674.5)
venous complications (671.0-671.9)
C&C Exclusions: See 648.5
AHA: 3Q 1998, 11

5 **648.7 Bone and joint disorders of back, pelvis, and lower limbs** ♀M
[0-4]
(✖ is only valid for fifth-digit "0")
Conditions classifiable to 720-724, and those classifiable to 711-719 or 725-738 specified as affecting the lower limbs

5 648.8 Abnormal glucose tolerance ♀M
[0-4] (✖ is only valid for fifth-digit "0")
Conditions classifiable to 790.21-790.29
Gestational diabetes
Use additional code, if applicable, for associated long-term (current) insulin use (V58.67)
AHA: 3Q 1991, 5; For Code 648.83: 4Q 2004, 56

5 648.9 Other current conditions classifiable elsewhere ♀M
[0-4] (✖ is only valid for fifth-digit "0")
Conditions classifiable to 440-459
Nutritional deficiencies [conditions classifiable to 260-269]
C&C Exclusions: 674.50, 674.51, 674.52, 674.53, 674.54
AHA: 3Q 2006, 14; 4Q 2004, 88; Nov-Dec 1987, 10; For Code 648.91: 1Q 2002, 14; For Code 648.93: 4Q 2004, 90

4 649 Other conditions or status of the mother complicating pregnancy, childbirth, or the puerperium
Requires fifth digit; valid digits are in [brackets] under each code. See beginning of section 640-649 for definitions.

5 649.0 Tobacco use disorder complicating pregnancy, childbirth, or the puerperium ♀M
[0-4] (✖ is only valid for fifth-digit "0")
Smoking complicating pregnancy, childbirth, or the puerperium
C&C Exclusions: 634.00, 634.01, 634.02, 634.10, 634.11, 634.12, 634.20, 634.21, 634.22, 634.30, 634.31, 634.32, 634.40, 634.41, 634.42, 634.50, 634.51, 634.52, 634.60, 634.61, 634.62, 634.70, 634.71, 634.72, 634.80, 634.81, 634.82, 634.90, 634.91, 634.92, 639.0, 639.1, 639.2, 639.3, 639.4, 639.5, 639.6, 639.8, 639.9, 640.00, 640.01, 640.03, 640.80, 640.81, 640.83, 640.90, 640.91, 640.93, 641.00, 641.01, 641.03, 641.10, 641.11, 641.13, 641.30, 641.31, 641.33, 641.80, 641.81, 641.83, 641.90, 641.91, 641.93, 642.40, 642.41, 642.42, 642.43, 642.44, 642.50, 642.51, 642.52, 642.53, 642.54, 642.60, 642.61, 642.62, 642.63, 642.64, 642.70, 642.71, 642.72, 642.73, 642.74, 644.00, 644.03, 644.10, 644.13, 646.60, 646.61, 646.62, 646.63, 646.64, 646.70, 646.71, 646.73, 647.30, 647.31, 647.32, 647.33, 647.34, 647.40, 647.41, 647.42, 647.43, 647.44, 648.00, 648.01, 648.02, 648.03, 648.04, 648.20, 648.21, 648.22, 648.23, 648.24, 648.30, 648.31, 648.32, 648.33, 648.34, 648.50, 648.51, 648.52, 648.53, 648.54, 648.60, 648.61, 648.62, 648.63, 648.64, 659.30, 659.31, 659.33, 665.00, 665.01, 665.03, 665.10, 665.11, 666.32, 666.34, 668.00, 668.01, 668.02, 668.03, 668.04, 668.10, 668.11, 668.12, 668.13, 668.14, 668.20, 668.21, 668.22, 668.23, 668.24, 668.80, 668.81, 668.82, 668.83, 668.84, 668.90, 668.91, 668.92, 668.93, 668.94, 669.10, 669.11, 669.12, 669.13, 669.14, 669.30, 669.32, 669.34, 670.00, 670.02, 670.04, 671.20, 671.21, 671.22, 671.23, 671.24, 671.30, 671.31, 671.33, 671.40, 671.42, 671.44, 673.00, 673.01, 673.02, 673.03, 673.04, 673.10, 673.11, 673.12, 673.13, 673.14, 673.20, 673.21, 673.22, 673.23, 673.24, 673.30, 673.31, 673.32, 673.33, 673.34, 673.80, 673.81, 673.82, 673.83, 673.84, 674.00, 674.01, 674.02, 674.03, 674.04, 674.10, 674.12, 674.20, 674.22, 674.24, 674.50, 674.51, 674.52, 674.53, 674.54, 675.10, 675.11, 675.12

5 649.1 Obesity complicating pregnancy, childbirth, or the puerperium ♀M
[0-4] (✖ is only valid for fifth-digit "0")
Use additional code to identify the obesity (278.00-278.01)
C&C Exclusions: See 649.0

5 649.2 Bariatric surgery status complicating pregnancy, childbirth, or the puerperium ♀M
[0-4] (✖ is only valid for fifth-digit "0")
Gastric banding status complicating pregnancy, childbirth, or the puerperium
Gastric bypass status for obesity complicating pregnancy, childbirth, or the puerperium
Obesity surgery status complicating pregnancy, childbirth, or the puerperium
C&C Exclusions: See 649.0

5 649.3 Coagulation defects complicating pregnancy, childbirth, or the puerperium ♀M
[0-4] (✖ is only valid for fifth-digit "0")
Conditions classifiable to 286
Use additional code to identify the specific coagulation defect (286.0-286.9)
Excludes *coagulation defects causing antepartum hemorrhage (641.3)*
postpartum coagulation defects (666.3)
C&C Exclusions: See 649.0

5 649.4 Epilepsy complicating pregnancy, childbirth, or the puerperium ♀M
[0-4] (✖ is only valid for fifth-digit "0")
Conditions classifiable to 345
Use additional code to identify the specific type of epilepsy (345.00-345.91)
Excludes *eclampsia (642.6)*
C&C Exclusions: See 649.0

5 649.5 Spotting complicating pregnancy ♀M
[0,1,3] (✖ is only valid for fifth-digit "0")
Excludes *antepartum hemorrhage (641.0-641.9)*
hemorrhage in early pregnancy (640.0-640.9)
C&C Exclusions: See 649.0

5 649.6 Uterine size date discrepancy ♀M
[0-4] (✖ is only valid for fifth-digit "0")
C&C Exclusions: See 649.0

NORMAL DELIVERY, AND OTHER INDICATIONS FOR CARE IN PREGNANCY, LABOR, AND DELIVERY (650-659)

The following fifth-digit subclassification is for use with categories 651-659 to denote the current episode of care:

0 unspecified as to episode of care or not applicable
1 delivered, with or without mention of antepartum condition
2 delivered, with mention of postpartum complication
3 antepartum condition or complication
4 postpartum condition or complication

650 Normal delivery ♀M
Delivery requiring minimal or no assistance, with or without episiotomy, without fetal manipulation [e.g., rotation version] or instrumentation [forceps] of a spontaneous, cephalic, vaginal, full-term, single, live-born infant. This code is for use as a single diagnosis code and is not to be used with any other code in the range 630-676.
Use additional code to indicate outcome of delivery (V27.0)
Excludes *breech delivery (assisted) (spontaneous) NOS (652.2)*
delivery by vacuum extractor, forceps, cesarean section, or breech extraction, without specified complication (669.5-669.7)
AHA: 2Q 2002, 10; 3Q 2001, 12; 3Q 2000, 5; 4Q 1995, 28, 59

4 651 Multiple gestation
Requires fifth digit; valid digits are in [brackets] under each code. See beginning of section 650-659 for definitions.

5 651.0 Twin pregnancy ♀M
[0,1,3] (✖ is only valid for fifth-digit "0")
AHA: For Code 651.03: 3Q 2006, 16

5 651.1 Triplet pregnancy ♀M
[0,1,3] (✖ is only valid for fifth-digit "0")

5 651.2 Quadruplet pregnancy ♀M
[0,1,3] (✖ is only valid for fifth-digit "0")

5 651.3 Twin pregnancy with fetal loss and retention of one fetus ♀M
[0,1,3] (✖ is only valid for fifth-digit "0")

5 651.4 Triplet pregnancy with fetal loss and retention of one or more fetus(es) ♀M
[0,1,3] (✖ is only valid for fifth-digit "0")

5 651.5 Quadruplet pregnancy with fetal loss and retention of one or more fetus(es) ♀M
[0,1,3] (✖ is only valid for fifth-digit "0")

❺ **651.6 Other multiple pregnancy with fetal loss and retention of one or more fetus(es)** ♀M
[0,1,3] (✖ is only valid for fifth-digit "0")

❺ **651.7 Multiple gestation following (elective) fetal reduction** ♀M
[0,1,3] Fetal reduction of multiple fetuses reduced to single fetus
AHA: For Code 651.71: 4Q 2005, 81; For Code 651.73: 3Q 2006, 17-18

❺ **651.8 Other specified multiple gestation** ♀M
[0,1,3] (✖ is only valid for fifth-digit "0")

✖❺ **651.9 Unspecified multiple gestation** ♀M
[0,1,3]

❹ **652 Malposition and malpresentation of fetus**
Requires fifth digit; valid digits are in [brackets] under each code. See beginning of section 650-659 for definitions.
Code first any associated obstructed labor (660.0)

❺ **652.0 Unstable lie** ♀M
[0,1,3] (✖ is only valid for fifth-digit "0")

❺ **652.1 Breech or other malpresentation successfully converted to cephalic presentation** ♀M
[0,1,3] (✖ is only valid for fifth-digit "0")
Cephalic version NOS

❺ **652.2 Breech presentation without mention of version** ♀M
[0,1,3] (✖ is only valid for fifth-digit "0")
Breech delivery (assisted) (spontaneous) NOS
Buttocks presentation
Complete breech
Frank breech
Excludes *footling presentation (652.8)*
incomplete breech (652.8)

❺ **652.3 Transverse or oblique presentation** ♀M
[0,1,3] (✖ is only valid for fifth-digit "0")
Oblique lie
Transverse lie
Excludes *transverse arrest of fetal head (660.3)*

❺ **652.4 Face or brow presentation** ♀M
[0,1,3] (✖ is only valid for fifth-digit "0")
Mentum presentation

❺ **652.5 High head at term** ♀M
[0,1,3] (✖ is only valid for fifth-digit "0")
Failure of head to enter pelvic brim

❺ **652.6 Multiple gestation with malpresentation of one fetus or more** ♀M
[0,1,3] (✖ is only valid for fifth-digit "0")

❺ **652.7 Prolapsed arm** ♀M
[0,1,3] (✖ is only valid for fifth-digit "0")

❺ **652.8 Other specified malposition or malpresentation** ♀M
[0,1,3] (✖ is only valid for fifth-digit "0")
Compound presentation

✖❺ **652.9 Unspecified malposition or malpresentation** ♀M
[0,1,3]

❹ **653 Disproportion**
Requires fifth digit; valid digits are in [brackets] under each code. See beginning of section 650-659 for definitions.
Code first any associated obstructed labor (660.1)

❺ **653.0 Major abnormality of bony pelvis, not further specified** ♀M
[0,1,3] (✖ is only valid for fifth-digit "0")
Pelvic deformity NOS

❺ **653.1 Generally contracted pelvis** ♀M
[0,1,3] (✖ is only valid for fifth-digit "0")
Contracted pelvis NOS

❺ **653.2 Inlet contraction of pelvis** ♀M
[0,1,3] (✖ is only valid for fifth-digit "0")
Inlet contraction (pelvis)

❺ **653.3 Outlet contraction of pelvis** ♀M
[0,1,3] (✖ is only valid for fifth-digit "0")
Outlet contraction (pelvis)

❺ **653.4 Fetopelvic disproportion** ♀M
[0,1,3] (✖ is only valid for fifth-digit "0")
Cephalopelvic disproportion NOS
Disproportion of mixed maternal and fetal origin, with normally formed fetus

❺ **653.5 Unusually large fetus causing disproportion** ♀M
[0,1,3] (✖ is only valid for fifth-digit "0")
Disproportion of fetal origin with normally formed fetus
Fetal disproportion NOS
Excludes *that when the reason for medical care was concern for the fetus (656.6)*

❺ **653.6 Hydrocephalic fetus causing disproportion** ♀M
[0,1,3] (✖ is only valid for fifth-digit "0")
Excludes *that when the reason for medical care was concern for the fetus (655.0)*

❺ **653.7 Other fetal abnormality causing disproportion** ♀M
[0,1,3] (✖ is only valid for fifth-digit "0")
Conjoined twins
Fetal:
- ascites
- hydrops
- myelomeningocele
- sacral teratoma
- tumor

❺ **653.8 Disproportion of other origin** ♀M
[0,1,3] (✖ is only valid for fifth-digit "0")
Excludes *shoulder (girdle) dystocia (660.4)*

✖❺ **653.9 Unspecified disproportion** ♀M
[0,1,3]

❹ **654 Abnormality of organs and soft tissues of pelvis**
Requires fifth digit; valid digits are in [brackets] under each code. See beginning of section 650-659 for definitions.
Includes the listed conditions during pregnancy, childbirth, or the puerperium
Excludes ▶*trauma to perineum and vulva complicating current delivery (664.0-664.9)*◀
Code first any associated obstructed labor (660.2)

❺ **654.0 Congenital abnormalities of uterus** ♀M
[0-4] (✖ is only valid for fifth-digit "0")
Double uterus
Uterus bicornis

❺ **654.1 Tumors of body of uterus** ♀M
[0-4] (✖ is only valid for fifth-digit "0")
Uterine fibroids

❺ **654.2 Previous cesarean delivery** ♀M
[0,1,3] (✖ is only valid for fifth-digit "0")
Uterine scar from previous cesarean delivery
AHA: 1Q 1992, 8

❺ **654.3 Retroverted and incarcerated gravid uterus** ♀M
[0-4] (✖ is only valid for fifth-digit "0")

❺ **654.4 Other abnormalities in shape or position of gravid uterus and of neighboring structures** ♀M
[0-4] (✖ is only valid for fifth-digit "0")
Cystocele
Pelvic floor repair
Pendulous abdomen
Prolapse of gravid uterus
Rectocele
Rigid pelvic floor

❺ **654.5 Cervical incompetence** ♀M
[0-4] (✖ is only valid for fifth-digit "0")
Presence of Shirodkar suture with or without mention of cervical incompetence

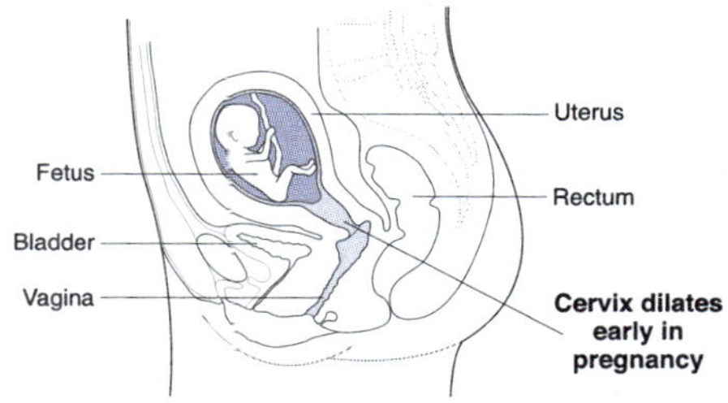

A Adult (15+ years) M Maternity (12-55 years) N Newborn (0 years) P Pediatric (0-17 years) ♂ Male ♀ Female ❷ Medicare Secondary Payer

654.6 Other congenital or acquired abnormality of cervix
[0-4]
(✖ is only valid for fifth-digit "0")
Cicatricial cervix
Polyp of cervix
Previous surgery to cervix
Rigid cervix (uteri)
Stenosis or stricture of cervix
Tumor of cervix

654.7 Congenital or acquired abnormality of vagina
[0-4]
(✖ is only valid for fifth-digit "0")
Previous surgery to vagina
Septate vagina
Stenosis of vagina (acquired) (congenital)
Stricture of vagina
Tumor of vagina

654.8 Congenital or acquired abnormality of vulva
[0-4]
(✖ is only valid for fifth-digit "0")
▶Anal sphincter tear (healed) (old) complicating delivery◀
Fibrosis of perineum
Persistent hymen
Previous surgery to perineum or vulva
Rigid perineum
Tumor of vulva
Excludes ▶*anal sphincter tear (healed) (old) not associated with delivery (569.43)*◀
varicose veins of vulva (671.1)
AHA: 1Q 2003, 14

✖ **654.9 Other and unspecified**
[0-4]
Uterine scar NEC

655 Known or suspected fetal abnormality affecting management of mother
Requires fifth digit; valid digits are in [brackets] under each code. See beginning of section 650-659 for definitions.
Includes the listed conditions in the fetus as a reason for observation or obstetrical care of the mother, or for termination of pregnancy
AHA: 3Q 1990, 4

655.0 Central nervous system malformation in fetus
[0,1,3]
(✖ is only valid for fifth-digit "0")
Fetal or suspected fetal:
anencephaly
hydrocephalus
spina bifida (with myelomeningocele)

655.1 Chromosomal abnormality in fetus
[0,1,3]
(✖ is only valid for fifth-digit "0")

655.2 Hereditary disease in family possibly affecting fetus
[0,1,3]
(✖ is only valid for fifth-digit "0")

655.3 Suspected damage to fetus from viral disease in the mother
[0,1,3]
(✖ is only valid for fifth-digit "0")
Suspected damage to fetus from maternal rubella

655.4 Suspected damage to fetus from other disease in the mother
[0,1,3]
(✖ is only valid for fifth-digit "0")
Suspected damage to fetus from maternal:
alcohol addiction
listeriosis
toxoplasmosis

655.5 Suspected damage to fetus from drugs
[0,1,3]
(✖ is only valid for fifth-digit "0")

655.6 Suspected damage to fetus from radiation
[0,1,3]
(✖ is only valid for fifth-digit "0")

655.7 Decreased fetal movements
[0,1,3]
(✖ is only valid for fifth-digit "0")
AHA: 4Q 1997, 41

655.8 Other known or suspected fetal abnormality, not elsewhere classified
[0,1,3]
(✖ is only valid for fifth-digit "0")
Suspected damage to fetus from:
environmental toxins
intrauterine contraceptive device
AHA: For Code 655.83: 3Q 2006, 16-18

✖ **655.9 Unspecified**
[0,1,3]

656 Other fetal and placental problems affecting management of mother
Requires fifth digit; valid digits are in [brackets] under each code. See beginning of section 650-659 for definitions.

656.0 Fetal-maternal hemorrhage
[0,1,3]
(✖ is only valid for fifth-digit "0")
Leakage (microscopic) of fetal blood into maternal circulation

656.1 Rhesus isoimmunization
[0,1,3]
(✖ is only valid for fifth-digit "0")
Anti-D [Rh] antibodies
Rh incompatibility

656.2 Isoimmunization from other and unspecified blood-group incompatibility
[0,1,3]
(✖ is only valid for fifth-digit "0")
ABO isoimmunization
AHA: 4Q 2006, 135

656.3 Fetal distress
[0,1,3]
(✖ is only valid for fifth-digit "0")
Fetal metabolic acidemia
Excludes *abnormal fetal acid-base balance (656.8)*
abnormality in fetal heart rate or rhythm (659.7)
fetal bradycardia (659.7)
fetal tachycardia (659.7)
meconium in liquor (656.8)
AHA: Nov-Dec 1986, 4

656.4 Intrauterine death
[0,1,3]
(✖ is only valid for fifth-digit "0")
Fetal death:
NOS
after completion of 22 weeks' gestation
late
Missed delivery
Excludes *missed abortion (632)*

656.5 Poor fetal growth
[0,1,3]
(✖ is only valid for fifth-digit "0")
"Light-for-dates"
"Placental insufficiency"
"Small-for-dates"

656.6 Excessive fetal growth
[0,1,3]
(✖ is only valid for fifth-digit "0")
"Large-for-dates"

656.7 Other placental conditions
[0,1,3]
(✖ is only valid for fifth-digit "0")
Abnormal placenta
Placental infarct
Excludes *placental polyp (674.4)*
placentitis (658.4)

656.8 Other specified fetal and placental problems
[0,1,3]
(✖ is only valid for fifth-digit "0")
Abnormal acid-base balance
Intrauterine acidosis
Lithopedian
Meconium in liquor

656.9 Unspecified fetal and placental problem
[0,1,3]
(✖ is only valid for fifth-digit "0")

657 Polyhydramnios
[0,1,3]
(✖ is only valid for fifth-digit "0")
Hydramnios
Requires fifth digit; valid digits are in [brackets] under each code. See beginning of section 650-659 for definitions.
Use 0 as fourth digit for category 657
AHA: 4Q 1991, 26; For Code 657.03: 3Q 2006, 16

❹ **658 Other problems associated with amniotic cavity and membranes**
Requires fifth digit; valid digits are in [brackets] under each code. See beginning of section 650-659 for definitions.
Excludes *amniotic fluid embolism (673.1)*

❺ **658.0 Oligohydramnios** ♀M
[0,1,3] (✖ is only valid for fifth-digit "0")
Oligohydramnios without mention of rupture of membranes
DEF: Lack of amniotic fluid in the womb.
AHA: For Code 658.03: 3Q 2006, 16

❺ **658.1 Premature rupture of membranes** ♀M
[0,1,3] (✖ is only valid for fifth-digit "0")
Rupture of amniotic sac less than 24 hours prior to the onset of labor
AHA: For Code 658.13: 1Q 2001, 5; 4Q 1998, 77

❺ **658.2 Delayed delivery after spontaneous or unspecified rupture of membranes** ♀M
[0,1,3] (✖ is only valid for fifth-digit "0")
Prolonged rupture of membranes NOS
Rupture of amniotic sac 24 hours or more prior to the onset of labor

❺ **658.3 Delayed delivery after artificial rupture of membranes** ♀M
[0,1,3] (✖ is only valid for fifth-digit "0")

❺ **658.4 Infection of amniotic cavity** ♀M
[0,1,3] (✖ is only valid for fifth-digit "0")
Amnionitis
Chorioamnionitis
Membranitis
Placentitis

❺ **658.8 Other** ♀M
[0,1,3] (✖ is only valid for fifth-digit "0")
Amnion nodosum
Amniotic cyst

✖❺ **658.9 Unspecified** ♀M
[0,1,3]

❹ **659 Other indications for care or intervention related to labor and delivery, not elsewhere classified**
Requires fifth digit; valid digits are in [brackets] under each code. See beginning of section 650-659 for definitions.

❺ **659.0 Failed mechanical induction** ♀M
[0,1,3] (✖ is only valid for fifth-digit "0")
Failure of induction of labor by surgical or other instrumental methods

❺ **659.1 Failed medical or unspecified induction** ♀M
[0,1,3] (✖ is only valid for fifth-digit "0")
Failed induction NOS
Failure of induction of labor by medical methods, such as oxytocic drugs

❺ **659.2 Maternal pyrexia during labor, unspecified** ♀M
[0,1,3] (✖ is only valid for fifth-digit "0")

❺ **659.3 Generalized infection during labor** ♀M
[0,1,3] (✖ is only valid for fifth-digit "0")
Septicemia during labor

❺ **659.4 Grand multiparity** ♀M
[0,1,3] (✖ is only valid for fifth-digit "0")
Excludes *supervision only, in pregnancy (V23.3)*
without current pregnancy (V61.5)

❺ **659.5 Elderly primigravida** ♀M
[0,1,3] (✖ is only valid for fifth-digit "0")
First pregnancy in a woman who will be 35 years of age or older at expected date of delivery
Excludes *supervision only, in pregnancy (V23.81)*
AHA: 3Q 2001, 12

❺ **659.6 Elderly multigravida** ♀M
[0,1,3] (✖ is only valid for fifth-digit "0")
Second or more pregnancy in a woman who will be 35 years of age or older at expected date of delivery
Excludes *elderly primigravida (659.5)*
supervision only, in pregnancy (V23.82)
AHA: 3Q 2001, 12

❺ **659.7 Abnormality in fetal heart rate or rhythm** ♀M
[0,1,3]
Depressed fetal heart tones
Fetal:
bradycardia
tachycardia
Fetal heart rate decelerations
Non-reassuring fetal heart rate or rhythm
AHA: 4Q 1998, 48

❺ **659.8 Other specified indications for care or intervention related to labor and delivery** ♀M
[0,1,3] (✖ is only valid for fifth-digit "0")
Pregnancy in a female less than 16 years of age at expected date of delivery
Very young maternal age
AHA: 3Q 2001, 12

✖❺ **659.9 Unspecified indication for care or intervention related to labor and delivery** ♀M
[0,1,3]

COMPLICATIONS OCCURRING MAINLY IN THE COURSE OF LABOR AND DELIVERY (660-669)

The following fifth-digit subclassification is for use with categories 660-669 to denote the current episode of care:

0 **unspecified as to episode of care or not applicable**
1 **delivered, with or without mention of antepartum condition**
2 **delivered, with mention of postpartum complication**
3 **antepartum condition or complication**
4 **postpartum condition or complication**

❹ **660 Obstructed labor**
Requires fifth digit; valid digits are in [brackets] under each code. See beginning of section 660-669 for definitions.
AHA: 3Q 1995, 10

❺ **660.0 Obstruction caused by malposition of fetus at onset of labor** ♀M
[0,1,3] (✖ is only valid for fifth-digit "0")
Any condition classifiable to 652, causing obstruction during labor
Use additional code from 652.0-652.9 to identify condition

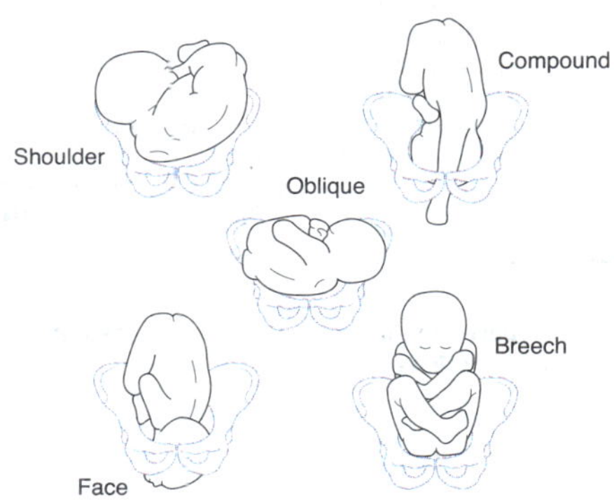

❺ **660.1 Obstruction by bony pelvis** ♀M
[0,1,3] (✖ is only valid for fifth-digit "0")
Any condition classifiable to 653, causing obstruction during labor
Use additional code from 653.0-653.9 to identify condition

❺ **660.2 Obstruction by abnormal pelvic soft tissues** ♀M
[0,1,3] (✖ is only valid for fifth-digit "0")
Prolapse of anterior lip of cervix
Any condition classifiable to 654, causing obstruction during labor
Use additional code from 654.0-654.9 to identify condition

5 660.3 Deep transverse arrest and persistent occipitoposterior position ♀ M
[0,1,3] (✖ is only valid for fifth-digit "0")

5 660.4 Shoulder (girdle) dystocia ♀ M
[0,1,3] (✖ is only valid for fifth-digit "0")
Impacted shoulders
DEF: Shoulders of the fetus becomes caught in the pelvis during delivery.

5 660.5 Locked twins ♀ M
[0,1,3] (✖ is only valid for fifth-digit "0")

5 660.6 Failed trial of labor, unspecified ♀ M
[0,1,3] (✖ is only valid for fifth-digit "0")
Failed trial of labor, without mention of condition or suspected condition

5 660.7 Failed forceps or vacuum extractor, unspecified ♀ M
[0,1,3] (✖ is only valid for fifth-digit "0")
Application of ventouse or forceps, without mention of condition

5 660.8 Other causes of obstructed labor ♀ M
[0,1,3] (✖ is only valid for fifth-digit "0")
Use additional code to identify condition
AHA: 4Q 2004, 88

5 660.9 Unspecified obstructed labor ♀ M
[0,1,3] (✖ is only valid for fifth-digit "0")
Dystocia:
- NOS
- fetal NOS
- maternal NOS

4 661 Abnormality of forces of labor
Requires fifth digit; valid digits are in [brackets] under each code. See beginning of section 660-669 for definitions.

5 661.0 Primary uterine inertia ♀ M
[0,1,3] (✖ is only valid for fifth-digit "0")
Failure of cervical dilation
Hypotonic uterine dysfunction, primary
Prolonged latent phase of labor

5 661.1 Secondary uterine inertia ♀ M
[0,1,3] (✖ is only valid for fifth-digit "0")
Arrested active phase of labor
Hypotonic uterine dysfunction, secondary

5 661.2 Other and unspecified uterine inertia ♀ M
[0,1,3] (✖ is only valid for fifth-digit "0")
▶ Atony of uterus without hemorrhage◀
Desultory labor
Irregular labor
Poor contractions
Slow slope active phase of labor
Excludes *▶ atony of uterus with hemorrhage (666.1)◀*
▶ postpartum atony of uterus without hemorrhage (669.8)◀

5 661.3 Precipitate labor ♀ M
[0,1,3] (✖ is only valid for fifth-digit "0")

5 661.4 Hypertonic, incoordinate, or prolonged uterine contractions ♀ M
[0,1,3] (✖ is only valid for fifth-digit "0")
Cervical spasm
Contraction ring (dystocia)
Dyscoordinate labor
Hourglass contraction of uterus
Hypertonic uterine dysfunction
Incoordinate uterine action
Retraction ring (Bandl's) (pathological)
Tetanic contractions
Uterine dystocia NOS
Uterine spasm

✖ 5 661.9 Unspecified abnormality of labor ♀ M
[0,1,3]

4 662 Long labor
Requires fifth digit; valid digits are in [brackets] under each code. See beginning of section 660-669 for definitions.

5 662.0 Prolonged first stage ♀ M
[0,1,3] (✖ is only valid for fifth-digit "0")

5 662.1 Prolonged labor, unspecified ♀ M
[0,1,3] (✖ is only valid for fifth-digit "0")

5 662.2 Prolonged second stage ♀ M
[0,1,3] (✖ is only valid for fifth-digit "0")

5 662.3 Delayed delivery of second twin, triplet, etc. ♀ M
[0,1,3] (✖ is only valid for fifth-digit "0")

4 663 Umbilical cord complications
Requires fifth digit; valid digits are in [brackets] under each code. See beginning of section 660-669 for definitions.

5 663.0 Prolapse of cord ♀ M
[0,1,3] (✖ is only valid for fifth-digit "0")
Presentation of cord
DEF: Umbilical cord enters the birth canal before the fetus during labor.

5 663.1 Cord around neck, with compression ♀ M
[0,1,3] (✖ is only valid for fifth-digit "0")
Cord tightly around neck

5 663.2 Other and unspecified cord entanglement, with compression ♀ M
[0,1,3] (✖ is only valid for fifth-digit "0")
Entanglement of cords of twins in mono-amniotic sac
Knot in cord (with compression)

5 663.3 Other and unspecified cord entanglement, without mention of compression ♀ M
[0,1,3] (✖ is only valid for fifth-digit "0")
AHA: For Code 663.31: 2Q 2003, 9

5 663.4 Short cord ♀ M
[0,1,3] (✖ is only valid for fifth-digit "0")

5 663.5 Vasa previa ♀ M
[0,1,3] (✖ is only valid for fifth-digit "0")

5 663.6 Vascular lesions of cord ♀ M
[0,1,3] (✖ is only valid for fifth-digit "0")
Bruising of cord
Hematoma of cord
Thrombosis of vessels of cord

5 663.8 Other umbilical cord complications ♀ M
[0,1,3] (✖ is only valid for fifth-digit "0")
Velamentous insertion of umbilical cord

✖ 5 663.9 Unspecified umbilical cord complication ♀ M
[0,1,3]

4 664 Trauma to perineum and vulva during delivery
Requires fifth digit; valid digits are in [brackets] under each code. See beginning of section 660-669 for definitions.
Includes damage from instruments
that from extension of episiotomy
AHA: 1Q 1992, 11; Nov-Dec 1984, 10

5 664.0 First-degree perineal laceration ♀ M
[0,1,4] (✖ is only valid for fifth-digit "0")
Perineal laceration, rupture, or tear involving:
- fourchette
- hymen
- labia
- skin
- vagina
- vulva

5 664.1 Second-degree perineal laceration ♀ M
[0,1,4] (✖ is only valid for fifth-digit "0")
Perineal laceration, rupture, or tear (following episiotomy) involving:
- pelvic floor
- perineal muscles
- vaginal muscles

Excludes *that involving anal sphincter (664.2)*

664.2 Third-degree perineal laceration ♀M
[0,1,4] (✖ is only valid for fifth-digit "0")
Perineal laceration, rupture, or tear (following episiotomy) involving:
anal sphincter
rectovaginal septum
sphincter NOS
Excludes ▶*anal sphincter tear during delivery not associated with third-degree perineal laceration (664.6)*◀
that with anal or rectal mucosal laceration (664.3)

664.3 Fourth-degree perineal laceration ♀M
[0,1,4] (✖ is only valid for fifth-digit "0")
Perineal laceration, rupture, or tear as classifiable to 664.2 and involving also:
anal mucosa
rectal mucosa

✖ **664.4 Unspecified perineal laceration** ♀M
[0,1,4]
Central laceration
AHA: 1Q 1992, 8

664.5 Vulval and perineal hematoma ♀M
[0,1,4] (✖ is only valid for fifth-digit "0")
AHA: Nov-Dec 1984, 10

● **664.6 Anal sphincter tear complicating delivery, not associated with third-degree perineal laceration** ♀M
[0,1,4] (✖ is only valid for fifth-digit "0")
Excludes *third-degree perineal laceration (664.2)*

664.8 Other specified trauma to perineum and vulva ♀M
[0,1,4] (✖ is only valid for fifth-digit "0")

✖ **664.9 Unspecified trauma to perineum and vulva** ♀M
[0,1,4]

665 Other obstetrical trauma
Requires fifth digit; valid digits are in [brackets] under each code. See beginning of section 660-669 for definitions.
Includes damage from instruments

665.0 Rupture of uterus before onset of labor ♀M
[0,1,3] (✖ is only valid for fifth-digit "0")
C&C Exclusions: 646.80, 646.81, 646.82, 646.83, 646.84, 646.90, 646.91, 646.93, 648.90, 648.91, 648.92, 648.93, 648.94, 650, 655.70, 655.71, 655.73, 665.00, 665.01, 665.03, 665.10, 665.11, 665.50, 665.51, 665.54, 665.80, 665.81, 665.82, 665.83, 665.84, 665.90, 665.91, 665.92, 665.93, 665.94, 669.40, 669.41, 669.42, 669.43, 669.44, 669.80, 669.81, 669.82, 669.83, 669.84, 669.90, 669.91, 669.92, 669.93, 669.94

665.1 Rupture of uterus during labor ♀M
[0,1] (✖ is only valid for fifth-digit "0")
Rupture of uterus NOS
C&C Exclusions: See 665.0

665.2 Inversion of uterus ♀M
[0,2,4] (✖ is only valid for fifth-digit "0")

665.3 Laceration of cervix ♀M
[0,1,4] (✖ is only valid for fifth-digit "0")

665.4 High vaginal laceration ♀M
[0,1,4] (✖ is only valid for fifth-digit "0")
Laceration of vaginal wall or sulcus without mention of perineal laceration

665.5 Other injury to pelvic organs ♀M
[0,1,4] (✖ is only valid for fifth-digit "0")
Injury to:
bladder
urethra
AHA: Mar-Apr 1987, 10

665.6 Damage to pelvic joints and ligaments ♀M
[0,1,4] (✖ is only valid for fifth-digit "0")
Avulsion of inner symphyseal cartilage
Damage to coccyx
Separation of symphysis (pubis)
AHA: Nov-Dec 1984, 12

665.7 Pelvic hematoma ♀M
[0-2,4] (✖ is only valid for fifth-digit "0")
Hematoma of vagina

665.8 Other specified obstetrical trauma ♀M
[0-4] (✖ is only valid for fifth-digit "0")

✖ **665.9 Unspecified obstetrical trauma** ♀M
[0-4]

666 Postpartum hemorrhage
Requires fifth digit; valid digits are in [brackets] under each code. See beginning of section 660-669 for definitions.
AHA: 1Q 1988, 14

666.0 Third-stage hemorrhage ♀M
[0,2,4] (✖ is only valid for fifth-digit "0")
Hemorrhage associated with retained, trapped, or adherent placenta
Retained placenta NOS

666.1 Other immediate postpartum hemorrhage ♀M
[0,2,4] (✖ is only valid for fifth-digit "0")
Atony of uterus with hemorrhage
Hemorrhage within the first 24 hours following delivery of placenta
▶ Postpartum atony of uterus with hemorrhage◀
Postpartum hemorrhage (atonic) NOS
Excludes *atony of uterus without hemorrhage (▶661.2◀)*
▶ *postpartum atony of uterus without hemorrhage (669.8)*◀

666.2 Delayed and secondary postpartum hemorrhage ♀M
[0,2,4] (✖ is only valid for fifth-digit "0")
Hemorrhage:
after the first 24 hours following delivery
associated with retained portions of placenta or membranes
Postpartum hemorrhage specified as delayed or secondary
Retained products of conception NOS, following delivery

666.3 Postpartum coagulation defects ♀M
[0,2,4] (✖ is only valid for fifth-digit "0")
Postpartum:
afibrinogenemia
fibrinolysis
C&C Exclusions: (for codes 666.32, 666.34) 646.80, 646.81, 646.82, 646.83, 646.84, 646.90, 646.91, 646.93, 648.90, 648.91, 648.92, 648.93, 648.94, 650, 666.00, 666.02, 666.04, 666.10, 666.12, 666.14, 666.20, 666.22, 666.24, 666.30, 666.32, 666.34, 669.40, 669.41, 669.42, 669.43, 669.44, 669.80, 669.81, 669.82, 669.83, 669.84, 669.90, 669.91, 669.92, 669.93, 669.94

667 Retained placenta without hemorrhage
Requires fifth digit; valid digits are in [brackets] under each code. See beginning of section 660-669 for definitions.
AHA: 1Q 1988, 14

667.0 Retained placenta without hemorrhage ♀M
[0,2,4] (✖ is only valid for fifth-digit "0")
Placenta accreta without hemorrhage
Retained placenta:
NOS without hemorrhage
total without hemorrhage

667.1 Retained portions of placenta or membranes, without hemorrhage ♀M
[0,2,4] (✖ is only valid for fifth-digit "0")
Retained products of conception following delivery, without hemorrhage

A Adult (15+ years) M Maternity (12-55 years) N Newborn (0 years) P Pediatric (0-17 years) ♂ Male ♀ Female Medicare Secondary Payer

❹ 668 Complications of the administration of anesthetic or other sedation in labor and delivery

Use additional code(s) to further specify complication

Requires fifth digit; valid digits are in [brackets] under each code. See beginning of section 660-669 for definitions.

Includes complications arising from the administration of a general or local anesthetic, analgesic, or other sedation in labor and delivery

Excludes *reaction to spinal or lumbar puncture (349.0)*
spinal headache (349.0)

❺ 668.0 Pulmonary complications ♀M
[0-4]
(✖ is only valid for fifth-digit "0")
Inhalation [aspiration] of stomach contents or secretions following anesthesia or other sedation in labor or delivery
Mendelson's syndrome following anesthesia or other sedation in labor or delivery
Pressure collapse of lung following anesthesia or other sedation in labor or delivery
C&C Exclusions: 646.80, 646.81, 646.82, 646.83, 646.84, 646.90, 646.91, 646.93, 648.90, 648.91, 648.92, 648.93, 648.94, 650, 668.00, 668.01, 668.02, 668.03, 668.04, 669.40, 669.41, 669.42, 669.43, 669.44, 669.80, 669.81, 669.82, 669.83, 669.84, 669.90, 669.91, 669.92, 669.93, 669.94

❺ 668.1 Cardiac complications ♀M
[0-4]
(✖ is only valid for fifth-digit "0")
Cardiac arrest or failure following anesthesia or other sedation in labor and delivery
C&C Exclusions: 646.80, 646.81, 646.82, 646.83, 646.84, 646.90, 646.91, 646.93, 648.90, 648.91, 648.92, 648.93, 648.94, 650, 668.10, 668.11, 668.12, 668.13, 668.14, 669.40, 669.41, 669.42, 669.43, 669.44, 669.80, 669.81, 669.82, 669.83, 669.84, 669.90, 669.91, 669.92, 669.93, 669.94

❺ 668.2 Central nervous system complications ♀M
[0-4]
(✖ is only valid for fifth-digit "0")
Cerebral anoxia following anesthesia or other sedation in labor and delivery
C&C Exclusions: 646.80, 646.81, 646.82, 646.83, 646.84, 646.90, 646.91, 646.93, 648.90, 648.91, 648.92, 648.93, 648.94, 650, 668.20, 668.21, 668.22, 668.23, 668.24, 669.40, 669.41, 669.42, 669.43, 669.44, 669.80, 669.81, 669.82, 669.83, 669.84, 669.90, 669.91, 669.92, 669.93, 669.94

❺ 668.8 Other complications of anesthesia or other sedation in labor and delivery ♀M
[0-4]
(✖ is only valid for fifth-digit "0")
C&C Exclusions: 646.80, 646.81, 646.82, 646.83, 646.84, 646.90, 646.91, 646.93, 648.90, 648.91, 648.92, 648.93, 648.94, 650, 668.80, 668.81, 668.82, 668.83, 668.84, 668.90, 668.91, 668.92, 668.93, 668.94, 669.40, 669.41, 669.42, 669.43, 669.44, 669.80, 669.81, 669.82, 669.83, 669.84, 669.90, 669.91, 669.92, 669.93, 669.94
AHA: 2Q 1999, 9

✖❺ 668.9 Unspecified complication of anesthesia and other sedation ♀M
[0-4]
C&C Exclusions: See 668.8

❹ 669 Other complications of labor and delivery, not elsewhere classified

Requires fifth digit; valid digits are in [brackets] under each code. See beginning of section 660-669 for definitions.

❺ 669.0 Maternal distress ♀M
[0-4]
(✖ is only valid for fifth-digit "0")
Metabolic disturbance in labor and delivery

❺ 669.1 Shock during or following labor and delivery ♀M
[0-4]
(✖ is only valid for fifth-digit "0")
Obstetric shock
C&C Exclusions: 646.80, 646.81, 646.82, 646.83, 646.84, 646.90, 646.91, 646.93, 648.90, 648.91, 648.92, 648.93, 648.94, 650, 669.10, 669.11, 669.12, 669.13, 669.14, 669.40, 669.41, 669.42, 669.43, 669.44, 669.80, 669.81, 669.82, 669.83, 669.84, 669.90, 669.91, 669.92, 669.93, 669.94

❺ 669.2 Maternal hypotension syndrome ♀M
[0-4]
(✖ is only valid for fifth-digit "0")

❺ 669.3 Acute renal failure following labor and delivery ♀M
[0,2,4]
(✖ is only valid for fifth-digit "0")
C&C Exclusions: 646.80, 646.81, 646.82, 646.83, 646.84, 646.90, 646.91, 646.93, 648.90, 648.91, 648.92, 648.93, 648.94, 650, 669.30, 669.31, 669.32, 669.33, 669.34, 669.40, 669.41, 669.42, 669.43, 669.44, 669.80, 669.81, 669.82, 669.83, 669.84, 669.90, 669.91, 669.92, 669.93, 669.94

❺ 669.4 Other complications of obstetrical surgery and procedures ♀M
[0-4]
(✖ is only valid for fifth-digit "0")
Cardiac:
arrest following cesarean or other obstetrical surgery or procedure, including delivery NOS
failure following cesarean or other obstetrical surgery or procedure, including delivery NOS
Cerebral anoxia following cesarean or other obstetrical surgery or procedure, including delivery NOS
Excludes *complications of obstetrical surgical wounds (674.1-674.3)*
C&C Exclusions: 674.50, 674.51, 674.52, 674.53, 674.54

❺ 669.5 Forceps or vacuum extractor delivery without mention of indication ♀M
[0,1]
(✖ is only valid for fifth-digit "0")
Delivery by ventouse, without mention of indication

❺ 669.6 Breech extraction, without mention of indication ♀M
[0,1]
(✖ is only valid for fifth-digit "0")
Excludes *breech delivery NOS (652.2)*

❺ 669.7 Cesarean delivery, without mention of indication ♀M
[0,1]
(✖ is only valid for fifth-digit "0")
AHA: For Code 669.71: 1Q 2001, 11

❺ 669.8 Other complications of labor and delivery ♀M
[0-4]
(✖ is only valid for fifth-digit "0")
C&C Exclusions: See 669.4
AHA: 4Q 2006, 135

✖❺ 669.9 Unspecified complication of labor and delivery ♀M
[0-4]
C&C Exclusions: See 669.4

❹ ❺ Additional Digit Required ✖ Nonspecific PDx ⊘ Unacceptable PDx ✚ Manifestation Code ▶◀ Revised Text ● New Code ▲ Revised Code

COMPLICATIONS OF THE PUERPERIUM (670-677)

Note: Categories 671 and 673-676 include the listed conditions even if they occur during pregnancy or childbirth.

The following fifth-digit subclassification is for use with categories 670-676 to denote the current episode of care:

- **0 unspecified as to episode of care or not applicable**
- **1 delivered, with or without mention of antepartum condition**
- **2 delivered, with mention of postpartum complication**
- **3 antepartum condition or complication**
- **4 postpartum condition or complication**

❹ **670 Major puerperal infection** ♀M
[0,2,4]

Requires fifth digit; valid digits are in [brackets] under each code. See beginning of section 670-676 for definitions.

(✖ is only valid for fifth-digit "0")

❺ Use 0 as fourth-digit for category 670

Puerperal:
- endometritis
- fever (septic)
- pelvic:
  - cellulitis
  - sepsis
- peritonitis
- pyemia
- salpingitis
- septicemia

Excludes *infection following abortion (639.0)*
minor genital tract infection following delivery (646.6)
puerperal fever NOS (672)
puerperal pyrexia NOS (672)
puerperal pyrexia of unknown origin (672)
urinary tract infection following delivery (646.6)

C&C Exclusions: 646.80, 646.81, 646.82, 646.83, 646.84, 646.90, 646.91, 646.93, 648.90, 648.91, 648.92, 648.93, 648.94, 650, 669.40, 669.41, 669.42, 669.43, 669.44, 669.80, 669.81, 669.82, 669.83, 669.84, 669.90, 669.91, 669.92, 669.93, 669.94, 670.00, 670.02, 670.04

AHA: 4Q 1991, 26; 2Q 1991, 7

❹ **671 Venous complications in pregnancy and the puerperium**

Requires fifth digit; valid digits are in [brackets] under each code. See beginning of section 670-676 for definitions.

❺ **671.0 Varicose veins of legs** ♀M
[0-4]
(✖ is only valid for fifth-digit "0")
Varicose veins NOS

❺ **671.1 Varicose veins of vulva and perineum** ♀M
[0-4]
(✖ is only valid for fifth-digit "0")

❺ **671.2 Superficial thrombophlebitis** ♀M
[0-4]
(✖ is only valid for fifth-digit "0")
Thrombophlebitis (superficial)
C&C Exclusions: 646.80, 646.81, 646.82, 646.83, 646.84, 646.90, 646.91, 646.93, 648.90, 648.91, 648.92, 648.93, 648.94, 650, 669.40, 669.41, 669.42, 669.43, 669.44, 669.80, 669.81, 669.82, 669.83, 669.84, 669.90, 669.91, 669.92, 669.93, 669.94, 671.20, 671.21, 671.22, 671.23, 671.24, 671.30, 671.31, 671.33, 671.40, 671.42, 671.44, 671.50, 671.51, 671.52, 671.53, 671.54, 671.80, 671.81, 671.82, 671.83, 671.84, 671.90, 671.91, 671.92, 671.93, 671.94

❺ **671.3 Deep phlebothrombosis, antepartum** ♀M
[0,1,3]
(✖ is only valid for fifth-digit "0")
Deep-vein thrombosis, antepartum
C&C Exclusions: See 671.2

❺ **671.4 Deep phlebothrombosis, postpartum** ♀M
[0,2,4]
(✖ is only valid for fifth-digit "0")
Deep-vein thrombosis, postpartum
Pelvic thrombophlebitis, postpartum
Phlegmasia alba dolens (puerperal)
C&C Exclusions: See 671.2

❺ **671.5 Other phlebitis and thrombosis** ♀M
[0-4]
(✖ is only valid for fifth-digit "0")
Cerebral venous thrombosis
Thrombosis of intracranial venous sinus

❺ **671.8 Other venous complications** ♀M
[0-4]
(✖ is only valid for fifth-digit "0")
Hemorrhoids

✖❺ **671.9 Unspecified venous complication** ♀M
[0-4]
Phlebitis NOS
Thrombosis NOS

❹ **672 Pyrexia of unknown origin during the puerperium** ♀M
[0,2,4]
(✖ is only valid for fifth-digit "0")
❺ Use 0 as fourth-digit for category 672
Postpartum fever NOS
Puerperal fever NOS
Puerperal pyrexia NOS
Requires fifth digit; valid digits are in [brackets] under each code. See beginning of section 670-676 for definitions.
AHA: 4Q 1991, 26

❹ **673 Obstetrical pulmonary embolism**

Requires fifth digit; valid digits are in [brackets] under each code. See beginning of section 670-676 for definitions.

Includes pulmonary emboli in pregnancy, childbirth, or the puerperium, or specified as puerperal

Excludes *embolism following abortion (639.6)*

❺ **673.0 Obstetrical air embolism** ♀M
[0-4]
(✖ is only valid for fifth-digit "0")
C&C Exclusions: 646.80, 646.81, 646.82, 646.83, 646.84, 646.90, 646.91, 646.93, 648.90, 648.91, 648.92, 648.93, 648.94, 650, 669.40, 669.41, 669.42, 669.43, 669.44, 669.80, 669.81, 669.82, 669.83, 669.84, 669.90, 669.91, 669.92, 669.93, 669.94, 673.00, 673.01, 673.02, 673.03, 673.04, 673.10, 673.11, 673.12, 673.13, 673.14, 673.20, 673.21, 673.22, 673.23, 673.24, 673.30, 673.31, 673.32, 673.33, 673.34, 673.80, 673.81, 673.82, 673.83, 673.84

❺ **673.1 Amniotic fluid embolism** ♀M
[0-4]
(✖ is only valid for fifth-digit "0")
C&C Exclusions: See 673.0

❺ **673.2 Obstetrical blood-clot embolism** ♀M
[0-4]
(✖ is only valid for fifth-digit "0")
Puerperal pulmonary embolism NOS
C&C Exclusions: See 673.0
AHA: For Code 673.24: 1Q 2005, 6

❺ **673.3 Obstetrical pyemic and septic embolism** ♀M
[0-4]
(✖ is only valid for fifth-digit "0")
C&C Exclusions: See 673.0

❺ **673.8 Other pulmonary embolism** ♀M
[0-4]
(✖ is only valid for fifth-digit "0")
Fat embolism
C&C Exclusions: See 673.0

❹ **674 Other and unspecified complications of the puerperium, not elsewhere classified**

Requires fifth digit; valid digits are in [brackets] under each code. See beginning of section 670-676 for definitions.

❺ **674.0 Cerebrovascular disorders in the puerperium** ♀M
[0-4]
(✖ is only valid for fifth-digit "0")
Any condition classifiable to 430-434, 436-437 occurring during pregnancy, childbirth, or the puerperium, or specified as puerperal
Excludes *intracranial venous sinus thrombosis (671.5)*
C&C Exclusions: 646.80, 646.81, 646.82, 646.83, 646.84, 646.90, 646.91, 646.93, 648.90, 648.91, 648.92, 648.93, 648.94, 650, 669.40, 669.41, 669.42, 669.43, 669.44, 669.80, 669.81, 669.82, 669.83, 669.84, 669.90, 669.91, 669.92, 669.93, 669.94, 674.00, 674.01, 674.02, 674.03, 674.04, 674.50, 674.51, 674.52, 674.53, 674.54

❺ **674.1 Disruption of cesarean wound** ♀ M
[0,2,4]
(✖ is only valid for fifth-digit "0")
Dehiscence or disruption of uterine wound
Excludes *uterine rupture before onset of labor (665.0)*
uterine rupture during labor (665.1)
C&C Exclusions: (for codes 674.10, 674.12) 646.80, 646.81, 646.82, 646.83, 646.84, 646.90, 646.91, 646.93, 648.90, 648.91, 648.92, 648.93, 648.94, 650, 669.40, 669.41, 669.42, 669.43, 669.44, 669.80, 669.81, 669.82, 669.83, 669.84, 669.90, 669.91, 669.92, 669.93, 669.94, 674.10, 674.34

❺ **674.2 Disruption of perineal wound** ♀ M
[0,2,4]
(✖ is only valid for fifth-digit "0")
Breakdown of perineum
Disruption of wound of:
episiotomy
perineal laceration
Secondary perineal tear
C&C Exclusions: See 674.1
AHA: For Code 674.24: 1Q 1997, 9

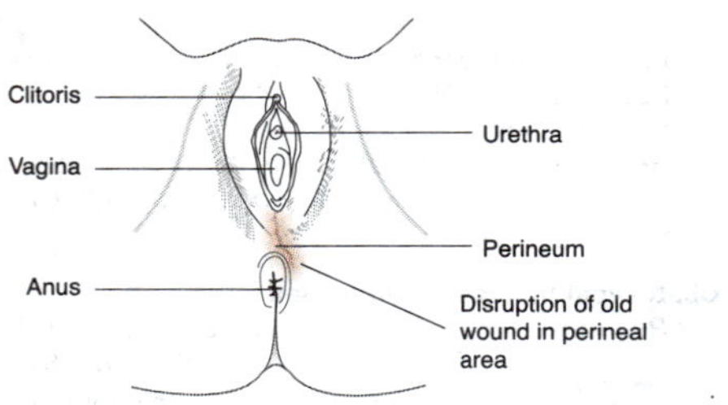

❺ **674.3 Other complications of obstetrical surgical wounds** ♀ M
[0,2,4]
(✖ is only valid for fifth-digit "0")
Hematoma of cesarean section or perineal wound
Hemorrhage of cesarean section or perineal wound
Infection of cesarean section or perineal wound
Excludes *damage from instruments in delivery (664.0-665.9)*
AHA: 2Q 1991, 7

❺ **674.4 Placental polyp** ♀ M
[0,2,4]
(✖ is only valid for fifth-digit "0")

❺ **674.5 Peripartum cardiomyopathy** ♀ M
[0-4]
(✖ is only valid for fifth-digit "0")
Postpartum cardiomyopathy
C&C Exclusions: 674.00, 674.01, 674.02, 674.03, 674.04, 674.50, 674.51, 674.52, 674.53, 674.54
AHA: 4Q 2003, 65

❺ **674.8 Other** ♀ M
[0,2,4]
(✖ is only valid for fifth-digit "0")
Hepatorenal syndrome, following delivery
Postpartum:
subinvolution of uterus
uterine hypertrophy
AHA: 3Q 1998, 16

✖❺ **674.9 Unspecified** ♀ M
[0,2,4]
Sudden death of unknown cause during the puerperium

❹ **675 Infections of the breast and nipple associated with childbirth**
Requires fifth digit; valid digits are in [brackets] under each code. See beginning of section 670-676 for definitions.
Includes the listed conditions during pregnancy, childbirth, or the puerperium

❺ **675.0 Infections of nipple** ♀ M
[0-4]
(✖ is only valid for fifth-digit "0")
Abscess of nipple

❺ **675.1 Abscess of breast** ♀ M
[0-4]
(✖ is only valid for fifth-digit "0")
Abscess:
mammary
subareolar
submammary
Mastitis:
purulent
retromammary
submammary
C&C Exclusions: (for codes 675.10-675.12) 646.80, 646.81, 646.82, 646.83, 646.84, 646.90, 646.91, 646.93, 648.90, 648.91, 648.92, 648.93, 648.94, 650, 669.40, 669.41, 669.42, 669.43, 669.44, 669.80, 669.81, 669.82, 669.83, 669.84, 669.90, 669.91, 669.92, 669.93, 669.94, 675.00, 675.01, 2, 675.03, 675.04, 675.10, 675.11, 675.12, 675.13, 675.14, 675.20, 675.21, 675.22, 675.23, 675.24, 675.80, 675.81, 675.82, 675.83, 675.84, 675.90, 675.91, 675.92, 675.93, 675.94

❺ **675.2 Nonpurulent mastitis** ♀ M
[0-4]
(✖ is only valid for fifth-digit "0")
Lymphangitis of breast
Mastitis:
NOS
interstitial
parenchymatous

❺ **675.8 Other specified infections of the breast and nipple** ♀ M
[0-4]
(✖ is only valid for fifth-digit "0")

❺ **675.9 Unspecified infection of the breast and nipple** ♀ M
[0-4]
(✖ is only valid for fifth-digit "0")

❹ **676 Other disorders of the breast associated with childbirth and disorders of lactation**
Requires fifth digit; valid digits are in [brackets] under each code. See beginning of section 670-676 for definitions.
Includes the listed conditions during pregnancy, the puerperium, or lactation

❺ **676.0 Retracted nipple** ♀ M
[0-4]
(✖ is only valid for fifth-digit "0")

❺ **676.1 Cracked nipple** ♀ M
[0-4]
(✖ is only valid for fifth-digit "0")
Fissure of nipple

❺ **676.2 Engorgement of breasts** ♀ M
[0-4]
(✖ is only valid for fifth-digit "0")

❺ **676.3 Other and unspecified disorder of breast** ♀ M
[0-4]
(✖ is only valid for fifth-digit "0")

❺ **676.4 Failure of lactation** ♀ M
[0-4]
(✖ is only valid for fifth-digit "0")
Agalactia

❺ **676.5 Suppressed lactation** ♀ M
[0-4]
(✖ is only valid for fifth-digit "0")

❺ **676.6 Galactorrhea** ♀ M
[0-4]
(✖ is only valid for fifth-digit "0")
Excludes *galactorrhea not associated with childbirth (611.6)*

❺ **676.8 Other disorders of lactation** ♀ M
[0-4]
(✖ is only valid for fifth-digit "0")
Galactocele

✖❺ **676.9 Unspecified disorder of lactation** ♀ M
[0-4]

✖ **677 Late effect of complication of pregnancy, childbirth, and the puerperium** ♀
Note: This category is to be used to indicate conditions in 632-648.9 and 651-676.9 as the cause of the late effect, themselves classifiable elsewhere. The "late effects" include conditions specified as such, or as sequelae, which may occur at any time after the puerperium.
Code first any sequelae
AHA: 1Q 1997, 9; 4Q 1994, 42

12. DISEASES OF THE SKIN AND SUBCUTANEOUS TISSUE (680-709)

INFECTIONS OF SKIN AND SUBCUTANEOUS TISSUE (680-686)

Excludes *certain infections of skin classified under "Infectious and Parasitic Diseases," such as:*
erysipelas (035)
erysipeloid of Rosenbach (027.1)
herpes:
simplex (054.0-054.9)
zoster (053.0-053.9)
molluscum contagiosum (078.0)
viral warts (078.1)

❹ **680 Carbuncle and furuncle**
Includes boil
furunculosis

680.0 Face
Ear [any part]
Face [any part, except eye]
Nose (septum)
Temple (region)
Excludes *eyelid (373.13)*
lacrimal apparatus (375.31)
orbit (376.01)

C&C Exclusions: 017.00, 017.01, 017.02, 017.03, 017.04, 017.05, 017.06, 017.90, 017.91, 017.92, 017.93, 017.94, 017.95, 017.96, 040.82, 040.89, 041.00, 041.01, 041.02, 041.03, 041.04, 041.05, 041.09, 041.10, 041.11, 041.19, 041.2, 041.3, 041.4, 041.5, 041.6, 041.7, 041.81, 041.82, 041.83, 041.84, 041.85, 041.86, 041.89, 041.9, 680.0, 680.8, 680.9, 686.00, 686.01, 686.09, 686.1, 686.8, 686.9, 705.83, 709.8, V09.0, V09.1, V09.2, V09.3, V09.4, V09.50, V09.51, V09.6, V09.70, V09.71, V09.80, V09.81, V09.90, V09.91

680.1 Neck
C&C Exclusions: 017.00, 017.01, 017.02, 017.03, 017.04, 017.05, 017.06, 017.90, 017.91, 017.92, 017.93, 017.94, 017.95, 017.96, 040.82, 040.89, 041.00, 041.01, 041.02, 041.03, 041.04, 041.05, 041.09, 041.10, 041.11, 041.19, 041.2, 041.3, 041.4, 041.5, 041.6, 041.7, 041.81, 041.82, 041.83, 041.84, 041.85, 041.86, 041.89, 041.9, 680.1, 680.8, 680.9, 686.00, 686.01, 686.09, 686.1, 686.8, 686.9, 705.83, 709.8, V09.0, V09.1, V09.2, V09.3, V09.4, V09.50, V09.51, V09.6, V09.70, V09.71, V09.80, V09.81, V09.90, V09.91

680.2 Trunk
Abdominal wall
Back [any part, except buttocks]
Breast
Chest wall
Flank
Groin
Pectoral region
Perineum
Umbilicus
Excludes *buttocks (680.5)*
external genital organs:
female (616.4)
male (607.2, 608.4)

C&C Exclusions: 017.00, 017.01, 017.02, 017.03, 017.04, 017.05, 017.06, 017.90, 017.91, 017.92, 017.93, 017.94, 017.95, 017.96, 040.82, 040.89, 041.00, 041.01, 041.02, 041.03, 041.04, 041.05, 041.09, 041.10, 041.11, 041.19, 041.2, 041.3, 041.4, 041.5, 041.6, 041.7, 041.81, 041.82, 041.83, 041.84, 041.85, 041.86, 041.89, 041.9, 680.2, 680.8, 680.9, 686.00, 686.01, 686.09, 686.1, 686.8, 686.9, 705.83, 709.8, V09.0, V09.1, V09.2, V09.3, V09.4, V09.50, V09.51, V09.6, V09.70, V09.71, V09.80, V09.81, V09.90, V09.91

680.3 Upper arm and forearm
Arm [any part, except hand]
Axilla
Shoulder

C&C Exclusions: 017.00, 017.01, 017.02, 017.03, 017.04, 017.05, 017.06, 017.90, 017.91, 017.92, 017.93, 017.94, 017.95, 017.96, 040.82, 040.89, 041.00, 041.01, 041.02, 041.03, 041.04, 041.05, 041.09, 041.10, 041.11, 041.19, 041.2, 041.3, 041.4, 041.5, 041.6, 041.7, 041.81, 041.82, 041.83, 041.84, 041.85, 041.86, 041.89, 041.9, 680.3, 680.8, 680.9, 686.00, 686.01, 686.09, 686.1, 686.8, 686.9, 705.83, 709.8, V09.0, V09.1, V09.2, V09.3, V09.4, V09.50, V09.51, V09.6, V09.70, V09.71, V09.80, V09.81, V09.90, V09.91

680.4 Hand
Finger [any]
Thumb
Wrist

C&C Exclusions: 017.00, 017.01, 017.02, 017.03, 017.04, 017.05, 017.06, 017.90, 017.91, 017.92, 017.93, 017.94, 017.95, 017.96, 040.82, 040.89, 041.00, 041.01, 041.02, 041.03, 041.04, 041.05, 041.09, 041.10, 041.11, 041.19, 041.2, 041.3, 041.4, 041.5, 041.6, 041.7, 041.81, 041.82, 041.83, 041.84, 041.85, 041.86, 041.89, 041.9, 680.4, 680.8, 680.9, 686.00, 686.01, 686.09, 686.1, 686.8, 686.9, 705.83, 709.8, V09.0, V09.1, V09.2, V09.3, V09.4, V09.50, V09.51, V09.6, V09.70, V09.71, V09.80, V09.81, V09.90, V09.91

680.5 Buttock
Anus
Gluteal region

C&C Exclusions: 017.00, 017.01, 017.02, 017.03, 017.04, 017.05, 017.06, 017.90, 017.91, 017.92, 017.93, 017.94, 017.95, 017.96, 040.82, 040.89, 041.00, 041.01, 041.02, 041.03, 041.04, 041.05, 041.09, 041.10, 041.11, 041.19, 041.2, 041.3, 041.4, 041.5, 041.6, 041.7, 041.81, 041.82, 041.83, 041.84, 041.85, 041.86, 041.89, 041.9, 680.5, 680.8, 680.9, 686.00, 686.01, 686.09, 686.1, 686.8, 686.9, 705.83, 709.8, V09.0, V09.1, V09.2, V09.3, V09.4, V09.50, V09.51, V09.6, V09.70, V09.71, V09.80, V09.81, V09.90, V09.91

680.6 Leg, except foot
Ankle
Hip
Knee
Thigh

C&C Exclusions: 017.00, 017.01, 017.02, 017.03, 017.04, 017.05, 017.06, 017.90, 017.91, 017.92, 017.93, 017.94, 017.95, 017.96, 040.82, 040.89, 041.00, 041.01, 041.02, 041.03, 041.04, 041.05, 041.09, 041.10, 041.11, 041.19, 041.2, 041.3, 041.4, 041.5, 041.6, 041.7, 041.81, 041.82, 041.83, 041.84, 041.85, 041.86, 041.89, 041.9, 680.6, 680.8, 680.9, 686.00, 686.01, 686.09, 686.1, 686.8, 686.9, 705.83, 709.8, V09.0, V09.1, V09.2, V09.3, V09.4, V09.50, V09.51, V09.6, V09.70, V09.71, V09.80, V09.81, V09.90, V09.91

680.7 Foot
Heel
Toe

C&C Exclusions: 017.00, 017.01, 017.02, 017.03, 017.04, 017.05, 017.06, 017.90, 017.91, 017.92, 017.93, 017.94, 017.95, 017.96, 040.82, 040.89, 041.00, 041.01, 041.02, 041.03, 041.04, 041.05, 041.09, 041.10, 041.11, 041.19, 041.2, 041.3, 041.4, 041.5, 041.6, 041.7, 041.81, 041.82, 041.83, 041.84, 041.85, 041.86, 041.89, 041.9, 680.7, 680.8, 680.9, 686.00, 686.01, 686.09, 686.1, 686.8, 686.9, 705.83, 709.8, V09.0, V09.1, V09.2, V09.3, V09.4, V09.50, V09.51, V09.6, V09.70, V09.71, V09.80, V09.81, V09.90, V09.91

680.8 Other specified sites
Head [any part, except face]
Scalp
Excludes *external genital organs:*
female (616.4)
male (607.2, 608.4)

C&C Exclusions: 017.00, 017.01, 017.02, 017.03, 017.04, 017.05, 017.06, 017.90, 017.91, 017.92, 017.93, 017.94, 017.95, 017.96, 040.82, 040.89, 041.00, 041.01, 041.02, 041.03, 041.04, 041.05, 041.09, 041.10, 041.11, 041.19, 041.2, 041.3, 041.4, 041.5, 041.6, 041.7, 041.81, 041.82, 041.83, 041.84, 041.85, 041.86, 041.89, 041.9, 680.8, 680.9, 686.00, 686.01, 686.09, 686.1, 686.8, 686.9, 705.83, 709.8, V09.0, V09.1, V09.2, V09.3, V09.4, V09.50, V09.51, V09.6, V09.70, V09.71, V09.80, V09.81, V09.90, V09.91

✖ **680.9 Unspecified site**
Boil NOS
Carbuncle NOS
Furuncle NOS

C&C Exclusions: See 680.8

❹ **681 Cellulitis and abscess of finger and toe**
Includes that with lymphangitis
Use additional code to identify organism, such as Staphylococcus (041.1)

AHA: 2Q 1991, 5; Jan-Feb 1987, 12

❺ **681.0 Finger**

681.00 Cellulitis and abscess, unspecified

681.01 Felon
Pulp abscess
Whitlow
Excludes *herpetic whitlow (054.6)*

DEF: Painful, pus-filled infection of a fingertip.

681.02 Onychia and paronychia of finger
Panaritium of finger
Perionychia of finger

DEF: Onychia: inflammation of the matrix of the fingernail, secreting pus and causing the nail to fall out.

DEF: Paronychia: inflammation and breakdown of the cuticle tissue around the nail.

❺ **681.1 Toe**

681.10 Cellulitis and abscess, unspecified
AHA: 1Q 2005, 14

681.11 Onychia and paronychia of toe
Panaritium of toe
Perionychia of toe

✖ **681.9 Cellulitis and abscess of unspecified digit**
Infection of nail NOS

❹ **682 Other cellulitis and abscess**
Includes abscess (acute) (with lymphangitis) except of finger or toe
cellulitis (diffuse) (with lymphangitis) except of finger or toe
lymphangitis, acute (with lymphangitis) except of finger or toe
Use additional code to identify organism, such as Staphylococcus (041.1)
Excludes *lymphangitis (chronic) (subacute) (457.2)*

AHA: 2Q 1991, 5; Jan-Feb 1987, 12; Sep-Oct 1985, 10

682.0 Face
Cheek, external
Chin
Forehead
Nose, external
Submandibular
Temple (region)
Excludes *ear [any part] (380.10-380.16)*
eyelid (373.13)
lacrimal apparatus (375.31)
lip (528.5)
mouth (528.3)
nose (internal) (478.1)
orbit (376.01)

C&C Exclusions: 017.00, 017.01, 017.02, 017.03, 017.04, 017.05, 017.06, 017.90, 017.91, 017.92, 017.93, 017.94, 017.95, 017.96, 040.89, 041.00, 041.01, 041.02, 041.03, 041.04, 041.05, 041.09, 041.10, 041.11, 041.19, 041.2, 041.3, 041.4, 041.5, 041.6, 041.7, 041.81, 041.82, 041.83, 041.84, 041.85, 041.86, 041.89, 041.9, 682.0, 682.8, 682.9, 686.00, 686.01, 686.09, 686.1, 686.8, 686.9, 705.83, 709.8, V09.0, V09.1, V09.2, V09.3, V09.4, V09.50, V09.51, V09.6, V09.70, V09.71, V09.80, V09.81, V09.90, V09.91

682.1 Neck

C&C Exclusions: 017.00, 017.01, 017.02, 017.03, 017.04, 017.05, 017.06, 017.90, 017.91, 017.92, 017.93, 017.94, 017.95, 017.96, 040.89, 041.00, 041.01, 041.02, 041.03, 041.04, 041.05, 041.09, 041.10, 041.11, 041.19, 041.2, 041.3, 041.4, 041.5, 041.6, 041.7, 041.81, 041.82, 041.83, 041.84, 041.85, 041.86, 041.89, 041.9, 682.1, 682.8, 682.9, 686.00, 686.01, 686.09, 686.1, 686.8, 686.9, 705.83, 709.8, V09.0, V09.1, V09.2, V09.3, V09.4, V09.50, V09.51, V09.6, V09.70, V09.71, V09.80, V09.81, V09.90, V09.91

682.2 Trunk
Abdominal wall
Back [any part, except buttock]
Chest wall
Flank
Groin
Pectoral region
Perineum
Umbilicus, except newborn
Excludes *anal and rectal regions (566)*
breast:
NOS (611.0)
puerperal (675.1)
external genital organs:
female (616.3-616.4)
male (604.0, 607.2, 608.4)
umbilicus, newborn (771.4)

C&C Exclusions: 017.00, 017.01, 017.02, 017.03, 017.04, 017.05, 017.06, 017.90, 017.91, 017.92, 017.93, 017.94, 017.95, 017.96, 040.89, 041.00, 041.01, 041.02, 041.03, 041.04, 041.05, 041.09, 041.10, 041.11, 041.19, 041.2, 041.3, 041.4, 041.5, 041.6, 041.7, 041.81, 041.82, 041.83, 041.84, 041.85, 041.86, 041.89, 041.9, 682.2, 682.8, 682.9, 686.00, 686.01, 686.09, 686.1, 686.8, 686.9, 705.83, 709.8, V09.0, V09.1, V09.2, V09.3, V09.4, V09.50, V09.51, V09.6, V09.70, V09.71, V09.80, V09.81, V09.90, V09.91

AHA: 4Q 1998, 42

682.3 Upper arm and forearm
Arm [any part, except hand]
Axilla
Shoulder
Excludes *hand (682.4)*

C&C Exclusions: 017.00, 017.01, 017.02, 017.03, 017.04, 017.05, 017.06, 017.90, 017.91, 017.92, 017.93, 017.94, 017.95, 017.96, 040.89, 041.00, 041.01, 041.02, 041.03, 041.04, 041.05, 041.09, 041.10, 041.11, 041.19, 041.2, 041.3, 041.4, 041.5, 041.6, 041.7, 041.81, 041.82, 041.83, 041.84, 041.85, 041.86, 041.89, 041.9, 682.3, 682.8, 682.9, 686.00, 686.01, 686.09, 686.1, 686.8, 686.9, 705.83, 709.8, V09.0, V09.1, V09.2, V09.3, V09.4, V09.50, V09.51, V09.6, V09.70, V09.71, V09.80, V09.81, V09.90, V09.91

AHA: 2Q 2003, 7

682.4 Hand, except fingers and thumb
Wrist
Excludes *finger and thumb (681.00-681.02)*
C&C Exclusions: 017.00, 017.01, 017.02, 017.03, 017.04, 017.05, 017.06, 017.90, 017.91, 017.92, 017.93, 017.94, 017.95, 017.96, 040.89, 041.00, 041.01, 041.02, 041.03, 041.04, 041.05, 041.09, 041.10, 041.11, 041.19, 041.2, 041.3, 041.4, 041.5, 041.6, 041.7, 041.81, 041.82, 041.83, 041.84, 041.85, 041.86, 041.89, 041.9, 682.4, 682.8, 682.9, 686.00, 686.01, 686.09, 686.1, 686.8, 686.9, 705.83, 709.8, V09.0, V09.1, V09.2, V09.3, V09.4, V09.50, V09.51, V09.6, V09.70, V09.71, V09.80, V09.81, V09.90, V09.91

682.5 Buttock
Gluteal region
Excludes *anal and rectal regions (566)*
C&C Exclusions: 017.00, 017.01, 017.02, 017.03, 017.04, 017.05, 017.06, 017.90, 017.91, 017.92, 017.93, 017.94, 017.95, 017.96, 040.89, 041.00, 041.01, 041.02, 041.03, 041.04, 041.05, 041.09, 041.10, 041.11, 041.19, 041.2, 041.3, 041.4, 041.5, 041.6, 041.7, 041.81, 041.82, 041.83, 041.84, 041.85, 041.86, 041.89, 041.9, 682.5, 682.8, 682.9, 686.00, 686.01, 686.09, 686.1, 686.8, 686.9, 705.83, 709.8, V09.0, V09.1, V09.2, V09.3, V09.4, V09.50, V09.51, V09.6, V09.70, V09.71, V09.80, V09.81, V09.90, V09.91

682.6 Leg, except foot
Ankle
Hip
Knee
Thigh
C&C Exclusions: 017.00, 017.01, 017.02, 017.03, 017.04, 017.05, 017.06, 017.90, 017.91, 017.92, 017.93, 017.94, 017.95, 017.96, 040.89, 041.00, 041.01, 041.02, 041.03, 041.04, 041.05, 041.09, 041.10, 041.11, 041.19, 041.2, 041.3, 041.4, 041.5, 041.6, 041.7, 041.81, 041.82, 041.83, 041.84, 041.85, 041.86, 041.89, 041.9, 682.6, 682.8, 682.9, 686.00, 686.01, 686.09, 686.1, 686.8, 686.9, 705.83, 709.8, V09.0, V09.1, V09.2, V09.3, V09.4, V09.50, V09.51, V09.6, V09.70, V09.71, V09.80, V09.81, V09.90, V09.91
AHA: 3Q 2004, 5; 4Q 2003, 108

682.7 Foot, except toes
Heel
Excludes *toe (681.10-681.11)*
C&C Exclusions: 017.00, 017.01, 017.02, 017.03, 017.04, 017.05, 017.06, 017.90, 017.91, 017.92, 017.93, 017.94, 017.95, 017.96, 040.89, 041.00, 041.01, 041.02, 041.03, 041.04, 041.05, 041.09, 041.10, 041.11, 041.19, 041.2, 041.3, 041.4, 041.5, 041.6, 041.7, 041.81, 041.82, 041.83, 041.84, 041.85, 041.86, 041.89, 041.9, 682.7, 682.8, 682.9, 686.00, 686.01, 686.09, 686.1, 686.8, 686.9, 705.83, 709.8, V09.0, V09.1, V09.2, V09.3, V09.4, V09.50, V09.51, V09.6, V09.70, V09.71, V09.80, V09.81, V09.90, V09.91

682.8 Other specified sites
Head [except face]
Scalp
Excludes *face (682.0)*
C&C Exclusions: 017.00, 017.01, 017.02, 017.03, 017.04, 017.05, 017.06, 017.90, 017.91, 017.92, 017.93, 017.94, 017.95, 017.96, 040.89, 041.00, 041.01, 041.02, 041.03, 041.04, 041.05, 041.09, 041.10, 041.11, 041.19, 041.2, 041.3, 041.4, 041.5, 041.6, 041.7, 041.81, 041.82, 041.83, 041.84, 041.85, 041.86, 041.89, 041.9, 682.8, 682.9, 686.00, 686.01, 686.09, 686.1, 686.8, 686.9, 705.83, 709.8, V09.0, V09.1, V09.2, V09.3, V09.4, V09.50, V09.51, V09.6, V09.70, V09.71, V09.80, V09.81, V09.90, V09.91

✖ **682.9 Unspecified site**
Abscess NOS
Cellulitis NOS
Lymphangitis, acute NOS
Excludes *lymphangitis NOS (457.2)*
C&C Exclusions: See 682.8

683 Acute lymphadenitis
Abscess (acute) lymph gland or node, except mesenteric
Adenitis, acute lymph gland or node, except mesenteric
Lymphadenitis, acute lymph gland or node, except mesenteric
Use additional code to identify organism such as Staphylococcus (041.1)
Excludes *enlarged glands NOS (785.6)*
lymphadenitis:
chronic or subacute, except mesenteric (289.1)
mesenteric (acute) (chronic) (subacute) (289.2)
unspecified (289.3)

Lymphadenitis

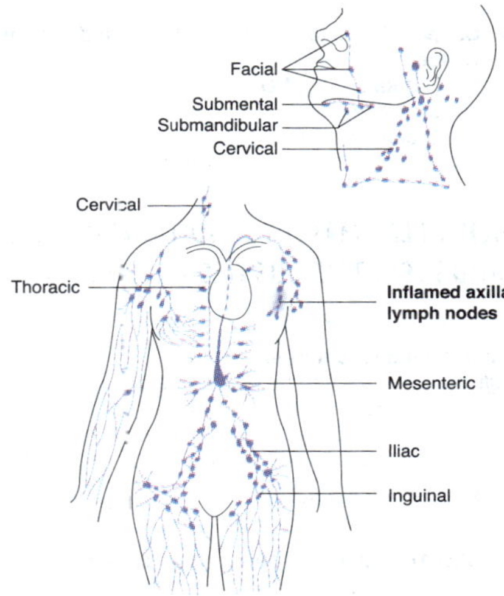

684 Impetigo
Impetiginization of other dermatoses
Impetigo (contagiosa) [any site] [any organism]:
bullous
circinate
neonatorum
simplex
Pemphigus neonatorum
Excludes *impetigo herpetiformis (694.3)*
DEF: Bacterial skin infection in children; small pustules form over a reddish rash and burst, leaving an itchy, yellow crust over the affected area.
C&C Exclusions: 684, 686.00, 686.01, 686.09, 686.1, 686.8, 686.9, 709.8

❹ **685 Pilonidal cyst**
Includes fistula, coccygeal or pilonidal
sinus, coccygeal or pilonidal
DEF: An abscessed sinus tract draining to the surface and located in the tailbone area, often associated with ingrown hairs.

685.0 With abscess
C&C Exclusions: 685.0, 685.1, 709.8

685.1 Without mention of abscess

❹ **686 Other local infections of skin and subcutaneous tissue**
Use additional code to identify any infectious organism (041.0-041.8)

❺ **686.0 Pyoderma**
Dermatitis:
purulent
septic
suppurative

✖ **686.00 Pyoderma, unspecified**

686.01 Pyoderma gangrenosum
AHA: 4Q 1997, 42

686.09 Other pyoderma

686.1 Pyogenic granuloma
Granuloma:
septic
suppurative
telangiectaticum
Excludes *pyogenic granuloma of oral mucosa (528.9)*

686.8 Other specified local infections of skin and subcutaneous tissue
Bacterid (pustular)
Dermatitis vegetans
Ecthyma
Perlèche
Excludes *dermatitis infectiosa eczematoides (690.8)*
panniculitis (729.30-729.39)

✖ **686.9 Unspecified local infection of skin and subcutaneous tissue**
Fistula of skin NOS
Skin infection NOS
Excludes *fistula to skin from internal organs - see Alphabetic Index*

OTHER INFLAMMATORY CONDITIONS OF SKIN AND SUBCUTANEOUS TISSUE (690-698)

Excludes *panniculitis (729.30-729.39)*

④ **690 Erythematosquamous dermatosis**
Excludes *eczematous dermatitis of eyelid (373.31)*
parakeratosis variegata (696.2)
psoriasis (696.0-696.1)
seborrheic keratosis (702.11-702.19)

⑤ **690.1 Seborrheic dermatitis**
AHA: 4Q 1995, 58

690.10 Seborheic dermatitis, unspecified
Seborrheic dermatitis NOS

690.11 Seborrhea capitis P
Cradle cap

690.12 Seborrheic infantile dermatitis P

690.18 Other seborrheic dermatitis

690.8 Other erythematosquamous dermatosis

④ **691 Atopic dermatitis and related conditions**

691.0 Diaper or napkin rash
Ammonia dermatitis
Diaper or napkin:
dermatitis
erythema
rash
Psoriasiform napkin eruption

691.8 Other atopic dermatitis and related conditions
Atopic dermatitis
Besnier's prurigo
Eczema:
atopic
flexural
intrinsic (allergic)
Neurodermatitis:
atopic
diffuse (of Brocq)

A chronic inflammation of the skin

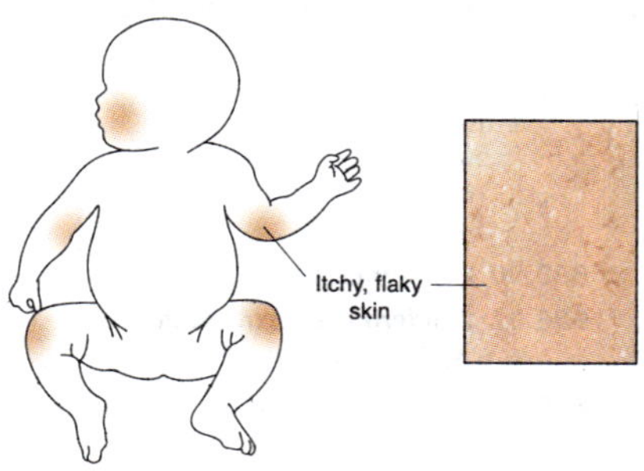

④ **692 Contact dermatitis and other eczema**
Includes dermatitis:
NOS
contact
occupational
venenata
eczema (acute) (chronic):
NOS
allergic
erythematous
occupational
Excludes *allergy NOS (995.3)*
contact dermatitis of eyelids (373.32)
dermatitis due to substances taken internally (693.0-693.9)
eczema of external ear (380.22)
perioral dermatitis (695.3)
urticarial reactions (708.0-708.9, 995.1)

692.0 Due to detergents

692.1 Due to oils and greases

692.2 Due to solvents
Dermatitis due to solvents of:
chlorocompound group
cyclohexane group
ester group
glycol group
hydrocarbon group
ketone group

692.3 Due to drugs and medicines in contact with skin
Dermatitis (allergic) (contact) due to:
arnica
fungicides
iodine
keratolytics
mercurials
neomycin
pediculocides
phenols
scabicides
any drug applied to skin
Dermatitis medicamentosa due to drug applied to skin
Use additional E code to identify drug
Excludes *allergy NOS due to drugs (995.27)*
dermatitis due to ingested drugs (693.0)
dermatitis medicamentosa NOS (693.0)

692.4 Due to other chemical products
Dermatitis due to:
acids
adhesive plaster
alkalis
caustics
dichromate
insecticide
nylon
plastic
rubber
AHA: 2Q 1989, 16

692.5 Due to food in contact with skin
Dermatitis, contact, due to:
cereals
fish
flour
fruit
meat
milk
Excludes *dermatitis due to:*
dyes (692.89)
ingested foods (693.1)
preservatives (692.89)

692.6 Due to plants [except food]
Dermatitis due to:
lacquer tree [Rhus verniciflua]
poison:
ivy [Rhus toxicodendron]
oak [Rhus diversiloba]
sumac [Rhus venenata]
vine [Rhus radicans]
primrose [Primula]
ragweed [Senecio jacobae]
other plants in contact with the skin
Excludes *allergy NOS due to pollen (477.0)*
nettle rash (708.8)

5 **692.7 Due to solar radiation**
Excludes *sunburn due to other ultraviolet radiation exposure (692.82)*

692.70 Unspecified dermatitis due to sun

692.71 Sunburn
First degree sunburn
Sunburn NOS
AHA: 4Q 2001, 47

692.72 Acute dermatitis due to solar radiation
Acute solar skin damage NOS
Berloque dermatitis
Photoallergic response
Phototoxic response
Polymorphous light eruption
Use additional E code to identify drug, if drug induced
Excludes *sunburn (692.71, 692.76-692.77)*

692.73 Actinic reticuloid and actinic granuloma

692.74 Other chronic dermatitis due to solar radiation
Chronic solar skin damage NOS
Solar elastosis
Excludes *actinic [solar] keratosis (702.0)*

692.75 Disseminated superficial actinic porokeratosis (DSAP)
AHA: 4Q 2000, 43

692.76 Sunburn of second degree
AHA: 4Q 2001, 47

692.77 Sunburn of third degree
AHA: 4Q 2001, 47

692.79 Other dermatitis due to solar radiation
Hydroa aestivale
Photodermatitis (due to sun)
Photosensitiveness (due to sun)
Solar skin damage NOS

5 **692.8 Due to other specified agents**

692.81 Dermatitis due to cosmetics

692.82 Dermatitis due to other radiation
Infrared rays
Light, except from sun
Radiation NOS
Tanning bed
Ultraviolet rays, except from sun
X-rays
Excludes *that due to solar radiation (692.70-692.79)*
AHA: 4Q 2001, 47; 3Q 2000, 5

692.83 Dermatitis due to metals
Jewelry

692.84 Due to animal (cat) (dog) dander
Due to animal (cat) (dog) hair

692.89 Other
Dermatitis due to:
cold weather
dyes
hot weather
preservatives
Excludes *allergy (NOS) (rhinitis) due to animal hair or dander (477.2)*
allergy to dust (477.8)
sunburn (692.71, 692.76-692.77)

692.9 Unspecified cause
Dermatitis:
NOS
contact NOS
venenata NOS
Eczema NOS

4 **693 Dermatitis due to substances taken internally**
Excludes *adverse effect NOS of drugs and medicines (995.20)*
allergy NOS (995.3)
contact dermatitis (692.0-692.9)
urticarial reactions (708.0-708.9, 995.1)

693.0 Due to drugs and medicines
Dermatitis medicamentosa NOS
Use additional E code to identify drug
Excludes *that due to drugs in contact with skin (692.3)*

693.1 Due to food

693.8 Due to other specified substances taken internally

693.9 Due to unspecified substance taken internally
Excludes *dermatitis NOS (692.9)*

4 **694 Bullous dermatoses**

694.0 Dermatitis herpetiformis
Dermatosis herpetiformis
Duhring's disease
Hydroa herpetiformis
Excludes *dermatitis herpetiformis:*
juvenile (694.2)
senile (694.5)
herpes gestationis (646.8)

694.1 Subcorneal pustular dermatosis
Sneddon-Wilkinson disease or syndrome

694.2 Juvenile dermatitis herpetiformis
Juvenile pemphigoid

694.3 Impetigo herpetiformis

694.4 Pemphigus
Pemphigus:
NOS
erythematosus
foliaceus
malignant
vegetans
vulgaris
Excludes *pemphigus neonatorum (684)*
DEF: Chronic, relapsing, autoimmune blistering diseases of the skin and mucous membranes with autoantibodies against epidermal cells.
C&C Exclusions: 694.4, 694.5, 694.6, 694.8, 694.9, 709.8

694.5 Pemphigoid
Benign pemphigus NOS
Bullous pemphigoid
Herpes circinatus bullosus
Senile dermatitis herpetiformis
C&C Exclusions: See 694.4

5 **694.6 Benign mucous membrane pemphigoid**
Cicatricial pemphigoid
Mucosynechial atrophic bullous dermatitis

694.60 Without mention of ocular involvement

694.61 With ocular involvement
Ocular pemphigus

694.8 Other specified bullous dermatoses
Excludes *herpes gestationis (646.8)*

✖ **694.9 Unspecified bullous dermatoses**

4 **695 Erythematous conditions**

695.0 Toxic erythema
Erythema venenatum
C&C Exclusions: 695.0, 695.1, 695.2, 695.3, 695.4, 709.8

695.1 Erythema multiforme
Erythema iris
Herpes iris
Lyell s syndrome
Scalded skin syndrome
Stevens-Johnson syndrome
Toxic epidermal necrolysis

695.2 Erythema nodosum
Excludes *tuberculous erythema nodosum (017.1)*

695.3 Rosacea
Acne:
- erythematosa
- rosacea

Perioral dermatitis
Rhinophyma

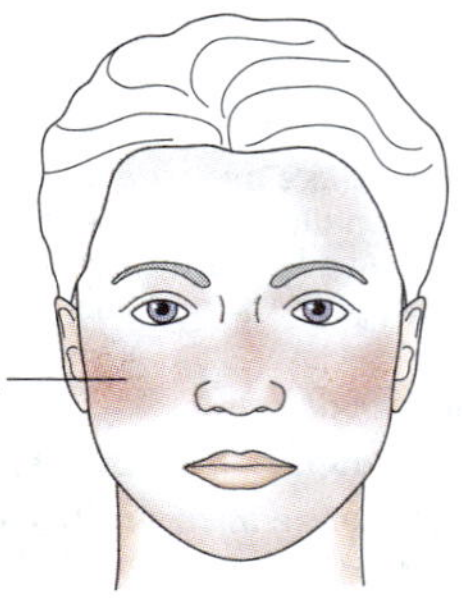

695.4 Lupus erythematosus
Lupus:
- erythematodes (discoid)
- erythematosus (discoid), not disseminated

Excludes *lupus (vulgaris) NOS (017.0)*
systemic [disseminated] lupus erythematosus (710.0)

5 **695.8 Other specified erythematous conditions**

695.81 Ritter's disease
Dermatitis exfoliativa neonatorum
DEF: Infectious viral skin disease affecting young children, causing large sections of skin to peel away leaving raw, exposed areas prone to infection.

695.89 Other
Erythema intertrigo
Intertrigo
Pityriasis rubra (Hebra)
Excludes *mycotic intertrigo (111.0-111.9)*
AHA: Sep-Oct 1986, 10

695.9 Unspecified erythematous condition
Erythema NOS
Erythroderma (secondary)

4 **696 Psoriasis and similar disorders**

696.0 Psoriatic arthropathy
C&C Exclusions: 015.80, 015.81, 015.82, 015.83, 015.84, 015.85, 015.86, 015.90, 015.91, 015.92, 015.93, 015.94, 015.95, 015.96, 017.90, 017.91, 017.92, 017.93, 017.94, 017.95, 017.96, 036.82, 056.71, 098.50, 098.51, 098.59, 098.89, 696.0, 711.00, 711.01, 711.02, 711.03, 711.04, 711.05, 711.06, 711.07, 711.08, 711.09, 711.10, 711.11, 711.12, 711.13, 711.14, 711.15, 711.16, 711.17, 711.18, 711.19, 711.20, 711.21, 711.22, 711.23, 711.24, 711.25, 711.26, 711.27, 711.28, 711.29, 711.30, 711.31, 711.32, 711.33, 711.34, 711.35, 711.36, 711.37, 711.38, 711.39, 711.40, 711.41, 711.42, 711.43, 711.44, 711.45, 711.45, 711.46, 711.47, 711.48, 711.49, 711.50, 711.51, 711.52, 711.53, 711.54, 711.55, 711.56, 711.57, 711.58, 711.59, 711.60, 711.61, 711.62, 3, 711.64, 711.65, 711.66, 711.67, 711.68, 711.69, 711.70, 711.71, 711.72, 711.73, 711.74, 711.75, 711.76, 711.77, 711.78, 711.79, 711.80, 711.81, 711.82, 711.83, 711.84, 711.85, 711.86, 711.87, 711.88, 711.89, 711.90, 711.91, 711.92, 711.93, 711.94, 711.95, 711.96, 711.97, 711.98, 711.99, 712.10, 712.11, 712.12, 712.13, 712.14, 712.15, 712.16, 712.17, 712.18, 712.19, 712.20, 712.21, 712.22, 712.23, 712.24, 712.25, 712.26, 712.27, 712.28, 712.29, 712.30, 712.31, 712.32, 712.33, 712.34, 712.35, 712.36, 712.37, 712.38, 712.39, 712.80, 712.81, 712.82, 712.83, 712.84, 712.85, 712.86, 712.87, 712.88, 712.89, 712.90, 712.91, 712.92, 712.93, 712.94, 712.95, 712.96, 712.97, 712.98, 712.99, 713.0, 713.1, 713.2, 713.3, 713.4, 713.5, 713.6, 713.7, 713.8, 714.0, 715.00, 715.09, 715.10, 715.18, 715.20, 715.21, 715.22, 715.23, 715.24, 715.25, 715.26, 715.27, 715.28, 715.30, 715.31, 715.32, 715.33, 715.34, 715.35, 715.36, 715.37, 715.38, 715.80, 715.89, 715.90,1, 715.92, 715.93, 715.94, 715.95, 715.96, 715.97, 715.98, 716.00, 716.01, 716.02, 716.03, 716.04, 716.05, 716.06, 716.07, 716.08, 716.09, 716.10, 716.11, 716.12, 716.13, 716.14, 716.15, 716.16, 716.17, 716.18, 716.19, 716.20, 716.21, 716.22, 716.23, 716.24, 716.25, 716.26, 716.27, 716.28, 716.29, 716.30, 716.31, 716.32, 716.33, 716.34, 716.35, 716.36, 716.37, 716.38, 716.39, 716.40, 716.41, 716.42, 716.43, 716.44, 716.45, 716.46, 716.47, 716.48, 716.49, 716.50, 716.51, 716.52, 716.53, 716.54, 716.55, 716.56, 716.57, 716.58, 716.59, 716.60, 716.61, 716.62, 716.63, 716.64, 716.65, 716.66, 716.67, 716.68, 716.80, 716.81, 716.82, 716.83. 716.84. 716.85, 716.86, 716.87, 716.88, 716.89, 716.90, 716.91, 716.92, 716.93, 716.94, 716.95, 716.96, 716.97, 716.98, 716.99, 718.00, 718.01, 718.02, 718.03, 718.04, 718.05, 718.07, 718.08, 719.00, 719.01, 719.02, 719.03, 719.04, 719.05, 719.06, 719.07, 719.08, 719.09, 719.10, 719.18, 719.19, 719.20, 719.21, 719.22, 719.23, 719.24, 719.25, 719.26, 719.27, 719.28, 719.29, 719.30, 719.31, 719.32, 719.33, 719.34, 719.35, 719.36, 719.37, 719.38, 719.39, 719.40, 719.41, 719.42, 719.43, 719.44, 719.45, 719.46, 719.47, 719.48, 719.49, 719.50, 719.51, 719.52, 719.53, 719.54, 719.55, 719.56, 719.57, 719.58, 719.59, 719.60, 719.61, 719.62, 719.63, 719.64, 719.65, 719.66, 719.67, 719.68, 719.70, 719.75, 719.76, 719.77, 719.78, 719.79, 719.80, 719.81, 719.82, 719.83. 719.84, 719.85, 719.86, 719.87, 719.88, 719.89, 719.90, 719.91, 719.92, 719.93, 719.94, 719.95, 719.96, 719.97, 719.98, 719.99

696.1 Other psoriasis
Acrodermatitis continua
Dermatitis repens
Psoriasis:
- NOS
- any type, except arthropathic

Excludes *psoriatic arthropathy (696.0)*

696.2 Parapsoriasis
Parakeratosis variegata
Parapsoriasis lichenoides chronica
Pityriasis lichenoides et varioliformis

696.3 Pityriasis rosea
Pityriasis circinata (et maculata)

696.4 Pityriasis rubra pilaris
Devergie's disease
Lichen ruber acuminatus
Excludes *pityriasis rubra (Hebra) (695.89)*
DEF: Rare skin condition of red-orange, scaly patches spreading over the body, thickened palms and soles, and rough, dry plugs within the rash.

696.5 Other and unspecified pityriasis
Pityriasis:
- NOS
- alba
- streptogenes

Excludes *pityriasis:*
- *simplex (690.18)*
- *versicolor (111.0)*

696.8 Other

4 **697 Lichen**
Excludes *lichen:*
- *obtusus corneus (698.3)*
- *pilaris (congenital) (757.39)*
- *ruber acuminatus (696.4)*
- *sclerosus et atrophicus (701.0)*
- *scrofulosus (017.0)*
- *simplex chronicus (698.3)*
- *spinulosus (congenital) (757.39)*
- *urticatus (698.2)*

697.0 Lichen planus
Lichen:
- planopilaris
- ruber planus

697.1 Lichen nitidus
Pinkus' disease

697.8 Other lichen, not elsewhere classified
Lichen:
- ruber moniliforme
- striata

697.9 Lichen, unspecified

❹ 698 Pruritus and related conditions
Excludes *pruritus specified as psychogenic (306.3)*

698.0 Pruritus ani
Perianal itch

DEF: Severe itching of the perianal region.

698.1 Pruritus of genital organs

698.2 Prurigo
Lichen urticatus
Prurigo:
NOS
Hebra's
mitis
simplex
Urticaria papulosa (Hebra)
Excludes *prurigo nodularis (698.3)*

DEF: Chronic inflammatory skin disease featuring blistering papules and severe itching.

698.3 Lichenification and lichen simplex chronicus
Hyde's disease
Neurodermatitis (circumscripta) (local)
Prurigo nodularis
Excludes *neurodermatitis, diffuse (of Brocq) (691.8)*

698.4 Dermatitis factitia [artefacta]
Dermatitis ficta
Neurotic excoriation
Use additional code to identify any associated mental disorder

698.8 Other specified pruritic conditions
Pruritus:
hiemalis
senilis
Winter itch

698.9 Unspecified pruritic disorder
Itch NOS
Pruritus NOS

OTHER DISEASES OF SKIN AND SUBCUTANEOUS TISSUE (700-709)

Excludes *conditions confined to eyelids (373.0-374.9)*
congenital conditions of skin, hair, and nails (757.0-757.9)

700 Corns and callosities
Callus
Clavus

❹ 701 Other hypertrophic and atrophic conditions of skin
Excludes *dermatomyositis (710.3)*
hereditary edema of legs (757.0)
scleroderma (generalized) (710.1)

701.0 Circumscribed scleroderma
Addison's keloid
Dermatosclerosis, localized
Lichen sclerosus et atrophicus
Morphea
Scleroderma, circumscribed or localized

701.1 Keratoderma, acquired
Acquired:
ichthyosis
keratoderma palmaris et plantaris
Elastosis perforans serpiginosa
Hyperkeratosis:
NOS
follicularis in cutem penetrans
palmoplantaris climacterica
Keratoderma:
climactericum
tylodes, progressive
Keratosis (blennorrhagica)
Excludes *Darier's disease [keratosis follicularis] (congenital) (757.39)*
keratosis:
arsenical (692.4)
gonococcal (098.81)

AHA: 4Q 1994, 48

701.2 Acquired acanthosis nigricans
Keratosis nigricans

701.3 Striae atrophicae
Atrophic spots of skin
Atrophoderma maculatum
Atrophy blanche (of Milian)
Degenerative colloid atrophy
Senile degenerative atrophy
Striae distensae

701.4 Keloid scar
Cheloid
Hypertrophic scar
Keloid

701.5 Other abnormal granulation tissue
Excessive granulation

701.8 Other specified hypertrophic and atrophic conditions of skin
Acrodermatitis atrophicans chronica
Atrophia cutis senilis
Atrophoderma neuriticum
Confluent and reticulate papillomatosis
Cutis laxa senilis
Elastosis senilis
Folliculitis ulerythematosa reticulata
Gougerot-Carteaud syndrome or disease

✖ 701.9 Unspecified hypertrophic and atrophic conditions of skin
Atrophoderma

❹ 702 Other dermatoses
Excludes *carcinoma in situ (232.0-232.9)*

702.0 Actinic keratosis
AHA: 1Q 1992, 18

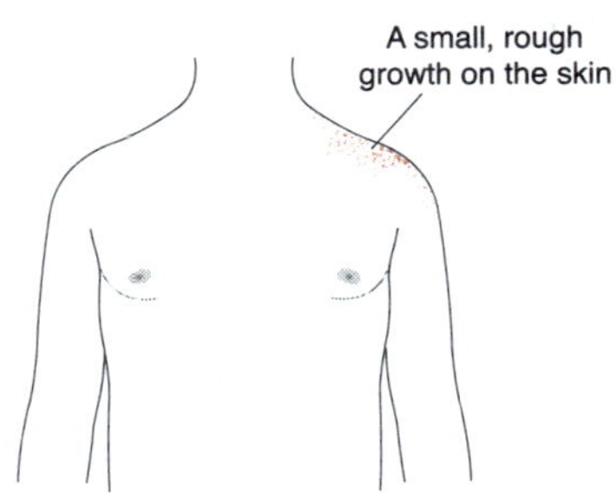

❺ 702.1 Seborrheic keratosis

702.11 Inflamed seborrheic keratosis
AHA: 4Q 1994, 48

702.19 Other seborrheic keratosis
Seborrheic keratosis NOS

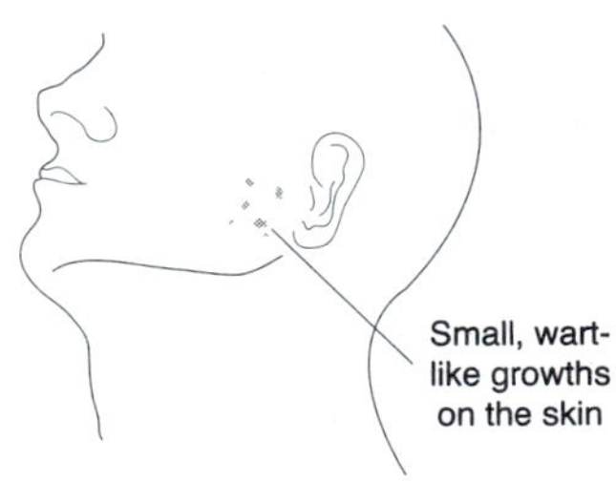

702.8 Other specified dermatoses

4 703 Diseases of nail

Excludes *congenital anomalies (757.5)*
onychia and paronychia (681.02, 681.11)

703.0 Ingrowing nail

Ingrowing nail with infection
Unguis incarnatus
Excludes *infection, nail NOS (681.9)*

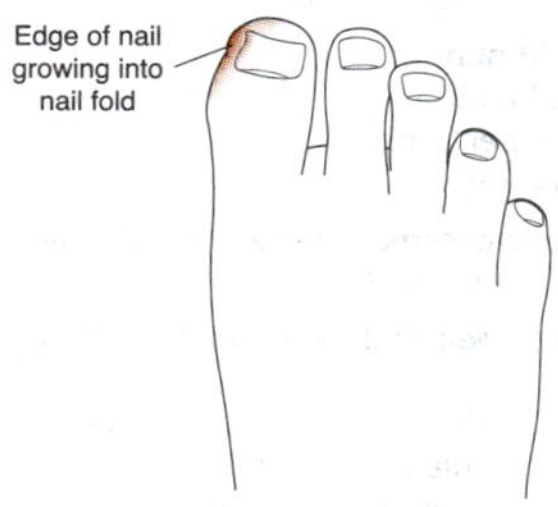

703.8 Other specified diseases of nail

Dystrophia unguium
Hypertrophy of nail
Koilonychia
Leukonychia (punctata) (striata)
Onychauxis
Onychogryposis
Onycholysis

703.9 Unspecified disease of nail

4 704 Diseases of hair and hair follicles

Excludes *congenital anomalies (757.4)*

5 704.0 Alopecia

Excludes *madarosis (374.55)*
syphilitic alopecia (091.82)

704.00 Alopecia, unspecified

Baldness
Loss of hair

704.01 Alopecia areata

Ophiasis

704.02 Telogen effluvium

704.09 Other

Folliculitis decalvans
Hypotrichosis:
  NOS
  postinfectional NOS
Pseudopelade

704.1 Hirsutism

Hypertrichosis:
  NOS
  lanuginosa, acquired
Polytrichia
Excludes *hypertrichosis of eyelid (374.54)*

DEF: Excess amounts of body hair.

704.2 Abnormalities of the hair

Atrophic hair
Clastothrix
Fragilitas crinium
Trichiasis:
  NOS
  cicatrical
Trichorrhexis (nodosa)
Excludes *trichiasis of eyelid (374.05)*

704.3 Variations in hair color

Canities (premature)
Grayness, hair (premature)
Heterochromia of hair
Poliosis:
  NOS
  circumscripta, acquired

704.8 Other specified diseases of hair and hair follicles

Folliculitis:
  NOS
  abscedens et suffodiens
  pustular
Perifolliculitis:
  NOS
  capitis abscedens et suffodiens
  scalp
Sycosis:
  NOS
  barbae [not parasitic]
  lupoid
  vulgaris

✖ 704.9 Unspecified disease of hair and hair follicles

4 705 Disorders of sweat glands

705.0 Anhidrosis

Hypohidrosis
Oligohidrosis

DEF: Inability to sweat; results in overheating in high temperatures or during exertion.

705.1 Prickly heat

Heat rash
Miliaria rubra (tropicalis)
Sudamina

DEF: Inflammatory heat rash caused by obstruction of the sweat glands with resultant skin rash of small clusters of red pimples on the skin.

5 705.2 Focal hyperhidrosis

Excludes *generalized (secondary) hyperhidrosis (780.8)*

705.21 Primary focal hyperhidrosis

Focal hyperhidrosis NOS
Hyperhidrosis NOS
Hyperhidrosis of:
  axilla
  face
  palms
  soles

AHA: 4Q 2004, 91

705.22 Secondary focal hyperhidrosis

Frey's syndrome

AHA: 4Q 2004, 91

5 705.8 Other specified disorders of sweat glands

705.81 Dyshidrosis

Cheiropompholyx
Pompholyx

705.82 Fox-Fordyce disease

705.83 Hidradenitis

Hidradenitis suppurativa

705.89 Other

Bromhidrosis
Chromhidrosis
Granulosis rubra nasi
Urhidrosis
Excludes *generalized hyperhidrosis (780.8)*
hidrocystoma (216.0-216.9)

✖ 705.9 Unspecified disorder of sweat glands

Disorder of sweat glands NOS

4 706 Diseases of sebaceous glands

706.0 Acne varioliformis

Acne:
  frontalis
  necrotica

706.1 Other acne

Acne:
  NOS
  conglobata
  cystic
  pustular
  vulgaris
Blackhead
Comedo
Excludes *acne rosacea (695.3)*

706.2 Sebaceous cyst
Atheroma, skin
Keratin cyst
Wen

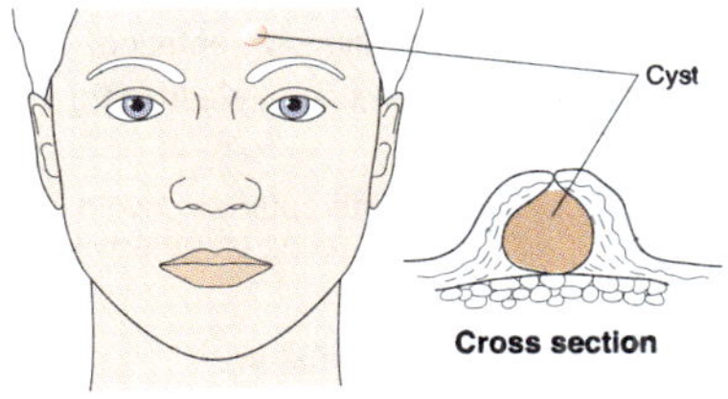

706.3 Seborrhea
Excludes *seborrhea:*
capitis (690.11)
sicca (690.18)
seborrheic:
dermatitis (690.10)
keratosis (702.11-702.19)

706.8 Other specified diseases of sebaceous glands
Asteatosis (cutis)
Xerosis cutis

✖ **706.9 Unspecified disease of sebaceous glands**

❹ **707 Chronic ulcer of skin**
Includes non-infected sinus of skin
non-healing ulcer
Excludes *specific infections classified under "Infectious and Parasitic Diseases" (001.0-136.9)*
varicose ulcer (454.0, 454.2)
AHA: 4Q 2004, 92

❺ **707.0 Decubitus ulcer**
Bed sore
Decubitus ulcer [any site]
Plaster ulcer
Pressure ulcer
AHA: 1Q 2004, 14; 4Q 2003, 110; 4Q 1999, 20; 1Q 1996, 15; 3Q 1990, 15; Nov-Dec 1987, 9

✖ **707.00 Unspecified site**
C&C Exclusions: 707.0, 707.8, 707.9, 709.8

707.01 Elbow
C&C Exclusions: See 707.00

707.02 Upper back
Shoulder blades
C&C Exclusions: See 707.00

707.03 Lower back
Sacrum
C&C Exclusions: See 707.00
AHA: 1Q 2005, 16

Sacral decubitus ulcer

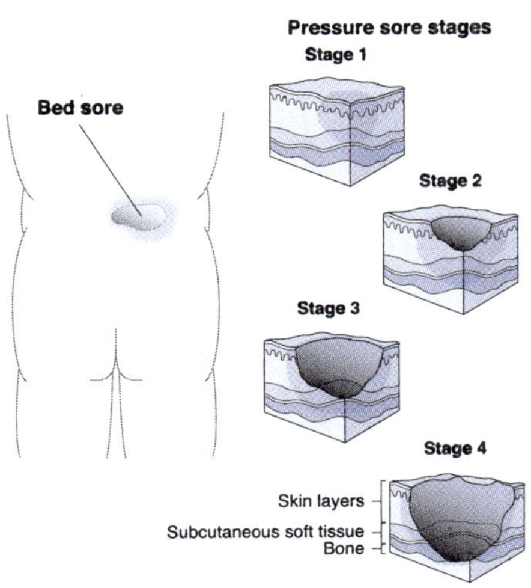

707.04 Hip
C&C Exclusions: See 707.00

707.05 Buttock
C&C Exclusions: See 707.00

707.06 Ankle
C&C Exclusions: See 707.00

707.07 Heel
C&C Exclusions: See 707.00
AHA: 1Q 2005, 16

707.09 Other site
Head
C&C Exclusions: See 707.00

❺ **707.1 Ulcer of lower limbs, except decubitus**
Ulcer, chronic, of lower limb:
neurogenic of lower limb
trophic of lower limb
Code, if applicable, any causal condition first:
atherosclerosis of the extremities with ulceration (440.23)
chronic venous hypertension with ulcer (459.31)
chronic venous hypertension with ulcer and inflammation (459.33)
diabetes mellitus (250.80-250.83)
postphlebitic syndrome with ulcer (459.11)
postphlebitic syndrome with ulcer and inflammation (459.13)
AHA: 4Q 2000, 44; 4Q 1999, 15

✖ **707.10 Ulcer of lower limb, unspecified**
C&C Exclusions: 707.10, 707.11,707.12, 707.13, 707.14, 707.15, 707.19, 707.8, 707.9, 709.8
AHA: 3Q 2004, 5; 4Q 2002, 43

707.11 Ulcer of thigh
C&C Exclusions: See 707.10

707.12 Ulcer of calf
C&C Exclusions: See 707.10

707.13 Ulcer of ankle
C&C Exclusions: See 707.10

707.14 Ulcer of heel and midfoot
Plantar surface of midfoot
C&C Exclusions: See 707.10

707.15 Ulcer of other part of foot
Toes
C&C Exclusions: See 707.10

707.19 Ulcer of other part of lower limb
C&C Exclusions: See 707.10

707.8 Chronic ulcer of other specified sites
Ulcer, chronic, of other specified sites:
neurogenic of other specified sites
trophic of other specified sites
C&C Exclusions: 707.10, 707.11,707.12, 707.13, 707.14, 707.15, 707.19

✖ **707.9 Chronic ulcer of unspecified site**
Chronic ulcer NOS
Trophic ulcer NOS
Tropical ulcer NOS
Ulcer of skin NOS
C&C Exclusions: See 707.8

4 708 Urticaria

Excludes *edema:*
angioneurotic (995.1)
Quincke's (995.1)
hereditary angioedema (277.6)
urticaria:
giant (995.1)
papulosa (Hebra) (698.2)
pigmentosa (juvenile) (congenital) (757.33)

708.0 Allergic urticaria

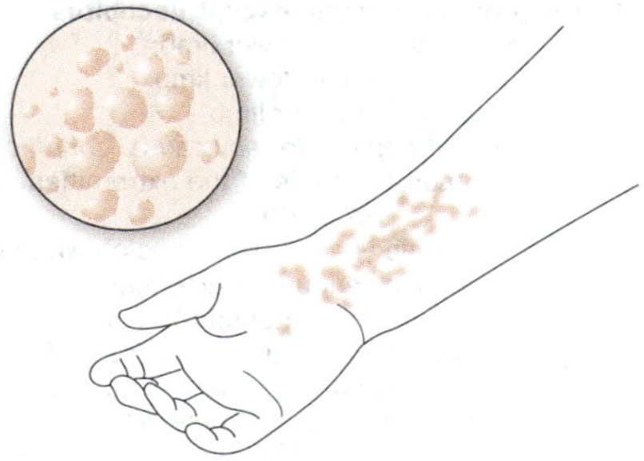

708.1 Idiopathic urticaria

708.2 Urticaria due to cold and heat
Thermal urticaria

708.3 Dermatographic urticaria
Dermatographia
Factitial urticaria

708.4 Vibratory urticaria

708.5 Cholinergic urticaria
DEF: Hives that occur in response to a rise in body temperature, such as from exercise, stress, or overheating.

708.8 Other specified urticaria
Nettle rash
Urticaria:
chronic
recurrent periodic

708.9 Urticaria, unspecified
Hives NOS

4 709 Other disorders of skin and subcutaneous tissue

5 709.0 Dyschromia

Excludes *albinism (270.2)*
pigmented nevus (216.0-216.9)
that of eyelid (374.52-374.53)

DEF: Disorder of skin pigmentation.

709.00 Dyschromia, unspecified

709.01 Vitiligo
DEF: White patches devoid of pigmentation appearing on otherwise normal skin.

709.09 Other

709.1 Vascular disorders of skin
Angioma serpiginosum
Purpura (primary) annularis telangiectodes

709.2 Scar conditions and fibrosis of skin
Adherent scar (skin)
Cicatrix
Disfigurement (due to scar)
Fibrosis, skin NOS
Scar NOS
Excludes *keloid scar (701.4)*

AHA: Nov-Dec 1984, 19

709.3 Degenerative skin disorders
Calcinosis:
circumscripta
cutis
Colloid milium
Degeneration, skin
Deposits, skin
Senile dermatosis NOS
Subcutaneous calcification

709.4 Foreign body granuloma of skin and subcutaneous tissue
Excludes *residual foreign body without granuloma of skin and subcutaneous tissue (729.6)*
that of muscle (728.82)

709.8 Other specified disorders of skin
Epithelial hyperplasia
Menstrual dermatosis
Vesicular eruption

C&C Exclusions: 707.10, 707.11,707.12, 707.13, 707.14, 707.15, 707.19

AHA: Nov-Dec 1987, 6

709.9 Unspecified disorder of skin and subcutaneous tissue
Dermatosis NOS

13. DISEASES OF THE MUSCULOSKELETAL SYSTEM AND CONNECTIVE TISSUE (710-739)

The following fifth-digit subclassification is for use with categories 711-712, 715-716, 718-719, and 730:

- **0 site unspecified**
- **1 shoulder region**
  - Acromioclavicular joint(s)
  - Clavicle
  - Glenohumeral joint(s)
  - Scapula
  - Sternoclavicular joint(s)
- **2 upper arm**
  - Elbow joint
  - Humerus
- **3 forearm**
  - Radius
  - Ulna
  - Wrist joint
- **4 hand**
  - Carpus
  - Metacarpus
  - Phalanges [fingers]
- **5 pelvic region and thigh**
  - Buttock
  - Femur
  - Hip (joint)
- **6 lower leg**
  - Fibula
  - Knee joint
  - Patella
  - Tibia
- **7 ankle and foot**
  - Ankle joint
  - Digits [toes]
  - Metatarsus
  - Phalanges, foot
  - Tarsus
  - Other joints in foot
- **8 other specified sites**
  - Head
  - Neck
  - Ribs
  - Skull
  - Trunk
  - Vertebral column
- **9 multiple sites**

ARTHROPATHIES AND RELATED DISORDERS (710-719)

Excludes *disorders of spine (720.0-724.9)*

❹ 710 Diffuse diseases of connective tissue

Includes all collagen diseases whose effects are not mainly confined to a single system

Excludes *those affecting mainly the cardiovascular system, i.e., polyarteritis nodosa and allied conditions (446.0-446.7)*

710.0 Systemic lupus erythematosus

Disseminated lupus erythematosus
Libman-Sacks disease
Use additional code to identify manifestation, as:
endocarditis (424.91)
nephritis (583.81)
chronic (582.81)
nephrotic syndrome (581.81)

Excludes *lupus erythematosus (discoid) NOS (695.4)*

C&C Exclusions: 710.0

AHA: 2Q 2003, 7-8; 2Q 1997, 8

710.1 Systemic sclerosis

Acrosclerosis
CRST syndrome
Progressive systemic sclerosis
Scleroderma
Use additional code to identify manifestation, as:
lung involvement (517.2)
myopathy (359.6)

Excludes *circumscribed scleroderma (701.0)*

C&C Exclusions: 710.1

AHA: 1Q 1988, 6

710.2 Sicca syndrome

Keratoconjunctivitis sicca
Sjögren's disease

710.3 Dermatomyositis

Poikilodermatomyositis
Polymyositis with skin involvement

C&C Exclusions: 710.3

710.4 Polymyositis

C&C Exclusions: 710.4

710.5 Eosinophilia myalgia syndrome

Toxic oil syndrome
Use additional E code to identify drug, if drug induced

C&C Exclusions: 292.0, 292.1, 292.2, 292.81, 292.82, 292.83, 292.84, 292.89, 292.9, 293.0, 293.1, 293.81, 293.82, 293.83, 293.84, 293.89, 293.9, 710.5

AHA: 4Q 1992, 21

710.8 Other specified diffuse diseases of connective tissue

Multifocal fibrosclerosis (idiopathic) NEC
Systemic fibrosclerosing syndrome

C&C Exclusions: 710.8

AHA: Mar-Apr 1987, 12

710.9 Unspecified diffuse connective tissue disease

Collagen disease NOS

❹ 711 Arthropathy associated with infections

Includes arthritis associated with conditions classifiable below
arthropathy associated with conditions classifiable below
polyarthritis associated with conditions classifiable below
polyarthropathy associated with conditions classifiable below

Excludes *rheumatic fever (390)*

AHA: 1Q 1992, 17

The following fifth-digit subclassification is for use with category 711; valid digits are in [brackets] under each code. See list at beginning of chapter for definitions:

- **0 site unspecified**
- **1 shoulder region**
- **2 upper arm**
- **3 forearm**
- **4 hand**
- **5 pelvic region and thigh**
- **6 lower leg**
- **7 ankle and foot**
- **8 other specified sites**
- **9 multiple sites**

❺ 711.0 Pyogenic arthritis
[0-9]

Arthritis or polyarthritis (due to):
coliform [Escherichia coli]
Hemophilus influenzae [H. influenzae]
pneumococcal
Pseudomonas
staphylococcal
streptococcal
Pyarthrosis
Use additional code to identify infectious organism (041.0-041.8)

DEF: Joint inflammation resulting from infectious bacteria, causing joint pain and warm to the touch swelling, chills, and fever.

C&C Exclusions: (for codes 711.00, 711.08-711.09) 015.80, 015.81, 015.82, 015.83, 015.84, 015.85, 015.86, 015.90, 015.91, 015.92, 015.93, 015.94, 015.95, 015.96, 017.90, 017.91, 017.92, 017.93, 017.94, 017.95, 017.96, 036.82, 056.71, 098.50, 098.51, 098.59, 098.89, 711.00, 711.01, 711.02, 711.03, 711.04, 711.05, 711.06, 711.07, 711.08, 711.09, 711.10, 711.11, 711.12, 711.13, 711.14, 711.15, 711.16, 711.17, 711.18, 711.19, 711.20, 711.21, 711.22, 711.23, 711.24, 711.25, 711.26, 711.27, 711.28, 711.29, 711.30, 711.31, 711.32, 711.33, 711.34, 711.35, 711.36, 711.37, 711.38, 711.39, 711.40, 711.41, 711.42, 711.43, 711.44, 711.45, 711.45, 711.46, 711.47, 711.48, 711.49, 711.50, 711.51, 711.52, 711.53, 711.54, 711.55, 711.56, 711.57, 711.58, 711.59, 711.60, 711.61, 711.62, 711.63, 711.64, 711.65, 711.66, 711.67, 711.68, 711.69, 711.70, 711.71, 711.72, 711.73, 711.74, 711.75, 711.76, 711.77, 711.78, 711.79, 711.80, 711.81, 711.82, 711.83,

711.84, 711.85, 711.86, 711.87, 711.88, 711.89, 711.90, 711.91, 711.92, 711.93, 711.94, 711.95, 711.96, 711.97, 711.98, 711.99, 712.10, 712.11, 712.12, 712.13, 712.14, 712.15, 712.16, 712.17, 712.18, 712.19, 712.20, 712.21, 712.22, 712.23, 712.24, 712.25, 712.26, 712.27, 712.28, 712.29, 712.30, 712.31, 712.32, 712.33, 712.34, 712.35, 712.36, 712.37, 712.38, 712.39, 712.80, 712.81, 712.82, 712.83, 712.84, 712.85, 712.86, 712.87, 712.88, 712.89, 712.90, 712.91, 712.92, 712.93, 712.94, 712.95, 712.96, 712.97, 712.98, 712.99, 713.0, 713.1, 713.2, 713.3, 713.4, 713.5, 713.6, 713.7, 713.8, 714.0, 715.00, 715.09, 715.10, 715.18, 715.20, 715.21, 715.22, 715.23, 715.24, 715.25, 715.26, 715.27, 715.28, 715.30, 715.31, 715.32, 715.33, 715.34, 715.35, 715.36, 715.37, 715.38, 715.80, 715.89, 715.90,1, 715.92, 715.93, 715.94, 715.95, 715.96, 715.97, 715.98, 716.00, 716.01, 716.02, 716.03, 716.04, 716.05, 716.06, 716.07, 716.08, 716.09, 716.10, 716.11, 716.12, 716.13, 716.14, 716.15, 716.16, 716.17, 716.18, 716.19, 716.20, 716.21, 716.22, 716.23, 716.24, 716.25, 716.26, 716.27, 716.28, 716.29, 716.30, 716.31, 716.32, 716.33, 716.34, 716.35, 716.36, 716.37, 716.38, 716.39, 716.40, 716.41, 716.42, 716.43, 716.44, 716.45, 716.46, 716.47, 716.48, 716.49, 716.50, 716.51, 716.52, 716.53, 716.54, 716.55, 716.56, 716.57, 716.58, 716.59, 716.60, 716.61, 716.62, 716.63, 716.64, 716.65, 716.66, 716.67, 716.68, 716.80, 716.81, 716.82, 716.83. 716.84, 716.85, 716.86, 716.87, 716.88, 716.89, 716.90, 716.91, 716.92, 716.93, 716.94, 716.95, 716.96, 716.97, 716.98, 716.99, 718.00, 718.01, 718.02, 718.03, 718.04, 718.05, 718.07, 718.08, 719.00, 719.01, 719.02, 719.03, 719.04, 719.05, 719.06, 719.07, 719.08, 719.09, 719.10, 719.18, 719.19, 719.20, 719.21, 719.22, 719.23, 719.24, 719.25, 719.26, 719.27, 719.28, 719.29, 719.30, 719.31, 719.32, 719.33, 719.34, 719.35, 719.36, 719.37, 719.38, 719.39, 719.40, 719.41, 719.42, 719.43, 719.44, 719.45, 719.46, 719.47, 719.48, 719.49, 719.50, 719.51, 719.52, 719.53, 719.54, 719.55, 719.56, 719.57, 719.58, 719.59, 719.60, 719.61, 719.62, 719.63, 719.64, 719.65, 719.66, 719.67, 719.68, 719.70, 719.75, 719.76, 719.77, 719.78, 719.79, 719.80, 719.81, 719.82, 719.83. 719.84, 719.85, 719.86, 719.87, 719.88, 719.89, 719.90, 719.91, 719.92, 719.93, 719.94, 719.95, 719.96, 719.97, 719.98, 719.99

C&C Exclusions: (for code 711.01) 015.80, 015.81, 015.82, 015.83, 015.84, 015.85, 015.86, 015.90, 015.91, 015.92, 015.93, 015.94, 015.95, 015.96, 017.90, 017.91, 017.92, 017.93, 017.94, 017.95, 017.96, 036.82, 056.71, 098.50, 098.51, 098.59, 098.89, 711.00, 711.01, 711.08, 711.09, 711.10, 711.11, 711.18, 711.19, 711.20, 711.21, 711.28, 711.29, 711.30, 711.31, 711.38, 711.39, 711.40, 711.41, 711.48, 711.49, 711.50, 711.51, 711.58, 711.59, 711.60, 711.61, 711.68, 711.69, 711.70, 711.71, 711.78, 711.79, 711.80, 711.81, 711.88, 711.89, 711.90, 711.91, 711.98, 711.99, 712.10, 712.11, 712.18, 712.19, 712.20, 712.21, 712.28, 712.29, 712.30, 712.31, 712.38, 712.39, 712.80, 712.81, 712.88, 712.89, 712.90, 712.91, 712.98, 712.99, 713.0, 713.1, 713.2, 713.3, 713.4, 713.5, 713.6, 713.7, 713.8, 714.0, 715.00, 715.09, 715.10, 715.11, 715.18, 715.20, 715.21, 715.28, 715.30, 715.31, 715.38, 715.80, 715.89, 715.90,1, 715.98, 716.00, 716.01, 716.08, 716.09, 716.10, 716.11, 716.18, 716.19, 716.20, 716.21, 716.28, 716.29, 716.30, 716.31, 716.38, 716.39, 716.40, 716.41, 716.48, 716.49, 716.50, 716.51, 716.58, 716.59, 716.60, 716.61, 716.68, 716.80, 716.81, 716.88, 716.89, 716.90, 716.91, 716.98, 716.99, 718.00, 718.01, 718.08, 719.00, 719.01, 719.08, 719.09, 719.10, 719.11, 719.18, 719.19, 719.20, 719.21, 719.28, 719.29, 719.30, 719.31, 719.38, 719.39, 719.40, 719.41, 719.48, 719.49, 719.50, 719.51, 719.58, 719.59, 719.60, 719.61, 719.68, 719.70, 719.78, 719.79, 719.80, 719.81, 719.88, 719.89, 719.90, 719.91, 719.98, 719.99

C&C Exclusions: (for code 711.02) 015.80, 015.81, 015.82, 015.83, 015.84, 015.85, 015.86, 015.90, 015.91, 015.92, 015.93, 015.94, 015.95, 015.96, 017.90, 017.91, 017.92, 017.93, 017.94, 017.95, 017.96, 036.82, 056.71, 098.50, 098.51, 098.59, 098.89, 711.00, 711.02, 711.08, 711.09, 711.10, 711.12, 711.18, 711.19, 711.20, 711.22, 711.28, 711.29, 711.30, 711.32, 711.38, 711.39, 711.40, 711.42, 711.48, 711.49, 711.50, 711.52, 711.58, 711.59, 711.60, 711.62, 711.68, 711.69, 711.70, 711.72, 711.78, 711.79, 711.80, 711.82, 711.88, 711.89, 711.90, 711.92, 711.98, 711.99, 712.10, 712.12, 712.18, 712.19, 712.20, 712.22, 712.28, 712.29, 712.30, 712.32, 712.38, 712.39, 712.80, 712.82, 712.88, 712.89, 712.90, 712.92, 712.98, 712.99, 713.0, 713.1, 713.2, 713.3, 713.4, 713.5, 713.6, 713.7, 713.8, 714.0, 715.00, 715.09, 715.10, 715.12, 715.18, 715.20, 715.22, 715.28, 715.30, 715.32, 715.38, 715.80, 715.89, 715.90,1, 715.98, 716.00, 716.02, 716.08, 716.09, 716.10, 716.12, 716.18, 716.19, 716.20, 716.22, 716.28, 716.29, 716.30, 716.32, 716.38, 716.39, 716.40, 716.42, 716.48, 716.49, 716.50, 716.52, 716.58, 716.59, 716.60, 716.62, 716.68, 716.80, 716.82, 716.88, 716.89, 716.90, 716.92, 716.98, 716.99, 718.00, 718.02, 718.08, 719.00, 719.02, 719.08, 719.09, 719.10, 719.12, 719.18, 719.19, 719.20, 719.22, 719.28, 719.29, 719.30, 719.32, 719.38, 719.39, 719.40, 719.42, 719.48, 719.49, 719.50, 719.52, 719.58, 719.59, 719.60, 719.62, 719.68, 719.70, 719.78, 719.79, 719.80, 719.82, 719.88, 719.89, 719.90, 719.92, 719.98, 719.99

C&C Exclusions: (for code 711.03) 015.80, 015.81, 015.82, 015.83, 015.84, 015.85, 015.86, 015.90, 015.91, 015.92, 015.93, 015.94, 015.95, 015.96, 017.90, 017.91, 017.92, 017.93, 017.94, 017.95, 017.96, 036.82, 056.71, 098.50, 098.51, 098.59, 098.89, 711.00, 711.03, 711.08, 711.09, 711.10, 711.13, 711.18, 711.19, 711.20, 711.23, 711.28, 711.29, 711.30, 711.33, 711.38, 711.39, 711.40, 711.43, 711.48, 711.49, 711.50, 711.53, 711.58, 711.59, 711.60, 711.63, 711.68, 711.69, 711.70, 711.73, 711.78, 711.79, 711.80, 711.83, 711.88, 711.89, 711.90, 711.93, 711.98, 711.99, 712.10, 712.13, 712.18, 712.19, 712.20, 712.23, 712.28, 712.29, 712.30, 712.33, 712.38, 712.39, 712.80, 712.83, 712.88, 712.89, 712.90, 712.93, 712.98, 712.99, 713.0, 713.1, 713.2, 713.3, 713.4, 713.5, 713.6, 713.7, 713.8, 714.0, 715.00, 715.09, 715.10, 715.13, 715.18, 715.20, 715.23, 715.28, 715.30, 715.33, 715.38, 715.80, 715.89, 715.90,1, 715.98, 716.00, 716.03, 716.08, 716.09, 716.10, 716.13, 716.18, 716.19, 716.20, 716.23, 716.28, 716.29, 716.30, 716.33, 716.38, 716.39, 716.40, 716.43, 716.48, 716.49, 716.50, 716.53, 716.58, 716.59, 716.60, 716.63, 716.68, 716.80, 716.83, 716.88, 716.89, 716.90, 716.93, 716.98, 716.99, 718.00, 718.03, 718.08, 719.00, 719.03, 719.08, 719.09, 719.10, 719.13, 719.18, 719.19, 719.20, 719.23, 719.28, 719.29, 719.30, 719.33, 719.38, 719.39, 719.40, 719.43, 719.48, 719.49, 719.50, 719.53, 719.58, 719.59, 719.60, 719.63, 719.68, 719.70, 719.78, 719.79, 719.80, 719.83, 719.88, 719.89, 719.90, 719.93, 719.98, 719.99

C&C Exclusions: (for code 711.04) 015.80, 015.81, 015.82, 015.83, 015.84, 015.85, 015.86, 015.90, 015.91, 015.92, 015.93, 015.94, 015.95, 015.96, 017.90, 017.91, 017.92, 017.93, 017.94, 017.95, 017.96, 036.82, 056.71, 098.50, 098.51, 098.59, 098.89, 711.00, 711.04, 711.08, 711.09, 711.10, 711.14, 711.18, 711.19, 711.20, 711.24, 711.28, 711.29, 711.30, 711.34, 711.38, 711.39, 711.40, 711.44, 711.48, 711.49, 711.50, 711.54, 711.58, 711.59, 711.60, 711.64, 711.68, 711.69, 711.70, 711.74, 711.78, 711.79, 711.80, 711.84, 711.88, 711.89, 711.90, 711.94, 711.98, 711.99, 712.10, 712.14, 712.18, 712.19, 712.20, 712.24, 712.28, 712.29, 712.30, 712.34, 712.38, 712.39, 712.80, 712.84, 712.88, 712.89, 712.90, 712.94, 712.98, 712.99, 713.0, 713.1, 713.2, 713.3, 713.4, 713.5, 713.6, 713.7, 713.8, 714.0, 715.00, 715.09, 715.10, 715.14, 715.18, 715.20, 715.24, 715.28, 715.30, 715.34, 715.38, 715.80, 715.89, 715.90,1, 715.98, 716.00, 716.04, 716.08, 716.09, 716.10, 716.14, 716.18, 716.19, 716.20, 716.24, 716.28, 716.29, 716.30, 716.34, 716.38, 716.39, 716.40, 716.44, 716.48, 716.49, 716.50, 716.54, 716.58, 716.59, 716.60, 716.64, 716.68, 716.80, 716.84, 716.88, 716.89, 716.90, 716.94, 716.98, 716.99, 718.00, 718.04, 718.08, 719.00, 719.04, 719.08, 719.09, 719.10, 719.14, 719.18, 719.19, 719.20, 719.24, 719.28, 719.29, 719.30, 719.34, 719.38, 719.39, 719.40, 719.44, 719.48, 719.49, 719.50, 719.54, 719.58, 719.59, 719.60, 719.64, 719.68, 719.70, 719.78, 719.79, 719.80, 719.84, 719.88, 719.89, 719.90, 719.94, 719.98, 719.99

C&C Exclusions: (for code 711.05) 015.80, 015.81, 015.82, 015.83, 015.84, 015.85, 015.86, 015.90, 015.91, 015.92, 015.93, 015.94, 015.95, 015.96, 017.90, 017.91, 017.92, 017.93, 017.94, 017.95, 017.96, 036.82, 056.71, 098.50, 098.51, 098.59, 098.89, 711.00, 711.05, 711.08, 711.09, 711.10, 711.15, 711.18, 711.19, 711.20, 711.25, 711.28, 711.29, 711.30, 711.35, 711.38, 711.39, 711.40, 711.45, 711.48, 711.49, 711.50, 711.55, 711.58, 711.59, 711.60, 711.65, 711.68, 711.69, 711.70, 711.75, 711.78, 711.79, 711.80, 711.85, 711.88, 711.89, 711.90, 711.95, 711.98, 711.99, 712.10, 712.15, 712.18, 712.19, 712.20, 712.25, 712.28, 712.29, 712.30, 712.35, 712.38, 712.39, 712.80, 712.85, 712.88, 712.89, 712.90, 712.95, 712.98, 712.99, 713.0, 713.1, 713.2, 713.3, 713.4, 713.5, 713.6, 713.7, 713.8, 714.0, 715.00, 715.09, 715.10, 715.15, 715.18, 715.20, 715.25, 715.28, 715.30, 715.35, 715.38, 715.80, 715.89, 715.90,1, 715.98, 716.00, 716.05, 716.08, 716.09, 716.10, 716.15, 716.18, 716.19, 716.20, 716.25, 716.28, 716.29, 716.30, 716.35, 716.38, 716.39, 716.40, 716.45, 716.48, 716.49, 716.50, 716.55, 716.58, 716.59,

716.60, 716.65, 716.68, 716.80, 716.85, 716.88, 716.89, 716.90, 716.95, 716.98, 716.99, 718.00, 718.05, 718.08, 719.00, 719.05, 719.08, 719.09, 719.10, 719.15, 719.18, 719.19, 719.20, 719.25, 719.28, 719.29, 719.30, 719.35, 719.38, 719.39, 719.40, 719.45, 719.48, 719.49, 719.50, 719.55, 719.58, 719.59, 719.60, 719.65, 719.68, 719.70, 719.78, 719.79, 719.80, 719.85, 719.88, 719.89, 719.90, 719.95, 719.98, 719.99

C&C Exclusions: (for code 711.06) 015.80, 015.81, 015.82, 015.83, 015.84, 015.85, 015.86, 015.90, 015.91, 015.92, 015.93, 015.94, 015.95, 015.96, 017.90, 017.91, 017.92, 017.93, 017.94, 017.95, 017.96, 036.82, 056.71, 098.50, 098.51, 098.59, 098.89, 711.00, 711.06, 711.08, 711.09, 711.10, 711.16, 711.18, 711.19, 711.20, 711.26, 711.28, 711.29, 711.30, 711.36, 711.38, 711.39, 711.40, 711.46, 711.48, 711.49, 711.50, 711.56, 711.58, 711.59, 711.60, 711.66, 711.68, 711.69, 711.70, 711.76, 711.78, 711.79, 711.80, 711.86, 711.88, 711.89, 711.90, 711.96, 711.98, 711.99, 712.10, 712.16, 712.18, 712.19, 712.20, 712.26, 712.28, 712.29, 712.30, 712.36, 712.38, 712.39, 712.80, 712.86, 712.88, 712.89, 712.90, 712.96, 712.98, 712.99, 713.0, 713.1, 713.2, 713.3, 713.4, 713.5, 713.6, 713.7, 713.8, 714.0, 715.00, 715.09, 715.10, 715.16, 715.18, 715.20, 715.26, 715.28, 715.30, 715.36, 715.38, 715.80, 715.89, 715.90,1, 715.98, 716.00, 716.06, 716.08, 716.09, 716.10, 716.16, 716.18, 716.19, 716.20, 716.26, 716.28, 716.29, 716.30, 716.36, 716.38, 716.39, 716.40, 716.46, 716.48, 716.49, 716.50, 716.56, 716.58, 716.59, 716.60, 716.66, 716.68, 716.80, 716.86, 716.88, 716.89, 716.90, 716.96, 716.98, 716.99, 718.00, 718.06, 718.08, 719.00, 719.06, 719.08, 719.09, 719.10, 719.16, 719.18, 719.19, 719.20, 719.26, 719.28, 719.29, 719.30, 719.36, 719.38, 719.39, 719.40, 719.46, 719.48, 719.49, 719.50, 719.56, 719.58, 719.59, 719.60, 719.66, 719.68, 719.70, 719.78, 719.79, 719.80, 719.86, 719.88, 719.89, 719.90, 719.96, 719.98, 719.99

C&C Exclusions: (for code 711.07) 015.80, 015.81, 015.82, 015.83, 015.84, 015.85, 015.86, 015.90, 015.91, 015.92, 015.93, 015.94, 015.95, 015.96, 017.90, 017.91, 017.92, 017.93, 017.94, 017.95, 017.96, 036.82, 056.71, 098.50, 098.51, 098.59, 098.89, 711.00, 711.07, 711.08, 711.09, 711.10, 711.17, 711.18, 711.19, 711.20, 711.27, 711.28, 711.29, 711.30, 711.37, 711.38, 711.39, 711.40, 711.47, 711.48, 711.49, 711.50, 711.57, 711.58, 711.59, 711.60, 711.67, 711.68, 711.69, 711.70, 711.77, 711.78, 711.79, 711.80, 711.87, 711.88, 711.89, 711.90, 711.97, 711.98, 711.99, 712.10, 712.17, 712.18, 712.19, 712.20, 712.27, 712.28, 712.29, 712.30, 712.37, 712.38, 712.39, 712.80, 712.87, 712.88, 712.89, 712.90, 712.97, 712.98, 712.99, 713.0, 713.1, 713.2, 713.3, 713.4, 713.5, 713.6, 713.7, 713.8, 714.0, 715.00, 715.09, 715.10, 715.17, 715.18, 715.20, 715.27, 715.28, 715.30, 715.36, 715.38, 715.80, 715.89, 715.90,1, 715.98, 716.00, 716.07, 716.08, 716.09, 716.10, 716.17, 716.18, 716.19, 716.20, 716.27, 716.28, 716.29, 716.30, 716.37, 716.38, 716.39, 716.40, 716.47, 716.48, 716.49, 716.50, 716.57, 716.58, 716.59, 716.60, 716.67, 716.68, 716.80, 716.87, 716.88, 716.89, 716.90, 716.97, 716.98, 716.99, 718.00, 718.07, 718.08, 719.00, 719.07, 719.08, 719.09, 719.10, 719.17, 719.18, 719.19, 719.20, 719.27, 719.28, 719.29, 719.30, 719.37, 719.38, 719.39, 719.40, 719.47, 719.48, 719.49, 719.50, 719.57, 719.58, 719.59, 719.60, 719.67, 719.68, 719.70, 719.78, 719.79, 719.80, 719.87, 719.88, 719.89, 719.90, 719.97, 719.98, 719.99

AHA: 1Q 1992, 16; 1Q 1991, 15

+⑤ ***711.1 Arthropathy associated with Reiter's disease and nonspecific urethritis***
[0-9]

Code first underlying disease, as:
nonspecific urethritis (099.4)
Reiter's disease (099.3)

+⑤ ***711.2 Arthropathy in Behçet's syndrome***
[0-9]

Code first underlying disease (136.1)

+⑤ ***711.3 Postdysenteric arthropathy***
[0-9]

Code first underlying disease, as:
dysentery (009.0)
enteritis, infectious (008.0-009.3)
paratyphoid fever (002.1-002.9)
typhoid fever (002.0)

Excludes *salmonella arthritis (003.23)*

+⑤ ***711.4 Arthropathy associated with other bacterial diseases***
[0-9]

Code first underlying disease, as:
diseases classifiable to 010-040, 090-099, except as in 711.1, 711.3, and 713.5
leprosy (030.0-030.9)
tuberculosis (015.0-015.9)

Excludes *gonococcal arthritis (098.50)*
meningococcal arthritis (036.82)

+⑤ ***711.5 Arthropathy associated with other viral diseases***
[0-9]

Code first underlying disease, as:
diseases classifiable to 045-049, 050-079, 480, 487
O'nyong nyong (066.3)

Excludes *that due to rubella (056.71)*

+⑤ ***711.6 Arthropathy associated with mycoses***
[0-9]

Code first underlying disease (110.0-118)

C&C Exclusions: (for codes 711.60, 711.68-711.69) See 711.0
C&C Exclusions: (for code 711.61) See 711.01
C&C Exclusions: (for code 711.62) See 711.02
C&C Exclusions: (for code 711.63) See 711.03
C&C Exclusions: (for code 711.64) See 711.04
C&C Exclusions: (for code 711.65) See 711.05
C&C Exclusions: (for code 711.66) See 711.06
C&C Exclusions: (for code 711.67) See 711.07

+⑤ ***711.7 Arthropathy associated with helminthiasis***
[0-9]

Code first underlying disease, as:
filariasis (125.0-125.9)

+⑤ ***711.8 Arthropathy associated with other infectious and parasitic diseases***
[0-9]

Code first underlying disease, as:
diseases classifiable to 080-088, 100-104, 130-136

Excludes *arthropathy associated with sarcoidosis (713.7)*

AHA: 4Q 1991, 15; 3Q 1990, 14

⑤ **711.9 Unspecified infective arthritis**
[0-9]

Infective arthritis or polyarthritis (acute) (chronic) (subacute) NOS

④ **712 Crystal arthropathies**

Includes crystal-induced arthritis and synovitis
Excludes *gouty arthropathy (274.0)*

The following fifth-digit subclassification is for use with category 712; valid digits are in [brackets] under each code. See list at beginning of chapter for definitions:

- **0** **site unspecified**
- **1** **shoulder region**
- **2** **upper arm**
- **3** **forearm**
- **4** **hand**
- **5** **pelvic region and thigh**
- **6** **lower leg**
- **7** **ankle and foot**
- **8** **other specified sites**
- **9** **multiple sites**

+⑤ ***712.1 Chondrocalcinosis due to dicalcium phosphate crystals***
[0-9]

Chondrocalcinosis due to dicalcium phosphate crystals (with other crystals)
Code first underlying disease (275.49)

+⑤ ***712.2 Chondrocalcinosis due to pyrophosphate crystals***
[0-9]

Code first underlying disease (275.49)

+⑤ ***712.3 Chondrocalcinosis, unspecified***
[0-9]

Code first underlying disease (275.49)

⑤ **712.8 Other specified crystal arthropathies**
[0-9]

⑤ **712.9 Unspecified crystal arthropathy**
[0-9]

❹ 713 Arthropathy associated with other disorders classified elsewhere

Includes arthritis associated with conditions classifiable below
arthropathy associated with conditions classifiable below
polyarthritis associated with conditions classifiable below
polyarthropathy associated with conditions classifiable below

+ *713.0 Arthropathy associated with other endocrine and metabolic disorders*

Code first underlying disease, as:
acromegaly (253.0)
hemochromatosis (275.0)
hyperparathyroidism (252.00-252.08)
hypogammaglobulinemia (279.00-279.09)
hypothyroidism (243-244.9)
lipoid metabolism disorder (272.0-272.9)
ochronosis (270.2)

Excludes arthropathy associated with:
amyloidosis (713.7)
crystal deposition disorders, except gout (712.1-712.9)
diabetic neuropathy (713.5)
gouty arthropathy (274.0)

+ *713.1 Arthropathy associated with gastrointestinal conditions other than infections*

Code first underlying disease, as:
regional enteritis (555.0-555.9)
ulcerative colitis (556)

+ *713.2 Arthropathy associated with hematological disorders*

Code first underlying disease, as:
hemoglobinopathy (282.4-282.7)
hemophilia (286.0-286.2)
leukemia (204.0-208.9)
malignant reticulosis (202.3)
multiple myelomatosis (203.0)

Excludes arthropathy associated with Henoch-Schönlein purpura (713.6)

+ *713.3 Arthropathy associated with dermatological disorders*

Code first underlying disease, as:
erythema multiforme (695.1)
erythema nodosum (695.2)

Excludes psoriatic arthropathy (696.0)

+ *713.4 Arthropathy associated with respiratory disorders*

Code first underlying disease, as:
diseases classifiable to 490-519

Excludes arthropathy associated with respiratory infections (711.0, 711.4-711.8)

+ *713.5 Arthropathy associated with neurological disorders*

Charcôt's arthropathy associated with diseases classifiable elsewhere
Neuropathic arthritis associated with diseases classifiable elsewhere

Code first underlying disease, as:
neuropathic joint disease [Charcot's joints]:
NOS (094.0)
diabetic (250.6)
syringomyelic (336.0)
tabetic [syphilitic] (094.0)

+ *713.6 Arthropathy associated with hypersensitivity reaction*

Code first underlying disease, as:
Henoch (-Schönlein) purpura (287.0)
serum sickness (999.5)

Excludes allergic arthritis NOS (716.2)

+ *713.7 Other general diseases with articular involvement*

Code first underlying disease, as:
amyloidosis (277.30-277.39)
familial Mediterranean fever (277.31)
sarcoidosis (135)

AHA: 2Q 1997, 12

+ *713.8 Arthropathy associated with other conditions classifiable elsewhere*

Code first underlying disease, as:
conditions classifiable elsewhere except as in 711.1-711.8, 712, and 713.0-713.7

❹ 714 Rheumatoid arthritis and other inflammatory polyarthropathies

Excludes rheumatic fever (390)
rheumatoid arthritis of spine NOS (720.0)

AHA: 2Q 1995, 3

714.0 Rheumatoid arthritis

Arthritis or polyarthritis:
atrophic
rheumatic (chronic)

Use additional code to identify manifestation, as:
myopathy (359.6)
polyneuropathy (357.1)

Excludes juvenile rheumatoid arthritis NOS (714.30)

DEF: Autoimmune systemic disease causing chronic joint inflammation, destruction, and functional disability.

AHA: 2Q 2006, 20; 1Q 1990, 5

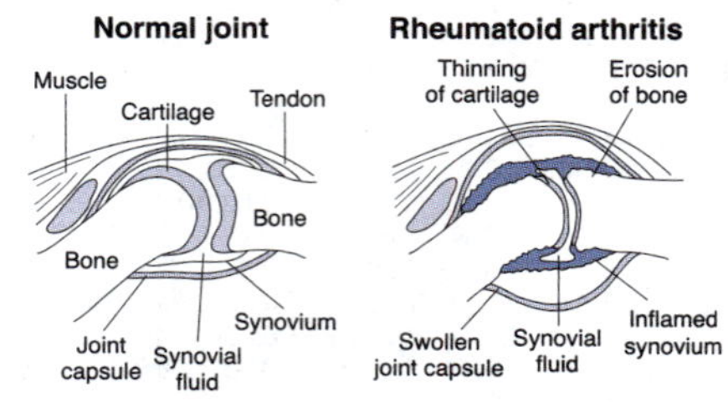

714.1 Felty's syndrome

Rheumatoid arthritis with splenoadenomegaly and leukopenia

DEF: Atypical form of rheumatoid arthritis presenting with fever, enlarged spleen, recurring infections, and decreased white cell count.

C&C Exclusions: 036.82, 056.71, 711.00, 711.01, 711.02, 711.03, 711.04, 711.05, 711.06, 711.07, 711.08, 711.09, 711.10, 711.11, 711.12, 711.13, 711.14, 711.15, 711.16, 711.17, 711.18, 711.19, 711.20, 711.21, 711.22, 711.23, 711.24, 711.25, 711.26, 711.27, 711.28, 711.29, 711.30, 711.31, 711.32, 711.33, 711.34, 711.35, 711.36, 711.37, 711.38, 711.39, 711.40, 711.41, 711.42, 711.43, 711.44, 711.45, 711.45, 711.46, 711.47, 711.48, 711.49, 711.50, 711.51, 711.52, 711.53, 711.54, 711.55, 711.56, 711.57, 711.58, 711.59, 711.60, 711.61, 711.62, 3, 711.64, 711.65, 711.66, 711.67, 711.68, 711.69, 711.70, 711.71, 711.72, 711.73, 711.74, 711.75, 711.76, 711.77, 711.78, 711.79, 711.80, 711.81, 711.82, 711.83, 711.84, 711.85, 711.86, 711.87, 711.88, 711.89, 711.90, 711.91, 711.92, 711.93, 711.94, 711.95, 711.96, 711.97, 711.98, 711.99, 712.10, 712.11, 712.12, 712.13, 712.14, 712.15, 712.16, 712.17, 712.18, 712.19, 712.20, 712.21, 712.22, 712.23, 712.24, 712.25, 712.26, 712.27, 712.28, 712.29, 712.30, 712.31, 712.32, 712.33, 712.34, 712.35, 712.36, 712.37, 712.38, 712.39, 712.80, 712.81, 712.82, 712.83, 712.84, 712.85, 712.86, 712.87, 712.88, 712.89, 712.90, 712.91, 712.92, 712.93, 712.94, 712.95, 712.96, 712.97, 712.98, 712.99, 713.0, 713.1, 713.2, 713.3, 713.4, 713.5, 713.6, 713.7, 713.8, 714.0, 714.1, 714.2, 714.30, 714.31, 714.32, 714.33, 714.4, 715.00, 715.09, 715.10, 715.18, 715.20, 715.21, 715.22, 715.23, 715.24, 715.25, 715.26, 715.27, 715.28, 715.30, 715.31, 715.32, 715.33, 715.34, 715.35, 715.36, 715.37, 715.38, 715.80, 715.89, 715.90,1, 715.92, 715.93, 715.94, 715.95, 715.96, 715.97, 715.98, 716.00, 716.01, 716.02, 716.03, 716.04, 716.05, 716.06, 716.07, 716.08, 716.09, 716.10, 716.11, 716.12, 716.13, 716.14, 716.15, 716.16, 716.17, 716.18, 716.19, 716.20, 716.21, 716.22, 716.23, 716.24, 716.25, 716.26, 716.27, 716.28, 716.29, 716.30, 716.31, 716.32, 716.33, 716.34, 716.35, 716.36, 716.37, 716.38, 716.39, 716.40, 716.41, 716.42, 716.43, 716.44, 716.45, 716.46, 716.47, 716.48, 716.49, 716.50, 716.51, 716.52, 716.53, 716.54, 716.55, 716.56, 716.57, 716.58, 716.59, 716.60, 716.61, 716.62, 716.63, 716.64, 716.65, 716.66, 716.67, 716.68, 716.80, 716.81, 716.82, 716.83. 716.84, 716.85, 716.86, 716.87, 716.88, 716.89, 716.90, 716.91, 716.92, 716.93, 716.94, 716.95, 716.96, 716.97, 716.98, 716.99, 718.00, 718.01, 718.02, 718.03, 718.04, 718.05, 718.07, 718.08, 719.00, 719.01, 719.02, 719.03, 719.04, 719.05, 719.06, 719.07, 719.08, 719.09, 719.10, 719.18, 719.19, 719.20, 719.21, 719.22, 719.23, 719.24, 719.25, 719.26, 719.27, 719.28, 719.29, 719.30, 719.31, 719.32, 719.33, 719.34, 719.35, 719.36, 719.37, 719.38, 719.39, 719.40,

719.41, 719.42, 719.43, 719.44, 719.45, 719.46, 719.47, 719.48, 719.49, 719.50, 719.51, 719.52, 719.53, 719.54, 719.55, 719.56, 719.57, 719.58, 719.59, 719.60, 719.61, 719.62, 719.63, 719.64, 719.65, 719.66, 719.67, 719.68, 719.70, 719.75, 719.76, 719.77, 719.78, 719.79, 719.80, 719.81, 719.82, 719.83, 719.84, 719.85, 719.86, 719.87, 719.88, 719.89, 719.90, 719.91, 719.92, 719.93, 719.94, 719.95, 719.96, 719.97, 719.98, 719.99

714.2 Other rheumatoid arthritis with visceral or systemic involvement

Rheumatoid carditis

C&C Exclusions: See 714.1

⑤ **714.3 Juvenile chronic polyarthritis**

714.30 Polyarticular juvenile rheumatoid arthritis, chronic or unspecified

Juvenile rheumatoid arthritis NOS
Still's disease

C&C Exclusions: See 714.1

714.31 Polyarticular juvenile rheumatoid arthritis, acute

C&C Exclusions: See 714.1

714.32 Pauciarticular juvenile rheumatoid arthritis

C&C Exclusions: See 714.1

714.33 Monoarticular juvenile rheumatoid arthritis

C&C Exclusions: See 714.1

714.4 Chronic postrheumatic arthropathy

Chronic rheumatoid nodular fibrositis
Jaccoud's syndrome

⑤ **714.8 Other specified inflammatory polyarthropathies**

714.81 Rheumatoid lung

Caplan's syndrome
Diffuse interstitial rheumatoid disease of lung
Fibrosing alveolitis, rheumatoid

714.89 Other

✖ **714.9 Unspecified inflammatory polyarthropathy**

Inflammatory polyarthropathy or polyarthritis NOS

Excludes *polyarthropathy NOS (716.5)*

④ **715 Osteoarthrosis and allied disorders**

Note: Localized, in the subcategories below, includes bilateral involvement of the same site.

Includes arthritis or polyarthritis:
degenerative
hypertrophic
degenerative joint disease
osteoarthritis

Excludes *Marie-Strümpell spondylitis (720.0)*
osteoarthrosis [osteoarthritis] of spine (721.0-721.9)

The following fifth-digit subclassification is for use with category 715; valid digits are in [brackets] under each code. See list at beginning of chapter for definitions:

- **0 site unspecified**
- **1 shoulder region**
- **2 upper arm**
- **3 forearm**
- **4 hand**
- **5 pelvic region and thigh**
- **6 lower leg**
- **7 ankle and foot**
- **8 other specified sites**
- **9 multiple sites**

⑤ **715.0 Osteoarthrosis, generalized**
[0,4,9]

Degenerative joint disease, involving multiple joints
Primary generalized hypertrophic osteoarthrosis

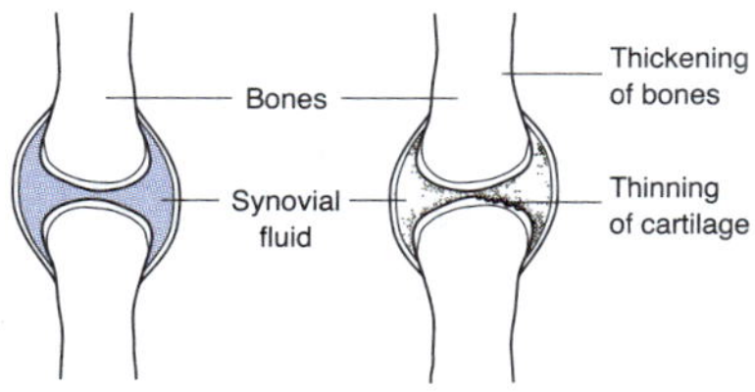

Normal **Osteoarthrosis**

⑤ **715.1 Osteoarthrosis, localized, primary**
[0-8]

Localized osteoarthropathy, idiopathic

⑤ **715.2 Osteoarthrosis, localized, secondary**
[0-8]

Coxae malum senilis

⑤ **715.3 Osteoarthrosis, localized, not specified whether primary or secondary**
[0-8]

Otto's pelvis

AHA: For Code 715.35: 3Q 2004, 12; 2Q 2004, 15; For Code 715.36: 4Q 2003, 118; 2Q 1995, 5

⑤ **715.8 Osteoarthrosis involving, or with mention of more than one site, but not specified as generalized**
[0,9]

⑤ **715.9 Osteoarthrosis, unspecified whether generalized or localized**
[0-8]

(✖ is only valid for fifth-digit "0")

AHA: For Code 715.90: 2Q 1997, 12

④ **716 Other and unspecified arthropathies**

Excludes *cricoarytenoid arthropathy (478.79)*

AHA: 2Q 1995, 3

The following fifth-digit subclassification is for use with category 716; valid digits are in [brackets] under each code. See list at beginning of chapter for definitions:

- **0 site unspecified**
- **1 shoulder region**
- **2 upper arm**
- **3 forearm**
- **4 hand**
- **5 pelvic region and thigh**
- **6 lower leg**
- **7 ankle and foot**
- **8 other specified sites**
- **9 multiple sites**

⑤ **716.0 Kaschin-Beck disease**
[0-9]

Endemic polyarthritis

⑤ **716.1 Traumatic arthropathy**
[0-9]

AHA: For Code 716.11: 1Q 2002, 9

⑤ **716.2 Allergic arthritis**
[0-9]

Excludes *arthritis associated with Henoch-Schönlein purpura or serum sickness (713.6)*

⑤ **716.3 Climacteric arthritis** ♀
[0-9]

Menopausal arthritis

⑤ **716.4 Transient arthropathy**
[0-9]

Excludes *palindromic rheumatism (719.3)*

⑤ **716.5 Unspecified polyarthropathy or polyarthritis**
[0-9]

⑤ **716.6 Unspecified monoarthritis**
[0-8]

Coxitis

⑤ **716.8 Other specified arthropathy**
[0-9]

⑤ **716.9 Arthropathy, unspecified**
[0-9]

Arthritis, (acute) (chronic) (subacute)
Arthropathy, (acute) (chronic) (subacute)
Articular rheumatism, (chronic)
Inflammation of joint, NOS

4 717 Internal derangement of knee

Includes degeneration of articular cartilage or meniscus of knee
rupture, old of articular cartilage or meniscus of knee
tear, old of articular cartilage or meniscus of knee

Excludes *acute derangement of knee (836.0-836.6)*
ankylosis (718.5)
contracture (718.4)
current injury (836.0-836.6)
deformity (736.4-736.6)
recurrent dislocation (718.3)

717.0 Old bucket handle tear of medial meniscus
Old bucket handle tear of unspecified cartilage

717.1 Derangement of anterior horn of medial meniscus

717.2 Derangement of posterior horn of medial meniscus

717.3 Other and unspecified derangement of medial meniscus
Degeneration of internal semilunar cartilage

5 717.4 Derangement of lateral meniscus

717.40 Derangement of lateral meniscus, unspecified

717.41 Bucket handle tear of lateral meniscus

717.42 Derangement of anterior horn of lateral meniscus

717.43 Derangement of posterior horn of lateral meniscus

717.49 Other

717.5 Derangement of meniscus, not elsewhere classified
Congenital discoid meniscus
Cyst of semilunar cartilage
Derangement of semilunar cartilage NOS

717.6 Loose body in knee
Joint mice, knee
Rice bodies, knee (joint)

717.7 Chondromalacia of patella
Chondromalacia patellae
Degeneration [softening] of articular cartilage of patella
AHA: Mar-Apr 1985, 14; Nov-Dec 1984, 9

5 717.8 Other internal derangement of knee

717.81 Old disruption of lateral collateral ligament

717.82 Old disruption of medial collateral ligament

717.83 Old disruption of anterior cruciate ligament

717.84 Old disruption of posterior cruciate ligament

717.85 Old disruption of other ligaments of knee
Capsular ligament of knee

717.89 Other
Old disruption of ligaments of knee NOS

✖ 717.9 Unspecified internal derangement of knee
Derangement NOS of knee

4 718 Other derangement of joint

Excludes *current injury (830.0-848.9)*
jaw (524.60-524.69)

The following fifth-digit subclassification is for use with category 718; valid digits are in [brackets] under each code. See list at beginning of chapter for definitions:

0 site unspecified
1 shoulder region
2 upper arm
3 forearm
4 hand
5 pelvic region and thigh
6 lower leg
7 ankle and foot
8 other specified sites
9 multiple sites

5 718.0 Articular cartilage disorder
[0-5,7-9]
Meniscus:
disorder
rupture, old
tear, old
Old rupture of ligament(s) of joint NOS

Excludes *articular cartilage disorder:*
in ochronosis (270.2)
knee (717.0-717.9)
chondrocalcinosis (275.49)
metastatic calcification (275.40)

5 718.1 Loose body in joint
[0-5,7-9]
Joint mice

Excludes *knee (717.6)*

AHA: For Code 718.17: 2Q 2001, 15

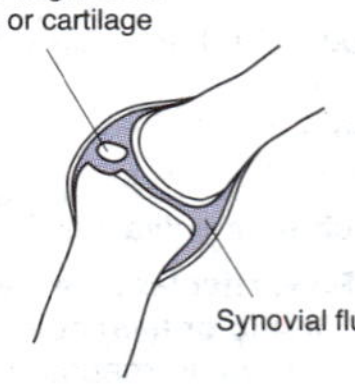

5 718.2 Pathological dislocation
[0-9]
Dislocation or displacement of joint, not recurrent and not current

5 718.3 Recurrent dislocation of joint
[0-9]
AHA: Nov-Dec 1987, 7

5 718.4 Contracture of joint
[0-9]
(✖ is only valid for fifth-digit "9")
AHA: 4Q 1998, 40

5 718.5 Ankylosis of joint
[0-9]
(✖ is only valid for fifth-digit "0")
Ankylosis of joint (fibrous) (osseous)

Excludes *spine (724.9)*
stiffness of joint without mention of ankylosis (719.5)

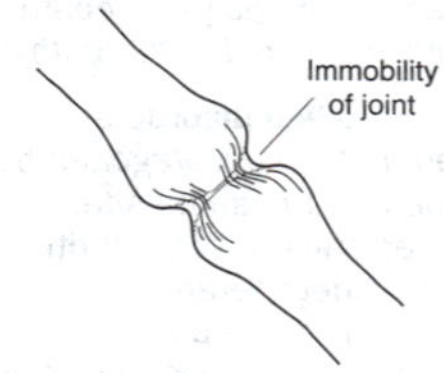

5 718.6 Unspecified intrapelvic protrusion of acetabulum
[0,5]
Protrusio acetabuli, unspecified

5 718.7 Developmental dislocation of joint
[0-9]
(✖ is only valid for fifth-digit "0")

Excludes *congenital dislocation of joint (754.0-755.8)*
traumatic dislocation of joint (830-839)

AHA: 4Q 2001, 48

5 718.8 Other joint derangement, not elsewhere classified
[0-9]
Flail joint (paralytic)
Instability of joint

Excludes *deformities classifiable to 736 (736.0-736.9)*

AHA: For Code 718.81: 2Q 2000, 14

5 718.9 Unspecified derangement of joint
[0-5,7-9]

Excludes *knee (717.9)*

4 5 Additional Digit Required ✖ Nonspecific PDx ⊘ Unacceptable PDx ✚ Manifestation Code ►◄ Revised Text ● New Code ▲ Revised Code

❹ **719 Other and unspecified disorders of joint**
Excludes *jaw (524.60-524.69)*

The following fifth-digit subclassification is for use with codes 719.0-719.6, 719.8-719.9; valid digits are in [brackets] under each code. See list at beginning of chapter for definitions:

- **0** **site unspecified**
- **1** **shoulder region**
- **2** **upper arm**
- **3** **forearm**
- **4** **hand**
- **5** **pelvic region and thigh**
- **6** **lower leg**
- **7** **ankle and foot**
- **8** **other specified sites**
- **9** **multiple sites**

❺ **719.0 Effusion of joint**
[0-9]
Hydrarthrosis
Swelling of joint, with or without pain
Excludes *intermittent hydrarthrosis (719.3)*

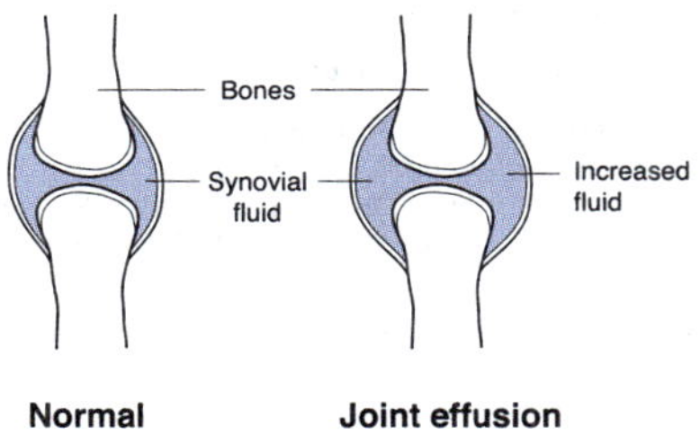

❺ **719.1 Hemarthrosis**
[0-9]
Excludes *current injury (840.0-848.9)*

❺ **719.2 Villonodular synovitis**
[0-9]

❺ **719.3 Palindromic rheumatism**
[0-9]
Hench-Rosenberg syndrome
Intermittent hydrarthrosis

❺ **719.4 Pain in joint**
[0-9]
Arthralgia
AHA: For Code 719.46: 1Q 2001, 3

❺ **719.5 Stiffness of joint, not elsewhere classified**
[0-9]

❺ **719.6 Other symptoms referable to joint**
[0-9]
Joint crepitus
Snapping hip
AHA: 1Q 1994, 15

719.7 Difficulty in walking
Excludes *abnormality of gait (781.2)*
C&C Exclusions: 696.0, 711.00, 711.01, 711.02, 711.03, 711.04, 711.05, 711.06, 711.07, 711.08, 711.09, 711.60, 711.61, 711.62, 3, 711.64, 711.65, 711.66, 711.67, 711.68, 711.69, 714.1, 714.2, 714.30, 714.31, 714.32, 714.33
AHA: 2Q 2004, 15; 4Q 2003, 66

❺ **719.8 Other specified disorders of joint**
[0-9]
Calcification of joint
Fistula of joint
Excludes *temporomandibular joint-pain-dysfunction syndrome [Costen's syndrome] (524.60)*

❺ **719.9 Unspecified disorder of joint**
[0-9]

DORSOPATHIES (720-724)

Excludes *curvature of spine (737.0-737.9)*
osteochondrosis of spine (juvenile) (732.0)
adult (732.8)

❹ **720 Ankylosing spondylitis and other inflammatory spondylopathies**

720.0 Ankylosing spondylitis
Rheumatoid arthritis of spine NOS
Spondylitis:
Marie-Strümpell
rheumatoid

720.1 Spinal enthesopathy
Disorder of peripheral ligamentous or muscular attachments of spine
Romanus lesion

720.2 Sacroiliitis, not elsewhere classified
Inflammation of sacroiliac joint NOS

❺ **720.8 Other inflammatory spondylopathies**

+ ***720.81 Inflammatory spondylopathies in diseases classified elsewhere***
Code first underlying disease, as:
tuberculosis (015.0)

720.89 Other

720.9 Unspecified inflammatory spondylopathy
Spondylitis NOS

❹ **721 Spondylosis and allied disorders**
AHA: 2Q 1989, 14

721.0 Cervical spondylosis without myelopathy
Cervical or cervicodorsal:
arthritis
osteoarthritis
spondylarthritis

721.1 Cervical spondylosis with myelopathy
Anterior spinal artery compression syndrome
Spondylogenic compression of cervical spinal cord
Vertebral artery compression syndrome
DEF: Abnormal wear and chronic degeneration of the vertebrae and cartilage in the neck, compressing a nerve root.

721.2 Thoracic spondylosis without myelopathy
Thoracic:
arthritis
osteoarthritis
spondylarthritis

721.3 Lumbosacral spondylosis without myelopathy
Lumbar or lumbosacral:
arthritis
osteoarthritis
spondylarthritis
AHA: 4Q 2002, 107

❺ **721.4 Thoracic or lumbar spondylosis with myelopathy**

721.41 Thoracic region
Spondylogenic compression of thoracic spinal cord

721.42 Lumbar region
Spondylogenic compression of lumbar spinal cord

721.5 Kissing spine
Baastrup's syndrome

721.6 Ankylosing vertebral hyperostosis

721.7 Traumatic spondylopathy
Kümmell's disease or spondylitis

721.8 Other allied disorders of spine

❺ **721.9 Spondylosis of unspecified site**

721.90 Without mention of myelopathy
Spinal:
arthritis (deformans) (degenerative) (hypertrophic)
osteoarthritis NOS
Spondylarthrosis NOS

721.91 With myelopathy
Spondylogenic compression of spinal cord NOS

4 **722 Intervertebral disc disorders**
AHA: 1Q 1988, 10

722.0 Displacement of cervical intervertebral disc without myelopathy
Neuritis (brachial) or radiculitis due to displacement or rupture of cervical intervertebral disc
Any condition classifiable to 722.2 of the cervical or cervicothoracic intervertebral disc

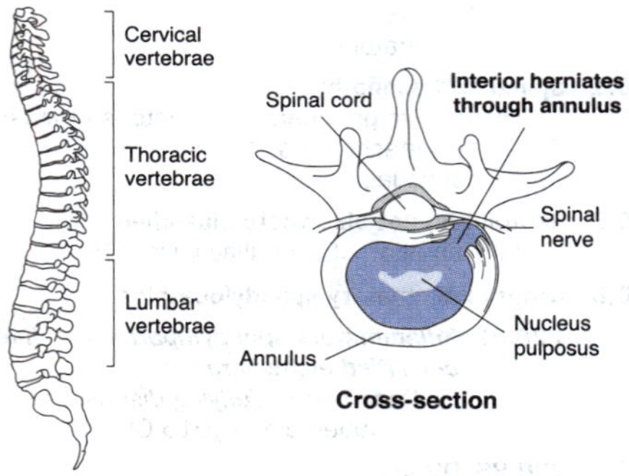

5 **722.1 Displacement of thoracic or lumbar intervertebral disc without myelopathy**

722.10 Lumbar intervertebral disc without myelopathy
Lumbago or sciatica due to displacement of intervertebral disc
Neuritis or radiculitis due to displacement or rupture of lumbar intervertebral disc
Any condition classifiable to 722.2 of the lumbar or lumbosacral intervertebral disc
AHA: 1Q 2007, 9; 3Q 2003, 12; 1Q 2003, 7; 4Q 2002, 107

722.11 Thoracic intervertebral disc without myelopathy
Any condition classifiable to 722.2 of thoracic intervertebral disc

722.2 Displacement of intervertebral disc, site unspecified, without myelopathy
Discogenic syndrome NOS
Herniation of nucleus pulposus NOS
Intervertebral disc NOS:
- extrusion
- prolapse
- protrusion
- rupture

Neuritis or radiculitis due to displacement or rupture of intervertebral disc

5 **722.3 Schmorl's nodes**

✖ **722.30 Unspecified region**

722.31 Thoracic region

722.32 Lumbar region

722.39 Other

722.4 Degeneration of cervical intervertebral disc
Degeneration of cervicothoracic intervertebral disc

5 **722.5 Degeneration of thoracic or lumbar intervertebral disc**

722.51 Thoracic or thoracolumbar intervertebral disc

722.52 Lumbar or lumbosacral intervertebral disc
AHA: 2Q 2006, 18; 4Q 2004, 133

722.6 Degeneration of intervertebral disc, site unspecified
Degenerative disc disease NOS
Narrowing of intervertebral disc or space NOS

5 **722.7 Intervertebral disc disorder with myelopathy**

✖ **722.70 Unspecified region**

722.71 Cervical region

722.72 Thoracic region

722.73 Lumbar region

5 **722.8 Postlaminectomy syndrome**
AHA: Jan-Feb 1987, 7

✖ **722.80 Unspecified region**
C&C Exclusions: 722.51, 722.52, 722.6, 722.70, 722.71, 722.72, 722.73, 722.80, 722.81, 722.82, 722.83, 722.90, 722.91, 722.92, 722.93

722.81 Cervical region
C&C Exclusions: See 722.80

722.82 Thoracic region
C&C Exclusions: See 722.80

722.83 Lumbar region
C&C Exclusions: See 722.80
AHA: 2Q 1997, 15

5 **722.9 Other and unspecified disc disorder**
Calcification of intervertebral cartilage or disc
Discitis

✖ **722.90 Unspecified region**
AHA: Nov-Dec 1984, 19

722.91 Cervical region

722.92 Thoracic region

722.93 Lumbar region

4 **723 Other disorders of cervical region**
Excludes conditions due to:
intervertebral disc disorders (722.0-722.9)
spondylosis (721.0-721.9)

AHA: 3Q 1994, 14; 2Q 1989, 14

723.0 Spinal stenosis of cervical region
AHA: 4Q 2003, 101

723.1 Cervicalgia
Pain in neck

723.2 Cervicocranial syndrome
Barré-Liéou syndrome
Posterior cervical sympathetic syndrome

723.3 Cervicobrachial syndrome (diffuse)
AHA: Nov-Dec 1985, 12

723.4 Brachia neuritis or radiculitis NOS
Cervical radiculitis
Radicular syndrome of upper limbs
C&C Exclusions: 722.6, 722.70, 722.71, 722.80, 722.81, 722.90, 722.91, 723.0, 723.1, 723.2, 723.3, 723.4, 723.5, 723.6, 723.7, 723.8, 723.9

723.5 Torticollis, unspecified
Contracture of neck
Excludes
congenital (754.1)
due to birth injury (767.8)
hysterical (300.11)
ocular torticollis (781.93)
psychogenic (306.0)
spasmodic (333.83)
traumatic, current (847.0)

DEF: Spasmodic contraction of the neck muscles causing limited neck motion and head positioned to one side.
C&C Exclusions: 053.71, 722.6, 722.70, 722.71, 722.80, 722.81, 722.90, 722.91, 723.0, 723.1, 723.2, 723.3, 723.4, 723.5, 723.6, 723.7, 723.8, 723.9
AHA: 2Q 2001, 21; 1Q 1995, 7

723.6 Panniculitis specified as affecting neck

723.7 Ossification of posterior longitudinal ligament in cervical region

723.8 Other syndromes affecting cervical region
Cervical syndrome NEC
Klippel's disease
Occipital neuralgia
AHA: 1Q 2000, 7

✖ **723.9 Unspecified musculoskeletal disorders and symptoms referable to neck**
Cervical (region) disorder NOS

724 Other and unspecified disorders of back

Excludes *collapsed vertebra (code to cause, e.g., osteoporosis, 733.00-733.09)*
conditions due to:
intervertebral disc disorders (722.0-722.9)
spondylosis (721.0-721.9)

AHA: 2Q 1989, 14

724.0 Spinal stenosis, other than cervical

724.00 Spinal stenosis, unspecified region

724.01 Thoracic region

724.02 Lumbar region

AHA: 1Q 2007, 10, 20-21; 4Q 1999, 13

724.09 Other

724.1 Pain in thoracic spine

724.2 Lumbago

Low back pain
Low back syndrome
Lumbalgia

AHA: Nov-Dec 1985, 12

724.3 Sciatica

Neuralgia or neuritis of sciatic nerve

Excludes *specified lesion of sciatic nerve (355.0)*

DEF: Severe pain in the sciatic nerve running down the lower back through the leg; usually resulting from nerve compression or pinching.

AHA: 2Q 1989, 12

724.4 Thoracic or lumbosacral neuritis or radiculitis, unspecified

Radicular syndrome of lower limbs

AHA: 2Q 1999, 3

724.5 Backache, unspecified

Vertebrogenic (pain) syndrome NOS

724.6 Disorders of sacrum

Ankylosis, lumbosacral or sacroiliac (joint)
Instability, lumbosacral or sacroiliac (joint)

724.7 Disorders of coccyx

724.70 Unspecified disorder of coccyx

724.71 Hypermobility of coccyx

724.79 Other

Coccygodynia

724.8 Other symptoms referable to back

Ossification of posterior longitudinal ligament NOS
Panniculitis specified as sacral or affecting back

724.9 Other unspecified back disorders

Ankylosis of spine NOS
Compression of spinal nerve root NEC
Spinal disorder NOS

Excludes *sacroiliitis (720.2)*

RHEUMATISM, EXCLUDING THE BACK (725-729)

Includes disorders of muscles and tendons and their attachments, and of other soft tissues

725 Polymyalgia rheumatica

726 Peripheral enthesopathies and allied syndromes

Note: Enthesopathies are disorders of peripheral ligamentous or muscular attachments.

Excludes *spinal enthesopathy (720.1)*

726.0 Adhesive capsulitis of shoulder

726.1 Rotator cuff syndrome of shoulder and allied disorders

726.10 Disorders of bursae and tendons in shoulder region, unspecified

Rotator cuff syndrome NOS
Supraspinatus syndrome NOS

AHA: 2Q 2001, 11

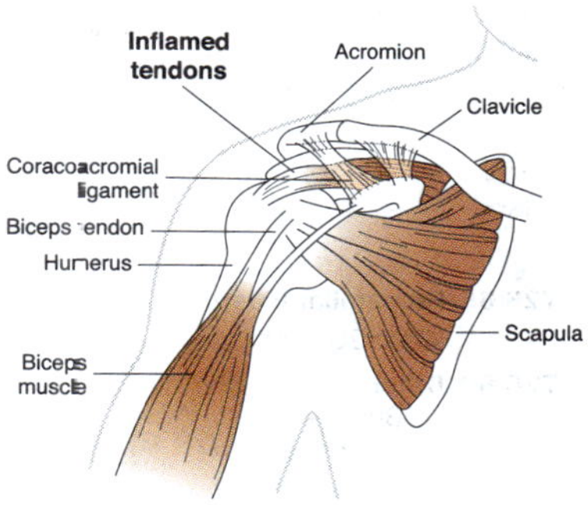

726.11 Calcifying tendinitis of shoulder

726.12 Bicipital tenosynovitis

726.19 Other specified disorders

Excludes *complete rupture of rotator cuff, nontraumatic (727.61)*

726.2 Other affections of shoulder region, not elsewhere classified

Periarthritis of shoulder
Scapulohumeral fibrositis

726.3 Enthesopathy of elbow region

726.30 Enthesopathy of elbow, unspecified

726.31 Medial epicondylitis

726.32 Lateral epicondylitis

Epicondylitis NOS
Golfers' elbow
Tennis elbow

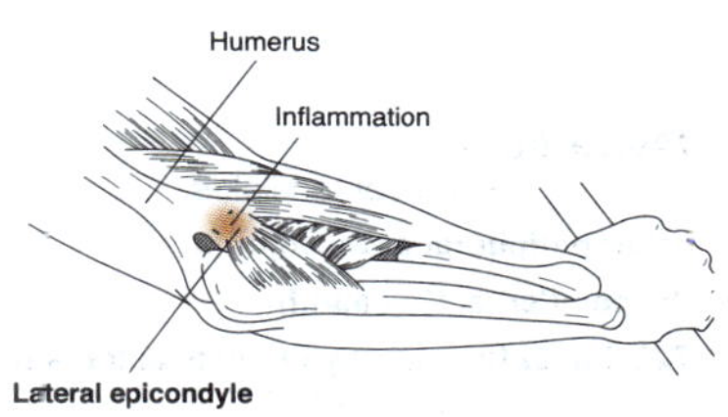

726.33 Olecranon bursitis

Bursitis of elbow

726.39 Other

726.4 Enthesopathy of wrist and carpus

Bursitis of hand or wrist
Periarthritis of wrist

726.5 Enthesopathy of hip region

Bursitis of hip
Gluteal tendinitis
Iliac crest spur
Psoas tendinitis
Trochanteric tendinitis

726.6 Enthesopathy of knee

726.60 Enthesopathy of knee, unspecified

Bursitis of knee NOS

726.61 Pes anserinus tendinitis or bursitis

726.62 Tibial collateral ligament bursitis

Pellegrini-Stieda syndrome

726.63 Fibular collateral ligament bursitis

726.64 Patellar tendinitis

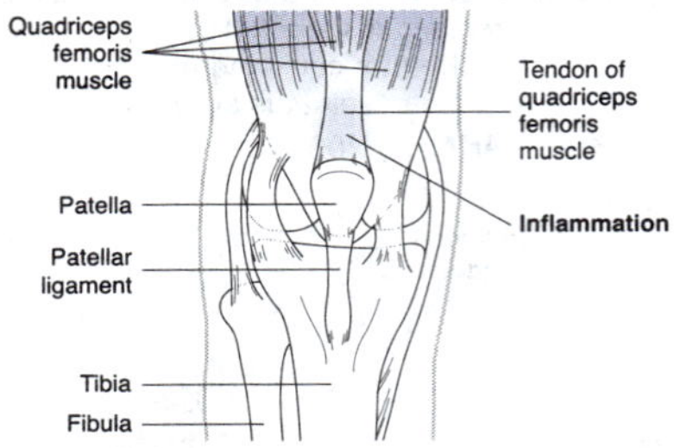

726.65 Prepatellar bursitis
AHA: 2Q 2006, 15

726.69 Other
Bursitis:
infrapatellar
subpatellar

❺ **726.7 Enthesopathy of ankle and tarsus**

726.70 Enthesopathy of ankle and tarsus, unspecified
Metatarsalgia NOS
Excludes *Morton's metatarsalgia (355.6)*

726.71 Achilles bursitis or tendinitis

726.72 Tibialis tendinitis
Tibialis (anterior) (posterior) tendinitis

726.73 Calcaneal spur

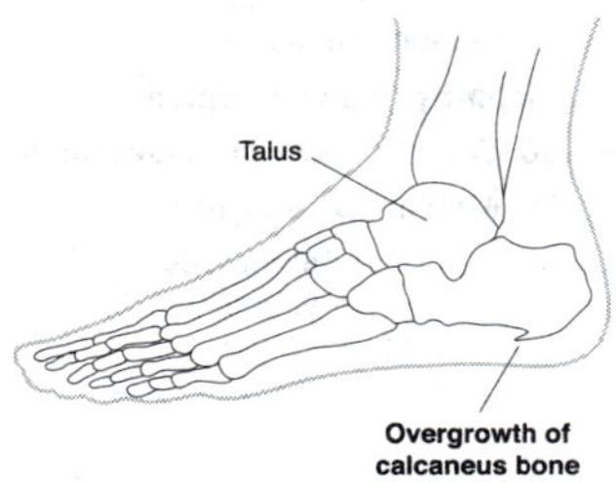

726.79 Other
Peroneal tendinitis

726.8 Other peripheral enthesopathies

❺ **726.9 Unspecified enthesopathy**

726.90 Enthesopathy of unspecified site
Capsulitis NOS
Periarthritis NOS
Tendinitis NOS

726.91 Exostosis of unspecified site
Bone spur NOS
AHA: 2Q 2001, 15

❹ **727 Other disorders of synovium, tendon, and bursa**

❺ **727.0 Synovitis and tenosynovitis**

727.00 Synovitis and tenosynovitis, unspecified
Synovitis NOS
Tenosynovitis NOS

✚ ***727.01 Synovitis and tenosynovitis in diseases classified elsewhere***
Code first underlying disease, as:
tuberculosis (015.0-015.9)
Excludes *crystal-induced (275.49)*
gonococcal (098.51)
gouty (274.0)
syphilitic (095.7)

727.02 Giant cell tumor of tendon sheath

727.03 Trigger finger (acquired)

727.04 Radial styloid tenosynovitis
de Quervain's disease

727.05 Other tenosynovitis or hand and wrist

727.06 Tenosynovitis of foot and ankle

727.09 Other

727.1 Bunion

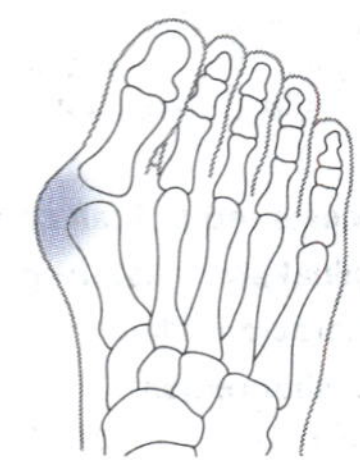

727.2 Specific bursitides often of occupational origin
Beat:
elbow
hand
knee
Chronic crepitant synovitis of wrist
Miners':
elbow
knee

727.3 Other bursitis
Bursitis NOS
Excludes *bursitis:*
gonococcal (098.52)
subacromial (726.19)
subcoracoid (726.19)
subdeltoid (726.19)
syphilitic (095.7)
"frozen shoulder" (726.0)

❺ **727.4 Ganglion and cyst of synovium, tendon, and bursa**

727.40 Synovial cyst, unspecified
Excludes *that of popliteal space (727.51)*
AHA: 2Q 1997, 6

727.41 Ganglion of joint

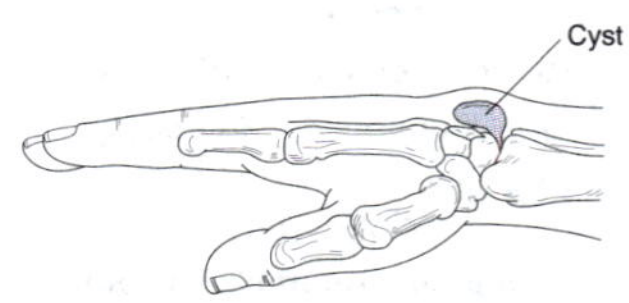

727.42 Ganglion of tendon sheath

727.43 Ganglion, unspecified

727.49 Other
Cyst of bursa

❺ **727.5 Rupture of synovium**

727.50 Rupture of synovium, unspecified

727.51 Synovial cyst of popliteal space
Baker's cyst (knee)

727.59 Other

❺ **727.6 Rupture of tendon, nontraumatic**

727.60 Nontraumatic rupture of unspecified tendon

727.61 Complete rupture of rotator cuff

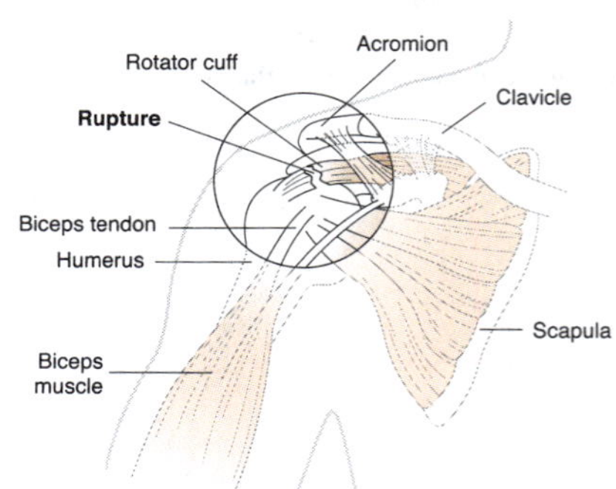

727.62 Tendons of biceps (long head)

727.63 Extensor tendons of hand and wrist

727.64 Flexor tendons of hand and wrist

727.65 Quadriceps tendon

727.66 Patellar tendon

727.67 Achilles tendon

727.68 Other tendons of foot and ankle

727.69 Other

5 **727.8 Other disorders of synovium, tendon, and bursa**

727.81 Contracture of tendon (sheath)
Short Achilles tendon (acquired)

727.82 Calcium deposits in tendon and bursa
Calcification of tendon NOS
Calcific tendinitis NOS
Excludes *peripheral ligamentous or muscular attachments (726.0-726.9)*

727.83 Plica syndrome
Plica knee
AHA: 4Q 2000, 44

727.89 Other
Abscess of bursa or tendon
Excludes *xanthomatosis localized to tendons (272.7)*
AHA: 2Q 1989, 15

727.9 Unspecified disorder of synovium, tendon, and bursa

4 **728 Disorders of muscle, ligament, and fascia**
Excludes *enthesopathies (726.0-726.9)*
muscular dystrophies (359.0-359.1)
myoneural disorders (358.00-358.9)
myopathies (359.2-359.9)
old disruption of ligaments of knee (717.81-717.89)

728.0 Infective myositis
Myositis:
purulent
suppurative
Excludes *myositis:*
epidemic (074.1)
interstitial (728.81)
myoneural disorder (358.00-358.9)
syphilitic (095.6)
tropical (040.81)
C&C Exclusions: 567.31, 728.0, 728.11, 728.12, 728.13, 728.19, 728.2, 728.3, 728.81, 728.86, 728.88

5 **728.1 Muscular calcification and ossification**

728.10 Calcification and ossification, unspecified
Massive calcification (paraplegic)

728.11 Progressive myositis ossificans
C&C Exclusions: 567.31, 728.88

728.12 Traumatic myositis ossificans
Myositis ossificans (circumscripta)
C&C Exclusions: See 728.11

728.13 Postoperative heterotopic calcification
C&C Exclusions: See 728.11

728.19 Other
Polymyositis ossificans
C&C Exclusions: See 728.11

728.2 Muscular wasting and disuse atrophy, not elsewhere classified
Amyotrophia NOS
Myofibrosis
Excludes *neuralgic amyotrophy (353.5)*
pelvic muscle wasting and disuse atrophy (618.83)
progressive muscular atrophy (335.0-335.9)
C&C Exclusions: See 728.11

728.3 Other specific muscle disorders
Arthrogryposis
Immobility syndrome (paraplegic)
Excludes *arthrogryposis multiplex congenita (754.89)*
stiff-man syndrome (333.91)
C&C Exclusions: See 728.11

728.4 Laxity of ligament

728.5 Hypermobility syndrome

728.6 Contracture of palmar fascia A
Dupuytren's contracture

5 **728.7 Other fibromatoses**

728.71 Plantar fascial fibromatosis
Contracture of plantar fascia
Plantar fasciitis (traumatic)

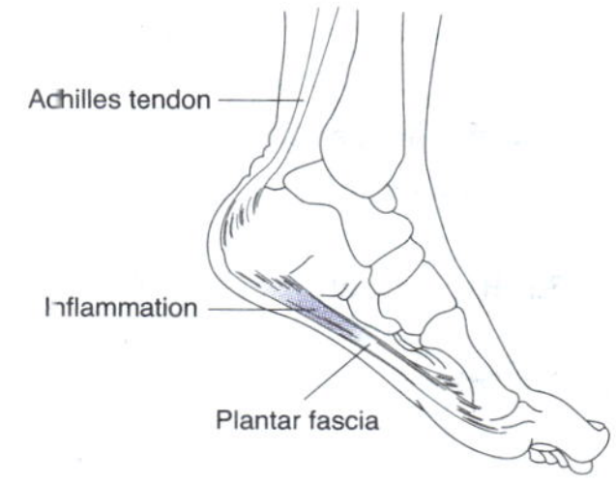

728.79 Other
Garrod's or knuckle pads
Nodular fasciitis
Pseudosarcomatous Fibromatosis (proliferative) (subcutaneous)

5 **728.8 Other disorders of muscle, ligament, and fascia**

728.81 Interstitial myositis
C&C Exclusions: 567.31

728.82 Foreign body granuloma of muscle
Talc granuloma of muscle

728.83 Rupture of muscle, nontraumatic

728.84 Diastasis of muscle
Diastatsis recti (abdomen)
Excludes *diastatsis recti complicating pregnancy, labor, and delivery (665.8)*

728.85 Spasm of muscle

728.86 Necrotizing fasciitis
Use additional code to identify:
infectious organism (041.00-041.89)
gangrene (785.4), if applicable
C&C Exclusions: 567.31, 728.0, 728.11, 728.12, 728.13, 728.19, 728.2, 728.3, 728.82, 728.86
AHA: 4Q 1995, 54

728.87 Muscle weakness (generalized)
Excludes *generalized weakness (780.79)*
AHA: 1Q 2005, 13; 4Q 2003, 66

728.88 Rhabdomyolysis
C&C Exclusions: 728.88
AHA: 4Q 2003, 66

728.89 Other
Eosinophilic fasciitis
Use additional E code to identify drug, if drug induced
AHA: 3Q 2006, 13; 3Q 2002, 28; 2Q 2001, 14-15

✖ **728.9 Unspecified disorder of muscle, ligament, and fascia**
AHA: 4Q 1988, 11

❹ **729 Other disorders of soft tissues**

Excludes *acroparesthesia (443.89)*
carpal tunnel syndrome (354.0)
disorders of the back (720.0-724.9)
entrapment syndromes (354.0-355.9)
palindromic rheumatism (719.3)
periarthritis (726.0-726.9)
psychogenic rheumatism (306.0)

729.0 Rheumatism, unspecified and fibrositis

729.1 Mylagia and myositis, unspecified
Fibromyositis NOS

729.2 Neuralgia, neuritis, and radiculitis, unspecified
Excludes *brachial radiculitis (723.4)*
cervical radiculitis (723.4)
lumbosacral radiculitis (724.4)
mononeuritis (354.0-355.9)
radiculitis due to intervertebral disc involvement (722.0-722.2,722.7)
sciatica (724.3)

❺ **729.3 Panniculitis, unspecified**

729.30 Panniculitis, unspecified site
Weber-Christian disease

729.31 Hypertrophy of fat pad, knee
Hypertrophy of infrapatellar fat pad

729.39 Other site
Excludes *panniculitis specified as (affecting):*
back (724.8)
neck (723.6)
sacral (724.8)

729.4 Fasciitis, unspecified
Excludes *necrotizing fasciitis (728.86)*
nodular fasciitis (728.79)

AHA: 2Q 1994, 13

729.5 Pain in limb

729.6 Residual foreign body in soft tissue
Excludes *foreign body granuloma:*
muscle (728.82)
skin and subcutaneous tissue (709.4)

❺ **729.7 Nontraumatic compartment syndrome**
Excludes *compartment syndrome NOS (958.90)*
traumatic compartment syndrome (958.90-958.99)

729.71 Nontraumatic compartment syndrome of upper extremity
Nontraumatic compartment syndrome of shoulder, arm, forearm, wrist, hand and fingers

AHA: 4Q 2006, 102

729.72 Nontraumatic compartment syndrome of lower extremity
Nontraumatic compartment syndrome of hip, buttock, thigh, leg, foot and toes

729.73 Nontraumatic compartment syndrome of abdomen

729.79 Nontraumatic compartment syndrome of other sites

❺ **729.8 Other musculoskeletal symptoms referable to limbs**

729.81 Swelling of limb
AHA: 4Q 1988, 6

729.82 Cramp

729.89 Other
Excludes *abnormality of gait (781.2)*
tetany (781.7)
transient paralysis of limb (781.4)

AHA: 4Q 1988, 12

729.9 Other and unspecified disorders of soft tissue
Polyalgia

OSTEOPATHIES, CHONDROPATHIES, AND ACQUIRED MUSCULOSKELETAL DEFORMITIES (730-739)

❹ **730 Osteomyelitis, periostitis, and other infections involving bone**

Excludes *jaw (526.4-526.5)*
petrous bone (383.2)

Use additional code to identify organism, such as Staphylococcus (041.1)

AHA: 4Q 1997, 43

The following fifth-digit subclassification is for use with category 730; valid digits are in [brackets] under each code. See list at beginning of chapter for definitions:

0 site unspecified
1 shoulder region
2 upper arm
3 forearm
4 hand
5 pelvic region and thigh
6 lower leg
7 ankle and foot
8 other specified sites
9 multiple sites

❺ **730.0 Acute osteomyelitis**
[0-9]
(✖ is only valid for fifth-digit "0")
Abscess of any bone except accessory sinus, jaw, or mastoid
Acute or subacute osteomyelitis, with or without mention of periostitis
Use additional code to identify major osseous defect, if applicable (731.3)

C&C Exclusions: (For codes 730.00, 730.09) 015.50, 015.51, 015.52, 015.53, 015.54, 015.55, 015.56, 015.70, 015.71, 015.72, 015.73, 015.74, 015.75, 015.76, 015.90, 015.91, 015.92, 015.93, 015.94, 015.95, 015.96, 017.90, 017.91, 017.92, 017.93, 017.94, 017.95, 017.96, 730.00, 730.01, 730.02, 730.03, 730.04, 730.05, 730.06, 730.07, 730.08, 730.09, 730.10, 730.11, 730.12, 730.13, 730.14, 730.15, 730.16, 730.17, 730.18, 730.19, 730.20, 730.21, 730.22, 730.23, 730.24, 730.25, 730.26, 730.27, 730.28, 730.29, 730.30, 730.31, 730.32, 730.33, 730.34, 730.35, 730.36, 730.37, 730.38, 730.39, 730.80, 730.81, 730.82, 730.83, 730.84, 730.85, 730.86, 730.87, 730.88, 730.89, 730.90, 730.91, 730.92, 730.93, 730.94, 730.95, 730.96, 730.97, 730.98, 730.99

C&C Exclusions: (for code 730.01) 015.50, 015.51, 015.52, 015.53, 015.54, 015.55, 015.56, 015.70, 015.71, 015.72, 015.73, 015.74, 015.75, 015.76, 015.90, 015.91, 015.92, 015.93, 015.94, 015.95, 015.96, 017.90, 017.91, 017.92, 017.93, 017.94, 017.95, 017.96, 730.00, 730.08, 730.09, 730.10, 730.11, 730.18, 730.19, 730.20, 730.21, 730.28, 730.29, 730.30, 730.31, 730.38, 730.39, 730.80, 730.81, 730.88, 730.89, 730.90, 730.91, 730.98, 730.99

C&C Exclusions: (for code 730.02) 015.50, 015.51, 015.52, 015.53, 015.54, 015.55, 015.56, 015.70, 015.71, 015.72, 015.73, 015.74, 015.75, 015.76, 015.90, 015.91, 015.92, 015.93, 015.94, 015.95, 015.96, 017.90, 017.91, 017.92, 017.93, 017.94, 017.95, 017.96, 730.00, 730.08, 730.09, 730.10, 730.12, 730.18, 730.19, 730.20, 730.22, 730.28, 730.29, 730.30, 730.32, 730.38, 730.39, 730.80, 730.82, 730.88, 730.89, 730.90, 730.92, 730.98, 730.99

C&C Exclusions: (for code 730.03) 015.50, 015.51, 015.52, 015.53, 015.54, 015.55, 015.56, 015.70, 015.71, 015.72, 015.73, 015.74, 015.75, 015.76, 015.90, 015.91, 015.92, 015.93, 015.94, 015.95, 015.96, 017.90, 017.91, 017.92, 017.93, 017.94, 017.95, 017.96, 730.00, 730.08, 730.09, 730.10, 730.13, 730.18, 730.19, 730.20, 730.23, 730.28, 730.29, 730.30, 730.33, 730.38, 730.39, 730.80, 730.83, 730.88, 730.89, 730.90, 730.93, 730.98, 730.99

C&C Exclusions: (for code 730.04) 015.50, 015.51, 015.52, 015.53, 015.54, 015.55, 015.56, 015.70, 015.71, 015.72, 015.73, 015.74, 015.75, 015.76, 015.90, 015.91, 015.92, 015.93, 015.94, 015.95, 015.96, 017.90, 017.91, 017.92, 017.93, 017.94, 017.95, 017.96, 730.00, 730.08, 730.09, 730.10, 730.14, 730.18, 730.19, 730.20, 730.24, 730.28, 730.29, 730.30, 730.34, 730.38, 730.39, 730.80, 730.84, 730.88, 730.89, 730.90, 730.94, 730.98, 730.99

C&C Exclusions: (for code 730.05) 015.50, 015.51, 015.52, 015.53, 015.54, 015.55, 015.56, 015.70, 015.71, 015.72, 015.73, 015.74, 015.75, 015.76, 015.90, 015.91, 015.92, 015.93, 015.94, 015.95, 015.96, 017.90, 017.91, 017.92, 017.93, 017.94, 017.95, 017.96, 730.00, 730.08, 730.09, 730.10, 730.15, 730.18, 730.19, 730.20, 730.25, 730.28,

730.29, 730.30, 730.35, 730.38, 730.39, 730.80, 730.85, 730.88, 730.89, 730.90, 730.95, 730.98, 730.99
C&C Exclusions: (for code 730.06) 015.50, 015.51, 015.52, 015.53, 015.54, 015.55, 015.56, 015.70, 015.71, 015.72, 015.73, 015.74, 015.75, 015.76, 015.90, 015.91, 015.92, 015.93, 015.94, 015.95, 015.96, 017.90, 017.91, 017.92, 017.93, 017.94, 017.95, 017.96, 730.00, 730.08, 730.09, 730.10, 730.16, 730.18, 730.19, 730.20, 730.26, 730.28, 730.29, 730.30, 730.36, 730.38, 730.39, 730.80, 730.86, 730.88, 730.89, 730.90, 730.96, 730.98, 730.99
C&C Exclusions: (for code 730.07) 015.50, 015.51, 015.52, 015.53, 015.54, 015.55, 015.56, 015.70, 015.71, 015.72, 015.73, 015.74, 015.75, 015.76, 015.90, 015.91, 015.92, 015.93, 015.94, 015.95, 015.96, 017.90, 017.91, 017.92, 017.93, 017.94, 017.95, 017.96, 730.00, 730.08, 730.09, 730.10, 730.17, 730.18, 730.19, 730.20, 730.27, 730.28, 730.29, 730.30, 730.37, 730.38, 730.39, 730.80, 730.87, 730.88, 730.89, 730.90, 730.97, 730.98, 730.99
C&C Exclusions: (for code 730.08) 015.00, 015.01, 015.02, 015.03, 015.04, 015.05, 015.06, 015.50, 015.51, 015.52, 015.53, 015.54, 015.55, 015.56, 015.70, 015.71, 015.72, 015.73, 015.74, 015.75, 015.76, 015.90, 015.91, 015.92, 015.93, 015.94, 015.95, 015.96, 017.90, 017.91, 017.92, 017.93, 017.94, 017.95, 017.96, 730.00, 730.01, 730.02, 730.03, 730.04, 730.05, 730.06, 730.07, 730.08, 730.09, 730.10, 730.11, 730.12, 730.13, 730.14, 730.15, 730.16, 730.17, 730.18, 730.19, 730.20, 730.21, 730.22, 730.23, 730.24, 730.25, 730.26, 730.27, 730.28, 730.29, 730.30, 730.31, 730.32, 730.33, 730.34, 730.35, 730.36, 730.37, 730.38, 730.39, 730.80, 730.81, 730.82, 730.83, 730.84, 730.85, 730.86, 730.87, 730.88, 730.89, 730.90, 730.91, 730.92, 730.93, 730.94, 730.95, 730.96, 730.97, 730.98, 730.99

AHA: For Code 730.06: 1Q 2002, 4; For Code 730.07: 1Q 2004, 14

5 **730.1 Chronic osteomyelitis**
[0-9]
(✖ is only valid for fifth-digit "0")
Brodie's abscess
Chronic or old osteomyelitis, with or without mention of periostitis
Sclerosing osteomyelitis of Garré
Sequestrum of bone
Use additional code to identify major osseous defect, if applicable (731.3)
Excludes *aseptic necrosis of bone (733.40-733.49)*
AHA: For Code 730.17: 3Q 2000, 4

5 **730.2 Unspecified osteomyelitis**
[0-9]
(✖ is only valid for fifth-digit "0")
Osteitis or osteomyelitis NOS, with or without mention of periostitis
Use additional code to identify major osseous defect, if applicable (731.3)

5 **730.3 Periostitis without mention of osteomyelitis**
[0-9]
(✖ is only valid for fifth-digit "0")
Abscess of periosteum, without mention of osteomyelitis
Periostosis, without mention of osteomyelitis
Excludes *that in secondary syphilis (091.61)*

+5 ***730.7 Osteopathy resulting from poliomyelitis***
[0-9]
Code first underlying disease (045.0-045.9)

+5 ***730.8 Other infections involving bone in disease classified elsewhere***
[0-9]
Code first underlying disease, as:
tuberculosis (015.0-015.9)
typhoid fever (002.0)
Excludes *syphilitis of bone NOS (095.5)*
C&C Exclusions: (For codes 730.80, 730.89) See 730.00
C&C Exclusions: (for code 730.81) See 730.01
C&C Exclusions: (for code 730.82) See 730.02
C&C Exclusions: (for code 730.83) See 730.03
C&C Exclusions: (for code 730.84) See 730.04
C&C Exclusions: (for code 730.85) See 730.05
C&C Exclusions: (for code 730.86) See 730.06
C&C Exclusions: (for code 730.87) See 730.07
C&C Exclusions: (for code 730.88) See 730.08
AHA: 2Q 1997, 16; 3Q 1991, 10

✖5 **730.9 Unspecified infection of bone**
[0-9]
C&C Exclusions: (For codes 730.90, 730.99) See 730.00
C&C Exclusions: (for code 730.91) See 730.01
C&C Exclusions: (for code 730.92) See 730.02
C&C Exclusions: (for code 730.93) See 730.03
C&C Exclusions: (for code 730.94) See 730.04
C&C Exclusions: (for code 730.95) See 730.05
C&C Exclusions: (for code 730.96) See 730.06
C&C Exclusions: (for code 730.97) See 730 07
C&C Exclusions: (for code 730.98) See 730 08

4 **731 Osteitis deformans and osteopathies associated with other disorders classified elsewhere**

731.0 Osteitis deformans without mention of bone tumor
Paget's disease of bone

+ ***731.1 Osteitis deformans in diseases classified elsewhere***
Code first underlying disease, as:
malignant neoplasm of bone (170.0-170.9)

731.2 Hypertrophic pulmonary osteoarthropathy
Bamberger-Marie disease

731.3 Major osseous defects
Code first underlying disease, if known, such as:
aseptic necrosis (733.40-733.49)
malignant neoplasm of bone (170 0-170.9)
osteomyelitis (730.00-730.29)
osteoporosis (▶733.00-733.09◀)
peri-prosthetic osteolysis (996.45)
AHA: 4Q 2006, 103-104

+ ***731.8 Other bone involvement in diseases classified elsewhere***
Code first underlying disease, as:
diabetes mellitus (250.8)
Use additional code to specify bone condition, such as:
acute osteomyelitis (730.00-730 09)
AHA: 1Q 2004, 14; 4Q 1997, 43; 2Q 1997, 16

4 **732 Osteochondropathies**

732.0 Juvenile osteochondrosis of spine
Juvenile osteochondrosis (of):
marginal or vertebral ephiphysis (of Scheurermann)
spine NOS
Vertebral epiphysitis
Excludes *adolescent postural kyphosis (737.0)*

732.1 Juvenile osteochondrosis of hip and pelvis
Coxa plana
Ischiopubic synchondrosis (of van Neck)
Osteochondrosis (juvenile) of:
acetabulum
head of femur (of Legg-Calvé-Perthes)
iliac crest (of Buchanan)
symphysis pubis (of Pierson)
Pseudocoxalgia

732.2 Nontraumatic slipped upper femoral epiphysis
Slipped upper femoral epiphysis NOS

732.3 Juvenile osteochondrosis of upper extremity
Osteochondrosis (juvenile) of:
capitulum of humerus (of Panner)
carpal lunate (of Kienbock)
hand NOS
head of humerus (of Haas)
heads of metacarpas (of Mauclaire)
lower ulna (of Burns)
radial head (of Brailsford)
upper extremity NOS

732.4 Juvenile osteochondrosis of lower extremity, excluding foot
Osteochondrosis (juvenile) of:
lower extremity NOS
primary patellar center (of Köhler)
proximal tibia (of Blount)
secondary patellar center (of Sinding-Larsen)
tibial tubercle (of Osgood-Schlatter)
Tibia vara

732.5 Juvenile osteochondrosis of foot
Calcaneal apophysitis
Epiphysitis, os calcis
Osteochondrosis (juvenile) of:
astragalus (of Diaz)
calcaneum (of Sever)
foot NOS
metatarsal:
second (of Freilberg)
fifth (of Iselin)
os tibiale externum (of Haglund)
tarsal navicular (of Köhler)

732.6 Other juvenile osteochondrosis
Apophysitis specified as juvenile, of other site, or site NOS
Epiphysitis specified as juvenile, of other site, or site NOS
Osteochondritis specified as juvenile, of other site, or site NOS
Osteochondrosis specified as juvenile, of other site, or site NOS

732.7 Osteochondritis dissecans

732.8 Other specified forms of osteochondropathy
Adult osteochondrosis of spine

732.9 Unspecified osteochondropathy
Apophysitis:
NOS
not specified as adult or juvenile, of unspecified site
Epiphysitis:
NOS
not specified as adult or juvenile, of unspecified site
Osteochondritis:
NOS
not specified as adult or juvenile, of unspecified site
Osteochondrosis:
NOS
not specified as adult or juvenile, of unspecified site

❹ **733 Other disorders of bone and cartilage**
Excludes *bone spur (726.91)*
cartilage of, or loose body in, joint (717.0-717.9, 718.0-718.9)
giant cell granuloma of jaw (526.3)
osteitis fibrosa cystica generalisata (252.01)
osteomalacia (268.2)
polyostotic fibrous dysplasia of bone (756.54)
prognathism, retrognathism (524.1)
xanthomatosis localized to bone (272.7)

❺ **733.0 Osteoporosis**
Use additional code to identify major osseous defect, if applicable (731.3)

733.00 Osteoporosis, unspecified
Wedging of vertebra NOS
AHA: 1Q 2007, 22; 3Q 2001, 19; 2Q 1998, 12

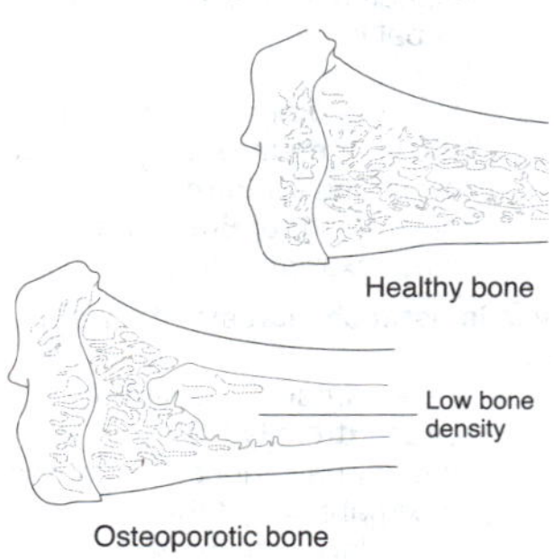

733.01 Senile osteoporosis
Postmenopausal osteoporosis
AHA: 1Q 2007, 5, 6

733.02 Idiopathic osteoporosis

733.03 Disuse osteoporosis

733.09 Other
Drug-induced osteoporosis
Use additional E code to identify drug

❺ **733.1 Pathologic fracture**
Spontaneous fracture
Excludes *stress fracture (733.93-733.95)*
traumatic fractures (800-829)
AHA: 4Q 1993, 25; Nov-Dec 1986, 10; Nov-Dec 1985, 16

✖ **733.10 Pathologic fracture, unspecified site**
C&C Exclusions: 733.10, 733.11, 733.12, 733.13, 733.14, 733.15, 733.16, 733.19, 733.93, 733.94, 733.95

733.11 Pathologic fracture of humerus
C&C Exclusions: See 733.10

733.12 Pathologic fracture of distal radius and ulna
Wrist NOS
C&C Exclusions: See 733.10

733.13 Pathologic fracture of vertebrae
Collapse of vertebra NOS
C&C Exclusions: See 733.10
AHA: 1Q 2007, 5, 6, 22; 3Q 1999, 5

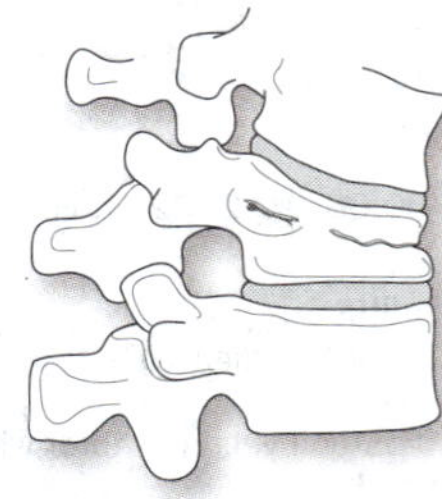

733.14 Pathologic fracture of neck of femur
Femur NOS
Hip NOS
C&C Exclusions: See 733.10
AHA: 1Q 2001, 1; 1Q 1996, 16

733.15 Pathologic fracture of other specified part of femur
C&C Exclusions: See 733.10
AHA: 2Q 1998, 12

733.16 Pathologic fracture of tibia and fibula
Ankle NOS
C&C Exclusions: See 733.10

733.19 Pathologic fracture of other specified site
C&C Exclusions: See 733.10

❺ **733.2 Cyst of bone**

733.20 Cyst of bone (localized), unspecified

733.21 Solitary bone cyst
Unicameral bone cyst

733.22 Aneurysmal bone cyst

733.29 Other
Fibrous dysplasia (monostotic)
Excludes *cyst of jaw (526.0-526.2, 526.89)*
osteitis fibrosa cystica (252.01)
polyostotic fibrous dysplasia of bone (756.54)

733.3 Hyperostosis of skull
Hyperostosis interna frontalis
Leontiasis ossium

❺ **733.4 Aseptic necrosis of bone**
Use additional code to identify major osseous defect, if applicable (731.3)
Excludes *osteochondropathies (732.0-732.9)*

✖ **733.40 Aseptic necrosis of bone, site unspecified**

733.41 Head of humerus

733.42 Head and neck of femur
Femur NOS
Excludes *Legg-Calvé-Perthes disease (732.1)*

733.43 Medial femoral condyle

733.44 Talus

● **733.45 Jaw**
Use additional E code to identify drug, if drug-induced
Excludes *osteoradionecrosis of jaw (526.89)*
DEF: The death of jaw bone tissue that can develop where the jaw fails to heal from minor trauma, such as a tooth extraction that exposes the bone.

733.49 Other

733.5 Osteitis condensans
Piriform sclerosis of ilium

733.6 Tietze's disease
Costochondral junction syndrome
Costochondritis

733.7 Algoneurodystrophy
Disuse atrophy of bone
Sudeck's atrophy

⑤ **733.8 Malunion and nonunion of fracture**
AHA: 2Q 1994, 5

733.81 Malunion of fracture
C&C Exclusions: 733.81, 733.82

733.82 Nonunion of fracture
Pseudoarthrosis (bone)
C&C Exclusions: See 733.81

⑤ **733.9 Other and unspecified disorders of bone and cartilage**

✖ **733.90 Disorder of bone and cartilage, unspecified**

733.91 Arrest of bone development or growth
Epiphyseal arrest

733.92 Chondromalacia
Chondromalacia:
NOS
localized, except patella
systemic
tibial plateau
Excludes *chondromalacia of patella (717.7)*
DEF: Joint cartilage softens and degenerates, causing tenderness, pain, and a grinding sensation.

733.93 Stress fracture of tibia or fibula
Stress reaction of tibia or fibula
C&C Exclusions: 733.10, 733.11, 733.12, 733.13, 733.14, 733.15, 733.16, 733.19, 733.93, 733.94, 733.95, 805.8, 805.9, 806.00, 806.01, 806.02, 806.03, 806.04, 806.05, 806.06, 806.07, 806.08, 806.09, 806.10, 806.11, 806.12, 806.13, 806.14, 806.15, 806.16, 806.17, 806.18, 806.19, 806.20, 806.21, 806.22, 806.23, 806.24, 806.25, 806.26, 806.27, 806.28, 806.29, 806.30, 806.31, 806.32, 806.33, 806.34, 806.35, 806.36, 806.37, 806.38, 806.39, 806.4, 806.5, 806.60, 806.61, 806.62, 806.69, 806.70, 806.71, 806.72, 806.79, 806.8, 806.9, 808.0, 808.2, 808.3, 808.43, 808.49, 808.51, 808.52, 808.53, 808.59, 808.8, 808.9, 820.00, 820.01, 820.02, 820.03, 820.09, 820.10, 820.11, 820.12, 820.13, 820.19, 820.20, 820.21, 820.22, 820.30, 820.31, 820.32, 820.8, 820.9, 821.00, 821.01, 821.10, 821.11
AHA: 4Q 2001, 48

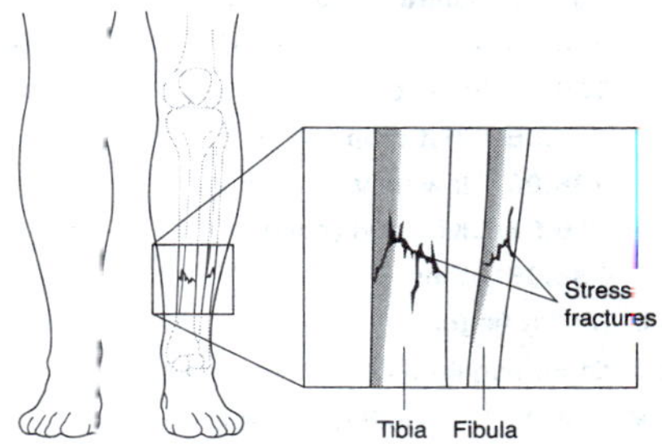

733.94 Stress fracture of the metatarsals
Stress reaction of metatarsals
C&C Exclusions: See 733.93
AHA: 4Q 2001, 48

733.95 Stress fracture of other bone
Stress reaction of other bone
C&C Exclusions: See 733.93
AHA: 4Q 2001, 48

733.99 Other
Diaphysitis
Hypertrophy of bone
Relapsing polychondritis
AHA: Jan-Feb 1987, 14

734 Flat foot
Pes planus (acquired)
Talipes planus (acquired)
Excludes *congenital (754.61)*
rigid flat foot (754.61)
spastic (everted) flat foot (754.61)

④ **735 Acquired deformities of toe**
Excludes *congenital (754.60-754.69, 755.65-755.66)*

735.0 Hallux valgus (acquired)

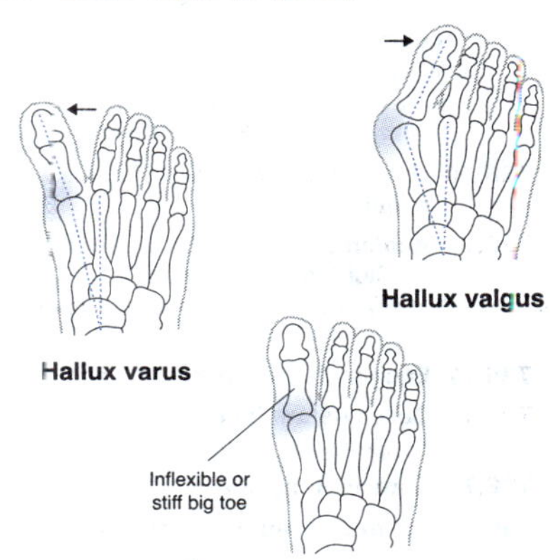

735.1 Hallux varus (acquired)
DEF: The big toe is pointed away from the rest of the toes.

735.2 Hallux rigidus

735.3 Hallux malleus

735.4 Other hammer toe (acquired)

735.5 Claw toe (acquired)

735.8 Other acquired deformities of toe

✖ **735.9 Unspecified acquired deformity of toe**

❹ **736 Other acquired deformities of limbs**
Excludes *congenital (754.3-755.9)*

❺ **736.0 Acquired deformities of forearm, excluding fingers**

✖ **736.00 Unspecified deformity**
Deformity of elbow, forearm, hand, or wrist (acquired) NOS

736.01 Cubitus valgus (acquired)

736.02 Cubitus varus (acquired)

736.03 Valgus deformity of wrist (acquired)

736.04 Varus deformity of wrist (acquired)

736.05 Wrist drop (acquired)

736.06 Claw hand (acquired)

736.07 Club hand (acquired)

736.09 Other

736.1 Mallet finger

❺ **736.2 Other acquired deformities of finger**

✖ **736.20 Unspecified deformity**
Deformity of finger (acquired) NOS

736.21 Boutonniere deformity

736.22 Swan-neck deformity

736.29 Other
Excludes *trigger finger (727.03)*
AHA: 2Q 2005, 7; 2Q 1989, 13

❺ **736.3 Acquired deformities of hip**

✖ **736.30 Unspecified deformity**
Deformity of hip (acquired) NOS

736.31 Coxa valga (acquired)

736.32 Coxa vara (acquired)

736.39 Other
AHA: 2Q 1991, 18

❺ **736.4 Genu valgum or varum (acquired)**

736.41 Genu valgum (acquired)
DEF: Deformity in which the knees are abnormally close together and the ankles are far apart when standing erect.

736.42 Genu varum (acquired)

736.5 Genu recurvatum (acquired)

736.6 Other acquired deformities of knee
Deformity of knee (acquired) NOS

❺ **736.7 Other acquired deformities of ankle and foot**
Excludes *deformities of toe (acquired) (735.0-735.9)*
pes planus (acquired) (734)

✖ **736.70 Unspecified deformity of ankle and foot, acquired**

736.71 Acquired equinovarus deformity
Clubfoot, acquired
Excludes *clubfoot not specified as acquired (754.5-754.7)*

736.72 Equinus deformity of foot, acquired

736.73 Cavus deformity of foot
Excludes *that with claw foot (736.74)*

736.74 Claw foot, acquired

736.75 Cavovarus deformity of foot, acquired

736.76 Other calcaneus deformity

736.79 Other
Acquired:
pes not elsewhere classified
talipes not elsewhere classified

❺ **736.8 Acquired deformities of other parts of limbs**

736.81 Unequal leg length (acquired)

736.89 Other
Deformity (acquired):
arm or leg, not elsewhere classified
shoulder

✖ **736.9 Acquired deformity of limb, site unspecified**

❹ **737 Curvature of spine**
Excludes *congenital (754.2)*

737.0 Adolescent postural kyphosis
Excludes *osteochondrosis of spine (juvenile) (732.0)*
adult (732.8)

❺ **737.1 Kyphosis (acquired)**

737.10 Kyphosis (acquired) (postural)

737.11 Kyphosis due to radiation

737.12 Kyphosis, postlaminectomy
AHA: Jan-Feb 1987, 7

737.19 Other
Excludes *that associated with conditions classifiable elsewhere (737.41)*
AHA: 1Q 2007, 21

❺ **737.2 Lordosis (acquired)**

737.20 Lordosis (acquired) (postural)

737.21 Lordosis, postlaminectomy

737.22 Other postsurgical lordosis

737.29 Other
Excludes *that associated with conditions classifiable elsewhere (737.42)*

❺ **737.3 Kyphoscoliosis and scoliosis**

737.30 Scoliosis [and kyphoscoliosis], idiopathic
AHA: 3Q 2003, 19

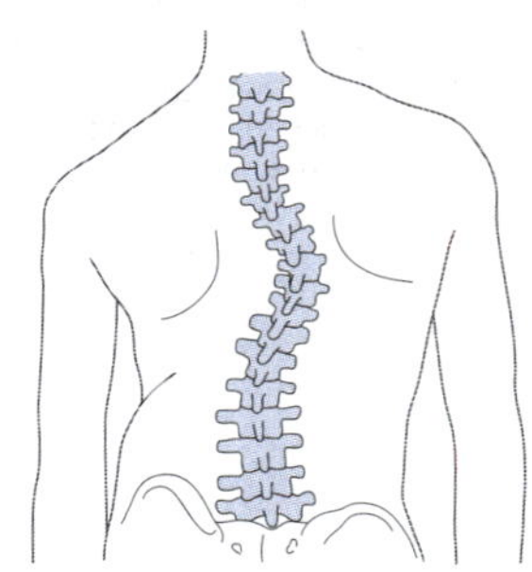

737.31 Resolving infantile idiopathic scoliosis

737.32 Progressive infantile idiopathic scoliosis
AHA: 3Q 2002, 12

737.33 Scoliosis due to radiation

737.34 Thoracogenic scoliosis

737.39 Other
Excludes *that associated with conditions classifiable elsewhere (737.43)*
that in kyphoscoliotic heart disease (416.1)
AHA: 2Q 2002, 16

737.4 Curvature of spine associated with other conditions
Code first associated condition, as:
Charcôt-Marie-Tooth disease (356.1)
mucopolysaccharidosis (277.5)
neurofibromatosis (237.7)
osteitis deformans (731.0)
osteitis fibrosa cystica (252.01)
osteoporosis (733.00-733.09)
poliomyelitis (138)
tuberculosis [Pott's curvature] (015.0)

+ ***737.40 Curvature of spine, unspecified***

+ ***737.41 Kyphosis***

+ ***737.42 Lordosis***

+ ***737.43 Scoliosis***

737.8 Other curvatures of spine

737.9 Unspecified curvature of spine
Curvature of spine (acquired) (idiopathic) NOS
Hunchback, acquired
Excludes *deformity of spine NOS (738.5)*

738 Other acquired deformity
Excludes *congenital (754.0-756.9, 758.0-759.9)*
dentofacial anomalies (524.0-524.9)

738.0 Acquired deformity of nose
Deformity of nose (acquired)
Overdevelopment of nasal bones
Excludes *deflected or deviated nasal septum (470)*

738.1 Other acquired deformity of head

738.10 Unspecified deformity

738.11 Zygomatic hyperplasia

738.12 Zygomatic hypoplasia

738.19 Other specified deformity
AHA: 1Q 2006, 2; 2Q 2003, 13

738.2 Acquired deformity of neck

738.3 Acquired deformity of chest and rib
Deformity:
chest (acquired)
rib (acquired)
Pectus:
carinatum, acquired
excavatum, acquired

738.4 Acquired spondylolisthesis
Degenerative spondylolisthesis
Spondylolysis, acquired
Excludes *congenital (756.12)*
AHA: 1Q 2007, 10

738.5 Other acquired deformity of back or spine
Deformity of spine NOS
Excludes *curvature of spine (737.0-737.9)*

738.6 Acquired deformity of pelvis
Pelvic obliquity
Excludes *intrapelvic protrusion of acetabulum (718.6)*
that in relation to labor and delivery (653.0-653.4, 653.8-653.9)

738.7 Cauliflower ear

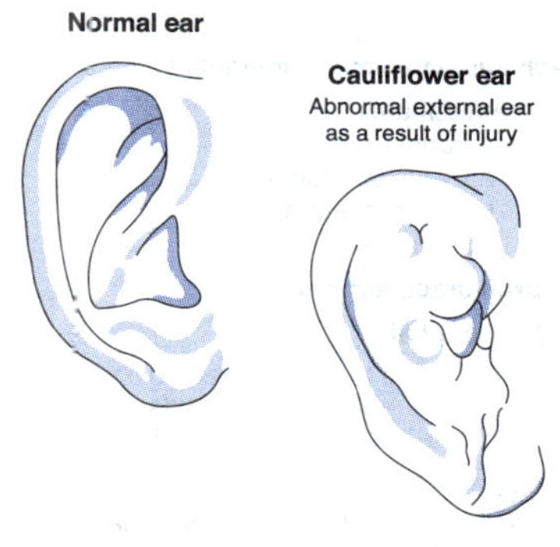

738.8 Acquired deformity of other specified site
Deformity of clavicle
AHA: 2Q 2001, 15

738.9 Acquired deformity of unspecified site

739 Nonallopathic lesions, not elsewhere classified
Includes segmental dysfunction
somatic dysfunction

739.0 Head region
Occipitocervical region

739.1 Cervical region
Cervicothoracic region

739.2 Thoracic region
Thoracolumbar region

739.3 Lumbar region
Lumbosacral region

739.4 Sacral region
Sacrococcygeal region
Sacroiliac region

739.5 Pelvic region
Hip region
Pubic region

739.6 Lower extremities

739.7 Upper extremities
Acromioclavicular region
Sternoclavicular region

739.8 Rib cage
Costochondral region
Costovertebral region
Sternochondral region

739.9 Abdomen and other
AHA: 2Q 1989, 14

14. CONGENITAL ANOMALIES (740-759)

❹ 740 Anencephalus and similar anomalies

740.0 Anencephalus
Acrania
Amyelencephalus
Hemianencephaly
Hemicephaly

740.1 Craniorachischisis

740.2 Iniencephaly
DEF: Neural tube birth defect in which the fetal head is severely bent backwards, the neck is usually absent, and other severe birth defects are present.

❹ 741 Spina bifida
Excludes *spina bifida occulta (756.17)*
AHA: 3Q 1994, 7

The following fifth-digit subclassification is for use with category 741:
0 unspecified region
1 cervical region
2 dorsal (thoracic) region
3 lumbar region

❺ 741.0 With hydrocephalus
(✖ is only valid for fifth-digit "0")
Arnold-Chiari syndrome, type II
Chiari malformation, type II
Any condition classifiable to 741.9 with any condition classifiable to 742.3
C&C Exclusions: 741.00, 741.01, 741.02, 741.03, 741.90, 741.91, 741.92, 741.93, 742.59, 742.8, 742.9, 759.7, 759.81, 759.82, 759.83, 759.89
AHA: 4Q 1997, 51; 4Q 1994, 37; Sep-Oct 1987, 10

❺ 741.9 Without mention of hydrocephalus
(✖ is only valid for fifth-digit "0")
Hydromeningocele (spinal)
Hydromyelocele
Meningocele (spinal)
Meningomyelocele
Myelocele
Myelocystocele
Rachischisis
Spina bifida (aperta)
Syringomyelocele
C&C Exclusions: See 741.0

❹ 742 Other congenital anomalies of nervous system
Excludes *congenital central alveolar hypoventilation syndrome (327.25)*

742.0 Encephalocele
Encephalocystocele
Encephalomyelocele
Hydroencephalocele
Hydromeningocele, cranial
Meningocele, cerebral
Meningoencephalocele
DEF: Part of the cranial contents protrudes through a defect in the skull.
AHA: 4Q 1994, 37

742.1 Microcephalus
Hydromicrocephaly
Micrencephaly

742.2 Reduction deformities of brain
Absence of part of brain
Agenesis of part of brain
Agyria
Aplasia of part of brain
Arhinencephaly
Holoprosencephaly
Hypoplasia of part of brain
Microgyria
AHA: 3Q 2003, 15; 4Q 1994, 37

742.3 Congenital hydrocephalus
Aqueduct of Sylvius:
  anomaly
  obstruction, congenital
  stenosis
Atresia of foramina of Magendie and Luschka
Hydrocephalus in newborn
Excludes *hydrocephalus:*
  acquired (331.3-331.4)
  due to congenital toxoplasmosis (771.2)
  with any condition classifiable to 741.9 (741.0)
AHA: 4Q 2005, 83

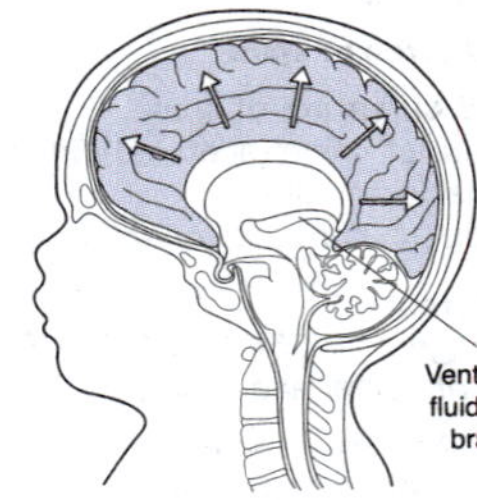

742.4 Other specified anomalies of brain
Congenital cerebral cyst
Macroencephaly
Macrogyria
Megalencephaly
Multiple anomalies of brain NOS
Porencephaly
Ulegyria
AHA: 1Q 1999, 9; 3Q 1992, 12

❺ 742.5 Other specified anomalies of spinal cord

742.51 Diastematomyelia

742.53 Hydromyelia
Hydrorhachis

742.59 Other
Amyelia
Atelomyelia
Congenital anomaly of spinal meninges
Defective development of cauda equina
Hypoplasia of spinal cord
Myelatelia
Myelodysplasia
AHA: 2Q 1991, 14; 1Q 1989, 10

742.8 Other specified anomalies of nervous system
Agenesis of nerve
Displacement of brachial plexus
Familial dysautonomia
Jaw-winking syndrome
Marcus-Gunn syndrome
Riley-Day syndrome
Excludes *neurofibromatosis (237.7)*

✖ 742.9 Unspecified anomaly of brain, spinal cord, and nervous system
Anomaly of brain, nervous system, and spinal cord
Congenital, of brain, nervous system, and spinal cord:
  disease of brain, nervous system, and spinal cord
  lesion of brain, nervous system, and spinal cord
Deformity of brain, nervous system, and spinal cord

❹ 743 Congenital anomalies of eye

❺ 743.0 Anophthalmos

743.00 Clinical anophthalmos, unspecified
Agenesis
Anophthalmos NOS
Congenital absence of eye

743.03 Cystic eyeball, congenital

743.06 Cryptophthalmos

743.1 Microphthalmos
Dysplasia of eye
Hypoplasia of eye
Rudimentary eye

743.10 Microphthalmos, unspecified

743.11 Simple microphthalmos

743.12 Microphthalmos associated with other anomalies of eye and adnexa

743.2 Buphthalmos
Glaucoma:
congenital
newborn
Hydrophthalmos
Excludes *glaucoma of childhood (365.14)*
traumatic glaucoma due to birth injury (767.8)

743.20 Buphthalmos, unspecified

743.21 Simple buphthalmos

743.22 Buphthalmos associated with other ocular anomalies
Keratoglobus, congenital, associated with buphthalmos
Megalocornea associated with buphthalmos

743.3 Congenital cataract and lens anomalies
Excludes *infantile cataract (366.00-366.09)*

743.30 Congenital cataract, unspecified

743.31 Capsular and subcapsular cataract

743.32 Cortical and zonular cataract

743.33 Nuclear cataract

743.34 Total and subtotal cataract, congenital

743.35 Congenital aphakia
Congenital absence of lens

743.36 Anomalies of lens shape
Microphakia
Spherophakia

743.37 Congenital ectopic lens

743.39 Other

743.4 Coloboma and other anomalies of anterior segment

743.41 Anomalies of corneal size and shape
Microcornea
Excludes *that associated with buphthalmos (743.22)*

743.42 Corneal opacities, interfering with vision, congenital

743.43 Other corneal opacities, congenital

743.44 Specified anomalies of anterior chamber, chamber angle, and related structures
Anomaly:
Axenfeld's
Peters'
Rieger's

743.45 Aniridia
DEF: Underdeveloped or completely absent iris.
AHA: 3Q 2002, 20

743.46 Other specified anomalies of iris and ciliary body
Anisocoria, congenital
Atresia of pupil
Coloboma of iris
Corectopia

743.47 Specified anomalies of sclera

743.48 Multiple and combined anomalies of anterior segment

743.49 Other

743.5 Congenital anomalies of posterior segment

743.51 Vitreous anomalies
Congenital vitreous opacity

743.52 Fundus coloboma

743.53 Chorioretinal degeneration, congenital

743.54 Congenital folds and cysts of posterior segment

743.55 Congenital macular changes

743.56 Other retinal changes, congenital
AHA: 3Q 1999, 12

743.57 Specified anomalies of optic disc
Coloboma of optic disc (congenital)

743.58 Vascular anomalies
Congenital retinal aneurysm

743.59 Other

743.6 Congenital anomalies of eyelids, lacrimal system, and orbit

743.61 Congenital ptosis
DEF: Congenital drooping of the upper eyelid.

743.62 Congenital deformities of eyelids
Ablepharon
Absence of eyelid
Accessory eyelid
Congenital:
ectropion
entropion
AHA: 1Q 2000, 22

743.63 Other specified congenital anomalies of eyelid
Absence, agenesis, of cilia

743.64 Specified congenital anomalies of lacrimal gland

743.65 Specified congenital anomalies of lacrimal passages
Absence, agenesis of:
lacrimal apparatus
punctum lacrimale
Accessory lacrimal canal

743.66 Specified congenital anomalies of orbit

743.69 Other
Accessory eye muscles

743.8 Other specified anomalies of eye
Excludes *congenital nystagmus (379.51)*
ocular albinism (270.2)
optic nerve hypoplasia (377.43)
retinitis pigmentosa (362.74)

743.9 Unspecified anomaly of eye
Congenital:
anomaly NOS of eye [any part]
deformity NOS of eye [any part]

744 Congenital anomalies of ear, face, and neck
Excludes *anomaly of:*
cervical spine (754.2, 756.10-756.19)
larynx (748.2-748.3)
nose (748.0-748.1)
parathyroid gland (759.2)
thyroid gland (759.2)
cleft lip (749.10-749.25)

744.0 Anomalies of ear causing impairment of hearing
Excludes *congenital deafness without mention of cause (380.0-389.9)*

744.00 Unspecified anomaly of ear with impairment of hearing

744.01 Absence of external ear
Absence of:
auditory canal (external)
auricle (ear) (with stenosis or atresia of auditory canal)

744.02 Other anomalies of external ear with impairment of hearing
Atresia or stricture of auditory canal (external)

744.03 Anomaly of middle ear, except ossicles
Atresia or stricture of osseous meatus (ear)

744.04 Anomalies of ear ossicles
Fusion of ear ossicles

744.05 Anomalies of inner ear
Congenital anomaly of:
membranous labyrinth
organ of Corti

744.09 Other
Absence of ear, congenital

744.1 Accessory auricle
Accessory tragus
Polyotia
Preauricular appendage
Supernumerary:
ear
lobule

❺ **744.2 Other specified anomalies of ear**
Excludes *that with impairment of hearing (744.00-744.09)*

744.21 Absence of ear lobe, congenital

744.22 Macrotia

744.23 Microtia

744.24 Specified anomalies of Eustachian tube
Absence of Eustachian tube

744.29 Other
Bat ear
Darwin's tubercle
Pointed ear
Prominence of auricle
Ridge ear
Excludes *preauricular sinus (744.46)*

744.3 Unspecified anomaly of ear
Congenital:
anomaly NOS of ear, NEC
deformity NOS of ear, NEC

❺ **744.4 Branchial cleft cyst or fistula, preauricular sinus**

744.41 Branchial cleft sinus or fistula
Branchial:
sinus (external) (internal)
vestige

744.42 Branchial cleft cyst

744.43 Cervical auricle

744.46 Preauricular sinus or fistula

744.47 Preauricular cyst

744.49 Other
Fistula (of):
auricle, congenital
cervicoaural

744.5 Webbing of neck
Pterygium colli
DEF: A thick flap of skin extending from the side of the neck to the shoulder, often in concert with other birth defects.

❺ **744.8 Other specified anomalies of face and neck**

744.81 Macrocheilia
Hypertrophy of lip, congenital
DEF: Abnormally large lips.

744.82 Microcheilia

744.83 Macrostomia

744.84 Microstomia
DEF: Abnormally small mouth.

744.89 Other
Excludes *congenital fistula of lip (750.25)*
musculoskeletal anomalies (754.0-754.1, 756.0)

✖ **744.9 Unspecified anomalies of face and neck**
Congenital:
anomaly NOS of face [any part] or neck [any part]
deformity NOS of face [any part] or neck [any part]

❹ **745 Bulbus cordis anomalies and anomalies of cardiac septal closure**

745.0 Common truncus
Absent septum between aorta and pulmonary artery
Aortic septal defect
Common aortopulmonary trunk
Communication (abnormal) between aorta and pulmonary artery
Persistent truncus arteriosus
C&C Exclusions: 429.71, 429.79, 745.0, 745.10, 745.11, 745.12, 745.19, 745.2, 745.3, 745.4, 745.5, 745.60, 745.61, 745.69, 745.7, 745.8, 745.9, 746.89, 746.9, 747.83, 747.89, 747.9, 759.7, 759.81, 759.82, 759.83, 759.89

❺ **745.1 Transposition of great vessels**

745.10 Complete transposition of great vessels
Transposition of great vessels:
NOS
classical
C&C Exclusions: See 745.0

745.11 Double outlet right ventricle
Dextratransposition of aorta
Incomplete transposition of great vessels
Origin of both great vessels from right ventricle
Taussig-Bing syndrome or defect
C&C Exclusions: See 745.0

745.12 Corrected transposition of great vessels
C&C Exclusions: See 745.0

745.19 Other
C&C Exclusions: See 745.0

745.2 Tetralogy of Fallot
Fallot's pentalogy
Ventricular septal defect with pulmonary stenosis or atresia, dextraposition of aorta, and hypertrophy of right ventricle
Excludes *Fallot's triad (746.09)*

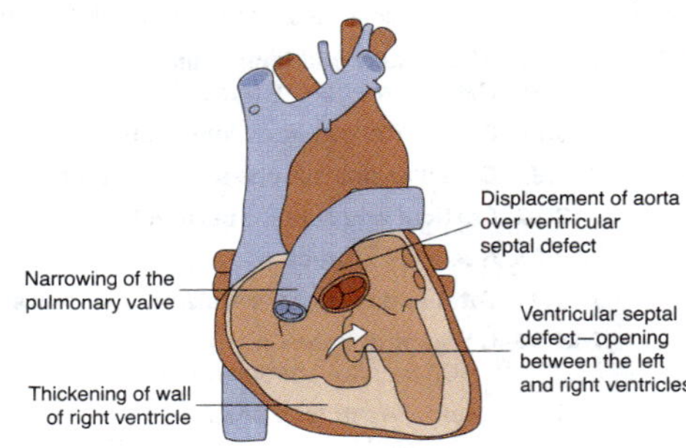

745.3 Common ventricle
Cor triloculare biatriatum
Single ventricle
DEF: No septum or membrane is present dividing the right ventricle from the left ventricle.
C&C Exclusions: See 745.0

745.4 Ventricular septal defect
Eisenmenger's defect or complex
Gerbode defect
Interventricular septal defect
Left ventricular-right atrial communication
Roger's disease
Excludes *common atrioventricular canal type (745.69)*
single ventricle (745.3)
C&C Exclusions: See 745.0

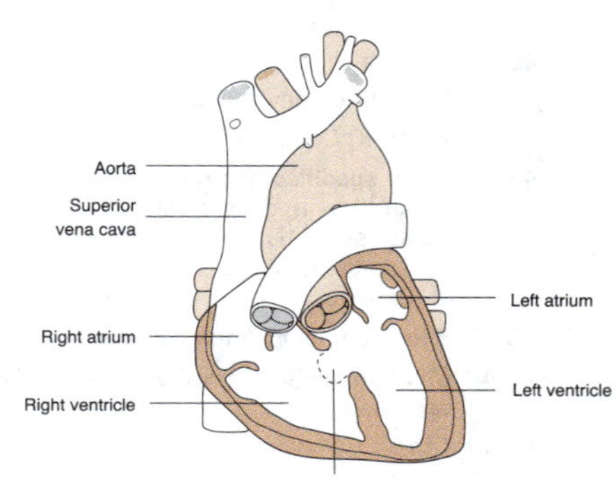

Abnormality of the membrane that divides the right and left heart ventricles

❹ ❺ Additional Digit Required ✖ Nonspecific PDx ⊘ Unacceptable PDx ✚ Manifestation Code ►◄ Revised Text ● New Code ▲ Revised Code

745.5 Ostium secundum type atrial septal defect
Defect:
atrium secundum
fossa ovalis
Lutembacher's syndrome
Patent or persistent:
foramen ovale
ostium secundum

⑤ **745.6 Endocardial cushion defects**

745.60 Endocardial cushion defect, unspecified type
C&C Exclusions: See 745.0

745.61 Ostium primum defect
Persistent ostium primum

745.69 Other
Absence of atrial septum
Atrioventricular canal type ventricular septal defect
Common atrioventricular canal
Common atrium
C&C Exclusions: See 745.0

745.7 Cor biloculare
Absence of atrial and ventricular septa
C&C Exclusions: See 745.0

745.8 Other

✖ **745.9 Unspecified defect of septal closure**
Septal defect NOS

④ **746 Other congenital anomalies of heart**
Excludes *endocardial fibroelastosis (425.3)*

⑤ **746.0 Anomalies of pulmonary valve**
Excludes *infundibular or subvalvular pulmonic stenosis (746.83)*
tetralogy of Fallot (745.2)

746.00 Pulmonary valve anomaly, unspecified

746.01 Atresia, congenital
Congenital absence of pulmonary valve
C&C Exclusions: 746.00, 746.01, 746.02, 746.09, 746.89, 746.9, 747.83, 747.89, 747.9, 759.7, 759.81, 759.82, 759.83, 759.89

746.02 Stenosis, congenital
C&C Exclusions: See 746.01

746.09 Other
Congenital insufficiency of pulmonary valve
Fallot's triad or trilogy

746.1 Tricuspid atresia and stenosis, congenital
Absence of tricuspid valve
C&C Exclusions: 746.1, 746.2, 746.3, 746.4, 746.5, 746.6, 746.7, 746.89, 746.9, 747.83, 747.89, 747.9, 759.7, 759.81, 759.82, 759.83, 759.89

746.2 Ebstein's anomaly
C&C Exclusions: See 746.1

746.3 Congenital stenosis of aortic valve
Congenital aortic stenosis
Excludes *congenital:*
subaortic stenosis (746.81)
supravalvular aortic stenosis (747.22)
C&C Exclusions: See 746.1
AHA: 4Q 1988, 8

746.4 Congenital insufficiency of aortic valve
Bicuspid aortic valve
Congenital aortic insufficiency
C&C Exclusions: See 746.1

746.5 Congenital mitral stenosis
Fused commissure of mitral valve
Parachute deformity of mitral valve
Supernumerary cusps of mitral valve
C&C Exclusions: See 746.1

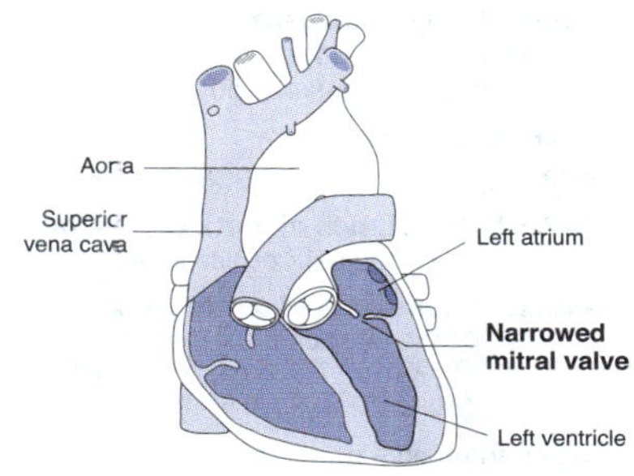

746.6 Congenital mitral insufficiency
C&C Exclusions: See 746.1

746.7 Hypoplastic left heart syndrome
Atresia, or marked hypoplasia, of aortic orifice or valve, with hypoplasia of ascending aorta and defective development of left ventricle (with mitral valve atresia)
C&C Exclusions: See 746.1

⑤ **746.8 Other specified anomalies of heart**

746.81 Subaortic stenosis
C&C Exclusions: 746.81, 746.82, 746.83, 746.84, 746.89, 746.9, 747.83, 747.89, 747.9, 759.7, 759.81, 759.82, 759.83, 759.89

746.82 Cor triatriatum
DEF: The heart has three atrial chambers with the left atrium divided into two segments.
C&C Exclusions: See 746.81

746.83 Infundibular pulmonic stenosis
Subvalvular pulmonic stenosis
C&C Exclusions: See 746.81

746.84 Obstructive anomalies of heart, NEC
Uhl's disease
C&C Exclusions: See 746.81

746.85 Coronary artery anomaly
Anomalous origin or communication of coronary artery
Arteriovenous malformation of coronary artery
Coronary artery:
absence
arising from aorta or pulmonary trunk
single
AHA: Nov-Dec 1985, 3

746.86 Congenital heart block
Complete or incomplete atrioventricular [AV] block
C&C Exclusions: 746.86, 746.89, 746.9, 747.83, 747.89, 747.9, 759.7, 759.81, 759.82, 759.83, 759.89

746.87 Malposition of heart and cardiac apex
Abdominal heart
Dextrocardia
Ectopia cordis
Levocardia (isolated)
Mesocardia
Excludes *dextrocardia with complete transposition of viscera (759.3)*

746.89 Other
Atresia of cardiac vein
Congenital:
cardiomegaly
diverticulum, left ventricle
pericardial defect
Hypoplasia of cardiac vein
AHA: 3Q 2000, 3; 1Q 1999, 11; Jan-Feb 1985, 3

✖ **746.9 Unspecified anomaly of heart**
Congenital:
anomaly of heart NOS
heart disease NOS

❹ **747 Other congenital anomalies of circulatory system**

747.0 Patent ductus arteriosus
Patent ductus Botalli
Persistent ductus arteriosus

❺ **747.1 Coarctation of aorta**
AHA: 1Q 1999, 11; 4Q 1988, 8

747.10 Coarctation of aorta (preductal) (postductal)
Hypoplasia of aortic arch

747.11 Interruption of aortic arch
C&C Exclusions: 747.10, 747.11, 747.20, 747.21, 747.22, 747.83, 747.89, 747.9, 759.7, 759.81, 759.82, 759.83, 759.89

❺ **747.2 Other anomalies of aorta**

747.20 Anomaly of aorta, unspecified

747.21 Anomalies of aortic arch
Anomalous origin, right subclavian artery
Dextraposition of aorta
Double aortic arch
Kommerell's diverticulum
Overriding aorta
Persistent:
convolutions, aortic arch
right aortic arch
Vascular ring
Excludes *hypoplasia of aortic arch (747.10)*
AHA: 1Q 2003, 15

747.22 Atresia and stenosis of aorta
Absence of aorta
Aplasia of aorta
Hypoplasia of aorta
Stricture of aorta
Supra (valvular)-aortic stenosis
Excludes *congenital aortic (valvular) stenosis or stricture, so stated (746.3)*
hypoplasia of aorta in hypoplastic left heart syndrome (746.7)
C&C Exclusions: See 747.11

747.29 Other
Aneurysm of sinus of Valsalva
Congenital:
aneurysm of aorta
dilation of aorta

747.3 Anomalies of pulmonary artery
Agenesis of pulmonary artery
Anomaly of pulmonary artery
Atresia of pulmonary artery
Coarctation of pulmonary artery
Hypoplasia of pulmonary artery
Pulmonary arteriovenous aneurysm
Stenosis of pulmonary artery
AHA: 1Q 1994, 15; 4Q 1988, 8

❺ **747.4 Anomalies of great veins**

747.40 Anomaly of great veins, unspecified
Anomaly NOS of:
pulmonary veins
vena cava

747.41 Total anomalous pulmonary venous connection
Total anomalous pulmonary venous return [TAPVR]:
subdiaphragmatic
supradiaphragmatic

747.42 Partial anomalous pulmonary venous connection
Partial anomalous pulmonary venous return

747.49 Other anomalies of great veins
Absence of vena cava (inferior) (superior)
Congenital stenosis of vena cava (inferior) (superior)
Persistent:
left posterior cardinal vein
left superior vena cava
Scimitar syndrome
Transposition of pulmonary veins NOS

747.5 Absence or hypoplasia of umbilical artery
Single umbilical artery

❺ **747.6 Other anomalies of peripheral vascular system**
Absence of artery or vein, NEC
Anomaly of artery or vein, NEC
Atresia of artery or vein, NEC
Arteriovenous aneurysm (peripheral)
Arteriovenous malformation of the peripheral vascular system
Congenital:
aneurysm (peripheral)
phlebectasia
stricture, artery
varix
Multiple renal arteries
Excludes *anomalies of:*
cerebral vessels (747.81)
pulmonary artery (747.3)
congenital retinal aneurysm (743.58)
hemangioma (228.00-228.09)
lymphangioma (228.1)

✖ **747.60 Anomaly of the peripheral vascular system, unspecified site**

747.61 Gastrointestinal vessel anomaly
AHA: 3Q 1996, 10

747.62 Renal vessel anomaly

747.63 Upper limb vessel anomaly

747.64 Lower limb vessel anomaly

747.69 Anomalies of other specified sites of peripheral vascular system

❺ **747.8 Other specified anomalies of circulatory system**

747.81 Anomalies of cerebrovascular system
Arteriovenous malformation of brain
Cerebral arteriovenous aneurysm, congenital
Congenital anomalies of cerebral vessels
Excludes *ruptured cerebral (arteriovenous) aneurysm (430)*

747.82 Spinal vessel anomaly
Arteriovenous malformation of spinal vessel
AHA: 3Q 1995, 5

747.83 Persistent fetal circulation N
Persistent pulmonary hypertension
Primary pulmonary hypertension of newborn
C&C Exclusions: 429.71, 429.79, 745.0, 745.10, 745.11, 745.12, 745.19, 745.2, 745.3, 745.4, 745.5, 745.60, 745.69, 745.7, 746.01, 746.02, 746.1, 746.2, 746.3, 746.4, 746.5, 746.6, 746.6, 746.7, 746.81, 746.82, 746.83, 746.84, 746.86, 746.89, 746.9, 747.11, 747.22, 747.83, 747.89, 747.9, 759.7, 759.81, 759.82, 759.83, 759.89
AHA: 4Q 2002, 62

747.89 Other
Aneurysm, congenital, specified site not elsewhere classified
Excludes *congenital aneurysm:*
coronary (746.85)
peripheral (747.6)
pulmonary (747.3)
retinal (743.58)
AHA: 4Q 2002, 63

747.9 Unspecified anomaly of circulatory system

④ 748 Congenital anomalies of respiratory system

Excludes *congenital central alveolar hypoventilation syndrome (327.25)*
congenital defect of diaphragm (756.6)

748.0 Choanal atresia

Atresia of nares (anterior) (posterior)
Congenital stenosis of nares (anterior) (posterior)

DEF: Fetal nasal airways are obstructed by membranous or bony tissue; infant is unable to breathe and nurse simultaneously.

748.1 Other anomalies of nose

Absent nose
Accessory nose
Cleft nose
Congenital:
- deformity of nose
- notching of tip of nose
- performation of wall of nasal sinus

Deformity of wall of nasal sinus

Excludes *congenital deviation of nasal septum (754.0)*

748.2 Web of larynx

Web of larynx:
- NOS
- glottic
- subglottic

748.3 Other anomalies of larynx, trachea, and bronchus

Absence or agenesis of:
- bronchus
- larynx
- trachea

Anomaly (of):
- cricoid cartilage
- epiglottis
- thyroid cartilage
- tracheal cartilage

Atresia (of):
- epiglottis
- glottis
- larynx
- trachea

Cleft thyroid, cartilage, congenital
Congenital:
- dilation, trachea
- stenosis:
  - larynx
  - trachea
- tracheocele

Diverticulum:
- bronchus
- trachea

Fissure of epiglottis
Laryngocele
Posterior cleft of cricoid cartilage (congenital)
Rudimentary tracheal bronchus
Stridor, laryngeal, congenital

AHA: 1Q 1999, 14

748.4 Congenital cystic lung

Disease, lung:
- cystic, congenital
- polycystic, congenital

Honeycomb lung, congenital

Excludes *acquired or unspecified cystic lung (518.89)*

C&C Exclusions: 748.4, 748.5, 748.60, 748.61, 748.69, 748.8, 748.9

748.5 Agenesis, hypoplasia, and dysplasia of lung

Absence of lung (fissures) (lobe)
Aplasia of lung
Hypoplasia of lung (lobe)
Sequestration of lung

C&C Exclusions: See 748.4

⑤ 748.6 Other anomalies of lung

748.60 Anomaly of lung, unspecified

748.61 Congenital bronchiectasis

C&C Exclusions: 079.82, 480.3, 494.0, 494.1, 496, 506.1, 506.4, 506.9, 748.61

748.69 Other

Accessory lung (lobe)
Azygos lobe (fissure), lung

748.8 Other specified anomalies of respiratory system

Abnormal communication between pericardial and pleural sacs
Anomaly, pleural folds
Atresia of nasopharynx
Congenital cyst of mediastinum

✖ 748.9 Unspecified anomaly of respiratory system

Anomaly of respiratory system NOS

④ 749 Cleft palate and cleft lip

⑤ 749.0 Cleft palate

✖ 749.00 Cleft palate, unspecified

749.01 Unilateral, complete

749.02 Unilateral, incomplete

Cleft uvula

749.03 Bilateral, complete

749.04 Bilateral, incomplete

⑤ 749.1 Cleft lip

Cheiloschisis
Congenital fissure of lip
Harelip
Labium leporinum

✖ 749.10 Cleft lip, unspecified

749.11 Unilateral, complete

749.12 Unilateral, incomplete

749.13 Bilateral, complete

749.14 Bilateral, incomplete

⑤ 749.2 Cleft palate with cleft lip

Cheilopalatoschisis

749.20 Cleft palate with cleft lip, unspecified

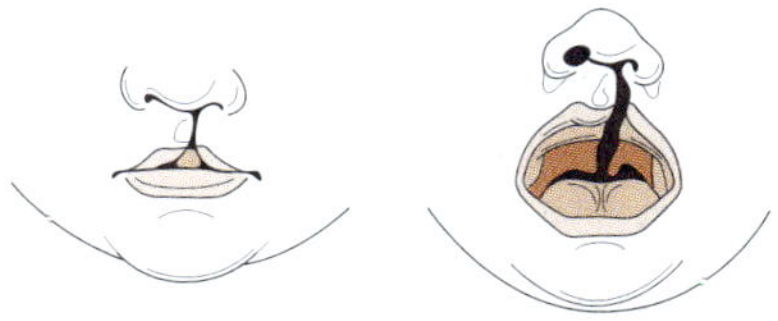

749.21 Unilateral, complete

749.22 Unilateral, incomplete

749.23 Bilateral, complete

AHA: 1Q 1996, 14

749.24 Bilateral, incomplete

749.25 Other combinations

④ 750 Other congenital anomalies of upper alimentary tract

Excludes *dentofacial anomalies (524.0-524.9)*

750.0 Tongue tie

Ankyloglossia

⑤ 750.1 Other anomalies of tongue

750.10 Anomaly of tongue, unspecified

750.11 Aglossia

DEF: Congenital absence of the tongue.

750.12 Congenital adhesions of tongue

750.13 Fissure of tongue

Bifid tongue
Double tongue

750.15 Macroglossia

Congenital hypertrophy of tongue

750.16 Microglossia

Hypoplasia of tongue

750.19 Other

⑤ 750.2 Other specified anomalies of mouth and pharynx

750.21 Absence of salivary gland

750.22 Accessory salivary gland

750.23 Atresia, salivary gland

Imperforate salivary duct

750.24 Congenital fistula of salivary gland

750.25 Congenital fistula of lip
Congenital (mucus) lip pits

750.26 Other specified anomalies of mouth
Absence of uvula

750.27 Diverticulum of pharynx
Pharyngeal pouch

750.29 Other specified anomalies of pharynx
Imperforate pharynx

750.3 Tracheoesophageal fistula, esophageal atresia and stenosis
Absent esophagus
Atresia of esophagus
Congenital:
- esophageal ring
- stenosis of esophagus
- stricture of esophagus

Congenital fistula:
- esophagobronchial
- esophagotracheal

Imperforate esophagus
Webbed esophagus

750.4 Other specified anomalies of esophagus
Dilatation, congenital, of esophagus
Displacement, congenital, of esophagus
Diverticulum of esophagus
Duplication of esophagus
Giant esophagus
Esophageal pouch
Excludes *congenital hiatus hernia (750.6)*
AHA: Jan-Feb 1985, 3

750.5 Congenital hypertrophic pyloric stenosis
Congenital or infantile:
- constriction of pylorus
- hypertrophy of pylorus
- spasm of pylorus
- stenosis of pylorus
- stricture of pylorus

750.6 Congenital hiatus hernia
Displacement of cardia through esophageal hiatus
Excludes *congenital diaphragmatic hernia (756.6)*

750.7 Other specified anomalies of stomach
Congenital:
- cardiospasm
- hourglass stomach

Displacement of stomach
Diverticulum of stomach, congenital
Duplication of stomach
Megalogastria
Microgastria
Transposition of stomach

750.8 Other specified anomalies of upper alimentary tract

✖ **750.9 Unspecified anomaly of upper alimentary tract**
Congenital:
- anomaly NOS of upper alimentary tract [any part, except tongue]
- deformity NOS of upper alimentary tract [any part, except tongue]

❹ **751 Other congenital anomalies of digestive system**

751.0 Meckel's diverticulum
Meckel's diverticulum (displaced) (hypertrophic)
Persistent:
- omphalomesenteric duct
- vitelline duct

AHA: 1Q 2004, 10

751.1 Atresia and stenosis of small intestine P
Atresia of:
- duodenum
- ileum
- intestine NOS

Congenital:
- absence of small intestine or intestine NOS
- obstruction of small intestine or intestine NOS
- stenosis of small intestine or intestine NOS
- stricture of small intestine or intestine NOS

Imperforate jejunum

751.2 Atresia and stenosis of large intestine, rectum, and anal canal P
Absence:
- anus (congenital)
- appendix, congenital
- large instestine, congenital
- rectum

Atresia of:
- anus
- colon
- rectum

Congenital or infantile:
- obstruction of large intestine
- occlusion of anus
- stricture of anus

Imperforate:
- anus
- rectum

Stricture of rectum, congenital
AHA: 2Q 1998, 16

751.3 Hirschsprung's disease and other congenital functional disorders of colon
Aganglionosis
Congenital dilation of colon
Congenital megacolon
Marcrocolon

751.4 Anomalies of intestinal fixation
Congenital adhesions:
- omental, anomalous
- peritoneal

Jackson's membrane
Malrotation of colon
Rotation of cecum or colon:
- failure of
- incomplete
- insufficient

Universal mesentery

751.5 Other anomalies of intestine
Congenital diverticulum, colon
Dolichocolon
Duplication of:
- anus
- appendix
- cecum
- intestine

Ectopic anus
Megaloappendix
Megaloduodenum
Microcolon
Persistent cloaca
Transposition of:
- appendix
- colon
- intestine

AHA: 3Q 2002, 11; 3Q 2001, 8

❺ **751.6 Anomalies of gallbladder, bile ducts, and liver**

751.60 Unspecified anomaly of gallbladder, bile ducts, and liver

751.61 Biliary atresia P
Congenital:
- absence of bile duct (common) or passage
- hypoplasia of bile duct (common) or passage
- obstruction of bile duct (common) or passage
- stricture of bile duct (common) or passage

AHA: Sep-Oct 1987, 8

751.62 Congenital cystic disease of liver
Congenital polycystic disease of liver
Fibrocystic disease of liver

751.69 Other anomalies of gallbladder, bile ducts, and liver
Absence of:
gallbladder, congenital
liver (lobe)
Accessory:
hepatic ducts
liver
Congenital:
choledochal cyst
hepatomegaly
Duplication of:
biliary duct
cystic duct
gallbladder
liver
Floating:
gallbladder
liver
Intrahepatic gallbladder
AHA: Sep-Oct 1987, 8

751.7 Anomalies of pancreas
Absence of pancreas
Accessory pancreas
Agenesis of pancreas
Annular pancreas
Ectopic pancreatic tissue
Hypoplasia of pancreas
Pancreatic heterotopia
Excludes *diabetes mellitus:*
congenital (250.0-250.9)
neonatal (775.1)
fibrocystic disease of pancreas (277.00-277.09)

751.8 Other specified anomalies of digestive system
Absence (complete) (partial) of alimentary tract NOS
Duplication of digestive organs NOS
Malposition, congenital of digestive organs NOS
Excludes *congenital diaphragmatic hernia (756.6)*
congenital hiatus hernia (750.6)

✖ **751.9 Unspecified anomaly of digestive system**
Congenital:
anomaly NOS of digestive system NOS
deformity NOS of digestive system NOS

❹ **752 Congenital anomalies of genital organs**
Excludes *syndromes associated with anomalies in the number and form of chromosomes (758.0-758.9)*
testicular feminization syndrome (259.5)

752.0 Anomalies of ovaries ♀
Absence, congenital, of ovary
Accessory ovary
Ectopic ovary
Streak of ovary

❺ **752.1 Anomalies of fallopian tubes and broad ligaments**

752.10 Unspecified anomaly of fallopian tubes and broad ligaments ♀

752.11 Embryonic cyst of fallopian tubes and broad ligaments ♀
Cyst:
epoophoron
fimbrial
parovarian
AHA: Sep-Oct 1985, 13

752.19 Other ♀
Absence of fallopian tube or broad ligament
Accessory fallopian tube or broad ligament
Atresia of fallopian tube or broad ligament

752.2 Doubling of uterus ♀
Didelphic uterus
Doubling of uterus [any degree] (associated with doubling of cervix and vagina)

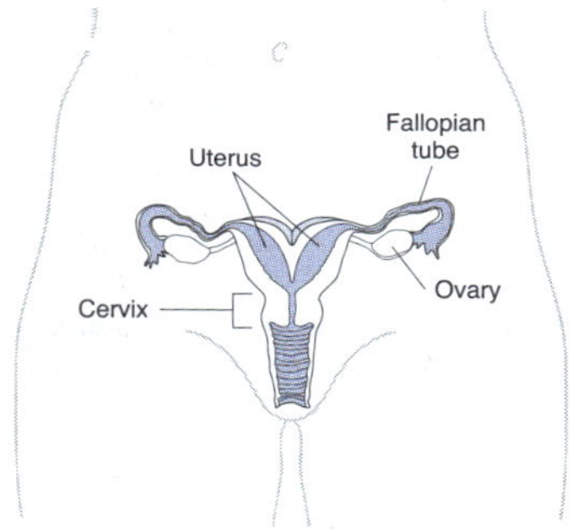

752.3 Other anomalies of uterus ♀
Absence, congenital, of uterus
Agenesis of uterus
Aplasia of uterus
Bicornuate uterus
Uterus unicornis
Uterus with only one functioning horn
AHA: 3Q 2006, 18

❺ **752.4 Anomalies of cervix, vagina, and external female genitalia**

752.40 Unspecified anomaly of cervix, vagina, and external female genitalia ♀

752.41 Embryonic cyst of cervix, vagina, and external female genitalia ♀
Cyst of:
canal of Nuck, congenital
Gartner's duct
vagina, embryonal
vulva, congenital

752.42 Imperforate hymen ♀

752.49 Other anomalies of cervix, vagina, and external female genitalia ♀
Absence of cervix, clitoris, vagina, or vulva
Agenesis of cervix, clitoris, vagina, or vulva
Congenital stenosis or stricture of:
cervical canal
vagina
Excludes *double vagina associated with total duplication (752.2)*
AHA: 3Q 2006, 18

❺ **752.5 Undescended and retractile testicle**
AHA: 4Q 1996, 33

752.51 Undescended testis ♂
Cryptorchism
Ectopic testis

752.52 Retractile testis ♂

❺ **752.6 Hypospadias and epispadias and other penile anomalies**
AHA: 4Q 1996, 34-35

752.61 Hypospadias ♂
AHA: 4Q 2003, 67-68; 3Q 1997, 6

752.62 Epispadias ♂
Anaspadias

752.63 Congenital chordee ♂

752.64 Micropenis ♂

752.65 Hidden penis ♂

752.69 Other penile anomalies ♂

752.7 Indeterminate sex and pseudohermaphroditism
Gynandrism
Hermaphroditism
Ovotestis
Pseudohermaphroditism (male) (female)
Pure gonadal dysgenesis
Excludes *pseudohermaphroditism:*
female, with adrenocortical disorder (255.2)
male, with gonadal disorder (257.8)
with specified chromosomal anomaly (758.0-758.9)
testicular feminization syndrome (259.5)

5 **752.8 Other specified anomalies of genital organs**
Excludes *congenital hydrocele (778.6)*
penile anomalies (752.61-752.69)
phimosis or paraphimosis (605)

752.81 Scrotal transposition ♂
C&C Exclusions: 597.0, 599.4, 614.0, 614.3, 614.5, 615.0, 616.3, 616.4, 620.7
AHA: 4Q 2003, 67-68

752.89 Other specified anomalies of genital organs
Absence of:
prostate
spermatic cord
vas deferens
Anorchism
Aplasia (congenital) of:
prostate
round ligament
testicle
Atresia of:
ejaculatory duct
vas deferens
Fusion of testes
Hypoplasia of testis
Monorchism
Polyorchism
C&C Exclusions: See 752.81

✖ **752.9 Unspecified anomaly of genital organs**
Congenital:
anomaly NOS of genital organ, NEC
deformity NOS of genital organ, NEC

4 **753 Congenital anomalies of urinary system**

753.0 Renal agenesis and dysgenesis
Atrophy of kidney:
congenital
infantile
Congenital absence of kidney(s)
Hypoplasia of kidney(s)
C&C Exclusions: 585.1, 585.2, 585.3, 585.4, 585.5, 585.6, 585.9, 599.60, 599.69

5 **753.1 Cystic kidney disease**
Excludes *acquired cyst of kidney (593.2)*
AHA: 4Q 1990, 3

✖ **753.10 Cystic kidney disease, unspecified**
C&C Exclusions: See 753.0

753.11 Congenital single renal cyst
C&C Exclusions: See 753.0

✖ **753.12 Polycystic kidney, unspecified type**
C&C Exclusions: See 753.0

753.13 Polycystic kidney, autosomal dominant
C&C Exclusions: See 753.0

753.14 Polycystic kidney, autosomal recessive
C&C Exclusions: See 753.0

753.15 Renal dysplasia
C&C Exclusions: See 753.0

753.16 Medullary cystic kidney
Nephronopthisis
C&C Exclusions: See 753.0

753.17 Medullary sponge kidney
C&C Exclusions: See 753.0

753.19 Other specified cystic kidney disease
Multicystic kidney
C&C Exclusions: See 753.0

5 **753.2 Obstructive defects of renal pelvis and ureter**
AHA: 4Q 1996, 35

✖ **753.20 Unspecified obstructive defect of renal pelvis and ureter**
C&C Exclusions: See 753.0

753.21 Congenital obstruction of ureteropelvic junction
C&C Exclusions: See 753.0

753.22 Congenital obstruction of ureterovesical junction
Adynamic ureter
Congenital hydroureter
C&C Exclusions: See 753.0

753.23 Congenital ureterocele
C&C Exclusions: See 753.0

753.29 Other
C&C Exclusions: See 753.0

753.3 Other specified anomalies of kidney
Accessory kidney
Congenital:
calculus of kidney
displaced kidney
Discoid kidney
Double kidney with double pelvis
Ectopic kidney
Fusion of kidneys
Giant kidney
Horseshoe kidney
Hyperplasia of kidney
Lobulation of kidney
Malrotation of kidney
Trifid kidney (pelvis)
C&C Exclusions: See 753.0
AHA: 1Q 2007, 23

753.4 Other specified anomalies of ureter
Absent ureter
Accessory ureter
Deviaton of ureter
Displaced ureteric orifice
Double ureter
Ectopic ureter
Implantation, anomalous, of ureter
C&C Exclusions: 599.60, 599.69

753.5 Exstrophy of urinary bladder
Ectopia vesicae
Extroversion of bladder
C&C Exclusions: See 753.4

753.6 Atresia and stenosis of urethra and bladder neck
Congenital obstruction:
bladder neck
urethra
Congenital stricture of:
urethra (valvular)
urinary meatus
vesicourethral orifice
Imperforate urinary meatus
Impervious urethra
Urethral valve formation
C&C Exclusions: See 753.4

753.7 Anomalies of urachus
Cyst (of) urachus
Fistula (of) urachus
Patent (of) urachus
Persistent umbilical sinus
C&C Exclusions: See 753.4

753.8 Other specified anomalies of bladder and urethra
Absence, congenital of:
bladder
urethra
Accessory:
bladder
urethra
Congenital:
diverticulum of bladder
hernia of bladder
Congenital prolapse of:
bladder (mucosa)
urethra
Congenital urethrorectal fistula
Double:
urethra
urinary meatus
C&C Exclusions: See 753.4

✖ **753.9 Unspecified anomaly of urinary system**
Congenital:
anomaly NOS of urinary system [any part, except urachus]
deformity NOS of urinary system [any part, except urachus]
C&C Exclusions: See 753.0

❹ **754 Certain congenital musculoskeletal deformities**
Includes nonteratogenic deformities which are considered to be due to intrauterine malposition and pressure

754.0 Of skull, face, and jaw
Asymmetry of face
Compression facies
Depressions in skull
Deviation of nasal septum, congenital
Dolichocephaly
Plagiocephaly
Potter's facies
Squashed or bent nose, congenital
Excludes *dentofacial anomalies (524.0-524.9)*
syphilitic saddle nose (090.5)

754.1 Of sternocleidomastoid muscle
Congenital sternomastoid torticollis
Congenital wryneck
Contracture of sternocleidomastoid (muscle)
Sternomastoid tumor

754.2 Of spine
Congenital postural:
lordosis
scoliosis

❺ **754.3 Congenital dislocation of hip**

754.30 Congenital dislocation of hip, unilateral
Congenital dislocation of hip NOS

754.31 Congenital dislocation of hip, bilateral

754.32 Congenital subluxation of hip, unilateral
Congenital flexion deformity, hip or thigh
Predislocation status of hip at birth
Preluxation of hip, congenital

754.33 Congenital subluxation of hip, bilateral

754.35 Congenital dislocation of one hip with subluxation of other hip

❺ **754.4 Congenital genu recurvatum and bowing of long bones of leg**

754.40 Genu recurvatum

754.41 Congenital dislocation of knee (with genu recurvatum)

754.42 Congenital bowing of femur

754.43 Congenital bowing of tibia and fibula

754.44 Congenital bowing of unspecified long bones of leg

❺ **754.5 Varus deformities of feet**
Excludes *acquired (736.71, 736.75, 736.79)*

754.50 Talipes varus
Congenital varus deformity of foot, unspecified
Pes varus

754.51 Talipes equinovarus
Equinovarus (congenital)

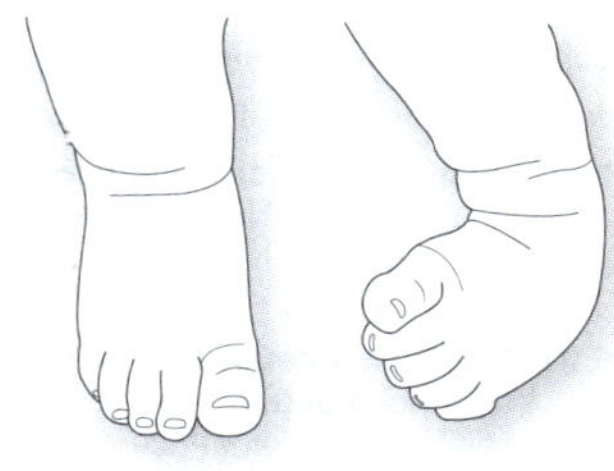

754.52 Metatarsus primus varus

754.53 Metatarsus varus

754.59 Other
Talipes calcaneovarus

❺ **754.6 Valgus deformities of feet**
Excludes *valgus deformity of foot (acquired) (736.79)*

754.60 Talipes valgus
Congenital valgus deformity of foot, unspecified

754.61 Congenital pes planus
Congenital rocker bottom flat foot
Flat foot, congenital
Excludes *pes planus (acquired) (734)*

754.62 Talipes calcaneovalgus

754.69 Other
Talipes:
equinovalgus
planovalgus

❺ **754.7 Other deformities of feet**
Excludes *acquired (736.70-736.79)*

754.70 Talipes, unspecified
Congenital deformity of foot NOS

754.71 Talipes cavus
Cavus foot (congenital)

754.79 Other
Asymmetric talipes
Talipes:
calcaneus
equinus

❺ **754.8 Other specified nonteratogenic anomalies**

754.81 Pectus excavatum
Congenital funnel chest

754.82 Pectus carinatum
Congenital pigeon chest [breast]

754.89 Other
Club hand (congenital)
Congenital:
deformity of chest wall
dislocation of elbow
Generalized flexion contractures of lower limb joints, congenital
Spade-like hand (congenital)

❹ **755 Other congenital anomalies of limbs**
Excludes *those deformities classifiable to 754.0-754.8*

❺ **755.0 Polydactyly**
DEF: An extra number of digits on a hand or foot.

755.00 Polydactyly, unspecified digits
Supernumerary digits

755.01 Of fingers
Accessory fingers

755.02 Of toes
Accessory toes

❺ **755.1 Syndactyly**
Symphalangy
Webbing of digits

755.10 Of multiple and unspecified sites

755.11 Of fingers without fusion of bone

755.12 Of fingers with fusion of bone

755.13 Of toes without fusion of bone

755.14 Of toes with fusion of bone

5 **755.2 Reduction deformities of upper limb**

755.20 Unspecified reduction deformity of upper limb
Ectromelia NOS of upper limb
Hemimelia NOS of upper limb
Shortening of arm, congenital

755.21 Transverse deficiency of upper limb
Amelia of upper limb
Congenital absence of:
fingers, all (complete or partial)
forearm, including hand and fingers
upper limb, complete
Congenital amputation of upper limb
Transverse hemimelia of upper limb

755.22 Longitudinal deficiency of upper limb, NEC
Phocomelia NOS of upper limb
Rudimentary arm

755.23 Longitudinal deficiency, combined, involving humerus, radius, and ulna (complete or incomplete)
Congenital absence of arm and forearm (complete or incomplete) with or without metacarpal deficiency and/or phalangeal deficiency, incomplete
Phocomelia, complete, of upper limb

755.24 Longitudinal deficiency, humeral, complete or partial (with or without distal deficiencies, incomplete)
Congenital absence of humerus (with or without absence of some [but not all] distal elements)
Proximal phocomelia of upper limb

755.25 Longitudinal deficiency, radioulnar, complete or partial (with or without distal deficiencies, incomplete)
Congenital absence of radius and ulna (with or without absence of some [but not all] distal elements)
Distal phocomelia of upper limb

755.26 Longitudinal deficiency, radial, complete or partial (with or without distal deficiencies, incomplete)
Agenesis of radius
Congenital absence of radius (with or without absence of some [but not all] distal elements)

755.27 Longitudinal deficiency, ulnar, complete or partial (with or without distal deficiencies, incomplete)
Agenesis of ulna
Congenital absence of ulna (with or without absence of some [but not all] distal elements)

755.28 Longitudinal deficiency, carpals or metacarpals, complete or partial (with or without incomplete phalangeal deficiency)

755.29 Longitudinal deficiency, phalanges, complete or partial
Absence of finger, congenital
Aphalangia of upper limb, terminal, complete or partial
Excludes *terminal deficiency of all five digits (755.21)*
transverse deficiency of phalanges (755.21)

5 **755.3 Reduction deformities of lower limb**

755.30 Unspecified reduction deformity of lower limb
Ectromelia NOS of lower limb
Hemimelia NOS of lower limb
Shortening of leg, congenital

755.31 Transverse deficiency of lower limb
Amelia of lower limb
Congenital absence of:
foot
leg, including foot and toes
lower limb, complete
toes, all, complete
Transverse hemimelia of lower limb

755.32 Longitudinal deficiency of lower limb, NEC
Phocomelia NOS of lower limb

755.33 Longitudinal deficiency, combined, involving femur, tibia, and fibula (complete or incomplete)
Congenital absence of thigh and (lower) leg (complete or incomplete) with or without metacarpal deficiency and/or phalangeal deficiency, incomplete
Phocomelia, complete, of lower limb

755.34 Longitudinal deficiency, femoral, complete or partial (with or without distal deficiencies, incomplete)
Congenital absence of femur (with or without absence of some [but not all] distal elements)
Proximal phocomelia of lower limb

755.35 Longitudinal deficiency, tibiofibular, complete or partial (with or without distal deficiencies, incomplete)
Congenital absence of tibia and fibula (with or without absence of some [but not all] distal elements)
Distal phocomelia of lower limb

755.36 Longitudinal deficiency, tibia, complete or partial (with or without distal deficiencies, incomplete)
Agenesis of tibia
Congenital absence of tibia (with or without absence of some [but not all] distal elements)

755.37 Longitudinal deficiency, fibular, complete or partial (with or without distal deficiencies, incomplete)
Agenesis of fibula
Congenital absence of fibula (with or without absence of some [but not all] distal elements)

755.38 Longitudinal deficiency, tarsals or metatarsals, complete or partial (with or without incomplete phalangeal deficiency)

755.39 Longitudinal deficiency, phalanges, complete or partial
Absence of toe, congenital
Aphalangia of lower limb, terminal, complete or partial
Excludes *terminal deficiency of all five digits (755.31)*
transverse deficiency of phalanges (755.31)

755.4 Reduction deformities, unspecified limb
Absence, congenital (complete or partial) of limb NOS
Amelia of unspecified limb
Ectromelia of unspecified limb
Hemimelia of unspecified limb
Phocomelia of unspecified limb

5 **755.5 Other anomalies of upper limb, including shoulder girdle**

755.50 Unspecified anomaly of upper limb

755.51 Congenital deformity of clavicle

755.52 Congenital elevation of scapula
Sprengel's deformity

755.53 Radioulnar synostosis

755.54 Madelung's deformity

755.55 Acrocephalosyndactyly
Apert's syndrome

755.56 Accessory carpal bones

755.57 Macrodactylia (fingers)

755.58 Cleft hand, congenital
Lobster-claw hand

755.59 Other
Cleidocranial dysostosis
Cubitus:
  valgus, congenital
  varus, congenital
Excludes *club hand (congenital) (754.89)*
congenital dislocation of elbow (754.89)

❺ **755.6 Other anomalies of lower limb, including pelvic girdle**

755.60 Unspecified anomaly of lower limb

755.61 Coxa valga, congenital

755.62 Coxa vara, congenital

755.63 Other congenital deformity of hip (joint)
Congenital anteversion of femur (neck)
Excludes *congenital dislocation of hip (754.30-754.35)*
AHA: 1Q 1994, 15; Sep-Oct 1984, 15

755.64 Congenital deformity of knee (joint)
Congenital:
  absence of patella
  genu valgum [knock-knee]
  genu varum [bowleg]
Rudimentary patella

755.65 Macrodactylia of toes

755.66 Other anomalies of toes
Congenital:
  hallux valgus
  hallux varus
  hammer toe

755.67 Anomalies of foot, NEC
Astragaloscaphoid synostosis
Calcaneonavicular bar
Coalition of calcaneus
Talonavicular synostosis
Tarsal coalitions

755.69 Other
Congenital:
  angulation of tibia
  deformity (of):
    ankle (joint)
    sacroiliac (joint)
  fusion of sacroiliac joint

755.8 Other specified anomalies of unspecified limb

✖ **755.9 Unspecified anomaly of unspecified limb**
Congenital:
  anomaly NOS of unspecified limb
  deformity NOS of unspecified limb
Excludes *reduction deformity of unspecified limb (755.4)*

❹ **756 Other congenital musculoskeletal anomalies**
Excludes *those deformities classifiable to 754.0-754.8*

756.0 Anomalies of skull and face bones
Absence of skull bones
Acrocephaly
Congenital deformity of forehead
Craniosynostosis
Crouzon's disease
Hypertelorism
Imperfect fusion of skull
Oxycephaly
Platybasia
Premature closure of cranial sutures
Tower skull
Trigonocephaly
Excludes *acrocephalosyndactyly [Apert's syndrome] (755.55)*
dentofacial anomalies (524.0-524.9)
skull defects associated with brain anomalies, such as:
  anencephalus (740.0)
  encephalocele (742.0)
  hydrocephalus (742.3)
  microcephalus (742.1)
AHA: 3Q 1998, 9; 3Q 1996, 15

❺ **756.1 Anomalies of spine**

756.10 Anomaly of spine, unspecified

756.11 Spondylolysis, lumbosacral region
Prespondylolisthesis (lumbosacral)

756.12 Spondylolisthesis

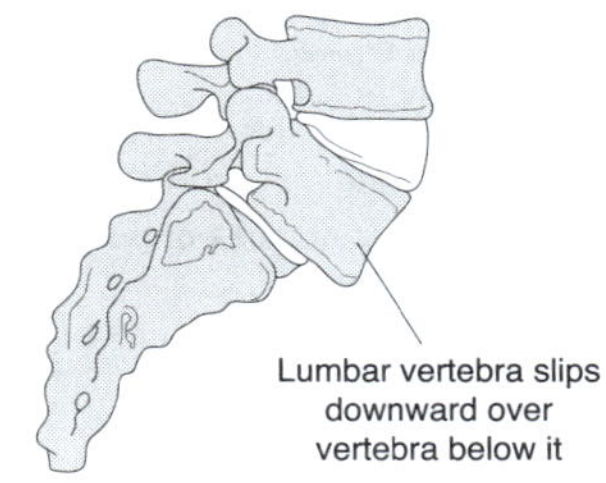

756.13 Absence of vertebra, congenital

756.14 Hemivertebra

756.15 Fusion of spine [vertebra], congenital

756.16 Klippel-Feil syndrome

756.17 Spina bifida occulta
Excludes *spina bifida (aperta) (741.0-741.9)*

756.19 Other
Platyspondylia
Supernumerary vertebra

756.2 Cervical rib
Supernumerary rib in the cervical region

756.3 Other anomalies of ribs and sternum
Congenital absence of:
  rib
  sternum
Congenital:
  fissure of sternum
  fusion of ribs
Sternum bifidum
Excludes *nonteratogenic deformity of chest wall (754.81-754.89)*

756.4 Chondrodystrophy
Achondroplasia
Chondrodystrophia (fetalis)
Dyschondroplasia
Enchondromatosis
Ollier's disease
Excludes ►*congenital myotonic chondrodystrophy (359.23)*◄
lipochondrodystrophy [Hurler's syndrome] (277.5)
Morquio's disease (277.5)
AHA: 2Q 2002, 16; Sep-Oct 1987, 10

❺ **756.5 Osteodystrophies**

756.50 Osteodystrophy, unspecified

756.51 Osteogenesis imperfecta
Fragilitas ossium
Osteopsathyrosis

756.52 Osteopetrosis

756.53 Osteopoikilosis

756.54 Polyostotic fibrous dysplasia of bone

756.55 Chondroectodermal dysplasia
Ellis-van Creveld syndrome

756.56 Multiple epiphyseal dysplasia

756.59 Other
Albright (-McCune)-Sternberg syndrome

756.6 Anomalies of diaphragm
Absence of diaphragm
Congenital hernia:
  diaphragmatic
  foramen of Morgagni
Eventration of diaphragm
Excludes *congenital hiatus hernia (750.6)*

5 756.7 Anomalies of abdominal wall

✖ 756.70 Anomaly of abdominal wall, unspecified

756.71 Prune belly syndrome
Eagle-Barrett syndrome
Prolapse of bladder mucosa
AHA: 4Q 1997, 44

756.79 Other congenital anomalies of abdominal wall
Exomphalos
Gastroschisis
Omphalocele
Excludes *umbilical hernia (551-553 with .1)*

5 756.8 Other specified anomalies of muscle, tendon, fascia, and connective tissue

756.81 Absence of muscle and tendon
Absence of muscle (pectoral)

756.82 Accessory muscle

756.83 Ehlers-Danlos syndrome

756.89 Other
Amyotrophia congenita
Congenital shortening of tendon
AHA: 3Q 1999, 16

756.9 Other and unspecified anomalies of musculoskeletal system
Congenital:
anomaly NOS of musculoskeletal system, NEC
deformity NOS of musculoskeletal system, NEC

4 757 Congenital anomalies of the integument
Includes anomalies of skin, subcutaneous tissue, hair, nails, and breast
Excludes *hemangioma (228.00-228.09)*
pigmented nevus (216.0-216.9)

757.0 Hereditary edema of legs
Congenital lymphedema
Hereditary trophedema
Milroy's disease

757.1 Ichthyosis congenita
Congenital ichthyosis
Harlequin fetus
Ichthyosiform erythroderma

757.2 Dermatoglyphic anomalies
Abnormal palmar creases

5 757.3 Other specified anomalies of skin

757.31 Congenital ectodermal dysplasia

757.32 Vascular hamartomas
Birthmarks
Port-wine stain
Strawberry nevus

757.33 Congenital pigmentary anomalies of skin
Congenital poikiloderma
Urticaria pigmentosa
Xeroderma pigmentosum
Excludes *albinism (270.2)*

757.39 Other
Accessory skin tags, congenital
Congenital scar
Epidermolysis bullosa
Keratoderma (congenital)
Excludes *pilonidal cyst (685.0-685.1)*

757.4 Specified anomalies of hair
Congenital:
alopecia
atrichosis
beaded hair
hypertrichosis
monilethrix
Persistent lanugo

757.5 Specified anomalies of nails
Anonychia
Congenital:
clubnail
koilonychia
leukonychia
onychauxis
pachyonychia

757.6 Specified anomalies of breast
Absent breast or nipple
Accessory breast or nipple
Supernumerary breast or nipple
Hypoplasia of breast
Excludes *absence of pectoral muscle (756.81)*

757.8 Other specified anomalies of the integument

✖ 757.9 Unspecified anomaly of the integument
Congenital:
anomaly NOS of integument
deformity NOS of integument

4 758 Chromosomal anomalies
Use additional codes for conditions associated with the chromosomal anomalies
Includes syndromes associated with anomalies in the number and form of chromosomes

758.0 Down's syndrome
Mongolism
Translocation Down's syndrome
Trisomy:
21 or 22
G

758.1 Patau's syndrome
Trisomy:
13
D1

758.2 Edward's syndrome
Trisomy:
18
E3

5 758.3 Autosomal deletion syndromes

758.31 Cri-du-chat syndrome
Deletion 5p

758.32 Velo-cardio-facial syndrome
Deletion 22q11.2

758.33 Other microdeletions
Miller-Dieker syndrome
Smith-Magenis syndrome

758.39 Other autosomal deletions

758.4 Balanced autosomal translocation in normal individual

758.5 Other conditions due to autosomal anomalies
Accessory autosomes NEC

758.6 Gonadal dysgenesis
Ovarian dysgenesis
Turner's syndrome
XO syndrome
Excludes *pure gonadal dysgenesis (752.7)*

758.7 Klinefelter's syndrome ♂
XXY syndrome

5 758.8 Other conditions due to chromosome anomalies

758.81 Other conditions due to sex chromosome anomalies

758.89 Other

758.9 Conditions due to anomaly of unspecified chromosome

4 759 Other and unspecified congenital anomalies

759.0 Anomalies of spleen
Aberrant spleen
Absent spleen
Accessory spleen
Congenital splenomegaly
Ectopic spleen
Lobulation of spleen

759.1 Anomalies of adrenal gland
Aberrant adrenal gland
Absent adrenal gland
Accessory adrenal gland
Excludes *adrenogenital disorders (255.2)*
congenital disorders of steroid metabolism (255.2)

759.2 Anomalies of other endocrine glands
Absent parathyroid gland
Accessory thyroid gland
Persistent thyroglossal or thyrolingual duct
Thyroglossal (duct) cyst
Excludes *congenital:*
goiter (246.1)
hypothyroidism (243)

759.3 Situs inversus
Situs inversus or transversus:
abdominalis
thoracis
Transposition of viscera:
abdominal
thoracic
Excludes *dextrocardia without mention of complete transposition (746.87)*

DEF: Congenital disorder in which the position of all major organs in the chest and abdomen are reversed horizontally.

759.4 Conjoined twins
Craniopagus
Dicephalus
Pygopagus
Thoracopagus
Xiphopagus

759.5 Tuberous sclerosis
Bourneville's disease
Epiloia

759.6 Other hamartoses, NEC
Syndrome:
Peutz-Jeghers
Sturge-Weber (-Dimitri)
von Hippel-Lindau
Excludes *neurofibromatosis (237.7)*
AHA: 3Q 1992, 12

759.7 Multiple congenital anomalies, so described
Congenital:
anomaly, multiple NOS
deformity, multiple NOS

5 **759.8 Other specified anomalies**
AHA: Sep-Oct 1987, 9; Sep-Oct 1985, 11

759.81 Prader-Willi syndrome
DEF: Defect of the 15th chromosome resulting in short stature, mental retardation, obesity, and insufficient sex organs.

759.82 Marfan syndrome
AHA: 3Q 1993, 11

759.83 Fragile X syndrome
AHA: 4Q 1994, 41

759.89 Other
Congenital malformation syndromes affecting multiple systems, NEC
Laurence-Moon-Biedl syndrome
AHA: 3Q 2006, 21; 2Q 2005, 17; 2Q 2004, 12; 1Q 2001, 3; 3Q 1999, 17-18; 3Q 1998, 8

✖ **759.9 Congenital anomaly, unspecified**

15. CERTAIN CONDITIONS ORIGINATING IN THE PERINATAL PERIOD (760-779)

Includes conditions which have their origin in the perinatal period, before birth through the first 28 days after birth, even though death or morbidity occurs later

Use additional code(s) to further specify condition

MATERNAL CAUSES OF PERINATAL MORBIDITY AND MORTALITY (760-763)

AHA: 3Q 1990, 5; 2Q 1989, 14

4 **760 Fetus or newborn affected by maternal conditions which may be unrelated to present pregnancy**
Includes the listed maternal conditions only when specified as a cause of mortality or morbidity of the fetus or newborn
Excludes *maternal endocrine and metabolic disorders affecting fetus or newborn (775.0-775.9)*
AHA: 1Q 1994, 8; 2Q 1992, 12; Nov-Dec 1984, 11

✖ **760.0 Maternal hypertensive disorders**
Fetus or newborn affected by maternal conditions classifiable to 642

✖ **760.1 Maternal renal and urinary tract diseases**
Fetus or newborn affected by maternal conditions classifiable to 580-599

✖ **760.2 Maternal infections**
Fetus or newborn affected by maternal infectious disease classifiable to 001-136 and 487, but fetus or newborn not manifesting that disease
Excludes *congenital infectious diseases (771.0-771.8)*
maternal genital tract and other localized infections (760.8)

✖ **760.3 Other chronic maternal circulatory and respiratory diseases**
Fetus or newborn affected by chronic maternal conditions classifiable to 390-459, 490-519, 745-748

✖ **760.4 Maternal nutritional disorders**
Fetus or newborn affected by:
maternal disorders classifiable to 260-269
maternal malnutrition NOS
Excludes *fetal malnutrition (764.10-764.29)*

✖ **760.5 Maternal injury**
Fetus or newborn affected by maternal conditions classifiable to 800-995

✖ **760.6 Surgical operation on mother**
Excludes *cesarean section for present delivery (763.4)*
damage to placenta from amniocentesis, cesarean section, or surgical induction (762.1)
previous surgery to uterus or pelvic organs (763.89)

5 **760.7 Noxious influences affecting fetus or newborn via placenta or breast milk**
Fetus or newborn affected by noxious substance transmitted via placenta or breast milk
Excludes *anesthetic and analgesic drugs administered during labor and delivery (763.5)*
drug withdrawal syndrome in newborn (779.5)
AHA: 3Q 1991, 21

✖ **760.70 Unspecified noxious substance**
Fetus or newborn affected by:
Drug NEC

760.71 Alcohol
Fetal alcohol syndrome

✖ **760.72 Narcotics**

✖ **760.73 Hallucinogenic agents**

✖ **760.74 Anti-infectives**
Antibiotics
Antifungals

760.75 Cocaine
AHA: 3Q 1994, 6; 2Q 1992, 12; 4Q 1991, 26

760.76 Diethylstilbestrol [DES]
AHA: 4Q 1994, 45

760.77 Anticonvulsants N
Carbamazepine
Phenobarbital
Phenytoin
Valproic acid
AHA: 4Q 2005, 82

760.78 Antimetabolic agents N
Methotrexate
Retinoic acid
Statins
AHA: 4Q 2005, 82-83

✖ **760.79 Other**
Fetus or newborn affected by:
immune sera transmitted via placenta or breast milk
medicinal agents NEC transmitted via placenta or breast milk
toxic substance NEC transmitted via placenta or breast milk

✖ **760.8 Other specified maternal conditions affecting fetus or newborn**
Maternal genital tract and other localized infection affecting fetus or newborn, but fetus or newborn not manifesting that disease
Excludes *maternal urinary tract infection affecting fetus or newborn (760.1)*

✖ **760.9 Unspecified maternal condition affecting fetus or newborn**

④ **761 Fetus or newborn affected by maternal complications of pregnancy**
Includes the listed maternal conditions only when specified as a cause of mortality or morbidity of the fetus or newborn

✖ **761.0 Incompetent cervix**

✖ **761.1 Premature rupture of membranes**

✖ **761.2 Oligohydramnios**
Excludes *that due to premature rupture of membranes (761.1)*
DEF: Inadequate amount of amniotic fluid in the womb affecting the fetus.

✖ **761.3 Polyhydramnios**
Hydramnios (acute) (chronic)
DEF: Excessive amount of amniotic fluid in the womb affecting the fetus.

✖ **761.4 Ectopic pregnancy**
Pregnancy:
abdominal
intraperitoneal
tubal

✖ **761.5 Multiple pregnancy**
Triplet (pregnancy)
Twin (pregnancy)

✖ **761.6 Maternal death**

✖ **761.7 Malpresentation before labor**
Breech presentation before labor
External version before labor
Oblique lie before labor
Transverse lie before labor
Unstable lie before labor

✖ **761.8 Other specified maternal complications of pregnancy affecting fetus or newborn**
Spontaneous abortion, fetus

✖ **761.9 Unspecified maternal complication of pregnancy affecting fetus or newborn**

④ **762 Fetus or newborn affected by complications of placenta, cord, and membranes**
Includes the listed maternal conditions only when specified as a cause of mortality or morbidity in the fetus or newborn
AHA: 1Q 1994, 8

762.0 Placenta previa N

762.1 Other forms of placental separation and hemorrhage N
Abruptio placentae
Antepartum hemorrhage
Damage to placenta from amniocentesis, cesarean section, or surgical induction
Maternal blood loss
Premature separation of placenta
Rupture of marginal sinus

762.2 Other and unspecified morphological and functional abnormalities of placenta N
Placental:
dysfunction
infarction
insufficiency

762.3 Placental transfusion syndromes N
Placental and cord abnormality resulting in twin-to-twin or other transplacental transfusion
Use additional code to indicate resultant condition in fetus or newborn:
fetal blood loss (772.0)
polycythemia neonatorum (776.4)

762.4 Prolapsed cord N
Cord presentation

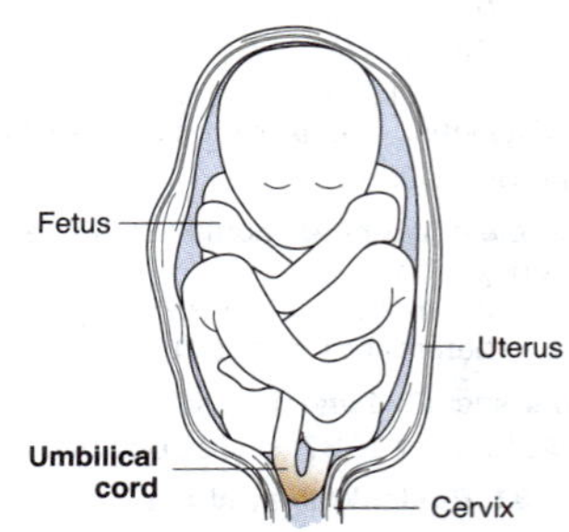

762.5 Other compression of umbilical cord N
Cord around neck
Entanglement of cord
Knot in cord
Torsion of cord
AHA: 2Q 2003, 9

762.6 Other and unspecified conditions of umbilical cord N
Short cord
Thrombosis of umbilical cord
Varices of umbilical cord
Vasa previa
Velamentous insertion of umbilical cord
Excludes *infection of umbilical cord (771.4)*
single umbilical artery (747.5)

762.7 Chorioamnionitis N
Amnionitis
Membranitis
Placentitis

762.8 Other specified abnormalities of chorion and amnion N

✖ **762.9 Unspecified abnormality of chorion and amnion** N

④ **763 Fetus or newborn affected by other complications of labor and delivery**
Includes the listed conditions only when specified as a cause of mortality or morbidity in the fetus or newborn
AHA: 1Q 1994, 8

✖ **763.0 Breech delivery and extraction** N

763.1 Other malpresentation, malposition, and disproportion during labor and delivery N
Fetus or newborn affected by:
- abnormality of bony pelvis
- contracted pelvis
- persistent occipitoposterior position
- shoulder presentation
- transverse lie
- conditions classifiable to 652, 653, and 660

763.2 Forceps delivery N
Fetus or newborn affected by forceps extraction

763.3 Delivery by vacuum extractor N

763.4 Cesarean delivery N
Excludes *placental separation or hemorrhage from cesarean section (762.1)*

763.5 Maternal anesthesia and analgesia N
Reactions and intoxications from maternal opiates and tranquilizers during labor and delivery
Excludes *drug withdrawal syndrome in newborn (779.5)*

763.6 Precipitate delivery N
Rapid second stage

763.7 Abnormal uterine contractions N
Fetus or newborn affected by:
- contraction ring
- hypertonic labor
- hypotonic uterine dysfunction
- uterine inertia or dysfunction
- conditions classifiable to 661, except 661.3

763.8 Other specified complications of labor and delivery affecting fetus or newborn
AHA: 4Q 1998, 46

763.81 Abnormality in fetal heart rate or rhythm before the onset of labor N

763.82 Abnormality in fetal heart rate or rhythm during labor N
AHA: 4Q 1998, 46

763.83 Abnormality in fetal heart rate or rhythm, unspecified as to time of onset N

763.84 Meconium passage during delivery N
Excludes *meconium aspiration (770.11, 770.12)*
meconium staining (779.84)
AHA: 4Q 2005, 83

763.89 Other specified complications of labor and delivery affecting fetus or newborn N
Fetus or newborn affected by:
- abnormality of maternal soft tissues
- destructive operation on live fetus to facilitate delivery
- induction of labor (medical)
- previous surgery to uterus or pelvic organs
- other conditions classifiable to 650-669
- other procedures used in labor and delivery

763.9 Unspecified complication of labor and delivery affecting fetus or newborn N

OTHER CONDITIONS ORIGINATING IN THE PERINATAL PERIOD (764-779)

The following fifth-digit subclassification is for use with category 764 and codes 765.0 and 765.1 to denote birthweight:

0 unspecified [weight]
1 less than 500 grams
2 500-749 grams
3 750-999 grams
4 1,000-1,249 grams
5 1,250-1,499 grams
6 1,500-1,749 grams
7 1,750-1,999 grams
8 2,000-2,499 grams
9 2,500 grams and over

764 Slow fetal growth and fetal malnutrition
Requires fifth digit. See beginning of section 764-779 for codes and definitions.
AHA: 3Q 2004, 4; 4Q 2002, 63; 1Q 1994, 8; 2Q 1991, 19; 2Q 1989, 15

764.0 "Light-for-dates" without mention of fetal malnutrition N
Infants underweight for gestational age
"Small-for-dates"

764.1 "Light-for-dates" with signs of fetal malnutrition N
Infants "light-for-dates" classifiable to 764.0, who in addition show signs of fetal malnutrition, such as dry peeling skin and loss of subcutaneous tissue

764.2 Fetal malnutrition without mention of "light-for-dates" N
Infants, not underweight for gestational age, showing signs of fetal malnutrition, such as dry peeling skin and loss of subcutaneous tissue
Intrauterine malnutrition

764.9 Fetal growth retardation, unspecified N
Intrauterine growth retardation
AHA: For Code 764.97: 1Q 1997, 6

765 Disorders relating to short gestation and low birthweight
Requires fifth digit. See beginning of section 764-779 for codes and definitions.
Includes the listed conditions, without further specification, as causes of mortality, morbidity, or additional care, in fetus or newborn
AHA: 1Q 1997, 6; 1Q 1994, 8; 2Q 1991, 19; 2Q 1989, 15

765.0 Extreme immaturity N
Note: *Usually implies a birthweight of less than 1,000 grams*
Use additional code for weeks of gestation (765.20-765.29)
C&C Exclusions: (for codes 765.01-765.08) 764.00, 764.01, 764.02, 764.03, 764.04, 764.05, 764.06, 764.07, 764.08, 764.09, 764.10, 764.11, 764.12, 764.13, 764.14, 764.15, 764.16, 764.17, 764.18, 764.19, 764.20, 764.21, 764.22, 764.23, 764.24, 764.25, 764.26, 764.27, 764.28, 764.29, 764.90, 764.91, 764.92, 764.93, 764.94, 764.95, 764.96, 764.97, 764.98, 764.99, 765.00, 765.01, 765.02, 765.03, 765.04, 765.05, 765.06, 765.07, 765.08, 765.09, 765.10, 765.11, 765.12, 765.13, 765.14, 765.15, 765.16, 765.17, 765.18, 765.19, 765.20, 765.21, 765.22, 765.23, 765.24, 765.25, 765.26, 765.27, 765.28, 765.29

765.1 Other preterm infants N
Note: *Usually implies birthweight of 1,000-2,499 grams*
Prematurity NOS
Prematurity or small size, not classifiable to 765.0 or as "light-for-dates" in 764
Use additional code for weeks of gestation (765.20-765.29)
AHA: 3Q 2004, 4; 4Q 2002, 63; For Code 765.10: 1Q 1994, 14; For Code 765.17: 1Q 1997, 6; For Code 765.18: 4Q 2002, 64

765.2 Weeks of gestation
AHA: 3Q 2004, 4; 4Q 2002, 63

765.20 Unspecified weeks of gestation N
C&C Exclusions: 765.01, 765.02, 765.03, 765.04, 765.05, 765.06, 765.07, 765.08

765.21 Less than 24 weeks of gestation N
C&C Exclusions: See 765.20

765.22 24 completed weeks of gestation N
C&C Exclusions: See 765.20

765.23 25-26 completed weeks of gestation N
C&C Exclusions: See 765.20

765.24 27-28 completed weeks of gestation N
C&C Exclusions: See 765.20

765.25 29-30 completed weeks of gestation N
C&C Exclusions: See 765.20

765.26 31-32 completed weeks of gestation N
C&C Exclusions: See 765.20

765.27 33-34 completed weeks of gestation N
C&C Exclusions: See 765.20

765.28 35-36 completed weeks of gestation N
C&C Exclusions: See 765.20
AHA: 4Q 2002, 64

765.29 37 or more completed weeks of gestation N
C&C Exclusions: See 765.20

4 **766 Disorders relating to long gestation and high birthweight**
Includes the listed conditions, without further specification, as causes of mortality, morbidity, or additional care, in fetus or newborn

766.0 Exceptionally large baby N
Note: *Usually implies a birthweight of 4,500 grams or more.*

766.1 Other "heavy-for-dates" infants N
Other fetus or infant "heavy-" or "large-for-dates" regardless of period of gestation

5 **766.2 Late infant, not "heavy-for-dates"**
AHA: 4Q 2003, 69

766.21 Post-term infant N
Infant with gestation period over 40 completed weeks to 42 completed weeks
AHA: 2Q 2006, 13

766.22 Prolonged gestation of infant N
Infant with gestation period over 42 completed weeks
Postmaturity NOS
AHA: 2Q 2006, 13

4 **767 Birth trauma**

767.0 Subdural and cerebral hemorrhage N
Subdural and cerebral hemorrhage, whether described as due to birth trauma or to intrapartum anoxia or hypoxia
Subdural hematoma (localized)
Tentorial tear
Use additional code to identify cause
Excludes *intraventricular hemorrhage (772.10-772.14)*
subarachnoid hemorrhage (772.2)
C&C Exclusions: 767.0, 767.11, 767.8, 767.9, 779.81, 779.82, 779.89

5 **767.1 Injuries to scalp**
AHA: 4Q 2003, 69

767.11 Epicranial subaponeurotic hemorrhage (massive) N
Subgaleal hemorrhage
C&C Exclusions: 767.11

767.19 Other injuries to scalp N
Caput succedaneum
Cephalhematoma
Chignon (from vacuum extraction)

767.2 Fracture of clavicle N

767.3 Other injuries to skeleton N
Fracture of:
- long bones
- skull

Excludes *congenital dislocation of hip (754.30-754.35)*
fracture of spine, congenital (767.4)

767.4 Injury to spine and spinal cord N
Dislocation of spine or spinal cord due to birth trauma
Fracture of spine or spinal cord due to birth trauma
Laceration of spine or spinal cord due to birth trauma
Rupture of spine or spinal cord due to birth trauma

767.5 Facial nerve injury N
Facial palsy

767.6 Injury to brachial plexus N
Palsy or paralysis:
- brachial
- Erb (-Duchenne)
- Klumpke (-Déjérine)

767.7 Other cranial and peripheral nerve injuries N
Phrenic nerve paralysis

767.8 Other specified birth trauma N
Eye damage
Hematoma of:
- liver (subcapsular)
- testes
- vulva

Rupture of:
- liver
- spleen

Scalpel wound
Traumatic glaucoma
Excludes *hemorrhage classifiable to 772.0-772.9*
C&C Exclusions: See 767.11

✖ **767.9 Birth trauma, unspecified** N
Birth injury NOS
C&C Exclusions: See 767.11

4 **768 Intrauterine hypoxia and birth asphyxia**
Use only when associated with newborn morbidity classifiable elsewhere
Excludes *acidemia NOS of newborn (775.81)*
acidosis NOS of newborn (775.81)
cerebral ischemia NOS (779.2)
hypoxia NOS of newborn (770.88)
mixed metabolic and respiratory acidosis of newborn (775.81)
respiratory arrest of newborn (770.87)
AHA: 4Q 1992, 20

768.0 Fetal death from asphyxia or anoxia before onset of labor or at unspecified time N

768.1 Fetal death from asphyxia or anoxia during labor N

768.2 Fetal distress before onset of labor, in liveborn infant N
Fetal metabolic acidemia before onset of labor, in liveborn infant

768.3 Fetal distress first noted during labor and delivery, in liveborn infant N
Fetal metabolic acidemia first noted during labor and delivery, in liveborn infant

768.4 Fetal distress, unspecified as to time of onset, in liveborn infant N
Fetal metabolic acidemia unspecified as to time of onset, in liveborn infant
AHA: Nov-Dec 1986, 10

768.5 Severe birth asphyxia N
Birth asphyxia with neurologic involvement
Excludes *hypoxic-ischemic encephalopathy (HIE) (768.7)*
C&C Exclusions: 768.5, 768.6, 768.9, 769, 770.0, 770.12, 770.14, 770.16, 770.18, 770.2, 770.3, 770.4, 770.5, 770.6, 770.7, 770.81, 770.82, 770.83, 770.84, 770.86, 770.89, 770.9, 779.81, 779.82, 779.89
AHA: Nov-Dec 1986, 3

768.6 Mild or moderate birth asphyxia N
Other specified birth asphyxia (without mention of neurologic involvement)
Excludes *hypoxic-ischemic encephalopathy (HIE) (768.7)*
C&C Exclusions: See 768.5
AHA: Nov-Dec 1986, 3

768.7 Hypoxic-ischemic encephalopathy (HIE) N
C&C Exclusions: See 768.5

✖ **768.9 Unspecified birth asphyxia in liveborn infant** N
Anoxia NOS, in liveborn infant
Asphyxia NOS, in liveborn infant
C&C Exclusions: See 768.5

769 Respiratory distress syndrome N
Cardiorespiratory distress syndrome of newborn
Hyaline membrane disease (pulmonary)
Idiopathic respiratory distress syndrome [IRDS or RDS] of newborn
Pulmonary hypoperfusion syndrome
Excludes *transient tachypnea of newborn (770.6)*
C&C Exclusions: See 768.5
AHA: 1Q 1989, 10; Nov-Dec 1986, 6

❹ **770 Other respiratory conditions of fetus and newborn**

770.0 Congenital pneumonia N
Infective pneumonia acquired prenatally
Excludes *pneumonia from infection acquired after birth (480.0-486)*
C&C Exclusions: See 768.5
AHA: 1Q 2005, 10

❺ **770.1 Fetal and newborn aspiration**
Excludes *aspiration of postnatal stomach contents (770.85, 770.86)*
meconium passage during delivery (763.84)
meconium staining (779.84)
AHA: 4Q 2005, 1983

✖ **770.10 Fetal and newborn aspiration, unspecified** N
C&C Exclusions: See 768.5

770.11 Meconium aspiration without respiratory symptoms N
Meconium aspiration NOS
C&C Exclusions: See 768.5

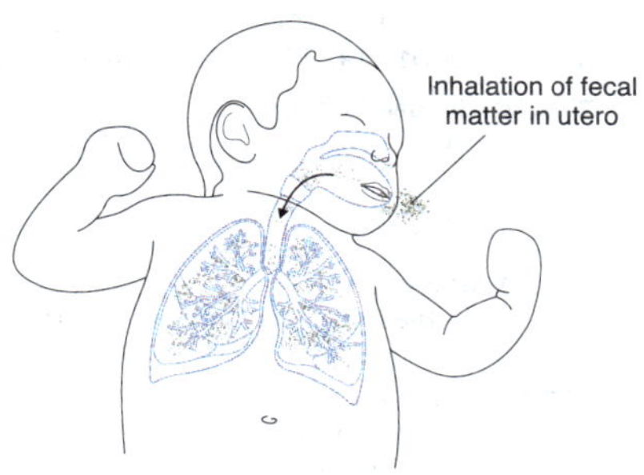

770.12 Meconium aspiration with respiratory symptoms N
Meconium aspiration pneumonia
Meconium aspiration pneumonitis
Meconium aspiration syndrome NOS
Use additional code to identify any secondary pulmonary hypertension (416.8) if applicable
C&C Exclusions: See 768.5

770.13 Aspiration of clear amniotic fluid without respiratory symptoms N
Aspiration of clear amniotic fluid NOS
C&C Exclusions: See 768.5

770.14 Aspiration of clear amniotic fluid with respiratory symptoms N
Aspiration of clear amniotic fluid with pneumonia
Aspiration of clear amniotic fluid with pneumonitis
Use additional code to identify any secondary pulmonary hypertension (416.8), if applicable
C&C Exclusions: See 768.5

770.15 Aspiration of blood without respiratory symptoms N
Aspiration of blood NOS
C&C Exclusions: See 768.5

770.16 Aspiration of blood with respiratory symptoms N
Aspiration of blood with pneumonia
Aspiration of blood with pneumonitis
Use additional code to identify any secondary pulmonary hypertension (416.8), if applicable
C&C Exclusions: See 768.5

770.17 Other fetal and newborn aspiration without respiratory symptoms N
C&C Exclusions: See 768.5

770.18 Other fetal and newborn aspiration with respiratory symptoms N
Other aspiration pneumonia
Other aspiration pneumonitis
Use additional code to identify any secondary pulmonary hypertension (416.8), if applicable
C&C Exclusions: See 768.5

770.2 Interstitial emphysema and related conditions N
Pneumomediastinum originating in the perinatal period
Pneumopericardium originating in the perinatal period
Pneumothorax originating in the perinatal period
C&C Exclusions: See 768.5

770.3 Pulmonary hemorrhage N
Hemorrhage:
alveolar (lung) originating in the perinatal period
intra-alveolar (lung) originating in the perinatal period
massive pulmonary originating in the perinatal period
C&C Exclusions: See 768.5

770.4 Primary atelectasis N
Pulmonary immaturity NOS
C&C Exclusions: See 768.5

770.5 Other and unspecified atelectasis N
Atelectasis:
NOS originating in the perinatal period
partial originating in the perinatal period
secondary originating in the perinatal period
Pulmonary collapse originating in the perinatal period
C&C Exclusions: See 768.5

770.6 Transitory tachypnea of newborn N
Idiopathic tachypnea of newborn
Wet lung syndrome
Excludes *respiratory distress syndrome (769)*
C&C Exclusions: See 768.5
AHA: 4Q 1995, 4; 1Q 1994, 12; 3Q 1993, 7; 1Q 1989, 10; Nov-Dec 1986, 6

770.7 Chronic respiratory disease arising in the perinatal period
Bronchopulmonary dysplasia
Interstitial pulmonary fibrosis of prematurity
Wilson-Mikity syndrome
C&C Exclusions: See 768.5
AHA: 2Q 1991, 19; Nov-Dec 1986, 11

❺ **770.8 Other respiratory problems after birth**
Excludes *mixed metabolic and respiratory acidosis of newborn (775.81)*
AHA: 4Q 2002, 65; 2Q 1998, 10; 2Q 1996, 10

770.81 Primary apnea of newborn N
Apneic spells of newborn NOS
Essential apnea of newborn
Sleep apnea of newborn
C&C Exclusions: 768.5, 769, 770.0, 770.12, 770.14, 770.16, 770.18, 770.2, 770.3, 770.4, 770.5, 770.6, 770.7, 770.84, 770.86

770.82 Other apnea of newborn N
Obstructive apnea of newborn
C&C Exclusions: See 770.81

770.83 Cyanotic attacks of newborn N
C&C Exclusions: See 770.81

770.84 Respiratory failure of newborn N
Excludes *respiratory distress syndrome (769)*
C&C Exclusions: See 768.5

A Adult (15+ years) M Maternity (12-55 years) N Newborn (0 years) P Pediatric (0-17 years) ♂ Male ♀ Female ❷ Medicare Secondary Payer

770.85 Aspiration of postnatal stomach contents without respiratory symptoms N
Aspiration of postnatal stomach contents NOS
C&C Exclusions: See 770.81
AHA: 4Q 2005, 83

770.86 Aspiration of postnatal stomach contents with respiratory symptoms N
Aspiration of postnatal stomach contents with pneumonia
Aspiration of postnatal stomach contents with pneumonitis
Use additional code to identify any secondary pulmonary hypertension (416.8) if applicable
C&C Exclusions: See 770.81
AHA: 4Q 2005, 83

770.87 Respiratory arrest of newborn N

770.88 Hypoxemia of newborn N
Hypoxia NOS, in liveborn infant

770.89 Other respiratory problems after birth N
C&C Exclusions: See 770.81

✖ **770.9 Unspecified respiratory condition of fetus and newborn** N
C&C Exclusions: See 770.81

④ **771 Infections specific to the perinatal period**
Includes infections acquired before or during birth or via the umbilicus or during the first 28 days after birth
Excludes *congenital pneumonia (770.0)*
congenital syphilis (090.0-090.9)
▶ *infant botulism (040.41)*◀
maternal infectious disease as a cause of mortality or morbidity in fetus or newborn, but fetus or newborn not manifesting the disease (760.2)
ophthalmia neonatorum due to gonococcus (098.40)
other infections not specifically classified to this category
AHA: Nov-Dec 1985, 4

771.0 Congenital rubella N
Congenital rubella pneumonitis
C&C Exclusions: 771.0, 771.1, 771.2, 779.81, 779.82, 779.89

771.1 Congenital cytomegalovirus infection N
Congenital cytomegalic inclusion disease
C&C Exclusions: See 771.0

771.2 Other congenital infections N
Congenital:
herpes simplex
listeriosis
malaria
toxoplasmosis
tuberculosis

771.3 Tetanus neonatorum N
Tetanus omphalitis
Excludes *hypocalcemic tetany (775.4)*
C&C Exclusions: 771.3, 779.81, 779.82, 779.89

771.4 Omphalitis of the newborn N
Infection:
navel cord
umbilical stump
Excludes *tetanus omphalitis (771.3)*
C&C Exclusions: 771.81, 771.83

771.5 Neonatal infective mastitis N
Excludes *noninfective neonatal mastitis (778.7)*
C&C Exclusions: See 771.4

771.6 Neonatal conjunctivitis and dacryocystitis N
Ophthalmia neonatorum NOS
Excludes *ophthalmia neonatorum due to gonococcus (098.40)*
C&C Exclusions: See 771.4

771.7 Neonatal Candida infection N
Neonatal moniliasis
Thrush in newborn
C&C Exclusions: See 771.4

⑤ **771.8 Other infection specific to the perinatal period**
Use additional code to identify organism (041.00-041.9)
AHA: 4Q 2002, 66

771.81 Septicemia [sepsis] of newborn N
C&C Exclusions: 771.4, 771.5, 771.6, 771.7, 771.81, 771.82, 771.83, 771.89, 776.0, 776.1, 776.2, 776.3, 776.4, 776.5, 776.6, 776.7, 776.8, 776.9, 779.81, 779.82, 779.83, 779.89

771.82 Urinary tract infection of newborn N
C&C Exclusions: See 771.4

771.83 Bacteremia of newborn N
C&C Exclusions: See 771.81

771.89 Other infections specific to the perinatal period N
Intra-amniotic infection of fetus NOS
Infection of newborn NOS
C&C Exclusions: See 771.4

④ **772 Fetal and neonatal hemorrhage**
Excludes *hematological disorders of fetus and newborn (776.0-776.9)*

772.0 Fetal blood loss N
Fetal blood loss from:
cut end of co-twin's cord
placenta
ruptured cord
vasa previa
Fetal exsanguination
Fetal hemorrhage into:
co-twin
mother's circulation
C&C Exclusions: 772.10, 772.11, 772.12, 772.13, 772.14, 779.7

⑤ **772.1 Intraventricular hemorrhage**
Intraventricular hemorrhage from any perinatal cause
AHA: 4Q 2001, 49; 3Q 1992, 8; 4Q 1988, 8

✖ **772.10 Unspecified grade** N
C&C Exclusions: 772.0, 772.10, 772.11, 772.12, 772.13, 772.14, 772.2, 772.8, 772.9, 776.0, 776.1, 776.2, 776.3, 776.4, 776.5, 776.6, 776.7, 776.8, 776.9, 779.7, 779.81, 779.82, 779.89

772.11 Grade I N
Bleeding into germinal matrix
C&C Exclusions: See 772.10

772.12 Grade II N
Bleeding into ventricle
C&C Exclusions: See 772.10

772.13 Grade III N
Bleeding with enlargement of ventricle
C&C Exclusions: See 772.10

772.14 Grade IV N
Bleeding into cerebral cortex
C&C Exclusions: See 772.10

772.2 Subarachnoid hemorrhage N
Subarachnoid hemorrhage from any perinatal cause
Excludes *subdural and cerebral hemorrhage (767.0)*
C&C Exclusions: 772.0, 772.10, 772.11, 772.12, 772.13, 772.14, 772.2, 772.8, 772.9, 776.0, 776.1, 776.2, 776.3, 776.4, 776.5, 776.6, 776.7, 776.8, 776.9, 779.7, 779.81, 779.82, 779.89

772.3 Umbilical hemorrhage after birth N
Slipped umbilical ligature

772.4 Gastrointestinal hemorrhage N
Excludes *swallowed maternal blood (777.3)*
C&C Exclusions: 772.0, 772.4, 772.5, 772.8, 772.9, 776.0, 776.1, 776.2, 776.3, 776.4, 776.5, 776.6, 776.7, 776.8, 776.9, 779.81, 779.82, 779.89

772.5 Adrenal hemorrhage N
C&C Exclusions: See 772.4

772.6 Cutaneous hemorrhage N
Bruising in fetus or newborn
Ecchymoses in fetus or newborn
Petechiae in fetus or newborn
Superficial hematoma in fetus or newborn

772.8 Other specified hemorrhage of fetus or newborn N
Excludes *hemorrhagic disease of newborn (776.0)*
pulmonary hemorrhage (770.3)
C&C Exclusions: 772.10, 772.11, 772.12, 772.13, 772.14, 779.7

772.9 Unspecified hemorrhage of newborn N
C&C Exclusions: See 772.8

773 Hemolytic disease of fetus or newborn, due to isoimmunization

773.0 Hemolytic disease due to Rh isoimmunization N
Anemia due to RH:
antibodies
isoimmunization
maternal/fetal incompatibility
Erythroblastosis (fetalis) due to RH:
antibodies
isoimmunization
maternal/fetal incompatibility
Hemolytic disease (fetus) (newborn) due to RH:
antibodies
isoimmunization
maternal/fetal incompatibility
Jaundice due to RH:
antibodies
isoimmunization
maternal/fetal incompatibility
Rh hemolytic disease
Rh isoimmunization
C&C Exclusions: 773.0, 773.1, 773.2,773.3, 773.4, 773.5, 779.81, 779.82, 779.89

773.1 Hemolytic disease due to ABO isoimmunization N
ABO hemolytic disease
ABO isoimmunization
Anemia due to ABO:
antibodies
isoimmunization
maternal/fetal incompatibility
Erythroblastosis (fetalis) due to ABO:
antibodies
isoimmunization
maternal/fetal incompatibility
Hemolytic disease (fetus) (newborn) due to ABO:
antibodies
isoimmunization
maternal/fetal incompatibility
Jaundice due to ABO:
antibodies
isoimmunization
maternal/fetal incompatibility
C&C Exclusions: See 773.0
AHA: 3Q 1992, 8

773.2 Hemolytic disease due to other and unspecified isoimmunization N
Erythroblastosis (fetalis) (neonatorum) NOS
Hemolytic disease (fetus) (newborn) NOS
Jaundice or anemia due to other and unspecified blood-group incompatibility
C&C Exclusions: See 773.0
AHA: 1Q 1994, 13

773.3 Hydrops fetalis due to isoimmunization N
Use additional code, if desired, to identify type of isoimmunization (773.0-773.2)
C&C Exclusions: See 773.0

773.4 Kernicterus due to isoimmunization N
Use additional code, if desired, to identify type of isoimmunization (773.0-773.2)
DEF: Serious form of jaundice caused by destruction of the infant's red blood cells by the mother's immune system.
C&C Exclusions: See 773.0

773.5 Late anemia due to isoimmunization N

774 Other perinatal jaundice

+ ***774.0 Perinatal jaundice from hereditary hemolytic anemias*** N
Code first underlying disease (282.0-282.9)
C&C Exclusions: 774.0, 774.1, 774.2, 774.30, 774.31, 774.39, 774.4, 774.5, 774.6, 774.7, 779.81, 779.82, 779.89

774.1 Perinatal jaundice from other excessive hemolysis N
Fetal or neonatal jaundice from:
bruising
drugs or toxins transmitted from mother
infection
polycythemia
swallowed maternal blood
Use additional code to identify cause
Excludes *jaundice due to isoimmunization (773.0-773.2)*
C&C Exclusions: See 774.0

774.2 Neonatal jaundice associated with preterm delivery N
Hyperbilirubinemia of prematurity
Jaundice due to delayed conjugation associated with preterm delivery
C&C Exclusions: See 774.0
AHA: 3Q 1991, 21

774.3 Neonatal jaundice due to delayed conjugation from other causes

774.30 Neonatal jaundice due to delayed conjugation, cause unspecified N
C&C Exclusions: See 774.0

+ ***774.31 Neonatal jaundice due to delayed conjugation in diseases classified elsewhere*** N
Code first underlying diseases, as:
congenital hypothyroidism (243)
Crigler-Najjar syndrome (277.4)
Gilbert's syndrome (277.4)
C&C Exclusions: See 774.0

774.39 Other N
Jaundice due to delayed conjugation from causes, such as:
breast milk inhibitors
delayed development of conjugating system
C&C Exclusions: See 774.0

774.4 Perinatal jaundice due to hepatocellular damage N
Fetal or neonatal hepatitis
Giant cell hepatitis
Inspissated bile syndrome
C&C Exclusions: See 774.0

+ ***774.5 Perinatal jaundice from other causes*** N
Code first underlying cause, as:
congenital obstruction of bile duct (751.61)
galactosemia (271.1)
mucoviscidosis (277.00-277.09)
C&C Exclusions: See 774.0

774.6 Unspecified fetal and neonatal jaundice N
Icterus neonatorum
Neonatal hyperbilirubinemia (transient)
Physiologic jaundice NOS in newborn
Excludes *that in preterm infants (774.2)*
AHA: 1Q 1994, 13; 2Q 1989, 15

774.7 Kernicterus not due to isoimmunization N
Bilirubin encephalopathy
Kernicterus of newborn NOS
Excludes *kernicterus due to isoimmunization (773.4)*
C&C Exclusions: See 774.0

775 Endocrine and metabolic disturbances specific to the fetus and newborn
Includes transitory endocrine and metabolic disturbances caused by the infant's response to maternal endocrine and metabolic factors, its removal from them, or its adjustment to extrauterine existence

775.0 Syndrome of "infant of a diabetic mother" N
Maternal diabetes mellitus affecting fetus or newborn (with hypoglycemia)
AHA: 1Q 2004, 7-8; 3Q 1991, 5

775.1 Neonatal diabetes mellitus N
Diabetes mellitus syndrome in newborn infant
C&C Exclusions: 775.0, 775.1, 775.2, 775.3, 775.4, 775.5, 775.6, 775.7, 775.8, 775.9, 779.81, 779.82, 779.89
AHA: 3Q 1991, 6

775.2 Neonatal myasthenia gravis N
C&C Exclusions: See 775.1

775.3 Neonatal thyrotoxicosis N
Neonatal hyperthyroidism (transient)
DEF: Abnormally high levels of thyroid hormone in the neonate.
C&C Exclusions: See 775.1

775.4 Hypocalcemia and hypomagnesemia of newborn N
Cow's milk hypocalcemia
Hypocalcemic tetany, neonatal
Neonatal hypoparathyroidism
Phosphate-loading hypocalcemia
C&C Exclusions: See 775.1

775.5 Other transitory neonatal electrolyte disturbances N
Dehydration, neonatal
C&C Exclusions: See 775.1
AHA: 1Q 2005, 9

775.6 Neonatal hypoglycemia N
Excludes *infant of mother with diabetes mellitus (775.0)*
C&C Exclusions: See 775.1
AHA: 1Q 1994, 8

775.7 Late metabolic acidosis of newborn N
C&C Exclusions: See 775.1

5 **775.8 Other neonatal endocrine and metabolic disturbances**

775.81 Other acidosis of newborn N
Acidemia NOS of newborn
Acidosis of newborn NOS
Mixed metabolic and respiratory acidosis of newborn

775.89 Other neonatal endocrine and metabolic disturbances N
Amino-acid metabolic disorders described as transitory

✖ **775.9 Unspecified endocrine and metabolic disturbances specific to the fetus and newborn** N

4 **776 Hematological disorders of fetus and newborn**
Includes disorders specific to the fetus or newborn

776.0 Hemorrhagic disease of newborn N
Hemorrhagic diathesis of newborn
Vitamin K deficiency of newborn
Excludes *fetal or neonatal hemorrhage (772.0-772.9)*
C&C Exclusions: 771.81, 771.83, 772.10, 772.11, 772.12, 772.13, 772.14, 776.0, 776.1, 776.2, 776.3, 776.4, 776.5, 776.6, 776.7, 776.8, 776.9, 779.7, 779.81, 779.82, 779.89

776.1 Transient neonatal thrombocytopenia N
Neonatal thrombocytopenia due to:
exchange transfusion
idiopathic maternal thrombocytopenia
isoimmunization
C&C Exclusions: See 776.0

776.2 Disseminated intravascular coagulation in newborn N
C&C Exclusions: See 776.0

776.3 Other transient neonatal disorders of coagulation N
Transient coagulation defect, newborn
C&C Exclusions: See 776.0

776.4 Polycythemia neonatorum N
Plethora of newborn
Polycythemia due to:
donor twin transfusion
maternal-fetal transfusion
DEF: Abnormally increased number of red blood cells in the neonate's bloodstream.
C&C Exclusions: 771.81, 771.83, 772.10, 772.11, 772.12, 772.13, 772.14, 779.7

776.5 Congenital anemia N
Anemia following fetal blood loss
Excludes *anemia due to isoimmunization (773.0-773.2, 773.5)*
hereditary hemolytic anemias (282.0-282.9)
C&C Exclusions: See 776.5

776.6 Anemia of prematurity N
C&C Exclusions: See 776.5

776.7 Transient neonatal neutropenia N
Isoimmune neutropenia
Maternal transfer neutropenia
Excludes *congenital neutropenia (nontransient) (288.01)*
C&C Exclusions: See 776.5

776.8 Other specified transient hematological disorders N
C&C Exclusions: See 776.5

✖ **776.9 Unspecified hematological disorder specific to fetus or newborn** N
C&C Exclusions: See 776.5

4 **777 Perinatal disorders of digestive system**
Includes disorders specific to the fetus and newborn
Excludes *intestinal obstruction classifiable to 560.0-560.9*

777.1 Meconium obstruction N
Congenital fecaliths
Delayed passage of meconium
Meconium ileus NOS
Meconium plug syndrome
Excludes *meconium ileus in cystic fibrosis (277.01)*
DEF: Dark green feces that comprises a newborns first bowel movement blocking the intestine.
C&C Exclusions: 777.1, 777.2, 777.3, 777.4, 777.5, 777.6, 777.8, 777.9, 779.81, 779.82, 779.89

777.2 Intestinal obstruction due to inspissated milk N
C&C Exclusions: See 777.1

777.3 Hematemesis and melena due to swallowed maternal blood N
Swallowed blood syndrome in newborn
Excludes *that not due to swallowed maternal blood (772.4)*

777.4 Transitory ileus of newborn N
Excludes *Hirschsprung's disease (751.3)*

777.5 Necrotizing enterocolitis in fetus or newborn N
Pseudomembranous enterocolitis in newborn
C&C Exclusions: See 777.1

777.6 Perinatal intestinal perforation N
Meconium peritonitis
C&C Exclusions: See 777.1

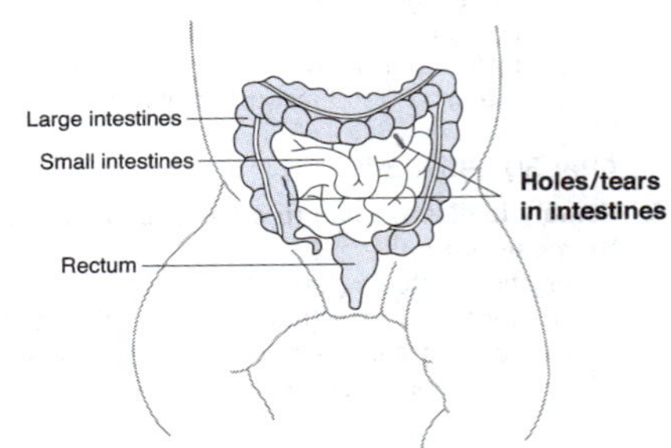

777.8 Other specified perinatal disorders of digestive system N

✖ **777.9 Unspecified perinatal disorder of digestive system** N

4 **778 Conditions involving the integument and temperature regulation of fetus and newborn**

778.0 Hydrops fetalis not due to isoimmunization N
Idiopathic hydrops
Excludes *hydrops fetalis due to isoimmunization (773.3)*
C&C Exclusions: 778.0, 779.81, 779.82, 779.89

778.1 Sclerema neonatorum N

778.2 Cold injury syndrome of newborn N

778.3 Other hypothermia of newborn N

778.4 Other disturbances of temperature regulation of newborn N
Dehydration fever in newborn
Environmentally induced pyrexia
Hyperthermia in newborn
Transitory fever of newborn

778.5 Other and unspecified edema of newborn N
Edema neonatorum

778.6 Congenital hydrocele
Congenital hydrocele of tunica vaginalis

778.7 Breast engorgement in newborn N
Noninfective mastitis of newborn
Excludes *infective mastitis of newborn (771.5)*

778.8 Other specified conditions involving the integument of fetus and newborn N
Urticaria neonatorum
Excludes *impetigo neonatorum (684)*
pemphigus neonatorum (684)

✖ **778.9 Unspecified condition involving the integument and temperature regulation of fetus and newborn** N

4 **779 Other and ill-defined conditions originating in the perinatal period**

779.0 Convulsions in newborn N
Fits in newborn
Seizures in newborn
C&C Exclusions: 779.0, 779.1, 779.81, 779.82, 779.89, 780.32
AHA: Nov-Dec 1994, 11

779.1 Other and unspecified cerebral irritability in newborn N
C&C Exclusions: See 779.0

779.2 Cerebral depression, coma, and other abnormal cerebral signs N
Cerebral ischemia NOS of newborn
CNS dysfunction in newborn NOS
Excludes *cerebral ischemia due to birth trauma (767.0)*
intrauterine cerebral ischemia (768.2-768.9)
intraventricular hemorrhage (772.10-772.14)

779.3 Feeding problems in newborn N
Regurgitation of food in newborn
Slow feeding in newborn
Vomiting in newborn
C&C Exclusions: 779.3
AHA: 2Q 1989, 15

779.4 Drug reactions and intoxications specific to newborn N
Gray syndrome from chloramphenicol administration in newborn
Excludes *fetal alcohol syndrome (760.71)*
reactions and intoxications from maternal opiates and tranquilizers (763.5)
C&C Exclusions: 779.4, 779.5

779.5 Drug withdrawal syndrome in newborn N
Drug withdrawal syndrome in infant of dependent mother
Excludes *fetal alcohol syndrome (760.71)*
AHA: 3Q 1994, 6

779.6 Termination of pregnancy (fetus) N
Fetal death due to:
induced abortion
termination of pregnancy
Excludes *spontaneous abortion (fetus) (761.8)*

779.7 Periventricular leukomalacia
C&C Exclusions: 772.0, 772.10, 772.11, 772.12, 772.13, 772.14, 772.2, 772.8, 772.9, 776.0, 776.1, 776.2, 776.3, 776.4, 776.5, 776.6, 776.7, 776.8, 776.9, 779.7, 779.81, 779.82, 779.89
AHA: 4Q 2001, 50-51

5 **779.8 Other specified conditions originating in the perinatal period**
AHA: 4Q 2002, 67; 1Q 1994, 15

779.81 Neonatal bradycardia N
Excludes *abnormality in fetal heart rate or rhythm complicating labor and delivery (763.81-763.83)*
bradycardia due to birth asphyxia (768.5-768.9)
DEF: Abnormally slow newborn heartbeat.
C&C Exclusions: 765.01, 765.02, 765.03, 765.04, 765.05, 765.06, 765.07, 765.08, 767.0, 767.11, 768.5, 769, 770.0, 770.12, 770.14, 770.16, 770.18, 770.2, 770.3, 770.4, 770.5, 770.6, 770.7, 770.84, 770.86, 771.0, 771.1, 771.3, 771.81, 771.83, 772.10, 772.11, 772.12, 772.13, 772.14, 772.2, 772.4, 772.5, 773.0, 773.1, 773.2, 773.3, 773.4, 774.0, 774.1, 774.2, 774 30, 774.31, 774.39, 774.4, 774.5, 774.7, 775.1, 775.2, 775.3, 775.4, 775.5, 775.6, 775.7, 776.0, 776.1, 776.2, 776.3, 777.1, 777.2, 777.5, 777.6, 778.0, 779.0, 779.1, 779.7

779.82 Neonatal tachycardia N
Excludes *abnormality in fetal heart rate or rhythm complicating labor and delivery (763.81-763.83)*
C&C Exclusions: See 779.81

779.83 Delayed separation of umbilical cord N
C&C Exclusions: See 779.81
AHA: 4Q 2003, 71

779.84 Meconium staining N
Excludes *meconium aspiration (770.11, 770.12)*
meconium passage during delivery (763.84)
C&C Exclusions: See 779.81
AHA: 4Q 2005, 83, 88

779.85 Cardiac arrest of newborn N
C&C Exclusions: See 779.81

779.89 Other specified conditions originating in the perinatal period N
Use additional code to specify condition
C&C Exclusions: See 779.81
AHA: 1Q 2006, 18; 1Q, 2005 ,9

✖ **779.9 Unspecified condition originating in the perinatal period** N
Congenital debility NOS
Stillbirth NEC

Certain Conditions Originating in the Perinatal Period

778.5 – 779.9

16. SYMPTOMS, SIGNS, AND ILL-DEFINED CONDITIONS (780-799)

This section includes symptoms, signs, abnormal results of laboratory or other investigative procedures, and ill-defined conditions regarding which no diagnosis classifiable elsewhere is recorded.

Signs and symptoms that point rather definitely to a given diagnosis are assigned to some category in the preceding part of the classification. In general, categories 780-796 include the more ill-defined conditions and symptoms that point with perhaps equal suspicion to two or more diseases or to two or more systems of the body, and without the necessary study of the case to make a final diagnosis. Practically all categories in this group could be designated as "not otherwise specified," or as "unknown etiology," or as "transient." The Alphabetic Index should be consulted to determine which symptoms and signs are to be allocated here and which to more specific sections of the classification; the residual subcategories numbered .9 are provided for other relevant symptoms which cannot be allocated elsewhere in the classification.

The conditions and signs or symptoms included in categories 780-796 consist of: (a) cases for which no more specific diagnosis can be made even after all facts bearing on the case have been investigated; (b) signs or symptoms existing at the time of initial encounter that proved to be transient and whose causes could not be determined; (c) provisional diagnoses in a patient who failed to return for further investigation or care; (d) cases referred elsewhere for investigation or treatment before the diagnosis was made; (e) cases in which a more precise diagnosis was not available for any other reason; (f) certain symptoms which represent important problems in medical care and which it might be desired to classify in addition to a known cause.

SYMPTOMS (780-789)

AHA: 1Q 1991, 12; 2Q 1990, 3; 2Q 1990, 5; 2Q 1990, 15; Mar-Apr 1985, 3

④ **780 General symptoms**

⑤ **780.0 Alteration of consciousness**

Excludes *coma:*
diabetic (250.2-250.3)
hepatic (572.2)
originating in the perinatal period (779.2)

AHA: 4Q 1992, 20

780.01 Coma

C&C Exclusions: 070.00, 070.01, 070.02, 070.03, 070.10, 070.11, 070.12, 070.13, 070.20, 070.21, 070.22, 070.23, 070.30, 070.31, 070.32, 070.33, 070.41, 070.42, 070.43, 070.44, 070.49, 070.51, 070.52, 070.53, 070.54, 070.59, 070.6, 070.9, 250.00, 250.01, 250.02, 250.03, 250.10, 250.11, 250.12, 250.13, 250.20, 250.21, 250.22, 250.23, 250.30, 250.31, 250.32, 250.33, 250.40, 250.41, 250.42, 250.43, 250.50, 250.51, 250.52, 250.53, 250.60, 250.61, 250.62, 250.63, 250.70, 250.71, 250.72, 250.73, 250.80, 250.81, 250.82, 250.83, 250.90, 250.91, 250.92, 250.93, 251.0, 251.1, 251.2, 251.3, 348.8, 348.9, 349.89, 349.9, 430, 431, 432.0, 432.1, 432.9, 575.2, 780.01, 780.02, 780.03, 780.09, 780.2, 780.4, 780.91, 780.92, 780.99, 799.8, 800.00, 800.01, 800.02, 800.03, 800.04, 800.05, 800.06, 800.09, 800.10, 800.11, 800.12, 800.13, 800.14, 800.15, 800.16, 800.19, 800.20, 800.21, 800.22, 800.23, 800.24, 800.25, 800.26, 800.29, 800.30, 800.31, 800.32, 800.33, 800.34, 800.35, 800.36, 800.39, 800.40, 800.41, 800.42, 800.43, 800.44, 800.45, 800.46, 800.49, 800.50, 800.51, 800.52, 800.53, 800.54, 800.55, 800.56, 800.59, 800.60, 800.61, 800.62, 800.63, 800.64, 800.65, 800.66, 800.69, 800.70, 800.71, 800.72, 800.73, 800.74, 800.75, 800.76, 800.79, 800.80, 800.81, 800.82, 800.83, 800.84, 800.85, 800.86, 800.89, 800.90, 800.91, 800.92, 800.93, 800.94, 800.95, 800.96, 800.99, 801.00, 801.01, 801.02, 801.03, 801.04, 801.05, 801.06, 801.09, 801.10, 801.11, 801.12, 801.13, 801.14, 801.15, 801.16, 801.19, 801.20, 801.21, 801.22, 801.23, 801.24, 801.25, 801.26, 801.29, 801.30, 801.31, 801.32, 801.33, 801.34, 801.35, 801.36, 801.39, 801.40, 801.41, 801.42, 801.43, 801.44, 801.45, 801.46, 801.49, 801.50, 801.51, 801.52, 801.53, 801.54, 801.55, 801.56, 801.59, 801.60, 801.61, 801.62, 801.63, 801.64, 801.65, 801.66, 801.69, 801.70, 801.71, 801.72, 801.73, 801.74, 801.75, 801.76, 801.79, 801.80, 801.81, 801.82, 801.83, 801.84, 801.85, 801.86, 801.89, 801.90, 801.91, 801.92, 801.93, 801.94, 801.95, 801.96, 801.99, 803.00, 803.01, 803.02, 803.03, 803.04, 803.05, 803.06, 803.09, 803.10, 803.11, 803.12, 803.13, 803.14, 803.15, 803.16, 803.19, 803.20, 803.21, 803.22, 803.23, 803.24, 803.25, 803.26, 803.29, 803.30, 803.31, 803.32, 803.33, 803.34, 803.35, 803.36, 803.39, 803.40, 803.41, 803.42, 803.43, 803.44, 803.45, 803.46, 803.49, 803.50, 803.51, 803.52, 803.53, 803.54, 803.55, 803.56, 803.59, 803.60, 803.61, 803.62, 803.63, 803.64, 803.65, 803.66, 803.69, 803.70, 803.71, 803.72, 803.73, 803.74, 803.75, 803.76, 803.79, 803.80, 803.81, 803.82, 803.83, 803.84, 803.85, 803.86, 803.89, 803.90, 803.91, 803.92, 803.93, 803.94, 803.95, 803.96, 803.99, 804.00, 804.01, 804.02, 804.03, 804.04, 804.05, 804.06, 804.09, 804.10, 804.11, 804.12, 804.13, 804.14, 804.15, 804.16, 804.19, 804.20, 804.21, 804.22, 804.23, 804.24, 804.25, 804.26, 804.29, 804.30, 804.31, 804.32, 804.33, 804.34, 804.35, 804.36, 804.39, 804.40, 804.41, 804.42, 804.43, 804.44, 804.45, 804.46, 804.49, 804.50, 804.51, 804.52, 804.53, 804.54, 804.55, 804.56, 804.59, 804.60, 804.61, 804.62, 804.63, 804.64, 804.65, 804.66, 804.69, 804.70, 804.71, 804.72, 804.73, 804.74, 804.75, 804.76, 804.79, 804.80, 804.81, 804.82, 804.83, 804.84, 804.85, 804.86, 804.89, 804.90, 804.91, 804.92, 804.93, 804.94, 804.95, 804.96, 850.0, 850.1, 850.2, 850.3, 850.5, 850.9, 851.00, 851.01, 851.02, 851.03, 851.04, 851.05, 851.06, 851.09, 851.10, 851.11, 851.12, 851.13, 851.14, 851.15, 851.16, 851.19, 851.20, 851.21, 851.22, 851.23, 851.24, 851.25, 851.26, 851.29, 851.30, 851.31, 851.32, 851.33, 851.34, 851.35, 851.36, 851.39, 851.40, 851.41, 851.42, 851.43, 851.44, 851.45, 851.46, 851.49, 851.50, 851.51, 851.52, 851.53, 851.54, 851.55, 851.56, 851.59, 851.60, 851.61, 851.62, 851.63, 851.64, 851.65, 851.66, 851.69, 851.70, 851.71, 851.72, 851.73, 851.74, 851.75, 851.76, 851.79, 851.80, 851.81, 851.82, 851.83, 851.84, 851.85, 851.86, 851.89, 851.90, 851.91, 851.92, 851.93, 851.94, 851.95, 851.96, 851.99, 852.00, 852.01, 852.02, 852.03, 852.04, 852.05, 852.06, 852.09, 852.10, 852.11, 852.12, 852.13, 852.14, 852.15, 852.16, 852.19, 852.21, 852.22, 852.23, 852.24, 852.25, 852.26, 852.29, 852.30, 852.31, 852.32, 852.33, 852.34, 852.35, 852.36, 852.39, 852.40, 852.41, 852.42, 852.43, 852.44, 852.45, 852.46, 852.49, 852.50, 852.51, 852.52, 852.53, 852.54, 852.55, 852.56, 852.59, 853.00, 853.01, 853.02, 853.03, 853.04, 853.05, 853.06, 853.09, 853.10, 853.11, 853.12, 853.13, 853.14, 853.15, 853.16, 853.19, 854.00, 854.01, 854.02, 854.03, 854.04, 854.05, 854.06, 854.09, 854.10, 854.11, 854.12, 854.13, 854.14, 854.15, 854.16, 854.19

AHA: 3Q 1996, 16

780.02 Transient alteration of awareness

780.03 Persistent vegetative state

C&C Exclusions: See 780.01

780.09 Other

Drowsiness
Semicoma
Somnolence
Stupor
Unconsciousness

780.1 Hallucinations

Hallucinations:
NOS
auditory
gustatory
olfactory
tactile

Excludes *those associated with mental disorders, as functional psychoses (295.0-298.9)*
organic brain syndromes (290.0-294.9, 310.0-310.9)
visual hallucinations (368.16)

C&C Exclusions: 780.1, 780.4, 780.91, 780.92, 780.99, 799.8

780.2 Syncope and collapse
Blackout
Fainting
(Near) (Pre)syncope
Vasovagal attack
Excludes *carotid sinus syncope (337.0)*
heat syncope (992.1)
neurocirculatory asthenia (306.2)
orthostatic hypotension (458.0)
shock NOS (785.50)

DEF: Fainting and collapse due to a lack of blood flow to the brain.

AHA: 1Q 2002, 6; 3Q 2000, 12; 3Q 1995, 14; Nov-Dec 1985, 12

5 **780.3 Convulsions**
Excludes *convulsions:*
epileptic (345.10-345.91)
in newborn (779.0)

AHA: 2Q 1997, 8; 1Q 1997, 12; 3Q 1994, 9; 1Q 1993, 24; 4Q 1992, 23; Nov-Dec 1987, 12

✖ **780.31 Febrile convulsions (simple), unspecified**
Febrile seizure NOS
C&C Exclusions: 345.00, 345.01, 345.10, 345.11, 345.2, 345.3, 345.40, 345.41, 345.50, 345.51, 345.60, 345.61, 345.70, 345.71, 345.80, 345.81, 345.90, 345.91, 348.8, 348.9, 349.89, 349.9, 779.0, 779.1, 780.31, 780.32, 780.39, 780.91, 780.92, 780.99, 799.8
AHA: 4Q 1997, 45

780.32 Complex febrile convulsions
Febrile seizures:
atypical
complex
complicated
Excludes *status epilepticus (345.3)*
C&C Exclusions: See 780.31

780.39 Other convulsions
Convulsive disorder NOS
Fits NOS
Recurrent convulsions NOS
▶ Seizure NOS◀
C&C Exclusions: See 780.31
AHA: 4Q 2004, 51; 1Q 2003, 7; 2Q 1999, 17; 4Q 1998, 39

780.4 Dizziness and giddiness
Light-headedness
Vertigo NOS
Excludes *Ménière's disease and other specified vertiginous syndromes (386.0-386.9)*

AHA: 2Q 2003, 11; 3Q 2000, 12; 2Q 1997, 9; 2Q 1991, 17

5 **780.5 Sleep disturbances**
Excludes *circadian rhythm sleep disorders (327.30-327.39)*
organic hypersomnia (327.10-327.19)
organic insomnia (327.00-327.09)
organic sleep apnea (327.20-327.29)
organic sleep related movement disorders (327.51-327.59)
parasomnias (327.40-327.49)
that of nonorganic origin (307.40-307.49)

AHA: 4Q 2005, 59

780.50 Sleep disturbance, unspecified

✖ **780.51 Insomnia with sleep apnea, unspecified**

✖ **780.52 Insomnia, unspecified**

✖ **780.53 Hypersomnia with sleep apnea, unspecified**
AHA: 1Q 1993, 28; Nov-Dec 1985, 4

✖ **780.54 Hypersomnia, unspecified**

✖ **780.55 Disruption of 24 hour sleep wake cycle, unspecified**

780.56 Dysfunctions associated with sleep stages or arousal from sleep

✖ **780.57 Unspecified sleep apnea**
AHA: 1Q 2001, 6; 1Q 1997, 5; 1Q 1993, 28

✖ **780.58 Sleep related movement disorder, unspecified**
Excludes *restless legs syndrome (333.94)*
AHA: 4Q 2004, 1995

780.59 Other

780.6 Fever
Chills with fever
Fever NOS
Fever of unknown origin (FUO)
Hyperpyrexia NOS
Pyrexia NOS
Pyrexia of unknown origin
Code first underlying condition when associated fever is present, such as with:
leukemia (codes from categories 204-208)
neutropenia (288.00-288.09)
sickle-cell disease (282.60-282.69)
Excludes *pyrexia of unknown origin (during):*
in newborn (778.4)
labor (659.2)
the puerperium (672)

AHA: 3Q 2005, 16; 3Q 2000, 13; 4Q 1999, 26; 2Q 1991, 8

5 **780.7 Malaise and fatigue**
Excludes *debility, unspecified (799.3)*
fatigue (during):
combat (308.0-308.9)
heat (992.6)
pregnancy (646.8)
neurasthenia (300.5)
senile asthenia (797)

AHA: 4Q 1988, 12; Mar-Apr 1987, 8

780.71 Chronic fatigue syndrome

✖ **780.79 Other malaise and fatigue**
Asthenia NOS
Lethargy
Postviral (asthenic) syndrome
Tiredness
AHA: 4Q 2004, 78; 1Q 2000, 6; 4Q 1999, 26

780.8 Generalized hyperhidrosis
Diaphoresis
Excessive sweating
Secondary hyperhidrosis
Excludes *focal (localized) (primary) (secondary) hyperhidrosis (705.21-705.22)*
Frey's syndrome (705.22)

5 **780.9 Other general symptoms**
Excludes *hypothermia:*
NOS (accidental) (991.6)
due to anesthesia (995.89)
of newborn (778.2-778.3)
memory disturbance as part of a pattern of mental disorder

AHA: 4Q 2002, 67; 4Q 1999, 10; 3Q 1993, 11; Nov-Dec 1985, 12

780.91 Fussy infant (baby) P
C&C Exclusions: 040.82, 440.24, 780.01, 780.03, 780.1, 780.31, 780.32, 780.39, 781.7, 785.4, 785.50, 785.51, 785.52, 785.59, 786.3, 788.20, 788.29, 789.5, 790.7, 791.1, 791.3, 799.01, 799.02, 799.1, 799.4

780.92 Excessive crying of infant (baby) N
Excludes *excessive crying of child, adolescent or adult (780.95)*
C&C Exclusions: See 780.91

780.93 Memory loss
Amnesia (retrograde)
Memory loss NOS
Excludes *mild memory disturbance due to organic brain damage (310.1)*
transient global amnesia (437.7)
C&C Exclusions: See 780.91
AHA: 4Q 2003, 71

780.94 Early satiety
C&C Exclusions: See 780.91
AHA: 4Q 2003, 72

Symptoms, Signs, and Ill-Defined Conditions 780.2 – 780.94

A Adult (15+ years) M Maternity (12-55 years) N Newborn (0 years) P Pediatric (0-17 years) ♂ Male ♀ Female 2 Medicare Secondary Payer

780.95 Excessive crying of child, adolescent, or adult
Excludes *excessive crying of infant (baby) (780.92)*
C&C Exclusions: See 780.91
AHA: 4Q 2005, 89

780.96 Generalized pain
Pain NOS
C&C Exclusions: See 780.91

780.97 Altered mental status
Change in mental status
Excludes *altered level of consciousness (780.01-780.09)*
altered mental status due to known condition - code to condition
delirium NOS (780.09)
C&C Exclusions: See 780.91
AHA: 4Q 2006, 108

780.99 Other general symptoms
Chill(s) NOS
Hypothermia, not associated with low environmental temperature
C&C Exclusions: See 780.91
AHA: 4Q 2003, 103

④ **781 Symptoms involving nervous and musculoskeletal systems**
Excludes *depression NOS (311)*
disorders specifically relating to:
back (724.0-724.9)
hearing (388.0-389.9)
joint (718.0-719.9)
limb (729.0-729.9)
neck (723.0-723.9)
vision (368.0-369.9)
pain in limb (729.5)

781.0 Abnormal involuntary movements
Abnormal head movements
Fasciculation
Spasms NOS
Tremor NOS
Excludes *abnormal reflex (796.1)*
chorea NOS (333.5)
infantile spasms (345.60-345.61)
spastic paralysis (342.1, 343.0-344.9)
specified movement disorders classifiable to 333 (333.0-333.9)
that of nonorganic origin (307.2-307.3)

781.1 Disturbances of sensation of smell and taste
Anosmia
Parageusia
Parosmia

781.2 Abnormality of gait
Gait:
ataxic
paralytic
spastic
staggering
Excludes *ataxia:*
NOS (781.3)
locomotor (progressive) (094.0)
difficulty in walking (719.7)
AHA: 2Q 2005, 6; 2Q 2004, 15

781.3 Lack of coordination
Ataxia NOS
Muscular incoordination
Excludes *ataxic gait (781.2)*
cerebellar ataxia (334.0-334.9)
difficulty in walking (719.7)
vertigo NOS (780.4)
AHA: 4Q 2004, 51; 3Q 1997, 12

781.4 Transient paralysis of limb
Monoplegia, transient NOS
Excludes *paralysis (342.0-344.9)*

781.5 Clubbing of fingers

781.6 Meningismus
Dupre's syndrome
Meningism
AHA: 3Q 2000, 13; Jan-Feb 1987, 7

781.7 Tetany
Carpopedal spasm
Excludes *tetanus neonatorum (771.3)*
tetany:
hysterical (300.11)
newborn (hypocalcemic) (775.4)
parathyroid (252.1)
psychogenic (306.0)
DEF: Calcium imbalance causing severe muscle spasms.
C&C Exclusions: 037, 332.0, 332.1, 333.0, 333.1, 333.2, 333.3, 333.4, 333.5, 333.6, 333.7, 333.81, 333.82, 333.83, 333.84, 333.89, 333.90, 333.91, 333.92, 333.93, 333.99, 334.0, 334.1, 334.2, 334.3, 334.4, 342.10, 342.11, 342.12, 771.3, 780.91, 780.92, 780.99, 781.7, 799.8

781.8 Neurologic neglect syndrome
Asomatognosia
Hemi-akinesia
Hemi-inattention
Hemispatial neglect
Left-sided neglect
Sensory extinction
Sensory neglect
Visuospatial neglect
AHA: 4Q 1994, 37

⑤ **781.9 Other symptoms involving nervous and musculoskeletal systems**
AHA: 4Q 2000, 45

781.91 Loss of height
Excludes *osteoporosis (733.00-733.09)*

781.92 Abnormal posture

781.93 Ocular torticollis
AHA: 4Q 2002, 68

781.94 Facial weakness
Facial droop
Excludes *facial weakness due to late effect of cerebrovascular accident (438.83)*
AHA: 4Q 2003, 72

781.99 Other symptoms involving nervous and musculoskeletal systems

④ **782 Symptoms involving skin and other integumentary tissue**
Excludes *symptoms relating to breast (611.71-611.79)*

782.0 Disturbance of skin sensation
Anesthesia of skin
Burning or prickling sensation
Hyperesthesia
Hypoesthesia
Numbness
Paresthesia
Tingling

782.1 Rash and other nonspecific skin eruption
Exanthem
Excludes *vesicular eruption (709.8)*

782.2 Localized superficial swelling, mass, or lump
Subcutaneous nodules
Excludes *localized adiposity (278.1)*

782.3 Edema
Anasarca
Dropsy
Localized edema NOS
Excludes *ascites (▶789.51-789.59◀)*
edema of:
newborn NOS (778.5)
pregnancy (642.0-642.9, 646.1)
fluid retention (276.6)
hydrops fetalis (773.3, 778.0)
hydrothorax (511.8)
nutritional edema (260, 262)
AHA: 2Q 2000, 18

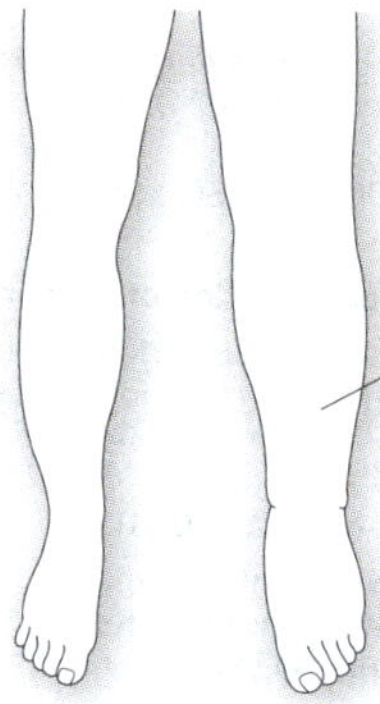

782.4 Jaundice, unspecified, not of newborn
Cholemia NOS
Icterus NOS
Excludes *jaundice in newborn (774.0-774.7)*
due to isoimmunization (773.0-773.2, 773.4)

✖ **782.5 Cyanosis**
Excludes *newborn (770.83)*
DEF: Bluish tint of the skin from lack of oxygen.

❺ **782.6 Pallor and flushing**

✖ **782.61 Pallor**
DEF: Excessive paleness of the skin, especially the face.

✖ **782.62 Flushing**
Excessive blushing

782.7 Spontaneous ecchymoses
Petechiae
Excludes *ecchymosis in fetus or newborn (772.6)*
purpura (287.0-287.9)

782.8 Changes in skin texture
Induration of skin
Thickening of skin

782.9 Other symptoms involving skin and integumentary tissues

❹ **783 Symptoms concerning nutrition, metabolism, and development**

783.0 Anorexia
Loss of appetite
Excludes *anorexia nervosa (307.1)*
loss of appetite of nonorganic origin (307.59)

783.1 Abnormal weight gain
Excludes *excessive weight gain in pregnancy (646.1)*
obesity (278.00)
morbid (278.01)

❺ **783.2 Abnormal loss of weight and underweight**
Use additional code to identify Body Mass Index (BMI), if known (V85.0-V85.54)
AHA: 4Q 2000, 45

783.21 Loss of weight
AHA: 4Q 2005, 96

783.22 Underweight
AHA: 4Q 2005, 96

783.3 Feeding difficulties and mismanagement
Feeding problem (elderly) (infant)
Excludes *feeding disturbance or problems:*
in newborn (779.3)
of nonorganic origin (307.50-307.59)
AHA: 3Q 1997, 12

❺ **783.4 Lack of expected normal physiological development in childhood**
Excludes *delay in sexual development and puberty (259.0)*
gonadal dysgenesis (758.6)
pituitary dwarfism (253.3)
slow fetal growth and fetal malnutrition (764.00-764.99)
specific delays in mental development (315.0-315.9)
AHA: 4Q 2000, 45; 3Q 1997, 4

✖ **783.40 Lack of normal physiological development, unspecified**
Inadequate development
Lack of development

783.41 Failure to thrive P
Failure to gain weight
AHA: 1Q 2003, 12

783.42 Delayed milestones P
Late talker
Late walker

783.43 Short stature
Growth failure
Growth retardation
Lack of growth
Physical retardation

783.5 Polydipsia
Excessive thirst

783.6 Polyphagia
Excessive eating
Hyperalimentation NOS
Excludes *disorders of eating of nonorganic origin (307.50-307.59)*

783.7 Adult failure to thrive A

783.9 Other symptoms concerning nutrition, metabolism, and development
Hypometabolism
Excludes *abnormal basal metabolic rate (794.7)*
dehydration (276.51)
other disorders of fluid, electrolyte, and acid-base balance (276.0-276.9)
AHA: 2Q 2004, 3

❹ **784 Symptoms involving head and neck**
Excludes *encephalopathy NOS (348.30)*
specific symptoms involving neck classifiable to 723 (723.0-723.9)

784.0 Headache
Facial pain
Pain in head NOS
Excludes *atypical face pain (350.2)*
migraine (346.0-346.9)
tension headache (307.81)
AHA: 2Q 2006, 18; 3Q 2000, 13; 1Q 1990, 4; 3Q 1992, 14

784.1 Throat pain
Excludes *dysphagia (▶787.20-787.29◀)*
neck pain (723.1)
sore throat (462)
chronic (472.1)

784.2 Swelling, mass, or lump in head and neck
Space-occupying lesion, intracranial NOS
AHA: 1Q 2003, 8

784.3 Aphasia
Excludes *aphasia due to late effects of cerebrovascular disease (438.11)*
developmental aphasia (315.31)
AHA: 4Q 2004, 78; 4Q 1998, 87; 3Q 1997, 12

A Adult (15+ years) M Maternity (12-55 years) N Newborn (0 years) P Pediatric (0-17 years) ♂ Male ♀ Female ❷ Medicare Secondary Payer

❺ **784.4 Voice disturbance**

784.40 Voice disturbance, unspecified

784.41 Aphonia
Loss of voice

784.49 Other
Change in voice
Dysphonia
Hoarseness
Hypernasality
Hyponasality

784.5 Other speech disturbance
Dysarthria
Dysphasia
Slurred speech
Excludes *stammering and stuttering (307.0)*
that of nonorganic origin (307.0, 307.9)

❺ **784.6 Other symbolic dysfunction**
Excludes *developmental learning delays (315.0-315.9)*

784.60 Symbolic dysfunction, unspecified

784.61 Alexia and dyslexia
Alexia (with agraphia)

784.69 Other
Acalculia
Agnosia
Agraphia NOS
Apraxia

784.7 Epistaxis
Hemorrhage from nose
Nosebleed
AHA: 3Q 2004, 7

784.8 Hemorrhage from throat
Excludes *hemoptysis (786.3)*

❺ **784.9 Other symptoms involving head and neck**

784.91 Postnasal drip

784.99 Other symptoms involving head and neck
Choking sensation
▶ Feeling of foreign body in throat◀
Halitosis
Mouth breathing
Sneezing
▶ Excludes *foreign body in throat (933.0)*◀

❹ **785 Symptoms involving cardiovascular system**
Excludes *heart failure NOS (428.9)*

785.0 Tachycardia, unspecified
Rapid heart beat
Excludes *neonatal tachycardia (779.82)*
paroxysmal tachycardia (427.0-427.2)
AHA: 2Q 2003, 11

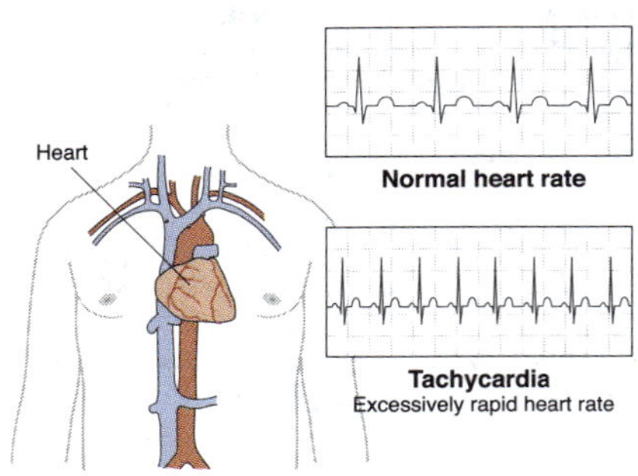

785.1 Palpitations
Awareness of heart beat
Excludes *specified dysrhythmias (427.0-427.9)*
DEF: Sensation of feeling the heart beat.

785.2 Undiagnosed cardiac murmurs
Heart murmur NOS
AHA: 4Q 1992, 16

785.3 Other abnormal heart sounds
Cardiac dullness, increased or decreased
Friction fremitus, cardiac
Precordial friction

785.4 Gangrene
Gangrene:
NOS
spreading cutaneous
Gangrenous cellulitis
Phagedena
Code first any associated underlying condition
Excludes *gangrene of certain sites - see Alphabetic Index*
gangrene with atherosclerosis of the extremities (440.24)
gas gangrene (040.0)
C&C Exclusions: 440.24, 780.91, 780.92, 780.99, 785.4, 799.8
AHA: 1Q 2004, 14; 3Q 1991, 12; 3Q 1990, 15; Mar-Apr 1986, 12

❺ **785.5 Shock without mention of trauma**

785.50 Shock, unspecified
Failure of peripheral circulation
C&C Exclusions: 040.82, 780.91, 780.92, 780.99, 785.50, 785.51, 785.52, 785.59, 785.9, 799.8
AHA: 2Q 1996, 10

785.51 Cardiogenic shock
C&C Exclusions: See 785.50
AHA: 3Q 2005, 14

✚ ***785.52 Septic shock***
Endotoxic
Gram-negative
Code first:
systemic inflammatory response syndrome due to infectious process with organ dysfunction (995.92)
C&C Exclusions: See 785.50
AHA: 2Q 2005, 18-19; 4Q 2003, 73, 79

785.59 Other
Shock:
hypovolemic
Excludes *shock (due to):*
anesthetic (995.4)
anaphylactic (995.0)
due to serum (999.4)
electric (994.8)
following abortion (639.5)
lightning (994.0)
obstetrical (669.1)
postoperative (998.0)
traumatic (958.4)
C&C Exclusions: See 785.50
AHA: 2Q 2000, 3

785.6 Enlargement of lymph nodes
Lymphadenopathy
"Swollen glands"
Excludes *lymphadenitis (chronic) (289.1-289.3)*
acute (683)

785.9 Other symptoms involving cardiovascular system
Bruit (arterial)
Weak pulse
C&C Exclusions: 040.82, 785.52

❹ **786 Symptoms involving respiratory system and other chest symptoms**

❺ **786.0 Dyspnea and respiratory abnormalities**

786.00 Respiratory abnormality, unspecified

786.01 Hyperventilation
Excludes *hyperventilation, psychogenic (306.1)*

786.02 Orthopnea
DEF: Difficulty breathing while lying down, necessitating sleeping propped up or in a chair.

786.03 Apnea
Excludes *apnea of newborn (770.81, 770.82)*
sleep apnea (780.51, 780.53, 780.57)
DEF: Temporary cessation of breathing.
C&C Exclusions: 518.81, 518.82, 518.83, 518.84, 519.8, 519.9, 786.03, 786.04, 799.1
AHA: 4Q 1998, 50

786.04 Cheyne-Stokes respiration
C&C Exclusions: 518.81, 518.82, 518.83, 518.84, 519.8, 519.9, 786.04, 786.04, 799.1
AHA: 4Q 1998, 50

786.05 Shortness of breath
AHA: 4Q 1999, 25; 1Q 1999, 6; 4Q 1998, 50

786.06 Tachypnea
Excludes *transitory tachypnea of newborn (770.6)*
AHA: 4Q 1998, 50

786.07 Wheezing
Excludes *asthma (493.00-493.92)*
AHA: 4Q 1998, 50

786.09 Other
Respiratory:
distress
insufficiency
Excludes *respiratory distress:*
following trauma and surgery (518.5)
newborn (770.89)
syndrome (newborn) (769)
adult (518.5)
respiratory failure (518.81, 518.83-518.84)
newborn (770.84)
AHA: 4Q 2005, 90; 2Q 1998, 10; 1Q 1997, 7; 1Q 1990, 9

786.1 Stridor
Excludes *congenital laryngeal stridor (748.3)*

786.2 Cough
Excludes *cough:*
psychogenic (306.1)
smokers' (491.0)
with hemorrhage (786.3)
AHA: 4Q 1999, 26

786.3 Hemoptysis
Cough with hemorrhage
Pulmonary hemorrhage NOS
Excludes *pulmonary hemorrhage of newborn (770.3)*
DEF: Coughing up blood or bloody mucous.
C&C Exclusions: 780.91, 780.92, 780.99, 786.3, 786.4, 786.9, 799.8
AHA: 2Q 2006, 17; 4Q 1990, 26

786.4 Abnormal sputum
Abnormal:
amount of sputum
color of sputum
odor of sputum
Excessive sputum

5 **786.5 Chest pain**

786.50 Chest pain, unspecified
AHA: 1Q 2007, 19; 2Q 2006, 8; 1Q 2003, 6; 1Q 2002, 4; 4Q 1999, 25

786.51 Precordial pain

786.52 Painful respiration
Pain:
anterior chest wall
pleuritic
Pleurodynia
Excludes *epidemic pleurodynia (074.1)*
AHA: Nov-Dec 1984, 17

786.59 Other
Discomfort in chest
Pressure in chest
Tightness in chest
Excludes *pain in breast (611.71)*
AHA: 1Q 2002, 6

786.6 Swelling, mass, or lump in chest
Excludes *lump in breast (611.72)*

786.7 Abnormal chest sounds
Abnormal percussion, chest
Friction sounds, chest
Rales
Tympany, chest
Excludes *wheezing (786.07)*

786.8 Hiccough
Excludes *psychogenic hiccough (306.1)*

786.9 Other symptoms involving respiratory system and chest
Breath-holding spell

4 **787 Symptoms involving digestive system**
Excludes *constipation (564.0-564.9)*
pylorospasm (537.81)
congenital (750.5)

5 **787.0 Nausea and vomiting**
Emesis
Excludes *hematemesis NOS (578.0)*
vomiting:
bilious, following gastrointestinal surgery (564.3)
cyclical (536.2)
psychogenic (306.4)
excessive, in pregnancy (643.0-643.9)
habit (536.2)
of newborn (779.3)
psychogenic NOS (307.54)
AHA: Mar-Apr 1985, 11

787.01 Nausea with vomiting
AHA: 1Q 2003, 5

787.02 Nausea alone
AHA: 3Q 2000, 12; 2Q 1997, 9

787.03 Vomiting alone

787.1 Heartburn
Pyrosis
Waterbrash
Excludes *dyspepsia or indigestion (536.8)*
AHA: 2Q 2001, 6

5 **787.2 Dysphagia**
▶ *Code first, if applicable, dysphagia due to late effect of cerebrovascular accident (438.82)*◀
AHA: 4Q 2003, 103, 109; 2Q 2001, 4

● **787.20 Dysphagia, unspecified**
Difficulty in swallowing NOS

● **787.21 Dysphagia, oral phase**

● **787.22 Dysphagia, oropharyngeal phase**

● **787.23 Dysphagia, pharyngeal phase**

● **787.24 Dysphagia, pharyngoesophageal phase**

● **787.29 Other dysphagia**
Cervical dysphagia
Neurogenic dysphagia

787.3 Flatulence, eructation, and gas pain
Abdominal distention (gaseous)
Bloating
Tympanites (abdominal) (intestinal)
Excludes *aerophagy (306.4)*

787.4 Visible peristalsis
Hyperperistalsis

787.5 Abnormal bowel sounds
Absent bowel sounds
Hyperactive bowel sounds

787.6 Incontinence of feces
Encopresis NOS
Incontinence of sphincter ani
Excludes *that of nonorganic origin (307.7)*
AHA: 1Q 1997, 9

787.7 Abnormal feces
Bulky stools
Excludes *abnormal stool content (792.1)*
melena:
NOS (578.1)
newborn (772.4, 777.3)

❺ **787.9 Other symptoms involving digestive system**
Excludes *gastrointestinal hemorrhage (578.0-578.9)*
intestinal obstruction (560.0-560.9)
specific functional digestive disorders:
esophagus (530.0-530.9)
stomach and duodenum (536.0-536.9)
those not elsewhere classified (564.0-564.9)

787.91 Diarrhea
Diarrhea NOS
AHA: 4Q 1995, 54

787.99 Other
Change in bowel habits
Tenesmus (rectal)

❹ **788 Symptoms involving urinary system**
Excludes *hematuria (599.7)*
nonspecific findings on examination of the urine (791.0-791.9)
small kidney of unknown cause (589.0-589.9)
uremia NOS (586)
urinary obstruction (599.60-599.69)

788.0 Renal colic
Colic (recurrent) of:
kidney
ureter
AHA: 3Q 2004, 8

788.1 Dysuria
Painful urination
Strangury
C&C Exclusions: 599.60, 599.69

❺ **788.2 Retention of urine**
Code, if applicable, any causal condition first, such as:
hyperplasia of prostate (600.0-600.9 with fifth-digit 1)

788.20 Retention of urine, unspecified
C&C Exclusions: 274.11, 344.61, 593.3, 593.4, 593.5, 596.0, 596.4, 596.51, 596.52, 596.53, 596.54, 596.55, 596.59, 596.8, 596.9, 599.6, 600.1, 600.2, 600.3, 600.9, 601.1, 601.2, 601.3, 601.4, 601.8, 601.9, 602.0, 602.1, 602.2, 602.3, 602.8, 602.9, 753.0, 753.10, 753.11, 753.12, 753.13, 753.14, 753.15, 753.16, 753.17, 753.19, 753.20, 753.21, 753.22, 753.23, 753.29, 753.3, 753.4, 753.5, 753.6, 753.7, 753.8, 753.9, 780.91, 780.92, 780.99, 788.20, 788.21, 788.29, 788.60, 788.61, 788.69, 788.9, 799.8
AHA: 4Q 2006, 95; 2Q 2004, 18; 3Q 2003, 12-13; 1Q 2003, 6; 3Q 1996, 10

788.21 Incomplete bladder emptying

788.29 Other specified retention of urine
C&C Exclusions: See 788.20

❺ **788.3 Urinary incontinence**
Excludes *that of nonorganic origin (307.6)*
Code, if applicable, any causal condition first, such as:
congenital ureterocele (753.23)
hyperplasia of prostate (600.0-600.9 with fifth-digit 1)
genital prolapse (618.00-618.9)
AHA: 4Q 1992, 22

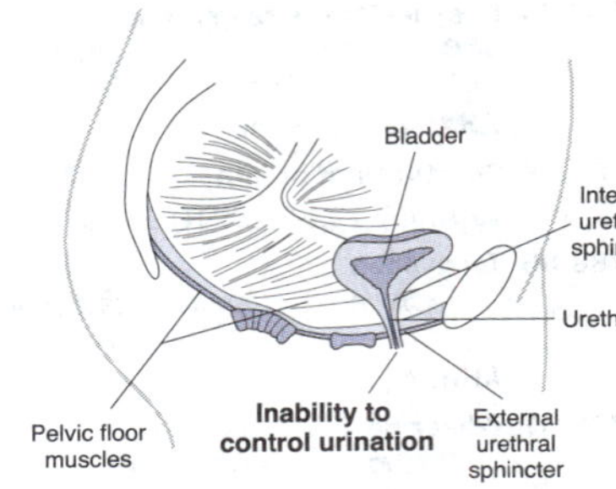

✖ **788.30 Urinary incontinence, unspecified**
Enuresis NOS

788.31 Urge incontinence
DEF: Inability to control urination after the urge to urinate.
AHA: 1Q 2000, 19

788.32 Stress incontinence, male ♂
Excludes *stress incontinence, female (625.6)*

788.33 Mixed incontinence (female) (male)
Urge and stress

788.34 Incontinence without sensory awareness

788.35 Post-void dribbling

788.36 Nocturnal enuresis

788.37 Continuous leakage

788.38 Overflow incontinence

788.39 Other urinary incontinence

❺ **788.4 Frequency of urination and polyuria**
Code, if applicable, any causal condition first, such as:
hyperplasia of prostate (600.0-600.9 with fifth-digit 1)

788.41 Urinary frequency
Frequency of micturition

788.42 Polyuria

788.43 Nocturia

788.5 Oliguria and anuria
Deficient secretion of urine
Suppression of urinary secretion
Excludes *that complicating:*
abortion (634-638 with .3, 639.3)
ectopic or molar pregnancy (639.3)
pregnancy, childbirth, or the puerperium (642.0-642.9, 646.2)

❺ **788.6 Other abnormality of urination**
Code, if applicable, any causal condition first, such as:
hyperplasia of prostate (600.0-600.9 with fifth-digit 1)

788.61 Splitting of urinary stream
Intermittent urinary stream

788.62 Slowing of urinary stream
Weak stream

788.63 Urgency of urination
Excludes *urge incontinence (788.31, 788.33)*
C&C Exclusions: 788.20, 788.29
AHA: 4Q 2003, 74

788.64 Urinary hesitancy
DEF: Difficulty starting urination.
C&C Exclusions: See 788.63

788.65 Straining on urination
C&C Exclusions: See 788.63

788.69 Other

788.7 Urethral discharge
Penile discharge
Urethrorrhea

788.8 Extravasation of urine

788.9 Other symptoms involving urinary system
Extrarenal uremia
Vesical:
pain
tenesmus
AHA: 1Q 2005, 12; 4Q 1988, 1

❹ **789 Other symptoms involving abdomen and pelvis**
Excludes *symptoms referable to genital organs:*
female (625.0-625.9)
male (607.0-608.9)
psychogenic (302.70-302.79)

The following fifth-digit subclassification is to be used for codes 789.0, 789.3, 789.4, 789.6
- **0 unspecified site**
- **1 right upper quadrant**
- **2 left upper quadrant**
- **3 right lower quadrant**
- **4 left lower quadrant**
- **5 periumbilic**
- **6 epigastric**
- **7 generalized**
- **9 other specified site**
  multiple sites

❺ **789.0 Abdominal pain**
Colic:
NOS
infantile
Cramps, abdominal
Excludes *renal colic (788.0)*
(✖ is only valid for fifth-digit "0")
AHA: 1Q 1995, 3; For Code 789.06: 1Q 2002, 5

789.1 Hepatomegaly
Enlargement of liver

789.2 Splenomegaly
Enlargement of spleen

❺ **789.3 Abdominal or pelvic swelling, mass, or lump**
(✖ is only valid for fifth-digit "0")
Diffuse or generalized swelling or mass:
abdominal NOS
umbilical
Excludes *abdominal distention (gaseous) (787.3)*
ascites (▶789.51-789.59◀)

❺ **789.4 Abdominal rigidity**
(✖ is only valid for fifth-digit "0")

❺ **789.5 Ascites**
Fluid in peritoneal cavity
C&C Exclusions: 780.91, 780.92, 780.99, 789.30, 789.31, 789.32, 789.33, 789.34, 789.35, 789.36, 789.37, 789.39, 789.40, 789.41, 789.42. 789.43. 789.44, 789.45, 789.46, 789.47, 789.49, 789.5, 789.9, 799.8
AHA: 2Q 2005, 8; 4Q 1989, 11

●✚ ***789.51 Malignant ascites***
Code first malignancy, such as:
malignant neoplasm of ovary (183.0)
secondary malignant neoplasm of retroperitoneum and peritoneum (197.6)
DEF: Abnormal accumulation of fluid containing cancer cells in the peritoneal cavity, usually from metastatic spread of a malignancy.

●✖ **789.59 Other ascites**

❺ **789.6 Abdominal tenderness**
(✖ is only valid for fifth-digit "0")
Rebound tenderness

789.9 Other symptoms involving abdomen and pelvis
Umbilical:
bleeding
discharge

NONSPECIFIC ABNORMAL FINDINGS (790-796)

AHA: 2Q 1990, 16

❹ **790 Nonspecific findings on examination of blood**
Excludes *abnormality of:*
platelets (287.0-287.9)
thrombocytes (287.0-287.9)
white blood cells (288.00-288.9)

❺ **790.0 Abnormality of red blood cells**
Excludes *anemia:*
congenital (776.5)
newborn, due to isoimmunization (773.0-773.2, 773.5)
of premature infant (776.6)
other specified types (280.0-285.9)
hemoglobin disorders (282.5-282.7)
polycythemia:
familial (289.6)
neonatorum (776.4)
secondary (289.0)
vera (238.4)
AHA: 4Q 2000, 46

790.01 Precipitous drop in hematocrit
Drop in hematocrit

✖ **790.09 Other abnormality of red blood cells**
Abnormal red cell morphology NOS
Abnormal red cell volume NOS
Anisocytosis
Poikilocytosis

✖ **790.1 Elevated sedimentation rate**

❺ **790.2 Abnormal glucose**
Excludes *diabetes mellitus (250.00-250.93)*
dysmetabolic syndrome X (277.7)
gestational diabetes (648.8)
glycosuria (791.5)
hypoglycemia (251.2)
that complicating pregnancy, childbirth, or the puerperium (648.8)
AHA: 4Q 2003, 74; 3Q 1991, 5

790.21 Impaired fasting glucose
Elevated fasting glucose

790.22 Impaired glucose tolerance test (oral)
Elevated glucose tolerance test

790.29 Other abnormal glucose
Abnormal glucose NOS
Abnormal non-fasting glucose
Hyperglycemia NOS
Pre-diabetes NOS
AHA: 2Q 2005, 21

790.3 Excessive blood level of alcohol
Elevated blood-alcohol
AHA: Sep-Oct 1986, 3

✖ **790.4 Nonspecific elevation of levels of transaminase or lactic acid dehydrogenase [LDH]**

✖ **790.5 Other nonspecific abnormal serum enzyme levels**
Abnormal serum level of:
acid phosphatase
alkaline phosphatase
amylase
lipase
Excludes *deficiency of circulating enzymes (277.6)*

Symptoms, Signs, and Ill-Defined Conditions

788.65 – 790.5

✖ **790.6 Other abnormal blood chemistry**

Abnormal blood levels of:
- cobalt
- copper
- iron
- lead
- lithium
- magnesium
- mineral
- zinc

Excludes *abnormality of electrolyte or acid-base balance (276.0-276.9)*
hypoglycemia NOS (251.2)
lead poisoning (984.0-984.9)
specific finding indicating abnormality of:
amino-acid transport and metabolism (270.0-270.9)
carbohydrate transport and metabolism (271.0-271.9)
lipid metabolism (272.0-272.9)
uremia NOS (586)

AHA: 4Q 1988, 1

790.7 Bacteremia

Excludes *bacteremia of newborn (771.83)*
septicemia (038)

Use additional code to identify organism (041)

C&C Exclusions: 780.91, 780.92, 780.99, 790.7, 790.8, 790.91, 790.92, 790.93, 790.94, 790.99, 799.8

AHA: 2Q 2003, 7; 4Q 1993, 29; 3Q 1988, 12

790.8 Viremia, unspecified

AHA: 4Q 1988, 10

❺ **790.9 Other nonspecific findings on examination of blood**

AHA: 4Q 1993, 29

✖ **790.91 Abnormal arterial blood gases**

DEF: Abnormal oxygen or carbon dioxide content in the arterial bloodstream.

✖ **790.92 Abnormal coagulation profile**

Abnormal or prolonged:
- bleeding time
- coagulation time
- partial thromboplastin time [PTT]
- prothrombin time [PT]

Excludes *coagulation (hemorrhagic) disorders (286.0-286.9)*

790.93 Elevated prostate specific antigen [PSA] ♂ A

790.94 Euthyroid sick syndrome

AHA: 4Q 1997, 45

790.95 Elevated C-reactive protein (CRP)

✖ **790.99 Other**

AHA: 2Q 2003, 14

❹ **791 Nonspecific findings on examination of urine**

Excludes *hematuria NOS (599.7)*
specific findings indicating abnormality of:
amino-acid transport and metabolism (270.0-270.9)
carbohydrate transport and metabolism (271.0-271.9)

791.0 Proteinuria

Albuminuria
Bence-Jones proteinuria

Excludes *postural proteinuria (593.6)*
that arising during pregnancy or the puerperium (642.0-642.9, 646.2)

AHA: 3Q 1991, 8

791.1 Chyluria

Excludes *filarial (125.0-125.9)*

C&C Exclusions: 780.91, 780.92, 780.99, 791.1, 791.9, 799.8

791.2 Hemoglobinuria

791.3 Myoglobinuria

C&C Exclusions: 780.91, 780.92, 780.99, 791.2, 791.3, 791.9, 799.8

791.4 Biliuria

791.5 Glycosuria

Excludes *renal glycosuria (271.4)*

791.6 Acetonuria

Ketonuria

791.7 Other cells and casts in urine

791.9 Other nonspecific findings on examination of urine

Crystalluria
Elevated urine levels of:
- 17-ketosteroids
- catecholamines
- indolacetic acid
- vanillylmandelic acid [VMA]

Melanuria

AHA: 1Q 2005, 12

❹ **792 Nonspecific abnormal findings in other body substances**

Excludes *that in chromosomal analysis (795.2)*

792.0 Cerebrospinal fluid

792.1 Stool contents

Abnormal stool color
Fat in stool
Mucus in stool
Occult blood
Pus in stool

Excludes *blood in stool [melena] (578.1)*
newborn (772.4, 777.3)

AHA: 2Q 1992, 9

792.2 Semen ♂

Abnormal spermatozoa

Excludes *azoospermia (606.0)*
oligospermia (606.1)

792.3 Amniotic fluid ♀ M

AHA: Nov-Dec 1986, 4

792.4 Saliva

Excludes *that in chromosomal analysis (795.2)*

792.5 Cloudy (hemodialysis) (peritoneal) dialysis effluent

✖ **792.9 Other nonspecific abnormal findings in body substances**

Peritoneal fluid
Pleural fluid
Synovial fluid
Vaginal fluids

❹ **793 Nonspecific abnormal findings on radiological and other examination of body structure**

Includes nonspecific abnormal findings of:
- thermography
- ultrasound examination [echogram]
- x-ray examination

Excludes *abnormal results of function studies and radioisotope scans (794.0-794.9)*

793.0 Skull and head

Excludes *nonspecific abnormal echoencephalogram (794.01)*

793.1 Lung field

Coin lesion (of) lung
Shadow (of) lung

793.2 Other intrathoracic organ

Abnormal:
- echocardiogram
- heart shadow
- ultrasound cardiogram

Mediastinal shift

793.3 Biliary tract

Nonvisualization of gallbladder

793.4 Gastrointestinal tract

793.5 Genitourinary organs

Filling defect:
- bladder
- kidney
- ureter

AHA: 4Q 2000, 46

793.6 Abdominal area, including retroperitoneum

793.7 Musculoskeletal system

⑤ **793.8 Breast**
AHA: 4Q 2001, 51

✖ **793.80 Abnormal mammogram, unspecified**

793.81 Mammographic microcalcification
Excludes *mammographic calcification (793.89)*
mammographic calculus (793.89)

793.89 Other abnormal findings on radiological examination of breast
Mammographic calcification
Mammographic calculus

⑤ **793.9 Other**
Excludes *abnormal finding by radioisotope localization of placenta (794.9)*

793.91 Image test inconclusive due to excess body fat
Use additional code to identify Body Mass Index (BMI), if known (V85.0-V85.54)
AHA: 4Q 2006, 110

793.99 Other nonspecific abnormal findings on radiological and other examinations of body structure
Abnormal:
placental finding by x-ray or ultrasound method
radiological findings in skin and subcutaneous tissue

④ **794 Nonspecific abnormal results of function studies**
Includes radioisotope:
scans
uptake studies
scintiphotography

⑤ **794.0 Brain and central nervous system**

794.00 Abnormal function study, unspecified

794.01 Abnormal echoencephalogram

794.02 Abnormal electroencephalogram [EEG]

794.09 Other
Abnormal brain scan

⑤ **794.1 Peripheral nervous system and special senses**

794.10 Abnormal response to nerve stimulation, unspecified

794.11 Abnormal retinal function studies
Abnormal electroretinogram [ERG]

794.12 Abnormal electro-oculogram [EOG]

794.13 Abnormal visually evoked potential

794.14 Abnormal oculomotor studies

794.15 Abnormal auditory function studies
AHA: 1Q 2004, 15-16

794.16 Abnormal vestibular function studies

794.17 Abnormal electromyogram [EMG]
Excludes *that of eye (794.14)*

794.19 Other

794.2 Pulmonary
Abnormal lung scan
Reduced:
ventilatory capacity
vital capacity

⑤ **794.3 Cardiovascular**

794.30 Abnormal function study, unspecified

794.31 Abnormal electrocardiogram [ECG] [EKG]
Excludes *long QT syndrome (426.82)*

794.39 Other
Abnormal:
ballistocardiogram
phonocardiogram
vectorcardiogram

794.4 Kidney
Abnormal renal function test

794.5 Thyroid
Abnormal thyroid:
scan
uptake

794.6 Other endocrine function study

794.7 Basal metabolism
Abnormal basal metabolic rate [BMR]

794.8 Liver
Abnormal liver scan

794.9 Other
Bladder
Pancreas
Placenta
Spleen

④ **795 Other and nonspecific abnormal cytological, histological, immunological and DNA test findings**
Excludes *nonspecific abnormalities of red blood cells (790.01-790.09)*

⑤ **795.0 Abnormal Papanicolaou smear of cervix and cervical HPV**
Abnormal cervical cytology
Abnormal thin preparation smear of cervix
Excludes *carcinoma in-situ of cervix (223.1)*
cervical intraepithelial-neoplasia I (CIN I) (622.11)
cervical intraepithelial-neoplasia II (CIN II) (622.12)
cervical intraepithelial-neoplasia III (CIN III) (233.1)
dysplasia (histologically confirmed) of cervix (uteri) NOS (622.10)
mild dysplasia (histologically confirmed) (622.11)
moderate dysplasia (histologically confirmed) (622.12)
severe dysplasia (histologically confirmed) (233.1)
AHA: 4Q 2002, 69

✖ **795.00 Abnormal glandular Papanicolaou smear of cervix** ♀
Atypical endocervical cells NOS
Atypical endometrial cells NOS
Atypical glandular cells NOS

795.01 Papanicolaou smear of cervix with atypical squamous cells of undetermined significance (ASC-US) ♀
AHA: 2Q 2006, 3

795.02 Papanicolaou smear of cervix with atypical squamous cells cannot exclude high grade squamous intraepithelial lesion (ASC-H) ♀

795.03 Papanicolaou smear of cervix with low grade squamous intraepithelial lesion (LGSIL) ♀

795.04 Papanicolaou smear of cervix with high grade squamous intraepithelial lesion (HGSIL) ♀

795.05 Cervical high risk human papillomavirus (HPV) DNA test positive ♀

795.06 Papanicolaou smear of cervix with cytologic evidence of malignancy ♀

795.08 Unsatisfactory smear ♀
Inadequate sample
AHA: 2Q 2006, 4

795.09 Other abnormal Papanicolaou smear of cervix and cervical HPV ♀
Cervical low risk human papillomavirus (HPV) DNA test positive
Use additional code for associated human papillomavirus (079.4)
Excludes *encounter for Papanicolaou cervical smear to confirm findings of recent normal smear following initial abnormal smear (V72.32)*

795.1 Nonspecific abnormal Papanicolaou smear of other site

795.2 Nonspecific abnormal findings on chromosomal analysis
Abnormal karyotype

❺ **795.3 Nonspecific positive culture findings**
Positive culture findings in:
nose
sputum
throat
wound
Excludes that of:
blood (790.7-790.8)
urine (791.9)

795.31 Nonspecific positive findings for anthrax
Positive findings by nasal swab
AHA: 4Q 2002, 70

795.39 Other nonspecific positive culture findings

✖ **795.4 Other nonspecific abnormal histological findings**

795.5 Nonspecific reaction to tuberculin skin test without active tuberculosis
Abnormal result of Mantoux test
PPD positive
Tuberculin (skin test):
positive
reactor

795.6 False positive serological test for syphilis
False positive Wassermann reaction

❺ **795.7 Other nonspecific immunological findings**
Excludes *abnormal tumor markers (795.81-795.89)*
elevated prostate specific antigen [PSA] (790.93)
elevated tumor associated antigens (795.81-795.89)
isoimmunization, in pregnancy (656.1-656.2)
affecting fetus or newborn (773.0-773.2)
AHA: 2Q 1993, 6

795.71 Nonspecific serologic evidence of human immunodeficiency virus [HIV]
Inconclusive human immunodeficiency virus [HIV] test (adult) (infant)
Note: This code is ONLY to be used when a test finding is reported as nonspecific. Asymptomatic positive findings are coded to V08. If any HIV infection symptom or condition is present, see code 042. Negative findings are not coded.
Excludes *acquired immunodeficiency syndrome [AIDS] (042)*
asymptomatic human immunodeficiency virus, [HIV] infection status (V08)
HIV infection, symptomatic (042)
human immunodeficiency virus [HIV] disease (042)
positive (status) NOS (V08)
AHA: 2Q 2004, 11; 1Q 1993, 21; 1Q 1993, 22; 2Q 1992, 11; Jul-Aug 1987, 24

795.79 Other and unspecified nonspecific immunological findings
Raised antibody titer
Raised level of immunoglobulins

❺ **795.8 Abnormal tumor markers**
Elevated tumor associated antigens [TAA]
Elevated tumor specific antigens [TSA]
Excludes *elevated prostate specific antigen [PSA] (790.93)*

795.81 Elevated carcinoembryonic antigen [CEA]

795.82 Elevated cancer antigen 125 [CA 125] ♀

795.89 Other abnormal tumor markers

❹ **796 Other nonspecific abnormal findings**

796.0 Nonspecific abnormal toxicological findings
Abnormal levels of heavy metals or drugs in blood, urine, or other tissue
Excludes *excessive blood level of alcohol (790.3)*
AHA: 1Q 1997, 16

796.1 Abnormal reflex

796.2 Elevated blood pressure reading without diagnosis of hypertension
Note: This category is to be used to record an episode of elevated blood pressure in a patient in whom no formal diagnosis of hypertension has been made, or as an incidental finding.
AHA: 2Q 2003, 11; 3Q 1990, 4; Jul-Aug 1984, 12

796.3 Nonspecific low blood pressure reading

✖ **796.4 Other abnormal clinical findings**
AHA: 1Q 1997, 16

796.5 Abnormal finding on antenatal screening ♀ M
AHA: 4Q 1997, 46

796.6 Abnormal findings on neonatal screening N
Excludes *nonspecified serologic evidence of human immunodeficiency virus [HIV] (795.71)*
AHA: 4Q 2004, 99

✖ **796.9 Other**

ILL-DEFINED AND UNKNOWN CAUSES OF MORBIDITY AND MORTALITY (797-799)

797 Senility without mention of psychosis
Old age
Senescence
Senile asthenia
Senile:
debility
exhaustion
Excludes *senile psychoses (290.0-290.9)*

❹ **798 Sudden death, cause unknown**

798.0 Sudden infant death syndrome P
Cot death
Crib death
Sudden death of nonspecific cause in infancy
C&C Exclusions: 799.01, 799.02

⃠ **798.1 Instantaneous death**

⃠ **798.2 Death occurring in less than 24 hours from onset of symptoms, not otherwise explained**
Death known not to be violent or instantaneous, for which no cause could be discovered
Died without sign of disease

⃠ **798.9 Unattended death**
Death in circumstances where the body of the deceased was found and no cause could be discovered
Found dead

❹ **799 Other ill-defined and unknown causes of morbidity and mortality**

❺ **799.0 Asphyxia and hypoxemia**
Excludes *asphyxia and hypoxemia (due to):*
carbon monoxide (986)
hypercapnia (786.09)
inhalation of food or foreign body (932-934.9)
newborn (768.0-768.9)
traumatic (994.7)

799.01 Asphyxia
C&C Exclusions: 799.01, 799.02, 799.1
AHA: 4Q 2005, 90

799.02 Hypoxemia
C&C Exclusions: See 799.01
AHA: 799.02

799.1 Respiratory arrest
Cardiorespiratory failure
Excludes *cardiac arrest (427.5)*
failure of peripheral circulation (785.50)
respiratory distress:
NOS (786.09)
acute (518.82)
following trauma or surgery (518.5)
newborn (770.89)
syndrome (newborn) (769)
adult (following trauma or surgery) (518.5)
other (518.82)
respiratory failure (518.81, 518.83-518.84)
newborn (770.84)
respiratory insufficiency (786.09)
acute (518.82)
C&C Exclusions: 518.81, 518.82, 518.83, 518.84, 780.91, 780.92, 780.99, 798.0, 799.0, 799.01, 799.02, 799.1, 799.8

799.2 Nervousness
"Nerves"

✖ **799.3 Debility, unspecified**
Excludes *asthenia (780.79)*
nervous debility (300.5)
neurasthenia (300.5)
senile asthenia (797)

799.4 Cachexia
Wasting disease
Code first underlying condition, if known
C&C Exclusions: 780.91, 780.92, 780.99, 799.3, 799.4, 799.8
AHA: 3Q 2006, 15; 3Q 1990, 17

⑤ **799.8 Other ill-defined conditions**

799.81 Decreased libido A
Decreased sexual desire
Excludes *psychosexual dysfunction with inhibited sexual desire (302.71)*
C&C Exclusions: 040.82, 440.24, 780.01, 780.03, 780.1, 780.31, 780.32, 780.39, 781.7, 785.4, 785.50, 785.51, 785.52, 785.59, 786.3, 788.20, 788.29, 789.5, 790.7, 791.1, 791.3, 799.01, 799.02, 799.1, 799.4
AHA: 4Q 2003, 75

✖ **799.89 Other ill-defined conditions**
C&C Exclusions: See 799.81

✖ **799.9 Other unknown and unspecified cause**
Undiagnosed disease, not specified as to site or system involved
Unknown cause of morbidity or mortality
AHA: 1Q 1998, 4; 1Q 1990, 20

17. INJURY AND POISONING (800-999)

Use E code(s) to identify the cause and intent of the injury or poisoning (E800-E999)
Note:

1. *The principle of multiple coding of injuries should be followed wherever possible. Combination categories for multiple injuries are provided for use when there is insufficient detail as to the nature of the individual conditions, or for primary tabulation purposes when it is more convenient to record a single code; otherwise, the component injuries should be coded separately.*

   Where multiple sites of injury are specified in the titles, the word "with" indicates involvement of both sites, and the word "and" indicates involvement of either or both sites. The word "finger" includes thumb.

2. *Categories for "late effect" of injuries are to be found at 905-909.*

FRACTURES (800-829)

Excludes *malunion (733.81)*
nonunion (733.82)
pathologic or spontaneous fracture (733.10-733.19)
stress fracture (733.93-733.95)

The terms "condyle," "coronoid process," "ramus," and "symphysis" indicate the portion of the bone fractured, not the name of the bone involved.

The descriptions "closed" and "open" used in the fourth-digit subdivisions include the following terms:
closed (with or without delayed healing):
comminuted
depressed
elevated
fissured
fracture NOS
greenstick
impacted
linear
simple
slipped epiphysis
spiral
open (with or without delayed healing):
compound
infected
missile
puncture
with foreign body

Note *A fracture not indicated as closed or open should be classified as closed.*

AHA: 4Q 1990, 26; 3Q 1990, 5, 13; 2Q 1990, 7; 2Q 1989, 15; Sep-Oct 1985, 3

FRACTURE OF SKULL (800-804)

The following fifth-digit subclassification is for use with the appropriate codes in categories 800, 801 803, and 804:
✖ **0 unspecified state of consciousness**
1 with no loss of consciousness
2 with brief [less than one hour] loss of consciousness
3 with moderate [1-24 hours] loss of consciousness
4 with prolonged [more than 24 hours] loss of consciousness and return to pre-existing conscious level
5 with prolonged [more than 24 hours] loss of consciousness, without return to pre-existing conscious level
Use fifth-digit 5 to designate when a patient is unconscious and dies before regaining consciousness, regardless of the duration of the loss of consciousness
✖ **6 with loss of consciousness of unspecified duration**
✖ **9 with concussion, unspecified**

Injury and Poisoning 799.1 – 799.9

❹ **800 Fracture of vault of skull**

Requires fifth digit. See beginning of section 800-804 for codes and definitions.

Includes frontal bone
parietal bone

AHA: 4Q 1996, 36

❺ **800.0 Closed without mention of intracranial injury** ❷

C&C Exclusions: 800.00, 800.01, 800.02, 800.03, 800.04, 800.05, 800.06, 800.09, 800.10, 800.11, 800.12, 800.13, 800.14, 800.15, 800.16, 800.19, 800.20, 800.21, 800.22, 800.23, 800.24, 800.25, 800.26, 800.29, 800.30, 800.31, 800.32, 800.33, 800.34, 800.35, 800.36, 800.39, 800.40, 800.41, 800.42, 800.43, 800.44, 800.45, 800.46, 800.49, 800.50, 800.51, 800.52, 800.53, 800.54, 800.55, 800.56, 800.59, 800.60, 800.61, 800.62, 800.63, 800.64, 800.65, 800.66, 800.69, 800.70, 800.71, 800.72, 800.73, 800.74, 800.75, 800.76, 800.79, 800.80, 800.81, 800.82, 800.83, 800.84, 800.85, 800.86, 800.89, 800.90, 800.91, 800.92, 800.93, 800.94, 800.95, 800.96, 800.99, 801.00, 801.01, 801.02, 801.03, 801.04, 801.05, 801.06, 801.09, 801.10, 801.11, 801.12, 801.13, 801.14, 801.15, 801.16, 801.19, 801.20, 801.21, 801.22, 801.23, 801.24, 801.25, 801.26, 801.29, 801.30, 801.31, 801.32, 801.33, 801.34, 801.35, 801.36, 801.39, 801.40, 801.41, 801.42, 801.43, 801.44, 801.45, 801.46, 801.49, 801.50, 801.51, 801.52, 801.53, 801.54, 801.55, 801.56, 801.59, 801.60, 801.61, 801.62, 801.63, 801.64, 801.65, 801.66, 801.69, 801.70, 801.71, 801.72, 801.73, 801.74, 801.75, 801.76, 801.79, 801.80, 801.81, 801.82, 801.83, 801.84, 801.85, 801.86, 801.89, 801.90, 801.91, 801.92, 801.93, 801.94, 801.95, 801.96, 801.99, 803.00, 803.01, 803.02, 803.03, 803.04, 803.05, 803.06, 803.09, 803.10, 803.11, 803.12, 803.13, 803.14, 803.15, 803.16, 803.19, 803.20, 803.21, 803.22, 803.23, 803.24, 803.25, 803.26, 803.29, 803.30, 803.31, 803.32, 803.33, 803.34, 803.35, 803.36, 803.39, 803.40, 803.41, 803.42, 803.43, 803.44, 803.45, 803.46, 803.49, 803.50, 803.51, 803.52, 803.53, 803.54, 803.55, 803.56, 803.59, 803.60, 803.61, 803.62, 803.63, 803.64, 803.65, 803.66, 803.69, 803.70, 803.71, 803.72, 803.73, 803.74, 803.75, 803.76, 803.79, 803.80, 803.81, 803.82, 803.83, 803.84, 803.85, 803.86, 803.89, 803.90, 803.91, 803.92, 803.93, 803.94, 803.95, 803.96, 803.99, 804.00, 804.01, 804.02, 804.03, 804.04, 804.05, 804.06, 804.09, 804.10, 804.11, 804.12, 804.13, 804.14, 804.15, 804.16, 804.19, 804.20, 804.21, 804.22, 804.23, 804.24, 804.25, 804.26, 804.29, 804.30, 804.31, 804.32, 804.33, 804.34, 804.35, 804.36, 804.39, 804.40, 804.41, 804.42, 804.43, 804.44, 804.45, 804.46, 804.49, 804.50, 804.51, 804.52, 804.53, 804.54, 804.55, 804.56, 804.59, 804.60, 804.61, 804.62, 804.63, 804.64, 804.65, 804.66, 804.69, 804.70, 804.71, 804.72, 804.73, 804.74, 804.75, 804.76, 804.79, 804.80, 804.81, 804.82, 804.83, 804.84, 804.85, 804.86, 804.89, 804.90, 804.91, 804.92, 804.93, 804.94, 804.95, 804.96, 804.99, 829.0, 829.1, 850.0, 850.11, 850.12, 850.2, 850.3, 850.5, 850.9, 851.00, 851.01, 851.02, 851.03, 851.04, 851.05, 851.06, 851.09, 851.10, 851.11, 851.12, 851.13, 851.14, 851.15, 851.16, 851.19, 851.20, 851.21, 851.22, 851.23, 851.24, 851.25, 851.26, 851.29, 851.30, 851.31, 851.32, 851.33, 851.34, 851.35, 851.36, 851.39, 851.40, 851.41, 851.42, 851.43, 851.44, 851.45, 851.46, 851.49, 851.50, 851.51, 851.52, 851.53, 851.54, 851.55, 851.56, 851.59, 851.60, 851.61, 851.62, 851.63, 851.64, 851.65, 851.66, 851.69, 851.70, 851.71, 851.72, 851.73, 851.74, 851.75, 851.76, 851.79, 851.80, 851.81, 851.82, 851.83, 851.84, 851.85, 851.86, 851.89, 851.90, 851.91, 851.92, 851.93, 851.94, 851.95, 851.96, 851.99, 852.00, 852.01, 852.02, 852.03, 852.04, 852.05, 852.06, 852.09, 852.10, 852.11, 852.12, 852.13, 852.14, 852.15, 852.16, 852.19, 852.21, 852.22, 852.23, 852.24, 852.25, 852.26, 852.29, 852.30, 852.31, 852.32, 852.33, 852.34, 852.35, 852.36, 852.39, 852.40, 852.41, 852.42, 852.43, 852.44, 852.45, 852.46, 852.49, 852.50, 852.51, 852.52, 852.53, 852.54, 852.55, 852.56, 852.59, 853.00, 853.01, 853.02, 853.03, 853.04, 853.05, 853.06, 853.09, 853.10, 853.11, 853.12, 853.13, 853.14, 853.15, 853.16, 853.19, 854.00, 854.01, 854.02, 854.03, 854.04, 854.05, 854.06, 854.09, 854.10, 854.11, 854.12, 854.13, 854.14, 854.15, 854.16, 854.19, 873.8, 873.9, 879.8, 879.9, 905.0, 925.1, 925.2, 929.0, 929.9, 958.8, 959.01, 959.09, 959.8, 959.9

❺ **800.1 Closed with cerebral laceration and contusion** ❷

C&C Exclusions: See 800.0

❺ **800.2 Closed with subarachnoid, subdural, and extradural hemorrhage** ❷

C&C Exclusions: See 800.0

❺ **800.3 Closed with other and unspecified intracranial hemorrhage** ❷

C&C Exclusions: See 800.0

❺ **800.4 Closed with intracranial injury of other and unspecified nature** ❷

C&C Exclusions: See 800.0

❺ **800.5 Open without mention of intracranial injury** ❷

C&C Exclusions: See 800.0

❺ **800.6 Open with cerebral laceration and contusion** ❷

C&C Exclusions: See 800.0

❺ **800.7 Open with subarachnoid, subdural, and extradural hemorrhage** ❷

C&C Exclusions: See 800.0

❺ **800.8 Open with other and unspecified intracranial hemorrhage** ❷

C&C Exclusions: See 800.0

❺ **800.9 Open with intracranial injury of other and unspecified nature** ❷

C&C Exclusions: See 800.0

❹ **801 Fracture of base of skull**

Requires fifth digit. See beginning of section 800-804 for codes and definitions.

Includes fossa:
anterior
middle
posterior
occiput bone
orbital roof
sinus:
ethmoid
frontal
sphenoid bone
temporal bone

AHA: 4Q 1996, 36

❺ **801.0 Closed without mention of intracranial injury** ❷

C&C Exclusions: See 800.0

❺ **801.1 Closed with cerebral laceration and contusion** ❷

C&C Exclusions: See 800.00

Base of skull fracture

Exterior view

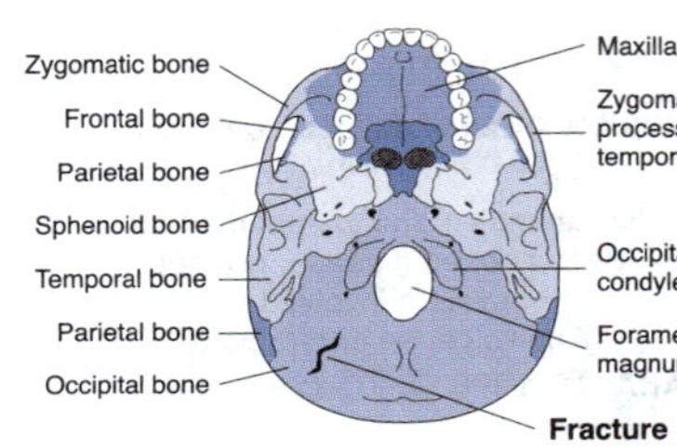

❺ **801.2 Closed with subarachnoid, subdural, and extradural hemorrhage** ❷

C&C Exclusions: See 800.0

AHA: 4Q 1996, 36

❺ **801.3 Closed with other and unspecified intracranial hemorrhage** ❷

C&C Exclusions: See 800.0

❺ **801.4 Closed with intracranial injury of other and unspecified nature** ❷

C&C Exclusions: See 800.0

❺ **801.5 Open without mention of intracranial injury** ❷

C&C Exclusions: See 800.0

❺ **801.6 Open with cerebral laceration and contusion** ❷

C&C Exclusions: See 800.0

❺ **801.7 Open with subarachnoid, subdural, and extradural hemorrhage** ❷

C&C Exclusions: See 800.0

❺ **801.8 Open with other and unspecified intracranial hemorrhage** ❷

C&C Exclusions: See 800.0

❺ **801.9 Open with intracranial injury of other and unspecified nature** ❷
C&C Exclusions: See 800.0

❹ **802 Fracture of face bones**
AHA: 4Q 1996, 36

802.0 Nasal bones, closed ❷

802.1 Nasal bones, open ❷
C&C Exclusions: 800.00, 800.01, 800.02, 800.03, 800.04, 800.05, 800.06, 800.09, 800.10, 800.11, 800.12, 800.13, 800.14, 800.15, 800.16, 800.19, 800.20, 800.21, 800.22, 800.23, 800.24, 800.25, 800.26, 800.29, 800.30, 800.31, 800.32, 800.33, 800.34, 800.35, 800.36, 800.39, 800.40, 800.41, 800.42, 800.43, 800.44, 800.45, 800.46, 800.49, 800.50, 800.51, 800.52, 800.53, 800.54, 800.55, 800.56, 800.59, 800.60, 800.61, 800.62, 800.63, 800.64, 800.65, 800.66, 800.69, 800.70, 800.71, 800.72, 800.73, 800.74, 800.75, 800.76, 800.79, 800.80, 800.81, 800.82, 800.83, 800.84, 800.85, 800.86, 800.89, 800.90, 800.91, 800.92, 800.93, 800.94, 800.95, 800.96, 800.99, 801.00, 801.01, 801.02, 801.03, 801.04, 801.05, 801.06, 801.09, 801.10, 801.11, 801.12, 801.13, 801.14, 801.15, 801.16, 801.19, 801.20, 801.21, 801.22, 801.23, 801.24, 801.25, 801.26, 801.29, 801.30, 801.31, 801.32, 801.33, 801.34, 801.35, 801.36, 801.39, 801.40, 801.41, 801.42, 801.43, 801.44, 801.45, 801.46, 801.49, 801.50, 801.51, 801.52, 801.53, 801.54, 801.55, 801.56, 801.59, 801.60, 801.61, 801.62, 801.63, 801.64, 801.65, 801.66, 801.69, 801.70, 801.71, 801.72, 801.73, 801.74, 801.75, 801.76, 801.79, 801.80, 801.81, 801.82, 801.83, 801.84, 801.85, 801.86, 801.89, 801.90, 801.91, 801.92, 801.93, 801.94, 801.95, 801.96, 801.99, 802.0, 802.1, 803.00, 803.01, 803.02, 803.03, 803.04, 803.05, 803.06, 803.09, 803.10, 803.11, 803.12, 803.13, 803.14, 803.15, 803.16, 803.19, 803.20, 803.21, 803.22, 803.23, 803.24, 803.25, 803.26, 803.29, 803.30, 803.31, 803.32, 803.33, 803.34, 803.35, 803.36, 803.39, 803.40, 803.41, 803.42, 803.43, 803.44, 803.45, 803.46, 803.49, 803.50, 803.51, 803.52, 803.53, 803.54, 803.55, 803.56, 803.59, 803.60, 803.61, 803.62, 803.63, 803.64, 803.65, 803.66, 803.69, 803.70, 803.71, 803.72, 803.73, 803.74, 803.75, 803.76, 803.79, 803.80, 803.81, 803.82, 803.83, 803.84, 803.85, 803.86, 803.89, 803.90, 803.91, 803.92, 803.93, 803.94, 803.95, 803.96, 803.99, 804.00, 804.01, 804.02, 804.03, 804.04, 804.05, 804.06, 804.09, 804.10, 804.11, 804.12, 804.13, 804.14, 804.15, 804.16, 804.19, 804.20, 804.21, 804.22, 804.23, 804.24, 804.25, 804.26, 804.29, 804.30, 804.31, 804.32, 804.33, 804.34, 804.35, 804.36, 804.39, 804.40, 804.41, 804.42, 804.43, 804.44, 804.45, 804.46, 804.49, 804.50, 804.51, 804.52, 804.53, 804.54, 804.55, 804.56, 804.59, 804.60, 804.61, 804.62, 804.63, 804.64, 804.65, 804.66, 804.69, 804.70, 804.71, 804.72, 804.73, 804.74, 804.75, 804.76, 804.79, 804.80, 804.81, 804.82, 804.83, 804.84, 804.85, 804.86, 804.89, 804.90, 804.91, 804.92, 804.93, 804.94, 804.95, 804.96, 804.99, 829.0, 829.1, 850.0, 850.11, 850.12, 850.2, 850.3, 850.5, 850.9, 851.00, 851.01, 851.02, 851.03, 851.04, 851.05, 851.06, 851.09, 851.10, 851.11, 851.12, 851.13, 851.14, 851.15, 851.16, 851.19, 851.20, 851.21, 851.22, 851.23, 851.24, 851.25, 851.26, 851.29, 851.30, 851.31, 851.32, 851.33, 851.34, 851.35, 851.36, 851.39, 851.40, 851.41, 851.42, 851.43, 851.44, 851.45, 851.46, 851.49, 851.50, 851.51, 851.52, 851.53, 851.54, 851.55, 851.56, 851.59, 851.60, 851.61, 851.62, 851.63, 851.64, 851.65, 851.66, 851.69, 851.70, 851.71, 851.72, 851.73, 851.74, 851.75, 851.76, 851.79, 851.80, 851.81, 851.82, 851.83, 851.84, 851.85, 851.86, 851.89, 851.90, 851.91, 851.92, 851.93, 851.94, 851.95, 851.96, 851.99, 852.00, 852.01, 852.02, 852.03, 852.04, 852.05, 852.06, 852.09, 852.10, 852.11, 852.12, 852.13, 852.14, 852.15, 852.16, 852.19, 852.21, 852.22, 852.23, 852.24, 852.25, 852.26, 852.29, 852.30, 852.31, 852.32, 852.33, 852.34, 852.35, 852.36, 852.39, 852.40, 852.41, 852.42, 852.43, 852.44, 852.45, 852.46, 852.49, 852.50, 852.51, 852.52, 852.53, 852.54, 852.55, 852.56, 852.59, 853.00, 853.01, 853.02, 853.03, 853.04, 853.05, 853.06, 853.09, 853.10, 853.11, 853.12, 853.13, 853.14, 853.15, 853.16, 853.19, 854.00, 854.01, 854.02, 854.03, 854.04, 854.05, 854.06, 854.09, 854.10, 854.11, 854.12, 854.13, 854.14, 854.15, 854.16, 854.19, 873.8, 873.9, 879.8, 879.9, 905.0, 925.1, 925.2, 929.0, 929.9, 958.8, 959.01, 959.09, 959.8, 959.9

❺ **802.2 Mandible, closed**
Inferior maxilla
Lower jaw (bone)

802.20 Unspecified site ❷
C&C Exclusions: 800.00, 800.01, 800.02, 800.03, 800.04, 800.05, 800.06, 800.09, 800.10, 800.11, 800.12, 800.13, 800.14, 800.15, 800.16, 800.19, 800.20, 800.21, 800.22, 800.23, 800.24, 800.25, 800.26, 800.29, 800.30, 800.31, 800.32, 800.33, 800.34, 800.35, 800.36, 800.39, 800.40, 800.41, 800.42, 800.43, 800.44, 800.45, 800.46, 800.49, 800.50, 800.51, 800.52, 800.53, 800.54, 800.55, 800.56, 800.59, 800.60, 800.61, 800.62, 800.63, 800.64, 800.65, 800.66, 800.69, 800.70, 800.71, 800.72, 800.73, 800.74, 800.75, 800.76, 800.79, 800.80, 800.81, 800.82, 800.83, 800.84, 800.85, 800.86, 800.89, 800.90, 800.91, 800.92, 800.93, 800.94, 800.95, 800.96, 800.99, 801.00, 801.01, 801.02, 801.03, 801.04, 801.05, 801.06, 801.09, 801.10, 801.11, 801.12, 801.13, 801.14, 801.15, 801.16, 801.19, 801.20, 801.21, 801.22, 801.23, 801.24, 801.25, 801.26, 801.29, 801.30, 801.31, 801.32, 801.33, 801.34, 801.35, 801.36, 801.39, 801.40, 801.41, 801.42, 801.43, 801.44, 801.45, 801.46, 801.49, 801.50, 801.51, 801.52, 801.53, 801.54, 801.55, 801.56, 801.59, 801.60, 801.61, 801.62, 801.63, 801.64, 801.65, 801.66, 801.69, 801.70, 801.71, 801.72, 801.73, 801.74, 801.75, 801.76, 801.79, 801.80, 801.81, 801.82, 801.83, 801.84, 801.85, 801.86, 801.89, 801.90, 801.91, 801.92, 801.93, 801.94, 801.95, 801.96, 801.99, 802.20, 802.21, 802.22, 3, 4,802.25,802.26, 802.27, 802.28, 802.29, 802.30, 802.31, 802.32, 802.33, 802.34, 802.35, 802.36, 802.37, 802.38, 802.39, 802.4, 802.5, 803.00, 803.01, 803.02, 803.03, 803.04, 803.05, 803.06, 803.09, 803.10, 803.11, 803.12, 803.13, 803.14, 803.15, 803.16, 803.19, 803.20, 803.21, 803.22, 803.23, 803.24, 803.25, 803.26, 803.29, 803.30, 803.31, 803.32, 803.33, 803.34, 803.35, 803.36, 803.39, 803.40, 803.41, 803.42, 803.43, 803.44, 803.45, 803.46, 803.49, 803.50, 803.51, 803.52, 803.53, 803.54, 803.55, 803.56, 803.59, 803.60, 803.61, 803.62, 803.63, 803.64, 803.65, 803.66, 803.69, 803.70, 803.71, 803.72, 803.73, 803.74, 803.75, 803.76, 803.79, 803.80, 803.81, 803.82, 803.83, 803.84, 803.85, 803.86, 803.89, 803.90, 803.91, 803.92, 803.93, 803.94, 803.95, 803.96, 803.99, 804.00, 804.01, 804.02, 804.03, 804.04, 804.05, 804.06, 804.09, 804.10, 804.11, 804.12, 804.13, 804.14, 804.15, 804.16, 804.19, 804.20, 804.21, 804.22, 804.23, 804.24, 804.25, 804.26, 804.29, 804.30, 804.31, 804.32, 804.33, 804.34, 804.35, 804.36, 804.39, 804.40, 804.41, 804.42, 804.43, 804.44, 804.45, 804.46, 804.49, 804.50, 804.51, 804.52, 804.53, 804.54, 804.55, 804.56, 804.59, 804.60, 804.61, 804.62, 804.63, 804.64, 804.65, 804.66, 804.69, 804.70, 804.71, 804.72, 804.73, 804.74, 804.75, 804.76, 804.79, 804.80, 804.81, 804.82, 804.83, 804.84, 804.85, 804.86, 804.89, 804.90, 804.91, 804.92, 804.93, 804.94, 804.95, 804.96, 804.99, 829.0, 829.1, 830.0, 830.1, 850.0, 850.11, 850.12, 850.2, 850.3, 850.5, 850.9, 851.00, 851.01, 851.02, 851.03, 851.04, 851.05, 851.06, 851.09, 851.10, 851.11, 851.12, 851.13, 851.14, 851.15, 851.16, 851.19, 851.20, 851.21, 851.22, 851.23, 851.24, 851.25, 851.26, 851.29, 851.30, 851.31, 851.32, 851.33, 851.34, 851.35, 851.36, 851.39, 851.40, 851.41, 851.42, 851.43, 851.44, 851.45, 851.46, 851.49, 851.50, 851.51, 851.52, 851.53, 851.54, 851.55, 851.56, 851.59, 851.60, 851.61, 851.62, 851.63, 851.64, 851.65, 851.66, 851.69, 851.70, 851.71, 851.72, 851.73, 851.74, 851.75, 851.76, 851.79, 851.80, 851.81, 851.82, 851.83, 851.84, 851.85, 851.86, 851.89, 851.90, 851.91, 851.92, 851.93, 851.94, 851.95, 851.96, 851.99, 852.00, 852.01, 852.02, 852.03, 852.04, 852.05, 852.06, 852.09, 852.10, 852.11, 852.12, 852.13, 852.14, 852.15, 852.16, 852.19, 852.21, 852.22, 852.23, 852.24, 852.25, 852.26, 852.29, 852.30, 852.31, 852.32, 852.33, 852.34, 852.35, 852.36, 852.39, 852.40, 852.41, 852.42, 852.43, 852.44, 852.45, 852.46, 852.49, 852.50, 852.51, 852.52, 852.53, 852.54, 852.55, 852.56, 852.59, 853.00, 853.01, 853.02, 853.03, 853.04, 853.05, 853.06, 853.09, 853.10, 853.11, 853.12,

853.13, 853.14, 853.15, 853.16, 853.19, 854.00, 854.01, 854.02, 854.03, 854.04, 854.05, 854.06, 854.09, 854.10, 854.11, 854.12, 854.13, 854.14, 854.15, 854.16, 854.19, 873.8, 873.9, 879.8, 879.9, 905.0, 925.1, 925.2, 929.0, 929.9, 958.8, 959.01, 959.09, 959.8, 959.9

802.21 Condylar process ❷
C&C Exclusions: See 802.20

802.22 Subcondylar ❷
C&C Exclusions: See 802.20

802.23 Coronoid process ❷
C&C Exclusions: See 802.20

802.24 Ramus, unspecified ❷
C&C Exclusions: See 802.20

802.25 Angle of jaw ❷
C&C Exclusions: See 802.20

802.26 Symphysis of body ❷
C&C Exclusions: See 802.20

802.27 Alveolar border of body ❷
C&C Exclusions: See 802.20

802.28 Body, other and unspecified ❷
C&C Exclusions: See 802.20

802.29 Multiple sites ❷
C&C Exclusions: See 802.20

❺ **802.3 Mandible, open**

802.30 Unspecified site ❷
C&C Exclusions: See 802.20

802.31 Condylar process ❷
C&C Exclusions: See 802.20

802.32 Subcondylar ❷
C&C Exclusions: See 802.20

802.33 Coronoid process ❷
C&C Exclusions: See 802.20

802.34 Ramus, unspecified ❷
C&C Exclusions: See 802.20

802.35 Angle of jaw ❷
C&C Exclusions: See 802.20

802.36 Symphysis of body ❷
C&C Exclusions: See 802.20

802.37 Alveolar border of body ❷
C&C Exclusions: See 802.20

802.38 Body, other and unspecified ❷
C&C Exclusions: See 802.20

802.39 Multiple sites ❷
C&C Exclusions: See 802.20

802.4 Malar and maxillary bones, closed ❷
Superior maxilla
Upper jaw (bone)
Zygoma
Zygomatic arch
C&C Exclusions: See 802.20

802.5 Malar and maxillary bones, open ❷
C&C Exclusions: See 802.20

802.6 Orbital floor (blow-out), closed ❷
C&C Exclusions: 800.00, 800.01, 800.02, 800.03, 800.04, 800.05, 800.06, 800.09, 800.10, 800.11, 800.12, 800.13, 800.14, 800.15, 800.16, 800.19, 800.20, 800.21, 800.22, 800.23, 800.24, 800.25, 800.26, 800.29, 800.30, 800.31, 800.32, 800.33, 800.34, 800.35, 800.36, 800.39, 800.40, 800.41, 800.42, 800.43, 800.44, 800.45, 800.46, 800.49, 800.50, 800.51, 800.52, 800.53, 800.54, 800.55, 800.56, 800.59, 800.60, 800.61, 800.62, 800.63, 800.64, 800.65, 800.66, 800.69, 800.70, 800.71, 800.72, 800.73, 800.74, 800.75, 800.76, 800.79, 800.80, 800.81, 800.82, 800.83, 800.84, 800.85, 800.86, 800.89, 800.90, 800.91, 800.92, 800.93, 800.94, 800.95, 800.96, 800.99, 801.00, 801.01, 801.02, 801.03, 801.04, 801.05, 801.06, 801.09, 801.10, 801.11, 801.12, 801.13, 801.14, 801.15, 801.16, 801.19, 801.20, 801.21, 801.22, 801.23, 801.24, 801.25, 801.26, 801.29, 801.30, 801.31, 801.32, 801.33, 801.34, 801.35, 801.36, 801.39, 801.40, 801.41, 801.42, 801.43, 801.44, 801.45, 801.46, 801.49, 801.50, 801.51, 801.52, 801.53, 801.54, 801.55, 801.56, 801.59, 801.60, 801.61, 801.62, 801.63, 801.64, 801.65, 801.66, 801.69, 801.70, 801.71, 801.72, 801.73, 801.74, 801.75, 801.76, 801.79, 801.80, 801.81, 801.82, 801.83, 801.84, 801.85, 801.86, 801.89, 801.90, 801.91, 801.92, 801.93, 801.94, 801.95, 801.96, 801.99, 802.6, 802.7, 802.8, 802.9, 803.00, 803.01, 803.02, 803.03, 803.04, 803.05, 803.06, 803.09, 803.10, 803.11, 803.12, 803.13, 803.14, 803.15, 803.16, 803.19, 803.20, 803.21, 803.22, 803.23, 803.24, 803.25, 803.26, 803.29, 803.30, 803.31, 803.32, 803.33, 803.34, 803.35, 803.36, 803.39, 803.40, 803.41, 803.42, 803.43, 803.44, 803.45, 803.46, 803.49, 803.50, 803.51, 803.52, 803.53, 803.54, 803.55, 803.56, 803.59, 803.60, 803.61, 803.62, 803.63, 803.64, 803.65, 803.66, 803.69, 803.70, 803.71, 803.72, 803.73, 803.74, 803.75, 803.76, 803.79, 803.80, 803.81, 803.82, 803.83, 803.84, 803.85, 803.86, 803.89, 803.90, 803.91, 803.92, 803.93, 803.94, 803.95, 803.96, 803.99, 804.00, 804.01, 804.02, 804.03, 804.04, 804.05, 804.06, 804.09, 804.10, 804.11, 804.12, 804.13, 804.14, 804.15, 804.16, 804.19, 804.20, 804.21, 804.22, 804.23, 804.24, 804.25, 804.26, 804.29, 804.30, 804.31, 804.32, 804.33, 804.34, 804.35, 804.36, 804.39, 804.40, 804.41, 804.42, 804.43, 804.44, 804.45, 804.46, 804.49, 804.50, 804.51, 804.52, 804.53, 804.54, 804.55, 804.56, 804.59, 804.60, 804.61, 804.62, 804.63, 804.64, 804.65, 804.66, 804.69, 804.70, 804.71, 804.72, 804.73, 804.74, 804.75, 804.76, 804.79, 804.80, 804.81, 804.82, 804.83, 804.84, 804.85, 804.86, 804.89, 804.90, 804.91, 804.92, 804.93, 804.94, 804.95, 804.96, 804.99, 829.0, 829.1, 850.0, 850.11, 850.12, 850.2, 850.3, 850.5, 850.9, 851.00, 851.01, 851.02, 851.03, 851.04, 851.05, 851.06, 851.09, 851.10, 851.11, 851.12, 851.13, 851.14, 851.15, 851.16, 851.19, 851.20, 851.21, 851.22, 851.23, 851.24, 851.25, 851.26, 851.29, 851.30, 851.31, 851.32, 851.33, 851.34, 851.35, 851.36, 851.39, 851.40, 851.41, 851.42, 851.43, 851.44, 851.45, 851.46, 851.49, 851.50, 851.51, 851.52, 851.53, 851.54, 851.55, 851.56, 851.59, 851.60, 851.61, 851.62, 851.63, 851.64, 851.65, 851.66, 851.69, 851.70, 851.71, 851.72, 851.73, 851.74, 851.75, 851.76, 851.79, 851.80, 851.81, 851.82, 851.83, 851.84, 851.85, 851.86, 851.89, 851.90, 851.91, 851.92, 851.93, 851.94, 851.95, 851.96, 851.99, 852.00, 852.01, 852.02, 852.03, 852.04, 852.05, 852.06, 852.09, 852.10, 852.11, 852.12, 852.13, 852.14, 852.15, 852.16, 852.19, 852.21, 852.22, 852.23, 852.24, 852.25, 852.26, 852.29, 852.30, 852.31, 852.32, 852.33, 852.34, 852.35, 852.36, 852.39, 852.40, 852.41, 852.42, 852.43, 852.44, 852.45, 852.46, 852.49, 852.50, 852.51, 852.52, 852.53, 852.54, 852.55, 852.56, 852.59, 853.00, 853.01, 853.02, 853.03, 853.04, 853.05, 853.06, 853.09, 853.10, 853.11, 853.12, 853.13, 853.14, 853.15, 853.16, 853.19, 854.00, 854.01, 854.02, 854.03, 854.04, 854.05, 854.06, 854.09, 854.10, 854.11, 854.12, 854.13, 854.14, 854.15, 854.16, 854.19, 873.8, 873.9, 879.8, 879.9, 905.0, 925.1, 925.2, 929.0, 929.9, 958.8, 959.01, 959.09, 959.8, 959.9

802.7 Orbital floor (blow-out), open ❷
C&C Exclusions: See 802.6

802.8 Other facial bones, closed ❷
Alveolus
Orbit:
NOS
part other than roof or floor
Palate

Excludes *orbital:*
floor (802.6)
roof (801.0-801.9)

C&C Exclusions: See 802.6

802.9 Other facial bones, open ❷
C&C Exclusions: See 802.6

❹ **803 Other and unqualified skull fractures**

Requires fifth digit. See beginning of section 800-804 for codes and definitions.

Includes skull NOS
skull multiple NOS

AHA: 4Q 1996, 36

❺ **803.0 Closed without mention of intracranial injury** ❷
C&C Exclusions: 800.00, 800.01, 800.02, 800.03, 800.04, 800.05, 800.06, 800.09, 800.10, 800.11, 800.12, 800.13, 800.14, 800.15, 800.16, 800.19, 800.20, 800.21, 800.22, 800.23, 800.24, 800.25, 800.26, 800.29, 800.30, 800.31, 800.32, 800.33, 800.34, 800.35, 800.36, 800.39, 800.40, 800.41, 800.42, 800.43, 800.44, 800.45, 800.46, 800.49, 800.50, 800.51, 800.52, 800.53, 800.54, 800.55, 800.56, 800.59, 800.60, 800.61, 800.62, 800.63, 800.64, 800.65, 800.66, 800.69, 800.70, 800.71, 800.72, 800.73, 800.74, 800.75, 800.76, 800.79, 800.80, 800.81, 800.82, 800.83, 800.84, 800.85, 800.86, 800.89, 800.90, 800.91, 800.92,

800.93, 800.94, 800.95, 800.96, 800.99, 801.00, 801.01, 801.02, 801.03, 801.04, 801.05, 801.06, 801.09, 801.10, 801.11, 801.12, 801.13, 801.14, 801.15, 801.16, 801.19, 801.20, 801.21, 801.22, 801.23, 801.24, 801.25, 801.26, 801.29, 801.30, 801.31, 801.32, 801.33, 801.34, 801.35, 801.36, 801.39, 801.40, 801.41, 801.42, 801.43, 801.44, 801.45, 801.46, 801.49, 801.50, 801.51, 801.52, 801.53, 801.54, 801.55, 801.56, 801.59, 801.60, 801.61, 801.62, 801.63, 801.64, 801.65, 801.66, 801.69, 801.70, 801.71, 801.72, 801.73, 801.74, 801.75, 801.76, 801.79, 801.80, 801.81, 801.82, 801.83, 801.84, 801.85, 801.86, 801.89, 801.90, 801.91, 801.92, 801.93, 801.94, 801.95, 801.96, 801.99, 803.00, 803.01, 803.02, 803.03, 803.04, 803.05, 803.06, 803.09, 803.10, 803.11, 803.12, 803.13, 803.14, 803.15, 803.16, 803.19, 803.20, 803.21, 803.22, 803.23, 803.24, 803.25, 803.26, 803.29, 803.30, 803.31, 803.32, 803.33, 803.34, 803.35, 803.36, 803.39, 803.40, 803.41, 803.42, 803.43, 803.44, 803.45, 803.46, 803.49, 803.50, 803.51, 803.52, 803.53, 803.54, 803.55, 803.56, 803.59, 803.60, 803.61, 803.62, 803.63, 803.64, 803.65, 803.66, 803.69, 803.70, 803.71, 803.72, 803.73, 803.74, 803.75, 803.76, 803.79, 803.80, 803.81, 803.82, 803.83, 803.84, 803.85, 803.86, 803.89, 803.90, 803.91, 803.92, 803.93, 803.94, 803.95, 803.96, 803.99, 804.00, 804.01, 804.02, 804.03, 804.04, 804.05, 804.06, 804.09, 804.10, 804.11, 804.12, 804.13, 804.14, 804.15, 804.16, 804.19, 804.20, 804.21, 804.22, 804.23, 804.24, 804.25, 804.26, 804.29, 804.30, 804.31, 804.32, 804.33, 804.34, 804.35, 804.36, 804.39, 804.40, 804.41, 804.42, 804.43, 804.44, 804.45, 804.46, 804.49, 804.50, 804.51, 804.52, 804.53, 804.54, 804.55, 804.56, 804.59, 804.60, 804.61, 804.62, 804.63, 804.64, 804.65, 804.66, 804.69, 804.70, 804.71, 804.72, 804.73, 804.74, 804.75, 804.76, 804.79, 804.80, 804.81, 804.82, 804.83, 804.84, 804.85, 804.86, 804.89, 804.90, 804.91, 804.92, 804.93, 804.94, 804.95, 804.96, 804.99, 829.0, 829.1, 850.0, 850.11, 850.12, 850.2, 850.3, 850.5, 850.9, 851.00, 851.01, 851.02, 851.03, 851.04, 851.05, 851.06, 851.09, 851.10, 851.11, 851.12, 851.13, 851.14, 851.15, 851.16, 851.19, 851.20, 851.21, 851.22, 851.23, 851.24, 851.25, 851.26, 851.29, 851.30, 851.31, 851.32, 851.33, 851.34, 851.35, 851.36, 851.39, 851.40, 851.41, 851.42, 851.43, 851.44, 851.45, 851.46, 851.49, 851.50, 851.51, 851.52, 851.53, 851.54, 851.55, 851.56, 851.59, 851.60, 851.61, 851.62, 851.63, 851.64, 851.65, 851.66, 851.69, 851.70, 851.71, 851.72, 851.73, 851.74, 851.75, 851.76, 851.79, 851.80, 851.81, 851.82, 851.83, 851.84, 851.85, 851.86, 851.89, 851.90, 851.91, 851.92, 851.93, 851.94, 851.95, 851.96, 851.99, 852.00, 852.01, 852.02, 852.03, 852.04, 852.05, 852.06, 852.09, 852.10, 852.11, 852.12, 852.13, 852.14, 852.15, 852.16, 852.19, 852.21, 852.22, 852.23, 852.24, 852.25, 852.26, 852.29, 852.30, 852.31, 852.32, 852.33, 852.34, 852.35, 852.36, 852.39, 852.40, 852.41, 852.42, 852.43, 852.44, 852.45, 852.46, 852.49, 852.50, 852.51, 852.52, 852.53, 852.54, 852.55, 852.56, 852.59, 853.00, 853.01, 853.02, 853.03, 853.04, 853.05, 853.06, 853.09, 853.10, 853.11, 853.12, 853.13, 853.14, 853.15, 853.16, 853.19, 854.00, 854.01, 854.02, 854.03, 854.04, 854.05, 854.06, 854.09, 854.10, 854.11, 854.12, 854.13, 854.14, 854.15, 854.16, 854.19, 873.8, 873.9, 879.8, 879.9, 905.0, 925.1, 925.2, 929.0, 929.9, 958.8, 959.01, 959.09, 959.8, 959.9

5 **803.1 Closed with cerebral laceration and contusion** ❷
C&C Exclusions: See 803.0

5 **803.2 Closed with subarachnoid, subdural, and extradural hemorrhage** ❷
C&C Exclusions: See 803.0

5 **803.3 Closed with other and unspecified intracranial hemorrhage** ❷
C&C Exclusions: See 803.0

5 **803.4 Closed with intracranial injury of other and unspecified nature** ❷
C&C Exclusions: See 803.0

5 **803.5 Open without mention of intracranial injury** ❷
C&C Exclusions: See 803.0

5 **803.6 Open with cerebral laceration and contusion** ❷
C&C Exclusions: See 803.0

5 **803.7 Open with subarachnoid, subdural, and extradural hemorrhage** ❷
C&C Exclusions: See 803.0

5 **803.8 Open with other and unspecified intracranial hemorrhage** ❷
C&C Exclusions: See 803.0

5 **803.9 Open with intracranial injury of other and unspecified nature** ❷
C&C Exclusions: See 803.0

4 **804 Multiple fractures involving skull or face with other bones**
Requires fifth digit. See beginning of section 800-804 for codes and definitions.
AHA: 4Q 1996, 36

5 **804.0 Closed without mention of intracranial injury** ❷
C&C Exclusions: See 803.0

5 **804.1 Closed with cerebral laceration and contusion** ❷
C&C Exclusions: See 803.0

5 **804.2 Closed with subarachnoid, subdural, and extradural hemorrhage** ❷
C&C Exclusions: See 803.0

5 **804.3 Closed with other and unspecified intracranial hemorrhage** ❷
C&C Exclusions: See 803.0

5 **804.4 Closed with intracranial injury of other and unspecified nature** ❷
C&C Exclusions: See 803.0

5 **804.5 Open without mention of intracranial injury** ❷
C&C Exclusions: See 803.0

5 **804.6 Open with cerebral laceration and contusion** ❷
C&C Exclusions: See 803.0

5 **804.7 Open with subarachnoid, subdural, and extradural hemorrhage** ❷
C&C Exclusions: See 803.0

5 **804.8 Open with other and unspecified intracranial hemorrhage** ❷
C&C Exclusions: See 803.0

5 **804.9 Open with intracranial injury of other and unspecified nature** ❷
C&C Exclusions: See 803.0

FRACTURE OF NECK AND TRUNK (805-809)

4 **805 Fracture of vertebral column without mention of spinal cord injury**

Includes: neural arch
spine
spinous process
transverse process
vertebra

The following fifth-digit subclassification is for use with codes 805.0-805.1:

- **0** cervical vertebra, unspecified level
- **1** first cervical vertebra
- **2** second cervical vertebra
- **3** third cervical vertebra
- **4** fourth cervical vertebra
- **5** fifth cervical vertebra
- **6** sixth cervical vertebra
- **7** seventh cervical vertebra
- **8** multiple cervical vertebrae

5 **805.0 Cervical, closed** ❷
Atlas
Axis
C&C Exclusions: 805.00, 805.01, 805.02, 805.03, 805.04, 805.05, 805.06, 805.07, 805.08, 805.10, 805.11, 805.12, 805.13, 805.14, 805.15, 805.16, 805.17, 805.18, 805.8, 805.9, 806.00, 806.01, 806.02, 806.03, 806.04, 806.05, 806.06, 806.07, 806.08, 806.09, 806.10, 806.11, 806.12, 806.13, 806.14, 806.15, 806.16, 806.17, 806.18, 806.19, 806.8, 806.9, 829.0, 829.1, 839.00, 839.01, 839.02, 839.03, 839.04, 839.05, 839.06, 839.07, 839.08, 839.10, 839.11, 839.12, 839.13, 839.14, 839.15, 839.16, 839.17, 839.18, 839.40, 839.49, 839.50, 839.59, 839.69, 839.79, 839.8, 839.9, 847.0, 847.9, 848.8, 848.9, 879.8, 879.9, 905.1, 926.11, 929.0, 929.9, 952.00, 952.01, 952.02, 952.03, 952.04, 952.05, 952.06, 952.07, 952.08, 952.09, 952.8, 952.9, 958.8, 959.1, 959.8, 959.9

5 **805.1 Cervical, open** ❷
C&C Exclusions: (for codes 805.10-805.18) See 805.0

805.2 Dorsal [thoracic], closed ❷
C&C Exclusions: 805.2, 805.3, 805.8, 805.9, 806.20, 806.21, 806.22, 806.23, 806.24, 806.25, 806.26, 806.27, 806.28, 806.29, 806.30, 806.31, 806.32, 806.33, 806.34, 806.35, 806.36, 806.37, 806.38, 806.39, 806.8, 806.9, 829.0, 829.1, 839.21, 839.31, 839.40, 839.49, 839.50, 839.59, 839.69, 839.79, 839.8, 839.9, 847.1, 847.9, 848.8, 848.9, 879.8, 879.9, 905.1, 926.11, 929.0, 929.9, 952.10, 952.11, 952.12, 952.13, 952.14, 952.15, 952.16, 952.17, 952.18, 952.19, 952.8, 952.9, 958.8, 959.1, 959.8, 959.9

805.3 Dorsal [thoracic], open ❷
C&C Exclusions: See 805.3

805.4 Lumbar, closed ❷
C&C Exclusions: 805.4, 805.5, 805.8, 805.9, 806.4, 806.5, 806.8, 806.9, 829.0, 829.1, 839.20, 839.30, 839.40, 839.49, 839.50, 839.59, 839.69, 839.79, 839.8, 839.9, 847.2, 847.9, 848.8, 848.9, 879.8, 879.9, 905.1, 926.11, 929.0, 929.9, 952.2, 952.8, 952.9, 958.8, 959.1, 959.8, 959.9
AHA: 1Q 2007, 8; 4Q 1999, 12

805.5 Lumbar, open ❷
C&C Exclusions: See 805.4

805.6 Sacrum and coccyx, closed ❷
C&C Exclusions: 805.6, 805.7, 805.8, 805.9, 806.60, 806.61, 806.62, 806.69, 806.70, 806.71, 806.72, 806.79, 806.8, 806.9, 829.0, 829.1, 839.40, 839.41, 839.42, 839.49, 839.50, 839.51, 839.52, 839.59, 839.69, 839.79, 839.8, 839.9, 846.0, 846.1, 846.2, 846.3, 846.8, 846.9, 847.3, 847.4, 847.9, 848.5, 848.8, 848.9, 879.8, 879.9, 905.1, 926.11, 929.0, 929.9, 952.3, 952.8, 952.9, 958.8, 959.1, 959.8, 959.9

805.7 Sacrum and coccyx, open ❷
C&C Exclusions: See 805.6

805.8 Unspecified, closed ❷
C&C Exclusions: 733.10, 733.11, 733.12, 733.13, 733.14, 733.15, 733.16, 733.19, 733.93, 733.94, 733.95, 805.00, 805.01, 805.02, 805.03, 805.04, 805.05, 805.06, 805.07, 805.08, 805.10, 805.11, 805.12, 805.13, 805.14, 805.15, 805.16, 805.17, 805.18, 805.8, 805.9, 806.00, 806.01, 806.02, 806.03, 806.04, 806.05, 806.06, 806.07, 806.08, 806.09, 806.10, 806.11, 806.12, 806.13, 806.14, 806.15, 806.16, 806.17, 806.18, 806.19, 806.20, 806.21, 806.22, 806.23, 806.24, 806.25, 806.26, 806207, 806.28, 806.29, 806.30, 806.31, 806.32, 806.33, 806.34, 806.35, 806.36, 806.37, 806.38, 806.39, 806.4, 806.5, 806.60, 806.61, 806.62, 806.69, 806.70, 806.71, 806.72, 806.79, 806.8, 806.9, 829.0, 829.1, 839.00, 839.01, 839.02, 839.03, 839.04, 839.05, 839.06, 839.07, 839.08, 839.10, 839.11, 839.12, 839.13, 839.14, 839.15, 839.16, 839.17, 839.18, 839.20, 839.21, 839.30, 839.31, 839.40, 839.41, 839.42, 839.49, 839.50, 839.51, 839.52, 839.59, 839.69, 839.79, 839.8, 839.9, 846.0, 846.1, 846.2, 846.3, 846.8, 846.9, 847.0, 847.1, 847.2, 847.3, 847.4, 847.9, 848.5, 848.8, 848.9, 879.8, 879.9, 905.1, 926.11, 929.0, 929.9, 952.00, 952.01, 952.02, 952.03, 952.04, 952.05, 952.06, 952.07, 952.08, 952.09, 952.8, 952.9, 958.8, 959.1, 959.8, 959.9

805.9 Unspecified, open ❷
C&C Exclusions: See 805.8

❹ **806 Fracture of vertebral column with spinal cord injury**

Includes any condition classifiable to 805 with:
- complete or incomplete transverse lesion (of cord)
- hematomyelia

injury to:
- cauda equina
- nerve

paralysis
paraplegia
quadriplegia
spinal concussion

❺ **806.0 Cervical, closed**

806.00 C_1-C_4 level with unspecified spinal cord injury ❷
Cervical region NOS with spinal cord injury NOS
C&C Exclusions: 733.10, 733.11, 733.12, 733.13, 733.14, 733.15, 733.16, 733.19, 733.93, 733.94, 733.95, 805.00, 805.01, 805.02, 805.03, 805.04, 805.05, 805.06, 805.07, 805.08, 805.10, 805.11, 805.12, 805.13, 805.14, 805.15, 805.16, 805.17, 805.18, 805.8, 805.9, 806.00, 806.01, 806.02, 806.03, 806.04, 806.05, 806.06, 806.07, 806.08, 806.09, 806.10, 806.11, 806.12, 806.13, 806.14, 806.15, 806.16, 806.17, 806.18, 806.19, 806.8, 806.9, 829.0, 829.1, 839.00, 839.01, 839.02, 839.03, 839.04, 839.05, 839.06, 839.07, 839.08, 839.10, 839.11, 839.12, 839.13, 839.14, 839.15, 839.16, 839.17, 839.18, 839.40, 839.49, 839.50, 839.59, 839.69, 839.79, 839.8, 839.9, 847.9, 848.8, 848.9, 879.8, 879.9, 905.1, 926.11, 929.0, 929.9, 952.00, 952.01, 952.02, 952.03, 952.04, 952.05, 952.06, 952.07, 952.08, 952.09, 952.8, 952.9, 958.8, 959.1, 959.8, 959.9

806.01 C_1-C_4 level with complete lesion of cord ❷
C&C Exclusions: See 806.00

806.02 C_1-C_4 level with anterior cord syndrome ❷
C&C Exclusions: See 806.00

806.03 C_1-C_4 level with central cord syndrome ❷
C&C Exclusions: See 806.00

806.04 C_1-C_4 level with other specified spinal cord injury ❷
C_1-C_4 level with:
- incomplete spinal cord lesion NOS
- posterior cord syndrome

C&C Exclusions: See 806.00

806.05 C_5-C_7 level with unspecified spinal cord injury ❷
C&C Exclusions: See 806.00

806.06 C_5-C_7 level with complete lesion of cord ❷
C&C Exclusions: See 806.00

806.07 C_5-C_7 level with anterior cord syndrome ❷
C&C Exclusions: See 806.00

806.08 C_5-C_7 level with central cord syndrome ❷
C&C Exclusions: See 806.00

806.09 C_5-C_7 level with other specified spinal cord injury ❷
C_5-C_7 level with:
- incomplete spinal cord lesion NOS
- posterior cord syndrome

C&C Exclusions: See 806.00

❺ **806.1 Cervical, open**

806.10 C_1-C_4 level with unspecified spinal cord injury ❷
C&C Exclusions: See 806.00

806.11 C_1-C_4 level with complete lesion of cord ❷
C&C Exclusions: See 806.00

806.12 C_1-C_4 level with anterior cord syndrome ❷
C&C Exclusions: See 806.00

806.13 C_1-C_4 level with central cord syndrome ❷
C&C Exclusions: See 806.00

806.14 C_1-C_4 level with other specified spinal cord injury ❷
C_1-C_4 level with:
- incomplete spinal cord lesion NOS
- posterior cord syndrome

C&C Exclusions: See 806.00

806.15 C_5-C_7 level with unspecified spinal cord injury ❷
C&C Exclusions: See 806.00

806.16 C_5-C_7 level with complete lesion of cord ❷
C&C Exclusions: See 806.00

806.17 C_5-C_7 level with anterior cord syndrome ❷
C&C Exclusions: See 806.00

806.18 C_5-C_7 level with central cord syndrome ❷
C&C Exclusions: See 806.00

806.19 C_5-C_7 level with other specified spinal cord injury ❷
C_5-C_7 level with:
- incomplete spinal cord lesion NOS
- posterior cord syndrome

C&C Exclusions: See 806.00

❺ **806.2 Dorsal [thoracic], closed**

806.20 T_1-T_6 level with unspecified spinal cord injury ❷
Thoracic region NOS with spinal cord injury NOS
C&C Exclusions: 733.10, 733.11, 733.12, 733.13, 733.14, 733.15, 733.16, 733.19, 733.93, 733.94, 733.95, 805.2, 805.3, 805.8, 805.9, 806.20, 806.21, 806.22, 806.23, 806.24, 806.25, 806.26, 806.27, 806.28, 806.29, 806.30, 806.31, 806.32, 806.33, 806.34, 806.35, 806.36, 806.37, 806.38, 806.39, 806.8, 806.9, 829.0, 829.1, 839.21, 839.31, 839.40, 839.49, 839.50, 839.59, 839.69, 839.79, 839.8, 839.9, 847.1, 847.9, 848.8, 848.9, 879.8, 879.9, 905.1, 926.11, 929.0, 929.9, 952.10, 952.11, 952.12, 952.13, 952.14, 952.15, 952.16, 952.17, 952.18, 952.19, 952.8, 952.9, 958.8, 959.1, 959.8, 959.9

806.21 T_1-T_6 level with complete lesion of cord ❷
C&C Exclusions: See 806.20

806.22 T_1-T_6 level with anterior cord syndrome ❷
C&C Exclusions: See 806.20

806.23 T_1-T_6 level with central cord syndrome ❷
C&C Exclusions: See 806.20

806.24 T_1-T_6 level with other specified spinal cord injury ❷
T_1-T_6 level with:
incomplete spinal cord lesion NOS
posterior cord syndrome
C&C Exclusions: See 806.20

806.25 T_7-T_{12} level with unspecified spinal cord injury ❷
C&C Exclusions: See 806.20

806.26 T_7-T_{12} level with complete lesion of cord ❷
C&C Exclusions: See 806.20

806.27 T_7-T_{12} level with anterior cord syndrome ❷
C&C Exclusions: See 806.20

806.28 T_7-T_{12} level with central cord syndrome ❷
C&C Exclusions: See 806.20

806.29 T_7-T_{12} level with other specified spinal cord injury ❷
T_7-T_{12} level with:
incomplete spinal cord lesion NOS
posterior cord syndrome
C&C Exclusions: See 806.20

❺ **806.3 Dorsal [thoracic], open**

806.30 T_1-T_6 level with unspecified spinal cord injury ❷
C&C Exclusions: See 806.20

806.31 T_1-T_6 level with complete lesion of cord ❷
C&C Exclusions: See 806.20

806.32 T_1-T_6 level with anterior cord syndrome ❷
C&C Exclusions: See 806.20

806.33 T_1-T_6 level with central cord syndrome ❷
C&C Exclusions: See 806.20

806.34 T_1-T_6 level with other specified spinal cord injury ❷
T_1-T_6 level with:
incomplete spinal cord lesion NOS
posterior cord syndrome
C&C Exclusions: See 806.20

806.35 T_7-T_{12} level with unspecified spinal cord injury ❷
C&C Exclusions: See 806.20

806.36 T_7-T_{12} level with complete lesion of cord ❷
C&C Exclusions: See 806.20

806.37 T_7-T_{12} level with anterior cord syndrome ❷
C&C Exclusions: See 806.20

806.38 T_7-T_{12} level with central cord syndrome ❷
C&C Exclusions: See 806.20

806.39 T_7-T_{12} level with other specified spinal cord injury ❷
T_7-T_{12} level with:
incomplete spinal cord lesion NOS
posterior cord syndrome
C&C Exclusions: See 806.20

806.4 Lumbar, closed ❷
C&C Exclusions: 733.10, 733.11, 733.12, 733.13, 733.14, 733.15, 733.16, 733.19, 733.93, 733.94, 733.95, 805.4, 805.5, 805.8, 805.9, 806.4, 806.5, 806.8, 806.9, 829.0, 829.1, 839.20, 839.30, 839.40, 839.49, 839.50, 839.59, 839.69, 839.79, 839.8, 839.9, 847.2, 847.9, 848.8, 848.9, 879.8, 879.9, 905.1, 926.11, 929.0, 929.9, 952.2, 952.8, 952.9, 958.8, 959.1, 959.8, 959.9
AHA: 4Q 1999, 11, 13

806.5 Lumbar, open ❷
C&C Exclusions: See 806.4

❺ **806.6 Sacrum and coccyx, closed**

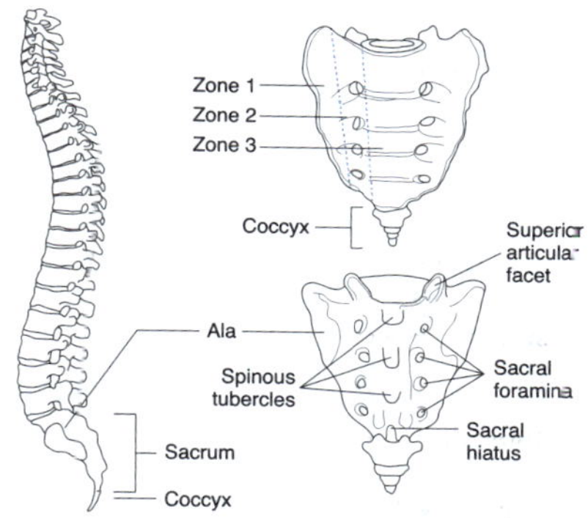

806.60 With unspecified spinal cord injury ❷
C&C Exclusions: 733.10, 733.11, 733.12, 733.13, 733.14, 733.15, 733.16, 733.19, 733.93, 733.94, 733.95, 805.6, 805.7, 805.8, 805.9, 806.60, 806.61, 806.62, 806.69, 806.70, 806.71, 806.72, 806.79, 806.8, 806.9, 829.0, 829.1, 839.40, 839.41, 839.42, 839.49, 839.50, 839.51, 839.52, 839.59, 839.69, 839.79, 839.8, 839.9, 846.0, 846.1, 846.2, 846.3, 846.8, 846.9, 847.0, 847.3, 847.4, 847.9, 848.5, 848.8, 848.9, 879.8, 879.9, 905.1, 926.11, 929.0, 929.9, 952.3, 952.8, 952.9, 958.8, 959.1, 959.8, 959.9

806.61 With complete cauda equina lesion ❷
C&C Exclusions: See 806.60

806.62 With other cauda equina injury ❷
C&C Exclusions: See 806.60

806.69 With other spinal cord injury ❷
C&C Exclusions: See 806.60

❺ **806.7 Sacrum and coccyx, open**

806.70 With unspecified spinal cord injury ❷
C&C Exclusions: See 806.60

806.71 With complete cauda equina lesion ❷
C&C Exclusions: See 806.60

806.72 With other cauda equina injury ❷
C&C Exclusions: See 806.60

806.79 With other spinal cord injury ❷
C&C Exclusions: See 806.60

806.8 Unspecified, closed ❷
C&C Exclusions: 733.10, 733.11, 733.12, 733.13, 733.14, 733.15, 733.16, 733.19, 733.93, 733.94, 733.95, 805.00, 805.01, 805.02, 805.03, 805.04, 805.05, 805.06, 805.07, 805.08, 806.00, 806.01, 806.02, 806.03, 806.04, 806.05, 806.06, 806.07, 806.08, 806.09, 829.0, 829.1, 839.00, 839.01, 839.02, 839.03, 839.04, 839.05, 839.06, 839.07, 839.08, 839.10, 839.11, 839.12, 839.13, 839.14, 839.15, 839.16, 839.17, 839.18, 839.20, 839.21, 839.30, 839.31, 839.40, 839.41, 839.42, 839.49, 839.50, 839.51, 839.52, 839.59, 839.69, 839.79, 839.8, 839.9, 846.0, 846.1, 846.2, 846.3, 846.8, 846.9, 847.0, 847.1, 847.2, 847.3, 847.4, 847.9, 848.5, 848.8, 848.9, 879.8, 879.9, 905.1, 926.11, 929.0, 929.9, 952.00, 952.01, 952.02, 952.03, 952.04, 952.05, 952.06, 952.07, 952.08, 952.09, 952.8, 952.9, 958.8, 959.1, 959.8, 959.9

806.9 Unspecified, open ❷
C&C Exclusions: See 806.8

④ 807 Fracture of rib(s), sternum, larynx, and trachea

The following fifth-digit subclassification is for use with codes 807.0-807.1:

- **0** rib(s), unspecified
- **1** one rib
- **2** two ribs
- **3** three ribs
- **4** four ribs
- **5** five ribs
- **6** six ribs
- **7** seven ribs
- **8** eight or more ribs
- **9** multiple ribs, unspecified

⑤ 807.0 Rib(s), closed②

C&C Exclusions: **(for codes 807.04-807.09)** 807.00, 807.01, 807.02, 807.03, 807.04, 807.05, 807.06, 807.07, 807.08, 807.09, 807.10, 807.11, 807.12, 807.13, 807.14, 807.15, 807.16, 807.17, 807.18, 807.19, 807.4, 819.0, 819.1, 828.0, 828.1, 829.0, 829.1, 848.8, 848.9, 879.8, 879.9, 929.0, 929.9, 958.8, 959.8, 959.9

⑤ 807.1 Rib(s), open②

C&C Exclusions: See 807.0

807.2 Sternum, closed②

C&C Exclusions: 807.2, 807.3, 807.4, 829.0, 829.1, 848.8, 848.9, 879.8, 879.9, 929.0, 929.9, 958.8, 959.8, 959.9

807.3 Sternum, open②

C&C Exclusions: See 807.2

807.4 Flail chest②

DEF: Multiple fractures of the ribs and sternum causing the entire ribcage to become unstable, threatening the organs in the chest cavity.

C&C Exclusions: 807.00, 807.01, 807.02, 807.03, 807.04, 807.05, 807.06, 807.07, 807.08, 807.09, 807.10, 807.11, 807.12, 807.13, 807.14, 807.15, 807.16, 807.17, 807.18, 807.19, 807.2, 807.3, 807.4, 829.0, 829.1, 848.8, 848.9, 879.8, 879.9, 929.0, 929.9, 958.8, 959.8, 959.9

807.5 Larynx and trachea, closed②

Hyoid bone
Thyroid cartilage
Trachea

C&C Exclusions: 807.5, 807.6, 829.0, 829.1, 848.8, 848.9, 879.8, 879.9, 929.0, 929.9, 958.8, 959.8, 959.9

807.6 Larynx and trachea, open②

C&C Exclusions: See 807.5

④ 808 Fracture of pelvis

808.0 Acetabulum, closed

C&C Exclusions: 733.10, 733.11, 733.12, 733.13, 733.14, 733.15, 733.16, 733.19, 733.93, 733.94, 733.95, 808.0, 808.1, 808.43, 808.49, 808.53, 808.59, 808.8, 808.9, 809.0, 809.1, 829.0, 829.1, 835.00, 835.01, 835.02, 835.03, 835.10, 835.11, 835.12, 835.13, 843.0, 843.1, 843.8, 843.9, 846.0, 846.1, 846.2, 846.3, 846.8, 846.9, 848.5, 848.8, 848.9, 879.8, 879.9, 929.0, 929.9, 958.8, 959.6, 959.8, 959.9

808.1 Acetabulum, open

C&C Exclusions: 808.0, 808.1, 808.43, 808.49, 808.53, 808.59, 808.8, 808.9, 809.0, 809.1, 829.0, 829.1, 835.00, 835.01, 835.02, 835.03, 835.10, 835.11, 835.12, 835.13, 843.0, 843.1, 843.8, 843.9, 846.0, 846.1, 846.2, 846.3, 846.8, 846.9, 848.5, 848.8, 848.9, 879.8, 879.9, 929.0, 929.9, 958.8, 959.6, 959.8, 959.9

808.2 Pubis, closed

C&C Exclusions: 733.10, 733.11, 733.12, 733.13, 733.14, 733.15, 733.16, 733.19, 733.93, 733.94, 733.95, 808.2, 808.3, 808.43, 808.49, 808.53, 808.59, 808.8, 808.9, 809.0, 809.1, 829.0, 829.1, 835.00, 835.01, 835.02, 835.03, 835.10, 835.11, 835.12, 835.13, 843.0, 843.1, 843.8, 843.9, 846.0, 846.1, 846.2, 846.3, 846.8, 846.9, 848.5, 848.8, 848.9, 879.8, 879.9, 929.0, 929.9, 958.8, 959.6, 959.8, 959.9

808.3 Pubis, open

C&C Exclusions: See 808.2

⑤ 808.4 Other specified part, closed

808.41 Ilium

808.42 Ischium

808.43 Multiple pelvic fractures with disruption of pelvic circle

C&C Exclusions: 733.10, 733.11, 733.12, 733.13, 733.14, 733.15, 733.16, 733.19, 733.93, 733.94, 733.95, 808.0, 808.1, 808.2, 808.3, 808.41, 808.42, 808.43, 808.49, 808.51, 808.52, 808.53, 808.59, 808.8, 808.9, 809.0, 809.1, 829.0, 829.1, 835.00, 835.01, 835.02, 835.03, 835.10, 835.11, 835.12, 835.13, 843.0, 843.1, 843.8, 843.9, 846.0, 846.1, 846.2, 846.3, 846.8, 846.9, 848.5, 848.8, 848.9, 879.8, 879.9, 929.0, 929.9, 958.8, 959.6, 959.8, 959.9

808.49 Other

Innominate bone
Pelvic rim

C&C Exclusions: See 808.43

⑤ 808.5 Other specified part, open

808.51 Ilium

C&C Exclusions: 733.10, 733.11, 733.12, 733.13, 733.14, 733.15, 733.16, 733.19, 733.93, 733.94, 733.95, 808.41, 808.43, 808.49, 808.51, 808.53, 808.59, 808.8, 808.9, 809.0, 809.1, 829.0, 829.1, 835.00, 835.01, 835.02, 835.03, 835.10, 835.11, 835.12, 835.13, 843.0, 843.1, 843.8, 843.9, 846.0, 846.1, 846.2, 846.3, 846.8, 846.9, 848.5, 848.8, 848.9, 879.8, 879.9, 929.0, 929.9, 958.8, 959.6, 959.8, 959.9

808.52 Ischium

C&C Exclusions: 733.10, 733.11, 733.12, 733.13, 733.14, 733.15, 733.16, 733.19, 733.93, 733.94, 733.95, 808.42, 808.43, 808.49, 808.52, 808.53, 808.59, 808.8, 808.9, 809.0, 809.1, 829.0, 829.1, 835.00, 835.01, 835.02, 835.03, 835.10, 835.11, 835.12, 835.13, 843.0, 843.1, 843.8, 843.9, 846.0, 846.1, 846.2, 846.3, 846.8, 846.9, 848.5, 848.8, 848.9, 879.8, 879.9, 929.0, 929.9, 958.8, 959.6, 959.8, 959.9

808.53 Multiple pelvic fractures with disruption of pelvic circle

C&C Exclusions: 733.10, 733.11, 733.12, 733.13, 733.14, 733.15, 733.16, 733.19, 733.93, 733.94, 733.95, 808.0, 808.1, 808.2, 808.3, 808.41, 808.42, 808.43, 808.49, 808.51, 808.52, 808.53, 808.59, 808.8, 808.9, 809.0, 809.1, 829.0, 829.1, 835.00, 835.01, 835.02, 835.03, 835.10, 835.11, 835.12, 835.13, 843.0, 843.1, 843.8, 843.9, 846.0, 846.1, 846.2, 846.3, 846.8, 846.9, 848.5, 848.8, 848.9, 879.8, 879.9, 929.0, 929.9, 958.8, 959.6, 959.8, 959.9

808.59 Other

C&C Exclusions: See 808.53

808.8 Unspecified, closed

C&C Exclusions: See 808.53

808.9 Unspecified, open

C&C Exclusions: See 808.53

④ 809 Ill-defined fractures of bones of trunk

Includes bones of trunk with other bones except those of skull and face
multiple bones of trunk

Excludes *multiple fractures of:*
pelvic bones alone (808.0-808.9)
ribs alone (807.0-807.1, 807.4)
ribs or sternum with limb bones (819.0-819.1, 828.0-828.1)
skull or face with other bones (804.0-804.9)

809.0 Fracture of bones of trunk, closed

809.1 Fracture of bones of trunk, open

FRACTURE OF UPPER LIMB (810-819)

④ **810 Fracture of clavicle**

Includes: collar bone
interligamentous part of clavicle

The following fifth-digit subclassification is for use with category 810:
- 0 **unspecified part**
  Clavicle NOS
- 1 **sternal end of clavicle**
- 2 **shaft of clavicle**
- 3 **acromial end of clavicle**

⑤ **810.0 Closed** ②

⑤ **810.1 Open** ②

④ **811 Fracture of scapula**

Includes: shoulder blade

The following fifth-digit subclassification is for use with category 811:
- 0 **unspecified part**
- 1 **acromial process**
  Acromion (process)
- 2 **coracoid process**
- 3 **glenoid cavity and neck of scapula**
- 9 **other**

⑤ **811.0 Closed** ②

⑤ **811.1 Open** ②

④ **812 Fracture of humerus**

⑤ **812.0 Upper end, closed**

812.00 Upper end, unspecified part
Proximal end
Shoulder

812.01 Surgical neck
Neck of humerus NOS

812.02 Anatomical neck

812.03 Greater tuberosity

812.09 Other
Head
Upper epiphysis

⑤ **812.1 Upper end, open**

812.10 Upper end, unspecified part

812.11 Surgical neck

812.12 Anatomical neck

812.13 Greater tuberosity

812.19 Other

⑤ **812.2 Shaft or unspecified part, closed**

812.20 Unspecified part of humerus
Humerus NOS
Upper arm NOS

812.21 Shaft of humerus
AHA: 4Q 2005, 129; 3Q 1999, 14

⑤ **812.3 Shaft or unspecified part, open**

812.30 Unspecified part of humerus

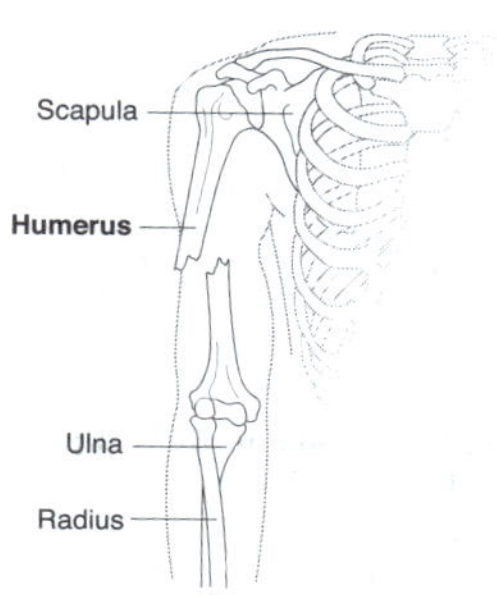

812.31 Shaft of humerus

⑤ **812.4 Lower end, closed**
Distal end of humerus
Elbow

812.40 Lower end, unspecified part

812.41 Supracondylar fracture of humerus
DEF: Fracture of the part of the upper arm interfacing with the elbow.

812.42 Lateral condyle
External condyle

812.43 Medial condyle
Internal epicondyle

812.44 Condyle(s), unspecified
Articular process NOS
Lower epiphysis

812.49 Other
Multiple fractures of lower end
Trochlea

⑤ **812.5 Lower end, open**

812.50 Lower end, unspecified part

812.51 Supracondylar fracture of humerus

812.52 Lateral condyle

812.53 Medial condyle

812.54 Condyle(s), unspecified

812.59 Other

④ **813 Fracture of radius and ulna**

⑤ **813.0 Upper end, closed**
Proximal end

813.00 Upper end of forearm, unspecified

813.01 Olecranon process of ulna

813.02 Coronoid process of ulna

813.03 Monteggia's fracture

813.04 Other and unspecified fractures of proximal end of ulna (alone)
Multiple fractures of ulna, upper end

813.05 Head of radius

813.06 Neck of radius

813.07 Other and unspecified fractures of proximal end of radius (alone)
Multiple fractures of radius, upper end

813.08 Radius with ulna, upper end [any part]

⑤ **813.1 Upper end, open**

813.10 Upper end of forearm, unspecified

813.11 Olecranon process of ulna

813.12 Coronoid process of ulna

813.13 Monteggia's fracture

813.14 Other and unspecified fractures of proximal end of ulna (alone)

813.15 Head of radius

813.16 Neck of radius

813.17 Other and unspecified fractures of proximal end of radius (alone)

813.18 Radius with ulna, upper end [any part]

⑤ **813.2 Shaft, closed**

813.20 Shaft, unspecified

813.21 Radius (alone)

813.22 Ulna (alone)

813.23 Radius with ulna

⑤ **813.3 Shaft, open**

813.30 Shaft, unspecified

813.31 Radius (alone)

813.32 Ulna (alone)

813.33 Radius with ulna

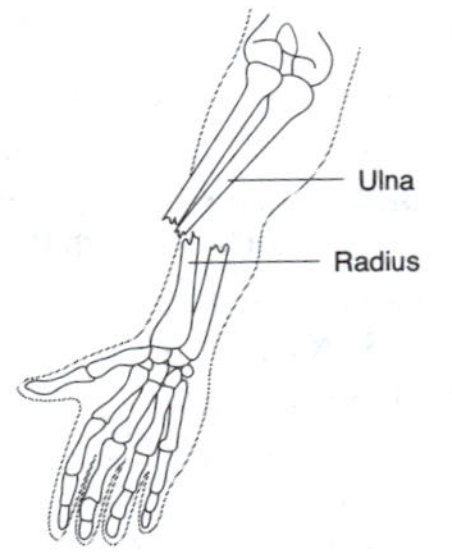

813.4 Lower end, closed
Distal end

813.40 Lower end of forearm, unspecified

813.41 Colles' fracture
Smith's fracture
DEF: Break in the lower end of the radius at the wrist, often caused by breaking a fall with an extended, outstretched hand.

813.42 Other fractures of distal end of radius (alone)
Dupuytren's fracture, radius
Radius, lower end

813.43 Distal end of ulna (alone)
Ulna:
head
lower end
lower epiphysis
styloid process

813.44 Radius with ulna, lower end
AHA: 1Q 2007, 7

813.45 Torus fracture of radius
AHA: 4Q 2002, 70

813.5 Lower end, open

813.50 Lower end of forearm, unspecified

813.51 Colles' fracture

813.52 Other fractures of distal end of radius (alone)

813.53 Distal end of ulna (alone)

813.54 Radius with ulna, lower end

813.8 Unspecified part, closed

813.80 Forearm, unspecified

813.81 Radius (alone)
AHA: 2Q 1998, 19

813.82 Ulna (alone)

813.83 Radius with ulna

813.9 Unspecified part, open

813.90 Forearm, unspecified

813.91 Radius (alone)

813.92 Ulna (alone)

813.93 Radius with ulna

814 Fracture of carpal bone(s)

The following fifth-digit subclassification is for use with category 814:
- **0 carpal bone, unspecified**
  Wrist NOS
- **1 navicular [scaphoid] of wrist**
- **2 lunate [semilunar] bone of wrist**
- **3 triquetral [cuneiform] bone of wrist**
- **4 pisiform**
- **5 trapezium bone [larger multangular]**
- **6 trapezoid bone [smaller multangular]**
- **7 capitate bone [os magnum]**
- **8 hamate [unciform] bone**
- **9 other**

814.0 Closed

814.1 Open

815 Fracture of metacarpal bone(s)
Includes: hand [except finger]
metacarpus

The following fifth-digit subclassification is for use with category 815:
- **0 metacarpal bone(s), site unspecified**
- **1 base of thumb [first] metacarpal**
  Bennett's fracture
- **2 base of other metacarpal bone(s)**
- **3 shaft of metacarpal bone(s)**
- **4 neck of metacarpal bone(s)**
- **9 multiple sites of metacarpus**

815.0 Closed

815.1 Open

816 Fracture of one or more phalanges of hand
Includes: finger(s)
thumb

The following fifth-digit subclassification is for use with category 816:
- **0 phalanx or phalanges, unspecified**
- **1 middle or proximal phalanx or phalanges**
- **2 distal phalanx or phalanges**
- **3 multiple sites**

816.0 Closed

816.1 Open
AHA: For Code 816.12: 4Q 2003, 77

817 Multiple fractures of hand bones
Includes: metacarpal bone(s) with phalanx or phalanges of same hand

817.0 Closed

817.1 Open

818 Ill-defined fractures of upper limb
Includes: arm NOS
multiple bones of same upper limb
Excludes: *multiple fractures of:*
metacarpal bone(s) with phalanx or phalanges (817.0-817.1)
phalanges of hand alone (816.0-816.1)
radius with ulna (813.0-813.9)

818.0 Closed

818.1 Open

819 Multiple fractures involving both upper limbs, and upper limb with rib(s) and sternum
Includes: arm(s) with rib(s) or sternum
both arms [any bones]

819.0 Closed

819.1 Open

FRACTURE OF LOWER LIMB (820-829)

820 Fracture of neck of femur

820.0 Transcervical fracture, closed

820.00 Intracapsular section, unspecified
C&C Exclusions: 733.10, 733.11, 733.12, 733.13, 733.14, 733.15, 733.16, 733.19, 733.93, 733.94, 733.95, 820.00, 820.01, 820.02, 820.03, 820.09, 820.10, 820.11, 820.12, 820.13, 820.19, 820.20, 820.21, 820.22, 820.30, 820.31, 820.32, 820.8, 820.9, 821.00, 821.01, 821.10, 821.11, 821.20, 821.21, 821.22, 821.23, 821.29, 821.30, 821.31, 821.32, 821.33, 821.39, 827.0, 827.1, 828.0, 828.1, 829.0, 829.1, 843.0, 843.1, 843.8, 843.9, 848.8, 848.9, 879.8, 879.9, 929.0, 929.9, 958.8, 959.6, 959.8, 959.9

820.01 Epiphysis (separation) (upper)
Transepiphyseal
C&C Exclusions: See 820.00

820.02 Midcervical section
Transcervical NOS
C&C Exclusions: See 820.00
AHA: 3Q 2003, 12

820.03 Base of neck
Cervicotrochanteric section
C&C Exclusions: See 820.00

820.09 Other
Head of femur
Subcapital
C&C Exclusions: See 820.00

❺ **820.1 Transcervical fracture, open**

820.10 Intracapsular section, unspecified
C&C Exclusions: See 820.00

820.11 Epiphysis (separation) (upper)
C&C Exclusions: See 820.00

820.12 Midcervical section

820.13 Base of neck

820.19 Other

❺ **820.2 Pertrochanteric fracture, closed**

820.20 Trochanteric section, unspecified
Trochanter:
NOS
greater
lesser

820.21 Intertrochanteric section

820.22 Subtrochanteric section

❺ **820.3 Pertrochanteric fracture, open**

820.30 Trochanteric section, unspecified

820.31 Intertrochanteric section

820.32 Subtrochanteric section

820.8 Unspecified part of neck of femur, closed
Hip NOS
Neck of femur NOS

820.9 Unspecified part of neck of femur, open

Femur fracture

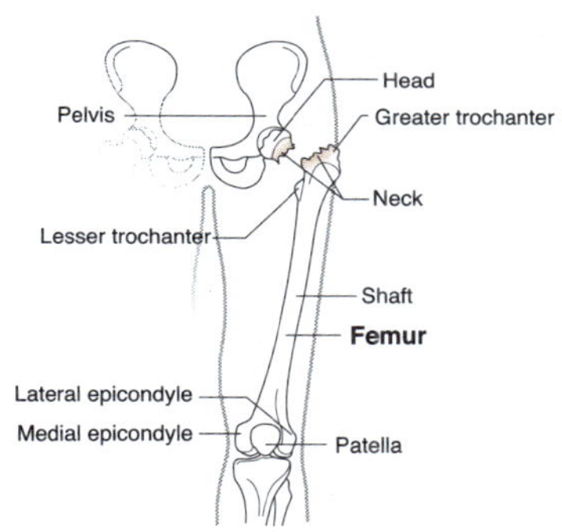

❹ **821 Fracture of other and unspecified parts of femur**

❺ **821.0 Shaft or unspecified part, closed**

821.00 Unspecified part of femur
Thigh
Upper leg
Excludes *hip NOS (820.8)*

821.01 Shaft
AHA: 1Q 2007, 4; 1Q 1999, 5

❺ **821.1 Shaft or unspecified part, open**

821.10 Unspecified part of femur

821.11 Shaft

❺ **821.2 Lower end, closed**
Distal end

821.20 Lower end, unspecified part

821.21 Condyle, femoral

821.22 Epiphysis, lower (separation)

821.23 Supracondylar fracture of femur

821.29 Other
Multiple fractures of lower end

❺ **821.3 Lower end, open**

821.30 Lower end, unspecified part

821.31 Condyle, femoral

821.32 Epiphysis, lower (separation)

821.33 Supracondylar fracture of femur

821.39 Other

❹ **822 Fracture of patella**

822.0 Closed

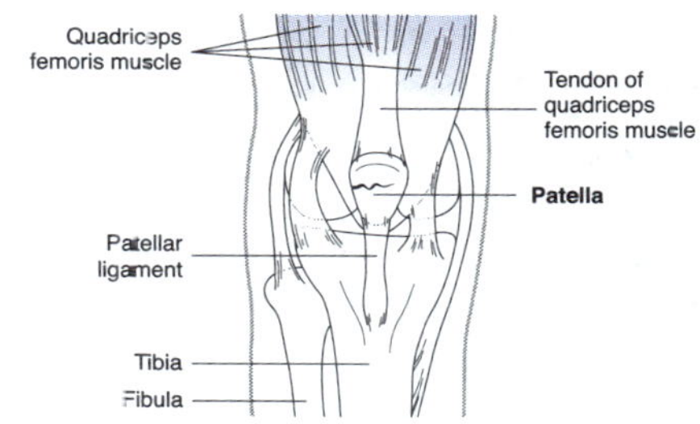

822.1 Open

❹ **823 Fracture of tibia and fibula**
Excludes *Dupuytren's fracture (824.4-824.5)*
ankle (824.4-824.5)
radius (813.42, 813.52)
Pott's fracture (824.4-824.5)
that involving ankle (824.0-824.9)

The following fifth-digit subclassification is for use with category 823:
0 tibia alone
1 fibula alone
2 fibula with tibia

❺ **823.0 Upper end, closed**
Head
Proximal end
Tibia:
condyles
tuberosity

❺ **823.1 Upper end, open**

❺ **823.2 Shaft, closed**

❺ **823.3 Shaft, open**

❺ **823.4 Torus fracture**
AHA: 4Q 2002, 70

❺ **823.8 Unspecified part, closed**
Lower leg NOS
AHA: For Code 823.82: 1Q 1997, 8

❺ **823.9 Unspecified part, open**

❹ **824 Fracture of ankle**

824.0 Medial malleolus, closed
Tibia involving:
ankle
malleolus
AHA: 1Q 2004, 9

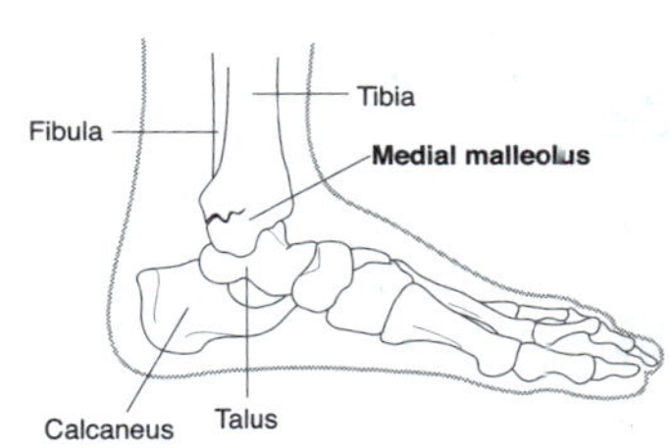

824.1 Medial malleolus, open

824.2 Lateral malleolus, closed
Fibula involving:
ankle
malleolus
AHA: 2Q 2002, 3

824.3 Lateral malleolus, open

824.4 Bimalleolar, closed
Dupuytren's fracture, fibula
Pott's fracture

824.5 Bimalleolar, open

824.6 Trimalleolar, closed
Lateral and medial malleolus with anterior or posterior lip of tibia

824.7 Trimalleolar, open

824.8 Unspecified, closed
Ankle NOS
AHA: 3Q 2000, 12

824.9 Unspecified, open

❹ **825 Fracture of one or more tarsal and metatarsal bones**

825.0 Fracture of calcaneus, closed
Heel bone
Os calcis

825.1 Fracture of calcaneus, open

❺ **825.2 Fracture of other tarsal and metatarsal bones, closed**

825.20 Unspecified bone(s) of foot [except toes]
Instep

825.21 Astragalus
Talus

825.22 Navicular [scaphoid], foot

825.23 Cuboid

825.24 Cuneiform, foot

825.25 Metatarsal bone(s)

825.29 Other
Tarsal with metatarsal bone(s) only
Excludes *calcaneus (825.0)*

❺ **825.3 Fracture of other tarsal and metatarsal bones, open**

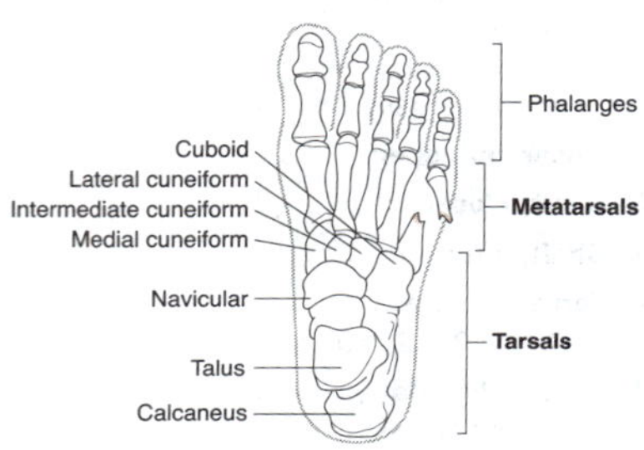

825.30 Unspecified bone(s) of foot [except toes]

825.31 Astragalus

825.32 Navicular [scaphoid], foot

825.33 Cuboid

825.34 Cuneiform, foot

825.35 Metatarsal bone(s)

825.39 Other

❹ **826 Fracture of one or more phalanges of foot**
Includes toe(s)

826.0 Closed

826.1 Open

❹ **827 Other, multiple, and ill-defined fractures of lower limb**
Includes leg NOS
multiple bones of same lower limb
Excludes *multiple fractures of:*
ankle bones alone (824.4-824.9)
phalanges of foot alone (826.0-826.1)
tarsal with metatarsal bones (825.29, 825.39)
tibia with fibula (823.0-823.9 with fifth-digit 2)

827.0 Closed

827.1 Open

❹ **828 Multiple fractures involving both lower limbs, lower with upper limb, and lower limb(s) with rib(s) and sternum**
Includes arm(s) with leg(s) [any bones]
both legs [any bones]
leg(s) with rib(s) or sternum

828.0 Closed ❷

828.1 Open ❷

❹ **829 Fracture of unspecified bones**

✖ **829.0 Unspecified bone, closed**

✖ **829.1 Unspecified bone, open**
AHA: 3Q 1990, 12

DISLOCATION (830-839)

Includes displacement
subluxation

Excludes *congenital dislocation (754.0-755.8)*
pathological dislocation (718.2)
recurrent dislocation (718.3)

The descriptions "closed" and "open," used in the fourth-digit subdivisions, include the following terms:

closed:
complete
dislocation NOS
partial
simple
uncomplicated

open:
compound
infected
with foreign body

Note: *A dislocation not indicated as closed or open should be classified as closed.*

❹ **830 Dislocation of jaw**
Includes jaw (cartilage) (meniscus)
mandible
maxilla (inferior)
temporomandibular (joint)

830.0 Closed dislocation

830.1 Open dislocation

❹ **831 Dislocation of shoulder**
Excludes *sternoclavicular joint (839.61, 839.71)*
sternum (839.61, 839.71)

The following fifth-digit subclassification is for use with category 831:

0 shoulder, unspecified
Humerus NOS
1 anterior dislocation of humerus
2 posterior dislocation of humerus
3 inferior dislocation of humerus
4 acromioclavicular (joint)
Clavicle
9 other
Scapula

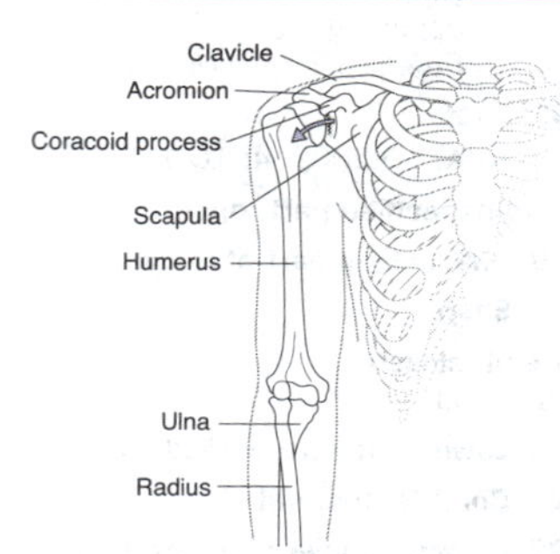

❺ **831.0 Closed dislocation**

❺ **831.1 Open dislocation**

❹ 832 Dislocation of elbow

The following fifth-digit subclassification is for use with category 832:
- **0 elbow, unspecified**
- **1 anterior dislocation of elbow**
- **2 posterior dislocation of elbow**
- **3 medial dislocation of elbow**
- **4 lateral dislocation of elbow**
- **9 other**

❺ 832.0 Closed dislocation

❺ 832.1 Open dislocation

❹ 833 Dislocation of wrist

The following fifth-digit subclassification is for use with category 833:
- **0 wrist, unspecified part**
  - Carpal (bone)
  - Radius, distal end
- **1 radioulnar (joint), distal**
- **2 radiocarpal (joint)**
- **3 midcarpal (joint)**
- **4 carpometacarpal (joint)**
- **5 metacarpal (bone), proximal end**
- **9 other**
  - Ulna, distal end

❺ 833.0 Closed dislocation

❺ 833.1 Open dislocation

❹ 834 Dislocation of finger

Includes finger(s)
phalanx of hand
thumb

The following fifth-digit subclassification is for use with category 834:
- **0 finger, unspecified part**
- **1 metacarpophalangeal (joint)**
  - Metacarpal (bone), distal end
- **2 interphalangeal (joint), hand**

❺ 834.0 Closed dislocation

❺ 834.1 Open dislocation

❹ 835 Dislocation of hip

The following fifth-digit subclassification is for use with category 835:
- **0 dislocation of hip, unspecified**
- **1 posterior dislocation**
- **2 obturator dislocation**
- **3 other anterior dislocation**

❺ 835.0 Closed dislocation

❺ 835.1 Open dislocation

❹ 836 Dislocation of knee

Excludes *dislocation of knee:*
old or pathological (718.2)
recurrent (718.3)
internal derangement of knee joint (717.0-717.5, 717.8-717.9)
old tear of cartilage or meniscus of knee (717.0-717.5, 717.8-717.9)

836.0 Tear of medial cartilage or meniscus of knee, current
Bucket handle tear:
NOS current injury
medial meniscus current injury

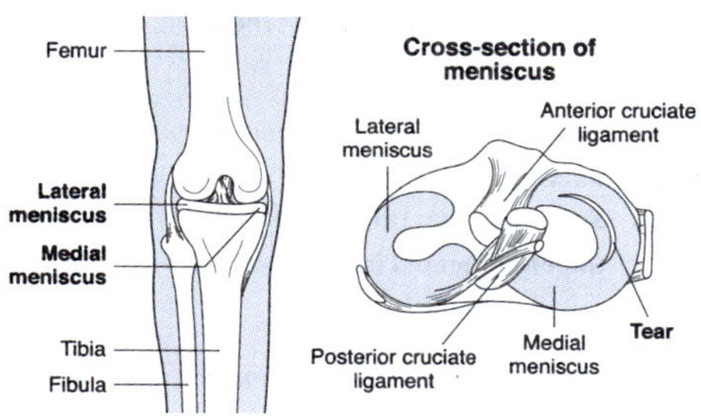

836.1 Tear of lateral cartilage or meniscus of knee, current

836.2 Other tear of cartilage or meniscus of knee, current
Tear of:
cartilage (semilunar) current injury, not specified as medial or lateral
meniscus current injury, not specified as medial or lateral

836.3 Dislocation of patella, closed

836.4 Dislocation of patella, open

❺ 836.5 Other dislocation of knee, closed

836.50 Dislocation of knee, unspecified

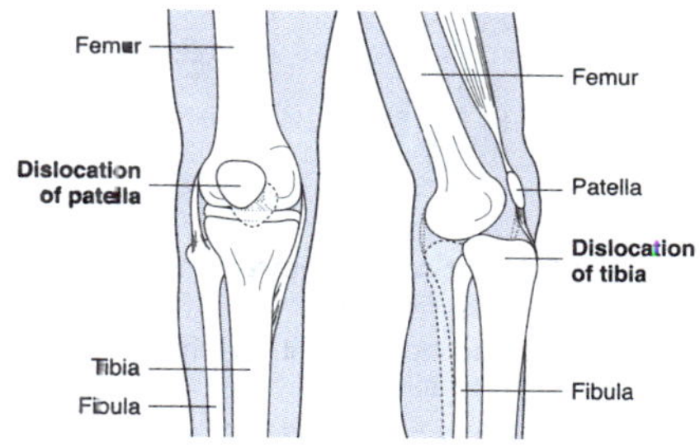

836.51 Anterior dislocation of tibia, proximal end
Posterior dislocation of femur, distal end

836.52 Posterior dislocation of tibia, proximal end
Anterior dislocation of femur, distal end

836.53 Medial dislocation of tibia, proximal end

836.54 Lateral dislocation of tibia, proximal end

836.59 Other

❺ 836.6 Other dislocation of knee, open

836.60 Dislocation of knee, unspecified

836.61 Anterior dislocation of tibia, proximal end

836.62 Posterior dislocation of tibia, proximal end

836.63 Medial dislocation of tibia, proximal end

836.64 Lateral dislocation of tibia, proximal end

836.69 Other

❹ 837 Dislocation of ankle

Includes astragalus
fibula, distal end
navicular, foot
scaphoid, foot
tibia, distal end

837.0 Closed dislocation

837.1 Open dislocation

❹ 838 Dislocation of foot

The following fifth-digit subclassification is for use with category 838:
- **0 foot, unspecified**
- **1 tarsal (bone), joint unspecified**
- **2 midtarsal (joint)**
- **3 tarsometatarsal (joint)**
- **4 metatarsal (bone), joint unspecified**
- **5 metatarsophalangeal (joint)**
- **6 interphalangeal (joint), foot**
- **9 other**
  - Phalanx of foot
  - Toe(s)

❺ 838.0 Closed dislocation

❺ 838.1 Open dislocation

Injury and Poisoning

832 – 838.1

④ 839 Other, multiple, and ill-defined dislocations

⑤ 839.0 Cervical vertebra, closed
Cervical spine
Neck

839.00 Cervical vertebra, unspecified ②
C&C Exclusions: 805.00, 805.01, 805.02, 805.03, 805.04, 805.05, 805.06, 805.07, 805.08, 805.10, 805.11, 805.12, 805.13, 805.14, 805.15, 805.16, 805.17, 805.18, 806.00, 806.01, 806.02, 806.03, 806.04, 806.05, 806.06, 806.07, 806.08, 806.09, 806.10, 806.11, 806.12, 806.13, 806.14, 806.15, 806.16, 806.17, 806.18, 806.19, 806.8, 806.9, 839.00, 839.01, 839.02, 839.03, 839.04, 839.05, 839.06, 839.07, 839.08, 839.10, 839.11, 839.12, 839.13, 839.14, 839.15, 839.16, 839.17, 839.18, 847.0, 848.8, 848.9, 879.8, 879.9, 929.0, 929.9, 952.00, 952.01, 952.02, 952.03, 952.04, 952.05, 952.06, 952.07, 952.08, 952.09, 958.8, 959.8, 959.9

839.01 First cervical vertebra ②
C&C Exclusions: See 839.00

839.02 Second cervical vertebra ②
C&C Exclusions: See 839.00

839.03 Third cervical vertebra ②
C&C Exclusions: See 839.00

839.04 Fourth cervical vertebra ②
C&C Exclusions: See 839.00

839.05 Fifth cervical vertebra ②
C&C Exclusions: See 839.00

839.06 Sixth cervical vertebra ②
C&C Exclusions: See 839.00

839.07 Seventh cervical vertebra ②
C&C Exclusions: See 839.00

839.08 Multiple cervical vertebrae ②
C&C Exclusions: See 839.00

⑤ 839.1 Cervical vertebra, open

839.10 Cervical vertebra, unspecified ②
C&C Exclusions: See 839.00

839.11 First cervical vertebra ②
C&C Exclusions: See 839.00

839.12 Second cervical vertebra ②
C&C Exclusions: See 839.00

839.13 Third cervical vertebra ②
C&C Exclusions: See 839.00

839.14 Fourth cervical vertebra ②
C&C Exclusions: See 839.00

839.15 Fifth cervical vertebra ②
C&C Exclusions: See 839.00

839.16 Sixth cervical vertebra ②
C&C Exclusions: See 839.00

839.17 Seventh cervical vertebra ②
C&C Exclusions: See 839.00

839.18 Multiple cervical vertebrae ②
C&C Exclusions: See 839.00

⑤ 839.2 Thoracic and lumbar vertebra, closed

839.20 Lumbar vertebra ②

839.21 Thoracic vertebra ②
Dorsal [thoracic] vertebra

⑤ 839.3 Thoracic and lumbar vertebra, open

839.30 Lumbar vertebra ②

839.31 Thoracic vertebra ②

⑤ 839.4 Other vertebra, closed

839.40 Vertebra, unspecified site
Spine NOS

839.41 Coccyx

839.42 Sacrum
Sacroiliac (joint)

839.49 Other

⑤ 839.5 Other vertebra, open

839.50 Vertebra, unspecified site

839.51 Coccyx

839.52 Sacrum

839.59 Other

⑤ 839.6 Other location, closed

839.61 Sternum
Sternoclavicular joint

839.69 Other
Pelvis

⑤ 839.7 Other location, open

839.71 Sternum ②

839.79 Other ②

✖ 839.8 Multiple and ill-defined, closed ②
Arm
Back
Hand
Multiple locations, except fingers or toes alone
Other ill-defined locations
Unspecified location

✖ 839.9 Multiple and ill-defined, open ②

SPRAINS AND STRAINS OF JOINTS AND ADJACENT MUSCLES (840-848)

Includes avulsion of joint capsule, ligament, muscle, tendon
hemarthrosis of joint capsule, ligament, muscle, tendon
laceration of joint capsule, ligament, muscle, tendon
rupture of joint capsule, ligament, muscle, tendon
sprain of joint capsule, ligament, muscle, tendon
strain of joint capsule, ligament, muscle, tendon
tear of joint capsule, ligament, muscle, tendon

Excludes *laceration of tendon in open wounds (880-884 and 890-894 with .2)*

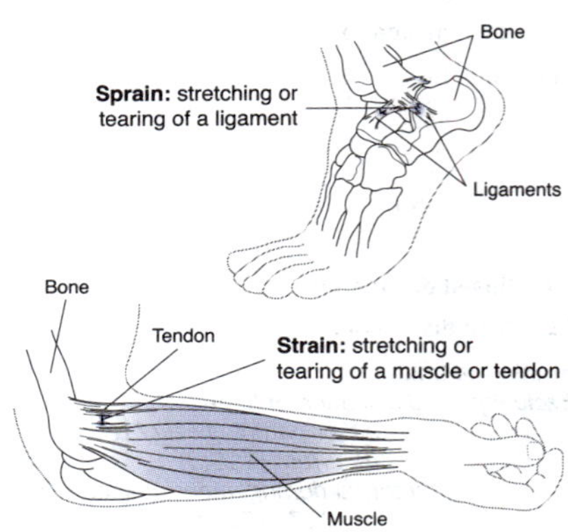

④ 840 Sprains and strains of shoulder and upper arm

840.0 Acromioclavicular (joint) (ligament)

840.1 Coracoclavicular (ligament)

840.2 Coracohumeral (ligament)

840.3 Infraspinatus (muscle) (tendon)

840.4 Rotator cuff (capsule)
Excludes *complete rupture of rotator cuff, nontraumatic (727.61)*

840.5 Subscapularis (muscle)

840.6 Supraspinatus (muscle) (tendon)

840.7 Superior glenoid labrum lesion
SLAP lesion
AHA: 4Q 2001, 52

840.8 Other specified sites of shoulder and upper arm

✖ 840.9 Unspecified site of shoulder and upper arm
Arm NOS
Shoulder NOS

❹ 841 Sprains and strains of elbow and forearm

841.0 Radial collateral ligament

841.1 Ulnar collateral ligament

841.2 Radiohumeral (joint)

841.3 Ulnohumeral (joint)

841.8 Other specified sites of elbow and forearm

✖ 841.9 Unspecified site of elbow and forearm
Elbow NOS

❹ 842 Sprains and strains of wrist and hand

❺ 842.0 Wrist

842.00 Unspecified site

842.01 Carpal (joint)

842.02 Radiocarpal (joint) (ligament)

842.09 Other
Radioulnar joint, distal

❺ 842.1 Hand

842.10 Unspecified site

842.11 Carpometacarpal (joint)

842.12 Metacarpophalangeal (joint)

842.13 Interphalangeal (joint)

842.19 Other
Midcarpal (joint)

❹ 843 Sprains and strains of hip and thigh

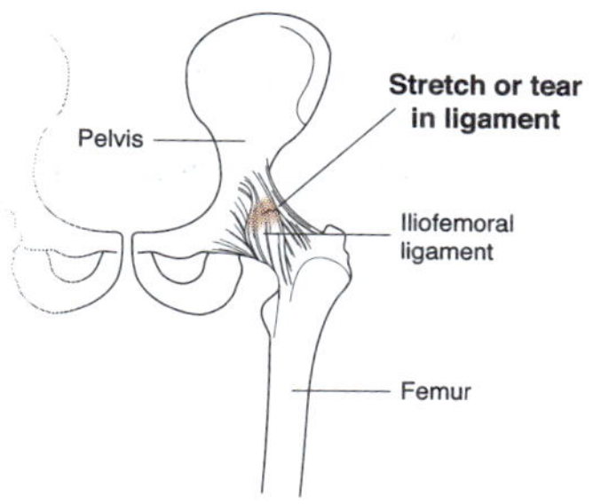

843.0 Iliofemoral (ligament)

843.1 Ischiocapsular (ligament)

843.8 Other specified sites of hip and thigh

✖ 843.9 Unspecified site of hip and thigh
Hip NOS
Thigh NOS

❹ 844 Sprains and strains of knee and leg

844.0 Lateral collateral ligament of knee

844.1 Medial collateral ligament of knee

844.2 Cruciate ligament of knee

844.3 Tibiofibular (joint) (ligament), superior

844.8 Other specified sites of knee and leg

844.9 Unspecified site of knee and leg
Knee NOS
Leg NOS

❹ 845 Sprains and strains of ankle and foot

❺ 845.0 Ankle

845.00 Unspecified site
AHA: 2Q 2002, 3

845.01 Deltoid (ligament), ankle
Internal collateral (ligament), ankle

845.02 Calcaneofibular (ligament)

845.03 Tibiofibular (ligament), distal
AHA: 1Q 2004, 9

845.09 Other
Achilles tendon

❺ 845.1 Foot

845.10 Unspecified site

845.11 Tarsometatarsal (joint) (ligament)

845.12 Metatarsophalangeal (joint)

845.13 Interphalangeal (joint), toe

845.19 Other

❹ 846 Sprains and strains of sacroiliac region

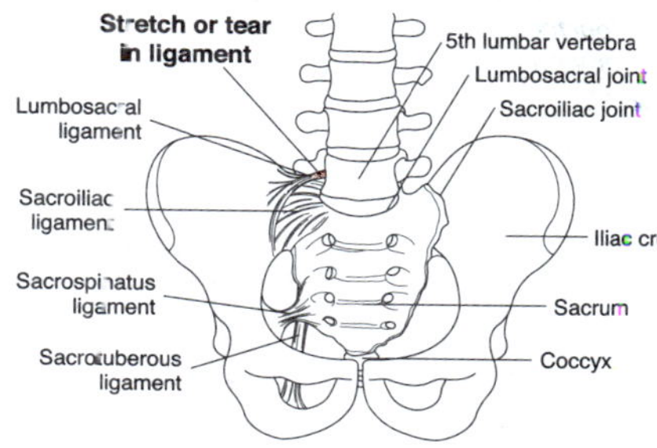

846.0 Lumbosacral (joint) (ligament)

846.1 Sacroiliac ligament

846.2 Sacrospinatus (ligament)

846.3 Sacrotuberous (ligament)

846.8 Other specified sites of sacroiliac region

✖ 846.9 Unspecified site of sacroiliac region

❹ 847 Sprains and strains of other and unspecified parts of back
Excludes *lumbosacral (846.0)*

847.0 Neck ❷
Anterior longitudinal (ligament), cervical
Atlanto-axial (joints)
Atlanto-occipital (joints)
Whiplash injury
Excludes *neck injury NOS (959.09)*
thyroid region (848.2)

847.1 Thoracic

847.2 Lumbar

847.3 Sacrum
Sacrococcygeal (ligament)

847.4 Coccyx

✖ 847.9 Unspecified site of back
Back NOS

❹ 848 Other and ill-defined sprains and strains

848.0 Septal cartilage of nose

848.1 Jaw
Temporomandibular (joint) (ligament)

848.2 Thyroid region
Cricoarytenoid (joint) (ligament)
Cricothyroid (joint) (ligament)
Thyroid cartilage

848.3 Ribs
Chondrocostal (joint) without mention of injury to sternum
Costal cartilage without mention of injury to sternum

❺ 848.4 Sternum

848.40 Unspecified site

848.41 Sternoclavicular (joint) (ligament)

848.42 Chondrosternal (joint)

848.49 Other
Xiphoid cartilage

848.5 Pelvis
Symphysis pubis
Excludes *that in childbirth (665.6)*

848.8 Other specified sites of sprains and strains

✖ 848.9 Unspecified site of sprain and strain

INTRACRANIAL INJURY, EXCLUDING THOSE WITH SKULL FRACTURE (850-854)

Excludes *intracranial injury with skull fracture (800-801 and 803-804, except .0 and .5)*
open wound of head without intracranial injury (870.0-873.9)
skull fracture alone (800-801 and 803-804 with .0, .5)

Note: The description "with open intracranial wound," used in the fourth-digit subdivisions, includes those specified as open or with mention of infection or foreign body.

AHA: 1Q 1993, 22

The following fifth-digit subclassification is for use with categories 851-854:

- **0** **unspecified state of consciousness**
- **1** **with no loss of consciousness**
- **2** **with brief [less than one hour] loss of consciousness**
- **3** **with moderate [1-24 hours] loss of consciousness**
- **4** **with prolonged [more than 24 hours] loss of consciousness and return to pre-existing conscious level**
- **5** **with prolonged [more than 24 hours] loss of consciousness without return to pre-existing conscious level**
  Use fifth-digit 5 to designate when a patient is unconscious and dies before regaining consciousness, regardless of the duration of the loss of consciousness
- **6** **with loss of consciousness of unspecified duration**
- **9** **with concussion, unspecified**

❹ 850 Concussion

Includes commotio cerebri

Excludes *concussion with:*
cerebral laceration or contusion (851.0-851.9)
cerebral hemorrhage (852-853)
head injury NOS (959.01)

AHA: 2Q 1996, 6; 4Q 1990, 24

850.0 With no loss of consciousness ❷

Concussion with mental confusion or disorientation, without loss of consciousness

C&C Exclusions: 800.00, 800.01, 800.02, 800.03, 800.04, 800.05, 800.06, 800.09, 800.10, 800.11, 800.12, 800.13, 800.14, 800.15, 800.16, 800.19, 800.20, 800.21, 800.22, 800.23, 800.24, 800.25, 800.26, 800.29, 800.30, 800.31, 800.32, 800.33, 800.34, 800.35, 800.36, 800.39, 800.40, 800.41, 800.42, 800.43, 800.44, 800.45, 800.46, 800.49, 800.50, 800.51, 800.52, 800.53, 800.54, 800.55, 800.56, 800.59, 800.60, 800.61, 800.62, 800.63, 800.64, 800.65, 800.66, 800.69, 800.70, 800.71, 800.72, 800.73, 800.74, 800.75, 800.76, 800.79, 800.80, 800.81, 800.82, 800.83, 800.84, 800.85, 800.86, 800.89, 800.90, 800.91, 800.92, 800.93, 800.94, 800.95, 800.96, 800.99, 801.00, 801.01, 801.02, 801.03, 801.04, 801.05, 801.06, 801.09, 801.10, 801.11, 801.12, 801.13, 801.14, 801.15, 801.16, 801.19, 801.20, 801.21, 801.22, 801.23, 801.24, 801.25, 801.26, 801.29, 801.30, 801.31, 801.32, 801.33, 801.34, 801.35, 801.36, 801.39, 801.40, 801.41, 801.42, 801.43, 801.44, 801.45, 801.46, 801.49, 801.50, 801.51, 801.52, 801.53, 801.54, 801.55, 801.56, 801.59, 801.60, 801.61, 801.62, 801.63, 801.64, 801.65, 801.66, 801.69, 801.70, 801.71, 801.72, 801.73, 801.74, 801.75, 801.76, 801.79, 801.80, 801.81, 801.82, 801.83, 801.84, 801.85, 801.86, 801.89, 801.90, 801.91, 801.92, 801.93, 801.94, 801.95, 801.96, 801.99, 803.00, 803.01, 803.02, 803.03, 803.04, 803.05, 803.06, 803.09, 803.10, 803.11, 803.12, 803.13, 803.14, 803.15, 803.16, 803.19, 803.20, 803.21, 803.22, 803.23, 803.24, 803.25, 803.26, 803.29, 803.30, 803.31, 803.32, 803.33, 803.34, 803.35, 803.36, 803.39, 803.40, 803.41, 803.42, 803.43, 803.44, 803.45, 803.46, 803.49, 803.50, 803.51, 803.52, 803.53, 803.54, 803.55, 803.56, 803.59, 803.60, 803.61, 803.62, 803.63, 803.64, 803.65, 803.66, 803.69, 803.70, 803.71, 803.72, 803.73, 803.74, 803.75, 803.76, 803.79, 803.80, 803.81, 803.82, 803.83, 803.84, 803.85, 803.86, 803.89, 803.90, 803.91, 803.92, 803.93, 803.94, 803.95, 803.96, 803.99, 804.00, 804.01, 804.02, 804.03, 804.04, 804.05, 804.06, 804.09, 804.10, 804.11, 804.12, 804.13, 804.14, 804.15, 804.16, 804.19, 804.20, 804.21, 804.22, 804.23, 804.24, 804.25, 804.26, 804.29, 804.30, 804.31, 804.32, 804.33, 804.34, 804.35, 804.36, 804.39, 804.40, 804.41, 804.42, 804.43, 804.44, 804.45, 804.46, 804.49, 804.50, 804.51, 804.52, 804.53, 804.54, 804.55, 804.56, 804.59, 804.60, 804.61, 804.62, 804.63, 804.64, 804.65, 804.66, 804.69, 804.70, 804.71, 804.72, 804.73, 804.74, 804.75, 804.76, 804.79, 804.80, 804.81, 804.82, 804.83, 804.84, 804.85, 804.86, 804.89, 804.90, 804.91, 804.92, 804.93, 804.94, 804.95, 804.96, 804.99, 850.0, 850.11, 850.12, 850.2, 850.3, 850.5, 850.9, 851.00, 851.01, 851.02, 851.03, 851.04, 851.05, 851.06, 851.09, 851.10, 851.11, 851.12, 851.13, 851.14, 851.15, 851.16, 851.19, 851.20, 851.21, 851.22, 851.23, 851.24, 851.25, 851.26, 851.29, 851.30, 851.31, 851.32, 851.33, 851.34, 851.35, 851.36, 851.39, 851.40, 851.41, 851.42, 851.43, 851.44, 851.45, 851.46, 851.49, 851.50, 851.51, 851.52, 851.53, 851.54, 851.55, 851.56, 851.59, 851.60, 851.61, 851.62, 851.63, 851.64, 851.65, 851.66, 851.69, 851.70, 851.71, 851.72, 851.73, 851.74, 851.75, 851.76, 851.79, 851.80, 851.81, 851.82, 851.83, 851.84, 851.85, 851.86, 851.89, 851.90, 851.91, 851.92, 851.93, 851.94, 851.95, 851.96, 851.99, 852.00, 852.01, 852.02, 852.03, 852.04, 852.05, 852.06, 852.09, 852.10, 852.11, 852.12, 852.13, 852.14, 852.15, 852.16, 852.19, 852.21, 852.22, 852.23, 852.24, 852.25, 852.26, 852.29, 852.30, 852.31, 852.32, 852.33, 852.34, 852.35, 852.36, 852.39, 852.40, 852.41, 852.42, 852.43, 852.44, 852.45, 852.46, 852.49, 852.50, 852.51, 852.52, 852.53, 852.54, 852.55, 852.56, 852.59, 853.00, 853.01, 853.02, 853.03, 853.04, 853.05, 853.06, 853.09, 853.10, 853.11, 853.12, 853.13, 853.14, 853.15, 853.16, 853.19, 854.00, 854.01, 854.02, 854.03, 854.04, 854.05, 854.06, 854.09, 854.10, 854.11, 854.12, 854.13, 854.14, 854.15, 854.16, 854.19, 873.8, 873.9, 879.8, 879.9, 905.0, 925.1, 925.2, 929.0, 929.9, 958.8, 959.01, 959.09, 959.8, 959.9

❺ 850.1 With brief loss of consciousness

Loss of consciousness for less than one hour

AHA: 4Q 2003, 76; 1Q 1999, 10; 2Q 1992, 5

850.11 With loss of consciousness of 30 minutes or less ❷

C&C Exclusions: 430, 431, 432.0, 432.1, 436, 780.01, 780.03, 800.00, 800.01, 800.02, 800.03, 800.04, 800.05, 800.06, 800.09, 800.10, 800.11, 800.12, 800.13, 800.14, 800.15, 800.16, 800.19, 800.20, 800.21, 800.22, 800.23, 800.24, 800.25, 800.26, 800.29, 800.30, 800.31, 800.32, 800.33, 800.34, 800.35, 800.36, 800.39, 800.40, 800.41, 800.42, 800.43, 800.44, 800.45, 800.46, 800.49, 800.50, 800.51, 800.52, 800.53, 800.54, 800.55, 800.56, 800.59, 800.60, 800.61, 800.62, 800.63, 800.64, 800.65, 800.66, 800.69, 800.70, 800.71, 800.72, 800.73, 800.74, 800.75, 800.76, 800.79, 800.80, 800.81, 800.82, 800.83, 800.84, 800.85, 800.86, 800.89, 800.90, 800.91, 800.92, 800.93, 800.94, 800.95, 800.96, 800.99, 801.00, 801.01, 801.02, 801.03, 801.04, 801.05, 801.06, 801.09, 801.10, 801.11, 801.12, 801.13, 801.14, 801.15, 801.16, 801.19, 801.20, 801.21, 801.22, 801.23, 801.24, 801.25, 801.26, 801.29, 801.30, 801.31, 801.32, 801.33, 801.34, 801.35, 801.36, 801.39, 801.40, 801.41, 801.42, 801.43, 801.44, 801.45, 801.46, 801.49, 801.50, 801.51, 801.52, 801.53, 801.54, 801.55, 801.56, 801.59, 801.60, 801.61, 801.62, 801.63, 801.64, 801.65, 801.66, 801.69, 801.70, 801.71, 801.72, 801.73, 801.74, 801.75, 801.76, 801.79, 801.80, 801.81, 801.82, 801.83, 801.84, 801.85, 801.86, 801.89, 801.90, 801.91, 801.92, 801.93, 801.94, 801.95, 801.96, 801.99, 802.1, 802.20, 802.21, 802.22, 802.23, 802.24, 802.25, 802.26, 802.27, 802.28, 802.29, 802.30, 802.31, 802.32, 802.33, 802.34, 802.35, 802.36, 802.37, 802.38, 802.39, 802.4, 802.5, 802.6, 802.7, 802.8, 802.9, 803.00, 803.01, 803.02, 803.03, 803.04, 803.05, 803.06, 803.09, 803.10, 803.11, 803.12, 803.13, 803.14, 803.15, 803.16, 803.19, 803.20, 803.21, 803.22, 803.23, 803.24, 803.25, 803.26, 803.29, 803.30, 803.31, 803.32, 803.33, 803.34, 803.35, 803.36, 803.39, 803.40, 803.41, 803.42, 803.43, 803.44, 803.45, 803.46, 803.49, 803.50, 803.51, 803.52, 803.53, 803.54, 803.55, 803.56, 803.59, 803.60, 803.61, 803.62, 803.63, 803.64, 803.65, 803.66, 803.69, 803.70, 803.71, 803.72, 803.73, 803.74, 803.75, 803.76, 803.79, 803.80, 803.81, 803.82, 803.83, 803.84, 803.85, 803.86, 803.89, 803.90, 803.91, 803.92, 803.93, 803.94, 803.95, 803.96, 803.99, 804.00, 804.01, 804.02, 804.03, 804.04, 804.05, 804.06, 804.09, 804.10, 804.11, 804.12, 804.13, 804.14,

804.15, 804.16, 804.19, 804.20, 804.21, 804.22, 804.23, 804.24, 804.25, 804.26, 804.29, 804.30, 804.31, 804.32, 804.33, 804.34, 804.35, 804.36, 804.39, 804.40, 804.41, 804.42, 804.43, 804.44, 804.45, 804.46, 804.49, 804.50, 804.51, 804.52, 804.53, 804.54, 804.55, 804.56, 804.59, 804.60, 804.61, 804.62, 804.63, 804.64, 804.65, 804.66, 804.69, 804.70, 804.71, 804.72, 804.73, 804.74, 804.75, 804.76, 804.79, 804.80, 804.81, 804.82, 804.83, 804.84, 804.85, 804.86, 804.89, 804.90, 804.91, 804.92, 804.93, 804.94, 804.95, 804.96, 804.99, 850.0, 850.11, 850.12, 850.2, 850.3, 850.5, 850.9, 851.00, 851.01, 851.02, 851.03, 851.04, 851.05, 851.06, 851.09, 851.10, 851.11, 851.12, 851.13, 851.14, 851.15, 851.16, 851.19, 851.20, 851.21, 851.22, 851.23, 851.24, 851.25, 851.26, 851.29, 851.30, 851.31, 851.32, 851.33, 851.34, 851.35, 851.36, 851.39, 851.40, 851.41, 851.42, 851.43, 851.44, 851.45, 851.46, 851.49, 851.50, 851.51, 851.52, 851.53, 851.54, 851.55, 851.56, 851.59, 851.60, 851.61, 851.62, 851.63, 851.64, 851.65, 851.66, 851.69, 851.70, 851.71, 851.72, 851.73, 851.74, 851.75, 851.76, 851.79, 851.80, 851.81, 851.82, 851.83, 851.84, 851.85, 851.86, 851.89, 851.90, 851.91, 851.92, 851.93, 851.94, 851.95, 851.96, 851.99, 852.00, 852.01, 852.02, 852.03, 852.04, 852.05, 852.06, 852.09, 852.10, 852.11, 852.12, 852.13, 852.14, 852.15, 852.16, 852.19, 852.21, 852.22, 852.23, 852.24, 852.25, 852.26, 852.29, 852.30, 852.31, 852.32, 852.33, 852.34, 852.35, 852.36, 852.39, 852.40, 852.41, 852.42, 852.43, 852.44, 852.45, 852.46, 852.49, 852.50, 852.51, 852.52, 852.53, 852.54, 852.55, 852.56, 852.59, 853.00, 853.01, 853.02, 853.03, 853.04, 853.05, 853.06, 853.09, 853.10, 853.11, 853.12, 853.13, 853.14, 853.15, 853.16, 853.19, 854.00, 854.01, 854.02, 854.03, 854.04, 854.05, 854.06, 854.09, 854.10, 854.11, 854.12, 854.13, 854.14, 854.15, 854.16, 854.19

850.12 With loss of consciousness from 31 minutes to 59 minutes ❷
C&C Exclusions: See 850.11

850.2 With moderate loss of consciousness ❷
Loss of consciousness for 1-24 hours
C&C Exclusions: See 850.0

850.3 With prolonged loss of consciousness and return to pre-existing conscious level ❷
Loss of consciousness for more than 24 hours with complete recovery
C&C Exclusions: See 850.0

850.4 With prolonged loss of consciousness, without return to pre-existing conscious level ❷
C&C Exclusions: See 850.0

850.5 With loss of consciousness of unspecified duration ❷
C&C Exclusions: See 850.0

850.9 Concussion, unspecified ❷
C&C Exclusions: See 850.0

❹ **851 Cerebral laceration and contusion**
Requires fifth digit. See beginning of section 850-854 for codes and definitions.
AHA: 4Q 1996, 36; 1Q 1993, 22; 4Q 1990, 24

❺ **851.0 Cortex (cerebral) contusion without mention of open intracranial wound** ❷
C&C Exclusions: See 850.0

❺ **851.1 Cortex (cerebral) contusion with open intracranial wound** ❷
C&C Exclusions: See 850.0
AHA: 1Q 1992, 9

❺ **851.2 Cortex (cerebral) laceration without mention of open intracranial wound** ❷
C&C Exclusions: See 850.0

❺ **851.3 Cortex (cerebral) laceration with open intracranial wound** ❷
C&C Exclusions: See 850.0

❺ **851.4 Cerebellar or brain stem contusion without mention of open intracranial wound** ❷
C&C Exclusions: See 850.0

❺ **851.5 Cerebellar or brain stem contusion with open intracranial wound** ❷
C&C Exclusions: See 850.0

❺ **851.6 Cerebellar or brain stem laceration without mention of open intracranial wound** ❷
C&C Exclusions: See 850.0

❺ **851.7 Cerebellar or brain stem laceration with open intracranial wound** ❷
C&C Exclusions: See 850.0

❺ **851.8 Other and unspecified cerebral laceration and contusion, without mention of open intracranial wound** ❷
Brain (membrane) NOS
C&C Exclusions: See 850.0
AHA: 4Q 1996, 37

❺ **851.9 Other and unspecified cerebral laceration and contusion, with open intracranial wound** ❷
C&C Exclusions: See 850.0

❹ **852 Subarachnoid, subdural, and extradural hemorrhage, following injury**
Requires fifth digit. See beginning of section 850-854 for codes and definitions.
Excludes cerebral contusion or laceration (with hemorrhage) (851.0-851.9)

❺ **852.0 Subarachnoid hemorrhage following injury without mention of open intracranial wound** ❷
Middle meningeal hemorrhage following injury
C&C Exclusions: See 850.0

❺ **852.1 Subarachnoid hemorrhage following injury with open intracranial wound** ❷
C&C Exclusions: See 850.0

❺ **852.2 Subdural hemorrhage following injury without mention of open intracranial wound** ❷
C&C Exclusions: (for code 852.20) 800.00, 800.01, 800.02, 800.03, 800.04, 800.05, 800.06, 800.09, 800.10, 800.11, 800.12, 800.13, 800.14, 800.15, 800.16, 800.19, 800.20, 800.21, 800.22, 800.23, 800.24, 800.25, 800.26, 800.29, 800.30, 800.31, 800.32, 800.33, 800.34, 800.35, 800.36, 800.39, 800.40, 800.41, 800.42, 800.43, 800.44, 800.45, 800.46, 800.49, 800.50, 800.51, 800.52, 800.53, 800.54, 800.55, 800.56, 800.59, 800.60, 800.61, 800.62, 800.63, 800.64, 800.65, 800.66, 800.69, 800.70, 800.71, 800.72, 800.73, 800.74, 800.75, 800.76, 800.79, 800.80, 800.81, 800.82, 800.83, 800.84, 800.85, 800.86, 800.89, 800.90, 800.91, 800.92, 800.93, 800.94, 800.95, 800.96, 800.99, 801.00, 801.01, 801.02, 801.03, 801.04, 801.05, 801.06, 801.09, 801.10, 801.11, 801.12, 801.13, 801.14, 801.15, 801.16, 801.19, 801.20, 801.21, 801.22, 801.23, 801.24, 801.25, 801.26, 801.29, 801.30, 801.31, 801.32, 801.33, 801.34, 801.35, 801.36, 801.39, 801.40, 801.41, 801.42, 801.43, 801.44, 801.45, 801.46, 801.49, 801.50, 801.51, 801.52, 801.53, 801.54, 801.55, 801.56, 801.59, 801.60, 801.61, 801.62, 801.63, 801.64, 801.65, 801.66, 801.69, 801.70, 801.71, 801.72, 801.73, 801.74, 801.75, 801.76, 801.79, 801.80, 801.81, 801.82, 801.83, 801.84, 801.85, 801.86, 801.89, 801.90, 801.91, 801.92, 801.93, 801.94, 801.95, 801.96, 801.99, 803.00, 803.01, 803.02, 803.03, 803.04, 803.05, 803.06, 803.09, 803.10, 803.11, 803.12, 803.13, 803.14, 803.15, 803.16, 803.19, 803.20, 803.21, 803.22, 803.23, 803.24, 803.25, 803.26, 803.29, 803.30, 803.31, 803.32, 803.33, 803.34, 803.35, 803.36, 803.39, 803.40, 803.41, 803.42, 803.43, 803.44, 803.45, 803.46, 803.49, 803.50, 803.51, 803.52, 803.53, 803.54, 803.55, 803.56, 803.59, 803.60, 803.61, 803.62, 803.63, 803.64, 803.65, 803.66, 803.69, 803.70, 803.71, 803.72, 803.73, 803.74, 803.75, 803.76, 803.79, 803.80, 803.81, 803.82, 803.83, 803.84, 803.85, 803.86, 803.89, 803.90, 803.91, 803.92, 803.93, 803.94, 803.95, 803.96, 803.99, 804.00, 804.01, 804.02, 804.03, 804.04, 804.05, 804.06, 804.09, 804.10, 804.11, 804.12, 804.13, 804.14, 804.15, 804.16, 804.19, 804.20, 804.21, 804.22, 804.23, 804.24, 804.25, 804.26, 804.29, 804.30, 804.31, 804.32, 804.33, 804.34, 804.35, 804.36, 804.39, 804.40, 804.41, 804.42, 804.43, 804.44, 804.45, 804.46, 804.49, 804.50, 804.51, 804.52, 804.53, 804.54, 804.55, 804.56, 804.59, 804.60, 804.61, 804.62, 804.63, 804.64, 804.65, 804.66, 804.69, 804.70, 804.71, 804.72, 804.73, 804.74, 804.75, 804.76, 804.79, 804.80, 804.81, 804.82, 804.83, 804.84, 804.85, 804.86, 804.89, 804.90, 804.91, 804.92, 804.93, 804.94, 804.95, 804.96, 804.99, 850.0, 850.11, 850.12, 850.2, 850.3, 850.5, 850.9, 851.00, 851.01, 851.02, 851.03, 851.04, 851.05, 851.06, 851.09, 851.10, 851.11, 851.12, 851.13,

851.14, 851.15, 851.16, 851.19, 851.20, 851.21, 851.22, 851.23, 851.24, 851.25, 851.26, 851.29, 851.30, 851.31, 851.32, 851.33, 851.34, 851.35, 851.36, 851.39, 851.40, 851.41, 851.42, 851.43, 851.44, 851.45, 851.46, 851.49, 851.50, 851.51, 851.52, 851.53, 851.54, 851.55, 851.56, 851.59, 851.60, 851.61, 851.62, 851.63, 851.64, 851.65, 851.66, 851.69, 851.70, 851.71, 851.72, 851.73, 851.74, 851.75, 851.76, 851.79, 851.80, 851.81, 851.82, 851.83, 851.84, 851.85, 851.86, 851.89, 851.90, 851.91, 851.92, 851.93, 851.94, 851.95, 851.96, 851.99, 852.00, 852.01, 852.02, 852.03, 852.04, 852.05, 852.06, 852.09, 852.10, 852.11, 852.12, 852.13, 852.14, 852.15, 852.16, 852.19, 852.20, 852.21, 852.22, 852.23, 852.24, 852.25, 852.26, 852.29, 852.30, 852.31, 852.32, 852.33, 852.34, 852.35, 852.36, 852.39, 852.40, 852.41, 852.42, 852.43, 852.44, 852.45, 852.46, 852.49, 852.50, 852.51, 852.52, 852.53, 852.54, 852.55, 852.56, 852.59, 853.00, 853.01, 853.02, 853.03, 853.04, 853.05, 853.06, 853.09, 853.10, 853.11, 853.12, 853.13, 853.14, 853.15, 853.16, 853.19, 854.00, 854.01, 854.02, 854.03, 854.04, 854.05, 854.06, 854.09, 854.10, 854.11, 854.12, 854.13, 854.14, 854.15, 854.16, 854.19, 873.8, 873.9, 879.8, 879.9, 905.0, 925.1, 925.2, 929.0, 929.9, 958.8, 959.01, 959.09, 959.8, 959.9

C&C Exclusions: (for codes 852.21-852.29) 800.00, 800.01, 800.02, 800.03, 800.04, 800.05, 800.06, 800.09, 800.10, 800.11, 800.12, 800.13, 800.14, 800.15, 800.16, 800.19, 800.20, 800.21, 800.22, 800.23, 800.24, 800.25, 800.26, 800.29, 800.30, 800.31, 800.32, 800.33, 800.34, 800.35, 800.36, 800.39, 800.40, 800.41, 800.42, 800.43, 800.44, 800.45, 800.46, 800.49, 800.50, 800.51, 800.52, 800.53, 800.54, 800.55, 800.56, 800.59, 800.60, 800.61, 800.62, 800.63, 800.64, 800.65, 800.66, 800.69, 800.70, 800.71, 800.72, 800.73, 800.74, 800.75, 800.76, 800.79, 800.80, 800.81, 800.82, 800.83, 800.84, 800.85, 800.86, 800.89, 800.90, 800.91, 800.92, 800.93, 800.94, 800.95, 800.96, 800.99, 801.00, 801.01, 801.02, 801.03, 801.04, 801.05, 801.06, 801.09, 801.10, 801.11, 801.12, 801.13, 801.14, 801.15, 801.16, 801.19, 801.20, 801.21, 801.22, 801.23, 801.24, 801.25, 801.26, 801.29, 801.30, 801.31, 801.32, 801.33, 801.34, 801.35, 801.36, 801.39, 801.40, 801.41, 801.42, 801.43, 801.44, 801.45, 801.46, 801.49, 801.50, 801.51, 801.52, 801.53, 801.54, 801.55, 801.56, 801.59, 801.60, 801.61, 801.62, 801.63, 801.64, 801.65, 801.66, 801.69, 801.70, 801.71, 801.72, 801.73, 801.74, 801.75, 801.76, 801.79, 801.80, 801.81, 801.82, 801.83, 801.84, 801.85, 801.86, 801.89, 801.90, 801.91, 801.92, 801.93, 801.94, 801.95, 801.96, 801.99, 803.00, 803.01, 803.02, 803.03, 803.04, 803.05, 803.06, 803.09, 803.10, 803.11, 803.12, 803.13, 803.14, 803.15, 803.16, 803.19, 803.20, 803.21, 803.22, 803.23, 803.24, 803.25, 803.26, 803.29, 803.30, 803.31, 803.32, 803.33, 803.34, 803.35, 803.36, 803.39, 803.40, 803.41, 803.42, 803.43, 803.44, 803.45, 803.46, 803.49, 803.50, 803.51, 803.52, 803.53, 803.54, 803.55, 803.56, 803.59, 803.60, 803.61, 803.62, 803.63, 803.64, 803.65, 803.66, 803.69, 803.70, 803.71, 803.72, 803.73, 803.74, 803.75, 803.76, 803.79, 803.80, 803.81, 803.82, 803.83, 803.84, 803.85, 803.86, 803.89, 803.90, 803.91, 803.92, 803.93, 803.94, 803.95, 803.96, 803.99, 804.00, 804.01, 804.02, 804.03, 804.04, 804.05, 804.06, 804.09, 804.10, 804.11, 804.12, 804.13, 804.14, 804.15, 804.16, 804.19, 804.20, 804.21, 804.22, 804.23, 804.24, 804.25, 804.26, 804.29, 804.30, 804.31, 804.32, 804.33, 804.34, 804.35, 804.36, 804.39, 804.40, 804.41, 804.42, 804.43, 804.44, 804.45, 804.46, 804.49, 804.50, 804.51, 804.52, 804.53, 804.54, 804.55, 804.56, 804.59, 804.60, 804.61, 804.62, 804.63, 804.64, 804.65, 804.66, 804.69, 804.70, 804.71, 804.72, 804.73, 804.74, 804.75, 804.76, 804.79, 804.80, 804.81, 804.82, 804.83, 804.84, 804.85, 804.86, 804.89, 804.90, 804.91, 804.92, 804.93, 804.94, 804.95, 804.96, 804.99, 850.0, 850.11, 850.12, 850.2, 850.3, 850.5, 850.9, 851.00, 851.01, 851.02, 851.03, 851.04, 851.05, 851.06, 851.09, 851.10, 851.11, 851.12, 851.13, 851.14, 851.15, 851.16, 851.19, 851.21, 851.22, 851.23, 851.24, 851.25, 851.26, 851.29, 851.30, 851.31, 851.32, 851.33, 851.34, 851.35, 851.36, 851.39, 851.40, 851.41, 851.42, 851.43, 851.44, 851.45, 851.46, 851.49, 851.50, 851.51, 851.52, 851.53, 851.54, 851.55, 851.56, 851.59, 851.60, 851.61, 851.62, 851.63, 851.64, 851.65, 851.66, 851.69, 851.70, 851.71, 851.72, 851.73, 851.74, 851.75, 851.76, 851.79, 851.80, 851.81, 851.82, 851.83, 851.84, 851.85, 851.86, 851.89, 851.90, 851.91, 851.92, 851.93, 851.94, 851.95, 851.96, 851.99, 852.00, 852.01, 852.02, 852.03, 852.04, 852.05, 852.06, 852.09, 852.10, 852.11, 852.12, 852.13, 852.14, 852.15, 852.16, 852.19, 852.21, 852.22, 852.23, 852.24, 852.25, 852.26, 852.29, 852.30, 852.31, 852.32, 852.33, 852.34, 852.35, 852.36, 852.39, 852.40, 852.41, 852.42, 852.43, 852.44, 852.45, 852.46, 852.49, 852.50, 852.51, 852.52, 852.53, 852.54, 852.55, 852.56, 852.59, 853.00, 853.01, 853.02, 853.03, 853.04, 853.05, 853.06, 853.09, 853.10, 853.11, 853.12, 853.13, 853.14, 853.15, 853.16, 853.19, 854.00, 854.01, 854.02, 854.03, 854.04, 854.05, 854.06, 854.09, 854.10, 854.11, 854.12, 854.13, 854.14, 854.15, 854.16, 854.19, 873.8, 873.9, 879.8, 879.9, 905.0, 925.1, 925.2, 929.0, 929.9, 958.8, 959.01, 959.09, 959.8, 959.9

AHA: 4Q 1996, 43

5 **852.3 Subdural hemorrhage following injury with open intracranial wound** 2

C&C Exclusions: See 852.21-852.29

5 **852.4 Extradural hemorrhage following injury without mention of open intracranial wound** 2

Epidural hematoma following injury

C&C Exclusions: See 852.21-852.29

5 **852.5 Extradural hemorrhage following injury with open intracranial wound** 2

C&C Exclusions: See 852.21-852.29

4 **853 Other and unspecified intracranial hemorrhage following injury**

Requires fifth digit. See beginning of section 850-854 for codes and definitions.

5 **853.0 Without mention of open intracranial wound** 2

Cerebral compression due to injury
Intracranial hematoma following injury
Traumatic cerebral hemorrhage

C&C Exclusions: See 852.21-852.29

AHA: 3Q 1990, 14

5 **853.1 With open intracranial wound** 2

C&C Exclusions: See 852.21-852.29

4 **854 Intracranial injury of other and unspecified nature**

Requires fifth digit. See beginning of section 850-854 for codes and definitions.

Includes injury:
- brain NOS
- cavernous sinus
- intracranial

Excludes *any condition classifiable to 850-853*
head injury NOS (959.01)

AHA: 1Q 1999, 10; 2Q 1992, 6

5 **854.0 Without mention of open intracranial wound** 2

C&C Exclusions: See 852.21-852.29

AHA: For Code 854.00: 2Q 2005, 6

5 **854.1 With open intracranial wound** 2

C&C Exclusions: See 852.21-852.29

INTERNAL INJURY OF THORAX, ABDOMEN, AND PELVIS (860-869)

Includes
- blast injuries of internal organs
- blunt trauma of internal organs
- bruise of internal organs
- concussion injuries (except cerebral) of internal organs
- crushing of internal organs
- hematoma of internal organs
- laceration of internal organs
- puncture of internal organs
- tear of internal organs
- traumatic rupture of internal organs

Excludes
- *concussion NOS (850.0-850.9)*
- *flail chest (807.4)*
- *foreign body entering through orifice (930.0-939.9)*
- *injury to blood vessels (901.0-902.9)*

Note: *The description "with open wound," used in the fourth-digit subdivisions, includes those with mention of infection or foreign body.*

4 **860 Traumatic pneumothorax and hemothorax**

AHA: 2Q 1993, 4

860.0 Pneumothorax without mention of open wound into thorax 2

C&C Exclusions: 860.0, 860.1, 860.2, 860.3, 860.4, 860.5, 861.20, 861.21, 861.22, 861.30, 861.31, 861.32, 862.29, 862.39, 862.8, 862.9, 875.0, 875.1, 879.8, 879.9, 929.0, 929.9, 958.7, 958.8, 959.8, 959.9

860.1 Pneumothorax with open wound into thorax 2

C&C Exclusions: See 860.0

4 5 Additional Digit Required ✖ Nonspecific PDx ⊘ Unacceptable PDx ✚ Manifestation Code ►◄ Revised Text ● New Code ▲ Revised Code

860.2 Hemothorax without mention of open wound into thorax ❷
C&C Exclusions: See 860.0

860.3 Hemothorax with open wound into thorax ❷
C&C Exclusions: See 860.0

860.4 Pneumohemothorax without mention of open wound into thorax ❷
C&C Exclusions: See 860.0

860.5 Pneumohemothorax with open wound into thorax ❷
C&C Exclusions: See 860.0

❹ **861 Injury to heart and lung**
Excludes *injury to blood vessels of thorax (901.0-901.9)*

❺ **861.0 Heart, without mention of open wound into thorax**
AHA: 1Q 1992, 9

861.00 Unspecified injury ❷
C&C Exclusions: 861.00, 861.01, 861.02, 861.03, 861.10, 861.11, 861.12, 861.13, 862.29, 862.39, 862.8, 862.9, 875.0, 875.1, 879.8, 879.9, 929.0, 929.9, 958.7, 958.8, 959.8, 959.9

861.01 Contusion ❷
Cardiac contusion
Myocardial contusion
C&C Exclusions: See 861.00

861.02 Laceration without penetration of heart chambers ❷
C&C Exclusions: See 861.00

861.03 Laceration with penetration of heart chambers ❷
C&C Exclusions: See 861.00

❺ **861.1 Heart, with open wound into thorax**

861.10 Unspecified injury ❷
C&C Exclusions: See 861.00

861.11 Contusion ❷
C&C Exclusions: See 861.00

861.12 Laceration without penetration of heart chambers ❷
C&C Exclusions: See 861.00

861.13 Laceration with penetration of heart chambers ❷
C&C Exclusions: See 861.00

❺ **861.2 Lung, without mention of open wound into thorax**

861.20 Unspecified injury ❷
C&C Exclusions: 861.20, 861.21, 861.22, 861.30, 861.31, 861.32, 862.29, 862.39, 862.8, 862.9, 875.0, 875.1, 879.8, 879.9, 929.0, 929.9, 958.7, 958.8, 959.8, 959.9

861.21 Contusion ❷
C&C Exclusions: See 861.20

861.22 Laceration ❷
C&C Exclusions: See 861.20

❺ **861.3 Lung, with open wound into thorax**

861.30 Unspecified injury ❷
C&C Exclusions: See 861.20

861.31 Contusion ❷
C&C Exclusions: See 861.20

861.32 Laceration ❷
C&C Exclusions: See 861.20

❹ **862 Injury to other and unspecified intrathoracic organs**
Excludes *injury to blood vessels of thorax (901.0-901.9)*

862.0 Diaphragm, without mention of open wound into cavity

862.1 Diaphragm, with open wound into cavity
C&C Exclusions: 862.0, 862.1, 862.29, 862.39, 862.8, 862.9, 875.0, 875.1, 879.8, 879.9, 929.0, 929.9, 958.7, 958.8, 959.8, 959.9

❺ **862.2 Other specified intrathoracic organs, without mention of open wound into cavity**

862.21 Bronchus
C&C Exclusions: 862.21, 862.29, 862.31, 862.39, 862.8, 862.9, 875.0, 875.1, 879.8, 879.9, 929.0, 929.9, 958.7, 958.8, 959.8, 959.9

862.22 Esophagus
C&C Exclusions: 862.22, 862.29, 862.32, 862.39, 862.8, 862.9, 875.0, 875.1, 879.8, 879.9, 929.0, 929.9, 958.7, 958.8, 959.8, 959.9

862.29 Other
Pleura
Thymus gland
C&C Exclusions: 862.29, 862.39, 862.8, 862.9, 875.0, 875.1, 879.8, 879.9, 929.0, 929.9, 958.7, 958.8, 959.8, 959.9

❺ **862.3 Other specified intrathoracic organs, with open wound into cavity**

862.31 Bronchus

862.32 Esophagus

862.39 Other

862.8 Multiple and unspecified intrathoracic organs, without mention of open wound into cavity ❷
Crushed chest
Multiple intrathoracic organs

862.9 Multiple and unspecified intrathoracic organs, with open wound into cavity

❹ **863 Injury to gastrointestinal tract**
Excludes *anal sphincter laceration during delivery (664.2)*
bile duct (868.0-868.1 with fifth-digit 2)
gallbladder (868.0-868.1 with fifth-digit 2)

863.0 Stomach, without mention of open wound into cavity ❷

863.1 Stomach, with open wound into cavity ❷
C&C Exclusions: 863.0, 863.1, 863.80, 863.89, 863.90, 863.99, 868.00, 868.03, 868.04, 868.09, 868.10, 868.13, 868.14, 868.19, 869.0, 869.1, 879.2, 879.3, 879.4, 879.5, 879.6, 879.7, 879.8, 879.9, 929.0, 929.9, 958.8, 959.8, 959.9

❺ **863.2 Small intestine, without mention of open wound into cavity**

863.20 Small intestine, unspecified site ❷

863.21 Duodenum ❷

863.29 Other ❷

❺ **863.3 Small intestine, with open wound into cavity**

863.30 Small intestine, unspecified site ❷
C&C Exclusions: 863.20, 863.21, 863.29, 863.30, 863.31, 863.39, 863.80, 863.89, 863.90, 863.99, 868.00, 868.03, 868.04, 868.09, 868.10, 868.13, 868.14, 868.19, 869.0, 869.1, 879.2, 879.3, 879.4, 879.5, 879.6, 879.7, 879.8, 879.9, 929.0, 929.9, 958.8, 959.8, 959.9

863.31 Duodenum ❷
C&C Exclusions: 863.21, 863.31, 863.39, 863.80, 863.89, 863.90, 863.99, 868.00, 868.03, 868.04, 868.09, 868.10, 868.13, 868.14, 868.19, 869.0, 869.1, 879.2, 879.3, 879.4, 879.5, 879.6, 879.7, 879.8, 879.9, 929.0, 929.9, 958.8, 959.8, 959.9

863.39 Other ❷
C&C Exclusions: See 863.30

❺ **863.4 Colon or rectum, without mention of open wound into cavity**

863.40 Colon, unspecified site ❷

863.41 Ascending [right] colon ❷

863.42 Transverse colon ❷

863.43 Descending [left] colon ❷

863.44 Sigmoid colon ❷

863.45 Rectum ❷

863.46 Multiple sites in colon and rectum ❷

863.49 Other ❷

❺ **863.5 Colon or rectum, with open wound into cavity**

863.50 Colon, unspecified site ❷
C&C Exclusions: 863.40, 863.41, 863.42, 863.43, 863.44, 863.45, 863.46, 863.49, 863.50, 863.51, 863.52, 863.53, 863.54, 863.55, 863.56, 863.59, 863.80, 863.89, 863.90, 863.99, 868.00, 868.03, 868.04, 868.09, 868.10, 868.13, 868.14, 868.19, 869.0, 869.1, 879.2, 879.3, 879.4, 879.5, 879.6, 879.7, 879.8, 879.9, 929.0, 929.9, 958.8, 959.8, 959.9

863.51 **Ascending [right] colon**
C&C Exclusions: See 863.50

863.52 **Transverse colon**
C&C Exclusions: See 863.50

863.53 **Descending [left] colon**
C&C Exclusions: See 863.50

863.54 **Sigmoid colon**
C&C Exclusions: See 863.50

863.55 **Rectum**
C&C Exclusions: See 863.50

863.56 **Multiple sites in colon and rectum**
C&C Exclusions: See 863.50

863.59 **Other**
C&C Exclusions: See 863.50

863.8 **Other and unspecified gastrointestinal sites, without mention of open wound into cavity**

863.80 **Gastrointestinal tract, unspecified site**

863.81 **Pancreas, head**

863.82 **Pancreas, body**

863.83 **Pancreas, tail**

863.84 **Pancreas, multiple and unspecified sites**

863.85 **Appendix**

863.89 **Other**
Intestine NOS

863.9 **Other and unspecified gastrointestinal sites, with open wound into cavity**

863.90 **Gastrointestinal tract, unspecified site**
C&C Exclusions: 863.80, 863.81, 863.82, 863.83, 863.84, 863.89, 863.90, 863.91, 863.92, 863.93, 863.94, 863.99, 868.00, 868.03, 868.04, 868.09, 868.10, 868.13, 868.14, 868.19, 869.0, 869.1, 879.2, 879.3, 879.4, 879.5, 879.6, 879.7, 879.8, 879.9, 929.0, 929.9, 958.8, 959.8, 959.9

863.91 **Pancreas, head**
C&C Exclusions: 863.80, 863.81, 863.82, 863.83, 863.84, 863.91, 863.92, 863.93, 863.94, 863.99, 868.00, 868.03, 868.04, 868.09, 868.10, 868.13, 868.14, 868.19, 869.0, 869.1, 879.2, 879.3, 879.4, 879.5, 879.6, 879.7, 879.8, 879.9, 929.0, 929.9, 958.8, 959.8, 959.9

863.92 **Pancreas, body**
C&C Exclusions: See 863.91

863.93 **Pancreas, tail**
C&C Exclusions: See 863.91

863.94 **Pancreas, multiple and unspecified sites**
C&C Exclusions: See 863.91

863.95 **Appendix**
C&C Exclusions: 863.80, 863.85, 863.95, 863.99, 868.00, 868.03, 868.04, 868.09, 868.10, 868.13, 868.14, 868.19, 869.0, 869.1, 879.2, 879.3, 879.4, 879.5, 879.6, 879.7, 879.8, 879.9, 929.0, 929.9, 958.8, 959.8, 959.9

863.99 **Other**
C&C Exclusions: 863.80, 863.99, 868.00, 868.03, 868.04, 868.09, 868.10, 868.13, 868.14, 868.19, 869.0, 869.1, 879.2, 879.3, 879.4, 879.5, 879.6, 879.7, 879.8, 879.9, 929.0, 929.9, 958.8, 959.8, 959.9

864 **Injury to liver**

The following fifth-digit subclassification is for use with category 864:
- 0 **unspecified injury**
- 1 **hematoma and contusion**
- 2 **laceration, minor**
  Laceration involving capsule only, or without significant involvement of hepatic parenchyma [i.e., less than 1 cm deep]
- 3 **laceration, moderate**
  Laceration involving parenchyma but without major disruption of parenchyma [i.e., less than 10 cm long and less than 3 cm deep]
- 4 **laceration, major**
  Laceration with significant disruption of hepatic parenchyma [i.e., 10 cm long and 3 cm deep]
  Multiple moderate lacerations, with or without hematoma
  Stellate lacerations of liver
- 5 **laceration, unspecified**
- 9 **other**

864.0 **Without mention of open wound into cavity**
C&C Exclusions: 863.80, 863.99, 864.00, 864.01, 864.02, 864.03, 864.04, 864.05, 864.09, 864.10, 864.11, 864.12, 864.13, 864.14, 864.15, 864.19, 868.00, 868.03, 868.04, 868.09, 868.10, 868.13, 868.14, 868.19, 869.0, 869.1, 879.2, 879.3, 879.4, 879.5, 879.6, 879.7, 879.8, 879.9, 929.0, 929.9, 958.8, 959.8, 959.9

864.1 **With open wound into cavity**
C&C Exclusions: See 864.0

865 **Injury to spleen**

The following fifth-digit subclassification is for use with category 865:
- 0 **unspecified injury**
- 1 **hematoma without rupture of capsule**
- 2 **capsular tears, without major disruption of parenchyma**
- 3 **laceration extending into parenchyma**
- 4 **massive parenchymal disruption**
- 9 **other**

865.0 **Without mention of open wound into cavity**
C&C Exclusions: 865.00, 865.01, 865.02, 865.03, 865.04, 865.09, 865.10, 865.11, 865.12, 865.13, 865.14, 865.19, 868.00, 868.03, 868.04, 868.09, 868.10, 868.13, 868.14, 868.19, 869.0, 869.1, 879.2, 879.3, 879.4, 879.5, 879.6, 879.7, 879.8, 879.9, 929.0, 929.9, 958.8, 959.8, 959.9

865.1 **With open wound into cavity**
C&C Exclusions: See 865.0

866 **Injury to kidney**

The following fifth-digit subclassification is for use with category 866:
- 0 **unspecified injury**
- 1 **hematoma without rupture of capsule**
- 2 **laceration**
- 3 **complete disruption of kidney parenchyma**

866.0 **Without mention of open wound into cavity**
C&C Exclusions: 866.00, 866.01, 866.02, 866.03, 866.10, 866.11, 866.12, 866.13, 868.00, 868.03, 868.04, 868.09, 868.10, 868.13, 868.14, 868.19, 869.0, 869.1, 879.2, 879.3, 879.4, 879.5, 879.6, 879.7, 879.8, 879.9, 929.0, 929.9, 958.8, 959.8, 959.9

866.1 **With open wound into cavity**
C&C Exclusions: See 866.0

867 **Injury to pelvic organs**
Excludes *injury during delivery (664.0-665.9)*

867.0 **Bladder and urethra, without mention of open wound into cavity**
C&C Exclusions: 867.0, 867.1, 867.6, 867.7, 867.8, 867.9, 866.03, 868.00, 868.03, 868.04, 868.09, 868.10, 868.13, 868.14, 868.19, 869.0, 869.1, 879.2, 879.3, 879.4, 879.5, 879.6, 879.7, 879.8, 879.9, 929.0, 929.9, 958.8, 959.8, 959.9
AHA: Nov-Dec 1985, 15

867.1 **Bladder and urethra, with open wound into cavity**
C&C Exclusions: See 867.0

867.2 Ureter, without mention of open wound into cavity ❷
C&C Exclusions: 867.2, 867.3, 867.6, 867.7, 867.8, 867.9, 866.03, 868.00, 868.03, 868.04, 868.09, 868.10, 868.13, 868.14, 868.19, 869.0, 869.1, 879.2, 879.3, 879.4, 879.5, 879.6, 879.7, 879.8, 879.9, 929.0, 929.9, 958.8, 959.8, 959.9

867.3 Ureter, with open wound into cavity ❷
C&C Exclusions: See 867.2

867.4 Uterus, without mention of open wound into cavity ♀ ❷
C&C Exclusions: 867.4, 867.5, 867.6, 867.7, 867.8, 867.9, 866.03, 868.00, 868.03, 868.04, 868.09, 868.10, 868.13, 868.14, 868.19, 869.0, 869.1, 879.2, 879.3, 879.4, 879.5, 879.6, 879.7, 879.8, 879.9, 929.0, 929.9, 958.8, 959.8, 959.9

867.5 Uterus, with open wound into cavity ♀ ❷
C&C Exclusions: See 867.4

867.6 Other specified pelvic organs, without mention of open wound into cavity ❷
Fallopian tube
Ovary
Prostate
Seminal vesicle
Vas deferens
C&C Exclusions: 867.6, 867.7, 867.8, 867.9, 866.03, 868.00, 868.03, 868.04, 868.09, 868.10, 868.13, 868.14, 868.19, 869.0, 869.1, 879.2, 879.3, 879.4, 879.5, 879.6, 879.7, 879.8, 879.9, 929.0, 929.9, 958.8, 959.8, 959.9

867.7 Other specified pelvic organs, with open wound into cavity ❷
C&C Exclusions: See 867.6

✖ **867.8 Unspecified pelvic organ, without mention of open wound into cavity** ❷
C&C Exclusions: See 867.6

✖ **867.9 Unspecified pelvic organ, with open wound into cavity** ❷
C&C Exclusions: See 867.6

❹ **868 Injury to other intra-abdominal organs**

The following fifth-digit subclassification is for use with category 868:
- **0** **unspecified intra-abdominal organ**
- **1** **adrenal gland**
- **2** **bile duct and gallbladder**
- **3** **peritoneum**
- **4** **retroperitoneum**
- **9** **other and multiple intra-abdominal organs**

❺ **868.0 Without mention of open wound into cavity** ❷
(✖ is only valid for fifth-digit "0")
C&C Exclusions: (for codes 868.00, 868.03-868.09) 868.00, 868.03, 868.04, 868.09, 868.10, 868.13, 868.14, 868.19, 869.0, 869.1, 879.2, 879.3, 879.4, 879.5, 879.6, 879.7, 879.8, 879.9, 929.0, 929.9, 958.8, 959.8, 959.9
C&C Exclusions: (for code 868.01) 868.00, 868.01, 868.03, 868.04, 868.09, 868.10, 868.11, 868.13, 868.14, 868.19, 869.0, 869.1, 879.2, 879.3, 879.4, 879.5, 879.6, 879.7, 879.8, 879.9, 929.0, 929.9, 958.8, 959.8, 959.9
C&C Exclusions: (for code 868.02) 868.00, 868.02, 868.03, 868.04, 868.09, 868.10, 868.13, 868.14, 868.19, 869.0, 869.1, 879.2, 879.3, 879.4, 879.5, 879.6, 879.7, 879.8, 879.9, 929.0, 929.9, 958.8, 959.8, 959.9

❺ **868.1 With open wound into cavity** ❷
(✖ is only valid for fifth-digit "0")
C&C Exclusions: (for codes 868.10, 868.13-868.19) See 868.00
C&C Exclusions: (for code 868.11) See 868.01
C&C Exclusions: (for code 868.12) 868.00, 868.03, 868.04, 868.09, 868.10, 868.12, 868.13, 868.14, 868.19, 869.0, 869.1, 879.2, 879.3, 879.4, 879.5, 879.6, 879.7, 879.8, 879.9, 929.0, 929.9, 958.8, 959.8, 959.9

❹ **869 Internal injury to unspecified or ill-defined organs**
Includes internal injury NOS
multiple internal injury NOS

869.0 Without mention of open wound into cavity ❷
C&C Exclusions: See 868.0

869.1 With open wound into cavity ❷
C&C Exclusions: See 868.0
AHA: 2Q 1989, 15

OPEN WOUNDS (870-897)

Includes animal bite
avulsion
cut
laceration
puncture wound
traumatic amputation

Excludes *burn (940.0-949.5)*
crushing (925-929.9)
puncture of internal organs (860.0-869.1)
superficial injury (910.0-919.9)
that incidental to:
dislocation (830.0-839.9)
fracture (800.0-829.1)
internal injury (860.0-869.1)
intracranial injury (851.0-854.1)

Note: The description "complicated" used in the fourth-digit subdivisions includes those with mention of delayed healing, delayed treatment, foreign body, or infection.

Use additional code to identify infection
AHA: 4Q 2001, 52

OPEN WOUND OF HEAD, NECK, AND TRUNK (870-879)

❹ **870 Open wound of ocular adnexa**

870.0 Laceration of skin of eyelid and periocular area

870.1 Laceration of eyelid, full-thickness, not involving lacrimal passages

870.2 Laceration of eyelid involving lacrimal passages

870.3 Penetrating wound of orbit, without mention of foreign body
C&C Exclusions: 870.0, 870.1, 870.2, 870.3, 870.4, 870.9, 871.0, 871.1, 871.2, 871.3, 871.4, 871.5, 871.6, 871.7, 871.9, 879.8, 879.9, 929.0, 958.8, 959.8, 959.9

870.4 Penetrating wound of orbit with foreign body
Excludes *retained (old) foreign body in orbit (376.6)*
C&C Exclusions: See 870.3

870.8 Other specified open wounds of ocular adnexa
C&C Exclusions: See 870.3

870.9 Unspecified open wound of ocular adnexa
C&C Exclusions: See 870.3

❹ **871 Open wound of eyeball**
Excludes *2nd cranial nerve [optic] injury (950.0-950.9)*
3rd cranial nerve [oculomotor] injury (951.0)

871.0 Ocular laceration without prolapse of intraocular tissue
C&C Exclusions: See 870.3
AHA: 3Q 1996, 7

871.1 Ocular laceration with prolapse or exposure of intraocular tissue
C&C Exclusions: See 870.3

871.2 Rupture of eye with partial loss of intraocular tissue
C&C Exclusions: See 870.3

871.3 Avulsion of eye
Traumatic enucleation
C&C Exclusions: See 870.3

871.4 Unspecified laceration of eye
C&C Exclusions: See 870.3

871.5 Penetration of eyeball with magnetic foreign body
Excludes *retained (old) magnetic foreign body in globe (360.50-360.59)*

871.6 Penetration of eyeball with (nonmagnetic) foreign body
Excludes *retained (old) (nonmagnetic) foreign body in globe (360.60-360.69)*

871.7 Unspecified ocular penetration

871.9 Unspecified open wound of eyeball
C&C Exclusions: See 870.3

❹ **872 Open wound of ear**

❺ **872.0 External ear, without mention of complication**

872.00 External ear, unspecified site

872.01 Auricle, ear
Pinna

872.02 Auditory canal

872.1 External ear, complicated

872.10 External ear, unspecified site

872.11 Auricle, ear

872.12 Auditory canal

872.6 Other specified parts of ear, without mention of complication

872.61 Ear drum
Drumhead
Tympanic membrane

872.62 Ossicles

872.63 Eustachian tube

872.64 Cochlea

872.69 Other and multiple sites

872.7 Other specified parts of ear, complicated

872.71 Ear drum

872.72 Ossicles
C&C Exclusions: 872.00, 872.01, 872.02, 872.10, 872.11, 872.12, 872.61, 872.62, 872.63, 872.64, 872.69, 872.71, 872.72, 872.73, 872.74, 872.79, 872.8, 872.9, 879.8, 879.9, 929.0, 958.8, 959.8, 959.9

872.73 Eustachian tube
C&C Exclusions: See 872.72

872.74 Cochlea
C&C Exclusions: See 872.72

872.79 Other and multiple sites

872.8 Ear, part unspecified, without mention of complication
Ear NOS

872.9 Ear, part unspecified, complicated

873 Other open wound of head

873.0 Scalp, without mention of complication

873.1 Scalp, complicated

873.2 Nose, without mention of complication

873.20 Nose, unspecified site

873.21 Nasal septum

873.22 Nasal cavity

873.23 Nasal sinus

873.29 Multiple sites

873.3 Nose, complicated

873.30 Nose, unspecified site

873.31 Nasal septum

873.32 Nasal cavity

873.33 Nasal sinus
C&C Exclusions: 873.20, 873.21, 873.22, 873.23, 873.29, 873.30, 873.31, 873.32, 873.33, 873.39, 879.8, 879.9, 929.0, 958.8, 959.8, 959.9

873.39 Multiple sites

873.4 Face, without mention of complication

873.40 Face, unspecified site

873.41 Cheek

873.42 Forehead
Eyebrow
AHA: 4Q 1996, 43

873.43 Lip

873.44 Jaw

873.49 Other and multiple sites

873.5 Face, complicated

873.50 Face, unspecified site

873.51 Cheek

873.52 Forehead

873.53 Lip

873.54 Jaw

873.59 Other and multiple sites

873.6 Internal structures of mouth, without mention of complication

873.60 Mouth, unspecified site

873.61 Buccal mucosa

873.62 Gum (alveolar process)

873.63 Tooth (broken) (fractured) (due to trauma)
Excludes *cracked tooth (521.81)*
AHA: 1Q 2004, 17

873.64 Tongue and floor of mouth

873.65 Palate

873.69 Other and multiple sites

873.7 Internal structures of mouth, complicated

873.70 Mouth, unspecified site

873.71 Buccal mucosa

873.72 Gum (alveolar process)

873.73 Tooth (broken) (fractured) (due to trauma)
Excludes *cracked tooth (521.81)*
AHA: 1Q 2004, 17

873.74 Tongue and floor of mouth

873.75 Palate

873.79 Other and multiple sites

873.8 Other and unspecified open wound of head without mention of complication
Head NOS
C&C Exclusions: 850.11, 850.12

873.9 Other and unspecified open wound of head, complicated
C&C Exclusions: 847.0, 850.11, 850.12, 873.40, 873.41, 873.42, 873.43, 873.44, 873.49, 873.50, 873.51, 873.52, 873.53, 873.54, 873.59, 873.60, 873.61, 873.62, 3, 873.64, 873.65, 873.69, 873.70, 873.71, 873.72, 3, 873.74, 873.75, 873.79, 873.9, 874.8, 874.9, 879.8, 879.9, 929.0, 929.9, 958.8, 959.8, 959.9

874 Open wound of neck

874.0 Larynx and trachea, without mention of complication

874.00 Larynx with trachea
C&C Exclusions: 847.0, 874.00, 874.01, 874.02, 874.10, 874.11, 874.12, 874.8, 874.9, 879.8, 879.9, 929.0, 929.9, 958.8, 959.8, 959.9

874.01 Larynx
C&C Exclusions: See 874.00

874.02 Trachea
C&C Exclusions: See 874.00

874.1 Larynx and trachea, complicated

874.10 Larynx with trachea
C&C Exclusions: See 874.00

874.11 Larynx
C&C Exclusions: See 874.00

874.12 Trachea
C&C Exclusions: See 874.00

874.2 Thyroid gland, without mention of complication

874.3 Thyroid gland, complicated
C&C Exclusions: 847.0, 874.2, 874.3, 874.8, 874.9, 879.8, 879.9, 929.0, 929.9, 958.8, 959.8, 959.9

874.4 Pharynx, without mention of complication
Cervical esophagus

874.5 Pharynx, complicated

874.8 Other and unspecified parts, without mention of complication
Nape of neck
Supraclavicular region
Throat NOS

874.9 Other and unspecified parts, complicated

4 875 Open wound of chest (wall)
Excludes *open wound into thoracic cavity (860.0-862.9)*
traumatic pneumothorax and hemothorax (860.1, 860.3, 860.5)
AHA: 3Q 1993, 17

875.0 Without mention of complication
C&C Exclusions: 847.1, 862.29, 862.39, 862.8, 862.9, 875.0, 875.1, 879.8, 879.9, 929.0, 929.9, 958.8, 959.8, 959.9

875.1 Complicated
C&C Exclusions: See 875.0

4 876 Open wound of back
Includes loin
lumbar region
Excludes *open wound into thoracic cavity (860.0-862.9)*
traumatic pneumothorax and hemothorax (860.1, 860.3, 860.5)

876.0 Without mention of complication

876.1 Complicated

4 877 Open wound of buttock
Includes sacroiliac region

877.0 Without mention of complication

877.1 Complicated

4 878 Open wound of genital organs (external), including traumatic amputation
Excludes *injury during delivery (664.0-665.9)*
internal genital organs (867.0-867.9)

878.0 Penis, without mention of complication ♂

878.1 Penis, complicated ♂

878.2 Scrotum and testes, without mention of complication ♂

878.3 Scrotum and testes, complicated ♂

878.4 Vulva, without mention of complication ♀
Labium (majus) (minus)

878.5 Vulva, complicated ♀

878.6 Vagina, without mention of complication ♀

878.7 Vagina, complicated ♀

878.8 Other and unspecified parts, without mention of complication

878.9 Other and unspecified parts, complicated

4 879 Open wound of other and unspecified sites, except limbs

879.0 Breast, without mention of complication

879.1 Breast, complicated

879.2 Abdominal wall, anterior, without mention of complication
Abdominal wall NOS
Epigastric region
Hypogastric region
Pubic region
Umbilical region
AHA: 2Q 1991, 22

879.3 Abdominal wall, anterior, complicated

879.4 Abdominal wall, lateral, without mention of complication
Flank
Groin
Hypochondrium
Iliac (region)
Inguinal region

879.5 Abdominal wall, lateral, complicated

879.6 Other and unspecified parts of trunk, without mention of complication
Pelvic region
Perineum
Trunk NOS

879.7 Other and unspecified parts of trunk, complicated

879.8 Open wound(s) (multiple) of unspecified site(s) without mention of complication
Multiple open wounds NOS
Open wound NOS
C&C Exclusions: 850.11, 850.12

879.9 Open wound(s) (multiple) of unspecified site(s), complicated
C&C Exclusions: See 879.8

OPEN WOUND OF UPPER LIMB (880-887)

AHA: Nov-Dec 1985, 5

4 880 Open wound of shoulder and upper arm

The following fifth-digit subclassification is for use with category 880:
0 **shoulder region**
1 **scapular region**
2 **axillary region**
3 **upper arm**
9 **multiple sites**

5 880.0 Without mention of complication

5 880.1 Complicated
AHA: For code 880.13: 2Q 2006, 7

5 880.2 With tendon involvement

4 881 Open wound of elbow, forearm, and wrist

The following fifth-digit subclassification is for use with category 881:
0 **forearm**
1 **elbow**
2 **wrist**

5 881.0 Without mention of complication

5 881.1 Complicated

5 881.2 With tendon involvement

4 882 Open wound of hand except finger(s) alone

882.0 Without mention of complication

882.1 Complicated

882.2 With tendon involvement

4 883 Open wound of finger(s)
Includes fingernail
thumb (nail)

883.0 Without mention of complication

883.1 Complicated

883.2 With tendon involvement

4 884 Multiple and unspecified open wound of upper limb
Includes arm NOS
multiple sites of one upper limb
upper limb NOS

884.0 Without mention of complication

884.1 Complicated

884.2 With tendon involvement

4 885 Traumatic amputation of thumb (complete) (partial)
Includes thumb(s) (with finger(s) of either hand)

885.0 Without mention of complication
AHA: 1Q 2003, 7

885.1 Complicated

4 886 Traumatic amputation of other finger(s) (complete) (partial)
Includes finger(s) of one or both hands, without mention of thumb(s)

886.0 Without mention of complication

886.1 Complicated

4 887 Traumatic amputation of arm and hand (complete) (partial)

887.0 Unilateral, below elbow, without mention of complication 2
C&C Exclusions: 880.00, 880.01, 880.02, 880.03, 880.09, 881.00, 881.01, 881.02, 881.03, 881.09, 881.20, 881.21, 881.22, 881.23, 881.29, 881.00, 881.01, 881.02, 881.10, 881.11, 881.12, 881.20, 881.21, 881.22, 882.0, 882.1, 882.2, 883.0, 883.1, 883.2, 884.0, 884.1, 884.2, 885.0, 885.1, 886.0, 886.1, 887.0, 887.1, 887.2, 887.3, 887.4, 887.5, 887.6, 887.7, 929.0, 929.9, 958.8, 959.8, 959.9

887.1 Unilateral, below elbow, complicated 2
C&C Exclusions: See 887.0

887.2 Unilateral, at or above elbow, without mention of complication ❷
C&C Exclusions: See 887.0

887.3 Unilateral, at or above elbow, complicated ❷
C&C Exclusions: See 887.0

887.4 Unilateral, level not specified, without mention of complication ❷
C&C Exclusions: See 887.0

887.5 Unilateral, level not specified, complicated ❷
C&C Exclusions: See 887.0

887.6 Bilateral [any level], without mention of complication ❷
One hand and other arm
C&C Exclusions: See 887.0

887.7 Bilateral [any level], complicated ❷
C&C Exclusions: See 887.0

OPEN WOUND OF LOWER LIMB (890-897)

AHA: Nov-Dec 1985, 5

❹ **890 Open wound of hip and thigh**

890.0 Without mention of complication

890.1 Complicated

890.2 With tendon involvement

❹ **891 Open wound of knee, leg [except thigh], and ankle**
Includes leg NOS
multiple sites of leg, except thigh
Excludes that of thigh (890.0-890.2)
with multiple sites of lower limb (894.0-894.2)

891.0 Without mention of complication

891.1 Complicated

891.2 With tendon involvement

❹ **892 Open wound of foot except toe(s) alone**
Includes heel

892.0 Without mention of complication

892.1 Complicated

892.2 With tendon involvement

❹ **893 Open wound of toe(s)**
Includes toenail

893.0 Without mention of complication

893.1 Complicated

893.2 With tendon involvement

❹ **894 Multiple and unspecified open wound of lower limb**
Includes lower limb NOS
multiple sites of one lower limb, with thigh

894.0 Without mention of complication

894.1 Complicated

894.2 With tendon involvement

❹ **895 Traumatic amputation of toe(s) (complete) (partial)**
Includes toe(s) of one or both feet

895.0 Without mention of complication

895.1 Complicated

❹ **896 Traumatic amputation of foot (complete) (partial)**

896.0 Unilateral, without mention of complication ❷
C&C Exclusions: 890.0, 890.1, 890.2, 891.0, 891.1, 891.2, 892.0, 892.1, 892.2, 893.0, 893.1, 893.2, 894.0, 894.1, 894.2, 895.0, 895.1, 896.0, 896.1, 896.2, 896.3, 897.0, 897.1, 897.2, 897.3, 897.4, 897.5, 897.6, 897.7, 929.0, 929.9, 958.8, 959.8, 959.9

896.1 Unilateral, complicated ❷
C&C Exclusions: See 896.0

896.2 Bilateral, without mention of complication ❷
Excludes one foot and other leg (897.6-897.7)
C&C Exclusions: See 896.0

896.3 Bilateral, complicated ❷
C&C Exclusions: See 896.0

❹ **897 Traumatic amputation of leg(s) (complete) (partial)**

897.0 Unilateral, below knee, without mention of complication ❷
C&C Exclusions: See 896.0

897.1 Unilateral, below knee, complicated ❷
C&C Exclusions: See 896.0

897.2 Unilateral, at or above knee, without mention of complication ❷
C&C Exclusions: See 896.0

897.3 Unilateral, at or above knee, complicated ❷
C&C Exclusions: See 896.0

897.4 Unilateral, level not specified, without mention of complication ❷
C&C Exclusions: See 896.0

897.5 Unilateral, level not specified, complicated ❷
C&C Exclusions: See 896.0

897.6 Bilateral [any level], without mention of complication ❷
One foot and other leg
C&C Exclusions: See 896.0

897.7 Bilateral [any level], complicated ❷
C&C Exclusions: See 896.0
AHA: 3Q 1990, 5

INJURY TO BLOOD VESSELS (900-904)

Includes arterial hematoma of blood vessel, secondary to other injuries, e.g., fracture or open wound
avulsion of blood vessel, secondary to other injuries, e.g., fracture or open wound
cut of blood vessel, secondary to other injuries, e.g., fracture or open wound
laceration of blood vessel, secondary to other injuries, e.g., fracture or open wound
rupture of blood vessel, secondary to other injuries, e.g., fracture or open wound
traumatic aneurysm or fistula (arteriovenous) of blood vessel, secondary to other injuries, e.g., fracture or open wound

Excludes accidental puncture or laceration during medical procedure (998.2)
intracranial hemorrhage following injury (851.0-854.1)

AHA: 3Q 1990, 5

❹ **900 Injury to blood vessels of head and neck**

❺ **900.0 Carotid artery**

900.00 Carotid artery, unspecified ❷
C&C Exclusions: 900.00, 900.82, 900.89, 900.9, 904.9, 929.0, 929.9, 958.8, 959.8, 959.9

900.01 Common carotid artery ❷
C&C Exclusions: See 900.00

900.02 External carotid artery ❷
C&C Exclusions: See 900.00

900.03 Internal carotid artery ❷
C&C Exclusions: See 900.00

900.1 Internal jugular vein ❷
C&C Exclusions: 900.82, 900.89, 900.9, 904.9, 929.0, 929.9, 958.8, 959.8, 959.9

❺ **900.8 Other specified blood vessels of head and neck**

900.81 External jugular vein ❷
Jugular vein NOS
C&C Exclusions: See 900.1

900.82 Multiple blood vessels of head and neck ❷
C&C Exclusions: See 900.1

900.89 Other ❷
C&C Exclusions: See 900.1

✖ **900.9 Unspecified blood vessel of head and neck** ❷
C&C Exclusions: See 900.1

❹ **901 Injury to blood vessels of thorax**
Excludes traumatic hemothorax (860.2-860.5)

901.0 Thoracic aorta
C&C Exclusions: 901.0, 904.9, 929.0, 929.9, 958.8, 959.8, 959.9

901.1 Innominate and subclavian arteries
C&C Exclusions: 901.1, 904.9, 929.0, 929.9, 958.8, 959.8, 959.9

901.2 Superior vena cava
C&C Exclusions: 901.2, 904.9, 929.0, 929.9, 958.8, 959.8, 959.9

901.3 Innominate and subclavian veins
C&C Exclusions: 901.3, 904.9, 929.0, 929.9, 958.8, 959.8, 959.9

5 **901.4 Pulmonary blood vessels**

901.40 Pulmonary vessel(s), unspecified

901.41 Pulmonary artery
C&C Exclusions: 901.40, 900.41, 904.9, 929.0, 929.9, 958.8, 959.8, 959.9

901.42 Pulmonary vein
C&C Exclusions: See 901.41

5 **901.8 Other specified blood vessels of thorax**

901.81 Intercostal artery or vein

901.82 Internal mammary artery or vein

901.83 Multiple blood vessels of thorax
C&C Exclusions: 904.9, 929.0, 929.9, 958.8, 959.8, 959.9

901.89 Other
Azygos vein
Hemiazygos vein

✖ **901.9 Unspecified blood vessel of thorax**

4 **902 Injury to blood vessels of abdomen and pelvis**

902.0 Abdominal aorta
C&C Exclusions: 902.0, 902.87, 902.89, 902.9, 904.9, 929.0, 929.9, 958.8, 959.8, 959.9

5 **902.1 Inferior vena cava**

902.10 Inferior vena cava, unspecified
C&C Exclusions: 902.10, 902.87, 902.89, 902.9, 904.9, 929.0, 929.9, 958.8, 959.8, 959.9

902.11 Hepatic veins
C&C Exclusions: 902.11, 902.87, 902.89, 902.9, 904.9, 929.0, 929.9, 958.8, 959.8, 959.9

902.19 Other
C&C Exclusions: 902.19, 902.87, 902.89, 902.9, 904.9, 929.0, 929.9, 958.8, 959.8, 959.9

5 **902.2 Celiac and mesenteric arteries**

902.20 Celiac and mesenteric arteries, unspecified
C&C Exclusions: 902.20, 902.87, 902.89, 902.9, 904.9, 929.0, 929.9, 958.8, 959.8, 959.9

902.21 Gastric artery

902.22 Hepatic artery
C&C Exclusions: 902.22, 902.87, 902.89, 902.9, 904.9, 929.0, 929.9, 958.8, 959.8, 959.9

902.23 Splenic artery
C&C Exclusions: 902.23, 902.87, 902.89, 902.9, 904.9, 929.0, 929.9, 958.8, 959.8, 959.9

902.24 Other specified branches of celiac axis
C&C Exclusions: 902.24, 902.87, 902.89, 902.9, 904.9, 929.0, 929.9, 958.8, 959.8, 959.9

902.25 Superior mesenteric artery (trunk)
C&C Exclusions: 902.25, 902.87, 902.89, 902.9, 904.9, 929.0, 929.9, 958.8, 959.8, 959.9

902.26 Primary branches of superior mesenteric artery
Ileo-colic artery
C&C Exclusions: 902.26, 902.87, 902.89, 902.9, 904.9, 929.0, 929.9, 958.8, 959.8, 959.9

902.27 Inferior mesenteric artery
C&C Exclusions: 902.27, 902.87, 902.89, 902.9, 904.9, 929.0, 929.9, 958.8, 959.8, 959.9

902.29 Other
C&C Exclusions: 902.29, 902.87, 902.89, 902.9, 904.9, 929.0, 929.9, 958.8, 959.8, 959.9

5 **902.3 Portal and splenic veins**

902.31 Superior mesenteric vein and primary subdivisions
Ileo-colic vein
C&C Exclusions: 902.31, 902.87, 902.89, 902.9, 904.9, 929.0, 929.9, 958.8, 959.8, 959.9

902.32 Inferior mesenteric vein
C&C Exclusions: 902.32, 902.87, 902.89, 902.9, 904.9, 929.0, 929.9, 958.8, 959.8, 959.9

902.33 Portal vein
C&C Exclusions: 902.33, 902.87, 902.89, 902.9, 904.9, 929.0, 929.9, 958.8, 959.8, 959.9

902.34 Splenic vein
C&C Exclusions: 902.34, 902.87, 902.89, 902.9, 904.9, 929.0, 929.9, 958.8, 959.8, 959.9

902.39 Other
Cystic vein
Gastric vein
C&C Exclusions: 902.39, 902.87, 902.89, 902.9, 904.9, 929.0, 929.9, 958.8, 959.8, 959.9

5 **902.4 Renal blood vessels**

902.40 Renal vessel(s), unspecified
C&C Exclusions: 902.40, 902.87, 902.89, 902.9, 904.9, 929.0, 929.9, 958.8, 959.8, 959.9

902.41 Renal artery
C&C Exclusions: 902.41, 902.87, 902.89, 902.9, 904.9, 929.0, 929.9, 958.8, 959.8, 959.9

902.42 Renal vein
C&C Exclusions: 902.42, 902.87, 902.89, 902.9, 904.9, 929.0, 929.9, 958.8, 959.8, 959.9

902.49 Other
Suprarenal arteries
C&C Exclusions: 902.49, 902.87, 902.89, 902.9, 904.9, 929.0, 929.9, 958.8, 959.8, 959.9

5 **902.5 Iliac blood vessels**

902.50 Iliac vessel(s), unspecified
C&C Exclusions: 902.50, 902.53, 902.54, 902.59, 902.87, 902.89, 902.9, 904.9, 929.0, 929.9, 958.8, 959.8, 959.9

902.51 Hypogastric artery
C&C Exclusions: 902.50, 902.59, 902.87, 902.89, 902.9, 904.9, 929.0, 929.9, 958.8, 959.8, 959.9

902.52 Hypogastric vein
C&C Exclusions: 902.52, 902.59, 902.87, 902.89, 902.9, 904.9, 929.0, 929.9, 958.8, 959.8, 959.9

902.53 Iliac artery
C&C Exclusions: 902.50, 902.53, 902.59, 902.87, 902.89, 902.9, 904.9, 929.0, 929.9, 958.8, 959.8, 959.9

902.54 Iliac vein
C&C Exclusions: 902.50, 902.54, 902.59, 902.87, 902.89, 902.9, 904.9, 929.0, 929.9, 958.8, 959.8, 959.9

902.55 Uterine artery ♀

902.56 Uterine vein ♀

902.59 Other
C&C Exclusions: See 902.50

5 **902.8 Other specified blood vessels of abdomen and pelvis**

902.81 Ovarian artery ♀

902.82 Ovarian vein ♀

902.87 Multiple blood vessels of abdomen and pelvis
C&C Exclusions: 902.87, 902.89, 902.9, 904.9, 929.0, 929.9, 958.8, 959.8, 959.9

902.89 Other

✖ **902.9 Unspecified blood vessel of abdomen and pelvis**

4 **903 Injury to blood vessels of upper extremity**

5 **903.0 Axillary blood vessels**

903.00 Axillary vessel(s), unspecified

903.01 Axillary artery

903.02 Axillary vein

903.1 Brachial blood vessels

903.2 Radial blood vessels

903.3 Ulnar blood vessels

903.4 Palmar artery

903.5 Digital blood vessels

903.8 Other specified blood vessels of upper extremity
Multiple blood vessels of upper extremity

Injury and Poisoning 901.1 – 903.8

✖ **903.9 Unspecified blood vessel of upper extremity**

❹ **904 Injury to blood vessels of lower extremity and unspecified sites**

904.0 Common femoral artery
Femoral artery above profunda origin

904.1 Superficial femoral artery

904.2 Femoral veins

904.3 Saphenous veins
Saphenous vein (greater) (lesser)

❺ **904.4 Popliteal blood vessels**

904.40 Popliteal vessel(s), unspecified

904.41 Popliteal artery

904.42 Popliteal vein

❺ **904.5 Tibial blood vessels**

904.50 Tibial vessel(s), unspecified

904.51 Anterior tibial artery

904.52 Anterior tibial vein

904.53 Posterior tibial artery

904.54 Posterior tibial vein

904.6 Deep plantar blood vessels

904.7 Other specified blood vessels of lower extremity
Multiple blood vessels of lower extremity

✖ **904.8 Unspecified blood vessel of lower extremity**

✖ **904.9 Unspecified site**
Injury to blood vessel NOS

LATE EFFECTS OF INJURIES, POISONINGS, TOXIC EFFECTS, AND OTHER EXTERNAL CAUSES (905-909)

Note: *These categories are to be used to indicate conditions classifiable to 800-999 as the cause of late effects, which are themselves classified elsewhere. The "late effects" include those specified as such, or as sequelae, which may occur at any time after the acute injury.*

❹ **905 Late effects of musculoskeletal and connective tissue injuries**
AHA: 1Q 1995, 10; 2Q 1994, 3

✖ **905.0 Late effect of fracture of skull and face bones**
Late effect of injury classifiable to 800-804
C&C Exclusions: 850.11, 850.12
AHA: 3Q 1997, 12

✖ **905.1 Late effect of fracture of spine and trunk without mention of spinal cord lesion**
Late effect of injury classifiable to 805, 807-809
AHA: 1Q 2007, 21

✖ **905.2 Late effect of fracture of upper extremities**
Late effect of injury classifiable to 810-819

✖ **905.3 Late effect of fracture of neck of femur**
Late effect of injury classifiable to 820

✖ **905.4 Late effect of fracture of lower extremities**
Late effect of injury classifiable to 821-827

✖ **905.5 Late effect of fracture of multiple and unspecified bones**
Late effect of injury classifiable to 828-829

✖ **905.6 Late effect of dislocation**
Late effect of injury classifiable to 830-839

✖ **905.7 Late effect of sprain and strain without mention of tendon injury**
Late effect of injury classifiable to 840-848, except tendon injury

✖ **905.8 Late effect of tendon injury**
Late effect of tendon injury due to:
open wound [injury classifiable to 880-884 with .2, 890-894 with .2]
sprain and strain [injury classifiable to 840-848]
AHA: 2Q 1989, 13, 15

✖ **905.9 Late effect of traumatic amputation**
Late effect of injury classifiable to 885-887, 895-897
Excludes *late amputation stump complication (997.60-997.69)*

❹ **906 Late effects of injuries to skin and subcutaneous tissues**

✖ **906.0 Late effect of open wound of head, neck, and trunk**
Late effect of injury classifiable to 870-879

✖ **906.1 Late effect of open wound of extremities without mention of tendon injury**
Late effect of injury classifiable to 880-884, 890-894 except .2

✖ **906.2 Late effect of superficial injury**
Late effect of injury classifiable to 910-919

✖ **906.3 Late effect of contusion**
Late effect of injury classifiable to 920-924

✖ **906.4 Late effect of crushing**
Late effect of injury classifiable to 925-929

✖ **906.5 Late effect of burn of eye, face, head, and neck**
Late effect of injury classifiable to 940-941
AHA: 4Q 2004, 76

✖ **906.6 Late effect of burn of wrist and hand**
Late effect of injury classifiable to 944
AHA: 4Q 1994, 22

✖ **906.7 Late effect of burn of other extremities**
Late effect of injury classifiable to 943 or 945
AHA: 4Q 1994, 22

✖ **906.8 Late effect of burns of other specified sites**
Late effect of injury classifiable to 942, 946-947
AHA: 4Q 1994, 22

✖ **906.9 Late effect of burn of unspecified site**
Late effect of injury classifiable to 948-949
AHA: 4Q 1994, 22

❹ **907 Late effects of injuries to the nervous system**

✖ **907.0 Late effect of intracranial injury without mention of skull fracture**
Late effect of injury classifiable to 850-854
AHA: 4Q 2003, 103; 3Q 1990, 14

✖ **907.1 Late effect of injury to cranial nerve**
Late effect of injury classifiable to 950-951

✖ **907.2 Late effect of spinal cord injury**
Late effect of injury classifiable to 806, 952
AHA: 4Q 2003, 103; 4Q 1998, 38

✖ **907.3 Late effect of injury to nerve root(s), spinal plexus(es), and other nerves of trunk**
Late effect of injury classifiable to 953-954

✖ **907.4 Late effect of injury to peripheral nerve of shoulder girdle and upper limb**
Late effect of injury classifiable to 955

✖ **907.5 Late effect of injury to peripheral nerve of pelvic girdle and lower limb**
Late effect of injury classifiable to 956

✖ **907.9 Late effect of injury to other and unspecified nerve**
Late effect of injury classifiable to 957

❹ **908 Late effects of other and unspecified injuries**

✖ **908.0 Late effect of internal injury to chest**
Late effect of injury classifiable to 860-862

✖ **908.1 Late effect of internal injury to intra-abdominal organs**
Late effect of injury classifiable to 863-866, 868

✖ **908.2 Late effect of internal injury to other internal organs**
Late effect of injury classifiable to 867 or 869

✖ **908.3 Late effect of injury to blood vessel of head, neck, and extremities**
Late effect of injury classifiable to 900, 903-904

✖ **908.4 Late effect of injury to blood vessel of thorax, abdomen, and pelvis**
Late effect of injury classifiable to 901-902

✖ **908.5 Late effect of foreign body in orifice**
Late effect of injury classifiable to 930-939

✖ **908.6 Late effect of certain complications of trauma**
Late effect of complications classifiable to 958

908.9 Late effect of unspecified injury
Late effect of injury classifiable to 959
AHA: 3Q 2000, 4

909 Late effects of other and unspecified external causes

909.0 Late effect of poisoning due to drug, medicinal or biological substance
Late effect of conditions classifiable to 960-979
Excludes *Late effect of adverse effect of drug, medicinal or biological substance (909.5)*
AHA: 4Q 2003, 103

909.1 Late effect of toxic effects of nonmedical substances
Late effect of conditions classifiable to 980-989

909.2 Late effect of radiation
Late effect of conditions classifiable to 990

909.3 Late effect of complications of surgical and medical care
Late effect of conditions classifiable to 996-999
AHA: 1Q 1993, 29

909.4 Late effect of certain other external causes
Late effect of conditions classifiable to 991-994

909.5 Late effect of adverse effect of drug, medicinal or biological substance
Excludes *late effect of poisoning due to drug, medicinal or biological substances (909.0)*
AHA: 4Q 1994, 48

909.9 Late effect of other and unspecified external causes

SUPERFICIAL INJURY (910-919)

Excludes *burn (blisters) (940.0-949.5)*
contusion (920-924.9)
foreign body:
granuloma (728.82)
inadvertently left in operative wound (998.4)
residual, in soft tissue (729.6)
insect bite, venomous (989.5)
open wound with incidental foreign body (870.0-897.7)

AHA: 2Q 1989, 15

910 Superficial injury of face, neck, and scalp except eye
Includes cheek
ear
gum
lip
nose
throat
Excludes *eye and adnexa (918.0-918.9)*

910.0 Abrasion or friction burn without mention of infection
910.1 Abrasion or friction burn, infected
910.2 Blister without mention of infection
910.3 Blister, infected
910.4 Insect bite, nonvenomous, without mention of infection
910.5 Insect bite, nonvenomous, infected
910.6 Superficial foreign body (splinter) without major open wound and without mention of infection
910.7 Superficial foreign body (splinter) without major open wound, infected
910.8 Other and unspecified superficial injury of face, neck, and scalp without mention of infection
910.9 Other and unspecified superficial injury of face, neck, and scalp, infected

911 Superficial injury of trunk
Includes abdominal wall
anus
back
breast
buttock
chest wall
flank
groin
interscapular region
labium (majus) (minus)
penis
perineum
scrotum
testis
vagina
vulva
Excludes *hip (916.0-916.9)*
scapular region (912.0-912.9)

911.0 Abrasion or friction burn without mention of infection
AHA: 3Q 2001, 10
911.1 Abrasion or friction burn, infected
911.2 Blister without mention of infection
911.3 Blister, infected
911.4 Insect bite, nonvenomous, without mention of infection
911.5 Insect bite, nonvenomous, infected
911.6 Superficial foreign body (splinter) without major open wound and without mention of infection
911.7 Superficial foreign body (splinter) without major open wound, infected
911.8 Other and unspecified superficial injury of trunk without mention of infection
911.9 Other and unspecified superficial injury of trunk, infected

912 Superficial injury of shoulder and upper arm
Includes axilla
scapular region

912.0 Abrasion or friction burn without mention of infection
912.1 Abrasion or friction burn, infected
912.2 Blister without mention of infection
912.3 Blister, infected
912.4 Insect bite, nonvenomous, without mention of infection
912.5 Insect bite, nonvenomous, infected
912.6 Superficial foreign body (splinter) without major open wound and without mention of infection
912.7 Superficial foreign body (splinter) without major open wound, infected
912.8 Other and unspecified superficial injury of shoulder and upper arm without mention of infection
912.9 Other and unspecified superficial injury of shoulder and upper arm, infected

913 Superficial injury of elbow, forearm, and wrist
913.0 Abrasion or friction burn without mention of infection
913.1 Abrasion or friction burn, infected
913.2 Blister without mention of infection
913.3 Blister, infected
913.4 Insect bite, nonvenomous, without mention of infection
913.5 Insect bite, nonvenomous, infected
913.6 Superficial foreign body (splinter) without major open wound and without mention of infection
913.7 Superficial foreign body (splinter) without major open wound, infected
913.8 Other and unspecified superficial injury of elbow, forearm, and wrist without mention of infection
913.9 Other and unspecified superficial injury of elbow, forearm, and wrist, infected

914 Superficial injury of hand(s) except finger(s) alone
914.0 Abrasion or friction burn without mention of infection
914.1 Abrasion or friction burn, infected
914.2 Blister without mention of infection

914.3 **Blister, infected**

914.4 **Insect bite, nonvenomous, without mention of infection**

914.5 **Insect bite, nonvenomous, infected**

914.6 **Superficial foreign body (splinter) without major open wound and without mention of infection**

914.7 **Superficial foreign body (splinter) without major open wound, infected**

914.8 **Other and unspecified superficial injury of hand without mention of infection**

914.9 **Other and unspecified superficial injury of hand, infected**

❹ 915 **Superficial injury of finger(s)**

Includes fingernail
thumb (nail)

915.0 **Abrasion or friction burn without mention of infection**

915.1 **Abrasion or friction burn, infected**

915.2 **Blister without mention of infection**

915.3 **Blister, infected**

915.4 **Insect bite, nonvenomous, without mention of infection**

915.5 **Insect bite, nonvenomous, infected**

915.6 **Superficial foreign body (splinter) without major open wound and without mention of infection**

915.7 **Superficial foreign body (splinter) without major open wound, infected**

915.8 **Other and unspecified superficial injury of fingers without mention of infection**
AHA: 3Q 2001, 10

915.9 **Other and unspecified superficial injury of fingers, infected**

❹ 916 **Superficial injury of hip, thigh, leg, and ankle**

916.0 **Abrasion or friction burn without mention of infection**

916.1 **Abrasion or friction burn, infected**

916.2 **Blister without mention of infection**

916.3 **Blister, infected**

916.4 **Insect bite, nonvenomous, without mention of infection**

916.5 **Insect bite, nonvenomous, infected**

916.6 **Superficial foreign body (splinter) without major open wound and without mention of infection**

916.7 **Superficial foreign body (splinter) without major open wound, infected**

916.8 **Other and unspecified superficial injury of hip, thigh, leg, and ankle without mention of infection**

916.9 **Other and unspecified superficial injury of hip, thigh, leg, and ankle, infected**

❹ 917 **Superficial injury of foot and toe(s)**

Includes heel
toenail

917.0 **Abrasion or friction burn without mention of infection**

917.1 **Abrasion or friction burn, infected**

917.2 **Blister without mention of infection**

917.3 **Blister, infected**

917.4 **Insect bite, nonvenomous, without mention of infection**

917.5 **Insect bite, nonvenomous, infected**

917.6 **Superficial foreign body (splinter) without major open wound and without mention of infection**

917.7 **Superficial foreign body (splinter) without major open wound, infected**

917.8 **Other and unspecified superficial injury of foot and toes without mention of infection**
AHA: 1Q 2003, 13

917.9 **Other and unspecified superficial injury of foot and toes, infected**
AHA: 1Q 2003, 13

❹ 918 **Superficial injury of eye and adnexa**

Excludes *burn (940.0-940.9)*
foreign body on external eye (930.0-930.9)

918.0 **Eyelids and periocular area**
Abrasion
Insect bite
Superficial foreign body (splinter)

918.1 **Cornea**
Corneal abrasion
Superficial laceration
Excludes *corneal injury due to contact lens (371.82)*

918.2 **Conjunctiva**

918.9 **Other and unspecified superficial injuries of eye**
Eye (ball) NOS

❹ 919 **Superficial injury of other, multiple, and unspecified sites**

Excludes *multiple sites classifiable to the same three-digit category (910.0-918.9)*

919.0 **Abrasion or friction burn without mention of infection**

919.1 **Abrasion or friction burn, infected**

919.2 **Blister without mention of infection**

919.3 **Blister, infected**

919.4 **Insect bite, nonvenomous, without mention of infection**

919.5 **Insect bite, nonvenomous, infected**

919.6 **Superficial foreign body (splinter) without major open wound and without mention of infection**

919.7 **Superficial foreign body (splinter) without major open wound, infected**

919.8 **Other and unspecified superficial injury without mention of infection**

919.9 **Other and unspecified superficial injury, infected**

CONTUSION WITH INTACT SKIN SURFACE (920-924)

Includes bruise without fracture or open wound
hematoma without fracture or open wound

Excludes *concussion (850.0-850.9)*
hemarthrosis (840.0-848.9)
internal organs (860.0-869.1)
that incidental to:
crushing injury (925-929.9)
dislocation (830.0-839.9)
fracture (800.0-829.1)
internal injury (860.0-869.1)
intracranial injury (850.0-854.1)
nerve injury (950.0-957.9)
open wound (870.0-897.7)

920 **Contusion of face, scalp, and neck except eye(s)**
Cheek
Ear (auricle)
Gum
Lip
Mandibular joint area
Nose
Throat

❹ 921 **Contusion of eye and adnexa**

921.0 **Black eye, NOS**

921.1 **Contusion of eyelids and periocular area**

921.2 **Contusion of orbital tissues**

921.3 **Contusion of eyeball**
AHA: Jul-Aug 1985, 16

✖ 921.9 **Unspecified contusion of eye**
Injury of eye NOS

❹ 922 **Contusion of trunk**

922.0 **Breast**

922.1 **Chest wall**

922.2 **Abdominal wall**
Flank
Groin

5 **922.3 Back**
AHA: 4Q 1996, 39

922.31 Back
Excludes *interscapular region (922.33)*

922.32 Buttock
AHA: 3Q 1999, 14

922.33 Interscapular region
Excludes *scapular region (923.01)*
DEF: Bruise on the region between the shoulder blades.

922.4 Genital organs
Labium (majus) (minus)
Penis
Perineum
Scrotum
Testis
Vagina
Vulva

922.8 Multiple sites of trunk

✖ **922.9 Unspecified part**
Trunk NOS

4 **923 Contusion of upper limb**

5 **923.0 Shoulder and upper arm**
923.00 Shoulder region
923.01 Scapular region
923.02 Axillary region
923.03 Upper arm
923.09 Multiple sites

5 **923.1 Elbow and forearm**
923.10 Forearm
923.11 Elbow

5 **923.2 Wrist and hand(s), except finger(s) alone**
923.20 Hand(s)
923.21 Wrist

923.3 Finger
Fingernail
Thumb (nail)

923.8 Multiple sites of upper limb

✖ **923.9 Unspecified part of upper limb**
Arm NOS

4 **924 Contusion of lower limb and of other and unspecified sites**

5 **924.0 Hip and thigh**
924.00 Thigh
924.01 Hip

5 **924.1 Knee and lower leg**
924.10 Lower leg
924.11 Knee

5 **924.2 Ankle and foot, excluding toe(s)**
924.20 Foot
Heel
924.21 Ankle

924.3 Toe
Toenail

924.4 Multiple sites of lower limb

924.5 Unspecified part of lower limb
Leg NOS

924.8 Multiple sites, not elsewhere classified
AHA: 1Q 2003, 7

✖ **924.9 Unspecified site**

CRUSHING INJURY (925-929)

Use additional code to identify any associated injuries, such as:
fractures (800-829)
internal injuries (860.0-869.1)
intracranial injury (850.0-854.1)

AHA: 4Q 2003, 77; 2Q 1993, 7

4 **925 Crushing injury of face, scalp, and neck**
Cheek
Ear
Larynx
Pharynx
Throat

925.1 Crushing injury of face and scalp 2
Cheek
Ear
C&C Exclusions: 850.11, 850.12, 873.8, 873.9, 905.0, 925.1, 925.2, 929.0, 929.9, 958.8, 959.01, 959.09, 959.8, 959.9

925.2 Crushing injury of neck 2
Larynx
Throat
Pharynx
C&C Exclusions: See 925.1

4 **926 Crushing injury of trunk**

926.0 External genitalia
Labium (majus) (minus)
Penis
Scrotum
Testis
Vulva

5 **926.1 Other specified sites**
926.11 Back
926.12 Buttock
926.19 Other
Breast

926.8 Multiple sites of trunk 2

✖ **926.9 Unspecified site**
Trunk NOS

4 **927 Crushing injury of upper limb**

5 **927.0 Shoulder and upper arm**
927.00 Shoulder region
927.01 Scapular region
927.02 Axillary region
927.03 Upper arm
927.09 Multiple sites

5 **927.1 Elbow and forearm**
927.10 Forearm
927.11 Elbow

5 **927.2 Wrist and hand(s), except finger(s) alone**
927.20 Hand(s)
927.21 Wrist

927.3 Finger(s)
AHA: 4Q 2003, 77

927.8 Multiple sites of upper limb

✖ **927.9 Unspecified site**
Arm NOS

4 **928 Crushing injury of lower limb**

5 **928.0 Hip and thigh**
928.00 Thigh
928.01 Hip

5 **928.1 Knee and lower leg**
928.10 Lower leg
928.11 Knee

5 **928.2 Ankle and foot, excluding toe(s) alone**
928.20 Foot
Heel
928.21 Ankle

928.3 **Toe(s)**

928.8 **Multiple sites of lower limb**

✖ 928.9 **Unspecified site**
Leg NOS

❹ 929 **Crushing injury of multiple and unspecified sites**

929.0 **Multiple sites, not elsewhere classified** ❷
C&C Exclusions: 850.11, 850.12, 929.0, 929.9, 958.8, 959.01, 959.09, 959.8, 959.9

✖ 929.9 **Unspecified site** ❷
C&C Exclusions: See 929.0

EFFECTS OF FOREIGN BODY ENTERING THROUGH ORIFICE (930-939)

Excludes *foreign body:*
granuloma (728.82)
inadvertently left in operative wound (998.4, 998.7)
in open wound (800-839, 851-897)
residual, in soft tissues (729.6)
superficial without major open wound (910-919 with .6 or .7)

❹ 930 **Foreign body on external eye**
Excludes *foreign body in penetrating wound of:*
eyeball (871.5-871.6)
retained (old) (360.5-360.6)
ocular adnexa (870.4)
retained (old) (376.6)

930.0 **Corneal foreign body**

930.1 **Foreign body in conjunctival sac**

930.2 **Foreign body in lacrimal punctum**

930.8 **Other and combined sites**

930.9 **Unspecified site**
External eye NOS

931 **Foreign body in ear**
Auditory canal
Auricle

932 **Foreign body in nose**
Nasal sinus
Nostril

❹ 933 **Foreign body in pharynx and larynx**

933.0 **Pharynx**
Nasopharynx
Throat NOS

933.1 **Larynx**
Asphyxia due to foreign body
Choking due to:
food (regurgitated)
phlegm

❹ 934 **Foreign body in trachea, bronchus, and lung**

934.0 **Trachea**

934.1 **Main bronchus**
AHA: 3Q 2002, 18

934.8 **Other specified parts**
Bronchioles
Lung

✖ 934.9 **Respiratory tree, unspecified**
Inhalation of liquid or vomitus, lower respiratory tract NOS

❹ 935 **Foreign body in mouth, esophagus, and stomach**

935.0 **Mouth**

935.1 **Esophagus**
AHA: 1Q 1988, 13

935.2 **Stomach**

936 **Foreign body in intestine and colon**

937 **Foreign body in anus and rectum**
Rectosigmoid (junction)

938 **Foreign body in digestive system, unspecified**
Alimentary tract NOS
Swallowed foreign body

❹ 939 **Foreign body in genitourinary tract**

939.0 **Bladder and urethra**

939.1 **Uterus, any part** ♀
Excludes *intrauterine contraceptive device:*
complications from (996.32, 996.65)
presence of (V45.51)

939.2 **Vulva and vagina** ♀

939.3 **Penis** ♂

✖ 939.9 **Unspecified site**

BURNS (940-949)

Includes burns from:
electrical heating appliance
electricity
flame
hot object
lightning
radiation
chemical burns (external) (internal)
scalds

Excludes *friction burns (910-919 with .0, .1)*
sunburn (692.71, 692.76-692.77)

AHA: 4Q 1994, 22; 2Q 1990, 7; 4Q 1988, 3; Mar-Apr 1986, 9

❹ 940 **Burn confined to eye and adnexa**

940.0 **Chemical burn of eyelids and periocular area**

940.1 **Other burns of eyelids and periocular area**

940.2 **Alkaline chemical burn of cornea and conjunctival sac**

940.3 **Acid chemical burn of cornea and conjunctival sac**

940.4 **Other burn of cornea and conjunctival sac**

940.5 **Burn with resulting rupture and destruction of eyeball**

940.9 **Unspecified burn of eye and adnexa**

❹ 941 **Burn of face, head, and neck**
Excludes *mouth (947.0)*
AHA: 4Q 1994, 22; Mar-Apr 1986, 9

The following fifth-digit subclassification is for use with category 941:
0 **face and head, unspecified site**
1 **ear [any part]**
2 **eye (with other parts of face, head, and neck)**
3 **lip(s)**
4 **chin**
5 **nose (septum)**
6 **scalp [any part]**
Temple (region)
7 **forehead and cheek**
8 **neck**
9 **multiple sites [except with eye] of face, head, and neck**

✖❺ 941.0 **Unspecified degree**

❺ 941.1 **Erythema [first degree]**
AHA: For Code 941.19: 3Q 2005, 10

❺ 941.2 **Blisters, epidermal loss [second degree]**

❺ 941.3 **Full-thickness skin loss [third degree NOS]**

❺ 941.4 **Deep necrosis of underlying tissues [deep third degree] without mention of loss of a body part**

❺ 941.5 **Deep necrosis of underlying tissues [deep third degree] with loss of a body part**

942 Burn of trunk
Excludes *scapular region (943.0-943.5 with fifth-digit 6)*
AHA: 4Q 1994, 22; Mar-Apr 1986, 9

The following fifth-digit subclassification is for use with category 942:
- **0 trunk, unspecified site**
- **1 breast**
- **2 chest wall, excluding breast and nipple**
- **3 abdominal wall**
  - Flank
  - Groin
- **4 back [any part]**
  - Buttock
  - Interscapular region
- **5 genitalia**
  - Labium (majus) (minus)
  - Penis
  - Perineum
  - Scrotum
  - Testis
  - Vulva
- **9 other and multiple sites of trunk**

942.0 Unspecified degree
942.1 Erythema [first degree]
942.2 Blisters, epidermal loss [second degree]
942.3 Full-thickness skin loss [third degree NOS]
942.4 Deep necrosis of underlying tissues [deep third degree] without mention of loss of a body part
942.5 Deep necrosis of underlying tissues [deep third degree] with loss of a body part

943 Burn of upper limb, except wrist and hand
AHA: 4Q 1994, 22; Mar-Apr 1986, 9

The following fifth-digit subclassification is for use with category 943:
- **0 upper limb, unspecified site**
- **1 forearm**
- **2 elbow**
- **3 upper arm**
- **4 axilla**
- **5 shoulder**
- **6 scapular region**
- **9 multiple sites of upper limb, except wrist and hand**

943.0 Unspecified degree
943.1 Erythema [first degree]
943.2 Blisters, epidermal loss [second degree]
943.3 Full-thickness skin loss [third degree NOS]
943.4 Deep necrosis of underlying tissues [deep third degree] without mention of loss of a body part
943.5 Deep necrosis of underlying tissues [deep third degree] with loss of a body part

944 Burn of wrist(s) and hand(s)

The following fifth-digit subclassification is for use with category 944:
- **0 hand, unspecified site**
- **1 single digit [finger (nail)] other than thumb**
- **2 thumb (nail)**
- **3 two or more digits, not including thumb**
- **4 two or more digits including thumb**
- **5 palm**
- **6 back of hand**
- **7 wrist**
- **8 multiple sites of wrist(s) and hand(s)**

944.0 Unspecified degree
944.1 Erythema [first degree]
944.2 Blisters, epidermal loss [second degree]
944.3 Full-thickness skin loss [third degree NOS]
944.4 Deep necrosis of underlying tissues [deep third degree] without mention of loss of a body part
944.5 Deep necrosis of underlying tissues [deep third degree] with loss of a body part

945 Burn of lower limb(s)
AHA: 4Q 1994, 22; Mar-Apr 1986, 9

The following fifth-digit subclassification is for use with category 945:
- **0 lower limb [leg], unspecified site**
- **1 toe(s) (nail)**
- **2 foot**
- **3 ankle**
- **4 lower leg**
- **5 knee**
- **6 thigh [any part]**
- **9 multiple sites of lower limb(s)**

945.0 Unspecified degree
945.1 Erythema [first degree]
945.2 Blisters, epidermal loss [second degree]
945.3 Full-thickness skin loss [third degree NOS]
945.4 Deep necrosis of underlying tissues [deep third degree] without mention of loss of a body part
945.5 Deep necrosis of underlying tissues [deep third degree] with loss of a body part

946 Burns of multiple specified sites
Includes burns of sites classifiable to more than one three-digit category in 940-945
Excludes *multiple burns NOS (949.0-949.5)*
AHA: 4Q 1994, 22; Mar-Apr 1986, 9

946.0 Unspecified degree
946.1 Erythema [first degree]
946.2 Blisters, epidermal loss [second degree]
946.3 Full-thickness skin loss [third degree NOS]
946.4 Deep necrosis of underlying tissues [deep third degree] without mention of loss of a body part
946.5 Deep necrosis of underlying tissues [deep third degree] with loss of a body part

947 Burn of internal organs
Includes burns from chemical agents (ingested)
AHA: 4Q 1994, 22; Mar-Apr 1986, 9

947.0 Mouth and pharynx
- Gum
- Tongue

947.1 Larynx, trachea, and lung
947.2 Esophagus
947.3 Gastrointestinal tract
- Colon
- Rectum
- Small intestine
- Stomach

947.4 Vagina and uterus ♀
947.8 Other specified sites
947.9 Unspecified site

Injury and Poisoning

942 – 947.9

Rule of Nines

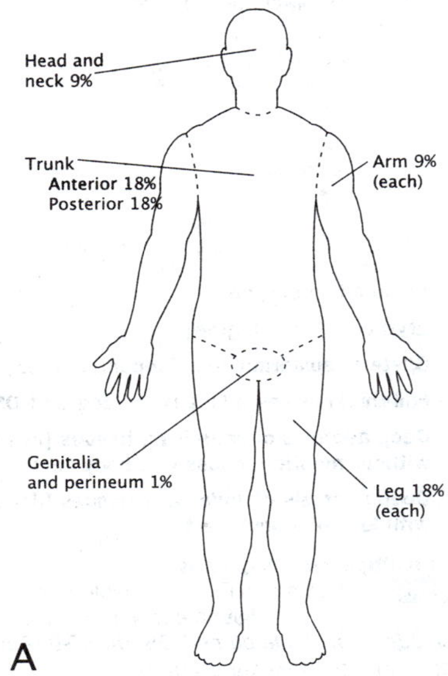

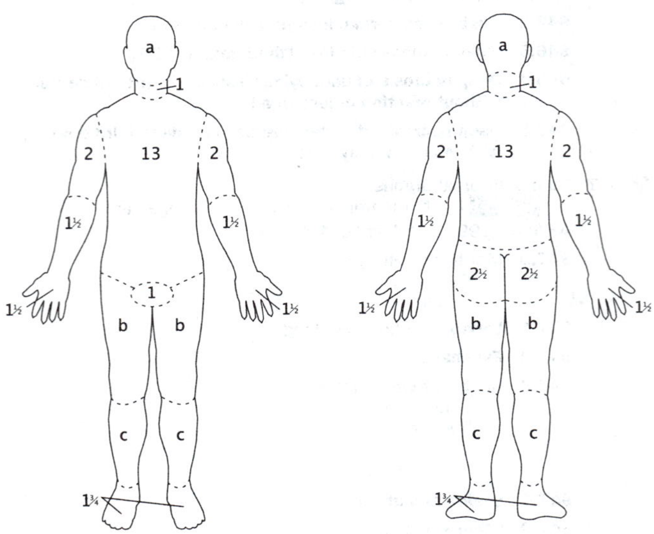

Anterior Posterior

Lund-Browder Chart

Relative percentage of body surface areas (% BSA) affected by growth

	0 yr	1yr	5yr	10yr	15+yr
a	9.5%	8.5%	6.5%	5.5%	4.5%
b	2.75%	3.25%	4%	4.25%	4.5%
c	2.5%	2.5%	2.75%	3%	3.25%

❹ **948 Burns classified according to extent of body surface involved**

Excludes *sunburn (692.71, 692.76-692.77)*

Note: This category is to be used when the site of the burn is unspecified, or with categories 940-947 when the site is specified.

AHA: 4Q 1994, 22; 4Q 1988, 3; Mar-Apr 1986, 9; Nov-Dec 1984, 13

The following fifth-digit subclassification is for use with category 948 to indicate the percent of body surface with third degree burn; valid digits are in [brackets] under each code:

- **0 less than 10 percent or unspecified**
- **1 10-19%**
- **2 20-29%**
- **3 30-39%**
- **4 40-49%**
- **5 50-59%**
- **6 60-69%**
- **7 70-79%**
- **8 80-89%**
- **9 90% or more of body surface**

❺ **948.0 Burn [any degree] involving less than 10 percent of body surface**
[0]

❺ **948.1 10-19 percent of body surface**
[0-1]

❺ **948.2 20-29 percent of body surface**
[0-2]

❺ **948.3 30-39 percent of body surface**
[0-3]

❺ **948.4 40-49 percent of body surface**
[0-4]

❺ **948.5 50-59 percent of body surface**
[0-5]

❺ **948.6 60-69 percent of body surface**
[0-6]

❺ **948.7 70-79 percent of body surface**
[0-7]

❺ **948.8 80-89 percent of body surface**
[0-8]

❺ **948.9 90 percent or more of body surface**
[0-9]

❹ **949 Burn, unspecified**

Includes burn NOS
multiple burns NOS

Excludes *burn of unspecified site but with statement of the extent of body surface involved (948.0-948.9)*

AHA: 4Q 1994, 22; Mar-Apr 1986, 9

✖ **949.0 Unspecified degree**

✖ **949.1 Erythema [first degree]**

✖ **949.2 Blisters, epidermal loss [second degree]**

✖ **949.3 Full-thickness skin loss [third degree NOS]**

✖ **949.4 Deep necrosis of underlying tissues [deep third degree] without mention of loss of a body part**

✖ **949.5 Deep necrosis of underlying tissues [deep third degree] with loss of a body part**

INJURY TO NERVES AND SPINAL CORD (950-957)

Includes division of nerve
lesion in continuity (with open wound)
traumatic neuroma (with open wound)
traumatic transient paralysis (with open wound)

Excludes *accidental puncture or laceration during medical procedure (998.2)*

❹ **950 Injury to optic nerve and pathways**

950.0 Optic nerve injury
Second cranial nerve

950.1 Injury to optic chiasm

950.2 Injury to optic pathways

950.3 Injury to visual cortex

950.9 Unspecified
Traumatic blindness NOS

④ **951 Injury to other cranial nerve(s)**

951.0 Injury to oculomotor nerve
Third cranial nerve

951.1 Injury to trochlear nerve
Fourth cranial nerve

951.2 Injury to trigeminal nerve
Fifth cranial nerve

951.3 Injury to abducens nerve
Sixth cranial nerve

951.4 Injury to facial nerve
Seventh cranial nerve

951.5 Injury to acoustic nerve
Auditory nerve
Eighth cranial nerve
Traumatic deafness NOS

951.6 Injury to accessory nerve
Eleventh cranial nerve

951.7 Injury to hypoglossal nerve
Twelfth cranial nerve

951.8 Injury to other specified cranial nerves
Glossopharyngeal [9th cranial] nerve
Olfactory [1st cranial] nerve
Pneumogastric [10th cranial] nerve
Traumatic anosmia NOS
Vagus [10th cranial] nerve

✖ **951.9 Injury to unspecified cranial nerve**

④ **952 Spinal cord injury without evidence of spinal bone injury**

⑤ **952.0 Cervical**

952.00 C_1-C_4 level with unspecified spinal cord injury
Spinal cord injury, cervical region NOS
C&C Exclusions: 805.00, 805.01, 805.02, 805.03, 805.04, 805.05, 805.06, 805.07, 805.08, 805.10, 805.11, 805.12, 805.13, 805.14, 805.15, 805.16, 805.17, 805.18, 805.8, 805.9, 806.00, 806.01, 806.02, 806.03, 806.04, 806.05, 806.06, 806.07, 806.08, 806.09, 806.10, 806.11, 806.12, 806.13, 806.14, 806.15, 806.16, 806.17, 806.18, 806.19, 806.8, 806.9, 839.00, 839.01, 839.02, 839.03, 839.04, 839.05, 839.06, 839.07, 839.08, 839.10, 839.11, 839.12, 839.13, 839.14, 839.15, 839.16, 839.17, 839.18, 839.40, 839.49, 839.50, 839.59, 839.69, 839.79, 839.8, 839.9, 847.9, 905.1, 926.11, 952.00, 952.01, 952.02, 952.03, 952.04, 952.05, 952.06, 952.07, 952.08, 952.09, 952.8, 952.9, 958.8, 959.1, 959.8, 959.9

952.01 C_1-C_4 level with complete lesion of spinal cord
C&C Exclusions: See 952.00

952.02 C_1-C_4 level with anterior cord syndrome
C&C Exclusions: See 952.00

952.03 C_1-C_4 level with central cord syndrome
C&C Exclusions: See 952.00

952.04 C_1-C_4 level with other specified spinal cord injury
Incomplete spinal cord lesion at C_1-C_4 level:
NOS
with posterior cord syndrome
C&C Exclusions: See 952.00

952.05 C_5-C_7 level with unspecified spinal cord injury
C&C Exclusions: See 952.00

952.06 C_5-C_7 level with complete lesion of spinal cord
C&C Exclusions: See 952.00

952.07 C_5-C_7 level with anterior cord syndrome
C&C Exclusions: See 952.00

952.08 C_5-C_7 level with central cord syndrome
C&C Exclusions: See 952.00

952.09 C_5-C_7 level with other specified spinal cord injury
Incomplete spinal cord lesion at C_5-C_7 level:
NOS
with posterior cord syndrome
C&C Exclusions: See 952.00

⑤ **952.1 Dorsal [thoracic]**

952.10 T_1-T_6 level with unspecified spinal cord injury
Spinal cord injury, thoracic region NOS
C&C Exclusions: 805.8, 805.9, 806.20, 806.21, 806.22, 806.23, 806.24, 806.25, 806.26, 806.27, 806.28, 806.29, 806.30, 806.31, 806.32, 806.33, 806.34, 806.35, 806.36, 806.37, 806.38, 806.39, 839.40, 839.49, 839.50, 839.59, 839.69, 839.79, 839.8, 839.9, 847.9, 905.1, 926.11, 952.10, 952.11, 952.12, 952.13, 952.14, 952.15, 952.16, 952.17, 952.18, 952.19, 952.8, 952.9, 958.8, 959.1, 959.8, 959.9

952.11 T_1-T_6 level with complete lesion of spinal cord
C&C Exclusions: See 952.10

952.12 T_1-T_6 level with anterior cord syndrome
C&C Exclusions: See 952.10

952.13 T_1-T_6 level with central cord syndrome
C&C Exclusions: See 952.10

952.14 T_1-T_6 level with other specified spinal cord injury
Incomplete spinal cord lesion at T_1-T_6 level:
NOS
with posterior cord syndrome
C&C Exclusions: See 952.10

952.15 T_7-T_{12} level with unspecified spinal cord injury
C&C Exclusions: See 952.10

952.16 T_7-T_{12} level with complete lesion of spinal cord
C&C Exclusions: See 952.10

952.17 T_7-T_{12} level with anterior cord syndrome
C&C Exclusions: See 952.10

952.18 T_7-T_{12} level with central cord syndrome
C&C Exclusions: See 952.10

952.19 T_7-T_{12} level with other specified spinal cord injury
Incomplete spinal cord lesion at T_7-T_{12} level:
NOS
with posterior cord syndrome
C&C Exclusions: See 952.10

952.2 Lumbar
C&C Exclusions: 805.8, 805.9, 806.4, 806.5, 839.40, 839.49, 839.50, 839.59, 839.69, 839.79, 839.8, 839.9, 847.2, 847.9, 905.1, 926.11, 929.0, 929.9, 952.2, 952.8, 952.9, 958.8, 959.1, 959.8, 959.9

952.3 Sacral
C&C Exclusions: 805.8, 805.9, 806.60, 806.61, 806.62, 806.69, 806.70, 806.71, 806.72, 806.79, 839.40, 839.49, 839.50, 839.59, 839.69, 839.79, 839.8, 839.9, 847.9, 905.1, 926.11, 929.0, 929.9, 952.3, 952.4, 952.8, 952.9, 958.8, 959.1, 959.8, 959.9

952.4 Cauda equina
C&C Exclusions: See 952.3

952.8 Multiple sites of spinal cord
C&C Exclusions: 805.8, 805.9, 839.40, 839.49, 839.50, 839.59, 839.69, 839.79, 839.8, 839.9, 847.9, 905.1, 926.11, 929.0, 929.9, 952.8, 952.9, 958.8, 959.1, 959.8, 959.9

✖ **952.9 Unspecified site of spinal cord**
C&C Exclusions: See 952.8

④ **953 Injury to nerve roots and spinal plexus**

953.0 Cervical root
C&C Exclusions: 953.8, 953.9, 958.8, 959.1, 959.8, 959.9

953.1 Dorsal root
C&C Exclusions: See 953.0

953.2 Lumbar root
C&C Exclusions: See 953.0

953.3 Sacral root
C&C Exclusions: See 953.0

953.4 Brachial plexus
C&C Exclusions: See 953.0

953.5 Lumbosacral plexus
C&C Exclusions: See 953.0

953.8 Multiple sites
C&C Exclusions: See 953.0

✖ **953.9 Unspecified site**
C&C Exclusions: See 953.0

④ 954 Injury to other nerve(s) of trunk, excluding shoulder and pelvic girdles

954.0 Cervical sympathetic

954.1 Other sympathetic
Celiac ganglion or plexus
Inferior mesenteric plexus
Splanchnic nerve(s)
Stellate ganglion

954.8 Other specified nerve(s) of trunk

✖ **954.9 Unspecified nerve of trunk**

④ 955 Injury to peripheral nerve(s) of shoulder girdle and upper limb

955.0 Axillary nerve

955.1 Median nerve

955.2 Ulnar nerve

955.3 Radial nerve

955.4 Musculocutaneous nerve

955.5 Cutaneous sensory nerve, upper limb

955.6 Digital nerve

955.7 Other specified nerve(s) of shoulder girdle and upper limb

955.8 Multiple nerves of shoulder girdle and upper limb

✖ **955.9 Unspecified nerve of shoulder girdle and upper limb**

④ 956 Injury to peripheral nerve(s) of pelvic girdle and lower limb

956.0 Sciatic nerve

956.1 Femoral nerve

956.2 Posterior tibial nerve

956.3 Peroneal nerve

956.4 Cutaneous sensory nerve, lower limb

956.5 Other specified nerve(s) of pelvic girdle and lower limb

956.8 Multiple nerves of pelvic girdle and lower limb

✖ **956.9 Unspecified nerve of pelvic girdle and lower limb**

④ 957 Injury to other and unspecified nerves

957.0 Superficial nerves of head and neck

957.1 Other specified nerve(s)

957.8 Multiple nerves in several parts
Multiple nerve injury NOS

✖ **957.9 Unspecified site**
Nerve injury NOS

CERTAIN TRAUMATIC COMPLICATIONS AND UNSPECIFIED INJURIES (958-959)

④ 958 Certain early complications of trauma
Excludes *adult respiratory distress syndrome (518.5)*
flail chest (807.4)
shock lung (518.5)
that occurring during or following medical procedures (996.0-999.9)

958.0 Air embolism
Pneumathemia
Excludes *that complicating:*
abortion (634-638 with .6, 639.6)
ectopic or molar pregnancy (639.6)
pregnancy, childbirth, or the puerperium (673.0)
C&C Exclusions: 958.0, 958.8, 959.8, 959.9, 997.91, 997.99, 998.81, 998.83, 998.89, 998.9, 999.1

958.1 Fat embolism
Excludes *that complicating:*
abortion (634-638 with .6, 639.6)
pregnancy, childbirth, or the puerperium (673.8)
C&C Exclusions: 958.1, 958.8, 959.8, 959.9, 997.91, 997.99, 998.81, 998.83, 998.89, 998.9

958.2 Secondary and recurrent hemorrhage
C&C Exclusions: 958.2, 958.8, 959.8, 959.9, 997.91, 997.99, 998.81, 998.83, 998.89, 998.9

958.3 Posttraumatic wound infection, not elsewhere classified
Excludes *infected open wounds - code to complicated open wound of site*
C&C Exclusions: 958.3, 958.8, 959.8, 959.9, 997.91, 997.99, 998.81, 998.83, 998.89, 998.9
AHA: 4Q 2001, 53; Sep-Oct 1985, 10

958.4 Traumatic shock ❷
Shock (immediate) (delayed) following injury
Excludes *shock:*
anaphylactic (995.0)
due to serum (999.4)
anesthetic (995.4)
electric (994.8)
following abortion (639.5)
lightning (994.0)
nontraumatic NOS (785.50)
obstetric (669.1)
postoperative (998.0)
C&C Exclusions: 958.4, 958.8, 959.8, 959.9, 997.91, 997.99, 998.81, 998.83, 998.89, 998.9

958.5 Traumatic anuria ❷
Crush syndrome
Renal failure following crushing
Excludes *that due to a medical procedure (997.5)*
C&C Exclusions: 958.5, 958.8, 959.8, 959.9, 997.91, 997.99, 998.81, 998.83, 998.89, 998.9

958.6 Volkmann's ischemic contracture
Posttraumatic muscle contracture

958.7 Traumatic subcutaneous emphysema
Excludes *subcutaneous emphysema resulting from a procedure (998.81)*
C&C Exclusions: 860.0, 860.1, 860.2, 860.3, 860.4, 860.5, 861.20, 861.21, 861.22, 861.30, 861.31, 861.32, 862.0, 862.1, 862.29, 862.31, 862.32, 862.39, 862.8, 862.9, 875.0, 875.1, 958.7, 958.8, 959.8, 959.9, 997.91, 997.99, 998.81, 998.83, 998.89, 998.9

958.8 Other early complications of trauma
C&C Exclusions: 850.11, 850.12, 958.8, 959.8, 959.9, 997.91, 997.99, 998.81, 998.83, 998.89, 998.9, 999.1
AHA: 2Q 1992, 13

⑤ 958.9 Traumatic compartment syndrome
Excludes *nontraumatic compartment syndrome (729.71-729.79)*

✖ **958.90 Compartment syndrome, unspecified**
C&C Exclusions: 800.00, 800.01, 800.02, 800.03, 800.04, 800.05, 800.06, 800.09, 800.10, 800.11, 800.12, 800.13, 800.14, 800.15, 800.16, 800.19, 800.20, 800.21, 800.22, 800.23, 800.24, 800.25, 800.26, 800.29, 800.30, 800.31, 800.32, 800.33, 800.34, 800.35, 800.36, 800.39, 800.40, 800.41, 800.42, 800.43, 800.44, 800.45, 800.46, 800.49, 800.50, 800.51, 800.52, 800.53, 800.54, 800.55, 800.56, 800.59, 800.60, 800.61, 800.62, 800.63, 800.64, 800.65, 800.66, 800.69, 800.70, 800.71, 800.72, 800.73, 800.74, 800.75, 800.76, 800.79, 800.80, 800.81, 800.82, 800.83, 800.84, 800.85, 800.86, 800.89, 800.90, 800.91, 800.92, 800.93, 800.94, 800.95, 800.96, 800.99, 801.00, 801.01, 801.02, 801.03, 801.04, 801.05, 801.06, 801.09, 801.10, 801.11, 801.12, 801.13, 801.14, 801.15, 801.16, 801.19, 801.20, 801.21, 801.22, 801.23, 801.24, 801.25, 801.26, 801.29, 801.30, 801.31, 801.32, 801.33, 801.34, 801.35, 801.36, 801.39, 801.40, 801.41, 801.42, 801.43, 801.44, 801.45, 801.46, 801.49, 801.50, 801.51, 801.52, 801.53, 801.54, 801.55, 801.56, 801.59, 801.60, 801.61, 801.62, 801.63, 801.64, 801.65, 801.66, 801.69, 801.70, 801.71, 801.72, 801.73, 801.74, 801.75, 801.76, 801.79, 801.80, 801.81, 801.82, 801.83, 801.84, 801.85, 801.86, 801.89, 801.90, 801.91, 801.92, 801.93, 801.94, 801.95, 801.96, 801.99, 802.1, 802.20, 802.21, 802.22, 802.23, 802.24, 802.25, 802.26, 802.27, 802.28, 802.29, 802.30, 802.31, 802.32, 802.33, 802.34, 802.35, 802.36, 802.37, 802.38, 802.39, 802.4, 802.5, 802.6, 802.7, 802.8, 802.9, 803.00, 803.01, 803.02, 803.03, 803.04, 803.05, 803.06, 803.09, 803.10, 803.11, 803.12, 803.13, 803.14, 803.15, 803.16, 803.19, 803.20, 803.21, 803.22, 803.23, 803.24, 803.25, 803.26, 803.29, 803.30, 803.31, 803.32, 803.33, 803.34, 803.35, 803.36, 803.39, 803.40, 803.41, 803.42, 803.43, 803.44, 803.45, 803.46,

803.49, 803.50, 803.51, 803.52, 803.53, 803.54, 803.55, 803.56, 803.59, 803.60, 803.61, 803.62, 803.63, 803.64, 803.65, 803.66, 803.69, 803.70, 803.71, 803.72, 803.73, 803.74, 803.75, 803.76, 803.79, 803.80, 803.81, 803.82, 803.83, 803.84, 803.85, 803.86, 803.89, 803.90, 803.91, 803.92, 803.93, 803.94, 803.95, 803.96, 803.99, 804.00, 804.01, 804.02, 804.03, 804.04, 804.05, 804.06, 804.09, 804.10, 804.11, 804.12, 804.13, 804.14, 804.15, 804.16, 804.19, 804.20, 804.21, 804.22, 804.23, 804.24, 804.25, 804.26, 804.29, 804.30, 804.31, 804.32, 804.33, 804.34, 804.35, 804.36, 804.39, 804.40, 804.41, 804.42, 804.43, 804.44, 804.45, 804.46, 804.49, 804.50, 804.51, 804.52, 804.53, 804.54, 804.55, 804.56, 804.59, 804.60, 804.61, 804.62, 804.63, 804.64, 804.65, 804.66, 804.69, 804.70, 804.71, 804.72, 804.73, 804.74, 804.75, 804.76, 804.79, 804.80, 804.81, 804.82, 804.83, 804.84, 804.85, 804.86, 804.89, 804.90, 804.91, 804.92, 804.93, 804.94, 804.95, 804.96, 804.99, 805.00, 805.01, 805.02, 805.03, 805.04, 805.05, 805.06, 805.07, 805.08, 805.10, 805.11, 805.12, 805.13, 805.14, 805.15, 805.16, 805.17, 805.18, 805.2, 805.3, 805.4, 805.5, 805.6, 805.7, 805.8, 805.9, 806.00, 806.01, 806.02, 806.03, 806.04, 806.05, 806.06, 806.07, 806.08, 806.09, 806.10, 806.11, 806.12, 806.13, 806.14, 806.15, 806.16, 806.17, 806.18, 806.19, 806.20, 806.21, 806.22, 806.23, 806.24, 806.25, 806.26, 806.27, 806.28, 806.29, 806.30, 806.31, 806.32, 806.33, 806.34, 806.35, 806.36, 806.37, 806.38, 806.39, 806.4, 806.5, 806.60, 806.61, 806.62, 806.69, 806.70, 806.71, 806.72, 806.79, 806.8, 806.9, 807.04, 807.05, 807.06, 807.07, 807.08, 807.09, 807.10, 807.11, 807.12, 807.13, 807.14, 807.15, 807.16, 807.17, 807.18, 807.19, 807.2, 807.3, 807.4, 807.5, 807.6, 808.0, 808.1, 808.2, 808.3, 808.43, 808.49, 808.51, 808.52, 808.53, 808.59, 808.8, 808.9, 820.00, 820.01, 820.02, 820.03, 820.09, 820.10, 820.11, 820.12, 820.13, 820.19, 820.20, 820.21, 820.22, 820.30, 820.31, 820.32, 820.8, 820.9, 821.00, 821.01, 821.10, 821.11, 839.00, 839.01, 839.02, 839.03, 839.04, 839.05, 839.06, 839.07, 839.08, 839.10, 839.11, 839.12, 839.13, 839.14, 839.15, 839.16, 839.17, 839.18, 850.0, 850.11, 850.12, 850.2, 850.3, 850.4, 850.5, 850.9, 851.00, 851.01, 851.02, 851.03, 851.04, 851.05, 851.06, 851.09, 851.10, 851.11, 851.12, 851.13, 851.14, 851.15, 851.16, 851.19, 851.20, 851.21, 851.22, 851.23, 851.24, 851.25, 851.26, 851.29, 851.30, 851.31, 851.32, 851.33, 851.34, 851.35, 851.36, 851.39, 851.40, 851.41, 851.42, 851.43, 851.44, 851.45, 851.46, 851.49, 851.50, 851.51, 851.52, 851.53, 851.54, 851.55, 851.56, 851.59, 851.60, 851.61, 851.62, 851.63, 851.64, 851.65, 851.66, 851.69, 851.70, 851.71, 851.72, 851.73, 851.74, 851.75, 851.76, 851.79, 851.80, 851.81, 851.82, 851.83, 851.84, 851.85, 851.86, 851.89, 851.90, 851.91, 851.92, 851.93, 851.94, 851.95, 851.96, 851.99, 852.00, 852.01, 852.02, 852.03, 852.04, 852.05, 852.06, 852.09, 852.10, 852.11, 852.12, 852.13, 852.14, 852.15, 852.16, 852.19, 852.20, 852.21, 852.22, 852.23, 852.24, 852.25, 852.26, 852.29, 852.30, 852.31, 852.32, 852.33, 852.34, 852.35, 852.36, 852.39, 852.40, 852.41, 852.42, 852.43, 852.44, 852.45, 852.46, 852.49, 852.50, 852.51, 852.52, 852.53, 852.54, 852.55, 852.56, 852.59, 853.00, 853.01, 853.02, 853.03, 853.04, 853.05, 853.06, 853.09, 853.10, 853.11, 853.12, 853.13, 853.14, 853.15, 853.16, 853.19, 854.00, 854.01, 854.02, 854.03, 854.04, 854.05, 854.06, 854.09, 854.10, 854.11, 854.12, 854.13, 854.14, 854.15, 854.16, 854.19, 860.0, 860.1, 860.2, 860.3, 860.4, 860.5, 861.01, 861.02, 861.03, 861.10, 861.11, 861.12, 861.13, 861.22, 861.30, 861.31, 861.32, 862.1, 862.21, 862.22, 862.29, 862.31, 862.32, 862.39, 862.9, 863.1, 863.30, 863.31, 863.39, 863.50, 863.51, 863.52, 863.53, 863.54, 863.55, 863.56, 863.59, 863.90, 863.91, 863.92, 863.93, 863.94, 863.95, 863.99, 864.00, 864.01, 864.02, 864.03, 864.04, 864.05, 864.09, 864.10, 864.11, 864.12, 864.13, 864.14, 864.15, 864.19, 865.00, 865.01, 865.02, 865.03, 865.04, 865.09, 865.10, 865.11, 865.12, 865.13, 865.14, 865.19, 866.00, 866.01, 866.02, 866.03, 866.10, 866.11, 866.12, 866.13, 867.0, 867.1, 867.2, 867.3, 867.4, 867.5, 867.6, 867.7, 867.8, 867.9, 868.00, 868.01, 868.02, 868.03, 868.04, 868.09, 868.10, 868.11, 868.12, 868.13, 868.14, 868.19, 869.0, 869.1, 870.3, 870.4, 870.8, 870.9, 871.0, 871.1, 871.2, 871.3, 871.4, 871.9, 872.72, 872.73, 872.74, 873.33, 873.9, 874.00, 874.01, 874.02, 874.10, 874.11, 874.12, 874.3, 874.5, 875.0, 875.1, 887.0, 887.1, 887.2, 887.3, 887.4, 887.5, 887.6, 887.7, 896.0, 896.1, 896.2, 896.3, 897.0, 897.1, 897.2, 897.3, 897.4, 897.5, 897.6, 897.7, 900.00, 900.01, 900.02, 900.03, 900.1, 900.81, 900.82, 900.89, 900.9, 901.0, 901.1, 901.2, 901.3, 901.41 901.42, 901.83, 902.0, 902.10, 902.11, 902.19, 902.20, 902.22, 902.23, 902.24, 902.25, 902.26, 902.27, 902.29, 902.31, 902.32, 902.33, 902.34, 902.39, 902.40, 902.41, 902.42, 902.49, 902.50, 902.51, 902.52, 902.53, 902.54, 902.59, 902.87, 925.1, 925.2, 929.0, 952.00, 952.01, 952.02, 952.03, 952.04, 952.05, 952.06, 952.07, 952.08, 952.09, 952.10, 952.11, 952.12, 952.13, 952.14, 952.15, 952.16, 952.17, 952.18, 952.19, 952.2, 952.3, 952.4, 952.8, 952.9, 953.0, 953.1, 953.2, 953.3, 953.4, 953.5, 953.8, 953.9, 958.0, 958.1, 958.2, 958.3, 958.4, 958.5, 958.7

958.91 Traumatic compartment syndrome of upper extremity

Traumatic compartment syndrome of shoulder, arm, forearm, wrist, hand, and fingers

C&C Exclusions: See 958.90

958.92 Traumatic compartment syndrome of lower extremity

Traumatic compartment syndrome of hip, buttock, thigh, leg, foot, and toes

C&C Exclusions: See 958.90

958.93 Traumatic compartment syndrome of abdomen

C&C Exclusions: See 958.90

AHA: 4Q 2006, 102

958.99 Traumatic compartment syndrome of other sites

C&C Exclusions: See 958.90

❹ 959 Injury, other and unspecified

Includes injury NOS

Excludes *injury NOS of:*
- *blood vessels (900.0-904.9)*
- *eye (921.0-921.9)*
- *internal organs (860.0-869.1)*
- *intracranial sites (854.0-854.1)*
- *nerves (950.0-951.9, 953.0-957.9)*
- *spinal cord (952.0-952.9)*

❺ 959.0 Head, face and neck

959.01 Head injury, unspecified ❷

Excludes *concussion (850.0-850.9)*
- *with head injury NOS (850.0-850.9)*

head injury NOS with loss of consciousness (850.1-850.5)

specified head injuries (850.0-854.1)

C&C Exclusions: 850.11, 850.12

AHA: 4Q 1997, 46

959.09 Injury of face and neck ❷

C&C Exclusions: See 959.01

AHA: 4Q 1997, 46

959.1 Trunk
Excludes *scapular region (959.2)*
AHA: 4Q 2003, 78; 1Q 1999, 10

959.11 Other injury of chest wall
C&C Exclusions: 805.00, 805.01, 805.02, 805.03, 805.04, 805.05, 805.06, 805.07, 805.08, 805.10, 805.11, 805.12, 805.13, 805.14, 805.15, 805.16, 805.17, 805.18, 805.2, 805.3, 805.4, 805.5, 805.6, 805.7, 805.8, 805.9, 806.00, 806.01, 806.02, 806.03, 806.04, 806.05, 806.06, 806.07, 806.08, 806.09, 806.10, 806.11, 806.12, 806.13, 806.14, 806.15, 806.16, 806.17, 806.18, 806.19, 806.20, 806.21, 806.22, 806.23, 806.24, 806.25, 806.26, 806.27, 806.28, 806.29, 806.30, 806.31, 806.32, 806.33, 806.34, 806.35, 806.36, 806.37, 806.38, 806.39, 806.4, 806.5, 806.60, 806.61, 806.62, 806.69, 806.70, 806.71, 806.72, 806.79, 806.8, 806.9, 952.00, 952.01, 952.02, 952.03, 952.04, 952.05, 952.06, 952.07, 952.08, 952.09, 952.10, 952.11, 952.12, 952.13, 952.14, 952.15, 952.16, 952.17, 952.18, 952.19, 952.2, 952.3, 952.4, 952.8, 952.9

959.12 Other injury of abdomen
C&C Exclusions: See 959.11

959.13 Fracture of corpus cavernosum penis ♂
C&C Exclusions: See 959.11

959.14 Other injury of external genitals
C&C Exclusions: See 959.11

959.19 Other injury of other sites of trunk
Injury of trunk NOS
C&C Exclusions: See 959.11

959.2 Shoulder and upper arm
Axilla
Scapular region

959.3 Elbow, forearm, and wrist
AHA: 1Q 1997, 8

959.4 Hand, except finger

959.5 Finger
Fingernail
Thumb (nail)

959.6 Hip and thigh
Upper leg

959.7 Knee, leg, ankle, and foot

959.8 Other specified sites, including multiple
Excludes *multiple sites classifiable to the same four-digit category (959.0-959.7)*
C&C Exclusions: 850.11, 850.12

✖ **959.9 Unspecified site**
C&C Exclusions: See 959.8

POISONING BY DRUGS, MEDICINAL AND BIOLOGICAL SUBSTANCES (960-979)

Includes overdose of these substances
wrong substance given or taken in error

Excludes *adverse effects ["hypersensitivity," "reaction," etc.] of correct substance properly administered. Such cases are to be classified according to the nature of the adverse effect, such as:*
adverse effect NOS (995.20)
allergic lymphadenitis (289.3)
aspirin gastritis (535.4)
blood disorders (280.0-289.9)
dermatitis:
contact (692.0-692.9)
due to ingestion (693.0-693.9)
nephropathy (583.9)
[The drug giving rise to the adverse effect may be identified by use of categories E930-E949.]
drug dependence (304.0-304.9)
drug reaction and poisoning affecting the newborn (760.0-779.9)
nondependent abuse of drugs (305.0-305.9)
pathological drug intoxication (292.2)

Use additional code to specify the effects of the poisoning
AHA: 2Q 1990, 11

960 Poisoning by antibiotics
Excludes *antibiotics:*
ear, nose, and throat (976.6)
eye (976.5)
local (976.0)

960.0 Penicillins
Ampicillin
Carbenicillin
Cloxacillin
Penicillin G

960.1 Antifungal antibiotics
Amphotericin B
Griseofulvin
Nystatin
Trichomycin
Excludes *preparations intended for topical use (976.0-976.9)*

960.2 Chloramphenicol group
Chloramphenicol
Thiamphenicol

960.3 Erythromycin and other macrolides
Oleandomycin
Spiramycin

960.4 Tetracycline group
Doxycycline
Minocycline
Oxytetracycline

960.5 Cephalosporin group
Cephalexin
Cephaloglycin
Cephaloridine
Cephalothin

960.6 Antimycobacterial antibiotics
Cycloserine
Kanamycin
Rifampin
Streptomycin

960.7 Antineoplastic antibiotics
Actinomycin such as:
Bleomycin
Cactinomycin
Dactinomycin
Daunorubicin
Mitomycin

960.8 Other specified antibiotics

✖ **960.9 Unspecified antibiotic**

961 Poisoning by other anti-infectives

Excludes anti-infectives:
ear, nose, and throat (976.6)
eye (976.5)
local (976.0)

961.0 Sulfonamides
Sulfadiazine
Sulfafurazole
Sulfamethoxazole

961.1 Arsenical anti-infectives

961.2 Heavy metal anti-infectives
Compounds of:
antimony
bismuth
lead
mercury
Excludes mercurial diuretics (974.0)

961.3 Quinoline and hydroxyquinoline derivatives
Chiniofon
Diiodohydroxyquin
Excludes antimalarial drugs (961.4)

961.4 Antimalarials and drugs acting on other blood protozoa
Chloroquine
Cycloguanil
Primaquine
Proguanil [chloroguanide]
Pyrimethamine
Quinine

961.5 Other antiprotozoal drugs
Emetine

961.6 Anthelmintics
Hexylresorcinol
Piperazine
Thiabendazole

961.7 Antiviral drugs
Methisazone
Excludes amantadine (966.4)
cytarabine (963.1)
idoxuridine (976.5)

961.8 Other antimycobacterial drugs
Ethambutol
Ethionamide
Isoniazid
Para-aminosalicylic acid derivatives
Sulfones

961.9 Other and unspecified anti-infectives
Flucytosine
Nitrofuran derivatives

962 Poisoning by hormones and synthetic substitutes

Excludes oxytocic hormones (975.0)

962.0 Adrenal cortical steroids
Cortisone derivatives
Desoxycorticosterone derivatives
Fluorinated corticosteroids

962.1 Androgens and anabolic congeners
Methandriol
Nandrolone
Oxymetholone
Testosterone

962.2 Ovarian hormones and synthetic substitutes
Contraceptives, oral
Estrogens
Estrogens and progestogens, combined
Progestogens

962.3 Insulins and antidiabetic agents
Acetohexamide
Biguanide derivatives, oral
Chlorpropamide
Glucagon
Insulin
Phenformin
Sulfonylurea derivatives, oral
Tolbutamide
AHA: Mar-Apr 1985, 8

962.4 Anterior pituitary hormones
Corticotropin
Gonadotropin
Somatotropin [growth hormone]

962.5 Posterior pituitary hormones
Vasopressin
Excludes oxytocic hormones (975.0)

962.6 Parathyroid and parathyroid derivatives

962.7 Thyroid and thyroid derivatives
Dextrothyroxin
Levothyroxine sodium
Liothyronine
Thyroglobulin

962.8 Antithyroid agents
Iodides
Thiouracil
Thiourea

962.9 Other and unspecified hormones and synthetic substitutes

963 Poisoning by primarily systemic agents

963.0 Antiallergic and antiemetic drugs
Antihistamines
Chlorpheniramine
Diphenhydramine
Diphenylpyraline
Thonzylamine
Tripelennamine
Excludes phenothiazine-based tranquilizers (969.1)

963.1 Antineoplastic and immunosuppressive drugs
Azathioprine
Busulfan
Chlorambucil
Cyclophosphamide
Cytarabine
Fluorouracil
Mercaptopurine
thio-TEPA
Excludes antineoplastic antibiotics (960.7)

963.2 Acidifying agents

963.3 Alkalizing agents

963.4 Enzymes, not elsewhere classified
Penicillinase

963.5 Vitamins, not elsewhere classified
Vitamin A
Vitamin D
Excludes nicotinic acid (972.2)
vitamin K (964.3)

963.8 Other specified systemic agents
Heavy metal antagonists

963.9 Unspecified systemic agent

964 Poisoning by agents primarily affecting blood constituents

964.0 Iron and its compounds
Ferric salts
Ferrous sulfate and other ferrous salts

964.1 Liver preparations and other antianemic agents
Folic acid

964.2 Anticoagulants
Coumarin
Heparin
Phenindione
Warfarin sodium

964.3 Vitamin K [phytonadione]

964.4 Fibrinolysis-affecting drugs
Aminocaproic acid
Streptodornase
Streptokinase
Urokinase

964.5 Anticoagulant antagonists and other coagulants
Hexadimethrine
Protamine sulfate

964.6 Gamma globulin

Injury and Poisoning 961 – 964.6

964.7 Natural blood and blood products
Blood plasma
Human fibrinogen
Packed red cells
Whole blood
Excludes *transfusion reactions (999.4-999.8)*

964.8 Other specified agents affecting blood constituents
Macromolecular blood substitutes
Plasma expanders

✖ **964.9 Unspecified agents affecting blood constituents**

④ **965 Poisoning by analgesics, antipyretics, and antirheumatics**
Use additional code to identify:
drug dependence (304.0-304.9)
nondependent abuse (305.0-305.9)

⑤ **965.0 Opiates and related narcotics**

965.00 Opium (alkaloids), unspecified

965.01 Heroin
Diacetylmorphine

965.02 Methadone

965.09 Other
Codeine [methylmorphine]
Meperidine [pethidine]
Morphine

965.1 Salicylates
Acetylsalicylic acid [aspirin]
Salicylic acid salts

965.4 Aromatic analgesics, not elsewhere classified
Acetanilid
Paracetamol [acetaminophen]
Phenacetin [acetophenetidin]

965.5 Pyrazole derivatives
Aminophenazone [aminopyrine]
Phenylbutazone

⑤ **965.6 Antirheumatics [antiphlogistics]**
Excludes *salicylates (965.1)*
steroids (962.0-962.9)

AHA: 4Q 1998, 50

965.61 Propionic acid derivatives
Fenoprofen
Flurbiprofen
Ibuprofen
Ketoprofen
Naproxen
Oxaprozin

AHA: 4Q 1998, 50

965.69 Other antirheumatics
Gold salts
Indomethacin

965.7 Other non-narcotic analgesics
Pyrabital

965.8 Other specified analgesics and antipyretics
Pentazocine

✖ **965.9 Unspecified analgesic and antipyretic**

④ **966 Poisoning by anticonvulsants and anti-Parkinsonism drugs**

966.0 Oxazolidine derivatives
Paramethadione
Trimethadione

966.1 Hydantoin derivatives
Phenytoin

966.2 Succinimides
Ethosuximide
Phensuximide

966.3 Other and unspecified anticonvulsants
Primidone
Excludes *barbiturates (967.0)*
sulfonamides (961.0)

966.4 Anti-Parkinsonism drugs
Amantadine
Ethopropazine [profenamine]
Levodopa [L-dopa]

④ **967 Poisoning by sedatives and hypnotics**
Use additional code to identify:
drug dependence (304.0-304.9)
nondependent abuse (305.0-305.9)

967.0 Barbiturates
Amobarbital [amylobarbitone]
Barbital [barbitone]
Butabarbital [butabarbitone]
Pentobarbital [pentobarbitone]
Phenobarbital [phenobarbitone]
Secobarbital [quinalbarbitone]
Excludes *thiobarbiturate anesthetics (968.3)*

967.1 Chloral hydrate group

967.2 Paraldehyde

967.3 Bromine compounds
Bromide
Carbromal (derivatives)

967.4 Methaqualone compounds

967.5 Glutethimide group

967.6 Mixed sedatives, not elsewhere classified

967.8 Other sedatives and hypnotics

✖ **967.9 Unspecified sedative or hypnotic**
Sleeping:
drug NOS
pill NOS
tablet NOS

④ **968 Poisoning by other central nervous system depressants and anesthetics**
Use additional code to identify:
drug dependence (304.0-304.9)
nondependent abuse (305.0-305.9)

968.0 Central nervous system muscle-tone depressants
Chlorphenesin (carbamate)
Mephenesin
Methocarbamol

968.1 Halothane

968.2 Other gaseous anesthetics
Ether
Halogenated hydrocarbon derivatives, except halothane
Nitrous oxide

968.3 Intravenous anesthetics
Ketamine
Methohexital [methohexitone]
Thiobarbiturates, such as thiopental sodium

968.4 Other and unspecified general anesthetics

968.5 Surface [topical] and infiltration anesthetics
Cocaine
Lidocaine [lignocaine]
Procaine
Tetracaine

AHA: 1Q 1993, 25

968.6 Peripheral nerve- and plexus-blocking anesthetics

968.7 Spinal anesthetics

968.9 Other and unspecified local anesthetics

④ **969 Poisoning by psychotropic agents**
Use additional code to identify:
drug dependence (304.0-304.9)
nondependent abuse (305.0-305.9)

969.0 Antidepressants
Amitriptyline
Imipramine
Monoamine oxidase [MAO] inhibitors

969.1 Phenothiazine-based tranquilizers
Chlorpromazine
Fluphenazine
Prochlorperazine
Promazine

969.2 Butyrophenone-based tranquilizers
Haloperidol
Spiperone
Trifluperidol

969.3 Other antipsychotics, neuroleptics, and major tranquilizers

969.4 Benzodiazepine-based tranquilizers
Chlordiazepoxide
Diazepam
Flurazepam
Lorazepam
Medazepam
Nitrazepam

969.5 Other tranquilizers
Hydroxyzine
Meprobamate

969.6 Psychodysleptics [hallucinogens]
Cannabis (derivatives)
Lysergide [LSD]
Marihuana (derivatives)
Mescaline
Psilocin
Psilocybin

969.7 Psychostimulants
Amphetamine
Caffeine
Excludes *central appetite depressants (977.0)*
AHA: 2Q 2003, 11

969.8 Other specified psychotropic agents

969.9 Unspecified psychotropic agent

970 Poisoning by central nervous system stimulants

970.0 Analeptics
Lobeline
Nikethamide

970.1 Opiate antagonists
Levallorphan
Nalorphine
Naloxone

970.8 Other specified central nervous system stimulants
AHA: 1Q 2005, 6

970.9 Unspecified central nervous system stimulant

971 Poisoning by drugs primarily affecting the autonomic nervous system

971.0 Parasympathomimetics [cholinergics]
Acetylcholine
Anticholinesterase:
organophosphorus
reversible
Pilocarpine

971.1 Parasympatholytics [anticholinergics and antimuscarinics] and spasmolytics
Atropine
Homatropine
Hyoscine [scopolamine]
Quaternary ammonium derivatives
Excludes *papaverine (972.5)*

971.2 Sympathomimetics [adrenergics]
Epinephrine [adrenalin]
Levarterenol [noradrenalin]

971.3 Sympatholytics [antiadrenergics]
Phenoxybenzamine
Tolazoline hydrochloride

971.9 Unspecified drug primarily affecting autonomic nervous system

972 Poisoning by agents primarily affecting the cardiovascular system

972.0 Cardiac rhythm regulators
Practolol
Procainamide
Propranolol
Quinidine
Excludes *lidocaine (968.5)*

972.1 Cardiotonic glycosides and drugs of similar action
Digitalis glycosides
Digoxin
Strophanthins

972.2 Antilipemic and antiarteriosclerotic drugs
Clofibrate
Nicotinic acid derivatives

972.3 Ganglion-blocking agents
Pentamethonium bromide

972.4 Coronary vasodilators
Dipyridamole
Nitrates [nitroglycerin]
Nitrites

972.5 Other vasodilators
Cyclandelate
Diazoxide
Papaverine
Excludes *nicotinic acid (972.2)*

972.6 Other antihypertensive agents
Clonidine
Guanethidine
Rauwolfia alkaloids
Reserpine

972.7 Antivaricose drugs, including sclerosing agents
Sodium morrhuate
Zinc salts

972.8 Capillary-active drugs
Adrenochrome derivatives
Metaraminol

972.9 Other and unspecified agents primarily affecting the cardiovascular system

973 Poisoning by agents primarily affecting the gastrointestinal system

973.0 Antacids and antigastric secretion drugs
Aluminum hydroxide
Magnesium trisilicate
AHA: 1Q 2003, 19

973.1 Irritant cathartics
Bisacodyl
Castor oil
Phenolphthalein

973.2 Emollient cathartics
Dioctyl sulfosuccinates

973.3 Other cathartics, including intestinal atonia drugs
Magnesium sulfate

973.4 Digestants
Pancreatin
Papain
Pepsin

973.5 Antidiarrheal drugs
Kaolin
Pectin
Excludes *anti-infectives (960.0-961.9)*

973.6 Emetics

973.8 Other specified agents primarily affecting the gastrointestinal system

973.9 Unspecified agent primarily affecting the gastrointestinal system

974 Poisoning by water, mineral, and uric acid metabolism drugs

974.0 Mercurial diuretics
Chlormerodrin
Mercaptomerin
Mersalyl

974.1 Purine derivative diuretics
Theobromine
Theophylline
Excludes *aminophylline [theophylline ethylenediamine] (975.7)*
caffeine (969.7)

974.2 Carbonic acid anhydrase inhibitors
Acetazolamide

974.3 Saluretics
Benzothiadiazides
Chlorothiazide group

974.4 Other diuretics
Ethacrynic acid
Furosemide

974.5 Electrolytic, caloric, and water-balance agents

974.6 Other mineral salts, not elsewhere classified

Injury and Poisoning
969.4 – 974.6

974.7 Uric acid metabolism drugs
Allopurinol
Colchicine
Probenecid

❹ **975 Poisoning by agents primarily acting on the smooth and skeletal muscles and respiratory system**

975.0 Oxytocic agents
Ergot alkaloids
Oxytocin
Prostaglandins

975.1 Smooth muscle relaxants
Adiphenine
Metaproterenol [orciprenaline]
Excludes *papaverine (972.5)*

975.2 Skeletal muscle relaxants

975.3 Other and unspecified drugs acting on muscles

975.4 Antitussives
Dextromethorphan
Pipazethate

975.5 Expectorants
Acetylcysteine
Guaifenesin
Terpin hydrate

975.6 Anti-common cold drugs

975.7 Antiasthmatics
Aminophylline [theophylline ethylenediamine]

975.8 Other and unspecified respiratory drugs

❹ **976 Poisoning by agents primarily affecting skin and mucous membrane, ophthalmological, otorhinolaryngological, and dental drugs**

976.0 Local anti-infectives and anti-inflammatory drugs

976.1 Antipruritics

976.2 Local astringents and local detergents

976.3 Emollients, demulcents, and protectants

976.4 Keratolytics, keratoplastics, other hair treatment drugs and preparations

976.5 Eye anti-infectives and other eye drugs
Idoxuridine

976.6 Anti-infectives and other drugs and preparations for ear, nose, and throat

976.7 Dental drugs topically applied
Excludes *anti-infectives (976.0)*
local anesthetics (968.5)

976.8 Other agents primarily affecting skin and mucous membrane
Spermicides [vaginal contraceptives]

✖ **976.9 Unspecified agent primarily affecting skin and mucous membrane**

❹ **977 Poisoning by other and unspecified drugs and medicinal substances**

977.0 Dietetics
Central appetite depressants

977.1 Lipotropic drugs

977.2 Antidotes and chelating agents, not elsewhere classified

977.3 Alcohol deterrents

977.4 Pharmaceutical excipients
Pharmaceutical adjuncts

977.8 Other specified drugs and medicinal substances
Contrast media used for diagnostic x-ray procedures
Diagnostic agents and kits

✖ **977.9 Unspecified drug or medicinal substance**

❹ **978 Poisoning by bacterial vaccines**

978.0 BCG

978.1 Typhoid and paratyphoid

978.2 Cholera

978.3 Plague

978.4 Tetanus

978.5 Diphtheria

978.6 Pertussis vaccine, including combinations with a pertussis component

978.8 Other and unspecified bacterial vaccines

978.9 Mixed bacterial vaccines, except combinations with a pertussis component

❹ **979 Poisoning by other vaccines and biological substances**
Excludes *gamma globulin (964.6)*

979.0 Smallpox vaccine

979.1 Rabies vaccine

979.2 Typhus vaccine

979.3 Yellow fever vaccine

979.4 Measles vaccine

979.5 Poliomyelitis vaccine

979.6 Other and unspecified viral and rickettsial vaccines
Mumps vaccine

979.7 Mixed viral-rickettsial and bacterial vaccines, except combinations with a pertussis component
Excludes *combinations with a pertussis component (978.6)*

979.9 Other and unspecified vaccines and biological substances

TOXIC EFFECTS OF SUBSTANCES CHIEFLY NONMEDICINAL AS TO SOURCE (980-989)

Excludes *burns from chemical agents (ingested) (947.0-947.9)*
localized toxic effects indexed elsewhere (001.0-799.9)
respiratory conditions due to external agents (506.0-508.9)

Use additional code to specify the nature of the toxic effect

❹ **980 Toxic effect of alcohol**

980.0 Ethyl alcohol
Denatured alcohol
Ethanol
Grain alcohol
Use additional code to identify any associated:
acute alcohol intoxication (305.0)
in alcoholism (303.0)
drunkenness (simple) (305.0)
pathological (291.4)

AHA: 3Q 1996, 16

980.1 Methyl alcohol
Methanol
Wood alcohol

980.2 Isopropyl alcohol
Dimethyl carbinol
Isopropanol
Rubbing alcohol

980.3 Fusel oil
Alcohol:
amyl
butyl
propyl

980.8 Other specified alcohols

✖ **980.9 Unspecified alcohol**

981 Toxic effect of petroleum products
Benzine
Gasoline
Kerosene
Paraffin wax
Petroleum:
ether
naphtha
spirit

❹ **982 Toxic effect of solvents other than petroleum based**

982.0 Benzene and homologues

982.1 Carbon tetrachloride

982.2 Carbon disulfide
Carbon bisulfide

982.3 Other chlorinated hydrocarbon solvents
Tetrachloroethylene
Trichloroethylene
Excludes *chlorinated hydrocarbon preparations other than solvents (989.2)*

982.4 Nitroglycol

982.8 Other nonpetroleum-based solvents
Acetone

❹ **983 Toxic effect of corrosive aromatics, acids, and caustic alkalis**

983.0 Corrosive aromatics
Carbolic acid or phenol
Cresol

983.1 Acids
Acid:
hydrochloric
nitric
sulfuric

983.2 Caustic alkalis
Lye
Potassium hydroxide
Sodium hydroxide

983.9 Caustic, unspecified

❹ **984 Toxic effect of lead and its compounds (including fumes)**
Includes that from all sources except medicinal substances

984.0 Inorganic lead compounds
Lead dioxide
Lead salts

984.1 Organic lead compounds
Lead acetate
Tetraethyl lead

984.8 Other lead compounds

✖ **984.9 Unspecified lead compound**

❹ **985 Toxic effect of other metals**
Includes that from all sources except medicinal substances

985.0 Mercury and its compounds
Minamata disease

985.1 Arsenic and its compounds

985.2 Manganese and its compounds

985.3 Beryllium and its compounds

985.4 Antimony and its compounds

985.5 Cadmium and its compounds

985.6 Chromium

985.8 Other specified metals
Brass fumes
Copper salts
Iron compounds
Nickel compounds
AHA: 1Q 1988, 5

✖ **985.9 Unspecified metal**

986 Toxic effect of carbon monoxide

❹ **987 Toxic effect of other gases, fumes, or vapors**

987.0 Liquefied petroleum gases
Butane
Propane

987.1 Other hydrocarbon gas

987.2 Nitrogen oxides
Nitrogen dioxide
Nitrous fumes

987.3 Sulfur dioxide

987.4 Freon
Dichloromonofluoromethane

987.5 Lacrimogenic gas
Bromobenzyl cyanide
Chloroacetophenone
Ethyliodoacetate

987.6 Chlorine gas

987.7 Hydrocyanic acid gas

987.8 Other specified gases, fumes, or vapors
Phosgene
Polyester fumes

987.9 Unspecified gas, fume, or vapor
AHA: 3Q 2005, 10

❹ **988 Toxic effect of noxious substances eaten as food**
Excludes *allergic reaction to food, such as:*
gastroenteritis (558.3)
rash (692.5, 693.1)
food poisoning (bacterial) (005.0-005.9)
toxic effects of food contaminants, such as:
aflatoxin and other mycotoxin (989.7)
mercury (985.0)

988.0 Fish and shellfish

988.1 Mushrooms

988.2 Berries and other plants

988.8 Other specified noxious substances eaten as food

✖ **988.9 Unspecified noxious substance eaten as food**

❹ **989 Toxic effect of other substances, chiefly nonmedicinal as to source**

989.0 Hydrocyanic acid and cyanides
Potassium cyanide
Sodium cyanide
Excludes *gas and fumes (987.7)*

989.1 Strychnine and salts

989.2 Chlorinated hydrocarbons
Aldrin
Chlordane
DDT
Dieldrin
Excludes *chlorinated hydrocarbon solvents (982.0-982.3)*

989.3 Organophosphate and carbamate
Carbaryl
Dichlorvos
Malathion
Parathion
Phorate
Phosdrin

989.4 Other pesticides, not elsewhere classified
Mixtures of insecticides

989.5 Venom
Bites of venomous snakes, lizards, and spiders
Tick paralysis

989.6 Soaps and detergents

989.7 Aflatoxin and other mycotoxin [food contaminants]

❺ **989.8 Other substances, chiefly nonmedicinal as to source**
AHA: 4Q 1995, 60

989.81 Asbestos
Excludes *asbestosis (501)*
exposure to asbestos (V15.84)

989.82 Latex

989.83 Silicone
Excludes *silicone used in medical devices, implants and grafts (996.00-996.79)*

989.84 Tobacco

989.89 Other

✖ **989.9 Unspecified substance, chiefly nonmedicinal as to source**

OTHER AND UNSPECIFIED EFFECTS OF EXTERNAL CAUSES (990-995)

990 Effects of radiation, unspecified
Complication of:
phototherapy
radiation therapy
Radiation sickness
Excludes *specified adverse effects of radiation. Such conditions are to be classified according to the nature of the adverse effect, as:*
burns (940.0-949.5)
dermatitis (692.7-692.8)
leukemia (204.0-208.9)
pneumonia (508.0)
sunburn (692.71, 692.76-692.77)
[The type of radiation giving rise to the adverse effect may be identified by use of the E codes.]

❹ **991 Effects of reduced temperature**

991.0 Frostbite of face

991.1 Frostbite of hand

991.2 Frostbite of foot

991.3 Frostbite of other and unspecified sites

991.4 Immersion foot
Trench foot

991.5 Chilblains
Erythema pernio
Perniosis

991.6 Hypothermia
Hypothermia (accidental)
Excludes *hypothermia following anesthesia (995.89)*
hypothermia not associated with low environmental temperature (780.99)

991.8 Other specified effects of reduced temperature

991.9 Unspecified effect of reduced temperature
Effects of freezing or excessive cold NOS

❹ **992 Effects of heat and light**
Excludes *burns (940.0-949.5)*
diseases of sweat glands due to heat (705.0-705.9)
malignant hyperpyrexia following anesthesia (995.86)
sunburn (692.71, 692.76-692.77)

992.0 Heat stroke and sunstroke
Heat apoplexy
Heat pyrexia
Ictus solaris
Siriasis
Thermoplegia

992.1 Heat syncope
Heat collapse
DEF: Prolonged heat exposure causing the patient to faint.

992.2 Heat cramps

992.3 Heat exhaustion, anhydrotic
Heat prostration due to water depletion
Excludes *that associated with salt depletion (992.4)*

992.4 Heat exhaustion due to salt depletion
Heat prostration due to salt (and water) depletion

992.5 Heat exhaustion, unspecified
Heat prostration NOS

992.6 Heat fatigue, transient

992.7 Heat edema

992.8 Other specified heat effects

✖ **992.9 Unspecified**

❹ **993 Effects of air pressure**

993.0 Barotrauma, otitic
Aero-otitis media
Effects of high altitude on ears

993.1 Barotrauma, sinus
Aerosinusitis
Effects of high altitude on sinuses

993.2 Other and unspecified effects of high altitude
Alpine sickness
Andes disease
Anoxia due to high altitude
Hypobaropathy
Mountain sickness
AHA: 3Q 1988, 4

993.3 Caisson disease
Bends
Compressed-air disease
Decompression sickness
Divers' palsy or paralysis

993.4 Effects of air pressure caused by explosion

993.8 Other specified effects of air pressure

✖ **993.9 Unspecified effect of air pressure**

❹ **994 Effects of other external causes**
Excludes *certain adverse effects not elsewhere classified (995.0-995.8)*

994.0 Effects of lightning
Shock from lightning
Struck by lightning NOS
Excludes *burns (940.0-949.5)*

994.1 Drowning and nonfatal submersion
Bathing cramp
Immersion
AHA: 3Q 1988, 4

994.2 Effects of hunger
Deprivation of food
Starvation

994.3 Effects of thirst
Deprivation of water

994.4 Exhaustion due to exposure

994.5 Exhaustion due to excessive exertion
Overexertion

994.6 Motion sickness
Air sickness
Seasickness
Travel sickness

994.7 Asphyxiation and strangulation
Suffocation (by):
bedclothes
cave-in
constriction
mechanical
plastic bag
pressure
strangulation
Excludes *asphyxia from:*
carbon monoxide (986)
inhalation of food or foreign body (932-934.9)
other gases, fumes, and vapors (987.0-987.9)

994.8 Electrocution and nonfatal effects of electric current
Shock from electric current
Excludes *electric burns (940.0-949.5)*

994.9 Other effects of external causes
Effects of:
abnormal gravitational [G] forces or states
weightlessness

4 995 Certain adverse effects not elsewhere classified
Excludes *complications of surgical and medical care (996.0-999.9)*

995.0 Other anaphylactic shock
Allergic shock NOS or due to adverse effect of correct medicinal substance properly administered
Anaphylactic reaction NOS or due to adverse effect of correct medicinal substance properly administered
Anaphylaxis NOS or due to adverse effect of correct medicinal substance properly administered
Excludes *anaphylactic reaction to serum (999.4)*
anaphylactic shock due to adverse food reaction (995.60-995.69)
Use additional E code to identify external cause, such as:
adverse effects of correct medicinal substance properly administered [E930-E949]
AHA: 4Q 1993, 30

995.1 Angioneurotic edema
Giant urticaria
Excludes *urticaria:*
due to serum (999.5)
other specified (698.2, 708.0-708.9, 757.33)

5 995.2 Other and unspecified adverse effect of drug, medicinal and biological substance
Adverse effect to correct medicinal substance properly administered
Allergic reaction to correct medicinal substance properly administered
Drug:
hypersensitivity NOS
reaction NOS
Hypersensitivity to correct medicinal substance properly administered
Idiosyncrasy due to correct medicinal substance properly administered
Excludes *pathological drug intoxication (292.2)*
AHA: 2Q 1997, 12; 3Q 1995, 13; 3Q 1992, 16

✖ **995.20 Unspecified adverse effect of unspecified drug, medicinal and biological substance**

995.21 Arthus phenomenon
Arthus reaction

✖ **995.22 Unspecified adverse effect of anesthesia**

✖ **995.23 Unspecified adverse effect of insulin**

995.27 Other drug allergy
Drug allergy NOS
Drug hypersensitivity NOS

✖ **995.29 Unspecified adverse effect of other drug, medicinal and biological substance**

995.3 Allergy, unspecified
Allergic reaction NOS
Hypersensitivity NOS
Idiosyncrasy NOS
Excludes *allergic reaction NOS to correct medicinal substance properly administered (995.27)*
allergy to existing dental restorative materials (525.66)
specific types of allergic reaction, such as:
allergic diarrhea (558.3)
dermatitis (691.0-693.9)
hayfever (477.0-477.9)

995.4 Shock due to anesthesia
Shock due to anesthesia in which the correct substance was properly administered
Excludes *complications of anesthesia in labor or delivery (668.0-668.9)*
overdose or wrong substance given (968.0-969.9)
postoperative shock NOS (998.0)
specified adverse effects of anesthesia classified elsewhere, such as:
anoxic brain damage (348.1)
hepatitis (070.0-070.9), etc.
unspecified adverse effect of anesthesia (995.22)
C&C Exclusions: 958.4, 995.4, 997.91, 997.99, 998.0, 998.11, 998.12, 998.13, 998.81, 998.83, 998.89, 998.9

5 995.5 Child maltreatment syndrome
Use additional code(s), if applicable, to identify any associated injuries
Use additional E code to identify:
nature of abuse (E960-E968)
perpetrator (E967.0-E967.9)
AHA: 1Q 1998, 11

✖ **995.50 Child abuse, unspecified** P

995.51 Child emotional/psychological abuse P
AHA: 4Q 1996, 38, 40

995.52 Child neglect (nutritional) P
Use additional code to identify intent of neglect (E904.0, E968.4)
AHA: 4Q 1996, 38, 40

995.53 Child sexual abuse P
AHA: 4Q 1996, 39, 40

995.54 Child physical abuse P
Battered baby or child syndrome
Excludes *shaken infant syndrome (995.55)*
AHA: 3Q 1999, 14; 4Q 1996, 39, 40

995.55 Shaken infant syndrome P
Use additional code(s) to identify any associated injuries
AHA: 4Q 1996, 40, 43

995.59 Other child abuse and neglect P
Multiple forms of abuse
Use additional code to identify intent of neglect (E904.0, E968.4)

5 995.6 Anaphylactic shock due to adverse food reaction
Anaphylactic shock due to nonpoisonous foods
DEF: Sudden, severe allergic reaction to food causing sharp decrease in blood pressure, fainting, swelling of respiratory passages, loss of consciousness, and death without epinephrine administration.
AHA: 4Q 1993, 30

995.60 Due to unspecified food

995.61 Due to peanuts

995.62 Due to crustaceans

995.63 Due to fruits and vegetables

995.64 Due to tree nuts and seeds

995.65 Due to fish

995.66 Due to food additives

995.67 Due to milk products

995.68 Due to eggs

995.69 Due to other specified food

995.7 Other adverse food reactions, not elsewhere classified
Use additional code to identify the type of reaction, such as:
hives (708.0)
wheezing (786.07)
Excludes *anaphylactic shock due to adverse food reaction (995.6)*
asthma (493.0, 493.9)
dermatitis due to food (693.1)
in contact with the skin (692.5)
gastroenteritis and colitis due to food (558.3)
rhinitis due to food (477.1)

5 995.8 Other specified adverse effects, not elsewhere classified

995.80 Adult maltreatment, unspecified A
Abused person NOS
Use additional code to identify:
any associated injury
nature of abuse (E960-E968)
perpetrator (E967.0-E967.9)
AHA: 4Q 1996, 41, 43

995.81 Adult physical abuse A
Battered:
man
person syndrome NEC
spouse
woman
Use additional code to identify:
any associated injury
nature of abuse (E960-E968)
perpetrator (E967.0-E967.9)
AHA: 4Q 1996, 42, 43

995.82 Adult emotional/psychological abuse A
Use additional E code to identify perpetrator (E967.0-E967.9)

995.83 Adult sexual abuse A
Use additional code to identify:
any associated injury
perpetrator (E967.0-E967.9)

995.84 Adult neglect (nutritional) A
Use additional code to identify:
intent of neglect (E904.0, E968.4)
perpetrator (E967.0-E967.9)

995.85 Other adult abuse and neglect A
Multiple forms of abuse and neglect
Use additional code to identify:
any associated injury
intent of neglect (E904.0, E968.4)
nature of abuse (E960-E968)
perpetrator (E967.0-E967.9)

995.86 Malignant hyperthermia
Malignant hyperpyrexia due to anesthesia
C&C Exclusions: 958.4, 995.4, 995.86, 997.91, 997.99, 998.0, 998.11, 998.12, 998.13, 998.81, 998.83, 998.89, 998.9
AHA: 4Q 1998, 51

995.89 Other
Hypothermia due to anesthesia
AHA: 2Q 2004, 18; 3Q 2003, 12

5 995.9 Systemic inflammatory response syndrome (SIRS)
AHA: 2Q 2004, 16; 4Q 2002, 71

995.90 Systemic inflammatory response syndrome, unspecified
SIRS NOS
C&C Exclusions: 003.1, 020.2, 036.2, 038.0, 038.10, 038.11, 038.19, 038.2, 038.3, 038.40, 038.41, 038.42, 038.43, 038.44, 038.49, 038.8, 038.9, 040.82, 040.89, 041.00, 041.01, 041.02, 041.03, 041.04, 041.05, 041.09, 041.10, 041.11, 041.19, 041.2, 041.3, 041.4, 041.5, 041.6, 041.7, 041.81, 041.82, 041.83, 041.84, 041.85, 041.86, 041.89, 041.9, 054.5, 139.8, 995.90, 995.91, 995.92, 995.93, 995.94, V09.0, V09.1, V09.2, V09.3, V09.4, V09.50, V09.51, V09.6, V09.70, V09.71, V09.80, V09.81, V09.90, V09.91

995.91 Sepsis
Systemic inflammatory response syndrome due to infectious process without acute organ dysfunction
Code first underlying infection
Excludes *sepsis with acute organ dysfunction (995.92)*
sepsis with multiple organ dysfunction (995.92)
severe sepsis (995.92)
C&C Exclusions: See 995.90
AHA: 2Q 2004, 16; 4Q 2003, 79

995.92 Severe sepsis
Sepsis with acute organ dysfunction
Sepsis with multiple organ dysfunction (MOD)
Systemic inflammatory response syndrome due to infectious process with acute organ dysfunction
Code first underlying infection
Use additional code to specify acute organ dysfunction, such as:
acute renal failure (584.5-584.9)
acute respiratory failure (518.81)
critical illness myopathy (359.81)
critical illness polyneuropathy (357.82)
disseminated intravascular coagulopathy (DIC) syndrome (286.6)
encephalopathy (348.31)
hepatic failure (570)
septic shock (785.52)
C&C Exclusions: See 995.90
AHA: 2Q 2005, 18-19; 1Q 2005, 7; 2Q 2004, 16; 4Q 2003, 73, 79

995.93 Systemic inflammatory response syndrome due to non-infectious process without acute organ dysfunction
Code first underlying conditions, such as:
acute pancreatitis (577.0)
trauma
Excludes *systemic inflammatory response syndrome due to noninfectious process with acute organ dysfunction (995.94)*
C&C Exclusions: See 995.90

995.94 Systemic inflammatory response syndrome due to noninfectious process with acute organ dysfunction
Code first underlying condition, such as:
acute pancreatitis (577.0)
trauma
Use additional code to specify acute organ dysfunction, such as:
acute renal failure (584.5-584.9)
acute respiratory failure (518.81)
critical illness myopathy (359.81)
critical illness polyneuropathy (357.82)
disseminated intravascular coagulopathy (DIC) syndrome (286.6)
encephalopathy (348.31)
hepatic failure (570)
Excludes *severe sepsis (995.92)*
C&C Exclusions: See 995.90
AHA: 4Q 2003, 76

COMPLICATIONS OF SURGICAL AND MEDICAL CARE, NOT ELSEWHERE CLASSIFIED (996-999)

Excludes *adverse effects of medicinal agents (001.0-799.9, 995.0-995.8)*
burns from local applications and irradiation (940.0-949.5)
complications of:
conditions for which the procedure was performed
surgical procedures during abortion, labor, and delivery (630-676.9)
poisoning and toxic effects of drugs and chemicals (960.0-989.9)
postoperative conditions in which no complications are present, such as:
artificial opening status (V44.0-V44.9)
closure of external stoma (V55.0-V55.9)
fitting of prosthetic device (V52.0-V52.9)
specified complications classified elsewhere:
anesthetic shock (995.4)
electrolyte imbalance (276.0-276.9)
postlaminectomy syndrome (722.80-722.83)
postmastectomy lymphedema syndrome (457.0)
postoperative psychosis (293.0-293.9)
any other condition classified elsewhere in the Alphabetic Index when described as due to a procedure

4 996 Complications peculiar to certain specified procedures
Includes complications, not elsewhere classified, in the use of artificial substitutes [e.g., Dacron, metal, Silastic, Teflon] or natural sources [e.g., bone] involving:
anastomosis (internal)
graft (bypass) (patch)
implant
internal device:
catheter
electronic
fixation
prosthetic
reimplant
transplant
Excludes *accidental puncture or laceration during procedure (998.2)*
complications of internal anastomosis of:
gastrointestinal tract (997.4)
urinary tract (997.5)
▶ *endosseous dental implant failures (525.71-525.79)*◀
▶ *intraoperative floppy iris syndrome (IFIS) (364.81)*◀
mechanical complication of respirator (V46.14)
other specified complications classified elsewhere, such as:
hemolytic anemia (283.1)
functional cardiac disturbances (429.4)
serum hepatitis (070.2-070.3)

AHA: 1Q 1994, 3

5 996.0 Mechanical complication of cardiac device, implant, and graft
Breakdown (mechanical)
Displacement
Leakage
Obstruction, mechanical
Perforation
Protrusion
AHA: 2Q 1993, 9

✖ **996.00 Unspecified device, implant, and graft** 2
C&C Exclusions: 996.00, 996.04, 996.57, 996.61, 996.62, 996.70, 996.71, 996.72, 996.73, 996.74, 997.91, 997.99, 998.81, 998.83, 998.89, 998.9

996.01 Due to cardiac pacemaker (electrode) 2
C&C Exclusions: 996.01, 996.57, 997.91, 997.99, 998.81, 998.83, 998.89, 998.9
AHA: 2Q 2006, 16; 2Q 1999, 11

996.02 Due to heart valve prosthesis 2
C&C Exclusions: 996.02, 996.57, 997.91, 997.99, 998.81, 998.83, 998.89, 998.9

996.03 Due to coronary bypass graft 2
Excludes *atherosclerosis of graft (414.02, 414.03)*
embolism [occlusion NOS] [thrombus] of graft (996.72)
C&C Exclusions: 996.03, 996.57, 997.91, 997.99, 998.81, 998.83, 998.89, 998.9
AHA: 2Q 1995, 17; Nov-Dec 1986, 5

996.04 Due to automatic implantable cardiac defibrillator 2
C&C Exclusions: 996.04, 996.57, 997.91, 997.99, 998.81, 998.83, 998.89, 998.9
AHA: 2Q 2005, 3

996.09 Other 2
C&C Exclusions: 996.09, 996.57, 997.91, 997.99, 998.81, 998.83, 998.89, 998.9
AHA: 2Q 1993, 9

996.1 Mechanical complication of other vascular device, implant, and graft 2
Mechanical complications involving:
aortic (bifurcation) graft (replacement)
arteriovenous:
dialysis catheter
fistula surgically created
shunt surgically created
balloon (counterpulsation) device, intra-aortic
carotid artery bypass graft
femoral-popliteal bypass graft
umbrella device, vena cava
Excludes *atherosclerosis of biological graft (440.30-440.32)*
embolism [occlusion NOS] [thrombus] of (biological) (synthetic) graft (996.74)
peritoneal dialysis catheter (996.56)
C&C Exclusions: 996.1, 996.57, 997.91, 997.99, 998.81, 998.83, 998.89, 998.9
AHA: 1Q 2006, 11; 2Q 2005, 8; 1Q 2002, 13; 1Q 1995, 3

996.2 Mechanical complication of nervous system device, implant, and graft 2
Mechanical complications involving:
dorsal column stimulator
electrodes implanted in brain [brain "pacemaker"]
peripheral nerve graft
ventricular (communicating) shunt
C&C Exclusions: 996.2, 996.57, 996.63, 996.75, 997.91, 997.99, 998.81, 998.83, 998.89, 998.9
AHA: 2Q 1999, 4; Sep-Oct 1987, 10

5 996.3 Mechanical complication of genitourinary device, implant, and graft
AHA: 3Q 2001, 13; Sep-Oct 1985, 3

✖ **996.30 Unspecified device, implant, and graft** 2
C&C Exclusions: 996.30, 996.57, 996.64, 996.65, 996.76, 997.91, 997.99, 998.81, 998.83, 998.89, 998.9

996.31 Due to urethral [indwelling] catheter 2

996.32 Due to intrauterine contraceptive device ♀ 2

996.39 Other 2
Cystostomy catheter
Prosthetic reconstruction of vas deferens
Repair (graft) of ureter without mention of resection
Excludes *complications due to:*
external stoma of urinary tract (997.5)
internal anastomosis of urinary tract (997.5)
C&C Exclusions: 996.39, 996.57, 996 64, 996.65, 996.76, 997.91, 997.99, 998.81, 998.83, 998.89, 998.9

996.4 Mechanical complication of internal orthopedic device, implant, and graft

Mechanical complications involving:
external (fixation) device utilizing internal screw(s), pin(s) or other methods of fixation
grafts of bone, cartilage, muscle, or tendon
internal (fixation) device such as nail, plate, rod, etc.

Use additional code to identify prosthetic joint with mechanical complication (V43.60-V43.69)

Excludes *complications of external orthopedic device, such as:*
pressure ulcer due to cast (707.00-707.09)

AHA: 4Q 2005, 91; 2Q 1999, 10; 2Q 1998, 19; 2Q 1996, 11; 3Q 1995, 16; Nov-Dec 1985, 11

996.40 Unspecified mechanical complication of internal orthopedic device, implant, and graft

C&C Exclusions: 996.40, 996.41, 996.42, 996.43, 996.44, 996.45, 996.46, 996.47, 996.49, 996.57, 996.60, 996.66, 996.67, 996.69, 996.70, 996.77, 996.78, 996.79

996.41 Mechanical loosening of prosthetic joint

Aseptic loosening

C&C Exclusions: See 996.40

AHA: 4Q 2005, 112

996.42 Dislocation of prosthetic joint

Instability of prosthetic joint
Subluxation of prosthetic joint

C&C Exclusions: See 996.40

996.43 Prosthetic joint implant failure

Breakage (fracture) of prosthetic joint

C&C Exclusions: See 996.40

996.44 Peri-prosthetic fracture around prosthetic joint

C&C Exclusions: See 996.40

AHA: 4Q 2005, 1993

996.45 Peri-prosthetic osteolysis

Use additional code to identify major osseous defect, if applicable (731.3)

C&C Exclusions: See 996.40

AHA: 4Q 2006, 103-104

996.46 Articular bearing surface wear of prosthetic joint

C&C Exclusions: See 996.40

996.47 Other mechanical complication of prosthetic joint implant

Mechanical complication of prosthetic joint NOS

C&C Exclusions: See 996.40

996.49 Other mechanical complication of other internal orthopedic device, implant, and graft

Excludes *mechanical complication of prosthetic joint implant (996.41-996.47)*

C&C Exclusions: See 996.40

996.5 Mechanical complication of other specified prosthetic device, implant, and graft

Mechanical complications involving:
nonabsorbable surgical material NOS
other graft, implant, and internal device, not elsewhere classified
prosthetic implant in:
bile duct
breast
chin
orbit of eye

AHA: 1Q 1998, 11

996.51 Due to corneal graft

C&C Exclusions: 996.51, 996.57, 997.91, 997.99

996.52 Due to graft of other tissue, not elsewhere classified

Skin graft failure or rejection

Excludes *failure of artificial skin graft (996.55)*
failure of decellularized allodermis (996.55)
sloughing of temporary skin allografts or xenografts (pigskin) - omit code

C&C Exclusions: 996.51, 996.52, 996.57, 997.91, 997.99

AHA: 1Q 1996, 10

996.53 Due to ocular lens prosthesis

Excludes *contact lenses - code to condition*

C&C Exclusions: 996.53, 996.57, 997.91, 997.99

AHA: 1Q 2000, 9

996.54 Due to breast prosthesis

Breast capsule (prosthesis)
Mammary implant

C&C Exclusions: 996.54, 996.57, 997.91, 997.99

AHA: 2Q 1998, 14; 3Q 1992, 4

996.55 Due to artificial skin graft and decellularized allodermis

Dislodgement
Displacement
Failure
Non-adherence
Poor incorporation
Shearing

C&C Exclusions: 996.52, 996.55, 996.56, 996.57, 996.59, 996.60, 996.68, 996.69, 996.70, 996.79, 997.91, 997.99

AHA: 4Q 1998, 52

996.56 Due to peritoneal dialysis catheter

Excludes *mechanical complication of arteriovenous dialysis catheter (996.1)*

C&C Exclusions: 996.56, 996.57, 996.59, 996.60, 996.68, 996.69, 996.70, 996.79, 997.91, 997.99

AHA: 4Q 1998, 54

996.57 Due to insulin pump

C&C Exclusions: 996.55, 996.56, 996.57, 996.59, 996.60, 996.61, 996.62, 996.63, 996.64, 996.65, 996.66, 996.67, 996.68, 996.69, 996.70, 996.71, 996.72, 996.73, 996.74, 996.75, 996.76, 996.77, 996.78, 996.79

AHA: 4Q 2003, 81-82

996.59 Due to other implant and internal device, not elsewhere classified

Nonabsorbable surgical material NOS
Prosthetic implant in:
bile duct
chin
orbit of eye

C&C Exclusions: 996.57, 996.59, 996.60, 996.68, 996.69, 996.70, 996.79, 997.91, 997.99

AHA: 2Q 1999, 13; 3Q 1994, 7

996.6 Infection and inflammatory reaction due to internal prosthetic device, implant, and graft

Infection (causing obstruction) due to (presence of) any device, implant, and graft classifiable to 996.0-996.5
Inflammation due to (presence of) any device, implant, and graft classifiable to 996.0-996.5
Use additional code to identify specified infections

AHA: 2Q 1989, 16; Jan-Feb 1987, 14

996.60 Due to unspecified device, implant and graft

C&C Exclusions: 996.57, 996.00, 996.01, 996.02, 996.03, 996.04, 996.09, 996.1, 996.2, 996.30, 996.39, 996.4, 996.51, 996.52, 996.53, 996.54, 996.55, 996.56, 996.59, 996.60, 996.61, 996.62, 996.63, 996.64, 996.65, 996.66, 996.67, 996.68, 996.69, 996.70, 996.71, 996.72, 996.73, 996.74, 996.75, 996.76, 996.77, 996.78, 996.79, 997.91, 997.99, 998.81, 998.83, 998.89, 998.9

996.61 Due to cardiac device, implant and graft
Cardiac pacemaker or defibrillator:
electrode(s), lead(s)
pulse generator
subcutaneous pocket
Coronary artery bypass graft
Heart valve prosthesis
C&C Exclusions: 996.57, 996.00, 996.01, 996.02, 996.03, 996.04, 996.09, 996.1, 996.52, 996.55, 996.56, 996.59, 996.60, 996.61, 996.62, 996.68, 996.69, 996.70, 996.71, 996.72, 996.73, 996.74, 996.79, 997.91, 997.99, 998.81, 998.83, 998.89, 998.9

996.62 Due to vascular device, implant and graft
Vascular catheter (arterial) (dialysis) (▶peripheral◀ venous)
▶ *Excludes* *infection due to:*◀
▶*central venous catheter (999.31)*◀
▶*Hickman catheter (999.31)*◀
▶*peripherally inserted central catheter (PICC) (999.31)*◀
▶*triple lumen catheter (999.31)*◀
C&C Exclusions: See 996.61
AHA: 2Q 2004, 16; 1Q 2004, 5; 4Q 2003, 107, 111; 2Q 2003, 7; 2Q 1994, 13

996.63 Due to nervous system device, implant and graft
Electrodes implanted in brain
Peripheral nerve graft
Spinal canal catheter
Ventricular (communicating) shunt (catheter)
C&C Exclusions: 996.57, 996.2, 996.52, 996.55, 996.56, 996.59, 996.60, 996.63, 996.68, 996.69, 996.70, 996.75, 996.79, 997.91, 997.99, 998.81, 998.83, 998.89, 998.9

996.64 Due to indwelling urinary catheter
Use additional code to identify specified infections, such as:
Cystitis (595.0-595.9)
Sepsis (038.0-038.9)
C&C Exclusions: 599.0, 996.30, 996.39, 996.56, 996.57, 996.59, 996.60, 996.64, 996.65, 996.68, 996.69, 996.70, 996.76, 996.79, 997.91, 997.99, 998.81, 998.83, 998.89, 998.9
AHA: 3Q 1993, 6

996.65 Due to other genitourinary device, implant and graft
Intrauterine contraceptive device
C&C Exclusions: 996.30, 996.39, 996.52, 996.55, 996.56, 996.57, 996.59, 996.60, 996.64, 996.65, 996.68, 996.69, 996.70, 996.76, 996.79, 997.91, 997.99, 998.81, 998.83, 998.89, 998.9
AHA: 1Q 2000, 15

996.66 Due to internal joint prosthesis
Use additional code to identify infected prosthetic joint (V43.60-V43.69)
C&C Exclusions: 996.40, 996.41, 996.42, 996.43, 996.44, 996.45, 996.46, 996.47, 996.49, 996.52, 996.55, 996.56, 996.57, 996.59, 996.60, 996.66, 996.67, 996.68, 996.69, 996.70, 996.77, 996.78, 996.79, 997.91, 997.99, 998.81, 998.83, 998.89, 998.9
AHA: 4Q 2005, 91, 113; 2Q 1991, 18

996.67 Due to other internal orthopedic device, implant and graft
Bone growth stimulator (electrode)
Internal fixation device (pin) (rod) (screw)
C&C Exclusions: See 996.66

996.68 Due to peritoneal dialysis catheter
Exit-site infection or inflammation
C&C Exclusions: 996.56, 996.57, 996.59, 996.60, 996.68, 996.69, 996.70, 996.79, 997.91, 997.99
AHA: 4Q 1998, 54

996.69 Due to other internal prosthetic device, implant, and graft
Breast prosthesis
Ocular lens prosthesis
Prosthetic orbital implant
C&C Exclusions: See 996.60
AHA: 4Q 2003, 108; 4Q 1998, 52

5 **996.7 Other complications of internal (biological) (synthetic) prosthetic device, implant, and graft**
Complication NOS due to (presence of) any device, implant, and graft classifiable to 996.0-996.5
Embolism due to (presence of) any device, implant, and graft classifiable to 996.0-996.5
Fibrosis due to (presence of) any device, implant, and graft classifiable to 996.0-996.5
Hemorrhage due to (presence of) any device, implant, and graft classifiable to 996.0-996.5
Occlusion NOS due to (presence of) any device, implant, and graft classifiable to 996.0-996.5
Pain due to (presence of) any device, implant, and graft classifiable to 996.0-996.5
Stenosis due to (presence of) any device, implant, and graft classifiable to 996.0-996.5
Thrombus due to (presence of) any device, implant, and graft classifiable to 996.0-996.5
Use additional code to identify complication, such as:
pain due to presence of device, implant or graft (338.18-338.19, 338.28-338.29)
Excludes *transplant rejection (996.8)*
AHA: 4Q 2005, 94; 1Q 1989, 9; Nov-Dec 1986, 5

✖ **996.70 Due to unspecified device, implant, and graft**
C&C Exclusions: See 996.60

996.71 Due to heart valve prosthesis
C&C Exclusions: 996.00, 996.02, 996.09, 996.1, 996.52, 996.55, 996.56, 996.57, 996.59, 996.60, 996.61, 996.62, 996.68, 996.69, 996.70, 996.71, 996.72, 996.73, 996.74, 996.79, 997.91, 997.99, 998.81, 998.83, 998.89, 998.9

996.72 Due to other cardiac device, implant, and graft
Cardiac pacemaker or defibrillator:
electrode(s), lead(s)
subcutaneous pocket
Coronary artery bypass (graft)
Excludes *occlusion due to atherosclerosis (414.00-414.07)*
C&C Exclusions: 996.00, 996.01, 996.02, 996.04, 996.09, 996.1, 996.52, 996.55, 996.56, 996.57, 996.59, 996.60, 996.61, 996.62, 996.68, 996.69, 996.70, 996.71, 996.72, 996.73, 996.74, 996.79, 997.91, 997.99, 998.81, 998.83, 998.89, 998.9
AHA: 3Q 2006, 8; 3Q 2001, 20

996.73 Due to renal dialysis device, implant, and graft
C&C Exclusions: 996.1, 996.52, 996.55, 996.56, 996.57, 996.59, 996.60, 996.68, 996.69, 996.70, 996.73, 996.79, 997.91, 997.99, 998.81, 998.83, 998.89, 998.9
AHA: 2Q 1991, 18

996.74 Due to vascular device, implant, and graft
Excludes *occlusion of biological graft due to atherosclerosis (440.30-440.32)*
C&C Exclusions: 996.00, 996.01, 996.02, 996.03, 996.04, 996.09, 996.1, 996.52, 996.55, 996.56, 996.57, 996.59, 996.60, 996.61, 996.62, 996.68, 996.69, 996.70, 996.71, 996.72, 996.73, 996.74, 996.79, 997.91, 997.99, 998.81, 998.83, 998.89, 998.9
AHA: 1Q 2003, 16-17

996.75 Due to nervous system device, implant, and graft
C&C Exclusions: 996.2, 996.52, 996.55, 996.56, 996.57, 996.59, 996.60, 996.63, 996.68, 996.69, 996.70, 996.75, 996.79, 997.91, 997.99, 998.81, 998.83, 998.89, 998.9

996.76 Due to genitourinary device, implant, and graft
C&C Exclusions: 996.30, 996.39, 996.52, 996.55, 996.56, 996.57, 996.59, 996.60, 996.64, 996.65, 996.68, 996.69, 996.70, 996.76, 996.79, 997.91, 997.99, 998.81, 998.83, 998.89, 998.9
AHA: 1Q 2000, 15

996.77 Due to internal joint prosthesis
▶ Use additional code to identify prosthetic joint (V43.60-V43.69)◀
C&C Exclusions: 996.40, 996.41, 996.42, 996.43, 996.44, 996.45, 996.46, 996.47, 996.49, 996.52, 996.55, 996.56, 996.57, 996.59, 996.60, 996.66, 996.67, 996.69, 996.70, 996.77, 996.78, 996.79, 997.91, 997.99, 998.81, 998.83, 998.89, 998.9
AHA: 4Q 2005, 91

996.78 Due to other internal orthopedic device, implant, and graft
C&C Exclusions: See 996.77
AHA: 2Q 2003, 14

996.79 Due to other internal prosthetic device, implant, and graft
C&C Exclusions: 996.00, 996.01, 996.02, 996.03, 996.04, 996.09, 996.1, 996.2, 996.30, 996.39, 996.4, 996.51, 996.52, 996.53, 996.54, 996.55, 996.56, 996.57, 996.59, 996.60, 996.61, 996.62, 996.63, 996.64, 996.65, 996.66, 996.67, 996.68, 996.69, 996.70, 996.71, 996.72, 996.73, 996.74, 996.75, 996.76, 996.77, 996.78, 996.79, 997.91, 997.99, 998.81, 998.83, 998.89, 998.9
AHA: 2Q 2004, 7; 1Q 2001, 8; 3Q 1995, 14; 3Q 1992, 4

5 **996.8 Complications of transplanted organ**
Transplant failure or rejection
Use additional code to identify nature of complication, such as:
Cytomegalovirus [CMV] infection (078.5)
AHA: 3Q 2001, 12; 3Q 1993, 3-4; 2Q 1993, 11; 1Q 1993, 24

✖ **996.80 Transplanted organ, unspecified**
C&C Exclusions: 996.57, 996.80, 996.87, 997.91, 997.99, V42.84

996.81 Kidney
C&C Exclusions: 996.81, 997.91, 997.99
AHA: 3Q 2003, 16; 3Q 1998, 6-7; 3Q 1994, 8; 2Q 1994, 9; 1Q 1993, 24

996.82 Liver
C&C Exclusions: 996.82, 997.91, 997.99
AHA: 3Q 2003, 17; 3Q 1998, 3-4

996.83 Heart
C&C Exclusions: 996.57, 996.83, 997.91, 997.99
AHA: 3Q 2003, 16; 4Q 2002, 53; 3Q 1998, 5

996.84 Lung
C&C Exclusions: 996.84, 997.91, 997.99
AHA: 2Q 2003, 12; 3Q 1998, 5

996.85 Bone marrow
Graft-versus-host disease (acute) (chronic)
C&C Exclusions: 996.85, 997.91, 997.99
AHA: 4Q 1990, 4

996.86 Pancreas
C&C Exclusions: 996.86, 997.91, 997.99

996.87 Intestine
C&C Exclusions: 996.80, 996.87, 997.91, 997.99, V42.0, V42.82, V42.83, V42.89, V43,2

996.89 Other specified transplanted organ
C&C Exclusions: 996.89, 997.91, 997.99, V42.84, V43.21, V43.22
AHA: 3Q 1994, 5

5 **996.9 Complications of reattached extremity or body part**

✖ **996.90 Unspecified extremity**
C&C Exclusions: 996.90, 997.91, 997.99, 998.81, 998.83, 998.89, 998.9

996.91 Forearm
C&C Exclusions: 996.91, 997.91, 997.99, 998.81, 998.83, 998.89, 998.9

996.92 Hand
C&C Exclusions: 996.92, 997.91, 997.99, 998.81, 998.83, 998.89, 998.9

996.93 Finger(s)
C&C Exclusions: 996.93, 997.91, 997.99, 998.81, 998.83, 998.89, 998.9

996.94 Upper extremity, other and unspecified
C&C Exclusions: 996.94, 997.91, 997.99, 998.81, 998.83, 998.89, 998.9

996.95 Foot and toe(s)
C&C Exclusions: 996.95, 997.91, 997.99, 998.81, 998.83, 998.89, 998.9

996.96 Lower extremity, other and unspecified
C&C Exclusions: 996.96, 997.91, 997.99, 998.81, 998.83, 998.89, 998.9

996.99 Other specified body part
C&C Exclusions: 996.99, 997.91, 997.99, 998.81, 998.83, 998.89, 998.9

4 **997 Complications affecting specified body systems, not elsewhere classified**
Use additional code to identify complication
Excludes *the listed conditions when specified as:*
causing shock (998.0)
complications of:
anesthesia:
adverse effect (001.0-799.9, 995.0-995.8)
in labor or delivery (668.0-668.9)
poisoning (968.0-969.9)
implanted device or graft (996.0-996.9)
obstetrical procedures (669.0-669.4)
reattached extremity (996.90-996.96)
transplanted organ (996.80-996.89)
AHA: 1Q 1994, 4; 1Q 1993, 26

5 **997.0 Nervous system complications**

✖ **997.00 Nervous system complication, unspecified**
C&C Exclusions: 997.00, 997.01, 997.02, 997.09, 997.91, 997.99, 998.81, 998.83, 998.89, 998.9

997.01 Central nervous system complication
Anoxic brain damage
Cerebral hypoxia
Excludes *cerebrovascular hemorrhage or infarction (997.02)*
C&C Exclusions: See 997.00
AHA: 1Q 2007, 22; 1Q 2006, 15

997.02 Iatrogenic cerebrovascular infarction or hemorrhage
Postoperative stroke
C&C Exclusions: See 997.00
AHA: 2Q 2004, 8; 4Q 1995, 57

997.09 Other nervous system complications
C&C Exclusions: See 997.00

997.1 Cardiac complications
Cardiac:
arrest during or resulting from a procedure
insufficiency during or resulting from a procedure
Cardiorespiratory failure during or resulting from a procedure
Heart failure during or resulting from a procedure
Excludes *the listed conditions as long-term effects of cardiac surgery or due to the presence of cardiac prosthetic device (429.4)*
C&C Exclusions: 997.1, 997.91, 997.99, 998.81, 998.83, 998.89, 998.9
AHA: 2Q 2002, 12

997.2 Peripheral vascular complications
Phlebitis or thrombophlebitis during or resulting from a procedure
Excludes *the listed conditions due to:*
implant or catheter device (996.62)
infusion, perfusion, or transfusion (999.2)
complications affecting blood vessels (997.71-997.79)
C&C Exclusions: 997.2, 997.71, 997.72, 997.79, 997.91, 997.99, 998.81, 998.83, 998.89, 998.9
AHA: 1Q 2003, 6; 3Q 2002, 24-26

997.3 Respiratory complications
Mendelson's syndrome resulting from a procedure
Pneumonia (aspiration) resulting from a procedure
Excludes *iatrogenic [postoperative] pneumothorax (512.1)*
iatrogenic pulmonary embolism (415.11)
Mendelson's syndrome in labor and delivery (668.0)
specified complications classified elsewhere, such as:
adult respiratory distress syndrome (518.5)
pulmonary edema, postoperative (518.4)
respiratory insufficiency, acute, postoperative (518.5)
shock lung (518.5)
tracheostomy complications (519.00-519.09)
transfusion related acute lung injury (TRALI) (518.7)
C&C Exclusions: 518.7, 997.3, 997.91, 997.99, 998.81, 998.83, 998.89, 998.9
AHA: 1Q 1997, 10; 2Q 1993, 3, 9; 4Q 1990, 25

997.4 Digestive system complications
Complications of:
intestinal (internal) anastomosis and bypass, not elsewhere classified, except that involving urinary tract
Hepatic failure specified as due to a procedure
Hepatorenal syndrome specified as due to a procedure
Intestinal obstruction NOS specified as due to a procedure
Excludes *gastrostomy complications (536.40-536.49)*
specified gastrointestinal complications classified elsewhere, such as:
blind loop syndrome (579.2)
colostomy or enterostomy complications (569.60-569.69)
gastrojejunal ulcer (534.0-534.9)
infection of esophagostomy (530.86)
infection of external stoma (569.61)
mechanical complication of esophagostomy (530.87)
pelvic peritoneal adhesions, female (614.6)
peritoneal adhesions (568.0)
peritoneal adhesions with obstruction (560.81)
postcholecystectomy syndrome (576.0)
postgastric surgery syndromes (564.2)
vomiting following gastrointestinal surgery (564.3)
C&C Exclusions: 536.40, 536.41, 536.42, 536.49, 997.4, 997.71, 997.91, 997.99, 998.81, 998.83, 998.9
AHA: 2Q 2001, 4-6; 3Q 1999, 4; 2Q 1999, 14; 3Q 1997, 7; 1Q 1997, 11; 2Q 1995, 7; 1Q 1993, 26; 3Q 1992, 15; 2Q 1989, 15; 1Q 1988, 14

997.5 Urinary complications
Complications of:
external stoma of urinary tract
internal anastomosis and bypass of urinary tract, including that involving intestinal tract
Oliguria or anuria specified as due to procedure
Renal:
failure (acute) specified as due to procedure
insufficiency (acute) specified as due to procedure
Tubular necrosis (acute) specified as due to procedure
Excludes *specified complications classified elsewhere, such as:*
postoperative stricture of:
ureter (593.3)
urethra (598.2)
C&C Exclusions: 997.5, 997.72, 997.91, 997.99, 998.81, 998.83, 998.9
AHA: 3Q 2003, 13; 3Q 1996, 10, 15; 4Q 1995, 73; 1Q 1992, 13; 2Q 1989, 16; Mar-Apr 1987, 10; Sep-Oct 1985, 3

5 **997.6 Amputation stump complication**
Excludes *admission for treatment for a current traumatic amputation - code to complicated traumatic amptutation*
phantom limb (syndrome) (353.6)
AHA: 4Q 1995, 82

997.60 Unspecified complication

997.61 Neuroma of amputation stump

997.62 Infection (chronic)
Use additional code to identify the organism
C&C Exclusions: 997.60, 997.62, 997.69, 997.91, 997.99, 998.81, 998.83, 998.9
AHA: 1Q 2005, 14; 4Q 1996, 46

997.69 Other
AHA: 1Q 2005, 15

5 **997.7 Vascular complications of other vessels**
Excludes *peripheral vascular complications (997.2)*

997.71 Vascular complications of mesenteric artery
C&C Exclusions: 536.40, 536.41, 536.42, 536.49, 569.62, 997.4, 997.71, 997.72, 997.79
AHA: 4Q 2001, 53

997.72 Vascular complications of renal artery
C&C Exclusions: 997.5, 997.71, 997.72, 997.79

997.79 Vascular complications of other vessels
C&C Exclusions: 997.2, 997.71, 997.72, 997.79

5 **997.9 Complications affecting other specified body systems, not elsewhere classified**
Excludes *specified complications classified elsewhere, such as:*
broad ligament laceration syndrome (620.6)
postartificial menopause syndrome (627.4)
postoperative stricture of vagina (623.2)

997.91 Hypertension
Excludes *essential hypertension (401.0-401.9)*
C&C Exclusions: 518.7, 996.40, 996.41, 996.42, 996.43, 996.44, 996.45, 996.46, 996.47, 996.49, 996.57, 996.87, 997.71, 997.72, 997.79, 997.91, 997.99, 998.31, 998.32, 998.81, 998.83, 998.9
AHA: 4Q 1995, 57

997.99 Other
Vitreous touch syndrome
C&C Exclusions: See 997.91
AHA: 2Q 1994, 12; 1Q 1994, 17

4 **998 Other complications of procedures, NEC**

998.0 Postoperative shock
Collapse NOS during or resulting from a surgical procedure
Shock (endotoxic) (hypovolemic) (septic) during or resulting from a surgical procedure
Excludes *shock:*
anaphylactic due to serum (999.4)
anesthetic (995.4)
electric (994.8)
following abortion (639.5)
obstetric (669.1)
traumatic (958.4)
C&C Exclusions: 958.4, 995.4, 997.91, 997.99, 998.0, 998.11, 998.12, 998.13, 998.81, 998.83, 998.89, 998.9

5 **998.1 Hemorrhage or hematoma or seroma complicating a procedure**

Excludes *hemorrhage, hematoma or seroma:*
complicating cesarean section or puerperal perineal wound (674.3)
due to implanted device or graft (996.70-996.79)

998.11 Hemorrhage complicating a procedure

C&C Exclusions: 456.0, 456.20, 530.81, 530.82, 530.83, 530.89, 531.00, 531.01, 531.20, 531.21, 531.40, 531.41, 531.60, 531.61, 532.00, 532.01, 532.20, 532.21, 532.40, 532.41, 532.60, 532.61, 533.00, 533.01, 533.20, 533.21, 533.40, 533.41, 533.60, 533.61, 534.00, 534.01, 534.20, 534.21, 534.40, 534.41, 534.61, 535.01, 535.11, 535.21, 535.31, 535.41, 535.51, 535.61, 537.83, 562.02, 562.03, 562.12, 562.13, 569.3, 569.85, 578.0, 578.1, 578.9, 772.4, 997.91, 997.99, 998.0, 998.11, 998.12, 998.13, 998.81, 998.89, 998.9

AHA: 3Q 2003, 13; 1Q 2003, 4; 4Q 1997, 52; 1Q 1997, 10

998.12 Hematoma complicating a procedure

C&C Exclusions: See 998.11

AHA: 3Q 2006, 12; 1Q 2003, 6; 3Q 2002, 24, 26

998.13 Seroma complicating a procedure

C&C Exclusions: See 998.11

AHA: 4Q 1996, 46; 1Q 1993, 26; 2Q 1992, 15; Sep-Oct 1987, 8

998.2 Accidental puncture or laceration during a procedure

Accidental perforation by catheter or other instrument during a procedure on:
blood vessel
nerve
organ

Excludes *iatrogenic [postoperative] pneumothorax (512.1)*
puncture or laceration caused by implanted device intentionally left in operation wound (996.0-996.5)
specified complications classified elsewhere, such as:
broad ligament laceration syndrome (620.6)
trauma from instruments during delivery (664.0-665.9)

C&C Exclusions: 997.91, 997.99, 998.2, 998.81, 998.83, 998.89, 998.9

AHA: 1Q 2006, 15; 3Q 2002, 24, 26; 3Q 1994, 6; 3Q 1990, 17, 18

5 **998.3 Disruption of operation wound**

Dehiscence of operation wound
Rupture of operation wound

Excludes *disruption of:*
amputation stump (997.69)
cesarean wound (674.1)
perineal wound, puerperal (674.2)

AHA: 4Q 2002, 73; 1Q 1993, 19

998.31 Disruption of internal operation wound

C&C Exclusions: 997.91, 997.99, 998.31, 998.32, 998.81, 998.83, 998.89, 998.9

998.32 Disruption of external operation wound

Disruption of operation wound NOS

C&C Exclusions: See 998.31

AHA: 1Q 2006, 8; 1Q 2005, 11; 4Q 2003, 104, 106

998.4 Foreign body accidentally left during a procedure

Adhesions due to foreign body accidentally left in operative wound or body cavity during a procedure
Obstruction due to foreign body accidentally left in operative wound or body cavity during a procedure
Perforation due to foreign body accidentally left in operative wound or body cavity during a procedure

Excludes *obstruction or perforation caused by implanted device intentionally left in body (996.0-996.5)*

C&C Exclusions: 997.91, 997.99, 998.4, 998.81, 998.83, 998.89, 998.9

AHA: 1Q 1989, 9

5 **998.5 Postoperative infection**

Excludes *bleb associated endophthalmitis (379.63)*
infection due to:
implanted device (996.60-996.69)
infusion, perfusion, or transfusion (▶999.31-999.39◀)
postoperative obstetrical wound infection (674.3)

998.51 Infected postoperative seroma

Use additional code to identify organism

C&C Exclusions: 997.91, 997.99, 998.51, 998.59, 998.81, 998.83, 998.89, 998.9

AHA: 4Q 1996, 46

998.59 Other postoperative infection

Abscess:
intra-abdominal postoperative
stitch postoperative
subphrenic postoperative
wound postoperative
Septicemia postoperative
Use additional code to identify infection

C&C Exclusions: See 998.51

AHA: 2Q 2006, 24; 4Q 2004, 76; 4Q 2003, 104, 106-107; 3Q 1998, 3; 3Q 1995, 5; 2Q 1995, 7; 3Q 1994, 6; 1Q 1993, 19; Jan-Feb 1987, 14

998.6 Persistent postoperative fistula

C&C Exclusions: 997.91, 997.99, 998.6, 998.81, 998.83, 998.89, 998.9

AHA: Jan-Feb 1987, 14

998.7 Acute reaction to foreign substance accidentally left during a procedure

Peritonitis:
aseptic
chemical

C&C Exclusions: 997.91, 997.99, 998.7, 998.81, 998.83, 998.89, 998.9

5 **998.8 Other specified complications of procedures, not elsewhere classified**

AHA: 4Q 1994, 46; 1Q 1989, 9

998.81 Emphysema (subcutaneous) (surgical) resulting from a procedure

C&C Exclusions: 518.7, 996.40, 996.41, 996.42, 996.43, 996.44, 996.45, 996.46, 996.47, 996.49, 996.57, 997.71, 997.72, 997.79, 998.31, 998.32,

998.82 Cataract fragments in eye following cataract surgery

998.83 Non-healing surgical wound

C&C Exclusions: 518.7, 996.40, 996.41, 996.42, 996.43, 996.44, 996.45, 996.46, 996.47, 996.49, 996.57, 997.71, 997.72, 997.79, 997.91, 997.99, 998.31, 998.32, 998.81, 998.83, 998.89, 998.9

AHA: 4Q 1996, 47

998.89 Other specified complications

C&C Exclusions: See 998.83

AHA: 3Q 2006, 9-10; 3Q 2005, 16; 3Q 1999, 13; 2Q 1998, 16

✖ **998.9 Unspecified complication of procedure, not elsewhere classified**
Postoperative complication NOS
Excludes *complication NOS of obstetrical surgery or procedure (669.4)*
C&C Exclusions: See 998.83
AHA: 4Q 1993, 37

❹ **999 Complications of medical care, not elsewhere classified**
▶ Use additional code, where applicable, to identify specific complication◀
Includes complications, not elsewhere classified, of:
dialysis (hemodialysis) (peritoneal) (renal)
extracorporeal circulation
hyperalimentation therapy
immunization
infusion
inhalation therapy
injection
inoculation
perfusion
transfusion
vaccination
ventilation therapy
Excludes *specified complications classified elsewhere such as:*
complications of implanted device (996.0-996.9)
contact dermatitis due to drugs (692.3)
dementia dialysis (294.8)
transient (293.9)
dialysis disequilibrium syndrome (276.0-276.9)
poisoning and toxic effects of drugs and chemicals (960.0-989.9)
postvaccinal encephalitis (323.51)
water and electrolyte imbalance (276.0-276.9)

999.0 Generalized vaccinia

999.1 Air embolism
Air embolism to any site following infusion, perfusion, or transfusion
Excludes *embolism specified as:*
complicating:
abortion (634-638 with .6, 639.6)
ectopic or molar pregnancy (639.6)
pregnancy, childbirth, or the puerperium (673.0)
due to implanted device (996.7)
traumatic (958.0)
C&C Exclusions: 958.0, 999.1

999.2 Other vascular complications
Phlebitis following infusion, perfusion, or transfusion
Thromboembolism following infusion, perfusion, or transfusion
Thrombophlebitis following infusion, perfusion, or transfusion
Excludes *the listed conditions when specified as:*
due to implanted device (996.61-996.62, 996.72-996.74)
postoperative NOS (997.2, 997.71-997.79)
C&C Exclusions: 999.2
AHA: 2Q 1997, 5

❺ **999.3 Other infection**
Infection following infusion, injection, transfusion, or vaccination
Sepsis following infusion, injection, transfusion, or vaccination
Septicemia following infusion, injection, transfusion, or vaccination
▶ Use additional code to identify the specified infection, such as:◀
▶ septicemia (038.0-038.9)◀
Excludes *the listed conditions when specified as:*
due to implanted device (996.60-996.69)
postoperative NOS (998.51-998.59)
C&C Exclusions: 999.3
AHA: 2Q 2001, 11-12; 2Q 1997, 5; Jan-Feb 1987, 14

● **999.31 Infection due to central venous catheter**
Catheter-related bloodstream infection (CRBSI)
Infection due to:
Hickman catheter
Peripherally inserted central catheter (PICC)
Triple lumen catheter
Excludes *infection due to:*
arterial catheter (996.62)
catheter NOS (996.69)
peripheral venous catheter (996.62)
urinary catheter (996.64)

● **999.39 Infection following other infusion, injection, transfusion, or vaccination**

999.4 Anaphylactic shock due to serum
Excludes *shock:*
allergic NOS (995.0)
anaphylactic:
NOS (995.0)
due to drugs and chemicals (995.0)
C&C Exclusions: 999.4

999.5 Other serum reaction
Intoxication by serum
Protein sickness
Serum rash
Serum sickness
Urticaria due to serum
Excludes *serum hepatitis (070.2-070.3)*
C&C Exclusions: 999.5

999.6 ABO incompatibility reaction
Incompatible blood transfusion
Reaction to blood group incompatibility in infusion or transfusion
C&C Exclusions: 999.6

999.7 Rh incompatibility reaction
Reactions due to Rh factor in infusion or transfusion
C&C Exclusions: 999.7

999.8 Other transfusion reaction
Septic shock due to transfusion
Transfusion reaction NOS
Excludes *postoperative shock (998.0)*
transfusion related acute lung injury (TRALI) (518.7)
C&C Exclusions: 999.8
AHA: 3Q 2000, 9

999.9 Other and unspecified complications of medical care, not elsewhere classified
Complications, not elsewhere classified, of:
electroshock therapy
inhalation therapy
ultrasound therapy
ventilation therapy
Unspecified misadventure of medical care
Excludes *unspecified complication of:*
phototherapy (990)
radiation therapy (990)
AHA: 2Q 2006, 25: 1Q 2003, 19; 2Q 1997, 5

SUPPLEMENTARY CLASSIFICATION OF FACTORS INFLUENCING HEALTH STATUS AND CONTACT WITH HEALTH SERVICES (V01-V86)

This classification is provided to deal with occasions when circumstances other than a disease or injury classifiable to categories 001-999 (the main part of ICD) are recorded as "diagnoses" or "problems." This can arise mainly in three ways:

a) When a person who is not currently sick encounters the health services for some specific purpose, such as to act as a donor of an organ or tissue, to receive prophylactic vaccination, or to discuss a problem which is in itself not a disease or injury. This will be a fairly rare occurrence among hospital inpatients, but will be relatively more common among hospital outpatients and patients of family practitioners, health clinics, etc.

b) When a person with a known disease or injury, whether it is current or resolving, encounters the health care system for a specific treatment of that disease or injury (e.g., dialysis for renal disease; chemotherapy for malignancy; cast change).

c) When some circumstance or problem is present which influences the person's health status but is not in itself a current illness or injury. Such factors may be elicited during population surveys, when the person may or may not be currently sick, or be recorded as an additional factor to be borne in mind when the person is receiving care for some current illness or injury classifiable to categories 001-999.

In the latter circumstances the V code should be used only as a supplementary code and should not be the one selected for use in primary, single cause tabulations. Examples of these circumstances are a personal history of certain diseases, or a person with an artificial heart valve in situ.

AHA: Jan-Feb, 1987, 8

PERSONS WITH POTENTIAL HEALTH HAZARDS RELATED TO COMMUNICABLE DISEASES (V01-V06)

Excludes *family history of infectious and parasitic diseases (V18.8)*
personal history of infectious and parasitic diseases (V12.0)

❹ **V01 Contact with or exposure to communicable diseases**

⊘ **V01.0 Cholera**
Conditions classifiable to 001

⊘ **V01.1 Tuberculosis**
Conditions classifiable to 010-018

⊘ **V01.2 Poliomyelitis**
Conditions classifiable to 045

⊘ **V01.3 Smallpox**
Conditions classifiable to 050

⊘ **V01.4 Rubella**
Conditions classifiable to 056

⊘ **V01.5 Rabies**
Conditions classifiable to 071

⊘ **V01.6 Venereal diseases**
Conditions classifiable to 090-099

❺ **V01.7 Other viral diseases**
Conditions classifiable to 042-078, and V08, except as above
AHA: 2Q 1992, 11

V01.71 Varicella

V01.79 Other viral diseases

❺ **V01.8 Other communicable diseases**
Conditions classifiable to 001-136, except as above
AHA: Jul-Aug, 1987, 24

⊘ **V01.81 Anthrax**
AHA: 4Q 2002, 70, 78

V01.82 Exposure to SARS-associated coronavirus
AHA: 4Q 2003, 46-47

V01.83 Escherichia coli (E. coli)

V01.84 Meningococcus

⊘ **V01.89 Other communicable diseases**

⊘ **V01.9 Unspecified communicable disease**

❹ **V02 Carrier or suspected carrier of infectious diseases**
AHA: 3Q 1995, 18; 3Q 1994, 4

⊘ **V02.0 Cholera**

⊘ **V02.1 Typhoid**

⊘ **V02.2 Amebiasis**

⊘ **V02.3 Other gastrointestinal pathogens**

⊘ **V02.4 Diphtheria**

❺ **V02.5 Other specified bacterial diseases**

⊘ **V02.51 Group B Streptococcus**
AHA: 3Q 2006, 14; 1Q 2002, 14; 4Q 1998, 56

⊘ **V02.52 Other Streptococcus**

⊘ **V02.59 Other specified bacterial diseases**
Meningococcal
Staphylococcal

❺ **V02.6 Viral hepatitis**

⊘ **V02.60 Viral hepatitis carrier, unspecified**
AHA: 4Q 1997, 47

⊘ **V02.61 Hepatitis B carrier**
AHA: 4Q 1997, 47

⊘ **V02.62 Hepatitis C carrier**
AHA: 4Q 1997, 47

⊘ **V02.69 Other viral hepatitis carrier**
AHA: 4Q 1997, 47

⊘ **V02.7 Gonorrhea**

⊘ **V02.8 Other venereal diseases**

⊘ **V02.9 Other specified infectious organism**
AHA: 3Q 1995, 18; 1Q 1993; 22; Jul-Aug, 1987, 24

❹ **V03 Need for prophylactic vaccination and inoculation against bacterial diseases**
Excludes *vaccination not carried out (V64.00-V64.09)*
vaccines against combinations of diseases (V06.0-V06.9)

⊘ **V03.0 Cholera alone**

⊘ **V03.1 Typhoid-paratyphoid alone [TAB]**

⊘ **V03.2 Tuberculosis [BCG]**

⊘ **V03.3 Plague**

⊘ **V03.4 Tularemia**

⊘ **V03.5 Diphtheria alone**

⊘ **V03.6 Pertussis alone**

⊘ **V03.7 Tetanus toxoid alone**

❺ **V03.8 Other specified vaccinations against single bacterial diseases**

⊘ **V03.81 Hemophilus influenza, type B [Hib]**

⊘ **V03.82 Streptococcus pneumoniae [pneumococcus]**

⊘ **V03.89 Other specified vaccination**
AHA: 2Q 2000, 9

⊘ **V03.9 Unspecified single bacterial disease**

❹ **V04 Need for prophylactic vaccination and inoculation against certain diseases**
Excludes *vaccines against combinations of diseases (V06.0-V06.9)*

⊘ **V04.0 Poliomyelitis**

⊘ **V04.1 Smallpox**

⊘ **V04.2 Measles alone**

⊘ **V04.3 Rubella alone**

⊘ **V04.4 Yellow fever**

⊘ **V04.5 Rabies**

⊘ **V04.6 Mumps alone**

⊘ **V04.7 Common cold**

❺ **V04.8 Other viral diseases**
AHA: 4Q 2003, 83

⊘ **V04.81 Influenza**

⊘ **V04.82 Respiratory syncytial virus (RSV)**

⊘ **V04.89 Other viral diseases**

A Adult (15+ years) M Maternity (12-55 years) N Neonates (0 years) P Pediatric (0-17 years) ♂ Male ♀ Female

V Codes

V05 Need for prophylactic vaccination and inoculation against single diseases
Excludes *vaccines against combinations of diseases (V06.0-V06.9)*

V05.0 Arthropod-borne viral encephalitis

V05.1 Other arthropod-borne viral diseases

V05.2 Leishmaniasis

V05.3 Viral hepatitis

V05.4 Varicella
Chicken pox

V05.8 Other specified disease
AHA: 1Q 2001, 4; 3Q 1991, 20

V05.9 Unspecified single disease

V06 Need for prophylactic vaccination and inoculation against combinations of diseases
Note: Use additional single vaccination codes from categories V03-V05 to identify any vaccinations not included in a combination code.

V06.0 Cholera with typhoid-paratyphoid [cholera TAB]

V06.1 Diphtheria-tetanus-pertussis, combined [DTP] [DTaP]
AHA: 4Q 2003, 83; 3Q 1998, 13

V06.2 Diphtheria-tetanus-pertussis with typhoid-paratyphoid [DTP+TAB]

V06.3 Diphtheria-tetanus-pertussis with poliomyelitis [DTP+polio]

V06.4 Measles-mumps-rubella [MMR]

V06.5 Tetanus-diphtheria [Td] [DT]
AHA: 4Q 2003, 83

V06.6 Streptococcus pneumoniae [pneumococcus] and influenza

V06.8 Other combinations
Excludes *multiple single vaccination codes (V03.0-V05.9)*
AHA: 1Q 1994, 19

V06.9 Unspecified combined vaccine

PERSONS WITH NEED FOR ISOLATION, OTHER POTENTIAL HEALTH HAZARDS AND PROPHYLACTIC MEASURES (V07-V09)

V07 Need for isolation and other prophylactic measures
Excludes *prophylactic organ removal (V50.41-V50.49)*

V07.0 Isolation
Admission to protect the individual from his surroundings or for isolation of individual after contact with infectious diseases

V07.1 Desensitization to allergens

V07.2 Prophylactic immunotherapy
Administration of:
antivenin
immune sera [gamma globulin]
RhoGAM
tetanus antitoxin

V07.3 Other prophylactic chemotherapy

V07.31 Prophylactic fluoride administration

V07.39 Other prophylactic chemotherapy
Excludes *maintenance chemotherapy following disease (V58.11)*

V07.4 Hormone replacement therapy (postmenopausal) ♀

V07.8 Other specified prophylactic measure
AHA: 1Q 1992, 11

V07.9 Unspecified prophylactic measure

V08 Asymptomatic human immunodeficiency virus [HIV] infection status
HIV positive NOS
Note: This code is ONLY to be used when NO HIV infection symptoms or conditions are present. If any HIV infection symptoms or conditions are present, see code 042.
Excludes *AIDS (042)*
human immunodeficiency virus [HIV] disease (042)
exposure to HIV (V01.79)
nonspecific serologic evidence of HIV (795.71)
symptomatic human immunodeficiency virus [HIV] infection (042)
AHA: 2Q 2004, 11; 2Q 1999, 8; 3Q 1995, 18

V09 Infection with drug-resistant microorganisms
Note: This category is intended for use as an additional code for infectious conditions classified elsewhere to indicate the presence of drug-resistance of the infectious organism.
AHA: 3Q 1jan-feb, 1987, 994, 4; 4Q 1993, 22

V09.0 Infection with microorganisms resistant to penicillins
Methicillin-resistant staphylococcus aureus (MRSA)
C&C Exclusions: 995.90, 995.91, 995.92, 995.93, 995.94
AHA: 2Q 2006, 16; 4Q 2003, 104, 106

V09.1 Infection with microorganisms resistant to cephalosporins and other B-lactam antibiotics
C&C Exclusions: See V09.0

V09.2 Infection with microorganisms resistant to macrolides
C&C Exclusions: See V09.0

V09.3 Infection with microorganisms resistant to tetracyclines
C&C Exclusions: See V09.0

V09.4 Infection with microorganisms resistant to aminoglycosides
C&C Exclusions: See V09.0

V09.5 Infection with microorganisms resistant to quinolones and fluoroquinolones

V09.50 Without mention of resistance to multiple quinolones and fluoroquinoles
C&C Exclusions: See V09.0

V09.51 With resistance to multiple quinolones and fluoroquinoles
C&C Exclusions: See V09.0

V09.6 Infection with microorganisms resistant to sulfonamides
C&C Exclusions: See V09.0

V09.7 Infection with microorganisms resistant to other specified antimycobacterial agents
Excludes *Amikacin (V09.4)*
Kanamycin (V09.4)
Streptomycin [SM] (V09.4)

V09.70 Without mention of resistance to multiple antimycobacterial agents
C&C Exclusions: See V09.0

V09.71 With resistance to multiple antimycobacterial agents
C&C Exclusions: See V09.0

V09.8 Infection with microorganisms resistant to other specified drugs
Vancomycin (glycopeptide) intermediate staphylococcus aureus (VISA/GISA)
Vancomycin (glycopeptide) resistant enterococcus (VRE)
Vancomycin (glycopeptide) resistant staphylococcus aureus (VRSA/GRSA)

V09.80 Without mention of resistance to multiple drugs
C&C Exclusions: See V09.0

V09.81 With resistance to multiple drugs
C&C Exclusions: See V09.0

V09.9 Infection with drug-resistant microorganisms, unspecified
Drug resistance NOS

V09.90 Without mention of multiple drug resistance
C&C Exclusions: See V09.0

V09.91 With multiple drug resistance
Multiple drug resistance NOS
C&C Exclusions: See V09.0

V05 – V09.91

PERSONS WITH POTENTIAL HEALTH HAZARDS RELATED TO PERSONAL AND FAMILY HISTORY (V10-V19)

Excludes *obstetric patients where the possibility that the fetus might be affected is the reason for observation or management during pregnancy (655.0-655.9)*

V10 Personal history of malignant neoplasm
AHA: 4Q 2002, 80; 4Q 1998, 69; 1Q 1995, 4; 3Q 1992, 5; 2Q 1990, 9; May-Jun, 1985, 10

V10.0 Gastrointestinal tract
History of conditions classifiable to 140-159

V10.00 Gastrointestinal tract, unspecified
V10.01 Tongue
V10.02 Other and unspecified oral cavity and pharynx
V10.03 Esophagus
V10.04 Stomach
V10.05 Large intestine
AHA: 3Q 1999, 7; 1Q 1995, 4
V10.06 Rectum, rectosigmoid junction, and anus
V10.07 Liver
V10.09 Other
AHA: 4Q 2003, 11

V10.1 Trachea, bronchus, and lung
History of conditions classifiable to 162

V10.11 Bronchus and lung
V10.12 Trachea

V10.2 Other respiratory and intrathoracic organs
History of conditions classifiable to 160, 161, 163-165

V10.20 Respiratory organ, unspecified
V10.21 Larynx
AHA: 4Q 2003, 108, 110
V10.22 Nasal cavities, middle ear, and accessory sinuses
V10.29 Other

V10.3 Breast
History of conditions classifiable to 174 and 175
AHA: 1Q 2007, 6; 2Q 2003, 5 ;4Q 2001, 66; 4Q 1998, 65; 4Q 1997, 50; 1Q 1991, 16; 1Q 1990, 21

V10.4 Genital organs
History of conditions classifiable to 179-187

V10.40 Female genital organ, unspecified ♀
V10.41 Cervix uteri ♀
V10.42 Other parts of uterus ♀
V10.43 Ovary ♀
V10.44 Other female genital organs ♀
V10.45 Male genital organ, unspecified ♂
V10.46 Prostate ♂
V10.47 Testis ♂
V10.48 Epididymis ♂
V10.49 Other male genital organs ♂

V10.5 Urinary organs
History of conditions classifiable to 188 and 189

V10.50 Urinary organ, unspecified
V10.51 Bladder
V10.52 Kidney
Excludes *renal pelvis (V10.53)*
AHA: 2Q 2004, 4
V10.53 Renal pelvis
AHA: 4Q 2001, 55
V10.59 Other

V10.6 Leukemia
Conditions classifiable to 204-208
Excludes *leukemia in remission (204-208)*
AHA: 2Q 1992, 13; 4Q 1991, 26; 4Q 1990, 3

V10.60 Leukemia, unspecified
V10.61 Lymphoid leukemia
V10.62 Myeloid leukemia
V10.63 Monocytic leukemia
V10.69 Other

V10.7 Other lymphatic and hematopoietic neoplasms
Conditions classifiable to 200-203
Excludes *listed conditions in 200-203 in remission*
AHA: May-Jun, 1985, 18

V10.71 Lymphosarcoma and reticulosarcoma
V10.72 Hodgkin's disease
V10.79 Other

V10.8 Personal history of malignant neoplasm of other sites
History of conditions classifiable to 170-173, 190-195

V10.81 Bone
AHA: 2Q 2003, 13
V10.82 Malignant melanoma of skin
V10.83 Other malignant neoplasm of skin
V10.84 Eye
V10.85 Brain
AHA: 1Q 2001, 6
V10.86 Other parts of nervous system
Excludes *peripheral, sympathetic, and parasympathetic nerves (V10.89)*
V10.87 Thyroid
V10.88 Other endocrine glands and related structures
V10.89 Other

V10.9 Unspecified personal history of malignant neoplasm

V11 Personal history of mental disorder

V11.0 Schizophrenia
Excludes *that in remission (295.0-295.9 with fifth-digit 5)*
V11.1 Affective disorders
Personal history of manic-depressive psychosis
Excludes *that in remission (296.0-296.6 with fifth-digit 5, 6)*
V11.2 Neurosis
V11.3 Alcoholism
V11.8 Other mental disorders
V11.9 Unspecified mental disorder

V12 Personal history of certain other diseases
AHA: 3Q 1992, 11

V12.0 Infectious and parasitic diseases
Excludes *personal history of infectious diseases specific to a body system*

V12.00 Unspecified infectious and parasitic disease
V12.01 Tuberculosis
V12.02 Poliomyelitis
V12.03 Malaria
V12.09 Other

V12.1 Nutritional deficiency
V12.2 Endocrine, metabolic, and immunity disorders
Excludes *history of allergy (V14.0-V14.9, V15.01-V15.09)*
V12.3 Diseases of blood and blood-forming organs
V12.4 Disorders of nervous system and sense organs

V12.40 Unspecified disorder of nervous system and sense organs
V12.41 Benign neoplasm of the brain
AHA: 4Q 1997, 48
V12.42 Infections of the central nervous system
Encephalitis
Meningitis
AHA: 4Q 2005, 95
V12.49 Other disorders of nervous system and sense organs
AHA: 4Q 1998, 59

❺ **V12.5 Diseases of circulatory system**
Excludes *old myocardial infarction (412)*
postmyocardial infarction syndrome (411.0)
AHA: 4Q 1995, 61

⊘ **V12.50 Unspecified circulatory disease**

⊘ **V12.51 Venous thrombosis and embolism**
Pulmonary embolism
AHA: 3Q 2006, 12; 4Q 2003, 108; 1Q 2002, 15

⊘ **V12.52 Thrombophlebitis**

●⊘ **V12.53 Sudden cardiac arrest**
Sudden cardiac death successfully resuscitated

●⊘ **V12.54 Transient ischemic attack (TIA), and cerebral infarction without residual deficits**
Prolonged reversible ischemic neurological deficit (PRIND)
Reversible ischemic neurologic deficit (RIND)
Stroke NOS without residual deficits
Excludes *late effects of cerebrovascular disease (438.0-438.9)*

⊘ **V12.59 Other**
AHA: 4Q 1999, 4; 4Q 1998, 88; 4Q 1997, 37

❺ **V12.6 Diseases of respiratory system**
Excludes *tuberculosis (V12.01)*

⊘ **V12.60 Unspecified disease of respiratory system**

⊘ **V12.61 Pneumonia (recurrent)**
AHA: 4Q 2005, 95

⊘ **V12.69 Other diseases of respiratory system**

❺ **V12.7 Diseases of digestive system**
AHA: 1Q 1995, 3; 2Q 1989, 16

⊘ **V12.70 Unspecified digestive disease**

⊘ **V12.71 Peptic ulcer disease**

⊘ **V12.72 Colonic polyps**
AHA: 3Q 2002, 15

⊘ **V12.79 Other**

❹ **V13 Personal history of other diseases**

❺ **V13.0 Disorders of urinary system**

⊘ **V13.00 Unspecified urinary disorder**

⊘ **V13.01 Urinary calculi**

⊘ **V13.02 Urinary (tract) infection**
AHA: 4Q 2005, 95

⊘ **V13.03 Nephrotic syndrome**
AHA: 4Q 2005, 95

⊘ **V13.09 Other**

⊘ **V13.1 Trophoblastic disease** ♀
Excludes *supervision during a current pregnancy (V23.1)*

❺ **V13.2 Other genital system and obstetric disorders**
Excludes *habitual aborter (646.3)*
without current pregnancy (▶629.81◀)
supervision during a current pregnancy of a woman with poor obstetric history (V23.0-V23.9)

⊘ **V13.21 Personal history of pre-term labor** ♀
Excludes *current pregnancy with history of pre-term labor (V23.41)*
AHA: 4Q 2002, 78

●⊘ **V13.22 Personal history of cervical dysplasia** ♀
Personal history of conditions classifiable to 622.10-622.12
Excludes *personal history of malignant neoplasm of cervix uteri (V10.41)*

⊘ **V13.29 Other genital system and obstetric disorders** ♀

⊘ **V13.3 Diseases of skin and subcutaneous tissue**

⊘ **V13.4 Arthritis**

⊘ **V13.5 Other musculoskeletal disorders**

❺ **V13.6 Congenital malformations**
AHA: 4Q 1998, 63

⊘ **V13.61 Hypospadias** ♂

⊘ **V13.69 Other congenital malformations**
AHA: 1Q 2004, 16

⊘ **V13.7 Perinatal problems**
Excludes *low birth weight status (V21.30-V21.35)*

⊘ **V13.8 Other specified diseases**

⊘ **V13.9 Unspecified disease**

❹ **V14 Personal history of allergy to medicinal agents**

⊘ **V14.0 Penicillin**

⊘ **V14.1 Other antibiotic agent**

⊘ **V14.2 Sulfonamides**

⊘ **V14.3 Other anti-infective agent**

⊘ **V14.4 Anesthetic agent**

⊘ **V14.5 Narcotic agent**

⊘ **V14.6 Analgesic agent**

⊘ **V14.7 Serum or vaccine**

⊘ **V14.8 Other specified medicinal agents**

⊘ **V14.9 Unspecified medicinal agent**

❹ **V15 Other personal history presenting hazards to health**

❺ **V15.0 Allergy, other than to medicinal agents**
Excludes *allergy to food substance used as base for medicinal agent (V14.0-V14.9)*
AHA: 4Q 2000, 42, 49

⊘ **V15.01 Allergy to peanuts**

⊘ **V15.02 Allergy to milk products**
Excludes *lactose intolerance (271.3)*
AHA: 1Q 2003, 12

⊘ **V15.03 Allergy to eggs**

⊘ **V15.04 Allergy to seafood**
Seafood (octopus) (squid) ink
Shellfish

⊘ **V15.05 Allergy to other foods**
Food additives
Nuts other than peanuts

⊘ **V15.06 Allergy to insects**
Bugs
Insect bites and stings
Spiders

⊘ **V15.07 Allergy to latex**
Latex sensitivity

⊘ **V15.08 Allergy to radiographic dye**
Contrast media used for diagnostic x-ray procedures

⊘ **V15.09 Other allergy, other than to medicinal agents**

⊘ **V15.1 Surgery to heart and great vessels**
Excludes *replacement by transplant or other means (V42.1-V42.2, V43.2-V43.4)*
AHA: 1Q 2004, 16

⊘ **V15.2 Surgery to other major organs**
Excludes *replacement by transplant or other means (V42.0-V43.8)*

⊘ **V15.3 Irradiation**
Previous exposure to therapeutic or other ionizing radiation

❺ **V15.4 Psychological trauma**
Excludes *history of condition classifiable to 290-316 (V11.0-V11.9)*

⊘ **V15.41 History of physical abuse**
Rape
AHA: 3Q 1999, 15

⊘ **V15.42 History of emotional abuse**
Neglect
AHA: 3Q 1999, 15

⊘ **V15.49 Other**
AHA: 3Q 1999, 15

V15.5 Injury

V15.6 Poisoning

V15.7 Contraception
 Excludes *current contraceptive management (V25.0-V25.4)*
 presence of intrauterine contraceptive device as incidental finding (V45.5)

5 V15.8 Other specified personal history presenting hazards to health
 AHA: 4Q 1995, 62

V15.81 Noncompliance with medical treatment
 AHA: 4Q 2006, 136; 2Q 2003, 7; 2Q 2001, 11-13; 2Q 1999, 17; 2Q 1997, 11; 1Q 1997, 12; 3Q 1996, 9

V15.82 History of tobacco use
 Excludes *tobacco dependence (305.1)*

V15.84 Exposure to asbestos

V15.85 Exposure to potentially hazardous body fluids

V15.86 Exposure to lead

V15.87 History of extracorporeal membrane oxygenation [ECMO]
 AHA: 4Q 2003, 84

V15.88 History of fall
 At risk for falling
 AHA: 4Q 2005, 95

V15.89 Other
 AHA: 1Q 1990, 21; Nov-Dec, 1984, 12

V15.9 Unspecified personal history presenting hazards to health

4 V16 Family history of malignant neoplasm

V16.0 Gastrointestinal tract
 Family history of condition classifiable to 140-159
 AHA: 1Q 1999, 4

V16.1 Trachea, bronchus, and lung
 Family history of condition classifiable to 162

V16.2 Other respiratory and intrathoracic organs
 Family history of condition classifiable to 160-161, 163-165

V16.3 Breast
 Family history of condition classifiable to 174
 AHA: 4Q 2004, 107; 2Q 2003, 4; 2Q 2000, 8; 1Q 1992, 11

5 V16.4 Genital organs
 Family history of condition classifiable to 179-187
 AHA: 4Q 1997, 48

V16.40 Genital organ, unspecified

V16.41 Ovary

V16.42 Prostate

V16.43 Testis

V16.49 Other
 AHA: 2Q 2006, 3

5 V16.5 Urinary organs
 Family history of condition classifiable to ▶188-◀189

V16.51 Kidney

● V16.52 Bladder

V16.59 Other

V16.6 Leukemia
 Family history of condition classifiable to 204-208

V16.7 Other lymphatic and hematopoietic neoplasms
 Family history of condition classifiable to 200-203

V16.8 Other specified malignant neoplasm
 Family history of other condition classifiable to 140-199

V16.9 Unspecified malignant neoplasm

4 V17 Family history of certain chronic disabling diseases

V17.0 Psychiatric condition
 Excludes *family history of mental retardation (V18.4)*

V17.1 Stroke (cerebrovascular)

V17.2 Other neurological diseases
 Epilepsy
 Huntington's chorea

V17.3 Ischemic heart disease

5 V17.4 Other cardiovascular diseases
 AHA: 1Q 2004, 6

● V17.41 Family history of sudden cardiac death (SCD)
 Excludes *family history of ischemic heart disease (V17.3)*
 family history of myocardial infarction (V17.3)

● V17.49 Family history of other cardiovascular diseases
 Family history of cardiovascular disease NOS

V17.5 Asthma

V17.6 Other chronic respiratory conditions

V17.7 Arthritis

5 V17.8 Other musculoskeletal diseases

V17.81 Osteoporosis
 AHA: 4Q 2005, 95

V17.89 Other musculoskeletal diseases

4 V18 Family history of certain other specific conditions

V18.0 Diabetes mellitus
 AHA: 1Q 2004, 8

5 V18.1 Other endocrine and metabolic diseases

● V18.11 Multiple endocrine neoplasia [MEN] syndrome

● V18.19 Other endocrine and metabolic diseases

V18.2 Anemia

V18.3 Other blood disorders

V18.4 Mental retardation

5 V18.5 Digestive disorders

V18.51 Colonic polyps
 Excludes *family history of malignant neoplasm of gastrointestinal tract (V16.0)*

V18.59 Other digestive disorders

5 V18.6 Kidney diseases

V18.61 Polycystic kidney

V18.69 Other kidney diseases

V18.7 Other genitourinary diseases

V18.8 Infectious and parasitic diseases

V18.9 Genetic disease carrier
 AHA: 4Q 2005, 95

4 V19 Family history of other conditions

V19.0 Blindness or visual loss

V19.1 Other eye disorders

V19.2 Deafness or hearing loss

V19.3 Other ear disorders

V19.4 Skin conditions

V19.5 Congenital anomalies

V19.6 Allergic disorders

V19.7 Consanguinity

V19.8 Other condition

PERSONS ENCOUNTERING HEALTH SERVICES IN CIRCUMSTANCES RELATED TO REPRODUCTION AND DEVELOPMENT (V20-V29)

4 V20 Health supervision of infant or child

V20.0 Foundling P

V20.1 Other healthy infant or child receiving care P
Medical or nursing care supervision of healthy infant in cases of:
maternal illness, physical or psychiatric
socioeconomic adverse condition at home
too many children at home preventing or interfering with normal care
AHA: 1Q 2000, 25; 3Q 1989, 14

V20.2 Routine infant or child health check P
Developmental testing of infant or child
Immunizations appropriate for age
Initial and subsequent routine newborn check
Routine vision and hearing testing
Excludes *special screening for developmental handicaps (V79.3)*
Use additional code(s) to identify:
special screening examination(s) performed (V73.0-V82.9)
AHA: 1Q 2004, 15

4 V21 Constitutional states in development

V21.0 Period of rapid growth in childhood

V21.1 Puberty

V21.2 Other adolescence

5 V21.3 Low birth weight status
Excludes *history of perinatal problems (V13.7)*
AHA: 4Q 2000, 51

V21.30 Low birth weight status, unspecified

V21.31 Low birth weight status, less than 500 grams

V21.32 Low birth weight status, 500-999 grams

V21.33 Low birth weight status, 1000-1499 grams

V21.34 Low birth weight status, 1500-1999 grams

V21.35 Low birth weight status, 2000-2500 grams

V21.8 Other specified constitutional states in development

V21.9 Unspecified constitutional state in development

4 V22 Normal pregnancy
Excludes *pregnancy examination or test, pregnancy unconfirmed (V72.40)*

V22.0 Supervision of normal first pregnancy ♀
AHA: 3Q 1999, 16

V22.1 Supervision of other normal pregnancy ♀
AHA: 3Q 1999, 16

V22.2 Pregnant state, incidental ♀
Pregnant state NOS

4 V23 Supervision of high-risk pregnancy
AHA: 1Q 1990, 10

V23.0 Pregnancy with history of infertility ♀ M

V23.1 Pregnancy with history of trophoblastic disease ♀ M
Pregnancy with history of:
hydatidiform mole
vesicular mole
Excludes *that without current pregnancy (V13.1)*

V23.2 Pregnancy with history of abortion ♀ M
Pregnancy with history of conditions classifiable to 634-638
Excludes *habitual aborter:*
care during pregnancy (646.3)
that without current pregnancy (▶629.81◀)

V23.3 Grand multiparity ♀ M
Excludes *care in relation to labor and delivery (659.4)*
that without current pregnancy (V61.5)

5 V23.4 Pregnancy with other poor obstetric history
Pregnancy with history of other conditions classifiable to 630-676

V23.41 Pregnancy with history of pre-term labor ♀ M
C&C Exclusions: V23.7, V23.81, V23.82, V23.83, V23.84, V23.89, V23.9
AHA: 4Q 2002, 79

V23.49 Pregnancy with other poor obstetric history ♀ M
C&C Exclusions: See V23.41

V23.5 Pregnancy with other poor reproductive history ♀ M
Pregnancy with history of stillbirth or neonatal death

V23.7 Insufficient prenatal care ♀ M
History of little or no prenatal care
C&C Exclusions: V22.0, V22.1, V22.2, V23.0, V23.1, V23.2, V23.3, V23.41, V23.49, V23.5, V23.7, V23.81, V23.82, V23.83, V23.84, V23.89, V23.9

5 V23.8 Other high-risk pregnancy
AHA: 4Q 1998, 56, 63

V23.81 Elderly primigravida ♀ M
First pregnancy in a woman who will be 35 years of age or older at expected date of delivery
Excludes *elderly primigravida complicating pregnancy (659.5)*
C&C Exclusions: See V23.7

V23.82 Elderly multigravida ♀ M
Second or more pregnancy in a woman who will be 35 years of age or older at expected date of delivery
Excludes *elderly multigravida complicating pregnancy (659.6)*
C&C Exclusions: See V23.7

V23.83 Young primigravida ♀ M
First pregnancy in a female less than 16 years old at expected date of delivery
Excludes *young primigravida complicating pregnancy (659.8)*
C&C Exclusions: See V23.7

V23.84 Young multigravida ♀ M
Second or more pregnancy in a female less than 16 years old at expected date of delivery
Excludes *young multigravida complicating pregnancy (659.8)*
C&C Exclusions: See V23.7

V23.89 Other high-risk pregnancy ♀ M
C&C Exclusions: See V23.7

V23.9 Unspecified high-risk pregnancy ♀ M
C&C Exclusions: See V23.7

4 V24 Postpartum care and examination

V24.0 Immediately after delivery ♀ M
Care and observation in uncomplicated cases
AHA: 3Q 2006, 11

V24.1 Lactating mother ♀
Supervision of lactation

V24.2 Routine postpartum follow-up ♀

4 V25 Encounter for contraceptive management
AHA: 4Q 1992, 24

5 V25.0 General counseling and advice

V25.01 Prescription of oral contraceptives ♀

V25.02 Initiation of other contraceptive measures
Fitting of diaphragm
Prescription of foams, creams, or other agents
AHA: 3Q 1997, 7

V25.03 Encounter for emergency contraceptive counseling and prescription
Encounter for postcoital contraceptive counseling and prescription
AHA: 4Q 2003, 84

● **V25.04 Counseling and instruction in natural family planning to avoid pregnancy**

V25.09 Other
Family planning advice

V25.1 Insertion of intrauterine contraceptive device ♀

V25.2 Sterilization
Admission for interruption of fallopian tubes or vas deferens

V25.3 Menstrual extraction ♀
Menstrual regulation

V25.4 Surveillance of previously prescribed contraceptive methods
Checking, reinsertion, or removal of contraceptive device
Repeat prescription for contraceptive method
Routine examination in connection with contraceptive maintenance
Excludes *presence of intrauterine contraceptive device as incidental finding (V45.5)*

V25.40 Contraceptive surveillance, unspecified

V25.41 Contraceptive pill ♀

V25.42 Intrauterine contraceptive device ♀
Checking, reinsertion, or removal of intrauterine device

V25.43 Implantable subdermal contraceptive ♀

V25.49 Other contraceptive method
AHA: 3Q 1997, 7

V25.5 Insertion of implantable subdermal contraceptive ♀
AHA: 3Q 1992, 9

V25.8 Other specified contraceptive management
Postvasectomy sperm count
Excludes *sperm count following sterilization reversal (V26.22)*
sperm count for fertility testing (V26.21)
AHA: 3Q 1996, 9

V25.9 Unspecified contraceptive management

V26 Procreative management

V26.0 Tuboplasty or vasoplasty after previous sterilization
AHA: 2Q 1995, 10

V26.1 Artificial insemination ♀

V26.2 Investigation and testing
Excludes *postvasectomy sperm count (V25.8)*
AHA: 4Q 2000, 56

V26.21 Fertility testing
Fallopian insufflation
Sperm count for fertility testing
Excludes *genetic counseling and testing (V26.31-V26.39)*

V26.22 Aftercare following sterilization reversal
Fallopian insufflation following sterilization reversal
Sperm count following sterilization reversal

V26.29 Other investigation and testing
AHA: 2Q 1996, 9; Nov-Dec, 1985, 15

V26.3 Genetic counseling and testing
Excludes *fertility testing (V26.21)*
nonprocreative genetic screening (V82.71, V82.79)
AHA: 4Q 2005, 96

V26.31 Testing of female for genetic disease carrier status ♀

V26.32 Other genetic testing of female ♀
Use additional code to identify habitual aborter (629.81, 646.3)

V26.33 Genetic counseling

V26.34 Testing of male for genetic disease carrier status ♂

V26.35 Encounter for testing of male partner of habitual aborter ♂

V26.39 Other genetic testing of male ♂

V26.4 General counseling and advice

● **V26.41 Procreative counseling and advice using natural family planning**

● **V26.49 Other procreative management counseling and advice**

V26.5 Sterilization status

V26.51 Tubal ligation status ♀
Excludes *infertility not due to previous tubal ligation (628.0-628.9)*

V26.52 Vasectomy status ♂

V26.8 Other specified procreative management

● **V26.81 Encounter for assisted reproductive fertility procedure cycle**
Patient undergoing in vitro fertilization cycle
Use additional code to identify the type of infertility
Excludes *pre-cycle diagnosis and testing – code to reason for encounter*

● **V26.89 Other specified procreative management**

V26.9 Unspecified procreative management

V27 Outcome of delivery
Note: *This category is intended for the coding of the outcome of delivery on the mother's record.*
AHA: 2Q 1991, 16

V27.0 Single liveborn ♀M
AHA: 4Q 2005, 81; 2Q 2003, 9; 2Q 2002, 10; 1Q 2001, 10; 3Q 2000, 5; 4Q 1998, 77; 4Q 1995, 59; 1Q 1992, 9

V27.1 Single stillborn ♀M

V27.2 Twins, both liveborn ♀M

V27.3 Twins, one liveborn and one stillborn ♀M

V27.4 Twins, both stillborn ♀M

V27.5 Other multiple birth, all liveborn ♀M

V27.6 Other multiple birth, some liveborn ♀M

V27.7 Other multiple birth, all stillborn ♀M

V27.9 Unspecified outcome of delivery ♀M

V28 Encounter for antenatal screening of mother
Excludes *abnormal findings on screening-code to findings*
AHA: 1Q 2004, 11

V28.0 Screening for chromosomal anomalies by amniocentesis ♀M

V28.1 Screening for raised alpha-fetoprotein levels in amniotic fluid ♀M

V28.2 Other screening based on amniocentesis ♀M

V28.3 Screening for malformation using ultrasonics ♀

V28.4 Screening for fetal growth retardation using ultrasonics ♀

V28.5 Screening for isoimmunization ♀

V28.6 Screening for Streptococcus B ♀M
AHA: 4Q 1997, 46

V28.8 Other specified antenatal screening ♀
AHA: 3Q 1999, 16

V28.9 Unspecified antenatal screening ♀

V29 Observation and evaluation of newborns for suspected condition not found
Note: *This category is to be used for newborns, within the neonatal period (the first 28 days of life), who are suspected of having an abnormal condition resulting from exposure from the mother or the birth process, but without signs or symptoms, and which, after examination and observation, is found not to exist.*
AHA: 1Q 2000, 25; 4Q 1994, 47; 1Q 1994, 9; 4Q 1992, 21

V29.0 Observation for suspected infectious condition N
AHA: 1Q 2001, 10

V29.1 Observation for suspected neurological condition N

V29.2 Observation for suspected respiratory condition N

⊘ **V29.3 Observation for suspected genetic or metabolic condition** N
AHA: 2Q 2005, 21; 4Q 1998, 59, 68

V29.8 Observation for other specified suspected condition N
AHA: 2Q 2003, 15

⊘ **V29.9 Observation for unspecified suspected condition** N
AHA: 1Q 2002, 6

LIVEBORN INFANTS ACCORDING TO TYPE OF BIRTH (V30-V39)

Note: *These categories are intended for the coding of liveborn infants who are consuming health care [e.g., crib or bassinet occupancy].*

AHA: 1Q 2001, 10

The following fourth-digit subdivisions are for use with categories V30-V39:

5 **.0 Born in hospital**
.1 Born before admission to hospital
.2 Born outside hospital and not hospitalized

The following two fifth-digits are for use with the fourth-digit .0, Born in hospital:

0 delivered without mention of cesarean delivery
1 delivered by cesarean delivery

4 **V30 Single liveborn** N
(⊘ is only valid for fourth-digit "2")
(N only applies to fourth-digits "0" and "1")
AHA: 2Q 2003, 9; 4Q 1998, 46, 59; 1Q 1994, 9; For Code V30.00: 1Q 2004, 8, 16; 4Q 2003, 68; For Code V30.01: 4Q 2005, 88; For Code V30.1: 3Q 2006, 10-11

4 **V31 Twin, mate liveborn** N
(⊘ is only valid for fourth-digit "2")
(N only applies to fourth-digits "0" and "1")
AHA: 3Q 1992, 10

4 **V32 Twin, mate stillborn** N
(⊘ is only valid for fourth-digit "2")
(N only applies to fourth-digits "0" and "1")

4 **V33 Twin, unspecified** N
(⊘ is only valid for fourth-digit "2")
(N only applies to fourth-digits "0" and "1")

4 **V34 Other multiple, mates all liveborn** N
(⊘ is only valid for fourth-digit "2")
(N only applies to fourth-digits "0" and "1")

4 **V35 Other multiple, mates all stillborn** N
(⊘ is only valid for fourth-digit "2")
(N only applies to fourth-digits "0" and "1")

4 **V36 Other multiple, mates live- and stillborn** N
(⊘ is only valid for fourth-digit "2")
(N only applies to fourth-digits "0" and "1")

4 **V37 Other multiple, unspecified** N
(⊘ is only valid for fourth-digit "2")
(N only applies to fourth-digits "0" and "1")

4 **V39 Unspecified** N
(⊘ is only valid for fourth-digits "1" & "2")
(N only applies to fourth-digits "0" and "1")

PERSONS WITH A CONDITION INFLUENCING THEIR HEALTH STATUS (V40-V49)

Note: *These categories are intended for use when these conditions are recorded as "diagnoses" or "problems."*

4 **V40 Mental and behavioral problems**
⊘ **V40.0 Problems with learning**
⊘ **V40.1 Problems with communication [including speech]**
⊘ **V40.2 Other mental problems**
⊘ **V40.3 Other behavioral problems**
⊘ **V40.9 Unspecified mental or behavioral problem**

4 **V41 Problems with special senses and other special functions**
⊘ **V41.0 Problems with sight**
⊘ **V41.1 Other eye problems**
⊘ **V41.2 Problems with hearing**
⊘ **V41.3 Other ear problems**
⊘ **V41.4 Problems with voice production**
⊘ **V41.5 Problems with smell and taste**
⊘ **V41.6 Problems with swallowing and mastication**
⊘ **V41.7 Problems with sexual function**
Excludes *marital problems (V61.10)*
psychosexual disorders (302.0-302.9)
⊘ **V41.8 Other problems with special functions**
⊘ **V41.9 Unspecified problem with special functions**

4 **V42 Organ or tissue replaced by transplant**
Includes homologous or heterologous (animal) (human) transplant organ status
AHA: 3Q 1998, 3-4

⊘ **V42.0 Kidney**
C&C Exclusions: 996.80, 996.81, 996.87, V42.0, V42.89, V42.9
AHA: 1Q 2003, 10; 3Q 2001, 12

⊘ **V42.1 Heart**
C&C Exclusions: 996.80, 996.83, 996.87, V42.1, V42.89, V42.9, V43.21, V43.22
AHA: 3Q 2003, 16; 3Q 2001, 13

⊘ **V42.2 Heart valve**
C&C Exclusions: 996.71, V42.2, V42.89, V42.9

⊘ **V42.3 Skin**
⊘ **V42.4 Bone**
⊘ **V42.5 Cornea**
⊘ **V42.6 Lung**
C&C Exclusions: 996.80, 996.84, 996.87, V42.6, V42.89, V42.9

⊘ **V42.7 Liver**
C&C Exclusions: 996.80, 996.82, 996.87, V42.7, V42.89, V42.9

5 **V42.8 Other specified organ or tissue**
AHA: 4Q 1998, 64; 4Q 1997, 49

⊘ **V42.81 Bone marrow**
C&C Exclusions: 996.80, 996.85, 996.87, V42.9

⊘ **V42.82 Peripheral stem cells**
C&C Exclusions: 996.80, 996.87, V42.9

⊘ **V42.83 Pancreas**
C&C Exclusions: 996.80, 996.86, 996.87, V42.83, V42.9
AHA: 1Q 2003, 10; 2Q 2001, 16

⊘ **V42.84 Intestines**
C&C Exclusions: 996.80, 996.89, V42.84, V42.9
AHA: 4Q 2000, 48, 50

⊘ **V42.89 Other**
C&C Exclusions: 996.80, 996.87, 996.89, V42.84, V42.89, V42.9

⊘ **V42.9 Unspecified organ or tissue**
C&C Exclusions: See V42.89

4 **V43 Organ or tissue replaced by other means**
Includes organ or tissue assisted by other means
replacement of organ by:
artificial device
mechanical device
prosthesis
Excludes *cardiac pacemaker in situ (V45.01)*
fitting and adjustment of prosthetic device (V52.0-V52.9)
renal dialysis status (V45.1)

⊘ **V43.0 Eye globe**
⊘ **V43.1 Lens**
Pseudophakos
AHA: 4Q 1998.65

5 **V43.2 Heart**
AHA: 4Q 2003, 85

⊘ **V43.21 Heart assist device**
C&C Exclusions: 996.80, 996.83, 996.87, V42.1, V43.21, V43.22

V43.22 **Fully implantable artificial heart**
C&C Exclusions: See V43.21

V43.3 **Heart valve**
AHA: 3Q 2006, 7; 3Q 2002, 13-14

V43.4 **Blood vessel**

V43.5 **Bladder**

V43.6 **Joint**
AHA: 4Q 2005, 91

V43.60 **Unspecified joint**

V43.61 **Shoulder**

V43.62 **Elbow**

V43.63 **Wrist**

V43.64 **Hip**
AHA: 3Q 2006, 4; 4Q 2005, 93, 112; 2Q 2004, 15

V43.65 **Knee**

V43.66 **Ankle**

V43.69 **Other**

V43.7 **Limb**

V43.8 **Other organ or tissue**

V43.81 **Larynx**
AHA: 4Q 1995, 55

V43.82 **Breast**
AHA: 4Q 1995, 55

V43.83 **Artificial skin**

V43.89 **Other**

V44 **Artificial opening status**
Excludes *artificial openings requiring attention or management (V55.0-V55.9)*

V44.0 **Tracheostomy**
AHA: 4Q 2003, 103, 107, 111; 1Q 2001, 6

V44.1 **Gastrostomy**
AHA: 4Q 2003, 103, 107-108, 110; 1Q 2001, 12; 3Q 1997, 12; 1Q 1993, 26

V44.2 **Ileostomy**

V44.3 **Colostomy**
AHA: 4Q 2003, 110

V44.4 **Other artificial opening of gastrointestinal tract**

V44.5 **Cystostomy**

V44.50 **Cystostomy, unspecified**

V44.51 **Cutaneous-vesicostomy**

V44.52 **Appendico-vesicostomy**

V44.59 **Other cystostomy**

V44.6 **Other artificial opening of urinary tract**
Nephrostomy
Ureterostomy
Urethrostomy

V44.7 **Artificial vagina**

V44.8 **Other artificial opening status**

V44.9 **Unspecified artificial opening status**

V45 **Other postprocedural states**
Excludes *aftercare management (V51-V58.9)*
malfunction or other complication – code to condition
AHA: 4Q 2003, 85

V45.0 **Cardiac device in situ**
Excludes *artificial heart (V43.22)*
heart assist device (V43.21)

V45.00 **Unspecified cardiac device**

V45.01 **Cardiac pacemaker**

V45.02 **Automatic implantable cardiac defibrillator**

V45.09 **Other specified cardiac device**
Carotid sinus pacemaker in situ

V45.1 **Renal dialysis status**
Hemodialysis status
Patient requiring intermittent renal dialysis
Peritoneal dialysis status
Presence of arterial-venous shunt (for dialysis)
Excludes *admission for dialysis treatment or session (V56.0)*
C&C Exclusions: 996.73, V45.1
AHA: 4Q 2006, 136; 4Q 2005, 96; 1Q 2004, 22-23; 2Q 2003, 7; 2Q 2001, 12-13

V45.2 **Presence of cerebrospinal fluid drainage device**
Cerebral ventricle (communicating) shunt, valve, or device in situ
Excludes *malfunction (996.2)*
AHA: 4Q 2003, 106

V45.3 **Intestinal bypass or anastomosis status**
Excludes: *bariatric surgery status (V45.86)*
gastric bypass status (V45.86)
obesity surgery status (V45.86)

V45.4 **Arthrodesis status**
AHA: Nov-Dec, 1984, 18

V45.5 **Presence of contraceptive device**
Excludes *checking, reinsertion, or removal of device (V25.42)*
complication from device (996.32)
insertion of device (V25.1)

V45.51 **Intrauterine contraceptive device** ♀

V45.52 **Subdermal contraceptive implant**

V45.59 **Other**

V45.6 **States following surgery of eye and adnexa**
Excludes *aphakia (379.31)*
artificial eye globe (V43.0)
AHA: 4Q 1998, 65; 4Q 1997, 49

V45.61 **Cataract extraction status**
Use additional code for associated artificial lens status (V43.1)

V45.69 **Other states following surgery of eye and adnexa**
AHA: 2Q 2001, 16; 1Q 1998, 10; 4Q 1997, 19

V45.7 **Acquired absence of organ**
AHA: 4Q 1998, 65; 4Q 1997, 50

V45.71 **Acquired absence of breast**
AHA: 4Q 2001, 66; 4Q 1997, 50

V45.72 **Acquired absence of intestine (large) (small)**

V45.73 **Acquired absence of kidney**

V45.74 **Other parts of urinary tract**
Bladder
AHA: 4Q 2000, 51

V45.75 **Stomach**
AHA: 4Q 2000, 51

V45.76 **Lung**
AHA: 4Q 2000, 51

V45.77 **Genital organs**
Excludes *female genital mutilation status (629 20-629.29)*
AHA: 1Q 2003, 13-14; 4Q 2000, 51

V45.78 **Eye**
AHA: 4Q 2000, 51

V45.79 **Other acquired absence of organ**
AHA: 4Q 2000, 51

V45.8 **Other postprocedural status**

V45.81 **Aortocoronary bypass status**
AHA: 4Q 2003, 105; 3Q 2001, 15; 3Q 1997, 16

V45.82 **Percutaneous transluminal coronary angioplasty status**

V45.83 **Breast implant removal status**
AHA: 4Q 1995, 55

V45.84 **Dental restoration status**
Dental crowns status
Dental fillings status
AHA: 4Q 2001, 54

V45.85 **Insulin pump status**

V45.86 Bariatric surgery status
Gastric banding status
Gastric bypass status for obesity
Obesity surgery status
Excludes *bariatric surgery status complicating pregnancy, childbirth, or the puerperium (649.2)*
intestinal bypass or anastomosis status (V45.3)

V45.89 Other
Presence of neuropacemaker or other electronic device
Excludes *artificial heart valve in situ (V43.3)*
vascular prosthesis in situ (V43.4)
AHA: 1Q 1995, 11

V46 Other dependence on machines

V46.0 Aspirator
C&C Exclusions: V46.13, V46.14

V46.1 Respirator [Ventilator]
Iron lung
AHA: 4Q 2005, 96; 4Q 2003, 103; 1Q 2001, 12; Jan-Feb, 1987, 73

V46.11 Dependence on respirator, status
C&C Exclusions: V46.0, V46.11, V46.12, V46.13, V46.14, V46.8, V46.9
AHA: 4Q 2004, 100

V46.12 Encounter for respirator dependence during power failure
C&C Exclusions: See V46.11
AHA: 4Q 2004, 100

V46.13 Encounter for weaning from respirator [ventilator]
C&C Exclusions: V46.11, V46.12, V46.13, V46.14

V46.14 Mechanical complication of respirator [ventilator]
Mechanical failure of respirator [ventilator]
C&C Exclusions: See V46.13

V46.2 Supplemental oxygen
Long-term oxygen therapy
C&C Exclusions: See V46.13
AHA: 4Q 2003, 108; 4Q 2002, 79

V46.8 Other enabling machines
Hyperbaric chamber
Possum [Patient-Operated-Selector-Mechanism]
Excludes *cardiac pacemaker (V45.0)*
kidney dialysis machine (V45.1)
C&C Exclusions: See V46.0

V46.9 Unspecified machine dependence
C&C Exclusions: See V46.0

V47 Other problems with internal organs

V47.0 Deficiencies of internal organs

V47.1 Mechanical and motor problems with internal organs

V47.2 Other cardiorespiratory problems
Cardiovascular exercise intolerance with pain (with):
at rest
less than ordinary activity
ordinary activity

V47.3 Other digestive problems

V47.4 Other urinary problems

V47.5 Other genital problems

V47.9 Unspecified

V48 Problems with head, neck, and trunk

V48.0 Deficiencies of head
Excludes *deficiencies of ears, eyelids, and nose (V48.8)*

V48.1 Deficiencies of neck and trunk

V48.2 Mechanical and motor problems with head

V48.3 Mechanical and motor problems with neck and trunk

V48.4 Sensory problem with head

V48.5 Sensory problem with neck and trunk

V48.6 Disfigurements of head

V48.7 Disfigurements of neck and trunk

V48.8 Other problems with head, neck, and trunk

V48.9 Unspecified problem with head, neck, or trunk

V49 Other conditions influencing health status

V49.0 Deficiencies of limbs

V49.1 Mechanical problems with limbs

V49.2 Motor problems with limbs

V49.3 Sensory problems with limbs

V49.4 Disfigurements of limbs

V49.5 Other problems of limbs

V49.6 Upper limb amputation status
AHA: 4Q 2005, 94; 4Q 1998, 42; 4Q 1994, 39

V49.60 Unspecified level

V49.61 Thumb

V49.62 Other finger(s)
AHA: 2Q 2005, 7

V49.63 Hand

V49.64 Wrist
Disarticulation of wrist

V49.65 Below elbow

V49.66 Above elbow
Disarticulation of elbow

V49.67 Shoulder
Disarticulation of shoulder

V49.7 Lower limb amputation status
AHA: 4Q 2005, 94; 4Q 1998, 42; 4Q 1994, 39

V49.70 Unspecified level

V49.71 Great toe

V49.72 Other toe(s)

V49.73 Foot

V49.74 Ankle
Disarticulation of ankle

V49.75 Below knee

V49.76 Above knee
Disarticulation of knee
AHA: 2Q 2005, 14

V49.77 Hip
Disarticulation of hip

V49.8 Other specified conditions influencing health status
AHA: 4Q 2000, 51

V49.81 Asymptomatic postmenopausal status (age-related) (natural) ♀ A
Excludes *menopausal and premenopausal disorders (627.0-627.9)*
postsurgical menopause (256.2)
premature menopause (256.31)
symptomatic menopause (627.0-627.9)
AHA: 4Q 2002, 79; 4Q 2000, 54

V49.82 Dental sealant status
AHA: 4Q 2001, 54

V49.83 Awaiting organ transplant status

V49.84 Bed confinement status
AHA: 4Q 2005, 96

● **V49.85 Dual sensory impairment**
Blindness with deafness
Combined visual hearing impairment
Code first:
hearing impairment (389.00-389.9)
visual impairment (369.00-369.9)

V49.89 Other specified conditions influencing health status
AHA: 4Q 2005, 94

V49.9 Unspecified

PERSONS ENCOUNTERING HEALTH SERVICES FOR SPECIFIC PROCEDURES AND AFTERCARE (V50-V59)

Note: *Categories V51-V58 are intended for use to indicate a reason for care in patients who may have already been treated for some disease or injury not now present, or who are receiving care to consolidate the treatment, to deal with residual states, or to prevent recurrence.*

Excludes *follow-up examination for medical surveillance following treatment (V67.0-V67.9)*

4 **V50 Elective surgery for purposes other than remedying health states**

V50.0 Hair transplant

V50.1 Other plastic surgery for unacceptable cosmetic appearance

Breast augmentation or reduction

Face-lift

Excludes *plastic surgery following healed injury or operation (V51)*

V50.2 Routine or ritual circumcision ♂

Circumcision in the absence of significant medical indication

⃠ **V50.3 Ear piercing**

5 **V50.4 Prophylactic organ removal**

Excludes *organ donations (V59.0-V59.9)*
therapeutic organ removal–code to condition

AHA: 4Q 1994, 44

V50.41 Breast

AHA: 4Q 2004, 107

V50.42 Ovary ♀

V50.49 Other

⃠ **V50.8 Other**

⃠ **V50.9 Unspecified**

V51 Aftercare involving the use of plastic surgery

Plastic surgery following healed injury or operation

Excludes *cosmetic plastic surgery (V50.1)*
plastic surgery as treatment for current injury - code to condition
repair of scar tissue - code to scar

4 **V52 Fitting and adjustment of prosthetic device and implant**

Includes removal of device

Excludes *malfunction or complication of prosthetic device (996.0-996.7)*
status only, without need for care (V43.0-V43.8)

AHA: 4Q 2005, 94; 4Q 1995, 55; 1Q 1990, 7

V52.0 Artificial arm (complete) (partial)

V52.1 Artificial leg (complete) (partial)

V52.2 Artificial eye

V52.3 Dental prosthetic device

V52.4 Breast prosthesis and implant ♀

Excludes *admission for breast implant insertion (V50.1)*

AHA: 4Q 1995, 80-81

V52.8 Other specified prosthetic device

AHA: 2Q 2002, 12, 16

⃠ **V52.9 Unspecified prosthetic device**

4 **V53 Fitting and adjustment of other device**

Includes removal of device
replacement of device

Excludes *status only, without need for care (V45.0-V45.8)*

5 **V53.0 Devices related to nervous system and special senses**

AHA: 4Q 1998, 66; 4Q 1997, 51

V53.01 Fitting and adjustment of cerebral ventricle (communicating) shunt

AHA: 4Q 1997, 51

V53.02 Neuropacemaker (brain) (peripheral nerve) (spinal cord)

V53.09 Fitting and adjustment of other devices related to nervous system and special senses

Auditory substitution device

Visual substitution device

AHA: 2Q 1999, 4

⃠ **V53.1 Spectacles and contact lenses**

⃠ **V53.2 Hearing aid**

5 **V53.3 Cardiac device**

Reprogramming

AHA: 3Q 1992, 3; 1Q 1990, 7; May-Jun, 1987, 8; Nov-Dec, 1984, 18

V53.31 Cardiac pacemaker

Excludes *mechanical complication of cardiac pacemaker (996.01)*

AHA: 1Q 2002, 3

V53.32 Automatic implantable cardiac defibrillator

AHA: 3Q 2005, 8

V53.39 Other cardiac device

⃠ **V53.4 Orthodontic devices**

⃠ **V53.5 Other intestinal appliance**

Excludes *colostomy (V55.3)*
ileostomy (V55.2)
other artifical opening of digestive tract (V55.4)

⃠ **V53.6 Urinary devices**

Urinary catheter

Excludes *cystostomy (V55.5)*
nephrostomy (V55.6)
ureterostomy (V55.6)
urethrostomy (V55.6)

⃠ **V53.7 Orthopedic devices**

Orthopedic:
brace
cast
corset
shoes

Excludes *other orthopedic aftercare (V54)*

⃠ **V53.8 Wheelchair**

5 **V53.9 Other and unspecified device**

AHA: 2Q 2003, 6

⃠ **V53.90 Unspecified device**

⃠ **V53.91 Fitting and adjustment of insulin pump**

Insulin pump titration

⃠ **V53.99 Other device**

4 **V54 Other orthopedic aftercare**

Excludes *fitting and adjustment of orthopedic devices (V53.7)*
malfunction of internal orthopedic device (996.40-996.49)
other complication of nonmechanical nature (996.60-996.79)

AHA: 3Q 1995, 3

5 **V54.0 Aftercare involving internal fixation device**

Excludes *malfunction of internal orthopedic device (996.40-996.49)*
other complication of nonmechanical nature (996.60-996.79)
removal of external fixation device (V54.89)

AHA: 4Q 2003, 87

V54.01 Encounter for removal of internal fixation device

V54.02 Encounter for lengthening/adjustment of growth rod

V54.09 Other aftercare involving internal fixation device

5 **V54.1 Aftercare for healing traumatic fracture**

Excludes: *aftercare for amputation stump (V54.89)*

AHA: 4Q 2002, 80

V54.10 Aftercare for healing traumatic fracture of arm, unspecified

V54.11 Aftercare for healing traumatic fracture of upper arm

V54.12 Aftercare for healing traumatic fracture of lower arm

AHA: 1Q 2007, 7

V54.13 Aftercare for healing traumatic fracture of hip

AHA: 4Q 2003, 103, 105; 2Q 2003, 16

A Adult (15+ years) M Maternity (12-55 years) N Neonates (0 years) P Pediatric (0-17 years) ♂ Male ♀ Female

V54.14 Aftercare for healing traumatic fracture of leg, unspecified

V54.15 Aftercare for healing traumatic fracture of upper leg

Excludes *aftercare for healing traumatic fracture of hip (V54.13)*

AHA: 3Q 2006, 6

V54.16 Aftercare for healing traumatic fracture of lower leg

V54.17 Aftercare for healing traumatic fracture of vertebrae

V54.19 Aftercare for healing traumatic fracture of other bone

AHA: 1Q 2005, 13; 4Q 2002, 80

5 **V54.2 Aftercare for healing pathologic fracture**

AHA: 4Q 2002, 80

V54.20 Aftercare for healing pathologic fracture of arm, unspecified

V54.21 Aftercare for healing pathologic fracture of upper arm

V54.22 Aftercare for healing pathologic fracture of lower arm

V54.23 Aftercare for healing pathologic fracture of hip

V54.24 Aftercare for healing pathologic fracture of leg, unspecified

V54.25 Aftercare for healing pathologic fracture of upper leg

Excludes *aftercare for healing pathologic fracture of hip (V54.23)*

V54.26 Aftercare for healing pathologic fracture of lower leg

V54.27 Aftercare for healing pathologic fracture of vertebrae

AHA: 1Q 2007, 6; 4Q 2003, 108

V54.29 Aftercare for healing pathologic fracture of other bone

AHA: 4Q 2002, 80

5 **V54.8 Other orthopedic aftercare**

AHA: 3Q 2001, 19; 4Q 1999, 5

V54.81 Aftercare following joint replacement

Use additional code to identify joint replacement site (V43.60-V43.69)

AHA: 3Q 2006, 4; 2Q 2004, 15; 4Q 2002, 80

V54.89 Other orthopedic aftercare

Aftercare for healing fracture NOS

⃠ **V54.9 Unspecified orthopedic aftercare**

4 **V55 Attention to artificial openings**

Includes adjustment or repositioning of catheter
closure
passage of sounds or bougies
reforming
removal or replacement of catheter
toilet or cleansing

Excludes *complications of external stoma (519.00-519.09, 569.60-569.69, 997.4, 997.5)*
status only, without need for care (V44.0-V44.9)

V55.0 Tracheostomy

V55.1 Gastrostomy

AHA: 4Q 1999, 9; 3Q 1997, 7-8; 1Q 1996, 14; 3Q 1995, 13

V55.2 Ileostomy

V55.3 Colostomy

AHA: 2Q 2005, 4; 3Q 1997, 9

V55.4 Other artificial opening of digestive tract

AHA: 2Q 2005, 14; 1Q 2003, 10

V55.5 Cystostomy

V55.6 Other artificial opening of urinary tract

Nephrostomy
Ureterostomy
Urethrostomy

V55.7 Artificial vagina

V55.8 Other specified artificial opening

⃠ **V55.9 Unspecified artificial opening**

4 **V56 Encounter for dialysis and dialysis catheter care**

Use additional code to identify the associated condition

Excludes *dialysis preparation - code to condition*

AHA: 4Q 1998, 66; 1Q 1993, 29

V56.0 Extracorporeal dialysis

Dialysis (renal) NOS

Excludes *dialysis status (V45.1)*

AHA: 4Q 2005, 79; 1Q 2004, 23; 4Q 2000, 40; 3Q 1998, 6; 2Q 1998, 20

V56.1 Fitting and adjustment of extracorporeal dialysis catheter

Removal or replacement of catheter
Toilet or cleansing
Use additional code for any concurrent extracorporeal dialysis (V56.0)

AHA: 2Q 1998, 20

⃠ **V56.2 Fitting and adjustment of peritoneal dialysis catheter**

Use additional code for any concurrent peritoneal dialysis (V56.8)

AHA: 4Q 1998, 55

5 **V56.3 Encounter for adequacy testing for dialysis**

AHA: 4Q 2000, 55

⃠ **V56.31 Encounter for adequacy testing for hemodialysis**

⃠ **V56.32 Encounter for adequacy testing for peritoneal dialysis**

Peritoneal equilibration test

V56.8 Other dialysis

Peritoneal dialysis

AHA: 4Q 1998, 55

4 **V57 Care involving use of rehabilitation procedures**

Use additional code to identify underlying condition

AHA: 3Q 2006, 3: 1Q 2002, 19; 3Q 1997, 12; 1Q 1990, 6; Sep-Oct 1986, 3

⃠ **V57.0 Breathing exercises**

⃠ **V57.1 Other physical therapy**

Therapeutic and remedial exercises, except breathing

AHA: 3Q 2006, 4; 2Q 2004, 15; 4Q 2002, 56; 4Q 1999, 5

5 **V57.2 Occupational therapy and vocational rehabilitation**

⃠ **V57.21 Encounter for occupational therapy**

AHA: 4Q 1999, 7

⃠ **V57.22 Encounter for vocational therapy**

⃠ **V57.3 Speech therapy**

AHA: 4Q 1997, 36

⃠ **V57.4 Orthoptic training**

5 **V57.8 Other specified rehabilitation procedure**

⃠ **V57.81 Orthotic training**

Gait training in the use of artificial limbs

⃠ **V57.89 Other**

Multiple training or therapy

AHA: 3Q 2006, 6; 4Q 2003, 105-106, 108; 2Q 2003, 16; 1Q 2002, 16; 3Q 2001, 21; 3Q 1997, 11-12; Sep-Oct 1986, 4

⃠ **V57.9 Unspecified rehabilitation procedure**

4 **V58 Encounter for other and unspecified procedures and aftercare**

Excludes *convalescence and palliative care (V66.0-V66.9)*

V58.0 Radiotherapy

Encounter or admission for radiotherapy

Excludes *encounter for radioactive implant – code to condition*
radioactive iodine therapy – code to condition

AHA: 3Q 1992, 5; 2Q 1990, 7; Jan-Feb, 1987, 13

V58.1 Encounter for antineoplastic chemotherapy and immunotherapy
Encounter or admission for chemotherapy
Excludes *chemotherapy and immunotherapy for nonneoplastic conditions – code to condition*
prophylactic chemotherapy against disease which has never been present (V03.0-V07.9)
AHA: 1Q 2004, 13; 2Q 2003, 16; 3Q 1993, 4; 2Q 1992, 6; 2Q 1991, 17; 2Q 1990, 7; Sep-Oct, 1984, 5

V58.11 Encounter for antineoplastic chemotherapy
AHA: 2Q 2006, 21; 4Q 2005, 98

V58.12 Encounter for antineoplastic immunotherapy
AHA: 4Q 2005, 98

V58.2 Blood transfusion, without reported diagnosis

V58.3 Attention to dressings and sutures
Change or removal of wound packing
Excludes: *attention to drains (V58.49)*
planned postoperative wound closure (V58.41)
AHA: 2Q 2005, 14

V58.30 Encounter for change or removal of nonsurgical wound dressing
Encounter for change or removal of wound dressing NOS

V58.31 Encounter for change or removal of surgical wound dressing

V58.32 Encounter for removal of sutures
Encounter for removal of staples

V58.4 Other aftercare following surgery
Note: Codes from this subcategory should be used in conjunction with other aftercare codes to fully identify the reason for the aftercare encounter.
Excludes *aftercare following sterilization reversal surgery (V26.22)*
attention to artificial openings (V55.0-V55.9)
orthopedic aftercare (V54.0-V54.9)
AHA: 4Q 1999, 9; Nov-Dec, 1987, 9

V58.41 Encounter for planned postoperative wound closure
Excludes *disruption of operative wound (998.3)*
encounter for dressings and suture aftercare (V58.30-V58.32)
AHA: 4Q 1999, 15

V58.42 Aftercare following surgery for neoplasm
Conditions classifiable to 140-239
AHA: 4Q 2002, 80

V58.43 Aftercare following surgery for injury and trauma
Conditions classifiable to 800-999
Excludes *aftercare for healing traumatic fracture (V54.10-V54.19)*
AHA: 4Q 2002, 80

V58.44 Aftercare following organ transplant
Use additional code to identify the organ transplanted (V42.0-V42.9)
AHA: 4Q 2004, 101

V58.49 Other specified aftercare following surgery
Change or removal of drains
AHA: 1Q 1996, 8-9

V58.5 Orthodontics
Excludes *fitting and adjustment of orthodontic device (V53.4)*

V58.6 Long-term (current) drug use
Excludes *drug abuse (305.00-305.93)*
drug dependence (304.00-304.93)
hormone replacement therapy (postmenopausal) (V07.4)
AHA: 4Q 2003, 85; 4Q 2002, 84; 3Q 2002, 15; 4Q 1995, 61

V58.61 Long-term (current) use of anticoagulants
Excludes *long-term (current) use of aspirin (V58.66)*
AHA: 3Q 2006, 13; 3Q 2004, 7; 4Q 2003, 108; 3Q 2002, 13-16; 1Q 2002, 15-16

V58.62 Long-term (current) use of antibiotics
AHA: 4Q 1998, 59

V58.63 Long-term (current) use of antiplatelets/antithrombotics
Excludes *long-term (current) use of aspirin (V58.66)*

V58.64 Long-term (current) use of non-steroidal anti-inflammatories (NSAID)
Excludes *long-term (current) use of aspirin (V58.66)*

V58.65 Long-term (current) use of steroids

V58.66 Long-term (current) use of aspirin
AHA: 4Q 2004, 102

V58.67 Long-term (current) use of insulin
AHA: 4Q 2004, 55-56, 103

V58.69 Long-term (current) use of other medications
▶Other◀ high-risk medications
AHA: 2Q 2004, 10; 1Q 2003, 11; 2Q 2000, 8; 3Q 1999, 13; 2Q 1999, 17; 1Q 1997, 12; 2Q 1996, 7

V58.7 Aftercare following surgery to specified body systems, not elsewhere classified
Note: Codes from this subcategory should be used in conjunction with other aftercare codes to fully identify the reason for the aftercare encounter.
Excludes *aftercare following organ transplant (V58.44)*
aftercare following surgery for neoplasm (V58.42)
AHA: 4Q 2003, 104; 4Q 2002, 80

V58.71 Aftercare following surgery of the sense organs, NEC
Conditions classifiable to 360-379, 380-389

V58.72 Aftercare following surgery of the nervous system, NEC
Conditions classifiable to 320-359
Excludes *aftercare following surgery to the sense organs, NEC (V58.71)*

V58.73 Aftercare following surgery of the circulatory system, NEC
Conditions classifiable to 390-459
AHA: 4Q 2003, 105

V58.74 Aftercare following surgery of the respiratory system, NEC
Conditions classifiable to 460-519

V58.75 Aftercare following surgery of the teeth, oral cavity and digestive system, NEC
Conditions classifiable to 520-579
AHA: 2Q 2005, 14

V58.76 Aftercare following surgery of the genitourinary system, NEC
Conditions classifiable to 580-629
Excludes *aftercare following sterilization reversal (V26.22)*
AHA: 1Q 2005, 11-12

V58.77 Aftercare following surgery of the skin and subcutaneous tissue, NEC
Conditions classifiable to 680-709

V58.78 Aftercare following surgery of the musculoskeletal system, NEC
Conditions classifiable to 710-739
Excludes ▶ *orthopedic aftercare (V54.01-V54.9)*◀

A Adult (15+ years) M Maternity (12-55 years) N Neonates (0 years) P Pediatric (0-17 years) ♂ Male ♀ Female

⑤ **V58.8 Other specified procedures and aftercare**

AHA: 4Q 1994, 45; 2Q 1994, 8

V58.81 Fitting and adjustment of vascular catheter

Removal or replacement of catheter
Toilet or cleansing

Excludes *complications of renal dialysis (996.73)*
complications of vascular catheter (996.74)
dialysis preparation – code to condition
encounter for dialysis (V56.0-V56.8)
fitting and adjustment of dialysis catheter (V56.1)

V58.82 Fitting and adjustment of non-vascular catheter NEC

Removal or replacement of catheter
Toilet or cleansing

Excludes *fitting and adjustment of peritoneal dialysis catheter (V56.2)*
fitting and adjustment of urinary catheter (V53.6)

V58.83 Encounter for therapeutic drug monitoring

Use additional code for any associated long-term (current) drug use (V58.61-V58.69)

Excludes *blood-drug testing for medicolegal reasons (V70.4)*

AHA: 2Q 2004, 10; 1Q 2004, 13; 4Q 2003, 85; 4Q 2002, 84; 3Q 2002, 13-16

V58.89 Other specified aftercare

AHA: 4Q 1998, 59

⊘ **V58.9 Unspecified aftercare**

④ **V59 Donors**

Excludes *examination of potential donor (V70.8)*
self-donation of organ or tissue - code to condition

AHA: 4Q 1995, 62; 1Q 1990, 10; Nov-Dec, 1984, 8

⑤ **V59.0 Blood**

⊘ **V59.01 Whole blood**

⊘ **V59.02 Stem cells**

⊘ **V59.09 Other**

V59.1 Skin

V59.2 Bone

V59.3 Bone marrow

V59.4 Kidney

V59.5 Cornea

V59.6 Liver

⑤ **V59.7 Egg (oocyte) (ovum)**

AHA: 4Q 2005, 99

⊘ **V59.70 Egg (oocyte) (ovum) donor, unspecified** ♀

⊘ **V59.71 Egg (oocyte) (ovum) donor, under age 35, anonymous recipient** ♀

Egg donor, under age 35 NOS

⊘ **V59.72 Egg (oocyte) (ovum) donor, under age 35, designated recipient** ♀

⊘ **V59.73 Egg (oocyte) (ovum) donor, age 35 and over, anonymous recipient** ♀

Egg donor, age 35 and over NOS

⊘ **V59.74 Egg (oocyte) (ovum) donor, age 35 and over, designated recipient** ♀

V59.8 Other specified organ or tissue

AHA: 3Q 2002, 20

V59.9 Unspecified organ or tissue

PERSONS ENCOUNTERING HEALTH SERVICES IN OTHER CIRCUMSTANCES (V60-V69)

④ **V60 Housing, household, and economic circumstances**

⊘ **V60.0 Lack of housing**

Hobos
Social migrants
Tramps
Transients
Vagabonds

⊘ **V60.1 Inadequate housing**

Lack of heating
Restriction of space
Technical defects in home preventing adequate care

⊘ **V60.2 Inadequate material resources**

Economic problem
Poverty NOS

⊘ **V60.3 Person living alone**

⊘ **V60.4 No other household member able to render care**

Person requiring care (has) (is):
family member too handicapped, ill, or otherwise unsuited to render care
partner temporarily away from home
temporarily away from usual place of abode

Excludes *holiday relief care (V60.5)*

⊘ **V60.5 Holiday relief care**

Provision of health care facilities to a person normally cared for at home, to enable relatives to take a vacation

⊘ **V60.6 Person living in residential institution**

Boarding school resident

⊘ **V60.8 Other specified housing or economic circumstances**

⊘ **V60.9 Unspecified housing or economic circumstance**

④ **V61 Other family circumstances**

Includes when these circumstances or fear of them, affecting the person directly involved or others, are mentioned as the reason, justified or not, for seeking or receiving medical advice or care

AHA: 1Q 1990, 9

⊘ **V61.0 Family disruption**

Divorce
Estrangement

⑤ **V61.1 Counseling for marital and partner problems**

Excludes *problems related to:*
psychosexual disorders (302.0-302.9)
sexual function (V41.7)

⊘ **V61.10 Counseling for marital and partner problems, unspecified**

Marital conflict
Marital relationship problem
Partner conflict
Partner relationship problem

⊘ **V61.11 Counseling for victim of spousal and partner abuse**

Excludes *encounter for treatment of current injuries due to abuse (995.80-995.85)*

⊘ **V61.12 Counseling for perpetrator of spousal and partner abuse**

⑤ **V61.2 Parent-child problems**

⊘ **V61.20 Counseling for parent-child problem, unspecified**

Concern about behavior of child
Parent-child conflict
Parent-child relationship problem

V61.21 Counseling for victim of child abuse

Child battering
Child neglect

Excludes *current injuries due to abuse (995.50-995.59)*

⊘ **V61.22 Counseling for perpetrator of parental child abuse**

Excludes *counseling for non-parental abuser (V62.83)*

V61.29 Other
Problem concerning adopted or foster child
AHA: 3Q 1999, 16

V61.3 Problems with aged parents or in-laws

V61.4 Health problems within family

V61.41 Alcoholism in family

V61.49 Other
Care of sick or handicapped person in family or household
Presence of sick or handicapped person in family or household

V61.5 Multiparity

V61.6 Illegitimacy or illegitimate pregnancy ♀ M

V61.7 Other unwanted pregnancy ♀ M

V61.8 Other specified family circumstances
Problems with family members NEC
Sibling relationship problem

V61.9 Unspecified family circumstance

V62 Other psychosocial circumstances
Includes those circumstances or fear of them, affecting the person directly involved or others, mentioned as the reason, justified or not, for seeking or receiving medical advice or care
Excludes *previous psychological trauma (V15.41-V15.49)*

V62.0 Unemployment
Excludes *circumstances when main problem is economic inadequacy or poverty (V60.2)*

V62.1 Adverse effects of work environment

V62.2 Other occupational circumstances or maladjustment
Career choice problem
Dissatisfaction with employment
Occupational problem

V62.3 Educational circumstances
Academic problem
Dissatisfaction with school environment
Educational handicap

V62.4 Social maladjustment
Acculturation problem
Cultural deprivation
Political, religious, or sex discrimination
Social:
isolation
persecution

V62.5 Legal circumstances
Imprisonment
Legal investigation
Litigation
Prosecution

V62.6 Refusal of treatment for reasons of religion or conscience

V62.8 Other psychological or physical stress, not elsewhere classified

V62.81 Interpersonal problems, not elsewhere classified
Relational problem NOS

V62.82 Bereavement, uncomplicated
Excludes *bereavement as adjustment reaction (309.0)*

V62.83 Counseling for perpetrator of physical/sexual abuse
Excludes *counseling for perpetrator of parental child abuse (V61.22)*
counseling for perpetrator of spousal and partner abuse (V61.12)

V62.84 Suicidal ideation
Excludes *suicidal tendencies (300.9)*
AHA: 4Q 2005, 96

V62.89 Other
Borderline intellectual functioning
Life circumstance problems
Phase of life problems
Religious or spiritual problem

V62.9 Unspecified psychosocial circumstance

V63 Unavailability of other medical facilities for care
AHA: 1Q 1991, 21

V63.0 Residence remote from hospital or other health care facility

V63.1 Medical services in home not available
Excludes *no other household member able to render care (V60.4)*
AHA: 4Q 2001, 67; 1Q 2001, 12

V63.2 Person awaiting admission to adequate facility elsewhere

V63.8 Other specified reasons for unavailability of medical facilities
Person on waiting list undergoing social agency investigation

V63.9 Unspecified reason for unavailability of medical facilities

V64 Persons encountering health services for specific procedures, not carried out

V64.0 Vaccination not carried out
AHA: 4Q 2005, 99

V64.00 Vaccination not carried out, unspecified reason

V64.01 Vaccination not carried out because of acute illness

V64.02 Vaccination not carried out because of chronic illness or condition

V64.03 Vaccination not carried out because of immune compromised state

V64.04 Vaccination not carried out because of allergy to vaccine or component

V64.05 Vaccination not carried out because of caregiver refusal
▶ Guardian refusal ◀
▶ Parent refusal ◀
AHA: 1Q 2007, 12

V64.06 Vaccination not carried out because of patient refusal

V64.07 Vaccination not carried out for religious reasons

V64.08 Vaccination not carried out because patient had disease being vaccinated against

V64.09 Vaccination not carried out for other reason

V64.1 Surgical or other procedure not carried out because of contraindication

V64.2 Surgical or other procedure not carried out because of patient's decision
AHA: 2Q 2001, 8

V64.3 Procedure not carried out for other reasons

V64.4 Closed surgical procedure converted to open procedure
AHA: 4Q 2003, 87; 4Q 1998, 68; 4Q 1997, 52

V64.41 Laparoscopic surgical procedure converted to open procedure

V64.42 Thoracoscopic surgical procedure converted to open procedure

V64.43 Arthroscopic surgical procedure converted to open procedure

V65 Other persons seeking consultation

V65.0 Healthy person accompanying sick person
Boarder

V65.1 Person consulting on behalf of another person
Advice or treatment for nonattending third party
Excludes *concern (normal) about sick person in family (V61.41-V61.49)*
AHA: 4Q 2003, 84

V65.11 Pediatric pre-birth visit for expectant mother ♀ M

⦸ **V65.19 Other person consulting on behalf of another person**

V65.2 Person feigning illness
Malingerer
Peregrinating patient
AHA: 3Q 1999, 20

⦸ **V65.3 Dietary surveillance and counseling**
Dietary surveillance and counseling (in):
NOS
colitis
diabetes mellitus
food allergies or intolerance
gastritis
hypercholesterolemia
hypoglycemia
obesity
Use additional code to identify Body Mass Index (BMI), if known (V85.0-V85.54)
AHA: 4Q 2005, 96

❺ **V65.4 Other counseling, not elsewhere classified**
Health:
advice
education
instruction
Excludes *counseling (for):*
contraception (V25.40-V25.49)
genetic (V26.31-V26.39)
on behalf of third party (V65.11, V65.19)
procreative management (▶V26.41-V26.49◀)

⦸ **V65.40 Counseling NOS**

⦸ **V65.41 Exercise counseling**

⦸ **V65.42 Counseling on substance use and abuse**

⦸ **V65.43 Counseling on injury prevention**

⦸ **V65.44 Human immunodeficiency virus [HIV] counseling**

⦸ **V65.45 Counseling on other sexually transmitted diseases**

⦸ **V65.46 Encounter for insulin pump training**

⦸ **V65.49 Other specified counseling**
AHA: 2Q 2000, 8

⦸ **V65.5 Person with feared complaint in whom no diagnosis was made**
Feared condition not demonstrated
Problem was normal state
"Worried well"

⦸ **V65.8 Other reasons for seeking consultation**
Excludes *specified symptoms*
AHA: 3Q 1992, 4

⦸ **V65.9 Unspecified reason for consultation**

❹ **V66 Convalescence and palliative care**

V66.0 Following surgery

V66.1 Following radiotherapy

V66.2 Following chemotherapy

V66.3 Following psychotherapy and other treatment for mental disorder

V66.4 Following treatment of fracture

⦸ **V66.5 Following other treatment**

V66.6 Following combined treatment

⦸ **V66.7 Encounter for palliative care**
End-of-life care
Hospice care
Terminal care
Code first underlying disease
AHA: 2Q 2005, 9; 4Q 2003, 107; 1Q 1998, 11; 4Q 1996, 47-48

⦸ **V66.9 Unspecified convalescence**
AHA: 4Q 1999, 8

❹ **V67 Follow-up examination**
Includes surveillance only following completed treatment
Excludes *surveillance of contraception (V25.40-V25.49)*
AHA: 2Q 2003, 5; 4Q 1994, 48

❺ **V67.0 Following surgery**
AHA: 4Q 2000, 56; 4Q 1998, 69; 4Q 1997, 50; 2Q 1995, 8; 1Q 1995, 4; 3Q 1992, 11

V67.00 Following surgery, unspecified

V67.01 Follow-up vaginal pap smear ♀
Vaginal pap smear, status-post hysterectomy for malignant condition
Use additional code to identify:
acquired absence of uterus (V45.77)
personal history of malignant neoplasm (V10.40-V10.44)
Excludes *vaginal pap smear status-post hysterectomy for non-malignant condition (V76.47)*

V67.09 Following other surgery
Excludes *sperm count following sterilization reversal (V26.22)*
AHA: 3Q 2003, 16; 3Q 2002, 15
sperm count for fertility testing (V26.21)

V67.1 Following radiotherapy

V67.2 Following chemotherapy
Cancer chemotherapy follow-up

V67.3 Following psychotherapy and other treatment for mental disorder

V67.4 Following treatment of healed fracture
Excludes *current (healing) fracture aftercare (V54.0-V54.9)*
AHA: 1Q 1990, 7

❺ **V67.5 Following other treatment**

V67.51 Following completed treatment with high-risk medication, not elsewhere classified
Excludes *Long-term (current) drug use (V58.61-V58.69)*
AHA: 1Q 1999, 5-6; 4Q 1995, 61; 1Q 1990, 18

V67.59 Other

V67.6 Following combined treatment

⦸ **V67.9 Unspecified follow-up examination**

❹ **V68 Encounters for administrative purposes**

❺ **V68.0 Issue of medical certificates**
Excludes *encounter for general medical examination (V70.0-V70.9)*

● ⦸ **V68.01 Disability examination**
Use additional code(s) to identify:
specific examination(s), screening and testing
performed (V72.0-V82.9)

● ⦸ **V68.09 Other issue of medical certificates**

⦸ **V68.1 Issue of repeat prescriptions**
Issue of repeat prescription for:
appliance
glasses
medications
Excludes *repeat prescription for contraceptives (V25.41-V25.49)*

⦸ **V68.2 Request for expert evidence**

❺ **V68.8 Other specified administrative purpose**

⦸ **V68.81 Referral of patient without examination or treatment**

⦸ **V68.89 Other**

⦸ **V68.9 Unspecified administrative purpose**

❹ **V69 Problems related to lifestyle**
AHA: 4Q 1994, 48

⦸ **V69.0 Lack of physical exercise**

V69.1 Inappropriate diet and eating habits
Excludes anorexia nervosa (307.1)
bulimia (783.6)
malnutrition and other nutritional deficiencies (260-269.9)
other and unspecified eating disorders (307.50-307.59)

V69.2 High-risk sexual behavior

V69.3 Gambling and betting
Excludes pathological gambling (312.31)

V69.4 Lack of adequate sleep
Sleep deprivation
Excludes insomnia (780.52)

V69.5 Behavioral insomnia of childhood P
AHA: 4Q 2005, 99

V69.8 Other problems related to lifestyle
Self-damaging behavior

V69.9 Problem related to lifestyle, unspecified

PERSONS WITHOUT REPORTED DIAGNOSIS ENCOUNTERED DURING EXAMINATION AND INVESTIGATION OF INDIVIDUALS AND POPULATIONS (V70-V82)

Note: *Nonspecific abnormal findings disclosed at the time of these examinations are classifiable to categories 790-796.*

V70 General medical examination
Use additional code(s) to identify any special screening examination(s) performed (V73.0-V82.9)

V70.0 Routine general medical examination at a health care facility
Health checkup
Excludes health checkup of infant or child (V20.2)
pre-procedural general physical examination (V72.83)

V70.1 General psychiatric examination, requested by the authority

V70.2 General psychiatric examination, other and unspecified

V70.3 Other medical examination for administrative purposes
General medical examination for:
admission to old age home
adoption
camp
driving license
immigration and naturalization
insurance certification
marriage
prison
school admission
sports competition
Excludes attendance for issue of medical certificates (V68.0)
pre-employment screening (V70.5)
AHA: 1Q 1990, 6

V70.4 Examination for medicolegal reasons
Blood-alcohol tests
Blood-drug tests
Paternity testing
Excludes examination and observation following:
accidents (V71.3, V71.4)
assault (V71.6)
rape (V71.5)

V70.5 Health examination of defined subpopulations
Armed forces personnel
Inhabitants of institutions
Occupational health examinations
Pre-employment screening
Preschool children
Prisoners
Prostitutes
Refugees
School children
Students

V70.6 Health examination in population surveys
Excludes special screening (V73.0-V82.9)

V70.7 Examination of participant in clinical trial
Examination of participant or control in clinical research
AHA: 2Q 2006, 6; 4Q 2001, 55

V70.8 Other specified general medical examinations
Examination of potential donor of organ or tissue

V70.9 Unspecified general medical examination

V71 Observation and evaluation for suspected conditions not found
Note: *This category is to be used when persons without a diagnosis are suspected of having an abnormal condition, without signs or symptoms, which requires study, but after examination and observation, is found not to exist. This category is also for use for administrative and legal observation status.*
AHA: 4Q 1994, 47; 2Q 1990, 5; Mar-Apr, 1987, 1

V71.0 Observation for suspected mental condition

V71.01 Adult antisocial behavior A
Dyssocial behavior or gang activity in adult without manifest psychiatric disorder

V71.02 Childhood or adolescent antisocial behavior
Dyssocial behavior or gang activity in child or adolescent without manifest psychiatric disorder

V71.09 Other suspected mental condition

V71.1 Observation for suspected malignant neoplasm

V71.2 Observation for suspected tuberculosis

V71.3 Observation following accident at work

V71.4 Observation following other accident
Examination of individual involved in motor vehicle traffic accident
AHA: 1Q 2006, 9

V71.5 Observation following alleged rape or seduction
Examination of victim or culprit

V71.6 Observation following other inflicted injury
Examination of victim or culprit

V71.7 Observation for suspected cardiovascular disease
AHA: 1Q 2004, 6; 3Q 1990, 10; Sep-Oct, 1987, 10

V71.8 Observation and evaluation for other specified suspected conditions
AHA: 4Q 2000, 54; 1Q 1990, 19

V71.81 Abuse and neglect
Excludes adult abuse and neglect (995.80-995.85)
child abuse and neglect (995.50-995.59)
AHA: 4Q 2000, 55

V71.82 Observation and evaluation for suspected exposure to anthrax
AHA: 4Q 2002, 70, 85

V71.83 Observation and evaluation for suspected exposure to other biological agent
AHA: 4Q 2003, 47

V71.89 Other specified suspected conditions
AHA: 2Q 2003, 15

V71.9 Observation for unspecified suspected condition
AHA: 1Q 2002, 6

V72 Special investigations and examinations
Includes routine examination of specific system
Excludes general medical examination (V70.0-70.4)
general screening examination of defined population groups (V70.5, V70.6, V70.7)
routine examination of infant or child (V20.2)
Use additional code(s) to identify any special screening examination(s) performed (V73.0-V82.9)

V72.0 Examination of eyes and vision
AHA: 1Q 2004, 15

V72.1 Examination of ears and hearing
AHA: 1Q 2004, 15

V72.11 Encounter for hearing examination following failed hearing screening

V72.12 Encounter for hearing conservation and treatment

A Adult (15+ years) M Maternity (12-55 years) N Neonates (0 years) P Pediatric (0-17 years) ♂ Male ♀ Female

V72.19 Other examination of ears and hearing

V72.2 Dental examination

V72.3 Gynecological examination
Excludes cervical Papanicolaou smear without general gynecological examination (V76.2)
routine examination in contraceptive management (V25.40-V25.49)

V72.31 Routine gynecological examination ♀
General gynecological examination with or without Papanicolaou cervical smear
Pelvic examination (annual) (periodic)
Use additional code to identify:
▶ human papillomavirus (HPV) screening (V73.81)◀
▶ routine vaginal Papanicolaou smear (V76.47)◀
AHA: 2Q 2006, 3; 4Q 2005, 98

V72.32 Encounter for Papanicolaou cervical smear to confirm findings of recent normal smear following initial abnormal smear ♀
AHA: 2Q 2006, 4

V72.4 Pregnancy examination or test

V72.40 Pregnancy examination or test, pregnancy unconfirmed ♀
Possible pregnancy, not (yet) confirmed
AHA: 4Q 2005, 98

V72.41 Pregnancy examination or test, negative result ♀

V72.42 Pregnancy examination or test, positive result ♀M

V72.5 Radiological examination, not elsewhere classified
Routine chest x-ray
Excludes examination for suspected tuberculosis (V71.2)
AHA: 1Q 1990, 19

V72.6 Laboratory examination
Excludes that for suspected disorder (V71.0-V71.9)
AHA: 2Q 2006, 4; 1Q 1990, 22

V72.7 Diagnostic skin and sensitization tests
Allergy tests
Skin tests for hypersensitivity
Excludes diagnostic skin tests for bacterial diseases (V74.0-V74.9)

V72.8 Other specified examinations

V72.81 Pre-operative cardiovascular examination
Pre-procedural cardiovascular examination

V72.82 Pre-operative respiratory examination
Pre-procedural respiratory examination
AHA: 3Q 1996, 14

V72.83 Other specified pre-operative examination
Other pre-procedural examination
Pre-procedural general physical examination
Excludes routine general medical examination (V70.0)
AHA: 3Q 1996, 14

V72.84 Pre-operative examination, unspecified
Pre-procedural examination, unspecified

V72.85 Other specified examination
AHA: 4Q 2005, 96; 1Q 2004, 12

V72.86 Encounter for blood typing

V72.9 Unspecified examination

V73 Special screening examination for viral and chlamydial diseases
AHA: 1Q 2004, 11

V73.0 Poliomyelitis

V73.1 Smallpox

V73.2 Measles

V73.3 Rubella

V73.4 Yellow fever

V73.5 Other arthropod-borne viral diseases
Dengue fever
Hemorrhagic fever
Viral encephalitis:
mosquito-borne
tick-borne

V73.6 Trachoma

V73.8 Other specified viral and chlamydial diseases

● V73.81 Human papillomavirus (HPV)

V73.88 Other specified chlamydial diseases

V73.89 Other specified viral diseases

V73.9 Unspecified viral and chlamydial disease

V73.98 Unspecified chlamydial disease

V73.99 Unspecified viral disease

V74 Special screening examination for bacterial and spirochetal diseases
Includes diagnostic skin tests for these diseases
AHA: 1Q 2004, 11

V74.0 Cholera

V74.1 Pulmonary tuberculosis

V74.2 Leprosy [Hansen's disease]

V74.3 Diphtheria

V74.4 Bacterial conjunctivitis

V74.5 Venereal disease
▶ Screening for bacterial and spirochetal sexually transmitted diseases◀
▶ Screening for sexually transmitted diseases NOS◀
Excludes ▶special screening for nonbacterial sexually transmitted diseases (V73.81-V73.89, V75.4, V75.8)◀

V74.6 Yaws

V74.8 Other specified bacterial and spirochetal diseases
Brucellosis
Leptospirosis
Plague
Tetanus
Whooping cough

V74.9 Unspecified bacterial and spirochetal disease

V75 Special screening examination for other infectious diseases
AHA: 1Q 2004, 11

V75.0 Rickettsial diseases

V75.1 Malaria

V75.2 Leishmaniasis

V75.3 Trypanosomiasis
Chagas' disease
Sleeping sickness

V75.4 Mycotic infections

V75.5 Schistosomiasis

V75.6 Filariasis

V75.7 Intestinal helminthiasis

V75.8 Other specified parasitic infections

V75.9 Unspecified infectious disease

V76 Special screening for malignant neoplasms
AHA: 1Q 2004, 11

V76.0 Respiratory organs

V76.1 Breast
AHA: 4Q 1998, 67

V76.10 Breast screening, unspecified

V76.11 Screening mammogram for high-risk patient ♀
AHA: 2Q 2003, 4

V76.12 Other screening mammogram
AHA: 2Q 2006, 10; 2Q 2003,3-4

V76.19 Other screening breast examination

V76.2 Cervix ♀
Routine cervical Papanicolaou smear
Excludes ▶*special screening for human papillomavirus (V73.81)*◀
that as part of a general gynecological examination (V72.31)

V76.3 Bladder

V76.4 Other sites

V76.41 Rectum

V76.42 Oral cavity

V76.43 Skin

V76.44 Prostate ♂

V76.45 Testis ♂

V76.46 Ovary ♀
AHA: 4Q 2000, 52

V76.47 Vagina ♀
Vaginal pap smear status-post hysterectomy for non-malignant condition
Use additional code to identify acquired absence of uterus (V45.77)
Excludes *vaginal pap smear status-post hysterectomy for malignant condition (V67.01)*
AHA: 4Q 2000, 52

V76.49 Other sites
AHA: 1Q 1999, 4

V76.5 Intestine
AHA: 4Q 2000, 52

V76.50 Intestine, unspecified

V76.51 Colon
Excludes *rectum (V76.41)*
AHA: 4Q 2001, 56

V76.52 Small intestine

V76.8 Other neoplasm

V76.81 Nervous system

V76.89 Other neoplasm

V76.9 Unspecified

V77 Special screening for endocrine, nutritional, metabolic, and immunity disorders
AHA: 1Q 2004, 11

V77.0 Thyroid disorders

V77.1 Diabetes mellitus

V77.2 Malnutrition

V77.3 Phenylketonuria [PKU]

V77.4 Galactosemia

V77.5 Gout

V77.6 Cystic fibrosis
Screening for mucoviscidosis

V77.7 Other inborn errors of metabolism

V77.8 Obesity

V77.9 Other and unspecified endocrine, nutritional, metabolic, and immunity disorders
AHA: 4Q 2000, 53

V77.91 Screening for lipoid disorders
Screening cholesterol level
Screening for hypercholesterolemia
Screening for hyperlipidemia

V77.99 Other and unspecified endocrine, nutritional, metabolic, and immunity disorders

V78 Special screening for disorders of blood and blood-forming organs
AHA: 1Q 2004, 11

V78.0 Iron deficiency anemia

V78.1 Other and unspecified deficiency anemia

V78.2 Sickle-cell disease or trait

V78.3 Other hemoglobinopathies

V78.8 Other disorders of blood and blood-forming organs

V78.9 Unspecified disorder of blood and blood-forming organs

V79 Special screening for mental disorders and developmental handicaps
AHA: 1Q 2004, 11

V79.0 Depression

V79.1 Alcoholism

V79.2 Mental retardation

V79.3 Developmental handicaps in early childhood

V79.8 Other specified mental disorders and developmental handicaps

V79.9 Unspecified mental disorder and developmental handicap

V80 Special screening for neurological, eye, and ear diseases
AHA: 1Q 2004, 11

V80.0 Neurological conditions

V80.1 Glaucoma

V80.2 Other eye conditions
Screening for:
cataract
congenital anomaly of eye
senile macular lesions
Excludes *general vision examination (V72.0)*

V80.3 Ear diseases
Excludes *general hearing examination (▶V72.11-V72.19◀)*

V81 Special screening for cardiovascular, respiratory, and genitourinary diseases
AHA: 1Q 2004, 11

V81.0 Ischemic heart disease

V81.1 Hypertension

V81.2 Other and unspecified cardiovascular conditions

V81.3 Chronic bronchitis and emphysema

V81.4 Other and unspecified respiratory conditions
Excludes *screening for:*
lung neoplasm (V76.0)
pulmonary tuberculosis (V74.1)

V81.5 Nephropathy
Screening for asymptomatic bacteriuria

V81.6 Other and unspecified genitourinary conditions

V82 Special screening for other conditions
AHA: 1Q 2004, 11

V82.0 Skin conditions

V82.1 Rheumatoid arthritis

V82.2 Other rheumatic disorders

V82.3 Congenital dislocation of hip

V82.4 Maternal postnatal screening for chromosomal anomalies ♀
Excludes *antenatal screening by amniocentesis (V28.0)*

V82.5 Chemical poisoning and other contamination
Screening for:
heavy metal poisoning
ingestion of radioactive substance
poisoning from contaminated water supply
radiation exposure

V82.6 Multiphasic screening

V82.7 Genetic screening
Excludes *genetic testing for procreative management (V26.31-▶V26.39◀)*

V82.71 Screening for genetic disease carrier status

V82.79 Other genetic screening

V82.8 Other specified conditions
AHA: 4Q 2000, 53

V82.81 Osteoporosis
Use additional code to identify:
hormone replacement therapy (postmenopausal) status (V07.4)
postmenopausal (natural) status (V49.81)
AHA: 4Q 2000, 54

V82.89 Other specified conditions

V82.9 Unspecified condition

GENETICS (V83-V84)

❹ **V83 Genetic carrier status**
AHA: 4Q 2002, 79; 4Q 2001, 54

❺ **V83.0 Hemophilia A carrier**
⊘ **V83.01 Asymptomatic hemophilia A carrier**
⊘ **V83.02 Symptomatic hemophilia A carrier**

❺ **V83.8 Other genetic carrier status**
⊘ **V83.81 Cystic fibrosis gene carrier**
⊘ **V83.89 Other genetic carrier status**

❹ **V84 Genetic susceptibility to disease**
Includes confirmed abnormal gene
Use additional code, if applicable, for any associated family history of the disease (V16-V19)
AHA: 4Q 2004, 106

❺ **V84.0 Genetic susceptibility to malignant neoplasm**
Code first, if applicable, any current malignant neoplasms (140.0-195.8, 200.0-208.9, 230.0-234.9)
Use additional code, if applicable, for any personal history of malignant neoplasm (V10.0-V10.9)

⊘ **V84.01 Genetic susceptibility to malignant neoplasm of breast**
AHA: 4Q 2004, 107
⊘ **V84.02 Genetic susceptibility to malignant neoplasm of ovary** ♀
⊘ **V84.03 Genetic susceptibility to malignant neoplasm of prostate** ♂
⊘ **V84.04 Genetic susceptibility to malignant neoplasm of endometrium** ♀
⊘ **V84.09 Genetic susceptibility to other malignant neoplasm**

❺ ⊘ **V84.8 Genetic susceptibility to other disease**
● ⊘ **V84.81 Genetic susceptibility to multiple endocrine neoplasia [MEN]**
● ⊘ **V84.89 Genetic susceptibility to other disease**

BODY MASS INDEX (V85)

❹ **V85 Body Mass Index [BMI]**
Kilograms per meters squared
Note: BMI adult codes are for use for persons over 20 years old
AHA: 4Q 2005, 97

⊘ **V85.0 Body Mass Index less than 19, adult** A
⊘ **V85.1 Body Mass Index between 19-24, adult** A

❺ **V85.2 Body Mass Index between 25-29, adult**
⊘ **V85.21 Body Mass Index 25.0-25.9, adult** A
⊘ **V85.22 Body Mass Index 26.0-26.9, adult** A
⊘ **V85.23 Body Mass Index 27.0-27.9, adult** A
⊘ **V85.24 Body Mass Index 28.0-28.9, adult** A
⊘ **V85.25 Body Mass Index 29.0-29.9, adult** A

❺ **V85.3 Body Mass Index between 30-39, adult**
⊘ **V85.30 Body Mass Index 30.0-30.9, adult** A
⊘ **V85.31 Body Mass Index 31.0-31.9, adult** A
⊘ **V85.32 Body Mass Index 32.0-32.9, adult** A
⊘ **V85.33 Body Mass Index 33.0-33.9, adult** A
⊘ **V85.34 Body Mass Index 34.0-34.9, adult** A
⊘ **V85.35 Body Mass Index 35.0-35.9, adult** A
⊘ **V85.36 Body Mass Index 36.0-36.9, adult** A
⊘ **V85.37 Body Mass Index 37.0-37.9, adult** A
⊘ **V85.38 Body Mass Index 38.0-38.9, adult** A
⊘ **V85.39 Body Mass Index 39.0-39.9, adult** A

⊘ **V85.4 Body Mass Index 40 and over, adult** A

❺ **V85.5 Body Mass Index, pediatric**
Note: BMI pediatric codes are for use for persons 2-20 years old. These percentiles are based on the growth charts published by the Centers for Disease Control and Prevention (CDC)
⊘ **V85.51 Body Mass Index, pediatric, less than 5th percentile for age** P
⊘ **V85.52 Body Mass Index, pediatric, 5th percentile to less than 85th percentile for age** P
⊘ **V85.53 Body Mass Index, pediatric, 85th percentile to less than 95th percentile for age** P
⊘ **V85.54 Body Mass Index, pediatric, greater than or equal to 95th percentile for age** P

ESTROGEN RECEPTOR STATUS (V86)

❹ **V86 Estrogen receptor status**
Code first malignant neoplasm of breast (174.0-174.9, 175.0-175.9)
⊘ **V86.0 Estrogen receptor positive status [ER+]**
⊘ **V86.1 Estrogen receptor negative status [ER-]**

SUPPLEMENTARY CLASSIFICATION OF EXTERNAL CAUSES OF INJURY AND POISONING (E800-E999)

This section is provided to permit the classification of environmental events, circumstances, and conditions as the cause of injury, poisoning, and other adverse effects. Where a code from this section is applicable, it is intended that it shall be used in addition to a code from one of the main chapters of ICD-9-CM, indicating the nature of the condition. Certain other conditions which may be stated to be due to external causes are classified in Chapters 1 to 16 of ICD-9-CM. For these, the "E" code classification should be used as an additional code for more detailed analysis.

Machinery accidents [other than those connected with transport] are classifiable to category E919, in which the fourth digit allows a broad classification of the type of machinery involved. If a more detailed classification of type of machinery is required, it is suggested that the "Classification of Industrial Accidents according to Agency," prepared by the International Labor Office, be used in addition; it is included in this publication.

Categories for "late effects" of accidents and other external causes are to be found at E929, E959, E969, E977, E989, and E999.

Definitions and examples related to transport accidents

(a) A **transport accident** (E800-E848) is any accident involving a device designed primarily for, or being used at the time primarily for, conveying persons or goods from one place to another.

Includes accidents involving:
- aircraft and spacecraft (E840-E845)
- watercraft (E830-E838)
- motor vehicle (E810-E825)
- railway (E800-E807)
- other road vehicles (E826-E829)

In classifying accidents which involve more than one kind of transport, the above order of precedence of transport accidents should be used.

Accidents involving agricultural and construction machines, such as tractors, cranes, and bulldozers, are regarded as transport accidents only when these vehicles are under their own power on a highway [otherwise the vehicles are regarded as machinery]. Vehicles which can travel on land or water, such as hovercraft and other amphibious vehicles, are regarded as watercraft when on the water, as motor vehicles when on the highway, and as off-road motor vehicles when on land, but off the highway.

Excludes *accidents:*
- *in sports which involve the use of transport but where the transport vehicle itself was not involved in the accident*
- *involving vehicles which are part of industrial equipment used entirely on industrial premises*
- *occurring during transportation but unrelated to the hazards associated with the means of transportation [e.g., injuries received in a fight on board ship; transport vehicle involved in a cataclysm such as an earthquake]*
- *to persons engaged in the maintenance or repair of transport equipment or vehicle not in motion, unless injured by another vehicle in motion*

(b) A **railway accident** is a transport accident involving a railway train or other railway vehicle operated on rails, whether in motion or not.

Excludes *accidents:*
- *in repair shops*
- *in roundhouse or on turntable*
- *on railway premises but not involving a train or other railway vehicle*

(c) A **railway train** or **railway vehicle** is any device with or without cars coupled to it, designed for traffic on a railway.

Includes interurban:
- electric car (operated chiefly on its own right-of-way, not open to other traffic)
- streetcar (operated chiefly on its own right-of-way, not open to other traffic)

railway train, any power [diesel] [electric] [steam]:
- funicular
- monorail or two-rail
- subterranean or elevated

other vehicle designed to run on a railway track

Excludes *interurban electric cars [streetcars] specified to be operating on a right-of-way that forms part of the public street or highway [definition (n)]*

(d) A **railway** or **railroad** is a right-of-way designed for traffic on rails, which is used by carriages or wagons transporting passengers or freight, and by other rolling stock, and which is not open to other public vehicular traffic

(e) A **motor vehicle accident** is a transport accident involving a motor vehicle. It is defined as a motor vehicle traffic accident or as a motor vehicle nontraffic accident according to whether the accident occurs on a public highway or elsewhere.

Excludes *injury or damage due to cataclysm*
injury or damage while a motor vehicle, not under its own power, is being loaded on, or unloaded from, another conveyance

(f) A **motor vehicle traffic accident** is any motor vehicle accident occurring on a public highway [i.e., originating, terminating, or involving a vehicle partially on the highway]. A motor vehicle accident is assumed to have occurred on the highway unless another place is specified, except in the case of accidents involving only off-road motor vehicles which are classified as nontraffic accidents unless the contrary is stated.

(g) A **motor vehicle nontraffic accident** is any motor vehicle accident which occurs entirely in any place other than a public highway.

(h) A **public highway [trafficway]** or **street** is the entire width between property lines [or other boundary lines] of every way or place, of which any part is open to the public for purposes of vehicular traffic as a matter of right or custom. A **roadway** is that part of the public highway designed, improved, and ordinarily used, for vehicular travel.

Includes approaches (public) to:
- docks
- public building
- station

Excludes *driveway (private)*
parking lot
ramp
roads in:
- *airfield*
- *farm*
- *industrial premises*
- *mine*
- *private grounds*
- *quarry*

E Codes

(i) A **motor vehicle** is any mechanically or electrically powered device, not operated on rails, upon which any person or property may be transported or drawn upon a highway. Any object such as a trailer, coaster, sled, or wagon being towed by a motor vehicle is considered a part of the motor vehicle.

Includes automobile [any type]
bus
construction machinery, farm and industrial machinery, steam roller, tractor, army tank, highway grader, or similar vehicle on wheels or treads, while in transport under own power
fire engine (motorized)
motorcycle
motorized bicycle [moped] or scooter
trolley bus not operating on rails
truck
van

Excludes *devices used solely to move persons or materials within the confines of a building and its premises, such as:*
building elevator
coal car in mine
electric baggage or mail truck used solely within a railroad station
electric truck used solely within an industrial plant
moving overhead crane

(j) A **motorcycle** is a two-wheeled motor vehicle having one or two riding saddles and sometimes having a third wheel for the support of a sidecar. The sidecar is considered part of the motorcycle.

Includes motorized:
bicycle [moped]
scooter
tricycle

(k) An **off-road motor vehicle** is a motor vehicle of special design, to enable it to negotiate rough or soft terrain or snow. Examples of special design are high construction, special wheels and tires, driven by treads, or support on a cushion of air.

Includes all terrain vehicle [ATV]
army tank
hovercraft, on land or swamp
snowmobile

(l) A **driver** of a motor vehicle is the occupant of the motor vehicle operating it or intending to operate it. A **motorcyclist** is the driver of a motorcycle. Other authorized occupants of a motor vehicle are **passengers**.

(m) An **other road vehicle** is any device, except a motor vehicle, in, on, or by which any person or property may be transported on a highway.

Includes animal carrying a person or goods
animal-drawn vehicle
animal harnessed to conveyance
bicycle [pedal cycle]
streetcar
tricycle (pedal)

Excludes *pedestrian conveyance [definition (q)]*

(n) A **streetcar** is a device designed and used primarily for transporting persons within a municipality, running on rails, usually subject to normal traffic control signals, and operated principally on a right-of-way that forms part of the traffic way. A trailer being towed by a streetcar is considered a part of the streetcar.

Includes interurban or intraurban electric or streetcar, when specified to be operating on a street or public highway
tram (car)
trolley (car)

(o) A **pedal cycle** is any road transport vehicle operated solely by pedals.

Includes bicycle
pedal cycle
tricycle

Excludes *motorized bicycle [definition (i)]*

(p) A **pedal cyclist** is any person riding on a pedal cycle or in a sidecar attached to such a vehicle.

(q) A **pedestrian conveyance** is any human powered device by which a pedestrian may move other than by walking or by which a walking person may move another pedestrian.

Includes baby carriage
coaster wagon
ice skates
perambulator
pushcart
pushchair
roller skates
scooter
skateboard
skis
sled
wheelchair

(r) A **pedestrian** is any person involved in an accident who was not at the time of the accident riding in or on a motor vehicle, railroad train, streetcar, animal-drawn or other vehicle, or on a bicycle or animal.

Includes person:
changing tire of vehicle
in or operating a pedestrian conveyance
making adjustment to motor of vehicle
on foot

(s) A **watercraft** is any device for transporting passengers or goods on the water.

(t) A **small boat** is any watercraft propelled by paddle, oars, or small motor, with a passenger capacity of less than ten.

Includes boat NOS
canoe
coble
dinghy
punt
raft
rowboat
rowing shell
scull
skiff
small motorboat

Excludes *barge*
lifeboat (used after abandoning ship)
raft (anchored) being used as a diving platform
yacht

(u) An **aircraft** is any device for transporting passengers or goods in the air.

Includes airplane [any type]
balloon
bomber
dirigible
glider (hang)
military aircraft
parachute

(v) A **commercial transport aircraft** is any device for collective passenger or freight transportation by air, whether run on commercial lines for profit or by government authorities, with the exception of military craft.

RAILWAY ACCIDENTS (E800-E807)

Note: *For definitions of railway accident and related terms see definitions (a) to (d).*

Excludes *accidents involving railway train and:*
aircraft (E840.0-E845.9)
motor vehicle (E810.0-E825.9)
watercraft (E830.0-E838.9)

The following fourth-digit subdivisions are for use with categories E800-E807 to identify the injured person:

.0 Railway employee
Any person who by virtue of his employment in connection with a railway, whether by the railway company or not, is at increased risk of involvement in a railway accident, such as:
catering staff of train
driver
guard
porter
postal staff on train
railway fireman
shunter
sleeping car attendant

.1 Passenger on railway
Any authorized person traveling on a train, except a railway employee.
Excludes: intending passenger waiting at station (.8)
unauthorized rider on railway vehicle (.8)

.2 Pedestrian
See definition (r)

.3 Pedal cyclist
See definition (p)

.8 Other specified person
Intending passenger or bystander waiting at station
Unauthorized rider on railway vehicle

.9 Unspecified person

❹ E800 Railway accident involving collision with rolling stock
Requires fourth digit. See beginning of section E800-E807 for codes and definitions.
Includes collision between railway trains or railway vehicles, any kind
collision NOS on railway
derailment with antecedent collision with rolling stock or NOS

❹ E801 Railway accident involving collision with other object
Requires fourth digit. See beginning of section E800-E807 for codes and definitions.
Includes collision of railway train with:
buffers
fallen tree on railway
gates
platform
rock on railway
streetcar
other nonmotor vehicle
other object
Excludes *collision with:*
aircraft (E840.0-E842.9)
motor vehicle (E810.0-E810.9, E820.0-E822.9)

❹ E802 Railway accident involving derailment without antecedent collision
Requires fourth digit. See beginning of section E800-E807 for codes and definitions.

❹ E803 Railway accident involving explosion, fire, or burning
Requires fourth digit. See beginning of section E800-E807 for codes and definitions.
Excludes *explosion or fire, with antecedent derailment (E802.0-E802.9)*
explosion or fire, with mention of antecedent collision (E800.0-E801.9)

❹ E804 Fall in, on, or from railway train
Requires fourth digit. See beginning of section E800-E807 for codes and definitions.
Includes fall while alighting from or boarding railway train
Excludes *fall related to collision, derailment, or explosion of railway train (E800.0-E803.9)*

❹ E805 Hit by rolling stock
Requires fourth digit. See beginning of section E800-E807 for codes and definitions.
Includes crushed by railway train or part
injured by railway train or part
killed by railway train or part
knocked down by railway train or part
run over by railway train or part
Excludes *pedestrian hit by object set in motion by railway train (E806.0-E806.9)*

❹ E806 Other specified railway accident
Requires fourth digit. See beginning of section E800-E807 for codes and definitions.
Includes hit by object falling in railway train
injured by door or window on railway train
nonmotor road vehicle or pedestrian hit by object set in motion by railway train
railway train hit by falling:
earth NOS
rock
tree
other object
Excludes *railway accident due to cataclysm (E908-E909)*

❹ E807 Railway accident of unspecified nature
Requires fourth digit. See beginning of section E800-E807 for codes and definitions.
Includes found dead on railway right-of-way NOS
injured on railway right-of-way NOS
railway accident NOS

MOTOR VEHICLE TRAFFIC ACCIDENTS (E810-E819)

Note: *For definitions of motor vehicle traffic accident, and related terms, see definitions (e) to (k).*
Excludes *accidents involving motor vehicle and aircraft (E840.0-E845.9)*

The following fourth-digit subdivisions are for use with categories E810-E819 to identify the injured person:

.0 Driver of motor vehicle other than motorcycle
See definition (l)

.1 Passenger in motor vehicle other than motorcycle
See definition (l)

.2 Motorcyclist
See definition (l)

.3 Passenger on motorcycle
See definition (l)

.4 Occupant of streetcar

.5 Rider of animal; occupant of animal-drawn vehicle

.6 Pedal cyclist
See definition (p)

.7 Pedestrian
See definition (r)

.8 Other specified person
Occupant of vehicle other than above
Person in railway train involved in accident
Unauthorized rider of motor vehicle

.9 Unspecified person

❹ E810 Motor vehicle traffic accident involving collision with train
Requires fourth digit. See beginning of section E810-E819 for codes and definitions.
Excludes *motor vehicle collision with object set in motion by railway train (E815.0-E815.9)*
railway train hit by object set in motion by motor vehicle (E818.0-E818.9)

❹ E811 Motor vehicle traffic accident involving re-entrant collision with another motor vehicle
Requires fourth digit. See beginning of section E810-E819 for codes and definitions.
Includes collision between motor vehicle which accidentally leaves the roadway then re-enters the same roadway, or the opposite roadway on a divided highway, and another motor vehicle
Excludes *collision on the same roadway when none of the motor vehicles involved have left and re-entered the roadway (E812.0-E812.9)*

④ E812 Other motor vehicle traffic accident involving collision with motor vehicle

Requires fourth digit. See beginning of section E810-E819 for codes and definitions.

Includes collision with another motor vehicle parked, stopped, stalled, disabled, or abandoned on the highway
motor vehicle collision NOS

Excludes *collision with object set in motion by another motor vehicle (E815.0-E815.9)*
re-entrant collision with another motor vehicle (E811.0-E811.9)

④ E813 Motor vehicle traffic accident involving collision with other vehicle

Requires fourth digit. See beginning of section E810-E819 for codes and definitions.

Includes collision between motor vehicle, any kind, and other road (nonmotor transport) vehicle, such as:
animal carrying a person
animal-drawn vehicle
pedal cycle
streetcar

Excludes *collision with:*
object set in motion by nonmotor road vehicle (E815.0-E815.9)
pedestrian (E814.0-E814.9)
nonmotor road vehicle hit by object set in motion by motor vehicle (E818.0-E818.9)

④ E814 Motor vehicle traffic accident involving collision with pedestrian

Requires fourth digit. See beginning of section E810-E819 for codes and definitions.

Includes collision between motor vehicle, any kind, and pedestrian
pedestrian dragged, hit, or run over by motor vehicle, any kind

Excludes *pedestrian hit by object set in motion by motor vehicle (E818.0-E818.9)*

④ E815 Other motor vehicle traffic accident involving collision on the highway

Requires fourth digit. See beginning of section E810-E819 for codes and definitions.

Includes collision (due to loss of control) (on highway) between motor vehicle, any kind, and:
abutment (bridge) (overpass)
animal (herded) (unattended)
fallen stone, traffic sign, tree, utility pole
guard rail or boundary fence
interhighway divider
landslide (not moving)
object set in motion by railway train or road vehicle (motor) (nonmotor)
object thrown in front of motor vehicle
other object, fixed, movable, or moving
safety island
temporary traffic sign or marker
wall of cut made for road

Excludes *collision with:*
any object off the highway (resulting from loss of control) (E816.0-E816.9)
any object which normally would have been off the highway and is not stated to have been on it (E816.0-E816.9)
motor vehicle parked, stopped, stalled, disabled, or abandoned on highway (E812.0-E812.9)
moving landslide (E909.2)
motor vehicle hit by object:
set in motion by railway train or road vehicle (motor) (nonmotor) (E818.0-E818.9)
thrown into or on vehicle (E818.0-E818.9)

④ E816 Motor vehicle traffic accident due to loss of control, without collision on the highway

Requires fourth digit. See beginning of section E810-E819 for codes and definitions.

Includes motor vehicle:
failing to make curve and:
colliding with object off the highway
overturning
stopping abruptly off the highway
going out of control (due to):
blowout and:
colliding with object off the highway
overturning
stopping abruptly off the highway
burst tire and:
colliding with object off the highway
overturning
stopping abruptly off the highway
driver falling asleep and:
colliding with object off the highway
overturning
stopping abruptly off the highway
driver inattention and:
colliding with object off the highway
overturning
stopping abruptly off the highway
excessive speed and:
colliding with object off the highway
overturning
stopping abruptly off the highway
failure of mechanical part and:
colliding with object off the highway
overturning
stopping abruptly off the highway

Excludes *collision on highway following loss of control (E810.0-E815.9)*
loss of control of motor vehicle following collision on the highway (E810.0-E815.9)

④ E817 Noncollision motor vehicle traffic accident while boarding or alighting

Requires fourth digit. See beginning of section E810-E819 for codes and definitions.

Includes fall down stairs of motor bus while boarding or alighting
fall from car in street while boarding or alighting
injured by moving part of the vehicle while boarding or alighting
trapped by door of motor bus boarding or alighting while boarding or alighting

④ E818 Other noncollision motor vehicle traffic accident

Requires fourth digit. See beginning of section E810-E819 for codes and definitions.

Includes accidental poisoning from exhaust gas generated by motor vehicle while in motion
breakage of any part of motor vehicle while in motion
collision of railway train or road vehicle except motor vehicle, with object set in motion by motor vehicle
explosion of any part of motor vehicle while in motion
fall, jump, or being accidentally pushed from motor vehicle while in motion
fire starting in motor vehicle while in motion
hit by object thrown into or on motor vehicle while in motion
injured by being thrown against some part of, or object in motor vehicle while in motion
injury from moving part of motor vehicle while in motion
object falling in or on motor vehicle while in motion
object thrown on motor vehicle while in motion
motor vehicle hit by object set in motion by railway train or road vehicle (motor) (nonmotor)
pedestrian, railway train, or road vehicle (motor) (nonmotor) hit by object set in motion by motor vehicle

Excludes *collision between motor vehicle and:*
object set in motion by railway train or road vehicle (motor) (nonmotor) (E815.0-E815.9)
object thrown towards the motor vehicle (E815.0-E815.9)
person overcome by carbon monoxide generated by stationary motor vehicle off the roadway with motor running (E868.2)

❹ E819 Motor vehicle traffic accident of unspecified nature

Requires fourth digit. See beginning of section E810-E819 for codes and definitions.

Includes motor vehicle traffic accident NOS
traffic accident NOS

MOTOR VEHICLE NONTRAFFIC ACCIDENTS (E820-E825)

Note: *For definitions of motor vehicle nontraffic accident and related terms see definition (a) to (k).*

Includes accidents involving motor vehicles being used in recreational or sporting activities off the highway
collision and noncollision motor vehicle accidents occurring entirely off the highway

Excludes *accidents involving motor vehicle and:*
aircraft (E840.0-E845.9)
watercraft (E830.0-E838.9)
accidents, not on the public highway, involving agricultural and construction machinery but not involving another motor vehicle (E919.0, E919.2, E919.7)

The following fourth-digit subdivisions are for use with categories E820-E825 to identify the injured person:

.0 Driver of motor vehicle other than motorcycle
See definition (l)
.1 Passenger in motor vehicle other than motorcycle
See definition (l)
.2 Motorcyclist
See definition (l)
.3 Passenger on motorcycle
See definition (l)
.4 Occupant of streetcar
.5 Rider of animal; occupant of animal-drawn vehicle
.6 Pedal cyclist
See definition (p)
.7 Pedestrian
See definition (r)
.8 Other specified person
Occupant of vehicle other than above
Person on railway train involved in accident
Unauthorized rider of motor vehicle
.9 Unspecified person

❹ E820 Nontraffic accident involving motor-driven snow vehicle

Requires fourth digit. See beginning of section E820-E825 for codes and definitions.

Includes breakage of part of motor-driven snow vehicle (not on public highway)
collision of motor-driven snow vehicle with:
animal (being ridden) (-drawn vehicle)
another off-road motor vehicle
other motor vehicle, not on public highway
railway train
other object, fixed or movable
fall from motor-driven snow vehicle (not on public highway)
hit by motor-driven snow vehicle (not on public highway)
injury caused by rough landing of motor-driven snow vehicle (after leaving ground on rough terrain)
overturning of motor-driven snow vehicle (not on public highway)
run over or dragged by motor-driven snow vehicle (not on public highway)

Excludes *accident on the public highway involving motor driven snow vehicle (E810.0-E819.9)*

❹ E821 Nontraffic accident involving other off-road motor vehicle

Requires fourth digit. See beginning of section E820-E825 for codes and definitions.

Includes breakage of part of off-road motor vehicle, except snow vehicle (not on public highway)
collision with:
animal (being ridden) (-drawn vehicle)
another off-road motor vehicle, except snow vehicle
other motor vehicle, not on public highway
other object, fixed or movable
fall from off-road motor vehicle, except snow vehicle (not on public highway)
hit by off-road motor vehicle, except snow vehicle (not on public highway)
overturning of off-road motor vehicle, except snow vehicle (not on public highway)
run over or dragged by off-road motor vehicle, except snow vehicle (not on public highway)
thrown against some part of or object in off-road motor vehicle, except snow vehicle (not on public highway)

Excludes *accident on public highway involving off-road motor vehicle (E810.0-E819.9)*
collision between motor driven snow vehicle and other off-road motor vehicle (E820.0-E820.9)
hovercraft accident on water (E830.0-E838.9)

❹ E822 Other motor vehicle nontraffic accident involving collision with moving object

Requires fourth digit. See beginning of section E820-E825 for codes and definitions.

Includes collision, not on public highway, between motor vehicle, except off-road motor vehicle and:
animal
nonmotor vehicle
other motor vehicle, except off-road motor vehicle
pedestrian
railway train
other moving object

Excludes *collision with:*
motor-driven snow vehicle (E820.0-E820.9)
other off-road motor vehicle (E821.0-E821.9)

❹ E823 Other motor vehicle nontraffic accident involving collision with stationary object

Requires fourth digit. See beginning of section E820-E825 for codes and definitions.

Includes collision, not on public highway, between motor vehicle, except off-road motor vehicle, and any object, fixed or movable, but not in motion

❹ E824 Other motor vehicle nontraffic accident while boarding and alighting

Requires fourth digit. See beginning of section E820-E825 for codes and definitions.

Includes fall while boarding or alighting from motor vehicle except off-road motor vehicle, not on public highway
injury from moving part of motor vehicle while boarding or alighting from motor vehicle except off-road motor vehicle, not on public highway
trapped by door of motor vehicle while boarding or alighting from motor vehicle except off-road motor vehicle, not on public highway

❹ E825 Other motor vehicle nontraffic accident of other and unspecified nature

Requires fourth digit. See beginning of section E820-E825 for codes and definitions.

Includes accidental poisoning from carbon monoxide generated by motor vehicle while in motion, not on public highway
breakage of any part of motor vehicle while in motion, not on public highway
explosion of any part of motor vehicle while in motion, not on public highway
fall, jump, or being accidentally pushed from motor vehicle while in motion, not on public highway
fire starting in motor vehicle while in motion, not on public highway
hit by object thrown into, towards, or on motor vehicle while in motion, not on public highway
injured by being thrown against some part of, or object in motor vehicle while in motion, not on public highway
injury from moving part of motor vehicle while in motion, not on public highway
object falling in or on motor vehicle while in motion, not on public highway
motor vehicle nontraffic accident NOS

Excludes fall from or in stationary motor vehicle (E884.9, E885.9)
overcome by carbon monoxide or exhaust gas generated by stationary motor vehicle off the roadway with motor running (E868.2)
struck by falling object from or in stationary motor vehicle (E916)

OTHER ROAD VEHICLE ACCIDENTS (E826-E829)

Note: Other road vehicle accidents are transport accidents involving road vehicles other than motor vehicles. For definitions of other road vehicle and related terms see definitions (m) to (o).

Includes accidents involving other road vehicles being used in recreational or sporting activities

Excludes collision of other road vehicle [any] with:
aircraft (E840.0-E845.9)
motor vehicle (E813.0-E813.9, E820.0-E822.9)
railway train (E801.0-E801.9)

The following fourth-digit subdivisions are for use with categories E826-E829 to identify the injured person:

.0 Pedestrian
See definition (r)
.1 Pedal cyclist
See definition (p)
.2 Rider of animal
.3 Occupant of animal-drawn vehicle
.4 Occupant of streetcar
.8 Other specified person
.9 Unspecified person

❹ E826 Pedal cycle accident
[0 - 9]

Requires fourth digit. See beginning of section E826-E829 for codes and definitions.

Includes breakage of any part of pedal cycle
collision between pedal cycle and:
animal (being ridden) (herded) (unattended)
another pedal cycle
nonmotor road vehicle, any
pedestrian
other object, fixed, movable, or moving, not set in motion by motor vehicle, railway train, or aircraft
entanglement in wheel of pedal cycle
fall from pedal cycle
hit by object falling or thrown on the pedal cycle
pedal cycle accident NOS
pedal cycle overturned

❹ E827 Animal-drawn vehicle accident
[0,2 - 4,8,9]

Requires fourth digit. See beginning of section E826-E829 for codes and definitions.

Includes breakage of any part of vehicle
collision between animal-drawn vehicle and:
animal (being ridden) (herded) (unattended)
nonmotor road vehicle, except pedal cycle
pedestrian, pedestrian conveyance, or pedestrian vehicle
other object, fixed, movable, or moving, not set in motion by motor vehicle, railway train, or aircraft
fall from animal-drawn vehicle
knocked down by animal-drawn vehicle
overturning of animal-drawn vehicle
run over by animal-drawn vehicle
thrown from animal-drawn vehicle

Excludes collision of animal-drawn vehicle with pedal cycle (E826.0-E826.9)

❹ E828 Accident involving animal being ridden
[0,2,4,8,9]

Requires fourth digit. See beginning of section E826-E829 for codes and definitions.

Includes collision between animal being ridden and:
another animal
nonmotor road vehicle, except pedal cycle, and animal-drawn vehicle
pedestrian, pedestrian conveyance, or pedestrian vehicle
other object, fixed, movable, or moving, not set in motion by motor vehicle, railway train, or aircraft
fall from animal being ridden
knocked down by animal being ridden
thrown from animal being ridden
trampled by animal being ridden
ridden animal stumbled and fell

Excludes collision of animal being ridden with:
animal-drawn vehicle (E827.0-E827.9)
pedal cycle (E826.0-E826.9)

E829 Other road vehicle accidents
[0,4,8,9]

Requires fourth digit. See beginning of section E826-E829 for codes and definitions.

Includes accident while boarding or alighting from:
- streetcar
- nonmotor road vehicle not classifiable to E826-E828

blow from object in:
- streetcar
- nonmotor road vehicle not classifiable to E826-E828

breakage of any part of:
- streetcar
- nonmotor road vehicle not classifiable to E826-E828

caught in door of:
- streetcar
- nonmotor road vehicle not classifiable to E826-E828

collision between streetcar or nonmotor road vehicle, except as in E826-E828, and:
- animal (not being ridden)
- another nonmotor road vehicle not classifiable to E826-E828
- pedestrian
- other object, fixed, movable, or moving, not set in motion by motor vehicle, railway train, or aircraft

derailment of:
- streetcar
- nonmotor road vehicle not classifiable to E826-E828

fall in, on, or from:
- streetcar
- nonmotor road vehicle not classifiable to E826-E828

fire in:
- streetcar
- nonmotor road vehicle not classifiable to E826-E828

nonmotor road vehicle accident NOS

streetcar accident NOS

Excludes *collision with:*
- *animal being ridden (E828.0-E828.9)*
- *animal-drawn vehicle (E827.0-E827.9)*
- *pedal cycle (E826.0-E826.9)*

WATER TRANSPORT ACCIDENTS (E830-E838)

Note: *For definitions of water transport accident and related terms see definitions (a), (s), and (t).*

Includes watercraft accidents in the course of recreational activities

Excludes *accidents involving both aircraft, including objects set in motion by aircraft, and watercraft (E840.0-E845.9)*

The following fourth-digit subdivisions are for use with categories E830-E838 to identify the injured person:

.0 Occupant of small boat, unpowered

.1 Occupant of small boat, powered
See definition (t)
Excludes: water skier (.4)

.2 Occupant of other watercraft - crew
Persons:
- engaged in operation of watercraft
- providing passenger services [cabin attendants, ship's physician, catering personnel]
- working on ship during voyage in other capacity [musician in band, operators of shops and beauty parlors]

.3 Occupant of other watercraft - other than crew
Passenger
Occupant of lifeboat, other than crew, after abandoning ship

.4 Water skier

.5 Swimmer

.6 Dockers, stevedores
Longshoreman employed on the dock in loading and unloading ships

.8 Other specified person
Immigration and custom officials on board ship
Person:
- accompanying passenger or member of crew
- visiting boat

Pilot (guiding ship into port)

.9 Unspecified person

E830 Accident to watercraft causing submersion

Requires fourth digit. See beginning of section E830-E838 for codes and definitions.

Includes submersion and drowning due to:
- boat overturning
- boat submerging
- falling or jumping from burning ship
- falling or jumping from crushed watercraft
- ship sinking
- other accident to watercraft

E831 Accident to watercraft causing other injury

Requires fourth digit. See beginning of section E830-E838 for codes and definitions.

Includes any injury, except submersion and drowning, as a result of an accident to watercraft
- burned while ship on fire
- crushed between ships in collision
- crushed by lifeboat after abandoning ship
- fall due to collision or other accident to watercraft
- hit by falling object due to accident to watercraft
- injured in watercraft accident involving collision
- struck by boat or part thereof after fall or jump from damaged boat

Excludes *burns from localized fire or explosion on board ship (E837.0-E837.9)*

④ E832 Other accidental submersion or drowning in water transport accident

Requires fourth digit. See beginning of section E830-E838 for codes and definitions.

Includes submersion or drowning as a result of an accident other than accident to the watercraft, such as:
fall:
from gangplank
from ship
overboard
thrown overboard by motion of ship
washed overboard

Excludes submersion or drowning of swimmer or diver who voluntarily jumps from boat not involved in an accident (E910.0-E910.9)

④ E833 Fall on stairs or ladders in water transport

Requires fourth digit. See beginning of section E830-E838 for codes and definitions.

Excludes fall due to accident to watercraft (E831.0-E831.9)

④ E834 Other fall from one level to another in water transport

Requires fourth digit. See beginning of section E830-E838 for codes and definitions.

Excludes fall due to accident to watercraft (E831.0-E831.9)

④ E835 Other and unspecified fall in water transport

Requires fourth digit. See beginning of section E830-E838 for codes and definitions.

Excludes fall due to accident to watercraft (E831.0-E831.9)

④ E836 Machinery accident in water transport

Requires fourth digit. See beginning of section E830-E838 for codes and definitions.

Includes injuries in water transport caused by:
deck machinery
engine room machinery
galley machinery
laundry machinery
loading machinery

④ E837 Explosion, fire, or burning in watercraft

Requires fourth digit. See beginning of section E830-E838 for codes and definitions.

Includes explosion of boiler on steamship
localized fire on ship

Excludes burning ship (due to collision or explosion) resulting in:
submersion or drowning (E830.0-E830.9)
other injury (E831.0-E831.9)

④ E838 Other and unspecified water transport accident

Requires fourth digit. See beginning of section E830-E838 for codes and definitions.

Includes accidental poisoning by gases or fumes on ship
atomic power plant malfunction in watercraft
crushed between ship and stationary object [wharf]
crushed between ships without accident to watercraft
crushed by falling object on ship or while loading or unloading
hit by boat while water skiing
struck by boat or part thereof (after fall from boat)
watercraft accident NOS

AIR AND SPACE TRANSPORT ACCIDENTS (E840-E845)

Note: *For definition of aircraft and related terms see definitions (u) and (v).*

The following fourth-digit subdivisions are for use with categories E840-E845 to identify the injured person:

.0 Occupant of spacecraft

.1 Occupant of military aircraft, any
Crew in military aircraft [air force] [army] [national guard] [navy]
Passenger (civilian) (military) in military aircraft [air force] [army] [national guard] [navy]
Troops in military aircraft [air force] [army] [national guard] [navy]
Excludes: *occupants of aircraft operated under jurisdiction of police departments (.5)*
parachutist (.7)

.2 Crew of commercial aircraft (powered) in surface-to-surface transport

.3 Other occupant of commercial aircraft (powered) in surface-to-surface transport
Flight personnel:
not part of crew
on familiarization flight
Passenger on aircraft (powered) NOS

.4 Occupant of commercial aircraft (powered) in surface-to-air transport
Occupant [crew] [passenger] of aircraft (powered) engaged in activities, such as:
aerial spraying (crops) (fire retardants)
air drops of emergency supplies
air drops of parachutists, except from military craft
crop dusting
lowering of construction material [bridge or telephone pole]
sky writing

.5 Occupant of other powered aircraft
Occupant [crew] [passenger] of aircraft [powered] engaged in activities, such as:
aerobatic flying
aircraft racing
rescue operation
storm surveillance
traffic surveillance
Occupant of private plane NOS

.6 Occupant of unpowered aircraft, except parachutist
Occupant of aircraft classifiable to E842

.7 Parachutist (military) (other)
Person making voluntary descent
Excludes *person making descent after accident to aircraft (.1-.6)*

.8 Ground crew, airline employee
Persons employed at airfields (civil) (military) or launching pads, not occupants of aircraft

.9 Other person

④ E840 Accident to powered aircraft at takeoff or landing

Requires fourth digit. See beginning of section E840-E845 for codes and definitions.

Includes collision of aircraft with any object, fixed, movable, or moving while taking off or landing
crash while taking off or landing
explosion on aircraft while taking off or landing
fire on aircraft while taking off or landing
forced landing

④ E841 Accident to powered aircraft, other and unspecified

Requires fourth digit. See beginning of section E840-E845 for codes and definitions.

Includes aircraft accident NOS
aircraft crash or wreck NOS
any accident to powered aircraft while in transit or when not specified whether in transit, taking off, or landing
collision of aircraft with another aircraft, bird, or any object, while in transit
explosion on aircraft while in transit
fire on aircraft while in transit

E842 Accident to unpowered aircraft
[6 - 9]

Requires fourth digit. See beginning of section E840-E845 for codes and definitions.

Includes any accident, except collision with powered aircraft, to:
- balloon
- glider
- hang glider
- kite carrying a person

hit by object falling from unpowered aircraft

E843 Fall in, on, or from aircraft
[0 - 9]

Requires fourth digit. See beginning of section E840-E845 for codes and definitions.

Includes accident in boarding or alighting from aircraft, any kind

fall in, on, or from aircraft [any kind], while in transit, taking off, or landing, except when as a result of an accident to aircraft

E844 Other specified air transport accidents
[0 - 9]

Requires fourth digit. See beginning of section E840-E845 for codes and definitions.

Includes hit by aircraft without accident to aircraft

hit by object falling from aircraft without accident to aircraft

injury by or from machinery on aircraft without accident to aircraft

injury by or from rotating propeller without accident to aircraft

injury by or from voluntary parachute descent without accident to aircraft

poisoning by carbon monoxide from aircraft while in transit without accident to aircraft

sucked into jet without accident to aircraft

any accident involving other transport vehicle (motor) (nonmotor) due to being hit by object set in motion by aircraft (powered)

Excludes *air sickness (E903)*

effects of:
- *high altitude (E902.0-E902.1)*
- *pressure change (E902.0-E902.1)*

injury in parachute descent due to accident to aircraft (E840.0-E842.9)

E845 Accident involving spacecraft
[0,8,9]

Requires fourth digit. See beginning of section E840-E845 for codes and definitions.

Includes launching pad accident

Excludes *effects of weightlessness in spacecraft (E928.0)*

VEHICLE ACCIDENTS NOT ELSEWHERE CLASSIFIABLE (E846-E848)

E846 Accidents involving powered vehicles used solely within the buildings and premises of industrial or commercial establishment

Accident to, on, or involving:
- battery-powered airport passenger vehicle
- battery-powered trucks (baggage) (mail)
- coal car in mine
- logging car
- self-propelled truck, industrial
- station baggage truck (powered)
- tram, truck, or tub (powered) in mine or quarry

Breakage of any part of vehicle

Collision with:
- pedestrian
- other vehicle or object within premises

Explosion of powered vehicle, industrial or commercial

Fall from powered vehicle, industrial or commercial

Overturning of powered vehicle, industrial or commercial

Struck by powered vehicle, industrial or commercial

Excludes *accidental poisoning by exhaust gas from vehicle not elsewhere classifiable (E868.2)*

injury by crane, lift (fork), or elevator (E919.2)

E847 Accidents involving cable cars not running on rails

Accident to, on, or involving:
- cable car, not on rails
- ski chair-lift
- ski-lift with gondola
- téléférique

Breakage of cable

Caught or dragged by cable car, not on rails

Fall or jump from cable car, not on rails

Object thrown from or in cable car not on rails

E848 Accidents involving other vehicles, not elsewhere classifiable

Accident to, on, or involving:
- ice yacht
- land yacht
- nonmotor, nonroad vehicle NOS

E849 Place of occurrence

Note: The following category is for use to denote the place where the injury or poisoning occurred.

E849.0 Home
- Apartment
- Boarding house
- Farm house
- Home premises
- House (residential)
- Noninstitutional place of residence
- Private:
  - driveway
  - garage
  - garden
  - home
  - walk
- Swimming pool in private house or garden
- Yard of home

Excludes *home under construction but not yet occupied (E849.3)*

institutional place of residence (E849.7)

E849.1 Farm
- buildings
- land under cultivation

Excludes *farm house and home premises of farm (E849.0)*

E849.2 Mine and quarry
- Gravel pit
- Sand pit
- Tunnel under construction

E849.3 Industrial place and premises
- Building under construction
- Dockyard
- Dry dock
- Factory:
  - building
  - premises
- Garage (place of work)
- Industrial yard
- Loading platform (factory) (store)
- Plant, industrial
- Railway yard
- Shop (place of work)
- Warehouse
- Workhouse

E849.4 Place for recreation and sport
Amusement park
Baseball field
Basketball court
Beach resort
Cricket ground
Fives court
Football field
Golf course
Gymnasium
Hockey field
Holiday camp
Ice palace
Lake resort
Mountain resort
Playground, including school playground
Public park
Racecourse
Resort NOS
Riding school
Rifle range
Seashore resort
Skating rink
Sports palace
Stadium
Swimming pool, public
Tennis court
Vacation resort
Excludes *that in private house or garden (E849.0)*

E849.5 Street and highway

E849.6 Public building
Building (including adjacent grounds) used by the general public or by a particular group of the public, such as:
airport
bank
cafe
casino
church
cinema
clubhouse
courthouse
dance hall
garage building (for car storage)
hotel
market (grocery or other commodity)
movie house
music hall
nightclub
office
office building
opera house
post office
public hall
radio broadcasting station
restaurant
school (state) (public) (private)
shop, commercial
station (bus) (railway)
store
theater
Excludes *home garage (E849.0)*
industrial building or workplace (E849.3)

E849.7 Residential institution
Children's home
Dormitory
Hospital
Jail
Old people's home
Orphanage
Prison
Reform School

E849.8 Other specified places
Beach NOS
Canal
Caravan site NOS
Derelict house
Desert
Dock
Forest
Harbor
Hill
Lake NOS
Mountain
Parking lot
Parking place
Pond or pool (natural)
Prairie
Public place NOS
Railway line
Reservoir
River
Sea
Seashore NOS
Stream
Swamp
Trailer court
Woods

E849.9 Unspecified place

ACCIDENTAL POISONING BY DRUGS, MEDICINAL SUBSTANCES, AND BIOLOGICALS (E850-E858)

Includes accidental overdose of drug, wrong drug given or taken in error, and drug taken inadvertently
accidents in the use of drugs and biologicals in medical and surgical procedures

Excludes *administration with suicidal or homicidal intent or intent to harm, or in circumstances classifiable to E980-E989 (E950.0-E950.5, E962.0, E980.0-E980.5)*
correct drug properly administered in therapeutic or prophylactic dosage, as the cause of adverse effect (E930.0-E949.9)

Note: See Alphabetic Index for more complete list of specific drugs to be classified under the fourth-digit subdivisions. The American Hospital Formulary numbers can be used to classify new drugs listed by the American Hospital Formulary Service (AHFS). See Appendix C.

❹ **E850 Accidental poisoning by analgesics, antipyretics, and antirheumatics**

E850.0 Heroin
Diacetylmorphine

E850.1 Methadone

E850.2 Other opiates and related narcotics
Codeine [methylmorphine]
Meperidine [pethidine]
Morphine
Opium (alkaloids)

E850.3 Salicylates
Acetylsalicylic acid [aspirin]
Amino derivatives of salicylic acid
Salicylic acid salts

E850.4 Aromatic analgesics, not elsewhere classified
Acetanilid
Paracetamol [acetaminophen]
Phenacetin [acetophenetidin]

E850.5 Pyrazole derivatives
Aminophenazone [amidopyrine]
Phenylbutazone

E850.6 Antirheumatics [antiphlogistics]
Gold salts
Indomethacin
Excludes *salicylates (E850.3)*
steroids (E858.0)

E850.7 Other non-narcotic analgesics
Pyrabital

E850.8 Other specified analgesics and antipyretics
Pentazocine

E850.9 Unspecified analgesic or antipyretic

E851 Accidental poisoning by barbiturates
Amobarbital [amylobarbitone]
Barbital [barbitone]
Butabarbital [butabarbitone]
Pentobarbital [pentobarbitone]
Phenobarbital [phenobarbitone]
Secobarbital [quinalbarbitone]
Excludes *thiobarbiturates (E855.1)*

❹ **E852 Accidental poisoning by other sedatives and hypnotics**

E852.0 Chloral hydrate group

E852.1 Paraldehyde

E852.2 Bromine compounds
Bromides
Carbromal (derivatives)

E852.3 Methaqualone compounds

E852.4 Glutethimide group

E852.5 Mixed sedatives, not elsewhere classified

E852.8 Other specified sedatives and hypnotics

E852.9 Unspecified sedative or hypnotic
Sleeping:
drug NOS
pill NOS
tablet NOS

❹ **E853 Accidental poisoning by tranquilizers**

E853.0 Phenothiazine-based tranquilizers
Chlorpromazine
Fluphenazine
Prochlorperazine
Promazine

E853.1 Butyrophenone-based tranquilizers
Haloperidol
Spiperone
Trifluperidol

E853.2 Benzodiazepine-based tranquilizers
Chlordiazepoxide
Diazepam
Flurazepam
Lorazepam
Medazepam
Nitrazepam

E853.8 Other specified tranquilizers
Hydroxyzine
Meprobamate

E853.9 Unspecified tranquilizer

❹ **E854 Accidental poisoning by other psychotropic agents**

E854.0 Antidepressants
Amitriptyline
Imipramine
Monoamine oxidase [MAO] inhibitors

E854.1 Psychodysleptics [hallucinogens]
Cannabis derivatives
Lysergide [LSD]
Marihuana (derivatives)
Mescaline
Psilocin
Psilocybin

E854.2 Psychostimulants
Amphetamine
Caffeine
Excludes *central appetite depressants (E858.8)*

E854.3 Central nervous system stimulants
Analeptics
Opiate antagonists

E854.8 Other psychotropic agents

❹ **E855 Accidental poisoning by other drugs acting on central and autonomic nervous system**

E855.0 Anticonvulsant and anti-Parkinsonism drugs
Amantadine
Hydantoin derivatives
Levodopa [L-dopa]
Oxazolidine derivatives [paramethadione]
[trimethadione]
Succinimides

E855.1 Other central nervous system depressants
Ether
Gaseous anesthetics
Halogenated hydrocarbon derivatives
Intravenous anesthetics
Thiobarbiturates, such as thiopental sodium

E855.2 Local anesthetics
Cocaine
Lidocaine [lignocaine]
Procaine
Tetracaine

E855.3 Parasympathomimetics [cholinergics]
Acetylcholine
Anticholinesterase:
organophosphorus
reversible
Pilocarpine

E855.4 Parasympatholytics [anticholinergics and antimuscarinics] and spasmolytics
Atropine
Homatropine
Hyoscine [scopolamine]
Quaternary ammonium derivatives

E855.5 Sympathomimetics [adrenergics]
Epinephrine [adrenalin]
Levarterenol [noradrenalin]

E855.6 Sympatholytics [antiadrenergics]
Phenoxybenzamine
Tolazoline hydrochloride

E855.8 Other specified drugs acting on central and autonomic nervous systems

E855.9 Unspecified drug acting on central and autonomic nervous systems

E856 Accidental poisoning by antibiotics

E857 Accidental poisoning by other anti-infectives

❹ **E858 Accidental poisoning by other drugs**

E858.0 Hormones and synthetic substitutes

E858.1 Primarily systemic agents

E858.2 Agents primarily affecting blood constituents

E858.3 Agents primarily affecting cardiovascular system

E858.4 Agents primarily affecting gastrointestinal system

E858.5 Water, mineral, and uric acid metabolism drugs

E858.6 Agents primarily acting on the smooth and skeletal muscles and respiratory system

E858.7 Agents primarily affecting skin and mucous membrane, ophthalmological, otorhinolaryngological, and dental drugs

E858.8 Other specified drugs
Central appetite depressants

E858.9 Unspecified drug

ACCIDENTAL POISONING BY OTHER SOLID AND LIQUID SUBSTANCES, GASES, AND VAPORS (E860-E869)

Note: *Categories in this section are intended primarily to indicate the external cause of poisoning states classifiable to 980-989. They may also be used to indicate external causes of localized effects classifiable to 001-799.*

❹ **E860 Accidental poisoning by alcohol, not elsewhere classified**

E860.0 Alcoholic beverages
Alcohol in preparations intended for consumption

E860.1 Other and unspecified ethyl alcohol and its products
Denatured alcohol
Ethanol NOS
Grain alcohol NOS
Methylated spirit

E860.2 Methyl alcohol
Methanol
Wood alcohol

E860.3 Isopropyl alcohol
Dimethyl carbinol
Isopropanol
Rubbing alcohol substitute
Secondary propyl alcohol

E860.4 Fusel oil
Alcohol:
amyl
butyl
propyl

E860.8 Other specified alcohols

E860.9 Unspecified alcohol

❹ **E861 Accidental poisoning by cleansing and polishing agents, disinfectants, paints, and varnishes**

E861.0 Synthetic detergents and shampoos

E861.1 Soap products

E861.2 Polishes

E861.3 Other cleansing and polishing agents
Scouring powders

E861.4 Disinfectants
Household and other disinfectants not ordinarily used on the person
Excludes *carbolic acid or phenol (E864.0)*

E861.5 Lead paints

E861.6 Other paints and varnishes
Lacquers
Oil colors
Paints, other than lead
White washes

E861.9 Unspecified

❹ **E862 Accidental poisoning by petroleum products, other solvents and their vapors, not elsewhere classified**

E862.0 Petroleum solvents
Petroleum:
ether
benzine
naphtha

E862.1 Petroleum fuels and cleaners
Antiknock additives to petroleum fuels
Gas oils
Gasoline or petrol
Kerosene
Excludes *kerosene insecticides (E863.4)*

E862.2 Lubricating oils

E862.3 Petroleum solids
Paraffin wax

E862.4 Other specified solvents
Benzene

E862.9 Unspecified solvent

❹ **E863 Accidental poisoning by agricultural and horticultural chemical and pharmaceutical preparations other than plant foods and fertilizers**
Excludes *plant foods and fertilizers (E866.5)*

E863.0 Insecticides of organochlorine compounds
Benzene hexachloride
Chlordane
DDT
Dieldrin
Endrine
Toxaphene

E863.1 Insecticides of organophosphorus compounds
Demeton
Diazinon
Dichlorvos
Malathion
Methyl parathion
Parathion
Phenylsulphthion
Phorate
Phosdrin

E863.2 Carbamates
Aldicarb
Carbaryl
Propoxur

E863.3 Mixtures of insecticides

E863.4 Other and unspecified insecticides
Kerosene insecticides

E863.5 Herbicides
2,4-Dichlorophenoxyacetic acid [2, 4-D]
2,4,5-Trichlorophenoxyacetic acid [2, 4, 5-T]
Chlorates
Diquat
Mixtures of plant foods and fertilizers with herbicides
Paraquat

E863.6 Fungicides
Organic mercurials (used in seed dressing)
Pentachlorophenols

E863.7 Rodenticides
Fluoroacetates
Squill and derivatives
Thallium
Warfarin
Zinc phosphide

E863.8 Fumigants
Cyanides
Methyl bromide
Phosphine

E863.9 Other and unspecified

❹ **E864 Accidental poisoning by corrosives and caustics, not elsewhere classified**
Excludes *those as components of disinfectants (E861.4)*

E864.0 Corrosive aromatics
Carbolic acid or phenol

E864.1 Acids
Acid:
hydrochloric
nitric
sulfuric

E864.2 Caustic alkalis
Lye

E864.3 Other specified corrosives and caustics

E864.4 Unspecified corrosives and caustics

❹ **E865 Accidental poisoning from poisonous foodstuffs and poisonous plants**
Includes any meat, fish, or shellfish
plants, berries, and fungi eaten as, or in mistake for food, or by a child
Excludes *anaphylactic shock due to adverse food reaction (995.60-995.69)*
food poisoning (bacterial) (005.0-005.9)
poisoning and toxic reactions to venomous plants (E905.6-E905.7)

E865.0 Meat

E865.1 Shellfish

E865.2 Other fish

E865.3 Berries and seeds

E865.4 Other specified plants

E865.5 Mushrooms and other fungi

E865.8 Other specified foods

E865.9 Unspecified foodstuff or poisonous plant

❹ **E866 Accidental poisoning by other and unspecified solid and liquid substances**
Excludes *these substances as a component of:*
medicines (E850.0-E858.9)
paints (E861.5-E861.6)
pesticides (E863.0-E863.9)
petroleum fuels (E862.1)

E866.0 Lead and its compounds and fumes

E866.1 Mercury and its compounds and fumes

E866.2 Antimony and its compounds and fumes

E866.3 Arsenic and its compounds and fumes

E866.4 Other metals and their compounds and fumes
Beryllium (compounds)
Brass fumes
Cadmium (compounds)
Copper salts
Iron (compounds)
Manganese (compounds)
Nickel (compounds)
Thallium (compounds)

E866.5 Plant foods and fertilizers
Excludes *mixtures with herbicides (E863.5)*

E866.6 Glues and adhesives

E866.7 Cosmetics

E866.8 Other specified solid or liquid substances

E866.9 Unspecified solid or liquid substance

E867 Accidental poisoning by gas distributed by pipeline
Carbon monoxide from incomplete combustion of piped gas
Coal gas NOS
Liquefied petroleum gas distributed through pipes (pure or mixed with air)
Piped gas (natural) (manufactured)

❹ **E868 Accidental poisoning by other utility gas and other carbon monoxide**

E868.0 Liquefied petroleum gas distributed in mobile containers
Butane or carbon monoxide from incomplete combustion of these gases
Liquefied hydrocarbon gas NOS or carbon monoxide from incomplete combustion of these gases
Propane or carbon monoxide from incomplete combustion of these gases

E868.1 Other and unspecified utility gas
Acetylene or carbon monoxide from incomplete combustion of these gases
Gas NOS used for lighting, heating, or cooking or carbon monoxide from incomplete combustion of these gases
Water gas or carbon monoxide from incomplete combustion of these gases

E868.2 Motor vehicle exhaust gas
Exhaust gas from:
farm tractor, not in transit
gas engine
motor pump
motor vehicle, not in transit
any type of combustion engine not in watercraft
Excludes *poisoning by carbon monoxide from:*
aircraft while in transit (E844.0-E844.9)
motor vehicle while in transit (E818.0-E818.9)
watercraft whether or not in transit (E838.0-E838.9)

E868.3 Carbon monoxide from incomplete combustion of other domestic fuels
Carbon monoxide from incomplete combustion of:
coal in domestic stove or fireplace
coke in domestic stove or fireplace
kerosene in domestic stove or fireplace
wood in domestic stove or fireplace
Excludes *carbon monoxide from smoke and fumes due to conflagration (E890.0-E893.9)*

E868.8 Carbon monoxide from other sources
Carbon monoxide from:
blast furnace gas
incomplete combustion of fuels in industrial use
kiln vapor

E868.9 Unspecified carbon monoxide

❹ **E869 Accidental poisoning by other gases and vapors**
Excludes *effects of gases used as anesthetics (E855.1, E938.2)*
fumes from heavy metals (E866.0-E866.4)
smoke and fumes due to conflagration or explosion (E890.0-E899)

E869.0 Nitrogen oxides

E869.1 Sulfur dioxide

E869.2 Freon

E869.3 Lacrimogenic gas [tear gas]
Bromobenzyl cyanide
Chloroacetophenone
Ethyliodoacetate

E869.4 Second-hand tobacco smoke

E869.8 Other specified gases and vapors
Chlorine
Hydrocyanic acid gas

E869.9 Unspecified gases and vapors

MISADVENTURES TO PATIENTS DURING SURGICAL AND MEDICAL CARE (E870-E876)

Excludes *accidental overdose of drug and wrong drug given in error (E850.0-E858.9)*
surgical and medical procedures as the cause of abnormal reaction by the patient, without mention of misadventure at the time of procedure (E878.0-E879.9)

❹ **E870 Accidental cut, puncture, perforation, or hemorrhage during medical care**

E870.0 Surgical operation

E870.1 Infusion or transfusion

E870.2 Kidney dialysis or other perfusion

E870.3 Injection or vaccination

E870.4 Endoscopic examination

E870.5 Aspiration of fluid or tissue, puncture, and catheterization
Abdominal paracentesis
Aspirating needle biopsy
Blood sampling
Lumbar puncture
Thoracentesis
Excludes *heart catheterization (E870.6)*

E870.6 Heart catheterization

E870.7 Administration of enema

E870.8 Other specified medical care

E870.9 Unspecified medical care

❹ **E871 Foreign object left in body during procedure**

E871.0 Surgical operation

E871.1 Infusion or transfusion

E871.2 Kidney dialysis or other perfusion

E871.3 Injection or vaccination

E871.4 Endoscopic examination

E871.5 Aspiration of fluid or tissue, puncture, and catheterization
Abdominal paracentesis
Aspiration needle biopsy
Blood sampling
Lumbar puncture
Thoracentesis
Excludes *heart catheterization (E871.6)*

E871.6 Heart catheterization

E871.7 Removal of catheter or packing

E871.8 Other specified procedures

E871.9 Unspecified procedure

❹ E872 Failure of sterile precautions during procedure

E872.0 Surgical operation

E872.1 Infusion or transfusion

E872.2 Kidney dialysis and other perfusion

E872.3 Injection or vaccination

E872.4 Endoscopic examination

E872.5 Aspiration of fluid or tissue, puncture, and catheterization

Abdominal paracentesis
Aspirating needle biopsy
Blood sampling
Lumbar puncture
Thoracentesis

Excludes *heart catheterization (E872.6)*

E872.6 Heart catheterization

E872.8 Other specified procedures

E872.9 Unspecified procedure

❹ E873 Failure in dosage

Excludes *accidental overdose of drug, medicinal or biological substance (E850.0-E858.9)*

E873.0 Excessive amount of blood or other fluid during transfusion or infusion

E873.1 Incorrect dilution of fluid during infusion

E873.2 Overdose of radiation in therapy

E873.3 Inadvertent exposure of patient to radiation during medical care

E873.4 Failure in dosage in electroshock or insulin-shock therapy

E873.5 Inappropriate [too hot or too cold] temperature in local application and packing

E873.6 Nonadministration of necessary drug or medicinal substance

E873.8 Other specified failure in dosage

E873.9 Unspecified failure in dosage

❹ E874 Mechanical failure of instrument or apparatus during procedure

E874.0 Surgical operation

E874.1 Infusion and transfusion

Air in system

E874.2 Kidney dialysis and other perfusion

E874.3 Endoscopic examination

E874.4 Aspiration of fluid or tissue, puncture, and catheterization

Abdominal paracentesis
Aspirating needle biopsy
Blood sampling
Lumbar puncture
Thoracentesis

Excludes *heart catheterization (E874.5)*

E874.5 Heart catheterization

E874.8 Other specified procedures

E874.9 Unspecified procedure

❹ E875 Contaminated or infected blood, other fluid, drug, or biological substance

Includes presence of:
bacterial pyrogens
endotoxin-producing bacteria
serum hepatitis-producing agent

E875.0 Contaminated substance transfused or infused

E875.1 Contaminated substance injected or used for vaccination

E875.2 Contaminated drug or biological substance administered by other means

E875.8 Other

E875.9 Unspecified

❹ E876 Other and unspecified misadventures during medical care

E876.0 Mismatched blood in transfusion

E876.1 Wrong fluid in infusion

E876.2 Failure in suture and ligature during surgical operation

E876.3 Endotracheal tube wrongly placed during anesthetic procedure

E876.4 Failure to introduce or to remove other tube or instrument

Excludes *foreign object left in body during procedure (E871.0-E871.9)*

E876.5 Performance of inappropriate operation

E876.8 Other specified misadventures during medical care

Performance of inappropriate treatment NEC

E876.9 Unspecified misadventure during medical care

SURGICAL AND MEDICAL PROCEDURES AS THE CAUSE OF ABNORMAL REACTION OF PATIENT OR LATER COMPLICATION, WITHOUT MENTION OF MISADVENTURE AT THE TIME OF PROCEDURE (E878-E879)

Includes procedures as the cause of abnormal reaction, such as:
displacement or malfunction of prosthetic device
hepatorenal failure, postoperative
malfunction of external stoma
postoperative intestinal obstruction
rejection of transplanted organ

Excludes *anesthetic management properly carried out as the cause of adverse effect (E937.0-E938.9)*
infusion and transfusion, without mention of misadventure in the technique of procedure (E930.0-E949.9)

❹ E878 Surgical operation and other surgical procedures as the cause of abnormal reaction of patient, or of later complication, without mention of misadventure at the time of operation

E878.0 Surgical operation with transplant of whole organ

Transplantation of:
heart
kidney
liver

E878.1 Surgical operation with implant of artificial internal device

Cardiac pacemaker
Electrodes implanted in brain
Heart valve prosthesis
Internal orthopedic device

E878.2 Surgical operation with anastomosis, bypass, or graft, with natural or artificial tissues used as implant

Anastomosis:
arteriovenous
gastrojejunal
Graft of blood vessel, tendon, or skin

Excludes *external stoma (E878.3)*

E878.3 Surgical operation with formation of external stoma

Colostomy
Cystostomy
Duodenostomy
Gastrostomy
Ureterostomy

E878.4 Other restorative surgery

E878.5 Amputation of limb(s)

E878.6 Removal of other organ (partial) (total)

E878.8 Other specified surgical operations and procedures

E878.9 Unspecified surgical operations and procedures

❹ E879 Other procedures, without mention of misadventure at the time of procedure, as the cause of abnormal reaction of patient, or of later complication

E879.0 Cardiac catheterization

E879.1 Kidney dialysis

E879.2 Radiological procedure and radiotherapy

Excludes *radio-opaque dyes for diagnostic x-ray procedures (E947.8)*

E879.3 Shock therapy

Electroshock therapy
Insulin-shock therapy

E879.4 Aspiration of fluid
Lumbar puncture
Thoracentesis

E879.5 Insertion of gastric or duodenal sound

E879.6 Urinary catheterization

E879.7 Blood sampling

E879.8 Other specified procedures
Blood transfusion

E879.9 Unspecified procedure

ACCIDENTAL FALLS (E880-E888)

Excludes *falls (in or from):*
burning building (E890.8, E891.8)
into fire (E890.0-E899)
into water (with submersion or drowning) (E910.0-E910.9)
machinery (in operation) (E919.0-E919.9)
on edged, pointed, or sharp object (E920.0-E920.9)
transport vehicle (E800.0-E845.9)
vehicle not elsewhere classifiable (E846-E848)

❹ **E880 Fall on or from stairs or steps**

E880.0 Escalator

E880.1 Fall on or from sidewalk curb
Excludes *fall from moving sidewalk (E885.9)*

E880.9 Other stairs or steps

❹ **E881 Fall on or from ladders or scaffolding**

E881.0 Fall from ladder

E881.1 Fall from scaffolding

E882 Fall from or out of building or other structure
Fall from:
balcony
bridge
building
flagpole
tower
turret
viaduct
wall
window
Fall through roof
Excludes *collapse of a building or structure (E916)*
fall or jump from burning building (E890.8, E891.8)

❹ **E883 Fall into hole or other opening in surface**
Includes fall into:
cavity
dock
hole
pit
quarry
shaft
swimming pool
tank
well
Excludes *fall into water NOS (E910.9)*
that resulting in drowning or submersion without mention of injury (E910.0-E910.9)

E883.0 Accident from diving or jumping into water [swimming pool]
Strike or hit:
against bottom when jumping or diving into water
wall or board of swimming pool
water surface
Excludes *diving with insufficient air supply (E913.2)*
effects of air pressure from diving (E902.2)

E883.1 Accidental fall into well

E883.2 Accidental fall into storm drain or manhole

E883.9 Fall into other hole or other opening in surface

❹ **E884 Other fall from one level to another**

E884.0 Fall from playground equipment
Excludes *recreational machinery (E919.8)*

E884.1 Fall from cliff

E884.2 Fall from chair

E884.3 Fall from wheelchair

E884.4 Fall from bed

E884.5 Fall from other furniture

E884.6 Fall from commode
Toilet

E884.9 Other fall from one level to another
Fall from:
embankment
haystack
stationary vehicle
tree

❹ **E885 Fall on same level from slipping, tripping, or stumbling**

E885.0 Fall from (nonmotorized) scooter

E885.1 Fall from roller skates
In-line skates

E885.2 Fall from skateboard

E885.3 Fall from skis

E885.4 Fall from snowboard

E885.9 Fall from other slipping, tripping, or stumbling
Fall on moving sidewalk

❹ **E886 Fall on same level from collision, pushing, or shoving, by or with other person**
Excludes *crushed or pushed by a crowd or human stampede (E917.1, E917.6)*

E886.0 In sports
Tackles in sports
Excludes *kicked, stepped on, struck by object, in sports (E917.0, E917.5)*

E886.9 Other and unspecified
Fall from collision of pedestrian (conveyance) with another pedestrian (conveyance)

E887 Fracture, cause unspecified

❹ **E888 Other and unspecified fall**
Accidental fall NOS
Fall on same level NOS

E888.0 Fall resulting in striking against sharp object
Use additional external cause code to identify object (E920)

E888.1 Fall resulting in striking against other object

E888.8 Other fall

E888.9 Unspecified fall
Fall NOS

ACCIDENTS CAUSED BY FIRE AND FLAMES (E890-E899)

Includes asphyxia or poisoning due to conflagration or ignition
burning by fire
secondary fires resulting from explosion

Excludes *arson (E968.0)*
fire in or on:
machinery (in operation) (E919.0-E919.9)
transport vehicle other than stationary vehicle (E800.0-E845.9)
vehicle not elsewhere classifiable (E846-E848)

❹ **E890 Conflagration in private dwelling**

Includes conflagration in:
apartment
boarding house
camping place
caravan
farmhouse
house
lodging house
mobile home
private garage
rooming house
tenement
conflagration originating from sources classifiable to E893-E898 in the above buildings

E890.0 Explosion caused by conflagration

E890.1 Fumes from combustion of polyvinylchloride [PVC] and similar material in conflagration

E890.2 Other smoke and fumes from conflagration
Carbon monoxide from conflagration in private building
Fumes NOS from conflagration in private building
Smoke NOS from conflagration in private building

E890.3 Burning caused by conflagration

E890.8 Other accident resulting from conflagration
Collapse of burning private building
Fall from burning private building
Hit by object falling from burning private building
Jump from burning private building

E890.9 Unspecified accident resulting from conflagration in private dwelling

❹ **E891 Conflagration in other and unspecified building or structure**

Conflagration in:
barn
church
convalescent and other residential home
dormitory of educational institution
factory
farm outbuildings
hospital
hotel
school
store
theater
Conflagration originating from sources classifiable to E893-E898, in the above buildings

E891.0 Explosion caused by conflagration

E891.1 Fumes from combustion of polyvinylchloride [PVC] and similar material in conflagration

E891.2 Other smoke and fumes from conflagration
Carbon monoxide from conflagration in building or structure
Fumes NOS from conflagration in building or structure
Smoke NOS from conflagration in building or structure

E891.3 Burning caused by conflagration

E891.8 Other accident resulting from conflagration
Collapse of burning building or structure
Fall from burning building or structure
Hit by object falling from burning building or structure
Jump from burning building or structure

E891.9 Unspecified accident resulting from conflagration of other and unspecified building or structure

E892 Conflagration not in building or structure

Fire (uncontrolled) (in) (of):
forest
grass
hay
lumber
mine
prairie
transport vehicle [any], except while in transit
tunnel

❹ **E893 Accident caused by ignition of clothing**

Excludes *ignition of clothing:*
from highly inflammable material (E894)
with conflagration (E890.0-E892)

E893.0 From controlled fire in private dwelling
Ignition of clothing from:
normal fire (charcoal) (coal) (electric) (gas) (wood) in:
brazier in private dwelling (as listed in E890)
fireplace in private dwelling (as listed in E890)
furnace in private dwelling (as listed in E890)
stove in private dwelling (as listed in E890)

E893.1 From controlled fire in other building or structure
Ignition of clothing from:
normal fire (charcoal) (coal) (electric) (gas) (wood) in:
brazier in other building or structure (as listed in E891)
fireplace in other building or structure (as listed in E891)
furnace in other building or structure (as listed in E891)
stove in other building or structure (as listed in E891)

E893.2 From controlled fire not in building or structure
Ignition of clothing from:
bonfire (controlled)
brazier fire (controlled), not in building or structure
trash fire (controlled)

Excludes *conflagration not in building (E892)*
trash fire out of control (E892)

E893.8 From other specified sources
Ignition of clothing from:
blowlamp
blowtorch
burning bedspread
candle
cigar
cigarette
lighter
matches
pipe
welding torch

E893.9 Unspecified source
Ignition of clothing (from controlled fire NOS) (in building NOS) NOS

E894 Ignition of highly inflammable material

Ignition of:
benzine (with ignition of clothing)
gasoline (with ignition of clothing)
fat (with ignition of clothing)
kerosene (with ignition of clothing)
paraffin (with ignition of clothing)
petrol (with ignition of clothing)

Excludes *ignition of highly inflammable material with:*
conflagration (E890.0-E892)
explosion (E923.0-E923.9)

E895 Accident caused by controlled fire in private dwelling
Burning by (flame of) normal fire (charcoal) (coal) (electric) (gas) (wood) in:
brazier in private dwelling (as listed in E890)
fireplace in private dwelling (as listed in E890)
furnace in private dwelling (as listed in E890)
stove in private dwelling (as listed in E890)
Excludes *burning by hot objects not producing fire or flames (E924.0-E924.9)*
ignition of clothing from these sources (E893.0)
poisoning by carbon monoxide from incomplete combustion of fuel (E867-E868.9)
that with conflagration (E890.0-E890.9)

E896 Accident caused by controlled fire in other and unspecified building or structure
Burning by (flame of) normal fire (charcoal) (coal) (electric) (gas) (wood) in:
brazier in other building or structure (as listed in E891)
fireplace in other building or structure (as listed in E891)
furnace in other building or structure (as listed in E891)
stove in other building or structure (as listed in E891)
Excludes *burning by hot objects not producing fire or flames (E924.0-E924.9)*
ignition of clothing from these sources (E893.1)
poisoning by carbon monoxide from incomplete combustion of fuel (E867-E868.9)
that with conflagration (E891.0-E891.9)

E897 Accident caused by controlled fire not in building or structure
Burns from flame of:
bonfire (controlled)
brazier fire (controlled), not in building or structure
trash fire (controlled)
Excludes *ignition of clothing from these sources (E893.2)*
trash fire out of control (E892)
that with conflagration (E892)

❹ **E898 Accident caused by other specified fire and flames**
Excludes *conflagration (E890.0-E892)*
that with ignition of:
clothing (E893.0-E893.9)
highly inflammable material (E894)

E898.0 Burning bedclothes
Bed set on fire NOS

E898.1 Other
Burning by:
blowlamp
blowtorch
candle
cigar
cigarette
fire in room NOS
lamp
lighter
matches
pipe
welding torch

E899 Accident caused by unspecified fire
Burning NOS

ACCIDENTS DUE TO NATURAL AND ENVIRONMENTAL FACTORS (E900-E909)

❹ **E900 Excessive heat**

E900.0 Due to weather conditions
Excessive heat as the external cause of:
ictus solaris
siriasis
sunstroke

E900.1 Of man-made origin
Heat (in):
boiler room
drying room
factory
furnace room
generated in transport vehicle
kitchen

E900.9 Of unspecified origin

❹ **E901 Excessive cold**

E901.0 Due to weather conditions
Excessive cold as the cause of:
chilblains NOS
immersion foot

E901.1 Of man-made origin
Contact with or inhalation of:
dry ice
liquid air
liquid hydrogen
liquid nitrogen
Prolonged exposure in:
deep freeze unit
refrigerator

E901.8 Other specified origin

E901.9 Of unspecified origin

❹ **E902 High and low air pressure and changes in air pressure**

E902.0 Residence or prolonged visit at high altitude
Residence or prolonged visit at high altitude as the cause of:
Acosta syndrome
Alpine sickness
altitude sickness
Andes disease
anoxia, hypoxia
barotitis, barodontalgia, barosinusitis, otitic barotrauma
hypobarism, hypobaropathy
mountain sickness
range disease

E902.1 In aircraft
Sudden change in air pressure in aircraft during ascent or descent as the cause of:
aeroneurosis
aviators' disease

E902.2 Due to diving
High air pressure from rapid descent in water as the cause of:
caisson disease
divers' disease
divers' palsy or paralysis
Reduction in atmospheric pressure while surfacing from deep water diving as the cause of:
caisson disease
divers' disease
divers' palsy or paralysis

E902.8 Due to other specified causes
Reduction in atmospheric pressure while surfacing from underground

E902.9 Unspecified cause

E903 Travel and motion

❹ **E904 Hunger, thirst, exposure, and neglect**
Excludes *any condition resulting from homicidal intent (E968.0-E968.9)*
hunger, thirst, and exposure resulting from accidents connected with transport (E800.0-E848)

E904.0 Abandonment or neglect of infants and helpless persons
Desertion of newborn
Exposure to weather conditions resulting from abandonment or neglect
Hunger or thirst resulting from abandonment or neglect
Inattention at or after birth
Lack of care (helpless person) (infant)
Excludes *criminal [purposeful] neglect (E968.4)*

E904.1 Lack of food
Lack of food as the cause of:
inanition
insufficient nourishment
starvation
Excludes *hunger resulting from abandonment or neglect (E904.0)*

E904.2 Lack of water
Lack of water as the cause of:
dehydration
inanition
Excludes *dehydration due to acute fluid loss (276.51)*

E904.3 Exposure (to weather conditions), not elsewhere classifiable
Exposure NOS
Humidity
Struck by hailstones
Excludes *struck by lightning (E907)*

E904.9 Privation, unqualified
Destitution

❹ **E905 Venomous animals and plants as the cause of poisoning and toxic reactions**
Includes chemical released by animal
insects
release of venom through fangs, hairs, spines, tentacles, and other venom apparatus
Excludes *eating of poisonous animals or plants (E865.0-E865.9)*

E905.0 Venomous snakes and lizards
Cobra
Copperhead snake
Coral snake
Fer de lance
Gila monster
Krait
Mamba
Rattlesnake
Sea snake
Snake (venomous)
Viper
Water moccasin
Excludes *bites of snakes and lizards known to be nonvenomous (E906.2)*

E905.1 Venomous spiders
Black widow spider
Brown spider
Tarantula (venomous)

E905.2 Scorpion

E905.3 Hornets, wasps, and bees
Yellow jacket

E905.4 Centipede and venomous millipede (tropical)

E905.5 Other venomous arthropods
Sting of:
ant
caterpillar

E905.6 Venomous marine animals and plants
Puncture by sea urchin spine
Sting of:
coral
jelly fish
nematocysts
sea anemone
sea cucumber
other marine animal or plant
Excludes *bites and other injuries caused by nonvenomous marine animal (E906.2-E906.8)*
bite of sea snake (venomous) (E905.0)

E905.7 Poisoning and toxic reactions caused by other plants
Injection of poisons or toxins into or through skin by plant thorns, spines, or other mechanisms
Excludes *puncture wound NOS by plant thorns or spines (E920.8)*

E905.8 Other specified

E905.9 Unspecified
Sting NOS
Venomous bite NOS

❹ **E906 Other injury caused by animals**
Excludes *poisoning and toxic reactions caused by venomous animals and insects (E905.0-E905.9)*
road vehicle accident involving animals (E827.0-E828.9)
tripping or falling over an animal (E885.9)

E906.0 Dog bite

E906.1 Rat bite

E906.2 Bite of nonvenomous snakes and lizards

E906.3 Bite of other animal except arthropod
Cats
Moray eel
Rodents, except rats
Shark

E906.4 Bite of nonvenomous arthropod
Insect bite NOS

E906.5 Bite by unspecified animal
Animal bite NOS

E906.8 Other specified injury caused by animal
Butted by animal
Fallen on by horse or other animal, not being ridden
Gored by animal
Implantation of quills of porcupine
Pecked by bird
Run over by animal, not being ridden
Stepped on by animal, not being ridden
Excludes *injury by animal being ridden (E828.0-E828.9)*

E906.9 Unspecified injury caused by animal

E907 Lightning
Excludes *injury from:*
fall of tree or other object caused by lightning (E916)
fire caused by lightning (E890.0-E892)

❹ **E908 Cataclysmic storms, and floods resulting from storms**
Excludes *collapse of dam or man-made structure causing flood (E909.3)*

E908.0 Hurricane
Storm surge
"Tidal wave" caused by storm action
Typhoon

E908.1 Tornado
Cyclone
Twisters

E908.2 Floods
Flash flood
Torrential rainfall
Excludes *collapse of dam or man-made structure causing flood (E909.3)*

E908.3 Blizzard (snow) (ice)

E908.4 Dust storm

E908.8 Other cataclysmic storms

E908.9 Unspecified cataclysmic storms, and floods resulting from storms
Storm NOS

❹ **E909 Cataclysmic earth surface movements and eruptions**

E909.0 Earthquakes

E909.1 Volcanic eruptions
Ash inhalation
Burns from lava

E909.2 Avalanche, landslide, or mudslide

E909.3 Collapse of dam or man-made structure

E909.4 Tidalwave caused by earthquake
Tidalwave NOS
Tsunami
Excludes *tidalwave caused by tropical storm (E908.0)*

E909.8 Other cataclysmic earth surface movements and eruptions

E909.9 Unspecified cataclysmic earth surface movements and eruptions

ACCIDENTS CAUSED BY SUBMERSION, SUFFOCATION, AND FOREIGN BODIES (E910-E915)

❹ E910 Accidental drowning and submersion

Includes immersion
swimmers' cramp

Excludes *diving accident (NOS) (resulting in injury except drowning) (E883.0)*
diving with insufficient air supply (E913.2)
drowning and submersion due to:
cataclysm (E908-E909)
machinery accident (E919.0-E919.9)
transport accident (E800.0-E845.9)
effect of high and low air pressure (E902.2)
injury from striking against objects while in running water (E917.2)

E910.0 While water-skiing

Fall from water skis with submersion or drowning

Excludes *accident to water-skier involving a watercraft and resulting in submersion or other injury (E830.4, E831.4)*

E910.1 While engaged in other sport or recreational activity with diving equipment

Scuba diving NOS
Skin diving NOS
Underwater spear fishing NOS

E910.2 While engaged in other sport or recreational activity without diving equipment

Fishing or hunting, except from boat or with diving equipment
Ice skating
Playing in water
Surfboarding
Swimming NOS
Voluntarily jumping from boat, not involved in accident, for swim NOS
Wading in water

Excludes *jumping into water to rescue another person (E910.3)*

E910.3 While swimming or diving for purposes other than recreation or sport

Marine salvage (with diving equipment)
Pearl diving (with diving equipment)
Placement of fishing nets (with diving equipment)
Rescue (attempt) of another person (with diving equipment)
Underwater construction or repairs (with diving equipment)

E910.4 In bathtub

E910.8 Other accidental drowning or submersion

Drowning in:
quenching tank
swimming pool

E910.9 Unspecified accidental drowning or submersion

Accidental fall into water NOS
Drowning NOS

E911 Inhalation and ingestion of food causing obstruction of respiratory tract or suffocation

Aspiration and inhalation of food [any] (into respiratory tract) NOS
Asphyxia by food [including bone, seed in food, regurgitated food]
Choked on food [including bone, seed in food, regurgitated food]
Compression of trachea by food lodged in esophagus
Interruption of respiration by food lodged in esophagus
Obstruction of pharynx by food (bolus)
Obstruction of respiration by food lodged in esophagus
Suffocation by food [including bone, seed in food, regurgitated food]

Excludes *injury, except asphyxia and obstruction of respiratory passage, caused by food (E915)*
obstruction of esophagus by food without mention of asphyxia or obstruction of respiratory passage (E915)

E912 Inhalation and ingestion of other object causing obstruction of respiratory tract or suffocation

Aspiration and inhalation of foreign body except food (into respiratory tract) NOS
Compression by foreign body in esophagus
Foreign object [bean] [marble] in nose
Interruption of respiration by foreign body in esophagus
Obstruction of pharynx by foreign body
Obstruction of respiration by foreign body in esophagus

Excludes *injury, except asphyxia and obstruction of respiratory passage, caused by foreign body (E915)*
obstruction of esophagus by foreign body without mention of asphyxia or obstruction in respiratory passage (E915)

❹ E913 Accidental mechanical suffocation

Excludes *mechanical suffocation from or by:*
accidental inhalation or ingestion of:
food (E911)
foreign object (E912)
cataclysm (E908-E909)
explosion (E921.0-E921.9, E923.0-E923.9)
machinery accident (E919.0-E919.9)

E913.0 In bed or cradle

Excludes *suffocation by plastic bag (E913.1)*

E913.1 By plastic bag

E913.2 Due to lack of air (in closed place)

Accidentally closed up in refrigerator or other airtight enclosed space
Diving with insufficient air supply

Excludes *suffocation by plastic bag (E913.1)*

E913.3 By falling earth or other substance

Cave-in NOS

Excludes *cave-in caused by cataclysmic earth surface movements and eruptions (E909.8)*
struck by cave-in without asphyxiation or suffocation (E916)

E913.8 Other specified means

Accidental hanging, except in bed or cradle

E913.9 Unspecified means

Asphyxia, mechanical NOS
Strangulation NOS
Suffocation NOS

E914 Foreign body accidentally entering eye and adnexa

Excludes *corrosive liquid (E924.1)*

E915 Foreign body accidentally entering other orifice

Excludes *aspiration and inhalation of foreign body, any, (into respiratory tract) NOS (E911-E912)*

OTHER ACCIDENTS (E916-E928)

E916 Struck accidentally by falling object

Collapse of building, except on fire
Falling:
rock
snowslide NOS
stone
tree
Object falling from:
machine, not in operation
stationary vehicle

Code first:
collapse of building on fire (E890.0-E891.9)
falling object in:
cataclysm (E908-E909)
machinery accidents (E919.0-E919.9)
transport accidents (E800.0-E845.9)
vehicle accidents not elsewhere classifiable (E846-E848)
object set in motion by:
explosion (E921.0-E921.9, E923.0-E923.9)
firearm (E922.0-E922.9)
projected object (E917.0-E917.9)

④ E917 Striking against or struck accidentally by objects or persons

Includes bumping into or against:
- object (moving) (projected) (stationary)
- pedestrian conveyance
- person

colliding with:
- object (moving) (projected) (stationary)
- pedestrian conveyance
- person

kicking against:
- object (moving) (projected) (stationary)
- pedestrian conveyance
- person

stepping on:
- object (moving) (projected) (stationary)
- pedestrian conveyance
- person

struck by:
- object (moving) (projected) (stationary)
- pedestrian conveyance
- person

Excludes *fall from:*
- *collision with another person, except when caused by a crowd (E886.0-E886.9)*
- *stumbling over object (E885.9)*

fall resulting in striking against object (E888.0-E888.1)

injury caused by:
- *assault (E960.0-E960.1, E967.0-E967.9)*
- *cutting or piercing instrument (E920.0-E920.9)*
- *explosion (E921.0-E921.9, E923.0-E923.9)*
- *firearm (E922.0-E922.9)*
- *machinery (E919.0-E919.9)*
- *transport vehicle (E800.0-E845.9)*
- *vehicle not elsewhere classifiable (E846-E848)*

E917.0 In sports without subsequent fall

Kicked or stepped on during game (football) (rugby)
Struck by hit or thrown ball
Struck by hockey stick or puck

E917.1 Caused by a crowd, by collective fear or panic without subsequent fall

Crushed by crowd or human stampede
Pushed by crowd or human stampede
Stepped on by crowd or human stampede

E917.2 In running water without subsequent fall

Excludes *drowning or submersion (E910.0-E910.9)*
that in sports (E917.0, E917.5)

E917.3 Furniture without subsequent fall

Excludes *fall from furniture (E884.2, E884.4-E884.5)*

E917.4 Other stationary object without subsequent fall

Bath tub
Fence
Lamp-post

E917.5 Object in sports with subsequent fall

Knocked down while boxing

E917.6 Caused by a crowd, by collective fear or panic with subsequent fall

E917.7 Furniture with subsequent fall

Excludes *fall from furniture (E884.2, E884.4-E884.5)*

E917.8 Other stationary object with subsequent fall

Bath tub
Fence
Lamp-post

E917.9 Other striking against with or without subsequent fall

E918 Caught accidentally in or between objects

Caught, crushed, jammed, or pinched in or between moving or stationary objects, such as:
- escalator
- folding object
- hand tools, appliances, or implements
- sliding door and door frame
- under packing crate
- washing machine wringer

Excludes *injury caused by:*
- *cutting or piercing instrument (E920.0-E920.9)*
- *machinery (E919.0-E919.9)*
- *transport vehicle (E800.0-E845.9)*
- *vehicle not elsewhere classifiable (E846-E848)*

struck accidentally by:
- *falling object (E916)*
- *object (moving) (projected) (E917.0-E917.9)*

④ E919 Accidents caused by machinery

Includes
- burned by machinery (accident)
- caught between machinery and other object
- caught in (moving parts of) machinery (accident)
- collapse of machinery (accident)
- crushed by machinery (accident)
- cut or pierced by machinery (accident)
- drowning or submersion caused by machinery (accident)
- explosion of, on, in machinery (accident)
- fall from or into moving part of machinery (accident)
- fire starting in or on machinery (accident)
- machinery accident NOS
- mechanical suffocation caused by machinery (accident)
- object falling from, on, in motion by machinery (accident)
- overturning of machinery (accident)
- pinned under machinery (accident)
- run over by machinery (accident)
- struck by machinery (accident)
- thrown from machinery (accident)

Excludes *accidents involving machinery, not in operation (E884.9, E916-E918)*

injury caused by:
- *electric current in connection with machinery (E925.0-E925.9)*
- *escalator (E880.0, E918)*
- *explosion of pressure vessel in connection with machinery (E921.0-E921.9)*
- *moving sidewalk (E885.9)*
- *poisoning by carbon monoxide generated by machine (E868.8)*
- *powered hand tools, appliances, and implements (E916-E918, E920.0-E921.9, E923.0-E926.9)*
- *transport vehicle accidents involving machinery (E800.0-E848.9)*

E919.0 Agricultural machines

Animal-powered agricultural machine
Combine
Derrick, hay
Farm machinery NOS
Farm tractor
Harvester
Hay mower or rake
Reaper
Thresher

Excludes *that in transport under own power on the highway (E810.0-E819.9)*
that being towed by another vehicle on the highway (E810.0-E819.9, E827.0-E827.9, E829.0-E829.9)
that involved in accident classifiable to E820-E829 (E820.0-E829.9)

E919.1 Mining and earth-drilling machinery
Bore or drill (land) (seabed)
Shaft hoist
Shaft lift
Under-cutter
Excludes *coal car, tram, truck, and tub in mine (E846)*

E919.2 Lifting machines and appliances
Chain hoist except in agricultural or mining operations
Crane except in agricultural or mining operations
Derrick except in agricultural or mining operations
Elevator (building) (grain) except in agricultural or mining operations
Forklift truck except in agricultural or mining operations
Lift except in agricultural or mining operations
Pulley block except in agricultural or mining operations
Winch except in agricultural or mining operations
Excludes *that being towed by another vehicle on the highway (E810.0-E819.9, E827.0-E827.9, E829.0-E829.9)*
that in transport under own power on the highway (E810.0-E819.9)
that involved in accident classifiable to E820-E829 (E820.0-E829.9)

E919.3 Metalworking machines
Abrasive wheel
Forging machine
Lathe
Mechanical shears
Metal:
- drilling machine
- milling machine
- power press
- rolling-mill
- sawing machine

E919.4 Woodworking and forming machines
Band saw
Bench saw
Circular saw
Molding machine
Overhead plane
Powered saw
Radial saw
Sander
Excludes *hand saw (E920.1)*

E919.5 Prime movers, except electrical motors
Gas turbine
Internal combustion engine
Steam engine
Water driven turbine
Excludes *that being towed by other vehicle on the highway (E810.0-E819.9, E827.0-E827.9, E829.0-E829.9)*
that in transport under own power on the highway (E810.0-E819.9)

E919.6 Transmission machinery
Transmission:
- belt
- cable
- chain
- gear
- pinion
- pulley
- shaft

E919.7 Earth moving, scraping, and other excavating machines
Bulldozer
Road scraper
Steam shovel
Excludes *that being towed by other vehicle on the highway (E810.0-E819.9)*
that in transport under own power on the highway (E810.0-E819.9)

E919.8 Other specified machinery
Machines for manufacture of:
- clothing
- foodstuffs and beverages
- paper

Printing machine
Recreational machinery
Spinning, weaving, and textile machines

E919.9 Unspecified machinery

❹ **E920 Accidents caused by cutting and piercing instruments or objects**
Includes accidental injury (by) object:
- edged
- pointed
- sharp

E920.0 Powered lawn mower

E920.1 Other powered hand tools
Any powered hand tool [compressed air] [electric] [explosive cartridge] [hydraulic power], such as:
- drill
- hand saw
- hedge clipper
- rivet gun
- snow blower
- staple gun

Excludes *band saw (E919.4)*
bench saw (E919.4)

E920.2 Powered household appliances and implements
Blender
Electric:
- beater or mixer
- can opener
- fan
- knife
- sewing machine

Garbage disposal appliance

E920.3 Knives, swords, and daggers

E920.4 Other hand tools and implements
Axe
Can opener NOS
Chisel
Fork
Hand saw
Hoe
Ice pick
Needle (sewing)
Paper cutter
Pitchfork
Rake
Scissors
Screwdriver
Sewing machine, not powered
Shovel

E920.5 Hypodermic needle
Contaminated needle
Needle stick

E920.8 Other specified cutting and piercing instruments or objects
Arrow
Broken glass
Dart
Edge of stiff paper
Lathe turnings
Nail
Plant thorn
Splinter
Tin can lid
Excludes *animal spines or quills (E906.8)*
flying glass due to explosion (E921.0-E923.9)

E920.9 Unspecified cutting and piercing instrument or object

❹ **E921 Accident caused by explosion of pressure vessel**
Includes accidental explosion of pressure vessels, whether or not part of machinery
Excludes *explosion of pressure vessel on transport vehicle (E800.0-E845.9)*

E921.0 Boilers

E921.1 Gas cylinders
Air tank
Pressure gas tank

E921.8 Other specified pressure vessels
Aerosol can
Automobile tire
Pressure cooker

E921.9 Unspecified pressure vessel

④ **E922 Accident caused by firearm and air gun missile**

E922.0 Handgun
Pistol
Revolver
Excludes *Verey pistol (E922.8)*

E922.1 Shotgun (automatic)

E922.2 Hunting rifle

E922.3 Military firearms
Army rifle
Machine gun

E922.4 Air gun
BB gun
Pellet gun

E922.5 Paintball gun

E922.8 Other specified firearm missile
Verey pistol [flare]

E922.9 Unspecified firearm missile
Gunshot wound NOS
Shot NOS

④ **E923 Accident caused by explosive material**

Includes flash burns and other injuries resulting from explosion of explosive material
ignition of highly explosive material with explosion

Excludes *explosion:*
in or on machinery (E919.0-E919.9)
on any transport vehicle, except stationary motor vehicle (E800.0-E848)
with conflagration (E890.0, E891.0, E892)
secondary fires resulting from explosion (E890.0-E899)

E923.0 Fireworks

E923.1 Blasting materials
Blasting cap
Detonator
Dynamite
Explosive [any] used in blasting operations

E923.2 Explosive gases
Acetylene
Butane
Coal gas
Explosion in mine NOS
Fire damp
Gasoline fumes
Methane
Propane

E923.8 Other explosive materials
Bomb
Explosion in munitions:
dump
factory
Explosive missile
Grenade
Mine
Shell
Torpedo

E923.9 Unspecified explosive material
Explosion NOS

④ **E924 Accident caused by hot substance or object, caustic or corrosive material, and steam**

Excludes *burning NOS (E899)*
chemical burn resulting from swallowing a corrosive substance (E860.0-E864.4)
fire caused by these substances and objects (E890.0-E894)
radiation burns (E926.0-E926.9)
therapeutic misadventures (E870.0-E876.9)

E924.0 Hot liquids and vapors, including steam
Burning or scalding by:
boiling water
hot or boiling liquids not primarily caustic or corrosive
liquid metal
steam
other hot vapor
Excludes *hot (boiling) tap water (E924.2)*

E924.1 Caustic and corrosive substances
Burning by:
acid [any kind]
ammonia
caustic oven cleaner or other substance
corrosive substance
lye
vitriol

E924.2 Hot (boiling) tap water

E924.8 Other
Burning by:
heat from electric heating appliance
hot object NOS
light bulb
steam pipe

E924.9 Unspecified

④ **E925 Accident caused by electric current**

Includes electric current from exposed wire, faulty appliance, high voltage cable, live rail, or open electric socket as the cause of:
burn
cardiac fibrillation
convulsion
electric shock
electrocution
puncture wound
respiratory paralysis

Excludes *burn by heat from electrical appliance (E924.8)*
lightning (E907)

E925.0 Domestic wiring and appliances

E925.1 Electric power generating plants, distribution stations, transmission lines
Broken power line

E925.2 Industrial wiring, appliances, and electrical machinery
Conductors
Control apparatus
Electrical equipment and machinery
Transformers

E925.8 Other electric current
Wiring and appliances in or on:
farm [not farmhouse]
outdoors
public building
residential institutions
schools

E925.9 Unspecified electric current
Burns or other injury from electric current NOS
Electric shock NOS
Electrocution NOS

④ **E926 Exposure to radiation**

Excludes *abnormal reaction to or complication of treatment without mention of misadventure (E879.2)*
atomic power plant malfunction in water transport (E838.0-E838.9)
misadventure to patient in surgical and medical procedures (E873.2-E873.3)
use of radiation in war operations (E996-E997.9)

E926.0 Radiofrequency radiation
Overexposure to:
microwave radiation from:
high-powered radio and television transmitters
industrial radiofrequency induction heaters
radar installations
radar radiation from:
high-powered radio and television transmitters
industrial radiofrequency induction heaters
radar installations
radiofrequency from:
high-powered radio and television transmitters
industrial radiofrequency induction heaters
radar installations
radiofrequency radiation [any] from:
high-powered radio and television transmitters
industrial radiofrequency induction heaters
radar installations

E926.1 Infra-red heaters and lamps
Exposure to infra-red radiation from heaters and lamps as the cause of:
blistering
burning
charring
inflammatory change
Excludes *physical contact with heater or lamp (E924.8)*

E926.2 Visible and ultraviolet light sources
Arc lamps
Black light sources
Electrical welding arc
Oxygas welding torch
Sun rays
Tanning bed
Excludes *excessive heat from these sources (E900.1-E900.9)*

E926.3 X-rays and other electromagnetic ionizing radiation
Gamma rays
X-rays (hard) (soft)

E926.4 Lasers

E926.5 Radioactive isotopes
Radiobiologicals
Radiopharmaceuticals

E926.8 Other specified radiation
Artificially accelerated beams of ionized particles generated by:
betatrons
synchrotrons

E926.9 Unspecified radiation
Radiation NOS

E927 Overexertion and strenuous movements
Excessive physical exercise
Overexertion (from):
lifting
pulling
pushing
Strenuous movements in:
recreational activities
other activities

❹ **E928 Other and unspecified environmental and accidental causes**

E928.0 Prolonged stay in weightless environment
Weightlessness in spacecraft (simulator)

E928.1 Exposure to noise
Noise (pollution)
Sound waves
Supersonic waves

E928.2 Vibration

E928.3 Human bite

E928.4 External constriction caused by hair

E928.5 External constriction caused by other object

● **E928.6 Environmental exposure to harmful algae and toxins**
Algae bloom NOS
Blue-green algae bloom
Brown tide
Cyanobacteria bloom
Florida red tide
Harmful algae bloom
Pfisteria piscicida
Red tide

E928.8 Other

E928.9 Unspecified accident
Accident NOS stated as accidentally inflicted
Blow NOS stated as accidentally inflicted
Casualty (not due to war) stated as accidentally inflicted
Decapitation stated as accidentally inflicted
Injury [any part of body, or unspecified] stated as accidentally inflicted, but not otherwise specified
Killed stated as accidentally inflicted, but not otherwise specified
Knocked down stated as accidentally inflicted, but not otherwise specified
Mangled stated as accidentally inflicted, but not otherwise specified
Wound stated as accidentally inflicted, but not otherwise specified
Excludes *fracture, cause unspecified (E887)*
injuries undetermined whether accidentally or purposely inflicted (E980.0-E989)

LATE EFFECTS OF ACCIDENTAL INJURY (E929)

Note: *This category is to be used to indicate accidental injury as the cause of death or disability from late effects, which are themselves classifiable elsewhere. The "late effects" include conditions reported as such or as sequelae, which may occur at any time after the acute accidental injury.*

❹ **E929 Late effects of accidental injury**
Excludes *late effects of:*
surgical and medical procedures (E870.0-E879.9)
therapeutic use of drugs and medicines (E930.0-E949.9)

E929.0 Late effects of motor vehicle accident
Late effects of accidents classifiable to E810-E825

E929.1 Late effects of other transport accident
Late effects of accidents classifiable to E800-E807, E826-E838, E840-E848

E929.2 Late effects of accidental poisoning
Late effects of accidents classifiable to E850-E858, E860-E869

E929.3 Late effects of accidental fall
Late effects of accidents classifiable to E880-E888

E929.4 Late effects of accident caused by fire
Late effects of accidents classifiable to E890-E899

E929.5 Late effects of accident due to natural and environmental factors
Late effects of accidents classifiable to E900-E909

E929.8 Late effects of other accidents
Late effects of accidents classifiable to E910-E928.8

E929.9 Late effects of unspecified accident
Late effects of accidents classifiable to E928.9

DRUGS, MEDICINAL AND BIOLOGICAL SUBSTANCES CAUSING ADVERSE EFFECTS IN THERAPEUTIC USE (E930-E949)

Includes correct drug properly administered in therapeutic or prophylactic dosage, as the cause of any adverse effect including allergic or hypersensitivity reactions
Excludes *accidental overdose of drug and wrong drug given or taken in error (E850.0-E858.9)*
accidents in the technique of administration of drug or biological substance such as accidental puncture during injection, or contamination of drug (E870.0-E876.9)
administration with suicidal or homicidal intent or intent to harm, or in circumstances classifiable to E980-E989 (E950.0-E950.5, E962.0, E980.0-E980.5)

Note: *See Alphabetic Index for more complete list of specific drugs to be classified under the fourth-digit subdivisions. The American Hospital Formulary numbers can be used to classify new drugs listed by the American Hospital Formulary Service (AHFS). See Appendix C.*

❹ Additional Digit Required ▶◀ Revised Text ● New Code ▲ Revised Code

❹ **E930 Antibiotics**

Excludes *that used as eye, ear, nose, and throat [ENT], and local anti-infectives (E946.0-E946.9)*

E930.0 Penicillins
Natural
Synthetic
Semisynthetic, such as:
ampicillin
cloxacillin
nafcillin
oxacillin

E930.1 Antifungal antibiotics
Amphotericin B
Griseofulvin
Hachimycin [trichomycin]
Nystatin

E930.2 Chloramphenicol group
Chloramphenicol
Thiamphenicol

E930.3 Erythromycin and other macrolides
Oleandomycin
Spiramycin

E930.4 Tetracycline group
Doxycycline
Minocycline
Oxytetracycline

E930.5 Cephalosporin group
Cephalexin
Cephaloglycin
Cephaloridine
Cephalothin

E930.6 Antimycobacterial antibiotics
Cycloserine
Kanamycin
Rifampin
Streptomycin

E930.7 Antineoplastic antibiotics
Actinomycins, such as:
Bleomycin
Cactinomycin
Dactinomycin
Daunorubicin
Mitomycin
Excludes *other antineoplastic drugs (E933.1)*

E930.8 Other specified antibiotics

E930.9 Unspecified antibiotic

❹ **E931 Other anti-infectives**

Excludes *ENT, and local anti-infectives (E946.0-E946.9)*

E931.0 Sulfonamides
Sulfadiazine
Sulfafurazole
Sulfamethoxazole

E931.1 Arsenical anti-infectives

E931.2 Heavy metal anti-infectives
Compounds of:
antimony
bismuth
lead
mercury
Excludes *mercurial diuretics (E944.0)*

E931.3 Quinoline and hydroxyquinoline derivatives
Chiniofon
Diiodohydroxyquin
Excludes *antimalarial drugs (E931.4)*

E931.4 Antimalarials and drugs acting on other blood protozoa
Chloroquine phosphate
Cycloguanil
Primaquine
Proguanil [chloroguanide]
Pyrimethamine
Quinine (sulphate)

E931.5 Other antiprotozoal drugs
Emetine

E931.6 Anthelmintics
Hexylresorcinol
Male fern oleoresin
Piperazine
Thiabendazole

E931.7 Antiviral drugs
Methisazone
Excludes *amantadine (E936.4)*
cytarabine (E933.1)
idoxuridine (E946.5)

E931.8 Other antimycobacterial drugs
Ethambutol
Ethionamide
Isoniazid
Para-aminosalicylic acid derivatives
Sulfones

E931.9 Other and unspecified anti-infectives
Flucytosine
Nitrofuran derivatives

❹ **E932 Hormones and synthetic substitutes**

E932.0 Adrenal cortical steroids
Cortisone derivatives
Desoxycorticosterone derivatives
Fluorinated corticosteroids

E932.1 Androgens and anabolic congeners
Nandrolone phenpropionate
Oxymetholone
Testosterone and preparations

E932.2 Ovarian hormones and synthetic substitutes
Contraceptives, oral
Estrogens
Estrogens and progestogens combined
Progestogens

E932.3 Insulins and antidiabetic agents
Acetohexamide
Biguanide derivatives, oral
Chlorpropamide
Glucagon
Insulin
Phenformin
Sulfonylurea derivatives, oral
Tolbutamide
Excludes *adverse effect of insulin administered for shock therapy (E879.3)*

E932.4 Anterior pituitary hormones
Corticotropin
Gonadotropin
Somatotropin [growth hormone]

E932.5 Posterior pituitary hormones
Vasopressin
Excludes *oxytocic agents (E945.0)*

E932.6 Parathyroid and parathyroid derivatives

E932.7 Thyroid and thyroid derivatives
Dextrothyroxine
Levothyroxine sodium
Liothyronine
Thyroglobulin

E932.8 Antithyroid agents
Iodides
Thiouracil
Thiourea

E932.9 Other and unspecified hormones and synthetic substitutes

❹ **E933 Primarily systemic agents**

E933.0 Antiallergic and antiemetic drugs
Antihistamines
Chlorpheniramine
Diphenhydramine
Diphenylpyraline
Thonzylamine
Tripelennamine
Excludes *phenothiazine-based tranquilizers (E939.1)*

E933.1 Antineoplastic and immunosuppressive drugs
Azathioprine
Busulfan
Chlorambucil
Cyclophosphamide
Cytarabine
Fluorouracil
Mechlorethamine hydrochloride
Mercaptopurine
Triethylenethiophosphoramide [thio-TEPA]
Excludes *antineoplastic antibiotics (E930.7)*

E933.2 Acidifying agents

E933.3 Alkalizing agents

E933.4 Enzymes, not elsewhere classified
Penicillinase

E933.5 Vitamins, not elsewhere classified
Vitamin A
Vitamin D
Excludes *nicotinic acid (E942.2)*
vitamin K (E934.3)

● **E933.6 Oral bisphosphonates**

● **E933.7 Intravenous bisphosphonates**

E933.8 Other systemic agents, not elsewhere classified
Heavy metal antagonists

E933.9 Unspecified systemic agent

❹ **E934 Agents primarily affecting blood constituents**

E934.0 Iron and its compounds
Ferric salts
Ferrous sulphate and other ferrous salts

E934.1 Liver preparations and other antianemic agents
Folic acid

E934.2 Anticoagulants
Coumarin
Heparin
Phenindione
Prothrombin synthesis inhibitor
Warfarin sodium

E934.3 Vitamin K [phytonadione]

E934.4 Fibrinolysis-affecting drugs
Aminocaproic acid
Streptodornase
Streptokinase
Urokinase

E934.5 Anticoagulant antagonists and other coagulants
Hexadimethrine bromide
Protamine sulfate

E934.6 Gamma globulin

E934.7 Natural blood and blood products
Blood plasma
Human fibrinogen
Packed red cells
Whole blood

E934.8 Other agents affecting blood constituents
Macromolecular blood substitutes

E934.9 Unspecified agent affecting blood constituents

❹ **E935 Analgesics, antipyretics, and antirheumatics**

E935.0 Heroin
Diacetylmorphine

E935.1 Methadone

E935.2 Other opiates and related narcotics
Codeine [methylmorphine]
Morphine
Opium (alkaloids)
Meperidine [pethidine]

E935.3 Salicylates
Acetylsalicylic acid [aspirin]
Amino derivatives of salicylic acid
Salicylic acid salts

E935.4 Aromatic analgesics, not elsewhere classified
Acetanilid
Paracetamol [acetaminophen]
Phenacetin [acetophenetidin]

E935.5 Pyrazole derivatives
Aminophenazone [aminopyrine]
Phenylbutazone

E935.6 Antirheumatics [antiphlogistics]
Gold salts
Indomethacin
Excludes *salicylates (E935.3)*
steroids (E932.0)

E935.7 Other non-narcotic analgesics
Pyrabital

E935.8 Other specified analgesics and antipyretics
Pentazocine

E935.9 Unspecified analgesic and antipyretic

❹ **E936 Anticonvulsants and anti-Parkinsonism drugs**

E936.0 Oxazolidine derivatives
Paramethadione
Trimethadione

E936.1 Hydantoin derivatives
Phenytoin

E936.2 Succinimides
Ethosuximide
Phensuximide

E936.3 Other and unspecified anticonvulsants
Beclamide
Primidone

E936.4 Anti-Parkinsonism drugs
Amantadine
Ethopropazine [profenamine]
Levodopa [L-dopa]

❹ **E937 Sedatives and hypnotics**

E937.0 Barbiturates
Amobarbital [amylobarbitone]
Barbital [barbitone]
Butabarbital [butabarbitone]
Pentobarbital [pentobarbitone]
Phenobarbital [phenobarbitone]
Secobarbital [quinalbarbitone]
Excludes *thiobarbiturates (E938.3)*

E937.1 Chloral hydrate group

E937.2 Paraldehyde

E937.3 Bromine compounds
Bromide
Carbromal (derivatives)

E937.4 Methaqualone compounds

E937.5 Glutethimide group

E937.6 Mixed sedatives, not elsewhere classified

E937.8 Other sedatives and hypnotics

E937.9 Unspecified
Sleeping:
- drug NOS
- pill NOS
- tablet NOS

❹ **E938 Other central nervous system depressants and anesthetics**

E938.0 Central nervous system muscle-tone depressants
Chlorphenesin (carbamate)
Mephenesin
Methocarbamol

E938.1 Halothane

E938.2 Other gaseous anesthetics
Ether
Halogenated hydrocarbon derivatives, except halothane
Nitrous oxide

E938.3 Intravenous anesthetics
Ketamine
Methohexital [methohexitone]
Thiobarbiturates, such as thiopental sodium

E938.4 Other and unspecified general anesthetics

E938.5 Surface and infiltration anesthetics
Cocaine
Lidocaine [lignocaine]
Procaine
Tetracaine

E938.6 Peripheral nerve- and plexus-blocking anesthetics

E938.7 Spinal anesthetics

E938.9 Other and unspecified local anesthetics

④ **E939 Psychotropic agents**

E939.0 Antidepressants
Amitriptyline
Imipramine
Monoamine oxidase [MAO] inhibitors

E939.1 Phenothiazine-based tranquilizers
Chlorpromazine
Fluphenazine
Phenothiazine
Prochlorperazine
Promazine

E939.2 Butyrophenone-based tranquilizers
Haloperidol
Spiperone
Trifluperidol

E939.3 Other antipsychotics, neuroleptics, and major tranquilizers

E939.4 Benzodiazepine-based tranquilizers
Chlordiazepoxide
Diazepam
Flurazepam
Lorazepam
Medazepam
Nitrazepam

E939.5 Other tranquilizers
Hydroxyzine
Meprobamate

E939.6 Psychodysleptics [hallucinogens]
Cannabis (derivatives)
Lysergide [LSD]
Marihuana (derivatives)
Mescaline
Psilocin
Psilocybin

E939.7 Psychostimulants
Amphetamine
Caffeine
Excludes *central appetite depressants (E947.0)*

E939.8 Other psychotropic agents

E939.9 Unspecified psychotropic agent

④ **E940 Central nervous system stimulants**

E940.0 Analeptics
Lobeline
Nikethamide

E940.1 Opiate antagonists
Levallorphan
Nalorphine
Naloxone

E940.8 Other specified central nervous system stimulants

E940.9 Unspecified central nervous system stimulant

④ **E941 Drugs primarily affecting the autonomic nervous system**

E941.0 Parasympathomimetics [cholinergics]
Acetylcholine
Anticholinesterase:
  organophosphorus
  reversible
Pilocarpine

E941.1 Parasympatholytics [anticholinergics and antimuscarinics] and spasmolytics
Atropine
Homatropine
Hyoscine [scopolamine]
Quaternary ammonium derivatives
Excludes *papaverine (E942.5)*

E941.2 Sympathomimetics [adrenergics]
Epinephrine [adrenalin]
Levarterenol [noradrenalin]

E941.3 Sympatholytics [antiadrenergics]
Phenoxybenzamine
Tolazoline hydrochloride

E941.9 Unspecified drug primarily affecting the autonomic nervous system

④ **E942 Agents primarily affecting the cardiovascular system**

E942.0 Cardiac rhythm regulators
Practolol
Procainamide
Propranolol
Quinidine

E942.1 Cardiotonic glycosides and drugs of similar action
Digitalis glycosides
Digoxin
Strophanthins

E942.2 Antilipemic and antiarteriosclerotic drugs
Cholestyramine
Clofibrate
Nicotinic acid derivatives
Sitosterols
Excludes *dextrothyroxine (E932.7)*

E942.3 Ganglion-blocking agents
Pentamethonium bromide

E942.4 Coronary vasodilators
Dipyridamole
Nitrates [nitroglycerin]
Nitrites
Prenylamine

E942.5 Other vasodilators
Cyclandelate
Diazoxide
Hydralazine
Papaverine

E942.6 Other antihypertensive agents
Clonidine
Guanethidine
Rauwolfia alkaloids
Reserpine

E942.7 Antivaricose drugs, including sclerosing agents
Monoethanolamine
Zinc salts

E942.8 Capillary-active drugs
Adrenochrome derivatives
Bioflavonoids
Metaraminol

E942.9 Other and unspecified agents primarily affecting the cardiovascular system

④ **E943 Agents primarily affecting gastrointestinal system**

E943.0 Antacids and antigastric secretion drugs
Aluminum hydroxide
Magnesium trisilicate

E943.1 Irritant cathartics
Bisacodyl
Castor oil
Phenolphthalein

E943.2 Emollient cathartics
Sodium dioctyl sulfosuccinate

E943.3 Other cathartics, including intestinal atonia drugs
Magnesium sulfate

E943.4 Digestants
Pancreatin
Papain
Pepsin

E943.5 Antidiarrheal drugs
Bismuth subcarbonate
Kaolin
Pectin
Excludes *anti-infectives (E930.0-E931.9)*

E943.6 Emetics

E943.8 Other specified agents primarily affecting the gastrointestinal system

E943.9 Unspecified agent primarily affecting the gastrointestinal system

E944 Water, mineral, and uric acid metabolism drugs

E944.0 Mercurial diuretics
Chlormerodrin
Mercaptomerin
Mercurophylline
Mersalyl

E944.1 Purine derivative diuretics
Theobromine
Theophylline
Excludes *aminophylline [theophylline ethylenediamine] (E945.7)*

E944.2 Carbonic acid anhydrase inhibitors
Acetazolamide

E944.3 Saluretics
Benzothiadiazides
Chlorothiazide group

E944.4 Other diuretics
Ethacrynic acid
Furosemide

E944.5 Electrolytic, caloric, and water-balance agents

E944.6 Other mineral salts, not elsewhere classified

E944.7 Uric acid metabolism drugs
Cinchophen and congeners
Colchicine
Phenoquin
Probenecid

E945 Agents primarily acting on the smooth and skeletal muscles and respiratory system

E945.0 Oxytocic agents
Ergot alkaloids
Prostaglandins

E945.1 Smooth muscle relaxants
Adiphenine
Metaproterenol [orciprenaline]
Excludes *papaverine (E942.5)*

E945.2 Skeletal muscle relaxants
Alcuronium chloride
Suxamethonium chloride

E945.3 Other and unspecified drugs acting on muscles

E945.4 Antitussives
Dextromethorphan
Pipazethate hydrochloride

E945.5 Expectorants
Acetylcysteine
Cocillana
Guaifenesin [glyceryl guaiacolate]
Ipecacuanha
Terpin hydrate

E945.6 Anti-common cold drugs

E945.7 Antiasthmatics
Aminophylline [theophylline ethylenediamine]

E945.8 Other and unspecified respiratory drugs

E946 Agents primarily affecting skin and mucous membrane, ophthalmological, otorhinolaryngological, and dental drugs

E946.0 Local anti-infectives and anti-inflammatory drugs

E946.1 Antipruritics

E946.2 Local astringents and local detergents

E946.3 Emollients, demulcents, and protectants

E946.4 Keratolytics, keratoplastics, other hair treatment drugs and preparations

E946.5 Eye anti-infectives and other eye drugs
Idoxuridine

E946.6 Anti-infectives and other drugs and preparations for ear, nose, and throat

E946.7 Dental drugs topically applied

E946.8 Other agents primarily affecting skin and mucous membrane
Spermicides

E946.9 Unspecified agent primarily affecting skin and mucous membrane

E947 Other and unspecified drugs and medicinal substances

E947.0 Dietetics

E947.1 Lipotropic drugs

E947.2 Antidotes and chelating agents, not elsewhere classified

E947.3 Alcohol deterrents

E947.4 Pharmaceutical excipients

E947.8 Other drugs and medicinal substances
Contrast media used for diagnostic x-ray procedures
Diagnostic agents and kits

E947.9 Unspecified drug or medicinal substance

E948 Bacterial vaccines

E948.0 BCG vaccine

E948.1 Typhoid and paratyphoid

E948.2 Cholera

E948.3 Plague

E948.4 Tetanus

E948.5 Diphtheria

E948.6 Pertussis vaccine, including combinations with a pertussis component

E948.8 Other and unspecified bacterial vaccines

E948.9 Mixed bacterial vaccines, except combinations with a pertussis component

E949 Other vaccines and biological substances
Excludes *gamma globulin (E934.6)*

E949.0 Smallpox vaccine

E949.1 Rabies vaccine

E949.2 Typhus vaccine

E949.3 Yellow fever vaccine

E949.4 Measles vaccine

E949.5 Poliomyelitis vaccine

E949.6 Other and unspecified viral and rickettsial vaccines
Mumps vaccine

E949.7 Mixed viral-rickettsial and bacterial vaccines, except combinations with a pertussis component
Excludes *combinations with a pertussis component (E948.6)*

E949.9 Other and unspecified vaccines and biological substances

SUICIDE AND SELF-INFLICTED INJURY (E950-E959)

Includes injuries in suicide and attempted suicide
self-inflicted injuries specified as intentional

E950 Suicide and self-inflicted poisoning by solid or liquid substances

E950.0 Analgesics, antipyretics, and antirheumatics

E950.1 Barbiturates

E950.2 Other sedatives and hypnotics

E950.3 Tranquilizers and other psychotropic agents

E950.4 Other specified drugs and medicinal substances

E950.5 Unspecified drug or medicinal substance

E950.6 Agricultural and horticultural chemical and pharmaceutical preparations other than plant foods and fertilizers

E950.7 Corrosive and caustic substances
Suicide and self-inflicted poisoning by substances classifiable to E864

E950.8 Arsenic and its compounds

E950.9 Other and unspecified solid and liquid substances

E951 Suicide and self-inflicted poisoning by gases in domestic use

E951.0 Gas distributed by pipeline

E951.1 Liquefied petroleum gas distributed in mobile containers

E951.8 Other utility gas

E952 Suicide and self-inflicted poisoning by other gases and vapors

E952.0 Motor vehicle exhaust gas

E952.1 Other carbon monoxide

E952.8 Other specified gases and vapors

E952.9 Unspecified gases and vapors

❹ **E953 Suicide and self-inflicted injury by hanging, strangulation, and suffocation**

E953.0 Hanging

E953.1 Suffocation by plastic bag

E953.8 Other specified means

E953.9 Unspecified means

E954 Suicide and self-inflicted injury by submersion [drowning]

❹ **E955 Suicide and self-inflicted injury by firearms, air guns and explosives**

E955.0 Handgun

E955.1 Shotgun

E955.2 Hunting rifle

E955.3 Military firearms

E955.4 Other and unspecified firearm
Gunshot NOS
Shot NOS

E955.5 Explosives

E955.6 Air gun
BB gun
Pellet gun

E955.7 Paintball gun

E955.9 Unspecified

E956 Suicide and self-inflicted injury by cutting and piercing instrument

❹ **E957 Suicide and self-inflicted injuries by jumping from high place**

E957.0 Residential premises

E957.1 Other man-made structures

E957.2 Natural sites

E957.9 Unspecified

❹ **E958 Suicide and self-inflicted injury by other and unspecified means**

E958.0 Jumping or lying before moving object

E958.1 Burns, fire

E958.2 Scald

E958.3 Extremes of cold

E958.4 Electrocution

E958.5 Crashing of motor vehicle

E958.6 Crashing of aircraft

E958.7 Caustic substances, except poisoning
Excludes *poisoning by caustic substance (E950.7)*

E958.8 Other specified means

E958.9 Unspecified means

E959 Late effects of self-inflicted injury
Note: This category is to be used to indicate circumstances classifiable to E950-E958 as the cause of death or disability from late effects, which are themselves classifiable elsewhere. The "late effects" include conditions reported as such or as sequelae which may occur at any time after the attempted suicide or self-inflicted injury.

HOMICIDE AND INJURY PURPOSELY INFLICTED BY OTHER PERSONS (E960-E969)

Includes injuries inflicted by another person with intent to injure or kill, by any means

Excludes *injuries due to:*
legal intervention (E970-E978)
operations of war (E990-E999)
terrorism (E979)

❹ **E960 Fight, brawl, rape**

E960.0 Unarmed fight or brawl
Beatings NOS
Brawl or fight with hands, fists, feet
Injured or killed in fight NOS
Excludes *homicidal:*
injury by weapons (E965.0-E966, E969)
strangulation (E963)
submersion (E964)

E960.1 Rape

E961 Assault by corrosive or caustic substance, except poisoning
Injury or death purposely caused by corrosive or caustic substance, such as:
acid [any]
corrosive substance
vitriol
Excludes *burns from hot liquid (E968.3)*
chemical burns from swallowing a corrosive substance (E962.0-E962.9)

❹ **E962 Assault by poisoning**

E962.0 Drugs and medicinal substances
Homicidal poisoning by any drug or medicinal substance

E962.1 Other solid and liquid substances

E962.2 Other gases and vapors

E962.9 Unspecified poisoning

E963 Assault by hanging and strangulation
Homicidal (attempt):
garrotting or ligature
hanging
strangulation
suffocation

E964 Assault by submersion [drowning]

❹ **E965 Assault by firearms and explosives**

E965.0 Handgun
Pistol
Revolver

E965.1 Shotgun

E965.2 Hunting rifle

E965.3 Military firearms

E965.4 Other and unspecified firearm

E965.5 Antipersonnel bomb

E965.6 Gasoline bomb

E965.7 Letter bomb

E965.8 Other specified explosive
Bomb NOS (placed in):
car
house
Dynamite

E965.9 Unspecified explosive

E966 Assault by cutting and piercing instrument
Assassination (attempt), homicide (attempt) by any instrument classifiable under E920
Homicidal:
cut any part of body
puncture any part of body
stab any part of body
Stabbed any part of body

❹ E967 Perpetrator of child and adult abuse
Note: selection of the correct perpetrator code is based on the relationship between the perpetrator and the victim.

E967.0 By father, stepfather, or boyfriend
Male partner of child's parent or guardian

E967.1 By other specified person

E967.2 By mother, stepmother, or girlfriend
Female partner of child's parent or guardian

E967.3 By spouse or partner
Abuse of spouse or partner by ex-spouse or ex-partner

E967.4 By child

E967.5 By sibling

E967.6 By grandparent

E967.7 By other relative

E967.8 By non-related caregiver

E967.9 By unspecified person

❹ E968 Assault by other and unspecified means

E968.0 Fire
Arson
Homicidal burns NOS
Excludes *burns from hot liquid (E968.3)*

E968.1 Pushing from a high place

E968.2 Striking by blunt or thrown object

E968.3 Hot liquid
Homicidal burns by scalding

E968.4 Criminal neglect
Abandonment of child, infant, or other helpless person with intent to injure or kill

E968.5 Transport vehicle
Being struck by other vehicle or run down with intent to injure
Pushed in front of, thrown from, or dragged by moving vehicle with intent to injure

E968.6 Air gun
BB gun
Pellet gun

E968.7 Human bite

E968.8 Other specified means

E968.9 Unspecified means
Assassination (attempt) NOS
Homicidal (attempt):
- injury NOS
- wound NOS

Manslaughter (nonaccidental)
Murder (attempt) NOS
Violence, non-accidental

E969 Late effects of injury purposely inflicted by other person
Note: This category is to be used to indicate circumstances classifiable to E960-E968 as the cause of death or disability from late effects, which are themselves classifiable elsewhere. The "late effects" include conditions reported as such, or as sequelae which may occur at any time after the injury purposely inflicted by another person.

LEGAL INTERVENTION (E970-E978)

Includes: injuries inflicted by the police or other law-enforcing agents, including military on duty, in the course of arresting or attempting to arrest lawbreakers, suppressing disturbances, maintaining order, and other legal action
legal execution

Excludes *injuries caused by civil insurrections (E990.0-E999)*

E970 Injury due to legal intervention by firearms
Gunshot wound
Injury by:
- machine gun
- revolver
- rifle pellet or rubber bullet
- shot NOS

E971 Injury due to legal intervention by explosives
Injury by:
- dynamite
- explosive shell
- grenade
- motor bomb

E972 Injury due to legal intervention by gas
Asphyxiation by gas
Injury by tear gas
Poisoning by gas

E973 Injury due to legal intervention by blunt object
Hit, struck by:
- baton (nightstick)
- blunt object
- stave

E974 Injury due to legal intervention by cutting and piercing instrument
Cut
Incised wound
Injured by bayonet
Stab wound

E975 Injury due to legal intervention by other specified means
Blow
Manhandling

E976 Injury due to legal intervention by unspecified means

E977 Late effects of injuries due to legal intervention
Note: This category is to be used to indicate circumstances classifiable to E970-E976 as the cause of death or disability from late effects, which are themselves classifiable elsewhere. The "late effects" include conditions reported as such, or as sequelae which may occur at any time after the injury due to legal intervention.

E978 Legal execution
All executions performed at the behest of the judiciary or ruling authority [whether permanent or temporary] as:
- asphyxiation by gas
- beheading, decapitation (by guillotine)
- capital punishment
- electrocution
- hanging
- poisoning
- shooting
- other specified means

TERRORISM (E979)

❹ E979 Terrorism
Injuries resulting from the unlawful use of force or violence against persons or property to intimidate or coerce a Government, the civilian population, or any segment thereof, in furtherance of political or social objective

E979.0 Terrorism involving explosion of marine weapons
Depth-charge
Marine mine
Mine NOS, at sea or in harbor
Sea-based artillery shell
Torpedo
Underwater blast

E979.1 Terrorism involving destruction of aircraft
Aircraft used as a weapon
Aircraft:
- burned
- exploded
- shot down

Crushed by falling aircraft

E979.2 Terrorism involving other explosions and fragments
Antipersonnel bomb
Blast NOS
Explosion (of):
artillery shell
breech-block
cannon block
mortar bomb
munitions being used in terrorism
NOS
Fragments from:
artillery shell
bomb
grenade
guided missile
land-mine
rocket
shell
shrapnel
Mine NOS

E979.3 Terrorism involving fires, conflagrations and hot substances
Burning building or structure:
collapse of
fall from
hit by falling object in
jump from
Conflagration NOS
Fire (causing):
asphyxia
burns
NOS
other injury
Melting of fittings and furniture in building
Petrol bomb
Smoldering building or structure

E979.4 Terrorism involving firearms
Bullet:
carbine
machine gun
pistol
rifle
rubber (rifle)
Pellets (shotgun)

E979.5 Terrorism involving nuclear weapons
Blast effects
Exposure to ionizing radiation from nuclear weapon
Fireball effects
Heat from nuclear weapon
Other direct and secondary effects of nuclear weapons

E979.6 Terrorism involving biological weapons
Anthrax
Cholera
Smallpox

E979.7 Terrorism involving chemical weapons
Gases, fumes, chemicals
Hydrogen cyanide
Phosgene
Sarin

E979.8 Terrorism involving other means
Drowning and submersion
Lasers
Piercing or stabbing instruments
Terrorism NOS

E979.9 Terrorism, secondary effects
Note: This code is for use to identify conditions occuring subsequent to a terrorist attack not those that are due to the initial terrorist attack
Excludes late effect of terrorist attack (E999.1)

INJURY UNDETERMINED WHETHER ACCIDENTALLY OR PURPOSELY INFLICTED (E980-E989)

Note: Categories E980-E989 are for use when it is unspecified or it cannot be determined whether the injuries are accidental (unintentional), suicide (attempted), or assault.

❹ E980 Poisoning by solid or liquid substances, undetermined whether accidentally or purposely inflicted

E980.0 Analgesics, antipyretics, and antirheumatics

E980.1 Barbiturates

E980.2 Other sedatives and hypnotics

E980.3 Tranquilizers and other psychotropic agents

E980.4 Other specified drugs and medicinal substances

E980.5 Unspecified drug or medicinal substance

E980.6 Corrosive and caustic substances
Poisoning, undetermined whether accidental or purposeful, by substances classifiable to E864

E980.7 Agricultural and horticultural chemical and pharmaceutical preparations other than plant foods and fertilizers

E980.8 Arsenic and its compounds

E980.9 Other and unspecified solid and liquid substances

❹ E981 Poisoning by gases in domestic use, undetermined whether accidentally or purposely inflicted

E981.0 Gas distributed by pipeline

E981.1 Liquefied petroleum gas distributed in mobile containers

E981.8 Other utility gas

❹ E982 Poisoning by other gases, undetermined whether accidentally or purposely inflicted

E982.0 Motor vehicle exhaust gas

E982.1 Other carbon monoxide

E982.8 Other specified gases and vapors

E982.9 Unspecified gases and vapors

❹ E983 Hanging, strangulation, or suffocation, undetermined whether accidentally or purposely inflicted

E983.0 Hanging

E983.1 Suffocation by plastic bag

E983.8 Other specified means

E983.9 Unspecified means

E984 Submersion [drowning], undetermined whether accidentally or purposely inflicted

❹ E985 Injury by firearms, air guns and explosives, undetermined whether accidentally or purposely inflicted

E985.0 Handgun

E985.1 Shotgun

E985.2 Hunting rifle

E985.3 Military firearms

E985.4 Other and unspecified firearm

E985.5 Explosives

E985.6 Air gun
BB gun
Pellet gun

E985.7 Paintball gun

E986 Injury by cutting and piercing instruments, undetermined whether accidentally or purposely inflicted

❹ E987 Falling from high place, undetermined whether accidentally or purposely inflicted

E987.0 Residential premises

E987.1 Other man-made structures

E987.2 Natural sites

E987.9 Unspecified site

E988 Injury by other and unspecified means, undetermined whether accidentally or purposely inflicted

E988.0 Jumping or lying before moving object

E988.1 Burns, fire

E988.2 Scald

E988.3 Extremes of cold

E988.4 Electrocution

E988.5 Crashing of motor vehicle

E988.6 Crashing of aircraft

E988.7 Caustic substances, except poisoning

E988.8 Other specified means

E988.9 Unspecified means

E989 Late effects of injury, undetermined whether accidentally or purposely inflicted

Note: This category is to be used to indicate circumstances classifiable to E980-E988 as the cause of death or disability from late effects, which are themselves classifiable elsewhere. The "late effects" include conditions reported as such or as sequelae which may occur at any time after injury, undetermined whether accidentally or purposely inflicted.

INJURY RESULTING FROM OPERATIONS OF WAR (E990-E999)

Includes injuries to military personnel and civilians caused by war and civil insurrections and occurring during the time of war and insurrection

Excludes accidents during training of military personnel, manufacture of war material and transport, unless attributable to enemy action

E990 Injury due to war operations by fires and conflagrations

Includes asphyxia, burns, or other injury originating from fire caused by a fire-producing device or indirectly by any conventional weapon

E990.0 From gasoline bomb

E990.9 From other and unspecified source

E991 Injury due to war operations by bullets and fragments

E991.0 Rubber bullets (rifle)

E991.1 Pellets (rifle)

E991.2 Other bullets

Bullet [any, except rubber bullets and pellets]:
- carbine
- machine gun
- pistol
- rifle
- shotgun

E991.3 Antipersonnel bomb (fragments)

E991.9 Other and unspecified fragments

Fragments from:
- artillery shell
- bombs, except antipersonnel
- grenade
- guided missile
- land mine
- rockets
- shell

Shrapnel

E992 Injury due to war operations by explosion of marine weapons

Depth charge
Marine mines
Mine NOS, at sea or in harbor
Sea-based artillery shell
Torpedo
Underwater blast

E993 Injury due to war operations by other explosion

Accidental explosion of munitions being used in war
Accidental explosion of own weapons
Air blast NOS
Blast NOS
Explosion NOS
Explosion of:
- artillery shell
- breech block
- cannon block
- mortar bomb

Injury by weapon burst

E994 Injury due to war operations by destruction of aircraft

Airplane:
- burned
- exploded
- shot down

Crushed by falling airplane

E995 Injury due to war operations by other and unspecified forms of conventional warfare

Battle wounds
Bayonet injury
Drowned in war operations

E996 Injury due to war operations by nuclear weapons

Blast effects
Exposure to ionizing radiation from nuclear weapons
Fireball effects
Heat
Other direct and secondary effects of nuclear weapons

E997 Injury due to war operations by other forms of unconventional warfare

E997.0 Lasers

E997.1 Biological warfare

E997.2 Gases, fumes, and chemicals

E997.8 Other specified forms of unconventional warfare

E997.9 Unspecified form of unconventional warfare

E998 Injury due to war operations but occurring after cessation of hostilities

Injuries due to operations of war but occurring after cessation of hostilities by any means classifiable under E990-E997

Injuries by explosion of bombs or mines placed in the course of operations of war, if the explosion occurred after cessation of hostilities

E999 Late effect of injury due to war operations and terrorism

Note: This category is to be used to indicate circumstances classifiable to E979, E990-E998 as the cause of death or disability from late effects, which are themselves classifiable elsewhere. The "late effects" include conditions reported as such or as sequelae which may occur at any time after injury resulting from operations of war or terrorism

E999.0 Late effects of injury due to war operations

E999.1 Late effects of injury due to terrorism

Official ICD-9-CM Government Appendices

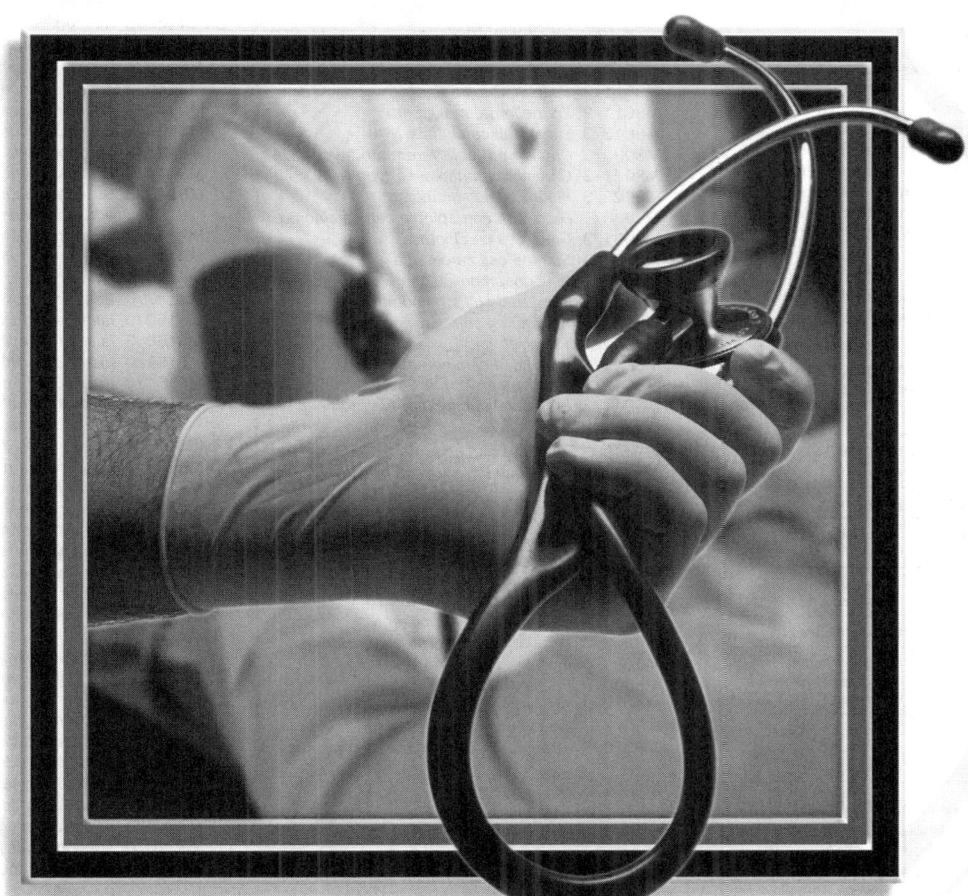

Morphology of Neoplasms

The World Health Organization has published an adaptation of the International Classification of Diseases for Oncology (ICD-O). It contains a coded nomenclature for the morphology of neoplasms, which is reproduced here for those who wish to use it in conjunction with Chapter 2 of the *International Classification of Diseases, 9th Revision, Clinical Modification.*

The morphology code numbers consist of five digits; the first four identify the histological type of the neoplasm and the fifth indicates its behavior. The one-digit behavior code is as follows:

- **/0 Benign**
- **/1 Uncertain whether benign or malignant**
  Borderline malignancy
- **/2 Carcinoma in situ**
  Intraepithelial
  Noninfiltrating
  Noninvasive
- **/3 Malignant, primary site**
- **/6 Malignant, metastatic site**
  Secondary site
- **/9 Malignant, uncertain whether primary or metastatic site**

In the nomenclature below, the morphology code numbers include the behavior code appropriate to the histological type of neoplasm, but this behavior code should be changed if other reported information makes this necessary. For example, "chordoma (M9370/3)" is assumed to be malignant; the term "benign chordoma" should be coded M9370/0. Similarly, "superficial spreading adenocarcinoma (M8143/3)" described as "noninvasive" should be coded M8143/2 and "melanoma (M8720/3)" described as "secondary" should be coded M8720/6.

The following table shows the correspondence between the morphology code and the different sections of Chapter 2:

Morphology Code Histology/Behavior			ICD-9-CM Chapter 2
Any	0	210-229	Benign neoplasms
M8000-M8004	1	239	Neoplasms of unspecified nature
M8010+	1	235-238	Neoplasms of uncertain behavior
Any	2	230-234	Carcinoma in situ
Any	3	140-195 200-208	Malignant neoplasms, stated or presumed to be primary
Any	6	196-198	Malignant neoplasms, stated or presumed to be secondary

The ICD-O behavior digit /9 is inapplicable in an ICD context, since all malignant neoplasms are presumed to be primary (/3) or secondary (/6) according to other information on the medical record.

Only the first-listed term of the full ICD-O morphology nomenclature appears against each code number in the list below. The ICD-9-CM Alphabetical Index (Volume 2), however, includes all the ICD-O synonyms as well as a number of other morphological names still likely to be encountered on medical records but omitted from ICD-O as outdated or otherwise undesirable

A coding difficulty sometimes arises where a morphological diagnosis contains two qualifying adjectives that have different code numbers. An example is "transitional cell epidermoid carcinomas." "Transitional cell carcinoma NOS" is M8120/3 and "epidermoid carcinoma NOS" is M8070/3. In such circumstances, the higher number (M8120/3 in this example) should be used, as it is usually more specific.

CODED NOMENCLATURE FOR MORPHOLOGY OF NEOPLASMS

M800 Neoplasms NOS
M8000/0 *Neoplasm, benign*
M8000/1 *Neoplasm, uncertain whether benign or malignant*
M8000/3 *Neoplasm, malignant*
M8000/6 *Neoplasm, metastatic*
M8000/9 *Neoplasm, malignant, uncertain whether primary or metastatic*
M8001/0 *Tumor cells, benign*
M8001/1 *Tumor cells, uncertain whether benign or malignant*
M8001/3 *Tumor cells, malignant*
M8002/3 *Malignant tumor, small cell type*
M8003/3 *Malignant tumor, giant cell type*
M8004/3 *Malignant tumor, fusiform cell type*

M801-M804 Epithelial neoplasms NOS
M8010/0 *Epithelial tumor, benign*
M8010/2 *Carcinoma in situ NOS*
M8010/3 *Carcinoma NOS*
M8010/6 *Carcinoma, metastatic NOS*
M8010/9 *Carcinomatosis*
M8011/0 *Epithelioma, benign*
M8011/3 *Epithelioma, malignant*
M8012/3 *Large cell carcinoma NOS*
M8020/3 *Carcinoma, undifferentiated type NOS*
M8021/3 *Carcinoma, anaplastic type NOS*
M8022/3 *Pleomorphic carcinoma*
M8030/3 *Giant cell and spindle cell carcinoma*
M8031/3 *Giant cell carcinoma*
M8032/3 *Spindle cell carcinoma*
M8033/3 *Pseudosarcomatous carcinoma*
M8034/3 *Polygonal cell carcinoma*
M8035/3 *Spheroidal cell carcinoma*
M8040/1 *Tumorlet*
M8041/3 *Small cell carcinoma NOS*
M8042/3 *Oat cell carcinoma*
M8043/3 *Small cell carcinoma, fusiform cell type*

M805-M808 Papillary and squamous cell neoplasms
M8050/0 *Papilloma NOS (except Papilloma of urinary bladder M8120/1)*
M8050/2 *Papillary carcinoma in situ*
M8050/3 *Papillary carcinoma NOS*
M8051/0 *Verrucous papilloma*
M8051/3 *Verrucous carcinoma NOS*
M8052/0 *Squamous cell papilloma*
M8052/3 *Papillary squamous cell carcinoma*
M8053/0 *Inverted papilloma*
M8060/0 *Papillomatosis NOS*
M8070/2 *Squamous cell carcinoma in situ NOS*
M8070/3 *Squamous cell carcinoma NOS*
M8070/6 *Squamous cell carcinoma, metastatic NOS*
M8071/3 *Squamous cell carcinoma, keratinizing type NOS*
M8072/3 *Squamous cell carcinoma, large cell, nonkeratinizing type*
M8073/3 *Squamous cell carcinoma, small cell, nonkeratinizing type*
M8074/3 *Squamous cell carcinoma, spindle cell type*
M8075/3 *Adenoid squamous cell carcinoma*
M8076/2 *Squamous cell carcinoma in situ with questionable stromal invasion*
M8076/3 *Squamous cell carcinoma, microinvasive*
M8080/2 *Queyrat's erythroplasia*
M8081/2 *Bowen's disease*
M8082/3 *Lymphoepithelial carcinoma*

M809-M811 Basal cell neoplasms
M8090/1 *Basal cell tumor*
M8090/3 *Basal cell carcinoma NOS*
M8091/3 *Multicentric basal cell carcinoma*
M8092/3 *Basal cell carcinoma, morphea type*
M8093/3 *Basal cell carcinoma, fibroepithelial type*
M8094/3 *Basosquamous carcinoma*
M8095/3 *Metatypical carcinoma*
M8096/0 *Intraepidermal epithelioma of Jadassohn*
M8100/0 *Trichoepithelioma*
M8101/0 *Trichofolliculoma*
M8102/0 *Tricholemmoma*
M8110/0 *Pilomatrixoma*

M812-M813 Transitional cell papillomas and carcinomas
M8120/0 *Transitional cell papilloma NOS*
M8120/1 *Urothelial papilloma*
M8120/2 *Transitional cell carcinoma in situ*
M8120/3 *Transitional cell carcinoma NOS*
M8121/0 *Schneiderian papilloma*
M8121/1 *Transitional cell papilloma, inverted type*
M8121/3 *Schneiderian carcinoma*
M8122/3 *Transitional cell carcinoma, spindle cell type*
M8123/3 *Basaloid carcinoma*
M8124/3 *Cloacogenic carcinoma*
M8130/3 *Papillary transitional cell carcinoma*

M814-M838 Adenomas and adenocarcinomas
M8140/0 *Adenoma NOS*
M8140/1 *Bronchial adenoma NOS*
M8140/2 *Adenocarcinoma in situ*
M8140/3 *Adenocarcinoma NOS*
M8140/6 *Adenocarcinoma, metastatic NOS*
M8141/3 *Scirrhous adenocarcinoma*
M8142/3 *Linitis plastica*
M8143/3 *Superficial spreading adenocarcinoma*
M8144/3 *Adenocarcinoma, intestinal type*
M8145/3 *Carcinoma, diffuse type*
M8146/0 *Monomorphic adenoma*
M8147/0 *Basal cell adenoma*
M8150/0 *Islet cell adenoma*
M8150/3 *Islet cell carcinoma*
M8151/0 *Insulinoma NOS*
M8151/3 *Insulinoma, malignant*
M8152/0 *Glucagonoma NOS*
M8152/3 *Glucagonoma, malignant*
M8153/1 *Gastrinoma NOS*
M8153/3 *Gastrinoma, malignant*
M8154/3 *Mixed islet cell and exocrine adenocarcinoma*
M8160/0 *Bile duct adenoma*
M8160/3 *Cholangiocarcinoma*
M8161/0 *Bile duct cystadenoma*
M8161/3 *Bile duct cystadenocarcinoma*
M8170/0 *Liver cell adenoma*
M8170/3 *Hepatocellular carcinoma NOS*
M8180/0 *Hepatocholangioma, benign*
M8180/3 *Combined hepatocellular carcinoma and cholangiocarcinoma*
M8190/0 *Trabecular adenoma*
M8190/3 *Trabecular adenocarcinoma*
M8191/0 *Embryonal adenoma*
M8200/0 *Eccrine dermal cylindroma*
M8200/3 *Adenoid cystic carcinoma*
M8201/3 *Cribriform carcinoma*
M8210/0 *Adenomatous polyp NOS*
M8210/3 *Adenocarcinoma in adenomatous polyp*
M8211/0 *Tubular adenoma NOS*
M8211/3 *Tubular adenocarcinoma*
M8220/0 *Adenomatous polyposis coli*
M8220/3 *Adenocarcinoma in adenomatous polyposis coli*
M8221/0 *Multiple adenomatous polyps*
M8230/3 *Solid carcinoma NOS*
M8231/3 *Carcinoma simplex*
M8240/1 *Carcinoid tumor NOS*
M8240/3 *Carcinoid tumor, malignant*
M8241/1 *Carcinoid tumor, argentaffin NOS*
M8241/3 *Carcinoid tumor, argentaffin, malignant*
M8242/1 *Carcinoid tumor, nonargentaffin NOS*
M8242/3 *Carcinoid tumor, nonargentaffin, malignant*
M8243/3 *Mucocarcinoid tumor, malignant*
M8244/3 *Composite carcinoid*
M8250/1 *Pulmonary adenomatosis*
M8250/3 *Bronchiolo-alveolar adenocarcinoma*
M8251/0 *Alveolar adenoma*

M8251/3 *Alveolar adenocarcinoma*
M8260/0 *Papillary adenoma NOS*
M8260/3 *Papillary adenocarcinoma NOS*
M8261/1 *Villous adenoma NOS*
M8261/3 *Adenocarcinoma in villous adenoma*
M8262/3 *Villous adenocarcinoma*
M8263/0 *Tubulovillous adenoma*
M8270/0 *Chromophobe adenoma*
M8270/3 *Chromophobe carcinoma*
M8280/0 *Acidophil adenoma*
M8280/3 *Acidophil carcinoma*
M8281/0 *Mixed acidophil-basophil adenoma*
M8281/3 *Mixed acidophil-basophil carcinoma*
M8290/0 *Oxyphilic adenoma*
M8290/3 *Oxyphilic adenocarcinoma*
M8300/0 *Basophil adenoma*
M8300/3 *Basophil carcinoma*
M8310/0 *Clear cell adenoma*
M8310/3 *Clear cell adenocarcinoma NOS*
M8311/1 *Hypernephroid tumor*
M8312/3 *Renal cell carcinoma*
M8313/0 *Clear cell adenofibroma*
M8320/3 *Granular cell carcinoma*
M8321/0 *Chief cell adenoma*
M8322/0 *Water-clear cell adenoma*
M8322/3 *Water-clear cell adenocarcinoma*
M8323/0 *Mixed cell adenoma*
M8323/3 *Mixed cell adenocarcinoma*
M8324/0 *Lipoadenoma*
M8330/0 *Follicular adenoma*
M8330/3 *Follicular adenocarcinoma NOS*
M8331/3 *Follicular adenocarcinoma, well differentiated type*
M8332/3 *Follicular adenocarcinoma, trabecular type*
M8333/0 *Microfollicular adenoma*
M8334/0 *Macrofollicular adenoma*
M8340/3 *Papillary and follicular adenocarcinoma*
M8350/3 *Nonencapsulated sclerosing carcinoma*
M8360/1 *Multiple endocrine adenomas*
M8361/1 *Juxtaglomerular tumor*
M8370/0 *Adrenal cortical adenoma NOS*
M8370/3 *Adrenal cortical carcinoma*
M8371/0 *Adrenal cortical adenoma, compact cell type*
M8372/0 *Adrenal cortical adenoma, heavily pigmented variant*
M8373/0 *Adrenal cortical adenoma, clear cell type*
M8374/0 *Adrenal cortical adenoma, glomerulosa cell type*
M8375/0 *Adrenal cortical adenoma, mixed cell type*
M8380/0 *Endometrioid adenoma NOS*
M8380/1 *Endometrioid adenoma, borderline malignancy*
M8380/3 *Endometrioid carcinoma*
M8381/0 *Endometrioid adenofibroma NOS*
M8381/1 *Endometrioid adenofibroma, borderline malignancy*
M8381/3 *Endometrioid adenofibroma, malignant*

M839-M842 Adnexal and skin appendage neoplasms

M8390/0 *Skin appendage adenoma*
M8390/3 *Skin appendage carcinoma*
M8400/0 *Sweat gland adenoma*
M8400/1 *Sweat gland tumor NOS*
M8400/3 *Sweat gland adenocarcinoma*
M8401/0 *Apocrine adenoma*
M8401/3 *Apocrine adenocarcinoma*
M8402/0 *Eccrine acrospiroma*
M8403/0 *Eccrine spiradenoma*
M8404/0 *Hidrocystoma*
M8405/0 *Papillary hydradenoma*
M8406/0 *Papillary syringadenoma*
M8407/0 *Syringoma NOS*
M8410/0 *Sebaceous adenoma*
M8410/3 *Sebaceous adenocarcinoma*
M8420/0 *Ceruminous adenoma*
M8420/3 *Ceruminous adenocarcinoma*

M843 Mucoepidermoid neoplasms

M8430/1 *Mucoepidermoid tumor*
M8430/3 *Mucoepidermoid carcinoma*

M844-M849 Cystic, mucinous, and serous neoplasms

M8440/0 *Cystadenoma NOS*
M8440/3 *Cystadenocarcinoma NOS*
M8441/0 *Serous cystadenoma NOS*
M8441/1 *Serous cystadenoma, borderline malignancy*
M8441/3 *Serous cystadenocarcinoma NOS*
M8450/0 *Papillary cystadenoma NOS*
M8450/1 *Papillary cystadenoma, borderline malignancy*
M8450/3 *Papillary cystadenocarcinoma NOS*
M8460/0 *Papillary serous cystadenoma NOS*
M8460/1 *Papillary serous cystadenoma, borderline malignancy*
M8460/3 *Papillary serous cystadenocarcinoma*
M8461/0 *Serous surface papilloma NOS*
M8461/1 *Serous surface papilloma, borderline malignancy*
M8461/3 *Serous surface papillary carcinoma*
M8470/0 *Mucinous cystadenoma NOS*
M8470/1 *Mucinous cystadenoma, borderline malignancy*
M8470/3 *Mucinous cystadenocarcinoma NOS*
M8471/0 *Papillary mucinous cystadenoma NOS*
M8471/1 *Papillary mucinous cystadenoma, borderline malignancy*
M8471/3 *Papillary mucinous cystadenocarcinoma*
M8480/0 *Mucinous adenoma*
M8480/3 *Mucinous adenocarcinoma*
M8480/6 *Pseudomyxoma peritonei*
M8481/3 *Mucin-producing adenocarcinoma*
M8490/3 *Signet ring cell carcinoma*
M8490/6 *Metastatic signet ring cell carcinoma*

M850-M854 Ductal, lobular, and medullary neoplasms

M8500/2 *Intraductal carcinoma, noninfiltrating NOS*
M8500/3 *Infiltrating duct carcinoma*
M8501/2 *Comedocarcinoma, noninfiltrating*
M8501/3 *Comedocarcinoma NOS*
M8502/3 *Juvenile carcinoma of the breast*
M8503/0 *Intraductal papilloma*
M8503/2 *Noninfiltrating intraductal papillary adenocarcinoma*
M8504/0 *Intracystic papillary adenoma*
M8504/2 *Noninfiltrating intracystic carcinoma*
M8505/0 *Intraductal papillomatosis NOS*
M8506/0 *Subareolar duct papillomatosis*
M8510/3 *Medullary carcinoma NOS*
M8511/3 *Medullary carcinoma with amyloid stroma*
M8512/3 *Medullary carcinoma with lymphoid stroma*
M8520/2 *Lobular carcinoma in situ*
M8520/3 *Lobular carcinoma NOS*
M8521/3 *Infiltrating ductular carcinoma*
M8530/3 *Inflammatory carcinoma*
M8540/3 *Paget's disease, mammary*
M8541/3 *Paget's disease and infiltrating duct carcinoma of breast*
M8542/3 *Paget's disease, extramammary (except Paget's disease of bone)*

M855 Acinar cell neoplasms

M8550/0 *Acinar cell adenoma*
M8550/1 *Acinar cell tumor*
M8550/3 *Acinar cell carcinoma*

M856-M858 Complex epithelial neoplasms

M8560/3 *Adenosquamous carcinoma*
M8561/0 *Adenolymphoma*
M8570/3 *Adenocarcinoma with squamous metaplasia*
M8571/3 *Adenocarcinoma with cartilaginous and osseous metaplasia*
M8572/3 *Adenocarcinoma with spindle cell metaplasia*
M8573/3 *Adenocarcinoma with apocrine metaplasia*
M8580/0 *Thymoma, benign*
M8580/3 *Thymoma, malignant*

M859-M867 Specialized gonadal neoplasms

M8590/1 *Sex cord-stromal tumor*
M8600/0 *Thecoma NOS*
M8600/3 *Theca cell carcinoma*
M8610/0 *Luteoma NOS*
M8620/1 *Granulosa cell tumor NOS*
M8620/3 *Granulosa cell tumor, malignant*
M8621/1 *Granulosa cell-theca cell tumor*
M8630/0 *Androblastoma, benign*
M8630/1 *Androblastoma NOS*
M8630/3 *Androblastoma, malignant*
M8631/0 *Sertoli-Leydig cell tumor*
M8632/1 *Gynandroblastoma*
M8640/0 *Tubular androblastoma NOS*
M8640/3 *Sertoli cell carcinoma*
M8641/0 *Tubular androblastoma with lipid storage*
M8650/0 *Leydig cell tumor, benign*
M8650/1 *Leydig cell tumor NOS*
M8650/3 *Leydig cell tumor, malignant*
M8660/0 *Hilar cell tumor*
M8670/0 *Lipid cell tumor of ovary*
M8671/0 *Adrenal rest tumor*

M868-M871 Paragangliomas and glomus tumors

M8680/1 *Paraganglioma NOS*
M8680/3 *Paraganglioma, malignant*
M8681/1 *Sympathetic paraganglioma*
M8682/1 *Parasympathetic paraganglioma*
M8690/1 *Glomus jugulare tumor*
M8691/1 *Aortic body tumor*
M8692/1 *Carotid body tumor*
M8693/1 *Extra-adrenal paraganglioma NOS*
M8693/3 *Extra-adrenal paraganglioma, malignant*
M8700/0 *Pheochromocytoma NOS*
M8700/3 *Pheochromocytoma, malignant*
M8710/3 *Glomangiosarcoma*
M8711/0 *Glomus tumor*
M8712/0 *Glomangioma*

M872-M879 Nevi and melanomas

M8720/0 *Pigmented nevus NOS*
M8720/3 *Malignant melanoma NOS*
M8721/3 *Nodular melanoma*
M8722/0 *Balloon cell nevus*
M8722/3 *Balloon cell melanoma*
M8723/0 *Halo nevus*
M8724/0 *Fibrous papule of the nose*
M8725/0 *Neuronevus*
M8726/0 *Magnocellular nevus*
M8730/0 *Nonpigmented nevus*
M8730/3 *Amelanotic melanoma*
M8740/0 *Junctional nevus*
M8740/3 *Malignant melanoma in junctional nevus*
M8741/2 *Precancerous melanosis NOS*
M8741/3 *Malignant melanoma in precancerous melanosis*
M8742/2 *Hutchinson's melanotic freckle*
M8742/3 *Malignant melanoma in Hutchinson's melanotic freckle*
M8743/3 *Superficial spreading melanoma*
M8750/0 *Intradermal nevus*
M8760/0 *Compound nevus*
M8761/1 *Giant pigmented nevus*
M8761/3 *Malignant melanoma in giant pigmented nevus*
M8770/0 *Epithelioid and spindle cell nevus*
M8771/3 *Epithelioid cell melanoma*
M8772/3 *Spindle cell melanoma NOS*
M8773/3 *Spindle cell melanoma, type A*
M8774/3 *Spindle cell melanoma, type B*
M8775/3 *Mixed epithelioid and spindle cell melanoma*
M8780/0 *Blue nevus NOS*
M8780/3 *Blue nevus, malignant*
M8790/0 *Cellular blue nevus*

M880 Soft tissue tumors and sarcomas NOS

M8800/0 *Soft tissue tumor, benign*
M8800/3 *Sarcoma NOS*
M8800/9 *Sarcomatosis NOS*
M8801/3 *Spindle cell sarcoma*

M8802/3 *Giant cell sarcoma (except of bone M9250/3)*
M8803/3 *Small cell sarcoma*
M8804/3 *Epithelioid cell sarcoma*

M881-M883 Fibromatous neoplasms
M8810/0 *Fibroma NOS*
M8810/3 *Fibrosarcoma NOS*
M8811/0 *Fibromyxoma*
M8811/3 *Fibromyxosarcoma*
M8812/0 *Periosteal fibroma*
M8812/3 *Periosteal fibrosarcoma*
M8813/0 *Fascial fibroma*
M8813/3 *Fascial fibrosarcoma*
M8814/3 *Infantile fibrosarcoma*
M8820/0 *Elastofibroma*
M8821/1 *Aggressive fibromatosis*
M8822/1 *Abdominal fibromatosis*
M8823/1 *Desmoplastic fibroma*
M8830/0 *Fibrous histiocytoma NOS*
M8830/1 *Atypical fibrous histiocytoma*
M8830/3 *Fibrous histiocytoma, malignant*
M8831/0 *Fibroxanthoma NOS*
M8831/1 *Atypical fibroxanthoma*
M8831/3 *Fibroxanthoma, malignant*
M8832/0 *Dermatofibroma NOS*
M8832/1 *Dermatofibroma protuberans*
M8832/3 *Dermatofibrosarcoma NOS*

M884 Myxomatous neoplasms
M8840/0 *Myxoma NOS*
M8840/3 *Myxosarcoma*

M885-M888 Lipomatous neoplasms
M8850/0 *Lipoma NOS*
M8850/3 *Liposarcoma NOS*
M8851/0 *Fibrolipoma*
M8851/3 *Liposarcoma, well differentiated type*
M8852/0 *Fibromyxolipoma*
M8852/3 *Myxoid liposarcoma*
M8853/3 *Round cell liposarcoma*
M8854/3 *Pleomorphic liposarcoma*
M8855/3 *Mixed type liposarcoma*
M8856/0 *Intramuscular lipoma*
M8857/0 *Spindle cell lipoma*
M8860/0 *Angiomyolipoma*
M8860/3 *Angiomyoliposarcoma*
M8861/0 *Angiolipoma NOS*
M8861/1 *Angiolipoma, infiltrating*
M8870/0 *Myelolipoma*
M8880/0 *Hibernoma*
M8881/0 *Lipoblastomatosis*

M889-M892 Myomatous neoplasms
M8890/0 *Leiomyoma NOS*
M8890/1 *Intravascular leiomyomatosis*
M8890/3 *Leiomyosarcoma NOS*
M8891/1 *Epithelioid leiomyoma*
M8891/3 *Epithelioid leiomyosarcoma*
M8892/1 *Cellular leiomyoma*
M8893/0 *Bizarre leiomyoma*
M8894/0 *Angiomyoma*
M8894/3 *Angiomyosarcoma*
M8895/0 *Myoma*
M8895/3 *Myosarcoma*
M8900/0 *Rhabdomyoma NOS*
M8900/3 *Rhabdomyosarcoma NOS*
M8901/3 *Pleomorphic rhabdomyosarcoma*
M8902/3 *Mixed type rhabdomyosarcoma*
M8903/0 *Fetal rhabdomyoma*
M8904/0 *Adult rhabdomyoma*
M8910/3 *Embryonal rhabdomyosarcoma*
M8920/3 *Alveolar rhabdomyosarcoma*

M893-M899 Complex mixed and stromal neoplasms
M8930/3 *Endometrial stromal sarcoma*
M8931/1 *Endolymphatic stromal myosis*
M8932/0 *Adenomyoma*
M8940/0 *Pleomorphic adenoma*
M8940/3 *Mixed tumor, malignant NOS*
M8950/3 *Mullerian mixed tumor*
M8951/3 *Mesodermal mixed tumor*
M8960/1 *Mesoblastic nephroma*
M8960/3 *Nephroblastoma NOS*
M8961/3 *Epithelial nephroblastoma*
M8962/3 *Mesenchymal nephroblastoma*
M8970/3 *Hepatoblastoma*
M8980/3 *Carcinosarcoma NOS*
M8981/3 *Carcinosarcoma, embryonal type*
M8982/0 *Myoepithelioma*
M8990/0 *Mesenchymoma, benign*
M8990/1 *Mesenchymoma NOS*
M8990/3 *Mesenchymoma, malignant*
M8991/3 *Embryonal sarcoma*

M900-M903 Fibroepithelial neoplasms
M9000/0 *Brenner tumor NOS*
M9000/1 *Brenner tumor, borderline malignancy*
M9000/3 *Brenner tumor, malignant*
M9010/0 *Fibroadenoma NOS*
M9011/0 *Intracanalicular fibroadenoma NOS*
M9012/0 *Pericanalicular fibroadenoma*
M9013/0 *Adenofibroma NOS*
M9014/0 *Serous adenofibroma*
M9015/0 *Mucinous adenofibroma*
M9020/0 *Cellular intracanalicular fibroadenoma*
M9020/1 *Cystosarcoma phyllodes NOS*
M9020/3 *Cystosarcoma phyllodes, malignant*
M9030/0 *Juvenile fibroadenoma*

M904 Synovial neoplasms
M9040/0 *Synovioma, benign*
M9040/3 *Synovial sarcoma NOS*
M9041/3 *Synovial sarcoma, spindle cell type*
M9042/3 *Synovial sarcoma, epithelioid cell type*
M9043/3 *Synovial sarcoma, biphasic type*
M9044/3 *Clear cell sarcoma of tendons and aponeuroses*

M905 Mesothelial neoplasms
M9050/0 *Mesothelioma, benign*
M9050/3 *Mesothelioma, malignant*
M9051/0 *Fibrous mesothelioma, benign*
M9051/3 *Fibrous mesothelioma, malignant*
M9052/0 *Epithelioid mesothelioma, benign*
M9052/3 *Epithelioid mesothelioma, malignant*
M9053/0 *Mesothelioma, biphasic type, benign*
M9053/3 *Mesothelioma, biphasic type, malignant*
M9054/0 *Adenomatoid tumor NOS*

M906-M909 Germ cell neoplasms
M9060/3 *Dysgerminoma*
M9061/3 *Seminoma NOS*
M9062/3 *Seminoma, anaplastic type*
M9063/3 *Spermatocytic seminoma*
M9064/3 *Germinoma*
M9070/3 *Embryonal carcinoma NOS*
M9071/3 *Endodermal sinus tumor*
M9072/3 *Polyembryoma*
M9073/1 *Gonadoblastoma*
M9080/0 *Teratoma, benign*
M9080/1 *Teratoma NOS*
M9080/3 *Teratoma, malignant NOS*
M9081/3 *Teratocarcinoma*
M9082/3 *Malignant teratoma, undifferentiated type*
M9083/3 *Malignant teratoma, intermediate type*
M9084/0 *Dermoid cyst*
M9084/3 *Dermoid cyst with malignant transformation*
M9090/0 *Struma ovarii NOS*
M9090/3 *Struma ovarii, malignant*
M9091/1 *Strumal carcinoid*

M910 Trophoblastic neoplasms
M9100/0 *Hydatidiform mole NOS*
M9100/1 *Invasive hydatidiform mole*
M9100/3 *Choriocarcinoma*
M9101/3 *Choriocarcinoma combined with teratoma*
M9102/3 *Malignant teratoma, trophoblastic*

M911 Mesonephromas
M9110/0 *Mesonephroma, benign*
M9110/1 *Mesonephric tumor*
M9110/3 *Mesonephroma, malignant*
M9111/1 *Endosalpingioma*

M912-M916 Blood vessel tumors
M9120/0 *Hemangioma NOS*
M9120/3 *Hemangiosarcoma*
M9121/0 *Cavernous hemangioma*
M9122/0 *Venous hemangioma*
M9123/0 *Racemose hemangioma*
M9124/3 *Kupffer cell sarcoma*
M9130/0 *Hemangioendothelioma, benign*
M9130/1 *Hemangioendothelioma NOS*
M9130/3 *Hemangioendothelioma, malignant*
M9131/0 *Capillary hemangioma*
M9132/0 *Intramuscular hemangioma*
M9140/3 *Kaposi's sarcoma*
M9141/0 *Angiokeratoma*
M9142/0 *Verrucous keratotic hemangioma*
M9150/0 *Hemangiopericytoma, benign*
M9150/1 *Hemangiopericytoma NOS*
M9150/3 *Hemangiopericytoma, malignant*
M9160/0 *Angiofibroma NOS*
M9161/1 *Hemangioblastoma*

M917 Lymphatic vessel tumors
M9170/0 *Lymphangioma NOS*
M9170/3 *Lymphangiosarcoma*
M9171/0 *Capillary lymphangioma*
M9172/0 *Cavernous lymphangioma*
M9173/0 *Cystic lymphangioma*
M9174/0 *Lymphangiomyoma*
M9174/1 *Lymphangiomyomatosis*
M9175/0 *Hemolymphangioma*

M918-M920 Osteomas and osteosarcomas
M9180/0 *Osteoma NOS*
M9180/3 *Osteosarcoma NOS*
M9181/3 *Chondroblastic osteosarcoma*
M9182/3 *Fibroblastic osteosarcoma*
M9183/3 *Telangiectatic osteosarcoma*
M9184/3 *Osteosarcoma in Paget's disease of bone*
M9190/3 *Juxtacortical osteosarcoma*
M9191/0 *Osteoid osteoma NOS*
M9200/0 *Osteoblastoma*

M921-M924 Chondromatous neoplasms
M9210/0 *Osteochondroma*
M9210/1 *Osteochondromatosis NOS*
M9220/0 *Chondroma NOS*
M9220/1 *Chondromatosis NOS*
M9220/3 *Chondrosarcoma NOS*
M9221/0 *Juxtacortical chondroma*
M9221/3 *Juxtacortical chondrosarcoma*
M9230/0 *Chondroblastoma NOS*
M9230/3 *Chondroblastoma, malignant*
M9240/3 *Mesenchymal chondrosarcoma*
M9241/0 *Chondromyxoid fibroma*

M925 Giant cell tumors
M9250/1 *Giant cell tumor of bone NOS*
M9250/3 *Giant cell tumor of bone, malignant*
M9251/1 *Giant cell tumor of soft parts NOS*
M9251/3 *Malignant giant cell tumor of soft parts*

M926 Miscellaneous bone tumors
M9260/3 *Ewing's sarcoma*
M9261/3 *Adamantinoma of long bones*
M9262/0 *Ossifying fibroma*

M927-M934 Odontogenic tumors
M9270/0 *Odontogenic tumor, benign*
M9270/1 *Odontogenic tumor NOS*
M9270/3 *Odontogenic tumor, malignant*
M9271/0 *Dentinoma*
M9272/0 *Cementoma NOS*
M9273/0 *Cementoblastoma, benign*
M9274/0 *Cementifying fibroma*
M9275/0 *Gigantiform cementoma*
M9280/0 *Odontoma NOS*
M9281/0 *Compound odontoma*
M9282/0 *Complex odontoma*
M9290/0 *Ameloblastic fibro-odontoma*
M9290/3 *Ameloblastic odontosarcoma*
M9300/0 *Adenomatoid odontogenic tumor*
M9301/0 *Calcifying odontogenic cyst*
M9310/0 *Ameloblastoma NOS*
M9310/3 *Ameloblastoma, malignant*
M9311/0 *Odontoameloblastoma*
M9312/0 *Squamous odontogenic tumor*
M9320/0 *Odontogenic myxoma*
M9321/0 *Odontogenic fibroma NOS*
M9330/0 *Ameloblastic fibroma*
M9330/3 *Ameloblastic fibrosarcoma*
M9340/0 *Calcifying epithelial odontogenic tumor*

M935-M937 Miscellaneous tumors
- M9350/1 *Craniopharyngioma*
- M9360/1 *Pinealoma*
- M9361/1 *Pineocytoma*
- M9362/3 *Pineoblastoma*
- M9363/0 *Melanotic neuroectodermal tumor*
- M9370/3 *Chordoma*

M938-M948 Gliomas
- M9380/3 *Glioma, malignant*
- M9381/3 *Gliomatosis cerebri*
- M9382/3 *Mixed glioma*
- M9383/1 *Subependymal glioma*
- M9384/1 *Subependymal giant cell astrocytoma*
- M9390/0 *Choroid plexus papilloma NOS*
- M9390/3 *Choroid plexus papilloma, malignant*
- M9391/3 Ependymoma NOS
- M9392/3 *Ependymoma, anaplastic type*
- M9393/1 *Papillary ependymoma*
- M9394/1 *Myxopapillary ependymoma*
- M9400/3 *Astrocytoma NOS*
- M9401/3 *Astrocytoma, anaplastic type*
- M9410/3 *Protoplasmic astrocytoma*
- M9411/3 *Gemistocytic astrocytoma*
- M9420/3 *Fibrillary astrocytoma*
- M9421/3 *Pilocytic astrocytoma*
- M9422/3 *Spongioblastoma NOS*
- M9423/3 *Spongioblastoma polare*
- M9430/3 *Astroblastoma*
- M9440/3 *Glioblastoma NOS*
- M9441/3 *Giant cell glioblastoma*
- M9442/3 *Glioblastoma with sarcomatous component*
- M9443/3 *Primitive polar spongioblastoma*
- M9450/3 *Oligodendroglioma NOS*
- M9451/3 *Oligodendroglioma, anaplastic type*
- M9460/3 *Oligodendroblastoma*
- M9470/3 *Medulloblastoma NOS*
- M9471/3 *Desmoplastic medulloblastoma*
- M9472/3 *Medullomyoblastoma*
- M9480/3 *Cerebellar sarcoma NOS*
- M9481/3 *Monstrocellular sarcoma*

M949-M952 Neuroepitheliomatous neoplasms
- M9490/0 *Ganglioneuroma*
- M9490/3 *Ganglioneuroblastoma*
- M9491/0 *Ganglioneuromatosis*
- M9500/3 *Neuroblastoma NOS*
- M9501/3 *Medulloepithelioma NOS*
- M9502/3 *Teratoid medulloepithelioma*
- M9503/3 *Neuroepithelioma NOS*
- M9504/3 *Spongioneuroblastoma*
- M9505/1 *Ganglioglioma*
- M9506/0 *Neurocytoma*
- M9507/0 *Pacinian tumor*
- M9510/3 *Retinoblastoma NOS*
- M9511/3 *Retinoblastoma, differentiated type*
- M9512/3 *Retinoblastoma, undifferentiated type*
- M9520/3 *Olfactory neurogenic tumor*
- M9521/3 *Esthesioneurocytoma*
- M9522/3 *Esthesioneuroblastoma*
- M9523/3 *Esthesioneuroepithelioma*

M953 Meningiomas
- M9530/0 *Meningioma NOS*
- M9530/1 *Meningiomatosis NOS*
- M9530/3 *Meningioma, malignant*
- M9531/0 *Meningotheliomatous meningioma*
- M9532/0 *Fibrous meningioma*
- M9533/0 *Psammomatous meningioma*
- M9534/0 *Angiomatous meningioma*
- M9535/0 *Hemangioblastic meningioma*
- M9536/0 *Hemangiopericytic meningioma*
- M9537/0 *Transitional meningioma*
- M9538/1 *Papillary meningioma*
- M9539/3 *Meningeal sarcomatosis*

M954-M957 Nerve sheath tumor
- M9540/0 *Neurofibroma NOS*
- M9540/1 *Neurofibromatosis NOS*
- M9540/3 *Neurofibrosarcoma*
- M9541/0 *Melanotic neurofibroma*
- M9550/0 *Plexiform neurofibroma*
- M9560/0 *Neurilemmoma NOS*
- M9560/1 *Neurinomatosis*
- M9560/3 *Neurilemmoma, malignant*
- M9570/0 *Neuroma NOS*

M958 Granular cell tumors and alveolar soft part sarcoma
- M9580/0 *Granular cell tumor NOS*
- M9580/3 *Granular cell tumor, malignant*
- M9581/3 *Alveolar soft part sarcoma*

M959-M963 Lymphomas, NOS or diffuse
- M9590/0 *Lymphomatous tumor, benign*
- M9590/3 *Malignant lymphoma NOS*
- M9591/3 *Malignant lymphoma, non Hodgkin's type*
- M9600/3 *Malignant lymphoma, undifferentiated cell type NOS*
- M9601/3 *Malignant lymphoma, stem cell type*
- M9602/3 *Malignant lymphoma, convoluted cell type NOS*
- M9610/3 *Lymphosarcoma NOS*
- M9611/3 *Malignant lymphoma, lymphoplasmacytoid type*
- M9612/3 *Malignant lymphoma, immunoblastic type*
- M9613/3 *Malignant lymphoma, mixed lymphocytic-histiocytic NOS*
- M9614/3 *Malignant lymphoma, centroblastic-centrocytic, diffuse*
- M9615/3 *Malignant lymphoma, follicular center cell NOS*
- M9620/3 *Malignant lymphoma, lymphocytic, well differentiated NOS*
- M9621/3 *Malignant lymphoma, lymphocytic, intermediate differentiation NOS*
- M9622/3 *Malignant lymphoma, centrocytic*
- M9623/3 *Malignant lymphoma, follicular center cell, cleaved NOS*
- M9630/3 *Malignant lymphoma, lymphocytic, poorly differentiated NOS*
- M9631/3 *Prolymphocytic lymphosarcoma*
- M9632/3 *Malignant lymphoma, centroblastic type NOS*
- M9633/3 *Malignant lymphoma, follicular center cell, noncleaved NOS*

M964 Reticulosarcomas
- M9640/3 *Reticulosarcoma NOS*
- M9641/3 *Reticulosarcoma, pleomorphic cell type*
- M9642/3 *Reticulosarcoma, nodular*

M965-M966 Hodgkin's disease
- M9650/3 *Hodgkin's disease NOS*
- M9651/3 *Hodgkin's disease, lymphocytic predominance*
- M9652/3 *Hodgkin's disease, mixed cellularity*
- M9653/3 *Hodgkin's disease, lymphocytic depletion NOS*
- M9654/3 *Hodgkin's disease, lymphocytic depletion, diffuse fibrosis*
- M9655/3 *Hodgkin's disease, lymphocytic depletion, reticular type*
- M9656/3 *Hodgkin's disease, nodular sclerosis NOS*
- M9657/3 *Hodgkin's disease, nodular sclerosis, cellular phase*
- M9660/3 *Hodgkin's paragranuloma*
- M9661/3 *Hodgkin's granuloma*
- M9662/3 *Hodgkin's sarcoma*

M969 Lymphomas, nodular or follicular
- M9690/3 *Malignant lymphoma, nodular NOS*
- M9691/3 *Malignant lymphoma, mixed lymphocytic-histiocytic, nodular*
- M9692/3 *Malignant lymphoma, centroblastic-centrocytic, follicular*
- M9693/3 *Malignant lymphoma, lymphocytic, well differentiated, nodular*
- M9694/3 *Malignant lymphoma, lymphocytic, intermediate differentiation, nodular*
- M9695/3 *Malignant lymphoma, follicular center cell, cleaved, follicular*
- M9696/3 *Malignant lymphoma, lymphocytic, poorly differentiated, nodular*
- M9697/3 *Malignant lymphoma, centroblastic type, follicular*
- M9698/3 *Malignant lymphoma, follicular center cell, noncleaved, follicular*

M970 Mycosis fungoides
- M9700/3 *Mycosis fungoides*
- M9701/3 *Sezary's disease*

M971-M972 Miscellaneous reticuloendothelial neoplasms
- M9710/3 *Microglioma*
- M9720/3 *Malignant histiocytosis*
- M9721/3 *Histiocytic medullary reticulosis*
- M9722/3 *Letterer-Siwe's disease*

M973 Plasma cell tumors
- M9730/3 *Plasma cell myeloma*
- M9731/0 *Plasma cell tumor, benign*
- M9731/1 *Plasmacytoma NOS*
- M9731/3 *Plasma cell tumor, malignant*

M974 Mast cell tumors
- M9740/1 *Mastocytoma NOS*
- M9740/3 *Mast cell sarcoma*
- M9741/3 *Malignant mastocytosis*

M975 Burkitt's tumor
- M9750/3 *Burkitt's tumor*

M980-M994 Leukemias
- M980 *Leukemias NOS*
- M9800/3 *Leukemia NOS*
- M9801/3 *Acute leukemia NOS*
- M9802/3 *Subacute leukemia NOS*
- M9803/3 *Chronic leukemia NOS*
- M9804/3 *Aleukemic leukemia NOS*

M981 Compound leukemias
- M9810/3 *Compound leukemia*

M982 Lymphoid leukemias
- M9820/3 *Lymphoid leukemia NOS*
- M9821/3 *Acute lymphoid leukemia*
- M9822/3 *Subacute lymphoid leukemia*
- M9823/3 *Chronic lymphoid leukemia*
- M9824/3 *Aleukemic lymphoid leukemia*
- M9825/3 *Prolymphocytic leukemia*

M983 Plasma cell leukemias
- M9830/3 *Plasma cell leukemia*

M984 Erythroleukemias
- M9840/3 *Erythroleukemia*
- M9841/3 *Acute erythremia*
- M9842/3 *Chronic erythremia*

M985 Lymphosarcoma cell leukemias
- M9850/3 *Lymphosarcoma cell leukemia*

M986 Myeloid leukemias
- M9860/3 *Myeloid leukemia NOS*
- M9861/3 *Acute myeloid leukemia*
- M9862/3 *Subacute myeloid leukemia*
- M9863/3 *Chronic myeloid leukemia*
- M9864/3 *Aleukemic myeloid leukemia*
- M9865/3 *Neutrophilic leukemia*
- M9866/3 *Acute promyelocytic leukemia*

M987 Basophilic leukemias
- M9870/3 *Basophilic leukemia*

M988 Eosinophilic leukemias
- M9880/3 *Eosinophilic leukemia*

M989 Monocytic leukemias
- M9890/3 *Monocytic leukemia NOS*
- M9891/3 *Acute monocytic leukemia*
- M9892/3 *Subacute monocytic leukemia*
- M9893/3 *Chronic monocytic leukemia*
- M9894/3 *Aleukemic monocytic leukemia*

M990-M994 Miscellaneous leukemias
- M9900/3 *Mast cell leukemia*
- M9910/3 *Megakaryocytic leukemia*
- M9920/3 *Megakaryocytic myelosis*
- M9930/3 *Myeloid sarcoma*
- M9940/3 *Hairy cell leukemia*

M995-M997 Miscellaneous myeloproliferative and lymphoproliferative disorders
- M9950/1 *Polycythemia vera*
- M9951/1 *Acute panmyelosis*
- M9960/1 *Chronic myeloproliferative disease*
- M9961/1 *Myelosclerosis with myeloid metaplasia*
- M9962/1 *Idiopathic thrombocythemia*
- M9970/1 *Chronic lymphoproliferative disease*

Appendix B was officially deleted October 1, 2004

Classification of Drugs by American Hospital Formulary Services List Number and Their ICD-9-CM Equivalents

The coding of adverse effects of drugs is keyed to the continually revised Hospital Formulary of the American Hospital Formulary Service (AHFS) published under the direction of the American Society of Hospital Pharmacists. The following section provides the ICD-9-CM diagnosis code for each AHFS list.

	AHFS List	ICD-9-CM Diagnosis Code
4:00	**ANTIHISTAMINE DRUGS**	963.0
8:00	**ANTI-INFECTIVE AGENTS**	
8:04	Amebacides	961.5
	hydroxyquinoline derivatives	961.3
	arsenical anti-infectives	961.1
8:08	Anthelmintics	961.6
	quinoline derivatives	961.3
8:12.04	Antifungal Antibiotics	960.1
	nonantibiotics	961.9
8:12.06	Cephalosporins	960.5
8:12.08	Chloramphenicol	960.2
8:12.12	The Erythromycins	960.3
8:12.16	The Penicillins	960.0
8:12.20	The Streptomycins	960.6
8:12.24	The Tetracyclines	960.4
8:12.28	Other Antibiotics	960.8
	antimycobacterial antibiotics	960.6
	macrolides	960.3
8:16	Antituberculars	961.8
	antibiotics	960.6
8:18	Antivirals	961.7
8:20	Plasmodicides (antimalarials)	961.4
8:24	Sulfonamides	961.0
8:26	The Sulfones	961.8
8:28	Treponemicides	961.2
8:32	Trichomonacides	961.5
	hydroxyquinoline derivatives	961.3
	nitrofuran derivatives	961.9
8:36	Urinary Germicides	961.9
	quinoline derivatives	961.3
8:40	Other Anti-Infectives	961.9
10:00	**ANTINEOPLASTIC AGENTS**	963.1
	antibiotics	960.7
	progestogens	962.2
12:00	**AUTONOMIC DRUGS**	
12:04	Parasympathomimetic (Cholinergic) Agents	971.0
12:08	Parasympatholytic (Cholinergic Blocking) Agents	971.1
12:12	Sympathomimetic (Adrenergic) Agents	971.2
12:16	Sympatholytic (Adrenergic Blocking) Agents	971.3
12:20	Skeletal Muscle Relaxants	975.2
	central nervous system muscle-tone depressants	968.0
16:00	**BLOOD DERIVATIVES**	964.7
20:00	**BLOOD FORMATION AND COAGULATION**	
20:04	Antianemia Drugs	964.1
20:04.04	Iron Preparations	964.0
20:04.08	Liver and Stomach Preparations	964.1
20:12.04	Anticoagulants	964.2
20:12.08	Antiheparin agents	964.5
20:12.12	Coagulants	964.5
20:12.16	Hemostatics	964.5
	capillary-active drugs	972.8
	fibrinolysis-affecting agents	964.4
	natural products	964.7
24:00	**CARDIOVASCULAR DRUGS**	
24:04	Cardiac Drugs	972.9
	cardiotonic agents	972.1
	rhythm regulators	972.0
24:06	Antilipemic Agents	972.2
	thyroid derivatives	962.7
24:08	Hypotensive Agents	972.6
	adrenergic blocking agents	971.3
	ganglion-blocking agents	972.3
	vasodilators	972.5
24:12	Vasodilating Agents	972.5
	coronary	972.4
	nicotinic acid derivatives	972.2
24:16	Sclerosing Agents	972.7
28:00	**CENTRAL NERVOUS SYSTEM DRUGS**	
28:04	General Anesthetics	968.4
	gaseous anesthetics	968.2
	halothane	968.1
	intravenous anesthetics	968.3
28:08	Analgesics and Antipyretics	965.9
	antirheumatics	965.6
	aromatic analgesics	965.4
	non-narcotics NEC	965.7
	opium alkaloids	965.00
	heroin	965.01
	methadone	965.02
	specified type NEC	965.09
	pyrazole derivatives	965.5
	salicylates	965.1
	specified type NEC	965.8
28:10	Narcotic Antagonists	970.1
28:12	Anticonvulsants	966.3
	barbiturates	967.0
	benzodiazepine-based tranquilizers	969.4
	bromides	967.3
	hydantoin derivatives	966.1
	oxazolidine derivative	966.0
	succinimides	966.2
28:16.04	Antidepressants	969.0
28:16.08	Tranquilizers	969.5
	benzodiazepine-based	969.4
	butyrophenone-based	969.2
	major NEC	969.3
	phenothiazine-based	969.1
28:16.12	Other Psychotherapeutic Agents	969.8
28:20	Respiratory and Cerebral Stimulants	970.9
	analeptics	970.0
	anorexigenic agents	977.0
	psychostimulants	969.7
	specified type NEC	970.8
28:24	Sedatives and Hypnotics	967.9
	barbiturates	967.0
	benzodiazepine-based tranquilizers	969.4
	chloral hydrate group	967.1
	glutethimide group	967.5
	intravenous anesthetics	968.3
	methaqualone	967.4
	paraldehyde	967.2
	phenothiazine-based tranquilizers	969.1
	specified type NEC	967.8
	thiobarbiturates	968.3
	tranquilizer NEC	969.5
36:00	**DIAGNOSTIC AGENTS**	977.8
40:00	**ELECTROLYTE, CALORIC, AND WATER BALANCE AGENTS NEC**	974.5
40:04	Acidifying Agents	963.2
40:08	Alkalinizing Agents	963.3
40:10	Ammonia Detoxicants	974.5
40:12	Replacement Solutions NEC	974.5
	plasma volume expanders	964.8
40:16	Sodium-Removing Resins	974.5
40:18	Potassium-Removing Resins	974.5
40:20	Caloric Agents	974.5
40:24	Salt and Sugar Substitutes	974.5
40:28	Diuretics NEC	974.4
	carbonic acid anhydrase inhibitors	974.2
	mercurials	974.0
	purine derivatives	974.1
	saluretics	974.3
40:36	Irrigating Solutions	974.5

Appendix C: Classification of Drugs by AHFS List

Appendix C: Classification of Drugs by AHFS List

40:40	Uricosuric Agents	974.7
44:00	**ENZYMES NEC**	963.4
	fibrinolysis-affecting agents	964.4
	gastric agents	973.4
48:00	**EXPECTORANTS AND COUGH PREPARATIONS**	
	antihistamine agents	963.0
	antitussives	975.4
	codeine derivatives	965.09
	expectorants	975.5
	narcotic agents NEC	965.09
52:00	**EYE, EAR, NOSE, AND THROAT PREPARATIONS**	
52:04	Anti-Infectives	
	ENT	976.6
	ophthalmic	976.5
52:04.04	Antibiotics	
	ENT	976.6
	ophthalmic	976.5
52:04.06	Antivirals	
	ENT	976.6
	ophthalmic	976.5
52:04.08	Sulfonamides	
	ENT	976.6
	ophthalmic	976.5
52:04.12	Miscellaneous Anti-Infectives	
	ENT	976.6
	ophthalmic	976.5
52:08	Anti-Inflammatory Agents	
	ENT	976.6
	ophthalmic	976.5
52:10	Carbonic Anhydrase Inhibitors	974.2
52:12	Contact Lens Solutions	976.5
52:16	Local Anesthetics	968.5
52:20	Miotics	971.0
52:24	Mydriatics	
	adrenergics	971.2
	anticholinergics	971.1
	antimuscarinics	971.1
	parasympatholytics	971.1
	spasmolytics	971.1
	sympathomimetics	971.2
52:28	Mouth Washes and Gargles	976.6
52:32	Vasoconstrictors	971.2
52:36	Unclassified Agents	
	ENT	976.6
	ophthalmic	976.5
56:00	**GASTROINTESTINAL DRUGS**	
56:04	Antacids and Absorbents	973.0
56:08	Anti-Diarrhea Agents	973.5
56:10	Antiflatulents	973.8
56:12	Cathartics NEC	973.3
	emollients	973.2
	irritants	973.1
56:16	Digestants	973.4
56:20	Emetics and Antiemetics	
	antiemetics	963.0
	emetics	973.6
56:24	Lipotropic Agents	977.1
60:00	**GOLD COMPOUNDS**	965.6
64:00	**HEAVY METAL ANTAGONISTS**	963.8
68:00	**HORMONES AND SYNTHETIC SUBSTITUTES**	
68:04	Adrenals	962.0
68:08	Androgens	962.1
68:12	Contraceptives	962.2
68:16	Estrogens	962.2
68:18	Gonadotropins	962.4
68:20	Insulins and Antidiabetic Agents	962.3
68:20.08	Insulins	962.3
68:24	Parathyroid	962.6
68:28	Pituitary	
	anterior	962.4
	posterior	962.5
68:32	Progestogens	962.2
68:34	Other Corpus Luteum Hormones	962.2
68:36	Thyroid and Antithyroid	
	antithyroid	962.8
	thyroid	962.7
72:00	**LOCAL ANESTHETICS NEC**	968.9
	topical (surface) agents	968.5
	infiltrating agents (intradermal) (sub-cutaneous) (submucosal)	968.5
	nerve blocking agents (peripheral) (plexus) (regional)	968.6
	spinal	968.7
76:00	**OXYTOCICS**	975.0
78:00	**RADIOACTIVE AGENTS**	990
80:00	**SERUMS, TOXOIDS, AND VACCINES**	
80:04	Serums	979.9
	immune globulin (gamma) (human)	964.6
80:08	Toxoids NEC	978.8
	diphtheria	978.5
	and tetanus	978.9
	with pertussis component	978.6
	tetanus	978.4
	and diphtheria	978.9
	with pertussis component	978.6
80:12	Vaccines NEC	979.9
	bacterial NEC	978.8
	with	
	other bacterial component	978.9
	pertussis component	978.6
	viral and rickettsial component	979.7
	rickettsial NEC	979.6
	with	
	bacterial component	979.7
	pertussis component	978.6
	viral component	979.7
	viral NEC	979.6
	with	
	bacterial component	979.7
	pertussis component	978.6
	rickettsial component	979.7
84:00	**SKIN AND MUCOUS MEMBRANE PREPARATIONS**	
84:04	Anti-Infectives	976.0
84:04.04	Antibiotics	976.0
84:04.08	Fungicides	976.0
84:04.12	Scabicides and Pediculicides	976.0
84:04.16	Miscellaneous Local Anti-Infectives	976.0
84:06	Anti-Inflammatory Agents	976.0
84:08	Antipruritics and Local Anesthetics	
	antipruritics	976.1
	local anesthetics	968.5
84:12	Astringents	976.2
84:16	Cell Stimulants and Proliferants	976.8
84:20	Detergents	976.2
84:24	Emollients, Demulcents, and Protectants	976.3
84:28	Keratolytic Agents	976.4
84:32	Keratoplastic Agents	976.4
84:36	Miscellaneous Agents	976.8
86:00	**SPASMOLYTIC AGENTS**	975.1
	antiasthmatics	975.7
	papaverine	972.5
	theophyllin	974.1
88:00	**VITAMINS**	
88:04	Vitamin A	963.5
88:08	Vitamin B Complex	963.5
	hematopoietic vitamin	964.1
	nicotinic acid derivatives	972.2
88:12	Vitamin C	963.5
88:16	Vitamin D	963.5
88:20	Vitamin E	963.5
88:24	Vitamin K Activity	964.3
88:28	Multivitamin Preparations	963.5
92:00	**UNCLASSIFIED THERAPEUTIC AGENTS**	977.8

Classification of Industrial Accidents According to Agency

Annex B to the Resolution concerning Statistics of Employment Injuries adopted by the Tenth International Conference of Labor Statisticians on 12 October 1962

1 MACHINES

11 Prime-Movers, except Electrical Motors
- 111 Steam engines
- 112 Internal combustion engines
- 119 Others

12 Transmission Machinery
- 121 Transmission shafts
- 122 Transmission belts, cables, pulleys, pinions, chains, gears
- 129 Others

13 Metalworking Machines
- 131 Power presses
- 132 Lathes
- 133 Milling machines
- 134 Abrasive wheels
- 135 Mechanical shears
- 136 Forging machines
- 137 Rolling-mills
- 139 Others

14 Wood and Assimilated Machines
- 141 Circular saws
- 142 Other saws
- 143 Molding machines
- 144 Overhand planes
- 149 Others

15 Agricultural Machines
- 151 Reapers (including combine reapers)
- 152 Threshers
- 159 Others

16 Mining Machinery
- 161 Under-cutters
- 169 Others

19 Other Machines Not Elsewhere Classified
- 191 Earth-moving machines, excavating and scraping machines, except means of transport
- 192 Spinning, weaving and other textile machines
- 193 Machines for the manufacture of foodstuffs and beverages
- 194 Machines for the manufacture of paper
- 195 Printing machines
- 199 Others

2 MEANS OF TRANSPORT AND LIFTING EQUIPMENT

21 Lifting Machines and Appliances
- 211 Cranes
- 212 Lifts and elevators
- 213 Winches
- 214 Pulley blocks
- 219 Others

22 Means of Rail Transport
- 221 Inter-urban railways
- 222 Rail transport in mines, tunnels, quarries, industrial establishments, docks, etc.
- 229 Others

23 Other Wheeled Means of Transport, Excluding Rail Transport
- 231 Tractors
- 232 Lorries
- 233 Trucks
- 234 Motor vehicles, not elsewhere classified
- 235 Animal-drawn vehicles
- 236 Hand-drawn vehicles
- 239 Others

24 Means of Air Transport

25 Means of Water Transport
- 251 Motorized means of water transport
- 252 Non-motorized means of water transport

26 Other Means of Transport
- 261 Cable-cars
- 262 Mechanical conveyors, except cable-cars
- 269 Others

3 OTHER EQUIPMENT

31 Pressure Vessels
- 311 Boilers
- 312 Pressurized containers
- 313 Pressurized piping and accessories
- 314 Gas cylinders
- 315 Caissons, diving equipment
- 319 Others

32 Furnaces, Ovens, Kilns
- 321 Blast furnaces
- 322 Refining furnaces
- 323 Other furnaces
- 324 Kilns
- 325 Ovens

33 Refrigerating Plants

34 Electrical Installations, Including Electric Motors, but Excluding Electric Hand Tools
- 341 Rotating machines
- 342 Conductors
- 343 Transformers
- 344 Control apparatus
- 349 Others

35 Electric Hand Tools

36 Tools, Implements, and Appliances, Except Electric Hand Tools
- 361 Power-driven hand tools, except electric hand tools
- 362 Hand tools, not power-driven
- 369 Others

37 Ladders, Mobile Ramps

38 Scaffolding

39 Other Equipment, Not Elsewhere Classified

4 MATERIALS, SUBSTANCES AND RADIATIONS

41 Explosives

42 Dusts, Gases, Liquids and Chemicals, Excluding Explosives
- 421 Dusts
- 422 Gases, vapors, fumes
- 423 Liquids, not elsewhere classified
- 424 Chemicals, not elsewhere classified

43 Flying Fragments

44 Radiations
- 441 Ionizing radiations
- 449 Others

49 Other Materials and Substances Not Elsewhere Classified

5 WORKING ENVIRONMENT

51 Outdoor
- 511 Weather
- 512 Traffic and working surfaces
- 513 Water
- 519 Others

52 Indoor
- 521 Floors
- 522 Confined quarters
- 523 Stairs
- 524 Other traffic and working surfaces
- 525 Floor openings and wall openings
- 526 Environmental factors (lighting, ventilation, temperature, noise, etc.)
- 529 Others

53 Underground
- 531 Roofs and faces of mine roads and tunnels, etc.
- 532 Floors of mine roads and tunnels, etc.
- 533 Working-faces of mines, tunnels, etc.
- 534 Mine shafts
- 535 Fire
- 536 Water
- 539 Others

6 OTHER AGENCIES, NOT ELSEWHERE CLASSIFIED

61 Animals
- 611 Live animals
- 612 Animals products

69 Other Agencies, Not Elsewhere Classified

7 AGENCIES NOT CLASSIFIED FOR LACK OF SUFFICIENT DATA

List of Three-Digit Categories

1. INFECTIOUS AND PARASITIC DISEASES

Intestinal infectious diseases (001-009)

001 Cholera
002 Typhoid and paratyphoid fevers
003 Other salmonella infections
004 Shigellosis
005 Other food poisoning (bacterial)
006 Amebiasis
007 Other protozoal intestinal diseases
008 Intestinal infections due to other organisms
009 Ill-defined intestinal infections

Tuberculosis (010-018)

010 Primary tuberculous infection
011 Pulmonary tuberculosis
012 Other respiratory tuberculosis
013 Tuberculosis of meninges and central nervous system
014 Tuberculosis of intestines, peritoneum, and mesenteric glands
015 Tuberculosis of bones and joints
016 Tuberculosis of genitourinary system
017 Tuberculosis of other organs
018 Miliary tuberculosis

Zoonotic bacterial diseases (020-027)

020 Plague
021 Tularemia
022 Anthrax
023 Brucellosis
024 Glanders
025 Melioidosis
026 Rat-bite fever
027 Other zoonotic bacterial diseases

Other bacterial diseases (030-041)

030 Leprosy
031 Diseases due to other mycobacteria
032 Diphtheria
033 Whooping cough
034 Streptococcal sore throat and scarlet fever
035 Erysipelas
036 Meningococcal infection
037 Tetanus
038 Septicemia
039 Actinomycotic infections
040 Other bacterial diseases
041 Bacterial infection in conditions classified elsewhere and of unspecified site

Human immunodeficiency virus (HIV) infection (042)

042 Human immunodeficiency virus [HIV] disease

Poliomyelitis and other non-arthropod-borne viral diseases of central nervous system (045-049)

045 Acute poliomyelitis
046 Slow virus infection of central nervous system
047 Meningitis due to enterovirus
048 Other enterovirus diseases of central nervous system
049 Other non-arthropod-borne viral diseases of central nervous system

Viral diseases accompanied by exanthem (050-057)

050 Smallpox
051 Cowpox and paravaccinia
052 Chickenpox
053 Herpes zoster
054 Herpes simplex
055 Measles
056 Rubella
057 Other viral exanthemata

Other human herpesvirus (058)

058 Other human herpesvirus

Arthropod-borne viral diseases (060-066)

060 Yellow fever
061 Dengue
062 Mosquito-borne viral encephalitis
063 Tick-borne viral encephalitis
064 Viral encephalitis transmitted by other and unspecified arthropods
065 Arthropod-borne hemorrhagic fever
066 Other arthropod-borne viral diseases

Other diseases due to viruses and Chlamydiae (070-079)

070 Viral hepatitis
071 Rabies
072 Mumps
073 Ornithosis
074 Specific diseases due to Coxsackie virus
075 Infectious mononucleosis
076 Trachoma
077 Other diseases of conjunctiva due to viruses and Chlamydiae
078 Other diseases due to viruses and Chlamydiae
079 Viral and chlamydial infection in conditions classified elsewhere and of unspecified site

Rickettsioses and other arthropod-borne diseases (080-088)

080 Louse-borne [epidemic] typhus
081 Other typhus
082 Tick-borne rickettsioses
083 Other rickettsioses
084 Malaria
085 Leishmaniasis
086 Trypanosomiasis
087 Relapsing fever
088 Other arthropod-borne diseases

Syphilis and other venereal diseases (090-099)

090 Congenital syphilis
091 Early syphilis, symptomatic
092 Early syphilis, latent
093 Cardiovascular syphilis
094 Neurosyphilis
095 Other forms of late syphilis, with symptoms
096 Late syphilis, latent
097 Other and unspecified syphilis
098 Gonococcal infections
099 Other venereal diseases

Other spirochetal diseases (100-104)

100 Leptospirosis
101 Vincent's angina
102 Yaws
103 Pinta
104 Other spirochetal infection

Mycoses (110-118)

110 Dermatophytosis
111 Dermatomycosis, other and unspecified
112 Candidiasis
114 Coccidioidomycosis
115 Histoplasmosis
116 Blastomycotic infection
117 Other mycoses
118 Opportunistic mycoses

Helminthiases (120-129)

120 Schistosomiasis [bilharziasis]
121 Other trematode infections
122 Echinococcosis
123 Other cestode infection
124 Trichinosis
125 Filarial infection and dracontiasis
126 Ancylostomiasis and necatoriasis
127 Other intestinal helminthiases
128 Other and unspecified helminthiases
129 Intestinal parasitism, unspecified

Other infectious and parasitic diseases (130-136)

130 Toxoplasmosis
131 Trichomoniasis
132 Pediculosis and phthirus infestation
133 Acariasis
134 Other infestation
135 Sarcoidosis
136 Other and unspecified infectious and parasitic diseases

Late effects of infectious and parasitic diseases (137-139)

137 Late effects of tuberculosis
138 Late effects of acute poliomyelitis
139 Late effects of other infectious and parasitic diseases

2. NEOPLASMS

Malignant neoplasm of lip, oral cavity, and pharynx (140-149)

140 Malignant neoplasm of lip
141 Malignant neoplasm of tongue
142 Malignant neoplasm of major salivary glands
143 Malignant neoplasm of gum
144 Malignant neoplasm of floor of mouth
145 Malignant neoplasm of other and unspecified parts of mouth
146 Malignant neoplasm of oropharynx
147 Malignant neoplasm of nasopharynx
148 Malignant neoplasm of hypopharynx
149 Malignant neoplasm of other and ill-defined sites within the lip, oral cavity, and pharynx

Malignant neoplasm of digestive organs and peritoneum (150-159)

150 Malignant neoplasm of esophagus
151 Malignant neoplasm of stomach
152 Malignant neoplasm of small intestine, including duodenum
153 Malignant neoplasm of colon
154 Malignant neoplasm of rectum, rectosigmoid junction, and anus
155 Malignant neoplasm of liver and intrahepatic bile ducts
156 Malignant neoplasm of gallbladder and extrahepatic bile ducts
157 Malignant neoplasm of pancreas
158 Malignant neoplasm of retroperitoneum and peritoneum
159 Malignant neoplasm of other and ill-defined sites within the digestive organs and peritoneum

Malignant neoplasm of respiratory and intrathoracic organs (160-165)

160 Malignant neoplasm of nasal cavities, middle ear, and accessory sinuses
161 Malignant neoplasm of larynx
162 Malignant neoplasm of trachea, bronchus, and lung
163 Malignant neoplasm of pleura
164 Malignant neoplasm of thymus, heart, and mediastinum
165 Malignant neoplasm of other and ill-defined sites within the respiratory system and intrathoracic organs

Malignant neoplasm of bone, connective tissue, skin, and breast (170-176)

170 Malignant neoplasm of bone and articular cartilage
171 Malignant neoplasm of connective and other soft tissue
172 Malignant melanoma of skin
173 Other malignant neoplasm of skin
174 Malignant neoplasm of female breast
175 Malignant neoplasm of male breast
176 Kaposi's sarcoma

Malignant neoplasm of genitourinary organs (179-189)

179 Malignant neoplasm of uterus, part unspecified
180 Malignant neoplasm of cervix uteri
181 Malignant neoplasm of placenta
182 Malignant neoplasm of body of uterus
183 Malignant neoplasm of ovary and other uterine adnexa
184 Malignant neoplasm of other and unspecified female genital organs

185 Malignant neoplasm of prostate
186 Malignant neoplasm of testis
187 Malignant neoplasm of penis and other male genital organs
188 Malignant neoplasm of bladder
189 Malignant neoplasm of kidney and other and unspecified urinary organs

Malignant neoplasm of other and unspecified sites (190-199)

190 Malignant neoplasm of eye
191 Malignant neoplasm of brain
192 Malignant neoplasm of other and unspecified parts of nervous system
193 Malignant neoplasm of thyroid gland
194 Malignant neoplasm of other endocrine glands and related structures
195 Malignant neoplasm of other and ill-defined sites
196 Secondary and unspecified malignant neoplasm of lymph nodes
197 Secondary malignant neoplasm of respiratory and digestive systems
198 Secondary malignant neoplasm of other specified sites
199 Malignant neoplasm without specification of site

Malignant neoplasm of lymphatic and hematopoietic tissue (200-208)

200 Lymphosarcoma and reticulosarcoma and other specified malignant tumors of lymphatic tissue
201 Hodgkin's disease
202 Other malignant neoplasm of lymphoid and histiocytic tissue
203 Multiple myeloma and immunoproliferative neoplasms
204 Lymphoid leukemia
205 Myeloid leukemia
206 Monocytic leukemia
207 Other specified leukemia
208 Leukemia of unspecified cell type

Benign neoplasms (210-229)

210 Benign neoplasm of lip, oral cavity, and pharynx
211 Benign neoplasm of other parts of digestive system
212 Benign neoplasm of respiratory and intrathoracic organs
213 Benign neoplasm of bone and articular cartilage
214 Lipoma
215 Other benign neoplasm of connective and other soft tissue
216 Benign neoplasm of skin
217 Benign neoplasm of breast
218 Uterine leiomyoma
219 Other benign neoplasm of uterus
220 Benign neoplasm of ovary
221 Benign neoplasm of other female genital organs
222 Benign neoplasm of male genital organs
223 Benign neoplasm of kidney and other urinary organs
224 Benign neoplasm of eye
225 Benign neoplasm of brain and other parts of nervous system
226 Benign neoplasm of thyroid glands
227 Benign neoplasm of other endocrine glands and related structures
228 Hemangioma and lymphangioma, any site
229 Benign neoplasm of other and unspecified sites

Carcinoma in situ (230-234)

230 Carcinoma in situ of digestive organs
231 Carcinoma in situ of respiratory system
232 Carcinoma in situ of skin
233 Carcinoma in situ of breast and genitourinary system
234 Carcinoma in situ of other and unspecified sites

Neoplasms of uncertain behavior (235-238)

235 Neoplasm of uncertain behavior of digestive and respiratory systems
236 Neoplasm of uncertain behavior of genitourinary organs
237 Neoplasm of uncertain behavior of endocrine glands and nervous system
238 Neoplasm of uncertain behavior of other and unspecified sites and tissues

Neoplasms of unspecified nature (239)

239 Neoplasms of unspecified nature

3. ENDOCRINE, NUTRITIONAL AND METABOLIC DISEASES, AND IMMUNITY DISORDERS

Disorders of thyroid gland (240-246)

240 Simple and unspecified goiter
241 Nontoxic nodular goiter
242 Thyrotoxicosis with or without goiter
243 Congenital hypothyroidism
244 Acquired hypothyroidism
245 Thyroiditis
246 Other disorders of thyroid

Diseases of other endocrine glands (250-259)

250 Diabetes mellitus
251 Other disorders of pancreatic internal secretion
252 Disorders of parathyroid gland
253 Disorders of the pituitary gland and its hypothalamic control
254 Diseases of thymus gland
255 Disorders of adrenal glands
256 Ovarian dysfunction
257 Testicular dysfunction
258 Polyglandular dysfunction and related disorders
259 Other endocrine disorders

Nutritional deficiencies (260-269)

260 Kwashiorkor
261 Nutritional marasmus
262 Other severe protein-calorie malnutrition
263 Other and unspecified protein-calorie malnutrition
264 Vitamin A deficiency
265 Thiamine and niacin deficiency states
266 Deficiency of B-complex components
267 Ascorbic acid deficiency
268 Vitamin D deficiency
269 Other nutritional deficiencies

Other metabolic disorders and immunity disorders (270-279)

270 Disorders of amino-acid transport and metabolism
271 Disorders of carbohydrate transport and metabolism
272 Disorders of lipoid metabolism
273 Disorders of plasma protein metabolism
274 Gout
275 Disorders of mineral metabolism
276 Disorders of fluid, electrolyte, and acid-base balance
277 Other and unspecified disorders of metabolism
278 Overweight, obesity and other hyperalimentation
279 Disorders involving the immune mechanism

4. DISEASES OF THE BLOOD AND BLOOD-FORMING ORGANS

Diseases of the blood and blood-forming organs (280-289)

280 Iron deficiency anemias
281 Other deficiency anemias
282 Hereditary hemolytic anemias
283 Acquired hemolytic anemias
284 Aplastic anemia and other bone marrow failure syndromes
285 Other and unspecified anemias
286 Coagulation defects
287 Purpura and other hemorrhagic conditions
288 Diseases of white blood cells
289 Other diseases of blood and blood-forming organs

5. MENTAL DISORDERS

Organic psychotic conditions (290-294)

290 Dementias
291 Alcohol-induced mental disorders
292 Drug-induced mental disorders
293 Transient mental disorders due to conditions classified elsewhere
294 Persistent mental disorders due to conditions classified elsewhere

Other psychoses (295-299)

295 Schizophrenic disorders
296 Episodic mood disorders
297 Delusional disorders
298 Other nonorganic psychoses
299 Pervasive developmental disorders

Neurotic disorders, personality disorders, and other nonpsychotic mental disorders (300-316)

300 Anxiety, dissociative and somatoform disorders
301 Personality disorders
302 Sexual and gender identity disorders
303 Alcohol dependence syndrome
304 Drug dependence
305 Nondependent abuse of drugs
306 Physiological malfunction arising from mental factors
307 Special symptoms or syndromes, not elsewhere classified
308 Acute reaction to stress
309 Adjustment reaction
310 Specific nonpsychotic mental disorders due to organic brain damage
311 Depressive disorder, not elsewhere classified
312 Disturbance of conduct, not elsewhere classified
313 Disturbance of emotions specific to childhood and adolescence
314 Hyperkinetic syndrome of childhood
315 Specific delays in development
316 Psychic factors associated with diseases classified elsewhere

Mental retardation (317-319)

317 Mild mental retardation
318 Other specified mental retardation
319 Unspecified mental retardation

6. DISEASES OF THE NERVOUS SYSTEM AND SENSE ORGANS

Inflammatory diseases of the central nervous system (320-326)

320 Bacterial meningitis
321 Meningitis due to other organisms
322 Meningitis of unspecified cause
323 Encephalitis, myelitis, and encephalomyelitis
324 Intracranial and intraspinal abscess
325 Phlebitis and thrombophlebitis of intracranial venous sinuses
326 Late effects of intracranial abscess or pyogenic infection

Organic sleep disorders (327)

327 Organic sleep disorders

Hereditary and degenerative diseases of the central nervous system (330-337)

330 Cerebral degenerations usually manifest in childhood
331 Other cerebral degenerations
332 Parkinson's disease
333 Other extrapyramidal disease and abnormal movement disorders
334 Spinocerebellar disease
335 Anterior horn cell disease
336 Other diseases of spinal cord
337 Disorders of the autonomic nervous system

Pain (338)

338 Pain, not elsewhere classified

Other disorders of the central nervous system (340-349)

340 Multiple sclerosis
341 Other demyelinating diseases of central nervous system
342 Hemiplegia and hemiparesis
343 Infantile cerebral palsy
344 Other paralytic syndromes
345 Epilepsy and recurrent seizures
346 Migraine

347 Cataplexy and narcolepsy
348 Other conditions of brain
349 Other and unspecified disorders of the nervous system

Disorders of the peripheral nervous system (350-359)

350 Trigeminal nerve disorders
351 Facial nerve disorders
352 Disorders of other cranial nerves
353 Nerve root and plexus disorders
354 Mononeuritis of upper limb and mononeuritis multiplex
355 Mononeuritis of lower limb
356 Hereditary and idiopathic peripheral neuropathy
357 Inflammatory and toxic neuropathy
358 Myoneural disorders
359 Muscular dystrophies and other myopathies

Disorders of the eye and adnexa (360-379)

360 Disorders of the globe
361 Retinal detachments and defects
362 Other retinal disorders
363 Chorioretinal inflammations and scars and other disorders of choroid
364 Disorders of iris and ciliary body
365 Glaucoma
366 Cataract
367 Disorders of refraction and accommodation
368 Visual disturbances
369 Blindness and low vision
370 Keratitis
371 Corneal opacity and other disorders of cornea
372 Disorders of conjunctiva
373 Inflammation of eyelids
374 Other disorders of eyelids
375 Disorders of lacrimal system
376 Disorders of the orbit
377 Disorders of optic nerve and visual pathways
378 Strabismus and other disorders of binocular eye movements
379 Other disorders of eye

Diseases of the ear and mastoid process (380-389)

380 Disorders of external ear
381 Nonsuppurative otitis media and Eustachian tube disorders
382 Suppurative and unspecified otitis media
383 Mastoiditis and related conditions
384 Other disorders of tympanic membrane
385 Other disorders of middle ear and mastoid
386 Vertiginous syndromes and other disorders of vestibular system
387 Otosclerosis
388 Other disorders of ear
389 Hearing loss

7. DISEASES OF THE CIRCULATORY SYSTEM

Acute rheumatic fever (390-392)

390 Rheumatic fever without mention of heart involvement
391 Rheumatic fever with heart involvement
392 Rheumatic chorea

Chronic rheumatic heart disease (393-398)

393 Chronic rheumatic pericarditis
394 Diseases of mitral valve
395 Diseases of aortic valve
396 Diseases of mitral and aortic valves
397 Diseases of other endocardial structures
398 Other rheumatic heart disease

Hypertensive disease (401-405)

401 Essential hypertension
402 Hypertensive heart disease
403 Hypertensive chronic kidney disease
404 Hypertensive heart and chronic kidney disease
405 Secondary hypertension

Ischemic heart disease (410-414)

410 Acute myocardial infarction
411 Other acute and subacute form of ischemic heart disease
412 Old myocardial infarction
413 Angina pectoris
414 Other forms of chronic ischemic heart disease

Diseases of pulmonary circulation (415-417)

415 Acute pulmonary heart disease
416 Chronic pulmonary heart disease
417 Other diseases of pulmonary circulation

Other forms of heart disease (420-429)

420 Acute pericarditis
421 Acute and subacute endocarditis
422 Acute myocarditis
423 Other diseases of pericardium
424 Other diseases of endocardium
425 Cardiomyopathy
426 Conduction disorders
427 Cardiac dysrhythmias
428 Heart failure
429 Ill-defined descriptions and complications of heart disease

Cerebrovascular disease (430-438)

430 Subarachnoid hemorrhage
431 Intracerebral hemorrhage
432 Other and unspecified intracranial hemorrhage
433 Occlusion and stenosis of precerebral arteries
434 Occlusion of cerebral arteries
435 Transcient cerebral ischemia
436 Acute but ill-defined cerebrovascular disease
437 Other and ill-defined cerebrovascular disease
438 Late effects of cerebrovascular disease

Diseases of arteries, arterioles, and capillaries (440-449)

440 Atherosclerosis
441 Aortic aneurysm and dissection
442 Other aneurysm
443 Other peripheral vascular disease
444 Arterial embolism and thrombosis
445 Atheroembolism
446 Polyarteritis nodosa and allied conditions
447 Other disorders of arteries and arterioles
448 Disease of capillaries
449 Septic arterial embolism

Diseases of veins and lymphatics, and other diseases of circulatory system (451-459)

451 Phlebitis and thrombophlebitis
452 Portal vein thrombosis
453 Other venous embolism and thrombosis
454 Varicose veins of lower extremities
455 Hemorrhoids
456 Varicose veins of other sites
457 Noninfectious disorders of lymphatic channels
458 Hypotension
459 Other disorders of circulatory system

8. DISEASES OF THE RESPIRATORY SYSTEM

Acute respiratory infections (460-466)

460 Acute nasopharyngitis [common cold]
461 Acute sinusitis
462 Acute pharyngitis
463 Acute tonsillitis
464 Acute laryngitis and tracheitis
465 Acute upper respiratory infections of multiple or unspecified sites
466 Acute bronchitis and bronchiolitis

Other diseases of upper respiratory tract (470-478)

470 Deviated nasal septum
471 Nasal polyps
472 Chronic pharyngitis and nasopharyngitis
473 Chronic sinusitis
474 Chronic disease of tonsils and adenoids
475 Peritonsillar abscess
476 Chronic laryngitis and laryngotracheitis
477 Allergic rhinitis
478 Other diseases of upper respiratory tract

Pneumonia and influenza (480-488)

480 Viral pneumonia
481 Pneumococcal pneumonia [Streptococcus pneumoniae pneumonia]
482 Other bacterial pneumonia
483 Pneumonia due to other specified organism
484 Pneumonia in infectious diseases classified elsewhere
485 Bronchopneumonia, organism unspecified
486 Pneumonia, organism unspecified
487 Influenza
488 Influenza due to identified avian influenza virus

Chronic obstructive pulmonary disease and allied conditions (490-496)

490 Bronchitis, not specified as acute or chronic
491 Chronic bronchitis
492 Emphysema
493 Asthma
494 Bronchiectasis
495 Extrinsic allergic alveolitis
496 Chronic airways obstruction, not elsewhere classified

Pneumoconioses and other lung diseases due to external agents (500-508)

500 Coalworkers' pneumoconiosis
501 Asbestosis
502 Pneumoconiosis due to other silica or silicates
503 Pneumoconiosis due to other inorganic dust
504 Pneumopathy due to inhalation of other dust
505 Pneumoconiosis, unspecified
506 Respiratory conditions due to chemical fumes and vapors
507 Pneumonitis due to solids and liquids
508 Respiratory conditions due to other and unspecified external agents

Other diseases of respiratory system (510-519)

510 Empyema
511 Pleurisy
512 Pneumothorax
513 Abscess of lung and mediastinum
514 Pulmonary congestion and hypostasis
515 Postinflammatory pulmonary fibrosis
516 Other alveolar and parietoalveolar pneumopathy
517 Lung involvement in conditions classified elsewhere
518 Other diseases of lung
519 Other diseases of respiratory system

9. DISEASES OF THE DIGESTIVE SYSTEM

Diseases of oral cavity, salivary glands, and jaws (520-529)

520 Disorders of tooth development and eruption
521 Diseases of hard tissues of teeth
522 Diseases of pulp and periapical tissues
523 Gingival and periodontal diseases
524 Dentofacial anomalies, including malocclusion
525 Other diseases and conditions of the teeth and supporting structures
526 Diseases of the jaws
527 Diseases of the salivary glands
528 Diseases of the oral soft tissues, excluding lesions specific for gingiva and tongue
529 Diseases and other conditions of the tongue

Diseases of esophagus, stomach, and duodenum (530-538)

530 Diseases of esophagus
531 Gastric ulcer
532 Duodenal ulcer
533 Peptic ulcer, site unspecified
534 Gastrojejunal ulcer
535 Gastritis and duodenitis
536 Disorders of function of stomach
537 Other disorders of stomach and duodenum

538 Gastrointestinal mucositis (ulcerative)

Appendicitis (540-543)

540 Acute appendicitis
541 Appendicitis, unqualified
542 Other appendicitis
543 Other diseases of appendix

Hernia of abdominal cavity (550-553)

550 Inguinal hernia
551 Other hernia of abdominal cavity, with gangrene
552 Other hernia of abdominal cavity, with obstruction, but without mention of gangrene
553 Other hernia of abdominal cavity without mention of obstruction or gangrene

Noninfective enteritis and colitis (555-558)

555 Regional enteritis
556 Ulcerative colitis
557 Vascular insufficiency of intestine
558 Other and unspecified noninfective gastroenteritis and colitis

Other diseases of intestines and peritoneum (560-569)

560 Intestinal obstruction without mention of hernia
562 Diverticula of intestine
564 Functional digestive disorders, not elsewhere classified
565 Anal fissure and fistula
566 Abscess of anal and rectal regions
567 Peritonitis and retroperitoneal infections
568 Other disorders of peritoneum
569 Other disorders of intestine

Other diseases of digestive system (570-579)

570 Acute and subacute necrosis of liver
571 Chronic liver disease and cirrhosis
572 Liver abscess and sequelae of chronic liver disease
573 Other disorders of liver
574 Cholelithiasis
575 Other disorders of gallbladder
576 Other disorders of biliary tract
577 Diseases of pancreas
578 Gastrointestinal hemorrhage
579 Intestinal malabsorption

10. DISEASES OF THE GENITOURINARY SYSTEM

Nephritis, nephrotic syndrome, and nephrosis (580-589)

580 Acute glomerulonephritis
581 Nephrotic syndrome
582 Chronic glomerulonephritis
583 Nephritis and nephropathy, not specified as acute or chronic
584 Acute renal failure
585 Chronic kidney disease (CKD)
586 Renal failure, unspecified
587 Renal sclerosis, unspecified
588 Disorders resulting from impaired renal function
589 Small kidney of unknown cause

Other diseases of urinary system (590-599)

590 Infections of kidney
591 Hydronephrosis
592 Calculus of kidney and ureter
593 Other disorders of kidney and ureter
594 Calculus of lower urinary tract
595 Cystitis
596 Other disorders of bladder
597 Urethritis, not sexually transmitted, and urethral syndrome
598 Urethral stricture
599 Other disorders of urethra and urinary tract

Diseases of male genital organs (600-608)

600 Hyperplasia of prostate
601 Inflammatory diseases of prostate
602 Other disorders of prostate
603 Hydrocele
604 Orchitis and epididymitis
605 Redundant prepuce and phimosis
606 Infertility, male
607 Disorders of penis
608 Other disorders of male genital organs

Disorders of breast (610-611)

610 Benign mammary dysplasias
611 Other disorders of breast

Inflammatory disease of female pelvic organs (614-616)

614 Inflammatory disease of ovary, fallopian tube, pelvic cellular tissue, and peritoneum
615 Inflammatory diseases of uterus, except cervix
616 Inflammatory disease of cervix, vagina, and vulva

Other disorders of female genital tract (617-629)

617 Endometriosis
618 Genital prolapse
619 Fistula involving female genital tract
620 Noninflammatory disorders of ovary, fallopian tube, and broad ligament
621 Disorders of uterus, not elsewhere classified
622 Noninflammatory disorders of cervix
623 Noninflammatory disorders of vagina
624 Noninflammatory disorders of vulva and perineum
625 Pain and other symptoms associated with female genital organs
626 Disorders of menstruation and other abnormal bleeding from female genital tract
627 Menopausal and postmenopausal disorders
628 Infertility, female
629 Other disorders of female genital organs

11. COMPLICATIONS OF PREGNANCY, CHILDBIRTH, AND THE PUERPERIUM

Ectopic and molar pregnancy (630-633)

630 Hydatidiform mole
631 Other abnormal product of conception
632 Missed abortion
633 Ectopic pregnancy

Other pregnancy with abortive outcome (634-639)

634 Spontaneous abortion
635 Legally induced abortion
636 Illegally induced abortion
637 Unspecified abortion
638 Failed attempted abortion
639 Complications following abortion and ectopic and molar pregnancies

Complications mainly related to pregnancy (640-649)

640 Hemorrhage in early pregnancy
641 Antepartum hemorrhage, abruptio placentae, and placenta previa
642 Hypertension complicating pregnancy, childbirth, and the puerperium
643 Excessive vomiting in pregnancy
644 Early or threatened labor
645 Late pregnancy
646 Other complications of pregnancy, not elsewhere classified
647 Infectious and parasitic conditions in the mother classifiable elsewhere but complicating pregnancy, childbirth, and the puerperium
648 Other current conditions in the mother classifiable elsewhere but complicating pregnancy, childbirth, and the puerperium
649 Other conditions or status of the mother complicating pregnancy, childbirth, or the puerperium

Normal delivery, and other indications for care in pregnancy, labor, and delivery (650-659)

650 Normal delivery
651 Multiple gestation
652 Malposition and malpresentation of fetus
653 Disproportion
654 Abnormality of organs and soft tissues of pelvis
655 Known or suspected fetal abnormality affecting management of mother
656 Other fetal and placental problems affecting management of mother
657 Polyhydramnios
658 Other problems associated with amniotic cavity and membranes
659 Other indications for care or intervention related to labor and delivery, not elsewhere classified

Complications occurring mainly in the course of labor and delivery (660-669)

660 Obstructed labor
661 Abnormality of forces of labor
662 Long labor
663 Umbilical cord complications
664 Trauma to perineum and vulva during delivery
665 Other obstetrical trauma
666 Postpartum hemorrhage
667 Retained placenta without hemorrhage
668 Complications of the administration of anesthetic or other sedation in labor and delivery
669 Other complications of labor and delivery not elsewhere classified

Complications of the puerperium (670-677)

670 Major puerperal infection
671 Venous complications in pregnancy and the puerperium
672 Pyrexia of unknown origin during the puerperium
673 Obstetrical pulmonary embolism
674 Other and unspecified complications of the puerperium, not elsewhere classified
675 Infections of the breast and nipple associated with childbirth
676 Other disorders of the breast associated with childbirth, and disorders of lactation
677 Late effect of complication of pregnancy, childbirth, and the puerperium

12. DISEASES OF THE SKIN AND SUBCUTANEOUS TISSUE

Infections of skin and subcutaneous tissue (680-686)

680 Carbuncle and furuncle
681 Cellulitis and abscess of finger and toe
682 Other cellulitis and abscess
683 Acute lymphadenitis
684 Impetigo
685 Pilonidal cyst
686 Other local infections of skin and subcutaneous tissue

Other inflammatory conditions of skin and subcutaneous tissue (690-698)

690 Erythematosquamous dermatosis
691 Atopic dermatitis and related conditions
692 Contact dermatitis and other eczema
693 Dermatitis due to substances taken internally
694 Bullous dermatoses
695 Erythematous conditions
696 Psoriasis and similar disorders
697 Lichen
698 Pruritus and related conditions

Other diseases of skin and subcutaneous tissue (700-709)

700 Corns and callosities
701 Other hypertrophic and atrophic conditions of skin
702 Other dermatoses
703 Diseases of nail
704 Diseases of hair and hair follicles
705 Disorders of sweat glands
706 Diseases of sebaceous glands
707 Chronic ulcer of skin
708 Urticaria
709 Other disorders of skin and subcutaneous tissue

13. DISEASES OF THE MUSCULOSKELETAL SYSTEM AND CONNECTIVE TISSUE

Arthropathies and related disorders (710-719)

710 Diffuse diseases of connective tissue
711 Arthropathy associated with infections
712 Crystal arthropathies
713 Arthropathy associated with other disorders classified elsewhere
714 Rheumatoid arthritis and other inflammatory polyarthropathies
715 Osteoarthrosis and allied disorders
716 Other and unspecified arthropathies
717 Internal derangement of knee
718 Other derangement of joint
719 Other and unspecified disorders of joint

Dorsopathies (720-724)

720 Ankylosing spondylitis and other inflammatory spondylopathies
721 Spondylosis and allied disorders
722 Intervertebral disc disorders
723 Other disorders of cervical region
724 Other and unspecified disorders of back

Rheumatism, excluding the back (725-729)

725 Polymyalgia rheumatica
726 Peripheral enthesopathies and allied syndromes
727 Other disorders of synovium, tendon, and bursa
728 Disorders of muscle, ligament, and fascia
729 Other disorders of soft tissues

Osteopathies, chondropathies, and acquired musculoskeletal deformities (730-739)

730 Osteomyelitis, periostitis, and other infections involving bone
731 Osteitis deformans and osteopathies associated with other disorders classified elsewhere
732 Osteochondropathies
733 Other disorders of bone and cartilage
734 Flat foot
735 Acquired deformities of toe
736 Other acquired deformities of limbs
737 Curvature of spine
738 Other acquired deformity
739 Nonallopathic lesions, not elsewhere classified

14. CONGENITAL ANOMALIES

Congential anomalies (740-759)

740 Anencephalus and similar anomalies
741 Spina bifida
742 Other congenital anomalies of nervous system
743 Congenital anomalies of eye
744 Congenital anomalies of ear, face, and neck
745 Bulbus cordis anomalies and anomalies of cardiac septal closure
746 Other congenital anomalies of heart
747 Other congenital anomalies of circulatory system
748 Congenital anomalies of respiratory system
749 Cleft palate and cleft lip
750 Other congenital anomalies of upper alimentary tract
751 Other congenital anomalies of digestive system
752 Congenital anomalies of genital organs
753 Congenital anomalies of urinary system
754 Certain congenital musculoskeletal deformities
755 Other congenital anomalies of limbs
756 Other congenital musculoskeletal anomalies
757 Congenital anomalies of the integument
758 Chromosomal anomalies
759 Other and unspecified congenital anomalies

15. CERTAIN CONDITIONS ORIGINATING IN THE PERINATAL PERIOD

Maternal causes of perinatal morbidity and mortality (760-763)

760 Fetus or newborn affected by maternal conditions which may be unrelated to present pregnancy
761 Fetus or newborn affected by maternal complications of pregnancy
762 Fetus or newborn affected by complications of placenta, cord, and membranes
763 Fetus or newborn affected by other complications of labor and delivery

Other conditions originating in the perinatal period (764-779)

764 Slow fetal growth and fetal malnutrition
765 Disorders relating to short gestation and unspecified low birthweight
766 Disorders relating to long gestation and high birthweight
767 Birth trauma
768 Intrauterine hypoxia and birth asphyxia
769 Respiratory distress syndrome
770 Other respiratory conditions of fetus and newborn
771 Infections specific to the perinatal period
772 Fetal and neonatal hemorrhage
773 Hemolytic disease of fetus or newborn, due to isoimmunization
774 Other perinatal jaundice
775 Endocrine and metabolic disturbances specific to the fetus and newborn
776 Hematological disorders of fetus and newborn
777 Perinatal disorders of digestive system
778 Conditions involving the integument and temperature regulation of fetus and newborn
779 Other and ill-defined conditions originating in the perinatal period

16. SYMPTOMS, SIGNS, AND ILL-DEFINED CONDITIONS

Symptoms (780-789)

780 General symptoms
781 Symptoms involving nervous and musculoskeletal systems
782 Symptoms involving skin and other integumentary tissue
783 Symptoms concerning nutrition, metabolism, and development
784 Symptoms involving head and neck
785 Symptoms involving cardiovascular system
786 Symptoms involving respiratory system and other chest symptoms
787 Symptoms involving digestive system
788 Symptoms involving urinary system
789 Other symptoms involving abdomen and pelvis

Nonspecific abnormal findings (790-796)

790 Nonspecific findings on examination of blood
791 Nonspecific findings on examination of urine
792 Nonspecific abnormal findings in other body substances
793 Nonspecific abnormal findings on radiological and other examination of body structure
794 Nonspecific abnormal results of function studies
795 Other and nonspecific abnormal cytological, histological, immunological and DNA test findings
796 Other nonspecific abnormal findings

Ill-defined and unknown causes of morbidity and mortality (797-799)

797 Senility without mention of psychosis
798 Sudden death, cause unknown
799 Other ill-defined and unknown causes of morbidity and mortality

17. INJURY AND POISONING

Fracture of skull (800-804)

800 Fracture of vault of skull
801 Fracture of base of skull
802 Fracture of face bones
803 Other and unqualified skull fractures
804 Multiple fractures involving skull or face with other bones

Fracture of spine and trunk (805-809)

805 Fracture of vertebral column without mention of spinal cord lesion
806 Fracture of vertebral column with spinal cord injury
807 Fracture of rib(s), sternum, larynx, and trachea
808 Fracture of pelvis
809 Ill-defined fractures of bones of trunk

Fracture of upper limb (810-819)

810 Fracture of clavicle
811 Fracture of scapula
812 Fracture of humerus
813 Fracture of radius and ulna
814 Fracture of carpal bone(s)
815 Fracture of metacarpal bone(s)
816 Fracture of one or more phalanges of hand
817 Multiple fractures of hand bones
818 Ill-defined fractures of upper limb
819 Multiple fractures involving both upper limbs, and upper limb with rib(s) and sternum

Fracture of lower limb (820-829)

820 Fracture of neck of femur
821 Fracture of other and unspecified parts of femur
822 Fracture of patella
823 Fracture of tibia and fibula
824 Fracture of ankle
825 Fracture of one or more tarsal and metatarsal bones
826 Fracture of one or more phalanges of foot
827 Other, multiple, and ill-defined fractures of lower limb
828 Multiple fractures involving both lower limbs, lower with upper limb, and lower limb(s) with rib(s) and sternum
829 Fracture of unspecified bones

Dislocation (830-839)

830 Dislocation of jaw
831 Dislocation of shoulder
832 Dislocation of elbow
833 Dislocation of wrist
834 Dislocation of finger
835 Dislocation of hip
836 Dislocation of knee
837 Dislocation of ankle
838 Dislocation of foot
839 Other, multiple, and ill-defined dislocations

Sprains and strains of joints and adjacent muscles (840-848)

840 Sprains and strains of shoulder and upper arm
841 Sprains and strains of elbow and forearm
842 Sprains and strains of wrist and hand
843 Sprains and strains of hip and thigh
844 Sprains and strains of knee and leg
845 Sprains and strains of ankle and foot
846 Sprains and strains of sacroiliac region
847 Sprains and strains of other and unspecified parts of back
848 Other and ill-defined sprains and strains

Intracranial injury, excluding those with skull fracture (850-854)

850 Concussion
851 Cerebral laceration and contusion
852 Subarachnoid, subdural, and extradural hemorrhage, following injury
853 Other and unspecified intracranial hemorrhage following injury
854 Intracranial injury of other and unspecified nature

Internal injury of thorax, abdomen, and pelvis (860-869)

860 Traumatic pneumothorax and hemothorax
861 Injury to heart and lung
862 Injury to other and unspecified intrathoracic organs
863 Injury to gastrointestinal tract
864 Injury to liver
865 Injury to spleen
866 Injury to kidney
867 Injury to pelvic organs
868 Injury to other intra-abdominal organs
869 Internal injury to unspecified or ill-defined organs

Open wound of head, neck, and trunk (870-879)

870 Open wound of ocular adnexa
871 Open wound of eyeball
872 Open wound of ear
873 Other open wound of head
874 Open wound of neck
875 Open wound of chest (wall)
876 Open wound of back
877 Open wound of buttock
878 Open wound of genital organs (external), including traumatic amputation
879 Open wound of other and unspecified sites, except limbs

Open wound of upper limb (880-887)

880 Open wound of shoulder and upper arm
881 Open wound of elbow, forearm, and wrist
882 Open wound of hand except finger(s) alone
883 Open wound of finger(s)
884 Multiple and unspecified open wound of upper limb
885 Traumatic amputation of thumb (complete) (partial)
886 Traumatic amputation of other finger(s) (complete) (partial)
887 Traumatic amputation of arm and hand (complete) (partial)

Open wound of lower limb (890-897)

890 Open wound of hip and thigh
891 Open wound of knee, leg [except thigh], and ankle
892 Open wound of foot except toe(s) alone
893 Open wound of toe(s)
894 Multiple and unspecified open wound of lower limb
895 Traumatic amputation of toe(s) (complete) (partial)
896 Traumatic amputation of foot (complete) (partial)
897 Traumatic amputation of leg(s) (complete) (partial)

Injury to blood vessels (900-904)

900 Injury to blood vessels of head and neck
901 Injury to blood vessels of thorax
902 Injury to blood vessels of abdomen and pelvis
903 Injury to blood vessels of upper extremity
904 Injury to blood vessels of lower extremity and unspecified sites

Late effects of injuries, poisonings, toxic effects, and other external causes (905-909)

905 Late effects of musculoskeletal and connective tissue injuries
906 Late effects of injuries to skin and subcutaneous tissues
907 Late effects of injuries to the nervous system
908 Late effects of other and unspecified injuries
909 Late effects of other and unspecified external causes

Superficial injury (910-919)

910 Superficial injury of face, neck, and scalp except eye
911 Superficial injury of trunk
912 Superficial injury of shoulder and upper arm
913 Superficial injury of elbow, forearm, and wrist
914 Superficial injury of hand(s) except finger(s) alone
915 Superficial injury of finger(s)
916 Superficial injury of hip, thigh, leg, and ankle
917 Superficial injury of foot and toe(s)
918 Superficial injury of eye and adnexa
919 Superficial injury of other, multiple, and unspecified sites

Contusion with intact skin surface (920-924)

920 Contusion of face, scalp, and neck except eye(s)
921 Contusion of eye and adnexa
922 Contusion of trunk
923 Contusion of upper limb
924 Contusion of lower limb and of other and unspecified sites

Crushing injury (925-929)

925 Crushing injury of face, scalp, and neck
926 Crushing injury of trunk
927 Crushing injury of upper limb
928 Crushing injury of lower limb
929 Crushing injury of multiple and unspecified sites

Effects of foreign body entering through orifice (930-939)

930 Foreign body on external eye
931 Foreign body in ear
932 Foreign body in nose
933 Foreign body in pharynx and larynx
934 Foreign body in trachea, bronchus, and lung
935 Foreign body in mouth, esophagus, and stomach
936 Foreign body in intestine and colon
937 Foreign body in anus and rectum
938 Foreign body in digestive system, unspecified
939 Foreign body in genitourinary tract

Burns (940-949)

940 Burn confined to eye and adnexa
941 Burn of face, head, and neck
942 Burn of trunk
943 Burn of upper limb, except wrist and hand
944 Burn of wrist(s) and hand(s)
945 Burn of lower limb(s)
946 Burns of multiple specified sites
947 Burn of internal organs
948 Burns classified according to extent of body surface involved
949 Burn, unspecified

Injury to nerves and spinal cord (950-957)

950 Injury to optic nerve and pathways
951 Injury to other cranial nerve(s)
952 Spinal cord injury without evidence of spinal bone injury
953 Injury to nerve roots and spinal plexus
954 Injury to other nerve(s) of trunk excluding shoulder and pelvic girdles
955 Injury to peripheral nerve(s) of shoulder girdle and upper limb
956 Injury to peripheral nerve(s) of pelvic girdle and lower limb
957 Injury to other and unspecified nerves

Certain traumatic complications and unspecified injuries (958-959)

958 Certain early complications of trauma
959 Injury, other and unspecified

Poisoning by drugs, medicinals and biological substances (960-979)

960 Poisoning by antibiotics
961 Poisoning by other anti-infectives
962 Poisoning by hormones and synthetic substitutes
963 Poisoning by primarily systemic agents
964 Poisoning by agents primarily affecting blood constituents
965 Poisoning by analgesics, antipyretics, and antirheumatics
966 Poisoning by anticonvulsants and anti-Parkinsonism drugs
967 Poisoning by sedatives and hypnotics
968 Poisoning by other central nervous system depressants and anesthetics
969 Poisoning by psychotropic agents
970 Poisoning by central nervous system stimulants
971 Poisoning by drugs primarily affecting the autonomic nervous system
972 Poisoning by agents primarily affecting the cardiovascular system
973 Poisoning by agents primarily affecting the gastrointestinal system
974 Poisoning by water, mineral, and uric acid metabolism drugs
975 Poisoning by agents primarily acting on the smooth and skeletal muscles and respiratory system
976 Poisoning by agents primarily affecting skin and mucous membrane, ophthalmological, otorhinolaryngological, and dental drugs
977 Poisoning by other and unspecified drugs and medicinals
978 Poisoning by bacterial vaccines
979 Poisoning by other vaccines and biological substances

Toxic effects of substances chiefly nonmedicinal as to source (980-989)

980 Toxic effect of alcohol
981 Toxic effect of petroleum products
982 Toxic effect of solvents other than petroleum-based
983 Toxic effect of corrosive aromatics, acids, and caustic alkalis
984 Toxic effect of lead and its compounds (including fumes)
985 Toxic effect of other metals
986 Toxic effect of carbon monoxide
987 Toxic effect of other gases, fumes, or vapors
988 Toxic effect of noxious substances eaten as food
989 Toxic effect of other substances, chiefly nonmedicinal as to source

Other and unspecified effects of external causes (990-995)

990 Effects of radiation, unspecified
991 Effects of reduced temperature
992 Effects of heat and light
993 Effects of air pressure
994 Effects of other external causes
995 Certain adverse effects, not elsewhere classified

Complications of surgical and medical care, not elsewhere classified (996-999)

996 Complications peculiar to certain specified procedures
997 Complications affecting specified body systems, not elsewhere classified
998 Other complications of procedures, NEC
999 Complications of medical care, not elsewhere classified

SUPPLEMENTARY CLASSIFICATION OF FACTORS INFLUENCING HEALTH STATUS AND CONTACT WITH HEALTH SERVICES

Persons with potential health hazards related to communicable diseases (V01-V06)

V01 Contact with or exposure to communicable diseases
V02 Carrier or suspected carrier of infectious diseases
V03 Need for prophylactic vaccination and inoculation against bacterial diseases
V04 Need for prophylactic vaccination and inoculation against certain diseases
V05 Need for other prophylactic vaccination and inoculation against single diseases
V06 Need for prophylactic vaccination and inoculation against combinations of diseases

Persons with need for isolation, other potential health hazards and prophylactic measures (V07-V09)

V07 Need for isolation and other prophylactic measures
V08 Asymptomatic human immunodeficiency virus [HIV] infection status
V09 Infection with drug-resistant microorganisms

Persons with potential health hazards related to personal and family history (V10-V19)

V10 Personal history of malignant neoplasm
V11 Personal history of mental disorder
V12 Personal history of certain other diseases
V13 Personal history of other diseases
V14 Personal history of allergy to medicinal agents
V15 Other personal history presenting hazards to health
V16 Family history of malignant neoplasm
V17 Family history of certain chronic disabling diseases
V18 Family history of certain other specific conditions
V19 Family history of other conditions

Persons encountering health services in circumstances related to reproduction and development (V20-V29)

V20 Health supervision of infant or child
V21 Constitutional states in development
V22 Normal pregnancy
V23 Supervision of high-risk pregnancy
V24 Postpartum care and examination
V25 Encounter for contraceptive management
V26 Procreative management
V27 Outcome of delivery
V28 Encounter for antenatal screening of mother
V29 Observation and evaluation of newborns and infants for suspected condition not found

Liveborn infants according to type of birth (V30-V39)

V30 Single liveborn
V31 Twin, mate liveborn
V32 Twin, mate stillborn
V33 Twin, unspecified
V34 Other multiple, mates all liveborn
V35 Other multiple, mates all stillborn
V36 Other multiple, mates live- and stillborn
V37 Other multiple, unspecified
V39 Unspecified

Persons with a condition influencing their health status (V40-V49)

V40 Mental and behavioral problems
V41 Problems with special senses and other special functions
V42 Organ or tissue replaced by transplant
V43 Organ or tissue replaced by other means
V44 Artificial opening status
V45 Other postsurgical states
V46 Other dependence on machines
V47 Other problems with internal organs
V48 Problems with head, neck, and trunk
V49 Other conditions influencing health status

Persons encountering health services for specific procedures and aftercare (V50-V59)

V50 Elective surgery for purposes other than remedying health states
V51 Aftercare involving the use of plastic surgery
V52 Fitting and adjustment of prosthetic device
V53 Fitting and adjustment of other device
V54 Other orthopedic aftercare
V55 Attention to artificial openings
V56 Encounter for dialysis and dialysis catheter care
V57 Care involving use of rehabilitation procedures
V58 Encounter for other and unspecified procedures and aftercare
V59 Donors

Persons encountering health services in other circumstances (V60-V69)

V60 Housing, household, and economic circumstances
V61 Other family circumstances
V62 Other psychosocial circumstances
V63 Unavailability of other medical facilities for care
V64 Persons encountering health services for specific procedures, not carried out
V65 Other persons seeking consultation
V66 Convalescence and palliative care
V67 Follow-up examination
V68 Encounters for administrative purposes
V69 Problems related to lifestyle

Persons without reported diagnosis encountered during examination and investigation of individuals and populations (V70-V82)

V70 General medical examination
V71 Observation and evaluation for suspected conditions not found
V72 Special investigations and examinations
V73 Special screening examination for viral and chlamydial diseases
V74 Special screening examination for bacterial and spirochetal diseases
V75 Special screening examination for other infectious diseases
V76 Special screening for malignant neoplasms
V77 Special screening for endocrine, nutritional, metabolic, and immunity disorders
V78 Special screening for disorders of blood and blood-forming organs
V79 Special screening for mental disorders and developmental handicaps
V80 Special screening for neurological, eye, and ear diseases
V81 Special screening for cardiovascular, respiratory, and genitourinary diseases
V82 Special screening for other conditions

Genetics (V83-V84)

V83 Genetic carrier status
V84 Genetic susceptibility to disease

Body Mass Index (V85)

V85 Body Mass Index [BMI]

Estrogen Receptor Status (V86)

V86 Estrogen receptor status

SUPPLEMENTARY CLASSIFICATION OF EXTERNAL CAUSES OF INJURY AND POISONING

Railway accidents (E800-E807)

E800 Railway accident involving collision with rolling stock
E801 Railway accident involving collision with other object
E802 Railway accident involving derailment without antecedent collision
E803 Railway accident involving explosion, fire, or burning
E804 Fall in, on, or from railway train
E805 Hit by rolling stock
E806 Other specified railway accident
E807 Railway accident of unspecified nature

Motor vehicle traffic accidents (E810-E819)

E810 Motor vehicle traffic accident involving collision with train
E811 Motor vehicle traffic accident involving re-entrant collision with another motor vehicle
E812 Other motor vehicle traffic accident involving collision with motor vehicle
E813 Motor vehicle traffic accident involving collision with other vehicle
E814 Motor vehicle traffic accident involving collision with pedestrian
E815 Other motor vehicle traffic accident involving collision on the highway
E816 Motor vehicle traffic accident due to loss of control, without collision on the highway
E817 Noncollision motor vehicle traffic accident while boarding or alighting
E818 Other noncollision motor vehicle traffic accident
E819 Motor vehicle traffic accident of unspecified nature

Motor vehicle nontraffic accidents (E820-E825)

E820 Nontraffic accident involving motor-driven snow vehicle
E821 Nontraffic accident involving other off-road motor vehicle
E822 Other motor vehicle nontraffic accident involving collision with moving object
E823 Other motor vehicle nontraffic accident involving collision with stationary object
E824 Other motor vehicle nontraffic accident while boarding and alighting
E825 Other motor vehicle nontraffic accident of other and unspecified nature

Other road vehicle accidents (E826-E829)

E826 Pedal cycle accident
E827 Animal-drawn vehicle accident
E828 Accident involving animal being ridden
E829 Other road vehicle accidents

Water transport accidents (E830-E838)

E830 Accident to watercraft causing submersion
E831 Accident to watercraft causing other injury
E832 Other accidental submersion or drowning in water transport accident
E833 Fall on stairs or ladders in water transport
E834 Other fall from one level to another in water transport
E835 Other and unspecified fall in water transport
E836 Machinery accident in water transport
E837 Explosion, fire, or burning in watercraft
E838 Other and unspecified water transport accident

Air and space transport accidents (E840-E845)

E840 Accident to powered aircraft at takeoff or landing
E841 Accident to powered aircraft, other and unspecified
E842 Accident to unpowered aircraft
E843 Fall in, on, or from aircraft
E844 Other specified air transport accidents
E845 Accident involving spacecraft

Vehicle accidents, not elsewhere classifiable (E846-E849)

E846 Accidents involving powered vehicles used solely within the buildings and premises of an industrial or commercial establishment
E847 Accidents involving cable cars not running on rails
E848 Accidents involving other vehicles, not elsewhere classifiable
E849 Place of occurrence

Accidental poisoning by drugs, medicinal substances, and biologicals (E850-E858)

E850 Accidental poisoning by analgesics, antipyretics, and antirheumatics
E851 Accidental-poisoning by barbiturates
E852 Accidental poisoning by other sedatives and hypnotics
E853 Accidental poisoning by tranquilizers
E854 Accidental poisoning by other psychotropic agents
E855 Accidental poisoning by other drugs acting on central and autonomic nervous systems
E856 Accidental poisoning by antibiotics
E857 Accidental poisoning by anti-infectives
E858 Accidental poisoning by other drugs

Accidental poisoning by other solid and liquid substances, gases, and vapors (E860-E869)

E860 Accidental poisoning by alcohol, not elsewhere classified
E861 Accidental poisoning by cleansing and polishing agents, disinfectants, paints, and varnishes
E862 Accidental poisoning by petroleum products, other solvents and their vapors, not elsewhere classified
E863 Accidental poisoning by agricultural and horticultural chemical and pharmaceutical preparations other than plant foods and fertilizers
E864 Accidental poisoning by corrosives and caustics, not elsewhere classified
E865 Accidental poisoning from poisonous foodstuffs and poisonous plants
E866 Accidental poisoning by other and unspecified solid and liquid substances
E867 Accidental poisoning by gas distributed by pipeline
E868 Accidental poisoning by other utility gas and other carbon monoxide
E869 Accidental poisoning by other gases and vapors

Misadventures to patients during surgical and medical care (E870-E876)

E870 Accidental cut, puncture, perforation, or hemorrhage during medical care
E871 Foreign object left in body during procedure
E872 Failure of sterile precautions during procedure
E873 Failure in dosage
E874 Mechanical failure of instrument or apparatus during procedure
E875 Contaminated or infected blood, other fluid, drug, or biological substance
E876 Other and unspecified misadventures during medical care

Surgical and medical procedures as the cause of abnormal reaction of patient or later complication, without mention of misadventure at the time of procedure (E878-E879)

E878 Surgical operation and other surgical procedures as the cause of abnormal reaction of patient, or of later complication, without mention of misadventure at the time of operation
E879 Other procedures, without mention of misadventure at the time of procedure, as the cause of abnormal reaction of patient, or of later complication

Accidental falls (E880-E888)

E880 Fall on or from stairs or steps
E881 Fall on or from ladders or scaffolding
E882 Fall from or out of building or other structure
E883 Fall into hole or other opening in surface
E884 Other fall from one level to another
E885 Fall on same level from slipping, tripping, or stumbling
E886 Fall on same level from collision, pushing or shoving, by or with other person
E887 Fracture, cause unspecified
E888 Other and unspecified fall

Accidents caused by fire and flames (E890-E899)

E890 Conflagration in private dwelling
E891 Conflagration in other and unspecified building or structure
E892 Conflagration not in building or structure
E893 Accident caused by ignition of clothing
E894 Ignition of highly inflammable material
E895 Accident caused by controlled fire in private dwelling
E896 Accident caused by controlled fire in other and unspecified building or structure
E897 Accident caused by controlled fire not in building or structure
E898 Accident caused by other specified fire and flames
E899 Accident caused by unspecified fire

Accidents due to natural and environmental factors (E900-E909)

E900 Excessive heat
E901 Excessive cold
E902 High and low air pressure and changes in air pressure
E903 Travel and motion
E904 Hunger, thirst, exposure, and neglect
E905 Venomous animals and plants as the cause of poisoning and toxic reactions
E906 Other injury caused by animals
E907 Lightning
E908 Cataclysmic storms, and floods resulting from storms
E909 Cataclysmic earth surface movements and eruptions

Accidents caused by submersion, suffocation, and foreign bodies (E910-E915)

E910 Accidental drowning and submersion
E911 Inhalation and ingestion of food causing obstruction of respiratory tract or suffocation
E912 Inhalation and ingestion of other object causing obstruction of respiratory tract or suffocation
E913 Accidental mechanical suffocation
E914 Foreign body accidentally entering eye and adnexa
E915 Foreign body accidentally entering other orifice

Other accidents (E916-E928)

E916 Struck accidentally by falling object
E917 Striking against or struck accidentally by objects or persons
E918 Caught accidentally in or between objects
E919 Accidents caused by machinery
E920 Accidents caused by cutting and piercing instruments or objects
E921 Accident caused by explosion of pressure vessel
E922 Accident caused by firearm and airgun missile
E923 Accident caused by explosive material
E924 Accident caused by hot substance or object, caustic or corrosive material, and steam
E925 Accident caused by electric current
E926 Exposure to radiation
E927 Overexertion and strenuous movements
E928 Other and unspecified environmental and accidental causes

Late effects of accidental injury (E929)

E929 Late effects of accidental injury

Drugs, medicinal and biological substances causing adverse effects in therapeutic use (E930-E949)

E930 Antibiotics
E931 Other anti-infectives
E932 Hormones and synthetic substitutes
E933 Primarily systemic agents
E934 Agents primarily affecting blood constituents
E935 Analgesics, antipyretics, and antirheumatics
E936 Anticonvulsants and anti-Parkinsonism drugs
E937 Sedatives and hypnotics
E938 Other central nervous system depressants and anesthetics
E939 Psychotropic agents
E940 Central nervous system stimulants
E941 Drugs primarily affecting the autonomic nervous system
E942 Agents primarily affecting the cardiovascular system
E943 Agents primarily affecting gastrointestinal system
E944 Water, mineral, and uric acid metabolism drugs
E945 Agents primarily acting on the smooth and skeletal muscles and respiratory system
E946 Agents primarily affecting skin and mucous membrane, ophthalmological, otorhinolaryngological, and dental drugs
E947 Other and unspecified drugs and medicinal substances
E948 Bacterial vaccines
E949 Other vaccines and biological substances

Suicide and self-inflicted injury (E950-E959)

E950 Suicide and self-inflicted poisoning by solid or liquid substances
E951 Suicide and self-inflicted poisoning by gases in domestic use
E952 Suicide and self-inflicted poisoning by other gases and vapors
E953 Suicide and self-inflicted injury by hanging, strangulation, and suffocation
E954 Suicide and self-inflicted injury by submersion [drowning]
E955 Suicide and self-inflicted injury by firearms, airguns and explosives
E956 Suicide and self-inflicted injury by cutting and piercing instruments
E957 Suicide and self-inflicted injuries by jumping from high place
E958 Suicide and self-inflicted injury by other and unspecified means
E959 Late effects of self-inflicted injury

Homicide and injury purposely inflicted by other persons (E960-E969)

E960 Fight, brawl, and rape
E961 Assault by corrosive or caustic substance, except poisoning
E962 Assault by poisoning
E963 Assault by hanging and strangulation
E964 Assault by submersion [drowning]
E965 Assault by firearms and explosives
E966 Assault by cutting and piercing instrument
E967 Perpetrator of child and adult abuse
E968 Assault by other and unspecified means
E969 Late effects of injury purposely inflicted by other person

Legal intervention (E970-E978)

E970 Injury due to legal intervention by firearms
E971 Injury due to legal intervention by explosives
E972 Injury due to legal intervention by gas
E973 Injury due to legal intervention by blunt object
E974 Injury due to legal intervention by cutting and piercing instruments
E975 Injury due to legal intervention by other specified means
E976 Injury due to legal intervention by unspecified means
E977 Late effects of injuries due to legal intervention
E978 Legal execution

Terrorism (E979)

E979 Terrorism

Injury undetermined whether accidentally or purposely inflicted (E980-E989)

E980 Poisoning by solid or liquid substances, undetermined whether accidentally or purposely inflicted
E981 Poisoning by gases in domestic use, undetermined whether accidentally or purposely inflicted
E982 Poisoning by other gases, undetermined whether accidentally or purposely inflicted
E983 Hanging, strangulation, or suffocation, undetermined whether accidentally or purposely inflicted
E984 Submersion [drowning], undetermined whether accidentally or purposely inflicted
E985 Injury by firearms, airguns and explosives, undetermined whether accidentally or purposely inflicted
E986 Injury by cutting and piercing instruments, undetermined whether accidentally or purposely inflicted
E987 Falling from high place, undetermined whether accidentally or purposely inflicted
E988 Injury by other and unspecified means, undetermined whether accidentally or purposely inflicted
E989 Late effects of injury, undetermined whether accidentally or purposely inflicted

Injury resulting from operations of war (E990-E999)

E990 Injury due to war operations by fires and conflagrations
E991 Injury due to war operations by bullets and fragments
E992 Injury due to war operations by explosion of marine weapons
E993 Injury due to war operations by other explosion
E994 Injury due to war operations by destruction of aircraft
E995 Injury due to war operations by other and unspecified forms of conventional warfare
E996 Injury due to war operations by nuclear weapons
E997 Injury due to war operations by other forms of unconventional warfare
E998 Injury due to war operations but occurring after cessation of hostilities
E999 Late effects of injury due to war operations and terrorism

Alphabetic Index to Procedures

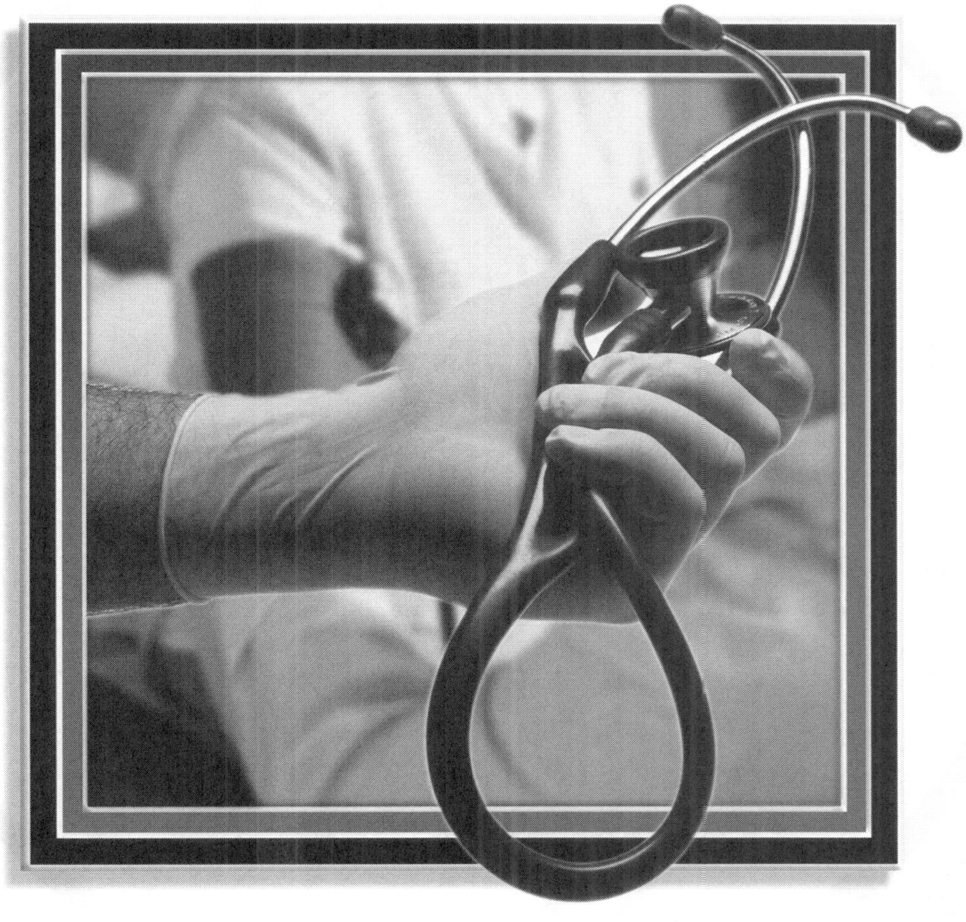

Volume 3

A

Abbe operation – Amputation

Amputation – *continued*
- carpals 84.03
- cervix 67.4
- Chopart's (midtarsal) 84.12
- clitoris 71.4
- Dieffenbach (hip disarticulation) 84.18
- Dupuytren's (shoulder disarticulation) 84.08
- ear, external 18.39
- elbow (disarticulation) 84.06
- finger, except thumb 84.01
  - thumb 84.02
- foot (middle) 84.12
- forearm 84.05
- forefoot 84.12
- forequarter 84.09
- Gordon-Taylor (hindquarter) 84.19
- Gritti-Stokes (knee disarticulation) 84.16
- Guyon (ankle) 84.13
- hallux 84.11
- hand 84.03
- Hey's (foot) 84.12
- hindquarter 84.19
- hip (disarticulation) 84.18
- humerus 84.07
- interscapulothoracic 84.09
- interthoracoscapular 84.09
- King-Steelquist (hindquarter) 84.19
- Kirk (thigh) 84.17
- knee (disarticulation) 84.16
- Kutler (revision of current traumatic amputation of finger) 84.01
- Larry (shoulder disarticulation) 84.08
- leg NEC 84.10
  - above knee (AK) 84.17
  - below knee (BK) 84.15
  - through
    - ankle (disarticulation) 84.13
    - femur (AK) 84.17
    - foot 84.12
    - hip (disarticulation) 84.18
    - tibia and fibula (BK) 84.15
- Lisfranc
  - foot 84.12
  - shoulder (disarticulation) 84.08
- Littlewood (forequarter) 84.09
- lower limb NEC (*see also* Amputation, leg) 84.10
- Mazet (knee disarticulation) 84.16
- metacarpal 84.03
- metatarsal 84.11
  - head (bunionectomy) 77.59
- metatarsophalangeal (joint) 84.11
- midtarsal 84.12
- nose 21.4
- penis (circle) (complete) (flap) (partial) (radical) 64.3
- Pirogoff's (ankle amputation through malleoli of tibia and fibula) 84.14
- ray
  - finger 84.01
  - foot 84.11
  - toe (metatarsal head) 84.11
- root (tooth) (apex) 23.73
  - with root canal therapy 23.72
- shoulder (disarticulation) 84.08
- Sorondo-Ferre (hindquarter) 84.19
- S.P. Rogers (knee disarticulation) 84.16
- supracondyler, above-knee 84.17
- supramalleolar, foot 84.14
- Syme's (ankle amputation through malleoli of tibia and fibula) 84.14
- thigh 84.17
- thumb 84.02
- toe (through metatarsophalangeal joint) 84.11
- transcarpal 84.03
- transmetatarsal 84.12
- upper limb NEC (*see also* Amputation, arm) 84.00
- wrist (disarticulation) 84.04

Amygdalohippocampotomy 01.39

Amygdalotomy 01.39

Analysis
- cardiac rhythm device (CRT-D) (CRT-P) (AICD) (pacemaker) – *see* Interrogation
- character 94.03
- gastric 89.39
- psychologic 94.31
- transactional
  - group 94.44
  - individual 94.39

Anastomosis
- abdominal artery to coronary artery 37.17
- accessory-facial nerve 04.72
- accessory-hypoglossal nerve 04.73
- anus (with formation of endorectal ileal pouch) 45.95
- aorta (descending)-pulmonary (artery) 39.0
- aorta-renal artery 39.24
- aorta-subclavian artery 39.22
- aortoceliac 39.26
- aorto(ilio)femoral 39.25
- aortomesenteric 39.26
- appendix 47.99
- arteriovenous NEC 39.29
  - for renal dialysis 39.27
- artery (suture of distal to proximal end) 39.31
  - with
    - bypass graft 39.29
      - extracranial-intracranial [EC-IC] 39.28
    - excision or resection of vessel – *see* Arteriectomy, with anastomosis, by site
  - revision 39.49
- bile ducts 51.39
- bladder NEC 57.88
  - with
    - isolated segment of intestine 57.87 *[45.50]*
      - colon (sigmoid) 57.87 *[45.52]*
      - ileum 57.87 *[45.51]*
    - open loop of ileum 57.87 *[45.51]*
  - to intestine 57.88
    - ileum 57.87 *[45.51]*
- bowel (*see also* Anastomosis, intestine) 45.90
- bronchotracheal 33.48
- bronchus 33.48
- carotid-subclavian artery 39.22
- caval-mesenteric vein 39.1
- caval-pulmonary artery 39.21
- cervicoesophageal 42.59
- colohypopharyngeal (intrathoracic) 42.55
  - antesternal or antethoracic 42.65
- common bile duct 51.39
- common pulmonary trunk and left atrium (posterior wall) 35.82
- cystic bile duct 51.39
- cystocolic 57.88
- epididymis to vas deferens 63.83
- esophagocolic (intrathoracic) NEC 42.56
  - with interposition 42.55
  - antesternal or antethoracic NEC 42.66
    - with interposition 42.65
- esophagocologastric (intrathoracic) 42.55
  - antesternal or antethoracic 42.65
- esophagoduodenal (intrathoracic) NEC 42.54
  - with interposition 42.53
- esophagoenteric (intrathoracic) NEC (*see also* Anastomosis, esophagus, to intestinal segment) 42.54
  - antesternal or antethoracic NEC (*see also* Anastomosis, esophagus, antesternal, to intestinal segment) 42.64
- esophagoesophageal (intrathoracic) 42.51
  - antesternal or antethoracic 42.61
- esophagogastric (intrathoracic) 42.52
  - antesternal or antethoracic 42.62
- esophagus (intrapleural) (intrathoracic) (retrosternal) NEC 42.59
  - with
    - gastrectomy (partial) 43.5
      - complete or total 43.99
    - interposition (of) NEC 42.58
      - colon 42.55
      - jejunum 42.53
      - small bowel 42.53
  - antesternal or antethoracic NEC 42.69
    - with
      - interposition (of) NEC 42.68
        - colon 42.65
        - jejunal loop 42.63
        - small bowel 42.63
      - rubber tube 42.68
    - to intestinal segment NEC 42.64
      - with interposition 42.68
      - colon NEC 42.66
        - with interposition 42.65
      - small bowel NEC 42.64
        - with interposition 42.63
  - to intestinal segment (intrathoracic) NEC 42.54
    - with interposition 42.58
    - antesternal or antethoracic NEC 42.64
      - with interposition 42.68
    - colon (intrathoracic) NEC 42.56
      - with interposition 42.55
      - antesternal or antethoracic 42.66
        - with interposition 42.65

Anastomosis – *continued*
- esophagus – *continued*
  - to intestinal segment – *continued*
    - small bowel NEC 42.54
      - with interposition 42.53
      - antesternal or antethoracic 42.64
        - with interposition 42.63
- facial-accessory nerve 04.72
- facial-hypoglossal nerve 04.71
- fallopian tube 66.73
  - by reanastomosis 66.79
- gallbladder 51.35
  - to
    - hepatic ducts 51.31
    - intestine 51.32
    - pancreas 51.33
    - stomach 51.34
- gastroepiploic artery to coronary artery 36.17
- hepatic duct 51.39
- hypoglossal-accessory nerve 04.73
- hypoglossal-facial nerve 04.71
- ileal loop to bladder 57.87 *[45.51]*
- ileoanal 45.95
- ileorectal 45.93
- inferior vena cava and portal vein 39.1
- internal mammary artery (to)
  - coronary artery (single vessel) 36.15
    - double vessel 36.16
  - myocardium 36.2
- intestine 45.90
  - large-to-anus 45.95
  - large-to-large 45.94
  - large-to-rectum 45.94
  - large-to-small 45.93
  - small-to-anus 45.95
  - small-to-large 45.93
  - small-to-rectal stump 45.92
  - small-to-small 45.91
- intrahepatic 51.79
- intrathoracic vessel NEC 39.23
- kidney (pelvis) 55.86
- lacrimal sac to conjunctiva 09.82
- left-to-right (systemic-pulmonary artery) 39.0
- lymphatic (channel) (peripheral) 40.9
- mesenteric-caval 39.1
- mesocaval 39.1
- nasolacrimal 09.81
- nerve (cranial) (peripheral) NEC 04.74
  - accessory-facial 04.72
  - accessory-hypoglossal 04.73
  - hypoglossal-facial 04.71
- pancreas (duct) (to) 52.96
  - bile duct 51.39
  - gall bladder 51.33
  - intestine 52.96
  - jejunum 52.96
  - stomach 52.96
- pleurothecal (with valve) 03.79
- portacaval 39.1
- portal vein to inferior vena cava 39.1
- pulmonary-aortic (Pott's) 39.0
- pulmonary artery and superior vena cava 39.21
- pulmonary-innominate artery (Blalock) 39.0
- pulmonary-subclavian artery (Blalock-Taussig) 39.0
- pulmonary vein and azygos vein 39.23
- pyeloileocutaneous 56.51
- pyeloureterovesical 55.86
- radial artery 36.19
- rectum, rectal NEC 48.74
  - stump to small intestine 45.92
- renal (pelvis) 55.86
  - vein and splenic vein 39.1
- renoportal 39.1
- salpingothecal (with valve) 03.79
- splenic to renal veins 39.1
- splenorenal (venous) 39.1
  - arterial 39.26
- subarachnoid-peritoneal (with valve) 03.71
- subarachnoid-ureteral (with valve) 03.72
- subclavian-aortic 39.22
- superior vena cava to pulmonary artery 39.21
- systemic-pulmonary artery 39.0
- thoracic artery (to)
  - coronary artery (single) 36.15
    - double 36.16
  - myocardium 36.2
- ureter (to) NEC 56.79
  - bladder 56.74
  - colon 56.71
  - ileal pouch (bladder) 56.51
  - ileum 56.71

- **Aortotomy** 38.04
- **Apexcardiogram** (with ECG lead) 89.57
- **Apheresis, therapeutic** – *see* category 99.7❹
- **Apicectomy**
  - lung 32.39 ▲
    - thoracoscopic 32.30 ●
  - petrous pyramid 20.59
  - tooth (root) 23.73
    - with root canal therapy 23.72
- **Apicoectomy** 23.73
  - with root canal therapy 23.72
- **Apicolysis** (lung) 33.39
- **Apicostomy, alveolar** 24.0
- **Aponeurectomy** 83.42
  - hand 82.33
- **Aponeurorrhaphy** (*see also* Suture, tendon) 83.64
  - hand (*see also* Suture, tendon, hand) 82.45
- **Aponeurotomy** 83.13
  - hand 82.11
- **Appendectomy** (with drainage) 47.09
  - incidental 47.19
    - laparoscopic 47.11
  - laparoscopic 47.01
- **Appendicectomy** (with drainage) 47.09
  - incidental 47.19
    - laparoscopic 47.11
  - laparoscopic 47.01
- **Appendicocecostomy** 47.91
- **Appendicoenterostomy** 47.91
- **Appendicolysis** 54.59
  - with appendectomy 47.09
    - laparoscopic 47.01
    - other 47.09
  - laparoscopic 54.51
- **Appendicostomy** 47.91
  - closure 47.92
- **Appendicotomy** 47.2
- **Application**
  - adhesion barrier substance 99.77
  - anti-shock trousers 93.58
  - arch bars (orthodontic) 24.7
    - for immobilization (fracture) 93.55
  - barrier substance, adhesion 99.77
  - Barton's tongs (skull) (with synchronous skeletal traction) 02.94
  - bone growth stimulator (surface) (transcutaneous) 99.86
  - bone morphogenetic protein (Infuse™)(OP-1™)(recombinant) (rhBMP) 84.52
  - Bryant's traction 93.44
    - with reduction of fracture or dislocation – *see* Reduction, fracture and Reduction, dislocation
  - Buck's traction 93.46
  - caliper tongs (skull) (with synchronous skeletal traction) 02.94
  - cast (fiberglass) (plaster) (plastic) NEC 93.53
    - with reduction of fracture or dislocation – *see* Reduction, fracture and Reduction, dislocation
    - spica 93.51
  - cervical collar 93.52
    - with reduction of fracture or dislocation – *see* Reduction, fracture and Reduction, dislocation
  - clamp, cerebral aneurysm (Crutchfield) (Silverstone) 39.51
  - croupette, croup tent 93.94
  - crown (artificial) 23.41
  - Crutchfield tongs (skull) (with synchronous skeletal traction) 02.94
  - Dunlop's traction 93.44
    - with reduction of fracture or dislocation – *see* Reduction, fracture and Reduction, dislocation
  - elastic stockings 93.59
  - electronic gaiter 93.59
  - external fixator device (bone) 78.10
    - carpal, metacarpal 78.14
    - clavicle 78.11
    - computer assisted (dependent) 84.73
    - femur 78.15
    - fibula 78.17
    - humerus 78.12
    - hybrid device or system 84.73
    - Ilizarov type 84.72
    - monoplanar system or device 84.71
    - patella 78.16
    - pelvic 78.19

Application – *continued*
  - external fixator device – *continued*
    - phalanges (foot) (hand) 78.19
    - radius 78.13
    - ring device or system 84.72
    - scapula 78.11
    - Sheffield type 84.72
    - specified site NEC 78.19
    - tarsal, metatarsal 78.18
    - thorax (ribs) (sternum) 78.11
    - tibia 78.17
    - ulna 78.13
    - vertebrae 78.19
  - forceps, with delivery – *see* Delivery, forceps
  - graft – *see* Graft
  - gravity (G-) suit 93.59
  - intermittent pressure device 93.59
  - Jewett extension brace 93.59
  - Jobst pumping unit (reduction of edema) 93.59
  - Lyman Smith traction 93.44
    - with reduction of fracture or dislocation – *see* Reduction, fracture and Reduction, dislocation
  - MAST (military anti-shock trousers) 93.58
  - Minerva jacket 93.52
  - minifixator device (bone) – *see* category 78.1❹
  - neck support (molded) 93.52
  - obturator (orthodontic) 24.7
  - orthodontic appliance (obturator) (wiring) 24.7
  - pelvic sling 93.44
  - with reduction of fracture or dislocation – *see* Reduction, fracture and Reduction, dislocation
  - peridontal splint (orthodontic) 24.7
  - plaster jacket 93.51
    - Minerva 93.52
  - pressure
    - dressing (bandage) (Gibney) (Robert Jones') (Shanz) 93.56
    - trousers (anti-shock) (MAST) 93.58
  - prosthesis for missing ear 18.71
  - Russell's traction 93.44
    - with reduction of fracture or dislocation – *see* Reduction, fracture and Reduction, dislocation
  - splint, for immobilization (plaster) (pneumatic) (tray) 93.54
    - with fracture reduction – *see* Reduction, fracture
  - stereotactic head frame 93.59
  - strapping (non-traction) 93.59
  - substance, adhesion barrier 99.77
  - Thomas collar 93.52
    - with reduction of fracture or dislocation – *see* Reduction, fracture and Reduction, dislocation
  - traction
    - with reduction of fracture or dislocation – *see* Reduction, fracture and Reduction, dislocation
    - adhesive tape (skin) 93.46
    - boot 93.46
    - Bryant's 93.44
    - Buck's 93.46
    - Cotrel's 93.42
    - Dunlop's 93.44
    - gallows 93.46
    - Lyman Smith 93.44
    - Russell's 93.44
    - skeletal NEC 93.44
      - intermittent 93.43
    - skin, limbs NEC 93.46
    - spinal NEC 93.42
      - with skull device (halo) (caliper) (Crutchfield) (Gardner-Wells) (Vinke) (tongs) 93.41
        - with synchronous insertion 02.94
    - Thomas' splint 93.45
  - Unna's paste boot 93.53
  - vasopneumatic device 93.58
  - Velpeau dressing 93.59
  - Vinke tongs (skull) (with synchronous skeletal traction) 02.94
  - wound dressing NEC 93.57
- **Aquapheresis** 99.78
- **Arc lamp** – *see* Photocoagulation
- **Arrest**
  - bone growth (epiphyseal) 78.20
    - by stapling – *see* Stapling, epiphyseal plate
    - femur 78.25
    - fibula 78.27
    - humerus 78.22
    - radius 78.23

Arrest – *continued*
  - bone growth – *continued*
    - tibia 78.27
    - ulna 78.23
  - cardiac, induced (anoxic) (circulatory) 39.63
  - circulatory, induced (anoxic) 39.63
  - hemorrhage – *see* Control, hemorrhage
- **Arslan operation** (fenestration of inner ear) 20.61
- **Arteriectomy** 38.60
  - with
    - anastomosis 38.30
      - abdominal 38.36
      - aorta (arch) (ascending) (descending) 38.34
      - head and neck NEC 38.32
      - intracranial NEC 38.31
      - lower limb 38.38
      - thoracic NEC 38.35
      - upper limb 38.33
    - graft replacement (interposition) 38.40
      - abdominal
        - aorta 38.44
      - aorta (arch) (ascending) (descending thoracic) (thoracic)
        - abdominal 38.44
        - thoracic 38.45
        - thoracoabdominal 38.45 *[38.44]*
      - head and neck NEC 38.42
      - intracranial NEC 38.41
      - lower limb 38.48
      - thoracic NEC 38.45
      - upper limb 38.43
  - abdominal 38.66
  - aorta (arch) (ascending) (descending) 38.64
  - head and neck NEC 38.62
  - intracranial NEC 38.61
  - lower-limb 38.68
  - thoracic NEC 38.65
  - upper limb 38.63
- **Arteriography** (contrast) (fluoroscopic) (retrograde) 88.40
  - by
    - radioisotope – *see* Scan, radioisotope
    - ultrasound (Doppler) – *see* Ultrasonography, by site
  - aorta (arch) (ascending) (descending) 88.42
  - basilar 88.41
  - brachial 88.49
  - carotid (internal) 88.41
  - cerebral (posterior circulation) 88.41
  - coronary (direct) (selective) NEC 88.57
    - double catheter technique (Judkins) (Ricketts and Abrams) 88.56
    - intra-operative fluorescence vascular 88.59 ●
    - single catheter technique (Sones) 88.55
  - Doppler (ultrasonic) – *see* Ultrasonography, by site
  - femoral 88.48
  - head and neck 88.41
  - intra-abdominal NEC 88.47
  - intrathoracic NEC 88.44
  - lower extremity 88.48
  - placenta 88.46
  - pulmonary 88.43
  - radioisotope – *see* Scan, radioisotope
  - renal 88.45
  - specified site NEC 88.49
  - SPY 88.59 ●
  - superior mesenteric artery 88.47
  - transfemoral 88.48
  - ultrasound – *see* Ultrasonography, by site
  - upper extremity 88.49
- **Arterioplasty** – *see* Repair, artery
- **Arteriorrhaphy** 39.31
- **Arteriotomy** 38.00
  - abdominal 38.06
  - aorta (arch) (ascending) (descending) 38.04
  - head and neck NEC 38.02
  - intracranial NEC 38.01
  - lower limb 38.08
  - thoracic NEC 38.05
  - upper limb 38.03
- **Arteriovenostomy** 39.29
  - for renal dialysis 39.27
- **Arthrectomy** 80.90
  - ankle 80.97
  - elbow 80.92
  - foot and toe 80.98
  - hand and finger 80.94
  - hip 80.95
  - intervertebral disc – *see* category 80.5❹
  - knee 80.96

Astragalectomy – Biopsy

Astragalectomy 77.98
Asymmetrogammagram – *see* Scan, radioisotope
Atherectomy
  cerebrovascular – *see* Angioplasty
  coronary – *see* Angioplasty
  peripheral 39.50
Atriocommissuropexy (mitral valve) 35.12
Atrioplasty NEC 37.99
  combined with repair of valvular and ventricular septal defects – *see* Repair, endocardial cushion defect
  septum (heart) NEC 35.71
Atrioseptopexy (*see also* Repair, atrial septal defect) 35.71
Atrioseptoplasty (*see also* Repair, atrial septal defect) 35.71
Atrioseptostomy (balloon) 35.41
Atriotomy 37.11
Atrioventriculostomy (cerebral-heart) 02.32
Attachment
  abutment (screw) for prosthetic ear device ●
    percutaneous 20.99 ●
  eye muscle
    orbicularis oculi to eyebrow 08.36
    rectus to frontalis 15.9
  pedicle (flap) graft 86.74
    hand 86.73
    lip 27.57
    mouth 27.57
  pharyngeal flap (for cleft palate repair) 27.62
    secondary or subsequent 27.63
  prosthetic ear device, abutment 20.99 ●
  retina – *see* Reattachment, retina
Atticoantrostomy (ear) 20.49
Atticoantrotomy (ear) 20.49
Atticotomy (ear) 20.23
Audiometry (Békésy 5-tone) (impedance) (stapedial reflex response) (subjective) 95.41
Augmentation
  bladder 57.87
  breast – *see* Mammoplasty, augmentation
  buttock ("fanny-lift") 86.89
  chin 76.68
  genioplasty 76.68
  mammoplasty – *see* Mammoplasty, augmentation
  outflow tract (pulmonary valve) (gusset type) 35.26
    in total repair of tetralogy of Fallot 35.81
  vocal cord(s) 31.0
Auriculectomy 18.39
Autograft – *see* Graft
Autologous – *see* Blood, transfusion
Autopsy 89.8
Autotransfusion (whole blood) 99.02 – *see* Blood, transfusion
Autotransplant, autotransplantation – *see also* Reimplantation
  adrenal tissue (heterotopic) (orthotopic) 07.45
  kidney 55.61
  lung – *see* Transplant, transplantation, lung 33.5❹
  ovary 65.72
    laparoscopic 65.75
  pancreatic tissue 52.81
  parathyroid tissue (heterotopic) (orthotopic) 06.95
  thyroid tissue (heterotopic) (orthotopic) 06.94
  tooth 23.5
Avulsion, nerve (cranial) (peripheral) NEC 04.07
  acoustic 04.01
  phrenic 33.31
  sympathetic 05.29
Azygography 88.63

B

Bacterial smear – *see* Examination, microscopic
Baffes operation (interatrial transposition of venous return) 35.91
Baffle, atrial or interatrial 35.91
Balanoplasty 64.69
Baldy-Webster operation (uterine suspension) 69.22
Ballistocardiography 89.59
Balloon
  angioplasty – *see* Angioplasty, balloon
  pump, intra-aortic 37.61
  systostomy (atrial) 35.41
Ball operation
  herniorrhaphy – *see* Repair, hernia, inguinal
  undercutting 40.92
Bandage 93.37
  elastic 93.56
Banding
  gastric 44.68
    vertical 44.68
  pulmonary artery 38.85
Bankhart operation (capsular repair into glenoid, for shoulder dislocation) 81.82
Bardenheurer operation (ligation of innominate artery) 38.85
Barium swallow 87.61
Barkan operation (goniotomy) 12.52
  with goniopuncture 12.53
Barr operation (transfer of tibialis posterior tendon) 83.75
Barsky operation (closure of cleft hand) 82.82
Basal metabolic rate 89.39
Basiotripsy 73.8
Bassett operation (vulvectomy with inguinal lymph node dissection) 71.5 *[40.3]*
Bassini operation – *see* Repair, hernia, inguinal
Batch-Spittler-McFaddin operation (knee disarticulation) 84.16
Batista operation (partial ventriculectomy) (ventricular reduction) (ventricular remodeling) 37.35
Bearing surface, hip
  ceramic-on-ceramic 00.76
  ceramic-on-polyethylene 00.77
  metal-on-metal 00.75
  metal on polyethylene 00.74
Beck operation
  aorta-coronary sinus shunt 36.39
  epicardial poudrage 36.39
Beck-Jianu operation (permanent gastrostomy) 43.19
Behavior modification 94.33
Bell-Beuttner operation (subtotal abdominal hysterectomy) 68.39
  laparoscopic 68.31
Belsey operation (esophagogastric sphincter) 44.65
Benenenti operation (rotation of bulbous urethra) 58.49
Berke operation (levator resection of eyelid) 08.33
Bicuspidization of heart valve 35.10
  aortic 35.11
  mitral 35.12
Bicycle dynamometer 93.01
Biesenberger operation (size reduction of breast, bilateral) 85.32
  unilateral 85.31
Bifurcation, bone (*see also* Osteotomy) 77.30
Bigelow operation (litholapaxy) 57.0
Bililite therapy (ultraviolet) 99.82
Billroth I operation (partial gastrectomy with gastroduodenostomy) 43.6
Billroth II operation (partial gastrectomy with gastrojejunostomy) 43.7
Binnie operation (hepatopexy) 50.69
Biofeedback, psychotherapy 94.39
Biopsy
  abdominal wall 54.22
  adenoid 28.11
  adrenal gland NEC 07.11
    closed 07.11
    open 07.12
    percutaneous (aspiration) (needle) 07.11
  alveolus 24.12
  anus 49.23
  appendix 45.26
  artery (any site) 38.21
  aspiration – *see* Biopsy, by site
  bile ducts 51.14
    closed (endoscopic) 51.14
    open 51.13
    percutaneous (needle) 51.12
  bladder 57.33
    closed 57.33
    open 57.34
    transurethral 57.33
  blood vessel (any site) 38.21
  bone 77.40
    carpal, metacarpal 77.44
    clavicle 77.41
    facial 76.11
    femur 77.45
    fibula 77.47
    humerus 77.42
    marrow 41.31
    patella 77.46
    pelvic 77.49
    phalanges (foot) (hand) 77.49
    radius 77.43
    scapula 77.41
    specified site NEC 77.49
    tarsal, metatarsal 77.48
    thorax (ribs) (sternum) 77.41
    tibia 77.47
    ulna 77.43
    vertebrae 77.49
  bowel – *see* Biopsy, intestine
  brain NEC 01.13
    closed 01.13
    open 01.14
    percutaneous (needle) 01.13
  breast 85.11
    blind 85.11
    closed 85.11
    open 85.12
    percutaneous (needle) (Vimm-Silverman) 85.11
  bronchus NEC 33.24
    brush 33.24
    closed (endoscopic) 33.24
    open 33.25
    washings 33.24
  bursa 83.21
  cardioesophageal (junction) 44.14
    closed (endoscopic) 44.14
    open 44.15
  cecum 45.25
    brush 45.25
    closed (endoscopic) 45.25
    open 45.26
  cerebral meninges NEC 01.11
    closed 01.11
    open 01.12
    percutaneous (needle) 01.11
  cervix (punch) 67.12
    conization (sharp) 67.2
  chest wall 34.23
  clitoris 71.11
  colon 45.25
    brush 45.25
    closed (endoscopic) 45.25
    open 45.26
  conjunctiva 10.21
  cornea 11.22
  cul-de-sac 70.23
  diaphragm 34.27
  duodenum 45.14
    brush 45.14
    closed (endoscopic) 45.14
    open 45.15
  ear (external) 18.12
    middle or inner 20.32
  endocervix 67.11
  endometrium NEC 68.16
    by
      aspiration curettage 69.59
      dilation and curettage 69.09
    closed (endoscopic) 68.16
    open 68.13
  epididymis 63.01
  esophagus 42.24
    closed (endoscopic) 42.24
    open 42.25
  extraocular muscle or tendon 15.01
  eye 16.23
    muscle (oblique) (rectus) 15.01
  eyelid 08.11
  fallopian tube 66.11
  fascia 83.21
  fetus 75.33
  gallbladder 51.12
    closed (endoscopic) 51.14
    open 51.13
    percutaneous (needle) 51.12
  ganglion (cranial) (peripheral) NEC 04.11
    closed 04.11
    open 04.12
    percutaneous (needle) 04.11
    sympathetic nerve 05.11

C

Change – *continued*
- pyelostomy catheter or tube 55.94
- tracheostomy tube 97.23
- ureterostomy catheter or tube 59.93
- urethral catheter, indwelling 57.95

Character analysis, psychologic 94.03
Charles operation (correction of lymphedema) 40.9
Charnley operation (compression arthrodesis)
- ankle 81.11
- hip 81.21
- knee 81.22

Cheatle-Henry operation – *see* Repair, hernia, femoral
Check
- automatic implantable cardioverter/defibrillator (AICD) (interrogation only) 89.49
- CRT-D (cardiac resynchronization defibrillator) (interrogation only) 89.49
- CRT-P (cardiac resynchronization pacemaker) (interrogation only) 89.45
- pacemaker, artificial (cardiac) (function) (interrogation only) (rate) 89.45
  - amperage threshold 89.48
  - artifact wave form 89.46
  - electrode impedance 89.47
  - voltage threshold 89.48
- vision NEC 95.09

Cheiloplasty 27.59
Cheilorrhaphy 27.51
Cheilostomatoplasty 27.59
Cheilotomy 27.0
Chemical peel, skin 86.24
Chemocauterization – *see also* Destruction, lesion, by site
- corneal epithelium 11.41
- palate 27.31

Chemodectomy 39.8
Chemoembolization 99.25
Chemolysis
- nerve (peripheral) 04.2
- spinal canal structure 03.8

Chemoneurolysis 04.2
Chemonucleolysis (nucleus pulposus) 80.52
Chemopallidectomy 01.42
Chemopeel (skin) 86.24
Chemosurgery
- esophagus 42.39
  - endoscopic 42.33
- Mohs' 86.24
- skin (superficial) 86.24
- stomach 43.49
  - endoscopic 43.41

Chemothalamectomy 01.41
Chemotherapy – *see also* Immunotherapy
- Antabuse 94.25
- for cancer NEC 99.25
  - brain wafer implantation 00.10
  - implantation of chemotherapeutic agent 00.10
  - interstitial implantation 00.10
  - intracavitary implantation 00.10
  - wafer chemotherapy 00.10
- lithium 94.22
- methadone 94.25
- palate (bony) 27.31

Chevalier-Jackson operation (partial laryngectomy) 30.29
Child operation (radical subtotal pancreatectomy) 52.53
Cholangiocholangiostomy 51.39
Cholangiocholecystocholedochectomy 51.22
Cholangio-enterostomy 51.39
Cholangiogastrostomy 51.39
Cholangiogram 87.54
- endoscopic retrograde (ERC) 51.11
- intraoperative 87.53
- intravenous 87.52
- percutaneous hepatic 87.51
- transhepatic 87.53

Cholangiography (*see also* Cholangiogram) 87.54
Cholangiojejunostomy (intrahepatic) 51.39
Cholangiopancreatography, endoscopic retrograde (ERCP) 51.10
Cholangiostomy 51.59
Cholangiotomy 51.59
Cholecystectomy (total) 51.22
- partial 51.21
  - laparoscopic 51.24
- total 51.22
  - laparoscopic 51.23

Cholecystenterorrhaphy 51.91
Cholecystocecostomy 51.32
Cholecystocholangiogram 87.59
Cholecystocolostomy 51.32
Cholecystoduodenostomy 51.32
Cholecystoenterostomy (Winiwater) 51.32
Cholecystogastrostomy 51.34
Cholecystogram 87.59
Cholecystoileostomy 51.32
Cholecystojejunostomy (Roux-en-Y) (with jejunojejunostomy) 51.32
Cholecystopancreatostomy 51.33
Cholecystopexy 51.99
Cholecystorrhaphy 51.91
Cholecystostomy NEC 51.03
- by trocar 51.02

Cholecystotomy 51.04
- percutaneous 51.01

Choledochectomy 51.63
Choledochoduodenostomy 51.36
Choledochoenterostomy 51.36
Choledochojejunostomy 51.36
Choledocholithotomy 51.41
- endoscopic 51.88

Choledocholithotripsy 51.41
- endoscopic 51.88

Choledochopancreatostomy 51.39
Choledochoplasty 51.72
Choledochorrhaphy 51.71
Choledochoscopy 51.11
Choledochostomy 51.51
Choledochotomy 51.51
Cholelithotomy 51.04
Chondrectomy 80.90
- ankle 80.97
- elbow 80.92
- foot and toe 80.98
- hand and finger 80.94
- hip 80.95
- intervertebral cartilage – *see* category 80.5❹
- knee (semilunar cartilage) 80.6
- nasal (submucous) 21.5
- semilunar cartilage (knee) 80.6
- shoulder 80.91
- specified site NEC 80.99
- spine – *see* category 80.5❹
- wrist 80.93

Chondroplasty – *see* Arthroplasty
Chondrosternoplasty (for pectus excavatum repair) 34.74
Chondrotomy (*see also* Division, cartilage) 80.40
- nasal 21.1

Chopart operation (midtarsal amputation) 84.12
Chordectomy, vocal 30.22
Chordotomy (spinothalmic) (anterior) (posterior) NEC 03.29
- percutaneous 03.21
- stereotactic 03.21

Ciliarotomy 12.55
Ciliectomy (ciliary body) 12.44
- eyelid margin 08.20

Cinch, cinching
- for scleral buckling (*see also* Buckling, scleral) 14.49
- ocular muscle (oblique) (rectus) 15.22
  - multiple (two or more muscles) 15.4

Cineangiocardiography (*see also* Angiocardiography) 88.50
Cineplasty, cineplastic prosthesis
- amputation – *see* Amputation
- arm 84.44
- biceps 84.44
- extremity 84.40
  - lower 84.48
  - upper 84.44
- leg 84.48

Cineradiograph – *see* Radiography
Cingulumotomy (brain) (percutaneous radiofrequency) 01.32
Circumcision (male) 64.0
- female 71.4

CISH (classic infrafascial SEMM hysterectomy) 68.31
Clagett operation (closure of chest wall following open flap drainage) 34.72
Clamp and cautery, hemorrhoids 49.43
Clamping
- aneurysm (cerebral) 39.51
- blood vessel – *see* Ligation, blood vessel
- ventricular shunt 02.43

Clavicotomy 77.31
- fetal 73.8

Claviculectomy (partial) 77.81
- total 77.91

Clayton operation (resection of metatarsal heads and bases of phalanges) 77.88
Cleaning, wound 96.59
Clearance
- bladder (transurethral) 57.0
- pelvic
  - female 68.8
  - male 57.71
- prescalene fat pad 40.21
- renal pelvis (transurethral) 56.0
- ureter (transurethral) 56.0

Cleidotomy 77.31
- fetal 73.8

Clipping
- aneurysm (basilar) (carotid) (cerebellar) (cerebellopontine) (communicating artery) (vertebral) 39.51
- arteriovenous fistula 39.53
- frenulum, frenum
  - labia (lips) 27.91
  - lingual (tongue) 25.91
- tip of uvula 27.72

Clitoridectomy 71.4
Clitoridotomy 71.4
Clivogram 87.02
Closure – *see also* Repair
- abdominal wall 54.63
  - delayed (granulating wound) 54.62
  - secondary 54.61
  - tertiary 54.62
- amputation stump, secondary 84.3
- aorticopulmonary fenestration (fistula) 39.59
- appendicostomy 47.92
- artificial opening
  - bile duct 51.79
  - bladder 57.82
  - bronchus 33.42
  - common duct 51.72
  - esophagus 42.83
  - gallbladder 51.92
  - hepatic duct 51.79
  - intestine 46.50
    - large 46.52
    - small 46.51
  - kidney 55.82
  - larynx 31.62
  - rectum 48.72
  - stomach 44.62
  - thorax 34.72
  - trachea 31.72
  - ureter 56.83
  - urethra 58.42
- atrial septal defect (*see also* Repair, atrial septal defect) 35.71
  - with umbrella device (King-Mills type) 35.52
  - combined with repair of valvular and ventricular septal defects – *see* Repair, endocardial cushion defect
- bronchostomy 33.42
- cecostomy 46.52
- cholecystostomy 51.92
- cleft hand 82.82
- colostomy 46.52
- cystostomy 57.82
- diastema (alveolar) (dental) 24.8
- disrupted abdominal wall (postoperative) 54.61
- duodenostomy 46.51
- encephalocele 02.12
- endocardial cushion defect (*see also* Repair, endocardial cushion defect) 35.73
- enterostomy 46.50
- esophagostomy 42.83
- fenestration
  - aorticopulmonary 39.59
  - septal, heart (*see also* Repair, heart, septum) 35.70
- filtering bleb, corneoscleral (postglaucoma) 12.66
- fistula
  - abdominothoracic 34.83
  - anorectal 48.73
  - anovaginal 70.73

Coagulation, electrocoagulation – Correction

❹ Fourth-Digit Required   *[code]* Manifestation Code   ►◄ Revised Text   ● New Line   ▲ Revised Code

Correction – Curettage

D

Curettage – Decortication

- **Destruction** – *continued*
  - lesion – *continued*
    - urethra (excisional) 58.39
      - endoscopic 58.31
    - uterus 68.29
  - nerve (cranial) (peripheral) (by cryoanalgesia) (by radiofrequency) 04.2
    - sympathetic, by injection of neurolytic agent 05.32
  - neuroma
    - acoustic 04.01
      - by craniotomy 04.01
      - by stereotactic radiosurgery 92.30
        - cobalt 60 92.32
        - linear accelerator (LINAC) 92.31
        - multi-source 92.32
        - particle beam 92.33
        - particulate 92.33
        - radiosurgery NEC 92.39
        - single source photon 92.31
    - cranial 04.07
    - Morton's 04.07
    - peripheral
      - Morton's 04.07
  - prostate (prostatic tissue)
    - by
      - cryotherapy 60.62
      - microwave 60.96
      - radiofrequency 60.97
    - transurethral microwave thermotherapy (TUMT) 60.96
    - transurethral needle ablation (TUNA) 60.97
    - TULIP (transurethral (ultrasound) guided laser induced prostatectomy) 60.21
    - TUMT (transurethral microwave thermotherapy) 60.96
    - TUNA (transurethral needle ablation) 60.97
  - semicircular canals, by injection 20.72
  - vestibule, by injection 20.72
- **Detachment, uterosacral ligaments** 69.3
- **Determination**
  - mental status (clinical) (medicolegal) (psychiatric) NEC 94.11
    - psychologic NEC 94.09
  - vital capacity (pulmonary) 89.37
- **Detorsion**
  - intestine (twisted) (volvulus) 46.80
    - large 46.82
      - endoscopic (balloon) 46.85
    - small 46.81
  - kidney 55.84
  - ovary 65.95
  - spermatic cord 63.52
    - with orchiopexy 62.5
  - testis 63.52
    - with orchiopexy 62.5
  - volvulus 46.80
    - endoscopic (balloon) 46.85
- **Detoxification therapy** 94.25
  - alcohol 94.62
    - with rehabilitation 94.63
    - combined alcohol and drug 94.68
      - with rehabilitation 94.69
  - drug 94.65
    - with rehabilitation 94.66
    - combined alcohol and drug 94.68
      - with rehabilitation 94.69
- **Devascularization, stomach** 44.99
- **Device**
  - CorCap™ 37.41
  - external fixator – *see* Fixator, external
- **Dewebbing**
  - esophagus 42.01
  - syndactyly (fingers) (toes) 86.85
- **Dextrorotation** – *see* Reduction, torsion
- **Dialysis**
  - hemodiafiltration, hemofiltration (extracorporeal) 39.95
  - kidney (extracorporeal) 39.95
  - liver 50.92
  - peritoneal 54.98
  - renal (extracorporeal) 39.95
- **Diaphanoscopy**
  - nasal sinuses 89.35
  - skull (newborn) 89.16
- **Diaphysectomy** – *see* category 77.8❹
- **Diathermy** 93.34
  - choroid – *see* Diathermy, retina
  - nasal turbinates 21.61
- **Diathermy** – *continued*
  - retina
    - for
      - destruction of lesion 14.21
      - reattachment 14.51
      - repair of tear 14.31
  - surgical – *see* Destruction, lesion, by site
  - turbinates (nasal) 21.61
- **Dickson operation** (fascial transplant) 83.82
- **Dickson-Diveley operation** (tendon transfer and arthrodesis to correct claw toe) 77.57
- **Dieffenbach operation** (hip disarticulation) 84.18
- **Dilation**
  - achalasia 42.92
  - ampulla of Vater 51.81
    - endoscopic 51.84
  - anus, anal (sphincter) 96.23
  - biliary duct
    - endoscopic 51.84
    - pancreatic duct 52.99
      - endoscopic 52.98
    - percutaneous (endoscopy) 51.98
    - sphincter
      - of Oddi 51.81
        - endoscopic 51.84
      - pancreatic 51.82
        - endoscopic 51.85
  - bladder 96.25
    - neck 57.92
  - bronchus 33.91
  - cervix (canal) 67.0
    - obstetrical 73.1
    - to assist delivery 73.1
  - choanae (nasopharynx) 29.91
  - colon (endoscopic) (balloon) 46.85
  - colostomy stoma 96.24
  - duodenum (endoscopic) (balloon) 46.85
  - endoscopic – *see* Dilation, by site
  - enterostomy stoma 96.24
  - esophagus (by bougie) (by sound) 42.92
  - fallopian tube 66.96
  - foreskin (newborn) 99.95
  - frontonasal duct 96.21
  - gastrojejunostomy site, endoscopic 44.22
  - heart valve – *see* Valvulotomy, heart
  - ileostomy stoma 96.24
  - ileum (endoscopic) (balloon) 46.85
  - intestinal stoma (artificial) 96.24
  - intestine (endoscopic) (balloon) 46.85
  - jejunum (endoscopic) (balloon) 46.85
  - lacrimal
    - duct 09.42
    - punctum 09.41
  - larynx 31.98
  - lymphatic structure(s) (peripheral) 40.9
  - nares 21.99
  - nasolacrimal duct (retrograde) 09.43
    - with insertion of tube or stent 09.44
  - nasopharynx 29.91
  - pancreatic duct 52.99
    - endoscopic 52.98
  - pharynx 29.91
  - prostatic urethra (transurethral) (balloon) 60.95
  - punctum, lacrimal papilla 09.41
  - pylorus
    - by incision 44.21
    - endoscopic 44.22
  - rectum 96.22
  - salivary duct 26.91
  - sphenoid ostia 22.52
  - sphincter
    - anal 96.23
    - cardiac 42.92
    - of Oddi 51.81
      - endoscopic 51.84
    - pancreatic 51.82
      - endoscopic 51.85
    - pylorus, endoscopic 44.22
      - by incision 44.21
  - Stenson's duct 26.91
  - trachea 31.99
  - ureter 59.8
    - meatus 56.91
  - ureterovesical orifice 59.8
  - urethra 58.6
    - prostatic (transurethral) (balloon) 60.95
  - urethrovesical junction 58.6
  - vagina (instrumental) (manual) NEC 96.16
  - vesical neck 57.92
  - Wharton's duct 26.91
- **Dilation** – *continued*
  - Wirsung's duct 52.99
    - endoscopic 52.98
- **Dilation and curettage, uterus** (diagnostic) 69.09
  - after
    - abortion 69.02
    - delivery 69.02
  - to terminate pregnancy 69.01
- **Diminution, ciliary body** 12.74
- **Disarticulation** 84.91
  - ankle 84.13
  - elbow 84.06
  - finger, except thumb 84.01
    - thumb 84.02
  - hip 84.18
  - knee 84.16
  - shoulder 84.08
  - thumb 84.02
  - toe 84.11
  - wrist 84.04
- **Discectomy** – *see* Diskectomy
- **Discission**
  - capsular membrane 13.64
  - cataract (Wheeler knife) (Ziegler knife) 13.2
    - congenital 13.69
    - secondary membrane 13.64
  - iris 12.12
  - lens (capsule) (Wheeler knife) (Ziegler knife) (with capsulotomy) 13.2
  - orbitomaxillary, radical 16.51
  - pupillary 13.2
  - secondary membrane (after cataract) 13.64
  - vitreous strands (posterior approach) 14.74
    - anterior approach 14.73
- **Discogram, diskogram** 87.21
- **Discolysis** (by injection) 80.52
- **Diskectomy** (discectomy)**, intervertebral** 80.51
  - with corpectomy 80.99
  - herniated (nucleus pulposus) 80.51
  - percutaneous 80.59
- **Dispensing** (with fitting)
  - contact lens 95.32
  - low vision aids NEC 95.33
  - spectacles 95.31
- **Disruption** ●
  - blood brain barrier via infusion [BBBD] 00.19 ●
- **Dissection** – *see also* Excision
  - aneurysm 38.60
  - artery-vein-nerve bundle 39.91
  - branchial cleft fistula or sinus 29.52
  - bronchus 32.1
  - femoral hernia 53.29
  - groin, radical 40.54
  - larynx block (en bloc) 30.3
  - mediastinum with pneumonectomy 32.59 ▲
    - thoracoscopic 32.50 ●
  - neck, radical 40.40
    - with laryngectomy 30.4
    - bilateral 40.42
    - unilateral 40.41
  - orbital fibrous bands 16.92
  - pterygium (with reposition) 11.31
  - radical neck – *see* Dissection, neck, radical
  - retroperitoneal NEC 59.00
  - thoracic structures (block) (en bloc) (radical) (brachial plexus, bronchus, lobe of lung, ribs, and sympathetic nerves) 32.6
  - vascular bundle 39.91
- **Distention, bladder** (therapeutic) (intermittent) 96.25
- **Diversion**
  - biliopancreatic (BPD) 43.7 *[45.51] [45.91]*
    - with duodenal switch 43.89 *[45.51] [45.91]*
  - urinary
    - cutaneous 56.61
    - ileal conduit 56.51
    - internal NEC 56.71
    - ureter to
      - intestine 56.71
      - skin 56.61
    - uretero-ileostomy 56.51
- **Diversional therapy** 93.81
- **Diverticulectomy**
  - bladder (suprapubic) 57.59
    - transurethral approach 57.49
  - duodenum 45.31
    - endoscopic 45.30
  - esophagus 42.31
    - endoscopic 42.33
  - esophagomyotomy 42.7

Diverticulectomy – Drainage

E

- **Electrogastrogram** 44.19
- **Electrokeratotomy** 11.49
- **Electrolysis**
  - ciliary body 12.71
  - hair follicle 86.92
  - retina (for)
    - destruction of lesion 14.21
    - reattachment 14.51
    - repair of tear 14.31
  - skin 86.92
  - subcutaneous tissue 86.92
- **Electromyogram, electromyography** (EMG) (muscle) 93.08
  - eye 95.25
  - urethral sphincter 89.23
- **Electronarcosis** 94.29
- **Electronic gaiter** 93.59
- **Electronystagmogram** (ENG) 95.24
- **Electro-oculogram** (EOG) 95.22
- **Electroresection** – *see also* Destruction, lesion, by site
  - bladder neck (transurethral) 57.49
  - esophagus 42.39
    - endoscopic 42.33
  - prostate (transurethral) 60.29
  - stomach 43.49
    - endoscopic 43.41
- **Electroretinogram** (ERG) 95.21
- **Electroshock therapy** (EST) 94.27
  - subconvulsive 94.26
- **Elevation**
  - bone fragments (fractured)
    - orbit 76.79
    - sinus (nasal)
      - frontal 22.79
      - maxillary 22.79
    - skull (with debridement) 02.02
    - spinal 03.53
  - pedicle graft 86.71
- **Elliot operation** (scleral trephination with iridectomy) 12.61
- **Ellis Jones operation** (repair of peroneal tendon) 83.88
- **Ellison operation** (reinforcement of collateral ligament) 81.44
- **Elmslie-Cholmeley operation** (tarsal wedge osteotomy) 77.28
- **Eloesser operation**
  - thoracoplasty 33.34
  - thoracostomy 34.09
- **Elongation** – *see* Lengthening
- **Embolectomy** 38.00
  - with endarterectomy – *see* Endarterectomy
  - abdominal
    - artery 38.06
    - vein 38.07
  - aorta (arch) (ascending) (descending) 38.04
  - arteriovenous shunt or cannula 39.49
  - bovine graft 39.49
  - head and neck NEC 38.02
  - intracranial NEC 38.01
  - lower limb
    - artery 38.08
    - vein 38.09
  - mechanical
    - endovascular
      - head and neck 39.74
  - pulmonary (artery) (vein) 38.05
  - thoracic NEC 38.05
  - upper limb (artery) (vein) 38.03
- **Embolization** (transcatheter)
  - adhesive (glue) 39.79
    - head and neck 39.72
  - arteriovenous fistula 39.53
    - endovascular 39.72
  - artery (selective) 38.80
    - by
      - endovascular approach 39.79
        - head and neck vessels 39.72
      - percutaneous transcatheter infusion 99.29
    - abdominal NEC 38.86
      - duodenal (transcatheter) 44.44
      - gastric (transcatheter) 44.44
      - renal (transcatheter) 38.86
    - aorta (arch) (ascending) (descending) 38.84
    - duodenal (transcatheter) 44.44
    - gastric (transcatheter) 44.44
    - head and neck NEC 38.82
    - intracranial NEC 38.81

Embolization – *continued*

  - artery – *continued*
    - lower limb 38.88
    - renal (transcatheter) 38.86
    - thoracic NEC 38.85
    - upper limb 38.83
  - AVM, intracranial, endovascular approach 39.72
  - carotid cavernous fistula 39.53
  - chemoembolization 99.25
  - coil, endovascular 39.79
    - head and neck 39.72
  - vein (selective) 38.80
    - by
      - endovascular approach 39.79
        - head and neck 39.72
    - abdominal NEC 38.87
      - duodenal (transcatheter) 44.44
      - gastric (transcatheter) 44.44
    - duodenal (transcatheter) 44.44
    - gastric (transcatheter) 44.44
- **Embryotomy** 73.8
- **EMG** – *see* Electromyogram
- **Emmet operation** (cervix) 67.61
- **Encephalocentesis** (*see also* Puncture) 01.09
  - fetal head, transabdominal 73.8
- **Encephalography** (cisternal puncture) (fractional) (lumbar) (pneumoencephalogram) 87.01
- **Encephalopuncture** 01.09
- **Encircling procedure** – *see also* Cerclage
  - sclera, for buckling 14.49
    - with implant 14.41
- **Endarterectomy** (gas) (with patch graft) 38.10
  - abdominal 38.16
  - aorta (arch) (ascending) (descending) 38.14
  - coronary artery – *see* category 36.0❹
    - open chest approach 36.03
  - head and neck NEC (open) 38.12

    Note – Also use 00.40, 00.41, 00.42, or 00.43 to show the total number of vessels treated. Use code 00.44 once to show procedure on a bifurcated vessel. In addition, use 00.45, 00.46, 00.47, or 00.48 to show the number of vascular stents inserted.

    - percutaneous approach, intracranial vessel(s) 00.62
    - percutaneous approach, precerebral (extracranial) vessel(s) 00.61
  - intracranial (open) NEC 38.11

    Note – Also use 00.40, 00.41, 00.42, or 00.43 to show the total number of vessels treated. Use code 00.44 once to show procedure on a bifurcated vessel. In addition, use 00.45, 00.46, 00.47, or 00.48 to show the number of vascular stents inserted

    - percutaneous approach, intracranial vessel(s) 00.62
  - lower limb 38.18
  - thoracic NEC 38.15
  - upper limb 38.13
- **Endoaneurysmorrhaphy** (*see also* Aneurysmorrhaphy) 39.52
  - by or with
    - endovascular graft
      - abdominal aorta 39.71
      - lower extremity artery(s) 39.79
      - thoracic aorta 39.73
      - upper extremity artery(s) 39.79
- **Endolymphatic** (-subarachnoid) **shunt** 20.71
- **Endometrectomy** (uterine) (internal) 68.29
  - bladder 57.59
  - cul-de-sac 70.32
- **Endoprosthesis**
  - bile duct 51.87
  - femoral head (bipolar) 81.52
- **Endoscopy**
  - with biopsy – *see* Biopsy, by site, closed
  - anus 49.21
  - biliary tract (operative) 51.11
    - by retrograde cholangiography (ERC) 51.11
    - by retrograde cholangiopancreatography (ERCP) 51.10
    - intraoperative 51.11
    - percutaneous (via T-tube or other tract) 51.98
      - with removal of common duct stones 51.96

Endoscopy – *continued*

  - bladder 57.32
    - through stoma (artificial) 57.31
  - bronchus NEC 33.23
    - with biopsy 33.24
    - fiberoptic 33.22
    - through stoma (artificial) 33.21
  - colon 45.23
    - through stoma (artificial) 45.22
    - transabdominal (operative) 45.21
  - cul-de-sac 70.22
  - ear 18.11
  - esophagus NEC 42.23
    - through stoma (artificial) 42.22
    - transabdominal (operative) 42.21
  - ileum 45.13
    - through stoma (artificial) 45.12
    - transabdominal (operative) 45.11
  - intestine NEC 45.24
    - large 45.24
      - fiberoptic (flexible) 45.23
      - through stoma (artificial) 45.22
      - transabdominal (intraoperative) 45.21
    - small 45.13
      - esophagogastroduodenosopy (EGD) 45.13
        - with closed biopsy 45.16
      - through stoma (artificial) 45.12
      - transabdominal (operative) 45.11
  - jejunum 45.13
    - through stoma (artificial) 45.12
    - transabdominal (operative) 45.11
  - kidney 55.21
  - larynx 31.42
    - through stoma (artificial) 31.41
  - lung – *see* Bronchoscopy
  - mediastinum (transpleural) 34.22
  - nasal sinus 22.19
  - nose 21.21
  - pancreatic duct 52.13
  - pelvis 55.22
  - peritoneum 54.21
  - pharynx 29.11
  - rectum 48.23
    - through stoma (artificial) 48.22
    - transabdominal (operative) 48 21
  - sinus, nasal 22.19
  - stomach NEC 44.13
    - through stoma (artificial) 44.12
    - transabdominal (operative) 44.11
  - thorax (transpleural) 34.21
  - trachea NEC 31.42
    - through stoma (artificial) 31.41
  - transpleural
    - mediastinum 34.22
    - thorax 34.21
  - ureter 56.31
  - urethra 58.22
  - uterus 68.12
  - vagina 70.21
- **Enema** (transanal) NEC 96.39
  - for removal of impacted feces 96.38
- **ENG** (electronystagmogram) 95.24
- **Enlargement**
  - aortic lumen, thoracic 38.14
  - atrial septal defect (pre-existing) 35.41
    - in repair of total anomalous pulmonary venous connection 35.82
  - eye socket 16.64
  - foramen ovale (pre-existing) 35.41
    - in repair of total anomalous pulmonary venous connection 35.82
  - intestinal stoma 46.40
    - large intestine 46.43
    - small intestine 46.41
  - introitus 96.16
  - orbit (eye) 16.64
  - palpebral fissure 08.51
  - punctum 09.41
  - sinus tract (skin) 86.89
- **Enterectomy** NEC 45.63
- **Enteroanastomosis**
  - large-to-large intestine 45.94
  - small-to-large intestine 45.93
  - small-to-small intestine 45.91
- **Enterocelectomy** 53.9
  - female 70.92
    - with graft or prosthesis 70 93 ●
  - vaginal 70.92
    - with graft or prosthesis 70.93 ●

Enterocentesis 45.00
duodenum 45.01
large intestine 45.03
small intestine NEC 45.02
Enterocholecystostomy 51.32
Enteroclysis (small bowel) 96.43
Enterocolectomy NEC 45.79
Enterocolostomy 45.93
Enteroentectropy 46.99
Enteroenterostomy 45.90
small-to-large intestine 45.93
small-to-small intestine 45.91
Enterogastrostomy 44.39
laparoscopic 44.38
Enterolithotomy 45.00
Enterolysis 54.59
laparoscopic 54.51
Enteropancreatostomy 52.96
Enterorrhaphy 46.79
large intestine 46.75
small intestine 46.73
Enterostomy NEC 46.39
cecum (*see also* Colostomy) 46.10
colon (transverse) (*see also* Colostomy) 46.10
loop 46.03
delayed opening 46.31
duodenum 46.39
loop 46.01
feeding NEC 46.39
percutaneous (endoscopic) 46.32
ileum (Brooke) (Dragstedt) 46.20
loop 46.01
jejunum (feeding) 46.39
loop 46.01
percutaneous (endoscopic) 46.32
sigmoid colon (*see also* Colostomy) 46.10
loop 46.03
transverse colon (*see also* Colostomy) 46.10
loop 46.03
Enterotomy 45.00
large intestine 45.03
small intestine 45.02
Enucleation – *see also* Excision, lesion, by site
cyst
broad ligament 69.19
dental 24.4
liver 50.29
ovarian 65.29
laparoscopic 65.25
parotid gland 26.29
salivary gland 26.29
skin 86.3
subcutaneous tissue 86.3
eyeball 16.49
with attachment of muscles 16.41
with implant (into Tenon's capsule) 16.42
EOG (electro-oculogram) 95.22
Epicardiectomy 36.39
Epididymectomy 63.4
with orchidectomy (unilateral) 62.3
bilateral 62.41
Epididymogram 87.93
Epididymoplasty 63.59
Epididymorrhaphy 63.81
Epididymotomy 63.92
Epididymovasostomy 63.83
Epiglottidectomy 30.21
Epikeratophakia 11.76
Epilation
eyebrow (forceps) 08.93
cryosurgical 08.92
electrosurgical 08.91
eyelid (forceps) NEC 08.93
cryosurgical 08.92
electrosurgical 08.91
skin 86.92
Epiphysiodesis – *see also* Arrest, bone growth – *see* category 78.2❹
Epiphysiolysis – *see also* Arrest, bone growth – *see* category 78.2❹
Epiploectomy 54.4
Epiplopexy 54.74
Epiplorrhaphy 54.74
Episioperineoplasty 71.79
Episioperineorrhaphy 71.71
obstetrical 75.69
Episioplasty 71.79
Episioproctotomy 73.6
Episiorrhaphy 71.71
following routine episiotomy – *see* Episiotomy for obstetrical laceration 75.69
Episiotomy (with subsequent episiorrhaphy) 73.6
high forceps 72.31
low forceps 72.1
mid forceps 72.21
nonobstetrical 71.09
outlet forceps 72.1
EPS (electrophysiologic stimulation)
as part of intraoperative testing - *omit code*
catheter based invasive electrophysiologic testing 37.26
device interrogation only without arrhythmia induction (bedside check) 89.45-89.49
noninvasive programmed electrical stimulation (NIPS) 37.20
Eptifibatide, infusion 99.20
Equalization, leg
lengthening – *see* category 78.3❹
shortening – *see* category 78.2❹
Equilibration (occlusal) 24.8
Equiloudness balance 95.43
ERC (endoscopic retrograde cholangiography) 51.11
ERCP (endoscopic retrograde cholangiopancreatography) 51.10
cannulation of pancreatic duct 52.93
ERG (electroretinogram) 95.21
ERP (endoscopic retrograde pancreatography) 52.13
Eruption, tooth, surgical 24.6
Erythrocytapheresis, therapeutic 99.73
Escharectomy 86.22
Escharotomy 86.09
Esophageal voice training (postlaryngectomy) 93.73
Esophagectomy 42.40
abdominothoracocervical (combined) (synchronous) 42.42
partial or subtotal 42.41
total 42.42
Esophagocologastrostomy (intrathoracic) 42.55
antesternal or antethoracic 42.65
Esophagocolostomy (intrathoracic) NEC 42.56
with interposition of colon 42.55
antesternal or antethoracic NEC 42.66
with interposition of colon 42.65
Esophagoduodenostomy (intrathoracic) NEC 42.54
with
complete gastrectomy 43.99
interposition of small bowel 42.53
Esophagoenterostomy (intrathoracic) NEC (*see also* Anastomosis, esophagus, to intestinal segment) 42.54
antesternal or antethoracic (*see also* Anastomosis, esophagus, antesternal, to intestinal segment) 42.64
Esophagoesophagostomy (intrathoracic) 42.51
antesternal or antethoracic 42.61
Esophagogastrectomy 43.99
Esophagogastroduodenoscopy (EGD) 45.13
with closed biopsy 45.16
through stoma (artificial) 45.12
transabdominal (operative) 45.11
Esophagogastromyotomy 42.7
Esophagogastropexy 44.65
Esophagogastroplasty 44.65
Esophagogastroscopy NEC 44.13
through stoma (artificial) 44.12
transabdominal (operative) 44.11
Esophagogastrostomy (intrathoracic) 42.52
with partial gastrectomy 43.5
antesternal or antethoracic 42.62
Esophagoileostomy (intrathoracic) NEC 42.54
with interposition of small bowel 42.53
antesternal or antethoracic NEC 42.64
with interposition of small bowel 42.63
Esophagojejunostomy (intrathoracic) NEC 42.54
with
complete gastrectomy 43.99
interposition of small bowel 42.53
antesternal or antethoracic NEC 42.64
with interposition of small bowel 42.63
Esophagomyotomy 42.7
Esophagoplasty NEC 42.89
Esophagorrhaphy 42.82
Esophagoscopy NEC 42.23
by incision (operative) 42.21
with closed biopsy 42.24
through stoma (artificial) 42.22
transabdominal (operative) 42.21
Esophagostomy 42.10
cervical 42.11
thoracic 42.19
Esophagotomy NEC 42.09
Estes operation (ovary) 65.72
laparoscopic 65.75
Estlander operation (thoracoplasty) 33.34
ESWL (extracorporeal shockwave lithotripsy) NEC 98.59
bile duct 98.52
bladder 98.51
gallbladder 98.52
kidney 98.51
Kock pouch (urinary diversion) 98.51
renal pelvis 98.51
specified site NEC 98.59
ureter 98.51
Ethmoidectomy 22.63
Ethmoidotomy 22.51
Evacuation
abscess – *see* Drainage, by site
anterior chamber (eye) (aqueous) (hyphema) 12.91
cyst – *see also* Excision, lesion, by site
breast 85.91
kidney 55.01
liver 50.29
hematoma – *see also* Incision, hematoma
obstetrical 75.92
incisional 75.91
hemorrhoids (thrombosed) 49.47
pelvic blood clot (by incision) 54.19
by
culdocentesis 70.0
culdoscopy 70.22
retained placenta
with curettage 69.02
manual 75.4
streptothrix from lacrimal duct 09.42
Evaluation (of)
audiological 95.43
cardiac rhythm device (CRT-D) (CRT-P) (AICD) (pacemaker) – *see* Interrogation
criminal responsibility, psychiatric 94.11
functional (physical therapy) 93.01
hearing NEC 95.49
orthotic (for brace fitting) 93.02
prosthetic (for artificial limb fitting) 93.03
psychiatric NEC 94.19
commitment 94.13
psychologic NEC 94.08
testimentary capacity, psychiatric 94.11
Evans operation (release of clubfoot) 83.84
Evisceration
eyeball 16.39
with implant (into scleral shell) 16.31
ocular contents 16.39
with implant (into scleral shell) 16.31
orbit (*see also* Exenteration, orbit) 16.59
pelvic (anterior) (posterior) (partial) (total) (female) 68.8
male 57.71
Evulsion
nail (bed) (fold) 86.23
skin 86.3
subcutaneous tissue 86.3
Examination (for)
breast
manual 89.36
radiographic NEC 87.37
thermographic 88.85
ultrasonic 88.73
cervical rib (by x-ray) 87.43
colostomy stoma (digital) 89.33
dental (oral mucosa) (peridontal) 89.31
radiographic NEC 87.12
enterostomy stoma (digital) 89.33
eye 95.09
color vision 95.06
comprehensive 95.02
dark adaptation 95.07
limited (with prescription of spectacles) 95.01
under anesthesia 95.04
fetus, intrauterine 75.35
general physical 89.7

- **Examination** (for) – *continued*
  - glaucoma 95.03
  - gynecological 89.26
  - hearing 95.47
  - microscopic (specimen) (of) 91.9❹

Note – Use the following fourth-digit subclassification with categories 90-91 to identify type of examination:

1	*bacterial smear*
2	*culture*
3	*culture and sensitivity*
4	*parasitology*
5	*toxicology*
6	*cell block and Papanicolaou smear*
9	*other microscopic examination*

- adenoid 90.3❹
- adrenal gland 90.1❹
- amnion 91.4❹
- anus 90.9❹
- appendix 90.9❹
- bile ducts 91.0❹
- bladder 91.3❹
- blood 90.5❹
- bone 91.5❹
  - marrow 90.6❹
- brain 90.0❹
- breast 91.6❹
- bronchus 90.4❹
- bursa 91.5❹
- cartilage 91.5❹
- cervix 91.4❹
- chest wall 90.4❹
- chorion 91.4❹
- colon 90.9❹
- cul-de-sac 91.1❹
- dental 90.8❹
- diaphragm 90.4❹
- duodenum 90.8❹
- ear 90.3❹
- endocrine gland NEC 90.1❹
- esophagus 90.8❹
- eye 90.2❹
- fallopian tube 91.4❹
- fascia 91.5❹
- female genital tract 91.4❹
- fetus 91.4❹
- gallbladder 91.0❹
- hair 91.6❹
- ileum 90.9❹
- jejunum 90.9❹
- joint fluid 91.5❹
- kidney 91.2❹
- large intestine 90.9❹
- larynx 90.3❹
- ligament 91.5❹
- liver 91.0❹
- lung 90.4❹
- lymph (node) 90.7❹
- meninges 90.0❹
- mesentery 91.1❹
- mouth 90.8❹
- muscle 91.5❹
- musculoskeletal system 91.5❹
- nails 91.6❹
- nerve 90.0❹
- nervous system 90.0❹
- nose 90.3❹
- omentum 91.1❹
- operative wound 91.7❹
- ovary 91.4❹
- pancreas 91.0❹
- parathyroid gland 90.1❹
- penis 91.3❹
- perirenal tissue 91.2❹
- peritoneum (fluid) 91.1❹
- periureteral tissue 91.2❹
- perivesical (tissue) 91.3❹
- pharynx 90.3❹
- pineal gland 90.1❹
- pituitary gland 90.1❹
- placenta 91.4❹
- pleura (fluid) 90.4❹
- prostate 91.3❹
- rectum 90.9❹
- retroperitoneum 91.1❹
- semen 91.3❹
- seminal vesicle 91.3❹
- sigmoid 90.9❹
- skin 91.6❹
- small intestine 90.9❹
- specified site NEC 91.8❹

- **Examination** (for) – *continued*
  - microscopic – *continued*
    - spinal fluid 90.0❹
    - spleen 90.6❹
    - sputum 90.4❹
    - stomach 90.8❹
    - stool 90.9❹
    - synovial membrane 91.5❹
    - tendon 91.5❹
    - thorax NEC 90.4❹
    - throat 90.3❹
    - thymus 90.1❹
    - thyroid gland 90.1❹
    - tonsil 90.3❹
    - trachea 90.4❹
    - ureter 91.2❹
    - urethra 91.3❹
    - urine 91.3❹
    - uterus 91.4❹
    - vagina 91.4❹
    - vas deferens 91.3❹
    - vomitus 90.8❹
    - vulva 91.4❹
  - neurologic 89.13
  - neuro-ophthalmology 95.03
  - ophthalmoscopic 16.21
  - panorex, mandible 87.12
  - pelvic (manual) 89.26
    - instrumental (by pelvimeter) 88.25
    - pelvimetric 88.25
  - physical, general 89.7
  - postmortem 89.8
  - rectum (digital) 89.34
    - endoscopic 48.23
      - through stoma (artificial) 48.22
      - transabdominal 48.21
  - retinal disease 95.03
  - specified type (manual) NEC 89.39
  - thyroid field, postoperative 06.02
  - uterus (digital) 68.11
    - endoscopic 68.12
  - vagina 89.26
    - endoscopic 70.21
  - visual field 95.05
- **Exchange transfusion** 99.01
  - intrauterine 75.2
- **Excision**
  - aberrant tissue – *see* Excision, lesion, by site of tissue origin
  - abscess – *see* Excision, lesion, by site
  - accessory tissue – *see also* Excision, lesion, by site of tissue origin
    - lung 32.29
      - endoscopic 32.28
      - thoracoscopic 32.20 ●
    - spleen 41.93
  - adenoids (tag) 28.6
    - with tonsillectomy 28.3
  - adenoma – *see* Excision, lesion, by site
  - adrenal gland (*see also* Adrenalectomy) 07.22
  - ampulla of Vater (with reimplantation of common duct) 51.62
  - anal papilla 49.39
    - endoscopic 49.31
  - aneurysm (arteriovenous) (*see also* Aneurysmectomy) 38.60
    - coronary artery 36.91
    - heart 37.32
    - myocardium 37.32
    - sinus of Valsalva 35.39
    - ventricle (heart) 37.32
  - anus (complete) (partial) 49.6
  - aortic subvalvular ring 35.35
  - apocrine gland 86.3
  - aponeurosis 83.42
    - hand 82.33
  - appendiceal stump 47.09
    - laparoscopic 47.01
  - appendices epiploicae 54.4
  - appendix – *see also* Appendectomy
    - epididymis 63.3
    - testis 62.2
  - arcuate ligament (spine) - *omit code*
  - arteriovenous fistula (*see also* Aneurysmectomy) 38.60
  - artery (*see also* Arteriectomy) 38.60
  - Baker's cyst, knee 83.39
  - Bartholin's gland 71.24
  - basal ganglion 01.59
  - bile duct 51.69
    - endoscopic 51.64
  - bladder – *see also* Cystectomy

- **Excision** – *continued*
  - bleb (emphysematous), lung 32.29
    - endoscopic 32.28
    - thoracoscopic 32.20 ●
  - blood vessel (*see also* Angiectomy) 38.60
  - bone (ends) (partial), except facial – *see* category 77.8❹
    - facial NEC 76.39
      - total 76.45
        - with reconstruction 76.44
    - for graft (autograft) (homograft) – *see* category 77.7❹
    - fragments (chips) (*see also* Incision, bone) 77.10
      - joint (*see also* Arthrotomy) 80.10
      - necrotic (*see also* Sequestrectomy, bone) 77.00
    - heterotopic, from
      - muscle 83.32
        - hand 82.22
      - skin 86.3
      - tendon 83.31
        - hand 82.21
    - mandible 76.31
      - with arthrodesis – *see* Arthrodesis
      - total 76.42
        - with reconstruction 76.41
    - spur – *see* Excision, lesion, bone
    - total, except facial – *see* category 77.9❹
      - facial NEC 76.45
        - with reconstruction 76.44
      - mandible 76.42
        - with reconstruction 76.41
  - brain 01.59
    - hemisphere 01.52
    - lobe 01.53
  - branchial cleft cyst or vestige 29.2
  - breast (*see also* Mastectomy) 85.41
    - aberrant tissue 85.24
    - accessory 85.24
    - ectopic 85.24
    - nipple 85.25
      - accessory 85.24
    - segmental 85.23
    - supernumerary 85.24
    - wedge 85.21
  - broad ligament 69.19
  - bronchogenic cyst 32.09
    - endoscopic 32.01
  - bronchus (wide sleeve) NEC 32.1
  - buccal mucosa 27.49
  - bulbourethral gland 58.92
  - bulbous tuberosities (mandible) (maxilla) (fibrous) (osseous) 24.31
  - bunion (*see also* Bunionectomy) 77.59
  - bunionette (with osteotomy) 77.54
  - bursa 83.5
    - hand 82.31
  - canal of Nuck 69.19
  - cardioma 37.33
  - carotid body (lesion) (partial) (total) 39.8
  - cartilage (*see also* Chondrectomy) 80.90
    - intervertebral – *see* category 80.5❹
    - knee (semilunar) 80.6
    - larynx 30.29
    - nasal (submucous) 21.5
  - caruncle, urethra 58.39
    - endoscopic 58.31
  - cataract (*see also* Extraction, cataract) 13.19
    - secondary membrane (after cataract) 13.65
  - cervical
    - rib 77.91
    - stump 67.4
  - cervix (stump) NEC 67.4
    - cold (knife) 67.2
    - conization 67.2
    - cryoconization 67.33
    - electroconization 67.32
  - chalazion (multiple) (single) 08.21
  - cholesteatoma – *see* Excision, lesion, by site
  - choroid plexus 02.14
  - cicatrix (skin) 86.3
  - cilia base 08.20
  - ciliary body, prolapsed 12.98
  - clavicle (head) (partial) 77.81
    - total (complete) 77.91
  - clitoris 71.4
  - coarctation of aorta (end-to-end anastomosis) 38.64
    - with
      - graft replacement (interposition) abdominal 38.44
        - thoracic 38.45
        - thoracoabdominal 38.45 *[38.44]*

- **Excision** – *continued*
  - lesion – *continued*
    - bone – *continued*
      - femur 77.65
      - fibula 77.67
      - humerus 77.62
      - jaw 76.2
        - dental 24.4
      - patella 77.66
      - pelvic 77.69
      - phalanges (foot) (hand) 77.69
      - radius 77.63
      - scapula 77.61
      - skull 01.6
      - specified site NEC 77.69
      - tarsal, metatarsal 77.68
      - thorax (ribs) (sternum) 77.61
      - tibia 77.67
      - ulna 77.63
      - vertebrae 77.69
    - brain (transtemporal approach) NEC 01.59
      - by stereotactic radiosurgery 92.30
        - cobalt 60 92.32
        - linear accelerator (LINAC) 92.31
        - multi-source 92.32
        - particle beam 92.33
        - particulate 92.33
        - radiosurgery NEC 92.39
        - single source photon 92.31
    - breast (segmental) (wedge) 85.21
    - broad ligament 69.19
    - bronchus NEC 32.09
      - endoscopic 32.01
    - cerebral (cortex) NEC 01.59
      - meninges 01.51
    - cervix (myoma) 67.39
    - chest wall 34.4
    - choroid plexus 02.14
    - ciliary body 12.44
    - colon 45.41
      - endoscopic NEC 45.43
        - polypectomy 45.42
    - conjunctiva 10.31
    - cornea 11.49
    - cranium 01.6
    - cul-de-sac (Douglas') 70.32
    - dental (jaw) 24.4
    - diaphragm 34.81
    - duodenum (local) 45.31
      - endoscopic 45.30
    - ear, external 18.29
      - radical 18.31
    - endometrium 68.29
    - epicardium 37.31
    - epididymis 63.3
    - epiglottis 30.09
    - esophagus NEC 42.32
      - endoscopic 42.33
    - eye, eyeball 16.93
      - anterior segment NEC 12.40
    - eyebrow (skin) 08.20
    - eyelid 08.20
      - by
        - halving procedure 08.24
        - wedge resection 08.24
      - major
        - full-thickness 08.24
        - partial-thickness 08.23
      - minor 08.22
    - fallopian tube 66.61
    - fascia 83.39
      - hand 82.29
    - groin region (abdominal wall) (inguinal) 54.3
      - skin 86.3
      - subcutaneous tissue 86.3
    - gum 24.31
    - heart 37.33
    - hepatic duct 51.69
    - inguinal canal 54.3
    - intestine
      - large 45.41
        - endoscopic NEC 45.43
          - polypectomy 45.42
      - small NEC 45.33
    - intracranial NEC 01.59
    - intranasal 21.31
    - intraspinal 03.4
    - iris 12.42
    - jaw 76.2
      - dental 24.4

- **Excision** – *continued*
  - lesion – *continued*
    - joint 80.80
      - ankle 80.87
      - elbow 80.82
      - foot and toe 80.88
      - hand and finger 80.84
      - hip 80.85
      - knee 80.86
      - shoulder 80.81
      - specified site NEC 80.89
      - spine 80.89
      - wrist 80.83
    - kidney 55.39
      - with partial nephrectomy 55.4
    - labia 71.3
    - lacrimal
      - gland (frontal approach) 09.21
      - passage 09.6
      - sac 09.6
    - larynx 30.09
    - ligament (joint) (*see also* Excision, lesion, joint) 80.80
      - broad 69.19
      - round 69.19
      - uterosacral 69.19
    - lip 27.43
      - by wide excision 27.42
    - liver 50.29
    - lung NEC 32.29
      - by lung volume reduction surgery 32.22
      - by wide excision 32.39 ▲
        - thoracoscopic 32.30 ●
      - endoscopic 32.28
      - thoracoscopic 32.20 ●
    - lymph structure(s) (channel) (vessel) NEC 40.29
      - node – *see* Excision, lymph, node
    - mammary duct 85.21
    - mastoid (bone) 20.49
    - mediastinum 34.3
    - meninges (cerebral) 01.51
      - spinal 03.4
    - mesentery 54.4
    - middle ear 20.51
    - mouth NEC 27.49
    - muscle 83.32
      - hand 82.22
      - ocular 15.13
    - myocardium 37.33
    - nail 86.23
    - nasal sinus 22.60
      - antrum 22.62
        - with Caldwell-Luc approach 22.61
        - specified approach NEC 22.62
      - ethmoid 22.63
      - frontal 22.42
      - maxillary 22.62
        - with Caldwell-Luc approach 22.61
        - specified approach NEC 22.62
      - sphenoid 22.64
    - nasopharynx 29.3❹
    - nerve (cranial) (peripheral) 04.07
      - sympathetic 05.29
    - nonodontogenic 24.31
    - nose 21.30
      - intranasal 21.31
      - polyp 21.31
      - skin 21.32
      - specified site NEC 21.32
    - odontogenic 24.4
    - omentum 54.4
    - orbit 16.92
    - ovary 65.29
      - by wedge resection 65.22
        - laparoscopic 65.24
      - that by laparoscope 65.25
    - palate (bony) 27.31
      - by wide excision 27.32
      - soft 27.49
    - pancreas (local) 52.22
      - endoscopic 52.21
    - parathyroid 06.89
    - parotid gland or duct NEC 26.29
    - pelvic wall 54.3
    - pelvirectal tissue 48.82
    - penis 64.2
    - pericardium 37.31
    - perineum (female) 71.3
      - male 86.3
    - periprostatic tissue 60.82
    - perirectal tissue 48.82

- **Excision** – *continued*
  - lesion – *continued*
    - perirenal tissue 59.91
    - peritoneum 54.4
    - perivesical tissue 59.91
    - pharynx 29.39
      - diverticulum 29.32
    - pineal gland 07.53
    - pinna 18.29
      - radical 18.31
    - pituitary (gland) (*see also* Hypophysectomy, partial) 07.63
      - by stereotactic radiosurgery 92.30
        - cobalt 60 92.32
        - linear accelerator (LINAC) 92.31
        - multi-source 92.32
        - particle beam 92.33
        - particulate 92.33
        - radiosurgery NEC 92.39
        - single source photon 92.31
    - pleura 34.59
    - pouch of Douglas 70.32
    - preauricular (ear) 18.21
    - presacral 54.4
    - prostate (transurethral) 60.61
    - pulmonary (fibrosis) 32.29
      - endoscopic 32.28
      - thoracoscopic 32.20 ●
    - rectovaginal septum 48.82
    - rectum 48.35
      - polyp (endoscopic) 48.36
    - retroperitoneum 54.4
    - salivary gland or duct NEC 26.29
      - en bloc 26.32
    - sclera 12.84
    - scrotum 61.3
    - sinus (nasal) – *see* Excision, lesion, nasal sinus
    - Skene's gland 71.3
    - skin 86.3
      - breast 85.21
      - nose 21.32
      - radical (wide) (involving underlying or adjacent structure) (with flap closure) 86.4
      - scrotum 61.3
    - skull 01.6
    - soft tissue NEC 83.39
      - hand 82.29
    - spermatic cord 63.3
    - sphincter of Oddi 51.62
      - endoscopic 51.64
    - spinal cord (meninges) 03.4
    - spleen (cyst) 41.42
    - stomach NEC 43.42
      - endoscopic 43.41
        - polyp 43.41
      - polyp (endoscopic) 43.41
    - subcutaneous tissue 86.3
      - breast 85.21
    - subgingival 24.31
    - sweat gland 86.3
    - tendon 83.39
      - hand 82.29
      - ocular 15.13
      - sheath 83.31
        - hand 82.21
    - testis 62.2
    - thorax 34.4
    - thymus
      - partial (open) (other) 07.81 ●
        - thoracoscopic 07.83 ●
      - total (open) (other) 07.82 ●
        - thoracoscopic 07.84 ●
    - thyroid 06.31
      - substernal or transsternal route 06.51
    - tongue 25.1
    - tonsil 28.92
    - trachea 31.5
    - tunica vaginalis 61.92
    - ureter 56.41
    - urethra 58.39
      - endoscopic 58.31
    - uterine ligament 69.19
    - uterosacral ligament 69.19
    - uterus 68.29
    - vagina 70.33
    - vein 38.60
      - abdominal 38.67
      - head and neck NEC 38.62
      - intracranial NEC 38.61
      - lower limb 38.69
      - thoracic NEC 38.65
      - upper limb 38.63

❹ Fourth-Digit Required   *[code]* Manifestation Code   ▶◀ Revised Text   ● New Line   ▲ Revised Code

- **Exploration** – *continued*
  - superficial fossa 86.09
  - tarsal tunnel 04.44
  - tendon (sheath) 83.01
    - hand 82.01
  - testes 62.0
  - thymus (gland) 07.92
    - field 07.91
    - thoracoscopic 07.95 ●
  - thyroid (field) (gland) (by incision) 06.09
    - postoperative 06.02
  - trachea (by incision) 31.3
    - endoscopic – *see* Tracheoscopy
  - tunica vaginalis 61.0
  - tympanum 20.09
    - transtympanic route 20.23
  - ureter (by incision) 56.2
    - endoscopic 56.31
  - urethra (by incision) 58.0
    - endoscopic 58.22
  - uterus (corpus) 68.0
    - cervix 69.95
    - digital 68.11
    - postpartal, manual 75.7
  - vagina (by incision) 70.14
    - endoscopic 70.21
  - vas deferens 63.6
  - vein 38.00
    - abdominal 38.07
    - head and neck NEC 38.02
    - intracranial NEC 38.01
    - lower limb 38.09
    - thoracic NEC 38.05
    - upper limb 38.03
  - vulva (by incision) 71.09
- **Exposure** – *see also* Incision, by site
  - tooth (for orthodontic treatment) 24.6
- **Expression, trachoma follicles** 10.33
- **Exsanguination transfusion** 99.01
- **Extension**
  - buccolabial sulcus 24.91
  - limb, forced 93.25
  - lingual sulcus 24.91
  - mandibular ridge 76.43
- **Exteriorization**
  - esophageal pouch 42.12
  - intestine 46.03
    - large 46.03
    - small 46.01
  - maxillary sinus 22.9
  - pilonidal cyst or sinus (open excision) (with partial closure) 86.21
- **Extirpation** – *see also* Excision, by site
  - aneurysm – *see* Aneurysmectomy
  - arteriovenous fistula – *see* Aneurysmectomy
  - lacrimal sac 09.6
  - larynx 30.3
    - with radical neck dissection (with synchronous thyroidectomy) (with synchronous tracheostomy) 30.4
  - nerve, tooth (*see also* Therapy, root canal) 23.70
  - varicose vein (peripheral) (lower limb) 38.59
    - upper limb 38.53
- **Extracorporeal**
  - circulation (regional), except hepatic 39.61
    - hepatic 50.92
    - percutaneous 39.66
  - hemodialysis 39.95
  - membrane oxygenation (ECMO) 39.65
  - photopheresis, therapeutic 99.88
  - shockwave lithotripsy (ESWL) NEC 98.59
    - bile duct 98.52
    - bladder 98.51
    - gallbladder 98.52
    - kidney 98.51
    - renal pelvis 98.51
    - specified site NEC 98.59
    - ureter 98.51
- **Extracranial-intracranial bypass [EC-IC]** 39.28
- **Extraction**
  - breech (partial) 72.52
    - with forceps to aftercoming head 72.51
    - total 72.54
      - with forceps to aftercoming head 72.53
  - cataract 13.19
    - after cataract (by)
      - capsulectomy 13.65
      - capsulotomy 13.64
      - discission 13.64
- **Extraction** – *continued*
  - cataract – *continued*
    - after cataract – *continued*
      - excision 13.65
      - iridocapsulectomy 13.65
      - mechanical fragmentation 13.66
      - needling 13.64
      - phacofragmentation (mechanical) 13.66
    - aspiration (simple) (with irrigation) 13.3
    - cryoextraction (intracapsular approach) 13.19
      - temporal inferior route (in presence of fistulization bleb) 13.11
    - curette evacuation (extracapsular approach) 13.2
    - emulsification (and aspiration) 13.41
    - erysiphake (intracapsular approach) 13.19
      - temporal inferior route (in presence of fistulization bleb) 13.11
    - extracapsular approach (with iridectomy) NEC 13.59
      - by temporal inferior route (in presence of fistulization bleb) 13.51
      - aspiration (simple) (with irrigation) 13.3
      - curette evacuation 13.2
      - emulsification (and aspiration) 13.41
      - linear extraction 13.2
      - mechanical fragmentation with aspiration by
        - posterior route 13.42
        - specified route NEC 13.43
      - phacoemulsification (ultrasonic) (with aspiration) 13.41
      - phacofragmentation (mechanical)
        - with aspiration by
          - posterior route 13.42
          - specified route NEC 13.43
        - ultrasonic (with aspiration) 13.41
      - rotoextraction (mechanical) with aspiration by
        - posterior route 13.42
        - specified route NEC 13.43
    - intracapsular (combined) (simple) (with iridectomy) (with suction) (with zonulolysis) 13.19
      - by temporal inferior route (in presence of fistulization bleb) 13.11
    - linear extraction (extracapsular approach) 13.2
    - phacoemulsification (and aspiration) 13.41
    - phacofragmentation (mechanical)
      - with aspiration by
        - posterior route 13.42
        - specified route NEC 13.43
      - ultrasonic 13.41
    - rotoextraction (mechanical)
      - with aspiration by
        - posterior route 13.42
        - specified route NEC 13.43
    - secondary membranous (after cataract) (by)
      - capsulectomy 13.65
      - capsulotomy 13.64
      - discission 13.64
      - excision 13.65
      - iridocapsulectomy 13.65
      - mechanical fragmentation 13.66
      - needling 13.64
      - phacofragmentation (mechanical) 13.66
  - common duct stones (percutaneous) (through sinus tract) (with basket) 51.96
  - foreign body – *see* Removal, foreign body
  - kidney stone(s), percutaneous 55.03
    - with fragmentation procedure 55.04
  - lens (eye) (*see also* Extraction, cataract) 13.19
  - Malström's 72.79
    - with episiotomy 72.71
  - menstrual, menses 69.6
  - milk from lactating breast (manual) (pump) 99.98
  - tooth (by forceps) (multiple) (single) NEC 23.09
    - with mucoperiosteal flap elevation 23.19
    - deciduous 23.01
    - surgical NEC (*see also* Removal, tooth, surgical) 23.19
  - vacuum, fetus 72.79
    - with episiotomy 72.71
  - vitreous (*see also* Removal, vitreous) 14.72

F

- **Face lift** 86.82
- **Facetectomy** 77.89
- **Facilitation, intraocular circulation** NEC 12.59
- **Failed** (trial) **forceps** 73.3
- **Family**
  - counselling (medical) (social) 94.49
  - therapy 94.42
- **Farabeuf operation** (ischiopubiotomy) 77.39
- **Fasanella-Servatt operation** (blepharoptosis repair) 08.35
- **Fasciaplasty** – *see* Fascioplasty
- **Fascia sling operation** – *see* Operation, sling
- **Fasciectomy** 83.44
  - for graft 83.43
    - hand 82.34
  - hand 82.35
    - for graft 82.34
  - palmar (release of Dupuytren's contracture) 82.35
- **Fasciodesis** 83.89
  - hand 82.89
- **Fascioplasty** (*see also* Repair, fascia) 83.89
  - hand (*see also* Repair, fascia, hand) 82.89
- **Fasciorrhaphy** – *see* Suture, fascia
- **Fasciotomy** 83.14
  - Dupuytren's 82.12
    - with excision 82.35
  - Dwyer 83.14
  - hand 82.12
  - Ober-Yount 83.14
  - orbital (*see also* Orbitotomy) 16.09
  - palmar (release of Dupuytren's contracture) 82.12
    - with excision 82.35
- **Fenestration**
  - aneurysm (dissecting), thoracic aorta 39.54
  - aortic aneurysm 39.54
  - cardiac valve 35.10
  - chest wall 34.01
  - ear
    - inner (with graft) 20.61
      - revision 20.62
    - tympanic 19.55
  - labyrinth (with graft) 20.61
  - Lempert's (endaural) 19.9
  - operation (aorta) 39.54
  - oval window, ear canal 19.55
  - palate 27.1
  - pericardium 37.12
  - semicircular canals (with graft) 20.61
  - stapes foot plate (with vein graft) 19.19
    - with incus replacement 19.11
  - tympanic membrane 19.55
  - vestibule (with graft) 20.61
- **Ferguson operation** (hernia repair) 53.00
- **Fetography** 87.81
- **Fetoscopy** 75.31
- **Fiberoscopy** – *see* Endoscopy, by site
- **Fibroidectomy, uterine** 68.29
- **Fick operation** (perforation of foot plate) 19.0
- **Filipuncture** (aneurysm) (cerebral) 39.52
- **Filleting**
  - hammer toe 77.56
  - pancreas 52.3
- **Filling, tooth** (amalgam) (plastic) (silicate) 23.2
  - root canal (*see also* Therapy, root canal) 23.70
- **Fimbriectomy** (*see also* Salpingectomy, partial) 66.69
  - Uchida (with tubal ligation) 66.32
- **Finney operation** (pyloroplasty) 44.29
- **Fissurectomy, anal** 49.39
  - endoscopic 49.31
  - skin (subcutaneous tissue) 49.04
- **Fistulectomy** – *see also* Closure, fistula, by site
  - abdominothoracic 34.83
  - abdominouterine 69.42
  - anus 49.12
  - appendix 47.92
  - bile duct 51.79
  - biliary tract NEC 51.79
  - bladder (transurethral approach) 57.84
  - bone (*see also* Excision, lesion, bone) 77.60
  - branchial cleft 29.52
  - bronchocutaneous 33.42
  - bronchoesophageal 33.42
  - bronchomediastinal 34.73
  - bronchopleural 34.73
  - bronchopleurocutaneous 34.73
  - bronchopleuromediastinal 34.73
  - bronchovisceral 33.42
  - cervicosigmoidal 67.62
  - cholecystogastroenteric 51.93
  - cornea 11.49

G

- **Graft, grafting** – *continued*
  - fascia 83.82
    - with hernia repair – *see* Repair, hernia
    - eyelid 08.32
    - hand 82.72
    - tarsal cartilage 08.69
  - fat pad NEC 86.89
    - with skin graft – *see* Graft, skin, full-thickness
  - flap (advanced) (rotating) (sliding) – *see also* Graft, skin, pedicle
    - tarsoconjunctival 08.64
  - hair-bearing skin 86.64
  - hand
    - fascia 82.72
    - free skin 86.62
    - muscle 82.72
    - pedicle (flap) 86.73
    - tendon 82.79
  - heart, for revascularization – *see* category 36.3❹
  - joint – *see* Arthroplasty
  - larynx 31.69
  - lip 27.56
    - full-thickness 27.55
  - lymphatic structure(s) (channel) (node) (vessel) 40.9
  - mediastinal fat to myocardium 36.39
  - meninges (cerebral) 02.12
  - mouth, except palate 27.56
    - full-thickness 27.55
  - muscle 83.82
    - hand 82.72
  - myocardium, for revascularization 36.39
  - nasolabial flaps 21.86
  - nerve (cranial) (peripheral) 04.5
  - nipple 85.86
  - nose 21.89
    - with
      - augmentation 21.85
      - rhinoplasty – *see* Rhinoplasty
      - total reconstruction 21.83
    - septum 21.88
    - tip 21.86
  - omentum 54.74
    - to myocardium 36.39
  - orbit (bone) (cartilage) (skin) 16.63
  - outflow tract (patch) (pulmonary valve) 35.26
    - in total repair of tetralogy of Fallot 35.81
  - ovary 65.92
  - palate 27.69
    - for cleft palate repair 27.62
  - pedicle – *see* Graft, skin, pedicle
  - penis (rib) (skin) 64.49
  - pigskin 86.65
  - pinch – *see* Graft, skin, free
  - pocket – *see* Graft, skin, pedicle
  - porcine 86.65
  - postauricular (Wolff) 18.79
  - razor – *see* Graft, skin, free
  - rope – *see* Graft, skin, pedicle
  - saphenous vein in aortocoronary bypass – *see* Bypass, aortocoronary
  - scrotum 61.49
  - skin (partial-thickness) (split-thickness) 86.69
    - amnionic membrane 86.66
    - auditory meatus (ear) 18.6
    - dermal-fat 86.69
      - for breast augmentation 85.50
    - dermal regenerative 86.67
    - ear
      - auditory meatus 18.6
      - postauricular 18.79
    - eyelid 08.61
    - flap – *see* Graft, skin, pedicle
    - free (autogenous) NEC 86.60
      - lip 27.56
        - thumb 86.62
          - for
            - pollicization 82.61
            - reconstruction 82.69
    - full-thickness 86.63
      - breast 85.83
      - hand 86.61
    - hair-bearing 86.64
      - eyelid or eyebrow 08.63
    - hand 86.62
      - full-thickness 86.61
    - heterograft 86.65
    - homograft 86.66
    - island flap 86.70
    - mucous membrane 86.69
      - eyelid 08.62
    - nose – *see* Graft, nose

- **Graft, grafting** – *continued*
  - skin – *continued*
    - pedicle (flap) (tube) 86.70
      - advancement 86.72
      - attachment to site (advanced) (double) (rotating) (sliding) 86.74
        - hand (cross finger) (pocket) 86.73
        - lip 27.57
        - mouth 27.57
        - thumb 86.73
          - for
            - pollicization 82.61
            - reconstruction NEC 82.69
      - breast 85.84
        - transverse rectus abdominis musculocutaneous (TRAM) 85.7
      - defatting 86.75
      - delayed 86.71
      - design and raising 86.71
      - elevation 86.71
      - preparation of (cutting) 86.71
      - revision 86.75
      - sculpturing 86.71
      - transection 86.71
      - transfer 86.74
      - trimming 86.71
    - postauricular 18.79
    - rotation flap 86.70
    - specified site NEC 86.69
      - full-thickness 86.63
  - tarsal cartilage 08.69
  - temporalis muscle to orbit 16.63
    - with exenteration of orbit 16.59
  - tendon 83.81
    - for joint repair – *see* Arthroplasty
    - hand 82.79
  - testicle 62.69
  - thumb (for reconstruction) NEC 82.69
  - tongue (mucosal) (skin) 25.59
  - trachea 31.79
  - tubular (tube) – *see* Graft, skin, pedicle
  - tunnel – *see* Graft, skin, pedicle
  - tympanum (*see also* Tympanoplasty) 19.4
  - ureter 56.89
  - vagina ●
    - biological 70.94 ●
    - synthetic 70.95 ●
  - vein (patch) 39.58
    - with
      - excision or resection of vessel – *see* Phlebectomy, with graft replacement
      - synthetic patch (Dacron) (Teflon) 39.57
      - tissue patch (vein) (autogenous) (homograft) 39.56
  - vermilion border (lip) 27.56
- **Grattage, conjunctiva** 10.31
- **Green operation** (scapulopexy) 78.41
- **Grice operation** (subtalar arthrodesis) 81.13
- **Grip, strength** 93.04
- **Gritti-Stokes operation** (knee disarticulation) 84.16
- **Gross operation** (herniorrhaphy) 53.49
- **Group therapy** 94.44
- **Guttering, bone** (*see also* Excision, lesion, bone) 77.60
- **Guyon operation** (amputation of ankle) 84.13

H

- **Hagner operation** (epididymotomy) 63.92
- **Halsted operation** – *see* Repair, hernia, inguinal
- **Hampton operation** (anastomosis small intestine to rectal stump) 45.92
- **Hanging hip operation** (muscle release) 83.19
- **Harelip operation** 27.54
- **Harrison-Richardson operation** (vaginal suspension) 70.77
  - with graft or prosthesis 70.78 ●
- **Hartmann resection** (of intestine) (with pouch) – *see* Colectomy, by site
- **Harvesting**
  - bone marrow 41.91
  - stem cells 99.79
- **Hauser operation**
  - achillotenotomy 83.11
  - bunionectomy with adductor tendon transfer 77.53
  - stabilization of patella 81.44
- **Heaney operation** (vaginal hysterectomy) 68.59
  - laparoscopically assisted (LAVH) 68.51
- **Hearing aid** (with battery replacement) 95.49
- **Hearing test** 95.47
- **Hegar operation** (perineorrhaphy) 71.79
- **Heine operation** (cyclodialysis) 12.55
- **Heineke-Mikulicz operation** (pyloroplasty) 44.29
- **Heller operation** (esophagomyotomy) 42.7
- **Hellstöm operation** (transplantation of aberrant renal vessel) 39.55
- **Hemicolectomy**
  - left 45.75
  - right (extended) 45.73
- **Hemicystectomy** 57.6
- **Hemigastrectomy** – *see* Gastrectomy
- **Hemiglossectomy** 25.2
- **Hemilaminectomy** (decompression) (exploration) 03.09
- **Hemilaryngectomy** (anterior) (lateral) (vertical) 30.1
- **Hemimandibulectomy** 76.31
- **Hemimastectomy** (radical) 85.23
- **Hemimaxillectomy** (with bone graft) (with prosthesis) 76.39
- **Heminephrectomy** 55.4
- **Hemipelvectomy** 84.19
- **Hemispherectomy** (cerebral) 01.52
- **Hemithyroidectomy** (with removal of isthmus) (with removal of portion of remaining lobe) 06.2
- **Hemodiafiltration** (extracorporeal) 39.95
- **Hemodialysis** (extracorporeal) 39.95
- **Hemodilution** 99.03
- **Hemofiltration** (extracorporeal) 39.95
- **Hemorrhage control** – *see* Control, hemorrhage
- **Hemorrhoidectomy** 49.46
  - by
    - cautery, cauterization 49.43
    - crushing 49.45
    - cryotherapy, cryosurgery 49.44
    - excision 49.46
    - injection 49.42
    - ligation 49.45
- **Hemostasis** – *see* Control, hemorrhage
- **Henley operation** (jejunal transposition) 43.81
- **Hepatectomy** (complete) (total) 50.4
  - partial or subtotal 50.22
- **Hepatic assistance, extracorporeal** 50.92
- **Hepaticocholangiojejunostomy** 51.37
- **Hepaticocystoduodenostomy** 51.37
- **Hepaticodochotomy** 51.59
- **Hepaticoduodenostomy** 51.37
- **Hepaticojejunostomy** 51.37
- **Hepaticolithectomy** 51.49
  - endoscopic 51.88
- **Hepaticolithotomy** 51.49
  - endoscopic 51.88
- **Hepaticostomy** 51.59
- **Hepaticotomy** 51.59
- **Hepatocholangiocystoduodenostomy** 51.37
- **Hepatocholedochostomy** 51.43
  - endoscopic 51.87
- **Hepatoduodenostomy** 50.69
- **Hepatogastrostomy** 50.69
- **Hepatojejunostomy** 50.69
- **Hepatolithotomy**
  - hepatic duct 51.49
  - liver 50.0
- **Hepatopexy** 50.69
- **Hepatorrhaphy** 50.61
- **Hepatostomy** (external) (internal) 50.69
- **Hepatotomy** (with packing) 50.0
- **Hernioplasty** – *see* Repair, hernia
- **Herniorrhaphy** – *see* Repair, hernia
- **Herniotomy** – *see* Repair, hernia
- **Heterograft** – *see* Graft
- **Heterotransplant, heterotransplantation** – *see* Transplant
- **Hey operation** (amputation of foot) 84.12
- **Hey-Groves operation** (reconstruction of anterior cruciate ligament) 81.45
- **Heyman operation** (soft tissue release for clubfoot) 83.84

Immunotherapy, antineoplastic – Implant, implantation

❹ Fourth-Digit Required | *[code]* Manifestation Code | ►◄ Revised Text | ● New Line | ▲ Revised Code

Implant, implantation – Implant, implantation

- **Implant, implantation** – *continued*
  - vitreous (silicone) 14.75
    - for retinal reattachment 14.41
      - with buckling 14.41
  - vocal cord(s) (paraglottic) 31.98
  - X Stop™ 84.80 ▲
- **Implosion** (psychologic desensitization) 94.33
- **Incision** (and drainage)
  - with
    - exploration – *see* Exploration
    - removal of foreign body – *see* Removal, foreign body
  - abdominal wall 54.0
    - as operative approach - *omit code*
  - abscess – *see also* Incision, by site
    - appendix 47.2
      - with appendectomy 47.09
        - laparoscopic 47.01
    - extraperitoneal 54.0
    - ischiorectal 49.01
    - lip 27.0
    - omental 54.19
    - perianal 49.01
    - perigastric 54.19
    - perisplenic 54.19
    - peritoneal NEC 54.19
      - pelvic (female) 70.12
    - retroperitoneal 54.0
    - sclera 12.89
    - skin 86.04
    - subcutaneous tissue 86.04
    - subdiaphragmatic 54.19
    - subhepatic 54.19
    - subphrenic 54.19
    - vas deferens 63.6
  - adrenal gland 07.41
  - alveolus, alveolar bone 24.0
  - antecubital fossa 86.09
  - anus NEC 49.93
    - fistula 49.11
    - septum 49.91
  - appendix 47.2
  - artery 38.00
    - abdominal 38.06
      - aorta (arch) (ascending) (descending) 38.04
    - head and neck NEC 38.02
    - intracranial NEC 38.01
    - lower limb 38.08
    - thoracic NEC 38.05
    - upper limb 38.03
  - atrium (heart) 37.11
  - auditory canal or meatus, external 18.02
  - auricle 18.09
  - axilla 86.09
  - Bartholin's gland or cyst 71.22
  - bile duct (with T or Y tube insertion) NEC 51.59
    - common (exploratory) 51.51
      - for
        - relief of obstruction NEC 51.42
        - removal of calculus 51.41
    - for
      - exploration 51.59
      - relief of obstruction 51.49
  - bladder 57.19
    - neck (transurethral) 57.91
    - percutaneous suprapubic (closed) 57.17
    - suprapubic NEC 57.18
  - blood vessel (*see also* Angiotomy) 38.00
  - bone 77.10
    - alveolus, alveolar 24.0
    - carpals, metacarpals 77.14
    - clavicle 77.11
    - facial 76.09
    - femur 77.15
    - fibula 77.17
    - humerus 77.12
    - patella 77.16
    - pelvic 77.19
    - phalanges (foot) (hand) 77.19
    - radius 77.13
    - scapula 77.11
    - skull 01.24
    - specified site NEC 77.19
    - tarsals, metatarsals 77.18
    - thorax (ribs) (sternum) 77.11
    - tibia 77.17
    - ulna 77.13
    - vertebrae 77.19
  - brain 01.39
    - cortical adhesions 02.91
  - breast (skin) 85.0
    - with removal of tissue expander 85.96

- **Incision** – *continued*
  - bronchus 33.0
  - buccal space 27.0
  - bulbourethral gland 58.91
  - bursa 83.03
    - hand 82.03
    - pharynx 29.0
  - carotid body 39.8
  - cerebral (meninges) 01.39
    - epidural or extradural space 01.24
    - subarachnoid or subdural space 01.31
  - cerebrum 01.39
  - cervix 69.95
    - to
      - assist delivery 73.93
      - replace inverted uterus 75.93
  - chalazion 08.09
    - with removal of capsule 08.21
  - cheek 86.09
  - chest wall (for extrapleural drainage) (for removal of foreign body) 34.01
    - as operative approach - *omit code*
  - common bile duct (for exploration) 51.51
    - for
      - relief of obstruction 51.42
      - removal of calculus 51.41
  - common wall between posterior left atrium and coronary sinus (with roofing of resultant defect with patch graft) 35.82
  - conjunctiva 10.1
  - cornea 11.1
    - radial (refractive) 11.75
  - cranial sinus 01.21
  - craniobuccal pouch 07.72
  - cul-de-sac 70.12
  - cyst
    - dentigerous 24.0
    - radicular (apical) (periapical) 24.0
  - Duhrssen's (cervix, to assist delivery) 73.93
  - duodenum 45.01
  - ear
    - external 18.09
    - inner 20.79
    - middle 20.23
  - endocardium 37.11
  - endolymphatic sac 20.79
  - epididymis 63.92
  - epidural space, cerebral 01.24
  - epigastric region 54.0
    - intra-abdominal 54.19
  - esophagus, esophageal NEC 42.09
    - web 42.01
  - exploratory – *see* Exploration
  - extradural space (cerebral) 01.24
  - extrapleural 34.01
  - eyebrow 08.09
  - eyelid 08.09
    - margin (trichiasis) 08.01
  - face 86.09
  - fallopian tube 66.01
  - fascia 83.09
    - with division 83.14
      - hand 82.12
    - hand 82.09
      - with division 82.12
  - fascial compartments, head and neck 27.0
  - fistula, anal 49.11
  - flank 54.0
  - furuncle – *see* Incision, by site
  - gallbladder 51.04
  - gingiva 24.0
  - gluteal 86.09
  - groin region (abdominal wall) (inguinal) 54.0
    - skin 86.09
    - subcutaneous tissue 86.09
  - gum 24.0
  - hair follicles 86.09
  - heart 37.10
    - valve – *see* Valvulotomy
  - hematoma – *see also* Incision, by site
    - axilla 86.04
    - broad ligament 69.98
    - ear 18.09
    - episiotomy site 75.91
    - fossa (superficial) NEC 86.04
    - groin region (abdominal wall) (inguinal) 54.0
      - skin 86.04
      - subcutaneous tissue 86.04
    - laparotomy site 54.12
    - mediastinum 34.1
    - perineum (female) 71.09
      - male 86.04

- **Incision** – *continued*
  - hematoma – *continued*
    - popliteal space 86.04
    - scrotum 61.0
    - skin 86.04
    - space of Retzius 59.19
    - subcutaneous tissue 86.04
    - vagina (cuff) 70.14
      - episotomy site 75.91
      - obstetrical NEC 75.92
  - hepatic ducts 51.59
  - hordeolum 08.09
  - hygroma – *see also* Incision, by site
    - cystic 40.0
  - hymen 70.11
  - hypochondrium 54.0
    - intra-abdominal 54.19
  - hypophysis 07.72
  - iliac fossa 54.0
  - infratemporal fossa 27.0
  - ingrown nail 86.09
  - intestine 45.00
    - large 45.03
    - small 45.02
  - intracerebral 01.39
  - intracranial (epidural space) (extradural space) 01.24
    - subarachnoid or subdural space 01.31
  - intraperitoneal 54.19
  - ischiorectal tissue 49.02
    - abscess 49.01
  - joint structures (*see also* Arthrotomy) 80.10
  - kidney 55.01
    - pelvis 55.11
  - labia 71.09
  - lacrimal
    - canaliculus 09.52
    - gland 09.0
    - passage NEC 09.59
    - punctum 09.51
    - sac 09.53
  - larynx NEC 31.3
  - ligamentum flavum (spine) - *omit code*
  - liver 50.0
  - lung 33.1
  - lymphangioma 40.0
  - lymphatic structure (channel) (node) (vessel) 40.0
  - mastoid 20.21
  - mediastinum 34.1
  - meibomian gland 08.09
  - meninges (cerebral) 01.31
    - spinal 03.09
  - midpalmar space 82.04
  - mouth NEC 27.92
    - floor 27.0
  - muscle 83.02
    - with division 83.19
      - hand 82.19
    - hand 82.02
      - with division 82.19
  - myocardium 37.11
  - nailbed or nailfold 86.09
  - nasolacrimal duct (stricture) 09.59
  - neck 86.09
  - nerve (cranial) (peripheral) NEC 04.04
    - root (spinal) 03.1
  - nose 21.1
  - omentum 54.19
  - orbit (*see also* Orbitotomy) 16.09
  - ovary 65.09
    - laparoscopic 65.01
  - palate 27.1
  - palmar space (middle) 82.04
  - pancreas 52.09
  - pancreatic sphincter 51.82
    - endoscopic 51.85
  - parapharyngeal (oral) (transcervical) 28.0
  - paronychia 86.09
  - parotid
    - gland or duct 26.0
    - space 27.0
  - pelvirectal tissue 48.81
  - penis 64.92
  - perianal (skin) (tissue) 49.02
    - abscess 49.01
  - perigastric 54.19
  - perineum (female) 71.09
    - male 86.09
  - peripheral vessels
    - lower limb
      - artery 38.08
      - vein 38.09

Incision – *continued*
  peripheral vessels – *continued*
    upper limb (artery) (vein) 38.03
  periprostatic tissue 60.81
  perirectal tissue 48.81
  perirenal tissue 59.09
  perisplenic 54.19
  peritoneum 54.95
    by laparotomy 54.19
    pelvic (female) 70.12
      male 54.19
  periureteral tissue 59.09
  periurethral tissue 58.91
  perivesical tissue 59.19
  petrous pyramid (air cells) (apex) (mastoid) 20.22
  pharynx, pharyngeal (bursa) 29.0
    space, lateral 27.0
  pilonidal sinus (cyst) 86.03
  pineal gland 07.52
  pituitary (gland) 07.72
  pleura NEC 34.09
  popliteal space 86.09
  postzygomatic space 27.0
  pouch of Douglas 70.12
  prostate (perineal approach) (transurethral
      approach) 60.0
  pterygopalatine fossa 27.0
  pulp canal (tooth) 24.0
  Rathke's pouch 07.72
  rectovaginal septum 48.81
  rectum 48.0
    stricture 48.91
  renal pelvis 55.11
  retroperitoneum 54.0
  retropharyngeal (oral) (transcervical) 28.0
  salivary gland or duct 26.0
  sclera 12.89
  scrotum 61.0
  sebaceous cyst 86.04
  seminal vesicle 60.72
  sinus – *see* Sinusotomy
  Skene's duct or gland 71.09
  skin 86.09
    with drainage 86.04
    breast 85.0
    cardiac pacemaker pocket, new site 37.79
    ear 18.09
    nose 21.1
    subcutaneous tunnel for pulse generator lead
        wire 86.99
      with initial procedure - *omit code*
    thalamic stimulator pulse generator pocket,
        new site 86.09
      with initial insertion of battery package - *omit
          code*
    tunnel, subcutaneous for pulse generator lead
        wire 86.99
      with initial procedure - *omit code*
  skull (bone) 01.24
  soft tissue NEC 83.09
    with division 83.19
      hand 82.19
    hand 82.09
      with division 82.19
  space of Retzius 59.19
  spermatic cord 63.93
  sphincter of Oddi 51.82
    endoscopic 51.85
  spinal
    cord 03.09
    nerve root 03.1
  spleen 41.2
  stomach 43.0
  stye 08.09
  subarachnoid space, cerebral 01.31
  subcutaneous tissue 86.09
    with drainage 86.04
    tunnel
      esophageal 42.86
        with anastomosis – *see* Anastomosis,
            esophagus, antesternal
      pulse generator lead wire 86.99
        with initial procedure - *omit code*
  subdiaphragmatic space 54.19
  subdural space, cerebral 01.31
  sublingual space 27.0
  submandibular space 27.0
  submaxillary 86.09
    with drainage 86.04
  submental space 27.0
  subphrenic space 54.19

Incision – *continued*
  supraclavicular fossa 86.09
    with drainage 86.04
  sweat glands, skin 86.04
  temporal pouches 27.0
  tendon (sheath) 83.01
    with division 83.13
      hand 82.11
    hand 82.01
    with division 82.11
  testis 62.0
  thenar space 82.04
  thymus ▶(open) (other)◀ 07.92
    thoracoscopic 07.95 ●
  thyroid (field) (gland) NEC 06.09
    postoperative 06.02
  tongue NEC 25.94
    for tongue tie 25.91
  tonsil 28.0
  trachea NEC 31.3
  tunica vaginalis 61.0
  umbilicus 54.0
  urachal cyst 54.0
  ureter 56.2
  urethra 58.0
  uterus (corpus) 68.0
    cervix 69.96
    for termination of pregnancy 74.91
    septum (congenital) 68.22
  uvula 27.71
  vagina (cuff) (septum) (stenosis) 70.14
    for
      incisional hematoma (episiotomy) 75.91
      obstetrical hematoma NEC 75.92
      pelvic abscess 70.12
  vas deferens 63.6
  vein 38.00
    abdominal 38.07
    head and neck NEC 38.02
    intracranial NEC 38.01
    lower limb 38.09
    thoracic NEC 38.05
    upper limb 38.03
  vertebral column 03.09
  vulva 71.09
    obstetrical 75.92
  web, esophageal 42.01
Incudectomy NEC 19.3
  with
    stapedectomy (*see also* Stapedectomy) 19.19
    tympanoplasty – *see* Tympanoplasty
Incudopexy 19.19
Incudostapediopexy 19.19
    with incus replacement 19.11
Indentation, sclera, for buckling (*see also* Buckling,
    scleral) 14.49
Indicator dilution flow measurement 89.68
Induction
  abortion
    by
      D and C 69.01
      insertion of prostaglandin suppository 96.49
      intra-amniotic injection (prostaglandin)
          (saline) 75.0
  labor
    medical 73.4
    surgical 73.01
      intra- and extra-amniotic injection 73.1
      stripping of membranes 73.1
Inflation
  belt wrap 93.99
  Eustachian tube 20.8
  fallopian tube 66.8
    with injection of therapeutic agent 66.95
Infolding, sclera, for buckling (*see also* Buckling,
    scleral) 14.49
Infraction, turbinates (nasal) 21.62
Infundibulectomy
  hypophyseal (*see also* Hypophysectomy, partial)
      07.63
  ventricle (heart) (right) 35.34
    in total repair of tetralogy of Fallot 35.81
Infusion (intra-arterial) (intravenous)
  with ●
    disruption of blood brain barrier [BBBD]
        00.19 ●
  Abciximab 99.20
  antibiotic
    oxazolidinone class 00.14

Infusion – *continued*
  antineoplastic agent (chemotherapeutic) 99.25
    biological response modifier [BRM] 99.28
    cintredekin besudotox 99.28
    high-dose interleukin-2 00.15
    low-dose interleukin-2 99.28
  biological response modifier [BRM], antineoplastic
      agent 99.28
    cintredekin besudotox 99.28
    high-dose interleukin-2 00.15
    low-dose interleukin-2 99.28
  cancer chemotherapy agent NEC 99.25
  cintredekin besudotox 99.28
  drotrecogin alfa (activated) 00.11
  electrolytes 99.18
  enzymes, thrombolytic (streptokinase) (tissue
      plasminogen activator) (TPA) (urokinase)
    direct coronary artery 36.04
    intravenous 99.10
  Eptifibatide 99.20
  gamma globulin 99.14 ●
  GP IIB/IIIa inhibitor 99.20
  hormone substance NEC 99.24
  human B-type natriuretic peptide (hBNP) 00.13
  immunosuppressive antibody therapy 00.18
  nesiritide 00.13
  neuroprotective agent 99.75
  nimodipine 99.75
  nutritional substance – *see* Nutrition
  platelet inhibitor
    direct coronary artery 36.04
    intravenous 99.20
  Proleukin (low-dose) 99.28
    high-dose 00.15
  prophylactic substance NEC 99.29
  radioimmunoconjugate 92.28
  radioimmunotherapy 92.28
  radioisotope (liquid brachytherapy) (liquid I-125)
      92.20
  recombinant protein 00.11
  reteplase 99.10
  therapeutic substance NEC 99.29
  thrombolytic agent (enzyme) (streptokinase)
      99.10
    with percutaneous transluminal angioplasty

Note – Also use 00.40, 00.41, 00.42, or 00.43 to show the total number of vessels treated.

      coronary 00.66
      non-coronary vessel(s) 39.50
        specified site NEC 39.50
    direct intracoronary artery 36.04
  tirofiban (HCL) 99.20
  vaccine
    tumor 99.28
  vasopressor 00.17
Injection (into) (hypodermically) (intramuscularly)
    (intravenously) (acting locally or systemically)
  Actinomycin D, for cancer chemotherapy 99.25
  adhesion barrier substance 99.77
  alcohol
    nerve – *see* Injection, nerve
    spinal 03.8
  anterior chamber, eye (air) (liquid) (medication)
      12.92
  antibiotic 99.21
    oxazolidinone class 00.14
  anticoagulant 99.19
  anti-D (Rhesus) globulin 99.11
  antidote NEC 99.16
  anti-infective NEC 99.22
  antineoplastic agent (chemotherapeutic) NEC
      99.25
    biological response modifier [BRM] 99.28
    cintredekin besudotox 99.28
    high-dose interleukin-2 00.15
    low-dose interleukin-2 99.28
  antivenin 99.16
  barrier substance, adhesion 99.77
  BCG
    for chemotherapy 99.25
    vaccine 99.33
  biological response modifier [BRM], antineoplastic
      agent 99.28
    cintredekin besudotox 99.28
    high-dose interleukin-2 00.15
    low-dose interleukin-2 99.28
  bone marrow 41.92
    transplant – *see* Transplant, bone, marrow

Injection – *continued*
breast (therapeutic agent) 85.92
inert material (silicone) (bilateral) 85.52
unilateral 85.51
bursa (therapeutic agent) 83.96
hand 82.94
cancer chemotherapeutic agent 99.25
caudal – *see* Injection, spinal
cintredekin besudotox 99.28
cortisone 99.23
costochondral junction 81.92
dinoprost-tromethine, intra-amniotic 75.0
disc, intervertebral (herniated) 80.52
ear, with alcohol 20.72
electrolytes 99.18
enzymes, thrombolytic (streptokinase) (tissue plasminogen activator) (TPA) (urokinase)
direct coronary artery 36.04
intravenous 99.10
epidural, spinal – *see* Injection, spinal
esophageal varices or blood vessel (endoscopic) (sclerosing agent) 42.33
Eustachian tube (inert material) 20.8
eye (orbit) (retrobulbar) 16.91
anterior chamber 12.92
subconjunctival 10.91
fascia 83.98
hand 82.96
gamma globulin 99.14
ganglion, sympathetic 05.39
ciliary 12.79
paravertebral stellate 05.39
gel, adhesion barrier – *see* Injection, adhesion barrier substance
globulin
anti-D (Rhesus) 99.11
gamma 99.14
Rh immune 99.11
heart 37.92
heavy metal antagonist 99.16
hemorrhoids (sclerosing agent) 49.42
hormone NEC 99.24
human B-type natriuretic peptide (hBNP) 00.13
immune sera 99.14
inert material – *see* Implant, inert material
inner ear, for destruction 20.72
insulin 99.17
intervertebral space for herniated disc 80.52
intra-amniotic
for induction of
abortion 75.0
labor 73.1
intrathecal – *see* Injection, spinal
joint (therapeutic agent) 81.92
temporomandibular 76.96
kidney (cyst) (therapeutic substance) NEC 55.96
larynx 31.0
ligament (joint) (therapeutic substance) 81.92
liver 50.94
lung, for surgical collapse 33.32
Methotrexate, for cancer chemotherapy 99.25
nerve (cranial) (peripheral) 04.80
agent NEC 04.89
alcohol 04.2
anesthetic for analgesia 04.81
for operative anesthesia - *omit code*
neurolytic 04.2
phenol 04.2
laryngeal (external) (recurrent) (superior) 31.91
optic 16.91
sympathetic 05.39
alcohol 05.32
anesthetic for analgesia 05.31
neurolytic agent 05.32
phenol 05.32
nesiritide 00.13
neuroprotective agent 99.75
nimodipine 99.75
orbit 16.91
pericardium 37.93
peritoneal cavity
air 54.96
locally-acting therapeutic substance 54.97
platelet inhibitor
direct coronary artery 36.04
intravenous 99.20
prophylactic substance NEC 99.29
prostate 60.92
radioimmunoconjugate 92.28
radioimmunotherapy 92.28
radioisotopes (intracavitary) (intravenous) 92.28
renal pelvis (cyst) 55.96

Injection – *continued*
retrobulbar (therapeutic substance) 16.91
for anesthesia - *omit code*
Rh immune globulin 99.11
RhoGAM 99.11
sclerosing agent NEC 99.29
esophageal varices (endoscopic) 42.33
hemorrhoids 49.42
pleura 34.92
treatment of malignancy (cytotoxic agent) 34.92 *[99.25]*
with tetracycline 34.92 *[99.21]*
varicose vein 39.92
vein NEC 39.92
semicircular canals, for destruction 20.72
silicone – *see* Implant, inert material
skin (sclerosing agent) (filling material) 86.02
soft tissue 83.98
hand 82.96
spinal (canal) NEC 03.92
alcohol 03.8
anesthetic agent for analgesia 03.91
for operative anesthesia - *omit code*
contrast material (for myelogram) 87.21
destructive agent NEC 03.8
neurolytic agent NEC 03.8
phenol 03.8
proteolytic enzyme (chymodiactin) (chymopapain) 80.52
saline (hypothermic) 03.92
steroid NEC 03.92
spinal nerve root (intrathecal) – *see* Injection, spinal
steroid NEC 99.23
subarachnoid, spinal – *see* Injection, spinal
subconjunctival 10.91
tendon 83.97
hand 82.95
testis 62.92
therapeutic agent NEC 99.29
thoracic cavity 34.92
thrombolytic agent (enzyme)(streptokinase) 99.10
with percutaneous transluminal angioplasty

Note – Also use 00.40, 00.41, 00.42, or 00.43 to show the total number of vessels treated.

coronary 00.66
non coronary vessels 39.50
specified site NEC 39.50
direct intracoronary artery 36.04
trachea 31.94
tranquilizer 99.26
tunica vaginalis (with aspiration) 61.91
tympanum 20.94
urethra (inert material)
for repair of urinary stress incontinence
collagen implant 59.72
endoscopic injection of implant 59.72
fat implant 59.72
polytef implant 59.72
vaccine
tumor 99.28
varices, esophagus (endoscopic) (sclerosing agent) 42.33
varicose vein (sclerosing agent) 39.92
esophagus (endoscopic) 42.33
vestibule, for destruction 20.72
vitreous substitute (silicone) 14.75
for reattachment of retina 14.59
vocal cords 31.0
Inlay, tooth 23.3
Inoculation
antitoxins – *see* Administration, antitoxins
toxoids – *see* Administration, toxoids
vaccine – *see* Administration, vaccine
Insemination, artificial 69.92
Insertion
airway
esophageal obturator 96.03
nasopharynx 96.01
oropharynx 96.02
Allen-Brown cannula 39.93
arch bars (orthodontic) 24.7
for immobilization (fracture) 93.55
atrial septal umbrella 35.52
Austin-Moore prosthesis 81.52
baffle, heart (atrial) (interatrial) (intra-atrial) 35.91
bag, cervix (nonobstetrical) 67.0
after delivery or abortion 75.8
to assist delivery or induce labor 73.1

Insertion – *continued*
Baker's (tube) (for stenting) 46.85
balloon
gastric 44.93
heart (pulsation-type) (Kantrowitz) 37.61
intestine (for decompression) (for dilation) 46.85
band (adjustable)
gastric, laparoscopic 44.95
Lap-Band™ 44.95
Barton's tongs (skull) (with synchronous skeletal traction) 02.94
bipolar endoprosthesis (femoral head) 81.52
Blakemore-Sengstaken tube 96.06
bone growth stimulator (invasive) (percutaneous) (semi-invasive) – *see* category 78.9❹
bone morphogenetic protein (Infuse™) (OP-1™) (recombinant) (rhBMP) 84.52
bone void filler 84.55
that with kyphoplasty 81.66
that with vertebroplasty 81.65
bougie, cervix, nonobstetrical 67.0
to assist delivery or induce labor 73.1
breast implant (for augmentation) (bilateral) 85.54
unilateral 85.53
bridge (dental) (fixed) 23.42
removable 23.43
bubble (balloon), stomach 44.93
caliper tongs (skull) (with synchronous skeletal traction) 02.94
cannula
Allen-Brown 39.93
for extracorporeal membrane oxygenation (ECMO) - *omit code*
nasal sinus (by puncture) 22.01
through natural ostium 22.02
pancreatic duct 52.92
endoscopic 52.93
vessel to vessel 39.93
cardiac resynchronization device
defibrillator (biventricular defibrillator) (BiV ICD) (BiV pacemaker with defibrillator) (BiV pacing with defibrillator) (CRT-D) (total system) (device and one or more leads) 00.51
left ventricular coronary venous lead only 00.52
pulse generator only 00.54
pacemaker (biventricular pacemaker) (BiV pacemaker) (CRT-P) (total system) (device and one or more leads) 00.50
left ventricular coronary venous lead only 00.52
pulse generator only 00.53
cardiac support device (CSD) (CorCap™) 37.41
carotid artery stent(s) (stent graft) 00.63

Note – Also use 00.40, 00.41, 00.42, or 00.43 to show the total number of vessels treated. Use code 00.44 once to show procedure on a bifurcated vessel. In addition, use 00.45, 00.46, 00.47, or 00.48 to show the number of vascular stents inserted.

catheter
abdomen of fetus, for intrauterine transfusion 75.2
anterior chamber (eye), for permanent drainage (glaucoma) 12.79
artery 38.91
bile duct(s) 51.59
common 51.51
endoscopic 51.87
endoscopic 51.87
bladder, indwelling 57.94
suprapubic 57.18
percutaneous (closed) 57.17
bronchus 96.05
with lavage 96.56
central venous NEC 38.93
for
hemodialysis 38.95
pressure monitoring 89.62
peripherally inserted central catheter (PICC) 38.93
chest 34.04
revision (with lysis of adhesions) 34.04
thoracoscopic 34.06 ●
thoracoscopic 34.06 ●
cranial cavity 01.26
placement via burr hole(s) 01.28

Insertion – *continued*
- catheter – *continued*
  - esophagus (nonoperative) 96.06
    - permanent tube 42.81
  - intercostal (with water seal), for drainage 34.04
    - revision (with lysis of adhesions) 34.04
      - thoracoscopic 34.06 ●
    - thoracoscopic 34.06 ●
  - intracerebral 01.26
    - placement via burr hole(s) 01.28
  - spinal canal space (epidural) (subarachnoid) (subdural) for infusion of therapeutic or palliative substances 03.90
  - Swan-Ganz (pulmonary) 89.64
  - transtracheal for oxygenation 31.99
  - vein NEC 38.93
    - for renal dialysis 38.95
- chest tube 34.04
  - thoracoscopic 34.06 ●
- choledochohepatic tube (for decompression) 51.43
  - endoscopic 51.87
- cochlear prosthetic device – *see* Implant, cochlear prosthetic device
- contraceptive device (intrauterine) 69.7
- CorCap™ 37.41
- cordis cannula 54.98
- coronary (artery)

> *Note – Also use 00.40, 00.41, 00.42, or 00.43 to show the total number of vessels treated. Use code 00.44 once to show procedure on a bifurcated vessel. In addition, use 00.45, 00.46, 00.47, or 00.48 to show the number of vascular stents inserted.*

  - stent, drug-eluting 36.07
  - stent, non-drug-eluting 36.06
- Crosby-Cooney button 54.98
- CRT-D (biventricular defibrillator) (BiV ICD) (BiV pacemaker with defibrillator) (BiV pacing with defibrillator) (cardiac resynchronization defibrillator) (device and one or more leads) 00.51
  - left ventricular coronary venous lead only 00.52
  - pulse generator only 00.54
- CRT-P (biventricular pacemaker) (BiV pacemaker) (cardiac resynchronization pacemaker) (device and one or more leads) 00.50
  - left ventricular coronary venous lead only 00.52
  - pulse generator only 00.53
- Crutchfield tongs (skull) (with synchronous skeletal traction) 02.94
- Davidson button 54.98
- denture (total) 99.97
- device
  - adjustable gastric band and port 44.95
  - bronchial device NOS 33.79
  - bronchial substance NOS 33.79
  - bronchial valve 33.71
  - cardiac resynchronization – *see* Insertion, cardiac resynchronization device
  - cardiac support device (CSD) 37.41
  - CorCap™ 37.41
  - epicardial support device 37.41
  - Lap-Band™ 44.95
  - left atrial appendage 37.90
  - left atrial filter 37.90
  - left atrial occluder 37.90
  - prosthetic cardiac support device 37.41
  - vascular access 86.07
  - ventricular support device 37.41
- diaphragm, vagina 96.17
- drainage tube
  - kidney 55.02
    - pelvis 55.12
  - renal pelvis 55.12
- Dynesys® 84.82 ▲
- elbow prosthesis (total) 81.84
  - revision 81.97
- electrode(s)
  - bone growth stimulator (invasive) (percutaneous) (semi-invasive) – *see* category 78.9❹
  - brain 02.93
    - depth 02.93
    - foramen ovale 02.93
    - sphenoidal 02.96
  - depth 02.93
  - foramen ovale 02.93
  - gastric 04.92

Insertion – *continued*
- electrode(s) – *continued*
  - heart (initial) (transvenous) 37.70
    - atrium (initial) 37.73
      - replacement 37.76
    - atrium and ventricle (initial) 37.72
      - replacement 37.76
    - epicardium (sternotomy or thoracotomy approach) 37.74
    - left ventricular coronary venous system 00.52
    - temporary transvenous pacemaker system 37.78
      - during and immediately following cardiac surgery 39.64
    - ventricle (initial) 37.71
      - replacement 37.76
  - intracranial 02.93
  - osteogenic (for bone growth stimulation) – *see* category 78.9❹
  - peripheral nerve 04.92
  - sacral nerve 04.92
  - sphenoidal 02.96
  - spine 03.93
- electroencephalographic receiver – *see* Implant, electroencephalographic receiver, by site
- electronic stimulator – *see* Implant, electronic stimulator, by site
- electrostimulator – *see* Implant, electronic stimulator, by site
- endograft(s), endovascular graft(s)
  - endovascular, abdominal aorta 39.71
  - endovascular, head and neck vessels 39.72
  - endovascular, other vessels (for aneurysm) 39.79
  - endovascular, thoracic aorta 39.73
- endoprosthesis
  - bile duct 51.87
  - femoral head (bipolar) 81.52
  - pancreatic duct 52.93
- epidural pegs 02.93
- external fixation device (bone) – *see* category 78.1❹
- facial bone implant (alloplastic) (synthetic) 76.92
- filling material, skin (filling of defect) 86.02
- filter
  - vena cava (inferior) (superior) (transvenous) 38.7
- fixator, mini device (bone) – *see* category 78.1❹
- frame (stereotactic)
  - for radiosurgery 93.59
- Gardner Wells tongs (skull) (with synchronous skeletal traction) 02.94
- gastric bubble (balloon) 44.93
- globe, into eye socket 16.69
- Greenfield filter 38.7
- halo device (skull) (with synchronous skeletal traction) 02.94
- Harrington rod – *see also* Fusion, spinal, by level
  - with dorsal, dorsolumbar fusion 81.05
- Harris pin 79.15
- heart
  - assist system – *see* Implant, heart assist system
  - cardiac support device (CSD) 37.41
  - circulatory assist system – *see* Implant, heart assist system
  - CorCap™ 37.41
  - epicardial support device 37.41
  - pacemaker – *see* Insertion, pacemaker, cardiac
  - prosthetic cardiac support device 37.41
  - pump (Kantrowitz) 37.62
  - valve – *see* Replacement, heart valve
  - ventricular support device 37.41
- hip prosthesis (partial) 81.52
  - revision NOS 81.53
    - acetabular and femoral components (total) 00.70
    - acetabular component only 00.71
    - acetabular liner and/or femoral head only 00.73
    - femoral component only 00.72
    - femoral head only and/or acetabular liner 00.73
    - partial
      - acetabular component only 00.71
      - acetabular liner and/or femoral head only 00.73
      - femoral component only 00.72
      - femoral head only and/or acetabular liner 00.73
    - total (acetabular and femoral components) 00.70

Insertion – *continued*
- hip prosthesis – *continued*
  - total 81.51
    - revision
      - acetabular and femoral components (total) 00.70
      - total (acetabular and femoral components) 00.70
- Holter valve 02.2
- Hufnagel valve – *see* Replacement, heart valve
- implant – *see* Insertion, prosthesis
- infusion pump 86.06
- interbody spinal fusion device 84.51
- intercostal catheter (with water seal), for drainage 34.04
  - revision (with lysis of adhesions) 34.04 ●
    - thoracoscopic 34.06 ●
- intra-arterial blood gas monitoring system 89.60
- intrauterine
  - contraceptive device 69.7
  - radium (intracavitary) 69.91
  - tamponade (nonobstetric) 69.91
- Kantrowitz
  - heart pump 37.62
  - pulsation balloon (phase-shift) 37.61
- keratoprosthesis 11.73
- King-Mills umbrella device (heart) 35.52
- Kirschner wire 93.44
  - with reduction of fracture or dislocation – *see* Reduction, fracture and Reduction, dislocation
- knee prosthesis (partial (total) 81.54
  - revision NOS 81.55
    - femoral component 00.82
    - partial
      - femoral component 00.82
      - patellar component 00.83
      - tibial component 00.81
      - tibial insert 00.84
    - patellar component 00.83
    - tibial component 00.81
    - tibial insert 00.84
    - total (all components) 00.80
- laminaria, cervix 69.93
- Lap-Band™ 44.95
- larynx, valved tube 31.75
- leads – *see* Insertion, electrode(s)
- lens, prosthetic (intraocular) 13.70
  - with cataract extraction, one-stage 13.71
  - secondary (subsequent to cataract extraction) 13.72
- limb lengthening device, internal, NOS 84.54
  - with kinetic distraction 84.53
- loop recorder 37.79
- M-Brace™ 84.82 ▲
- metal staples into epiphyseal plate (*see also* Stapling, epiphyseal plate) 78.20
- minifixator device (bone) – *see* category 78.1❹
- Mobitz-Uddin umbrella, vena cava 38.7
- mold, vagina 96.15
- Moore (cup) 81.52
- myringotomy device (button) (tube) 20.01
  - with intubation 20.01
- nasobiliary drainage tube (endoscopic) 51.86
- nasogastric tube
  - for
    - decompression, intestinal 96.07
    - feeding 96.6
- naso-intestinal tube 96.08
- nasolacrimal tube or stent 09.44
- nasopancreatic drainage tube (endoscopic) 52.97
- neuropacemaker – *see* Implant, neurostimulator, by site
- neurostimulator – *see* Implant, neurostimulator, by site
- non-coronary vessel
  - stent(s) (stent graft)

> *Note – Also use 00.40, 00.41, 00.42, or 00.43 to show the total number of vessels treated. Use code 00.44 once to show procedure on a bifurcated vessel. In addition, use 00.45, 00.46, 00.47, or 00.48 to show the number of vascular stents inserted.*

    - with angioplasty or atherectomy 39.50
    - with bypass - *omit code*
    - basilar 00.64
    - carotid 00.63
    - extracranial 00.64
    - intracranial 00.65

Insertion – Insertion

- **Insertion** – *continued*
  - non-coronary vessel – *continued*
    - stent(s) (stent graft) – *continued*
      - peripheral 39.90
        - bare, drug-coated 39.90
        - drug-eluting 00.55
      - vertebral 00.64
  - non-invasive (transcutaneous) (surface) stimulator 99.86
  - obturator (orthodontic) 24.7
  - ocular implant
    - with synchronous
      - enucleation 16.42
        - with muscle attachment to implant 16.41
      - evisceration 16.31
    - following or secondary to
      - enucleation 16.61
      - evisceration 16.61
  - Ommaya reservoir 02.2
  - orbital implant (stent) (outside muscle cone) 16.69
    - with orbitotomy 16.02
  - orthodontic appliance (obturator) (wiring) 24.7
  - outflow tract prosthesis (gusset type) (heart)
    - in
      - pulmonary valvuloplasty 35.26
      - total repair of tetralogy of Fallot 35.81
  - pacemaker
    - brain – *see* Implant, neurostimulator, brain
    - cardiac (device) (initial) (permanent) (replacement) 37.80
      - dual-chamber device (initial) 37.83
        - replacement 37.87
      - during and immediately following cardiac surgery 39.64
      - resynchronization (biventricular pacemaker) (BiV pacemaker) (CRT-P) (device)
        - device only (initial) (replacement) 00.53
        - total system (device and one or more leads) 00.50
        - transvenous lead into left ventricular coronary venous system 00.52
      - single-chamber device (initial) 37.81
        - rate responsive 37.82
        - replacement 37.85
          - rate responsive 37.86
      - temporary transvenous pacemaker system 37.78
        - during and immediately following cardiac surgery 39.64
    - carotid 39.8
    - gastric 04.92
    - heart – *see* Insertion, pacemaker, cardiac
    - intracranial – *see* Implant, neurostimulator, intracranial
    - neural – *see* Implant, neurostimulator, by site
    - peripheral nerve – *see* Implant, neurostimulator, peripheral nerve
    - spine – *see* Implant, neurostimulator, spine
  - pacing catheter – *see* Insertion, pacemaker, cardiac
  - pack
    - auditory canal, external 96.11
    - cervix (nonobstetrical) 67.0
      - after delivery or abortion 75.8
      - to assist delivery or induce labor 73.1
    - rectum 96.19
    - sella turcica 07.79
    - vagina (nonobstetrical) 96.14
      - after delivery or abortion 75.8
  - palatal implant 27.64
  - penile prosthesis (non-inflatable) (internal) 64.95
    - inflatable (internal) 64.97
  - peridontal splint (orthodontic) 24.7
  - peripheral blood vessel – *see* non-coronary
  - pessary
    - cervix 96.18
      - to assist delivery or induce labor 73.1
    - vagina 96.18
  - pharyngeal valve, artificial 31.75
  - port, vascular access 86.07
  - prostaglandin suppository (for abortion) 96.49
  - prosthesis, prosthetic device
    - acetabulum (partial) 81.52
      - hip 81.52
        - revision NOS 81.53
          - acetabular and femoral components (total) 00.70
          - acetabular component only 00.71
          - acetabular liner and/or femoral head only 00.73
          - femoral component only 00.72

- **Insertion** – *continued*
  - prosthesis, prosthetic device – *continued*
    - acetabulum – *continued*
      - hip – *continued*
        - revision – *continued*
          - femoral head only and/or acetabular liner 00.73
          - partial
            - acetabular component only 00.71
            - acetabular liner and/or femoral head only 00.73
            - femoral component only 00.72
            - femoral head only and/or acetabular liner 00.73
          - total (acetabular and femoral components) 00.70
      - revision 81.53
    - ankle (total) 81.56
    - arm (bioelectric) (cineplastic) (kineplastic) 84.44
    - biliary tract 51.99
    - breast (bilateral) 85.54
      - unilateral 85.53
    - cardiac support device (CSD) (CorCap™) 37.41
    - chin (polyethylene) (silastic) 76.68
    - elbow (total) 81.84
      - revision 81.97
    - extremity (bioelectric) (cineplastic) (kineplastic) 84.40
      - lower 84.48
      - upper 84.44
    - fallopian tube 66.93
    - femoral head (Austin-Moore) (bipolar) (Eicher) (Thompson) 81.52
    - hip (partial) 81.52
      - revision NOS 81.53
        - acetabular and femoral components (total) 00.70
        - acetabular component only 00.71
        - acetabular liner and/or femoral head only 00.73
        - femoral component only 00.72
        - femoral head only and/or acetabular liner 00.73
        - partial
          - acetabular component only 00.71
          - acetabular liner and/or femoral head only 00.73
          - femoral component only 00.72
          - femoral head only and/or acetabular liner 00.73
        - total (acetabular and femoral components) 00.70
      - total 81.51
        - revision
          - acetabular and femoral components (total) 00.70
          - total (acetabular and femoral components) 00.70
    - joint – *see* Arthroplasty
    - knee (partial) (total) 81.54
      - revision NOS 81.55
        - femoral component 00.82
        - partial
          - femoral component 00.82
          - patellar component 00.83
          - tibial component 00.81
          - tibial insert 00.84
        - patellar component 00.83
        - tibial component 00.81
        - tibial insert 00.84
        - total (all components) 00.80
    - leg (bioelectric) (cineplastic) (kineplastic) 84.48
    - lens 13.91
    - ocular (secondary) 16.61
      - with orbital exenteration 16.42
    - outflow tract (gusset type) (heart)
      - in
        - pulmonary valvuloplasty 35.26
        - total repair of tetralogy of Fallot 35.81
    - penis (internal) (noninflatable) 64.95
      - with
        - construction 64.43
        - reconstruction 64.44
      - inflatable (internal) 64.97
    - Rosen (for urinary incontinence) 59.79
    - shoulder
      - partial 81.81
      - revision 81.97
      - total 81.80

- **Insertion** – *continued*
  - prosthesis, prosthetic device – *continued*
    - spine
      - artificial disc, NOS 84.60
        - cervical 84.62
          - nucleus 84.61
          - partial 84.61
          - total 84.62
        - lumbar, lumbosacral 84.65
          - nucleus 84.64
          - partial 84.64
          - total 84.65
        - thoracic (partial) (total) 84.63
      - other device 84.59
    - testicular (bilateral) (unilateral) 62.7
    - toe 81.57
      - hallux valgus repair 77.59
    - vagina ●
      - synthetic 70.95 ●
  - pseudophakos (*see also* Insertion, lens) 13.70
  - pump, infusion 86.06
  - radioactive isotope 92.27
  - radium 92.27
  - radon seeds 92.27,
  - Reuter bobbin (with intubation) 20.01
  - Rickham reservoir 02.2
  - Rosen prosthesis (for urinary incontinence) 59.79
  - Scribner shunt 39.93
  - Sengstaken-Blakemore tube 96.06
  - sensor (lead)
    - intra-arterial, for continuous blood gas monitoring 89.60
    - intracardiac hemodynamic monitoring 00.56
  - sieve, vena cava 38.7
  - skeletal muscle stimulator 83.92
  - skull
    - plate 02.05
    - stereotactic frame 93.59
    - tongs (Barton) (caliper) (Garder Wells) (Vinke) (with synchronous skeletal traction) 02.94
  - spacer (cement) (joint) ▶(methylmethacrylate)◀ 84.56
    - spine 84.51
  - sphenoidal electrodes 02.96
  - spine
    - bone void filler
      - that with kyphoplasty 81.66
      - that with vertebroplasty 81.65
    - cage (BAK) 84.51
    - facet replacement device(s) 84.84 ●
    - interbody spinal fusion device 84.51
    - interspinous process decompression device 84.80 ▲
    - non-fusion stabilization device ▶– *see* category 84.8 ❹◀
    - pedicle-based dynamic stabilization device(s) 84.82 ●
    - posterior motion preservation device(s) – *see* category 84.8❹ ●
    - spacer 84.51
  - Spitz-Holter valve 02.2
  - Steinmann pin 93.44
    - with reduction of fracture or dislocation – *see* Reduction, fracture and Reduction, dislocation
  - stent(s) (stent graft)
    - artery (bare) (bonded) (drug coated) (non-drug-eluting)

> *Note – Also use 00.40, 00.41, 00.42, or 00.43 to show the total number of vessels treated. Use code 00.44 once to show procedure on a bifurcated vessel. In addition, use 00.45, 00.46, 00.47, or 00.48 to show the number of vascular stents inserted.*

      - basilar 00.64
      - carotid 00.63
      - cerebrovascular
        - cerebral (intracranial) 00.65
        - precerebral (extracranial) 00.64
          - carotid 00.63
      - coronary (bare) (bonded) (drug coated) (non-drug-eluting) 36.06
        - drug-eluting 36.07
      - extracranial 00.64
        - carotid 00.63
      - intracranial 00.65
      - non-coronary vessel
        - basilar 00.64
        - carotid 00.63
        - extracranial 00.64

Insertion – Intubation

❹ Fourth-Digit Required [code] Manifestation Code ▶◀ Revised Text ● New Line ▲ Revised Code

- **Intubation** – *continued*
  - lacrimal for
    - dilation 09.42
    - tear drainage, intranasal 09.81
  - larynx 96.05
  - nasobiliary (drainage) 51.86
  - nasogastric
    - for
      - decompression, intestinal 96.07
      - feeding 96.6
  - naso-intestinal 96.08
  - nasolacrimal (duct) (with irrigation) 09.44
  - nasopancreatic drainage (endoscopic) 52.97
  - respiratory tract NEC 96.05
  - small intestine (Miller-Abbott) 96.08
  - stomach (nasogastric) (for intestinal decompression) NEC 96.07
    - for feeding 96.6
  - trachea 96.04
  - ventriculocisternal 02.2
- **Invagination, diverticulum**
  - gastric 44.69
    - laparoscopic 44.68
  - pharynx 29.59
  - stomach 44.69
    - laparoscopic 44.68
- **Inversion**
  - appendix 47.99
  - diverticulum
    - gastric 44.69
      - laparoscopic 44.68
    - intestine
      - large 45.49
        - endoscopic 45.43
      - small 45.34
    - stomach 44.69
      - laparoscopic 44.68
  - tunica vaginalis 61.49
- **IOERT** (intra-operative electron radiation therapy) 92.41 ●
- **IOM** (intra-operative neurophysiologic monitoring) 00.94 ●
- **Ionization, medical** 99.27
- **Iontherapy** 99.27
- **Iontophoresis** 99.27
- **Iridectomy** (basal) (buttonhole) (optical) (peripheral) (total) 12.14
  - with
    - capsulectomy 13.65
    - cataract extraction – *see* Extraction, cataract
    - filtering operation (for glaucoma) NEC 12.65
    - scleral
      - fistulization 12.65
      - thermocauterization 12.62
      - trephination 12.61
- **Iridencleisis** 12.63
- **Iridesis** 12.63
- **Irido-capsulectomy** 13.65
- **Iridocyclectomy** 12.44
- **Iridocystectomy** 12.42
- **Iridodesis** 12.63
- **Iridoplasty** NEC 12.39
- **Iridosclerectomy** 12.65
- **Iridosclerotomy** 12.69
- **Iridotasis** 12.63
- **Iridotomy** 12.12
  - by photocoagulation 12.12
  - with transfixion 12.11
  - for iris bombé 12.11
  - specified type NEC 12.12
- **Iron lung** 93.99
- **Irradiation**
  - gamma, stereotactic 92.32
- **Irrigation**
  - anterior chamber (eye) 12.91
  - bronchus NEC 96.56
  - canaliculus 09.42
  - catheter
    - ureter 96.46
    - urinary, indwelling NEC 96.48
    - vascular 96.57
    - ventricular 02.41
    - wound 96.58
  - cholecystostomy 96.41
  - cornea 96.51
    - with removal of foreign body 98.21
  - corpus cavernosum 64.98
  - cystostomy 96.47
- **Irrigation** – *continued*
  - ear (removal of cerumen) 96.52
  - enterostomy 96.36
  - eye 96.51
    - with removal of foreign body 98.21
  - gastrostomy 96.36
  - lacrimal
    - canaliculi 09.42
    - punctum 09.41
  - muscle 83.02
    - hand 82.02
  - nasal
    - passages 96.53
    - sinus 22.00
  - nasolacrimal duct 09.43
    - with insertion of tube or stent 09.44
  - nephrostomy 96.45
  - peritoneal 54.25
  - pyelostomy 96.45
  - rectal 96.39
  - stomach 96.33
  - tendon (sheath) 83.01
    - hand 82.01
  - trachea NEC 96.56
  - traumatic cataract 13.3
  - tube
    - biliary NEC 96.41
    - nasogastric NEC 96.34
    - pancreatic 96.42
  - ureterostomy 96.46
  - ventricular shunt 02.41
  - wound (cleaning) NEC 96.59
- **Irving operation** (tubal ligation) 66.32
- **Irwin operation** (*see also* Osteotomy) 77.30
- **Ischiectomy** (partial) 77.89
  - total 77.99
- **Ischiopubiotomy** 77.39
- **Isolation**
  - after contact with infectious disease 99.84
  - ileal loop 45.51
  - intestinal segment or pedicle flap
    - large 45.52
    - small 45.51
- **Isthmectomy, thyroid** (*see also* Thyroidectomy, partial) 06.39

J

- **Jaboulay operation** (gastroduodenostomy) 44.39
  - laparoscopic 44.38
- **Janeway operation** (permanent gastrostomy) 43.19
- **Jatene operation** (arterial switch) 35.84
- **Jejunectomy** 45.62
- **Jejunocecostomy** 45.93
- **Jejunocholecystostomy** 51.32
- **Jejunocolostomy** 45.93
- **Jejunoileostomy** 45.91
- **Jejunojejunostomy** 45.91
- **Jejunopexy** 46.61
- **Jejunorrhaphy** 46.73
- **Jejunostomy** (feeding) 46.39
  - delayed opening 46.31
  - loop 46.01
  - percutaneous (endoscopic) (PEJ) 46.32
  - revision 46.41
- **Jejunotomy** 45.02
- **Johanson operation** (urethral reconstruction) 58.46
- **Jones operation**
  - claw toe (transfer of extensor hallucis longus tendon) 77.57
    - modified (with arthrodesis) 77.57
  - dacryocystorhinostomy 09.81
  - hammer toe (interphalangeal fusion) 77.56
  - modified (tendon transfer with arthrodesis) 77.57
  - repair of peroneal tendon 83.88
- **Joplin operation** (exostectomy with tendon transfer) 77.53

K

- **Kader operation** (temporary gastrostomy) 43.19
- **Kasai portoenterostomy** 51.37
- **Kaufman operation** (for urinary stress incontinence) 59.79
- **Kazanjiian operation** (buccal vestibular sulcus extension) 24.91
- **Kehr operation** (hepatopexy) 50.69
- **Keller operation** (bunionectomy) 77.59
- **Kelly** (-Kennedy) **operation** (urethrovesical plication) 59.3
- **Kelly-Stoeckel operation** (urethrovesical plication) 59.3
- **Kelotomy** 53.9
- **Keratectomy** (complete) (partial) (superficial) 11.49
  - for pterygium 11.39
    - with corneal graft 11.32
- **Keratocentesis** (for hyphema) 12.91
- **Keratomileusis** 11.71
- **Keratophakia** 11.72
- **Keratoplasty** (tectonic) (with autograft) (with homograft) 11.60
  - lamellar (nonpenetrating) (with homograft) 11.62
    - with autograft 11.61
  - penetrating (full-thickness) (with homograft) 11.64
    - with autograft 11.63
  - perforating – *see* Keratoplasty, penetrating
  - refractive 11.71
  - specified type NEC 11.69
- **Keratoprosthesis** 11.73
- **Keratotomy** (delimiting) (posterior) 11.1
  - radial (refractive) 11.75
- **Kerr operation** (low cervical cesarean section) 74.1
- **Kessler operation** (arthroplasty, carpometacarpal joint) 81.74
- **Kidner operation** (excision of accessory navicular bone) (with tendon transfer) 77.98
- **Killian operation** (frontal sinusotomy) 22.41
- **Kineplasty** – *see* Cineplasty
- **King-Steelquist operation** (hind-quarter amputation) 84.19
- **Kirk operation** (amputation through thigh) 84.17
- **Kock pouch**
  - bowel anastomosis - *omit code*
  - continent ileostomy 46.22
  - cutaneous uretero-ileostomy 56.51
  - ESWL (electrocorporeal shockwave lithotripsy) 98.51
  - removal, calculus 57.19
  - revision, cutaneous uretero-ileostomy 56.52
  - urinary diversion procedure 56.51
- **Kockogram** (ileal conduitogram) 87.78
- **Kockoscopy** 45.12
- **Kondoleon operation** (correction of lymphedema) 40.9
- **Krause operation** (sympathetic denervation) 05.29
- **Kroener operation** (partial salpingectomy) 66.69
- **Kroenlein operation** (lateral orbitotomy) 16.01
- **Kronig operation** (low cervical cesarean section) 74.1
- **Krunkenberg operation** (reconstruction of below-elbow amputation) 82.89
- **Kuhnt-Szymanowski operation** (ectropion repair with lid reconstruction) 08.44
- **Kyphoplasty** 81.66

L

- **Labbe operation** (gastrotomy) 43.0
- **Labiectomy** (bilateral) 71.62
  - unilateral 71.61
- **Labyrinthectomy** (transtympanic) 20.79
- **Labyrinthotomy** (transtympanic) 20.79
- **Ladd operation** (mobilization of intestine) 54.95
- **Lagrange operation** (iridosclerectomy) 12.65
- **Lambrinudi operation** (triple arthrodesis) 81.12
- **Laminectomy** (decompression) (for exploration) 03.09
  - as operative approach - *omit code*
  - with
    - excision of herniated intervertebral disc (nucleus pulposus) 80.51
    - excision of other intraspinal lesion (tumor) 03.4
  - reopening of site 03.02
- **Laminography** – *see* Radiography
- **Laminoplasty, expansile** 03.09
- **Laminotomy** (decompression) (for exploration) 03.09
  - as operative approach - *omit code*
  - reopening of site 03.02

- **Langenbeck operation** (cleft palate repair) 27.62
- **Laparoamnioscopy** 75.31
- **Laparorrhaphy** 54.63
- **Laparoscopy** 54.21
  - with
    - biopsy (intra-abdominal) 54.24
      - uterine ligaments 68.15
      - uterus 68.16
    - destruction of fallopian tubes – *see* Destruction, fallopian tube
- **Laparotomy** NEC 54.19
  - as operative approach - *omit code*
  - exploratory (pelvic) 54.11
  - reopening of recent operative site (for control of hemorrhage) (for exploration) (for incision of hematoma) 54.12
- **Laparotrachelotomy** 74.1
- **Lapidus operation** (bunionectomy with metatarsal osteotomy) 77.51
- **Larry operation** (shoulder disarticulation) 84.08
- **Laryngectomy**
  - with radical neck dissection (with synchronous thyroidectomy) (with synchronous tracheostomy) 30.4
  - complete (with partial laryngectomy) (with synchronous tracheostomy) 30.3
    - with radical neck dissection (with synchronous thyroidectomy) (with synchronous tracheostomy) 30.4
  - frontolateral partial (extended) 30.29
  - glottosupraglottic partial 30.29
  - lateral partial 30.29
  - partial (frontolateral) (glottosupraglottic) (lateral) (submucous) (supraglottic) (vertical) 30.29
  - radical (with synchronous thyroidectomy) (with synchronous tracheostomy) 30.4
  - submucous (partial) 30.29
  - supraglottic partial 30.29
  - total (with partial pharyngectomy) (with synchronous tracheostomy) 30.3
    - with radical neck dissection (with synchronous thyroidectomy) (with synchronous tracheostomy) 30.4
  - vertical partial 30.29
  - wide field 30.3
- **Laryngocentesis** 31.3
- **Laryngoesophagectomy** 30.4
- **Laryngofissure** 30.29
- **Laryngogram** 87.09
  - contrast 87.07
- **Laryngopharyngectomy** (with synchronous tracheostomy) 30.3
  - radical (with synchronous thyroidectomy) 30.4
- **Laryngopharyngoesophagectomy** (with synchronous tracheostomy) 30.3
  - with radical neck dissection (with synchronous thyroidectomy) 30.4
- **Laryngoplasty** 31.69
- **Laryngorrhaphy** 31.61
- **Laryngoscopy** (suspension) (through artificial stoma) 31.42
- **Laryngostomy** (permanent) 31.29
  - revision 31.63
  - temporary (emergency) 31.1
- **Laryngotomy** 31.3
- **Laryngotracheobronchoscopy** 33.23
  - with biopsy 33.24
- **Laryngotracheoscopy** 31.42
- **Laryngotracheostomy** (permanent) 31.29
  - temporary (emergency) 31.1
- **Laryngotracheotomy** (temporary) 31.1
  - permanent 31.29
- **Laser** – *see also* Coagulation, Destruction, and Photocoagulation by site
  - angioplasty, percutaneous transluminal 39.59
    - coronary – *see* Angioplasty, coronary
- **Lash operation**
  - internal cervical os repair 67.59
  - laparoscopic supracervical hysterectomy 68.31
- **LASIK** (Laser-assisted in situ keratomileusis) 11.71
- **Latzko operation**
  - cesarean section 74.2
  - colpocleisis 70.8
- **Lavage**
  - antral 22.00
  - bronchus NEC 96.56
    - diagnostic (endoscopic) bronchoalveolar lavage (BAL) 33.24
  - endotracheal 96.56
  - gastric 96.33
  - lung (total)(whole) 33.99
    - diagnostic (endoscopic) bronchoalveolar lavage (BAL) 33.24
  - nasal sinus(es) 22.00
    - by puncture 22.01
    - through natural ostium 22.02
  - peritoneal (diagnostic) 54.25
  - trachea NEC 96.56
- **Leadbetter operation** (urethral reconstruction) 58.46
- **Leadbetter-Politano operation** (ureteroneocystostomy) 56.74
- **LEEP** (loop electrosurgical excision procedure) of cervix 67.32
- **Le Fort operation** (colpocleisis) 70.8
- **LeMesurier operation** (cleft lip repair) 27.54
- **Lengthening**
  - bone (with bone graft) 78.30
    - femur 78.35
    - for reconstruction of thumb 82.69
    - specified site NEC 78.39 (*see also* category 78.3❹)
    - tibia 78.37
    - ulna 78.33
  - extraocular muscle NEC 15.21
    - multiple (two or more muscles) 15.4
  - fascia 83.89
    - hand 82.89
  - hamstring NEC 83.85
  - heel cord 83.85
  - leg
    - femur 78.35
    - tibia 78.37
  - levator palpebrae muscle 08.38
  - muscle 83.85
    - extraocular 15.21
      - multiple (two or more muscles) 15.4
    - hand 82.55
  - palate 27.62
    - secondary or subsequent 27.63
  - tendon 83.85
    - for claw toe repair 77.57
    - hand 82.55
- **Leriche operation** (periarterial sympathectomy) 05.25
- **Leucotomy, leukotomy** 01.32
- **Leukopheresis, therapeutic** 99.72
- **Lid suture operation** (blepharoptosis) 08.31
- **Ligation**
  - adrenal vessel (artery) (vein) 07.43
  - aneurysm 39.52
  - appendages, dermal 86.26
  - arteriovenous fistula 39.53
    - coronary artery 36.99
  - artery 38.80
    - abdominal 38.86
    - adrenal 07.43
    - aorta (arch) (ascending) (descending) 38.84
    - coronary (anomalous) 36.99
    - ethmoidal 21.04
    - external carotid 21.06
    - for control of epistaxis – *see* Control, epistaxis
    - head and neck NEC 38.82
    - intracranial NEC 38.81
    - lower limb 38.88
    - maxillary (transantral) 21.05
    - middle meningeal 02.13
    - thoracic NEC 38.85
    - thyroid 06.92
    - upper limb 38.83
  - atrium, heart 37.99
  - auricle, heart 37.99
  - bleeding vessel – *see* Control, hemorrhage
  - blood vessel 38.80
    - abdominal
      - artery 38.86
      - vein 38.87
    - adrenal 07.43
    - aorta (arch) (ascending) (descending) 38.84
    - esophagus 42.91
      - endoscopic 42.33
    - head and neck 38.82
    - intracranial NEC 38.81

- **Ligation** – *continued*
  - blood vessel – *continued*
    - lower limb
      - artery 38.88
      - vein 38.89
    - meningeal (artery) (longitudinal sinus) 02.13
    - thoracic NEC 38.85
    - thyroid 06.92
    - upper limb (artery) (vein) 38.83
  - bronchus 33.92
  - cisterna chyli 40.64
  - coronary
    - artery (anomalous) 36.99
    - sinus 36.39
  - dermal appendage 86.26
  - ductus arteriosus, patent 38.85
  - esophageal vessel 42.91
    - endoscopic 42.33
  - ethmoidal artery 21.04
  - external carotid artery 21.06
  - fallopian tube (bilateral) (remaining) (solitary) 66.39
    - by endoscopy (culdoscopy) (hysteroscopy) (laparoscopy) (peritoneoscopy) 66.29
    - with
      - crushing 66.31
        - by endoscopy (laparoscopy) 66.21
      - division 66.32
        - by endoscopy (culdoscopy) (laparoscopy) (peritoneoscopy) 66.22
      - Falope ring 66.39
        - by endoscopy (laparoscopy) 66.29
    - unilateral 66.92
  - fistula, arteriovenous 39.53
    - coronary artery 36.99
  - gastric
    - artery 38.86
    - varices 44.91
      - endoscopic 43.41
  - hemorrhoids 49.45
  - longitudinal sinus (superior) 02.13
  - lymphatic (channel) (peripheral) 40.9
    - thoracic duct 40.64
  - maxillary artery 21.05
  - meningeal vessel 02.13
  - spermatic
    - cord 63.72
      - varicocele 63.1
    - vein (high) 63.1
  - splenic vessels 38.86
  - subclavian artery 38.85
  - superior longitudinal sinus 02.13
  - supernumerary digit 86.26
  - thoracic duct 40.64
  - thyroid vessel (artery) (vein) 06.92
  - toes (supernumerary) 86.26
  - tooth 93.55
    - impacted 24.6
  - ulcer (peptic) (base) (bed) (bleeding vessel) 44.40
    - duodenal 44.42
    - gastric 44.41
  - ureter 56.95
  - varices
    - esophageal 42.91
      - endoscopic 42.33
    - gastric 44.91
      - endoscopic 43.41
    - peripheral vein (lower limb) 38.59
      - upper limb 38.53
  - varicocele 63.1
  - vas deferens 63.71
  - vein 38.80
    - abdominal 38.87
    - adrenal 07.43
    - head and neck NEC 38.82
    - intracranial NEC 38.81
    - lower limb 38.89
    - spermatic, high 63.1
    - thoracic NEC 38.85
    - thyroid 06.92
    - upper limb 38.83
    - varicose 38.50
      - abdominal 38.57
      - esophagus 42.91
        - endoscopic 42.33
      - gastric 44.91
        - endoscopic 43.41
      - head and neck 38.52
      - intracranial NEC 38.51
      - lower limb 38.59
      - stomach 44.91
      - thoracic NEC 38.55
      - upper limb 38.53

Langenbeck operation – Ligation

Ligation – *continued*
  vena cava, inferior 38.7
  venous connection between anomalous vein to
    left innominate vein 35.82
    superior vena cava 35.82
  wart 86.26
Light coagulation – *see* Photocoagulation
Lindholm operation (repair of ruptured tendon) 83.88
Lingulectomy, lung 32.39 ▲
Linton operation (varicose vein) 38.59
Lipectomy (subcutaneous tissue) (abdominal) (submental) 86.83
Liposuction 86.83
Lip reading training 95.49
Lip shave 27.43
Lisfranc operation
  foot amputation 84.12
  shoulder disarticulation 84.08
Litholapaxy, bladder 57.0
  by incision 57.19
Lithotomy
  bile passage 51.49
  bladder (urinary) 57.19
  common duct 51.41
    percutaneous 51.96
  gallbladder 51.04
  hepatic duct 51.49
  kidney 55.01
    percutaneous 55.03
  ureter 56.2
Lithotripsy
  bile duct NEC 51.49
    extracorporeal shockwave (ESWL) 98.52
  bladder 57.0
    with ultrasonic fragmentation 57.0 *[59.95]*
    extracorporeal shockwave (ESWL) 98.51
  extracorporeal shockwave (ESWL) NEC 98.59
    bile duct 98.52
    bladder (urinary) 98.51
    gallbladder 98.52
    kidney 98.51
    Kock pouch 98.51
    renal pelvis 98.51
    specified site NEC 98.59
    ureter 98.51
  gallbladder NEC 51.04
    endoscopic 51.88
    extracorporeal shockwave (ESWL) 98.52
  kidney 56.0
    extracorporeal shockwave (ESWL) 98.51
    percutaneous nephrostomy with fragmentation (laser) (ultrasound) 55.04
  renal pelvis 56.0
    extracorporeal shockwave (ESWL) 98.51
    percutaneous nephrostomy with fragmentation (laser) (ultrasound) 55.04
  ureter 56.0
    extracorporeal shockwave (ESWL) 98.51
Littlewood operation (forequarter amputation) 84.09
LLETZ (large loop excision of the transformation zone) of cervix 67.32
Lloyd-Davies operation (abdominoperineal resection) 48.5
Lobectomy
  brain 01.53
    partial 01.59
  liver (with partial excision of adjacent lobes) 50.3
  lung (complete) 32.49 ▲
    partial 32.39 ▲
      thoracoscopic 32.30 ●
    segmental (with resection of adjacent lobes) 32.49 ▲
      thoracoscopic 32.41 ●
    thoracoscopic 32.41 ●
  thyroid (total) (unilateral) (with removal of isthmus) (with removal of portion of remaining lobe) 06.2
    partial (*see also* Thyroidectomy, partial) 06.39
    substernal 06.51
    subtotal (*see also* Thyroidectomy, partial) 06.39
Lobotomy, brain 01.32
Localization, placenta 88.78
  by RISA injection 92.17
Longmire operation (bile duct anastomosis) 51.39
Loop ileal stoma (*see also* Ileostomy) 46.01
Loopogram 87.78
Looposcopy (ileal conduit) 56.35
Lord operation
  dilation of anal canal for hemorrhoids 49.49
  hemorrhoidectomy 49.49
  orchidopexy 62.5
Lower GI series (x-ray) 87.64
Lucas and Murray operation (knee arthrodesis with plate) 81.22
Lumpectomy
  breast 85.21
  specified site – *see* Excision, lesion, by site
Lymphadenectomy (simple) (*see also* Excision, lymph, node) 40.29
Lymphadenotomy 40.0
Lymphangiectomy (radical) (*see also* Excision, lymph, node, by site, radical) 40.50
Lymphangiogram
  abdominal 88.04
  cervical 87.08
  intrathoracic 87.34
  lower limb 88.36
  pelvic 88.04
  upper limb 88.34
Lymphangioplasty 40.9
Lymphangiorrhaphy 40.9
Lymphangiotomy 40.0
Lymphaticostomy 40.9
  thoracic duct 40.62
Lysis
  adhesions

Note: blunt – omit code
digital – omit code
manual – omit code
mechanical – omit code
without instrumentation – omit code

    abdominal 54.59
      laparoscopic 54.51
    appendiceal 54.59
      laparoscopic 54.51
    artery-vein-nerve bundle 39.91
    biliary tract 54.59
      laparoscopic 54.51
    bladder (neck) (intraluminal) 57.12
      external 59.11
        laparoscopic 59.12
      transurethral 57.41
    blood vessels 39.91
    bone – *see* category 78.4 ❹
    bursa 83.91
      by stretching or manipulation 93.28
      hand 82.91
    cartilage of joint 93.26
    chest wall 33.99
    choanae (nasopharynx) 29.54
    conjunctiva 10.5
    corneovitreal 12.34
    cortical (brain) 02.91
    ear, middle 20.23
    Eustachian tube 20.8
    extraocular muscle 15.7
    extrauterine 54.59
      laparoscopic 54.51
    eyelid 08.09
      and conjunctiva 10.5
    eye muscle 15.7
    fallopian tube 65.89
      laparoscopic 65.81
    fascia 83.91
      hand 82.91
        by stretching or manipulation 93.26
    gallbladder 54.59
      laparoscopic 54.51
    ganglion (peripheral) NEC 04.49
      cranial NEC 04.42
    hand 82.91
      by stretching or manipulation 93.26
    heart 37.10
    intestines 54.59
      laparoscopic 54.51
    iris (posterior) 12.33
      anterior 12.32
    joint (capsule) (structure) (*see also* Division, joint capsule) 80.40
    kidney 59.02
      laparoscopic 59.03
    labia (vulva) 71.01
    larynx 31.92

Lysis – *continued*
  adhesions – *continued*
    liver 54.59
      laparoscopic 54.51
    lung (for collapse of lung) 33.39
    mediastinum 34.99
    meninges (spinal) 03.6
      cortical 02.91
    middle ear 20.23
    muscle 83.91
      by stretching or manipulation 93.27
      extraocular 15.7
      hand 82.91
        by stretching or manipulation 93.26
    nasopharynx 29.54
    nerve (peripheral) NEC 04.49
      cranial NEC 04.42
      roots, spinal 03.6
      trigeminal 04.41
    nose, nasal 21.91
    ocular muscle 15.7
    ovary 65.89
      laparoscopic 65.81
    pelvic 54.59
      laparoscopic 54.51
    penile 64.93
    pericardium 37.12
    perineal (female) 71.01
    peripheral vessels 39.91
    perirectal 48.81
    perirenal 59.02
      laparoscopic 59.03
    peritoneum (pelvic) 54.59
      laparoscopic 54.51
    periureteral 59.02
      laparoscopic 59.03
    perivesical 59.11
      laparoscopic 59.12
    pharynx 29.54
    pleura (for collapse of lung) 33.39
    spermatic cord 63.94
    spinal (cord) (meninges) (nerve roots) 03.6
    spleen 54.59
      laparoscopic 54.51
    tendon 83.91
      by stretching or manipulation 93.27
      hand 82.91
        by stretching or manipulation 93.26
    thorax 34.99
    tongue 25.93
    trachea 31.92
    tubo-ovarian 65.89
      laparoscopic 65.81
    ureter 59.02
      with freeing or repositioning of ureter 59.02
      intraluminal 56.81
      laparoscopic 59.03
    urethra (intraluminal) 58.5
    uterus 54.59
      intraluminal 68.21
      laparoscopic 54.51
      peritoneal 54.59
        laparoscopic 54.51
    vagina (intraluminal) 70.13
    vitreous (posterior approach) 14.74
      anterior approach 14.73
    vulva 71.01
  goniosynechiae (with injection of air or liquid) 12.31
  synechiae (posterior) 12.33
    anterior (with injection of air or liquid) 12.32

M

Madlener operation (tubal ligation) 66.31
Magnet extraction
  foreign body
    anterior chamber, eye 12.01
    choroid 14.01
    ciliary body 12.01
    conjunctiva 98.22
    cornea 11.0
    eye, eyeball NEC 98.21
      anterior segment 12.01
      posterior segment 14.01
    intraocular (anterior segment) 12.01
    iris 12.01
    lens 13.01
    orbit 98.21
    retina 14.01

Magnet extraction – Meatoplasty

N

Neuroablation – Operation

❹ Fourth-Digit Required [code] Manifestation Code ►◄ Revised Text ● New Line ▲ Revised Code

Operation – *continued*
- palate NEC 27.99
- palpebral ligament sling 08.36
- Panas (linear proctotomy) 48.0
- Pancoast (division of trigeminal nerve at foramen ovale) 04.02
- pancreas NEC 52.99
- pantaloon (revision of gastric anastomosis) 44.5
- papillary muscle (heart) NEC 35.31
- Paquin (ureteroneocystostomy) 56.74
- parathyroid gland(s) NEC 06.99
- parotid gland or duct NEC 26.99
- Partsch (marsupialization of dental cyst) 24.4
- Pattee (auditory canal) 18.6
- Peet (splanchnic resection) 05.29
- Pemberton
  - osteotomy of ilium 77.39
  - rectum (mobilization and fixation for prolapse repair) 48.76
- penis NEC 64.98
- Pereyra (paraurethral suspension) 59.6
- pericardium NEC 37.99
- perineum (female) NEC 71.8
  - male NEC 86.99
- perirectal tissue NEC 48.99
- perirenal tissue NEC 59.92
- peritoneum NEC 54.99
- periurethral tissue NEC 58.99
- perivesical tissue NEC 59.92
- pharyngeal flap (cleft palate repair) 27.62
  - secondary or subsequent 27.63
- pharynx, pharyngeal (pouch) NEC 29.99
- pineal gland NEC 07.59
- Pinsker (obliteration of nasoseptal telangiectasia) 21.07
- Piper (forceps) 72.6
- Pirogoff (ankle amputation through malleoli of tibia and fibula) 84.14
- pituitary gland NEC 07.79
- plastic – *see* Repair, by site
- pleural cavity NEC 34.99
- Politano-Leadbetter (ureteroneocystostomy) 56.74
- pollicization (with nerves and blood supply) 82.61
- Polya (gastrectomy) 43.7
- Pomeroy (ligation and division of fallopian tubes) 66.32
- Poncet
  - lengthening of Achilles tendon 83.85
  - urethrostomy, perineal 58.0
- Porro (cesarean section) 74.99
- posterior chamber (eye) NEC 14.9
- Potts-Smith (descending aorta-left pulmonary artery anastomosis) 39.0
- Printen and Mason (high gastric bypass) 44.31
- prostate NEC (*see also* Prostatectomy) 60.69
  - specified type 60.99
- pterygium 11.39
  - with corneal graft 11.32
- Puestow (pancreaticojejunostomy) 52.96
- pull-through NEC 48.49
- pulmonary NEC 33.99
- push-back (cleft palate repair) 27.62
- Putti-Platt (capsulorrhaphy of shoulder for recurrent dislocation) 81.82
- pyloric exclusion 44.39
  - laparoscopic 44.38
- pyriform sinus NEC 29.99
- "rabbit ear" (anterior urethropexy) (Tudor) 59.79
- Ramadier (intrapetrosal drainage) 20.22
- Ramstedt (pyloromyotomy) (with wedge resection) 43.3
- Rankin
  - exteriorization of intestine 46.03
  - proctectomy (complete) 48.5
- Rashkind (balloon septostomy) 35.41
- Rastelli (creation of conduit between right ventricle and pulmonary artery) 35.92
  - in repair of
    - pulmonary artery atresia 35.92
    - transposition of great vessels 35.92
    - truncus arteriosus 35.83
- Raz-Pereyra procedure (bladder neck suspension) 59.79
- rectal NEC 48.99
- rectocele NEC 70.52
- re-entry (aorta) 39.54
- renal NEC 55.99
- respiratory (tract) NEC 33.99
- retina NEC 14.9
- Ripstein (repair of rectal prolapse) 48.75
- Rodney Smith (radical subtotal pancreatectomy) 52.53

Operation – *continued*
- Roux-en-Y
  - bile duct 51.36
  - cholecystojejunostomy 51.32
  - esophagus (intrathoracic) 42.54
  - gastroenterostomy 44.39
    - laparoscopic 44.38
  - gastrojejunostomy 44.39
    - laparoscopic 44.38
  - pancreaticojejunostomy 52.96
- Roux-Goldthwait (repair of patellar dislocation) 81.44
- Roux-Herzen-Judine (jejunal loop interposition) 42.63
- Ruiz-Mora (proximal phalangectomy for hammer toe) 77.99
- Russe (bone graft of scaphoid) 78.04
- Saemisch (corneal section) 11.1
- salivary gland or duct NEC 26.99
- Salter (innominate osteotomy) 77.39
- Sauer-Bacon (abdominoperineal resection) 48.5
- Schanz (femoral osteotomy) 77.35
- Schauta (-Amreich) (radical vaginal hysterectomy) 68.79
  - laparoscopic 68.71
- Schede (thoracoplasty) 33.34
- Scheie
  - cautery of sclera 12.62
  - sclerostomy 12.62
- Schlatter (total gastrectomy) 43.99
- Schroeder (endocervical excision) 67.39
- Schuchardt (nonobstetrical episiotomy) 71.09
- Schwartze (simple mastoidectomy) 20.41
- sclera NEC 12.89
- Scott
  - intestinal bypass for obesity 45.93
  - jejunocolostomy (bypass) 45.93
- scrotum NEC 61.99
- Seddon-Brooks (transfer of pectoralis major tendon) 83.75
- Semb (apicolysis of lung) 33.39
- seminal vesicle NEC 60.79
- Senning (correction of transposition of great vessels) 35.91
- Sever (division of soft tissue of arm) 83.19
- Sewell (heart) 36.2
- sex transformation NEC 64.5
- Sharrard (iliopsoas muscle transfer) 83.77
- shelf (hip arthroplasty) 81.40
- Shirodkar (encirclement suture, cervix) 67.59
- sigmoid NEC 46.99
- Silver (bunionectomy) 77.59
- Sistrunk (excision of thyroglossal cyst) 06.7
- Skene's gland NEC 71.8
- skin NEC 86.99
- skull NEC 02.99
- sling
  - eyelid
    - fascia lata, palpebral 08.36
    - frontalis fascial 08.32
    - levator muscle 08.33
    - orbicularis muscle 08.36
    - palpebrae ligament, fascia lata 08.36
    - tarsus muscle 08.35
  - fascial (fascia lata)
    - eye 08.32
    - for facial weakness (trigeminal nerve paralysis) 86.81
    - palpebral ligament 08.36
    - tongue 25.59
  - tongue (fascial) 25.59
  - urethra (suprapubic) 59.4
    - retropubic 59.5
  - urethrovesical 59.5
- Slocum (pes anserinus transfer) 81.47
- Sluder (tonsillectomy) 28.2
- Smith (open osteotomy of mandible) 76.62
- Smith-Peterson (radiocarpal arthrodesis) 81.25
- Smithwick (sympathectomy) 05.29
- Soave (endorectal pull-through) 48.41
- soft tissue NEC 83.99
  - hand 82.99
- Sonneberg (inferior maxillary neurectomy) 04.07
- Sorondo-Ferré (hindquarter amputation) 84.19
- Soutter (iliac crest fasciotomy) 83.14
- Spalding-Richardson (uterine suspension) 69.22
- spermatic cord NEC 63.99
- sphincter of Oddi NEC 51.89
- spinal (canal) (cord) (structures) NEC 03.99
- Spinelli (correction of inverted uterus) 75.93
- Spivack (permanent gastrostomy) 43.19
- spleen NEC 41.99

Operation – *continued*
- S.P. Rogers (knee disarticulation) 84.16
- Ssabanejew-Frank (permanent gastrostomy) 43.19
- Stacke (simple mastoidectomy) 20.41
- Stallard (conjunctivocystorhinostomy) 09.82
  - with insertion of tube or stent 09.83
- Stamm (-Kader) (temporary gastrostomy) 43.19
- Steinberg 44.5
- Steindler
  - fascia stripping (for cavus deformity) 83.14
  - flexorplasty (elbow) 83.77
  - muscle transfer 83.77
- sterilization NEC
  - female (*see also* specific operation) 66.39
  - male (*see also* Ligation, vas deferens) 63.70
- Stewart (renal plication with pyeloplasty) 55.87
- stomach NEC 44.99
- Stone (anoplasty) 49.79
- Strassman (metroplasty) 69.49
  - metroplasty (Jones modification) 69.49
  - uterus 68.22
- Strayer (gastrocnemius recession) 83.72
- stress incontinence – *see* Repair, stress incontinence
- Stromeyer-Little (hepatotomy) 50.0
- Strong (unbridling of celiac artery axis) 39.91
- Sturmdorf (conization of cervix) 67.2
- subcutaneous tissue NEC 86.99
- sublingual gland or duct NEC 26.99
- submaxillary gland or duct NEC 26.99
- Summerskill (dacryocystorhinostomy by intubation) 09.81
- Surmay (jejunostomy) 46.39
- Swenson
  - bladder reconstruction 57.87
  - proctectomy 48.49
- Swinney (urethral reconstruction) 58.46
- Syme
  - ankle amputation through malleoli of tibia and fibula 84.14
  - urethrotomy, external 58.0
- sympathetic nerve NEC 05.89
- Taarnhoj (trigeminal nerve root decompression) 04.41
- Tack (sacculotomy) 20.79
- Talma-Morison (omentopexy) 54.74
- Tanner (devascularization of stomach) 44.99
- TAPVC NEC 35.82
- tarsus NEC 08.99
  - muscle sling 08.35
- tendon NEC 83.99
  - extraocular NEC 15.9
  - hand NEC 82.99
- testis NEC 62.99
- tetralogy of Fallot
  - partial repair – *see* specific procedure
  - total (one-stage) 35.81
- Thal (repair of esophageal stricture) 42.85
- thalamus 01.41
  - by stereotactic radiosurgery 92.32
    - cobalt 60 92.32
    - linear accelerator (LINAC) 92.31
    - multi-source 92.32
    - particle beam 92.33
    - particulate 92.33
    - radiosurgery NEC 92.39
    - single source photon 92.31
- Thiersch
  - anus 49.79
  - skin graft 86.69
    - hand 86.62
- Thompson
  - cleft lip repair 27.54
  - correction of lymphedema 40.9
  - quadricepsplasty 83.86
  - thumb apposition with bone graft 82.69
- thoracic duct NEC 40.69
- thorax NEC 34.99
- Thorek (partial cholecystectomy) 51.21
- three-snip, punctum 09.51
- thymus NEC 07.99
  - thoracoscopic, NEC 07.98 ●
- thyroid gland NEC 06.98
- TKP (thermokeratoplasty) 11.74
- Tomkins (metroplasty) 69.49
- tongue NEC 25.99
  - flap, palate 27.62
  - tie 25.91
- tonsil NEC 28.99
- Torek (-Bevan) (orchidopexy) (first stage) (second stage) 62.5

- **Osteotomy** – *continued*
  - phalanges – *continued*
    - wedge 77.29
      - for repair of
        - bunion – *see* Bunionectomy
        - bunionette 77.54
        - hallux valgus – *see* Bunionectomy
  - radius 77.33
    - wedge 77.23
  - scapula 77.31
    - wedge 77.21
  - specified site NEC 77.39
    - wedge 77.29
  - tarsal 77.38
    - wedge 77.28
  - thorax (ribs) (sternum) 77.31
    - wedge 77.21
  - tibia 77.37
    - wedge 77.27
  - toe 77.39
    - for repair of
      - bunion – *see* Bunionectomy
      - bunionette 77.54
      - hallux valgus – *see* Bunionectomy
    - wedge 77.29
      - for repair of
        - bunion – *see* Bunionectomy
        - bunionette 77.54
        - hallux valgus – *see* Bunionectomy
  - ulna 77.33
    - wedge 77.23
  - vertebrae 77.39
    - wedge 77.29
- **Otonecrectomy** (inner ear) 20.79
- **Otoplasty** (external) 18.79
  - auditory canal or meatus 18.6
  - auricle 18.79
  - cartilage 18.79
    - reconstruction 18.71
  - prominent or protruding 18.5
- **Otoscopy** 18.11
- **Outfolding, sclera, for buckling** (*see also* Buckling, scleral) 14.49
- **Outfracture, turbinates** (nasal) 21.62
- **Output and clearance, circulatory** 92.05
- **Overdistension, bladder** (therapeutic) 96.25
- **Overlapping, sclera, for buckling** (*see also* Buckling, scleral) 14.49
- **Oversewing**
  - pleural bleb 32.21
  - ulcer crater (peptic) 44.40
    - duodenum 44.42
    - stomach 44.41
- **Oxford operation** (for urinary incontinence) 59.4
- **Oximetry**
  - fetal pulse 75.38
- **Oxygenation** 93.96
  - extracorporeal membrane (ECMO) 39.65
  - hyperbaric 93.95
    - wound 93.59
- **Oxygen therapy** (catalytic) (pump) 93.96
  - hyperbaric 93.95

P

- **Pacemaker**
  - cardiac (*see also* Insertion, pacemaker, cardiac
    - intraoperative (temporary)) 39.64
    - temporary (during and immediately following cardiac surgery) 39.64
- **Packing** – *see also* Insertion, pack
  - auditory canal 96.11
  - nose, for epistaxis (anterior) 21.01
    - posterior (and anterior) 21.02
  - rectal 96.19
  - sella turcica 07.79
  - vaginal 96.14
- **Palatoplasty** 27.69
  - for cleft palate 27.62
    - secondary or subsequent 27.63
- **Palatorrhaphy** 27.61
  - for cleft palate 27.62
- **Pallidectomy** 01.42
- **Pallidoansotomy** 01.42
- **Pallidotomy** 01.42
  - by stereotactic radiosurgery 92.32
    - cobalt 60 92.32
    - linear accelerator (LINAC) 92.31
    - multi-source 92.32
    - particle beam 92.33
    - particulate 92.33
    - radiosurgery NEC 92.39
    - single source photon 92.31
- **Panas operation** (linear proctotomy) 48.0
- **Pancoast operation** (division of trigeminal nerve at foramen ovale) 04.02
- **Pancreatectomy** (total) (with synchronous duodenectomy) 52.6
  - partial NEC 52.59
    - distal (tail) (with part of body) 52.52
    - proximal (head) (with part of body) (with synchronous duodenectomy) 52.51
    - radical 52.53
    - subtotal 52.53
  - radical 52.7
    - subtotal 52.53
- **Pancreaticocystoduodenostomy** 52.4
- **Pancreaticocystoenterostomy** 52.4
- **Pancreaticocystogastrostomy** 52.4
- **Pancreaticocystojejunostomy** 52.4
- **Pancreaticoduodenectomy** (total) 52.6
  - partial NEC 52.59
    - proximal 52.51
    - radical subtotal 52.53
  - radical (one-stage) (two-stage) 52.7
    - subtotal 52.53
- **Pancreaticoduodenostomy** 52.96
- **Pancreaticoenterostomy** 52.96
- **Pancreaticogastrostomy** 52.96
- **Pancreaticoileostomy** 52.96
- **Pancreaticojejunostomy** 52.96
- **Pancreatoduodenectomy** (total) 52.6
  - partial NEC 52.59
  - radical (one-stage) (two-stage) 52.7
    - subtotal 52.53
- **Pancreatogram** 87.66
  - endoscopic retrograde (ERP) 52.13
- **Pancreatolithotomy** 52.09
  - endoscopic 52.94
- **Pancreatotomy** 52.09
- **Pancreolithotomy** 52.09
  - endoscopic 52.94
- **Panendoscopy** 57.32
  - specified site, other than bladder – *see* Endoscopy, by site
  - through artificial stoma 57.31
- **Panhysterectomy** (abdominal) 68.49
  - laparoscopic 68.41
  - vaginal 68.59
    - laparoscopically assisted (LAVH) 68.51
- **Panniculectomy** 86.83
- **Panniculotomy** 86.83
- **Pantaloon operation** (revision of gastric anastomosis) 44.5
- **Papillectomy, anal** 49.39
  - endoscopic 49.31
- **Papillotomy** (pancreas) 51.82
  - endoscopic 51.85
- **Paquin operation** (ureteroneocystostomy) 56.74
- **Paracentesis**
  - abdominal (percutaneous) 54.91
  - anterior chamber, eye 12.91
  - bladder 57.11
  - cornea 12.91
  - eye (anterior chamber) 12.91
  - thoracic, thoracis 34.91
  - tympanum 20.09
    - with intubation 20.01
- **Parasitology** – *see* Examination, microscopic
- **Parathyroidectomy** (partial) (subtotal) NEC 06.89
  - complete 06.81
  - ectopic 06.89
  - global removal 06.81
  - mediastinal 06.89
  - total 06.81
- **Parenteral nutrition, total** 99.15
  - peripheral 99.15
- **Parotidectomy** 26.30
  - complete 26.32
  - partial 26.31
  - radical 26.32
- **Partsch operation** (marsupialization of dental cyst) 24.4
- **Passage** – *see* Insertion and Intubation
- **Passage of sounds, urethra** 58.6
- **Patch**
  - blood, spinal (epidural) 03.95
  - graft – *see* Graft
  - spinal, blood (epidural) 03.95
  - subdural, brain 02.12
- **Patellapexy** 78.46
- **Patellaplasty** NEC 78.46
- **Patellectomy** 77.96
  - partial 77.86
- **Pattee operation** (auditory canal) 18.6
- **Pectenotomy** (*see also* Sphincterotomy, anal) 49.59
- **Pedicle flap** – *see* Graft, skin, pedicle
- **Peet operation** (splanchnic resection) 05.29
- **PEG** (percutaneous endoscopic gastrostomy) 43.11
- **PEJ** (percutaneous endoscopic jejunostomy) 46.32
- **Pelvectomy, kidney** (partial) 55.4
- **Pelvimetry** 88.25
  - gynecological 89.26
- **Pelviolithotomy** 55.11
- **Pelvioplasty, kidney** 55.87
- **Pelviostomy** 55.12
  - closure 55.82
- **Pelviotomy** 77.39
  - to assist delivery 73.94
- **Pelvi-ureteroplasty** 55.87
- **Pemberton operation**
  - osteotomy of ilium 77.39
  - rectum (mobilization and fixation for prolapse repair) 48.76
- **Penectomy** 64.3
- **Pereyra operation** (paraurethral suspension) 59.6
- **Perforation**
  - stapes footplate 19.0
- **Perfusion** NEC 39.97
  - carotid artery 39.97
  - coronary artery 39.97
  - for
    - chemotherapy NEC 99.25
    - hormone therapy NEC 99.24
  - head 39.97
  - hyperthermic (lymphatic), localized region or site 93.35
  - intestine (large) (local) 46.96
    - small 46.95
  - kidney, local 55.95
  - limb (lower) (upper) 39.97
  - liver, localized 50.93
  - neck 39.97
  - subarachnoid (spinal cord) (refrigerated saline) 03.92
  - total body 39.96
- **Pericardiectomy** 37.31
- **Pericardiocentesis** 37.0
- **Pericardiolysis** 37.12
- **Pericardioplasty** 37.49
- **Pericardiorrhaphy** 37.49
- **Pericardiostomy** (tube) 37.12
- **Pericardiotomy** 37.12
- **Peridectomy** 10.31
- **Perilimbal suction** 89.11
- **Perimetry** 95.05
- **Perineoplasty** 71.79
- **Perineorrhaphy** 71.71
  - obstetrical laceration (current) 75.69
- **Perineotomy** (nonobstetrical) 71.09
  - to assist delivery – *see* Episiotomy
- **Periosteotomy** (*see also* Incision, bone) 77.10
  - facial bone 76.09
- **Perirectofistulectomy** 48.93
- **Peritectomy** 10.31
- **Peritomy** 10.1
- **Peritoneocentesis** 54.91
- **Peritoneoscopy** 54.21
- **Peritoneotomy** 54.19
- **Peritoneumectomy** 54.4
- **Phacoemulsification** (ultrasonic) (with aspiration) 13.41
- **Phacofragmentation** (mechanical) (with aspiration) 13.43
  - posterior route 13.42
  - ultrasonic 13.41

Phalangectomy – Polya operation

Q

R

- **Radiography** – *continued*
  - nasopharynx 87.09
  - neck NEC 87.09
  - nose 87.16
  - orbit 87.16
  - pelvis (skeletal) 88.26
    - pelvimetry 88.25
    - soft tissue 88.19
  - prostate NEC 87.92
  - retroperitoneum NEC 88.16
  - ribs 87.43
  - root canal 87.12
  - salivary gland 87.09
  - seminal vesicles NEC 87.92
  - shoulder (skeletal) 88.21
    - soft tissue 88.35
  - skeletal NEC 88.33
    - series (whole or complete) 88.31
  - skull (lateral, sagittal or tangential projection) NEC 87.17
  - spine NEC 87.29
    - cervical 87.22
    - lumbosacral 87.24
    - sacrococcygeal 87.24
    - thoracic 87.23
  - sternum 87.43
  - supraorbital area 87.16
  - symphysis menti 87.16
  - teeth NEC 87.12
    - full-mouth 87.11
  - thigh (skeletal) 88.27
    - soft tissue 88.37
  - thyroid region 87.09
  - tonsils and adenoids 87.09
  - trachea 87.49
  - ultrasonic – *see* Ultrasonography
  - upper arm (skeletal) 88.21
    - soft tissue 88.35
  - upper limb (skeletal) NEC 88.24
    - soft tissue NEC 88.35
  - urinary system NEC 87.79
  - uterus NEC 87.85
    - gravid 87.81
  - uvula 87.09
  - vas deferens NEC 87.95
  - wrist 88.23
  - zygomaticomaxillary complex 87.16
- **Radioimmunotherapy** 92.28
- **Radioisotope**
  - scanning – *see* Scan, radioisotope
  - therapy – *see* Therapy, radioisotope
- **Radiology**
  - diagnostic – *see* Radiography
  - therapeutic – *see* Therapy, radiation
- **Radiosurgery, stereotactic** 92.30
  - cobalt 60 92.32
  - linear accelerator (LINAC) 92.31
  - multi-source 92.32
  - particle beam 92.33
  - particulate 92.33
  - radiosurgery NEC 92.39
  - single source photon 92.31
- **Raising, pedicle graft** 86.71
- **Ramadier operation** (intrapetrosal drainage) 20.22
- **Ramisection** (sympathetic) 05.0
- **Ramstedt operation** (pyloromyotomy) (with wedge resection) 43.3
- **Range of motion testing** 93.05
- **Rankin operation**
  - exteriorization of intestine 46.03
  - proctectomy (complete) 48.5
- **Rashkind operation** (balloon septostomy) 35.41
- **Rastelli operation** (creation of conduit between right ventricle and pulmonary artery) 35.92
  - in repair of
    - pulmonary artery atresia 35.92
    - transposition of great vessels 35.92
    - truncus arteriosus 35.83
- **Raz-Pereyra procedure** (bladder neck suspension) 59.79
- **RCSA** (radical cryosurgical ablation) of prostate 60.62
- **Readjustment** – *see* Adjustment
- **Reamputation, stump** 84.3
- **Reanastomosis** – *see* Anastomosis
- **Reattachment**
  - amputated ear 18.72
  - ankle 84.27
- **Reattachment** – *continued*
  - arm (upper) NEC 84.24
  - choroid and retina NEC 14.59
    - by
      - cryotherapy 14.52
      - diathermy 14.51
      - electrocoagulation 14.51
      - photocoagulation 14.55
        - laser 14.54
        - xenon arc 14.53
  - ear (amputated) 18.72
  - extremity 84.29
    - ankle 84.27
    - arm (upper) NEC 84.24
    - fingers, except thumb 84.22
      - thumb 84.21
    - foot 84.26
    - forearm 84.23
    - hand 84.23
    - leg (lower) NEC 84.27
    - thigh 84.28
    - thumb 84.21
    - toe 84.25
    - wrist 84.23
  - finger 84.22
    - thumb 84.21
  - foot 84.26
  - forearm 84.23
  - hand 84.23
  - joint capsule (*see also* Arthroplasty) 81.96
  - leg (lower) NEC 84.27
  - ligament – *see also* Arthroplasty
    - uterosacral 69.22
  - muscle 83.74
    - hand 82.54
    - papillary (heart) 35.31
  - nerve (peripheral) 04.79
  - nose (amputated) 21.89
  - papillary muscle (heart) 35.31
  - penis (amputated) 64.45
  - retina (and choroid) NEC 14.59
    - by
      - cryotherapy 14.52
      - diathermy 14.51
      - electrocoagulation 14.51
      - photocoagulation 14.55
        - laser 14.54
        - xenon arc 14.53
  - tendon (to tendon) 83.73
    - hand 82.53
    - to skeletal attachment 83.88
      - hand 82.85
  - thigh 84.28
  - thumb 84.21
  - toe 84.25
  - tooth 23.5
  - uterosacral ligament(s) 69.22
  - vessels (peripheral) 39.59
    - renal, aberrant 39.55
  - wrist 84.23
- **Recession**
  - extraocular muscle 15.11
    - multiple (two or more muscles) (with advancement or resection) 15.3
  - gastrocnemius tendon (Strayer operation) 83.72
  - levator palpebrae (superioris) muscle 08.38
  - prognathic jaw 76.64
  - tendon 83.72
    - hand 82.52
- **Reclosure** – *see also* Closure
  - disrupted abdominal wall (postoperative) 54.61
- **Reconstruction** (plastic) – *see also* Construction and Repair, by site
  - alveolus, alveolar (process) (ridge) (with graft or implant) 24.5
  - artery (graft) – *see* Graft, artery
  - artificial stoma, intestine 46.40
  - auditory canal (external) 18.6
  - auricle (ear) 18.71
  - bladder 57.87
    - with
      - ileum 57.87 *[45.51]*
      - sigmoid 57.87 *[45.52]*
  - bone, except facial (*see also* Osteoplasty) 78.40
    - facial NEC 76.46
      - with total ostectomy 76.44
    - mandible 76.43
      - with total mandibulectomy 76.41
  - breast, total 85.7
  - bronchus 33.48
  - canthus (lateral) 08.59
- **Reconstruction** – *continued*
  - cardiac annulus 35.33
  - chest wall (mesh) (silastic) 34.79
  - cleft lip 27.54
  - conjunctival cul-de-sac 10.43
    - with graft (buccal mucous membrane) (free) 10.42
  - cornea NEC 11.79
  - diaphragm 34.84
  - ear (external) (auricle) 18.71
    - external auditory canal 18.6
    - meatus (new) (osseous skin-lined) 18.6
    - ossicles 19.3
    - prominent or protruding 18.5
  - eyebrow 08.70
  - eyelid 08.70
    - with graft or flap 08.69
      - hair follicle 08.63
      - mucous membrane 08.62
      - skin 08.61
      - tarsoconjunctival (one-stage) (two-stage) 08.64
    - full-thickness 08.74
      - involving lid margin 08.73
    - partial-thickness 08.72
      - involving lid margin 08.71
  - eye socket 16.64
    - with graft 16.63
  - fallopian tube 66.79
  - foot and toes (with fixation device) 81.57
    - with prosthetic implant 81.57
  - frontonasal duct 22.79
  - hip (total) (with prosthesis) 81.51
  - intraoral 27.59
  - joint – *see* Arthroplasty
  - lymphatic (by transplantation) 40.9
  - mandible 76.43
    - with total mandibulectomy 76.41
  - mastoid cavity 19.9
  - mouth 27.59
  - nipple NEC 85.87
  - nose (total) (with arm flap) (with forehead flap) 21.83
  - ossicles (graft) (prosthesis) NEC 19.3
    - with
      - stapedectomy 19.19
      - tympanoplasty 19.53
  - pelvic floor 71.79
  - penis (rib graft) (skin graft) (myocutaneous flap) 64.44
  - pharynx 29.4
  - scrotum (with pedicle flap) (with rotational flap) 61.49
  - skin (plastic) (without graft) NEC 86.89
    - with graft – *see* Graft, skin
  - subcutaneous tissue (plastic) (without skin graft) NEC 86.89
    - with graft – *see* Graft, skin
  - tendon pulley (with graft) (with local tissue) 83.83
    - for opponensplasty 82.71
    - hand 82.71
  - thumb (osteoplastic) (with bone graft) (with skin graft) 82.69
  - trachea (with graft) 31.75
  - umbilicus 53.49
  - ureteropelvic junction 55.87
  - urethra 58.46
  - vagina 70.62
    - with graft or prosthesis 70.64 ●
  - vas deferens, surgically divided 63.82
- **Recontour, gingiva** 24.2
- **Recreational therapy** 93.81
- **Rectectomy** (*see also* Resection, rectum) 48.69
- **Rectopexy** (Delorme) 48.76
  - abdominal (Ripstein) 48.75
- **Rectoplasty** 48.79
- **Rectorectostomy** 48.74
- **Rectorrhaphy** 48.71
- **Rectosigmoidectomy** (*see also* Resection, rectum) 48.69
  - transsacral 48.61
- **Rectosigmoidostomy** 45.94
- **Rectostomy** 48.1
  - closure 48.72
- **Red cell survival studies** 92.05
- **Reduction**
  - adipose tissue 86.83
  - batwing arms 86.83
  - breast (bilateral) 85.32
    - unilateral 85.31

Removal – *continued*
- cyst – *see also* Excision, lesion, by site
  - dental 24.4
  - lung 32.29
    - endoscopic 32.28
    - thoracoscopic 32.20 ●
- cystic duct remnant 51.61
- decidua (by)
  - aspiration curettage 69.52
  - curettage (D and C) 69.02
  - manual 75.4
- dental wiring (immobilization device) 97.33
  - orthodontic 24.8
- device (therapeutic) NEC 97.89
  - abdomen NEC 97.86
  - bronchus 33.78
    - valve 33.78
  - digestive system NEC 97.59
  - drainage – *see* Removal, tube
  - external fixation device 97.88
    - mandibular NEC 97.36
    - minifixator (bone) – *see* category 78.6❹
  - for musculoskeletal immobilization NEC 97.88
  - genital tract NEC 97.79
  - head and neck NEC 97.39
  - intrauterine contraceptive 97.71
  - spine 80.09
  - thorax NEC 97.49
  - trunk NEC 97.87
  - urinary system NEC 97.69
- diaphragm, vagina 97.73
- drainage device – *see* Removal, tube
- dye, spinal canal 03.31
- ectopic fetus (from) 66.02
  - abdominal cavity 74.3
  - extraperitoneal (intraligamentous) 74.3
  - fallopian tube (by salpingostomy) 66.02
    - by salpingotomy 66.01
    - with salpingectomy 66.62
  - intraligamentous 74.3
  - ovarian 74.3
  - peritoneal (following uterine or tubal rupture) 74.3
  - site NEC 74.3
  - tubal (by salpingostomy) 66.02
    - by salpingotomy 66.01
    - with salpingectomy 66.62
- electrodes
  - bone growth stimulator – *see* category 78.6❹
  - brain 01.22
    - depth 01.22
      - with synchronous replacement 02.93
    - foramen ovale 01.22
      - with synchronous replacement 02.93
    - sphenoidal - *omit code*
      - with synchronous replacement 02.96
  - cardiac pacemaker (atrial) (transvenous) (ventricular) 37.77
    - with replacement 37.76
  - carotid sinus 04.93 ●
    - with synchronous replacement 04.92 ●
  - depth 01.22
    - with synchronous replacement 02.93
  - epicardial (myocardial) 37.77
    - with replacement (by)
      - atrial and/or ventricular lead(s) (electrode) 37.76
      - epicardial lead 37.74
  - epidural pegs 01.22
    - with synchronous replacement 02.93
  - foramen ovale 01.22
    - with synchronous replacement 02.93
  - gastric 04.93
    - with synchronous replacement 04.92
  - intracranial 01.22
    - with synchronous replacement 02.93
  - peripheral nerve 04.93
    - with synchronous replacement 04.92
  - sacral nerve 04.93
  - sphenoidal - *omit code*
    - with synchronous replacement 02.96
  - spinal 03.94
    - with synchronous replacement 03.93
  - temporary transvenous pacemaker system - *omit code*
- electroencephalographic receiver (brain) (intracranial) 01.22
  - with synchronous replacement 02.93

Removal – *continued*
- electronic
  - stimulator – *see* Removal, neurostimulator, by site
    - bladder 57.98
    - bone 78.6❹
    - skeletal muscle 83.93
      - with synchronous replacement 83.92
    - ureter 56.94
- electrostimulator – *see* Removal, electronic, stimulator, by site
- embolus 38.00
  - with endarterectomy – *see* Endarterectomy
  - abdominal
    - artery 38.06
    - vein 38.07
  - aorta (arch) (ascending) (descending) 38.04
  - arteriovenous shunt or cannula 39.49
  - bovine graft 39.49
  - head and neck vessel
    - endovascular approach 39.74
    - open approach, intracranial vessels 38.01
    - open approach, other vessels of head and neck 38.02
  - intracranial vessel
    - endovascular approach 39.74
    - open approach, intracranial vessels 38.01
    - open approach, other vessels of head and neck 38.02
  - lower limb
    - artery 38.08
    - vein 38.09
  - pulmonary (artery) (vein) 38.05
  - thoracic vessel NEC 38.05
  - upper limb (artery) (vein) 38.03
- embryo – *see* Removal, ectopic fetus
- encircling tube, eye (episcleral) 14.6
- epithelial downgrowth, anterior chamber 12.93
- external fixation device 97.88
  - mandibular NEC 97.36
  - minifixator (bone) – *see* category 78.6❹
- extrauterine embryo – *see* Removal, ectopic fetus
- eyeball 16.49
  - with implant 16.42
    - with attachment of muscles 16.41
- fallopian tube – *see* Salpingectomy
- feces (impacted) (by flushing) (manual) 96.38
- fetus, ectopic – *see* Removal, ectopic fetus
- fingers, supernumerary 86.26
- fixation device
  - external 97.88
    - mandibular NEC 97.36
    - minifixator (bone) – *see* category 78.6❹
  - internal 78.60
    - carpal, metacarpal 78.64
    - clavicle 78.61
    - facial (bone) 76.97
    - femur 78.65
    - fibula 78.67
    - humerus 78.62
    - patella 78.66
    - pelvic 78.69
    - phalanges (foot) (hand) 78.69
    - radius 78.63
    - scapula 78.61
    - specified site NEC 78.69
    - tarsal, metatarsal 78.68
    - thorax (ribs) (sternum) 78.61
    - tibia 78.67
    - ulna 78.63
    - vertebrae 78.69
- foreign body NEC (*see also* Incision, by site) 98.20
  - abdominal (cavity) 54.92
    - wall 54.0
  - adenoid 98.13
    - by incision 28.91
  - alveolus, alveolar bone 98.22
    - by incision 24.0
  - antecubital fossa 98.27
    - by incision 86.05
  - anterior chamber 12.00
    - by incision 12.02
      - with use of magnet 12.01
  - anus (intraluminal) 98.05
    - by incision 49.93
  - artificial stoma (intraluminal) 98.18
  - auditory canal, external 18.02
  - axilla 98.27
    - by incision 86.05
  - bladder (without incision) 57.0
    - by incision 57.19

Removal – *continued*
- foreign body – *continued*
  - bone, except fixation device (*see also* Incision, bone) 77.10
    - alveolus, alveolar 98.22
      - by incision 24.0
  - brain 01.39
    - without incision into brain 01.24
  - breast 85.0
  - bronchus (intraluminal) 98.15
    - by incision 33.0
  - bursa 83.03
    - hand 82.03
  - canthus 98.22
    - by incision 08.51
  - cerebral meninges 01.31
  - cervix (intraluminal) NEC 98.16
    - penetrating 69.97
  - choroid (by incision) 14.00
    - with use of magnet 14.01
    - without use of magnet 14.02
  - ciliary body (by incision) 12.00
    - with use of magnet 12.01
    - without use of magnet 12.02
  - conjunctiva (by magnet) 98.22
    - by incision 10.0
  - cornea 98.21
    - by
      - incision 11.1
      - magnet 11.0
  - duodenum 98.03
    - by incision 45.01
  - ear (intraluminal) 98.11
    - with incision 18.09
  - epididymis 63.92
  - esophagus (intraluminal) 98.02
    - by incision 42.09
  - extrapleural (by incision) 34.01
  - eye, eyeball (by magnet) 98.21
    - anterior segment (by incision) 12.00
      - with use of magnet 12.01
      - without use of magnet 12.02
    - posterior segment (by incision) 14.00
      - with use of magnet 14.01
      - without use of magnet 14 02
    - superficial 98.21
  - eyelid 98.22
    - by incision 08.09
  - fallopian tube
    - by salpingostomy 66.02
    - by salpingotomy 66.01
  - fascia 83.09
    - hand 82.09
  - foot 98.28
  - gall bladder 51.04
  - groin region (abdominal wall) (inguinal) 54.0
  - gum 98.22
    - by incision 24.0
  - hand 98.26
  - head and neck NEC 98.22
  - heart 37.11
  - internal fixation device – *see* Removal, fixation device, internal
  - intestine
    - by incision 45.00
    - large (intraluminal) 98.04
      - by incision 45.03
    - small (intraluminal) 98.03
      - by incision 45.02
  - intraocular (by incision) 12.00
    - with use of magnet 12.01
    - without use of magnet 12.02
  - iris (by incision) 12.00
    - with use of magnet 12.01
    - without use of magnet 12.02
  - joint structures (*see also* Arthrotomy) 80.10
  - kidney (transurethral) (by endoscopy) 56.0
    - by incision 55.01
    - pelvis (transurethral) 56.0
      - by incision 55.11
  - labia 98.23
    - by incision 71.09
  - lacrimal
    - canaliculi 09.42
      - by incision 09.52
    - gland 09.3
      - by incision 09.0
    - passage(s) 09.49
      - by incision 09.59
    - punctum 09.41
      - by incision 09.51

Removal – *continued*
  foreign body – *continued*
    lacrimal – *continued*
      sac 09.49
        by incision 09.53
    large intestine (intraluminal) 98.04
      by incision 45.03
    larynx (intraluminal) 98.14
      by incision 31.3
    lens 13.00
      by incision 13.02
        with use of magnet 13.01
    liver 50.0
    lower limb, except foot 98.29
      foot 98.28
    lung 33.1
    mediastinum 34.1
    meninges (cerebral) 01.31
      spinal 03.01
    mouth (intraluminal) 98.01
      by incision 27.92
    muscle 83.02
      hand 82.02
    nasal sinus 22.50
      antrum 22.2
        with Caldwell-Luc approach 22.39
      ethmoid 22.51
      frontal 22.41
      maxillary 22.2
        with Caldwell-Luc approach 22.39
      sphenoid 22.52
    nerve (cranial) (peripheral) NEC 04.04
      root 03.01
    nose (intraluminal) 98.12
      by incision 21.1
    oral cavity (intraluminal) 98.01
      by incision 27.92
    orbit (by magnet) 98.21
      by incision 16.1
    palate (penetrating) 98.22
      by incision 27.1
    pancreas 52.09
    penis 98.24
      by incision 64.92
    pericardium 37.12
    perineum (female) 98.23
      by incision 71.09
      male 98.25
        by incision 86.05
    perirenal tissue 59.09
    peritoneal cavity 54.92
    perivesical tissue 59.19
    pharynx (intraluminal) 98.13
      by pharyngotomy 29.0
    pleura (by incision) 34.09
    popliteal space 98.29
      by incision 86.05
    rectum (intraluminal) 98.05
      by incision 48.0
    renal pelvis (transurethral) 56.0
      by incision 56.1
    retina (by incision) 14.00
      with use of magnet 14.01
      without use of magnet 14.02
    retroperitoneum 54.92
    sclera (by incision) 12.00
      with use of magnet 12.01
      without use of magnet 12.02
    scrotum 98.24
      by incision 61.0
    sinus (nasal) 22.50
      antrum 22.2
        with Caldwell-Luc approach 22.39
      ethmoid 22.51
      frontal 22.41
      maxillary 22.2
        with Caldwell-Luc approach 22.39
      sphenoid 22.52
    skin NEC 98.20
      by incision 86.05
    skull 01.24
      with incision into brain 01.39
    small intestine (intraluminal) 98.03
      by incision 45.02
    soft tissue NEC 83.09
      hand 82.09
    spermatic cord 63.93
    spinal (canal) (cord) (meninges) 03.01
    stomach (intraluminal) 98.03
      bubble (balloon) 44.94
      by incision 43.0

Removal – *continued*
  foreign body – *continued*
    subconjunctival (by magnet) 98.22
      by incision 10.0
    subcutaneous tissue NEC 98.20
      by incision 86.05
    supraclavicular fossa 98.27
      by incision 86.05
    tendon (sheath) 83.01
      hand 82.01
    testis 62.0
    thorax (by incision) 34.09
    thyroid (field) (gland) (by incision) 06.09
    tonsil 98.13
      by incision 28.91
    trachea (intraluminal) 98.15
      by incision 31.3
    trunk NEC 98.25
    tunica vaginalis 98.24
    upper limb, except hand 98.27
      hand 98.26
    ureter (transurethral) 56.0
      by incision 56.2
    urethra (intraluminal) 98.19
      by incision 58.0
    uterus (intraluminal) 98.16
    vagina (intraluminal) 98.17
      by incision 70.14
    vas deferens 63.6
    vitreous (by incision) 14.00
      with use of magnet 14.01
      without use of magnet 14.02
    vulva 98.23
      by incision 71.09
  gallstones
    bile duct (by incision) NEC 51.49
      endoscopic 51.88
    common duct (by incision) 51.41
      endoscopic 51.88
      percutaneous 51.96
    duodenum 45.01
    gallbladder 51.04
      endoscopic 51.88
      laparoscopic 51.88
    hepatic ducts 51.49
      endoscopic 51.88
    intestine 45.00
      large 45.03
      small NEC 45.02
    liver 50.0
  Gardner Wells tongs (skull) 02.95
    with synchronous replacement 02.94
  gastric band (adjustable), laparoscopic 44.97
  gastric bubble (balloon) 44.94
  granulation tissue – *see also* Excision, lesion, by site
    with repair – *see* Repair, by site
    cranial 01.6
    skull 01.6
  halo traction device (skull) 02.95
    with synchronous replacement 02.94
  heart assist system
    with replacement 37.63
    intra-aortic balloon pump (IABP) 97.44
    nonoperative 97.44
    open removal 37.64
    percutaneous external device 97.44
  hematoma – *see* Drainage, by site
  Hoffman minifixator device (bone) – *see* category 78.6❹
  hydatidiform mole 68.0
  impacted
    feces (rectum) (by flushing) (manual) 96.38
    tooth 23.19
      from nasal sinus (maxillary) 22.61
  implant
    breast 85.94
    cochlear prosthetic device 20.99
    cornea 11.92
    lens (prosthetic) 13.8
    middle ear NEC 20.99
    ocular 16.71
      posterior segment 14.6
    orbit 16.72
    retina 14.6
    tympanum 20.1
  implantable hemodynamic sensor (lead) and monitor device 37.79
  internal fixation device – *see* Removal, fixation device, internal
  intra-aortic balloon pump (IABP) 97.44
  intrauterine contraceptive device (IUD) 97.71

Removal – *continued*
  joint (structure) NOS 80.90
    ankle 80.97
    elbow 80.92
    foot and toe 80.98
    hand and finger 80.94
    hip 80.95
    knee 80.96
    other specified sites 80.99
    shoulder 80.91
    spine 80.99
    toe 80.98
    wrist 80.93
  Kantrowitz heart pump 37.64
    nonoperative 97.44
  keel (tantalum plate), larynx 31.98
  kidney – *see also* Nephrectomy
    mechanical 55.98
    transplanted or rejected 55.53
  laminaria (tent), uterus 97.79
  leads (cardiac) – *see* Removal, electrodes, cardiac pacemaker
  lesion – *see* Excision, lesion, by site
  ligamentum flavum (spine) - *omit code*
  ligature
    fallopian tube 66.79
    ureter 56.86
    vas deferens 63.84
  limb lengthening device, internal – *see* category 78.6❹
  loop recorder 86.05
  loose body
    bone – *see* Sequestrectomy, bone
    joint 80.10
    mesh (surgical) – *see* Removal, foreign body, by site
  lymph node – *see* Excision, lymph, node
  minifixator device (bone) – *see* category 78.6❹
    external fixation device 97.88
  Mulligan hood, fallopian tube 66.94
    with synchronous replacement 66.93
  muscle stimulator (skeletal) 83.93
    with replacement 83.92
  myringotomy device or tube 20.1
  nail (bed) (fold) 86.23
    internal fixation device – *see* Removal, fixation device, internal
  necrosis
    skin 86.28
      excisional 86.22
  neuropacemaker – *see* Removal, neurostimulator, by site
  neurostimulator
    electrodes
      brain 01.22
        with synchronous replacement 02.93
      carotid sinus 04.93 ●
        with synchronous replacement 04.92 ●
      gastric 04.93
        with synchronous replacement 04.92
      intracranial 01.22
        with synchronous replacement 02.93
      peripheral nerve 04.93
        with synchronous replacement 04.92
      sacral nerve 04.93
        with synchronous replacement 04.92
      spinal 03.94
        with synchronous replacement 03.93
    pulse generator (single array, dual array) 86.05
      with synchronous replacement 86.96
        dual array 86.95
          rechargeable 86.98
        single array 86.94
          rechargeable 86.97
  nonabsorbable surgical material NEC – *see* Removal, foreign body, by site
  odontoma (tooth) 24.4
  orbital implant 16.72
  osteocartilagenous loose body, joint structures (*see also* Arthrotomy) 80.10
  outer attic wall (middle ear) 20.59
  ovo-testis (unilateral) 62.3
    bilateral 62.41
  pacemaker
    brain (intracranial) – *see* Removal, neurostimulator
    cardiac (device) (initial) (permanent) 37.89
      with replacement
        dual-chamber device 37.87
        single-chamber device 37.85
          rate responsive 37.86

- **Removal** – *continued*
  - pacemaker – *continued*
    - cardiac – *continued*
      - electrodes (atrial) (transvenous) (ventricular) 37.77
        - with replacement 37.76
      - epicardium (myocardium) 37.77
        - with replacement (by)
          - atrial and/or ventricular lead(s) (electrode) 37.76
          - epicardial lead 37.74
      - temporary transvenous pacemaker system - *omit code*
    - intracranial – *see* Removal, neurostimulator
    - neural – *see* Removal, neurostimulator
    - peripheral nerve – *see* Removal, neurostimulator
    - spine – *see* Removal, neurostimulator
  - pack, packing
    - dental 97.34
    - intrauterine 97.72
    - nasal 97.32
    - rectum 97.59
    - trunk NEC 97.85
    - vagina 97.75
    - vulva 97.75
  - pantopaque dye, spinal canal 03.31
  - patella (complete) 77.96
    - partial 77.86
  - pectus deformity implant device 34.01
  - pelvic viscera, en masse (female) 68.8
    - male 57.71
  - pessary, vagina NEC 97.74
  - pharynx (partial) 29.33
  - phlebolith – *see* Removal, embolus
  - placenta (by)
    - aspiration curettage 69.52
    - D and C 69.02
    - manual 75.4
  - plaque, dental 96.54
  - plate, skull 02.07
    - with synchronous replacement 02.05
  - polyp – *see also* Excision, lesion, by site
    - esophageal 42.32
      - endoscopic 42.33
    - gastric (endoscopic) 43.41
    - intestine 45.41
      - endoscopic 45.42
    - nasal 21.31
  - prosthesis
    - bile duct 51.95
      - nonoperative 97.55
    - cochlear prosthetic device 20.99
    - dental 97.35
    - eye 97.31
    - facial bone 76.99
    - fallopian tube 66.94
      - with synchronous replacement 66.93
    - joint structures 80.00
      - with replacement – *see* Revision, joint replacement, by site ●
      - ankle 80.07
      - elbow 80.02
      - foot and toe 80.08
      - hand and finger 80.04
      - hip 80.05
      - knee 80.06
      - shoulder 80.01
      - specified site NEC 80.09
      - spine 80.09
      - wrist 80.03
    - lens 13.8
    - penis (internal) without replacement 64.96
    - Rosen (urethra) 59.99
    - testicular, by incision 62.0
    - urinary sphincter, artificial 58.99
      - with replacement 58.93
  - pseudophakos 13.8
  - pterygium 11.39
    - with corneal graft 11.32
  - pulse generator
    - cardiac pacemaker 37.86
    - cardioverter/defibrillator 37.79
    - neurostimulator – *see* Removal, neurostimulator, pulse generator
  - pump assist device, heart 37.64
    - with replacement 37.63
    - nonoperative 97.44
  - radioactive material – *see* Removal, foreign body, by site
  - redundant skin, eyelid 08.86

- **Removal** – *continued*
  - rejected organ
    - kidney 55.53
    - testis 62.42
  - reservoir, ventricular (Ommaya) (Rickham) 02.43
    - with synchronous replacement 02.42
  - retained placenta (by)
    - aspiration curettage 69.52
    - D and C 69.02
    - manual 75.4
  - retinal implant 14.6
  - Rheos™ carotid sinus baroreflex activation device 86.05 ●
  - rhinolith 21.31
  - rice bodies, tendon sheaths 83.01
    - hand 82.01
  - Roger-Anderson minifixator device (bone) – *see* category 78.6❹
  - root, residual (tooth) (buried) (retained) 23.11
  - Rosen prosthesis (urethra) 59.99
  - scleral buckle or implant 14.6
  - Scribner shunt 39.43
  - secondary membranous cataract (with iridectomy) 13.65
  - secundines (by)
    - aspiration curettage 69.52
    - D and C 69.02
    - manual 75.4
  - sequestrum – *see* Sequestrectomy
  - seton, anus 49.93
  - Shepard's tube (ear) 20.1
  - Shirodkar suture, cervix 69.96
  - shunt
    - arteriovenous 39.43
      - with creation of new shunt 39.42
    - lumbar-subarachnoid NEC 03.98
    - pleurothecal 03.98
    - salpingothecal 03.98
    - spinal (thecal) NEC 03.98
    - subarachnoid-peritoneal 03.98
    - subarachnoid-ureteral 03.98
  - silastic tubes
    - ear 20.1
    - fallopian tubes 66.94
      - with synchronous replacement 66.93
  - skin
    - necrosis or slough 86.28
      - excisional 86.22
      - superficial layer (by dermabrasion) 86.25
  - skull tongs 02.95
    - with synchronous replacement 02.94
  - spacer (cement) (joint) ▶(methylmethacrylate)◀ 84.57
  - splint 97.88
  - stent
    - bile duct 97.55
    - larynx 31.98
    - ureteral 97.62
    - urethral 97.65
  - stimoceiver – *see* Removal, neurostimulator
  - subdural
    - grids 01.22
    - strips 01.22
  - supernumerary digit(s) 86.26
  - suture(s) NEC 97.89
    - abdominal wall 97.83
    - by incision – *see* Incision, by site
    - genital tract 97.79
    - head and neck 97.38
    - thorax 97.43
    - trunk NEC 97.84
  - symblepharon – *see* Repair, symblepharon
  - temporary transvenous pacemaker system - *omit code*
  - testis (unilateral) 62.3
    - bilateral 62.41
    - remaining or solitary 62.42
  - thrombus 38.00
    - with endarterectomy – *see* Endarterectomy
    - abdominal
      - artery 38.06
      - vein 38.07
    - aorta (arch) (ascending) (descending) 38.04
    - arteriovenous shunt or cannula 39.49
    - bovine graft 39.49
    - coronary artery 36.09
    - head and neck vessel NEC 38.02
    - intracranial vessel NEC 38.01
    - lower limb
      - artery 38.08
      - vein 38.09
    - pulmonary (artery) (vein) 38.05

- **Removal** – *continued*
  - thrombus – *continued*
    - thoracic vessel NEC 38.05
    - upper limb (artery) (vein) 38.03
  - tissue expander (skin) NEC 86.05
    - breast 85.96
  - toes, supernumerary 86.26
  - tongs, skull 02.95
    - with synchronous replacement 02.94
  - tonsil tag 28.4
  - tooth (by forceps) (multiple) (single) NEC 23.09
    - deciduous 23.01
    - surgical NEC 23.19
      - impacted 23.19
      - residual root 23.11
      - root apex 23.73
        - with root canal therapy 23.72
  - trachoma follicles 10.33
  - T-tube (bile duct) 97.55
  - tube
    - appendix 97.53
    - bile duct (T-tube) NEC 97.55
    - cholecystostomy 97.54
    - cranial cavity 01.27
    - cystostomy 97.63
    - ear (button) 20.1
    - gastrostomy 97.51
    - large intestine 97.53
    - liver 97.55
    - mediastinum 97.42
    - nephrostomy 97.61
    - pancreas 97.56
    - peritoneum 97.82
    - pleural cavity 97.41
    - pyelostomy 97.61
    - retroperitoneum 97.81
    - small intestine 97.52
    - thoracotomy 97.41
    - tracheostomy 97.37
    - tympanostomy 20.1
    - tympanum 20.1
    - ureterostomy 97.62
  - ureteral splint (stent) 97.62
  - urethral sphincter, artificial 58.99
    - with replacement 58.93
  - urinary sphincter, artificial 58.99
    - with replacement 58.93
  - utricle 20.79
  - valve
    - vas deferens 63.85
    - ventricular (cerebral) 02.43
  - vascular graft or prosthesis 39.49
  - ventricular shunt or reservoir 02.43
    - with synchronous replacement 02.42
  - Vinke tongs (skull) 02.95
    - with synchronous replacement 02.94
  - vitreous (with replacement) 14.72
    - anterior approach (partial) 14.71
    - open sky technique 14.71
  - Wagner-Brooker minifixator device (bone) – *see* category 78.6❹
  - wiring, dental (immobilization device) 97.33
    - orthodontic 24.8
- **Renipuncture** (percutaneous) 55.92
- **Renogram** 92.03
- **Renotransplantation** NEC 55.69

  Note – To report donor source:
  cadaver 00.93
  live non-related donor 00.92
  live related donor 00.91
  live unrelated donor 00.92

- **Reopening** – *see also* Incision, by site
  - blepharorrhaphy 08.02
  - canthorrhaphy 08.02
  - cilia base 08.71
  - craniotomy or craniectomy site 01.23
  - fallopian tube (divided) 66.79
  - iris in anterior chambers 12.97
  - laminectomy or laminotomy site 03.02
  - laparotomy site 54.12
  - osteotomy site (*see also* Incision, bone) 77.10
    - facial bone 76.09
  - tarsorrhaphy 08.02
  - thoracotomy site (for control of hemorrhage) (for examination) (for exploration) 34.03
  - thyroid field wound (for control of hemorrhage) (for examination) (for exploration) (for removal of hematoma) 06.02
- **Repacking** – *see* Replacement, pack, by site

Removal – Repacking

Repair
  abdominal wall 54.72
  adrenal gland 07.44
  alveolus, alveolar (process) (ridge) (with graft) (with implant) 24.5
  anal sphincter 49.79
    artificial sphincter
      implantation 49.75
      revision 49.75
    laceration (by suture) 49.71
      obstetric (current) 75.62
        old 49.79
  aneurysm (false) (true) 39.52
    by or with
      clipping 39.51
      coagulation 39.52
      coil (endovascular approach) 39.79
        head and neck 39.72
      electrocoagulation 39.52
        excision or resection of vessel – *see also* Aneurysmectomy, by site
        with
          anastomosis – *see* Aneurysmectomy, with anastomosis, by site
          graft replacement – *see* Aneurysmectomy, with graft replacement, by site
      endovascular graft 39.79
        abdominal aorta 39.71
        head and neck 39.72
        lower extremity artery(s) 39.79
        thoracic aorta 39.73
        upper extremity artery(s) 39.79
      filipuncture 39.52
      graft replacement – *see* Aneurysmectomy, with graft replacement, by site
      ligation 39.52
      liquid tissue adhesive (glue) 39.79
        endovascular approach 39.79
          head and neck 39.72
      methyl methacrylate 39.52
        endovascular approach 39.79
          head and neck 39.72
      occlusion 39.52
        endovascular approach 39.79
          head and neck 39.72
      suture 39.52
      trapping 39.52
      wiring 39.52
      wrapping (gauze) (methyl methacrylate) (plastic) 39.52
    coronary artery 36.91
    heart 37.32
    sinus of Valsalva 35.39
    thoracic aorta (dissecting), by fenestration 39.54
  anomalous pulmonary venous connection (total)
    one-stage 35.82
    partial – *see* specific procedure
    total 35.82
  anus 49.79
    laceration (by suture) 49.71
      obstetric (current) 75.62
        old 49.79
  aorta 39.31
  aorticopulmonary window 39.59
  arteriovenous fistula 39.53
    by or with
      clipping 39.53
      coagulation 39.53
      coil (endovascular approach) 39.79
        head and neck vessels 39.72
      division 39.53
      excision or resection – *see also* Aneurysmectomy, by site
        with
          anastomosis – *see* Aneurysmectomy, with anastomosis, by site
          graft replacement – *see* Aneurysmectomy, with graft replacement, by site
      ligation 39.53
        coronary artery 36.99
      occlusion 39.53
        endovascular approach 39.79
          head and neck 39.72
      suture 39.53

Repair – *continued*
  artery NEC 39.59
    by
      endovascular approach
        abdominal aorta 39.71
        head and neck (embolization or occlusion) 39.72
        other repair (of aneurysm) 39.79
        percutaneous repair of intracranial vessel(s) (for stent insertion) 00.62

Note – Also use 00.40, 00.41, 00.42, or 00.43 to show the total number of vessels treated. Use code 00.44 once to show procedure on a bifurcated vessel. In addition, use 00.45, 00.46, 00.47, or 00.48 to show the number of vascular stents inserted.

        percutaneous repair of precerebral (extracranial) vessel(s) (for stent insertion) 00.61

Note – Also use 00.40, 00.41, 00.42, or 00.43 to show the total number of vessels treated. Use code 00.44 once to show procedure on a bifurcated vessel. In addition, use 00.45, 00.46, 00.47, or 00.48 to show the number of vascular stents inserted.

        thoracic aorta 39.73
      non-coronary percutaneous transluminal angioplasty or atherectomy

Note – Also use 00.40, 00.41, 00.42, or 00.43 to show the total number of vessels treated. Use code 00.44 once to show procedure on a bifurcated vessel. In addition, use 00.45, 00.46, 00.47, or 00.48 to show the number of vascular stents inserted.

        basilar 00.61
        carotid 00.61
        femoropopliteal 39.50
        iliac 39.50
        lower extremity NOS 39.50
        mesenteric 39.50
        renal 39.50
        upper extremity NOS 39.50
        vertebral 00.61
    with
      patch graft 39.58
        with excision or resection of vessel – *see* Arteriectomy, with graft replacement, by site
        synthetic (Dacron) (Teflon) 39.57
        tissue (vein) (autogenous) (homograft) 39.56
      suture 39.31
    coronary NEC 36.99
      by angioplasty – *see* Angioplasty, coronary
      by atherectomy – *see* Angioplasty, coronary
  artificial opening – *see* Repair, stoma
  atrial septal defect 35.71
    with
      prosthesis (open heart technique) 35.51
        closed heart technique 35.52
      tissue graft 35.61
    combined with repair of valvular and ventricular septal defects – *see* Repair, endocardial cushion defect
    in total repair of total anomalous pulmonary venous connection 35.82
  atrioventricular canal defect (any type) 35.73
    with
      prosthesis 35.54
      tissue graft 35.63
  bifid digit (finger) 82.89
  bile duct NEC 51.79
    laceration (by suture) NEC 51.79
      common bile duct 51.71
  bladder NEC 57.89
    exstrophy 57.86
    for stress incontinence – *see* Repair, stress incontinence
    laceration (by suture) 57.81
      obstetric (current) 75.61
        old 57.89
    neck 57.85
  blepharophimosis 08.59

Repair – *continued*
  blepharoptosis 08.36
    by
      frontalis muscle technique (with)
        fascial sling 08.32
        suture 08.31
    levator muscle technique 08.34
      with resection or advancement 08.33
    orbicularis oculi muscle sling 08.36
    tarsal technique 08.35
  blood vessel NEC 39.59
    with
      patch graft 39.58
        with excision or resection – *see* Angiectomy, with graft replacement
        synthetic (Dacron) (Teflon) 39.57
        tissue (vein) (autogenous) (homograft) 39.56
      resection – *see* Angiectomy
      suture 39.30
    coronary artery NEC 36.99
      by angioplasty – *see* Angioplasty, coronary
      by atherectomy – *see* Angioplasty, coronary
    peripheral vessel NEC 39.59
      by angioplasty 39.50

Note – Also use 00.40, 00.41, 00.42, or 00.43 to show the total number of vessels treated. Use code 00.44 once to show procedure on a bifurcated vessel. In addition, use 00.45, 00.46, 00.47, or 00.48 to show the number of vascular stents inserted.

      by atherectomy 39.50

Note – Also use 00.40, 00.41, 00.42, or 00.43 to show the total number of vessels treated. Use code 00.44 once to show procedure on a bifurcated vessel. In addition, use 00.45, 00.46, 00.47, or 00.48 to show the number of vascular stents inserted.

      by endovascular approach 39.79
  bone NEC – *see also* Osteoplasty – *see* category 78.4❹
    by synostosis technique – *see* Arthrodesis
    accessory sinus 22.79
    cranium NEC 02.06
      with
        flap (bone) 02.03
        graft (bone) 02.04
    for malunion, nonunion, or delayed union of fracture – *see* Repair, fracture, malunion or nonunion
    nasal 21.89
    skull NEC 02.06
      with
        flap (bone) 02.03
        graft (bone) 02.04
  bottle, hydrocele of tunica vaginalis 61.2
  brain (trauma) NEC 02.92
  breast (plastic) (*see also* Mammoplasty) 85.89
  broad ligament 69.29
  bronchus NEC 33.48
    laceration (by suture) 33.41
  bunionette (with osteotomy) 77.54
  canaliculus, lacrimal 09.73
  canthus (lateral) 08.59
  cardiac pacemaker NEC 37.89
    electrode(s) (lead) NEC 37.75
  cardioverter/defibrillator (automatic) pocket, (skin) (subcutaneous) 37.99
  cerebral meninges 02.12
  cervix 67.69
    internal os 67.59
      transabdominal 67.51
      transvaginal 67.59
    aceration (by suture) 67.61
      obstetric (current) 75.51
        old 67.69
  chest wall (mesh) (silastic) NEC 34.79
  chordae tendineae 35.32
  choroid NEC 14.9
    with retinal repair – *see* Repair, retina
  cisterna chyli 40.69
  claw toe 77.57
  cleft
    hand 82.82
    laryngotracheal 31.69
    lip 27.54
    palate 27.62
      secondary or subsequent 27.63
  coarctation of aorta – *see* Excision, coarctation of aorta

❹ Fourth-Digit Required *[code]* Manifestation Code ►◄ Revised Text ● New Line ▲ Revised Code

Repair – Repair

- **Revision** – *continued*
  - cholecystostomy 51.99
  - cleft palate repair 27.63
  - colostomy 46.43
  - conduit, urinary 56.52
  - cystostomy (stoma) 57.22
  - disc – *see* Revision, intervertebral disc
  - elbow replacement (prosthesis) 81.97
  - enterostomy (stoma) 46.40
    - large intestine 46.43
    - small intestine 46.41
  - enucleation socket 16.64
    - with graft 16.63
  - esophagostomy 42.83
  - exenteration cavity 16.66
    - with secondary graft 16.65
  - extraocular muscle surgery 15.6
  - fenestration, inner ear 20.62
  - filtering bleb 12.66
  - fixation device (broken) (displaced) (*see also* Fixation, bone, internal) 78.50
  - flap or pedicle graft (skin) 86.75
  - foot replacement (prosthesis) 81.59
  - gastric anastomosis (with jejunal interposition) 44.5
  - gastric band, laparoscopic 44.96
  - gastric port device
    - laparoscopic 44.96
  - gastroduodenostomy (with jejunal interposition) 44.5
  - gastrointestinal anastomosis (with jejunal interposition) 44.5
  - gastrojejunostomy 44.5
  - gastrostomy 44.69
    - laparoscopic 44.68
  - hand replacement (prosthesis) 81.97
  - heart procedure NEC 35.95
  - hip replacement NOS 81.53
    - acetabular and femoral components (total) 00.70
    - acetabular component only 00.71
    - acetabular liner and/or femoral head only 00.73
    - femoral component only 00.72
    - femoral head only and/or acetabular liner 00.73
    - partial
      - acetabular component only 00.71
      - acetabular liner and/or femoral head only 00.73
      - femoral component only 00.72
      - femoral head only and/or acetabular liner 00.73
    - total (acetabular and femoral components) 00.70
  - Holter (-Spitz) valve 02.42
  - ileal conduit 56.52
  - ileostomy 46.41
  - intervertebral disc, artificial (partial) (total) NOS 84.69
    - cervical 84.66
    - lumbar, lumbosacral 84.68
    - thoracic 84.67
  - jejunoileal bypass 46.93
  - jejunostomy 46.41
  - joint replacement
    - acetabular and femoral components (total) 00.70
    - acetabular component only 00.71
    - acetabular liner and/or femoral head only 00.73
    - ankle 81.59
    - elbow 81.97
    - femoral component only 00.72
    - femoral head only and/or acetabular liner 00.73
    - foot 81.59
    - hand 81.97
    - hip 81.53
      - acetabular and femoral components (total) 00.70
      - acetabular component only 00.71
      - acetabular liner and/or femoral head only 00.73
      - femoral component only 00.72
      - femoral head only and/or acetabular liner 00.73
      - partial
        - acetabular component only 00.71
        - acetabular liner and/or femoral head only 00.73
        - femoral component only 00.72

- **Revision** – *continued*
  - joint replacement – *continued*
    - hip – *continued*
      - partial – *continued*
        - femoral head only and/or acetabular liner 00.73
      - total (acetabular and femoral components) 00.70
    - knee replacement NOS 81.55
      - femoral component 00.82
      - partial
        - femoral component 00.82
        - patellar component 00.83
        - tibial component 00.81
        - tibial insert 00.84
      - patellar component 00.83
      - tibial component 00.81
      - tibial insert 00.84
      - total (all components) 00.80
    - lower extremity NEC 81.59
    - toe 81.59
    - upper extremity 81.97
    - wrist 81.97
  - knee replacement (prosthesis) NOS 81.55
    - femoral component 00.82
    - partial
      - femoral component 00.82
      - patellar component 00.83
      - tibial component 00.81
      - tibial insert 00.84
    - patellar component 00.83
    - tibial component 00.81
    - tibial insert 00.84
    - total (all components) 00.80
  - laryngostomy 31.63
  - lateral canthus 08.59
  - mallet finger 82.84
  - mastoid antrum 19.9
  - mastoidectomy 20.92
  - nephrostomy 55.89
  - neuroplasty 04.75
  - ocular implant 16.62
  - orbital implant 16.62
  - pocket
    - cardiac device (defibrillator) (pacemaker)
      - with initial insertion of cardiac device - *omit code*
      - new site (cardiac device pocket) (skin)(subcutaneous) 37.79
    - intracardiac hemodynamic monitoring 37.79
    - subcutaneous device pocket NEC
      - with initial insertion of generator or device - *omit code*
      - new site 86.09
    - thalamic stimulator pulse generator
      - with initial insertion of battery package - *omit code*
      - new site (skin)(subcutaneous) 86.09
  - previous mastectomy site – *see* categories 85.0-85.99
  - proctostomy 48.79
  - prosthesis
    - acetabular and femoral components (total) 00.70
    - acetabular component only 00.71
    - acetabular liner and/or femoral head only 00.73
    - ankle 81.59
    - breast 85.93
    - elbow 81.97
    - femoral component only 00.72
    - femoral head only and/or acetabular liner 00.73
    - foot 81.59
    - hand 81.97
    - heart valve (poppet) 35.95
    - hip 81.53
      - acetabular and femoral components (total) 00.70
      - acetabular component only 00.71
      - acetabular liner and/or femoral head only 00.73
      - femoral component only 00.72
      - femoral head only and/or acetabular liner 00.73
      - partial
        - acetabular component only 00.71
        - acetabular liner and/or femoral head only 00.73
        - femoral component only 00.72
        - femoral head only and/or acetabular liner 00.73

- **Revision** – *continued*
  - prosthesis – *continued*
    - hip – *continued*
      - total (acetabular and femoral components) 00.70
    - knee NOS 81.55
      - femoral component 00.82
      - partial
        - femoral component 00.82
        - patellar component 00.83
        - tibial component 00.81
        - tibial insert 00.84
      - patellar component 00.83
      - tibial component 00.81
      - tibial insert 00.84
      - total (all components) 00.80
    - lower extremity NEC 81.59
    - shoulder 81.97
    - spine ●
      - facet replacement device(s) 84.85 ●
      - interspinous process device(s) 84.81 ●
      - pedicle-based dynamic stabilization device(s) 84.83 ●
    - toe 81.59
    - upper extremity 81.97
    - wrist 81.97
  - ptosis overcorrection 08.37
  - pyelostomy 55.12
  - pyloroplasty 44.29
  - rhinoplasty 21.84
  - scar
    - skin 86.84
      - with excision 86.3
  - scleral fistulization 12.66
  - shoulder replacement (prosthesis) 81.97
  - shunt
    - arteriovenous (cannula) (for dialysis) 39.42
    - lumbar-subarachnoid NEC 03.97
    - peritoneojugular 54.99
    - peritoneovascular 54.99
    - pleurothecal 03.97
    - salpingothecal 03.97
    - spinal (thecal) NEC 03.97
    - subarachnoid-peritoneal 03.97
    - subarachnoid-ureteral 03.97
    - ventricular (cerebral) 02.42
    - ventriculoperitoneal
      - at peritoneal site 54.95
      - at ventricular site 02.42
  - stapedectomy NEC 19.29
    - with incus replacement (homograft) (prosthesis) 19.21
  - stoma
    - bile duct 51.79
    - bladder (vesicostomy) 57.22
    - bronchus 33.42
    - common duct 51.72
    - esophagus 42.89
    - gallbladder 51.99
    - hepatic duct 51.79
    - intestine 46.40
      - large 46.43
      - small 46.41
    - kidney 55.89
    - larynx 31.63
    - rectum 48.79
    - stomach 44.69
      - laparoscopic 44.68
    - thorax 34.79
    - trachea 31.74
    - ureter 56.62
    - urethra 58.49
  - tack operation 20.79
  - toe replacement (prosthesis) 81.59
  - tracheostomy 31.74
  - tunnel
    - pulse generator lead wire 86.99
      - with initial procedure - *omit code*
  - tympanoplasty 19.6
  - uretero-ileostomy, cutaneous 56.52
  - ureterostomy (cutaneous) (stoma) NEC 56.62
    - ileal 56.52
  - urethrostomy 58.49
  - urinary conduit 56.52
  - vascular procedure (previous) NEC 39.49
  - ventricular shunt (cerebral) 02.42
  - vesicostomy stoma 57.22
  - wrist replacement (prosthesis) 81.97
- **Rhinectomy** 21.4
- **Rhinocheiloplasty** 27.59
  - cleft lip 27.54

S

❹ Fourth-Digit Required *[code]* Manifestation Code ▶◀ Revised Text ● New Line ▲ Revised Code

Section – *continued*
  nerve (cranial) (peripheral) NEC 04.03
    acoustic 04.01
    spinal root (posterior) 03.1
    sympathetic 05.0
    trigeminal tract 04.02
  Saemisch (corneal) 11.1
  spinal ligament 80.49
    arcuate - *omit code*
    flavum - *omit code*
  tooth (impacted) 23.19
Seddon-Brooks operation (transfer of pectoralis major tendon) 83.75
Semb operation (apicolysis of lung) 33.39
Senning operation (correction of transposition of great vessels) 35.91
Separation
  twins (attached) (conjoined) (Siamese) 84.93
    asymmetrical (unequal) 84.93
    symmetrical (equal) 84.92
Septectomy
  atrial (closed) 35.41
    open 35.42
    transvenous method (balloon) 35.41
  submucous (nasal) 21.5
Septoplasty NEC 21.88
  with submucous resection of septum 21.5
Septorhinoplasty 21.84
Septostomy (atrial) (balloon) 35.41
Septotomy, nasal 21.1
Sequestrectomy
  bone 77.00
    carpals, metacarpals 77.04
    clavicle 77.01
    facial 76.01
    femur 77.05
    fibula 77.07
    humerus 77.02
    nose 21.32
    patella 77.06
    pelvic 77.09
    phalanges (foot) (hand) 77.09
    radius 77.03
    scapula 77.01
    skull 01.25
    specified site NEC 77.09
    tarsals, metatarsals 77.08
    thorax (ribs) (sternum) 77.01
    tibia 77.07
    ulna 77.03
    vertebrae 77.09
  nose 21.32
  skull 01.25
Sesamoidectomy 77.98
Setback, ear 18.5
Sever operation (division of soft tissue of arm) 83.19
Severing of blepharorrhaphy 08.02
Sewell operation (heart) 36.2
Sharrard operation (iliopsoas muscle transfer) 83.77
Shaving
  bone (*see also* Excision, lesion, bone) 77.60
  cornea (epithelium) 11.41
    for smear or culture 11.21
  patella 77.66
Shelf operation (hip arthroplasty) 81.40
Shirodkar operation (encirclement suture, cervix) 67.59
Shock therapy
  chemical 94.24
  electroconvulsive 94.27
  electrotonic 94.27
  insulin 94.24
  subconvulsive 94.26
Shortening
  bone (fusion) 78.20
    femur 78.25
    specified site NEC – *see* category 78.2
    tibia 78.27
    ulna 78.23
  endopelvic fascia 69.22
  extraocular muscle NEC 15.22
    multiple (two or more muscles) 15.4
  eyelid margin 08.71
  eye muscle NEC 15.22
    multiple (two or more muscles) (with lengthening) 15.4
  finger (macrodactyly repair) 82.83

Shortening – *continued*
  heel cord 83.85
  levator palpebrae muscle 08.33
  ligament – *see also* Arthroplasty
    round 69.22
    uterosacral 69.22
  muscle 83.85
    extraocular 15.22
      multiple (two or more muscles) 15.4
    hand 82.55
  sclera (for repair of retinal detachment) 14.59
    by scleral buckling (*see also* Buckling, scleral) 14.49
  tendon 83.85
    hand 82.55
  ureter (with reimplantation) 56.41
Shunt – *see also* Anastomosis and Bypass, vascular
  abdominovenous 54.94
  aorta-coronary sinus 36.39
  aorta (descending)-pulmonary (artery) 39.0
  aortocarotid 39.22
  aortoceliac 39.26
  aortofemoral 39.25
  aortoiliac 39.25
  aortoiliofemoral 39.25
  aortomesenteric 39.26
  aorto-myocardial (graft) 36.2
  aortorenal 39.24
  aortosubclavian 39.22
  apicoaortic 35.93
  arteriovenous NEC 39.29
    for renal dialysis (by)
      anastomosis 39.27
      external cannula 39.93
  ascending aorta to pulmonary artery (Waterston) 39.0
  axillary-femoral 39.29
  carotid-carotid 39.22
  carotid-subclavian 39.22
  caval-mesenteric 39.1
  corpora cavernosa-corpus spongiosum 64.98
  corpora-saphenous 64.98
  descending aorta to pulmonary artery (Potts-Smith) 39.0
  endolymphatic (-subarachnoid) 20.71
  endolymph-perilymph 20.71
  extracranial-intracranial (EC-IC) 39.28
  femoroperoneal 39.29
  femoropopliteal 39.29
  iliofemoral 39.25
  ilioiliac 39.25
  intestinal
    large-to-large 45.94
    small-to-large 45.93
    small-to-small 45.91
  left subclavian to descending aorta (Blalock-Park) 39.0
  left-to-right (systemic-pulmonary artery) 39.0
  left ventricle (heart) (apex) and aorta 35.93
  lienorenal 39.1
  lumbar-subarachnoid (with valve) NEC 03.79
  mesocaval 39.1
  peritoneal-jugular 54.94
  peritoneo-vascular 54.94
  peritoneovenous 54.94
  pleuroperitoneal 34.05
  pleurothecal (with valve) 03.79
  portacaval (double) 39.1
  portal-systemic 39.1
  portal vein to vena cava 39.1
  pulmonary-innominate 39.0
  pulmonary vein to atrium 35.82
  renoportal 39.1
  right atrium and pulmonary artery 35.94
  right ventricle and pulmonary artery (distal) 35.92
    in repair of
      pulmonary artery atresia 35.92
      transposition of great vessels 35.92
      truncus arteriosus 35.83
  salpingothecal (with valve) 03.79
  semicircular subarachnoid 20.71
  spinal (thecal) (with valve) NEC 03.79
    subarachnoid-peritoneal 03.71
    subarachnoid-ureteral 03.72
  splenorenal (venous) 39.1
    arterial 39.26
  subarachnoid-peritoneal (with valve) 03.71
  subarachnoid-ureteral (with valve) 03.72
  subclavian-pulmonary 39.0
  subdural-peritoneal (with valve) 02.34
  superior mesenteric-caval 39.1
  systemic-pulmonary artery 39.0

Shunt – *continued*
  transjugular intrahepatic portosystemic [TIPS] 39.1
  vena cava to pulmonary artery (Green) 39.21
  ventricular (cerebral) (with valve) 02.2
    to
      abdominal cavity or organ 02.34
      bone marrow 02.39
      cervical subarachnoid space 02.2
      circulatory system 02.32
      cisterna magna 02.2
      extracranial site NEC 02.39
      gallbladder 02.34
      head or neck structure 02.31
      intracerebral site NEC 02.2
      lumbar site 02.39
      mastoid 02.31
      nasopharynx 02.31
      thoracic cavity 02.33
      ureter 02.35
      urinary system 02.35
      venous system 02.32
  ventriculoatrial (with valve) 02.32
  ventriculocaval (with valve) 02.32
  ventriculocisternal (with valve) 02.2
  ventriculolumbar (with valve) 02.39
  ventriculomastoid (with valve) 02.31
  ventriculonasopharyngeal 02.31
  ventriculopleural (with valve) 02.33
Sialoadenectomy (parotid) (sublingual) (submaxillary) 26.30
  complete 26.32
  partial 26.31
  radical 26.32
Sialoadenolithotomy 26.0
Sialoadenotomy 26.0
Sialodochoplasty NEC 26.49
Sialogram 87.09
Sialolithotomy 26.0
Sieve, vena cava 38.7
Sigmoid bladder 57.87 *[45.52]*
Sigmoidectomy 45.76
Sigmoidomyotomy 46.91
Sigmoidopexy (Moschowitz) 46.63
Sigmoidoproctectomy (*see also* Resection, rectum) 48.69
Sigmoidoproctostomy 45.94
Sigmoidorectostomy 45.94
Sigmoidorrhaphy 46.75
Sigmoidoscopy (rigid) 48.23
  with biopsy 45.25
  flexible 45.24
  through stoma (artificial) 45.22
  transabdominal 45.21
Sigmoidosigmoidostomy 45.94
  proximal to distal segment 45.76
Sigmoidostomy (*see also* Colostomy) 46.10
Sigmoidotomy 45.03
Sign language 93.75
Silver operation (bunionectomy) 77.59
Sinogram
  abdominal wall 88.03
  chest wall 87.38
  retroperitoneum 88.14
Sinusectomy (nasal) (complete) (partial) (with turbinectomy) 22.60
  antrum 22.62
    with Caldwell-Luc approach 22.61
  ethmoid 22.63
  frontal 22.42
  maxillary 22.62
    with Caldwell-Luc approach 22.61
  sphenoid 22.64
Sinusotomy (nasal) 22.50
  antrum (intranasal) 22.2
    with external approach (Caldwell-Luc) 22.39
      radical (with removal of membrane lining) 22.31
  ethmoid 22.51
  frontal 22.41
  maxillary (intranasal) 22.2
    external approach (Caldwell-Luc) 22.39
      radical (with removal of membrane lining) 22.31
  multiple 22.53
  perinasal 22.50
  sphenoid 22.52

Section – Sinusotomy

❹ Fourth-Digit Required   *[code]* Manifestation Code   ►◄ Revised Text   ● New Line   ▲ Revised Code

❹ Fourth-Digit Required *[code]* Manifestation Code ▶◀ Revised Text ● New Line ▲ Revised Code

Thrombectomy – *continued*
  head and neck vessel NEC 38.02
  intracranial vessel NEC 38.01
  lower limb
    artery 38.08
    vein 38.09
  mechanical
    endovascular
      head and neck 39.74
  pulmonary vessel 38.05
  thoracic vessel NEC 38.05
  upper limb (artery) (vein) 38.03
Thromboendarterectomy 38.10
  abdominal 38.16
  aorta (arch) (ascending) (descending) 38.14
  coronary artery 36.09
    open chest approach 36.03
  head and neck NEC 38.12
  intracranial NEC 38.11
  lower limb 38.18
  thoracic NEC 38.15
  upper limb 38.13
Thymectomy 07.80
  partial ▶(open) (other)◀ 07.81
    thoracoscopic 07.83 ●
  total ▶(open) (other)◀ 07.82
    thoracoscopic 07.84 ●
  transcervical 07.99 ●
Thyrochondrotomy 31.3
Thyrocricoidectomy 30.29
Thyrocricotomy (for assistance in breathing) 31.1
Thyroidectomy NEC 06.39
  by mediastinotomy (*see also* Thyroidectomy, substernal) 06.50
  with laryngectomy – *see* Laryngectomy
  complete or total 06.4
    substernal (by mediastinotomy) (transsternal route) 06.52
    transoral route (lingual) 06.6
  lingual (complete) (partial) (subtotal) (total) 06.6
  partial or subtotal NEC 06.39
    with complete removal of remaining lobe 06.2
    submental route (lingual) 06.6
    substernal (by mediastinotomy) (transsternal route) 06.51
  remaining tissue 06.4
  submental route (lingual) 06.6
  substernal (by mediastinotomy) (transsternal route) 06.50
    complete or total 06.52
    partial or subtotal 06.51
  transoral route (lingual) 06.6
  transsternal route (*see also* Thyroidectomy, substernal) 06.50
  unilateral (with removal of isthmus) (with removal of portion of other lobe) 06.2
Thyroidorrhaphy 06.93
Thyroidotomy (field) (gland) NEC 06.09
  postoperative 06.02
Thyrotomy 31.3
  with tantalum plate 31.69
Tirofiban (HCL), **infusion** 99.20
Toilette
  skin – *see* Debridement, skin or subcutaneous tissue
  tracheostomy 96.55
Token economy (behavior therapy) 94.33
Tomkins operation (metroplasty) 69.49
Tomography – *see also* Radiography
  abdomen NEC 88.02
  cardiac 87.42
  computerized axial NEC 88.38
    abdomen 88.01
    bone 88.38
      quantitative 88.98
    brain 87.03
    head 87.03
    kidney 87.71
    skeletal 88.38
      quantitative 88.98
    thorax 87.41
  head NEC 87.04
  kidney NEC 87.72
  lung 87.42
  thorax NEC 87.42
Tongue tie operation 25.91
Tonography 95.26
Tonometry 89.11
Tonsillectomy 28.2
  with adenoidectomy 28.3
Tonsillotomy 28.0
Topectomy 01.32
Torek (-Bevan) **operation** (orchidopexy) (first stage) (second stage) 62.5
Torkildsen operation (ventriculocisternal shunt) 02.2
Torpin operation (cul-de-sac resection) 70.92
Toti operation (dacryocystorhinostomy) 09.81
Touchas operation 86.83
Touroff operation (ligation of subclavian artery) 38.85
Toxicology – *see* Examination, microscopic
TPN (total parenteral nutrition) 99.15
Trabeculectomy ab externo 12.64
Trabeculodialysis 12.59
Trabeculotomy ab externo 12.54
Trachelectomy 67.4
Trachelopexy 69.22
Tracheloplasty 67.69
Trachelorrhaphy (Emmet) (suture) 67.61
  obstetrical 75.51
Trachelotomy 69.95
  obstetrical 73.93
Tracheocricotomy (for assistance in breathing) 31.1
Tracheofissure 31.1
Tracheography 87.32
Tracheolaryngotomy (emergency) 31.1
  permanent opening 31.29
Tracheoplasty 31.79
  with artificial larynx 31.75
Tracheorrhaphy 31.71
Tracheoscopy NEC 31.42
  through tracheotomy (stoma) 31.41
Tracheostomy (emergency) (temporary) (for assistance in breathing) 31.1
  mediastinal 31.21
  permanent NEC 31.29
  revision 31.74
Tracheotomy (emergency) (temporary) (for assistance in breathing) 31.1
  permanent 31.29
Tracing, carotid pulse with ECG lead 89.56
Traction
  with reduction of fracture or dislocation – *see* Reduction, fracture and Reduction, dislocation
  adhesive tape (skin) 93.46
  boot 93.46
  Bryant's (skeletal) 93.44
  Buck's 93.46
  caliper tongs 93.41
    with synchronous insertion of device 02.94
  Cortel's (spinal) 93.42
  Crutchfield tongs 93.41
    with synchronous insertion of device 02.94
  Dunlop's (skeletal) 93.44
  gallows 93.46
  Gardner Wells 93.41
    with synchronous insertion of device 02.94
  halo device, skull 93.41
    with synchronous insertion of device 02.94
  Lyman Smith (skeletal) 93.44
  manual, intermittent 93.21
  mechanical, intermittent 93.21
  Russell's (skeletal) 93.44
  skeletal NEC 93.44
    intermittent 93.43
  skin, limbs NEC 93.46
  spinal NEC 93.42
    with skull device (halo) (caliper) (Crutchfield) (Gardner Wells) (Vinke) (tongs) 93.41
      with synchronous insertion of device 02.94
  Thomas' splint 93.45
  Vinke tongs 93.41
    with synchronous insertion of device 02.94
Tractotomy
  brain 01.32
  medulla oblongata 01.32
  mesencephalon 01.32
  percutaneous 03.21
  spinal cord (one-stage) (two-stage) 03.29
  trigeminal (percutaneous) (radiofrequency) 04.02
Training (for) (in)
  ADL (activities of daily living) 93.83
    for the blind 93.78
  ambulation 93.22
Training – *continued*
  braille 93.77
  crutch walking 93.24
  dyslexia 93.71
  dysphasia 93.72
  esophageal speech (postlaryngectomy) 93.73
  gait 93.22
  joint movements 93.14
  lip reading 93.75
  Moon (blind reading) 93.77
  orthoptic 95.35
  prenatal (natural childbirth) 93.37
  prosthetic or orthotic device usage 93.24
  relaxation 94.33
  speech NEC 93.75
    esophageal type 93.73
    for correction of defect 93.74
  use of lead dog for the blind 93.76
  vocational 93.85
TRAM (transverse rectus abdominis musculocutaneous) **flap of breast** 85.7
Transactional analysis
  group 94.44
  individual 94.39
Transection – *see also* Division
  artery (with ligation) (*see also* Division, artery) 38.80
    renal, aberrant (with reimplantation) 39.55
  bone (*see also* Osteotomy) 77.30
  fallopian tube (bilateral) (remaining) (solitary) 66.39
    by endoscopy 66.22
    unilateral 66.92
  isthmus, thyroid 06.91
  muscle 83.19
    eye 15.13
      multiple (two or more muscles) 15.3
    hand 82.19
  nerve (cranial) (peripheral) NEC 04.03
    acoustic 04.01
    root (spinal) 03.1
    sympathetic 05.0
    tracts in spinal cord 03.29
    trigeminal 04.02
    vagus (transabdominal) (*see also* Vagotomy) 44.00
  pylorus (with wedge resection) 43.3
  renal vessel, aberrant (with reimplantation) 39.55
  spinal
    cord tracts 03.29
    nerve root 03.1
  tendon 83.13
    hand 82.11
  uvula 27.71
  vas deferens 63.71
  vein (with ligation) (*see also* Division, vein) 38.80
    renal, aberrant (with reimplantation) 39.55
    varicose (lower limb) 38.59
Transfer, transference
  bone shaft, fibula into tibia 78.47
  digital (to replace absent thumb) 82.69
    finger (to thumb) (same hand) 82.61
      to
        finger, except thumb 82.81
        opposite hand (with amputation) 82.69 *[84.01]*
    toe (to thumb) (with amputation) 82.69 *[84.11]*
      to finger, except thumb 82.81 *[84.11]*
  fat pad NEC 86.89
    with skin graft – *see* Graft, skin, full-thickness
  finger (to replace absent thumb) (same hand) 82.61
    to
      finger, except thumb 82.81
      opposite hand (with amputation) 82.69 *[84.01]*
  muscle origin 83.77
    hand 82.58
  nerve (cranial) (peripheral) (radial anterior) (ulnar) 04.6
  pedicle graft 86.74
  pes anserinus (tendon) (repair of knee) 81.47
  tarsoconjunctival flap, from opposing lid 08.64
  tendon 83.75
    hand 82.56
    pes anserinus (repair of knee) 81.47
  toe-to-thumb (free) (pedicle) (with amputation) 82.69 *[84.11]*
Transfixion – *see also* Fixation
  iris (bombé) 12.11

Transfusion – Tympanotomy

U

V

Vasorrhaphy – Z-plasty

Tabular List Procedures

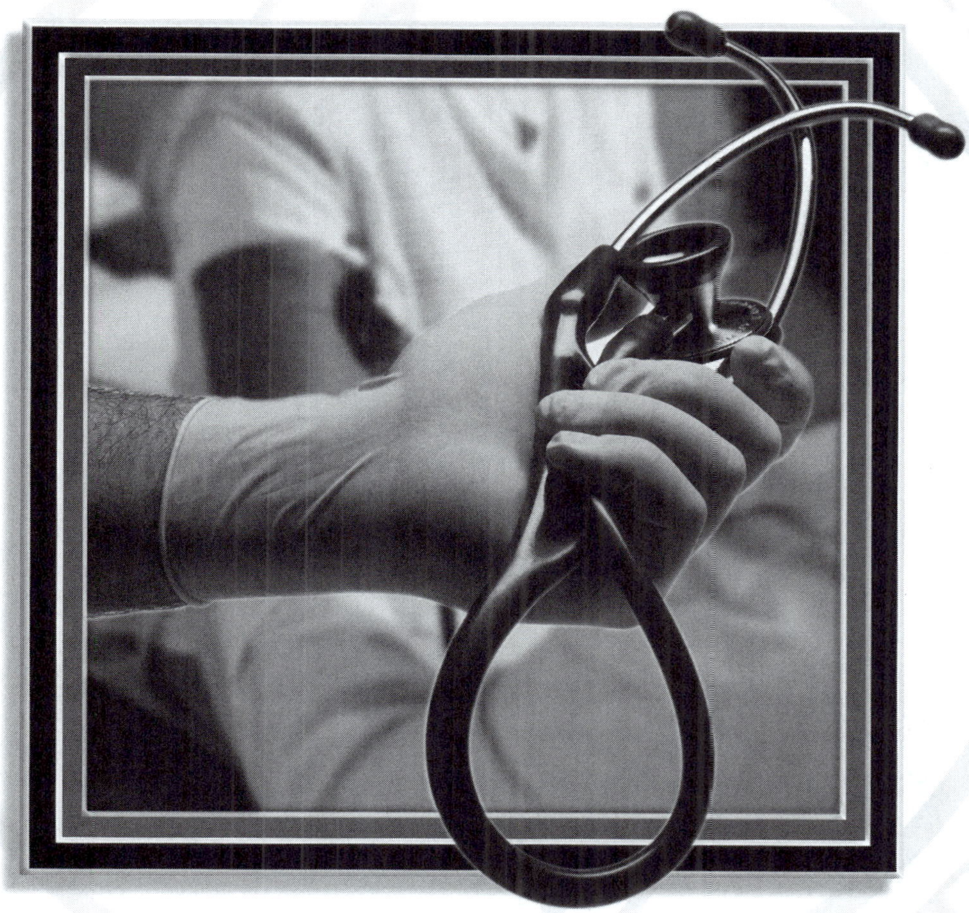

Volume 3

0. PROCEDURES AND INTERVENTIONS, NOT ELSEWHERE CLASSIFIED (00)

PROCEDURES AND INTERVENTIONS, NOT ELSEWHERE CLASSIFIED (00)

00.0 Therapeutic ultrasound
Excludes *diagnostic ultrasound (non-invasive) (88.71-88.79)*
intracardiac echography [ICE] (heart chamber(s)) (37.28)
intravascular imaging (adjunctive) (00.21-00.29)

00.01 Therapeutic ultrasound of vessels of head and neck
Anti-restenotic ultrasound
Intravascular non-ablative ultrasound
Excludes *diagnostic ultrasound of:*
eye (95.13)
head and neck (88.71)
that of inner ear (20.79)
ultrasonic:
angioplasty of non-coronary vessel (39.50)
embolectomy (38.01, 38.02)
endarterectomy (38.11, 38.12)
thrombectomy (38.01, 38.02)

DEF: Withdrawal of cerebrospinal fluid from the subarachnoid space via a needle inserted below the occipital bone at the back of the skull.

00.02 Therapeutic ultrasound of heart
Anti-restenotic ultrasound
Intravascular non-ablative ultrasound
Excludes *diagnostic ultrasound of heart (88.72)*
ultrasonic ablation of heart lesion (37.34)
ultrasonic angioplasty of coronary vessels (00.66, 36.09)

00.03 Therapeutic ultrasound of peripheral vascular vessels
Anti-restenotic ultrasound
Intravascular non-ablative ultrasound
Excludes *diagnostic ultrasound of peripheral vascular system (88.77)*
ultrasonic angioplasty of:
non-coronary vessel (39.50)

00.09 Other therapeutic ultrasound
Excludes *ultrasonic:*
fragmentation of urinary stones (59.95)
percutaneous nephrostomy with fragmentation (55.04)
physical therapy (93.35)
transurethral guided laser induced prostatectomy (TULIP) (60.21)

00.1 Pharmaceuticals

00.10 Implantation of chemotherapeutic agent
Brain wafer chemotherapy
Interstitial/ intracavitary
Excludes *injection or infusion of cancer chemotherapeutic substance (99.25)*

00.11 Infusion of drotrecogin alfa (activated)
Infusion of recombinant protein

00.12 Administration of inhaled nitric oxide
Nitric oxide therapy

00.13 Injection or infusion of nesiritide
Human B-type natriuretic peptide (hBNP)

00.14 Injection or infusion of oxazolidinone class of antibiotics
Linezolid injection

00.15 High-dose infusion interleukin-2 [IL-2]
Infusion (IV bolus, CIV) interleukin
Injection of aldesleukin
Excludes *low-dose infusion interleukin-2 (99.28)*

00.16 Pressurized treatment of venous bypass graft [conduit] with pharmaceutical substance
Ex-vivo treatment of vessel
Hyperbaric pressurized graft [conduit]

00.17 Infusion of vasopressor agent

00.18 Infusion of immunosuppressive antibody therapy
Monoclonal antibody therapy
Polyclonal antibody therapy
Includes ▶during induction phase of solid organ transplantation◀

00.19 Disruption of blood brain barrier via infusion [BBBD]
Infusion of substance to disrupt blood brain barrier
Code also chemotherapy (99.25)
Excludes *other perfusion (39.97)*

00.2 Intravascular imaging of blood vessels
Note: real-time imaging of lumen of blood vessel(s) using sound waves
Endovascular ultrasonography
Intravascular [ultrasound] imaging of blood vessels
Intravascular ultrasound (IVUS)
Code also any synchronous diagnostic or therapeutic procedures
Excludes *adjunct vascular system procedures, number of vessels treated (00.40-00.43)*
diagnostic procedures on blood vessels (38.21-38.29)
diagnostic ultrasound of peripheral vascular system (88.77)
magnetic resonance imaging (MRI) (88.91-88.97)
therapeutic ultrasound (00.01-00.09)

00.21 Intravascular imaging of extracranial cerebral vessels
Common carotid vessels and branches
Intravascular ultrasound (IVUS), extracranial cerebral vessels
Excludes *diagnostic ultrasound (non-invasive) of head and neck (88.71)*

00.22 Intravascular imaging of intrathoracic vessels
Aorta and aortic arch
Intravascular ultrasound (IVUS), intrathoracic vessels
Vena cava (superior)(inferior)
Excludes *diagnostic ultrasound (non-invasive) of other sites of thorax (88.73)*

00.23 Intravascular imaging of peripheral vessels
Imaging of:
vessels of arm(s)
vessels of leg(s)
Intravascular ultrasound (IVUS), peripheral vessels
Excludes *diagnostic ultrasound (non-invasive) of peripheral vascular system (88.77)*

00.24 Intravascular imaging of coronary vessels
Intravascular ultrasound (IVUS), coronary vessels
Excludes *diagnostic ultrasound (non-invasive) of heart (88.72)*
intracardiac echocardiography [ICE] (ultrasound of heart chamber(s)) (37.28)

00.25 Intravascular imaging of renal vessels
Intravascular ultrasound (IVUS), renal vessels
Renal artery
Excludes *diagnostic ultrasound (non-invasive) of urinary system (88.75)*

00.28 Intravascular imaging, other specified vessel(s)

00.29 Intravascular imaging, unspecified vessel(s)

00.3 Computer assisted surgery [CAS]
CT-free navigation
Image guided navigation (IGN)
Image guided surgery (IGS)
Imageless navigation
Code also any diagnostic or therapeutic procedure
Excludes *stereotactic frame application only (93.59)*

00.31 Computer assisted surgery with CT/CTA
AHA: 4Q 2004, 113

00.32 Computer assisted surgery with MR/MRA
AHA: 4Q 2004, 113

00.33 Computer assisted surgery with fluoroscopy

00.34 Imageless computer assisted surgery

00.35 Computer assisted surgery with multiple datasets

00.39 Other computer assisted surgery
Computer assisted surgery NOS

00.4 Adjunct vascular system procedures

Note: These codes can apply to both coronary and peripheral vessels. These codes are to be used in conjunction with other therapeutic procedure codes to provide additional information on the number of vessels upon which a procedure was performed and/or the number of stents inserted. As appropriate, code both the number of vessels operated on (00.40-00.43), and the number of stents inserted (00.45-00.48).

Code also any:

angioplasty or atherectomy (00.61-00.62, 00.66, 39.50)
endarterectomy (38.10-38.18)
insertion of vascular stent(s) (00.55, 00.63-00.65, 36.06-36.07, 39.90)
other removal of coronary artery obstruction (36.09)

00.40 Procedure on single vessel

Number of vessels, unspecified

Excludes *(aorto)coronary bypass (36.10-36.19)*
intravascular imaging of blood vessels (00.21-00.29)

AHA: 4Q 2005, 105

00.41 Procedure on two vessels

Excludes *(aorto) coronary bypass (36.10-36.19)*
intravascular imaging of blood vessels (00.21-00.29)

AHA: 4Q 2005, 103, 105

00.42 Procedure on three vessels

Excludes *(aorto) coronary bypass (36.10-36.19)*
intravascular imaging of blood vessels (00.21-00.29)

00.43 Procedure on four or more vessels

Excludes *(aorto) coronary bypass (36.10-36.19)*
intravascular imaging of blood vessels (00.21-00.29)

00.44 Procedure on vessel bifurcation

Note: This code is to be used to identify the presence of a vessel bifurcation; it does not describe a specific bifurcation stent. Use this code only once per operative episode, irrespective of the number of bifurcations in vessels.

00.45 Insertion of one vascular stent

Number of stents, unspecified

00.46 Insertion of two vascular stents

AHA: 4Q 2005, 105, 106

00.47 Insertion of three vascular stents

00.48 Insertion of four or more vascular stents

00.5 Other cardiovascular procedures

Pacemaker Implantation

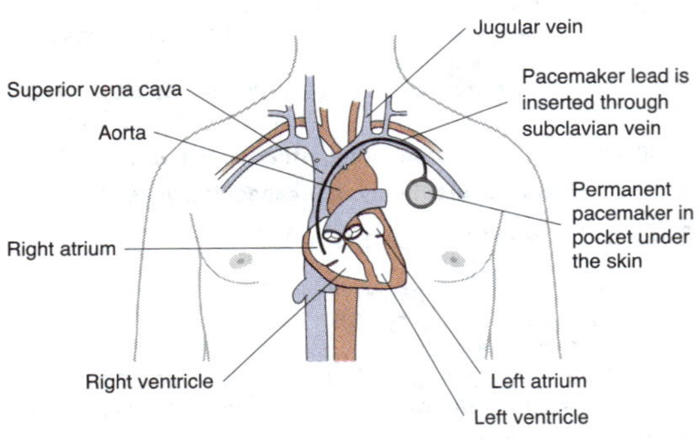

00.50 Implantation of cardiac resynchronization pacemaker without mention of defibrillation, total system [CRT-P]

Note: Device testing during procedure - omit code

Biventricular pacing without internal cardiac defibrillator
Biventricular pacemaker
BiV pacemaker
Implantation of cardiac resynchronization (biventricular) pulse generator pacing device, formation of pocket, transvenous leads including placement of lead into left ventricular coronary venous system, and intraoperative procedures for evaluation of lead signals.
That with CRT-P generator and one or more leads

Excludes *implantation of cardiac resynchronization defibrillator, total system [CRT-D] (00.51)*
insertion or replacement of any type pacemaker device (37.80-37.87)
replacement of cardiac resynchronization defibrillator pulse generator only [CRT-D](00.54)
replacement of cardiac resynchronization pacemaker pulse generator only [CRT-P](00.53)

AHA: 3Q 2005, 3-4, 7

00.51 Implantation of cardiac resynchronization defibrillator, total system [CRT-D]

Note: Device testing during procedure - omit code

BiV defibrillator
Biventricular defibrillator
Biventricular pacing with internal cardiac defibrillator
BiV ICD
BiV pacemaker with defibrillator
BiV pacing with defibrillator
Implantation of a cardiac resynchronization (biventricular) pulse generator with defibrillator [AICD], formation of pocket, transvenous leads, including placement of lead into left ventricular coronary venous system, intraoperative procedures for evaluation of lead signals, and obtaining defibrillator threshold measurements.
That with CRT-D generator and one or more leads

Excludes *implantation of cardiac resynchronization pacemaker, total system [CRT-P](00.50)*
implantation or replacement of automatic cardioverter/defibrillator, total system [AICD] (37.94)
replacement of cardiac resynchronization defibrillator pulse generator, only [CRT-D](00.54)

AHA: 3Q 2005, 3-4, 7, 9

00.52 Implantation or replacement of transvenous lead [electrode] into left ventricular coronary venous system

Excludes *implantation of cardiac resynchronization defibrillator, total system [CRT-D](00.51)*
implantation of cardiac resynchronization pacemaker, total system [CRT-P](00.50)
initial insertion of transvenous lead [electrode] (37.70-37.72)
replacement of transvenous atrial and/or ventricular lead(s) [electrodes] (37.76)

AHA: 3Q 2005, 4, 5

00.53 Implantation or replacement of cardiac resynchronization pacemaker pulse generator only [CRT-P]

Note: Device testing during procedure - omit code

Implantation of CRT-P device with removal of any existing CRT-P or other pacemaker device

Excludes *implantation of cardiac resynchronization pacemaker, total system [CRT-P] (00.50)*
implantation or replacement of cardiac resynchronization defibrillator pulse generator only [CRT-D](00.54)
insertion or replacement of any type pacemaker device (37.80-37.87)

AHA: 3Q 2005, 5

✖ **00.54 Implantation or replacement of cardiac resynchronization defibrillator pulse generator device only [CRT-D]**
Note: Device testing during procedure - omit code
Implantation of CRT-D device with removal of any existing CRT-D, CRT-P, pacemaker, or defibrillator device
Excludes *implantation of automatic cardioverter/ defibrillator pulse generator only (37.96)*
implantation of cardiac resynchronization defibrillator, total system [CRT-D] (00.51)
implantation or replacement of cardiac resynchronization pacemaker pulse generator only [CRT-P] (00.53)
AHA: 3Q 2005, 5

✓ **00.55 Insertion of drug-eluting peripheral vessel stent(s)**
Endograft(s)
Endovascular graft(s)
Stent grafts
Code also any:
angioplasty or atherectomy of other non-coronary vessels(s) (39.50)
number of vascular stents inserted (00.45-00.48)
number of vessels treated (00.40-00.43)
procedure on vessel bifurcation (00.44)
Excludes *drug-coated peripheral stents, e.g., heparin coated (39.90)*
insertion of cerebrovascular stent(s) (00.63-00.65)
insertion of drug-eluting coronary artery stent (36.07)
insertion of non-drug-eluting stent(s):
coronary artery (36.06)
peripheral vessel (39.90)
that for aneurysm repair (39.71-39.79)

✓ **00.56 Insertion or replacement of implantable pressure sensor (lead) for intracardiac hemodynamic monitoring**
Code also any associated implantation or replacement of monitor (00.57)
Excludes *circulatory monitoring (blood gas, arterial or venous pressure, cardiac output and coronary blood flow) (89.60-89.69)*

✓ **00.57 Implantation or replacement of subcutaneous device for intracardiac hemodynamic monitoring**
Implantation of monitoring device with formation of subcutaneous pocket and connection to intracardiac pressure sensor (lead)
Code also any associated insertion or replacement of implanted pressure sensor (lead) (00.56)

❹ **00.6 Procedures on blood vessels**

✓ **00.61 Percutaneous angioplasty or atherectomy of precerebral (extracranial) vessel(s)**
Basilar
Carotid
Vertebral
Code also any:
injection or infusion of thrombolytic agent (99.10)
number of vascular stents inserted (00.45-00.48)
number of vessels treated (00.40-00.43)
percutaneous insertion of carotid artery stent(s) (00.63)
percutaneous insertion of other precerebral artery stent(s) (00.64)
procedure on vessel bifurcation (00.44)
Excludes *angioplasty or atherectomy of other non-coronary vessel(s) (39.50)*
removal of cerebrovascular obstruction of vessel(s) by open approach (38.01-38.02, 38.11-38.12, 38.31-38.32, 38.41-38.42)

✓ **00.62 Percutaneous angioplasty or atherectomy of intracranial vessel(s)**
Code also any:
injection or infusion of thrombolytic agent (99.10)
number of vascular stents inserted (00.45-00.48)
number of vessels treated (00.40-00.43)
percutaneous insertion of intracranial stent(s) (00.65)
procedure on vessel bifurcation (00.44)
Excludes *angioplasty or atherectomy of other non-coronary vessel(s) (39.50)*
removal of cerebrovascular obstruction of vessel(s) by open approach (38.01-38.02, 38.11-38.12, 38.31-38.32, 38.41-38.42)

✖ **00.63 Percutaneous insertion of carotid artery stent(s)**
Includes the use of any embolic protection device, distal protection device, filter device, or stent delivery system
Non-drug-eluting stent
Code also any:
number of vascular stents inserted (00.45-00.48)
number of vessels treated (00.40-00.43)
percutaneous angioplasty or atherectomy of precerebral vessel(s) (00.61)
procedure on vessel bifurcation (00.44)
Excludes *angioplasty or atherectomy of other non-coronary vessel(s) (39.50)*
insertion of drug-eluting peripheral vessel stent(s) (00.55)

✖ **00.64 Percutaneous insertion of other precerebral (extracranial) artery stent(s)**
Includes the use of any embolic protection device, distal protection device, filter device, or stent delivery system
Basilar stent
Vertebral stent
Code also any:
number of vascular stents inserted (00.45-00.48)
number of vessels treated (00.40-00.43)
percutaneous angioplasty or atherectomy of precerebral vessel(s) (00.61)
procedure on vessel bifurcation (00.44)
Excludes *angioplasty or atherectomy of other non-coronary vessel(s) (39.50)*
insertion of drug-eluting peripheral vessel stent(s) (00.55)

✖ **00.65 Percutaneous insertion of intracranial vascular stent(s)**
Includes the use of any embolic protection device, distal protection device, filter device, or stent delivery system
Code also any:
number of vascular stents inserted (00.45-00.48)
number of vessels treated (00.40-00.43)
percutaneous angioplasty or atherectomy of intracranial vessel(s) (00.62)
procedure on vessel bifurcation (00.44)
Excludes *angioplasty or atherectomy of other non-coronary vessel(s) (39.50)*
insertion of drug-eluting peripheral vessel stent(s) (00.55)

✓ **00.66 Percutaneous transluminal coronary angioplasty [PTCA] or coronary atherectomy**
Balloon angioplasty of coronary artery
Coronary atherectomy
Percutaneous coronary angioplasty NOS
PTCA NOS
Code also any:
injection or infusion of thrombolytic agent (99.10)
insertion of coronary artery stent(s) (36.06-36.07)
intracoronary artery thrombolytic infusion (36.04)
number of vascular stents inserted (00.45-00.48)
number of vessels treated (00.40-00.43)
procedure on vessel bifurcation (00.44)
AHA: 4Q 2005, 103, 105, 106

00.7 Other hip procedures

00.70 Revision of hip replacement, both acetabular and femoral components
Total hip revision
Code also any:
removal of (cement) (joint) spacer (84.57)
type of bearing surface, if known (00.74-00.77)
Excludes *revision of hip replacement, acetabular component only (00.71)*
revision of hip replacement, femoral component only (00.72)
revision of hip replacement, Not Otherwise Specified (81.53)
revision with replacement of acetabular liner and/or femoral head only (00.73)
AHA: 4Q 2005, 113

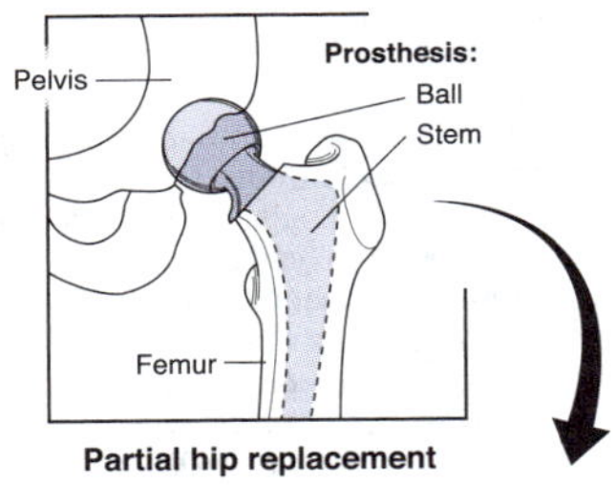

Partial hip replacement

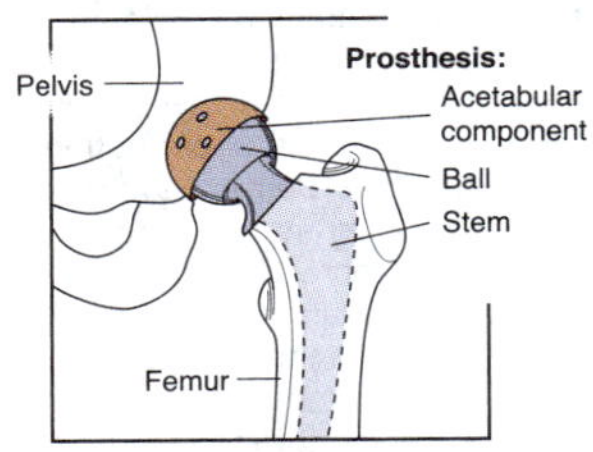

Total hip replacement

00.71 Revision of hip replacement, acetabular component
Partial, acetabular component only
That with:
exchange of acetabular cup and liner
exchange of femoral head
Code also any type of bearing surface, if known (00.74-00.77)
Excludes *revision of hip replacement, both acetabular and femoral components (00.70)*
revision of hip replacement, femoral component (00.72)
revision of hip replacement, Not Otherwise Specified (81.53)
revision with replacement of acetabular liner and/or femoral head only (00.73)
AHA: 4Q 2005, 112

00.72 Revision of hip replacement, femoral component
Partial, femoral component only
That with:
exchange of acetabular liner
exchange of femoral stem and head
Code also any type of bearing surface, if known (00.74-00.77)
Excludes *revision of hip replacement, acetabular component (00.71)*
revision of hip replacement, both acetabular and femoral components (00.70)
revision of hip replacement, not otherwise specified (81.53)
revision with replacement of acetabular liner and/or femoral head only (00.73)

00.73 Revision of hip replacement, acetabular liner and/or femoral head only
Code also any type of bearing surface, if known (00.74-00.77)

▲ **00.74 Hip bearing surface, metal-on-polyethylene**

▲ **00.75 Hip bearing surface, metal-on-metal**

▲ **00.76 Hip bearing surface, ceramic-on-ceramic**
AHA: 4Q 2005, 112

▲ **00.77 Hip bearing surface, ceramic-on-polyethylene**

00.8 Other knee and hip procedures
Note: *Report up to two components using 00.81-00.83 to describe revision of knee replacements. If all three components are revised, report 00.80.*

00.80 Revision of knee replacement, total (all components)
Replacement of femoral, tibial, and patellar components (all components)
Code also any removal of (cement) (joint) spacer (84.57)
Excludes *revision of only one or two components (tibial, femoral or patellar component) (00.81-00.84)*

00.81 Revision of knee replacement, tibial component
Replacement of tibial baseplate and tibial insert (liner)
Excludes *revision of knee replacement, total (all components) (00.80)*
AHA: 4Q 2005, 117

00.82 Revision of knee replacement, femoral component
That with replacement of tibial insert (liner)
Excludes *revision of knee replacement, total (all components) (00.80)*
AHA: 4Q 2005, 117

00.83 Revision of knee replacement, patellar component
Excludes *revision of knee replacement, total (all components) (00.80)*

00.84 Revision of total knee replacement, tibial insert (liner)
Replacement of tibial insert (liner)
Excludes *that with replacement of tibial component (tibial baseplate and liner) (00.81)*

00.85 Resurfacing hip, total, acetabulum and femoral head
Hip resurfacing arthroplasty, total

00.86 Resurfacing hip, partial, femoral head
Hip resurfacing arthroplasty, NOS
Hip resurfacing arthroplasty, partial, femoral head
Excludes *that with resurfacing of acetabulum (00.85)*

00.87 Resurfacing hip, partial, acetabulum
Hip resurfacing arthroplasty, partial, acetabulum
Excludes *that with resurfacing of femoral head (00.85)*

00.9 Other procedures and interventions

00.91 Transplant from live related donor
Code also organ transplant procedure

00.92 Transplant from live non-related donor
Code also organ transplant procedure
AHA: 4Q 2004, 117

00.93 Transplant from cadaver
Code also organ transplant procedure

● **00.94 Intra-operative neurophysiologic monitoring**
Includes *Cranial nerve, peripheral nerve and spinal cord testing performed intra-operatively*
Intra-operative neurophysiologic testing
IOM
Nerve monitoring
Neuromonitoring
Excludes *brain temperature monitoring (01.17)*
intracranial oxygen monitoring (01.16)
intracranial pressure monitoring (01.10)
plethysmogram (89.58)

1. OPERATIONS ON THE NERVOUS SYSTEM (01-05)

INCISION AND EXCISION OF SKULL, BRAIN, AND CEREBRAL MENINGES (01)

01.0 Cranial puncture

01.01 Cisternal puncture
Cisternal tap
Excludes *pneumocisternogram (87.02)*

01.02 Ventriculopuncture through previously implanted catheter
Puncture of ventricular shunt tubing

01.09 Other cranial puncture
Aspiration of:
subarachnoid space
subdural space
Cranial aspiration NOS
Puncture of anterior fontanel
Subdural tap (through fontanel)

01.1 Diagnostic procedures on skull, brain, and cerebral meninges

01.10 Intracranial pressure monitoring
Includes *insertion of catheter or probe for monitoring*

01.11 Closed [percutaneous] [needle] biopsy of cerebral meninges
Burr hole approach

01.12 Open biopsy of cerebral meninges
DEF: Removal of cerebral membrane tissue sample via open surgical incision.

01.13 Closed [percutaneous] [needle] biopsy of brain
Burr hole approach
Stereotactic method
AHA: Mar-Apr 1987, 9

01.14 Open biopsy of brain

01.15 Biopsy of skull

01.16 Intracranial oxygen monitoring
Includes *insertion of catheter or probe for monitoring*
partial pressure of brain oxygen ($PbtO_2$)

01.17 Brain temperature monitoring
Includes *insertion of catheter or probe for monitoring*

01.18 Other diagnostic procedures on brain and cerebral meninges
Excludes *▶brain temperature monitoring (01.17)◀*
cerebral:
arteriography (88.41)
thermography (88.81)
contrast radiogram of brain (87.01-87.02)
echoencephalogram (88.71)
electroencephalogram (89.14)
▶intracranial oxygen monitoring (01.16)◀
▶intracranial pressure monitoring (01.10)◀
microscopic examination of specimen from nervous system and of spinal fluid (90.01-90.09)
neurologic examination (89.13)
phlebography of head and neck (88.61)
pneumoencephalogram (87.01)
radioisotope scan:
cerebral (92.11)
head NEC (92.12)
tomography of head:
C.A.T. scan (87.03)
other (87.04)
AHA: 3Q 1998, 10

01.19 Other diagnostic procedures on skull
Excludes *transillumination of skull (89.16)*
x-ray of skull (87.17)

01.2 Craniotomy and craniectomy
Excludes *decompression of skull fracture (02.02)*
exploration of orbit (16.01-16.09)
that as operative approach - omit code
DEF: Craniotomy: Surgical incision into the skull.
Craniectomy: Surgical excision of a portion of the skull.

01.21 Incision and drainage of cranial sinus

01.22 Removal of intracranial neurostimulator lead(s)
Code also any removal of neurostimulator pulse generator (86.05)
Excludes *removal with synchronous replacement (02.93)*

01.23 Reopening of craniotomy site
DEF: Reopening a previous skull incision.

01.24 Other craniotomy
Cranial:
decompression
exploration
trephination
Craniotomy NOS
Craniotomy with removal of:
epidural abscess
extradural hematoma
foreign body of skull
Excludes *removal of foreign body with incision into brain (01.39)*
AHA: 2Q 1991, 14; Mar-Apr 1984, 20

01.25 Other craniectomy
Debridement of skull NOS
Sequestrectomy of skull
Excludes *debridement of compound fracture of skull (02.02)*
strip craniectomy (02.01)
DEF: Sequestrectomy of skull: Surgical removal of a piece of necrotic skull bone.
AHA: 1Q 2006, 6

01.26 Insertion of catheter(s) into cranial cavity or tissue
Code also any concomitant procedure (e.g. resection (01.59))
Excludes *placement of intracerebral catheter(s) via burr hole(s) (01.28)*
AHA: 4Q 2005, 118

01.27 Removal of catheter(s) from cranial cavity or tissue
AHA: 4Q 2005, 119

01.28 Placement of intracerebral catheter(s) via burr hole(s)
Convection enhanced delivery
Stereotactic placement of intracerebral catheter(s)
Code also infusion of medication
Excludes *insertion of catheter(s) into cranial cavity or tissue(s) (01.26)*

01.3 Incision of brain and cerebral meninges

01.31 Incision of cerebral meninges
Drainage of:
intracranial hygroma
subarachnoid abscess (cerebral)
subdural empyema

01.32 Lobotomy and tractotomy
Division of:
brain tissue
cerebral tracts
Percutaneous (radiofrequency) cingulotomy

01.39 Other incision of brain
Amygdalohippocampotomy
Drainage of intracerebral hematoma
Incision of brain NOS
Excludes *division of cortical adhesions (02.91)*

01.4 Operations on thalamus and globus pallidus

01.41 Operations on thalamus
Chemothalamectomy
Thalamotomy
Excludes *that by stereotactic radiosurgery (92.30-92.39)*
DEF: Chemothalamectomy: Destruction of tissue in the thalamus via chemical agent introduction.

✓ **01.42 Operations on globus pallidus**
Pallidoansectomy
Pallidotomy
Excludes *that by stereotactic radiosurgery (92.30-92.39)*

❹ **01.5 Other excision or destruction of brain and meninges**

✓ **01.51 Excision of lesion or tissue of cerebral meninges**
Decortication of (cerebral) meninges
Resection of (cerebral) meninges
Stripping of subdural membrane of (cerebral) meninges
Excludes *biopsy of cerebral meninges (01.11-01.12)*

✓ **01.52 Hemispherectomy**
DEF: Removal of one half of the brain.

✓ **01.53 Lobectomy of brain**
DEF: Removal of one lobe of the brain.

✓ **01.59 Other excision or destruction of lesion or tissue of brain**
Curettage of brain
Debridement of brain
Marsupialization of brain cyst
Transtemporal (mastoid) excision of brain tumor
Excludes *biopsy of brain (01.13-01.14)*
that by stereotactic radiosurgery (92.30-92.39)
AHA: 4Q 2005, 118; 3Q 1999, 7; 1Q 1999, 9; 3Q 1998, 12; 1Q 1998, 6-7; 4Q 1993, 33

✓ **01.6 Excision of lesion of skull**
Removal of granulation tissue of cranium
Excludes *biopsy of skull (01.15)*
sequestrectomy (01.25)

OTHER OPERATIONS ON SKULL, BRAIN, AND CEREBRAL MENINGES (02)

❹ **02.0 Cranioplasty**
Excludes *that with synchronous repair of encephalocele (02.12)*

✓ **02.01 Opening of cranial suture**
Linear craniectomy
Strip craniectomy
DEF: Opening the skull along a line of thin fibrous connective tissue uniting the skull bones.

✓ **02.02 Elevation of skull fracture fragments**
Debridement of compound fracture of skull
Decompression of skull fracture
Reduction of skull fracture
Code also any synchronous debridement of brain (01.59)
Excludes *debridement of skull NOS (01.25)*
removal of granulation tissue of cranium (01.6)

✓ **02.03 Formation of cranial bone flap**
Repair of skull with flap

✓ **02.04 Bone graft to skull**
Pericranial graft (autogenous) (heterogenous)

✓ **02.05 Insertion of skull plate**
Replacement of skull plate

✓ **02.06 Other cranial osteoplasty**
Repair of skull NOS
Revision of bone flap of skull
AHA: 1Q 2006, 7; 1Q 2005, 11; 3Q 1998, 9

✓ **02.07 Removal of skull plate**
Excludes *removal with synchronous replacement (02.05)*

❹ **02.1 Repair of cerebral meninges**
Excludes *marsupialization of cerebral lesion (01.59)*

✓ **02.11 Simple suture of dura mater of brain**
DEF: Suture of the outermost, fibrous layer covering the brain.

✓ **02.12 Other repair of cerebral meninges**
Closure of fistula of cerebrospinal fluid
Dural graft
Repair of encephalocele including synchronous cranioplasty
Repair of meninges NOS
Subdural patch

✓ **02.13 Ligation of meningeal vessel**
Ligation of:
longitudinal sinus
middle meningeal artery

✓ **02.14 Choroid plexectomy**
Cauterization of choroid plexus

✓ **02.2 Ventriculostomy**
Anastomosis of ventricle to:
cervical subarachnoid space
cisterna magna
Insertion of Holter valve
Ventriculocisternal intubation
DEF: An opening made in a cerebral ventricle; most often to treat hydrocephalus by draining cerebrospinal fluid.

❹ **02.3 Extracranial ventricular shunt**
Includes that with insertion of valve

✓ **02.31 Ventricular shunt to structure in head and neck**
Ventricle to nasopharynx shunt
Ventriculomastoid anastomosis

✓ **02.32 Ventricular shunt to circulatory system**
Ventriculoatrial anastomosis
Ventriculocaval shunt

✓ **02.33 Ventricular shunt to thoracic cavity**
Ventriculopleural anastomosis

✓ **02.34 Ventricular shunt to abdominal cavity and organs**
Ventriculocholecystostomy
Ventriculoperitoneostomy

✓ **02.35 Ventricular shunt to urinary system**
Ventricle to ureter shunt

✓ **02.39 Other operations to establish drainage of ventricle**
Ventricle to bone marrow shunt
Ventricular shunt to extracranial site NEC

❹ **02.4 Revision, removal, and irrigation of ventricular shunt**
Excludes *revision of distal catheter of ventricular shunt (54.95)*

✖ **02.41 Irrigation and exploration of ventricular shunt**
Exploration of ventriculoperitoneal shunt at ventricular site
Re-programming of ventriculoperitoneal shunt

✓ **02.42 Replacement of ventricular shunt**
Reinsertion of Holter valve
Replacement of ventricular catheter
Revision of ventriculoperitoneal shunt at ventricular site
AHA: Nov-Dec 1986, 8

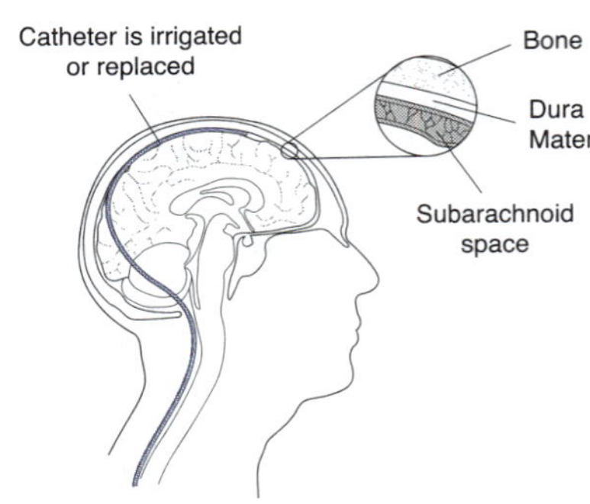

✓ **02.43 Removal of ventricular shunt**
AHA: Nov-Dec 1986, 8

02.9 Other operations on skull, brain, and cerebral meninges
Excludes operations on:
pineal gland (07.17, 07.51-07.59)
pituitary gland [hypophysis] (07.13-07.15, 07.61-07.79)

02.91 Lysis of cortical adhesions

02.92 Repair of brain

02.93 Implantation or replacement of intracranial neurostimulator lead(s)
Implantation, insertion, placement, or replacement of intracranial:
brain pacemaker [neuropacemaker]
depth electrodes
electroencephalographic receiver
epidural pegs
foramen ovale electrodes
intracranial electrostimulator
subdural grids
subdural strips
Code also any insertion of neurostimulator pulse generator (86.94-86.98)
AHA: 4Q 1997, 58; 4Q 1992, 28

02.94 Insertion or replacement of skull tongs or halo traction device
AHA: 3Q 2001, 8; 3Q 1996, 15

02.95 Removal of skull tongs or halo traction device

02.96 Insertion of sphenoidal electrodes
AHA: 4Q 1992, 28

02.99 Other
Excludes *chemical shock therapy (94.24)*
electroshock therapy:
subconvulsive (94.26)
other (94.27)

OPERATIONS ON SPINAL CORD AND SPINAL CANAL STRUCTURES (03)

Code also any application or administration of an adhesion barrier substance (99.77)

03.0 Exploration and decompression of spinal canal structures

03.01 Removal of foreign body from spinal canal

03.02 Reopening of laminectomy site

03.09 Other exploration and decompression of spinal canal
Decompression:
laminectomy
laminotomy
Expansile laminoplasty
Exploration of spinal nerve root
Foraminotomy
▶*Code also any synchronous insertion, replacement and revision of posterior spinal motion preservation device(s), if performed (84.80- 84.85)*◀
Excludes *drainage of spinal fluid by anastomosis (03.71-03.79)*
laminectomy with excision of intervertebral disc (80.51)
spinal tap (03.31)
that as operative approach - omit code
DEF: Foraminotomy: Surgical removal of the roof over the spinal nerve passageway for relieving nerve root compression.
AHA: 3Q 2004, 6-7; 4Q 2002, 109; 2Q 2002, 15; 4Q 1999, 13-14; 2Q 1997, 6; 2Q 1995, 9-10; 2Q 1990, 22

03.1 Division of intraspinal nerve root
Rhizotomy
DEF: Cutting the spinal nerve roots within the spinal canal for relieving pain or spastic paralysis.

03.2 Chordotomy
DEF: Interruption of the lateral spinothalamic tract of the spinal cord, commonly in the anterolateral quadrant, for relief of intractable pain.

03.21 Percutaneous chordotomy
Stereotactic chordotomy

03.29 Other chordotomy
Chordotomy NOS
Tractotomy (one-stage) (two-stage) of spinal cord
Transection of spinal cord tracts

03.3 Diagnostic procedures on spinal cord and spinal canal structures

03.31 Spinal tap
Lumbar puncture for removal of dye
Excludes *lumbar puncture for injection of dye [myelogram] (87.21)*
DEF: Needle insertion into the spinal subarachnoid space, usually between the 3rd and 4th lumbar vertebrae, to remove cerebrospinal fluid.

03.32 Biopsy of spinal cord or spinal meninges

03.39 Other diagnostic procedures on spinal cord and spinal canal structures
Excludes *microscopic examination of specimen from nervous system or of spinal fluid (90.01-90.09)*
x-ray of spine (87.21-87.29)

03.4 Excision or destruction of lesion of spinal cord or spinal meninges
Curettage of spinal cord or spinal meninges
Debridement of spinal cord or spinal meninges
Marsupialization of cyst of spinal cord or spinal meninges
Resection of spinal cord or spinal meninges
Excludes *biopsy of spinal cord or meninges (03.32)*
AHA: 3Q 1995, 5

03.5 Plastic operations on spinal cord structures

03.51 Repair of spinal meningocele
Repair of meningocele NOS
DEF: Correction of a hernial protrusion of spinal meninges through a vertebral column defect, most often in the thoracic or lumbar region.

03.52 Repair of spinal myelomeningocele

03.53 Repair of vertebral fracture
Elevation of spinal bone fragments
Reduction of fracture of vertebrae
Removal of bony spicules from spinal canal
Excludes *kyphoplasty (81.66)*
vertebroplasty (81.65)
AHA: 4Q 2004, 126

03.59 Other repair and plastic operations on spinal cord structures
Repair of:
diastematomyelia
spina bifida NOS
spinal cord NOS
spinal meninges NOS
vertebral arch defect
DEF: Repair of diastematomyelia: Surgical correction of an anomaly in which the spinal cord is split in half by a bony spicule or fibrous band.

03.6 Lysis of adhesions of spinal cord and nerve roots
AHA: 2Q 1998, 18

03.7 Shunt of spinal theca
Includes that with valve

03.71 Spinal subarachnoid-peritoneal shunt

03.72 Spinal subarachnoid-ureteral shunt

03.79 Other shunt of spinal theca
Lumbar-subarachnoid shunt NOS
Pleurothecal anastomosis
Salpingothecal anastomosis
AHA: 1Q 1997, 7

✖ **03.8 Injection of destructive agent into spinal canal**

Neurolytic Injection

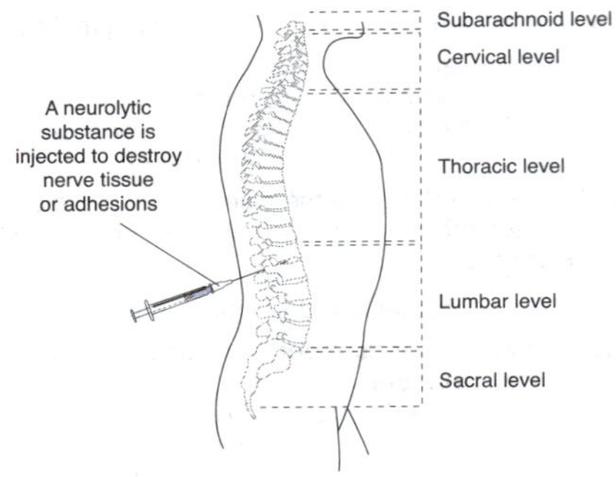

❹ **03.9 Other operations on spinal cord and spinal canal structures**

✖ **03.90 Insertion of catheter into spinal canal for infusion of therapeutic or palliative substances**
Insertion of catheter into epidural, subarachnoid, or subdural space of spine with intermittent or continuous infusion of drug (with creation of any reservoir)
Code also any implantation of infusion pump (86.06)

✖ **03.91 Injection of anesthetic into spinal canal for analgesia**
Excludes *that for operative anesthesia - omit code*
AHA: 3Q 2000, 15; 1Q 1999, 7-8; 2Q 1998, 18; Mar-Apr 1985, 15; Mar-Apr 1984, 20

✖ **03.92 Injection of other agent into spinal canal**
Intrathecal injection of steroid
Subarachnoid perfusion of refrigerated saline
Excludes *injection of:*
contrast material for myelogram (87.21)
destructive agent into spinal canal (03.8)
AHA: 2Q 2003, 6; 3Q 2000, 15; 2Q 1998, 18

✔ **03.93 Implantation or replacement of spinal neurostimulator lead(s)**
Code also any insertion of neurostimulator pulse generator (86.94-86.98)

✔ **03.94 Removal of spinal neurostimulator lead(s)**
Code also any removal of neurostimulator pulse generator (86.05)

✖ **03.95 Spinal blood patch**

✖ **03.96 Percutaneous denervation of facet**

✔ **03.97 Revision of spinal thecal shunt**
AHA: 2Q 1999, 4

✔ **03.98 Removal of spinal thecal shunt**

✔ **03.99 Other**
AHA: Mar-Apr 1985, 15; Mar-Apr 1984, 20

OPERATIONS ON CRANIAL AND PERIPHERAL NERVES (04)

❹ **04.0 Incision, division, and excision of cranial and peripheral nerves**
Excludes *opticociliary neurectomy (12.79)*
sympathetic ganglionectomy (05.21-05.29)

✔ **04.01 Excision of acoustic neuroma**
That by craniotomy
Excludes *that by stereotactic radiosurgery (92.30-92.39)*
DEF: Removal of a benign growth on the 8th cranial nerve, which runs from the brain to the inner ear.
AHA: 2Q 1995, 8; 4Q 1992, 26

✔ **04.02 Division of trigeminal nerve**
Retrogasserian neurotomy

✔ **04.03 Division or crushing of other cranial and peripheral nerves**
Excludes *that of:*
glossopharyngeal nerve (29.92)
laryngeal nerve (31.91)
nerves to adrenal glands (07.42)
phrenic nerve for collapse of lung (33.31)
vagus nerve (44.00-44.03)
AHA: 2Q 1998, 20

✔ **04.04 Other incision of cranial and peripheral nerves**

✔ **04.05 Gasserian ganglionectomy**
DEF: Excision of a ganglion on the sensory root of the fifth cranial nerve; also called trigeminal ganglion.

✔ **04.06 Other cranial or peripheral ganglionectomy**
Excludes *sympathetic ganglionectomy (05.21-05.29)*

✔ **04.07 Other excision or avulsion of cranial and peripheral nerves**
Curettage of peripheral nerve
Debridement of peripheral nerve
Excision of peripheral neuroma [Morton's]
Resection of peripheral nerve
Excludes *biopsy of cranial or peripheral nerve (04.11-04.12)*
AHA: 2Q 1995, 8; 4Q 1992, 26

❹ **04.1 Diagnostic procedures on peripheral nervous system**

✖ⓞ **04.11 Closed [percutaneous] [needle] biopsy of cranial or peripheral nerve or ganglion**

✔Ⓞ **04.12 Open biopsy of cranial or peripheral nerve or ganglion**

✔ **04.19 Other diagnostic procedures on cranial and peripheral nerves and ganglia**
Excludes *microscopic examination of specimen from nervous system (90.01-90.09)*
neurologic examination (89.13)

✖ **04.2 Destruction of cranial and peripheral nerves**
Destruction of cranial or peripheral nerves by:
cryoanalgesia
injection of neurolytic agent
radiofrequency
Radiofrequency ablation
AHA: 3Q 2002, 11; 4Q 1995, 74

✔ **04.3 Suture of cranial and peripheral nerves**

❹ **04.4 Lysis of adhesions and decompression of cranial and peripheral nerves**

✔ **04.41 Decompression of trigeminal nerve root**

✔ **04.42 Other cranial nerve decompression**
AHA: 3Q 2002, 13; Mar-Apr 1987, 8

✔ **04.43 Release of carpal tunnel**
DEF: Cutting of the transverse carpal ligament to release the compressed median nerve.

✔ **04.44 Release of tarsal tunnel**

✔ **04.49 Other peripheral nerve or ganglion decompression or lysis of adhesions**
Peripheral nerve neurolysis NOS
AHA: 2Q 1993, 8

✔ **04.5 Cranial or peripheral nerve graft**

✔ **04.6 Transposition of cranial and peripheral nerves**
Nerve transplantation

❹ **04.7 Other cranial or peripheral neuroplasty**

✔ **04.71 Hypoglossal-facial anastomosis**

✔ **04.72 Accessory-facial anastomosis**

✔ **04.73 Accessory-hypoglossal anastomosis**

✔ **04.74 Other anastomosis of cranial or peripheral nerve**

✔ **04.75 Revision of previous repair of cranial and peripheral nerves**

✔ **04.76 Repair of old traumatic injury of cranial and peripheral nerves**

✔ **04.79 Other neuroplasty**
AHA: 1Q 2006, 11

04.8 Injection into peripheral nerve
Excludes *destruction of nerve (by injection of neurolytic agent) (04.2)*

04.80 Peripheral nerve injection, not otherwise specified

04.81 Injection of anesthetic into peripheral nerve for analgesia
Excludes *that for operative anesthesia - omit code*
AHA: 1Q 2000, 7

04.89 Injection of other agent, except neurolytic
Excludes *injection of neurolytic agent (04.2)*

04.9 Other operations on cranial and peripheral nerves

04.91 Neurectasis
DEF: Operative stretching of a nerve or nerve trunk.

04.92 Implantation or replacement of peripheral neurostimulator lead(s)
Code also any insertion of neurostimulator pulse generator (86.94-86.98)
AHA: 2Q 2004, 7; 3Q 2001, 16; 2Q 2000, 22; 3Q 1996, 12

04.93 Removal of peripheral neurostimulator lead(s)
Code also any removal of neurostimulator pulse generator (86.05)
AHA: 3Q 2001, 16

04.99 Other

OPERATIONS ON SYMPATHETIC NERVES OR GANGLIA (05)

Excludes *paracervical uterine denervation (69.3)*

05.0 Division of sympathetic nerve or ganglion
Excludes *that of nerves to adrenal glands (07.42)*

05.1 Diagnostic procedures on sympathetic nerves or ganglia

05.11 Biopsy of sympathetic nerve or ganglion

05.19 Other diagnostic procedures on sympathetic nerves or ganglia

05.2 Sympathectomy
DEF: Cutting a malfunctioning sympathetic nerve pathway at a specified site.

05.21 Sphenopalatine ganglionectomy

05.22 Cervical sympathectomy

05.23 Lumbar sympathectomy

05.24 Presacral sympathectomy

05.25 Periarterial sympathectomy

05.29 Other sympathectomy and ganglionectomy
Excision or avulsion of sympathetic nerve NOS
Sympathetic ganglionectomy NOS
Excludes *biopsy of sympathetic nerve or ganglion (05.11)*
opticociliary neurectomy (12.79)
periarterial sympathectomy (05.25)
tympanosympathectomy (20.91)

05.3 Injection into sympathetic nerve or ganglion
Excludes *injection of ciliary sympathetic ganglion (12.79)*

05.31 Injection of anesthetic into sympathetic nerve for analgesia

05.32 Injection of neurolytic agent into sympathetic nerve
DEF: Destruction of a sympathetic nerve pathway via chemical introduction.

05.39 Other injection into sympathetic nerve or ganglion

05.8 Other operations on sympathetic nerves or ganglia

05.81 Repair of sympathetic nerve or ganglion

05.89 Other

05.9 Other operations on nervous system

2. OPERATIONS ON THE ENDOCRINE SYSTEM (06-07)

OPERATIONS ON THYROID AND PARATHYROID GLANDS (06)

Includes incidental resection of hyoid bone

06.0 Incision of thyroid field
Excludes *division of isthmus (06.91)*

06.01 Aspiration of thyroid field
Percutaneous or needle drainage of thyroid field
Excludes *aspiration biopsy of thyroid (06.11)*
drainage by incision (06.09)
postoperative aspiration of field (06.02)

06.02 Reopening of wound of thyroid field
Reopening of wound of thyroid field for:
control of (postoperative) hemorrhage
examination
exploration
removal of hematoma

06.09 Other incision of thyroid field
Drainage of hematoma by incision
Drainage of thyroglossal tract by incision
Exploration:
neck by incision
thyroid (field) by incision
Removal of foreign body by incision
Thyroidotomy NOS by incision
Excludes *postoperative exploration (06.02)*
removal of hematoma by aspiration (06.01)

06.1 Diagnostic procedures on thyroid and parathyroid glands

06.11 Closed [percutaneous] [needle] biopsy of thyroid gland
Aspiration biopsy of thyroid

06.12 Open biopsy of thyroid gland

06.13 Biopsy of parathyroid gland

06.19 Other diagnostic procedures on thyroid and parathyroid glands
Excludes *radioisotope scan of:*
parathyroid (92.13)
thyroid (92.01)
soft tissue x-ray of thyroid field (87.09)

06.2 Unilateral thyroid lobectomy
Complete removal of one lobe of thyroid (with removal of isthmus or portion of other lobe)
Hemithyroidectomy
Excludes *partial substernal thyroidectomy (06.51)*
DEF: Hemithyroidectomy: removal of one lobe of the thyroid gland.

06.3 Other partial thyroidectomy

06.31 Excision of lesion of thyroid
Excludes *biopsy of thyroid (06.11-06.12)*

06.39 Other
Isthmectomy
Partial thyroidectomy NOS
Excludes *partial substernal thyroidectomy (06.51)*
DEF: Isthmectomy: Excision of the middle portion of the thyroid.

06.4 Complete thyroidectomy
Excludes *complete substernal thyroidectomy (06.52)*
that with laryngectomy (30.3-30.4)

06.5 Substernal thyroidectomy

06.50 Substernal thyroidectomy, not otherwise specified

06.51 Partial substernal thyroidectomy

06.52 Complete substernal thyroidectomy

06.6 Excision of lingual thyroid
Excision of thyroid by:
submental route
transoral route

06.7 Excision of thyroglossal duct or tract

06.8 Parathyroidectomy
DEF: Removal of the parathyroid glands.

06.81 Complete parathyroidectomy

✖ Deleted Code ▼ Nonspecific O.R. Procedure ✔ Valid O.R. Procedure ✖ Non-O.R. Procedure ♂ Male ♀ Female

✓ **06.89 Other parathyroidectomy**
Parathyroidectomy NOS
Partial parathyroidectomy
Excludes *biopsy of parathyroid (06.13)*

❹ **06.9 Other operations on thyroid (region) and parathyroid**

✓ **06.91 Division of thyroid isthmus**
Transection of thyroid isthmus

✓ **06.92 Ligation of thyroid vessels**

✓ **06.93 Suture of thyroid gland**

✓ **06.94 Thyroid tissue reimplantation**
Autotransplantation of thyroid tissue

✓ **06.95 Parathyroid tissue reimplantation**
Autotransplantation of parathyroid tissue
AHA: 1Q 1995, 9

✓ **06.98 Other operations on thyroid glands**

✓ **06.99 Other operations on parathyroid glands**

OPERATIONS ON OTHER ENDOCRINE GLANDS (07)

Includes operations on:
adrenal glands
pineal gland
pituitary gland
thymus

Excludes *operations on:*
aortic and carotid bodies (39.8)
ovaries (65.0-65.99)
pancreas (52.01-52.99)
testes (62.0-62.99)

❹ **07.0 Exploration of adrenal field**
Excludes *incision of adrenal (gland) (07.41)*

✓▼ **07.00 Exploration of adrenal field, not otherwise specified**

✓ **07.01 Unilateral exploration of adrenal field**

✓ **07.02 Bilateral exploration of adrenal field**

❹ **07.1 Diagnostic procedures on adrenal glands, pituitary gland, pineal gland, and thymus**

✗❶ **07.11 Closed [percutaneous] [needle] biopsy of adrenal gland**

✓⓪ **07.12 Open biopsy of adrenal gland**

✓ **07.13 Biopsy of pituitary gland, transfrontal approach**

✓ **07.14 Biopsy of pituitary gland, transsphenoidal approach**
DEF: Removal of a sample of pituitary tissue through the sphenoid bone.

✓ **07.15 Biopsy of pituitary gland, unspecified approach**

✓ **07.16 Biopsy of thymus**

✓ **07.17 Biopsy of pineal gland**

✓ **07.19 Other diagnostic procedures on adrenal glands, pituitary gland, pineal gland, and thymus**
Excludes *microscopic examination of specimen from endocrine gland (90.11-90.19)*
radioisotope scan of pituitary gland (92.11)

❹ **07.2 Partial adrenalectomy**

✓ **07.21 Excision of lesion of adrenal gland**
Excludes *biopsy of adrenal gland (07.11-07.12)*

✓ **07.22 Unilateral adrenalectomy**
Adrenalectomy NOS
Excludes *excision of remaining adrenal gland (07.3)*
DEF: Removal of one adrenal gland.

✓ **07.29 Other partial adrenalectomy**
Partial adrenalectomy NOS
AHA: 2Q 2005, 5

✓ **07.3 Bilateral adrenalectomy**
Excision of remaining adrenal gland
Excludes *bilateral partial adrenalectomy (07.29)*

❹ **07.4 Other operations on adrenal glands, nerves, and vessels**

✓ **07.41 Incision of adrenal gland**
Adrenalotomy (with drainage)

✓ **07.42 Division of nerves to adrenal glands**

✓ **07.43 Ligation of adrenal vessels**

✓ **07.44 Repair of adrenal gland**

✓ **07.45 Reimplantation of adrenal tissue**
Autotransplantation of adrenal tissue

✓ **07.49 Other**

❹ **07.5 Operations on pineal gland**

✓ **07.51 Exploration of pineal field**
Excludes *that with incision of pineal gland (07.52)*

✓ **07.52 Incision of pineal gland**

✓ **07.53 Partial excision of pineal gland**
Excludes *biopsy of pineal gland (07.17)*

✓ **07.54 Total excision of pineal gland**
Pinealectomy (complete) (total)

✓ **07.59 Other operations on pineal gland**

❹ **07.6 Hypophysectomy**
DEF: Removal or destruction of the hypophysis, or pituitary gland.

✓ **07.61 Partial excision of pituitary gland, transfrontal approach**
Cryohypophysectomy, partial transfrontal approach
Division of hypophyseal stalk transfrontal approach
Excision of lesion of pituitary [hypophysis] transfrontal approach
Hypophysectomy, subtotal transfrontal approach
Infundibulectomy, hypophyseal transfrontal approach
Excludes *biopsy of pituitary gland, transfrontal approach (07.13)*

✓ **07.62 Partial excision of pituitary gland, transsphenoidal approach**
Excludes *biopsy of pituitary gland, transsphenoidal approach (07.14)*
AHA: 3Q 1992, 13

✓▼ **07.63 Partial excision of pituitary gland, unspecified approach**
Excludes *biopsy of pituitary gland NOS (07.15)*

✓ **07.64 Total excision of pituitary gland, transfrontal approach**
Ablation of pituitary by implantation (strontium-yttrium) (Y) transfrontal approach
Cryohypophysectomy, complete transfrontal approach

✓ **07.65 Total excision of pituitary gland, transsphenoidal approach**

✓ **07.68 Total excision of pituitary gland, other specified approach**

✓▼ **07.69 Total excision of pituitary gland, unspecified approach**
Hypophysectomy NOS
Pituitectomy NOS

❹ **07.7 Other operations on hypophysis**

✓ **07.71 Exploration of pituitary fossa**
Excludes *exploration with incision of pituitary gland (07.72)*

✓ **07.72 Incision of pituitary gland**
Aspiration of:
craniobuccal pouch
craniopharyngioma
hypophysis
pituitary gland
Rathke's pouch

✓ **07.79 Other**
Insertion of pack into sella turcica

❹ **07.8 Thymectomy**
DEF: Removal of the thymus gland.

✓▼ **07.80 Thymectomy, not otherwise specified**

▲✓ **07.81 Other partial excision of thymus**
▶Open partial excision of thymus◀
Excludes *biopsy of thymus (07.16)*
▶thoracoscopic partial excision of thymus (07.83)◀

▲✓ **07.82 Other total excision of thymus**
▶Open total excision of thymus◀
Excludes *▶thoracoscopic total excision of thymus (07.84)◀*

●✓ **07.83 Thoracoscopic partial excision of thymus**
Excludes *▶other partial excision of thymus (07.81)◀*

●✓ **07.84 Thoracoscopic total excision of thymus**
Excludes *▶other total excision of thymus (07.82)◀*

❹ Fourth Digit Required ⓪ Open Biopsy ❶ Closed Biopsy ▶◀ Revised Text ● New Code ▲ Revised Code

07.9 Other operations on thymus

07.91 Exploration of thymus field
Excludes *exploration with incision of thymus (07.92)*

07.92 Other incision of thymus
▶Open incision of thymus◀
Excludes *▶thoracoscopic incision of thymus (07.95)◀*

07.93 Repair of thymus

07.94 Transplantation of thymus

07.95 Thoracoscopic incision of thymus
Excludes *▶other incision of thymus (07.92)◀*

07.98 Other and unspecified thoracoscopic operations on thymus

07.99 Other and unspecified operations on thymus
▶Transcervical thymectomy◀
Excludes *▶other thoracoscopic operations on thymus (07.98)◀*

3. OPERATIONS ON THE EYE (08-16)

OPERATIONS ON EYELIDS (08)

Includes operations on the eyebrow

08.0 Incision of eyelid

08.01 Incision of lid margin

08.02 Severing of blepharorrhaphy
DEF: Release of sutures previously placed to shut the eyelids.

08.09 Other incision of eyelid

08.1 Diagnostic procedures on eyelid

08.11 Biopsy of eyelid

08.19 Other diagnostic procedures on eyelid

08.2 Excision or destruction of lesion or tissue of eyelid
Code also any synchronous reconstruction (08.61-08.74)
Excludes *biopsy of eyelid (08.11)*

08.20 Removal of lesion of eyelid, not otherwise specified
Removal of meibomian gland NOS

08.21 Excision of chalazion

08.22 Excision of other minor lesion of eyelid
Excision of:
verucca
wart

08.23 Excision of major lesion of eyelid, partial-thickness
Excision involving one-fourth or more of lid margin, partial-thickness

08.24 Excision of major lesion of eyelid, full-thickness
Excision involving one-fourth or more of lid margin, full-thickness
Wedge resection of eyelid

08.25 Destruction of lesion of eyelid

08.3 Repair of blepharoptosis and lid retraction
DEF: Repair of blepharoptosis: Correcting a drooping upper eyelid, usually by suturing or muscle sling.

08.31 Repair of blepharoptosis by frontalis muscle technique with suture

08.32 Repair of blepharoptosis by frontalis muscle technique with fascial sling

08.33 Repair of blepharoptosis by resection or advancement of levator muscle or aponeurosis

08.34 Repair of blepharoptosis by other levator muscle techniques

08.35 Repair of blepharoptosis by tarsal technique

08.36 Repair of blepharoptosis by other techniques
Correction of eyelid ptosis NOS
Orbicularis oculi muscle sling for correction of blepharoptosis

08.37 Reduction of overcorrection of ptosis

08.38 Correction of lid retraction

08.4 Repair of entropion or ectropion

08.41 Repair of entropion or ectropion by thermocauterization

08.42 Repair of entropion or ectropion by suture technique

08.43 Repair of entropion or ectropion with wedge resection

08.44 Repair of entropion or ectropion with lid reconstruction

08.49 Other repair of entropion or ectropion

08.5 Other adjustment of lid position

08.51 Canthotomy
Enlargement of palpebral fissure

08.52 Blepharorrhaphy
Canthorrhaphy
Tarsorrhaphy

08.59 Other
Canthoplasty NOS
Repair of epicanthal fold

08.6 Reconstruction of eyelid with flaps or grafts
Excludes *that associated with repair of entropion and ectropion (08.44)*

08.61 Reconstruction of eyelid with skin flap or graft

08.62 Reconstruction of eyelid with mucous membrane flap or graft

08.63 Reconstruction of eyelid with hair follicle graft

08.64 Reconstruction of eyelid with tarsoconjunctival flap
Transfer of tarsoconjunctival flap from opposing lid

08.69 Other reconstruction of eyelid with flaps or grafts

08.7 Other reconstruction of eyelid
Excludes *that associated with repair of entropion and ectropion (08.44)*

08.70 Reconstruction of eyelid, not otherwise specified
AHA: 2Q 1996, 11

08.71 Reconstruction of eyelid involving lid margin, partial-thickness

08.72 Other reconstruction of eyelid, partial-thickness

08.73 Reconstruction of eyelid involving lid margin, full-thickness

08.74 Other reconstruction of eyelid, full-thickness

08.8 Other repair of eyelid

08.81 Linear repair of laceration of eyelid or eyebrow

08.82 Repair of laceration involving lid margin, partial-thickness

08.83 Other repair of laceration of eyelid, partial-thickness

08.84 Repair of laceration involving lid margin, full-thickness

08.85 Other repair of laceration of eyelid, full-thickness

08.86 Lower eyelid rhytidectomy

08.87 Upper eyelid rhytidectomy
AHA: 2Q 1996, 11

08.89 Other eyelid repair
AHA: 1Q 2000, 22

08.9 Other operations on eyelids

08.91 Electrosurgical epilation of eyelid

08.92 Cryosurgical epilation of eyelid

08.93 Other epilation of eyelid

08.99 Other

OPERATIONS ON LACRIMAL SYSTEM (09)

09.0 Incision of lacrimal gland
Incision of lacrimal cyst (with drainage)

09.1 Diagnostic procedures on lacrimal system

09.11 Biopsy of lacrimal gland

09.12 Biopsy of lacrimal sac

09.19 Other diagnostic procedures on lacrimal system
Excludes *contrast dacryocystogram (87.05)*
soft tissue x-ray of nasolacrimal duct (87.09)

09.2 Excision of lesion or tissue of lacrimal gland

09.20 Excision of lacrimal gland, not otherwise specified

09.21 Excision of lesion of lacrimal gland
Excludes *biopsy of lacrimal gland (09.11)*

09.22 Other partial dacryoadenectomy
Excludes *biopsy of lacrimal gland (09.11)*

09.23 Total dacryoadenectomy
DEF: Complete excision of the lacrimal, or tear gland.

09.3 Other operations on lacrimal gland

09.4 Manipulation of lacrimal passage
Includes removal of calculus
that with dilation
Excludes *contrast dacryocystogram (87.05)*

09.41 Probing of lacrimal punctum

09.42 Probing of lacrimal canaliculi
DEF: Tear duct exploration using a small, flexible, tube-shaped probe.

09.43 Probing of nasolacrimal duct
Excludes *that with insertion of tube or stent (09.44)*

09.44 Intubation of nasolacrimal duct
Insertion of stent into nasolacrimal duct

09.49 Other manipulation of lacrimal passage

09.5 Incision of lacrimal sac and passages

09.51 Incision of lacrimal punctum
DEF: Cutting into the tear duct opening.

09.52 Incision of lacrimal canaliculi

09.53 Incision of lacrimal sac

09.59 Other incision of lacrimal passages
Incision (and drainage) of nasolacrimal duct NOS

09.6 Excision of lacrimal sac and passage
Excludes *biopsy of lacrimal sac (09.12)*

09.7 Repair of canaliculus and punctum
Excludes *repair of eyelid (08.81-08.89)*

09.71 Correction of everted punctum

09.72 Other repair of punctum

09.73 Repair of canaliculus

09.8 Fistulization of lacrimal tract to nasal cavity

09.81 Dacryocystorhinostomy [DCR]
DEF: Creation of drainage pathway for tears into the nose from the lacrimal sac.

09.82 Conjunctivocystorhinostomy
Conjunctivodacryocystorhinostomy [CDCR]
Excludes *that with insertion of tube or stent (09.83)*

09.83 Conjunctivorhinostomy with insertion of tube or stent

09.9 Other operations on lacrimal system

09.91 Obliteration of lacrimal punctum
DEF: Total destruction of the eyelid's tear duct opening.

09.99 Other
AHA: 2Q 1994, 11

OPERATIONS ON CONJUNCTIVA (10)

10.0 Removal of embedded foreign body from conjunctiva by incision
Excludes *removal of:*
embedded foreign body without incision (98.22)
superficial foreign body (98.21)

10.1 Other incision of conjunctiva

10.2 Diagnostic procedures on conjunctiva

10.21 Biopsy of conjunctiva

10.29 Other diagnostic procedures on conjunctiva

10.3 Excision or destruction of lesion or tissue of conjunctiva

10.31 Excision of lesion or tissue of conjunctiva
Excision of ring of conjunctiva around cornea
Excludes *biopsy of conjunctiva (10.21)*
AHA: 4Q 2000, 41; 3Q 1996, 7

10.32 Destruction of lesion of conjunctiva
Excludes *excision of lesion (10.31)*
thermocauterization for entropion (08.41)

10.33 Other destructive procedures on conjunctiva
Removal of trachoma follicles

10.4 Conjunctivoplasty

10.41 Repair of symblepharon with free graft
AHA: 3Q 1996, 7

10.42 Reconstruction of conjunctival cul-de-sac with free graft
Excludes *revision of enucleation socket with graft (16.63)*

10.43 Other reconstruction of conjunctival cul-de-sac
Excludes *revision of enucleation socket (16.64)*

10.44 Other free graft to conjunctiva

✔ **10.49 Other conjunctivoplasty**
Excludes *repair of cornea with conjunctival flap (11.53)*

✔ **10.5 Lysis of adhesions of conjunctiva and eyelid**
Division of symblepharon (with insertion of conformer)

✔ **10.6 Repair of laceration of conjunctiva**
Excludes *that with repair of sclera (12.81)*

❹ **10.9 Other operations on conjunctiva**

✔ **10.91 Subconjunctival injection**
AHA: 3Q 1996, 7

✔ **10.99 Other**

OPERATIONS ON CORNEA (11)

✔ **11.0 Magnetic removal of embedded foreign body from cornea**
Excludes *that with incision (11.1)*

✔ **11.1 Incision of cornea**
Incision of cornea for removal of foreign body

Removal of Corneal Foreign Body

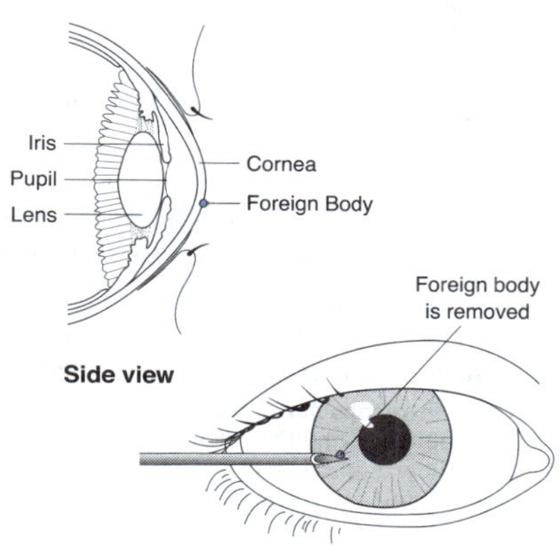

❹ **11.2 Diagnostic procedures on cornea**

✔ **11.21 Scraping of cornea for smear or culture**

✔ **11.22 Biopsy of cornea**

✔ **11.29 Other diagnostic procedures on cornea**

❹ **11.3 Excision of pterygium**

✔ **11.31 Transposition of pterygium**

✔ **11.32 Excision of pterygium with corneal graft**

✔ **11.39 Other excision of pterygium**

❹ **11.4 Excision or destruction of tissue or other lesion of cornea**

✔ **11.41 Mechanical removal of corneal epithelium**
That by chemocauterization
Excludes *that for smear or culture (11.21)*
AHA: 3Q 2002, 20

✔ **11.42 Thermocauterization of corneal lesion**

✔ **11.43 Cryotherapy of corneal lesion**

✔ **11.49 Other removal or destruction of corneal lesion**
Excision of cornea NOS
Excludes *biopsy of cornea (11.22)*

❹ **11.5 Repair of cornea**

✔ **11.51 Suture of corneal laceration**
AHA: 3Q 1996, 7

✔ **11.52 Repair of postoperative wound dehiscence of cornea**

✔ **11.53 Repair of corneal laceration or wound with conjunctival flap**

✔ **11.59 Other repair of cornea**

❹ **11.6 Corneal transplant**
Excludes *excision of pterygium with corneal graft (11.32)*

✔ **11.60 Corneal transplant, not otherwise specified**
Note. To report donor source - see codes 00.91-00.93
Keratoplasty NOS

✔ **11.61 Lamellar keratoplasty with autograft**

✔ **11.62 Other lamellar keratoplasty**
AHA: Sep-Oct 1985, 6

✔ **11.63 Penetrating keratoplasty with autograft**
Perforating keratoplasty with autograft

✔ **11.64 Other penetrating keratoplasty**
Perforating keratoplasty (with homograft)

✔ **11.69 Other corneal transplant**

❹ **11.7 Other reconstructive and refractive surgery on cornea**

✔ **11.71 Keratomileusis**

✔ **11.72 Keratophakia**
DEF: Implantation of a shaped portion of donor cornea beween recipient corneal layers to correct a refractive error.

✔ **11.73 Keratoprosthesis**

✔ **11.74 Thermokeratoplasty**

✔ **11.75 Radial keratotomy**

✔ **11.76 Epikeratophakia**

✔ **11.79 Other**

❹ **11.9 Other operations on cornea**

✔ **11.91 Tattooing of cornea**

✔ **11.92 Removal of artificial implant from cornea**

✔ **11.99 Other**
AHA: 3Q 2002, 20

OPERATIONS ON IRIS, CILIARY BODY, SCLERA, AND ANTERIOR CHAMBER (12)

Excludes *operations on cornea (11.0-11.99)*

❹ **12.0 Removal of intraocular foreign body from anterior segment of eye**

✔ **12.00 Removal of intraocular foreign body from anterior segment of eye, not otherwise specified**

✔ **12.01 Removal of intraocular foreign body from anterior segment of eye with use of magnet**

✔ **12.02 Removal of intraocular foreign body from anterior segment of eye without use of magnet**

❹ **12.1 Iridotomy and simple iridectomy**
Excludes *iridectomy associated with:*
cataract extraction (13.11-13.69)
removal of lesion (12.41-12.42)
scleral fistulization (12.61-12.69)

DEF: Iridotomy: Surgical incision into the iris.
Iridectomy: Surgical removal of part of the iris.

✔ **12.11 Iridotomy with transfixion**

✔ **12.12 Other iridotomy**
Corectomy
Discission of iris
Iridotomy NOS

✔ **12.13 Excision of prolapsed iris**

✔ **12.14 Other iridectomy**
Iridectomy (basal) (peripheral) (total)

❹ **12.2 Diagnostic procedures on iris, ciliary body, sclera, and anterior chamber**

✔ **12.21 Diagnostic aspiration of anterior chamber of eye**

✔ **12.22 Biopsy of iris**

✔ **12.29 Other diagnostic procedures on iris, ciliary body, sclera, and anterior chamber**

❹ **12.3 Iridoplasty and coreoplasty**

✔ **12.31 Lysis of goniosynechiae**
Lysis of goniosynechiae by injection of air or liquid

✓ **12.32 Lysis of other anterior synechiae**
Lysis of anterior synechiae:
NOS
by injection of air or liquid

✓ **12.33 Lysis of posterior synechiae**
Lysis of iris adhesions NOS

✓ **12.34 Lysis of corneovitreal adhesions**

✓ **12.35 Coreoplasty**
Needling of pupillary membrane

✓ **12.39 Other iridoplasty**

❹ **12.4 Excision or destruction of lesion of iris and ciliary body**

✓ **12.40 Removal of lesion of anterior segment of eye, not otherwise specified**

✓ **12.41 Destruction of lesion of iris, nonexcisional**
Destruction of lesion of iris by:
cauterization
cryotherapy
photocoagulation

✓ **12.42 Excision of lesion of iris**
Excludes *biopsy of iris (12.22)*

✓ **12.43 Destruction of lesion of ciliary body, nonexcisional**

✓ **12.44 Excision of lesion of ciliary body**

❹ **12.5 Facilitation of intraocular circulation**

✓ **12.51 Goniopuncture without goniotomy**

✓ **12.52 Goniotomy without goniopuncture**

✓ **12.53 Goniotomy with goniopuncture**

✓ **12.54 Trabeculotomy ab externo**

✓ **12.55 Cyclodialysis**
DEF: Creation of a path between the anterior chamber and suprachoroidal space.

✓ **12.59 Other facilitation of intraocular circulation**

❹ **12.6 Scleral fistulization**
Excludes *exploratory sclerotomy (12.89)*

✓ **12.61 Trephination of sclera with iridectomy**

✓ **12.62 Thermocauterization of sclera with iridectomy**

✓ **12.63 Iridencleisis and iridotasis**

✓ **12.64 Trabeculectomy ab externo**

✓ **12.65 Other scleral fistulization with iridectomy**

✓ **12.66 Postoperative revision of scleral fistulization procedure**
Revision of filtering bleb
Excludes *repair of fistula (12.82)*
AHA: 2Q 2001, 16

✓ **12.69 Other fistulizing procedure**
AHA: 3Q 1996, 4

❹ **12.7 Other procedures for relief of elevated intraocular pressure**

✓ **12.71 Cyclodiathermy**

✓ **12.72 Cyclocryotherapy**

✓ **12.73 Cyclophotocoagulation**

✓ **12.74 Diminution of ciliary body, not otherwise specified**

✓ **12.79 Other glaucoma procedures**
AHA: 2Q 1998, 16

❹ **12.8 Operations on sclera**
Excludes *those associated with:*
retinal reattachment (14.41-14.59)
scleral fistulization (12.61-12.69)

✓ **12.81 Suture of laceration of sclera**
Suture of sclera with synchronous repair of conjunctiva

✓ **12.82 Repair of scleral fistula**
Excludes *postoperative revision of scleral fistulization procedure (12.66)*

✓ **12.83 Revision of operative wound of anterior segment, not elsewhere classified**
Excludes *postoperative revision of scleral fistulization procedure (12.66)*

✓ **12.84 Excision or destruction of lesion of sclera**

✓ **12.85 Repair of scleral staphyloma with graft**

✓ **12.86 Other repair of scleral staphyloma**

✓ **12.87 Scleral reinforcement with graft**

✓ **12.88 Other scleral reinforcement**

✓ **12.89 Other operations on sclera**
Exploratory sclerotomy

❹ **12.9 Other operations on iris, ciliary body, and anterior chamber**

✓ **12.91 Therapeutic evacuation of anterior chamber**
Paracentesis of anterior chamber
Excludes *diagnostic aspiration (12.21)*

✓ **12.92 Injection into anterior chamber**
Injection of:
air into anterior chamber
liquid into anterior chamber
medication into anterior chamber
AHA: Mar-Apr 1984, 1

✓ **12.93 Removal or destruction of epithelial downgrowth from anterior chamber**
Excludes *that with iridectomy (12.41-12.42)*

✓ **12.97 Other operations on iris**

✓ **12.98 Other operations on ciliary body**

✓ **12.99 Other operations on anterior chamber**

OPERATIONS ON LENS (13)

❹ **13.0 Removal of foreign body from lens**
Excludes *removal of pseudophakos (13.8)*

✓ **13.00 Removal of foreign body from lens, not otherwise specified**

✓ **13.01 Removal of foreign body from lens with use of magnet**

✓ **13.02 Removal of foreign body from lens without use of magnet**

❹ **13.1 Intracapsular extraction of lens**
Code also any synchronous insertion of pseudophakos (13.71)

✓ **13.11 Intracapsular extraction of lens by temporal inferior route**

✓ **13.19 Other intracapsular extraction of lens**
Cataract extraction NOS
Cryoextraction of lens
Erysiphake extraction of cataract
Extraction of lens NOS

✓ **13.2 Extracapsular extraction of lens by linear extraction technique**

✓ **13.3 Extracapsular extraction of lens by simple aspiration (and irrigation) technique**
Irrigation of traumatic cataract

❹ **13.4 Extracapsular extraction of lens by fragmentation and aspiration technique**

✓ **13.41 Phacoemulsification and aspiration of cataract**
AHA: 3Q 1996, 4; 1Q 1994, 16

✓ **13.42 Mechanical phacofragmentation and aspiration of cataract by posterior route**
Code also any synchronous vitrectomy (14.74)

✓ **13.43 Mechanical phacofragmentation and other aspiration of cataract**

❹ **13.5 Other extracapsular extraction of lens**
Code also any synchronous insertion of pseudophakos (13.71)

✓ **13.51 Extracapsular extraction of lens by temporal inferior route**

✓ **13.59 Other extracapsular extraction of lens**

❹ **13.6 Other cataract extraction**
Code also any synchronous insertion of pseudophakos (13.71)

✓ **13.64 Discission of secondary membrane [after cataract]**
DEF: Cutting into or rupturing the fibrotic lens capsule that has developed following lens extraction.

✓ **13.65 Excision of secondary membrane [after cataract]**
Capsulectomy

✓ **13.66 Mechanical fragmentation of secondary membrane [after cataract]**

✓ **13.69 Other cataract extraction**

13.7 Insertion of prosthetic lens [pseudophakos]
Excludes *implantation of intraocular telescope prosthesis (13.91)*

13.70 Insertion of pseudophakos, not otherwise specified
AHA: Mar-Apr 1984, 1

13.71 Insertion of intraocular lens prosthesis at time of cataract extraction, one-stage
Code also synchronous extraction of cataract (13.11-13.69)
AHA: 3Q 1996, 4; Mar-Apr 1984, 1

13.72 Secondary insertion of intraocular lens prosthesis
AHA: Mar-Apr 1984, 1

13.8 Removal of implanted lens
Removal of pseudophakos

13.9 Other operations on lens
AHA: 1Q 2000, 9

13.90 Operation on lens, not elsewhere classified

13.91 Implantation of intraocular telescope prosthesis
Implantable miniature telescope
Includes removal of lens, any method
Excludes *secondary insertion of ocular implant (16.61)*

OPERATIONS ON RETINA, CHOROID, VITREOUS, AND POSTERIOR CHAMBER (14)

14.0 Removal of foreign body from posterior segment of eye
Excludes *removal of surgically implanted material (14.6)*

14.00 Removal of foreign body from posterior segment of eye, not otherwise specified

14.01 Removal of foreign body from posterior segment of eye with use of magnet

14.02 Removal of foreign body from posterior segment of eye without use of magnet

14.1 Diagnostic procedures on retina, choroid, vitreous, and posterior chamber

14.11 Diagnostic aspiration of vitreous

14.19 Other diagnostic procedures on retina, choroid, vitreous, and posterior chamber

14.2 Destruction of lesion of retina and choroid
Includes destruction of chorioretinopathy or isolated chorioretinal lesion
Excludes *that for repair of retina (14.31-14.59)*

14.21 Destruction of chorioretinal lesion by diathermy

14.22 Destruction of chorioretinal lesion by cryotherapy

14.23 Destruction of chorioretinal lesion by xenon arc photocoagulation

14.24 Destruction of chorioretinal lesion by laser photocoagulation

14.25 Destruction of chorioretinal lesion by photocoagulation of unspecified type

14.26 Destruction of chorioretinal lesion by radiation therapy

14.27 Destruction of chorioretinal lesion by implantation of radiation source

14.29 Other destruction of chorioretinal lesion
Destruction of lesion of retina and choroid NOS

14.3 Repair of retinal tear
Includes repair of retinal defect
Excludes *repair of retinal detachment (14.41-14.59)*

14.31 Repair of retinal tear by diathermy

14.32 Repair of retinal tear by cryotherapy

14.33 Repair of retinal tear by xenon arc photocoagulation

14.34 Repair of retinal tear by laser photocoagulation
AHA: 1Q 1994, 17

14.35 Repair of retinal tear by photocoagulation of unspecified type

14.39 Other repair of retinal tear

14.4 Repair of retinal detachment with scleral buckling and implant

14.41 Scleral buckling with implant
AHA: 3Q 1996, 6

14.49 Other scleral buckling
Scleral buckling with:
air tamponade
resection of sclera
vitrectomy
AHA: 1Q 1994, 16, 17

14.5 Other repair of retinal detachment
Includes that with drainage

14.51 Repair of retinal detachment with diathermy

14.52 Repair of retinal detachment with cryotherapy

14.53 Repair of retinal detachment with xenon arc photocoagulation

14.54 Repair of retinal detachment with laser photocoagulation
AHA: Nov-Dec 1987, 10

14.55 Repair of retinal detachment with photocoagulation of unspecified type

14.59 Other

14.6 Removal of surgically implanted material from posterior segment of eye

14.7 Operations on vitreous

14.71 Removal of vitreous, anterior approach
Open sky technique
Removal of vitreous, anterior approach (with replacement)

14.72 Other removal of vitreous
Aspiration of vitreous by posterior sclerotomy

14.73 Mechanical vitrectomy by anterior approach
AHA: 3Q 1996, 4

14.74 Other mechanical vitrectomy
Posterior approach
AHA: 3Q 1996, 5

14.75 Injection of vitreous substitute
Excludes *that associated with removal (14.71-14.72)*
AHA: 1Q 1998, 5; 3Q 1996, 5; 1Q 1994, 17

14.79 Other operations on vitreous
AHA: 3Q 1999, 12; 1Q 1999, 11; 1Q 1998, 5

14.9 Other operations on retina, choroid, and posterior chamber
AHA: 3Q 1996, 5

OPERATIONS ON EXTRAOCULAR MUSCLES (15)

15.0 Diagnostic procedures on extraocular muscles or tendons

15.01 Biopsy of extraocular muscle or tendon

15.09 Other diagnostic procedures on extraocular muscles and tendons

15.1 Operations on one extraocular muscle involving temporary detachment from globe

15.11 Recession of one extraocular muscle
AHA: 3Q 1996, 3

15.12 Advancement of one extraocular muscle

15.13 Resection of one extraocular muscle

15.19 Other operations on one extraocular muscle involving temporary detachment from globe
Excludes *transposition of muscle (15.5)*

15.2 Other operations on one extraocular muscle

15.21 Lengthening procedure on one extraocular muscle

15.22 Shortening procedure on one extraocular muscle

15.29 Other

15.3 Operations on two or more extraocular muscles involving temporary detachment from globe, one or both eyes
AHA: 3Q 1996, 3

15.4 Other operations on two or more extraocular muscles, one or both eyes

15.5 Transposition of extraocular muscles
Excludes *that for correction of ptosis (08.31-08.36)*

15.6 Revision of extraocular muscle surgery

✖ Deleted Code ▼ Nonspecific O.R. Procedure ✔ Valid O.R. Procedure ✖ Non-O.R. Procedure ♂ Male ♀ Female

✓ **15.7 Repair of injury of extraocular muscle**
Freeing of entrapped extraocular muscle
Lysis of adhesions of extraocular muscle
Repair of laceration of extraocular muscle, tendon, or Tenon's capsule

✓ **15.9 Other operations on extraocular muscles and tendons**

OPERATIONS ON ORBIT AND EYEBALL (16)

Excludes *reduction of fracture of orbit (76.78-76.79)*

❹ **16.0 Orbitotomy**

✓ **16.01 Orbitotomy with bone flap**
Orbitotomy with lateral approach

✓ **16.02 Orbitotomy with insertion of orbital implant**
Excludes *that with bone flap (16.01)*

✓ **16.09 Other orbitotomy**

✓ **16.1 Removal of penetrating foreign body from eye, not otherwise specified**
Excludes *removal of nonpenetrating foreign body (98.21)*

❹ **16.2 Diagnostic procedures on orbit and eyeball**

✗ **16.21 Ophthalmoscopy**

✓ **16.22 Diagnostic aspiration of orbit**

✓ **16.23 Biopsy of eyeball and orbit**

✓ **16.29 Other diagnostic procedures on orbit and eyeball**
Excludes *examination of form and structure of eye (95.11-95.16)*
general and subjective eye examination (95.01-95.09)
microscopic examination of specimen from eye (90.21-90.29)
objective functional tests of eye (95.21-95.26)
ocular thermography (88.82)
tonometry (89.11)
x-ray of orbit (87.14, 87.16)

❹ **16.3 Evisceration of eyeball**
DEF: Removal of the contents of the eyeball, leaving the sclera intact.

✓ **16.31 Removal of ocular contents with synchronous implant into scleral shell**

✓ **16.39 Other evisceration of eyeball**

❹ **16.4 Enucleation of eyeball**
DEF: Removal of the entire eyeball, requiring muscle and nerve detachment.

✓ **16.41 Enucleation of eyeball with synchronous implant into Tenon's capsule with attachment of muscles**
Integrated implant of eyeball

✓ **16.42 Enucleation of eyeball with other synchronous implant**

✓ **16.49 Other enucleation of eyeball**
Removal of eyeball NOS

❹ **16.5 Exenteration of orbital contents**
DEF: Removal of all contents within the bony orbital cavity.

✓ **16.51 Exenteration of orbit with removal of adjacent structures**
Radical orbitomaxillectomy

✓ **16.52 Exenteration of orbit with therapeutic removal of orbital bone**

✓ **16.59 Other exenteration of orbit**
Evisceration of orbit NOS
Exenteration of orbit with temporalis muscle transplant

❹ **16.6 Secondary procedures after removal of eyeball**
Excludes *that with synchronous:*
enucleation of eyeball (16.41-16.42)
evisceration of eyeball (16.31)

✓ **16.61 Secondary insertion of ocular implant**

✓ **16.62 Revision and reinsertion of ocular implant**

✓ **16.63 Revision of enucleation socket with graft**

✓ **16.64 Other revision of enucleation socket**

✓ **16.65 Secondary graft to exenteration cavity**

✓ **16.66 Other revision of exenteration cavity**

✓ **16.69 Other secondary procedures after removal of eyeball**

❹ **16.7 Removal of ocular or orbital implant**

✓ **16.71 Removal of ocular implant**

✓ **16.72 Removal of orbital implant**

❹ **16.8 Repair of injury of eyeball and orbit**

✓ **16.81 Repair of wound of orbit**
Excludes *reduction of orbital fracture (76.78-76.79)*
repair of extraocular muscles (15.7)

✓ **16.82 Repair of rupture of eyeball**
Repair of multiple structures of eye
Excludes *repair of laceration of:*
cornea (11.51-11.59)
sclera (12.81)

✓ **16.89 Other repair of injury of eyeball or orbit**

❹ **16.9 Other operations on orbit and eyeball**
Excludes *irrigation of eye (96.51)*
prescription and fitting of low vision aids (95.31-95.33)
removal of:
eye prosthesis NEC (97.31)
nonpenetrating foreign body from eye without incision (98.21)

✗ **16.91 Retrobulbar injection of therapeutic agent**
Excludes *injection of radiographic contrast material (87.14)*
opticociliary injection (12.79)

DEF: Injection into the area behind the eyeball.

✓ **16.92 Excision of lesion of orbit**
Excludes *biopsy of orbit (16.23)*

✓ **16.93 Excision of lesion of eye, unspecified structure**
Excludes *biopsy of eye NOS (16.23)*

✓ **16.98 Other operations on orbit**

✓ **16.99 Other operations on eyeball**

❹ Fourth Digit Required ⓞ Open Biopsy ⓒ Closed Biopsy ►◄ Revised Text ● New Code ▲ Revised Code

4. OPERATIONS ON THE EAR (18-20)

OPERATIONS ON EXTERNAL EAR (18)

Includes operations on:
external auditory canal
skin and cartilage of:
auricle
meatus

18.0 Incision of external ear
Excludes *removal of intraluminal foreign body (98.11)*

18.01 Piercing of ear lobe
Piercing of pinna

18.02 Incision of external auditory canal

18.09 Other incision of external ear
AHA: 1Q 2005, 18

18.1 Diagnostic procedures on external ear

18.11 Otoscopy

18.12 Biopsy of external ear

18.19 Other diagnostic procedures on external ear
Excludes *microscopic examination of specimen from ear (90.31-90.39)*

18.2 Excision or destruction of lesion of external ear

18.21 Excision of preauricular sinus
Radical excision of preauricular sinus or cyst
Excludes *excision of preauricular remnant [appendage] (18.29)*

18.29 Excision or destruction of other lesion of external ear
Cauterization of external ear
Coagulation of external ear
Cryosurgery of external ear
Curettage of external ear
Electrocoagulation of external ear
Enucleation of external ear
Excision of:
exostosis of external auditory canal
preauricular remnant [appendage]
Partial excision of ear
Excludes *biopsy of external ear (18.12)*
radical excision of lesion (18.31)
removal of cerumen (96.52)

18.3 Other excision of external ear
Excludes *biopsy of external ear (18.12)*

18.31 Radical excision of lesion of external ear
Excludes *radical excision of preauricular sinus (18.21)*

18.39 Other
Amputation of external ear
Excludes *excision of lesion (18.21-18.29, 18.31)*

18.4 Suture of laceration of external ear

18.5 Surgical correction of prominent ear
Ear:
pinning
setback

18.6 Reconstruction of external auditory canal
Canaloplasty of external auditory meatus
Construction [reconstruction] of external meatus of ear:
osseous portion
skin-lined portion (with skin graft)

18.7 Other plastic repair of external ear

18.71 Construction of auricle of ear
Prosthetic appliance for absent ear
Reconstruction:
auricle
ear

18.72 Reattachment of amputated ear

18.79 Other plastic repair of external ear
Otoplasty NOS
Postauricular skin graft
Repair of lop ear
AHA: 3Q 2003, 12

18.9 Other operations on external ear
Excludes *irrigation of ear (96.52)*
packing of external auditory canal (96.11)
removal of:
cerumen (96.52)
foreign body (without incision) (98.11)

RECONSTRUCTIVE OPERATIONS ON MIDDLE EAR (19)

19.0 Stapes mobilization
Division, otosclerotic:
material
process
Remobilization of stapes
Stapediolysis
Transcrural stapes mobilization
Excludes *that with synchronous stapedectomy (19.11-19.19)*

19.1 Stapedectomy
Excludes *revision of previous stapedectomy (19.21-19.29)*
stapes mobilization only (19.0)

DEF: Removal of the innermost ossicle in the middle ear, which connects with the oval window.

19.11 Stapedectomy with incus replacement
Stapedectomy with incus:
homograft
prosthesis

19.19 Other stapedectomy

19.2 Revision of stapedectomy

19.21 Revision of stapedectomy with incus replacement

19.29 Other revision of stapedectomy

19.3 Other operations on ossicular chain
Incudectomy NOS
Ossiculectomy NOS
Reconstruction of ossicles, second stage

19.4 Myringoplasty
Epitympanic, type I
Myringoplasty by:
cauterization
graft
Tympanoplasty (type I)
DEF: Reconstruction or plastic repair of the eardrum.

19.5 Other tympanoplasty

19.52 Type II tympanoplasty
Closure of perforation with graft against incus or malleus

19.53 Type III tympanoplasty
Graft placed in contact with mobile and intact stapes
AHA: Mar-Apr 1985, 15

19.54 Type IV tympanoplasty
Mobile footplate left exposed with air pocket between round window and graft

19.55 Type V tympanoplasty
Fenestra in horizontal semicircular canal covered by graft

19.6 Revision of tympanoplasty

19.9 Other repair of middle ear
Closure of mastoid fistula
Mastoid myoplasty
Obliteration of tympanomastoid cavity

OTHER OPERATIONS ON MIDDLE AND INNER EAR (20)

20.0 Myringotomy
DEF: Creating an opening in the eardrum by perforation or puncture.

20.01 Myringotomy with insertion of tube
Myringostomy

20.09 Other myringotomy
Aspiration of middle ear NOS

Deleted Code | Nonspecific O.R. Procedure | Valid O.R. Procedure | Non-O.R. Procedure | Male | Female

20.1 Removal of tympanostomy tube
AHA: 3Q 1994, 7; Nov-Dec 1987 9

20.2 Incision of mastoid and middle ear

20.21 Incision of mastoid

20.22 Incision of petrous pyramid air cells

20.23 Incision of middle ear
Atticotomy
Division of tympanum
Lysis of adhesions of middle ear
Excludes *division of otosclerotic process (19.0)*
stapediolysis (19.0)
that with stapedectomy (19.11-19.19)

20.3 Diagnostic procedures on middle and inner ear

20.31 Electrocochleography

20.32 Biopsy of middle and inner ear

20.39 Other diagnostic procedures on middle and inner ear
Excludes *auditory and vestibular function tests (89.13, 95.41-95.49)*
microscopic examination of specimen from ear (90.31-90.39)

20.4 Mastoidectomy
Code also any:
skin graft (18.79)
tympanoplasty (19.4-19.55)
Excludes *that with implantation of cochlear prosthetic device (20.96-20.98)*

DEF: Excision of the temporal bone protrusion behind the ear.

20.41 Simple mastoidectomy

20.42 Radical mastoidectomy

20.49 Other mastoidectomy
Atticoantrostomy
Mastoidectomy:
NOS
modified radical

20.5 Other excision of middle ear
Excludes *that with synchronous mastoidectomy (20.41-20.49)*

20.51 Excision of lesion of middle ear
Excludes *biopsy of middle ear (20.32)*

20.59 Other
Apicectomy of petrous pyramid
Tympanectomy

DEF: Tympanectomy: Removal of the eardrum.

20.6 Fenestration of inner ear

20.61 Fenestration of inner ear (initial)
Fenestration of:
labyrinth with graft (skin) (vein)
semicircular canals with graft (skin) (vein)
vestibule with graft (skin) (vein)
Excludes *that with tympanoplasty, type V (19.55)*

20.62 Revision of fenestration of inner ear

20.7 Incision, excision, and destruction of inner ear

20.71 Endolymphatic shunt

20.72 Injection into inner ear
Destruction by injection (alcohol):
inner ear
semicircular canals
vestibule

20.79 Other incision, excision, and destruction of inner ear
Decompression of labyrinth
Drainage of inner ear
Fistulization:
endolymphatic sac
labyrinth
Incision of endolymphatic sac
Labyrinthectomy (transtympanic)
Opening of bony labyrinth
Perilymphatic tap
Excludes *biopsy of inner ear (20.32)*

20.8 Operations on Eustachian tube
Catheterization of Eustachian tube
Inflation of Eustachian tube
Injection (Teflon paste) of Eustachian tube
Insufflation (boric acid-salicylic acid)
Intubation of Eustachian tube
Politzerization of Eustachian tube

20.9 Other operations on inner and middle ear

20.91 Tympanosympathectomy

20.92 Revision of mastoidectomy
AHA: 2Q 1998, 20

20.93 Repair of oval and round windows
Closure of fistula:
oval window
perilymph
round window

20.94 Injection of tympanum

20.95 Implantation of electromagnetic hearing device
Bone conduction hearing device
Excludes *cochlear prosthetic device (20.96-20.98)*
AHA: 4Q 1989, 5-7

20.96 Implantation or replacement of cochlear prosthetic device, not otherwise specified
Implantation of receiver (within skull) and insertion of electrode(s) in the cochlea
Includes mastoidectomy
Excludes *electromagnetic hearing device (20.95)*
AHA: 4Q 1989, 5-7

20.97 Implantation or replacement of cochlear prosthetic device, single channel
Implantation of receiver (within skull) and insertion of electrode in the cochlea
Includes mastoidectomy
Excludes *electromagnetic hearing device (20.95)*
AHA: 4Q 1989, 5-7

20.98 Implantation or replacement of cochlear prosthetic device, multiple channel
Implantation of receiver (within skull) and insertion of electrodes in the cochlea
Includes mastoidectomy
Excludes *electromagnetic hearing device (20.95)*
AHA: 4Q 1989, 5-7

20.99 Other operations on middle and inner ear
Repair or removal of cochlear prosthetic device (receiver) (electrode)
▶Attachment of percutaneous abutment (screw) for prosthetic device◀
Excludes *adjustment (external components) of cochlear prosthetic device (95.49)*
fitting of hearing aid (95.48)
AHA: 4Q 1989, 5-7

5. OPERATIONS ON THE NOSE, MOUTH, AND PHARYNX (21-29)

OPERATIONS ON NOSE (21)

Includes operations on:
bone of nose
skin of nose

❹ **21.0 Control of epistaxis**
DEF: Control of nasal bleeding.

✖ **21.00 Control of epistaxis, not otherwise specified**
✖ **21.01 Control of epistaxis by anterior nasal packing**
✖ **21.02 Control of epistaxis by posterior (and anterior) packing**
AHA: 1Q 1995, 5
✖ **21.03 Control of epistaxis by cauterization (and packing)**
✔ **21.04 Control of epistaxis by ligation of ethmoidal arteries**
✔ **21.05 Control of epistaxis by (transantral) ligation of the maxillary artery**
✔ **21.06 Control of epistaxis by ligation of the external carotid artery**
✔ **21.07 Control of epistaxis by excision of nasal mucosa and skin grafting of septum and lateral nasal wall**
✔ **21.09 Control of epistaxis by other means**

✖ **21.1 Incision of nose**
Chondrotomy
Incision of skin of nose
Nasal septotomy

❹ **21.2 Diagnostic procedures on nose**
✖ **21.21 Rhinoscopy**
DEF: Visual examination of the nasal passages via rhinoscope or speculum.
✖ **21.22 Biopsy of nose**
✖ **21.29 Other diagnostic procedures on nose**
Excludes *microscopic examination of specimen from nose (90.31-90.39)*
nasal:
function study (89.12)
x-ray (87.16)
rhinomanometry (89.12)

❹ **21.3 Local excision or destruction of lesion of nose**
Excludes *biopsy of nose (21.22)*
nasal fistulectomy (21.82)
✖ **21.30 Excision or destruction of lesion of nose, not otherwise specified**
✖ **21.31 Local excision or destruction of intranasal lesion**
Nasal polypectomy
✖ **21.32 Local excision or destruction of other lesion of nose**
AHA: 2Q 1989, 16

✔ **21.4 Resection of nose**
Amputation of nose

✔ **21.5 Submucous resection of nasal septum**

❹ **21.6 Turbinectomy**
✔ **21.61 Turbinectomy by diathermy or cryosurgery**
✔ **21.62 Fracture of the turbinates**
✔ **21.69 Other turbinectomy**
Excludes *turbinectomy associated with sinusectomy (22.31-22.39, 22.42, 22.60-22.64)*

❹ **21.7 Reduction of nasal fracture**
✖ **21.71 Closed reduction of nasal fracture**
✔ **21.72 Open reduction of nasal fracture**

❹ **21.8 Repair and plastic operations on the nose**
✖ **21.81 Suture of laceration of nose**
✔ **21.82 Closure of nasal fistula**
Nasolabial fistulectomy
Nasopharyngeal fistulectomy
Oronasal fistulectomy
✔ **21.83 Total nasal reconstruction**
Reconstruction of nose with:
arm flap
forehead flap
✔ **21.84 Revision rhinoplasty**
Rhinoseptoplasty
Twisted nose rhinoplasty
✔ **21.85 Augmentation rhinoplasty**
Augmentation rhinoplasty with:
graft
synthetic implant
✔ **21.86 Limited rhinoplasty**
Plastic repair of nasolabial flaps
Tip rhinoplasty
DEF: Plastic surgery of one specific area of the nose, such as the tip or the nasal folds around the nostrils.
✔ **21.87 Other rhinoplasty**
Rhinoplasty NOS
✔ **21.88 Other septoplasty**
Crushing of nasal septum
Repair of septal perforation
Excludes *septoplasty associated with submucous resection of septum (21.5)*
✔ **21.89 Other repair and plastic operations on nose**
Reattachment of amputated nose

❹ **21.9 Other operations on nose**
✖ **21.91 Lysis of adhesions of nose**
Posterior nasal scrub
✔ **21.99 Other**
Excludes *dilation of frontonasal duct (96.21)*
irrigation of nasal passages (96.53)
removal of:
intraluminal foreign body without incision (98.12)
nasal packing (97.32)
replacement of nasal packing (97.21)

OPERATIONS ON NASAL SINUSES (22)

❹ **22.0 Aspiration and lavage of nasal sinus**
✖ **22.00 Aspiration and lavage of nasal sinus, not otherwise specified**
✖ **22.01 Puncture of nasal sinus for aspiration or lavage**
✖ **22.02 Aspiration or lavage of nasal sinus through natural ostium**

❹ **22.1 Diagnostic procedures on nasal sinus**
✖⓿ **22.11 Closed [endoscopic] [needle] biopsy of nasal sinus**
✔⓪ **22.12 Open biopsy of nasal sinus**
✖ **22.19 Other diagnostic procedures on nasal sinuses**
Endoscopy without biopsy
Excludes *transillumination of sinus (89.35)*
x-ray of sinus (87.15-87.16)

✗ **22.2 Intranasal antrotomy**
Excludes *antrotomy with external approach (22.31-22.39)*

Maxillary Antrotomy

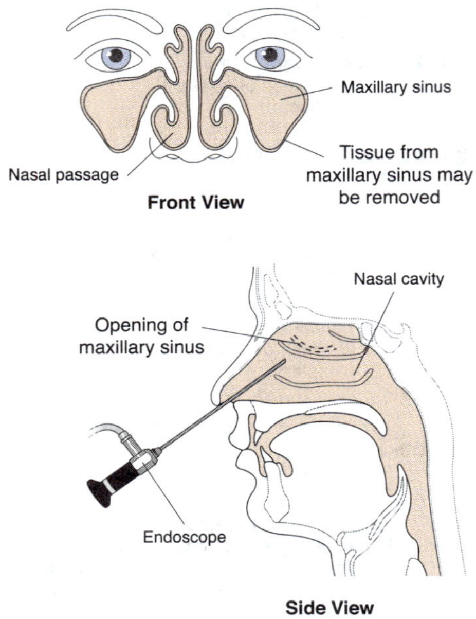

❹ **22.3 External maxillary antrotomy**

✓ **22.31 Radical maxillary antrotomy**
Removal of lining membrane of maxillary sinus using Caldwell-Luc approach

✓ **22.39 Other external maxillary antrotomy**
Exploration of maxillary antrum with Caldwell-Luc approach

❹ **22.4 Frontal sinusotomy and sinusectomy**

✓ **22.41 Frontal sinusotomy**
DEF: Incision into a frontal sinus, creating an opening.

✓ **22.42 Frontal sinusectomy**
Excision of lesion of frontal sinus
Obliteration of frontal sinus (with fat)
Excludes *biopsy of nasal sinus (22.11-22.12)*

❹ **22.5 Other nasal sinusotomy**

✓ **22.50 Sinusotomy, not otherwise specified**

✓ **22.51 Ethmoidotomy**

✓ **22.52 Sphenoidotomy**

✓ **22.53 Incision of multiple nasal sinuses**

❹ **22.6 Other nasal sinusectomy**
Includes that with incidental turbinectomy
Excludes *biopsy of nasal sinus (22.11-22.12)*

✓ **22.60 Sinusectomy, not otherwise specified**

✓ **22.61 Excision of lesion of maxillary sinus with Caldwell-Luc approach**

✓ **22.62 Excision of lesion of maxillary sinus with other approach**

✓ **22.63 Ethmoidectomy**
DEF: Removal of all or part of the mucosal lining and bones of the ethmoid sinuses.

✓ **22.64 Sphenoidectomy**

❹ **22.7 Repair of nasal sinus**

✓ **22.71 Closure of nasal sinus fistula**
Repair of oro-antral fistula

✓ **22.79 Other repair of nasal sinus**
Reconstruction of frontonasal duct
Repair of bone of accessory sinus

✓ **22.9 Other operations on nasal sinuses**
Exteriorization of maxillary sinus
Fistulization of sinus
Excludes *dilation of frontonasal duct (96.21)*

REMOVAL AND RESTORATION OF TEETH (23)

❹ **23.0 Forceps extraction of tooth**

✗ **23.01 Extraction of deciduous tooth**
DEF: Forceps removal of a baby tooth.

✗ **23.09 Extraction of other tooth**
Extraction of tooth NOS

❹ **23.1 Surgical removal of tooth**

✗ **23.11 Removal of residual root**

✗ **23.19 Other surgical extraction of tooth**
Odontectomy NOS
Removal of impacted tooth
Tooth extraction with elevation of mucoperiosteal flap

✗ **23.2 Restoration of tooth by filling**

✗ **23.3 Restoration of tooth by inlay**

❹ **23.4 Other dental restoration**

✗ **23.41 Application of crown**

✗ **23.42 Insertion of fixed bridge**

✗ **23.43 Insertion of removable bridge**

✗ **23.49 Other**

✗ **23.5 Implantation of tooth**

✗ **23.6 Prosthetic dental implant**
Endosseous dental implant

❹ **23.7 Apicoectomy and root canal therapy**

✗ **23.70 Root canal, not otherwise specified**

✗ **23.71 Root canal therapy with irrigation**

✗ **23.72 Root canal therapy with apicoectomy**

✗ **23.73 Apicoectomy**
DEF: Removal of the tip of a tooth root.

OTHER OPERATIONS ON TEETH, GUMS, AND ALVEOLI (24)

✗ **24.0 Incision of gum or alveolar bone**
Apical alveolotomy

❹ **24.1 Diagnostic procedures on teeth, gums, and alveoli**

✗ **24.11 Biopsy of gum**

✗ **24.12 Biopsy of alveolus**

✗ **24.19 Other diagnostic procedures on teeth, gums, and alveoli**
Excludes *dental:*
examination (89.31)
x-ray:
full-mouth (87.11)
other (87.12)
microscopic examination of dental specimen (90.81-90.89)

✓ **24.2 Gingivoplasty**
Gingivoplasty with bone or soft tissue graft

❹ **24.3 Other operations on gum**

✗ **24.31 Excision of lesion or tissue of gum**
Excludes *biopsy of gum (24.11)*
excision of odontogenic lesion (24.4)

✗ **24.32 Suture of laceration of gum**

✗ **24.39 Other**

✓ **24.4 Excision of dental lesion of jaw**
Excision of odontogenic lesion

✓ **24.5 Alveoloplasty**
Alveolectomy (interradicular) (intraseptal) (radical) (simple) (with graft or implant)
Excludes *biopsy of alveolus (24.12)*
en bloc resection of alveolar process and palate (27.32)

✗ **24.6 Exposure of tooth**

✖ **24.7 Application of orthodontic appliance**
Application, insertion, or fitting of:
arch bars
orthodontic obturator
orthodontic wiring
periodontal splint
Excludes *nonorthodontic dental wiring (93.55)*

✖ **24.8 Other orthodontic operation**
Closure of diastema (alveolar) (dental)
Occlusal adjustment
Removal of arch bars
Repair of dental arch
Excludes *removal of nonorthodontic wiring (97.33)*

❹ **24.9 Other dental operations**

✖ **24.91 Extension or deepening of buccolabial or lingual sulcus**

✖ **24.99 Other**
Excludes *dental:*
debridement (96.54)
examination (89.31)
prophylaxis (96.54)
scaling and polishing (96.54)
wiring (93.55)
fitting of dental appliance [denture] (99.97)
microscopic examination of dental specimen (90.81-90.89)
removal of dental:
packing (97.34)
prosthesis (97.35)
wiring (97.33)
replacement of dental packing (97.22)

OPERATIONS ON TONGUE (25)

❹ **25.0 Diagnostic procedures on tongue**

✖⓪ **25.01 Closed [needle] biopsy of tongue**

✔⓪ **25.02 Open biopsy of tongue**
Wedge biopsy

✖ **25.09 Other diagnostic procedures on tongue**

✔ **25.1 Excision or destruction of lesion or tissue of tongue**
Excludes *biopsy of tongue (25.01-25.02)*
frenumectomy:
labial (27.41)
lingual (25.92)
AHA: 2Q 2002, 5

✔ **25.2 Partial glossectomy**
DEF: Excision of part of the tongue.

✔ **25.3 Complete glossectomy**
Glossectomy NOS
Code also any neck dissection (40.40-40.42)

✔ **25.4 Radical glossectomy**
Code also any:
neck dissection (40.40-40.42)
tracheostomy (31.1-31.29)

❹ **25.5 Repair of tongue and glossoplasty**

✖ **25.51 Suture of laceration of tongue**

✔ **25.59 Other repair and plastic operations on tongue**
Fascial sling of tongue
Fusion of tongue (to lip)
Graft of mucosa or skin to tongue
Excludes *lysis of adhesions of tongue (25.93)*
AHA: 1Q 1997, 5

❹ **25.9 Other operations on tongue**

✖ **25.91 Lingual frenotomy**
Excludes *labial frenotomy (27.91)*

✖ **25.92 Lingual frenectomy**
Excludes *labial frenectomy (27.41)*

✖ **25.93 Lysis of adhesions of tongue**

✔ **25.94 Other glossotomy**

✔ **25.99 Other**

OPERATIONS ON SALIVARY GLANDS AND DUCTS (26)

Includes operations on:
lesser salivary gland and duct
parotid gland and duct
sublingual gland and duct
submaxillary gland and duct
Code also any neck dissection (40.40-40.42)

✖ **26.0 Incision of salivary gland or duct**

❹ **26.1 Diagnostic procedures on salivary glands and ducts**

✖⓪ **26.11 Closed [needle] biopsy of salivary gland or duct**

✔⓪ **26.12 Open biopsy of salivary gland or duct**

✖ **26.19 Other diagnostic procedures on salivary glands and ducts**
Excludes *x-ray of salivary gland (87.09)*

❹ **26.2 Excision of lesion of salivary gland**

✔ **26.21 Marsupialization of salivary gland cyst**

✔ **26.29 Other excision of salivary gland lesion**
Excludes *biopsy of salivary gland (26.11-26.12)*
salivary fistulectomy (26.42)

❹ **26.3 Sialoadenectomy**
DEF: Removal of a salivary gland.

✔▼ **26.30 Sialoadenectomy, not otherwise specified**

✔ **26.31 Partial sialoadenectomy**

✔ **26.32 Complete sialoadenectomy**
En bloc excision of salivary gland lesion
Radical sialoadenectomy

❹ **26.4 Repair of salivary gland or duct**

✔ **26.41 Suture of laceration of salivary gland**

✔ **26.42 Closure of salivary fistula**

✔ **26.49 Other repair and plastic operations on salivary gland or duct**
Fistulization of salivary gland
Plastic repair of salivary gland or duct NOS
Transplantation of salivary duct opening

❹ **26.9 Other operations on salivary gland or duct**

✖ **26.91 Probing of salivary duct**

✔ **26.99 Other**

OTHER OPERATIONS ON MOUTH AND FACE (27)

Includes operations on:
lips
palate
soft tissue of face and mouth, except tongue and gingiva
Excludes *operations on:*
gingiva (24.0-24.99)
tongue (25.01-25.99)

✔ **27.0 Drainage of face and floor of mouth**
Drainage of:
facial region (abscess)
fascial compartment of face
Ludwig's angina
Excludes *drainage of thyroglossal tract (06.09)*

✔ **27.1 Incision of palate**

❹ **27.2 Diagnostic procedures on oral cavity**

✔ **27.21 Biopsy of bony palate**

✔ **27.22 Biopsy of uvula and soft palate**

✖ **27.23 Biopsy of lip**

✖ **27.24 Biopsy of mouth, unspecified structure**

✖ **27.29 Other diagnostic procedures on oral cavity**
Excludes *soft tissue x-ray (87.09)*

❹ **27.3 Excision of lesion or tissue of bony palate**

✔ **27.31 Local excision or destruction of lesion or tissue of bony palate**
Local excision or destruction of palate by:
cautery
chemotherapy
cryotherapy
Excludes *biopsy of bony palate (27.21)*

✔ **27.32 Wide excision or destruction of lesion or tissue of bony palate**
En bloc resection of alveolar process and palate

❹ **27.4 Excision of other parts of mouth**

✖ **27.41 Labial frenectomy**
Excludes *division of labial frenum (27.91)*

✔ **27.42 Wide excision of lesion of lip**

✔ **27.43 Other excision of lesion or tissue of lip**

✔ **27.49 Other excision of mouth**
Excludes *biopsy of mouth NOS (27.24)*
excision of lesion of:
palate (27.31-27.32)
tongue (25.1)
uvula (27.72)
fistulectomy of mouth (27.53)
frenectomy of:
lip (27.41)
tongue (25.92)
AHA: 2Q 2005, 8-9

❹ **27.5 Plastic repair of mouth**
Excludes *palatoplasty (27.61-27.69)*

✖ **27.51 Suture of laceration of lip**

✖ **27.52 Suture of laceration of other part of mouth**

✔ **27.53 Closure of fistula of mouth**
Excludes *fistulectomy:*
nasolabial (21.82)
oro-antral (22.71)
oronasal (21.82)

✔ **27.54 Repair of cleft lip**

✔ **27.55 Full-thickness skin graft to lip and mouth**

✔ **27.56 Other skin graft to lip and mouth**

✔ **27.57 Attachment of pedicle or flap graft to lip and mouth**

✔ **27.59 Other plastic repair of mouth**

❹ **27.6 Palatoplasty**

✔ **27.61 Suture of laceration of palate**

✔ **27.62 Correction of cleft palate**
Correction of cleft palate by push-back operation
Excludes *revision of cleft palate repair (27.63)*

Palatoplasty

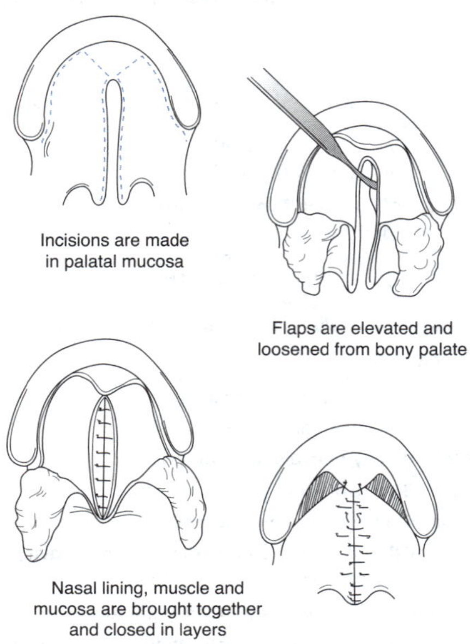

✔ **27.63 Revision of cleft palate repair**
Secondary:
attachment of pharyngeal flap
lengthening of palate
AHA: 1Q 1996, 14

✖ **27.64 Insertion of palatal implant**

✔ **27.69 Other plastic repair of palate**
Code also any insertion of palatal implant (27.64)
Excludes *fistulectomy of mouth (27.53)*
AHA: 3Q 1999, 22; 1Q 1997, 5

❹ **27.7 Operations on uvula**

✔ **27.71 Incision of uvula**

✔ **27.72 Excision of uvula**
Excludes *biopsy of uvula (27.22)*

✔ **27.73 Repair of uvula**
Excludes *that with synchronous cleft palate repair (27.62)*
uranostaphylorrhaphy (27.62)

✔ **27.79 Other operations on uvula**

❹ **27.9 Other operations on mouth and face**

✖ **27.91 Labial frenotomy**
Division of labial frenum
Excludes *lingual frenotomy (25.91)*

✔ **27.92 Incision of mouth, unspecified structure**
Excludes *incision of:*
gum (24.0)
palate (27.1)
salivary gland or duct (26.0)
tongue (25.94)
uvula (27.71)

✔ **27.99 Other operations on oral cavity**
Graft of buccal sulcus
Excludes *removal of:*
intraluminal foreign body (98.01)
penetrating foreign body from mouth without incision (98.22)

OPERATIONS ON TONSILS AND ADENOIDS (28)

✔ **28.0 Incision and drainage of tonsil and peritonsillar structures**
Drainage (oral) (transcervical) of:
parapharyngeal abscess
peritonsillar abscess
retropharyngeal abscess
tonsillar abscess

❹ **28.1 Diagnostic procedures on tonsils and adenoids**

✔ **28.11 Biopsy of tonsils and adenoids**

✔ **28.19 Other diagnostic procedures on tonsils and adenoids**
Excludes *soft tissue x-ray (87.09)*

✔ **28.2 Tonsillectomy without adenoidectomy**
AHA: 1Q 1997, 5; 2Q 1990, 23

✔ **28.3 Tonsillectomy with adenoidectomy**
AHA: 2Q 2005, 16

✔ **28.4 Excision of tonsil tag**

✔ **28.5 Excision of lingual tonsil**

✔ **28.6 Adenoidectomy without tonsillectomy**
Excision of adenoid tag

✔ **28.7 Control of hemorrhage after tonsillectomy and adenoidectomy**

❹ **28.9 Other operations on tonsils and adenoids**

✔ **28.91 Removal of foreign body from tonsil and adenoid by incision**
Excludes *that without incision (98.13)*

✔ **28.92 Excision of lesion of tonsil and adenoid**
Excludes *biopsy of tonsil and adenoid (28.11)*

✔ **28.99 Other**

OPERATIONS ON PHARYNX (29)

Includes operations on:
hypopharynx
nasopharynx
oropharynx
pharyngeal pouch
pyriform sinus

✓ **29.0 Pharyngotomy**
Drainage of pharyngeal bursa
Excludes *incision and drainage of retropharyngeal abscess (28.0)*
removal of foreign body (without incision) (98.13)
DEF: Incision into the pharynx.

❹ **29.1 Diagnostic procedures on pharynx**
✖ **29.11 Pharyngoscopy**
✖ **29.12 Pharyngeal biopsy**
Biopsy of supraglottic mass
✖ **29.19 Other diagnostic procedures on pharynx**
Excludes *x-ray of nasopharynx:*
contrast (87.06)
other (87.09)

✓ **29.2 Excision of branchial cleft cyst or vestige**
Excludes *branchial cleft fistulectomy (29.52)*

❹ **29.3 Excision or destruction of lesion or tissue of pharynx**
AHA: 2Q 1989, 18; Jan-Feb 1985, 4
✓ **29.31 Cricopharyngeal myotomy**
Excludes *that with pharyngeal diverticulectomy (29.32)*
✓ **29.32 Pharyngeal diverticulectomy**
✓ **29.33 Pharyngectomy (partial)**
Excludes *laryngopharyngectomy (30.3)*
DEF: Removal of a part of the pharynx.
✓ **29.39 Other excision or destruction of lesion or tissue of pharynx**

✓ **29.4 Plastic operation on pharynx**
Correction of nasopharyngeal atresia
Excludes *pharyngoplasty associated with cleft palate repair (27.62-27.63)*
AHA: 3Q 1999, 22; 1Q 1997, 5; Mar-Apr 1985, 12

❹ **29.5 Other repair of pharynx**
✓ **29.51 Suture of laceration of pharynx**
✓ **29.52 Closure of branchial cleft fistula**
✓ **29.53 Closure of other fistula of pharynx**
Pharyngoesophageal fistulectomy
✓ **29.54 Lysis of pharyngeal adhesions**
✓ **29.59 Other**
AHA: 2Q 1989, 18

❹ **29.9 Other operations on pharynx**
✖ **29.91 Dilation of pharynx**
Dilation of nasopharynx
✓ **29.92 Division of glossopharyngeal nerve**
✓ **29.99 Other**
Excludes *insertion of radium into pharynx and nasopharynx (92.27)*
removal of intraluminal foreign body (98.13)

6. OPERATIONS ON THE RESPIRATORY SYSTEM (30-34)

EXCISION OF LARYNX (30)

❹ **30.0 Excision or destruction of lesion or tissue of larynx**
✓ **30.01 Marsupialization of laryngeal cyst**
✓ **30.09 Other excision or destruction of lesion or tissue of larynx**
Stripping of vocal cords
Excludes *biopsy of larynx (31.43)*
laryngeal fistulectomy (31.62)
laryngotracheal fistulectomy (31.62)

✓ **30.1 Hemilaryngectomy**
DEF: Excision of one half of the larynx.

❹ **30.2 Other partial laryngectomy**
✓ **30.21 Epiglottidectomy**
✓ **30.22 Vocal cordectomy**
Excision of vocal cords
✓ **30.29 Other partial laryngectomy**
Excision of laryngeal cartilage

✓ **30.3 Complete laryngectomy**
Block dissection of larynx (with thyroidectomy) (with synchronous tracheostomy)
Laryngopharyngectomy
Excludes *that with radical neck dissection (30.4)*

✓ **30.4 Radical laryngectomy**
Complete [total] laryngectomy with radical neck dissection (with thyroidectomy) (with synchronous tracheostomy)

OTHER OPERATIONS ON LARYNX AND TRACHEA (31)

✖ **31.0 Injection of larynx**
Injection of inert material into larynx or vocal cords

✖ **31.1 Temporary tracheostomy**
Tracheotomy for assistance in breathing
AHA: 1Q 1997, 6

❹ **31.2 Permanent tracheostomy**
DEF: Creation of an opening in the anterior trachea with the insertion of a tube for long-term breathing assistance.
✓ **31.21 Mediastinal tracheostomy**
✓ **31.29 Other permanent tracheostomy**
Excludes *that with laryngectomy (30.3-30.4)*
AHA: 2Q 2005, 8-9; 2Q 2002, 6

✓ **31.3 Other incision of larynx or trachea**
Excludes *that for assistance in breathing (31.1-31.29)*

❹ **31.4 Diagnostic procedures on larynx and trachea**
✖ **31.41 Tracheoscopy through artificial stoma**
Excludes *that with biopsy (31.43-31.44)*
✖ **31.42 Laryngoscopy and other tracheoscopy**
Excludes *that with biopsy (31.43-31.44)*
✖ⓞ **31.43 Closed [endoscopic] biopsy of larynx**
✖ⓞ **31.44 Closed [endoscopic] biopsy of trachea**
✓ⓞ **31.45 Open biopsy of larynx or trachea**
✖ **31.48 Other diagnostic procedures on larynx**
Excludes *contrast laryngogram (87.07)*
microscopic examination of specimen from larynx (90.31-90.39)
soft tissue x-ray of larynx NEC (87.09)
✖ **31.49 Other diagnostic procedures on trachea**
Excludes *microscopic examination of specimen from trachea (90.41-90.49)*
x-ray of trachea (87.49)

✓ **31.5 Local excision or destruction of lesion or tissue of trachea**
Excludes *biopsy of trachea (31.44-31.45)*
laryngotracheal fistulectomy (31.62)
tracheoesophageal fistulectomy (31.73)

❹ **31.6 Repair of larynx**
✓ **31.61 Suture of laceration of larynx**

✓ **31.62 Closure of fistula of larynx**
Laryngotracheal fistulectomy
Take-down of laryngostomy

✓ **31.63 Revision of laryngostomy**

✓ **31.64 Repair of laryngeal fracture**

✓ **31.69 Other repair of larynx**
Arytenoidopexy
Graft of larynx
Transposition of vocal cords
Excludes *construction of artificial larynx (31.75)*

❹ **31.7 Repair and plastic operations on trachea**

✓ **31.71 Suture of laceration of trachea**

✓ **31.72 Closure of external fistula of trachea**
Closure of tracheotomy

✓ **31.73 Closure of other fistula of trachea**
Tracheoesophageal fistulectomy
Excludes *laryngotracheal fistulectomy (31.62)*

✓ **31.74 Revision of tracheostomy**

✓ **31.75 Reconstruction of trachea and construction of artificial larynx**
Tracheoplasty with artificial larynx

✓ **31.79 Other repair and plastic operations on trachea**

❹ **31.9 Other operations on larynx and trachea**

✓ **31.91 Division of laryngeal nerve**

✓ **31.92 Lysis of adhesions of trachea or larynx**

✗ **31.93 Replacement of laryngeal or tracheal stent**

✗ **31.94 Injection of locally-acting therapeutic substance into trachea**

✗ **31.95 Tracheoesophageal fistulization**

✓ **31.98 Other operations on larynx**
Dilation of larynx
Division of congenital web of larynx
Removal of keel or stent of larynx
Excludes *removal of intraluminal foreign body from larynx without incision (98.14)*

✓ **31.99 Other operations on trachea**
Excludes *removal of:*
intraluminal foreign body from trachea without incision (98.15)
tracheostomy tube (97.37)
replacement of tracheostomy tube (97.23)
tracheostomy toilette (96.55)

AHA: 1Q 1997, 14

EXCISION OF LUNG AND BRONCHUS (32)

Includes rib resection as operative approach
sternotomy as operative approach
sternum-splitting incision as operative approach
thoracotomy as operative approach

Code also any synchronous bronchoplasty (33.48)

❹ **32.0 Local excision or destruction of lesion or tissue of bronchus**
Excludes *biopsy of bronchus (33.24-33.25)*
bronchial fistulectomy (33.42)

AHA: 4Q 1988, 11

✗ **32.01 Endoscopic excision or destruction of lesion or tissue of bronchus**

✓ **32.09 Other local excision or destruction of lesion or tissue of bronchus**
Excludes *that by endoscopic approach (32.01)*

✓ **32.1 Other excision of bronchus**
Resection (wide sleeve) of bronchus
Excludes *radical dissection [excision] of bronchus (32.6)*

❹ **32.2 Local excision or destruction of lesion or tissue of lung**

●✓ **32.20 Thoracoscopic excision of lesion or tissue of lung**
Thoracoscopic wedge resection

✓ **32.21 Plication of emphysematous bleb**

✓ **32.22 Lung volume reduction surgery**
DEF: Removal of a portion(s) of lung tissue to reduce breathing effort in cases of emphysema.
AHA: 1Q 1997, 6; 4Q 1995, 64

✓ **32.23 Open ablation of lung lesion or tissue**

✓ **32.24 Percutaneous ablation of lung lesion or tissue**

✓ **32.25 Thoracoscopic ablation of lung lesion or tissue**
Excludes ▶*thoracoscopic excision of lesion or tissue of lung (32.20)*◀

✓▼ **32.26 Other and unspecified ablation of lung lesion or tissue**

✗ **32.28 Endoscopic excision or destruction of lesion or tissue of lung**
Excludes *ablation of lung lesion or tissue:*
open (32.23)
other (32.26)
percutanous (32.24)
thoracoscopic (32.25)
biopsy of lung (33.26-33.27)

✓ **32.29 Other local excision or destruction of lesion or tissue of lung**
Resection of lung:
NOS
wedge
Excludes *ablation of lung lesion or tissue:*
open (32.23)
other (32.26)
percutanous (32.24)
thoracoscopic (32.25)
biopsy of lung (33.26-33.27)
that by endoscopic approach (32.28)
▶*thoracoscopic excision of lesion or tissue of lung (32.20)*◀
wide excision of lesion of lung (32.3)

AHA: 3Q 1999, 3

❹ **32.3 Segmental resection of lung**
Partial lobectomy

●✓ **32.30 Thoracoscopic segmental resection of lung**

●✓ **32.39 Other and unspecified thoracoscopic segmental resection of lung**
Excludes ▶*thoracoscopic segmental resection of lung (32.30)*◀

❹ **32.4 Lobectomy of lung**
Lobectomy with segmental resection of adjacent lobes of lung
Excludes *that with radical dissection [excision] of thoracic structures (32.6)*

Lobectomy

Lungs are exposed and lobe is removed

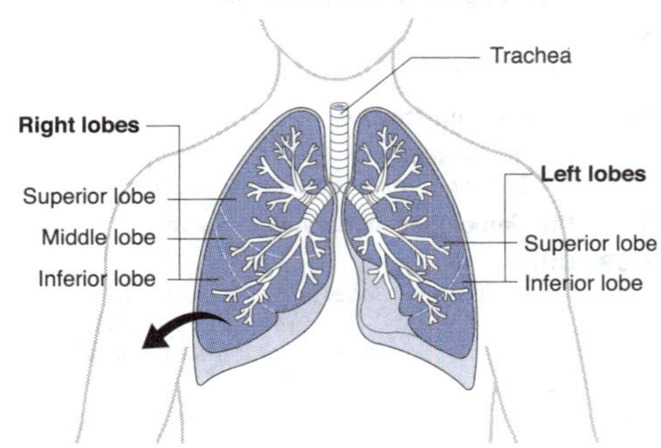

●✓ **32.41 Thoracoscopic lobectomy of lung**

●✓ **32.49 Other lobectomy of lung**
Excludes ▶*thoracoscopic lobectomy of lung (32.41)*◀

▲❹ **32.5 Pneumonectomy**
Excision of lung NOS
Pneumonectomy (with mediastinal dissection)
DEF: Removal of an entire lung.
AHA: 1Q 1999, 6

●✓ **32.50 Thoracoscopic pneumonectomy**

●✓ **32.59 Other and unspecified pneumonectomy**
▶Excludes *thoracoscopic pneumonectomy (32.50)*◀

✓ **32.6 Radical dissection of thoracic structures**
Block [en bloc] dissection of bronchus, lobe of lung, brachial plexus, intercostal structure, ribs (transverse process), and sympathetic nerves

✓ **32.9 Other excision of lung**
Excludes *biopsy of lung and bronchus (33.24-33.27)*
pulmonary decortication (34.51)

OTHER OPERATIONS ON LUNG AND BRONCHUS (33)

Includes rib resection as operative approach
sternotomy as operative approach
sternum-splitting incision as operative approach
thoracotomy as operative approach

✓ **33.0 Incision of bronchus**

✓ **33.1 Incision of lung**
Excludes *puncture of lung (33.93)*

④ **33.2 Diagnostic procedures on lung and bronchus**

●✓ **33.20 Thoracoscopic lung biopsy**
Excludes ▶*closed endoscopic biopsy of lung (33.27)*◀
▶*closed [percutaneous] [needle] biopsy of lung (33.26)*◀
▶*open biopsy of lung (33.28)*◀

✗ **33.21 Bronchoscopy through artificial stoma**
Excludes *that with biopsy (33.24, 33.27)*

✗ **33.22 Fiber-optic bronchoscopy**
Excludes *that with biopsy (33.24, 33.27)*
AHA: 1Q 2004, 4; Sep-Oct 1986, 11

✗ **33.23 Other bronchoscopy**
Excludes *that for:*
aspiration (96.05)
biopsy (33.24, 33.27)
AHA: 3Q 2002, 18; 1Q 1999, 6

✗⓪ **33.24 Closed [endoscopic] biopsy of bronchus**
Bronchoscopy (fiberoptic) (rigid) with:
brush biopsy of "lung"
brushing or washing for specimen collection
excision (bite) biopsy
Diagnostic bronchoalveolar lavage (BAL)
Excludes *closed biopsy of lung, other than brush biopsy of "lung" (33.26, 33.27)*
whole lung lavage (33.99)
AHA: 3Q 2004, 9; 3Q 2002, 16; 3Q 1991, 15

✓⓪ **33.25 Open biopsy of bronchus**
Excludes *open biopsy of lung (33.28)*

✗⓪ **33.26 Closed [percutaneous] [needle] biopsy of lung**
▶Fine needle aspiration (FNA) of lung◀
▶Transthoracic needle biopsy of lung (TTNB)◀
Excludes *endoscopic biopsy of lung (33.27)*
▶*thoracoscopic lung biopsy (33.20)*◀
AHA: 3Q 1992, 12-13

✓ **33.27 Closed endoscopic biopsy of lung**
Fiber-optic (flexible) bronchoscopy with fluoroscopic guidance with biopsy
Transbronchial lung biopsy
Excludes *brush biopsy of "lung" (33.24)*
percutaneous biopsy of lung (33.26)
▶*thoracoscopic lung biopsy (33.20)*◀
AHA: 3Q 2004, 9; 3Q 2002, 16; 3Q 1991, 15; Sep-Oct 1986, 11

✓⓪ **33.28 Open biopsy of lung**
AHA: 3Q 1999, 3; 3Q 1992, 12-13

✓ **33.29 Other diagnostic procedures on lung and bronchus**
Excludes *contrast bronchogram:*
endotracheal (87.31)
other (87.32)
lung scan (92.15)
magnetic resonance imaging (88.92)
microscopic examination of specimen from bronchus or lung (90.41-90.49)
routine chest x-ray (87.44)
ultrasonography of lung (88.73)
vital capacity determination (89.37)
x-ray of bronchus or lung NOS (87.49)

④ **33.3 Surgical collapse of lung**

✗ **33.31 Destruction of phrenic nerve for collapse of lung**

✗ **33.32 Artificial pneumothorax for collapse of lung**
Thoracotomy for collapse of lung

✗ **33.33 Pneumoperitoneum for collapse of lung**

✓ **33.34 Thoracoplasty**
DEF: Removal of several ribs to force the chest wall upon the lungs and achieve therapeutic lung collapse.

✓ **33.39 Other surgical collapse of lung**
Collapse of lung NOS

④ **33.4 Repair and plastic operation on lung and bronchus**

✓ **33.41 Suture of laceration of bronchus**

✓ **33.42 Closure of bronchial fistula**
Closure of bronchostomy
Fistulectomy:
bronchocutaneous
bronchoesophageal
bronchovisceral
Excludes *closure of fistula:*
bronchomediastinal (34.73)
bronchopleural (34.73)
bronchopleuromediastinal (34.73)

✓ **33.43 Closure of laceration of lung**

✓ **33.48 Other repair and plastic operations on bronchus**

✓ **33.49 Other repair and plastic operations on lung**
Excludes *closure of pleural fistula (34.73)*

④ **33.5 Lung transplant**
Note: To report donor source - see codes 00.91-00.93
Code also cardiopulmonary bypass [extracorporeal circulation] [heart-lung machine] (39.61)
Excludes *combined heart-lung transplantation (33.6)*

✓ **33.50 Lung transplantation, not otherwise specified**

✓ **33.51 Unilateral lung transplantation**

✓ **33.52 Bilateral lung transplantation**
Double-lung transplantation
En bloc transplantation
Code also cardiopulmonary bypass [extracorporeal circulation] [heart-lung machine] (39.61)

✓ **33.6 Combined heart-lung transplantation**
Note: To report donor source - see codes 00.91-00.93
Code also cardiopulmonary bypass [extracorporeal circulation] [heart-lung machine] (39.61)

④ **33.7 Endoscopic insertion, replacement and removal of therapeutic device or substances in bronchus or lung**
Biologic Lung Volume Reduction (BLVR)
Excludes *insertion of tracheobronchial stent (96.05)*

✗ **33.71 Endoscopic insertion or replacement of bronchial valve(s)**
Endobronchial airflow redirection valve
Intrabronchial airflow redirection valve

✗ **33.78 Endoscopic removal of bronchial device(s) or substances**

✗ **33.79 Endoscopic insertion of other bronchial device or substances**
Biologic Lung Volume Reduction NOS (BLVR)

④ **33.9 Other operations on lung and bronchus**

✗ **33.91 Bronchial dilation**
AHA: 1Q 1997, 14

✓ **33.92 Ligation of bronchus**

✓ **33.93 Puncture of lung**
Excludes *needle biopsy (33.26)*

✓ **33.98 Other operations on bronchus**
Excludes *bronchial lavage (96.56)*
removal of intraluminal foreign body from bronchus without incision (98.15)

✓ **33.99 Other operations on lung**
Whole lung lavage
Excludes *other continuous mechanical ventilation (96.70-96.72)*
respiratory therapy (93.90-93.99)
AHA: 3Q 2002, 17

OPERATIONS ON CHEST WALL, PLEURA, MEDIASTINUM, AND DIAPHRAGM (34)

Excludes *operations on breast (85.0-85.99)*

④ **34.0 Incision of chest wall and pleura**
Excludes *that as operative approach - omit code*

✗ **34.01 Incision of chest wall**
Extrapleural drainage
Excludes *incision of pleura (34.09)*
AHA: 3Q 2000, 12; 1Q 1992, 13

✓ **34.02 Exploratory thoracotomy**

✓ **34.03 Reopening of recent thoracotomy site**

✗ **34.04 Insertion of intercostal catheter for drainage**
Chest tube
Closed chest drainage
Revision of intercostal catheter (chest tube) (with lysis of adhesions)
Excludes ▶*thoracoscopic drainage of pleural cavity (34.06)*◀
AHA: 2Q 2003, 7; 2Q 1999, 12; 1Q 1999, 9; 1Q 1992, 12

✗ **34.05 Creation of pleuroperitoneal shunt**
AHA: 4Q 1994, 50

●✓ **34.06 Thoracoscopic drainage of pleural cavity**

✗ **34.09 Other incision of pleura**
Creation of pleural window for drainage
Intercostal stab
Open chest drainage
Excludes *thoracoscopy (34.21)*
thoracotomy for collapse of lung (33.32)
AHA: 3Q 2002, 22, 27; 1Q 1994, 7

✓ **34.1 Incision of mediastinum**
Excludes *mediastinoscopy (34.22)*
mediastinotomy associated with pneumonectomy (32.5)

④ **34.2 Diagnostic procedures on chest wall, pleura, mediastinum, and diaphragm**

●✓ **34.20 Thoracoscopic pleural biopsy**

✓ **34.21 Transpleural thoracoscopy**
AHA: 3Q 2002, 27

✓ **34.22 Mediastinoscopy**
Code also any lymph node biopsy (40.11)

✗ **34.23 Biopsy of chest wall**

▲✗ **34.24 Other pleural biopsy**
Excludes ▶*thoracoscopic pleural biopsy (34.20)*◀
AHA: 3Q 2002, 22, 27; 1Q 1992, 14

✗⓪ **34.25 Closed [percutaneous] [needle] biopsy of mediastinum**

✓Ⓞ **34.26 Open mediastinal biopsy**

✓ **34.27 Biopsy of diaphragm**

✓ **34.28 Other diagnostic procedures on chest wall, pleura, and diaphragm**
Excludes *angiocardiography (88.50-88.58)*
aortography (88.42)
arteriography of:
intrathoracic vessels NEC (88.44)
pulmonary arteries (88.43)
microscopic examination of specimen from chest wall, pleura, and diaphragm (90.41-90.49)
phlebography of:
intrathoracic vessels NEC (88.63)
pulmonary veins (88.62)
radiological examinations of thorax:
C.A.T. scan (87.41)
diaphragmatic x-ray (87.49)
intrathoracic lymphangiogram (87.34)
routine chest x-ray (87.44)
sinogram of chest wall (87.38)
soft tissue x-ray of chest wall NEC (87.39)
tomogram of thorax NEC (87.42)
ultrasonography of thorax (88.73)

✓ **34.29 Other diagnostic procedures on mediastinum**
Excludes *mediastinal:*
pneumogram (87.33)
x-ray NEC (87.49)

✓ **34.3 Excision or destruction of lesion or tissue of mediastinum**
Excludes *biopsy of mediastinum (34.25-34.26)*
mediastinal fistulectomy (34.73)

✓ **34.4 Excision or destruction of lesion of chest wall**
Excision of lesion of chest wall NOS (with excision of ribs)
Excludes *biopsy of chest wall (34.23)*
costectomy not incidental to thoracic procedure (77.91)
excision of lesion of:
breast (85.20-85.25)
cartilage (80.89)
skin (86.2-86.3)
fistulectomy (34.73)

④ **34.5 Pleurectomy**

✓ **34.51 Decortication of lung**
Excludes *thoracoscopic decortication of lung (34.52)*

●✓ **34.52 Thoracoscopic decortication of lung**

✓ **34.59 Other excision of pleura**
Excision of pleural lesion
Excludes *biopsy of pleura (34.24)*
pleural fistulectomy (34.73)

✓ **34.6 Scarification of pleura**
Pleurosclerosis
Excludes *injection of sclerosing agent (34.92)*

④ **34.7 Repair of chest wall**

✗ **34.71 Suture of laceration of chest wall**
Excludes *suture of skin and subcutaneous tissue alone (86.59)*

✗ **34.72 Closure of thoracostomy**

✓ **34.73 Closure of other fistula of thorax**
Closure of:
bronchopleural fistula
bronchopleurocutaneous fistula
bronchopleuromediastinal fistula

✓ **34.74 Repair of pectus deformity**
Repair of:
pectus carinatum (with implant)
pectus excavatum (with implant)
AHA: 2Q 2004, 6

✓ **34.79 Other repair of chest wall**
Repair of chest wall NOS
AHA: 2Q 2004, 6; Jan-Feb 1987, 13

34.8 Operations on diaphragm

34.81 Excision of lesion or tissue of diaphragm
Excludes *biopsy of diaphragm (34.27)*

34.82 Suture of laceration of diaphragm

34.83 Closure of fistula of diaphragm
Thoracicoabdominal fistulectomy
Thoracicogastric fistulectomy
Thoracicointestinal fistulectomy

34.84 Other repair of diaphragm
Excludes *repair of diaphragmatic hernia (53.7-53.82)*

34.85 Implantation of diaphragmatic pacemaker

34.89 Other operations on diaphragm

34.9 Other operations on thorax

34.91 Thoracentesis
DEF: Needle puncture of chest wall and pleural cavity for fluid aspiration.
AHA: Sep-Oct 1985, 6

34.92 Injection into thoracic cavity
Chemical pleurodesis
Injection of cytotoxic agent or tetracycline
Instillation into thoracic cavity
Requires additional code for any cancer chemotherapeutic substance (99.25)
Excludes *that for collapse of lung (33.32)*
AHA: 1Q 1992, 12; 2Q 1989, 17

34.93 Repair of pleura

34.99 Other
Excludes *removal of:*
mediastinal drain (97.42)
sutures (97.43)
thoracotomy tube (97.41)
AHA: 1Q 2000, 17; 1Q 1988, 9

7. OPERATIONS ON THE CARDIOVASCULAR SYSTEM (35-39)

OPERATIONS ON VALVES AND SEPTA OF HEART (35)

Includes sternotomy (median) (transverse) as operative approach
thoracotomy as operative approach
Code also cardiopulmonary bypass [extracorporeal circulation] [heart-lung machine] (39.61)

35.0 Closed heart valvotomy
Excludes *percutaneous (balloon) valvuloplasty (35.96)*

35.00 Closed heart valvotomy, unspecified valve

35.01 Closed heart valvotomy, aortic valve

35.02 Closed heart valvotomy, mitral valve

35.03 Closed heart valvotomy, pulmonary valve
AHA: Nov-Dec 1985, 10

35.04 Closed heart valvotomy, tricuspid valve

35.1 Open heart valvuloplasty without replacement
Includes open heart valvotomy
Code also cardiopulmonary bypass if performed [extracorporeal circulation] [heart-lung machine] (39.61)
Excludes *that associated with repair of:*
endocardial cushion defect (35.54, 35.63, 35.73)
valvular defect associated with atrial and ventricular septal defects (35.54, 35.63, 35.73)
percutaneous (balloon) valvuloplasty (35.96)

35.10 Open heart valvuloplasty without replacement, unspecified valve

35.11 Open heart valvuloplasty of aortic valve without replacement

35.12 Open heart valvuloplasty of mitral valve without replacement
AHA: 1Q 1997, 13

35.13 Open heart valvuloplasty of pulmonary valve without replacement

35.14 Open heart valvuloplasty of tricuspid valve without replacement

35.2 Replacement of heart valve
Includes excision of heart valve with replacement
Code also cardiopulmonary bypass [extracorporeal circulation] [heart-lung machine] (39.61)
Excludes *that associated with repair of:*
endocardial cushion defect (35.54, 35.63, 35.73)
valvular defect associated with atrial and ventricular septal defects (35.54, 35.63, 35.73)

35.20 Replacement of unspecified heart valve
Repair of unspecified heart valve with tissue graft or prosthetic implant

35.21 Replacement of aortic valve with tissue graft
Repair of aortic valve with tissue graft (autograft) (heterograft) (homograft)
AHA: 2Q 1997, 8

35.22 Other replacement of aortic valve
Repair of aortic valve with replacement:
NOS
prosthetic (partial) (synthetic) (total)
AHA: 1Q 1996, 11

35.23 Replacement of mitral valve with tissue graft
Repair of mitral valve with tissue graft (autograft) (heterograft) (homograft)

35.24 Other replacement of mitral valve
Repair of mitral valve with replacement:
NOS
prosthetic (partial) (synthetic) (total)
AHA: 4Q 1997, 55

✓ **35.25 Replacement of pulmonary valve with tissue graft**
Repair of pulmonary valve with tissue graft (autograft) (heterograft) (homograft)
AHA: 1Q 2004, 16; 2Q 1997, 8

✓ **35.26 Other replacement of pulmonary valve**
Repair of pulmonary valve with replacement:
NOS
prosthetic (partial) (synthetic) (total)

✓ **35.27 Replacement of tricuspid valve with tissue graft**
Repair of tricuspid valve with tissue graft (autograft) (heterograft) (homograft)

✓ **35.28 Other replacement of tricuspid valve**
Repair of tricuspid valve with replacement:
NOS
prosthetic (partial) (synthetic) (total)

❹ **35.3 Operations on structures adjacent to heart valves**
Code also cardiopulmonary bypass [extracorporeal circulation] [heart-lung machine] (39.61)

✓ **35.31 Operations on papillary muscle**
Division of papillary muscle
Reattachment of papillary muscle
Repair of papillary muscle

✓ **35.32 Operations on chordae tendineae**
Division of chordae tendineae
Repair of chordae tendineae

✓ **35.33 Annuloplasty**
Plication of annulus
DEF: Repair of a cardiac valve by tightening the circumference of its ring.
AHA: 1Q 1997, 13; 1Q 1988, 10

✓ **35.34 Infundibulectomy**
Right ventricular infundibulectomy

✓ **35.35 Operations on trabeculae carneae cordis**
Division of trabeculae carneae cordis
Excision of trabeculae carneae cordis
Excision of aortic subvalvular ring

✓ **35.39 Operations on other structures adjacent to valves of heart**
Repair of sinus of Valsalva (aneurysm)

❹ **35.4 Production of septal defect in heart**

✗ **35.41 Enlargement of existing atrial septal defect**
Rashkind procedure
Septostomy (atrial) (balloon)

✓ **35.42 Creation of septal defect in heart**
Blalock-Hanlon operation

❹ **35.5 Repair of atrial and ventricular septa with prosthesis**
Includes repair of septa with synthetic implant or patch
Code also cardiopulmonary bypass [extracorporeal circulation] [heart-lung machine] (39.61)

✓▼ **35.50 Repair of unspecified septal defect of heart with prosthesis**
Excludes *that associated with repair of:*
endocardial cushion defect (35.54)
septal defect associated with valvular defect (35.54)

✓ **35.51 Repair of atrial septal defect with prosthesis, open technique**
Atrioseptoplasty with prosthesis
Correction of atrial septal defect with prosthesis
Repair:
foramen ovale (patent)
with prosthesis ostium secundum defect with prosthesis
Excludes *that associated with repair of:*
atrial septal defect associated with valvular and ventricular septal defects (35.54)
endocardial cushion defect (35.54)

✓ **35.52 Repair of atrial septal defect with prosthesis, closed technique**
Insertion of atrial septal umbrella [King-Mills]
AHA: 2Q 2005, 17-18; 3Q 1998, 11

✓ **35.53 Repair of ventricular septal defect with prosthesis, open technique**
Correction of ventricular septal defect with prosthesis
Repair of supracristal defect with prosthesis
Excludes *that associated with repair of:*
endocardial cushion defect (35.54)
ventricular defect associated with valvular and atrial septal defects (35.54)

✓ **35.54 Repair of endocardial cushion defect with prosthesis**
Repair:
atrioventricular canal with prosthesis (grafted to septa)
ostium primum defect with prosthesis (grafted to septa)
valvular defect associated with atrial and ventricular septal defects with prosthesis (grafted to septa)
Excludes *repair of isolated:*
atrial septal defect (35.51-35.52)
valvular defect (35.20, 35.22, 35.24, 35.26, 35.28)
ventricular septal defect (35.53)

✓ **35.55 Repair of ventricular septal defect with prosthesis, closed technique**

❹ **35.6 Repair of atrial and ventricular septa with tissue graft**
Code also cardiopulmonary bypass [extracorporeal circulation] [heart-lung machine] (39.61)

✓▼ **35.60 Repair of unspecified septal defect of heart with tissue graft**
Excludes *that associated with repair of:*
endocardial cushion defect (35.63)
septal defect associated withvalvular defect (35.63)

✓ **35.61 Repair of atrial septal defect with tissue graft**
Atrioseptoplasty with tissue graft
Correction of atrial septal defect with tissue graft
Repair:
foramen ovale (patent) with tissue graft
ostium secundum defect with tissue graft
Excludes *that associated with repair of:*
atrial septal defect associated with valvular and ventricular septal defects (35.63)
endocardial cushion defect (35.63)

✓ **35.62 Repair of ventricular septal defect with tissue graft**
Correction of ventricular septal defect with tissue graft
Repair of supracristal defect with tissue graft
Excludes *that associated with repair of:*
endocardial cushion defect (35.63)
ventricular defect associate with valvular and atrial septal defects (35.63)

✓ **35.63 Repair of endocardial cushion defect with tissue graft**
Repair of:
atrioventricular canal with tissue graft
ostium primum defect with tissue graft
valvular defect associated with atrial and ventricular septal defects with tissue graft
Excludes *repair of isolated:*
atrial septal defect (35.61)
valvular defect (35.20-35.21, 35.23, 35.25, 35.27)
ventricular septal defect (35.62)

❹ **35.7 Other and unspecified repair of atrial and ventricular septa**
Code also cardiopulmonary bypass [extracorporeal circulation] [heart-lung machine] (39.61)

✓▼ **35.70 Other and unspecified repair of unspecified septal defect of heart**
Repair of septal defect NOS
Excludes *that associated with repair of:*
endocardial cushion defect (35.73)
septal defect associated with valvular defect (35.73)

✓ **35.71 Other and unspecified repair of atrial septal defect**
Repair NOS:
atrial septum
foramen ovale (patent)
ostium secundum defect
Excludes *that associated with repair of:*
atrial septal defect associated with valvular ventricular septal defects (35.73)
endocardial cushion defect (35.73)

✓ **35.72 Other and unspecified repair of ventricular septal defect**
Repair NOS:
supracristal defect
ventricular septum
Excludes *that associated with repair of:*
endocardial cushion defect (35.73)
ventricular septal defect associated with valvular and atrial septal defects (35.73)

✓ **35.73 Other and unspecified repair of endocardial cushion defect**
Repair NOS:
atrioventricular canal
ostium primum defect
valvular defect associated with atrial and ventricular septal defects
Excludes *repair of isolated:*
atrial septal defect (35.71)
valvular defect (35.20, 35.22, 35.24, 35.26, 35.28)
ventricular septal defect (35.72)

35.8 Total repair of certain congenital cardiac anomalies
Note: *For partial repair of defect [e.g. repair of atrial septal defect in tetralogy of Fallot] - code to specific procedure*

✓ **35.81 Total repair of tetralogy of Fallot**
One-stage total correction of tetralogy of Fallot with or without:
commissurotomy of pulmonary valve
infundibulectomy
outflow tract prosthesis
patch graft of outflow tract
prosthetic tube for pulmonary artery
repair of ventricular septal defect (with prosthesis)
take-down of previous systemic-pulmonary artery anastomosis

✓ **35.82 Total repair of total anomalous pulmonary venous connection**
One-stage total correction of total anomalous pulmonary venous connection with or without:
anastomosis between (horizontal) common pulmonary trunk and posterior wall of left atrium (side-to-side)
enlargement of foramen ovale
incision [excision] of common wall between posterior left atrium and coronary sinus and roofing of resultant defect with patch graft (synthetic)
ligation of venous connection (descending anomalous vein) (to left innominate vein) (to superior vena cava)
repair of atrial septal defect (with prosthesis)

✓ **35.83 Total repair of truncus arteriosus**
One-stage total correction of truncus arteriosus with or without:
construction (with aortic homograft) (with prosthesis) of a pulmonary artery placed from right ventricle to arteries supplying the lung
ligation of connections between aorta and pulmonary artery
repair of ventricular septal defect (with prosthesis)

✓ **35.84 Total correction of transposition of great vessels, not elsewhere classified**
Arterial switch operation [Jatene]
Total correction of transposition of great arteries at the arterial level by switching the great arteries, including the left or both coronary arteries, implanted in the wall of the pulmonary artery
Excludes *baffle operation [Mustard] [Senning] (35.91)*
creation of shunt between right ventricle and pulmonary artery [Rastelli] (35.92)

35.9 Other operations on valves and septa of heart
Code also cardiopulmonary bypass, if performed [extracorporeal circulation] [heart-lung machine] (39.61)

✓ **35.91 Interatrial transposition of venous return**
Baffle:
atrial
interatrial
Mustard's operation
Resection of atrial septum and insertion of patch to direct systemic venous return to tricuspid valve and pulmonary venousreturn to mitral valve

✓ **35.92 Creation of conduit between right ventricle and pulmonary artery**
Creation of shunt between right ventricle and (distal) pulmonary artery
Excludes *that associated with total repair of truncus arteriosus (35.83)*

✓ **35.93 Creation of conduit between left ventricle and aorta**
Creation of apicoaortic shunt
Shunt between apex of left ventricle and aorta

✓ **35.94 Creation of conduit between atrium and pulmonary artery**
Fontan procedure

✓ **35.95 Revision of corrective procedure on heart**
Replacement of prosthetic heart valve poppet
Resuture of prosthesis of:
septum
valve
Excludes *complete revision-code to specific procedure*
replacement of prosthesis or graft of:
septum (35.50-35.63)
valve (35.20-35.28)

✓ **35.96 Percutaneous valvuloplasty**
Percutaneous balloon valvuloplasty
AHA: 3Q 2004, 10

✓ **35.98 Other operations on septa of heart**

✓ **35.99 Other operations on valves of heart**

OPERATIONS ON VESSELS OF HEART (36)

Includes sternotomy (median) (transverse) as operative approach
thoracotomy as operative approach
Code also any:
cardiopulmonary bypass, if performed [extracorporeal circulation] [heart-lung machine] (39.61)
injection or infusion of platelet inhibitor (99.20)
injection or infusion of thrombolytic agent (99.10)

36.0 Removal of coronary artery obstruction and insertion of stent(s)
AHA: 2Q 1990, 24; Jul-Aug 1985, 8

✓ **36.03 Open chest coronary artery angioplasty**
Coronary (artery):
endarterectomy (with patch graft)
thromboendarterectomy (with patch graft)
Open surgery for direct relief of coronary artery obstruction
Code also any:
insertion of drug-eluting coronary stent(s) (36.07)
insertion of non-drug-eluting coronary stent(s) (36.06)
number of vascular stents inserted (00.45-00.48)
number of vessels treated (00.40-00.43)
procedure on vessel bifurcation (00.44)
Excludes *that with coronary artery bypass graft (36.10-36.19)*
AHA: 3Q 1993, 7

Operations on the Cardiovascular System 35.71 – 36.03

✖ **36.04 Intracoronary artery thrombolytic infusion**
That by direct coronary artery injection, infusion, or catheterization:
enzyme infusion
platelet inhibitor
Excludes *infusion of platelet inhibitor (99.20)*
infusion of thrombolytic agent (99.10)
that associated with any procedure in 36.03

✖ **36.06 Insertion of non-drug-eluting coronary artety stent(s)**
Bare stent(s)
Bonded stent(s)
Drug-coated stent(s), i.e. heparin coated
Endograft(s)
Endovascular graft(s)
Stent grafts
Code also any:
number of vascular stents inserted (00.45-00.48)
number of vessels treated (00.40-00.43)
open chest coronary artery angioplasty (36.03)
percutaneous transluminal coronary angioplasty [PTCA] or coronary atherectomy (00.66)
procedure on vessel bifurcation (00.44)
Excludes *insertion of drug-eluting coronary artery stent(s) (36.07)*

✔ **36.07 Insertion of drug-eluting coronary artery stent(s)**
Endograft(s)
Endovascular graft(s)
Stent graft(s)
Code also any:
number of vascular stents inserted (00.45-00.48)
number of vessels treated (00.40-00.43)
open chest coronary artery angioplasty (36.03)
percutaneous transluminal coronary angioplasty [PTCA] or coronary atherectomy (00.66)
procedure on vessel bifurcation (00.44)
Excludes *drug-coated stents, e.g., heparin coated (36.06)*
insertion of non-drug-eluting coronary artery stent(s) (36.06)
AHA: 4Q 2005, 105, 106

✔ **36.09 Other removal of coronary artery obstruction**
Coronary angioplasty NOS
Code also any:
number of vascular stents inserted (00.45-00.48)
number of vessels treated (00.40-00.43)
procedure on vessel bifurcation (00.44)
Excludes *that by open angioplasty (36.03)*
that by percutaneous transluminal coronary angioplasty [PTCA] or coronary atherectomy (00.66)

❹ **36.1 Bypass anastomosis for heart revascularization**
Note: Do not assign codes from series 00.40-00.43 with codes from series 36.10-36.19
Code also:
cardiopulmonary bypass [extracorporeal circulation] [heart-lung machine] (39.61)
pressurized treatment of venous bypass graft [conduit] with pharmaceutical substance, if performed (00.16)
AHA: 3Q 1993, 7; 2Q 1990, 24; 1Q 1989, 8

✔▼ **36.10 Aortocoronary bypass for heart revascularization, not otherwise specified**
Direct revascularization:
cardiac with catheter stent, prosthesis, or vein graft
coronary with catheter stent, prosthesis, or vein graft
heart muscle with catheter stent, prosthesis, or vein graft
myocardial with catheter stent, prosthesis, or vein graft
Heart revascularization NOS
AHA: 4Q 1989, 3-5

✔ **36.11 (Aorto)coronary bypass of one coronary artery**
AHA: 3Q 2002, 4-9; 2Q 1996, 6-8; 4Q 1989, 3-5

✔ **36.12 (Aorto)coronary bypass of two coronary arteries**
AHA: 3Q 2002, 4-9; 4Q 1999, 15-16; 2Q 1996, 6-8; 1Q 1991, 7-9; 4Q 1989, 3-5

✔ **36.13 (Aorto)coronary bypass of three coronary arteries**
AHA: 3Q 2002, 4-9; 2Q 1996, 6-8; 1Q 1991, 7-9; 4Q 1989, 3-5

✔ **36.14 (Aorto)coronary bypass of four or more coronary arteries**
AHA: 3Q 2002, 4-9; 2Q 1996, 6-8; 1Q 1991, 7-9; 4Q 1989, 3-5

✔ **36.15 Single internal mammary-coronary artery bypass**
Anastomosis (single):
mammary artery to coronary artery
thoracic artery to coronary artery
AHA: 3Q 2002, 4-9; 4Q 1999, 15-16; 2Q 1996, 6-8; 1Q 1991, 7-9; 3Q 1990, 12; 4Q 1989, 3-5

Coronary artery bypass

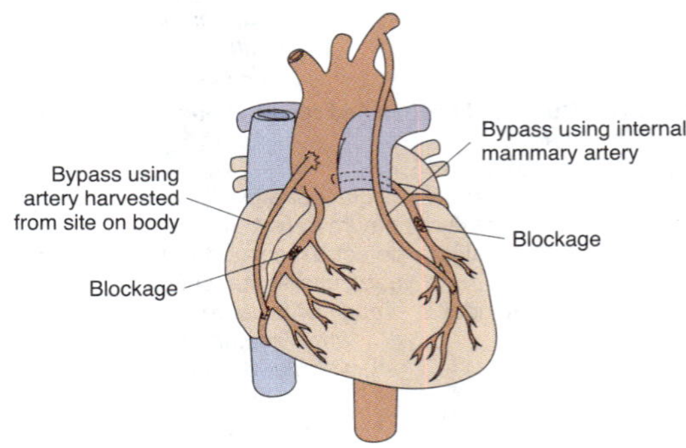

✔ **36.16 Double internal mammary-coronary artery bypass**
Anastomosis, double:
mammary artery to coronary artery
thoracic artery to coronary artery
AHA: 3Q 2002, 4-9; 2Q 1996, 6-8; 4Q 1989, 3-5

✔ **36.17 Abdominal-coronary artery bypass**
Anastomosis:
gastroepiploic-coronary artery
AHA: 3Q 1997, 13

✔ **36.19 Other bypass anastomosis for heart revascularization**
AHA: 2Q 1996, 6-8

✔ **36.2 Heart revascularization by arterial implant**
Implantation of:
aortic branches [ascending aortic branches] into heart muscle
blood vessels into myocardium
internal mammary artery [internal thoracic artery] into:
heart muscle
myocardium
ventricle
ventricular wall
Indirect heart revascularization NOS

❹ **36.3 Other heart revascularization**

✔ **36.31 Open chest transmyocardial revascularization**

✔ **36.32 Other transmyocardial revascularization**
AHA: 4Q 1998, 74

✔ **36.33 Endoscopic transmyocardial revascularization**
Robot-assisted transmyocardial revascularization
Thoracoscopic transmyocardial revascularization

✔ **36.34 Percutaneous transmyocardial revascularization**
Endovascular transmyocardial revascularization

✔ **36.39 Other heart revascularization**
Abrasion of epicardium
Cardio-omentopexy
Intrapericardial poudrage
Myocardial graft:
mediastinal fat
omentum
pectoral muscles

❹ **36.9 Other operations on vessels of heart**
Code also cardiopulmonary bypass [extracorporeal circulation] [heart-lung machine] (39.61)

✔ **36.91 Repair of aneurysm of coronary vessel**

✔ **36.99 Other operations on vessels of heart**
Exploration of coronary artery
Incision of coronary artery
Ligation of coronary artery
Repair of arteriovenous fistula
AHA: 3Q 2003, 18

OTHER OPERATIONS ON HEART AND PERICARDIUM (37)

Code also any injection or infusion of platelet inhibitor (99.20)

✖ **37.0 Pericardiocentesis**

❹ **37.1 Cardiotomy and pericardiotomy**
Code also cardiopulmonary bypass [extracorporeal circulation] [heart-lung machine] (39.61)

✔▼ **37.10 Incision of heart, not otherwise specified**
Cardiolysis NOS
DEF: Cardiolysis: surgical freeing of the heart and pericardium in adhesive mediastinopericarditis.

✔ **37.11 Cardiotomy**
Incision of:
- atrium
- endocardium
- myocardium
- ventricle

✔ **37.12 Pericardiotomy**
Pericardial window operation
Pericardiolysis
Pericardiotomy
DEF: Pericardial window: creation of an opening in the heart's lining for drainage.

❹ **37.2 Diagnostic procedures on heart and pericardium**

✖ **37.20 Noninvasive programmed electrical stimulation [NIPS]**
Excludes *that as part of intraoperative testing - omit code*
catheter based invasive electrophysiologic testing (37.26)
device interrogation only without arrhythmia induction (bedside check) (89.45-89.49)

✖ **37.21 Right heart cardiac catheterization**
Cardiac catheterization NOS
Excludes *that with catheterization of left heart (37.23)*
AHA: 3Q 2004, 10; 3Q 2003, 9; May-Jun 1987, 11; Sep-Oct 1985, 3; Jul-Aug 1984, 12

✖ **37.22 Left heart cardiac catheterization**
Excludes *that with catheterization of right heart (37.23)*
AHA: 3Q 2005, 15; 3Q 2004, 10; May-Jun 1987, 11; Sep-Oct 1985, 3

✖ **37.23 Combined right and left heart cardiac catheterization**
AHA: 2Q 2005, 17-18; 3Q 2004, 10; 1Q 2000, 20; 3Q 1998, 11; 1Q 1996, 7; May-Jun 1987, 11; Sep-Oct 1985, 3

✔ **37.24 Biopsy of pericardium**

✖ **37.25 Biopsy of heart**
AHA: 3Q 2003, 16; 3Q 1994, 7

✖ **37.26 Catheter based invasive electrophysiologic testing**
Electrophysiologic studies [EPS]
Code also any concomitant procedure
Excludes *that as part of intraoperative testing - omit code*
device interrogation only without arrhythmia induction (bedside check) (89.45-89.49)
His bundle recording (37.29)
noninvasive programmed electrical stimulation (NIPS) (37.20)
AHA: 3Q 2003, 23; 1Q 2002, 8; 1Q 1999, 3; 2Q 1997, 10; 3Q 1990, 12

✖ **37.27 Cardiac mapping**
Code also any concomitant procedure
Excludes *electrocardiogram (89.52)*
His bundle recording (37.29)

✖ **37.28 Intracardiac echocardiography**
Echocardiography of heart chambers
ICE
Code also any synchronous Doppler flow mapping (88.72)
Excludes *intravascular imaging of coronary vessels (intravascular ultrasound) (IVUS) (00.24)*
AHA: 4Q 2001, 62

✖ **37.29 Other diagnostic procedures on heart and pericardium**
Excludes *angiocardiography (88.50-88.58)*
cardiac function tests (89.41-89.69)
cardiovascular radioisotopic scan and function study (92.05)
coronary arteriography (88.55-88.57)
diagnostic pericardiocentesis (37.0)
diagnostic ultrasound of heart (88.72)
x-ray of heart (87.49)
AHA: Sep-Oct 1987, 3-5; Sep-Oct 1985, 3

❹ **37.3 Pericardiectomy and excision of lesion of heart**
Code also cardiopulmonary bypass [extracorporeal circulation] [heart-lung machine] (39.61)

✔ **37.31 Pericardiectomy**
Excision of:
- adhesions of pericardium constricting scar of:
  - epicardium
  - pericardium

✔ **37.32 Excision of aneurysm of heart**
Repair of aneurysm of heart

✔ **37.33 Excision or destruction of other lesion or tissue of heart, open approach**
Ablation of heart tissue (cryoablation) (electrocurrent) (laser) (microwave) (radiofrequency) (resection), open chest approach
Cox-maze procedure
Maze procedure
Modified maze procedure, transthoracic approach
Excludes *ablation, excision or destruction of lesion or tissue of heart, endovascular approach (37.34)*
DEF: Maze procedure: surgical division or destruction of aberrant conduction pathways in the heart between the sinoatrial node and atrioventricular node.
AHA: 4Q 2003, 93; 2Q 1994, 12

✔ **37.34 Excision or destruction of other lesion or tissue of heart, other approach**
Ablation of heart tissue (cryoablation) (electrocurrent) (laser) (microwave) (radiofrequency) (resection), via peripherally inserted catheter
Modified maze procedure, endovascular approach
AHA: 4Q 2003, 94; 1Q 2000, 20

✔ **37.35 Partial ventriculectomy**
Ventricular reduction surgery
Ventricular remodeling
Code also any synchronous:
- mitral valve repair (35.02, 35.12)
- mitral valve replacement (35.23-35.24)

AHA: 4Q 1997, 55

❹ **37.4 Repair of heart and pericardium**

✔ **37.41 Implantation of prosthetic cardiac support device around the heart**
Cardiac support device (CSD)
Epicardial support device
Fabric (textile) (mesh) device
Ventricular support device on surface of heart
Excludes *circulatory assist systems (37.61-37.68)*
Code also any:
- cardiopulmonary bypass [extracorporeal circulation] [heart-lung machine] if performed (39.61)
- mitral valve repair (35.02, 35.12)
- mitral valve replacement (35.23-35.24)
- transesophageal echocardiography (88.72)

AHA: 4Q 2005, 120

✔ **37.49 Other repair of heart and pericardium**

✖ Deleted Code ▼ Nonspecific O.R. Procedure ✔ Valid O.R. Procedure ✖ Non-O.R. Procedure ♂ Male ♀ Female

37.5 Heart replacement procedures

37.51 Heart transplantation

Excludes *combined heart-lung transplantation (33.6)*

AHA: 2Q 2005, 15

37.52 Implantation of total replacement heart system

Artificial heart

Implantation of fully implantable total replacement heart system, including ventriculectomy

Excludes *implantation of heart assist system [VAD](37.62, 37.65, 37.66)*

37.53 Replacement or repair of thoracic unit of total replacement heart system

Excludes *replacement and repair of heart assist system [VAD](37.63)*

37.54 Replacement of repair of other implantable component of total replacement heart system

Implantable battery

Implantable controller

Trancutaneous energy transfer [TET] device

Excludes *replacement and repair of heart assist system [VAD](37.63)*
replacement or repair of thoracic unit of total replacement heart system (37.53)

37.6 Implantation of heart and circulatory assist system

Excludes *implantation of prosthetic cardiac support system (37.41)*

37.61 Implant of pulsation balloon

AHA: 3Q 2005, 15

37.62 Insertion of non-implantable heart assist system

Insertion of heart assist system, NOS

Insertion of heart pump

Excludes *implantation of total replacement heart system (37.52)*
insertion of percutaneous external heart assist device (37.68)

AHA: 2Q 1990, 25

37.63 Repair of heart assist system

Replacement of parts of an existing ventricular assist device (VAD)

Excludes *replacement or repair of other implantable component of total replacement heart system [artificial heart](37.54)*
replacement or repair of thoracic unit of total replacement heart system [artificial heart](37.53)

37.64 Removal of heart assist system

Excludes *explantation [removal] of percutaneous external heart assist device (97.44)*
nonoperative removal of heart assist system (97.44)
that with replacement of implant (37.63)

37.65 Implant of external heart assist system

Note: *Device (outside the body but connected to heart) with external circulation and pump*

Includes open chest (sternotomy) procedure for cannulae attachments

Excludes *implant of pulsation balloon (37.61)*
implantation of total replacement heart system (37.52)
insertion of percutaneous external heart assist device (37.68)

37.66 Insertion of implantable heart assist system

Note: *Device directly connected to the heart and implanted in the upper left quadrant of peritoneal cavity*

Note: *This device can be used for either destination therapy (DT) or bridge-to-transplant (BTT)*

Axial flow heart assist system

Diagonal pump heart assist system

Left ventricular assist device (LVAD)

Pulsatile heart assist system

Right ventricular assist device (RVAD)

Rotary pump heart assist system

Transportable, implantable heart assist system

Ventricular assist device (VAD) not otherwise specified

Excludes *implant of pulsation balloon (37.61)*
implantation of total replacement heart system [artificial heart](37.52)
insertion of percutaneous external heart assist device (37.68)

AHA: 4Q 2003, 116; 1Q 1998, 8

37.67 Implantation of cardiomyostimulation system

Note: *Two-step open procedure consisting of transfer of one end of the latissimus dorsi muscle; wrapping it around the heart; rib resection; implantation of epicardial cardiac pacing leads into the right ventricle; tunneling and pocket creation for the cardiomyostimulator.*

AHA: 4Q 1998, 75

37.68 Insertion of percutaneous external heart assist device

Circulatory assist device

Extrinsic heart assist device

pVAD

Percutaneous heart assist device

Includes percutaneous [femoral] insertion of cannulae attachments

37.7 Insertion, revision, replacement, and removal of leads; insertion of temporary pacemaker system; or revision of cardiac device pocket

Code also any insertion and replacement of pacemaker device (37.80-37.87)

Excludes *implantation or replacement of transvenous lead [electrode] into left ventricular cardiac venous system (00.52)*

37.70 Initial insertion of lead [electrode], not otherwise specified

Excludes *insertion of temporary transvenous pacemaker system (37.78)*
replacement of atrial and/or ventricular lead(s) (37.76)

AHA: May-Jun 1987, 5, 7

37.71 Initial insertion of transvenous lead [electrode] into ventricle

Excludes *insertion of temporary transvenous pacemaker system (37.78)*
replacement of atrial and/or ventricular lead(s) (37.76)

AHA: Sep-Oct 1987, 12; May-Jun 1987, 4, 5, 7; Sep-Oct 1985, 3

37.72 Initial insertion of transvenous leads [electrodes] into atrium and ventricle

Excludes *insertion of temporary transvenous pacemaker system (37.78)*
replacement of atrial and/or ventricular lead(s) (37.76)

AHA: 2Q 1997, 4; Sep-Oct 1987, 12; May-Jun 1987, 4, 5, 7; Sep-Oct 1985, 3

37.73 Initial insertion of transvenous lead [electrode] into atrium

Excludes *insertion of temporary transvenous pacemaker system (37.78)*
replacement of atrial and/or ventricular lead(s) (37.76)

AHA: May-Jun 1987, 4, 5, 7

✔ **37.74 Insertion or replacement of epicardial lead [electrode] into epicardium**
Insertion or replacement of epicardial by:
sternotomy
thoracotomy
Excludes *replacement of atrial and/or ventricular lead(s) (37.76)*
AHA: 3Q 2005, 4, 6, 7; May-Jun 1987, 4, 5

✔ **37.75 Revision of lead [electrode]**
Repair of electrode [removal with re-insertion]
Repositioning of lead(s) (AICD) (cardiac device) (CRT-D) (CRT-P) (defibrillator) (pacemaker) (pacing) (sensing) [electrode]
Revision of lead NOS
Excludes *repositioning of temporary transvenous pacemaker system - omit code*
AHA: 3Q 2005, 8; 2Q 1999, 11

✔ **37.76 Replacement of transvenous atrial and/or ventricular lead(s) [electrode]**
Removal or abandonment of existing transvenous or epicardial lead(s) with transvenous lead(s) replacement
Excludes *replacement of epicardial lead [electrode] (37.74)*
AHA: 3Q 2005, 4; May-Jun 1987, 4

✔ **37.77 Removal of lead(s) [electrode] without replacement**
Removal:
epicardial lead (transthoracic approach)
transvenous lead(s)
Excludes *removal of temporary transvenous pacemaker system - omit code*
that with replacement of:
atrial and/or ventricular lead(s) [electrode] (37.76)
epicardial lead [electrode] (37.74)
AHA: May-Jun 1987, 5, 7

✖ **37.78 Insertion of temporary transvenous pacemaker system**
Excludes *intraoperative cardiac pacemaker (39.64)*
AHA: 4Q 1993, 33

✔ **37.79 Revision or relocation of cardiac device pocket**
Debridement and reforming pocket (skin and subcutaneous tissue)
Insertion of loop recorder
Relocation of pocket [creation of new pocket] pacemaker or CRT-P
Removal of cardiac device/pulse generator without replacement
Removal of the implantable hemodynamic pressure sensor (lead) and monitor device
Removal without replacement of cardiac resynchronization defibrillator device
Repositioning of implantable hemodynamic pressure sensor (lead) and monitor device
Repositioning of pulse generator
Revision of cardioverter/defibrillator (automatic) pocket
Revision of pocket for intracardiac hemodynamic monitoring
Revision or relocation of CRT-D pocket
Revision or relocation of pacemaker, defibrillator, or other implanted cardiac device pocket
Excludes *removal of loop recorder (86.05)*
AHA: 3Q 2005, 6; 2Q 1994, 10; May-Jun 1987, 6, 7

❹ **37.8 Insertion, replacement, removal, and revision of pacemaker device**
Note: *Device testing during procedure - omit code*
Code also any lead insertion, lead replacement, lead removal and/or lead revision (37.70-37.77)
Excludes *implantation of cardiac resynchronization pacemaker [CRT-P] (00.50)*
implantation or replacement of cardiac resynchronization pacemaker pulse generator only [CRT-P] (00.53)

✔ **37.80 Insertion of permanent pacemaker, initial or replacement, type of device not specified**
AHA: May-Jun 1987, 7

✖ **37.81 Initial insertion of single-chamber device, not specified as rate responsive**
Excludes *replacement of existing pacemaker device (37.85-37.87)*
AHA: May-Jun 1987, 4, 5

✖ **37.82 Initial insertion of single-chamber device, rate responsive**
Rate responsive to physiologic stimuli other than atrial rate
Excludes *replacement of existing pacemaker device (37.85-37.87)*
AHA: May-Jun 1987, 4, 5

✖ **37.83 Initial insertion of dual-chamber device**
Atrial ventricular sequential device
Excludes *replacement of existing pacemaker device (37.85-37.87)*
AHA: 2Q 1997, 4; May-Jun 1987, 4, 5

✔ **37.85 Replacement of any type pacemaker device with single-chamber device, not specified as rate responsive**
AHA: May-Jun 1987, 6

✔ **37.86 Replacement of any type of pacemaker device with single-chamber device, rate responsive**
Rate responsive to physiologic stimuli other than atrial rate
AHA: May-Jun 1987, 6

✔ **37.87 Replacement of any type pacemaker device with dual-chamber device**
Atrial ventricular sequential device
AHA: May-Jun 1987, 6

✔ **37.89 Revision or removal of pacemaker device**
Removal without replacement of cardiac resynchronization pacemaker device [CRT-P]
Repair of pacemaker device
Excludes *removal of temporary transvenous pacemaker system - omit code*
replacement of existing pacemaker device (37.85-37.87)
replacement of existing pacemaker device with CRT-P pacemaker device (00.53)
AHA: Nov-Dec 1986, 1; May-Jun 1987, 7

❹ **37.9 Other operations on heart and pericardium**

✖ **37.90 Insertion of left atrial appendage device**
Left atrial filter
Left atrial occluder
Transseptal catheter technique
AHA: 4Q 2004, 121-122

✔ **37.91 Open chest cardiac massage**
Excludes *closed chest cardiac massage (99.63)*

✖ **37.92 Injection of therapeutic substance into heart**

✖ **37.93 Injection of therapeutic substance into pericardium**

✔ **37.94 Implantation or replacement of automatic cardioverter/defibrillator, total system [AICD]**
Note: *Device testing during procedure - omit code*
Implantation of defibrillator with leads (epicardial patches), formation of pocket (abdominal fascia) (subcutaneous), any transvenous leads, intraoperative procedures for evaluation of lead signals, and obtaining defibrillator threshold measurements
Techniques:
lateral thoracotomy
medial sternotomy
subxiphoid procedure
Code also extracorporeal circulation, if performed (39.61)
Code also any concomitant procedure [e.g., coronary bypass] (36.00-36.19)
Excludes *implantation of cardiac resynchronization defibrillator, total system [CRT-D] (00.51)*
AHA: 1Q 1999, 3; 3Q 1990, 12; Sep-Oct 1987, 5

✔ **37.95 Implantation of automatic cardioverter/defibrillator lead(s) only**
AHA: 3Q 1990, 12

Operations on the Cardiovascular System 37.74 – 37.95

✖ Deleted Code ▼ Nonspecific O.R. Procedure ✔ Valid O.R. Procedure ✖ Non-O.R. Procedure ♂ Male ♀ Female

✓ 37.96 Implantation of automatic cardioverter/defibrillator pulse generator only

Note: Device testing during procedure - omit code

Excludes *implantation or replacement of cardiac resynchronization defibrillator, pulse generator device only [CRT-D] (00.54)*

AHA: 3Q 1990, 12

✓ 37.97 Replacement of automatic cardioverter/defibrillator lead(s) only

Excludes *replacement of epicardial lead [electrode] into epicardium (37.74)*
replacement of transvenous lead [electrode] into left ventricular coronary venous system (00.52)

AHA: 3Q 2005, 4; 3Q 1990, 12

✓ 37.98 Replacement of automatic cardioverter/defibrillator pulse generator only

Note: Device testing during procedure - omit code

Excludes *replacement of cardiac resynchronization defibrillator, pulse generator device only [CRT-D] (00.54)*

AHA: 1Q 1999, 3; 3Q 1990, 12

✓ 37.99 Other

Excludes *cardiac retraining (93.36)*
conversion of cardiac rhythm (99.60-99.69)
implantation of prosthetic cardiac support device (37.41)
insertion of left atrial appendage device (37.90)
maze procedure (Cox-maze), open (37.33)
maze procedure, endovascular approach (37.34)
repositioning of pulse generator (37.79)
revision of lead(s) (37.75)
revision or relocation of pacemaker, defibrillator or other implanted cardiac device pocket (37.79)

AHA: 3Q 2005, 5; 2Q 2005, 15; 1Q 1997, 12; 1Q 1994, 19; 3Q 1990, 12; 1Q 1989, 11; Nov-Dec 1985, 7

INCISION, EXCISION, AND OCCLUSION OF VESSELS (38)

Code also:
any application or administration of an adhesion barrier substance (99.77)
cardiopulmonary bypass [extracorporeal circulation] [heart-lung machine] (39.61)

Excludes *that of coronary vessels (00.66, 36.03, 36.04, 36.09, 36.10-36.99)*

The following fourth-digit subclassification is for use with appropriate categories in section 38.0, 38.1, 38.3, 38.5, 38.6, and 38.8 according to site. Valid fourth-digits are in [brackets] at the end of each code/description.

0 unspecified site

1 intracranial vessels
Cerebral (anterior) (middle)
Circle of Willis
Posterior communicating artery

2 other vessels of head and neck
Carotid artery (common) (external) (internal)
Jugular vein (external) (internal)

3 upper limb vessels
Axillary
Brachial
Radial
Ulnar

4 aorta

5 other thoracic vessels
Innominate
Pulmonary (artery) (vein)
Subclavian
Vena cava, superior

6 abdominal arteries
Celiac
Gastric
Hepatic
Iliac
Mesenteric
Renal
Splenic
Umbilical
Excludes *abdominal aorta (4)*

7 abdominal veins
Iliac
Portal
Renal
Splenic
Vena cava (inferior)

8 lower limb arteries
Femoral (common) (superficial)
Popliteal
Tibial

9 lower limb veins
Femoral
Popliteal
Saphenous
Tibial

❹✓ 38.0 Incision of vessel
[0-9]
(▼ is only valid for fourth-digit "0")
Embolectomy
Thrombectomy

Excludes *endovascular removal of obstruction from head and neck vessel(s) (39.74)*
puncture or catheterization of any:
artery (38.91, 38.98)
vein (38.92-38.95, 38.99)

AHA: For Code 38.02: 2Q 1998, 23; **For Codes 38.08 and 38.09**: 1Q 2003, 17

❹✓ 38.1 Endarterectomy
[0-6, 8]
(▼ is only valid for fourth-digit "0")
Endarterectomy with:
embolectomy
patch graft
temporary bypass during procedure
thrombectomy

Code also any:
number of vascular stents inserted (00.45-00.48)
number of vessels treated (00.40-00.43)
procedure on vessel bifurcation (00.44)

AHA: For Code 38.12: 1Q 2002, 10; 1Q 2000, 16; 2Q 1999, 5; 2Q 1995, 16

38.2 Diagnostic procedures on blood vessels
Excludes *adjunct vascular system procedures (00.40-00.43)*

38.21 Biopsy of blood vessel

38.22 Percutaneous angioscopy
Excludes *angioscopy of eye (95.12)*

38.29 Other diagnostic procedures on blood vessels
Excludes *blood vessel thermography (88.86)*
circulatory monitoring (89.61-89.69)
contrast:
angiocardiography (88.50-88.58)
arteriography (88.40-88.49)
phlebography (88.60-88.67)
impedance phlebography (88.68)
peripheral vascular ultrasonography (88.77)
plethysmogram (89.58)
AHA: 3Q 2000, 16; 1Q 1999, 6; Nov-Dec 1985, 9

38.3 Resection of vessel with anastomosis
[0-9] (▼ is only valid for fourth-digit "0")
Angiectomy
Excision of:
aneurysm (arteriovenous) with anastomosis
blood vessel (lesion) with anastomosis

Category 38.4 requires the use of one of the following fourth-digit subclassifications to identify site:
0 unspecified site
1 intracranial vessels
Cerebral (anterior) (middle)
Circle of Willis
Posterior communicating artery
2 other vessels of head and neck
Carotid artery (common) (external) (internal)
Jugular vein (external) (internal)
3 upper limb vessels
Axillary
Brachial
Radial
Ulnar
4 aorta, abdominal
Code also any thoracic vessel involvement (thoracoabdominal procedure) (38.45)
5 thoracic vessels
Aorta (thoracic)
Innominate
Pulmonary (artery) (vein)
Subclavian
Vena cava, superior
Code also any abdominal aorta involvement (thoracoabdominal procedure) (38.44)
6 abdominal arteries
Celiac
Gastric
Hepatic
Iliac
Mesenteric
Renal
Splenic
Umbilical
Excludes *abdominal aorta (4)*
7 abdominal veins
Iliac
Portal
Renal
Splenic
Vena cava (inferior)
8 lower limb arteries
Femoral (common) (superficial)
Popliteal
Tibial
9 lower limb veins
Femoral
Popliteal
Saphenous
Tibial

38.4 Resection of vessel with replacement
[0-9] (▼ is only valid for fourth-digit "0")
Angiectomy
Excision of:
aneurysm (arteriovenous) or blood vessel (lesion) with replacement
Partial resection with replacement
Excludes *endovascular repair of aneurysm (39.71-39.79)*
AHA: For Code 38.42: 2Q 1999, 5; **For Codes 38.44 and 38.45**: 3Q 1992, 10

38.5 Ligation and stripping of varicose veins
[0-3, 5, 7, 9] (▼ is only valid for fourth-digit "0")
Excludes *ligation of varices:*
esophageal (42.91)
gastric (44.91)
AHA: For Code 38.59: 2Q 1997, 7

38.6 Other excision of vessel
[0-9] (▼ is only valid for fourth-digit "0")
Excision of blood vessel (lesion) NOS
Excludes *excision of vessel for aortocoronary bypass (36.10-36.14)*
excision with:
anastomosis (38.30-38.39)
graft replacement (38.40-38.49)
implant (38.40-38.49)
AHA: For Code 38.68: 3Q 1990, 17

38.7 Interruption of the vena cava
Insertion of implant or sieve in vena cava
Ligation of vena cava (inferior) (superior)
Plication of vena cava
AHA: 2Q 1994, 9; Sep-Oct 1985, 5

38.8 Other surgical occlusion of vessels
[0-9] (▼ is only valid for fourth-digit "0")
Clamping of blood vessel
Division of blood vessel
Ligation of blood vessel
Occlusion of blood vessel
Excludes *adrenal vessels (07.43)*
esophageal varices (42.91)
gastric or duodenal vessel for ulcer (44.40-44.49)
gastric varices (44.91)
meningeal vessel (02.13)
percutaneous transcatheter infusion embolization (99.29)
spermatic vein for varicocele (63.1)
surgical occlusion of vena cava (38.7)
that for chemoembolization (99.25)
that for control of (postoperative) hemorrhage:
anus (49.95)
bladder (57.93)
following vascular procedure (39.41)
nose (21.00-21.09)
prostate (60.94)
tonsil (28.7)
thyroid vessel (06.92)
transcatheter (infusion) 99.29
AHA: For Code 38.85: 1Q 2003, 15; 1Q 1996, 7;
For Code 38.86: 1Q 2005, 14; Nov-Dec 1987, 4;
For Code 38.88: 2Q 1996, 5

38.9 Puncture of vessel
Excludes *that for circulatory monitoring (89.60-89.69)*

38.91 Arterial catheterization
AHA: 1Q 2005, 14; 1Q 1997, 4; 1Q 1995, 3; 2Q 1990, 23; 1Q 1988, 8

38.92 Umbilical vein catheterization

38.93 Venous catheterization, not elsewhere classified
Excludes *that for cardiac catheterization (37.21-37.23)*
that for renal dialysis (38.95)
AHA: 3Q 2000, 9; 2Q 1998, 24; 2Q 1996, 15; 1Q 1996, 3; 3Q 1991, 13; 2Q 1991, 15; 2Q 1990, 24; 3Q 1988, 13

38.94 Venous cutdown
AHA: May-Jun 1985, 20

Operations on the Cardiovascular System 38.2 – 38.94

✖ **38.95 Venous catheterization for renal dialysis**
Excludes *insertion of totally implantable vascular access device [VAD] (86.07)*
AHA: 3Q 1998, 13

✖ **38.98 Other puncture of artery**
Excludes *that for:*
arteriography (88.40-88.49)
coronary arteriography (88.55-88.57)

✖ **38.99 Other puncture of vein**
Phlebotomy
Excludes *that for:*
angiography (88.60-88.69)
extracorporeal circulation (39.61, 50.92)
injection or infusion of:
sclerosing solution (39.92)
therapeutic or prophylactic substance (99.11-99.29)
perfusion (39.96-39.97)
phlebography (88.60-88.69)
transfusion (99.01-99.09)
AHA: 4Q 1994, 50; 1Q 1988, 11

OTHER OPERATIONS ON VESSELS (39)

Excludes *those on coronary vessels (36.00-36.99)*

✔ **39.0 Systemic to pulmonary artery shunt**
Descending aorta-pulmonary artery anastomosis (graft)
Left to right anastomosis (graft)
Subclavian-pulmonary anastomosis (graft)
Code also cardiopulmonary bypass [extracorporeal circulation] [heart-lung machine] (39.61)

✔ **39.1 Intra-abdominal venous shunt**
Anastomosis:
mesocaval
portacaval
portal vein to inferior vena cava
splenic and renal veins
transjugular intrahepatic portosystemic shunt (TIPS)
Excludes *peritoneovenous shunt (54.94)*
AHA: 2Q 2002, 4; 4Q 1994, 50; 4Q 1993, 31; 2Q 1993, 8; Nov-Dec 1987, 4

❹ **39.2 Other shunt or vascular bypass**
Code also pressurized treatment of venous bypass graft [conduit] with pharmaceutical substance, if performed (00.16)

✔ **39.21 Caval-pulmonary artery anastomosis**
Code also cardiopulmonary bypass (39.61)

✔ **39.22 Aorta-subclavian-carotid bypass**
Bypass (arterial):
aorta to carotid and brachial
aorta to subclavian and carotid
carotid to subclavian

✔ **39.23 Other intrathoracic vascular shunt or bypass**
Intrathoracic (arterial) bypass graft NOS
Excludes *coronary artery bypass (36.10-36.19)*

✔ **39.24 Aorta-renal bypass**

✔ **39.25 Aorta-iliac-femoral bypass**
Bypass:
aortofemoral
aortoiliac
aortoiliac to popliteal
aortopopliteal
iliofemoral [iliac-femoral]
AHA: 1Q 2003, 16-17; 4Q 1990, 27; 1Q 1988, 10

✔ **39.26 Other intra-abdominal vascular shunt or bypass**
Bypass:
aortoceliac
aortic-superior mesenteric
common hepatic-common iliac-renal
Intra-abdominal arterial bypass graft NOS
Excludes *peritoneovenous shunt (54.94)*

✔ **39.27 Arteriovenostomy for renal dialysis**
Anastomosis for renal dialysis
Formation of (peripheral) arteriovenous fistula for renal [kidney] dialysis
Code also any renal dialysis (39.95)
AHA: 1Q 2006, 10-11; Sep-Oct 1985, 12; Jul-Aug 1984, 4

✔ **39.28 Extracranial-intracranial (EC-IC) vascular bypass**
AHA: 2Q 1992, 7; 4Q 1991, 22

✔ **39.29 Other (peripheral) vascular shunt or bypass**
Bypass (graft):
axillary-brachial
axillary-femoral [axillofemoral] (superficial)
brachial
femoral-femoral
femoroperoneal
femoropopliteal (arteries)
femorotibial (anterior) (posterior)
popliteal
vascular NOS
Excludes *peritoneovenous shunt (54.94)*
AHA: 1Q 2003, 17; 2Q 2002, 8; 1Q 2002, 13; Sep-Oct 1985, 13; Mar-Apr 1984, 20

❹ **39.3 Suture of vessel**
Repair of laceration of blood vessel
Excludes *any other vascular puncture closure device - omit code*
suture of aneurysm (39.52)
that for control of hemorrhage (postoperative):
anus (49.95)
bladder (57.93)
following vascular procedure (39.41)
nose (21.00-21.09)
prostate (60.94)
tonsil (28.7)

✔ **39.30 Suture of unspecified blood vessel**

✔ **39.31 Suture of artery**

✔ **39.32 Suture of vein**

❹ **39.4 Revision of vascular procedure**

✔ **39.41 Control of hemorrhage following vascular surgery**
Excludes *that for control of hemorrhage (post operative):*
anus (49.95)
bladder (57.93)
nose (21.00-21.09)
prostate (60.94)
tonsil (28.7)

✔ **39.42 Revision of arteriovenous shunt for renal dialysis**
Conversion of renal dialysis:
end-to-end anastomosis to end-to-side
end-to-side anastomosis to end-to-end
vessel-to-vessel cannula to arteriovenous shunt
Removal of old arteriovenous shunt and creation of new shunt
Excludes *replacement of vessel-to-vessel cannula (39.94)*
AHA: 4Q 1993, 33

✔ **39.43 Removal of arteriovenous shunt for renal dialysis**
Excludes *that with replacement [revision] of shunt (39.42)*

✔ **39.49 Other revision of vascular procedure**
Declotting (graft)
Revision of:
anastomosis of blood vessel
vascular procedure (previous)
AHA: 1Q 1997, 4; 2Q 1994, 15

❹ Fourth Digit Required Ⓞ Open Biopsy ⓿ Closed Biopsy ▶◀ Revised Text ● New Code ▲ Revised Code

❹ **39.5 Other repair of vessels**

✓ **39.50 Angioplasty or atherectomy of other non-coronary vessel(s)**
Percutaneous transluminal angioplasty (PTA) of non-coronary vessel:
lower extremity vessels
mesenteric artery
renal artery
upper extremity vessels
Code also any:
injection or infusion of thrombolytic agent (99.10)
insertion of non-coronary stent(s) or stent grafts(s) (39.90)
number of vascular stents inserted (00.45-00.48)
number of vessels treated (00.40-00.43)
procedure on vessel bifurcation (00.44)
Excludes *percutaneous angioplasty of atherectomy of precerebral or cerebral vessel(s) (00.61-00.62)*
AHA: 3Q 2003, 10; 1Q 2002, 13; 2Q 2000, 10; 2Q 2001, 23; 1Q 2000, 12; 2Q 1998, 17; 1Q 1997, 3; 4Q 1996, 6

Transluminal balloon angioplasty

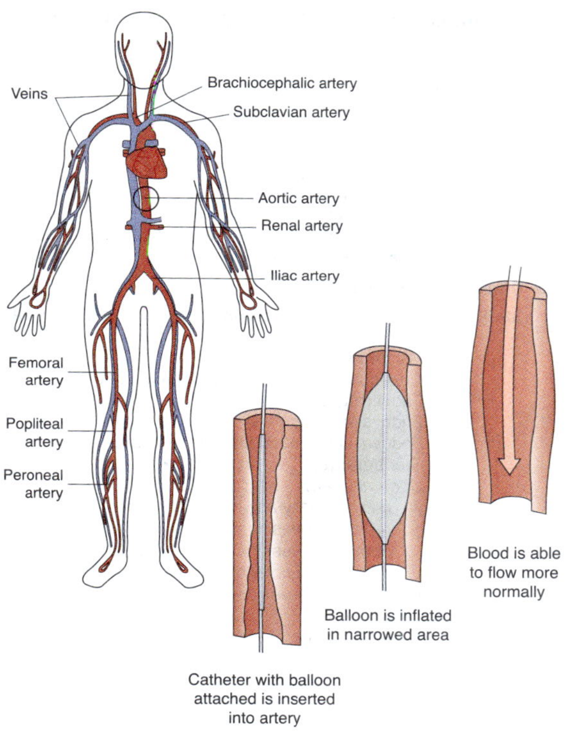

✓ **39.51 Clipping of aneurysm**
Excludes *clipping of arteriovenous fistula (39.53)*

✓ **39.52 Other repair of aneurysm**
Repair of aneurysm by:
coagulation
electrocoagulation
filipuncture
methyl methacrylate
suture
wiring
wrapping
Excludes *endovascular repair of aneurysm (39.71-39.79)*
re-entry operation (aorta) (39.54)
that with:
graft replacement (38.40-38.49)
resection (38.30-38.49, 38.60-38.69)
AHA: 3Q 2002, 25-26; 1Q 1999, 15-17; 1Q 1988, 10

✓ **39.53 Repair of arteriovenous fistula**
Embolization of carotid cavernous fistula
Repair of arteriovenous fistula by:
clipping
coagulation
ligation and division
Excludes *repair of :*
arteriovenous shunt for renal dialysis (39.42)
head and neck vessels, endovascular approach (39.72)
that with:
graft replacement (38.40-38.49)
resection (38.30-38.49, 38.60-38.69)
AHA: 1Q 2000, 8

✓ **39.54 Re-entry operation (aorta)**
Fenestration of dissecting aneurysm of thoracic aorta
Code also cardiopulmonary bypass [extracorporeal circulation] [heart-lung machine] (39.61)

✓ **39.55 Reimplantation of aberrant renal vessel**

✓ **39.56 Repair of blood vessel with tissue patch graft**
Excludes *that with resection (38.40-38.49)*
AHA: 1Q 2004, 16

✓ **39.57 Repair of blood vessel with synthetic patch graft**
Excludes *that with resection (38.40-38.49)*

✓ **39.58 Repair of blood vessel with unspecified type of patch graft**
Excludes *that with resection (38.40-38.49)*

✓ **39.59 Other repair of vessel**
Aorticopulmonary window operation
Arterioplasty NOS
Construction of venous valves (peripheral)
Plication of vein (peripheral)
Reimplantation of artery
Code also cardiopulmonary bypass [extracorporeal circulation] [heart-lung machine] (39.61)
Excludes *interruption of the vena cava (38.7)*
reimplantation of renal artery (39.55)
that with:
graft (39.56-39.58)
resection (38.30-38.49, 38.60-38.69)
AHA: 4Q 1993, 31; 2Q 1986, 17; Nov-Dec 1986, 8; Sep-Oct 1985, 5; Mar-Apr 1985, 15

❹ **39.6 Extracorporeal circulation and procedures auxiliary to heart surgery**

✖ **39.61 Extracorporeal circulation auxiliary to open heart surgery**
Artificial heart and lung
Cardiopulmonary bypass
Pump oxygenator
Excludes *extracorporeal hepatic assistance (50.92)*
extracorporeal membrane oxygenation [ECMO] (39.65)
hemodialysis (39.95)
percutaneous cardiopulmonary bypass (39.66)
AHA: 1Q 2004, 16; 3Q 2002, 5; 3Q 1990, 12; 2Q 1990, 24; 4Q 1997, 55; 2Q 1997, 8; 4Q 1996, 6-8; Nov-Dec 1985, 7; Jul-Aug 1985, 8

✖ **39.62 Hypothermia (systemic) incidental to open heart surgery**

✖ **39.63 Cardioplegia**
Arrest:
anoxic
circulatory

✖ **39.64 Intraoperative cardiac pacemaker**
Temporary pacemaker used during and immediately following cardiac surgery
AHA: 1Q 1989, 2; May-Jun 1987, 3

✖ **39.65 Extracorporeal membrane oxygenation [ECMO]**
Excludes *extracorporeal circulation auxiliary to open heart surgery (39.61)*
percutaneous cardiopulmonary bypass (39.66)
AHA: 2Q 1990, 23; 2Q 1989, 17; 4Q 1988, 5

39.66 Percutaneous cardiopulmonary bypass
Closed chest
Excludes extracorporeal circulation auxiliary to open heart surgery (39.61)
extracorporeal hepatic assistance (50.92)
extracorporeal membrane oxygenation [ECMO] (39.65)
hemodialysis (39.95)
AHA: 3Q 1996, 11

39.7 Endovascular repair of vessel
Endoluminal repair
Excludes angioplasty or atherectomy of other non-coronary vessel(s) (39.50)
insertion of non-drug-eluting peripheral vessel stent(s) (39.90)
other repair of aneurysm (39.52)
percutaneous insertion of carotid artery stent(s) (00.63)
percutaneous insertion of intracranial stent(s) (00.65)
percutaneous insertion of other precerebral artery stent(s) (00.64)
resection of abdominal aorta with replacement (38.44)
resection of lower limb arteries with replacement (38.48)
resection of thoracic aorta with replacement (38.45)
resection of upper limb vessels with replacement (38.43)

39.71 Endovascular implantation of graft in abdominal aorta
Endovascular repair of abdominal aortic aneurysm with graft
Stent graft(s)
AHA: 1Q 2002, 13; 4Q 2000, 63-64

39.72 Endovascular repair or occlusion of head and neck vessels
Coil embolization or occlusion
Endograft(s)
Endovascular graft(s)
Liquid tissue adhesive (glue) embolization or occlusion
Other implant or substance for repair, embolization or occlusion
That for repair of aneurysm, arteriovenous malformation [AVM] or fistula
Excludes mechanical thrombectomy of pre-cerebral and cerebral vessels (39.74)

39.73 Endovascular implantation of graft in thoracic aorta
Endograft(s)
Endovascular graft(s)
Endovascular repair of defect of thoracic aorta with graft(s) or device(s)
Stent graft(s) or device(s)
That for repair of aneurysm, dissection, or injury
Excludes fenestration of dissecting aneurysm of thoracic aorta (39.54)

39.74 Endovascular removal of obstruction from head and neck vessel(s)
Endovascular embolectomy
Endovascular thrombectomy of pre-cerebral and cerebral vessels
Mechanical embolectomy or thrombectomy
Code also:
any injection or infusion of thrombolytic agent (99.10)
number of vessels treated (00.40-00.43)
procedure on vessel bifurcation (00.44)
Excludes endarterectomy of intracranial vessels and other vessels of head and neck (38.11-38.12)
occlusive endovascular repair of head or neck vessels (39.72)
open embolectomy or thrombectomy (38.01-38.02)

39.79 Other endovascular repair (of aneurysm) of other vessels
Coil embolization or occlusion
Endograft(s)
Endovascular graft(s)
Liquid tissue adhesive (glue) embolization or occlusion
Other implant or substance for repair, embolization or occlusion
Excludes endovascular implantation of graft in thoracic aorta (39.73)
endovascular repair or occlusion of head and neck vessels (39.72)
insertion of drug-eluting peripheral vessel stent(s) (00.55)
insertion of non-drug-eluting peripheral vessel stent(s) (for other than aneurysm repair) (39.90)
non-endovascular repair of arteriovenous fistula (39.53)
other surgical occlusion of vessels-see category 38.8
percutaneous transcatheter infusion (99.29)
transcatheter embolization for gastric or duodenal bleeding (44.44)
AHA: 3Q 2001, 17-18; 4Q 2000, 64

39.8 Operations on carotid body, carotid sinus and other vascular bodies
Chemodectomy
Denervation of:
aortic body
carotid body
▶Electronic stimulator◀
Glomectomy, carotid
▶Implantation or replacement of carotid sinus baroreflex activation device◀
Excludes excision of glomus jugulare (20.51)
▶replacement of carotid sinus lead(s) only (04.92)◀

39.9 Other operations on vessels

39.90 Insertion of non-drug-eluting peripheral vessel stent(s)
Bare stent(s)
Bonded stent(s)
Drug-coated stent(s), i.e., heparin coated
Endograft(s)
Endovascular graft(s)
Endovascular recanalization techniques
Stent graft(s)
Code also any:
non-coronary angioplasty or atherectomy (39.50)
number of vascular stents inserted (00.45-00.48)
number of vessels treated (00.40-00.43)
procedure on vessel bifurcation (00.44)
Excludes insertion of drug-eluting peripheral vessel stent(s) (00.55)
percutaneous insertion of carotid artery stent(s) (00.63)
percutaneous insertion of intracranial artery stent(s) (00.65)
percutaneous insertion of other precerebral artery stent(s) (00.64)
that for aneurysm repair (39.71-39.79)
AHA: 2Q 2004, 101; 2Q 2001, 23; 1Q 2000, 12; 4Q 1996, 63

39.91 Freeing of vessel
Dissection and freeing of adherent tissue:
artery-vein-nerve bundle
vascular bundle
AHA: 3Q 2002, 13

39.92 Injection of sclerosing agent into vein
Excludes injection:
esophageal varices (42.33)
hemorrhoids (49.42)

39.93 Insertion of vessel-to-vessel cannula
Formation of:
arteriovenous:
fistula by external cannula
shunt by external cannula
Code also any renal dialysis (39.95)
AHA: 3Q 1988, 13; Sep-Oct 1985, 12

✓ **39.94 Replacement of vessel-to-vessel cannula**
Revision of vessel-to-vessel cannula

✖ **39.95 Hemodialysis**
Artificial kidney
Hemodiafiltration
Hemofiltration
Renal dialysis
Excludes *peritoneal dialysis (54.98)*
AHA: 1Q 2004, 22; 4Q 2003, 111; 2Q 2001, 12-14; 4Q 2000, 40; 2Q 1998, 20-21; Sep-Oct 1986, 11; May-Jun 1984, 3

✖ **39.96 Total body perfusion**
Code also substance perfused (99.21-99.29)

✖ **39.97 Other perfusion**
Perfusion NOS
Perfusion, local [regional] of:
carotid artery
coronary artery
head
lower limb
neck
upper limb
Code also substance perfused (99.21-99.29)
Excludes *perfusion of:*
kidney (55.95)
large intestine (46.96)
liver (50.93)
small intestine (46.95)
AHA: 3Q 1996, 11

✓ **39.98 Control of hemorrhage, not otherwise specified**
Angiotripsy
Control of postoperative hemorrhage NOS
Venotripsy
Excludes *control of hemorrhage (postoperative):*
anus (49.95)
bladder (57.93)
following vascular procedure (39.41)
nose (21.00-21.09)
prostate (60.94)
tonsil (28.7)
that by:
ligation (38.80-38.89)
suture (39.30-39.32)

✓ **39.99 Other operations on vessels**
Excludes *injection or infusion of therapeutic or prophylactic substance (99.11-99.29)*
transfusion of blood and blood components (99.01-99.09)
AHA: 1Q 1989, 11

8. OPERATIONS ON THE HEMIC AND LYMPHATIC SYSTEM (40-41)

OPERATIONS ON LYMPHATIC SYSTEM (40)

✓ **40.0 Incision of lymphatic structures**

④ **40.1 Diagnostic procedures on lymphatic structures**

✓ **40.11 Biopsy of lymphatic structure**
AHA: Jul-Aug 1984, 12

✓ **40.19 Other diagnostic procedures on lymphatic structures**
Excludes *lymphangiogram:*
abdominal (88.04)
cervical (87.08)
intrathoracic (87.34)
lower limb (88.36)
upper limb (88.34)
microscopic examination of specimen (90.71-90.79)
radioisotope scan (92.16)
thermography (88.89)

④ **40.2 Simple excision of lymphatic structure**
Excludes *biopsy of lymphatic structure (40.11)*

✓ **40.21 Excision of deep cervical lymph node**
AHA: 4Q 1999, 16

✓ **40.22 Excision of internal mammary lymph node**

✓ **40.23 Excision of axillary lymph node**
AHA: 2Q 2002, 7

✓ **40.24 Excision of inguinal lymph node**

✓ **40.29 Simple excision of other lymphatic structure**
Excision of:
cystic hygroma
lymphangioma
Simple lymphadenectomy
AHA: 1Q 1999, 6

✓ **40.3 Regional lymph node excision**
Extended regional lymph node excision
Regional lymph node excision with excision of lymphatic drainage area including skin, subcutaneous tissue, and fat
AHA: 2Q 1992, 7

④ **40.4 Radical excision of cervical lymph nodes**
Resection of cervical lymph nodes down to muscle and deep fascia
Excludes *that associated with radical laryngectomy (30.4)*

✓▼ **40.40 Radical neck dissection, not otherwise specified**

✓ **40.41 Radical neck dissection, unilateral**
AHA: 2Q 2005, 8-9; 2Q 1999, 6

✓ **40.42 Radical neck dissection, bilateral**

④ **40.5 Radical excision of other lymph nodes**
Excludes *that associated with radical mastectomy (85.45-85.48)*

✓▼ **40.50 Radical excision of lymph nodes, not otherwise specified**
Radical (lymph) node dissection NOS

✓ **40.51 Radical excision of axillary lymph nodes**

✓ **40.52 Radical excision of periaortic lymph nodes**

✓ **40.53 Radical excision of iliac lymph nodes**

✓ **40.54 Radical groin dissection**

✓ **40.59 Radical excision of other lymph nodes**
Excludes *radical neck dissection (40.40-40.42)*

④ **40.6 Operations on thoracic duct**

✓ **40.61 Cannulation of thoracic duct**

✓ **40.62 Fistulization of thoracic duct**

✓ **40.63 Closure of fistula of thoracic duct**

✓ **40.64 Ligation of thoracic duct**

✓ **40.69 Other operations on thoracic duct**

✓ **40.9 Other operations on lymphatic structures**
Anastomosis of peripheral lymphatics
Correction of lymphedema of limb, NOS
Dilation of peripheral lymphatics
Ligation of peripheral lymphatics
Obliteration of peripheral lymphatics
Reconstruction of peripheral lymphatics
Repair of peripheral lymphatics
Transplantation of peripheral lymphatics
Excludes *reduction of elephantiasis of scrotum (61.3)*

OPERATIONS ON BONE MARROW AND SPLEEN (41)

④ **41.0 Bone marrow or hematopoietic stem cell transplant**
Note: To report donor source - see codes 00.91-00.93
Excludes *aspiration of bone marrow from donor (41.91)*
AHA: 1Q 1991, 3; May-Jun 1985, 18

✓▼ **41.00 Bone marrow transplant, not otherwise specified**

✓ **41.01 Autologous bone marrow transplant without purging**
Excludes *that with purging (41.09)*
AHA: 4Q 1994, 52-53; 4Q 1990, 3

✓ **41.02 Allogeneic bone marrow transplant with purging**
Allograft of bone marrow with in vitro removal (purging) of T-cells

✓ **41.03 Allogeneic bone marrow transplant without purging**
Allograft of bone marrow NOS

✓ **41.04 Autologous hematopoietic stem cell transplant without purging**
Excludes *that with purging (41.07)*
AHA: 4Q 1994, 52-53

✓ **41.05 Allogeneic hematopoietic stem cell transplant without purging**
Excludes *that with purging (41.08)*
AHA: 4Q 1997, 56

✓ **41.06 Cord blood stem cell transplant**
AHA: 4Q 1997, 56

✓ **41.07 Autologous hematopoietic stem cell transplant with purging**
Cell depletion

✓ **41.08 Allogeneic hematopoietic stem cell transplant**
Cell depletion

✓ **41.09 Autologous bone marrow transplant with purging**
With extracorporeal purging of malignant cells from marrow
Cell depletion

✖ **41.1 Puncture of spleen**
Excludes *aspiration biopsy of spleen (41.32)*

✓ **41.2 Splenotomy**

④ **41.3 Diagnostic procedures on bone marrow and spleen**

✖ **41.31 Biopsy of bone marrow**

✖Ⓞ **41.32 Closed [aspiration] [percutaneous] biopsy of spleen**

✓Ⓞ **41.33 Open biopsy of spleen**

✖ **41.38 Other diagnostic procedures on bone marrow**
Excludes *microscopic examination of specimen from bone marrow (90.61-90.69)*
radioisotope scan (92.05)

✖ **41.39 Other diagnostic procedures on spleen**
Excludes *microscopic examination of specimen from spleen (90.61-90.69)*
radioisotope scan (92.05)

④ **41.4 Excision or destruction of lesion or tissue of spleen**
Code also any application or administration of an adhesion barrier substance (99.77)
Excludes *excision of accessory spleen (41.93)*

✓ **41.41 Marsupialization of splenic cyst**

✓ **41.42 Excision of lesion or tissue of spleen**
Excludes *biopsy of spleen (41.32-41.33)*

✓ **41.43 Partial splenectomy**

✓ **41.5 Total splenectomy**
Splenectomy NOS
Code also any application or administration of an adhesion barrier substance (99.77)
DEF: Complete removal of the spleen.

④ **41.9 Other operations on spleen and bone marrow**
Code also any application or administration of an adhesion barrier substance (99.77)

✖ **41.91 Aspiration of bone marrow from donor for transplant**
Excludes *biopsy of bone marrow (41.31)*
AHA: 1Q 1991, 3; Jan-Feb 1985, 15

✖ **41.92 Injection into bone marrow**
Excludes *bone marrow transplant (41.00-41.03)*
AHA: 3Q 1996, 17

✓ **41.93 Excision of accessory spleen**

✓ **41.94 Transplantation of spleen**

✓ **41.95 Repair and plastic operations on spleen**

✖ **41.98 Other operations on bone marrow**
AHA: 3Q 1994, 10

✓ **41.99 Other operations on spleen**

9. OPERATIONS ON THE DIGESTIVE SYSTEM (42-54)

OPERATIONS ON ESOPHAGUS (42)

④ **42.0 Esophagotomy**

✓ **42.01 Incision of esophageal web**

✓ **42.09 Other incision of esophagus**
Esophagotomy NOS
Excludes *esophagomyotomy (42.7)*
esophagostomy (42.10-42.19)

④ **42.1 Esophagostomy**
DEF: Creation of an artificial opening into the esophagus.

✓▼ **42.10 Esophagostomy, not otherwise specified**

✓ **42.11 Cervical esophagostomy**

✓ **42.12 Exteriorization of esophageal pouch**

✓ **42.19 Other external fistulization of esophagus**
Thoracic esophagostomy
Code also any resection (42.40-42.42)

④ **42.2 Diagnostic procedures on esophagus**

✓ **42.21 Operative esophagoscopy by incision**

✖ **42.22 Esophagoscopy through artificial stoma**
Excludes *that with biopsy (42.24)*

✖ **42.23 Other esophagoscopy**
Excludes *that with biopsy (42.24)*
AHA: 1Q 2000, 20; 3Q 1998, 11

Esophagoscopy

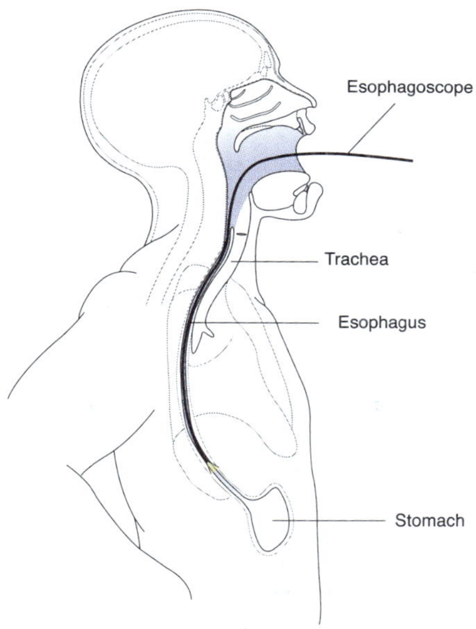

✖⓪ **42.24 Closed [endoscopic] biopsy of esophagus**
Brushing or washing for specimen collection
Esophagoscopy with biopsy
Suction biopsy of the esophagus
Excludes *esophagogastroduodenoscopy [EGD] with closed biopsy (45.16)*

✓⓪ **42.25 Open biopsy of esophagus**

✖ **42.29 Other diagnostic procedures on esophagus**
Excludes *barium swallow (87.61)*
esophageal manometry (89.32)
microscopic examination of specimen from esophagus (90.81-90.89)

④ **42.3 Local excision or destruction of lesion or tissue of esophagus**

✓ **42.31 Local excision of esophageal diverticulum**
AHA: Jan-Feb 1985, 4

✓ **42.32 Local excision of other lesion or tissue of esophagus**
Excludes *biopsy of esophagus (42.24-42.25)*
esophageal fistulectomy (42.84)

✖ **42.33 Endoscopic excision or destruction of lesion or tissue of esophagus**
Ablation of esophageal neoplasm by endoscopic approach
Control of esophageal bleeding by endoscopic approach
Esophageal polypectomy by endoscopic approach
Esophageal varices by endoscopic approach
Injection of esophageal varices by endoscopic approach
Excludes *biopsy of esophagus (42.24-42.25)*
fistulectomy (42.84)
open ligation of esophageal varices (42.91)
AHA: 1Q 2000, 20

✓ **42.39 Other destruction of lesion or tissue of esophagus**
Excludes *that by endoscopic approach (42.33)*

④ **42.4 Excision of esophagus**
Excludes *esophagogastrectomy NOS (43.99)*

✓▼ **42.40 Esophagectomy, not otherwise specified**

✓ **42.41 Partial esophagectomy**
Code also any synchronous:
anastomosis other than end-to-end (42.51-42.69)
esophagostomy (42.10-42.19)
gastrostomy (43.11-43.19)

✓ **42.42 Total esophagectomy**
Code also any synchronous:
gastrostomy (43.11-43.19)
interposition or anastomosis other than end-to-end (42.51-42.69)
Excludes *esophagogastrectomy (43.99)*
AHA: 4Q 1988, 11

④ **42.5 Intrathoracic anastomosis of esophagus**
Code also any synchronous:
esophagectomy (42.40-42.42)
gastrostomy (43.1)

✓ **42.51 Intrathoracic esophagoesophagostomy**

✓ **42.52 Intrathoracic esophagogastrostomy**

✓ **42.53 Intrathoracic esophageal anastomosis with interposition of small bowel**

✓ **42.54 Other intrathoracic esophagoenterostomy**
Anastomosis of esophagus to intestinal segment NOS

✓ **42.55 Intrathoracic esophageal anastomosis with interposition of colon**

✓ **42.56 Other intrathoracic esophagocolostomy**
Esophagocolostomy NOS

✓ **42.58 Intrathoracic esophageal anastomosis with other interposition**
Construction of artificial esophagus
Retrosternal formation of reversed gastric tube

✓ **42.59 Other intrathoracic anastomosis of esophagus**
AHA: 4Q 1988, 11

④ **42.6 Antesternal anastomosis of esophagus**
Code also any synchronous:
esophagectomy (42.40-42.42)
gastrostomy (43.1)

✓ **42.61 Antesternal esophagoesophagostomy**

✓ **42.62 Antesternal esophagogastrostomy**

✓ **42.63 Antesternal esophageal anastomosis with interposition of small bowel**

✓ **42.64 Other antesternal esophagoenterostomy**
Antethoracic:
esophagoenterostomy
esophagoileostomy
esophagojejunostomy

✓ **42.65 Antesternal esophageal anastomosis with interposition of colon**

✓ **42.66 Other antesternal esophagocolostomy**
Antethoracic esophagocolostomy

42.68 Other antesternal esophageal anastomosis with interposition

42.69 Other antesternal anastomosis of esophagus

42.7 Esophagomyotomy
AHA: Jan-Feb 1985, 4

42.8 Other repair of esophagus

42.81 Insertion of permanent tube into esophagus
AHA: 1Q 1997, 15

42.82 Suture of laceration of esophagus

42.83 Closure of esophagostomy
DEF: Closure of a previously created surgical opening in the esophagus.

42.84 Repair of esophageal fistula, not elsewhere classified
Excludes *repair of fistula:*
bronchoesophageal (33.42)
esophagopleurocutaneous (34.73)
pharyngoesophageal (29.53)
tracheoesophageal (31.73)

42.85 Repair of esophageal stricture

42.86 Production of subcutaneous tunnel without esophageal anastomosis

42.87 Other graft of esophagus
Excludes *antesternal esophageal anastomosis with interposition of:*
colon (42.65)
small bowel (42.63)
antesternal esophageal anastomosis with other interposition (42.68)
intrathoracic esophageal anastomosis with interposition of:
colon (42.55)
small bowel (42.53)
intrathoracic esophageal anastomosis with other interposition (42.58)

42.89 Other repair of esophagus

42.9 Other operations on esophagus

42.91 Ligation of esophageal varices
Excludes *that by endoscopic approach (42.33)*
AHA: Nov-Dec 1987, 4-5

42.92 Dilation of esophagus
Dilation of cardiac sphincter
Excludes *intubation of esophagus (96.03, 96.06-96.08)*

42.99 Other
Excludes *insertion of Sengstaken tube (96.06)*
intubation of esophagus (96.03, 96.06-96.08)
removal of intraluminal foreign body from esophagus without incision (98.02)
tamponade of esophagus (96.06)

INCISION AND EXCISION OF STOMACH (43)

Code also any application or administration of an adhesion barrier substance (99.77)

43.0 Gastrotomy
Excludes *gastrostomy (43.11-43.19)*
that for control of hemorrhage (44.49)
DEF: Incision of the stomach.

43.1 Gastrostomy
DEF: Creation of an artificial opening into the stomach to facilitate tube feeding.
AHA: Sep-Oct 1985, 5

43.11 Percutaneous [endoscopic] gastrostomy [PEG]
Percutaneous transabdominal gastrostomy
AHA: 2Q 1994, 10

43.19 Other gastrostomy
Excludes *percutaneous [endoscopic] gastrostomy [PEG] (43.11)*
AHA: 1Q 1992, 14; 3Q 1989, 14

43.3 Pyloromyotomy

43.4 Local excision or destruction of lesion or tissue of stomach

43.41 Endoscopic excision or destruction of lesion or tissue of stomach
Gastric polypectomy by endoscopic approach
Gastric varices by endoscopic approach
Excludes *biopsy of stomach (44.14-44.15)*
control of hemorrhage (44.43)
open ligation of gastric varices (44.91)
AHA: 3Q 1996, 10

43.42 Local excision of other lesion or tissue of stomach
Excludes *biopsy of stomach (44.14-44.15)*
gastric fistulectomy (44.62-44.63)
partial gastrectomy (43.5-43.89)

43.49 Other destruction of lesion or tissue of stomach
Excludes *that by endoscopic approach (43.41)*
AHA: Nov-Dec 1987, 5; Sep-Oct 1985, 6

43.5 Partial gastrectomy with anastomosis to esophagus
Proximal gastrectomy

43.6 Partial gastrectomy with anastomosis to duodenum
Billroth I operation
Distal gastrectomy
Gastropylorectomy

43.7 Partial gastrectomy with anastomosis to jejunum
Billroth II operation
AHA: 3Q 2003, 7

43.8 Other partial gastrectomy

43.81 Partial gastrectomy with jejunal transposition
Henley jejunal transposition operation
Code also any synchronous intestinal resection (45.51)

43.89 Other
Partial gastrectomy with bypass gastrogastrostomy
Sleeve resection of stomach
AHA: 3Q 2003, 6-8

43.9 Total gastrectomy
DEF: Removal of the entire stomach.

43.91 Total gastrectomy with intestinal interposition

43.99 Other total gastrectomy
Complete gastroduodenectomy
Esophagoduodenostomy with complete gastrectomy
Esophagogastrectomy NOS
Esophagojejunostomy with complete gastrectomy
Radical gastrectomy

OTHER OPERATIONS ON STOMACH (44)

Code also any application or administration of an adhesion barrier substance (99.77)

44.0 Vagotomy

44.00 Vagotomy, not otherwise specified
Division of vagus nerve NOS

44.01 Truncal vagotomy

44.02 Highly selective vagotomy
Parietal cell vagotomy
Selective proximal vagotomy

44.03 Other selective vagotomy

44.1 Diagnostic procedures on stomach

44.11 Transabdominal gastroscopy
Intraoperative gastroscopy
Excludes *that with biopsy (44.14)*

44.12 Gastroscopy through artificial stoma
Excludes *that with biopsy (44.14)*

44.13 Other gastroscopy
Excludes *that with biopsy (44.14)*
AHA: 1Q 1988, 15; Nov-Dec 1987, 5

44.14 Closed [endoscopic] biopsy of stomach
Brushing or washing for specimen collection
Excludes *esophagogastroduodenoscopy [EGD] with closed biopsy (45.16)*
AHA: 1Q 1988, 15; Nov-Dec 1987, 5

✓Ⓞ **44.15 Open biopsy of stomach**

✖ **44.19 Other diagnostic procedures on stomach**
Excludes *gastric lavage (96.33)*
microscopic examination of specimen from stomach (90.81-90.89)
upper GI series (87.62)

❹ **44.2 Pyloroplasty**

✓ **44.21 Dilation of pylorus by incision**

✖ **44.22 Endoscopic dilation of pylorus**
Dilation with balloon endoscope
Endoscopic dilation of gastrojejunostomy site
AHA: 2Q 2001, 17

✓ **44.29 Other pyloroplasty**
Pyloroplasty NOS
Revision of pylorus
AHA: 3Q 1999, 3

❹ **44.3 Gastroenterostomy without gastrectomy**
DEF: Gastroenterostomy: Creation of an artificial connection from the stomach to the intestines.

✓ **44.31 High gastric bypass**
Printen and Mason gastric bypass

✓ **44.32 Percutaneous [endoscopic] gastrojejunostomy**
Endoscopic conversion of gastrostomy to jejunostomy
PEG

✓ **44.38 Laparoscopic gastroenterostomy**
Bypass:
gastroduodenostomy
gastroenterostomy
gastrogastrostomy
Laparoscopic gastrojejunostomy without gastrectomy NEC
Excludes *gastroenterostomy, open approach (44.39)*

✓ **44.39 Other gastroenterostomy**
Bypass:
gastroduodenostomy
gastroenterostomy
gastrogastrostomy
Gastrojejunostomy without gastrectomy NOS
AHA: 3Q 2003, 6; 1Q 2001, 16

❹ **44.4 Control of hemorrhage and suture of ulcer of stomach or duodenum**

✓▼ **44.40 Suture of peptic ulcer, not otherwise specified**

✓ **44.41 Suture of gastric ulcer site**
Excludes *ligation of gastric varices (44.91)*

✓ **44.42 Suture of duodenal ulcer site**
AHA: Jan-Feb 1987, 11

✖ **44.43 Endoscopic control of gastric or duodenal bleeding**
AHA: 2Q 2004, 12; 2Q 1992, 17

✖ **44.44 Transcatheter embolization for gastric or duodenal bleeding**
Excludes *surgical occlusion of abdominal vessels (38.86-38.87)*

✖ **44.49 Other control of hemorrhage of stomach or duodenum**
That with gastrotomy

✓ **44.5 Revision of gastric anastomosis**
Closure of:
gastric anastomosis
gastroduodenostomy
gastrojejunostomy
Pantaloon operation

❹ **44.6 Other repair of stomach**

✓ **44.61 Suture of laceration of stomach**
Excludes *that of ulcer site (44.41)*

✖ **44.62 Closure of gastrostomy**
DEF: Closure of a previously created artificial opening in the stomach.

✓ **44.63 Closure of other gastric fistula**
Closure of:
gastrocolic fistula
gastrojejunocolic fistula

✓ **44.64 Gastropexy**

✓ **44.65 Esophagogastroplasty**
Belsey operation
Esophagus and stomach cardioplasty

✓ **44.66 Other procedures for creation of esophagogastric sphincteric competence**
Fundoplication
Gastric cardioplasty
Nissen's fundoplication
Restoration of cardio-esophageal angle
Excludes *that by laparoscopy (44.67)*
AHA: 2Q 2003, 12; 2Q 2001, 3-6; 3Q 1998, 10

✓ **44.67 Laparoscopic procedures for creation of esophagogastric sphincteric competence**
Fundoplication
Gastric cardioplasty
Nissen's fundoplication
Restoration of cardio-esophageal angle

✓ **44.68 Laparoscopic gastroplasty**
Banding
Silastic vertical banding
Vertical banded gastroplasty (VBG)
Code also any synchronous laparoscopic gastroenterostomy (44.38)
Excludes *insertion, laparoscopic adjustable gastric band (restrictive procedure) (44.95)*
other repair of stomach, open approach (44.61-44.65, 44.69)

✓ **44.69 Other**
Inversion of gastric diverticulum
Repair of stomach NOS
AHA: 3Q 2003, 8; 2Q 2001, 3; 3Q 1999, 3; Jul-Aug 1984, 13

❹ **44.9 Other operations on stomach**

✓ **44.91 Ligation of gastric varices**
Excludes *that by endoscopic approach (43.41)*

✓ **44.92 Intraoperative manipulation of stomach**
Reduction of gastric volvulus

✖ **44.93 Insertion of gastric bubble (balloon)**

✖ **44.94 Removal of gastric bubble (balloon)**

✓ **44.95 Laparoscopic gastric restrictive procedure**
Adjustable gastric band and port insertion
Excludes *laparoscopic gastroplasty (44.68)*
other repair of stomach (44.69)

✓ **44.96 Laparoscopic revision of gastric restrictive procedure**
Revision or replacement of:
adjustable gastric band
subcutaneous gastric port device

✓ **44.97 Laparoscopic removal of gastric restrictive device(s)**
Removal of either or both:
adjustable gastric band
subcutaneous port device
Excludes *nonoperative removal of gastric restrictive device(s) (97.86)*
open removal of gastric restrictive device(s) (44.99)

✓ **44.98 (Laparoscopic) adjustment of size of adjustable gastric restrictive device**
Infusion of saline for device tightening
Withdrawal of saline for device loosening
Code also any:
abdominal ultrasound (88.76)
abdominal wall fluoroscopy (88.09)
barium swallow (87.61)

Operations on the Digestive System 44.15 – 44.98

✖ Deleted Code ▼ Nonspecific O.R. Procedure ✓ Valid O.R. Procedure ✖ Non-O.R. Procedure ♂ Male ♀ Female

✓ **44.99 Other**
Excludes *change of gastrostomy tube (97.02)*
dilation of cardiac sphincter (42.92)
gastric:
cooling (96.31)
freezing (96.32)
gavage (96.35)
hypothermia (96.31)
lavage (96.33)
insertion of nasogastric tube (96.07)
irrigation of gastrostomy (96.36)
irrigation of nasogastric tube (96.34)
removal of:
gastrostomy tube (97.51)
intraluminal foreign body from stomach without incision (98.03)
replacement of:
gastrostomy tube (97.02)
(naso-)gastric tube (97.01)
AHA: 3Q 2004, 5; Nov-Dec 1987, 5

INCISION, EXCISION, AND ANASTOMOSIS OF INTESTINE (45)

Code also any application or administration of an adhesion barrier substance (99.77)

④ **45.0 Enterotomy**
Excludes *duodenocholedochotomy (51.41-51.42, 51.51)*
that for destruction of lesion (45.30-45.34)
that of exteriorized intestine (46.14, 46.24, 46.31)
DEF: Incision of the intestine.

✓▼ **45.00 Incision of intestine, not otherwise specified**

✓ **45.01 Incision of duodenum**

✓ **45.02 Other incision of small intestine**

✓ **45.03 Incision of large intestine**
Excludes *proctotomy (48.0)*

④ **45.1 Diagnostic procedures on small intestine**
Code also any laparotomy (54.11-54.19)

✓ **45.11 Transabdominal endoscopy of small intestine**
Intraoperative endoscopy of small intestine
Excludes *that with biopsy (45.14)*

✗ **45.12 Endoscopy of small intestine through artificial stoma**
Excludes *that with biopsy (45.14)*

✗ **45.13 Other endoscopy of small intestine**
Esophagogastroduodenoscopy [EGD]
Excludes *that with biopsy (45.14, 45.16)*
AHA: 3Q 2004, 5; Nov-Dec 1987, 5

✗⓿ **45.14 Closed [endoscopic] biopsy of small intestine**
Brushing or washing for specimen collection
Excludes *esophagogastroduodenoscopy [EGD] with closed biopsy (45.16)*

✓⓪ **45.15 Open biopsy of small intestine**
AHA: 2Q 2005, 12

✗ **45.16 Esophagogastroduodenoscopy [EGD] with closed biopsy**
Biopsy of one or more sites involving esophagus, stomach, and/or duodenum
AHA: 3Q 2005, 18; 2Q 2001, 9

✗ **45.19 Other diagnostic procedures on small intestine**
Excludes *microscopic examination of specimen from small intestine (90.91-90.99)*
radioisotope scan (92.04)
ultrasonography (88.74)
x-ray (87.61-87.69)

④ **45.2 Diagnostic procedures on large intestine**
Code also any laparotomy (54.11-54.19)

✓ **45.21 Transabdominal endoscopy of large intestine**
Intraoperative endoscopy of large intestine
Excludes *that with biopsy (45.25)*

✗ **45.22 Endoscopy of large intestine through artificial stoma**
Excludes *that with biopsy (45.25)*

✗ **45.23 Colonoscopy**
Flexible fiberoptic colonoscopy
Excludes *endoscopy of large intestine through artificial stoma (45.22)*
flexible sigmoidoscopy (45.24)
rigid proctosigmoidoscopy (48.23)
transabdominal endoscopy of large intestine (45.21)
AHA: 3Q 2005, 17, 18; Sep-Oct 1985, 5

✗ **45.24 Flexible sigmoidoscopy**
Endoscopy of descending colon
Excludes *rigid proctosigmoidoscopy (48.23)*

✗⓿ **45.25 Closed [endoscopic] biopsy of large intestine**
Biopsy, closed, of unspecified intestinal site
Brushing or washing for specimen collection
Colonoscopy with biopsy
Excludes *proctosigmoidoscopy with biopsy (48.24)*
AHA: 1Q 2003, 11

✓⓪ **45.26 Open biopsy of large intestine**

✗ **45.27 Intestinal biopsy, site unspecified**

✗ **45.28 Other diagnostic procedures on large intestine**

✗ **45.29 Other diagnostic procedures on intestine, site unspecified**
Excludes *microscopic examination of specimen (90.91-90.99)*
scan and radioisotope function study (92.04)
ultrasonography (88.74)
x-ray (87.61-87.69)

④ **45.3 Local excision or destruction of lesion or tissue of small intestine**

✗ **45.30 Endoscopic excision or destruction of lesion of duodenum**
Excludes *biopsy of duodenum (45.14-45.15)*
control of hemorrhage (44.43)
fistulectomy (46.72)

✓ **45.31 Other local excision of lesion of duodenum**
Excludes *biopsy of duodenum (45.14-45.15)*
fistulectomy (46.72)
multiple segmental resection (45.61)
that by endoscopic approach (45.30)

✓ **45.32 Other destruction of lesion of duodenum**
Excludes *that by endoscopic approach (45.30)*
AHA: Nov-Dec 1987, 5; Sep-Oct 1985, 6

✓ **45.33 Local excision of lesion or tissue of small intestine, except duodenum**
Excision of redundant mucosa of ileostomy
Excludes *biopsy of small intestine (45.14-45.15)*
fistulectomy (46.74)
multiple segmental resection (45.61)
AHA: Jan-Feb 1985, 3

✓ **45.34 Other destruction of lesion of small intestine, except duodenum**

④ **45.4 Local excision or destruction of lesion or tissue of large intestine**

✓ **45.41 Excision of lesion or tissue of large intestine**
Excision of redundant mucosa of colostomy
Excludes *biopsy of large intestine (45.25-45.27)*
endoscopic polypectomy of large intestine (45.42)
fistulectomy (46.76)
multiple segmental resection (45.71)
that by endoscopic approach (45.42-45.43)
AHA: Nov-Dec 1987, 11

✗ **45.42 Endoscopic polypectomy of large intestine**
Excludes *that by open approach (45.41)*
AHA: 2Q 2005, 17; 2Q 1990, 25

✗ **45.43 Endoscopic destruction of other lesion or tissue of large intestine**
Endoscopic ablation of tumor of large intestine
Endoscopic control of colonic bleeding
Excludes *endoscopic polypectomy of large intestine (45.42)*
AHA: 4Q 2002, 61

✓ **45.49 Other destruction of lesion of large intestine**
Excludes *that by endoscopic approach (45.43)*
AHA: Nov-Dec 1987, 11

❹ **45.5 Isolation of intestinal segment**
Code also any synchronous:
anastomosis other than end-to-end (45.90-45.94)
enterostomy (46.10-46.39)

✓ **45.50 Isolation of intestinal segment, not otherwise specified**
Isolation of intestinal pedicle flap
Reversal of intestinal segment

✓ **45.51 Isolation of segment of small intestine**
Isolation of ileal loop
Resection of small intestine for interposition
AHA: 2Q 2005, 12, 13; 3Q 2003, 7; 2Q 2003, 11; 3Q 2000, 7

✓ **45.52 Isolation of segment of large intestine**
Resection of colon for interposition

❹ **45.6 Other excision of small intestine**
Code also any synchronous:
anastomosis other than end-to-end (45.90-45.93, 45.95)
colostomy (46.10-46.13)
enterostomy (46.10-46.39)
Excludes *cecectomy (45.72)*
enterocolectomy (45.79)
gastroduodenectomy (43.6-43.99)
ileocolectomy (45.73)
pancreatoduodenectomy (52.51-52.7)

✓ **45.61 Multiple segmental resection of small intestine**
Segmental resection for multiple traumatic lesions of small intestine

✓ **45.62 Other partial resection of small intestine**
Duodenectomy
Ileectomy
Jejunectomy
Excludes *duodenectomy with synchronous pancreatectomy (52.51-52.7)*
resection of cecum and terminal ileum (45.72)
DEF: Ileectomy: Removal of the ileum, the distal portion of the small intestine.
AHA: 1Q 2004, 10; 1Q 2003, 18; Jan-Feb 1985, 3

✓ **45.63 Total removal of small intestine**

❹ **45.7 Partial excision of large intestine**
Code also any synchronous:
anastomosis other than end-to-end (45.92-45.94)
enterostomy (46.10-46.39)

✓ **45.71 Multiple segmental resection of large intestine**
Segmental resection for multiple traumatic lesions of large intestine

✓ **45.72 Cecectomy**
Resection of cecum and terminal ileum

✓ **45.73 Right hemicolectomy**
Ileocolectomy
Right radical colectomy
AHA: 3Q 1999, 10

✓ **45.74 Resection of transverse colon**

✓ **45.75 Left hemicolectomy**
Excludes *proctosigmoidectomy (48.41-48.69)*
second stage Mikulicz operation (46.04)

✓ **45.76 Sigmoidectomy**
AHA: 3Q 1989, 15

✓ **45.79 Other partial excision of large intestine**
Enterocolectomy NEC
AHA: 3Q 1997, 9-10; 2Q 1991, 16

Colectomy

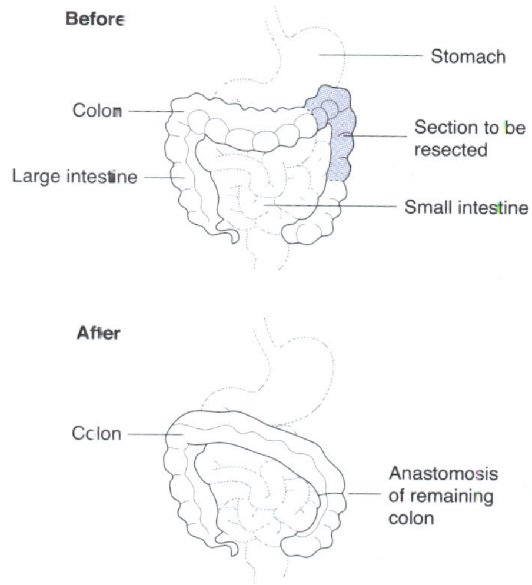

✓ **45.8 Total intra-abdominal colectomy**
Excision of cecum, colon, and sigmoid
Excludes *coloproctectomy (48.41-48.69)*

❹ **45.9 Intestinal anastomosis**
Code also any synchronous resection (45.31-45.8, 48.41-48.69)
Excludes *end-to-end anastomosis - omit code*

✓▼ **45.90 Intestinal anastomosis, not otherwise specified**

✓ **45.91 Small-to-small intestinal anastomosis**
AHA: 3Q 2003, 7

✓ **45.92 Anastomosis of small intestine to rectal stump**
Hampton procedure

✓ **45.93 Other small-to-large intestinal anastomosis**
AHA: 1Q 2003, 18; Nov-Dec 1986, 11

✓ **45.94 Large-to-large intestinal anastomosis**
Excludes *rectorectostomy (48.74)*
AHA: 3Q 1989, 15

✓ **45.95 Anastomosis to anus**
Formation of endorectal ileal pouch (H-pouch) (J-pouch) (S-pouch) with anastomosis of small intestine to anus
AHA: 2Q 2005, 13

OTHER OPERATIONS ON INTESTINE (46)

Code also any application or administration of an adhesion barrier substance (99.77)

❹ **46.0 Exteriorization of intestine**
Includes loop enterostomy
multiple stage resection of intestine

✓ **46.01 Exteriorization of small intestine**
Loop ileostomy

✓ **46.02 Resection of exteriorized segment of small intestine**

✓ **46.03 Exteriorization of large intestine**
Exteriorization of intestine NOS
First stage Mikulicz exteriorization of intestine
Loop colostomy

✓ **46.04 Resection of exteriorized segment of large intestine**
Resection of exteriorized segment of intestine NOS
Second stage Mikulicz operation

46.1 Colostomy
Code also any synchronous resection (45.49, 45.71-45.79, 45.8)
Excludes *loop colostomy (46.03)*
that with abdominoperineal resection of rectum (48.5)
that with synchronous anterior rectal resection (48.62)
DEF: Creation of an artificial opening from the large intestine to the external body surface.

46.10 Colostomy, not otherwise specified
46.11 Temporary colostomy
46.13 Permanent colostomy
46.14 Delayed opening of colostomy

46.2 Ileostomy
Code also any synchronous resection (45.34, 45.61-45.63)
Excludes *loop ileostomy (46.01)*

46.20 Ileostomy, not otherwise specified
46.21 Temporary ileostomy
46.22 Continent ileostomy
AHA: May-Jun 1985, 17
46.23 Other permanent ileostomy
46.24 Delayed opening of ileostomy

46.3 Other enterostomy
Code also any synchronous resection (45.61-45.8)

46.31 Delayed opening of other enterostomy
46.32 Percutaneous (endoscopic) jejunostomy [PEJ]
46.39 Other
Duodenostomy
Feeding enterostomy
AHA: 3Q 1989, 15

46.4 Revision of intestinal stoma

46.40 Revision of intestinal stoma, not otherwise specified
Plastic enlargement of intestinal stoma
Reconstruction of stoma of intestine
Release of scar tissue of intestinal stoma
Excludes *excision of redundant mucosa (45.41)*
46.41 Revision of stoma of small intestine
Excludes *excision of redundant mucosa (45.33)*
AHA: 2Q 2005, 11-12
46.42 Repair of pericolostomy hernia
46.43 Other revision of stoma of large intestine
Excludes *excision of redundant mucosa (45.41)*
AHA: 2Q 2002, 9

46.5 Closure of intestinal stoma
Code also any synchronous resection (45.34, 45.49, 45.61-45.8)

46.50 Closure of intestinal stoma, not otherwise specified
46.51 Closure of stoma of small intestine
46.52 Closure of stoma of large intestine
Closure or take-down of:
cecostomy
colostomy
sigmoidostomy
AHA: 2Q 2005, 5; 3Q 1997, 9-10; Nov-Dec 1987, 8

46.6 Fixation of intestine

46.60 Fixation of intestine, not otherwise specified
Fixation of intestine to abdominal wall
46.61 Fixation of small intestine to abdominal wall
Ileopexy
46.62 Other fixation of small intestine
Noble plication of small intestine
Plication of jejunum
46.63 Fixation of large intestine to abdominal wall
Cecocoloplicopexy
Sigmoidopexy (Moschowitz)
46.64 Other fixation of large intestine
Cecofixation
Colofixation

46.7 Other repair of intestine
Excludes *closure of:*
ulcer of duodenum (44.42)
vesicoenteric fistula (57.83)

46.71 Suture of laceration of duodenum
46.72 Closure of fistula of duodenum
46.73 Suture of laceration of small intestine, except duodenum
46.74 Closure of fistula of small intestine, except duodenum
Excludes *closure of:*
artificial stoma (46.51)
vaginal fistula (70.74)
repair of gastrojejunocolic fistula (44.63)
46.75 Suture of laceration of large intestine
46.76 Closure of fistula of large intestine
Excludes *closure of:*
gastrocolic fistula (44.63)
rectal fistula (48.73)
sigmoidovesical fistula (57.83)
stoma (46.52)
vaginal fistula (70.72-70.73)
vesicocolic fistula (57.83)
vesicosigmoidovaginal fistula (57.83)
AHA: 3Q 1999, 8
46.79 Other repair of intestine
Duodenoplasty
AHA: 3Q 2002, 11

46.8 Dilation and manipulation of intestine

46.80 Intra-abdominal manipulation of intestine, not otherwise specified
Correction of intestinal malrotation
Reduction of:
intestinal torsion
intestinal volvulus
intussusception
Excludes *reduction of intussusception with:*
fluoroscopy (96.29)
ionizing radiation enema (96.29)
ultrasonography guidance (96.29)
AHA: 4Q 1998, 82
46.81 Intra-abdominal manipulation of small intestine
AHA: Jan-Feb 1985, 3
46.82 Intra-abdominal manipulation of large intestine
46.85 Dilation of intestine
Dilation (balloon) of duodenum
Dilation (balloon) of jejunum
Endoscopic dilation (balloon) of large intestine
That through rectum or colostomy
AHA: 3Q 1989, 15

46.9 Other operations on intestines

46.91 Myotomy of sigmoid colon
DEF: Cutting of the muscle(s) of the sigmoid colon.
46.92 Myotomy of other parts of colon
46.93 Revision of anastomosis of small intestine
46.94 Revision of anastomosis of large intestine
46.95 Local perfusion of small intestine
Code also substance perfused (99.21-99.29)
46.96 Local perfusion of large intestine
Code also substance perfused (99.21-99.29)
46.97 Transplant of intestine
Note: To report donor source - see codes 00.91-00.93
AHA: 4Q 2000, 66

Fourth Digit Required | Open Biopsy | Closed Biopsy | ▶◀ Revised Text | ● New Code | ▲ Revised Code

✓ **46.99 Other**
Ileoentectropy
Excludes diagnostic procedures on intestine (45.11-45.29)
dilation of enterostomy stoma (96.24)
intestinal intubation (96.08)
removal of:
intraluminal foreign body from large intestine without incision (98.04)
intraluminal foreign body from small intestine without incision (98.03)
tube from large intestine (97.53)
tube from small intestine (97.52)
replacement of:
large intestine tube or enterostomy device (97.04)
small intestine tube or enterostomy device (97.03)
AHA: 3Q 1999, 11; 1Q 1989, 11

OPERATIONS ON APPENDIX (47)

Includes appendiceal stump
Code also any application or administration of an adhesion barrier substance (99.77)

④ **47.0 Appendectomy**
Excludes *incidental appendectomy, so described:*
laparoscopic (47.11)
other (47.19)
AHA: 3Q 1992, 12

✓ **47.01 Laparoscopic appendectomy**
AHA: 1Q 2001, 15; 4Q 1996, 64

✓ **47.09 Other appendectomy**
AHA: 4Q 1997, 52

④ **47.1 Incidental appendectomy**
AHA: Jul-Aug 1984, 12

✓ **47.11 Laparoscopic incidental appendectomy**

✓ **47.19 Other incidental appendectomy**
AHA: 4Q 1996, 65

✓ **47.2 Drainage of appendiceal abscess**
Excludes *that with appendectomy (47.0)*

④ **47.9 Other operations on appendix**

✓ **47.91 Appendicostomy**

✓ **47.92 Closure of appendiceal fistula**

✓ **47.99 Other**
Anastomosis of appendix
Excludes *diagnostic procedures on appendix (45.21-45.29)*
AHA: 3Q 2001, 16

OPERATIONS ON RECTUM, RECTOSIGMOID AND PERIRECTAL TISSUE (48)

Code also any application or administration of an adhesion barrier substance (99.77)

✓ **48.0 Proctotomy**
Decompression of imperforate anus
Panas' operation [linear proctotomy]
Excludes *incision of perirectal tissue (48.81)*
AHA: 3Q 1999, 8
DEF: Incision into the rectum.

✓ **48.1 Proctostomy**

④ **48.2 Diagnostic procedures on rectum, rectosigmoid and perirectal tissue**

✓ **48.21 Transabdominal proctosigmoidoscopy**
Intraoperative proctosigmoidoscopy
Excludes *that with biopsy (48.24)*

✗ **48.22 Proctosigmoidoscopy through artificial stoma**
Excludes *that with biopsy (48.24)*

✗ **48.23 Rigid proctosigmoidoscopy**
Excludes *flexible sigmoidoscopy (45.24)*
AHA: 1Q 2001, 8

✗ Ⓞ **48.24 Closed [endoscopic] biopsy of rectum**
Brushing or washing for specimen collection
Proctosigmoidoscopy with biopsy
AHA: 1Q 2003, 14

✓ Ⓞ **48.25 Open biopsy of rectum**

✗ **48.26 Biopsy of perirectal tissue**

✗ **48.29 Other diagnostic procedures on rectum, rectosigmoid and perirectal tissue**
Excludes *digital examination of rectum (89.34)*
lower GI series (87.64)
microscopic examination of specimen from rectum (90.91-90.99)

④ **48.3 Local excision or destruction of lesion or tissue of rectum**

✗ **48.31 Radical electrocoagulation of rectal lesion or tissue**

✗ **48.32 Other electrocoagulation of rectal lesion or tissue**
AHA: 2Q 1998, 18; Nov-Dec 1987, 11

✗ **48.33 Destruction of rectal lesion or tissue by laser**

✗ **48.34 Destruction of rectal lesion or tissue by cryosurgery**

✓ **48.35 Local excision of rectal lesion or tissue**
Excludes *biopsy of rectum (48.24-48.25)*
excision of perirectal tissue (48.82)
hemorrhoidectomy (49.46)
[endoscopic] polypectomy of rectum (48.36)
rectal fistulectomy (48.73)

✗ **48.36 [Endoscopic] polypectomy of rectum**
AHA: 4Q 1995, 65

④ **48.4 Pull-through resection of rectum**
Code also any synchronous anastomosis other than end-to-end (45.90, 45.92-45.95)

✓ **48.41 Soave submucosal resection of rectum**
Endorectal pull-through operation

✓ **48.49 Other pull-through resection of rectum**
Abdominoperineal pull-through
Altemeier operation
Swenson proctectomy
Excludes *Duhamel abdominoperineal pull through (48.65)*
AHA: 3Q 2001, 8; 2Q 1999, 13

✓ **48.5 Abdominoperineal resection of rectum**
Includes with synchronous colostomy
Combined abdominoendorectal resection
Complete proctectomy
Code also any synchronous anastomosis other than end-to-end (45.90, 45.92-45.95)
Excludes *Duhamel abdominoperineal pull-through (48.65)*
that as part of pelvic exenteration (68.8)
AHA: 2Q 1997, 5

④ **48.6 Other resection of rectum**
Code also any synchronous anastomosis other than end-to-end (45.90, 45.92-45.95)

✓ **48.61 Transsacral rectosigmoidectomy**

✓ **48.62 Anterior resection of rectum with synchronous colostomy**

✓ **48.63 Other anterior resection of rectum**
Excludes *that with synchronous colostomy (48.62)*
AHA: 1Q 1996, 9

✓ **48.64 Posterior resection of rectum**

✓ **48.65 Duhamel resection of rectum**
Duhamel abdominoperineal pull-through

✓ **48.69 Other**
Partial proctectomy
Rectal resection NOS
AHA: 2Q 2005, 13; Jan-Feb 1987, 11; Nov-Dec 1986, 11

④ **48.7 Repair of rectum**
Excludes *repair of:*
current obstetric laceration (75.62)
vaginal rectocele (70.50, 70.52)

✓ **48.71 Suture of laceration of rectum**

Operations on the Digestive System 46.99 – 48.71

✖ Deleted Code ▼ Nonspecific O.R. Procedure ✓ Valid O.R. Procedure ✗ Non-O.R. Procedure ♂ Male ♀ Female

✓ **48.72 Closure of proctostomy**

✓ **48.73 Closure of other rectal fistula**
Excludes *fistulectomy:*
perirectal (48.93)
rectourethral (58.43)
rectovaginal (70.73)
rectovesical (57.83)
rectovesicovaginal (57.83)

✓ **48.74 Rectorectostomy**
Rectal anastomosis NOS
▶ Stapled transanal rectal resection (STARR)◀

✓ **48.75 Abdominal proctopexy**
Frickman procedure
Ripstein repair of rectal prolapse

✓ **48.76 Other proctopexy**
Delorme repair of prolapsed rectum
Proctosigmoidopexy
Puborectalis sling operation
Excludes *manual reduction of rectal prolapse (96.26)*

✓ **48.79 Other repair of rectum**
Repair of old obstetric laceration of rectum
Excludes *anastomosis to:*
large intestine (45.94)
small intestine (45.92-45.93)
repair of:
current obstetrica laceration (75.62)
vaginal rectocele (70.50, 70.52)

❹ **48.8 Incision or excision of perirectal tissue or lesion**
Includes pelvirectal tissue
rectovaginal septum

✓ **48.81 Incision of perirectal tissue**
Incision of rectovaginal septum

✓ **48.82 Excision of perirectal tissue**
Excludes *perirectal biopsy (48.26)*
perirectofistulectomy (48.93)
rectal fistulectomy (48.73)

❹ **48.9 Other operations on rectum and perirectal tissue**

✓ **48.91 Incision of rectal stricture**

✓ **48.92 Anorectal myectomy**

✓ **48.93 Repair of perirectal fistula**
Excludes *that opening into rectum (48.73)*

✓ **48.99 Other**
Excludes *digital examination of rectum (89.34)*
dilation of rectum (96.22)
insertion of rectal tube (96.09)
irrigation of rectum (96.38-96.39)
manual reduction of rectal prolapse (96.26)
proctoclysis (96.37)
rectal massage (99.93)
rectal packing (96.19)
removal of:
impacted feces (96.38)
intraluminal foreign body from rectum without incision (98.05)
rectal packing (97.59)
transanal enema (96.39)

OPERATIONS ON ANUS (49)

Code also any application or administration of an adhesion barrier substance (99.77)

❹ **49.0 Incision or excision of perianal tissue**

✓ **49.01 Incision of perianal abscess**
AHA: 2Q 2005, 10

✓ **49.02 Other incision of perianal tissue**
Undercutting of perianal tissue
Excludes *anal fistulotomy (49.11)*

✗ **49.03 Excision of perianal skin tags**

✓ **49.04 Other excision of perianal tissue**
Excludes *anal fistulectomy (49.12)*
biopsy of perianal tissue (49.22)
AHA: 1Q 2001, 8

❹ **49.1 Incision or excision of anal fistula**
Excludes *closure of anal fistula (49.73)*

✓ **49.11 Anal fistulotomy**

✓ **49.12 Anal fistulectomy**

❹ **49.2 Diagnostic procedures on anus and perianal tissue**

✗ **49.21 Anoscopy**

✗ **49.22 Biopsy of perianal tissue**

✗ **49.23 Biopsy of anus**

✗ **49.29 Other diagnostic procedures on anus and perianal tissue**
Excludes *microscopic examination of specimen from anus (90.91-90.99)*

❹ **49.3 Local excision or destruction of other lesion or tissue of anus**
Anal cryptotomy
Cauterization of lesion of anus
Excludes *biopsy of anus (49.23)*
control of (postoperative) hemorrhage of anus (49.95)
hemorrhoidectomy (49.46)

✗ **49.31 Endoscopic excision or destruction of lesion or tissue of anus**

✓ **49.39 Other local excision or destruction of lesion or tissue of anus**
Excludes *that by endoscopic approach (49.31)*
AHA: 1Q 2001, 8

❹ **49.4 Procedures on hemorrhoids**

✗ **49.41 Reduction of hemorrhoids**

✗ **49.42 Injection of hemorrhoids**

✗ **49.43 Cauterization of hemorrhoids**
Clamp and cautery of hemorrhoids

✓ **49.44 Destruction of hemorrhoids by cryotherapy**

✓ **49.45 Ligation of hemorrhoids**

✓ **49.46 Excision of hemorrhoids**
Hemorrhoidectomy NOS

✗ **49.47 Evacuation of thrombosed hemorrhoids**

✓ **49.49 Other procedures on hemorrhoids**
Lord procedure

❹ **49.5 Division of anal sphincter**

✓ **49.51 Left lateral anal sphincterotomy**

✓ **49.52 Posterior anal sphincterotomy**

✓ **49.59 Other anal sphincterotomy**
Division of sphincter NOS

✓ **49.6 Excision of anus**

❹ **49.7 Repair of anus**
Excludes *repair of current obstetric laceration (75.62)*

✓ **49.71 Suture of laceration of anus**

✓ **49.72 Anal cerclage**

✓ **49.73 Closure of anal fistula**
Excludes *excision of anal fistula (49.12)*

✓ **49.74 Gracilis muscle transplant for anal incontinence**

✗ **49.75 Implantation or revision of artificial anal sphincter**
Removal with subsequent replacement
Replacement during same or subsequent operative episode

✗ **49.76 Removal of artificial anal sphincter**
Explantation or removal without replacement
Excludes *revision with implantation during same operative episode (49.75)*

✓ **49.79 Other repair of anal sphincter**
Repair of old obstetric laceration of anus
Excludes *anoplasty with synchronous hemorrhoidectomy (49.46)*
repair of current obstetric laceration (75.62)
AHA: 2Q 1998, 16; 1Q 1997, 9-10

❹ **49.9 Other operations on anus**
Excludes *dilation of anus (sphincter) (96.23)*

✓ **49.91 Incision of anal septum**

✓ **49.92 Insertion of subcutaneous electrical anal stimulator**

✓ **49.93 Other incision of anus**
Removal of:
foreign body from anus with incision
seton from anus
Excludes *anal fistulotomy (49.11)*
removal of intraluminal foreign body without incision (98.05)

✓ **49.94 Reduction of anal prolapse**
Excludes *manual reduction of rectal prolapse (96.26)*

✓ **49.95 Control of (postoperative) hemorrhage of anus**

✓ **49.99 Other**

OPERATIONS ON LIVER (50)

Code also any application or administration of an adhesion barrier substance (99.77)

✓ **50.0 Hepatotomy**
Incision of abscess of liver
Removal of gallstones from liver
Stromeyer-Little operation
DEF: Incision into the liver.

④ **50.1 Diagnostic procedures on liver**

✖ **50.11 Closed (percutaneous) [needle] biopsy of liver**
Diagnostic aspiration of liver
AHA: 3Q 2005, 24; 3Q 1994, 11; 4Q 1988, 12

Liver Biopsy

A tissue sample is taken for examination

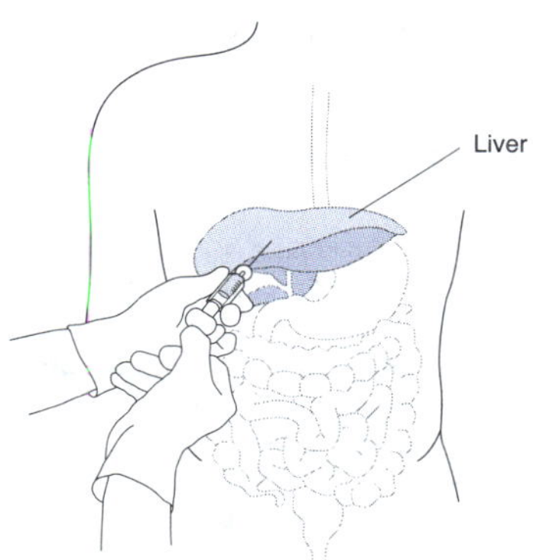

✓ **50.12 Open biopsy of liver**
Wedge biopsy
AHA: 3Q 2005, 24; 2Q 2005, 13; Jul-Aug 1984, 12

● ✖ **50.13 Transjugular liver biopsy**
Transvenous liver biopsy
Excludes *closed (percutaneous) [needle] biopsy of liver (50.11)*
laparoscopic liver biopsy (50.14)

● ✓ **50.14 Laparoscopic liver biopsy**
Excludes *closed (percutaneous) [needle] biopsy of liver (50.11)*
open biopsy of liver (50.12)
transjugular liver biopsy (50.13)

✓ **50.19 Other diagnostic procedures on liver**
Excludes ▶*laparoscopic liver biopsy (50.14)*◀
liver scan and radioisotope function study (92.02)
microscopic examination of specimen from liver (91.01-91.09)
▶*transjugular liver biopsy (50.13)*◀

④ **50.2 Local excision or destruction of liver tissue or lesion**

✓ **50.21 Marsupialization of lesion of liver**

✓ **50.22 Partial hepatectomy**
Wedge resection of liver
Excludes *biopsy of liver (50.11-50.12)*
hepatic lobectomy (50.3)

✓ **50.23 Open ablation of liver lesion or tissue**

✓ **50.24 Percutaneous ablation of liver lesion or tissue**

✓ **50.25 Laparoscopic ablation of liver lesion or tissue**

✓▼ **50.26 Other and unspecified ablation of liver lesion or tissue**

✓ **50.29 Other destruction of lesion of liver**
Cauterization of hepatic lesion
Enucleation of hepatic lesion
Evacuation of hepatic lesion
Excludes *ablation of liver lesion or tissue:*
laparoscopic (50.25)
open (50.23)
other (50.26)
percutaneous (50.24)
percutaneous aspiration of lesion (50.91)
AHA: 2Q 2003, 9

✓ **50.3 Lobectomy of liver**
Total hepatic lobectomy with partial excision of other lobe

✓ **50.4 Total hepatectomy**

④ **50.5 Liver transplant**
Note: To report donor source - see codes 00.91-00.93

✓ **50.51 Auxiliary liver transplant**
Auxiliary hepatic transplantation leaving patient's own liver in situ

✓ **50.59 Other transplant of liver**

④ **50.6 Repair of liver**

✓ **50.61 Closure of laceration of liver**

✓ **50.69 Other repair of liver**
Hepatopexy
DEF: Hepatopexy: Surgical fixation of the liver.

④ **50.9 Other operations on liver**
Excludes *lysis of adhesions (54.5)*

✖ **50.91 Percutaneous aspiration of liver**
Excludes *percutaneous biopsy (50.11)*

✖ **50.92 Extracorporeal hepatic assistance**
Liver dialysis
AHA: 2Q 2001, 21

✖ **50.93 Localized perfusion of liver**

✖ **50.94 Other injection of therapeutic substance into liver**

✖ **50.99 Other**

OPERATIONS ON GALLBLADDER AND BILIARY TRACT (51)

Includes operations on:
ampulla of Vater
common bile duct
cystic duct
hepatic duct
intrahepatic bile duct
sphincter of Oddi

Code also any application or administration of an adhesion barrier substance (99.77)

④ **51.0 Cholecystotomy and cholecystostomy**

✖ **51.01 Percutaneous aspiration of gallbladder**
Percutaneous cholecystotomy for drainage
That by: needle or catheter
Excludes *needle biopsy (51.12)*

✓ **51.02 Trocar cholecystostomy**
AHA: 3Q 1989, 18

✓ **51.03 Other cholecystostomy**

✓ **51.04 Other cholecystotomy**
Cholelithotomy NOS

④ **51.1 Diagnostic procedures on biliary tract**
Excludes *that for endoscopic procedures classifiable to 51.64, 51.84-51.88, 52.14, 52.21, 52.93-52.94, 52.97-52.98*

✖ **51.10 Endoscopic retrograde cholangiopancreatography [ERCP]**
Excludes *endoscopic retrograde:*
cholangiography [ERC] (51.11)
pancreatography [ERP] (52.13)
AHA: 4Q 2003, 118; 3Q 2003, 17; 1Q 2001, 8; 2Q 1999, 13

✖ Deleted Code ▼ Nonspecific O.R. Procedure ✓ Valid O.R. Procedure ✖ Non-O.R. Procedure ♂ Male ♀ Female

51.11 Endoscopic retrograde cholangiography [ERC]
Laparoscopic exploration of common bile duct
Excludes *endoscopic retrograde:*
cholangiopancreatography [ERCP] (51.10)
pancreatography [ERP] (52.13)
AHA: 1Q 1996, 11-12; 4Q 1988, 7; Nov-Dec 1987, 3

51.12 Percutaneous biopsy of gallbladder or bile ducts
Needle biopsy of gallbladder

51.13 Open biopsy of gallbladder or bile ducts

51.14 Other closed [endoscopic] biopsy of biliary duct or sphincter of Oddi
Brushing or washing for specimen collection
Closed biopsy of biliary duct or sphincter of Oddi by procedures classifiable to 51.10-51.11, 52.13

51.15 Pressure measurement of sphincter of Oddi
Pressure measurement of sphincter by procedures classifiable to 51.10-51.11, 52.13

51.19 Other diagnostic procedures on biliary tract
Excludes *biliary tract x-ray (87.51-87.59)*
microscopic examination of specimen from biliary tract (91.01-91.09)

51.2 Cholecystectomy

51.21 Other partial cholecystectomy
Revision of prior cholecystectomy
Excludes *that by laparoscope (51.24)*

51.22 Cholecystectomy
Excludes *laparoscopic cholecystectomy (51.23)*
DEF: Removal of the gallbladder.
AHA: 4Q 1997, 52; 2Q 1995, 11; 1Q 1993, 17; 4Q 1988, 7

51.23 Laparoscopic cholecystectomy
That by laser
AHA: 3Q 1998, 10; 1Q 1996, 11-12; 1Q 1993, 17

51.24 Laparoscopic partial cholecystectomy
AHA: 4Q 1996, 69

51.3 Anastomosis of gallbladder or bile duct
Excludes *resection with end-to-end anastomosis (51.61-51.69)*

51.31 Anastomosis of gallbladder to hepatic ducts

51.32 Anastomosis of gallbladder to intestine

51.33 Anastomosis of gallbladder to pancreas

51.34 Anastomosis of gallbladder to stomach

51.35 Other gallbladder anastomosis
Gallbladder anastomosis NOS

51.36 Choledochoenterostomy

51.37 Anastomosis of hepatic duct to gastrointestinal tract
Kasai portoenterostomy
AHA: 2Q 2002, 12

51.39 Other bile duct anastomosis
Anastomosis of bile duct NOS
Anastomosis of unspecified bile duct to:
intestine
liver
pancreas
stomach

51.4 Incision of bile duct for relief of obstruction

51.41 Common duct exploration for removal of calculus
Excludes *percutaneous extraction (51.96)*
AHA: 1Q 1996, 12; 4Q 1988, 7

51.42 Common duct exploration for relief of other obstruction
AHA: 3Q 1989, 18

51.43 Insertion of choledochohepatic tube for decompression
Hepatocholedochostomy
AHA: 3Q 1989, 18; 4Q 1988, 7

51.49 Incision of other bile ducts for relief of obstruction
AHA: 3Q 1989, 18

51.5 Other incision of bile duct
Excludes *that for relief of obstruction (51.41-51.49)*

51.51 Exploration of common duct
Incision of common bile duct
AHA: 2Q 1997, 16; 1Q 1996, 11-12

51.59 Incision of other bile duct
AHA: 2Q 1997, 16; 3Q 1989, 18

51.6 Local excision or destruction of lesion or tissue of biliary ducts and sphincter of Oddi
Code also anastomosis other than end-to-end (51.31, 51.36-51.39)
Excludes *biopsy of bile duct (51.12-51.13)*

51.61 Excision of cystic duct remnant
AHA: 3Q 1989, 18

51.62 Excision of ampulla of Vater (with reimplantation of common duct)

51.63 Other excision of common duct
Choledochectomy
Excludes *fistulectomy (51.72)*
DEF: Choledochectomy: Removal of a portion of the common bile duct.

51.64 Endoscopic excision or destruction of lesion of biliary ducts or sphincter of Oddi
Excision or destruction of lesion of biliary duct by procedures classifiable to 51.10-51.11, 52.13

51.69 Excision of other bile duct
Excision of lesion of bile duct NOS
Excludes *fistulectomy (51.79)*

51.7 Repair of bile ducts

51.71 Simple suture of common bile duct

51.72 Choledochoplasty
Repair of fistula of common bile duct

51.79 Repair of other bile ducts
Closure of artificial opening of bile duct NOS
Suture of bile duct NOS
Excludes *operative removal of prosthetic device (51.95)*

51.8 Other operations on biliary ducts and sphincter of Oddi

51.81 Dilation of sphincter of Oddi
Dilation of ampulla of Vater
Excludes *that by endoscopic approach (51.84)*

51.82 Pancreatic sphincterotomy
Incision of pancreatic sphincter
Transduodenal ampullary sphincterotomy
Excludes *that by endoscopic approach (51.85)*

51.83 Pancreatic sphincteroplasty

51.84 Endoscopic dilation of ampulla and biliary duct
Dilation of ampulla and biliary duct by procedures classifiable to 51.10-51.11, 52.13

51.85 Endoscopic sphincterotomy and papillotomy
Sphincterotomy and papillotomy by procedures classifiable to 51.10-51.11, 52.13
AHA: 4Q 2003, 118; 3Q 2003, 17; 2Q 1997, 7

51.86 Endoscopic insertion of nasobiliary drainage tube
Insertion of nasobiliary tube by procedures classifiable to 51.10-51.11, 52.13

51.87 Endoscopic insertion of stent (tube) into bile duct
Endoprosthesis of bile duct
Insertion of stent into bile duct by procedures classifiable to 51.10-51.11, 52.13
Excludes *nasobiliary drainage tube (51.86)*
replacement of stent (tube) (97.05)
AHA: 3Q 2003, 17

51.88 Endoscopic removal of stone(s) from biliary tract
Laparoscopic removal of stone(s) from biliary tract
Removal of biliary tract stone(s) by procedures classifiable to 51.10-51.11, 52.13
Excludes *percutaneous extraction of common duct stones (51.96)*
AHA: 2Q 2000, 11; 2Q 1997, 7

51.89 Other operations on sphincter of Oddi

Fourth Digit Required | Open Biopsy | Closed Biopsy | ►◄ Revised Text | ● New Code | ▲ Revised Code

④ **51.9 Other operations on biliary tract**

✓ **51.91 Repair of laceration of gallbladder**

✓ **51.92 Closure of cholecystostomy**

✓ **51.93 Closure of other biliary fistula**
Cholecystogastroenteric fistulectomy

✓ **51.94 Revision of anastomosis of biliary tract**

✓ **51.95 Removal of prosthetic device from bile duct**
Excludes *nonoperative removal (97.55)*

✖ **51.96 Percutaneous extraction of common duct stones**
AHA: 4Q 1988, 7

✖ **51.98 Other percutaneous procedures on biliary tract**
Percutaneous biliary endoscopy via existing T-tube or other tract for:
dilation of biliary duct stricture
exploration (postoperative)
removal of stone(s) except common duct stone
Percutaneous transhepatic biliary drainage
Excludes *percutaneous aspiration of gallbladder (51.01)*
percutaneous biopsy and/or collection of specimen by brushing or washing (51.12)
percutaneous removal of common duct stone(s) (51.96)
AHA: 1Q 1997, 14; 3Q 1989, 18; Nov-Dec 1987, 3

✓ **51.99 Other**
Insertion or replacement of biliary tract prosthesis
Excludes *biopsy of gallbladder (51.12-51.13)*
irrigation of cholecystostomy and other biliary tube (96.41)
lysis of peritoneal adhesions (54.5)
nonoperative removal of:
cholecystostomy tube (97.54)
tube from biliary tract or liver (97.55)

OPERATIONS ON PANCREAS (52)

Includes operations on pancreatic duct
Code also any application or administration of an adhesion barrier substance (99.77)

④ **52.0 Pancreatotomy**

✓ **52.01 Drainage of pancreatic cyst by catheter**

✓ **52.09 Other pancreatotomy**
Pancreatolithotomy
Excludes *drainage by anastomosis (52.4, 52.96)*
incision of pancreatic sphincte (51.82)
marsupialization of cyst (52.3)
DEF: Pancreatolithotomy: Incision into the pancreas with removal of stones.

④ **52.1 Diagnostic procedures on pancreas**

✖⓪ **52.11 Closed [aspiration] [needle] [percutaneous] biopsy of pancreas**

✓⓪ **52.12 Open biopsy of pancreas**

✖ **52.13 Endoscopic retrograde pancreatography [ERP]**
Excludes *endoscopic retrograde:*
cholangiography [ERC] (51.11)
cholangiopancreatography [ERCP] (51.10)
that for procedures classifiable to 51.14-51.15, 51.64, 51.84-51.88, 52.14, 52.21, 52.92-52.94, 52.97-52.98

✖ **52.14 Closed [endoscopic] biopsy of pancreatic duct**
Closed biopsy of pancreatic duct by procedures classifiable to 51.10-51.11, 52.13

✓ **52.19 Other diagnostic procedures on pancreas**
Excludes *contrast pancreatogram (87.66)*
endoscopic retrograde pancreatography [ERP] (52.13)
microscopic examination of specimen from pancreas (91.01-91.09)

④ **52.2 Local excision or destruction of pancreas and pancreatic duct**
Excludes *biopsy of pancreas (52.11-52.12, 52.14)*
pancreatic fistulectomy (52.95)

✖ **52.21 Endoscopic excision or destruction of lesion or tissue of pancreatic duct**
Excision or destruction of lesion or tissue of pancreatic duct by procedures classifiable to 51.10-51.11, 52.13

✓ **52.22 Other excision or destruction of lesion or tissue of pancreas or pancreatic duct**

✓ **52.3 Marsupialization of pancreatic cyst**
Excludes *drainage of cyst by catheter (52.01)*
DEF: Suturing the cut edges of an incised pancreatic cyst to create an open pouch for drainage and facilitate healing without excision.

✓ **52.4 Internal drainage of pancreatic cyst**
Pancreaticocystoduodenostomy
Pancreaticocystogastrostomy
Pancreaticocystojejunostomy

④ **52.5 Partial pancreatectomy**
Excludes *pancreatic fistulectomy (52.95)*

✓ **52.51 Proximal pancreatectomy**
Excision of head of pancreas (with part of body)
Proximal pancreatectomy with synchronous duodenectomy

✓ **52.52 Distal pancreatectomy**
Excision of tail of pancreas (with part of body)

✓ **52.53 Radical subtotal pancreatectomy**

✓ **52.59 Other partial pancreatectomy**

✓ **52.6 Total pancreatectomy**
Pancreatectomy with synchronous duodenectomy
AHA: 4Q 1996, 71

✓ **52.7 Radical pancreaticoduodenectomy**
One-stage pancreaticoduodenal resection with choledochojejunal anastomosis, pancreaticojejunal anastomosis, and gastrojejunostomy
Two-stage pancreaticoduodenal resection (first stage) (second stage)
Radical resection of the pancreas
Whipple procedure
Excludes *radical subtotal pancreatectomy (52.53)*
AHA: 1Q 2001, 13

④ **52.8 Transplant of pancreas**
Note: To report donor source - see codes 00.91-00.93

✓ **52.80 Pancreatic transplant, not otherwise specified**

✓ **52.81 Reimplantation of pancreatic tissue**

✓ **52.82 Homotransplant of pancreas**

✓ **52.83 Heterotransplant of pancreas**

✖ **52.84 Autotransplantation of cells of Islets of Langerhans**
Homotransplantation of islet cells of pancreas
AHA: 4Q 1996, 71

✖ **52.85 Allotransplantation of cells of Islets of Langerhans**
Heterotransplantation of islet cells of pancreas
AHA: 4Q 1996, 71

✖ **52.86 Transplantation of cells of Islets of Langerhans, not otherwise specified**

④ **52.9 Other operations on pancreas**

✓ **52.92 Cannulation of pancreatic duct**
Excludes *that by endoscopic approach (52.93)*

✖ **52.93 Endoscopic insertion of stent (tube) into pancreatic duct**
Insertion of cannula or stent into pancreatic duct by procedures classifiable to 51.10-51.11, 52.13
Excludes *endoscopic insertion of nasopancreatic drainage tube (52.97)*
replacement of stent (tube) (97.05)
AHA: 2Q 1997, 7

✖ **52.94 Endoscopic removal of stone(s) from pancreatic duct**
Removal of stone(s) from pancreatic duct by procedures classifiable to 51.10-51.11, 52.13

✓ **52.95 Other repair of pancreas**
Fistulectomy of pancreas
Simple suture of pancreas

✓ **52.96 Anastomosis of pancreas**
Anastomosis of pancreas (duct) to:
intestine
jejunum
stomach
Excludes *anastomosis to:*
bile duct (51.39)
gallbladder (51.33)

✗ **52.97 Endoscopic insertion of nasopancreatic drainage tube**
Insertion of nasopancreatic drainage tube by procedures classifiable to 51.10-51.11, 52.13
Excludes *drainage of pancreatic cyst by catheter (52.01)*
replacement of stent (tube) (97.05)

✗ **52.98 Endoscopic dilation of pancreatic duct**
Dilation of Wirsung's duct by procedures classifiable to 51.10-51.11, 52.13

✓ **52.99 Other**
Dilation of pancreatic [Wirsung's] duct by open approach
Repair of pancreatic [Wirsung's] duct by open approach
Excludes *irrigation of pancreatic tube (96.42)*
removal of pancreatic tube (97.56)

REPAIR OF HERNIA (53)

Includes hernioplasty
herniorrhaphy
Code also any application or administration of an adhesion barrier substance (99.77)
Excludes *manual reduction of hernia (96.27)*
AHA: 3Q 1994, 8

④ **53.0 Unilateral repair of inguinal hernia**

✓▼ **53.00 Unilateral repair of inguinal hernia, not otherwise specified**
Inguinal herniorrhaphy NOS
AHA: 3Q 2003, 10

✓ **53.01 Repair of direct inguinal hernia**
AHA: 4Q 1996, 66

✓ **53.02 Repair of indirect inguinal hernia**

✓ **53.03 Repair of direct inguinal hernia with graft or prosthesis**

✓ **53.04 Repair of indirect inguinal hernia with graft or prosthesis**

✓ **53.05 Repair of inguinal hernia with graft or prosthesis, not otherwise specified**

④ **53.1 Bilateral repair of inguinal hernia**

✓▼ **53.10 Bilateral repair of inguinal hernia, not otherwise specified**

✓ **53.11 Bilateral repair of direct inguinal hernia**

✓ **53.12 Bilateral repair of indirect inguinal hernia**

✓ **53.13 Bilateral repair of inguinal hernia, one direct and one indirect**

✓ **53.14 Bilateral repair of direct inguinal hernia with graft or prosthesis**

✓ **53.15 Bilateral repair of indirect inguinal hernia with graft or prosthesis**

✓ **53.16 Bilateral repair of inguinal hernia, one direct and one indirect, with graft or prosthesis**

✓ **53.17 Bilateral inguinal hernia repair with graft or prosthesis, not otherwise specified**

④ **53.2 Unilateral repair of femoral hernia**

✓ **53.21 Unilateral repair of femoral hernia with graft or prosthesis**

✓ **53.29 Other unilateral femoral herniorrhaphy**

④ **53.3 Bilateral repair of femoral hernia**

✓ **53.31 Bilateral repair of femoral hernia with graft or prosthesis**

✓ **53.39 Other bilateral femoral herniorrhaphy**

④ **53.4 Repair of umbilical hernia**
Excludes *repair of gastroschisis (54.71)*

▲✓ **53.41 Repair of umbilical hernia with graft or prosthesis**

✓ **53.49 Other umbilical herniorrhaphy**

④ **53.5 Repair of other hernia of anterior abdominal wall (without graft or prosthesis)**

✓ **53.51 Incisional hernia repair**
AHA: 3Q 2003, 6

✓ **53.59 Repair of other hernia of anterior abdominal wall**
Repair of hernia:
epigastric
hypogastric
spigelian
ventral
AHA: 3Q 2003, 7; 3Q 1996, 15

④ **53.6 Repair of other hernia of anterior abdominal wall with graft or prosthesis**

▲✓ **53.61 Incisional hernia repair with graft or prosthesis**
AHA: 3Q 2003, 11

▲✓ **53.69 Repair of other hernia of anterior abdominal wall with graft or prosthesis**

✓ **53.7 Repair of diaphragmatic hernia, abdominal approach**

④ **53.8 Repair of diaphragmatic hernia, thoracic approach**

✓ **53.80 Repair of diaphragmatic hernia with thoracic approach, not otherwise specified**
Thoracoabdominal repair of diaphragmatic hernia
AHA: Jan-Feb 1985, 4

✓ **53.81 Plication of the diaphragm**

✓ **53.82 Repair of parasternal hernia**

✓ **53.9 Other hernia repair**
Repair of hernia:
ischiatic
ischiorectal
lumbar
obturator
omental
retroperitoneal
sciatic
Excludes *relief of strangulated hernia with exteriorization of intestine (46.01, 46.03)*
repair of pericolostomy hernia (46.42)
repair of vaginal enterocele (70.92)

OTHER OPERATIONS ON ABDOMINAL REGION (54)

Includes operations on:
epigastric region
flank
groin region
hypochondrium
inguinal region
loin region
pelvic cavity
mesentery
omentum
peritoneum
retroperitoneal tissue space
Code also any application or administration of an adhesion barrier substance (99.77)
Excludes *hernia repair (53.00-53.9)*
obliteration of cul-de-sac (70.92)
retroperitoneal tissue dissection (59.00-59.09)
skin and subcutaneous tissue of abdominal wall (86.01-86.99)

✓ **54.0 Incision of abdominal wall**
Drainage of:
abdominal wall
extraperitoneal abscess
retroperitoneal abscess
Excludes *incision of peritoneum (54.95)*
laparotomy (54.11-54.19)

54.1 Laparotomy

DEF: Incision into the abdomen.

54.11 Exploratory laparotomy

Excludes *exploration incidental to intra abdominal surgery - omit code*

AHA: 3Q 1989, 14; 4Q 1988, 12; Jul-Aug 1984, 12

54.12 Reopening of recent laparotomy site

Reopening of recent laparotomy site for:
- control of hemorrhage
- exploration
- incision of hematoma

54.19 Other laparotomy

Drainage of intraperitoneal abscess or hematoma

Excludes *culdocentesis (70.0)*
drainage of appendiceal abscess (47.2)
exploration incidental to intra abdominal surgery - omit code
Ladd operation (54.95)
percutaneous drainage of abdomen (54.91)
removal of foreign body (54.92)

54.2 Diagnostic procedures of abdominal region

54.21 Laparoscopy

Peritoneoscopy

Excludes *laparoscopic cholecystectomy (51.23)*
that incidental to destruction of fallopian tubes (66.21-66.29)

54.22 Biopsy of abdominal wall or umbilicus

54.23 Biopsy of peritoneum

Biopsy of:
- mesentery
- omentum
- peritoneal implant

Excludes *closed biopsy of:*
- *omentum (54.24)*
- *peritoneum (54.24)*

Laparascopy with biopsy

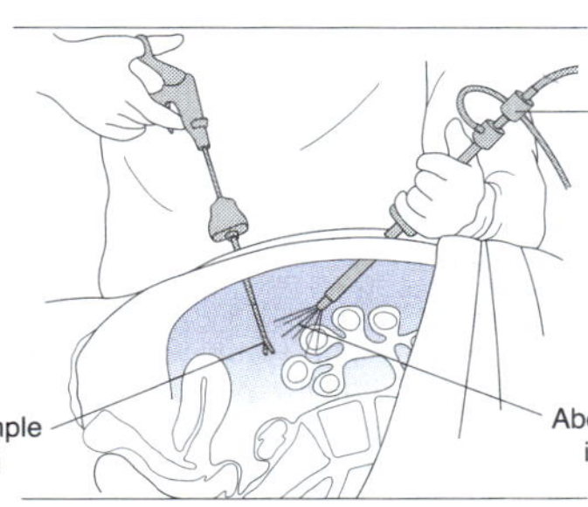

54.24 Closed [percutaneous] [needle] biopsy of intra-abdominal mass

Closed biopsy of:
- omentum
- peritoneal implant
- peritoneum

Excludes *that of:*
- *fallopian tube (66.11)*
- *ovary (65.11)*
- *uterine ligaments (68.15)*
- *uterus (68.16)*

AHA: 4Q 1997, 57

54.25 Peritoneal lavage

Diagnostic peritoneal lavage

Excludes *peritoneal dialysis (54.98)*

AHA: 2Q 1998, 19; 4Q 1993, 28

54.29 Other diagnostic procedures on abdominal region

Excludes *abdominal lymphangiogram (88.04)*
abdominal x-ray NEC (88.19)
angiocardiography of venae cava (88.51)
C.A.T. scan of abdomen (88.01)
contrast x-ray of abdominal cavity (88.11-88.15)
intra-abdominal arteriography NEC (88.47)
microscopic examination of peritoneal and retroperitoneal specimen (91.11-91.19)
phlebography of:
- *intra-abdominal vessels NEC (88.65)*
- *portal venous system (88.64)*

sinogram of abdominal wall (88.03)
soft tissue x-ray of abdominal wall NEC (88.09)
tomography of abdomen NEC (88.02)
ultrasonography of abdomen and retroperitoneum (88.76)

54.3 Excision or destruction of lesion or tissue of abdominal wall or umbilicus

Debridement of abdominal wall
Omphalectomy

Excludes *biopsy of abdominal wall or umbilicus (54.22)*
size reduction operation (86.83)
that of skin of abdominal wall (86.22, 86.26, 86.3)

DEF: Omphalectomy: Surgical removal of the umbilicus.

AHA: 1Q 1989, 11

54.4 Excision or destruction of peritoneal tissue

Excision of:
- appendices epiploicae
- falciform ligament
- gastrocolic ligament
- lesion of:
  - mesentery
  - omentum
  - peritoneum
- presacral lesion NOS
- retroperitoneal lesion NOS

Excludes *biopsy of peritoneum (54.23)*
endometrectomy of cul-de-sac (70.32)

AHA: Jan-Feb 1985, 3

54.5 Lysis of peritoneal adhesions

Freeing of adhesions of:
- biliary tract
- intestines
- liver
- pelvic peritoneum
- peritoneum
- spleen
- uterus

Excludes *lysis of adhesions of:*
- *bladder (59.11)*
- *fallopian tube and ovary:*
  - *laparoscopic (65.81)*
  - *other (65.89)*
- *kidney (59.02)*
- *ureter (59.02)*

AHA: 3Q 1994, 8; Jan-Feb 1985, 3

54.51 Laparoscopic lysis of peritoneal adhesions

AHA: 3Q 2003, 7; 4Q 1996, 65

54.59 Other lysis of peritoneal adhesions

AHA: 3Q 2003, 11; 4Q 1996, 66

54.6 Suture of abdominal wall and peritoneum

54.61 Reclosure of postoperative disruption of abdominal wall

54.62 Delayed closure of granulating abdominal wound

Tertiary subcutaneous wound closure

54.63 Other suture of abdominal wall

Suture of laceration of abdominal wall

Excludes *closure of operative wound - omit code*

54.64 Suture of peritoneum

Secondary suture of peritoneum

Excludes *closure of operative wound - omit code*

Operations on the Digestive System

54.1 – 54.64

✖ Deleted Code ▼ Nonspecific O.R. Procedure ✔ Valid O.R. Procedure ✖ Non-O.R. Procedure ♂ Male ♀ Female

❹ **54.7 Other repair of abdominal wall and peritoneum**

✓ **54.71 Repair of gastroschisis**
AHA: 2Q 2002, 9

✓ **54.72 Other repair of abdominal wall**

✓ **54.73 Other repair of peritoneum**
Suture of gastrocolic ligament

✓ **54.74 Other repair of omentum**
Epiplorrhaphy
Graft of omentum
Omentopexy
Reduction of torsion of omentum
Excludes *cardio-omentopexy (36.39)*

✓ **54.75 Other repair of mesentery**
Mesenteric plication
Mesenteropexy

❹ **54.9 Other operations of abdominal region**
Excludes *removal of ectopic pregnancy (74.3)*

✖ **54.91 Percutaneous abdominal drainage**
Paracentesis
Excludes *creation of cutaneoperitoneal fistula (54.93)*
AHA: 3Q 1999, 9; 2Q 1999, 14; 3Q 1998, 10; 1Q 1992, 14; 2Q 1990, 25

✓ **54.92 Removal of foreign body from peritoneal cavity**
AHA: 1Q 1989, 11

✓ **54.93 Creation of cutaneoperitoneal fistula**
AHA: 2Q 1995, 10; May-Jun 1984, 3

✓ **54.94 Creation of peritoneovascular shunt**
Peritoneovenous shunt
AHA: 1Q 1994, 4; 1Q 1988, 9; Sep-Oct 1985, 6

✓ **54.95 Incision of peritoneum**
Exploration of ventriculoperitoneal shunt at peritoneal site
Ladd operation
Revision of distal catheter of ventricular shunt
Revision of ventriculoperitoneal shunt at peritoneal site
Excludes *that incidental to laparotomy (54.11-54.19)*

✖ **54.96 Injection of air into peritoneal cavity**
Pneumoperitoneum
Excludes *that for:*
collapse of lung (33.33)
radiography (88.12-88.13, 88.15)

✖ **54.97 Injection of locally-acting therapeutic substance into peritoneal cavity**
Excludes *peritoneal dialysis (54.98)*

✖ **54.98 Peritoneal dialysis**
Excludes *peritoneal lavage (diagnostic) (54.25)*
AHA: 4Q 1993, 28; May-Jun 1984, 3

✖ **54.99 Other**
Excludes *removal of:*
abdominal wall suture (97.83)
peritoneal drainage device (97.82)
retroperitoneal drainage device (97.81)
AHA: 1Q, 1999, 4; Sep-Oct 1985, 6

10. OPERATIONS ON THE URINARY SYSTEM (55-59)

OPERATIONS ON KIDNEY (55)

Includes operations on renal pelvis
Code also any application or administration of an adhesion barrier substance (99.77)
Excludes *perirenal tissue (59.00-59.09, 59.21-59.29, 59.91-59.92)*

❹ **55.0 Nephrotomy and nephrostomy**
Excludes *drainage by:*
anastomosis (55.86)
aspiration (55.92)
incision of kidney pelvis (55.11-55.12)

✓ **55.01 Nephrotomy**
Evacuation of renal cyst
Exploration of kidney
Nephrolithotomy

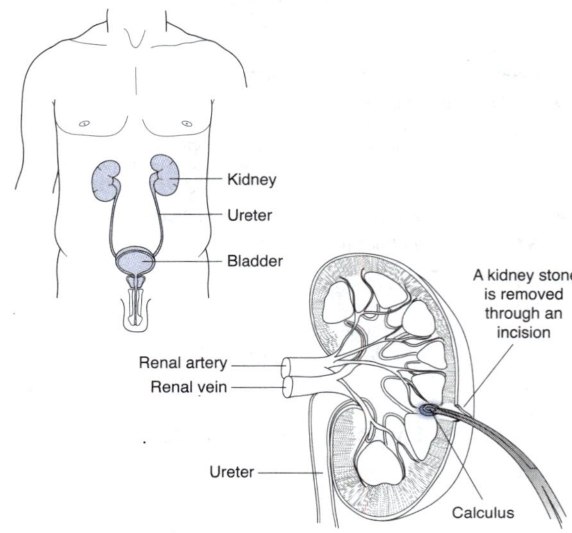

Cross-section of kidney

✓ **55.02 Nephrostomy**
AHA: 2Q 1997, 4

✓ **55.03 Percutaneous nephrostomy without fragmentation**
Nephrostolithotomy, percutaneous (nephroscopic)
Percutaneous removal of kidney stone(s) by:
basket extraction
forceps extraction (nephroscopic)
Pyelostolithotomy, percutaneous (nephroscopic)
With placement of catheter down ureter
Excludes *percutaneous removal by fragmentation (55.04)*
repeat nephroscopic removal during current episode (55.92)
AHA: 2Q 1996, 5

✓ **55.04 Percutaneous nephrostomy with fragmentation**
Percutaneous nephrostomy with disruption of kidney stone by ultrasonic energy and extraction (suction) through endoscope
With placement of catheter down ureter
With fluoroscopic guidance
Excludes *repeat fragmentation during current episode (59.95)*
AHA: 1Q 1989, 3; Sep-Oct 1986, 11

55.1 Pyelotomy and pyelostomy
Excludes *drainage by anastomosis (55.86)*
percutaneous pyelostolithotomy (55.03)
removal of calculus without incision (56.0)

55.11 Pyelotomy
Exploration of renal pelvis
Pyelolithotomy
DEF: Incision into the renal pelvis for exploration or stone removal.

55.12 Pyelostomy
Insertion of drainage tube into renal pelvis

55.2 Diagnostic procedures on kidney

55.21 Nephroscopy

55.22 Pyeloscopy

55.23 Closed [percutaneous] [needle] biopsy of kidney
Endoscopic biopsy via existing nephrostomy, nephrotomy, pyelostomy, or pyelotomy

55.24 Open biopsy of kidney

55.29 Other diagnostic procedures on kidney
Excludes *microscopic examination of specimen from kidney (91.21-91.29)*
pyelogram:
intravenous (87.73)
percutaneous (87.75)
retrograde (87.74)
radioisotope scan (92.03)
renal arteriography (88.45)
tomography:
C.A.T. scan (87.71)
other (87.72)

55.3 Local excision or destruction of lesion or tissue of kidney

55.31 Marsupialization of kidney lesion

55.32 Open ablation of renal lesion or tissue

55.33 Percutaneous ablation of renal lesion or tissue

55.34 Laparoscopic ablation of renal lesion or tissue

55.35 Other and unspecified ablation of renal lesion or tissue

55.39 Other local destruction or excision of renal lesion or tissue
Obliteration of calyceal diverticulum
Excludes *ablation of renal lesion or tissue:*
laparoscopic (55.34)
open (55.32)
other (55.35)
percutaneous (55.33)
biopsy of kidney (55.23-55.24)
partial nephrectomy (55.4)
percutaneous aspiration of kidney (55.92)
wedge resection of kidney (55.4)

55.4 Partial nephrectomy
Calycectomy
Wedge resection of kidney
Code also any synchronous resection of ureter (56.40-56.42)
DEF: Removal of a portion of one kidney.

55.5 Complete nephrectomy
Code also any synchronous excision of:
adrenal gland (07.21-07.3)
bladder segment (57.6)
lymph nodes (40.3, 40.52-40.59)

55.51 Nephroureterectomy
Nephroureterectomy with bladder cuff
Total nephrectomy (unilateral)
Excludes *removal of transplanted kidney (55.53)*
AHA: 2Q 2005, 5

55.52 Nephrectomy of remaining kidney
Removal of solitary kidney
Excludes *removal of transplanted kidney (55.53)*

55.53 Removal of transplanted or rejected kidney

55.54 Bilateral nephrectomy
Excludes *complete nephrectomy NOS (55.51)*

55.6 Transplant of kidney
Note: To report donor source - see codes 00.91-00.93

55.61 Renal autotransplantation

55.69 Other kidney transplantation
AHA: 4Q 2004, 117; 4Q 1996, 71

55.7 Nephropexy
Fixation or suspension of movable [floating] kidney

55.8 Other repair of kidney

55.81 Suture of laceration of kidney

55.82 Closure of nephrostomy and pyelostomy

55.83 Closure of other fistula of kidney

55.84 Reduction of torsion of renal pedicle

55.85 Symphysiotomy for horseshoe kidney

55.86 Anastomosis of kidney
Nephropyeloureterostomy
Pyeloureterovesical anastomosis
Ureterocalyceal anastomosis
Excludes *nephrocystanastomosis NOS (56.73)*

55.87 Correction of ureteropelvic junction

55.89 Other

55.9 Other operations on kidney
Excludes *lysis of perirenal adhesions (59.02)*

55.91 Decapsulation of kidney
Capsulectomy of kidney
Decortication of kidney

55.92 Percutaneous aspiration of kidney (pelvis)
Aspiration of renal cyst
Renipuncture
Excludes *percutaneous biopsy of kidney (55.23)*

55.93 Replacement of nephrostomy tube

55.94 Replacement of pyelostomy tube

55.95 Local perfusion of kidney

55.96 Other injection of therapeutic substance into kidney
Injection into renal cyst

55.97 Implantation or replacement of mechanical kidney

55.98 Removal of mechanical kidney

55.99 Other
Excludes *removal of pyelostomy or nephrostomy tube (97.61)*

OPERATIONS ON URETER (56)

Code also any application or administration of an adhesion barrier substance (99.77)

56.0 Transurethral removal of obstruction from ureter and renal pelvis
Removal of:
blood clot from ureter or renal pelvis without incision
calculus from ureter or renal pelvis without incision
foreign body from ureter or renal pelvis without incision
Excludes *manipulation without removal of obstruction (59.8)*
that by incision (55.11, 56.2)
transurethral insertion of ureteral stent for passage of calculus (59.8)
AHA: 1Q 1989, 1; Sep-Oct 1986, 11

56.1 Ureteral meatotomy

56.2 Ureterotomy
Incision of ureter for:
drainage
exploration
removal of calculus
Excludes *cutting of ureterovesical orifice (56.1)*
removal of calculus without incision (56.0)
transurethral insertion of ureteral stent for passage of calculus (59.8)
urinary diversion (56.51-56.79)
AHA: Sep-Oct 1986, 10; Mar-Apr 1985, 13

56.3 Diagnostic procedures on ureter

56.31 Ureteroscopy
AHA: Mar-Apr 1985, 13

56.32 Closed percutaneous biopsy of ureter
Excludes *endoscopic biopsy of ureter (56.33)*

✖ **56.33 Closed endoscopic biopsy of ureter**
Cystourethroscopy with ureteral biopsy
Transurethral biopsy of ureter
Ureteral endoscopy with biopsy through ureterotomy
Ureteroscopy with biopsy
Excludes *percutaneous biopsy of ureter (56.32)*

✔Ⓞ **56.34 Open biopsy of ureter**

✖ **56.35 Endoscopy (cystoscopy) (looposcopy)of ileal conduit**

✔ **56.39 Other diagnostic procedures on ureter**
Excludes *microscopic examination of specimen from ureter (91.21-91.29)*

❹ **56.4 Ureterectomy**
Code also anastomosis other than end-to-end (56.51-56.79)
Excludes *fistulectomy (56.84)*
nephroureterectomy (55.51-55.54)

✔▼ **56.40 Ureterectomy, not otherwise specified**

✔ **56.41 Partial ureterectomy**
Excision of lesion of ureter
Shortening of ureter with reimplantation
Excludes *biopsy of ureter (56.32-56.34)*

✔ **56.42 Total ureterectomy**

❹ **56.5 Cutaneous uretero-ileostomy**

✔ **56.51 Formation of cutaneous uretero-ileostomy**
Construction of ileal conduit
External ureteral ileostomy
Formation of open ileal bladder
Ileal loop operation
Ileoureterostomy (Bricker's) (ileal bladder)
Transplantation of ureter into ileum with external diversion
Excludes *closed ileal bladder (57.87)*
replacement of ureteral defect by ileal segment (56.89)
AHA: May-Jun 1985, 17

✔ **56.52 Revision of cutaneous uretero-ileostomy**
AHA: 3Q 1996, 15; 4Q 1988, 7

❹ **56.6 Other external urinary diversion**

✔ **56.61 Formation of other cutaneous ureterostomy**
Anastomosis of ureter to skin
Ureterostomy NOS
DEF: Ureterostomy: Creation of channel for urinary diversion to the skin with all or part of the ureter left intact.

✔ **56.62 Revision of other cutaneous ureterostomy**
Revision of ureterostomy stoma
Excludes *nonoperative removal of ureterostomy tube (97.62)*

❹ **56.7 Other anastomosis or bypass of ureter**
Excludes *ureteropyelostomy (55.86)*

✔ **56.71 Urinary diversion to intestine**
Anastomosis of ureter to intestine
Internal urinary diversion NOS
Code also any synchronous colostomy (46.10-46.13)
Excludes *external ureteral ileostomy (56.51)*

✔ **56.72 Revision of ureterointestinal anastomosis**
Excludes *revision of external ureteral ileostomy (56.52)*

✔ **56.73 Nephrocystanastomosis, not otherwise specified**

✔ **56.74 Ureteroneocystostomy**
Replacement of ureter with bladder flap
Ureterovesical anastomosis

✔ **56.75 Transureteroureterostomy**
Excludes *ureteroureterostomy associated with partial resection (56.41)*

✔ **56.79 Other**

❹ **56.8 Repair of ureter**

✔ **56.81 Lysis of intraluminal adhesions of ureter**
Excludes *lysis of periureteral adhesions (59.01-59.02)*
ureterolysis (59.01-59.02)

✔ **56.82 Suture of laceration of ureter**

✔ **56.83 Closure of ureterostomy**
DEF: Closure of a previously created channel for urinary diversion to the skin surface.

✔ **56.84 Closure of other fistula of ureter**

✔ **56.85 Ureteropexy**

✔ **56.86 Removal of ligature from ureter**

✔ **56.89 Other repair of ureter**
Graft of ureter
Replacement of ureter with ileal segment implanted into bladder
Ureteroplication

❹ **56.9 Other operations on ureter**

✖ **56.91 Dilation of ureteral meatus**

✔ **56.92 Implantation of electronic ureteral stimulator**

✔ **56.93 Replacement of electronic ureteral stimulator**

✔ **56.94 Removal of electronic ureteral stimulator**
Excludes *that with synchronous replacement (56.93)*

✔ **56.95 Ligation of ureter**

✔ **56.99 Other**
Excludes *removal of ureterostomy tube and ureteral catheter (97.62)*
ureteral catheterization (59.8)

OPERATIONS ON URINARY BLADDER (57)

Code also any application or administration of an adhesion barrier substance (99.77)
Excludes *perivesical tissue (59.11-59.29, 59.91-59.92)*
ureterovesical orifice (56.0-56.99)

✖ **57.0 Transurethral clearance of bladder**
Drainage of bladder without incision
Removal of:
blood clots from bladder without incision
calculus from bladder without incision
foreign body from bladder without incision
Excludes *that by incision (57.19)*
AHA: Sep-Oct 1986, 11

❹ **57.1 Cystotomy and cystostomy**
Excludes *cystotomy and cystostomy as operative approach - omit code*

✖ **57.11 Percutaneous aspiration of bladder**

✔ **57.12 Lysis of intraluminal adhesions with incision into bladder**
Excludes *transurethral lysis of intraluminal adhesions (57.41)*

✖ **57.17 Percutaneous cystostomy**
Closed cystostomy
Percutaneous suprapubic cystostomy
Excludes *removal of cystostomy tube (97.63)*
replacement of cystostomy tube (59.94)

✔ **57.18 Other suprapubic cystostomy**
Excludes *percutaneous cystostomy (57.17)*
removal of cystostomy tube (97.63)
replacement of cystostomy tube (59.94)

✔ **57.19 Other cystotomy**
Cystolithotomy
Excludes *percutaneous cystostomy (57.17)*
suprapubic cystostomy (57.18)
DEF: Cystolithotomy: Incision of the urinary bladder for removal of a calculus.
AHA: 4Q 1995, 73; Sep-Oct 1986, 11; Mar-Apr 1985, 13

❹ **57.2 Vesicostomy**
Excludes *percutaneous cystostomy (57.17)*
suprapubic cystostomy (57.18)

✔ **57.21 Vesicostomy**
Creation of permanent opening from bladder to skin using a bladder flap

✔ **57.22 Revision or closure of vesicostomy**
Excludes *closure of cystostomy (57.82)*

❹ **57.3 Diagnostic procedures on bladder**

✖ **57.31 Cystoscopy through artificial stoma**

✖ **57.32 Other cystoscopy**
Transurethral cystoscopy
Excludes *cystourethroscopy with ureteral biopsy (56.33)*
retrograde pyelogram (87.74)
that for control of hemorrhage (postoperative):
bladder (57.93)
prostate (60.94)
AHA: 1Q 2001, 14

✓ **57.33 Closed [transurethral] biopsy of bladder**

Cystourethroscopy with biopsy

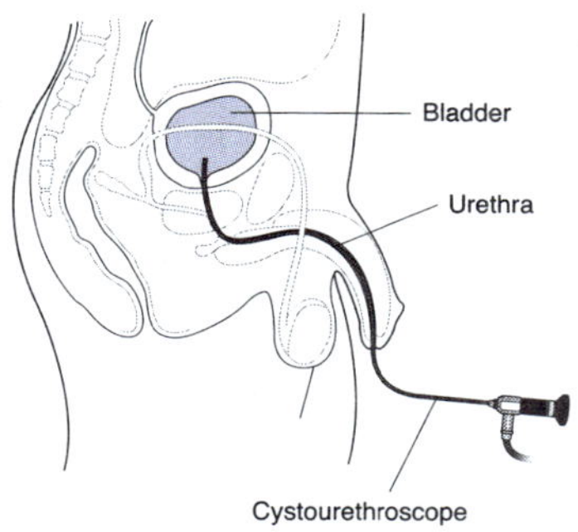

✓ **57.34 Open biopsy of bladder**
AHA: 2Q 2005, 12

✓ **57.39 Other diagnostic procedures on bladder**
Excludes *cystogram NEC (87.77)*
microscopic examination of specimen from bladder (91.31-91.39)
retrograde cystourethrogram (87.76)
therapeutic distention of bladder (96.25)

57.4 Transurethral excision or destruction of bladder tissue

✓ **57.41 Transurethral lysis of intraluminal adhesions**

✓ **57.49 Other transurethral excision or destruction of lesion or tissue of bladder**
Endoscopic resection of bladder lesion
Excludes *transurethral biopsy of bladder (57.33)*
transurethral fistulectomy (57.83-57.84)

57.5 Other excision or destruction of bladder tissue
Excludes *that with transurethral approach (57.41-57.49)*

✓ **57.51 Excision of urachus**
Excision of urachal sinus of bladder
Excludes *excision of urachal cyst of abdominal wall (54.3)*

✓ **57.59 Open excision or destruction of other lesion or tissue of bladder**
Endometrectomy of bladder
Suprapubic excision of bladder lesion
Excludes *biopsy of bladder (57.33-57.34)*
fistulectomy of bladder (57.83-57.84)

✓ **57.6 Partial cystectomy**
Excision of bladder dome
Trigonectomy
Wedge resection of bladder
DEF: Removal of a portion of the bladder.

57.7 Total cystectomy
Includes total cystectomy with urethrectomy

✓ **57.71 Radical cystectomy**
Pelvic exenteration in male
Removal of bladder, prostate, seminal vesicles, and fat
Removal of bladder, urethra, and fat in a female
Code also any:
lymph node dissection (40.3, 40.5)
urinary diversion (56.51-56.79)
Excludes *that as part of pelvic exenteration in female (68.8)*

✓ **57.79 Other total cystectomy**

57.8 Other repair of urinary bladder
Excludes *repair of:*
current obstetric laceration (75.61)
cystocele (70.50-70.51)
that for stress incontinence (59.3-59.79)

✓ **57.81 Suture of laceration of bladder**

✓ **57.82 Closure of cystostomy**

✓ **57.83 Repair of fistula involving bladder and intestine**
Rectovesicovaginal fistulectomy
Vesicosigmoidovaginal fistulectomy

✓ **57.84 Repair of other fistula of bladder**
Cervicovesical fistulectomy
Urethroperineovesical fistulectomy
Uterovesical fistulectomy
Vaginovesical fistulectomy
Excludes *vesicoureterovaginal fistulectomy (56.84)*

✓ **57.85 Cystourethroplasty and plastic repair of bladder neck**
Plication of sphincter of urinary bladder
V-Y plasty of bladder neck

✓ **57.86 Repair of bladder exstrophy**

✓ **57.87 Reconstruction of urinary bladder**
Anastomosis of bladder with isolated segment of ileum
Augmentation of bladder
Replacement of bladder with ileum or sigmoid [closed ileal bladder]
Code also resection of intestine (45.50-45.52)
AHA: 2Q 2005, 12, 13; 2Q 2003, 11; 3Q 2000, 7

✓ **57.88 Other anastomosis of bladder**
Anastomosis of bladder to intestine NOS
Cystocolic anastomosis
Excludes *formation of closed ilea bladder (57.87)*

✓ **57.89 Other repair of bladder**
Bladder suspension, not elsewhere classified
Cystopexy NOS
Repair of old obstetric laceration of bladder
Excludes *repair of current obstetric laceration (75.61)*
DEF: Cystopexy: Surgical fixation of the bladder to the abdominal wall.

57.9 Other operations on bladder

✓ **57.91 Sphincterotomy of bladder**
Division of bladder neck
AHA: 3Q 1994, 12; 2Q 1990, 26

✖ **57.92 Dilation of bladder neck**

✓ **57.93 Control of (postoperative) hemorrhage of bladder**

✖ **57.94 Insertion of indwelling urinary catheter**

✖ **57.95 Replacement of indwelling urinary catheter**

✓ **57.96 Implantation of electronic bladder stimulator**

✓ **57.97 Replacement of electronic bladder stimulator**

✓ **57.98 Removal of electronic bladder stimulator**
Excludes *that with synchronous replacement (57.97)*

✓ **57.99 Other**
Excludes *irrigation of:*
cystostomy (96.47)
other indwelling urinary catheter (96.48)
lysis of external adhesions (59.11)
removal of:
cystostomy tube (97.63)
other urinary drainage devic (97.64)
therapeutic distention of bladder (96.25)

OPERATIONS ON URETHRA (58)

Includes operations on:
bulbourethral gland [Cowper's gland]
periurethral tissue

Code also any application or administration of an adhesion barrier substance (99.77)

✓ **58.0 Urethrotomy**
Excision of urethral septum
Formation of urethrovaginal fistula
Perineal urethrostomy
Removal of calculus from urethra by incision
Excludes *drainage of bulbourethral gland or periurethral tissue (58.91)*
internal urethral meatotomy (58.5)
removal of urethral calculus without incision (58.6)

DEF: Incision of the urethra.

✓ **58.1 Urethral meatotomy**
Excludes *internal urethral meatotomy (58.5)*

❹ **58.2 Diagnostic procedures on urethra**

✖ **58.21 Perineal urethroscopy**

✖ **58.22 Other urethroscopy**

✖ **58.23 Biopsy of urethra**

✖ **58.24 Biopsy of periurethral tissue**

✖ **58.29 Other diagnostic procedures on urethra and periurethral tissue**
Excludes *microscopic examination of specimen from urethra (91.31-91.39)*
retrograde cystourethrogram (87.76)
urethral pressure profile (89.25)
urethral sphincter electromyogram (89.23)

❹ **58.3 Excision or destruction of lesion or tissue of urethra**
Excludes *biopsy of urethra (58.23)*
excision of bulbourethral gland (58.92)
fistulectomy (58.43)
urethrectomy as part of:
complete cystectomy (57.79)
pelvic evisceration (68.8)
radical cystectomy (57.71)

✖ **58.31 Endoscopic excision or destruction of lesion or tissue of urethra**
Fulguration of urethral lesion

✖ **58.39 Other local excision or destruction of lesion or tissue of urethra**
Excision of:
congenital valve of urethra
lesion of urethra
stricture of urethra
Urethrectomy
Excludes *that by endoscopic approach (58.31)*

❹ **58.4 Repair of urethra**
Excludes *repair of current obstetric laceration (75.61)*

✓ **58.41 Suture of laceration of urethra**

✓ **58.42 Closure of urethrostomy**

✓ **58.43 Closure of other fistula of urethra**
Excludes *repair of urethroperineovesical fistula (57.84)*

✓ **58.44 Reanastomosis of urethra**
Anastomosis of urethra

✓ **58.45 Repair of hypospadias or epispadias**
AHA: 3Q 1997, 6; 4Q 1996, 35

✓ **58.46 Other reconstruction of urethra**
Urethral construction

✓ **58.47 Urethral meatoplasty**

✓ **58.49 Other repair of urethra**
Benenenti rotation of bulbous urethra
Repair of old obstetric laceration of urethra
Urethral plication
Excludes *repair of:*
current obstetric laceration (75.61)
urethrocele (70.50-70.51)

✓ **58.5 Release of urethral stricture**
Cutting of urethral sphincter
Internal urethral meatotomy
Urethrolysis
AHA: 1Q 1997, 13

✖ **58.6 Dilation of urethra**
Dilation of urethrovesical junction
Passage of sounds through urethra
Removal of calculus from urethra without incision
Excludes *urethral calibration (89.29)*
AHA: 1Q 2001, 14; 1Q 1997, 13

❹ **58.9 Other operations on urethra and periurethral tissue**

✓ **58.91 Incision of periurethral tissue**
Drainage of bulbourethral gland

✓ **58.92 Excision of periurethral tissue**
Excludes *biopsy of periurethral tissue (58.24)*
lysis of periurethral adhesions:
laparoscopic (59.12)
other (59.11)

✓ **58.93 Implantation of artificial urinary sphincter [AUS]**
Placement of inflatable:
bladder sphincter
urethral sphincter
Removal with replacement of sphincter device [AUS]
With pump and/or reservoir

✓ **58.99 Other**
Removal of inflatable urinary sphincter without replacement
Repair of inflatable sphincter pump and/or reservoir
Surgical correction of hydraulic pressure of inflatable sphincter device
Excludes *removal of:*
intraluminal foreign body from urethra without incision (98.19)
urethral stent (97.65)
AHA: 4Q 1995, 72

OTHER OPERATIONS ON URINARY TRACT (59)

Code also any application or administration of an adhesion barrier substance (99.77)

❹ **59.0 Dissection of retroperitoneal tissue**

✓ **59.00 Retroperitoneal dissection, not otherwise specified**

✓ **59.02 Other lysis of perirenal or periureteral adhesions**
Excludes *that by laparoscope (59.03)*

✓ **59.03 Laparoscopic lysis of perirenal or periureteral adhesions**

✓ **59.09 Other incision of perirenal or periureteral tissue**
Exploration of perinephric area
Incision of perirenal abscess

❹ **59.1 Incision of perivesical tissue**

✓ **59.11 Other lysis of perivesical adhesions**

✓ **59.12 Laparoscopic lysis of perivesical adhesions**

✓ **59.19 Other incision of perivesical tissue**
Exploration of perivesical tissue
Incision of hematoma of space of Retzius
Retropubic exploration

❹ **59.2 Diagnostic procedures on perirenal and perivesical tissue**

✓ **59.21 Biopsy of perirenal or perivesical tissue**

✓ **59.29 Other diagnostic procedures on perirenal tissue, perivesical tissue, and retroperitoneum**
Excludes *microscopic examination of specimen from:*
perirenal tissue (91.21-91.29)
perivesical tissue (91.31-91.39)
retroperitoneum NEC (91.11-91.19)
retroperitoneal x-ray (88.14-88.16)

✓ **59.3 Plication of urethrovesical junction**
Kelly-Kennedy operation on urethra
Kelly-Stoeckel urethral plication

59.4 Suprapubic sling operation
Goebel-Frangenheim-Stoeckel urethrovesical suspension
Millin-Read urethrovesical suspension
Oxford operation for urinary incontinence
Urethrocystopexy by suprapubic suspension

59.5 Retropubic urethral suspension
Burch procedure
Marshall-Marchetti-Krantz operation
Suture of periurethral tissue to symphysis pubis
Urethral suspension NOS
AHA: 1Q 1997, 11

59.6 Paraurethral suspension
Pereyra paraurethral suspension
Periurethral suspension

59.7 Other repair of urinary stress incontinence

59.71 Levator muscle operation for urethrovesical suspension
Cystourethropexy with levator muscle sling
Gracilis muscle transplant for urethrovesical suspension
Pubococcygeal sling

59.72 Injection of implant into urethra and/or bladder neck
Collagen implant
Endoscopic injection of implant
Fat implant
Polytef implant
AHA: 4Q 1995, 72

59.79 Other
Anterior urethropexy
Repair of stress incontinence NOS
Tudor "rabbit ear" urethropexy
AHA: 2Q 2001, 20; 1Q 2000, 14-15, 19

59.8 Ureteral catheterization
Drainage of kidney by catheter
Insertion of ureteral stent
Ureterovesical orifice dilation
Code also any ureterotomy (56.2)
Excludes *that for:*
retrograde pyelogram (87.74)
transurethral removal of calculus or clot from ureter and renal pelvis (56.0)
AHA: 2Q 2005, 12, 13; 2Q 2003, 11; 3Q 2000, 7; 1Q 1989, 3; Sep-Oct 1986, 10

59.9 Other operations on urinary system
Excludes *nonoperative removal of therapeutic device (97.61-97.69)*

59.91 Excision of perirenal or perivesical tissue
Excludes *biopsy of perirenal or perivesical tissue (59.21)*

59.92 Other operations on perirenal or perivesical tissue

59.93 Replacement of ureterostomy tube
Change of ureterostomy tube
Reinsertion of ureterostomy tube
Excludes *nonoperative removal of ureterostomy tube (97.62)*

59.94 Replacement of cystostomy tube
Excludes *nonoperative removal of cystostomy tube (97.63)*

59.95 Ultrasonic fragmentation of urinary stones
Shattered urinary stones
Excludes *percutaneous nephrostomy with fragmentation (55.04)*
shock-wave disintegration (98.51)
AHA: 1Q 1989, 1; Sep-Oct 1986, 11

59.99 Other
Excludes *instillation of medication into urinary tract (96.49)*
irrigation of urinary tract (96.45-96.48)

11. OPERATIONS ON THE MALE GENITAL ORGANS (60-64)

OPERATIONS ON PROSTATE AND SEMINAL VESICLES (60)

Code also any application or administration of an adhesion barrier substance (99.77)
Includes operations on periprostatic tissue
Excludes *that associated with radical cystectomy (57.71)*

60.0 Incision of prostate ♂
Drainage of prostatic abscess
Prostatolithotomy
Excludes *drainage of periprostatic tissue only (60.81)*
DEF: Prostatolithotomy: Incision into the prostate for removal of a stone.

60.1 Diagnostic procedures on prostate and seminal vesicles

60.11 Closed [percutaneous] [needle] biopsy of prostate ♂
Approach:
transrectal
transurethral
Punch biopsy

60.12 Open biopsy of prostate ♂

60.13 Closed [percutaneous] biopsy of seminal vesicles ♂
Needle biopsy of seminal vesicles

60.14 Open biopsy of seminal vesicles ♂

60.15 Biopsy of periprostatic tissue ♂

60.18 Other diagnostic procedures on prostate and periprostatic tissue ♂
Excludes *microscopic examination of specimen from prostate (91.31-91.39)*
x-ray of prostate (87.92)

60.19 Other diagnostic procedures on seminal vesicles ♂
Excludes *microscopic examination of specimen from seminal vesicles (91.31-91.39)*
x-ray:
contrast seminal vesiculogram (87.91)
other (87.92)

60.2 Transurethral prostatectomy
Excludes *local excision of lesion of prostate (60.61)*
AHA: 3Q 1994, 12; 2Q 1994, 9; 3Q 1992, 13; Sep-Oct 1985, 10

60.21 Transurethral (ultrasound) guided laser induced prostatectomy (TULIP) ♂
Ablation (contact) (noncontact) by laser
AHA: 4Q 1995, 71

Transurethral resection of prostate

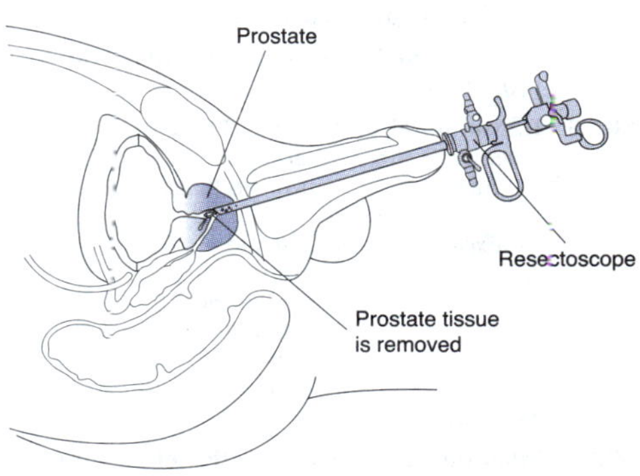

60.29 Other transurethral prostatectomy ♂
Excision of median bar by transurethral approach
Transurethral electrovaporization of prostrate (TEVAP)
Transurethral enucleative procedure
Transurethral prostatectomy NOS
Transurethral resection of prostate (TURP)
AHA: 3Q 1997, 3

✓ **60.3 Suprapubic prostatectomy ♂**
Transvesical prostatectomy
Excludes *local excision of lesion of prostate (60.61)*
radical prostatectomy (60.5)

✓ **60.4 Retropubic prostatectomy ♂**
Excludes *local excision of lesion of prostate (60.61)*
radical prostatectomy (60.5)

✓ **60.5 Radical prostatectomy ♂**
Prostatovesiculectomy
Radical prostatectomy by any approach
Excludes *cystoprostatectomy (57.71)*
AHA: 3Q 1993, 12

④ **60.6 Other prostatectomy**

✓ **60.61 Local excision of lesion of prostate ♂**
Excision of prostatic lesion by any approach
Excludes *biopsy of prostate (60.11-60.12)*

✓ **60.62 Perineal prostatectomy ♂**
Cryoablation of prostate
Cryoprostatectomy
Cryosurgery of prostate
Radical cryosurgical ablation of prostate (RCSA)
Excludes *local excision of lesion of prostate (60.61)*

✓ **60.69 Other ♂**

④ **60.7 Operations on seminal vesicles**

✖ **60.71 Percutaneous aspiration of seminal vesicle ♂**
Excludes *needle biopsy of seminal vesicle (60.13)*

✓ **60.72 Incision of seminal vesicle ♂**

✓ **60.73 Excision of seminal vesicle ♂**
Excision of Müllerian duct cyst
Spermatocystectomy
Excludes *biopsy of seminal vesicle (60.13-60.14)*
prostatovesiculectomy (60.5)

✓ **60.79 Other operations on seminal vesicles ♂**

④ **60.8 Incision or excision of periprostatic tissue**

✓ **60.81 Incision of periprostatic tissue ♂**
Drainage of periprostatic abscess

✓ **60.82 Excision of periprostatic tissue ♂**
Excision of lesion of periprostatic tissue
Excludes *biopsy of periprostatic tissue (60.15)*

④ **60.9 Other operations on prostate**

✖ **60.91 Percutaneous aspiration of prostate ♂**
Excludes *needle biopsy of prostate (60.11)*

✖ **60.92 Injection into prostate test link ♂**

✓ **60.93 Repair of prostate ♂**

✓ **60.94 Control of (postoperative) hemorrhage of prostate ♂**
Coagulation of prostatic bed
Cystoscopy for control of prostatic hemorrhage

✓ **60.95 Transurethral balloon dilation of the prostatic urethra ♂**
AHA: 4Q 1991, 23

✓ **60.96 Transurethral destruction of prostate tissue by microwave thermotherapy ♂**
Transurethral microwave thermotherapy (TUMT) of prostate
Excludes *Prostatectomy:*
other (60.61-60.69)
radical (60.5)
retropubic (60.4)
suprapubic (60.3)
transurethral (60.21-60.29)
AHA: 4Q 2000, 67

✓ **60.97 Other transurethral destruction of prostate tissue by other thermotherapy ♂**
Radiofrequency thermotherapy
Transurethral needle ablation (TUNA) of prostate
Excludes *Prostatectomy:*
other (60.61-60.69)
radical (60.5)
retropubic (60.4)
suprapubic (60.3)
transurethral (60.21-60.29)
AHA: 4Q 2000, 67

✓ **60.99 Other ♂**
Excludes *prostatic massage (99.94)*
AHA: 3Q 1990, 12

OPERATIONS ON SCROTUM AND TUNICA VAGINALIS (61)

✖ **61.0 Incision and drainage of scrotum and tunica vaginalis ♂**
Excludes *percutaneous aspiration of hydrocele (61.91)*

④ **61.1 Diagnostic procedures on scrotum and tunica vaginalis**

✖ **61.11 Biopsy of scrotum or tunica vaginalis ♂**

✖ **61.19 Other diagnostic procedures on scrotum and tunica vaginalis ♂**

✓ **61.2 Excision of hydrocele (of tunica vaginalis) ♂**
Bottle repair of hydrocele of tunica vaginalis
Excludes *percutaneous aspiration of hydrocele (61.91)*

✖ **61.3 Excision or destruction of lesion or tissue of scrotum ♂**
Fulguration of lesion of scrotum
Partial scrotectomy of scrotum
Reduction of elephantiasis of scrotum
Excludes *biopsy of scrotum (61.11)*
scrotal fistulectomy (61.42)

④ **61.4 Repair of scrotum and tunica vaginalis**

✖ **61.41 Suture of laceration of scrotum and tunica vaginalis ♂**

✓ **61.42 Repair of scrotal fistula ♂**

✓ **61.49 Other repair of scrotum and tunica vaginalis ♂**
Reconstruction with rotational or pedicle flaps

④ **61.9 Other operations on scrotum and tunica vaginalis**

✖ **61.91 Percutaneous aspiration of tunica vaginalis ♂**
Aspiration of hydrocele of tunica vaginalis

✓ **61.92 Excision of lesion of tunica vaginalis other than hydrocele ♂**
Excision of hematocele of tunica vaginalis

✓ **61.99 Other ♂**
Excludes *removal of foreign body from scrotum without incision (98.24)*

OPERATIONS ON TESTES (62)

✓ **62.0 Incision of testis ♂**

④ **62.1 Diagnostic procedures on testes**

✖ⓞ **62.11 Closed [percutaneous] [needle] biopsy of testis ♂**

✓Ⓞ **62.12 Open biopsy of testis ♂**

✓ **62.19 Other diagnostic procedures on testes ♂**

✓ **62.2 Excision or destruction of testicular lesion ♂**
Excision of appendix testis
Excision of cyst of Morgagni in the male
Excludes *biopsy of testis (62.11-62.12)*

✓ **62.3 Unilateral orchiectomy ♂**
Orchidectomy (with epididymectomy) NOS
DEF: Removal of one testis.

④ **62.4 Bilateral orchiectomy**
Male castration
Radical bilateral orchiectomy (with epididymectomy)
Code also any synchronous lymph node dissection (40.3, 40.5)
DEF: Surgical removal of both testes, resulting in castration.

✓ **62.41 Removal of both testes at same operative episode ♂**
Bilateral orchidectomy NOS

✓ **62.42 Removal of remaining testis ♂**
Removal of solitary testis

✓ **62.5 Orchiopexy ♂**
Mobilization and replacement of testis in scrotum
Orchiopexy with detorsion of testis
Torek (-Bevan) operation (orchidopexy) (first stage) (second stage)
Transplantation to and fixation of testis in scrotum

❹ **62.6 Repair of testes**
Excludes *reduction of torsion (63.52)*

✔ **62.61 Suture of laceration of testis** ♂

✔ **62.69 Other repair of testis** ♂
Testicular graft

✔ **62.7 Insertion of testicular prosthesis** ♂

❹ **62.9 Other operations on testes**

✖ **62.91 Aspiration of testis** ♂
Excludes *percutaneous biopsy of testis (62.11)*

✖ **62.92 Injection of therapeutic substance into testis** ♂

✔ **62.99 Other** ♂

OPERATIONS ON SPERMATIC CORD, EPIDIDYMIS, AND VAS DEFERENS (63)

❹ **63.0 Diagnostic procedures on spermatic cord, epididymis, and vas deferens**

✖ **63.01 Biopsy of spermatic cord, epididymis, or vas deferens** ♂

✔ **63.09 Other diagnostic procedures on spermatic cord, epididymis, and vas deferens** ♂
Excludes *contrast epididymogram (87.93)*
contrast vasogram (87.94)
other x-ray of epididymis and vas deferens (87.95)

✔ **63.1 Excision of varicocele and hydrocele of spermatic cord** ♂
High ligation of spermatic vein
Hydrocelectomy of canal of Nuck

✔ **63.2 Excision of cyst of epididymis** ♂
Spermatocelectomy

✔ **63.3 Excision of other lesion or tissue of spermatic cord and epididymis** ♂
Excision of appendix epididymis
Excludes *biopsy of spermatic cord or epididymis (63.01)*

✔ **63.4 Epididymectomy** ♂
Excludes *that synchronous with orchiectomy (62.3-62.42)*

❹ **63.5 Repair of spermatic cord and epididymis**

✔ **63.51 Suture of laceration of spermatic cord and epididymis** ♂

✖ **63.52 Reduction of torsion of testis or spermatic cord** ♂
Excludes *that associated with orchiopexy (62.5)*

✔ **63.53 Transplantation of spermatic cord** ♂

✔ **63.59 Other repair of spermatic cord and epididymis** ♂

✖ **63.6 Vasotomy** ♂
Vasostomy

❹ **63.7 Vasectomy and ligation of vas deferens**

✖ **63.70 Male sterilization procedure, not otherwise specified** ♂

✖ **63.71 Ligation of vas deferens** ♂
Crushing of vas deferens
Division of vas deferens

✖ **63.72 Ligation of spermatic cord** ♂

✖ **63.73 Vasectomy** ♂
AHA: 2Q 1998, 13

❹ **63.8 Repair of vas deferens and epididymis**

✔ **63.81 Suture of laceration of vas deferens and epididymis** ♂

✔ **63.82 Reconstruction of surgically divided vas deferens** ♂

✔ **63.83 Epididymovasostomy** ♂

✖ **63.84 Removal of ligature from vas deferens** ♂

✔ **63.85 Removal of valve from vas deferens** ♂

✔ **63.89 Other repair of vas deferens and epididymis** ♂

❹ **63.9 Other operations on spermatic cord, epididymis, and vas deferens**

✖ **63.91 Aspiration of spermatocele** ♂

✔ **63.92 Epididymotomy** ♂

✔ **63.93 Incision of spermatic cord** ♂

✔ **63.94 Lysis of adhesions of spermatic cord** ♂

✔ **63.95 Insertion of valve in vas deferens** ♂

✔ **63.99 Other** ♂

OPERATIONS ON PENIS (64)

Includes operations on:
corpora cavernosa
glans penis
prepuce

✔ **64.0 Circumcision** ♂

❹ **64.1 Diagnostic procedures on the penis**

✔ **64.11 Biopsy of penis** ♂

✖ **64.19 Other diagnostic procedures on penis** ♂

✔ **64.2 Local excision or destruction of lesion of penis** ♂
Excludes *biopsy of penis (64.11)*

✔ **64.3 Amputation of penis** ♂

❹ **64.4 Repair and plastic operation on penis**

✔ **64.41 Suture of laceration of penis** ♂

✔ **64.42 Release of chordee** ♂
AHA: 4Q 1996, 34

✔ **64.43 Construction of penis** ♂

✔ **64.44 Reconstruction of penis** ♂

✔ **64.45 Replantation of penis** ♂
Reattachment of amputated penis

✔ **64.49 Other repair of penis** ♂
Excludes *repair of epispadias and hypospadias (58.45)*

✔ **64.5 Operations for sex transformation, not elsewhere classified** ♂

❹ **64.9 Other operations on male genital organs**

✖ **64.91 Dorsal or lateral slit of prepuce** ♂

✔ **64.92 Incision of penis** ♂

✔ **64.93 Division of penile adhesions** ♂

✖ **64.94 Fitting of external prosthesis of penis** ♂
Penile prosthesis NOS

✔ **64.95 Insertion or replacement of non-inflatable penile prosthesis** ♂
Insertion of semi-rigid rod prosthesis into shaft of penis
Excludes *external penile prosthesis (64.94)*
inflatable penile prosthesis (64.97)
plastic repair, penis (64.43-64.49)
that associated with:
construction (64.43)
reconstruction (64.44)

✔ **64.96 Removal of internal prosthesis of penis** ♂
Removal without replacement of non-inflatable or inflatable penile prosthesis

✔ **64.97 Insertion or replacement of inflatable penile prosthesis** ♂
Insertion of cylinders into shaft of penis and placement of pump and reservoir
Excludes *external penile prosthesis (64.94)*
non-inflatable penile prosthesis (64.95)
plastic repair, penis (64.43-64.49)
AHA: 2Q 1990, 26

✔ **64.98 Other operations on penis** ♂
Corpora cavernosa-corpus spongiosum shunt
Corpora-saphenous shunt
Irrigation of corpus cavernosum
Excludes *removal of foreign body:*
intraluminal (98.19)
without incision (98.24)
stretching of foreskin (99.95)
AHA: 3Q 1992, 9

✔ **64.99 Other** ♂
Excludes *collection of sperm for artificial insemination (99.96)*

12. OPERATIONS ON THE FEMALE GENITAL ORGANS (65-71)

OPERATIONS ON OVARY (65)

Code also any application or administration of an adhesion barrier substance (99.77)

❹ **65.0 Oophorotomy**
Salpingo-oophorotomy

✓ **65.01 Laparoscopic oophorotomy** ♀

✓ **65.09 Other oophorotomy** ♀

❹ **65.1 Diagnostic procedures on ovaries**

✓ **65.11 Aspiration biopsy of ovary** ♀

✓ **65.12 Other biopsy of ovary** ♀

✓ **65.13 Laparoscopic biopsy of ovary** ♀
AHA: 4Q 1996, 67

✓ **65.14 Other laparoscopic diagnostic procedures on ovaries** ♀

✓ **65.19 Other diagnostic procedures on ovaries** ♀
Excludes *microscopic examination of specimen from ovary (91.41-91.49)*

❹ **65.2 Local excision or destruction of ovarian lesion or tissue**

✓ **65.21 Marsupialization of ovarian cyst** ♀
Excludes *that by laparoscope (65.23)*

✓ **65.22 Wedge resection of ovary** ♀
Excludes *that by laparoscope (65.24)*

✓ **65.23 Laparoscopic marsupialization of ovarian cyst** ♀

✓ **65.24 Laparoscopic wedge resection of ovary** ♀

✓ **65.25 Other laparoscopic local excision or destruction of ovary** ♀

✓ **65.29 Other local excision or destruction of ovary** ♀
Bisection of ovary
Cauterization of ovary
Partial excision of ovary
Excludes *biopsy of ovary (65.11-65.13)*
that by laparoscope (65.25)

❹ **65.3 Unilateral oophorectomy**
AHA: 3Q 1995, 15

✓ **65.31 Laparoscopic unilateral oophorectomy** ♀

✓ **65.39 Other unilateral oophorectomy** ♀
Excludes *that by laparoscope (65.31)*

❹ **65.4 Unilateral salpingo-oophorectomy**

✓ **65.41 Laparoscopic unilateral salpingo-oophorectomy** ♀
AHA: 4Q 1996, 67

✓ **65.49 Other unilateral salpingo-oophorectomy** ♀

❹ **65.5 Bilateral oophorectomy**

✓ **65.51 Other removal of both ovaries at same operative episode** ♀
Female castration
Excludes *that by laparoscope (65.53)*

✓ **65.52 Other removal of remaining ovary** ♀
Removal of solitary ovary
Excludes *that by laparoscope (65.54)*

✓ **65.53 Laparoscopic removal of both ovaries at same operative episode** ♀

✓ **65.54 Laparoscopic removal of remaining ovary** ♀

❹ **65.6 Bilateral salpingo-oophorectomy**

✓ **65.61 Other removal of both ovaries and tubes at same operative episode** ♀
Excludes *that by laparoscope (65.63)*
AHA: 4Q 1996, 65

✓ **65.62 Other removal of remaining ovary and tube** ♀
Removal of solitary ovary and tube
Excludes *that by laparoscope (65.64)*

✓ **65.63 Laparoscopic removal of both ovaries and tubes at same operative episode** ♀
AHA: 4Q 1996, 68

✓ **65.64 Laparoscopic removal of remaining ovary and tube** ♀

❹ **65.7 Repair of ovary**
Excludes *salpingo-oophorostomy (66.72)*

✓ **65.71 Other simple suture of ovary** ♀
Excludes *that by laparoscope (65.74)*

✓ **65.72 Other reimplantation of ovary** ♀
Excludes *that by laparoscope (65.75)*

✓ **65.73 Other salpingo-oophoroplasty** ♀
Excludes *that by laparoscope (65.76)*

✓ **65.74 Laparoscopic simple suture of ovary** ♀

✓ **65.75 Laparoscopic reimplantation of ovary** ♀

✓ **65.76 Laparoscopic salpingo-oophoroplasty** ♀

✓ **65.79 Other repair of ovary** ♀
Oophoropexy
DEF: Oophoropexy: Surgical fixation of an ovary to the abdominal wall.

❹ **65.8 Lysis of adhesions of ovary and fallopian tube**

✓ **65.81 Laparoscopic lysis of adhesions of ovary and fallopian tube** ♀
AHA: 4Q 1996, 67

✓ **65.89 Other lysis of adhesions of ovary and fallopian tube** ♀
Excludes *that by laparoscope (65.81)*

❹ **65.9 Other operations on ovary**

✓ **65.91 Aspiration of ovary** ♀
Excludes *aspiration biopsy of ovary (65.11)*

✓ **65.92 Transplantation of ovary** ♀
Excludes *reimplantation of ovary:*
laparoscopic (65.75)
other (65.72)

✓ **65.93 Manual rupture of ovarian cyst** ♀

✓ **65.94 Ovarian denervation** ♀

✓ **65.95 Release of torsion of ovary** ♀

✓ **65.99 Other** ♀
Ovarian drilling
AHA: Nov-Dec 1986, 9

OPERATIONS ON FALLOPIAN TUBES (66)

Code also any application or administration of an adhesion barrier substance (99.77)

❹ **66.0 Salpingotomy and salpingostomy**

✓ **66.01 Salpingotomy** ♀
DEF: Incision into a fallopian tube.

✓ **66.02 Salpingostomy** ♀

❹ **66.1 Diagnostic procedures on fallopian tubes**

✓ **66.11 Biopsy of fallopian tube** ♀

✓ **66.19 Other diagnostic procedures on fallopian tubes** ♀
Excludes *microscopic examination of specimen from fallopian tubes (91.41-91.49)*
radiography of fallopian tubes (87.82-87.83, 87.85)
Rubin's test (66.8)

❹ **66.2 Bilateral endoscopic destruction or occlusion of fallopian tubes**
Includes bilateral endoscopic destruction or occlusion of fallopian tubes by:
culdoscopy
endoscopy
hysteroscopy
laparoscopy
peritoneoscopy
endoscopic destruction of solitary fallopian tube

✓ **66.21 Bilateral endoscopic ligation and crushing of fallopian tubes** ♀

✓ **66.22 Bilateral endoscopic ligation and division of fallopian tubes** ♀

✓ **66.29 Other bilateral endoscopic destruction or occlusion of fallopian tubes** ♀

❹ **66.3 Other bilateral destruction or occlusion of fallopian tubes**
Includes destruction of solitary fallopian tube
Excludes *endoscopic destruction or occlusion of fallopian tubes (66.21-66.29)*

✓ **66.31 Other bilateral ligation and crushing of fallopian tubes** ♀

✓ **66.32 Other bilateral ligation and division of fallopian tubes** ♀
Pomeroy operation

✓ **66.39 Other bilateral destruction or occlusion of fallopian tubes** ♀
Female sterilization operation NOS

✓ **66.4 Total unilateral salpingectomy** ♀
DEF: Complete removal of one fallopian tube.

❹ **66.5 Total bilateral salpingectomy**
Excludes *bilateral partial salpingectomy for sterilization (66.39)*
that with oophorectomy (65.61-65.64)

✓ **66.51 Removal of both fallopian tubes at same operative episode** ♀

✓ **66.52 Removal of remaining fallopian tube** ♀
Removal of solitary fallopian tube

❹ **66.6 Other salpingectomy**
Includes salpingectomy by:
cauterization
coagulation
electrocoagulation
excision
Excludes *fistulectomy (66.73)*

✓ **66.61 Excision or destruction of lesion of fallopian tube** ♀
Excludes *biopsy of fallopian tube (66.11)*

✓ **66.62 Salpingectomy with removal of tubal pregnancy** ♀
Code also any synchronous oophorectomy (65.31, 65.39)
AHA: 3Q 1995, 15; Sep-Oct 1985, 14

✓ **66.63 Bilateral partial salpingectomy, not otherwise specified** ♀

✓ **66.69 Other partial salpingectomy** ♀

❹ **66.7 Repair of fallopian tube**

✓ **66.71 Simple suture of fallopian tube** ♀

✓ **66.72 Salpingo-oophorostomy** ♀

✓ **66.73 Salpingo-salpingostomy** ♀

✓ **66.74 Salpingo-uterostomy** ♀

✓ **66.79 Other repair of fallopian tube** ♀
Graft of fallopian tube
Reopening of divided fallopian tube
Salpingoplasty
DEF: Salpingoplasty: Plastic repair of a fallopian tube defect.
AHA: 2Q 1995, 10; May-Jun 1984, 3

✖ **66.8 Insufflation of fallopian tube** ♀
Insufflation of fallopian tube with:
air
dye
gas
saline
Rubin's test
Excludes *insufflation of therapeutic agent (66.95)*
that for hysterosalpingography (87.82-87.83)
AHA: 2Q 1990, 26

❹ **66.9 Other operations on fallopian tubes**

✖ **66.91 Aspiration of fallopian tube** ♀

✓ **66.92 Unilateral destruction or occlusion of fallopian tube** ♀
Excludes *that of solitary tube (66.21-66.39)*

✓ **66.93 Implantation or replacement of prosthesis of fallopian tube** ♀

✓ **66.94 Removal of prosthesis of fallopian tube** ♀

✓ **66.95 Insufflation of therapeutic agent into fallopian tubes** ♀

✓ **66.96 Dilation of fallopian tube** ♀

✓ **66.97 Burying of fimbriae in uterine wall** ♀

✓ **66.99 Other** ♀
Excludes *lysis of adhesions of ovary and tube*
laparoscopic (65.81)
other (65.89)
AHA: 2Q 1994, 11; Nov-Dec 1986, 9

OPERATIONS ON CERVIX (67)

Code also any application or administration of an adhesion barrier substance (99.77)

✖ **67.0 Dilation of cervical canal** ♀
Excludes *dilation and curettage (69.01-69.09)*
that for induction of labor (73.1)

❹ **67.1 Diagnostic procedures on cervix**

✓ **67.11 Endocervical biopsy** ♀
Excludes *conization of cervix (67.2)*

✓ **67.12 Other cervical biopsy** ♀
Punch biopsy of cervix NOS
Excludes *conization of cervix (67.2)*

✓ **67.19 Other diagnostic procedures on cervix** ♀
Excludes *microscopic examination of specimen from cervix (91.41-91.49)*

✓ **67.2 Conization of cervix** ♀
Excludes *that by:*
cryosurgery (67.33)
electrosurgery (67.32)

Cervical Conization

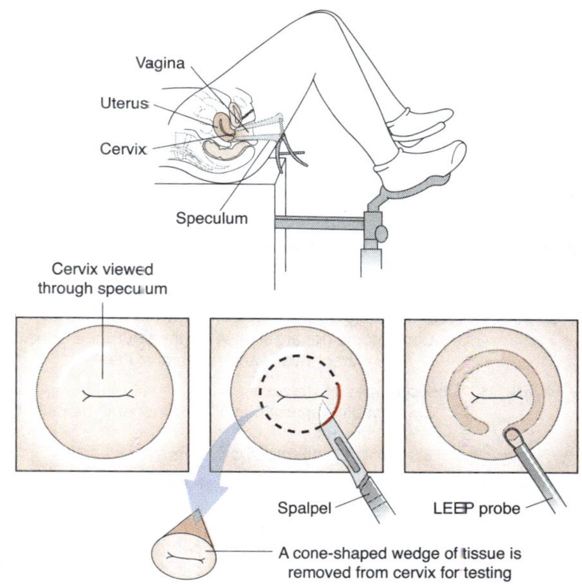

❹ **67.3 Other excision or destruction of lesion or tissue of cervix**

✓ **67.31 Marsupialization of cervical cyst** ♀

✓ **67.32 Destruction of lesion of cervix by cauterization** ♀
Electroconization of cervix
LEEP (loop electrosurgical excision procedure)
LLETZ (large loop excision of the transformation zone)
AHA: 1Q 1998, 3

✓ **67.33 Destruction of lesion of cervix by cryosurgery** ♀
Cryoconization of cervix

✓ **67.39 Other excision or destruction of lesion or tissue of cervix** ♀
Excludes *biopsy of cervix (67.11-67.12)*
cervical fistulectomy (67.62)
conization of cervix (67.2)

✓ **67.4 Amputation of cervix** ♀
Cervicectomy with synchronous colporrhaphy

67.5 Repair of internal cervical os
AHA: 4Q 2001, 63; 3Q 2000, 11

67.51 Transabdominal cerclage of cervix ♀

67.59 Other repair of internal cervical os ♀
Cerclage of isthmus uteri
McDonald operation
Shirodkar operation
Transvaginal cerclage
Excludes *laparoscopically assisted supracervical hysterectomy [LASH] (68.31)*
transabdominal cerclage of cervix (67.51)

67.6 Other repair of cervix
Excludes *repair of current obstetric laceration (75.51)*

67.61 Suture of laceration of cervix ♀

67.62 Repair of fistula of cervix ♀
Cervicosigmoidal fistulectomy
Excludes *fistulectomy:*
cervicovesical (57.84)
ureterocervical (56.84)
vesicocervicovaginal (57.84)

67.69 Other repair of cervix ♀
Repair of old obstetric laceration of cervix

OTHER INCISION AND EXCISION OF UTERUS (68)

Code also any application or administration of an adhesion barrier substance (99.77)

68.0 Hysterotomy ♀
Hysterotomy with removal of hydatidiform mole
Excludes *hysterotomy for termination of pregnancy (74.91)*

68.1 Diagnostic procedures on uterus and supporting structures

68.11 Digital examination of uterus ♀
Excludes *pelvic examination, so describe (89.26)*
postpartal manual exploration of uterine cavity (75.7)

68.12 Hysteroscopy ♀
Excludes *that with biopsy (68.16)*
AHA: 2Q 1990, 26

68.13 Open biopsy of uterus ♀
Excludes *closed biopsy of uterus(68.16)*

68.14 Open biopsy of uterine ligaments ♀
Excludes *closed biopsy of uterine ligaments (68.15)*

68.15 Closed biopsy of uterine ligaments ♀
Endoscopic (laparoscopy) biopsy of uterine adnexa, except ovary and fallopian tube

68.16 Closed biopsy of uterus ♀
Endoscopic (laparoscopy) hysteroscopy) biopsy of uterus
Excludes *open biopsy of uterus (68.13)*

68.19 Other diagnostic procedures on uterus and supporting structures ♀
Excludes *diagnostic:*
aspiration curettage (69.59)
dilation and curettage (69.09)
microscopic examination of specimen from uterus (91.41-91.49)
pelvic examination (89.26)
radioisotope scan of:
placenta (92.17)
uterus (92.19)
ultrasonography of uterus (88.78-88.79)
x-ray of uterus (87.81-87.89)

68.2 Excision or destruction of lesion or tissue of uterus

68.21 Division of endometrial synechiae ♀
Lysis of intraluminal uterine adhesions

68.22 Incision or excision of congenital septum of uterus ♀

68.23 Endometrial ablation ♀
Dilation and curettage
Hysteroscopic endometrial ablation
AHA: 4Q 1996, 68

68.29 Other excision or destruction of lesion of uterus ♀
Uterine myomectomy
Excludes *biopsy of uterus (68.13, 68.16)*
uterine fistulectomy (69.42)
DEF: Uterine myomectomy: Removal of a uterine leiomyoma.
AHA: 1Q 1996, 14

68.3 Subtotal abdominal hysterectomy

68.31 Laparoscopic supracervical hysterectomy [LSH] ♀
Classic infrafascial SEMM hysterectomy [CISH]
Laparoscopically assisted supracervical hysterectomy [LASH]
AHA: 4Q 2003, 98

68.39 Other and unspecified subtotal abdominal hysterectomy ♀
Supracervical hysterectomy
Excludes *classic infrafascial SEMM hysterectomy [CISH] (68.31)*
laparoscopic supracervical hysterectomy [LSH] (68.31)

68.4 Total abdominal hysterectomy
Hysterectomy:
extended
Code also any synchronous removal of tubes and ovaries (65.31-65.64)
Excludes *laparoscopic total abdominal hysterectomy (68.41)*
radical abdominal hysterectomy, any approach (68.61-68.69)
AHA: 4Q 1996, 65

68.41 Laparoscopic total abdominal hysterectomy ♀
Total laparoscopic hysterectomy [TLH]

68.49 Other and unspecified total abdominal hysterectomy ♀
Hysterectomy:
extended

68.5 Vaginal hysterectomy
Code also any synchronous:
removal of tubes and ovaries (65.31-65.64)
repair of cystocele or rectocele (70.50-70.52)
repair of pelvic floor (70.79)

68.51 Laparoscopically assisted vaginal hysterectomy (LAVH) ♀
AHA: 4Q 1996, 68

68.59 Other and unspecified vaginal hysterectomy ♀
Excludes *laparoscopically assisted vaginal hysterectomy (LAVH) (68.51)*
radical vaginal hysterectomy (68.7)

Vaginal hysterectomy

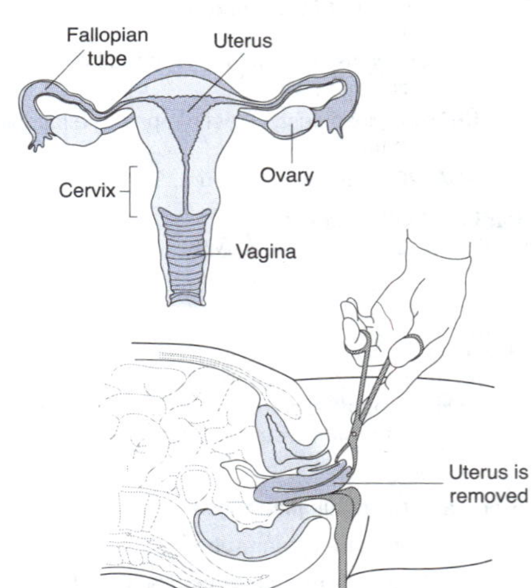

68.6 Radical abdominal hysterectomy
Modified radical hysterectomy
Wertheim's operation
Code also any synchronous:
lymph gland dissection (40.3, 40.5)
removal of tubes and ovaries (65.31-65.64)
Excludes *pelvic evisceration (68.8)*

68.61 Laparoscopic radical abdominal hysterectomy ♀
Laparoscopic modified radical hysterectomy
Total laparoscopic radical hysterectomy [TLRH]

68.69 Other and unspecified radical abdominal hysterectomy ♀
Modified radical hysterectomy
Wertheim's operation
Excludes *laparoscopic radical abdominal hysterectomy (68.61)*
laparoscopic total abdominal hysterectomy (68.41)

68.7 Radical vaginal hysterectomy
Schauta operation
Code also any synchronous:
lymph gland dissection (40.3, 40.5)
removal of tubes and ovaries (65.31-65.64)
Excludes *abdominal hysterectomy, any approach (68.31-68.39, 68.41-68.49, 68.61-68.69, 68.9)*

68.71 Laparoscopic radical vaginal hysterectomy [LRVH] ♀

68.79 Other and unspecified radical vaginal hysterectomy ♀
Hysterocolpectomy
Schauta operation

68.8 Pelvic evisceration ♀
Removal of ovaries, tubes, uterus, vagina, bladder, and urethra (with removal of sigmoid colon and rectum)
Code also any synchronous:
colostomy (46.12-46.13)
lymph gland dissection (40.3, 40.5)
urinary diversion (56.51-56.79)

68.9 Other and unspecified hysterectomy ♀
Hysterectomy NOS
Excludes *abdominal hysterectomy, any approach (68.31-68.39, 68.41-68.49, 68.61-68.69)*
vaginal hysterectomy, any approach (68.51-68.59, 68.71-68.79)

OTHER OPERATIONS ON UTERUS AND SUPPORTING STRUCTURES (69)

Code also any application or administration of an adhesion barrier substance (99.77)

69.0 Dilation and curettage of uterus
Excludes *aspiration curettage of uterus (69.51-69.59)*

69.01 Dilation and curettage for termination of pregnancy ♀

69.02 Dilation and curettage following delivery or abortion ♀
AHA: 3Q 1993, 6

69.09 Other dilation and curettage ♀
Diagnostic D and C
AHA: 1Q 1998, 4

69.1 Excision or destruction of lesion or tissue of uterus and supporting structures

69.19 Other excision or destruction of uterus and supporting structures ♀
Excludes *biopsy of uterine ligament (68.14)*

69.2 Repair of uterine supporting structures

69.21 Interposition operation ♀
Watkins procedure

69.22 Other uterine suspension ♀
Hysteropexy
Manchester operation
Plication of uterine ligament

69.23 Vaginal repair of chronic inversion of uterus ♀

69.29 Other repair of uterus and supporting structures ♀

69.3 Paracervical uterine denervation ♀

69.4 Uterine repair
Excludes *repair of current obstetric laceration (75.50-75.52)*

69.41 Suture of laceration of uterus ♀

69.42 Closure of fistula of uterus ♀
Excludes *uterovesical fistulectomy (57.84)*

69.49 Other repair of uterus ♀
Repair of old obstetric laceration of uterus

69.5 Aspiration curettage of uterus
Excludes *menstrual extraction (69.6)*

69.51 Aspiration curettage of uterus for termination of pregnancy ♀
Therapeutic abortion NOS

69.52 Aspiration curettage following delivery or abortion ♀

69.59 Other aspiration curettage of uterus ♀
AHA: 1Q 1998, 7

69.6 Menstrual extraction or regulation ♀

69.7 Insertion of intrauterine contraceptive device ♀

69.9 Other operations on uterus, cervix, and supporting structures
Excludes *obstetric dilation or incision of cervix (73.1, 73.93)*

69.91 Insertion of therapeutic device into uterus ♀
Excludes *insertion of:*
intrauterine contraceptive device (69.7)
laminaria (69.93)
obstetric insertion of bag, bougie, or pack (73.1)

69.92 Artificial insemination ♀

69.93 Insertion of laminaria ♀

69.94 Manual replacement of inverted uterus ♀
Excludes *that in immediate postpartal period (75.94)*

69.95 Incision of cervix ♀
Excludes *that to assist delivery (73.93)*

69.96 Removal of cerclage material from cervix ♀

69.97 Removal of other penetrating foreign body from cervix ♀
Excludes *removal of intraluminal foreign body from cervix (98.16)*

69.98 Other operations on supporting structures of uterus ♀
Excludes *biopsy of uterine ligament (68.14)*

69.99 Other operations on cervix and uterus ♀
Excludes *removal of:*
foreign body (98.16)
intrauterine contraceptive device (97.71)
obstetric bag, bougie, or pack (97.72)
packing (97.72)

OPERATIONS ON VAGINA AND CUL-DE-SAC (70)

Code also any application or administration of an adhesion barrier substance (99.77)

70.0 Culdocentesis ♀
AHA: 2Q 1990, 26

70.1 Incision of vagina and cul-de-sac

70.11 Hymenotomy ♀

70.12 Culdotomy ♀

70.13 Lysis of intraluminal adhesions of vagina ♀

70.14 Other vaginotomy ♀
Division of vaginal septum
Drainage of hematoma of vaginal cuff

70.2 Diagnostic procedures on vagina and cul-de-sac

70.21 Vaginoscopy ♀

70.22 Culdoscopy ♀

70.23 Biopsy of cul-de-sac ♀

70.24 Vaginal biopsy ♀

70.29 Other diagnostic procedures on vagina and cul-de-sac ♀

Deleted Code | Nonspecific O.R. Procedure | Valid O.R. Procedure | Non-O.R. Procedure | ♂ Male | ♀ Female

70.3 Local excision or destruction of vagina and cul-de-sac

70.31 Hymenectomy ♀
DEF: Excision of the hymen.

70.32 Excision or destruction of lesion of cul-de-sac ♀
Endometrectomy of cul-de-sac
Excludes *biopsy of cul-de-sac (70.23)*

70.33 Excision or destruction of lesion of vagina ♀
Excludes *biopsy of vagina (70.24)*
vaginal fistulectomy (70.72-70.75)

70.4 Obliteration and total excision of vagina ♀
Vaginectomy
Excludes *obliteration of vaginal vault (70.8)*
DEF: Vaginectomy: Compete removal of the vagina.

70.5 Repair of cystocele and rectocele

70.50 Repair of cystocele and rectocele ♀

70.51 Repair of cystocele ♀
Anterior colporrhaphy (with urethrocele repair)
AHA: Jul-Aug 1984, 20

70.52 Repair of rectocele ♀
Posterior colporrhaphy
Excludes ▶*STARR procedure (48.74)*◀
AHA: 1Q 2006, 12

● **70.53 Repair of cystocele and rectocele with graft or prosthesis ♀**
Use additional code for biological substance (70.94) or synthetic substance (70.95), if known

● **70.54 Repair of cystocele with graft or prosthesis ♀**
Anterior colporrhaphy (with urethrocele repair)
Use additional code for biological substance (70.94) or synthetic substance (70.95), if known

● **70.55 Repair of rectocele with graft or prosthesis ♀**
Posterior colporrhaphy
Use additional code for biological substance (70.94) or synthetic substance (70.95), if known

70.6 Vaginal construction and reconstruction

70.61 Vaginal construction ♀

70.62 Vaginal reconstruction ♀

● **70.63 Vaginal construction with graft or prosthesis ♀**
Use additional code for biological substance (70.94) or synthetic substance (70.95), if known
Excludes *vaginal construction (70.61)*

● **70.64 Vaginal reconstruction with graft or prosthesis ♀**
Use additional code for biological substance (70.94) or synthetic substance (70.95), if known
Excludes *vaginal reconstruction (70.62)*

70.7 Other repair of vagina
Excludes *lysis of intraluminal adhesions (70.13)*
repair of current obstetric laceration (75.69)
that associated with cervical amputation (67.4)

70.71 Suture of laceration of vagina ♀
AHA: Jul-Aug 1984, 20

70.72 Repair of colovaginal fistula ♀

70.73 Repair of rectovaginal fistula ♀

70.74 Repair of other vaginoenteric fistula ♀

70.75 Repair of other fistula of vagina ♀
Excludes *repair of fistula:*
rectovesicovaginal (57.83)
ureterovaginal (56.84)
urethrovaginal (58.43)
uterovaginal (69.42)
vesicocervicovaginal (57.84)
vesicosigmoidovaginal (57.83)
vesicoureterovaginal (56.84)
vesicovaginal (57.84)

70.76 Hymenorrhaphy ♀

70.77 Vaginal suspension and fixation ♀

● **70.78 Vaginal suspension and fixation with graft or prosthesis ♀**
Use additional code for biological substance (70.94) or synthetic substance (70.95), if known

70.79 Other repair of vagina ♀
Colpoperineoplasty
Repair of old obstetric laceration of vagina

70.8 Obliteration of vaginal vault ♀
LeFort operation
DEF: LeFort operation: Surgically uniting the anterior and posterior vaginal walls along the midline.
AHA: 4Q 1994, 54

70.9 Other operations on vagina and cul-de-sac

70.91 Other operations on vagina ♀
Excludes *insertion of:*
diaphragm (96.17)
mold (96.15)
pack (96.14)
pessary (96.18)
suppository (96.49)
removal of:
diaphragm (97.73)
foreign body (98.17)
pack (97.75)
pessary (97.74)
replacement of:
diaphragm (97.24)
pack (97.26)
pessary (97.25)
vaginal dilation (96.16)
vaginal douche (96.44)

70.92 Other operations on cul-de-sac ♀
Obliteration of cul-de-sac
Repair of vaginal enterocele
AHA: 4Q 1994, 54

● **70.93 Other operations on cul-de-sac with graft or prosthesis ♀**
Repair of vaginal enterocele with graft or prosthesis
Use additional code for biological substance (70.94) or synthetic substance (70.95), if known

● **70.94 Insertion of biological graft ♀**
Allogenic material or substance
Allograft
Autograft
Autologous material or substance
Heterograft
Xenogenic material or substance
Code first these procedures when done with graft or prosthesis: Other operations on cul-de-sac (70.93)
Repair of cystocele (70.54)
Repair of cystocele and rectocele (70.53)
Repair of rectocele (70.55)
Vaginal construction (70.63)
Vaginal reconstruction (70.64)
Vaginal suspension and fixation (70.78)

● **70.95 Insertion of synthetic graft or prosthesis ♀**
Artificial tissue
Code first these procedures when done with graft or prosthesis: Other operations on cul-de-sac (70.93)
Repair of cystocele (70.54)
Repair of cystocele and rectocele (70.53)
Repair of rectocele (70.55)
Vaginal construction (70.63)
Vaginal reconstruction (70.64)
Vaginal suspension and fixation (70.78)

OPERATIONS ON VULVA AND PERINEUM (71)

Code also any application or administration of an adhesion barrier substance (99.77)

71.0 Incision of vulva and perineum

71.01 Lysis of vulvar adhesions ♀

71.09 Other incision of vulva and perineum ♀
Enlargement of introitus NOS
Excludes *removal of foreign body without incision (98.23)*

71.1 Diagnostic procedures on vulva

71.11 Biopsy of vulva ♀

71.19 Other diagnostic procedures on vulva ♀

71.2 Operations on Bartholin's gland

- **71.21 Percutaneous aspiration of Bartholin's gland (cyst)** ♀
- **71.22 Incision of Bartholin's gland (cyst)** ♀
- **71.23 Marsupialization of Bartholin's gland (cyst)** ♀
- **71.24 Excision or other destruction of Bartholin's gland (cyst)** ♀
- **71.29 Other operations on Bartholin's gland** ♀

71.3 Other local excision or destruction of vulva and perineum ♀
Division of Skene's gland
Excludes *biopsy of vulva (71.11)*
vulvar fistulectomy (71.72)

71.4 Operations on clitoris ♀
Amputation of clitoris
Clitoridotomy
Female circumcision

71.5 Radical vulvectomy ♀
Code also any synchronous lymph gland dissection (40.3, 40.5)

71.6 Other vulvectomy

- **71.61 Unilateral vulvectomy** ♀
- **71.62 Bilateral vulvectomy** ♀
  Vulvectomy NOS

71.7 Repair of vulva and perineum
Excludes *repair of current obstetric laceration (75.69)*

- **71.71 Suture of laceration of vulva or perineum** ♀
- **71.72 Repair of fistula of vulva or perineum** ♀
  Excludes *repair of fistula:*
  urethroperineal (58.43)
  urethroperineovesical (57.84)
  vaginoperineal (70.75)
- **71.79 Other repair of vulva and perineum** ♀
  Repair of old obstetric laceration of vulva or perineum
  AHA: 1Q 1997, 9-10

71.8 Other operations on vulva ♀
Excludes *removal of:*
foreign body without incision (98.23)
packing (97.75)
replacement of packing (97.26)

71.9 Other operations on female genital organs ♀
AHA: 4Q 2004, 90; 1Q 2003, 13

13. OBSTETRICAL PROCEDURES (72-75)

FORCEPS, VACUUM, AND BREECH DELIVERY (72)

72.0 Low forceps operation ♀
Outlet forceps operation

72.1 Low forceps operation with episiotomy ♀
Outlet forceps operation with episiotomy

72.2 Mid forceps operation

- **72.21 Mid forceps operation with episiotomy** ♀
- **72.29 Other mid forceps operation** ♀

72.3 High forceps operation

- **72.31 High forceps operation with episiotomy** ♀
- **72.39 Other high forceps operation** ♀

72.4 Forceps rotation of fetal head ♀
DeLee maneuver
Key-in-lock rotation
Kielland rotation
Scanzoni's maneuver
Code also any associated forceps extraction (72.0-72.39)

72.5 Breech extraction

- **72.51 Partial breech extraction with forceps to aftercoming head** ♀
- **72.52 Other partial breech extraction** ♀
- **72.53 Total breech extraction with forceps to aftercoming head** ♀
- **72.54 Other total breech extraction** ♀

72.6 Forceps application to aftercoming head ♀
Piper forceps operation
Excludes *partial breech extraction with forceps to aftercoming head (72.51)*
total breech extraction with forceps to aftercoming head (72.53)

72.7 Vacuum extraction
Includes Malström's extraction

- **72.71 Vacuum extraction with episiotomy** ♀
- **72.79 Other vacuum extraction** ♀

72.8 Other specified instrumental delivery ♀

72.9 Unspecified instrumental delivery ♀

OTHER PROCEDURES INDUCING OR ASSISTING DELIVERY (73)

73.0 Artificial rupture of membranes

- **73.01 Induction of labor by artificial rupture of membranes** ♀
  Surgical induction NOS
  Excludes *artificial rupture of membranes after onset of labor (73.09)*
  AHA: 3Q 2000, 5
- **73.09 Other artificial rupture of membranes** ♀
  Artificial rupture of membranes at time of delivery

73.1 Other surgical induction of labor ♀
Induction by cervical dilation
Excludes *injection for abortion (75.0)*
insertion of suppository for abortion (96.49)

73.2 Internal and combined version and extraction

- **73.21 Internal and combined version without extraction** ♀
  Version NOS
- **73.22 Internal and combined version with extraction** ♀

73.3 Failed forceps ♀
Application of forceps without delivery
Trial forceps

73.4 Medical induction of labor ♀
Excludes *medication to augment active labor - omit code*

73.5 Manually assisted delivery

- **73.51 Manual rotation of fetal head** ♀

✖ Deleted Code ▼ Nonspecific O.R. Procedure ✔ Valid O.R. Procedure ✖ Non-O.R. Procedure ♂ Male ♀ Female

✖ **73.59 Other manually assisted delivery** ♀
Assisted spontaneous delivery
Credé maneuver
DEF: Crede' maneuver: Expressing the placenta by forcing the uterus down into the pelvis and squeezing the uterus from all sides so that its contents are expelled.
AHA: 4Q 1998, 76

✖ **73.6 Episiotomy** ♀
Episioproctotomy
Episiotomy with subsequent episiorrhaphy
Excludes *that with:*
high forceps (72.31)
low forceps (72.1)
mid forceps (72.21)
outlet forceps (72.1)
vacuum extraction (72.71)
AHA: 1Q 1992, 10

✖ **73.8 Operations on fetus to facilitate delivery** ♀
Clavicotomy on fetus
Destruction of fetus
Needling of hydrocephalic head

❹ **73.9 Other operations assisting delivery**

✖ **73.91 External version** ♀

✖ **73.92 Replacement of prolapsed umbilical cord** ♀

✖ **73.93 Incision of cervix to assist delivery** ♀
Dührssen's incisions

✓ **73.94 Pubiotomy to assist delivery** ♀
Obstetrical symphysiotomy
DEF: Separation of the pubic bone for obstetric reasons.

✓ **73.99 Other** ♀
Excludes *dilation of cervix, obstetrical to induce labor (73.1)*
insertion of bag or bougie to induce labor (73.1)
removal of cerclage material (69.96)

CESAREAN SECTION AND REMOVAL OF FETUS (74)

Code also any synchronous:
hysterectomy (68.3-68.4, 68.6, 68.8)
myomectomy (68.29)
sterilization (66.31-66.39, 66.63)

✓ **74.0 Classical cesarean section** ♀
Transperitoneal classical cesarean section

✓ **74.1 Low cervical cesarean section** ♀
Lower uterine segment cesarean section
AHA: 1Q, 2001, 11

✓ **74.2 Extraperitoneal cesarean section** ♀
Supravesical cesarean section

✓ **74.3 Removal of extratubal ectopic pregnancy** ♀
Removal of:
ectopic abdominal pregnancy
fetus from peritoneal or extraperitoneal cavity following uterine or tubal rupture
Excludes *that by salpingostomy (66.02)*
that by salpingotomy (66.01)
that with synchronous salpingectomy (66.62)
AHA: 4Q 1992, 25; 2Q 1990, 25, 27; 1Q 1989, 11; Sep-Oct 1985, 14

✓ **74.4 Cesarean section of other specified type** ♀
Peritoneal exclusion cesarean section
Transperitoneal cesarean section NOS
Vaginal cesarean section

❹ **74.9 Cesarean section of unspecified type**

✓ **74.91 Hysterotomy to terminate pregnancy** ♀
Therapeutic abortion by hysterotomy

✓ **74.99 Other cesarean section of unspecified type** ♀
Cesarean section NOS
Obstetrical abdominouterotomy
Obstetrical hysterotomy

OTHER OBSTETRIC OPERATIONS (75)

✖ **75.0 Intra-amniotic injection for abortion** ♀
Injection of:
prostaglandin for induction of abortion
saline for induction of abortion
Termination of pregnancy by intrauterine injection
Excludes *insertion of prostaglandin suppository for abortion (96.49)*

✖ **75.1 Diagnostic amniocentesis** ♀

✖ **75.2 Intrauterine transfusion** ♀
Exchange transfusion in utero
Insertion of catheter into abdomen of fetus for transfusion
Code also any hysterotomy approach (68.0)

❹ **75.3 Other intrauterine operations on fetus and amnion**
Code also any hysterotomy approach (68.0)

✖ **75.31 Amnioscopy** ♀
Fetoscopy
Laparoamnioscopy

✖ **75.32 Fetal EKG (scalp)** ♀

✖ **75.33 Fetal blood sampling and biopsy** ♀

✖ **75.34 Other fetal monitoring** ♀
Antepartum fetal nonstress test
Fetal monitoring, not otherwise specified
Excludes *fetal pulse oximetry (75.38)*

✖ **75.35 Other diagnostic procedures on fetus and amnion** ♀
Intrauterine pressure determination
Excludes *amniocentesis (75.1)*
diagnostic procedures on gravid uterus and placenta (87.81, 88.46, 88.78, 92.17)

✓ **75.36 Correction of fetal defect** ♀

✓ **75.37 Amnioinfusion** ♀
Code also injection of antibiotic (99.21)
DEF: Introduction or injection of solutions into the amnion.
AHA: 4Q 1998, 76

✖ **75.38 Fetal pulse oximetry**
Transcervical fetal oxygen saturation monitoring
Transcervical fetal SpO_2 monitoring
AHA: 4Q 2001, 64

✖ **75.4 Manual removal of retained placenta** ♀
Excludes *aspiration curettage (69.52)*
dilation and curettage (69.02)

❹ **75.5 Repair of current obstetric laceration of uterus**

✓▼ **75.50 Repair of current obstetric laceration of uterus, not otherwise specified** ♀

✓ **75.51 Repair of current obstetric laceration of cervix** ♀

✓ **75.52 Repair of current obstetric laceration of corpus uteri** ♀

❹ **75.6 Repair of other current obstetric laceration**

✓ **75.61 Repair of current obstetric laceration of bladder and urethra** ♀
AHA: 1Q 1992, 11

✖ **75.62 Repair of current obstetric laceration of rectum and sphincter ani** ♀
AHA: 1Q 1992, 11

✖ **75.69 Repair of other current obstetric laceration** ♀
Episioperineorrhaphy
Repair of:
pelvic floor
perineum
vagina
vulva
Secondary repair of episiotomy
Excludes *repair of routine episiotomy (73.6)*
AHA: 1Q 1992, 11

✖ **75.7 Manual exploration of uterine cavity, postpartum** ♀

✖ **75.8 Obstetric tamponade of uterus or vagina** ♀
Excludes *antepartum tamponade (73.1)*

75.9 Other obstetric operations

✖ **75.91 Evacuation of obstetrical incisional hematoma of perineum** ♀
Evacuation of hematoma of:
episiotomy
perineorrhaphy

✖ **75.92 Evacuation of other hematoma of vulva or vagina** ♀

✔ **75.93 Surgical correction of inverted uterus** ♀
Spintelli operation
Excludes *vaginal repair of chronic inversion of uterus (69.23)*

✖ **75.94 Manual replacement of inverted uterus** ♀

✔ **75.99 Other** ♀

14. OPERATIONS ON THE MUSCULOSKELETAL SYSTEM (76-84)

OPERATIONS ON FACIAL BONES AND JOINTS (76)

Excludes *accessory sinuses (22.00-22.9)*
nasal bones (21.00-21.99)
skull (01.01-02.99)

76.0 Incision of facial bone without division

✔ **76.01 Sequestrectomy of facial bone**
Removal of necrotic bone chip from facial bone

✔ **76.09 Other incision of facial bone**
Reopening of osteotomy site of facial bone
Excludes *osteotomy associated with orthognathic surgery (76.61-76.69)*
removal of internal fixation device (76.97)

76.1 Diagnostic procedures on facial bones and joints

✔ **76.11 Biopsy of facial bone**

✔ **76.19 Other diagnostic procedures on facial bones and joints**
Excludes *contrast arthrogram of temporomandibular joint (87.13)*
other x-ray (87.11-87.12, 87.14-87.16)
AHA: Nov-Dec 1987, 12

✔ **76.2 Local excision or destruction of lesion of facial bone**
Excludes *biopsy of facial bone (76.11)*
excision of odontogenic lesion (24.4)

76.3 Partial ostectomy of facial bone

✔ **76.31 Partial mandibulectomy**
Hemimandibulectomy
Excludes *that associated with temporomandibular arthroplasty (76.5)*
AHA: 2Q 2005, 8-9

Excision of bone

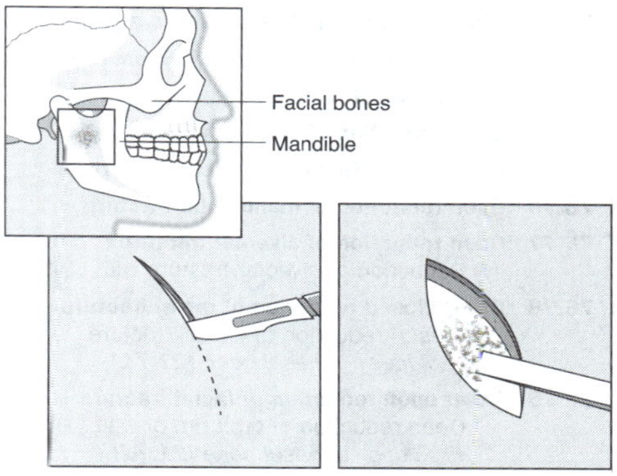

Incision is made

Abscessed or infected bone is excised

✔ **76.39 Partial ostectomy of other facial bone**
Hemimaxillectomy (with bone graft or prosthesis)
AHA: Jan-Feb 1987, 14

76.4 Excision and reconstruction of facial bones

✔ **76.41 Total mandibulectomy with synchronous reconstruction**

✔ **76.42 Other total mandibulectomy**

✔ **76.43 Other reconstruction of mandible**
Excludes *genioplasty (76.67-76.68)*
that with synchronous total mandibulectomy (76.41)
AHA: 2Q 2003, 13

✔ **76.44 Total ostectomy of other facial bone with synchronous reconstruction**
AHA: 3Q 1993, 6

✔ **76.45 Other total ostectomy of other facial bone**

✓ **76.46 Other reconstruction of other facial bone**
Excludes *that with synchronous total ostectomy (76.44)*

✓ **76.5 Temporomandibular arthroplasty**
AHA: 4Q 1999, 20

④ **76.6 Other facial bone repair and orthognathic surgery**
Code also any synchronous:
bone graft (76.91)
synthetic implant (76.92)
Excludes *reconstruction of facial bones (76.41-76.46)*

✓ **76.61 Closed osteoplasty [osteotomy] of mandibular ramus**
Gigli saw osteotomy

✓ **76.62 Open osteoplasty [osteotomy] of mandibular ramus**

✓ **76.63 Osteoplasty [osteotomy] of body of mandible**

✓ **76.64 Other orthognathic surgery on mandible**
Mandibular osteoplasty NOS
Segmental or subapical osteotomy
AHA: 2Q 2004, 9-10

✓ **76.65 Segmental osteoplasty [osteotomy] of maxilla**
Maxillary osteoplasty NOS

✓ **76.66 Total osteoplasty [osteotomy] of maxilla**

✓ **76.67 Reduction genioplasty**
Reduction mentoplasty

✓ **76.68 Augmentation genioplasty**
Mentoplasty:
NOS
with graft or implant

✓ **76.69 Other facial bone repair**
Osteoplasty of facial bone NOS

④ **76.7 Reduction of facial fracture**
Includes internal fixation
Code also any synchronous:
bone graft (76.91)
synthetic implant (76.92)
Excludes *that of nasal bones (21.71-21.72)*

✓▼ **76.70 Reduction of facial fracture, not otherwise specified**

✖ **76.71 Closed reduction of malar and zygomatic fracture**

✓ **76.72 Open reduction of malar and zygomatic fracture**

✖ **76.73 Closed reduction of maxillary fracture**

✓ **76.74 Open reduction of maxillary fracture**

✖ **76.75 Closed reduction of mandibular fracture**

✓ **76.76 Open reduction of mandibular fracture**

✓ **76.77 Open reduction of alveolar fracture**
Reduction of alveolar fracture with stabilization of teeth

✖ **76.78 Other closed reduction of facial fracture**
Closed reduction of orbital fracture
Excludes *nasal bone (21.71)*

✓ **76.79 Other open reduction of facial fracture**
Open reduction of orbit rim or wall
Excludes *nasal bone (21.72)*

④ **76.9 Other operations on facial bones and joints**

✓ **76.91 Bone graft to facial bone**
Autogenous graft to facial bone
Bone bank graft to facial bone
Heterogenous graft to facial bone

✓ **76.92 Insertion of synthetic implant in facial bone**
Alloplastic implant to facial bone

✖ **76.93 Closed reduction of temporomandibular dislocation**

✓ **76.94 Open reduction of temporomandibular dislocation**

✖ **76.95 Other manipulation of temporomandibular joint**

✖ **76.96 Injection of therapeutic substance into temporomandibular joint**

✓ **76.97 Removal of internal fixation device from facial bone**
Excludes *removal of:*
dental wiring (97.33)
external mandibular fixation device NEC (97.36)

✓ **76.99 Other**

INCISION, EXCISION, AND DIVISION OF OTHER BONES (77)

Excludes *laminectomy for decompression (03.09)*
operations on:
accessory sinuses (22.00-22.9)
ear ossicles (19.0-19.55)
facial bones (76.01-76.99)
joint structures (80.00-81.99)
mastoid (19.9-20.99)
nasal bones (21.00-21.99)
skull (01.01-02.99)

The following fourth-digit subclassification is for use with appropriate categories in section 77 to identify the site. Valid fourth-digit categories are in brackets under each code.

0 unspecified site
1 scapula, clavicle, and thorax [ribs and sternum]
2 humerus
3 radius and ulna
4 carpals and metacarpals
5 femur
6 patella
7 tibia and fibula
8 tarsals and metatarsals
9 other
Pelvic bones
Phalanges (of foot) (of hand)
Vertebrae

④✓ **77.0 Sequestrectomy**
[0-9] (▼ is only valid for fourth-digit "0")

④✓ **77.1 Other incision of bone without division**
[0-9]
Reopening of osteotomy site
Excludes *aspiration of bone marrow (41.31, 41.91)*
removal of internal fixation device (78.60-78.69)
AHA: For Code 77.17: 1Q 2002, 3

④✓ **77.2 Wedge osteotomy**
[0-9] (▼ is only valid for fourth-digit "4")
Excludes *that for hallux valgus (77.51)*

④✓ **77.3 Other division of bone**
[0-9]
Osteoarthrotomy
Excludes *clavicotomy of fetus (73.8)*
laminotomy or incision of vertebra (03.01-03.09)
pubiotomy to assist delivery (73.94)
sternotomy incidental to thoracic operation - omit code
DEF: Osteoarthrotomy: Excision of the articular end of a bone.

④✓ **77.4 Biopsy of bone**
[0-9]
AHA: For Code 77.45: 2Q 1998, 13

④ **77.5 Excision and repair of bunion and other toe deformities**

✓ **77.51 Bunionectomy with soft tissue correction and osteotomy of the first metatarsal**

✓ **77.52 Bunionectomy with soft tissue correction and arthrodesis**

✓ **77.53 Other bunionectomy with soft tissue correction**

✓ **77.54 Excision or correction of bunionette**
That with osteotomy

✓ **77.56 Repair of hammer toe**
Filleting of hammer toe
Fusion of hammer toe
Phalangectomy (partial) of hammer toe

✓ **77.57 Repair of claw toe**
Capsulotomy of claw toe
Fusion of claw toe
Phalangectomy (partial) of claw toe
Tendon lengthening of claw toe

✓ **77.58 Other excision, fusion and repair of toes**
Cockup toe repair
Overlapping toe repair
That with use of prosthetic materials

✓ **77.59 Other bunionectomy**
Resection of hallux valgus joint with insertion of prosthesis

77.6 Local excision of lesion or tissue of bone
[0-9]
(▼ is only valid for fourth-digit "0")
Excludes biopsy of bone (77.40-77.49)
debridement of compound fracture (79.60-79.69)

AHA: **For Code 77.61**: 3Q 2001, 9; **For Code 77.65**: 4Q 2004, 128-129; Sep-Oct 1985, 4; **For Code 77.67**: 1Q 2002, 3; 1Q 1999, 8; **For Code 77.69**: 2Q 2000, 18

77.7 Excision of bone for graft
[0-9]
(▼ is only valid for fourth-digit "0")

AHA: **For Code 77.71**: 3Q 2003, 19; **For Code 77.79**: 2Q 2003, 13; 4Q 2002, 109-110; 2Q 2002, 16; 2Q 2000, 12-13; 4Q 1999, 11-13; 2Q 1995, 9; 2Q 1994, 7

77.8 Other partial ostectomy
[0-9]
(▼ is only valid for fourth-digit "0")
Condylectomy
Excludes *amputation (84.00-84.19, 84.91)*
arthrectomy (80.90-80.99)
excision of bone ends associated with:
arthrodesis (81.00-81.29)
arthroplasty (81.31-81.87)
excision of cartilage (80.5-80.6, 80.80-80.99)
excision of head of femur with synchronous replacement (00.70-00.73, 81.51-81.53)
hemilaminectomy (03.01-03.09)
laminectomy (03.01-03.09)
ostectomy for hallux valgus (77.51-77.59)
partial amputation:
finger (84.01)
thumb (84.02)
toe (84.11)
resection of ribs incidental to thoracic operation - omit code
that incidental to other operation - omit code

DEF: Removal of a portion of a bone.

AHA: **For code 77.89**: 2Q 2002, 8

77.9 Total ostectomy
[0-9]
(▼ is only valid for fourth-digit "0")
Excludes *amputation of limb (84.00-84.19, 84.91)*
that incidental to other operation - omit code

OTHER OPERATIONS ON BONES, EXCEPT FACIAL BONES (78)

Excludes *operations on:*
accessory sinuses (22.00-22.9)
facial bones (76.01-76.99)
joint structures (80.00-81.99)
nasal bones (21.00-21.99)
skull (01.01-02.99)

The following fourth-digit subclassification is for use with categories in section 78 to identify the site. Valid fourth-digit categories are in [brackets] under each code.

0 unspecified site
1 scapula, clavicle, and thorax [ribs and sternum]
2 humerus
3 radius and ulna
4 carpals and metacarpals
5 femur
6 patella
7 tibia and fibula
8 tarsals and metatarsals
9 other
Pelvic bones
Phalanges (of foot) (of hand)
Vertebrae

78.0 Bone graft
[0-9]
(▼ is only valid for fourth-digit "0")
Bone:
bank graft
graft (autogenous) (heterogenous)
That with debridement of bone graft site (removal of sclerosed, fibrous or necrotic bone or tissue)
Transplantation of bone
Code also any excision of bone for graft (77.70-77.79)
Excludes *that for bone lengthening (78.30-78.39)*

AHA: 2Q 2002, 11; **For Code 78.05**: 2Q 1998, 13; 3Q 1994, 10; **For Code 78.07**: 2Q 1994, 4

78.1 Application of external fixator device
[0-9]
(▼ is only valid for fourth-digit "0")
Fixator with insertion of pins/wires/screws into bone
Code also any type of fixator device, if known (84.71-84.73)
Excludes *other immobilization, pressure, and attention to wound (93.51-93.59)*

AHA: **For Code 78.12**: 4Q 2005, 129

78.2 Limb shortening procedures
[0, 2-5, 7-9]
(▼ is only valid for fourth-digit "0")
Epiphyseal stapling
Open epiphysiodesis
Percutaneous epiphysiodesis
Resection/osteotomy

78.3 Limb lengthening procedures
[0, 2-5, 7-9]
(▼ is only valid for fourth-digit "0")
Bone graft with or without internal fixation devices or osteotomy
Distraction technique with or without corticotomy/osteotomy
Code also any application of an external fixation device (78.10-78.19)

78.4 Other repair or plastic operations on bone
[0-9]
(▼ is only valid for fourth-digit "0")
Other operation on bone NEC
Repair of malunion or nonunion fracture NEC
Excludes *application of external fixation device (78.10-78.19)*
limb lengthening procedures (78.30-78.39)
limb shortening procedures (78.20-78.29)
osteotomy (77.3)
reconstruction of thumb (82.61-82.69)
repair of pectus deformity (34.74)
repair with bone graft (78.00-78.09)

AHA: **For Code 78.41**: 2Q 2002, 16; **For Code 78.47**: 3Q 1991, 20; **For Code 78.49**: 3Q 2004, 9; 2Q 2003, 22; 3Q 2002, 12; 2Q 2002, 14-15; 4Q 1999, 22; 1Q 1997, 4

78.5 Internal fixation of bone without fracture reduction
[0-9]
(▼ is only valid for fourth-digit "0")
Internal fixation of bone (prophylactic)
Reinsertion of internal fixation device
Revision of displaced or broken fixation device
Excludes *arthroplasty and arthrodesis (81.00-81.85)*
bone graft (78.00-78.09)
limb shortening procedures (78.20-78.29)
that for fracture reduction (79.10-79.19, 79.30-79.59)

AHA: **For Code 78.59**: 3Q 2004, 7; 2Q 2003, 15; 4Q 1999, 13-14; 2Q 1999, 10-11; 3Q 1995, 12

78.6 Removal of implanted devices from bone
[0-9]
External fixator device (invasive)
Internal fixation device
Removal of bone growth stimulator (invasive)
Removal of internal limb lengthening device
Removal of pedicle screw(s) used in spinal fusion
Excludes *removal of cast, splint, and traction device (Kirschner wire) (Steinmann pin) (97.88)*
▶*removal of posterior spinal motion preservation (facet replacement, pedicle-based dynamic stabilization, interspinous process) device(s) (80.09)*◀
removal of skull tongs or halo traction device (02.95)

AHA: **For Code 78.65**: 1Q 1995, 10; **For Code 78.67**: 2Q 2003, 14; For Code 78.69: 4Q 2002, 110; 2Q 2000, 18; 1Q 2000, 15

78.7 Osteoclasis
[0-9]
(▼ is only valid for fourth-digit "0")

78.8 Diagnostic procedures on bone, not elsewhere classified
[0-9]
(▼ is only valid for fourth-digit "0")
Excludes *biopsy of bone (77.40-77.49)*
magnetic resonance imaging (88.94)
microscopic examination of specimen from bone (91.51-91.59)
radioisotope scan (92.14)
skeletal x-ray (87.21-87.29, 87.43, 88.21-88.33)
thermography (88.83)

78.9 Insertion of bone growth stimulator
[0-9] (▼ is only valid for fourth-digit "0")
Insertion of:
bone stimulator (electrical) to aid bone healing
osteogenic electrodes for bone growth stimulation
totally implanted device (invasive)
Excludes *non-invasive (transcutaneous) (surface) stimulator (99.86)*

REDUCTION OF FRACTURE AND DISLOCATION (79)

Includes application of cast or splint reduction with insertion of traction device (Kirschner wire) (Steinmann pin)

Code also any:
application of external fixator device (78.10-78.19)
type of fixator device, if known (84.71-84.73)

Excludes *external fixation alone for immobilization of fracture (93.51-93.56, 93.59)*
internal fixation without reduction of fracture (78.50-78.59)
operations on:
facial bones (76.70-76.79)
nasal bones (21.71-21.72)
orbit (76.78-76.79)
skull (02.02)
vertebrae (03.53)
removal of cast or splint (97.88)
replacement of cast or splint (97.11-97.14)
traction alone for reduction of fracture (93.41-93.46)

The following fourth-digit subclassification is for use with appropriate categories in section 79 to identify the site. Valid fourth-digit categories are in [brackets] under each code.
- **0 unspecified site**
- **1 humerus**
- **2 radius and ulna**
  Arm NOS
- **3 carpals and metacarpals**
  Hand NOS
- **4 phalanges of hand**
- **5 femur**
- **6 tibia and fibula**
  Leg NOS
- **7 tarsals and metatarsals**
  Foot NOS
- **8 phalanges of foot**
- **9 other specified bone**

79.0 Closed reduction of fracture without internal fixation
[0-9]
Excludes *that for separation of epiphysis (79.40-79.49)*
AHA: For Code 79.01: 4Q 2005, 129; **For Code 79.05**: 3Q 1989, 16; 4Q 1988, 11

79.1 Closed reduction of fracture with internal fixation
[0-9] (▼ is only valid for fourth-digit "0")
Excludes *that for separation of epiphysis (79.40-79.49)*
AHA: For Code 79.13: 2Q 1994, 4; **For Code 79.15**: 2Q 1994, 4; 1Q 1993, 24

79.2 Open reduction of fracture without internal fixation
[0-9] (▼ is only valid for fourth-digit "0")
Excludes *that for separation of epiphysis (79.50-79.59)*

79.3 Open reduction of fracture with internal fixation
[0-9] (▼ is only valid for fourth-digit "0")
Excludes *that for separation of epiphysis (79.50-79.59)*
AHA: For Code 79.35: 3Q 1994, 10; 2Q 1998, 13; 3Q 1994, 10; **For Code 79.36**: 2Q 1994, 3; For Code 79.37: 2Q 1994, 3

79.4 Closed reduction of separated epiphysis
[0-2, 5, 6, 9]
(▼ is only valid for fourth-digit "0")
Reduction with or without internal fixation

79.5 Open reduction of separated epiphysis
[0-2, 5, 6, 9]
(▼ is only valid for fourth-digit "0")
Reduction with or without internal fixation

79.6 Debridement of open fracture site
[0-9] (▼ is only valid for fourth-digit "0")
Debridement of compound fracture
AHA: For Code 79.64: 3Q 1995, 12

79.7 Closed reduction of dislocation
Includes closed reduction (with external traction device)
Excludes *closed reduction of dislocation of temporomandibular joint (76.93)*

- **79.70 Closed reduction of dislocation of unspecified site**
- **79.71 Closed reduction of dislocation of shoulder**
- **79.72 Closed reduction of dislocation of elbow**
- **79.73 Closed reduction of dislocation of wrist**
- **79.74 Closed reduction of dislocation of hand and finger**
- **79.75 Closed reduction of dislocation of hip**
- **79.76 Closed reduction of dislocation of knee**
  AHA: Nov-Dec 1986, 7
- **79.77 Closed reduction of dislocation of ankle**
- **79.78 Closed reduction of dislocation of foot and toe**
- **79.79 Closed reduction of dislocation of other specified sites**

79.8 Open reduction of dislocation
Includes open reduction (with internal and external fixation devices)
Excludes *open reduction of dislocation of temporomandibular joint (76.94)*

- ▼ **79.80 Open reduction of dislocation of unspecified site**
- **79.81 Open reduction of dislocation of shoulder**
- **79.82 Open reduction of dislocation of elbow**
- **79.83 Open reduction of dislocation of wrist**
- **79.84 Open reduction of dislocation of hand and finger**
- **79.85 Open reduction of dislocation of hip**
- **79.86 Open reduction of dislocation of knee**
- **79.87 Open reduction of dislocation of ankle**
- **79.88 Open reduction of dislocation of foot and toe**
- **79.89 Open reduction of dislocation of other specified sites**

79.9 Unspecified operation on bone injury
[0-9] (▼ is only valid for fourth-digit "0")

INCISION AND EXCISION OF JOINT STRUCTURES (80)

Includes operations on:
capsule of joint
cartilage
condyle
ligament
meniscus
synovial membrane

Excludes *cartilage of:*
ear (18.01-18.9)
nose (21.00-21.99)
temporomandibular joint (76.01-76.99)

The following fourth-digit subclassification is for use with appropriate categories in section 80 to identify the site:
- **0 unspecified site**
- **1 shoulder**
- **2 elbow**
- **3 wrist**
- **4 hand and finger**
- **5 hip**
- **6 knee**
- **7 ankle**
- **8 foot and toe**
- **9 other specified sites**
  Spine

80.0 Arthrotomy for removal of prosthesis
[0-9] (▼ is only valid for fourth-digit "0")
▶Includes removal of posterior spinal motion preservation (dynamic stabilization, facet replacement, interspinous process) device(s)◀
Code also any:
insertion of (cement) (joint) ▶(methylmethacrylate)◀ spacer (84.56)
removal of (cement) (joint) ▶ (methylmethacrylate)◀ spacer (84.57)
Excludes ▶ *removal of pedicle screws used in spinal fusion (78.69)*◀
AHA: For Code 80.05: 2Q 1991, 18; For Code 80.06: 2Q 1997, 10

❹✓**80.1 Other arthrotomy**
[0-9] (▼ is only valid for fourth-digit "0")
Arthrostomy
Excludes that for:
arthrography (88.32)
arthroscopy (80.20-80.29)
injection of drug (81.92)
operative approach - omit code
DEF: Arthrostomy: Creation of an opening into a joint.

❹✓**80.2 Arthroscopy**
[0-9] (▼ is only valid for fourth-digit "0")

❹✗ **80.3 Biopsy of joint structure**
[0-9]
Aspiration biopsy
AHA: For Code 80.39: 3Q 2005, 13, 14

❹✓**80.4 Division of joint capsule, ligament, or cartilage**
[0-9] (▼ is only valid for fourth-digit "0")
Goldner clubfoot release
Heyman-Herndon(-Strong) correction of metatarsus varus
Release of:
adherent or constrictive joint capsule
joint
ligament
Excludes *symphysiotomy to assist delivery (73.94)*
that for:
carpal tunnel syndrome (04.43)
tarsal tunnel syndrome (04.44)
AHA: For Code 80.49: 2Q 2002, 16

❹ **80.5 Excision or destruction of intervertebral disc**

✓ **80.50 Excision or destruction of intervertebral disc, unspecified**
Unspecified as to excision or destruction

✓ **80.51 Excision of intervertebral disc**
Code also any concurrent spinal fusion (81.00-81.09)
Diskectomy
Level:
cervical
thoracic
lumbar (lumbosacral)
Removal of herniated nucleus pulposus
That by laminotomy or hemilaminectomy
That with decompression of spinal nerve root at same level
Requires additional code for any concomitant decompression of spinal nerve root at different level from excision site
Excludes *intervertebral chemonucleolysis (80.52)*
laminectomy for exploration of intraspinal canal (03.09)
laminotomy for decompression of spinal nerve root only (03.09)
that for insertion of (non-fusion) spinal disc replacement device (84.60-84.69)
that with corpectomy (vertebral) (80.99)
AHA: 1Q 2006, 13; 3Q 2003, 12; 1Q 1996, 7; 2Q 1995, 9; 2Q 1990, 27; Sep-Oct 1986, 12

✗ **80.52 Intervertebral chemonucleolysis**
With aspiration of disc fragments
With diskography
Injection of proteolytic enzyme into intervertebral space (chymopapain)
Excludes *injection of anesthetic substance (03.91)*
injection of other substances (03.92)

✓ **80.59 Other destruction of intervertebral disc**
Destruction NEC
That by laser
AHA: 3Q 2002, 10; 1Q 1989, 11; 4Q 1988, 11

Percutaneous intradiscal electrothermal annuloplasty

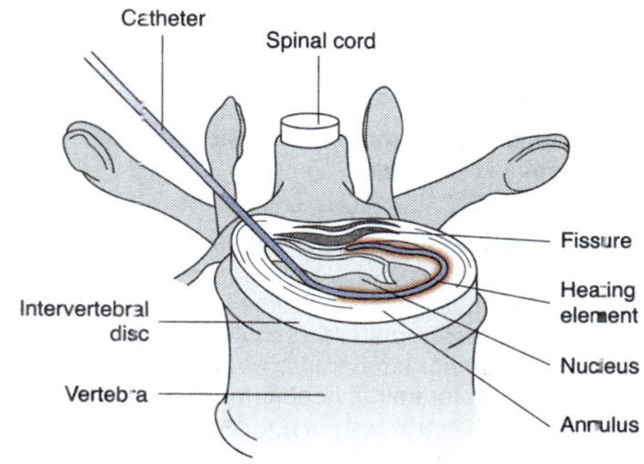

✓ **80.6 Excision of semilunar cartilage of knee**
Excision of meniscus of knee
AHA: 2Q 2003, 18; 3Q 2000, 4; 2Q 1996, 3; 1Q 1993, 23

❹✓**80.7 Synovectomy**
[0-9] (▼ is only valid for fourth-digit "0")
Complete or partial resection of synovial membrane
Excludes *excision of Baker's cyst (83.39)*
AHA: For Code 80.76: Jul-Aug 1984, 9

❹✓**80.8 Other local excision or destruction of lesion of joint**
[0-9] (▼ is only valid for fourth-digit "0")

❹✓**80.9 Other excision of joint**
[0-9] (▼ is only valid for fourth-digit "0")
Excludes *cheilectomy of joint (77.80-77.89)*
excision of bone ends (77.80-77.89)

REPAIR AND PLASTIC OPERATIONS ON JOINT STRUCTURES (81)

❹ **81.0 Spinal fusion**
Includes arthrodesis of spine with:
bone graft
internal fixation
Code also:
any insertion of interbody spinal fusion device (84.51)
any insertion of recombinant bone morphogenetic protein (84.52)
▶ any synchronous excision of (locally) harvested bone for graft (77.70-77.79)◀
the total number of vertebrae fused (81.62-81.64)
Excludes *correction of pseudarthrosis of spine (81.30-81.39)*
refusion of spine (81.30-81.39)
AHA: 4Q 2003, 99-100

✓▼ **81.00 Spinal fusion, not otherwise specified**

✓ **81.01 Atlas-axis spinal fusion**
Craniocervical fusion by anterior, transoral, or posterior technique
C_1-C_2 fusion by anterior, transoral, or posterior technique
Occiput C_2 fusion by anterior, transoral, or posterior technique

✓ **81.02 Other cervical fusion, anterior technique**
Arthrodesis of C_2 level or below:
anterior (interbody) technique
anterolateral technique
AHA: 4Q 2003, 101; 1Q 2001, 6; 1Q 1996, 6

✓ **81.03 Other cervical fusion, posterior technique**
Arthrodesis of C_2 level or below:
posterior (interbody) technique
posterolateral technique

✓ **81.04 Dorsal and dorsolumbar fusion, anterior technique**
Arthrodesis of thoracic or thoracolumbar region:
anterior (interbody) technique
anterolateral technique
AHA: 3Q 2003, 19

✓ **81.05 Dorsal and dorsolumbar fusion, posterior technique**
Arthrodesis of thoracic or thoracolumbar region:
posterior (interbody) technique
posterolateral technique
AHA: 2Q 2002, 16; 4Q 1999, 11

✓ **81.06 Lumbar and lumbosacral fusion, anterior technique**
Anterior lumbar interbody fusion (ALIF)
Arthrodesis of lumbar or lumbosacral region:
anterior (interbody) technique
anterolateral technique
AHA: 4Q 2002, 107; 4Q 1999, 11

✓ **81.07 Lumbar and lumbosacral fusion, lateral transverse process technique**
AHA: 4Q 2002, 109

✓ **81.08 Lumbar and lumbosacral fusion, posterior technique**
Arthrodesis of lumbar or lumbosacral region:
posterior (interbody) technique
posterolateral technique
Posterior lumbar interbody fusion (PLIF)
Transforaminal lumbar interbody fusion (TLIF)
AHA: 1Q 2006, 13; 4Q 2005, 123; 4Q 2002, 107-109; 2Q 2000, 12-13; 2Q 1995, 9

④ **81.1 Arthrodesis and arthroereisis of foot and ankle**
Includes arthrodesis of foot and ankle with:
bone graft
external fixation device
DEF: Arthrodesis: Surgical fixation of a joint.

✓ **81.11 Ankle fusion**
Tibiotalar fusion

✓ **81.12 Triple arthrodesis**
Talus to calcaneus and calcaneus to cuboid and navicular

✓ **81.13 Subtalar fusion**
Excludes *arthroereisis (81.18)*

✓ **81.14 Midtarsal fusion**

✓ **81.15 Tarsometatarsal fusion**

✓ **81.16 Metatarsophalangeal fusion**

✓ **81.17 Other fusion of foot**

✓ **81.18 Subtalar joint arthroereisis**

④ **81.2 Arthrodesis of other joint**
Includes arthrodesis with:
bone graft
external fixation device
excision of bone ends and compression

✓▼ **81.20 Arthrodesis of unspecified joint**

✓ **81.21 Arthrodesis of hip**

✓ **81.22 Arthrodesis of knee**

✓ **81.23 Arthrodesis of shoulder**

✓ **81.24 Arthrodesis of elbow**

✓ **81.25 Carporadial fusion**

✓ **81.26 Metacarpocarpal fusion**

✓ **81.27 Metacarpophalangeal fusion**

✓ **81.28 Interphalangeal fusion**

✓ **81.29 Arthrodesis of other specified joints**

④ **81.3 Refusion of spine**
Includes arthrodesis of spine with:
bone graft
internal fixation
correction of pseudarthrosis of spine
Code also:
any insertion of interbody spinal fusion device (84.51)
any insertion of recombinant bone morphogenetic protein (84.52)
▶ any synchronous excision of (locally) harvested bone for graft (77.70-77.79)◀
the total number of vertebrae fused (81.62-81.64)
AHA: 4Q 2003, 99; 4Q 2001, 64

✓▼ **81.30 Refusion of spine, not otherwise specified**

✓ **81.31 Refusion of atlas-axis spine**
Craniocervical fusion by anterior, transoral, or posterior technique
C_1-C_2 fusion by anterior, transoral, or posterior technique
Occiput C_2 fusion by anterior, transoral, or posterior technique

✓ **81.32 Refusion of other cervical spine, anterior technique**
Arthrodesis of C_2 level or below:
anterior (interbody) technique
anterolateral technique

✓ **81.33 Refusion of other cervical spine, posterior technique**
Arthrodesis of C_2 level or below:
posterior (interbody) technique
posterolateral technique

✓ **81.34 Refusion of dorsal and dorsolumbar spine, anterior technique**
Arthrodesis of thoracic or thoracolumbar region:
anterior (interbody) technique
anterolateral technique

✓ **81.35 Refusion of dorsal and dorsolumbar spine, posterior technique**
Anterior lumbar interbody fusion (ALIF)
Arthrodesis of thoracic or thoracolumbar region:
posterior (interbody) technique
posterolateral technique

✓ **81.36 Refusion of lumbar and lumbosacral spine, anterior technique**
Arthrodesis of lumbar or lumbosacral region:
anterior (interbody) technique
anterolateral technique

✓ **81.37 Refusion of lumbar and lumbosacral spine, lateral transverse process technique**

✓ **81.38 Refusion of lumbar and lumbosacral spine, posterior technique**
Arthrodesis of lumbar or lumbosacral region:
posterior (interbody) technique
posterolateral technique
Posterior lumbar interbody fusion (PLIF)
Transforaminal lumbar interbody fusion (TLIF)
AHA: 4Q 2002, 110

✓ **81.39 Refusion of spine, not elsewhere classified**

④ **81.4 Other repair of joint of lower extremity**
Includes arthroplasty of lower extremity with:
external traction or fixation
graft of bone (chips) or cartilage
internal fixation device

✓ **81.40 Repair of hip, not elsewhere classified**

✓ **81.42 Five-in-one repair of knee**
Medial meniscectomy, medial collateral ligament repair, vastus medialis advancement, semitendinosus advancement, and pes anserinus transfer

✓ **81.43 Triad knee repair**
Medial meniscectomy with repair of the anterior cruciate ligament and the medial collateral ligament
O'Donoghue procedure

✓ **81.44 Patellar stabilization**
Roux-Goldthwait operation for recurrent dislocation of patella

✓ **81.45 Other repair of the cruciate ligaments**
AHA: 1Q 1995, 8; Mar-Apr 1987, 12

✓ **81.46 Other repair of the collateral ligaments**
AHA: 1Q 1995, 8

✓ **81.47 Other repair of knee**
AHA: 2Q 2003, 18; 1Q 2000, 12-13; 2Q 1996, 3; 1Q 1995, 8; 3Q 1993, 5

✓ **81.49 Other repair of ankle**
AHA: 2Q 2001, 15; 3Q 2000, 4

81.5 Joint replacement of lower extremity
Includes arthroplasty of lower extremity with:
external traction or fixation
graft of bone (chips) or cartilage
internal fixation device or prosthesis

✓ **81.51 Total hip replacement**
Replacement of both femoral head and acetabulum by prosthesis
Total reconstruction of hip
Code also any type of bearing surface, if known (00.74▶00.77◀)
AHA: 4Q 2004, 113; 2Q 1991, 18; Sep-Oct 1985, 4

✓ **81.52 Partial hip replacement**
Bipolar endoprosthesis
Code also any type of bearing surface, if known (00.74▶00.77◀)
AHA: 2Q 1991, 18

✓ **81.53 Revision of hip replacement, not otherwise specified**
Revision of hip replacement, not specified as to components(s) replaced, (acetabular, femoral or both)
Code also any:
removal of (cement)(joint) spacer (84.57)
type of bearing surface, if known (00.74▶00.77◀)
Excludes *revision of hip replacement, components specified (00.70-00.73)*
AHA: 4Q 2005, 125; 3Q 1997, 12

✓ **81.54 Total knee replacement**
Bicompartmental
Tricompartmental
Unicompartmental (hemijoint)

✓ **81.55 Revision of knee replacement, not otherwise specified**
Code also any removal of (cement) spacer (84.57)
Excludes *arthrodesis of knee (81.22)*
revision of knee replacement, components specified (00.80-00.84)
AHA: 2Q 1997, 10

✓ **81.56 Total ankle replacement**

✓ **81.57 Replacement of joint of foot and toe**

✓ **81.59 Revision of joint replacement of lower extremity, not elsewhere classified**
AHA: Sep-Oct 1985, 4

81.6 Other procedures on spine
Note: Number of vertebrae:
The vertebral spine consists of 25 vertebrae in the following order and number:
Cervical: C_1 (atlas), C_2 (axis), C_3, C_4, C_5, C_6, C_7
Thoracic or Dorsal: T_1, T_2, T_3, T_4, T_5, T_6, T_7, T_8, T_9, T_{10}, T_{11}, T_{12}
Lumbar and Sacral: L_1, L_2, L_3, L_4, L_5, S_1
Coders should report only one code from the series 81.62 or 81.63 or 81.64 to show the total number of vertebrae fused on the patient.
Code also the level and approach of the fusion or refusion (81.00-81.08, 81.30-81.39)
AHA: 4Q 2003, 99-100

✓ **81.62 Fusion or refusion of 2-3 vertebrae**
AHA: 1Q 2006, 13; 4Q 2005, 123; 4Q 2003, 99-100

✓ **81.63 Fusion or refusion of 4-8 vertebrae**
AHA: 4Q 2003, 99-100

✓ **81.64 Fusion or refusion of 9 or more vertebrae**
AHA: 4Q 2003, 99-100

✓ **81.65 Vertebroplasty**
Injection of bone void filler (cement) (polymethylmethacrylate) (PMMA) into the diseased or fractured vertebral body
Excludes *kyphoplasty (81.66)*
AHA: 4Q 2004, 125-126

✓ **81.66 Kyphoplasty**
Insertion of inflatable balloon, bone tamp, or other device to create a cavity for partial restoration of height of diseased or fractured vertebral body prior to injection of bone void filler (cement) (polymethylmethacrylate) (PMMA)
Excludes *vertebroplasty (81.65)*
AHA: 4Q 2004, 125-126

81.7 Arthroplasty and repair of hand, fingers and wrist
Includes arthroplasty of hand and finger with:
external traction or fixation
graft of bone (chips) or cartilage
internal fixation device or prosthesis
Excludes *operations on muscle, tendon and fascia of hand (82.01-82.99)*

✓ **81.71 Arthroplasty of metacarpophalangeal and interphalangeal joint with implant**

✓ **81.72 Arthroplasty of metacarpophalangeal and interphalangeal joint without implant**

✓ **81.73 Total wrist replacement**

✓ **81.74 Arthroplasty of carpocarpal or carpometacarpal joint with implant**

✓ **81.75 Arthroplasty of carpocarpal or carpometacarpal joint without implant**
AHA: 3Q 1993, 8

✓ **81.79 Other repair of hand, fingers and wrist**

81.8 Arthroplasty and repair of shoulder and elbow
Includes arthroplasty of upper limb NEC with:
external traction or fixation
graft of bone (chips) or cartilage
internal fixation device or prosthesis

✓ **81.80 Total shoulder replacement**

✓ **81.81 Partial shoulder replacement**

✓ **81.82 Repair of recurrent dislocation of shoulder**
AHA: 3Q 1995, 15

✓ **81.83 Other repair of shoulder**
Revision of arthroplasty of shoulder
AHA: 1Q 2002, 9; 4Q 2001, 51; 2Q 2000, 14; 3Q 1993, 5

✓ **81.84 Total elbow replacement**

✓ **81.85 Other repair of elbow**

81.9 Other operations on joint structures

✖ **81.91 Arthrocentesis**
Joint aspiration
Excludes *that for:*
arthrography (88.32)
biopsy of joint structure 80.30-80.39)
injection of drug (81.92)

✖ **81.92 Injection of therapeutic substance into joint or ligament**
AHA: 2Q 2000, 14; 3Q 1989, 16

✓ **81.93 Suture of capsule or ligament of upper extremity**
Excludes *that associated with arthroplasty (81.71-81.75, 81.80-81.81, 81.84)*

✓ **81.94 Suture of capsule or ligament of ankle and foot**
Excludes *that associated with arthroplasty (81.56-81.59)*

✓ **81.95 Suture of capsule or ligament of other lower extremity**
Excludes *that associated with arthroplasty (81.51-81.55, 81.59)*

✓ **81.96 Other repair of joint**

✓ **81.97 Revision of joint replacement of upper extremity**
Partial
Removal of cement spacer
Total
AHA: 1Q 2004, 12

✓ **81.98 Other diagnostic procedures on joint structures**
Excludes *arthroscopy (80.20-80.29)*
biopsy of joint structure (80.30-80.39)
microscopic examination of specimen from joint (91.51-91.59)
thermography (88.83)
x-ray (87.21-87.29, 88.21-88.33)

✓ **81.99 Other**

✖ Deleted Code ▼ Nonspecific O.R. Procedure ✓ Valid O.R. Procedure ✖ Non-O.R. Procedure ♂ Male ♀ Female

OPERATIONS ON MUSCLE, TENDON, AND FASCIA OF HAND (82)

Includes operations on:
aponeurosis
synovial membrane (tendon sheath)
tendon sheath

❹ **82.0 Incision of muscle, tendon, fascia, and bursa of hand**

✔ **82.01 Exploration of tendon sheath of hand**
Incision of tendon sheath of hand
Removal of rice bodies in tendon sheath of hand
Excludes *division of tendon (82.11)*

✔ **82.02 Myotomy of hand**
Excludes *myotomy for division (82.19)*

✔ **82.03 Bursotomy of hand**

✖ **82.04 Incision and drainage of palmar or thenar space**

✔ **82.09 Other incision of soft tissue of hand**
Excludes *incision of skin and subcutaneous tissue alone (86.01-86.09)*
AHA: Nov-Dec 1987, 10

❹ **82.1 Division of muscle, tendon, and fascia of hand**

✔ **82.11 Tenotomy of hand**
Division of tendon of hand

✔ **82.12 Fasciotomy of hand**
Division of fascia of hand

✔ **82.19 Other division of soft tissue of hand**
Division of muscle of hand

❹ **82.2 Excision of lesion of muscle, tendon, and fascia of hand**

✔ **82.21 Excision of lesion of tendon sheath of hand**
Ganglionectomy of tendon sheath (wrist)

Removal of Wrist Ganglion

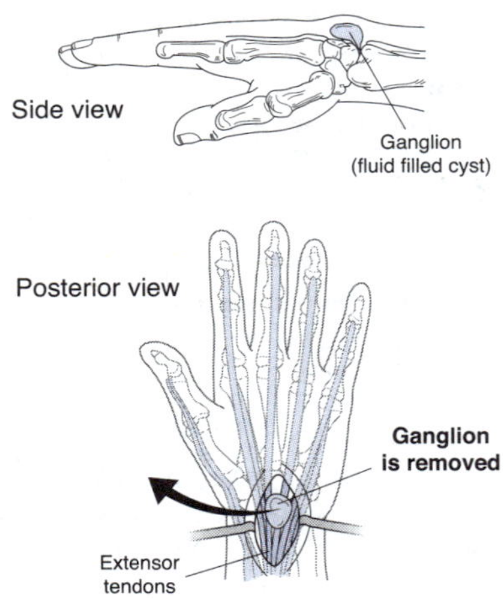

✔ **82.22 Excision of lesion of muscle of hand**

✔ **82.29 Excision of other lesion of soft tissue of hand**
Excludes *excision of lesion of skin and subcutaneous tissue (86.21-86.3)*

❹ **82.3 Other excision of soft tissue of hand**
Code also any skin graft (86.61-86.62, 86.73)
Excludes *excision of skin and subcutaneous tissue (86.21-86.3)*

✔ **82.31 Bursectomy of hand**

✔ **82.32 Excision of tendon of hand for graft**

✔ **82.33 Other tenonectomy of hand**
Tenosynovectomy of hand
Excludes *excision of lesion of:*
tendon (82.29)
sheath (82.21)
DEF: Tenonectomy: Removal of a portion of a tendon to shortening the length.
Tenosynovectomy: Removal or resection of a tendon sheath.

✔ **82.34 Excision of muscle or fascia of hand for graft**

✔ **82.35 Other fasciectomy of hand**
Release of Dupuytren's contracture
Excludes *excision of lesion of fascia (82.29)*

✔ **82.36 Other myectomy of hand**
Excludes *excision of lesion of muscle (82.22)*

✔ **82.39 Other excision of soft tissue of hand**
Excludes *excision of skin (86.21-86.3)*
excision of soft tissue lesion (82.29)

❹ **82.4 Suture of muscle, tendon, and fascia of hand**

✔ **82.41 Suture of tendon sheath of hand**

✔ **82.42 Delayed suture of flexor tendon of hand**

✔ **82.43 Delayed suture of other tendon of hand**

✔ **82.44 Other suture of flexor tendon of hand**
Excludes *delayed suture of flexor tendon of hand (82.42)*

✔ **82.45 Other suture of other tendon of hand**
Excludes *delayed suture of other tendon of hand (82.43)*

✔ **82.46 Suture of muscle or fascia of hand**

❹ **82.5 Transplantation of muscle and tendon of hand**

✔ **82.51 Advancement of tendon of hand**

✔ **82.52 Recession of tendon of hand**

✔ **82.53 Reattachment of tendon of hand**

✔ **82.54 Reattachment of muscle of hand**

✔ **82.55 Other change in hand muscle or tendon length**

✔ **82.56 Other hand tendon transfer or transplantation**
Excludes *pollicization of thumb (82.61)*
transfer of finger, except thumb (82.81)
AHA: 2Q 1999, 10; 4Q 1998, 40

✔ **82.57 Other hand tendon transposition**
AHA: 3Q 1993, 8; 1Q 1993, 28

✔ **82.58 Other hand muscle transfer or transplantation**

✔ **82.59 Other hand muscle transposition**

❹ **82.6 Reconstruction of thumb**
Includes digital transfer to act as thumb
Code also any amputation for digital transfer (84.01, 84.11)

✔ **82.61 Pollicization operation carrying over nerves and blood supply**
DEF: Surgical reconstruction and replacement of a thumb by transferring another digit, such as the index finger or big toe.

✔ **82.69 Other reconstruction of thumb**
"Cocked-hat" procedure [skin flap and bone]
Grafts:
bone to thumb
skin (pedicle) to thumb

❹ **82.7 Plastic operation on hand with graft or implant**

✔ **82.71 Tendon pulley reconstruction**
Reconstruction for opponensplasty

✔ **82.72 Plastic operation on hand with graft of muscle or fascia**

✔ **82.79 Plastic operation on hand with other graft or implant**
Tendon graft to hand
AHA: Jan-Feb 1987, 6

❹ **82.8 Other plastic operations on hand**

✔ **82.81 Transfer of finger, except thumb**
Excludes *pollicization of thumb (82.61)*
AHA: 2Q 2005, 7

✔ **82.82 Repair of cleft hand**

✔ **82.83 Repair of macrodactyly**

✔ **82.84 Repair of mallet finger**

✔ **82.85 Other tenodesis of hand**
Tendon fixation of hand NOS

✔ **82.86 Other tenoplasty of hand**
Myotenoplasty of hand

✔ **82.89 Other plastic operations on hand**
Plication of fascia
Repair of fascial hernia
Excludes *that with graft or implant (82.71-82.79)*

82.9 Other operations on muscle, tendon, and fascia of hand
Excludes *diagnostic procedures on soft tissue of hand (83.21-83.29)*

82.91 Lysis of adhesions of hand
Freeing of adhesions of fascia, muscle, and tendon of hand
Excludes *decompression of carpal tunnel (04.43)*
that by stretching or manipulation only (93.26)

82.92 Aspiration of bursa of hand

82.93 Aspiration of other soft tissue of hand
Excludes *skin and subcutaneous tissue (86.01)*

82.94 Injection of therapeutic substance into bursa of hand

82.95 Injection of therapeutic substance into tendon of hand

82.96 Other injection of locally-acting therapeutic substance into soft tissue of hand
Excludes *subcutaneous or intramuscular injection (99.11-99.29)*

82.99 Other operations on muscle, tendon, and fascia of hand

OPERATIONS ON MUSCLE, TENDON, FASCIA, AND BURSA, EXCEPT HAND (83)

Includes operations on:
aponeurosis
synovial membrane of bursa and tendon sheaths
tendon sheaths
Excludes *diaphragm (34.81-34.89)*
hand (82.01-82.99)
muscles of eye (15.01-15.9)

83.0 Incision of muscle, tendon, fascia, and bursa

83.01 Exploration of tendon sheath
Incision of tendon sheath
Removal of rice bodies from tendon sheath

83.02 Myotomy
Excludes *cricopharyngeal myotomy (29.31)*
AHA: 2Q 1989, 18

83.03 Bursotomy
Removal of calcareous deposit of bursa
Excludes *aspiration of bursa (percutaneous) (83.94)*

83.09 Other incision of soft tissue
Incision of fascia
Excludes *incision of skin and subcutaneous tissue alone (86.01-86.09)*

83.1 Division of muscle, tendon, and fascia

83.11 Achillotenotomy
DEF: Surgical cutting of the Achilles tendon.

83.12 Adductor tenotomy of hip

83.13 Other tenotomy
Aponeurotomy
Division of tendon
Tendon release
Tendon transection
Tenotomy for thoracic outlet decompression

83.14 Fasciotomy
Division of fascia
Division of iliotibial band
Fascia stripping
Release of Volkmann's contracture by fasciotomy
AHA: 3Q 1998, 8

83.19 Other division of soft tissue
Division of muscle
Muscle release
Myotomy for thoracic outlet decompression
Myotomy with division
Scalenotomy
Transection of muscle
DEF: Scalenotomy: Division of the scalene muscles to restrict respiratory activity of the upper thorax.

83.2 Diagnostic procedures on muscle, tendon, fascia, and bursa, including that of hand

83.21 Biopsy of soft tissue
Excludes *biopsy of chest wall (34.23)*
biopsy of skin and subcutaneous tissue (86.11)

83.29 Other diagnostic procedures on muscle, tendon, fascia, and bursa, including that of hand
Excludes *microscopic examination of specimen (91.51-91.59)*
soft tissue x-ray (87.09, 87.38-87.39, 88.09, 88.35, 88.37)
thermography of muscle (88.84)

83.3 Excision of lesion of muscle, tendon, fascia, and bursa
Excludes *biopsy of soft tissue (83.21)*

83.31 Excision of lesion of tendon sheath
Excision of ganglion of tendon sheath, except of hand

83.32 Excision of lesion of muscle
Excision of:
heterotopic bone
muscle scar for release of Volkmann's contracture
myositis ossificans

83.39 Excision of lesion of other soft tissue
Excision of Baker's cyst
Excludes *bursectomy (83.5)*
excision of lesion of skin and subcutaneous tissue (86.3)
synovectomy (80.70-80.79)
AHA: 2Q 2005, 3-4; Q2 1997, 6

83.4 Other excision of muscle, tendon, and fascia

83.41 Excision of tendon for graft

83.42 Other tenonectomy
Excision of:
aponeurosis
tendon sheath
Tenosynovectomy

83.43 Excision of muscle or fascia for graft

83.44 Other fasciectomy

83.45 Other myectomy
Debridement of muscle NOS
Scalenectomy
AHA: 1Q 1999, 8-9

83.49 Other excision of soft tissue

83.5 Bursectomy
AHA: 2Q 1999, 10-11

83.6 Suture of muscle, tendon, and fascia

83.61 Suture of tendon sheath

83.62 Delayed suture of tendon

83.63 Rotator cuff repair
AHA: 1Q 2006, 6; 2Q 1993, 8

83.64 Other suture of tendon
Achillorrhaphy
Aponeurorrhaphy
Excludes *delayed suture of tendon (83.62)*

83.65 Other suture of muscle or fascia
Repair of diastasis recti

83.7 Reconstruction of muscle and tendon
Excludes *reconstruction of muscle and tendon associated with arthroplasty*

83.71 Advancement of tendon

83.72 Recession of tendon

83.73 Reattachment of tendon

83.74 Reattachment of muscle

83.75 Tendon transfer or transplantation

83.76 Other tendon transposition

83.77 Muscle transfer or transplantation
Release of Volkmann's contracture by muscle transplantation

83.79 Other muscle transposition

✖ Deleted Code ▼ Nonspecific O.R. Procedure ✔ Valid O.R. Procedure ✖ Non-O.R. Procedure ♂ Male ♀ Female

83.8 Other plastic operations on muscle, tendon, and fascia
Excludes *plastic operations on muscle, tendon, and fascia associated with arthroplasty*

83.81 Tendon graft

83.82 Graft of muscle or fascia
AHA: 3Q 2001, 9

83.83 Tendon pulley reconstruction

83.84 Release of clubfoot, not elsewhere classified
Evans operation on clubfoot

83.85 Other change in muscle or tendon length
Hamstring lengthening
Heel cord shortening
Plastic achillotenotomy
Tendon plication

83.86 Quadricepsplasty

83.87 Other plastic operations on muscle
Musculoplasty
Myoplasty
AHA: 1Q 1997, 9-10

83.88 Other plastic operations on tendon
Myotenoplasty
Tendon fixation
Tenodesis
Tenoplasty
DEF: Tenodesis: Fixing the end of a tendon to a bone.

83.89 Other plastic operations on fascia
Fascia lengthening
Fascioplasty
Plication of fascia

83.9 Other operations on muscle, tendon, fascia, and bursa
Excludes *nonoperative:*
manipulation (93.25-93.29)
stretching (93.27-93.29)

83.91 Lysis of adhesions of muscle, tendon, fascia, and bursa
Excludes *that for tarsal tunnel syndrome (04.44)*

83.92 Insertion or replacement of skeletal muscle stimulator
Implantation, insertion, placement, or replacement of skeletal muscle:
electrodes
stimulator
AHA: 2Q 1999, 10

83.93 Removal of skeletal muscle stimulator

83.94 Aspiration of bursa

83.95 Aspiration of other soft tissue
Excludes *that of skin and subcutaneous tissue (86.01)*

83.96 Injection of therapeutic substance into bursa

83.97 Injection of therapeutic substance into tendon

Injection into Tendon

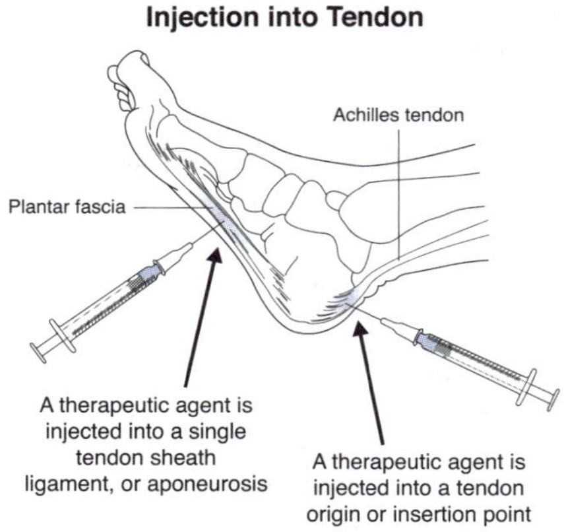

83.98 Injection of locally-acting therapeutic substance into other soft tissue
Excludes *subcutaneous or intramuscular injection (99.11-99.29)*

83.99 Other operations on muscle, tendon, fascia, and bursa
Suture of bursa

OTHER PROCEDURES ON MUSCULOSKELETAL SYSTEM (84)

84.0 Amputation of upper limb
Excludes *revision of amputation stump (84.3)*

84.00 Upper limb amputation, not otherwise specified
Closed flap amputation of upper limb NOS
Kineplastic amputation of upper limb NOS
Open or guillotine amputation of upper limb NOS
Revision of current traumatic amputation of upper limb NOS

84.01 Amputation and disarticulation of finger
Excludes *ligation of supernumerary finger (86.26)*

84.02 Amputation and disarticulation of thumb

84.03 Amputation through hand
Amputation through carpals

84.04 Disarticulation of wrist

84.05 Amputation through forearm
Forearm amputation

84.06 Disarticulation of elbow

84.07 Amputation through humerus
Upper arm amputation

84.08 Disarticulation of shoulder

84.09 Interthoracoscapular amputation
Forequarter amputation

84.1 Amputation of lower limb
Excludes *revision of amputation stump (84.3)*

84.10 Lower limb amputation, not otherwise specified
Closed flap amputation of lower limb NOS
Kineplastic amputation of lower limb NOS
Open or guillotine amputation of lower limb NOS
Revision of current traumatic amputation of lower limb NOS

84.11 Amputation of toe
Amputation through metatarsophalangeal joint
Disarticulation of toe
Metatarsal head amputation
Ray amputation of foot (disarticulation of the metatarsal head of the toe extending across the forefoot just proximal to the metatarsophalangeal crease)
Excludes *ligation of supernumerary toe (86.26)*
AHA: 2Q 2005, 7; 4Q 1999, 19

84.12 Amputation through foot
Amputation of forefoot
Amputation through middle of foot
Chopart's amputation
Midtarsal amputation
Transmetatarsal amputation (amputation of the forefoot, including all the toes)
Excludes *Ray amputation of foot (84.11)*
DEF: Chopart's amputation: amputation of the forefoot, with retention of the calcaneus, talus, and other tarsal parts.
AHA: 4Q 1999, 19

84.13 Disarticulation of ankle

84.14 Amputation of ankle through malleoli of tibia and fibula

84.15 Other amputation below knee
Amputation of leg through tibia and fibula NOS

84.16 Disarticulation of knee
Batch, Spitler, and McFaddin amputation
Mazet amputation
S.P. Roger's amputation

84.17 Amputation above knee
Amputation of leg through femur
Amputation of thigh
Conversion of below-knee amputation into above-knee amputation
Supracondylar above-knee amputation
AHA: 1Q 2005, 16; 3Q 2003, 14; 1Q 1995, 10; 4Q 1988, 12

84.18 Disarticulation of hip

84.19 Abdominopelvic amputation
Hemipelvectomy
Hindquarter amputation

84.2 Reattachment of extremity

84.21 Thumb reattachment

84.22 Finger reattachment

84.23 Forearm, wrist, or hand reattachment

84.24 Upper arm reattachment
Reattachment of arm NOS

84.25 Toe reattachment

84.26 Foot reattachment

84.27 Lower leg or ankle reattachment
Reattachment of leg NOS
AHA: 1Q 1995, 8

84.28 Thigh reattachment

84.29 Other reattachment

84.3 Revision of amputation stump
Reamputation of stump
Secondary closure of stump
Trimming of stump
Excludes *revision of current traumatic amputation [revision by further amputation of current injury] (84.00-84.19, 84.91)*
AHA: 1Q 2005, 15

84.4 Implantation or fitting of prosthetic limb device

84.40 Implantation or fitting of prosthetic limb device, not otherwise specified

84.41 Fitting of prosthesis of upper arm and shoulder

84.42 Fitting of prosthesis of lower arm and hand

84.43 Fitting of prosthesis of arm, not otherwise specified

84.44 Implantation of prosthetic device of arm

84.45 Fitting of prosthesis above knee

84.46 Fitting of prosthesis below knee

84.47 Fitting of prosthesis of leg, not otherwise specified

84.48 Implantation of prosthetic device of leg

84.5 Implantation of other musculoskeletal devices and substances
Excludes *insertion of (non-fusion) spinal disc replacement device (84.60-84.69)*

84.51 Insertion of interbody spinal fusion device
Insertion of:
cages (carbon, ceramic, metal, plastic or titanium)
interbody fusion cage
synthetic cages or spacers
threaded bone dowels
Code also refusion of spine (81.30-81.39)
Code also spinal fusion (81.00-81.08)
AHA: 4Q 2005, 123; 1Q 2004, 21; 4Q 2002, 109-110

84.52 Insertion of recombinant bone morphogenetic protein
rhBMP
That via collagen sponge, coral, ceramic and other carriers
Code also primary procedure performed:
fracture repair (79.00-79.99)
spinal fusion (81.00-81.08)
spinal refusion (81.30-81.39)
AHA: 4Q 2002, 110

84.53 Implantation of internal limb lengthening device with kinetic distraction
Code also limb lengthening procedure (78.30-78.39)

84.54 Implantation of other internal limb lengthening device
Implantation of internal limb lengthening device, not otherwise specified (NOS)
Code also limb lengthening procedure (78.30-78.39)

84.55 Insertion of bone void filler
Insertion of:
acrylic cement (PMMA)
bone void cement
calcium based bone void filler
polymethylmethacrylate (PMMA)
Excludes *that with kyphoplasty (81.66)*
that with vertebroplasty (81.65)
AHA: 4Q 2004, 128-129

84.56 Insertion of (cement) spacer
Insertion of joint ▶(methylmethacrylate)◀ spacer

84.57 Removal of (cement) spacer
Removal of joint ▶(methylmethacrylate)◀ spacer
AHA: 4Q 2005, 125

~~**84.58 Implantation of interspinous process decompression device**~~

84.59 Insertion of other spinal devices
Excludes ▶*initial insertion of pedicle screws with spinal fusion-omit code*
insertion of facet replacement device(s) (84.84)
insertion of interspinous process device(s) (84.80)
insertion of pedicle-based dynamic stabilization device(s) (84.82)◀

84.6 Replacement of spinal disc
Includes non-fusion arthroplasty of the spine with insertion of artificial disc prosthesis

84.60 Insertion of spinal disc prosthesis, not otherwise specified
Replacement of spinal disc, NOS
Includes diskectomy (discectomy)

84.61 Insertion of partial spinal disc prosthesis, cervical
Nuclear replacement device, cervical
Partial artificial disc prosthesis (flexible), cervical
Replacement of nuclear disc (nucleus pulposus), cervical
Includes diskectomy (discectomy)

84.62 Insertion of total spinal disc prosthesis, cervical
Replacement of cervical spinal disc, NOS
Replacement of total spinal disc, cervical
Total artificial disc prosthesis (flexible), cervical
Includes diskectomy (discectomy)

84.63 Insertion of spinal disc prosthesis, thoracic
Artificial disc prosthesis (flexible), thoracic
Replacement of thoracic spinal disc, partial or total
Includes diskectomy (discectomy)

84.64 Insertion of partial spinal disc prosthesis, lumbosacral
Nuclear replacement device, lumbar
Partial artificial disc prosthesis (flexible), lumbar
Replacement of nuclear disc (nucleus pulposus), lumbar
Includes diskectomy (discectomy)

84.65 Insertion of total spinal disc prosthesis, lumbosacral
Replacement of lumbar spinal disc, NOS
Replacement of total spinal disc, lumbar
Total artificial disc prosthesis (flexible), lumbar
Includes diskectomy (discectomy)
AHA: 4Q 2004, 133

84.66 Revision or replacement of artificial spinal disc prosthesis, cervical
Removal of (partial) (total) spinal disc prosthesis with synchronous insertion of new (partial) (total) spinal disc prosthesis, cervical
Repair of previously inserted spinal disc prosthesis, cervical

84.67 Revision or replacement of artificial spinal disc prosthesis, thoracic
Removal of (partial) (total) spinal disc prosthesis with synchronous insertion of new (partial) (total) spinal disc prosthesis, thoracic
Repair of previously inserted spinal disc prosthesis, thoracic

84.68 Revision or replacement of artificial spinal disc prosthesis, lumbosacral
Removal of (partial) (total) spinal disc prosthesis with synchronous insertion of new (partial) (total) spinal disc prosthesis, lumbosacral
Repair of previously inserted spinal disc prosthesis, lumbosacral

84.69 Revision or replacement of artificial spinal disc prosthesis, not otherwise specified
Removal of (partial) (total) spinal disc prosthesis with synchronous insertion of new (partial) (total) spinal disc prosthesis
Repair of previously inserted spinal disc prosthesis

✖ Deleted Code ▼ Nonspecific O.R. Procedure ✔ Valid O.R. Procedure ✖ Non-O.R. Procedure ♂ Male ♀ Female

❹ **84.7 Adjunct codes for external fixator devices**
Code also any primary procedure performed:
application of external fixator device (78.10, 78.12-78.13, 78.15, 78.17-78.19)
reduction of fracture and dislocation (79.00-79.89)

✖ **84.71 Application of external fixator device, monoplanar system**
Excludes *other hybrid device or system (84.73)*
ring device or system (84.72)
AHA: 4Q 2005, 129

✖ **84.72 Application of external fixator device, ring system**
Ilizarov type
Sheffield type
Excludes *monoplanar device or system (84.71)*
other hybrid device or system (84.73)

✖ **84.73 Application of hybrid external fixator device**
Computer (assisted) (dependent) external fixator device
Hybrid system using both ring and monoplanar devices
Excludes *monoplanar device or system, when used alone (84.71)*
ring device or system, when used alone (84.72)

●❹ **84.8 Insertion, replacement and revision of posterior spinal motion preservation device(s)**
Dynamic spinal stabilization device(s)
Includes any synchronous facetectomy (partial, total) performed at the same level
Code also any synchronous surgical decompression (foraminotomy, laminectomy, laminotomy), if performed (03.09)
Excludes *fusion of spine (81.00 – 81.08, 81.30-81.39)*
insertion of artificial disc prosthesis (84.60-84.69)
insertion of interbody spinal fusion device (84.51)

●✔ **84.80 Insertion or replacement of interspinous process device(s)**
Interspinous process decompression device(s)
Interspinous process distraction device(s)
Excludes *insertion or replacement of facet replacement device (84.84)*
insertion or replacement of pedicle-based dynamic stabilization device (84.82)

●✔ **84.81 Revision of interspinous process device(s)**
Repair of previously inserted interspinous process device(s)
Excludes *revision of facet replacement device(s) (84.85)*
revision of pedicle-based dynamic stabilization device (84.83)

●✔ **84.82 Insertion or replacement of pedicle-based dynamic stabilization device(s)**
Excludes *initial insertion of pedicle screws with spinal fusion – omit code*
insertion or replacement of facet replacement device(s) (84.84)
insertion or replacement of interspinous process device(s) (84.80)
replacement of pedicle screws used in spinal fusion (78.59)

●✔ **84.83 Revision of pedicle-based dynamic stabilization device(s)**
Repair of previously inserted pedicle-based dynamic stabilization device(s)
Excludes *removal of pedicle screws used in spinal fusion (78.69)*
replacement of pedicle screws used in spinal fusion (78.59)
revision of facet replacement device(s) (84.85)
revision of interspinous process device(s) (84.81)

●✔ **84.84 Insertion or replacement of facet replacement device(s)**
Facet arthroplasty
Excludes *initial insertion of pedicle screws with spinal fusion – omit code*
insertion or replacement of interspinous process device(s) (84.80)
insertion or replacement of pedicle-based dynamic stabilization device(s) (84.82)
replacement of pedicle screws used in spinal fusion (78.59)

●✔ **84.85 Revision of facet replacement device(s)**
Repair of previously inserted facet replacement device(s)
Excludes *removal of pedicle screws used in spinal fusion (78.69)*
replacement of pedicle screws used in spinal fusion (78.59)
revision of interspinous process device(s) (84.81)
revision of pedicle-based dynamic stabilization device(s) (84.83)

❹ **84.9 Other operations on musculoskeletal system**
Excludes *nonoperative manipulation (93.25-93.29)*

✔ **84.91 Amputation, not otherwise specified**

✔ **84.92 Separation of equal conjoined twins**

✔ **84.93 Separation of unequal conjoined twins**
Separation of conjoined twins NOS

✔ **84.99 Other**

15. OPERATIONS ON THE INTEGUMENTARY SYSTEM (85-86)

OPERATIONS ON THE BREAST (85)

Includes operations on the skin and subcutaneous tissue of:
- breast female or male
- previous mastectomy site female or male

revision of previous mastectomy site

✖ **85.0 Mastotomy**
Incision of breast (skin)
Mammotomy
Excludes *aspiration of breast (85.91)*
removal of implant (85.94)
AHA: 1Q 2004, 3; 2Q 1990, 27

❹ **85.1 Diagnostic procedures on breast**

✖⓪ **85.11 Closed [percutaneous] [needle] biopsy of breast**
AHA: 2Q 2000, 10; 3Q 1989, 17

✔⓪ **85.12 Open biopsy of breast**
AHA: 3Q 1989, 17; Mar-Apr 1986, 11

✖ **85.19 Other diagnostic procedures on breast**
Excludes *mammary ductogram (87.35)*
mammography NEC (87.37)
manual examination (89.36)
microscopic examination of specimen (91.61-91.69)
thermography (88.85)
ultrasonography (88.73)
xerography (87.36)

❹ **85.2 Excision or destruction of breast tissue**
Excludes *mastectomy (85.41-85.48)*
reduction mammoplasty (85.31-85.32)

✔ **85.20 Excision or destruction of breast tissue, not otherwise specified**

Breast Tissue Ablation

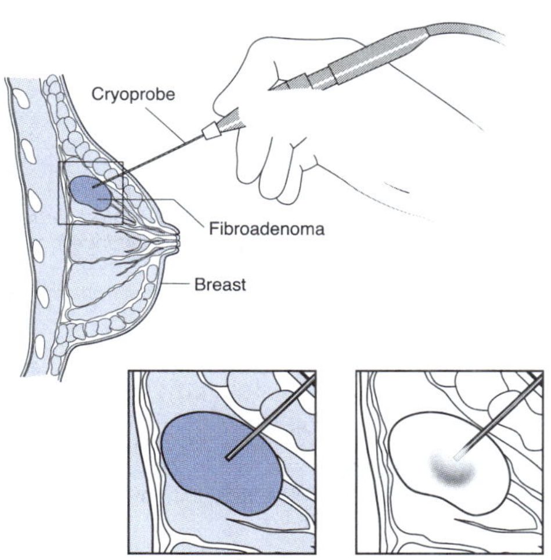

Cryoprobe is placed within the fibroadenoma under ultrasound

Cryoprobe initiates freezing

✔ **85.21 Local excision of lesion of breast**
Lumpectomy
Removal of area of fibrosis from breast
Excludes *biopsy of breast (85.11-85.12)*
AHA: 2Q 1990, 27; 3Q 1989, 17; Mar-Apr 1986, 11; Sep-Oct 1985, 12

✔ **85.22 Resection of quadrant of breast**
AHA: Sep-Oct 1985, 12

✔ **85.23 Subtotal mastectomy**
Excludes *quadrant resection (85.22)*
AHA: 2Q 1992, 7; Sep-Oct 1985, 12

✔ **85.24 Excision of ectopic breast tissue**
Excision of accessory nipple

✔ **85.25 Excision of nipple**
Excludes *excision of accessory nipple (85.24)*

❹ **85.3 Reduction mammoplasty and subcutaneous mammectomy**
AHA: 4Q 1995, 79-80

✔ **85.31 Unilateral reduction mammoplasty**
Unilateral:
amputative mammoplasty
size reduction mammoplasty

✔ **85.32 Bilateral reduction mammoplasty**
Amputative mammoplasty
Reduction mammoplasty (for gynecomastia)

✔ **85.33 Unilateral subcutaneous mammectomy with synchronous implant**
Excludes *that without synchronous implant (85.34)*

✔ **85.34 Other unilateral subcutaneous mammectomy**
Removal of breast tissue with preservation of skin and nipple
Subcutaneous mammectomy NOS

✔ **85.35 Bilateral subcutaneous mammectomy with synchronous implant**
Excludes *that without synchronous implant (85.36)*

✔ **85.36 Other bilateral subcutaneous mammectomy**

❹ **85.4 Mastectomy**

✔ **85.41 Unilateral simple mastectomy**
Mastectomy:
NOS
complete

✔ **85.42 Bilateral simple mastectomy**
Bilateral complete mastectomy

✔ **85.43 Unilateral extended simple mastectomy**
Extended simple mastectomy NOS
Modified radical mastectomy
Simple mastectomy with excision of regional lymph nodes
AHA: 3Q 1991, 24; 2Q 1991, 21

✔ **85.44 Bilateral extended simple mastectomy**
AHA: 3Q 1991, 24; 2Q 1991, 21

✔ **85.45 Unilateral radical mastectomy**
Excision of breast, pectoral muscles, and regional lymph nodes [axillary, clavicular, supraclavicular]
Radical mastectomy NOS
AHA: 2Q 1991, 21

✔ **85.46 Bilateral radical mastectomy**
AHA: 2Q 1991, 21

✔ **85.47 Unilateral extended radical mastectomy**
Excision of breast, muscles, and lymph nodes [axillary, clavicular, supraclavicular, internal mammary, and mediastinal]
Extended radical mastectomy NOS

✔ **85.48 Bilateral extended radical mastectomy**

❹ **85.5 Augmentation mammoplasty**
Excludes *that associated with subcutaneous mammectomy (85.33, 85.35)*

✔ **85.50 Augmentation mammoplasty, not otherwise specified**

✖ **85.51 Unilateral injection into breast for augmentation**
AHA: 3Q 1997, 12

✖ **85.52 Bilateral injection into breast for augmentation**
Injection into breast for augmentation NOS

✔ **85.53 Unilateral breast implant**
AHA: 2Q 2000, 18; 2Q 1998, 14

✔ **85.54 Bilateral breast implant**
Breast implant NOS

✔ **85.6 Mastopexy**

✔ **85.7 Total reconstruction of breast**
AHA: 4Q 1995, 77; 3Q 1991, 27

85.8 Other repair and plastic operations on breast
Excludes that for:
augmentation (85.50-85.54)
reconstruction (85.7)
reduction (85.31-85.32)

85.81 Suture of laceration of breast

85.82 Split-thickness graft to breast
AHA: 4Q 1995, 77

85.83 Full-thickness graft to breast
AHA: 4Q 1995, 77

85.84 Pedicle graft to breast
AHA: 4Q 1995, 77

85.85 Muscle flap graft to breast
AHA: 4Q 1995, 77

85.86 Transposition of nipple
AHA: 4Q 1995, 78

85.87 Other repair or reconstruction of nipple
AHA: 4Q 1995, 78

85.89 Other mammoplasty

85.9 Other operations on the breast

85.91 Aspiration of breast
Excludes *percutaneous biopsy of breast (85.11)*

85.92 Injection of therapeutic agent into breast
Excludes *that for augmentation of breast (85.51-85.52)*

85.93 Revision of implant of breast
AHA: 2Q 1998, 14; 4Q 1995, 76

85.94 Removal of implant of breast
AHA: 3Q 1992, 4; 2Q 1998, 14

85.95 Insertion of breast tissue expander
Insertion (soft tissue) of tissue expander (one or more) under muscle or platysma to develop skin flaps for donor use

85.96 Removal of breast tissue expander
AHA: 2Q 2000, 18; 4Q 1995, 78

85.99 Other
AHA: Nov-Dec 1987, 10

OPERATIONS ON SKIN AND SUBCUTANEOUS TISSUE (86)

Includes operations on:
hair follicles
male perineum
nails
sebaceous glands
subcutaneous fat pads
sudoriferous glands
superficial fossae

Excludes those on skin of:
anus (49.01-49.99)
breast (mastectomy site) (85.0-85.99)
ear (18.01-18.9)
eyebrow (08.01-08.99)
eyelid (08.01-08.99)
female perineum (71.01-71.9)
lips (27.0-27.99)
nose (21.00-21.99)
penis (64.0-64.99)
scrotum (61.0-61.99)
vulva (71.01-71.9)

86.0 Incision of skin and subcutaneous tissue

86.01 Aspiration of skin and subcutaneous tissue
Aspiration of:
abscess of nail, skin, or subcutaneous tissue
hematoma of nail, skin, or subcutaneous tissue
seroma of nail, skin, or subcutaneous tissue
AHA: 3Q 1989, 16

86.02 Injection or tattooing of skin lesion or defect
Injection of filling material
Insertion of filling material
Pigmenting of skin of filling material

86.03 Incision of pilonidal sinus or cyst
Excludes *marsupialization (86.21)*

86.04 Other incision with drainage of skin and subcutaneous tissue
Excludes drainage of:
fascial compartments of face and mouth (27.0)
palmar or thenar space 82.04)
pilonidal sinus or cyst 86.03)
AHA: 4Q 2004, 76

86.05 Incision with removal of foreign body or device from skin and subcutaneous tissue
Removal of carotid sinus baroreflex activation device
Removal of loop recorder
Removal of neurostimulator pulse generator (single array, dual array)
Removal of tissue expander(s) from skin or soft tissue other than breast tissue
Excludes *removal of foreign body without incision (98.20-98.29)*
AHA: Nov-Dec 1987, 10; Nov-Dec 1986, 9

86.06 Insertion of totally implantable infusion pump
Code also any associated catheterization
Excludes *insertion of totally implantable vascular access device (86.07)*
AHA: 2Q 1999, 4; 4Q 1990, 14

86.07 Insertion of totally implantable vascular access device [VAD]
Totally implanted port
Excludes *insertion of totally implantable infusion pump (86.06)*
AHA: 1Q 2001, 13; 1Q 1996, 3; 2Q 1994, 11; 3Q 1991, 13; 4Q 1990, 15

86.09 Other incision of skin and subcutaneous tissue
Creation of thalamic stimulator pulse generator pocket, new site
Escharotomy
Exploration:
sinus tract, skin
superficial fossa
Relocation of subcutaneous device pocket NEC
Reopening subcutaneous pocket for device revision without replacement
Undercutting of hair follicle
Excludes *creation of loop recorder pocket, new site and insertion/relocation of device (37.79)*
creation of pocket for implantable, patient-activated cardiac event recorder and insertion/relocation of device (37.79)
removal of catheter from cranial cavity (01.27)
that of:
cardiac pacemaker pocket, new site (37.79)
fascial compartments of face and mouth (27.0)
AHA: 1Q 2005, 17; 4Q 2000, 68; 4Q 1999, 21; 4Q 1997, 57; 3Q 1989, 17; Nov-Dec 1986, 1; Nov-Dec 1984, 6

86.1 Diagnostic procedures on skin and subcutaneous tissue

86.11 Biopsy of skin and subcutaneous tissue

86.19 Other diagnostic procedures on skin and subcutaneous tissue
Excludes *microscopic examination of specimen from skin and subcutaneous tissue (91.61-91.79)*

86.2 Excision or destruction of lesion or tissue of skin and subcutaneous tissue

86.21 Excision of pilonidal cyst or sinus
Marsupialization of cyst
Excludes *incision of pilonidal cyst or sinus (86.03)*

✔ **86.22 Excisional debridement of wound, infection, or burn**
Removal by excision of:
devitalized tissue
necrosis
slough
Excludes *debridement of:*
abdominal wall (wound) (54.3)
bone (77.60-77.69)
muscle (83.45)
of hand (82.36)
nail (bed) (fold) (86.27)
nonexcisional debridement of wound, infection, or burn (86.28)
open fracture site (79.60-79.69)
pedicle or flap graft (86.75)
AHA: 1Q 2005, 14-15; 4Q 2004, 138; 3Q 2002, 23; 1Q 1999, 8-9; 2Q 1992, 17; 3Q 1991, 18; 3Q 1989, 16; 4Q 1988, 5; Nov-Dec 1986, 1

✖ **86.23 Removal of nail, nail bed, or nail fold**

✖ **86.24 Chemosurgery of skin**
Chemical peel of skin

✔ **86.25 Dermabrasion**
That with laser
Excludes *dermabrasion of wound to remove embedded debris (86.28)*

✖ **86.26 Ligation of dermal appendage**
Excludes *excision of preauricular appendage (18.29)*

✖ **86.27 Debridement of nail, nail bed, or nail fold**
Removal of:
necrosis
slough
Excludes *removal of nail, nail bed, or nail fold (86.23)*

✖ **86.28 Nonexcisional debridement of wound, infection or burn**
Debridement NOS
Maggot therapy
Removal of devitalized tissue, necrosis and slough by such methods as:
brushing
irrigation (under pressure)
scrubbing
washing
Water scalpel (jet)
AHA: 1Q 2005, 14-15; 2Q 2004, 5; 4Q 2003, 110; 2Q 2003, 15; 3Q 2002, 23; 2Q 2001, 18; 3Q 1991, 18; 4Q 1988, 5

✖ **86.3 Other local excision or destruction of lesion or tissue of skin and subcutaneous tissue**
Destruction of skin by:
cauterization
cryosurgery
fulguration
laser beam
That with Z-plasty
Excludes *adipectomy (86.83)*
biopsy of skin (86.11)
wide or radical excision of skin (86.4)
Z-plasty without excision (86.84)
AHA: 1Q 1996, 15; 3Q 1995, 14; 2Q 1990, 27; 1Q 1989, 12

✔ **86.4 Radical excision of skin lesion**
Wide excision of skin lesion involving underlying or adjacent structure
Code also any lymph node dissection (40.3-40.5)

④ **86.5 Suture or other closure of skin and subcutaneous tissue**

✖ **86.51 Replantation of scalp**

✖ **86.59 Closure of skin and subcutaneous tissue of other sites**
Adhesives (surgical) (tissue)
Staples
Sutures
Excludes *application of adhesive strips (butterfly) - omit code*
AHA: 4Q 1999, 23

④ **86.6 Free skin graft**
Includes excision of skin for autogenous graft
Excludes *construction or reconstruction of:*
penis (64.43-64.44)
trachea (31.75)
vagina (70.61►70.64◄)

✔▼ **86.60 Free skin graft, not otherwise specified**

✔ **86.61 Full-thickness skin graft to hand**
Excludes *heterograft (86.65)*
homograft (86.66)

✔ **86.62 Other skin graft to hand**
Excludes *heterograft (86.65)*
homograft (86.66)

✔ **86.63 Full-thickness skin graft to other sites**
Excludes *heterograft (86.65)*
homograft (86.66)

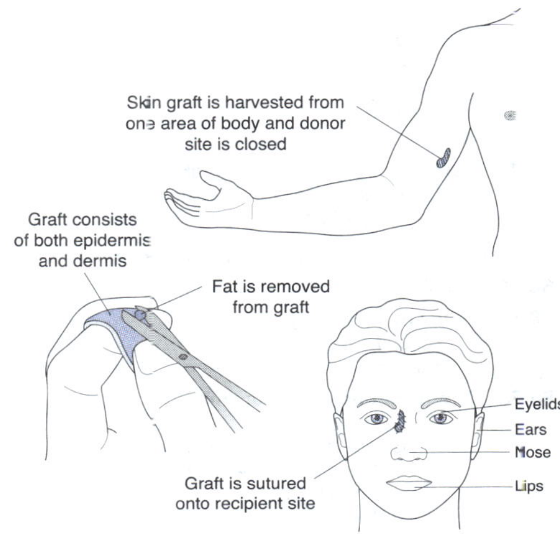

✖ **86.64 Hair transplant**
Excludes *hair follicle transplant to eyebrow or eyelash (08.63)*

✔ **86.65 Heterograft to skin**
Pigskin graft
Porcine graft
Excludes *application of dressing only (93.57)*

✔ **86.66 Homograft to skin**
Graft to skin of:
amnionic membrane from donor
skin from donor

✔ **86.67 Dermal regenerative graft**
Artificial skin, NOS
Creation of "neodermis"
Decellularized allodermis
Integumentary matrix implants
Prosthetic implant of dermal layer of skin
Regenerate dermal layer of skin
Excludes *heterograft to skin (86.65)*
homograft to skin (86.66)
AHA: 4Q 1998, 77-79

✔ **86.69 Other skin graft to other sites**
Excludes *heterograft (86.65)*
homograft (86.66)
AHA: 4Q 1999, 15

④ **86.7 Pedicle grafts or flaps**
Excludes *construction or reconstruction of:*
penis (64.43-64.44)
trachea (31.75)
vagina (70.61-70.6►4◄)

✔▼ **86.70 Pedicle or flap graft, not otherwise specified**

✖ Deleted Code ▼ Nonspecific O.R. Procedure ✔ Valid O.R. Procedure ✖ Non-O.R. Procedure ♂ Male ♀ Female

✓ **86.71 Cutting and preparation of pedicle grafts or flaps**
Elevation of pedicle from its bed
Flap design and raising
Partial cutting of pedicle or tube
Pedicle delay
Excludes *pollicization or digital transfer (82.61, 82.81)*
revision of pedicle (86.75)
AHA: 4Q 2001, 66

✓ **86.72 Advancement of pedicle graft**
AHA: 3Q 1999, 9-10

✓ **86.73 Attachment of pedicle or flap graft to hand**
Excludes *pollicization or digital transfer (82.61, 82.81)*

✓ **86.74 Attachment of pedicle or flap graft to other sites**
Attachment by:
advanced flap
double pedicled flap
pedicle graft
rotating flap
sliding flap
tube graft
AHA: 3Q 1999, 9-10

✓ **86.75 Revision of pedicle or flap graft**
Debridement of pedicle or flap graft
Defatting of pedicle or flap graft

❹ **86.8 Other repair and reconstruction of skin and subcutaneous tissue**

✓ **86.81 Repair for facial weakness**

✓ **86.82 Facial rhytidectomy**
Face lift
Excludes *rhytidectomy of eyelid (08.86-08.87)*

✓ **86.83 Size reduction plastic operation**
Liposuction
Reduction of adipose tissue of:
abdominal wall (pendulous)
arms (batwing)
buttock
thighs (trochanteric lipomatosis)
Excludes *breast (85.31-85.32)*

✓ **86.84 Relaxation of scar or web contracture of skin**
Z-plasty of skin
Excludes *Z-plasty with excision of lesion (86.3)*

✓ **86.85 Correction of syndactyly**

✓ **86.86 Onychoplasty**

✓ **86.89 Other repair and reconstruction of skin and subcutaneous tissue**
Excludes *mentoplasty (76.67-76.68)*
AHA: 4Q 2002, 107; 1Q 2000, 26; 2Q 1998, 20; 2Q 1993, 11

❹ **86.9 Other operations on skin and subcutaneous tissue**

✓ **86.91 Excision of skin for graft**
Excision of skin with closure of donor site
Excludes *that with graft at same operative episode (86.60-86.69)*

✖ **86.92 Electrolysis and other epilation of skin**
Excludes *epilation of eyelid (08.91-08.93)*

✓ **86.93 Insertion of tissue expander**
Insertion (subcutaneous) (soft tissue) of expander (one or more) in scalp (subgaleal space), face, neck, trunk except breast, and upper and lower extremities for development of skin flaps for donor use
Excludes *flap graft preparation (86.71)*
tissue expander, breast (85.95)

✓ **86.94 Insertion or replacement of single array neurostimulator pulse generator, not specified as rechargeable**
Pulse generator (single array, single channel) for intracranial, spinal, and peripheral neurostimulator
Code also any associated lead implantation (02.93, 03.93, 04.92)
Excludes *insertion or replacement of single array rechargeable neurostimulator pulse generator (86.97)*
AHA: 4Q 2004, 135

✓ **86.95 Insertion or replacement of dual array neurostimulator pulse generator, not specified as rechargeable**
Pulse generator (dual array, dual channel) for intracranial, spinal, and peripheral neurostimulator
Code also any associated lead implantation (02.93, 03.93, 04.92)
Excludes *insertion or replacement of dual array rechargeable neurostimulator pulse generator (86.98)*

✓ **86.96 Insertion or replacement of other neurostimulator pulse generator**
Code also any associated lead implantation (02.93, 03.93, 04.92)
Excludes *insertion of dual array neurostimulator pulse generator (86.95, 86.98)*
insertion of single array neurostimulator pulse generator (86.94, 86.97)

✓ **86.97 Insertion or replacement of single array rechargeable neurostimulator pulse generator**
Rechargeable pulse generator (single array, single channel) for intracranial, spinal, and peripheral neurostimulator
Code also any associated lead implantation (02.93, 03.93, 04.92)

✓ **86.98 Insertion or replacement of dual array rechargeable neurostimulator pulse generator**
Rechargeable pulse generator (dual array, dual channel) for intracranial, spinal, and peripheral neurostimulator
Code also any associated lead implantation (02.93, 03.93, 04.92)

✖ **86.99 Other**
Excludes *removal of sutures from:*
abdomen (97.83)
head and neck (97.38)
thorax (97.43)
trunk NEC (97.84)
wound catheter:
irrigation (96.58)
replacement (97.15)
AHA: Nov-Dec 1986, 1

16. MISCELLANEOUS DIAGNOSTIC AND THERAPEUTIC PROCEDURES (87-99)

DIAGNOSTIC RADIOLOGY (87)

87.0 Soft tissue x-ray of face, head, and neck
Excludes *angiography (88.40-88.68)*

87.01 Pneumoencephalogram

87.02 Other contrast radiogram of brain and skull
Pneumocisternogram
Pneumoventriculogram
Posterior fossa myelogram

87.03 Computerized axial tomography of head
C.A.T. scan of head
AHA: 3Q 2005, 13; 3Q 1999, 7

87.04 Other tomography of head

87.05 Contrast dacryocystogram

87.06 Contrast radiogram of nasopharynx

87.07 Contrast laryngogram

87.08 Cervical lymphangiogram

87.09 Other soft tissue x-ray of face, head, and neck
Noncontrast x-ray of:
adenoid
larynx
nasolacrimal duct
nasopharynx
salivary gland
thyroid region
uvula
Excludes *x-ray study of eye (95.14)*

87.1 Other x-ray of face, head, and neck
Excludes *angiography (88.40-88.68)*

87.11 Full-mouth x-ray of teeth

87.12 Other dental x-ray
Orthodontic cephalogram or cephalometrics
Panorex examination of mandible
Root canal x-ray

87.13 Temporomandibular contrast arthrogram

87.14 Contrast radiogram of orbit

87.15 Contrast radiogram of sinus

87.16 Other x-ray of facial bones
X-ray of:
frontal area
mandible
maxilla
nasal sinuses
nose
orbit
supraorbital area
symphysis menti
zygomaticomaxillary complex

87.17 Other x-ray of skull
Lateral projection of skull
Sagittal projection
Tangential projection

87.2 X-ray of spine

87.21 Contrast myelogram

87.22 Other x-ray of cervical spine

87.23 Other x-ray of thoracic spine

87.24 Other x-ray of lumbosacral spine
Sacrococcygeal x-ray

87.29 Other x-ray of spine
Spinal x-ray NOS

87.3 Soft tissue x-ray of thorax
Excludes *angiocardiography (88.50-88.58)*
angiography (88.40-88.68)

87.31 Endotracheal bronchogram

87.32 Other contrast bronchogram
Transcricoid bronchogram

87.33 Mediastinal pneumogram

87.34 Intrathoracic lymphangiogram

87.35 Contrast radiogram of mammary ducts

87.36 Xerography of breast

87.37 Other mammography
AHA: 3Q 1989, 17

87.38 Sinogram of chest wall
Fistulogram of chest wall

87.39 Other soft tissue x-ray of chest wall

87.4 Other x-ray of thorax
Excludes *angiocardiography (88.50-88.58)*
angiography (88.40-88.68)

87.41 Computerized axial tomography of thorax
C.A.T. scan of thorax
Crystal linea scan of x-ray beam of thorax
Electronic substraction of thorax
Photoelectric response of thorax
Tomography with use of computer, x-rays, and camera of thorax

87.42 Other tomography of thorax
Cardiac tomogram

87.43 X-ray of ribs, sternum, and clavicle
Examination for:
cervical rib
fracture

87.44 Routine chest x-ray, so described
X-ray of chest NOS

87.49 Other chest x-ray
X-ray of:
bronchus NOS
diaphragm NOS
heart NOS
lung NOS
mediastinum NOS
trachea NOS

87.5 Biliary tract x-ray

87.51 Percutaneous hepatic cholangiogram
AHA: 2Q 1990, 28; Nov-Dec 1987, 3

87.52 Intravenous cholangiogram

87.53 Intraoperative cholangiogram
AHA: 1Q 1996, 11-12

87.54 Other cholangiogram

87.59 Other biliary tract x-ray
Cholecystogram

87.6 Other x-ray of digestive system

87.61 Barium swallow

87.62 Upper GI series

87.63 Small bowel series

87.64 Lower GI series

87.65 Other x-ray of intestine

87.66 Contrast pancreatogram
AHA: Nov-Dec 1987, 3

87.69 Other digestive tract x-ray

87.7 X-ray of urinary system
Excludes *angiography of renal vessels (88.45. 88.65)*

87.71 Computerized axial tomography of kidney
C.A.T. scan of kidney

87.72 Other nephrotomogram

87.73 Intravenous pyelogram
Diuretic infusion pyelogram

87.74 Retrograde pyelogram

87.75 Percutaneous pyelogram

87.76 Retrograde cystourethrogram

87.77 Other cystogram

87.78 Ileal conduitogram

87.79 Other x-ray of the urinary system
KUB x-ray

✖ Deleted Code ▼ Nonspecific O.R. Procedure ✔ Valid O.R. Procedure ✖ Non-O.R. Procedure ♂ Male ♀ Female

❹ **87.8 X-ray of female genital organs**

✖ **87.81 X-ray of gravid uterus** ♀
Intrauterine cephalometry by x-ray

✖ **87.82 Gas contrast hysterosalpingogram** ♀

✖ **87.83 Opaque dye contrast hysterosalpingogram** ♀

✖ **87.84 Percutaneous hysterogram** ♀

✖ **87.85 Other x-ray of fallopian tubes and uterus** ♀

✖ **87.89 Other x-ray of female genital organs** ♀

❹ **87.9 X-ray of male genital organs**

✖ **87.91 Contrast seminal vesiculogram** ♂

✖ **87.92 Other x-ray of prostate and seminal vesicles** ♂

✖ **87.93 Contrast epididymogram** ♂

✖ **87.94 Contrast vasogram** ♂

✖ **87.95 Other x-ray of epididymis and vas deferens** ♂

✖ **87.99 Other x-ray of male genital organs** ♂

OTHER DIAGNOSTIC RADIOLOGY AND RELATED TECHNIQUES (88)

❹ **88.0 Soft tissue x-ray of abdomen**
Excludes *angiography (88.40-88.68)*

✖ **88.01 Computerized axial tomography of abdomen**
C.A.T. scan of abdomen
Excludes *C.A.T. scan of kidney (87.71)*
AHA: 2Q 1998, 14

✖ **88.02 Other abdomen tomography**
Excludes *nephrotomogram (87.72)*

✖ **88.03 Sinogram of abdominal wall**
Fistulogram of abdominal wall

✖ **88.04 Abdominal lymphangiogram**

✖ **88.09 Other soft tissue x-ray of abdominal wall**

❹ **88.1 Other x-ray of abdomen**

✖ **88.11 Pelvic opaque dye contrast radiography**

✖ **88.12 Pelvic gas contrast radiography**
Pelvic pneumoperitoneum

✖ **88.13 Other peritoneal pneumogram**

✖ **88.14 Retroperitoneal fistulogram**

✖ **88.15 Retroperitoneal pneumogram**

✖ **88.16 Other retroperitoneal x-ray**

✖ **88.19 Other x-ray of abdomen**
Flat plate of abdomen
AHA: 3Q 1999, 9

❹ **88.2 Skeletal x-ray of extremities and pelvis**
Excludes *contrast radiogram of joint (88.32)*

✖ **88.21 Skeletal x-ray of shoulder and upper arm**

✖ **88.22 Skeletal x-ray of elbow and forearm**

✖ **88.23 Skeletal x-ray of wrist and hand**

✖ **88.24 Skeletal x-ray of upper limb, not otherwise specified**

✖ **88.25 Pelvimetry**

✖ **88.26 Other skeletal x-ray of pelvis and hip**

✖ **88.27 Skeletal x-ray of thigh, knee, and lower leg**

✖ **88.28 Skeletal x-ray of ankle and foot**

✖ **88.29 Skeletal x-ray of lower limb, not otherwise specified**

❹ **88.3 Other x-ray**

✖ **88.31 Skeletal series**
X-ray of whole skeleton

✖ **88.32 Contrast arthrogram**
Excludes *that of temporomandibular joint (87.13)*

✖ **88.33 Other skeletal x-ray**
Excludes *skeletal x-ray of:*
extremities and pelvis 88.21-88.29)
face, head, and neck (87.11-87.17)
spine (87.21-87.29)
thorax (87.43)

✖ **88.34 Lymphangiogram of upper limb**

✖ **88.35 Other soft tissue x-ray of upper limb**

✖ **88.36 Lymphangiogram of lower limb**

✖ **88.37 Other soft tissue x-ray of lower limb**
Excludes *femoral angiography (88.48, 88.66)*

✖ **88.38 Other computerized axial tomography**
C.A.T. scan NOS
Excludes *C.A.T. scan of:*
abdomen (88.01)
head (87.03)
kidney (87.71)
thorax (87.41)
AHA: 3Q 2005, 13, 14

✖ **88.39 X-ray, other and unspecified**

❹ **88.4 Arteriography using contrast material**
Note: The fourth-digit subclassification identifies the site to be viewed, not the site of injection.
Includes angiography of arteries
arterial puncture for injection of contrast material
radiography of arteries (by fluoroscopy)
retrograde arteriography
Excludes *arteriography using:*
radioisotopes or radionuclides (92.01-92.19)
ultrasound (88.71-88.79)
fluorescein angiography of eye (95.12)

✖ **88.40 Arteriography using contrast material, unspecified site**
AHA: Nov-Dec 1985, 14

✖ **88.41 Arteriography of cerebral arteries**
Angiography of:
basilar artery
carotid (internal)
posterior cerebral circulation
vertebral artery
AHA: 1Q 2000, 16; 1Q 1999, 6; 1Q 1997, 3; 2Q 1995, 12; Nov-Dec 1985, 14

✖ **88.42 Aortography**
Arteriography of aorta and aortic arch
AHA: 1Q 1999, 17; May-Jun 1987, 11; Nov-Dec 1985, 14

✖ **88.43 Arteriography of pulmonary arteries**
AHA: May-Jun 1987, 11; Nov-Dec 1985, 14

✖ **88.44 Arteriography of other intrathoracic vessels**
Excludes *angiocardiography (88.50-88.58)*
arteriography of coronary arteries (88.55-88.57)
AHA: May-Jun 1987, 11; Nov-Dec 1985, 14

✖ **88.45 Arteriography of renal arteries**
AHA: Nov-Dec 1985, 14

✖ **88.46 Arteriography of placenta** ♀
Placentogram using contrast material
AHA: Nov-Dec 1985, 14

✖ **88.47 Arteriography of other intra-abdominal arteries**
AHA: 4Q 1990, 22; Nov-Dec 1985, 14; Sep-Oct 1985, 5

✖ **88.48 Arteriography of femoral and other lower extremity arteries**
AHA: 3Q 2003, 10; 1Q 2003, 17; 2Q 1996, 5; Nov-Dec 1985, 14; Sep-Oct 1985, 5

✖ **88.49 Arteriography of other specified sites**
AHA: Nov-Dec 1985, 14

❹ **88.5 Angiocardiography using contrast material**
Includes arterial puncture and insertion of arterial catheter for injection of contrast material
cineangiocardiography
selective angiocardiography
Code also synchronous cardiac catheterization (37.21-37.23)
Excludes *angiography of pulmonary vessels (88.43, 88.62)*

✖ **88.50 Angiocardiography, not otherwise specified**
AHA: May-Jun 1987, 11

✖ **88.51 Angiocardiography of venae cavae**
Inferior vena cavography
Phlebography of vena cava (inferior) (superior)
AHA: May-Jun 1987, 11

✖ **88.52 Angiocardiography of right heart structures**
Angiocardiography of:
pulmonary valve
right atrium
right ventricle (outflow tract)
Excludes ▶*intra-operative fluorescence vascular angiography (88.59)*◀
that combined with left heart angiocardiography (88.54)
AHA: May-Jun 1987, 11

✖ **88.53 Angiocardiography of left heart structures**
Angiocardiography of:
aortic valve
left atrium
left ventricle (outflow tract)
Excludes ▶*intra-operative fluorescence vascular angiography (88.59)*◀
that combined with right heart angiocardiography (88.54)
AHA: 4Q 2005, 69; 3Q 2005, 15; 1Q 2000, 20; 4Q 1988, 4; May-Jun 1987, 11

✖ **88.54 Combined right and left heart angiocardiography**
Excludes ▶*intra-operative fluorescence vascular angiography (88.59)*◀
AHA: May-Jun 1987, 11

✖ **88.55 Coronary arteriography using a single catheter**
Coronary arteriography by Sones technique
Direct selective coronary arteriography using a single catheter
Excludes ▶*intra-operative fluorescence vascular angiography (88.59)*◀
AHA: 3Q 2002, 20; 3Q 1992, 10; May-Jun 1987, 11

✖ **88.56 Coronary arteriography using two catheters**
Coronary arteriography by:
Judkins technique
Ricketts and Abrams technique
Direct selective coronary arteriography using two catheters
Excludes ▶*intra-operative fluorescence vascular angiography (88.59)*◀
AHA: 1Q 2000, 20; 3Q 1992, 10; May-Jun 1987, 11

✖ **88.57 Other and unspecified coronary arteriography**
Coronary arteriography NOS
Excludes ▶*intra-operative fluorescence vascular angiography (88.59)*◀
AHA: 4Q 2005, 69; 3Q 2005, 15; 2Q 2005, 17-18; 3Q 1992, 10; May-Jun 1987, 11

✖ **88.58 Negative-contrast cardiac roentgenography**
Cardiac roentgenography with injection of carbon dioxide
AHA: May-Jun 1987, 11

● ✖ **88.59 Intra-operative fluorescence vascular angiography**
Intraoperative laser arteriogram (SPY)
SPY arteriogram
SPY arteriography

④ **88.6 Phlebography**
Note: The fourth-digit subclassification (88.60-88.67) identifies the site to be viewed, not the site of injection.
Includes angiography of veins
radiography of veins (by fluoroscopy)
retrograde phlebography
venipuncture for injection of contrast material
venography using contrast material
Excludes *angiography using:*
radioisotopes or radionuclides (92.01-92.19)
ultrasound (88.71-88.79)
fluorescein angiography of eye (95.12)

✖ **88.60 Phlebography using contrast material, unspecified site**

✖ **88.61 Phlebography of veins of head and neck using contrast material**

✖ **88.62 Phlebography of pulmonary veins using contrast material**

✖ **88.63 Phlebography of other intrathoracic veins using contrast material**

✖ **88.64 Phlebography of the portal venous system using contrast material**
Splenoportogram (by splenic arteriography)

✖ **88.65 Phlebography of other intra-abdominal veins using contrast material**
AHA: 3Q 2000, 9

✖ **88.66 Phlebography of femoral and other lower extremity veins using contrast material**

✖ **88.67 Phlebography of other specified sites using contrast material**

✖ **88.68 Impedance phlebography**

④ **88.7 Diagnostic ultrasound**
Includes echography
non-invasive ultrasound
ultrasonic angiography
ultrasonography
Excludes *intravascular imaging (adjunctive) (IVUS) (00.21-00.29)*
therapeutic ultrasound (00.01-00.09)

✖ **88.71 Diagnostic ultrasound of head and neck**
Determination of midline shift of brain
Echoencephalography
Excludes *eye (95.13)*
AHA: 1Q 2002, 10; 1Q 1992, 11

✖ **88.72 Diagnostic ultrasound of heart**
Echocardiography
Transesophageal echocardiography
Excludes *echocardiography of heart chambers (37.28)*
intracardiac echocardiography (ICE) (37.28)
intravascular (IVUS) imaging of coronary vessels (00.24)
AHA: 3Q 2005, 15; 2Q 2005, 17-18; 4Q 2004, 121-122; 1Q 2004, 16; 1Q 2000, 20; 3Q 1998, 11

✖ **88.73 Diagnostic ultrasound of other sites of thorax**
Aortic arch ultrasonography
Breast ultrasonography
Lung ultrasonography

✖ **88.74 Diagnostic ultrasound of digestive system**

✖ **88.75 Diagnostic ultrasound of urinary system**

✖ **88.76 Diagnostic ultrasound of abdomen and retroperitoneum**
AHA: 2Q 1999, 14

✖ **88.77 Diagnostic ultrasound of peripheral vascular system**
Deep vein thrombosis ultrasonic scanning
Excludes *adjunct vascular system procedures (00.40-00.43)*
AHA: 4Q 1999, 17; 1Q 1999, 10-11

✖ **88.78 Diagnostic ultrasound of gravid uterus** ♀
Intrauterine cephalometry:
echo
ultrasonic
Placental localization by ultrasound

✖ **88.79 Other diagnostic ultrasound**
Ultrasonography of:
multiple sites
nongravid uterus
total body

④ **88.8 Thermography**

✖ **88.81 Cerebral thermography**

✖ **88.82 Ocular thermography**

✖ **88.83 Bone thermography**
Osteoarticular thermography

✖ **88.84 Muscle thermography**

✖ **88.85 Breast thermography**

✖ **88.86 Blood vessel thermography**
Deep vein thermography

✖ **88.89 Thermography of other sites**
Lymph gland thermography
Thermography NOS

④ **88.9 Other diagnostic imaging**

✖ **88.90 Diagnostic imaging, not elsewhere classified**

88.91 Magnetic resonance imaging of brain and brain stem
Excludes *intraoperative magnetic resonance imaging (88.96)*
real-time magnetic resonance imaging (88.96)

88.92 Magnetic resonance imaging of chest and myocardium
For evaluation of hilar and mediastinal lymphadenopathy

88.93 Magnetic resonance imaging of spinal canal
Spinal cord levels:
- cervical
- thoracic
- lumbar (lumbosacral)

Spinal cord
Spine

88.94 Magnetic resonance imaging of musculoskeletal
Bone marrow blood supply
Extremities (upper) (lower)

88.95 Magnetic resonance imaging of pelvis, prostate, and bladder

88.96 Other intraoperative magnetic resonance imaging
iMRI
Real-time magnetic resonance imaging
AHA: 4Q 2002, 111

88.97 Magnetic resonance imaging of other and unspecified sites
Abdomen
Eye orbit
Face
Neck

88.98 Bone mineral density studies
Dual photon absorptiometry
Quantitative computed tomography (CT) studies
Radiographic densitometry
Single photon absorptiometry

INTERVIEW, EVALUATION, CONSULTATION, AND EXAMINATION (89)

89.0 Diagnostic interview, consultation, and evaluation
Excludes *psychiatric diagnostic interview (94.11-94.19)*

89.01 Interview and evaluation, described as brief
Abbreviated history and evaluation

89.02 Interview and evaluation, described as limited
Interval history and evaluation

89.03 Interview and evaluation, described as comprehensive
History and evaluation of new problem

89.04 Other interview and evaluation

89.05 Diagnostic interview and evaluation, not otherwise specified

89.06 Consultation, described as limited
Consultation on a single organ system

89.07 Consultation, described as comprehensive

89.08 Other consultation

89.09 Consultation, not otherwise specified

89.1 Anatomic and physiologic measurements and manual examinations-nervous system and sense organs
Excludes *ear examination (95.41-95.49)*
eye examination (95.01-95.26)
the listed procedures when done as part of a general physical examination (89.7)

89.10 Intracarotid amobarbital test
Wada test

89.11 Tonometry

89.12 Nasal function study
Rhinomanometry

89.13 Neurologic examination

89.14 Electroencephalogram
Excludes *that with polysomnogram (89.17)*
AHA: 3Q 2005, 13

89.15 Other nonoperative neurologic function tests
AHA: 3Q 1995, 5; 2Q 1991, 14; Jan-Feb 1987, 16

89.16 Transillumination of newborn skull

89.17 Polysomnogram
Sleep recording

89.18 Other sleep disorder function tests
Multiple sleep latency test [MSLT]

89.19 Video and radio-telemetered electroencephalographic monitoring
Radiographic EEG monitoring
Video EEG monitoring
AHA: 1Q 1992, 17; 2Q 1991, 14

89.2 Anatomic and physiologic measurements and manual examinations-genitourinary system
Excludes *the listed procedures when done as part of a general physical examination (89.7)*

89.21 Urinary manometry
Manometry through:
- indwelling ureteral catheter
- nephrostomy
- pyelostomy
- ureterostomy

89.22 Cystometrogram
AHA: 2Q 1990, 27

Cystometrogram

An electronic device is inserted into the bladder to measure the pressure of urine in the lower urinary system.

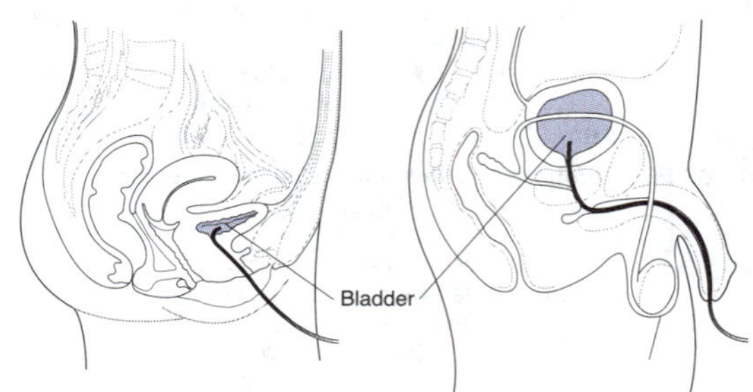

Female Male

89.23 Urethral sphincter electromyogram
AHA: 2Q 1990, 27

89.24 Uroflowmetry [UFR]
AHA: 2Q 1990, 27

89.25 Urethral pressure profile [UPP]
AHA: 2Q 1990, 27

89.26 Gynecological examination ♀
Pelvic examination

89.29 Other nonoperative genitourinary system measurements
Bioassay of urine
Renal clearance
Urine chemistry

89.3 Other anatomic and physiologic measurements and manual examinations
Excludes *the listed procedures when done as part of a general physical examination (89.7)*

89.31 Dental examination
Oral mucosal survey
Periodontal survey

89.32 Esophageal manometry
AHA: 3Q 1996, 13

89.33 Digital examination of enterostomy stoma
Digital examination of colostomy stoma

89.34 Digital examination of rectum

89.35 Transillumination of nasal sinuses

89.36 Manual examination of breast

89.37 Vital capacity determination

89.38 Other nonoperative respiratory measurements
Plethysmography for measurement of respiratory function
Thoracic impedance plethysmography
AHA: Sep-Oct 1987, 6

Fourth Digit Required | Open Biopsy | Closed Biopsy | ▶◀ Revised Text | ● New Code | ▲ Revised Code

✖ **89.39 Other nonoperative measurements and examinations**
14 C-Urea breath test
Basal metabolic rate [BMR]
Gastric:
analysis
function NEC
Excludes *body measurement (93.07)*
cardiac tests (89.41-89.69)
fundus photography (95.11)
limb length measurement (93.06)
AHA: 2Q 2001, 9; 3Q 2000, 9; 3Q 1996, 13; 1Q 1994, 18

④ **89.4 Cardiac stress tests, pacemaker and defibrillator checks**

✖ **89.41 Cardiovascular stress test using treadmill**
AHA: 1Q 1988, 11

✖ **89.42 Masters' two-step stress test**
AHA: 1Q 1988, 11

✖ **89.43 Cardiovascular stress test using bicycle ergometer**
AHA: 1Q 1988, 11

✖ **89.44 Other cardiovascular stress test**
Thallium stress test with or without transesophageal pacing

✖ **89.45 Artificial pacemaker rate check**
Artificial pacemaker function check NOS
Bedside device check of pacemaker or cardiac resynchronization pacemaker [CRT-P]
Interrogation only without arrhythmia induction
Excludes *catheter based invasive electrophysiologic testing (37.26)*
non-invasive programmed electrical stimulation [NIPS] (arrhythmia induction) (37.20)
AHA: 1Q 2002, 4

✖ **89.46 Artificial pacemaker artifact wave form check**

✖ **89.47 Artificial pacemaker electrode impedance check**

✖ **89.48 Artificial pacemaker voltage or amperage threshold check**

✖ **89.49 Automatic implantable cardioverter/defibrillator (AICD) check**
Bedside check of an AICD or cardiac resynchronization defibrillator [CRT-D]
Checking pacing thresholds of device
Interrogation only without arrhythmia induction
Excludes *catheter based invasive electrophysiologic testing (37.26)*
non-invasive programmed electrical stimulation [NIPS] (arrhythmia induction) (37.20)
AHA: 4Q 2004, 136

④ **89.5 Other nonoperative cardiac and vascular diagnostic procedures**
Excludes *fetal EKG (75.32)*

✖ **89.50 Ambulatory cardiac monitoring**
Analog devices [Holter-type]
AHA: 4Q 1999, 21; 4Q 1991, 23

✖ **89.51 Rhythm electrocardiogram**
Rhythm EKG (with one to three leads)

✖ **89.52 Electrocardiogram**
ECG NOS
EKG (with 12 or more leads)
AHA: 1Q 1988, 11; Sep-Oct 1987, 6

✖ **89.53 Vectorcardiogram (with ECG)**

✖ **89.54 Electrographic monitoring**
Telemetry
Excludes *ambulatory cardiac monitoring (89.50)*
electrographic monitoring during surgery - omit code
AHA: 4Q 1991, 23; 1Q 1988, 11; Jul-Aug 1984, 12

✖ **89.55 Phonocardiogram with ECG lead**

✖ **89.56 Carotid pulse tracing with ECG lead**
Excludes *oculoplethysmography (89.58)*

✖ **89.57 Apexcardiogram (with ECG lead)**
AHA: Jan-Feb 1987, 16

✖ **89.58 Plethysmogram**
Penile plethysmography with nerve stimulation
Excludes *plethysmography (for):*
measurement of respiratory function (89.38)
thoracic impedance (89.38)
AHA: Sep-Oct 1987, 6

✖ **89.59 Other nonoperative cardiac and vascular measurements**
AHA: 3Q 2005, 21; 3Q 2003, 23; 2Q 1992, 12

④ **89.6 Circulatory monitoring**
Excludes *electrocardiographic monitoring during surgery - omit code*
implantation or replacement of subcutaneous device for intracardiac hemodynamic monitoring (00.57)
insertion or replacement of implantable pressure sensor (lead) for intracardiac hemodynamic monitoring (00.56)

✔ **89.60 Continuous intra-arterial blood gas monitoring**
Insertion of blood gas monitoring system and continuous monitoring of blood gases through an intra-arterial sensor

✖ **89.61 Systemic arterial pressure monitoring**

✖ **89.62 Central venous pressure monitoring**

✖ **89.63 Pulmonary artery pressure monitoring**
Excludes *pulmonary artery wedge monitoring (89.64)*

✖ **89.64 Pulmonary artery wedge monitoring**
Pulmonary capillary wedge [PCW] monitoring
Swan-Ganz catheterization

✖ **89.65 Measurement of systemic arterial blood gases**
Excludes *continuous intra-arterial blood gas monitoring (89.60)*

✖ **89.66 Measurement of mixed venous blood gases**

✖ **89.67 Monitoring of cardiac output by oxygen consumption technique**
Fick method

✖ **89.68 Monitoring of cardiac output by other technique**
Cardiac output monitor by thermodilution indicator

✖ **89.69 Monitoring of coronary blood flow**
Coronary blood flow monitoring by coincidence counting technique

✖ **89.7 General physical examination**

✖ **89.8 Autopsy**

MICROSCOPIC EXAMINATION-I (90)

The following fourth-digit subclassification is for use with categories in section 90 to identify type of examination:
1 **bacterial smear**
2 **culture**
3 **culture and sensitivity**
4 **parasitology**
5 **toxicology**
6 **cell block and Papanicolaou smear**
9 **other microscopic examination**

④ ✖ **90.0 Microscopic examination of specimen from nervous system and of spinal fluid**

④ ✖ **90.1 Microscopic examination of specimen from endocrine gland, not elsewhere classified**

④ ✖ **90.2 Microscopic examination of specimen from eye**

④ ✖ **90.3 Microscopic examination of specimen from ear, nose, throat, and larynx**

④ ✖ **90.4 Microscopic examination of specimen from trachea, bronchus, pleura, lung, and other thoracic specimen, and of sputum**

④ ✖ **90.5 Microscopic examination of blood**

④ ✖ **90.6 Microscopic examination of specimen from spleen and of bone marrow**

④ ✖ **90.7 Microscopic examination of specimen from lymph node and of lymph**

90.8 Microscopic examination of specimen from upper gastrointestinal tract and of vomitus

90.9 Microscopic examination of specimen from lower gastrointestinal tract and of stool

MICROSCOPIC EXAMINATION-II (91)

The following fourth-digit subclassification is for use with categories in section 91 to identify type of examination

1 **bacterial smear**
2 **culture**
3 **culture and sensitivity**
4 **parasitology**
5 **toxicology**
6 **cell block and Papanicolaou smear**
9 **other microscopic examination**

91.0 Microscopic examination of specimen from liver, biliary tract, and pancreas

91.1 Microscopic examination of peritoneal and retroperitoneal specimen

91.2 Microscopic examination of specimen from kidney, ureter, perirenal and periureteral tissue

91.3 Microscopic examination of specimen from bladder, urethra, prostate, seminal vesicle, perivesical tissue, and of urine and semen

91.4 Microscopic examination of specimen from female genital tract ♀
Amnionic sac
Fetus

91.5 Microscopic examination of specimen from musculoskeletal system and of joint fluid
Microscopic examination of:
bone
bursa
cartilage
fascia
ligament
muscle
synovial membrane
tendon

91.6 Microscopic examination of specimen from skin and other integument
Microscopic examination of:
hair
nails
skin
Excludes *mucous membrane-code to organ site that of operative wound (91.70-91.79)*

91.7 Microscopic examination of specimen from operative wound

91.8 Microscopic examination of specimen from other site

91.9 Microscopic examination of specimen from unspecified site

NUCLEAR MEDICINE (92)

92.0 Radioisotope scan and function study

92.01 Thyroid scan and radioisotope function studies
Iodine-131 uptake
Protein-bound iodine
Radio-iodine uptake

92.02 Liver scan and radioisotope function study

92.03 Renal scan and radioisotope function study
Renal clearance study

92.04 Gastrointestinal scan and radioisotope function study
Radio-cobalt B_{12} Schilling test
Radio-iodinated triolein study

92.05 Cardiovascular and hematopoietic scan and radioisotope function study
Bone marrow scan or function study
Cardiac output scan or function study
Circulation time scan or function study
Radionuclide cardiac ventriculogram scan or function study
Spleen scan or function study
AHA: 2Q 1992, 7; 1Q 1988, 11

92.09 Other radioisotope function studies

92.1 Other radioisotope scan

92.11 Cerebral scan
Pituitary

92.12 Scan of other sites of head
Excludes *eye (95.16)*

92.13 Parathyroid scan

92.14 Bone scan

92.15 Pulmonary scan

92.16 Scan of lymphatic system

92.17 Placental scan ♀

92.18 Total body scan

92.19 Scan of other sites

92.2 Therapeutic radiology and nuclear medicine
Excludes *that for:*
ablation of pituitary gland (07.64-07.69)
destruction of chorioretinal lesion (14.26-14.27)

92.20 Infusion of liquid brachytherapy radioisotope
I-125 radioisotope
Intracavitary brachytherapy
Includes removal of radioisotope
AHA: 4Q 2005, 119

92.21 Superficial radiation
Contact radiation [up to 150 KVP]

92.22 Orthovoltage radiation
Deep radiation [200-300 KVP]

92.23 Radioisotopic teleradiotherapy
Teleradiotherapy using:
cobalt-60
iodine-125
radioactive cesium

92.24 Teleradiotherapy using photons
Megavoltage NOS
Supervoltage NOS
Use of:
Betatron
linear accelerator

92.25 Teleradiotherapy using electrons
Beta particles
Excludes *intra-operative electron radiation therapy (92.41)*

92.26 Teleradiotherapy of other particulate radiation
Neutrons
Protons NOS

92.27 Implantation or insertion of radioactive elements
Code also incision of site
Intravascular brachytherapy
Excludes *infusion of liquid brachytherapy radioisotope (92.20)*
AHA: 1Q 2004, 4; 1Q 2000, 11-12; 3Q 1994, 11; 1Q 1998, 4

92.28 Injection or instillation of radioisotopes
Injection or infusion of radioimmunoconjugate
Intracavitary injection or instillation
Intravenous injection or instillation
Iodine-131 [I-131] tositumomab
Radioimmunotherapy
Ytrium-90 [Y-90] ibritumomab tiuxetan
Excludes *infusion of liquid brachytherapy radioisotope (92.20)*

92.29 Other radiotherapeutic procedure
AHA: 2Q 1994, 10

92.3 Stereotactic radiosurgery
Code also stereotactic head frame application (93.59)
Excludes *stereotactic biopsy*

92.30 Stereotactic radiosurgery, not otherwise specified

92.31 Single source photon radiosurgery
High energy x-rays
Linear accelerator (LINAC)

✖ **92.32 Multi-source photon radiosurgery**
Cobalt 60 radiation
Gamma irradiation
AHA: 4Q 2004, 113

✖ **92.33 Particulate radiosurgery**
Particle beam radiation (cyclotron)
Proton accerlerator

✖ **92.39 Stereotactic radiosurgery, not elsewhere classified**

●④ **92.4 Intra-operative radiation procedures**

●✖ **92.41 Intra-operative electron radiation therapy**
IOERT
That using a mobile linear accelerator

PHYSICAL THERAPY, RESPIRATORY THERAPY, REHABILITATION, AND RELATED PROCEDURES (93)

④ **93.0 Diagnostic physical therapy**

✖ **93.01 Functional evaluation**

✖ **93.02 Orthotic evaluation**

✖ **93.03 Prosthetic evaluation**

✖ **93.04 Manual testing of muscle function**
AHA: Jan-Feb 1987, 16

✖ **93.05 Range of motion testing**
AHA: Jan-Feb 1987, 16; Nov-Dec 1986, 7

✖ **93.06 Measurement of limb length**

✖ **93.07 Body measurement**
Girth measurement
Measurement of skull circumference

✖ **93.08 Electromyography**
Excludes *eye EMG (95.25)*
that with polysomnogram (89.17)
urethral sphincter EMG (89.23)
AHA: Jan-Feb 1987, 16

✖ **93.09 Other diagnostic physical therapy procedure**

④ **93.1 Physical therapy exercises**

✖ **93.11 Assisting exercise**
Excludes *assisted exercise in pool (93.31)*

✖ **93.12 Other active musculoskeletal exercise**

✖ **93.13 Resistive exercise**

✖ **93.14 Training in joint movements**

✖ **93.15 Mobilization of spine**

✖ **93.16 Mobilization of other joints**
Excludes *manipulation of temporomandibular joint (76.95)*

✖ **93.17 Other passive musculoskeletal exercise**

✖ **93.18 Breathing exercise**

✖ **93.19 Exercise, not elsewhere classified**

④ **93.2 Other physical therapy musculoskeletal manipulation**

✖ **93.21 Manual and mechanical traction**
Excludes *skeletal traction (93.43-93.44)*
skin traction (93.45-93.46)
spinal traction (93.41-93.42)

✖ **93.22 Ambulation and gait training**

✖ **93.23 Fitting of orthotic device**

✖ **93.24 Training in use of prosthetic or orthotic device**
Training in crutch walking

✖ **93.25 Forced extension of limb**

✖ **93.26 Manual rupture of joint adhesions**
AHA: Nov-Dec 1986, 7

✖ **93.27 Stretching of muscle or tendon**
AHA: Nov-Dec 1986, 7

✖ **93.28 Stretching of fascia**
AHA: Nov-Dec 1986, 7

✖ **93.29 Other forcible correction of deformity**
AHA: Nov-Dec 1986, 7; Nov-Dec 1985, 11

④ **93.3 Other physical therapy therapeutic procedures**

✖ **93.31 Assisted exercise in pool**

✖ **93.32 Whirlpool treatment**

✖ **93.33 Other hydrotherapy**

✖ **93.34 Diathermy**

✖ **93.35 Other heat therapy**
Acupuncture with smouldering moxa
Hot packs
Hyperthermia NEC
Infrared irradiation
Moxibustion
Paraffin bath
Excludes *hyperthermia for treatment of cancer (99.85)*

✖ **93.36 Cardiac retraining**

✖ **93.37 Prenatal training**
Training for natural childbirth

✖ **93.38 Combined physical therapy without mention of the components**

✖ **93.39 Other physical therapy**
AHA: 2Q 2005, 6-7; 4Q 2003, 105-110; 3Q 1997, 12; 3Q 1991, 15

④ **93.4 Skeletal traction and other traction**

✖ **93.41 Spinal traction using skull device**
Traction using:
caliper tongs
Crutchfield tongs
halo device
Vinke tongs
Excludes *insertion of tongs or halo traction device (02.94)*
AHA: 3Q 2001, 8; 3Q 1996, 15; 2Q 1994, 3

✖ **93.42 Other spinal traction**
Cotrel's traction
Excludes *cervical collar (93.52)*

✖ **93.43 Intermittent skeletal traction**

✖ **93.44 Other skeletal traction**
Bryant's traction
Dunlop's traction
Lyman Smith traction
Russell's traction
DEF: Russell's traction: traction applied via a sling beneath the knee that is connected to an overhead pulley.

✖ **93.45 Thomas' splint traction**

✖ **93.46 Other skin traction of limbs**
Adhesive tape traction
Boot traction
Buck's traction
Gallows traction

④ **93.5 Other immobilization, pressure, and attention to wound**
Excludes external fixator device (84.71-84.73)
wound cleansing (96.58-96.59)

✖ **93.51 Application of plaster jacket**
Excludes *Minerva jacket (93.52)*

✖ **93.52 Application of neck support**
Application of:
cervical collar
Minerva jacket
molded neck support

✖ **93.53 Application of other cast**

✖ **93.54 Application of splint**
Plaster splint
Tray splint
Excludes *periodontal splint (24.7)*

✖ **93.55 Dental wiring**
Excludes *that for orthodontia (24.7)*

✖ **93.56 Application of pressure dressing**
Application of:
Gibney bandage
Robert Jones' bandage
Shanz dressing

✖ **93.57 Application of other wound dressing**
Porcine wound dressing
AHA: 3Q 2002, 23

✖ **93.58 Application of pressure trousers**
Application of:
anti-shock trousers
MAST trousers
vasopneumatic device
AHA: 3Q 1996, 13

✖ **93.59 Other immobilization, pressure, and attention to wound**
Elastic stockings
Electronic gaiter
Intermittent pressure device
Oxygenation of wound (hyperbaric)
Stereotactic head frame application
Strapping (non-traction)
Velpeau dressing
AHA: 3Q 1999, 7; 1Q 1999, 12-13; 1Q 1991, 11; 1Q 1989, 12; 4Q 1988, 11

④ **93.6 Osteopathic manipulative treatment**

✖ **93.61 Osteopathic manipulative treatment for general mobilization**
General articulatory treatment

✖ **93.62 Osteopathic manipulative treatment using high-velocity, low-amplitude forces**
Thrusting forces

✖ **93.63 Osteopathic manipulative treatment using low-velocity, high-amplitude forces**
Springing forces

✖ **93.64 Osteopathic manipulative treatment using isotonic, isometric forces**

✖ **93.65 Osteopathic manipulative treatment using indirect forces**

✖ **93.66 Osteopathic manipulative treatment to move tissue fluids**
Lymphatic pump

✖ **93.67 Other specified osteopathic manipulative treatment**

④ **93.7 Speech and reading rehabilitation and rehabilitation of the blind**

✖ **93.71 Dyslexia training**

✖ **93.72 Dysphasia training**

✖ **93.73 Esophageal speech training**

✖ **93.74 Speech defect training**

✖ **93.75 Other speech training and therapy**
AHA: 4Q 2003, 106, 109; 4Q 1997, 36; 3Q 1997, 12

✖ **93.76 Training in use of lead dog for the blind**

✖ **93.77 Training in braille or Moon**

✖ **93.78 Other rehabilitation for the blind**

④ **93.8 Other rehabilitation therapy**

✖ **93.81 Recreation therapy**
Diversional therapy
Play therapy
Excludes *play psychotherapy (94.36)*

✖ **93.82 Educational therapy**
Education of bed-bound children
Special schooling for the handicapped

✖ **93.83 Occupational therapy**
Daily living activities therapy
Excludes *training in activities of daily living for the blind (93.78)*
AHA: 2Q 2005, 6-7; 3Q 1997, 12

✖ **93.84 Music therapy**

✖ **93.85 Vocational rehabilitation**
Sheltered employment
Vocational:
assessment
retraining
training

✖ **93.89 Rehabilitation, not elsewhere classified**
AHA: 2Q 2005, 6-7

④ **93.9 Respiratory therapy**
Excludes *insertion of airway (96.01-96.05)*
other continuous mechanical ventilation (96.70-96.72)

✖ **93.90 Continuous positive airway pressure [CPAP]**
Bi-level airway pressure
Non-invasive positive pressure (NIPPV)
AHA: 3Q 2004, 3; 1Q 2002, 12-13; 3Q 1998, 14; 4Q 1991, 21

✖ **93.91 Intermittent positive pressure breathing [IPPB]**
AHA: 4Q 1991, 21

✖ **93.93 Nonmechanical methods of resuscitation**
Artificial respiration
Manual resuscitation
Mouth-to-mouth resuscitation
AHA: 2Q 2003, 17

✖ **93.94 Respiratory medication administered by nebulizer**
Mist therapy

✖ **93.95 Hyperbaric oxygenation**
Excludes *oxygenation of wound (93.59)*

✖ **93.96 Other oxygen enrichment**
Catalytic oxygen therapy
Cytoreductive effect
Oxygenators
Oxygen therapy
Excludes *oxygenation of wound (93.59)*

✖ **93.97 Decompression chamber**

✖ **93.98 Other control of atmospheric pressure and composition**
Antigen-free air conditioning
Helium therapy
Excludes *inhaled nitric oxide therapy (INO) (00.12)*
AHA: 1Q 2002, 14

✖ **93.99 Other respiratory procedures**
Continuous negative pressure ventilation [CNP]
Postural drainage
AHA: 4Q 2003, 107; 3Q 1999, 11; 4Q 1991, 21

PROCEDURES RELATED TO THE PSYCHE (94)

④ **94.0 Psychologic evaluation and testing**

✖ **94.01 Administration of intelligence test**
Administration of:
Stanford-Binet
Wechsler Adult Intelligence Scale
Wechsler Intelligence Scale for Children

✖ **94.02 Administration of psychologic test**
Administration of:
Bender Visual-Motor Gestalt Test
Benton Visual Retention Test
Minnesota Multiphasic Personality Inventory
Wechsler Memory Scale

✖ **94.03 Character analysis**

✖ **94.08 Other psychologic evaluation and testing**

✖ **94.09 Psychologic mental status determination, not otherwise specified**

④ **94.1 Psychiatric interviews, consultations, and evaluations**

✖ **94.11 Psychiatric mental status determination**
Clinical psychiatric mental status determination
Evaluation for criminal responsibility
Evaluation for testimentary capacity
Medicolegal mental status determination
Mental status determination NOS

✖ **94.12 Routine psychiatric visit, not otherwise specified**

✖ **94.13 Psychiatric commitment evaluation**
Pre-commitment interview

✖ **94.19 Other psychiatric interview and evaluation**
Follow-up psychiatric interview NOS

④ **94.2 Psychiatric somatotherapy**

✖ **94.21 Narcoanalysis**
Narcosynthesis

✖ **94.22 Lithium therapy**

✖ **94.23 Neuroleptic therapy**

✖ **94.24 Chemical shock therapy**

✖ **94.25 Other psychiatric drug therapy**

✖ **94.26 Subconvulsive electroshock therapy**

✖ **94.27 Other electroshock therapy**
Electroconvulsive therapy (ECT)
EST

✖ **94.29 Other psychiatric somatotherapy**

❹ **94.3 Individual psychotherapy**

✖ **94.31 Psychoanalysis**

✖ **94.32 Hypnotherapy**
Hypnodrome
Hypnosis

✖ **94.33 Behavior therapy**
Aversion therapy
Behavior modification
Desensitization therapy
Extinction therapy
Relaxation training
Token economy

✖ **94.34 Individual therapy for psychosexual dysfunction**
Excludes *that performed in group setting (94.41)*

✖ **94.35 Crisis intervention**

✖ **94.36 Play psychotherapy**

✖ **94.37 Exploratory verbal psychotherapy**

✖ **94.38 Supportive verbal psychotherapy**

✖ **94.39 Other individual psychotherapy**
Biofeedback

❹ **94.4 Other psychotherapy and counselling**

✖ **94.41 Group therapy for psychosexual dysfunction**

✖ **94.42 Family therapy**

✖ **94.43 Psychodrama**

✖ **94.44 Other group therapy**

✖ **94.45 Drug addiction counselling**

✖ **94.46 Alcoholism counselling**
AHA: Jul-Aug 1985, 15

✖ **94.49 Other counselling**

❹ **94.5 Referral for psychologic rehabilitation**

✖ **94.51 Referral for psychotherapy**

✖ **94.52 Referral for psychiatric aftercare:**
That in:
halfway house
outpatient (clinic) facility

✖ **94.53 Referral for alcoholism rehabilitation**

✖ **94.54 Referral for drug addiction rehabilitation**

✖ **94.55 Referral for vocational rehabilitation**

✖ **94.59 Referral for other psychologic rehabilitation**

❹ **94.6 Alcohol and drug rehabilitation and detoxification**

✖ **94.61 Alcohol rehabilitation**

✖ **94.62 Alcohol detoxification**

✖ **94.63 Alcohol rehabilitation and detoxification**

✖ **94.64 Drug rehabilitation**

✖ **94.65 Drug detoxification**

✖ **94.66 Drug rehabilitation and detoxification**

✖ **94.67 Combined alcohol and drug rehabilitation**

✖ **94.68 Combined alcohol and drug detoxification**

✖ **94.69 Combined alcohol and drug rehabilitation and detoxification**

OPHTHALMOLOGIC AND OTOLOGIC DIAGNOSIS AND TREATMENT (95)

❹ **95.0 General and subjective eye examination**

✖ **95.01 Limited eye examination**
Eye examination with prescription of spectacles

✖ **95.02 Comprehensive eye examination**
Eye examination covering all aspects of the visual system

✖ **95.03 Extended ophthalmologic work-up**
Examination (for):
glaucoma
neuro-ophthalmology
retinal disease

✓ **95.04 Eye examination under anesthesia**
Code also type of examination

✖ **95.05 Visual field study**

✖ **95.06 Color vision study**

✖ **95.07 Dark adaptation study**

✖ **95.09 Eye examination, not otherwise specified**
Vision check NOS

❹ **95.1 Examinations of form and structure of eye**

✖ **95.11 Fundus photography**

✖ **95.12 Fluorescein angiography or angioscopy of eye**

✖ **95.13 Ultrasound study of eye**

✖ **95.14 X-ray study of eye**

✖ **95.15 Ocular motility study**

✖ **95.16 P32 and other tracer studies of eye**

❹ **95.2 Objective functional tests of eye**
Excludes *that with polysomnogram (89.17)*

✖ **95.21 Electroretinogram [ERG]**

✖ **95.22 Electro-oculogram [EOG]**

✖ **95.23 Visual evoked potential [VEP]**

✖ **95.24 Electronystagmogram [ENG]**

✖ **95.25 Electromyogram of eye [EMG]**

✖ **95.26 Tonography, provocative tests, and other glaucoma testing**

❹ **95.3 Special vision services**

✖ **95.31 Fitting and dispensing of spectacles**

✖ **95.32 Prescription, fitting, and dispensing of contact lens**

✖ **95.33 Dispensing of other low vision aids**

✖ **95.34 Ocular prosthetics**

✖ **95.35 Orthoptic training**

✖ **95.36 Ophthalmologic counselling and instruction**
Counselling in:
adaptation to visual loss
use of low vision aids

❹ **95.4 Nonoperative procedures related to hearing**

✖ **95.41 Audiometry**
Békésy 5-tone audiometry
Impedance audiometry
Stapedial reflex response
Subjective audiometry
Tympanogram

✖ **95.42 Clinical test of hearing**
Tuning fork test
Whispered speech test

✖ **95.43 Audiological evaluation**
Audiological evaluation by:
Bárány noise machine
blindfold test
delayed feedback
masking
Weber lateralization

✖ **95.44 Clinical vestibular function tests**
Thermal test of vestibular function

✖ **95.45 Rotation tests**
Bárány chair

✖ **95.46 Other auditory and vestibular function tests**

✖ **95.47 Hearing examination, not otherwise specified**

✖ **95.48 Fitting of hearing aid**
Excludes *implantation of electromagnetic hearing device (20.95)*
AHA: 4Q 1989, 5

✖ Deleted Code ▼ Nonspecific O.R. Procedure ✓ Valid O.R. Procedure ✖ Non-O.R Procedure ♂ Male ♀ Female

✖ **95.49 Other nonoperative procedures related to hearing**
Adjustment (external components) of cochlear prosthetic device

NONOPERATIVE INTUBATION AND IRRIGATION (96)

❹ **96.0 Nonoperative intubation of gastrointestinal and respiratory tracts**

✖ **96.01 Insertion of nasopharyngeal airway**

✖ **96.02 Insertion of oropharyngeal airway**

✖ **96.03 Insertion of esophageal obturator airway**

✖ **96.04 Insertion of endotracheal tube**
AHA: 3Q 2005, 10, 11; 2Q 2005, 20

✖ **96.05 Other intubation of respiratory tract**
Excludes *endoscopic insertion or replacement of bronchial device or substance (33.71, 33.79)*
AHA: 1Q 1997, 14

✖ **96.06 Insertion of Sengstaken tube**
Esophageal tamponade
AHA: Nov-Dec 1987, 4

✖ **96.07 Insertion of other (naso-)gastric tube**
Intubation for decompression
Excludes *that for enteral infusion of nutritional substance (96.6)*
AHA: 1Q 1988, 6-7

✖ **96.08 Insertion of (naso-)intestinal tube**
Miller-Abbott tube (for decompression)
AHA: 1Q 1988, 6-7

✖ **96.09 Insertion of rectal tube**
Replacement of rectal tube

❹ **96.1 Other nonoperative insertion**
Excludes *nasolacrimal intubation (09.44)*

✖ **96.11 Packing of external auditory canal**

✖ **96.14 Vaginal packing** ♀

✖ **96.15 Insertion of vaginal mold** ♀

✖ **96.16 Other vaginal dilation** ♀

✖ **96.17 Insertion of vaginal diaphragm** ♀

✖ **96.18 Insertion of other vaginal pessary** ♀

✖ **96.19 Rectal packing**

❹ **96.2 Nonoperative dilation and manipulation**

✖ **96.21 Dilation of frontonasal duct**

✖ **96.22 Dilation of rectum**

✖ **96.23 Dilation of anal sphincter**

✖ **96.24 Dilation and manipulation of enterostomy stoma**

✖ **96.25 Therapeutic distention of bladder**
Intermittent distention of bladder

✖ **96.26 Manual reduction of rectal prolapse**

✖ **96.27 Manual reduction of hernia**

✖ **96.28 Manual reduction of enterostomy prolapse**
AHA: Nov-Dec 1987, 11

✖ **96.29 Reduction of intussusception of alimentary tract**
With:
- fluoroscopy
- ionizing radiation enema
- ultrasonography guidance

Hydrostatic reduction
Pneumatic reduction
Excludes *intra-abdominal manipulation of intestine, not otherwise specified (46.80)*
AHA: 4Q 1998, 82

❹ **96.3 Nonoperative alimentary tract irrigation, cleaning, and local instillation**

✖ **96.31 Gastric cooling**
Gastric hypothermia

✖ **96.32 Gastric freezing**

✖ **96.33 Gastric lavage**
AHA: Nov-Dec 1987, 4

✖ **96.34 Other irrigation of (naso-)gastric tube**

✖ **96.35 Gastric gavage**

✖ **96.36 Irrigation of gastrostomy or enterostomy**

✖ **96.37 Proctoclysis**

✖ **96.38 Removal of impacted feces**
Removal of impaction:
by flushing manually

✖ **96.39 Other transanal enema**
Rectal irrigation
Excludes *reduction of intussusception of alimentary tract by ionizing radiation enema (96.29)*

❹ **96.4 Nonoperative irrigation, cleaning, and local instillation of other digestive and genitourinary organs**

✖ **96.41 Irrigation of cholecystostomy and other biliary tube**

✖ **96.42 Irrigation of pancreatic tube**

✖ **96.43 Digestive tract instillation, except gastric gavage**

✖ **96.44 Vaginal douche** ♀

✖ **96.45 Irrigation of nephrostomy and pyelostomy**

✖ **96.46 Irrigation of ureterostomy and ureteral catheter**

✖ **96.47 Irrigation of cystostomy**

✖ **96.48 Irrigation of other indwelling urinary catheter**

✖ **96.49 Other genitourinary instillation**
Insertion of prostaglandin suppository
AHA: 1Q 2001, 5

❹ **96.5 Other nonoperative irrigation and cleaning**

✖ **96.51 Irrigation of eye**
Irrigation of cornea
Excludes *irrigation with removal of foreign body (98.21)*

✖ **96.52 Irrigation of ear**
Irrigation with removal of cerumen

✖ **96.53 Irrigation of nasal passages**

✖ **96.54 Dental scaling, polishing, and debridement**
Dental prophylaxis
Plaque removal

✖ **96.55 Tracheostomy toilette**

✖ **96.56 Other lavage of bronchus and trachea**
Excludes *diagnostic bronchoalveolar lavage (BAL)(33.24)*
whole lung lavage (33.99)
AHA: 3Q 2002, 18

✖ **96.57 Irrigation of vascular catheter**
AHA: 3Q 2003, 5

✖ **96.58 Irrigation of wound catheter**

✖ **96.59 Other irrigation of wound**
Wound cleaning NOS
Excludes *debridement (86.22, 86.27-86.28)*
AHA: Sep-Oct 1985, 7

✖ **96.6 Enteral infusion of concentrated nutritional substances**

❹ 96.7 Other continuous mechanical ventilation

Includes
Endotracheal respiratory assistance
Intermittent mandatory ventilation [IMV]
Positive end expiratory pressure [PEEP]
Pressure support ventilation [PSV]
That by tracheostomy
Weaning of an intubated (endotracheal tube) patient

Excludes
bi-level ▶positive◀ airway pressure ▶BiPAP◀ (93.90)
continuous negative pressure ventilation [CNP] (iron lung) (cuirass) (93.99)
continuous positive airway pressure [CPAP] (93.90)
intermittent positive pressure breathing [IPPB] (93.91)
non-invasive positive pressure (NIPPV) (93.90)
that by face mask (93.90-93.99)
that by nasal cannula (93.90-93.99)
that by nasal catheter (93.90-93.99)

Code also any associated:
endotracheal tube insertion (96.04)
tracheostomy (31.1-31.29)

Note: Endotracheal Intubation:
To calculate the number of hours (duration) of continuous mechanical ventilation during a hospitalization, begin the count from the start of the (endotracheal) intubation. The duration ends with (endotracheal) extubation.

If a patient is intubated prior to admission, begin counting the duration from the time of the admission. If a patient is transferred (discharged) while intubated, the duration would end at the time of transfer (discharge).

For patients who begin on (endotracheal) intubation and subsequently have a tracheostomy performed for mechanical ventilation, the duration begins with the (endotracheal) intubation and ends when the mechanical ventilation is turned off (after the weaning period).

Tracheostomy:
To calculate the number of hours of continuous mechanical ventilation during a hospitalization, begin counting the duration when mechanical ventilation is started. The duration ends when the mechanical ventilator is turned off (after the weaning period).

If a patient has received a tracheostomy prior to admission and is on mechanical ventilation at the time of admission, begin counting the duration from the time of admission. If a patient is transferred (discharged) while still on mechanical ventilation via tracheostomy, the duration would end at the time of the transfer (discharge).

✖ **96.70 Continuous mechanical ventilation of unspecified duration**
Mechanical ventilation NOS
AHA: 3Q 2004, 3; 2Q 1992, 13-14; 4Q 1991, 21

✖ **96.71 Continuous mechanical ventilation for less than 96 consecutive hours**
AHA: 3Q 2005, 10, 11; 3Q 2004, 3; 2Q 1992, 13-14; 4Q 1991, 21

✖ **96.72 Continuous mechanical ventilation for 96 consecutive hours or more**
AHA: 2Q 2005, 20; 3Q 2004, 3; 2Q 1992, 13-14; 4Q 1991, 21

REPLACEMENT AND REMOVAL OF THERAPEUTIC APPLIANCES (97)

❹ 97.0 Nonoperative replacement of gastrointestinal appliance

✖ **97.01 Replacement of (naso-)gastric or esophagostomy tube**

✖ **97.02 Replacement of gastrostomy tube**
AHA: 1Q 1997, 11

✖ **97.03 Replacement of tube or enterostomy device of small intestine**
AHA: 1Q 2003, 10

✖ **97.04 Replacement of tube or enterostomy device of large intestine**

✖ **97.05 Replacement of stent (tube) in biliary or pancreatic duct**
AHA: 2Q 1999, 13

❹ 97.1 Nonoperative replacement of musculoskeletal and integumentary system appliance

✖ **97.11 Replacement of cast on upper limb**

✖ **97.12 Replacement of cast on lower limb**

✖ **97.13 Replacement of other cast**

✖ **97.14 Replacement of other device for musculoskeletal immobilization**

✖ **97.15 Replacement of wound catheter**

✖ **97.16 Replacement of wound packing or drain**
Excludes *repacking of:*
dental wound (97.22)
vulvar wound (97.26)

❹ 97.2 Other nonoperative replacement

✖ **97.21 Replacement of nasal packing**

✖ **97.22 Replacement of dental packing**

✖ **97.23 Replacement of tracheostomy tube**
AHA: Nov-Dec 1987, 11

✖ **97.24 Replacement and refitting of vaginal diaphragm** ♀

✖ **97.25 Replacement of other vaginal pessary** ♀

✖ **97.26 Replacement of vaginal or vulvar packing or drain** ♀

✖ **97.29 Other nonoperative replacements**
AHA: 3Q 1999, 9; 3Q 1998, 12; Mar-Apr 1985, 11

❹ 97.3 Nonoperative removal of therapeutic device from head and neck

✖ **97.31 Removal of eye prosthesis**
Excludes *removal of ocular implant (16.71)*
removal of orbital implant (16.72)

✖ **97.32 Removal of nasal packing**

✖ **97.33 Removal of dental wiring**

✖ **97.34 Removal of dental packing**

✖ **97.35 Removal of dental prosthesis**

✖ **97.36 Removal of other external mandibular fixation device**

✖ **97.37 Removal of tracheostomy tube**

✖ **97.38 Removal of sutures from head and neck**

✖ **97.39 Removal of other therapeutic device from head and neck**
Excludes *removal of skull tongs (02.94)*

❹ 97.4 Nonoperative removal of therapeutic device from thorax

✖ **97.41 Removal of thoracotomy tube or pleural cavity drain**
AHA: 1Q 1999, 9

✖ **97.42 Removal of mediastinal drain**

✖ **97.43 Removal of sutures from thorax**

✖ **97.44 Nonoperative removal of heart assist system**
Explantation [removal] of circulatory assist device
Explantation [removal] of percutaneous external heart assist device
Intra-aortic balloon pump [IABP]
Removal of extrinsic heart assist device
Removal of pVAD
Removal of percutaneous heart assist device
AHA: 4Q 2001, 65

✖ **97.49 Removal of other device from thorax**
Excludes *▶Endoscopic removal of bronchial device(s) or substances (33.78)◀*
AHA: Nov-Dec 1986, 9

❹ 97.5 Nonoperative removal of therapeutic device from digestive system

✖ **97.51 Removal of gastrostomy tube**

✖ **97.52 Removal of tube from small intestine**

✖ **97.53 Removal of tube from large intestine or appendix**

✖ **97.54 Removal of cholecystostomy tube**

✖ **97.55 Removal of T-tube, other bile duct tube, or liver tube**
Removal of bile duct stent
AHA: 1Q 2001, 8

✖ **97.56 Removal of pancreatic tube or drain**

✖ **97.59 Removal of other device from digestive system**
Removal of rectal packing

97.6 Nonoperative removal of therapeutic device from urinary system

97.61 Removal of pyelostomy and nephrostomy tube

97.62 Removal of ureterostomy tube and ureteral catheter

97.63 Removal of cystostomy tube

97.64 Removal of other urinary drainage device
Removal of indwelling urinary catheter

97.65 Removal of urethral stent

97.69 Removal of other device from urinary system

97.7 Nonoperative removal of therapeutic device from genital system

97.71 Removal of intrauterine contraceptive device ♀

97.72 Removal of intrauterine pack ♀

97.73 Removal of vaginal diaphragm ♀

97.74 Removal of other vaginal pessary ♀

97.75 Removal of vaginal or vulvar packing ♀

97.79 Removal of other device from genital tract
Removal of sutures

97.8 Other nonoperative removal of therapeutic device

97.81 Removal of retroperitoneal drainage device

97.82 Removal of peritoneal drainage device
AHA: 2Q 1990, 28; Sep-Oct 1986, 12

97.83 Removal of abdominal wall sutures

97.84 Removal of sutures from trunk, not elsewhere classified

97.85 Removal of packing from trunk, not elsewhere classified

97.86 Removal of other device from abdomen

97.87 Removal of other device from trunk

97.88 Removal of external immobilization device
Removal of:
brace
cast
splint

97.89 Removal of other therapeutic device

NONOPERATIVE REMOVAL OF FOREIGN BODY OR CALCULUS (98)

98.0 Removal of intraluminal foreign body from digestive system without incision
Excludes *removal of therapeutic device (97.51-97.59)*

98.01 Removal of intraluminal foreign body from mouth without incision

98.02 Removal of intraluminal foreign body from esophagus without incision

98.03 Removal of intraluminal foreign body from stomach and small intestine without incision

98.04 Removal of intraluminal foreign body from large intestine without incision

98.05 Removal of intraluminal foreign body from rectum and anus without incision

98.1 Removal of intraluminal foreign body from other sites without incision
Excludes *removal of therapeutic device (97.31-97.49, 97.61-97.89)*

98.11 Removal of intraluminal foreign body from ear without incision

98.12 Removal of intraluminal foreign body from nose without incision

98.13 Removal of intraluminal foreign body from pharynx without incision

98.14 Removal of intraluminal foreign body from larynx without incision

98.15 Removal of intraluminal foreign body from trachea and bronchus without incision
▶Excludes *Endoscopic removal of bronchial device(s) or substances (33.78)*◀

98.16 Removal of intraluminal foreign body from uterus without incision ♀
Excludes *removal of intrauterine contraceptive device (97.71)*

98.17 Removal of intraluminal foreign body from vagina without incision ♀

98.18 Removal of intraluminal foreign body from artificial stoma without incision

98.19 Removal of intraluminal foreign body from urethra without incision

98.2 Removal of other foreign body without incision
Excludes *removal of intraluminal foreign body (98.01-98.19)*

98.20 Removal of foreign body, not otherwise specified

98.21 Removal of superficial foreign body from eye without incision

98.22 Removal of other foreign body without incision from head and neck
Removal of embedded foreign body from eyelid or conjunctiva without incision

98.23 Removal of foreign body from vulva without incision ♀

98.24 Removal of foreign body from scrotum or penis without incision ♂

98.25 Removal of other foreign body without incision from trunk except scrotum, penis, or vulva

98.26 Removal of foreign body from hand without incision
AHA: Nov-Dec 1987, 10

98.27 Removal of foreign body without incision from upper limb, except hand

98.28 Removal of foreign body from foot without incision

98.29 Removal of foreign body without incision from lower limb, except foot

98.5 Extracorporeal shockwave lithotripsy [ESWL]
Disintegration of stones by extracorporeal induced shockwaves
Lithotriptor tank procedure
That with insertion of stent

98.51 Extracorporeal shockwave lithotripsy [ESWL] of the kidney, ureter and/or bladder
AHA: 4Q 1995, 73 ; 1Q 1989, 2

98.52 Extracorporeal shockwave lithotripsy [ESWL] of the gallbladder and/or bile duct

98.59 Extracorporeal shockwave lithotripsy of other sites

OTHER NONOPERATIVE PROCEDURES (99)

99.0 Transfusion of blood and blood components
Use additional code for that done via catheter or cutdown (38.92-38.94)

99.00 Perioperative autologous transfusion of whole blood or blood components
Intraoperative blood collection
Postoperative blood collection
Salvage
AHA: 4Q 1995, 69

99.01 Exchange transfusion
Transfusion:
exsanguination
replacement
AHA: 2Q 1989, 15

99.02 Transfusion of previously collected autologous blood
Blood component
AHA: 1Q 1990, 10; Jul-Aug 1985, 16

99.03 Other transfusion of whole blood
Transfusion:
blood NOS
hemodilution
NOS

99.04 Transfusion of packed cells

99.05 Transfusion of platelets
Transfusion of thrombocytes

99.06 Transfusion of coagulation factors
Transfusion of antihemophilic factor

✖ **99.07 Transfusion of other serum**
Transfusion of plasma
Excludes *injection [transfusion] of:*
antivenin (99.16)
gamma globulin (99.14)
AHA: Nov-Dec 1985, 14

✖ **99.08 Transfusion of blood expander**
Transfusion of Dextran

✖ **99.09 Transfusion of other substance**
Transfusion of:
blood surrogate
granulocytes
Excludes *transplantation [transfusion] of bone marrow (41.0)*

❹ **99.1 Injection or infusion of therapeutic or prophylactic substance**
Includes injection or infusion given:
hypodermically acting locally or systemically
intramuscularly acting locally or systemically
intravenously acting locally or systemically

✖ **99.10 Injection or infusion of thrombolytic agent**
Alteplase
Anistreplase
Reteplase
Streptokinase
Tenecteplase
Tissue plasminogen activator (TPA)
Urokinase
Excludes *aspirin - omit code*
GP IIB/IIIa platelet inhibitor (99.20)
heparin (99.19)
warfarin - omit code
AHA: 4Q 2005, 103; 2Q 2001, 7; 4Q 1998, 83

✖ **99.11 Injection of Rh immune globulin**
Injection of:
Anti-D (Rhesus) globulin
RhoGAM

✖ **99.12 Immunization for allergy**
Desensitization

✖ **99.13 Immunization for autoimmune disease**

▲✖ **99.14 Injection or infusion of gamma globulin**
Injection of immune sera

✖ **99.15 Parenteral infusion of concentrated nutritional substances**
Hyperalimentation
Peripheral parenteral nutrition [PPN]
Total parenteral nutrition [TPN]

✖ **99.16 Injection of antidote**
Injection of:
antivenin
heavy metal antagonist

✖ **99.17 Injection of insulin**

✖ **99.18 Injection or infusion of electrolytes**

✖ **99.19 Injection of anticoagulant**
Excludes *infusion of drotrecogin alfa (activated)(00.11)*

❹ **99.2 Injection or infusion of other therapeutic or prophylactic substance**
Includes injection or infusion given:
hypodermically acting locally or systemically
intramuscularly acting locally or systemically
intravenously acting locally or systemically
Use additional code for:
injection (into):
breast (85.92)
bursa (82.94, 83.96)
intraperitoneal (cavity) (54.97)
intrathecal (03.92)
joint (76.96, 81.92)
kidney (55.96)
liver (50.94)
orbit (16.91)
other sites - *see* Alphabetic Index
perfusion:
NOS (39.97)
intestine (46.95, 46.96)
kidney (55.95)
liver (50.93)
total body (39.96)

✖ **99.20 Injection or infusion of platelet inhibitor**
Glycoprotein IIB/IIIa inhibitor
GP IIB/IIIa inhibitor
GP IIB-IIIa inhibitor
Excludes *infusion of heparin (99.19)*
injection or infusion of thrombolytic agent (99.10)
AHA: 4Q 2002, 114; 4Q 1998, 84

✖ **99.21 Injection of antibiotic**
Excludes *injection or infusion of oxazolidinone class of antibiotics (00.14)*
AHA: 3Q 1992, 6; 2Q 1990, 24; 3Q 1989, 16; Mar-Apr 1987, 9

✖ **99.22 Injection of other anti-infective**
Excludes *injection or infusion of oxazolidinone class of antibiotics (00.14)*

✖ **99.23 Injection of steroid**
Injection of cortisone
Subdermal implantation of progesterone
AHA: 3Q 2000, 15; 1Q 1999, 8; 3Q 1996, 7; 3Q 1992, 9; Sep-Oct 1985, 7

Insertion of implantable contraceptive capsules

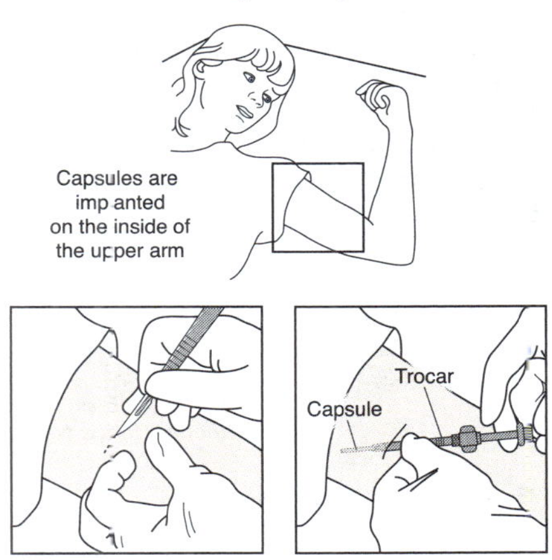

Small incision is made
Capsules are inserted using a trocar

✖ **99.24 Injection of other hormone**
AHA: 1Q 2006, 9; 3Q 1992, 9

✖ **99.25 Injection or infusion of cancer chemotherapeutic substance**
▶ Use additional code for disruption of blood brain barrier, if performed [BBBD] (00.19)◀
Chemoembolization
Injection or infusion of antineoplastic agent
Excludes *immunotherapy, antineoplastic (00.15, 99.28)*
implantation of chemotherapeutic agent (00.10)
injection of radioisotope (92.28)
injection or infusion of biological response modifier [BRM] as an antineoplastic agent (99.28)
AHA: 2Q 2003, 6; 4Q 2002, 93; 1Q 1998, 6; 3Q 1996, 11; 2Q 1992, 7; 1Q 1992, 12

✖ **99.26 Injection of tranquilizer**

✖ **99.27 Iontophoresis**

✖ **99.28 Injection or infusion of biological response modifier [BRM] as an antineoplastic agent**
Immunotherapy, antineoplastic
Interleukin therapy
Low-dose interleukin-2 (IL-2) therapy
Tumor vaccine
Includes infusion of cintredekin besudotox
Excludes *high-dose infusion interleukin-2 [IL-2] (00.15)*
AHA: 2Q 1999, 8; 2Q 1998, 12; 4Q 1994, 51

✖ **99.29 Injection or infusion of other therapeutic or prophylactic substance**
Excludes *administration of neuroprotective agent (99.75)*
immunization (99.31-99.59)
▶ *infusion of blood brain barrier disruption substance (00.19)*◀
injection of sclerosing agent into:
esophageal varices (42.33)
hemorrhoids (49.42)
veins (39.92)
injection or infusion of:
human B-type natriuretic peptide (hBNP)(00.13)
inesiritide (00.13)
platelet inhibitor (99.20)
thrombolytic agent (99.10)
AHA: 1Q 2000, 8; 2Q 1998, 23-24; 1Q 1998, 5; 1Q 1997, 3-4; 2Q 1990, 24; 2Q 1989, 17; Nov-Dec 1987, 4-5; Jul-Aug 1984, 12

④ **99.3 Prophylactic vaccination and inoculation against certain bacterial diseases**

✖ **99.31 Vaccination against cholera**

✖ **99.32 Vaccination against typhoid and paratyphoid fever**
Administration of TAB vaccine

✖ **99.33 Vaccination against tuberculosis**
Administration of BCG vaccine

✖ **99.34 Vaccination against plague**

✖ **99.35 Vaccination against tularemia**

✖ **99.36 Administration of diphtheria toxoid**
Excludes *administration of:*
diphtheria antitoxin (99.58)
diphtheria-tetanus-pertussis, combined (99.39)

✖ **99.37 Vaccination against pertussis**
Excludes *administration of diphtheria tetanus-pertussis, combined (99.39)*

✖ **99.38 Administration of tetanus toxoid**
Excludes *administration of:*
diphtheria-tetanus-pertussis, combined (99.39)
tetanus antitoxin (99.56)

✖ **99.39 Administration of diphtheria-tetanus-pertussis, combined**

④ **99.4 Prophylactic vaccination and inoculation against certain viral diseases**

✖ **99.41 Administration of poliomyelitis vaccine**

✖ **99.42 Vaccination against smallpox**

✖ **99.43 Vaccination against yellow fever**

✖ **99.44 Vaccination against rabies**

✖ **99.45 Vaccination against measles**
Excludes *administration of measles-mumps-rubella vaccine (99.48)*

✖ **99.46 Vaccination against mumps**
Excludes *administration of measles-mumps-rubella vaccine (99.48)*

✖ **99.47 Vaccination against rubella**
Excludes *administration of measles-mumps-rubella vaccine (99.48)*

✖ **99.48 Administration of measles-mumps-rubella vaccine**

④ **99.5 Other vaccination and inoculation**

✖ **99.51 Prophylactic vaccination against the common cold**

✖ **99.52 Prophylactic vaccination against influenza**

✖ **99.53 Prophylactic vaccination against arthropod-borne viral encephalitis**

✖ **99.54 Prophylactic vaccination against other arthropod-borne viral diseases**

✖ **99.55 Prophylactic administration of vaccine against other diseases**
Vaccination against:
anthrax
brucellosis
Rocky Mountain spotted fever
Staphylococcus
Streptococcus
typhus
AHA: 2Q 2000, 9; 1Q 1994, 19; 4Q 1993, 24

✖ **99.56 Administration of tetanus antitoxin**

✖ **99.57 Administration of botulism antitoxin**

✖ **99.58 Administration of other antitoxins**
Administration of:
diphtheria antitoxin
gas gangrene antitoxin
scarlet fever antitoxin

✖ **99.59 Other vaccination and inoculation**
Vaccination NOS
Excludes *injection of:*
gamma globulin (99.14)
Rh immune globulin (99.11)
immunization for:
allergy (99.12)
autoimmune disease (99.13)

④ **99.6 Conversion of cardiac rhythm**
Excludes *open chest cardiac:*
electric stimulation (37.91)
massage (37.91)

✖ **99.60 Cardiopulmonary resuscitation, not otherwise specified**
AHA: 1Q 1994, 16

✖ **99.61 Atrial cardioversion**

✖ **99.62 Other electric countershock of heart**
Cardioversion:
NOS
external
Conversion to sinus rhythm
Defibrillation
External electrode stimulation

✖ **99.63 Closed chest cardiac massage**
Cardiac massage NOS
Manual external cardiac massage

✖ **99.64 Carotid sinus stimulation**

✖ **99.69 Other conversion of cardiac rhythm**
AHA: 4Q 1988, 11

④ **99.7 Therapeutic apheresis or other injection, administration, or infusion of other therapeutic or prophylactic substance**

✖ **99.71 Therapeutic plasmapheresis**
Excludes *extracorporeal immunoadsorption [ECI] (99.76)*

✖ **99.72 Therapeutic leukopheresis**
Therapeutic leukocytapheresis

✖ **99.73 Therapeutic erythrocytapheresis**
Therapeutic erythropheresis
AHA: 1Q 1994, 20

✖ **99.74 Therapeutic plateletpheresis**

✔ **99.75 Administration of neuroprotective agent**

✔ **99.76 Extracorporeal immunoadsorption**
Removal of antibodies from plasma with protein A columns

✔ **99.77 Application or administration of adhesion barrier substance**

✖ **99.78 Aquapheresis**
Plasma water removal
Ultrafiltration [for water removal]
Excludes *hemodiafiltration (39.95)*
hemodialysis (39.95)
therapeutic plasmapheresis (99.71)

✖ **99.79 Other**
Apheresis (harvest) of stem cells
AHA: 1Q 2006, 13; 1Q 2005, 16

④ 99.8 Miscellaneous physical procedures

✖ **99.81 Hypothermia (central) (local)**
Excludes *gastric cooling (96.31)*
gastric freezing (96.32)
that incidental to open heart surgery (39.62)

✖ **99.82 Ultraviolet light therapy**
Actinotherapy

✖ **99.83 Other phototherapy**
Phototherapy of the newborn
Excludes *extracorporeal photochemotherapy (99.88)*
photocoagulation of retinal lesion (14.23-14.25, 14.33-14.35, 14.53-14.55)
AHA: 2Q 1989, 15

✖ **99.84 Isolation**
Isolation after contact with infectious disease
Protection of individual from his surroundings
Protection of surroundings from individual

✖ **99.85 Hyperthermia for treatment of cancer**
Hyperthermia (adjunct therapy) induced by microwave, ultrasound, low energy radio frequency, probes (interstitial), or other means in the treatment of cancer
Code also any concurrent chemotherapy or radiation therapy
AHA: 3Q 1996, 11

✖ **99.86 Non-invasive placement of bone growth stimulator**
Transcutaneous (surface) placement of pads or patches for stimulation to aid bone healing
Excludes *insertion of invasive or semi invasive bone growth stimulators (device) (percutaneous electrodes) (78.90-78.99)*

✖ **99.88 Therapeutic photopheresis**
Extracorporeal photochemotherapy
Extracorporeal photopheresis
Excludes *other phototherapy (99.83)*
ultraviolet light therapy (99.82)
AHA: 2Q 1999, 7

④ 99.9 Other miscellaneous procedures

✖ **99.91 Acupuncture for anesthesia**

✖ **99.92 Other acupuncture**
Excludes *that with smouldering moxa (93.35)*

✖ **99.93 Rectal massage (for levator spasm)**

✖ **99.94 Prostatic massage** ♂

✖ **99.95 Stretching of foreskin** ♂

✖ **99.96 Collection of sperm for artificial insemination** ♂

✖ **99.97 Fitting of denture**

✖ **99.98 Extraction of milk from lactating breast** ♀

✖ **99.99 Other**
Leech therapy

Notes

Notes

Notes

Notes

Notes

Notes

Notes